Principles of
Addiction Medicine
Third Edition

Allan W. Graham, M.D., FACP, FASAM
Terry K. Schultz, M.D., FASAM
Michael F. Mayo-Smith, M.D., M.P.H.
Richard K. Ries, M.D.
Bonnie B. Wilford

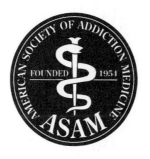

American Society of Addiction Medicine, Inc.
Chevy Chase, Maryland
2003

Published by the American Society of Addiction Medicine, Inc.

4601 North Park Avenue, Suite 101
Chevy Chase, Maryland 20815
U.S.A.

Telephone 301/656-3920
Telefax 301/656-3815
E-mail@asam.org

Principles of Addiction Medicine is a publication of the American Society of Addiction Medicine (ASAM). ASAM is a national medical specialty society of physicians who are concerned about alcoholism and other drug dependencies, and who care for persons affected by those illnesses. For information about ASAM's programs, policies and publications, contact the American Society of Addiction Medicine, 4601 North Park Ave., Suite 101, Chevy Chase, MD 20815.

First Edition 1994
Second Edition 1998
Third Edition 2003

Library of Congress Cataloging in Publication Data:

Principles of addiction medicine / edited by
    Allan W. Graham, Terry K. Schultz, Michael F. Mayo-Smith, Richard K. Ries,
    Bonnie B. Wilford — 3rd ed.
             p.cm.
    Includes bibliographical references and index.
    ISBN 1-880425-08-4
    1. Substance abuse. 2. Substance abuse—treatment.
    3. Substance abuse—diagnosis. 4. Addiction medicine
    I. Graham, Allan W. II. Schultz, Terry K.
    III. Mayo-Smith, Michael F. IV. Ries, Richard K.
    V. Wilford, Bonnie B.
    [DNLM: 1. Substance abuse.   WM 270 S941]
    RC564._____ 2003
    ISBN 1-880425-08-4

Medicine is an ever-changing science. As new research and clinical experience broaden our knowledge, changes in diagnosis and treatment are required. The Editors and publisher of this work have made every effort to ensure that the clinical recommendations and drug dosages described herein are accurate and in accord with the standards accepted at the time of publication. Readers are advised, however, that changes may occur in recommended practices as new research emerges.

Printed in the United States of America.
First Printing 2003
Second Printing 2004

ISBN: 1-880425-08-4

SENIOR EDITORS

Allan W. Graham, M.D., FACP, FASAM
Chemical Dependency Treatment Services
Kaiser Permanente
Denver, Colorado

Terry K. Schultz, M.D., FASAM
Chemical Dependency Treatment Services
Kaiser Permanente
Fairfax, Virginia

EDITORS

Michael F. Mayo-Smith, M.D., M.P.H.
Veterans Affairs Medical Center
Manchester, New Hampshire, and
Harvard Medical School
Boston, Massachusetts

Richard K. Ries, M.D.
Department of Psychiatry and Behavioral Sciences
University of Washington
Seattle, Washington

ASSOCIATE EDITOR

Bonnie B. Wilford
Center for Health Services
and Outcomes Research
Arlington, Virginia

FOR THE AMERICAN SOCIETY OF ADDICTION MEDICINE

President
Lawrence S. Brown, Jr., M.D., M.P.H., FASAM

Immediate Past President
Marc Galanter, M.D., FASAM

Chair, Publications Committee
Elizabeth F. Howell, M.D., FASAM

Executive Vice President and CEO
Eileen McGrath, J.D.

Preface to the Third Edition

The Third Edition of ASAM's *Principles of Addiction Medicine* is the product of intensive collaboration among a large number of clinicians, researchers, and scholars, many of whom are affiliated with the American Society of Addiction Medicine (ASAM), the National Institute on Alcohol Abuse and Alcoholism (NIAAA), and the National Institute on Drug Abuse (NIDA). As editors, we wish to thank our colleagues for their work, their wisdom, and their devotion in developing this textbook. The central goal of the book is to improve the medical care given to patients with addictive disorders. With the publication of the Third Edition, we believe that we have refined and enriched the definition of addiction medicine, described its neuroscientific foundations, and reviewed the most effective techniques and concepts essential to its practice.

This edition is based on the solid foundation established with the First Edition of *Principles*, edited by Drs. Norman Miller and Martin Doot, and the Second Edition, edited by Drs. Allan W. Graham and Terry K. Schultz. Like those earlier works, the Third Edition has benefited from generous gifts of time and expertise by ASAM members, by fellow physicians from a variety of specialties, and by our colleagues in the related disciplines of psychology, sociology, epidemiology, and the basic sciences. Without their support, the textbook would not have been possible. The text also has benefited from expansion of the panel of Editors with the appointment of Drs. Michael F. Mayo-Smith and Richard K. Ries.

The scientific understanding of addiction and the clinical practice of addiction medicine have advanced dramatically in the years since *Principles* first was published. Accordingly, the Third Edition has been completely revised and updated to reflect the rapidly expanding knowledge base. The Editors are confident that *Principles* will be useful to physicians who specialize in the practice of addiction medicine. Beyond that, we hope that the book will prove useful to physicians in primary care and other medical specialties, as well as to the professionals in many disciplines who care for patients with addictive disorders.

Some persons opening this book may ask, "What is addiction medicine and what makes it different from other fields of practice?" Addiction medicine is an interdisciplinary practice which specializes in the identification and treatment of persons whose disorders are caused or exacerbated by the use of addictive substances. Such substances have the unique property of promoting continued use in a compulsive manner despite adverse consequences to the user. In our society, the most notable offending substances are nicotine, alcohol, opiates, stimulant drugs, and marijuana. The services most commonly offered by specialists in addiction medicine are:

- Management of withdrawal from addictive substances;

- Consultation with other physicians concerning identification, intervention, and management of patients in hospital or office practice whose disorders are directly linked to use of these substances;

- Facilitation of patient engagement in treatment programs designed to reduce the progression of the patient's substance-related problems;

- Development of outcomes-based treatment programs for such patients;

- Environmental modifications so as to alter the social, behavioral, and pharmacologic inputs that support the continuation of substance abuse and dependence; and

- Research into the genetic and neurobiologic aspects of addiction, with the ultimate goal of developing improved methods of prevention, early intervention, and treatment (behavioral and pharmacologic) of addictive disorders.

We are grateful to ASAM and its Board of Directors for affording us the privilege of guiding this work to completion. We also express special thanks

i

to Dr. Dorynne Czechowicz of NIDA and Dr. Raye Z. Litten of NIAAA for helping us in many ways. Lastly, we are indebted to our Associate Editor, Bonnie Wilford, whose expertise as both editor and specialist in the field of addiction medicine has served us well throughout this endeavor.

We welcome readers' comments, recommendations, criticisms, and engagement, for the field of addiction medicine is evolving rapidly and all of us are responsible for nurturing its growth.

The Editors:

Allan W. Graham, M.D., FACP, FASAM
Terry K. Schultz, M.D., FASAM
Michael F. Mayo-Smith, M.D., M.P.H.
Richard K. Ries, M.D.

Contents

© 2003, AMERICAN SOCIETY OF ADDICTION MEDICINE

SECTION

1 | # Basic Science and Core Concepts

Section Coordinator

Terry K. Schultz, M.D., FASAM

Contributors

Rosa M. Crum, M.D., M.H.S.
Departments of Epidemiology, Psychiatry
   and Mental Hygiene
Welch Center for Prevention,
   Epidemiology and Clinical Research
The Johns Hopkins Medical Institutions
Baltimore, Maryland

Enoch Gordis, M.D.
Former Director
National Institute on Alcohol Abuse and Alcoholism
National Institutes of Health
Bethesda, Maryland

Alan I. Leshner, Ph.D.
President, American Academy
   for the Advancement of Science, and
Former Director
National Institute on Drug Abuse
National Institutes of Health
Bethesda, Maryland

Eric J. Nestler, M.D., Ph.D.
Department of Psychiatry and
Center for Basic Neuroscience
The University of Texas
Southwestern Medical Center
Dallas, Texas

Terry K. Schultz, M.D., FASAM
Chemical Dependency Treatment Service
Kaiser Permanente
Fairfax, Virginia

George E. Vaillant, M.D.
Professor of Psychiatry
Harvard Medical School, and
Division of Psychiatry
Brigham & Women's Hospital
Boston, Massachusetts

Roy A. Wise, Ph.D.
Behavioral Neuroscience Branch
Intramural Research Program
National Institute on Drug Abuse
National Institutes of Health
Bethesda, Maryland

Chapter 1

Natural History of Addiction and Pathways to Recovery

George E. Vaillant, M.D.

Why Does Addiction Begin?
Why Does Addiction Persist?
Why Does Addiction Cease?

Addiction is a medical disorder with a complex etiology, multiple manifestations of illness, and a varied clinical course. Nevertheless, it may be viewed as a discrete disorder with a discernible natural history. Unlike most medical disorders, however, the risk factors for the onset of addiction are surprisingly independent of the risk factors militating against eventual recovery. The major reason for this paradox is that high severity of addiction is associated with both the best and the worst long-term outcomes.

Longitudinal, prospective studies are better suited for analyzing the natural history of addiction (Vaillant, 1988) than are cross-sectional or retrospective studies. In part, this difference is because schedules of reinforcement are important in determining the effects of drugs on behavior (Morse & Kelleher, 1970). Long-term followup helps to clarify the regular sequence of events or schedules under which drugs of abuse are sought and to promote an understanding of the facets of an addict's life that facilitate recovery.

For the purposes of this chapter, the term "addiction" will encompass "substance dependence," as specified in the criteria of the *Diagnostic and Statistical Manual of Mental Disorders, 4th Edition* (*DSM-IV*) of the American Psychiat-ric Association (1994). For heuristic purposes, the chapter will divide addiction (substance dependence) into two broad facets: (1) addiction without significant premorbid psychiatric comorbidity—of which nicotine and alcohol dependence are examples—and (2) addiction that results in part from efforts at self-medication due to premorbid psychiatric comorbidity—of which heroin and polydrug abuse are examples. In order to address these two facets of addiction, the chapter will contrast alcohol and heroin addiction.

Alcoholism differs from heroin dependence in many ways. First, alcoholism generally develops slowly over a person's lifetime; it can begin at any age; and it often occurs in individuals who have little premorbid psychosocial pathology. Heroin dependence, by contrast, usually begins in young adults who have comorbid personality disorders and/or depression. Such differences arise, in part, because alcohol—like gambling and smoking—is highly addicting but a very poor anodyne. In contrast, heroin—like cocaine—relieves, over the short term, multiple sources of pain. Chronic alcoholism, however, exerts greater long-term effects on the central nervous system than does heroin use. Thus, chronic alcoholism often creates the illusion that it is the result rather than the cause of psychopathology.

TABLE 1.   Risk Factors for Addiction
In the agent:
■ Availability
■ Cost
■ Rapidity with which the agent reaches the brain
■ Efficacy of the agent as a tranquilizer.
In the environment:
■ Occupation
■ Peer group
■ Culture
■ Social instability.
In the host:
■ Genetic predisposition
■ Multiproblem family
■ Comorbid psychiatric disorder.

In order to describe the natural history of any medical disorder, three questions must be addressed: Why does it begin? Why does it persist? Why does it cease?

WHY DOES ADDICTION BEGIN?

To understand the natural history of any disorder, the major etiologic factors must be kept in mind. To do this, the critical and interactive roles played by host *and* agent *and* environment must be known. When the agent causing the addiction is readily accessible (that is, inexpensive and/or available at sales outlets that are numerous and often open), or when an agent is available in rapid-acting forms, then abuse will increase. Drug abuse may increase whenever the host is demoralized, ignorant of healthy social drug use, or susceptible to the influence of peers who are heavily involved in drug use; or when the host has a high genetic predisposition to abuse the agent or to antisocial personality; or when the host is poorly socialized into the culture or is in pain. In all of these situations, addiction may increase. Finally, addiction will increase whenever the environment makes the agent the recreational drug of choice, or fails to structure healthy drug use practices, or places no taboos on abuse, or is dysfunctional. Thus, understanding the cause and course of addiction requires knowledge of genetics, behavioral psychology, sociology, and economics, as well as pharmacology and psychopathology.

Characteristics of the Agent. An important factor in addiction, of course, is the fact that addictive agents produce physiological and psychological habituation. But addiction is far more complicated than mere pharmacology. Thus, the first risk factor to be considered is the *availability* of the agent (see Table 1). Availability has more to do with climate, economics and politics than with pharmacology. In 18th century London, for example, the advent of cheap gin as a means of economically disposing of excess grain led to an epidemic of alcoholism of devastating proportions. In contrast, alcohol abuse is rare in countries with grain shortages. This effect is seen most clearly in Moslem countries, where availability of alcohol is restricted not only by religious law and the availability of alternative mood-altering drugs, such as cannabis, but also by agricultural and climatic patterns that inhibit the production of crops from which alcohol may be produced cheaply.

In another example, the availability of cheap heroin grown in nearby Burma and Thailand led to an epidemic of heroin abuse among American troops in Vietnam, even though they lacked other risk factors. In contrast, shipping restrictions imposed during World War II virtually abolished heroin use in New York City during that period, even among previously intractable addicts who had many risk factors.

A second etiologic factor in addiction is *cost*. The ratio of heroin to cocaine abuse is at least partially a function of relative cost. The prevalence of alcoholism bears a direct relationship to per capita consumption of alcohol, and per capita consumption of alcohol bears a direct relationship to cost. Thus, to the extent that social policy affects price structure, these factors also influence alcohol abuse. However, as Moore and Gerstein (1981) have demonstrated convincingly, controlling alcohol abuse by manipulating social policy is a very difficult process.

A third factor affecting the likelihood of addiction is the *rapidity with which the agent reaches the brain*. Cultural patterns that encourage consumption of low-proof alcoholic beverages and that create social norms in which alcohol is consumed only with food—which delays its absorption into the bloodstream—reduce the likelihood of alcohol dependence. In contrast, drinking practices that encourage ingestion of high-proof alcohol in the absence of food (for example, in bars) increase the likelihood of alcohol dependence. As other examples, consider that, other factors being equal, use of intravenous short-acting heroin leads to dependence far more rapidly than does oral ingestion of long-acting methadone. Or that rapid-acting pentobarbital and alprazolam (Xanax®) are more addicting than slow-acting phenobarbital and chlordiazepoxide (Librium®).

A fourth risk factor is the agent's *efficacy as a tranquilizer*. Heroin produces effective relief of pain, anger, insomnia, hunger, and depression. Thus, heroin is an excellent agent for self-medication. In contrast, alcohol—even at low doses—interferes with sleep architecture, makes depression worse, and is little better than placebo (c.f. barbiturates) in the management of anxiety. (Alcohol is a tranquilizer only to the degree that it reduces guilt, produces muscle relaxation, and alters psychological state.) Thus, contrary to popular belief, self-medication rarely is a major etiological factor in alcohol dependence.

Characteristics of the Environment. Environment is very important as a source of both risk for and protection from addiction. Thus, *occupation* is a fifth contributing factor. Especially dangerous are occupations that break down the time-dependent rituals that help to prevent "social" drugs from being consumed around the clock. Occupations such as bartending and the diplomatic service put individuals in close contact with alcohol during most of the day. Solitary occupations, such as journalism, which deprive an individual of the structure of the work day (and unemployment, of course), also are associated with increased rates of alcoholism. Prostitution, with its accompanying danger, pain, and shame, is associated with opiate use to make the profession bearable.

A sixth source of risk is the individual's *peer group*. The choice of recreational drug—and thus, the rate of addiction—among adolescents and young adults is almost as susceptible to peer fashion as is clothing or music. On the one hand, a common reason for men to shift from a pattern of heavy, prealcoholic drinking to "social" drinking is marriage and its effect on social network. On the other hand, marriage to an alcoholic mate puts the nonalcoholic spouse at risk. Despite a vast theoretical literature implicating nonalcoholic spouses as the cause of their partners' alcohol abuse, however, prospective studies indicate that alcoholic spouses create unhappy marriages far more often than unhappy marriages create alcoholic spouses. Studies of the children of alcoholic step-parents and adoptive parents suggest that alcohol abuse usually is not environmentally transmitted from parent to child.

Culture is a seventh factor in the risk for addiction. Illegal drugs of abuse often are preferred in deviant subcultures and remain taboo among the law-abiding. For example,

passage of the Harrison Narcotic Act in 1914 motivated recovery among the majority of medically addicted morphine addicts in the United States, but had little effect on hitherto legal heroin abuse in the New York underworld. In one study that held constant other risk factors such as availability and cost, alcohol dependence was five times less common in men of Italian and other Southern European descent than in Anglo-American ethnic groups (Vaillant, 1995). Such differences can be attributed, at least in part, to variations in cultural attitudes toward alcohol consumption (Heath, 1975; Greely & McReady, 1980). For example, in the traditional Italian culture, alcohol usually is consumed with meals and, although social alcohol consumption is taught to children, intoxication is proscribed for adults. Conversely, American mores forbid children to learn social consumption of alcohol, drinking often occurs in bars apart from food and, in adults, intoxication historically has been considered humorous or "manly."

An eighth risk factor for addiction is *social instability*, which not only breaks down environmental controls for safe use of the agent, but has a powerful effect on self-care. One need only examine the interface between Western industrialized cultures and those of developing countries to appreciate that societal change and alcohol abuse often go hand in hand. Epidemics of alcoholism may be seen in the aboriginal communities at the fringes of modern Australian cities, at the interface of Native American communities and White settlements, and in the new African cities, with their sudden mix of tribal and European ways. All offer grim testimony that, for individuals to learn the safe use of potentially addicting substances, the host must painstakingly evolve societal rituals to constrain abuse. By contrast, very stable, homogeneous, integrated communities (for example, Moslem, Hasid, Mormon) increase host resistance to drug use as well as abuse. Stable communities value state change less than do communities in transition.

Characteristics of the Host. The host characteristics leading to vulnerability to use of alcohol and of heroin are very different. Thus, the ninth risk factor for addiction, *genetic predisposition*, is important for alcoholism, but twin and cross-fostering studies have not clearly implicated genetic factors in heroin addiction.

Sensitivity to the effects of alcohol serves as a protective factor for many persons (Schuckit, 1995) and facilitates sustained social use of a highly addicting substance. Early studies hypothesized that unstable childhoods with broken homes and inconsistent upbringing were a cause of future alcoholism (McCord & McCord, 1960; Robins, 1966), but more recent studies (Vaillant, 1995) have found that such association is present only when a child raised in an alcoholic family also is biologically related to the alcoholic family member.

Regular use of illegal opiates almost invariably progresses to physiological dependence. In contrast, heavy medicinal use of legally prescribed opiates often can be abandoned once the reason for the prescription ceases to exist, without the user experiencing marked craving or relapse to drug use. Such differential rates of addiction appear to lie in the host rather than the drug.

Such predisposition brings us to the tenth risk factor: *dysfunctional, multiproblem families*. Multiproblem families are an etiologic factor in delinquency of all kinds, including illegal and polydrug abuse. Many studies describe heroin addicts as coming from broken homes in which maternal supervision and affection in the preschool years was inadequate, where the father was absent, where there was little family cohesion, and where there often was parent-child cultural disparity. Few heroin addicts have regular work histories before addiction. In short, the heroin addict initiates his or her drug-seeking behavior because he or she has had very little opportunity to engage in competing forms of activity, rather than because morphine or heroin *per se* is a powerful reinforcer. These rather sweeping generalizations have been documented by comparing delinquents and addicts with nondelinquent and nonaddict controls who were matched for variables such as social class, place of residence, intelligence, and ethnic background (Glueck & Glueck, 1950; Chein, Gerard et al., 1964; Vaillant, 1966b). Being raised in a multiproblem family not only predisposes such individuals to illegal behavior, but also to the use of agents such as heroin, which pharmacologically reduce suffering.

If genetic factors are controlled for, however, multiproblem families are less important in the etiology of alcohol dependence. Many American soldiers in Vietnam became dependent on the readily available, inexpensive pure heroin for environmental reasons, but those who persisted in using heroin on their return to the States tended to be those with host vulnerabilities such as unstable childhoods and prior polydrug abuse (Robins, 1974).

An 11th major risk factor in host vulnerability to addiction is *comorbid psychiatric disorder*. Host resistance to heroin dependence and/or polydrug abuse is reduced by many Axis I disorders, including depression and anxiety,

and by Axis II disorders, particularly antisocial and borderline personality disorders. In the etiology of heroin abuse (and of alcoholism associated with polydrug abuse), antisocial personality is an important factor. In contrast, although many delinquents abuse alcohol as part of their antisocial behavior, and some will become alcoholic, the majority of alcoholics are not sociopathic except as a result of their addiction.

The common comorbidity of alcoholism and depression (Merikangas & Gelernter, 1990) has led to a belief that individuals abuse alcohol in order to self-medicate their depression. However, prospective study of the natural history of alcoholism shows that comorbid depression usually is a consequence rather than a cause of alcoholism (Vaillant, 1995). First, the children of alcoholics often are at environmental risk for depressive disorder by virtue of being raised in a dysfunctional family. They also are genetically predisposed to alcoholism. Second, the rate of alcoholism among manic-depressive patients, who (according to the self-medication hypothesis) should be using alcohol frequently, is not higher than the rate among other psychiatric patients (Woodruff, Guze et al., 1973; Morrison, 1974). Third, biochemical tests that can distinguish between genetically determined (primary) and environmentally determined (secondary) depression have found that depressed alcoholics resemble patients with evidence of environmentally induced depression rather than depressed patients with a family history of depression (Schlesser, Winokur et al., 1980). Fourth, although depression and alcoholism may run in the same families, multigenerational studies have documented that the family linkages for each disorder are genetically separate (Weissman, Gershon et al., 1984; Merikangas & Gelernter, 1990). Fifth, in clinical studies, the use of antidepressants to treat patients with both alcoholism and depression did not alter the course of the alcoholism; however, abstinence from alcohol in such patients did alleviate their depression (Brown, Irwin et al., 1988; Dorus, Ostrow et al., 1989).

Three psychiatric disorders do seem to contribute to the risk for alcoholism: antisocial personality disorder, panic disorder, and attention deficit hyperactivity disorder.

At the risk of oversimplification: culture, genes, social networks, and sociopathy all play major roles in the facets of substance abuse that are epitomized by alcohol abuse; sociopathy, dysfunctional childhoods, social alienation, rapidity of action, and psychiatric comorbidity all play major roles in substance abuse that is epitomized by heroin dependence. In any single individual, these two etiological clusters may overlap.

Women develop alcoholism for the same reasons as men: premorbid antisocial personality, hyperactivity (Glenn & Parsons, 1989), peers (especially spouses) who drink heavily, genetic predisposition, work environments conducive to heavy drinking, and being raised in cultures that forbid drinking, yet encourage drunkenness. Statistically, a woman who develops alcoholism usually manifests more risk factors than an alcoholic man (Svanum & McAdoo, 1991; Blume, 1986).

WHY DOES ADDICTION PERSIST?

Addiction is a disorder marked by remission, relapse, and, often, premature death. Because alcohol or heroin consumption by the addict—like food consumption by the obese—waxes and wanes from month to month, studies that examine the same subjects over decades are required to clarify the natural history of the disorder. Such longitudinal studies support the finding that, unlike most medical disorders, severity ("hitting bottom") in an addict can paradoxically facilitate a favorable prognosis. As a result, the 11 risk factors enumerated here are *not* statistically correlated with long-term prognosis (Vaillant, 1988, 1995). Over a lifetime, except for an earlier mean age of onset, the natural history of the heroin subtype of substance abuse does not reveal a worse prognosis than the alcohol subtype. In short-term studies, however, this paradox is less readily apparent. In clinical studies of addiction, good motivation, the presence of social resources, marital and employment stability, and lack of criminality all predict a good short-term prognosis.

During young adulthood, the course of addiction—like that of multiple sclerosis—often is progressive; after age 40, however, it may stabilize. (Chronic obesity and cigarette consumption are familiar examples of eventual stabilization.) The same leveling-off may be seen in heroin and alcohol abuse. Thus, addiction—whether to legal drugs like tobacco or to illegal ones like crack cocaine—often evolves into stable, lifelong abstinence.

Addicts with a progressive course either continue to abuse substances, despite a worsening of their problems, or they become stably abstinent, usually in response to the very severity of their addiction. As will be discussed below, however, such abstinence does not occur by chance or because the addict has "burned out," any more than heavy smokers just grow "tired" or "mature out" of cigarette use. Surprisingly, no significant differences have been found in terms of

the severity of the dependence that would distinguish individuals whose addiction progresses from those who achieve stable abstinence. Indeed, in alcohol abuse, greater severity of dependence actually is associated with a greater likelihood of stable abstinence (Vaillant, 1995).

Women with alcoholism are prone to a more fulminant clinical course than are men (Fillmore, 1987). This may be because the net effect of having more risk factors, greater shame, and thus more denial, as well as greater difficulty in obtaining treatment, puts women at risk for more rapid progression of alcohol-related complications. Alcoholic women are more likely than men to die from cirrhosis and violence; in general, they experience more medical complications from alcohol abuse than men (Ashley, Olin et al., 1977; Blume, 1986). Indeed, women who die from alcoholism and its direct sequelae do so an estimated 11 years earlier than their male counterparts (Krasner, Davis et al., 1977).

In most long-term studies, the prevalence of addiction declines steadily after age 40 (Vaillant, 1988). For example, examination of the long-term studies illustrated in Table 2 shows that among alcoholics followed for several decades, or until they were approximately 60 years old, only a third of the patients still were alcohol-dependent at the end of the period of observation (Vaillant, 1995). Few returned to stable asymptomatic drinking, but death and stable abstinence both contributed equally to the observed decline. Several studies indicate that about 2% of all alcoholics achieve stable abstinence each year, with or without treatment. Although not as well documented, similar patterns are seen for heroin abuse (Vaillant, 1988) and tobacco dependence. However, a recent 33-year followup of 242 surviving male heroin addicts (of an original cohort of 581) suggests that after 20 years, stable abstinence ceased to occur and thereafter, chronic heroin use stopped only when the subject died (Hser, Hoffman et al., 2001).

In most alcoholic individuals, the progression from social drinking to alcohol abuse to alcohol dependence occurs gradually, generally over a period of 3 to 15 years. Dependence occurs somewhat more rapidly in women than in men. In persons with higher educational levels and in men from stable families, progression to alcohol dependence occurs more slowly. Some individuals drink asymptomatically for as long as 20 or 30 years before developing alcohol abuse, and such abuse may never progress to severe dependence. Conversely, antisocial adolescent males exhibit a much more rapid onset of alcoholism, with clear physiological dependence occurring within two to five years. (It must be

TABLE 2.   Twelve Long-term Followup Studies of Alcohol Abuse

Study and nature of sample	Nature of treatment	Type and length of follow-up	Size of original sample	Attrition (%)		Number of survivors followed	Outcome for survivors (%)		
				Lost or refused	Dead		Abstinent	Asymptomatic drinkers[a]	Still alcoholic
Sundby 1967 Clinic; poor prognosis; all classes; ages 30–55	Nonspecific	Record search 20–35 years	1722	2	62	632	64		36
Goodwin, Crane & Guze 1971 Prison; alcoholic only by history; ages 20–35	Nonspecific	Interviews 8 years	c. 111	13	5	93	8	33	59
Lundquist 1973 Inpatient; good prognosis; middle class; ages 30–55	1–4 weeks in hospital	Interviews 9 years	200	0	23	155	37		63
Vaillant 1983 Inpatient; poor prognosis; men and women; ages 30–50	Detoxification; AA oriented; follow-up	Interviews 18 years	106	6	27	71	39	6	55
Ojesjo 1981 Community; good prognosis; age Σ 46	Nonspecific	Interviews 15 years	96	0	26	71	32		68
Vaillant 1996 Community; good prognosis; men; ages 10–20	Nonspecific	Questionnaire/Interviews 40–50 years	207	11	23	137	29	23	48
Marshall, Edwards & Taylor 1994; alcohol dependent men	Same as above	Interviews 20 years	99	2	43	54	44	30	26
Nordstrom and Berglund 1987 alcohol-dependent men age ca. 32; 70% excellent post-hospital adjustment	Inpatient treatment	Interviews 21 ± 4 years	105	21	NA	84	18	26	56
O'Connor and Daly 1985 men; voluntary first admission; age ca. 48	Inpatient treatment	Questionnaire 20 years	133	30	40	40	67	15	18
Smith et al. 1983 alcohol-dependent women; age ca. 44	Inpatient treatment	Interviews 11 years	103	11[a]	31	61	41[b]		59[b]
Langle et al. 1993 alcohol-dependent men and women; age ca. 38	Inpatient treatment	Interviews 10 years	96	5	22	70	70		30
Cross et al. 1990 men and women; age ca. 48	Inpatient treatment plus AA	Questionnaire 10 years	200	21	22	114	76		24

a. Percent of asymptomatic drinkers is high because it reflects point prevalence. Such outcomes were very unstable over time.
b. Estimated; text not clear.

TABLE 3. Mortality in Prospective Studies of Alcoholism

Sample	Deaths in total sample	fo/fe[a]	Number of deaths from selected causes					
			Cardio-vascular	fo/fe	Cirrhosis	fo/fe	Accident/murder/suicide	fo/fe
Sundby, 1967	1061	2	117	1.6	20	10	149	5
Schmidt & deLint, 1972	738	2	258	2	66	12	140	4
Pell & D'Alonzo, 1973	102	3	41	3	11	—	4	—
Nicholls, Edwards & Kyle, 1974	309	2.7	71	2	9	23	83	17
Polich, Armor & Braiker, 1981	111	3	23	1.2	8	8	37	10
Marshall, Edwards & Taylor, 1994	46	3.6	13	—	4	—	6	—
Vaillant[b]	80	2	23	1.4	7	6	21	10
Brenner, 1967	217	3	52	1.8	37	10	44	6
Berglund, 1985	497	2.5	144	1.5	21	4	171	8.5

a. Rate of observed deaths among alcoholics divided by rate of expected deaths in the population or of observed deaths in controls, controlling for age.
b. Unpublished current data from the 206 alcohol abusing men in the 2 cohorts described in Vaillant (1995).

appreciated, however, that pharmacological tolerance, like high blood pressure or obesity, is a matter of arbitrary definition rather than an unambiguous state, like pregnancy.)

Early onset antisocial alcoholics with alcoholic fathers are called type 2 and late-onset alcoholics are called type 1, with a postulated underlying genetic distinction (Cloninger, Sigvardsson et al., 1988). This distinction, however, probably is an artifact of the fact that type 2 alcoholics may be premorbidly antisocial because of their dysfunctional family environments and thus demonstrate the fulminant alcoholic course for environmental rather than genetic reasons.

Drug addiction profoundly hastens mortality, with cigarette smoking the most frequent cause of death. Roughly a third of alcoholics die before their 60th birthdays and, as Tables 2 and 3 illustrate, the mortality rate of alcoholics at any age is two or three times that of the nonalcoholic population. As Table 3 illustrates, most of the premature deaths are from suicide, unintentional injuries, and heart disease. Half of Hser's original sample of heroin abusers died before age 60; this was three times the expected mortality, with overdose, cirrhosis, homicide, suicide, and traumatic injury accounting for 60% of the deaths (Hser, Hoffman et al., 2001). Surprisingly, HIV/AIDS accounted for only 1% of the deaths. In their multi-decade followup studies of heroin addicts, O'Donnell (1969) and Vaillant (1973) also found

death rates almost three times those expected, and a similar pattern of unnatural deaths.

To summarize, possible long-term outcomes of substance abuse include stable abstinence, a return to controlled asymptomatic use, continued abuse, and premature death. In part, outcome depends on habit strength which, in turn, is determined by the duration and severity of dependence. Thus, in adolescents, excessive drinking that meets *DSM-IV* criteria for substance dependence can evolve into a life-long pattern of moderate consumption. After several years, however, such plasticity becomes increasingly rare (Jessor, 1987; Fillmore, 1987). For example, in an eight-year followup study, one third of felons under age 30 who met the criteria for alcoholism successfully returned to asymptomatic drinking (Goodwin, Crane et al., 1971). In contrast, long-term followup studies of Harvard graduates and inner-city males who were abusing alcohol at age 40 found that eventual return to asymptomatic drinking rarely was successful. The difference is that a young felon can meet the diagnostic criteria for alcoholism with far less chronicity and dependence than can a middle-aged prosecutor.

WHY DOES ADDICTION CEASE?

Detoxification, while often life-saving and useful in providing an opportunity for education, in itself rarely alters the natural history of addiction. Three useful analogous situations are going on a successful six-week diet, going to the hospital for diabetic acidosis, and stopping smoking for Lent. All are examples of detoxifications that, however successful, do not affect the natural history of a disorder. Table 4 summarizes two longitudinal studies of addiction which suggest that, for both alcohol and heroin dependence, detoxification is associated with relapse rates so high that they have little bearing on the natural history of the disorder. The findings in Table 4 are consistent with many other studies that have found that single episodes of detoxification have little long-term effect on addiction (Lindstrom, 1992).

There are many reasons why this is so. First, detoxification addresses only the problem of physiologic dependence. It ignores the underlying, inadvertently reinforced behaviors implicit in the multifactorial etiology of addiction, as discussed earlier. Second, with chronic use, narcotics may provide little or no conscious gratification (similarly, later in an alcoholic's drinking career, alcohol consumption produces more dysphoria than it relieves [McNamee, Mendelson et al., 1968]). Thus, once dependence is established, the reinforcing properties of drug self-administration serve in large part to avoid the discomfort of real or imagined withdrawal. Over time, craving and withdrawal symptoms become maintained by many nonpharmacological reinforcers. Friends and holidays, pubs and bierstuben, rituals of injection and syringes, all acquire reinforcing properties and become unconscious stimuli for relapse.

Third, even withdrawal symptoms themselves are not simple physiologic responses to the withdrawal of biologically active substances. Withdrawal symptoms, too, are under considerable control of schedules of behavior and past experience. The withdrawal symptoms of monkeys can be relieved effectively by injections of saline, if the saline is administered in settings in which morphine was given in the past (Thompson & Schuster, 1964). On research wards, men who have been abstinent for months can experience acute craving and signs of withdrawal (for example, lacrimation, runny nose, and gooseflesh) while watching another addict receive an injection of narcotics.

The converse also is true. If morphine-addicted monkeys are given nalorphine, withdrawal symptoms are abruptly precipitated. When morphine-satiated monkeys are given saline instead of nalorphine, withdrawal symptoms still occur (Goldberg & Schuster, 1966). Studies in humans suggest that the memory of mental discomfort that, in the past, was relieved by opiates can evoke conditioned

TABLE 4. Relative Efficacy of Different Modes of Treatment

	Known "treatment" exposures	% Followed by 1 year of abstinence
100 Heroin Addicts (followed 20 years)		
Hospital Detoxification	361	3
Short Imprisonment	363	3
Prison and > 1 year of Parole	34	71
Methadone Maintenance	15	67
100 Alcoholics (followed 8 years)		
Hospital Detoxification	c. 1500	3
300 + Visits to AA	19	74

SOURCE: Vaillant GE (1988). What can long-term follow-up teach us about relapse and prevention of relapse in addiction? *British Journal of Addiction* 83:1147-1157.

withdrawal signs (Dole & Nyswander, 1965). Conversely, in a highly structured laboratory setting (for example, Sobell & Sobell, 1983; Merry, 1966), active alcoholics who had binged uncontrollably in community settings could drink alcohol in moderation. In short, the sources of relapse or non-relapse depend on environmental cues as much as they do on pharmacologic determinants and conscious motivation.

Fourth, as is implicit in the *DSM-IV* definition of substance dependence, over time drug addiction assumes the characteristics of a career. In someone whose daily life lacks the pattern provided by a job, addiction imposes a very definite and gratifying, if rather stereotyped, pattern of behavior. Having been adolescent "misfits"—both in school and in street gangs—some heroin addicts finally achieve a means of social reinforcement. Thus, drug addiction provides an ersatz occupation, but a very absorbing one. In similar fashion, Hodgson and colleagues (1978) noted that alcohol dependence can be defined by the degree to which alcohol-seeking and consumption become the individual's most salient and preoccupying source of gratification.

To summarize, many of the reinforcing consequences and antecedents of drug addiction have no direct pharmacologic basis. For a given individual, the temporal pattern of drug use may be maintained almost entirely by secondary reinforcers. It is not surprising, then, that addicts, upon release from weeks of inpatient treatment, can relapse into substance abuse within a few months despite firm conscious resolutions to the contrary. Not only does a history of poorly patterned social behavior contribute to the initiation of addiction, but the substitute behavioral patterns that evolve as a result of addiction become strongly associated with relapse. What is needed is for addicts to alter their whole pattern of living.

No known "cure" exists for alcohol, tobacco, or heroin dependence. Some addicts appear to recover completely without clinical treatment, while others experience an inexorably fatal course even with extensive clinical treatment. The natural history of addiction is more likely to be affected by informal, even inadvertent, relapse prevention than it is by many clinical treatment regimens.

First, as already noted, the control that a drug exerts over an individual's behavior depends only modestly on its pharmacologic properties (Marlatt & Rohsenow, 1980). Thus, to focus too closely on detoxification is to miss the forest for the trees. Second, to a remarkable degree, relapse to drugs is independent of conscious free will and motivation. Finally, most clinical studies of substance abuse have been too brief to clarify the recovery process. On the one hand, it has been demonstrated repeatedly that a majority of treated addicts will function better and use less drugs in a given month after treatment than in a month immediately prior to admission. This is because, as with any chronic illness with a fluctuating course, hospitalization usually is sought during clinical nadirs; thus, seeming improvements post-treatment may be less hopeful than they appear. On the other hand, also due to probability, most clinical studies are overweighted with chronically relapsing patients. Thus, post-treatment failures are not as common as they appear.

Recovery from addiction can occur in two ways: stable abstinence (the only "cure" for two-pack-a-day cigarette smokers) or a less stable return to controlled asymptomatic use (the only "cure" for obesity). Stable abstinence, like "recovery" after surgery for cancer, is an actuarial term. As with many forms of cancer, remissions of less than two years often are transient. On the other hand, if abstinence lasts for more than five years, there is a greater probability for cancer patients, for heroin addicts (Hser, Hoffman et al., 2001), and for alcoholics (Vaillant, 1996) that the remission will be permanent.

Stable abstinence depends on relapse prevention, not detoxification. Relapse prevention most often is achieved through a strict but gratifying regimen to which the patient voluntarily consents and that consistently alters his or her behavior in the community over time. Perhaps the clearest example of such a regimen is the return of practice privileges to addicted physicians on condition that they agree to undergo random supervised urine testing and attend support groups. Stable abstinence thus requires both carrot and stick.

Often, successful regimens leading to abstinence are not a result of intentional clinical treatment programs. Such regimens can be identified by conducting community studies of the natural history of addicts who recover and those who do not. The critical ingredients appear to include abstinence that (1) occurs in the community and lasts for years rather than months, (2) is the product of compulsory supervision or experiencing a consistently aversive experience related to alcohol or drug use, (3) involves finding a substitute activity to compete with substance use, (4) requires developing a new drug-free social network, and (5) includes membership in a self-help group (through which one may discover a sustained source of hope, inspiration, and self-esteem in religion or Alcoholics Anonymous [AA]). In their extensive review of the literature on remission from abuse of tobacco, food, opiates, and alcohol, Stall and Biernacki (1986) identified the same five factors, all of which serve to alter behavior over time and all of which are independent of conscious motivation.

Prolonged Extinction of Secondary Reinforcers. In order to be stable, abstinence must be maintained for years in settings that closely resemble those in which drugs were consumed in the past. One reason that supervised abstinence (whether under parole, disulfiram, or AA) (see Table 4) may be more enduring than voluntary abstinence achieved after formal treatment or during geographic "cures" is that supervised community abstinence occurs in the presence of many secondary reinforcers (other addicts, drug sellers, community stressors, and the like). When secondary reinforcers continue to be present, but in the absence of pharmacologic reinforcement, the reinforcers lose their effectiveness in controlling the addict's behavior.

Compulsory Supervision. As Table 4 suggests, external interventions that restructure the patient's life in the community—such as parole, methadone maintenance, and AA—often are associated with sustained abstinence. The analogy between the treatment of addiction and that of diabetes is helpful. The diabetic patient's control over his or her illness must take place in the community through modification of lifestyle and, often, lifelong habits, as well as consistent use of prescribed medications. Relapse always is possible and will power, alone, is all too fallible. In diabetes, such conscious awareness of relapse is maintained by daily rituals like urine testing and dietary restrictions and substitutions. Compulsory supervision is not successful if it only punishes; instead, it should focus on altering the individual's schedule of reinforcement and providing alternative sources of gratification. For example, in the studies described in Table 4, parole required weekly proof of employment by heroin addicts who previously were convinced that they could not hold a job. Parole-enforced work provided structure to the recovering addict's life, and such structure interferes with addiction. In addition, parole—like disulfiram and painful alcohol-induced medical complaints—provided an external reminder of the consequences of relapse. Finally, parole also altered old social networks and thus removed another common factor in relapse.

Compulsory abstinence from alcohol is similarly reinforced by events contingent on alcohol use that systematically and negatively alter the consequences of alcohol consumption. These events, rather than "will power" or warnings about liver disease (which is painless in onset), remind the alcoholic that alcohol is an "enemy." Such contingent events may be medical consequences (for example, painful stomach problems exacerbated by alcohol consumption), or legal consequences (such as probation), or even chemicals (such as disulfiram [Antabuse®]).

Substitute Dependencies. Principles of behavior modification help to explain why substitute dependencies (that is, competing behaviors) are useful in altering the recovering person's behavior. The importance of providing competing behaviors in preventing relapse is illustrated by the failure of disulfiram administration alone to prove more effective than placebo in facilitating long-term abstinence from alcohol use. Disulfiram reinforces abstinence from alcohol use, but it does not provide a competing behavior. Substitute dependencies can take many different forms, ranging from the somewhat maladaptive (for example, chain smoking, compulsive working, or gambling) to the clinically designed (such as learning to sip a glass of soda at cocktail parties or becoming "addicted" to attending a methadone maintenance clinic).

New Social Networks. Formation of stable new social relationships often is associated with remission (Vaillant, 1988). New social networks help to extinguish many of the secondary reinforcers associated with relapse. Therapeutic communities and AA "home groups" offer perhaps the best example of such networks. Such communities do not ask the recovering individual to bond to family members, whose presence may induce shame, or to non-addicts with whom they cannot identify. Rather, they ask him or her to bond with a group of companions whose only novel characteristic is that they do not use alcohol or drugs. It is especially valuable for the recovering individual to associate with people they have not hurt in the past. This is true in part because shame and guilt are among the few dysphoric emotions that are relieved by alcohol. Thus, studies suggest that while marital therapy is good for family stability and communication, it has little effect on the long-term outcome of alcohol treatment (Orford & Edwards, 1977).

Inspirational Group Membership. In *The Varieties of Religious Experience,* William James (1902) articulated the close relationship between religious conversion and recovery from intractable addiction. Miller and C'de Baca (2001) have furthered developed this concept. Sudden "conversion" to abstinence also is triggered through what Knupfer (1972) called "strangely trivial" but significant accidents. Instead of being miraculous, however, such "conversion" experiences often have been incubating for some time. Always the psychic task of successful treatment is to transmute the addict's mind set so that the beloved drug is transformed from friend to foe. Both evangelical religious involvement and participation in groups like AA can effect such conversion. Enhanced hope and/or self-esteem assists addicts in maintaining abstinence. Intense religious involvement also provides group forgiveness and relieves feelings of shame over past relapses (which can fuel future relapses). Membership in such groups also provides a "new nonstigmatized identity," which is cited as important by Stall and Biernacki (1986).

AA and inspirational residential communities provide the other three ingredients found in naturalistic studies of relapse prevention: compulsory supervision, substitute dependencies, and a non-addicted, non-delinquent, non-guilt-inducing social network. As Table 4 suggests, stably abstinent individuals are more likely to attend AA meetings regularly than are those who relapse (Vaillant, 1995). Although it is not entirely clear whether AA attendance is a cause or a consequence of abstinence, the strong association between AA participation and abstinence cannot be attributed to premorbid social stability (Vaillant, Clark et al., 1983) or even to prior motivation for abstinence (Miller et al., 1992) or to the lack of severity of alcoholism (Vaillant, 1996; Timko, Moos et al., 1999). However, followup of the Project MATCH clients offers perhaps the best evidence yet that AA is at least as effective as cognitive-behavioral therapy or motivational interviewing (Project MATCH, 1999).

Increasingly, the five factors described above are becoming the basis of clinical relapse prevention programs. Methadone maintenance programs can provide not only compulsory supervision by requiring random urine screens but also a direct substitute for heroin. Court-mandated commitment to therapeutic communities also effects sustained alterations in community behavior through compulsory supervision, substitute dependency, self-esteem building, and drug-free social networks. The same principles also apply to abstinence-focused cognitive-behavioral techniques. In addition to providing positive feedback in response to successful abstinence and facilitating the recall of alcohol-related negative experiences, cognitive-behavioral programs often encourage the recovering individual to develop a plan to stop drinking that enlists the help of others, incorporates ways to recognize an imminent relapse, identifies substitutes for drinking, and establishes social supports to help reinforce sobriety (Marlatt & Gordon, 1985).

Abstinence. Although many highly regarded treatment programs consider sustained abstinence the only desirable outcome, the effects of abstinence on the alcoholic's physical and psychological well-being rarely have been examined over prolonged periods of time. Certainly, abstinence does not automatically restore an alcoholic's physical and psychological health. Prospective studies of community samples (Vaillant, 1995) have noted that abstinence, if maintained for more than three years, improved the psychological health and quality of life of securely abstinent alcoholics, but such beneficial effects of abstinence may take several years to develop. For example, divorce and depression are common among newly abstinent alcoholics who must readjust to their familial responsibilities and occupational roles. In some studies, the short-term death rate among abstinent alcoholics was similar to that among progressive alcoholics. Kurtines and colleagues (1978) found that newly abstinent alcoholics were "less normal" on several measures of psychological functioning than were alcoholics who had been abstinent for more than four years. Thus, abstinence should not be considered in isolation but within a context of overall social rehabilitation that may require years to achieve.

Return to Asymptomatic Drinking. A few addicts with atypical course either maintain a relatively stable pattern of intermittent substance abuse without dependence from a young age, or they return to controlled use of the substance that they once abused. In general, such atypical addicts have fewer drug-related problems and do not develop physiological dependence. They also experience a later onset and manifest fewer risk factors.

Several studies of less than two years' duration have suggested that the natural history of alcohol dependence includes not only abstinence but also a return to asymptomatic or "controlled" drinking (Edwards & Grant, 1980; Sobell & Sobell, 1983). Compared with individuals who remained alcoholic or who became abstinent, the alcoholic careers of such controlled drinkers were significantly less symptomatic, and the presence of physiological dependence was extremely rare. Proponents likened such outcomes to situations in which individuals with high blood pressure or diabetes learned to control their illness through lifestyle changes and diet alone.

More prolonged followup, however, has demonstrated that, even in these selected individuals, return to controlled drinking is a very unstable outcome (Edwards, 1985; Pendery, Maltzman et al., 1982; Miller et al., 1992). In one study, by age 60, only 6 of 42 men once classified as stable asymptomatic drinkers still qualified as such (Vaillant, 1995); the others had relapsed, become stably abstinent, left the study, or been reclassified as not meeting the criteria for alcohol abuse. Similarly, Helzer and colleagues (1985) found that among 1,289 clinically treated alcoholics, fewer than 2% returned to asymptomatic drinking for more than two years.

In summary, when clinicians plan interventions, they must determine where patients are in the natural history of their disorder. In the initial phases of the treatment career of any alcoholic, a trial of return to controlled drinking almost always is worth the effort (Sanchez-Craig & Lei, 1986). Once such efforts have been documented to fail, clinician and patient can focus on abstinence as the goal of choice.

CONCLUSIONS

On the one hand, we must cease to conceptualize addiction as simply a more or less voluntary use of a psychoactive drug in order to provide self-medication, self-indulgence, or the relief of physiologic withdrawal symptoms. Instead, it is more accurate to conceive of addiction as a career—that is, as a whole constellation of conditioned, unconscious behaviors more akin to destructive fingernail biting than to self-medication. When addiction is viewed as a loss of behavioral plasticity, the importance of behavior modification techniques becomes clear. With this understanding, clinicians can understand why abstinence, parole, methadone maintenance, and AA may be superior to insight, conventional detoxification, disulfiram, and scripted admonitions to "cut down." Sustained community interventions serve to impose a structure on the recovering person's life. Such structure interferes with unconscious drug-seeking behavior based on conditioned withdrawal symptoms and secondary reinforcers.

On the other hand, the natural history of chronic substance dependence also must evoke our compassion. Active substance dependence produces enormous suffering. To deny palliation through short-term treatment because we are not always certain that such an intervention will alter the natural history of the illness is as inhumane as denying short-term palliation to patients with multiple sclerosis and diabetes because such treatment does not alter the natural history of their diseases. First, if detoxification does not always cure, it does reduce mortality and suffering. Second, no matter how refractory addiction seems, addicts should not be excluded from medical insurance coverage, from treatment by emergency departments and/or detoxification centers, or from shelters for those who are homeless. One of the great lessons to be learned from prolonged followup of addicts is that stable remission may occur among the most unlikely prospects.

Finally, many controlled cost-benefit studies conclude that the expense of providing treatment is more than recovered through declines in medical care utilization, in lost time from work, and in reduced health benefit costs. Thus, to understand the natural history of addiction, we must consider more than substance use.

REFERENCES

American Psychiatric Association (1994). *Diagnostic and Statistical Manual of Mental Disorders, 4th Edition (DSM-IV).* Washington, DC: American Psychiatric Press.

Ashley MJ, Olin JS, le Riche WH et al. (1977). Morbidity in alcoholics: Evidence for accelerated development of physical disease in women. *Archives of Internal Medicine* 137:883-887.

Berglund M (1985). Cerebral dysfunction in alcoholism related to mortality and long-term social adjustment. *Alcoholism: Clinical & Experimental Research* 9:153-157.

Blume SB (1986). Women and alcohol: A review. *Journal of the American Medical Association* 256:1467-1470.

Brenner B (1967). Alcoholism and fatal accidents. *Quarterly Journal of Studies on Alcohol* 28:517-528.

Brown SA, Irwin M & Schuckit MA (1988). Changes in depression among abstinent alcoholics. *Journal of Studies on Alcohol* 49:412-417.

Chein I, Gerard D, Lee R et al. (1964). *The Road to H.* New York, NY: Basic Books.

Cloninger CR, Sigvardsson S & Bohman M (1988). Childhood personality predicts alcohol abuse in young adults. *Alcoholism: Clinical & Experimental Research* 12(4):494-505.

Cros GM et al. (1990). Alcoholism treatment: A ten-year follow-up study. *Alcoholism: Clinical & Experimental Research* 14:169-173.

Dole VP & Nyswander M (1965). A medical treatment for diacetylmorphine (heroin) addiction. *Journal of the American Medical Association* 193:646-650.

Dorus W, Ostrow DG, Anton R et al. (1989). Lithium treatment of depressed and nondepressed alcoholics. *Journal of the American Medical Association* 162:1646-1652.

Edwards G (1985). A later follow-up of a classic case series: D.L. Davies' (1962) report and its significance for the present. *Journal of Studies on Alcohol* 46:181-190.

Edwards G & Grant M, eds. (1980). *Alcoholism Treatment in Transition.* London, England: Croom Helm.

Fillmore KM (1987). Women's drinking across adult life course as compared to men's: A longitudinal and cohort analysis. *British Journal of Addiction* 82:801-812.

Glenn SW & Parsons OA (1989). Alcohol abuse and familial alcoholism: Psychosocial correlates in men and women. *Journal of Studies on Alcohol* 50:116-127.

Glueck S & Glueck E (1950). *Unraveling Juvenile Delinquency.* New York, NY: Commonwealth Fund.

Goldberg S & Schuster CR (1966). Classic conditioning of the morphine withdrawal syndrome. *Federation Proceedings* 25:261.

Goodwin DW, Crane JB & Guze SB (1971). Felons who drink: An 8-year follow-up. *Quarterly Journal of Studies on Alcohol* 32:136-147.

Greely A & McReady WC (1980). *Ethnic Drinking Subcultures.* New York, NY: Praeger.

Heath DB (1975). A critical review of ethnographic studies of alcohol use. In RJ Gibbins et al. (eds.) *Research Advances in Alcohol and Drug Problems, 2nd Edition.* New York, NY: John Wiley & Sons.

Helzer JE, Robins LN, Taylor JR et al. (1985). The extent of long-term moderate drinking among alcoholics discharged from medical and psychiatric treatment facilities. *New England Journal of Medicine* 312(26):1678-1685.

Hodgson RT, Stockwell T, Rankin H et al. (1978). Alcohol dependence: The concept, its utility and measurement. *British Journal of Addiction* 73:339-342.

Hser Y-I, Hoffman V, Grella GE et al. (2001). A 33-year follow-up of narcotics addicts. *Archives of General Psychiatry* 58:503-508.

James W (1902). *The Varieties of Religious Experience.* London, England: Longmans Green.

Jessor R (1987). Problem-behavior theory, psychosocial development and adolescent problem drinking. *British Journal of Addiction* 82:331-342.

Jones KR & Vischi TR (1979). Impact of drug abuse and mental health on treatment of medical care utilization. *Medical Care* 17(Suppl):1-81.

Krasner N, Davis M, Portmann B et al. (1977). Changing pattern of alcohol liver disease in Great Britain: Relation to sex and signs of autoimmunity. *British Medical Journal* 1:1497-1500.

Knupfer G (1972). Ex-problem drinkers. In M Roff, L Tobins & M Pollack (eds.) *Life History Research and Psychopathology.* Minneapolis, MN: University of Minnesota Press, 256-280.

Kurtines WM, Ball LR & Wood GH (1978). Personality characteristics of long-term recovered alcoholics: A comparative analysis. *Journal of Consulting and Clinical Psychology* 46:971-977.

Langle G et al. (1993). Ten years after—The post-treatment course of alcoholism. *European Psychiatry* 8:95-100.

Lindström L (1992). *Managing Alcoholism.* Oxford, England: Oxford University Press.

Lundquist GAR (1973). Alcohol dependence. *Acta Psychiatrica Scandinavica* 49:332-340.

Mann RE, Smart R, Anglin L et al. (1991). Reductions in cirrhosis deaths in the United States: Associations with per capita consumption and AA membership. *Journal of Studies on Alcohol* 52:361-365.

Marlatt GA & Gordon JR, eds. (1985). *Relapse Prevention: Maintenance Strategies in the Treatment of Addictive Behaviors.* New York, NY: Guilford Press.

Marlatt G & Rohsenow DJ (1980). Cognitive processes in alcohol use: Expectancy and the balanced placebo design. In NK Mello (ed.) *Advances in Substance Abuse: Behavioral and Biological Research.* Greenwich, CT: JAI Press.

Marshall EJ, Edwards G & Taylor C (1994). Mortality in men with drinking problems: A 20 year follow-up. *Addiction* 89.

McCord W & McCord J (1960). *Origins of Alcoholism.* Stanford, CA: Stanford University Press.

McNamee HB, Mendelson JH & Mello NK (1968). Experimental analysis of drinking patterns of alcoholics, concurrent psychiatric observations. *American Journal of Psychiatry* 124:1063-1069.

Merikangas KR & Gelernter CS (1990). Comorbidity for alcoholism and depression. *Psychiatric Clinics of North America* 13:613-632.

Merry J (1966). The loss of control myth. *Lancet* 1:1257-1258.

Miller WR et al. (1992). Long-term follow-up of behavioral self-control training. *Journal of Studies on Alcohol* 53:249-261.

Miller WR & C'de Baca J (2001). *Quantum Change.* New York, NY: Guilford Press.

Moore NIH & Gerstein DR, eds. (1981). *Alcohol and Public Policy: Beyond the Shadow of Prohibition.* Washington, DC: National Academy Press.

Morrison JR (1974). Bipolar affective disorder and alcoholism. *American Journal of Psychiatry* 131:1130-1133.

Morse WH & Kelleher RT (1970). Schedules as fundamental determinants of behavior. In WN Schoenfeld (ed.) *The Theory of Reinforcement Schedules.* New York, NY: Appleton-Century-Crofts.

Mottin JL (1973). Drug induced attenuation of alcohol consumption. *Quarterly Journal of Studies on Alcohol* 34:444-472.

Nicholls P, Edwards G & Kyle E (1974). A study of alcoholics admitted to four hospitals, II: General and cause-specific mortality during follow-up. *Quarterly Journal of Studies on Alcohol* 35:841-855.

Nordstrom G & Berglund M (1987). Type 1 and Type 2 alcoholics (Cloninger and Bohman) have different patterns of successful long-term adjustment. *British Journal of Addiction* 82:761-769.

O'Connor A & Daly J (1985). Alcoholics: A twenty year follow-up study. *British Journal of Psychiatry* 146:645-647.

O'Donnell JA (1969). *Narcotic Addicts in Kentucky (U.S. Public Health Service Pub. No. 1881).* Washington, DC: U.S. Government Printing Office.

Ojesjo L (1981). Long-term outcome in alcohol abuse and alcoholism among males in the Lundby general population, Sweden. *British Journal of Addiction* 76(4):391-400.

Orford J & Edwards G (1977). *Alcoholism.* Oxford, England: Oxford University Press.

Pell S & D'Alonzo CA (1973). A five year mortality study of alcoholics. *Journal of Occupational Medicine* 15:120-125.

Pendery ML, Maltzman IM & West LJ (1982). Controlled drinking by alcoholics? New findings and a reevaluation of a major affirmative study. *Science* 217:169-175.

Polich JM, Armor J & Braiker HB (1981). *The Course of Alcoholism.* New York, NY: John Wiley & Sons.

Project MATCH Research Group (Babor TF, Miller WR, DiClemente C et al., eds.) (1999). Comments on Project MATCH: Matching alcohol treatments to client heterogeneity. *Addiction* 94:31-69.

Reiff S, Griffith B, Forsythe AB et al. (1981). Utilization of medical services by alcoholics participating in a health maintenance organization outpatient treatment program: Three year follow-up. *Alcoholism: Clinical & Experimental Research* 5:559-562.

Robins LN (1966). *Deviant Children Grown Up: A Sociological and Psychiatric Study of Sociopathic Personality.* Baltimore. MD: Williams & Wilkins.

Robins LN (1974). The Vietnam drug user returns. In *Special Action Office Monograph Series A (No. 2).* Washington, DC: U.S. Government Printing Office.

Sanchez-Craig M & Lei H (1986). Disadvantages to imposing the goal of abstinence on problem drinkers: An empirical study. *British Journal of Addiction* 81:505-512.

Schlesser MA, Winokur G & Sherman BM (1980). Hypothalamic-pituitary-adrenal axis activity in depressive illness. *Archives of General Psychiatry* 37:737-743.

Schmidt W & deLint J (1972). Causes of death of alcoholics. *Quarterly Journal of Studies on Alcohol* 33:171-185.

Schuckit MA (1995). A long-term study of sons of alcoholics. *Alcohol Health & Research World* 19(3):172-175.

Smith EM, Cloninger CR & Bradford S (1983). Predictors of mortality in alcoholic women: A prospective follow-up study. *Alcoholism: Clinical & Experimental Research* 7:237-243.

Sobell MB & Sobell L (1983). *The Behavioral Treatment of Alcohol Problems.* New York, NY: Plenum Press.

Stall R & Biemacki P (1986). Spontaneous remission from the problematic use of substances: An inductive model derived from a comparative analysis of the alcohol, opiate, tobacco and food/obesity literatures. *International Journal of the Addictions* 21:1-23.

Sundby P (1967). *Alcoholism and Mortality.* Oslo, Norway: Universitets Forlaget.

Svanum S & McAdoo WG (1991). Parental alcoholism: An examination of male and female alcoholics in treatment. *Journal of Studies on Alcohol* 52:127-132.

Thompson T & Schuster CR (1964). Morphine self-administration, food reinforce, and avoidance behaviors in rhesus monkeys. *Psychopharmacologia* 5:87-94.

Timko C, Moos RH, Finney JW et al. (1999). Long-term treatment careers and outcomes of previously untreated alcoholics. *Journal of Studies on Alcohol* 60:437-447.

Vaillant GE (1966b). A 12 year follow-up of New York narcotic addicts, III. Some social and psychiatric characteristics. *Archives of General Psychiatry* 15:599-609.

Vaillant GE (1973). A 20 year follow-up of New York narcotic addicts. *Archives of General Psychiatry* 29:237-241.

Vaillant GE (1996). A long-term follow-up of male alcohol abuse. *Archives of General Psychiatry* 53:243-249.

Vaillant GE (1988). What can long-term follow-up teach us about relapse and prevention of relapse in addiction? *British Journal of Addiction* 83:1147-1157.

Vaillant GE (1995). *Natural History of Alcoholism, Revisited.* Cambridge, MA: Harvard University Press.

Vaillant GE, Clark W, Cyrus C et al. (1983). The natural history of alcoholism: An eight year follow-up. *American Journal of Medicine* 75:455-466.

Weissman MM, Gershon ES, Kidd KK et al. (1984). Psychiatric disorders in the relatives of probands with affective disorders. *Archives of General Psychiatry* 41:13-21.

Woodruff RA, Guze SB, Clayton PJ et al. (1973). Alcoholism and depression. *Archives of General Psychiatry* 28:97-100.

Chapter 2

The Epidemiology of Addictive Disorders

Rosa M. Crum, M.D., M.H.S.

Some Epidemiologic Principles
Prevalence of Alcohol Disorders
Incidence of Alcohol Disorders
Prevalence of Drug Use Disorders
Incidence of Drug Use Disorders
Correlates and Suspected Risk Factors
Comorbidity of Alcohol and Drug Addiction

This chapter is organized to cover several areas. First, epidemiologic terms and types of epidemiologic studies are discussed. Second, the literature regarding prevalence and incidence rates of alcohol and drug use disorders is reviewed. The remainder of the chapter is devoted to discussing some of the correlates and risk factors associated with alcohol and drug use disorders.

SOME EPIDEMIOLOGIC PRINCIPLES

Epidemiology "is concerned with the patterns of disease occurrence in human populations and of the factors that influence those patterns" (Lilienfeld & Lilienfeld, 1980). Some basic terms used in epidemiology deserve attention in this chapter, because they are important to understanding the literature and some of the studies reported here. *Prevalence* generally is taken to represent the ratio of the total number of cases of a particular disease, divided by the total number of individuals in a particular population at a specific time. *Incidence* refers to the rate of occurrence of new cases of a disease, divided by the total number at risk for the disorder during a specified period of time (Mausner & Kramer, 1985). Prevalence takes into account both the in-

cidence and duration of a disease, because it depends not only on the proportion of newly developed cases over time, but also on the length of time the disease exists in the population. In turn, the duration of the disorder is affected by the degree of recovery and death from the disease. Incidence generally is taken to represent the risk of disease, whereas prevalence is an indicator of the public health burden the disease imposes on the community (Mausner & Kramer, 1985).

The strength of association between a particular characteristic and the development of disease generally is represented by the *relative risk,* or the estimated relative risk (often called the odds ratio). The relative risk measures the incidence of disease among those with a particular characteristic (such as family history of alcohol addiction), divided by the incidence of disease among those without exposure to that characteristic. If there is no difference in the incidence rates among those with and without the characteristic, the ratio is equal to one. A relative risk greater than one indicates an increased risk of disease associated with a given characteristic. A relative risk less than one signifies a lower risk, which may indicate a protective effect associated with the characteristic.

Excellent detailed discussions of epidemiologic studies can be found elsewhere (Gordis, 2000; Lilienfeld, 1994; Mausner & Kramer, 1985). For the purposes of this chapter, epidemiologic studies can be divided into two types: (1) observational or (2) experimental. Observational studies may include cross-sectional, case-control, or cohort studies. In cross-sectional studies or surveys, individuals are assessed (by interview or physical examination, for example) at a particular point in time (Mausner & Kramer, 1985). Analytic studies usually are classified as case-control (retrospective) or cohort (longitudinal, prospective). Analytic studies generally test a hypothesis of a suspected association between a particular exposure (risk factor) and a disease.

In all observational studies, the investigator observes the study participants and gathers information for analysis (Mausner & Kramer, 1985). In contrast, experimental studies, such as randomized clinical trials, are designed by the investigator, study groups are selected, and often an intervention (such as a new type of treatment) is given to one group of participants. The study participants are followed and the outcomes of each group are measured and compared.

PREVALENCE OF ALCOHOL DISORDERS

Several major surveys in the U.S. and internationally have assessed the prevalence of addiction. Comparison of these studies sometimes is difficult because they employ different definitions of addiction. Recent surveys have used structured interviews according to criteria that have become universally recognized, such as the *Diagnostic and Statistical Manual of Mental Disorders* (APA, 2000), now in a revised fourth edition, and the *International Classification of Diseases*, now in its 10th revision (WHO, 1992).

The earliest survey to assess the epidemiology of psychiatric and substance use disorders in the United States using a structured psychiatric interview was the National Institute of Mental Health's Epidemiologic Catchment Area (ECA) study (Eaton & Kessler, 1985; Eaton, Kramer et al., 1989b; Robins & Regier, 1991). Baseline interviews for this study were conducted between 1980 and 1984, when collaborators in the ECA assessed a probability sample of more then 20,000 adult participants in five metropolitan areas of the United States. Using the Diagnostic Interview Schedule (DIS) (Robins, Helzer et al., 1981), diagnoses of substance abuse and dependence were assessed according to criteria from the *Diagnostic and Statistical Manual of Mental Disorders, 3rd Edition* (*DSM-III*; American Psychiatric Association, 1980). Overall rates of alcohol disorders in the ECA survey data were 13.5% for lifetime prevalence, 4.8% for six-month prevalence, and 2.8% for one-month prevalence (Regier, Farmer et al., 1990). However, stratification by gender revealed large rates for men compared with those for women. Lifetime prevalence for men was found to be 23.8%, with a one-year prevalence rate of 11.9% (Helzer, Burnam et al., 1991). For women, the lifetime prevalence for an alcohol disorder was 4.7%, with a one-year prevalence rate of 2.2% (Helzer, Burnam et al., 1991). ECA survey results consistently showed higher lifetime, one-year and one-month prevalence rates for men than for women across all age and racial groups (Helzer, Burnam et al., 1991).

More recent studies have identified alcohol use disorders according to the criteria of the revised third (*DSM-IIIR*) and fourth (*DSM-IV*) editions of the *Diagnostic and Statistical Manuals of Mental Disorders* (APA, 1987, 1994). Findings from the National Comorbidity Survey (NCS), completed in 1990-1992, which used *DSM-IIIR* criteria for abuse and dependence and a modified version of the Composite International Diagnostic Interview (CIDI), yielded higher lifetime and 12-month prevalence estimates than previously had been reported. Lifetime prevalence for alcohol abuse without dependence among males was found to be 12.5%, and among females was 6.4%. Lifetime prevalence of alcohol dependence was 20.1% for males and 8.2% for females. Twelve-month prevalence estimates from the National Comorbidity Survey also were higher for alcohol abuse without dependence (3.4% for males and 1.6% for females), and alcohol dependence (10.7% for males, and 3.7% for females) (Kessler, McGonagle et al., 1994; Kessler, Crum et al., 1997). Analyses of the NCS also have revealed that approximately a third of adolescent drinkers will transition to alcohol abuse or dependence (Warner, Canino et al., 2001).

Data from the 1992 National Longitudinal Alcohol Epidemiologic Survey (NLAES), sponsored by the National Institute on Alcohol Abuse and Alcoholism, provided lifetime and 12-month estimates of alcohol use disorders based on *DSM-IV* criteria (Grant, 1997; Grant, Harford et al., 1994). Twelve-month prevalence of alcohol abuse from the NLAES was found to be 4.7% among men and 1.5% among women (Grant, Harford et al., 1994). For alcohol dependence, the estimates were 6.3% for men and 2.6% for women (Grant, 1997). Lifetime prevalence of alcohol dependence in the NLAES was 13.3% overall. Prevalence estimates for *DSM-IV* alcohol dependence also have been provided by the 1990 U.S. National Alcohol Survey (Caetano & Tam, 1995). Twelve-month prevalence findings from this survey are close to those from the NLAES (5.7% among men, and 2.2% among women).

Most studies have found that the prevalence of alcohol disorders is highest among young adults. For example, prevalence rates for the lifetime, year, and month all are highest among the ECA survey participants, who are between the ages of 18 and 45. Rates tend to drop among older cohorts (Helzer, Burnam et al., 1991).

Some of the differences in estimates across surveys may be due to differences in the diagnostic instruments used to assess alcohol use disorder criteria, the version of the Diagnostic and Statistical Manual that prevailed at the time the survey was completed, the size of the survey sample, and the locale of the survey participants (nationally representative samples versus individual communities), as well as specific characteristics of the populations surveyed, including the age range of study participants. For example, the National Comorbidity Survey included a relatively younger population (persons aged 15 to 54 years) than some other surveys. Recently, Narrow and colleagues have provided revised prevalence estimates, based on data from both the ECA and NCS, by focusing on clinical significance criteria among cases from both surveys that met diagnostic criteria (Narrow, Rae et al., 2002). When the clinical significance criteria were used, disparities between the two surveys were attenuated. For example, the revised one-year prevalence of alcohol disorders among adults aged 18 to 54 was estimated to be 6.5% once the clinical significance criteria were applied. A total of 1.7% of those aged 18 and over had clinically significant drug abuse or dependence in the preceding year.

INCIDENCE OF ALCOHOL DISORDERS

Data from the Swedish Lundby study provide one of the few estimates of incidence of alcoholism over a prolonged followup period (Ojesjo, Hagnell et al., 1982). The Lundby community was interviewed for the first time in 1947, re-interviewed in 1957 (with 1% lost to followup), and then examined again in 1972 (Ojesjo, Hagnell et al., 1982; Ojesjo, 1980; Hagnell, 1966). Of the 1,877 participants in the original survey, 98% of those still alive in 1972 were re-interviewed. The investigators found that, among males, the overall age-adjusted annual incidence of alcoholism was

0.3%. They further found a general decline in incidence with age, with a sharp drop in incidence of alcohol disorders among men, beginning in their thirties (Ojesjo, Hagnell et al., 1982). The highest annual incidence for any type of alcohol disorder among men—0.67% annual incidence—was found among the youngest age group: those 10 to 19 years of age (Ojesjo, Hagnell et al., 1982). Of the 925 women examined in the Lundby community in 1972, only three were identified as having an alcohol disorder (Ojesjo, 1980).

Fillmore examined longitudinal data from population-based U.S. samples and also found that incidence rates of problem drinking generally were lower for women than for men, and that incidence rates for both men and women declined with age (Fillmore, 1987a; Fillmore, 1987b). However, Fillmore's data also showed different patterns of drinking by gender. For example, women tended to develop problems associated with drinking later in life than men, and women were found to have higher rates of remission across all age groups than did men (Fillmore, 1987b).

Data from the ECA surveys on the incidence of DIS-identified alcohol disorders are consistent with other studies (Eaton, Kramer et al., 1989a). The estimated annual incidence of DIS-defined alcohol disorders among men was highest for the youngest age group (those aged 18 to 29: 5.8 per 100 person years) and decreased with age, with an overall annual incidence of 3.7 per 100 person years for men. For women, incidence also decreased with age, with an overall incidence of 0.6 per 100 person years. The peak incidence in women also was among those 18 to 29 years of age (1.1 per 100 person years) (Eaton, Kramer et al., 1989a).

PREVALENCE OF DRUG USE DISORDERS

Although several surveys have assessed the epidemiology of drug use in the United States, there are relatively few population-based studies that have examined the prevalence and/or incidence of drug use disorders or drug addiction. Analysis of the ECA surveys yields an overall lifetime prevalence of drug abuse and dependence of 6.2% (Anthony & Helzer, 1991). As discussed with regard to alcohol disorders, men generally have a higher lifetime prevalence of illicit drug use and illicit drug use disorders (Robins, Helzer et al., 1984). Lifetime prevalence of illicit drug use disorders in the overall study population was 7.7% for men and 4.8% for women. However, among drug users, lifetime prevalence differed little by gender (for male users, lifetime prevalence was 21%, while for female users it was 19%) (Anthony & Helzer, 1991).

More recent data on the prevalence of illicit drug use disorders has been provided by findings from the National Comorbidity Survey (Kessler, McGonagle et al., 1994). In that survey, the lifetime prevalence of drug abuse without dependence was found to be 5.4% among males and 3.5% among females. The estimates for lifetime prevalence of drug dependence were 9.2% for males and 5.9% for females. The NCS also yielded results for 12-month prevalence: for drug abuse without dependence, the estimates were 1.3% among males and 0.3% among females; for drug dependence, 3.8% of the males and 1.9% of the females met the criteria. The data showed that close to half of adolescent drug users developed drug abuse or dependence (Warner, Canino et al., 2001).

Lifetime prevalence estimates of drug dependence from the NLAES (Grant, 1996) were reported to be 3.7% among men and 2.2% among women. In this survey as well, there was no overall gender difference in lifetime prevalence of dependence among drug users (which was 18.8% for men and 18.4% among women). The one-year prevalence of illicit drug disorders tended to be higher for men than for women and decreased steadily with age (Grant, 1996; Anthony & Helzer, 1991).

The prevalence of nicotine dependence recently has been reported from two surveys. Lifetime prevalence, estimated from the NCS, has been reported to be 24% (Breslau, Johnson, et al., 2001). Kandel and colleagues used three aggregated surveys from the National Household Surveys on Drug Abuse to provide estimates of last-year prevalence of specific drugs (alcohol, nicotine, marijuana, and cocaine) in the population surveyed, which included adolescents aged 12 and older (Kandel, Chen et al., 1997). In that population, estimates of last-year dependence were highest among nicotine users (28.0% overall), and lowest among alcohol users (5.2%).

INCIDENCE OF DRUG USE DISORDERS

There is a relative paucity of information regarding the incidence of drug use disorders as a group, with even less information available for specific drugs. From the ECA data, it is clear that the incidence of illicit drug use disorders is greater for men than for women across the entire lifespan (Eaton, Kramer et al., 1989a). In the ECA study, the estimated annual incidence was 1.09 per 100 person-years of risk (Eaton, Kramer et al., 1989a). For men, the estimated

annual incidence for drug abuse/dependence was 1.66 per 100 person-years of risk, while for women, the estimated annual incidence was 0.66 per 100 person-years of risk. As was the case for alcohol-related disorders, the highest incidence for both men and women was found in the 18- to 29-year-old age group; this dropped sharply after young adulthood. The incidence of drug use disorders was zero among persons 65 years of age and older (Eaton, Kramer et al., 1989a).

CORRELATES AND SUSPECTED RISK FACTORS

A number of correlates and suspected risk factors for alcohol and drug use disorders have been examined. These are discussed in this section for both alcohol and drugs, because the suspected risk factors are similar, and there are many findings in common. This section is restricted to a discussion of a selection of personal or individual characteristics that have been found to be associated with drug and alcohol addiction. The discussion is by no means exhaustive and reviews only a fraction of the investigations in this area.

Gender. As discussed earlier, alcohol disorders and alcohol-related problems are more common among men than among women. This consistent finding has been shown in a number of cross-sectional surveys in the United States and in other countries (Kessler, McGonagle et al., 1994; Kessler, Crum et al., 1997; Grant, Harford et al., 1994; Grant, 1997; Caetano & Tam, 1995; Helzer, Burnam et al., 1991; Robins, Helzer et al., 1984; Ojesjo, 1980), as well as in prospective studies (Fillmore, 1987b; Eaton, Kramer et al., 1989a). Women drinkers are less likely to transition to alcohol dependence, or to have persistent dependence once it develops (Grant, 1997). Differences in prevalence and incidence between men and women have been attributed to a number of factors. Cultural norms, societal standards, as well as body size and differences in the metabolism of alcohol all may contribute to the finding that women appear to use less alcohol and to have lower rates of alcohol addiction. As reviewed in detail by Greenfield (2002), survey data over the past 20 years provides evidence that the prevalence of alcohol use disorders among women may be increasing, perhaps as the result of changes in drinking patterns. Some hypothesize that changes in patterns of drinking among women may be a result of deviations from traditional female social roles, or related to changes brought about by the increased number of women in the labor force, as well as the combined input of home and work environments

(Parker & Harford, 1992; Hall, 1992). Many characteristics (such as marital status, full-time employment, ethnicity, age, occupation, and educational level), as well as the occurrence of other life events and the presence of other psychopathology (such as depression), may play a role in gender variability with respect to alcohol consumption and the development of alcohol disorders (Gorman, 1988; Wilsnack, Klassen et al., 1991). In their review, Wilsnack and Wilsnack (1995) assessed drinking and problem drinking among women in the United States. They found that certain subgroups of women were more likely to have adverse drinking consequences and higher rates of heavy drinking patterns. These included younger women, those in non-traditional jobs, and unmarried women cohabiting with a partner. In some subpopulations, there may be a strong association between physical and sexual violence and alcohol use disorders (Lown & Vega, 2001). A history of childhood sexual abuse also has been found to be a potential predictor of women's increased risk for alcohol and drug use disorders (Wilsnack, Vogeltanz et al., 1997). However, the relationship of childhood sexual abuse to alcohol disorders among women is complex, and may involve a number of other family characteristics (Fleming, Mullen et al., 1998).

There also are gender differences with respect to illicit drug disorders. As discussed for alcohol, males (boys and men) generally are more likely to use illicit drugs (Anthony & Helzer, 1991; Johnston, O'Malley et al., 1992) and they have a higher prevalence of drug use disorders than do women (Anthony & Helzer, 1991). The social or cultural restrictions that were mentioned as possible explanations for the reduced prevalence of alcohol use among women also may apply to some types of illicit drug use. However, some (Grant, 1996) but not all data (Warner, Kessler et al., 1995) show that among drug users, the proportion of men and women who develop dependence is similar.

Several studies that have used large community surveys to evaluate particular types of illicit substances have found differences by gender. For example, Adams and Gfroerer (1991) examined characteristics associated with the development of cocaine dependence, using data from the National Household Surveys on Drug Abuse. Some sociodemographic characteristics, as well as factors related to drug use (route of administration, and frequency and length of cocaine use) were found to account for the different rates at which male and female cocaine users progressed to co-caine dependence (Adams & Gfroerer, 1991). More recently, Kandel, Chen et al. (1997) analyzed data from the National Household Surveys on Drug Abuse and found that men had significantly higher prevalence rates of alcohol and marijuana dependence within the preceding year, but that women had significantly higher prevalence rates of nicotine dependence. Moreover, there is evidence that violence associated with drug use differs by gender. In one study examining cocaine use and violence, it was found that among those reporting violent events, men who regularly used cocaine were more likely to have perpetrated violent crimes, while women who regularly used cocaine were more likely to have been victims of violence (Goldstein, Bellucci et al., 1991).

Age. Prevalence rates for alcohol disorders is lower among older adults (Helzer, Burnam et al., 1991; Narrow, Rae et al., 2002; Grant, 1997; Kandel, Chen et al., 1997). This may occur for a number of reasons. Because the measure of prevalence is dependent on the incidence as well as the duration of the disease (Mausner & Kramer, 1985; Lilienfeld & Lilienfeld, 1980), alcoholism may be less prevalent among the elderly because (1) the incidence decreases over the lifespan, or (2) the duration of the disorder is reduced, or (3) some combination of the two factors is in effect. If the duration of the disorder is reduced, it may be a result of an increase in remission with age, or a reduction in survival. In other words, with age, prevalence may be reduced because fewer individuals develop the disease, because the addiction problems have resolved, or because addicted individuals die earlier. Explanations for a decreased prevalence with age also may include (1) a reduced tolerance to alcohol with age (Vestal, McGuire et al., 1977); (2) poorer recall among older adults; or (3) a cohort effect (Helzer, Burnam et al., 1991). Further, the means by which alcohol disorders are identified in young adults may not be relevant to the elderly (Graham, 1986), with the result that alcohol problems and disorders may be under-recognized in older adults (Graham, 1986; Blow, 2000). Surveys that include only household participants may miss many with alcohol disorders who reside in nursing homes; also, older community residents with alcohol disorders may be less willing to participate in household surveys. Although longitudinal analyses show declines in the proportion of older adults who consume alcohol (Adams, Garry et al., 1990), problems related to alcohol use among the elderly may occur at lower levels of consumption, and older adults with alcohol use disorders may be at greater risk for comorbid problems (Dufour & Fuller, 1995; Liberto, Oslin et al., 1992).

The age of onset of alcohol use has been investigated as a predictor of subsequent alcohol abuse and dependence (DeWit, Adlaf et al., 2000; Grant & Dawson, 1997; Grant, Stinson et al., 2001). In general, the earlier the age of first use, the greater the risk for the development of an alcohol use disorder. In addition, early drinking onset is associated with elevated risk of alcohol-related injuries (Hingson, Heeren et al., 2000), motor vehicle accidents (Hingson, Heeren et al., 2002), and physical violence after drinking (Hingson, Heeren et al., 2001). Moreover, early onset drug use is associated with an increased risk for the development of drug use disorders, as well as alcohol dependence (Grant & Dawson, 1998). Smoking at an early age has been identified as a predictor of drinking, and also increases the risk for transition to alcohol abuse and dependence and is associated with greater severity of alcohol use disorders if they do develop (Grant, 1998).

As with alcohol disorders, age correlates with the occurrence of drug use disorders. The highest prevalence and incidence rates for illicit drug disorders are found among individuals in late adolescence and young adulthood (Anthony & Helzer, 1991). Beyond the fact that incidence is low among older adults, and that survival may be decreased for drug addicts as they age, other factors also may be involved. Prevalence may be lower among older adults because of a cohort effect. Exposure and availability of illicit drugs differs by birth cohort. For example, the current cohort of older adults had no access to crack cocaine in their youth. When evaluating changes in the frequency of a disorder (in this case, drug and alcohol addiction), distinctions need to be made between changes that uniformly occur for all age groups during a particular historical period (period effect), changes that occur with age as the individual matures (age effect), and a cohort effect that reflects differences in disease rate for individuals born in different years (O'Malley, Bachman et al., 1988; Kleinbaum, Kupper et al., 1982). Recent analyses show that patterns of addiction have changed and show a greater prevalence of alcohol and illicit drug dependence among cohorts born since World War II (Grant, 1997, 1996; Warner, Kessler et al., 1995). Similarly, the risk of nicotine dependence is greatest among smokers in the most recent birth cohorts (Breslau, Johnson et al., 2001).

Race and Ethnicity. Information on the relationship between alcohol and illicit drug disorders and racial and ethnic background is complex and sometimes conflicting. Some of the inconsistent findings result from the relative paucity of data involving ethnic and racial groups, the classifications used to group ethnic minorities, the social acceptability of drinking and drug use practices in different groups, and the relationship of socioeconomic status and the availability of health care to ethnic minority populations.

The onset of alcohol disorders appears to begin at later ages among African Americans, and a greater proportion of African Americans tend to be abstainers relative to Caucasians (Helzer, Burnam et al., 1991; Caetano & Herd, 1984). However, compared with Caucasians, African Americans tend to suffer more severe medical consequences, such as relatively high mortality rates associated with cirrhosis (Ronan, 1986, 1987). The elevated rates may be related to issues of socioeconomic status, cultural environment, and access to health care (Herd, 1990; Otten, 1990). Not infrequently, when measures of socioeconomic status (such as household residence or educational level) are taken into account, differences between ethnic minorities and Caucasians are minimized (Crum, Bucholz et al., 1992). Although African Americans and Hispanics are less likely than Caucasians to use alcohol in their lifetimes, they are more likely to have persistent or chronic alcohol dependence once the disorder develops (Grant, 1997).

Differences in drinking patterns vary across Hispanic ethnic subgroups, and variations may reflect factors such as degree of acculturation, country of national origin, and generational status or time since immigration (Caetano & Raspberry, 2000; Zayas, Rojas et al., 1998; Caetano, 1988, 1987; Epstein, Botvin et al., 2001; Polednak, 1997). For example, in one study, Mexican Americans were more likely to report problems with alcohol, and were more liberal in their acceptance of drinking, than other Hispanic groups (Caetano, 1988). Caetano also found that Hispanic Americans (particularly Hispanic women) who were acculturated to U.S. society tended to drink more and were classified more frequently as heavy drinkers (Caetano, 1987). Trend analysis of drinking patterns among racial subgroups found that, between 1984 and 1992, heavy drinking decreased among white men but not among African American or Hispanic men. In addition, abstention rates remained essentially unchanged among Hispanic women, but increased in all other subgroups (Caetano & Kaskutas, 1995).

Asian Americans generally are believed to have some of the lowest levels of alcohol consumption and lowest rates of alcohol disorders. There is some evidence that this is the result of the discomfort that occurs with the physiological effects of the flushing response present in many individuals of this ethnic background (Suddendorf, 1989), because of variations in the aldehyde dehydrogenase gene (Luczak, Elvine-Kreis et al., 2002; Wall, Shea et al., 2001; McCarthy, Wall et al., 2000; Higuchi, Matsushita et al., 1995). There also is evidence that genetic heterogeneity may explain differences in rates of alcoholism among certain subgroups (Hsu, Loh et al., 1996). However, as with Hispanic Americans, the Asian American population is composed of many subgroups with different backgrounds and cultural drinking practices (Nemoto, Aoki et al., 1999). Some data provide evidence that prevalence rates differ among various groups of Asian Americans, and that some rates of heavy drinking may not be substantially different from those for the U.S. population as a whole (Chi, Lubben et al., 1989).

Native Americans historically have had high death rates from alcohol-related disorders (Gilliland, Becker et al., 1995; Rhoades, Hammond et al., 1987; Christian, DuFour et al., 1989). However, it is not accurate to generalize to all Native American populations, as drinking practices are quite varied across tribal groups, and cultural factors as well as socioeconomic factors play a role (Rhoades, Hammond et al., 1987; Christian, DuFour et al., 1989).

Patterns of drug use and drug disorders also vary by racial-ethnic group (Anthony & Helzer, 1991; Warner, Kessler et al., 1995). However, less information is available for drug addiction than for alcoholism among different ethnic populations. Data from the NCS and the NLAES show that whites are more likely than African Americans or Hispanics to use drugs, but are less likely to have persistent dependence once the disorder develops (Grant, 1996; Warner, Kessler et al., 1995). More recently, data from the National Household Surveys of Drug Abuse showed that, among those who smoked in the preceding year, whites have the highest probability of developing nicotine dependence and, among those who used cocaine in the preceding year, African Americans are more likely to be dependent on cocaine (Kandel, Chen et al., 1997). As with alcohol disorders, there are differences among subgroups of ethnic minorities, and factors such as degree of acculturation are associated with the prevalence of drug disorders (Burnam, Hough et al., 1987; Gfroerer & De La Rosa, 1993). It also has been shown that the relationship of risk factors to drug use among adolescents (such as low family

pride, depressed mood, and low self-esteem) also differ by ethnic group (Vega, Zimmerman et al., 1993).

The evaluation of race and its association with addiction is complex. As stated in the discussion on alcohol disorders, when examining illicit drug use patterns among different ethnic groups, it is important to consider socioeconomic characteristics (Herd, 1994). One study found that, although national survey data indicated a higher prevalence of crack cocaine smoking among some ethnic minorities, when area of neighborhood residence was taken into account, differences in the prevalence of drug use between racial groups were attenuated (Lillie-Blanton, Anthony et al., 1993).

Family History. Alcohol disorders cluster in families. Twin studies (Heath, Bucholz et al., 1997; Prescott & Kendler, 1999; Kendler, Heath et al., 1992; Kendler, Neale et al., 1994; Hrubec & Omenn, 1981; Kaprio, Koskenvuo et al., 1987), adoption and cross-fostering studies (Cloninger, 1981; Goodwin, Schulsinger et al., 1973; Sigvardsson, Bohman et al., 1996; Yates, Cadoret et al., 1996), studies involving genetically selected animal models (Chester, Price et al., 2002; Dolney, Szalai et al., 2001; Gerlai, Lahav et al., 2000; He, Nebert et al., 1997), segregation analysis (Aston & Hill, 1990), and allelic association (Blum, Noble et al., 1990) have attempted to answer the question of whether such familial relationships are the result of genetic transmission or a shared environment. There also have been a number of investigations of physiological and biochemical markers associated with alcoholism (Froehlich, Zink et al., 2000; Wall, Peterson et al., 1997; Borras, Coutelle et al., 2000; Begleiter & Projesz, 1988; Rausch, Monteiro et al., 1991; Bailly, Vignau et al., 1993). Studies examining familial patterns of alcoholism have demonstrated a possible genetic relationship. However, many individuals whose parents drink do not become alcoholic themselves (West & Prinz, 1987; Ohannessian & Hesselbrook, 1993), and many who develop alcohol disorders do not have a family history of alcoholism (Cotton, 1979; Schuckit, 1983). Clearly, environmental influences also play a significant role (Kendler, Gardner et al., 1997; Chilcoat, Dishion et al., 1995).

Studies to assess the relationship of genetic liability to drug use disorders have shown evidence for heritability involving nicotine (Kendler, Thornton et al., 2000; Kendler, Neale et al., 1999), caffeine (Kendler & Prescott, 1999), cannabis (Kendler, Neale et al., 2002), as well as illicit drugs such as cocaine, hallucinogens, stimulants, and opiates (Tsuang, Lyons et al., 1996; van den Bree, Johnson et al.,

1998; Kendler, Karkowski et al., 2000; Kendler & Prescott, 1998; Pickens & Svikis, 1988; Cadoret, Yates et al., 1995). Moreover, recent assessments of the liability for more than one substance use disorder (True, Xian et al., 1999; True, Health et al., 1999; Hettema, Corey et al., 1999) have found evidence indicating common genetic vulnerabilities among some diagnoses such as alcohol and nicotine dependence (True, Xian et al., 1999). Recent analyses also have examined the associations of genetic liability to drug disorders with personality traits such as antisocial traits (Jang, Vernon et al., 2000) behavioral undercontrol (Slutske, Health et al., 2002), and risk taking (Miles, van den Bree et al., 2001). Many of these studies have provided evidence for the importance of familial and potentially genetic mechanisms in the development of drug disorders.

Employment Status and Occupation. Employment, or working for pay, also is related to the prevalence of alcohol disorders (Helzer, Burnam et al., 1991). For example, McCord found that alcoholics were more frequently unable to work on a regular basis than those who were not alcoholic (McCord & McCord, 1962). Similarly, study results from the ECA have reported that individuals who were unemployed six months or more in the preceding five years had higher prevalence rates of alcoholism (Helzer, Burnam et al., 1991), and greater risk for development of alcohol disorders (Crum, Bucholz et al., 1992). However, working relatively long work hours may increase alcohol and drug use among adolescents (McMorris & Uggen, 2000; Valois, Dunham et al., 1999). An assessment of recent trends in drinking-related problems from survey data taken in 1984 and in 1990 found that there were significant increases in reports of two or more social consequences of drinking among the unemployed (Midanik & Clark, 1995). In addition, the prevalence of alcohol disorders differs by type of occupation. For example, higher rates of alcohol addiction have been found among those in occupations typically associated with laborers, "blue collar" occupations, or those in lower socioeconomic levels (Olkinoura, 1984; Roberts & Lee, 1993). There also is evidence that the relationship of employment status with the frequency of alcohol-related health problems is different for men than for women (Lahelma, Kangas et al., 1995). Analyses of the ECS surveys also have provided evidence that the effect of alcoholism on lower income status may occur as a result of the indirect and direct effects the disorder has on educational achievement and marriage (Mullahy & Sindelar, 1994).

Unlike alcohol disorders, data from the ECA survey did not show an appreciable association of unemployment with illicit drug disorders (Anthony & Helzer, 1991). However, there was a tendency for employed men with illicit drug disorders to have lower income (Anthony & Helzer, 1991). Further, as with alcoholism, there appear to be differences in the prevalence of illicit drug disorders and cigarette smoking associated with specific occupations (Anthony, Eaton et al., 1992; Bang & Kim, 2001). Yet, with few exceptions (including Claussen, 1999; Dooley & Prause, 1997), it is not possible to know which developed first; that is, whether lack of employment led to heavy drinking or drug use, or whether alcohol or drug problems resulted in job loss, inability to obtain work, or selection into a particular type of occupation.

Marital Status. Marital status also has been found to be related to the occurrence of alcohol disorders and drinking behavior, but these relationships are complex (Prescott & Kendler, 2001; Power, Rodgers et al., 1999). Alcohol and drug addiction may predate the time that individuals make decisions about marriage, and problems associated with drinking and drug use may be the reason some individuals remain single, or become separated or divorced. Data from the ECA surveys showed that individuals in stable marriages had the lowest lifetime prevalence of alcoholism (8.9%), as opposed to cohabiting adults who had never been married (29.2%) (Helzer, Burnam et al., 1991). Longitudinal analyses also show that cohabiting women may be at elevated risk for heavy drinking (Wilsnack & Wilsnack, 1995). Chilcoat and Breslau (1996) found that the incidence of alcohol disorder symptoms was higher among single or divorced participants than in those who were married. There also is evidence that the risk of problem drinking is higher for women with spouses or partners who drink heavily (Wilsnack & Wilsnack, 1995), and that the quality of marital relationships may vary as a function of the presence of current heavy drinking (McLeod, 1993). Recent prospective data (Prescott & Kendler, 2001; Curran, Muthen et al., 1998) indicate that the time of transition to one's first marriage is associated with reduced drinking.

Lifetime prevalence rates of illicit drug disorders also have been found to vary appreciably by marital status. Anthony and Helzer found that, for both men and women and generally across all ages, individuals who lived with a significant other but had never married had the highest lifetime prevalence of drug disorders. Cohabiting unmarried men had a 30.2% lifetime prevalence of an illicit drug disorder, compared to a 3.6% prevalence for married men. Cohabiting women had a lifetime prevalence of 19.9%, compared to 1.8% among women with a stable marital history (Anthony & Helzer, 1992). Lack of marital stability and the periods of transition to and from marriage or divorce appear to influence substance use, treatment outcomes, and drug-related mortality (Fu & Goldman, 2000; Hartmann, Sullivan et al., 1991; Curran, Muthen et al., 1998; Westhuis, Gwaltney et al., 2001; Kallan, 1998). Moreover, the severity of alcohol and drug use affect marital functioning and are associated with the risk of partner violence (Chermack, Fuller et al., 2000; Mudar, Leonard et al., 2001). However, as recently reviewed by Epstein and McCrady (2000), couples treatment of alcohol and drug disorders may achieve improvements in marital functioning and substance use.

Educational Level. Studies of the relationship between educational level and the development of alcoholism often have yielded conflicting results, yet educational level often is included as part of broader sociodemographic or social-class characteristics. Heavier consumption patterns frequently have been found among those with lower educational levels (Droomers, Schrijvers et al., 1999). Moreover, studies using prospective data have shown that dropping out of high school or leaving college early is associated with an increased risk of alcohol abuse and dependence in adulthood (Crum, Bucholz et al., 1992; Crum, Helzer et al., 1993). Analyses of inner city school children also have provided evidence suggesting that poor educational achievement and some early school behaviors are associated with risk for alcohol use disorders (Crum, Ensminger et al., 1998). Academic competence has been reported to be important in studies of risk factors for problem drinking behavior among adolescents (Harrison & Luxenberg, 1995; Thomas, 1993; Thomas & Hsiu, 1993). The relationship between educational attainment and alcohol misuse may differ by race (Paschall, Flewelling et al., 2000).

Lifetime prevalence of drug disorders also varies by educational level. Using data from the ECA surveys, Anthony and Helzer showed that for men and women of all ages, lifetime prevalence of illicit drug disorders was highest for those who dropped out of high school, and for those who entered college but failed to earn a degree (Anthony & Helzer, 1991). Analyses of the National Household Surveys on Drug Abuse found that use of tobacco and illicit drugs was highest among high school dropouts (Gfroerer, Greenblatt et al., 1997). Eggert and Herting (1993) found that high-risk youth (defined as adolescents with a history of school problems and/or school dropout) had greater adverse consequences from drug use as well as greater access to drugs relative to students considered low-risk (those defined as typical high-school students). Performance on some achievement tests was different and lower for substance-abusing adolescents than for a comparison group of student controls (Braggio, Pishkin et al., 1993). Moreover, a prospective analysis of high school seniors has provided evidence of an association between poor educational achievement and substance use following high school (Schulenberg, Bachman et al., 1994).

COMORBIDITY OF ALCOHOL AND DRUG ADDICTION

Cross-sectional survey data and clinical studies have indicated that individuals who have one alcohol or drug disorder often have another substance use diagnosis (see Regier, Farmer et al., 1990; Clark, Pollock et al., 1997). Other psychopathologies (such as affective disorders, schizophrenic disorders, and anxiety disorders) also frequently co-occur with addictions (Regier, Farmer et al., 1990; Farrell, Howes et al., 2001). Using data from the ECA surveys, Regier and colleagues found that, among individuals with a drug disorder, the lifetime prevalence of an alcohol disorder was 47%, and the lifetime prevalence of a psychiatric disorder was 53%. Among those with an alcohol disorder, 37% had a current or prior psychiatric disorder, and lifetime prevalence for a drug disorder was 21% (Regier, Farmer et al., 1990). Analyses of lifetime diagnoses of alcohol abuse and dependence from the National Comorbidity Survey also found that individuals with a lifetime history of alcohol abuse or dependence frequently had a history of another psychiatric or substance use disorder (Kessler, Crum et al., 1997). In addition, past psychiatric and substance use disorders may be stronger predictors of alcohol dependence than alcohol abuse.

Few population-based studies allow a prospective examination of comorbid relationships (for example, Gilman & Abraham, 2001). The ECA data set is one that provides some of this information. For example, there is evidence that the incidence of alcohol abuse and dependence may be elevated among individuals who have other psychopathologies, including illicit drug diagnoses (Crum, Helzer et al., 1993); anxiety disorders and alcohol dependence may have a bidirectional causal relationship (Kushner, Sher et al., 1999); and cocaine use may be associated with the develop-

---

ment of several psychiatric conditions (Anthony & Petronis, 1991).

In studying the stages of drug use among adolescents and young adults, a pattern of drug use progression has been described that begins with the use of tobacco and/or alcohol, progresses to marijuana, and then to the use of other illicit drugs (Kandel, 1975; Donovan & Jessor, 1983). For example, among most cocaine and crack users, marijuana use is an antecedent. Recent evidence supports gender differences with regard to the significant role of the early use of alcohol for young men and cigarettes for young women (Kandel & Yamaguchi, 1993). Further, there may be differences by gender with respect to the pathways that lead to substance use disorders, as well as in the type and severity of comorbid psychopathologies (Luthar, Cushing et al., 1996).

As more information becomes available from longitudinal studies, it will be possible to better assess these temporal relationships. In addition, future investigations into the age of onset and the progression of symptoms will provide valuable information for clinical treatment, as well as a better understanding of potential etiologic relationships.

CONCLUSIONS

This chapter has attempted to summarize a sampling of major findings in epidemiologic studies of alcohol and drug addiction. In contrast to clinical practice, or basic science and laboratory research, epidemiology is a study of populations. As discussed in detail by Kleinbaum and colleagues, it is through this study of populations that epidemiologic research aims to describe the health status and distribution of disease in populations, as well as to identify risk factors and potential etiologic agents of disease, which may enable us to better predict and prevent disease (Kleinbaum, Kupper et al., 1982). These basic principles have been extended to the epidemiology of drug and alcohol addiction, with the ultimate goals of improving understanding of etiologic mechanisms, identifying targets for intervention, and reducing the prevalence of addictive disorders.

ACKNOWLEDGMENT: This work was supported by a Scientist Development Award for Clinicians from the National Institute on Alcohol Abuse and Alcoholism (AA00168).

REFERENCES

Adams EH & Gfroerer J (1991). Risk of cocaine abuse and dependence. In S Schober & C Schade (eds.) *The Epidemiology of Cocaine Use and Abuse (NIDA Research Monograph 110).* Rockville, MD: National Institute on Drug Abuse, 253-262.

Adams WL, Garry PJ, Rhyne R et al. (1990). Alcohol intake in the healthy elderly. Changes with age in a cross-sectional and longitudinal study. *Journal of the American Geriatric Society* 38:211-216.

American Psychiatric Association (APA) (1980). *Diagnostic and Statistical Manual of Mental Disorders, 3rd Edition (DSM-III).* Washington, DC: American Psychiatric Press.

American Psychiatric Association (APA) (1987). *Diagnostic and Statistical Manual of Mental Disorders, 3rd Edition, Revised (DSM-IIIR).* Washington, DC: American Psychiatric Press.

American Psychiatric Association (APA) (1994). *Diagnostic and Statistical Manual of Mental Disorders, 4th Edition (DSM-IV).* Washington, DC: American Psychiatric Press.

American Psychiatric Association (APA) (2000). *Diagnostic and Statistical Manual of Mental Disorders, 4th Edition, Text Revision.* Washington, DC: American Psychiatric Press.

Anthony JC, Eaton WW, Mandell W et al. (1992). Psychoactive drug dependence and abuse: More common in some occupations than others? *Journal of Employee Assistance Research* 1(1):148-186.

Anthony JC & Helzer JE (1991). Syndromes of drug abuse and dependence. In LN Robins & DA Regier (eds.) *Psychiatric Disorders in America.* New York, NY: The Free Press/Macmillan, 116-154.

Anthony JC & Petronis KR (1991). Epidemiologic evidence on suspected associations between cocaine use and psychiatric disturbances. In S Schober & C Schade (eds.) *The Epidemiology of Cocaine Use and Abuse (NIDA Research Monograph 110).* Rockville, MD: National Institute on Drug Abuse, 71-94.

Aston CE & Hill SY (1990). Segregation analysis of alcoholism in families ascertained through a pair of male alcoholics. *American Journal of Human Genetics* 46:879-887.

Bailly D, Vignau J, Racadot N et al. (1993). Platelet serotonin levels in alcoholic patients: Changes related to physiological and pathological factors. *Psychiatry Research* 47(1):57-88.

Bang KM & Kim JH (2001). Prevalence of cigarette smoking by occupation and industry in the United States. *American Journal of Industrial Medicine* 40(3):233-239.

Begleiter H & Porjesz B (1988). Potential biological markers in individuals at high risk for developing alcoholism. *Alcoholism: Clinical & Experimental Research* 12(4):488-493.

Blow FC (2000). Treatment of older women with alcohol problems: Meeting the challenge for a special population. *Alcoholism: Clinical & Experimental Research* 24:1257-1266.

Blum K, Noble EP, Sheridan PJ et al. (1990). Allelic association of human dopamine D_2 receptor gene in alcoholism. *Journal of the American Medical Association* 263(15):2055-2060.

Borras E, Coutelle C, Rosell A et al. (2000). Genetic polymorphism of alcohol dehydrogenase in Europeans: The ADH2*2 allele decreases the risk for alcoholism and is associated with ADH3*. *Hepatology* 31(4):984-989.

Braggio JT, Pishkin V, Gameros TA et al. (1993). Academic achievement in substance-abusing and conduct-disordered adolescents. *Journal of Clinical Psychology* 49(2):282-291.

Breslau N, Johnson EO, Hiripi E et al. (2001). Nicotine dependence in the United States: Prevalence, trends, and smoking persistence. *Archives of General Psychiatry* 58(9):810-816.

Burnam MA, Hough RL, Karno M et al. (1987). Acculturation and lifetime prevalence of psychiatric disorders among Mexican Americans in Los Angeles. *Journal of Health and Social Behavior* 28:89-102.

Cadoret RJ, Yates, WR, Troughton E et al. (1995). Adoption study demonstrating two genetic pathways to drug abuse. *Archives of General Psychiatry* 52(1):42-52.

Caetano R (1987). Acculturation and drinking patterns among U.S. Hispanics. *British Journal of Addiction* 82:789-799.

Caetano R (1988). Alcohol use among Hispanic groups in the United States. *American Journal of Drug and Alcohol Abuse* 14(3):293-308.

Caetano R & Herd D (1984). Black drinking practices in Northern California. *American Journal of Drug and Alcohol Abuse* 10(4):571-587.

Caetano R & Kaskutas LA (1995). Changes in drinking patterns among Whites, Blacks and Hispanics, 1984-1992. *Journal of Studies on Alcohol* 56:558-565.

Caetano R & Raspberry K (2000). Drinking and DSM-IV alcohol and drug dependence among white and Mexican-American DUI offenders. *Journal of Studies on Alcohol* 61:420-426.

Caetano R & Tam TW (1995). Prevalence and correlates of DSM-IV and ICD-10 alcohol dependence: 1990 U.S. National Alcohol Survey. *Alcohol & Alcoholism* 30(2):177-186.

Chermack ST, Fuller BE & Blow FC (2000). Predictors of expressed partner and non-partner violence among patients in substance abuse treatment. *Drug and Alcohol Dependence* 58(1-2):43-54.

Chester JA, Price CS & Froehlich JC (2002). Inverse genetic association between alcohol preference and severity of alcohol withdrawal in two sets of rat lines selected for the same phenotype. *Alcoholism: Clinical & Experimental Research* 26(1):19-27.

Chi I, Lubben JE & Kitano HHL (1989). Differences in drinking behavior among three Asian American groups. *Journal of Studies on Alcohol* 50(1):15-23.

Chilcoat HD, Dishion TJ & Anthony JC (1995). Parent monitoring and the incidence of drug sampling in urban elementary school children. *American Journal of Epidemiology* 141(1):25-31.

Chilcoat HD & Breslau N (1996). Alcohol disorders in young adulthood: Effects of transitions into adult roles. *Journal of Health and Social Behavior* 37(4):339-349.

Christian CM, Dufour M & Bertolucci D (1989). Differential alcohol-related mortality among American Indian Tribes in Oklahoma, 1968-1978. *Social Science and Medicine* 28(3):275-284.

Clark DB, Pollock N, Buckstein OG et al. (1997). Gender and comorbid psychopathology in adolescents with alcohol dependence. *Journal of the American Academy of Child and Adolescent Psychiatry* 36(9):1195-1203.

Claussen B (1999). Alcohol disorders and re-employment in a 5-year follow-up of long-term unemployed. *Addiction* 94(1):133-138.

Cloninger CR, Bohman M & Sigvardsson S (1981). Inheritance of alcohol abuse: Cross-fostering analysis of adopted men. *Archives of General Psychiatry* 38:861-868.

Cotton NS (1979). The familial incidence of alcoholism. A review. *Journal of Studies on Alcohol* 40(1):89-116.

Crum RM, Bucholz KK, Helzer JE et al. (1992). The risk of alcohol abuse and dependence in adulthood: The association with educational level. *American Journal of Epidemiology* 135(9):989-999.

Crum RM, Ensminger ME, Ro M et al. (1998). The association of educational achievement and school dropout with risk of alcoholism: A twenty-five-year prospective study of inner-city children. *Journal of Studies on Alcohol* 59:318-326.

Crum RM, Helzer JE & Anthony JC (1993). Level of education and alcohol abuse and dependence in adulthood: A further inquiry. *American Journal of Public Health* 83(6):830-837.

Curran PJ, Muthen BO & Harford TC (1998). The influence of changes in marital status on developmental trajectories of alcohol use in young adults. *Journal of Studies on Alcohol* 59(6):647-658.

DeWit DJ, Adlaf EM, Offord DR et al. (2000). Age at first alcohol use: A risk factor for the development of alcohol disorders. *American Journal of Psychiatry* 157:745-750.

Dolney DE, Szalai G, Duester G et al. (2001). Molecular analysis of genetic differences among inbred mouse strains controlling tissue expression pattern of alcohol dehydrogenase 4. *Gene* 267(2):145-156.

Dooley D & Prause J (1997). Effect of favorable employment change on alcohol abuse: One- and five-year follow-ups in the National Longitudinal Survey of Youth. *American Journal of Community Psychology* 25(6):787-807.

Donovan JE & Jessor R (1983). Problem drinking and the dimension of involvement with drugs. A Guttman Scalogram Analysis of adolescent drug use. *American Journal of Public Health* 73(5):543-551.

Dufour M & Fuller RK (1995). Alcohol in the elderly. *Annual Review of Medicine* 46:123-132.

Droomers M, Schrijvers CT, Stronks K et al. (1999). Educational differences in excessive alcohol consumption: The role of psychosocial and material stressors. *Preventive Medicine* 29(1):1-10.

Eaton WW & Kessler LG (1985). *Epidemiologic Field Methods in Psychiatry. The NIMH Epidemiologic Catchment Area Program.* Orlando, FL: Academic Press, Inc.

Eaton WW, Kramer M, Anthony JC et al. (1989a). The incidence of specific DIS/DSM-III mental disorders: Data from the NIMH Epidemiologic Catchment Area Program. *Acta Psychiatrica Scandinavica* 79:163-178.

Eaton WW, Kramer M, Anthony JC et al. (1989b). Conceptual and methodological problems in estimation of the incidence of mental disorders from field survey data. In Cooper B & Helgason T (eds.) *Epidemiology and the Prevention of Mental Disorders* (World Psychiatric Association). New York, NY: Routledge, 108-127.

Eggert LL & Herting JR (1993). Drug involvement among potential dropouts and "typical" youth. *Journal of Drug Education* 23(1):31-55.

Epstein EE & McCrady BS (1998). Behavioral couples treatment of alcohol and drug use disorders: Current status and innovations. *Clinical Psychology Review* 18(6):689-711.

Epstein JA, Botvin GJ & Diaz T (2001). Alcohol use among Dominican and Puerto Rican adolescents residing in New York City: Role of Hispanic group and gender. *Journal of Developmental and Behavioral Pediatrics* 22:113-118.

Farrell M, Howes S, Bebbington P et al. (2001). Nicotine, alcohol and drug dependence and psychiatric comorbidity. Results of a national household survey. *British Journal of Psychiatry* 179:432-437.

Fillmore KM (1987a). Prevalence, incidence and chronicity of drinking patterns and problems among men as a function of age: A longitudinal and cohort analysis. *British Journal of Addiction* 82:77-83.

Fillmore KM (1987b). Women's drinking across the adult life course as compared to men's. *British Journal of Addiction* 82:801-811.

Fleming J, Mullen PE, Sibthorpe B et al. (1998). The relationship between childhood sexual abuse and alcohol abuse in women—A case-control study. *Addiction* 93:1787-1798.

Froehlich JC, Zink RW, Li TK et al. (2000). Analysis of heritability of hormonal responses to alcohol in twins: Beta-endorphin as a potential biomarker of genetic risk for alcoholism. *Alcoholism: Clinical & Experimental Research* 24(3)265-277.

Fu H & Goldman N (2000). The association between health-related behaviours and the risk of divorce in the USA. *Journal of Biosocial Science* 32(1):63-88.

Gerlai R, Lahav M, Guo S et al. (2000). Drinks like a fish: Zebra fish (Danio rerio) as a behavior genetic model to study alcohol effects. *Pharmacology, Biochemistry, and Behavior* 67(4)773-782.

Gilliland FD, Becker TM, Samet JM et al. (1995). Trends in alcohol-related mortality among New Mexico's American Indians, Hispanics, and non-Hispanic whites. *Alcoholism: Clinical & Experimental Research* 19:1572-1577.

Gilman SE & Abraham HD (2001). A longitudinal study of the order of onset of alcohol dependence and major depression. *Drug and Alcohol Dependence* 63(3):277-286.

Gfroerer J & De La Rosa M (1993). Protective and risk factors associated with drug use among Hispanic youth. *Journal of Addictive Diseases* 12(2):87-107.

Gfroerer JC, Greenblatt JC & Wright DA (1997). Substance use in the US college-age population: Differences according to educational status and living arrangement. *American Journal of Public Health* 87(1):62-65.

Goldstein PJ, Bellucci PA, Spunt BJ et al. (1991). Frequency of cocaine use and violence: A comparison between men and women. In S Schober & C Schade (eds.) *The Epidemiology of Cocaine Use and Abuse (NIDA Research Monograph 110)*. Rockville, MD: National Institute on Drug Abuse, 113-138.

Goodwin DW, Schulsinger F, Hermansen L et al. (1973). Alcohol problems in adoptees raised apart from alcoholic biological parents. *Archives of General Psychiatry* 28:238-243.

Gordis E (2000). *Epidemiology, 2nd Ed.* Philadelphia, PA: W.B. Saunders.

Gorman DM (1988). Employment, stressful life events and the development of alcohol dependence. *Drug and Alcohol Dependence* 22:151-159.

Graham K (1986). Identifying and measuring alcohol abuse among the elderly: Serious problems with existing instrumentation. *Journal of Studies on Alcohol* 47(4):322-326.

Grant BF (1996). Prevalence and correlates of drug use and DSM-IV drug dependence in the United States: Results of the National Longitudinal Alcohol Epidemiologic Survey. *Journal of Substance Abuse* 8(2):195-210.

Grant BF (1997). Prevalence and correlates of alcohol use and DSM-IV alcohol dependence in the United States: Results of the National Longitudinal Alcohol Epidemiologic Survey. *Journal of Studies on Alcohol* 58(5):464-473.

Grant BF (1998). Age at smoking onset and its association with alcohol consumption and DSM-IV alcohol abuse and dependence: Results from the National Longitudinal Alcohol Epidemiologic Survey. *Journal of Substance Abuse* 10:59-73.

Grant BF & Dawson DA (1997). Age at onset of alcohol use and its association with DSM-IV alcohol abuse and dependence: Results from the National Longitudinal Alcohol Epidemiologic Survey. *Journal of Substance Abuse* 9:103-110.

Grant BF & Dawson DA (1998). Age of onset of drug use and its association with DSM-IV drug abuse and dependence: Results from the National Longitudinal Alcohol Epidemiologic Survey. *Journal of Substance Abuse* 10:163-173.

Grant BF, Harford TC, Dawson DA et al. (1994). Prevalence of DSM-IV alcohol abuse and dependence: United States, 1992. *Alcohol Health & Research World* 18(3):243-248.

Grant BF, Stinson FS & Harford TC (2001). Age at onset of alcohol use and DSM-IV alcohol abuse and dependence: A 12-year follow-up. *Journal of Substance Abuse* 13:493-504.

Greenfield SF (2002). Women and alcohol use disorders. *Harvard Review of Psychiatry* 10:76-85.

Hagnell O (1966). *A Prospective Study of the Incidence of Mental Disorder*. Lund, Sweden: Svenska Bokforlaget.

Hall EM (1992). Double exposure: The combined impact of the home and work environments on psychosomatic strain in Swedish women and men. *International Journal of Health Services* 22(2):239-260.

Harrison PA & Luxenberg M (1995). Comparisons of alcohol and other drug problems among Minnesota adolescents in 1989 and 1992. *Archives of Pediatric and Adolescent Medicine* 149:137-144.

Hartmann DJ, Sullivan WP & Wolk JL (1991). A state-wide assessment: Marital stability and client outcomes. *Drug and Alcohol Dependence* 29(1):27-38.

He XX, Nebert DW, Vasiliou V et al. (1997). Genetic differences in alcohol drinking preferences between inbred strains of mice. *Pharmacogenetics* 7(3):223-233.

Heath AC, Bucholz KK, Madden PA et al. (1997). Genetic and environmental contributions to alcohol dependence risk in a national twin sample: Consistency of findings in women and men. *Psychological Medicine* 27(6):1381-1396.

Helzer JE, Burnam A & McEvoy LT (1991). Alcohol abuse and dependence. In LN Robins & DA Regier (eds.) *Psychiatric Disorders in America: The Epidemiologic Catchment Area Study*. New York, NY: The Free Press/MacMillan, Inc., 81-115.

Herd D (1990). Subgroup differences in drinking patterns among black and white men: Results from a national survey. *Journal of Studies on Alcohol* 51(3):221-232.

Herd D (1994). Predicting drinking problems among black and white men: Results from a national survey. *Journal of Studies on Alcohol* 55:61-71.

Hettema JM, Corey LA & Kendler KS (1999). A multivariate genetic analysis of the use of tobacco, alcohol, and caffeine in a population based sample of male and female twins. *Drug and Alcohol Dependence* 57(1):69-78.

Higuchi S, Matsushita S, Murayama M et al. (1995). Alcohol and aldehyde dehydrogenase polymorphisms and the risk for alcoholism.
American Journal of Psychiatry 152(8): 1219-1221.

Hingson RW, Heeren T, Jamanka A et al. (2000). Age of drinking onset
and unintentional injury involvement after drinking. *Journal of the
American Medical Association* 284:1527-1533.

Hingson R, Heeren T, Levenson S et al. (2002). Age of drinking onset,
driving after drinking, and involvement in alcohol related motor-ve-
hicle crashes. *Accident; Analysis and Prevention* 34:85-92.

Hingson R, Heeren T & Zakocs R (2001). Age of drinking onset and involvement in physical fights after drinking. *Pediatrics* 108:872-827.

Holck SE, Warren CW, Smith JC et al. (1984). Alcohol consumption among
Mexican American and Anglo women: Results of a survey along the
U.S.-Mexico border. *Journal of Studies on Alcohol* 45(2):149-154.

Hrubec Z & Omenn GS (1981). Evidence of genetic predisposition to
alcoholic cirrhosis and psychosis: Twin concordances for alcoholism
and its biological end points by zygosity among male veterans. *Alcoholism: Clinical & Experimental Research* 5(2):207-215.

Hsu YP, Loh EW, Chen WJ et al. (1996). Association of monoamine oxidase A alleles with alcoholism among male Chinese in Taiwan.
American Journal of Psychiatry 153(9):1209-1211.

Jang KL, Vernon PA & Livesley WJ (2000). Personality disorder traits,
family environment, and alcohol misuse: A multivariate behavioral
genetic analysis. *Addiction* 95(6):873-888.

Jessor R & Jessor SL (1977). *Problem Behavior and Psychosocial Development: A Longitudinal Study of Youth.* New York, NY: Academic
Press.

Johnston LD, O'Malley PM & Bachman JG (1992). *Smoking, Drinking,
and Illicit Drug Use among American Secondary School Students,
College Students, and Young Adults, 1975-1991; Vol. I, Secondary
School Students.* Rockville, MD: National Institute on Drug Abuse.

Kallan JE (1998). Drug abuse-related mortality in the United States: Patterns and correlates. *American Journal of Drug and Alcohol Abuse*
24(1):103-117.

Kandel D (1975). Stages in adolescent involvement in drug use. *Science*
190:912-914.

Kandel D, Chen K, Warner LA et al. (1997). Prevalence and demographic
correlates of symptoms of last year dependence on alcohol, nicotine,
marijuana and cocaine in the U.S. population. *Drug and Alcohol
Dependence* 44:11-29.

Kandel D & Yamaguchi K (1993). From beer to crack: Developmental
patterns of drug involvement. *American Journal of Public Health*
83(6):851-855.

Kaprio J, Koskenvuo M, Langinvainio H et al. (1987). Genetic influences
on use and abuse of alcohol: A study of 5638 adult Finnish
twin brothers. *Alcoholism: Clinical & Experimental Research*
11(4):349-356.

Kellam SG, Brown CH, Rubin BR et al. (1983). Paths leading to teenage
psychiatric symptoms and substance use: Developmental epidemiological studies in Woodlawn. In SB Guze, FJ Earls & JE Barrett (eds.)
Childhood Psychopathology and Development. New York, NY: Raven
Press.

Kendler KS, Gardner CO & Prescott CA (1997). Religion, psychopathology, and substance use and abuse; A multimeasure, genetic-
epidemiologic study. *American Journal of Psychiatry* 154(3):322-
329.

Kendler KS, Heath AC, Neale MC et al. (1992). A population-based twin
study of alcoholism in women. *Journal of the American Medical
Association* 268(14):1877-1882.

Kendler KS, Karkowski LM, Neale MC et al. (2000). Illicit psychoactive
substance use, heavy use, abuse, and dependence in a US-popula-
tion-based sample of male twins. *Archives of General Psychiatry*
57(3):261-269.

Kendler KS, Neale MC, Heath AC et al. (1994). A twin-family study
of alcoholism in women. *American Journal of Psychiatry*
151(5):707-715.

Kendler KS, Neale MC, Sullivan P et al. (1999). A population-based twin
study in women of smoking initiation and nicotine dependence. *Psychological Medicine* 29(2):299-308.

Kendler KS, Neale MC, Thornton LM et al. (2002). Cannabis use in the
last year in a US national sample of twin and sibling pairs. *Psychological Medicine* 32(3):551-554.

Kendler KS & Prescott CA (1999). Caffeine intake, tolerance, and withdrawal in women: A population-based twin study. *American Journal
of Psychiatry* 156(2):223-228.

Kendler KS & Prescott CA (1998). Cocaine use, abuse and dependence in
a population-based sample of female twins. *British Journal of Psychiatry* 173:345-350.

Kendler KS, Thornton LM & Pedersen NL (2000). Tobacco consumption
in Swedish twins reared apart and reared together. *Archives of General Psychiatry* 57(9):886-892.

Kessler RC, Crum RM, Warner LA et al. (1997). Lifetime co-occurrence
of DSM-IIIR alcohol abuse and dependence with other psychiatric
disorders in the National Comorbidity Survey. *Archives of General
Psychiatry* 54(4):313-321.

Kessler RC, McGonagle KA, Zhao S et al. (1994). Lifetime and 12-month
prevalence of DSM-IIIR psychiatric disorders in the United States.
Archives of General Psychiatry 51:8-19.

Kleinbaum DG, Kupper LL & Morgenstern H (1982). *Epidemiologic
Research.* New York, NY: Van Nostrand Reinhold.

Kushner MG, Sher KJ & Erickson DJ (1999). Prospective analysis of the
relation between DSM-III anxiety disorders and alcohol use disorders. *American Journal of Psychiatry* 156(5):723-732.

Lahelma E, Kangas R & Manderbacka K (1995). Drinking and unemployment: Contrasting patterns among men and women. *Drug and
Alcohol Dependence* 37:71-82.

Liberto JG, Oslin DW & Ruskin PE (1992). Alcoholism in older persons:
A review of the literature. *Hospital & Community Psychiatry*
43(10):975-984.

Lilienfeld DE (1994). *Foundations of Epidemiology, 3rd Ed.* New York,
NY: Oxford University Press.

Lilienfeld AM & Lilienfeld DE (1980). *Foundations of Epidemiology,
2nd Ed.* New York, NY: Oxford University Press.

Lillie-Blanton M, Anthony JC & Schuster CR (1993). Probing the meaning of racial/ethnic group comparisons in crack cocaine smoking.
Journal of the American Medical Association 269(8):993-997.

Lown AE & Vega WA (2001). Alcohol abuse or dependence among Mexican American women who report violence. *Alcoholism: Clinical &
Experimental Research* 25:1479-1986.

Luthar SS, Cushing G & Rounsaville BJ (1996). Gender differences among
opioid abusers: Pathways to disorder and profiles of psychopathology. *Drug and Alcohol Dependence* 43(3):179-189.

Luczak SE, Elvine-Kreis B, Shea SH et al. (2002). Genetic risk for alcoholism relates to level of response to alcohol in Asian American men and women. *Journal of Studies on Alcohol* 63:74-82.

Mausner JS & Kramer S (1985). *Mausner and Bahn Epidemiology: An Introductory Text*. Philadelphia, PA: W.B. Saunders.

McCarthy DM, Wall TL, Brown SA et al. (2000). Integrating biological and behavioral factors in alcohol use risk: The role of ALDH2 status and alcohol expectancies in a sample of Asian Americans. *Experimental and Clinical Psychopharmacology* 8:168-175.

McCord W & McCord J (1962). A longitudinal study of the personality of alcoholics. In DJ Pittman & CR Snyder (eds.) *Society, Culture, and Drinking Patterns*. New York, NY: John Wiley & Sons, 413-430.

McLeod JD (1993). Spouse concordance for alcohol dependence and heavy drinking: Evidence from a community sample. *Alcoholism: Clinical & Experimental Research* 17(6):1146-1155.

McMorris BJ & Uggen C (2000). Alcohol and employment in the transition to adulthood. *Journal of Health and Social Behavior* 41(3):276-294.

Midanik LT & Clark WB (1995). Drinking-related problems in the United States: Description and trends, 1984-1990. *Journal of Studies on Alcohol* 56:395-402.

Miles DR, van den Bree MB, Gupman AE et al. (2001). A twin study on sensation seeking, risk taking behavior and marijuana use. *Drug and Alcohol Dependence* 62(1): 57-68.

Mudar P, Leonard KE & Soltysinski K (2001). Discrepant substance use and marital functioning in newlywed couples. *Journal of Consulting Clinical Psychology* 69(1):130-134.

Mullahy J & Sindelar JL (1994). Alcoholism and income: The role of indirect effects. *The Milbank Quarterly* 72(2):359-375.

Narrow WE, Rae DS, Robins LN et al. (2002). Revised prevalence estimates of mental disorders in the United States. Using a clinical significance criterion to reconcile 2 surveys' estimates. *Archives of General Psychiatry* 59:115-123.

Nemoto T, Aoki B, Huang K et al. (1999). Drug use behaviors among Asian drug users in San Francisco. *Addictive Behaviors* 24:823-838.

Ohannessian CM & Hesselbrock VM (1993). The influence of perceived social support on the relationship between family history of alcoholism and drinking behaviors. *Addiction* 88(12):1651-1658.

Ojesjo L (1980). Prevalence of known and hidden alcoholism in the revisited Lundby population. *Social Psychiatry* 15:81-90.

Ojesjo L, Hagnell O & Lanke J (1982). Incidence of alcoholism among men in the Lundby Community Cohort, Sweden, 1957-1972. *Journal of Studies on Alcohol* 43(11):1190-1198.

Olkinuora M (1984). Alcoholism and occupation. *Scandinavian Journal of Work Environment and Health* 10:511-515.

O'Malley PM, Bachman JG & Johnston LD (1988). Period, age and cohort effects on substance use among young Americans: A decade of change, 1976-1986. *American Journal of Public Health* 78(10):1315-1321.

Otten MC, Teutsch SM, Williamson DF et al. (1990). The effect of known risk factors on the excess mortality of black adults in the United States. *Journal of the American Medical Association* 263(6):845-850.

Parker DA & Harford TC (1992). Gender-role attitudes, job competition and alcohol consumption among women and men. *Alcoholism: Clinical & Experimental Research* 16(2):159-165.

Paschall MJ, Flewelling RL & Faulkner DL (2000). Alcohol misuse in young adulthood: Effects of race, educational attainment, and social context. *Substance Use & Misuse* 35(11):1485-1506.

Pickens RW & Svikis DS (1988). *Biological Vulnerability to Drug Abuse (NIDA Research Monograph 89)* Rockville, MD: National Institute on Drug Abuse.

Polednak AP (1997). Gender and acculturation in relation to alcohol use among Hispanic (Latino) adults in two areas of the northeastern United States. *Substance Use & Misuse* 32:1513-1524.

Power C, Rodgers B & Hope S (1999). Heavy alcohol consumption and marital status: Disentangling the relationship in a national study of young adults. *Addiction* 94(10):1477-1487.

Prescott CA & Kendler KS (1999). Genetic and environmental contributions to alcohol abuse and dependence in a population-based sample of male twins. *American Journal of Psychiatry* 156(1):34-40.

Prescott CA & Kendler KS (2001). Associations between marital status and alcohol consumption in a longitudinal study of female twins. *Journal of Studies on Alcohol* 62(5):589-604.

Rausch JL, Monteiro MG & Schuckit MA (1991). Platelet serotonin uptake in men with family histories of alcoholism. *Neuropsychopharmacology* 4(2):83-86.

Regier DA, Farmer ME, Rae DS et al. (1990). Co-morbidity of mental disorders with alcohol and other drug abuse: Results from the Epidemiologic Catchment Area (ECA) Study. *Journal of the American Medical Association* 264(19):2511-2518.

Rhoades ER, Hammond J, Welty TK et al. (1987). The Indian burden of illness and future health interventions. *Public Health Reports* 102(4):361-368.

Roberts RE & Lee ES (1993). Occupation and the prevalence of major depression, alcohol, and drug abuse in the United States. *Environmental Research* 61(2):266-278.

Robins LN, Helzer JE, Croughan J et al. (1981). National Institute of Mental Health Diagnostic Interview Schedule. *Archives of General Psychiatry* 38:381-389.

Robins LN, Helzer JE, Weissman MM et al. (1984). Lifetime prevalence of specific psychiatric disorders in three sites. *Archives of General Psychiatry* 41:949-958.

Robins LN & Regier DA (1991). *Psychiatric Disorders in America: The Epidemiologic Catchment Area Study*. New York, NY: The Free Press, Macmillan, Inc.

Ronan L (1986-87). Alcohol-related health risks among Black Americans. *Alcohol Health & Research World* 11(2):36-39, 65.

Schuckit MA (1983). Alcoholic men with no alcoholic first-degree relatives. *American Journal of Psychiatry* 140(4):439-443.

Schulenberg J, Bachman JG, O'Malley PM et al. (1994). High school educational success and subsequent substance use: A panel analysis following adolescents into young adulthood. *Journal of Health and Social Behavior* 35:45-62.

Sigvardsson S, Bohman M, Cloninger CR (1996). Replication of the Stockholm Adoption Study of alcoholism. *Archives of General Psychiatry* 53(8):681-687.

Slutske WS, Heath AC, Madden PA et al. (2002). Personality and the genetic risk for alcohol dependence. *Journal of Abnormal Psychology* 111(1):124-133.

Suddendorf RF (1989). Research on alcohol metabolism among Asians and its implications for understanding causes of alcoholism. *Public Health Reports* 104(6):615-620.

Thomas BS (1993). Drug use in a small Midwestern community and relationships to selected characteristics. *Journal of Drug Education* 23:247-258.

Thomas BS & Hsiu LT (1993). The role of selected risk factors in predicting adolescent drug use and its adverse consequences. *International Journal of the Addictions* 28:1549-1563.

True WR, Heath AC, Scherrer JF et al. (1999). Interrelationship of genetic and environmental influences on conduct disorder and alcohol and marijuana dependence symptoms. *American Journal of Medical Genetics* 88(4):391-397.

True WR, Xian H, Scherrer JF et al. (1999). Common genetic vulnerability for nicotine and alcohol dependence in men. *Archives of General Psychiatry* 56(7):655-661.

Tsuang MT, Lyons MJ, Eisen SA et al. (1996). Genetic influences on DSM-IIIR drug abuse and dependence: A study of 3,372 twin pairs. *American Journal of Medical Genetics* 67(5):473-477.

Valois RF, Dunham AC, Jackson KL et al. (1999). Association between employment and substance abuse behaviors among public high school adolescents. *Journal of Adolescent Health* 25(4):256-263.

van den Bree MB, Johnson EO et al. (1998). Genetic and environmental influences on drug use and abuse/dependence in male and female twins. *Drug and Alcohol Dependence* 52(3):231-241.

Vega WA, Zimmerman RS, Warheit GJ et al. (1993). Risk factors for early adolescent drug use in four ethnic and racial groups. *American Journal of Public Health* 83(2):185-189.

Vestal RE, McGuire EA, Tobin JD et al. (1977). Aging and ethanol metabolism. *Clinical Pharmacology & Therapeutics* 21(3):343-354.

Wall TL, Peterson CM, Peterson KP et al. (1997). Alcohol metabolism in Asian American men with genetic polymorphisms of aldehyde dehydrogenase. *Annals of Internal Medicine* 127(5):376-379.

Wall TL, Shea SH, Chan KK et al. (2001). A genetic association with the development of alcohol and other substance use behavior in Asian Americans. *Journal of Abnormal Psychology* 11:173-178.

Warner LA, Canino G & Colón HM (2001). Prevalence and correlates of substance use disorders among older adolescents in Puerto Rico and the United States: A cross-cultural comparison. *Drug and Alcohol Dependence* 63:229-243.

Warner LA, Kessler RC, Hughes M et al. (1995). Prevalence and correlates of drug use and dependence in the United States. Results from the National Comorbidity Survey. *Archives of General Psychiatry* 52(3):219-229.

West MO & Prinz RJ (1987). Parental alcoholism and childhood psychopathology. *Psychological Bulletin* 102(2):204-218.

Westhuis DJ, Gwaltney L & Hayashi R (2001). Outpatient cocaine abuse treatment: Predictors of success. *Journal of Drug Education* 31(2):171-183.

Wilsnack SC, Klassen AD, Schur BE et al. (1991). Predicting onset and chronicity of women's problem drinking: A five-year longitudinal analysis. *American Journal of Public Health* 81:305-318.

Wilsnack SC, Vogeltanz ND, Klassen AD et al. (1997). Childhood sexual abuse and women's substance abuse: National survey findings. *Journal of Studies on Alcohol* 58(3):264-271.

Wilsnack SC & Wilsnack RW (1995). Drinking and problem drinking in U.S. women. In M Galanter (ed.) *Recent Developments in Alcoholism Volume 12: Women and Alcoholism.* New York, NY: Plenum Press.

World Health Organization (WHO) (1992). *The ICD-10 Classification of Mental and Behavioural Disorders.* Geneva, Switzerland: The Organization.

Yates WR, Cadoret RJ, Troughton E et al. (1996). An adoption study of DSM-IIIR alcohol and drug dependence severity. *Drug and Alcohol Dependence* 41(1):9-15.

Zayas LH, Rojas M & Malgady RG (1998). Alcohol and drug use, and depression among Hispanic men in early adulthood. *American Journal of Community Psychology* 26:425-438.

| Chapter 3 | # Understanding Alcoholism: Insights from the Research |

Enoch Gordis, M.D.

The Problem of Alcoholism
Major Conceptual Advances
The Promise of Research

Alcoholism, like many other serious diseases, results from the interaction of complex biological and behavioral systems. Understanding the systems involved in the development of alcoholism and its consequences, how individual components of biological and behavioral systems interact to produce disease, and how to interrupt this process to prevent disease and reduce harm are the major goals of alcohol research. This is no simple task. It is, however, a very necessary one: it is no more likely that alcoholism will yield to one type of intervention or one type of treatment than it is that all cancers will respond to the same regimen of chemotherapy or radiation. Moreover, in today's health care environment, demands by managed care organizations, other third-party payers, state funding agencies, and the Congress for accountability require the same type of safety and efficacy evidence for the treatment of alcoholism as that required for all other illnesses. We may believe we know "what works," but it is the evidence of efficacy that will bring financial and patient support.

Today's alcohol researchers are working at the cutting edge of science in many different areas, seeking answers to the most perplexing questions facing the alcoholism field.

This overview of the science of alcoholism discusses some of the major conceptual advances in alcohol research that have occurred over the past several decades, highlights research progress toward answering the basic questions about alcoholism, and provides some thoughts about scientific advances that are just over the horizon.

THE PROBLEM OF ALCOHOLISM

Alcoholism is one of the nation's most serious and persistent health problems. Approximately two-thirds of all American adults (aged 18 and older) drink an alcoholic beverage during the course of a year (Midanik & Room, 1992). At least 13.8 million American adults develop problems from drinking (Grant, Harford et al., 1994). Young people, for whom alcohol remains the number one drug of abuse, also are at risk for developing alcohol-related problems. Recently published data from the National Longitudinal Alcohol Epidemiologic Survey sponsored by the National Institute on Alcohol Abuse and Alcoholism (NIAAA), which assesses lifetime risk for alcohol use disorders, provides convincing evidence that the younger an individual is when he or she begins drinking, the greater is his or her chance of subsequently developing a clinically diagnosable alcohol use disorder. For example, individuals who begin drinking before age 15 are four times more likely to develop alcohol dependence during their lifetimes than those who begin drinking at age 21 (Grant & Dawson, 1997). The reasons for this association are not yet understood, but researchers are beginning to address this issue. In one recent study, investigators examined whether the association between age of drinking onset and later alcoholism was caused, in part, by a genetic risk for developing a broad range of behavioral problems, including alcoholism, rather than a risk that is specific to alcohol problems (McGue, Iacono et al., 2001). This research is important to the design of prevention efforts because it will permit more precise identification of behaviors that must be targeted to reduce the risk for developing alcohol use problems over the lifespan.

Health problems caused by alcohol use include damage to the brain, liver, gastrointestinal tract, and heart. The relative risk for many alcohol-related illnesses rises in parallel with the quantity of alcohol consumed each day (Boffeta & Garfinkel, 1990). Other consequences of alcohol use include motor vehicle crashes and other injuries, domestic violence, neglect of work and family, and costs to society associated with police, courts, jails, and unemployment. Altogether, the consequences of alcohol abuse and dependence are estimated to cost the nation almost $100 billion (NIAAA, 1997a) and more than 100,000 deaths a year (NIAAA, 1993).

MAJOR CONCEPTUAL ADVANCES
Several conceptual breakthroughs have been instrumental in advancing the study and understanding of alcoholism. These involve the acceptance of alcoholism as a disease; the demonstration that a significant portion of vulnerability to alcoholism is inherited; the application of neuroscience to understanding drinking and the phenomenon of addiction; the study of mental processes involved in alcohol use, abuse, and dependence; new insights into how alcohol causes organ damage; the demonstration that prevention can be studied rigorously; and new approaches to treatment.

Alcoholism as a Disease. The acceptance of alcoholism as a medical disorder is the conceptual advance that has most influenced the direction and shape of alcoholism research. This concept has evolved progressively and with considerable controversy over the past 20 years (Jaffe, 1993). Competing views have included the idea of alcoholism as a symptom of psychological maladjustment or as the arbitrarily delineated upper end of a continuum of drinking (Keller,

1990). The disease concept defines alcoholism as an independent disorder characterized by a craving for alcohol—a dependence, or addiction. As such, it is distinguished from drinking that is merely heavy, problematic, ill advised, or socially unacceptable. Many alcohol-related problems result from misuse of alcohol by persons who are not alcoholic. Nevertheless, the disease concept has sharpened the focus of alcohol research and is helping to remove the stigma from this major chronic disorder.

Gene Involvement in Vulnerability. In the 1970s, rigorous scientific research began to explore the reasons for the common observation that alcoholism runs in families. The question was, "Does this familial transmission occur through exposure to the environment, or through the inheritance of genes, or both?" Adoption and twin studies provided the first evidence of a genetic component of the risk for alcoholism. This conceptual advance has led to an explosion in human and animal genetic work that promises to lead to the development of new treatments and better-focused prevention efforts for those who are most at risk for developing the disease of alcoholism. Exactly what is inherited is not yet known. Among the possibilities are differences in a number of biological and psychological reactions to alcohol use, including temperament, initial sensitivity to the rewarding or aversive qualities of alcohol, ability to develop tolerance after repeated exposure, rates and routes of alcohol metabolism, taste preferences, signaling from peripheral sites to the brain after drinking alcohol, and ability to relate memories of drinking experiences to the outcome of such experiences (expectancies). It is very possible that when we find the genes for the vulnerability to alcoholism, they could code for many functions. For example, reduced sensitivity to alcohol in the young has been shown to predict later alcoholism (Schuckit & Smith, 1996). This sensitivity could be inherited. We also are learning more about how protection against developing alcoholism also may be genetically determined. Such is the case of the Asian "flushing" enzyme, which now is known to result from a mutation in the gene for the enzyme aldehyde dehydrogenase. Absence of the enzyme protects somewhat against developing alcoholism simply because the first exposure of an individual with this enzyme to alcohol is so noxious.

Neurosciences Applied to Drinking and Addiction. The application of neuroscience techniques to alcoholism research has led to an increased understanding of how alcohol's actions in the brain are related to the phenomenon of addiction, including how alcohol affects gene proteins and second messengers and expression of those substances. New imaging techniques have permitted alcohol neuroscientists to study alcohol's effects on the brain in ways not possible just a decade ago. The puzzling question of how alcohol—a substance that permeates every part of the body, every cell, and distributes in all body water—can have such specific action in the brain is being examined. Research into craving, the prelude to relapse, is yielding important information about the brain mechanisms involved in this phenomenon. This conceptual advance has led to the development of new pharmacotherapies for alcoholism, such as naltrexone and acamprosate, and to the possibility of developing "designer" medications targeted at specific alcohol actions.

Mental Processes Involved in Alcohol Use, Abuse, and Dependence. Another conceptual advance is the acceptance of mental processes in alcohol addiction. This advance has led to increasing emphasis by investigators on the importance of understanding the cognitive processes involved in alcoholism, as well as the biology of alcoholism. As Y. Dudai, the Israeli neuroscientist, has said, "Psychologists must remember that beyond the behavior is a brain, and the biologist must remember that the animal behaved prior to homogenization!" Acceptance of this concept has stimulated important research into effects that result from alcohol use because of the drinker's expectations of how he or she will feel, rather than the pharmacological actions of alcohol. It also has led to studies investigating whether craving exists intrinsically or depends on cues from the environment.

Alcohol's Effects on the Body. Investigating the toxicology of alcohol, or the damage to the body caused by alcohol use, is one of the oldest areas of alcohol research. In addition to understanding what damage occurs (for example, alcoholic cirrhosis), scientists are investigating how, and the mechanisms by which, such damage occurs. The demonstration that alcohol use potentially benefits health also has helped advance the study of alcohol's effects on the body. Increased understanding of alcohol's action on various body systems has led to a new understanding of withdrawal and how to safely detoxify patients, discovery of the mechanisms involved in alcoholic liver damage, and recognition of the effects of low doses of alcohol on the fetus. Over the past few years, research has flourished on the toxic effects of alcohol on different receptor systems, such as N-methyl-D-aspartate (NMDA), or nitric oxide, and especially of the elaborate cytokine network that has been shown to be involved in alcohol's toxic effects in the liver.

Determining how alcohol affects the body both positively and negatively will help researchers to develop medications and other therapies to prevent or limit the damage that alcohol causes and will help clinicians to provide more accurate advice to their patients about the risks and benefits of alcohol use.

Prevention Can Be Studied Rigorously. The demonstration that approaches to preventing alcohol abuse and alcoholism, including social and regulatory policies, can be studied rigorously is a welcome occurrence in the alcohol field. This conceptual advance has stimulated a substantial amount of research seeking to define what programs work best with various populations to prevent alcohol-related problems. The findings from prevention research, applied to various public policies, already have been shown to save lives. New approaches to school-based and community-based prevention also are demonstrating that well-planned prevention programs that build on rigorously studied and validated models can significantly reduce the magnitude and extent of our nation's alcohol-related problems.

New Approaches to Treatment. A major change in the alcohol field is the growing acceptance of the need for alcohol treatment research. Today, many alcoholism treatment professionals—including physicians, social workers, nurses, and counselors—expect to have access to scientifically validated screening, assessment, diagnostic, and treatment tools. Managed care and other determiners of health care policies also demand good data. These and other factors have combined to support the need for alcoholism treatment research. This conceptual advance has led to two important developments. First is the rigorous analysis of things that have been done for a very long time, as in subjecting traditional treatment approaches to modern clinical trial research. Second is the development of new verbal treatments (such as brief intervention) and new pharmacotherapies (such as naltrexone in the United States and acamprosate in Europe).

THE PROMISE OF RESEARCH

Alcohol research has one fundamental purpose: to develop the knowledge necessary to effectively prevent and treat alcohol abuse and alcoholism and the consequences of those disorders. From its modest beginnings a quarter century ago, NIAAA's alcohol research enterprise has expanded to a broad-based program of biomedical and behavioral research in areas such as the epidemiology of alcohol use, abuse, and dependence; alcohol's effects on the brain; the genetics of alcoholism; alcohol's effects on health; the effects of public policies on preventing alcohol use disorders; and clinical trials to develop or evaluate promising therapies. Whether research involves understanding the basic mechanisms of alcohol action or the development of a diagnostic manual for use by clinicians, the science of alcoholism is guided by the "promise of research"—that each new discovery made by alcohol researchers will move the field closer to the goal of helping those with alcohol-related problems. The highlights of alcohol research discussed below demonstrate how very far alcohol research has progressed toward fulfilling this promise.

The Genetics of Alcoholism. There is ample evidence that a significant portion of the vulnerability to alcoholism is inherited. Genetics researchers are engaged in identifying the genes that confer this vulnerability and in developing ways to apply this information to clinical populations. The task is difficult because alcoholism is considered to be a polygenic disorder that is related to many different genes, each of which contributes only a portion of the vulnerability. The search for the relevant genes is being pursued in several settings.

Collaborative Project on the Genetics of Alcoholism: One important research enterprise is the Collaborative Study on the Genetics of Alcoholism (COGA), a multisite study at six centers. COGA investigators have interviewed hundreds of probands and families, developed a complex computerized pedigree database, and applied statistical genetics and molecular biology techniques to "informative" families. Phenotypic markers shown previously to be relevant to alcohol are incorporated into the study, including biochemical markers, evoked potential responses, and tests of initial sensitivity to alcohol. (Initial sensitivity to alcohol has been shown to be a strong predictor of later alcoholism [Schuckit & Smith, 1996], suggesting the possibility of a biological marker for identifying individuals, as well as groups, who are at greatest risk of developing alcoholism.)

COGA scientists have located chromosomal "hot spots"—areas of potential linkage to alcohol dependence—on chromosomes 1, 2, and 7 (Reich, Edenberg et al., 1998), the suggestion of protective factors by possible linkage on chromosome 4 for resilience to alcoholism (Reich, Edenberg et al., 1998), and recently, evidence for a link between alcoholism and depression on chromosome 1 (Nurnberger, Foroud et al, 2001). Locations of the genes involved in the expression of evoked potential responses, a high-risk marker for alcoholism, have been tentatively identified (Begleiter, Porjesz et al., 1998). These findings bring us a step closer

to finding the specific genes underlying the genetic vulnerability to this chronic disorder.

Animal Genetics: The alcohol research field has been a leader in developing animal models for medical inquiry. Many rat and mouse strains have been selectively bred for sensitivity to various effects of alcohol. The development of such strains demonstrates that the selected trait is, to some extent, genetically determined. Studies in selectively bred strains have shown that tolerance and dependence probably are not controlled by the same mechanism, because it is possible to alter alcohol tolerance without affecting alcohol dependence. Similarities between the mouse and human genome give hope that animal work will provide clues that will accelerate the search for alcohol-related genes in humans. Even lower organisms, such as Drosophila (fruit fly) and invertebrates (such as the nematode), which have neural and other systems that are homologous to those in mammals, are teaching us much about the genetics of alcohol use problems. For example, Drosophila is a model system of mammalian development and behavior. Using this model, investigators identified genetic mutations associated with increased or decreased sensitivity to alcohol (Moore, DeZazzo et al., 1998).

Scientists also are using animals to identify the location of genes responsible for the genetically influenced traits that are thought to underlie responses to alcohol. These are known as "quantitative traits." More than one gene influences the magnitude of a trait. A section of DNA on a chromosome that is thought to influence a quantitative trait is known as a quantitative trait loci (QTL). Using powerful genetic analysis techniques, researchers can locate and measure the effects of a single QTL on a trait, or phenotype, and ultimately gain knowledge of the complex physiologic underpinnings of alcohol-related behavior. For example, scientists have identified two loci—*Alcp*1 and *Alcp*2—that appear to have significant gender-specific effects on alcohol consumption in mice (Melo, Shendure et al., 1995). This finding suggests that preference for alcohol—a quantitative trait—may be controlled by different genetic mechanisms in males and females.

Molecular genetic techniques, which permit highly selective breeding of mice that express different receptor subtypes on their neurons, are providing a wealth of information about the effects of alcohol on the brain. Animal models that are devoted to alcohol drinking preferences and methodologies in genetic "knock-out" technology and transgenetics all contribute to an understanding of why some individuals are more vulnerable than others to developing alcoholism. There now are more than 20 gene knock-out and transgenic animals that model different aspects of alcohol-related behavior. This is allowing alcohol researchers to learn about the circuits that control drinking and affect alcohol consumption.

Other powerful tools for investigating the link between biology and behavior are microarrays. The long-term adaptation of the brain's neurons to alcohol may result, in part, from changes in gene function (Miles, 1995). Because alcohol is known to affect gene expression (Bachtell, Wang et al., 1999), activity can be tracked to determine how genes associated with alcohol-induced effects are expressed. Tracking the activity of a single gene takes time; given the large number of genes that may be involved in producing alcohol's effects, the task of linking specific genes to particular effects may be formidable. Microarrays permit the simultaneous study of many genes (up to 10,000 at a time) and provide scientists with new power to understand changes in gene expression that relate to the vulnerability to alcoholism. As more researchers begin to employ this technique, it may become possible to identify virtually every gene and its protein that play a significant role in alcohol-related behavior.

Gene-Environment Interactions: Although a significant portion of the vulnerability to development of alcoholism is inherited, ample research indicates that both biological and nonbiological factors influence drinking behavior. For example, although it can be predicted that an Asian individual who inherits an $ALDH_2$ (aldehyde dehydrogenase) mutation will be much less likely to develop alcoholism than an individual who does not inherit this mutation, more precise prediction of outcome requires additional knowledge of that individual's cultural context and alcohol-specific expectancies. In recent years, alcohol researchers have begun to test and apply models that emphasize the process by which environmental factors can transform heritable characteristics to promote or impede the expression of alcohol problems and the reciprocal influence that biological and nonbiological factors impose over time.

An example of this type of research is the now-classic adoption studies (Cloninger, Bohman et al., 1981), which have identified two alcoholism subtypes that differ in inheritance patterns as well as other characteristics. Type 1 alcoholism, which affects both men and women, requires the presence of a specific genetic background as well as certain environmental factors (such as low socioeconomic status

of the father). Mild or severe alcohol abuse, adult onset of the disease, a loss of control over drinking, and guilt and fear about alcohol dependence characterize this alcoholism subtype. Individuals with this type of alcoholism generally exhibit high harm avoidance and low novelty-seeking personality traits, and drink primarily to relieve anxiety.

In contrast, type 2 alcoholism, which occurs more commonly in men than in women, primarily requires a genetic predisposition, with environmental factors playing only a minor role in its development. Type 2 alcoholism is associated with early onset (before age 25) of both alcohol abuse and criminal behavior and an inability to abstain from alcohol. Type 2 alcoholics exhibit high novelty-seeking personality characteristics and consume alcohol primarily to induce euphoria (Cloninger, Sigvardsson et al., 1996).

Characterizing the specific environmental factors that play a role in the etiology of alcoholism is emerging as a fundamental research issue. Predisposing genetic factors may remain dormant in the absence of environmental cues. On the other hand, given certain environmental factors, alcoholism may develop in the absence of genetic predisposition. Consequently, it is important not only to identify the principal environmental factors involved in the development of alcoholism, but also to understand the manner and extent to which they interact with genetic factors. Greater knowledge of these factors and their contribution to alcohol problems will facilitate the design of prevention and early intervention strategies that focus on environmental risk factors for alcohol abuse and alcoholism.

Alcohol and the Brain. The actions of alcohol that cause intoxication, reinforce drinking behavior, and lead to addiction are based principally in the brain. Alcohol investigators are working vigorously to understand the mechanisms in the brain by which alcohol produces these effects. For example, several lines of investigation using animal models have helped scientists to discover two factors—reinforcement and cellular adaptation—that may explain alcohol-dependent behavior. Alcohol is considered to be reinforcing because the ingestion of alcohol, or withdrawal from chronic long-term alcohol use, or sometimes just the sight or smell of an alcoholic drink, increases the probability that an individual will drink. One explanation for reinforcement is that alcohol appears to interact with the brain's reward system, thus stimulating continued use: this is called "positive reinforcement." Relief of abstinence, or negative reinforcement, is another possible mechanism. For example, alcohol-dependent rats undergoing withdrawal have been shown to perform lever press responses for alcohol in an apparent attempt to alleviate withdrawal symptoms (Schulteis, Hyytia et al., 1996). Thus, "negative reinforcement" also may contribute to continued drinking; its precise mechanism is a subject of current investigation.

When alcohol is chronically present, some neurons seem to adapt to this physiological change by enhancing or reducing their response to normal stimuli. This adaptation is hypothesized to lead to the development of tolerance and dependence. A primary question under investigation is the mechanism of cellular adaptation to the long-term presence of alcohol. One successful approach to exploring cellular adaptation is through molecular genetic studies. Scientists have uncovered evidence that alcohol can cause changes in cellular communication and functioning by directly influencing the function of specific genes. Sophisticated genetic mapping techniques and related technology may pinpoint exactly which genes are involved. Researchers then can selectively investigate the effects of alcohol on specific receptor constituents by directly manipulating genetic material. Data obtained from studies such as these will provide major advances in understanding the process of cellular adaptation to alcohol and thus provide clues about the mechanisms of alcohol dependence, tolerance, and withdrawal.

Investigators also have evidence that the cellular adaptive changes that occur with alcohol exposure can alter the degree of reinforcement experienced. Thus, adaptation and reinforcement, acting in concert, determine an individual's short-term or acute response to alcohol as well as the long-term or chronic craving for alcohol that characterizes dependence. Some adaptive changes may be permanent and are hypothesized to produce the persistent sense of discomfort during abstinence that can trigger relapse. Relapse is very common among recovering alcoholics, so understanding the mechanisms that cause or promote relapse is critical to treating alcohol dependence. Clarification of these processes will enable scientists to develop specifically designed medications and may lead to the design of effective treatment strategies tailored to individual physiology and psychology.

Because alcohol bathes every cell in the body, the challenge is to sort out the critical effects that cause uncontrolled drinking in the face of negative consequences, as well as how alcohol causes brain damage. Following the discovery of complex cell membranes, neuroscientists began probing the ways in which the brain controls thinking, behavior,

movement, and other key bodily functions. Current research strongly suggests that alcohol affects multiple neurotransmitter systems in the brain. The specific neurotransmitters involved in the behavioral aspects of alcoholism, the mode of release, and the corresponding receptors involved in these effects now are under investigation.

Molecular biological experiments using animal research techniques—such as chimeric proteins, deletion mutations, and site-directed mutagenesis—have identified regions of proteins in the brain that appear to be involved in alcohol's actions. For example, one neurotransmitter that appears to have particular importance for explaining alcohol's action is gamma-aminobutyric acid (GABA). Using these techniques, scientists have determined the specific region of one GABA receptor subunit that mediates alcohol's sedative action (Mihic, Ye et al., 1997). Additional animal studies are enhancing scientists' understanding of which subunit assemblies of GABA receptors are most sensitive to alcohol. Continuing work in this area will help to determine the molecular nature of the presumed ethanol binding sites, perhaps leading to new diagnostic tools for predicting an individual's vulnerability to developing alcoholism and to new medications for treating the disease.

Health Effects of Alcohol Use. Research over the past 25 years has brought about an increasing awareness of alcohol's medical effects and the mechanisms by which these effects occur. There also is growing research evidence that alcohol may have certain beneficial effects. These damaging and protective effects, the mechanisms by which the damage or protection occurs, and the risks and benefits alcohol poses to particular individuals currently are under study.

The Liver: Liver damage may be among the most serious consequences of alcohol abuse. Heavy alcohol use can cause liver inflammation and progressive liver scarring (fibrosis or cirrhosis). Among the mechanisms thought to contribute to liver damage are the release of cytokines, which are substances with inflammatory, fibrogenic, and cell growth-promoting properties, and the formation of free radicals, which are reactive oxygen molecules that can interact with proteins, lipids, and DNA, causing damage or death to liver cells. Acetaldehyde, a principal metabolite of alcohol, can form adducts by reacting with cellular proteins, potentially resulting in direct damage to liver cells or stimulation of inflammatory autoimmune reactions in liver tissues. Acetaldehyde protein adducts also may stimulate liver cell collagen synthesis, a process thought to contribute to fibrosis and cirrhosis. A promising approach to preventing fibrosis involves administration of polyunsaturated soybean lecithin, which may promote the breakdown of hepatic collagen.

Cardiovascular System: Alcohol use can contribute to heart and cardiovascular disease. Heavy alcohol consumption can interfere with the mechanical functions of the heart and may cause progressive functional changes and tissue damage, leading to cardiomyopathy and heart failure. Excessive alcohol consumption also is associated with high blood pressure and an increased risk for coronary artery disease and stroke. However, light to moderate drinking appears to be beneficial in preventing coronary artery disease, perhaps by elevating blood levels of high-density lipoprotein or by inhibiting clotting processes that contribute to atherosclerosis and thrombosis.

Neuropsychological Disorders: Alcohol-associated neuropsychological disorders typically involve damage to the limbic system, the diencephalon, and the frontal cerebral cortex of the brain. Among the problems resulting from this damage are deficits in short-term memory, disruption of cognitive and motor functioning, reduced perceptual abilities, and emotional and personality changes. With advances in brain and functional imaging techniques and the development of neurocognitive tests, researchers hope to identify connections between alcohol-associated structural and metabolic changes in the brain and alcohol-associated impairment in mental processes.

Endocrine System: A variety of studies show that alcohol interferes with normal endocrine system activities. Excessive alcohol use may profoundly impair reproductive development and function in both women and men. In postmenopausal women, low-level alcohol consumption may enhance estrogen production, which in turn may provide protection from osteoporosis as well as from coronary heart disease. In premenopausal women, chronic heavy drinking can contribute to many reproductive disorders, including problems with the menstrual cycle, early menopause, and increased risk of spontaneous abortions. Some of these problems have been observed in women classified as social drinkers (two or more standard drinks a day). Women who drink at these levels also may increase their risk for breast cancer.

Chronic alcohol exposure may alter the secretion patterns of growth hormone. Consequences of this disruption include numerous metabolic and endocrine changes, because growth hormone regulates levels of other growth stimula-

tors as well as alcohol- and steroid-metabolizing enzymes. In addition, alcohol withdrawal induces marked elevations in glucocorticoid stress hormones. Glucocorticoids in excess may be neurotoxic; thus, glucocorticoid elevations may contribute to the behavioral and neurological changes observed in withdrawal.

Immune System: In healthy individuals, the complex network of lymphoid cells and regulatory cytokines that compose the immune system efficiently detects and eliminates potential pathogens. Alcohol consumption, particularly of a chronic or abusive nature, depresses the immune system by altering the function, regulation, and distribution of lymphoid cells. The result may be immune system dysfunction and an increased susceptibility to infectious disease and cancer. Immunological abnormalities observed with long-term alcohol abuse in humans also include autoimmune processes that damage liver tissues.

Fetal Alcohol Syndrome: Fetal alcohol syndrome (FAS) is a severe alcohol-induced birth defect, consisting of mild facial anomalies, growth retardation, and severe impairment of the central nervous system. The behavioral and neurological problems associated with prenatal alcohol exposure in the absence of other indications of FAS are termed "alcohol-related neurodevelopmental disorder" (ARND).

Children with FAS and ARND often are described as hyperactive, impulsive, and having short attention spans. Maladaptive behaviors are common and include poor judgment, failure to consider the consequences of one's actions, and difficulty perceiving social cues. Studies indicate that the deficits associated with FAS are pervasive and long-lasting and have a marked effect on an individual's ability to live independently. Although many of the physical characteristics of FAS become less prominent after puberty, the intellectual problems endure, while the behavioral, emotional, and social problems become more pronounced. Findings from some (but not all) studies of the relationship of quantity, frequency, timing, and pattern of maternal drinking to infant and child outcomes have revealed an association between prenatal alcohol exposure and growth deficits at birth. However, the timing of alcohol exposure, the dose-response, and the effect of maternal drinking patterns at particular stages of fetal development have not yet been defined.

Progress has been made in research aimed at understanding the basic mechanisms involved in the neurobiological damage that occurs in alcohol-exposed fetuses and in developing potential new therapies to prevent such damage. For example, rather than a generalized impairment of mental functioning, studies show that some neurobehavioral functions are consistently impaired while others are not (Janzen, Nanson et al., 1995; Mattson, Riley et al., 1996; Olson, Feldman et al., 1998; Mattson & Riley, 1998). Researchers investigating why this is so are learning about the routes by which alcohol causes damage to the fetus. For example, within the fetus, embryonic cells destined to become brain neurons grow in number, move to their ultimate locations, and mature into a wide variety of functionally distinct neuronal cell types, eventually forming connections with other brain cells in a predetermined pattern. Alcohol metabolism is associated with increased susceptibility to cell damage caused by free radicals, which can kill sensitive populations of brain cells at critical times of development in the first trimester of pregnancy (Cartwright & Smith, 1995; Chen & Sulik, 1996).

Alcohol or the products of its metabolism also may interfere with brain development by altering the production or function of natural regulatory substances that help to promote the orderly growth and differentiation of neurons (Michaelis & Michaelis, 1994). Research using animals or cell cultures show that many of alcohol's adverse effects on brain cells can be prevented by treatments aimed at restoring the balance of regulatory substances upset by alcohol (Luo, West et al., 1997; Tajuddin & Druse, 1999). Promising results have been obtained in similar experiments by administering substances (such as antioxidants) that help protect cells against damage induced by free radicals (Heaton, Mitchell et al., 2000). This mechanism is only one of several that may contribute to alcohol-related fetal injury. Further research is needed to determine if such an approach is both effective and safe in humans during pregnancy.

Alcohol-Related Trauma: Alcohol use and abuse can have adverse effects on a wide variety of behaviors, with serious consequences for persons of all ages and backgrounds and for the health and well-being of society. Motor vehicle crashes, falls, fires, and drownings cause more than 75% of deaths from unintentional injuries (NIAAA, 1997b), and alcohol use has been associated with a large percentage of deaths from these causes. Alcohol use also has been linked with high-risk sexual behaviors, as well as with family and marital violence, homicide, and suicide.

Researchers have theorized that alcohol and injury may interact in two ways. First, the context and the place in which an individual consumes alcohol may result in an increased risk of injury. For example, drinking in bars where the risk of assault may be high increases an individual's exposure to hazardous circumstances. Second, direct biological effects of alcohol may lead to injury by interfering with the individual's perception of and responsiveness to potential hazards. The consequences of alcohol's direct biological effects are apparent in the large proportion of motor vehicle-related injuries and deaths that are associated with alcohol.

Motor vehicle crashes are the leading cause of death for Americans under the age of 35, and alcohol use plays a significant role in these deaths. On a positive note, research shows that drinking and driving in the United States has decreased over the past decade, especially among young drivers. The proportion of all traffic fatalities that are related to alcohol use has decreased. The overall percentage of drivers with a positive blood alcohol content (BAC) among all drivers surveyed on weekend nights also has decreased. In addition, crash statistics and driver surveys both show reductions in the proportion of drivers with BACs of 0.10 percent or higher, with the largest reductions found in drivers younger than age 21 (Voas, Wells et al., 1997; NHTSA, 2000). Strategies to reduce drinking and driving may be a significant factor in these reductions. For example, the National Highway Traffic Safety Administration (NHTSA) estimates that raising the minimum legal drinking age to 21 has reduced traffic fatalities involving 18- to 20-year-old drivers by 13% and has saved an estimated 19,121 lives since 1975. Zero-tolerance laws, which set the legal BAC limit for drivers younger than age 21 at 0.00 or 0.02 percent, have been associated with 20% reductions in the proportion of drinking drivers under the age of 21 who are involved in fatal crashes (Voas, Lange et al., 1998) and in the proportion of single-vehicle, nighttime fatal crashes among drivers younger than age 21 (Hingson, Heeren et al., 1994).

Intervening with individuals who have been injured as a result of their drinking may prove a useful clinical strategy to reduce problem drinking. In one recent study, emergency room patients injured in alcohol-related crashes were found to have an increased motivation to change their drinking behavior (DiClemente, Bellino et al., 1999). Emergency room interventions also have been shown to reduce subsequent drinking and re-admission for traumatic injuries (Gentilello, Rivara et al., 1999), as well as drinking and driving, traffic violations, alcohol-related injuries, and alcohol-related problems among 18- and 19-year-olds (Monti, Colby et al., 1999).

Direct associations between alcohol use and other types of injury, such as those associated with aircraft crashes, fires and burns, boating accidents, and violence, are less clear. For example, although associations have been observed between alcohol use by pilots and reduced aircraft safety, these findings must be interpreted with caution because many of the data are based on individual case reports rather than on epidemiologic studies. However, simulated flight experiments clearly show that pilot planning, performance, and vigilance are impaired by the acute and hangover effects of alcohol.

Data from numerous studies support a strong relationship between alcohol and various types of violence, including homicides, suicides, and spousal abuse. For example, a review of investigations examining the link between alcohol and homicide found that, in most studies, more than 60% of persons who committed homicides were drinking at the time of the offense (NIAAA, 1997c). Alcohol use also may increase the risk of becoming a victim of violence and of sustaining injury due to violence. One study has found that emergency room patients who were injured in violent events were twice as likely to have consumed alcohol than were patients whose injuries were unrelated to violence (NIAAA, 1997d). However, the presence of alcohol in violent episodes does not mean that alcohol itself causes violent behavior. Rather, alcohol is likely to be only one of many factors that interact to precipitate violent behavior in some individuals.

Finally, alcohol use is thought to play a role in many risk-taking or sensation-seeking behaviors. For example, research has correlated drinking with high-risk sexual behaviors (those that contribute to the spread of sexually transmitted diseases such as HIV/AIDS). Understanding the role of alcohol in high-risk sexual behavior is of great concern, particularly in view of survey results showing that individuals who meet the diagnostic criteria for alcohol dependence or abuse or who are heavy or binge drinkers have an increased risk of exposure to human immunodeficiency virus and of developing AIDS (NIAAA, 1997d).

Preventing Alcohol-Related Problems. Historically, programs to prevent alcohol abuse and alcoholism have relied almost exclusively on educational approaches. During the past 10 to 15 years, there has been increasing interest in research into strategies aimed at preventing alcohol problems by altering the social, legal, and economic context in which drinking occurs (Holder & Wallack, 1986).

Prevention encompasses activities or actions ranging from those affecting the whole population through social and regulatory controls to those affecting specific groups (such as adolescents) or individuals. Many of these activities overlap. For example, health warning labels, a product of legislation (social and regulatory control), also are educational. The good news is that, using contemporary tools of science, prevention can be rigorously studied with meaningful results that are generalizable to other populations. Current research evidence shows that some prevention efforts are effective, while others have little or no effect. Having this knowledge will help local communities, the states, and others who have made significant investments in prevention develop or refine existing programs to achieve their desired objectives.

Although prevention research is difficult to do, because investigators have little control over activities in the community that may affect outcomes, important results have been obtained in well-designed studies. For example, research has confirmed that young lives can be saved by raising the legal drinking age to 21 (Voas, Lange et al., 1998; O'Malley & Wagenaar, 1991; Wagenaar, 1986) and setting the maximum blood alcohol limit in young drivers to .02% ("zero tolerance") (Hingson, Heeren et al., 1994). School-based programs closely linked to other community activities also have been shown to reduce drinking among preadolescents.

The past few years have seen tremendous progress in specifying and estimating a number of important economic relationships connected to alcohol use. For example, historical analysis (Cook, 1981) and computer modeling (Chaloupka, 1993) indicate that highway deaths and cirrhosis deaths have varied inversely with the price of beverage alcohol and that even heavy drinkers drink less in response to increases in alcohol price. Moreover, overall consumption of beer, wine, and distilled spirits declines in response to increases in the prices or taxes associated with those beverages. But this research also suggests that the small proportion of drinkers with the highest consumption levels may be much less sensitive to price changes than are drinkers who consume at more moderate levels. Obviously, the issues involved in using price or tax policy to address alcohol problems are complex; they involve not just science but economic, social, and political issues as well. Science can contribute to this policy debate, but it is only one of many viewpoints that must be considered (Kenkel & Manning, 1996).

Treating Alcohol Abuse and Alcoholism. The principal goal of alcoholism treatment is to help alcoholics maintain sobriety. Research progress has been made in developing both behavioral strategies and medications, such as naltrexone, to help achieve this goal. These two classes of treatment strategies are not competitive. Rather, research suggests that pharmacologic agents may be combined with verbal therapy to improve treatment outcomes.

Traditional behavioral therapies include exposure to Alcoholics Anonymous, use of disulfiram, group therapy, didactic sessions about alcoholism, teaching about alcoholism as a disease, vocational counseling, or family therapy. Other therapies include behavior modification approaches, which emphasize coping skills and techniques patients can use to recognize and manage situations that allegedly are stressful and trigger relapse. A third approach, especially suggested for the less dependent, is minimal intervention, which involves instructing the patient about the consequences of drinking, recommending abstinence or reducing drinking, and then leaving the patient to his or her own devices without extensive repeated treatment sessions.

Many of the behavioral treatments that have been used in treating alcoholism evolved informally and are based on clinical judgment and anecdotal information about what works best. Only during the past decade have modern standards of evaluating treatment outcomes—involving the use of controls, blinding, and random assignment of subjects—been used to evaluate existing alcoholism treatments. For example, although disulfiram has been used to treat alcoholism since 1949, it was not until 1986 that the efficacy of this medication was subjected to research methods. An individual taking disulfiram experiences uncomfortable physical reactions (such as nausea, vomiting, and facial flushing) if he or she drinks alcohol. It was presumed that an individual taking disulfiram would avoid alcohol rather than experience these decidedly unpleasant reactions. However, in a large, multisite, double-blind controlled clinical trial conducted by the Department of Veterans Affairs, researchers found that disulfiram alone did not improve abstinence; rather, patients who wanted to drink simply stopped taking the medication or drank in spite of the aversive reaction (Fuller, Branchey et al., 1986). However, patients who remained in the study and continued to take their disulfiram exhibited fewer drinking days. This research demonstrated the importance of ensuring medication compliance in disulfiram treatment.

A significant advance in understanding what works in alcoholism treatment resulted from a large multisite clinical trial (Project MATCH) initiated by NIAAA. The hypothesis—that patients who are appropriately matched to treatments will show better outcomes than those who are unmatched or mismatched—is well founded in medicine, behavioral science, and alcoholism treatment. The findings from Project MATCH, however, challenge this notion. In this trial, three specific treatment approaches were evaluated: Twelve Step Facilitation, Cognitive-Behavioral Coping Skills Therapy, and Motivational Enhancement. Project MATCH did not find any decisive match (although patients with low psychiatric severity did better with Twelve Step Facilitation therapy than with cognitive-behavioral therapy), leading investigators to speculate that patient-treatment matching does not substantially alter treatment outcome. Treatment in all three approaches resulted in substantial reductions in drinking, with reductions sustained over a 12-month period. Alcoholism treatment also was found to result in reductions in alcohol-related problems, other drug use problems, and depression, and improvements in liver functioning. These findings are good news for treatment providers and for patients, who can have confidence that any one of the treatments tested, if well delivered, represents the state of the art in behavioral therapies.

Although psychological therapies can help many alcohol-dependent persons reduce their drinking and maintain abstinence, these approaches alone are not effective for some patients. Thus, developing effective pharmacotherapies for alcoholism treatment has become a top priority of alcohol research. Studies are under way to determine how alcoholism treatment medications work, the potential therapeutic value of using pharmacotherapies over a longer period of time, and which patients are most likely to benefit from new pharmacological treatments. To find better treatments, researchers are looking for new pharmacotherapies that target the mechanisms of the addiction itself. New knowledge about the brain processes underlying addiction is aiding scientists in this search. For example, drugs that interfere with the reward properties of alcohol may be found to block the phenomenon of craving and become a valuable adjunct to alcoholism treatment. With a more precise understanding of the physiology of alcohol withdrawal, new drugs may be developed that allow improved medical management of the withdrawal syndrome or reduce the potential for development of *delirium tremens*. Science also may provide a better understanding of how the withdrawal experience affects both subsequent drinking and the potential for effective treatment. Using pharmacotherapies that control specific clinical features of alcoholism (such as craving), in combination with traditional behavioral and verbal therapies, has the potential to greatly enhance treatment outcomes.

Although we are far from having the proverbial "magic bullet" for treating alcoholism (and, given the complexity of the disease, it is doubtful that science ever will discover one medication to treat all forms of alcohol dependence), we already have begun to see the fruits of neuroscience research translated into medications that are available as adjuncts to behavioral therapy for the treatment of alcoholism. Key among these medications has been naltrexone. A product of neuroscience research, the opiate antagonist naltrexone is the first medication approved to help patients maintain sobriety after detoxification from alcohol since disulfiram was approved in 1949. Studies have shown that, when used in combination with verbal therapy, naltrexone prevents relapse better than standard verbal therapy alone (Volpicelli, Alterman et al., 1992; O'Malley, Jaffe et al., 1992, 1996).

The European-developed compound acamprosate also should receive approval by the U.S. Food and Drug Administration in the near future. Both medications have been found to reduce craving in alcoholics with varying degrees of success. A variety of other promising medications also are being tested, including the opiate antagonist nalmefene.

Combining behavioral therapies with pharmacotherapies is likely to be the next important advance in alcoholism treatment. This coupling of verbal with pharmacological approaches may produce profound changes in the way we view and treat alcoholism. For example, one therapy might continue to function even if the other fails, each therapy might increase the efficacy of the other, or verbal and pharmacological therapy might act on the same neural circuits. The last is an especially intriguing possibility for which there already is some evidence in another field. In a study of obsessive-compulsive disorder, positron emission tomography (PET) scans of patients before and after behavioral treatment were compared with PET scans of patients before and after pharmacological treatment. Changes in the scans of patients who had responded to the behavioral treatment resembled changes in patients who had responded to the pharmacological treatment (Baxter, Schwartz et al., 1992). Project COMBINE, a new large-scale randomized study supported by NIAAA, will take advantage of the knowledge learned from Project MATCH to further explore the coupling of verbal and pharmacological therapies. In Project COMBINE, mixed pharmacological and behavioral approaches will be evaluated in an effort to determine what combinations work best in the treatment of alcohol dependence.

Refined therapies will benefit many people. For alcohol-dependent individuals, who face the realistic fear of relapse, improved interventions can abate and, optimally, prevent relapse occurrences and halt continuing disease that ultimately can lead to death. For society, which bears the weight of the enormous economic and social costs of problem drinking, improved treatment strategies that heighten the potential for long-term abstinence can lessen this burden and enhance the quality of civic life. New therapies promise to reduce the billions of dollars lost annually from reduced workplace productivity, alcohol-related injuries and illnesses, and alcohol-related premature deaths. Further, more effective treatments can reduce the frequency of the various social tragedies associated with alcohol abuse, including motor vehicle crashes, falls, drownings, fires and burns, crime, and family violence.

CONCLUSIONS

The science of alcoholism has made much progress since the early years, when neither scientists nor the alcohol field believed that research into the causes and consequences of alcohol abuse and alcoholism was necessary. As we move into the 21st century, there will be many challenges—and many opportunities—for further scientific progress. Each step toward solving the currently unanswerable questions is a step toward a future in which alcohol-related problems yield to effective, science-based prevention and treatment, and the burden of alcohol abuse and alcoholism on individuals, families, communities, and nations is diminished.

ACKNOWLEDGMENT: The author wishes to acknowledge the outstanding assistance of Brenda G. Hewitt in the development and preparation of this manuscript.

REFERENCES

Bachtell RK, Wang YM, Freeman P et al. (1999). Alcohol drinking produces brain-region selective changes in expression of inducible transport factors. *Brain Research* 847(2):157-165.

Baxter LR, Schwartz JM, Bergman KS et al. (1992). Caudate glucose metabolic rate changes with both drug and behavior therapy for obsessive-compulsive disorder. *Archives of General Psychiatry* 49:681-689.

Begleiter H, Porjesz B, Reich T et al. (1998). Quantitative trait loci analysis of human event-related brain potentials: P3 voltage. *Electroencephalography and Clinical Neurophysiology* 108(3):244-250.

Boffeta P & Garfinkel L (1990). Alcohol drinking and mortality among men enrolled in an American Cancer Society Prospective Study. *Epidemiology* 1(5):342-348.

Cartwright MM & Smith SM (1995). Increased cell death and reduced neural crest cell numbers in ethanol-exposed embryos: Partial basis for the fetal alcohol syndrome. *Alcoholism: Clinical & Experimental Research* 19:378-386.

Chaloupka FJ (1993). Effects of price on alcohol-related problems. *Alcohol Health & Research World* 17:46-53.

Chen S & Sulik KK (1996). Free radicals and ethanol-induced cytotoxicity in neural crest cells. *Alcoholism: Clinical & Experimental Research* 20:1071-1076.

Cloninger CR, Bohman M & Sigvardsson S (1981). Inheritance of alcohol abuse. *Archives of General Psychiatry* 38:861-868.

Cloninger CR, Sigvardsson S & Bohman M (1996). Type I and Type II alcoholism: An update. *Alcohol Health & Research World* 20(1):30-35.

Cook PJ (1981). The effect of liquor taxes on drinking, cirrhosis, and auto accidents. In MH Moore & DR Gerstein (eds.) *Alcohol and Public Policy: Beyond the Shadow of Prohibition*. Washington, DC: National Academy Press, 255-297.

DiClemente CC, Bellino LE & Neavins TM (1999). Motivation for change and alcoholism treatment. *Alcohol Research & Health* 23(2):86-92.

Fuller RK, Branchey L, Brightwell DR et al. (1986). Disulfiram treatment of alcoholism. *Journal of the American Medical Association* 256:1449-1455.

Gentilello LM, Rivara FP, Donovan DM et al. (1999). Alcohol interventions in a trauma center as a means of reducing the risk of injury recurrence. *Annals of Surgery* 230(4):473-483.

Grant BF & Dawson DA (1997). Age at onset of alcohol use and its association with *DSM-IV* alcohol abuse and dependence: Results from the National Longitudinal Alcohol Epidemiologic Survey. *Journal of Substance Abuse* 9:103-110.

Grant BF, Harford TC, Dawson DA et al. (1994). Prevalence of *DSM-IV* alcohol abuse and dependence—United States, 1992. *Alcohol Health & Research World* 183:243-248.

Heaton MB, Mitchell JJ & Paiva M (2000). Amelioration of ethanol-induced neurotoxicity in the neonatal rat central nervous system by antioxidant therapy. *Alcoholism: Clinical & Experimental Research* 24(4):512-518.

Hingson R, Heeren T & Winter M (1994). Lower legal blood alcohol limits for young drivers. *Public Health Reports* 109:736-744.

Holder HD & Wallack L (1986). Contemporary perspectives for preventing alcohol problems: An empirically-derived model. *Journal of Public Health Policy* 7(3):324-339.

Jaffe JH (1993). The concept of dependence: Historical reflections. *Alcohol Health & Research World* 17(3):188-189.

Janzen LA, Nanson JL & Block GW (1995). Neuropsychological evaluation of preschoolers with fetal alcohol syndrome. *Neurotoxicology and Teratology* 17(3):273-279.

Keller M (1990). *Models of Alcoholism: From Days of Old to Nowadays*. Piscataway, NJ: Rutgers Center of Alcohol Studies.

Kenkel D & Manning W (1996). Perspectives on alcohol taxation. *Alcohol Health & Research World* 20(4):230-238.

Luo J, West JR & Pantazis NJ (1997). Nerve growth factor and basic fibroblast growth factor protect rat cerebellar granule cells in culture against ethanol-induced cell death. *Alcoholism: Clinical & Experimental Research* 21(6):1108-1120.

Mattson SN, & Riley EP (1998) A review of the neurobehavioral deficits in children with fetal alcohol syndrome or prenatal exposure to alcohol. *Alcoholism: Clinical & Experimental Research* 22(2):279-294.

Mattson SN, Riley EP, Delis DC et al. (1996). Verbal learning and memory in children with fetal alcohol syndrome. *Alcoholism: Clinical & Experimental Research* 20(5):810-816.

McGue M, Iacono WG, Legrand LE et al. (2001). Origins and consequences of age at first drink. I. Associations with substance-use disorders, disinhibitory behavior and psychopathology, and P3 amplitude. *Alcoholism: Clinical & Experimental Research* 25(8):1156-1165.

Melo JA, Shendure J, Pociask K et al. (1995). Identification of sex-specific quantitative trait loci controlling alcohol preference in C57BL/6 mice. *Journal of Nature Genetics* 13:147-153.

Michaelis EK & Michaelis ML (1994). Cellular and molecular bases of alcohol's teratogenic effects. *Alcohol Health & Research World* 18(1):17-21.

Midanik LT & Room R (1992). The epidemiology of alcohol consumption. *Alcohol Health & Research World* 16(3):183-190.

Mihic SJ, Ye Q, Wick MJ et al. (1997). Sites of alcohol and volatile anaesthetic action on GABA sub A and glycine receptors. *Nature* 389(6649):385-389.

Miles MF (1995). Alcohol's effects on gene expression. *Alcohol Health & Research World* 19(3):237-243.

Monti PM, Colby SM, Barnett NP et al. (1999). Brief intervention for harm reduction with alcohol-positive older adolescents in a hospital emergency department. *Journal of Consulting and Clinical Psychology* (6):989-994.

Moore MS, DeZazzo J, Luk AY et al. (1998). Ethanol intoxication in Drosophila: Genetic and pharmacological evidence for regulation by the cAMP signaling pathway. *Cell* 93(6):997-1007.

National Highway Traffic Safety Administration (NHTSA) (2000). *Traffic Safety Facts 1999: Alcohol*. Washington, DC: NHTSA.

National Institute on Alcohol Abuse and Alcoholism (NIAAA) (1993). *Eighth Special Report to the U.S. Congress on Alcohol and Health* (Publication No. 94-3699). Bethesda, MD: NIAAA, National Institutes of Health, 13.

National Institute on Alcohol Abuse and Alcoholism (NIAAA) (1997a). *Ninth Special Report to the U.S. Congress on Alcohol and Health* (Publication No. 97-4017). Bethesda, MD: NIAAA, National Institutes of Health, 388.

National Institute on Alcohol Abuse and Alcoholism (NIAAA) (1997b). *Ninth Special Report to the U.S. Congress on Alcohol and Health* (Publication No. 97-4017). Bethesda, MD: NIAAA, National Institutes of Health, 247.

National Institute on Alcohol Abuse and Alcoholism (NIAAA) (1997c). *Ninth Special Report to the U.S. Congress on Alcohol and Health* (Publication No. 97-4017). Bethesda, MD: NIAAA, National Institutes of Health, 259.

National Institute on Alcohol Abuse and Alcoholism (NIAAA) (1997d). *Ninth Special Report to the U.S. Congress on Alcohol and Health* (Publication No. 97-4017). Bethesda, MD: NIAAA, National Institutes of Health, 267.

Nurnberger JI Jr, Foroud T, Flury L et al. (2001). Evidence for a locus on chromosome 1 that influences vulnerability to alcoholism and affective disorder. *American Journal of Psychiatry* 158(5):718-24.

Olson HC, Feldman JJ, Streissguth AP et al. (1998). Neuropsychological deficits in adolescents with fetal alcohol syndrome: Clinical findings. *Alcoholism: Clinical & Experimental Research* 22(9):1998-2012.

O'Malley SS, Jaffe AJ, Chang G et al. (1992). Naltrexone and coping skills therapy for alcohol dependence: A controlled study. *Archives of General Psychiatry* 49:881-887.

O'Malley SS, Jaffe AJ, Chang G et al. (1996). Six-month follow-up of naltrexone and psychotherapy for alcohol dependence. *Archives of General Psychiatry* 53:217-224.

O'Malley PM & Wagenaar AC (1991). Effects of minimum drinking age laws on alcohol use, related behaviors, and traffic crash involvement among American youth: 1976–1987. *Journal of Studies on Alcohol* 52:478-491.

Reich T, Edenberg H, Goate A et al. (1998). A genome-wide search for genes affecting the risk for alcohol dependence. *American Journal of Medical Genetics (Neuropsychiatric Genetics)* 81:207-215.

Schuckit MA & Smith TL (1996). 8-year follow-up of 450 sons of alcoholic and control subjects. *Archives of General Psychiatry* 53(3):202-210.

Schulteis G, Hyytia P, Heinrichs SC et al. (1996). Effects of chronic ethanol exposure on oral self-administration of ethanol or saccharin by Wistar rats. *Alcoholism: Clinical & Experimental Research* 20(1):164-171.

Tajuddin NF & Druse MJ (1999). In utero ethanol exposure decreased the density of serotonin neurons: Maternal ipsapirone treatment exerted a protective effect. *Developmental Brain Research* 117(1): 91-97.

Voas RB, Lange JE & Tippetts (1998). Enforcement of the zero tolerance law in California: A missed opportunity? In *42nd Annual Proceedings: Association for the Advancement of Automotive Medicine.* Des Plaines, IL: AAAM.

Voas RB, Wells JK, Lestina DC et al. (1997). Drinking and driving in the U.S.: The 1996 National Roadside Survey. *National Highway Traffic Safety Administration Traffic Task No. 152.* Arlington, VA: Insurance Institute for Highway Safety.

Volpicelli JR, Alterman AI, Hayashida M et al. (1992). Naltrexone in the treatment of alcohol dependence. *Archives of General Psychiatry* 49(11):876-880.

Wagenaar AC (1986). Preventing highway crashes by raising the legal minimum age for drinking: The Michigan experience 6 years later. *Journal of Safety Research* 17:101-109.

| Chapter 4 | # Understanding Drug Addiction: Insights from the Research |

Alan I. Leshner, Ph.D.

The Mind and the Brain
Basic Research
Treatment Research
Future Research Issues

The American public is beginning to shed long-standing myths that drug addiction is a moral problem or character fault brought on by lack of willpower. Now, for the first time, there is evidence to confirm this actual turning point in attitude.

A recent public opinion survey (Harvard University & The Robert Wood Johnson Foundation, 2000) shows broad understanding of the addiction-as-brain disease concept, in that 74% of Americans believe that addicts can stop using drugs, but that to do so they need help from professionals or organizations outside their families. By "help," 65% said they meant treatment by health care professionals.

The survey results also show that the public recognizes the concept of relapse in addiction treatment. Although most of those surveyed said they believe that treatment can be successful, three out of four also said that drug addicts need to try more than once to stop for good. Recognition of the cycle of relapse during treatment builds on the fact that one out of two Americans told pollsters they personally know someone who received addiction treatment and that, of those, two of three said that the treatment was somewhat (33%) or very (31%) successful. These survey results are most heartening: the first preliminary evidence that the American public is beginning to recognize the reality about addiction.

That reality, based on almost three decades of research, is that drug addiction is without doubt a brain disease—a disease that disrupts the mechanisms responsible for generating, modulating, and controlling cognitive, emotional, and social behavior. In the same way that many other diseases and disorders once thought to be caused by psychological problems or stress, such as ulcers (NIH, 1994) and schizophrenia (Barondes, Alberts et al., 1997), have been shown to have a physical origin, drug addiction also has been shown to be a disease with a physical basis. However, because of misconceptions about the brain, behavior, and mind, and the resulting societal and cultural biases, there is a "disconnect" between the scientific data and public perceptions (and, in many cases, professional perceptions) about the nature of addiction and its appropriate treatment.

Although the victims of almost all diseases are viewed with compassion and sympathy, those suffering from most brain diseases have not been so fortunate. Malfunction of the kidneys is equated with kidney disease. But malfunction of the brain is equated with being different, eccentric, or crazy. Not very long ago, those with mental illnesses were shunned and mistreated, shipped off to asylums—to Bedlam—where their antics provided entertainment for visitors. The public could not understand why someone with depression was emotionally and physically paralyzed or why a person with schizophrenia heard voices or saw apparitions. In the absence of knowledge, these conditions were attributed to other-worldly causes, ranging from weak will to poor parenting. Modern science has shown, of course, that depression and schizophrenia are physical disorders of the brain that manifest themselves—as do all brain diseases and disorders, including autism, stroke, obsessive-compulsive disorder, mania, anorexia, and drug addiction—in behavior. The function of the brain is to generate, mediate, and modify behavior—to produce the mind. Drug addiction alters the functioning of the brain and thus changes the mind.

The brain of someone addicted to drugs is a changed brain; it is qualitatively different from that of a normal person in fundamental ways, including gene expression (Liu, Nickolenko et al., 1994; Daunais & McGinty, 1995; Konradi, Leveque et al., 1996; Curran, Akil et al., 1996), glucose utilization (Volkow, Gillespie et al., 1996; London, Cascella et al., 1990), and responsiveness to environmental cues (O'Brien, Childress et al., 1993; Kilgus & Pumariega, 1994; Luborsky, McKay et al., 1995). Whether these changes produce physical or psychological addiction, as viewed in a classical sense, is unimportant. What is critical is that drugs change the brain and thereby produce uncontrollable, compulsive drug-seeking and use—the essence of addiction.

A New Paradigm. To create a new paradigm of how addiction develops, it would be helpful to use an analogy to cardiovascular disease and high cholesterol. Although the victim of a heart attack or stroke could be said to bring the disease on him- or herself through diet and other lifestyle behaviors, once diagnosed, the disease is treated, not its long-distant origins. In this more productive concept, it makes little difference whether a disease is brought on by excessive exposure to fat or to abused drugs; one changes the functioning of the arteries and the heart, the other changes the functioning of the brain. Both require treatment.

It is interesting to note that opiate (Pert & Snyder, 1973) and lipoprotein (Brown & Goldstein, 1976) receptors were identified at approximately the same time. How different the reaction to diseases that act through these two similar classes of receptors! On the one hand, following a massive research effort, extraordinarily effective cholesterol-lowering drugs were developed to treat heart disease (Hebert, Gaziano et al., 1997). These drugs are used extensively by physicians and accepted by the public. On the other hand, until recently there was little interest in developing medications to treat addiction and poor acceptance by physicians and patients of those already approved.

Society has viewed addicts as being responsible for their problems. In some sense that is true. Initial drug use is a voluntary behavior. However, over time, users lose control over their drug use and become addicted. To deal with their addiction effectively requires a shift away from blaming them and exhorting them to change their evil ways, and toward treating them. The focus must change from "who is at fault" to "what to do about the problem."

Most drug addicts would prefer to stop using drugs. That stopping proves so difficult is, in itself, a demonstration of the reality of the disease. Consider one of the most common addictions, to tobacco. More than half of tobacco smokers who have cardiovascular disease and are told that continued smoking will lead to an early death are unable to quit. It is not that most smokers are weak-willed, but that nicotine has changed the brains of smokers so that they cannot stop. The smoker has a disease that does not allow him to stop.

THE MIND AND THE BRAIN

To come to terms with the problems of mental diseases in general and drug addiction in particular, the mind-brain dualism of our scientific and philosophical heritage must be discarded. This separation has little heuristic or practical value in light of modern scientific discoveries. Mind and behavior do not exist without brain activity; although the exact mechanisms have yet to be specified, it is obvious that cognition, emotion, learning, and memory all emanate from cohesive brain activity. Absent such activity, there is disordered behavior and loss of mind.

This reality is confronted daily by countless families across the country who are caring for elderly parents with Alzheimer's disease. The body is there—it consumes oxygen, metabolizes sugar, disposes of waste—but the person is gone because the brain no longer works properly.

Alzheimer's disease is an extreme case of a loss of cognitive function and the global deterioration of mind. It is easily recognized for what it is: a brain disease. Other brain diseases can produce more specific effects: hallucinations, seizures, mania, depression. Although the survey cited earlier suggests that progress has been made in changing public attitudes, the public and, to some extent, the health professions need to appreciate more fully the fact that changes in the brain lead to behavioral diseases and that addiction is just another such disease.

The repeated administration of certain drugs causes changes in the functioning of the brain and thus leads to addiction. Almost all psychoactive drugs activate the mesolimbic dopamine system (Koob, 1996), an area of the brain thought to mediate reward and appetitive behaviors. Although defining the precise mechanisms is the target of an intense research effort, it is known that repeated self-administration of drugs produces a qualitative change in the way the brain functions. The affected individual has an intense need for, and focus on, repeating the drug experience. But there comes a point (as is the case when a depressed person becomes clinically depressed) at which the drug user becomes an addict. At that point, it appears that a figurative "switch" has been thrown and the individual suffers a significant loss of his or her ability to make free choices about continued use of drugs.

Just as depression is more than a lot of sadness, drug addiction is more than a lot of drug use. The addict cannot voluntarily move back and forth between abuse and addiction because the addicted brain is, in fact, different in its neurobiology from the nonaddicted brain.

Addiction thus is not a matter of moral weakness or lack of will. Rather, it occurs when a drug seizes control of an individual's brain, thereby usurping first the mind, and then the life. The functioning of those parts of the brain that normally allow the exercise of choice is disrupted. In a way, drugs do to the brain what HIV does to the immune system: they attack the very cells that could stop the disease process—in the case of addiction, the cells that allow individuals to regulate and control behavior.

Unfortunately, it is easier to accept the concept of a brain disease when it involves motor function rather than behavior. Drug-addicted patients should not be seen as weak-willed if they are unable to stop using drugs. Both the Parkinson's patient and the drug addict are suffering from dysfunctions of the dopamine system—the manifestations of one are primarily motor and those of the other primarily behavioral, but both are brain diseases.

To authenticate the chronic relapsing disease model, researchers recently documented striking similarities between drug addiction and three common chronic diseases: type 2 diabetes, hypertension, and asthma. A literature review compared the diagnoses, heritability, etiology (genetic and environmental factors), pathophysiology, and response to treatments (adherence and relapse) of drug addiction as compared to those factors for type 2 diabetes, hypertension, and asthma. The review found that genetic heritability, personal choice, and environment are comparably involved in the etiology and course of all of these disorders. The researchers confirmed that drug addiction produces significant and lasting changes in brain chemistry and function. Medication adherence and relapse rates are similar across all four illnesses (although no effective medication was yet available for treating stimulant or marijuana dependence). They concluded that addiction should be considered a long-term disease, just like the chronic conditions of diabetes, hypertension, and asthma. Moreover, drug addiction should be insured, treated, and evaluated like other chronic illnesses (McClellan, Lewis et al., 2000).

BASIC RESEARCH

Chapters in this text amply demonstrate the great strides that have been made in our basic understanding of drug addiction and its underlying mechanisms. Over the past 30 years, scientists have identified the primary receptors for every major class of abused drug, identified their genetic code, and cloned the receptors (NIDA, 1994, 1996; Kilty, Lorang et al., 1991; Matsuda, Lolait et al., 1990; Chen, Mestek et al., 1993). They have mapped the locations of those receptors in the brain and determined the neurotransmitter systems involved (Koob, 1992; Self, in press; IOM, 1996); demonstrated the activation of these areas during addiction, withdrawal, and craving (Grant, London et al., 1996; Volkow, Ding et al., 1996a); identified and separated the mechanisms underlying drug-seeking behavior and physical dependence (Wise & Bozarth, 1985; Maldonado, Saiardi et al., 1997); developed animal models for drug self-administration (Koob, 1995); and, most important of all, demonstrated that the mesolimbic dopamine system is the primary site of the dysfunction caused by abused drugs (Koob, 1992; Schulties & Koob, 1994; Wise, 1996).

A number of discoveries demonstrate the exciting possibilities of current research. With knowledge about the gene that codes for the dopamine transporter—the primary target for cocaine—a strain of mice was developed in which this important protein was disabled or "knocked out" (Giros, Jaber et al., 1996). The animals' response to cocaine thus was altered both physiologically and behaviorally. Although knocking out the dopamine transporter may well have affected other neurotransmitter systems, such as serotonin, this study nevertheless demonstrates that the dopamine transporter is an important mechanism through which cocaine exerts its influence on the brain.

Another significant study (Self, Barnhart et al., 1996) investigated the potential role of D_1 and D_2 dopamine receptors. Using compounds that stimulate either the D_1 or the D_2 receptor, this study involved rats that were allowed to self-administer cocaine for two hours, followed by two hours of saline, during which time self-administration diminished or ceased. The subsequent administration of a D_2 agonist led to a dramatic resumption of cocaine-seeking, whereas the D_1 agonist had virtually no effect. In a second study, pretreatment with a D_1 receptor agonist suppressed cocaine-seeking, whereas the D_2 agonist increased it. This dissociation between the action of D_1 and D_2 receptors opens up a potential line of research for targeting new treatment drugs.

While much addiction research focuses on the role of dopamine, studies indicate that humans are differentially susceptible to dopamine and that nature endows humans with differing levels of dopamine. For example, a deficiency of dopamine in the brain may explain why some individuals engage in pathological overeating, resulting in severe obesity (Wang, Volkow et al., 2001). Studies show that several neurotransmitter systems other than dopamine may be involved. Animal research suggests that both dopamine and serotonin transporters play a role in cocaine's pleasure response. And studies with opiates, cocaine, amphetamine, and alcohol demonstrate that a complex phenomenon known as the "glutamate cascade" is involved in drug addiction, playing a role in drug tolerance, sensitization, dependence, and neurotoxicity. Recent research into the acute reinforcing effects of drugs of abuse in the brain's amygdala indicates involvement by multiple neurotransmitter systems: dopamine, opioid peptides, serotonin, GABA, and glutamate (Koob, 2000). Researchers are seeking a better understanding of the multifaceted actions and interactions among various brain-altering circuits and systems.

Addictive behaviors may be mediated by both positive and negative reinforcing events, such as withdrawal. Rodriguez de Fonseca and colleagues (1997) studied commonalities underlying the withdrawal effects of drugs of abuse. They found that corticotrophin-releasing factor—a hormone that generally is associated with stress response and also appears to be involved in the mediation of the negative reinforcing events associated with withdrawal from alcohol, cocaine, and opiates—also was elevated in the limbic system after withdrawal from marijuana. The fact that these disparate drugs all cause a similar reaction in the same neural circuitry raises the possibility that all of the drugs, over time, act cumulatively as contributors to the development of brain dysfunction and drug addiction.

Self-administration of abused drugs bypasses the cognitive "filters" that are part of normal brain homeostatic function and artificially and powerfully stimulates the mesolimbic dopamine system. This leads to maladaptive, pathological brain function. For reasons not yet understood, the cognitive world of the addict changes. Everything becomes focused on drugs: thinking about them, talking about them, obtaining them, and using them. Most people would attribute this obsession with drugs to "psychological" processes. A more likely explanation is that it reflects an underlying change in the relative functioning of various cognitive and reward centers in the brain. The mechanisms that normally override or suppress the activity of the mesolimbic dopamine system are unable to do so in the face of massive "artificial" drug stimulation. It is as if someone receiving direct electrical stimulation of the right-arm dorsal root fibers is told to stop feeling the sensation of tingling or pain in the affected limb. No matter how strong the individual's "will," the person is unable to do so. Similarly, the repeated stimulation of the mesocortical limbic dopamine system by abused drugs eventually leads to a change in the brain, to the "addiction switch" being turned on, with a consequent loss of control, irrespective of the will of the individual. Author Samuel Taylor Coleridge expressed this idea most eloquently: "My case is a species of madness, only that it is a derangement of the Volition, and not of the intellectual faculties."

Emerging Research Opportunities. As the body of knowledge about addiction continues to grow, so too do research approaches. Several areas of drug addiction and neuroscience research involve emerging concepts that promise exciting avenues for future studies. One of these uses brain-imaging techniques to provide dramatic documentation that drugs of abuse effectively usurp the brain's motivational systems. For example, a study shows that the limbic regions of the brain, where cocaine is thought to produce its pleasurable effects by disrupting normal dopamine functioning, also are activated when subjects with a history of cocaine use view videotapes containing drug-associated cues in the form of cocaine-related scenes. Other studies suggest that this cocaine craving does not merely involve the brain's reward circuits, but that it takes over these sites and essentially rewrites normal preferences. Yet another study shows how the brain's motivational systems can be usurped, indicating that cues related to normal human pleasures, such as sex, also can activate the same sites in the brain (Childress, 1999; Garavan, Pankiewicz et al., 2000).

A mounting body of evidence shows that chronic use of MDMA or "Ecstasy" may cause brain damage in humans, and that such damage may last for many years, perhaps permanently. MDMA-related brain damage is well documented in animal studies. MDMA creates feelings of euphoria through a massive release of the brain chemical serotonin. Research shows that, over time, this release can lead to a loss of brain cells known as serotonin transporters. Studies show that MDMA-related brain damage in nonhuman primates persists for seven to eight years (Hatzidimitriou, McCann et al., 1999). Researchers have found that MDMA use in humans is associated with verbal and visual memory problems in individuals who had not used the drug for at least two weeks (Bolla, McCann et al., 1998). Researchers see a relationship between the quantity of MDMA consumed and the severity of the brain damage to memory and learning capabilities (McCann, Szabo et al., 2001). How long the brain damage persists in humans, and whether it is reversible, is not yet known, but given the popularity of MDMA and the widespread misconception that it is "harmless," the long-range implications are critical.

Another promising concept to be pursued offers hope of finding ways to block or actually to reverse some of the brain damage wreaked by certain psychostimulants. One such stimulant, methamphetamine, may damage the brain in several ways, including impairing blood flow, producing harmful free radicals, and causing damage to brain cells. Recent research suggests that brain damage from methamphetamine use, as measured in reduced levels of dopamine transporter cells and glucose metabolism, may be reversed over time after use of the drug stops, thus allowing recovery of brain function. A study using positron emission tomography (PET) found that, in a small group of methamphetamine users, dopamine transporter levels increased significantly (16%-19%) after protracted abstinence (less than six months of abstinence versus 12 to 17 months of abstinence) (Volkow et al., 2001). However, the indicated reversal of brain damage was not supported by subjects' scores on mental performance tests. The results suggest that, because the neuropsychological tests did not improve to the same extent as the restoration of dopamine transporter levels, the increases of transporter levels were not sufficient for complete functional recovery or that functional recovery may require additional time. Further, the study showed that potential for recovery from brain damage is associated with both severity and duration of drug abuse. Obviously, much more research is needed, but any evidence of recovery from brain damage is encouraging.

TREATMENT RESEARCH

Current research on the neurobehavioral bases of drug addiction is creating a better understanding and appreciation of the uses of older therapies and a greater recognition of opportunities to develop new ones. Most importantly, this knowledge has shown that drug addiction is a treatable disease.

As noted earlier, the fact that addiction is the result of repeated self-administration of drugs should cause those who suffer from this disease to become objects of derision and contempt, unworthy of sympathy. As with many preventable and treatable diseases—AIDS, heart disease, and emphysema, to name a few—the focus must be on caring for afflicted individuals without allowing public attitudes toward addiction to affect acceptance of proven treatments.

Methadone Maintenance. Research shows that methadone maintenance produces significant medical and public health benefits. Methadone is longer acting than heroin and can serve to stabilize brain function, perhaps by stopping the rapid cycling and stimulation of the mesolimbic dopamine system. Because methadone is not injected, the spread of AIDS is curtailed (Metzger, Woody et al., 1993). Children born to methadone-maintained women are much healthier at birth than children born to heroin addicts (Jarvis & Schnoll, 1994). The methadone model now is widely accepted for the treatment of nicotine addiction. (No one suggests that the use of alternative nicotine delivery systems constitutes the substitution of one addiction for another; such delivery systems are seen as part of a comprehensive plan to get people to stop smoking. So too with methadone.)

Beyond methadone, other pharmacologic therapies, such as LAAM and (as soon as it is approved) buprenorphine, should provide physicians with a variety of medications that can be tailored to the needs of individual patients.

New Treatment Approaches. A brain disease model of addiction requires a broadened search for new treatment modalities. It is essential to study ways to prevent abused drugs from ever reaching the brain, possibly through

Mecamylamine?

immunization (Carrera, Ashley et al., 1995) or by modification of the blood-brain barrier. It also is necessary to discover mechanisms to block abused drugs from affecting brain function indirectly. For example, cocaine may act, in part, through its local anesthetic and vasoconstrictive actions. Perhaps the very earliest phase of the cocaine "rush" is the result of a relative shutdown in cortical function, which releases subcortical structures from tonic inhibitory influences. Consideration also must be given to the possibility that some of the effects of abused drugs result from a generalized diffusion of neurotransmitters.

Medications: Replacement therapies, antagonist therapy (such as naltrexone and mecamylamine), and other techniques to block abused drug-receptor coupling serve a valuable function in stabilizing patients and helping them to reduce or eliminate drug use. In addition to directly targeting the drug molecule and its receptor, new medical interventions designed to restore normal brain function (including gene-based therapies) should be explored. Ideally, such medications would affect higher-level brain systems; they would not necessarily be drug-specific.

Greater consideration should be given to the mechanisms underlying drug craving, relapse, and environmental triggers, which probably involve much more complex mechanisms than simple models of changed neurotransmitter synthesis, altered receptor sensitivity, and up/down-regulation of receptors. Basic research is needed on the homeostatic mechanisms that regulate the interplay between cortical and subcortical structures in the mediation of emotions, memory, and learning. For example, drug experiences are difficult, if not impossible, to forget. The persistence of drug-related memory and its ability to evoke past drug experiences appear to be comparable to the power of olfactory memory—an intriguing finding in that olfaction is a chemical sense that bypasses thalamic systems used by other senses and has inputs directly to the limbic system.

Medications that act on other brain systems (for example, glutamatergic or GABAergic) that also are implicated in the effects of drugs of abuse are another area for development of pharmacotherapies. Methods of delivering psychotherapeutics so that they are active only in specific brain regions may be even more important. The future of medications development for the treatment of all brain diseases lies in therapeutics that do not necessarily target a specific disease but rather target a specific neurotransmitter system in a particular nucleus in the brain. Using available research findings and new diagnostic tests, the skilled clinician then will be able to prescribe medications to regulate brain function and return it to a degree of normalcy.

Because abused drugs act on the same parts of the brain that allow feelings of pleasure, the challenge is to develop medications that can negate the acute and chronic effects of drugs without blocking the ability to enjoy a romantic dinner, a walk on the beach, or a drive in a new car. Fortunately, the exquisite technologies made available by the fields of molecular biology and neuroscience and the computer-assisted development and design of medications that have a specific structure provide the tools that are needed to meet this challenge.

Basic Studies: In addition to medications development, more basic research is required. One exciting area is the neurocognitive aspects of drug addiction. What are the neural bases of just saying "no"? What are the neural bases of making a resolution? Many people have tried to diet. They get up in the morning determined to eat lightly, cut down on calories, and exercise at the end of the day. And they truly believe they can and will follow such a regimen. During the day, however, stress builds, fatigue develops, mood changes, and the diet is viewed as less important than it was in the morning. Would-be dieters think: "I will start tomorrow, I really will." And they truly believe they will. Studies are needed to identify the brain systems that mediate changes in the cognitive importance a given individual attaches to various activities, thereby modifying his or her behavior according to mood and affective states.

Studies also are needed to investigate the neural mechanisms that mediate "moral fiber" when there is a conflict between needs or desires and intellect. These are not simple issues. In the past, they have been thought of only in psychological terms and have been addressed only with psychological interventions and theories; now, however, we know that neural systems must be involved. That knowledge is crucial to the development of new technologies that will enable individuals to be more resolute in modulating any number of behaviors, including drug use.

Another important and frequently overlooked cognitive aspect of drug addiction involves self-recognition and acceptance of the existence of disease. Drug addicts typically lose their health, families, and careers, yet still deny they have a problem. They believe that they can stop at any time. The ability to suppress external reality and to deny disease is not unique to drug addicts and is present in other brain diseases (Cutting, 1978). Addicts, however, represent a unique part of the spectrum and should be the subject of neurocognitive research into denial.

Combined Pharmacological and Behavioral Treatments: The treatment of drug addiction requires both behavioral and pharmacological interventions. There is little value in thinking about behavioral therapies as opposed to or in contrast with pharmacological therapies. Drug addiction, like other brain diseases, occurs in a social, environmental, and historical context. The brain functions in response to internal and external chemical cues and in response to feedback and stimulation from the behaviors it produces. The brain produces behaviors, and evidence from studies of obsessive-compulsive disorder (Schwartz, 1996; Baxter, 1992) indicates that behavioral therapies can produce changes in the brain. The task for treatment is to reverse, or at least to compensate for, the qualitative brain changes that characterize addiction.

Combinations of pharmacological and behavioral treatments for addictive disorders appear to be more beneficial than either component alone (Stitzer & Walsh, 1997). This benefit is seen in other diseases as well. For example, cholesterol levels can be dramatically reduced through a regimen that combines diet and exercise with cholesterol-lowering drugs. In treating patients with high cholesterol and other chronic conditions, the health professional must determine the best combination of therapies to meet the health needs of the patient, based on availability of services, costs, severity of illness, and other risk factors. A similar model, which tailors pharmacological and behavioral treatment approaches to the needs of an addicted patient, is critical for success.

Drug addiction is a brain disease, so brain normalization through pharmacological and behavioral techniques should be the ultimate goal of treatment. There will be no "magic bullet" to treat or cure addiction. However, pharmacotherapies should be of value in treating the direct acute and chronic brain effects of abused drugs. The success of selective serotonergic reuptake blockers in treating a variety of mental diseases that once were thought to require years of intense psychotherapy offers the hope that addiction medications more effective than those that currently can be imagined may one day be developed. Nevertheless, medications will be only part of the treatment armamentarium. Because of the complexity of addiction and its sequelae, it is likely that many—if not all—addicts will require and benefit from a combination of pharmacological and behavioral interventions. For many addicts, the behav-

ioral interventions employed will have to address at least two sets of problems, and thus will need to incorporate at least two types of therapy. One involves a cognitive approach that will help patients reframe how they relate to and view the world. This would, of necessity, include deconditioning of the environmental cues that elicit drug craving. The other approach is social rehabilitation. Efforts to treat any disease, be it cancer, stroke, or addiction, often overlook the impact of disease on the person. The cancer patient must learn to live with fear, uncertainty, and anxiety; the stroke patient must accommodate to a loss of function and mental capacity; and the addict must overcome the dysfunction caused by addiction. Those who have lived an addict's life often need professional assistance in learning how to live effectively in the non-drug using world.

The importance of psychosocial interventions in the treatment of addiction has been demonstrated in a dose-response study (McLellan, Arndt et al., 1993). Patients in a methadone maintenance program were assigned to three levels of therapy: minimum services (no regular counseling), standard services (regular counseling), and enhanced services (regular counseling plus on-site medical and psychiatric care, family therapy, and employment counseling). None of the subjects receiving minimum services achieved 16 weeks of opiate-free urine samples, whereas 28% of the subjects receiving standard services did so, as did 55% of the subjects receiving enhanced services. Moreover, longer term followup indicated that the more intense the services, the better the outcome on a variety of important measures, including drug use, employment, and criminal activity. In short, the more intense the psychosocial intervention, the more effective is the pharmacological intervention.

The efficacy of new treatments for drug addiction has been demonstrated primarily in specialized research settings, with somewhat limited patient populations. There has been a need to evaluate new treatments in multisite clinical trials to determine their effectiveness across a range of community-based treatment settings and diverse patient populations and then to facilitate the transfer of results to the treatment community. To blend strategies and advances of drug abuse researchers with those of treatment practitioners, the National Institute on Drug Abuse (NIDA) has created the National Drug Abuse Treatment Clinical Trials Network (CTN). At various sites, the CTN tests the efficacy of behavioral, pharmacological, and integrated treatment interventions and seeks to bring effective therapies to treatment providers and their patients.

FUTURE RESEARCH ISSUES

The overall picture of drug abuse in the United States is constantly changing. As quickly as researchers develop a clear understanding of certain drug use patterns and gain some control over existing drug problems, newer and more dangerous substances seem to emerge. Similar to the way a virus mutates, both regional and national drug abuse patterns are constantly reshaping and rarely remain static. Tried and true prevention and treatment approaches may not work with many of these new drugs. For example, drugs such as MDMA, which acts as both a hallucinogen and a stimulant, require new prevention and treatment approaches, as does the unique stimulant methamphetamine. By carefully monitoring these shifting drug trends, NIDA is poised to use the power of scientific research and its application to avert emerging drug problems before they become national epidemics. This area will continue to be a high priority for NIDA.

Radically different mind-altering drugs and technologies may emerge in the 21st century. For example, it is not too soon to consider the possibility that a technique will be developed to use short-term genetic manipulation of brain cells as a new form of drug abuse and addiction; theoretically, a man-made psychoactive "virus" could be created that would carry instructions to alter neurotransmitter systems and produce entirely novel phenomenal and euphoric states. The potential for genetic manipulation of behavior will make current biomedical ethical issues pale in comparison.

Questions will arise about the abuse of personality-altering drugs, performance-enhancing drugs, cognition-enhancing drugs, anti-aging drugs, and growth-stimulating drugs. Experience shows that certain drugs, such as LSD, are uniquely rewarding to humans, perhaps because of their unusual cognitive and perceptual effects. The use of LSD has been reported to produce "psychological dependence," a term that conveys ignorance of the underlying physiology. Studies are needed to determine whether the reinforcing effects of LSD ultimately operate through some pathway to the mesolimbic dopamine system, or whether there are other reward pathways and systems subserving higher mental processes such as curiosity or the appreciation of beauty.

The time to start thinking about such issues and society's response to them is now.

CONCLUSIONS: THE FINAL FRONTIER

The disease of addiction begins in the brain, which is the target organ for abused drugs. Within that structure, abused drugs affect specific sites and initiate the cascade of events that can lead from casual drug use to addiction. Unraveling the disease of addiction will require a comprehensive understanding of how a drug occupies a receptor; how the act of occupying a receptor triggers a response in the cell, leading to an electrical impulse; and how that electrical impulse travels through the brain, integrating with other electrical signals emanating from structures responsible for various functions—including learning, memory and forgetting, cognition, attention, and social behavior—and ultimately leads to the qualitative changes that characterize addiction. Drugs change the brain, possibly forever. They leave something behind that can be exorcised only by knowledge gained through the power of science. As Cocteau wrote: "There exists, therefore, outside alkaloids and habit, a sense for opium, an intangible habit which lives on, despite the recasting of the organism. The dead drug leaves a ghost behind. At certain hours it haunts the house."

The 20th century opened with a golden age in the physical sciences and closed with a golden age in the biological sciences. Nowhere is this more true than in neurobiology. Incredible progress has been made in understanding brain and behavior, prompting radical changes in the conception and treatment of a variety of diseases previously thought to be little more than weaknesses or bad habits. The specification of the precise anatomical, biochemical, and physiological mechanisms that direct how the brain works, with the concomitant ability to change those mechanisms, will challenge society as never before. It will be a revolution more profound than those created by Copernicus, Newton, and Einstein: they gave us only time and space. Genetic research is determining the nature of man. In the 21st century, brain research will determine the nature of mind.

REFERENCES

Barondes SH, Alberts BM, Andreasen NC et al. (1997). Workshop on schizophrenia. *Proceedings of the National Academy of Sciences* 94(5):1612-1614.

Baxter LR Jr. (1992). Caudate glucose metabolic rate changes with both drug and behavior therapy for obsessive-compulsive disorder. *Archives of General Psychiatry* 49(9):681-689.

Bolla KI, McCann UD & Ricaurte GA (1998). Memory impairment in abstinent MDMA ("ecstasy") users. *Neurology* 51:1532-1537.

Brown MS & Goldstein JL (1976). Receptor-mediated control of cholesterol metabolism. *Science* 191(4223):150-154.

Carrera MR, Ashley JA, Parsons LH et al. (1995). Suppression of psychoactive effects of cocaine by active immunization. *Nature* 378(6558):727-730.

Chen Y, Mestek A, Liu J et al. (1993). Molecular cloning and functional expression of a mu-opioid receptor from rat brain. *Molecular Pharmacology* 44(1):8-12.

Childress AR et al. (1999). Limbic activation during cue-induced cocaine craving. *American Journal of Psychiatry* 156(1):11-18.

Curran EJ, Akil H & Watson SJ (1996) Psychomotor stimulant- and opiate-induced c-fos mRNA expression patterns in the rat forebrain: Comparisons between acute drug treatment and a drug challenge in sensitized animals. *Neurochemical Research* 21(11):1425-1435.

Cutting J (1978). Study of anosognosia. *Journal of Neurology, Neurosurgery and Psychiatry* 41(6):548-555.

Daunais JB & McGinty JF (1995). Cocaine binges differentially alter striatal preprodynorphin and zif/268 mRNAs. *Brain Research and Molecular Brain Research* 29(2):201-210.

Garavan H, Pankiewicz J, Bloom A et al. (2000). Cue-induced cocaine craving: Neuroanatomical specificity for drug users and drug stimuli. *American Journal of Psychiatry* 157(11):1789-1798

Giros B, Jaber M, Jones SR et al. (1996). Hyperlocomotion and indifference to cocaine and amphetamine in mice lacking the dopamine transporter. *Nature* 379:606-612.

Grant S, London ED, Newlin DB et al. (1996). Activation of memory circuits during cue-elicited cocaine craving. *Proceedings of the National Academy of Sciences* 93(21):12040-12045.

Harvard School of Public Health & Robert Wood Johnson Foundation (2000). Report on public attitudes toward illegal drug use and drug treatment (telephone survey of 1,012 adults conducted by International Communications Research), unpublished slide presentation.

Hatzidimitriou G, McCann UD & Ricaurte GA (1999). Altered serotonin innervation patterns in the forebrain of monkeys treated with MDMA seven years previously: Factors influencing abnormal recovery. *Journal of Neuroscience* 191(12):5096-5107.

Hebert PR, Gaziano JM, Chan KS et al. (1997). Cholesterol lowering with statin drugs, risk of stroke, and total mortality. An overview of randomized trials. *Journal of the American Medical Association* 278(4):313-321.

Institute of Medicine (IOM) (1996). *Pathways of Addiction: Opportunities in Drug Abuse Research.* Washington, DC: National Academy Press.

Jarvis MA & Schnoll SH (1994). Methadone treatment during pregnancy. *Journal of Psychoactive Drugs* 26(2):155-161.

Kilgus MD & Pumariega AJ (1994). Experimental manipulation of cocaine craving by videotaped environmental cues. *Southern Medical Journal* 87(11):1138-1140.

Kilty JE, Lorang D & Amara SG (1991). Cloning and expression of a cocaine-sensitive rat dopamine transporter. *Science* 254(5031):578-579.

Konradi C, Leveque JC & Hyman SE (1996). Amphetamine and dopamine-induced immediate early gene expression in striatal neurons depends on postsynaptic NMDA receptors and calcium. *Journal of Neuroscience* 16(13):4231-4239.

Koob GF (1992). Drugs of abuse: Anatomy, pharmacology, and function of reward pathways. *Trends in Pharmacological Sciences* 13(5):177-184.

Koob GF (1995). Animal models of drug addiction. In FE Bloom & DJ Kupfer (eds.) *Psychopharmacology: The Fourth Generation of Progress.* New York, NY: Raven Press, 759-772.

Koob GF (1996). Drug addiction: The Yin and Yang of hedonic homeostasis. *Neuron* 16(5):893-896.

Koob GF (2000). Neurobiology of addiction. Toward the development of new therapies. *Annals of the New York Academy of Sciences* 909:170-185.

Liu J, Nickolenko J & Sharp FR (1994). Morphine induces c-fos and junB in striatum and nucleus accumbens via D1 and N-methyl-D-aspartate receptors. *Proceedings of the National Academy of Sciences* 91(18):8537-8541.

London E, Cascella NG, Wong DF et al. (1990). Cocaine-induced reduction of glucose utilization in human brain. A study using positron emission tomography and [fluorine 18]-fluorodeoxyglucose. *Archives of General Psychiatry* 47(6):567-574.

Luborsky L, McKay J, Mercer D et al. (1995). To use or to refuse cocaine—The deciding factors. *Journal of Substance Abuse* 7(3):293-310.

Maldonado R, Saiardi A, Valverde O et al. (1997). Absence of opiate rewarding effects in mice lacking dopamine D2 receptors. *Nature* 1388(6642):586-589.

Matsuda LA, Lolait SJ, Brownstein MJ et al. (1990). Structure of cannabinoid receptor and functional expression of the cloned cDNA. *Nature* 346(6284):561-564.

McCann UD, Szabo Z, Scheffel U et al. (in press). Positron emission tomographic evidence of toxic effect of MDMA ("ecstasy") on brain serotonin neurons in humans beings.

McLellan AT, Arndt IO, Metzger DS et al. (1993). The effects of psychosocial services in substance abuse treatment. *Journal of the American Medical Association* 269(15):1953-1959.

McClellan AT, Lewis DC, O'Brien CP et al. (2000). Drug dependence, a chronic medical illness: Implications for treatment, insurance, and outcomes evaluation. *Journal of the American Medical Association* 284(13):1689-1695.

Metzger DS, Woody GE, McLellan AT et al. (1993). Human immunodeficiency virus seroconversion among intravenous drug users in and out-of-treatment: An 18-month prospective follow-up. *Journal of Acquired Immunodeficiency Syndromes* 6(9):1049-1056.

National Institutes of Health (NIH) (1994). Helicobacter pylori in peptic ulcer disease. *NIH Consensus Statement* 12(1):1-23.

National Institute on Drug Abuse (NIDA) (1994). *Drug Abuse and Drug Abuse Research: The Third Triennial Report to Congress From the Secretary, Department of Health and Human Services.* Bethesda, MD: NIDA, National Institutes of Health.

National Institute on Drug Abuse (NIDA) (1996). *Drug Abuse and Drug Abuse Research: The Fourth Triennial Report to Congress From the Secretary, Department of Health and Human Services.* Bethesda, MD: NIDA, National Institutes of Health.

O'Brien CP, Childress AR, McLellan AT et al. (1993). Developing treatments that address classical conditioning. *NIDA Research Monograph 135.* Rockville, MD: National Institute on Drug Abuse, 71-91.

Pert CB & Snyder SH (1973). Opiate receptor: Demonstration in nervous tissue. *Science* 179(77):1011-1014.

Rigotti NA, Singer DE, Mulley AG Jr et al. (1991). Smoking cessation following admission to a coronary care unit. *Journal of General Internal Medicine* 6(4):305-311.

Rodriguez de Fonseca F, Carrera MRA, Navarro M et al. (1997). Activation of corticotropin-releasing factor in the limbic system during cannabinoid withdrawal. *Science* 276(5321): 2050-2054.

Schulties G & Koob G (1994). Dark side of drug dependence. *Nature* 371(6493):108-109.

Schwartz JM (1996). Systematic changes in cerebral glucose metabolic rate after successful behavior modification treatment of obsessive-compulsive disorder. *Archives of General Psychiatry* 53(2):109-113.

Self DW (in press). The Neurobiology of Relapse. In *Handbook of Drug Abuse*. New York, NY: CRC Press.

Self DW, Barnhart WJ, Lehman DA et al. (1996). Opposite modulation of cocaine-seeking behavior by D_1- and D_2-like dopamine receptor agonists. *Science* 271(5255):1586-1589.

Sora I, Wichems C, Takahashi N et al. (1998). Cocaine reward models: Conditioned place preference can be established in dopamine- and in serotonin-transporter knockout mice. *Proceedings of the National Academy of Sciences* 95(13):7699-7704.

Stitzer ML & Walsh SL (1997). Psychostimulant abuse: The case for combined behavioral and pharmacological treatments. *Pharmacology, Biochemistry and Behavior* 57(3):457-470.

Volkow ND, Ding Y, Fowler JS et al. (1996). Cocaine addiction: Hypothesis derived from imaging studies with PET. *Journal of Addictive Diseases* 15(4):55-71.

Volkow ND, Gillespie H, Mullani N et al. (1996). Brain glucose metabolism in chronic marijuana users at baseline and during marijuana intoxication. *Psychiatry Research: Neuro-imaging* 67:29-38.

Volkow ND et al. (in press). Loss of dopamine transporters in methamphetamine abusers recovers with protracted abstinence. *Journal of Neuroscience*.

Wang GJ, Volkow ND, Logan J et al. (2001). Brain dopamine and obesity. *Lancet* 357(9253):354-357.

Wise RA (1996). Addictive drugs and brain stimulation reward. *Annual Review of Neuroscience* 19:319-340.

Wise RA & Bozarth MA (1985). Brain mechanisms of drug reward and euphoria. *Psychiatric Medicine* 3(4):445-460.

Chapter 5

Brain Reward Circuitry: Insights from Unsensed Incentives

Roy A. Wise, Ph.D.

Anatomy of Drug Reward
Reward and Compulsion
Reward Receipt and Reward Prediction

The discovery by Olds and Milner (1954) that rats would learn to work for direct electrical stimulation of the brain initiated the search for the anatomical circuitry through which the normal pleasures of life establish habits that come to dominate the behavior of higher animals. It soon became apparent that lateral hypothalamic brain stimulation was not only rewarding; it was also drive inducing (Olds & Olds, 1965; Coons, Levak et al., 1965; Glickman & Schiff, 1967). Electrical stimulation of reward-related structures thus became a tool to identify anatomical substrates presumed to participate in natural motivation (Mendelson & Chorover,1965; MacDonnell & Flynn, 1966a, 1966b; Wise, 1974) and reward (Olds & Olds, 1963; German & Bowden, 1974; Routtenberg, 1976). Inasmuch as the reward of direct brain stimulation was not detected by sight, sound, taste, smell, or touch, it provided an unsensed incentive with some degree of anatomical specificity. Intravenous (Weeks, 1962; Thompson & Schuster,1964; Deneau, Yanagita et al., 1969) and intracranial (Olds, Yuwiler et al., 1964; Phillips & LePiane, 1980; Bozarth & Wise, 1981)

drug reinforcement soon offered an unsensed incentive with neurochemical specificity. These two techniques subsequently have been used extensively to characterize brain reward circuitry with respect to both its anatomy and neurochemistry. Because these laboratory incentives are not detected in the external world of the animal, they also reveal important insights into behavior motivated by natural rewards. The present paper comprises three sections. The first characterizes the elements of brain reward circuitry that have been identified by central drug injections and intracranial stimulation and that offer our best clues as to the trigger zones at which addictive drugs initiate their habit-forming actions. The second discusses possible explanations for the fact that drug reward and brain stimulation reward establish seemingly more compulsive habits than do the natural pleasures of life. The final section illustrates—again, by contrasting sensed and unsensed incentives—the fuzziness of the distinction between the "receipt" of reward and the prediction of reward.

ANATOMY OF DRUG REWARD

While there is much to learn about which dopamine neurons play roles in incentive motivation and reinforcement and there is much more to learn about the afferents to and the efferents from those dopamine neurons, a good deal is known about the brain structures and receptor subtypes at which addictive drugs trigger their habit-forming actions. This information comes in large part from studies involving intracranial drug injections that are reviewed below. The guiding assumption of such studies is that the relevant receptors for drug reward are to be found at sites where the lowest doses of microinjected drugs are rewarding. This is a fair assumption so long as care is taken to sample enough injection sites to ensure that the site of action is at the site of microinjection. The minimum controls for ensuring the validity of this assumption are "geologic" controls; unless one can demonstrate that similar injections in the regions bounding the putative site of action are not rewarding, one can never be sure that the drug is not spreading to act at a distance (Routtenberg, 1972; Wise & Hoffman, 1992). Of particular danger with hydraulic injections is that the drug spreads up the cannula shaft to a distant site of action or to the ventricular system (a pressure sink that is frequently penetrated by injection cannulae). The dangers of such spread are well illustrated by studies of the dipsogenic actions of carbachol (Routtenberg & Simpson, 1974) and angiotensin (Johnson & Epstein, 1975).

The Mesolimbic Dopamine System. A number of drugs are rewarding when injected into the nucleus accumbens, where they act at mesolimbic dopamine terminals. Amphetamine, a dopamine releaser, is self-administered (Hoebel, Monaco et al., 1983) and establishes conditioned place preferences (Carr & White, 1983) when injected into this region. Amphetamine injections into this region also potentiate (summate with) the rewarding effects of lateral hypothalamic brain stimulation (Colle & Wise, 1988). The dopamine uptake inhibitors nomifensine and cocaine also are self-administered into nucleus accumbens; injections into the shell are effective, whereas injections into the more dorsal and lateral core are not (Carlezon, Devine et al., 1995). Nomifensine also potentiates lateral hypothalamic brain stimulation reward by its action in this region (Carlezon & Wise, 1996b).

Cholinergic agents are rewarding when injected into the ventral tegmental area (VTA). Cytisine, a nicotinic agonist, induces conditioned place preference when injected into the VTA but not when injected just dorsal to it (Museo & Wise,

1994). The cholinergic agonist carbachol causes conditioned place preference when injected into the VTA (Yeomans, Kofman et al., 1985). Carbachol and the acetylcholinesterase inhibitor neostigmine are self-administered into the VTA; posterior VTA injections are most effective, and injections dorsal or lateral to the VTA are ineffective (Ikemoto & Wise, 2002). Low doses of carbachol are effective in producing conditioned place preferences when injected into the posterior but not the anterior VTA and not dorsal to the posterior VTA (Ikemoto & Wise, 2002). Carbachol activates both muscarinic and nicotinic receptors, and each type of receptor is expressed by dopaminergic neurons (Clarke & Pert, 1985; Weiner, Levey et al., 1990) and appears to contribute to carbachol's rewarding (Ikemoto & Wise, 2002) and reward-enhancing (Yeomans & Baptista, 1997) effects in this region.

Rewarding hypothalamic brain stimulation appears to depend on trans-synaptically induced release of acetylcholine in the VTA (Yeomans, Kofman et al., 1985). The axons of the mesolimbic dopamine system have high thresholds, and very few are directly activated, at traditional stimulation parameters, by rewarding hypothalamic stimulation (Yeomans, 1989; Murray & Shizgal, 1994). The bulk of the "first-stage" hypothalamic reward fibers—the reward-relevant portion of the medial forebrain bundle that is directly depolarized by cathodal current in the lateral hypothalamic medial forebrain bundle—are thought to be caudally projecting fibers (Bielajew & Shizgal, 1986) with refractory periods in the range of 0.4 to 2.5 ms (Yeomans, 1979; Bielajew, LaPointe et al., 1982; Gratton & Wise, 1985) and conduction velocities in the range of 2 to 8 m/s (Bielajew & Shizgal, 1982; Murray & Shizgal, 1994). At least the major portion of these fibers is thought to synapse in the pedunculopontine or latero-dorsal tegmental nucleus, the cholinergic efferents of which relay their message back to the VTA (Yeomans, Mathur et al., 1993). Hypothalamic brain stimulation reward elevates acetylcholine levels in the VTA (Rada, Mark et al., 2000), where injections of muscarinic blockers elevate reward thresholds (Yeomans, Kofman et al., 1985; Kofman, McGlynn et al., 1990; Yeomans & Baptista, 1997). Conversely, VTA injections of acetylcholine decrease the threshold for hypothalamic brain stimulation reward (Redgrave & Horrell, 1976). The VTA cholinergic contribution to brain stimulation reward appears to involve the activation of the mesolimbic dopamine system at M5 muscarinic receptors expressed by the dopaminergic neurons of this region (Yeomans, Takeuchi et al., 2000; Yeomans, Forster et al., 2001; Forster, Yeomans et al., 2002).

Mesolimbic Afferents. Opiates appear to have their strongest rewarding effects through afferents to the mesolimbic dopamine system. Mu and delta opioids are self-administered into the region of the mesolimbic dopamine cell bodies of the VTA (Bozarth & Wise, 1981; Welzl, Kuhn et al., 1989; Devine & Wise, 1994; David, Durkin et al., 2002). The selective mu agonist DAMGO is effective at two orders of magnitude lower doses than the selective delta agonist DPDPE (Devine & Wise, 1994); the two activate the mesolimbic dopamine system with the same relative potencies (Devine, Leone et al., 1993). The presumed mechanism of action of mu opioids in this region involves disinhibition of the dopamine system by inhibition of nearby GABAergic neurons that normally hold their dopaminergic neighbors under inhibitory control (Johnson & North, 1992). GABAergic agents themselves also are self-administered into the VTA (Ikemoto, Murphy et al., 1997c, 1998b; David, Durkin et al.,1997). The GABA$_A$ antagonists picrotoxin and bicuculline are self-administered into the anterior VTA, while, somewhat surprisingly, the GABA$_A$ agonist muscimol is self-administered into the posterior VTA; co-infusion of muscimol antagonizes the rewarding effects of anterior VTA picrotoxin injections, and, conversely, co-infusion of picrotoxin antagonizes the rewarding effects of posterior VTA muscimol injections. Self-administration of the GABA$_A$ antagonists, at least, is thought to be dopamine dependent (Ikemoto, Kohl et al., 1997b; David, Durkin et al., 1997). The mechanisms for these effects are not yet completely clear, because GABA$_A$ receptors are expressed not only by VTA dopamine neurons (Sugita, Johnson et al., 1992) but also by the GABAergic neurons that normally inhibit the dopamine neurons (Rick & Lacey, 1994).

Microinjections of dopamine D1 antagonists in the VTA attenuate the rewarding effects of intravenous cocaine (Ranaldi & Wise, 2001), presumably by blocking the effects of dendritically released dopamine on either GABAergic (Starr, 1987; Cameron & Williams, 1993) or glutamatergic (Kalivas & Duffy, 1995) inputs to the region. Glutamatergic input to the VTA appears to offer an important link in the brain's reward circuitry. VTA glutamate inputs arise from cortical sites including the frontal cortex. Rats will lever-press for injections of phencyclidine and other NMDA antagonists into the frontal cortex (Carlezon & Wise, 1996a), and direct electrical stimulation in this region is also rewarding (Routtenberg & Sloan, 1972; Corbett, Silva et al.,

1985). Such stimulation causes glutamate release in the VTA; blockade of ionotropic glutamate receptors in VTA blocks the rewarding effects of such stimulation as well as the ability of such stimulation to elevate nucleus accumbens dopamine levels (You, Tzschentki et al., 1998).

Mesolimbic Efferents. The mesolimbic dopamine system synapses on the shafts of the dendritic spines of GABA-containing medium spiny neurons of nucleus accumbens (Bouyer, Park et al., 1984). The medium spiny neurons express both D1-type and D2-type dopamine receptors (Surmeier, Song et al., 1996), though the D1-type receptors are largely restricted to a subpopulation of medium spiny neurons expressing dynorphin and substance P and projecting to the zona reticulata of the substantia nigra, whereas the D2-type receptors are largely restricted to a subpopulation of medium spiny neurons expressing enkephalin and projecting primarily to the pallidum (Gerfen, 1992). A third subpopulation of medium spiny neurons coexpresses substance P and enkephalin and similarly coexpresses both D1-type and D2-type dopamine receptors (Surmeier, Song et al., 1996; Aizman, Brismar et al., 2000); the projection of this subpopulation is not known. Rats do not self-administer either selective D1 or D2 agonists by themselves but do self-administer a mixture of the two (Ikemoto, Glazier et al., 1997a). It is tempting to suppose that they self-administer the mixture because of its actions on the subpopulation expressing both receptor subtypes, but most behavioral effects of dopaminergic agonists require cooperativity between the two receptor subtypes (Woolverton, 1986; Walters, Bergstrom et al., 1987; Clark & White, 1987), and it is not clear that all such effects depend on only the subpopulation expressing both receptors.

Glutamatergic inputs from a variety of cortical sources synapse on the heads of medium spiny neurons in nucleus accumbens, and antagonists of the NMDA-type glutamate receptor are self-administered into this region. The rewarding effects of phencyclidine and other NMDA antagonists are localized to the nucleus accumbens shell; injections in the core are not effective (Carlezon & Wise, 1996a). Unlike the rewarding effects of the dopamine uptake inhibitor nomifensine and despite the fact that phencyclidine is, like nomifensine (but at higher concentrations), a dopamine uptake inhibitor (Gerhardt, Pang et al., 1987), the effects of self-administered doses of nucleus accumbens phencyclidine and other NMDA antagonists are not antagonized by dopamine receptor blockers (Carlezon & Wise, 1996a). Nucleus accumbens injections of phencyclidine and other

NMDA antagonists also potentiate lateral hypothalamic brain stimulation reward (Carlezon & Wise, 1996b).

Opiates, too, are self-administered into nucleus accumbens. Morphine (Olds, 1982; David & Cazala, 2000) and the mixed mu-delta agonist methionine enkephalin (Goeders, Lane et al., 1984) are each effective, while the selective mu agonist endomorphin-1 is not (Zangen, Ikemo et al., 2002). While opiates in nucleus accumbens induce locomotion, their dopamine-independent actions in nucleus accumbens require an order of magnitude higher doses than do their dopamine-dependent actions in the ventral tegmental area (Kalivas, Widerlov et al., 1983). Interestingly, the locomotor stimulant effects of opioids in nucleus accumbens are enhanced by treatments that cause dopamine depletion or block dopamine receptor function in this region (Stinus, Winnock et al., 1985; Stinus, Nadaud et al., 1986).

Finally, rats self-administer the cholinergic agonist carbachol into nucleus accumbens (Ikemoto, Glazier et al., 1998a). Cholinergic interneurons are sparse in this region (they comprise less than 2% of all striatal neurons), but they branch profusely and innervate the medium spiny neurons of this region (Walaas & Fonnum, 1979; Phelps, Houser et al., 1985).

The medium spiny neurons of nucleus accumbens are the output neurons of this region; they may be viewed as a final common path for the currently identified portions of drug reward circuitry. It would appear to be depression of medium spiny neuron output—direct inhibition in the case of dopamine agonists or opiates and inhibition of excitatory input in the case of NMDA antagonists—that is common to these various drug rewards. It is not clear whether all or merely a subset of medium spiny neurons contributes to reward function.

REWARD AND COMPULSION

The defining property of rewards or "reinforcers" is that they "stamp in" (Thorndike, 1898) learned associations (Pavlov, 1928) and response habits (Thorndike 1898, 1933; Skinner, 1933). The distinction between a habit and an addiction has never been a clean distinction (West, 1992; Robinson & Pritchard, 1995; Stolerman & Jarvis, 1995). With the failure of traditional dependence theory to provide a definition of addiction that covers the cases of stimulants like cocaine and nicotine (Jaffe, 1985; Wise, 1988), the current distinction between a habit and an addiction is that an addiction is a compulsive habit maintained despite harmful consequences (Jaffe, 1985; Leshner, 1999; McLellan, Lewis et al., 2000). Inasmuch as it is as difficult to objectively define compulsion as it is to define addiction, the distinction between a simple habit and a compulsive habit seems more likely to be a quantitative than a qualitative distinction. Nonetheless, the attempt to characterize the mechanisms responsible for the transition from a simple habit to a compulsive habit has led to a major thrust of current work on addiction: the search for neuroadaptations that can explain the transition from habit to compulsion (e.g., Nestler, 1992, 2001; Robinson & Berridge, 1993, 2000; White & Kalivas, 1998; Berke & Hyman, 2000; Laakso, Mohn et al., 2002). The unsensed incentives of brain stimulation and intravenous drugs establish self-administration habits sufficiently compulsive as to qualify as addictions and offer potential insights into the neuroadaptations involved in reinforcement and addiction.

Unsensed incentives can establish very compulsive habits of seeking and ingesting. Rats will work continuously—lever-pressing at rates of several thousand responses per hour—for days to obtain direct electrical stimulation of the lateral hypothalamus and related brain regions (Olds, 1958b; Annau, Heffner et al., 1974). They do so to the exclusion of other behaviors, starving themselves for the opportunity to self-stimulate if food and stimulation are concurrently available for only a limited portion of each day (Routtenberg & Lindy, 1965). Once experienced with the stimulation, rats will cross electrified grids to gain access to the lever, accepting higher shock to obtain stimulation than they are willing to accept to obtain food (even when deprived for 24 hours [Olds, 1959]). The most obvious hypotheses as to why brain stimulation reward is so effective are (1) that they activate the reward pathway directly, bypassing synaptic barriers in sensory pathways (Wise, 1987); (2) that they activate the reward pathway powerfully, directly depolarizing a population of reward fibers within a radius of 0.25 to 0.5 mm (Fouriezos & Wise, 1984); and (3) that they do so with no delay of reinforcement (even a delay of 1 second between the lever-press and the delivery of reward can dramatically reduce reward effectiveness [Black et al., 1985; Fouriezos & Randall, 1997]). Rats and monkeys will work similarly compulsively for intravenous stimulants; if given unlimited access, they will self-administer intravenous injections of these drugs to the point of severe weight loss and death

(Johanson, Balster et al., 1976; Bozarth & Wise, 1985). What begins as a tentative response tendency becomes a compulsive habit very quickly.

In the case of brain stimulation reward, the habit of self-administration appears to become compulsive almost immediately. The first few lever-presses that result in lateral or posterior hypothalamic stimulation are, of course, accidental. However, rats begin to respond in a focused and frenetic fashion after as few as two or three earned stimulations (Olds, 1958a). That the behavior is locked in so quickly raises serious questions as to whether any of the known neuroadaptations associated with addiction (see, for example, Nestler, 1992, 2001; Robinson & Berridge, 1993, 2000; White & Kalivas, 1998; Berke & Hyman, 2000; Hyman & Malenka, 2001)—above and beyond the neuroadaptations involved in laying down a memory trace for past drug experience—could be a necessary condition for the development of a compulsive habit from a simple habit.

In the case of self-administration of intravenous stimulants or opiates, the compulsive nature of the early response habit is less dramatic. Rats appear to pursue intravenous heroin compulsively after as little as a single earned injection, but they tend to respond at rates of only two or three responses per hour because of apparent satiety (Wise, Leone et al., 1995a). Unlike brain stimulation reward, which is usually terminated abruptly 200 to 500 ms after its onset, drug reward decays slowly, usually by first-order kinetics. (When trains of rewarding brain stimulation reward are delivered with the slow rise and decay times of rewarding drug injections, brain stimulation, too, produces periods of satiety [Lepore & Franklin, 1992].) While animals frequently learn to respond for intravenous cocaine in the first hour or two of opportunity, the development of compulsive responding is less rapid with this drug than with heroin. Short-latency repetition of the instrumental task is infrequent in the early days of training. For example, a typical case involved an animal that responded for 1 mg/kg injections at intervals of between 14 and 55 minutes in the first four-hour session. In the second session, the animal began responding more regularly, with inter-response intervals of 6 to 13 minutes after three longer latencies at the beginning of the session. By the fourth day, the animal was responding at 6 ± 2 minute intervals. This degree of regularity of responding is itself an indication of compulsive behavior and is sufficient to allow confident prediction that if unlimited drug access is continued, the animal will self-administer

it to the point of self-induced starvation and death (Bozarth & Wise, 1985). Thus, where compulsiveness is demonstrated in tens of seconds by animals lever-pressing for brain stimulation reward and in tens of minutes in animals lever-pressing for intravenous heroin reward, it is demonstrated more on the order of days with intravenous cocaine or amphetamine self-administration. Nonetheless, one must wonder, even with cocaine and amphetamine reward, how much neuroadaptation could have taken place before the habit was stamped in to the point of compulsion.

The classic explanation for addiction is, first, that initial "recreational" use of a drug causes compensatory physiological adaptations to the drug that render the addicted brain different from the non-addicted brain and that require the user to escalate intake in order to maintain the desired effect of the drug. In this view, the neuroadaptations are thought to explain the transition from recreational to compulsive drug use. From this perspective, it should not be necessary for the animal to self-administer the drug in order to develop the adaptations that establish compulsion. Rather, compulsive self-administration should develop quickly after sufficient pre-exposure to induce the hypothesized adaptations. This prediction does not stand up very well against the facts. For example, there have been countless failed attempts to establish compulsive alcohol consumption in rodents by first establishing alcohol dependence (Lester, 1966; Falk, Samson et al., 1972; Mello, 1973; Cicero, 1980). Some success seems possible if extreme measures are taken, but it appears that alcohol must be established as a reinforcer *before* dependence is induced if dependence is to augment intake in such cases (Roberts, Heyser et al., 2000). Opiate dependence, too, seems not a sufficient condition for establishing compulsive opiate self-administration: it has been estimated that fewer than 0.01% of patients receiving chronic opiates passively are at risk for subsequent addiction (Woods, 1990). Finally, addiction involves compulsive *habits* of drug self-administration. Subjects receiving drug passively do not build up the motor memories for the skilled acts of the drug-taking ritual or the procedures of drug procurement. It is the ex-user returning on the train to the place where he or she has self-administered the drug, not the ex-patient returning on the train to the hospital where he or she was treated, who experiences drug cravings and conditioned withdrawal symptoms (O'Brien, Childress et al., 1998).

Early addiction theories focused on autonomic withdrawal symptoms as evidence for the critical physiological

---

adaptations that were the basis of compulsive drug taking; these symptoms are now known not to be necessary for compulsive drug seeking (Deneau, Yanagita et al., 1969; Woods & Schuster, 1971; Bozarth & Wise, 1984; Woods,1990). Current attention focuses instead on neuroadaptations within the brain circuitry of reward itself (Koob & Bloom, 1988; Nestler, 1992; White & Kalivas,1998; Berke & Hyman, 2000; Nestler, 2001). Neuroadaptations within the reward circuitry, though having no overt signs, could alter drug responsiveness and thus alter drug intake. This notion is supported by findings that thresholds for brain stimulation reward are higher in animals withdrawn from various drugs of abuse (Leith & Barrett, 1976; Kokkinidis, Zacharko et al., 1980; Kokkinidis & McCarter, 1990; Frank, Martz et al., 1988; Schulteis, Markou et al., 1995; Watkins, Stinus et al., 2000). While animals that are allowed to earn moderate doses of intravenous drugs for short periods each day tend to regulate their drug intake (Pickens & Thompson, 1968; Gerber & Wise, 1989; Wise, Leone et al., 1995a; Wise, Newton et al., 1995b; Ranaldi, Pocock et al., 1999), animals that are given access to high doses for long periods can show escalation (Ahmed & Koob, 1998) and dysregulation (Tornatzky & Miczek, 2000) of intake. One hypothesis is that prolonged high doses destabilize the mechanisms by which animals regulate limited-access drug intake (Koob & Le Moal, 2001) and that when pushed too far they, like other stress mechanisms (Sterling & Eyer, 1988; Schulkin, McEwen et al., 1994), never return fully to normal. The clearest correlate of drug satiety is dopamine level in nucleus accumbens (Wise, Leone et al., 1995a; Wise, Newton et al., 1995b; Ranaldi & Wise, 2001).

Animals that are given repeated intermittent experimenter-administered doses of opiates or psychomotor stimulants become sensitized to these drugs, showing increased responsiveness to their locomotor stimulating (Downs & Eddy, 1932; Segal & Mandell,1974; Bartoletti, Gaiardi et al., 1983; Kalivas & Duffy, 1987) and rewarding (Lett, 1989; Piazza, Deminiere et al., 1990; Horger, Shelton et al., 1990; Shippenberg & Heidbreder, 1995; Vezina, Pierre et al., 1999) effects. This sensitization is long lasting and appears to involve enhanced responsiveness of the mesolimbic dopamine system or its synaptic targets (Wolf, White et al., 1993; Paulson & Robinson, 1995; Heidbreder, Thompson et al., 1996; Nestler, 2001). Just as desensitization or tolerance of the reward circuitry has been offered as an explanation of escalating and compulsive drug seeking (Koob, 1996), so has its opposite, sensitization or "reverse-

tolerance," been suggested to underlie the compulsive drug seeking of addiction (Robinson & Berridge, 2000).

While it is clearly the case that brain changes associated with tolerance and dependence and brain changes associated with sensitization can develop under the right circumstances, what remains to be determined is the degree to which either of these changes is necessary for motivational habits to become compulsive. The rapid onset of compulsive self-stimulation would seem to preclude any of these drug-induced long-term neuroadaptations as a necessary condition for compulsive drug seeking. Indeed, given the strong dosing regimens that have been used to demonstrate reliable neuroadaptations, one might ask the opposite question: is, perhaps, compulsive drug seeking a necessary precursor for the development of neuroadaptations in animals not subjected to experimenter-administered drugs? Similarly, one might ask if other motivational compulsions, such as compulsive eating, compulsive sexual activity, or compulsive gambling, are likely to affect the nervous system strongly enough to produce any of the neuroadaptations associated with drugs of abuse. One direction that is just beginning to be explored is whether any of the known neuroadaptations can be established with the minimal drug treatments necessary before drug self-administration becomes compulsive or, for that matter, before animals become behaviorally sensitized to the drugs. A second fact that is just beginning to receive attention is that increases in the tendency for compulsive drug-seeking behavior can grow in the absence of drug-seeking opportunity; indeed, drug seeking can be many times stronger a few weeks (Shalev, Morales et al., 2001) or a few months (Grimm, Hope et al., 2001) after the last exposure to drug. A third interesting direction is the study of the effects of drug exposure on other motivated behaviors (Mitchell & Stewart, 1990; Harmer & Phillips, 1998; Fiorino & Phillips, 1999; Taylor & Horger, 1999). While sensed incentives may not activate the brain strongly enough to sensitize it to drugs, drug incentives may activate it strongly enough to sensitize the brain to more natural (and modest) sensed incentives.

The alternative to the view that drug-induced neuroadaptations make drug-seeking compulsive is that the neuroadaptations that differentiate the addicted from the non-addicted brain are the neuroadaptations associated with the learning of the drug-seeking habit. The memory of early drug experiences is stamped in by the same reinforcement process that stamps in the ordinary habits via weaker incentives. This hypothesis offers a potential explanation of the compulsiveness not only of drug self-administration, where neuroadaptations have been demonstrated (Robinson, Gorny et al., 2001), but also of intracranial self-stimulation, where they have not. It is possible that the neuroadaptations of addiction are merely the neuroadaptations of habit formation, stamped in more strongly by drug rewards that can elevate nucleus accumbens dopamine levels three- to fivefold more than by conventional rewards that tend to elevate dopamine by a factor of 1.5 or 2 (Hernandez & Hoebel, 1988; Fiorino, Coury et al., 1997; Bassareo & Di Chiara, 1999).

REWARD RECEIPT AND REWARD PREDICTION

Comparison of the sensed rewards of food, water, and sexual interaction with the unsensed laboratory rewards of brain stimulation and intravenous and intracranial drugs illustrates the difficulty in distinguishing the actual receipt of reward from the receipt of sensory information that reward is coming (prediction of reward). How can one single out a specific event that constitutes the receipt of reward? In the case of a food reward, is the reward received when we see it, touch it, or taste it? This question is not so easily answered as common sense would have us believe.

Rewards are, in the simplest terms, the environmental incentives we tend to approach (Schneirla, 1959). More precisely, they are the environmental incentives we return to after having previously contacted them. It is the return to a reward previously experienced that is the essence of habit and addiction. This is easily understood when the reward is localized in space by one or more of the senses. Consider the case of food reward, however. Once the animal has tasted a sweet substance, it will return to it again and again. However, the return to a previously experienced reward involves the return to reward-associated landmarks as much as it involves return to the reward itself. The animal only finds the reward by approaching the environmental stimuli that point to the location of the reward. As the animal becomes experienced at foraging for food, it identifies and is guided by more and more distal stimuli that, sequentially, help the animal reach the food. Thus, the animal might first learn the smell of a given food and begin to follow the odor trail. Next, the animal might learn the sight of the plants that give off the odor in question and learn to follow the sight path until reaching the odor trail. Finally, the animal might learn the sound of the waterfall that is near the visible landmarks and follow the sound until the landmarks are visible, the sight line until the odor trail is

sensed, and then the odor to the ripe and tasty portion of the plant. The sounds, sights, and smells associated with the food are clearly predictors of reward, and the efficiency of the animal increases with the identification of more and more distal predictors of reward, predictors that guide the foraging and that are important for the "error signals" that guide *corrections* to the foraging path.

If the sound, sight, and smell of food are predictors of reward, what is the "receipt" of reward? The widespread assumption is that the taste of a sweet substance (when hungry) or a salty substance (when sodium deficient) constitutes the receipt of reward. In the case of unsensed incentives—brain stimulation reward or intravenous or intracranial drug reward, for example—it is a much more central event that constitutes the receipt of reward. These rewards do not activate any of the five senses (except taste, eventually, when drugs diffuse from the blood to the saliva and reach the taste buds). Yet they have the critical attribute of all rewards; they, by association, establish otherwise neutral stimuli in the environment as things to be approached. The animal trained to lever-press for brain stimulation is guided first by visual stimuli (the sight of the distal lever) and then by tactile stimuli; the stimulation itself has no locus in space. Should we then consider the taste of sweet food simply another sensory predictor of the central process that really constitutes the rewarding event? In part to separate the subjective and sensory experience of reward from the central events that are critical to habit formation, psychologists have come to use Pavlov's term "reinforcement" in preference to the lay term "reward" (Wise, 1989). Is taste merely a predictor of food reinforcement?

The term "reinforcement" was first used by Pavlov (in 1903; cited in Pavlov, 1928) to refer to the strengthening of the association between a conditioned stimulus and its unconditioned partner. Pavlov pointed out that the effectiveness of a conditioned stimulus would extinguish if not reinforced by occasional repeat pairings with its associated unconditioned stimulus. By reinforcement he meant something akin to the "stamping in" of stimulus-response associations first discussed by Thorndike (1898). Skinner (1933) and Thorndike (1933) adopted the term reinforcement to the stamping in of response habits (1937); Skinner (1937) posited two forms of reinforcement, one associated with the stamping in of stimulus-stimulus (Pavlovian) associations and one associated with the stamping in of instrumental behavior (which he called "operant" behavior). The brain mechanism of "stamping in" is, of course, the brain mechanism of learning and memory formation, and its locus in the case of habit learning and the question of whether the stamping in of stimulus-stimulus associations involves different structures than the stamping in of response-consequence associations remain matters of speculation (see, for example, White, 1996).

The clearest illustration of the reinforcement process is the stamping in of memory that occurs when a reinforcer such as brain stimulation (Huston & Mueller, 1978) or sucrose (Messier & White, 1984) is given, independent of the animal's performance, following an unrelated learning experience. Post-trial reinforcers (and stressors) improve consolidation of memories for immediately previous events. This post-trial consolidation of learning and memory has been suggested as the essential mechanism of reinforcement, not only the reinforcement of stimulus-stimulus (Pavlovian) associations but also the reinforcement of habit-learning (Landauer, 1969; Pfaff, 1969).

The stamping in of food-rewarded memories appears to depend critically on postingestional consequences of food. If animals are given neutrally flavored foods and each is accompanied by an intragastric glucose load, the animals learn flavor preferences that are proportional to the associated glucose load (Le Magnen, 1959). It takes three or four days of exposure to learn these preferences, similar to the time it takes for vitamin-deficient rats to learn preferences for flavors associated with the missing vitamin (Harris, Clay et al., 1933). Thus, it would appear that the most fundamental event in the identification of sweet taste with food reward is the stamping in of the memory for ingesting sweet substances by some postingestional consequence of those substances. That is to say, the reinforcement process begins some significant time after the taste of the food; the taste of food is, like the smell and sight of food and the sounds that precede the delivery of food, a predictor of reward and not the primary reward itself.

While animals will learn habits that are rewarded by saccharin, a non-nutritive sweet substance (Sheffield & Roby, 1950), post-trial saccharin is very ineffective, relative to equally preferred concentrations of sucrose, in stamping in post-trial memories (Messier & White, 1984). Moreover, the rewarding effects of saccharin have been demonstrated only in animals that have a history of reinforcement by sweet substances with nutritive value. The first of these in a mammal's life is mother's milk, and rodents begin learning milk-rewarded habits from the first postnatal day (Johanson

& Hall, 1979). In all probability, then, the sweet taste of saccharin is a *conditioned* reinforcer, as are most predictors of reward. Consider, for example, the winning of a lottery. The excitement of reward is experienced at the announcement of the winning number and the receipt of the check, not at the postingestional receipt of the food that the money eventually buys.

This is, perhaps, best illustrated with the unsensed rewards of brain stimulation and drugs. Here, the animal has only the reward-associated lever or cue light to approach; the reward itself is not sensed peripherally, either by the distance senses of sight, hearing, and smell or by the proximal senses of taste and touch. Here, the receipt of reward is concurrent with the illumination of the cue light and the click of the relay; these are synonymous with the receipt of reward if not the perceived rewarding events themselves, at least for laboratory rats.

This is an interesting issue because of the work of Schultz and colleagues, showing that the dopamine system—clearly critical for reward function—becomes increasingly responsive to reward predictors and seemingly unresponsive to the reward "itself." Unit recordings in the awake animal present a complex and interesting picture of dopaminergic responsiveness to rewards. When food reward is first earned or discovered, midbrain dopaminergic neurons respond with short-latency phasic bursts of firing (Ljungberg, Apicella et al., 1992; Schultz, Apicella et al., 1993; Mirenowicz & Schultz, 1994). In experiments where juice near the animal's mouth was the incentive, the neurons appeared to respond to the taste of the juice (Schultz, Apicella et al., 1993; Mirenowicz & Schultz, 1994). With repeated testing, however, this phasic response becomes associated with stimuli that predict the presentation of the incentive. In experiments where a small piece of apple was the incentive, the neurons came to respond to the sight of the apple or the click of the latch to the door that hid the apple (Ljungberg, Apicella et al., 1992). As the neurons began to respond to the distant signals of the rewarding event, they ceased responding to the proximal (taste) cue (Ljungberg, Apicella et al., 1992; Mirenowicz & Schultz, 1994). In these studies, dopamine neurons were seen as responding to primary rewards "only when the reward occurs unpredictably, either outside of a task or during learning. By contrast, a fully predicted reward does not elicit a response in dopamine neurons, and the response is transferred to the earliest conditioned, reward-predicting stimulus" (Schultz, 1997). This interpretation has been the focus of several recent attempts to understand the role of dopamine in motivated behavior (Schultz et al., 1997; Schultz & Dickinson, 2000; O'Doherty, Deichmann et al., 2002; Schultz, 2002).

What are the lessons from studies of unsensed incentives for the question of whether dopamine is important for the prediction rather than the receipt of reward? The first lesson is that what we tend to designate as the receipt of reward might more accurately be designated as simply a more proximal predictor of reward. Human exultation, if it were objectively studied, would underscore the fact that it is the receipt of reward predictors that arouse us most. In the human situation, it is such things as the receipt of money, the receipt of the promise of an assignation, or the receipt of an invitation to compete in the finals of an athletic tournament that elicits the explosive "Yes!" and that marks, as much as anything, the emotional excitement of "receiving" reward. These things are clearly rewards, but they are conditioned rewards, not primary rewards; they are rewarding only because of previous learning. These are rewards because of their association with things to come; they are rewards because they predict—just as sweet taste predicts the stamping in of memory by postingestional glucose—something more closely linked to the survival of the individual and the species.

In the case of intravenous or intracranial drug reward, the sensed incentives—sight of the lever or cue light—are learned incentives that arrive tens of seconds or perhaps minutes (Heron, Costentin et al., 1994; Stathis, Scheffel et al., 1995; Kiyatkin, Kiyatkin et al., 2000) before a drug such as cocaine can significantly elevate extracellular dopamine. Thus, contact with the approached incentive does not mark the receipt of the *primary* reward. The sight of the lighted cue light signals the receipt of the secondary (learned) incentive just as does the sight of the distant apple. The click of the lever is no more or less the receipt of cocaine reward than is the click of Ljungberg et al.'s (1992) door the receipt of apple reward. That is to say, in each case the click may be what the subject is "waiting for" but it—like the taste of the apple itself—is only a predictor of the reinforcer, the event that stamps in memory (Landauer, 1969; Pfaff, 1969; Huston, Mondadori et al., 1974; Messier & White, 1984).

CONCLUSIONS

The mesolimbic dopamine system, its cholinergic input from the brainstem, its glutamatergic input from cortical struc-

FIGURE 1. Selected Elements and Connectivity of Brain Reward Circuitry

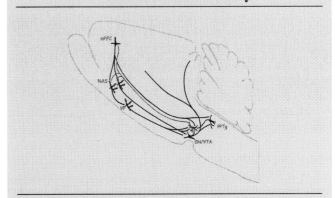

Amphetamine and cocaine are rewarding because they act at the dopamine transporter to elevate nucleus accumbens (NAS) dopamine levels; nicotine is rewarding because of actions on nicotinic cholinergic receptors, expressed at both the cell bodies and the terminals of the mesolimbic system, that result in elevated dopamine release in NAS. Dopamine in NAS inhibits the output neurons of NAS. The normal cholinergic input to these receptors in the VTA is from the pedunculopontine tegmental nucleus (PPTg) and the latero-dorsal pontine tegmental nucleus; these nuclei send branching projections to several basal forebrain targets (not shown). Rewarding electrical stimulation of the lateral hypothalamus is thought to be rewarding because it activates fibers to PPTg. The excitatory amino acid (glutamate) projections of medial prefrontal cortex (mPFC) are in grey. Projections from this and other cortical areas that receive mesolimbic dopamine input (amygdala, hippocampus) also project to NAS; amygdala also projects to the substantia nigra and ventral tegmental area (SNMA). Phencyclidine is rewarding because it blocks NMDA-type glutamate receptors in NAS and mPFC. Blockade of NMDA receptors in NAS reduces the excitatory input to the GABAergic output neurons. Electrical stimulation of mPFC is rewarding because it causes glutamate release in VTA and dopamine release in NAS. Two subsets of GABAergic projection neurons exit NAS; one projects to the ventral pallidum (VP) and the other to the SN/VTA. GABAergic neurons in VP also project to SNMA. Most of the GABAergic projection to SN synapses again on GABAergic neurons; these, in turn, project to the pedunculo-pontine tegmental nucleus, the deep layers of the superior colliculus, and the dorsomedial thalamus. Heroin and morphine have two rewarding actions: inhibition of GABAergic cells that normally hold the mesolimbic dopamine system under inhibitory control (thus morphine disinhibits the dopamine system) and inhibition of output neurons in NAS. Ethanol and cannabis act by unknown mechanisms to increase the firing of the mesolimbic dopamine system and are apparently rewarding for that reason. The habit-forming effects of barbiturates and benzodiazepines appear to be triggered at one or more of the GABAergic links in the circuitry, not necessarily through feedback links to the dopamine system. Caffeine appears to be rewarding through some independent circuitry.

tures including the medial and occipital prefrontal cortex and amygdala, its GABAergic inputs from striatal sources, and, finally, its GABAergic efferents in nucleus accumbens (and their glutamatergic inputs from cortical structures) comprise a major portion of the endogenous circuitry through which the pleasures of the flesh come to shape the habits of animal life (Figure 1). The proximity of the mesolimbic system to the nigro-striatal dopamine system— a system widely identified with motor function—has suggested this system to be an interface between motivational and motor mechanisms (Nauta & Domesick, 1978; Mogenson, Jones et al., 1980). The rewarding effects of food, water, sexual interaction, lateral hypothalamic brain stimulation, and most drugs of abuse can be eliminated by lesions or blockade of the output neurons of nucleus accumbens or of their dopaminergic input. This system is activated trans-synaptically by the normal pleasures of life but can be activated directly by the laboratory rewards of intravenous drugs or electrical or chemical brain stimulation.

The activation of this system somehow serves to establish the response habits that are followed reliably by such activation, presumably by augmenting the consolidation—by "stamping in"—the still-active memory traces of the exteroceptive (reward-associated) and interoceptive (response feedback) stimuli that led to the behavior that preceded activation of the system. This stamping in is not done by the sensory events by which we identify rewards so much as by the postsynaptic—and sometimes postingestional—consequences of those sensory events. The sensations of reward are varied; most rewards or incentives can be at least partially identified with both the distal senses of vision, audition, and olfaction and the contact senses of touch and taste. However, laboratory rewards that do not activate any of the five senses can directly activate the system even more strongly than can the natural pleasures of life. Thus, the five senses themselves are responsible not for the receipt of reward but rather the prediction of the stamping-in process. Indeed, the mesolimbic dopamine system is excited as much or more by the distant sensory message that guarantees a reward or incentive is coming as by the contact sense message that a reward has arrived. This raises the possibility that the neural circuitry of learned habits is not only stamped in after rewards are received but is also primed by the stimuli that predict that rewards are coming.

ACKNOWLEDGMENTS: The author thanks Yavin Shaham for comments on an earlier draft. Reprinted by permission of Elsevier Science from Wise A (2002). Brain reward circuitry: Insights from unsensed incentives (Review). Neuron 36:229-240. *Copyright 2002, Cell Press, Oxford, England.*

REFERENCES

Ahmed SH & Koob GF (1998). Transition from moderate to excessive drug intake: Change in hedonic set point. *Science* 282:298-300.

Aizman O, Brismar H, Uhlen P et al. (2000). Anatomical and physiological evidence for D1 and D2 dopamine receptor colocalization in neostriatal neurons. *Nature Neuroscience* 3:226-230.

Annau Z, Heffner R & Koob GF (1974). Electrical self-stimulation of single and multiple loci: Long term observations. *Physiology and Behavior* 13:281-290.

Bartoletti M, Gaiardi M, Gubellini G et al. (1983). Long-term sensitization to the excitatory effects of morphine. A motility study in post-dependent rats. *Neuropharmacology* 22:1193-1196.

Bassareo V & Di Chiara G (1999). Modulation of feeding-induced activation of mesolimbic dopamine transmission by appetitive stimuli and its relation to motivational state. *European Journal of Neuroscience* 11:4389-4397.

Berke JD & Hyman SE (2000). Addiction, dopamine, and the molecular mechanisms of memory. *Neuron* 25:515-532.

Bielajew C & Shizgal P (1982). Behaviorally derived measures of conduction velocity in the substrate for rewarding medial forebrain bundle stimulation. *Brain Research* 237:107-119.

Bielajew C & Shizgal P (1986). Evidence implicating descending fibers in self-stimulation of the medial forebrain bundle. *Journal of Neuroscience* 6:919-929.

Bielajew C, LaPointe M, Kiss L et al. (1982). Absolute and relative refractory periods of the substrates for lateral hypothalamic and ventral midbrain self-stimulation. *Physiology and Behavior* 28:125-132.

Black J, Belluzzi J & Stein L (1985). Reinforcement delay of one second severely impairs acquisition of brain self-stimulation. *Brain Research* 359:113-119.

Bouyer JJ, Park DH, Joh TH et al. (1984). Chemical and structural analysis of the relation between cortical inputs and tyrosine hydroxylase-containing terminals in rat neostriatum. *Brain Research* 302:267-275.

Bozarth MA & Wise RA (1981). Intracranial self-administration of morphine into the ventral tegmental area in rats. *Life Sciences* 28:551-555.

Bozarth MA & Wise RA (1984). Anatomically distinct opiate receptor fields mediate reward and physical dependence. *Science* 224:516-517.

Bozarth MA & Wise RA (1985). Toxicity associated with long-term intravenous heroin and cocaine self-administration in the rat. *Journal of the American Medical Association* 254:81-83.

Cameron DL & Williams JT (1993). Dopamine D1 receptors facilitate transmitter release. *Nature* 366:344-347.

Carlezon WA Jr & Wise RA (1996a). Rewarding actions of phencyclidine and related drugs in nucleus accumbens shell and frontal cortex. *Journal of Neuroscience* 16:3112-3122.

Carlezon WA Jr & Wise RA (1996b). Microinjections of phencyclidine (PCP) and related drugs into nucleus accumbens shell potentiate lateral hypothalamic brain stimulation reward. *Psychopharmacology (Berl.)* 128:413-420.

Carlezon WA Jr, Devine DP & Wise RA (1995). Habit-forming actions of nomifensine in nucleus accumbens. *Psychopharmacology (Berl.)* 122:194-197.

Carr GD & White NM (1983). Conditioned place preference from intra-accumbens but not intra-caudate amphetamine injections. *Life Sciences* 33:2551-2557.

Cicero TJ (1980). Animal models of alcoholism. In K Eriksson, JD Sinclair & K Kiianmaa (eds.) *Animal Models in Alcohol Research*. New York, NY: Academic Press, 99-118.

Clarke PBS & Pert A (1985). Autoradiographic evidence for nicotine receptors on nigrostriatal and mesolimbic dopaminergic neurons. *Brain Research* 348:355 358.

Clark D & White FJ (1987). Review: D1 dopamine receptor–The search for a function: A critical evaluation of the D1/D2 dopamine receptor classification and its function implications. *Synapse* 1:347-388.

Colle LM & Wise RA (1988). Effects of nucleus accumbens amphetamine on lateral hypothalamic brain stimulation reward. *Brain Research* 459:361-368.

Coons EE, Levak M & Miller NE (1965). Lateral hypothalamus: Learning of food-seeking response motivated by electrical stimulation. *Science* 150:1320-1321.

Corbett D, Silva LR & Stellar JR (1985). An investigation of the factors affecting development of frontal cortex self-stimulation. *Physiology and Behavior* 34:89-95.

David V & Cazala P (2000). Anatomical and pharmacological specificity of the rewarding effect elicited by microinjections of morphine into the nucleus accumbens of mice. *Psychopharmacology (Berl.)* 150:24-34.

David V, Durkin TP & Cazala P (1997). Self-administration of the GABA$_A$ antagonist bicuculline into the ventral tegmental area in mice: Dependence on D2 dopaminergic mechanisms. *Psychopharmacology (Berl.)* 130:85-90.

David V, Durkin TP & Cazala P (2002). Differential effects of the dopamine D(2)/D(3) receptor antagonist sulpiride on self-administration of morphine into the ventral tegmental area or the nucleus accumbens. *Psychopharmacology (Berl.)* 160:307-317.

Deneau G, Yanagita T & Seevers MH (1969). Self-administration of psychoactive substances by the monkey: A measure of psychological dependence. *Psychopharmacologia* 16:30-48.

Devine DP & Wise RA (1994). Self-administration of morphine, DAMGO, and DPDPE into the ventral tegmental area of rats. *Journal of Neuroscience* 14:1978-1984.

Devine DP, Leone P, Pocock D et al. (1993). Differential involvement of ventral tegmental mu, delta and kappa opioid receptors in modulation of basal mesolimbic dopamine release: In vivo microdialysis studies. *Journal of Pharmacology and Experimental Therapeutics* 266, 1236-1246.

Downs AW & Eddy NB (1932). The effect of repeated doses of cocaine on the dog. *Journal of Pharmacology and Experimental Therapeutics* 46:195-198.

Folk JL, Samson HM & Winger G (1972). Behavioural maintenance of high concentrations of blood ethanol and physical dependence in the rat. *Science* 177:811-813.

Fiorino DF & Phillips AG (1999). Facilitation of sexual behavior in male rats following d-amphetamine-induced behavioral sensitization. *Psychopharmacology (Berl.)* 142:200-208.

Fiorino DF, Coury A & Phillips AG (1997). Dynamic changes in nucleus accumbens dopamine efflux during the Coolidge effect in male rats. *Journal of Neuroscience* 17:4849-4855.

Forster GL, Yeomans JS, Takeuchi J et al. (2002). M5 muscarinic receptors are required for prolonged accumbal dopamine release after electrical stimulation of the pons in mice. *Journal of Neuroscience* 22:RC190.

Fouriezos G & Randall D (1997). The cost of delaying rewarding brain stimulation. *Behavioral Brain Research* 87:111-113.

Fouriezos G & Wise RA (1984). Current-distance relation for rewarding brain stimulation. *Behavioral Brain Research* 14:85-89.

Frank RA, Martz S & Pommering T (1988). The effect of chronic cocaine on self-stimulation train-duration thresholds. *Pharmacology, Biochemistry and Behavior* 29, 755-758.

Gerber GJ & Wise RA (1989). Pharmacological regulation of intravenous cocaine and heroin self-administration in rats: A variable dose paradigm. *Pharmacology, Biochemistry and Behavior* 32:527-531.

Gerfen CR (1992). The neostriatal mosaic: Multiple levels of compartmental organization. *Trends in Neurosciences* 15:133-139.

Gerhardt GA, Pang K & Rose GM (1987). In viva electrochemical demonstration of the presynaptic actions of phencyclidine in rat caudate nucleus. *Journal of Pharmacology and Experimental Therapeutics* 241:714-721.

German DC & Bowden DM (1974). Catecholamine systems as the neural substrate for intracranial self-stimulation: A hypothesis. *Brain Research* 73:381-419.

Glickman SE & Schiff BB (1967). A biological theory of reinforcement. *Psychological Review* 74:81-109.

Goeders NE, Lane JD & Smith JE (1984). Self-administration of methionine enkephalin into the nucleus accumbens. *Pharmacology, Biochemistry and Behavior* 20:451-455.

Gratton A & Wise RA (1985). Hypothalamic reward mechanism: Two first-stage fiber populations with a cholinergic component. *Science* 227:545-548.

Grimm JW, Hope BT, Wise RA et al. (2001). Incubation of cocaine craving during withdrawal. *Nature* 412:141-142.

Harmer CJ & Phillips GD (1998). Enhanced appetitive conditioning following repeated pretreatment with d-amphetamine. *Behavioural Pharmacology* 9:299-308.

Harris LJ, Clay J, Hargreaves FJ et al. (1933). Appetite and choice of diet: The ability of the vitamin B deficient rat to discriminate between diets containing and lacking the vitamin. *Proceedings of the Royal Society of London. Series B: Biological Sciences* 113:161-190.

Heidbreder CA, Thompson AC & Shippenberg TS (1996). Role of extracellular dopamine in the initiation and long-term expression of behavioral sensitization to cocaine. *Journal of Pharmacology and Experimental Therapeutics* 278:490-502.

Hernandez L & Hoebel BG (1988). Food reward and cocaine increase extracellular dopamine in the nucleus accumbens as measured by microdialysis. *Life Sciences* 42:1705-1712.

Heron C, Costentin J & Bonnet JJ (1994). Evidence that pure uptake inhibitors including cocaine interact slowly with the dopamine neuronal carrier. *European Journal of Pharmacology* 264:391-398.

Hoebel BG, Monaco AP, Hernandez L et al. (1983). Self-injection of amphetamine directly into the brain. *Psychopharmacology (Berl.)* 81:158-163.

Horger BA, Shelton K & Schenk S (1990). Preexposure sensitizes rats to the rewarding effects of cocaine. *Pharmacology, Biochemistry and Behavior* 37:707-711.

Huston JP & Mueller CC (1978). Enhanced passive avoidance learning and appetitive T-maze learning with post-trial rewarding hypothalamic stimulation. *Brain Research Bulletin* 3:265-270.

Huston JP, Mondadori C & Waser PG (1974). Facilitation of learning by reward of post-trial memory processes. *Experientia* 30:1038-1040.

Hyman SE & Malenka RC (2001). Addiction and the brain: The neurobiology of compulsion and its persistence. *Nature Review. Neuroscience* 2:695-703.

Ikemoto S & Wise RA (in press 2002). Rewarding effects of carbachol and neostigmine in the posterior ventral tegmental area. *Journal of Neuroscience.*

Ikemoto S, Glazier BS, Murphy JM et al. (1997a). Role of dopamine D_1 and D_2 receptors in the nucleus accumbens in mediating reward. *Journal of Neuroscience* 17:8580-8587.

Ikemoto S, Kohl RR & McBride WJ (1997b). GABA(A) receptor blockade in the anterior ventral tegmental area increases extracellular levels of dopamine in the nucleus accumbens of rats. *Journal of Neurochemistry* 69:137-143.

Ikemoto S, Murphy JM & McBride WJ (1997c). Self-infusion of $GABA_A$ antagonists directly into the ventral tegmental area and adjacent regions. *Behavioral Neuroscience* 111:369-380.

Ikemoto S, Glazier BS, Murphy JM et al. (1998a). Rats self-administer carbachol directly into the nucleus accumbens. *Physiology and Behavior* 63:811-814.

Ikemoto S, Murphy JM & McBride WJ (1998b). Regional differences within the rat ventral tegmental area for muscimol self-infusions. *Pharmacology, Biochemistry and Behavior* 61:87-92.

Jaffe JH (1985). Drug addiction and drug abuse. In AG Gilman & LS Goodman (eds.) *The Pharmacological Basis of Therapeutics.* New York, NY: Macmillan, 532-581.

Johanson LB & Hall WG (1979). Appetitive learning in 1-day-old rat pups. *Science* 205:419-421.

Johanson CE, Bolster RL & Bonese K (1976). Self-administration of psychomotor stimulant drugs: The effects of unlimited access. *Pharmacology, Biochemistry and Behavior* 4:45-51.

Johnson AK & Epstein AN (1975). The cerebral ventricles as the avenue for the dipsogenic action of intracranial angiotensin. *Brain Research* 86:399-418.

Johnson SW & North RA (1992). Opioids excite dopamine neurons by hyperpolarization of local interneurons. *Journal of Neuroscience* 12:483-488.

Kalivas PW & Duffy P (1987). Sensitization to repeated morphine injection in the rat: Possible involvement of A10 dopamine neurons. *Journal of Pharmacology and Experimental Therapeutics* 241:204-212.

Kalivas PW & Duffy P (1995). D1 receptors modulate glutamate transmission in the ventral tegmental area. *Journal of Neuroscience* 15:53795388.

Kalivas PW, Widerlov E, Stanley D et al. (1983). Enkephalin action on the mesolimbic system: A dopamine-dependent and a dopamine-independent increase in locomotor activity. *Journal of Pharmacology and Experimental Therapeutics* 227:229-237.

Kiyatkin EA, Kiyatkin DE & Rebec GV (2000). Phasic inhibition of dopamine uptake in nucleus accumbens induced by intravenous cocaine in freely behaving rats. *Neuroscience* 98:729-741.

Koob GF (1996). Drug addiction: The yin and yang of hedonic homeostasis. *Neuron* 16:893-896.

Koob GF & Bloom FE (1988). Cellular and molecular mechanisms of drug dependence. *Science* 242:715-723.

Koob GF & Le Moal M (2001). Drug addiction, dysregulation of reward, and allostasis. *Neuropsychopharmacology* 24:97-129.

Kofman O, McGlynn SM, Olmstead MC et al. (1990). Differential effects of atropine, procaine and dopamine in the rat ventral tegmentum on lateral hypothalamic rewarding brain stimulation. *Behavioural Brain Research* 38:55-68.

Kokkinidis L & McCarter BD (1990). Postcocaine depression and sensitization of brain-stimulation reward: Analysis of reinforcement and performance effects. *Pharmacology, Biochemistry and Behavior* 36:463-471.

Kokkinidis L, Zacharko RM & Predy PA (1980). Post-amphetamine depression of self-stimulation responding from the substantia nigra: Reversal by tricyclic antidepressants. *Pharmacology, Biochemistry and Behavior* 13:379-383.

Laakso A, Mohn AR, Gainetdinov RR et al. (2002). Experimental genetic approaches to addiction. *Neuron* 36:213-228.

Landauer TK (1969). Reinforcement as consolidation. *Psychological Review* 76:82-96.

Leith NJ & Barrett RJ (1976). Amphetamine and the reward system: Evidence for tolerance and post-drug depression. *Psychopharmacologia* 46:19-25.

Le Magnen J (1959). Effets des administrations post-prandiales de glucose sur l'établissement des appétits. *Comptes Rendus des Seances ce la Societe de Biologie (Paris)* 153:212-215.

Lepore M & Franklin KBJ (1992). Modelling drug kinetics with brain stimulation: Dopamine antagonists increase self-stimulation. *Pharmacology, Biochemistry and Behavior* 41:489-496.

Leshner AI (1999). Science-based views of drug addiction and its treatment. *Journal of the American Medical Association* 282:1314-1316.

Lester D (1966). Self-selection of alcohol by animals, human variation and the etiology of alcoholism: A critical review. *Quarterly Journal of Studies on Alcohol* 27:395-438.

Lett BT (1989). Repeated exposures intensify rather than diminish the rewarding effects of amphetamine, morphine, and cocaine. *Psychopharmacology (Berl.)* 98:357-362.

Ljungberg T, Apicella P & Schultz W (1992). Responses of monkey dopamine neurons during learning of behavioral reactions. *Journal of Neurophysiology* 67:145-163.

MacDonnell MF & Flynn JP (1966a). Sensory control of hypothalamic attack. *Animal Behavior* 14:399-405.

MacDonnell MF & Flynn JP (1966b). Control of sensory fields by stimulation of hypothalamus. *Science* 152:1046-1048.

McLellan AT, Lewis DC, O'Brien CP et al. (2000). Drug dependence, a chronic medical illness: Implications for treatment, insurance, and outcomes evaluation. *Journal of the American Medical Association* 284:1689-1695.

Mello NK (1973). A review of methods to induce alcohol addiction in animals. *Pharmacology, Biochemistry and Behavior* 1:89-101.

Mendelson J & Chorover SL (1965). Lateral hypothalamic stimulation in satiated rats: T-maze learning for food. *Science* 149:559-561.

Messier C & White NM (1984). Contingent and non-contingent actions of sucrose and saccharin reinforcers: Effects on taste preference and memory. *Physiology and Behavior* 32:195-203.

Mirenowicz J & Schultz W (1994). Importance of unpredictedness for reward responses in primate dopamine neurons. *Journal of Neurophysiology* 72:1024-1027.

Mitchell JB & Stewart J (1990). Facilitation of sexual behaviors in the male rat in the presence of stimuli previously paired with systemic injections of morphine. *Pharmacology, Biochemistry and Behavior* 35:367-372.

Mogenson GJ, Jones DL & Yim CY (1980). From motivation to action: Functional interface between the limbic system and the motor system. *Progress in Neurobiology* 14:69-97.

Murray B & Shizgal P (1994). Evidence implicating both slow- and fast-conducting fibers in the rewarding effect of medial forebrain bundle stimulation. *Behavioural Brain Research* 63:47-60.

Museo E & Wise RA (1994). Place preference conditioning with ventral tegmental injections of cytisine. *Life Sciences* 55:1179-1186.

Nauta WJH & Domesick VB (1978). Crossroads of limbic and striatal circuitry: Hypothalamo-nigral connections. In KE Livingston & O Hornykiewicz (eds.) *Limbic Mechanisms.* New York, NY: Plenum Press, 75-93.

Nestler EJ (1992). Molecular mechanisms of drug addiction. *Journal of Neuroscience* 12:2439-2450.

Nestler EJ (2001). Molecular basis of long-term plasticity underlying addiction. *Nature Review. Neuroscience* 2:119-128.

O'Brien CP, Childress AR, Ehrman R et al. (1998). Conditioning factors in drug abuse: Can they explain compulsion? *Journal of Psychopharmacology* 12:15-22.

O'Doherty JP, Deichmann R, Critchley HD et al. (2002). Neural responses during anticipation of a primary taste reward. *Neuron* 33:815-826.

Olds J (1958a). Self-stimulation of the brain. *Science* 127:315-324.

Olds J (1958b). Satiation effects in self-stimulation of the brain. *Journal of Comparative Physiology and Psychology* 51:675-678.

Olds J (1959). Self-stimulation experiments and differentiated reward systems. In H Jasper, LD Proctor, RS Knighton et al. (eds.) *Reticular Formation of the Brain.* Boston, MA: Little, Brown & Company, 671-687.

Olds ME (1982). Reinforcing effects of morphine in the nucleus accumbens. *Brain Research* 237:429-440.

Olds J & Milner PM (1954). Positive reinforcement produced by electrical stimulation of septal area and other regions of rat brain. *Journal of Comparative Physiology and Psychology* 47:419-427.

Olds ME & Olds J (1963). Approach-avoidance analysis of rat diencephalon. *Journal of Comparative Neurology* 120:259-295.

Olds J & Olds ME (1965). Drives, rewards, and the brain. In TM Newcombe (ed.) *New Directions in Psychology.* New York, NY: Holt, Rinehart and Winston, 327-410.

Olds J, Yuwiler A, Olds ME et al. (1964). Neurohumors in hypothalamic substrates of reward. *American Journal of Physiology* 207:242-254.

Paulson PE & Robinson TE (1995). Amphetamine-induced time-dependent sensitization of dopamine neurotransmission in the dorsal and ventral striatum: A microdialysis study in behaving rats. *Synapse* 19:56-65.

Pavlov LP (1928). *Lectures on Conditioned Reflexes.* New York, NY: International Publishers.

Pfaff D (1969). Parsimonious biological models of memory and reinforcement. *Psychological Review* 76:70-81.

Phelps PE, Houser CR & Vaughn JE (1985). Immunocytochemical localization of choline acetyltransferase within the rat neostriatum: A correlated light and electron microscopic study of cholinergic neurons and synapses. *Journal of Comparative Neurology* 238:286-307.

Phillips AG & LePiane FG (1980). Reinforcing effects of morphine microinjection into the ventral tegmental area. *Pharmacology, Biochemistry and Behavior* 12:965-968.

Piazza PV, Deminiere JM, Le Moal M et al. (1990). Stress- and pharmacologically-induced behavioral sensitization increases vulnerability to acquisition of amphetamine self-administration. *Brain Research* 514:22-26.

Pickens R & Thompson T (1968). Cocaine-reinforced behavior in rats: Effects of reinforcement magnitude and fixed-ratio size. *Journal of Pharmacology and Experimental Therapeutics* 161:122-129.

Rada PV, Mark GP, Yeomans JJ et al. (2000). Acetylcholine release in ventral tegmental area by hypothalamic self-stimulation, eating, and drinking. *Pharmacology, Biochemistry and Behavior* 65:375-379.

Ranaldi R & Wise RA (2001). Blockade of D1 dopamine receptors in the ventral tegmental area decreases cocaine reward: Possible role for dendritically released dopamine. *Journal of Neuroscience* 21:58415846.

Ranaldi R, Pocock D, Zereik R et al. (1999). Dopamine fluctuations in the nucleus accumbens during maintenance, extinction, and reinstatement of intravenous D-amphetamine self-administration. *Journal of Neuroscience* 19:4102-4109.

Redgrave P & Horrell RI (1976). Potentiation of central reward by localized perfusion of acetylcholine and 6-hydroxytryptamine. *Nature* 262:305-307.

Rick CE & Lacey MG (1994). Rat substantia nigra pars reticulata neurons are topically inhibited via GABA$_A$, but not GABA$_B$, receptors in vitro. *Brain Research* 659:133-137.

Roberts AJ, Heyser CJ, Cole M et al. (2000). Excessive ethanol drinking following a history of dependence: Animal model of allostasis. *Neuropsychopharmacology* 22:581-594.

Robinson TE & Berridge KC (1993). The neural basis of drug craving: An incentive-sensitization theory of addiction. *Brain Research Review* 18:247-292.

Robinson TE & Berridge KC (2000). The psychology and neurobiology of addiction: An incentive-sensitization view. *Addiction* 95(Suppl 2):S91-S117.

Robinson JH & Pritchard WS (1995). Differentiating habits and addictions: The evidence that nicotine is not "addictive." In PBS Clarke, M Quik, F Adlkofer et al. (eds.) *Effects of Nicotine on Biological Systems II.* Basel, Switzerland: Birkhauser Verlag, 273-278.

Robinson TE, Gorny G, Milton E et al. (2001). Cocaine self-administration alters the morphology of dendrites and dendritic spines in the nucleus accumbens and neocortex. *Synapse* 39:257-266.

Routtenberg A (1972). Intracranial chemical injection and behavior: A critical review. *Behavioral Biology* 7:601-641.

Routtenberg A (1976). Self-stimulation pathways: Origins and terminations—A three-stage technique. In A Wauquier & ET Rolls (eds.) *Brain-Stimulation Reward.* New York, NY: Elsevier, 31-39.

Routtenberg A & Lindy J (1965). Effects of the availability of rewarding septal and hypothalamic stimulation on bar pressing for food under conditions of deprivation. *Journal of Comparative Physiology and Psychology* 1:158-161.

Routtenberg A & Simpson JB (1974). Carbachol-induced drinking at ventricular and subfornical organ sites. *Life Sciences* 10:481-490.

Routtenberg A & Sloan M (1972). Self-stimulation in the frontal cortex of Rattus norvegicus. *Behavioral Biology* 7:567-572.

Schneirla TC (1959). An evolutionary and developmental theory of biphasic processes underlying approach and withdrawal. In MR Jones (ed.) *Nebraska Symposium on Motivation.* Lincoln, NB: University of Nebraska Press, 1-42.

Schulkin J, McEwen BS & Gold PW (1994). Allostasis, amygdala, and anticipatory angst. *Neuroscience and Biobehavioral Reviews* 18:385-396.

Schulteis G, Markou A, Cole M et al. (1995). Decreased brain reward produced by ethanol withdrawal. *Proceedings of the National Academy of Sciences* 92:5880-5884.

Schultz W (1997). Dopamine neurons and their role in reward mechanisms. *Current Opinion in Neurobiology* 7:191-197.

Schultz W (2002). Getting formal with dopamine and reward. *Neuron* 36:241-263.

Schultz W & Dickinson A (2000). Neuronal coding of prediction errors. *Annual Review of Neuroscience* 23:473-500.

Schultz W, Apicella P & Ljungberg T (1993). Responses of monkey dopamine neurons to reward and conditioned stimuli during successive steps of learning a delayed response task. *Journal of Neuroscience* 13:900-913.

Schultz W, Dayan P & Montague PR (1997). A neural substrate of prediction and reward. *Science* 275:1593-1599.

Segal DS & Mandell AJ (1974). Long-term administration of d-amphetamine: Progressive augmentation of motor activity and stereotypy. *Pharmacology, Biochemistry and Behavior* 2:249-255.

Shalev U, Morales M, Hope B et al. (2001). Time-dependent changes in extinction behavior and stress-induced reinstatement of drug seeking following withdrawal from heroin in rats. *Psychopharmacology (Berl.)* 156:98-107.

Sheffield FD & Roby TB (1950). Reward value of a non-nutritive sweet taste. *Journal of Comparative Physiology and Psychology* 43:471-481.

Shippenberg TS & Heidbreder C (1995). Sensitization to the conditioned rewarding effects of cocaine: Pharmacological and temporal characteristics. *Journal of Pharmacology and Experimental Therapeutics* 273:808-815.

Skinner BF (1933). The rate of establishment of a discrimination. *Journal of General Psychology* 9:302-350.

Skinner BF (1937). Two types of conditioned reflex: A reply to Konorski and Miller. *Journal of General Psychology* 16:272-279.

Starr M (1987). Opposing roles of dopamine D1 and D2 receptors in nigral gamma-[3H]aminobutyric acid release? *Journal of Neurochemistry* 49:1042-1049.

Stathis M, Scheffel U, Lever SZ et al. (1995). Rate of binding of various inhibitors at the dopamine transporter in vivo. *Psychopharmacology (Berl.)* 119:376-384.

Sterling P & Eyer J (1988). Allostasis: A new paradigm to explain arousal pathology. In S Fisher & J Reason (eds.) *Handbook of Life Stress, Cognition and Health.* New York, NY: John Wiley & Sons, 629-649.

Stinus L, Winnock M & Kelley AE (1985). Chronic neuroleptic treatment and mesolimbic dopamine deprivation induce behavioural supersensitivity to opiates. *Psychopharmacology (Berl.)* 85:323-328.

Stinus L, Nadaud D, Jauregui J et al. (1986). Chronic treatment with five different neuroleptics elicits behavioral supersensitivity to opiate infusion into the nucleus accumbens. *Biological Psychiatry* 21:34-48.

Stolerman LP & Jarvis MJ (1995). The scientific case that nicotine is addictive. *Psychopharmacology (Berl.)* 117:2-10.

Sugita S, Johnson SW & North RA (1992). Synaptic inputs to $GABA_A$ and $GABA_B$ receptors originate from discrete afferent neurons. *Neuroscience Letters* 134:207-211.

Surmeier DJ, Song WJ & Yan Z (1996). Coordinated expression of dopamine receptors in neostriatal medium spiny neurons. *Journal of Neuroscience* 16:6579-6591.

Taylor JR & Horger BA (1999). Enhanced responding for conditioned reward produced by infra-accumbens amphetamine is potentiated after cocaine sensitization. *Psychopharmacology (Berl.)* 142:31-40.

Thompson T & Schuster CR (1964). Morphine self-administration, food-reinforced, and avoidance behaviors in rhesus monkeys. *Psychopharmacologia* 5:87.

Thorndike EL (1898). Animal intelligence: An experimental study of the associative processes in animals. *Psychology Monograph* 8:1-109.

Thorndike EL (1933). A theory of the action of the after-effects of a connection upon it. *Psychological Review* 40:434-439.

Tornatzky W & Miczek K (2000). Cocaine self-administration "binges": Transition from behavioral and autonomic regulation toward homeostatic dysregulation in rats. *Psychopharmacology (Berl.)* 148:289-298.

Vezina P, Pierre PJ & Lorrain DS (1999). The effect of previous exposure to amphetamine on drug-induced locomotion and self-administration of a low dose of the drug. *Psychopharmacology (Berl.)* 147:125-134.

Walaas L & Fonnum F (1979). The distribution and origin of glutamate decarboxylase and choline acetyltransferase in ventral pallidum and other basal forebrain regions. *Brain Research* 177:325-336.

Walters JR, Bergstrom EA, Carlson JH et al. (1987). D_1 dopamine receptor activation required for post-synaptic expression of D_2 agonist effects. *Science* 236:719-722.

Watkins SS, Stinus L, Koob GF et al. (2000). Reward and somatic changes during precipitated nicotine withdrawal in rats: Centrally and peripherally mediated effects. *Journal of Pharmacology and Experimental Therapeutics* 292:1053-1064.

Weeks JR (1962). Experimental morphine addiction: Method for automatic intravenous injections in unrestrained rats. *Science* 143:143-144.

Weiner DM, Levey AL & Brann MR (1990). Expression of muscarinic acetylcholine and dopamine receptor mRNAs in rat basal ganglia. *Proceedings of the National Academy of Sciences* 87:7050-7054.

Welzl H, Kuhn G & Huston JP (1989). Self-administration of small amounts of morphine through glass micropipettes into the ventral tegmental area of the rat. *Neuropharmacology* 28:1017-1023.

West R (1992). Nicotine addiction: A re-analysis of the arguments. *Psychopharmacology (Berl.)* 108:408-410.

White NM (1996). Addictive drugs as reinforcers: Multiple partial actions on memory systems. *Addiction* 91:921-949.

White FJ & Kalivas PW (1998). Neuroadaptations involved in amphetamine and cocaine addiction. *Drug and Alcohol Dependence* 51:141-153.

Wise RA (1974). Lateral hypothalamic electrical stimulation: does it make animals 'hungry'? *Brain Research* 67:187-209.

Wise RA (1987). Intravenous drug self-administration: A special case of positive reinforcement. In MA Bozarth (ed.) *Methods of Assessing the Reinforcing Properties of Abused Drugs.* New York, NY: Springer-Verlag, 117-141.

Wise RA (1988). The neurobiology of craving; Implications for understanding and treatment of addiction. *Journal of Abnormal Psychology* 97:118-132.

Wise RA (1989). The brain and reward. In JM Liebman & SJ Cooper (eds.) *The Neuropharmacological Basis of Reward.* Oxford, England: Oxford University Press, 377-424.

Wise RA & Hoffman DC (1992). Localization of drug reward mechanisms by intracranial injections. *Synapse* 10:247-263.

Wise RA, Leone P, Rivest R et al. (1995a). Elevations of nucleus accumbens dopamine and DOPAC levels during intravenous heroin self-administration. *Synapse* 21:140-148.

Wise RA, Newton P, Leeb K et al. (1995b). Fluctuations in nucleus accumbens dopamine concentration during intravenous cocaine self-administration in rats. *Psychopharmacology (Berl.)* 120:10-20.

Wolf ME, White FJ, Nassar R et al. (1993). Differential development of autoreceptor subsensitivity and enhanced dopamine release during amphetamine sensitization. *Journal of Pharmacology and Experimental Therapeutics* 264:249-255.

Woods JH (1990). Abuse liability and the regulatory control of therapeutic drugs: Untested assumptions. *Drug and Alcohol Dependence* 25:229-233.

Woods JH & Schuster CR (1971). Opiates as reinforcing stimuli. In T Thompson & R Pickens (eds.) *Stimulus Properties of Drugs.* New York, NY: Appleton-Century-Crofts, 163-175.

Woolverton WL (1986). Effects of a D_1 and a D_2 dopamine antagonist on the self-administration of cocaine and piribedil by rhesus monkeys. *Pharmacology, Biochemistry and Behavior* 24:531-535.

Yeomans JS (1979). Absolute refractory periods of self-stimulation neurons. *Physiology and Behavior* 22:911-919.

Yeomans JS (1989). Two substrates for medial forebrain bundle self-stimulation: Myelinated axons and dopamine axons. *Neuroscience and Biobehavior Review* 13:91-98.

Yeomans JS & Baptista M (1997). Both nicotinic and muscarinic receptors in ventral tegmental area contribute to brain-stimulation reward. *Pharmacology, Biochemistry and Behavior* 57:915-921.

Yeomans JS, Kofman O & McFarlane V (1985). Cholinergic involvement in lateral hypothalamic rewarding brain stimulation. *Brain Research* 329:19-26.

Yeomans JS, Mathur A & Tampakeras M (1993). Rewarding brain stimulation: Role of tegmental cholinergic neurons that activate dopamine neurons. *Behavioral Neuroscience* 107:1077-1087.

Yeomans JS, Takeuchi J, Baptista M et al. (2000). Brain-stimulation reward thresholds raised by an antisense oligonucleotide for the M5 muscarinic receptor infused near dopamine cells. *Journal of Neuroscience* 20:8861-8867.

Yeomans JS, Forster G & Blaha C (2001). M5 muscarinic receptors are needed for slow activation of dopamine neurons and for rewarding brain stimulation. *Life Sciences* 68:2449-2456.

You Z-B, Tzschentke TM, Brodin E et al. (1998). Electrical stimulation of the prefrontal cortex increases cholecystokinin, glutamate, and dopamine release in the nucleus accumbens: An in vivo microdialysis study in freely moving rats. *Journal of Neuroscience* 18:6492-6500.

Zangen A, Ikemo S & Wise RA (in press 2002). Rewarding and psychomotor stimulant effects of endomorphin-1: Anterior-posterior differences within the ventral tegmental area and lack of effect in nucleus accumbens. *Journal of Neuroscience.*

| Chapter 6 | # From Neurobiology to Treatment: Progress Against Addiction |

Eric J. Nestler, M.D., Ph.D.

Blockade of Drug Targets
Mimicry of Drug Action
Blockade of the Addiction Process

In terms of lost lives and productivity, drug addiction remains one of the most serious threats to our nation's public health. Addiction can be defined as the loss of control over drug use, or the compulsive seeking and taking of drug regardless of the consequences. Available treatments for addiction remain inadequately effective for most individuals. Consequently, there is intense interest in better understanding the neurobiology of addiction in the hope that such knowledge will lead eventually to more effective treatments.

Diverse types of chemicals—drugs of abuse—cause addiction. Such drugs share no similarities in chemical structure, and yet they produce similar behavioral syndromes—addiction. Considerable progress has been made in understanding how drugs of abuse cause addiction. The initial protein targets for almost all drugs of abuse are known (Table 1) (Nestler, 2001). Also, several circuits in the brain, containing these drug targets, are known to mediate the addicting actions of drugs of abuse (Nestler, 2001; Koob, Sanna et al., 1998; Wise, 1998; Everitt & Wolf, 2002). Most attention has been given to the nucleus accumbens (also called the ventral striatum) and its dopaminergic input from the ventral tegmental area of the midbrain as key substrates

for these drug effects. Other brain regions interact with this circuit, including the amygdala, prefrontal and other limbic cortical regions, hippocampus, and hypothalamus, to name a few.

These brain structures represent reward pathways, which are very old from an evolutionary point of view and which presumably evolved to mediate an individual's response to natural rewards, such as food, sex, and social interaction. Drugs of abuse activate these reward pathways, in the absence of natural rewards, with a force and persistence that is not seen under normal conditions (Nestler, 2001; Koob, Sanna et al., 1998; Wise, 1998; Everitt & Wolf, 2002). Over time, repeated drug exposure causes adaptations in the brain's reward pathways, which seem to have two major consequences. First, during periods of active drug use or shortly after ceasing drug intake, the ability of natural rewards to activate the reward pathways is diminished, and the individual experiences depressed motivation and mood. Taking more drug is the quickest, easiest way for an addict to feel "normal" again. Second, drug use causes long-lasting memories related to the drug experience, such that even after prolonged periods of withdrawal (months, years), stressful events or exposure to drug-associated cues

TABLE 1.	Initial Targets of Drugs of Abuse
Drug	**Target**
Opiates	Agonist at μ, δ, and κ opioid receptors[a]
Cocaine	Indirect agonist at dopamine receptors by inhibiting dopamine transporters[b]
Amphetamine	Indirect agonist at dopamine receptors by stimulating dopamine release[b]
Ethanol	Facilitates $GABA_A$ receptor and inhibits NMDA glutamate receptor function[c]
Nicotine	Agonist at nicotine acetylcholine receptors
Cannabinoids	Agonist at CB_1 and CB_2 cannabinoid receptors[d]
Phencyclidine (PCP)	Antagonist at NMDA glutamate receptors
Hallucinogens	Partial agonist at $5HT_{2A}$ serotonin receptors
Inhalants	Unknown

[a] Activity at μ (and possibly) δ receptors mediates the addicting actions of opiates; kappa receptors mediate aversive actions.

[b] Cocaine and amphetamine exert analogous actions on serotonergic and noradrenergic systems, which may also contribute to the addicting effects of these drugs.

[c] Ethanol affects several other ligand-gated channels, and at higher concentrations, voltage-gated channels as well. In addition, ethanol is reported to influence many other neurotransmitter systems.

[d] Activity at CB_1 receptors mediates the addicting actions of cannabinoids; CB_2 receptors are expressed in the periphery only. Proposed endogenous ligands for the CB_1 receptor include the arachidonic acid metabolites, anandamide and 2-arachidonylglycerol.

can trigger intense craving, and in many cases relapse, in part by activating the brain's reward pathways. Roughly half the risk for addiction is genetic. A great deal of effort is aimed at identifying the specific genes involved and the mechanisms by which diverse non-genetic factors influence the development of an addictive disorder.

Addiction should be viewed as distinct from physical dependence, wherein individuals become physically sick when drug administration ceases (Nestler, 2001; O'Brien, 1997). Physical dependence *per se* is neither necessary nor sufficient to cause addiction: some drugs of abuse do not cause physical dependence, and some medications used in general medicine cause physical dependence but are not addicting. Moreover, physical dependence and withdrawal syndromes are largely mediated by different CNS regions than those important for addiction. Nevertheless, much of the clinical progress in the addiction field has come from improved methods of treating the physical dependence and severe withdrawal syndromes associated with opiates and alcohol (O'Brien, 1997). Knowledge of opiate action on opioid receptors at a cellular level led to the development of several medications now used to treat opiate withdrawal. Clonidine, an alpha$_2$-adrenergic agonist, produces cellular effects similar to opioid receptor activation, and was later shown to dampen many of the physical signs and symptoms of opiate withdrawal in humans (Aghajanian, 1978; Gold, Redmond et al., 1978). By combining clonidine with naltrexone, an opioid receptor antagonist, or with buprenorphine, an opioid receptor partial agonist, it is now possible to detoxify a patient from opiates over a few days with relatively minor distress (O'Brien, 1997). This is in striking contrast to the extremely painful "cold turkey" method that characterized opiate detoxification a generation ago. Similarly, based on the knowledge that benzodiazepines, like alcohol, facilitate gamma-aminobutyric acid ($GABA_A$) receptor function, benzodiazepines are now used routinely to prevent the life-threatening sequelae of alcohol withdrawal (O'Brien, 1997).

The impact of these advances, however, is limited because treatment of physical dependence and withdrawal does not target the core clinical symptoms of addiction, namely, drug craving and relapse to drug use even after prolonged abstinence. Unfortunately, treatment of the core symptoms of addiction has proved much more difficult than treatment of physical withdrawal syndromes.

BLOCKADE OF DRUG TARGETS

Approaches pursued to date can be divided into several categories, including blockade of drug targets, mimicry of drug action, and blockade of the addiction process (Figure 1) (O'Brien, 1997). The most straightforward strategy is to block the drug from getting to its target. Such a treatment agent should have the additional requirement of not affecting that target on its own. The best example of this approach is naltrexone (O'Brien, 1997). In theory, naltrexone is inactive in the absence of an opiate, but blocks the ability of opiates to produce their many effects, including addiction. Indeed, naltrexone can be used to treat opiate addiction,

FIGURE 1.   General Strategies Used to Treat Drug Addiction or Associated Physical Withdrawal Syndromes

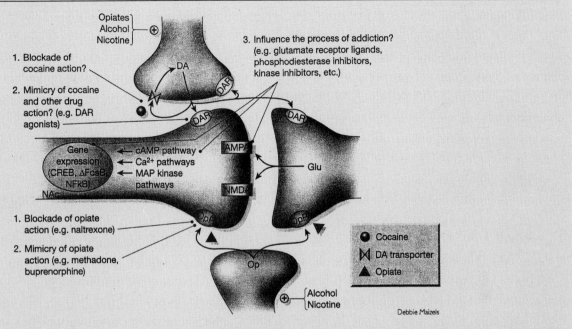

A dendritic spine of a nucleus accumbens (NAc) neuron and its innervation by terminals of glutamatergic (Glu), dopaminergic (DA), and opioidergic (Op) neurons are shown. 1. One approach is to block the ability of a drug to reach its initial protein target: for example, naltrexone's antagonism of opioid receptors (OR) or a hypothetical drug that interferes with cocaine's actions on the dopamine transporter. Not depicted is the use of immunological methods (such as a cocaine or nicotine vaccine) to prevent a drug from entering the brain. 2. A second approach is to mimic drug action: for example, sustained activation of OR by methadone, or activation of DA receptors (DAR) by various agonists or partial agonists. 3: A third approach is to influence the process of addiction: for example, via perturbation of Glu receptors (AMPA, NMDA) or a host of post-receptor signaling proteins (such as those involved in the CAMP, calcium and MAP kinase pathways and in the regulation of gene expression—ΔFosB, CREB or NFκB) that have been implicated in addiction (Nestler, 2001; Hyman & Malenka, 2001).

but its use has limitations. Naltrexone is not inactive in the absence of exogenous opiates. This is because the drug blocks the actions of the body's endogenous opioid peptides (enkephalin, dynorphin, endorphin), and this can cause negative emotional effects (such as depressed mood), which reduce patient compliance. As a result, naltrexone is mostly effective for highly "motivated" addicts whose employment can be used to coerce compliance. Based on animal studies showing that alcohol's and nicotine's addicting actions are mediated in part via activation of endogenous opioidergic neurons (Figure 1), naltrexone has been used to treat addiction to these drugs as well. Although some efficacy has been observed clinically, the effects of naltrexone are relatively small in magnitude (Krystal, Cramer et al., 2001).

A related approach with cocaine or other stimulants (amphetamine, methamphetamine) has not yet been effective. The most important mechanism of action of cocaine is inhibition of presynaptic dopamine transporters (Figure 1). The goal for treatment would be to prevent cocaine's binding to the transporter without affecting the transporter's normal functioning. Despite intense effort, suitable molecules have not to date been developed and validated. An alternative to such a "cocaine antagonist" is the "cocaine vaccine," which would block cocaine's entry into the brain through immunological approaches. By immunizing with cocaine coupled to a carrier, it has been possible to generate immunity in animals (Kantak, Collins et al., 2001). When the animals are subsequently challenged with cocaine, the drug's clearance is increased, its penetration into the brain is decreased, and its behavioral effects are attenuated. Cocaine vaccines are now in clinical development and could prove useful, but there are several potential drawbacks. First, cocaine already has a very short half-life. It is not clear whether increased clearance made possible by active immunity would have a functionally meaningful effect in humans. Second, a cocaine vaccine would not be active against other stimulants, and addicts could rapidly switch to another drug. The use of a cocaine vaccine also raises important ethical considerations, such as the potential loss of privacy (the presence of such antibodies would "mark" an addict) and whether the vaccine should be voluntary (Cohen, 1997). Similar efforts are under way to generate a vaccine toward nicotine, which is currently in early clinical trials.

MIMICRY OF DRUG ACTION

Contrary to efforts to block drug effects, there has been considerable interest and progress in treating addiction by mimicking drug action (O'Brien, 1997). This approach is based on the notion that blocking drug targets, as mentioned earlier, would leave the addict with an altered, addicted brain and the intense drug craving it produces. In contrast, by activating drug targets, it might be possible to partially alleviate this drug craving and allow the brain to slowly recover. A critical aspect of this approach, and presumably of brain recovery, is to use long-acting medications that would do more than simply mimic a drug of abuse; they would need to do so in a sustained manner, and thereby avoid the rapid on and off phases of repeated drug exposure. Although the effectiveness of drug mimicry has been documented clinically, it is poorly understood at the neurobiological level.

The best-established example of this approach is methadone, a particularly long-acting opioid receptor agonist. The only difference between methadone and other opiates is its long half-life, which means that, at the proper dose, addicts on methadone have a low level of sustained activation of opioid receptors. This enables addicts to avoid the daily extremes of highs upon drug administration and withdrawal as the drug effects wear off. This, in turn, enables an addict to return to a more normal life of steady work and social interactions. Decades of experience have documented the safety and efficacy of methadone and another long-acting opioid agonist, LAAM (levo-alpha-acetylmethadol), in the treatment of a subset of opiate addicts, although it is difficult to predict which individuals will respond (National Consensus Development Panel, 1998; Kreek, 2000). A variation in this theme is the use of buprenorphine (Ling, Charuvastra et al., 1998). As a high-affinity partial agonist, buprenorphine binds to opioid receptors and produces a mild agonist effect. Higher doses of the drug do not produce stronger effects because the ability of buprenorphine to activate the receptor is intrinsically low. However, buprenorphine, bound to the receptor at high affinity, can block the effects of opiate drugs of abuse, which limits an addict's attempts to obtain a drug high during treatment. Despite the clear utility of this general approach, there remains significant concern and skepticism toward methadone and related treatments, because the addict is still being exposed to opiates and may be vulnerable to some of the deleterious effects of these drugs.

Another example of the mimicry approach is the use of nicotine patches or chewing gum to treat tobacco addiction. The resulting sustained release of low levels of nicotine can dampen craving for cigarettes in some patients long enough to help the individuals quit smoking (Silagy, Lancaster et al., 2001). However, such approaches are not effective in most smokers, perhaps because of the very stable nicotine-induced changes in the brain that sustain the addiction. Perhaps agonists selective for particular nicotinic cholinergic receptors in the brain that mediate nicotine addiction would be more effective than low levels of nicotine itself, although this is speculative.

Mentioned briefly above is the important role of dopamine in drug addiction. Stimulation of dopaminergic transmission in the nucleus accumbens and elsewhere seems to be the most important mechanism of stimulant action and contributes to the actions of other drugs of abuse as well (Koob, Sanna et al., 1998; Wise, 1998) (Figure 1). Thus, activation of opioid, cholinergic or cannabinoid receptors increases dopaminergic transmission in these brain regions. Based on this knowledge, there has been intense effort to use dopamine receptor antagonists and agonists in the treatment of addiction. The goal is to develop agents that regulate the general process of addiction, which might be equally effective for all drugs of abuse. Use of dopamine antagonists is based on the notion that inhibition of drug effects would limit drug use, whereas use of dopamine agonists is based on the notion that mimicry of drug effects would be more efficacious. The former approach has not been promising. Although dopamine receptor antagonists can block acute drug effects, there is no evidence that they limit drug craving or self-administration. They may even make animals and humans more sensitive to drugs of abuse via adaptive increases in dopamine receptor signaling efficacy. In contrast, there is some promise for the use of D_1 receptor agonists and D_2 receptor partial agonists, which dampen cocaine craving and relapse in animal models (Pulvirenti & Koob, 1994; Self, Barnhart et al., 1996). Studies in humans are a high priority, but are limited by the lack of availability of suitable compounds for human use.

BLOCKADE OF THE ADDICTION PROCESS

A great deal has been learned over the past decade about the changes that drugs of abuse cause in the brain's reward pathways to produce addiction (Nestler, 2001; Hyman & Malenka, 2001). Current research aims to exploit this information for the development of more effective treatments. However, efforts in this realm are almost entirely speculative and must be viewed with skepticism. It is clear, for example, that glutamatergic circuits are crucial for the normal activity of the nucleus accumbens and ventral tegmental area. Moreover, drugs of abuse alter levels or activity of glutamate receptors within these regions (Everitt & Wolf, 2002; Carlezon, Haile et al., 2000; Nicola, Surmeier et al., 2000; Cornish & Kalivas, 2001; Ungless, Whistler et al., 2001; Self, 2002). This raises the possibility, untested to date in humans, that drugs aimed at these receptors might be of use in the treatment of addiction. Given the prominent role of glutamatergic mechanisms in learning and memory, and increasing evidence that important aspects of addiction can be viewed as a form of memory, it is possible that glutamatergic agents, given in conjunction with behavioral therapies, might be most efficacious at fundamentally altering addictive behavior (Nestler, 2001; Hyman & Malenka, 2001; Self, 2002; Hutcheson, Everitt et al., 2001; Shalev, Morales et al., 2001; Shaham, Erb et al., 2000). In a similar way, numerous other neurotransmitter, neuropeptide, and neurotrophic factor systems are altered by drugs of abuse and, in turn, modulate drug effects in laboratory animals: GABA, neuropeptide Y (NPY), corticotropin releasing factor (CRF), serotonin, norepinephrine, melanocortins, and brain-derived neurotrophic factor (BDNF), to name a few. As these effects are better defined in animal models, and putative treatment agents suitable for human investigation are developed, these various mechanisms can be tested in clinical populations.

Drug addiction also involves adaptations at post-receptor, intracellular signaling cascades, including alterations in gene expression (Nestler, 2001; Hyman & Malenka, 2001).

Moreover, modification of particular signaling proteins can have dramatic effects on an animal's responses to drugs of abuse. Examples include several proteins that regulate the function of G protein-coupled receptors: G proteins, G protein receptor kinases (GRKs), arrestins, and RGS (regulators of G protein signaling) proteins (Nestler, 2001; Bohn, Gainetdinov et al., 2000; Potenza & Nestler, 1999). Because the acute targets of many drugs of abuse are G protein-coupled receptors, it is possible that agents affecting these modulatory proteins could exert interesting functional effects on the receptor systems so as to treat aspects of addiction. Similarly, given the evidence for an important role of the cyclic adenosine monophosphate (cAMP) pathway in addiction, and of the transcription factor ΔFosB (Nestler, Barrot et al., 2001), it is conceivable that novel agents directed against protein components of these pathways (such as phosphodiesterase inhibitors, which would enhance cAMP function) might warrant investigation as clinical treatments. Such efforts should, of course, focus on subtypes of these various intracellular signaling proteins that are highly enriched in the brain's reward pathways and would therefore represent potentially viable drug targets.

One of the central problems in approaching addiction is that truly effective treatments are not yet available. Thus, it is impossible to know what types of treatment are theoretically possible. For example, before the advent of antidepressant medications, there was considerable debate about the nature and magnitude of improvement possible with chemical treatments. By analogy, the drug abuse field now aims to identify medications that dampen drug craving or reward without interfering with motivation for natural rewards. Only as putative treatment agents are developed and tested in animals and humans will insight into the feasibility of this aim become available.

Perhaps an even greater obstacle in the development of new treatments for addiction is the relative lack of interest by the pharmaceutical industry. This problem is due to many factors, including the perceived stigma of dealing with addicts as well as the presumption that markets for addiction treatment agents might be too small. The latter would seem to represent a major miscalculation by the industry. Experience tells us that the size of many markets only becomes apparent when truly effective treatments are available. The antidepressants, now a worldwide market of over $10 billion, are a case in point. By analogy, treatment agents that can correct compulsive behavior toward drug rewards, if they can be developed, would represent enormous successes, given their potential to treat not only drug addictions, but addictions to non-drug stimuli, such as gambling, food, and sex, which may be mediated by similar mechanisms. Such treatments could be highly successful and offer dramatic improvement in public health.

ACKNOWLEDGMENTS: Preparation of this review was supported by grants from the National Institute on Drug Abuse. Reprinted by permission of the publisher from Nestler EJ (2002). From neurobiology to treatment: Progress against addiction. Nature Neuroscience *5(Suppl):1076-1079. Copyright 2002, Nature Neuroscience, New York, NY.*

REFERENCES

Aghajanian GK (1978). Tolerance of locus coeruleus neurones to morphine and suppression of withdrawal response by clonidine. *Nature* 276:186-188.

Bohn LM, Gainetdinov RR, Lin ET et al. (2000). Mu-opioid receptor desensitization by beta-arrestin-2 determines morphine tolerance but not dependence. *Nature* 408:720-723.

Carlezon WA Jr, Haile CN, Neve R et al. (2000). Distinct sites of opiate reward and aversion within the midbrain identified using a herpes simplex virus (HSV) vector expressing G1uR1. *Journal of Neuroscience* 20:RC62.

Cohen PJ (1997). Immunization for prevention and treatment of cocaine abuse: Legal and ethical implications. *Drug and Alcohol Dependence* 48:167-174.

Cornish JL & Kalivas PW (2001). Cocaine sensitization and craving: Differing roles for dopamine and glutamate in the nucleus accumbens. *Journal of Addictive Diseases* 20:43-54.

Everitt BJ & Wolf ME (2002). Psychomotor stimulant addiction: A neural systems perspective. *Journal of Neuroscience* 22:3312-3320.

Gold MS, Redmond DE Jr & Kleber HD (1978). Clonidine blocks acute opiate-withdrawal symptoms. *Lancet* 2:599-602.

Hutcheson DM, Everitt BJ, Robbins TW et al. (2001). The role of withdrawal in heroin addiction: Enhances reward or promotes avoidance? *Nature Neuroscience* 4:943-947.

Hyman SE & Malenka RC (2001). Addiction and the brain: The neurobiology of compulsion and its persistence. *Nature Reviews. Neuroscience* 2:695-703.

Kantak KM, Collins SL, Bond J et al. (2001). Time course of changes in cocaine self-administration behavior in rats during immunization with the cocaine vaccine IPC-1010. *Psychopharmacology* 153:334-340.

Koob GE, Sanna PP & Bloom EE (1998). Neuroscience of addiction. *Neuron* 21:467-476.

Kreek MJ (2000). Methadone-related opioid agonist pharmacotherapy for heroin addiction. History, recent molecular and neurochemical research and future in mainstream medicine. *Annals of the New York Academy of Sciences* 909:186-216.

Krystal JH, Cramer JA, Krol WE et al. (2001). Veterans Affairs Naltrexone Cooperative Study 425 Group. Naltrexone in the treatment of alcohol dependence. *New England Journal of Medicine* 345:1734-1739.

Ling W, Charuvastra C, Collins JF et al. (1998). Buprenorphine maintenance treatment of opiate dependence: A multicenter, randomized clinical trial. *Addiction* 93:475-486.

National Consensus Development Panel (1998). Effective medical treatment of opiate addiction. *Journal of the American Medical Association* 280:1936-1943.

Nestler EJ (2001). Molecular basis of neural plasticity underlying addiction. *Nature Reviews. Neuroscience* 2:119-128.

Nestler EJ, Barrot M & Self SW (2001). ΔFosB: A molecular switch for addiction. *Proceedings of the National Academy of Sciences* 98:11042-11046.

Nicola SM, Surmeier J & Malenka RC (2000). Dopaminergic modulation of neuronal excitability in the striatum and nucleus accumbens. *Annual Review of Neuroscience* 23:185-215.

O'Brien CP (1997). A range of research-based pharmacotherapies for addiction. *Science* 278:66-70.

Potenza MN & Nestler EJ (1999). Effects of RGS proteins on the functional response of the mu opioid receptor in a melanophore-based assay. *Journal of Pharmacology and Experimental Therapeutics* 291:482-491.

Pulvirenti L & Koob GR (1994). Dopamine receptor agonists, partial agonists and psychostimulant addiction. *Trends in Pharmacological Sciences* 15:374-379.

Self DW (2002). Where's the excitement in psychostimulant sensitization? *Neuropsychopharmacology* 26:14-17.

Self DW, Barnhart WJ, Lehman DA et al. (1996). Opposite modulation of cocaine-seeking behavior by D_1-like and D_2-like dopamine receptor agonists. *Science* 271:1586-1589.

Shaham Y, Erb S & Stewart J (2000). Stress-induced relapse to heroin and cocaine seeking in rats: A review. *Brain Research Reviews* 33:13-33.

Shalev U, Morales M, Hope B et al. (2001). Time-dependent changes in extinction behavior and stress-induced reinstatement of drug seeking following withdrawal from heroin in rats. *Psychopharmacology* 156:98-107.

Silagy C, Lancaster T, Stead L et al. (2001). Nicotine replacement therapy for smoking cessation. *Cochrane Database of Systematic Reviews* 3:CD000146.

Ungless MA, Whistler JL, Malenka RC et al. (2001). Single cocaine exposure in vivo induces long-term potentiation in dopamine neurons. *Nature* 411:583-587.

Wise RA (1998). Drug-activation of brain reward pathways. *Drug and Alcohol Dependence* 51:13-22.

SECTION 2 | Pharmacology

Section Coordinators
Lori D. Karan, M.D., FACP, FASAM
David R. Pating, M.D.

Contributors

Robert L. Balster, Ph.D.
Professor of Pharmacology and Toxicology
Medical College of Virginia
Virginia Commonwealth University
Richmond, Virginia

Neal Benowitz, M.D.
Professor and Chair
Division of Clinical Pharmacology
  and Experimental Therapeutics
University of California, San Francisco
San Francisco, California

William C. Bobo, M.D.
Staff Psychiatrist
U.S. Naval Hospital
Jacksonville, Florida

Lisa Borg, M.D.
The Laboratory of the Biology of the Addictive Diseases
The Rockefeller University, and
Associate Physician
The Rockefeller University Hospital
New York, New York

Allison L. Chausmer, Ph.D.
Department of Psychiatry and Behavioral Science
Johns Hopkins University School of Medicine
Baltimore, Maryland

Jennifer L. Cornish, Ph.D.
Intramural Research Program
National Institute on Drug Abuse
National Institutes of Health
Baltimore, Maryland

Debrah S. Cowley, M.D.
Professor of Psychiatry
Department of Psychiatry and Behavioral Sciences
University of Washington
Seattle, Washington

John A. Dani, Ph.D.
Professor, Division of Neuroscience
Baylor College of Medicine
Houston, Texas

Edward F. Domino, M.D.
Professor of Pharmacology
University of Michigan
Ann Arbor, Michigan

Gannt P. Galloway, Pharm.D.
Chief of Pharmacologic Research
Haight Ashbury Free Clinics, Inc.
San Francisco, California

Richard A. Glennon, Ph.D.
Professor of Medicinal Chemistry
Medical College of Virginia
Virginia Commonwealth University
Richmond, Virginia

David A. Gorelick, M.D., Ph.D.
Chief, Clinical Pharmacology Section
Intramural Research Program
National Institute on Drug Abuse
National Institutes of Health, and
Adjunct Professor of Psychiatry
University of Maryland School of Medicine
Baltimore, Maryland

Roland R. Griffiths, Ph.D.
Professor, Departments of Psychiatry and Neuroscience
Johns Hopkins University School of Medicine
Baltimore, Maryland

Jonathan C. Jackson, M.D.
David Grant Medical Center
Travis Air Force Base, California

Steven M. Juergens, M.D., FASAM
Assistant Clinical Professor of Psychiatry
University of Washington, and
Medical Director, Virginia Mason
  Outpatient Chemical Dependency Program
Seattle, Washington

Laura M. Juliano, Ph.D.
Department of Psychology
American University
Washington, D.C.

Lori D. Karan, M.D., FACP, FASAM
Assistant Adjunct Professor
Department of Clinical Pharmacology
University of California, San Francisco
San Francisco, California

Mary Jeanne Kreek, M.D.
Professor and Head
The Laboratory of the Biology of the Addictive Diseases
The Rockefeller University, and
Senior Physician
The Rockefeller University Hospital
New York, New York

Scott E. Lukas, Ph.D.
Director, Behavioral Psychopharmacology Research Laboratory
Associate Professor of Psychiatry (Pharmacology)
McLean Hospital/Harvard Medical School
Belmont, Massachusetts

Billy R. Martin, Ph.D.
Professor of Pharmacology and Toxicology
Medical College of Virginia
Virginia Commonwealth University
Richmond, Virginia

John Mendelson, M.D.
Associate Clinical Professor of Psychiatry and Medicine
Drug Dependence Research Center
University of California, San Francisco
San Francisco, California

Shannon C. Miller, M.D., CMRO
Assistant Professor of Psychiatry
Wright State University
Wright Patterson Air Force Base, Ohio

David R. Pating, M.D.
Assistant Clinical Professor of Psychiatry
University of California, San Francisco, and
Chief of Addiction Medicine
Kaiser Permanente Medical Center
San Francisco, California

Sandra P. Welch, Ph.D.
Professor of Pharmacology and Toxicology
Medical College of Virginia
Virginia Commonwealth University
Richmond, Virginia

John J. Woodward, Ph.D.
Professor, Department of Physiology and Neuroscience
    and Department of Psychiatry
Center for Drug and Alcohol Programs
Medical University of South Carolina
Charleston, South Carolina

Anne Zajicek, M.D., Pharm.D.
Office of Clinical Pharmacology
Center for Drug Evaluation and Research
Food and Drug Administration
Rockville, Maryland

| Chapter 1 | # Pharmacokinetic and Pharmacodynamic Principles |

Lori D. Karan, M.D., FACP, FASAM
Anne Zajicek, M.D., Pharm.D.
David R. Pating, M.D.

Pharmacology is the study of drugs. Historically, drugs have been impure mixtures of components derived from plants and animals, whose composition was little understood. In contrast, today's drugs are highly formulated chemicals that are intended to specifically target pathogenesis as well as to maximize safety, convenience, and therapeutic efficacy. Illicit drugs are used for their mood-altering effects and often contain adulterants. Advances in pharmacology further our knowledge of both licit and illicit drugs.

Pharmacokinetics describes the movement of a drug within the body, and especially how a drug's concentration in blood, body fluids, and tissues varies over time. A drug's concentration is determined by factors that influence its absorption, distribution, metabolism, elimination, and excretion. An understanding of pharmacokinetics is important because the magnitude of a drug's pharmacologic effect depends on the concentration of drug at its site of action.

The study of the biochemical and physiologic effects of drugs and their mechanisms of action is termed *pharmacodynamics*. While pharmacokinetics can be explained as "what the body does to the drug," pharmacodynamics can be thought of as "what the drug does to the body."

As our knowledge of systems, circuits, receptors, and intracellular pathways advances, so does our ability to intervene pharmacotherapeutically. The chapters in this section summarize our advancing state of knowledge in these areas.

PHARMACOKINETICS

Absorption. Psychoactive drugs can be inhaled (glue, solvents, amyl nitrate), smoked (nicotine, marijuana, freebase cocaine), sniffed intranasally (cocaine, heroin), taken orally (ethanol, caffeine, amphetamines, barbiturates, opiates), administered intravenously (heroin, cocaine), or injected subcutaneously. Occasionally, such drugs are taken transdermally (fentanyl and nicotine patches), intramuscularly, sublingually, or rectally (Figure 1).

The more rapidly a psychoactive drug is delivered to its site of action in the central nervous system, the greater is its reinforcing effect. Smoked and inhaled drugs bypass the venous system and thus have the most rapid rate of delivery. Absorption of inhaled drug depends on the physical characteristics of the drug, including its volatility, particle size, and lipid solubility (Meng, Lichtman et al., 1997). Drugs that reach the alveoli of the lungs have rapid access

FIGURE 1. Venous Drug Concentrations After Different Routes of Administration

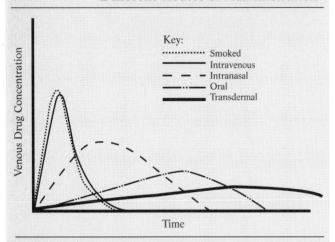

Key:
.... Smoked
———— Intravenous
– – – – Intranasal
—·—·— Oral
▬▬▬▬ Transdermal

Venous Drug Concentration

Time

Comparison of Rates of Delivery of Smoked, Intravenous, Intranasal, Oral, and Transdermally Applied Drug.

to the bloodstream through closely applied capillary alveolar surfaces (Figure 2). Because a large portion of the cardiac output passes through the pulmonary circulation, the delivery of drug from the alveoli to the brain is enhanced.

In contrast to inhaled drugs, different factors affect the rate of absorption for orally administered drugs. These factors include (1) the pharmaceutical properties of the oral dosage form, (2) the pH of gastric contents (drugs can be destroyed by extreme acid or basic conditions), (3) gastric emptying time (except dumping; faster gastric emptying time results in more rapid delivery to the small intestine, the site of absorption), (4) intestinal transit time (for drugs absorbed in the small intestine, there is an increased rate of absorption with a faster intestinal transit time), unless saturation occurs, (5) integrity of intestinal epithelium, and (6) the presence of food (which decreases the interaction time between the drug and the intestinal villi) (Caviness, MacKichan et al., 1987).

With illicit drugs, dose often is difficult to determine because of the presence of adulterants in the preparations, as well as imprecise measurement of the amount consumed (as compared to the quantity of active ingredients in prescription medications, which is known precisely).

Bioavailability is defined as the fraction of unchanged drug that reaches the systemic circulation after administration by any route. The *bioavailability factor (F)* takes into account the portion of the administered dose that is able to enter the circulation unchanged. For intravenously administered drugs, F=1.0 (100%). Bioavailability depends on a given drug's site-specific membrane permeability and its first-pass metabolism.

First-pass metabolism is the metabolism that occurs before a drug reaches the systemic circulation. Examples of drugs that show strong first-pass effects include morphine, methylphenidate, and desipramine. First-pass metabolism is particularly important for drugs administered by oral and deep rectal routes. Following absorption across the gut wall, the portal blood delivers the drug to the liver before it enters into the systemic circulation. The liver can excrete the drug in the bile, and the drug can undergo enterohepatic recirculation. Metabolism by the gut and liver can significantly reduce a drug's bioavailable fraction.

First-pass metabolism is relatively unimportant for drugs administered through the intravenous, sublingual, intramuscular, subcutaneous, and transdermal routes. This is because drugs administered by these routes enter the general circulation directly.

Drugs must pass through biological membranes to be absorbed. With passive diffusion, biologic membranes are more permeable to lipid soluble and uncharged molecules. Some drugs have diminished absorption because of a reverse transporter associated with p-glycoprotein. This reverse transporter actively pumps drug out of the gut wall cells back into the gut lumen. When p-glycoprotein is inhibited, increased drug absorption results.

Some food and drug interactions alter first-pass metabolism and absorption from the intestinal wall. For example, components of grapefruit juice and other foods that either inhibit or induce intestinal wall CYP3A4 or p-glycoprotein can lead to altered bioavailability of drugs that are substrates for this cytochrome (Dresser, Spence et al., 2000). Also, the nonselective monoamine oxidase inhibitors (MAOIs) such as phenelzine and tranylcypromine (Parnate®)—and, to a much lesser extent, the MAO B inhibitor selegiline (Eldepryl®) and the reversible MAOI moclobemide—inhibit MAO A in the intestinal wall and liver. This inhibition diminishes the first-pass metabolism of tyramine, which is present in cheeses and various foods (Garner, Shulman et al., 1996). When tyramine, an indirect-acting sympathomimetic amine, reaches the systemic circulation, it can produce increased release of norepinephrine from the sympathetic postganglionic neurons; this, in turn, can result in a severe pressor response and hypertensive crisis.

Upon absorption, when drug concentrations are graphed against time, a peak drug concentration (C_{max}) is reached at T_{max}. The trough concentration is C_{min}. The area under the concentration-time curve (AUC) is a measure of drug exposure that can be calculated (as the sum of trapezoids) and quantified.

Hastening gastric emptying can help to achieve a more rapid drug effect without altering bioavailability. Gastric emptying can be hastened by taking a drug on an empty stomach with at least 200 mL water and remaining in an upright position. Food, recumbency, heavy exercise, and drugs that slow gastric emptying (such as narcotics, anticholinergic drugs, and antacids) can result in later and lower peak concentrations of the index drug.

If the rate but not the extent of absorption is diminished, then the peak concentration decreases, the trough concentration increases, and the area under the curve is unchanged. The average steady-state concentration is unchanged, and there is no need to adjust the dose of a given drug to achieve therapeutic drug levels. In contrast, if the rate of absorption is unchanged but the extent of absorption is diminished, then both the peak and trough concentrations will be less. The area under the curve will decrease. Because the average steady-state concentration also will be diminished, a dose adjustment will be needed to achieve the therapeutic drug level (Figure 3). Therefore, when dosing prescribed drugs, a change in the rate of drug absorbed generally has less clinical significance than a change in the extent of drug absorbed.

Distribution. Once absorbed, a drug is distributed to the various organs of the body. Distribution is influenced by how well each organ is perfused with blood, the organ's size, binding of the drug within the blood and in the tissues, and the permeability of tissue membranes (Rowland & Tozer, 1995).

Distribution in the body can be understood by using a single "well-stirred" compartment, multiple compartments, or a model-independent approach. The single compartment model assumes spontaneous equilibration of the drug between tissues and blood; it can be used when experimental data plotted on a logarithmic scale of drug concentration versus time yields a straight line with a declining slope.

In multi-compartment models, spontaneous equilibration of the drug between the tissues and blood is not assumed, and the drug may be eliminated from one of several compartments. In a multi-compartment model, the number of compartments required equals the number

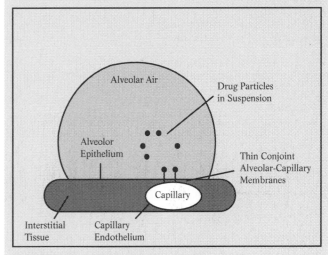

FIGURE 2.   Rapid Access of Drug Particles From Alveolar Air to Capillaries

Alveolar Air

Drug Particles in Suspension

Alveolor Epithelium

Thin Conjoint Alveolar-Capillary Membranes

Capillary

Interstitial Tissue

Capillary Endothelium

SOURCE: Morgan JP (1994). Principles of pharmacology. In NS Miller (ed.) *Principles of Addiction Medicine*. Chevy Chase, MD: American Society of Addiction Medicine, 2.

of exponential terms needed to describe the experimentally derived plasma concentration time curve (Figure 4). Thus, a two-compartment model is best described by a bi-exponential equation, with constants used to describe the average transfer rate between compartments. For instance, a two-compartment model might include a central compartment and a tissue or peripheral compartment. Although drug distribution within a compartment is not homogenous, and the concentrations of drug within and among such tissues may be quite variable, tissues of a compartment are grouped together because the time to achieve distribution equilibrium in such tissues is similar. Thus, the mathematically derived compartments may not be physiologically representative (Rowland & Tozer, 1995). Also, calculations involved in multi-compartment models use differential equations and can become quite complex.

More recently, model-independent pharmacokinetic analysis has been developed as a simpler alternative to multi-compartmental modeling. Noncompartmental pharmacokinetic analysis focuses on the average time drug molecules are in the body and uses calculations derived from a moment curve, which plots the product of concentration and time versus time alone.

FIGURE 3.   Comparison of C_{max}, T_{max}, and AUC When There Is Either a Decreased Rate of Absorption or a Decreased Extent of Absorption

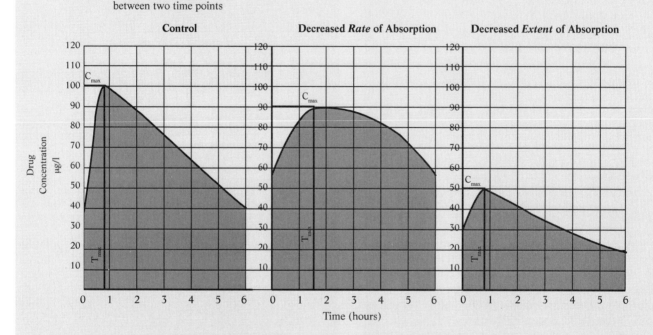

Key:
C_{max} = peak concentration
T_{max} = time when peak concentration is reached
AUC_{t_2,t_1} = area under the curve between two time points

When there is a decreased *rate* of absorption, AUC is unchanged, T_{max} is delayed, and drug dosage should not require alteration. When there is a decreased *extent* of absorption, AUC is diminished, T_{max} is unchanged, and drug dosage may need to be adjusted.

SOURCE: Modified from Caviness MD, MacKichan J, Bottorff M et al. (1987). *Therapeutic Drug Monitoring: A Guide to Clinical Application.* Irving, TX: Abbott Laboratories, Diagnostics Division, 20.

When a drug distributes into all of the body compartments and tissues, it is said to distribute into an apparent *volume of distribution* (V_d). This volume has no direct physical equivalent because it describes the amount of serum, plasma, or blood that would be required to account for all drug in the body if the entire dose of that drug were spread uniformly throughout. V_d can be thought of as the amount of drug in the body (D=dose) divided by the concentration of drug (C) in the plasma, or

$$V_d = \frac{D}{C}$$

Drugs with a small V_d are confined primarily to the intravascular space of approximately 5L. The drugs may be tightly bound to plasma proteins, or they may have a high molecular weight (large proteins, dextrans, and so forth). Drugs can have large V_d values up to 50,000 L if they are highly bound to tissue sites or are lipophilic.

Drugs with a large V_d thus partition into fat and bind to tissue. The volume of distribution and the fraction of unbound drug are terms that help quantify drug distribution. Acidic drugs commonly bind to albumin, the most abundant plasma protein. Drugs that bind primarily to albumin include barbiturates, benzodiazepines, and phenytoin.

Basic drugs often bind to alpha$_1$-acid glycoprotein and to lipoproteins. Methadone is an example of a drug that primarily binds to alpha$_1$-acid glycoprotein, whereas amitriptyline and nortriptyline bind primarily to lipoproteins. Other binding proteins include gamma-globulin, transcortin, fibrinogen, and thyroid-binding globulin.

Several comparisons between albumin and alpha$_1$-acid glycoprotein can be made (Israili & Dayton, 2001). Albumin, which is synthesized by the liver, can be decreased, especially with chronic illness and renal failure. Alpha$_1$-acid glycoprotein, which is an acute phase reactant produced by the liver, is relatively unaffected by chronic renal failure. Alpha$_1$-acid glycoprotein increases with chronic inflammatory disease, acute trauma, and stress. Alpha$_1$-acid glycoprotein levels vary relative to their total amount more than those of albumin. Also, alpha$_1$-acid glycoprotein (0.8 g/100 mL) is saturated much more readily than albumin (4.0 g/100 mL) because it is present in lower amounts.

The activity of a drug depends not on its total quantity, but on the concentration of free drug at its site of action. This free concentration is clinically relevant for drugs such as phenytoin, warfarin, and thyroxine, which are more than 90% bound to plasma proteins.

The rate of blood flow delivered to specific organs and tissues is important. Well-perfused tissues can receive large quantities of drug, provided that the drug can cross the membranes or other barriers present between the plasma and tissue. In contrast, poorly perfused tissues, such as fat, receive drug at a slow rate. This action explains why the concentration of drug in fat can continue to increase long after the concentration in plasma has begun to decrease.

Most psychoactive drugs enter the brain because they are highly lipid soluble. The blood-brain barrier hinders the ability of non-lipid-soluble drugs to reach the brain tissue by diffusion (Dziegielewska & Saunders, 2002). Unlike the fenestrated capillaries found throughout the body, which allow movement of molecules less than 25,000 daltons, the endothelial cells lining brain capillaries have tight junctions and do not permit these small molecules to pass through. Without fenestrations, drugs must cross the two membranes of the endothelial cell by passive diffusion in order to enter the brain. The blood-brain barrier limits the admittance of many drugs to the brain. However, for some compounds, specific active transport systems exist. These active transport systems enable glucose, amino acids, amines, purines, nucleosides, and organic acids to gain access to the brain. In contrast, p-glycoprotein is an efflux carrier present in the

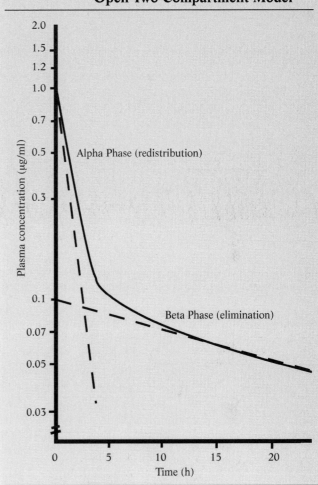

FIGURE 4.   Plot of Log Concentration Versus Time for Drug Disposition Characteristics Consistent With an Open Two-Compartment Model

brain capillary endothelial cell, which bars the drug from translocating across the endothelial cell and actively exports the drug out of the brain.

It is important to note where the blood-brain barrier exists. The blood-brain barrier is found throughout the brain and spinal cord at all regions central to the arachnoid membrane, except for the floor of the hypothalamus and the area postrema, including the chemoreceptor trigger zone (where direct-acting chemicals can provoke vomiting).

Metabolism. Metabolism is the process by which lipophilic drugs and foods are mostly transformed to more polar

---

FIGURE 5.   Cytochrome P450 Oxidation and NADPH-Cytochrome P450 Reductase

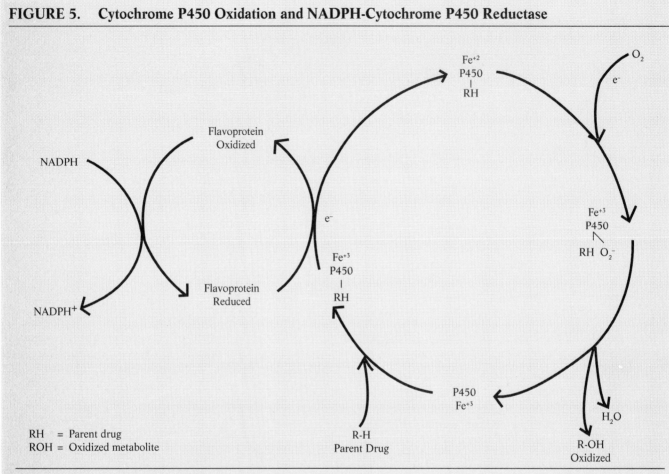

RH = Parent drug
ROH = Oxidized metabolite

SOURCE: Modified from Correia MA (2001). Drug transformation. In B Katzung (ed.) *Basic and Clinical Pharmacology, 8th Edition.* New York, NY: Lange Medical Books/McGraw-Hill, 53.

products that are more readily eliminated. Compared with the parent drug, drug metabolites usually have a diminished volume of distribution and diminished ability to penetrate cellular membranes. Not all metabolites are inactive or nontoxic; some biotransformation products have enhanced activity or toxic properties, including mutagenicity, teratogenicity, and carcinogenicity. Active metabolites need to be considered when assessing a drug's total activity. Also, scientists have made use of inherent drug-metabolizing enzymes to optimize drug delivery by designing pharmacologically inactive prodrugs that are converted *in vivo* to pharmacologically active molecules. One example of a prodrug is levodopa, which (after crossing the blood-brain barrier) is converted in the basal ganglia to dopamine.

Drugs can be metabolized by Phase One and/or Phase Two reactions. Phase One reactions are nonsynthetic reactions in which the drug is chemically altered and oxidized. Phase Two reactions are synthetic reactions in which the drug is conjugated with another moiety, such as glucuronide. Phase One reactions often provide the active site for Phase Two reactions, but occasionally a Phase Two conjugate becomes a substrate for a Phase One oxidation. Examples of nonsynthetic reactions include the oxidation of phenobarbital, amphetamine, meperidine, and codeine by microsomal enzymes. Examples of synthetic reactions include the glucuronidation of morphine and meprobamate, acetylation of clonazepam and mescaline, and methylation of dopamine and epinephrine. In each case, the drug is made more polar to facilitate elimination.

The enzymes that metabolize drugs do so for a wide variety of moieties. Oxidations can take place by cytochrome P450-dependent and independent mechanisms. The name cytochrome P450 is derived from the spectral properties of this hemoprotein. In its reduced (ferrous) form, it binds carbon monoxide to produce a complex that absorbs light maximally at 450 nm. Cytochrome P450-dependent oxidations include aromatic (phenytoin, amphetamine) and aliphatic (pentobarbital, meprobamate) hydroxylations, epoxidation, and oxidative dealkylation (morphine, caffeine, codeine), deamination (amphetamine), desulfuration (thiopental), and dechlorination. Cytochrome P450-independent oxidations include dehydrogenations (ethanol); azo, nitro, and carbonyl reductions (methadone and naloxone); and ester and amide hydrolyses (Correia, 2001).

Cytochrome-dependent microsomal drug oxidation requires cytochrome P450, cytochrome P450 reductase, nicotinamide adenine dinucleotide phosphate (NADPH), and molecular oxygen. During a typical reaction, one molecule of oxygen is consumed (reduced) per substrate molecule, with one oxygen atom appearing in the product and the other in the form of water (Figure 5). The potent oxidizing properties of this activated oxygen permit oxidation of a large number of substrates. These structurally unrelated compounds, which serve as substrates for this system, share in their high lipid solubility.

Many isoforms of cytochrome P450 have been identified. Of these, CYP1A2, CYP2A6, CYP2C9, CYP2D6, CYP2E1, and CYP3A4 are responsible for catalyzing the bulk of the hepatic drug and xenobiotic metabolism. It is noteworthy that CYP3A4 alone is responsible for metabolizing more than 60% of clinically prescribed drugs. Examples of drugs that are metabolized by CYP3A4 include diazepam (Valium®), tetrahydrocannabinol, indinavir (Crixivan®) and saquinavir (Fortovase®) (protease inhibitors used to treat HIV).

Many drugs, foods, and environmental chemicals can induce and/or inhibit the activity of the cytochromes, speeding up or slowing down their own metabolism. Each cytochrome isozyme responds differently to specific exogenous chemicals. For example, CYP1A1 is induced by polycyclic aromatic hydrocarbons, including benzo[α]pyrene contained in cigarette smoke. Noninvasive markers are being developed to assess the activity of these cytochrome isozymes, including caffeine

for CYP1A2, coumarin for CYP2A6, dextromethorphan for CYP2D6, and erythomycin for CYP3A4 (Correia, 2001; Zhu, Ou-Yang et al., 2001).

The new discipline of pharmacogenetics aims to elucidate cytochrome and other drug-metabolizing enzyme polymorphisms, the degrees of expression of these polymorphisms, and the functional significance of such expression. Understanding these polymorphisms can help to explain individual differences in drug response. For instance, slow metabolizers of a drug may have a relative deficiency of specific enzyme responsible for the drug's metabolism. Such poor metabolizers may experience increased side effects of specific drugs at lower drug doses.

Persons who experience adverse drug reactions at lower drug doses may be protected from developing addiction. Higuchi and colleagues (1992) found that Japanese men and women who had the "Asian" type of inactive aldehyde dehydrogenase-2 (ALDH2) drank significantly less alcohol than did those with the active "Caucasian" ALDH2. The Japanese with inactive ALDH2 displayed facial flushing and experienced less pleasurable feelings when they were exposed to alcohol. Tyndale and colleagues (1997) showed that a sample of Caucasians who inherited two nonfunctional alleles for CYP2D6 were less likely to become dependent on oral opiates (estimated odds ratio >7). Those researchers were among the first to postulate the existence of "pharmacogenetic protection factors" that diminish vulnerability to addiction.

Scientists, physicians, and pharmaceutical manufacturers also are interested in pharmacogenetics. Drug manufacturers would like to prevent adverse drug effects in consumers. One idea to help prevent adverse effects to drugs is to develop a registry that identifies persons lacking specific metabolic enzymes and cytochromes. Given a choice of medications, it would be better to choose a therapeutic regimen that does not require metabolism for a person deficient in such mechanisms (Wrighton, VandenBranden et al., 1996).

In addition to issues related to metabolism of single drugs, there also are concerns about interactions between multiple drugs. Drug interactions may take place during metabolism at the level of the cytochromes. For example, a significant drug interaction has been reported between methadone and ciprofloxacin (Cipro®), a quinolone antibiotic useful against many gram-negative infections (Herrlin, Segerdahl et al., 2000). Because methadone is metabolized by the cytochrome P450 isozymes CYP1A2, CYP2D6, and

FIGURE 6.   Achievement of Average Steady-State Concentration Occurs in 4 to 5 Half-lives

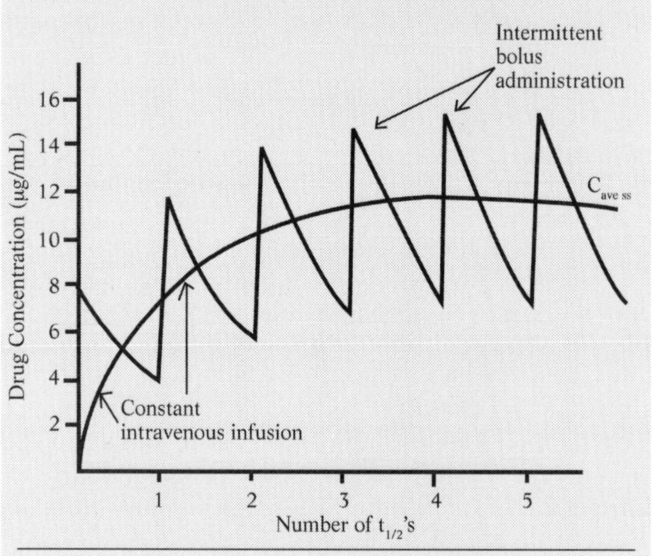

but these changes are not uniform among the liver enzyme classes (Blaschke, in press; Blaschke, 1977).

Although drug metabolism occurs largely in the liver, most other tissues and organs, including the lungs, gastrointestinal tract, skin, and kidneys, carry out varying degrees of drug metabolism. Understanding brain metabolism can be especially important in understanding the activity of psychoactive drugs. Many P450 cytochromes have been shown to catalyze the metabolism of neurosteroids as well as psychoactive drugs such as neuroleptics and antidepressants. Alcohol produces a three- to five-fold increase in the level of brain P450 and induces CYP2C, CYP2E1, and CYP4A (Warner, Stromstedt et al., 1993). P450s in other brain areas are induced by different factors; for example, levels of CYP2C and CYP4A influence the activity of neurotransmitters such as dopamine, which use fatty acid metabolites as intracellular mediators.

Novel brain CYPs, such as 5α-androstane-3β, 17β-diol hydroxylase, CYP7B, and CYP2D4, continue to be discovered. Because the level of CYPs in the brain is approximately 0.5% to 2% of that in the liver, and brain CYP isoenzymes are of different types than those found in the liver, brain CYPs appear to be locally active, but contribute little to overall pharmacokinetics of drugs in the body. (Hedlund, Gustafsson et al., 2001). The regulation of cytochrome P450 isozyme expression in the brain and elsewhere is being studied.

Elimination/Excretion. *Elimination* refers to disappearance of the parent and/or active molecule from the bloodstream or body, which can occur by metabolism and/or excretion. *Excretion* is the process of removing a compound from the body without chemically changing that compound. Drugs can be excreted through the urine or feces, exhaled through the lungs, or secreted through sweat or salivary glands.

The term *clearance* (Cl) represents the theoretical volume of blood or plasma that is completely cleared of drug in a given period of time (Winter, 1990). It is calculated as follows:

$$\frac{\text{Dose}}{\text{AUC}} = k_{el} \times V$$

Clearance is a *rate* whose units are volume over time. Because it is a rate, clearance is not an indicator of the amount of drug that is being removed.

The factors that determine hepatic clearance are hepatic blood flow (Q), the fraction of drug that is unbound (f_{ub}),

CYP3A4, and ciprofloxacin can inhibit CYP1A2 and CYP3A4 activity up to 65%, this enzyme inhibition can result in significantly elevated methadone levels, respiratory depression, and a clinical opioid overdose. Close medication monitoring is needed for patients prescribed both ciprofloxacin and methadone.

Drug interactions also can cause altered *biotransformation*. When cocaine is used in conjunction with ethanol, the pharmacologic effect of cocaine is both prolonged and enhanced (Andrews, 1997). A carboxylesterase catalyzes an ethyl transesterification of cocaine to cocaethylene, which is biologically active. In addition, ethanol inhibits cocaine metabolism. The increased levels of cocaine and cocaethylene can contribute to the prolonged and enhanced effects of cocaine.

Liver disease has many pharmacokinetic implications. The direction and quantity of these effects can change with the extent and course of illness. Reductions in liver blood flow, shunting of blood, alterations in plasma proteins and bile flow, and dysfunction of hepatocytes could be associated with the pathologic process. Drug bioavailability increases as first-pass metabolism decreases. The fraction of unbound drug could be altered. Modifications in the number and activity of metabolizing enzymes can take place,

FIGURE 7.   Graphs of First-Order and Zero-Order Elimination Kinetics on Regular and Semilog Plots

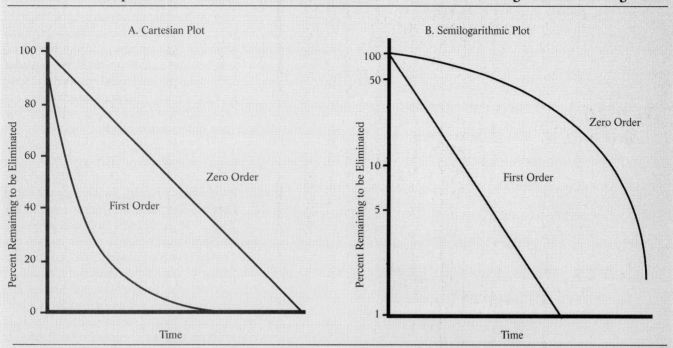

SOURCE: Modified from Rowland M & Tozer TN, eds. (1995). *Clinical Pharmacokinetics: Concepts and Applications, 3rd Edition*. Baltimore, MD: Williams & Wilkins, 35.

and the drug's intrinsic clearance (Cl_{int}). The intrinsic clearance is a measure of the liver's ability to metabolize the drug. These terms are related by the following equation:

$$Cl_{hep} = \frac{Q\, f_{ub}\, Cl_{int}}{Q + f_{ub}\, Cl_{int}}$$

If the intrinsic clearance of an unbound drug is very small, the metabolic capacity of the liver, rather than hepatic blood flow, becomes the major determinant of hepatic clearance. If the intrinsic clearance of an unbound drug is very large, blood flow to the liver becomes rate-limiting.

The total clearance for a drug is the sum of its renal and nonrenal clearances. A convenient method to determine a given drug's renal clearance is to quantify the amount of drug excreted unchanged in the urine during a given time interval and to divide this value by the area under the plasma concentration versus time curve (AUC) for the same time interval (t_2-t_1). The equation for this determination is as follows:

$$Cl_R = \frac{C_{ur} \times V}{AUC_{t_2 - t_1}}$$

Here, C_{ur} is the drug concentration excreted in the urine collected during the time interval ($t_2 - t_1$), and V is the urine volume collected. Nonrenal clearance then is determined as the difference between the total and the renal clearances.

The *half-life* ($t_{1/2}$) of a drug is a measure of time required for a drug to arrive at or decay from steady state. This measure is such that 1 half-life represents a 50% change, and 2, 3, 4, and 5 half-lives represent 75%, 87.5%, 93.7%, and 96.8% changes, respectively.

Drugs that have dose-independent (first-order) disposition and elimination characteristics reach a steady-state concentration in 4 to 5 half-lives (Figure 6). In this case, the time to reach steady state depends on the duration of the half-life, whereas the amount of drug in the body at steady state will depend on the frequency of drug administration and its dose.

A drug's half-life ($t_{1/2}$) depends on its volume of distribution (V_d) and its clearance (Cl). This relationship can be written as follows:

$$t_{1/2} = \frac{0.693 \times V_d}{Cl}$$

FIGURE 8.   Extrapolating the Decrease in Blood Alcohol Concentration From Two Prior Readings

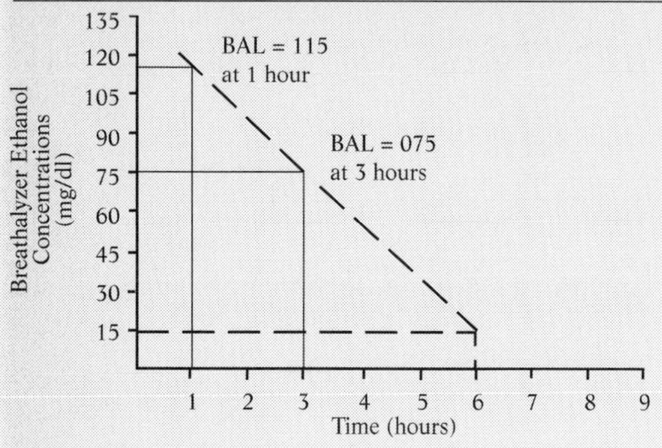

$$\text{slope} = \frac{115 - 75}{2} = \frac{40}{2} = 20 \text{ mg/dl/h}$$

expect at   4 hrs. BAL to be 55 mg/dl
5 hrs. BAL to be 35 mg/dl
6 hrs. BAL to be 15 mg/dl

The constant 0.693 in this equation is derived as an approximation of the natural logarithm of two [ln(2)]. Because drug elimination can be described by an exponential process, the time taken for a two-fold decrease can be shown to be proportional to ln(2) (Holford, 2001).

Half-life is dependent on clearance and volume of distribution. For example, as clearance decreases because of a disease process, half-life would be expected to increase. However, this reciprocal relationship occurs only when the disease process does not also change the drug's volume of distribution. A classic example occurs with diazepam. Because the volume of distribution of diazepam increases to the same proportion with age, the clearance remains essentially unchanged (Klotz, Avant et al., 1975).

Thus, one cannot make assumptions about the volume of distribution or clearance of a drug based solely on knowledge of its half-life. If the half-life of a drug is lengthened, the clearance can be increased, decreased, or unchanged, depending on corresponding changes in the volume of distribution. In addition, because $k_{el} = Cl/V_d$, the preceding equation can be written as $k_{el} = 0.693/t_{1/2}$, where k_{el} is a percentage of drug in the body that is eliminated per unit of time.

Most drugs display *first-order elimination* kinetics. When first-order kinetics are graphed, there is an exponential decay in the rate of elimination of the drug so that the concentration of drug in the body diminishes logarithmically over time (Figure 7). The *fraction* or *percentage* of the total amount of drug present in the body that is removed at any one time remains constant and is independent of dose. Given these relationships, a drug's plasma concentration can be calculated if its initial concentration, elimination half-life, and elapsed time are known:

$$C_t = C_o e^{-(k_{el}t)}$$

In contrast, drugs with *zero-order elimination* kinetics eliminate a constant amount of drug (rather than a constant fraction of drug). In most cases, the maximal rate of metabolism and/or elimination is due to the saturation of a key enzyme. Clearance then varies with the concentration of the drug, according to the Michaelis Menton equation. Because the half-life depends on the variable clearance, it too is not constant. Therefore, half-life is not particularly useful for drugs eliminated by zero-order kinetics. Ethanol, phenytoin, and salicylic acid are prominent examples of drugs that display zero-order kinetics. Ethanol is eliminated at a constant rate no matter how much drug is in the system. With the use of regular graph paper, one can determine future alcohol concentrations at specific times by extrapolating a line from two data points, as shown in Figure 8.

According to multi-compartmental modeling, a drug can have multiple half-lives rather than a single half-life. The terminal half-life is the most important, as it characterizes the elimination rate from the body. The other half-lives (alpha, beta, and so forth) can represent a combination of absorption, redistribution, and/or elimination.

Model independent pharmacokinetics uses the concept of the mean residence time (MRT) to determine an elimination half-life without attention to the different phases. The mean residence time is the average amount of time a molecule resides in the body and is calculated as the area under the moment curve (AUMC) divided by the area under the concentration versus time curve (AUC), or:

$$MRT = \frac{AUMC}{AUC}$$

The area under the momentum curve (AUMC) is derived from a plot of concentration multiplied by time (c x t) on the y axis, versus time (t) on the x axis (Figure 9).

Therapeutics Based on Pharmacokinetic Calculations. Pharmacokinetics explores the relationship between drug dose and the time-varying concentration of drug at its site(s) of action. When pharmacokinetic equations are used to make therapeutic calculations, half-life can be used to determine the dosing interval, clearance to determine the dosing rate, the volume of distribution to determine the loading dose, and bioavailability to determine the dose adjustment.

A rational dosage regimen is based on the assumption that there is a target concentration that will produce a desired therapeutic effect. This target drug concentration falls within a therapeutic range whose lower bounds are a minimal therapeutic concentration and whose upper bounds are a minimum toxic concentration. Pharmacokinetic computations can be used to achieve such a dosage regimen.

First, a *maintenance dose* can be calculated as a product of the dosing rate and dosing interval, as follows:

$$\text{Maintenance dose} = \text{Dosing rate} \times \text{Dosing interval}$$

In a steady state, the dosing rate is primarily determined by the clearance of a drug. Because a *steady state* (ss) is reached when the rate of drug acquisition into the body is equal to the rate of its elimination:

At steady-state, rate in = rate out:

$$\text{Bioavailability} \times \frac{\text{dosing}}{\text{rate}} = \text{clearance} \times \frac{\text{desired}}{\text{plasma}}_{\text{concentration}} = \frac{\text{rate}}{\text{of}}_{\text{elimination}}$$

$$F \times \frac{\text{dose}}{\text{dosage interval}} = Cl \times Cp^{ss}$$

Rearranging the terms, the dosing rate can be calculated if the clearance, target concentration of the drug in plasma, and its bioavailability are known:

$$\frac{\text{Dosing}}{\text{rate}} = \text{clearance} \times \frac{\begin{array}{c}\text{desired steady}\\\text{state plasma}\\\text{concentration}\end{array}}{\text{bioavailability}} = \frac{Cl \times Cp^{ss}}{F}$$

The units (volume/time) should be consistent for the variables in the calculations.

When it is essential to produce a therapeutic concentration of a drug quickly, a loading dose (D_1) may be given:

$$\begin{array}{c}\textit{Loading}\\\textit{dose}\end{array} = \frac{\begin{array}{c}\text{volume}\\\text{of}\\\text{distribution}\end{array} \times \frac{\begin{array}{c}\text{desired}\\\text{plasma}\\\text{concentration}\end{array}}{\text{bioavailability}} = \frac{V_d \times Cp}{F}$$

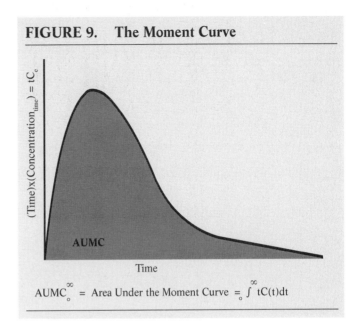

FIGURE 9.   The Moment Curve

$$\text{AUMC}_o^\infty = \text{Area Under the Moment Curve} = \int_o^\infty tC(t)dt$$

A loading dose may be needed at the onset of therapy, especially if a drug's volume of distribution is large. Note that clearance does not enter into this calculation. If an incremental *loading dose* is needed, then the formula is as follows:

$$\text{Incremental loading dose} = \frac{V_d \times (C_{p\ desired} - C_{p\ initial})}{F}$$

As illustrated in Table 1, pharmacokinetic principles can be used to help practitioners attain target drug concentrations in their patients. A protocol designed by Holford (2001) uses these calculations to individualize and adjust drug dosage. It has the following steps:

1. Choose the target concentration.

2. Predict V_d and Cl according to standard population values, with adjustments for factors such as weight and renal function.

3. Administer a loading dose or maintenance dose calculated by using target concentration, V_d, and Cl.

4. Measure the patient's response and drug concentration.

5. Revise V_d and/or Cl according to the measured concentration.

6. Repeat steps 3 to 5, adjusting the predicted dose to achieve the target concentration.

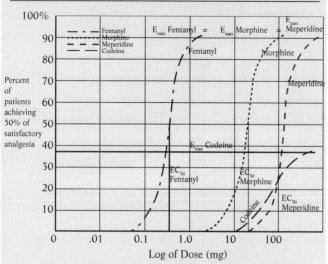

FIGURE 10. Dose Response Curves of Some Opioids

Fentanyl has a lower EC_{50} than morphine, and is more potent than morphine. Both fentanyl and morphine have a higher E_{max} than codeine, and are more efficacious than codeine. Meperidine is less potent than morphine but more efficacious than codeine.

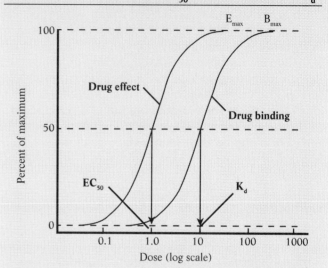

FIGURE 11. Spare Receptors Are Present When the EC_{50} Is Less Than the K_d

A system is said to have spare receptors when the activation of fewer than 50% of the receptors achieves 50% of maximal effect.

SOURCE: Modified from Katzung BG & Masters SB (2002). Pharmacodynamics. In *Katzung & Trevor's Pharmacology Examination and Board Review.* New York, NY: Lange Medical Books/McGraw-Hill, 13.

In the preceding discussion, the estimates of dosing rate and average steady-state concentration (calculated by using clearance) are independent of any specific pharmacokinetic model. In contrast, the determination of the maximum and minimum steady-state concentrations require further pharmacokinetic assumptions. The accumulation factor assumes that the drug follows a one-compartment body model, and the peak concentration assumes that the absorption rate is more rapid than the elimination rate (Holford, 2001).

PHARMACODYNAMICS

The study of pharmacodynamics is the study of the biochemical and physiologic effects of drugs on the body. This study includes an understanding of dose-response phenomena, the mechanisms of drug action, and the body's regulatory response to this activity. Drugs act on receptors to modulate specific intrinsic physiologic functions. The receptors and their associated effector and transducer proteins coordinate signals from multiple ligands with the metabolic activities of the cell to act as integrators of this information. A few

drugs affect the body's physiologic functions by changing the environment of the cells rather than acting directly through cellular receptors. They include ammonium chloride, used to acidify the urine; antacids, used to neutralize gastric acidity; and sodium bicarbonate.

Drugs can interact with receptors through covalent, ionic, hydrogen, van der Waals, and/or hydrophobic bonding. Examples of highly reactive covalent bond-forming drugs are the DNA-alkylating agents used in cancer chemotherapy to disrupt cell division, and HIV-RNA nucleoside reverse transcriptase inhibitors. The duration of action of drugs that bind covalently is frequently, but not necessarily, prolonged. The duration of interactions for drugs that bond noncovalently to their receptor varies with the affinity of the drug for that receptor. Noncovalent interactions of high-affinity drugs can appear largely irreversible.

Most drugs act through electrostatic and/or hydrophobic bonds that require a very precise fit of the drug to the receptor. Drugs have selectivity when they bind to a few types of receptors more tightly than to others and when these receptors control discrete physiologic processes. Scientists are working to discover subtypes of receptors and to delineate structure-function relationships of their components, as well as their anatomy, circuitry, and regulation. Medications development aims to use this knowledge to better target new drug therapies.

When the response of a particular receptor-effector system is measured against increasing concentrations of drug, a graded dose-response graph is attained (Figure 10). When drug dose is plotted on a logarithmic scale, a sigmoidal curve often results, permitting mathematical manipulation of the results. The *maximal efficacy* of a drug occurs at E_{max}, its maximal effect. Efficacy is determined mainly by the nature of the receptor and its associated effector system. In contrast, potency is primarily determined by the affinity of the receptor for the drug. *Potency* denotes the amount of drug needed to produce a given effect. The concentration of the drug needed to produce 50% maximal effect occurs at EC_{50}; the more potent the drug, the smaller the dose required to achieve maximal effect. In general, low potency is important only if the drug needs to be administered in undesirably large amounts. Because drug doses are readily adjusted, it is the maximal efficacy that is more often clinically relevant.

A similar sigmoidal curve is attained when the percentage of receptors that bind a drug is plotted against log drug concentration. Here, the concentration at which 50% of the receptors are bound is denoted K_d, and the maximum number of receptors bound are termed B_{max}. Both "dose-response" and "dose-receptor bound" graphs have a linear or nearly linear middle segment, indicating a first-order process. As the concentration of drug increases, a constant proportion of the drug binds to the receptor, causing a proportionate drug effect.

Spare receptors are said to exist if the maximal drug response is less than the maximal occupation of the receptors. This determination is made by comparing the concentration for 50% of maximal effect with the concentration of 50% of maximal binding K_d. If the EC_{50} is less than the K_d, spare receptors are said to be present (Figure 11). The presence of spare receptors does not alter the maximal biological response, but it does increase the sensitivity to the drug ligand. This relationship occurs because drug-receptor interactions are more likely to appear when there are proportionately more available receptors.

When the log dose of a drug is plotted against the cumulative percentage of a population responding to a specified

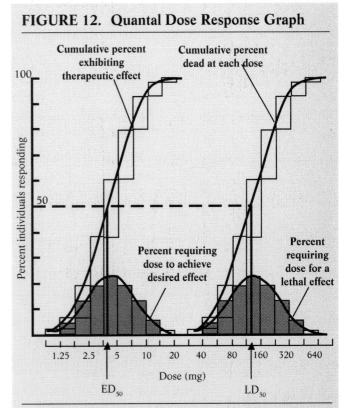

FIGURE 12.   Quantal Dose Response Graph

SOURCE: Modified from Bourne HR & Zastrow M (2001). Drug receptors and pharmacodynamics. In BG Katzung (ed.) *Basic & Clinical Pharmacology, 8th Edition*. New York, NY: Lange Medical Books/ McGraw-Hill, 29.

drug response, a quantal dose-response graph is achieved (Figure 12). The results of animal experiments can be plotted in this manner to discern the *median effective dose* (ED_{50}), *median toxic dose* (TD_{50}), and *median lethal dose* (LD_{50}). The *therapeutic index* is defined as the ratio of the TD_{50} to the ED_{50}. Because it is unethical to design experiments using a full range of drug doses to determine these indices in humans, the range of therapeutic drug concentrations and the margin of safety are estimated more broadly through extrapolation from animal studies, human drug trials, and clinical experience. In practice, both the risks and benefits of prescribing a medication are taken into account when making therapeutic decisions. Judgment about the clinically acceptable risk of toxicity often is influenced by the severity of the disease being treated.

Drugs can bind to receptors at the same site or at a different site than the endogenous compound that physi-

FIGURE 13. Full Agonist, Partial Agonist, and Competitive and Noncompetitive Antagonists

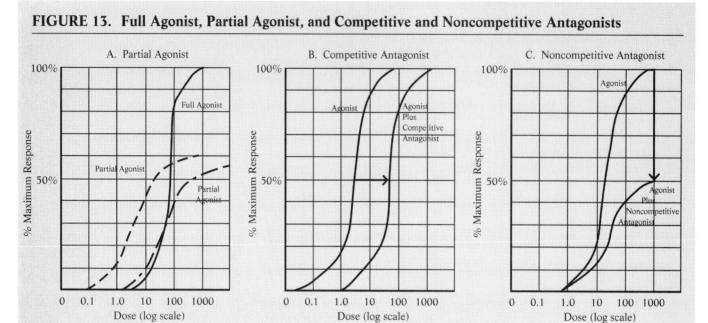

A. No matter how much the dose is increased, a partial agonist always will have a lower maximal efficiency (E_{max}). A partial agonist may be more potent, less potent, or equally potent as the agonist. In this example, both partial agonists decrease E_{max}. However, one partial agonist is more potent, and the other partial agonist is equipotent, when compared to the full agonist. B. If there are no spare receptors, competitive agonists increase the EC_{50} but do not alter the other E_{max}. C. Non-competitive antagonists decrease the E_{max}.

SOURCE: Modified from Katzung BG & Masters SB (2002). Pharmacodynamics. In *Katzung & Trevor's Pharmacology Examination and Board Review*. New York, NY: Lange Medical Books/McGraw-Hill, 13.

ologically activates that receptor. Those ligands that bind to a different site on the receptor allosterically alter the magnitude of the signal generated when the endogenous agent also binds to its site.

An *agonist* is a drug capable of fully activating the effector system when it binds to the receptor. *Partial agonists* produce less than the full effect when they have saturated the receptors and there are no spare receptors. In the case of spare receptors, when the partial agonist produces a maximal biologic response, it occupies a larger percentage of receptors than the full agonist. In the presence of a full agonist, a partial agonist acts as an inhibitor (Figure 13).

Buprenorphine is an example of a highly potent mu opioid receptor partial agonist. The drug has a high affinity for mu receptors, and displaces morphine, methadone, and other full opiate agonists from these receptors. In contrast to the full agonists, however, increases in buprenorphine dose may result in a longer duration of action, but do not

result in increased pharmacologic effects. Higher doses of buprenorphine can be given without respiratory depression. The partial agonist properties of buprenorphine may precipitate withdrawal in individuals who have a high level of physical dependence on opioids.

Antagonists are compounds that inhibit or block receptor activity. Pharmacologic antagonists can have little intrinsic activity of their own. *Competitive antagonists* compete with the agonist for reversible binding to the same receptor site. If there are no spare receptors, competitive antagonists displace the log concentration-effect curve for the agonist to higher concentrations, increasing EC_{50} but not altering the E_{max}. Adding agonist can overcome competitive antagonism by displacing the antagonist molecules from the vicinity of the receptor site. A *noncompetitive antagonist* is not capable of being reversed by excess agonist. With noncompetitive antagonists, there is a decrease in the agonist-induced E_{max}. If there are spare receptors, the curve also may be shifted to the right, requiring higher agonist concentrations to obtain maximal effect. The potency of some antagonists, particularly those that act by inhibiting the activity of an enzyme, often are expressed as an I_{50} value, which is the concentration of antagonist needed to elicit a 50% inhibition of enzyme activity.

Two other mechanisms exist by which an antagonist may act. Some physiologic antagonists bind to different receptors than the drug they inhibit to produce an effect that is the opposite of the agonist drug. Other chemical antagonists interact directly with the drug itself to prevent it from reaching its target, rather than interacting with the receptor. Examples of chemical antagonists include chelating agents and the new catalytic antibodies that are being developed as vaccines against specific addicting drugs such as cocaine and nicotine. *Inverse agonists* stabilize the receptor in its inactive conformation and inhibit activity at that receptor (Figure 14).

Agents that work at gamma-aminobutyric acid (GABA)-gated chloride ion channels illustrate this spectrum of drug activity. The endogenous agonist, GABA, acts at this receptor to produce inhibitory, hyperpolarizing postsynaptic potentials. Depending on variations in receptor structure and location in the central nervous system, this activity produces an assortment of sedative, anxiolytic, and anticonvulsant effects. Both barbiturates and benzodiazepines are pharmaceutical agonists that act at the GABA receptor. Binding of each of these drugs to the GABA receptor complex occurs at distinct sites and allosterically facilitates the activity of GABA to open the chloride-ion channel. Benzodiazepines increase the frequency of GABA-mediated chloride ion channel opening, whereas barbiturates increase the *duration* of this opening (Trevor & Way, 2001). Bicuculline, a competitive antagonist of GABA, binds selectively to the GABA site, interfering with GABA binding to that site. In contrast, picrotoxin, a noncompetitive antagonist of GABA, binds to the barbiturate site on the receptor, blocking the channel directly. Beta-carboline is an inverse agonist that allosterically reduces chlorideion conductance and increases excitability and irritability of the central nervous system; in fact, beta-carboline has no therapeutic use and can precipitate panic attacks. Flumazenil, an allosteric blocker at the benzodiazepine site that lacks intrinsic activity, has therapeutic utility in treating benzodiazepine overdose. Flumazenil also blocks beta-carboline activity, although it does not antagonize the actions of ethanol or barbiturates.

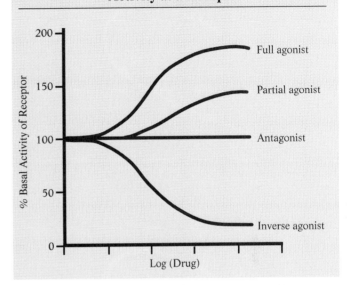

FIGURE 14.   Full Agonist, Partial Agonist, Antagonist, and Inverse Agonist Compared According to Basal Activity at a Receptor

Some drugs, depending on their concentrations, act as mixed agonists and antagonists. Mixed opioid agonist-antagonists have been developed in an attempt to produce analgesia with drugs that have less addictive potential and less respiratory depression. For example, nalbuphine (Nubain®) and butorphanol (Stadol®) are competitive mu receptor antagonists that exert their analgesic actions by acting as agonists at kappa receptors. Although each of these drugs has a place in the therapeutic armamentarium, unfortunately, each is dependence-producing and associated with adverse effects, especially at higher doses.

RELATING PHARMACOKINETICS AND PHARMACODYNAMICS

When drugs are administered to patients, the pharmacodynamic response can vary over the dose interval. If the drug effect continues to increase even after the drug concentration in the circulation begins to decline, *hysteresis* is said to occur. Hysteresis is graphed as a *counterclockwise* deviation from linearity when drug effect is monitored over time, first for rising and then for falling drug concentrations. However, if the drug effect is diminished at the same drug concentration as that concentration begins to decline, *proteresis* is said to occur. In contrast to hysteresis, proteresis

FIGURE 15.   Hysteresis and Proteresis

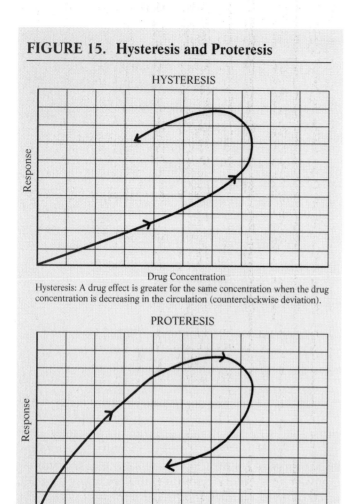

HYSTERESIS

Hysteresis: A drug effect is greater for the same concentration when the drug concentration is decreasing in the circulation (counterclockwise deviation).

PROTERESIS

Proteresis: A drug effect is lesser for the same concentration when the drug concentration is decreasing in the circulation (clockwise deviation).

is graphed as a *clockwise* deviation from linearity when drug effect is monitored over time for both rising and falling drug concentrations (Figure 15). An example of proteresis occurs when, during an evening of drinking alcohol, an individual feels more intoxicated at a blood alcohol level of 60 mg/dl on the way up the concentration curve than at the same blood alcohol level as the concentration is declining. Hysteresis can reflect acute sensitization, and proteresis can reflect acute tolerance because of changes in receptor activity and other feedback mechanisms. However, other processes may also be possible. For example, hysteresis can represent delayed access of a drug molecule to its site of action, the presence of active metabolites, or deviations in

equilibration because of the arterial versus venous site from which blood is sampled (Sitar, 2000).

Tolerance and sensitization reflect changes in the way the body responds to a drug *when it is used repeatedly.* Tolerance is the reduction in response to a drug after its repeated administration. Tolerance shifts the dose-response curve to the right, requiring higher doses than the initial doses to achieve the same effect. Sensitization indicates an increase in drug response after its repeated administration. Sensitization shifts the dose-response curve to the left, so that repeated doses cause a greater effect than that seen with the initial dose.

Tolerance and sensitization develop more readily to some drug effects than to other effects of the same drug. For example, tolerance to the euphoria produced by cocaine occurs much more rapidly than does tolerance to its cardiovascular effects. The discrepancy between tolerance to the "rush" experienced by drug users and tolerance to a drug's cardiovascular and respiratory effects can be an important cause of mortality in the user who overdoses. Also, chronic opiate users often have constipation and constricted pupils even though they no longer feel "high" after taking their drug. Differential toxicity can be explained by the dissimilar rates of drug tolerance that occur in diverse organ systems in individuals with unlike host characteristics.

Rodents experience sensitization, evidenced by an increase in locomotion, after being exposed to intermittent repeated doses of cocaine or amphetamine. In one study (Kalivas & Duffy, 1990), this increase in behavioral activity was linked to an increase in dopamine levels in the extracellular fluid of the nucleus accumbens. Rats given repeated daily intraperitoneal cocaine injections (10 mg/kg) for seven days had higher levels of dopamine detected by microdialysis on the seventh day than on the first day. Sensitization can be a phenomenon underlying chronic stimulant psychosis and/or alcohol withdrawal seizures.

There are several mechanisms by which tolerance can occur. *Pharmacokinetic tolerance* most often occurs as a consequence of increased metabolism of a drug after its repeated administration, resulting in less drug available at the receptor for drug activity. For example, the microsomal ethanol metabolizing system, which usually is not important in metabolizing ethanol, can be induced by prolonged ethanol exposure. *Pharmacodynamic tolerance* refers to the adaptive changes in receptor density, efficiency of receptor coupling, and/or signal transduction pathways that occur after repeated drug exposure. This mechanism is fur-

---

Table 1.   **An Example Using Pharmacokinetic Calculations: Determination of a Loading Dose, the Expected Resulting Plasma Concentration, an Infusion Rate, and an Incremental Loading Dose**

M.B. is a 4-year-old African American child, weighing 15 kg, who is to receive intravenous phenobarbital to treat his seizure disorder. The $t_{1/2}$ for phenobarbital is 48 hours. Given a V_d of 0.5 L/kg and a desired steady-state concentration (Cp_{ss}) between 15 and 40 mg/L, calculate an appropriate dosage regimen.

What loading dose would you recommend to achieve a concentration of 30 mg/L?

$C_{p\ desired}$ = 30 mg/L

V_d = 0.5 L/kg x 15 kg = 7.5 L

Loading dose = D = C_o x V_d = 30 mg/L x 7.5 L = 225 mg

If no further doses are given, what is the expected plasma concentration at 24 hours?

K_{el} = 0.693/$t_{1/2}$ = 0.693/48 h = 0.015/h

C_{24h} = C_o $e^{-(kt)}$ = 30 mg/l [$e^{-(.015/h)(24\ h)}$] = 20.9 mg/l

What is the infusion rate if M.B. were to be maintained at the 30 mg/L concentration level?

Cl = k_{el} x V_d = (0.015/h) x (7.5 L) = 0.113 L/h

Infusion rate = K_o = dosing rate = $\dfrac{Cl\ x\ Cp^{ss}}{F}$

$= \dfrac{(0.113\ \frac{L}{H}\ x\ 30\ mg/L)}{1}$ = 3.4 mg/h

M.B. is not responding to a Cp^{ss} of 30 mg/L. You consider increasing his Cp^{ss} to 45 mg/L before adding another medication. To achieve this, what incremental loading dose would you now order?

Incremental loading dose = $\dfrac{V_d\ x\ Cp^{ss}}{F}$

$= \dfrac{V_d\ x\ (C_{desired} - C_{current})}{F}$

$= \dfrac{7.5\ L\ (\frac{45\ mg}{L} - \frac{30\ mg}{L})}{1}$

= 7.5 L x 15 mg/L = 112.5 mg

---

ther discussed in the chapters that follow. *Learned tolerance* refers to a reduction in the effects of a drug because of compensatory mechanisms that are learned. A common example of learned tolerance is the ability for roofers and workers at heights to walk in a straight line despite motor impairment from alcohol intoxication. *Conditioned tolerance*, which is a subset of learned tolerance, occurs when specific environmental cues such as sights, smells, or circumstances are paired with drug administration so that, when the drug is taken in the presence of the specific environmental cue, a state of expectation occurs. With expectation, the drug effect may be experienced before the drug is taken—and an adaptive response may be learned (O'Brien, 2001). A powerful example of conditioned tolerance occurred in a study when rats died after being given a dose of opiates to which they previously had been tolerant. The deaths occurred when the rats were put in an unusual environment instead of the home cage where they were used to receiving the drug (Siegel, Hinson et al., 1982).

Cross-tolerance occurs when tolerance to the repeated use of a specific drug in a given category is generalized to other drugs in that same structural and mechanistic category. The cross-tolerance that occurs between alcohol, barbiturates, and benzodiazepines can be used to facilitate the smooth weaning of a patient from their drug of dependence during detoxification (see Section 5).

Physical dependence is a state that develops as a result of the adaptation produced by resetting homeostatic mechanisms after repeated drug use. Withdrawal signs and symptoms can occur in a physically dependent person when

---

drug administration is abruptly stopped. Withdrawal symptoms reflect the interactions of numerous neurocircuits and organ systems. Patients who take prescribed medications for appropriate medical indications can show tolerance, physical dependence, and withdrawal if the drug is stopped abruptly, even though they do not exhibit the compulsive drug use and negative consequences characteristic of drug addiction (O'Brien, 2001). The hypertensive rebound that occurs in patients when chronic administration of beta-adrenergic receptor blockers is abruptly discontinued is but one example of this phenomena.

CONCLUSIONS

This chapter is an introduction to the pharmacologic principles that underlie the use of drugs for both therapeutic and non-therapeutic purposes. Pharmacokinetics, the study of how the concentration of a drug in the body varies over time, was discussed according to the processes of absorption, distribution, metabolism, elimination, and excretion. Tools to quantitatively compare pharmacodynamic interactions between drugs, receptors, and their effectors were introduced along with a classification for drug activity. Finally, both pharmacokinetic and pharmacodynamic considerations were taken into account to present the topics of hysteresis, tolerance, sensitization, and physical dependence.

The following chapters in this section will elaborate on the pharmacology of individual mood and mind-altering chemicals and their drug classes.

NOTE: The views expressed in this chapter are those of the authors and do not represent the official policy of the U.S. Food and Drug Administration. No official support of or endorsement by the FDA is intended or should be inferred.

REFERENCES

Andrews P (1997). Cocaethylene toxicity. *Journal of Addictive Diseases* 16(3):75-84.

Blaschke TF (1977). Protein binding and kinetics of drugs in liver diseases. *Clinical Pharmacokinetics* 2(1):32-44.

Blaschke TF (in press). Effect of liver disease on dose optimization. *International Congress Series*.

Caviness MD, MacKichan J, Bottorff M et al. (1987). *Therapeutic Drug Monitoring: A Guide to Clinical Application*. Irving, TX: Abbott Laboratories, Diagnostics Division, 20.

Correia MA (2001). Drug biotransformation. In BG Katzung (ed.) *Basic and Clinical Pharmacology, 5th Edition*. San Mateo, CA: Appleton & Lange, 50-61.

Dresser GK, Spence JD & Bailey DG (2000). Pharmacokinetic-pharmacodynamic consequences and clinical relevance of cytochrome P450 3A4 inhibition. *Clinical Pharmacokinetics* 38(1):41-57.

Dziegielewska KM & Sunders NR (2002). The ins and outs of brain-barrier mechanisms. *Trends in Neurosciences* 25(2):69-70.

Garner DM, Shulman KI, Walker SE et al. (1996). The making of a user friendly MAOI diet. *Journal of Clinical Psychiatry* 61(2):145-146.

Hedlulnd E, Gustafsson JA & Warner M (2001). Cytochrome P450 in the brain: A review. *Current Drug Metabolism* 2(3):245-263.

Herrlin K, Segerdahl M, Gustafsson LL et al. (2000). Methadone, ciprofloxacin, and adverse drug reactions. *Lancet* 356:2069-2070.

Higuchi S, Muramatsu T, Shigemori K et al. (1992). The relationship between low K_m aldehyde dehydrogenase phenotype and drinking behavior in Japanese. *Journal of Studies on Alcohol* 53:170-175.

Holford NGH (2001a). Pharmacokinetics and pharmacodynamics: Rational dosing and the time course of drug action. In BG Katzung (ed.) *Basic & Clinical Pharmacology, 8th Edition*. New York, NY: Lange Medical Books/McGraw-Hill, 40.

Israili ZH & Dayton PG (2001). Human alpha-1-glycoprotein and its interactions with drugs. *Drug Metabolism Reviews* 33(2):161-235.

Kalivas PW & Duffy P (1990). Effect of acute and daily cocaine treatment on extracellular dopamine in the nucleus accumbens. *Synapse* 5:48-58.

Klotz U, Avant GR, Hoyumpa A et al. (1975). The effects of age and liver disease on the disposition and elimination of diazepam in adult man. *Journal of Clinical Investigation* 55:347-359.

Meng Y, Lichtman AH, Bridgen DT et al. (1997). Inhalation studies with drugs of abuse. In RS Rapaka, N Chiang & BR Martin (eds.) *Pharmacokinetics, Metabolism, and Pharmaceutics of Drugs of Abuse (NIDA Research Monograph 173)*. Rockville, MD: National Institute on Drug Abuse, 203.

O'Brien CP (2001). Drug addiction and drug abuse. In JG Hardman, LE Limbird & AG Gilman (eds.) *Goodman and Gilman's The Pharmacologic Basis of Therapeutics, 10th Edition*. New York, NY: McGraw-Hill, 625.

Rowland M & Tozer TN, eds. (1995). *Clinical Pharmacokinetics: Concepts and Applications, 3rd Edition*. Baltimore, MD: Williams & Wilkins.

Siegel S, Hinson RE, Krank MD et al. (1982). Heroin "overdose" death: The contribution of drug-associated environmental cues. *Science* 216:436-437.

Sitar DS (2000). Clinical pharmacokinetics and pharmacodynamics. In SG Carruthers, BB Hoffman, KL Melmon et al. (eds.) *Melmon and Morrelli's Clinical Pharmacology, 4th Edition*. New York, NY: McGraw-Hill, 1219.

Trevor AJ & Way WL (2001). Sedative-hypnotic drugs. In BG Katzung (ed.) *Basic & Clinical Pharmacology, 8th Edition*. New York, NY: Lange Medical Books/McGraw-Hill, 370.

Tyndale RF, Droll KP & Sellers EM (1997). Genetically deficient CYP2D6 metabolism provides protection against oral opiate dependence. *Pharmacogenetics* 7(5):375-379.

Warner M, Stromstedt M, Wyss A et al. (1993). Regulation of cytochrome P450 in the central nervous system. *Journal of Steroid Biochemistry and Molecular Biology* 47(1-6):191-194.

Winter ME (1990). *Basic Clinical Pharmacokinetics, 2nd Edition*. Vancouver, WA: Applied Therapeutics.

Wrighton SA, VandenBranden M & Ring BJ (1996). The human drug metabolizing cytochromes P450. *Journal of Pharmacokinetics and Biopharmaceutics* 24(5):461-473.

Zhu B, Ou-Yang DS, Xiao-Ping C et al., (2001). Assessment of cytochrome P450 activity by a five-drug cocktail approach. *Clinical Pharmacology and Therapeutics* 70:455-461.

| Chapter 2 | # The Pharmacology of Alcohol |

John J. Woodward, Ph.D.

Drugs in the Class
Absorption and Metabolism
Pharmacologic Actions
Mechanisms of Action
Addiction Liability
Toxicity/Adverse Effects
Genetic Contributions to Alcoholism and Alcohol Abuse

This chapter reviews the mechanisms and sites of action of alcohol on the brain. The past 10 years have seen tremendous advances in understanding alcohol's effects on brain function, in large part because of the use of molecular biology techniques that permit the expression and study of specific neuronal proteins. It is now well established that a major site of action for alcohol in the brain is the large family of ligand-gated and voltage-gated ion channels. These ion channels are essential in generating and transmitting electrical activity in the brain. Results of these studies have led to a view that alcohol, like other drugs of abuse, does show specificity and selectivity of action, especially at concentrations associated with intoxication and sedation.

However, alcohol still must be considered a wide-spectrum drug in that there are multiple proteins from different gene families that are affected by alcohol. Thus, the intoxicating effects of alcohol likely are mediated by different proteins than those that underlie alcohol's rewarding effects or those involved in alcohol withdrawal.

Understanding how these multiple effects combine in some individuals to produce the complex behavioral disorder known as alcoholism is one of the great challenges of alcohol research. This chapter presents an overview of our current understanding of alcohol as an addictive drug. Readers interested in this area are encouraged to consult several excellent summaries on this topic published under the auspices of the National Institute on Alcohol Abuse and Alcoholism, which supports much of the research on alcohol in the United States (U.S. Public Health Service [USPHS], 2000; Noronha, Eckhardt et al., 2000).

Note that the terms "alcohol" and "ethanol" are used more or less interchangeably throughout the chapter.

DRUGS IN THE CLASS

Alcohol is one of the oldest used and abused substances. It is second only to caffeine in incidence of use, and its manufacture, distribution, and sale are of major economic importance. Despite its pervasive and apparently acceptable use in nearly all segments of American society, annual alcohol-related costs in terms of lost productivity and health care are estimated at $185 billion and are expected to increase in future years (USPHS, 2000). Although problem drinking and alcoholism are viewed by a growing number of Americans as legitimate health problems that deserve all of the resources that the medical community can command, relatively few effective pharmacotherapies are available for alcoholism and alcohol abuse. Advances in understanding alcohol's effects on fundamental cellular processes have yielded several promising areas for drug development that may help reduce the incidence of relapse in alcoholic patients.

Types of Alcoholism. Clinical studies of alcohol abuse and alcoholism have led to the classification of two types of alcoholism, based on the appearance of certain alcohol-related problems and the degree of expression of certain personality traits, including novelty seeking, harm avoidance, and reward dependence (Cloninger, 1987). *Type 1* alcoholism accounts for about 75% of male alcoholics and is characterized by the following factors: (1) onset of alcohol-related problems after the age of 25, (2) a low degree of spontaneous alcohol-seeking behavior and alcohol-related fighting, (3) psychological dependence, coupled with guilt and fear about alcohol dependence, and (4) a low degree of novelty-seeking and a high degree of harm avoidance and reward dependence. *Type 2* alcoholism involves a much smaller subset of alcoholics, whose characteristics are essentially the opposite of those listed for type 1 alcoholism. They include infrequent feelings of guilt and fear about alcohol dependence and a low degree of harm avoidance.

ABSORPTION AND METABOLISM

Alcohol is a small, water-soluble molecule that is rapidly and efficiently absorbed into the bloodstream from the stomach, small intestine, and colon. The rate of absorption depends on the gastric emptying time and can be delayed by the presence of food in the small intestine. Once in the bloodstream, alcohol is rapidly distributed throughout the body and gains access to all tissues, including the fetus in pregnant women.

Alcohol is metabolized primarily in the liver by the actions of alcohol dehydrogenase (ADH) and mixed function oxidases such as P450IIE1 (CYP2E1). Levels of CYP2E1 may be increased in chronic drinkers. ADH converts alcohol to acetaldehyde, which subsequently can be converted to acetate by the actions of acetaldehyde dehydrogenase (ALDH). Small amounts of alcohol can be excreted by the lungs. The odor of the breath is not a reliable indicator of alcohol consumption, because it is due not to alcohol vapor but to impurities in the alcoholic beverage.

The rate of alcohol metabolism by ADH is relatively constant, as the enzyme is saturated at relatively low blood alcohol levels and thus exhibits zero order kinetics (constant amount oxidized per unit of time). Alcohol metabolism is proportional to body weight (and probably liver weight) and averages approximately one ounce of pure alcohol per three hours in adults. Thus, the time for an individual to become sober after even moderate intake of alcohol can be substantial. At present, there do not appear to be any effective "alcohol antagonists" (amethystic agents) that can quickly reverse the intoxicating effects of alcohol, although such an agent is the object of research (reviewed in Litten & Allen, 1991). The lack of such a substance is undoubtedly due to the myriad interactions between alcohol and the cellular processes that control neuronal activity (as reviewed below). Some candidates for the role of amethystic agent include the opiate antagonist naloxone (Narcan®), which may reverse ethanol-induced respiratory depression, and the experimental benzodiazepine RO 15-4513, which has been reported to reverse some of the signs of alcohol intoxication in certain strains of rats. The clinical utility of such an agent in the treatment of life-threatening alcohol intoxication notwithstanding, there are moral, ethical, and medical concerns to be considered in the development of such a drug, because it probably would not reduce the toxicity associated with the chronic ingestion of alcohol.

PHARMACOLOGIC ACTIONS

Central Nervous System. Acutely, alcohol acts as a central nervous system (CNS) depressant. At higher blood levels, it acts as a sedative-hypnotic, although the quality of sleep often is reduced after alcohol intake. In patients with sleep apnea, alcohol increases the frequency and severity of apneic episodes and the resulting hypoxia. Alcohol potentiates the sedative-hypnotic properties of both benzodiazepines and barbiturates, probably reflecting common mechanisms of action for these substances. Acute alcohol intoxication is not always associated with sedation or coma; indeed, some intoxicated individuals display violent behavior that requires administration of other sedative or antipsychotic agents. The use of these agents with a severely intoxicated individual must be approached cautiously to prevent respiratory failure.

Acute alcohol ingestion usually produces a feeling of warmth as cutaneous blood flow is increased and is accompanied by a reduction in core body temperature. Gastric secretions usually are increased, although the characteristics of these secretions depend on the concentration of alcohol ingested, with high concentrations (>20%) inhibiting secretions. Continual ingestion of high concentrations of alcohol can lead to erosive gastritis, which can limit absorption of nutrients and vitamins. These nutritional deficiencies are associated with several serious neurologic and mental disorders, including brain damage, memory loss, sleep disturbances, and psychoses such as Wernicke's and Korsakoff's. Finally, acute and chronic ingestion of alcohol decreases sexual responsiveness in both men and women.

Behavioral Pharmacology. A widely accepted tenet of addiction research is that addictive substances, by definition, engender actions that promote further drug-seeking behavior. This concept of positive reinforcement suggests that a positive reward is obtained after ingestion of an addictive substance, such as alcohol, and that the desire to re-experience the reward leads to more drinking. However, evidence suggests that alcohol's reinforcing properties may be more of a reflection of its anti-anxiety properties. Certainly, these two mechanisms of reinforcement are not mutually exclusive and probably coexist to a greater or lesser degree in individuals addicted to alcohol.

Animal and human studies have suggested that the biochemical substrates for the reinforcing properties of alcohol and other drugs of abuse involve discrete neuronal pathways in the brain, including the dopaminergic projections to the mesolimbic areas of the forebrain (as reviewed in Koob, Roberts et al., 1998). These neurons originate in the ventral tegmental area (VTA) and project to discrete areas of the forebrain, including the nucleus accumbens, olfactory tubercle, frontal cortex, amygdala, and the septal area. These areas of the cortex are thought to be involved in translating emotion into action through the activation of motor pathways. Thus, they may be important in initiating and sustaining drug-seeking behavior. Lesions of these discrete brain areas in experimental animals reduce motor activity in response to novel environmental stimuli, food presentation, and other factors that normally increase locomotor activity in animals without lesions. Conversely, direct injection of dopamine and compounds with dopamine agonist-like properties, such as amphetamine and cocaine, into these areas stimulates locomotor activity. The effects are blocked by prior administration of selective dopamine antagonists. Thus, a "dopamine hypothesis" has emerged, which asserts that all addictive drugs either directly or indirectly increase dopaminergic activity in the mesolimbic areas of the forebrain (Di Chiara, Imperato et al., 1988). This hypothesis is undoubtedly a simplification of a very complex behavior, but it has an impressive amount of experimental data to support it.

The reinforcing properties of alcohol may involve modulation of mesolimbic dopaminergic neurotransmission by several mechanisms that, in the final result, enhance the synaptic concentrations of dopamine in key mesolimbic cortical regions. This modulation is suggested by the locomotor-enhancing effects in animals given low doses of alcohol, which are accompanied by increases in extracellular levels of dopamine as determined by *in vivo* microdialysis in the nucleus accumbens (Imperato & Di Chiara, 1986). In addition, dopamine levels (estimated from dopamine metabolite measurements) after alcohol ingestion are higher in animals genetically selected for alcohol preference over non-preferring strains, again suggesting a dopamine involvement in the reinforcing properties of alcohol (Fadda, Mosca et al., 1989; Khatib, Murphy et al., 1988).

Weiss and colleagues (1992) carried out a series of elegant studies using *in vivo* microdialysis to monitor extracellular dopamine levels in rats trained to self-administer alcohol. The results of these experiments showed that the self-administration of alcohol in rats was accompanied by significant dose-dependent increases in extracellular dopamine levels in the nucleus accumbens. In addition, dopamine levels were elevated to a greater extent in alcohol-preferring strains of rats (compared with non-preferring strains), even though total alcohol consumption over the test period was nearly identical in both strains. These results suggest that the alcohol-preferring strains are sensitized to the dopamine-enhancing effects of alcohol compared with non-preferring strains and that this sensitization may be important in determining the degree of alcohol preference in these animals. A fascinating finding of the studies was the significant increase in dopamine found only in the alcohol-preferring strains during the 15-minute waiting period that preceded alcohol self-administration. This finding suggests that the expected reward that the ingestion of alcohol may provide is sufficient to enhance activity in the pathway. Thus, the genetic differences in this pathway may contribute to the motivational factors that drive alcohol-seeking behavior in certain individuals.

Recent studies with human alcoholics have examined the neurobehavioral aspects of alcohol abuse, using drug discrimination procedures similar to those used in animal studies. In the studies, human alcoholics are asked to rate the effects produced by a variety of drugs in terms of their similarity to

TABLE 1.   Molecular Properties of Alcohol-Sensitive Ion Channels

Neurotransmitter Agonist or Activator	Channel Name	Subunit Families	Brain Subtypes	Major Permeant Ions	Alcohol Effect (Acute)
GABA	$GABA_A$	$\alpha,\beta,\gamma,\delta,\rho$	$\alpha 1/\beta 1/\gamma 2$	Cl^-	Enhance/Inhibit (ρ)
Glycine	Glycine	α,β	$\alpha 1/\beta 1$	Cl^-	Enhance
Acetylcholine ($\alpha 7$)	nAchR	α,β	$\alpha 4\beta 2$, $\alpha 7$-9	Na^+	Enhance/Inhibit
Serotonin	$5HT_3$	$5HT_{3a,b}$	$5HT_3$	Na^+	Enhance
ATP	$P2_X$	$P2_{X1-4, Z}$	$P_{2X2/3}$	Na^+	Inhibit
Glutamate	NMDA	NR1, NR2A-D	NR1/2A/2B	Ca^{++}/Na^+	Inhibit
Glutamate	Non-NMDA	GluR1-7	GluR2/3	Na^+/Ca^{++}	Inhibit
Voltage-gated	BK_{Ca}	α,β_{1-4}	α, α/β	K^+	Enhance
Voltage-gated	L,N,P,Q,T	α (S,C,D) β,γ,δ	Multiple	Ca^{++}	Inhibit

Ion channels are listed according to their natural agonist or mode of activation. Subunit families represent those found in the brain and spinal cord. Brain subtypes are examples of subunit combinations commonly thought to be expressed by brain neurons. Alcohol's effect is based on electrophysiologic responses to acutely administered alcohol to recombinant or native receptor combination. GABA, gamma-aminobutyric acid; $5HT_3$, 5-hydroxytryptamine; ATP, adenosine triphosphate; NMDA, N-methyl-D-aspartate.

those produced by alcohol. For example, studies by Krystal and colleagues (1998) showed that ketamine, a dissociative anesthetic that blocks the N-methyl-D-aspartate (NMDA) subtype of glutamate receptors, induces ethanol-like effects in recently detoxified alcoholics. These effects were dose dependent: At low doses, they mimicked the effects of one to two standard drinks of alcohol, whereas higher doses produced effects similar to those of eight to nine drinks. Interestingly, the effects of ketamine that were ethanol-like were associated with the descending phase of blood alcohol concentration associated with ethanol-induced sedation.

Other human clinical studies have implicated neurotransmitters such as gamma-aminobutyric acid (GABA), serotonin, and the opiates in mediating the rewarding and craving aspects of alcohol action. Such human studies are important in the context of understanding the underlying causes of alcohol abuse because alcohol, unlike most drugs of abuse, interacts with a wide variety of molecular and cellular processes to produce its pharmacologic, physiologic, and psychological effects.

MECHANISMS OF ACTION

The cellular and molecular actions of alcohol have been pursued with intense interest since the studies of the German scientists Meyer and Overton, who suggested in the early 1900s that ethanol and other higher chain alcohols produce their effects by altering the lipid environment of cell membranes. The relevance of the membrane-disordering action of ethyl alcohol as it relates to its profound behavioral effects is controversial.

Numerous studies have shown ethyl alcohol does indeed induce measurable changes in brain membrane fluidity. However, these changes are relatively modest, require rather high concentrations, and are less than the effects produced by a change in temperature of 1°C. to 2°C. that, by itself, is not associated with behavioral signs of intoxication (reviewed in Forman & Miller, 1989). This finding does not exclude the possibility that specific areas of certain neuronal membranes, such as those directly in contact with membrane-spanning receptors or ion channels, may be especially sensitive to perturbation by alcohol, but there is little compelling evidence to suggest that this is true.

The next likely target for alcohol is membrane-bound and intracellular proteins. Although there is no evidence of a specific receptor for alcohol, it is important to remember that alcohol does interact rather selectively with the enzyme ADH in a classic enzyme-substrate complex, suggesting that such an interaction might occur with important brain proteins that could alter their function. As shown in Table 1, many ligand-gated ion channels and some voltage-activated channels form a large subset of proteins that are uniquely sensitive to behaviorally relevant concentrations of alcohol.

These proteins all function as gates or pores that allow the passage of certain ions into and out of neurons on binding of the appropriate neurotransmitter. The presence of a specific neurotransmitter-binding site whose occupation is required for activation and opening of the ion channel distinguishes these proteins from the other major class of ion channels, which are activated solely by changes in membrane potential.

Two distinct classes of ligand-gated ion channels appear to be particularly important as targets for the actions of alcohol in the brain. These ion channels can be classified as inhibitory and include the GABA$_A$ receptor and strychnine-sensitive glycine receptor and excitatory that are composed of glutamate-activated channels (NMDA and non-NMDA), acetylcholine-activated nicotinic receptors, adenosine triphosphate (ATP)-gated channels, and the 5-hydroxytryptamine (5-HT$_3$) subtype of serotonin receptors. Activation of the GABA$_A$ and glycine receptors by their respective neurotransmitters usually results in hyperpolarization of neurons because of the inward flux of negatively charged chloride ions. This result makes the cell less likely to reach the threshold membrane potential required for firing. The NMDA receptor and non-NMDA glutamate receptors gate the inward flux of sodium and calcium on binding of the endogenous neurotransmitters glutamate or aspartate and thus are considered an excitatory receptor that leads to depolarization of neuronal membranes. In brain neurons, the NMDA receptor is especially important be-

cause it has a high permeability to calcium that is a trigger for many intracellular processes. The non-NMDA class of glutamate receptors (called the AMPA/kainate receptors in recognition of their selective agonists) and the 5-HT$_3$ subtype of serotonin receptors are much less permeable to calcium, and most of their current is carried by sodium ions.

Most ligand-gated ion channels are made up of several subunits that assemble to form the functional ion channel. These receptors contain an extracellular domain that recognizes the neurotransmitter and a membrane-associated domain that forms the ion channel through which the ions flow in or out of the neuron. In a current model of ion channel structure based on the proposed organization of the muscle-type nicotinic acetylcholine receptor, most ligand-gated ion channels are thought to be tetrameric or pentameric in structure, with the subunits arranged in a circle surrounding a central ion pore (Figure 1).

For the GABA$_A$, glycine, and 5-HT$_3$ receptors, each subunit has four sections that span the membrane (TMI-TMIV) and that are connected by short and long loops of amino acids (Figure 1). Intracellular loop number 2, which connects transmembrane sections numbers 3 and 4, is particularly important because it contains specific sequences that are recognized as targets for kinases and other modifying proteins. Phosphorylation is a powerful means of controlling the activity of various receptor proteins and may play an important role in determining the sensitivity of certain ion channels to the actions of alcohol. The proposed structure of the glutamate family of ligand-gated channels is somewhat different in that the TMII domain does not completely traverse the membrane, but forms a hairpin loop (Figure 1). This formation places the C-terminus of the subunit inside the neuron where it is subject to regulation by phosphorylation and other cellular processes.

In functional ion channels of all types, all of the TMII domains appear to face each other and make up the central ion pore. The ion selectivity of the particular channel is determined largely by the sequence of amino acids in TMII, although, in glutamate receptors, amino acids from other TM domains contribute to pore formation. The successful cloning and expression of ion channel subunits in experimental systems has greatly enhanced our understanding of the function of these receptors and has allowed for a detailed examination of their sensitivity to alcohol. A brief review of the effects of alcohol on each of these important ion channels follows.

FIGURE 1.   Proposed Organization of Ligand-Gated Ion Channels

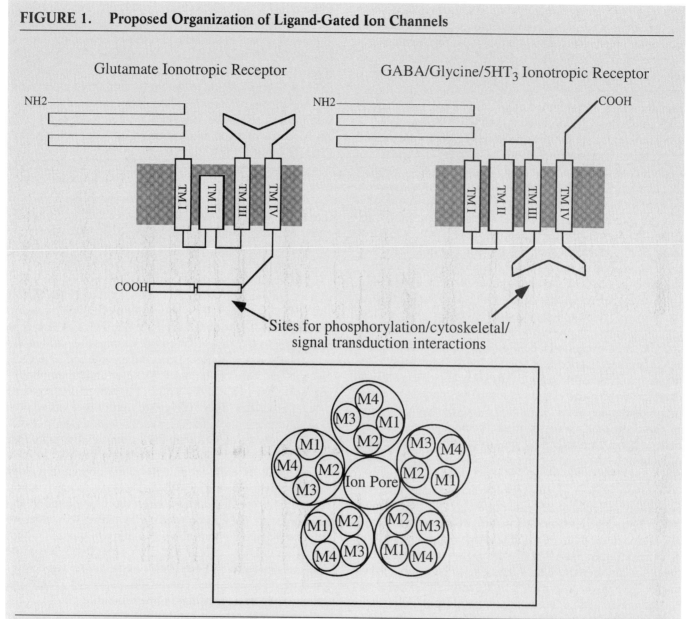

This figure shows the proposed arrangement of 4 membrane-spanning regions (TMI-TMIV) for glutamatergic and nicotinic, GABAergic, glycinergic, and serotonergic receptors. Note the hairpin structure of the TMII domain of the glutamate receptor, which alters the location of the extracellular and intracellular loops as compared with the other receptors. Sites for phosphorylation by intracellular kinases are shown. The insert shows a cross-section of a functional ligand-gated channel composed of 5 subunits. Note how the transmembrane regions (M2) face one another and form the central ion pore.

GABA_A and Glycine Receptors. As shown in Table 1, there are distinct families of subunits that make up GABA_A and glycine receptors. Each class of subunits may have multiple members that differ slightly in their sequence and function. Different subunit combinations can give rise to a variety of GABA$_A$ and glycine receptors that show variable sensitivity to pharmacologic agents, including alcohol. Alcohol generally enhances GABA$_A$ and glycine receptor function, although GABA$_A$ P receptors are inhibited by alcohol. Through use of the oocyte expression system, alcohol was shown to enhance the GABA$_A$ currents in receptors containing the γ2L variant of the GABA receptor, along with alpha and beta subunits (Wafford, Burnett et al., 1991; Wafford & Whiting, 1992). This variant contains an additional eight amino acids that introduce a site for phosphorylation of the receptor by protein kinase C. Omission of the γ2L subunit or even substitution of other gamma subunits (including the γ2 short variant) resulted in cells that did not show significant potentiation of the GABA-induced currents by alcohol. Despite these intriguing results, subsequent studies have shown that γ2L expression is not sufficient in itself to confer sensitivity to alcohol. In addition, knock-out mice lacking this subunit show normal sensitivity to alcohol, although their responsiveness to benzodiazepines is enhanced (Homanics, Harrison et al., 1999; Quinlan, Firestone et al., 2000).

It has been shown that the potentiating effects of alcohol on GABA$_A$ and glycine receptor function can be dramatically altered by single amino acid substitutions within the transmembrane domains of the alpha or beta subunits. In these studies, replacement of a serine in the TMII domain of these subunits by an isoleucine abolished the potentiating effects of alcohol on GABA$_A$ or glycine receptor currents (Mihic, Ye et al., 1997). Subsequent studies by this group and others have shown that the site may be involved in mediating the effects of some volatile anesthetics on GABA$_A$ and glycine receptor function (Mascia, Machu et al., 1996). It is unclear whether this amino acid is part of an alcohol-binding site because this mutation also increased the apparent affinity of the receptor for GABA, thus eliminating alcohol's action on GABA efficacy.

A variable distribution or expression of GABA$_A$ subunits that show variable alcohol sensitivity could dictate to some extent the degree of sensitivity of various individuals to alcohol. Several lines of alcohol-preferring rats have shown to have a greater density of GABAergic terminals in the nucleus accumbens than nonalcohol-preferring strains (Hwang, Lumeng et al., 1990). This finding suggests that enhanced GABAergic function is linked with preference for alcohol in a brain region that has been shown to be an important site for the reinforcing actions of alcohol. Thus,

enhanced GABA$_A$ function by alcohol may in some way lead to the increases in dopamine in the nucleus accumbens that are associated with self-administration of alcohol in rats. The generation of transgenic animals expressing ethanol-insensitive GABA$_A$ receptor subunits may help refine that actions of alcohol require enhanced GABAergic function. GABA$_A$ receptors show changes after chronic alcohol exposure, with some subunits showing decreases and others showing decreases or no change (reviewed in Grobin, Papadeas et al., 2000). Whether these changes are related to the development of tolerance to the various CNS effects of alcohol has not been established.

NMDA Receptors. NMDA receptors are calcium-permeable ion channels that require both glutamate and glycine for activation. The amino acid-binding sites on the receptor are contributed by two different subunits, NR1 and NR2 (Figure 2). Antagonism of either of these two sites is sufficient to completely block the ion flux that normally follows receptor activation.

Receptor activity is inhibited by other drugs, such as ketamine, phencyclidine, and MK-801, which bind in the channel pore and block ion flux.

At the molecular level, NMDA receptors are composed of multiple subunits (NR1, NR2A-D) that co-assemble to form functional channels (Figure 2). NR1 subunits exist as a family of eight splice variants generated by alternative splice of one N-terminal cassette and two intracellular C-terminal cassettes (Figure 2). The presence of one or more of the NR1 and NR2 subunits in a single receptor complex confers unique biophysical and pharmacologic properties to the NMDA receptor (Watkins & Collingridge, 1994). NMDA receptors have large intracellular C-termini that interact with a variety of important proteins that regulate receptor phosphorylation and clustering to important signaling complexes (Figure 2). Non-NMDA receptors are made up of multiple subunits as well (GluR1-7), and specific combinations of subunits also yield receptors with distinct properties. Changes in the expression of these subunits either during development or as a result of disease or drug exposure can alter neuronal excitability and plasticity.

NMDA receptors expressed in neurons are readily antagonized by alcohol at concentrations associated with intoxication and sedation (10 to 100 mM) (Lovinger, White et al., 1989; Hoffman, Moses et al., 1989; Woodward & Gonzales, 1990; Gonzales & Woodward, 1990). Differences in the sensitivity to alcohol's inhibitory effects are observed between different brain regions (Simson, Griwell

FIGURE 2.   Topologic Organization and Interaction of NMDA Receptor Subunits With Intracellular Cytoskeletal and Signaling Proteins

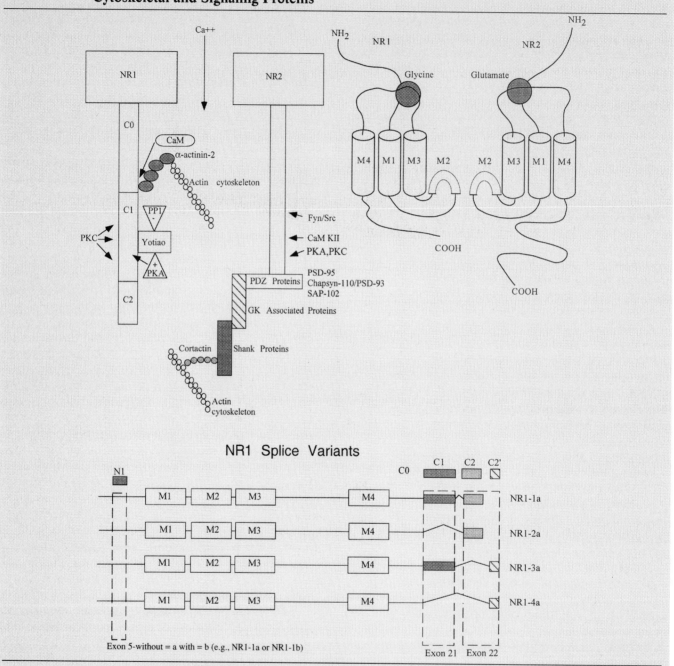

The top right panel shows the two major subunits of the NMDA receptor, NR1 and NR2, and the binding sites for glycine and glutamate, respectively. The top left panel illustrates some of the interactions between the intracellular C-termini of NR1 and NR2 subunits, various intracellular proteins, and the actin cytoskeleton. The bottom panel shows the diversity of NR1 subunits that can be obtained by alternative splicing of the N1, C1, and C2 cassettes.

et al., 1991; Gothert & Fink, 1989; Gonzales & Woodward, 1990; Woodward & Gonzales, 1990). Part of this difference may result from differential expression of NMDA subunits, as alcohol's inhibition of recombinant NMDA receptors (Figure 3) is influenced by the subunits expressed (Kuner, Schoepfer et al., 1993; Masood, Wu et al., 1994; Mirshahi & Woodward, 1995; Lovinger, 1995; Smothers, Clayton et al., 2001) as well as by phosphorylation and cytoskeletal interactions (Anders, Blevins et al., 1999, 2000).

The situation with the non-NMDA glutamate receptor is similar, although there is some controversy over whether non-NMDA receptors expressed in brain neurons are as sensitive to alcohol as the NMDA subtype. Overall, alcohol's blockade of the activation of excitatory NMDA and non-NMDA receptors is likely to be important in mediating the intoxicating and sedative effects of alcohol. The antagonism of NMDA receptors by alcohol may be involved in its rewarding properties because NMDA receptors are thought to be important in regulating the release of dopamine in mesolimbic areas such as the nucleus accumbens. For example, with the use of microdialysis techniques, NMDA antagonists were shown to increase levels of dopamine in the nucleus accumbens (Youngren, Daly et al., 1993). These results suggest that glutamate may exert an inhibitory control over dopamine release by NMDA receptors. Thus, alcohol may produce increases in accumbens dopamine by its inhibitory actions on NMDA receptors. In animal studies designed to evaluate the subjective effects of ethanol on behavior, NMDA antagonists can produce ethanol-appropriate lever response in rats trained to discriminate ethanol from saline (Colombo & Grant, 1992). These results suggest that alcohol does behave as an NMDA antagonist in the intact animal.

NMDA receptors are altered during chronic exposure to alcohol and appear to be important in mediating some of the signs of alcohol withdrawal. It has been demonstrated in cultured neurons that chronic exposure to alcohol increases the density of MK-801 binding sites (Iorio, Reinlib et al., 1992), suggesting that neurons may compensate for the acute inhibitory actions of alcohol on NMDA receptor function by increasing the density of these receptors. This up-regulation of receptor density is a common response of many cell and tissue types to the prolonged presence of receptor antagonists. Because NMDA itself can induce seizure activity in animals, increased numbers of NMDA receptors after chronic alcohol exposure may underlie the increased susceptibility of animals and humans to seizures during abrupt withdrawal from alcohol. Experiments with mice show that NMDA-induced seizure activity was elevated in mice made dependent on alcohol and that the NMDA antagonist MK-801 could reduce the severity of these seizures during withdrawal (Grant, Valverius et al., 1990). More recent studies have suggested that the enhancement in NMDA receptor function after chronic alcohol may involve changes in the expression pattern of specific NMDA receptor subunits (Blevins, Mirshahi et al., 1995; Follesa & Ticku, 1995; Snell, Nunley et al., 1996).

Chronic exposure to alcohol was shown to increase the density of binding sites for dihydropyridine-sensitive, voltage-sensitive calcium channels (Dolin, Little et al., 1987; Messing, Carpenter et al., 1986). These and other voltage-sensitive calcium channels are inhibited by acute alcohol, although less potently than NMDA-stimulated calcium flux (Leslie, Barr et al., 1983). Increased activation of these channels during withdrawal from chronic alcohol might contribute to seizure activity and the general enhancement of neuronal activity that accompanies withdrawal.

5-HT$_3$ Receptors. The 5-HT$_3$ receptor is a ligand-gated ion channel activated by serotonin and is permeable primarily to monovalent cations, such as sodium and potassium. In cultured neurons, low doses of alcohol potentiated the currents elicited by activation of the 5-HT$_3$ receptor (Lovinger & White, 1991). In behavioral studies involving both rats and pigeons, 5-HT$_3$ receptor antagonists blocked the animal's ability to discriminate ethanol from saline, suggesting that alcohol's acute actions on 5-HT$_3$ receptors may underlie some of the subjective effects of alcohol (Grant & Barrett, 1991).

Acetylcholine Nicotinic Receptors. Acetylcholine activates a variety of ligand-gated ion channels that are expressed in brain neurons and that are related to the nicotinic receptor expressed at the neuromuscular junction. Alcohol has been shown either to potentiate or inhibit acetylcholine-induced currents in cultured neurons (Aistrup, Marszalec et al., 1999) or expressed in oocytes (Cardoso, Brozowski et al., 1999). This biphasic effect appears to result from expression of different subtypes of nicotinic receptors by brain neurons that show a differential response to ethanol. Thus, heteromeric nicotinic receptors composed of alpha/beta subunits appear to be potentiated by ethanol, whereas homomeric receptors composed only of alpha subunits (α7, for example) are inhibited by ethanol (Cardoso, Brozowski et al., 1999). It is not yet clear how the different effects of ethanol on neuronal nicotinic receptors are manifested at the behavioral level.

FIGURE 3. **Inhibition of Recombinant NMDA Receptor Function by Alcohol**

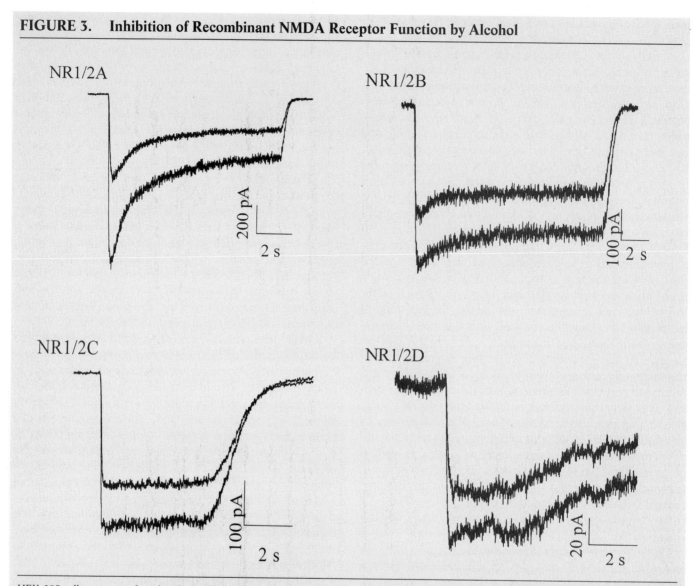

HEK 293 cells were transfected with the NR1-1a subunit and various NR2 subunits, and currents were recorded by using whole-cell patch clamp electrophysiology. The larger trace in each pair represents the current produced by application of glutamate and glycine. Note the extensive degree of desensitization in NR1/2A receptors as compared with other combinations. The smaller trace in each pair represents the current elicited by glutamate and glycine in the presence of 100 mM alcohol.

Other Ion Channels. Calcium-activated potassium channels (BK channels), those gated by ATP (P2X), and some voltage-sensitive calcium channels are affected by alcohol. BK channel activity is enhanced by alcohol, and this enhancement may contribute to the inhibition of vasopressin release from neurohypophysial terminals and the resulting diuresis that accompanies alcohol ingestion (Dopico, Chu et al., 1999). Alcohol inhibits the function of native and some subtypes of recombinant ATP-gated purinergic receptors (Li, Peoples et al., 1994; Xiong, Li et al., 2000; Koles, Wirkner et al., 2000). Similarly, some types of voltage-gated calcium channels (L, N, and P/Q) are inhibited by alcohol, and L-type channels appear to be up-regulated by chronic alcohol exposure (Walter & Messing, 1999).

Pharmacologic Studies Implicating Other Neurotransmitter Systems. Much of our working knowledge of alcohol's effects on neuronal function comes from studies that have examined the effects of alcohol on various neurotransmitter systems, as well as the ability of known pharmacologic agents to mediate alcohol drinking behavior. These studies are important because they may provide new leads to follow in our attempt to understand how alcohol's addictive properties are produced at the molecular and cellular level. A brief review of this literature is presented here.

Adenosine: Adenosine is a major inhibitory neurotransmitter in the brain and may serve as an endogenous anti-epileptic because of its ability to inhibit neuronal function. Alcohol has been shown to inhibit the function of one type of adenosine transporter, leading to increased extracellular adenosine levels (Diamond, Nagy et al., 1991). Increased synaptic concentrations of adenosine may contribute to some of the effects of acute and chronic alcohol. Adenosine interacts with two receptors: A1, which is coupled to inhibition of adenylate cyclase, and A2, which is coupled to the stimulation of adenylate cyclase. In cultured cells that express only the A2 receptor, alcohol increases extracellular adenosine, which leads to receptor-stimulated increases in the second messenger cyclic adenosine monophosphate (AMP) within the cells.

Chronic exposure of these cells to alcohol results in desensitization, such that adenosine stimulation leads to smaller increases in cyclic AMP (cAMP) within the cell. This desensitization is associated with a reduction in the amount of the stimulatory guanosine triphosphate-binding protein GαS, which couples various receptors to the stimulation of cAMP production. This reduction in GαS results in a heterologous form of desensitization, thereby reducing the effectiveness not only of adenosine but also of other neurotransmitters, which act via GαS to increase cAMP levels. The importance of this finding as it relates to alcohol addiction is unknown, but may be important, because regulation of intracellular cAMP levels by a whole variety of neurotransmitters and neuromodulators is important for regulating neuronal activity. Although these studies were performed by using a transformed neural cell line, it was found that adenosine-stimulated increases in cAMP in blood lymphocytes taken from actively drinking alcoholics were reduced by approximately 76%. These data from alcoholics support the laboratory findings and suggest that chronic alcohol use may desensitize receptor-coupled cAMP-mediated signal transduction in a variety of cell types. More work is needed to understand how these changes may influence drinking behavior.

Dopamine: As mentioned earlier in this chapter, increases in mesolimbic dopamine are thought to be associated with the reinforcing effects of many drugs of abuse, including alcohol. Electrophysiologic studies have demonstrated that alcohol increases the firing of dopamine-containing neurons, which arise in the VTA and project to the nucleus accumbens and other mesolimbic areas (Brodie, Shefner et al., 1990). The mechanism underlying this effect of alcohol is not precisely known, but appears to involve a direct effect of alcohol on VTA neurons (Brodie, Pesold et al., 1999). Interestingly, the sensitivity of VTA neurons to alcohol-induced excitation is lower in mice that show a higher voluntary consumption of alcohol, suggesting that the animals consume more alcohol to sufficiently activate a dopaminergic reward pathway (Brodie & Appel, 2000). Alcohol was shown to directly enhance the basal efflux of dopamine from striatal slices, although the concentrations required for this effect are very high (Snape & Engel, 1988).

Another approach that was used to increase the understanding of the role of dopamine in alcohol addiction involves pharmacologic agonists and antagonists that directly interact with dopamine receptors. Studies using dopamine receptor antagonists to probe the reinforcing properties of alcohol were limited in some cases by the nonspecific motor effects of these drugs. The use of dopamine agonists to mimic the effects of alcohol provided some indirect evidence that dopamine may be involved in alcohol-drinking behavior in animals. The long-acting dopamine agonist bromocriptine (Parlodel®), administered systemically, shifted the animal's preference from alcohol to water, especially in those strains of rats that show alcohol preference (Weiss, Mitchiner et al., 1990). Similar findings were demonstrated with another dopamine agonist, apomorphine. These results suggested that administration of direct dopamine agonists reduced the need for alcohol's dopamine-enhancing activity in these animals, such that the "reward state" was achieved at lower alcohol levels. These studies provide compelling but indirect evidence that alcohol's addictive properties involve alterations in mesolimbic dopamine and offer possible sites of action for drug-based therapies.

Opioids: The involvement of endogenous opioids (endorphins and enkephalins) in alcohol addiction is suggested by several lines of research. One of the first links between alcohol and opioids was suggested by the finding that acetaldehyde could undergo a metabolic reaction with monoamines to form compounds (tetrahydrisoquinolines or TIQs) that were structurally related to morphine (Davis & Walsh, 1970). TIQs were shown to elicit alcohol-drinking behavior and alcohol preference even after cessation of TIQ administration (Meyers, 1989). This hypothesis, although attractive, remains controversial because of the inability to replicate some of these findings and the demonstration that TIQ formation *in vivo* could be accounted by dietary factors rather than direct effects of alcohol (Collins, 1988). Alcohol was shown to increase the release of certain opioids (such as beta endorphin) from rat pituitary glands, as well as to increase blood levels of beta endorphins in humans (Gianoulakis & Barcomb, 1987; Gianoulakis, 1989). If alcohol drinking is mediated in part by opioids, then selective opioid antagonists should inhibit alcohol-drinking behavior. Naloxone and naltrexone (ReVia®), both opioid antagonists, were shown to reduce alcohol intake, although large doses were required to produce these effects (Altshuler, Phillips et al., 1980; Sandi, Borell et al., 1988). Moreover, opiate antagonists reduce consumption of a wide variety of foods and of water (Hynes, Gallagher et al., 1981) and were found not to alter the alcohol preference of rats bred for this trait (Weiss, Mitchiner et al., 1990). Other studies found that these opiate antagonists reduced alcohol preference, although differences in the methods used to determine these effects may underlie the apparent discrepancies.

Serotonin: Electrophysiologic studies have demonstrated that alcohol enhances cation conductance through 5-HT$_3$ receptors (Lovinger & White, 1991). These alterations could have important consequences, depending on the location of these receptors and the extent to which they are potentiated. Serotonin interacts with a number of 5-HT-specific receptors that are coupled to various signal transduction pathways. The direct effects of alcohol on these receptor systems are not as well characterized. However, there is a fairly large amount of literature describing the effects on alcohol-drinking behavior of various drugs that modulate serotonergic tone. 5-HT and 5-HT-metabolite levels are reduced in the cerebrospinal fluid of many alcohol abusers, suggesting that reduced 5-HT levels or a reduction in 5-HT-mediated neurotransmission may predispose certain people to uncontrollable drinking behavior (reviewed in Sellers, Higgins et al., 1992).

It has been suggested that similar deficiencies in 5-HT neurotransmission underlie the development of a variety of other disorders, including bulimia and obsessive-compulsive behavior, which are characterized by a loss of behavioral control. This hypothesis is supported by studies in which certain pharmacologic agents that enhance 5-HT neurotransmission (such as selective-uptake inhibitors) appear to be therapeutically effective in the treatment of these disorders. Similarly, these agents (such as zimeldine, fluoxetine [Prozac®], and sertraline [Zoloft®]) were also shown to decrease alcohol intake in both animals and humans. It should be noted that the magnitude of these effects is small (<20%) and is confounded by the finding that increasing synaptic concentrations of 5-HT is associated with reductions in food intake, suggesting that the effect of these drugs on alcohol intake may be nonselective. However, the involvement of the serotonergic system in modulating drinking behavior is supported by a report that showed that alcohol consumption was increased in genetic knock-out mice lacking the 5-HT1b receptor (Crabbe, Phillips et al., 1996). Food and water consumption were normal in these animals, and the animals were less sensitive to the ataxic effects of alcohol. These types of studies in which specific receptor subunits can be deleted from the animal genome may help unravel the importance of various neurotransmitter systems in alcohol's actions on brain and behavior.

Neuroimaging Studies. A variety of brain imaging techniques have been applied to the study of alcoholism and alcohol abuse (reviewed in Sullivan, 2000). These techniques include computed tomography, magnetic resonance imaging (MRI), single photon emission computed tomography (SPECT), and positron emission tomography (PET). Imaging studies of human alcoholics have found increases in cortical cerebrospinal fluid in both gray and white matter, distinct from that found in other neuropsychiatric disorders such as schizophrenia and Alzheimer's disease. When corrected for age-related changes in these parameters, the frontal lobes and cerebellar gray matter are particularly sensitive to alcohol-induced damage. MRI studies have shown that volume deficits are found in anterior but not posterior hippocampus and that these deficits were more severe in patients who displayed symptoms of memory loss and possible Korsakoff's syndrome. Prenatal as well as adult exposure to alcohol was shown to disrupt and reduce the area of the corpus callosum. Functional imaging techniques were used to study alcohol-related changes in brain function. These techniques monitor the levels of certain metabolites (N-acetyl-aspartate and myo-inositol) that may give useful information as to the integrity and functional status of the cells of the brain. Results from these studies show improvements in neuronal integrity and energy status during abstinence in recently detoxified alcoholics. PET studies have been used to monitor brain glucose metabolism and have shown reduced brain glucose metabolism in alcoholics compared with control subjects. PET studies have shown that brain glucose metabolism increases 16 to 30 days after withdrawal, consistent with improvements in neuronal integrity measured by MRI. SPECT studies can detect changes in cerebral blood flow and have shown that alcoholics may have low perfusion of frontal lobe areas. PET, SPECT, and functional MRI have been used to measure activation of specific brain areas during certain types of cognitive testing, thus allowing one to map specific activities to selected brain structures. Recent imaging studies in human drug addicts and alcoholics showed that specific brain areas are involved in the craving for alcohol and other drugs of abuse (reviewed in Hommer, 1999). For example, cocaine users watching cocaine-related videotapes showed increased blood flow in the amygdala, dorsal lateral frontal cortex, and anterior cingulate cortex and decreased blood flow in the caudate nucleus. Imaging studies in human alcoholics are few and are not as conclusive as those with cocaine, although changes in blood flow in the caudate nucleus were observed.

ADDICTION LIABILITY

Chronic exposure to alcohol in both animals and man induces changes in alcohol sensitivity that can be manifested as sensitization, tolerance, and dependence.

Sensitization. Sensitization is defined as an increase in the pharmacologic and physiologic response to a drug after repeated exposures. These phenomena are best characterized by drugs of abuse such as cocaine, in which changes occur in dopaminergic signaling in the neurons of the VTA. Sensitization to the locomotor effects of alcohol have been reported, but this effect is strain- and species-dependent. Another form of sensitization is characterized by an increase in the severity and intensity of withdrawal signs after multiple episodes of alcohol intoxication and withdrawal (Becker & Hale, 1993). This form of sensitization has been suggested to be similar to the kindling phenomena observed after repeated brain seizures and may involve some of the same mechanisms that are related to cellular adaptation to impaired neuronal signaling.

Tolerance and Dependence. Tolerance is manifested as a reduced sensitivity to alcohol and is subdivided into

several forms, depending on the specific action being measured. For example, concentrations of alcohol required to produce sedation may increase in individuals or animals given alcohol chronically. In human alcoholics, tolerance to the sedative and even lethal effects of alcohol can be profound. Dependence is defined as the occurrence of symptoms that appear after the cessation of alcohol drinking. These symptoms include both physical (tremors, convulsions) and psychological (negative emotions) components. At the cellular level, tolerance and dependence can develop so that the effects of alcohol on ion channel function may be diminished in animals chronically exposed to alcohol. As mentioned in the earlier section, adaptation to alcohol may involve changes in subunit expression and phosphorylation state of the ion channel as cells attempt to adapt to the chronic presence of alcohol.

Craving and Relapse: A main feature of human alcoholism is the strong desire or "craving" for alcohol in subjects under treatment for alcohol abuse. Bouts of heavy drinking often follow periods of abstinence even when the symptoms of alcohol withdrawal have long subsided. This occurrence suggests that prolonged alcohol abuse may involve long-lasting or permanent changes in brain systems that alter a person's responsiveness to alcohol. An animal model of craving and relapse has been established that involves depriving animals of alcohol after periods of voluntary consumption. In most cases, animals display a robust increase in alcohol consumption after deprivation, and this effect is characterized by not only higher rates of drinking but also increased preference for solutions containing higher ethanol concentrations. In addition, this deprivation effect on subsequent drinking persists for very long periods of abstinence (up to 9 months), suggesting irreversible changes in mechanisms regulating drinking behavior. These models have obvious importance with respect to testing pharmacologic treatments that may reduce the increase in alcohol consumption after long periods of deprivation. Several studies have shown that drugs such as acamprosate (calcium N-acetylhomotaurine) may reduce or reverse the increase in ethanol intake produced by periods of forced deprivation (Spanagel & Zieglgansberger, 1997). Although the mechanism of action underlying this effect is not well understood, it raises the possibility of developing pharmacologic treatments that are effective in reducing the incidence and severity of relapse among human alcoholics.

Withdrawal. Dependence is an important factor in continued drinking by an alcoholic because cessation of alcohol drinking induces unpleasant and occasionally life-threatening symptoms of withdrawal.

TOXICITY/ADVERSE EFFECTS

Neurotoxicity. Brain dysfunction after heavy drinking is widespread, and it is estimated that alcohol-induced dementia is the second leading cause of adult dementia in the United States, behind Alzheimer's disease. Studies of alcoholic brains show that heavy drinking causes noticeable changes in brain structure. These changes include enlarged cerebral ventricles and sulci, which are paralleled by decreases in overall brain density. Although heavy drinking is associated with loss of neurons in most areas of the brain, certain regions—such as the frontal cortex—are particularly susceptible to alcohol-induced cell loss. Such neuron loss may underlie the changes in cognitive and emotional behaviors observed in alcoholics.

Although a lifetime of heavy drinking long has been known to produce substantial changes in brain neuron density, recent data obtained in animal studies suggest that episodes of heavy drinking, or binges, are effective in causing neuron loss. This loss is particularly important as the incidence of heavy binge drinking among high-school and college-aged men and women appears to have increased.

The mechanisms underlying ethanol-induced neurotoxicity are not completely understood. There is a consensus that some forms of ethanol-induced damage may arise from over-activation of NMDA receptors during ethanol withdrawal. Thus, chronic exposure of neurons to ethanol induces an up-regulation in the functional status of the NMDA receptor that is revealed during ethanol withdrawal (Chandler, Newson et al., 1993). It is not completely clear whether enhanced NMDA receptor function, which usually follows chronic ethanol ingestion, is due to increases in NMDA receptor subunit protein or whether there is a redistribution of these receptors from nonsynaptic to synaptic sites. In either case, in the absence of ethanol, enhanced receptor activation by glutamate may lead to above-normal production of cellular signals that contribute to cell death.

In other cases of ethanol-induced neurotoxicity, it appears that a non–NMDA-mediated mechanism is at work. In an acute binge model of alcohol intoxication, rats given large doses of alcohol over a three- to four-day period show pronounced loss of neurons in specific brain areas, including the entorhinal cortex and dentate gyrus. The toxic actions of ethanol were not blocked by NMDA antagonists, but were attenuated by the diuretic furosemide (Lasix®), suggesting other pathways for ethanol-induced brain damage (Collins, Zhou et al., 1998).

Effects on Major Organ Systems. Alcohol affects nearly all tissue and organ systems studied, and heavy drinkers show damage to tissues such as brain, liver, and heart, as well as increased susceptibility to some diseases and increased skeletal fragility. Evidence suggests that alcohol may slightly enhance a woman's risk of developing breast cancer. Despite the negative effects, beneficial effects of moderate alcohol intake have been demonstrated. These include a reduced risk of coronary heart disease in individuals classified as light to moderate drinkers. Two factors that are important in determining whether alcohol drinking is associated with positive or negative effects are how an individual drinks and for how long. Most beneficial effects of alcohol are associated with light to moderate drinking, consisting of two or fewer drinks per day for men and one or less per day for women. These amounts are well below those experienced by alcohol abusers or alcoholics, who may consume more than 10 to 12 drinks per day. At higher levels, significant toxicity develops in most tissues, including the brain.

Teratogenicity. Heavy alcohol use during pregnancy can lead to a variety of birth defects and alterations in normal growth and development of the newborn. Fetal alcohol syndrome (FAS) consists of a variety of characteristic symptoms in newborns exposed to alcohol *in utero*. One in three infants born to alcoholic mothers displays symptoms of FAS, including CNS dysfunction, such as low IQ and microcephaly; delayed growth; and facial abnormalities, among others. FAS generally is associated with heavy drinking, especially early in pregnancy, although it is not known if there is any safe lower limit for alcohol consumption (for a detailed discussion, see Section 10).

GENETIC CONTRIBUTIONS TO ALCOHOLISM AND ALCOHOL ABUSE

Studies involving twins and their families, and the sons and daughters of alcoholics, suggest that an individual's vulnerability to alcohol has a genetic component. For example, studies by Schuckit (1991) examined the acute effects of alcohol on sons of alcoholic fathers and sons of nonalcoholic fathers. Both groups were given an alcohol-containing beverage or a placebo and used a self-rating scale to describe their feelings of drunkenness, dizziness, drug effect, sleepiness, and other subjective characteristics after the alcohol beverage challenge. Sons of alcoholic fathers consistently scored themselves lower than sons of nonalcoholic fathers on these measures of acute alcohol effects. In separate studies involving sons and daughters of alcoholic and nonalcoholic fathers, similar results were found when measurements of body sway or ataxia were measured after the alcohol challenge. These results suggest that sons of alcoholic fathers experience a less intense reaction to alcohol than sons of nonalcoholic fathers, which could be related to the future risk of developing alcoholism in these men.

Results from twin studies demonstrated a substantial heritability to alcoholism (up to 50%) in both men and women. However, the genes that are responsible for a predisposition to alcoholism have not been identified. Genetic linkage and association studies have suggested that there are multiple genes, located on various chromosomes, that influence susceptibility to alcoholism. Candidates for these genes include enzymes that are involved in the metabolism of alcohol, as well as those that may be involved in mediating alcohol's acute effects on brain function, such as specific ion channel subunits.

Studies of ADH and ALDH variants suggest that genetically determined differences in metabolic or other key biochemical processes may play a role in the development of alcohol addiction in certain individuals. For example, about half of all persons of Japanese ancestry have a variant of the mitochondrial form of ALDH, which is less able to metabolize acetaldehyde (Goedde, Harada et al., 1979; Harada, Agarwal et al., 1980; Teng, 1981). Levels of acetaldehyde in these persons after ingestion of alcohol may be 10 times higher than in an individual with the normal mitochondrial variant of ALDH. In such persons, even small amounts of alcohol can produce the so-called "alcohol flush reaction," which consists of facial flushing, vasodilation, tachycardia, and headaches. Nausea, vomiting, edema, and hypotension can occur at higher levels of alcohol consumption. These symptoms resemble those seen after ingestion of alcohol in patients taking disulfiram (Antabuse®), which inhibits the actions of ALDH.

Interestingly, the presence of this less-efficient ALDH isozyme appears to have a significant effect on drinking behavior. The presence of the ALDH variant is associated with lower drinking frequencies and amounts of alcohol consumed, suggesting that the ALDH variant is protective against heavy drinking and alcoholism. Conversely, the ALDH variant is rare in Japanese alcoholics with alcoholic liver disease (Harada, Agarwal et al., 1983). Other studies extended the findings to populations of Taiwanese and Chinese ancestry (Thomasson, Mai et al., 1989). An ALDH variant that reduces the individual's ability to metabolize acetaldehyde has not yet been detected in populations of European descent. Women generally have been found to possess less gastric mucosal ADH activity than do men (Frezza, Di Padova et al., 1990). This occurrence results in significantly higher blood alcohol levels after alcohol ingestion in women; even more, in fact, than would be expected based solely on differences in liver weight. This finding may contribute to an enhanced vulnerability of women to the acute and chronic effects of alcohol.

The search for genes that contribute to alcohol vulnerability is intensifying, as the results of the human genome project are made available and new techniques for analyzing changes in gene expression are developed. Researchers long have used animal models to examine the influence of genetics on alcohol sensitivity and have used selective breeding to generate strains of mice and rats that respond differently to alcohol. These studies are useful because humans and rodents share most of their genes and respond to alcohol in similar ways, suggesting that it may be possible to identify genes that contribute to alcohol sensitivity by using selected lines of animals. In addition, recent advances in gene detection techniques such as those used in DNA microarray analysis allow for investigators to examine what gene products are altered in various disease states or after chronic drug or alcohol exposure. The ability to monitor changes in the levels of thousands of gene products simultaneously may lead to identification of a gene profile that can identify those individuals who are most at risk of developing alcohol-related problems.

CONCLUSIONS

It is clear that, over the past 10 to 20 years, a great deal of progress has been made in understanding the sites and mechanisms of alcohol's effects on the brain. A consensus is emerging that ligand-gated ion channels represent a likely site for the acute effects of alcohol on neuronal function. Adaptation of neurons to the continued presence of alcohol may involve changes in the expression and distribution of these ion channel subunits and their downstream signaling processes and thus result in a permanently altered neuropsychologic state in some individuals, which is defined as alcoholism. More work is needed with transgenic animals that overexpress ion channels with altered alcohol sensitivity to better understand the correlation between these channels and alcohol's behavioral effects. For example, if ion channels gated by glutamate, GABA, acetylcholine, and serotonin represent primary targets of alcohol action, how do these effects influence behaviors such as reward, craving, and reinforcement, which appear to involve complex neurocircuitry and multiple neurotransmitters such as dopamine, opioids, and serotonin?

Other areas that need attention include elucidating the normal physiologic processes that operate in nonalcoholics in response to food and other reinforcers, as well as what is different in alcoholics that drives their excessive drinking. More work is needed to bridge the gap between single cell and recombinant receptor studies and those performed in whole animals so that alcohol's actions on neuronal signaling in intact circuits can be determined. Better use of brain imaging techniques in conjunction with electrophysiologic recording would improve our understanding of the neural regions that are involved in mediating the various behaviors associated with alcohol abuse and alcoholism.

ACKNOWLEDGMENTS: Development of this chapter was supported by grants RO1-AA09986 and KO2-AA00238 from the National Institute on Alcohol Abuse and Alcoholism.

REFERENCES

Aistrup GL, Marszalec W & Narahashi T (1999). Ethanol modulation of nicotinic acetylcholine receptor currents in cultured cortical neurons. *Molecular Pharmacology* 55:39-49.

Altshuler HL, Phillips PE & Feinhandler DA (1980). Alterations of ethanol self-administration by naltrexone. *Life Sciences* 26:679-688.

Anders DL, Blevins T, Smothers CT et al. (2000). Reduced ethanol inhibition of N-methyl-D-aspartate receptors by deletion of the NR1 C0 domain or over-expression of alpha-actinin-2 proteins. *Journal of Biological Chemistry* 275:15019-15024.

Anders DL, Blevins T, Sutton G et al. (1999). Fyn tyrosinekinase reduces the ethanol inhibition of recombinant NR1/NR2A but not NR1/NR2B receptors expressed in HEK cells. *Journal of Neurochemistry* 72:1389-1393.

Becker HC & Hale RL (1993). Repeated episodes of ethanol withdrawal potentiate the severity of subsequent withdrawal seizures: An animal model of alcohol withdrawal. *Alcoholism: Clinical & Experimental Research* 17:94-98.

Blevins T, Mirshahi T & Woodward JJ (1995). Increased agonist and antagonist sensitivity of N-methyl-D-aspartate stimulated calcium flux in cultured neurons following chronic ethanol exposure. *Neuroscience Letters* 200:214-218.

Brodie MS & Appel SB (2000). Dopaminergic neurons in the ventral tegmental area of C57BL/6J and DBA/2J mice differ in sensitivity to ethanol excitation. *Alcoholism: Clinical & Experimental Research* 24:1120-1124.

Brodie MS, Pesold C & Appel SB (1999). Ethanol directly excites dopaminergic ventral tegmental area reward neurons. *Alcoholism: Clinical & Experimental Research* 23:1848-1852.

Brodie MS, Shefner SA & Dunwiddie TV (1990). Ethanol increases the firing rate of dopamine neurons of the rat ventral tegmental area in vitro. *Brain Research* 508:65-69.

Cardoso RA, Brozowski SJ, Chavez-Noriega LE et al. (1999). Effects of ethanol on recombinant human neuronal nicotinic acetylcholine receptors expressed in Xenpus oocytes. *Journal of Pharmacology and Experimental Therapeutics* 289:774-780.

Chandler LJ, Newsom H, Sumners C et al. (1993). Chronic ethanol exposure potentiates NMDA excitotoxicity in cerebral cortical neurons. *Journal of Neurochemistry* 60:1578-1581.

Cloninger CR (1987). Neurogenetic adaptive mechanisms in alcoholism. *Science* 236:410-416.

Collins MA (1988). Acetaldehyde and its condensation products as markers in alcoholism. In M Galanter (ed.) *Recent Developments in Alcoholism*, Vol. 6. New York, NY: Plenum Press, 387-403.

Collins MA, Zhou JY & Neafsey EJ (1998). Brain damage due to episodic alcohol exposure in vivo and in vitro: Furosemide neuroprotection implicates edema-based mechanism. *FASEB Journal* 12:221-230.

Colombo G & Grant KA (1992). NMDA receptor complex antagonists have ethanol-like discriminative stimulus effects. *Annals of the New York Academy of Sciences* 654:421-423.

Crabbe JC, Phillips TJ, Feller DJ et al. (1996). Elevated alcohol consumption in null mutant mice lacking 5-HT1b serotonin receptors. *Nature Genetics* 14:98-101.

Davis VE & Walsh MJ (1970). Alcohol, amines, and alkaloids: A possible biochemical basis for alcohol addiction. *Science* 167:1005-1007.

Diamond I, Nagy L, Mochly-Rosen D et al. (1991). The role of adenosine and adenosine transport in ethanol-induced cellular tolerance and dependence: Possible biologic and genetic markers of alcoholism. *Annals of the New York Academy of Sciences* 625:473-487.

Di Chiara G, Imperato A & Mulas A (1988). Preferential stimulation of dopamine release in mesolimbic systems: A common feature of drugs of abuse. In M Sandler, C Feuerstein & B Scatton (eds.) *Neurotransmitter Interactions in the Basal Ganglia*. New York, NY: Raven Press, 171-182.

Dolin S, Little H, Hudspith M et al. (1987). Increased dihydropyridine-sensitive calcium channels in rat brain may underlie ethanol physical dependence. *Neuropharmacology* 26:275-279.

Dopico AM, Chu B, Lemos JR et al. (1999). Alcohol modulation of calcium-activated potassium channels. *Neurochemistry International* 35:103-106.

Fadda F, Mosca E, Colombo G et al. (1989). Effects of spontaneous ingestion of ethanol on brain dopamine metabolism. *Life Science* 44:281-287.

Follesa P & Ticku MK (1995). Chronic ethanol treatment differentially regulates NMDA receptor subunit mRNA expression in rat brain. *Molecular Brain Research* 29:99-105.

Forman SA & Miller KW (1989). Molecular sites of anesthetic action in postsynaptic nicotinic membranes. *Trends in Pharmacological Science* 10:447-452.

Frezza M, Di Padova C, Pozzato G et al. (1990). High blood alcohol levels in women: The role of decreased gastric alcohol dehydrogenase activity and first-pass metabolism. *New England Journal of Medicine* 322:95-99.

Gianoulakis C (1989). The effect of ethanol on the biosynthesis and regulation of opioid peptides. *Experientia* 45:428-435.

Gianoulakis C & Barcomb A (1987). Effect of acute ethanol in vivo and in vitro on the beta endorphin system in the rat. *Life Science* 40:19-28.

Goedde HW, Harada S & Agarwal DP (1979). Racial differences in alcohol sensitivity: A new hypothesis. *Human Genetics* 51:331-334.

Gonzales RA & Woodward JJ (1990). Ethanol inhibits N-methyl-D-aspartate-stimulated [³H]norepinephrine release from rat cortical slices. *Journal of Pharmacology and Experimental Therapeutics* 252:1138-1144.

Gothert M & Fink K (1989). Inhibition of N-methyl-D-aspartate (NMDA)- and L-glutamate-induced noradrenaline and acetylcholine release in the rat brain by ethanol. *Naunyn-Schmiedeberg's Archives of Pharmacology* 340:516-521.

Grant KA & Barrett JE (1991). Blockade of the discriminative stimulus effects of ethanol with 5-HT3 receptor antagonists. *Pyschopharmacology* (Berl.) 104:451-456.

Grant KA, Valverius P, Hudspith M et al. (1990). Ethanol withdrawal seizures and the NMDA receptor complex. *European Journal of Pharmacology* 176:289-296.

Grobin AC, Papadeas ST & Morrow AL (2000). Regional variations in the effects of chronic ethanol administration on GABAA receptor expression: Potential mechanisms. *Neurochemistry International* 37:453-461.

Harada S, Agarwal DP & Goedde HW (1980). Electrophoretic and biochemical studies of human acetaldehyde dehydrogenase isozymes in various tissues. *Life Science* 26:1773-1780.

Harada S, Agarwal DP, Goedde HW et al. (1983). Aldehyde dehydrogenase isoenzyme variation and alcoholism in Japan. *Pharmacology, Biochemistry and Behavior* 18(Suppl 1):151-153.

Hoffman PL, Moses F & Tabakoff B (1989). Selective inhibition by ethanol of glutamate-stimulated cyclic GMP production in primary cultures of cerebellar granule cells. *Neuropharmacology* 28:1239-1243.

Homanics GE, Harrison NL, Quinlan JJ et al. (1999). Normal electrophysiological and behavioral responses to ethanol in mice lacking the long splice variant of the gamma2 subunit of the gamma-aminobutyrate type A receptor. *Neuropharmacology* 38:253-65.

Hommer DW (1999). Functional imaging of craving. *Alcohol Research & Health* 23:187-196.

Hwang BH, Lumeng L, Wu JY et al. (1990). Increased number of GABAergic terminals in the nucleus accumbens is associated with alcohol preference in rats. *Alcoholism: Clinical & Experimental Research* 14:503-507.

Hynes MA, Gallagher M & Yacos KV (1981). Systemic and intraventricular naloxone administration: Effects on food and water intake. *Behavioral and Neural Biology* 32:334-342.

Imperato A & Di Chiara G (1986). Preferential stimulation of dopamine release in the nucleus accumbens of freely moving rats by ethanol. *Journal of Pharmacology and Experimental Therapeutics* 239:219-239.

Iorio KR, Reinlib L, Tabakoff B et al. (1992). Chronic exposure of cerebellar granule cells to ethanol results in increased N-methyl-D-aspartate receptor function. *Molecular Pharmacology* 41:1142-1148.

Khatib SA, Murphy JM & McBride WJ (1988). Biochemical evidence for activation of specific monoamine pathways by ethanol. *Alcohol* 5:295-299.

Koles L, Wirkner K, Furst S et al. (2000). Tricholorethanol inhibits ATP-induced membrane currents in cultured HEK 293-hP2X3 cells. *European Journal of Pharmacology* 409:R3-R5.

Koob GF, Roberts AJ, Schulteis G et al. (1998). Neurocircuitry targets in ethanol reward and dependence. *Alcoholism: Clinical & Experimental Research* 22:3-9.

Krystal JH, Petrakis IL, Webb E et al. (1998). Dose-related ethanol-like effects of the NMDA antagonist, ketamine, in recently detoxified alcoholics. *Archives of General Psychiatry* 55:354-360.

Kuner T, Schoepfer R & Korpi ER (1993). Ethanol inhibits glutamate-induced currents in heteromeric NMDA receptor subtypes. *Neuroreport* 5:297-300.

Leslie SW, Barr E, Chandler J et al. (1983). Inhibition of fast- and slow-phase depolarization-dependent synaptosomal calcium uptake by ethanol. *Journal of Pharmacology and Experimental Therapeutics* 225:571-575.

Li C, Peoples RW & Weight FF (1994). Alcohol action on a neuronal membrane receptor: Evidence for a direct interaction with the receptor protein. *Proceedings of the National Academy of Sciences* 91:8200-8204.

Litten RZ & Allen JP (1991). Pharmacotherapies for alcoholism: Promising agents and clinical issues. *Alcoholism: Clinical & Experimental Research* 15:620-633.

Lovinger DM (1995). Developmental decrease in ethanol inhibition of N-methyl-D-aspartate receptors in rat neocortical neurons: Relation to the actions of ifenprodil. *Journal of Pharmacology and Experimental Therapeutics* 274:164-172.

Lovinger DM & White G (1991). Ethanol potentiation of 5-hydroxytryptamine₃ receptor-mediated ion current in neuroblastoma cells and isolated adult mammalian neurons. *Molecular Pharmacology* 40:263-270.

Lovinger DM, White G & Weight FF (1989). Ethanol inhibits NMDA activated ion current in hippocampal neurons. *Science* 243:1721-1724.

Mascia MP, Machu TK & Harris RA (1996). Enhancement of homomeric glycine receptor function by long-chain alcohols and anesthetics. *British Journal of Pharmacology* 119:1331-1336.

Masood K, Wu C, Brauneis U et al. (1994). Differential ethanol sensitivity of recombinant N-methyl-D-aspartate receptor subunits. *Molecular Pharmacology* 45:324-329.

Messing RO, Carpenter CL, Diamond I et al. (1986). Ethanol regulates calcium channels in clonal neural cells. *Proceedings of the National Academy of Sciences* 83:6213-6215.

Meyers RD (1989). Isoquinolines, beta-carbolines and alcohol drinking: Involvement of opioid and dopaminergic mechanisms. *Experientia* 45:436-443.

Mihic SJ, Ye Q, Wick MJ et al. (1997). Sites of alcohol and volatile anaesthetic action on GABA(A) and glycine receptors. *Nature* 389:385-389.

Mirshahi T & Woodward JJ (1995). Ethanol sensitivity of heteromeric NMDA receptors: Effects of subunit assembly, glycine and NMDAR1 Mg2+-insensitive mutants. *Neuropharmacology* 34:347-355.

Noronha A, Eckhardt M & Warren K, eds. (2000). *Review of NIAAA's Neuroscience and Behavioral Research Portfolio (Research Monograph 34)*. Rockville, MD: National Institute on Alcohol Abuse and Alcoholism.

Quinlan JJ, Firestone LL & Homanics GE (2000). Mice lacking the long splice variant of the gamma 2 subunit of the GABA(A) receptor are more sensitive to benzodiazepines. *Pharmacology, Biochemistry and Behavior* 66:371-374.

Sandi C, Borell J & Gusaz C (1988). Naloxone decreases ethanol consumption within a free choice paradigm in rats. *Pharmacology, Biochemistry and Behavior* 29:39-43.

Schuckit MA (1991). A longitudinal study of children of alcoholics. *Recent Developments in Alcoholism* 9:5-19.

Sellers EM, Higgins GA & Sobell MB (1992). 5-HT and alcohol abuse. *Trends in Pharmacological Science* 13:69-75.

Simson PE, Criswell HE & Breese GR (1991). Inhibition of NMDA-evoked electrophysiological activity by ethanol in selected brain regions: Evidence for ethanol-sensitive and ethanol-insensitive NMDA-evoked responses. *Brain Research* 607:9-16.

Smothers CT, Clayton R, Blevins T et al. (2001). Ethanol sensitivity of recombinant human N-methyl-D-aspartate receptors. *Neurochemistry International* 38:333-340.

Snape BM & Engel JA (1988). Ethanol enhances the calcium-dependent stimulus-induced release of endogenous dopamine from slices of rat striatum and nucleus accumbens in vitro. *Neuropharmacology* 27:1097-1101.

Snell LD, Nunley KR, Lickteig RL et al. (1996). Regional and subunit specific changes in NMDA receptor mRNA and immunoreactivity in mouse brain following chronic ethanol ingestion. *Molecular Brain Research* 40:71-78.

Spanagel R & Zieglgansberger W (1997). Anti-craving compounds for ethanol: New pharmacological tools for studying addictive processes. *Trends in Pharmacological Sciences* 18:54-59.

Sullivan EV (2000). Human brain vulnerability to alcoholism: Evidence from neuroimaging studies. In A Noronha, M Eckhardt & K Warren (eds.) *Review of NIAAA's Neuroscience and Behavioral Research Portfolio (Research Monograph 34)*. Rockville, MD: National Institute on Alcohol Abuse and Alcoholism, 473-508.

Teng YS (1981). Human liver aldehyde dehydrogenase in Chinese and Asiatic Indians: Gene deletion and its possible implications in alcohol metabolism. *Biochemical Genetics* 19:107-114.

Thomasson HR, Mai XL, Crabb DW et al. (1989). Aldehyde dehydrogenase deficiency: Relationship of aldehyde dehydrogenase-2 genotype with risk for alcoholism in Taiwanese. *Clinical Research* 37:898A.

U.S. Public Health Service (USPHS) (2000). *Tenth Special Report to the U.S. Congress on Alcohol and Health*. Washington, DC: Department of Health and Human Services.

Wafford KA, Burnett DM, Leidenheimer NJ et al. (1991). Ethanol sensitivity of the GABAa receptor expressed in Xenopus oocytes requires 8 amino acids contained in the gamma 2L subunit of the receptor complex. *Neuron* 7:27-33.

Wafford KA & Whiting PJ (1992). Ethanol potentiation of GABAa receptors requires phosphorylation of the alternatively spliced variant of the g2 subunit. *FEBS Letters* 313:113-117.

Walter HJ & Messing RO (1999). Regulation of neuronal voltage-gated calcium channels by ethanol. *Neurochemistry International* 35:95-101.

Watkins JC & Collingridge GL, eds. (1994). *The NMDA Receptor*. Oxford, England: IRL Press.

Weiss F, Hurd YL, Ungerstedt U et al. (1992). Neurochemical correlates of cocaine and ethanol self-administration. *Annals of the New York Academy of Sciences* 654:220-241.

Weiss F, Mitchiner M, Bloom FE et al. (1990). Free-choice responding for ethanol versus water in alcohol-preferring (P) and unselected Wistar rats is differentially altered by naloxone, bromocriptine and methysergide. *Psychopharmacology* 101:178-186.

Woodward JJ & Gonzales RA (1990). Ethanol inhibition of N-methyl-D-aspartate-stimulated endogenous dopamine release from rat striatal slices: Reversal by glycine. *Journal of Neurochemistry* 54:712-715.

Xiong K, Li C & Weight FF (2000). Inhibition by ethanol of rat P2X4 receptors expressed in Xenopus oocytes. *British Journal of Pharmacology* 130:1394-1398.

Youngren KD, Daly DA & Moghaddam B (1993). Distinct actions of endogenous excitatory amino acids on the outflow of dopamine in the nucleus accumbens. *Journal of Pharmacology and Experimental Therapeutics* 264:289-293.

Chapter 3

The Pharmacology of Benzodiazepines and Other Sedative-Hypnotics

Steven M. Juergens, M.D., FASAM
Debra S. Cowley, M.D.

Drugs in the Class
Absorption and Metabolism
Pharmacologic Actions
Mechanisms of Action
Addiction Liability
Toxicity/Adverse Effects
Future Research Directions

Sedatives, hypnotics, and anxiolytic drugs—all central nervous system (CNS) depressants—traditionally are used to reduce anxiety and/or induce sleep. Bromide was introduced as a sedative in the 1850s, barbiturates in the early 1900s, benzodiazepines in the early 1960s, and non-benzodiazepine omega-1 agonist hypnotics in the 1990s. Critical examination of their use continues, with particular attention to concerns about dependence and addiction.

DRUGS IN THE CLASS

The benzodiazepines and the non-benzodiazepine omega-1 agonists are the primary focus of this chapter, as they have largely supplanted the barbiturate and barbiturate-like sedative-hypnotics. The chapter focuses mostly on the pharmacology of benzodiazepines, but briefly reviews other sedative-hypnotics (including barbiturates, meprobamate, chloryl hydrate, and glutethimide), whose use has diminished and whose clinical applications have become less relevant. This chapter also discusses buspirone and some newer novel non-benzodiazepine sedative-hypnotics.

Benzodiazepines. The core structure of benzodiazepines consists of a benzene ring fused to a 7-membered 1,4 diazepine ring, hence the name. Almost all have a 5-aryl substituent ring. They differ from one another in the chemical nature of the substituent groups at positions 1, 2, 3, and 4 (of the diazepine ring), position 7 (of the benzene ring), and position 2' (of the 5-aryl substituent ring).

Benzodiazepines are used clinically for their anxiolytic and sedative-hypnotic effects. (Their use in alcohol withdrawal is covered in Section 5.) They also are used as anticonvulsants and muscle relaxants (uses that will not be reviewed here).

Panic Disorder: Panic disorder responds to benzodiazepines, with alprazolam (Xanax®) the drug most extensively studied, although it appears that many benzodiazepines can be effective in short-term treatment if they are given in adequate doses (Moller, 1999). The usual dose is the equivalent of 2 to 6 mg of alprazolam daily. Selective serotonin reuptake inhibitors (SSRIs) generally are seen as first-line pharmacotherapy for panic disorder, but a combination of a benzodiazepine and an antidepressant or even benzodiazepine alone often is used (Uhlenhuth, Balter et al., 1998). Benzodiazepines have a rapid onset of action compared with antidepressants. However, they do not treat the comorbid depression that can develop with panic disorder, and there is concern about dependence and withdrawal. Research indicates that maintenance therapy does not lead to tolerance requiring increasing doses of benzodiazepines, even with the use of high-potency benzodiazepines. Over time, the benzodiazepine dose usually is decreased, and completion of long-term maintenance is strongly associated with remission.

Generalized Anxiety Disorder: Benzodiazepines are used for the treatment of generalized anxiety disorder (GAD). GAD is a diagnosis with poor interrater reliability, often coexists with other anxiety and affective disorders, and can be diagnosed in patients with subsyndromal forms of other psychiatric disorders, or addictive disorder or withdrawal states (Cowley & Dunner, 1991; Janicek, 1999a). Benzodiazepines are indicated for severe generalized anxiety when immediate symptom relief is necessary. Because short-acting, high-potency benzodiazepines (such as alprazolam) prompt more interdose rebound and dependency, long-acting, low-potency benzodiazepines (such as chlordiazepoxide [Librium®], 25 to 75 mg/day) are preferred. They are best used for exacerbations of anxiety (usually for one to four weeks) rather than for continuous use (Maxmen & Ward, 1995).

Atypical Depression: Benzodiazepines often are combined with antidepressants to achieve initial symptom relief in patients with depression and anxiety. Clonazepam (Klonopin®) augmentation of fluoxetine (Prozac®) was superior to fluoxetine alone in the first three weeks of treatment for major depression (Smith, Londborg et al., 1998). Alprazolam and lorazepam (Ativan®) were shown to be effective in outpatient treatment of mild depression, but benzodiazepines are not considered a primary pharmacologic treatment, as they are ineffective in more severe depressions and carry risks of dependence and of exacerbation of depressive symptoms (Laakmann, Faltermaier-Temizel et al., 1996).

Premenstrual Syndrome: Patients with premenstrual syndrome (late luteal phase disorder) can be helped with intermittent use of alprazolam premenstrually (Freeman, Rickels et al., 1995).

Psychoses: Benzodiazepines are used as an adjunct to typical antipsychotic agents in treating patients with schizophrenia and active psychotic symptomatology who do not respond satisfactorily to antipsychotics alone (Wasserf, Dott et al., 1999) and as an adjunct in patients with manic bipolar disorders (Post, Frye et al., 1998).

Insomnia: Benzodiazepine hypnotics are used for transient insomnia, prescribed at the lowest effective dose (for example, flurazepam [Dalmane®], 15 mg or triazolam [Halcion®], 0.125 mg) in a time-limited fashion, usually for two weeks. A recent review of the literature indicated that benzodiazepines are associated with an insignificant decrease in sleep latency compared with placebo, but their effect on overall sleep duration is more marked (approximately one hour) and perhaps clinically meaningful. Rebound insomnia (intense worsening of sleep above baseline levels, after withdrawal of the benzodiazepine), daytime drowsiness, dizziness or lightheadedness, and cognitive impairment were reported (Holbrook, Crowther et al., 2000).

Tolerance to benzodiazepines' sedative effects develops within two to four weeks, especially with the short half-life agents (American Psychiatric Association, 1990). Rebound insomnia develops after short-term use and can lead to patients asking to continue the benzodiazepine for sleep, which should be avoided. Tapering the hypnotic can attenuate the symptoms of rebound insomnia.

Other Sleep Disorders: Clonazepam is the treatment of choice for rapid eye movement (REM) behavior disorders (Schenck & Mahowald, 1996b). Periodic limb movements during sleep and restless leg syndrome can be treated with benzodiazepines, but dopaminergic drugs, including levodopa and dopaminergic agonists, are the current first-line treatment (Wetter & Pollmacher, 1997).

Other Indications: Other uses for benzodiazepines include catatonia (lorazepam 1 to 2 mg intramuscularly) and acute aggression (lorazepam 1 to 2 mg orally or infusion every hour until calm) (Maxmen & Ward, 1995). Social phobia can be treated by benzodiazepines (clonazepam 0.5 to 3 mg daily), but SSRI antidepressants are the drugs of choice to begin treatment (Stein, Liebowitz et al., 1998).

Misuse: The misuse of benzodiazepines can develop when patients are maintained on higher doses and/or for a longer term than is necessary. Lack of a clear diagnosis, without defined measures of benefit and projected time course of treatment, can lead to indiscriminate use. Once begun, a cycle of dependence, withdrawal, continued treatment, and further dependence can develop, with many patients unable to withdraw completely from the benzodiazepine (Rickels, Schweizer et al., 1993).

Another concern is the population of patients with polydrug and alcohol addictions who have anxiety symptoms and phobias. Because of poor history-taking or lack of recognition of addiction, such patients sometimes are given benzodiazepines, posing the significant risk that they will become addicted to the benzodiazepines, relapse to their drug of choice, and/or have a more difficult withdrawal.

In prescribing benzodiazepines, the physician needs to weigh carefully the potential therapeutic benefit against the risks of dependence, acute and chronic toxicity, and addiction. In most cases, use should be short term and at the lowest effective dose. Longer term use should be reevaluated at regular intervals to ensure that continued use of the benzodiazepine is appropriate. DuPont (1990) has elucidated a checklist for use in making this determination. He emphasizes the need to evaluate whether the diagnosis, distress, and disability warrant use; whether the benzodiazepine is providing a positive therapeutic response, with appropriate doses and no other drug or alcohol addiction; whether there is no evidence of any benzodiazepine-induced adverse effects; and whether a family member or significant other can confirm the effectiveness of the drug use and the lack of impairment or addiction.

The best means of avoiding dependence associated with long-term use involves: (1) regular treatment monitoring, (2) use of the lowest possible dose compatible with achieving the desired therapeutic effect, (3) use of intermittent and flexible dosing schedules rather than a fixed regimen, and (4) gradual dose reduction (Janicak, 1999b). Many patients may do better with antidepressant medications such as venlafaxine (Effexor®; Gelenberg, Lydiard et al., 1999), paroxetine (Paxil®; Rocca, Fonzo et al., 1997), other antianxiety medications such as buspirone (BuSpar®), or other forms of psychosocial intervention, such as cognitive-behavioral therapy, than with benzodiazepines. In fact, the pharmacologic first-line treatment for GAD now is antidepressants or buspirone.

Identification of problems is easier in patients who use benzodiazepines in the context of addiction to multiple drugs and/or alcohol, or if there is clear escalation of the dose. It is more difficult to assess appropriateness of use in patients who use the drug at therapeutic doses. Adverse effects (such as memory difficulties, psychomotor effects, benzodiazepine-induced depression or anxiety, behavioral disinhibition, or sleep disturbances) can be subtle, unobtrusive, or attributed to other causes, so that the physician, family, friends, or patient are not aware that these problems are caused by the drug.

When prescribing benzodiazepines, a process of informed consent should take place, including a discussion with the patient about the rationale for prescribing the medication, the expected duration of treatment, effects of the drugs on memory and psychomotor function (including concerns about driving), and the potential for development of tolerance and dependence. If use of a benzodiazepine is contemplated in a patient who is recovering from alcohol or other drug addiction, a consultation with an expert in addiction medicine clearly is indicated.

It should be noted that, despite the concerns discussed above, most patients who are prescribed benzodiazepines who do not have a history of addictive disorder do not escalate the dose, even with prolonged treatment. There are patients whose anxiety disorders are undermedicated with benzodiazepines as a result of physician concerns about tolerance and dependence and who thus gain only partial therapeutic effects from these medications.

Barbiturates and Barbiturate-Like Drugs. Except for the anticonvulsant actions of phenobarbital and its congeners, the barbiturate and other barbiturate-like sedative-hypnotics, with the partial exception of meprobamate, have similar properties. All have a low therapeutic index and low selectivity, so that the therapeutic effect of sedation or anxiolysis is accompanied by CNS depression with little or no analgesia. Other disadvantages compared with the benzodiazepines are that barbiturates and barbiturate-like drugs induce hepatic enzymes, causing more drug interactions; produce more tolerance, physiologic impairment, and toxic reactions; have a greater liability for development of dependence; and are more dangerous in overdose. Acute intoxication produces respiratory depression and hypotension. The withdrawal syndrome following chronic use can be severe and life-threatening (Kisnad, 1990; Charney, Mihic et al., 2001).

Unfortunately, evidence suggests an increase in the use of barbiturate and barbiturate-like sedative-hypnotics and problems with using these and older, less effective, and more hazardous substitute medications (such as phenothiazines and antihistamines) in locales where the benzodiazepines have come under more stringent regulation (Weintraub, Singh et al., 1991; Woods, 1998).

For years, the barbiturates were used extensively as sedative-hypnotic drugs, but they have been largely replaced by the much safer benzodiazepines. They can produce all degrees of depression of the CNS, from mild sedation to general anesthesia. Their antianxiety effects are not equal to those of the benzodiazepines, especially in relation to the degree of sedation produced.

Pentobarbital, secobarbital, and butabarbital are used as sedatives, and butalbital is marketed in combination with analgesic agents. They are classified as short- to intermediate-acting barbiturates. However, the half-life of these drugs (from 15 to 80 hours) is such that none has an elimination half-life short enough for elimination to be virtually complete in 24 hours, so the drug will accumulate during repetitive administration. These are the most frequently abused barbiturates and have a higher liability for abuse than do the benzodiazepines. Phenobarbital is a long-acting barbiturate (with a half-life of 80 to 120 hours) that is used predominantly for treatment of seizure disorders, and abuse of it is relatively uncommon. Ultrashort-acting agents such as thiopental or methohexital are used as anesthetics. Anesthetic doses of barbiturates attenuate cerebral edema resulting from surgery, head injury, or cerebral ischemia. Amobarbital has been administered into the carotid artery before neurosurgery as a means of identifying the dominant cerebral hemisphere for speech. Rarely, the barbiturates may be used for psychiatric diagnostic interviews (narcoanalysis).

Barbiturates combine with other CNS depressants to cause severe CNS depressant effects, with alcohol being the most common offender. The greatest number of drug interactions results from induction of hepatic microsomal enzymes and the accelerated disappearance of many drugs and endogenous substances. For example, the enhanced metabolism of oral contraceptives may result in unwanted pregnancy.

Glutethimide. Glutethimide is a sedative-hypnotic drug with abuse liability and severity of withdrawal symptoms equal to those of barbiturates. The pharmacology of glutethimide is like the barbiturates, but it also exhibits pronounced anticholinergic activity. It is erratically absorbed and is 95% metabolized in the liver, with a half-life of 5 to 22 hours, and induces hepatic enzymes. With therapeutic doses, rare toxic effects consist of "hangover," excitement, blurred vision, gastric irritation, and headache. In acute intoxication, the symptoms are similar to barbiturate poisoning with somewhat less severe respiratory depression. However, the antimuscarinic actions cause xerostomia, ileus, atony of the urinary bladder, and long-lasting mydriasis and hyperpyrexia, which can persist for hours after the patient has regained consciousness. In some cases, there can be tonic muscle spasms, twitching, and even convulsions. A dose of 5 g will produce severe intoxication, while the lethal dose is between 10 and 20 g (Rall, 1990).

Choral Hydrate. Choral hydrate is a sedative hypnotic and is rapidly reduced to the active compound, trichloro-ethanol, largely by hepatic alcohol dehydrogenase. Trichloro-ethanol probably is responsible for chloral hydrate's pharmacologic effects. Trichlorethanol is conjugated with glucuronic acid and excreted mostly into the urine. The plasma half-life is 4 to 12 hours. Trichlorethanol exerts barbiturate-like effects on the gamma-aminobutyric acid-A ($GABA_A$) receptor channel.

Chloral hydrate is irritating to the skin and mucous membranes, which gives rise to an unpleasant taste, epigastric distress, nausea, and occasional vomiting, especially if the drug is insufficiently diluted or taken on an empty stomach. Choral hydrate and alcohol in combination is the "Mickey Finn" of detective novel fame.

The effects of overdose resemble acute barbiturate intoxication, although chloral hydrate can cause icterus. The withdrawal syndrome is similar to barbiturate withdrawal. Chronic users of chloral hydrate may exhibit sudden acute intoxication, which can be fatal. This intoxication results either from an overdose or from a failure of the detoxification mechanism secondary to hepatic damage (Rall, 1990).

Meprobamate. Introduced in 1955 as an antianxiety agent, meprobamate also is used as a sedative-hypnotic. Abuse has continued despite a decrease in the clinical use of the drug. The pharmacologic properties of meprobamate resemble those of the benzodiazepines. Like benzodiazepines, meprobamate can release suppressed behaviors in animals at doses that cause little impairment of locomotor activity, and it does not cause anesthesia. However, unlike the benzodiazepines, ingestion of large doses of meprobamate alone can cause severe or even fatal respiratory depression, hypotension, shock, and heart failure.

Meprobamate is well absorbed, with peak levels at one to three hours, and is metabolized in the liver, principally to a side-chain hydroxy derivative and a glucuronide. An important aspect of intoxication with meprobamate is the formation of gastric bezoars, consisting of undissolved meprobamate tablets, so that treatment may require endoscopy and mechanical removal of the bezoar.

Carisprodol (Soma®), a skeletal muscle relaxant whose active metabolite is meprobamate, also has abuse potential and is a street drug. Meprobamate is preferred to the benzodiazepines in persons with a history of drug abuse. A withdrawal syndrome after long-term use can occur with anxiety, insomnia, tremor, and, frequently, hallucinations. Generalized seizures can occur (Charney, Mihic et al., 2001).

Buspirone (BuSpar®). An azapirone, buspirone is a non-benzodiazepine anxiolytic and a partial 5-HT1A receptor agonist. It has been shown to be superior to placebo and is as effective as benzodiazepines for GAD (Rickels, Schweizer et al., 1988). It has a relatively slow onset of action (two to three weeks), does not cause memory impairment or psychomotor deficits, does not potentiate the central nervous effects of alcohol, causes no withdrawal symptoms, and—despite the slower onset of action—is comparable to the benzodiazepines in the treatment of anxiety. It does not have abuse potential. It is useful only when taken regularly for several weeks. It is not helpful in treating an acute anxiety episode and has no immediate effect after a single tablet. It has demonstrated antidepressant properties in double-blind studies, but has not been shown to be effective for panic attacks. It does not block benzodiazepine withdrawal symptoms (Lader & Olafide, 1987). Buspirone undergoes extensive metabolism with hydroxylation and dealkylation in the liver being the major pathways. Interactions with other coadministered drugs seem to be minimal (Chouinard, Lefko-Singh et al., 1999).

A study of anxious alcoholics who received weekly relapse prevention therapy in addition to buspirone found buspirone superior to placebo in the reduction of anxiety, retention in treatment, reduction of drinking days at followup, and delayed return to heavy drinking (Kranzler, Burleson et al., 1994). However, in patients with GAD who had a recent previous history of benzodiazepine treatment, there were greater discontinuation rates, more adverse events, and less efficacy compared with patients treated with buspirone who had no recent or remote benzodiazepine treatment (DeMartinis, Rynn et al., 2000).

Novel Non-Benzodiazepine Hypnotics. Zolpidem (Ambien®), an imadozopyridine, and Zaleplon (Sonata®), a pyrazolopyrimidine, are non-benzodiazepine hypnotics with rapid onset (within one hour), short duration of action, and short half-lives (zolpidem, 2.5 hours; zaleplon, 1 hour). Their actions are mediated at the omega-1 benzodiazepine receptor subtype. Both have a dose range of 5 to 20 mg, with 5 mg the starting dose in older adults or persons with medical disorders. Both appear to be relatively safe in older adults, especially compared with longer acting benzodiazepine hypnotics (Ancoli-Israel, 2000). Both are extensively metabolized in the liver, eliminated by renal excretion, and appear to have no active metabolites (Darcourt, Pringuey et al., 1999; Hurst & Noble, 1999). Both potentiate psychomotor impairment with alcohol. Zolpidem is the most commonly prescribed hypnotic in the United States. Zaleplon was approved for use by the U.S. Food and Drug Administration (FDA) in August 1999. Like benzodiazepines, both zolpidem and zaleplon are classified as Schedule IV controlled substances under the federal Controlled Substances Act.

While benzodiazepines decrease the time to onset of sleep (sleep latency), prolong the first two stages of sleep, and shorten stages 3 and 4 (deep sleep) and REM sleep, zaleplon and zolpidem, at recommended doses, decrease sleep latency with little effect on sleep stages (*The Medical Letter*, 1999; Kupfer & Reynolds, 1997). In a large four-week study, both agents significantly and consistently reduced sleep latency. Zolpidem increased sleep duration and sleep quality more consistently than zaleplon. Rebound insomnia and withdrawal symptoms were shown to occur with zolpidem but not with zaleplon at therapeutic doses (Elie, Ruther et al., 1999). However, other studies of zolpidem 10 mg for 28 days produced only minimal rebound insomnia (Ware, Walsh et al.,1997).

Zolpidem alone appears not to show a significant degree of toxicity in overdose. However, in combination with other drugs, zolpidem can cause coma, and respiratory depression can occur and can be fatal (Darcourt, Pringuey et al., 1999). There is limited experience with overdose of zaleplon, although no deaths have been reported at doses up to 100 mg (*The Medical Letter*, 1999). The benzodiazepine receptor antagonist flumazenil (Romazicon®) appears to be an effective antidote to zolpidem and zaleplon (Darcourt, Pringuey et al., 1999; Hurst & Noble, 1999).

Compared with temazepam (Restoril®) and triazolam in healthy subjects, zolpidem produces similar impairment of learning, recall, and performance as well as estimates of drug effects. None of the hypnotics were noted to be reinforcing (Rush & Griffiths, 1996). Zolpidem 15 mg impaired coordinative, reactive, and cognitive skills at 1 and 3.5 hours more clearly than diazepam (Valium®) 15 mg, oxazepam (Serax®) 30 mg, zopiclone 7.5 mg (a non-benzodiazepine sedative-hypnotic not available in the United States), and ethanol. Some performance measures were impaired for up to five hours by zolpidem. All these agents impaired learning and memory, but diazepam and zolpidem had a more negative effect than the others (Mattila, Vanakoski et al., 1998). However, in an evaluation of studies of cognitive function and next-day performance that compared zolpidem 5 to 10 mg with other sedative-hypnotics, zolpidem appeared to induce minimal next-day effects. Next-day impairment has been reported in doses above the therapeutic range (Darcourt, Pringuey et al., 1999).

Zaleplon 10 mg produced no decrements in psychomotor performance, memory, or learning compared with placebo at 1.25 hours after administration, although zolpidem 10 mg and triazolam 0.25 mg did. The test scores for those taking doses of 10 and 20 mg at 8.25 hours after administration were no different from placebo, but cognitive impairment was demonstrated in those administered triazolam 0.25 mg and zolpidem 20 mg at that time (Troy, Lucki et al., 2000). Zaleplon 10 mg was free of residual hypnotic or sedative effects when administered nocturnally as little as two hours before waking in healthy subjects, whereas residual effects of zolpidem 10 mg still were apparent on objective assessments up to five hours after nocturnal administration (Danjou, Paty et al., 1999).

Rush (1998) reviewed the behavioral pharmacology of zolpidem relative to benzodiazepines in humans and nonhumans and concluded that zolpidem is similar to benzodiazepines in terms of its reinforcing effects, abuse potential, subject-rated effects (in individuals with and without a history of drug or ethanol abuse), and performance-impairing effects (alone and in combination with alcohol). Some evidence suggests the tolerance and dependence-producing effects may be less than those of benzodiazepines, although there are few appropriate studies of the issue. Isolated cases of abuse and withdrawal symptoms are reported with zolpidem (Cavallaro, Regazzetti et al., 1993; Gericke & Ludolph, 1994).

Zaleplon at high doses (25, 50, and 75 mg), triazolam (0.25, 0.5, and 0.75 mg), and placebo were compared for abuse potential and behavioral effects. Zaleplon and triazolam produced comparable dose-dependent decrements on several performance tasks. Subject-rated measures that reflect abuse potential (for example, drug liking, good effects, and monetary street value) suggested that zaleplon and triazolam were comparable (Rush, Frey et al., 1999).

Minimal interactions have been reported with zolpidem and other drugs; however, it has been reported to affect the C_{max} and clearance of chlorpromazine (Thorazine®) and to decrease metabolism of the antiviral agent ritonavir (Norvir®) (Chouinard, Lefko-Singh et al., 1999). Because CYP3A4 has been reported to play an important role in metabolism of zolpidem and zaleplon, drugs that inhibit or induce this isozyme can affect their serum concentrations as with benzodiazepines. For example, rifampin (Rifadin®) decreased zaleplon serum concentrations by about 80%, and cimetidine (Tagamet®), which inhibits aldehyde oxidase and—to a lesser extent—CYP3A4, increased serum concentrations of zaleplon by about 85% (*The Medical Letter*, 1999).

Zopiclone (Imovane®), available only in Europe and Canada, is a non-benzodiazepine that binds to a site close to, but not directly on, the benzodiazepine-binding site of the $GABA_A$ receptor. It is short to intermediate acting, with a half-life ranging from 3.5 to 6.5 hours, and it has no active metabolites. It demonstrates improvements in sleep in patients with insomnia similar to those seen with benzodiazepines. Impaired psychomotor performance comparable to temazepam and nitrazepam is seen in the morning after a nighttime dose. It causes memory impairment in the first few hours after use, but there are no clear morning-after effects. There is rebound insomnia when discontinued. Dependence and withdrawal have been reported in patients with a history of addictive disorders (Wagner, Wagner et al., 1998).

ABSORPTION AND METABOLISM

Pharmacokinetics. The pharmacokinetic properties of the sedative-hypnotics are important considerations in evaluating their addiction potential. Pharmacokinetic properties of benzodiazepines (as well as barbiturate and barbiturate-like drugs) that can contribute to their abuse liability and persistent self-administration are summarized in Table 1. Drugs that are rapidly absorbed, are potent positive reinforcers, or that cause the development of physical dependence and withdrawal symptoms have the greatest potential for abuse and addiction.

Metabolism. The rate of elimination after multiple doses is related to the elimination half-life of the parent drug and its metabolites (Table 3). In benzodiazepines with a shorter elimination half-life and little accumulation (that is, lorazepam and alprazolam), there is a greater chance of developing withdrawal or rebound symptoms if doses are missed, spaced too far apart, or abruptly discontinued, so that continued use may be related to this negatively reinforcing quality (Cowley, Roy-Byrne et al., 1991).

Absorption. The rapidity of absorption of benzodiazepines from the gastrointestinal tract is an important determinant of the rate at which these compounds enter the CNS. Gastric emptying can be slowed by anticholinergic agents and even by food. Tablets are more rapidly absorbed than capsules. The most rapidly absorbed benzodiazepines (such as diazepam) may produce more euphoria and be more reinforcing than others, whereas a drug that is absorbed more slowly, such as oxazepam or temazepam,

FIGURE 1.   The Structure of Benzodiazepines

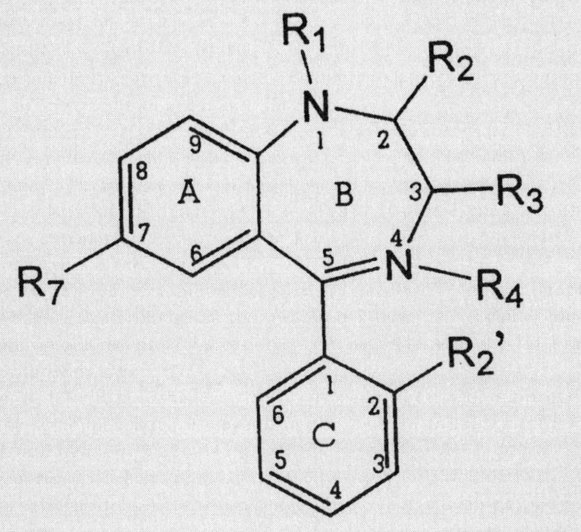

has a longer latency period before its effect is perceptible and produces a lower peak, so it is perceived as less intense and more gradual. The drug can be modified by gastric acid to affect absorption (for example, clorazepate is a prodrug modified by acid hydrolysis in the stomach to form desmethyldiazepam, which then is absorbed with a fast onset of action). Only lorazepam currently is available in a form suitable for sublingual administration, but the absorption rate is not different from oral administration (Roache, 1990; Chouinard, Lefko-Singh et al, 1999).

Chlordiazepoxide, diazepam, lorazepam, and midazolam are formulated to be administered intramuscularly. Chlordiazepoxide can precipitate locally and is slowly and poorly absorbed, while diazepam is absorbed in a variable and unpredictable manner (Greenblatt, Shader et al., 1983). There is little experience with midazolam except for preanesthetic use. The rates of absorption and peak plasma levels with intramuscular lorazepam and midazolam are higher than for oral administration (Chouinard, Lefko-Singh et al., 1999).

All benzodiazepines are highly lipophilic and thus rapidly enter brain tissue. Nevertheless, differences in lipophilicity can produce significant differences in onset of action and reinforcing effects. The more highly lipophilic benzodiazepines, such as diazepam (Table 1), are rapidly distributed to peripheral tissue and have high volumes of distribution. After single doses, the duration of action is shorter than one would predict from the time that it takes the drug to be metabolized to inactive conjugated forms (Chouinard, Lefko-Singh et al., 1999; Cowley, Roy-Byrne et al., 1991), and this short duration of action can be reinforcing as well.

To be excreted in the urine, benzodiazepines first must be conjugated in the liver to form pharmacologically inactive, water-soluble glucuronide metabolites (Chouinard, Lefko-Singh et al., 1999).

On the basis of the common R-group substituents, five chemical types of benzodiazepines have been defined and their metabolism described. First, 2-keto compounds (clorazepate [Tranxene®], chlordiazepoxide [Libritabs®], diazepam, halazepam, prazepam, flurazepam) all are metabolized to desmethyldiazepam. Benzodiazepines in this class are oxidized in the liver before they can be conjugated and tend to have long half-lives, as desmethyldiazepam has a 30- to 200-hour half-life, with the length increasing with age. Second, 3-hydroxy compounds (lorazepam, oxazepam, temazepam) are active compounds with shorter half-lives, which are rapidly metabolized by direct conjugation with a glucuronide radical and which do not generate active metabolites. Age, drug interactions, or liver function do not affect the metabolism. Third, triazolo (alprazolam, triazolam, estazolam [ProSom®]) and, fourth, imidazo (midazolam [Versed®]) compounds have short half-lives and are transformed into hydroxylated compounds before conjugation, but these hydroxylated intermediates, although quite active, are conjugated rapidly and do not accumulate. Fifth, 7-nitro compounds (clonazepam) are active, have long half-lives, have no active metabolites, and are metabolized by nitroreduction. In each subgroup, the metabolism by the liver is similar, so the half-lives are within similar ranges. However, even benzodiazepines with very similar chemical structures can differ significantly in their potency, rate of absorption, lipophilicity, and other important parameters (Chouinard, Lefko-Singh et al., 1999; Maxmen & Ward, 1995).

Important Drug Interactions. All benzodiazepines have additive CNS effects with other sedative drugs. The processes of oxidation and nitroreduction are mediated by the hepatic cytochrome P450 (CYP) system, which can be impaired in old age and in patients with significant hepatic cirrhosis. The metabolism of benzodiazepines (except the 3-hydroxy compounds) is catalyzed primarily by CYP3A3/4 isoenzyme. At high concentrations, diazepam is catalyzed

TABLE 1. Pharmacokinetic Properties of Benzodiazepines

Generic Name	Dosage Equivalent (mg)	Onset of Action	Relative Lipo-philicity	Active Substance	Elimination Half-life (hours)[a]	Metabolism
Clonazepam (Klonopin®)	0.25 mg	Intermediate	+½	Clonazepam	18-50	Oxidation, Nitroeduction
Alprazolam (Xanax®)	0.5 mg	Intermediate	+++	Alprazolam Alphahydroxy-alprozelam	6-20 6-10	Oxidation
Triazolam (Halcion®)	0.5 mg	Fast	+++	Triazolam	1.7-3.0	Oxidation
Lorazepam (Ativan®)	1.0 mg	Intermediate	++	Lorazepam	10-20	Conjugation
Estazolam (ProSom®)	2.0 mg	Intermediate	0	Estazolam	8-24	Oxidation
Diazepam (Valium® and others)	5.0 mg	Fast	+++++	Diazepam Desmethyldiazepam	30-100 30-200	Oxidation
Clorazepate[b] (Tranxene®)	7.5 mg	Fast	++++	Desmethyldiazepam[c] Oxazepam	30-200 3-11	Oxidation
Chlordiazepoxide (Librium® and others)	10.0 mg	Intermediate	++	Chlordiazepoxide Desmthlchlori-diazepoxide Demoxepam Desmthyldiazepam	5-100 18 14-95 30-200	Oxidation
Oxazepam (Serax®)	15.0 mg	Slow	++	Oxazepam	3-21	Conjugation
Flurazepam (Dalmane®)	30.0 mg	Fast		Flurazepam Hydroxyethyl-flurazepam Desalkylflurazepam[c]	0.5-3.5 1-4 48-120	Oxidation
Temazepam (Restoril®)	30.0 mg	Slow	+++	Temazepam	10-12	Conjugation
Quazepam (Doral®)	30.0 mg	Fast	+++++	Quazepam Oxyoquazepam Desalkylflurazepam[c]	20-120	Oxidation
Buspirone (BuSpar®)	15.0-30.0 mg (usual dose)	Rapid peak; very slow onset (>7 da)		1-Pyrimidinyl-piperazine	2-11	
Zolpidem (Ambien®)	10.0 mg	Rapid		Zolpidem	2.5	Oxidation
Zaleplon (Sonata®)	10.0 mg	Rapid		Zaleplon	1	Oxidation

[a] Elimination represents the total for all active metabolites.
[b] Clorazepate is a prodrug that is converted in the stomach to desmthyldiazepam, the active substance in the blood.
[c] Desalkylflurazepam is identical to N-desalkyl-2-oxoquozepam.

SOURCES: Adapted from Cowley DS, Roy-Byrne PP & Greenblatt, 1991; Maxmen JG & Ward NG, 1995; Chouinard G, Lefko-Singh K & Teboul E, 1999; and The Medical Letter, 1999.

by CYP3A3/4, while at low concentrations, CYP2C19 mainly is involved. SSRIs, nefazodone (Serzone®), the antimycotics ketoconazole (Nizoral®) and intraconazole, macrolide antibiotics such as erythromycin, cimetidine, omeprazole (Prilosec®), ritonavir, and grapefruit juice all can inhibit CYP3A4 and increase benzodiazepine levels (Chouinard, Lefko-Singh et al., 1999; Tanaka, 1999; Greenblatt, Von Moltke et al., 1999). In the case of high-dose therapy and overdose, they can lead to toxicity or delayed recovery.

Regarding the SSRIs, paroxetine (Paxil®) and citalopram (Celexa®) are unlikely to cause interactions with benzodiazepines, and sertraline (Zoloft®) inhibits these enzymes only mildly to moderately at usual therapeutic doses, so the potential for interaction is low (Sproule, Naranjo et al., 1997).

MECHANISMS OF ACTION

GABA is the primary inhibitory neurotransmitter within the mammalian CNS. Indeed, 20% to 30% of all synapses within the mammalian brain are thought to be GABAergic. GABA mediates its effects by activating two types of receptors, GABA$_A$ receptors and GABA$_B$ receptors. GABA$_B$ receptors are related structurally to the glutamate receptor and will not be discussed here. Benzodiazepines act by binding to specific recognition sites on GABA$_A$ receptors. Barbiturates, alcohol, picrotoxin, zolpidem, zaleplon, the volatile anesthetics such as halothane, and agents such as etomidate are thought to mediate their effect partially, if not completely, through the GABA$_A$ receptor (Figure 2) (Whiting, Bonnert et al., 1999). Benzodiazepines act only by potentiating the effects of GABA at the GABA$_A$ receptors and have no action independent of GABA.

GABA$_A$ receptors are ligand-gated ion channels that mediate synaptic inhibition in the brain. The conformation of the GABA receptor changes when it binds to GABA, increasing chloride conductance and thus hyperpolarizing the postsynaptic membrane. GABA$_A$ receptors assemble as pentameric, transmembrane glycoprotein complexes consisting of various combinations of 16 genetically distinct peptide subunits of several major classes (alpha, beta, gamma, delta, epsilon, pi, rho), with various isoforms within each subunit class (for example, alpha$_1$ to alpha$_6$). Most GABA receptors consist of alpha, beta, or gamma subunits. The subunit composition in a particular brain region or cell

TABLE 2.   Kinetics and Abuse Potential

Properties That Increase Potency as a Reinforcer
High intrinsic pharmacologic activity of drug
Rapid absorption
Rapid entry into specific brain regions
High oral bioavailability
Low protein binding
Short half-life
Small volume of distribution
High clearance.

Factors That Promote Physical Dependence
High intrinsic pharmacologic activity of drug
Cumulative drug load (dose, frequency, duration of treatment)
Small volume of distribution
Long half-life
Low clearance.

Factors That Promote Appearance of the Withdrawal Syndrome
High intrinsic pharmacologic activity of drug
Short half-life
High clearance
Rapid exit from specific brain regions
Small volume of distribution.

SOURCE: Reprinted with permission from Coppell HD, Sellers EM & Busto U (1986). Benzodiazepines as drugs of abuse and dependence. In HD Cappell, FG Blaser, Y Israel, H Halant & W Schmidt (eds.) *Recent Advances in Alcohol and Drug Problems, Vol. 9.* New York, NY: Plenum Press, 63.

type determines the pharmacologic and functional properties of GABA$_A$ receptors (Weinberger, 2001). Probably more than 500 distinct GABA$_A$ receptor subtypes exist in the brain (Sieghart, 2000).

To form an active GABA binding site, combinations of alpha and beta subunits are necessary. To bind benzodiazepines, these receptors require alpha and gamma subunits, and the alpha isoforms have to be type 1, 2, 3, or 5. Classic benzodiazepines exhibit comparable affinities for all these GABA$_A$ receptors (Sieghart, 2000; Weinberger, 2001).

Recent studies of genetic mutations of the alpha subunits in mice have shown that alpha$_1$ subunits, which are expressed abundantly throughout the cerebral cortex, are critical for mediating the sedative, amnesic, possibly ataxic, and, to a lesser extent, anticonvulsant effects of benzodia-

FIGURE 2. **Diagrammatic representation of a prototypic GABA$_A$ receptor, showing the putative localization of the binding sites of the agonist and various modulatory agents.**

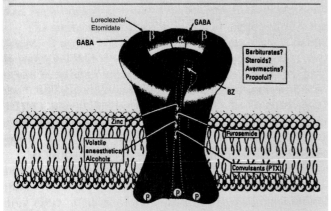

BZ = benzodiazepine; PTX = picrotoxin. The locations of binding sites for barbiturates, steroids, avermectins, and propofol remain unclear. The P in a circle represents the phosphorylation sites located on the cytoplasmic domain between TM3 and TM4 of the alpha, beta, and gamma subunits.

SOURCE: Reprinted with permission from Whiting PJ, Bonnert TP, McKenzie RM et al. (1999). Molecular and functional diversity of the expanding GABA$_A$ receptor gene family. *Annals of the New York Academy of Sciences* 868:648.

zepines. Agents that bind specifically to alpha$_1$ subunits, such as zolpidem, have no effects in animals in which the alpha$_1$ subunit is made to be insensitive. In contrast, alpha$_2$ subunits, which are expressed in the hippocampus, amygdala, and cortex on the initial axonal segments of pyramidal neurons, are most likely involved primarily in the antianxiety effects of benzodiazepines. The alpha$_3$ and alpha$_5$ subunits most likely are involved in the other actions of the benzodiazepines (Weinberger, 2001).

Endogenous benzodiazepines such as diazepam and nordiazepam (as well as other benzodiazepine-like compounds termed "endozepines," which are not halogenated) have been found in human blood and brain. They are present only in trace amounts, but are increased in patients with cirrhosis and can be a factor in hepatic encephalopathy. The source is unknown, but they are in vegetables and medicinal plants such as camomile, or can be synthesized by intestinal bacteria (Baraldi, Avallone et al., 2000).

Benzodiazepine receptors are distinctly linked with the GABA$_A$ receptors. GABA can enhance the binding of benzodiazepines to the benzodiazepine receptor by increasing benzodiazepine affinity (the "GABA shift"), and benzodiazepines can increase the binding of GABA and the frequency of GABA-induced chloride channel opening (Roy-Byrne & Nutt, 1991).

Barbiturates are positive modulators of GABA$_A$ receptors by binding to an undefined site on the GABA complex to interact with GABA in a concentration-dependent manner. Most drugs that affect the GABA$_A$ receptor do not directly affect channel conductance, but instead allosterically modify the effect of GABA on the dynamics of channel opening. Benzodiazepines increase the frequency of channel openings induced by GABA. In contrast, the alteration of the GABA$_A$/chloride channel state produced by barbiturates is distinct from the alteration produced by benzodiazepines and is antagonized by picrotoxin (Ito, Suzuki et al., 1996).

Alcohol potentiates GABA on receptors with the alpha$_2$ subunit, increasing the flow of chloride ions, causing sedation and psychomotor problems. At higher concentrations (>250 mg/dL), alcohol has a direct action on the receptor, causing a prolonged opening of the chloride channel that is GABA-independent. This prolonged opening also is true of barbiturates but not benzodiazepines. This difference in mechanism of action explains why alcohol and barbiturates are much more toxic in overdose, as the chloride influx results in paralysis of the neurons responsible for respiratory drive (Nutt, 1999).

The concept of benzodiazepine agonists, antagonists, and inverse agonists has evolved from the complex interaction of benzodiazepines with the GABA$_A$ receptors. Agonists include the commonly used benzodiazepines (alprazolam, diazepam), which increase the affinity of GABA for its receptor and thus augment GABA-mediated inhibition (Zorumski & Isenberg, 1991). Benzodiazepine antagonists (such as flumazenil) have no intrinsic activity, but block the effects of both agonists and inverse agonists by competitive receptor binding (Roy-Byrne & Nutt, 1991). The inverse agonists (such as beta-carboline-3-carboxylic acid ethyl ester [B-CCE]) have the opposite action of the benzodiazepines, decreasing GABA-mediated chloride responses, thereby increasing arousal and activation and promoting seizures by increasing neuronal excitability (Roy-Byrne & Nutt, 1991; Zorumski & Isenberg, 1991).

With chronic administration of benzodiazepines, evidence exists that changes in gene expression and consequent $GABA_A$ receptor function can be responsible for tolerance and low-level, long-term withdrawal symptoms (Sanger, Benavides et al., 1994; Roy-Byrne & Nutt, 1991; Morrow, 1995).

ADDICTION LIABILITY

Reinforcing Effects. The addiction liability of sedatives, hypnotics, and anxiolytics can be assessed by examining the reinforcing effects of these drugs. There is a good correspondence between those drugs that maintain self-administration behavior in laboratory animals; those that produce self-administration, choice, and subjective drug liking in drug abusers; and those that are actually abused by drug abusers (Griffths & Weerts, 1997). Griffiths and Weerts (1997) have reviewed the data about benzodiazepine self-administration in humans and laboratory animals and found that benzodiazepines are reinforcing in laboratory animals by oral, intravenous, and intragastric routes of administration.

In humans, benzodiazepines are reinforcers in subjects with histories of drug abuse but not in subjects who do not have histories of moderate drinking, anxiety, or insomnia. They are reinforcers in subjects with histories of moderate social alcohol drinking and, although not investigated prospectively, there is a suggestion that a history of low-frequency recreational drug use that does not meet the diagnostic criteria for abuse and dependence is associated with benzodiazepine reinforcement. Abstinent alcoholics and children of alcoholics (Ciraulo & Sarid-Segal, 1991; Ciraulo, Sarid-Segal et al., 1996) have reinforcing responses to benzodiazepines. Benzodiazepines can function as reinforcers in anxious and insomniac subjects.

Benzodiazepines are more likely to function as reinforcers when the study design allows the subjects to control the time and total dose that is self-administered. For example, studies that provide subjects with multiple opportunities to self-administer small doses of benzodiazepine generally show greater preference for the drug. The reinforcing effects of benzodiazepines can be determined by the behavioral requirements after drug ingestion; for example, they are more reinforcing before subjects engage in a relaxing task and are not reinforcing before a task requiring vigilance (Silverman, Kirby et al., 1994). Rapid onset of drug effect enhances the reinforcing efficacy of benzodiazepines. One example is a study (Mumford, Evans et al., 1995) that found immediate-release alprazolam was more reinforcing than extended-release alprazolam in subjects with a history of drug abuse.

Benzodiazepines are less reinforcing and have a lower abuse potential than several barbiturates (amobarbital, pentobarbital, secobarbital) and older generation sedative-hypnotics (glutethimide, meprobamate, methaqualone). Barbiturates, meprobamate, and methaqualone appear to have more euphoric or reinforcing properties than benzodiazepines (Roache & Meisch, 1995)

Benzodiazepines vary in abuse liability based on differential subjective effects. Diazepam, lorazepam, triazolam, flunitrazepam, and alprazolam have relatively high abuse liability, whereas oxazepam, halazepam, clorazepate, prazepam, and chlordiazepoxide do not. The speed of onset of pleasurable effects is an important factor in addiction potential (Roache & Meisch, 1995; Mintzer & Griffiths, 1998).

Tolerance. Effects of chronic benzodiazepine administration have been examined in both preclinical and human studies. Animals and humans chronically exposed to benzodiazepines display time-dependent decreases in benzodiazepine effects or tolerance. Tolerance is a commonly encountered phenomenon in the clinical use of sedative-hypnotics. The neurochemical basis of tolerance remains unclear, but may involve changes in benzodiazepine receptor binding, receptor densities, receptor subunit composition, brain GABA levels, or glutaminergic function (Pratt, Brett et al., 1998; Fujita, Woods et al., 1999). Changes can be regionally specific or vary with the particular sedative-hypnotic. For example, receptor binding changes appear to vary in time course and regional specificity within the CNS with different benzodiazepines (Miller, Woolverton et al., 1989).

Tolerance develops at varying rates for different behavioral effects. In animals, tolerance occurs rapidly to sedative and psychomotor effects of benzodiazepines, less rapidly to anticonvulsant effects, slowly to anxiolytic effects, and perhaps not at all to increased motor activity induced by low doses (File, 1985; Nutt, 1990). Strain differences in the extent of tolerance to different benzodiazepine actions suggest a possible genetic contribution to the development of tolerance (File, 1983). A similar genetically determined pattern of sensitivity and tolerance to these agents in humans might place some individuals at higher risk of developing tolerance with chronic use.

Differential tolerance to varying benzodiazepine effects is seen in humans. As in animals, sedative and psychomotor effects diminish first (Smith & Kroboth, 1987; Van Laar, Volkerts et al., 1992), with tolerance to impairment of driving ability observed after the first few weeks of treatment. However, benzodiazepine effects on memory and anxiety persist despite chronic use (Lader & File, 1987; Lucki, Rickels et al., 1986). The lack of tolerance to anxiolytic actions of benzodiazepines seen in most anxious patients (Rickels, Case et al., 1983), as well as the observation that anxious patients without a history of addictive disorder rarely escalate doses or overuse these medications (Woods, Katz et al., 1988), form the basis of their successful clinical use.

Several studies have examined the effects of long-term therapeutic use of benzodiazepines. In a double-blind study of 106 patients with panic disorder treated for 8 months with alprazolam, imipramine, or placebo, patients treated with alprazolam showed persistent improvement at a mean dose of 5.6 mg/day, without escalation of dose over the course of the trial (Rickels & Schweizer, 1998). Naturalistic followup studies of chronically treated patients with panic disorder have observed stable or gradually decreasing benzodiazepine doses over time, without loss of efficacy (Nagy, Krystal et al., 1989; Worthington, Pollack et al., 1998). However, Allen and colleagues (1991), in an eight-week trial of alprazolam for panic and agoraphobia, noted continuing impairments in word recall throughout the study. Pomara and colleagues (1998), in a study examining effects of acute doses of alprazolam or lorazepam after three weeks of treatment in older adult patients, noted only partial tolerance to memory effects and continued impairment on a discriminant reaction time task. Thus, although anxiolytic efficacy is maintained without dose escalation in selected (nonsubstance abusing) patients, lack of tolerance to memory effects can be a significant drawback of chronic treatment.

Individual benzodiazepines display different rates of tolerance with respect to sedative effects. For example, chronic users (1 to 20 years) of lorazepam showed tolerance to sedative effects of the drug compared with healthy controls, whereas chronic users of temazepam did not (van Stevenick, Wallnofer et al., 1997). A meta-analysis of sleep laboratory studies (Soldatos, Dikeos et al., 1999) showed the clear development of tolerance and rebound insomnia on withdrawal with triazolam, but significantly less tolerance with midazolam or zolpidem. Of note, in 170 patients with severe sleep disorders (chronic, severe insomnia, rest-less legs/periodic limb movement disorder, sleepwalking, sleep terrors, REM behavior disorder), 146 patients (86%) responded well to benzodiazepines, and 136 were able to maintain therapeutic efficacy with these agents over a mean of 3.5 years without dose escalation (Schenck & Mahowald, 1996b). Of note, however, 4% of patients suffered a relapse to substance use disorders or misused their medications.

Overall, then, patients treated with benzodiazepines for anxiety or specific sleep disorders often are able to maintain therapeutic effects without apparent tolerance, as measured by dose escalation. Nevertheless, only partial tolerance to memory and some psychomotor effects are of concern in chronically treated patients and certain individuals, especially those with a history of addictive disorder, who are at higher risk for tolerance, escalating doses, and misusing medications with chronic treatment.

Of note, barbiturate and benzodiazepine sedative-hypnotics display cross-tolerance with ethanol and other sedative-hypnotic agents (Khanna, Kalant et al., 1998). Although zolpidem and zaleplon are thought to confer less risk of tolerance with chronic use, few long-term studies have specifically addressed this issue.

Dependence. The physical dependence and withdrawal liability of the benzodiazepines is a deterrent to their therapeutic use. Physical dependence contributes to addiction potential because of the negative reinforcement of withdrawal and often is a major factor in patients' unsuccessful efforts to discontinue benzodiazepine use.

Data about benzodiazepine dependence in clinical settings are surprisingly inadequate. Reports document populations of benzodiazepine-addicted patients, largely from hospitals and addiction treatment centers (Busto, Romach et al., 1996; Finlayson & Davis, 1994). Survey data give evidence of a large number of persons engaged in long-term use of benzodiazepines and a significant amount of abuse/nonmedical use, but it is difficult to translate that into estimates of addiction (Griffiths & Weerts, 1997).

Two patterns of problematic benzodiazepine use have been described: (1) nonmedical use for the purpose of getting high (recreational abuse) and (2) long-term drug-taking by patients for a duration that is inconsistent with accepted medical practice (chronic quasitherapeutic use). The recreational abuser uses benzodiazepines to become intoxicated in an intermittent or chronic pattern of high doses, often in a pattern of polydrug abuse. The source of the drug often is illicit, and the incidence is relatively small, given the rate of widespread legitimate medical use, but it is similar to rates of abuse of other illicit substances such as opioids or cocaine.

Chronic quasitherapeutic users often are older, may or may not have a history of alcohol or drug abuse, or may have a chronic pain problem. The motive for use is symptomatic relief, and patients may report unsuccessful efforts to cut down use or to relieve or avoid withdrawal. The incidence of such quasitherapeutic use is unknown, but is estimated to be relatively common, as long-term use of benzodiazepines accounts for most sales of the drug, although the efficacy of long-term use is uncertain. Therapeutic doses typically are used, and the source of the drug usually is licit, although it can involve patient deception to obtain the drug—for example, through contact with multiple physicians (Griffiths & Weerts, 1997). Both groups have significant psychiatric morbidity (Busto, Romach et al., 1996; Finlayson & Davis, 1994).

Withdrawal. The benzodiazepine withdrawal syndrome is similar to that produced by barbiturates and barbiturate-like sedative-hypnotics; it can be described as of the sedative-hypnotic type (Roache, 1990). However, distinguishing between withdrawal and rebound anxiety can be difficult. Withdrawal is defined by "new" time-limited symptoms that are not part of the original anxiety state and that begin and end depending on the pharmacokinetics of the particular benzodiazepine; relapse is defined as reemergence of the original anxiety state; and rebound is defined as an increase in anxiety that is above original baseline levels and that can be a combination of relapse and withdrawal (Roy-Byrne, 1991).

With abrupt discontinuation, symptoms begin the day after with short and intermediate half-life drugs, within three to eight days of cessation of long-acting benzodiazepines, and are most severe between the second and 18th day after cessation of drug use, again depending on half-life (Busto, Sellars et al., 1986).

With gradual taper, the withdrawal syndrome is the most severe in the last quarter of the taper with short half-life benzodiazepines, but it is the most severe in the first week of abstinence in those using long half-life benzodiazepines. For the most part, the withdrawal syndrome remits by three to five weeks after the taper. However, isolated symptoms such as tinnitus can persist for months (Schweizer, Rickels et al., 1990; Rickels, Schweizer et al., 1993).

Common symptoms of withdrawal include anxiety, irritability, insomnia, fatigue, headache, muscle twitching or aching, tremor, shakiness, sweating, dizziness, and con tration difficulties—all symptoms common in anxie Symptoms that are more likely to represent withdrawal rather than a return or exacerbation of the original anxiety are nausea, loss of appetite, depression, derealization, increased sensory perception (smell, light, taste, touch), and an abnormal perception of movement (Roy-Byrne, 1991). Seizures, persistent tinnitus, delirium, confusion, and psychotic symptoms have been reported, but are uncommon (APA, 1990). Depression, mania, and obsessive-compulsive disorder are reported to have been triggered by withdrawal as well (Roy-Byrne, 1991).

The majority (more than 90%) of long-term users of benzodiazepines (that is, those who have used longer than 8 months to a year) experience withdrawal symptoms, whether withdrawn slowly or rapidly (Rickels, Schweizer et al., 1990, 1993; Schweizer, Rickels et al., 1990). Gradual taper of alprazolam after long-term treatment of panic disorder results in significant rebound of panic and anxiety symptoms, exceeding pretreatment levels in 50% to 90% of patients (Rickels, Schweizer et al., 1993). Withdrawal does not appear to worsen if the benzodiazepine is used for longer than a year, suggesting that there is a threshold duration of treatment, beyond which further drug exposure has little pharmacologic influence on the withdrawal experience (Schweizer, Rickels et al., 1990; Rickels, Schweizer et al., 1990).

For anxiety problems that are treated with benzodiazepines for two weeks or less, there are few withdrawal symptoms. With eight weeks of use in patients with generalized disorder, there can be mild and manageable withdrawal symptoms. In patients with short-term use, prior benzodiazepine use does not appear to affect withdrawal (Rickels & Freeman, 2000), as compared with longer periods of use, in which prior benzodiazepine use is associated with more severe withdrawal problems (Rickels, Schweizer et al., 1988).

The inability of patients on long-term benzodiazepines to discontinue use because of withdrawal is a concern. Even with a slow withdrawal procedure over 30 days, more than a third of subjects are unable to discontinue the drug (Schweizer, Rickels et al., 1990; Rickels, Schweizer et al., 1993). However, it may be that slowing the taper significantly (that is, taper the first 50% in two to four weeks and then maintain the reduced dose for several months before finally completing the taper) and using agents such as carbamazepine (Tegretol®), imipramine (Tofranil®),

®), and trazodone (Desyrel®) to help
ine discontinuation would increase the
s, DeMartinis et al., 1999, 2000). If
per off benzodiazepines, about three-
benzodiazepines three years later.
However, in patients whose taper attempt is unsuccessful
but whose intake is reduced by 50%, there was only a 39%
success rate of being without a benzodiazepine three years
later. Among patients who refused to participate in a taper
program, all but 14% used benzodiazepines daily. Patients
who were able to remain off benzodiazepines for three years
had a significantly lower level of anxiety and depression compared with patients who continued to use benzodiazepines
over the three-year period (Rickels, Case et al., 1991).

Cognitive behavior therapy is very effective in easing
benzodiazepine discontinuation and preventing relapse to
panic disorder. Reduction in the fear of anxiety symptoms
is the best prediction of a patient's ability to achieve and
maintain drug abstinence (Bruce, Spiegel et al., 1995).

Some of the more consistent pharmacologic variables
predicting withdrawal severity and the inability to discontinue benzodiazepines are (1) higher daily dose of
benzodiazepine (or higher plasma level), (2) short benzodiazepine half-life, (3) longer duration of daily benzodiazepine
therapy, and (4) more rapid rate of taper (especially the final 50% of the taper). Patient variables include (1) diagnosis
of panic disorder but not GAD, (2) higher pretaper levels
of anxiety and depression, (3) concomitant alcohol and/or
substance dependence or abuse, and (4) higher levels of
personality psychopathology (for example, neuroticism,
dependency) (Rickels, DeMartinis et al., 1999). Nonpharmacologic variables contribute almost as much to withdrawal severity and discontinuation problems as pharmacologic variables. The severity of the withdrawal experience
does not correlate significantly with the inability of the patient to taper off the benzodiazepine successfully. Patients
with personality disorders are sensitive to even minor cues
of withdrawal symptoms and tend to drop out in the early
phases of the benzodiazepine taper (before the severe withdrawal symptoms occur), never giving the taper a chance
(Rickels, DeMartinis et al., 1999).

Benzodiazepine half-life is more important for abrupt
(Rickels, Schweizer et al., 1990) than for gradual discontinuation (Schweizer, Rickels et al., 1990). Withdrawal reactions
appear to be most severe with the quickly eliminated, high-
potency benzodiazepines (for example, alprazolam, lorazepam,
triazolam); intermediate with quickly eliminated low-potency
(oxazepam) and slowly eliminated, high-potency benzodiazepines (clonazepam); and mildest with slowly eliminated,
low-potency benzodiazepines (diazepam, clorazepate, chlordiazepoxide) (Wolf & Griffiths, 1991).

TOXICITY/ADVERSE EFFECTS

Effects on Memory. Most studies demonstrate that benzodiazepines impair recall of new information (anterograde
amnesia). This impairment apparently occurs when the
benzodiazepine disrupts the process through which
information is transferred from temporary, short-term
memory to longer term memory storage (the consolidation
phase) (APA, 1990). Anterograde amnesia is more likely
with increased dose, faster absorption, intravenous administration, and use of higher potency benzodiazepines.
Tolerance to anterograde amnesia occurs, but is not complete. The severity of the amnestic effects is correlated with
the peak plasma benzodiazepine levels (King 1992; Buffett-
Jerrott, Stewart et al., 1999). Older adults are more sensitive
to the effects of benzodiazepines on memory.

The increased sensitivity of older adults may be due, in
part, to a lower baseline performance, so that an equal decre-
ment in memory is more noticeable and has more serious
consequences (APA, 1990). In older adults, benzodiazepines
are the drugs that most commonly exacerbate underlying
dementia and can cause excess morbidity. The cognitive
impairment often appears to develop insidiously as a "late
complication" of a drug initially prescribed at a younger
age. Some patients can be given other drugs to treat side
effects of the benzodiazepines; that is, neuroleptics given to
patients who develop confusion while on benzodiazepines.

Patients have a significant improvement in measures of
memory and cognitive functioning after discontinuation of
benzodiazepines. Family and staff members note that older
adult patients who discontinue benzodiazepines are brighter,
more energetic, less dysphoric, and substantially more in-
tellectually alert than while on the drug (Salzman, Fisher et
al., 1992).

Benzodiazepine-induced memory problems can be unrecognized by patients, family, or clinicians, and the true
incidence is unknown. People experiencing such memory
problems can conclude that nothing worth remembering
had happened if they are unable to recall events. In older
adults, memory problems can be blamed on aging rather
than on the benzodiazepine.

Cognitive Effects. Benzodiazepines impair cognitive
and motor functioning with acute and chronic dosing, al-

though the effects of chronic administration are not consistent from person to person and can depend on dose and time of drug administration. Sedation, drowsiness, ataxia, incoordination, vertigo, and dizziness are common side effects related to dose and individual susceptibility. Tolerance to these effects develops, although it may not be complete (APA, 1990). Impaired visual spatial ability and sustained attention have been found in long-term benzodiazepine users, and patients often are unaware of their reduced ability (Golombeck, Moodley et al., 1988). Being an older adult, using alcohol, using high doses of benzodiazepine, and taking other drugs such as anticholinergics are associated with increased sensitivity to cognitive and psychomotor effects (APA, 1990).

Patients with evidence of impaired cognitive functions while on long-term benzodiazepine therapy have been shown to improve in these functions when benzodiazepines therapy is discontinued. Compared with patients who were unable to taper off benzodiazepines, the successfully tapered patients were more alert, more relaxed, and less anxious, and that change was accompanied by improved psychomotor functions (Rickels, Lucki et al., 1999). However, there is concern that some patients withdrawn from long-term therapeutic benzodiazepine use do not have full recovery of cognitive function (Tata, Rollings et al., 1994).

Psychomotor Effects. Benzodiazepines impair skills of importance to driving. Epidemiologic evidence shows an increased risk of motor vehicle crashes in younger and older benzodiazepine users (Ray, Purushottam et al., 1993). In older users, the annual rate of involvement in injurious crashes is up to 1.5 to 2 times higher than nonusers and increases as a function of the prescribed dose (Ray, Purushottam et al., 1993). Long half-life benzodiazepines are implicated most often (Thomas, 1998; Hemmelgarn, Suissa et al., 1997).

In older persons, there is evidence that current use of long and short half-life benzodiazepines increases the risk of falls (Leipzig, Cummings et al., 1999) and femur fracture (Herings, Stricker et al., 1995). The risk of falls leading to femur fracture is dose dependent, irrespective of elimination half-life or type of use (intermittent or continuous). There is a high relative risk among patients prescribed benzodiazepines for the first time, among those continually exposed whose dose is increased, and among those who concomitantly use several benzodiazepines (Herings, Stricker et al., 1995). The timing of peak levels appears to be important. In older patients, short half-life benzodiazepines have significant incapacitating psychomotor effects in the first few hours after drug administration, which puts them at risk of falling if the benzodiazepine is used as a hypnotic should they need to void or get out of bed for any reason (Fisch, Bakir et al., 1990).

The use of benzodiazepines in the first weeks after stroke has detrimental effects on recovery of motor function, and their routine use in these patients should be avoided (Goldstein & Study Investigators, 1995).

Teratogenicity and Fetal Effects. Considerable controversy exists about the use of benzodiazepines by pregnant women. Bergman and colleagues (1992) found that 2% of pregnant women receiving Medicaid benefits filled one or more prescriptions for benzodiazepines during pregnancy. There is inadvertent exposure of the fetus to benzodiazepines in the first trimester, as about half the pregnancies in the United States are unintended (Skrabanek, 1992).

A meta-analysis of studies that examined the teratogenicity of benzodiazepines (Dolovich, Addis et al., 1998) found that pooled data from cohort studies showed no association between fetal exposure to benzodiazepines and the risk of major malformations or oral cleft. However, a small but significantly increased risk of oral cleft was seen, according to data from the available case-control studies. Benzodiazepines did not seem to be major human teratogens, but it was recommended that, until further research is reported, level 2 ultrasonography should be used to rule out visible forms of oral cleft if the mother had taken benzodiazepines in the first trimester.

A syndrome of dysmorphic features, growth aberrations, and abnormalities of the CNS has been reported in infants who were exposed to benzodiazepines during pregnancy (Laegreid, Olegard et al., 1989, 1990), but this syndrome has not been confirmed by others, and alternative causes of these abnormalities have been suggested (Dolovich, Addis et al., 1998). Lower birth weight in babies with maternal use of benzodiazepines has been reported (Laegreid, Hagbert et al., 1992). Sedation and withdrawal has been shown in infants of mothers taking benzodiazepines up to term (Bergman, Rosa et al., 1992; Laegreid, Hagberg et al.,1992).

Other Psychopathology. Behavioral disinhibition reactions with various benzodiazepines can occur. Usually, these are associated with higher doses and higher pretreatment levels of hostility (Rothschild, 1992). The use of benzodiazepines also is associated with the development of delirium in postoperative patients (Marcantonio, Juarez et al., 1994).

Studies show that significant anxiety and depressive symptoms remain in many long-term benzodiazepine users while they are using benzodiazepines. However, patients who are able to withdraw successfully from long-term benzodiazepine treatment have significantly improved levels of anxiety and depression compared with pretaper baseline (Schweizer, Rickels et al., 1990; Rickels, Lucki et al., 1999); this implies that benzodiazepines can worsen depression and anxiety long term. Some patients on low daily doses of benzodiazepines may be in a constant mild withdrawal state. Depression and interdose anxiety have been reported to emerge with benzodiazepine therapy (APA, 1990). Deterioration in mood and social behavior in subjects taking benzodiazepines has been noted by raters but not the subjects themselves, so negative effects may be difficult to elicit by self-report (Griffiths, Bigelow et al., 1983).

Benzodiazepines can be a complicating factor in those patients with past or current addictive disorders. Benzodiazepine abuse and dependence appear more frequently among alcoholics and drug abusers compared with the population that does not have a history of addictive disorders (Woods, 1998). The development of alcohol or other drug addiction after primary benzodiazepine dependence, although reported less often than the reverse, has been observed (Wolf, Grohmann et al., 1989). High-dose benzodiazepine use has been correlated with alcohol dependence as well as a greater number of cigarettes and amount of caffeine consumed compared with low-dose benzodiazepine users and control subjects (Lekka, Paschalis et al., 1997).

Benzodiazepines are commonly used in suicide attempts. Although benzodiazepines are safer than barbiturates, there can be completed suicides with overdoses of benzodiazepines alone (Drummer & Ransom, 1996) or in combination with alcohol or other drugs (Ekkedahl, Lowenhielm et al., 1994; Serfaty & Masterton, 1993). In long-term followup, the risk of suicide in patients who have been hospitalized for dependence on prescribed narcotics and sedatives is very high (Aggulander, Brandt et al., 1994). In opiate addicts, deaths have been linked to the concomitant use of buprenorphine (Buprenex®) and benzodiazepines, most likely related to respiratory depression (Reynaud, Petit et al., 1998).

Substantial social and occupational impairment also have been associated with benzodiazepine addiction (Juergens & Morse, 1988).

Benzodiazepine use is a risk factor for pulmonary aspiration in neurologically impaired long-term care patients (Pick, McDonald et al., 1996), and aspiration, as well as respiratory depression, can be a cause of death in benzodiazepine overdoses (Drummer & Ranson, 1996). Benzodiazepines are contraindicated in patients who have sleep apnea or significant respiratory disease because of the risk of respiratory depression.

The high rate of withdrawal symptoms and difficulties with benzodiazepine discontinuation also must be seen as an adverse consequence of their use.

Victimization can occur with the use of many drugs and alcohol, but benzodiazepines and other sedative-hypnotics often have been implicated. Robbery and sexual assault (including "date rape") have been associated with the involuntary and voluntary use of benzodiazepines, often with the use of other drugs or alcohol (Boussairi, Dupeyron et al., 1996; Calhoun, Wesson et al., 1996). Flunitrazepam (Rohypnol®) is a rapid-onset, intermediate-acting, highly potent (10 times more potent than diazepam) hypnotic benzodiazepine that has never been marketed in the United States, but has been smuggled into the country. Its abuse and alleged use to facilitate date rape have attracted much attention. However, it is not clear that it poses a greater public health risk than other benzodiazepines (Woods, 1998; Simmons & Cupp, 1998).

FUTURE RESEARCH DIRECTIONS

Although benzodiazepines provide rapid onset of anxiolytic and sedative effects, and are safer than barbiturate and barbiturate-like sedative-hypnotics, their use is limited by concerns about adverse effects, including tolerance and dependence. Future research elucidating the mechanisms by which benzodiazepines produce their various effects and the relationship between $GABA_A$ receptor subunit composition and benzodiazepine actions may allow targeted drug development of benzodiazepine receptor ligands that are selective for desired therapeutic effects but without unwanted psychomotor impairment, cognitive effects, or tolerance and dependence. Aims of such research would include the development of selective nonsedating anxiolytics and of hypnotics with somewhat longer half-lives than zolpidem and zaleplon to address middle insomnia and early morning awakening. The efficacy of buspirone, a non-benzodiazepine anxiolytic that does not act at the $GABA_A$ receptor, suggests that it may be possible to develop anxiolytic agents with novel mechanisms of action. Increased understanding of interindividual differences in benzodiazepine effects can help to identify in advance those individuals who are at highest and lowest risk of specific adverse effects of benzodiazepines. Finally, further research about the mechanisms underlying tolerance, dependence, and addiction with benzodiazepines may allow prevention of these phenomena during benzodiazepine treatment.

CONCLUSIONS

Benzodiazepines are potentially addicting drugs that are used routinely in medical and psychiatric practice. They are very effective in producing rapid anxiolysis and sedation. However, close monitoring of their use by a physician is necessary, because the potential for occurrence of physical dependence, adverse effects, and addiction must be weighed and respected. The novel non-benzodiazepine sedatives have some distinct properties and benefits, but whether they will be linked to the side effects and concerns of benzodiazepines is yet to be determined.

REFERENCES

Aggulander C, Brandt L & Allebeck P (1994). Suicide and psychopathology in 1,537 patients dependent on prescribed psychoactive medications: Stockholm, Sweden. *American Journal on Addictions* 3:236-240.

Allen D, Curran HV & Lader M (1991). The effects of repeated doses of clomipramine and alprazolam on physiological, psychomotor, and cognitive functions in normal subjects. *European Journal of Clinical Pharmacology* 40:355-362.

American Psychiatric Association (1990). *Task Force Report on Benzodiazepines*. Washington, DC: The Association.

Ancoli-Israel S (2000). Insomnia in the elderly: A review for the primary care practitioner. *Sleep* 23(Suppl 1):S23-S38.

Baraldi M, Avallone R, Corsi L et al. (2000). Endogenous benzodiazepines. *Therapie* 55:143-146.

Bergman U, Rosa FW, Baum C et al. (1992). Effects of exposure to benzodiazepine during fetal life. *Lancet* 340:694-696.

Boussairi A, Dupeyron JP, Hernandez B et al. (1996). Urine benzodiazepine screening of involuntarily drugged and robbed or raped patients. *Clinical Toxicology* 34(6):721-724.

Bruce TJ, Spiegel DA, Gregg SF et al. (1995). Predictors of alprazolam discontinuation with and without cognitive behavior therapy in panic disorder. *American Journal of Psychiatry* 152:1156-1160.

Buffet-Jerrott SE, Stewart SH, Bird S et al. (1999). An examination of differences in the time course of oxazepam's effects on implicit vs. explicit memory. *Journal of Psychopharmacology* 12:338-347.

Busto UE, Romach MK & Sellers EM (1996). Multiple drug use and psychiatric comorbidity in patients admitted to the hospital with severe benzodiazepine dependence. *Journal of Clinical Psychopharmacology* 16:51-57.

Busto U, Sellars EM, Naranjo CA et al. (1986a). Patterns of benzodiazepine abuse and dependence. *British Journal of Addictions* 81:87-94.

Busto U, Sellars EM, Naranjo CA et al. (1986b). Withdrawal reactions after long-term therapeutic use of benzodiazepines. *New England Journal of Medicine* 315:854-589.

Calhoun SR, Wesson DA, Galloway GP et al. (1996). Abuse of flunitrazepam (Rohypnol) and other benzodiazepines in Austin and South Texas. *Journal of Psychoactive Drugs* 28(2):183-189.

Cavallaro R, Regazzetti MG, Cavelli G et al. (1993). Tolerance and withdrawal with zolpidem [letter]. *Lancet* 342:868-869.

Charney DS, Mihic SJ & Harris RA (2001). Hypnotics and sedatives. In JG Hardman & LE Limbird (eds.) *Goodman and Gillman's The Pharmacological Basis of Therapeutics, 10th Edition*. New York, NY: McGraw-Hill, 399-427.

Chouninard G, Lefko-Singh K & Teboul E (1999). Metabolism of anxiolytics and hypnotics: Benzodiazepines, buspirone, zopiclone, and zolpidem. *Cellular and Molecular Neurobiology* 19:533-552.

Ciraulo DA & Sarid-Segal O (1991). Benzodiazepines: Abuse liability. In PP Roy-Byrne & DS Cowley (eds.) *Benzodiazepines in Clinical Practice: Risks and Benefits*. Washington, DC: American Psychiatric Press, 157-174.

Ciraulo DA, Sarid-Segal O, Knapp C et al. (1996). Liability to alprazolam abuse in daughters of alcoholics. *American Journal of Psychiatry* 153:956-958.

Cowley DS & Dunner DL (1991). Benzodiazepines in anxiety and depression. In PP Roy-Byrne & DS Cowley (eds.) *Benzodiazepines in Clinical Practice: Risks and Benefits*. Washington, DC: American Psychiatric Press, 37-56.

Cowley DS, Roy-Byrne PP & Greenblatt DJ (1991). Benzodiazepines: Pharmacokinetics and pharmacodynamics. In PP Roy-Byrne & DS Cowley (eds.) *Benzodiazepines in Clinical Practice: Risks and Benefits*. Washington, DC: American Psychiatric Press, 21-32.

Danjou P, Paty I, Fruncillo R et al. (1999). A comparison of residual effects of zaleplon and zolpidem following administration 5 to 2 h before awakening. *British Journal of Clinical Pharmacology* 48:367-374.

Darcourt G, Pringuey D, Salliere D et al. (1999). The safety and tolerability of zolpidem—An update. *Journal of Psychopharmacology* 13:81-93.

DeMartinis N, Rynn M, Rickels K et al. (2000). Prior benzodiazepine use and buspirone response in the treatment of generalized anxiety disorder. *Journal of Clinical Psychiatry* 61:91-94.

Dolovich LR, Addis A, Vaillancourt JMR et al. (1998). Benzodiazepine use in pregnancy and major malformations or oral cleft: Meta-analysis of cohort and case-control studies. *British Medical Journal* 317:839-843.

Drummer O & Ranson DL (1996). Sudden death and benzodiazepines. *American Journal of Forensic Medicine and Pathology* 17:336-342.

DuPont RL (1990). A practical approach to benzodiazepine discontinuation. *Journal of Psychiatric Research* 24:81-90.

Ekedahl AM, Lowenhielm P, Nimeus A et al. (1994). Medicine self-poisoning and the sources of the drugs in Lund, Sweden. *Acta Psychiatrica Scandinavica* 89:255-261.

Elie R, Ruther E, Farr I et al. (1999). Sleep latency is shortened during 4 weeks of treatment with zalepon, a novel nonbenzodiazepine hypnotic. *Journal of Clinical Psychiatry* 60:536-544.

File SE (1983). Strain differences in mice in the development of tolerance to the anti-pentylenetetrazole effects of diazepam. *Neuroscience Letters* 42:95-98.

File SE (1985). Tolerance to the behavioral actions of benzodiazepines. *Neuroscience and Biobehavioral Reviews* 9:113-121.

Finlayson RE & Davis LJ (1994). Prescription drug dependence in the elderly population: Demographic and clinical features of 100 patients. *Mayo Clinic Proceedings* 69:1137-1145.

Fisch HU, Bakir G, Karlaganis G et al. (1990). Excessive motor impairment two hours after triazolam in the elderly. *European Journal of Clinical Pharmacology* 38:229-232.

Freeman EW, Rickels K, Sondheimer SJ et al. (1995). A double-blind trial of oral progesterone alprazolam and placebo in treatment of severe premenstrual syndrome. *Journal of the American Medical Association* 274:51-57.

Fujita M, Woods SW, Verhoeff NP et al. (1999). Changes of benzodiazepine receptors during chronic benzodiazepine administration in humans. *European Journal of Pharmacology* 368:161-172.

Gelenberg AJ (1994). Buspirone: Seven-year update. *Journal of Clinical Psychiatry* 55:222-229.

Gelenberg AJ, Lydiard RB, Rudolph RL et al. (2000). Efficacy of venlafaxine extended-release capsules in nondepressed outpatients with generalized anxiety disorder: A 6-month randomized controlled trail. *Journal of the American Medical Association* 283:3082-3088.

Gericke CA & Ludolph AD (1994). Chronic abuse of zolpidem. *Journal of the American Medical Association* 272:1721-1722.

Goldstein LB and the Sygen in Acute Stroke Study Investigators (1995). Common drugs may influence motor recovery after stroke. *Neurology* 45:865-871.

Golombeck S, Moodley P & Lader M (1988). Cognitive impairment in long-term benzodiazepine users. *Psychology in Medicine* 18:365-374.

Greenblatt DJ, Shader RI & Abernethy DR (1983). Current status of benzodiazepines (first of two parts). *New England Journal of Medicine* 309:354-358.

Greenblatt DJ, Von Moltke LL, Daily JP et al. (1999). Extensive impairment of triazolam and alprazolam clearance by short-term low-dose ritonavir: The clinical dilemma of concurrent inhibition and induction. *Journal of Clinical Psychopharmacology* 19:293-296.

Griffiths RR, Bigelow GE & Liebson I (1983). Differential effects of diazepam and pentobarbital on mood and behavior. *Archives of General Psychiatry* 40:865-873.

Griffiths RR & Weerts EM (1997). Benzodiazepine self-administration in humans and laboratory animals—Implications for problems of long-term use and abuse. *Psychopharmacology* 134:1-37.

Hemmelgarn B, Suissa S, Huang A et al. (1997). Benzodiazepine use and the risk of motor vehicle crash in the elderly. *Journal of the American Medical Association* 278:27-31.

Herings RMC, Stricker BH, de Boer A et al. (1995). Benzodiazepines and the risk of falling leading to femur fractures: Dosage more important than elimination half-life. *Archives of Internal Medicine* 144:1801-1807.

Holbrook AM, Crowther R, Lotter A et al. (2000). Meta-analysis of benzodiazepine use in the treatment of insomnia. *Canadian Medical Association* 162:225-233.

Hurst M & Nobel S (1999). Zaleplon. *Central Nervous System Drugs* 11:387-392.

Ito T, Suzuki T, Wellman SE et al. (1996). Pharmacology of barbiturate tolerance/dependence: GABA$_A$ receptors and molecular aspects. *Life Sciences* 59:169-195.

Janicak PG (1999a). Indications for antianxiety and sedative-hypnotic agents. In PG Janicak (ed.) *Handbook of Psychopharmacotherapy.* Baltimore, MD: Lippincott Williams & Wilkins, 253-258.

Janicak PG (1999b). Treatment with antianxiety and sedative-hypnotic agents. In PG Janicak (ed.) *Handbook of Psychopharmacotherapy.* Baltimore, MD: Lippincott Williams & Wilkins, 259-289.

Juergens SM & Morse RM (1988). Alprazolam dependence in seven patients. *American Journal of Psychiatry* 1455:625-627.

Kan CC, Treteler MHM & Zitman FG (1997). High prevalence of benzodiazepine dependence in out-patient users, based on the DSM-III-R and ICD-10 criteria. *Acta Psychiatrica Scandinavica* 96:85-93.

Khanna JM, Kalant H, Chau A et al. (1998). Rapid tolerance and cross-tolerance to motor impairment effects of benzodizepines, barbiturates, and ethanol. *Pharmacology, Biochemistry and Behavior* 59:511-519.

King DJ (1992). Benzodiazepines, amnesia and sedation: Theoretical and clinical issues and controversies. *Human Psychopharmacology* 7:79-87.

Kisnad H (1990). Sedative-Hypnotics (not including benzodiazepines). In NS Miller (ed.) *Comprehensive Handbook of Drug and Alcohol Addiction.* New York, NY: Marcel Dekker, 477-502.

Kranzler HR, Burleson JA, Del Bocca FK et al. (1994). Buspirone treatment of anxious alcoholics: A placebo-controlled trial. *Archives of General Psychiatry* 51:720-731.

Kupfer DJ & Reynolds CF (1997). Management of insomnia. *New England Journal of Medicine* 336:341-346.

Laakmann G, Faltermaier-Temizel, Bossert-Zaudig S et al. (1996). Are benzodiazepines antidepressants? [letter]. *Psychopharmacology* 124:291-292.

Lader M & File S (1987). The biological basis of benzodiazepine dependence. *Psychological Medicine* 17:539-547.

Lader MM & Olafide D (1987). A comparison of buspirone and placebo in relieving benzodiazepine withdrawal symptoms. *Journal of Clinical Psychopharmacology* 7:11-15.

Laegreid L, Hagberg G & Lundberg A (1992). The effect of benzodiazepines on the fetus and the newborn. *Neuropediatrics* 23:18-23.

Laegreid L, Olegard R, Conradi N et al. (1990). Congenital malformations and maternal consumption of benzodiazepines: A case-control study. *Developmental Medicine and Child Neurology* 32:432-441.

Laegreid L, Olegard R, Wahlstrom J et al. (1989). Teratogenic effects of benzodiazepine use during pregnancy. *Journal of Pediatrics* 114:126-131.

Leipzig RM, Cummings RG & Tinetti ME (1999). Drugs and falls in older people: A systematic review and meta-analysis: I. Psychotropic drugs. *Journal of the American Geriatric Society* 47:30-39.

Lekka NP, Paschalis C & Beratis S (1997). Nicotine, caffeine, and alcohol use in high- and low-dose benzodiazepines. *Drug and Alcohol Dependence* 45:207-212.

Lucki I, Rickels K & Geller AM (1986). Chronic use of benzodiazepines and psychomotor and cognitive test performance. *Psychopharmacology* 88:426-433.

Marcantonio ER, Juarez G, Goldman L et al. (1996). The relationship of postoperative delirium with psychoactive medications. *Journal of the American Medical Association* 272:1518-1522.

Mattila MJ, Vanokoski J, Kalska H et al. (1998). Effects of alcohol, zolpidem, and some other sedatives and hypnotics on human performance and memory. *Pharmacology Biochemistry and Behavior* 59:917-203.

Maxmen JS & Ward NG (1995). Antianxiety agents. In JS Maxmen & NG Ward (eds.) *Psychotropic Drugs Fast Facts, 2nd Edition.* New York, NY: W.W. Norton & Company, 255-312.

Medical Letter, The (1999). Zolpidem for insomnia. *The Medical Letter on Drugs and Therapeutics* 41:93-94.

Miller LG, Woolverton S, Greenblatt DJ et al. (1989). Chronic benzodiazepine administration. IV. Rapid development of tolerance and receptor down-regulation associated with alprazolam administration. *Biochemical Pharmacology* 38:3773-3777.

Mintzer MZ & Griffiths RR (1998). Flunitrazepam and triazolam: A comparison of behavioral effects and abuse liability. *Drug and Alcohol Dependence* 53: 49-66.

Moller HJ (1999). Effectiveness and safety of benzodiazepines. *Journal of Clinical Psychopharmacology* 19(Suppl 2):2S-11S.

Morrow AL (1995). Regulation of GABA$_A$ receptor function and gene expression in the central nervous system. *International Review of Neurobiology* 38:1-41.

Mumford GK, Evans SM, Fleishaker JC et al. (1995). Alprazolam absorption kinetics affects abuse liability. *Clinical Pharmacology and Therapeutics* 57:356-365.

Nagy LM, Krystal JH, Woods SW et al. (1989). Clinical and medication outcome after short-term alprazolam and behavioral group treatment in panic disorder. *Archives of General Psychiatry* 46:993-999.

Nutt D (1990). Pharmacological mechanisms of benzodiazepine withdrawal. *Journal of Psychiatric Research* 24(Suppl 2):105-110.

Nutt D (1999). Alcohol and the brain. *British Journal of Psychiatry* 175:114-119.

Pick N, McDonald A, Bennett N et al. 91996). Pulmonary aspiration in a long-term care setting: Clinical and laboratory observations and an analysis of risk factors. *Journal of the American Geriatric Society* 44:763-768.

Pomara N, Tun H, DaSilva D et al. (1998). The acute and chronic performance effects of alprazolam and lorazepam in the elderly: Relationship to duration of treatment and self-rated sedation. *Psychopharmacology Bulletin* 34:139-154.

Post RM, Frye MA, Denicoff KD et al. (1998). Beyond lithium in the treatment of bipolar illness. *Neuropsychopharmacology* 19:206-219.

Pratt JA, Breett RR & Laurie DJ (1994). Benzodiazepine dependence: From neural circuits to gene expression. *Pharmacology, Biochemistry and Behavior* 59:925-934.

Rall TW (1990). Hypnotics and sedatives: Ethanol. In AG Gilman, TW Rall, AS Nies et al. (eds.) *Goodman and Gilman's The Pharmacological Basis of Therapeutics, 8th Edition.* New York, NY: Pergamon Press, 345-382.

Ray WA, Purushottam BT & Shorr RI (1993). Medications and the older driver. *Clinics in Geriatric Medicine* 9:413-438.

Reynaud M, Petit G, Potard D et al. (1998). Six deaths linked to concomitant use of buprenorphine and benzodiazepines. *Addiction* 93(9):1385-1392.

Rickels K, Case GW, Downing RW et al. (1983). Long-term diazepam therapy and clinical outcome. *Journal of the American Medical Association* 250:767-771.

Rickels K, Case WG, Schweizer E et al. (1991). Long-term benzodiazepine users 3 years after participation in a discontinuation program. *American Journal of Psychiatry* 148:757-761.

Rickels K, DeMartinis N, Garcia-Espana F et al. (2000). Imipramine and vuspirone in treatment of patients with generalized anxiety disorder who are discontinuing long-term benzodiazepine therapy. *American Journal of Psychiatry* 157:1973-1979.

Rickels K, DeMartinis N, Rynn M et al. (1999). Pharmacologic strategies for discontinuing benzodiazepine treatment. *Journal of Clinical Psychopharmacology* 19(suppl 2):12S-16S.

Rickels K & Freeman EW (2000). Prior benzodiazepine exposure and benzodiazepine treatment outcome. *Journal of Clinical Psychiatry* 61:409-413.

Rickels K, Lucki I, Schweizer E et al. (1999). Psychomotor performance of long-term benzodiazepine users before, during, and after benzodiazepine discontinuation. *Journal of Clinical Psychopharmacology* 19:107-113.

Rickels K & Schweizer E (1998). Panic disorder: Long-term pharmacotherapy and discontinuation. *Journal of Clinical Psychopharmacology* 18:(supp 2):12S-18S.

Rickels K, Schweizer E, Case G et al. (1990). Long-term therapeutic use of benzodiazepines: I. Effects of abrupt discontinuation. *Archives of General Psychiatry* 47:899-907.

Rickels K, Schweizer E, Csanalosi I et al. (1988). Long-term treatment of anxiety and risk of withdrawal: Prospective comparison of clorazepate and buspirone. *Archives of General Psychiatry* 45:444-450.

Rickels K, Schweizer E, Weiss S et al. (1993). Maintenance drug treatment for panic disorder. II. Short- and long-term outcome after drug taper. *Archives of General Psychiatry* 50:61-68.

Roache JD (1990). Addiction potential of benzodiazepines and non-benzodiazepine anxiolytics. In CK Erickson, MA Javors & WW Morgan (eds.) *Addiction Potential of Abused Drugs and Drug Classes.* Binghamton, NY: Haworth Press, 103-128.

Roache JD & Meisch RA (1995). Findings from self-administration research on the addition potential of benzodiazepines. *Psuchiatric Annals* 25: 153-157.

Rocca P, Fonzo V Scotta M et al. 91997). Paroxetine efficacy in the treatment of generalized anxiety disorder. *Acta Psychiatrica Scandinavia* 95:444-450.

Rothschild AJ (1992). Disinhibition, amnestic reactions, and other adverse reactions secondary to triazolam: A review of the literature. *Journal of Clinical Psychiatry* 53(12 Suppl):69-79.

Roy-Byrne PP (1991). Benzodiazepines: Dependence and withdrawal. In PP Roy-Byrne & DS Cowley (eds.) *Benzodiazepines in Clinical Practice: Risks and Benefits.* Washington, DC: American Psychiatric Press, 133-153.

Roy-Byrne PP & Nutt DJ (1991). Benzodiazepines biological mechanisms. In PP Roy-Byrne & DS Cowley (eds.) *Benzodiazepines in Clinical Practice: Risks and Benefits.* Washington, DC: American Psychiatric Press, 5-18.

Rush CR (1998). Behavioral pharmacology of zolpidem relative to benzodiazepines: A review. *Pharmacology, Biochemistry and Behavior* 61:253-269.

Rush CR, Frey JM & Griffiths RR (1999). Zaleplon and triazolam in humans: Acute behavioral effects and abuse potential. *Psychopharmacology* 145:39-51.

Rush CR & Griffiths RR (1996). Zolpidem, triazolam, and temazepam: Behavioral and subject-rated effects in normal volunteers. *Journal of Clinical Psychopharmacology* 16:146-157.

Salzman C, Fisher J, Nobel K et al. (1992). Cognitive improvement following benzodiazepine discontinuation in elderly nursing home residents. *International Journal of Geriatric Psychiatry* 7:89-93.

Sanger DJ, Benavides J, Perrault G et al. (1994). Recent developments in the behavioral pharmacology of benzodiazepine (omega) receptors: Evidence for the functional significance of receptor subtypes. *Neuroscience and Biobehavioral Reviews* 18:355-372.

Schenck CH & Mahowald MW (1996a). Long-term, nightly benzodiazepine treatment of injurious parasomnias and other disorders of disrupted nocturnal sleep in 170 adults. *American Journal of Medicine* 100:33-337.

Schenck CH & Mahowald MW (1996b). REM sleep parasomnias. *Neurologic Clinics* 14:697-720.

Schweizer E, Rickels K, Case G et al. (1990). Long-term therapeutic use of benzodiazepines: II. Effects of gradual taper. *Archives of General Psychiatry* 47:908-915.

Serfaty M & Masterton G (1993). Fatal poisonings attributed to benzodiazepines in Britain during the 1980s. *British Journal of Psychiatry* 163:386-393.

Sieghart W (2000). Unraveling the function of GABA-A receptor subtypes. *Trends in Pharmacological Sciences* 21:411-413.

Silverman K, Kirby KD & Griffiths RR (1994). Modulation of drug reinforcement by behavioral requirements following drug ingestion. *Psychopharmacology* 114:243-247.

Simmons MM & Cupp MJ (1998). Use and abuse of flunitrazepam. *Annals of Pharmacology* 32:117-118.

Skrabanek P (1992). Smoking and statistical overkill. *Lancet* 340:1208-1209.

Smith RB & Kroboth PD (1987). Influence of dosing regimens on alprazolam and metabolic serum concentrations and tolerance to sedative and psychomotor effects. *Psychopharmacology* 93:105-112.

Smith WT, Londborg PD, Glaudin V et al. (1998). Short-term augmentation of fluoxetine with clonazepam in the treatment of depression: A double-blind study. *American Journal of Psychiatry* 155:1339-1345.

Soldatos CR, Dikeos DG & Whitehead A (1999). Tolerance and rebound insomnia with rapidly eliminated hypnotics: A meta-analysis of sleep laboratory studies. *International Clinical Psychopharmacology* 14:287-303.

Sproule BA, Naranjo CA, Bremner KE et al. (1997). Selective serotonin reuptake inhibitors and CNS drug interactions. A critical review of the evidence. *Clinical Pharmacokinetics* 33:454-457.

Stein MR, Liebowitz MR, Lydiard RB et al. (1998). Paroxetine treatment of generalized social phobia (social anxiety disorder): A randomized controlled trial. *Journal of the American Medical Association* 280:708-713.

Tanaka E (1999). Clinically significant pharmacokinetic drug interaction with benzodiazepines. *Journal of Clinical Pharmacology and Therapeutics* 24:347-355.

Tata PR, Rollings J, Collins M et al. (1994). Lack of cognitive recovery following withdrawal from long-term benzodiazepine use. *Psychological Medicine* 24:203-213.

Thomas RE (1998). Benzodiazepine use and motor vehicle accidents: Systematic review of reported association. *Canadian Family Physician* 44:799-808.

Troy SM, Lucki I, Unruh MA et al. (2000). Comparison of the effects of zaleplon, zolpidem, and triazolam on memory, learning and psychomotor performance. *Journal of Clinical Psychopharmacology* 20:328-337.

Uhlenhuth EH, Balter MB, Ban TA et al. (1998). International study of expert judgment on therapeutic use of benzodiazepines and other psychotherapeutic medications: V. Treatment strategies in panic disorder, 1992-1997. *Journal of Clinical Psychopharmacology* 18(Suppl 2):17S-31S.

Van Laar MW, Volkerts ER & Van Willigenburg APP (1992). *Journal of Clinical Psychopharmacology* 12:86-95.

van Stevenick AL, Wallnofer AE, Schoemaker RC et al. (1997). A study of the effects of long-term use on individual sensitivity to temazepam and lorazepam in a clinical population. *British Journal of Clinical Pharmacology* 44:267-275.

Wagner J, Wagner ML & Hening WA (1998). Beyond benzodiazepines: Alternative pharmacology agents for the treatment of insomnia. *Annals of Pharmacotherapy* 32:680-691.

Ware JC, Walsh JK, Scharf MB et al. (1997). Minimal rebound insomnia after treatment with 10-mg zolpidem. *Clinical Neuropharmacology* 20:116-125.

Wasserf AA, Dott SG, Haris A et al. (1999). Critical review of GABA-ergic drugs in the treatment of schizophrenia. *Journal of Clinical Psychopharmacology* 19:206-219.

Weinberger DR (2001). Anxiety at the frontier of molecular medicine. *New England Journal of Medicine* 344:1247-1249.

Weintraub M, Singh S, Byrne L et al. (1991). Consequences of the New York State triplicate benzodiazepine prescription regulation. *Journal of the American Medical Association* 266:2392-2397.

Wetter TC & Pollmacher T (1997). Restless legs and periodic leg movements in sleep syndromes. *Journal of Neurology* 244(Suppl 1):S37-S45.

Whiting PJ, Bonnert TP, McKenzie RM et al. (1999). Molecular and functional diversity of the expanding GABA-A receptor gene family. *Annals of the New York Academy of Sciences* 868:645-653.

Wolf B & Griffiths RR (1991). Physical dependence on benzodiazepines: Differences within the class. *Drug and Alcohol Dependence* 29:153-156.

Wolf B, Grohmann R, Biber PM et al. (1989). Benzodiazepine abuse and dependence in psychiatric inpatients. *Pharmacopsychiatry* 22:54-60.

Woods JH (1998). Problems and opportunities in regulation of benzodiazepines. *Journal of Clinical Pharmacology* 38:773-782.

Woods JH, Katz JL & Winger G (1988). Use and abuse of benzodiazepines: Issues relevant to prescribing. *Journal of the American Medical Association* 260:3476-3480.

Worthington JJ 3d, Pollack MH, Otto MW et al. (1998). Long-term experience with clonazepam in patients with a primary diagnosis of panic disorder. *Psychophamacology Bulletin* 34:199-205.

Zorumski CF & Isenberg KE (1991). Insights into the structure and function of GABA-benzodiazepine receptor: Ion channels and psychiatry. *American Journal of Psychiatry* 148:162-173.

Gamma-hydroxybutyrate (GHB): A New Drug of Abuse

GANTT P. GALLOWAY, PHARM.D.

Gamma-hydroxybutyrate (GHB) is a simple, 4-carbon molecule that originally was synthesized in an effort to find an orally active gamma-aminobutyric acid (GABA)ergic agent. Although structurally similar to GABA, GHB appears to be a neurotransmitter in its own right (Cash, 1994). GHB has been used as a general anesthetic, to induce seizures in animal models of epilepsy and, more recently, in the treatment of narcolepsy and alcohol and opiate dependence (Galloway, Frederick-Osborne et al., 2000). Narcolepsy is the only indication for which GHB is approved in the United States.

Reports of abuse of GHB date to the early 1990s. Initially used by bodybuilders who believed it would increase circulating levels of growth hormones, the drug's hypnotic and euphoric properties rapidly became apparent and contributed to its popularity. The desired effects of GHB resemble those of alcohol and include relaxation, disinhibition, and euphoria.

GHB is inexpensive and readily available at some nightclubs and "rave" parties. It typically is sold as "GHB," "G," or "liquid Ecstasy." GHB almost always is sold in aqueous solution (which has a salty taste). It may have a variable concentration or measured inaccurately. This undoubtedly contributes to the high incidence of adverse effects.

The Internet has been a source of information promoting GHB, as well as a venue through simple kits for the manufacture of GHB can be purchased. In response to increasing legal restrictions on the purchase of GHB, many users have switched to gamma-butyrolactone (GBL, G, "lactone," "Renewtrient," "Blue Nitro") and 1,4-butanediol (BD, G, "1, 4B," "Pro-G," "Thunder"), both of which are converted to GHB in the body.

ADDICTION LIABILITY

Physical dependence and addiction have been reported with GHB, GBL, and BD (Galloway, Frederick et al., 1994; McDaniel & Miotto, 2001). It is important to note that our knowledge of the nature and treatment of dependence on these drugs comes from a relatively small number of case reports and one survey. Frequent (that is, at least four times a day) use seems to be required for physical dependence.

The withdrawal syndrome may be mild, involving insomnia, agitation, anxiety, and limited sympathetic arousal or severe. It also may involve agitation, delirium, and psychosis (McDaniel & Miotto, 2001). Onset of withdrawal occurs within six hours, peaks in approximately one day, and may last up to two weeks. The severity of withdrawal may progress rapidly, as from mild to severe within one hour.

Of the many medications that have been used to treat GHB withdrawal, the most experience is with benzodiazepines, which may need to be given in extraordinarily high doses and may not ameliorate delirium (McDaniel & Miotto, 2001; Dyer, Roth et al., 2001). Antipsychotics appear to be less effective than benzodiazepines, while limited data suggest that pentobarbital may be effective for the full range of withdrawal symptoms (Sivilotti, Burns et al., 2001). Delirium, psychosis, and use of high doses of benzodiazepines or barbiturates all are indications for inpatient hospitalization.

TOXICITY/ADVERSE EFFECTS

GHB has a narrow therapeutic window and users frequently experience adverse effects, including dizziness, nausea, vomiting, decreased respiratory effort, and coma (Chin, Sporer et al., 1998; Miotto, Darakjian et al., 2001). Other sedative-hypnotics, notably alcohol, may act additively with GHB with respect to these adverse effects.

The half-life of GHB is approximately 20 minutes. Patients may make a surprisingly rapid transition from apneic and comatose to alert and eager to terminate medical care.

REFERENCES

Cash CD (1994). Gamma-hydroxybutyrate: An overview of the pros and cons for it being a neurotransmitter and/or a useful therapeutic agent. *Neuroscience and Biobehavioral Reviews* 18(2):291-304.

Chin RL, Sporer KA, Cullison B et al. (1998). Clinical course of gamma-hydroxybutyrate overdose. *Annals of Emergency Medicine* 31(6):716-722.

Dyer J, Roth B & Hyma BA (2001). Gamma-hydroxybutyrate withdrawal syndrome. *Annals of Emergency Medicine* 37:147-153.

Galloway GP, Frederick SL & Staggers F Jr (1994). Physical dependence on sodium oxybate. *Lancet* 343(8888):57.

Galloway GP, Frederick-Osborne SL, Seymour R et al. (2000). Abuse and therapeutic potential of gamma-hydroxybutyric acid. *Alcohol* 20(3):263-269.

McDaniel CH & Miotto KA (2001). Gamma hydroxybutyrate (GHB) and gamma butyrolactone (GBL) withdrawal: Five case studies. *Journal of Psychoactive Drugs* 33(2):143-149.

Miotto K, Darakjian J, Basch J et al. (2001). Gamma-hydroxybutyric acid: Patterns of use, effects and withdrawal. *American Journal on Addictions* 10(3):232-241.

Sivilotti ML, Burns MJ, Aaron CK et al. (2001). Pentobarbital for severe gamma-butyrolactone withdrawal. *Annals of Emergency Medicine* 38(6):660-665.

Chapter 4

The Pharmacology of Opioids

Lisa Borg, M.D.
Mary Jeanne Kreek, M.D.

Drugs in the Class
Pharmacokinetics and Metabolism
Pharmacologic Actions
Neurobiology
Future Research Directions

Three principal opioid receptors are found in the central nervous system (CNS): mu, kappa, and delta. Opioids are considered to include the natural opiates (drugs derived from opium) and their manmade congeners, which are the agonist and antagonist drugs with mostly morphine-like activity (primarily at the mu opioid receptor), as well as other naturally occurring endogenous opioid peptides, which also are active at opioid receptors (Borg & Kreek, 1998). The genes for each of these three receptors have been cloned in humans as well as in rodent species (see LaForge, Yuferov et al., 2000).

This chapter reviews the pharmacology and neurobiology of five exogenous opioids that are particularly significant in the area of opioid addiction and its pharmacotherapy: heroin, morphine, methadone, levo-alpha-acetylmethadol (LAAM), and buprenorphine.

DRUGS IN THE CLASS

Heroin. Diacetylmorphine, or heroin, is synthetically derived from the natural opioid, morphine. In large part because of its rapid onset of action and very short half-life, heroin is a popular drug of abuse. Heroin is absorbed most efficiently when used intravenously, but the drug increasingly is used intranasally, mainly because of users' desire to reduce the risk of HIV-1 transmission from injection drug use and because of the wider availability of high-purity heroin (around 70% purity in certain geographic regions, as compared with less than 30% purity in recent years) (Frank, 2000).

Heroin is biotransformed rapidly to monoacetylmorphine and then metabolized, mostly to morphine.

Morphine and Synthetic Compounds. Morphine has a longer half-life (around two to four hours in humans) and high potency. It is prescribed primarily as an analgesic.

Modifications of the chemical structure of the morphine molecule at the 3, 6, and 17 position produce other compounds, including agonists such as morphine-6-glucuronide (M6G), which is a major pharmacologically active metabolite of morphine. Synthetic compounds include hydrocodone (Vicodin®) and oxycodone (OxyContin®) and the fentanyl compounds (as well as heroin). Synthetics also include antagonists such as naloxone (Narcan®), naltrexone (ReVia®), and nalmefene (Revex®); as well as partial agonists such as buprenorphine (Buprenex®) (Reisine & Pasternak, 1996).

Methadone and LAAM. Methadone is a synthetic, orally administered, long-acting, pure opioid agonist that first was studied and used in the mid-1960s. It was approved by the U.S. Food and Drug Administration (FDA) in 1972 as an effective chronic treatment for heroin addiction. LAAM is a synthetic, longer-acting (48 hours) congener of methadone that also is orally effective. LAAM first was studied in the 1970s for the treatment of heroin addiction and approved in 1993 by the FDA as a pharmacotherapy for opioid addiction.

The stereochemistry of the methadone molecule determines its activity, in that *l*-methadone has up to 50 times more analgesic activity than the *d*-isomer, as well as the potential to produce respiratory depression.

Epidemiology. It is estimated that 2.7 million persons in the United States have used heroin at some point in their lives, with about 1 million actually addicted to the drug (according to the definitions contained in federal guidelines). At present, 179,000 patients in the United States are enrolled in methadone maintenance programs, with an additional 5,000 enrolled in LAAM maintenance as treatment for their opioid or heroin addiction. A comparable number are in treatment in other countries (Kreek & Vocci, in press 2002).

The pharmacology of opioids is of particular relevance to the treatment of addictive disorders, given reports of recent increases in the abuse of illicit opioids, as well as illicit use of prescribed opioid medications (WWW.NIDA.NIH.GOV, 2002).

PHARMACOKINETICS AND METABOLISM
Heroin (Diacetylmorphine). Diacetylmorphine first was synthesized in 1874, then produced in 1898 by the Bayer company and marketed under the name "heroin." Heroin is more water soluble and also more potent than morphine (Sawynok, 1986). It is synthesized from morphine by acetylation at both the 3 and 6 position. Heroin is metabolized in humans by deacetylation to 6-mono-acetylmorphine and then further metabolized to morphine (Kamendulis, Brzezinski et al., 1996).

Heroin is not available for any therapeutic use in the United States. It is prescribed in a few other countries as a pain medication or for use in the management of heroin addiction.

Well-designed studies of heroin pharmacokinetics in humans have been performed (Kaiko, Wallenstein et al., 1981; Inturrisi, Schultz et al., 1983; Inturrisi, Max et al., 1984; Cone, Holicky et al., 1993; Kamendulis, Brzezinski

et al., 1996; Skopp, Ganssmann et al., 1997). Measures of pain relief that compare heroin with morphine given intramuscularly in patients with cancer showed that heroin was about two times as potent as morphine, with faster onset of peak mood effect (an average of 1.2 ± 0.10 versus 1.8 ± 0.13 hours, respectively); however, it has less sustained effect (Kaiko, Wallenstein et al., 1981). Heroin apparently is a lipid-soluble prodrug that lacks intrinsic opioid activity, exerting its effect after metabolism to 6-acetylmorphine and morphine (Inturrisi, Schultz et al., 1983), as shown by opiate binding studies in rat brain. More recent studies in mice, involving the use of antisense probes, have shown a lack of cross-tolerance to morphine by M6G, heroin, and 6-acetylmorphine, along with strain differences in sensitivity to morphine, M6G, and heroin. This finding has been hypothesized by some to suggest the possibility that heroin and 6-acetylmorphine can act through different receptor systems, such as through splice variants or through linkage to different signal transduction systems (Rossi, Brown et al., 1996). Heroin, 6-acetylmorphine, and M6G all can elicit analgesia in some mice that are insensitive to morphine because of genetic deletions of the mu opioid receptor (Schuller, King et al., 1999), but not in most other knockout mice (Loh, Liu et al., 1998; Kitanaka, Sora et al., 1998; Matthes, Maldonado et al., 1996).

Heroin has an average half-life in blood of three minutes after intravenous administration. When heroin is given as an infusion to patients with chronic pain, the onset of pain relief after 15 and 45 minutes occurs with the presence of heroin and 6-acetylmorphine in the blood, before the appearance of morphine (Inturrisi, Max et al., 1984). Oral heroin has complete first-pass metabolism, first to 6-acetylmorphine and then to morphine (Inturrisi, Max et al., 1984); however, both heroin and morphine have very limited systemic bioavailability when given orally, in comparison to methadone and LAAM. The blood clearance of heroin (2,134 mL/minute) is greater than the upper range of hepatic blood flow in humans (1,500 mL/minute). This indicates that organs other than the liver likely are involved in the biotransformation and removal of heroin. These may include the gastrointestinal (GI) wall and the kidney (Inturrisi, Max et al., 1984), as well as blood esterases such as pseudo-cholinesterase (Kamendulis, Brzezinski et al., 1996). The half-life of 6-acetylmorphine in humans appears to be less than one hour (Skopp, Ganssmann et al., 1997). In comparing sublingual to oral absorption, the more lipid-soluble drugs (including methadone and heroin) are absorbed to the greatest degree, regardless of concentration of opioid, with increased absorption producing higher potential systemic bioavailability of the opioid (Weinberg, Inturrisi et al., 1988).

In humans, the pharmacokinetic profile of intranasal heroin appears to be comparable to that of heroin given by intramuscular administration (Cone, Holicky et al., 1993; Skoop, Ganssmann et al., 1997). The use of intranasal heroin produces peak blood levels of heroin or 6-acetylmorphine within five minutes, which is comparable to the time course after the intramuscular route of administration, with about half the relative potency in terms of behavioral and physiologic effects (Cone, Holicky et al., 1993).

Further research needs to be done on the role of 6-acetylmorphine (administered directly) in relation to the pharmacokinetics of parenteral heroin, particularly its onset of action and potency as compared with morphine.

Morphine. Morphine is largely selective for the mu opioid receptor at lower doses and is the opioid agonist that is considered the drug of choice for the treatment of cancer pain. Morphine is biotransformed mainly by hepatic glucuronidation to the major but inactive metabolite morphine-3-glucuronide (M3G) and the other biologically active M6G compound.

The pharmacokinetics of morphine and its metabolites vary, depending on the route of administration. Plasma concentration of morphine given orally every four hours to cancer patients with chronic pain demonstrated a significant, linear correlation between dose and mean plasma level by radioimmunoassay (RIA) with low cross-reactivity. However, considerable variation was found in individual plasma measures of morphine during the same dose intervals, possibly related to rapid absorption and short elimination half-life (Neumann, Henriksen et al., 1982).

The clinical effects of morphine may be partially the result of the active metabolite M6G, with greater M6G/morphine ratios after oral versus intravenous administration (Osborne, Joel et al., 1988; Hasselström & Säwe 1993). Much of morphine analgesia may be derived from the M6G metabolite (Osborne, Joel et al., 1988; Portenoy, Thaler et al., 1992), although unmetabolized morphine can have higher affinity for mu receptors, as demonstrated in mouse brain studies (Paul, Standifer et al., 1989). The half-life of morphine ($t_{1/2}$) is almost comparable when given by different routes: 1.4 ± 0.44 hours with oral dosing versus 1.7 ± 0.8 hours when given intravenously (Osborne, Joel et al., 1990), with a plasma half-life of about two hours when given by intramuscular or subcutaneous routes (Reisine & Pasternak, 1996). Sublingual, buccal, and sustained-release buccal morphine are absorbed more slowly (Osborne, Joel et al., 1990). The difference in oral/parenteral potency of morphine of 1:3 may be due to differences in the amounts of morphine in the blood, because the ratios of M6G/M3G for a dose administered by either route are approximately the same (4.4:3.0), according to one report (Hasselström & Säwe, 1993). Transdermal absorption is relatively poor (Westerling, Hoglund et al., 1994) because of the low lipophilicity of morphine; this is true of sublingual absorption of morphine (18% to 22%) as well (Weinberg, Inturrisi et al., 1988). Rectal dosing produces less metabolites, probably because of bypassed hepatic biotransformation, and greater intersubject variability (Babul & Darke, 1993).

Morphine is metabolized mostly in the liver, with prolonged clearance because of enterohepatic cycling with oral dosing (Westerling, Frigen et al., 1993; Hasselström & Säwe, 1993; Mazoit, Sandouk et al.,1990). In the setting of chronic liver disease, morphine oxidation is more affected than glucuronidation. One study in humans (Hasselström, Eriksson et al., 1990) showed increased oral bioavailblity and a prolonged elimination half-life in patients with cirrhosis who received morphine orally and intravenously. Use of lower doses or longer dosing intervals is recommended to minimize the risk of accumulation of morphine when chronic liver disease is present, particularly with repeated dosing (Tegeder, Lotsch et al., 1999).

At 24 hours, more than 90% of morphine has been excreted in urine. M6G elimination seems to be closely tied to renal function (Osborne, Joel et al., 1988), so accumulation of metabolite can occur. With renal compromise, less than 10% of morphine and its metabolites are excreted in feces; therefore, morphine should be used with great caution in patients with renal disease (unlike methadone, which can be given relatively safely in these patients [see the discussion of methadone metabolism, following]). The effect of renal failure on the disposition of morphine and its metabolites was observed by investigators using RIA techniques and was not observed when investigators used more specific chromatography assays (Chan & Matzke, 1987). Earlier disposition studies using nonspecific RIAs show much higher (3- to 16-fold) morphine concentrations than that obtained by using a highly specific RIA for morphine, with less than 0.2% cross-reactivity with M6G and M3G (Got, Baud et al., 1994).

Aging also affects morphine pharmacokinetics. For example, the higher sensitivity of older adults to the analgesic properties of morphine may be related in part to altered pharmacokinetics. For example, there is a 50% reduction in total apparent volume of distribution because of lowered central and peripheral kinetic compartment volumes, along with higher calculated peripheral morphine measures after 10 mg/70 kg given intravenously (Owen, Sitar et al., 1983).

Methadone. Methadone first was synthesized by Bayer as an analgesic in Germany in the late 1930s, but was not studied in the U.S. until it was brought to the United States by the government after World War II. Initially used in the treatment of chronic pain, methadone has been used primarily as a treatment for heroin addiction since the early 1960s, when it was found to be quite effective, as it meets the two important criteria for a medication for the treatment of addiction: high systemic bioavailability (>90%) with oral administration and long apparent half-life with long-term administration.

Pharmacokinetic studies have shown that oral methadone has a delayed onset of action, with peak plasma levels achieved by two to four hours and sustained over a 24-hour dosing period (Änggaard, Gunne et al., 1974; Dole & Kreek, 1973; Inturrisi & Verebely, 1972a, 1972b; Kreek, 1973a, 1973b; Kreek, Schecter et al., 1974; Kling, Carson et al., 2000). Moreover, the mean plasma apparent terminal half-life of racemic *d,l*-methadone in human subjects, as used for therapeutics in the United States, is around 24 hours. Further studies using stable isotopes have shown that the *l*-enantiomer has a half-life of 36 hours (Hachey, Kreek et al., 1977; Kreek, Hachey et al., 1979; Nakamura, Hachey et al., 1982).

When taken on a chronic basis, methadone is stored and accumulates mostly in liver tissue (Kreek, Oratz et al., 1978). Methadone plasma levels are kept relatively constant because of the slow release of unmetabolized methadone into the blood, which extends the apparent terminal half-life. Methadone is more than 90% plasma protein bound, both to albumin and all globulins (Kreek, Gutjahr et al., 1976; Pond, Kreek et al., 1985). Methadone is relatively lipid soluble, with 34% to 75% absorption when given sublingually, depending on the pH (Weinberg, Inturrisi et al., 1988).

These pharmacokinetic studies help explain why methadone maintenance is effective as a once-daily, orally administered pharmacotherapy for heroin addiction (Dole, Nyswander et al., 1966) and why methadone is very different from heroin and morphine, both of which have a relatively rapid onset and offset of effect and short duration of action. The long half-life of methadone must be considered when beginning methadone treatment (usually starting with a 20 to 40 mg daily dose), because it can result in accumulation in plasma, with sedation and respiratory depression. Thus dosages must be increased slowly, usually by 10 mg every four to seven days. It is not yet fully understood why some patients in methadone maintenance experience symptoms of opioid abstinence despite adequate dose (80 to 120 mg) and apparent therapeutic blood levels of 250 to 400 ng/mL (Borg, Ho et al., 1995; Wolff, Hay et al., 1991, 1993). These symptoms may be due to pharmacodynamic factors that are not yet well understood or to other factors such as concomitant illness, psychological factors, or "rapid metabolism" related to individual genetic differences of the cytochrome P450-related enzyme system (Eap, Broly et al., 2001; Leavitt, Shinderman et al., 2000). Methadone levels in the cerebrospinal fluid peak three to eight hours after methadone dosing (Rubenstein, Kreek et al., 1978).

Methadone is biotransformed in the liver by the cytochrome P450-related enzymes (primarily by the 3A4 and, to a lesser extent, the 2D6 and 1A2 systems) to two N-demethylated biologically inactive metabolites, which undergo additional oxidative metabolism (Änggaard, Gunne et al., 1974; Kreek, Garfield et al., 1976; Kreek, Gutjahr et al., 1976; Sullivan, Smits et al., 1972). Methadone is excreted nearly equally in urine and feces (Kreek, Bencsath et al., 1980, 1983; Kreek, Schecter et al., 1980).

In patients with renal disease, methadone can be cleared almost entirely by the GI tract, unlike morphine and many other opiates. This fecal route reduces potential toxicity by preventing accumulation (Bowen, Smit et al., 1978; Kreek, Bencsath et al., 1980, 1983; Kreek, Gutjahr et al., 1976, 1978; Kreek, Schecter et al., 1980). Therefore, methadone can be given safely to patients with chronic renal disease because it is excreted by the feces as an alternative to renal excretion, unlike morphine (see the preceding discussion of morphine). Less than 1% of unmetabolized methadone is removed in dialysis, probably because of its extensive plasma protein binding and the small degree to which methadone is actually present in the blood (rather than stored in the liver) at any one point (Kreek, Schecter et al., 1980). Patients with severe long-standing liver disease have decreased methadone metabolism and thus slower metabolic clearance of methadone, yet lower than expected plasma methadone levels as a result of lower hepatic reservoirs of methadone because of reduced function or liver size. Methadone disposition is relatively normal in patients with mild to moderate liver impairment (Kreek, Bencsath et al., 1980, 1983; Kreek, Kalisman et al., 1980; Kreek, Oratz et al., 1978; Novick, Kreek et al., 1981, 1985).

Other drugs can interact with methadone because of their effects on hepatic enzymes in the cytochrome P450-related enzyme system. Metabolism of methadone is increased with the concurrent use of rifampin (Rifadin®) and phenytoin (Dilantin®) (Kreek, Garfield et al., 1976; Kreek, Gutjahr et al., 1976; Tong, Pond et al., 1981) and, probably, barbiturates.

Disulfiram (Antabuse®), when used as a treatment for alcohol and cocaine abuse, has been shown to inhibit cytochrome P450-related enzymes (McCance-Katz, Kosten et al., 1998). However, the metabolic interaction between methadone and disulfiram has been rigorously studied, with measurements over a 24 hour/day period, first using disulfiram alone and then using disulfiram with methadone. These investigations demonstrated that there is no interaction between these two agents (Tong, Pond et al., 1981).

It has been documented that there can be drug interactions between methadone and antiretroviral medications used to treat HIV-1 (reviewed in Borg & Kreek, 1995; Gourevitch & Friedland, 2000), which can affect concentrations of methadone (such as nevirapine [Viramune®]) or the HIV-related medication (such as zidovudine or AZT®). Another important potential drug-drug interaction through the hepatic cytochrome P450-related system is inhibition by ciprofloxacin (Cipro®) of CYP1A2 and CYP3A4 (Herrlin, Segerdahl et al., 2000). CYP1A2 and CYP3A4 are two of the three hepatic microsomal systems that have been found to be involved in the metabolism of methadone (along with CYP2D6), resulting in increased methadone levels.

The selective serotonin reuptake inhibitor fluvoxamine (Luvox®) can inhibit the cytochrome P450 system, posing a potential for methadone toxicity (Bertschy, Baumann et al., 1994); however, no such toxicity ever has been observed. Methadone levels are not significantly affected by the regular consumption of up to four alcoholic drinks per day (Kreek, 1978b, 1981, 1984, 1988, 1990), but with heavier long-term alcohol use, methadone biotransformation can be accelerated (when alcohol is not actually present, but enzymes have been induced) or slowed (when alcohol is present at >150 mg/dL and enzymes are occupied), depending on the blood levels of alcohol and their effect on hepatic enzymes. Greater methadone biotransformation is found several hours after chronic heavy alcohol use (when ethanol levels have diminished), resulting in decreased methadone in the blood. It may be that less methadone biotransformation secondary to hepatic enzyme competition occurs after similar excessive ethanol use, when blood measures of ethanol are still very elevated (>150 mg/dL), with resultant increases in levels of methadone.

LAAM. LAAM was synthesized and initially studied as a possible analgesic and addiction treatment from the late 1940s to the early 1950s (Bockmuhl & Erhart, 1948; Eddy, May et al., 1952; Fraser & Isbell, 1951, 1952; Keats & Beecher, 1952; Sung & Way, 1954, as cited in Kreek, 1996). LAAM is a congener of methadone that was approved in 1993 by the FDA for use in the treatment of heroin addiction. It shares with methadone the properties of long duration of effect (48 hours versus 24 hours for methadone), oral effectiveness (Kaiko & Inturrisi, 1973; Kreek, 1973b, 1978a; Levine, Zaks et al., 1973), and functioning as a pure opioid agonist, active mostly at the mu opioid receptor. Like methadone, LAAM achieves steady-state perfusion of mu opioid receptors. Unlike methadone, LAAM has active metabolites that are produced after initial oxidative metabolism by cytochrome P450-related enzymes (mostly the 3A4 subtype) to two principal active metabolites produced by N-demethylation: first, noracetylmethadol (norLAAM), and then dinoracetylmethadol (dinorLAAM), both of which are found in the urine along with LAAM (Billings, McMahon et al., 1974; Kiang, Campos-Flor et al., 1981; Sullivan, Due et al., 1973; Sung & Way, 1954; Moody, Alburges et al., 1997; Borg, Ho et al., 2002).

NorLAAM and dinorLAAM probably account in part for the prolonged duration of action of LAAM, because those metabolites accumulate with chronic administration. In addition, LAAM and its metabolites bind to tissue proteins (Henderson, Wilson et al., 1976).

The clearance of norLAAM and LAAM is similar, whereas the clearance of dinorLAAM is more prolonged than that of its parent compound. Pharmacokinetic studies of LAAM in humans that have been reviewed and accepted by the FDA have shown the apparent beta-terminal half-life of LAAM to be about 2.5 days, compared to two days for norLAAM and four days for the dinorLAAM metabolite (Abramowic, 1994; Blaine & Renault, 1976; Henderson, Wilson et al. 1976; Kaiko & Inturrisi, 1975; Misra & Mule, 1975; ORLAAM® package insert, 2000).

In one study (Kaiko & Inturrisi, 1975), the peak pharmacologic effect of LAAM as measured by amount of pupillary constriction occurred at eight hours, then diminished at a rate most like that of norLAAM metabolism. Kinetic studies of norLAAM and dinorLAAM directly administered in humans have not yet been done. Recent treatment studies (Borg, Ho et al., 2002) examined the pharmacokinetics of LAAM in a population of individuals in recovery from heroin addiction; they found that norLAAM is very active but that its half-life is not as long as had been thought, which may account for the withdrawal symptoms that patients often experience toward the end of the 72-hour dosing interval.

Because of the metabolism of LAAM by cytochrome P450 system-related microsomal enzymes to norLAAM and dinorLAAM, drug interactions can occur. Some medications (such as rifampin) tend to induce this enzyme system, as does the presence of long-term alcohol abuse. In their presence, LAAM can be metabolized faster than in control subjects, as has been shown to occur with methadone (Kreek, 1990; Kreek, Garfield et al., 1976; Kreek, Gutjahr et al., 1976; Tong, Pond et al., 1981). Increased biotransformation of LAAM could accelerate the production of norLAAM and dinorLAAM, which may affect the steady state perfusion of opioid receptors. LAAM metabolism theoretically could be retarded if hepatic drug metabolism is diminished, as occurs in the presence of very large quantities of either ethanol or perhaps with large doses of benzodiazepines, or with intake of cimetidine (Tagamet®). Although the actual occurrence of such possible drug interactions and their effects have not yet been demonstrated, it appears that, like methadone, the cytochrome P450 (3A4) microsomal enzyme system has a major role in the metabolism of LAAM and norLAAM (Moody, Alburges et al., 1997). Recently, several cases have been reported of increased QT intervals on electrocardiogram that may have been caused by LAAM. On the other hand, they may have been the result of preexisting cardiac disease or unknown drug interactions. Nevertheless, they resulted in a product warning in the United States and removal of the product in some other countries (Kreek & Vocci, 2003).

Buprenorphine. Buprenorphine (Buprenex®, Subutex®, Suboxone®) is a synthetic, primarily mu opioid receptor-directed partial agonist. Its chemical structure is that of an oripavine with a C_7 side chain, which contains a tert-butyl group. Norbuprenorphine is a major metabolite of buprenorphine in both humans and rats, with activity at the mu opioid receptor as well (Huang, Kehner et al., 2001). The metabolism of buprenorphine to norbuprenorphine appears to occur by dealkylation in the cytochrome P450-related enzyme 3A4 system, of which buprenorphine itself is a weak inhibitor (Kobayashi, Yamamoto et al., 1998; Ibrahim, Wilson et al., 2000).

Initially developed as an analgesic, buprenorphine has been shown in most studies to be as effective as morphine in many situations and more potent when given by parenteral administration. It is a mu opioid receptor partial agonist (with some modest kappa-opioid receptor activity). It has a long duration of action, not because of its pharmacokinetic profile but because of its very slow dissociation from receptors. Two important properties of buprenorphine are (1) its apparent lower severity of withdrawal signs and symptoms on cessation, compared with heroin, methadone, and possibly LAAM, and (2) its reduced potential to produce lethal overdose in opiate-naive or nontolerant persons because of its partial agonist properties.

Given intravenously to humans, buprenorphine has an apparent beta-terminal plasma half-life of about three to five hours (Kuhlman, Lalani et al., 1996). When given orally, it is relatively ineffective because of its "first pass" metabolism (Cone, Gorodetzky et al., 1984; Kreek, 1996), that is, rapid biotransformation, probably by the intestinal mucosa and especially by the liver. However, the very long-acting properties of buprenorphine (24 to 48 hours) when it is administered on a chronic basis are the result of its sustained mu opioid receptor occupancy. Sublingual preparations of buprenorphine can be liquid or tablet, both of which require about 120 minutes for time-to-peak. However, one study found that peak plasma concentrations of the sublingual tablet were 55% of the concentrations produced by equivalent doses of the sublingual liquid. In addition, the mean area under the curve (AUC) for the sublingual tablet was approximately 64% of the mean liquid AUC (Schuh & Johanson, 1999).

Buprenorphine is a partial agonist; that is, it has a "ceiling effect": doses in humans greater than 24 or 32 mg have no greater opioid agonist effect, but in humans (unlike rodents) do not act as antagonists. Thus, buprenorphine is better characterized as a partial agonist, with 16 mg buprenorphine SL similar in efficacy to 60 mg methadone.

Positron emission tomography studies found that mu opioid receptor occupancy was lowered by only 19% to 32% in 14 subjects who were maintained long term on daily doses of methadone, ranging from 30 to 90 mg/day (Kling, Carson et al., 2000). In contrast, it has been shown that, during buprenorphine treatment, mu opioid receptor occupancy was 36% to 50% after administration of 2 mg sublingual doses daily and 79% to 95% at 16 mg after 10 days of stabilization on each dose in four subjects (Zubieta, Greenwald et al., 2000). These findings have potential implications for the differences in effect on normal physiology between the two drugs.

After reports of intravenous buprenorphine abuse in several countries, buprenorphine has been developed for use in the United States as a combined preparation with naloxone. In this formulation, naloxone will not precipitate withdrawal when taken orally or sublingually because of the limited oral bioavailability of naloxone. It will, however, precipitate acute opioid withdrawal and block the euphoric effects of buprenorphine when used intravenously (Kreek, 1996; Harris, Jones et al., 2000).

PHARMACOLOGIC ACTIONS

The pharmacodynamics of the clinically important mu opioid receptor agonists are wide ranging, with the most pronounced effects produced in the CNS and the GI tract. The mechanism of action for all five of the clinically relevant opioids described here is at the mu opioid receptor, in which they act preferentially as agonists (except for buprenorphine, which is a partial mu opioid agonist with high affinity at the opioid receptor). The mu opioid receptor is part of the family of seven transmembrane-spanning G protein-coupled receptors. The effects of opioids on their function is partially mediated by changes in adenylyl cyclase activity, with resultant effects on cyclic adenosine 3'5' monophosphate, or cAMP (Dhawan, Cesselin et al., 1996).

The medical safety of long-term methadone maintenance treatment has been studied both prospectively and retrospectively (Kreek, 1973a). The mu opioid agonists affect every organ system, with tolerance developing at different rates to each effect. The primary actions of the mu opioid agonists depend on dose and chronicity of use. In the treatment of illicit opioid dependence or pain with prescribed opiates, proper dosing (titrated to the tolerance of the individual patient) is essential to avoid CNS depression. The precise, pure neuronal and molecular mechanisms of physical tolerance are not known at this time (Kreek, 2002).

However, it has been shown in studies of the *d* (R-) enantiomer of methadone (which is relatively inactive at the mu opioid receptor) that this isomer has modest N-methyl-D-aspartate antagonist activity, which attenuates the development of morphine tolerance in rodents but does not affect physical dependence (Davis & Inturrisi, 1999). Tolerance to the different effects of methadone occurs at different time points, with persistence (after at least three years of chronic treatment) of increased sweating and constipation (Kreek, 1973a), as well as a persistence of the pulsatile increase in prolactin entrained to the peak level of methadone, which occurs approximately two to four hours after daily administration.

CNS effects of opioids include analgesia, sleepiness, mood changes, and impaired mentation. With the use of oral methadone, analgesia occurs at 30 to 60 minutes, at a usual oral dose for analgesia in an unexposed (opioid-naive) individual at 2.5 to 15 mg. The analgesic effect of a single methadone dose is equivalent to morphine, but its cumulative effects occur over time. The euphoria produced by the mu opioid agonists apparently are mediated in part by the ventral tegmentum, where opioid agonist-mediated inhibition of GABAergic neurons results in disinhibition and thus activation of dopamine neurons extending to the nucleus accumbens. Norepinephrine-secreting cells in the locus ceruleus appear to play an important role in opioid withdrawal, whereas both serotonin and dopamine exert effects on dependence and craving.

Prudent dosing is important, as diminished respiration occurs with opioids until tolerance develops. This is partially because of a direct effect on the brainstem. Reduced response to carbon dioxide of centers in the pons and medulla can lead to CO_2 retention. Initially there is depressed cough (which is mediated by the medulla), as well as nausea and vomiting, which is mediated by the area postrema of the medulla and which disappear with the development of tolerance. Constriction of the pupil is the result of parasympathetic nerve excitation. In opioid overdose, convulsions can occur, probably because of inhibition of the release of gamma-aminobutyric acid in the CNS.

Short-acting opiates such as heroin and morphine have neuroendocrine effects, such as reductions in gonadotropin-releasing hormone and corticotropin-releasing factor, which leads to lowered luteinizing hormone and follicle-stimulating hormone, accompanied by decreases in adrenocorticotropic hormone (ACTH) and beta-endorphin, as well as testosterone and cortisol (Kreek, Borg et al., 2002). Chronic administration of long-acting opioids (such as methadone) leads to tolerance to effects on hypothalamic-releasing factors, with resumption of normal menses and return of plasma levels of testosterone to normal after one year, as well as return to normal levels and activity of anterior pituitary-derived ACTH and beta-endorphin and normal ACTH stimulation. In humans, prolactin release is under tonic inhibition by dopaminergic tone. With the use of short-acting opiates, there is a prompt increase in the release of prolactin because of an abrupt lowering of dopamine levels in the tuberoinfundibular dopaminergic system. With chronic methadone treatment, there is some tolerance to this response but not complete tolerance, because of the lowering of dopamine that is still present. The metyrapone test blocks 11-beta-hydroxylation of cortisol in the adrenal cortex. Heroin reduces the normal stress response to this test. However, a normal response is restored with methadone. With heroin use, thyroid levels are elevated because of raised thyroid-binding globulin; thus, there are increased measures of thyroid without abnormal function. Hypothalamus and pituitary effects of opioids can produce antidiuretic and heat regulation changes.

In the cardiovascular system, opioids cause peripheral vasodilatation, decreased peripheral resistance, reduced baroreceptor reflexes, histamine release, and decreased reflex vasoconstriction caused by raised PCO_2. In the stomach, hydrochloric acid secretion is inhibited and somatostatin release from the pancreas is elevated. Acetylcholine release from the GI tract is inhibited and motility is slowed, as is absorption of drugs. The presence of increased feeding also has been noted. Biliary, pancreatic, and intestinal secretions may be reduced and digestion in the small intestine slowed. In the large intestine, there is reduced propulsion and higher tone.

Immunologic effects also occur. The short-acting opioids such as morphine reduce rosettes formed by human T lymphocytes. Morphine reduces cytotoxic activity of natural killer cells and increases growth of implanted tumors. Beta-endorphin increases cytotoxic action of human monocytes *in vitro*, and enhances recruitment of precursor cells to the killer cell population. With the use of methadone, absolute numbers of T cells, T-cell subsets, B cells, and quantitative immunoglobulins are restored to normal, with normal natural killer cell activity (Novick, Ochshorn et al., 1989). These indices are abnormal with the use of heroin, possibly because of mediation through the neuroendocrine

system, as cortisol suppresses many parameters of immune function.

Studies in rodents have shown that long-term administration of opiates produces marked changes (that is, enhancement) in sensitivity to the aversive effects of opiate antagonists—effects that appear to be localized to the nucleus accumbens and central nucleus of the amygdala (Kreek & Koob, 1998)

NEUROBIOLOGY

Mechanisms of Action and Neuroadaptation. Morphine acutely inhibits adenylyl cyclase in the locus ceruleus, leading to inhibition of the cAMP-dependent cascade. With long-term morphine treatment, this initial inhibition results in a compensating increase of adenylyl cyclase and increase in the cAMP-dependent cascade. This compensation includes increases in protein kinase A, phosphorylated proteins, and cAMP-dependent response element binding (CREB) protein. Chronic morphine treatment has been reported to produce an uncoupling of the mu opioid receptor and its G-protein coupled inwardly rectifying potassium channels, which has been shown to cause reduced maximal outward current and reduced efficiency, with decreased opioid potency (Kreek, 2002).

The specific neuronal and molecular basis of opioid tolerance and dependence remains unclear. Specific opiate receptors first were documented in 1973; at this point in time, all have been cloned. They have been shown to be part of the G-protein coupled group of seven transmembrane receptors. Studies have shown varied results in opioid receptor binding and density with chronic mu opioid agonist administration. Effects can be mediated by receptor internalization or signal transduction, mostly through G-protein coupling (see LaForge, Yuferov et al., 2000). Neuroadaptation with sensitization as well as neurotoxicity do not occur with clinically used opioids in humans.

Human Molecular Genetics. Among the major factors contributing to vulnerability to the development of addiction are genetic factors that probably involve specific alleles of multiple genes that act to increase or reduce vulnerability to addiction. Because the mu opioid receptor is the primary site of action for heroin, it is notable that five single nucleotide polymorphisms have been identified in the coding region of the human mu opioid receptor gene (Bond, LaForge et al., 1998). Three of these five single nucleotide polymorphisms lead to amino acid changes, and two (the A118G and the C17T variants) have very high allelic frequencies: 2% to more than 40% in various populations). On the basis of association studies, the A118G variant can confer some protection against opiate dependency in certain population subsets but increases vulnerability in others. The C17T variant, on the other hand, may have some association with opiate dependence, although significant associations have not been confirmed.

Binding studies have shown that exogenous ligands, including methadone and morphine, bind threefold more tightly to the A118G variant than to the prototype receptor. Functional studies have shown that the endogenous opioid beta-endorphin produces three times more potent activation of one of the two major signal transduction systems when bound to the A118G variant. Further studies are under way to examine binding and function in the C17T variant.

Human Neurobiology. Atypical response to stress and stressors (as demonstrated by changes in hypothalamic-pituitary-adrenal (HPA) axis function) have been shown in heroin addicts during induction into methadone treatment, with normalization of response after stabilization on a steady dose of methadone. During cycles of heroin addiction, there is a flattened circadian rhythm of levels of glucocorticoids. During opiate withdrawal, there are increased levels of glucocorticoids, ACTH, and beta-endorphin. However, with steady-state methadone treatment, both circadian rhythms and plasma levels of the HPA axis normalize, as do responses to chemically induced stress to the HPA axis by using the compound metyrapone, which blocks the final step of cortisol synthesis and thus removes the normal tonic inhibition of the HP part of the stress-responsive axis by cortisol (Schluger, Borg et al., 2001). These studies suggest that, with the use of heroin, the addicted individual may be seeking suppression of atypical (either endogenous or drug-induced) hyperresponsivity to stress and stressors, and that the long-acting opioid methadone gradually produces normal responsivity of the stress-responsive systems. In addition, a recent imaging study using positron emission tomography has shown only 19% to 32% greater occupancy of opiate receptors in specific brain areas that are related to pain and analgesia as well as addiction (caudate, putamen, amygdala, anterior cingulate cortex, and thalamus) during steady-dose methadone maintenance treatment compared with normal volunteers (Kling, Carson et al., 2000). The presence of these unoccupied receptors helps to explain how physiologic systems dependent on mu opioid receptor activation, which are disrupted during cycles of heroin abuse, can become normalized during methadone maintenance treatment. Few

studies to date have examined the neuroendocrine status of patients treated with LAAM (Mendelson, Inturrisi et al., 1975; Mendelson, Ellingboe et al., 1984; Borg, Ho et al., 2002).

FUTURE RESEARCH DIRECTIONS

In the area of opioid agonist treatment pharmacology, more rigorous studies of complex drug interactions with methadone and other medications are needed, including studies of medications for patients with comorbid conditions such as HIV-1, hepatitis C virus, and psychiatric illnesses.

From a broader perspective, integration of basic science information at the molecular and animal level with clinical research and observation should be pursued. This research should include further elucidation of the differences in the stress-responsive HPA axis in persons maintained on long-acting opioid agonist pharmacotherapy, as with methadone or LAAM, as compared with normal subjects, including areas such as possible gender differences and possible effects of polysubstance abuse.

Further exploration of genetic factors that can interact (protect from or predispose to) opioid addiction and integration of these genetic factors with the neuroendocrine findings can be valuable in increasing our understanding of neurobiologic differences that may predispose at-risk individuals to opioid addiction.

Finally, studies conducted since the mid-1980s have demonstrated that many patients are able to be treated for heroin addiction with methadone maintenance in a private practice setting with properly trained physicians. There are two principal models for this type of treatment. The best studied model, known as medical maintenance, is one in which patients already maintained on chronic opioid agonist pharmacotherapy at conventional methadone maintenance clinics are transferred to office-based treatment, where they are seen at least monthly (Novick, Pascarelli et al., 1988). These subjects must meet specific criteria, including abstinence from illicit substances for a specific period ranging from months to years, reliable employment or domestic responsibilities, and a good record of adherence to conventional treatment. The studies, which have been conducted in different cities (New York, Baltimore, Chicago, and New Haven), report good outcomes as measured by high treatment retention and low relapse rates (Novick, Joseph et al. 1990, 1994; Novick & Joseph, 1991; Salsitz, Joseph et al., 2000; Schwartz, Brooner et al., 1999; Senay, Barthwell et al., 1993; Fiellin, O'Connor et al., 2001).

Another experimental model currently under review involves direct admission of opioid-dependent subjects to office-based treatment with buprenorphine and naloxone. Such subjects are inducted to buprenorphine maintenance pharmacotherapy in the primary care or private office setting (O'Connor, Oliveto et al., 1998; Casadonte, Walsh et al., 2001). In one 12-week study, 46 heroin-dependent patients were randomly assigned to either a primary care clinic for addicted patients or a traditional methadone clinic. While higher retention and lower rates of opioid use were seen in the patients treated in the primary care setting (O'Connor, Oliveto et al., 1998), further followup studies are ongoing and have not yet been reported.

REFERENCES

Abramowic M (1994). LAAM: A long-acting methadone for treatment of heroin addiction. *Medical Letter on Drugs and Therapeutics* 36:52.

Änggaard E, Gunne L-M, Holmstrand J et al. (1974). Disposition of methadone in methadone maintenance. *Clinical Pharmacology and Therapeutics* 17:258-266.

Babul N & Darke AC (1993). Disposition of morphine and its glucuronide metabolites after oral and rectal administration: Evidence of route specificity. *Clinical Pharmacology and Therapeutics* 54:286-292.

Bertschy G, Baumann P, Eap CB et al. (1994). Probable metabolic interaction between methadone and fluvoxamine in addict patients. *Therapeutic Drug Monitoring* 16:42-45.

Billings RE, McMahon RE & Blake DA (1974). L-acetylmethadol (LAAM) treatment of opiate dependence: Plasma and urine levels of two pharmacologically active metabolites. *Life Sciences* 14:1437-1446.

Blaine JD & Renault P, eds. (1976). *Rx 3x a Week LAAM: Alternative to Methadone (NIDA Research Monograph No. 8)*. Rockville, MD: National Institute on Drug Abuse.

Bockmuhl M & Erhart G (1948). Spasmolytic and analgesic compounds.1. *Justus Liebigs Annalen der Chemie* 561:52-85.

Bond C, LaForge KS, Tian M et al. (1998). Single-nucleotide polymorphism in the human mu opioid receptor gene alters beta-endorphin binding and activity: Possible implications for opiate addiction. *Proceedings of the National Academy of Sciences* 95:9608-9613.

Borg L & Kreek MJ (1995). Clinical problems associated with interactions between methadone pharmacotherapy and medications used in the treatment of HIV-positive and AIDS patients. *Current Opinion in Psychiatry* 8:199-202.

Borg L & Kreek MJ (1998). Pharmacology of opiates. In R Tarter et al. (eds.) *Handbook of Substance Abuse: Neurobehavioral Pharmacology*. New York, NY: Plenum Press, 331-341.

Borg L, Ho A, Peters JE et al. (1995). Availability of reliable serum methadone determination for management of symptomatic patients. *Journal of Addictive Diseases* 14:83-96.

Borg L, Ho A, Wells JH et al. (2002). The use of levo-alpha-acetylmethadol (LAAM) in methadone patients who have not achieved heroin abstinence. *Journal of Addictive Diseases* 21:13-22.

Bowen DV, Smit ALC & Kreek MJ (1978). Fecal excretion of methadone and its metabolites in man: Application of GC-MS. In NR Daly (ed.) *Advances in Mass Spectrometry*. Philadelphia, PA: Heyden & Son, 1634-1639.

Casadonte P, Walsh R, Vocci F et al. (2001). Treatment of opioid dependence with buprenorphine naloxone in a solo private psychiatry practice. *Drug and Alcohol Dependence* 63(Suppl 1):92.

Chan GLC & Matzke GR (1987). Effects of renal insufficiency on the pharmacokinetics and pharmacodynamics of opioid analgesics. *Drug Intelligence and Clinical Pharmacy* 21:773-783.

Cone EJ, Gorodetzky CW, Yousefnejad D et al. (1984). The metabolism and excretion of buprenorphine in humans. *Drug Metabolism and Disposition* 12:577-581.

Cone EJ, Holicky BA, Grant TM et al. (1993). Pharmacokinetics and pharmacodynamics of intranasal "snorted" heroin. *Journal of Analytical Toxicology* 17:327-337.

Davis AM & Inturrisi CE (1999). D-methadone blocks morphine tolerance and N-methyl-D-aspartate-induced hyperalgesia. *Journal of Pharmacology and Experimental Therapeutics* 289:1048-1053.

Dhawan BN, Cesselin F, Raghubir R et al. (1996). International Union of Pharmacology. XII. Classification of opioid receptors. *Pharmacological Reviews* 48:567-592.

Dole VP & Kreek MJ (1973). Methadone plasma level: Sustained by a reservoir of drug in tissue. *Proceedings of the National Academy of Sciences* 70:10.

Dole VP, Nyswander ME & Kreek MJ (1966). Narcotic blockade. *Archives of Internal Medicine* 118:304-309.

Eap CB, Broly F, Mino A et al. (2001). Cytochrome P450 2D6 genotype and methadone steady-state concentrations. *Journal of Clinical Psychopharmacology* 21:229-234.

Eddy NB, May EL & Mosettig E (1952). Chemistry and pharmacology of the methadols and acetylmethadols. *Journal of Organic Chemistry* 17:321-326.

Fiellin DA, O'Connor PG, Chawarski M et al. (2001). Methadone maintenance in primary care: A randomized controlled trial. *Journal of the American Medical Association* 286:1724-1731.

Frank B (2000). An overview of heroin trends in New York City: Past, present and future. *Mount Sinai Journal of Medicine* 67:340-346.

Fraser HF & Isbell H (1951). Addiction potentialities of isomers of 6-dimethylamino-4-4-diphenyl-3 acetyoxy-heptane (acetylmethadol). *Journal of Pharmacology and Experimental Therapeutics* 101:12.

Fraser HF & Isbell H (1952). Actions and addiction liabilities of alpha-acetylmethadols in man. *Journal of Pharmacology and Experimental Therapeutics* 105:210-215.

Got P, Baud FJ, Sandouk P et al. (1994). Morphine disposition in opiate-intoxicated patients: Relevance of nonspecific opiate immunoassays. *Journal of Analytical Toxicology* 18:189-194.

Gourevitch MN & Friedland GH (2000). Interactions between methadone and medications used to treat HIV infection: A review. *Mount Sinai Journal of Medicine* 67:429-426.

Hachey DL, Kreek MJ & Mattson DH (1977). Quantitative analysis of methadone in biological fluids using deuterium-labelled methadone and GLC-chemical-ionization mass spectrometry. *Journal of Pharmaceutical Sciences* 66:1579-1582.

Harris DS, Jones RT, Welm S et al. (2000). Buprenorphine and naloxone co-administration in opiate-dependent patients stabilized on sublingual buprenorphine. *Drug and Alcohol Dependence* 61:85-94.

Harte EH, Gutjahr CL & Kreek MJ (1976). Long-term persistence of *dl*-methadone in tissues. *Clinical Research* 24:623A.

Hasselström J & Säwe J (1993). Morphine pharmacokinetics and metabolism in humans: Enterohepatic cycling and relative contribution of metabolites to active opioid concentrations. *Clinical Pharmacokinetics* 24:344-354.

Hasselström J, Eriksson S, Persson A et al. (1990). The metabolism and bioavailability of morphine in patients with severe liver cirrhosis. *British Journal of Pharmacology* 29:289-297.

Henderson GL, Wilson K & Lau DHM (1976). Plasma levo-alpha-acetylmethadol (LAAM) after acute and chronic administration. *Clinical Pharmacology and Therapeutics* 21:16-25.

Herrlin K, Segerdahl M, Gustafsson LL et al. (2000). Methadone, ciprofloxacin and adverse drug reactions [letter]. *Lancet* 356: 2069-2070.

Huang P, Kehner GB, Cowan A et al. (2001) Comparison of pharmacological activities of buprenorphine and norbuprenorphine: Norbuprenorphine is a potent opioid agonist. *Journal of Pharmacology and Experimental Therapeutics* 297:688-695.

Ibrahim RB, Wilson JG, Thorsby ME et al. (2000). Effects of buprenorphine on CYP3A activity in rat and human liver microsomes. *Life Sciences* 66:1293-1298.

Inturrisi CE & Verebely K (1972a). A gas-liquid chromatographic method for the quantitative determination of methadone in human plasma and urine. *Journal of Chromatography* 65:361-369.

Inturrisi CE & Verebely K (1972b). The levels of methadone in the plasma in methadone maintenance. *Clinical Pharmacology and Therapeutics* 13:633-637.

Inturrisi CE, Max MB, Foley KM et al. (1984). The pharmacokinetics of heroin in patients with chronic pain. *New England Journal of Medicine* 310:1213-1217.

Inturrisi CE, Schultz M, Shin S et al. (1983). Evidence from opiate binding that heroin acts through its metabolites. *Life Sciences* 33(Suppl 1):773-776.

Kaiko RF & Inturrisi CE (1973). A gas-liquid chromatographic method for the quantitative determination of acetylmethadol and its metabolites in human urine. *Journal of Chromatography* 82:315-321.

Kaiko RF & Inturrisi CE (1975). Disposition of acetylmethadol in relation to pharmacologic action. *Clinical Pharmacology and Therapeutics* 18:96-103.

Kaiko RF, Wallenstein SL, Rogers AG et al. (1981). Analgesic and mood effects of heroin and morphine in cancer patients with postoperative pain. *New England Journal of Medicine* 304:1501-1505.

Kamendulis LM, Brzezinski MR, Pindel EV et al. (1996). Metabolism of cocaine and heroin is catalyzed by the same human liver carboxylesterases. *Journal of Pharmacology and Experimental Therapeutics* 279:713-717.

Keats AS & Beecher HK (1952). Analgesic activity and toxic effects of acetylmethadol isomers in man. *Journal of Pharmacology and Experimental Therapeutics* 105:210-215.

Kiang C-H, Campos-Flor S & Inturrisi CE (1981). Determination of acetylmethadol and metabolites by use of high-performance liquid chromatography. *Journal of Chromatography* 222:81-93.

Kitanaka N, Sora I, Kinsey S et al. (1998) No heroin or morphine 6-beta-glucuronide analgesia in mu-opioid receptor knockout mice *European Journal of Pharmacology* 355:R1-R3.

Kling MA, Carson RE, Borg L et al. (2000). Opioid receptor imaging with positron emission tomography and [^{18}F]cyclofoxyl in long-term, methadone-treated former heroin addicts. *Journal of Pharmacology and Experimental Therapeutics* 295:1070-1076.

Kobayishi K, Yamamoto T, Chiba K et al. (1998). Human buprenorphine N-dealkylation is catalyzed by cytochrome P450 3A4. *Drug Metabolism and Disposition* 26:818-821.

Kreek MJ (1973a). Medical safety and side effects of methadone in tolerant individuals. *Journal of the American Medical Association* 223:665-668.

Kreek MJ (1973b). Plasma and urine levels of methadone. *New York State Journal of Medicine* 73:2773-2777.

Kreek MJ (1978a). Medical complications in methadone patients. *Annals of the New York Academy of Sciences* 311:110-134.

Kreek MJ (1978b). Effects of drugs and alcohol on opiate disposition and action. In MW Adler et al. (eds.) *Factors Affecting the Action of Narcotics*. New York, NY: Raven Press, 717-739.

Kreek MJ (1981). Metabolic interactions between opiates and alcohol. *Annals of the New York Academy of Sciences* 362:36-49.

Kreek MJ (1984). Opioid interactions with alcohol. *Journal of Addictive Diseases* 3:35-46.

Kreek MJ (1988). Opiate-ethanol interactions: Implications for the biological basis and treatment of combined addictive diseases. In LS Harris (ed.) *Problems of Drug Dependence, 1987; Proceedings of the 49th Annual Scientific Meeting of the Committee on Problems of Drug Dependence*. Rockville, MD: National Institute on Drug Abuse, 428-439.

Kreek MJ (1990). Drug interactions in humans related to drug abuse and its treatment. *Modern Methods in Pharmacology* 6:265-282.

Kreek MJ (1996). Long-term pharmacotherapy for opiate (primarily heroin) addiction: Opiate antagonists and partial agonists. In CR Schuster & MK Kuhar (eds.) *Pharmacological Aspects of Drug Dependence: Toward an Integrated Neurobehavioral Approach*. Berlin, Germany: Springer-Verlag, 563-592.

Kreek MJ (2002). Molecular and cellular neurobiology and pathophysiology of opiate addiction. In KL Davis et al. (eds.) *Neuropsychopharmacology: The Fifth Generation of Progress*. Philadelphia, PA: Lippincott Williams & Wilkins, 1491-1506.

Kreek MJ, Bencsath FA & Field FH (1980). Effects of liver disease on urinary excretion of methadone and metabolites in maintenance patients: Quantitation by direct probe chemical ionization mass spectrometry. *Biomedical Mass Spectrometry* 7:385-395.

Kreek MJ, Bencsath FA, Fanizza A et al. (1983). Effects of liver disease on fecal excretion of methadone and its unconjugated metabolites in maintenance patients: Quantitation by direct probe chemical ionization mass spectrometry. *Biomedical Mass Spectrometry* 10:544-549.

Kreek MJ, Borg L, Zhou Y et al. (2002). Relationships between endocrine functions and substance abuse syndromes: Heroin and related short-acting opiates in addiction contrasted with methadone and other long-acting opioid agonists used in pharmacotherapy of addiction. In D Pfaff (ed.) *Hormones, Brain and Behavior*. San Diego, CA: Academic Press, 781-830.

Kreek MJ, Garfield JW, Gutjahr CL et al. (1976). Rifampin-induced methadone withdrawal. *New England Journal of Medicine* 294:1104-1106.

Kreek MJ, Gutjahr CL, Garfield JW et al. (1976). Drug interactions with methadone. *Annals of the New York Academy of Science* 281:350-374.

Kreek MJ, Gutjahr CL, Bowen DV et al. (1978). Fecal excretion of methadone and its metabolites: A major pathway of elimination in man. In A Schecter, H Alksne, & E Kaufman (eds.) *Critical Concerns in the Field of Drug Abuse: Proceedings of the Third National Drug Abuse Conference*. New York, NY: Marcel Dekker, 1206-1210.

Kreek MJ, Hachey DL & Klein PD (1979). Stereoselective disposition of methadone in man. *Life Sciences* 24:925-932.

Kreek MJ, Kalisman M, Irwin M et al. (1980). Biliary secretion of methadone and methadone metabolites in man. *Research Communications in Chemical Pathology and Pharmacology* 29:67-78.

Kreek M & Koob GF (1998). Drug dependence: Stress and dysregulation of brain reward pathways. *Drug and Alcohol Dependence* 51:23-47.

Kreek MJ, Oratz M & Rothschild MA (1978). Hepatic extraction of long and short-acting narcotics in the isolated perfused rabbit liver. *Gastroenterology* 75:88-94.

Kreek MJ, Schecter A, Gutjahr CL et al. (1980). Methadone use in patients with chronic renal disease. *Drug and Alcohol Dependence* 5:197-205.

Kreek MJ, Schecter A, Gutjahr CL et al. (1974). Analyses of methadone and other drugs in maternal and neonatal body fluids: Use in evaluation of symptoms in a neonate of mother maintained on methadone. *American Journal of Drug and Alcohol Abuse* 1:409-419.

Kreek MJ & Vocci FJ (2003). History and current status of opioid maintenance treatments: Blending conference session. *Journal of Substance Abuse Treatment* 23:93-105.

Kuhlman JJ, Lalani S, Magluilo J et al. (1996). Human pharmacokinetics of intravenous, sublingual and buccal buprenorphine. *Journal of Analytical Toxicology* 20:369-378.

LaForge KS, Yuferov V & Kreek MJ (2000). Opioid receptor and peptide gene polymorphisms: Potential implications for addictions. *European Journal of Pharmacology* 410:249-268.

Leavitt SB, Shinderman M, Maxwell S et al. (2000). When "enough" is not enough: New perspectives on optimal methadone maintenance dose. *Mount Sinai Journal of Medicine* 67:404-411.

Levine R, Zaks A, Fink M et al. (1973). Levomethadyl acetate: Prolonged duration of opioid effects, including cross tolerance to heroin in man. *Journal of the American Medical Association* 226:316-318.

Loh HH, Liu H-C, Cavalli A et al. (1998). Mu opioid receptor knockout in mice: Effects on ligand-induced analgesia and morphine lethality. *Molecular Brain Research* 54:321-326.

Matthes HW, Maldonado R, Simonin F et al. (1996). Loss of morphine-induced analgesia, reward effect and withdrawal symptoms in mice lacking the mu-opioid–receptor gene. *Nature* 383:819-823.

Mazoit JX, Sandouk P, Scherrmann J-P et al. (1990). Extrahepatic metabolism of morphine occurs in humans. *Clinical Pharmacology and Therapeutics* 4:613-618.

McCance-Katz EF, Kosten TR & Jatlow P (1998). Disulfiram effects on acute cocaine administration. *Drug and Alcohol Dependence* 52:27-39.

Mendelson JH, Ellingboe J, Judson BA et al. (1984). Plasma testosterone and luteinizing hormone concentrations during levo-alpha-acetylmethadol maintenance and withdrawal. *Clinical Pharmacology and Therapeutics* 15:545-547.

Mendelson JH, Inturrisi CE, Renault P et al. (1975). Effects of acetylmethadol on plasma testosterone. *Clinical Pharmacology and Therapeutics* 35:371-374.

Misra AL & Mule SJ (1975). L-alpha-acetylmethadol (LAAM) pharmacokinetics and metabolism: Current status. *American Journal of Drug and Alcohol Abuse* 2:301-305.

Moody DE, Alburges ME, Parker RJ et al. (1997). The involvement of cytochrome P450 3A4 in the N-demethylation of L-alpha-acetylmethadol (LAAM), norLAAM and methadone. *Drug Metabolism and Disposition* 25:1347-1353.

Nakamura K, Hachey DL, Kreek MJ et al. (1982). Quantitation of methadone enantiomers in humans using stable isotope-labeled [2H3]-, [2H5]-, and [2H8] methadone. *Journal of Pharmaceutical Sciences* 71:39-43.

National Institute on Drug Abuse (2002). Available at WWW.NIDA.NIH.GOV. In Zickler P (2001). NIDA scientific panel reports on prescription drug misuse and abuse. *NIDA Notes* 16; Mathias R (2000) Cocaine, marijuana, and heroin abuse up, methamphetamine abuse down *NIDA Notes* 15. Accessed 6/18/02.

Neumann PB, Henriksen H, Grosman N et al. (1982). Plasma morphine concentrations during chronic oral administration in patients with cancer pain. *Pain* 13:247-252.

Novick DM & Joseph H (1991). Medical maintenance: The treatment of chronic opiate dependence in general medical practice. *Journal of Substance Abuse Treatment* 8:233-239.

Novick DM, Joseph H, Croxson TS et al. (1990). Absence of antibody to human immunodeficiency virus in long-term, socially rehabilitated methadone maintenance patients. *Archives of Internal Medicine* 150:97-99.

Novick DM, Joseph H, Salsitz EA et al. (1994). Outcomes of treatment of socially rehabilitated methadone maintenance patients in physicians offices (medical maintenance). *Journal of General Internal Medicine* 33:235-245.

Novick DM, Kreek MJ, Fanizza AM et al. (1981). Methadone disposition in patients with chronic liver disease. *Clinical Pharmacology and Therapeutics* 30:353-362.

Novick DM, Kreek MJ, Arns PA et al. (1985). Effect of severe alcoholic liver disease on the disposition of methadone in maintenance patients. *Alcoholism: Clinical & Experimental Research* 9:349-354.

Novick DM, Ochshorn M, Ghali V et al. (1989). Natural killer cell activity and lymphocyte subsets in parenteral heroin abusers and long-term methadone maintenance patients. *Journal of Pharmacology and Experimental Therapeutics* 250:606-610.

Novick DM, Pascarelli EF, Joseph H et al. (1988). Methadone maintenance patients in general medical practice: A preliminary report. *Journal of the American Medical Association* 259:3299-3302.

O'Connor PG, Oliveto AH, Shi JM et al. (1998). A randomized trial of buprenorphine maintenance for heroin dependence in a primary care clinic for substance users versus a methadone clinic. *American Journal of Medicine* 105:100-105.

ORLAAM® drug information (2000). Levomethadyl acetate hydrochloride oral solution [Package insert].

Osborne R, Joel S, Trew D et al. (1988). Analgesic activity of morphine-6-glucuronide [letter]. *Lancet* 1:828.

Osborne R, Joel S, Trew D et al. (1990). Morphine and metabolite behavior after different routes of morphine administration: Demonstration of the importance of the active metabolite morphine-6-glucuronide. *Clinical Pharmacology and Therapeutics* 47:12-19.

Owen JA, Sitar DS, Berger L et al. (1983). Age-related morphine kinetics. *Clinical Pharmacology and Therapeutics* 34:364-368.

Paul D, Standifer KM, Inturrisi CE et al. (1989). Pharmacological characterization of morphine-6-glucuronide, a very potent morphine metabolite. *Journal of Pharmacology and Experimental Therapeutics* 251:477-483.

Pond SM, Kreek MJ, Tong TG et al. (1985). Altered methadone pharmacokinetics in methadone-maintained pregnant women. *Journal of Pharmacology and Experimental Therapeutics* 233:1-6.

Portenoy RK, Thaler HT, Inturrisi CE et al. (1992). The metabolite morphine-6-glucuronide contributes to the analgesia produced by morphine infusion in patients with pain and normal renal function. *Clinical Pharmacology and Therapeutics* 51:422-431.

Reisine T & Pasternak G (1996). Opioid analgesics and antagonists. In JG Hardman, AG Gilman & LE Limbird (eds.) *Goodman and Gilman's The Pharmacological Basis of Therapeutics, 9th Edition.* New York, NY: McGraw-Hill, 521-555.

Rossi GC, Brown GP, Leventhal L et al. (1996). Novel receptor mechanisms for heroin and morphine-6-glucuronide analgesia. *Neuroscience Letters* 216:1-4.

Rubenstein RB, Kreek MJ, Mbawa N et al. (1978). Human spinal fluid methadone levels. *Drug and Alcohol Dependence* 3:103-106.

Salsitz EA, Joseph H, Frank B et al. (2000). Methadone medical maintenance (MMM): Treating chronic opioid dependence in private medical practice—A summary report (1983-1998). *Mount Sinai Journal of Medicine* 67:388-397.

Sawynok J (1986). The therapeutic use of heroin: A review of the pharmacological literature. *Canadian Journal of Physiology and Pharmacology* 64:1-6.

Schluger JH, Borg L, Ho A et al. (2001). Altered HPA axis responsivity to metyrapone testing in methadone maintained former heroin addicts with ongoing cocaine addiction. *Neuropsychopharmacology* 24:568-575.

Schuh KJ & Johanson C-E (1999). Pharmacokinetic comparison of the buprenorphine sublingual liquid and tablet. *Drug and Alcohol Dependence* 56:55-60.

Schuller AGP, King MA, Zhang J et al. (1999). Retention of heroin and morphine 6-beta-glucuronide analgesia in a new line of mice lacking exon 1 of MOR-1. *Nature Neuroscience* 2:151-156.

Schwartz RP, Brooner RK, Montoya ID et al. (1999). A 12-year follow-up of a methadone medical maintenance program. *American Journal on Addictions* 8:293-299.

Senay EC, Barthwell AG, Marks R et al. (1993). Medical maintenance: A pilot study. *Journal of Addictive Diseases* 12:59-76.

Skopp G, Ganssmann B, Cone EJ et al. (1997). Plasma concentrations of heroin and morphine-related metabolites after intranasal and intramuscular administration. *Journal of Analytical Toxicology* 21:105-111.

Sullivan HR, Due SL & McMahon RE (1973). Metabolism of alpha-*l*-methadol: N-acetylation, a new metabolic pathway. *Research Communications in Chemical Pathology and Pharmacology* 6:1072-1078.

Sullivan HR, Smits SE, Due SL et al. (1972). Metabolism of *d*-methadone: Isolation and identification of analgesically active metabolites. *Life Sciences* 11:1093-1104.

Sung C-Y & Way EL (1954). The fate of the optical isomers of alpha-acetylmethadol. *Journal of Pharmacology and Experimental Therapeutics* 110:260-270.

Tegeder I, Lotsch J & Geisslinger G (1999). Pharmacokinetics of opioids in liver disease. *Clinical Pharmacokinetics* 37:17-40.

Tong TG, Pond SM, Kreek MJ et al. (1981). Phenytoin-induced methadone withdrawal. *Annals of Internal Medicine* 94:349-351.

Weinberg DSA, Inturrisi CE, Reidenberg B et al. (1988). Sublingual absorption of selected opioid analgesics. *Clinical Pharmacology and Therapeutics* 44:335-342.

Westerling D, Frigen L & Hogland P (1993). Morphine pharmacokinetics and effects on salivation and continuous reaction times in healthy volunteers. *Therapeutic Drug Monitoring* 15:364-374.

Westerling D, Hoglund P, Lundin S et al. (1994). Transdermal administration of morphine to healthy subjects. *British Journal of Clinical Pharmacology* 37:571-576.

Wolff K, Hay A & Raistrick D (1991). High-dose methadone and the need for drug measurements. *Clinical Chemistry* 37:1651-1654.

Wolff K, Hay AWM, Raistrick D et al. (1993). Steady-state pharmacokinetics of methadone in opioid addicts. *European Journal of Clinical Pharmacology* 44:189-194.

Zubieta J-K, Greenwald MK, Lombardi U et al. (2000). Buprenorphine-induced changes in mu-opioid receptor availability in male heroin-dependent volunteers: A preliminary study. *Neuropsychopharmacology* 23:326-334.

Dextromethorphan As A Drug of Abuse

William C. Bobo, M.D.

Shannon C. Miller, M.D., CMRO

Jonathan C. Jackson, M.D.

Dextromethorphan (DM) is an antitussive medication used in more than 140 over-the-counter cough remedies. At indicated doses, DM inhibits medullary cough centers to approximately the same extent as opiate alkaloids such as codeine, but without other opioid effects such as analgesia, CNS depression, and respiratory suppression. As such, its efficacy and safety for indicated use are well established. At excessive doses, however, a well-characterized toxic syndrome may emerge (despite early reports indicating a total lack of CNS effects, including abuse potential). Such effects, interestingly, are seen not only in cases of accidental overdose, but also in the context of intentional overdose and recreational use.

POTENTIAL FOR ABUSE

Reports of high-dose DM abuse have appeared sporadically over the past 30 years. In spite of this lengthy history, the potential public health effects of DM abuse have not been fully appreciated. Nevertheless, there is a growing consensus that DM carries a significant abuse potential and that abuse of this seemingly benign pharmaceutical has become increasingly popular among adolescents and young adults. As one indication of the latter, the National Clearinghouse on Alcohol and Drug Information (NCADI) recently added DM to its list of abusable dissociative agents, placing it alongside more notorious agents such as ketamine and PCP.

Surprisingly little empirical data are available to characterize the scope of DM abuse. The published literature consists largely of case reports. It appears that the drug has become especially popular among adolescents, and it is likely that the social impact of the problem has yet to be fully appreciated. Reasons for this are varied and complex. Because large epidemiologic studies or trend analyses are lacking, it is not clear who is at increased risk for DM abuse or what non-demographic predisposing factors are operative in identifying potential abusers.

Also, there seem to be relatively few deterrents to abuse of DM, thus furthering its appeal among prospective and active users. For example, those who experiment with DM have access to an inexpensive and licit pharmaceutical product that is available over the counter to any age group. Because pharmaceutical companies produce the drug, abusers may believe that it has a higher safety profile than illicit drugs such as heroin or cocaine, or even legal substances such as nicotine and alcohol (both of which are accompanied by warnings from the Surgeon General). Use of DM also may engender less social disapproval than, for example, abuse of crack cocaine, which has a clearly negative social connotation. DM is not among the substances routinely tested for in urinary or serologic toxicology screens, and the legal consequences of a drug screen that is positive for DM are questionable at best, as individuals who test positive could claim that they are self-medicating for a cough.

DISSOCIATIVE EFFECTS

Those abusing DM may experience euphoria, dissociation, and hallucinosis—similar to that encountered with well-established agents such as PCP or ketamine—within 15 to 30 minutes of ingestion. Other reported effects include increased perceptual awareness, altered time perception, hyperexcitability, pressure of thought, and disorientation.

The DM "high" may last from three to six hours. Such effects require the ingestion of large amounts of the substance, with doses estimated as ranging from 300 to 1,800 mg/kg (or more than 100 times the amount in a normal prescribed dose). This translates to over four ounces of DM-containing cough syrup, prompting some abusers to ingest the drug in a concentrated powder form (which is reported to be available for purchase on the street and on the Internet). Coricidin® HBP Cough and Cold (which has the street name "C-C-C" or "triple Cs") has become popular among DM users, as it contains the highest concentration of DM per dosage unit on the market: 30 mg DM. The metabolic byproduct of DM, dextrorphan (DOR), is similar to PCP with respect to its antagonist activity at the NMDA receptor.

In general, psychoactive effects are seen in patients who have adequate amounts of the enzyme subfamily responsible for DM's metabolic conversion to DOR, while those who lack sufficient amounts (referred to as phenotypic "poor metabolizers") are better protected against DM-induced psychomimesis.

DM AND THE DRUG CULTURE

As with the better-known drugs of abuse, users of DM have developed a social culture around the drug over the past 30 years. Popular street names include "DM," "DXM," "DMX," "Skittles," "Vitamin D," "Dex," "Tussin," or "Robo." Numerous Internet sites dedicated to the misuse of DM further this cultural movement by explaining how to acquire the drug (either directly through mail order or via simple chemical extraction). The sites also warn abusers of potential drug-drug interactions and other safety concerns. Many such sites employ a scientific lexicon and may even refer to articles in the medical literature and in established databases, thus assuming an air of scientific legitimacy.

DM has been distributed at dance parties referred to as "raves," which are characterized by the open use and sale of psychoactive agents. At high doses, DM has been used as an adulterating agent for the club drug MDMA (as when DM is combined with MDMA to enhance the latter agent's dissociative effects). Internet sites also display the artwork of artists who use DM to "enhance their creative expression" (in ways similar to the early users of LSD and other hallucinogens). Moreover, Internet sites advertise several so-called "DXM-enhanced" musical artists such as "DXM" and "Sigma" (a name chosen because of DM's activity at sigma-type opiate receptors in the brain).

Because DM has many characteristics that make it an attractive choice for abuse, particularly by adolescents, clinicians should be educated about this drug of abuse and future studies should focus on its epidemiology and prevention.

REFERENCES

Bern JL & Peck R (1992). Dextromethorphan: An overview of safety issues. *Drug Safety* 7:190-199.

Cranston JW & Yoast R (1999). Abuse of dextromethorphan. *Archives of Family Medicine* 8:99-100.

Darboe MN (1996). Abuse of dextromethorphan-based cough syrup as a substitute for licit and illicit drugs: A theoretical framework. *Adolescence* 31:239-245.

National Institute on Drug Abuse (NIDA) (1999). Executive summary: Other drugs. In *Epidemiologic Trends in Drug Abuse, Vol. 1. Proceedings of the Community Epidemiology Work Group*. Bethesda, MD: NIDA, National Institutes of Health.

National Institute on Drug Abuse (NIDA) (2002). Hallucinogens and dissociative drugs, including LSD, PCP, ketamine and dextromethorphan. *NIDA Research Report*. Available at WWW.NIDA.NIH.GOV/ RESEARCHREPORTS/HALLUCINOGENS.HTML.

Nicholson KL, Hayes BA & Balster RL (1999). Evaluation of the reinforcing properties and phencyclidine-like discriminative stimulus effects of dextrorphan in rats and rhesus monkeys. *Psychopharmacology* 146:49-59.

Nordt SP (1998). DXM: A new drug of abuse? *Annals of Emergency Medicine* 31:794-795.

Pender ES & Parks BR (1991). Toxicology with dextromethorphan-containing preparations: A literature review and report of two additional cases. *Pediatric Emergency Care* 7:163-167.

Wolfe TR & Caravati EM (1995). Massive dextromethorphan ingestion and abuse. *American Journal of Emergency Medicine* 13:174-176.

| Chapter 5 | # The Pharmacology of Cocaine, Amphetamines, and Other Stimulants |

David A. Gorelick, M.D., Ph.D.
Jennifer L. Cornish, Ph.D.

Stimulants are a class of drugs that stimulate activity in the central and sympathetic peripheral nervous systems, chiefly by enhancing neurotransmitter activity at catecholaminergic synapses.

DRUGS IN THE CLASS

Naturally occurring stimulants, such as cocaine (Figure 1) and ephedra, have been used in traditional medicine for thousands of years. More than a dozen synthetic stimulants, such as the amphetamines, have been introduced into medicine over the past century. Most of these are variants of the basic phenethylamine chemical structure, which is shared by the endogenous catecholamine neurotransmitters norepinephrine and dopamine (Figure 2).

All stimulants share the same range of psychological and physiological effects, while differing in potency and pharmacokinetic characteristics. This chapter reviews the history, epidemiology, clinical pharmacology, neurobiology, and abuse liability of cocaine, amphetamines, and other stimulants currently abused or available for medical use. Caffeine, the most widely used stimulant, is considered separately in Chapter 6. 3,4-Methylenedioxymethamphetamine (MDMA, "Ecstasy"), a structural analogue of methamphetamine with both stimulant and hallucinogenic characteristics, is considered separately at the end of this chapter.

History. Naturally occurring plant alkaloids have been used for their central nervous system (CNS) stimulant properties for thousands of years (Karch, 1996). Chinese medicine has used the herbal preparation ma-huang (ephedra) for at least 5,000 years. Chewing of coca leaves has been prevalent in the Andean regions of South America for at least 2,000 years (Karch, 1998). Coca leaves and pottery images of figures with bulging cheeks (presumably wads of coca leaf) have been found in 1,400-year-old Peruvian burial sites. The Spanish conquerors of South America found coca leaf chewing common in the Andean regions and noted its association with increased energy and decreased need for food and sleep. They did not discourage the practice, which continues to this day and is legal in Bolivia and Peru (Montoya & Chilcoat, 1996).

Coca received little attention in Europe until the second half of the nineteenth century. In 1860, a German graduate student, Albert Niemann, reported as part of his doctoral thesis the isolation of cocaine as the active ingredient of coca leaf. This discovery helped generate the popularity of cocaine-containing products throughout

FIGURE 1.   Chemical Structures of Cocaine, Mazindol, and Methylphenidate

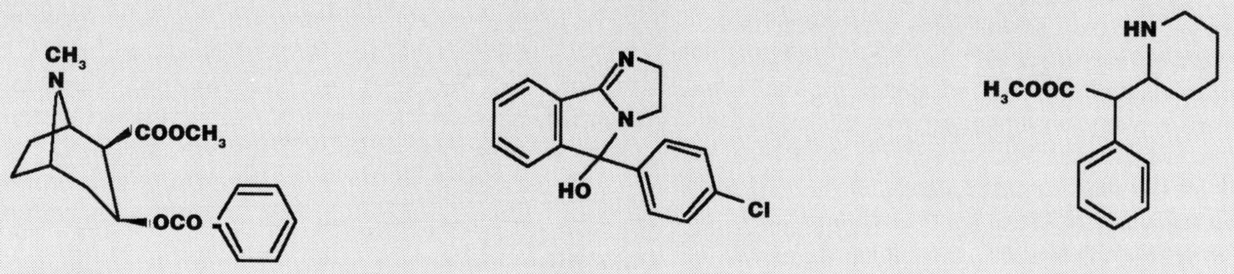

Europe and North America. Cocaine-containing wines, such as Vin Mariani (containing 6 to 8 mg of cocaine per ounce), were widely advertised and endorsed by prominent political and cultural figures. A nonalcoholic beverage (containing 4.5 mg of cocaine per 6 ounces) was introduced in 1886 and quickly became one of the world's most popular soft drinks: Coca-Cola®. A fluid extract of coca for medical use (containing 0.5 mg of cocaine per ml) appeared in the U.S. Pharmacopeia in 1882. The first specific use of cocaine in medicine came in 1884, when the German ophthalmologist Koller discovered its efficacy as a local anesthetic during surgery. In the same year, Sigmund Freud published his monograph *Uber Coca*, describing the first systematic study of cocaine's psychological effects (albeit with a sample of one, himself) and suggesting its use as a treatment for morphine addiction.

With widespread use of cocaine came increasing reports of adverse effects. The first report of cocaine-associated cardiac arrest and stroke was published in 1886. By 1903, cocaine had been removed from Coca-Cola. In 1914, the Harrison Narcotic Act banned cocaine from over-the-counter (OTC) medications, beverages, and foods in the United States, restricting its use to prescription drugs. For the next 50 years, cocaine remained largely out of public view and medical attention, except for limited use as a local anesthetic.

Synthetic stimulants first appeared with the synthesis of amphetamine in 1887 (by Edeleau) and of methamphetamine in 1919. These attracted little attention until amphetamine became popular as an OTC bronchodilator (in the Benzedrine® inhaler) in the early 1930s. By 1933, its CNS stimulant properties were recognized, leading to its use for weight loss, narcolepsy, depression, and childhood hyperactivity. Amphetamine's advantages also were recognized by stimulant abusers. It largely replaced cocaine in illicit use because of its low cost, ready availability, and longer duration of action. This growing abuse pattern led to a switch in 1937 from OTC to prescription-only status.

During World War II, amphetamine was widely used by the Allied and Axis countries to enhance the performance of troops and factory workers. After the war, widespread abuse in Japan and Sweden of large leftover stockpiles led to tight restrictions on amphetamine manufacture and dispensing. In response to increasing rates of intravenous abuse of amphetamine extracted from Benzedrine inhalers, the U.S. Food and Drug Administration (FDA) banned the inhalers in 1959. With passage of the Controlled Substances Act (CSA) in 1970, cocaine, amphetamine, and methamphetamine were placed in Schedule II because they have high potential for abuse and accepted medical use only with severe restrictions. As recognition of their abuse potential grew, the number of prescription stimulants available in the United States declined from 65 (marketed by 40 different companies) in 1970 to eight (marketed by six companies) in 1995 (Masand & Tesar, 1996).

Epidemiology. There are substantial geographic and sociodemographic differences in the epidemiology of stimulant use (Anthony & Helzer, 1995; U.N. Drug Control Program, 2000). Cocaine use is most prevalent in the Western Hemisphere, with some use in Western Europe, and little or no use in Africa and Asia. Amphetamine misuse is most prevalent in Oceania, East and Southeast Asia, and

Western Europe, with some use in North and Central America and little or no use elsewhere. These patterns may reflect availability and access, because the only source of cocaine is the Andean region of South America, while amphetamines can be readily synthesized anywhere.

Oral use of cocaine has a long cultural tradition and is legal in Bolivia and Peru. Surveys have found lifetime prevalence of coca leaf use up to 90% in Bolivia and 30% in Peru (Montoya & Chilcoat, 1996). Purified cocaine, suitable for intravenous, smoked, or intranasal administration, is illegal in all Andean countries. The lifetime prevalence of such cocaine use is similar to that reported in North America.

A detailed view of stimulant epidemiology in the United States comes from two annual national surveys conducted by the Substance Abuse and Mental Health Services Administration (SAMHSA). The National Household Survey on Drug Abuse (NHSDA) surveys a representative sample of household residents 12 years and older that is sufficiently large to generate valid population estimates of drug use. NHSDA data may tend to underestimate overall drug use because the survey sample does not include some groups in which drug use is likely to be higher, such as persons in correctional settings, homeless persons, hospital patients, and residential college students. The NHSDA does include nonmedical use of prescription drugs, but does not measure use of OTC medications or drugs considered dietary supplements, such as caffeine (see Chapter 6).

Information on adverse consequences of stimulant use comes from the Drug Abuse Warning Network (DAWN). DAWN is a nationwide survey of about 500 hospital emergency departments, in which data are collected on patient visits associated with the use of illegal drugs or nonmedical use of prescription and OTC medications. DAWN also surveys about 140 medical examiners in 40 metropolitan areas for data on deaths (other than those due to homicide or AIDS) associated with medications or illegal drugs.

According to the NHSDA data, cocaine is the second most widely used illegal drug in the United States, after marijuana. Cocaine use in the United States peaked during the mid-1980s, then declined about 50% to stable levels throughout the 1990s. The 2000 NHSDA estimated that 24.9 million Americans (11.2% of the U.S. population ≥12 years old) had used cocaine at some time during their lifetimes (about one-fifth by smoking "crack" cocaine); 3.3 million (1.5%) had used cocaine within the preceding year; and 1.2 million (0.7%) had used cocaine within the preceding month, which NHSDA classifies as current use (265,000

by smoking "crack" cocaine) (Office of Applied Studies, 2001b).

An estimated 770,000 Americans met the *DSM-IV* criteria of the American Psychiatric Association (1994) for cocaine dependence in 1999. Earlier community-based interview surveys had estimated a 0.2% lifetime prevalence of cocaine abuse (by *DSM-III* criteria) during the early 1980s (Anthony & Helzer, 1990) and 2.7% lifetime prevalence of cocaine dependence (*DSM-IIIR* criteria) during the early 1990s (Anthony, Warner et al., 1994). In 2000, about 270 metric tons of illegal cocaine were used in the U.S., on which users spent about $35 billion (Rhodes, Layne et al., 2000).

Cocaine use occurs in all segments of American society, but is substantially more prevalent in certain population groups. Data from the 2000 NHSDA suggest that the most likely cocaine user is an unemployed man in his early 20s, living in a large city on the West Coast, who is a high school dropout, smokes cigarettes, and drinks alcohol heavily. Lifetime and current cocaine use are at least 50% more prevalent among men than women.

Cocaine use also varies widely by age. Current use rates are lowest in early adolescents (0.1% to 0.2% in 12- to 14-year-olds), peak from ages 19 to 23 (2.1% in 20-year-olds), and decline to unmeasurable levels after age 54. A similar pattern holds for lifetime use. In 2000, an estimated 144,000 persons 65 years or older (0.5%) reported lifetime use of cocaine. Native Americans and Alaska Natives have the highest rate of cocaine use of any racial/ethnic group, with 1.4% reporting current use and 16.4% reporting lifetime use in 2000. Cocaine use is about twice as common in persons without a high school diploma as in those with at least some college education, and at least three times more common in persons who are unemployed than in those who are employed full-time, students, retired, or disabled.

Cocaine use is highly associated with legal substance use and with psychiatric syndromes. Cigarette smokers or heavy alcohol drinkers are each at least 10 times more likely to use cocaine than are nonsmokers or moderate (nonbinge) drinkers. Current cocaine users are twice as likely to have symptoms of depressive or anxiety disorders than are nonusers (Kandel, Huang et al., 2001).

Cocaine use varies by geographic location. The highest rates of current and lifetime use are found in the Pacific region of the United States (0.9% and 16.5%, respectively), while the lowest rates of use are found in the South (0.4% and 9.2%). Cocaine use is about twice as common in large urban areas than it is in rural areas.

Nonmedical use of prescription stimulants (other than cocaine) peaked in the United States at 2.7 million current users (1.3% of the population) in 1985. The number declined to 960,000 current users (0.6% of the population) by 1990 and remained below one million throughout the decade. The number of persons who initiated nonmedical stimulant use peaked in 1974 at 735,000, with a mean age at first use of 19.6 years. Initiation rates then declined to a low of 194,000 in 1991 (mean age at first use: 18.1 years), before rising again to 646,000 in 1999 (mean age of first use: 19.6 years). The 2000 NHSDA estimated that 14.7 million Americans (6.6% of the U.S. population ≥12 years old) were nonmedical users of stimulants other than cocaine at some time during their lifetimes; 2.1 million (0.9%) had used such stimulants within the preceding year; and 788,000 were current users (0.4%).

An estimated 278,000 Americans met psychiatric criteria (*DSM-IV*) for noncocaine stimulant dependence in 1999. Earlier community-based surveys had estimated a 1.7% lifetime prevalence of noncocaine stimulant dependence (*DSM-III* criteria) during the early 1980s (Anthony & Helzer, 1990) and early 1990s (Anthony, Warner et al., 1994).

The most commonly misused prescription stimulant is methamphetamine. The 2000 NHSDA estimated that 8.8 million Americans (4.0% of population) were lifetime methamphetamine users; 1.0 million (0.5%) had used methamphetamine within the past year; and 387,000 (0.2%) were current users (Office of Applied Studies, 2001b). In 2000, about 15 million metric tons of methamphetamine were used in the United States, on which users spent about $5.4 billion (Rhodes, Layne et al., 2000). Methamphetamine use is confined almost entirely to the western two-thirds of the United States, with very little use reported on the East Coast, even in cities with high rates of cocaine use.

Stimulant use often is associated with adverse consequences. In the 2000 DAWN survey, cocaine was the drug associated most often with visits to hospital emergency departments, with 174,896 visits (29.06% of all visits)—almost twice as often as the next two most common drugs, heroin/morphine (16.17% of visits) and marijuana (16.03%) (Office of Applied Studies, 2001a). Amphetamine was ranked 10th (2.69% of visits), methamphetamine 12th (2.25%), OTC stimulants 31st (0.65%), and methylphenidate 43rd (0.25%). Cocaine was the drug most often reported by those 26 years and older; it ranked second, behind marijuana, among those 18 to 25 years old, and fifth among those 6 to 17 years old. Amphetamine and metham-

phetamine were in the top 15 in all age groups, except for methamphetamine in those 35 years and older.

Cocaine was the drug most commonly reported in all racial/ethnic groups and by both genders. Almost three-quarters of cocaine users who visited emergency departments also were using other substances, including alcohol (46.3%), marijuana (19.0%), opiates (17.7%), and benzodiazepines (6.3%). This also was true of amphetamine and methylphenidate users. However, the majority of methamphetamine and OTC stimulant users were not using any other drug.

Cocaine was the drug most often associated with deaths investigated by medical examiners in 1999, being mentioned 4,864 times (41.75% of all deaths) (Office of Applied Studies, 2000). Methamphetamine ranked 5th (5.92% of deaths), amphetamine 11th (3.88%), OTC stimulants 28th (1.34%), and phentermine 64th (0.19%). Cocaine was the drug most often reported by those 26 years and older, second (behind heroin/morphine) among those 18 to 25 years old, and third (behind heroin/morphine and marijuana) among those 6 to 17 years old. Cocaine was the drug most commonly reported for African American and female decedents and second (behind heroin/morphine) among white, Hispanic, and male decedents.

Only a minority of stimulant users appear to seek drug abuse treatment. While there were an estimated 770,000 cocaine-dependent persons and 1.1 million weekly users in 1999, only 228,206 persons who reported cocaine as their primary drug of abuse were admitted to publicly funded substance abuse treatment programs in that year, out of more than 1.5 million admissions overall (Treatment Episode Data Set [TEDS]; Office of Applied Studies, 2001c). About three-quarters of patients admitted using smoked cocaine (as compared to about one-quarter cocaine smokers among the general population of cocaine users). Another 57,834 patients were admitted for primary methamphetamine use, 13,730 for use of other amphetamines, and 821 for other stimulant use. The majority of cocaine abusers were African American (51.4%), while the majority of methamphetamine/amphetamine abusers were white (79.1%). The peak age group among patients was 30 to 39 years—substantially older than the 19- to 23-year-old peak age among cocaine users in the general population.

PREPARATIONS AND USES
Plant-Derived Stimulants. Several naturally occurring, plant-derived stimulants are widely available for traditional

oral use in many areas of the world. These include cocaine (in South America), ephedra (in North America and East Asia), and khat (in East Africa and Arabia). (Caffeine, the most widely used stimulant, is addressed in Chapter 6.) Such use often is culturally sanctioned and may not be associated with abuse or dependence. Use of more potent formulations (for example, the extracted active chemical) or more rapidly acting routes of administration has significant abuse potential and is illegal even where oral formulations are allowed.

Cocaine: Cocaine is an alkaloid with a tropane ester chemical structure (Figure 1) similar to that of scopolamine and other plant alkaloids. It occurs in leaves of the coca bush, *Erythroxylon coca*, which grows at altitudes of 1,500 to 6,000 feet in the Andean region of South America. The leaf contains cocaine (0.2% to 1%) and more than a dozen other tropane alkaloids (such as benzoylecgonine, methylecgonine, ecgnonine, and cinnamoylcocaine), most of which are of unknown pharmacologic activity. Another *Erythroxylon* species, *E. novogranatense*, contains lesser amounts of cocaine and greater levels of other alkaloids (Moore & Casale, 1994). Cocaine exists as two stereoisomers: naturally occurring (-)-cocaine and (+)-cocaine, which has less affinity for the dopamine transporter and is relatively inactive *in vivo* because of its very rapid metabolism by butyrylcholinesterase (Fowler, Volkow et al., 2001).

About 870 square miles of coca were cultivated in Bolivia, Colombia, and Peru in 1999. This resulted in net production of about 230,000 metric tons of coca leaf (U.S. Department of State, 2000), most destined for export. Domestic use of oral cocaine is legal in these countries, usually as coca tea or by chewing the leaves. Coca leaves typically are chewed in conjunction with lime or plant ash, which alkalinizes the saliva and thus enhances absorption of the cocaine. Cocaine is legally available in the United States only as a 4% or 10% injectable solution (or powder for reconstitution) or viscous liquid for use as a local or topical anesthetic. Legal cocaine preparations rarely are diverted for misuse.

Illicit cocaine is smuggled into the United States specifically for abuse purposes from its countries of origin. An estimated 259 metric tons of cocaine, with a retail value of about $35 billion, entered the United States in 2000 (ONDCP, 2002). Based on samples seized by law enforcement agencies, the average wholesale (dealer) and retail (user) prices for cocaine in 2000 were $51 and $212 per gram, respectively (ONDCP, 2002).

Preparation of illicit cocaine begins with crushing the coca leaves and heating it in an organic solvent (often kerosene) to extract and partially purify the cocaine (Bono, 1998). After several more extraction and filtering steps, the coca paste (now 80% to 90% pure) is heated in an organic solvent (often ether or acetone) with concentrated acid to convert it to salt form. The salt is readily converted back to the base by heating it in an organic solvent at basic pH. This process is known as "freebasing," and was practiced by cocaine users during the 1980s, before cocaine base (or "freebase") was widely available on the retail street market. "Crack" as a street name for base cocaine reportedly derives from the crackling sound made during this process.

Cocaine is available for street use in two forms: base and salt (Hatsukami & Fischman, 1996; Karch, 1996). These have different physical properties, which favor different routes of administration. The base has a relatively low melting point (98° C.) and vaporizes before substantial pyrolytic destruction has occurred. This allows cocaine base to be smoked, although the majority of the cocaine may be in the form of small particles (< 5 microns) that reach the alveoli, rather than true cocaine vapor (Snyder, Wood et al., 1988). Cocaine base is relatively insoluble in water (alcohol:water solubility ratio of 100:1), making it difficult to dissolve for injection purposes. In contrast, cocaine salt does not melt at less than 195° C., so that heating it for smoking results in destruction of most of the cocaine. However, cocaine salt is highly water soluble (alcohol:water solubility ratio of 1:8), making it easy to dissolve for injection purposes and facilitating absorption across mucus membranes. Regardless of the chemical form or route of administration, the cocaine molecule exerts the same actions once it reaches the brain or other target organ (Hatsukami & Fischman, 1996).

The average purity of seized cocaine samples is around 60% (ONDCP, 2002). Diluents are added (that is, the cocaine is "cut") to enhance dealer profits. Diluents include both inert fillers that look like cocaine (such as dextrose, lactose, mannitol, or starch) and active chemicals that either mimic the local anesthetic effect of cocaine (such as benzocaine, lidocaine, or procaine) or provide some psychoactive effect (such as ephedrine, amphetamine, caffeine, or PCP) (Bono, 1998; Shesser, Jotte et al., 1991). Street cocaine also may contain contaminants from the preparation process (such as benzene, acetone, or sodium bicarbonate) (Shesser, Jotte et al., 1991). Street amphetamines generally

FIGURE 2. Chemical Structures of Endogenous Catecholamine Neurotransmitters (Dopamine, Norepinephrine) and Phenethylamine Stimulant Drugs

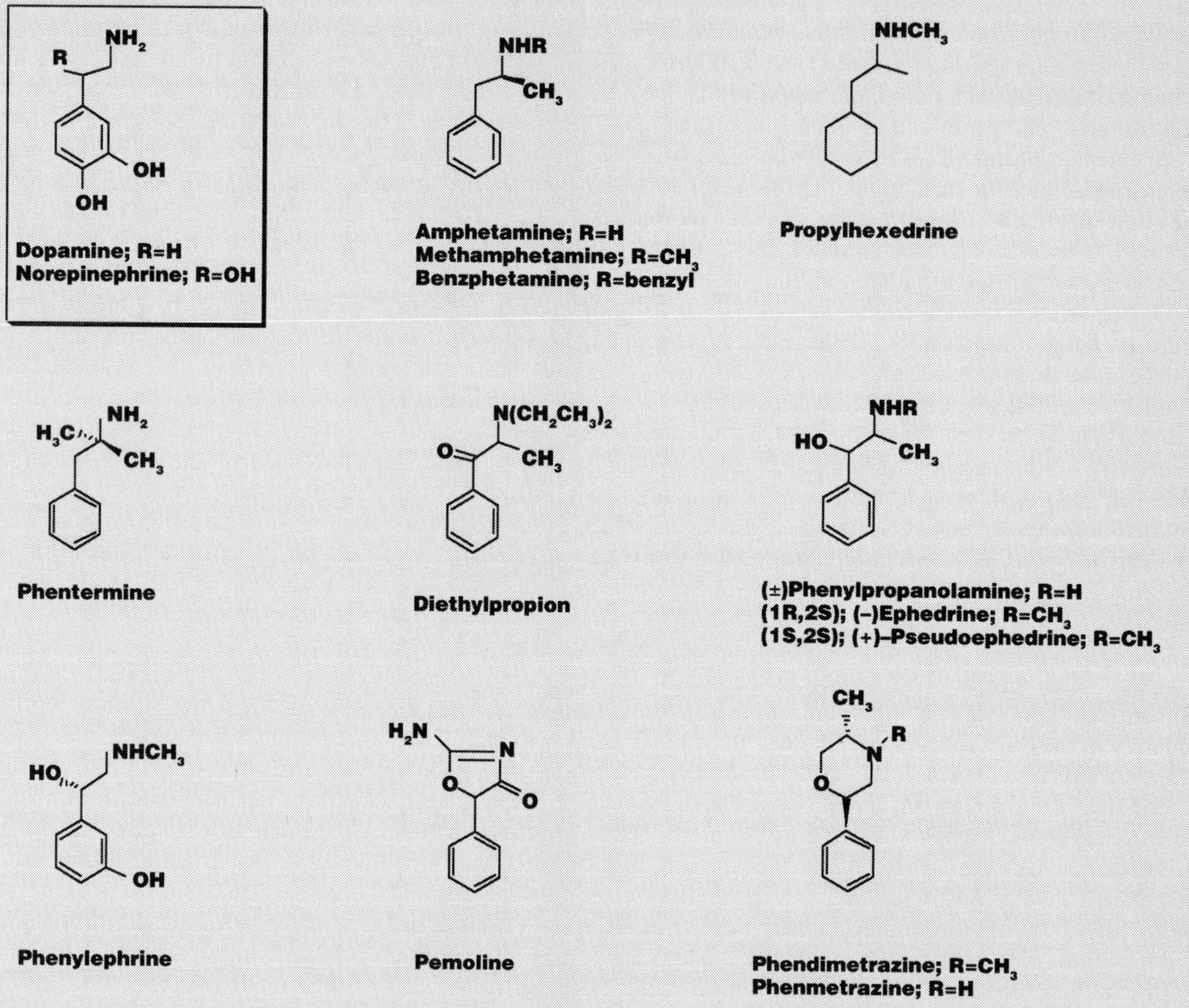

Dopamine; R=H
Norepinephrine; R=OH

Amphetamine; R=H
Methamphetamine; R=CH₃
Benzphetamine; R=benzyl

Propylhexedrine

Phentermine

Diethylpropion

(±)Phenylpropanolamine; R=H
(1R,2S); (–)Ephedrine; R=CH₃
(1S,2S); (+)–Pseudoephedrine; R=CH₃

Phenylephrine

Pemoline

Phendimetrazine; R=CH₃
Phenmetrazine; R=H

are purer than street cocaine; the only common diluents are other stimulants (Renfroe & Messinger, 1985).

Ephedra: Ephedrine and pseudoephedrine are naturally occurring alkaloids with a phenethylamine chemical structure (Figure 2) that are found in several Ephedraceae species (especially *Ephedra sinica, E. equisetina*, and *E. gerardiana*) (Karch, 1996). Ephedra is a preparation of dried young branches of *Ephedra* species, typically containing at least 1% ephedrine. This may be converted into a capsule, tincture, liquid extract, or tea. Ephedra products are widely used in East Asia and North America; they appear in the pharmacopoeias of China, Japan, and Germany.

Under the Dietary Supplement Health and Education Act of 1994, these products are not closely regulated by the FDA, and so they vary widely in purity and potency in the United States. Ephedra products often are advertised as legal versions of or alternatives to the more strictly regulated manufactured stimulants. They may appeal to consumers as safer than synthetic stimulants because they are "natural" or "herbal." Synthetic ephedrine and pseudoephedrine also are available as tablets or capsules (see below).

Ephedra alkaloids have the same range of psychological and physiological effects as do cocaine and amphetamines (Karch, 1996). There is limited evidence of their efficacy for weight loss in obese individuals (Yanovski & Yanovski, 2002). Ephedra use has been associated with severe cardiovascular and CNS effects, including death (Haller & Benowitz, 2000).

Khat: Khat is the common term for preparations of the *Catha edulis* plant, which is native to East Africa (Sudan to Madagascar) and the southern Arabian peninsula (Yemen) (Karch, 1996). Fresh khat leaves contain at least two stimulant alkaloids with phenethylamine chemical structures: cathinone (present at 1% to 3%) and cathine (norpseudoephedrine). Pure cathinone is a Schedule I controlled substance; cathine is in Schedule IV. The potent (Schedule I) cathinone congener methcathinone ("CAT"), known as ephedrone in Europe, is clandestinely synthesized from ephedrine or pseudoephedrine (Bono, 1998). Both cathinone and methcathinone inhibit the presynaptic neuronal dopamine and serotonin transporters with a potency similar to that of amphetamines (see Neurotransmitters, below) (Fleckenstein, Gibb et al., 2000).

Khat use has been a widely accepted social custom for centuries, apparently predating the use of coffee (caffeine). The leaves are used in the same way as coca leaves in South America, that is, chewed and kept in the cheek for several hours. Less often, the leaves are brewed into tea or crushed with honey to make a paste. Moderate use reduces fatigue and appetite. Compulsive use may result in manic behavior or psychotic symptoms such as paranoia or hallucinations. The extent of abuse or dependence is unclear. Khat loses much of its potency within two days of harvesting, as cathinone is converted to the much less potent cathine. Some khat use is found among immigrant communities in Europe, but there appears to be negligible use of khat in the United States. Methcathinone is widely abused in Russia and the Baltic area.

Little is known about the long-term toxicity of khat use. It has been associated with oral cancers, and with mutagenesis, teratogenesis, and embryotoxicity in rodent studies (Li & Lin, 1998).

Synthetic Stimulants. More than a dozen synthetic stimulant medications are legally available in the United States, either by prescription (Table 1) or over the counter (Table 2). Most represent variations on the basic phenethylamine structure (Figure 2). Common trade and street names, schedules, clinical uses (FDA-approved and otherwise), and typical doses are listed in Tables 1 and 2.

All stimulants, other than cocaine, are legally sold for oral use in tablet, capsule, or liquid form. Several prescription stimulants are available in extended or sustained-release formulations. Some OTC stimulants also are available in aerosolized formulations for nasal inhalation (insufflation) for use as decongestants. Phenylephrine is available as a sterile solution for parenteral administration to treat hypotension.

Synthetic stimulants typically are abused by the oral or intravenous route. Amphetamines, especially highly pure crystallized methamphetamine ("ice"), may be used intranasally or smoked, as is cocaine. Some abused synthetic stimulants, such as methylphenidate, are diverted from legitimate sources and thus are of known content and purity. If oral administration is not intended, the original tablet or capsule may be crushed or opened to allow the drug to be taken intranasally or mixed with water for injection. In contrast, amphetamines, especially methamphetamine, usually are synthesized in clandestine laboratories directly for illicit use. This can be done with standard chemical reactions applied to legally available precursors. For example, methamphetamine (desoxyephedrine) can be made by reducing ephedrine or pseudoephedrine. For this reason, single-transaction retail purchases of products containing ephedrine or pseudoephedrine are limited to 24 g under the Comprehensive Methamphetamine Control Act of 1996 (Public Law 104-237). Federal law enforcement agents seized 1,756 kg of methamphetamine and 2,155 clandestine methamphetamine laboratories in 2000, the vast majority in the western two-thirds of the United States (Drug Enforcement Administration, 2001).

Stimulants with a phenylisopropylamine structure (such as amphetamine, methamphetamine, ephedrine, pseudoephedrine, and phenylpropanolamine) have a chiral (stereoisomeric) center at the alpha-carbon atom (Figure 2),

TABLE 1. Stimulants Available by Prescription in the United States

Drug	Trade Names	Street Names	CSA Schedule	Indications	Typical Oral Dose (mg/day)
Amphetamine	Adderall,® Dexedrine,® Dextrostat®	Amp, Bennies, Dex, Black beauties	II	ADHD, Narcolepsy, Weight control, Depression*	5-60 5-60 5-60
Benzphetamine	Didrex®		III	Weight control	25-150
Cocaine		Coke, Crack, Flake, Snow	II	Local anesthetic	(topical solution)
Diethylpropion	Tenuate®		IV	Weight control	75-100
Mazindol	Sanorex,® Mazanor®		IV	Weight control	1-3
Methamphetamine	Adipex,® Desoxyn,® Methedrine®	Ice, Meth, Speed, Crank, Crystal	II	ADHD, Weight control	5-40 10-15
Methylphenidate	Ritalin®	Rits, Vitamin R	II	ADHD, Narcolepsy	10-60 10-60
Pemoline	Cylert®		IV	ADHD, Narcolepsy*	56-112 56-112
Phendimetrazine	Bontril,® Plegine®		III	Weight control	35-105
Phenmetrazine	Preludin®		II	Weight control	25-75
Phentermine	Adipex-P,® Fastin,® Ionamin®		IV	Weight control	15-90

* Not labeled for this indication by the U.S. Food & Drug Administration
CSA = Federal Controlled Substances Act
ADHD = attention deficit/hyperactivity disorder

and so exist in two (or more) stereoisomer forms that differ in pharmacodynamic and pharmacokinetic properties (Baselt, 1999; Cho & Melega, 2002). The *d*- or S-(+) isomer generally has three to five times the CNS activity and about one-third the half-life of the *l*- or R-(-) isomer. The *l*-isomers have more peripheral alpha-adrenergic activity. For example, *d*-methamphetamine is a potent CNS stimulant, while *l*-methamphetamine (*l*-desoxyephedrine)

has been used as a decongestant (as in the Vicks® nasal inhaler) (Ellenhorn, Schonwald et al., 1997). Methylphenidate also exists in four stereoisomeric forms, of which the *d*-threo enantiomer is the active one (Ding, Fowler et al., 1997).

Clinical Uses. Cocaine is used clinically only as a local or topical anesthetic, chiefly for eye, ear, nose, or throat surgery or procedures. Other prescription stimulants generally are used for one of several FDA-approved indications: attention deficit/hyperactivity disorder (ADHD) in both children (Greenhill, Halperin et al., 1999; Kimko, Cross et al., 1999) and adults (Higgins, 1999), narcolepsy (ASDA Standards of Practice Committee, 1994) and excessive daytime sleepiness (Nishino & Mignot, 1999), and appetite suppression to promote weight loss in exogenous obesity (Bray, 1999; Yanovski & Yanovski, 2002) (Table 1).

OTC stimulants generally are used for decongestion and bronchodilation in the treatment of asthma, upper respiratory infections, allergic rhinitis, sinusitis, or bronchitis, and for appetite suppression to promote weight loss in exogenous obesity (both of which are FDA-approved indications) (Table 2). Parenteral phenylephrine also is approved by the FDA as an adjunct to prolong the duration of spinal anesthesia, to terminate paroxysmal supraventricular tachycardia (probably indirectly by stimulation of arterial baroreceptors), and for immediate, short-term treatment of hypotension (especially when due to anesthesia, drugs, or hypersensitivity reactions).

In addition to their FDA-approved indications, oral stimulants have a long history of accepted clinical use for other indications. Amphetamines, methylphenidate, and pemoline are used as quick acting (two- to three-day), short-term antidepressants in persons who are elderly, medically ill, HIV-infected, or those with neurological conditions such as stroke or traumatic brain injury, especially those who cannot tolerate the side effects of standard antidepressants (Challman & Lipsky, 2000; Masand & Tesar, 1996; Wagner & Rabkin, 2000). Such patients may exhibit apathy, fatigue, and psychomotor retardation, rather than a full-blown classic depressive syndrome. Often, it is unclear whether the beneficial effect of stimulants in such patients is due to the drugs' activating effects or to true antidepressant actions (Glenn, 1998). Stimulants also have been used to augment the response to standard antidepressants. Amphetamines, methylphenidate, and mazindol have been used to potentiate opiate analgesia and to counteract opiate-induced sedation and respiratory suppression, thus allowing larger doses of opiates to be used (Corey, Heck et al., 1999; Dalal & Melzack, 1998; Masand & Tesar, 1996). Cocaine has been used for this purpose as part of Brompton's cocktail (with alcohol and an opiate) in the treatment of cancer pain. Ephedrine and phenylephrine still are used parenterally to counteract hypotension associated with spinal anesthesia (especially in obstetrical and urologic surgery)

(Karch, 1996). Most other clinical uses of stimulants for their pressor effect have been superceded by more selective agents.

There is no evidence that medical use of stimulants at therapeutic doses in appropriately diagnosed patients leads to stimulant abuse or significantly lowers the seizure threshold, although most data come from case series and anecdotal experience, rather than controlled trials (Masand & Tesar, 1996). Recent prospective, longitudinal studies in children being treated for ADHD found a decreased risk of developing substance abuse in those receiving stimulants (Biederman, Wilens et al., 1999; Vitiello, 2001). Because ADHD itself is a potent risk factor for developing substance abuse, these findings may reflect the beneficial effect of successful ADHD treatment with stimulants.

Nonmedical Use, Abuse, and Dependence. Oral stimulants (both prescription and OTC) have been widely used in work, school, military, and sports settings, often without medical supervision, for their alerting, antifatigue, sleep-suppressing, and performance-enhancing properties (Akerstedt & Ficca, 1997). Use in the U.S. military has declined more than 80% over the past two decades, largely as the result of a comprehensive antidrug policy that includes mandatory urine drug testing (Bray, Sanchez et al., 1999). In 1998, 0.9% of U.S. military personnel had used cocaine or other stimulants within the preceding 12 months—substantially less than among the general population of similar age and gender. Use by other occupational groups, such as long-distance truck drivers and night-shift workers, remains problematic.

The stimulants' antifatigue and sleep-suppression effects have been well demonstrated in laboratory and field studies. Enhancement of cognitive and psychomotor performance is more difficult to demonstrate in controlled studies, and occurs more robustly in persons who already are fatigued or sleep-deprived. Amphetamines are used by athletes in endurance sports such as cycling because they enhance anaerobic performance (George, 2000). Stimulants of all types (illicit, prescription, and OTC) are banned by the International Olympic Committee and many other sports organizations (Segura, 1998).

All stimulants have a potential for misuse, abuse, and dependence, varying only in their potency. Cocaine, amphetamine, and methamphetamine have high abuse potential, as reflected in their placement in Schedule II. Community-based interview surveys suggest that up to one in six persons who use cocaine and one in nine who use

TABLE 2. Stimulants Available as Over-the-Counter Preparations in the United States

Drug	Trade Names	Indications	Typical Oral Dose (mg/day)
Caffeine	(various)	Weight control, alertness	50-250
Ephedrine	Marax,® Quadrinal®	Decongestant, bronchodilation	50-100
Phenylephrine	Comhist,® Dristan,® Neo-Synephrine®	Decongestant	40-60
Phenylpropanolamine*	Comtrex,® Triaminic® Acutrim,® Dexatrim®	Decongestant, weight control	150
Pseudoephedrine	Sudafed,® Sine-Aid®	Decongestant	90-240
Propylhexedrine	Benzedrex,® Dristan,® Obesin®	Decongestant, weight control	50-150

* Withdrawn from the U.S. market in October 2000.

prescription stimulants for other than medical purposes will become dependent (Anthony, Warner et al., 1994). Even higher rates are found in treatment-seeking populations: up to four-fifths of those who have used cocaine several times and up to half of those who have used amphetamines become dependent (Woody, Cottler et al., 1993). Heavier users and those who use the intravenous and smoked forms are more likely to become dependent than are lighter users or those who use the intranasal and oral forms (Gorelick, 1992; Gossop, Griffiths et al., 1994; Woody, Cottler et al., 1993). However, even lower potency stimulants in Schedule IV, such as pemoline and phentermine, or OTC stimulants such as ephedrine, pseudoephedrine, and phenylpropanolamine, have been misused and abused (Tinsley & Watkins, 1998).

Studies of drug use by pairs of fraternal (dizygotic) and identical (monozygotic) twins suggest less of a genetic influence on initiation of stimulant use than on stimulant abuse and dependence (Kendler, 2001). Family environment (including religious and social factors) has the strongest influence on initial use, while genetic factors are more important for the development of abuse or dependence once use has begun (heritabilities generally >60%). Efforts to identify a specific gene or genes responsible for stimulant dependence have not been successful. The most widely studied gene, for the dopamine D_2 receptor, has yielded inconsistent results in association studies (Sery, Vojtova et al., 2001).

The greater abuse liability of intravenous and smoked (as opposed to oral and intranasal) routes of administration is considered to be attributable to their faster rate of drug delivery to the brain (6 to 8 seconds, in the case of smoking), resulting in a faster onset of psychological effects (Gorelick, 1998; Volkow, Fowler et al., 1999a). This faster onset is associated with a more intense pleasurable response and greater abuse liability (the so-called "rate hypothesis" of psychoactive drug action).

Stimulants are used in a variety of patterns (Levin, Hess et al., 1993; Myers, Rohsenow et al., 1995). "Binge" use involves short periods of heavy use (for example, on weekends or after payday), separated by longer periods of little or no use. Others may use frequently for an extended period until their finances are exhausted or their access to drug is interrupted. A small number of users may use low doses daily without dose escalation over time. (Some of these users may be self-medicating an underlying neuropsychiatric disorder such as ADHD or narcolepsy.) Typical cocaine doses are 12 to 15 g orally (coca leaf chewing), 20 to 100 mg intranasally, 10 to 50 mg intravenously, and 50 to 200 mg smoked.

High rates of stimulant abuse have been documented in persons involved with the criminal justice system. National surveys of state and federal prisoners in 1997 found that 14.8% and 9.3%, respectively, had used cocaine at the time of their offense, while 4.2% and 4.1% had used other stimulants (Bureau of Justice Statistics, 1999). Urine drug testing of male adult arrestees in 27 major U.S. cities in 2000 found one-sixth to one-half (median 30%) positive for cocaine and, in Western cities, up to one-quarter positive for methamphetamine (as compared with none in East Coast cities) (National Institute of Justice, 2001). These high occurrence rates suggest an association between stimulant use and crime, violence, and aggression. There are several potential causal mechanisms for this association, including behaviors associated with the illegal manufacture, distribution, and marketing of drugs, behaviors associated with users obtaining drug (or the money to buy drug), or a direct pharmacologic effect of stimulants on behavior (Giannini, Miller et al., 1993; Licata, Taylor et al., 1993; Miller, Gold et al., 1991). The association also may reflect the co-occurrence of stimulant use and antisocial personality disorder (which is associated with high rates of criminal behavior).

Low doses of stimulants do increase aggressive behavior in human laboratory models of aggression (as evidenced by willingness to administer electric shock, for example) (Licata, Taylor et al., 1993). Numerous case reports document violent behavior due to stimulant-induced irritability, paranoia, or frank psychosis (Fukushima, 1994).

Unintended use of cocaine may occur in persons who swallow the drug in their possession to avoid arrest or prosecution ("body stuffers") or who swallow large quantities to transport it without detection by law enforcement authorities ("body packers," "mules") (Sporer & Firestone, 1997). The drug may be wrapped in plastic bags, balloons, condoms, paper, aluminum foil, or a combination. If the wrapper fails, the carrier may be exposed suddenly to large doses of cocaine in the gastrointestinal tract, resulting in severe acute cocaine intoxication.

Stimulants often are used in combination with other drugs, either concurrently or sequentially. Concurrent use of a stimulant and an opiate, sometimes in the same injecting syringe, is considered by many users to provide a qualitatively better subjective effect ("high") than either drug alone (Grella, Anglin et al., 1997; Kreek, 1997). Concurrent intravenous use of cocaine plus heroin is termed "speedballing," and is common even among patients in drug abuse treatment. Combined use of oral amphetamine plus an oral opiate (such as codeine) also is common. Human experimental studies suggest that the acute psychological effects of cocaine are somewhat enhanced with concurrent administration of cocaine and an opiate (Foltin & Fischman, 1996). Other drugs sometimes used concurrently with smoked cocaine include phencyclidine (PCP), marijuana, or tobacco (Gorelick, Simmons et al., 1997). CNS depressant drugs such as alcohol, benzodiazepines, opiates, and marijuana often are used following cocaine use to temper unpleasant effects of cocaine intoxication (such as anxiety, paranoia, restlessness) and/or to relieve symptoms of cocaine withdrawal.

PHARMACOKINETICS

Absorption and Distribution. Route of administration has a major effect on the pharmacokinetic characteristics of stimulants (Cone, Tsadik et al., 1998). Smoked stimulants (such as cocaine base or methamphetamine) are rapidly absorbed through the lungs and probably reach the brain in 6 to 8 seconds. Thus, the onset and peak effect occur within minutes of administration. As the stimulant redistributes from the brain, there is a rapid decline in effect. Intravenous administration produces peak brain uptake in four to seven minutes, based on positron emission tomography (PET) studies with radiolabeled cocaine (Telang, Volkow et al., 1999). Greatest cocaine uptake occurs in the striatum (caudate, putamen, and nucleus accumbens) and least uptake in the orbital cortex and cerebellum. Clearance to half-peak brain levels requires 17 to 30 minutes and is fastest in the orbital cortex, thalamus, and cerebellum and slowest in the striatum. The rapid offset following rapid onset often is experienced as a "crash" by users of smoked or intravenous stimulants. Heavy cocaine users have about 20% less brain cocaine uptake than do healthy nonusers (Volkow, Wang et al., 1996). The mechanism of this difference is not known, but could be related to differences in plasma protein binding or permeability of the blood-brain barrier.

Intranasal and oral stimulants have a slower absorption and onset of effect (30 to 45 minutes), a longer peak effect, and a more gradual decline from peak. The peak intensity of effect is weaker than with smoked or intravenous administration because less active drug reaches its site of action in the brain. Coca leaf chewing produces less than half the peak cocaine plasma concentrations of an equivalent dose of intranasal cocaine (Jenkins & Cone, 1998). However, even a single oral dose of cocaine (such as 2 mg in a cup of coca tea) may yield detectable urine

TABLE 3.   Pharmacokinetic Parameters of Oral Stimulants

Drug	T_{max} (h)	$T_{1/2}$ (h)	Vd (L/kg)	pKa	Fb
Amphetamine	2-4	7-34*	3.2-5.6	9.9	0.16
Benzphetamine				6.6	
Chlorphentermine	4	35-44	3.0	9.6	
Cocaine	1	.75-1.5	1.2-1.9		
Diethylpropion		2.5			
Ephedrine	1	5-7.5		9.6	
Mazindol	1	33-55			
Methamphetamine	1-3	6-15*	3-7	9.9	0.1-0.2
Methylphenidate	1-3	2.4-4.2	11-33	8.8	0.15
Pemoline	1-3.5	11	0.22-0.59	10.5	0.3
Phendimetrazine	1			7.6	
Phenmetrazine	2	8		8.5	
Phentermine	4	19-24	3-4	10.1	
Phenylephrine	1	2-3	5	8.8	
Phenylpropanolamine	1-2	3-4.4	4.5	9.1	
Propylhexedrine				10.4	
Pseudoephedrine	2-3	3-16*		9.7	

SOURCE: Baselt, 1999.

T_{max} = time of maximum plasma concentration (in hours)
$T_{1/2}$ = half-life (in hours)
Vd = apparent volume of distribution (in liters per kg of body weight)
pKa = acid dissociation constant (= pH at which drug is 50% ionized)
Fb = fraction of bound drug

* urine pH-dependent: lower pH equals shorter half-life

concentrations of cocaine metabolites (Jackson, Saady et al., 1991; Kavanagh, Maijub et al., 1992). Pharmacokinetic parameters for oral stimulants are given in Table 3.

Cocaine is well absorbed through mucus membranes and also is absorbed through intact skin or by passive inhalation of smoked cocaine or aerosolized particles (Cone, Yousefnejad et al., 1995; Kavanagh, Maijub et al., 1992; Le, Taylor et al., 1992). Passive exposure can result in adverse medical effects in infants (Mott, Packer et al., 1994; Mirchandani, Mirchandani et al., 1991) and detectable urine concentrations of cocaine metabolites in medical and laboratory personnel (Bruns, Zieske et al., 1994; Le, Taylor et al., 1992). In many cases, these concentrations are too low to trigger a positive result on routine urine drug testing.

Stimulants distribute into most tissues of the body. Cocaine is rapidly taken up into the heart, kidney, adrenal glands, and liver (Fowler, Volkow et al., 2001). In addition to blood and urine, cocaine and its hydrolytic metabolites, amphetamines, phentermine, and ephedrine and its analogues appear in hair (Nakahara, 1999), sweat (Kidwell, Holland et al., 1998; Skopp & Potsch, 1999), saliva (Kidwell, Holland et al., 1998; Skopp & Potsch, 1999), and breast milk (AAP Committee on Drugs, 2001; Nice, Snyder et al., 2000), and cross the placenta to appear in meconium (Ostrea, 1999). Analysis of these tissues and fluids is used for drug detection in workplace, legal, and treatment settings (Caplan & Goldberger, 2001).

Metabolism. In humans (and other primates), 95% of cocaine is metabolized by hydrolysis of ester bonds to ecgonine methylester (by the action of carboxyesterases in the liver and butyrylcholinesterase in the liver, plasma, brain, lung, and other tissues) and to benzoylecgonine (spontaneously at physiological temperature and pH) (Cone, 1995; Jenkins & Cone, 1998; Warner & Norman, 2000). The remaining 5% of cocaine is N-demethylated to norcocaine by the liver cytochrome P450 microsomal enzyme system. This is the predominant metabolic pathway in rodents. Norcocaine has some pharmacologic actions similar to those of cocaine, and is hepatotoxic. This may account for the significant hepatotoxicity of cocaine in rodents, which is not found in primates. Cocaine's hydrolytic metabolites appear to be much less active pharmacologically, although this has not been well studied (Gorelick, 1997).

Amphetamines are metabolized in the liver via three different pathways: deamination to inactive metabolites, oxidation to norephedrine and other active metabolites, and para-hydroxylation to active metabolites (Jenkins & Cone, 1998). Amphetamine itself is the initial metabolite of methamphetamine.

When cocaine is smoked, a pyrolysis product is formed (anhydroecgonine methylester), the presence of which indicates that this route of administration was used (Cone, Tsadik et al., 1998; Jenkins & Cone, 1998).

Elimination. Stimulants and their metabolites are largely eliminated in the urine (Baselt, 1999; Jenkins & Cone, 1998). Benzoylecgonine is the cocaine metabolite found in highest concentration in urine for several days after cocaine use. It is this substance, rather than the parent drug cocaine, that actually is measured in routine urine drug tests for cocaine. Urinary elimination of amphetamines is highly pH dependent. Acidification of the urine substantially increases excretion and may halve the half-life (Jenkins & Cone, 1998). Conversely, alkalinization of the urine can reduce excretion to negligible levels. This fact is exploited by drug users who take large doses of sodium bicarbonate to prolong the action of amphetamines and reduce the amount present in the urine for detection by drug tests (Braithwaite, Jarvie et al., 1995).

Drug Interactions. The primary drug interaction of stimulants that is of clinical concern is with other stimulants or with other medications that also enhance catecholamine activity (Masand & Tesar, 1996). Such interactions risk overstimulation of the sympathetic nervous system, with possible cardiac arrhythmia, hypertension, seizure, cardiovascular collapse, and death. The major potential for interaction is presented by monoamine oxidase inhibitors (MAOIs), which are used as antidepressants. MAOIs enhance catecholamine activity by inhibiting a major metabolic pathway for catecholamines. Potent prescription stimulants such as amphetamine and methamphetamine should not be used within two weeks of MAOI use.

Stimulants should be used cautiously in conjunction with tricyclic antidepressants, many of which block presynaptic reuptake of catecholamines. Such antidepressants also may potentiate the effects of amphetamines by enhancing their GI absorption and slowing their hepatic metabolism.

When cocaine is used in combination with alcohol, a new compound, cocaethylene, is formed by transesterification (Jenkins & Cone, 1998). Cocaethylene blocks the dopamine transporter with an affinity similar to that of cocaine (Katz, Izenwasser et al., 2000) and has pharmacologic actions similar to, but less potent than, those of cocaine, with a longer half-life (Cami, Farre et al., 1998; Hart, Jatlow et al., 2000). Formation of cocaethylene may contribute to more severe or longer lasting toxic effects of cocaine when it is used along with alcohol.

PHARMACOLOGIC ACTIONS

Central Nervous System. *Intoxication:* All stimulants produce a similar range of psychological, behavioral, and physiological effects, with the intensity and duration depending on potency, dose, route of administration, and duration of use. The initial effects—usually desired—include increased energy, alertness, and sociability; elation or euphoria;

and decreased fatigue, need for sleep, and appetite. The intense pleasurable feeling has been described as a "total body orgasm" (Angrist, 1987). These effects may occur after 5 to 20 mg of oral amphetamine, methamphetamine, or methylphenidate; 100 to 200 mg of oral cocaine; 40 to 100 mg of intranasal cocaine; or 15 to 25 mg of IV or smoked cocaine (Angrist, 1987; Baselt, 2001; Fischman & Foltin, 1998). Such single oral doses of stimulants improve cognitive and psychomotor performance in subjects whose performance has been impaired by fatigue, sleep deprivation, or alcohol, especially in tasks that require focused and sustained attention (vigilance) (Baselt, 2001; Heishman, 1998). There is less consistent evidence that stimulants are of any benefit in subjects who are fully alert and attentive or engaged in tasks involving learning, memory, or problem solving.

With increasing potency, dose, duration of use, or a more efficient route of administration, stimulant effects often progress to include dysphoric effects such as anxiety, irritability, panic attacks, interpersonal sensitivity, hypervigilance, suspiciousness, paranoia, grandiosity, impaired judgment, and psychotic symptoms such as delusions and hallucinations. Among nontreatment-seeking users, 10% to 40% may have sleep disturbance and weight loss (due to appetite suppression), and up to a quarter may experience severe paranoia and/or hallucinations (Hando, Topp et al., 1997; Williamson, Gossop et al., 1997). In some case series, more than half of chronic cocaine and amphetamine users report psychotic symptoms (Cubells, McCance-Katz et al., 2000; Hall, Hando et al., 1996; Satel, Southwick et al., 1991c; Serper, Chou et al., 1999), but this may reflect selection bias among users who come to medical or research attention.

Patients with stimulant psychosis may closely resemble those with acute schizophrenia (Harris & Batki, 2000)—perhaps not surprising, given that both conditions share the presumed pathophysiology of excessive brain dopamine activity (Ellison, 1994). Cocaine-induced psychosis may differ from acute schizophrenic psychosis in being marked by less thought disorder and bizarre delusions and fewer negative symptoms such as alogia and inattention (Serper, Chou et al., 1999). Stimulant-induced hallucinations may be auditory, visual, or somatosensory (Cubells, McCance-Katz et al., 2000). Tactile hallucinations are especially typical of stimulant psychosis, and include the sensation of something crawling under the skin ("formication").

Parallel behavioral effects include restlessness, agitation, tremor, dyskinesia, and repetitive or stereotyped behaviors such as picking at the skin or foraging for drug ("punding," "hung-up activity") (Rosse, Fay-McCarthy et al., 1993). Associated physiological effects include tachycardia, pupil dilation, diaphoresis, and nausea, reflecting stimulation of the sympathetic nervous system. Criteria for the psychiatric diagnosis of stimulant intoxication are given in Section 5 (APA, 2000).

Cocaine and the more potent synthetic stimulants (such as amphetamines) produce these adverse effects at readily available doses by any route of administration. Less potent oral stimulants may require chronic, high dose use or diversion to intravenous use to cause these effects. Even OTC stimulants have been associated with severe psychological effects, abuse, and dependence.

There is wide individual variability in the response to stimulants. The reasons are poorly understood, but presumably are related to differences in genetics, psychological characteristics (including personality traits), previous drug experience, the setting in which the drug is taken, and the existence of psychiatric or medical comorbidities (Angrist, 1987; Laviola, Adriani et al., 1999; LeSage, Stafford et al., 1999). Identical twins are highly concordant in their response to single doses of stimulants, suggesting an important genetic component. In animals, response to stimulants appears to be under polygenic control, with independent genetic influences on responses to cocaine or amphetamine (Elmer, Miner et al., 1998). In rats, behavioral response to cocaine shows a negative correlation with baseline brain dopamine concentrations and a positive correlation with the increase in dopamine concentration elicited by a cocaine challenge (Gardner, 2000).

Individual differences in tolerance and sensitization to stimulants (see Neuroadaptations, below) may account for the poor correlation between stimulant plasma concentrations and toxic effects (Angrist, 1987; Blaho, Logan et al., 2000). Fatal cases of amphetamine or cocaine intoxication may present with 100-fold differences in plasma stimulant concentration (Karch, 1996).

Chronic Effects: Chronic cocaine or amphetamine abuse is associated with cognitive impairment that may persist for at least several weeks of abstinence (Rogers & Robbins, 2001). Most affected are visuo-motor performance, attention, and verbal memory. Several studies have found abnormalities of behavioral regulation and risk-reward decisionmaking. This type of impairment is associated with lesions of the frontal cortex, a brain area that shows decreased regional blood flow and metabolic activity in abstinent cocaine abusers.

Chronic amphetamine or methamphetamine use (either oral or intravenous) can cause a psychotic syndrome (with paranoia and hallucinations) that may persist for years after the last drug use, even in persons with no personal or family history of psychiatric disorder (Flaum & Schultz, 1996; Yui, Ishiguro et al., 1998). Methamphetamine psychosis may be associated with focal perfusion deficits in the frontal, parietal, and temporal lobes of the cerebral cortex (Buffenstein, Heaster et al., 1999). Psychotic flashbacks have been reported in methamphetamine abusers up to two years after their last drug use, and often are precipitated by threatening experiences (Yui, Ishiguro et al., 1998). A persisting psychosis after cocaine use has not been reported, except in patients with an underlying psychiatric disorder (such as schizophrenia or bipolar disorder) (Satel, Seibyl et al., 1991b).

Withdrawal: Cessation of stimulant use may result in a withdrawal syndrome that does not have prominent physiological features and is not life-threatening (Coffey, Dansky et al., 2000; Cottler, Shillington et al., 1993; Lago & Kosten, 1994). Withdrawal symptoms generally are the opposite of those associated with stimulant intoxication and include depressed mood, anhedonia (inability to experience pleasure), fatigue, difficulty concentrating, increased sleep (including REM sleep), and increased appetite. Criteria for the psychiatric diagnosis of stimulant withdrawal are discussed in Section 5 (APA, 2000).

An early report of cocaine withdrawal among 30 outpatients described a complex triphasic syndrome lasting several months. This finding has not been replicated in subsequent inpatient or outpatient studies (Coffey, Dansky et al., 2000; Lago & Kosten, 1994; Satel, Price et al., 1991a). Several studies of inpatients undergoing cocaine withdrawal found a monotonic decline in symptoms over one to two weeks. Treatment of stimulant withdrawal is reviewed in Section 5.

Rodents undergoing cocaine or amphetamine withdrawal after a period of chronic drug exposure tend to show biphasic changes in the brain: initial increases in extracellular dopamine concentrations and expression of dopamine transporter and kappa and mu opiate receptors, followed by decreases in these variables (Pilotte, 1997; Sharpe, Pilotte et al., 2000). The few human studies on cocaine withdrawal do not find consistent changes in peripheral markers of dopamine activity, as in plasma concentrations of dopamine metabolites or of prolactin (a hormone under dopamine control) (Kuhar & Pilotte, 1996; Wu, Bell et al., 1997). Human brain imaging studies suggest a modest increase in dopamine transporter binding during early cocaine withdrawal (using SPECT) (Malison, Best et al., 1998), followed by a decrease after 11 to 30 days of abstinence (using PET) (Wu, Bell et al., 1997). This pattern is consistent with most, but not all, postmortem studies of cocaine users (Little, McLaughlin et al., 1998).

Behavioral Pharmacology: Cocaine, amphetamines, cathinone, ephedrine, and most other stimulants that have been tested in animals consistently produce increased motor activity, repetitive stereotyped behavior, drug discrimination, and evidence of reinforcing effects (such as drug self-administration and conditioned place preference) (Glennon, 1999; Kollins, MacDonald et al., 2001; Preston & Walsh, 1998). Animals allowed free access to stimulants often self-administer in a "binge-abstinence" pattern: periods of high levels of drug intake (producing stereotyped behavior, hyperactivity, decreased eating and little sleep), alternating with periods of abstinence, during which behavior returns to normal (Gardner, 2000; LeSage, Stafford et al., 1999). Animals given unlimited access to stimulants may self-administer to the point of death during a binge period. The rewarding effect of stimulants in animals is influenced by the same factors as are other drug and natural reinforcers; for example, the dose of drug available, the schedule of reinforcement, the animal's past history of development and drug exposure, and the current environment and condition of the animal. Stimulant self-administration is reduced by increased work requirements, availability of an alternative potent reinforcer, or the concurrent presence of punishment (as by electric shock), and increased by food deprivation or stress (Bergman & Katz, 1998; LeSage, Stafford et al., 1999).

Animals undergoing enforced abstinence after a period of stimulant self-administration initially increase their responding in an apparent attempt to obtain drug, but eventually extinguish their drug-seeking behavior (Gardner, 2000). However, they will promptly resume drug-seeking behavior if given a single "priming" dose of the drug or exposed to drug-associated stimuli or stress (such as electric foot shock). This reinstatement of drug-seeking behavior has been considered an animal model of relapse to drug use after treatment.

Stimulants produce a distinctive set of subjective psychological effects (including euphoria, drug liking, increased energy, and increased alertness) in humans under controlled double-blind experimental conditions (Heishman & Henningfield, 1991; Kollins, MacDonald et al., 2001).

d-Amphetamine, benzphetamine, cocaine, ephedrine, mazindol, methylphenidate, phenmetrazine, and phenylpropanolamine are readily distinguished from placebo or sedative drugs, but often are not distinguished from each other when equipotent doses are given.

Other Effects on the Central Nervous System: Stimulant euphoria is associated with transient increases in EEG alpha activity, followed by longer-lasting increases in beta activity (Lukas & Renshaw, 1998). Stimulant use by any route of administration is associated with seizures, even in persons without a pre-existing seizure disorder (Boghdadi & Henning, 1997; Brust, 1998; Neiman, Haapaniemi et al., 2000). These can occur with the first use and most often are single, generalized tonic-clonic seizures, although multiple seizures and status epilepticus can occur. Most cocaine-associated seizures occur within 90 minutes of drug use, during the time of peak plasma concentration.

Cocaine use is associated with cerebral vasoconstriction, cerebrovascular disease, and stroke (Boghdadi & Henning, 1997; Brust, 1998; Kaufman, Levin et al., 2001; Neiman, Haapaniemi et al., 2000). Hemorrhagic stroke appears more common in intranasal or intravenous users, while ischemic stroke is more common in smokers.

Neurologic symptoms usually appear within three hours of drug use, although a minority of patients may be asymptomatic for up to 24 hours. An underlying cerebrovascular abnormality (such as arterial aneurysm or arteriovenous malformation) probably increases the risk of cocaine-associated stroke, but the majority of such stroke patients do not have any cerebrovascular risk factors. The OTC stimulant phenylpropanolamine, marketed as a decongestant and appetite suppressant, was associated with a significant risk of hemorrhagic stroke in a recent case-control study, even in patients who used it at recommended doses (Kernan, Viscoli et al., 2000). This finding led the FDA to remove phenylpropanolamine from the U.S. market in October 2000.

Stimulant use is associated with a variety of movement disorders, presumably as the result of increased dopamine activity in the basal ganglia and other brain areas that control movement (Angrist, 1987; Boghdadi & Henning, 1997; Warner, 1993). Such disorders include repetitive stereotyped behaviors (such as repeated dismantling of objects, cleaning, doodling, and searching for imaginary objects), acute dystonic reactions, choreoathetosis and akathisia (so-called "crack dancers"), buccolingual dyskinesias ("twisted mouth" or "boca torcida"), and exacerbation of Tourette's syndrome and tardive dyskinesia. Cocaine users are at increased risk of acute dystonic reactions to the use of neuroleptic (antipsychotic) medications (van Harten, van Trier et al., 1998).

Cardiovascular System. Stimulants act acutely on the cardiovascular system both directly (by increasing adrenergic activity at sympathetic nerve terminals) and via the CNS to increase heart rate, blood pressure, and systemic vascular resistance (Boghdadi & Henning, 1997; Ghuran & Nolan, 2000; Lange & Hillis, 2001). Cocaine-induced increases in heart rate and blood pressure are significantly correlated with increases in plasma norepinephrine and epinephrine concentrations (Sofuoglu, Nelson et al., 2001), suggesting mediation by increased activity of the sympathetic nervous system. The mechanism may be prolonged blockade of norepinephrine transporters in the heart (Fowler, Volkow et al., 2001), amplifying the action of endogenous norepinephrine. Cocaine-induced tachycardia is blocked by beta-adrenergic receptor blockade (propranolol), but not by muscarinic receptor blockade (atropine) (Vongpatanasin, Mansour et al., 1999), further suggesting a sympathetic role.

The resulting increase in myocardial oxygen demand, often accompanied by decreased coronary blood flow (from vasospasm and vasoconstriction), may cause acute myocardial infarction, even in young persons without atherosclerosis. This process may be promoted by cocaine-induced increases in circulating activated platelets, platelet aggregation, and thromboxane synthesis. Cocaine use is a factor in about one-quarter of nonfatal heart attacks in persons younger than 45 years (Qureshi, Suri et al., 2001). Frequent cocaine users are up to seven times more likely to have a nonfatal heart attack than are nonusers (Qureshi, Suri et al., 2001).

Cocaine use is associated with cardiac arrhythmias (such as ventricular tachycardia or fibrillation) and sudden death (Boghdadi & Henning, 1997; Ghuran & Nolan, 2000; Lange & Hillis, 2001). The mechanisms include blockade of myocyte sodium channels (resulting in impaired cardiac conduction and areas of localized conduction block) and increased concentration of plasma norepinephrine (which sensitizes the myocardium).

Chronic cocaine use is associated with cardiomyopathy and myocarditis (Boghdadi & Henning, 1997; Ghuran & Nolan, 2000). Case series of asymptomatic cocaine abusers have found up to half with echocardiographic abnormalities such as left ventricular hypertrophy and abnormal segmental wall motion. Cocaine-associated cases of dilated cardiomyopathy and myocardial fibrosis may be due to direct toxic effects of high concentrations of circulating norepinephrine. Cocaine-associated myocarditis (whose acute symptoms may mimic myocardial infarction) may be a direct toxic effect of cocaine or a hypersensitivity effect. Autopsy series of current cocaine users have found myocarditis in up to 20%.

Other Organ Systems. No large surveys or prospective studies have comprehensively evaluated the natural history of stimulant use or the frequency of adverse effects. Existing knowledge derives largely from case reports or case series of persons who come to medical attention. In the absence of experimental data, it may be difficult to determine the extent to which an observed adverse effect is the result of a direct action on the affected organ or tissue, an indirect action, an effect of a street drug contaminant, or secondary to other factors that are part of a drug-using lifestyle, such as needle sharing, malnutrition, use of other substances, and the like. The most relevant indirect action of cocaine in producing adverse effects in many organs and tissues is ischemia and infarction. These result from several mechanisms, including vasoconstriction, vasospasm, damage to endothelium, and increased clotting as the result of increased number of circulating activated platelets, enhanced platelet aggregation, and increased thromboxane synthesis (Boghdadi & Henning, 1997). These mechanisms often reinforce each other: for example, vasospasm may damage endothelium, endothelial damage increases thromboxane synthesis, and thromboxane causes platelet aggregation and vasoconstriction.

Adverse effects of stimulant use on particular organ systems often depend on the route of administration. For example, smoked stimulants produce lung toxicity not found with other routes, injection use is associated with infectious diseases such as HIV and hepatitis C, and intranasal use is associated with damage to the nasal septum.

Pulmonary: Smoked cocaine produces both acute and chronic pulmonary toxicity (Haim, Lippmann et al., 1995; Tashkin, 2001). Acute respiratory symptoms may develop in up to half of users within minutes to several hours after smoking. Symptoms include productive cough, shortness of breath, wheezing, chest pain, hemoptysis, and exacerbation of asthma. More severe, and rarer, acute effects include pulmonary edema, pulmonary hemorrhage, pneumothorax, pneumomediastinum, and thermal airway injury. Pulmonary edema also has been reported after intravenous cocaine use. Chronic cocaine smoking has been associated in case

reports with pulmonary and peripheral eosinophilia, interstitial pneumonitis, and bronchiolitis obliterans. The pathophysiology of these adverse effects is not definitively understood, but presumably involves a combination of direct damage by cocaine or inhaled microparticles to the alveolar-capillary membrane, vasoconstriction and damage to the pulmonary vascular bed, and/or interstitial disease.

The long-term effect of cocaine smoking on pulmonary function remains unclear (Haim, Lippmann et al., 1995; Tashkin, 2001). Standard pulmonary function tests (spirometry) have been normal in most studies. Some studies have found increased alveolar epithelial permeability and moderately decreased (up to 20%) pulmonary diffusion capacity among cocaine smokers without acute symptoms, while other studies have found normal function. The attribution of these abnormalities to cocaine use is confounded by the fact that the vast majority of cocaine-smoking subjects also were smokers of tobacco and/or marijuana.

Renal: Stimulants have little direct toxic effect on the kidneys. Acute renal failure can occur as a result of renal ischemia or infarction, malignant hypertension, or rhabdomyolysis (see Musculoskeletal, below) (Boghdadi & Henning, 1997; Nzerue, Hewan-Lowe et al., 2000). Release of myoglobin during rhabdomyolysis may cause renal tubular obstruction or direct myoglobin damage to renal tubules. Intrarenal arterial constriction with resulting renal medullary ischemia also may contribute to renal tubular damage.

Gastrointestinal: Cocaine reduces gastric motility and delays gastric emptying, in part by affecting medullary centers that regulate these functions (Boghdadi & Henning, 1997). The major gastrointestinal effects of cocaine use are due to vasoconstriction and ischemia: gastroduodenal ulceration and perforation, intestinal infarction and perforation, and ischemic colitis (Boghdadi & Henning, 1997; Warner, 1993). The distribution of cocaine-associated ulcers is primarily in the greater curvature and prepyloric region of the stomach, pyloric canal, and first portion of the duodenum, whereas peptic ulcers occur primarily in the duodenal bulb. Concealing cocaine by swallowing large packets ("body packing") may result in severe acute toxicity if the wrapping deteriorates and allows cocaine into the gastrointestinal tract (Warner, 1993).

Liver: Cocaine is hepatotoxic in rodents, presumably because of oxidative metabolism to norcocaine by the cytochrome P450 microsomal enzyme system in the liver, with further transformation to reactive hepatotoxic compounds

TABLE 4. Neuropharmacologic Actions of Selected Stimulants

	Catecholamines		Serotonin		MAO Inhibition	Na Channel Blockade
	Reuptake Blockade	Presynaptic Release	Reuptake Blockade	Presynaptic Release		
Amphetamine	++	+++	+	+	+	0
Cocaine	+++	+	+++	+	0	+++
Ephedrine*	+	++	0	0	0	0
Mazindol	+++	0	+	0	0	0
Methamphetamine	++	+++	+	+++	+	0
Methylphenidate	+++	0	+	0	0	0
Pemoline	+	+	0	0	?	0
Phentermine	+	++	0	0	+	0

* Also direct agonist at adrenergic (norepinephrine) receptors
MAO = monoamine oxidase

SOURCES: Rothman, Baumann et al., 2001; Boja & Meil, 1998.

such as N-hydroxynorcocaine (Warner, 1993). This is a very minor metabolic pathway in humans (see Metabolism, above). There is no direct evidence that cocaine is hepatotoxic in humans. Liver abnormalities reported in case series of cocaine users can be accounted for by viral hepatitis from injection drug use, alcoholic liver disease, or other consequences of a drug-using lifestyle.

Pemoline has been associated with hepatocellular toxicity, sometimes resulting in fulminant liver failure and death (Karch, 1996; Marotta & Roberts, 1998). This has led to pemoline's exclusion as a first-line agent in the treatment of ADHD.

Endocrine: Acute cocaine use activates the hypothalamic-pituitary-adrenal (HPA) axis, stimulating secretion of epinephrine, corticotropin-releasing hormone (CRH), ACTH, and cortisol (Mello & Mendelson, 1997; Warner, 1993; Warner, Greene et al., 1998). Acute cocaine use decreases plasma prolactin concentrations in cocaine-naive individuals, presumably because of increased dopamine activity (dopamine inhibits prolactin release from the pituitary). Chronic cocaine users may have increased, normal, or decreased prolactin levels, and usually do not show changes in response to acute cocaine. Acute cocaine use increases plasma luteinizing hormone, but chronic cocaine users have normal levels of testosterone, cortisol, luteinizing hormone, and thyroid hormones. A blunted thyroid-stimulating hormone response to thyroid-releasing hormone stimulation has been reported in one study, but has not been replicated. Cocaine use is associated with increased risk of diabetic ketoacidosis, either because of poor treatment adherence or acute stimulation of the HPA (Warner, Greene et al., 1998).

Musculoskeletal: Stimulants may cause rhabdomyolysis by several different mechanisms: a direct toxic effect causing myofibrillar degeneration (probably rare except at very high doses), indirectly by vasoconstriction of intramuscular arteries resulting in ischemia, and secondary to stimulant-induced hyperthermia or seizures (Boghdadi & Henning, 1997; Warner, 1993). Up to one-third of patients with rhabdomyolysis will develop acute renal failure, sometimes accompanied by disseminated intravascular coagulation and liver damage. This syndrome often is fatal.

Head and Neck: Common head and neck complications of cocaine use depend on the route of administration (Boghdadi & Henning, 1997; Warner, 1993). Intranasal cocaine use ("snorting") is associated with chronic rhinitis, perforated nasal septum, oropharyngeal ulcers, and osteolytic sinusitis, presumably due to vasoconstriction and resulting ischemic necrosis. Changes in the sense of smell are rare, even in heavy users with intranasal damage (Gordon, Moran et al., 1990). Oral cocaine use is associated with gingival ulceration and erosion of dental enamel (Warner, 1993). In South America, chronic coca leaf chewing has been associated with mild epithelial changes, but no evidence of premalignant or malignant lesions (Hamner & Villegas, 1969). The observed changes may result from the alkaline ash usually chewed with the leaves to enhance cocaine extraction, rather than from the cocaine itself.

Cocaine use by any route of administration may reduce salivary secretions (xerostomia) and cause bruxism (Pallasch & Joseph, 1987).

Sexual Function: Stimulants are commonly thought of as an aphrodisiac, but actually may impair sexual function, especially with chronic use (Angrist, 1987; Hando, Topp et al., 1997; Macdonald, Waldorf et al., 1988; Warner, 1993). Some users report greater sexual arousal and prolonged stamina, sometimes to the point of compulsive sexuality. Others report inhibited sexual desire and function (the latter sometimes are associated with higher doses or more prolonged use). The most common form of impairment in males is delayed or inhibited ejaculation. Several cases of priapism have been reported. Women may develop irregular menses.

Reproductive, Fetal, and Neonatal Health: Prescription stimulants, including cocaine and amphetamines, are classified by the FDA in pregnancy category C, meaning that risk cannot be ruled out because human studies are lacking. One exception is diethylpropion, which is category B (no evidence of risk in humans).

Prenatal (*in utero*) exposure to cocaine, amphetamines, or methylphenidate has been associated with reduced gestation period, vaginal bleeding, abruptio placenta, placenta previa, premature rupture of membranes, decreased head circumference, low birth weight, autonomic instability, decreased ability to deal with stressful situations, and attention deficits (Bishai & Koren, 1999; Debooy, Seshia et al., 1993; Eyler & Behnke, 1999; Johnson & Leff, 1999; Plessinger, 1998). Usually, it is difficult in these studies to distinguish a direct effect of the stimulant from the effects of concomitant factors frequently present in drug users, such as other drug use (including alcohol, nicotine, and opiates), poor nutrition, and lack of prenatal care. The importance of concomitant factors is underscored by studies in which participation in prenatal care is associated with better outcomes even when stimulant use continues (Schama, Howell et al., 1998). Rodent and monkey studies, in which confounding factors can be excluded, show few direct adverse effects of prenatal exposure to cocaine (Schama, Howell et al., 1998).

The long-term effects of prenatal exposure to stimulants also are unclear (Lester, 2000). Earlier concerns over substantial cognitive and behavioral problems in children of cocaine-using mothers have not been confirmed in well-controlled, prospective studies (Schama, Howell et al., 1998). Subtler cognitive problems, as with habituation, have been noted in such children and require further study.

In animal models, fetal cocaine exposure produces abnormalities in the cytoarchitecture of the neocortex, particularly the dopamine terminal regions of the anterior cingulate and the medial prefrontal cortices. The anterior cingulate cortex also shows increased activity of gamma-aminobutyric acid (GABA) neurons and a functional uncoupling of D_1 dopamine receptors from second messenger systems (Gs) (Levitt, 1998).

Cocaine, amphetamines, phentermine, ephedrine, pseudoephedrine, and phenylpropanolamine are known to appear in breast milk (AAP Committee on Drugs, 2001; Nice, Snyder et al., 2000). Cocaine and amphetamines may cause irritability, sleep disturbance, and tremors in the infant. Phenylpropanolamine may decrease milk volume in the mother. Medical use by the mother of other prescription and OTC stimulants in appropriate doses usually does not have clinically significant adverse effects on nursing infants.

NEUROBIOLOGY

Mechanisms of Action. *Neurotransmitters*: All stimulants act to enhance monoamine (dopamine, norepinephrine, and serotonin) activity in the central and peripheral nervous systems (Table 4). Potent stimulants, such as cocaine, amphetamines, mazindol, and methylphenidate, do this

FIGURE 3. Mechanism of Action of Amphetamine and Cocaine at Dopamine Synapse

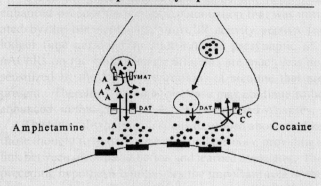

Diagram of a dopamine synapse, showing the mechanism of action of amphetamine (As; left side) and cocaine (Cs; right side). Amphetamine acts as a false substrate for the dopamine transporter (DAT) in the presynaptic nerve membrane, being taken up by the DAT from the synaptic cleft into the cytosol in exchange for release of dopamine (black circles) into the synaptic cleft. In addition, amphetamine, unlike cocaine, is a substrate for the intracellular vesicular monoamine transporter (VMAT), being taken up by the VMAT from the cytosol into the vesicle. This action results in release of dopamine from the vesicle into the cytosol, thus making more dopamine available for release from the presynaptic nerve cell into the synaptic cleft.

Cocaine blocks the uptake of dopamine by DAT from the synaptic cleft, but is not itself transported.

These effects of amphetamine and cocaine result in more dopamine being available to cross the synaptic cleft and bind to postsynaptic dopamine receptors (black bars).

Cocaine and amphetamine have similar actions at presynaptic norepinephrine and serotonin transporters.

indirectly by acting on membrane reuptake pumps (transporters) for monoamines (Figure 3) (Rothman, Baumann et al., 2001; White & Kalivas, 1998). These transporters at presynaptic nerve endings carry monoamine neurotransmitters from the synaptic cleft back into the nerve ending, thus ending their synaptic activity. Cocaine, mazindol, and methylphenidate block this transport, thus allowing more neurotransmitter to remain active at the synapse. Amphetamines and phentermine act as false substrates for the transporter. They are taken up into the presynaptic nerve ending, in exchange for neurotransmitter released back into the synapse. Once inside the nerve ending, amphetamines are taken up into the intracellular vesicles that store monoamines within the presynaptic ending. They foster release of neurotransmitter from the vesicles into the cytosol, thereby making more neurotransmitter available for presynaptic release (Boja & Meil, 1998). This effect depends on action at the vesicular monoamine transporter (VMAT), an action not shared by cocaine. Knock-out mice lacking half the genes for the VMAT show more locomotor stimulation in response to amphetamine than do wild-type (normal) mice, but find amphetamine less rewarding and do not show behavioral sensitization to amphetamine, although they do to cocaine (Uhl, Li et al., 2000).

Less potent stimulants (for example, OTC decongestants) act directly by binding to and activating norepinephrine receptors. Ephedrine, pseudoephedrine, phenylephrine, and phenylpropanolamine are more effective at alpha-adrenergic receptors, which mediate vasoconstriction (hence their use as decongestants and antihypotensive agents). Ephedrine also has some action at beta-adrenergic receptors, which mediate bronchodilation.

Dopamine: Cocaine, amphetamines, and mazindol enhance synaptic dopamine activity by acting at presynaptic membrane dopamine transporters, as described above (Table 4). Cocaine appears to bind at a site different from that at which dopamine and several other transport inhibitors bind (Izenwasser, 1998), but at the same (or a similar) site to that at which methylphenidate binds (Volkow, Wang et al., 1999b). This may explain why some other inhibitors (such as nomifensine and tricyclic antidepressants) do not have the same rewarding effects and abuse liability as does cocaine (Izenwasser, 1998).

Acute administration of cocaine or amphetamine in rodents transiently increases extracellular dopamine concentrations, especially in the shell of the nucleus accumbens, and increases dopamine D_1 receptor density in the striatum. Repeated administration of cocaine or amphetamine increases D_1 receptor sensitivity in the nucleus accumbens, but has variable effects on other dopamine receptor measures (Pierce & Kalivas, 1997).

Postmortem studies of human brain suggest that cocaine abusers have decreased dopamine levels in the frontal cortex (Little, Patel et al., 1996), normal levels of dopamine receptor binding (Meador-Woodruff, Little et al., 1995), and increased dopamine transporter binding in striatum, in conjunction with decreased transporter protein and messenger RNA levels (Letchworth, Nader et al., 2001; Little, McLaughlin et al., 1998; Wilson, Levey et al., 1996). *In vivo* human studies using PET suggest that cocaine users have decreased dopamine D_2 binding in striatum and frontal cortex and normal levels of dopamine transporter binding (Volkow, Fowler et al., 1999a). In contrast, methamphetamine abusers have increased D_1 receptors in the nucleus accumbens (Worsley, Moszczynsky et al., 2000) and decreased dopamine transporter density in nucleus accumbens, striatum, and prefrontal cortex (Sekine, Iyo et al., 2001).

Several lines of evidence from animal studies suggest that it is the increased synaptic dopamine activity in the mesocorticolimbic reward circuit that mediates the behavioral effects of stimulants (Gardner, 2000; Koob, 1999). Fluctuations in extracellular dopamine concentrations and neuronal firing in the nucleus accumbens parallel cocaine self-administration. The potency of cocaine analogues and other stimulants for being self-administered or producing cocaine-like discriminative stimuli is highly correlated with their potency for binding to the dopamine transporter, but not with their binding to other monoamine transporters or receptors (Cook, Carroll et al., 2001; Katz, Izenwasser et al., 2000; Kuhar, Ritz et al., 1991). Conversely, animals with lesions of this dopaminergic circuit (but not of other neurotransmitter systems) will not self-administer cocaine or amphetamine (Koob, 1999; Wise, 1998). Selective blockade of the dopamine transporter reduces cocaine self-administration (Dworkin, Lambert et al., 1998).

Dopamine D_1 and D_3 receptors appear to play reciprocal roles in the behavioral effects of stimulants. Blockade of D_1 receptors in regions of the brain reward circuit (for example, the shell of the nucleus accumbens or ventral tegmental area) reduces the rewarding effects of cocaine or amphetamine in the rat, as does stimulation of D_3 receptors (Koob, 1999; Pierre & Vezina, 1998; Ranaldi & Wise, 2001). Knock-out mice that lack the D_1 receptor no longer show a locomotor response to cocaine, while D_3 knock-out mice show enhanced responses to cocaine or amphetamine (Zhang & Xu, 2001).

Recent studies with genetically engineered knock-out mice complicate, but do not contradict, the dopamine hypothesis of stimulant behavioral effects. Knock-out mice that lack the gene for the dopamine transporter no longer respond to cocaine or amphetamine with increased motor activity (Giros, Jaber et al., 1996; Spielewoy, Biala et al., 2001), decreased sleep (Wisor, Nishino et al., 2001), or increased extracellular dopamine concentrations in the striatum (Rocha, Fumagalli et al., 1998). However, such mice still self-administer cocaine (Rocha, Fumagalli et al., 1998) and still prefer to spend time in an environment previously associated with cocaine or methylphenidate

(conditioned place preference) (Sora, Wichems et al., 1998). These findings seem to cast doubt on the importance of the dopamine transporter for stimulant reward, and suggest a pharmacologic dissociation between the rewarding and other behavioral effects of stimulants.

A possible explanation is that the norepinephrine transporter has taken over the function of the missing dopamine transporters in regulating synaptic dopamine concentrations (Carboni, Spielewoy et al., 2001; Moron, Brockington et al., 2002). The norepinephrine transporter has a greater affinity for dopamine than does the dopamine transporter, and can transport dopamine, as well as norepinephrine, *in vivo*. In mice lacking the dopamine transporter, blockade of the norepinephrine transporter by either cocaine or a selective norepinephrine transporter inhibitor (nisoxetine) reduces dopamine uptake and increases extracellular dopamine concentration.

Evidence from human brain imaging studies using PET or single photon emission computed tomography (SPECT) is largely consistent with an important role for dopamine in the acute psychological effects of stimulants. The acute positive psychological response (euphoria or "high") to intravenous cocaine or methylphenidate correlates in time course and intensity with drug concentration in the brain, with dopamine transporter occupancy (in the case of cocaine) (Malison, Best et al., 1995; Volkow, Wang et al., 1997a), and with extracellular dopamine release in the striatum (as measured by displacement from dopamine receptors) (Schlaepfer, Pearlson et al., 1997; Volkow, Fowler et al., 1999a). One exception to this pattern is a finding that intravenous methylphenidate decreased dopamine release in the striatum of drug users, while increasing it in the thalamus (an effect not seen in nondrug-using control subjects) (Volkow, Wang et al., 1997b).

Clinical evidence is not as supportive of an important role for dopamine activity in stimulant effects. Schizophrenic patients taking antipsychotic (neuroleptic) medication (which are potent dopamine D_2 receptor antagonists), at doses which well control their schizophrenic symptoms, still experience the psychoactive effects of cocaine and frequently abuse it (Buckley, 1998). Experimental attempts to block the acute psychological effects of cocaine or amphetamine with antipsychotic medication or by blocking dopamine and norepinephrine synthesis with the tyrosine hydroxylase inhibitor alpha-methyl-p-tyrosine have not been successful (Brauer & de Wit, 1997; Kuhar, Ritz et al., 1991; Stine, Krystal et al., 1997). These failures may have been due to the inability of subjects to tolerate sufficient doses of medication to influence the cocaine's effects. PET studies estimate that occupancy of at least half of brain dopamine transporter sites is sufficient to produce pleasurable cocaine effects ("high") (Volkow, Wang et al., 1997a).

Norepinephrine: Cocaine, amphetamines, mazindol, phentermine, and ephedrine enhance synaptic norepinephrine activity by acting at the presynaptic membrane norepinephrine transporter, as described above (Table 4). Consistent with this synaptic action, intravenous cocaine increases plasma norepinephrine and epinephrine concentrations within minutes of injection (Sofuoglu, Nelson et al., 2001). There is a significant positive correlation between potency of norepinephrine release (measured *in vitro*) and the oral stimulant dose that produces stimulant-like subjective effects in humans, suggesting a role for norepinephrine in the psychological effects of stimulants (Rothman, Baumann et al., 2001). Knock-out mice lacking the norepinephrine transporter are supersensitive to the locomotor stimulation produced by cocaine or amphetamine (Xu, Gainetdinov et al., 2000) and still find cocaine rewarding (Uhl, Hall et al., 2002).

Ephedrine, pseudoephedrine, phenylephrine, and other direct-acting stimulants are agonists at alpha-adrenergic norepinephrine receptors. The effect of chronic administration of stimulants on adrenoreceptor subtypes has not been well studied.

Serotonin: Cocaine, amphetamines, and mazindol enhance synaptic serotonin activity by acting at the presynaptic membrane serotonin transporter, as described above (see Table 4). Acute cocaine administration increases extracellular serotonin concentrations in the striatum and ventral tegmental area and reduces firing of serotonin neurons in the dorsal raphe (Cunningham, Bradberry et al., 1996). The latter action probably is mediated by negative feedback from stimulation of 5-HT$_{1A}$ autoreceptors. Chronic cocaine exposure upregulates the sensitivity of 5-HT$_{1A}$ receptors, enhancing the ability of serotonin to inhibit medium spiny neurons of the striatum (Pierce & Kalivas, 1997). Repeated cocaine administration also reduces serotonin concentrations in the frontal cortex of rats (Egan, Wing et al., 1994). Human cocaine users have normal 5-HT$_2$ receptor availability in brain (Wang, Volkow et al., 1995).

The role that serotonin plays in stimulant reward is unclear. Knock-out mice lacking the serotonin transporter still find cocaine rewarding (conditioned place preference) (Sora, Wichems et al., 1998), while double knock-out mice

lacking both the dopamine and serotonin transporters do not (Sora, Hall et al., 2001). Knock-out mice lacking both the norepinephrine and serotonin transporters show increased sensitivity to cocaine reward (Uhl, Hall et al., 2002). These findings suggest a permissive, but not obligatory, role for the serotonin transporter in cocaine reward.

Activation of 5-HT$_3$ receptors enhances the effects of cocaine on dopamine release in the nucleus accumbens and the locomotor response to cocaine or methamphetamine, but reduces the rewarding effect (conditioned place preference) of cocaine—another example of pharmacologic dissociation between locomotor and reward effects of stimulants (Allan, Galindo et al., 2001). 5-HT$_3$ receptor antagonism also reduces the rewarding effect of cocaine, methamphetamine, or mazindol, as well as the effect of cocaine or mazindol on dopamine release in the nucleus accumbens and of cocaine, amphetamine, or mazindol on locomotor activity (Allan, Galindo et al., 2001; Kankaanpaa, Meririnne et al., 2002). Activation of 5-HT$_{1B}$ receptors enhances cocaine self-administration (Parsons, Weiss et al., 1998), while knock-out mice lacking 5-HT$_{1B}$ receptors also show increased cocaine self-administration and enhanced locomotor response to cocaine (Castanon, Scearce-Levie et al., 2000). However, wild-type mice treated with a 5-HT$_{1B}$ receptor antagonist show normal cocaine reward but decreased locomotor response. These apparently contradictory findings suggest a complicated modulatory role for serotonin in stimulant reward and a different role in stimulant motor activation.

Human studies using nonselective serotonin manipulations also provide an inconsistent picture. Enhancement of synaptic serotonin activity with another type of serotonin transporter blocker (selective serotonin reuptake inhibitor [SSRI] antidepressants), activation of serotonin receptors with a partial agonist, or depletion of serotonin levels (via a tryptophan-free diet) all are reported to reduce the acute subjective effects ("high," craving) of cocaine (Buydens-Branchey, Branchey et al., 1997; Walsh & Cunningham, 1997). A postmortem study of human brain found higher serotonin levels in the frontal cortex among cocaine users than among matched controls (Little, Patel et al., 1996). Clarification of the role of serotonin in stimulant reward must await the development for human use of selective agonists and antagonists at the more than dozen known serotonin receptor subtypes.

Endogenous Opiates: Stimulants do not directly interact with opiate receptors, but do influence endogenous opiate (endorphin) systems in the brain. In rats, single doses of cocaine or amphetamine increase extracellular endorphin levels in the nucleus accumbens (Olive, Koenig et al., 2001) and enkephalin and dynorphin mRNA levels in striatum (Hurd & Herkenham, 1992). The mechanism does not appear to be direct activation of endorphin-containing neurons, but may be indirect via other neurotransmitters that influence endorphin release, such as dopamine and serotonin. Repeated cocaine administration, especially in an intermittent "binge" pattern, increases brain mu and kappa opiate receptor binding in rodents, with no change in delta opiate receptors (Unterwald, 2001). Human cocaine users show increased mu opiate receptor binding in some brain regions with PET scanning, and this increased binding correlates with self-reported cocaine craving (Zubieta, Gorelick et al., 1996). Postmortem brains from fatal cocaine overdose victims show increased kappa opiate receptor binding in limbic areas (Staley, Rothman et al., 1997).

Animal studies suggest that brain kappa opiate systems have an influence on cocaine effects. In general, activation of endogenous kappa opiate receptor systems (such as by administration of the endogenous ligand dynorphin) reduces behavioral and neuropharmacological effects of stimulants (Shippenberg, Chefer et al., 2001). These findings have stimulated research on kappa opiate receptor ligands as possible treatment for stimulant addiction.

Glutamate: The acute administration of cocaine increases glutamate release in the ventral tegmental area, nucleus accumbens, and striatum, while acute administration of methamphetamine reduces glutamate release in these regions (Zhang, Loonam et al., 2001). The chronic administration of cocaine enhances the expression of several types of glutamate receptor, N-methyl-D-aspartate (NMDAR1), AMPA (GluR1), and metabotropic mGluR5, while decreasing another type (GluR4) (Vanderschuren & Kalivas, 2000). Knock-out mice lacking the mGluR5 receptor do not self-administer cocaine or show increased locomotor activity in response to cocaine (Chiamulera, Epping-Jordan et al., 2001), suggesting the importance of this glutamate receptor in mediating cocaine's behavioral effects.

A growing body of evidence suggests that glutamate plays an important role in relapse to cocaine or amphetamine abuse. Withdrawal from chronic cocaine or amphetamine exposure significantly alters brain glutamate receptor density in rodents. Readministration of the stimulant leads to a marked increase in extracellular glutamate levels and changes in glutamate receptor function in the nucleus accumbens that are absent after acute administration of the drug (Pierce & Kalivas, 1997). A recent hypothesis proposes that the chronic administration of cocaine or amphetamine leads to the recruitment of cortical glutamatergic neurotransmission in the nucleus accumbens as a consequence of associations with the drug-taking environment. Thus, an environmental stimulus may evoke drug-seeking behavior through enhanced glutamate transmission, independent of dopamine neurotransmission. In the nucleus accumbens, the role of dopamine in producing drug-seeking behavior may be secondary to glutamate neurotransmission (Cornish & Kalivas, 2001). Sensitized locomotor activity in response to repeated stimulant administration is blocked by the peripheral administration of glutamatergic antagonists (Gaytan, Nason et al., 2000a; Vanderschuren & Kalivas, 2000).

Acetylcholine: Cocaine blocks neuronal nicotinic acetylcholine (ACh) receptors with an affinity similar to that for blocking voltage-gated sodium channels (Francis, Vazquez et al., 2000) and increases extracellular ACh release in the rat nucleus accumbens (Mark, Hajnal et al., 1999). Presynaptic ACh receptors modulate activity of dopamine projections from the ventral tegmental area to the nucleus accumbens, which may account for nicotine enhancement of cocaine or methylphenidate-stimulated dopamine release in the nucleus accumbens (Gerasimov, Franceschi et al., 2000). Cocaine also blocks muscarinic ACh receptors in the brain and on cardiac myocytes (Sharkey, Ritz et al., 1988; Xiao & Morgan, 1998), resulting in decreased potassium current. This action may contribute to cardiac arrhythmias.

Other Actions: Some stimulants have additional neuropharmacological actions (Table 4). Amphetamines and phentermine inhibit monoamine oxidase (MAO), which also would increase catecholamine activity. This action probably is not significant at the drug concentrations achieved with typical therapeutic or abused doses (Rothman & Baumann, 2000). Cocaine is unique in also blocking voltage-gated membrane sodium ion channels. This action accounts for its effect as a local anesthetic, and may contribute to cardiac arrhythmias.

Signal Transduction. When monoamine neurotransmitters such as dopamine activate their membrane receptors on the nerve cell surface, they trigger a cascade of intracellular chemical events (Gelowitz & Berger, 2001; Nestler, 2001). The neurotransmitter receptors are coupled to G-proteins, which regulate adenylyl cyclase activity to alter levels of cyclic 3',5'-adenosine monophosphate (cAMP), a "second messenger." Cyclic AMP, in turn, regulates the activity of protein kinases, phospholipases, and other intracellular enzymes. These enzymes regulate various intracellular processes, including the activity of transcription factors that regulate gene transcription by binding to specific DNA sequences in the regulatory regions of genes (see Gene Expression, below). Stimulants up-regulate the cAMP pathway in neurons of the brain reward circuit (such as the nucleus accumbens) by increasing activity of adenylyl cyclase, resulting in increased activity of intracellular enzymes such as protein kinase A and phospholipase A and of transcription factors such as cAMP response element-binding protein (CREB). Activation of adenylyl cyclase appears to increase the behavioral response to stimulants, while its inhibition reduces the response. Changes to these pathways from chronic exposure to stimulants may mediate tolerance and sensitization (see Neuroadaptation, below).

The most extensively studied signal transduction pathways engaged by stimulant administration are those associated with dopamine receptor activation. Chronic cocaine administration enhances sensitivity of dopamine D_1 receptor function, which activates the cAMP pathway and increases protein kinase A activity. In contrast, the sensitivity of dopamine D_2 receptors is attenuated through a reduction in levels of its coupled inhibitory G-proteins (Gi/Go) and subsequent decrease in cAMP formation and protein kinase A activity. In rats trained to self-administer cocaine, the activation of protein kinase A decreases the reinforcing effects of cocaine, suggesting up-regulated cAMP activity as a mechanism for tolerance to cocaine (Self, Genova et al., 1998). Chronic methylphenidate administration down-regulates protein kinase A activity and inhibits dopamine-stimulated adenylyl cyclase activity (Crawford, McDougall et al., 1998).

Gene Expression. Acute administration of stimulants (such as cocaine, amphetamine, and methylphenidate) to rodents promptly activates (within minutes to hours) several "immediate early" genes in the brain, such as c-fos and c-jun (Kuhar, Joyce et al., 2001; Nestler, 2001; Torres & Horowitz, 1999). The protein products of these genes appear to be nuclear transcription factors that regulate gene expression. Repeated administration of stimulants results in a tolerance to the gene activation effect and, in some cases, to a down-regulation of the gene product.

Chronic stimulant administration leads to accumulation of long-lasting Fos-related antigens (FRAs), such as ΔFosB (Nestler, 2001; Nestler, Barrot et al., 2001), a transcription factor involved in modulating gene expression (for example, of AMPA-type glutamate receptor subunits). FRAs enhance the behavioral response to cocaine and may mediate the development of sensitization (see Neuroadaptation, below). FRAs interact with other immediate early gene products to form other transcription factors that reduce the behavioral response to cocaine and may mediate the development of tolerance. Enhanced ΔFosB expression is associated with sensitization to the locomotor and reinforcing effects of cocaine in rodents, suggesting an important role for this transcription factor in the behavioral effects of stimulants. Repeated cocaine administration also leads to up-regulation of NAC-1 in the nucleus accumbens. NAC-1 mediates interactions among gene transcription regulators and may serve as a compensatory mechanism in the sensitization process to repeated cocaine administration (Vanderschuren & Kalivas, 2000).

Administration of cocaine or amphetamine to rodents leads within one hour to the appearance of cocaine and amphetamine-regulated transcript (CART) peptide in brain regions associated with memory and reward (for example, the hippocampus, nucleus accumbens, amygdala, and striatum) (Yermolaieva, Chen et al., 2001). The function of CART peptide remains unknown, but it has some of the localization and pharmacologic properties of a neurotransmitter or neuromodulator. CART peptide is found in vesicles within presynaptic axon terminals, inhibits voltage-dependent intracellular calcium signaling, and attenuates the effect of cocaine on such calcium signaling in hippocampal neurons.

Neural Circuits and Systems. Animal studies suggest that the rewarding effects of stimulants (and most other abused drugs) are mediated by a neural circuit involving connections among the ventral tegmental area (VTA) of the midbrain, the ventral prefrontal cortex (PFC), and the limbic regions of the basal forebrain sometimes called the "extended amygdala" (including the medial amygdala, medial ventral pallidum, and shell of the nucleus accumbens) (Cornish & Kalivas, 2001; Koob, 1999; McFarland & Kalivas, 2001; Wise, 1998). The VTA sends dopaminergic projections to the PFC, nucleus accumbens, and ventral pallidum. In return, it receives inhibitory GABAergic input from the ventral pallidum and nucleus accumbens, and excitatory glutamatergic input from the PFC. The PFC also sends glutamatergic input to the nucleus accumbens. The nucleus accumbens and ventral pallidum have reciprocal dopaminergic connections.

The nucleus accumbens and PFC appear to be the key sites for stimulant reward (Gardner, 2000; Wise, 1998). In rodents, selective dopamine lesions or administration of dopamine receptor blockers in the nucleus accumbens, but not in other sites, abolish the rewarding effects of cocaine or amphetamine. Rodents will self-administer amphetamine directly into the nucleus accumbens or PFC and cocaine directly into the PFC, but not into other brain sites. Cocaine administration into the PFC increases dopamine turnover in the nucleus accumbens. The relationship between cocaine self-administration and extracellular dopamine concentration in the nucleus accumbens also suggests a key role for this site (Gardner, 2000). A period of cocaine self-administration increases tonic concentrations of extracellular dopamine, with each individual dose producing a time-locked phasic increase. The subsequent decline in dopamine concentration predicts the self-administration of the next dose. Overall, the animal appears to be titrating extracellular dopamine concentration in the nucleus accumbens to maintain an increase above baseline concentration.

The evidence for brain localization of stimulant effects in humans is very limited, but somewhat consistent with the animal studies. Brain imaging studies using PET, SPECT, or functional magnetic resonance imaging (fMRI) have found stimulant-induced changes in blood flow or metabolic rate in a variety of brain regions, including cortex, striatum, and amygdala (Kilts, Schweitzer et al., 2001; London, Bonson et al., 1999). Exposure to cocaine-associated stimuli that elicit cocaine craving has been associated with increased blood flow or metabolic activity in the prefrontal cortex, amygdala, and anterior cingulate gyrus (Childress, Mozley et al., 1999). A postmortem study of methamphetamine users found significantly decreased concentrations of G-protein only in the nucleus accumbens (McLeman, Warsh et al., 2000).

Neuroadaptation. Repeated exposure to stimulants results in two distinct neuroadaptations: sensitization (increased drug response) and tolerance (decreased drug response) (Koob, 1996; Schenk & Partridge, 1997). Sensitization tends to result from initial low-dose, intermittent exposure, while tolerance tends to result from more frequent, high-dose, or long-term exposure. The precise pharmacologic, neurobiological, and behavioral factors that determine sensitization and tolerance are not well understood. There is growing evidence that the development of sensitization or tolerance depends on the balance of activity of gene transcription factors induced by the cAMP intracellular second messenger cascade (see Signal Transduction and Gene Expression, above).

Sensitization: Sensitization is the phenomenon whereby prior low-intensity, intermittent (rather than continuous) exposure to a drug results in an enhanced response to a later exposure. Sensitization is the opposite of tolerance and thus sometimes is termed "reverse tolerance."

Stimulants such as amphetamines or cocaine robustly produce sensitization in rodents, typically observed as a progressive increase in locomotor activity or stereotyped behavior with succeeding drug doses (Robinson & Berridge, 2000). Sensitization occurs not only to behavioral responses, but also to changes in EEG power spectrum (Ferger, Stahl et al., 1996) and HPA axis activation (Vanderschuren, Schmidt et al., 1999). Sensitization may occur after a single drug exposure (Vanderschuren, Schmidt et al., 1999) and last for months. There is cross-sensitization among stimulants, so that previous exposure to amphetamine enhances the response to cocaine (Bonate, Swann et al., 1997). However, there is some evidence of neuropharmacologic differences in the sensitization process induced by cocaine, amphetamine, and methylphenidate (Gaytan, Yang et al., 2000b; Vanderschuren & Kalivas, 2000).

Behavioral sensitization has two temporally distinct phases: *initiation* or *induction* and *expression*. A combination of environmental and pharmacologic factors influence both phases (Ohmori, Abekawa et al., 2000; Robinson, Browman et al., 1998). Sensitization may be influenced by circadian rhythm (Gaytan, Lewis et al., 1999) and by the animal's prior drug experience in the environment in which the drug is administered (so-called "context-specific" or "conditioned" sensitization). Neurotransmitter action and gene expression are essential in the development of sensitization. Behavioral sensitization to stimulants is reduced or absent in the presence of a dopamine D_1 receptor or NMDA-type glutamate receptor antagonist (Gelowitz & Berger, 2001; Gaytan, Nason et al., 2000a) or in knock-out mice that lack the dopamine transporter (Spielewoy, Biala et al., 2001). Activation of adenylyl cyclase or induction of fos-related antigens such as ΔFosB enhances the response to subsequent stimulant doses, while inhibition of adenylyl cyclase, activation of protein kinase A, or induction of CREB reduces stimulant response (Gelowitz & Berger, 2001; Nestler, 2001). Conversely, inhibition of protein kinase A or reduction of CREB activity enhances the stimulant response (Nestler, 2001; Walters & Blendy, 2001). Neurotrophic factors in the brain also influence sensitization, although their exact role remains unclear (Flores, Samaha et al., 2000; Pierce & Bari, 2001).

Kindling is a process by which low-intensity, intermittent electrical or chemical stimulation of neurons results in a progressive increase in cellular response to subsequent stimulation. Kindling has been considered the neurophysiological process mediating the sensitization that occurs following repeated stimulant administration. Both processes are dependent on neuroadaptations in glutamate systems (McNamara, 1995).

Behavioral sensitization to stimulants has been suggested as a mechanism for drug craving and relapse (Kalivas, Pierce et al., 1998) and for stimulant-induced psychosis (Post & Weiss, 1988). Neither has been directly demonstrated in humans. Several retrospective evaluations of patients presenting with stimulant-induced psychosis found that psychotic symptoms were more severe than during prior episodes of use, or were elicited at lower doses that previously had not caused such symptoms (Bartlett, Hallin et al., 1997; Little & Romans, 1993). This pattern is consistent with sensitization, that is, an enhanced response to the drug after prior exposure.

Attempts to demonstrate sensitization prospectively in humans have yielded inconsistent results. Two studies using intravenous cocaine in experienced cocaine users failed to show sensitization after one or four prior cocaine exposures (Gorelick & Rothman, 1997), as did a study using oral cocaine (Walsh, Haberny et al., 2000). However, another study using oral cocaine did find significant sensitization to cocaine's cardiovascular effects, but not to its psychological effects (Kollins & Rush, 2002). Several studies using oral amphetamine or methamphetamine also failed to show sensitization in subjects with histories of stimulant use (Comer, Hart et al., 2001; Wachtel & de Wit, 1999). Three recent studies in research volunteers with no prior stimulant use did show sensitization to psychological and physiological (eye blink rate) responses after two or three prior oral amphetamine exposures (Strakowski, Sax et al., 2001). The failure to show sensitization in other studies may have been due to the prior stimulant exposure of most subjects, resulting in sensitization already having occurred (that is, a "ceiling" effect) (Gorelick & Rothman, 1997).

Tolerance: Tolerance to the behavioral (including reinforcing, appetite-suppressing) effects of stimulants has been demonstrated in animals after high-dose, frequent, or continuous administration (Angrist, 1987; Hammer, Egilmez et al., 1997; King, Xiong et al., 1999; Schenk & Partridge, 1997). Tolerance to cardiovascular, hyperthermic, and lethal effects occurs even more quickly, sometimes after just one or two exposures (Angrist, 1987; Tella, Schindler et al., 1999). Stimulant tolerance dissipates after 7 to 14 days of no exposure (Hammer, Egilmez et al., 1997; King, Xiong et al., 1999; Tella, Schindler et al., 1999). There is significant cross-tolerance among various stimulants, but not between stimulants and other drug groups, such as opiates (Woolverton & Weiss, 1998).

Stimulant tolerance is pharmacodynamic (that is, due to adaptive changes in the brain) rather than pharmacokinetic; chronic stimulant exposure does not cause substantial changes in stimulant pharmacokinetics (Hammer, Egilmez et al., 1997). Development of behavioral tolerance is associated with attenuation of the dopamine response to stimulants, decreased activation of immediate early genes, and increased activity of the signal transduction pathway involving protein kinase A and the gene transcription factor CREB (Hammer, Egilmez et al., 1997; Nestler, 2001).

In clinical use, tolerance to stimulants develops differentially to various effects. Patients typically become tolerant to the appetite-suppressing effects within several weeks of daily use, while the beneficial effects in narcolepsy or ADHD remain over months of treatment (Angrist, 1987). In human laboratory studies, tolerance to psychological, cardiovascular, and neuroendocrine effects of cocaine and amphetamines may develop after several doses (Comer, Hart et al., 2001; Mendelson, Sholar et al., 1998; Ward, Haney et al., 1997). There is some evidence that tolerance to cardiovascular effects develops more quickly and completely than does tolerance to psychological effects (Perez-Reyes, White et al., 1991; Ward, Haney et al., 1997). Rapid tolerance to adverse effects presumably allows binge users to take large cumulative doses of stimulants (Cho, Melega et al., 2001).

Neurotoxicity. In animal studies, cocaine and methylphenidate do not produce appreciable neurotoxicity of dopamine or serotonin neurons (Fleckenstein, Gibb et al., 2000; Yuan, McCann et al., 1997). In contrast, high doses of amphetamine or methamphetamine produce substantial dopamine and serotonin neurotoxicity, possibly through interference with monoamine transport and increased production of reactive oxygen species. Such neurotoxicity in human users has not been conclusively demonstrated. Chronic methamphetamine or methcathinone users have reduced density of dopamine transporters in the brain (measured by PET scanning) for at least three years after last use (McCann, Wong et al., 1998), but there is evidence of recovery after a year of abstinence (Volkow, Chang et al., 2001). Thus, it is not clear whether the loss of transporters represents a reversible physiological response (downregulation) to chronic stimulant exposure or a true loss of dopamine nerve endings. Postmortem brain studies in methamphetamine abusers are more consistent with the former alternative. Their findings of decreased dopamine synthesis and dopamine transporter function, but intact vesicular transporter function, suggest that dopamine nerve terminals and the intracellular storage vesicles they contain remain intact (Cho & Melega, 2002).

Cocaine has caused DNA synthesis inhibition and cell death of brain neurons in rodents (Li & Lin, 1998), but the clinical relevance of these findings is unknown.

FUTURE RESEARCH DIRECTIONS

Future research at both preclinical and clinical levels is needed to increase understanding of the mechanisms of stimulant addiction and to develop more effective prevention and treatment approaches.

Productive areas for preclinical research include the neurochemical mechanisms that underlie stimulant sensitization and tolerance, the role of glutamate and other nondopamine neurotransmitter systems in modulating the dopamine reward circuit, the intracellular signaling cascades triggered by stimulant attachment to membrane binding sites, and the role of various genes and gene transcription factors in stimulant action.

Productive areas for clinical research include the genetic, hormonal, psychological, and environmental factors that influence response to stimulants and the progression to stimulant addiction, and the development of effective treatments for stimulant addiction and its medical consequences.

REFERENCES

Akerstedt T & Ficca G (1997). Alertness-enhancing drugs as a countermeasure to fatigue in irregular work hours. *Chronobiology International* 14(2):145-158.

Allan AM, Galindo R, Chynoweth J et al. (2001). Conditioned place preference for cocaine is attenuated in mice over-expressing the 5-HT$_3$ receptor. *Psychopharmacology* 158:18-27.

American Academy of Pediatrics (AAP), Committee on Drugs (2001). The transfer of drugs and other chemicals into human milk. *Pediatrics* 108(3):776-789.

American Psychiatric Association (APA) (2000). *Diagnostic and Statistical Manual of Mental Disorders, 4th Edition (DSM-IV)*. Washington, DC: American Psychiatric Press.

American Sleep Disorders Association (ASDA), Standards of Practice Committee (1994). Practice parameters for the use of stimulants in the treatment of narcolepsy. *Sleep* 17(4):348-351.

Angrist B (1987). Clinical effects of central nervous system stimulants: A selective update. In J Engel, L Oreland, DH Ingvar et al. (eds.) *Brain Reward Systems and Abuse*. New York, NY: Raven Press, 109-127.

Anthony JC & Helzer JE (1990). Syndromes of drug abuse and dependence. In LN Robins & DA Regier (eds.) *Psychiatric Disorders in America*. New York, NY: The Free Press, 116-154.

Anthony JC & Helzer JE (1995). Epidemiology of drug dependence. In MT Tsuang, M Tohen & GEP Zahner (eds.) *Textbook in Psychiatric Epidemiology*. New York, NY: Wiley-Liss, 361-406.

Anthony JC, Warner LA & Kessler RC (1994). Comparative epidemiology of dependence on tobacco, alcohol, controlled substances, and inhalants: Basic findings from the National Comorbidity Survey. *Experimental and Clinical Psychopharmacology* 2:244-268.

Bartlett E, Hallin A, Chapman B et al. (1997). Selective sensitization to the psychosis-inducing effects of cocaine: A possible marker for addiction relapse vulnerability? *Neuropsychopharmacology* 16(1):77-82.

Baselt RC (1999). *Disposition of Toxic Drugs and Chemicals in Man, 5th Edition*. Foster City, CA: Chemical Toxicology Institute.

Baselt RC (2001). *Drug Effects on Psychomotor Performance*. Foster City, CA: Biomedical Publications.

Bergman J & Katz JL (1998). Behavioral pharmacology of cocaine and the determinants of abuse liability. In ST Higgins & JL Katz (eds.) *Cocaine Abuse: Behavior, Pharmacology, and Clinical Applications*. San Diego, CA: Academic Press, 51-79.

Biederman J, Wilens T, Mick E et al. (1999). Pharmacotherapy of attention-deficit/hyperactivity disorder reduces risk for substance use disorder. *Pediatrics* 104(2):e20.

Bishai R & Koren G (1999). Maternal and obstetric effects of prenatal drug exposure. *Clinics in Perinatology* 26(1):75-86.

Blaho K, Logan B, Winbery S et al. (2000). Blood cocaine and metabolite concentrations, clinical findings, and outcome of patients presenting to an ED. *American Journal of Emergency Medicine* 18(5):593-598.

Boghdadi MS & Henning RJ (1997). Cocaine: Pathophysiology and clinical toxicology. *Heart & Lung* 26:466-483.

Boja JW & Meil WM (1998). The dopamine transporter and addiction. In SB Karch (ed.) *Drug Abuse Handbook*. Boca Raton, FL: CRC Press, 397-412.

Bonate PL, Swann A & Silverman PB (1997). Context-dependent cross-sensitization between cocaine and amphetamine. *Life Sciences* 60(1):PL1-PL7.

Bono JP (1998). Criminalistics—Introduction to controlled substances. In SB Karch (ed.) *Drug Abuse Handbook*. Boca Raton, FL: CRC Press, 1-75.

Braithwaite RA, Jarvie DR, Minty PSB et al. (1995). Screening for drugs of abuse. I: Opiates, amphetamines and cocaine. *Annals of Clinical Biochemistry* 32:123-153.

Brauer LH & de Wit H (1997). High dose pimozide does not block amphetamine-induced euphoria in normal volunteers. *Pharmacology, Biochemistry and Behavior* 56:265-272.

Bray GA (1999). Drug treatment of obesity. *Bailliere's Clinical Endocrinology and Metabolism* 13:131-148.

Bray RM, Sanchez RP, Ornstein ML et al. (1999). *Highlights: 1998 Department of Defense Survey of Health Related Behaviors Among Military Personnel.* Available at: www.tricare.osd.mil/analysis/surveys/98survey/survey5.html#5.

Bruns AD, Zieske LA & Jacobs AJ (1994). Analysis of the cocaine metabolite in the urine of patients and physicians during clinical use. *Otolaryngology-Head & Neck Surgery* 111(6):722-726.

Brust JCM (1998). Acute neurologic complications of drug and alcohol abuse. *Neurologic Clinics of North America* 16(2):503-519.

Buckley PF (1998). Substance abuse in schizophrenia: A review. *Journal of Clinical Psychiatry* 59:26-30.

Buffenstein A, Heaster J & Ko P (1999). Chronic psychotic illness from methamphetamine. *American Journal of Psychiatry* 156(4):662.

Bureau of Justice Statistics (1999). *Substance Abuse and Treatment, State and Federal Prisoners, 1997* (NCJ 172871). Washington, DC: U.S. Department of Justice.

Buydens-Branchey L, Branchey M, Fergeson P et al. (1997). Craving for cocaine in addicted users: Role of serotonergic mechanisms. *American Journal of Addictions* 6:65-73.

Cami J, Farre M, Gonzalez ML et al. (1998). Cocaine metabolism in humans after use of alcohol. Clinical and research implications. *Recent Developments in Alcoholism* 14:437-455.

Caplan YH & Goldberger BA (2001). Alternative specimens for workplace drug testing. *Journal of Analytical Toxicology* 25(5): 396-399.

Carboni E, Spielewoy C, Vacca C et al. (2001). Cocaine and amphetamine increase extracellular dopamine in the nucleus accumbens of mice lacking the dopamine transporter gene. *Journal of Neuroscience* 21:1-4.

Castanon N, Scearce-Levie K, Lucas JJ et al. (2000). Modulation of the effects of cocaine by 5-HT1B receptors: A comparison of knockouts and antagonists. *Pharmacology, Biochemistry and Behavior* 67:559-566.

Challman TD & Lipsky JJ (2000). Methylphenidate: Its pharmacology and uses. *Mayo Clinic Proceedings* 75:711-721.

Chiamulera C, Epping-Jordan MP, Zocchi A et al. (2001). Reinforcing and locomotor stimulant effects of cocaine are absent in mGluR5 null mutant mice. *Nature Neuroscience* 4(9):873-874.

Childress AR, Mozley PD, McElgin W et al. (1999). Limbic activation during cue-induced cocaine craving. *American Journal of Psychiatry* 156:11-18.

Cho AK & Melega WP (2002). Patterns of methamphetamine abuse and their consequences. *Journal of Addictive Diseases* 21:21-34.

Cho AK, Melega WP, Kuczenski R et al. (2001). Relevance of pharmacokinetic parameters in animal models of methamphetamine abuse. *Synapse* 39:161-166.

Coffey SF, Dansky BS, Carrigan MH et al. (2000). Acute and protracted cocaine abstinence in an outpatient population: A prospective study of mood, sleep and withdrawal symptoms. *Drug and Alcohol Dependence* 59:277-286.

Comer SD, Hart CL, Ward AS et al. (2001). Effects of repeated oral methamphetamine administration in humans. *Psychopharmacology* 155:397-404.

Cone EJ (1995). Pharmacokinetics and pharmacodynamics of cocaine. *Journal of Analytical Toxicology* 19:459-478.

Cone EJ, Tsadik A, Oyler J et al. (1998). Cocaine metabolism and urinary excretion after different routes of administration. *Therapeutic Drug Monitoring* 20:556-560.

Cone EJ, Yousefnejad D, Hillsgrove MJ et al. (1995). Passive inhalation of cocaine. *Journal of Analytical Toxicology* 19:399-411.

Cook CD, Carroll FI & Beardsley PM (2001). Cocaine-like discriminative stimulus effects of novel cocaine and 3-phenyltropane analogs in the rat. *Psychopharmacology* 159:58-63.

Corey PJ, Heck AM & Weathermon RA (1999). Amphetamines to counteract opioid-induced sedation. *Annals of Pharmacotherapy* 33:1362-1366.

Cornish JL & Kalivas PW (2001). Cocaine sensitization and craving: Differing roles for dopamine and glutamate in the nucleus accumbens. *Journal of Addictive Diseases* 20:43-54.

Cottler LB, Shillington AM, Compton WM III et al. (1993). Subjective reports of withdrawal among cocaine users: Recommendations for *DSM-IV. Drug and Alcohol Dependence* 33:97-104.

Crawford CA, McDougall SA, Meier TL et al. (1998). Repeated methylphenidate treatment induces behavioral sensitization and decreases protein kinase A and dopamine-stimulated adenylyl cyclase activity in the dorsal striatum. *Psychopharmacology* 136:34-43.

Cubells JF, McCance-Katz EF, Grieg T et al. (2000). Phenotypic assessment of cocaine-induced paranoia and psychotic symptoms (CIPPS). *Biological Psychiatry* 47(Suppl):167S-168S.

Cunningham KA, Bradberry CW, Chang AS et al. (1996). The role of serotonin in the actions of psychostimulants: Molecular and pharmacological analyses. *Behavioural Brain Research* 73: 93-102.

Dalal S & Melzack R (1998). Potentiation of opioid analgesia by psychostimulant drugs: A review. *Journal of Pain & Symptom Management* 16(4):245-253.

Debooy VD, Seshia MM, Tenenbein M et al. (1993). Intravenous pentazocine and methylphenidate abuse during pregnancy: Maternal lifestyle and infant outcome. *American Journal of Diseases in Children* 147:1062-1065.

Ding Y-S, Fowler JS, Volkow ND et al. (1997). Chiral drugs: Comparison of the pharmacokinetics of [^{11}C]d-threo and l-threo-methylphenidate in the human and baboon brain. *Psychopharmacology* 131:71-78.

Dworkin SI, Lambert P, Sizemore GM et al. (1998). RTI-113 administration reduces cocaine self-administration at high occupancy of dopamine transporter. *Synapse* 30:49-55.

Egan MF, Wing L, Li R et al. (1994). Effects of chronic cocaine treatment on rat brain: Long-term reduction in frontal cortical serotonin. *Biological Psychiatry* 36:637-640.

Ellenhorn MJ, Schonwald S, Ordog G et al. (1997). *Ellenhorn's Medical Toxicology: Diagnosis and Treatment of Human Poisoning, 2nd Edition.* Baltimore, MD: Williams & Wilkins.

Ellison G (1994). Stimulant-induced psychosis, the dopamine theory of schizophrenia, and the habenula. *Brain Research Reviews* 19: 223-239.

Elmer GI, Miner LL & Pickens RW (1998). The contribution of genetic factors in cocaine and other drug abuse. In ST Higgins & JL Katz (eds.) *Cocaine Abuse: Behavior, Pharmacology, and Clinical Applications.* San Diego, CA: Academic Press, 289-311.

Eyler FD & Behnke M (1999). Early development of infants exposed to drugs prenatally. *Clinics in Perinatology* 26(1):107-150.

Ferger B, Stahl D & Kuschinsky K (1996). Effects of cocaine on the EEG power spectrum of rats are significantly altered after its repeated administration: Do they reflect sensitization phenomena? *Naunyn Schmiedebergs Archives of Pharmacology* 353:545-551.

Fischman MW & Foltin RW (1998). Cocaine self-administration research: Implications for rational pharmacotherapy. In ST Higgins & JL Katz (eds.) *Cocaine Abuse: Behavior, Pharmacology, and Clinical Applications*. San Diego, CA: Academic Press, 181-207.

Flaum M & Schultz SK (1996). When does amphetamine-induced psychosis become schizophrenia? *American Journal of Psychiatry* 153(6):812-815.

Fleckenstein AE, Gibb JW & Hanson GR (2000). Differential effects of stimulants on monoaminergic transporters: Pharmacological consequences and implications for neurotoxicity. *European Journal of Pharmacology* 406:1-13.

Flores C, Samaha A-N & Stewart J (2000). Requirement of endogenous basic fibroblast growth factor for sensitization to amphetamine. *Journal of Neuroscience* 20(RC55):1-5.

Foltin RW & Fischman MW (1996). Effects of methadone or buprenorphine maintenance on the subjective and reinforcing effects of intravenous cocaine in humans. *Journal of Pharmacology and Experimental Therapeutics* 278:1153-1164.

Fowler JS, Volkow ND, Wang G-J et al. (2001). [¹¹]Cocaine: PET studies of cocaine pharmacokinetics, dopamine transporter availability and dopamine transporter occupancy. *Nuclear Medicine & Biology* 28:561-572.

Francis MM, Vazquez RW, Papke RL et al. (2000). Subtype-selective inhibition of neuronal nicotinic acetylcholine receptors by cocaine is determined by the alpha4 and beta4 subunits. *Molecular Pharmacology* 58:109-119.

Fukushima A (1994). Criminal responsibility in amphetamine psychosis. *Japanese Journal of Psychiatry & Neurology* 48(Suppl):1-4.

Gardner EL (2000). What we have learned about addiction from animal models of drug self-administration. *American Journal on Addictions* 9:285-313.

Gaytan O, Lewis C, Swann A et al. (1999). Diurnal differences in amphetamine sensitization. *European Journal of Pharmacology* 374:1-9.

Gaytan O, Nason R, Alagugurusamy R et al. (2000). MK-801 blocks the development of sensitization to the locomotor effects of methylphenidate. *Brain Research Bulletin* 51:485-492.

Gaytan O, Yang P, Swann A et al. (2000). Diurnal differences in sensitization to methylphenidate. *Brain Research* 864:24-39.

Gelowitz DL & Berger SP (2001). Signal transduction mechanisms and behavioral sensitization to stimulant drugs: An overview of cAMP and PLA₂. *Journal of Addictive Diseases* 20:33-42.

George AJ (2000). Central nervous system stimulants. *Bailliere's Clinical Endocrinology and Metabolism* 14(1):79-88.

Gerasimov MR, Franceschi M, Volkow ND et al. (2000). Synergistic interactions between nicotine and cocaine or methylphenidate depend on the dose of dopamine transporter inhibitor. *Synapse* 38(4):432-437.

Ghuran A & Nolan J (2000). Recreational drug misuse: Issues for the cardiologist. *Heart* 83:627-633.

Giannini AJ, Miller NS, Loiselle RH et al. (1993). Cocaine-associated violence and relationship to route of administration. *Journal of Substance Abuse Treatment* 10:67-69.

Giros B, Jaber M, Jones SR et al. (1996). Hyperlocomotion and indifference to cocaine and amphetamine in mice lacking the dopamine transporter. *Nature* 379:606-612.

Glenn MB (1998). Methylphenidate for cognitive and behavioral dysfunction after traumatic brain injury. *Journal of Head Trauma & Rehabilitation* 13(5):87-90.

Glennon RA (1999). Arylalkylamine drugs of abuse: An overview of drug discrimination studies. *Pharmacology, Biochemistry and Behavior* 64(2):251-256.

Gordon AS, Moran DT, Jafek BW et al. (1990). The effect of chronic cocaine abuse on human olfaction. *Archives of Otolaryngology & Head & Neck Surgery* 116:1415-1418.

Gorelick DA (1992). Progression of dependence in male cocaine addicts. *American Journal of Drug and Alcohol Abuse* 18:13-19.

Gorelick DA (1997). Enhancing cocaine metabolism with butyrylcholinesterase as a treatment strategy. *Drug and Alcohol Dependence* 48:159-165.

Gorelick DA (1998). The rate hypothesis and agonist substitution approaches to cocaine abuse treatment. In DS Goldstein, G Eisenhofer & R McCarty (eds.) *Catecholamines: Bridging Basic Science with Clinical Medicine*. San Diego, CA: Academic Press, 995-997.

Gorelick DA & Rothman RB (1997). Stimulant sensitization in humans. *Biological Psychiatry* 42:230-231.

Gorelick DA, Simmons MS, Carriero N et al. (1997). Characteristics of smoked drug use among cocaine smokers. *American Journal on Addictions* 6:237-245.

Gossop M, Griffiths P, Powis B et al. (1994). Cocaine: Patterns of use, route of administration, and severity of dependence. *British Journal of Psychiatry* 164:660-664.

Greenhill LL, Halperin JM & Abikoff H (1999). Stimulant medications. *Journal of the American Academy of Child and Adolescent Psychiatry* 38(5):503-512.

Grella CE, Anglin MD & Wugalter SE (1997). Patterns and predictors of cocaine and crack use by clients in standard and enhanced methadone maintenance treatment. *American Journal of Drug and Alcohol Abuse* 23:15-42.

Haim DY, Lippmann ML, Goldberg SK et al. (1995). The pulmonary complications of crack cocaine: A comprehensive review. *Chest* 107:233-240.

Hall W, Hando J, Darke S et al. (1996). Psychological morbidity and route of administration among amphetamine users in Sydney, Australia. *Addiction* 91(1):81-87.

Haller CA & Benowitz NL (2000). Adverse cardiovascular and central nervous system events associated with dietary supplements containing ephedra alkaloids. *New England Journal of Medicine* 343(25):1833-1838.

Hammer RP Jr, Egilmez Y & Emmett-Oglesby MW (1997). Neural mechanisms of tolerance to the effects of cocaine. *Behavioural Brain Research* 84:225-239.

Hamner JE 3rd & Villegas OL (1969). The effect of coca leaf chewing on the buccal mucosa of Aymara and Quechua Indians in Bolivia. *Oral Surgery, Oral Medicine, Oral Pathology* 28:287-295.

Hando J, Topp L & Hall W (1997). Amphetamine-related harms and treatment preferences of regular amphetamine users in Sydney, Australia. *Drug and Alcohol Dependence* 46:105-113.

Harris D & Batki SL (2000). Stimulant psychosis: Symptom profile and acute clinical course. *American Journal on Addictions* 9(1):28-37.

Hart CL, Jatlow P, Sevarino KA et al. (2000). Comparison of intravenous cocaethylene and cocaine in humans. *Psychopharmacology* 149(2):153-162.

Hatsukami DK & Fischman MW (1996). Crack cocaine and cocaine hydrochloride: Are the differences myth or reality? *Journal of the American Medical Association* 276(19):1580-1588.

Heishman SJ (1998). Effects of abused drugs on human performance: Laboratory assessment. In SB Karch (ed.) *Drug Abuse Handbook*. Boca Raton, FL: CRC Press, 206-235.

Heishman SJ & Henningfield JE (1991). Discriminative stimulus effects of *d*-amphetamine, methylphenidate, and diazepam in humans. *Psychopharmacology* 103:436-442.

Higgins ES (1999). A comparative analysis of antidepressants and stimulants for the treatment of adults with attention-deficit hyperactivity disorder. *Journal of Family Practice* 48(1):15-20.

Hurd YL & Herkenham M (1992). Influence of a single injection of cocaine, amphetamine or GBR 12909 on mRNA expression of striatal neuropeptides. *Molecular Brain Research* 16:97-104.

Izenwasser S (1998). Basic pharmacological mechanisms of cocaine. In ST Higgins & JL Katz (eds.) *Cocaine Abuse: Behavior, Pharmacology, and Clinical Applications*. San Diego, CA: Academic Press, 1-20.

Jackson GF, Saady JJ & Poklis A (1991). Urinary excretion of benzoylecgonine following ingestion of health Inca tea. *Forensic Science International* 49:57-64.

Jenkins AJ & Cone EJ (1998). Pharmacokinetics: Drug absorption, distribution, and elimination. In SB Karch (ed.) *Drug Abuse Handbook*. Boca Raton, FL: CRC Press, 151-201.

Johnson JL & Leff M (1999). Children of substance abusers: Overview of research findings. *Pediatrics* 103:1085-1099.

Kalivas PW, Pierce RC, Cornish J et al. (1998). A role for sensitization in craving and relapse in cocaine addiction. *Journal of Psychopharmacology* 12(1):49-53.

Kandel DB, Huang FY & Davies M (2001). Comorbidity between patterns of substance use dependence and psychiatric syndromes. *Drug and Alcohol Dependence* 64(2):233-241.

Kankaanpaa A, Meririnne E & Seppala T (2002). 5-HT$_3$ receptor antagonist MDL 72222 attenuates cocaine- and mazindol-, but not methylphenidate-induced neurochemical and behavioral effects in the rat. *Psychopharmacology* 159:341-350.

Karch SB (1996). *The Pathology of Drug Abuse, 2nd Edition*. Boca Raton, FL: CRC Press.

Karch SB (1998). *A Brief History of Cocaine* Boca Raton, FL: CRC Press.

Katz JL, Izenwasser S & Terry P (2000). Relationships among dopamine transporter affinities and cocaine-like discriminative-stimulus effects. *Psychopharmacology* 148:90-98.

Kaufman MJ, Levin JM, Maas LC et al. (2001). Cocaine-induced cerebral vasoconstriction differs as a function of sex and menstrual cycle phase. *Biological Psychiatry* 49:774-781.

Kavanagh KT, Maijub AG & Brown JR (1992). Passive exposure to cocaine in medical personnel and its effect on urine drug screening tests. *Otolaryngology, Head, & Neck Surgery* 107:363-366.

Kendler KS (2001). Twin studies of psychiatric illness: An update. *Archives of General Psychiatry* 58:1005-1014.

Kernan WN, Viscoli CM, Brass LM et al. (2000). Phenylpropanolamine and the risk of hemorrhagic stroke. *New England Journal of Medicine* 343(25):1826-1832.

Kidwell DA, Holland JC & Athanaselis S (1998). Testing for drugs of abuse in saliva and sweat. *Journal of Chromatography B* 713:111-135.

Kilts CD, Schweitzer JB, Quinn CK et al. (2001). Neural activity related to drug craving in cocaine addiction. *Archives of General Psychiatry* 58:334-341.

Kimko HC, Cross JT & Abernethy DR (1999). Pharmacokinetics and clinical effectiveness of methylphenidate. *Clinical Pharmacokinetics* 37(6):457-470.

King GR, Xiong Z & Ellinwood EH Jr (1999). Withdrawal from continuous cocaine administration: Time dependent changes in accumbens 5-HT3 receptor function and behavioral tolerance. *Psychopharmacology* 142:352-359.

Kollins SH, MacDonald EK & Rush CR (2001). Assessing the abuse potential of methylphenidate in nonhuman and human subjects. A review. *Pharmacology, Biochemistry and Behavior* 68:611-627.

Kollins SH & Rush CR (2002). Sensitization to the cardiovascular but not subject-rated effects of oral cocaine in humans. *Biological Psychiatry* 51(2):143-150.

Koob GF (1996). Drug addiction: The yin and yang of hedonic homeostasis. *Neuron* 16:893-896.

Koob GF (1999). The role of the striatopallidal and extended amygdala systems in drug addiction. *Annals of the New York Academy of Sciences* 877:445-460.

Kreek MJ (1997). Opiate and cocaine addictions: Challenge for pharmacotherapies. *Pharmacology, Biochemistry and Behavior* 57:551-569.

Kuhar MJ, Joyce A & Dominguez G (2001). Genes in drug abuse. *Drug and Alcohol Dependence* 62:157-162.

Kuhar MJ & Pilotte NS (1996). Neurochemical changes in cocaine withdrawal. *Trends in Pharmacological Science* 17:260-264.

Kuhar MJ, Ritz MC & Boja JW (1991). The dopamine hypothesis of the reinforcing properties of cocaine. *Trends in Neuroscience* 14:299-302.

Lago JA & Kosten TR (1994). Stimulant withdrawal. *Addiction* 89:1477-1481.

Lange RA & Hillis LD (2001). Cardiovascular complications of cocaine use. *New England Journal of Medicine* 345(5):351-358.

Laviola G, Adriani W, Terranova ML et al. (1999). Psychobiological risk factors for vulnerability to psychostimulants in human adolescents and animal models. *Neuroscience & Biobehavioral Reviews* 23:993-1010.

Le SD, Taylor RW, Vidal D et al. (1992). Occupational exposure to cocaine involving crime lab personnel. *Journal of Forensic Sciences* 37(4):959-968.

LeSage MG, Stafford D & Glowa JR (1999). Preclinical research on cocaine self-administration: Environmental determinants and their interaction with pharmacological treatment. *Neuroscience & Biobehavioral Reviews* 23:717-741.

Lester BM (2000). Prenatal cocaine exposure and child outcome: A model for the study of the infant at risk. *Israel Journal of Psychiatry & Related Sciences* 37(3):223-235.

Letchworth SR, Nader MA, Smith HR et al. (2001). Progression of changes in dopamine transporter binding site density as a result of cocaine self-administration in rhesus monkeys. *Journal of Neuroscience* 21:2799-2807.

Levin FR, Hess JM, Gorelick DA et al. (1993). Patterns of cocaine use among cocaine-dependent outpatients. *American Journal on Addictions* 2(2):109-115.

Levitt P (1998). Prenatal effects of drugs of abuse on brain development. *Drug and Alcohol Dependence* 51:109-125.

Li J-H & Lin L-F (1998). Genetic toxicology of abused drugs: A brief review. *Mutagenesis* 13(6):557-565.

Licata A, Taylor S, Berman M et al. (1993). Effects of cocaine on human aggression. *Pharmacology, Biochemistry and Behavior* 45:549-552.

Little JD & Romans SE (1993). Psychosis following readministration of diethyl proprion: A possible role for kindling? *International Clinical Psychopharmacology* 8:67-70.

Little KY, McLaughlin DP, Zhang L et al. (1998). Brain dopamine transporter messenger RNA and binding sites in cocaine users. *Archives of General Psychiatry* 55:793-799.

Little KY, Patel UN, Clark TB et al. (1996). Alteration of brain dopamine and serotonin levels in cocaine users: A preliminary report. *American Journal of Psychiatry* 153(9):1216-1218.

London ED, Bonson KR, Ernst M et al. (1999). Brain imaging studies of cocaine abuse: Implications for medication development. *Critical Reviews in Neurobiology* 13:227-242.

Lukas SE & Renshaw PF (1998). Cocaine effects on brain function. In ST Higgins & JL Katz (eds.) *Cocaine Abuse: Behavior, Pharmacology, and Clinical Applications*. San Diego, CA: Academic Press, 265-287.

Macdonald PT, Waldorf D, Reinarman C et al. (1988). Heavy cocaine use and sexual behavior. *Journal of Drug Issues* 18(3):437-455.

Malison RT, Best SE, van Dyck CH et al. (1998). Elevated striatal dopamine transporters during acute cocaine abstinence as measured by [^{123}I]-CIT SPECT. *American Journal of Psychiatry* 155:832-834.

Malison RT, Best SE, Wallace EA et al. (1995). Euphorigenic doses of cocaine reduce [^{123}I]beta-CIT SPECT measures of dopamine transporter availability in human cocaine addicts. *Psychopharmacology* 122:358-362.

Mark GP, Hajnal A, Kinney AE et al. (1999). Self-administration of cocaine increases the release of acetylcholine to a greater extent than response-independent cocaine in the nucleus accumbens of rats. *Psychopharmacology* 143(1):47-53.

Marotta PJ & Roberts EA (1998). Pemoline hepatotoxicity in children. *Journal of Pediatrics* 132:894-897.

Masand PS & Tesar GE (1996). Use of stimulants in the medically ill. *Psychiatric Clinics of North America* 19(3):515-547.

McCann UD, Wong DF, Yokoi F et al. (1998). Reduced striatal dopamine transporter density in abstinent methamphetamine and methcathinone users: Evidence from positron emission tomography studies with [^{11}C]WIN-35,428. *Journal of Neuroscience* 18(20):8417-8422.

McFarland K & Kalivas PW (2001). The circuitry mediating cocaine-induced reinstatement of drug-seeking behavior. *Journal of Neuroscience* 21:8655-8663.

McLeman ER, Warsh JJ, Ang L et al. (2000). The human nucleus accumbens is highly susceptible to G protein down-regulation by methamphetamine and heroin. *Journal of Neurochemistry* 74:2120-2126.

McNamara JO (1995). Analyses of the molecular basis of kindling development. *Psychiatry & Clinical Neuroscience* 49:S175-S178.

Meador-Woodruff JH, Little KY, Damask SP et al. (1995). Effects of cocaine on D3 and D4 expression in the human striatum. *Biological Psychiatry* 38:263-266.

Mello NK & Mendelson JH (1997). Cocaine's effects on neuroendocrine systems: Clinical and preclinical studies. *Pharmacology, Biochemistry and Behavior* 57(3):571-599.

Mendelson JH, Sholar M, Mello NK et al. (1998). Cocaine tolerance: Behavioral, cardiovascular, and neuroendocrine function in men. *Neuropsychopharmacology* 18:263-271.

Miller NS, Gold MS & Mahler JC (1991). Violent behaviors associated with cocaine use: Possible pharmacological mechanisms. *International Journal of the Addictions* 26(10):1077-1088.

Mirchandani HG, Mirchandani IH, Hellman F et al. (1991). Passive inhalation of free-base cocaine ('crack') smoke by infants. *Archives of Pathology & Laboratory Medicine* 115:494-498.

Montoya ID & Chilcoat HD (1996). Epidemiology of coca derivatives use in the Andean Region: A tale of five countries. *Substance Use & Misuse* 31(10):1227-1240.

Moore JM & Casale JF (1994). In-depth chromatographic analyses of illicit cocaine and its precursor, coca leaves. *Journal of Chromatography A* 674:165-205.

Moron JA, Brockington A, Wise RA et al. (2002). Dopamine uptake through the norepinephrine transporter in brain regions with low levels of the dopamine transporter: Evidence from knock-out mouse lines. *Journal of Neuroscience* 22:389-395.

Mott SH, Packer RJ & Soldin SJ (1994). Neurologic manifestations of cocaine exposure in childhood. *Pediatrics* 93(4):557-560.

Myers MG, Rohsenow DJ, Monti PM et al. (1995). Patterns of cocaine use among individuals in substance abuse treatment. *American Journal of Drug and Alcohol Abuse* 21(2):223-231.

Nakahara Y (1999). Hair analysis for abused and therapeutic drugs. *Journal of Chromatography B* 733(1-2):161-180.

National Institute of Justice (2001). *ADAM Preliminary 2000 Findings on Drug Use and Drug Markets—Adult Male Arrestees* (NCJ 189101). Washington, DC, U.S. Department of Justice.

Neiman J, Haapaniemi HM & Hillbom M (2000). Neurological complications of drug abuse: Pathophysiological mechanisms. *European Journal of Neurology* 7:595-606.

Nestler EJ (2001). Molecular neurobiology of addiction. *American Journal on Addictions* 10:201-217.

Nestler EJ, Barrot M & Self DW (2001). ΔFosB: A sustained molecular switch for addiction. *Proceedings of the National Academy of Sciences of the United States of America* 98:11042-11046.

Nice FJ, Snyder JL & Kotansky BC (2000). Breastfeeding and over-the-counter medications. *Journal of Human Lactation* 16(4):319-331.

Nishino S & Mignot E (1999). Drug treatment of patients with insomnia and excessive daytime sleepiness: Pharmacokinetic considerations. *Clinical Pharmacokinetics* 37(4):305-330.

Nzerue CM, Hewan-Lowe K & Riley LJ Jr (2000). Cocaine and the kidney: A synthesis of pathophysiologic and clinical perspectives. *American Journal of Kidney Diseases* 35(5):783-795.

Office of Applied Studies (2000). *DAWN Annual Medical Examiner Data 1999*. Rockville, MD: Substance Abuse and Mental Health Services Administration.

Office of Applied Studies (2001a). *DAWN Detailed Emergency Department Tables 2000*. Rockville, MD: Substance Abuse and Mental Health Services Administration.

Office of Applied Studies (2001b). *Summary of Findings From the 2000 National Household Survey on Drug Abuse.* Rockville, MD: Substance Abuse and Mental Health Services Administration.

Office of Applied Studies (2001c). *Treatment Episode Data Set (TEDS): 1994-1999, National Admissions to Substance Abuse Treatment Services* (DHHS Publication [SMA] 01-3550). Rockville, MD: Substance Abuse and Mental Health Services Administration.

Office of National Drug Control Policy (ONDCP) (2002). *National Drug Control Strategy: 2002.* Washington, DC: Executive Office of the President, The White House.

Ohmori T, Abekawa T, Ito K et al. (2000). Context determines the type of sensitized behaviour: A brief review and a hypothesis on the role of environment in behavioural sensitization. *Behavioural Pharmacology* 11(3-4):211-221.

Olive MF, Koenig HN, Nannini MA et al. (2001). Stimulation of endorphin neurotransmission in the nucleus accumbens by ethanol, cocaine, and amphetamine. *Journal of Neuroscience* 21:1-5.

Ostrea EM Jr (1999). Testing for exposure to illicit drugs and other agents in the neonate: A review of laboratory methods and the role of meconium analysis. *Current Problems in Pediatrics* 29(2):37-56.

Pallasch TJ & Joseph CE (1987). Oral manifestations of drug abuse. *Journal of Psychoactive Drugs* 19(4):375-377.

Parsons LH, Weiss F & Koob GF (1998). Serotonin$_{1B}$ receptor stimulation enhances cocaine reinforcement. *Journal of Neuroscience* 18:10078-10089.

Perez-Reyes M, White WR, McDonald SA et al. (1991). Clinical effects of daily methamphetamine administration. *Clinical Neuropharmacology* 14(4):352-358.

Pierce RC & Bari AA (2001). The role of neurotrophic factors in psychostimulant-induced behavioral and neuronal plasticity. *Reviews of Neuroscience* 12(2):95-110.

Pierce RC & Kalivas PW (1997). A circuitry model of the expression of behavioral sensitization to amphetamine-like psychostimulants. *Brain Research Reviews* 25:192-216.

Pierre PJ & Vezina P (1998). D$_1$ dopamine receptor blockade prevents the facilitation of amphetamine self-administration induced by prior exposure to the drug. *Psychopharmacology* 138:159-166.

Pilotte NS (1997). Neurochemistry of cocaine withdrawal. *Current Opinion in Neurology* 10:534-538.

Plessinger MA (1998). Prenatal exposure to amphetamines: Risks and adverse outcomes in pregnancy. *Obstetrics & Gynecology Clinics of North America* 25(1):119-138.

Post RM & Weiss SRB (1988). Stimulant-induced behavioral sensitization: A model for neuroleptic nonresponsiveness. In P Simon, P Soubrie & D Wildlocer (eds.) *Animal Models of Psychiatric Disorders.* Basel, Switzerland: S Karger, 52-60.

Preston KL & Walsh SL (1998). Evaluating abuse liability: Methods and predictive value. In SB Karch (ed.) *Drug Abuse Handbook.* Boca Raton, FL: CRC Press, 276-306.

Qureshi AI, Suri FK, Guterman LR et al. (2001). Cocaine use and the likelihood of nonfatal myocardial infarction and stroke. *Circulation* 103:502-506.

Ranaldi R & Wise RA (2001). Blockade of D$_1$ dopamine receptors in the ventral tegmental area decreases cocaine reward: Possible role for dendritically released dopamine. *Journal of Neuroscience* 21(15):5841-5846.

Renfroe CL & Messinger TA (1985). Street drug analysis: An eleven year perspective on illicit drug alteration. *Seminars in Adolescent Medicine* 1(4):247-257.

Rhodes W, Layne M, Johnston P et al. (2000). *What America's Users Spend on Illegal Drugs: 1988-1998.* Washington, DC: U.S. Office of National Drug Control Policy.

Robinson TE & Berridge KC (2000). The psychology and neurobiology of addiction: An incentive-sensitization view. *Addiction* 95:S91-S117.

Robinson TE, Browman KE, Crombag HS et al. (1998). Modulation of the induction or expression of psychostimulant sensitization by the circumstances surrounding drug administration. *Neuroscience & Biobehavioral Reviews* 22(2):347-354.

Rocha BA, Fumagalli F, Gainetdinov RR et al. (1998). Cocaine self-administration in dopamine-transporter knockout mice. *Nature Neuroscience* 1:132-137.

Rogers RD & Robbins TW (2001). Investigating the neurocognitive deficits associated with chronic drug misuse. *Current Opinion in Neurobiology* 11:250-257.

Rosse RB, Fay-McCarthy M, Collins JP Jr et al. (1993). Transient compulsive foraging behavior associated with crack cocaine use. *American Journal of Psychiatry* 150(1):155-156.

Rothman RB & Baumann MH (2000). Neurochemical mechanisms of phentermine and fenfluramine: Therapeutic and adverse effects. *Drug Development Research* 51:52-65.

Rothman RB, Baumann MH, Dersch CM et al. (2001). Amphetamine-type central nervous system stimulants release norepinephrine more potently than they release dopamine and serotonin. *Synapse* 39:32-41.

Satel SL, Price LH, Palumbo JM et al. (1991a). Clinical phenomenology and neurobiology of cocaine abstinence: A prospective inpatient study. *American Journal of Psychiatry* 148:1712-1716.

Satel SL, Seibyl JP & Charney DS (1991b). Prolonged cocaine psychosis implies underlying major psychopathology. *Journal of Clinical Psychiatry* 52(8):349-350.

Satel SL, Southwick SM & Gawin FH (1991c). Clinical features of cocaine-induced paranoia. *American Journal of Psychiatry* 148(4):495-498.

Schama KF, Howell LL & Byrd LD (1998). Prenatal exposure to cocaine. In ST Higgins & JL Katz (eds.) *Cocaine Abuse: Behavior, Pharmacology, and Clinical Applications.* San Diego, CA: Academic Press, 159-179.

Schenk S & Partridge B (1997). Sensitization and tolerance in psychostimulant self-administration. *Pharmacology, Biochemistry and Behavior* 57(3):543-550.

Schlaepfer TE, Pearlson GD, Wong DF et al. (1997). PET study of competition between intravenous cocaine and [^{11}C]raclopride at dopamine receptors in human subjects. *American Journal of Psychiatry* 154:1209-1213.

Segura J (1998). Summary of International Olympic Committee regulations. In SB Karch (ed.) *Drug Abuse Handbook.* Boca Raton, FL: CRC Press, 720-726.

Sekine Y, Iyo M, Ouchi Y et al. (2001). Methamphetamine-related psychiatric symptoms and reduced brain dopamine transporters studied with PET. *American Journal of Psychiatry* 158(8):1206-1214.

Self DW, Genova LM, Hope BT et al. (1998). Involvement of cAMP-dependent protein kinase in the nucleus accumbens in cocaine self-administration and relapse of cocaine-seeking behavior. *Journal of Neuroscience* 18:1848-1859.

Serper MR, Chou JC, Allen MH et al. (1999). Symptomatic overlap of cocaine intoxication and acute schizophrenia at emergency presentation. *Schizophrenia Bulletin* 25(2):387-394.

Sery O, Vojtova V & Zvolsky P (2001). The association study of DRD2, ACE and AGT gene polymorphisms and methamphetamine dependence. *Physiological Research* 50:43-50.

Sharkey J, Ritz MC, Schenden JA et al. (1988). Cocaine inhibits muscarinic cholinergic receptors in heart and brain. *Journal of Pharmacology and Experimental Therapeutics* 246:1048-1052.

Sharpe LG, Pilotte NS, Shippenberg TS et al. (2000). Autoradiographic evidence that prolonged withdrawal from intermittent cocaine reduces mu-opioid receptor expression in limbic regions of the rat brain. *Synapse* 37:292-297.

Shesser R, Jotte R & Olshaker J (1991). The contribution of impurities to the acute morbidity of illegal drug use. *American Journal of Emergency Medicine* 9:336-342.

Shippenberg TS, Chefer VI, Zapata A et al. (2001). Modulation of the behavioral and neurochemical effects of psychostimulants by κ-opioid receptor systems. *Annals of New York Academy of Sciences* 937:50-73.

Skopp G & Potsch L (1999). Perspiration versus saliva—Basic aspects concerning their use in roadside drug testing. *International Journal of Legal Medicine* 112(4):213-221.

Snyder CA, Wood RW, Graefe JF et al. (1988). "Crack smoke" is a respirable aerosol of cocaine base. *Pharmacology, Biochemistry and Behavior* 29(1):93-95.

Sofuoglu M, Nelson D, Babb DA et al. (2001). Intravenous cocaine increases plasma epinephrine and norepinephrine in humans. *Pharmacology, Biochemistry and Behavior* 68:455-459.

Sora I, Hall FS, Andrews AM et al. (2001). Molecular mechanisms of cocaine reward: Combined dopamine and serotonin transporter knockouts eliminate cocaine place preference. *Proceedings of the National Academy of Sciences of the United States of America* 98(9):5300-5305.

Sora I, Wichems C, Takahashi N et al. (1998). Cocaine reward models: Conditioned place preference can be established in dopamine- and in serotonin-transporter knockout mice. *Proceedings of the National Academy of Sciences of the United States of America* 95:7699-7704.

Spielewoy C, Biala G, Roubert C et al. (2001). Hypolocomotor effects of acute and daily *d*-amphetamine in mice lacking the dopamine transporter. *Psychopharmacology* 159(1):2-9.

Sporer KA & Firestone J (1997). Clinical course of crack cocaine body stuffers. *Annals of Emergency Medicine* 29:596-601.

Staley JK, Rothman RB, Rice KC et al. (1997). κ₂ Opioid receptors in limbic areas of the human brain are upregulated by cocaine in fatal overdose victims. *Journal of Neuroscience* 17:8225-8233.

Stine SM, Krystal JH, Petrakis IL et al. (1997). Effect of alpha-methyl-para-tyrosine on response to cocaine challenge. *Biological Psychiatry* 42:181-190.

Strakowski SM, Sax KW, Rosenberg HL et al. (2001). Human response to repeated low-dose d-amphetamine. *Neuropsychopharmacology* 25:548-554.

Tashkin DP (2001). Airway effects of marijuana, cocaine, and other inhaled illicit agents. *Current Opinion in Pulmonary Medicine* 7:43-61.

Telang FW, Volkow ND, Levy A et al. (1999). Distribution of tracer levels of cocaine in the human brain as assessed with averaged [^{11}C]cocaine images. *Synapse* 31:290-296.

Tella SR, Schindler CW & Goldberg SR (1999). Cardiovascular responses to cocaine self-administration: Acute and chronic tolerance. *European Journal of Pharmacology* 383:57-68.

Tinsley JA & Watkins DD (1998). Over-the-counter stimulants: Abuse and addiction. *Mayo Clinic Proceedings* 73:977-982.

Torres G & Horowitz JM (1999). Drugs of abuse and brain gene expression. *Psychosomatic Medicine* 61:630-650.

U.S. Department of State (2000). *International Narcotics Control Strategy Report*. Washington, DC: U.S. Department of State.

U.S. Drug Enforcement Administration (2001). *Federalwide Drug Seizure System, 1989-2001*. Washington, DC: U.S. Drug Enforcement Administration.

Uhl GR, Hall FS & Sora I (2002). Cocaine, reward, movement and monoamine transporters. *Molecular Psychiatry* 7:21-26.

Uhl GR, Li S, Takahashi N et al. (2000). The VMAT2 gene in mice and humans: Amphetamine responses, locomotion, cardiac arrhythmias, aging, and vulnerability to dopaminergic toxins. *FASEB Journal* 14:2459-2465.

United Nations Drug Control Program (2000). *Global Illicit Drug Trends 2000*. New York, NY: United Nations.

Unterwald EM (2001). Regulation of opioid receptors by cocaine. *Annals of New York Academy of Sciences* 937:74-92.

van Harten PN, van Trier JCAM, Horwitz EH et al. (1998). Cocaine as a risk factor for neuroleptic-induced acute dystonia. *Journal of Clinical Psychiatry* 59:128-130.

Vanderschuren LJMJ & Kalivas PW (2000). Alterations in dopaminergic and glutamatergic transmission in the induction and expression of behavioral sensitization: A critical review of preclinical studies. *Psychopharmacology* 151:99-120.

Vanderschuren LJMJ, Schmidt ED, De Vries TJ et al. (1999). A single exposure to amphetamine is sufficient to induce long-term behavioral, neuroendocrine, and neurochemical sensitization in rats. *Journal of Neuroscience* 19(21):9579-9586.

Vitiello B (2001). Long-term effects of stimulant medications on the brain: Possible relevance to the treatment of attention deficit hyperactivity disorder. *Journal of Child and Adolescent Psychopharmacology* 11(1):25-34.

Volkow ND, Chang L, Wang G-J et al. (2001). Loss of dopamine transporters in methamphetamine abusers recovers with protracted abstinence. *Journal of Neuroscience* 21(23):9414-9418.

Volkow ND, Fowler JS & Wang G-J (1999a). Imaging studies on the role of dopamine in cocaine reinforcement and addiction in humans. *Journal of Psychopharmacology* 13:337-345.

Volkow ND, Wang G-J, Fischman MW et al. (1997a). Relationship between subjective effects of cocaine and dopamine transporter occupancy. *Nature* 386:827-830.

Volkow ND, Wang G-J, Fowler JS et al. (1996). Cocaine uptake is decreased in the brain of detoxified cocaine abusers. *Neuropsychopharmacology* 14(3):159-168.

Volkow ND, Wang G-J, Fowler JS et al. (1999b). Methylphenidate and cocaine have similar in vivo potency to block dopamine transporters in the human brain. *Life Sciences* 65:PL7-PL12.

Volkow ND, Wang G-J, Fowler JS et al. (1997b). Decreased striatal dopaminergic responsiveness in detoxified cocaine-dependent subjects. *Nature* 386:830-833.

Vongpatanasin W, Mansour Y, Chavoshan B et al. (1999). Cocaine stimulates the human cardiovascular system via a central mechanism of action. *Circulation* 100:497-502.

Wachtel SR & de Wit H (1999). Subjective and behavioral effects of repeated *d*-amphetamine in humans. *Behavioural Pharmacology* 10(3):271-281.

Wagner GJ & Rabkin R (2000). Effects of dextroamphetamine on depression and fatigue in men with HIV: A double-blind, placebo-controlled trial. *Journal of Clinical Psychiatry* 61:436-440.

Walsh SL & Cunningham KA (1997). Serotonergic mechanisms involved in the discriminative stimulus, reinforcing and subjective effects of cocaine. *Psychopharmacology* 130:41-58.

Walsh SL, Haberny KA & Bigelow GE (2000). Modulation of intravenous cocaine effects by chronic oral cocaine in humans. *Psychopharmacology* 150:361-373.

Walters CL & Blendy JA (2001). Different requirements for cAMP response element binding protein in positive and negative reinforcing properties of drugs of abuse. *Journal of Neuroscience* 21:9438-9444.

Wang G-J, Volkow ND, Logan J et al. (1995). Serotonin 5-HT$_2$ receptor availability in chronic cocaine abusers. *Life Sciences* 56:PL299-PL303.

Ward AS, Haney M, Fischman MW et al. (1997). Binge cocaine self-administration in humans: Intravenous cocaine. *Psychopharmacology* 132:375-381.

Warner A & Norman AB (2000). Mechanisms of cocaine hydrolysis and metabolism in vitro and in vivo: A clarification. *Therapeutic Drug Monitoring* 22:266-270.

Warner EA (1993). Cocaine abuse. *Annals of Internal Medicine* 119:226-235.

Warner EA, Greene GS, Buchsbaum MS et al. (1998). Diabetic ketoacidosis associated with cocaine use. *Archives of Internal Medicine* 158:1799-1802.

White FJ & Kalivas PW (1998). Neuroadaptations involved in amphetamine and cocaine addiction. *Drug and Alcohol Dependence* 51:141-153.

Williamson S, Gossop M, Powis B et al. (1997). Adverse effects of stimulant drugs in a community sample of drug users. *Drug and Alcohol Dependence* 44:87-94.

Wilson JM, Levey AI, Bergeron C et al. (1996). Striatal dopamine, dopamine transporter, and vesicular monoamine transporter in chronic cocaine users. *Annals of Neurology* 40:428-439.

Wise RA (1998). Drug-activation of brain reward pathways. *Drug and Alcohol Dependence* 51:13-22.

Wisor JP, Nishino S, Sora I et al. (2001). Dopaminergic role in stimulant-induced wakefulness. *Journal of Neuroscience* 21(5):1787-1794.

Woody GE, Cottler LB & Cacciola J (1993). Severity of dependence: Data from the DSM-IV field trials. *Addiction* 88:1573-1579.

Woolverton WL & Weiss SRB (1998). Tolerance and sensitization to cocaine: An integrated view. In ST Higgins & JL Katz (eds.) *Cocaine Abuse: Behavior, Pharmacology, and Clinical Applications.* San Diego, CA: Academic Press, 107-134.

Worsley JN, Moszczynska A, Falardeau P et al. (2000). Dopamine D1 receptor protein is elevated in nucleus accumbens of human, chronic methamphetamine users. *Molecular Psychiatry* 5:664-672.

Wu JC, Bell K, Najafi A et al. (1997). Decreasing striatal 6-FDOPA uptake with increasing duration of cocaine withdrawal. *Neuropsychopharmacology* 17:402-409.

Xiao Y-F & Morgan JP (1998). Cocaine blockade of the acetylcholine-activated muscarinic K+ channel in ferret cardiac myocytes. *Journal of Pharmacology and Experimental Therapeutics* 284(1):10-18.

Xu F, Gainetdinov RR, Wetsel WC et al. (2000). Mice lacking the norepinephrine transporter are supersensitive to psychostimulants. *Nature Neuroscience* 3:465-471.

Yanovski SZ & Yanovski JA (2002). Drug therapy: Obesity. *New England Journal of Medicine* 346:591-602.

Yermolaieva O, Chen J, Couceyro PR et al. (2001). Cocaine- and amphetamine-regulated transcript peptide modulation of voltage-gated Ca^{2+} signaling in hippocampal neurons. *Journal of Neuroscience* 21(19):7474-7480.

Yuan J, McCann U & Ricaurte G (1997). Methylphenidate and brain dopamine neurotoxicity. *Brain Research* 767:172-175.

Yui K, Ishiguro T, Goto K et al. (1998). Factors affecting the development of spontaneous recurrence of methamphetamine psychosis. *Acta Psychiatrica Scandinavica* 97:220-227.

Zhang J & Xu M (2001). Toward a molecular understanding of psychostimulant actions using genetically engineered dopamine receptor knockout mice as model systems. *Journal of Addictive Diseases* 20:7-18.

Zhang Y, Loonam TM, Noailles PA et al. (2001). Comparison of cocaine- and methamphetamine-evoked dopamine and glutamate overflow in somatodendritic and terminal field regions of the rat brain during acute, chronic, and early withdrawal conditions. *Annals of the New York Academy of Sciences* 937:93-120.

Zubieta JK, Gorelick DA, Stauffer R et al. (1996). Increased mu opioid receptor binding detected by PET in cocaine-dependent men is associated with cocaine craving. *Nature Medicine* 2:1225-1229.

MDMA (Ecstasy): Clinical Perspectives

JOHN MENDELSOHN, M.D.

Methylenedioxymethamphetamine (MDMA, also known as "Ecstasy" or "X") is a synthetic phenethylamine that has emerged as a major drug of abuse in the United States and worldwide. In the United States, epidemiological estimates are that 7.2% of adults between the ages of 19 and 28 have tried MDMA. In a perhaps more ominous development, 1% of 12th graders report having used MDMA more than 10 times in the preceding year (Johnston, O'Malley et al., 2001). Worldwide, epidemics of MDMA are occurring in Europe (particularly in England and in Switzerland), in Israel, and in parts of Southeast Asia.

MDMA initially was not a drug of abuse. Rather, Pfizer synthesized it in 1914, and psychotherapists used it in the early 1970s to increase feelings of empathy and decrease barriers to therapeutic progress. Currently there is no accepted therapeutic use of MDMA (although some clinical trials are under way). Abuse is primarily by young people, often while dancing.

MECHANISMS OF ACTION

Once in the brain, MDMA binds to the serotonin transporter with micromolar affinities. However, the drug activates several other brain neurochemical systems, with micro- to millimolar affinities for $\alpha 2$ adrenergic receptors, 5-HT$_2$ receptors (the possible source of hallucinogenic effects), muscarinic and histaminic receptors.

The pharmacokinetics of MDMA are complex. MDMA usually is taken orally, and absorption is rapid, with peak plasma levels occurring between one and two hours after dosing. The drug is distributed primarily to lipophilic tissues, such as the brain, and elimination is via the liver and kidney. MDMA probably is metabolized by cytochrome P450-2D6, but it is unclear if this is the only isoform responsible for elimination. MDMA has a chiral center, and the drug usually is taken as the racemate.

Biodisposition of MDMA is both stereoselective and nonlinear. The S-enantiomer (which is thought to be the psychopharmacologically active) has a more rapid clearance and a shorter half-life than the R-enantiomer. If users take repeated, closely spaced doses of MDMA in pursuit of the effects of the S-enantiomer, accumulation of the R-enantiomer may occur.

Biodisposition is nonlinear, with MDMA appearing to inhibit its own metabolism. Therefore, small increases in the dose of MDMA can produce large increases in plasma concentration. Thus, stereoselective and nonlinear kinetics may contribute to the toxicity of MDMA.

ADDICTION LIABILITY

Although MDMA is widely abused, reports of dependence and addiction have been relatively rare. However, recent data suggest that MDMA dependence may become a significant public health issue. For example, in a survey of Australian polydrug users, 35% had used MDMA in a binge pattern (defined as three days' consecutive use without sleep), 42% reported Ecstasy-related occupational impairments, and 15% sought treatment for Ecstasy-related problems.

The withdrawal syndrome for MDMA is not well defined, but probably is similar to that seen with amphetamines and cocaine. Finally, MDMA overdoses are well documented and have been associated with a wide range of morbidities, including death.

TOXICITY/ADVERSE EFFECTS

In animal species, from rodents to primates, MDMA produces a lifelong depletion of serotonergic axons (but not their cell bodies). The loss of axons can be substantial and has functional consequences, with up to 80% depletions in levels of brain serotonin, 5-HIAA (the primary serotonin metabolite), and tryptophan hydroxlase (the enzyme that synthesizes serotonin). Despite these profound neurotoxic effects, there are no detectable behavioral abnormalities in these animals. The cause of the neurotoxicity is unclear, but it may be due to a reactive metabolite of MDMA or neuronal energy exhaustion induced by the drug. There is no easy explanation for the discordance between anatomical and neurochemical findings and the observed behavior, but perhaps this is because the serotonergic cell bodies are spared or the available behavioral measures are relatively insensitive to serotonin depletion.

In humans, studies have shown that MDMA use is associated with behavioral changes that include increased depression, anxiety, anger, hostility, impulsiveness, and sensation- and novelty-seeking. These changes are subtle and may precede MDMA use. They are seen only with sophisticated neuropsychological testing, but they are accompanied by alterations in serotonergic functioning as measured with PET scanning. Despite this worrisome data, to date there are no obvious impairments in regular or casual MDMA users, and most individuals who have tried MDMA seem to lead fairly normal lives.

The controversy over neurotoxicity really is about the future. If subtle but measurable behavioral changes occur in young MDMA users and the serotonergic "axotomy" induced by MDMA is lifelong, what will happen as the users age? Will there be more depression and earlier dementia in MDMA users? Currently, authoritative answers to these questions do not exist, but form the basis of many investigators' serious concerns about MDMA use and abuse.

MDMA dramatically increases heart rate, blood pressure, and myocardial oxygen consumption but, in general, these effects are well tolerated by the predominantly young drug users. One important difference between the effects of MDMA and endogenous sympathetic stimulation of the heart is that MDMA does not increase inotropy; for a given heart rate and blood pressure, MDMA produces more wall stress (and oxygen consumption) than exercise or intravenous infusions of dobutamine. The lack of inotropy may result in imbalances between myocardial oxygen supply and demand and thus could be responsible for some of the puzzling cardiovascular catastrophes associated with MDMA use.

In laboratory studies and in surveys of users, MDMA produces pleasurable, even potentially beneficial effects, including increased perceived closeness to others, empathy, and insight. Unfortunately, even if MDMA has some salutary effects, it produces a host of toxic events. However, the severity and persistence of these events are yet to be determined; this clearly is an important topic for future research. The increasing popularity of the drug suggests that addiction, dependence, and long-term consequences will emerge and require a medical response. Clinicians should familiarize themselves with this agent in expectation of future problems.

REFERENCES

Cami J, Farre M, Mas M et al. (2000). Human pharmacology of 3,4-methylenedioxymethamphetamine ("ecstasy"): Psychomotor performance and subjective effects. *Journal of Clinical Psychopharmacology* 20:455-466.

Harris D, Baggott M, Mendelson JH et al. (in press, 2002). Psychological and hormonal effects of 3,4-Methylenedioxymethamphetamine (MDMA) in humans. *Psychopharmacology*.

Johnston LD, O'Malley PM & Bachman JG (2001). *Monitoring the Future: National Survey Results on Drug Use, 1975-2000. Volume I: Secondary School Students.* Bethesda, MD: National Institute on Drug Abuse.

Lester SJ, Baggott M, Welm S et al. (2000). Cardiovascular effects of 3,4-methylenedioxymethamphetamine. A double-blind, placebo-controlled trial. *Annals of Internal Medicine* 133:969-973.

Topp L, Hando J, Dillon P et al. (1999). Ecstasy use in Australia: Patterns of use and associated harm. *Drug and Alcohol Dependence* June 1;55(1-2):105-115.

Vollenweider FX, Gamma A, Liechti M et al. (1998). Psychological and cardiovascular effects and short-term sequelae of MDMA ("Ecstasy") in MDMA-naive healthy volunteers [see comments]. *Neuropsychopharmacology* 19:241-251.

| Chapter 6 | # Caffeine: Pharmacology and Clinical Effects |

Roland R. Griffiths, Ph.D.
Laura M. Juliano, Ph.D.
Allison L. Chausmer, Ph.D.

Drugs in the Class
Absorption and Metabolism
Mechanisms of Action
Effects on Major Organ Systems
Behavioral Effects in Animals
Effects on Human Performance
Subjective Effects
Discriminative Stimulus Effects
Reinforcing Effects

Caffeine Tolerance
Caffeine Intoxication
Anxiety and Caffeine
Sleep and Caffeine
Caffeine Withdrawal
Caffeine Dependence
Heritability of Caffeine Use Problems
Associations With Other Drugs of Dependence
Clinical Implications and Treatment
Addiction Liability

Caffeine, which is a member of the methylxanthine class of alkaloids, is the most widely used mood-altering drug in the world. More than 60 species of caffeine-containing plants have been identified. The most widely consumed are coffee, tea, cola nut, cocao pod, guarana, and maté (Gilbert, 1984).

DRUGS IN THE CLASS

Caffeine is the common name for 1,3,7-trimethylxanthine (Figure 1). The structurally related dimethylxanthines, theophylline and theobromine, also are found in a variety of plants. Caffeine is a weakly basic alkaloid. The free base is a bitter white powder that is moderately soluble in water (21.7 mg/ml) (Budavari, O'Neil et al., 1996).

Clinically available pharmaceutical preparations of caffeine include caffeine anhydrous, caffeine sodium benzoate, and citrated caffeine.

Common Sources of Caffeine. Table 1 shows the range of caffeine content in common foods and medications, as well as estimated "typical" caffeine content of these products. Of the three major dietary sources of caffeine, servings of tea and soft drinks usually contain about one-half to one-third the amount of caffeine in a serving of coffee.

A significant problem in estimating caffeine exposure occurs because of the wide differences in the amount of caffeine delivered in common foods, as well as significant differences in common serving sizes (cf. Table 1). For example, the amount of caffeine in a serving of coffee may vary over a 10-fold range, from as little as 20 mg for a small 5-ounce cup of instant coffee to 300 mg for a large 12-ounce cup of strong drip coffee. A similar 10-fold variation may occur with soft drinks, with a small glass of one of the weaker cola drinks containing as little as 12 mg of caffeine, in con-

FIGURE 1. The Chemical Structure of Caffeine

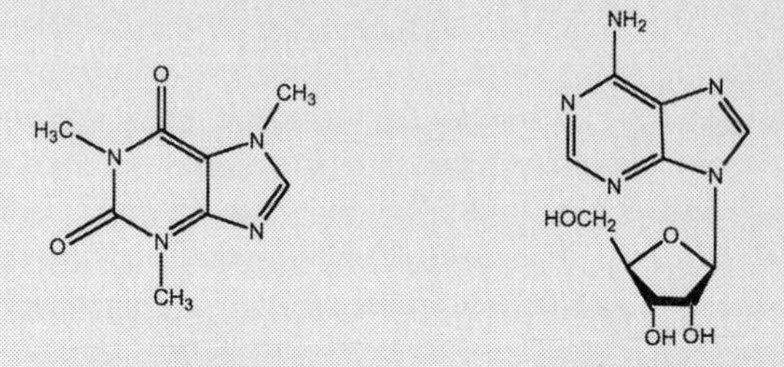

CAFFEINE
(an adenosine receptor antagonist)

ADENOSINE
(an endogenous neuromodulator)

The chemical structures of caffeine (1,3,7-trimethylxanthine) and adenosine. Adenosine is an endogenous neuromodulator that has structural similarities to caffeine. Most of the physiological effects of caffeine, including the CNS stimulant effects, probably are mediated through adenosine receptor antagonism.

trast to about 120 mg from a 20-ounce bottle of one of the stronger colas.

Although most people are aware that coffee, tea, and most cola beverages contain caffeine, there are several sources of caffeine about which there is less awareness. In the United States, about 70% of all soft drinks consumed contain caffeine (Beverage Digest Company, 1999). A number of non-cola drinks (such as root beer, orange soda, cream soda, and lemon-lime drinks) contain caffeine in amounts similar to those in the cola drinks. Some, but not all, coffee ice creams and yogurts deliver a significant dose of caffeine. Although chocolate milk, cocoa, and milk chocolate candy also contain caffeine, the dose delivered in a usual serving generally is below the threshold for readily detectable mood and behavioral effects (<10 mg). The one exception is that a serving of dark or bitter chocolate candy may contain about 30 mg of caffeine.

Popular over-the-counter (OTC) medications containing caffeine include the stimulants NoDoz® (100 and 200 mg/tablet) and Vivarin® (200 mg/tablet); the analgesics Excedrin® (130 mg/2 tablets), Anacin® (64 mg/2 tablets), and Midol Menstrual® (120 mg/2 tablets); and the weight-loss supplements Metabolife 365® (80 mg/2 tablets) and Diet Fuel® (200mg/3 capsules).

History. Cultivation of tea in China, coffee in Ethiopia, and cocoa pod in South America date back to time immemorial (Hattox, 1985; Weinberg & Bealer, 2001). Recorded use of tea dates back at least 2,000 years in China (Hara, Luo et al., 1995). About 600 years ago, the use of coffee spread from Ethiopia to Yemen (Hattox, 1985), and about 500 years ago, the use of cocao spread from Mexico to Spain (Weinberg & Bealer, 2001). With the development of world trade in the 17th and 18th centuries, the use of caffeinated foods spread rapidly from their points of geographic origin, despite unsuccessful attempts to restrict or eliminate the use of these caffeine-containing foods, based on economic, religious, medical, or political grounds (Austin, 1979; Pendergrast, 1999; Weinberg & Bealer, 2001).

Although difficult to imagine in the context of the present culture, in which caffeine products are widely and freely used, the ancient spread of caffeinated foods and the substantial economic and social effects they engendered have many parallels in the contemporary growth of the international trade in cocaine. Numerous failed efforts to eliminate the use of caffeine-containing foods have been documented worldwide (in Arabia, Turkey, England, France, and Prussia, among others). In America, the protest of a British tax on tea became a symbolic focal point for revolution, resulting in the famous "Boston tea party," during which containers of tea were thrown into the Boston harbor in 1773. In the aftermath, the Continental Congress passed a resolution against tea consumption and, over the course of a few years, America was transformed from a predominantly tea-drinking society to one in which coffee was the caffeinated beverage of choice (Pendergrast, 1999).

Coffee has become a major agricultural import into the United States, second only after oil in the total value of imported goods (Gilbert, 1984). In addition to the wide availability of coffee and tea, the last 100 years have seen the development of flavored carbonated beverages ("soft drinks") as a commercially successful alternative for the delivery of caffeine (Pendergrast, 1993).

Epidemiology. Today, consumption of caffeine is almost universal, with only alcohol consumption coming close in popularity (Gilbert, 1984). Dietary survey studies in North America indicate that weekly or more frequent consumption of caffeine-containing foods occurs in 80% to 90% of children and adults (Gilbert, 1984; Hughes & Oliveto, 1997). Figure 2 depicts recent trends in annual per capita consumption of the three major sources of dietary caffeine in the United States: coffee, tea, and soft drinks. Over the 31 years shown, consumption of carbonated soft drinks has more than doubled, increasing from 24 to 49 gallons per capita, while coffee consumption decreased by 25%, from

TABLE 1.   Typical Caffeine Content of Common Foods and Medications

Substance	Serving Size (volume or weight)	Caffeine Content (range)	Caffeine Content (typical)
Coffee			
Brewed/Drip	6 oz	77-150 mg	100 mg
Instant	6 oz	20-130 mg	70 mg
Espresso	1 oz	30-50 mg	40 mg
Decaffeinated	6 oz	2-9 mg	4 mg
Tea			
Brewed	6 oz	30-90 mg	40 mg
Instant	6 oz	10-35 mg	30 mg
Canned or Bottled	12 oz	8-32 mg	20 mg
Caffeinated Soft Drinks	12 oz	22-71 mg	40 mg
Caffeinated Water	16.9 oz	50-125 mg	100 mg
Cocoa/Hot Chocolate	6 oz	2-10 mg	7 mg
Chocolate Milk	6 oz	2-7 mg	4 mg
Coffee Ice Cream or Yogurt	1 cup (8 oz)	8-85 mg	50 mg
Chocolate Bar			
Milk Chocolate	1.5 oz	2-10 mg	10 mg
Dark Chocolate	1.5 oz	5-35 mg	30 mg
Caffeinated Gum	1 stick	50 mg	50 mg
Caffeine-Containing OTC Products			
Analgesics	2 tablets	64-130 mg	64 or 130 mg
Stimulants	1 tablet	75-350 mg	100 or 200 mg
Weight-loss Products	2-3 tablets	80-200 mg	80-200 mg
Sports Nutrition	2 tablets	200 mg	200 mg

1 fluid oz = 30 ml; 1 oz weight = 28 g; Serving sizes are based on commonly consumed portions, typical container sizes, or pharmaceutical instructions.

SOURCES: Data are from Barone & Roberts (1996), Carriollo & Benitez (2000), Amurol Confections Company (personal communication) and the web sites for the National Soft Drink Association (2001), National Coffee Association (2001), Center for Science and the Public Interest (2001), Hershey Foods (2001), Lindt & Sprüngli AG (2001), and Twinlab Corporation (2001).

33 to 26 gallons per person. Tea consumption increased only modestly over this time period. A survey of the general population showed that the prevalence of weekly use of coffee, soft drinks, and tea was 62%, 47%, and 24%, respectively (Hughes & Oliveto, 1997). Among those who had ever used caffeine, 14% had stopped caffeine use altogether, citing concern about health and unpleasant side effects.

Mean daily intake of caffeine for adult consumers in the United States has been estimated to be about 280 mg, with higher intakes estimated for consumers in the United Kingdom and Denmark (Barone & Roberts, 1996).

Therapeutic Uses. As a mild central nervous system (CNS) stimulant, caffeine is widely used to restore behavior that has been degraded by fatigue (Penetar, McCann et al., 1994; Patat, Rosenzweig et al., 2000). Caffeine also is commonly used in the treatment of pain of various origins (cf. Sawynok, 1995; James, 1997). Not surprisingly, caffeine alone is the most effective treatment for caffeine withdrawal headache (Dreisbach & Pfeiffer, 1943; Griffiths & Woodson, 1988a), with prophylactic caffeine administration recognized as an effective treatment for post-surgical withdrawal headaches (Fennelly, Galletly et al., 1991; Nikolajsen, Larsen et al., 1994; Hampl, Schneider et al., 1995). Caffeine also is used in the treatment of post-dural puncture headache following lumbar puncture or spinal anesthesia, although its efficacy may be due in part to suppression of caffeine withdrawal (James, 1997; Yucel, Ozyalcin et al., 1999). Caffeine in combination with ergotamine is used in treatment of migraine headache (Sawynok, 1995). Finally, because evidence suggests that caffeine functions as an analgesic adjuvant (Laska, Sunshine et al., 1984), it is combined with commonly used analgesics such as aspirin and acetaminophen in a wide range of OTC and prescription analgesic products.

Administered intravenously or orally, caffeine is efficacious as a respiratory stimulant in treating apnea in neonates and infants (James, 1997; Tobias, 2000). Intravenous caffeine has been administered prior to electroconvulsive therapy (ECT) for the treatment of severe depression and other serious psychiatric disorders (James, 1997). Although caffeine has been shown to lengthen the duration of seizures, the therapeutic merits of caffeine augmentation of ECT are unclear (Rosenquist, McCall et al., 1994; Kelsey & Grossberg, 1995). Because caffeine is known to have both lipolytic and thermogenic effects, it sometimes is used for weight loss. Modest effects of caffeine-ephedrine combinations on weight loss appear to be greater than the effects of either drug alone (James, 1997). Caffeine has been used to prevent postprandial reductions in blood pressure in elderly persons (Hesseltine, el-Jabri et al., 1991), although studies have questioned the clinical relevance of this effect (Lipsitz, Jansen et al., 1994). Because caffeine is ergogenic and has been shown to increase speed and/or power output in simulated race conditions, it often is used to facilitate athletic performance (Graham, 2001).

ABSORPTION AND METABOLISM

Routes of Administration. By far the most common route of administration of caffeine is oral. Caffeine sometimes is

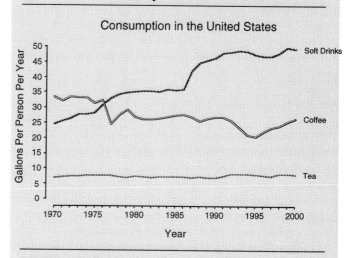

FIGURE 2. Annual Per Capita Consumption in the U.S. of the Three Major Dietary Sources of Caffeine

SOURCE: U.S. Department of Agriculture, 2002.

Annual per capita consumption in the U.S. of the three major dietary sources of caffeine: coffee, tea, and soft drinks (that is, flavored carbonated beverages).

administered intravenously in the treatment of post-surgical headache, neonatal apnea, and to enhance electroconvulsive therapy. Caffeine in combination with ergotamine also sometimes is administered rectally via suppository (Caferot®) for the treatment of migraine headaches. Topical administration of caffeine has been used in neonates (Amato, Isenschmid et al., 1991).

Absorption and Distribution. Caffeine is rapidly and completely absorbed after oral administration, with peak levels reached in 30 to 45 minutes (Mumford, Benowitz et al., 1996; Liguori, Hughes et al., 1997b). Caffeine absorption from soft drinks containing sugar and from chocolate may be somewhat slower, with peak levels attained at 60 to 120 minutes (Marks & Kelly, 1973; Mumford, Benowitz et al., 1996; Liguori, Hughes et al., 1997b). Caffeine is readily distributed throughout the body, with concentrations in blood correlating strongly with those in saliva, breast milk, amniotic fluid, fetal tissue, semen, and the brain (James, 1997). Binding to plasma proteins is estimated to range between 10% and 35% (Denaro & Benowitz, 1991). Caffeine concentrations in saliva, which often exceed 75% of plasma concentrations (Cook, Tallent et al., 1976; Zylber-

Katz, Granit et al., 1984) are used as a noninvasive alternative to serum monitoring.

Metabolism. Caffeine metabolism is complex, with more than 25 metabolites identified in humans (Carrillo & Benitez, 2000). The primary metabolic pathways involve the P-450 liver enzyme system, which is responsible for the demethylation of caffeine to three biologically active dimethylxanthines: paraxanthine, theobromine, and theophylline, which account for 80%, 10%, and 4% of caffeine metabolism, respectively (Denaro & Benowitz, 1991). The large amounts of paraxanthine, coupled with the demonstration of similar sympathomimetic effects of paraxanthine and caffeine (Benowitz, Jacob et al., 1995), suggest that paraxanthine needs to be considered in understanding the clinical pharmacology of caffeine. Substantial differences between species in primary metabolic pathways and in rates of elimination underscore the need for caution when generalizing findings from animal studies to humans (Bonati, Latini et al., 1985).

Individual Differences in Caffeine Elimination. On average, caffeine half-life is four to six hours; however, there are wide individual differences in rates of caffeine elimination, with half-lives varying more than 10-fold in healthy subjects (Denaro & Benowitz, 1991). An important implication of the central role of P450 in metabolizing caffeine is that drugs or conditions that affect this metabolic system also significantly alter caffeine elimination. Caffeine's half-life is prolonged by liver disease (Denaro & Benowitz, 1991). Although caffeine half-life does not differ between younger and older adults (Blanchard & Sawers, 1983), caffeine half-life is markedly increased in premature and full-term newborns (in whom the half-life is 80 to 100 hours) because liver enzyme capacity is not completely developed until about six months of age (Aranda, Cook et al., 1979; Parsons & Neims, 1981). Cigarette smoking, which induces liver enzymes, decreases caffeine half-life by as much as 50% (Parsons & Neims, 1978; May, Jarboe et al., 1982).

Numerous compounds have been shown to inhibit caffeine metabolism, including high doses of caffeine itself, oral contraceptive steroids, cimetidine, some quinoline antibiotics, fluvoxamine, and mexiletine (Denaro, Brown et al., 1990; Carrillo & Benitez, 2000). Caffeine inhibits the metabolism of the antipsychotic clozapine and the bronchodilator theophylline to an extent that might be clinically significant (Carrillo & Benitez, 2000; Hagg, Spigset et al., 2000). Caffeine half-life increases markedly toward the end of pregnancy (Aldridge, Bailey et al., 1981).

MECHANISMS OF ACTION

Molecular Sites of Action. Three primary sites of action for caffeine have been proposed: mobilization of calcium, inhibition of phosphodiesterase activity, and blockade of adenosine receptors (Daly, 1993). There are data suggesting that some of the cardiac and respiratory effects of caffeine may be mediated by inhibition of phosphodiesterase (Daly, 1993; Howell, 1993; Howell & Landrum, 1997). However, intracellular calcium release and inhibition of phosphodiesterase generally occur at caffeine concentrations considerably above those attained during usual human caffeine consumption. In contrast, adenosine antagonism occurs at physiologically relevant concentrations. These observations have led increasingly to the conclusion that antagonism of adenosine receptors is the primary cellular mechanism underlying most of the physiological effects of caffeine, including its centrally mediated mood- and performance-stimulating effects (Daly, 1993; Fredholm, Bättig et al., 1999).

Competitive Antagonism of Adenosine Receptors. Caffeine, which is structurally related to adenosine (Figure 1), is a competitive antagonist at A_1 and A_{2A} receptors, which are tonically activated at basal adenosine concentrations (Fredholm, Bättig et al., 1999). Thus, caffeine produces a range of central and peripheral effects that are opposite those of adenosine. For example, in the central nervous system, adenosine decreases spontaneous electrical activity, inhibits neurotransmitter release, has anticonvulsant activity, and depresses locomotor activity and operant response rates. In the periphery, adenosine constricts bronchial smooth muscle, produces negative inotropic/chronotropic effects on the heart, and inhibits lipolysis, renin release, and gastric secretions. All of these effects are opposite those that are produced by caffeine (Daly, 1993; Garrett & Griffiths, 1997). Moreover, the behavioral stimulant effects of caffeine in rodents and non-human primates correlate with caffeine's ability to antagonize adenosine receptors (Snyder, Katims et al., 1981; Howell, Coffin et al., 1997). These stimulant effects are abolished in A_{2A} receptor knock-out mice (El Yacoubi, Ledent et al., 2000), suggesting that adenosine receptor antagonism plays a critical role in the stimulant effects of caffeine.

Effects on Neurotransmitters. Preclinical studies have shown that caffeine affects turnover or levels of a range of neurotransmitters in the central nervous system; such neurotransmitters include norepinephrine, dopamine, serotonin, acetylcholine, GABA, and glutamate (Shi, Nikodijevic et al., 1993; Daly, 1993). A probable mechanism for some of these effects is that caffeine blocks basal levels of adenosine at A_1 receptors, which tonically inhibit neurotransmitter release (Daly, 1993). The release of norepinephrine, in particular, has been suggested as a mechanism underlying caffeine's stimulant effects (Daly, 1993), and some data suggest that the discriminative effects of caffeine are mediated in part by an alpha adrenergic mechanism (Holtzman, 1986).

Dopaminergic Effects. Considerable evidence suggests that some of the behavioral effects of caffeine are mediated by dopaminergic mechanisms. It is well established that caffeine enhances dopaminergic activity by competitive antagonism of A_{2A}, and possibly A_1, receptors that are co-localized and functionally interact with dopamine receptors (Fredholm, Bättig et al., 1999). As a competitive antagonist at adenosine receptors, caffeine is believed to produce its stimulant behavioral effects by removing the negative modulatory effects of adenosine from dopamine receptors, thus stimulating dopaminergic activity. Evidence for this mechanism is particularly compelling for blockade of A_{2A} receptors in the striatum (Fredholm, Bättig et al., 1999).

Consistent with the *in vitro* data, preclinical behavioral studies show that caffeine produces behavioral effects similar to classic dopaminergically mediated stimulants such as cocaine and amphetamine, including increased locomotor activity, increased rotational behavior in 6-hydroxydopamine lesioned rats, stimulant-like discriminative stimulus effects, and self-injection. Moreover, caffeine potentiates the effects of dopaminergically mediated drugs on locomotor activity, rotational behavior, drug discrimination, and self-injection. Finally, some of caffeine's effects on these behaviors can be blocked by dopamine receptor antagonists (Garrett & Griffiths, 1997; Fredholm, Bättig et al., 1999; Powell, Koppelman et al., 1999; Green & Schenk, 2002).

EFFECTS ON MAJOR ORGAN SYSTEMS

Cardiovascular. At moderate dietary dose levels, caffeine produces increases in blood pressure and tends to have no effect on or to reduce heart rate in humans (Rush, Sullivan et al., 1995; James, 1997). Although the magnitude of caffeine-induced blood pressure increases is small, some recent studies suggest that it may be clinically significant in individuals with borderline hypertension (James, 1997; Nurminen, Niittynen et al., 1999; Hartley, Sung et al., 2000; Lovallo, al'Absi et al., 2000). Coffee has been shown to contain lipids that significantly raise total and LDL cholesterol levels in humans. Decaffeination does not remove these lipids. Although paper-filtered and instant coffee contain low levels of the lipids, high levels are delivered in espresso, French press, mocha, Turkish, and boiled coffee (Urgert & Katan, 1997).

Gastrointestinal. Caffeine stimulates gastric acid secretion (Cohen & Booth, 1975), although the exacerbation of gastroesophageal reflux by coffee probably is due to coffee constituents other than caffeine (Wendl, Pfeiffer et al., 1994). Caffeine is a colonic stimulant, with caffeinated coffee producing colonic motor activity stimulation similar to that produced by a meal (Rao, Welcher et al., 1998).

Renal and Urinary. Caffeine is a diuretic, increasing urine volume 30% or more for several hours after ingestion (Wemple, Lamb et al., 1997). Caffeine also has been shown to increase detrusor pressure on the bladder in patients with complaints of urinary urgency and confirmed detrusor instability (Creighton & Stanton, 1990). Chronic caffeine consumption has been shown to contribute to urinary incontinence in psychogeriatric patients (James, Sawczuk et al., 1989). Lithium toxicity may occur after caffeine withdrawal due to decreased renal clearance of lithium (Carrillo & Benitez, 2000).

Respiratory. Like theophylline, caffeine is a bronchodilator at high doses (Becker, Simons et al., 1984; Duffy & Phillips, 1991). Caffeine also is a respiratory stimulant (Pianosi, Grondin et al., 1994), a characteristic that has been used therapeutically in the treatment of apnea in neonates and infants (James, 1997; Tobias, 2000).

Musculoskeletal. Caffeine is ergogenic in most exercise situations, with activity mediated by various mechanisms, including effects on muscle contractility (Tarnopolsky & Cupido, 2000).

Hormonal. Caffeine increases plasma epinephrine, norepinephrine, renin, and free fatty acids, particularly in nontolerant individuals (Patwardhan, Desmond et al., 1980; Robertson, Wade et al., 1981; Benowitz, Jacob et al., 1995). Caffeine also has been shown to increase ACTH and cortisol (Lovallo, al'Absi et al., 1996; Lin, Uhde et al., 1997; al'Absi, Lovallo et al., 1998).

Reproductive. Although the physiological mechanism is not clear, recent studies and a meta-analysis of previous studies suggest that maternal caffeine use increases the rate of spontaneous abortion (James, 1997; Fernandes, Sabharwal et al., 1998; Klebanoff, Levine et al., 1999; Cnattingius, Signorello et al., 2000; Wen, Shu et al., 2001).

BEHAVIORAL EFFECTS IN ANIMALS

Stimulant Motor Activity. Acute caffeine produces biphasic effects on spontaneous motor activity in rodents, with moderate doses (for example, 10 to 30 mg/kg) increasing, and higher doses decreasing, overall activity. A similar inverted U-shaped function is shown on rotational behavior in rodents (Garrett & Holtzman, 1994, 1996; Fredholm, Bättig et al., 1999). Caffeine potentiates the stimulatory effects of psychomotor stimulants on motor activity and rotational behavior (Garrett & Griffiths, 1997; Gasior, Jaszyna et al., 2000).

Drug Discrimination. Drug discrimination procedures in animals provide information analogous to subjective effect measures in humans. In the discrimination paradigm, animals typically are trained to make one response after administration of drug (such as caffeine) and another response after administration of vehicle. The extent to which a novel drug occasions drug-appropriate responding (that is, generalization) provides a measure of the similarity between the training stimulus and the test stimulus. As with motor activity, the discriminative dose effects of caffeine are biphasic. Stimulant drugs such as cocaine and d-amphetamine occasion responding in animals trained to low and moderate doses of caffeine (10 to 30 mg/kg) (Holtzman, 1986; Mumford & Holtzman, 1991).

Although caffeine does not usually occasion drug-appropriate responding in animals trained with other behavioral stimulants alone, caffeine potentiates the discriminative effects of subthreshold doses of the training drug in cocaine and amphetamine-trained rats (Garrett & Griffiths, 1997). The discriminative stimulus effects of high caffeine doses appear to be qualitatively different than the discriminative stimulus effects of low caffeine training doses, with only theophylline occasioning drug-appropriate responding (Mumford & Holtzman, 1991).

Reinforcement. The reinforcing efficacy of a drug refers to the relative effectiveness in establishing or maintaining drug self-administration behavior. Intravenous drug self-injection in laboratory animals is often regarded as providing the most direct and unequivocal assessment of a drug's reinforcing effect. With this procedure, animals are given access to a lever, responding on which results in a drug injection. The ability of the injection to reinforce behavior is assessed by examining the establishment or maintenance of responding. Eight of 10 studies that have examined caffeine self-injection have demonstrated that caffeine can function as a reinforcer (cf. Griffiths & Mumford, 1995;

Fredholm, Bättig et al., 1999). Most of these studies demonstrated caffeine self-injection in all animals; however, some studies showed that only a subset of animals (25% to 33%) self-injected caffeine. A sporadic pattern of caffeine self-injection, which is characterized by periods of relatively high rates of intake alternating irregularly with periods of low intake, has been reported in three studies with nonhuman primates which examined self-injection over an extended period of consecutive days (Deneau, Yanigita et al., 1969; Griffiths, Brady et al., 1979; Griffiths & Mumford, 1995). These intravenous self-injection studies show that caffeine can function as a reinforcer under some conditions. However, the inconsistent results across animals and studies contrast with the results reported with the classic abused stimulants (such as amphetamine and cocaine), which have more consistently been shown to maintain intravenous self-injection across a wide range of species and conditions (Griffiths, Brady et al., 1979).

The variation in results with caffeine is analogous to that which has been reported in self-injection studies with nicotine: nicotine has not reliably maintained self-injection across animals and studies (Goldberg & Henningfield, 1988; Dworkin, Vrana et al., 1993).

Conditioned place preference procedures provide an indirect approach to assessing the reinforcing effects of drugs. With this procedure, animals initially are administered a drug when confined in a distinctive compartment. During subsequent testing, when animals may move between compartments, the relative time spent in the drug-paired compartment provides an indirect measure of reinforcing effect. Studies in rats have shown that low doses of caffeine produce conditioned place preference, while higher doses produce clear place avoidance (Brockwell, Eikelboom et al., 1991; Patkina & Zvartau, 1998; Bedingfield, King et al., 1998). These biphasic dose effects of caffeine are similar to the biphasic effects on other preclinical and clinical measures. Similar to the self-injection data, a direct comparison of place preference between caffeine and cocaine suggests that cocaine has greater reinforcing effects (Patkina & Zvartau, 1998).

As with preclinical data on locomotor and discriminative performance, there is evidence from studies of drug reinforcement that caffeine increases the effects of dopaminergically mediated stimulants. Low doses of caffeine and cocaine produced additive effects on measures of conditioned place preference (Bedingfield, King et al., 1998). Intravenous self-injection studies show that caffeine increases low rates of cocaine self-injection, enhances the rate of acquisition of cocaine self-injection, and reinstates previous cocaine self-administration behavior (Comer & Carroll, 1996; Fredholm, Bättig et al., 1999; Schenk & Partridge, 1999; Kuzmin, Johansson et al., 1999, 2000). Whether such caffeine-induced enhancements reflect interactions with cocaine reinforcement *per se* is unclear (Kuzmin, Johansson et al., 2000).

Tolerance. Tolerance refers to an acquired change in responsiveness of an individual as a result of exposure to drug, such that an increased dose of drug is necessary to produce the same degree of response, or that less effect is produced by the same dose of drug. Seventeen studies have demonstrated the development of caffeine tolerance across different species (such as mice, rats, and monkeys) and a wide range of experimental measures (for example, locomotor activity, schedule-controlled responding, reinforcement thresholds for electrical brain stimulation, caffeine-induced seizure thresholds, and discriminative responding in caffeine-trained animals) (cf. Griffiths & Mumford, 1996; Fredholm, Bättig et al., 1999; Powell, Iuvone et al., 2001).

Caffeine tolerance has been most widely studied with regard to its locomotor stimulant effect in rats. Studies have shown that such tolerance is rapid, usually insurmountable, and exhibits cross-tolerance to other methylxanthines, but not to other nonmethylxanthine psychomotor stimulants such as *d*-amphetamine and methylphenidate (Holtzman, 1983; Finn & Holtzman, 1987, 1988; Holtzman & Finn, 1988).

Tolerance to other effects of caffeine (such as the discriminative stimulus effects) may develop more slowly, suggesting that different mechanisms may be operative for different behaviors (Holtzman & Finn, 1988). Although changes in various neurotransmitter receptors have been demonstrated following chronic caffeine administration, the neurochemical mechanism(s) underlying caffeine tolerance remain unclear (Shi, Nikodijevic et al., 1993; Holtzman, Mante et al., 1991; Johansson, Georgiev et al., 1997; Fredholm, Bättig et al., 1999; Powell, Iuvone et al., 2001).

Physical Dependence. Physical dependence is manifested by time-limited biochemical, physiological and behavioral disruptions (that is, a withdrawal syndrome) on termination of chronic or repeated drug administration. Of the 11 reports of caffeine withdrawal in laboratory animals (mice, rats, cats, and monkeys) (cf. Griffiths & Mumford, 1996; Fredholm, Bättig et al., 1999), most have documented substantial behavioral disruptions following cessation of chronic caffeine dosing (for example, 50% to 80% reductions in spontaneous locomotor activity, or 20% to 50% reductions in operant responding). Similar to human studies, the severity of withdrawal in laboratory animals is a function of the caffeine maintenance dose, with maximal withdrawal effects occurring on the first or second day of caffeine withdrawal (Holtzman, 1983; Finn & Holtzman, 1986). It has been speculated—and there is some evidence to support the notion—that increased functional tissue sensitivity to endogenous adenosine is the mechanism underlying some caffeine withdrawal effects (von Borstel, Wurtman et al., 1983; Hirsh, 1984; Ahlijanian & Takemori, 1986).

EFFECTS ON HUMAN PERFORMANCE

A large number of studies have examined the effects of caffeine on human performance. The most consistent generality to emerge is that caffeine reliably reduces decrements in performances on a variety of tasks when those decrements are the result of reduced alertness (for example, under conditions of sleep deprivation, fatigue, or prolonged vigilance) (cf. Weiss & Laties, 1962; James, 1997; van der Stelt & Snel, 1998). Results of most studies of caffeine on performance have been quite inconsistent.

Typically, studies have compared the effects of caffeine and placebo on performance of subjects who abstained from caffeine, usually overnight. Although the results are variable (James, 1997; van der Stelt & Snel, 1998), authors have reported that, compared to placebo, caffeine may improve reaction time, tapping speed, vigilance, attention, and psychomotor performance (Rogers & Dernoncourt, 1998). Likewise, a growing literature on the effects of caffeine on exercise performance suggests that, relative to placebo, caffeine can increase endurance for long-term (30 to 60 minutes) exercise and can improve speed and/or power output in simulated race conditions (Spriet, 1995; Graham, 2001).

A dilemma in interpreting the effects of caffeine on performance is that almost all of these studies have been confounded by caffeine withdrawal. Thus, improvements in performance after caffeine relative to placebo may simply reflect a restoration of deficits caused by withdrawal (James, 1997; Rogers & Dernoncourt, 1998; Rogers, 2000). Although some investigators recently have attempted to address this issue (Warburton, 1995; Smith, 1998), an unequivocal study should involve biologically verified caffeine abstinence for at least a week before testing (James, 1997).

The only study to include such a condition showed performance decrements during acute abstinence, but failed to demonstrate performance benefits of caffeine (James, 1998). Based on the preclinical literature, which clearly documents the behavioral stimulant effects of caffeine, it seems quite likely that caffeine will be shown to enhance human performance on some types of tasks in non-tolerant individuals. However, at present it is not clear to what extent performance enhancement commonly perceived and reported by regular caffeine consumers after their first morning dose of caffeine is due to true improvement over caffeine-free baseline levels, compared to a caffeine-induced restoration of performance that has been degraded by caffeine withdrawal after overnight abstinence.

SUBJECTIVE EFFECTS IN HUMANS

"Subjective effects" refer to drug-induced changes in an individual's experiences or feelings that cannot be measured directly by an observer. Subjective effects most often are assessed via self-report instruments that are given after double-blind administration of drug. Many human laboratory studies on caffeine have included questionnaires pertaining to caffeine's subjective effects, and so a substantial amount of data has been acquired across a number of caffeine vehicles (such as capsules, coffee, tea, soft drinks, and other beverages). The qualitative subjective effects of caffeine are dose-dependent, with low dietary doses producing mostly positive effects (such as increased feelings of well-being and energetic arousal) and higher doses leading to predominantly "dysphoric" effects (Griffiths & Mumford, 1995).

Positive Subjective Effects. Human laboratory studies have demonstrated that single low to moderate doses of caffeine can produce a number of positive subjective effects. Table 2 lists the various types of positive subjective effects that have been reported in 10 double-blind placebo-controlled studies with caffeine. Caffeine has been shown to result in ratings that indicate increased well-being, happiness, energetic arousal, alertness, and sociability. Although caffeine-induced positive effects have not been observed consistently across all experimental studies (James, 1997), factors that increase the likelihood of positive effects have been identified (Griffiths & Mumford, 1995). First, the positive subjective effects of caffeine most often are demonstrated at low doses, or doses in the range of typical dietary consumption (for example, 20 to 200 mg). Although there appear to be wide individual differences in sensitivity to

---

TABLE 2.   Positive Subjective Effects of Caffeine After Low to Intermediate Doses (18 to 178 mg)

- Increased sense of wellbeing
- Increased energy/active/vigor
- Increased alertness/clear headedness
- Improved concentration
- Increased self-confidence
- Increased motivation for work
- Increased desire to talk/sociability
- Decreased sleepiness
- Decreased muzzy; not clear-headed.

NOTE: Subjective dimensions significantly affected in double-blind placebo controlled studies: cf. Leathwood & Pollet, 1983; Lieberman, Wurtman et al., 1987; Griffiths, Evans et al., 1990a; Silverman & Griffiths, 1992; Mumford, Evans et al., 1994; Silverman, Mumford & Griffiths, 1994; Robelin & Rogers, 1998; Liguori, Grass & Hughes, 1999; Smit & Rogers, 2000; Watson, Lunt et al., 2000.

---

caffeine, it is clear that the dysphoric/anxiogenic subjective effects of caffeine emerge at higher doses (Chait & Griffiths, 1983; Griffiths & Woodson, 1988b). Second, most studies that have demonstrated positive subjective effects of caffeine have had participants abstain from caffeine prior to testing (often through overnight abstinence). Third, individuals or populations in which caffeine functions as a reinforcer (as demonstrated by caffeine chosen over placebo in blind choice tests) tend to report greater positive effects from caffeine (Griffiths & Mumford, 1995). Although physical dependence and withdrawal may augment the perceived pleasurable effects of caffeine, positive mood effects have been demonstrated in non-habitual users and those maintained on a caffeine-free diet, as well as under conditions of minimal deprivation (Silverman & Griffiths, 1992; Mumford, Evans et al., 1994; Silverman, Mumford et al., 1994; James, 1998).

The overall profile of positive subjective effects of low to moderate doses of caffeine is qualitatively similar to those produced by *d*-amphetamine and cocaine (including increases in energy, alertness, and sociability). Unlike *d*-amphetamine and cocaine, caffeine is more likely to produce dysphoria/anxiety with increased dose (Chait & Griffiths, 1983; Chait & Johanson, 1988).

Negative Subjective Effects. In general, acute doses of caffeine greater than 200 mg are more likely to be associated with negative subjective effects, such as increases in anxiety, nervousness, jitteriness, upset stomach, and "bad effects" (Goldstein, Kaizer et al., 1969; Evans & Griffiths, 1991; Griffiths & Mumford, 1995; Liguori, Grass et al., 1999). Individual differences in sensitivity and tolerance seem to play an important role in the likelihood and severity of negative subjective effects. Individuals with panic disorder and generalized anxiety disorder, as well as nonclinical populations with higher anxiety sensitivity, tend to be particularly sensitive to the anxiogenic effects of caffeine at high doses (Boulenger, Uhde et al., 1984; Bruce, Scott et al., 1992; Charney, Heninger et al., 1985; Telch, Silverman et al., 1996). Although high-dose subjective effects of caffeine show some overlap with the subjective effects of *d*-amphetamine, caffeine produces greater negative effects (such as anxiety) and fewer positive effects (such as positive mood) (Chait & Griffiths, 1983; Chait & Johanson, 1988). In most cases, the negative subjective effects of caffeine are relatively mild and short-lived. However, acute and/or chronic use of caffeine, especially in very high doses, can cause distress and discrete psychopathology, as discussed below.

DISCRIMINATIVE STIMULUS EFFECTS

In the drug discrimination paradigm, subjects are trained to respond differentially after administration of different drugs that are given under double-blind conditions. In the typical two-response drug-versus-placebo procedure, subjects are reinforced (usually with money) for making one response (for example, a correct verbal or written drug identification response: "I received Drug A") after double-blind administration of one drug condition on one day, and an alternative response (for example: "I received Drug B") after the other drug condition on another day. A testing phase often is instituted after discrimination training in order to determine how individuals respond to various doses of the drug or another drug (that is, was the test drug "like" or "unlike" the training dose?). In addition, subjects often are asked to report subjective effects as well as the basis on which they made the discrimination. Although the measurement of subjective effects and discriminative stimulus effects are methodologically independent operations, which theoretically could provide totally independent data, research across a range of compounds, including caffeine, has demonstrated an impressive covariation between these measures (cf. Griffiths & Mumford, 1996).

More than 80% of subjects acquired a caffeine versus placebo discrimination in the seven discrimination studies published to date (cf. Griffiths & Mumford, 1996). Doses at which the initial discrimination was acquired have ranged between 100 and 320 mg. Once acquired, the discrimination performance has been very stable over sessions.

Very low caffeine doses (<20 mg) produce discriminative and performance effects. Studies that have explicitly trained discrimination of progressively lower caffeine doses have shown that caffeine doses as low as 1.8 to 10 mg can be reliably discriminated by some subjects (Griffiths, Evans et al., 1990a; Silverman & Griffiths, 1992; Mumford, Evans et al., 1994). In those studies, 70% of subjects detected 56 mg or less, while about 35% detected 18 mg or less. Studies documenting that caffeine can produce reliable discriminative effects at very low doses are consistent with a recent study showing that 12.5 mg of caffeine produced significant increases in behavioral performance (Smit & Rogers, 2000).

Discriminative Effects of Caffeine Relative to Other Stimulant Drugs. Several drug discrimination studies demonstrate the similarities and differences between caffeine and other stimulant drugs. In one study, both caffeine and *d*-amphetamine produced dose-related increases in drug-appropriate responding in drug abusing subjects who were trained to discriminate cocaine from placebo (Oliveto, McCance-Katz et al., 1998). These findings are consistent with a previous study (Rush, Sullivan et al., 1995) of drug abusers, which showed that intravenous caffeine produced dose-related increases in the frequency of stimulant identifications (that is, like cocaine or *d*-amphetamine) on a Pharmacological Class Identification questionnaire. However, another study failed to show this effect (Garrett & Griffiths, 2001).

Other discrimination studies (Oliveto, Bickel et al., 1992, 1993) showed that the stimulants methylphenidate and theophylline tended to produce caffeine-appropriate responding in subjects trained to discriminate caffeine from placebo; in contrast, the sedative drugs triazolam and buspirone produced predominantly placebo-appropriate responding. Another study concluded that 100 and 300 mg caffeine produced dose-related partial generalization to *d*-amphetamine in subjects trained in a *d*-amphetamine versus placebo discrimination (Chait & Johanson, 1988). Despite these documented similarities in the discriminative effects of caffeine and other stimulants, one study has shown that subjects can be trained to discriminate reliably between caffeine and d-amphetamine (Heishman, Taylor et al., 1992).

REINFORCING EFFECTS

Drug reinforcement is defined by the ability of a drug to maintain drug self-administration or choice behavior. The circumstantial evidence for caffeine as a reinforcer is compelling: it is the most widely self-administered mood-altering drug in the world. Historically, repeated efforts to restrict or eliminate consumption of caffeinated foods have been completely unsuccessful. As reviewed in detail elsewhere (Griffiths & Mumford, 1995), nine blinded studies provide unequivocal evidence of the reinforcing effects of caffeine (Griffiths, Bigelow et al., 1986a, 1986b, 1989; Griffiths & Woodson, 1988b; Hughes, Higgins et al., 1991; Hughes, Hunt et al., 1992; Hughes, Oliveto et al., 1992a; Oliveto, Hughes et al., 1992; Silverman, Mumford et al., 1994).

The present section updates that review based on an additional eight recent studies that provide information about the reinforcing effects of caffeine (Evans, Critchfield et al., 1994; Mitchell, de Wit et al., 1995; Hughes, Oliveto et al., 1995; Hale, Hughes et al., 1995; Liguori, Hughes et al., 1997c; Liguori & Hughes, 1997; Schuh & Griffiths, 1997; Garrett & Griffiths, 1998). These studies demonstrated caffeine reinforcement under double-blind conditions with various subject populations (moderate and heavy adult and adolescent caffeine users; individuals with and without histories of alcohol or drug abuse), using a variety of different methodological approaches (variations on both choice and ad libitum self-administration procedures), when caffeine was available in different vehicles (coffee, soft drinks, or capsules), when subjects did and did not have immediate past histories of chronic caffeine exposure, and in the context of different behavioral requirements after drug ingestion (vigilance versus relaxation activities).

Incidence of Reinforcement. The overall incidence of caffeine reinforcement in normal caffeine users is 40% (50 of 125 subjects, based on the seven publications that provide this information) (cf. Griffiths & Woodson, 1988b; Hughes, Oliveto et al., 1993; Evans, Critchfield et al., 1994; Silverman, Mumford et al., 1994; Hale, Hughes et al., 1995; Liguori, Hughes et al., 1997c; Liguori & Hughes, 1997). A substantially higher incidence of caffeine reinforcement in normal subjects (82% and 100%) has been demonstrated

in studies that involved repeated exposure to the caffeine and placebo test conditions before reinforcement testing (Evans, Critchfield et al., 1994), or that involved repeated exposure plus the requirement that subjects engage in a vigilance task after drug administration (Silverman, Mumford et al., 1994). Subjects with histories of heavy caffeine use and abuse of alcohol or other drugs have shown a higher incidence of caffeine reinforcement (100% of 20 subjects) (Griffiths, Bigelow et al., 1986a, 1986b, 1989), compared to normal subjects (40%).

Subjective Effects Covary With Caffeine Reinforcement. Studies repeatedly have demonstrated that qualitative ratings of subjective effects have covaried with measures of reinforcement or choice (Griffiths & Mumford, 1995). An example is provided from a choice study (Evans & Griffiths, 1992), which assessed the subjective effects of placebo and caffeine on forced-exposure days preceding choice days. When the subjective effect data were retrospectively categorized into caffeine choosers and nonchoosers, a face-valid profile of changes in subjective effects emerged: (1) choosers showed "positive" subjective effects of caffeine relative to placebo (for example, increased alertness, contentedness, energy, and liking); (2) nonchoosers showed "negative" effects of caffeine relative to placebo (for example, increased anxiety, mood disturbance, or jitteriness); and (3) choosers showed "negative" effects of placebo (for example, increased headache and fatigue).

Effects of Dose on Reinforcement. Caffeine reinforcement appears to be an inverted U-shaped function of dose. Doses as low as 25 mg per cup of coffee and 33 mg per serving of soft drink have been shown to function as reinforcers when subjects could repeatedly self-administer those doses within a day (Hughes, Hunt et al., 1992; Hughes, Oliveto et al., 1995; Liguori, Hughes et al., 1997c). Doses above 50 or 100 mg tend to decrease choice or self-administration (Griffiths, Bigelow et al., 1986b; Griffiths & Woodson, 1988b; Stern, Chait et al., 1989; Hughes, Hunt et al., 1992), with relatively high doses of caffeine (for example, 400 or 600 mg) producing significant caffeine avoidance (Griffiths & Woodson, 1988b).

Physical Dependence Potentiates Reinforcement. It is clear that avoidance of abstinence-associated withdrawal symptoms plays a central role in the reinforcing effects of caffeine among regular caffeine consumers. This relationship has been shown in retrospective questionnaire studies (Goldstein & Kaizer, 1969) and in experimental studies that have used indirect (Yeomans, Spetch et al., 1998; Yeomans,

Jackson et al., 2000) and direct (Griffiths, Bigelow et al., 1986a; Hughes, Oliveto et al., 1993; Schuh & Griffiths, 1997; Liguori & Hughes, 1997; Garrett & Griffiths, 1998) behavioral measures of caffeine reinforcement. For example, Hughes and colleagues (1993) showed that moderate caffeine consumers who reported caffeine withdrawal symptoms (headache, drowsiness) after drinking decaffeinated coffee were more than twice as likely to show caffeine reinforcement. In studies that prospectively manipulated caffeine physical dependence, subjects chose caffeine more than twice as often when they were physically dependent than when they were not physically dependent (Griffiths, Bigelow et al., 1986a; Garrett & Griffiths, 1998).

Caffeine and Conditioned Flavor Preference. In addition to the studies providing direct behavioral assessments of caffeine reinforcement, a series of recent studies by Rogers and colleagues used a conditioned flavor preference paradigm to provide indirect indicators of caffeine reinforcement. In the studies, moderate consumers of caffeine were repeatedly exposed over days to a novel flavored drink paired with either caffeine or placebo. Relative to subjects who received the placebo-paired drink, subjects who received the caffeine-paired drink rated the drink as more pleasant (Richardson, Rogers et al., 1996; Yeomans, Spetch et al., 1998) or more preferred (Rogers, Richardson et al., 1995). Analysis of data over days showed that subjects who received the caffeine-paired drink significantly increased ratings of pleasantness, while subjects receiving placebo-paired drinks showed significantly decreased ratings of pleasantness (Yeomans, Spetch et al., 1998; Yeomans, Jackson et al., 2000). In the natural environment, the development of such conditioned flavor preferences over many days of self-administration seems likely to play an important role in development of strong consumer preferences for specific types or even brands of caffeine-containing beverages.

CAFFEINE TOLERANCE

"Tolerance" refers to an acquired decrease in responsiveness to a drug as the result of drug exposure. Tolerance to caffeine can be expected to vary with caffeine dose, dose frequency, number of doses, and the individual's elimination rate (Shi, Benowitz et al., 1993). As in the animal laboratory, development of tolerance to caffeine in humans has been clearly demonstrated; however, quantitative parametric information is quite fragmentary (cf. Griffiths & Mumford, 1996; Fredholm, Bättig et al., 1999). As described below, several studies have shown that, when very high doses

of caffeine (750 to 1200 mg/day throughout the day) are administered daily, "complete" tolerance (that is, caffeine effects no longer are different from baseline or placebo) can occur on some, but not all, measures. It should be noted, however, that at lower doses (similar to those usually consumed in the natural environment), complete tolerance does not occur.

Tolerance to the subjective effects of caffeine was clearly demonstrated in a study in which two groups of subjects received either caffeine (300 mg TID) or placebo (TID) for 18 consecutive days (Evans & Griffiths, 1992). During the last 14 days of chronic dosing, the caffeine and placebo groups did not differ meaningfully on ratings of mood and subjective effects. Moreover, after chronic dosing, caffeine (300 mg BID) produced significant subjective effects (including increases in ratings of tension-anxiety, jittery/nervous/shaky, active/stimulated/energetic, and strength of drug effect) in the chronic placebo group but not in the chronic caffeine group, suggesting the development of "complete" tolerance at these high doses.

Two studies provided some experimental evidence for caffeine tolerance to sleep disruption by demonstrating decreases in caffeine-induced disruption of objective measures of sleep after caffeine dosing of 250 mg BID for two days (Zwyghuizen-Doorenbos, Roehrs et al., 1990) or 400 mg TID for seven days (Bonnet & Arand, 1992). By day 7 in the latter study, a number of sleep measures no longer were different from baseline, suggesting the development of complete tolerance. However, the authors point out that sleep efficiency remained below 90%, suggesting some continuing sleep disruption even after seven days of caffeine consumption.

In addition to the three studies that demonstrated tolerance to centrally mediated caffeine effects, there is good evidence that repeated daily caffeine administration produces decreased responsiveness to physiological effects of caffeine, including diuresis, parotid gland salivation, increased metabolic rate (oxygen consumption), increased blood pressure, increased plasma norepinephrine and epinephrine, and increased plasma renin activity (cf. Griffiths & Mumford, 1996). Several studies (Robertson, Wade et al., 1981; Ammon, Bieck et al., 1983; Denaro, Brown et al., 1991) have demonstrated complete tolerance to blood pressure and other cardiovascular and physiological responses with repeated daily caffeine administration (for example, tolerance to 250 mg TID in one to four days; Robertson, Wade et al., 1981). Despite substantial tolerance development to cardiovascular effects at very high doses, caffeine as usually consumed is considered a risk factor in hypertension-prone individuals (Green, Kirby et al., 1996; Nurminen, Niittynen et al., 1999).

CAFFEINE INTOXICATION

The potential for caffeine intoxication to cause clinically significant distress is reflected by its inclusion as a diagnosis in the *DSM-IV* of the American Psychiatric Association (1994) and the *ICD-10* of the World Health Organization (1992a, 1992b).

Caffeine intoxication long has been recognized as a discrete syndrome associated with excessive caffeine use. In fact, reports of caffeine intoxication can be found in the medical literature dating back to the 1800s (cf. Strain & Griffiths, 1997). "Caffeinism" is an older term that has been used to describe the toxic effects of caffeine that result from acute or chronic use (Greden, 1981; *DSM-IIIR*, APA, 1987).

Diagnostic Criteria for Intoxication. Caffeine intoxication currently is defined by a number of symptoms and clinical features that emerge in response to recent consumption of caffeine. As listed in Table 3, common features of caffeine intoxication include nervousness (anxiety), restlessness, insomnia, gastrointestinal upset, tremors, tachycardia, and psychomotor agitation. In addition, there have been reports of patients with caffeine intoxication experiencing fever, irritability, tremors, sensory disturbances, tachypnea, and headaches (cf. Strain & Griffiths, 1997).

There have been no studies comparing the relative importance of the various *DSM-IV* criteria to the diagnosis of caffeine intoxication. However, in a study of general hospital patients, the symptoms most often associated with caffeine use were diuresis, insomnia, withdrawal headache, diarrhea, anxiety, tachycardia, and tremulousness (Victor, Lubsesky et al., 1981). Unlike many other drugs of dependence, but similar to nicotine, the high-dose intoxicating effects of caffeine are not usually sought out by users. High-dose caffeine toxicity very rarely is fatal. However, caffeine can be lethal at very high doses (for example, 5 to 10 g) and there is documentation of suicide by caffeine overdose (Serafin, 1996; Bryant, 1981).

Although *DSM-IV* diagnostic guidelines (Table 3) suggest that diagnosis should depend on the recent daily consumption of at least 250 mg of caffeine, the equivalent of just two and a half cups of brewed coffee, intoxication usually involves much higher doses (>500 mg) (Greden &

TABLE 3.   DSM Criteria for Caffeine Intoxication

A. Recent consumption of caffeine, usually in excess of 250 mg (for example, more than 2 to 3 cups of brewed coffee).

B. Five (or more) of the following signs, developing during, or shortly after, caffeine use:

    (1)   Restlessness
    (2)   Nervousness
    (3)   Excitement
    (4)   Insomnia
    (5)   Flushed face
    (6)   Diuresis
    (7)   Gastrointestinal disturbance
    (8)   Muscle twitching
    (9)   Rambling flow of thought and speech
    (10) Tachycardia or cardiac arrhythmia
    (11) Periods of inexhaustibility
    (12) Psychomotor agitation.

C. The symptoms in Criterion B cause clinically significant distress or impairment in social, occupational, or other important areas of functioning.

D. The symptoms are not due to a general medical condition and are not better accounted for by another mental disorder (*e.g.*, an Anxiety Disorder).

SOURCE: American Psychiatric Association (1994). *Diagnostic and Statistical Manual of Mental Disorders, 4th Edition (DSM-IV)*. Washington, DC: American Psychiatric Press.

Pomerleau, 1995). However, differences in individual sensitivity and tolerance are likely to influence the dose response. For example, an individual with high sensitivity and little tolerance might show signs and symptoms of caffeine intoxication in response to doses of caffeine much lower than those of a regular user.

Little is known about who may be most vulnerable to caffeine intoxication. Because caffeine intoxication is directly related to excess caffeine ingestion, any individual who consumes caffeine in large excess of his or her typical consumption may be at risk. Subgroups that have been identified as consuming large amounts of caffeine relative to the general population include psychiatric patients, prisoners, smokers, alcoholics, and individuals with eating disorders (cf. Strain & Griffiths, 1997). It has been noted that caffeine intoxication can occur in someone who has been using caffeine for many years without apparent problems (Greden & Pomerleau, 1995).

Treatment providers should be familiar with the signs and symptoms of caffeine intoxication. Such intoxication should be ruled out in the differential diagnosis of psychiatric disorders such as panic disorder, generalized anxiety disorder, sleep disorder, mania, and other substance abuse and substance withdrawal. Because many features of caffeine intoxication overlap with those of other medical and psychiatric disorders, identifying recent ingestion of excess caffeine is critical in diagnosing caffeine intoxication. Serum or saliva assays can be used to verify caffeine use.

Management of Intoxication. Caffeine intoxication usually resolves rapidly (consistent with caffeine's half-life of four to six hours) and appears to have no long-lasting consequences. Treatment may consist of short-term management and support of the patient for the time that it takes symptoms to resolve spontaneously. The patient who frequently consumes excessive amounts of caffeine and experiences repeated episodes of caffeine intoxication may benefit from education and behavior modification strategies (see the section on Clinical Implications and Treatment).

Very few studies have examined the incidence and prevalence of caffeine intoxication in the general population. Although many users may experience the negative effects of caffeine on occasion, caffeine intoxication serious enough to come to clinical attention is considered relatively rare (Strain & Griffiths, 2000). A random digit telephone survey found that 7% of current caffeine users met *DSM-IV* criteria for caffeine intoxication by reporting use of more than 250 mg, five or more symptoms, and symptoms that interfered with their functioning at work, school, or home (Hughes, Oliveto et al., 1998). Prior studies that have used ambiguous criteria and have focused on special populations (such as psychiatric patients or college students) have reported caffeine intoxication rates ranging from 2% to 19% (see Strain & Griffiths, 1997).

ANXIETY AND CAFFEINE

Acute doses of caffeine (generally, >200 mg) have been shown to increase anxiety ratings in non-clinical populations (Goldstein, Kaizer et al., 1969; Chait & Griffiths, 1983; Stern, Chait et al., 1989; Nickell & Uhde, 1994/1995). Higher doses have been shown to induce unequivocal panic attacks in some normal subjects (Uhde, 1990; Nickell &

Uhde, 1994/1995; Telch, Silverman et al., 1996; Lin, Uhde et al., 1997). Individuals who score higher on baseline measures of anxiety are less likely to choose caffeine over placebo in blind choice procedures (Evans & Griffiths, 1992; Griffiths & Woodson, 1988b).

Individuals with anxiety disorders appear to be particularly sensitive to the effects of caffeine. When individuals with panic disorder are asked about their responses to caffeine, they report greater anxiety than do respondents in matched control groups (Boulenger, Uhde et al., 1984; Lee, Cameron et al., 1985). Experimental studies have demonstrated that caffeine exacerbates anxiety symptoms in individuals with generalized anxiety disorder (Bruce, Scott et al., 1992) and panic disorder (Beck & Berisford, 1992; Charney, Heninger et al., 1985; Newman, Stein et al., 1992) to a greater extent than in healthy control subjects. Surveys have found that individuals with anxiety disorders tend to report lower levels of caffeine consumption relative to controls (Lee, Cameron et al., 1985; Lee, Flegel et al., 1988; Uhde, 1990; Rihs, Müller et al., 1996).

Caffeine-Induced Anxiety Disorder. Caffeine-induced anxiety disorder is a diagnosis included in the *DSM-IV* (APA, 1994). This disorder is characterized by prominent anxiety, panic attacks, or obsessions or compulsions that are related etiologically to caffeine use. Although the symptoms of caffeine-induced anxiety disorder may meet full criteria for a *DSM* anxiety disorder (such as panic disorder or generalized anxiety disorder), one need not meet all diagnostic criteria in order to qualify for a diagnosis of caffeine-induced anxiety disorder. There is no research examining this disorder, although studies have examined the relationship between caffeine and anxiety (as reviewed above). Clinical features of caffeine-induced anxiety have been described (Greden, 1974; Uhde, 1990). The diagnosis requires that the anxiety symptoms comprising the disorder must be caused by caffeine and be greater than what would be expected during caffeine intoxication or withdrawal. Because diagnosing caffeine-induced anxiety disorder depends on demonstrating that caffeine is linked to the anxiety symptoms, a trial of caffeine abstinence (and subsequent symptom remission) may be used to confirm the diagnosis. Although highly anxious individuals tend to be more likely to limit their caffeine use, not all individuals with anxiety problems naturally avoid caffeine, and some may fail to recognize the role that caffeine is playing in their anxiety symptoms. For example, Bruce and Lader (1989) found that instructions to cease caffeine use for one week led to significant improvements in more than half of individuals who presented for treatment at an anxiety disorders clinic and some required no further treatment.

SLEEP AND CAFFEINE

It is widely accepted that caffeine affects sleep. Numerous studies have shown that caffeine increases wakefulness and reduces decrements in performance under conditions of sleep deprivation (Snel, 1993; Wright, Badia et al., 1997; Reyner & Horne, 2000; Patat, Rosenzweig et al., 2000). Because of its ability to cause insomnia, sleep researchers have used caffeine as a challenge agent in order to study insomnia in healthy volunteers (Okuma, Matsuoka et al, 1982; Alford, Bhatti et al., 1996). Caffeine's effects on sleep appear to be determined by a variety of factors, including dose, the time between caffeine ingestion and attempted sleep, and individual differences in sensitivity and/or tolerance to caffeine (Snel, 1993).

The effects of caffeine on sleep are dose-dependent, with higher doses showing greater disruption on a number of sleep quality measures (Karacan, Thornby et al., 1976; Alford, Bhatti et al., 1996; Hindmarch, Rigney et al., 2000). Caffeine administered immediately prior to bedtime or throughout the day has been shown to delay sleep onset, reduce total sleep time, alter the normal stages of sleep, and decrease the reported quality of sleep (cf. Snel, 1993; Alford, Bhatti et al., 1996; Hindmarch, Rigney et al., 2000). There is less evidence to suggest that caffeine taken early in the day negatively affects nighttime sleep (Snel, 1993). However, a recent study found that caffeine (200 mg) taken at 7:10 in the morning produced small but significant effects on the following night's total sleep time, sleep efficiency, and electroencephalography (EEG) power spectra (Landolt, Werth et al., 1995).

Caffeine-induced sleep disturbance is greatest among individuals who are not regular caffeine users (Colton, Gosselin et al., 1968; Snel, 1993). It is not clear whether this difference is due to acquired pharmacologic tolerance or to a preexisting population difference in sensitivity to caffeine (Goldstein, 1964; Goldstein, Warren et al., 1965; Snel, 1993). Although there is evidence for some tolerance to the sleep-disrupting effects of caffeine (Bonnet & Arand, 1992; Zwyghuizen-Doorenbol, Roehrs et al., 1990), complete tolerance may not occur and thus habitual caffeine consumers remain vulnerable to caffeine-induced sleep problems (Goldstein, 1964; Goldstein, Warren et al., 1965).

In addition to caffeine's well-documented ability to disrupt sleep, a few studies have shown that caffeine withdrawal after acute abstinence from chronic caffeine can increase sleep duration and quality (Goldstein, Warren et al., 1965; James, 1998).

Caffeine-Induced Sleep Disorder. Caffeine-induced sleep disorder is a diagnosis included in the *DSM-IV* (APA, 1994). The disorder is characterized by a prominent disturbance of sleep that is related etiologically to caffeine use. Caffeine use most often is associated with insomnia; however, cases of caffeine causing excessive sleepiness also have been reported (Regestein, 1989). Like caffeine-induced anxiety disorder, caffeine-induced sleep disorder is diagnosed when symptoms of a sleep disturbance are greater than would be expected during caffeine intoxication or caffeine withdrawal.

There is little information about the incidence or prevalence of caffeine-induced sleep disorder. As discussed earlier, it appears that sleep disturbances due to caffeine are more likely to occur in individuals who are not regular caffeine consumers; nevertheless, complete tolerance to the effects of caffeine on sleep probably does not occur even among heavy caffeine users. Such heavy users may be vulnerable to, but relatively unaware of, the disruptive effects of caffeine on sleep because the pattern develops slowly. In elderly persons, occult caffeine consumption in the form of caffeine-containing analgesic medications may lead to sleep problems (Brown, Salive et al., 1995). Because diagnosing caffeine-induced sleep disorder depends on demonstrating that caffeine is linked to the sleep disturbance, a trial of caffeine abstinence (and subsequent symptom remission) may be used to confirm the diagnosis.

CAFFEINE WITHDRAWAL

The caffeine withdrawal syndrome has been well-characterized in humans. Fifty-three case reports and experimental studies previously were reviewed by Griffiths & Mumford (1995). This chapter updates their review by incorporating an additional 31 recent studies that provide information about caffeine withdrawal (Bruce, Scott et al., 1991; Weber, Ereth et al., 1993; Strain, Mumford et al., 1994; Lane, 1994; Nikolajsen, Larsen et al., 1994; Brauer, Buican et al., 1994; Höfer & Bättig, 1994a, 1994b; Reeves, Struve et al., 1995; Mitchell, de Wit et al., 1995; Streufert, Pogash et al., 1995; Hampl, Schneider et al., 1995; Richardson, Rogers et al., 1995; Lader, Cardwell et al., 1996; Comer, Haney et

...indworth et al., 1997; Hamill & Levin, ...man et al., 1997; Goldstein & Wallace, ...riffiths, 1997; Lane, 1997; Phillips-Bute ...ine & Phillips-Bute, 1998; James, 1998; ...t al., 1998; Bernstein, Carroll et al., 1998b; Garrett & ...hs, 1998; Dews, Curtis et al., 1999; Evans & Griffiths, 1999; Jones, Herning et al., 2000; Watson, Lunt et al., 2000). Although most research on withdrawal has been performed with adults, there is evidence that children also experience withdrawal effects during caffeine abstinence (Bernstein, Carroll et al., 1998; Goldstein & Wallace, 1997; Hale, Hughes et al., 1995).

Signs and Symptoms. The most commonly reported withdrawal symptom is headache, often described as being gradual in development and diffuse, and sometimes as throbbing and severe (Griffiths & Woodson, 1988a; Strain, Mumford et al., 1994; Lader, Cardwell et al., 1996). Other symptoms, in roughly descending order of prominence, are fatigue (fatigue, lethargy, sluggishness); sleepiness/drowsiness (sleepy, drowsy, yawning); difficulty concentrating (muzzy); work difficulty (decreased motivation for tasks/work); irritability (irritable, cross, miserable, decreased well-being/contentedness); depression (depressed mood); anxiety (anxious, nervous); influenza-like symptoms (nausea/vomiting, muscle aches/stiffness, hot and cold spells, heavy feelings in arms or legs).

In addition to these symptoms, caffeine withdrawal may produce impairment in psychomotor, vigilance, and cognitive performance, increases in cerebral blood flow, and changes in quantitative EEG activity. The observation that withdrawal symptoms such as fatigue or drowsiness can occur in absence of a headache indicates that such symptoms are not merely an epiphenomenon of headache (Griffiths & Woodson, 1988a; Griffiths, Evans et al., 1990b; Streufert, Pogash et al., 1995; Garrett & Griffiths, 1998; Phillips-Bute & Lane, 1998; Jones, Herning et al., 2000).

Dosing Parameters. *Caffeine Maintenance Dose*: The incidence (Goldstein & Kaizer, 1969; Goldstein, Kaizer et al., 1969; Galletly, Fennelly et al., 1989; Fennelly, Galletly et al., 1991; Weber, Ereth et al., 1993; Nikolajsen, Larsen et al., 1994) and severity (cf. Griffiths & Woodson, 1988a; Lader, Cardwell et al., 1996) of caffeine withdrawal are an increasing function of daily self-reported caffeine dose. However, this relationship between caffeine dose and withdrawal appears to be relatively weak because it has not been consistently demonstrated across studies (Verhoeff & Millar, 1990; Hughes, Oliveto et al., 1993; Höfer & Bättig, 1994a),

and some studies have shown no or only very mild withdrawal after stopping high doses of caffeine (Griffiths, Bigelow et al., 1986a; Strain, Mumford et al., 1994).

The only study to manipulate caffeine maintenance dose experimentally found that withdrawal severity increased progressively across three caffeine maintenance doses (100, 300, and 600 mg/day), with significantly greater withdrawal demonstrated at 600 mg/day than at 100 mg/day (Evans & Griffiths, 1999). This study and a previous study (Griffiths, Evans et al., 1990b) also demonstrated that significant caffeine withdrawal occurred after abstinence from a dose as low as 100 mg/day, which is the caffeine equivalent of one cup of brewed coffee or two to three 12-ounce servings of a caffeinated soft drink.

Duration of Exposure: Caffeine withdrawal has been shown to occur after relatively short-term exposure to daily caffeine (Dreisbach & Pfeiffer, 1943; Griffiths, Bigelow et al., 1986a; Evans & Griffiths, 1999). One study showed that significant withdrawal occurred after only three consecutive days of 300 mg/day caffeine, with somewhat greater severity shown after 7 and 14 consecutive days of exposure (Evans & Griffiths, 1999). Another study showed that caffeine withdrawal headache occurred in three individuals who normally abstained from caffeinated beverages, but were given 600 to 750 mg/day caffeine for six or seven days (Dreisbach & Pfeiffer, 1943).

Within-Day Frequency of Exposure: One study showed that the range and severity of caffeine withdrawal symptoms did not differ when 300 mg of caffeine was taken as a single dose in the morning, versus 100 mg taken at three time points across the day (Evans & Griffiths, 1999). Thus, although caffeine is eliminated relatively quickly, its mean half-life of four to six hours apparently is long enough to maintain significant caffeine exposure even under a once-a-day dosing regimen.

Caffeine Suppression of Withdrawal: Even low doses of caffeine are capable of suppressing caffeine withdrawal. One study showed that when individuals were maintained on 300 mg caffeine/day and tested with a range of lower doses (200, 100, 50, 25, and 0 mg/day), a substantial reduction in caffeine dose (100 mg/day or less) was necessary for the manifestation of caffeine withdrawal (Evans & Griffiths, 1999). Interestingly, even a mere 25 mg/day was sufficient to suppress significant caffeine withdrawal headache. The observation that low doses of caffeine suppress withdrawal is consistent with a recent study, which found that 12.5 mg of caffeine produced performance enhancement in a group of caffeine users who had been abstinent overnight, but not in a group that consumed very low levels of caffeine (Smit & Rogers, 2000). One implication of these findings is that a substantial percentage reduction in caffeine consumption is necessary to elicit the full caffeine withdrawal syndrome.

Incidence of Withdrawal. Blind experimental studies in healthy normal caffeine users who abstained for 24 hours indicate that the incidence of headache is about 50% (ranging from 30% to 86%) (Dreisbach & Pfeiffer, 1943; Griffiths, Evans et al., 1990b; van Dusseldorp & Katan, 1990; Silverman, Evans et al., 1992; Hughes, Oliveto et al., 1993; Lader, Cardwell et al., 1996; Höfer & Battig, 1994a; James, 1998). A similar incidence of headache has been reported in studies of subjects specifically selected for reporting problems with caffeine use or withdrawal (Strain, Mumford et al., 1994; Dews, Curtis et al., 1999). Not surprisingly, when all withdrawal symptoms are considered, the incidence of caffeine withdrawal is higher (ranging from 39% to 100%) (Griffiths, Evans et al., 1990b; Hughes, Oliveto et al., 1993; Strain, Mumford et al., 1994; Lader, Cardwell et al., 1996; Dews, Curtis et al., 1999).

Retrospective studies have been conducted to determine the frequency of caffeine withdrawal in the general population. In a population-based random digit dial telephone survey (Hughes, Oliveto et al., 1998), 44% of caffeine users reported having stopped or reduced caffeine use for at least 24 hours in the preceding year. Of those, 41% reported that they experienced at least one *DSM-IV* defined caffeine withdrawal symptom. Among individuals who stopped caffeine use in an attempt at permanent abstinence, at least 71% reported experiencing *DSM-IV* symptoms, and 24% reported having headache plus other symptoms that interfered with performance. The percentage of those endorsing individual symptoms is shown in Figure 3.

In another study that surveyed callers about participation in a clinical research trial, only 11% of caffeine users endorsed that they had problems or symptoms on stopping caffeine in the past, with 25% of this group reporting that the symptoms were severe enough to interfere with normal activity (Dews, Curtis et al., 1999). However, the number of individuals who actually abstained from caffeine was not determined, nor was it determined whether significant underreporting of symptoms occurred because of the desire to participate in a research trial.

Such studies may underestimate the true rate of caffeine withdrawal. Many caffeine consumers may be unaware of their physical dependence on caffeine because their frequent habitual consumption precludes a period of sustained abstinence. Moreover, it has been demonstrated that as little as 25 mg of caffeine is sufficient to suppress withdrawal (Evans & Griffiths, 1999). Thus, even small amounts of caffeine that are unknowingly consumed on their reported "caffeine-free" days may result in underestimates of the occurrence of withdrawal. Finally, caffeine withdrawal symptoms (headache, nausea, muscle aches) may be attributed incorrectly to other causes or ailments (viral infection).

Severity of Withdrawal. When signs or symptoms of caffeine withdrawal occur, their severity can vary from mild to extreme. At its worst, caffeine withdrawal repeatedly has been shown to produce clinically significant distress or impairment in daily functioning and, on rare occasions, to be totally incapacitating (Kingdon, 1833; Bridge, 1893; Dreisbach & Pfeiffer, 1943; Goldstein & Kaizer, 1969; Cobbs, 1982; Greden, Victor et al., 1980; Rainey, 1985; Griffiths, Evans et al., 1990b; Silverman, Evans et al., 1992; Strain, Mumford et al., 1994; Lader, Cardwell et al., 1996). For example, in a double-blind caffeine-withdrawal evaluation (Strain, Mumford et al., 1994), 73% of individuals who met criteria for *DSM-IV* substance dependence on caffeine reported functional impairment in normal activities during an experimental withdrawal phase. Examples of functional impairment included missed work, costly mistakes at work, inability to care for children, and inability to complete schoolwork.

The proportion of regular caffeine users who are at risk for severe functional impairment during caffeine withdrawal is difficult to estimate. One blind study (Dreisbach & Pfeiffer, 1943) conducted in a relatively unselected group of graduate and medical students reported "headache as extreme in severity as the subjects had ever experienced" upon blind withdrawal of caffeine. This extreme headache occurred in 55% of 38 trials in 22 subjects. Another study (Silverman, Evans et al., 1992) tested 62 individuals from the general community with mean caffeine intake of 235 mg/day. The study involved double-blind caffeine abstinence under conditions that obscured that the purpose of the study was to investigate caffeine. During withdrawal, 52% reported moderate to severe headache, and 8% to 11% showed abnormally high scores on standardized depression, anxiety, and fatigue scales. This incidence of moderate to severe caffeine-withdrawal headache is similar to that reported in other studies of healthy subjects (Lader, Cardwell et al., 1996; Couturier, Laman et al., 1997). In the double-

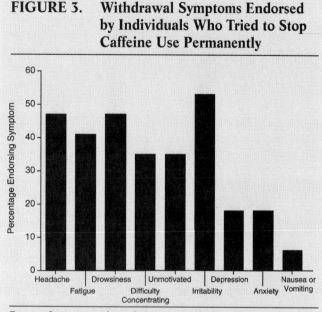

FIGURE 3.   Withdrawal Symptoms Endorsed by Individuals Who Tried to Stop Caffeine Use Permanently

Data are from a general population survey (Hughes, Oliveto et al., 1998). Bars show percentage of individuals endorsing the symptoms.

blind study by Lader and colleagues, 45% of subjects with a mean caffeine intake of 360 mg/day experienced a "diffuse, throbbing headache." Twenty-eight percent of those reporting headache also reported nausea and sickness.

Another study (Dews, Curtis et al., 1999) evaluated the incidence of functional impairment during abrupt caffeine withdrawal in a group of 18 subjects who reported mild or severe problems or symptoms when previously stopping caffeine. The study found that 33% of subjects spontaneously reported caffeine withdrawal symptoms, while 22% showed substantial decreases in their ratings of daily functioning (in work and leisure activities). However, the authors note that none of the subjects reported "incapacitating" symptoms. Although totally incapacitating symptoms of caffeine withdrawal (such as complete inability to work or going to bed because of symptoms misattributed to illness) have been documented (Bridge, 1893; Silverman, Evans et al., 1992; Strain, Mumford et al., 1994), the rate appears low and thus may be undetected with a sample size of only 18 subjects. The authors also commented that the frequency and severity of caffeine withdrawal symptoms are lower than reported in previous studies. Possible reasons for this discrepancy include: (1) caffeine withdrawal symptoms were

not assessed directly, but rather were inferred from spontaneous written comments in a "remarks" section of the questionnaire that asked about daily functioning; (2) subjects completed all questionnaires outside of the laboratory under unmonitored and unstructured conditions, reporting to the laboratory only at weekly intervals; (3) subjects consumed relatively low doses of caffeine immediately prior to abstinence (mean=231 mg/day); and (4) biological verification of caffeine abstinence was questionable (sample collection was not observed, data were reported only on the first morning of abstinence, and the lower limits of caffeine detection in the assay would have been unable to detect use of a small dose of caffeine sufficient caffeine to significantly suppress caffeine withdrawal).

Individual Differences. There are substantial differences within and across individuals with regard to the incidence and/or severity of caffeine withdrawal. As discussed above, only about 50% of regular caffeine consumers report headache after any single episode of caffeine abstinence. One study that examined repeated abstinence trials clearly documented differences within and across subjects: one subject never showed caffeine withdrawal headache, some subjects showed consistent headaches, while others reported headaches on some trials but not other trials (Griffiths, Evans et al., 1990b). A second study, which analyzed the effects of repeated abstinence trials, found that at least 36% of subjects who showed statistically significant elevations in headache failed to report this effect consistently across repeated trials (Hughes, Oliveto et al., 1993). Little is known about the determinants of these differences.

Time Course of Withdrawal. The caffeine withdrawal syndrome follows an orderly time course, as shown in Figure 4. Onset usually occurs 12 to 24 hours after the last dose of caffeine, although onset as late as 36 hours has been documented (cf. Griffiths & Woodson, 1988a; Griffiths, Evans et al., 1990b). Peak withdrawal intensity generally occurs 20 to 48 hours after the last dose (Griffiths & Woodson, 1988a; Griffiths, Evans et al., 1990b; Höfer & Bättig, 1994a). The duration of withdrawal usually is described as ranging between two and seven days (Griffiths, Bigelow et al., 1986a; Griffiths, Evans et al., 1990b; van Dusseldorp & Katan, 1990; Evans & Griffiths, 1992; Höfer & Bättig, 1994a), although longer durations have been reported (Griffiths, Bigelow et al., 1986a; Griffiths, Evans et al., 1990b; Richardson, Rogers et al., 1995).

Diagnostic Criteria for Withdrawal. The potential for caffeine withdrawal to cause clinically significant distress or impairment in function is reflected in its inclusion as an official diagnosis in the *ICD-10* (WHO, 1992a, 1992b) and as a proposed diagnosis in the *DSM-IV* (APA, 1994). (The 1994 DSM Work Group included caffeine withdrawal as a proposed diagnosis rather than an official diagnosis to encourage further research on the range and specificity of caffeine withdrawal symptoms [Hughes, 1994].) As reviewed above, the research literature on caffeine withdrawal has almost doubled since 1994, and now provides a sound empirical basis for a diagnosis of caffeine withdrawal.

As described in Table 4, the proposed criteria for a *DSM-IV* research diagnosis of caffeine withdrawal require the presence of headache and one or more of the following: marked fatigue or drowsiness, marked anxiety or depression, nausea or vomiting.

These criteria are very conservative because they exclude cases in which withdrawal headache is not accompanied by other symptoms and cases in which symptoms are experienced without headache. They also exclude several withdrawal symptoms that have been documented repeatedly in recent studies: difficulty concentrating, irritability, and work difficulty (such as decreased motivation for tasks/work).

The only study to evaluate the incidence of caffeine withdrawal using the criteria for the *DSM-IV* research diagnosis was a random-digit telephone survey of the general population (Hughes, Oliveto et al., 1998). That study found that 11% of those who had given up or reduced caffeine use in the past year met criteria for caffeine withdrawal. Notably, among the subgroup of individuals who reported trying to stop caffeine use permanently, 24% met criteria for the diagnosis (see Figure 3 for withdrawal symptoms).

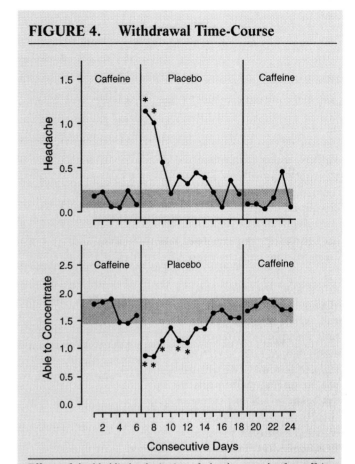

FIGURE 4.   Withdrawal Time-Course

Effects of double-blind substitution of placebo capsules for caffeine capsules (100 mg/day). Asterisks show which placebo days are significantly different from the initial caffeine period. Data are from Griffiths, Evans et al. (1990b).

CAFFEINE DEPENDENCE

In the terminology of the *DSM-IV*, "substance dependence" is characterized by a cluster of cognitive, behavioral, and physiological symptoms indicating that the individual continues use of a substance despite significant substance-related problems (APA, 1994). The clinical diagnosis of substance dependence encompasses several features, which may or may not include physical dependence (as evidenced by withdrawal). The *ICD-10* recognizes a diagnosis of substance dependence due to caffeine (WHO, 1992a, 1992b). Despite the fact that the *DSM-IV* uses very similar criteria for making a diagnosis of substance dependence, caffeine dependence is not presently included in *DSM-IV* and it is explicitly stated that "a diagnosis of substance dependence can be applied to every class of substance except caffeine." The rationale for excluding caffeine dependence from the *DSM-IV* was that, although caffeine withdrawal had been documented, there was no available database pertaining to other important features of substance dependence, such as inability to stop use and continued use despite harm (Hughes, Oliveto et al., 1992b; Hughes, 1994).

More recently, three studies have identified adults and adolescents who report problematic caffeine consumption and fulfill the *DSM-IV* criteria for substance dependence on caffeine. In one study (Strain, Mumford et al., 1994), 16 of 99 individuals who self-identified as having psychological or physical dependence on caffeine met the *DSM-IV*

TABLE 4.   Proposed DSM Criteria for Caffeine Withdrawal

A. Prolonged daily use of caffeine.

B. Abrupt cessation of caffeine use, or reduction in the amount of caffeine used, closely followed headache and one (or more) of the following symptoms:

   (1)   Marked fatigue or drowsiness
   (2)   Marked anxiety or depression
   (3)   Nausea or vomiting.

C. The symptoms in criterion B cause clinically significant distress or impairment in social, occupational, or other important areas of functioning.

D. The symptoms are not due to the direct physiological effects of a general medical condition (*e.g.*, migraine, viral illness) and are not better accounted for by another medical disorder.

SOURCE: American Psychiatric Association (1994). *Diagnostic and Statistical Manual of Mental Disorders, 4th Edition (DSM-IV).* Washington, DC: American Psychiatric Press.

criteria for substance dependence on caffeine when four of the seven *DSM-IV* criteria that seemed most applicable to caffeine were assessed. Criteria used for making the diagnosis and rates of endorsement were: withdrawal (94%), use continued despite knowledge of a persistent or recurrent physical or psychological problem that is likely to have been caused or exacerbated by caffeine use (94%), persistent desire or unsuccessful efforts to cut down or control caffeine use (81%), and tolerance (75%). Median daily caffeine intake of those fulfilling a caffeine dependence diagnosis was 357 mg, with a range of 129 to 2,548. The preferred vehicle was almost equally divided between soft drinks and coffee. Interestingly, although there were few concurrent psychiatric disorders in this population, 57% had a past diagnosis of alcohol abuse or dependence.

Using the same four *DSM-IV* criteria, another study identified adolescents who met diagnostic criteria for caffeine dependence (Bernstein, Carroll et al., 2002; Oberstar, Bernstein et al., 2002). The third study was a random-digit dial telephone survey of the general population in which all seven *DSM-IV* substance dependence criteria were assessed

(Hughes, Oliveto et al., 1998). Thirty percent of 162 caffeine users (222 mg/day) fulfilled diagnostic criteria for caffeine dependence by endorsing three or more of the seven criteria. When the restrictive set of four criteria (described above) were used, only 9% were considered caffeine dependent. The most commonly reported symptom (56%) was persistent desire or unsuccessful efforts to reduce or control caffeine use (see Figure 5).

The *DSM-IV* diagnostic studies by Strain and colleagues and Bernstein and colleagues can be considered a series of case reports documenting that caffeine can produce a substance dependence disorder. The study by Hughes and colleagues suggests that the prevalence of the disorder in the general population is not trivial. The validity of the diagnosis is suggested by two studies that prospectively demonstrated that the severity of caffeine withdrawal (Strain, Mumford et al., 1994) and the incidence of caffeine reinforcement (Liguori & Hughes, 1997) was greater in individuals who fulfilled diagnostic criteria for caffeine dependence. However, the clinical and research utility of the diagnosis remains to be determined.

Clearly, additional research is needed to characterize more fully the prevalence of the disorder, the extent of clinically significant distress experienced, the prognosis if the disorder is untreated, and the relationship of the disorder to problems with other abused substances. For research purposes, a section for the diagnosis of caffeine dependence according to *DSM-IV* or *ICD-10* criteria is now available on the Composite International Diagnostic Interview—Substance Abuse Module (CIDI-SAM), which is a reliable and valid structured interview focused on substance use disorders (Cottler, Robins et al., 1989; Compton, Cottler et al., 1996).

HERITABILITY OF CAFFEINE USE PROBLEMS

Genetic factors have been shown to account for individual variability in the use and effects of caffeine. Several twin studies comparing monozygotic and dizygotic twins found that the heritability of coffee consumption ranged from 36% to 51% (cf. Swan, Carmelli et al., 1996; Kendler & Prescott, 1999). A study of male twins also showed heritability of heavy coffee use (>5 cups/day) to be 51% (Swan, Carmelli et al., 1997). A recent detailed analysis of caffeine use in female twins found that total caffeine consumption, heavy use (> 625 mg/day), caffeine tolerance, caffeine withdrawal, and caffeine intoxication also had a greater co-occurrence in monozygotic twins than dizygotic twins, with heritabilities between 35% and 77% (Kendler & Prescott, 1999).

Interestingly, three additional twin studies using multivariate structural equation modeling of caffeine use, cigarette smoking, and alcohol use concluded that a common genetic factor (polysubstance use) underlies the use of these three substances, with 28% to 41% of the heritable effects of caffeine use (or heavy use) shared with alcohol and smoking (Swan, Carmelli et al., 1996, 1997; Hettema, Corey et al., 1999). The conclusion that a common factor underlies joint use of caffeine, cigarettes, and alcohol is consistent with findings of a study by Kozlowski, Henningfield et al., (1993) on the co-occurrence of substance use among drug abusers. They found that severity of alcoholism was directly related to use of caffeine and cigarettes, and they concluded that dependence on caffeine, nicotine, and alcohol may be governed by the same factors.

These results in humans are consistent with previous research with inbred mice demonstrating genetic differences in responses to caffeine (Seale, Johnson et al., 1985; Logan, Seale et al., 1986). As a whole, these data on the genetics of use vulnerability underscore the fact that caffeine use problems have an underlying biological basis, part of which is shared with other commonly abused substances.

ASSOCIATIONS WITH OTHER DRUGS OF DEPENDENCE

In addition to the twin studies and the population-based study suggesting that common factors underlie the use of caffeine, nicotine, and alcohol, a substantial body of research also documents associations between caffeine use and individual drugs of dependence.

Nicotine and Cigarette Smoking. Epidemiologic studies have shown that cigarette smokers consume more caffeine than do nonsmokers (Istvan & Matarazzo, 1984; Swanson, Lee et al., 1994). This finding is consistent with the observation previously discussed, that cigarette smoking increases the rate of caffeine elimination (Parson & Neims, 1978; May, Jarboe et al., 1982). Although coffee drinking and cigarette smoking also tend to covary temporally within individuals (Emurian, Nellis et al., 1982; Lane, 1996), caffeine administration does not reliably increase cigarette smoking (Chait & Griffiths, 1983), suggesting that the coffee-smoking interaction is not controlled by the pharmacologic effects of caffeine alone. A recent series of preclinical studies showed that chronic exposure to caffeine facilitated acquisition of nicotine self-administration and produced alterations in

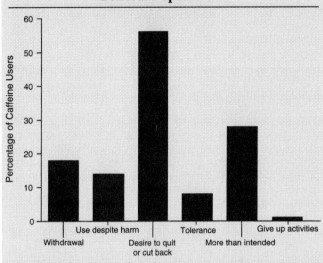

FIGURE 5.   DSM-IV Dependence Criteria Endorsed in a Survey of the General Population

DSM-IV criteria for Substance Dependence endorsed by caffeine users in a survey of the general population. One of the criteria (a great deal of time spent in activities necessary to use the substance) is omitted because it is not clinically meaningful with caffeine. Data are from Hughes, Oliveto et al. (1998).

brain dopaminergic activity consistent with caffeine enhancing the reinforcing effects of nicotine (Shoaib, Swanner et al., 1999; Gasior, Jaszyna et al., 2000; Tanda & Goldberg, 2000).

Several studies have shown that abstinence from cigarette smoking can produce substantial increases in blood levels of caffeine in heavy consumers of caffeine, presumably as the result of reversal of cigarette-smoking induced caffeine metabolism (Brown, Jacob et al., 1988; Benowitz, Hall et al., 1989). Although it has been speculated that such an effect might make smoking cessation attempts more difficult, the clinical significance has not been demonstrated (Oliveto, Hughes et al., 1991; Hughes & Oliveto, 1993; Swanson, Lee et al., 1994).

Alcohol. Heavy use and clinical dependence on alcohol is associated with heavy use and clinical dependence on caffeine (Istvan & Matsarazzo, 1984; Kozlowski, Henningfield et al., 1993; Hughes, Oliveto et al., 2000). One study reported substantial increases in caffeine consumption following alcohol detoxification in alcoholics (Aubin, Laureaux et al., 1999). A study of individuals who met the *DSM-IV* diagnostic criteria for substance dependence on caffeine found that almost 60% had a past diagnosis of alcohol abuse or dependence (Strain, Mumford et al., 1994).

It is common clinical lore that caffeine can reverse the impairing effects of alcohol. There has been some speculation that a mechanism underlying such an effect is caffeine antagonism of adenosine-mediated alcohol effects (cf. Fredholm, Bättig et al., 1999). Although some animal and human studies show that caffeine can reduce alcohol sedation and impairment, a number of studies contradict that finding (Rush, Higgins et al., 1993; Hasenfratz, Buzzini et al., 1994; White, 1994; Liguori & Robinson, 2001). The available data suggest that such interactive effects generally are incomplete and inconsistent across different types of behavioral and subjective measures.

Benzodiazepines. Benzodiazepines are used widely in the treatment of anxiety, panic, and insomnia. Both animal and human studies suggest a mutually antagonistic relationship between caffeine and benzodiazepines (cf. White, 1994). Although it is possible that this interaction occurs at the benzodiazepine receptor, the lack of uniform antagonism across measures suggests that the effect is functional in nature (Roache & Griffiths, 1987; Oliveto, Bickel et al., 1997; White, 1994). Interestingly, although individuals with anxiety disorders tend to report lower levels of caffeine consumption than do controls (Lee, Cameron et al., 1985; Lee, Flegel et al., 1988; Uhde, 1990; Rihs, Müller et al., 1996), one study reported that a greater proportion of heavy caffeine consumers also use benzodiazepine tranquilizers (Greden, Procter et al., 1981). An important clinical implication is that the role of caffeine should be carefully evaluated in the treatment of anxiety, panic, or insomnia with benzodiazepines.

Cocaine. Cocaine users report using more caffeine than do caffeine consumers in the general population; however, the prevalence of caffeine use among cocaine users is lower (Budney, Higgins et al., 1993). Interestingly, caffeine-using cocaine users reported using cocaine less frequently than did cocaine users who did not use caffeine regularly (Budney, Higgins et al., 1993). Preclinical studies show that caffeine increases acquisition of cocaine self-administration, reinstates self-administration behavior previously maintained by cocaine, and potentiates the stimulant and discriminative stimulus effects of cocaine (cf. Garrett & Griffiths, 1997).

In human experimental studies, oral caffeine increases drug-appropriate responding in individuals trained to discriminate cocaine (Oliveto, McCance-Katz et al., 1998). Intravenous caffeine administration produced a significant increase in craving for cocaine in cocaine abusers (Rush, Sullivan et al., 1995); however, a study involving oral administration of caffeine in coffee showed no such effect (Liguori, Hughes et al., 1997a). The subjective effects of intravenous caffeine were identified as cocaine-like in one study (Rush, Sullivan et al., 1995), but not another (Garrett & Griffiths, 2001). Overall, although intriguing interactions between caffeine and cocaine effects have been documented, the clinical significance remains to be determined.

CLINICAL IMPLICATIONS AND TREATMENT

Differential Diagnosis. Given the wide range of symptoms produced by caffeine use, intoxication, and withdrawal, caffeine use should be assessed routinely as part of a patient's medical and psychiatric history.

Caffeine use or intoxication can mimic or exacerbate symptoms of a variety of medical and psychiatric conditions, such as generalized anxiety disorder, panic disorder, mania, amphetamine or cocaine intoxication, primary insomnia, medication-induced side effects, arrhythmia, gastroesophageal reflux, hyperthyroidism, and pheochromocytoma. Caffeine use should be considered in the diagnosis of patients presenting with common symptoms such as anxiety, insomnia, panic attacks, palpitations, tachycardia, or gastrointestinal disturbance. Likewise, caffeine withdrawal can completely mimic or exacerbate migraine and other headache disorders, viral illnesses, and other drug withdrawal states such as amphetamine or cocaine withdrawal. Caffeine withdrawal should be evaluated in individuals presenting with headaches, fatigue, mood disturbances, or impaired concentration.

Medication Interactions. Benzodiazepine-like drugs, including diazepam, alprazolam, triazolam, and zolpidem, are widely used in the treatment of anxiety, panic, and insomnia. Because animal and human studies suggest a mutually antagonistic relationship between caffeine and benzodiazepines (White, 1994), the role of caffeine should be carefully evaluated when using benzodiazepines to treat patients with anxiety, panic, or insomnia.

Caffeine inhibits the metabolism of the antipsychotic clozapine to an extent that might be clinically significant.

Because caffeine and theophylline mutually inhibit each other's metabolism, caffeine consumption during theophylline therapy should be monitored.

Finally, lithium toxicity may occur after caffeine withdrawal due to decreased renal clearance of lithium (cf. Carrillo & Benitez, 2000).

Short-Term Abstinence for Medical Procedures. Patients often are asked to stop food and fluids before certain blood tests, surgeries, or procedures such as endoscopies, colonoscopies, and cardiac catherizations. Whether patients scheduled to undergo such procedures could be allowed caffeine supplements to avoid the symptoms of withdrawal should be considered. Caffeine withdrawal has been identified as a significant cause of postoperative headaches, the risk of which can be reduced if regular caffeine users are given caffeine on the day of the surgical procedure (Galletly, Fennelly et al., 1989; Fennelly, Galletly et al., 1991; Weber, Ereth et al., 1993; Nikolajsen, Larsen et al., 1994; Weber, Klindworth et al., 1997).

Medically Indicated Long-Term Abstinence. The majority of habitual caffeine consumers experience no clinically significant problems as a result of their caffeine use. Long-term reduction or elimination of caffeine intake should be advised for patients who have a caffeine-related clinical diagnosis (such as caffeine intoxication, caffeine-induced anxiety disorder, caffeine-induced sleep disorder, caffeine withdrawal, or caffeine dependence) or when it is suspected that caffeine is mimicking or exacerbating psychiatric or medical conditions or interfering with the efficacy of medications (as with benzodiazepines or clozapine). Long-term caffeine reduction or abstinence also may be recommended to pregnant women.

Strategies for Reduction or Elimination of Caffeine. There have been few evaluations of strategies to reduce or eliminate caffeine use. A scheduled caffeine reduction program is believed to help attenuate withdrawal symptoms, although there is no systematic research to determine the most efficacious reduction schedule. Indeed, there have been very few evaluations of strategies to reduce or eliminate caffeine use.

Several studies with heavy caffeine consumers demonstrated the efficacy of a structured caffeine reduction treatment program ("caffeine fading") in achieving substantial reductions in consumption (Foxx & Rubinoff, 1979; Bernard, Dennehy et al., 1981; James, Stirling et al., 1985; James, Paull et al., 1988). One of these studies found that a four-week structured caffeine fading schedule was more ef-fective than self-guided reduction (James, Stirling et al., 1985). However, little is known about the long-term efficacy of these procedures (James, Paull et al., 1988). There are no reports on treatment interventions for individuals who would like to eliminate caffeine completely.

In the absence of empirically validated treatments for problematic caffeine use, a reasonable approach would be to use behavior modification strategies that are effective in treating other drugs of dependence (such as education, behavioral substitution, coping suggestions, self-monitoring, and reinforcement for abstinence). Many individuals may not be knowledgeable about sources of caffeine in their diets, so education and history-taking are likely to be important components of treatment. It has been suggested that a caffeine-free trial should be recommended to individuals who are resistant to the idea that caffeine is contributing to their problems (Greden & Walters, 1992).

The clinician should anticipate that withdrawal symptoms may thwart quit attempts. One rationale for the caffeine fading approach is that withdrawal symptoms may be avoided or attenuated. No data about the probability of relapse are available, although relapse after caffeine reduction has been reported (Greden & Pomerleau, 1995; James, Paull et al., 1988). Practical guidelines for reducing or eliminating caffeine use include the following:

- Educate the patient about sources of caffeine. For example, some individuals may not be aware that caffeine is present in non-cola soft drinks or OTC analgesics.

- Have the patient self-monitor caffeine consumption, using a food diary, for one week.

- Identify all sources of caffeine and calculate the total caffeine consumption in mg.

- Present caffeine cessation as a temporary trial to patients who are resistant to treatment or who appear to have a caffeine-related disorder, but do not believe that caffeine is the cause of their complaints.

- Generate a graded reduction ("fading") schedule with the patient. A reasonable decrease would be 10% to 25% of the usual dose every couple of days.

- Help the patient identify a non-caffeinated substitute for their usual caffeine-containing beverage. If the patient is a coffee drinker, have him or her begin by mixing decaffeinated and caffeinated coffee, then progressively increase the percentage of decaffeinated coffee until the desired level is achieved. If the patient consumes soft drinks, ask him or her to alternate between caffeinated and caffeine-free soft drinks, or to mix the two until the caffeinated soft drink is reduced or eliminated.

■ Discuss the possibility of relapse with the patient. Discuss triggers (antecedent conditions) for caffeine use and offer suggestions for coping with situations that pose a high risk of relapse.

■ Suggest that the patient continue to self-monitor his or her caffeine consumption.

ADDICTION LIABILITY

Given that caffeine is the most widely used mood-altering drug in the world, that some users report difficulty quitting, and that abrupt abstinence can produce clinically significant functional impairment, it is not surprising that it is periodically labeled as a drug of abuse or addiction (Gilbert, 1973; Austin, 1979). Objections to considering caffeine to be a classic drug of addiction include the observations that caffeine is used by most people in our society, that it has subtle psychological effects that are socially acceptable, that the harmful effects of excess use are largely transient, and that overuse of any food substance can be harmful. However, definitions of what constitutes a drug of addiction can be controversial, as indicated by the debate as to whether nicotine should be considered a drug of addiction (Robinson & Prichard, 1992a, 1992b; West, 1992).

Psychiatric Approach. One approach to considering whether it is meaningful to consider caffeine a drug of addiction is to evaluate the effects of caffeine from a psychiatric perspective. A number of studies have shown that some individuals fulfill criteria (of the *ICD-10* and *DSM-IV*) for a psychiatric diagnosis of substance dependence on caffeine by endorsing diagnostic items including withdrawal, continued use despite persistent or recurrent physical or psychological problems that are likely to have been caused or exacerbated by caffeine use, and persistent desire or unsuccessful efforts to cut down or control caffeine use.

Although the World Health Organization (*ICD-10*) recognizes the diagnosis of substance dependence on caffeine, the American Psychiatric Association (*DSM-IV*) currently explicitly excludes caffeine because of an insufficient database documenting clinical features of caffeine dependence (Hughes, Oliveto et al., 1992b; Hughes, 1994). However, a recent population-based survey study showed that a substantial portion of caffeine users (9% or more) may fulfill *DSM-IV* criteria for substance dependence on caffeine, with more than half reporting desire or unsuccessful efforts to stop caffeine use (Hughes, Oliveto et al., 1998).

Reinforcement/Adverse Effects Analysis. Another approach is to consider a reinforcement/adverse effects analysis (cf. Griffiths, Lamb et al., 1985). This model is useful in explaining societal perceptions of the relative abuse liability of a range of psychotropic drugs. In this framework, drugs of abuse or addiction have two defining characteristics: They have reinforcing effects, and their use leads to adverse effects (that is, they have the capacity to harm the individual or society). The relative abuse potential of a drug can be considered to be a multiplicative function of the degree of reinforcing effect and the degree of adverse effect.

With regard to reinforcing effects, the animal and human studies reviewed in this chapter demonstrate that caffeine can function as a reinforcer under certain conditions. Studies in which laboratory animals learn to self-inject caffeine indicate that, like nicotine, caffeine functions as a reinforcer under a more limited range of conditions than classic psychomotor stimulant drugs of abuse such as cocaine. In humans, self-administration and choice studies clearly demonstrate modest reinforcing effects of low and moderate doses of caffeine and suggest that such effects may be potentiated by physical dependence on caffeine.

With regard to adverse effects, a balanced discussion is beyond the scope of this chapter and has been the focus of several scholarly books (Spiller, 1984; James, 1991, 1997; Garattini, 1993). The adverse health effects of caffeine use reviewed in this chapter include caffeine intoxication, caffeine withdrawal, caffeine-induced sleep disorder, and caffeine-induced anxiety disorder. Medical and psychiatric conditions for which caffeine use often is thought to be contraindicated include generalized anxiety disorder, panic disorder, primary insomnia, gastroesophageal reflux, and pregnancy. In addition, the modest pressor effects of caffeine and the potent cholesterol-raising components of unfiltered coffee have raised concerns about the role of caffeine and coffee in cardiovascular disease (cf. James, 1997). Importantly, however, and in contrast to many classic drugs of abuse, significant health risk from nonreversible pathological consequences of caffeine use (including cancer, heart disease, and reproductive disorders) has not been demonstrated conclusively.

This reinforcement/adverse effects analysis indicates that caffeine does indeed have the two defining characteristics of drugs of abuse. However, the modest reinforcing effects and modest adverse effects documented to date suggest that caffeine has a low abuse liability relative to classic drugs of abuse. This analysis also predicts that if future research were to demonstrate conclusively that life-threatening health risks are associated with caffeine, societal perceptions of the abuse liability of caffeine would be increased substantially, as has been the case with nicotine over the past few decades.

ACKNOWLEDGMENT: Preparation of this chapter was supported, in part, by U.S. Public Health Service grants R01 DA03890 and R01 DA01147 from the National Institute on Drug Abuse.

REFERENCES

Ahlijanian MK & Takemori AE (1986). Cross-tolerance studies between caffeine and (--) – N⁶–(Phenylisopropy)-adenosine (PIA) in mice. *Life Sciences* 38:577-588.

al'Absi M, Lovallo WR, McKey B et al. (1998). Hypothalamic-pituitary-adrenocortical responses to psychological stress and caffeine in men at high and low risk for hypertension. *Psychosomatic Medicine* 60(4):521-527.

Aldridge A, Bailey J & Neims AH (1981). The disposition of caffeine during and after pregnancy. *Seminars in Perinatology* 5(4):310-314.

Alford C, Bhatti J, Leigh T et al. (1996). Caffeine-induced sleep disruption: Effects on waking the following day and its reversal with an hypnotic. *Human Psychopharmacology* 11:185-198.

Amato M, Isenschmid M & Huppi P (1991). Percutaneous caffeine application in the treatment of neonatal apnoea. *European Journal of Pediatrics* 150(8):592-594.

American Psychiatric Association (APA) (1987). *Diagnostic and Statistical Manual of Mental Disorders, 3rd Edition, Revised.* Washington, DC: American Psychiatric Press.

American Psychiatric Association (APA) (1994). *Diagnostic and Statistical Manual of Mental Disorders, 4th Edition (DSM-IV).* Washington, DC: American Psychiatric Press.

Ammon HPT, Bieck PR, Mandalaz D et al. (1983). Adaptation of blood pressure to continuous heavy coffee drinking in young volunteers: A double-blind crossover study. *British Journal of Clinical Pharmacology* 15:701-706.

Aranda JV, Cook CE, Gorman W et al. (1979). Pharmacokinetic profile of caffeine in the premature newborn infant with apnea. *Journal of Pediatrics* 94(4):663-668.

Aubin H-J, Laureaux C, Tilikete S et al. (1999). Changes in cigarette smoking and coffee drinking after alcohol detoxification in alcoholics. *Addiction* 94(3):411-416.

Austin GA (1979). Perspectives on the history of psychoactive substance use. In *NIDA Research Issues, Vol. 24.* Rockville, MD: National Institute on Drug Abuse, 50-66.

Barone JJ & Roberts HR (1996). Caffeine consumption. *Food Chemistry and Toxicology* 34(1):119-129.

Beck JG & Berisford MA (1992). The effects of caffeine on panic patients: Response components of anxiety. *Behavior Therapy* 23:405-422.

Becker AB, Simons KJ, Gillespie CA et al. (1984). The bronchodilator effects and pharmacokinetics of caffeine in asthma. *New England Journal of Medicine* 310(12):743-746.

Bedingfield JB, King DA & Holloway FA (1998). Cocaine and caffeine: Conditioned place preference, locomotor activity, and additivity. *Pharmacology, Biochemistry and Behavior* 61(3):291-296.

Benowitz NL, Hall SM & Modin G (1989). Persistent increase in caffeine concentrations in people who stop smoking. *British Medical Journal* 298:1075-1076.

Benowitz NL, Jacob P III, Mayan H et al. (1995). Sympathomimetic effects of paraxanthine and caffeine in humans. *Clinical Pharmacology and Therapeutics* 58:684-691.

Bernard ME, Dennehy S & Keefauver LW (1981). Behavioral treatment of excessive coffee and tea drinking: A case study and partial replication. *Behavior Therapy* 12:543-548.

Bernstein GA, Carroll M, Thuras PD et al. (2002). Caffeine dependence in teenagers. *Drug and Alcohol Dependence* 66:1-6.

Bernstein GA, Carroll ME, Dean NW et al. (1998). Caffeine withdrawal in normal school-age children. *Journal of the American Academy of Child and Adolescent Psychiatry* 37(8):858-865.

Beverage Digest Company (1999). *Beverage Digest Fact Book 1999.* Bedford Hills, NY: Beverage Digest Co.

Blanchard J & Sawers SJA (1983). Comparative pharmacokinetics of caffeine in young and elderly men. *Journal of Pharmacokinetics and Biopharmaceutics* 11(2):109-126.

Bonati M, Latini R, Tognoni G et al. (1984-1985). Interspecies comparison of in vivo caffeine pharmacokinetics in man, monkey, rabbit, rat, and mouse. *Drug Metabolism Reviews* 15(7):1355-1383.

Bonnet MH & Arand DL (1992). Caffeine use as a model of acute and chronic insomnia. *Sleep* 15(6):526-536.

Boulenger J-P, Uhde TW, Wolff EA III et al. (1984). Increased sensitivity to caffeine in patients with panic disorders. *Archives of General Psychiatry* 41(11):1067-1071.

Brauer LH, Buican B & de Wit H (1994). Effects of caffeine deprivation on taste and mood. *Behavioural Pharmacology* 5:111-118.

Bridge N (1893). Coffee-drinking as a frequent cause of disease. *Transactions of the Associations of American Physicians* 8:281-288.

Brockwell NT, Eikelboom R & Beninger RJ (1991). Caffeine-induced place and taste conditioning: Production of dose-dependent preference and aversion. *Pharmacology Biochemistry and Behavior* 38:513-517.

Brown CR, Jacob P III, Wilson M et al. (1988). Changes in rate and pattern of caffeine metabolism after cigarette abstinence. *Clinical Pharmacology and Therapeutics* 43(5):488-491.

Brown SL, Salive ME, Pahor M et al. (1995). Occult caffeine as a source of sleep problems in an older population. *Journal of the American Geriatrics Society* 43:860-864.

Bruce M, Scott N, Shine P (1991). Caffeine withdrawal: A contrast of withdrawal symptoms in normal subjects who have abstained from caffeine for 24 hours and for 7 days. *Journal of Psychopharmacology* 5(2):129-134.

Bruce M, Scott N, Shine P et al. (1992). Anxiogenic effects of caffeine in patients with anxiety disorders. *Archives of General Psychiatry* 49:867-869.

Bruce MS & Lader M (1989). Caffeine abstention in the management of anxiety disorders. *Psychological Medicine* 19:211-214.

Bryant J (1981). Suicide by ingestion of caffeine. *Archives of Pathology and Laboratory Medicine* 105:685-686.

Budavari S, O'Neil MJ, Smith A et al., eds. (1996). *The Merck Index*. Whitehouse Station, NJ: Merck Research Laboratories.

Budney AJ, Higgins ST, Hughes JR et al. (1993). Nicotine and caffeine use in cocaine-dependent individuals. *Journal of Substance Abuse* 5(2):117-130.

Carrillo JA & Benitez J (2000). Clinically significant pharmacokinetic interactions between dietary caffeine and medications. *Clinical Pharmacokinetics* 39(2):127-153.

Chait LD & Griffiths RR (1983). Effects of caffeine on cigarette smoking and subjective response. *Clinical Pharmacology and Therapeutics* 34(5):612-622.

Chait LD & Johanson CE (1988). Discriminative stimulus effects of caffeine and benzphetamine in amphetamine-trained volunteers. *Psychopharmacology* 96:302-308.

Charney DS, Heninger GR & Jatlow PI (1985). Increased anxiogenic effects of caffeine in panic disorders. *Archives of General Psychiatry* 42:233-243.

Cnattingius S, Signorello LB, Annerén G et al. (2000). Caffeine intake and the risk of first-trimester spontaneous abortion. *New England Journal of Medicine* 343:1839-1845.

Cobbs LW (1982). Lethargy, anxiety, and impotence in a diabetic. *Hospital Practice* 17(8):67,70,73.

Cohen S & Booth Jr GH (1975). Gastric acid secretion and lower-esophageal-sphincter pressure in response to coffee and caffeine. *New England Journal of Medicine* 293(18):897-899.

Colton T, Gosselin RE & Smith RP (1968). The tolerance of coffee drinkers to caffeine. *Clinical Pharmacology and Therapeutics* 9(1):31-39.

Comer SD & Carroll ME (1996). Oral caffeine pretreatment produced modest increases in smoked cocaine self-administration in rhesus monkeys. *Psychopharmacology* 126:281-285.

Comer SD, Haney M, Foltin RW et al. (1997). Effects of caffeine withdrawal on humans living in a residential laboratory. *Experimental and Clinical Psychopharmacology* 5(4):399-403.

Compton WM, Cottler LB, Dorsey KB et al. (1996). Comparing assessments of DSM-IV substance dependence disorders using CIDI-SAM and SCAN. *Drug and Alcohol Dependence* 41:179-187.

Cook CE, Tallent CR, Amerson EW et al. (1976). Caffeine in plasma and saliva by a radioimmunoassay procedure. *Journal of Pharmacology and Experimental Therapeutics* 199(3):679-686.

Cottler LB, Robins LN & Helzer JE (1989). The reliability of the CIDI-SAM: A comprehensive substance abuse interview. *British Journal of Addiction* 84(7):801-814.

Couturier EGM, Laman DM, van Duijn MAJ et al. (1997). Influence of caffeine withdrawal on headache and cerebral blood flow velocities. *Cephalalgia* 17:188-190.

Creighton SM & Stanton SL (1990). Caffeine: Does it affect your bladder? *British Journal of Urology* 66:613-614.

Daly JW (1993). Mechanism of action of caffeine. In S Garattini (ed.) *Caffeine, Coffee and Health*. New York, NY: Raven Press, 97-150.

Denaro CP & Benowitz NL (1991). Caffeine metabolism: Disposition in liver disease and hepatic-function testing. In RR Watson (ed.) *Drug and Alcohol Abuse Reviews, Vol. 2: Liver Pathology and Alcohol*. Totowa, NJ: The Humana Press, Inc., 513-539.

Denaro CP, Brown CR, Jacob III P et al. (1991). Effects of caffeine with repeated dosing. *European Journal of Clinical Pharmacology* 40:273-278.

Denaro CP, Brown CR, Wilson M et al. (1990). Dose-dependency of caffeine metabolism with repeated dosing. *Clinical Pharmacology and Therapeutics* 48:277-285.

Deneau G, Yanagita T & Seevers MH (1969). Self-administration of psychoactive substances by the monkey: A measure of psychological dependence. *Psychopharmacologia* 16:30-48.

Dews PB, Curtis GL, Hanford KJ et al. (1999). The frequency of caffeine withdrawal in a population-based survey and in a controlled, blinded pilot experiment. *Journal of Clinical Pharmacology* 39:1221-1232.

Dreisbach RH & Pfeiffer C (1943). Caffeine-withdrawal headache. *Journal of Laboratory and Clinical Medicine* 28:1212-1219.

Duffy P & Phillips YY (1991). Caffeine consumption decreases the response to bronchoprovocation challenge with dry gas hyperventilation. *Chest* 99(6):1374-1377.

Dworkin SI, Vrana SL, Broadbent J et al. (1993). Comparing the reinforcing effects of nicotine, caffeine, methylphenidate and cocaine. *Medicinal Chemistry Research* 2:593-602.

El Yacoubi M, Ledent C, Ménard J-F et al. (2000). The stimulant effects of caffeine on locomotor behaviour in mice are mediated through its blockade of adenosine A_{2A} receptors. *British Journal of Pharmacology* 129:1463-1473.

Emurian HH, Nellis MJ, Brady JV et al. (1982). Event time-series relationship between cigarette smoking and coffee drinking. *Addictive Behaviors* 7(4):441-444.

Evans SM, Critchfield TS & Griffiths RR (1994). Caffeine reinforcement demonstrated in a majority of moderate caffeine users. *Behavioural Pharmacology* 5:231-238.

Evans SM & Griffiths RR (1992). Caffeine tolerance and choice in humans. *Psychopharmacology* 108:51-59.

Evans SM & Griffiths RR (1999). Caffeine withdrawal: A parametric analysis of caffeine dosing conditions. *Journal of Pharmacology and Experimental Therapeutics* 289(1):285-294.

Evans SM & Griffiths RR (1991). Dose-related caffeine discrimination in normal volunteers: Individual differences in subjective effects and self-reported cues. *Behavioural Pharmacology* 2:345-356.

Fennely M, Galletly DC & Puride GI (1991). Is caffeine withdrawal the mechanism of postoperative headache? *Anesthesia and Analgesia* 72:449-453.

Fernandes O, Sabharwal M, Smiley T et al. (1998). Moderate to heavy caffeine consumption during pregnancy and relationship to spontaneous abortion and abnormal fetal growth: A meta-analysis. *Reproductive Toxicology* 12(4):435-444.

Finn IB & Holtzman SG (1987). Pharmacologic specificity of tolerance to caffeine-induced stimulation of locomotor activity. *Psychopharmacology* 93:428-434.

Finn IB & Holtzman SG (1988). Tolerance and cross-tolerance to theophylline-induced stimulation of locomotor activity in rats. *Life Sciences* 42:2475-2482.

Finn IB & Holtzman SG (1986). Tolerance to caffeine-induced stimulation of locomotor activity in rats. *Journal of Pharmacology and Experimental Therapeutics* 238:542-546.

Foxx RM & Rubinoff A (1979). Behavioral treatment of caffeinism: Reducing excessive coffee drinking. *Journal of Applied Behavior Analysis* 12(3):335-344.

Fredholm BB, Bättig K, Holmén J et al. (1999). Actions of caffeine in the brain with special reference to factors that contribute to its widespread use. *Pharmacological Reviews* 51(1):83-133.

Galletly DC, Fennelly M & Whitwam JG (1989). Does caffeine withdrawal contribute to post anaesthetic morbidity? *Lancet* 10(1):1335.

Garattini S, ed. (1993). *Caffeine, Coffee, and Health.* New York, NY: Raven Press, Ltd.

Garrett BE & Griffiths RR (1997). The role of dopamine in the behavioral effects of caffeine in animals and humans. *Pharmacology, Biochemistry and Behavior* 57(3):533-541.

Garrett BE & Griffiths RR (1998). Physical dependence increases the relative reinforcing effects of caffeine versus placebo. *Psychopharmacology* 139:195-202.

Garrett BE & Griffiths RR (2001). Intravenous nicotine and caffeine: Subjective and physiological effects in cocaine abusers. *Journal of Pharmacology and Experimental Therapeutics* 296(2):486-494.

Garrett BE & Holtzman SG (1994). Caffeine cross-tolerance to selective dopamine D_1 and D_2 receptor agonists but not to their synergistic interaction. *European Journal of Pharmacology* 262:65-75.

Garrett BE & Holtzman SG (1996). Comparison of the effects of prototypical behavioral stimulants on locomotor activity and rotational behavior in rats. *Pharmacology, Biochemistry and Behavior* 54(2):469-477.

Gasior M, Jaszyna M, Peters J et al. (2000). Changes in the ambulatory activity and discriminative stimulus effects of psychostimulant drugs in rats chronically exposed to caffeine: Effect of caffeine dose. *Journal of Pharmacology and Experimental Therapeutics* 295(3):1101-1111.

Gilbert RM (1973). Caffeine as a drug of abuse. In RJ Gibbins, Y Israel, H Kalant et al. (eds.) *Research Advances in Alcohol and Drug Problems.* New York, NY: John Wiley & Sons, 49-176.

Gilbert RM (1984). Caffeine consumption. In GA Spiller (ed.) *The Methylxanthine Beverages and Foods: Chemistry, Consumption, and Health Effects.* New York, NY: Alan R. Liss, Inc., 185-213.

Goldberg SR & Henningfield JE (1988). Reinforcing effects of nicotine in humans and experimental animals responding under intermittent schedules of IV drug injection. *Pharmacology Biochemistry and Behavior* 30:227-234.

Goldstein A (1964). Wakefulness caused by caffeine. *Archiv fur Experimentelle Pathologic und Pharmakologic* 248:269-278.

Goldstein A & Kaizer S (1969). Psychotropic effects of caffeine in man. III. A questionnaire survey of coffee drinking and its effects in a group of housewives. *Clinical Pharmacology and Therapeutics* 10(4):477-488.

Goldstein A, Kaizer S & Whitby O (1969). Psychotropic effects of caffeine in man. IV. Quantitative and qualitative differences associated with habituation to coffee. *Clinical Pharmacology and Therapeutics* 10:489-497.

Goldstein A & Wallace ME (1997). Caffeine dependence in school children? *Experimental and Clinical Psychopharmacology* 5(4):388-392.

Goldstein A, Warren R & Kaizer S (1965). Psychotropic effects of caffeine in man. I. Individual differences in sensitivity to caffeine-induced wakefulness. *Journal of Pharmacology and Experimental Therapeutics* 149(1):156-159.

Graham TE (2001). Caffeine and exercise: Metabolism, endurance and performance. *Sports Medicine* 31(11):785-807.

Greden JF (1974). Anxiety of caffeinism: A diagnostic dilemma. *American Journal of Psychiatry* 131(10):1089-1092.

Greden JF (1981). Caffeinism and caffeine withdrawal. In JH Lowinson & P Ruiz (eds.) *Substance Abuse: Clinical Problems and Perspectives.* Baltimore, MD: Lippincott Williams & Wilkins, 274-286.

Greden JF & Pomerleau OF (1995). Caffeine-related disorders and nicotine-related disorders. In HI Kaplan & BJ Sadock (eds.) *Comprehensive Textbook of Psychiatry/VI.* Baltimore, MD: Williams & Wilkins, 799-810.

Greden JF, Procter A & Victor B (1981). Caffeinism associated with greater use of other psychotropic agents. *Comprehensive Psychiatry* 22(6):565-571.

Greden JF & Walters A (1992). Caffeine. In JH Lowinson, P Ruiz, RB Millman & JG Langrod (eds.) *Substance Abuse: A Comprehensive Textbook, 3rd Edition.* Baltimore, MD: Williams & Wilkins, 357-370.

Greden JF, Victor BS, Fontaine P et al. (1980). Caffeine-withdrawal headache: A clinical profile. *Psychosomatics* 21(5):411-418.

Green PJ, Kirby R & Suls J (1996). The effects of caffeine on blood pressure and heart rate: A review. *Annals of Behavior Medicine* 18(3):201-216.

Green TA & Schenk S (2002). Dopaminergic mechanism for caffeine-produced cocaine-seeking in rats. *Neuropsychopharmacology* 26(4):422-430.

Griffiths RR, Bigelow GE & Liebson IA (1986a). Human coffee drinking: Reinforcing and physical dependence producing effects of caffeine. *Journal of Pharmacology and Experimental Therapeutics* 239(2):416-425.

Griffiths RR, Bigelow GE & Liebson IA (1989). Reinforcing effects of caffeine in coffee and capsules. *Journal of the Experimental Analysis of Behavior* 52:127-140.

Griffiths RR, Bigelow GE, Liebson IA et al. (1986a). Human coffee drinking: Manipulation of concentration and caffeine dose. *Journal of the Experimental Analysis of Behavior* 45:133-148.

Griffiths RR, Brady JV & Bradford LD (1979). Predicting the abuse liability of drugs with animal drug self-administration procedures: Psychomotor stimulants and hallucinogens. In T Thompson & PB Dews (eds.) *Advances in Behavioral Pharmacology, Vol. 2.* New York, NY: Academic Press, 163-208.

Griffiths RR, Evans SM, Heishman SJ et al. (1990a). Low-dose caffeine discrimination in humans. *Journal of Pharmacology and Experimental Therapeutics* 252:970-978.

Griffiths RR, Evans SM, Heishman SJ et al. (1990b). Low-dose caffeine physical dependence in humans. *Journal of Pharmacology and Experimental Therapeutics* 255:1123-1132.

Griffiths RR, Lamb RJ, Ator NA et al. (1985). Relative abuse liability of triazolam: Experimental assessment in animals and humans. *Neuroscience and Biobehavioral Reviews* 9:133-151.

Griffiths RR & Mumford GK (1995). Caffeine—A drug of abuse? In FE Bloom & DJ Kupfer (eds.) *Psychopharmacology: The Fourth Generation of Progress.* New York, NY: Raven Press, Ltd., 1699-1713.

Griffiths RR & Mumford GK (1996). Caffeine reinforcement, discrimination, tolerance and physical dependence in laboratory animals and humans. In CR Schuster & MJ Kuhars (eds.) *Pharmacological Aspects of Drug Dependence: Toward an Integrated Neurobehavioral Approach* (Handbook of Experimental Pharmacology, Vol. 118). Heidelberg, Germany: Springer-Verlag, 315-341.

Griffiths RR & Woodson PP (1988a). Caffeine physical dependence: A review of human and laboratory animal studies. *Psychopharmacology* 94:437-451.

Griffiths RR & Woodson PP (1988b). Reinforcing effects of caffeine in humans. *Journal of Pharmacology and Experimental Therapeutics* 246:21-29.

Hagg S, Spigset O, Mjorndal T et al. (2000). Effect of caffeine on clozapine pharmacokinetics in healthy volunteers. *British Journal of Clinical Pharmacology* 49(1):59-63.

Hale KL, Hughes JR, Oliveto AH et al. (1995). Caffeine self-administration and subjective effects in adolescents. *Experimental and Clinical Psychopharmacology* 3(4):364-370.

Hamill NJ & Levin RJ (1997). Caffeine withdrawal after head and neck surgery. *Otolaryngology and Head and Neck Surgery* 117:S179-S181.

Hampl KF, Schneider MC, Ruttimann U et al. (1995). Perioperative administration of caffeine tablets for prevention of postoperative headaches. *Canadian Journal of Anaesthesia* 42(9):789-792.

Hara Y, Luo S-J, Wickremasinghe RL et al. (1995). III. Tea-producing countries. *Food Reviews International* 11(3):381-407.

Hartley TR, Sung BH, Pincomb GA et al. (2000). Hypertension risk status and effect of caffeine on blood pressure. *Hypertension* 36:137-141.

Hasenfratz M, Buzzini P, Cheda P et al. (1994). Temporal relationships of the effects of caffeine and alcohol on rapid information processing. *Pharmacopsychoecologia* 7:87-96.

Hattox RS (1985). *Coffee and Coffeehouses: The Origins of a Social Beverage in the Medieval Near East*. Seattle, WA: University of Washington Press.

Heishman SJ, Taylor RC, Goodman ML et al. (1992). Discriminative stimulus effects of d-amphetamine, caffeine, and mazindol in humans. *Pharmacology Biochemistry and Behavior* 46:502-503.

Heseltine D, el-Jabri M, Ahmed F et al. (1991). The effect of caffeine on postprandial blood pressure in the frail elderly. *Postgraduate Medical Journal* 67(788):543-547.

Hettema JM, Corey LA & Kendler KS (1999). A multivariate genetic analysis of the use of tobacco, alcohol, and caffeine in a population based sample of male and female twins. *Drug and Alcohol Dependence* 57:69-78.

Hindmarch I, Rigney U, Stanley N et al. (2000). A naturalistic investigation of the effects of day-long consumption of tea, coffee and water on alertness, sleep onset and sleep quality. *Psychopharmacology* 149:203-216.

Hirsh K (1984). Central nervous system pharmacology of the dietary methylxanthines. In GA Spiller (ed.) *The Methylxanthine Beverages and Foods: Chemistry, Consumption, and Health Effects*. New York, NY: Liss, 235-301.

Höfer I & Bättig K (1994a). Cardiovascular, behavioral, and subjective effects of caffeine under field conditions. *Pharmacology Biochemistry and Behavior* 48(4):899-908.

Höfer I & Bättig K (1994b). Psychophysiological effects of switching to caffeine tablets or decaffeinated coffee under field conditions. *Pharmacopsychoecologia* 7:169-177.

Holtzman SG (1983). Complete, reversible, drug-specific tolerance to stimulation of locomotor activity by caffeine. *Life Sciences* 33:779-787.

Holtzman SG (1986). Discriminative stimulus properties of caffeine in the rat: Noradrenergic mediation. *Journal of Pharmacology and Experimental Therapeutics* 239(3):706-714.

Holtzman SG & Finn IB (1988). Tolerance to behavioral effects of caffeine in rats. *Pharmacology Biochemistry and Behavior* 29:411-418.

Holtzman SG, Mante S & Minneman KP (1991). Role of adenosine receptors in caffeine tolerance. *Journal of Pharmacology and Experimental Therapeutics* 256:62-68.

Howell LL (1993). Comparative effects of caffeine and selective phosphodiesterase inhibitors on respiration and behavior in rhesus monkeys. *Journal of Pharmacology and Experimental Therapeutics* 266:894-902.

Howell LL, Coffin VL & Spealman RD (1997). Behavioral and physiological effects of xanthines in nonhuman primates. *Psychopharmacology* 129:1-14.

Howell LL & Landrum AM (1997). Effects of chronic caffeine administration on respiration and schedule-controlled behavior in rhesus monkeys. *Journal of Pharmacology and Experimental Therapeutics* 283(1):190-199.

Hughes JR (1994). Caffeine withdrawal, dependence, and abuse. *Diagnostic and Statistical Manual of Mental Disorders, 4th Edition*. Washington, DC: American Psychiatric Press, 129-134.

Hughes JR, Higgins ST, Bickel WK et al. (1991). Caffeine self-administration, withdrawal, and adverse effects among coffee drinkers. *Archives of General Psychiatry* 48:611-617.

Hughes JR, Hunt WK, Higgins ST et al. (1992). Effect of dose on the ability of caffeine to serve as a reinforcer in humans. *Behavioural Pharmacology* 3:211-218.

Hughes JR & Oliveto AH (1997). A systematic survey of caffeine intake in Vermont. *Experimental and Clinical Psychopharmacology* 5(4):393-398.

Hughes JR & Oliveto AH (1993). Coffee and alcohol intake as predictors of smoking cessation and tobacco withdrawal. *Journal of Substance Abuse* 5(3):305-310.

Hughes JR, Oliveto AH, Bickel WK et al. (1993). Caffeine self-administration and withdrawal: Incidence, individual differences and interrelationships. *Drug and Alcohol Dependence* 32:239-246.

Hughes JR, Oliveto AH, Bickel WK et al. (1992a). Caffeine self-administration and withdrawal in soda drinkers. *Journal of Addictive Diseases* 4:178.

Hughes JR, Oliveto AH, Bickel WR et al. (1995). The ability of low doses of caffeine to serve as reinforcers in humans: A replication. *Experimental and Clinical Psychopharmacology* 3(4):358-363.

Hughes JR, Oliveto AH, Helzer JE et al. (1992b). Should caffeine abuse, dependence, or withdrawal be added to DSM-IV and ICD-10? *American Journal of Psychiatry* 149(1):33-40.

Hughes JR, Oliveto AH, Liguori A et al. (1998). Endorsement of DSM-IV dependence criteria among caffeine users. *Drug and Alcohol Dependence* 52:99-107.

Hughes JR, Oliveto AH & MacLaughlin M (2000). Is dependence on one drug associated with dependence on other drugs? The cases of alcohol, caffeine and nicotine. *American Journal on Addictions* 9:196-201.

Istvan J & Matarazzo JD (1984). Tobacco, alcohol, and caffeine use: A review of their interrelationships. *Psychological Bulletin* 95(2):301-326.

James JE (1991). *Caffeine and Health.* San Diego, CA: Academic Press Inc.

James JE (1997). *Understanding Caffeine.* Thousand Oaks, CA: Sage Publications, Inc.

James JE (1998). Acute and chronic effects of caffeine on performance, mood, headache, and sleep. *Neuropsychobiology* 38:32-41.

James JE, Paull I, Cameron-Traub E et al. (1988). Biochemical validation of self-reported caffeine consumption during caffeine fading. *Journal of Behavioral Medicine* 11(1):15-30.

James JE, Sawczuk D & Merrett S (1989). The effect of chronic caffeine consumption on urinary incontinence in psychogeriatric inpatients. *Psychology and Health* 3:297-305.

James JE, Stirling KP & Hampton BAM (1985). Caffeine fading: Behavioral treatment of caffeine abuse. *Behavior Therapy* 16:15-27.

Johansson B, Georgiev V, Lindström K et al. (1997). A_1 and A_{2A} adenosine receptors and A_1 mRNA in mouse brain: Effect of long-term caffeine treatment. *Brain Research* 762:153-164.

Jones HE, Herning RI, Cadet JL et al. (2000). Caffeine withdrawal increases cerebral blood flow velocity and alters quantitative electroencephalography (EEG) activity. *Psychopharmacology* 147:371-377.

Karacan I, Thornby JI, Anch MA et al. (1976). Dose-related sleep disturbances induced by coffee and caffeine. *Clinical Pharmacology and Therapeutics* 20(6):682-689.

Kelsey MC & Grossberg GT (1995). Safety and efficacy of caffeine-augmented ECT in elderly depressives: A retrospective study. *Journal of Geriatric Psychiatry and Neurology* 8(3):168-172.

Kendler KS & Prescott CA (1999). Caffeine intake, tolerance, and withdrawal in women: A population-based twin study. *American Journal of Psychiatry* 156:223-228.

Kingdon (1833). Effects of tea and coffee drinking. *Lancet* II:47-48.

Klebanoff MA, Levine RJ, DerSimonian R et al. (1999). Maternal serum paraxanthine, a caffeine metabolite, and the risk of spontaneous abortion. *New England Journal of Medicine* 341(22):1639-1644.

Kozlowski LT, Henningfield JE, Keenan RM et al. (1993). Patterns of alcohol, cigarette, and caffeine and other drug use in two drug abusing populations. *Journal of Substance Abuse Treatment* 10:171-179.

Kuzmin A, Johansson B, Semenova S et al. (2000). Differences in the effect of chronic and acute caffeine on self-administration of cocaine in mice. *European Journal of Neuroscience* 12:3026-3032.

Kuzmin A, Johansson B, Zvartau EE et al. (1999). Caffeine, acting on adenosine A_1 receptors, prevents the extinction of cocaine-seeking behavior in mice. *Journal of Pharmacology and Experimental Therapeutics* 290(2):535-542.

Lader M, Cardwell C, Shine P et al. (1996). Caffeine withdrawal symptoms and rate of metabolism. *Journal of Psychopharmacology* 10(2):110-118.

Landolt H-P, Werth E, Borbély AA et al. (1995). Caffeine intake (200 mg) in the morning affects human sleep and EEG power spectra at night. *Brain Research* 675:67-74.

Lane JD (1996). Association of coffee drinking with cigarette smoking in the natural environment. *Experimental and Clinical Psychopharmacology* 4(4):409-412.

Lane JD (1997). Effects of brief caffeinated-beverage deprivation on mood, symptoms, and psychomotor performance. *Pharmacology Biochemistry and Behavior* 58(1):203-208.

Lane JD (1994). Neuroendocrine responses to caffeine in the work environment. *Psychosomatic Medicine* 546:267-270.

Lane JD & Phillips-Bute BG (1998). Caffeine deprivation affects vigilance performance and mood. *Physiology and Behavior* 65(1):171-175.

Laska EM, Sunshine A, Mueller F et al. (1984). Caffeine as an analgesic adjuvant. *Journal of the American Medical Association* 251(13):1711-1718.

Leathwood PD & Pollet P (1983). Diet-induced mood changes in normal populations. *Journal of Psychiatric Research* 17:147-154.

Lieberman HR, Wurtman RJ, Emde GG et al. (1987). The effects of caffeine and aspirin on mood and performance. *Journal of Clinical Psychopharmacology* 7:315-320.

Lee MA, Cameron OG & Greden JF (1985). Anxiety and caffeine consumption in people with anxiety disorders. *Psychiatry Research* 15:211-217.

Lee MA, Flegel P, Greden JF et al. (1988). Anxiogenic effects of caffeine on panic and depressed patients. *American Journal of Psychiatry* 145(5):632-635.

Liguori A, Grass JA & Hughes JR (1999). Subjective effects of caffeine among introverts and extroverts in the morning and evening. *Experimental and Clinical Psychopharmacology* 7(3):244-249.

Liguori A & Hughes JR (1997). Caffeine self-administration in humans: 2. A within-subjects comparison of coffee and cola vehicles. *Experimental and Clinical Psychopharmacology* 5(3):295-303.

Liguori A, Hughes JR, Goldberg K et al. (1997a). Subjective effects of oral caffeine in formerly caffeine-dependent humans. *Drug and Alcohol Dependence* 49:17-24.

Liguori A, Hughes JR & Grass JA (1997b). Absorption and subjective effects of caffeine from coffee, cola and capsules. *Pharmacology Biochemistry and Behavior* 58(3):721-726.

Liguori A, Hughes JR & Oliveto AH (1997c). Caffeine self-administration in humans: 1. Efficacy of cola vehicle. *Experimental and Clinical Psychopharmacology* 5(3):286-294.

Liguori A & Robinson JH (2001). Caffeine antagonism of alcohol-induced driving impairment. *Drug and Alcohol Dependence* 63(2):123-129.

Lin AS, Uhde TW, Slate SO et al. (1997). Effects of intravenous caffeine administered to healthy males during sleep. *Depression and Anxiety* 5(1):21-28.

Lipsitz LA, Jansen RW, Connelly CM et al. (1994). Haemodynamic and neurohumoral effects of caffeine in elderly patients with symptomatic postprandial hypotension: A double-blind, randomized, placebo-controlled study. *Clinical Science* 87(2):259-267.

Logan L, Seale TW & Carney JM (1986). Inherent differences in sensitivity to methylxanthines among inbred mice. *Pharmacology Biochemistry and Behavior* 24(5):1281-1286.

Lovallo WR, al'Absi M, Pincomb GA et al. (2000). Caffeine, extended stress, and blood pressure in borderline hypertensive men. *International Journal of Behavioral Medicine* 7(2):183-188.

Marks V & Kelly JF (1973). Absorption of caffeine from tea, coffee, and coca cola. *Lancet* 14;1(7807):827.

May DC, Jarboe CH, VanBakel AB et al. (1982). Effects of cimetidine on caffeine disposition in smokers and nonsmokers. *Clinical Pharmacology and Therapeutics* 31(5):656-661.

Mester R, Toren P, Mizrachi I et al. (1995). Caffeine withdrawal increases lithium blood levels. *Biological Psychiatry* 37(5):348-350.

Mitchell SH, de Wit H & Zacny JP (1995). Caffeine withdrawal symptoms and self-administration following caffeine deprivation. *Pharmacology Biochemistry and Behavior* 51(4):941-945.

Mumford GK, Benowitz NL, Evans SM et al. (1996). Absorption rate of methylxanthines following capsules, cola and chocolate. *European Journal of Clinical Pharmacology* 51:319-325.

Mumford GK, Evans SM, Kaminski BJ et al. (1994). Discriminative stimulus and subjective effects of theobromine and caffeine in humans. *Psychopharmacology* 115:1-8.

Mumford GK & Holtzman SG (1991). Qualitative differences in the discriminative stimulus effects of low and high doses of caffeine in the rat. *Journal of Pharmacology and Experimental Therapeutics* 258:857-865.

Newman F, Stein MB, Trettau JR et al. (1992). Quantitative electroencephalographic effects of caffeine in panic disorder. *Psychiatry Research: Neuroimaging* 45:105-113.

Nickell PV & Uhde TW (1994/1995). Dose-response effects of intravenous caffeine in normal volunteers. *Anxiety* 1:161-168.

Nikolajsen L, Larsen KM & Kierkegaard O (1994). Effect of previous frequency of headache, duration of fasting and caffeine abstinence on perioperative headache. *British Journal of Anaesthesia* 72(3):295-297.

Nurminen M-L, Nittynen L, Korpela R et al. ((1999). Coffee, caffeine and blood pressure: A critical review. *European Journal of Clinical Nutrition* 53:831-839.

Oberstar JV, Bernstein GA & Thuras PD (2002). Caffeine use and dependence in adolescents: One-year follow-up. *Journal of Child and Adolescent Psychopharmacology* 12(2):127-135.

Okuma T, Matsuoka H, Matsue Y et al. (1982). Model insomnia by methylphenidate and caffeine and use in the evaluation of temazepam. *Psychopharmacology* 76:201-208.

Oliveto AH, Bickel WK, Hughes JR et al. (1992). Caffeine drug discrimination in humans: Acquisition, specificity and correlation with self-reports. *Journal of Pharmacology and Experimental Therapeutics* 261:885-894.

Oliveto AH, Bickel WK, Hughes JR et al. (1997). Functional antagonism of the caffeine-discriminative stimulus by triazolam in humans. *Behavioural Pharmacology* 8(2-3):124-138.

Oliveto AH, Bickel WK, Hughes JR et al. (1993). Pharmacological specificity of the caffeine discriminative stimulus in humans: Effects of theophylline, methylphenidate and buspirone. *Behavioural Pharmacology* 4:237-246.

Oliveto AH, Hughes JR, Higgins ST et al. (1992). Forced-choice versus free-choice procedures: Caffeine self-administration in humans. *Psychopharmacology* 109:85-91.

Oliveto AH, Hughes JR, Terry SY et al. (1991). Effects of caffeine on tobacco withdrawal. *Clinical Pharmacology and Therapeutics* 50:157-164.

Oliveto AH, McCance-Katz E, Singha A et al. (1998). Effects of *d*-amphetamine and caffeine in humans under a cocaine discrimination procedure. *Behavioural Pharmacology* 9:207-217.

Parsons WD & Neims AH (1978). Effect of smoking on caffeine clearance. *Clinical Pharmacology Therapeutics* 24(1):40-45.

Parsons WD & Neims AH (1981). Brief clinical and laboratory observations: Prolonged half-life of caffeine in healthy term newborn infants. *Journal of Pediatrics* 98(4):640-641.

Patat A, Rosenzweig P, Enslen M et al. (2000). Effects of a new slow release formulation of caffeine on EEG, psychomotor and cognitive functions in sleep-deprived subjects. *Human Psychopharmacology Clinical and Experimental* 15:153-170.

Patkina NA & Zvartau EE (1998). Caffeine place conditioning in rats: Comparison with cocaine and ethanol. *European Neuropsychopharmacology* 8:287-291.

Patwardhan RV, Desmond PV, Johnson RF et al. (1980). Effects of caffeine on plasma free fatty acids, urinary catecholamines, and drug binding. *Clinical Pharmacology and Therapeutics* 28(3):398-403.

Pendergrast M (1993). *For God, Country and Coca-Cola: The Unauthorized History of the Great American Soft Drink and the Company that Makes It.* New York, NY: Charles Scribner's Sons.

Pendergrast M (1999). *Uncommon Grounds: The History of Coffee and How It Transformed Our World.* New York, NY: Basic Books.

Penetar DM, McCann U, Thorne D et al. (1994). Effects of caffeine on cognitive performance, mood, and alertness in sleep-deprived humans. In BM Marriott (ed.) *Food Components to Enhance Performance: An Evaluation of Potential Performance-Enhancing Food Components for Operational Rations (Committee on Military Nutrition Research, Food and Nutrition Board, Institute of Medicine).* Washington, DC: National Academy Press, 407-431.

Phillips-Bute BG & Lane JD (1998). Caffeine withdrawal symptoms following brief caffeine deprivation. *Physiology and Behavior* 63(1):35-39.

Pianosi P, Grondin D, Desmond K et al. (1994). Effect of caffeine on the ventilatory response to inhaled carbon dioxide. *Respiration Physiology* 95(3):311-320.

Powell KR, Iuvone PM & Holtzman SG (2001). The role of dopamine in the locomotor stimulant effects and tolerance to these effects of caffeine. *Pharmacology Biochemistry and Behavior* 69(1-2):59-70.

Powell KR, Koppelman LF & Holtzman SG (1999). Differential involvement of dopamine in mediating the discriminative stimulus effects of low and high doses of caffeine in rats. *Behavioural Pharmacology* 10:707-716.

Rainey JT (1985). Headache related to chronic caffeine addiction. *Texas Dental Journal* 102(7):29-30.

Rao SSC, Welcher K, Zimmerman B et al. (1998) Is coffee a colonic stimulant? *European Journal of Gastroenterology and Hepatology* 10:113-118.

Reeves RR, Struve FA, Patrick G et al. (1995). Topographic quantitative EEG measures of alpha and theta power changes during caffeine withdrawal: Preliminary findings from normal subjects. *Clinical Electroencephalography* 26(3):154-162.

Regestein QR (1989). Pathologic sleepiness induced by caffeine. *American Journal of Medicine* 87(5):586-588.

Reyner LA & Horne JA (2000). Early morning driver sleepiness: Effectiveness of 200 mg caffeine. *Psychophysiology* 37:251-256.

Richardson NJ, Rogers PJ & Elliman NA (1996). Conditioned flavour preferences reinforced by caffeine consumed after lunch. *Physiology and Behavior* 60(1):257-263.

Richardson NJ, Rogers PJ, Elliman NA et al. (1995). Mood and performance effects of caffeine in relation to acute and chronic caffeine deprivation. *Pharmacology Biochemistry and Behavior* 52(2):313-320.

Rihs M, Müller C & Baumann P (1996). Caffeine consumption in hospitalized psychiatric patients. *European Archives of Psychiatry and Clinical Neuroscience* 246:83-92.

Rizzo AA, Stamps LE & Fehr LA (1988). Effects of caffeine withdrawal on motor performance and heart rate changes. *International Journal of Psychophysiology* 6:9-14.

Roache JD & Griffiths RR (1987). Interactions of diazepam and caffeine: Behavioral and subjective dose effects in humans. *Pharmacology Biochemistry and Behavior* 26(4):801-812.

Robelin M & Rogers PJ (1998). Mood and psychomotor performance effects of the first, but not of subsequent, cup-of-coffee equivalent doses of caffeine consumed after overnight caffeine abstinence. *Behavioural Pharmacology* 9(7):611-618.

Robertson D, Wade D, Workman R et al. (1981). Tolerance to the humoral and hemodynamic effects of caffeine in man. *Journal of Clinical Investigation* 67(4):1111-1117.

Robinson JH & Pritchard WS (1992a). The role of nicotine in tobacco use. *Psychopharmacology* 108:397-407.

Robinson JH & Pritchard WS (1992b). The meaning of addiction: Reply to West. *Psychopharmacology* 108:411-416.

Rogers PJ (2000). Why we drink caffeine-containing beverages, and the equivocal benefits of regular caffeine intake for mood and cognitive performance. In TH Parliment, C-T Ho & P Schieberle (eds.) *Caffeinated Beverages: Health Benefits, Physiological Effects, and Chemistry.* ACS Symposium Series No. 754. Washington DC: American Chemical Society, 37-45.

Rogers PJ & Dernoncourt C (1998). Regular caffeine consumption: A balance of adverse and beneficial effects for mood and psychomotor performance. *Pharmacology Biochemistry and Behavior* 59(4):1039-1045.

Rogers PJ, Richardson NJ & Elliman NA (1995). Overnight caffeine abstinence and negative reinforcement of preference for caffeine-containing drinks. *Psychopharmacology* 120:457-462.

Rosenquist PB, McCall WV, Farah A et al. (1994). Effects of caffeine pretreatment on measures of seizure impact. *Convulsive Therapy* 10(2):181-185.

Rush CR, Higgins ST, Hughes JR et al. (1993). Acute behavioral and cardiac effects of alcohol and caffeine, alone and in combination, in humans. *Behavioural Pharmacology* 4:562-572.

Rush CR, Sullivan JT & Griffiths RR (1995). Intravenous caffeine in stimulant drug abusers: Subjective reports and physiological effects. *Journal of Pharmacology and Experimental Therapeutics* 273(1):351-358.

Sawynok J (1995). Pharmacological rationale for the clinical use of caffeine. *Drugs* 49(1):37-50.

Schenk S & Partridge B (1999). Cocaine-seeking produced by experimenter-administered drug injections: Dose-effect relationships in rats. *Psychopharmacology* 147:285-290.

Schuh KJ & Griffiths RR (1997). Caffeine reinforcement: The role of withdrawal. *Psychopharmacology* 130:320-326.

Seale TW, Johnson P, Roderick TH et al. (1985). A single gene difference determines relative susceptibility to caffeine-induced lethality in SWR and CBA inbred mice. *Pharmacology Biochemistry and Behavior* 23:275-278.

Serafin WE (1996). Drugs used in the treatment of asthma. In MJ Wonsiewicz & P McCurdy (eds.) *The Pharmacological Basis of Therapeutics.* Hightstown, NJ: McGraw-Hill Publishers, 659-682.

Shi D, Nikodijevic O, Jacobson KA et al. (1993). Chronic caffeine alters the density of adenosine, adrenergic, cholinergic, GABA, and serotonin receptors and calcium channels in mouse brain. *Cellular and Molecular Neurobiology* 13(3):247-261.

Shi J, Benowitz NL, Denaro CP et al. (1993). Pharmacokinetic-pharmacodynamic modeling of caffeine: Tolerance to pressor effects. *Clinical Pharmacology and Therapeutics* 53:6-14.

Shoaib M, Swanner LS, Yasar S et al. (1999). Chronic caffeine exposure potentiates nicotine self-administration in rats. *Psychopharmacology* 142:327-333.

Silverman K, Evans SM, Strain EC et al. (1992). Withdrawal syndrome after the double-blind cessation of caffeine consumption. *New England Journal of Medicine* 327:1109-1114.

Silverman K & Griffiths RR (1992). Low-dose caffeine discrimination and self-reported mood effects in normal volunteers. *Journal of the Experimental Analysis of Behavior* 57:91-107.

Silverman K, Mumford GK & Griffiths RR (1994). Enhancing caffeine reinforcement by behavioral requirements following drug ingestion. *Psychopharmacology* 114:424-432.

Smit HJ & Rogers PJ (2000). Effects of low doses of caffeine on cognitive performance, mood, and thirst in low and higher caffeine consumers. *Psychopharmacology* 152:167-173.

Smith AP (1998). Effects of caffeine on attention: Low levels of arousal. In J Snel & MM Lorist (eds.) *Nicotine, Caffeine, and Social Drinking.* Amsterdam, The Netherlands: Harwood Academic Publishers, 215-227.

Snel J (1993). Coffee and caffeine sleep and wakefulness. In S Garattini (ed.) *Caffeine, Coffee, and Health.* New York, NY: Raven Press, Ltd., 255-290.

Snyder SH, Katims JJ, Annau A et al. (1981). Adenosine receptors in the central nervous system: Relationship to the central actions of methylxanthines. *Life Sciences* 28:2083-2097.

Spiller GA, ed. (1984). *The Methylxanthine Beverages and Foods: Chemistry, Consumption, and Health Effects.* New York, NY: Alan R. Liss, Inc.

Spriet LL (1995). Caffeine and performance. *International Journal of Sport Nutrition* 5:584-599.

Stern KN, Chait LD & Johanson CE (1989). Reinforcing and subjective effects of caffeine in normal human volunteers. *Psychopharmacology* 98:81-88.

Strain EC & Griffiths RR (1997). Caffeine. In A Tasman, J Kay & JA Lieberman (eds.) *Psychiatry, Volume I.* Philadelphia, PA: W. B. Saunders Company, 779-794.

Strain EC & Griffiths RR (2000). Caffeine-related disorders. In BJ Sadock & VA Sadock (eds.) *Comprehensive Textbook of Psychiatry/VII, Volume 1.* Philadelphia, PA: Lippincott Williams & Wilkins, 982-990.

Strain EC, Mumford GK, Silverman K et al. (1994). Caffeine dependence syndrome. Evidence from case histories and experimental evaluations. *Journal of the American Medical Association* 272(13):1043-1048.

Streufert S, Pogash R, Miller J et al. (1995). Effects of caffeine deprivation on complex human functioning. *Psychopharmacology* 118:377-384.

Swan GE, Carmelli D & Cardon LR (1996). The consumption of tobacco, alcohol, and coffee in caucasian male twins: A multivariate genetic analysis. *Journal of Substance Abuse* 8(1):19-31.

Swan GE, Carmelli D & Cardon LR (1997). Heavy consumption of cigarettes, alcohol and coffee in male twins. *Journal of Studies on Alcohol* 58(2):182-190.

Swanson JA, Lee JW & Hopp JW (1994). Caffeine and nicotine: A review of their joint use and possible interactive effects in tobacco withdrawal. *Addictive Behaviors* 19(3):229-256.

Tanda G & Goldberg SR (2000). Alteration of the behavioral effects of nicotine by chronic caffeine exposure. *Pharmacology Biochemistry and Behavior* 66(1):47-64.

Tarnopolsky M & Cupido C (2000). Caffeine potentiates low frequency skeletal muscle force in habitual and nonhabitual caffeine consumers. *Journal of Applied Physiology* 89:1719-1724.

Telch MJ, Silverman A & Schmidt NB (1996). Effects of anxiety sensitivity and perceived control on emotional responding to caffeine challenge. *Journal of Anxiety Disorders* 10(1):21-35.

Tobias JD (2000). Caffeine in the treatment of apnea associated with respiratory syncytial virus infection in neonates and infants. *Southern Medical Journal* 93(3):294-296.

Uhde TW (1990). Caffeine provocation of panic: A focus on biological mechanisms. In JC Ballenger (ed.) *Neurobiology of Panic Disorder.* New York, NY: Alan R. Liss, Inc., 219-242.

Urgert R & Katan MB (1997). The cholesterol-raising factor from coffee beans. *Annual Review of Nutrition* 17:305-324.

U.S. Department of Agriculture, Economic Research Service (2002). *Food Consumption, Prices, and Expenditures, 1970-2000.* Washington, DC: The Department.

van de Stelt O & Snel J (1998). Caffeine and human performance. In J Snel & MM Lorist (eds.) *Nicotine, Caffeine and Social Drinking.* Amsterdam, The Netherlands: Harwood Academic Publishers, 167-183.

van der Stelt O & Snel J (1993). Effects of caffeine on human information processing: A cognitive-energetic approach. In S Garattini (ed.) *Caffeine, Coffee and Health.* New York, NY: Raven Press, Ltd., 291-316.

van Dusseldrop M & Katan MB (1990). Headache caused by caffeine withdrawal among moderate coffee drinkers switched from ordinary to decaffeinated coffee: A 12 week double blind trial. *British Medical Journal* 300:1558-1559.

Verhoeff FH & Millar JM (1990). Does caffeine contribute to postoperative morbidity? *Lancet* 8:632.

Victor BS, Lubetsky M & Greden JF (1981). Somatic manifestations of caffeinism. *Journal of Clinical Psychiatry* 42:185-188.

von Borstel RW, Wurtman RJ & Conlay LA (1983). Chronic caffeine consumption potentiates the hypotensive action of circulating adenosine. *Life Sciences* 32:1151-1158.

Warburton DM (1995). Effects of caffeine on cognition and mood without caffeine abstinence. *Psychopharmacology* 119:66-70.

Watson JM, Lunt MJ, Morris S et al. (2000). Reversal of caffeine withdrawal by ingestion of a soft beverage. *Pharmacology Biochemistry and Behavior* 66(1):15-18.

Weber JG, Ereth MH & Danielson DR (1993). Perioperative ingestion of caffeine and postoperative headache. *Mayo Clinic Proceedings* 68:842-845.

Weber JG, Klindworth JT, Arnold JJ et al. (1997). Prophylactic intravenous administration of caffeine and recovery after ambulatory surgical procedures. *Mayo Clinic Proceedings* 72:621-626.

Weinberg BA & Bealer BK (2001). *The World of Caffeine: The Science and Culture of the World's Most Popular Drug.* New York, NY: Routledge.

Weiss B & Laties VG (1962). Enhancement of human performance by caffeine and the amphetamines. *Pharmacological Reviews* 14:1-36.

Wemple RD, Lamb DR & McKeever KH (1997). Caffeine vs. caffeine-free sports drinks: Effects on urine production at rest and during prolonged exercise. *International Journal of Sports Medicine* 18(1):40-46.

Wen W, Shu XO, Jacobs DR et al. (2001). The associations of maternal caffeine consumption and nausea with spontaneous abortion. *Epidemiology* 12:38-42.

Wendl B, Pfeiffer A, Pehl C et al. (1994). Effect of decaffeination of coffee or tea on gastro-esophageal reflux. *Alimentary Pharmacology and Therapeutics* 8:283-287.

West R (1992) Nicotine addiction: A re-analysis of the arguments. *Psychopharmacology* 108:408-410.

White JM (1994). Behavioral effects of caffeine coadministered with nicotine, benzodiazepines and alcohol. *Pharmacopsychoecologia* 7:119-126.

World Health Organization (1992a). *The ICD-10 Classification of Mental and Behavioural Disorders: Clinical Descriptions and Diagnostic Guidelines.* Geneva, Switzerland: World Health Organization, 70-83.

World Health Organization (1992b). *International Statistical Classification of Diseases and Related Health Problems, 10th Revision, Vol. 1.* Geneva, Switzerland: World Health Organization, 320-324.

Wright Jr. KP, Badia P, Myers BL et al. (1997). Combination of bright light and caffeine as a countermeasure for impaired alertness and performance during extended sleep deprivation. *Journal of Sleep Research* 6:26-35.

Yeomans MR, Jackson A, Lee MD et al. (2000). Expression of flavour preferences conditioned by caffeine is dependent on caffeine deprivation state. *Psychopharmacology* 150:208-215.

Yeomans MR, Spetch H & Rogers PJ (1998). Conditioned flavour preference negatively reinforced by caffeine in human volunteers. *Psychopharmacology* 137:401-409.

Yucel A, Ozyalcin S, Talu GK et al. (1999). Intravenous administration of caffeine sodium benzoate for postdural puncture headache. *Regional Anesthesia and Pain Medicine* 24(1):51-54.

Zwyghuizen-Doorenbos A, Roehrs TA, Lipschutz L et al. (1990). Effects of caffeine on alertness. *Psychopharmacology* 100:36-39.

Zylber-Katz E, Granit L & Levy M (1984). Relationship between caffeine concentrations in plasma and saliva. *Clinical Pharmacology and Therapeutics* 36(1):133-137.

The Pharmacology of Nicotine and Tobacco

Chapter 7

Lori D. Karan, M.D., FACP, FASAM
John A. Dani, Ph.D.
Neal Benowitz, M.D.

Drugs in the Class
Pharmacokinetics
Pharmacologic Actions
Neurobiologic Mechanisms of Action
Systemic Toxicity

Understanding the pharmacology of nicotine is important in devising effective interventions for smoking cessation and in developing nicotine as a therapeutic agent. This chapter examines the pharmacology of nicotine as it is present in tobacco and as an agent by itself. First, the absorption, distribution, metabolism, and elimination of nicotine are described. Discussions follow of the actions of nicotine, issues of tolerance and dependence, and the neuroscience underpinning nicotine's activity on circuits, receptors, and cells. Finally, the metabolic and toxic effects of using nicotine and tobacco are described.

This chapter is dedicated to the memory of John Slade, M.D., FASAM, founder of the ASAM Nicotine Dependence Committee, leader, mentor, and friend. John demonstrated that cigarettes were nicotine delivery devices, and he challenged tobacco advertising locally, nationally, and internationally. He pioneered the treatment of nicotine addiction during chemical dependency treatment, helped write the seminal analyses of the Brown & Williamson documents, and made possible FDA's quest to gain regulatory authority over tobacco. John created opportunities, fostered credibility and advocacy, influenced our thinking, and touched our souls. We dedicate our continued work to the memory of John's quiet wit and steadfast determination.

DRUGS IN THE CLASS

Nicotine, the addictive component of tobacco, is responsible for the compulsive use of tobacco in cigarettes, bidis, cigars, pipes, snuff, and chewing tobacco. Nicotine replacement medications, which are used to facilitate smoking cessation, include nicotine polacrilex gum, transdermal patches, nasal spray, inhalers, buccal lozenges and oral nicotine solutions. Nicotine and its analogs are being investigated as potential therapeutic agents for ulcerative colitis, Parkinson's disease, Alzheimer's disease, attention deficit/hyperactivity disorder (ADHD), schizophrenia, anxiety, depression, obesity, sleep apnea, and Tourette's syndrome (Karan, 1993).

PHARMACOKINETICS

Absorption, Distribution, Metabolism, and Elimination. Nicotine is a tertiary amine that consists of a pyridine and a pyrrolidine ring. There are two stereoisomers of nicotine. (S)-nicotine is the active isomer that binds to nicotinic cholinergic receptors, and is found in tobacco. (R)-nicotine is a weak agonist at cholinergic receptors. During smoking, some racemization takes place, and small quantities of (R)-nicotine are found in cigarette smoke.

The absorption of nicotine depends on its pH. Below pH 6, smoke contains less than 1% unprotonated (free) nicotine. As the pH rises, so does the proportion of unprotonated nicotine. At pH 7.26, 15% of the nicotine is unprotonated, increasing to 50% at pH 8. Unprotonated nicotine is present mainly in the vapor phase of the smoke, whereas protonated nicotine is bound within particles in the smoke aerosol (Zevin & Benowitz, 1998).

Unprotonated nicotine is absorbed through the mucous membranes of the oral and nasal cavities (Benowitz, 1988; DHHS, 1988; Henningfield, Radzius et al., 1990). Tobacco products such as cigars, many pipe tobaccos, snuffs, and chewing tobaccos present nicotine either as an un-ionized (unprotonated), vaporized component of smoke or as an alkaline solution of nicotine. Tobacco smoke with pH levels above 6.2 contains increasing amounts of free ammonia, nitrates that are partially reduced to ammonia during smoking, and other volatile basic components (Hoffmann & Hoffmann, 1997).

Because alkaline smoke is irritating to the pharynx, it is harsh and difficult to inhale. Therefore, smoke from cigarettes and from some pipe tobaccos has an acidic pH. The ionized nicotine in such smoke is largely dissolved in the aerosol droplets. Once small droplets of tar-containing nicotine are inhaled and deposited in small airways and alveoli, the protonated nicotine is buffered to a physiologic pH and absorbed. Inhaled nicotine avoids first-pass metabolism. It is quickly delivered from the large surface area of the alveoli and circulation in the lung to the arterial bloodstream and then to the tissues and the nicotinic receptors in the brain. Nicotine reaches the brain in approximately 10 to 19 seconds after inhalation. The brain is exposed to high peak levels of nicotine, so that the arterial levels of nicotine after cigarette smoking exceed venous levels by two- to six-fold (Henningfield, Stapleton et al., 1993; Gourlay & Benowitz, 1997). The rapid, finely tuned access of smoked nicotine to central nicotinic receptors is fundamental to the enhanced capacity of cigarette smoking (compared to other forms of nicotine delivery) to cause addiction.

The smoking process allows precise dose titration so that the smoker can obtain the desired effects. Smokers can alter their puff volume, the number of puffs they take from a cigarette, the intensity of puffing, and the depth to which they inhale. Smokers also can block the ventilation holes of the filter with their fingers or their lips. Because of the complexity of smoking, the exact dose of nicotine cannot be accurately predicted from the nicotine content of the tobacco or a cigarette's machine-rated yield (Benowitz, Hall et al., 1983). Individuals smoke in ways that largely compensate for the engineering tricks that reduce the amount of nicotine deposited on a filter pad in a smoking machine.

Nicotine is absorbed across the skin. "Green tobacco sickness," an occupational illness among tobacco croppers and harvesters, results from an accumulation of toxic levels of transdermally absorbed nicotine (Boylan, Brandt et al., 1993). Cases of poisoning have occurred following skin contact with pesticides containing nicotine. The design of the nicotine patches is based on a controlled delivery rate of much smaller fixed dosages of nicotine through the skin (Jarvik & Henningfield, 1993; Rose, Herskovic et al., 1985).

Nicotine is poorly absorbed from the stomach because of the acidity of the gastric fluid, but it is well absorbed in the small intestine, which has a more alkaline pH and a large surface area. When nicotine is administered in capsules, peak concentrations are reached in just over an hour. Nicotine undergoes first-pass metabolism; its oral bioavailability is approximately 45% (Benowitz, Porchet et al., 1990).

After it is absorbed, nicotine enters the bloodstream. Nicotine has a volume of distribution of 180 L, with less than 5% binding to plasma proteins. Nicotine crosses the placenta freely and has been found in the amniotic fluid and in the umbilical cord blood of neonates. Nicotine also is found in breast milk at concentrations approximately twice those found in blood.

Nicotine obtained from tobacco reaches high initial concentrations in the arterial blood, lung, and brain; subsequently, it is distributed to storage adipose and muscle tissue. The average steady-state concentration of nicotine in the body tissues is 2.6 times the average steady-state concentration of nicotine in the blood (Benowitz, Porchet et al., 1990). The distribution half-life of approximately eight minutes, rather than the elimination half-life of two hours, determines the time course of nicotine's actions on the central nervous system (CNS).

Based on a half-life of two hours, nicotine accumulates over six to eight hours (3 to 4 half-lives) of regular smoking and persists for six to eight hours (3 to 4 half-lives) after smoking ceases. Steady-state plasma nicotine levels, which plateau in the early afternoon, typically range between 10 and 50 ng/mL. The increment in blood nicotine concentration after smoking a single cigarette ranges from 5 to 30 ng/mL, depending on how the cigarette is smoked (Benowitz, Porchet et al., 1989). Peak blood concentrations of

FIGURE 1.   Mean Blood Concentrations of Nicotine

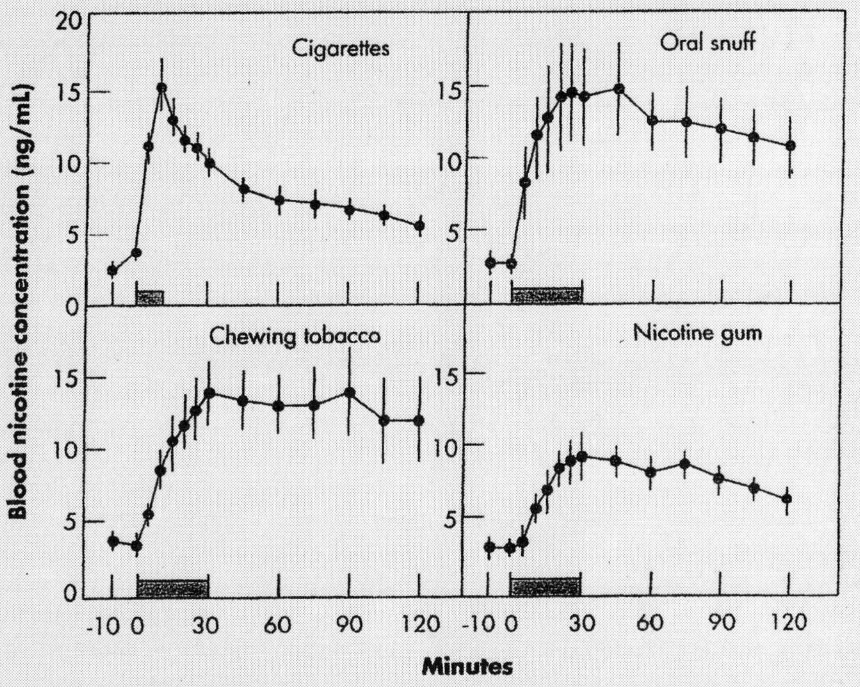

Mean blood concentrations of nicotine in 10 subjects who smoked cigarettes for 9 minutes (1.3 cigarettes), used oral snuff (2.5 g), used chewing tobacco (mean, 7.9 g), and chewed nicotine gum (two 2-mg pieces). Shaded bars above the time axis indicate the period of exposure to tobacco or nicotine gum.

nicotine are similar for cigar smokers, users of snuff, chewers of tobacco, and those who smoke cigarettes, although the rate of rise of nicotine concentrations is slower for the nonsmoking methods of tobacco use (Figure 1). Individual smokers seem to manipulate their nicotine intake to maintain a consistent level of nicotine from day to day (Benowitz, Jacob et al., 1982; Benowitz, Zevin et al., 1997). Intra-individual differences in maintenance plasma nicotine levels are much less pronounced than inter-individual differences.

Smoking represents a multiple-dosing situation, with considerable accumulation of nicotine in the body tissues while smoking. Nicotine persists in the body around the clock. Peaks and troughs in blood nicotine concentrations follow each cigarette but, as the day progresses for the regular smoker, trough levels rise and it is felt that the influence of the peak levels becomes less important. Tolerance occurs, so that the effects of individual cigarettes tend to lessen throughout the day. Overnight abstinence allows consider-

able resensitization (Figure 2). However, full resensitization requires days, weeks, or longer.

Nicotine is extensively metabolized, primarily in the liver and to a lesser extent in the lung and in the brain. About 70% to 80% of nicotine is metabolized to cotinine, which is further metabolized to trans 3' hydroxycotinine, the major nicotine metabolite found in the urine, as well as cotinine methonium ion, 5' hydroxycotinine, and cotinine-N-oxide. Only 17% of cotinine is excreted unchanged in the urine (Benowitz, Kuyt et al., 1983). CYP 2A6 is primarily responsible for both the C-oxidation of nicotine to cotinine and for the oxidation of cotinine to trans 3' hydroxycotinine. Nicotine, cotinine, and trans 3' hydroxycotinine are further metabolized by glucuronidation. The metabolites of nicotine are not believed to be highly psychoactive.

Renal clearance accounts for 2% to 35% of total nicotine clearance. The renal clearance of unchanged nicotine increases in acidic urine and decreases in alkaline urine.

Cigars and Smokeless Tobacco

According to data from the National Household Survey on Drug Abuse (SAMHSA, 2001), an estimated 65.5 million Americans age 12 and older (29.3%) reported current use of a tobacco product in 2000. An estimated 55.7 million (24.9%) smoked cigarettes, while 10.7 million (4.8%) smoked cigars, 7.6 million (3.4%) used smokeless tobacco (chewing tobacco and oral snuff), and 2.1 million (1.0%) smoked tobacco in pipes.

CIGARS

A typical cigarette contains approximately 0.5 to 1.0 g of tobacco and approximately 8 to 12 mg nicotine, of which most smokers absorb about 1 to 3 mg nicotine. The pH of tobacco smoke from cigarettes generally is between 5.5 and 6. In contrast, there are a wide variety of cigars. In 1996, the U.S. Department of the Treasury defined a cigar as "any roll of tobacco wrapped in leaf tobacco or in any substance containing tobacco." Cigars vary in size from small bidis to large premium cigars, and contain 0.5 g to more than 20 g of tobacco and 10 mg to more than 400 mg nicotine (Henningfield, Hariharan et al., 1996). The pH of tobacco smoke from cigars varies between 6.2 and 8.2. The protonated nicotine in the particulate phase of acidic cigar smoke is absorbable by inhalation, whereas the unprotonated nicotine in the vapor phase of basic cigar smoke is absorbable through the mucosa of the mouth, nose, and throat. Cigar smokers vary in the amount of smoke that they inhale. Former cigarette smokers tend to inhale more than cigar smokers who have not previously smoked cigarettes.

Whereas the cigarette usually is smoked in seven to eight minutes, smoking a cigar can take as long as 60 to 90 minutes. Most cigars do not have filters. As a result, cigars and smokeless tobacco are in direct contact with the buccal mucosa. The process of holding an unlit cigar in the mouth can contribute to the total daily nicotine intake of some cigar smokers. An individual might achieve an equivalent level of nicotine exposure from one to two cigars per day as from a pack or more of cigarettes (NCI, 1998).

Large cigars, in part because of the low porosity of the cigar binder and wrapper, produce more carbon monoxide, nitrogen oxides, and carcinogenic N-nitrosamines in mainstream smoke per gram of tobacco burned than do cigarettes. Free ammonia in cigar smoke contributes to the pungent smell of a burning cigar. Although cigars generate similar amounts of environmental tobacco smoke (ETS) per minute as cigarettes, they contribute a total amount of ETS that is much greater than that of a single cigarette because they burn for a longer duration.

SMOKELESS TOBACCO

Users of smokeless tobacco suffer abrasions to and staining of the teeth, loss of tooth structure, and dental caries because irritating juices from chewing and dipping tobacco are in contact with the gums, cheeks, and/or lips for prolonged periods of time (NCI, 1992). Gingival recession and leukoplakia also can occur. In the range of 3% to 5% of cases of leukoplakia progress to oral cancer.

Smokeless tobacco is associated with cancer of the pharynx, larynx, and esophagus. Cancer caused by smokeless tobacco is believed to result from the presence of N-nitrosamines, 4-(methylnitrosamino)1-(3-pyridyl)-1-bitanone, N-nitrosonormicotine, and 12-O-tetradecanoylphhorbol-13 acetate, a tumor promoter. Swedish snuff contains levels of tobacco-specific nitrosamines as low as 2.8 μg/g of dried tobacco, whereas Skoal® contains 64.0 μg nitrosamines per gram of dried tobacco, and Copenhagen® contains 41.1 μg nitrosamines per gram of dried tobacco. American snuff has higher levels of bacterial activity leading to the formation of nitrosamines because it generally is fermented and shipped without refrigeration (Fairclough, 2001). With regular use of smokeless tobacco, blood levels of nicotine rise slowly and maintain a consistent level during the day because of the prolonged contact of tobacco with the oral cavity.

REFERENCES

Fairclough G (2001). Health officials criticize snuff makers for allowing high levels of carcinogens. *Wall Street Journal* August 21; A3-A6.

Henningfield JE, Hariharan M & Kozlowski LT (1996). Nicotine content and health risks of cigars. *Journal of the American Medical Association* 276(23):1857-1858.

National Cancer Institute (NCI) (1998). *Cigars: Health Effects and Trends (NIH Smoking and Tobacco Control Monograph 9).* Bethesda, MD: National Institutes of Health.

National Cancer Institute (NCI) (1992). *Smokeless Tobacco or Health: An International Perspective (NIH Smoking and Tobacco Control Monograph 2).* Bethesda, MD: National Institutes of Health.

Substance Abuse and Mental Health Services Administration (SAMHSA) (2001). *National Household Survey on Drug Abuse, 2000.* Rockville, MD: SAMHSA, U.S. Department of Health and Human Services.

Cotinine excretion is influenced less by urinary pH than nicotine because it occurs primarily in the unionized form within physiologic pH. Other metabolites of nicotine also appear in the urine.

Investigators are beginning to explore ethnic differences in nicotine metabolism. For example, recent research (Perez-Stable, Herrera et al., 1998) has demonstrated that persons of African descent have a 30% higher intake of nicotine per cigarette, and that they clear nicotine and cotinine more slowly than do Caucasians. The slower nicotine clearance is due to the less rapid oxidative metabolism of nicotine to cotinine, presumably via cytochrome P450-2A6. A population subgroup of African descent form nicotine N-glucuronide more slowly than do Caucasians (Benowitz, Perez-Stable et al., 1999). Along with the potential role of smoking mentholated cigarettes, these findings may help to explain why black men have a higher incidence of mortality from lung cancer than do white men.

In another study (Benowitz, Perez-Stable et al., 2002), Chinese Americans had both a lower nicotine intake per cigarette and smoked fewer cigarettes per day than did Caucasians. Chinese Americans also metabolized nicotine and cotinine more slowly than did Caucasians or Hispanic Americans. Because nicotine intake per cigarette is a marker for tobacco smoke per cigarette, these findings may help to clarify why Chinese American smokers have lower rates of lung cancer than either African Americans or Caucasians.

Indeed, ethnic variations in the amount of nicotine intake per cigarette, the number of cigarettes smoked, and the metabolism of nicotine may elucidate the basis for population-based differences in the incidence and prevalence of progression from nicotine use to addiction, as well as the associated tobacco-related risk of disease.

Monitoring Exposure to Nicotine and Tobacco. Blood, salivary, and plasma cotinine are commonly used biochemical markers of nicotine intake. Other measures of smoking include expired carbon monoxide concentrations, blood carboxyhemoglobin concentrations, and plasma or salivary thiocyanate concentrations. Anabasine and anatabine are being developed as indicators of tobacco use in individuals who are concurrently using nicotine medications.

The 18-hour half-life of cotinine lends it to being used as a plasma and salivary marker of nicotine intake. Salivary cotinine concentrations correlate well with blood cotinine concentrations (r=0.82 to 0.90) (Jarvis, Tunstall-Pedoe et al., 1984). The cotinine level produced by a single cigarette is 8 to 10 ng/mL. It takes several hours for the cotinine to peak after a cigarette is smoked. A cotinine value of greater than 14 ng/mL typically is used to determine smoking. A smoker with a plasma cotinine concentration of 100 ng/mL would have an estimated intake of 8 mg nicotine per day, which corresponds to smoking approximately a half pack of cigarettes per day. Cotinine blood levels average about 250 to 300 ng/mL in regular smokers, but range from 10 to 900 ng/mL (Benowitz, Porchet et al., 1990). Because of individual variability in the fractional conversion of nicotine to cotinine and in the rate of elimination of cotinine itself, blood levels of cotinine are not perfect quantitative markers of nicotine intake in individual smokers, but are useful in studying populations of smokers. Cotinine levels may persist for up to seven days after cessation of habitual smoking.

CO Breathalyzers® are a relatively inexpensive way to help motivate smokers to quit smoking and to monitor for relapse. Breath measurements of expired air that contain more than 10 to 12 ppm carbon monoxide (CO) usually indicate recent tobacco smoking. Elevated CO levels in the absence of smoking may be the result of exposure to environmental pollutants, such as faulty gas boilers, car exhausts, and smog. Some newer monitors correct for the CO in ambient air. Another potential source of error occurs when persons of African or Asian descent, or those among the 6% of Caucasians who are lactose intolerant, exhale hydrogen after ingesting milk. Several monitors misinterpret this exhaled hydrogen as CO (McNeill, Owen et al., 1990). Breath CO has a relatively short half-life and should be below cutoff levels after not smoking for 8 to 12 hours.

Hydrogen cyanide is inhaled as a combustion product of nitrogen-containing compounds. It is metabolized in the body from thiosulfate to thiocyanate, which can be detected in the blood and saliva (Tsuge, Kataoka et al., 2000). Thiocyanate levels also may be affected by consumption of common foods (such as almonds, tapioca, cabbage, broccoli, and cauliflower), and these levels can vary from one person to the next. Assays of thiocyanate are insensitive to low amounts of smoking, and thiocyanate levels can remain elevated for up to 14 days after smoking has ceased (DHHS, 1988). CO and cotinine levels generally are preferred to thiocyanate levels in the assessment of smoking.

Drug Interactions With Nicotine and Tobacco. Smoking is well known to accelerate the metabolism of many drugs, particularly those metabolized by CYP1A2. It is difficult to know which of the 3,000 components of cigarette smoke are responsible for changes in drug metabolism, although it is likely that polycyclic aromatic hydrocarbons have an important role. Cigarette smoking induces the metabolism of theophylline, propranolol, flecainide, tacrine, caffeine, clozapine, imipramine, haloperidol, oxazepam, pentazocine, phenacetin, lidocaine, and estradiol. When smokers stop smoking, as often occurs during hospitalization for an acute illness, the doses of these medications may need to be adjusted to avoid toxicity.

Several pharmacodynamic interactions arise between cigarette smoking and other drugs. Cigarette smoking results in faster clearance of heparin, possibly because of smoking-related activation of thrombosis, with enhanced heparin binding to antithrombin III. Cigarette smoking and oral contraceptives interact synergistically to increase the risk of stroke and premature myocardial infarction in women. Cigarettes appear to enhance the procoagulant effect of estrogens. For this reason, oral contraceptives are relatively contraindicated in women who smoke cigarettes. Also, the stimulant actions of nicotine inhibit reductions in blood pressure and heart rate from beta-blockers. Smoking results in less sedation from benzodiazepines and less analgesia from some opioids. Smoking adversely effects mucosal aggressive and protective factors and impairs the therapeutic effects of histamine H2-receptor antagonists. Cutaneous vasoconstriction by nicotine can slow the rate of absorption of subcutaneously administered insulin.

PHARMACOLOGIC ACTIONS

Central Nervous System. Nicotine has a complex dose-response relationship (Benowitz, 1988). At low doses (like those achieved by smoking a cigarette), nicotine acts on the sympathetic nervous system to acutely increase blood pressure, heart rate, and cardiac output and to cause cutaneous vasoconstriction. At higher doses, nicotine produces ganglionic stimulation and the release of adrenal catecholamines. At extremely high doses, nicotine causes hypotension and slowing of the heart rate, possibly via peripheral ganglionic blockade and/or vagal afferent nerve stimulation. Because of the development of tolerance, chronic nicotine exposure in and of itself does not cause hypertension.

Nicotine causes muscle relaxation by stimulating discharge of the Renshaw cells and/or pulmonary afferent nerves, while inhibiting the activity of motor neurons.

Psychoactive Effects. The primary CNS effects of nicotine in smokers are arousal, relaxation (particularly in stressful situations), and enhancement of mood, attention, and reaction time, with improvement in performance of some behavioral tasks. Some or all of these effects may result from the relief of withdrawal symptoms in addicted smokers rather than as a direct enhancing effect. Spilich and colleagues (1992) conducted a series of tests of cognitive performance on nonsmokers, deprived smokers, and smokers who had just smoked. They found that on simple tasks, smoking enhanced performance, but on more difficult tasks, smokers who had just smoked performed significantly worse than nonsmokers. Smoking may simply reverse the effects of abstinence, rather than offer an advantage by relieving stress and improving cognition. Parrott and Kaye (1999) compared self-rated feelings of stress, arousal, pleasure, and evaluations of cognitive failure in 25 cigarette smokers, 25 temporarily abstaining smokers, and 25 nonsmokers. The abstaining smokers reported significantly worse psychological states on every assessment measure than did the nonsmokers and nondeprived smokers, who did not differ from each other. The investigators concluded that smokers need regular doses of nicotine to feel normal rather than to enhance their capabilities.

The psychoactive effects of nicotine and tobacco are determined not only by the route and speed of drug administration and the pharmacokinetic parameters that determine the concentration at receptor sites over time, but also by a variety of host and environmental factors. The magnitude of nicotine's subjective effects may depend on the predrug subjective state, level of activity, genetic predisposition, history and/or current intake of other drugs, expectancy of the individual, and other situational factors.

Nicotine's effects are baseline dependent. Low-activity rats become more active on exposure to nicotine, whereas the reverse occurs in high-activity rats (Rosecrans, 1995). Similarly, electroencephalograms of humans have shown that nicotine has stimulant-like effects during quiet conditions but minimal effects during high-noise conditions (Gilbert, Estes et al., 1997).

Nicotine's ability to cause stimulation when smoked at a low level of arousal (such as fatigue) and to affect relaxation when smoked at a high level of arousal (such as anxiety) underlies its reinforcing effects under a range of conditions (Grobe & Perkins, 2000). Smokers increase their smoking under both low- and high-arousal conditions (Parrott, 1998; Rose, Ananda et al., 1983). Subtle stimulation and/or relaxation effects may be thought beneficial by users who would like to fine-tune their disposition at a given time. The subtle modulatory effects preferred by tobacco users are in stark contrast to the flagrant intoxicating effects desired by some users of alcohol and other psychoactive substances.

Several studies have shown gender differences in nicotine responsiveness. Women have less sensitivity to changes in nicotine dose during nicotine discrimination experiments, and they may not benefit as much as men from nicotine replacement therapy during smoking cessation (Perkins, 1999). However, women may be influenced more by non-nicotine stimuli, such as the olfactory and taste attributes of cigarette smoke, indicating greater conditioned reinforcement (Perkins, Gerlach et al., 2001).

Genetic Predisposition. Monozygotic twins are more similar than dizygotic twins with respect to smoking behavior (Cederlof, Friberg et al., 1977), and this similarity occurs even when the monozygotic twins are reared apart (Raaschou-Nielsen, 1960; Shields, 1962). Data derived from large cohorts of the Swedish and Finnish twin registries support estimates that 53% of the total variance (range, 28% to 84%) of smoking can be attributed to genetic effects (Kaprio, Koskenvuo et al., 1981). When twin pairs from the National Academy of Sciences-National Research Council registry were studied, heritability estimates for smoking, alcohol use, and coffee consumption (after adjustment for covariance with the other substances) were 42%, 30%, and 44%, respectively (Carmelli, Swan et al., 1990). Animal studies show that genetics mediate differences in sensitivity to nicotine (Mohammed, 2000). Different mice strains react differently to nicotine, self-administer nicotine to different extents (Robinson, Marks et al., 1996), differ in the ability to develop tolerance, and have different numbers of nicotine receptor-binding sites (Tritto, Stitzel et al., 2002).

Psychiatric Comorbidity. Patients with psychiatric disorders—particularly schizophrenia, depression, and ADHD—have a higher prevalence of cigarette smoking than the population as a whole. Clinical experience shows that this group of patients has difficulty in stopping smoking, often experiencing profound depression. Nicotine is a potential treatment for Tourette's syndrome (Shytle, Baker et al., 2000), and either nicotine or the components of cigarette smoke (particularly the components that inhibit monoamine oxidase B, thus inhibiting the degradation of dopamine in the CNS) seem to be protective toward the development of Parkinson's disease and, possibly, Alzheimer's disease (Newhause & Whitehouse, 2000).

Among schizophrenic patients, 70% to 88% are smokers (Dalack, Healy et al., 1998). Schizophrenic patients have diminished sensory gating to repeated stimuli, which can be measured by their failure to inhibit the P50 auditory event-evoked response (Adler, Hoffer et al., 1993). Nicotine and clozapine, but not haloperidol, reverse this abnormality. Nicotine also reverses some of the haloperidol dose-related impairments on a variety of cognitive tasks (Levin, Wilson et al., 1996) and relieves some of the negative symptoms (such as blunted affect, emotional withdrawal, and lack of spontaneity and flow of conversation) that occur with schizophrenia. Genetic linkage in schizophrenic families supports a role for the α7 nicotinic receptor subunit, with linkage at the α7 locus on chromosome 15 (Leonard, Adler et al., 2001). These data suggest a shared underlying neurobiology for both cigarette smoking and schizophrenia. Through an increased understanding of this neurobiology, scientists hope to target new treatments for both disorders.

Among adult smokers, the presence of ADHD has been found to be associated with early initiation of regular cigarette smoking, even when investigators controlled for confounding variables such as socioeconomic status, IQ, and psychiatric comorbidity (Milberger, Biederman et al., 1997). The rates of nicotine dependence are substantially higher among adults with ADHD (40%) than in the general population (26%) (Sullivan & Rudnik-Levin, 2001). Nicotine administered through transdermal patches does improve the attentional symptoms of ADHD (Levin, Conners et al., 1996). However, patients with adult ADHD do not exhibit the inhibitory deficit of P50 prepulse inhibition that is seen in patients with schizophrenia (Olincy, Ross et al., 2000). Therefore, nicotine addiction and ADHD may share an underlying neurobiology, but this is thought to be different from that for schizophrenia.

Population-based Epidemiologic Catchment Area studies (Glassman, Helzer et al., 1990) found a prevalence of depression of 6.6% among subjects who had ever smoked daily, compared to 2.9% in those who had never smoked. Other reports confirm that the prevalence of smoking in individuals with major depression is twice that observed in the general population. Breslau and colleagues (1993) interviewed 995 young adults aged 21 to 30 years, repeating the interviews 14 months later. She found that subjects with a history of depression progressed to nicotine dependence more readily than did subjects who did not have a

FIGURE 2. **A Simulation of Plasma Nicotine Concentration Throughout the Day in Relation to Psychoactive Effect**

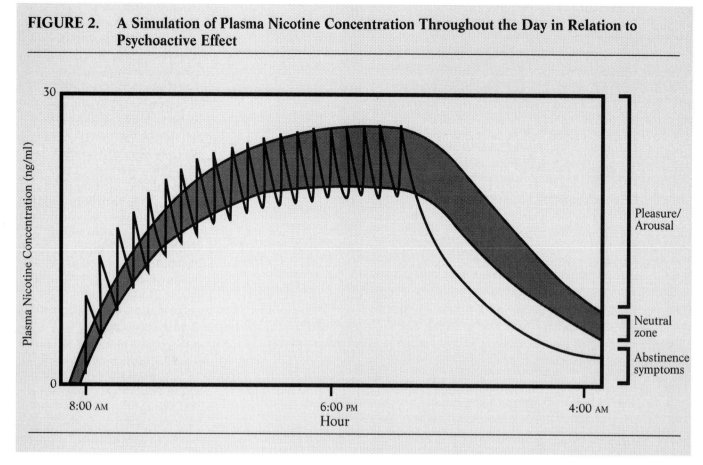

history of major depression (odds ratio: 2.06; 95% confidence interval: 1.21 to 3.49). In a study of 1,566 twins, Kendler and colleagues (1993) found that the best statistical fit for the data supported a model with common risk factors for both depression and cigarette smoking, rather than a causal relationship between the two. Smokers with a history of depression who stop smoking are at risk of developing more severe withdrawal symptoms, have poorer outcomes, and are more likely to experience a depressive episode, especially during the first three months after stopping smoking (Glassman, 1993).

Discrimination and Self-Administration. Squirrel monkeys, rats, and even mice are able to distinguish the subjective effects of nicotine and nicotine analogs from drugs of other classes. This effect is attenuated when the animals are pretreated with mecamylamine, a centrally acting nicotinic receptor antagonist, but not when they are pretreated with hexamethonium, an antagonist that does not enter the brain.

Models of nicotine self-administration demonstrate the drug's reinforcing properties. Although animals will self-administer nicotine, the environment, dose, and timing of the reinforcement schedule are more critical with nicotine than with cocaine. Using intermittent rather than fixed-ratio schedules of reinforcement and adjusting the nicotine dose to 30 μg per kg of body weight enabled the development of a model of nicotine self-administration (Nowak, 1994).

Human volunteers will lever-press for intravenous nicotine (DHHS, 1988). They experience intravenous nicotine as pleasurable, and subjects who have experience with a variety of other drugs indicate that the feelings are similar to those evoked by cocaine. Human smokers regulate the nicotine levels that they self-administer. For example, they block the ventilation holes on the cigarette filter, puff harder, inhale more deeply, and smoke more frequently when smoking "light" cigarettes. Also, if smokers are pretreated with mecamylamine, they smoke more to overcome the blocking effects of this antagonist (Rose, Behm et al., 2001).

Human smokers associate the irritant effects of nicotine on the tissues of the mouth and throat with the desired psychoactive effects achieved by smoking a cigarette in a process termed "secondary reinforcement." Experienced smokers can use the tissue irritant effects to assess how much nicotine they are receiving when smoking (Rose, Behm et al., 1993). Research also has demonstrated a short-term reduction in cigarette craving when the sensory input from tobacco smoke is simulated with ascorbic acid (Levin, Behm et al., 1993) or black pepper extract (Rose & Behm, 1994). Products that replicate the taste, flavor, throat, and chest sensations of cigarette smoking and/or the sensorimotor handling of a cigarette may reduce craving and some of the symptoms of nicotine withdrawal. Some of these products are being developed as smoking cessation aids.

Dependence, Tolerance, and Withdrawal. Most tobacco use can be understood as the controlled, orderly ingestion of nicotine to achieve particular pharmacologic effects (DHHS, 1988). Such use was recognized as addiction by early European observers. Indeed, in 1622, Sir Francis Bacon observed that "The use of tobacco . . . conquers men with a certain secret pleasure so that those who have once become accustomed thereto can hardly be restrained therefrom."

Dependence and Tolerance: According to the *Diagnostic and Statistical Manual of Mental Disorders, 4th Edition* (*DSM-IV*; American Psychiatric Association, 1994), substance dependence, including nicotine dependence, is "a maladaptive pattern of substance use, leading to clinically significant impairment or distress, as manifested by three (or more) of the following, occurring at any time in the same 12-month period: (1) tolerance; (2) withdrawal; (3) the substance is often taken in larger amounts or over a longer period than was intended; (4) there is a persistent desire or unsuccessful efforts to cut down or control substance use; (5) a great deal of time is spent in activities necessary to obtain the substance, or recover from its effects; (6) important social, occupational, or recreational activities are given up or reduced because of substance use; and (7) the substance use is continued despite knowledge of having a persistent or recurrent physical or psychological problem that is likely to have been caused or exacerbated by the substance."

The addiction liability of tobacco results from a complex interplay of environmental, host (genetic vulnerability), and agent (psychopharmacologic properties of the drug) factors. Environmental factors are thought to be of major importance in explaining the ubiquity of nicotine use compared with other drugs.

Environmental factors also are thought to be of major importance. Although only one in four adults smokes, cigarettes are second only to soft drinks and newspapers as the nation's most widely available consumer product. There are more than a million retail outlets for tobacco products. In 1999 (the first year in which advertising and promotional expenditures were affected by the tobacco industry's Master Settlement Agreement with the Attorneys General of 46 states), the five largest cigarette manufacturers spent $8.24 billion, a 22% increase over the $6.73 billion spent on advertising and promotion in 1998 (FTC, 2001). Much cigarette advertising employs imagery that capitalizes on the disparity between the ideal and actual self, implying that smoking can close the gap (DHHS, 1994). Family and peers also affect the likelihood that an individual will take up regular tobacco use. Those who begin smoking in adolescence have more friends who smoke and score more highly on scales of rebelliousness and independence (Mittelmark, Murray et al., 1987). Many of the environmental factors that interact with agent and host to produce nicotine addiction are potential opportunities for policy change to control the epidemic (DHHS, 1994; Fisher, Lichtenstein et al., 1993).

The development of nicotine addiction has some unique characteristics when compared with the development of addiction to alcohol, heroin, and cocaine. Nicotine obtained through chewing tobacco and cigarettes often precedes the use of other drugs. The earlier the age at which use begins, the more difficult it is for the user to quit. Whereas one often thinks of initial drug use as occurring in mid-adolescence, in fact many persons have been exposed to nicotine *in utero* as a result of smoking by their mothers (Weissman, Warner et al., 1999). Nicotine exposure alters the number of nicotine receptor numbers and influences their function. In smokers who progress to chronic use, tolerance develops rapidly to the headache, dizziness, nausea, and dysphoria associated with the first cigarette. However, tolerance is far from complete; the ingestion of as little as 50% more than the usual dose can result in those symptoms (Collins, 1990). Chronic use is associated with the regular ingestion of quantities far larger than those used initially, even though consumption levels typically remain steady for many years once addiction has been established. Animal studies

New Tobacco Products and Nicotine Delivery Devices

A variety of new tobacco products and nicotine delivery devices are being test marketed in the United States and abroad. These products are designed to have "reduced risk." However, since a 2001 United States Supreme Court decision holding that the U.S. Food and Drug Administration (FDA) does not have jurisdiction over tobacco products, scientists fear that monitoring advertising claims will be suboptimal and that consumers will use these products with the illusion that they are safe. Independent peer-reviewed research to inform the public is needed immediately.

Over the past decade, health claims have been made about "light" cigarettes. Unfortunately, the lower nicotine delivery from light cigarettes causes smokers to take more frequent and deeper puffs. No evidence exists that smoking light cigarettes reduces the risk of either COPD or lung cancer.

American Spirit® cigarettes boast additive-free and, in some cases, organically grown tobacco. However, this brand contains higher nicotine and tar levels because the cigarettes contain only leaf tobacco (Fairclough, 2001b). Many consumers mistakenly believe that most of the toxic substances in cigarette smoke are due to pesticides and manufacturing additives rather than the byproducts of the combustion of tobacco itself. No evidence exists that smoking additive-free cigarettes is associated with less smoking-related morbidity and mortality than smoking traditional cigarettes.

One innovation shared by both R.J. Reynolds' Eclipse® and Philip Morris' Accord® is to heat rather than to burn tobacco. The object is to reduce combustion and diminish the level of carcinogens and oxidant gases. Accord has its own puff-activated lighter, whereas Eclipse uses a carbon fuel element that is conventionally lighted. Eclipse contains an aerosol-generating chamber that is composed of shredded reconstituted tobacco with greater than 50% glycerine encased in glass fiber insulation inside an aluminum foil liner. When burned, both Eclipse and Accord produce a vapor but no sidestream smoke. The nicotine delivery of Eclipse, as tested using standard smoking machine parameters, is similar to that of an "ultra light" cigarette. However, when smokers compensate to increase their nicotine intake, they puff harder and increase their nicotine and carbon monoxide (CO) exposure. Moreover, there is a problem with Eclipse in that the glass particles are inhaled (Pauly, Lee et al., 1998). In U.S. market tests, Eclipse was rejected because it was difficult to light, draw, tell when completed, and extinguish. Eclipse continues to be marketed overseas, and its future development in those markets is difficult to ascertain.

Star Scientific, Inc., and Brown & Williamson are test-marketing Advance® cigarettes. The Star-cure® processing reduces tobacco-specific nitrosamine content by 70%, and the Trionic® filter reduces many toxins, including hydrogen cyanide, formaldehyde, benzene, and acrolein. Vector Tobacco, Ltd., is developing a cigarette that contains genetically modified tobacco lacking a key gene for nicotine synthesis (Shield, 2002). Vector can market this product as a nonaddictive way to enjoy smoking, thus avoiding claims that might prompt FDA intervention (for example, that the cigarettes are an aid smoking cessation).

Several brands of snuff and smokeless, spitless tobacco packets or sachets are being developed with specially cured and/or processed tobacco that contains lower levels of nitrosamines and other toxins. These smoke-free products are being marketed as ways to enjoy tobacco in places where smoking is prohibited.

A heated debate over harm reduction approaches to tobacco use is ongoing. While it is acknowledged that the health risks incurred by addicted smokers should be reduced as much as possible, the public health community fears that the health claims made by these products will discourage tobacco cessation efforts (IOM, 2001).

REFERENCES

Fairclough G (2001b). Tobacco titans bid for "organic" cigarette maker. *Wall Street Journal* August 21; B1-B4.

Institute of Medicine (IOM) (2001). Clearing the smoke. *Assessing the Science Base for Tobacco Harm Reduction*. Washington, DC: National Academy Press.

Pauly JL, Lee HJ, Hurley EL et al. (1998). Glass fiber contamination of cigarette filters: An additional health risk to the smoker? *Cancer Epidemiology, Biomarkers and Prevention* 7:967-979.

Shield M (2002). New tobacco products: Truth and consequences. *TRDRP Newsletter* 5(1):7-15.

demonstrate that tolerance to nicotine is long lasting. Tolerance is regarded as a clinical manifestation of neural adaptation to nicotine, and the extent to which changes in nicotinic receptors, signaling, and circuits are reversible and/or irreversible is being actively researched.

As a method of ingestion, inhaling nicotine through cigarettes is similar to "freebasing." Rapid absorption through the lung, with distribution into the arterial blood and brain, enables its quick action. Smokers can adjust their puffs to get a desired dose with a rapid effect, so that cigarettes are a very user-friendly drug delivery device. Smokers can use nicotine to stimulate or relax themselves and fine-tune their moods within seconds of puffing on a cigarette.

If a cigarette provides approximately 10 puffs, then a person who smokes 20 cigarettes (1 pack) per day is taking 200 doses of nicotine daily. No other drug, even cocaine, is dosed that frequently. Conditioned cues become established 200 to 400 times a day, beginning at an early age. Desiring a cigarette becomes associated with everyday events such as driving a car, finishing a meal, talking on the telephone, waking from sleep, and taking a break. Tobacco users link the need to modulate their moods with smoking. The subliminal imagery promoted by cigarette advertising adds to this expectation. Thus, a person who begins smoking a pack of cigarettes a day at age 17 would experience 724,000 doses of nicotine-conditioned internal emotional states and external cues by the age of 27. The quantity and power of this conditioning is unique to cigarette smoking, and it is one of the reasons that smokers find cigarette smoking so difficult to quit.

Although conditioning is a critical element of addiction to tobacco products, conditioning loses its power without the presence of an active drug. Hence, nicotine-free cigarettes have not succeeded in the marketplace. Nicotine is the psychoactive component of tobacco products that causes persons to continue to smoke despite harmful physiologic and social consequences. However, it is the CO, other gasses, and components of tar that cause most of the cardiovascular, pulmonary, and oncologic morbidity and mortality.

The regular use of tobacco commonly leads to its compulsive use. Addicted smokers often recall rummaging through drawers, making special trips to stores, and engaging in other extraordinary maneuvers to find a cigarette when one is needed. Because of their capacity for fine-tuning, smokers count on smoking a cigarette to awaken them, take a break, or calm themselves. Persons who quit cigarettes

have to learn to rely on their own internal resources rather than on a cigarette for emotional modulation.

Current definitions, measures, and models of nicotine addiction are limited in that they do not adequately explain or predict degrees of nicotine dependence. Typologies such as the Horn-Waingrow Reasons for Smoking (RFS) scale (Ikard, Green et al., 1969) are intuitively appealing because they aim for differentiated and individualized treatment for smoking cessation. The RFS motives include stimulation, pleasure, sensorimotor manipulation, negative affect reduction, habit, and psychological addiction (craving). However, at best there has been little agreement as to the questionnaire's validity coefficients (Tate & Stanton, 1990), and its clinical utility remains unproved (Shiffman, 1998).

There have been attempts to correlate the severity of nicotine addiction with factors such as the duration of smoking, potency of cigarettes, puff frequency, puff duration, and inhalation volume. However, these items have only weakly correlated with biochemical measures, and they have not predicted the intensity and extent of withdrawal symptoms (Heatherton, Koslowski et al., 1991). The *DSM-IV* is useful diagnostically, but it was not designed as a quantitative tool to measure the severity of nicotine addiction. The Fagerström Tolerance Questionnaire (FTQ) (Fagerström, 1978) is one of the most universally accepted measures of the severity of nicotine dependence. Some studies show a relationship between the Fagerström questionnaire and the ability to achieve tobacco cessation (see Section 6).

Evidence that nicotine is one of the most addicting drugs is found in the high rate of relapse among individuals who try to quit smoking. For example, population surveys consistently find that up to 75% of adults who smoke want to stop (DHHS, 1988). About a third actually try to stop each year, but only a small number (less than 3%) succeed. Among persons who experience myocardial infarctions, laryngectomies, COPD, and other medical sequelae of smoking, 50% or more revert to cigarette use within days or weeks after leaving the hospital (DHHS, 1988). As discussed earlier, factors that contribute to the profoundly addictive quality of nicotine include the early onset of drug use with neuroadaptation, the capability of the drug to subtly stimulate or relax and moderate mood, its rapid onset of action, its ability to allow for self-titration, its short and frequent dosing interval, and its pairing to multiple conditioned cues that are intertwined with daily life events. In addition, the cigarette's role in oral gratification, sensorimotor handling, and advertising-invoked changes in self-image, as well as nicotine's ability to cause weight loss, contribute to continued tobacco use.

Withdrawal: Tobacco use is sustained by the need to prevent the symptoms of nicotine withdrawal. These symptoms vary, but include craving for nicotine, irritability and frustration or anger, anxiety, depression, difficulty concentrating, restlessness, and increased appetite. Performance measures such as reaction time and attention are impaired during withdrawal. While these symptoms often are distressing and can be disruptive to interpersonal functioning, they are not in themselves life-threatening. Most acute withdrawal symptoms reach maximum intensity at 24 to 48 hours after cessation and then gradually diminish over a period of a few weeks. However, some (including dysphoria, mild depression, and anhedonia) may persist for months. The extinction of conditioned cues requires months to years. That nicotine itself is responsible for the withdrawal symptoms is supported by the appearance of similar symptoms with the sudden withdrawal from the use of chewing tobacco, snuff, or nicotine gum, and relief of those symptoms provided by nicotine. Abstinent smokers gain an average of 2 to 3 kg during the first year after they stop smoking.

Nicotine withdrawal is best understood as a process of reversing neuronal adaptation. The next section discusses the neurobiologic mechanisms that underlie nicotine's actions. The anatomy and physiology of nicotinic receptors in the CNS are introduced, followed by a discussion of the neurotransmitters and circuitry involved. Finally, a model is proposed to account for human smoking behavior.

NEUROBIOLOGIC MECHANISMS OF ACTION

Nicotinic Acetylcholine Receptors. Nicotinic acetylcholine receptors (nAChRs) belong to a superfamily of ligand-gated ion channels that includes gamma-aminobutyric acid (GABA$_A$), glycine, and 5-hydroxytryptamine (5-HT$_3$) serotonin receptors. The most basic conformational states of a nAChR channel are the closed state at rest, the open state, and the desensitized state (Dani, 2001; Lena & Changeux, 1998). Acetylcholine (ACh) released from cholinergic terminals and nicotine obtained exogenously from tobacco are agonists capable of stabilizing the open conformation of the nAChR channel. Upon binding ACh, the nAChR ion channel is stabilized in the open conformation for several milliseconds. Then the open pore of the receptor/channel complex closes to a resting state or closes to a desensitized state that is unresponsive to ACh or other agonists for many milliseconds or longer. While open, nAChRs conduct cations that cause a local depolarization of the membrane and produce an intracellular ionic signal. Although sodium and potassium ions carry most of the current through nAChR channels, calcium also can make a small but significant contribution.

The structure of the nicotinic receptor-channel complex arises from five polypeptide subunits assembled like staves of a barrel around a central water-filled core (Cooper, Couturier et al., 1991). Various subunit combinations produce many different nAChR types. On the basis of pharmacology, physiologic function, and evolutionary considerations, three functional classes of nAChRs are recognized: muscle nAChRs (which are not discussed here), neuronal nAChRs formed from alpha-beta combinations (α2 to α6 and β2 to β4), and homomeric neuronal nAChRs subunits (α7 to α9). In the third classification, only homomeric α7 is widely distributed in the mammalian CNS. This classification scheme is not perfect because evidence suggests that subunits of the separate classes are capable of combining to form nAChRs, but such combinations may be rare in biology (Girod, Crabtree et al., 1999). According to evidence gained from the heterologous expression of nAChR subunits, the following conclusion can be drawn: a limited number of subunit combinations are favored, but more rare combinations are possible.

Some general rules can be applied when trying to simplify the influence of particular subunits. Most nAChRs in the mammalian brain contain either α4β2 or α7. The α4β2* nAChRs constitute most of the high-affinity binding sites for nicotine. The next most common type of nAChR in the brain contains the α7 subunit, most likely in a homomeric form. The α7* nAChRs have a lower affinity for nicotine, a high calcium permeability, rapid activation and desensitization kinetics, and are inhibited by alpha-bungarotoxin and methyllycaconitine. In contrast, α4β2* nAChRs have slower kinetics and lower calcium permeability.

Neurobiology of the Cholinergic Systems. Cholinergic neurons serve diverse roles in the CNS and peripheral nervous system. The most highly studied vertebrate cholinergic synapse is the neuromuscular junction formed between a motor neuron located in the spinal cord and a skeletal muscle. That synapse provides the best example of fast, excitatory, nicotinic synaptic transmission. When an action potential arrives at the presynaptic terminal of the motor neuron, it releases ACh, which diffuses across the synaptic cleft and activates nAChRs on the postsynaptic muscle, initiating the excitation-contraction process.

Fast nicotinic synaptic transmission is seen throughout the mammalian autonomic nervous system, which is primarily an involuntary effector system that controls visceral functions. Cholinergic neurons serve in motor nuclei of the brainstem and throughout the autonomic nervous system. The preganglionic neurons of both the sympathetic and the parasympathetic branches of the autonomic nervous system release ACh onto postsynaptic, ganglionic, and neuronal nAChRs. The preganglionic neurons of the sympathetic branch originate in the spinal cord and synapse onto paravertebral ganglia that run in a chain along the spinal cord. The postganglionic sympathetic neurons are mostly noradrenergic. Preganglionic neurons of the parasympathetic branch originate in the brainstem and send long myelinated fibers out to the parasympathetic ganglia located in or near the effector organs. The parasympathetic postganglionic neurons are mainly cholinergic, releasing ACh onto muscarinic (not nicotinic) AChRs.

Cholinergic neurons also project throughout the CNS, providing diffuse, sparse innervation to practically all of the brain (Woolf, 1991). In general, a relatively few cholinergic neurons make sparse projections that reach broad areas. Thus, the activity of a rather small number of cholinergic neurons can influence diverse and relatively large neuronal structures. The cholinergic cell bodies are located in a loosely contiguous axis that runs from the striatum and basal forebrain nuclei of the telencephalon, continuing sparsely through the diencephalon and to the pontomesencephalic tegmentum, medullary tegmentum, and cranial nerve nuclei of the brainstem. Although cholinergic neurons are distributed along the axis from the basal telencephalon to the spinal cord and brainstem, two major cholinergic projection subsystems can be identified. One cholinergic system arises from neurons in the basal forebrain and makes broad projections throughout the cortex and hippocampus. The second arises in the pedunculopontine tegmentum and the laterodorsal pontine tegmentum, providing widespread innervation mainly to the thalamus and midbrain areas, as well as descending innervation that reaches to the brainstem.

The situation in the striatum is somewhat different, in that cholinergic interneurons within the striatum provide very rich local innervation (Zhou, Liang et al., 2001).

Despite the relatively sparse innervation in the CNS, cholinergic activity influences a wide variety of behaviors.

By acting initially on nAChRs, nicotine or nicotinic cholinergic innervation can increase arousal, heighten attention, influence stages of sleep, produce states of euphoria, decrease fatigue, decrease anxiety, act centrally as an analgesic, and influence a number of cognitive functions. It is thought that cholinergic systems affect discriminatory processes by increasing the signal-to-noise ratio and helping to evaluate the significance and relevance of stimuli.

Nicotinic Mechanisms in the CNS. The most widely observed synaptic role of nAChRs in the mammalian CNS is to influence neurotransmitter release (Dani, 2001; Jones, Sudweeks et al., 1999; McGehee & Role, 1995; Wonnacott, 1997). Presynaptic nAChRs are thought to initiate a calcium signal that boosts the release of neurotransmitters. Exogenous application of nicotinic agonists can enhance, and nicotinic antagonists often can diminish, the release of ACh, dopamine, norepinephrine, serotonin, GABA, and glutamate. In many cases, the $\alpha7^*$ nAChRs, which are highly calcium permeable, mediate the increased release of neurotransmitter, but in other cases different nAChR types are involved.

Fast nicotinic synaptic transmission in the mammalian CNS exists, but it is not the predominant mediator of excitatory synaptic transmission (Alkondon, Pereira et al., 1998). Because nicotinic synapses have a low density, they are difficult to detect experimentally in brain preparations. Where it has been reported, fast nicotinic transmission is a minor component of the excitatory input, which is overwhelmingly glutamatergic. Although direct nicotinic excitation of a neuron usually does not predominate, it can influence the excitability of a group of neurons because of the broad cholinergic projections into an area. Thus, beyond their specific roles at discreet synapses, nAChRs also modulate neuronal circuits in a broader sense.

Nicotinic AChRs also have roles during development and neuronal plasticity (Broide & Leslie, 1999; Dani, Ji et al., 2001; Role & Berg, 1996). The density of nAChRs varies during the course of development, and nAChRs can contribute to activity-dependent calcium signals. Nicotinic regulatory, plasticity, and developmental influences are particularly important when considering the etiology of disease. Biological changes that inappropriately alter nicotinic mechanisms could immediately influence the release of many neurotransmitters and alter circuit excitability. Moreover, nicotinic dysfunction could have long-term developmental consequences that are expressed later in life.

In summary, the tremendous diversity of nAChRs provides the flexibility necessary for them to play multiple, varied roles. Broad, sparse cholinergic projections ensure that nicotinic mechanisms modulate the neuronal excitability of relatively wide circuits. Although fast nicotinic transmission is not the predominant driving force, it can contribute excitatory input to many synapses at one time. Presynaptic and preterminal nAChRs modulate the release of many neurotransmitters.

Nicotine's Influence on Dopaminergic Neurons. Much evidence supports the theory that nicotine is the major addictive component of tobacco (Balfour, Wright et al., 2000; Dani & Heinemann, 1996; Dani & De Biasi, 2001; Di Chiara, 2000). Under controlled laboratory conditions, nicotine reinforces intravenous self-administration and elicits place preference on the part of animals and humans. In addition, nicotine cessation produces a withdrawal syndrome with both somatic and affective symptoms, which are relieved by nicotine replacement.

The addiction process acts on cellular and molecular mechanisms that normally operate in the brain. Long-term exposure to an addictive drug produces neuroadaptations that often are homeostatic reactions to abnormal stimulation by the drug (Koob & Le Moal, 2001). For example, chronic exposure to nicotine results in an increased number of nAChRs, and that change is likely to be a homeostatic response arising from increased nAChR desensitization (Buisson & Bertrand, 2001). Neuroadaptations often are invoked to explain tolerance, sensitization, and dependence, but those changes are less able to explain the long-lasting cravings that arise after years of abstinence. Cravings and relapse often are linked to the people, context, and cues associated with the initial drug use. Repeated use of the addictive drug reinforces associated factors that are consistently a part of the drug experience, and eventually those factors become independent motivators for continued use. Associative learning arises as addictive drugs initiate, influence, and alter normal neuronal mechanisms (Berke & Hyman, 2000; Dani, Ji et al., 2001; Di Chiara, 1999; Wise, 2000). It is hypothesized that addictive drugs remodel circuits of the brain that normally participate in the complex process of reinforcing rewarding behaviors.

Of the many psychopharmacologic factors that contribute to addiction, dopaminergic systems have received much attention (Balfour, Wright et al., 2000; Berke & Hyman,

2000; Dani, Ji et al., 2001; Dani & De Biasi, 2001; Di Chiara, 1999; Wise, 2000). The roles of the dopaminergic systems are not completely understood, but it is clear that they do participate in arousal, cognition, and motor function. Addiction research has focused on dopamine's complex participation in the processes associated with reinforcing behaviors that lead to reward. Although many areas of the brain participate, the mesocorticolimbic dopamine (DA) system serves a vital role in the acquisition of behaviors that are inappropriately reinforced by addictive drugs. An important dopaminergic pathway originates in the ventral tegmental area (VTA) of the midbrain and projects to the prefrontal cortex, as well as the limbic and striatal structures, including the nucleus accumbens. A role for the mesocorticolimbic DA system in nicotine addiction is supported by a number of findings. For example, blocking DA release in the nucleus accumbens with antagonists or lesions reduces nicotine self-administration in rodents (Corrigall, 1999; Corrigall, Franklin et al., 1992).

More sophisticated theories of how DA participates in the reinforcement of rewarding behaviors have evolved during the past few years. DA concentrations in the nucleus accumbens are not directly related to reward. More likely, the DA signal conveys novelty and reward expectation, or it serves to indicate the deviation of the environmental input from the animal's expectations, which were constructed by experience (Schultz, Dayan et al., 1997). DA thus can participate in the ongoing associative learning of adaptive behaviors as an animal continually updates a construct of environmental saliency.

Nicotine Activates and Desensitizes nAChRs on Mesocorticolimbic Neurons. In rat brain slices, it has been shown that the concentration of nicotine obtained from tobacco can activate and desensitize nAChRs on VTA dopamine neurons and thereby potently modulate the firing of VTA neurons (Dani, Ji et al., 2001; Mansvelder & McGehee, 2000; Picciotto, Zoli et al., 1998; Pidoplichko, DeBiasi et al., 1997). Although intensive research on this topic still is under way, a tenable hypothesis of the cellular and synaptic events occurring in the midbrain dopamine area can be summarized as follows.

Nicotine that arrives in the brain reaches nAChRs at many different locations, including those at both presynaptic and postsynaptic (or somal) locations. On the dopamine neuron's cell bodies and postsynaptically, most of the nAChRs contain $\alpha 4\beta 2^*$ subunits that have a high affinity for nicotine. The $\alpha 4\beta 2^*$ nAChR type also predominates

---

FIGURE 3. A Simplified Cycle for Continued Tobacco Use, Based on Nicotine's Cellular Actions

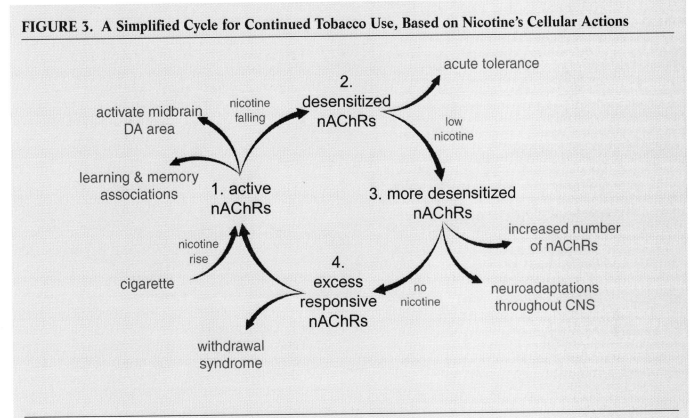

The nAChRs are initially and transiently activated when nicotine first arrives. The desensitization of the receptors follows as the concentration of nicotine slowly decreases. The increased number of nAChRs and the neuroadaptations are hypothesized to develop after chronic use of nicotine.

---

presynaptically on inhibitory GABAergic neurons innervating this area. However, mainly $\alpha7^*$ nAChRs, which have a low affinity for nicotine, are located on the presynaptic terminals of excitatory glutamatergic afferents into this midbrain area. This arrangement of the nAChRs is hypothesized to underlie their enhancement of excitatory synaptic potentiation (Dani, Ji et al., 2001; Mansvelder & McGehee, 2000).

Synaptic potentiation arises when excitatory presynaptic activity (glutamate release) is coincident in time with a strong postsynaptic response. The postsynaptic response is a depolarization that relieves the Mg^{2+} block of the N-methyl-D-aspartate (NMDA) subtype of glutamate receptors, enabling those receptors to mediate a sufficiently large Ca^{2+} signal to initiate the intracellular events leading to synaptic potentiation. While the length of time that a synapse

is potentiated can vary, in some cases it is long-lasting. Synaptic plasticity of this kind is thought to be among the processes that underlie learning and memory.

When nicotine first arrives in the midbrain dopamine area, it excites nAChRs, particularly the high-affinity $\alpha4\beta2^*$ nAChRs and, to a lesser degree, the $\alpha7^*$ nAChRs. Activation of the presynaptic nAChRs enhances the release of GABA and glutamate. Also at this time, the postsynaptic (and somal) $\alpha4\beta2^*$ nAChRs contribute to the depolarization of the dopamine neurons, helping NMDA receptors to participate in glutamatergic synaptic potentiation. After the initial exposure to nicotine, there is significant desensitization of the high-affinity $\alpha4beta2^*$ receptors. Consequently, the presynaptic enhancement of inhibitory GABA transmission ceases because the $\alpha4\beta2^*$ nAChRs desensitize. Therefore, the GABAergic inhibition of the dopamine neurons is decreased because any afferent cholinergic activity that normally boosted GABA release no longer can act on the $\alpha4\beta2*$ receptors.

Glutamatergic excitation of the dopamine neurons is enhanced because the synaptic potentiation that was initiated by the transient $\alpha4\beta2*$ nAChR activity persists for longer time periods. In addition, the presynaptic $\alpha7*$ nAChRs on the glutamatergic afferents are much less desensitized by the low concentrations of nicotine that are present. Therefore, glutamate release may continue to be enhanced, in that glutamate acts at potentiated synapses.

The types of synaptic plasticity described above are like those thought to underlie learning and memory, providing a link between nicotine addiction and learned associates. The preceding hypothesis emphasizes the important role of the mesocorticolimbic dopamine neurons in the addiction process. Other circuitry throughout the brain certainly is involved in the rewarding effects, neuroadaptations, and learned or associative behaviors linked with nicotine addiction. For example, multiple forms of synaptic plasticity in the hippocampus are influenced by nAChR activity (Ji, Lape et al., 2001).

Mechanisms such as those described here may be pertinent to suggestions that cigarette smoking is a gateway to illegal drug use. When data from 17,809 respondents who completed the 1994 National Household Survey on Drug Abuse were adjusted for age, race, and gender, it was found that those who had smoked cigarettes were far more likely to use cocaine (odds ratio [OR]=7.5; 95% confidence interval [CI], 5.7-9.9), crack (OR=13.9; 95% CI: 7.9-24.5), heroin (OR=16.0; 95% CI: 6.8-37.9), and marijuana (OR=7.3; 95% CI, 6.2-8.7) (Lai, Lai et al., 2000).

Hypotheses to Extrapolate the Cellular Results to Smokers. On the basis of the cellular studies of nAChR activation and desensitization, it is possible to infer some of the effects of smoking a cigarette, which delivers about 50 to 300 nM nicotine to the brain (Gourlay & Benowitz, 1997; Rose, Behm et al., 1999). Initially, the brain is free of nicotine and the nAChRs should be responding normally to cholinergic synaptic activity. When nicotine first arrives, nAChRs are activated, causing the neurons to depolarize and fire action potentials. This process occurs throughout the brain, with multiple consequences (Figure 3). Dopamine neurons are activated, contributing to the increase in dopamine that has been detected in the nucleus accumbens. Present theories hold that these neuronal events reinforce the behaviors that produced the dopamine release. Thus,

smoking and associated behaviors, whether incidental or meaningful, are reinforced (in a type of learning process). As the nicotine from the cigarette lingers, desensitization of nAChRs begins. This process decreases the effect obtained by smoking more than a few cigarettes in a row. However, the desensitization process is not complete and, in fact, there is considerable variability in desensitization of the various nAChR types, leading to significant differences in the level of desensitization even when comparing similar, neighboring neurons.

Nicotinic receptor desensitization has other effects (Dani, Radcliffe et al., 2000). Because the delivery and removal of ACh at synapses normally is very rapid, desensitization usually is not thought to be important in the CNS. When nicotine obtained from tobacco is present, however, the high affinity nicotine sites (including $\alpha4\beta2*$ nAChRs) are more likely to desensitize. The nAChRs at rapidly firing cholinergic synapses are even more likely to desensitize. At those cholinergic synapses, nAChRs experience repeated exposures to synaptic ACh and are exposed to nicotine from the cigarette. The combination of agonist exposures increases the probability that nAChRs at active cholinergic synapses will enter desensitization. Thus, smoking will turn down the gain for information arriving via nicotinic cholinergic synapses because fewer nAChRs will be able to respond to the released ACh. In summary, nicotine not only sends inappropriate information through the mesocorticolimbic dopamine system, but it also decreases the amplitude for normal nicotinic cholinergic information processing.

Another important piece of information about long-term nicotine exposure is that it causes an increase in the number of nAChRs in brains of humans, rats, and mice (Buisson & Bertrand, 2001). This increase affects mainly the high-affinity nicotinic receptors. Evidence indicates that the increase in nAChRs occurs because long exposures to nicotine cause nAChRs to enter states of desensitization more often. In those desensitized conformations, the nAChRs are turned over more slowly in the cell membrane. Therefore, following long periods (months or years) of exposure to smoking, nAChRs enter the desensitized state more often, eventually leading to an overall increase in number. Along with other factors that alter excitation and inhibition of dopamine neurons, this increase in the number of nAChRs can contribute to nicotine sensitization.

When nicotine is removed from the brain, some of the excess nAChRs recover from desensitization, resulting in an excess excitability of the nicotinic cholinergic systems of smokers. This hyperexcitability at cholinergic synapses could contribute to the unrest and agitation that contribute to the smoker's motivation for the next cigarette, which "medicates" the smoker by desensitizing the excess number of nAChRs back toward a more normal level.

Taken together, this information supports speculation as to a common pattern of cigarette smoking. Most smokers report that the first cigarette of the day is the most pleasurable. After a night of abstinence, nicotine concentrations in the brain are at their lowest level. Thus, smoking the first cigarette most strongly activates nAChRs, possibly causing the largest activity of the midbrain dopamine areas and contributing to the most pleasurable effect (Figure 3, Step 1). After a few cigarettes, there is significant (albeit incomplete) desensitization, causing some acute tolerance and less effect from additional cigarettes (Figure 3, Step 2). The process of activation and desensitization affects different nAChR types differently and influences synaptic plasticity, contributing to the long-term changes associated with addiction. When smoking continues for long periods of time, the nicotinic system undergoes neuroadaptations, including an increase in the number of high-affinity nAChRs (Figure 3, Step 3). Cigarettes are smoked throughout the day, driven by smaller, variable rewards and by the agitation arising, in part, from the excess nAChRs and hyperexcitability at cholinergic synapses experienced during abstinence (Figure 3, Step 4).

Often, episodes of cigarette smoking are separated by hours of abstinence. During that time, nicotine levels drop and some nAChRs recover from desensitization. Smokers often report that cigarettes smoked during the day help them to focus and relax so that they can work more efficiently. As an individual smokes several times during the course of a day, the background level of nicotine slowly increases. Therefore, a smoker experiences some exposure to nicotine throughout the day, ensuring that some types of nAChRs visit states of desensitization. These episodes of nAChR desensitization ensure that the number of nAChRs becomes and remains elevated. If nicotine is avoided for a few weeks, the number of nAChRs returns to the lower value seen in nonsmokers. The process of quitting then would be well under way.

However, most attempts to quit fail, and the explanation for this is a very active area of research. Over years of smoking, neuroadaptations occur and long-term synaptic changes result in learned behaviors, some of which are associated with smoking and some with the context in which smoking takes place. Because these behaviors are reinforced by repeated variable reinforcements from cigarettes and linked sensory cues, the desire for cigarettes extinguishes slowly and sometimes incompletely. Craving for cigarettes may be experienced even years after having quit.

To be sure, nicotine and the addiction process have many complex components that were not discussed here or that are not yet known. Nicotine obtained from tobacco bathes the whole brain. Because cholinergic projections and nAChRs are so widely distributed in the brain, it is difficult to imagine all the processes that are influenced. Despite recent progress, there is much to be learned about nicotine addiction.

SYSTEMIC TOXICITY

Particulate and Gaseous Components of Tobacco Smoke. Although it is nicotine that causes addiction, there are other components in the particulate and gaseous phases of tobacco smoke that are primarily responsible for human morbidity and mortality. Cigarette smoke is composed of volatile and particulate phases. The volatile phase accounts for about 95% of the weight of the cigarette, while the particulate phase composes the other 5%. There are about 3,500 different compounds in the particulate phase. The "tar" in a cigarette is composed of the particulate matter minus its alkaloid and water content. Tar contains many carcinogens, including polynuclear aromatic hydrocarbons, N-nitrosamines, and aromatic amines. The particulate phase consists of the pharmacologically active alkaloids, nornicotine, anabasine, anatabine, myosmene, and nicotyrine, in addition to nicotine. Assays for some of these alkaloids are being developed as biomarkers of tobacco use and exposure to secondhand smoke. The volatile phase of cigarette smoke contains more than 500 gaseous compounds, including nitrogen, CO, carbon dioxide, ammonia, hydrogen cyanide, and benzene.

Cardiovascular, Pulmonary, and Oncologic Toxicities. When they light up, smokers are exposed to more than 4,000 different chemicals, including at least 50 known carcinogens. The increased risk of cardiovascular disease among cigarette smokers likely is related to exposure to oxidant gases and CO, as well as hydrogen cyanide, carbon disulfide, cadmium, and zinc (Hoffman, Djordjevic et al., 1997). Although CO reduces oxygen delivery to the heart, oxidant gases may be responsible for endothelial dysfunction, platelet activation, thrombosis, and coronary vasoconstriction.

Cigarette smoking has significant detrimental effects on both the structure and function of the lung. Cigarette smoking causes an imbalance between proteolytic and antiproteolytic forces in the lung and heightens airway responsiveness. Chronic obstructive lung diseases are linked with exposure to tar, nitrogen oxides, hydrogen cyanide, and volatile aldehydes, enhanced by inducers of superoxide and H_2O_2 (Hoffman, Djordjevic et al., 1997).

The agents contributing most significantly to lung cancer are the carcinogenic polynuclear aromatic hydrocarbons (PAHs) and the tobacco-specific N-nitrosamines, followed by polonium-210 and volatile aldehydes. Catechol, the weakly acidic agents, volatile aldehydes, and nitrogen oxides that can serve as precursors in the exogenous and endogenous formation of N-nitrosamines enhance tobacco smoke-induced tumorigenesis (Hoffman, Djordjevic et al., 1997). New research suggests that individuals who later develop lung cancer have greater biological susceptibility to tobacco carcinogens while exposure is ongoing. Active smokers with elevated levels of DNA damage from PAHs in their white blood cells (DNA adducts) are three times more likely to be diagnosed with lung cancer 1 to 13 years later than are smokers with lower adduct concentrations (OR, 2.98; 95% CI, 1.05-8.42; $p=0.04$) (Tang, Phillips et al., 2001). As with other tobacco-related diseases, the risk of cancer of the mouth, larynx, esophagus, lung, stomach, pancreas, kidney, urinary bladder, and uterine cervix is directly related to the intensity and duration of exposure to cigarette smoke.

Other Physiologic Effects and Toxicities. Cigarette smoking is associated with skin changes, including yellow-staining of fingers, vasospasm and obliteration of small skin vessels, precancerous and squamous cell carcinomas on the lips and oral mucosa, and enhanced facial skin wrinkling. Tobacco smoke and exposure to ultraviolet A radiation each cause wrinkle formation. When excessive sun exposure (>2 hours/day) and heavy smoking (>35 pack years) occur together, the risk of developing wrinkles is 11.4 times higher than that of nonsmokers and those with less sun exposure at the same age (Yin, Morita et al., 2001). The induction of matrix metalloproteinase-1 (MMP-1), mediated by reactive oxygen species (especially in persons with low glutathione content fibroblasts), is thought to be an important mechanism underlying premature skin aging caused by cigarette smoking and exposure to ultraviolet A radiation.

Christen and colleagues (1992) demonstrated that current smokers of 20 or more cigarettes per day had statistically significant increases in nuclear sclerosis (relative risk, 2.24; 95% CI, 1.47-3.41; $p<0.001$) and posterior subcapsular cataracts (relative risk, 3.17; 95% CI, 1.81-5.53; $p\leq0.001$) compared with individuals who never smoked. After adjusting for age and average number of cigarettes smoked per day, Weintraub and colleagues (2002) found a 20% lower risk of cataracts in former smokers who had quit smoking 25 or more years previously, but the risk did not decrease to the level observed among subjects who never smoked. Current smokers of more than 20 cigarettes per day also have an increased risk of age-related macular degeneration (Christen, Glynn et al., 1996).

Although the role of nicotine versus tobacco and the mechanism are not clear, cigarette smoking in women is associated with lower levels of estrogen, earlier menopause, and increased risk of osteoporosis. The alkaloids in tobacco smoke diminish estrogen formation by inhibiting an aromatase enzyme in granulosa cells or placental tissue (Barbieri, McShane et al., 1986).

In men, smoking is believed to affect penile erection through the impairment of endothelium-dependent smooth muscle relaxation. Smoking also doubles the likelihood of moderate or complete erectile dysfunction associated with other risk factors, such as coronary artery disease and hypertension. Because the prevalence of erectile dysfunction in former smokers is no different from that in individuals who never smoked, erectile dysfunction may improve with smoking cessation (McVary, Carrier et al., 2001).

Nicotine causes both appetite suppression and an increase in metabolic rate. Smokers weigh an average 2.7 to 4.5 kg (6 to 10 lbs.) less than nonsmokers. With smoking cessation, individuals typically crave sweets and miss handling the cigarette and oral gratification. Individuals who stop smoking typically gain weight to approximately the levels of never smokers in the 6 to 12 months following smoking cessation (Perkins, 1993).

Through release of catecholamines, nicotine increases lipolysis and releases free fatty acids, which are taken up by the liver (Hellerstein, Benowitz et al., 1994). This could contribute to the increase in very low-density lipoprotein and low-density lipoprotein and the decrease in high-density lipoprotein seen in smokers.

Cigarette smoking decreases the mucous bicarbonate barrier in the stomach and reduces the production of endogenous prostaglandins in the gastric mucosa. Smoking is associated with increased proliferation of *Helicobacter py-*

lori, delayed healing, and recurrence of ulcers (Rhodes, Green et al., 1998).

Tobacco and Pregnancy. Compared with nonsmoking women, the relative risk of having a low birthweight infant is nearly doubled in women who smoke during pregnancy, and the relative risks of spontaneous abortion and perinatal and neonatal mortality are increased by about a third (Walsh, 1994). The components of tobacco smoke responsible for obstetric and fetal problems have not been definitively identified. CO clearly is detrimental, as it markedly reduces the oxygen-carrying capacity of fetal hemoglobin.

New research (Wang, Zuckerman et al., 2002) suggests that the magnitude of the effect of smoking in lowering birthweight is due, at least in part, to an interaction between maternal smoking and the metabolic genes CYP1A1 and GSTT1. The study by Wang and colleagues found that infants born to smoking mothers who had metabolic genes absent in CYP1A1 Aa and aa (heterozygous and homozygous variant types) and GSTT1 absent genotypes had greater reductions in birthweight than did infants born to smoking mothers who had the metabolic genes CYP1A1 AA (homozygous wild type) or GSTT1 genotype. The CYP1A1 gene is a phase 1 enzyme relevant to the metabolism of chemicals in cigarette smoke, and GSTT1 present is a phase 2 metabolic enzyme that assists the conjugation of chemicals into more polar, easily excreted substances. Future research will need to confirm this genetic-environmental interaction and look further for other candidate loci (Vogler & Kozlowski, 2002).

In the developing fetus, nicotine can arrest neuronal replication and differentiation, and can contribute to sudden infant death syndrome (Slotkin, 1998). Nicotine prematurely activates nicotinic cholinergic receptors in the fetal brain, resulting in abnormalities of cell proliferation and differentiation that lead to shortfalls in cell numbers and eventually to altered synaptic activity. Comparable alterations occur in peripheral autonomic pathways, and are hypothesized to lead to increased susceptibility to hypoxia-induced brain damage, perinatal mortality, and sudden infant death (Benowitz, 1991). (Also see Section 10.)

Environmental Tobacco Smoke (ETS). ETS or secondhand smoke is the complex mixture formed by the escaping smoke of a burning tobacco product, as well as smoke that is exhaled by a smoker. Sidestream smoke contains higher concentrations of some toxins than does mainstream smoke. As ETS combines with other constituents in the ambient air and ages, its characteristics may

TABLE 1.   Selected Health Problems Related to Tobacco Use

Toxic to the User*
- Cardiovascular
  - Coronary heart disease
  - Cerebrovascular accidents
  - Peripheral vascular disease
    - Burger's disease
    - Impaired wound healing
- Chronic obstructive pulmonary disease
  - Chronic bronchitis
  - Emphysema
- Respiratory infections
  - Pneumonia
  - Bronchitis
  - Asthma
- Cancer
  - Oropharyngeal
  - Laryngeal
  - Esophageal
  - Lung
  - Bladder
  - Pancreatic
  - Colon
- Peptic ulcer disease
- Reproductive disorders
  - Impotence (men)
  - Reduced fertility (women)
  - Impaired ability to sustain lactation (women)
  - Early menopause (women)
- Vision
  - Cataracts
  - Macular degeneration
- Oral
  - Staining of teeth
  - Gum recession and loss of teeth
- Immune Suppression
- Earlier development of pneumonia in HIV-infected persons
- Reduced athletic performance
- Impaired cognitive performance
- Skin wrinkling
- Fatal fires

Toxic to Infants and Children
- Miscarriage
- Low birthweight infants
- Bronchitis and pneumonia
- Middle ear effusions
- Asthma

*Toxic to persons near the user as well, although the relative degree of risk may be less.

change (NCI, 1999). Exposure to ETS can be assessed through the measurement of indoor air concentrations of smoke constituents, calculated on volumes, ventilation, and other variables; measured with environmental and personal monitors; or determined by using biomarkers in the saliva, urine, and blood.

Exposure to ETS is causally associated with acute and chronic coronary heart disease, lung cancer, nasal sinus cancer, and eye and nasal irritation in adults. ETS is causally associated with asthma, chronic respiratory symptoms, and acute lower respiratory tract infections such as bronchitis and pneumonia in children. ETS also is causally associated with low birth weight and sudden infant death syndrome in infants (NCI, 1999). Young children's exposure to tobacco smoke comes mainly from smokers in the home, especially parents. Maternal smoking has the greatest effect on children's measured cotinine levels. Additional contributors include paternal smoking, smoking by other household members, and smoking by child care personnel.

Repace and colleagues (1996) estimated that an average salivary cotinine level of 0.4 ng/mL corresponds to an increased lifetime mortality risk of 1/1,000 for lung cancer and 1/100 for heart disease. Assuming a prevalence of 28% for unrestricted smoking in the workplace, passive smoking would yield 4,000 heart disease deaths and 400 lung cancer deaths annually. Therefore, Repace and colleagues estimated that more than 95% of ETS-exposed office workers exceeded the significant risk level for heart disease mortality and more than 60% exceeded the significant risk level for lung cancer mortality established by the Occupational Safety and Health Administration (Repace, Jinot et al., 1997).

Morbidity and Mortality. The cumulative result of these health effects, according to the Centers for Disease Control and Prevention (2002), is that each pack of cigarettes sold in the United States costs the nation an estimated $7.18 in medical care expenditures and lost productivity. A study of deaths related to smoking, years of life lost, and economic costs found that smoking continues to be a leading cause of preventable death in the United States, accounting for an estimated 402,374 premature deaths annually from 1995 through 1999. This includes 148,605 deaths (36.9%) from cardiovascular causes, 155,761 deaths (38.7%) from cancer, and 98,008 deaths (24.3%) from nonmalignant pulmonary disease (CDC, 2002). On average, adult men and women smokers lost 13.2 and 14.5 years of life, respectively. In contrast, the annual mortality attributable to

passive smoking between 1995 and 1999 was estimated at 39,060 deaths, including 35,053 from cardiovascular diseases, 3,000 from lung cancer, and 1,007 from perinatal conditions (CDC, 2002). These data qualify tobacco products by a large margin as the leading cause of preventable death. Table 1 lists a variety of health problems caused by or highly associated with tobacco products for consumers and for those around consumers. Stopping tobacco use slows down or reverses many of these problems (DHHS, 1990).

Tobacco and Other Addictions. Tobacco also synergizes with alcohol in causing a number of medical complications. Persons with alcohol problems are far more likely to smoke, and to smoke heavily, than are non-alcoholics (Hurt, Eberman et al., 1993). Smoking and heavy drinking, in combination, are associated with substantially increased rates of oral and esophageal cancers (DHHS, 1982; Blot, McLaughlin et al., 1988), pancreatitis (Pitchumoni, Jain et al., 1988), and cirrhosis (Klatsky & Armstrong, 1992). Finally, as long as cigarettes are designed so that they smolder when they fall lit into folds of upholstered furniture, alcohol use will continue to combine synergistically with smoking in causing household fires that claim more than 1,000 deaths per year among children and adults (McGuire, 1989).

Persons recovering from other substance use disorders often die from tobacco-related illnesses. In a landmark population-based retrospective cohort study by Hurt and colleagues (1996), death certificates were examined for 214 of 854 persons who were admitted between 1972 and 1983 to an inpatient program for the treatment of alcoholism and other non-nicotine drugs of dependence. Of the deaths reported, 50.9% were caused by tobacco use, while 34.1% were attributable to alcohol use. The cumulative 20-year mortality was 48.1% versus an expected 18.5% for a demographically matched control population ($p<0.001$).

Benefits of Cessation. The good news is that smoking cessation has benefits for smokers of all ages. The immediately decreased risk of death in those who stop smoking may reflect a decrease in blood coagulability, improved tissue oxygenation, and reduced predisposition to cardiac arrhythmias. Among former smokers, the reduced risk of death compared with continuing smokers begins shortly after quitting and continues for at least 10 to 15 years. After 10 to 15 years' abstinence, the risk of all-cause mortality returns nearly to that of persons who never smoked (DHHS, 1990). Chapters in Sections 6 and 7 describe pharmacologic and behavioral interventions to achieve tobacco cessation.

REFERENCES

Adler LE, Hoffer LD, Wiser A et al. (1993). Normalization of auditory physiology by cigarette smoking in schizophrenic patients. *American Journal of Psychiatry* 150:1856-1861.

Alkondon M, Pereira EF & Albuquerque EX (1998). Alpha-bungarotoxin- and methyllycaconitine-sensitive nicotinic receptors mediate fast synaptic transmission in interneurons of rat hippocampal slices. *Brain Research* 810:257-263.

American Psychiatric Association (APA) (1994). *Diagnostic and Statistical Manual, 4th Edition (DSM-IV)*. Washington, DC: American Psychiatric Press.

Balfour DJ, Wright AE, Benwell ME et al. (2000). The putative role of extra-synaptic mesolimbic dopamine in the neurobiology of nicotine dependence. *Behavioural Brain Research* 113:73-83.

Barbieri RL, McShane PM & Ryan KJ (1986). Constitutents of cigarette smoke inhibit human granulose cell aromatase. *Fertility and Sterility* 46:232-236.

Benowitz NL (1988). Pharmacologic aspects of cigarette smoking and nicotine addiction. *New England Journal of Medicine* 319:1318-1330.

Benowitz NL, Hall SM, Herning RI et al. (1983). Smokers of low-yield cigarettes do not consume less nicotine. *New England Journal of Medicine* 309:139-142.

Benowitz NL, Jacob P III, Jones RT et al. (1982). Interindividual variability in the metabolism and cardiovascular effects of nicotine in man. *Journal of Pharmacology and Experimental Therapeutics* 268:296-303.

Benowitz NL, Kuyt F, Jacob P III et al. (1983). Cotinine disposition and effects. *Clinical Pharmacology and Therapeutics* 309:1399-1142.

Benowitz NL, Perez-Stable EJ, Fong I et al. (1999). Ethnic differences in N-glucuronidation of nicotine and cotinine. *Journal of Pharmacology and Experimental Therapeutics* 291:1196-1203.

Benowitz NL, Perez-Stable EJ, Herrera B et al. (2002). Slower metabolism and reduced intake of nicotine from cigarette smoking in Chinese-Americans. *Journal of the National Cancer Institute* 94(2):108-115.

Benowitz NL, Porchet H & Jacob P III (1989). Nicotine dependence and tolerance in man: Pharmacokinetic and pharmacodynamic investigations. *Progress in Brain Research* 79:279-287.

Benowitz NL, Porchet H & Jacob P III (1990). Pharmacokinetics, metabolism, and pharmacodynamics of nicotine. In S Wonnacott, MAH Russell & IP Stolerman (eds.) *Nicotine Psychopharmacology: Molecular, Cellular, and Behavioural Aspects*. New York, NY: Oxford University Press, 112-157.

Benowitz NL, Zevin S & Jacob P III (1997). Sources of variability in nicotine and cotinine levels with use of nicotine nasal spray, transdermal nicotine, and cigarette smoking. *British Journal of Clinical Pharmacology* 43:259-267.

Berke JD & Hyman SE (2000). Addiction, dopamine, and the molecular mechanisms of memory. *Neuron* 25:515-532.

Blot WJ, McLaughlin JK, Winn DM et al. (1988). Smoking and drinking in relation to oral and pharyngeal cancer. *Cancer Research* 48:3282-3287.

Boylan B, Brandt V, Muehlbauer J et al. (1993). Green tobacco sickness in tobacco harvesters—Kentucky, 1992. *Morbidity and Mortality Weekly Reports* 42:237-240.

Breslau N, Kilbey MM & Andreski P (1993). Nicotine dependence and major depression: New evidence from a prospective investigation. *Archives of General Psychiatry* 50:31-35.

Broide RS & Leslie FM (1999). The alpha7 nicotinic acetylcholine receptor in neuronal plasticity. *Molecular Neurobiology* 20:1-16.

Buisson B & Bertrand D (2001). Chronic exposure to nicotine upregulates the human (alpha)4((beta)2 nicotinic acetylcholine receptor function. *Journal of Neuroscience* 21:1819-1829.

Carmelli D, Swan GE, Robinette D et al. (1990). Heritability of substance use in the NAS-NRC Twin Registry. *Acta Geneticae Medicae et Gemellologiae (Roma)* 39:91-98.

Cederlof R, Friberg L & Lundman T (1977). The interactions of smoking, environment, and heredity and their implications for disease etiology. A report of epidemiological studies in the Swedish twin registries. *Acta Medica Scandinavica Supplement* 612:1-128.

Center for Disease Control and Prevention (CDC) (2002). Annual smoking-attributable mortality, years of potential life lost, and economic costs—United States, 1995-1999. *Morbidity and Mortality Weekly Reports* 51(14):300-303 .

Christen WG, Glynn RJ, Manson JE et al. (1996). A prospective study of cigarette smoking and risk of age-related macular degeneration in men. *Journal of the American Medical Association* 276(14):1178-1179.

Christen WG, Manson JE, Seddon JM et al. (1992). A prospective study of cigarette smoking and risk of cataract in men. *Journal of the American Medical Association* 268(8):989-993.

Collins AC (1990). An analysis of the addiction liability of nicotine. In CK Erikson, MA Javors & WW Morgan (eds.) *Addiction Potential of Abused Drugs and Drug Classes*. New York, NY: Haworth Press, 83-103.

Cooper E, Couturier S & Ballivet M (1991). Pentameric structure and subunit stoichiometry of a neuronal acetylcholine receptor. *Nature* 350:235-238.

Corrigall WA (1999). Nicotine self-administration in animals as a dependence model. *Nicotine and Tobacco Research* 1(1):11-20.

Corrigall WA, Franklin KB, Coen KM et al. (1992). The mesolimbic dopaminergic system is implicated in the reinforcing effects of nicotine. *Psychopharmacology (Berlin)* 107:285-289.

Dalack GW, Healy DJ & Meador-Woodruff JH (1998). Nicotine dependence in schizophrenia: clinical phenomena and laboratory findings. *American Journal of Psychiatry* 155:1490-1501.

Dani JA (2001). Overview of nicotinic receptors and their roles in the central nervous system. *Biological Psychiatry* 49:166-174.

Dani JA & De Biasi M (2001). Cellular mechanisms of nicotine addiction. *Pharmacology, Biochemistry and Behavior* 70:439-446.

Dani JA & Heinemann S (1996). Molecular and cellular aspects of nicotine abuse. *Neuron* 16:905-908.

Dani JA, Ji D & Zhou F-M (2001). Nicotinic mechanisms in synaptic plasticity of nicotine addiction. *Neuron* 31:349-352.

Dani JA, Radcliffe KA & Pidoplichko VI (2000). Variations in desensitization of nicotinic acetylcholine receptors from hippocampus and midbrain dopamine areas. *European Journal of Pharmacology* 393:31-38.

Di Chiara G (2000). Role of dopamine in the behavioural actions of nicotine related to addiction. *European Journal of Pharmacology* 393:295-314.

Fagerström KO (1978). Measuring degree of physical dependence to tobacco smoking with reference to individualization of treatment. *Addictive Behaviors* 3:235-241.

Fairclough G (2001a). Health officials criticize snuff makers for allowing high levels of carcinogens. *Wall Street Journal*. August 21;A3, A6.

Fairclough G (2001b). Tobacco titans bid for 'organic' cigarette maker. *Wall Street Journal* B1, B4.

Federal Trade Commission (FTC) (2001). Federal Trade Commission Cigarette Report for 1999. Washington, DC: Government Printing Office, 1-26.

Fisher EB, Lichtenstein E & Haire-Joshu D (1993). Multiple determinants of tobacco use and cessation. In CT Orleans & J Slade (eds.) *Nicotine Addiction: Principles and Management*. New York, NY: Oxford University Press, 59-88.

Gilbert DG, Estes SL & Welser R (1997). Does noise stress modulate effects of smoking nicotine?: Mood, vigilance, and EEG responses. *Psychopharmacology* 129:382-389.

Girod R, Crabtree G, Ernstrom G et al. (1999). Heteromeric complexes of alpha 5 and/or alpha 7 subunits. Effects of calcium and potential role in nicotine-induced presynaptic facilitation. *Annals of the New York Academy of Science* 868:578-590.

Glassman AH (1993). Cigarette smoking: Implications for psychiatric illness. *American Journal of Psychiatry* 150:546-553.

Glassman AH, Helzer JE, Covey LS et al. (1990). Smoking, smoking cessation, and major depression. *Journal of the American Medical Association* 264(12):1546-1549.

Gourlay SG & Benowitz NL (1997). Arteriovenous differences in plasma concentrations of nicotine and catecholamines and related cardiovascular effects after smoking, nicotine nasal spay, and intravenous nicotine. *Clinical Pharmacology and Therapeutics* 62:453-463.

Grobe JE & Perkins KA (2000). Behavioral factors influencing the effects of nicotine. In M Piasecki & P Newhause (eds.) *Nicotine: Neurotropic and Neurotoxic Effects*. Washington, DC: American Psychiatric Press, 59-81.

Heatherton TF, Koslowski LT, Frecker RC et al. (1991). The Fagerström Test for Nicotine Dependence: A revision of the Fagerström Tolerance Questionnaire. *British Journal of Addiction* 86(9):11199-1127.

Hellerstein MK, Benowitz NL, Neese RA et al. (1994). Effects of cigarette smoking and its cessation on lipid metabolism and energy expenditure in heavy smokers. *Journal of Clinical Investigation* 93:265-272.

Henningfield JE, Radzius A, Cooper TM et al. (1990). Drinking coffee and carbonated beverages blocks absorption of nicotine from nicotine polacrilex gum. *Journal of the American Medical Association* 264:1560-1564.

Henningfield JE, Stapleton JM, Benowitz NL et al. (1993). Higher levels of nicotine in arterial than in venous blood after cigarette smoking. *Drug Alcohol Dependence* 33:23-29.

Hoffmann D & Hoffmann I (1997). The changing cigarette, 1950-1995. *Journal of Toxicology and Environmental Health* 50:307-364.

Hoffmann D, Djordjevic MV & Hoffmann I (1997). The changing cigarette. *Preventive Medicine* 26:427-434.

Hurt RD, Eberman KM, Slade J et al. (1993). Treating nicotine dependence in patients with other addictive disorders. In CT Orleans & J Slade (eds.) *Nicotine Addiction: Principles and Management*. New York, NY: Oxford University Press, 310-326.

Hurt RD, Offord KP, Croghan IT et al. (1996). Mortality following inpatient addictions treatment: Role of tobacco use in a community-based cohort. *Journal of the American Medical Association* 275(14):1097-1103.

Ikard FF, Green D & Horn D (1969). A scale to differentiate between types of smoking as related to the management of affect. *International Journal of the Addictions* 4:649-659.

Institute of Medicine (IOM) (2001). Clearing the smoke. *Assessing the Science Base for Tobacco Harm Reduction*. Washington, DC: National Academy Press.

Jarvik ME & Henningfield JE (1993). Pharmacological adjuncts for the treatment of tobacco dependence. In CT Orleans & J Slade (eds.) *Nicotine Addiction: Principles and Management*. New York, NY: Oxford University Press, 245-261.

Jarvik ME, Tunstall-Pedoe H, Feyerabend C et al. (1984). Biochemical markers of smoke absorption and self-reported exposure to passive smoking. *Journal Epidemiology and Community Health* 48:335-339.

Ji D, Lape R & Dani JA (2001). Timing and location of nicotinic activity enhances or depresses hippocampal synaptic plasticity. *Neuron* 31:131-141.

Jones S, Sudweeks S & Yakel JL (1999). Nicotinic receptors in the brain: Correlating physiology with function. *Trends in Neurosciences* 22:555-561.

Kaprio J, Koskenvuo M & Sarna S (1981). Cigarette smoking, use of alcohol, and leisure time physical activity among same-sexed adult male twins. In L Gedda, P Parise & WE Nance (eds.) *Twin Research 3: Part C, Epidemiological and Clinical Studies*. New York, NY: Wiley Liss, 37-46.

Karan LD (1993). Nicotine as a potential therapeutic agent: An overview and clinical perspective. *Medicinal Chemistry Research* 2:514-521

Kendler KS, Neale MC, MacLean CJ et al. (1993). Smoking and major depression: A causal analysis. *Archives of General Psychiatry* 50:36-43.

Klatsky AL & Armstrong MA (1992). Alcohol, smoking, coffee, and cirrhosis. *American Journal of Epidemiology* 136:1248-1257.

Koob GF & Le Moal M (2001). Drug addiction, dysregulation of reward, and allostasis. *Neuropsychopharmacology* 24:97-129.

Lai S, Lai H, Page JB et al. (2000). The association between cigarette smoking and drug abuse in the United States. *Journal of Addictive Diseases* 19(4):11-24.

Lena C & Changeux JP (1998). Allosteric nicotinic receptors, human pathologies. *Journal of Physiology (Paris)* 92:63-74.

Leonard S, Adler LE, Benhammou K et al. (2001). Smoking and mental illness. *Pharmacology, Biochemistry, and Behavior* 70(4):561-570.

Levin ED, Behm F, Carnahan E et al. (1993). Clinical trials using ascorbic acid aerosol to aid smoking cessation. *Drug and Alcohol Dependence* 33(3):211-223.

Levin ED, Conners CK, Sparrow E et al. (1996). Nicotine effects on adults with attention-deficit/hyperactivity disorder. *Psychopharmacology* 123(1):55-63.

Levin ED, Wilson W, Rose JE et al. (1996). Nicotine-haloperidol interactions and cognitive performance in schizphrenics. *Neuropsychopharmacology* 15:429-436.

Mansvelder HD & McGehee DS (2000). Long-term potentiation of excitatory inputs to brain reward areas by nicotine. *Neuron* 27:349-357.

McGehee DS & Role LW (1995). Physiological diversity of nicotinic acetylcholine receptors expressed by vertebrate neurons. *Annual Review of Physiology* 57:521-546.

McGuire A (1989). Fires, cigarettes and advocacy. *Law, Medicine and Health Care* 17:73-77.

McNeill AD, Owen LA, Belcher M et al. (1990). Abstinence from smoking and expired-air carbon monoxide levels: Lactose intolerance as a possible source of error. *American Journal of Public Health.* 80(9):1114-1115.

McVary KT, Carrier S, Wessells H et al. (2001). Smoking and erectile dysfunction: Evidence based analysis. *Journal of Urology* 166(5):1624-1632.

Milberger S, Biederman J, Faraone SV et al. (1997). ADHD is associated with early initiation of cigarette smoking in children and adolescents. *Journal of the American Academy of Child and Adolescent Psychiatry* 36(1):37-44.

Mittelmark MB, Murray DM, Luepker RV et al. (1987). Prediction experimentation with cigarettes: The childhood antecedents of smoking study (CASS). *American Journal of Public Health* 77(2):206-208.

Mohammed AH (2000). Genetic dissection of nicotine-related behaviour: A review of animal studies. *Behavioural Brain Research* 113(1-2):35-41.

National Cancer Institute (NCI) (1992). *Smokeless Tobacco or Health: An International Perspective* (NIH Smoking and Tobacco Control Monograph 2). Bethesda, MD: National Institutes of Health.

National Cancer Institute (NCI) (1998). *Cigars: Health Effects and Trends* (NIH Smoking and Tobacco Control Monograph 9). Bethesda, MD: National Institutes of Health.

National Cancer Institute (NCI) (1999). *Health Effects of Exposure to Environmental Tobacco Smoke: The Report of the California Environmental Protection Agency* (Smoking and Tobacco Control Monograph 10). Bethesda, MD: National Institutes of Health, ES 1-9.

Newhause PA & Whitehouse PJ (2000). Nicotinic cholinergic systems in Alzeheimer's and Parkinson's diseases. In M Piasecki & P Newhause (eds.) *Nicotine: Neurotropic and Neurotoxic Effects.* Washington, DC: American Psychiatric Press, 149-181.

Nowak R (1994). Key study unveiled-11 years late. *Science* 264:196-197.

Olincy A, Ross RG, Harris JG et al. (2000). The P50 auditory event-evoked potential in adult attention-deficit disorder: Comparison with schizophrenia. *Biological Psychiatry* 47(11):969-977.

Parrott AC (1998). Nesbitt's paradox resolved? Stress and arousal modulation during cigarette smoking. *Addiction* 93:27-39.

Parrott AC & Kaye FJ (1999). Daily uplifts, hassles, stresses and cognitive failures: In cigarette smokers, abstaining smokers, and non-smokers. *Behavioral Pharmacology* 10(6-7):639-646.

Pauly JL, Lee HJ, Hurley EL et al. (1998). Glass fiber contamination of cigarette filters: An additional health risk to the smoker? *Cancer Epidemiology, Biomarkers and Prevention* 7:967-979.

Perez-Stable DJ, Herrera B, Jacob P III et al. (1998). Nicotine metabolism and intake in black and white smokers. *Journal of the American Medical Association* 280(2):152-156.

Perkins KA (1993). Weight gain following smoking cessation. *Journal of Consulting and Clinical Psychology* 61:768-777.

Perkins KA (1999). Nicotine discrimination in men and women. *Pharmacology, Biochemistry and Behavior* 64(2):295-299.

Perkins KA, Gerlach D, Vender J et al. (2001). Sex differences in the subjective and reinforcing effects of visual and olfactory cigarette smoke stimuli. *Nicotine & Tobacco Research* 3(2):141-150.

Picciotto MR, Zoli M, Rimondini R et al. (1998). Acetylcholine receptors containing the beta2 subunit are involved in the reinforcing properties of nicotine. *Nature* 391:173-177.

Pidoplichko VI, DeBiasi M, Williams JT et al. (1997). Nicotine activates and desensitizes midbrain dopamine neurons. *Nature* 390:401-404.

Pitchumoni CS, Jain NK, Lowenfels AB et al. (1988). Chronic cyanide poisoning: Unifying concept for alcoholic and tropical pancreatitis. *Pancreas* 3:220-222.

Raaschou-Nielsen E (1960). Smoking habits in twins. *Danish Medical Bulletin* 7:82-88.

Repace JL, Jinot J, Bayard S et al. (1997). Air nicotine and saliva cotinine as indicators of workplace passive smoking exposure and risk. *Risk Analysis* 18(1):71-83.

Rhodes J, Green J & Thomas G (1998). Nicotine and the gastrointestinal tract. In N Benowitz (ed.) *Nicotine Safety and Toxicity.* New York, NY: Oxford University Press, 161-166.

Robinson SF, Marks MJ & Collins AC (1996). Inbred mouse strains vary in oral self-selection of nicotine. *Psychopharmacology* 124(4):332-339.

Role LW & Berg DK (1996). Nicotinic receptors in the development and modulation of CNS synapses. *Neuron* 16:1077-1085.

Rose JE & Behm FM (1994). Inhalation of vapor from black pepper extract reduces smoking withdrawal symptoms. *Drug and Alcohol Dependence* 34(3):225-229.

Rose JE, Ananda S & Jarvik ME (1983). Cigarette smoking during anxiety-provoking and monotonous tasks. *Addictive Behaviors* 8:353-359.

Rose JE, Behm FM & Levin ED (1993). Role of nicotine dose and sensory cues in the regulation of smoke intake. *Pharmacology, Biochemistry and Behavior* 44(4):891-900.

Rose JE, Behm FM & Westman EC (2001). Acute effects of nicotine and mecamylamine on tobacco withdrawal symptoms, cigarette reward and ad lib smoking. *Pharmacology, Biochemistry and Behavior* 68(2):187-197.

Rose JE, Behm FM, Westman EC et al. (1999). Arterial nicotine kinetics during cigarette smoking and intravenous nicotine administration: Implications for addiction. *Drug and Alcohol Dependence* 56:99-107.

Rose JE, Herskovic JE, Trilling Y et al. (1985). Transdermal nicotine reduces cigarette craving and nicotine preference. *Clinical Pharmacology and Therapeutics* 38(4):450-456.

Rosecrans JA (1995). The psychopharmacological basis of nicotine's differential effects on individual subject variability in the rat. *Behavioral Genetics* 25(2):187-196.

Schultz W, Dayan P & Montague PR (1997). A neural substrate of prediction and reward. *Science* 275:1593-1599.

Shields J (1962). *Monozygotic Twins Brought Up Apart and Brought Up Together.* New York, NY: Oxford University Press.

Shiffman S (1988). Behavioral assessment. In DM Donovan & GA Marlatt (eds.) *Assessment of Addictive Behaviors.* New York, NY: Guilford Press, 139-188.

Shytle RD, Baker M, Silver AA et al. (2000). Smoking nicotine and movement disorders. In M Piasecki & P Newhause (eds.) *Nicotine: Neurotropic and Neurotoxic Effects.* Washington, DC: American Psychiatric Press, 183-202.

Slotkin TA (1998). Fetal nicotine or cocaine exposure: Which one is worse? *Journal of Pharmacology and Experimental Therapeutics* 285(3):931-945.

Spilich GJ, June L & Renner J (1992). Cigarette smoking and cognitive performance. *British Journal of Addiction* 87:1313-1326.

Substance Abuse and Mental Health Administration (SAMHSA) (2001). *Summary of Findings from the 2000 National Household Survey on Drug Abuse.* Rockville, MD: SAMHSA, Office of Applied Studies.

Sullivan MA & Rudnik-Levin F (2001). Attention deficit/hyperactivity disorder and substance abuse. Diagnostic and therapeutic considerations. *Annals of the New York Academy of Sciences* 931:251-270.

Tang D, Phillips DH, Stampfer M et al. (2001). Association between carcinogen-DNA adducts in white blood cells and lung cancer risk in the Physicians' Health Study. *Cancer Research* 61(18):6708-6712.

Tate JC & Stanton AL (1990). Assessment of the validity of the Reasons for Smoking Scale. *Addictive Behaviors* 15:129-135.

Tritto T, Stitzel JA, Marks MJ et al. (2002). Variability in response to nicotine in the LS x SS RI strains: Potential role of polymorphism in alpha 4 and alpha 6 nicotinic receptor genes. *Pharmacogenetics* 12(3):197-208.

Tsuge K, Katoaoka M & Seto Y (2000). Cyanide and thiocyanate levels in blood and saliva of healthy adult volunteers. *Journal of Health Science* 46(5):343-350.

U.S. Department of Health and Human Services (USDHHS) (1982). *The Health Consequences of Smoking: Cancer. A Report of the Surgeon General.* Rockville, MD: Office on Smoking and Health.

U.S. Department of Health and Human Services (USDHHS) (1988). *The Health Consequences of Smoking: Nicotine Addiction: A Report of the Surgeon General.* Rockville, MD: Office on Smoking and Health.

U.S. Department of Health and Human Services (USDHHS) (1990). *The Health Benefits of Smoking Cessation: A Report of the Surgeon General.* Rockville, MD: Office on Smoking and Health.

U.S. Department of Health and Human Services (USDHHS) (1994). *Preventing Tobacco Use Among Young People: A Report of the Surgeon General.* Rockville, MD: Office on Smoking and Health.

Vogler GP & Kozlowski LT (2002). Differential influence of maternal smoking on infant birth weight: Gene-environment interaction and targeted intervention. *Journal of the American Medical Association* 280(2):241-242.

Walsh RA (1994). Effects of maternal smoking on adverse pregnancy outcomes: Examination of the criteria of causation. *Human Biology* 66(6):1059-1092.

Wang X, Zuckerman B, Pearson C et al. (2002). Maternal cigarette smoking, metabolic gene polymorphism, and infant birth weight. *Journal of the American Medical Association* 287:195-202.

Weintraub JM, Willett WC, Rosner B et al. (2002). Smoking cessation and risk of cataract extraction among US women and men. *American Journal of Epidemiology* 155(1):72-79.

Weissman MM, Warner V, Wickramaratne PJ et al. (1999). Maternal smoking during pregnancy and psychopathology in offspring followed to adulthood. *Journal of the American Academy of Child and Adolescent Psychiatry* 38(7):892-899.

Wise RA (2000). Addiction becomes a brain disease. *Neuron* 26:27-33.

Wonnacott S (1997). Presynaptic nicotinic ACh receptors. *Trends in Neurosciences* 20:92-98.

Woolf NJ (1991). Cholinergic systems in mammalian brain and spinal cord. *Progress in Neurobiology* 37:475-524.

Yin L, Morita A & Tsuji T (2001). Skin aging induced by ultraviolet exposure and tobacco smoking: Evidence from epidemiological and molecular studies. *Photodermatology, Photoimmunology and Photomedicine* 17(4):178-183.

Zevin S & Benowitz NL (1998). Pharmacokinetics and pharmacodynamics of nicotine. In M Piasecki & P Newhause (eds.) *Nicotine: Neurotropic and Neurotoxic Effects.* Washington, DC: American Psychiatric Press, 37-57.

Zhou FM, Liang Y & Dani JA (2001). Endogenous nicotinic cholinergic activity regulates dopamine release in the striatum. *Nature Neuroscience* 4:1224-1229.

| Chapter 8 | # The Pharmacology of Marijuana |

Sandra P. Welch, Ph.D.
Billy R. Martin, Ph.D.

Drugs in the Class
Absorption and Metabolism
Pharmacologic Actions
Mechanisms of Action
Addiction Liabiity
Toxicity/Adverse Effects
Future Research Directions

Cannabis sativa, obtained from hemp plants, is among the oldest and most widely used drugs in the world (Harris, Dewey et al., 1977). A recent review elegantly summarizes the chemistry and uses of the hemp plant throughout history (Mechoulam & Hanus, 2000).

DRUGS IN THE CLASS

THC, the major psychoactive ingredient in marijuana, first was isolated and purified in 1965 (Mechoulam & Gaoni, 1965). This important discovery was the first step in elucidating the site and mechanism of action of the cannabinoids—the term for all compounds that are structurally related to THC. More than 400 chemicals are synthesized from the hemp plant, approximately 60 of which are cannabinoids. The knowledge of cannabinoid pharmacology has expanded significantly over the past decade to include the discovery of naturally occurring cannabinoids (endocannabinoids or endogenous cannabinoids) in most species, as well as two major receptors for the cannabinoids: CB_1 and CB_2. Knowledge of the pharmacology of the cannabinoids and endocannabinoids represents a work in progress, as research provides an ever-expanding view of their mechanism of action and biological functions.

History. Cannabis use dates back more than 12,000 years (Abel, 1979) and is believed to have started in central Asia and continued to flourish in Southeast Asia and India. It was used by the ancient Chinese and Greeks to make clothes and rope from hemp. It is believed that cannabis was introduced into the Americas in the 1600s by the English settlers and Spanish conquistadors. Cannabis was cultivated early in American history for its fiber. Medicinally, it long has been used in China, India, the Middle East, South America, and South Africa. The earliest references to its medicinal uses date from 2700 BC (Grinspoon & Bakalar, 1993). Uses in ancient China included treatment for constipation, malaria, rheumatic pains, and female disorders. The euphoric properties were discovered in India around 2000 BC, and cannabis was recommended for reducing fevers, producing sleep, stimulating the appetite, relieving headaches, and curing venereal diseases (Mechoulam & Feigenbaum, 1987).

Epidemiology. In the United States, recreational use of cannabis began to surge in the 1930s during the Prohibition era. Although cannabis was recognized as an official drug and was listed in the *U.S. Pharmacopoeia* from 1850 until 1942, its medical use was essentially abolished in 1937 with enactment of the Marijuana Tax Act. A dramatic increase in cannabis use was observed during the 1960s, which led to extensive research in the field of cannabinoid pharmacology.

The Community Epidemiology Work Group (CEWG), sponsored by the National Institute on Drug Abuse (NIDA), reported that in several cities the use of marijuana, as quantified by arrests and emergency department admissions, recently has stabilized after an increase throughout the 1990s (CEWG, 2000). However, CEWG reports on some major cities indicate increased prevalence of use, particularly among the 18- to 25-year-old population. The number of reports of marijuana use based on criminal court cases remains high and, in male arrestees, is higher than for any other drug of abuse, including crack cocaine. Among drug-related admissions to emergency departments, marijuana ranked ahead of alcohol (the second most prevalent drug detected) and cocaine (the third most frequently detected drug). NIDA data (2000) show that concurrent alcohol use was detected in 23% to 79% of marijuana users, depending on geographic area. In addition, the CEWG reported that an increase in the use of "blunts" (empty cigarette wrappers into which marijuana is inserted) has contributed to the combination of marijuana with other drugs of abuse such as PCP (phencyclidine, a hallucinogen), the most prevalent additive. In sum, the use of marijuana remains prevalent throughout the country.

Moreover, the increased potency of newer hydroponically grown strains has led to an increase in total delta-9-tetrahydrocannabinol (THC) content that is predicted to increase the prevalence of dependence.

Therapeutic Use. In 1842, O'Shaughnessy, an army physician in India, published a review on the uses of cannabis in treating various medical conditions (O'Shaughnessy, 1842). Interestingly, several of these early references to the medical uses of marijuana include disease states on which research continues today (Hollister, 2001; Russo, 2001). Several recent reviews of the medicinal uses of marijuana have alluded to O'Shaughnessy's early review. Recently, the medicinal uses of cannabis in Azerbaijan, as described in medieval texts from as early as the 9th century AD, have been reviewed, and uses for the drug in modern medicine based on folkloric uses have been proposed (reviewed in Mechoulam & Harrus, 2000).

Current interest in the medicinal effects of cannabinoids stems almost entirely from reports by individuals who have self-medicated with cannabis (Grinspoon & Bakalar, 1993), as well as recent reports of preclinical trials in nonhuman subjects. The medical profession has not enthusiastically endorsed cannabis use for almost any disorder, although numerous clinical trials have been conducted with THC and its synthetic derivatives. Often these data are used to justify the use of cannabis. However, it is inappropriate to justify the use of cannabis on the basis of controlled clinical trials conducted with THC because of the vast differences between smoked cannabis and the ingestion of a pure synthetic compound. In addition, cannabis smoke has the potential for producing health problems. Therapeutic agents need to be efficacious, have an acceptable safety margin, and should be administered in a set dosage formulation of consistent composition. Smoked cannabis fails to meet these basic requirements. Administration of smoked cannabis, or THC alone, by other novel routes of administration could be justified if the patient were refractory to other medications or if the basic tenants of an effective therapeutic agent could be satisfied by altering the route of administration or the cannabinoid agent administered.

Proposed Indications. Therapeutic uses for cannabis have been anecdotally reported for thousands of years. Only recently have several uses described in folk medicine been formally evaluated. The most intense interest has been directed toward the prevention of weight loss in AIDS patients, management of pain, prevention of emesis, control of glaucoma, and control of movement disorders. The use of smoked cannabis remains both politically and scientifically controversial. The issue certainly will remain the subject of debate even when controlled clinical studies are completed. The availability of synthetic THC in capsule form provides an alternative to the smoked plant material.

The potential for development of alternative methods of drug delivery using either pure THC or one of the newer THC derivatives may obviate the problems and the controversial nature of the use of the smoked plant material. Those advocating the use of cannabis for medicinal purposes argue that THC is delivered more effectively in smoke, that cannabis is less expensive than THC, and that cannabis produces few if any harmful effects. All are issues that eventually must be addressed in the development of a novel route for administration of the pure THC or a THC derivative. In addition, more data describing the role or roles of the endocannabinoid system in the etiology of disease states, coupled with the pharmacologic activity of the endocannabinoids administered exogenously, have opened a new and exciting area for the development of potential therapeutic agents.

Antiemetic Effect: Marketed for oral administration, dronabinol (Marinol®) is a Schedule III drug under the federal Controlled Substances Act. It currently is used as an appetite stimulant in AIDS-wasting patients and as an antiemetic for cancer chemotherapy. THC has antiemetic effects superior to those of placebo in chemotherapy patients who are experiencing moderate emesis, and THC is approximately equivalent in potency to prochlorperazine (Compazine®) in most studies (Sallan, Cronin et al., 1980). However, Gralla and colleagues (1984) found metoclopramide (Reglan®) to be more efficacious in controlling emesis in patients receiving cisplatin. Synthetic analogs of THC, such as nabilone, have been tested in clinical trials for their antiemetic potency in cancer patients who are receiving chemotherapy and have been found to be effective in alleviating nausea and vomiting (Razdan, Howes et al., 1983).

Although THC has side effects (psychotropic effects and sedation), its efficacy as an antiemetic treatment led to its approval in the United States for this indication. Clinical trials were conducted in which oral dronabinol (Marinol®) and smoked cannabis were compared. In a random-order crossover study, 35% of the patients preferred oral dronabinol, 20% preferred smoked cannabis, and the remainder had no preference. In an open study of patients who were refractory to antiemetic agents and were given smoked cannabis (Vinciguerra, Moore et al., 1988), 25% dropped out because of dissatisfaction, 24% rated cannabis "very effective," 35% "moderately effective," and 16% "ineffective." Almost all patients reported sedation, dry mouth, and dizziness.

Appetite Stimulation and Cachexia: Smoked cannabis stimulates appetite—an effect that has led to efforts to use cannabis for disorders involving loss of appetite and body weight, such as that associated with AIDS. AIDS patients have lobbied to make cannabis available to those suffering from cachexia or body wasting related to HIV infection. THC was approved in the early 1990s for this indication. Clinical trials indicate some improvement in appetite, slight increases in caloric intake, and weight gain in AIDS patients who use THC (Plasse, Krasnow et al., 1991). However, given animal studies indicating that cannabinoids adversely affect the immune system, the use of THC in those whose immune systems already are compromised by HIV

disease poses an ethical dilemma. Although Marinol/marijuana use was associated with declining health in patients undergoing antiretroviral therapies, all clinical indicators of pancreatitis improved (Whitfield, Bechtel et al., 1997). In those AIDS patients with the lowest CD4[+] counts, use of Marinol/marijuana did not appear to cause harm, and the long-term, safe use of THC for anorexia associated with weight loss in patients with AIDS was reported (Beal, Olson et al., 1997). The question of the efficacy of the smoked cannabis as therapy must be demonstrated in controlled clinical studies, and efforts must be made to determine whether it offers advantages over oral THC. It is likely that guidelines will need to be formulated to guide use in all patients, rather than limited use in the late stages of the disease.

Recent studies have provided additional insights into the role of the endogenous cannabinoid system in controlling food intake—a role that it appears to play from birth. Newborn mice given the cannabinoid antagonist SR141716A fail to suckle, lose weight, and die if not rescued through administration of THC or endocannabinoids such as 2-AG (Fride, Ginzburg et al., 2001). In these animal studies, at least, the cannabinoid system appears to play a critical role in early development. Similarly, it has been shown that administering anandamide to rats increases their appetites and induces overeating after satiation (Williams & Kirkham, 1999).

Because cannabinoid receptors and the endocannabinoids are present in the hypothalamus, it is logical that the endocannabinoid system can regulate food intake, although until recently it was not known how such an effect occurs. Recently, it was shown that CB$_1$ receptor knockout mice eat less than their wild-type littermates, and endocannabinoids in the hypothalamus can tonically activate CB$_1$ receptors to maintain food intake. The mechanism by which endocannabinoids appear to regulate food intake involves modulation of leptin, the major signaling peptide through which the hypothalamus senses satiety. Defects in the leptin/endocannabinoid interplay have been proposed to underlie obesity in genetically obese rats and may underlie obesity in humans (Di Marzo, Goparaju et al., 2001). Conversely, a clinically relevant effect of the cannabinoid antagonist has been reported: SR141716A significantly reduces food intake. These results have been reported in animal studies and, more recently, in human clinical trials, in which significant weight loss has been reported. Such results afford important new insights into the role of endocannabinoids in regulating appetite and suggest novel possibilities for treating a variety of eating disorders.

Anticonvulsant Effect: The therapeutic potential of cannabis as an anticonvulsant was demonstrated in the 1940s when children, poorly controlled on conventional anticonvulsant medications, improved after the use of cannabis. In rodent models, THC produces both convulsant and anticonvulsant effects. Cannabidiol, a natural component of cannabis with practically no cannabis-like psychoactivity, has demonstrated some moderate anticonvulsant activity in animals (Karler & Turkanis, 1981). Nevertheless, interest in cannabidiol for human use has waned, mainly because of its low efficacy. However, the recent observation that CB_1-receptor knock-out mice are prone to seizures (Zimmer, Zimmer et al., 2000) has rekindled interest in cannabidiol for the control of seizure activity.

Neurologic and Movement Disorders: Numerous anecdotal reports suggest that smoked cannabis is effective in relieving spasticity arising from multiple sclerosis and spinal cord injury. However, few controlled studies have compared the effectiveness of either cannabis or THC with other therapies. Recently, Di Marzo's research group (Baker, Pryce et al., 2001) demonstrated that increasing the concentration of endogenous cannabinoids 2-AG and palmitoylethanolamide, an anandamide (AEA) derivative, can reduce spasticity in multiple sclerosis in animal models. In addition, endocannabinoid tone appears to play a critical role in the modulation of basal ganglia-mediation of the spasticity in Parkinson's disease (Di Marzo, Bisogno et al., 2000). This recent work opens up a new area for increased research involving the role of the endocannabinoids in neuromuscular and neurodegenerative diseases.

Analgesia: Recent studies summarize the extensive evaluation of the analgesic and antinociceptive effects of the cannabinoids (Martin & Lichtman, 1998) and the neural substrates mediating such responses (Walker, Hohmann et al., 1999). Early experiments to evaluate the analgesic effects of the cannabinoids dealt mainly with an examination of the effects of THC, the principal active ingredient in cannabis. Studies in human subjects indicate that, at oral doses of 10 and 20 mg/kg, THC is no more effective than codeine as an analgesic, while producing a significant degree of dysphoric side effects (Noyes, Brunk et al., 1975). When tested after intravenous administration to human dental patients, THC produced antinociception that was accompanied by dysphoria and anxiety (Raft, Gregg et al.,

1977). Thus it appears that THC analgesia could be elicited only at doses producing other behavioral side effects. In addition, THC appears to be no more potent than the more commonly used opioid analgesics.

Cannabinoids are active as analgesic drugs when administered to laboratory animals by several routes of administration (Yaksh, 1981; Gilbert, 1981; Lichtman & Martin, 1991a, 1991b; Welch & Stevens, 1992; Welch, Dunlow et al., 1995). Early studies by Sofia and colleagues (1973) and by Moss and Johnson (1980) established that oral THC is effective in the rat paw pressure test. Similarly, it has been shown that the synthetic cannabinoid WINN 55,212-2 alleviates the pain associated with sciatic nerve constriction in rats (Herzberg, Eliav et al. 1997) and capsaicin-induced hyperalgesia in rats (Li, Daughters et al., 1999) and in rhesus monkeys (Ko & Woods, 1999). Cannabinoid-induced antinociception appears to be produced by the inhibition of wide dynamic range neurons in the spinal cord dorsal horn (Hohmann, Tsou et al., 1999). The endogenous cannabinoid system appears to be an active component of chronic pain, in that the CB_1 antagonist SR141716A has been shown to produce hyperalgesia in rats (Strangman, Patrick et al., 1998; Martin, Loo et al., 1999) and mice (Richardson, Aanonsen et al., 1997, 1998).

Recently, the interaction of cannabinoids with opioids has been extensively reviewed (Manzanares, Corchero et al., 1999). Cannabinoids produce antinociception by interaction with endogenous kappa opioids, such as dynorphins, in the spinal cord (intrathecally administered) (Smith & Dewey, 1993). THC releases endogenous dynorphin A (1-17), as well as leucine enkephalin—another endogenous opioid—in the spinal cord (Mason & Welch, 1999a, 1999b). As animals become tolerant to THC, dynorphin A release is elicited only by very high doses. Thus, tolerance to THC involves a reduction in the release of dynorphin A (Mason & Welch, 1999b). The kappa opioid-receptor antagonist, nor-binaltorphimine (nor-BNI), blocks THC-induced (intrathecal) antinociception, but does not block catalepsy, hypothermia, or hypoactivity (Smith & Dewey, 1993; Pugh, Abood et al., 1995). Data on the lack of nor-BNI block of certain cannabinoid actions were the first indication that not all the behavioral effects of the cannabinoids are mediated through a single mechanism.

It is unlikely that either THC-induced antinociception or tolerance is totally due to dynorphin release. The events that precede and follow dynorphin release, and which are likely to modulate dynorphin release, have not yet been characterized. Cannabinoid-induced release of dynorphin most likely is a modulator of other downstream systems (possibly decreasing Substance P release or CGRP release), which culminate in antinociception on administration of cannabinoids. Substance P and related neurokinins are major mediators of nociceptive transmission in the spinal cord (Nishiyama, Kwak et al., 1995). Morphine and other opioids, as well as endogenous opioids, have been shown to decrease the release of Substance P (reviewed in Gao & Peet, 1999; Dray & Rang, 1998). In addition, it has been shown that chronic THC treatment increases Substance P and enkephalin mRNAs concurrently in the same neurons in the caudate.

Cannabinoid receptors co-localize with Substance P receptors in the striatum (Mailleux & Vanderhaeghen, 1992, 1994), providing additional evidence for the interactions of the two systems. Recently, it was demonstrated that in CB_1 knock-out mice, brain levels of Substance P, dynorphin, and enkephalin are significantly increased. Thus, it is likely that the CB_1 receptor plays a role in the tonic regulation of these peptides (Zimmer, Zimmer et al., 1999). In summary, THC-induced release of endogenous kappa opioid peptides plays a role in the production of THC-induced antinociception. The interaction of cannabinoids and opioids with similar downstream mediators of nociceptive transmission, such as Substance P, provides evidence that it may be possible to enhance antinociception and analgesia through opioid/THC interactions without augmenting the side effects of either individual agent.

Recent work with dynorphin, enkephalin, and mu opioid receptor knock-out mice suggests that the antinociceptive effects of THC are attenuated (Zimmer, Valjent et al., 2001). One explanation could be the functional coupling of the gamma/kappa and gamma/delta receptors, which can lead to enhanced antinociceptive effects of opioids by the cannabinoids. The release of leucine enkephalin is a critical factor in THC/morphine enhancement. Prevention of the metabolism of dynorphin A (1-17) to dynorphin (1-8) or to leucine enkephalin prevents the enhancement of morphine-induced antinociception by the THC (Pugh, Smith et al., 1996). In CB_1 knock-out mice, the reinforcing effects of opioids are decreased (Ledent, Valverde et al., 1999). Increases in prodynorphin and proenkephalin mRNA (precursors of dynorphins and enkephalins) after exposure to THC have been shown (Corchero, Avila et al., 1997). It is significant that the lack of behavioral tolerance to the combination of THC and morphine is accompanied by pre-

vention of the development of biochemical correlates of tolerance observed with either drug alone, as quantified by changes in opioid and cannabinoid receptor proteins using Western immunoblotting techniques (Cichewicz, Haller et al., 2001). Thus, an important potential clinical ramification of these studies is the understanding that combination cannabinoid/opioid treatment produces effective antinociception with reduced development of tolerance and, most likely, dependence.

In summary, cannabinoids produce antinociception by interfacing with the opioid system in the control of pain. The mechanisms that underlie such an interaction between the two systems are not known but clearly involve the release of endogenous opioids by cannabinoids, particularly dynorphins. Subsequent attenuation of Substance P release by both the opioids and cannabinoids clearly is possible. The clinical implications of the interplay of the cannabinoid and opioid systems may lead investigators to an increased therapeutic potential for the drugs used in combination.

Glaucoma: Although there is some variability among studies, most show that smoking cannabis lowers intraocular pressure to a significant degree. The synthetic cannabinoid, nabilone, is marketed in Europe for the treatment of glaucoma. However, evidence is lacking that cannabis is capable of lowering intraocular pressure sufficiently to prevent optic nerve damage. The necessity of smoking cannabis or the systemic administration of synthetic cannabinoids for beneficial effects has tempered enthusiasm for its use in glaucoma.

One of the major drawbacks of cannabis is that it must be smoked at relatively short intervals to depress intraocular pressure. One study reports on a topical preparation of cannabis that is effective for glaucoma and is marketed as Canasol in Jamaica (Noyes, Brunk et al., 1975). However, at present no evidence is available that cannabis or THC is more effective than other agents in controlling glaucoma or that cannabis is effective in patients who are refractory to current therapies. Development of a cannabinoid derivative that is effective topically could be beneficial in that it would most likely exert its effects through a mechanism distinct from that of current medications.

ABSORPTION AND METABOLISM

Preparations. The concentration of THC varies across the three most common forms of cannabis: marijuana, hashish, and hash oil. Marijuana is prepared from the dried flowering tops and leaves of the harvested plant. However, potency varies among the upper leaves, lower leaves, stems, and seeds. THC concentrations in marijuana containing mostly leaves and stems ranges from 0.5% to 5%. However, the "sinsemilla," the flowering tops from unfertilized female plants, can have THC concentrations of 7% to 14%. Hashish, which is composed of dried cannabis resin and compressed flowers, typically has a THC content ranging from 2% to 8%. Hash oil, which is obtained by extracting THC from hashish (or marijuana) with an organic solvent, is a highly potent substance with a THC concentration of 15% to 50%. Fiber-type cannabis has a low THC content (typically less than 0.4%) coupled with a high cannabidiol content.

Kinetics. The most common route of administration is smoking marijuana as a hand-rolled "joint" the size of a cigarette or larger, often with tobacco added to assist burning. A typical joint contains 0.5 to 1.0 g cannabis and varies in THC from 5 to 150 mg (typically between 1% and 15%). The actual amount of THC delivered in the smoke has been estimated at 20% to 70% (Hawks, 1982). Only a small amount of smoked cannabis (2 to 3 mg available THC) is required to produce a brief pleasurable high for the occasional user. A water pipe known as a "bong" is a popular implement for all cannabis preparations because water cools the hot smoke and less drug is lost through sidestream smoke.

Smokers generally inhale and hold their breath to increase absorption of THC in the lungs, where the blood supply is extensive. Thus, inhalation produces the most rapid onset and intense "high" of the major routes of administration.

Marijuana and hashish also can by taken orally in food products. However, the onset of the psychoactive effects is slow (about an hour), and absorption is erratic. The kinetics of oral absorption leads to a slower onset but also a longer duration of action. The high is of lesser intensity, but lasts longer. Human studies typically employ THC doses of 10, 20, and 25 mg orally as low, medium, and high doses (Perez-Reyes, Di Guiseppi et al., 1982).

THC is insoluble in water. Therefore, little or no drug is actually present in THC extracts that are injected intravenously.

THC is metabolized to the active metabolite, 11-OH-THC, which is unlikely to contribute significantly to drug's pharmacologic effect because of its rapid conversion to an inactive metabolite that serves as the primary urinary marker for detecting cannabis use. THC can be deposited in fatty tissues for long periods of time after use. However, no evidence shows that THC exerts a deleterious effect when slowly released from fat tissues. The relationship between blood levels of THC and pharmacologic effects is not linear, which makes it difficult to predict impairment related to THC use. Approximately 45 minutes after use, a linear relationship between blood concentrations and pharmacologic effects appears; this can be modelled mathematically to estimate the time elapsed since marijuana use (Huestis, Henningfield et al., 1992a, 1992b).

PHARMACOLOGIC ACTIONS

Psychomotor Effects. Object distance and outlines often are distorted after smoked cannabis use, as are the ability to discriminate shapes and to make rapid critical judgments (Isbell, Gorodetzsky et al., 1967; Adams, Brown et al., 1975). Other observations include slowed reaction time and information processing, impaired perceptual-motor coordination and motor performance, impaired short-term memory, attention, signal detection, tracking behavior, and slowed time perception (Chait & Pierri, 1992). Because the use of marijuana with alcohol is prevalent (CEWG, 2000), the additive effects of such drugs on performance tasks such as driving should be emphasized in educational programs (Klonoff, 1974; Sharma & Moskowitz, 1972). However, studies of the effects of cannabis alone on driving performance have found at most minor impairments (Sutton, 1983). Eye-tracking performance is disrupted by THC smoking in human subjects, but the residual effects of a single marijuana cigarette on eye-tracking performance are minimal after 24 hours (Fant, Heishman et al., 1998).

The effects of cannabis on psychomotor tasks generally is dose-related (Chait & Pierri, 1992). The effects generally are larger, more consistent, and of increased persistence in difficult tasks that involve sustained attention (Hansteen, Miller et al., 1976; Smiley & Moskowitz, 1986).

Behavioral Effects. Cannabis use has been associated with reports of an "amotivational syndrome." However, there is little scientific evidence to support the existence of such a syndrome (Kolansky & Moore,1971; Millman & Sbriglio,1986). Studies to date have been narrow in scope and small in number (Hollister, 1986; Dornbush,1974; Negrete, 1983). An increased risk of quitting high school and increased job turnover in young adults has been shown, but such studies fail to account for the initial aspirations and goal orientation of the study participants.

Cognitive Effects. Marijuana use is associated with subtle decrements in cognition and memory, as evidenced in alterations in memory, attention, and integration of complex information (Page, Fletcher et al., 1988; Solowij, Miche et al., 1995). Decreases in short-term (new) memory have been observed (Voth, 1980). Other behaviors altered are time and space perception and sense of self ("depersonalization") (Mathew, Wilson et al., 1993). Pope and Todd-Yurgelun (1996) were able to associate heavy marijuana use with residual effects on memory and learning, thus implicating even short-term heavy use with persistent plasticity changes in memory. The longer cannabis is used, the more pronounced the cognitive impairment. However, no evidence suggests that marijuana use produces cognitive impairments like those found in chronic heavy alcohol users (Hall, 1995). In addition, evidence of brain damage from chronic cannabis use is equivocal (Hall, 1995; Co, Goodwin et al., 1977; Kuehnle, Mendelson et al., 1977). Recent evidence indicates that the endocannabinoid system is a selective and rapid modulator of hippocampal synapse function from effects on neurotransmitter release (Wilson, Kunos et al., 2001). In addition, the cannabinoid analog WINN 55212-2, as well as THC and the endocannabinoid AEA, block the formation of new synapses in rat hippocampal cells in culture (Kim & Thayer, 2001). Changes in the plasticity of the hippocampal system can explain memory deficits observed in THC users and abusers.

THC may have more pronounced effects on cognition if an individual simultaneously uses other drugs. For example, it has been shown that THC decreases cognition profoundly and in a synergistic manner if it is used concurrently with MDMA, also known as "Ecstasy" (Croft, Mackay et al., 2001). Given the polypharmacy that accompanies much THC use, it is possible that other drugs of abuse would have a similar effect in combination with THC.

MECHANISMS OF ACTION

The effects of THC are due to both peripheral and central nervous system (CNS) activity. Behavioral effects are characterized at low doses as a mixture of depression and stimulation and, at higher doses, as predominantly CNS depression (Dewey, 1986), leading to hyperreflexia. Cannabinoids generally cause a reduction in spontaneous locomotor activity and a decrease in response rates. They impair learning and memory in rodents and nonhuman primates. Other effects that have been shown in the mouse include hypothermia (Compton, Rice et al., 1993), immobility (catalepsy), and antinociception. These comprise the "tetrad" of tests for cannabinoid activity (Martin, 1985).

The mechanisms that underlie the other effects of the cannabinoids as tested in the tetrad have been shown to be sensitive to pertussis toxin (Lichtman, Meng et al., 1996) and thus probably are mediated by G-protein activation.

Neurobiology. *Cannabinoid Receptors:* THC is the prototypical cannabinoid and major psychoactive component in marijuana. THC is a noncrystalline, waxy-liquid substance at room temperature. The pharmacologic activity of THC is stereoselective, with the (-)-trans isomer having 6 to 100 times more potency than the (+)-trans isomer, depending on the pharmacologic test (Dewey, Martin et al., 1984). In more recent studies, the enantio-purity of THC analogs synthesized in the Mechoulam laboratory have been shown to have greater than 1,000-fold stereoselectivity (Martin, Balster et al., 1991). Initially, it was thought that because of the lipophilic nature of THC and its central depressant effects, cannabinoids mediated their actions through the disruption of membrane ordering, similar to the mechanism of general anesthetics (Paton & Pertwee, 1972; Lawrence & Gill, 1975). *In vitro* studies revealed a distinct relationship between cannabinoid interaction with attenuation of G-protein-mediated cAMP production and its behavioral effects (Howlett, 1984; Howlett, Qualy et al., 1986; Howlett, Johnson et al., 1988; Howlett, Evans et al., 1992). The enantioselectivity of THC reinforced the hypothesis that cannabinoids are receptor-mediated (Mechoulam, Feigenbaum et al., 1988).

Definitive evidence for a specific cannabinoid receptor became apparent when the receptor was cloned (Matsuda, Lolait et al., 1990; Munro, Thomas et al., 1993) from a rat brain library and had homology with other receptors that interacted with G proteins in the cell membrane. The mRNA distribution of the receptor clone paralleled that of the cannabinoid receptor. Confirmation of the identity of the clone occurred when adenylyl cyclase was inhibited on exposure to THC in cells transfected with the clone. The human cannabinoid receptor subsequently was cloned and found to have almost identical homology to the rat receptor (Gerard, Mollerearu et al., 1991). The cannabinoid CB_1 receptor, a saturable binding site for which cannabinoids possess high affinity, has been identified primarily in tissues of CNS origin (Devane, Dysarz et al., 1988; Matsuda, Lolait et al., 1990). A splice variant of the cannabinoid CB_1 receptor, the cannabinoid CB$_{1A}$ receptor, has been characterized (Shire, Cariollon et al., 1995). However, no pharmacologic relevance has been attributed to this splice variant.

A cannabinoid antagonist for the CB$_1$ receptor, SR141716A, has been described (Rinaldi-Carmona, Barth et al., 1994) and appears to selectively attenuate cannabinoid CB$_1$ receptor-mediated activity *in vivo* and *in vitro* (Wiley, Barrett et al., 1995; Wiley, Lowe et al., 1995; Collins, Pertwee et al., 1995).

The CB$_2$ receptor first was identified on splenic macrophages (Munro, Thomas et al., 1993). Although a specific antagonist for the CB$_2$ receptor has been discovered (SR144528) (Rinaldi-Carmona, Barth et al., 1998), the physiologic role of the CB$_2$ receptors in the spleen and at other peripheral sites remains elusive. Even though the CB$_1$ and CB$_2$ receptors share only 40% homology, THC has similar binding affinity for both receptor subtypes. Ledent and colleagues (1999), using CB$_1$-receptor knock-out mice, demonstrated that the main pharmacologic responses to THC, as well as the addictive properties of cannabinoids, are almost completely mediated by the CB$_1$ receptor. It has been suggested that CB$_1$ receptors are required for the development of dependence to cannabinoids.

Endocannabinoids: AEA was the first endogenous ligand (endocannabinoid) for the cannabinoid receptor to be discovered (Devane, Hanus et al., 1992). The behavioral effects of AEA are comparable to those of other psychoactive cannabinoids, and cross-tolerance with other cannabinoids has been demonstrated (Smith, Welch et al., 1994; Fride & Mechoulam, 1993; Pertwee, Stevenson et al., 1993; Welch, Dunlow et al., 1995; Vogel, Barg et al., 1993; Felder, Briley et al., 1993). AEA is but one of a family of arachidonic acid derivatives that have cannabinoid effects (reviewed in Di Marzo, 1998; Childers & Breivogel, 1998; Mechoulam & Hanus, 2000). Another major endocannabinoid is 2-arachidonoylglycerol (2-AG), which was discovered by Mechoulam and colleagues (1995) in canine gut. In addition, a variety of endogenous substances known as "entourage proteins" were shown to be released with and to protect the degradation of 2-AG (Ben-Shabat, Fride et al., 1998). 2-AG levels are higher in the brain than are those of AEA. The nature of such a distinct difference in concentrations is yet to be determined (Sugiura, Kondo et al., 1995; Kempe, Hsu et al., 1996).

After the initial discovery of the endocannabinoids, several synthetic pathways for AEA and 2-AG were proposed. Initially, it was thought that the condensation of arachidonic acid with ethanolamine could result in AEA (Deutsch & Chin, 1993; Hillard, Wilkison et al., 1995; Ueda, Kurahashi et al., 1995). However, the concentrations of reactants would have had to be in the high micromolar range for such an effect. An alternative mechanism was proposed by DiMarzo and colleagues (1994). The hydrolysis by phospholipase D of arachidonylethanolamide from a precursor N-acylphosphatidylethanolamine was demonstrated in cultured neurons.

The mechanisms underlying uptake of AEA and its metabolism to free arachidonic acid and ethanolamine have been determined (Deutsch &Chin, 1993; DiMarzo, Fontana et al., 1994; Koutek, Prestwich et al., 1994; Ueda, Kurahashi et al., 1995). AEA is taken up into cells by a putative AEA transporter, which transports 2-AG into cells (Piomelli, Beltramo et al., 1999) and is thought to be the first step in the termination of activity of both endocannabinoids (Beltramo, Steall et al., 1997; Piomelli, Beltramo et al., 1999). An AEA transporter inhibitor, AM404, has been synthesized (Beltramo, Stella et al., 1997). A fatty acid amide hydrolase, FAAH, was found in membrane fractions from brain (Desarnaud, Cades et al., 1995; Hillard, Wilkison et al., 1995; Ueda, Kurahashi et al., 1995) and later cloned (Cravatt, Giang et al., 1996). FAAH has been shown to degrade intracellular AEA. FAAH hydrolyzes 2-AG, but the reaction proceeds to completion at least four times faster than with AEA (Goparaju et al., 1998). An alternative metabolic pathway for AEA, which has been less studied, involves cytochrome P450s and results in epoxides or hydroxylated eicosanoids (Bornheim, Kim et al., 1995). The function of such prostanoids is not known.

A number of FAAH inhibitors were synthesized, and the structure-activity relationships for the endocannabinoid interactions with both the transporter and with FAAH recently were reviewed (Reggio & Traore, 2000). Recent work indicates that the FAAH-induced regulation of AEA may be the key regulator of AEA levels and, thus, AEA signaling pathways. In FAAH knock-out mice, pain sensation is significantly reduced—an effect correlated with increased AEA levels. Thus, the authors propose that FAAH may be the target for increased research and pharmaceutical interventions into the functions of the endocannabinoid system and its tonic control of pain perception (Cravatt, Demarest et al., 2001).

Intracellular Mechanisms of Action. It is now well recognized that THC and other cannabinoids produce their psychoactive effects through binding to CB$_1$ receptors. Investigations using CB$_1$ knock-out mice have provided evidence that the activation of CB$_1$ receptors is necessary for the elicitation of antinociception, decreased spontaneous activity, and other psychopharmacologic effects (Ledent, Valverde et al., 1999; Zimmer, Zimmer et al., 1999; Buckley, McCoy et al., 2000). Considerable evidence indicates that CB$_1$ receptors are coupled to G-proteins, some of which are Gi/Go and others that are Gs. Activation of the Gi/Go proteins leads to an inhibition of adenylyl cyclase, whereas activation of the Gs proteins by psychoactive cannabinoids leads to an activation of adenylyl cyclase (Howlett, 1995). These results may explain the bidirectional aspects of many of the CNS effects of the cannabinoids, but this is yet to be proved. One example of the bidirectional effects is the ability of THC, synthetic cannabinoids, and the endocannabinoids either to stimulate or to inhibit nitrous oxide formation. More than 80% of transmitters and hormones—including opioid and cannabinoid receptors—produce their biological effects via G-protein-coupled receptors (GPCRs) (Birnbaumer, Abramowitz et al., 1990). G-proteins transduce extracellular receptor activation into an intracellular response by effectors, including adenylyl cyclase, ion channels, and phospholipases (Gilman 1987; Birnbaumer, Abramowitz et al., 1990; Brown & Birnbaumer, 1990) that regulate neuronal activity and genetic expression.

The receptor-G-protein activation cycle has been characterized in detail (Gilman 1987; Birnbaumer, Abramowitz et al., 1990). The functional activity of GPCRs can be measured directly by using receptor-stimulated binding of the hydrolysis-resistant GTP analog, [^{35}S]GTPgS, in membranes and tissue sections (Sim, Selley et al., 1995). These studies have shown cannabinoid receptor-stimulated G-proteins in brain regions that contain cannabinoid receptors (Sim, Selley et al., 1995, 1996). Previous studies using agonist-stimulated [^{35}S]GTPgS binding have demonstrated cannabinoid receptor-activated G-proteins in membrane homogenates and sections of brain from mouse (Sim-Selley, Brunk et al., 2001), rat (Sim, Selley et al., 1995), guinea pig (Sim & Childers 1997), and Cynomolgus monkey. The receptor specificity of agonist-stimulated [^{35}S]GTPgS binding has been confirmed by demonstrating (1) specific anatomical localization corresponding to appropriate receptor distribution, (2) antagonist reversibility of the response, and (3) concentration dependent and saturable nature of stimulation (Sim, Selley et al., 1995). In addition, agonist-stimulated [^{35}S]GTPgS binding has allowed the investigation of desensitization of cannabinoid (Sim, Selley et al., 1996) receptors after chronic agonist treatment; receptor efficiency (defined as the ratio of activated G-protein to receptor B$_{max}$) (Sim, Selley et al., 1996), and agonist efficacy (maximal stimulation) (Sim, Selley et al., 1996; Selley, Sim et al., 1997).

Considerable literature is available on the important role of protein phosphorylation in the mechanism of action of GPCRs and, even more importantly, on the role of protein phosphorylation in the development of tolerance and dependence to opioids and cannabinoids (Bernstein & Welch, 1998; Smith, Welch et al., 1994). MAPK, which is modulated by CB$_1$ receptor activation, catalyzes protein phosphorylation (Bouaboula, Poinot-Chzel et al., 1995), and this effect, coupled with the inhibition of cAMP-dependent PKA, is the basis of a number of cannabinoid actions. MAPK activation by cannabinoids can occur independently from inhibition of PKA or be due at least in part to inhibition of cAMP formation. It has been proposed that the inhibition of adenylyl cyclase and PKA may be involved in the CB$_1$-induced activation of focal adhesion kinases (FAK+) in hippocampal slices—an effect suggested to lead to modulation by cannabinoids of synaptic plasticity and learning processes (Derkinderen, Toutant et al., 1996). These effects of cannabinoids on multiple families of kinases suggest the importance of alterations in protein phosphorylation in the mechanism of action of cannabinoids.

Other systems of cannabinoid receptor signal transduction pathways have been proposed. Some studies show that cannabinoids activate the inositol phospholipid pathway. This pathway involves the receptor activation of a G protein, which in turn activates phospholipase C. Phospholipase C cleaves phosphatidylinositol-bisphosphate (PIP2) into inositol-triphosphate (IP3) and diacylglycerol (DAG). DAG activates protein kinase C (PKC), while IP3 triggers calcium release from intracellular stores (Chaudry, Thompson et al. 1988). It has been shown that cannabinoids increase the activity of brain PKC *in vitro* (Hillard & Auchampach, 1994), phosphorylating the CB$_1$ receptor with PKC attenuates and P/Q-type calcium currents and the inwardly rectifying potassium currents after cannabinoid receptor activation (Zamponi, Bourinett et al., 1997; Garcia, Brown et al., 1998). Therefore, cannabinoid-induced activation of PKC decreases neuronal excitability and synaptic activity. It has been shown electrophysiologically that cannabinoids inhibit an omega conotoxin-sensitive, high voltage-activated N-type calcium channel (Caufield & Brown, 1992; Mackie & Hille, 1992). Cannabinoids were reported to enhance the low-voltage A-type potassium channels (Deadwyler, Hampson et al., 1993).

The CB_2 receptor is coupled to the G_i protein and inhibits adenylyl cyclase (Felder, Joyce et al., 1995). However, evidence exists that the CB_2 receptor is not coupled to phospholipase C or phospholipase D signal transduction pathways, mobilization of intracellular Ca^{2+} stores, and does not inhibit voltage-gated Ca^{2+} currents or activate inwardly rectifying potassium channels (Felder, Joyce et al., 1995).

The mechanism of action of endocannabinoids recently was reviewed (Howlett & Mukhopadhyay, 2000). The endocannabinoids bind both CB_1 and CB_2 receptors and produce effects on transduction pathways similar to those of the cannabinoids. That is, the endocannabinoids decrease cAMP by inhibition of adenylyl cyclase, activation of MAPK, and modulation of calcium currents. In addition, olvanil, an endocannabinoid, was shown by DiMarzo (1998) to interact with the vanilloid receptor. The vanilloid receptor, VR1, is widely distributed in the brain and spinal cord, is heat-activated, and is activated by the application of capsaicin (an ingredient in hot chili peppers). VR1 activation gates calcium entry to cells, particularly sensory neurons (Szallasi & Blumberg, 1999). AEA activation of VR1-mediated cardiovascular processes has been shown (Zygmunt, Petersson et al., 1999.) Thus, the interactions with VR1 appear to be unique to the endocannabinoids, rather than the exogenous or synthetic cannabinoids, and may indicate a role for endocannabinoids in the modulation of pain and cardiovascular responses independent of CB receptor activation.

Other non-CB_1/non-CB_2-mediated effects of endocannabinoids recently were reported. These include the presence of AEA-induced antinociception in CB_1 knock-out mice (mice devoid of the CB_1 receptor) and the absence of blockade of the effects of AEA and certain other endocannabinoids by SR141716A (Breivogel, Griffin et al., 2001).

In summary, considerable strides have been made in understanding cannabinoid receptor pharmacology because of the identification of specific receptor agonists and antagonists, as well as the elucidation of endogenous cannabinoids and the pathways of their synthesis and degradation. The use of novel biochemical techniques, such as the quantitation of G-protein coupling to receptors and subsequent modulation of intracellular second messengers and enzyme systems, has contributed to the understanding of cannabinoid receptor-mediated intracellular systems. Given the wide array of effects produced by cannabinoids, in addition to effects of the drugs that appear CB independent, it is becoming apparent that another cannabinoid receptor may exist.

ADDICTION LIABILITY

Dependence on marijuana is associated with a gradual increase in use, but withdrawal from the drug is difficult to demonstrate. The most common complaints are of anxiety and mental clouding, which are unlikely to be reported.

A combination of THC and alcohol in humans can result in increased levels of THC because of ethanol-induced increases in THC absorption, resulting in enhanced subjective effects on mood. It has been proposed that the effects of alcohol on THC may enhance the abuse of those drugs in combination (Lukas & Orozco, 2001). In addition, chronic administration of THC produces sensitization to the effects of amphetamine and heroin in rats. Interestingly, the rats most profoundly affected by the THC sensitization were those "high-responding" rats subject to high intrinsic levels of drug-seeking behavior. Although the data are preliminary, they could indicate a propensity of THC to increase drug seeking in individuals who are particularly sensitive or vulnerable to addictive behaviors (Lamarque, Taghzouti et al., 2001). The acute euphoric effects of THC in human studies appear to be due to CB_1 receptor activation and blocked by the CB_1 antagonist, SR141716A (Huestis, Gorelick et al., 2001).

Tolerance. Tolerance develops to the pharmacologic effects of cannabinoids in a variety of animal species, including pigeons, rodents, dogs, monkeys, and rabbits. Tolerance has occurred to antinociception, anticonvulsant activity, catalepsy, depression of locomotor activity, hypothermia, hypotension, corticosteroid release, ataxia in dogs, and schedule-controlled behavior. In mice, tolerance has been shown to occur to most THC-induced behaviors.

The precise mechanism of the development of tolerance is unknown. Most of the research efforts to date have been directed toward receptor regulation by evaluation of receptor inactivation or desensitization, or on decreased receptor number (down-regulation). In addition, tertiary signaling processes and plasticity of other neurotransmitter/neuromodulatory systems have been evaluated, such as those described for the endogenous opioid system. Desensitization can involve a conformation change in the receptor, internalization of the receptor, uncoupling of the receptor from G-proteins, or a combination of such processes. The process of down-regulation includes loss of receptors from the membrane as evidenced by a decrease in receptor number in binding assays and/or changes in messenger RNA (mRNA) and protein levels for such receptors. There is little evidence that chronic administration of cannabinoids alters disposition or metabolism of cannabinoids in the brain or periphery (Oviedo, Glowa et al., 1993), suggesting that tolerance is pharmacodynamic in nature rather than a consequence of reduced bioavailability. In autoradiographic studies, it was shown that binding to the CB receptor was decreased, with no apparent regional selectivity, suggesting a lack of involvement of neural circuitry, second messengers, or other intervening variables that might lead to differential effects. The reductions appear to be receptor mediated. In chronically treated animals, a decrease in receptor number rather than a change in affinity was observed (Oviedo, Glowa et al., 1993). Thus, there is not likely to be a conformational change in the receptor in chronically treated animals.

The cannabinoid receptor is rapidly internalized after binding of an agonist. The internalization appears to occur through clathrin-coated pits and is reversible after short treatment (<15 minutes), but not after long treatment (>90 minutes). Internalization is not blocked by pretreatment with pertussis toxin and/or cholera toxin, suggesting activation of G proteins is not required for internalization. This pathway appears similar to that of the beta-2-adrenergic receptor (beta-AR) (Hsieh, Brown et al., 1999). Receptor internalization is highly dependent on kinase-induced phosphorylation. The decreased responsiveness of the beta-AR after stimulation with a near saturating concentration of ligand appears to be caused by rapid cAMP-dependent protein kinase A (PKA) and G-protein-coupled protein kinase (GRK) phosphorylation. GRK phosphorylation, in turn, promotes beta-arrestin binding and receptor internalization (Seibold, January et al., 1998). There is indirect evidence that a variety of kinases, not just PKA and GRK, could be involved in the development of tolerance to cannabinoids.

In non-tolerant animals, acute administration of THC or anandamide decreases cAMP formation by inhibiting adenylyl cyclase. This reduction in cAMP formation decreases the likelihood that PKA will be activated. The injection of the PKA inhibitor KT-5720 does not affect the antinociceptive potency of THC. These results suggest that adenylyl cyclase is not constitutively active in sites mediat-

ing antinociception in non-tolerant animals. Homologous desensitization to the inhibition of cAMP accumulation occurs during chronic cannabinoid exposure (Dill & Howelett, 1988). In rats, chronic exposure enhances the adenylyl cyclase pathway, as shown by the significant increase in cAMP levels and PKA activity in the same areas that CB_1 receptor down-regulation is observed (cerebellum, striatum, and cortex) (Rubino, Vigano et al., 2000). During tolerance, CB_1 receptors lose the ability to inhibit adenylyl cyclase, either through desensitization or switching to Gs-protein stimulation. Thus, the adenylyl cyclase cascade appears to become constitutively active during tolerance. In support of this, KT-5720 completely reversed THC-induced tolerance (Rubino, Vigano et al., 2000).

Under conditions of acute cannabinoid exposure, CB_1 and CB_2 receptors are G-protein coupled to $G_{i/o}$ proteins that, when activated by phosphorylation, inhibit the activity of adenylyl cyclase (Howlett & Fleming, 1984). However, on agonist binding, the alpha subunit disassociates from the beta/gamma subunit of the G-protein (Childers & Deadwyler, 1996). The beta/gamma subunit has been linked to stimulation of other cellular events such as the activation of Src tyrosine kinase (TK), one of numerous types of TKs. G-protein-coupled receptors interact with TKs in intracellular signaling subsequently involving mitogen-activated protein kinase (MAPK). Src TK has been shown to activate the factor, Ras, that can activate MAPK. It has been demonstrated that CB_1-receptor activation stimulates MAPK (Rinaldi-Carmona, Barth et al., 1998; Bouaboula, Poinot-Chzel et al., 1995). The Src TK inhibitor PP1 (Daub, Wallasch et al.,1997) has been tested in mice. In non-tolerant mice, PP1 had no effect on the antinociceptive potency of THC. However, PP1 completely reversed THC tolerance.

It has been shown that AEA and THC increase the activity of brain protein kinase C (PKC) *in vitro* (Hillard & Auchampach, 1994). AEA appears to act by increasing phosphatidylserine-induced PKC activation, as well as acting at the diacylglycerol site on PKC. Because PKC plays a part in activating MAPK, it is possible that PKC activators (phorbol esters) and PKC inhibitors modulate the antinociceptive effects of THC and the endocannabinoids. PKC appears to directly affect CB_1 receptors. Phosphorylation of the CB_1 receptor with PKC suppresses the modulation of calcium channels by cannabinoids (Garcia, Brown et al., 1998). However, application of neurotransmitters that stimulate the PI cascade and activate PKC restore the neuronal excitability and synaptic activity inhibited by cannabinoids.

In summary, desensitization has been shown to occur after repeated administration of cannabinoids. The process of desensitization appears to mimic that of the beta-adrenergic receptor and involves several kinase phosphorylation steps and possibly the constitutive activation of several of the kinases.

Down-regulation of cannabinoid receptors after tolerance to cannabinoids is an area of research in which several inconsistencies exist. Abood and colleagues (1993) found no alterations in cannabinoid receptor mRNA or protein levels in mouse whole brain homogenates after a chronic injection paradigm sufficient to induce 27-fold tolerance in a behavioral assay. However, the possibility remains that in distinct brain regions receptor mRNA and protein levels are altered, and, by measuring whole brain homogenates, these changes would not be apparent. Conversely, Oviedo and colleagues (1993) observed dose-dependent alterations in the cannabinoid receptor number and affinity in rat brain regions by using autoradiography, and a decrease in mRNA for the CB_1 receptor was noted in the caudate (Rubino, Vigano et al., 2000). Down-regulation of receptors after chronic THC in rat was likewise observed in striatum and nigrostriatal and mesolimbic areas in another study (Rodriguez de Fonseca, Gorriti et al., 1994). Conversely, tolerance to THC in the vas deferens model did not involve an alteration in the number of cannabinoid receptors (Pertwee & Griffin, 1995).

A bidirectional cross-tolerance is noted between the kappa opioids and THC that implies a common mechanism of tolerance can underlie both classes of drugs (Rowen, Embrey et al. 1988). Kappa opioid receptor antisense administration blocks the antinociceptive effects of THC. Another mechanism of tolerance that must not be discounted is the role of the G protein subunit, $G_{i2\alpha}$, which appears to be involved in opioid-induced tolerance. Antisense specific for the $G_{i2\alpha}$ subunit blocks morphine-induced antinociception and to different degrees blocks the effects of different kappa agonists. Therefore, alterations in G proteins, or an uncoupling at the receptor, could account for cannabinoid-induced tolerance by the interaction of the cannabinoids with kappa opioids (Rowen, Embrey et al., 1998).

In summary, despite research reports to the contrary, marijuana use still is considered by many to be a "safe" drug (CEWG, 2000). Marijuana has all of the properties consistent with a drug that is reinforcing, including a fast onset after inhalation, high lipophilicity, and rapid entry to brain and spinal cord sites. Its long half-life and euphoric activity enhance the potential for physical dependence.

Newer forms of cannabis have higher levels of THC, which makes the drug's effects increasingly rewarding. In addition, most of the chemical entities present in cannabis, as well as the pyrolysis (burning) products, have not been evaluated for either psychoactive or toxicologic properties. Thus, the effects of prolonged drug use are difficult to predict, although clearly, neurochemical changes are observed on tolerance and dependence to THC.

Dependence. Animals develop tolerance to the effects of THC on repeated exposure. Human chronic heavy cannabis users develop tolerance to the drug's subjective and cardiovascular effects and experience withdrawal symptoms on abrupt cessation of use (Jones, Benowitz et al., 1976). Clinical and epidemiologic evidence indicates that a cannabis dependence syndrome occurs in heavy chronic users, as exhibited by a lack of control over use and continued use of the drug despite adverse personal consequences (Roffman, Stephens et al., 1988). The cannabis dependence syndrome is analogous to the alcohol dependence syndrome, but the clinical features of cannabis dependence need to be better defined. The risk of becoming dependent on cannabis probably is more like the risk for alcohol than for nicotine or the opioids, with around 10% of those who ever use cannabis eventually meeting the criteria for dependence (Hall, 1995). Kandel and Raveis (1989) estimated the risk of dependence among near daily cannabis users (according to approximated *DSM-III* criteria) at one in three.

In animal studies, withdrawal symptoms after chronic administration of cannabinoids have not been detected in the absence of precipitation of withdrawal. A few reports noted that abrupt cessation of cannabinoids produces certain behavioral changes, which include increased grooming and motor activity, aggression, and susceptibility to electroshock-induced convulsions. However, the development of a specific cannabinoid antagonist (Rinaldi-Carmona, Barth et al., 1994) led to the demonstration that a withdrawal syndrome could be elicited in animals treated chronically with THC. Studies in rats and mice chronically injected or infused with THC and then challenged with the antagonist SR 141716A elicited behavioral signs such as head shakes, facial tremors, tongue rolling, biting, wet-dog shakes, eyelid ptosis, facial rubbing, paw treading, retropulsion, immobility, ear twitch, chewing, licking, stretching, and arched back (Tsou, Patrick et al., 1995; Aceto, Scates et al., 1995). Subsequently, Aceto and colleagues (2001) observed spontaneous withdrawal after abrupt cessation of chronic treatment with the synthetic cannabinoid, WINN 55,212. Those studies provided convincing evidence that cannabinoids can produce dependence in animals.

In addition, several studies have linked withdrawal from cannabinoids with the opioid system. It appears that the opioid/endogenous opioid system can play a modulatory role in the severity of cannabinoid withdrawal signs, because cannabinoid withdrawal is lessened in mu opioid receptor knock-out mice and proenkephalin knock-out mice. Conversely, in CB_1 knock-out mice, the withdrawal effects from morphine are reduced (Ledent, Valverde et al., 1999). However, the relationship between these animal models and the abuse pattern of cannabinoids in humans remains to be understood in terms of the neuronal systems that subserve the cannabis withdrawal syndrome. Manipulation of these systems can provide a means for treating individuals who seek assistance in terminating their marijuana use.

Withdrawal. Marijuana abstinence has been monitored in some studies in humans (Mendelson, Meyer et al., 1972; Mendelson, Mello et al., 1984) and includes effects that are typically the opposite of those produced by the drug, such as insomnia, anorexia, anxiety, irritability, depression, and tremor. Cessation of drug use results in a time course of effects that peaks at 10 hours and is observed for five days. Similar effects were observed by Mendelson and colleagues (1984) after administration of a dose of THC of 3.2 mg/kg for three weeks. In animal studies, marijuana is self-administered and acts by reward neuroanatomy similar to those of other drugs of abuse (Gardner & Lowinson, 1991). Although it is difficult to establish self-administration paradigms for THC, rats have been observed to self-administer the THC analog, WINN 55,212-2 (Fattore, Cossu et al., 2001). It appears that the self-administration of THC and WINN 55,212-2 can be abolished by the administration of the CB_1 antagonist, SR141716A. Thus, as with many other pharmacologic effects of THC (Zimmer, Zimmer et al., 1999), the drug's abuse potential appears at this point to be mediated by CB_1 receptor activation.

Induction of Other Drug Use. Cannabis use typically precedes involvement with other drugs such as stimulants (Donovan & Jessor, 1983), yet there is no scientific evidence of a neurobiologic basis for such a "gateway" effect. The effect may be due to the increased opportunity of cannabis users to associate with users of other types of drugs or group peer pressure to use other drugs (Baumrind, 1983; Goode, 1974).

TOXICITY/ADVERSE EFFECTS

Psychopathology. Marijuana users frequently report euphoria, hunger, and relaxation—and, less often, panic, anxiety, nausea, and dizziness. In rare instances, marijuana may increase paranoia (Naditch, 1974). These effects most often are reported by naive users or patients receiving THC therapeutically who are unfamiliar with the drug's effects. Discussions of potential effects can reduce the intensity of such experiences. Experienced users rarely report these effects. Some evidence indicates that large doses of THC can produce psychosis, which remits rapidly on abstinence from cannabis (Chopra & Smith, 1974). It has been suggested that schizophrenia can be induced by chronic cannabinoid use. However, definitive evidence is lacking that cannabis use leads to schizophrenia that would not have occurred in the absence of such use (Der, Gupta et al., 1990).

Effects on Major Organ Systems. *Respiratory:* The major adverse health effect associated with marijuana smoking is damage to the respiratory system, although the major adverse effect perceived by patients treated with THC alone is dysphoria. Many of the same mutagens and carcinogens in nicotine cigarettes are found in marijuana smoke (Sherman, Aberland et al., 1997). In addition, marijuana smoking results in increased airway resistance and decreased pulmonary function (Tashkin, Shapiro et al., 1976; Tilles, Goldenheim et al., 1986; Henderson, Tennant et al., 1972; Mendelson, Meyer et al., 1972). Chronic heavy cannabis smoking impairs the functioning of the large airways and probably causes symptoms of chronic bronchitis, such as coughing, sputum, and wheezing (Bloom, Kaltenborn et al., 1987; Tashkin, Wu et al., 1988; Tashkin, 1990).

Concurrent use of tobacco by marijuana smokers increases the risk of lung cancers or lung injury (Gil, Kelp et al., 1995). No differences were seen between cannabis and tobacco smokers in the prevalence of these symptoms. Lung function tests showed significantly poorer functioning and significantly greater abnormalities in small airways among tobacco smokers (regardless of concomitant cannabis use), whereas marijuana smokers showed poorer large airways functioning than non-marijuana smokers (regardless of concomitant tobacco use). Many such effects are not reversed on abstinence (Tashkin, Shapiro et al., 1976). Given the qualitative similarity between tobacco and cannabis smoke (Tashkin, Wu et al., 1988), it is likely that chronic cannabis use predisposes individuals to develop respiratory cancer (Tashkin, 1993). However, there is no controlled evidence showing a higher rate of respiratory cancers among cannabis smokers (Bloom, Kaltenborn et al., 1987; Tashkin, Wu, et al., 1988; Tashkin, 1990). However, there is evidence that chronic cannabis smoking can produce histopathologic changes in lung tissue of the type that precede the development of lung cancer in tobacco smokers (Fligiel, Venkat et al., 1988).

Immunologic: The existence of the CB_2 receptor that is expressed on cells of the immune system has led to the hypothesis that the cannabinoid system plays a significant role in immune modulation. Immunomodulatory effects of THC on macrophage function are abolished in CB_2 knock-out mice shown to be devoid of CB_2 receptors (Buckley, McCoy et al., 2000). In addition, it has been shown that CB_2-induced modulation of certain second messenger pathways, such as those involving cyclic adenosine monophosphate (cAMP), is critical for the gene regulation of immune cells, possibly by the decreased production of various chemokines such as interleukin 1 (Condie, Herring et al, 1996), leading to immune suppression. Immune suppression by THC results in protective effects on pancreatic beta cells in an experimental model of autoimmune diabetes. However, such work is confounded by other data indicating a potential stimulation of immune responses by lymphocyte activation (Kaminski, Koh et al., 1994). Thus, cannabinoid use to decrease inflammation (Mechoulam, 1986) could be accompanied by an increase in viral infections (Klein, Newton et al., 1998b). Overall, it is apparent that THC decreases macrophage function (McCoy, Matveyeva et al., 1999) and natural killer cell activity (Klein, Newton et al. 1998a). It has been reported that THC increases HIV-1 host infection in cell lines (Noe, Newton et al., 2001). Thus, the effects of cannabinoid activation or endocannabinoid activation of the immune system are complex, but numerous studies are in agreement that host resistance is impaired by THC administration (Friedman, Klein et al., 1995; Cabral & Dove-Pettit, 1998; Klein, Newton et al. 1998b). For a recent review of immune function and the cannabinoid system, see Berdyshev (2000).

The adverse effects of cannabis use on immune effects in human studies are equivocal (Hollister, 1992). No epidemiologic evidence is available to demonstrate increased rates of infectious disease among chronic heavy cannabis users (Coates, Farewell et al., 1990). However, one cannot exclude the possibility that chronic heavy cannabis use produces minor impairments in immunity that might tend to increase the rate of common bacterial and viral illnesses among chronic cannabis users (Polen, Sidney et al., 1993).

Cardiovascular: Numerous recent publications indicate a renewal of interest in the cardiovascular effects of the cannabinoids and the role endocannabinoid tone plays in cardiac function. It had previously been reported that marijuana increases heart rate and produces orthostatic hypotension in some individuals (Galanter, Weingartner et al., 1973), which can worsen cardiac conditions and increase hypertension. Direct stimulation of the cardiac pacemaker by marijuana leads to an increase in heart rate, making the drug less safe in cardiac patients (Beaconsfield, Ginsburg et al., 1972; Tashkin, Scares et al., 1978). In healthy young users, such cardiovascular effects are unlikely to be of clinical significance (Hall, 1995). Similar studies have indicated that THC and its analogs have profound hypotensive and bradycardic effects in rats, which are mediated by the CB_1 receptor. However, recent evidence indicates that endocannabinoids are involved in peripheral regulation of vascular tone and have potent hemodynamic effects, such as hypotension and bradycardia (reviewed in Kunos, Jarai et al., 2000). The critical therapeutic role of reversing the endocannabinoid effects in such states as endotoxic and hemorrhagic shock may lead to alternative therapies for such conditions.

Reproductive: THC has been shown to alter pituitary hormones. In particular, THC has inhibitory effects on pituitary luteinizing hormone, prolactin, and growth hormone, but little effect on the secretion of follicle-stimulating hormone (Wenger, Toth et al., 1995). Recent work indicates that the cannabinoid analog WINN 55,212-2-induced modulation of pituitary hormones occurs by the CB_1 receptor, particularly in the anterior lobe of the pituitary—the site at which growth hormone and prolactin are released (inhibited by the WINN 55,212-2) in normal and hyperactive pituitary states (Pagotto, Marsicano et al., 2001).

Marijuana can disrupt the female reproductive system and induce galactorrhea (Cohen, 1985). Animal studies using CB_1 and CB_2 knock-out mice indicate that the endocannabinoid system plays a role in the development and implantation of the embryo by synchronizing its developmental stage to the receptive stage for implantation in the uterus. Such studies suggest that far more research is needed to determine the role of the endocannabinoid system in reproduction and potential adverse effects of THC use on pregnancy (Paria, Song et al., 2001).

Studies of smoking marijuana during pregnancy are unclear as to the effects on the fetus because of polypharmacy, which often is observed with marijuana smokers. However, women who smoke marijuana during pregnancy often have children with low birth weights, possibly because of a shorter gestation (Tennes, 1984). The lipid solubility of THC allows for rapid transit to the fats in breast milk, where it has been shown to accumulate and be passed to the newborn (Fehr & Kalant, 1983).

In male animals, chronic administration of high doses of THC disrupts reproductive function, reducing the secretion of testosterone, sperm production, motility, and viability. However, evidence of THC-induced abnormalities in reproduction in human males has not been demonstrated conclusively (Mendelson & Mello, 1984).

Overall, the effects of THC on reproduction and fetal development are areas of research wrought with difficulties, in part because of the polypharmacy of most cannabis users, as well as the large number of confounding variables, such as diet, age, and health status, that have not been well controlled in many studies.

FUTURE RESEARCH DIRECTIONS

Cannabinoids are an ancient class of compounds with a rich history of anecdotal uses for both recreational and therapeutic purposes. It is only within the past decade that the mechanisms underlying cannabinoid actions have been described, aided by the discovery of receptors, antagonists for those receptors, and new transgenic technology in which the receptors are genetically "removed" from an animal. Despite all the advances in the pharmacology of the cannabinoids, considerable controversies remain as to the potential uses of these drugs for a variety of disease states, as well as the route of administration of the active agent, THC, and other cannabinoid compounds.

As was evident from the ancient sources, cannabinoids appear to have a variety of potentially useful therapeutic effects. The problem that will need to be addressed by future research is how to develop a cannabinoid agent devoid of undesirable side effects. The hypothesis that the CB_1 and CB_2 receptors may not be the only cannabinoid receptors is supported by several lines of research indicating non-CB_1, non-CB_2 effects of the drugs (Breivogel, Griffin et al., 2001).

If such novel cannabinoid receptors exist, they certainly will become therapeutic targets by which the multiplicity of the cannabinoid effects can be separated. In addition, increasing knowledge of the endocannabinoid system's role in tonic regulation of analgesia, cognition, food intake, and cardiovascular tone indicate that possible analogs of the endocannabinoids, or modulators of endocannabinoid pathways, may be targets for drug development. The goal of novel therapeutic interventions will be to decease the potential for tolerance and dependence to the cannabinoid drugs.

In summary, the cannabinoids are a class of drugs with a diverse profile of pharmacologic activities, including the unwanted side effects of tolerance and dependence. The endocannabinoids and cannabinoid receptors are highly conserved phylogenically.

Researchers now confront the task of determining the reasons for the preservation of the cannabinoid system through both invertebrate and vertebrate evolution and the roles that receptors, known and yet to be found, play in diseases, including addictive behaviors.

REFERENCES

Abel EL (1979). *A Comprehensive Guide to the Cannabis Literature.* Westport, CT: Greenwood Press.

Abood ME, Sauss C, Fan F et al. (1993). Development of behavioral tolerance to delta 9-THC without alteration of cannabinoid receptor binding or mRNA levels in whole brain. *Pharmacology, Biochemistry and Behavior* 46(3):575-579.

Aceto MD, Scates SM, Lowe JA et al. (1995). Cannabinoid precipitated withdrawal by the selective cannabinoid receptor antagonist, SR 141716A. *European Journal of Pharmacology* 282(1-3):R1-2.

Aceto MD, Scates SM & Martin BB (2001). Spontaneous and precipitated withdrawal with a synthetic cannabinoid, WIN 55212-2. *European Journal of Pharmacology* 416(1-2):75-81.

Adams AJ, Brown B & Flom MC (1975). Alcohol and marijuana effects on static visual acuity. *American Journal of Optometry and Physiological Optics* 52:729-735.

Adams IB, Ryan W & Singer M (1995). Evaluation of the cannabinoid receptor binding and the in vivo activities for the anandamide analog. *Journal of Pharmacology and Experimental Therapeutics* 273:1172-1182.

Baker D, Pryce G, Croxford JL et al. (2001). Endocannabinoids control spasticity in a multiple sclerosis model. *FASEB Journal* 15(2):300-302.

Baumrind D (1983). Specious causal attributions in the social sciences: The reformulated stepping-stone theory of heroin use as exemplar. *Journal of Personality and Social Psychology* 45(6):1289-1298.

Beaconsfield P, Ginsburg I & Rainsbury R (1972). Marijuana smoking: Cardiovascular effects in man and possible mechanisms. *New England Journal of Medicine* 287:209-212.

Beal JE, Olson R, Lefkowitz L et al. (1997). Long-term efficacy and safety of dronabinol for acquired immunodeficiency syndrome-associated anorexia. *Journal of Pain Symptom Management* 14(1):7-14.

Beltramo M, Stella N, Calignano A et al. (1997). Functional role of high-affinity anandamide transport, as revealed by selective inhibition. *Science* 277(5329):1094-1097.

Ben-Shabat S, Fride E, Sheskin T et al. (1998). An entourage effect: Inactive endogenous fatty acid glycerol esters enhance 2-arachidonoyl-glycerol cannabinoid activity. *European Journal of Pharmacology* 353(1):23-31.

Berdyshev EV (2000). Cannabinoid receptors and the regulation of immune response. *Chemistry and Physics of Lipids* 108(1-2):169-190.

Bernstein MA & Welch SP (1998). mu-Opioid receptor down-regulation and cAMP-dependent protein kinase phosphorylation in a mouse model of chronic morphine tolerance. *Molecular Brain Research* 55(2):237-242.

Birnbaumer L, Abramowitz J & Brown AM (1990). Receptor-effector coupling by G proteins. *Biochemica et Biophysica Acta* 1031:163-224.

Bloom JW, Kaltenborn WT, Paoletti P et al. (1987). Respiratory effects of non-tobacco cigarettes. *British Medical Journal* (Clinical Research Edition) 295(6612):1516-1518.

Bornheim LM, Kim KY, Chen B et al. (1995). Microsomal cytochrome P450-mediated liver and brain anandamide metabolism. *Biochemical Pharmacology* 50:677-686.

Bouaboula M, Poinot-Chzel C, Bourrie B et al. (1995). Activation of mitogen-activated protein kinases by stimulation of the central cannabinoid receptor CB1. *Biochemical Journal* 312:637-641.

Breivogel CS, Griffin G, Di Marzo V et al. (2001). Evidence for a new G protein-coupled cannabinoid receptor in mouse brain. *Molecular Pharmacology* 60(1):155-163.

Brown AM & Birnbaumer L (1990). Ionic channels and their regulation by G protein subunits. *Annual Review of Physiology* 52:197-213.

Buckley NE, McCoy KL, Mezey E et al. (2000). Immunomodulation by cannabinoids is absent in mice deficient for the cannabinoid CB(2) receptor. *European Journal of Pharmacology* 396(2-3):141-149.

Cabral GA & Dove Pettit DA (1998). Drugs and immunity: Cannabinoids and their role in decreased resistance to infectious disease. *Journal of Neuroimmunology* 83(1-2):116-123.

Campbell FA, Tramer MR, Carroll D et al. (2001). Are cannabinoids an effective and safe treatment option in the management of pain? A qualitative systematic review. *British Medical Journal* 323(7303):13-16.

Caufield MP & Brown DA (1992). Cannabinoid receptor agonists inhibit Ca Current in NG108-15 neuroblastoma cells via a pertussis toxin sensitive mechanism. *British Journal of Pharmacology* 106:231-232.

Community Epidemiology Work Group (CEWG) (2000). *Proceedings of the Community Epidemiology Work Group: Epidemiologic Trends in Drug Abuse, Vol. 1*. Bethesda, MD: National Institute on Drug Abuse.

Chait LD & Pierri J (1992). Effects of smoked marijuana on human performance: A critical review. In L Murphy & A Bartke (eds.) *Marijuana/Cannabinoids Neurobiology and Neurophysiology*. Boca Raton, FL: CRC, 387-424.

Chaudry A, Thompson RH, Rubin RP et al. (1988). Relationship between delta-9-tetrahydrocannabinol-induced arachidonic acid release and secretagogue-evoked phosphoinositide breakdown and Ca^{2+} mobilization of exocrine pancreas. *Molecular Pharmacology* 34:543-548.

Childers SR & Breivogel CS (1998). Cannabis and endogenous cannabinoid systems. *Drug and Alcohol Dependence* 51(1-2):173-187.

Childers SR & Deadwyler SA (1996). Role of cyclic AMP in the actions of cannabinoid receptors. *Biochemical Pharmacology* 52(6):819-827.

Chopra GS & Smith JW (1974). Psychotic reactions following cannabis use in East Indians. *Archives of General Psychiatry* 30(1):24-27.

Cichewicz DL, Haller VL & Welch SP (2001). Changes in opioid and cannabinoid receptor protein following short-term combination treatment with delta(9)-tetrahydrocannabinol and morphine. *Journal of Pharmacology and Experimental Therapeutics* 297(1):121-127.

Co BT, Goodwin DW, Gado M et al. (1977). Absence of cerebral atrophy in chronic cannabis users. Evaluation by computerized transaxial tomography. *Journal of the American Medical Association* 237(12):1229-1230.

Coates RA, Farewell VT, Raboud J et al. (1990). Cofactors of progression to acquired immunodeficiency syndrome in a cohort of male sexual contacts of men with human immunodeficiency virus disease. *American Journal of Epidemiology* 132(4):717-722.

Cohen S (1985). Marijuana and reproductive functions. *Drug Abuse and Alcoholism News* 13:1.

Collins DR, Pertwee RG & Davies SN (1995). Prevention by the cannabinoid antagonist, SR141716A, of cannabinoid-mediated blockade of long-term potentiation in the rat hippocampal slice. *British Journal of Pharmacology* 115:869-870.

Compton DR, Rice KC, De Costa BR et al. (1993). Cannabinoid structure-activity relationships: Correlation of receptor bonding and in-vivo activities. *Journal of Pharmacology and Experimental Therapeutics* 265:218-226.

Condie R, Herring A, Koh WS et al. (1996). Cannabinoid inhibition of adenylate cyclase-mediated signal transduction and interleukin 2 (IL-2) expression in the murine T-cell line, EL4.IL-2. *Journal of Biological Chemistry* 271(22):13175-13183.

Corchero J, Avila MA, Fuentes JA et al. (1997). Delta-9-tetrahydrocannabinol increases prodynorphin and proenkephalin gene expression in the spinal cord of the rat. *Life Sciences* 61:PL39-43.

Cravatt BF, Demarest K, Patricelli MP et al. (2001). Supersensitivity to anandamide and enhanced endogenous cannabinoid signaling in mice lacking fatty acid amide hydrolase. *Proceedings of the National Academy of Sciences* 98(16):9371-9376.

Cravatt BF, Giang DK, Mayfield SP et al. (1996). Molecular characterization of an enzyme that degrades neuromodulatory fatty-acid amides. *Nature* 384(6604):83-87.

Croft RJ, Mackay AJ, Mills AT et al. (2001). The relative contributions of ecstasy and cannabis to cognitive impairment. *Psychopharmacology* (Berlin) 153(3):373-379.

Daub H, Wallasch C, Lankenau A et al. (1997). Signal characteristics of G protein-transactivated EGF receptor. *EMBO Journal* 16(23):7032-7044.

Deadwyler SA, Hampson R E, Bennett BA et al. (1993). Cannabinoids modulate potassium current in cultured hippocampal neurons. *Receptors and Channels* 1:121-134.

Der G, Gupta S & Murray RM (1990). Is schizophrenia disappearing? *Lancet* 335(8688):513-516.

Derkinderen P, Toutant M, Burgaya F et al. (1996). Regulation of a neuronal form of focal adhesion kinase by anandamide. *Science* 273(5282):1719-1722.

Desarnaud F, Cadas H & Piomelli D (1995). Anandamide amidohydrolase activity in rat brain microsomes: Identification and partial characterization. *Journal of Biological Chemistry* 270:6030-6035.

Deutsch DG & Chin SA (1993). Enzymatic synthesis and degradation of anandamide, a cannabinoid receptor agonist. *Biochemical Pharmacology* 46:791-796.

Devane WA, Dysarz FA 3rd, Johnson MR et al. (1988). Determination and characterization of a cannabinoid receptor in rat brain. *Molecular Pharmacology* 34:605-613.

Devane WA, Hanus L, Breuer A et al. (1992). Isolation and structure of a brain constituent that binds to the cannabinoid receptor. *Science* 258:1946-1949.

Dewey WL (1986). Cannabinoid pharmacology. *Pharmacology Review* 38:151-175.

Dewey WL, Martin BR & May EL (1984). Cannabinoid stereoisomers: Pharmacological effects. In DF Smith (ed.) *CRC Handbook of Stereoisomers: Drugs in Psychopharmacology*. CRC Press, 317-326.

Dill JA & Howlett AC (1988). Regulation of adenylate cyclase by chronic exposure to cannabimimetic drugs. *Journal of Pharmacology and Experimental Therapeutics* 244(3):1157-1163.

Di Marzo V (1998). Endocannabinoids and other fatty acid derivatives with cannabimimetic properties: Biochemistry and possible physiopathological relevance. *Biochima et Biophysica Acta* 1392(2-3):153-175.

Di Marzo V, Bisogno T & De Petrocellis L (2000). Endocannabinoids: New targets for drug development. *Current Pharmaceutical Design* 6(13):1361-1380.

Di Marzo V, Fontana A, Cadas H et al. (1994). Formation and inactivation of endogenous cannabinoid anandamide in central neurons. *Nature* 372(6507):686-691.

Di Marzo V, Goparaju SK, Wang L et al. (2001). Leptin-regulated endocannabinoids are involved in maintaining food intake. *Nature* 410(6830):822-825.

Donovan JE & Jessor R (1983). Problem drinking and the dimension of involvement with drugs: A Guttman scalogram analysis of adolescent drug use. *American Journal of Public Health* 73(5):543-552.

Dornbush RL (1974). Marijuana and memory: Effects of smoking on storage. *Annals of the New York Academy of Sciences* 36(1):94-100.

Dray A & Rang H (1998). The how and why of chronic pain states and the what of new analgesia therapies. *Trends in Neurosciences* 21:315-317.

Fant RV, Heishman SJ, Bunker EB et al. (1998). Acute and residual effects of marijuana in humans. *Pharmacology, Biochemistry and Behavior* 60(4):777-784.

Fattore L, Cossu G, Martellotta CM et al. (2001). Intravenous self-administration of the cannabinoid CB1 receptor agonist WIN 55,212-2 in rats. *Psychopharmacology* (Berlin) 156(4):410-416.

Fehr KO & Kalant H (1983). *Addiction Research Foundation/World Health Organization Meeting on Adverse Health and Behavioral Consequences of Cannabis Use*. Toronto, Ontario: Addiction Research Foundation.

Felder CC, Briley EM, Axelrod J et al. (1993). Anandamide, an endogenous cannabimimetic eicosanoid, binds to the cloned human cannabinoids receptor and stimulates receptor-mediated signal transduction. *Cell Biology* 90:7656-7660.

Felder CC, Joyce KE, Briley EM et al. (1995). Comparison of the pharmacology and signal transduction of the human cannabinoid CB1 and CB2 receptors. *Molecular Pharmacology* 48(3):443-450.

Fligiel SE, Venkat H, Gong H et al. (1988). Bronchial pathology in chronic marijuana smokers: A light and electron microscopic study. *Journal of Psychoactive Drugs* 20(1):33-42.

Fride E, Ginzburg Y, Breuer A et al. (2001). Critical role of the endogenous cannabinoid system in mouse pup suckling and growth. *European Journal of Pharmacology* 419(2-3):207-214.

Fride E & Mechoulam R (1993). Pharmacological activity of the cannabinoid receptor agonist, anandamide, a brain constituent. *European Journal of Pharmacology* 231:313-314.

Friedman H, Klein TW, Newton C et al. (1995). Marijuana, receptors and immunomodulation. *Advances in Experimental Medicine and Biology* 373:103-113.

Galanter M, Weingartner H & Vaughn TB (1973). Delta-9-tetrahydrocannabinol and natural marihuana: A controlled comparison. *Archives of General Psychiatry* 28:278-281.

Gao Z & Peet NP (1999). Recent advances in neurokinin receptor antagonists. *Current Medicinal Chemistry* 6:375-388.

Garcia DE, Brown S, Hille B et al. (1998). Protein kinase C disrupts cannabinoid actions by phosphorylation of the CB1 cannabinoid receptor. *Journal of Neuroscience* 18(8):2834-2841.

Gardner EL & Lowinson JH (1991). Marijuana's interaction with brain reward systems: Update 1991. *Pharmacology, Biochemistry and Behavior* 40:571-580.

Gerard CM, Mollerearu C, Vasart G et al. (1991). Molecular cloning of a human cannabinoid receptor which is also expressed in testis. *Biochemistry Journal* 279:129-134.

Gil E, Kelp E, Webber M et al. (1995). Acute and chronic effects of marijuana smoking on pulmonary alveolar permeability. *Life Sciences* 56:2193-2199.

Gilbert PE (1981). A comparison of THC, nantradol, nabilone, and morphine in the chronic spinal dog. *Journal of Clinical Pharmacology* 21:311S-319S.

Gilman AG (1987). G proteins: Transducers of receptor-generated signals. *Annual Review of Biochemistry* 56:615-649.

Goode E (1974). The criminogenics of marijuana. *Addictive Diseases* 1(3):297-322.

Gralla RJ, Tyson LB, Bordin LA et al. (1984). Antiemetic therapy: A review of recent studies and a report of a random assignment trial comparing metoclopramide with delta-9-tetrahydrocannabinol. *Cancer Treatment Reports* 68(1):163-172.

Grinspoon L & Bakalar JB (1993). *Marihuana: The Forbidden Medicine*. New Haven, CT: Yale University Press.

Hall W (1995). The health risks of cannabis. *Australian Family Physician* 24(7):1237-1240.

Hansteen RW, Miller RD, Lonero L et al. (1976). Effects of cannabis and alcohol on automobile driving and psychomotor tracking. *Annals of the New York Academy of Sciences* 282:240-256.

Harris LS, Dewey WL & Rasdan RK (1977). Cannabis: Its chemistry, pharmacology and toxicology. In WR Martin (ed.) *Handbook of Experimental Pharmacology*. New York, NY: Springer-verlag, 371-429.

Hawks RL (1982). The constituents of cannabis and the disposition and metabolism of cannabinoids. *Analysis of Cannabinoids in Biological Fluids (NIDA Research Monograph 42)*. Rockville, MD: National Institute on Drug Abuse, 125-137.

Henderson RL, Tennant FS & Guerry R (1972). Respiratory manifestations of hashish smoking. *Archives of Otolaryngology* 92:248-251.

Herzberg U, Eliav E, Bennett GJ et al. (1997). The analgesic effects of R(+)-WIN 55,212-2 mesylate, a high affinity cannabinoid agonist, in a rat model of neuropathic pain. *Neuroscience Letters* 221:157-160.

Hillard CJ & Auchampach A (1994). In vitro activation of brain protein kinase C by the cannabinoids. *Biochimica et Biophysica Acta* 1220:163-170.

Hillard C J, Wilkison DM, Edgemond WS et al. (1995). Characterization of the kinetics and distribution of N-arachidonylethanolamine (anandamide) hydrolysis by rat brain. *Biochimica et Biophysica Acta* 1257:249-256.

Hohmann AG, Tsou K & Walker JM (1999). Cannabinoid suppression of noxious heat-evoked activity in wide dynamic range neurons in the lumbar dorsal horn of the rat. *Journal of Neurophysiology* 81(2):575-583.

Hollister AS (1992). Orthostatic hypotension. Causes, evaluation, and management. *Western Journal of Medicine* 157(6):652-657.

Hollister LE (1986). Health aspects of cannabis. *Pharmacology Review* 38:1-20.

Hollister LE (2000). An approach to the medical marijuana controversy. *Drug and Alcohol Dependence* 58(1-2):3-7.

Howlett AC (1984). Inhibition of neuroblastoma adenylate cyclase by cannabinoid and nantradol compounds. *Life Sciences* 35:1803-1810.

Howlett AC (1995). Pharmacology of cannabinoid receptors. *Annual Review of Pharmacology and Toxicology* 35:607-634.

Howlett AC, Evans DM & Houston DB (1992). The cannabinoid receptor. In L Murphy & A Bartke (ed.) *Marijuana/Cannabinoids: Neurobiology and Neurophysiology*. Boca Raton, FL: CRC Press, 35-72.

Howlett AC & Fleming RM (1984). Cannabinoid inhibition of adenylate cyclase. Pharmacology of the response in neuroblastoma cell membranes. *Molecular Pharmacology* 26(3):532-538.

Howlett AC, Johnson MR, Melvin LS et al. (1988). Nonclassical cannabinoid analgetics inhibit adenylate cyclase: Development of a cannabinoid receptor model. *Molecular Pharmacology* 33:297-302.

Howlett AC & Mukhopadhyay S (2000). Cellular signal transduction by anandamide and 2-arachidonoylglycerol. *Chemistry and Physics of Lipids* 108(1-2):53-70.

Howlett AC, Qualy JM & Khachatrian LL (1986). Involvement of Gi in the inhibition of adenylate cyclase by cannabimimetic drugs. *Molecular Pharmacology* 29:307-313.

Hsieh C, Brown S, Derleth C et al. (1999). Internalization and recycling of the CB1 cannabinoid receptor. *Journal of Neurochemistry* 73(2):493-501.

Huestis MA, Gorelick DA, Heishman SJ et al. (2001). Blockade of effects of smoked marijuana by the CB1-selective cannabinoid receptor antagonist SR141716. *Archives of General Psychiatry* 58(4):322-328.

Huestis MA, Henningfield JE & Cone EJ (1992a). Blood cannabinoids. I. Absorption of THC and formation of 11-OH-THC and THCCOOH during and after smoking marijuana. *Journal of Analytical Toxicology* 16(5):276-282.

Huestis MA, Henningfield JE & Cone EJ (1992b). Blood cannabinoids. II. Models for the prediction of time of marijuana exposure from plasma concentrations of delta 9-tetrahydrocannabinol (THC) and 11-nor-9-carboxy-delta 9-tetrahydrocannabinol (THCCOOH). *Journal of Analytical Toxicology* 16(5):283-290.

Isbell H, Gorodetzsky CW & Jasinski DR (1967). Effects of (-) trans-tetrahydrocannabinol in man. *Psychopharmacologia* 11:184-188.

Jarai Z, Wagner JA, Goparaju SK et al. (2000). Cardiovascular effects of 2-arachidonoyl glycerol in anesthetized mice. *Hypertension* 35(2):679-684.

Jones RT (1976). *Marihuana Research Findings: 1976 (NIDA Research Monograph 14)*. Rockville, MD: National Institute on Drug Abuse, 128-178.

Jones RT, Benowitz N & Bachman J (1976). Clinical studies of cannabis tolerance and dependence. *Annals of the New York Academy of Sciences* 282:221-239.

Kaminski NE, Koh WS, Yang KH et al. (1994). Suppression of the humoral immune response by cannabinoids is partially mediated through inhibition of adenylate cyclase by a pertussis toxin-sensitive G-protein coupled mechanism. *Biochemical Pharmacology* 48(10):1899-1908.

Kandel DB & Raveis VH (1989). Cessation of illicit drug use in young adulthood. *Archives of General Psychiatry* 46(2):109-116.

Karler R & Turkanis SA (1981). The cannabinoids as potential antiepileptics. *Journal of Clinical Pharmacology* 21(8-9 Suppl): 437S-448S.

Kempe K, Hsu FF, Bohrer A et al. (1996). Isotope dilution mass spectrometric measurements indicate that arachidonylethanolamide, the proposed endogenous ligand of the cannabinoid receptor, accumulates in rat brain tissue post mortem but is contained at low levels in or is absent from fresh tissue. *Journal of Biological Chemistry* 271:17287-17295.

Kim DJ & Thayer SA (2000). Activation of CB1 cannabinoid receptors inhibits neurotransmitter release from identified synaptic sites in rat hippocampal cultures. *Brain Research* 852(2):398-405.

Klein TW, Newton C & Friedman H (1998a). Cannabinoid receptors and the cytokine network. *Advances in Experimental Medicine and Biology* 437:215-222.

Klein TW, Newton C & Friedman H (1998b). Cannabinoid receptors and immunity. *Immunology Today* 19(8):373-381.

Klonoff H (1974). Marijuana and driving in real-life situations. *Science* 317-324.

Ko MC & Woods JH (1999). Local administration of delta-9-tetrahydrocannabinol attenuates capsaicin-induced thermal nociception in rhesus monkeys: A peripheral cannabinoid action. *Psychopharmacology* 143:322-326.

Kolansky H & Moore WT (1971). Effects of marihuana on adolescents and young adults. *Journal of the American Medical Association* 216(3):486-492.

Koutek B, Prestwich GD, Howlett AC et al. (1994). Inhibitors of arachidonoyl ethanolamide hydrolysis. *Journal of Biological Chemistry* 269:22937-22940.

Kuehnle J, Mendelson JH, Davis KR et al. (1977). Computed tomographic examination of heavy marijuana smokers. *Journal of the American Medical Association* 237(12):1231-1232.

Kunos G, Jarai Z, Varga K et al. (2000). Cardiovascular effects of endocannabinoids—The plot thickens. *Prostaglandins & Other Lipid Mediators* 61(1-2):71-84.

Lawrence DK & Gill EW (1975). Tile effects of delta 1-tetrahydrocannabinol and other cannabinoids on spin-labeled liposomes and their relationship to mechanisms of general anesthesia. *Molecular Pharmacology* 1: 595-602.

Lamarque S, Taghzouti K & Simon H (2001). Chronic treatment with delta-9-tetrahydrocannabinol enhances the locomotor response to amphetamine and heroin. Implications for vulnerability to drug addiction. *Neuropharmacology* 41(1):118-129.

Ledent C, Valverde O, Cossu G et al. (1999). Unresponsiveness to cannabinoids and reduced addictive effects of opiates in CB1 receptor knockout mice. *Science* 283:401-404.

Levitt M (1982). Nabilone vs. placebo in the treatment of chemotherapy-induced nausea and vomiting in cancer patients. *Cancer Treatment Reviews* 9(Suppl B):49-53.

Li J, Daughters RS, Bullis C et al. (1999). The cannabinoid receptor agonist WIN 55,212-2 mesylate blocks the development of hyperalgesia produced by capsaicin in rats. *Pain* 81(1-2):25-33.

Lichtman AH & Martin BR (1991a). Spinal and supraspinal mechanisms of cannabinoid-induced antinociception. *Journal of Pharmacology and Experimental Therapeutics* 258:517-523.

Lichtman AH & Martin BR (1991b). Cannabinoid-induced antinociception is mediated by a spinal alpha2-noradrenergic mechanism. *Brain Research* 559:309-314.

Lichtman AH, Meng Y & Martin BR (1996). Inhalation exposure to volatilized opioids produces antinociception in mice. *Journal of Pharmacology and Experimental Therapeutics* 279:69-76.

Lichtman AH, Poklis JL, Poklis A et al. (2001). The pharmacological activity of inhalation exposure to marijuana smoke in mice. *Drug and Alcohol Dependence* 63(2):107-116.

Lukas SE & Orozco S (2001). Ethanol increases plasma delta-9-tetrahydrocannabinol (THC) levels and subjective effects after marihuana smoking in human volunteers. *Drug and Alcohol Dependence* 64(2):143-149.

Mackie K & Hille B (1992). Cannabinoids inhibit N-type calcium channels in neuroblastoma-glioma cells. *Proceedings of the National Academy of Sciences* 89:3825-3829.

Mailleux P & Vanderhaeghen JJ (1992). Localization of cannabinoid receptor in the human developing and adult basal ganglia. Higher levels in the striatonigral neurons. *Neuroscience Letters* 148(1-2):173-176.

Mailleux P & Vanderhaeghen JJ (1994). Delta-9-tetrahydrocannabinol regulates substance P and enkephalin mRNAs levels in the caudate-putamen. *European Journal of Pharmacology* 267(1):R1-3.

Manzanares J, Corchero J, Romero J et al. (1999). Pharmacological and biochemical interactions between opioids and cannabinoids. *Trends in Pharmacological Sciences* 20:287-294.

Martin BR (1985). Characterization of the antinociceptive activity of intravenously administered delta-9-tetrahydrocannabinol in mice. In DJ Harvey (ed.) *Marihuana '84, Proceedings of the Oxford Symposium on Cannabis*. Oxford, England: IRL Press, 685-692.

Martin BR & Lichtman AH (1998). Cannabinoid transmission and pain perception. *Neurobiology of Disease* 5(6 Pt B):447-461.

Martin BR, Balster RL, Razdan RK et al. (1991). Behavioral comparisons of the stereoisomers of tetrahydrocannabinols. *Life Sciences* 29:565-574.

Martin BR, Compton DR, Prescott WR et al. (1995). Pharmacological evaluation of dimethylheptyl analogs of delta 9-THC: Reassessment of the putative three-point cannabinoid-receptor interaction. *Drug and Alcohol Dependence* 37(3):231-240.

Martin WJ, Loo CM & Basbaum AI (1999). Spinal cannabinoids are antiallodynic in rats with persistent inflammation. *Pain* 82(2):199-205.

Mason DL & Welch SP (1999a). A diminution of 9-tetrahydrocannabinol modulation of dynorphin A-(1-17) in conjunction with tolerance development. *European Journal of Pharmacology* 381:105-111.

Mason DJ & Welch SP (1999b). Cannabinoid modulation of dynorphin A: Correlation to cannabinoid-induced antinociception. *European Journal of Pharmacology* 378:237-248.

Mathew RJ, Wilson WH, Humphreys D et al. (1993). Depersonalization after marijuana smoking. *Biological Psychiatry* 33:431-441.

Matsuda LA, Lolait SJ, Brownstein MJ et al. (1990). Structure of a cannabinoid receptor and functional expression of the cloned cDNA. *Nature* 346:561-564.

McCoy KL, Matveyeva M, Carlisle SJ et al. (1999). Cannabinoid inhibition of the processing of intact lysozyme by macrophages: Evidence for CB2 receptor participation. *Journal of Pharmacology and Experimental Therapeutics* 289(3):1620-1625.

Mechoulam R (1986). The pharmacohistory of Cannabis sativa. In R Mechoulam (ed.) *Cannabinoids as Therapeutic Agents*. Boca Raton, FL: CRC Press, 1-9.

Mechoulam R, Ben-Shabat S, Hanus L et al. (1995). Identification of an endogenous 2-monoglyceride, present in canine gut, that binds to cannabinoid receptors. *Biochemical Pharmacology* 50:83-90.

Mechoulam R & Feigenbaum JJ (1987). Towards cannabinoid drugs. *Progress in Medicinal Chemistry* 24:159-207.

Mechoulam R, Feigenbaum JJ, Lander N et al. (1988). Enantiomeric cannabinoids: Stereospecificity of psychotropic activity. *Experientia* 44:762-764.

Mechoulam R & Gaoni Y (1965). A total synthesis of dl-D^1-tetrahydrocannabinol, the active constituent of hashish. *Journal of the American Chemical Society* 87:3273-3275.

Mechoulam R & Hanus L (2000). A historical overview of chemical research on cannabinoids. *Chemistry and Physics of Lipids* 108:1-13.

Mendelson JH & Mello NK (1984). Effects of marijuana on neuroendocrine hormones in human males and females. *Effect of Marijuana on Pregnancy and Fetal Development in the Human (NIDA Research Monograph 44)*. Rockville, MD: National Institute on Drug Abuse, 97-114.

Mendelson JH, Mello NK & Lex BW (1984). Marijuana withdrawal syndrome in a woman. *American Journal of Psychiatry* 141:1289-1290.

Mendelson JH, Meyer RE & Rossi AM (1972). Behavioral and biological concomitants of chronic marihuana smoking by heavy and casual users. In *Marijuana: A Signal of Misunderstanding (Technical Papers, Vol. 1)*. Rockville, MD: National Institute on Drug Abuse, 68-246.

Millman RB & Sbriglio R (1986). Patterns of use and psychopathology in chronic marijuana users. *Psychiatric Clinics of North America* 9(3):533-545.

Moss DE & Johnson RL (1980). Tonic analgesic effects of delta 9-tetrahydrocannabinol as measured with the formalin test. *European Journal of Pharmacology* 61(3):313-315.

Munro S, Thomas KL & Abu-Shaar M (1993). Molecular characterization of a peripheral receptor for cannabinoids. *Nature* 365:61-65.

Naditch MP (1974). Acute adverse reactions to psychoactive drugs, drug usage and psychopathology. *Journal of Abnormal Psychology* 83:394-403.

Negrete JC (1983). Effect of cannabis use on health. *Acta Psiquiatrica y Psicologica de America Latina* 29(4):267-276.

Nishiyama K, Kwak S, Murayama S et al. (1995). Substance P is a possible neurotransmitter in the rat spinothalamic tract. *Neuroscience Research* 21(3):261-266.

Noe SN, Newton C, Widen R, Friedman H & Klein TW (2001). Modulation of cb1 mrna upon activation of murine splenocytes. *Advances in Experimental Medicine and Biology* 493:215-221.

Noyes R Jr., Brunk SF, Avery S et al. (1975). The analgesic properties of delta-9-tetrahydrocannabinol and codeine. *Clinical Pharmacology and Therapeutics* 18(1):84-89.

O'Shaughnessy WB (1842). On the preparation of Indian hemp or gunjah. *Transcripts of Medical Physicians Society, Bombay* 8:421-461.

Oviedo A, Glowa J & Herkenham M (1993). Chronic cannabinoid administration alters cannabinoid receptor binding in rat brain: A quantitative autoradiographic study. *Brain Research* 9;616(1-2):293-302.

Page JB, Fletcher J & True WR (1988). Psychosociocultural perspectives on chronic cannabis use: The Costa Rican follow-up. *Journal of Psychoactive Drugs* 20(1):57-65.

Pagotto U, Marsicano G, Fezza F et al. (2001). Normal human pituitary gland and pituitary adenomas express cannabinoid receptor type 1 and synthesize endogenous cannabinoids: First evidence for a direct role of cannabinoids on hormone modulation at the human pituitary level. *Journal of Clinical Endocrinology and Metabolism* 86(6):2687-2696.

Paria BC, Song H & Dey SK (2001). Implantation: Molecular basis of embryo-uterine dialogue. *International Journal of Developmental Biology* 45(3 Spec No):597-605.

Paton WD & Pertwee RG (1972). Effect of cannabis and certain of its constituents on pentobarbitone sleeping times and phenazone metabolism. *British Journal of Pharmacology* 44:250-261.

Perez-Reyes M, Di Guiseppi S, Davis KH et al. (1982). Comparison of effects of marihuana cigarettes to three different potencies. *Clinical Pharmacology and Therapeutics* 31(5):617-624.

Pertwee RG & Griffin G (1995). A preliminary investigation of the mechanisms underlying cannabinoid tolerance in the mouse vas deferens. *European Journal of Pharmacology* 272(1):67-72.

Pertwee RG, Stevenson LA & Griffin G (1993). Cross-tolerance between delta-9-THC and the cannabimimetic agents, CP 55,940, WIN 55,212-2 and anandamide. *British Journal of Pharmacology* 110:1483-1490.

Plasse TF, Gorter RW, Krasnow SH et al. (1991). Recent clinical experience with dronabinol. *Pharmacology, Biochemistry and Behavior* 40:695-700.

Piomelli D, Beltramo M, Glasnapp S et al. (1999). Structural determinants for recognition and translocation by the anandamide transporter. *Proceedings of the National Academy of Sciences* 96(10):5802-5807.

Polen MR, Sidney S, Tekawa IS et al. (1993). Health care use by frequent marijuana smokers who do not smoke tobacco. *Western Journal of Medicine* 158:596-601.

Pope HG & Todd-Yurgelun D (1996). The residual cognitive effects of heavy marijuana use in college students. *Journal of the American Medical Association* 275:521-527.

Pugh GJ, Abood ME & Welch SP (1995). Antisense oligonucleotides to the kappa-1 receptor block the antinociceptive effects of delta-9-THC in the spinal cord. *Brain Research* 689:157-158.

Pugh GJ, Smith PB, Dombrowski DS et al. (1996). The role of endogenous opioids in enhancing the antinociception produced by the combination of delta-9-THC and morphine in the spinal cord. *Journal of Pharmacology and Experimental Therapeutics* 279:608-616.

Raft D, Gregg J, Ghia J et al. (1977). Effects of intravenous tetrahydrocannabinol on experimental and surgical pain. Psychological correlates of the analgesic response. *Clinical Pharmacology and Therapeutics* 21(1):26-33.

Razdan RK, Howes JF & Pars HG (1983). Development of orally active cannabinoids for the treatment of glaucoma. *Problems of Drug Dependence, 1982 (NIDA Research Monograph 43)*. Rockville, MD: National Institute on Drug Abuse, 157-163.

Reggio PH & Traore H (2000). Conformational requirements for endocannabinoid interaction with the cannabinoid receptors, the anandamide transporter and fatty acid amidohydrolase. *Chemistry and Physics of Lipids* 108(1-2):15-35.

Richardson J, Aanonsen L & Hargreaves KM (1997). SR141716A, A cannabinoid receptor antagonist, produces hyperalgesia in untreated mice. *European Journal of Pharmacology* 319:3R-5R.

Richardson JD, Aanonsen L & Hargreaves KM (1998). Antihyperalgesic effects of spinal cannabinoids. *European Journal of Pharmacology* 345(2):145-153.

Rinaldi-Carmona M, Barth F, Heaulme M et al. (1994). SR141716A, a potent and selective antagonist of the cannabinoid receptor. *FEBS Letters* 350:240-244.

Rinaldi-Carmona M, Barth F, Millan J et al. (1998). SR 144528, the first potent and selective antagonist of the CB2 cannabinoid receptor. *Journal of Pharmacology and Experimental Therapeutics* 284:644-650.

Rodriguez de Fonseca F, Gorriti MA, Fernandez-Ruiz JJ et al. (1994). Downregulation of rat brain cannabinoid binding sites after chronic delta 9-tetrahydrocannabinol treatment. *Pharmacology, Biochemistry and Behavior* 47(1):33-40.

Roffman RA, Stephens RS, Simpson EE et al. (1988). Treatment of marijuana dependence: Preliminary results. *Journal of Psychoactive Drugs* 20(1):129-137.

Rowen DW, Embrey JP, Moore CH et al. (1998). Antisense oligodeoxynucleotides to the kappa1 receptor enhance delta9-THC-induced antinociceptive tolerance. *Pharmacology, Biochemistry and Behavior* 59(2):399-404.

Rubino T, Vigano D, Massi P et al. (2000). Chronic delta-9-tetrahydrocannabinol treatment increases cAMP levels and cAMP-dependent protein kinase activity in some rat brain regions. *Neuropharmacology* 39(7):1331-1336.

Russo E (2001). Cannabinoids in pain management. Study was bound to conclude that cannabinoids had limited efficacy. *British Medical Journal* 323(7323):1249-1251.

Sallan SE, Cronin C, Zelen M et al. (1980). Antiemetics in patients receiving chemotherapy for cancer: A randomized comparison of delta-9-tetrahydrocannabinol and prochlorperazine. *New England Journal of Medicine* 302(3):135-138.

Seibold A, January BG, Friedman J et al. (1998). Desensitization of beta2-adrenergic receptors with mutations of the proposed G protein-coupled receptor kinase phosphorylation sites. *Journal of Biological Chemistry* 273(13):7637-7642.

Selley DE, Rorrer WK, Breivogel CS et al. (2001). Agonist efficacy and receptor efficiency in heterozygous CB1 knockout mice: Relationship of reduced CB1 receptor density to G-protein activation. *Journal of Neurochemistry* 77(4):1048-1057.

Selley DE, Sim LJ, Xiao R et al. (1997). Mu opioid receptor-stimulated [^{35}S]GTPgS binding in rat thalamus and cultured cell lines: Signal transduction mechanisms underlying agonist efficacy. *Molecular Pharmacology* 51:87-96.

Sharma S & Moskowitz H (1972). Effect of marihuana on the visual autokinetic phenomenon. *Perceptual and Motor Skills* 35:891-894.

Sherman MP, Aberland EE, Wong VZ et al. (1997). Effects of smoking marijuana, tobacco or cocaine alone or in combination on DNA damage in human alveolar macrophages. *Life Sciences* 56:2301-2307.

Shire D, Carillon C, Kaghad M et al. (1995). An amino-terminal variant of the central cannabinoid receptor resulting from alternative splicing. *Journal of Biological Chemistry* 270: 3726-3731.

Sim LJ & Childers SR (1997). Anatomical distribution of mu, delta, and kappa opioid- and nocioception/orphanin FQ-stimulated [35S]guanylyl-5'-O-(gamma-thio)-triphosphate binding in guinea pig brain. *Journal of Comparative Neurology* 386(4):562-572.

Sim LJ, Selley DE & Childers SR (1995). In vitro autoradiography of receptor-activated G-proteins in rat brain by agonist-stimulated guanylyl 5'-[_-[^{35}S]thio]-triphosphate binding. *Proceedings of the National Academy of Sciences* 92:7242-7246.

Sim LJ, Selley DE, Xiao R et al. (1996). Differences in G-protein activation by mu and delta opioid, and cannabinoid, receptors in rat striatum. *European Journal of Pharmacology* 307:95-107.

Sim-Selley LJ, Brunk LK & Selley DE (2001). Inhibitory effects of SR141716A on G-protein activation in rat brain. *European Journal of Pharmacology* 414(2-3):135-143.

Smith FL & Dewey WL (1993). Endogenous dynorphin modulates calcium-mediated antinociception in mice. *Pharmacology, Biochemistry and Behavior* 45(2):383-391.

Smith PB, Welch SP & Martin BR (1994). Interactions between Δ^9-tetrahydrocannabinol and kappa opioids in mice. *Journal of Pharmacology and Experimental Therapeutics* 268:1382-1387.

Smiley A & Moskowitz H (1986). Effects of long-term administration of buspirone and diazepam on driver steering control. *American Journal of Medicine* 31:80(3B):22-29.

Sofia RD, Nalepa SD, Harakal JJ et al. (1973). Anti-edema and analgesic properties of delta-9-tetrahydrocannabinol (THC). *Journal of Pharmacology and Experimental Therapeutics* 186:646-655.

Solowij N, Miche PT & Fox AM (1995). Differential impairments of selective attention due to frequency and duration of cannabis use. *Biological Psychiatry* 37:731-739.

Strangman NM, Patrick SL, Hohmann AG et al. (1998). Evidence for a role of endogenous cannabinoids in the modulation of acute and tonic pain sensitivity. *Brain Research* 813(2):323-328.

Sugiura T, Kondo S, Sukagawa A et al. (1995). 2-arachidonoylglycerol: A possible endogenous cannabinoid receptor ligand in brain. *Biochemical and Biophysical Research Communications* 215:89-97.

Sutton LR (1983). The effects of alcohol, marihuana and their combination on driving ability. *Journal of Studies on Alcohol* 44(3):438-445.

Szallasi A & Blumberg PM (1999). Vanilloid (Capsaicin) receptors and mechanisms. *Pharmacological Review* 51(2):159-212.

Tashkin DP (1990). Pulmonary complications of smoked substance abuse. *Western Journal of Medicine* 152(5):525-530.

Tashkin DP (1993). Is frequent marijuana smoking harmful to health? *Western Journal of Medicine* 158(6):635-637.

Tashkin DP, Scares JR, Hepler RS et al. (1978). Cannabis 1978. *Annals of Internal Medicine* 89:539-549.

Tashkin DP, Shapiro BJ, Lee EY et al. (1976). Subacute effects of heavy marijuana smoking pulmonary function in healthy young mates. *New England Journal of Medicine* 294:125-129.

Tashkin DP, Wu TC & Djahed B (1988). Acute and chronic effects of marijuana smoking compared with tobacco smoking on blood carboxyhemoglobin levels. *Journal of Psychoactive Drugs* 20(1):27-31.

Tennes K (1984). Effect of marijuana on pregnancy and fetal development in the human. In MC Braude & JP Ludford (eds.) *Marijuana Effects on the Endocrine and Reproductive Systems (NIDA Research Monograph 44).* Rockville, MD: National Institute on Drug Abuse, 115-123.

Tilles DS, Goldenheim PD & Johnson DC (1986). Marijuana smoking as cause of reduction in single-breath carbon monoxide diffusing capacity. *American Journal of Medicine* 80:601-606.

Tsou K, Patrick SL & Walker JM (1995). Physical withdrawal in rats tolerant to delta 9-tetrahydrocannabinol precipitated by a cannabinoid receptor antagonist. *European Journal of Pharmacology* 280(3):R13-15.

Ueda N, Kurahashi Y, Yamamoto S et al. (1995). Partial purification and characterization of the porcine brain enzyme hydrolyzing and synthesizing anandamide. *Journal of Biological Chemistry* 270:23823-23827.

Vinciguerra V, Moore T & Brennan E (1988). Inhalation marijuana as an antiemetic for cancer chemotherapy. *New York State Journal of Medicine* 88(10):525-527.

Vogel Z, Barg J, Levy R et al. (1993). Anandamide, a brain endogenous compound, interacts specifically with cannabinoid receptors and inhibits adenylate cyclase. *Journal of Neurochemistry* 61:352-355.

Voth HM (1980). The future of America. *Military Medicine* 145(3):169-175.

Walker JM, Hohmann AG, Martin WJ et al. (1999). The neurobiology of cannabinoid analgesia. *Life Sciences* 65(6-7):665-673.

Welch SP (1997). Characterization of anandamide-induced tolerance: Comparison to delta 9-THC-induced interactions with dynorphinergic systems. *Drug and Alcohol Dependence* 45:39-45.

Welch SP, Dunlow LD & Patrick GS (1995). Characterization of anandamide- and fluoroanandamide-induced antinociception and cross-tolerance to delta-9-THC following intrathecal administration to mice: Blockade of delta-9-THC-induced antinociception. *Journal of Pharmacology and Experimental Therapeutics* 273:1235-1244.

Welch SP, Huffman JW & Lowe J (1998). Differential blockade of the antinociceptive effects of centrally administered cannabinoids by SR141716A. *Journal of Pharmacology and Experimental Therapeutics* 286:1301-1308.

Welch SP & Stevens DL (1992). Antinociceptive activity of intrathecally administered cannabinoids alone, and in combination with morphine, in mice. *Journal of Pharmacology and Experimental Therapeutics* 262:10-18.

Wenger T, Toth BE & Martin BR (1995). Effects of anandamide (endogenous cannabinoid) on the anterior pituitary hormone secretion in adult ovariectomized rats. *Life Sciences* 56:2057-2063.

Whitfield RM, Bechtel LM & Starich GH (1997). The impact of ethanol and Marinol/marijuana usage on HIV+/AIDS patients undergoing azidothymidine, azidothymidine/dideoxycytidine, or dideoxyinosine therapy. *Alcoholism: Clinical & Experimental Research* 21(1):122-127.

Wiley JL, Barrett RL, Lowe J et al. (1995). Discriminative effects of CP 55,940 and structurally dissimilar cannabinoids in rats. *Neuropharmacology* 34:669-676.

Wiley JL, Lowe JA, Balster RL et al. (1995). Discriminative stimulus effect of delta-9-tetrahydrocannabinol in rats and rhesus monkeys. *Journal of Pharmacology and Experimental Therapeutics* 275:1-6.

Williams CM & Kirkham TC (1999). Anandamide induces overeating: Mediation by central cannabinoid (CB1) receptors. *Psychopharmacology* (Berlin) 143(3):315-317.

Wilson RI, Kunos G & Nicoll RA (2001). Presynaptic specificity of endocannabinoid signaling in the hippocampus. *Neuron* 31(3):453-462.

Yamaguchi K & Kandel DB (1984). Patterns of drug use from adolescence to young adulthood: II. Sequences of progression. *American Journal of Public Health* 74(7):668-672.

Yaksh TL (1981). The antinociceptive effects of the intrathecally administered levonantradol and desacetyllevonantradol in the rat. *Journal of Clinical Pharmacology* 21:334S-340S.

Zamponi GW, Bourinett E, Nelson D et al. (1997). Crosstalk between G-proteins and protein kinase C mediated by the calcium channel $\alpha 1$ subunit. *Nature* 385:442-446.

Zimmer A, Valjent E, Konig M et al. (2001). Absence of delta-9-tetrahydrocannabinol dysphoric effects in dynorphin-deficient mice. *Journal of Neuroscience* 21(23):9499-9505.

Zimmer A, Zimmer AM, Hohmann AG et al. (1999). Increased mortality, hypoactivity, and hypoalgesia in cannabinoid CB1 receptor knockout mice. *Proceedings of the National Academy of Sciences* 96(10):5780-5785.

Zygmunt PM, Petersson J, Andersson DA et al. (1999). Vanilloid receptors on sensory nerves mediate the vasodilator action of anandamide. *Nature* 400(6743):452-457.

Chapter 9

The Pharmacology of Serotonergic Hallucinogens and "Designer Drugs"

Richard A. Glennon, Ph.D.

Drugs in the Class
Absorption and Metabolism
Pharmacologic Actions
Mechanisms of Action
Addiction Liability
Toxicity/Adverse Effects

One of the largest categories of abusable drugs is the "classical hallucinogens" (Glennon, 1998). Because these agents are believed to act as agonists at serotonin receptors, they also are termed "serotonergic hallucinogens"—a subcategory of hallucinogens that includes several groups of agents.

Structural modification of these hallucinogens has been shown to result in so-called "designer drugs," which either retain hallucinogenic properties, show diminished hallucinogenic character, or display a novel action with or without hallucinogenic character.

DRUGS IN THE CLASS

Serotonergic (or "classical") hallucinogens are those hallucinogens that possess an arylethylamine skeleton of the indolealkylamine type or phenylalkylamine type. Most of these agents have not been thoroughly investigated in humans, but many have seen at least some human evaluation (Jacob & Shulgin, 1994; Shulgin & Shulgin, 1991, 1997). Agents from this class do not necessarily produce identical effects. However, all have been shown to bind at 5-HT$_2$ receptors, and, where they have been investigated, all (ex-

cept beta-carboline derivatives) have been demonstrated to behave as 5-HT$_2$ agonists or partial agonists. Nearly all examples of serotonergic hallucinogens described herein have been examined in tests of stimulus generalization using animals trained to discriminate 1-(2,5-dimethoxy-4-methylphenyl)-2-aminopropane (DOM) from vehicle. For these agents, a significant correlation exists between stimulus generalization potency and human hallucinogenic potency.

Serotonergic hallucinogens fall into two structural categories: the indolealkylamines and the phenylalkylamines, referred to collectively as arylalkylamines. The indolealkylamines are further divided into the tryptamines (amine-substituted or N-alkyltryptamines, and alpha-alkyltryptamines), the ergolines (or lysergamides), and, possibly, the beta-carbolines. The phenylalkylamines consist of the phenylethylamines and the phenylisopropylamines.

Common drugs in this class include lysergic acid diethylamide (LSD), mescaline, peyote, psilocybin (the active ingredient in mushrooms), harmaline (a hallucinogen used in some South American countries), and certain so-called "designer drugs" that are related to 1-(3,4-methylenedioxyphenyl)-2-aminopropane (MDA) and that possess hallucinogenic and/or stimulant-like properties.

Indolealkylamines.
Alkyltryptamines (such as DMT, Psilocin, psylocybin, and "shrooms"): In the general structure, *R* and *R'* typically are methyl or a small alkyl group, and *X* is H or methoxy (Figure 1).

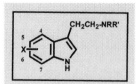

Figure 1

One of the best investigated hallucinogens is N,N-dimethyltryptamine (DMT) (Table 1), which is considered the prototype of this subclass of agents. DMT is a naturally occurring substance, but is readily synthesized in the laboratory. Its actions are characterized by a rapid onset (typically <5 minutes) and short duration of action (about 30 minutes). DMT-like agents possess a characteristically unpleasant odor, particularly when freebased or smoked. DMT, like some other members of this family, is not orally active, but generally is administered by inhalation, by smoking, and—less frequently—by injection. The corresponding secondary amine (N-monomethyltryptamine) and primary amine (tryptamine) are not known to be hallucinogenic, most likely because they are not sufficiently lipophilic to readily penetrate the blood-brain barrier, and because what little does get into the brain is rapidly metabolized by monoamine oxidase. Other tertiary amine derivatives, such as N-ethyl-N-methyltryptamine, N,N-diethyltryptamine(DET), N,N-di-*n*-propyltryptamine (DPT), and some secondary amines, also are hallucinogenic in humans (Shulgin & Shulgin, 1997). If the N-alkyl or N,N-dialkyl substituents are sufficiently bulky and lipophilic, these tryptamines can be orally active (see Table 1).

Relatively few aryl-substituted tryptamine analogs have been systematically explored, but substitution in the benzenoid ring can enhance or diminish potency, depending on the specific nature and location of the substituents. Some of the more frequently encountered derivatives of DMT, their common names, and their approximate human potency are shown in Table 1.

N,N-Dimethylserotonin (bufotenine, 5-OH DMT) might be a weak hallucinogen, but the results of human studies are controversial. With its polar hydroxyl group, bufotenine likely does not readily penetrate the blood-brain barrier and produces considerable peripheral effects (facial flushing, cardiovascular actions), which prevent evaluation of an extended dose range. O-Methylation of bufotenine decreases its polarity and results in 5-OMe DMT, one of the more potent N-alkylated tryptamines. 5-OMe DMT is a naturally occurring substance and is a constituent of a number of plants and grasses. Bufotenine and 5-OMe DMT are found in the skin of certain frogs and can be responsible for the phenomenon of "toad licking." Psilocin is 4-hydroxy DMT; with a polar hydroxyl group like bufotenine, psilocin might not have been expected to enter the brain. Yet, it is hallucinogenic. Although there is no documented support for the concept, it has been speculated that the 4-hydroxyl group forms a hydrogen bond with the terminal amine and that this reduces polarity just enough that psilocin penetrates the blood-brain barrier. Psilocin and its phosphate ester, psilocybin, are widely found in certain species of mushrooms and have given rise to the terms "shrooms" and "shrooming."

There are no reports that 6-methoxy DMT or 7-methoxy DMT is hallucinogenic. It is quite difficult to make strict human potency comparisons within this series because of the varied routes of administration employed (Table 1). In drug discrimination studies using DOM-trained animals (Table 1), generalization potency follows the order of 5-OMe DMT > 4-OMe DMT > DMT. 6- and 7-OMe DMT failed to substitute for DOM.

Alpha-Alkyltryptamines: Hallucinogenic alpha-alkyltryptamines typically possess an alpha-methyl group (R=methyl) and *X* is hydrogen or methoxy at the 4- or 5-position (Figure 2); 2 optical isomers are possible. Tryptamine is not hallucinogenic, but introduction of an alpha-methyl group seems to enhance lipophilicity and to protect against metabolism, with the result

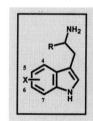

Figure 2

that alpha-methyltryptamine (alpha-MeT; Table 1) is at least twice as potent as DMT and is orally active (Murphree, Dippy et al., 1961). In general, alpha-methyltryptamines, where they have been investigated, have been found to be somewhat more potent than their corresponding DMT counterparts. Otherwise, their structure-activity relationships (SARs) are essentially the same as those of the DMT analogs. For example, in animal studies, racemic 5-methoxy-alpha-methyltryptamine (5-OMe αMeT) is about twice as potent as 5-OMe DMT (Table 1). Where they have been investigated, the *S*(+)-isomers of alpha-methyltryptamines have been found to be more potent than their *R*(-)-enantiomers. Homologation of the alpha-methyl group to an alpha-ethyl group affords alpha-ethyltryptamines; alpha-ethyltryptamine will be discussed in the section below on designer drugs.

TABLE 1.   Examples of Indolealkylamine Hallucinogens and Related Compounds

Agent	Common Name	R'/R"	R	X	Approximate DOM Stimulus Generalization Potency (μ mol/kg)[a]	Approximate Human Hallucinogenic Dose (mg)[b]
Tryptamine		-H/-H	-H	-H	Inactive	Inactive
α-Methyltryptamine	α-MeT	-H/-H	-Me	-H	15	5-20 (s); 15-30 (po)
N,N-Dimethyltryptamine	DMT	-Me/-Me	-H	-H	26	60-100 (s); 4-30 (iv)
N,N-Diethyltryptamine	DET	-Et/-Et	-H	-H	10	50-100 (po)
N,N-Dipropyltryptamine	DPT	-Pr/-Pr	-H	-H	8	100-250 (po)
N,N-Diisopropyltryptamine	DIPT	-iPr/-iPr	-H	-H	9	25-100 (po)
4-Hydroxy DMT	Psilocin	-Me/-Me	-H	4-OH	—	10-20 (po)
4-Methoxy DMT	4-OMe DMT	-Me/-Me	-H	4-OMe	12	Unknown
5-Hydroxy DMT	Bufotenine	-Me/-Me	-H	5-OH	Inactive	Unknown
5-Methoxy DMT	5-OMe DMT	-Me/-Me	-H	5-OMe	4	6-20 (s); 2-3 (iv)
(±)5-Methocy α-MeT	5-OMe α-MeT	-H/-H	-Me	5-OMe	2	2.5-4.5 (po)

[a]Drug discrimination data, transformed to approximate μ mol/kg dose, from Glennon (1989, 1991).
[b]Data primarily from Shulgin and colleagues (Jacob & Shulgin, 1994; Shulgin & Shulgin, 1997).
Key: s = smoked; po = oral; iv = intravenous.

Ergolines or Lysergamides (for example, LSD, acid, "blotter"): (+)LSD (Figure 3; R=R'=Et) is perhaps the best known, and one of the most potent, of the classical hallucinogens. Although LSD itself is not naturally occurring, many related ergolines and synthetic precursors are found in nature. In terms of potency, LSD is active at total human doses of 100 to 200 μg or less. Although numerous derivatives of LSD are possible, relatively few have been investigated in humans. Some work has been reported on the SAR of LSD (Pfaff, Huang et al., 1994; Siva Sankar, 1975).

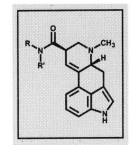

Figure 3

No hallucinogen has been as extensively studied in animals or humans as LSD (reviewed in Hoffer & Osmond, 1967; Siva Sankar, 1975). Its actions in humans can be divided into three major categories: perceptual (altered shapes and colors, heightened sense of hearing), psychic (alterations in mood, depersonalization, visual hallucinations, altered sense of time), and somatic (nausea, blurred vision, dizziness). In terms of principal effects, there seem to be few differences among LSD, psilocybin, and mescaline.

Although LSD has been sold on the clandestine market in tablet form, it is not uncommon to find this material available on "blotter paper" because of its high potency (Pellerin, 1998). A sheet of porous paper is impregnated with a solution of LSD, and the sheet later is cut to afford the desired dose.

Beta-carbolines (for example, harmaline, harmine): The beta-carbolines represent an interesting and controversial class of agents, which generally are referred to as the "harmala alkaloids." Several are naturally occurring. In South America, beta-carbolines are found in certain vines and lianas (*Banisteriopsis caapi*). In the Old World, beta-carbolines are found as constituents of Syrian Rue (*Pegnum harmala*). Naturally occurring harmala alkaloids can have a double-bond at the C_1-N_2 position or at both the C_1-N_2 and C_3-C_4 positions; X generally is hydrogen or a 7-methoxy group (Figure 4). South American Indians use beta-carbolines to prepare a variety of concoctions and snuffs—the most notable of which is Ayahuasca—for their hallucinogenic and visionary healing properties. Based on the number of reports that have appeared, there is little question that such concoctions are psychoactive; however, the plant preparations usually consist of admixtures in which indolealkylamines such as DMT or 5-OMe DMT sometimes have been identified.

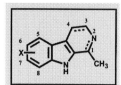

Figure 4

Some beta-carbolines possess activity as monoamine oxidase (MAO) inhibitors, and it has been suggested that the MAO inhibitory effect of the beta-carbolines simply potentiates the effect of any indolealkylamine hallucinogen present in the admixture by interfering with its metabolism. Studies with individual beta-carbolines, especially under carefully controlled clinical settings, have been very few. The most commonly occurring beta-carbolines are harmine, harmaline, and tetrahydroharmine. Evidence suggests that harmine and harmaline are hallucinogenic in humans (with potencies not greater than that of DMT) (Naranjo, 1967, 1973). Harmaline has seen some limited experimental application as an adjunct to psychotherapy (Naranjo, 1973). Like other classical hallucinogens, certain beta-carbolines bind at 5-HT$_{2A}$ receptors (Glennon, Dukat et al., 2000) and, in animal studies, DOM-stimulus generalization occurs to harmaline (Grella, Dukat et al., 1998). However, none of the beta-carbolines examined produced the type of 5-HT$_{2A}$ agonist effects (phosphoinositol hydrolysis) that are com-

mon to other classical hallucinogens (Glennon, Dukat et al., 2000); hence, they cannot yet be formally classified as serotonergic hallucinogens. Moreover, an ibogaine stimulus, but not an LSD stimulus, generalizes to certain of these beta-carbolines (Helsley, Rabin et al., 1998; Helsley, Fiorella et al., 1998). In any event, over the past decade or so, beta-carbolines have begun to make an appearance in clandestine markets. They have been referred to as fantasy-enhancing agents (Naranjo, 1973) and have the potential to serve as templates for the development of novel designer drugs. Because relatively little is known about these agents, there is increased interest in their investigation.

Phenylalkylamines. *Phenylethylamines (for example, mescaline, peyote):* Phenylethylamines (Figure 5) and phenylisopropylamines (Figure 6), collectively referred to as phenylalkylamines, represent the largest group of serotonergic hallucinogens (Glennon, 1996; Shulgin & Shulgin, 1997). The phenylethylamines are the alpha-*des*methyl counterparts of the phenylisopropylamines; as with the indolealkylamines, the presence of the alpha-methyl group increases an agent's lipophilicity and reduces its susceptibility to metabolism. As a consequence, the phenylethylamine hallucinogens typically produce effects that are qualitatively similar to those of their corresponding phenylisopropylamines, but usually are several-fold less potent.

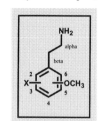

Figure 5

Phenylethylamine counterparts of weak phenylisopropylamines might be inactive. Literally hundreds of analogs have been examined in human and animal studies (Shulgin & Shulgin, 1991). Phenylethylamine hallucinogens generally possess at least two methoxy substituents, and X can be either another methoxy group or a non-methoxy group. Some hallucinogenic phenylisopropylamines are described as possessing some stimulant characteristics, which can be minimized or altogether absent in the corresponding phenylethylamines. At the alpha-position, the phenylisopropylamines possess a chiral center that is absent in the phenylethylamines. Otherwise, the SARs of the two groups of agents are relatively similar. Consequently, the phenylethylamines will not be discussed here in detail; see Shulgin and Shulgin (1991) for an extended discussion of phenylethylamine hallucinogens.

One of the best recognized and oldest known phenylethylamine hallucinogens is mescaline. A constituent of peyote (and other) cactus, mescaline is a relatively weak hallucinogenic agent (total oral human dose is approximately 350 mg). Like many of the hallucinogens, mescaline is classified as a Schedule I substance under the federal Controlled Substances Act; however, the use of peyote in certain Native American religious practices is legally sanctioned.

Phenylisopropylamines (such as DOM, DOB, DMA, MDA): Structural modification of mescaline and related substances by introduction of an alpha-methyl group and by deletion and/or rearrangement of the position of its methoxy groups results in a series of agents known as the phenylisopropyla-mine hallucinogens. Numerous names and terminologies have been used to describe these phenyl-isopropylamine hallucinogens (Shulgin & Shulgin, 1991), but one of the more common and readily applied nomenclatures is that associated with the number and location of methoxy groups in the molecule. Analogs with two methoxy groups are called DMAs (dimethoxy analogs), whereas analogs with three methoxy groups are called trimethoxy analogs, or TMAs. For example, introduction of an alpha-methyl group to mescaline results in 3,4,5-TMA.

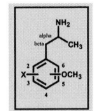

Figure 6

There are three possible monomethoxyphenylisopropylamines: the *ortho*-methoxy analog OMA, the *meta*-methoxy analog MMA, and the *para*-methoxy analog PMA (Table 2). Although PMA is classified as a Schedule I substance, none of these three analogs has been demonstrated to be hallucinogenic in humans. PMA possesses weak central stimulant actions, acts as a 5-HT-releasing agent, and has been found on the clandestine market; several deaths have been attributed to PMA overdose within the past few years. PMA is discussed below in the section on designer drugs.

There are six isomeric DMA analogs. These analogs have not been thoroughly investigated in humans, and few produce DOM-like stimulus effects in animals (Table 2). None is more potent than DOM. One of the more potent positional isomers, and one that has been evaluated in humans, is 1-(2,5-dimethoxyphenyl)-2-aminopropane or 2,5-DMA (sometimes referred to simply as "DMA"). There are six different TMA analogs (Table 2). Most show some activity, but the 2,4,5-timethoxy analog 2,4,5-TMA is the most potent of the series. Most of the trimethoxy analogs are recognized by DOM-trained animals, but none is more potent than DOM itself (Glennon, 1991, 1996). The presence of the 2,5-methoxy substitution pattern in 2,5-DMA and 2,4,5-TMA might be noted.

Replacement of the 4-methoxy group of 2,4,5-TMA with a methyl group results in DOM or 1-(2,5-dimethoxy-4-methylphenyl)-2-aminopropane. Perhaps for no other reason than its frequency of occurrence in the scientific literature, DOM represents the prototype member of this family of agents. Increasing the length of this 4-methyl group to an ethyl or *n*-propyl group (that is, DOET and DOPR, respectively) results in enhanced potency on a molar basis. Further extension of the alkyl chain results in decreased potency or loss of action. Substitution at the 4-position by electron-withdrawing groups, particularly those with hydrophobic character, results in active agents such as DOB (Table 2).

DOB is quite potent and has been misrepresented on the clandestine market as LSD both in tablet and "blotter" form.

When optical isomers have been examined, activity resides primarily with the *R*(-)isomer; the *S*(+)isomers typically are less active, inactive, or have received little study. For example, although not well investigated, it appears that *R*(-)DOM and *R*(-)DOB show activity at total human doses of about 4 mg and 1 mg, respectively. Animal studies (drug discrimination studies) show that, for all of the phenylisopropylamine hallucinogens, the R(-)isomers are more potent than their S(+)isomers by severalfold. N-monomethylation reduces potency or abolishes activity; for example, the N-monomethyl analogs of DOM and DOB are about one-tenth as potent as their primary amine counterparts. SARs for the DOM-like actions of phenylisopropylamines have been summarized (Glennon, 1996; Nichols & Glennon, 1984).

MDA or 1-(3,4-methylenedioxyphenyl)-2-aminopropane was popular during the 1960s, when it was known on the street as the "Love Drug"; MDA seems to be gaining in popularity once again. MDA is structurally distinct from many of the other hallucinogenic phenylisopropylamines by virtue of its lack of methoxy groups. It might be viewed as an analog of 3,4-DMA in which the two methoxy groups have been "connected" through a common carbon atom. MDA has been reported to produce effects in humans akin to a combination of cocaine and LSD. MDA produces both amphetamine-like and DOM-like stimulus effects in animals; further, animals trained to discriminate MDA recognize central stimulants (such as amphetamine and cocaine) as well as classical hallucinogens (such as LSD, mescaline, and

TABLE 2.   Examples of Psychoactive Phenylisopropylamines and Related Agents

Agent	R2	R3	R4	R5	R6	DOM-Stimulus Generalization Potency (μmol/kg)[a]	Approximate Human Hallucinogenic Dose (mg)[b]
Amphetamine	-H	-H	-H	-H	-H	NSG	NH
OMA	-OMe	-H	-H	-H	-H	NSG	NH
MMA	-H	-OMe	-H	-H	-H	NSG	NH
PMA	-H	-H	-OMe	-H	-H	NSG	NH
2,3-DMA	-OMe	-OMe	-H	-H	-H	NSG	(?)
2,4-DMA	-OMe	-H	-OMe	-H	-H	21.0	>60 (?)
2,5-DMA	-OMe	-H	-H	-OMe	-H	23.8	120 (80-160)
2,5-DMA, R(-)-	-OMe	-H	-H	-OMe	-H	14.0	(?)
2,6-DMA	-OMe	-H	-H	-H	-OMe	NSG	(?)
3,4-DMA	-H	-OMe	-OMe	-H	-H	NSG	>500 (?)
3,5-DMA	-H	-OMe	-H	-OMe	-H	NSG	>500 (?)
2,3,4-TMA	-OMe	-OMe	-OMe	-H	-H	29.8	>100 (?)
2,3,5-TMA	-OMe	-OMe	-H	-OMe	-H	63.0	>80 (?)
2,3,6-TMA	-OMe	-OMe	-H	-H	-OMe	—	>30 (?)
2,4,5-TMA	-OMe	-H	-OMe	-OMe	-H	13.7	30 (20-40)
2,4,6-TMA	-OMe	-H	-OMe	-H	-OMe	13.9	38 (25-50)
3,4,5-TMA	-H	-OMe	-OMe	-OMe	-H	24.2	175 (100-250)
MEM	-OMe	-H	-OC$_2$H$_5$	-OMe	-H	22.9	35 (20-50)
DOM	-OMe	-H	-CH$_3$	-OMe	-H	1.8	7 (3-10)
DOM, R(-)-	-OMe	-H	-CH$_3$	-OMe	-H	0.9	(?)
DOM, S(+)-	-OMe	-H	-CH$_3$	-OMe	-H	6.9	(?)
DOET	-OMe	-H	-C$_2$H$_5$	-OMe	-H	0.9	4 (2-6)
DOPR	-OMe	-H	-nC$_3$H$_7$	-OMe	-H	0.9	4 (2.5-5)
DOBU	-OMe	-H	-nC$_4$H$_9$	-OMe	-H	3.2	(?)
DOAM	-OMe	-H	-nC$_5$H$_{11}$	-OMe	-H	NSG	(?)
DON	-OMe	-H	-NO$_2$	-OMe	-H	2.7	4 (3-4.5)
DOC	-OMe	-H	-Cl	-OMe	-H	1.2	2.5 (1.5-3)
DOB	-OMe	-H	-Br	-OMe	-H	0.6	2 (1-3)
DOB, R(-)-	-OMe	-H	-Br	-OMe	-H	0.3	1.0-1.5 (?)
DOI	-OMe	-H	-I	-OMe	-H	1.2	2.5 (1.5-3)
DOOC	-OMe	-H	-COOH	-OMe	-H	NSG	(?)
DOOH	-OMe	-H	-OH	-OMe	-H	NSG	(?)

[a]Drug discrimination data represent ED50 values and are from Glennon (1989, 1991, 1996). NSG, no stimulus generalization (that is, the agent did not produce DOM-like stimulus effects).

[b]Data are primarily from Shulgin and co-workers (Jacob & Shulgin, 1994; Shulgin & Shulgin, 1991). Where a dose range was reported in the original literature, the arithmetic mean is also provided here to facilitate comparison and the original range is given in parenthesis; the values should not be taken as a measure of precision. In fact, doses are approximate and no implication is made that the different agents produce an identical effect. Key: NH indicates that the material has not been reported to be hallucinogenic, (?) indicates that the material has not been well investigated or that its actions or potency are essentially unknown.

DOM) (Young & Glennon, 1996). The hallucinogenic qualities of MDA reside primarily in it R(-)isomer, whereas the S(+)isomer seems primarily responsible for its stimulant character.

Table 2 provides a comparison of the approximate human doses of various phenylisopropylamines when administered by the oral route. These agents represent a mere sampling of the agents that have been examined (Shulgin & Shulgin, 1991); using only those functional groups shown in the table, imagine how many different analogs are possible on the basis of structural rearrangement. There is no reason to suspect that each of these agents produces identical effects. In fact, the actions of some of these agents have been reported to be quite unique and range from hallucinations and closed-eye imagery to intellectual and sensory enhancement to erotic arousal (Shulgin & Shulgin, 1991).

Designer Drugs. Application of drug design concepts by clandestine chemists results in what are termed "designer drugs," or *controlled substance analogs.* Recently, it seems that almost any new agent appearing on the street is referred to as a "designer drug," whether or not it is a novel entity. To illustrate, DOB is a potent hallucinogen; removal of the alpha-methyl group of DOB should, according to established SARs, result in a phenylethylamine analog that retains—although with severalfold reduced potency—the actions of DOB. Its effects in humans might not be identical with those of DOB, but significant similarities should exist. Even though alpha-*des*methyl DOB was known in the scientific literature, it has made an appearance on the clandestine market as "Nexus" or "2-CB." As expected, the agent is hallucinogenic and is somewhat less potent than DOB.

Aryl-unsubstituted phenylisopropylamine is known as amphetamine. That is, removal of the 4-methyl group and the two methoxy groups of DOM results not in a hallucinogenic agent but in a central stimulant: amphetamine. Even though there is significant structural similarity between DOM and its stripped-down analog (amphetamine), they differ dramatically in their actions in animals and in humans. Actually, amphetamine is rather unusual in that few phenylisopropylamines retain its central stimulant character and very few analogs retain a level of the potency similar to that of amphetamine.

One of the best known examples of an analog that retains potent stimulant properties is the N-monomethyl analog of amphetamine, or methamphetamine (Figure 7

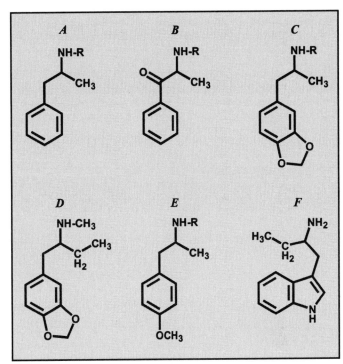

FIGURE 7. Chemical structures of *A*: amphetamine and methamphetamine (R = -H and -CH₃, respectively), *B*: cathinone and methcathinone ((R = -H and -CH₃, respectively), *C*: MDA and MDMA (R= -H and -CH₃, respectively), *D*: MBDB, *E*: PMA and PMMA (R= -H and -CH₃, respectively), and *F*: α-ethyltryptamine.

shows its chemical structure). Nevertheless, structural variation of amphetamine can result in controlled substance analogs. For example, cathinone is the beta-keto analog of amphetamine; cathinone is a naturally occurring substance (a constituent of khat) that retains central stimulant character. N-Monomethylation of cathinone results in methcathinone or ephedrone ("CAT"; Figure 7)—a potent stimulant and drug of abuse. Structurally, methcathinone is to cathinone what methamphetamine is to amphetamine. In this manner, designer drugs have appeared that are structurally related to either the hallucinogens or stimulants. In many instances, their actions are what might have been expected on the basis of published SARs.

Not all designer drugs result in actions that are entirely predictable. One of the most popular of such agents is MDMA (Figure 7) or N-methyl-1-(3,4-methylenedioxyphenyl)-2-aminopropane (also called "Ecstasy," "XTC," "Adam," "X,"or "e"). MDMA is the N-monomethyl analog of MDA. On the basis of established SARs, it might be expected that

N-monomethylation of a phenylisopropylamine stimulant would enhance the amphetamine-like stimulant actions of MDA, whereas the same structural modification would diminish its hallucinogenic or DOM-like action. Although this appears to be the case, what emerged was an agent that, in addition to its stimulant character, also possesses an empathogenic action (producing increased empathy and sociability, as well as enhanced feelings of well-being). MDMA was used for several years as an adjunct to psychotherapy and then as a recreational drug before its emergency scheduling under the federal Controlled Substances Act as a Schedule I substance. This agent has been extensively investigated; while studies show that both optical isomers are active, the S(+)isomer is the more active (Nichols & Oberlender, 1989). A structurally related, but less popular, agent is its N-ethyl homolog MDE ("Eve"). The consensus today is that MDMA probably is an empathogen with amphetamine-like stimulant side effects. Homologation of the alpha-methyl group of phenylisopropylamine stimulants and hallucinogens typically diminishes their potency or abolishes their activity; however, the alpha-ethyl analog of MDMA, MBDB or N-methyl-1-(3,4-methylenedioxyphenyl)-2-aminobutane (Figure 7), retains MDMA-like actions, but lacks amphetamine-like central stimulant character (Nichols, 1986; Oberlender & Nichols, 1990).

In recent times, agents such as MDA, PMA, PMMA (see below), and others have been represented and sold as MDMA on the illicit drug market. Possibly because of the adverse cardiovascular effects associated with PMA or its potential neurotoxicity (Steele, Katz et al., 1992), there is growing concern among MDMA users about the authenticity of the drugs they use. Test kits and assays have been developed so that users can, at least to some extent, validate the authenticity of the substances.

An agent closely related in structure to MDMA is PMMA or N-methyl-1-(4-methoxyphenyl)-2-aminopropane (Figure 1). PMMA is a hybrid structure of two phenylisopropylamine stimulants: PMA and methamphetamine. Surprisingly, in contradiction to established stimulant SARs, PMMA lacks significant central stimulant actions. Unlike PMA and methamphetamine, PMMA is not recognized by (+)amphetamine-trained animals. PMMA has seen little human evaluation (Shulgin & Shulgin, 1991). Because PMMA is structurally related to metabolites of MDMA, it was examined in MDMA-trained animals; PMMA substituted for and was several-fold more potent than MDMA. PMMA has been suggested to be the structural parent of

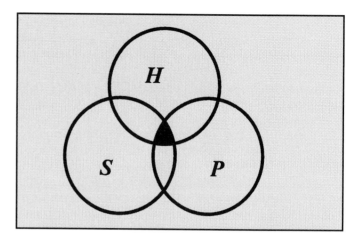

FIGURE 8. Venn diagram showing a relationship between the stimulus properties of hallucinogens (H), stimulants (S) and PMMA-like agents (P) (adapted from Glennon, Young et al., 1997). Some agents produce only one of the three possible effects, whereas other agents can produce multiple effects, such as stimulant and PMMA-like effects, that are best represented by the S/P intersect.

MDMA-like agents. Like MDMA, PMMA has been reported to produce neurotoxic effects in animals (Steele, Katz et al., 1992). Animals have been trained to discriminate PMMA from vehicle, and PMMA stimulus generalization occurs to (±)MDMA, S(+)MDMA, S(+)MBDB, R(-)MBDB, S(+)3,4-DMA, and R(-)3,4-DMA but not to DOM, (+)amphetamine, R(-)MDMA, or R(-)PMMA (Rangisetty, Bondarev et al., 2001). These results, coupled with the earlier discussion of MDMA, suggest that phenylisopropylamines might not be best described as being merely central stimulants or hallucinogens, but as possessing yet a third action that needs to be accounted for. This third type of effect, shared by PMMA and MBDB in animal studies, is one that requires further clinical investigation.

On the basis of drug discrimination studies, it has been proposed that phenylalkylamines with abuse potential can produce one or more of at least three distinct stimulus effects in animals: a hallucinogenic or DOM-like effect (H), a central stimulant or (+)amphetamine-like effect (S), and a PMMA-like effect (P) (Figure 8). This relationship is illustrated in Figure 2. Compounds such as DOM fall into the H category of the Venn diagram, whereas (+)amphetamine serves as the prototype of the S agents. The P category is typified by PMMA and MBDB. MDMA produces both PMMA-like and amphetamine-like effects and would fall into the S-P intersect. MDA has been shown to possess MDMA-like actions in addition to the hallucinogenic and stimulant actions described earlier. Hence, R(-)MDA falls into the *H-P* intersect, and S(+)MDA falls into the *S-P* intersect. Racemic MDA (that is, the combination of MDA optical isomers commonly encountered on the clandestine market) actually falls into the common intersect (shaded area of Figure 2) because it produces all three types of stimulus effects (Glennon & Young, 2002). Other agents recently demonstrated to produce a PMMA-like stimulus effect include R(-)PMA ("chicken powder," "white mitsubishi," "death"), and 4-MTA or 1-(4-methylthio)-phenylisopropylamine ("flatliners," "golden eagles") (Dukat, Young et al., 2002). It must be emphasized that this proposal was developed on the basis of animal studies; although it appears to describe the human actions of the agents, additional work, particularly in a clinical setting, obviously will be required to further substantiate the model. Nevertheless, the classification scheme suggests that there will be three different SARs and three different mechanisms of action. Certain agents, because they fall into more than one category, can represent mechanistic and structure-activity composites. The same can be said of indolealkylamine designer drugs; indeed, it may be the particular "mix" of actions that makes certain designer drugs attractive as drugs of abuse.

Recent evidence suggests that alpha-ethyltryptamine (alpha-ET, alpha-EtT, AET, "ET"; Figure 1) represents a novel agent of abuse that possesses several kinds of actions. alpha-ET was briefly marketed in the early 1960s as an antidepressant, but was withdrawn shortly after its introduction. alpha-ET acts as an MAO inhibitor, but it has been shown that alpha-ET is hallucinogenic in humans and also behaves as a central stimulant (Hoffer & Osmond, 1967; Murphree, Dippy et al., 1961). Until recently, an evaluation of the two optical isomers of alpha-ET had not been reported. It has now been shown that S(+)alpha-ET produces both DOM- and PMMA-like effects but not (+)amphetamine-like effects, whereas R(-)alpha-ET produces (+)amphetamine- and PMMA-like effects but not DOM-like effects; both optical isomers of alpha-ET produce MDMA-like actions (Glennon, 1999). The last is consistent with the mention of alpha-ET being sold as a substitute for MDMA (Martinez & Geyer, 1997). In the classification scheme shown in Figure 2, S(+)alpha-ET might best be described as falling into the *H-P* intersect, whereas R(-)alpha-ET falls into the *S-P* intersect.

Certain designer drugs, then, behave like serotonergic hallucinogens and hence involve a serotonergic mechanism. Others might produce more than one effect; that is, certain agents (for example, MDA) possess hallucinogenic character but also produce other effects. Evidence exists for the involvement of other serotonin receptor subpopulations in the actions of designer drugs. For example, as discussed below, the 5-HT_{1A} agonist 8-OH DPAT seems to potentiate the effect of DOM. In addition, 8-OH DPAT and both its optical isomers substitute for MDMA in animals trained to discriminate MDMA from vehicle (Glennon & Young, 2000). As a consequence, because MDMA and serotonergic hallucinogens sometimes are used in combination at "raves" for a heightened drug effect (a process known as "flipping" or "candy-flipping"), it has been suggested that this phenomenon may, at least in part, involve both a 5-HT_2 and a 5-HT_{1A} mechanism.

ABSORPTION AND METABOLISM

Few detailed studies have been conducted on the human metabolism of hallucinogenic agents. Simple indolealkylamines such as DMT and 5-OMe DMT undergo multiple routes of metabolism, including N-demethylation, cyclization to tetrahydro-beta-carbolines, and N-oxidation; however, their major route of metabolism is via oxidative deamination by monoamine oxidase (Barker, Littlefield-Chabaud et al., 2001). Substituted derivatives such as psilocybin also are hydrolyzed to psilocin, whereas certain methoxy derivatives might be O-demethylated. Most metabolic studies on LSD were conducted some time ago, when analytical techniques were not as refined as they are today. This fact, coupled with the small drug doses necessary to produce behavioral effects, has created some controversy about the exact structures of LSD metabolites formed after pharmacologically relevant LSD doses. A discussion of early studies is provided by Siva Sankar (1975).

Detailed investigations of the metabolism of phenylalkylamine hallucinogens also are lacking, but most phenylalkylamines are believed to be substrates for monoamine oxidase and cytochrome P450. DOM is one of the better investigated hallucinogens. The S(+)-isomer of DOM is metabolized more rapidly than its R(-)-enantiomer, and the aromatic methyl group is oxidized to the corresponding hydroxymethyl and, subsequently, carboxylate derivatives. DOM also is O-demethylated by rabbit liver homogenates to afford its 2-O-demethylated, 5-O-demethylated and 2,5-di-O-demethylated products (Zweig & Castagnoli, 1977). It has been suggested that the latter metabolite might undergo oxidation to a quinone and behave as a neurotoxin *in vivo* (Zweig & Castagnoli, 1977).

Various hallucinogenic and nonhallucinogenic phenyl-isopropylamines are substrates and/or inhibitors of human cytochrome P450 (CYP2D6) and their SARs have been investigated; methylenedioxy analogs, such as MDA and MDMA, display particularly high affinity for the enzyme (Wu, Otton et al., 1997).

Recent interest in MDMA has led to extensive investigations of its metabolism. One of the major metabolites of MDMA is its N-desmethyl analog, MDA. The methylenedioxy rings both of MDMA and MDA are attacked by cytochrome P450 to give ring-opened products: HHMA (N-methyl-3,4-dihydroxyamphetamine) and HHA (3,4-dihydroxyamphetamine), respectively. These dihydroxy compounds are O-methylated, primarily to HMMA (N-methyl-4-hydroxy-3-methoxyamphetamine) and HMA (4-hydroxy-3-methoxyamphetamine) (see Maurer, Bickeboeller-Friedrich et al., 2000, for a detailed description of the metabolism of MDA, MDMA, and the MDMA homologs MDE and MBDB, as well as the specific cyptochrome P450 isozymes involved in their metabolism). The major human urinary MDMA metabolite is HHMA (Segura, Ortuno et al., 2001).

PHARMACOLOGIC ACTIONS

Although the effects of various indolealkylamine hallucinogens are not necessarily identical, descriptions of DMT and psilocybin intoxication provide some idea of the actions associated with agents of this type. For example, recent studies suggest that intravenous administration of 0.3 mg/kg DMT produces a spectrum of "psychedelic" effects, including an abstract, rapidly moving, intensely colored, kaleidoscopic display of visual effects, transient anxiety, elation, and euphoria. On the other hand, cognition was relatively unimpaired, and there was a heightening of evaluative processes (Strassman, Qualls et al., 1996). Similar doses of DMT also produced increased heart rate and blood pressure, elevated prolactin and cortisol levels, and hyperthermia (Strassman, Qualls et al., 1996 and references therein). Psilocybin (0.25 mg/kg, orally) produced a psychotic syndrome that included disturbances of emotion and sensory perception, difficulty in thinking and reality appraisal, and loss of ego boundaries. Symptoms appeared 20 to 30 minutes after administration, peaked after another 30 to 40 minutes, and completely subsided after five or six hours. During the peak period, perceptual alterations included auditory and visual hallucinations ranging from illusions to complex scenery hallucinations (Vollenweider, Vontobel et al., 1999). Because of the rapid hydrolysis of psilocybin to

psilocin in humans (Hasler, Bourquin et al., 1997), it is quite likely that the effects observed after administration of the former are due to psilocin.

In general, the serotonergic hallucinogens produce alterations in thought, mood, and perception. Somewhat distinct from these effects are the actions of MDMA. Indeed, the designer drugs do not represent a homogeneous class of agents; that is, certain designer drugs are hallucinogens, some are stimulants, others are empathogens, and yet others can be of mixed action. Few of the designer drugs have been investigated in detail. However, several clinical investigations of MDMA have been reported; in them, MDMA has been found to produce a rather unique spectrum of effects that would not be considered "hallucinogenic" in nature. For example, the acute effects of MDMA include extroversion, heightened mood (heightened sense of confidence and well-being), dry mouth and increased thirst, difficulty in concentrating, impaired balance, dizziness, jaw clenching, lack of appetite, and restlessness (Liechti, Saur et al., 2000). Perceptual changes induced by MDMA are modest and consist primarily of intensification of tactile, visual, and acoustic perception and exclude hallucinations (Liechti, Saur et al., 2000).

MECHANISMS OF ACTION

An argument can be made that human subjects are best suited to provide the most reliable assessment of the actions and potency of hallucinogenic agents. Unfortunately, extensive human data, particularly data from well-controlled clinical studies with large subject populations, are available for only a very few agents (for example, LSD, DMT, and mescaline). The information available for most agents is derived from studies that involved limited subject populations and/or from studies that investigated only few drug doses, with or without proper controls. Some of what is known, and often cited, comes from anecdotal reports, from which even the identity or purity of the test material could not be authenticated. Today, for example, an enormous amount of anecdotal information on the human effects of hallucinogenic agents can be found on the Internet (Halpern & Pope, 2001), but such information (although it should not be ignored) must be considered in the proper context.

Very few clinical studies with psychotomimetic agents were sanctioned after the early 1960s. Although some limited human evaluation has resumed within the past decade (Strassman, 1996; Strassman, Qualls et al., 1996;

Vollenweider, Vollenweider-Scherpenhuyzen et al., 1998), for a period of about 30 years, information on hallucinogenic substances relied heavily on the use of animal studies, as it does today. Many attempts have been made to develop animal models of hallucinogenic activity but, to date, no single animal model accounts for the actions of these agents as a class (reviewed in Glennon, 1992). In contrast, one animal procedure that has found considerable application in the classification of hallucinogenic agents is the drug discrimination paradigm, which uses mostly rats as test subjects (reviewed in Glennon, Jarbe et al., 1991).

In a two-lever operant (or, less commonly, some other behavioral) procedure, animals can be trained to recognize or discriminate the stimulus effects of a specific training drug from vehicle. Once animals have reliably learned the stimulus, tests of *substitution* or *stimulus generalization* can be conducted. That is, novel agents can be administered to the trained animals; it is thought that if there is similarity between the constellation of effects produced by the training drug and the novel agent, the animals will respond on the training-drug-appropriate lever. In other words, animals trained to a specific training drug will respond in like manner when administered a novel agent that produces similar effects. The results can be quantitative as well as qualitative and, where substitution occurs, an estimation of potency (that is, an ED50 value) can be calculated.

This procedure does not represent a general model of hallucinogenic activity. In fact, the drug discrimination paradigm has seen broad application in the investigation of a wide variety of centrally acting agents and drugs of abuse (Colpaert & Slangen, 1982; Glennon, Jarbe et al., 1991). The procedure, although somewhat labor intensive, is very robust, and results generally are highly reproducible from laboratory to laboratory. With this procedure, large numbers of animals can be used, numerous drugs and drug doses can be evaluated, testing parameters can be widely manipulated, and mechanistic studies can be conducted. Many types of hallucinogens and psychoactive agents have been used as training drugs, and the results of such studies have contributed to the categorization of these agents. Animals can differentiate the effects of these agents, and it is presumed that they may be able to distinguish drug effects much in the same way that humans do. Animals trained to discriminate LSD, for example, do not recognize (substitute for, generalize to) phencyclidine (PCP), just as animals trained to discriminate PCP do not recognize LSD. Neither LSD- nor PCP-trained animals recognize tetrahydrocannabinol.

LSD-trained animals, however, recognize mescaline, DOM, and certain other hallucinogens. LSD and DOM have seen the most extensive application as training drugs for investigations of mechanism of action, classification, and SARs of hallucinogenic agents (Appel, White et al., 1982; Glennon, 1991, 1999). Through use of this technique, it has been possible to identify what are termed the "classical hallucinogens"—agents that share common (although not necessarily identical) stimulus character and that probably act by a shared mechanism of action (Glennon, 1999).

Knowledge about this class of drugs thus suffers from the conundrum that on the one hand, there are extensive, carefully controlled results from animal studies (in which something other than "hallucinogenic activity" *per se* was measured), whereas on the other hand, human data (which in theory should be the most reliable) are relatively scarce. Fortunately, for a number of classical hallucinogens, drug discrimination data have been shown to be significantly correlated with human hallucinogenic potency (Glennon, 1996).

LSD was one of the first hallucinogens to be investigated mechanistically; another agent to see extensive investigation is mescaline. Interestingly, from a potency perspective, these agents represent opposites. Over the years, LSD has been proposed to produce its hallucinogenic effects by numerous mechanisms and, in fact, some of the effects produced by LSD likely involve multiple mechanisms. That is, LSD binds with high affinity at many different receptor populations and acts as an agonist at some, an antagonist at others, and as a partial agonist at yet others. For many years, it was supposed that mescaline might be acting by a dopaminergic or adrenergic mechanism because of its structural similarity to dopamine and norepinephrine. As early as the late 1950s, it was speculated that LSD might be working through a serotonergic mechanism because of its structural resemblance to 5-HT (reviewed in Wooley, 1962). Significant experimental evidence supported this claim. However, there was controversy as to whether LSD is a serotonergic agonist or antagonist. Moreover, subsequent studies showed that seven populations of 5-HT receptors exist (that is, 5-HT_1 to 5-HT_7) and that several are composed of subpopulations. It now has been demonstrated that the serotonergic hallucinogens bind at 5-HT_2 receptors and behave as agonists (Glennon, 1996).

With the development of 5-HT_2-selective antagonists, it was demonstrated that several of these antagonists (for example, ketanserin and pirenperone) were particularly effective in blocking the stimulus effects of DOM, and/or of DOM-stimulus generalization to other hallucinogens such as LSD, in tests of stimulus antagonism. It was later shown that the classical hallucinogens bind at 5-HT$_2$ serotonin receptors and that their receptor affinities are significantly correlated with both their DOM-stimulus generalization potencies and their human hallucinogenic potencies (reviewed in Glennon, 1996). Today, the classical hallucinogens are thought to produce their effect by acting as agonists at 5-HT$_2$ receptors in the brain—the 5-HT$_2$ hypothesis of hallucinogen action. Radiolabeled analogs of DOB and its iodinated counterpart DOI (for example, [^{3}H]DOB, [^{125}I]DOI) currently are available for the investigation of 5-HT$_2$ pharmacology.

More recently, it was demonstrated that 5-HT$_2$ receptors actually represent a family of 5-HT receptors consisting of 5-HT$_{2A}$, 5-HT$_{2B}$, and 5-HT$_{2C}$ receptor subpopulations. Fewer than three dozen arylalkylamines have been compared, but it appears that they show little selectivity for one subpopulation over the others (Nelson, Lucaites et al., 1999). Various pharmacologic studies with selective antagonists (Ismaiel, De Los Angeles et al., 1993; Nelson, Lucaites et al., 1999; Schreiber, Brocco et al., 1994) or studies using antagonist correlation analysis (Fiorella, Rabin et al., 1995), however, suggest that the 5-HT$_{2A}$ subtype plays a predominant role in the behavioral actions of these agents. Although 5-HT$_{2A}$ receptors might be responsible for the actions that the classical hallucinogens have in common, it may be that other neurochemical mechanisms account for their differences. For example, LSD is a very promiscuous agent that binds with high affinity at many receptor populations for which most other classical hallucinogens show little to no affinity. Many of the indolealkylamines bind with high affinity at multiple populations of 5-HT receptors, and some display comparable or higher affinity at those receptors (for example, 5-HT$_{1A}$, h5-HT$_{1D}$, 5-HT$_6$) than they do at 5-HT$_{2A}$ receptors. The phenylalkylamines are quite selective for 5-HT$_2$ receptors, but display little selectivity for the 3 5-HT$_2$ subpopulations. Some beta-carbolines, although they bind at 5-HT$_2$ receptors (Glennon, Dukat et al., 2000), possess activity as MAO inhibitors (Hoffer & Osmond, 1967); alpha-ET is an MAO inhibitor (Hoffer & Osmond, 1967). Thus, these differences might account for their somewhat different actions.

Other neurotransmitter mechanisms also may contribute to the actions of the hallucinogens. For example, although DOM does not bind at 5-HT$_{1A}$ receptors, the 5-HT$_{1A}$ agonist 8-hydroxy-2-(N,N-di-*n*-propylamino)tetralin (8-OH DPAT) can enhance the stimulus potency of DOM (Glennon, 1996). In similar fashion, PCP, which does not bind at 5-HT$_{2A}$ receptors, potentiates the actions of DOM (Rabin, Doat et al., 2000). Interaction of hallucinogens with 5-HT$_{2A}$ receptors thus may be too simplistic an explanation to account for all the actions of the serotonergic hallucinogens. However, the one feature that all these hallucinogens have in common (that is, the common component hypothesis) is that they bind at 5-HT$_{2A}$ receptors.

Although the 5-HT$_2$ hypothesis of classical hallucinogen action was first proposed in 1984 (Glennon, Titeler et al., 1984), it was not for another 15 years that clinical results in support of the hypothesis would become available. Volenweider and colleagues (1998) subsequently demonstrated that the 5-HT$_2$ antagonist ketanserin dose dependently antagonizes the psychotomimetic effects of psylocibin in healthy human volunteers.

MDMA is not usually considered to produce hallucinogenic effects. However, MDMA is metabolized, at least in part, to MDA, and MDA is a weak hallucinogenic agent. Consistent with this concept, MDMA has been reported to produce "slight hallucinogen-like effects," consisting of increased vividness of perception, including an intensification of colors and tactile awareness (Liechti, Saur et al., 2000). These MDMA-induced perceptual alterations, as well as the hyperthermic actions of MDMA—hyperthermia also being a consequence of 5-HT$_2$ agonism (Glennon, 1992)—were attenuated by pretreatment of human volunteers with ketanserin (Liechti, Saur et al., 2000).

ADDICTION LIABILITY

Although relatively few studies have been conducted, serotonergic hallucinogens are not generally considered to possess amphetamine-like or cocaine-like reinforcing properties on the basis of self-administration studies. There are a few exceptions, notably MDMA and MDA. MDMA is self-administered by nonhuman primates (Beardsley, Balster et al., 1986; Lamb & Griffiths, 1987) and produces conditioned place preference in rats (Marona-Lewicka, Rhee et al., 1996). MDA is self-administered by baboons (Griffiths, Winger et al., 1976) and rats (Markert & Roberts, 1991), but is about 20 to 30 times less potent than (+)amphetamine (Griffiths, Winger et al., 1976). Perhaps these agents stand apart from most other serotonergic hallucinogens because MDMA is metabolized, at least to some extent, to MDA, and both MDMA and MDA have been demonstrated to possess amphetaminergic character. Referring to Figure 8, agents classified as hallucinogens (that is, those falling into the "*H*" category) likely lack reinforcing properties, whereas those classified as "*S*" (for example, amphetamine and methamphetamine) are reinforcing. Because the "*S-P*"-type agents MDA and MDMA are reinforcing, although somewhat less so than amphetamine, this category of agents also might be associated with reinforcing properties. A recent interesting, and concerning, finding is that preexposure to MDMA facilitates acquisition of cocaine self-administration in rats, leading to speculation that MDMA users might be at risk for developing psychomotor stimulant abuse (Fletcher, Robinson et al., 2001).

TOXICITY/ADVERSE EFFECTS

MDMA is one of the first phenylalkylamines shown to produce neurotoxic effects in animals and has become a major target of investigation. The neurotoxicity of MDMA and other phenylalkylamines has been reviewed (Curran, 2000; Gibb, Johnson et al., 1997; Kalant, 2001; Morgan, 2000; Seiden & Sabol, 1996). High-dose MDMA users, in particular, run a significant risk of persistent cognitive impairment and disturbances of affect and personality (Morgan, 2000). The possibility cannot be excluded that these sequellae might be a result of the neurotoxic actions of MDMA. MDMA has been shown to destroy brain serotonin neurons in animals by creating long-lasting decrements in the number of axon terminals, decreasing the major metabolite of serotonin—5-hydroxyindoleacetic acid (5-HIAA), and interfering with the rate-limiting 5-HT biosynthetic enzyme tryptophan hydroxylase and the 5-HT reuptake transporter (SERT). Studies with humans also indicate that some MDMA users may have selective decrements in cerebrospinal 5-HIAA and SERT levels and that humans with a history of MDMA use show lasting decrements in global brain transporter binding (Ricaurte, McCann et al., 2000). It has been suggested that reactive metabolites (Bai, Jones et al., 2001) of MDA and MDMA, such as HHMA (Segura, Ortuno et al., 2001), or free radicals derived from MDMA, might play important roles in producing the neurotoxic effect.

ACKNOWLEDGMENT: Work from the author's laboratory was supported by U.S. Public Health Service grants DA 01642 and DA-09153.

REFERENCES

Appel JB, White FJ & Holohean AM (1982). Analyzing mechanism(s) of hallucinogenic drug action with drug discrimination procedures. *Neuroscience and Biobehavioral Reviews* 6(4):529-536.

Bai F, Jones DC, Lau SS et al. (2001). Serotonergic neurotoxicity of 3,4-(±)-methylenedioxyamphetamine and 3,4-(±)-methylenedioxymethamphetamine (ecstasy) is potentiated by inhibition of gamma-glutamyl transpeptidase. *Chemical Research in Toxicology* 14(7):863-870.

Barker SA, Littlefield-Chabaud MA & David C (2001). Distribution of the hallucinogens N,N-dimethyltryptamine and 5-methoxy-N,N-dimethyltryptamine in rat brain following intraperitoneal injection: Application of a new solid-phase extraction LC-APcI-MS-MS-isotope dilution method. *Journal of Chromatography; B. Biomedical Scientific Applications* 751(1):37-47.

Beardsley PM, Balster RL & Harris LS (1986). Self-administration of methylenedioxymethamphetamine (MDMA) by rhesus monkeys. *Drug and Alcohol Dependence* 18:149-157.

Brimblecombe RW & Pinder RM (1975). *Hallucinogenic Agents.* Bristol, England: Wright-Scientechnica.

Colpaert FC & Slangen JL, eds. (1982). *Drug Discrimination: Applications in CNS Pharmacology.* Amsterdam, The Netherlands: Elsevier.

Curran HV (2000). Is MDMA ('Ecstasy') neurotoxic in humans? An overview of evidence and of methodological problems in research. *Neuropsychobiology* 42:34-41.

Dukat M, Young R & Glennon RA (2002). Effect of PMA optical isomers and 4-MTA in PMMA-trained rats. *Pharmacology Biochemistry and Behavior* 72:299-305.

Fiorella D, Rabin RA & Winter JC (1995). The role of the 5-HT$_{2A}$ and 5-HT$_{2C}$ receptors in the stimulus effects of hallucinogenic drugs. I: Antagonist correlation analysis. *Psychopharmacology* (Berl) 121(3):347-356.

Fletcher PJ, Robinson SR & Slippoy DL (2001). Pre-exposure to (±)3,4-methylenedioxymethamphetamine (MDMA) facilitates acquisition of intravenous cocaine self-administration in rats. *Neuropsychopharmacology* 25:195-203.

Gibb JW, Johnson M, Elayan I et al. (1997). Neurotoxicity of amphetamines and their metabolites. In RS Rapaka, N Chiang & BR Martin (eds.) *Pharmacokinetics, Metabolism, and Pharmaceutics of Drugs of Abuse (NIDA Research Monograph 173).* Rockville, MD: National Institute on Drug Abuse, 128-145.

Glennon RA (1989). Synthesis and evaluation of amphetamine analogs. In M Klein, F Sapienza, H McClain et al. (eds.) *Clandestinely Produced Drugs, Analogues, and Precursors.* Washington DC: U.S. Department of Justice, Drug Enforcement Administration, 39-65.

Glennon RA (1991). Discriminative stimulus properties of hallucinogens and related designer drugs. In RA Glennon, TUC Jarbe & J Frankenheim (eds.) *Drug Discrimination: Applications to Drug Abuse Research (NIDA Research Monograph 116).* Rockville, MD: National Institute on Drug Abuse, 25-44.

Glennon RA (1992). Animal models for assessing hallucinogenic agents. In AA Boulton, GB Baker & PH Wu (eds.) *Animal Models of Drug Addiction.* Totowa, NJ: Humana Press, 345-381.

Glennon RA (1996). Classical hallucinogens. In CR Schuster & MJ Kuhar (eds.) *Pharmacological Aspects of Drug Dependence.* Berlin, Germany: Springer, 343-371.

Glennon RA (1998). Pharmacology of hallucinogens. In RE Tarter, RA Ammerman & PJ Ott (eds.) *Handbook of Substance Abuse. Neurobehavioral Pharmacology.* New York, NY: Plenum Press, 217-227.

Glennon RA (1999). Arylalkylamine drugs of abuse: An overview of drug discrimination studies. *Pharmacology, Biochemistry and Behavior* 64:251-256.

Glennon RA, Dukat M, Grella B et al. (2000). Binding of beta-carbolines and related agents at serotonin (5-HT$_2$ and 5-HT$_{1A}$), dopamine (D$_2$) and benzodiazepine receptors. *Drug and Alcohol Dependence* 60:121-132.

Glennon RA, Jarbe TUC & Frankenheim J, eds. (1991). *Drug Discrimination: Applications to Drug Abuse Research (NIDA Research Monograph 116).* Rockville, MD: National Institute on Drug Abuse.

Glennon RA, Titeler M & McKenney JD (1984). Evidence for 5-HT$_2$ involvement in the mechanism of action of hallucinogenic agents. *Life Sciences* 35:2505-2511.

Glennon RA & Young R (2002). Effect of 1-(3,4-methylenedioxyphenyl)-2-aminopropane and its optical isomers in PMMA-trained rats. *Pharmacology, Biochemistry and Behavior* 72:379-387.

Glennon RA & Young R (2000). MDMA stimulus generalization to the 5-HT$_{1A}$ serotonin agonist 8-hydroxy-2-(di-*n*-propylamino)tetralin. *Pharmacology, Biochemistry and Behavior* 66(3):483-488.

Glennon RA, Young R, Dukat M et al. (1997). Initial characterization of PMMA as a discriminative stimulus. *Pharmacology Biochemistry and Behavior* 57:151-158.

Grella B, Dukat M, Young R et al. (1998). Investigation of hallucinogenic and related beta-carbolines. *Drug and Alcohol Dependence* 50:99-107.

Griffiths RR, Winger G, Brady JV et al. (1976). Comparison of behavior maintained by infusions of eight phenylethylamines in baboons. *Psychopharmacologia* 24:251-258.

Halpern JH & Pope HG Jr (2001). Hallucinogens on the internet: A vast new source of underground drug information. *American Journal of Psychiatry* 158(3):481-483.

Hasler P, Bourquin D, Brenneisen R et al. (1997). Determination of psilocin and 4-hydroxyindole-3-acetic acid in plasma by HPLC-ECD and pharmacokinetic profiles or oral and intravenous psilocybin in man. *Pharmaceutica Acta Helvetica* 72:175-184.

Helsley S, Fiorella D, Rabin RA et al. (1998). A comparison of N,N-dimethyl tryptamine, harmaline, and selected congeners in rats trained with LSD as a discriminative stimulus. *Progress in Neuropsychopharmacology and Biological Psychiatry* 22(4):649-663.

Helsley S, Rabin RA & Winter JC (1998). The effects of beta-carbolines in rats trained with ibogaine as discriminative stimulus. *European Journal of Pharmacology* 345(2):139-143.

Hoffer A & Osmond H (1967). *The Hallucinogens.* New York, NY: Academic Press.

Hollister LE (1968). *Chemical Psychoses.* Springfield, IL: Charles C. Thomas.

Ismaiel AM, De Los Angeles J, Teitler M et al. (1993). Antagonism of 1-(2,5-dimethoxy-4-methylphenyl)-2-aminopropane stimulus with a newly identified 5-HT$_2$- versus 5-HT$_{1C}$-selective antagonist. *Journal of Medicinal Chemistry* 36:2519-2525.

Jacob P III & Shulgin AT (1994). Structure-activity relationships of classical hallucinogens and their analogs. In LC Lin & RA Glennon (eds.) *Hallucinogens: An Update (NIDA Research Monograph 146).* Rockville, MD: National Institute on Drug Abuse, 74-91.

Jacobs BL, ed. (1984). *Hallucinogens: Neurochemical, Behavioral, and Clinical Perspectives.* New York, NY: Raven Press.

Kalant H (2001). The pharmacology and toxicology of "ecstasy" (MDMA) and related drugs. *Canadian Medical Association Journal* 165:917-928.

Lamb R & Griffiths RR (1987). Self-injections of d-3,4-methylenedioxymethamphetamine (MDMA) in the baboon. *Psychopharmacology* 91:268-272.

Liechti ME, Saur MR, Gamma A et al. (2000). Psychological and physiological effects of MDMA ("Ecstasy") after pretreatment with the 5-HT2 antagonist ketanserin in healthy humans. *Neuropsychopharmacology* 23:396-404.

Lin JC & Glennon RA, eds. (1994). *Hallucinogens: An Update (NIDA Research Monograph 146).* Rockville, MD: National Institute on Drug Abuse.

Markert LE & Roberts DCS (1991). 3,4-Methylenedioxy amphetamine (MDA) self-administration and neurotoxicity. *Pharmacology, Biochemistry and Behavior* 39:569-574.

Marona-Lewicka D, Rhee GS, Sprague JE et al. (1996). Reinforcing effects of serotonin-releasing amphetamine derivatives. *Pharmacology, Biochemistry and Behavior* 53:99-105.

Martinez DL & Geyer MA (1997). Characterization of the disruptions of prepulse inhibition and habituation of startle induced by alpha-ethyltryptamine. *Neuropsychopharmacology* 16:246-255.

Maurer HH, Bickeboeller-Friedrich J, Kraemer T et al. (2000). Toxicokinetics and analytical toxicology of amphetamine-derived designer drugs ('Ecstasy'). *Toxicology Letters* 112-113:133-142.

Morgan MJ (2000). Ecstasy (MDMA): A review of its possible persistent psychological effects. *Psychopharmacology* 152:230-248.

Murphree HB, Dippy RH, Jenney EH et al. (1961). Effects in normal man of alpha-methyltryptamine and alpha-ethyltryptamine. *Clinical Pharmacology and Therapeutics* 2:722-726.

Naranjo C (1967). Psychotropic properties of harmala alkaloids. In DK Efron, B Holmstedt & NS Kline (eds.) *Ethnopharmacologic Search for Psychoactive Drugs.* Washington DC: U.S. Government Printing Office, 385-391.

Naranjo C (1973). *The Healing Journey.* New York, NY: Pantheon Books.

Nelson DL, Lucaites VL, Wainscot DB et al. (1999). Comparisons of hallucinogenic phenylisopropylamine binding affinities at cloned human 5-HT$_{2A}$, 5-HT$_{2B}$, and 5-HT$_{2C}$ receptors. *Naunyn-Schmiedeberg's Archives of Pharmacology* 359:1-6.

Nichols DE (1986). Differences between the mechanism of action of MDMA, MBDB, and the classical hallucinogens: Identification of a new therapeutic class: Entactogens. *Journal of Psychoactive Drugs* 18:305-313.

Nichols DE & Glennon RA (1984). Medicinal chemistry and structure-activity relationships of hallucinogens. In BL Jacobs (ed.) *Hallucinogens: Neurochemical, Behavioral, and Clinical Perspectives.* New York, NY: Raven Press, 95-142.

Nichols DE & Oberlender R (1989). Structure-activity relationships of MDMA-like substances. In K Ashgar & E De Souza (eds.) *Pharmacology and Toxicology of Amphetamine and Related Designer Drugs (NIDA Research Monograph 94).* Rockville, MD: National Institute on Drug Abuse, 1-29.

Oberlender R & Nichols DE (1990). (+)N-Methyl-1-(1,3-benzodioxol-5-yl)-2-butanamine as a discriminative stimulus in studies of 3,4-methylenedioxyamphetamine-like behavioral activity. *Journal of Pharmacology and Experimental Therapeutics* 255:1098-1106.

Pellerin C (1998). *Trips.* New York, NY: Seven Stories Press.

Pfaff RC, Huang X, Marona-Lewicka D et al. (1994). Lysergamides revisited. In JC Lin & RA Glennon (eds.) *Hallucinogens: An Update (NIDA Research Monograph 146).* Rockville, MD: National Institute on Drug Abuse, 52-73.

Rabin RA, Doat M & Winter JC (2000). Role of serotonergic 5-HT$_{2A}$ receptors in the psychotomimetic actions of phencyclidine. *International Journal of Neuropsychopharmacology* 3:333-338.

Rangisetty JB, Bondarev ML, Chang-Fong J et al. (2001). PMMA-stimulus generalization to the optical isomers of MBDB and 3,4-DMA. *Pharmacology, Biochemistry and Behavior* 69:261-267.

Ricaurte GA, McCann UD, Szabo Z et al. (2000). Toxicodynamics and long-term toxicity of the recreational drug, 3,4-methylenedioxymethamphetamine (MDMA, "Ecstasy"). *Toxicology Letters* 112-113:143-146.

Schreiber R, Brocco M & Millan MJ (1994). Blockade of the discriminative stimulus effects of DOI by MDL 100,907 and the "atypical" antipsychotics, clozapine and risperidone. *European Journal of Pharmacology* 264(1):99-102.

Schuster CR & Kuhar MJ, eds. (1996). *Pharmacological Aspects of Drug Dependence.* Berlin, Germany: Springer.

Segura M, Ortuno J, Farre M et al. (2001). 3,4-Dihydroxymethamphetamine (HHMA). A major in vivo 3,4-methylenedioxymethamphetamine (MDMA) metabolite in humans. *Chemical Research in Toxicology* 14:1203-1208.

Seiden LS & Sabol KE (1996). Methamphetamine and methylenedioxymethamphetamine: Possible mechanisms of cell destruction. In MD Majewska (ed.) *Neuropathology and Neurotoxicity Associated with Cocaine/Stimulant Abuse (NIDA Research Monograph 163).* Rockville, MD: National Institute on Drug Abuse, 251-276.

Shulgin AT & Shulgin A (1991). *Pihkal.* Berkeley, CA: Transform Press.

Shulgin AT & Shulgin A (1997). *Tihkal.* Berkeley, CA: Transform Press.

Siva Sankar DV, ed. (1975). *LSD–A Total Study.* Westbury, NY: PJD Press.

Steele TD, Katz JL & Ricaurte GA (1992). Evaluation of the neurotoxicity of N-methyl-1-(4-methoxyphenyl)-2-aminopropane (para-methoxymethamphetamine, PMMA). *Brain Research* 589(2):349-352.

Strassman RJ (1996). Human psychopharmacology of N,N-dimethyltryptamine. *Behavioral Brain Research* 73(1-2):121-124.

Strassman RJ, Qualls CR & Berg LM (1996). Differential tolerance to biological and subjective effects of four closely spaced doses of N,N-dimethyltryptamine in humans. *Biological Psychiatry* 39(9):784-795.

Vollenweider FX, Vollenweider-Scherpenhuyzen MF, Babler A et al. (1998). Psylocybin induces schizophrenia-like psychosis in humans via a serotonin-2 agonist action. *Neuroreport* 9:3897-3902.

Vollenweider FX, Vontobel P, Hell D et al. (1999). 5-HT modulation of dopamine release in basal ganglia in psilocybin-induced psychosis in man—A PET study with [^{11}C]raclopride. *Neuropsychopharmacology* 20:425-433.

Wooley DW (1962). *The Biochemical Bases of Psychoses.* New York, NY: John Wiley & Sons.

Wu D, Otton V, Inaba T et al. (1997). Interactions of amphetamine analogs with human liver CYP2D6. *Biochemical Pharmacology* 53:1605-1612.

Young R & Glennon RA (1996). A three-lever operant procedure differentiates the stimulus effects of R(-)-MDA from S(+)-MDA. *Journal of Pharmacology and Experimental Therapeutics* 276:594-601.

Zweig JS & Castagnoli N (1977). In vitro O-demethylation of the psychotomimetic amine 1-(2,5-dimethoxy-4-methylphenyl)-2-aminopropane. *Journal of Medicinal Chemistry* 20:414-419.

Lysergic Acid Diethylamide (LSD) and Other Classical Psychedelics

Gantt P. Galloway, Pharm.D.

Commonly used classical psychedelics are lysergic acid diethylamide ("LSD," "acid"), psilocybin-containing mushrooms ("shrooms"), and 2,5-dimethoxy-4-bromo-phenethylamine ("2C-B," "Nexus"). Of these, LSD is the most potent, most readily available, and least expensive. For these reasons, it also is the most often misrepresented as other psychedelics.

ADDICTION LIABILITY

The addiction liability of these drugs appears to be extremely low, with essentially no one presenting to addiction treatment for such dependence. In fact, the more salient issue is the potential efficacy of psychedelics in the treatment of drug and alcohol dependence. Data suggesting that psychedelic-assisted psychotherapy is effective in the treatment of addictive disease date to the 1950s, but conclusive evidence is lacking (Grinspoon & Bakalar, 1997; Mangini, 1998).

Recent attention has focused on the African psychedelic ibogaine, which is used in a few treatment programs outside the United States (Mash, Kovera et al., 2000). In addition to the psychological mechanisms postulated for other classical psychedelics—enhanced insight and personality restructuring—ibogaine reportedly prevents withdrawal symptoms from, and craving for, drugs of abuse (notably opiates). However, the safety and efficacy of psychedelics in the treatment of addiction have not been rigorously evaluated, so they cannot be recommended for use outside of research protocols.

TOXICITY/ADVERSE EFFECTS

Classical psychedelics have a high margin of safety with respect to adverse physical effects, but acute adverse psychiatric effects do occur, notably anxiety and disorientation. Conditions leading to these adverse effects are unpredictable, but are more likely to occur in inexperienced users, with higher doses, and in environments with abundant stimuli or that users find unfamiliar or distressing. Most patients with these symptoms can be treated effectively with "talk-down" therapy, which involves minimizing stimulation (dim lighting, low noise level, minimal foot traffic) and providing nonjudgmental support.

Individuals who experience an intense psychedelic reaction may not recall that they are under the influence of a drug or may not remember that the effects are time-limited. A reminder of the external, transitory cause of their distress may be salutary. If talk-down therapy does not provide sufficient relief of symptoms, intramuscular administration of 2 mg haloperidol and 2 mg lorazepam, along with continued nonjudgmental support, has been reported to be effective (Miller, Gay et al., 1992).

Use of psychedelics does not seem to be associated with a significantly increased risk of persistent psychosis (Strassman, 1984) or cognitive impairment (Halpern & Pope, 1999). However, hallucinogen persisting perception disorder (HPPD) does occur rarely after use of classical psychedelics (Abraham & Aldridge, 1993). HPPD is characterized by visual distortions reminiscent of those seen while under the influence of psychedelics, may have a delayed onset after the last use of a psychedelic, and may either resolve in weeks or persist for decades. Anxiety can precipitate or worsen symptoms of HPPD, and HPPD symptoms can cause anxiety. Limited data suggest that selective serotonin reuptake inhibitors can be useful in the treatment of HPPD (Young, 1997).

REFERENCES

Abraham H & Aldridge A (1993). Adverse consequences of lysergic acid diethylamide. *Addiction* 88:1327-1334.

Grinspoon L & Bakalar B (1997). *Psychedelic Drugs Reconsidered*. New York, NY: The Lindesmith Center.

Halpern J & Pope H (1999). Do hallucinogens cause residual neuropsychological toxicity? *Drug and Alcohol Dependence* 53:247-256.

Mangini M (1998). Treatment of alcoholism using psychedelic drugs: A review of the program of research. *Journal of Psychoactive Drugs* 30(4):381-418.

Mash D, Kovera C, Pablo J et al. (2000). Ibogaine: Complex pharmacokinetics, concerns for safety, and preliminary efficacy measures. *Annals of the New York Academy of Sciences* 914:394-401.

Miller P, Gay G, Ferris KC et al. (1992). Treatment of acute, adverse psychedelic reactions: "I've tripped and I can't get down." *Journal of Psychoactive Drugs* 24(3):277-279.

Strassman R (1984). Adverse reactions to psychedelic drugs: A review of the literature. *Journal of Nervous and Mental Disorders* 172:577-595.

Young C (1997). Sertraline treatment of hallucinogen persisting perception disorder. *Journal of Clinical Psychiatry* 58:85.

Chapter 10

The Pharmacology of NMDA Antagonists: Psychotomimetics and Dissociative Anesthetics

Edward F. Domino, M.D.

Drugs in the Class
Absorption and Metabolism
Pharmacologic Actions
Mechanisms of Action
Addiction Liability
Toxicity/Adverse Effects

A number of heterogeneous chemicals are antagonists of the N-methyl-D-aspartate (NMDA) receptor subtype of the major excitatory neurotransmitter, glutamic acid, in the brain. These substances include various arylcyclohexylamines (of which phencyclidine and ketamine are best known), dizocilpine (MK-801), and—perhaps surprisingly—the gaseous anesthetic, nitrous oxide. Ketamine and nitrous oxide are used clinically in animals and humans as anesthetics.

Most of the known NMDA antagonists are drugs of abuse when used in subanesthetic doses/concentrations. Subanesthetic doses of phencyclidine and ketamine induce a psychotomimetic state, which resembles many of the signs and symptoms of schizophrenia. Nitrous oxide or "laughing gas" has not yet been classified as a psychotomimetic. Its euphoric and dysphoric properties have been known for more than 200 years but have not been well studied by psychiatrists.

This chapter reviews the known pharmacology of these diverse substances, which have multiple mechanisms of action, primarily including NMDA receptor antagonism.

DRUGS IN THE CLASS

The chemical structures of abused arylcyclohexylamines are shown in Figure 1. Phencyclidine and ketamine are the principal abused compounds. Gas chromatographic-mass spectrometric assays are needed to positively identify each specific arylcyclohexylamine, and they may not be easily available to the clinician.

Therapeutic Use and Misuse. The discovery of phencyclidine, or PCP, has been well documented by those involved with its development (Domino, 1981a). The drug was developed as an intravenous anesthetic. The unique anesthesia it produced was complicated by a prolonged emergence delirium; this quickly led to its demise as a clinically useful agent. Phencyclidine caused symptoms of sensory deprivation, which is an excellent drug model of schizophrenia. Its trade name was Sernyl® or Sernylan®. Years later, phencyclidine was rediscovered by the drug abuse community in the form of "PCP," "Angel Dust," "Hog," and "Crystal" (Domino, 1981b).

The desirable anesthetic properties of Sernyl were retained in the short-acting arylcyclohexylamine derivative

FIGURE 1. Chemical Structures of Abused Arylcyclohexylamines

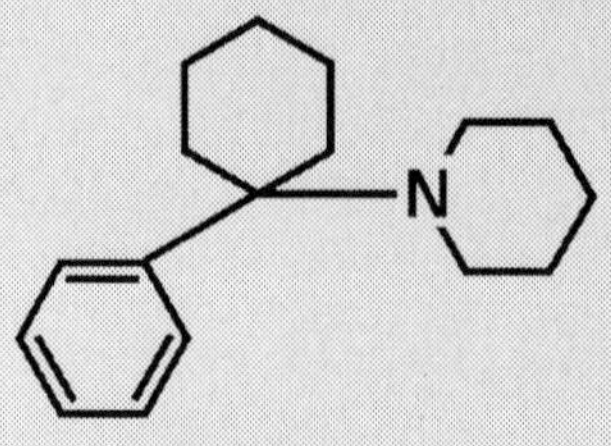

Phencyclidine (PCP)
1-(phenylcyclohexyl) piperidine

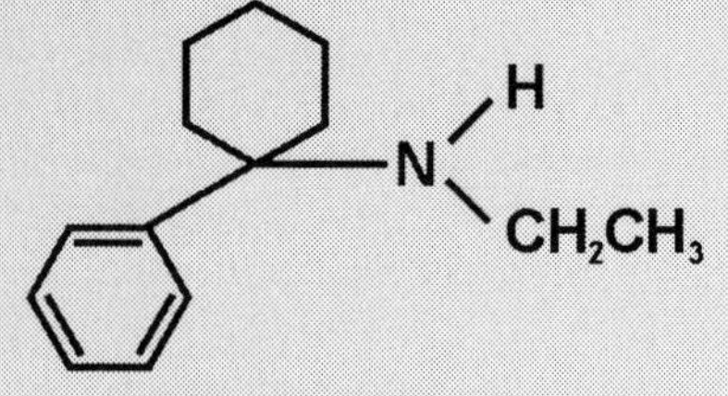

Cyclohexamine (PCE)
N-ethyl-1-phenylcyclohexylamine
(CI-400)

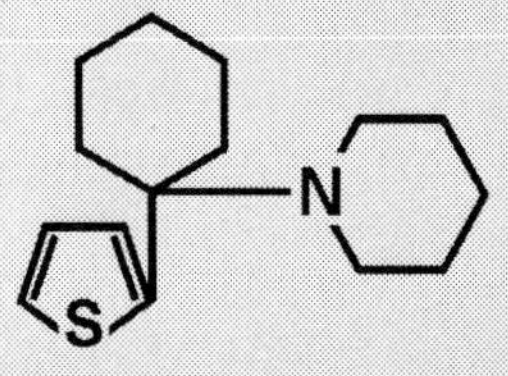

TCP
1-(1-2-thienylcyclohexyl) piperidine

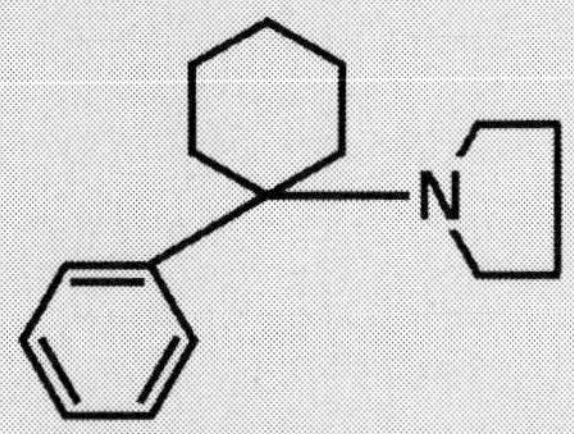

PHP
1-(1-phenylcyclohexyl) pyrrolidine

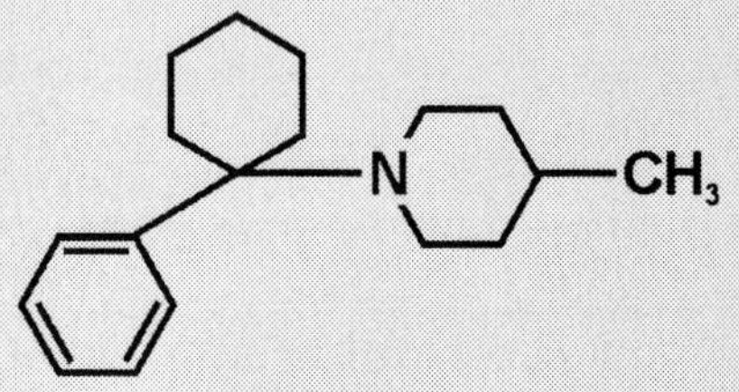

4-Methyl pip PCP
1-(phenylcyclohexyl)-4-methylpiperidine

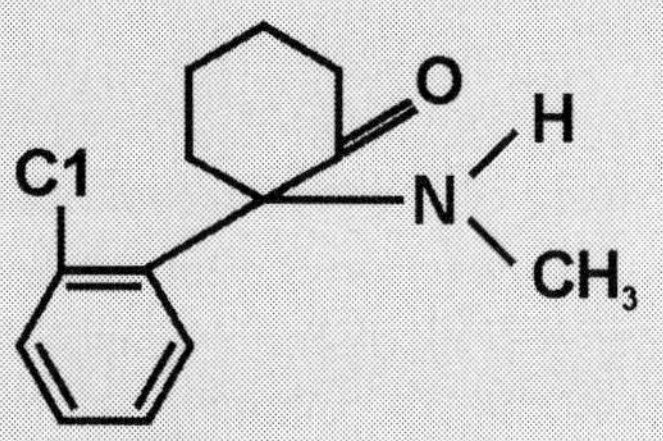

Ketamine
1-(o-chlorophenyl)-2-methylamine
cyclohexanone (CI-581)

ketamine (Ketalar®), which produced a much briefer emergence delirium. The term "dissociative anesthetic" was coined to emphasize that the anesthetized patient was "disconnected" from his or her environment. Ketamine subsequently was discovered by the drug abuse community, where it is known as "K," "Super K," "Special K," and "Cat Valium." Phencyclidine has been placed in Schedule I of the federal Controlled Substance Act, and ketamine in Schedule II. Several other arylcyclohexylamines available in illicit trade also are Schedule I substances.

Arylcyclohexylamine abuse occurs primarily in large metropolitan areas. Because the drugs are easy to synthesize, they are relatively inexpensive substitutes for many street drugs. The user may not realize that he or she has used an arylcyclohexylamine, because the drugs frequently are misrepresented as LSD, amphetamine, or synthetic marijuana.

Nitrous oxide has been known for more than 226 years. It is widely used today in anesthesia. In addition, its recreational use as "laughing gas" has been well described since it first was discovered.

Ketamine and nitrous oxide still are used in humans as anesthetic agents. Ketamine is used in circumstances in which other anesthetic agents are relatively contraindicated. In contrast, nitrous oxide is widely used today as part of the mixture of anesthetics used to achieve "balanced anesthesia."

In contrast to the arylcyclohexylamines, MK-801 (dizocilpine) was developed as an anticonvulsant (Troupin, Mendius et al., 1986) and subsequently was used as a brain protective agent; however, it was discarded because of its PCP-like effects (Piercey, Hoffman et al., 1988). Clinical trials of MK-801 have been extremely limited, and the results are not publicly available. Very little is known of its properties in humans.

The desirable "brain protective" properties of NMDA antagonists have been pursued slightly by the pharmaceutical industry in developing relatively weak derivatives of amantadine, dextromethorphan, and other so-called sigma agonists and antagonists. For example, amantadine is an antiviral agent used in the prophylaxis and therapy of influenza A. Patients with Parkinson's disease who took amantadine reported that it improved their motor symptoms. The mechanism of action of amantadine is unclear, but may include dopamine release or blockade of its reuptake and possible muscarinic anticholinergic action. Amantadine and a related compound, memantadine, have been shown to be NMDA receptor antagonists (Stoof, Booij et al., 1992), but are relatively weak and do not appear to be abused.

Dextromethorphan is an antitussive agent. When taken in very large amounts, it produces dysphoric mental effects that can be related to its weak NMDA antagonistic properties.

ABSORPTION AND METABOLISM

Baselt (2000) summarized much of the known data on the blood concentrations, pharmacokinetics biotransformation, and toxicity of the arylcyclohexylamines phencyclidine and ketamine. The pharmacokinetics of phencyclidine in humans never have been well studied with small psychoactive doses using modern methods. Blood phencyclidine concentrations from 7 to 240 ng/mL (mean, 75) were found in arrested persons intoxicated in public or driving under its influence. The blood/plasma concentration ratio is 1. The plasma $t_{1/2}$ of phencyclidine has been reported to vary from 7 to 46 hours, suggesting that dose and/or the alpha and beta $t_{1/2}$s are involved. Terminal gamma $t_{1/2}$s of one to four

days have been reported in cases of severe phencyclidine poisoning. Phencyclidine is biotransformed in the liver to several metabolites and excreted in the urine as both free and glucuronide conjugates. Acidification of the urine increases its renal clearance, as expected, because phencyclidine is a base.

Ketamine exists as the (S)- and (R)-enantiomers in combination, which is how it usually is available in the United States. (S)-Ketamine *in vitro* has a lower inhibition constant for the NMDA receptor and a higher one for the sigma-binding site than does (R)-ketamine. (S)-Ketamine is available as the preferred intravenous anesthetic, especially in Germany, and there is some evidence of its superior analgesic potency. From a practical clinical point of view, the separate enantiomers have properties that are grossly similar to those of the racemic mixture. Thus, the pharmacology of ketamine is that of the mixture. The fact that ketamine is more lipophilic than phencyclidine accounts for its rapid onset, short anesthetic duration of action, and shorter period of emergence delirium. Plasma concentrations of ketamine vary widely depending on the dose, route, and time elapsed since administration. Anesthetic doses produce plasma or serum concentrations of 1 to 6.3 ng/mL.

Nonanesthetic psychoactive blood concentrations of ketamine are in the low nanogram per milliliter range. Ketamine has at least two plasma $t_{1/2}$s when it is given intravenously: a beta $t_{1/2}$ of three to four hours has been reported, but it has a much shorter alpha $t_{1/2}$ of about seven minutes because of rapid redistribution. As used in general anesthesia, an intravenous dose of 2.0 mg/kg produces rapid induction. This dose produces an onset in 30 seconds, with the coma lasting for 8 to 10 minutes. The intramuscular injection of ketamine has a latency of three to five minutes and a duration of 10 to 20 minutes or more, depending on the dose administered.

PHARMACOLOGIC ACTIONS

Arylcyclohexylamines (PCP, ketamine). Depending on the dose and specific arylcyclohexylamine ingested, patients present with widely different neurologic and psychiatric signs and symptoms. These signs and symptoms can be subdivided into three major clinical pictures, including (1) confusion, delirium, and psychosis; (2) semicoma and coma; and (3) coma with seizures. One can observe patients becoming progressively more obtunded and eventually comatose—or the reverse when the patient is emerging from

TABLE 1.   Dose-Related Effects of Phencyclidine in Normal Subjects

Total dose by IV infusion: mg/kg:	1 mg 0.014	2 mg 0.03	7 mg 0.10	7-10 mg	14 mg 0.20	17.5 mg 0.25	35 mg 0.50	70 mg 1.0
Acute effects								
Subjective effects	+	+						
Nystagmus			+					
Gait ataxia			+					
Increased blood pressure			+					
Confusional state				+				
Theta slowing (EEG)			−	±	+	+	+	+
Anesthesia-Analgesia (loss of consciousness, no response to painful or auditory stimuli)					−			
Amnesia						+	+	+
Purposeless movements (state of agitation)							+	
Muscle rigidity and extensor posturing (severe rigidity and catatonia)								+
Seizure activity								+
Respiration depression								−

SOURCE: Data summarized by Burns & Lerner in Domino EF, ed. (1981). *Phencyclidine: Historical and Current Perspectives.* Ann Arbor, MI: NPP Books, 450.

coma and showing emergence delirium. Table 1 lists the various clinical correlates of phencyclidine signs and symptoms at different blood levels.

Most phencyclidine abusers do not grossly overdose themselves to the point of semicoma and coma. Hence, most patients intoxicated with phencyclidine show a clinical picture of confusion, delirium, and psychosis.

When ketamine first was developed as a general anesthetic, the early clinical trials found that about a third of patients experienced an obvious emergence delirium. Why only 33% rather than 100% of patients given ketamine showed a delirium or psychosis remains unexplained, but suggests important preoperative and postoperative medications, dosage, environmental, and psychologic or genetic factors. Schizophrenic patients appear to be much more susceptible to a prolonged psychotic episode related to phencyclidine than do other individuals. In addition, environmental and genetic factors influence phencyclidine biotransformation in animals and humans.

After the initial induction dose, an intravenous drip of 15 to 30 μg/kg per minute (or about 1 to 2 μg/kg per hour) provides adequate amnesia and analgesia, in combination with $N_2O:O_2$ and a skeletal muscle relaxant. Muscle relaxants are necessary for intubation and for maintenance, because ketamine causes no relaxation of the jaw and other skeletal musculature; rather, it increases muscle tone. Abnormal jerky muscle movements of the extremities can occur during anesthesia or coma. Diazepam (Valium®) 0.3 to 0.5 mg/kg given intravenously reduces the occurrence of jerky muscle movements. Both agents should be given only when persons are competent to maintain an airway.

During and after slow intravenous administration of 2.0 mg/kg ketamine, the following sequence of eye signs is observed: blinking, staring, closure of lids, nystagmus, strabismus, and loss of lid reflex. Initially, when the patient falls into a dissociative or cataleptic state, the eyelids are widely open, and horizontal or vertical nystagmus is seen. Later on, the eyeballs become centrally fixed in a gaze.

During this stage, both somatosensory and visual stimulation elicits evoked potentials in the cortex. This finding supports the contention that the patient's brain cannot interpret the afferent impulses because of the disruption of the normal connections of sensory cortex with the associated areas. Such eye signs are differentiated from those caused by other intravenous and inhalational anesthetics or coma-producing substances by the fact that the eyes remain open during the course of anesthesia (after a transient closure immediately after induction), despite coma and adequate analgesia. The difficulty of relying on the eye signs of anesthesia to determine anesthetic or coma depth is one of the major disadvantages of ketamine as an anesthetic agent.

Ketamine induces coma in a dose-dependent manner. A minimum of 0.5 mg/kg intravenous is necessary to induce coma for approximately 1.5 minutes. A dose of 1.0 mg/kg induces coma for approximately 5.8 minutes, whereas a dose of 2.0 mg/kg induces coma for approximately 10 minutes. (It should be noted that these doses and approximate durations of coma are after intravenous administration for anesthesia purposes and not as abused by lay persons.)

Persons who abuse ketamine may use a variety of routes of administration, and general anesthesia obviously is not the object of their use. Rather, it is the low-dose mental state that ketamine induces that is considered reinforcing by substance abusers. The one exception to the low-dose use of ketamine is when it is given in large doses surreptitiously to an unsuspecting person as one of the "date rape" drugs.

MECHANISMS OF ACTION

The mechanism of action of arylcyclohexylamines on NMDA receptors of glutamic acid first was described by Lodge and colleagues (Anis, Berry et al., 1983). Other investigators suggested different mechanisms of action involving biogenic amines and sigma-binding sites (Tadimeti, Rao et al., 1989; Rao, Kim et al., 1989, 1990; Rabin, Doat et al., 2000). However, noncompetitive blockade of NMDA receptors is the primary mechanism of action of low concentrations of these agents. This important conclusion had a major effect on the role of glutamic acid in the complex disorders of human schizophrenias (Kornhuber, Kornhuber et al., 1986; Kornhuber, Mack-Burkhardt et al., 1989; Javitt & Zukin, 1991; Vollenweider, 1992, 1994; Vollenweider, Antonini et al., 1992; Vollenweider, Leenders et al., 1997a, 1997b). Krystal and colleagues (1994, 1998a, 1998b, 1999, 2000)

have been especially active in studying ketamine and possible antagonists in human volunteers. They have reviewed the promise and pitfalls of the use of NMDA antagonists as a model of schizophrenia (Abi-Saab, D'Souza et al., 1998). Moreover, understanding the role of glycine and other agonists in modulating NMDA-receptor function has led to possible novel therapeutic approaches to schizophrenia.

The fact that nitrous oxide is an NMDA antagonist has been another major advance in our knowledge, as described by Olney and colleagues (Jevtovic-Todorovic, Todorovic et al., 1998; Jevtovic-Todorovic, Benshoff et al., 2000; Mennerick, Jevtovic-Todorovic et al., 1998), and has stimulated much new thinking (de Lima, Hatch et al., 2000; Franks & Lieb, 1998; Maze & Fujinaga, 2000).

ADDICTION LIABILITY

Why substances such as phencyclidine, and now ketamine, are reinforcing is difficult to understand except in the context of individuals who wish to experience the feelings of floating in space, temporary schizophrenia, sensory isolation, mental distortions, and so forth. A recent book by Jansen (2001) provides insight into why some persons find these agents reinforcing and others have bad experiences, as well as the influence of doses and routes of administration. There is much misrepresentation of ketamine for other substances of abuse, such as MDMA.

Neuroadaption and Sensitization. Rats show marked behavioral sensitization to both phencyclidine and MK-801 with asymmetric cross-sensitization (Xu & Domino, 1994a, 1994b, 1999). However, the significance of this phenomenon for humans is unknown. Whether individuals who abuse phencyclidine or ketamine show enhanced psychotomimetic effects over time needs to be studied.

TOXICITY/ADVERSE EFFECTS

Neurotoxicity. Since the 1970s, when Olney described its neurotoxic effects, glutamic acid excess has been a target for finding brain-protective agents. NMDA antagonists have remarkable effects on brain neurons (Allen, Iverson et al., 1990), including toxicity (Olney, Labruyere et al., 1991), which can be reduced or prevented (Olney, Labruyere et al., 1991). These agents induce significant vesicular changes in rat brain posterior cingulate retrosplenial neurons. Not all species of animals evidence these changes. The relationship of such neurotoxicity to humans who use or abuse NMDA antagonists is as yet unclear. The fact that such neurotoxic changes can be reduced by pretreatments with benzodiazepines is noteworthy, involving a gamma-aminobutyric acid (GABA) mechanism of decreased recurrent inhibition. Phencyclidine analogs inhibit NMDA release of GABA from cultured neurons (Drejer & Honoré, 1987). Persons who abuse arylcyclohexylamines and nitrous oxide obviously should be warned that some animal data indicate these agents produce microscopic neurotoxic changes whose long-term consequences and significance for humans is unknown and needs more research.

Intoxication and Overdose. Although a preliminary diagnosis of arylcyclohexylamine intoxication can be made on the basis of history, clinical signs, and symptoms, only a drug-positive blood or urine specimen will unequivocally establish it. A large variety of different chemical assays are available, but the best still is gas chromatography-mass spectrometry. The brain wave changes induced by arylcyclohexylamines are unusual, and an electroencephalogram can be helpful if the patient is cooperative or comatose. Serum skeletal creatinine phosphokinase levels are increased, and the urine can contain myoglobin because of rhabdomyolysis.

The first step in the differential diagnosis of arylcyclohexylamine intoxication must be on the basis of whether the patient is in coma with or without seizures, emerging from coma, descending into coma, or in a psychotic state. Obviously, the patient in coma—with or without seizures—has a differential diagnosis that includes all other causes of coma and seizures. Again, history and laboratory analysis are crucial.

Psychotic manifestations of arylcyclohexylamine poisoning can be confused with catatonic schizophrenia, an acute toxic psychosis induced with other hallucinogens, and various acute organic brain syndromes. Arylcyclohexylamine intoxication readily induces nystagmus, an organic brain syndrome, as well as cardiovascular and renal complications that are seldom, if ever, seen with other psychiatric syndromes. Body image loss (especially numbness of the entire body), feelings of being in outer space, and relatively rare visual hallucinations suggest arylcyclohexylamine abuse as opposed to use of hallucinogens such as LSD or related agents.

Antidote Therapy. Attempts to block the action of phencyclidine at its binding site with the derivative metaphit have provided basic science evidence of a possible antagonist, which, unfortunately, has not led to a clinically useful antidote. The "naloxone" of arylcyclohexylamines has not been found. Therefore, treatment is symptomatic. Comatose patients should be closely observed for airway, breathing, and cardiovascular status and treated accordingly. All catatonic or comatose patients should have an intravenous line for receiving appropriate fluids. Naloxone (Narcan®) and glucose do not antagonize arylcyclohexylamine-induced depression, but can be useful to rule out opioid overdose or insulin coma. Seizures are best treated with benzodiazepines, but dosage should be reasonably small so as not to deepen central nervous system depression. Urinary acidification does eliminate basic compounds such as arylcyclohexylamine, but the amount excreted usually is not very large compared with the amount ingested. Ammonium chloride 1 to 2 g every six hours to reduce urine pH to about 5.0 and forced diuresis with furosemide (Lasix®) can be used. Systemic acidosis enhances urinary myoglobin excretion and causes kidney damage, so the issue of skeletal muscle injury and its hazards must be taken into account. Activated charcoal, in a dose of 1 gm/kg every two to four hours given shortly after oral arylcyclohexylamine, reduces absorption.

Psychological symptoms are best treated by appropriate psychological techniques without any pharmacotherapy. Neuroleptics that reduce its biotransformation are contraindicated until the arylcyclohexlamine is out of the body. Reports have appeared that the long-acting arylcyclohexylamines (such as phencyclidine) can persist in some tissues, such as fat, or in cerebrospinal fluid for weeks. Benzodiazepines can be helpful in managing extremely anxious or disturbed patients. Restraints are contraindicated in view of possible enhanced rhabdomyolysis, unless such patients are a great danger to themselves or others. Phencyclidine-intoxicated patients can have long-term residual psychological and psychiatric symptoms that require extensive psychological, psychiatric, and possibly pharmacologic therapy. Such patients can continue to show symptoms of psychosis or depression and should be treated accordingly. High-potency antipsychotics or antidepressants then may be indicated.

Attenuation and/or modulation of the neuropsychiatric symptoms of ketamine has been reported for the anticonvulsant lamotrigine (Lamictal®) (Anand, Charney et al., 2000; Charney, Charney et al., 2000), the antipsychotic haloperidol (Haldol®) (Krystal, D'Souza et al., 1999), and the GABA agonist lorazepam (Ativan®) (Krystal, Karper et al., 1998a). However, no specific antagonist is available, and the physician must pick and choose therapies based on symptom reduction. In the case of short-acting psychotomimetics such as ketamine, the passage of time often is the patient's best treatment modality, so long as he or she is placed in a safe and secure supportive environment. Followup referral for expert assessment and treatment is essential once the patient is coherent and recovered to his or her preintoxication status.

REFERENCES

Abi-Saab WM, D'Souza DC, Moghaddam B et al. (1998). The NMDA antagonist model for schizophrenia: Promise and pitfalls. *Pharmacopsychiatry* 31(Suppl2):104-109.

Allen HL, Iversen LL, Olney JW et al. (1990). Phencyclidine, dizocilpine, and cerebrocortical neurons. *Science* 247:221.

Anand A, Charney DS, Oren DA et al. (2000). Attenuation of the neuro-psychiatric effects of ketamine with lamotrigine. *Archives of General Psychiatry* 57:270-276.

Anis NA, Berry SC, Burton NR et al. (1983). The dissociative anesthetics, ketamine and phencyclidine selectively reduce excitation of central mammalian neurons by N-methyl-D-aspartate. *British Journal of Pharmacology* 79:565-575.

Baselt RC (2000). *Disposition of Toxic Drugs and Chemicals in Man.* Foster City, CA: Chemical Toxicology Institute, 456-458, 676-679.

Charney AA, Charney DS, Oren DA et al. (2000). Attenuation of the neuropsychiatric effects of ketamine with lamotrigine: Support for hyperglutamatergic effects of N-methyl-D-aspartate receptor antagonists. *Archives of General Psychiatry* 57(3):270-276.

de Lima J, Hatch D & Torsney C (2000). Nitrous oxide analgesia—A 'sting in the tail'. *Anaesthesia* 55(9):932-933.

Domino EF, ed. (1981a). *Phencyclidine: Historical and Current Perspectives.* Ann Arbor, MI: NPP Books.

Domino EF (1981b). From Sernyl to angel dust: The return of PCP. *University of Michigan Medical Center Journal* XLVII:1-5.

Drejer J & Honoré T (1987). Phencyclidine analogues inhibit NMDA-stimulated [³H]GABA release from cultured cortex neurons. *European Journal of Pharmacology* 143:287-290.

Franks NP & Lieb WR (1998). A serious target for laughing gas. *Nature Medicine* 4(4):383-384.

Jansen K (2001). *Ketamine: Dreams and Realities.* Sarasota, FL: Multidisciplinary Association for Psychedelic Studies (MAPS).

Javitt DC & Zukin SR (1991). Recent advances in the phencyclidine model of schizophrenia. *American Journal of Psychiatry* 148:1301-1308.

Jevtovic-Todorovic V, Benshoff N & Olney JW (2000). Ketamine potentiates cerebrocortical damage induced by the common anesthetic agent nitrous oxide in adult rats. *British Journal of Pharmacology* 130:1692-1698.

Jevtovic-Todorovic V, Todorovic SM, Mennerick S et al. (1998). Nitrous oxide (laughing gas) is an NMDA antagonist, neuroprotectant and neurotoxin. *Nature Medicine* 4(4):460-463.

Kornhuber ME, Kornhuber J, Zettlmeibl H et al. (1986). Phencyclidin und das glutamaterge System. *Biologische Psychiatrie* 176-180.

Kornhuber J, Mack-Burkhardt F & Riederer P et al. (1989). [³H]MK-801 binding sites in postmortem brain regions of schizophrenic patients. *Journal of Neural Transmission* 77:231-236.

Krystal JH, Bennet A, Abi-Saab D et al. (2000). Dissociation of ketamine effects on rule acquisition and rule implementation: Possible relevance to NMDA receptor contribution to executive cognitive function. *Biological Psychiatry* 47(2):137-143.

Krystal JH, D'Souza DC, Karper LP et al. (1999). Interactive effects of subanesthetic ketamine and haloperidol in healthy humans. *Psychopharmacology* 145(2):193-204.

Krystal JH, Karper LP, Bennett A et al. (1998a). Interactive effects of subanesthetic ketamine and subhypnotic lorazepam in humans. *Psychopharmacology* 135(3):213-229.

Krystal JH, Karper LP, Seibyl JP et al. (1994). Subanesthetic effects of the noncompetitive NMDA antagonist, ketamine, in humans. Psychotomimetic, perceptual, cognitive, and neuroendocrine responses. *Archives of General Psychiatry* 51(3):199-214.

Krystal JH, Petrakis IL, Webb E et al. (1998). Dose-related ethanol-like effects of the NMDA antagonist, ketamine, in recently detoxified alcoholics. *Archives of General Psychiatry* 55(4):354-360.

Maze M & Fujinaga M (2000). Recent advances in understanding the actions and toxicity of nitrous oxide [editorial]. *Anaesthesia* 55:311-314.

Mennerick S, Jevtovic-Todorovic V, Todorovic SM et al. (1998). Effect of nitrous oxide on excitatory and inhibitory synaptic transmission in hippocampal cultures. *Journal of Neuroscience* 18(23):9716-9726.

Olney JW, Labruyere J & Price MT (1989). Phencyclidine, dizocilpine, and cerebrocortical neurons. *Science* 244:1360-1362.

Olney JW, Labruyere J, Wang G et al. (1991). NMDA antagonists neurotoxicity: Mechanism and prevention. *Science* 254:1515-1518.

Piercey MF, Hoffman WE & Kaczkofsky P (1988). Functional evidence for PCP-like effects of the anti-stroke candidate MK-801. *Psychopharmacology* 96:561-562.

Rabin RA, Doat M & Winter JC (2000). Role of serotonergic 5-HT$_{2A}$ receptors in the psychotomimetic actions of phencyclidine. *International Journal of Neuropsychopharmacology* 3:333-338.

Rao TS, Kim S, Lehmann J et al. (1989). Differential effects of phencyclidine (PCP) and ketamine on mesocortical and mesostriatal dopamine release in vivo. *Life Sciences* 45:1065-1072.

Rao TS, Kim HS, Lehmann J et al. (1990). Interactions of phencyclidine receptor agonist MK-801 with dopaminergic system: Regional studies in the rat. *Journal of Neurochemistry* 54:1157-1162.

Stoof JC, Booij J & Drukarch B (1992). Amantadine as N-methyl-D-aspartic acid receptor antagonist: New possibilities for therapeutic application? *Clinical Neurology and Neurosurgery* 94:S4-S6.

Tadimeti S, Rao HS, Kim JL et al. (1989). Differential effects of phencyclidine (PCP) and ketamine on mesocortical and mesostriatal dopamine release in vivo. *Life Sciences* 45:1065-1072.

Troupin AS, Mendius JR, Cheng F et al. (1986). MK-801. In BS Meldrum & RJ Porter (eds.) *Epilepsy.* London, England: John Libbey & Co, 191-201.

Vollenweider FX (1992). The use of psychotomimetics in schizophrenia research with special emphasis on the PCP/ketamine model psychosis. *Sucht* 38:398-409.

Vollenweider FX (1994). Evidence for a cortical-subcortical imbalance of sensory information processing during altered states of consciousness using positron emission tomography and [18F]fluorodeoxyglucose. In A Pletscher & A Ladewig (eds.) *50 Years of LSD—Current Status and Perspectives of Hallucinogens*. New York, NY: Parthenon Publishing Group, 67-86.

Vollenweider FX, Antonini A, Angst J et al. (1992). Zerebraler energiemetabolismus *(PET/FDG)* bei gesunden probanden während ketamin- und psilocybin-induzierten modell-psychosen. *Fortschrift Neurologie Psychiatiarie* 60:103.

Vollenweider FX, Leenders KL, Øye I et al. (1997a). Differential psychopathology and patterns of cerebral glucose utilization produced by (S)- and (R)-ketamine in healthy volunteers using positron emission tomography (PET). *European Neuropsychopharmacology* 7(1):25-38.

Vollenweider FX, Leenders KL, Scharfetter C et al. (1997b). Metabolic hyperfrontality and psychopathology in the ketamine model of psychosis using positron emission tomography (PET). *European Neuropsychopharmacology* 7(1):9-24.

Xu X & Domino EF (1994a). Phencyclidine-induced behavioral sensitization. *Pharmacology, Biochemistry and Behavior* 47:603-608.

Xu X & Domino EF (1994b). Asymmetric cross-sensitization to the locomotor stimulant effects of phencyclidine and MK-801. *Neurochemistry International* 25:155-159.

Xu X & Domino EF (1999). A further study on asymmetric cross-sensitization between MK-801 and phencyclidine-induced ambulatory activity. *Pharmacology, Biochemistry and Behavior* 63:413-416.

<table>
<tr><td>Chapter 11</td><td># The Pharmacology of Inhalants</td></tr>
</table>

Robert L. Balster, Ph.D.

Abused inhalants comprise a staggeringly large array of individual chemicals and chemical mixtures. They often are classified by chemical name (for example, toluene, nitrous oxide), by intended use (anesthetic, solvent, adhesive, fuel, and the like), or by form (gas, vapor, or aerosol). This uncertainty as to how to subclassify inhalants has led to some disorder in the field and in difficulty comparing prevalence figures from one survey to another.

DRUGS IN THE CLASS

With other drugs of abuse, it has proved most useful for addiction medicine to classify the substances primarily on the basis of shared pharmacologic and behavioral effects rather than by structure, source, or form. It would be desirable if the same could be done for inhalants (Balster, 1998). The problem is that there is not sufficient knowledge of the effects of inhalants to make very fine distinctions among them. In addition, the toxicologic effects of these compounds differ, and these differences do not necessarily follow classifications based on acute abuse-related pharmacologic and behavioral effects. Nonetheless, three subdivisions of abused inhalants are useful, as shown in Table 1. The rationale for

this subclassification has been presented elsewhere (Balster, 1998), and is summarized below.

Volatile Alkyl Nitrites. The prototypic alkyl nitrite is amyl nitrite, used medically as a vasodilator for treatment of angina. Amyl nitrite is available as a volatile liquid in ampules that are broken open and the vapor inhaled. At one time, the ampules were available over the counter, and abusers would "pop" them open—hence the name "poppers." When amyl nitrite was brought under prescription control by the U.S. Food and Drug Administration (FDA), retailers made products from other alkyl nitrites with names such as "Locker Room" (nitrites smell like a locker room), "Rush," "Hardware," and "Climax." The latter connote their use in the context of sexual activity, particularly by homosexual men familiar with the ability of these products to increase tumescence and relax smooth muscle. As of this writing, cyclohexyl nitrite appears to be the most easily obtained volatile nitrite, for reasons described below. Very little is known about the safety of these products.

Relatively little research has been done to determine the mechanisms of action for the abuse-related effects of volatile nitrites. It is clear from animal studies that they do not produce acute intoxications similar to those of abused solvents such as toluene and trichloroethane (Rees, Knisely et al., 1987). It seems likely that they are abused because of their ability to produce syncope secondary to venous pooling in the periphery and because of their effects on tumescence and smooth muscles. The attractiveness of syncope as a drug effect might be questioned until one recalls that even children like to hold their breath or twirl around until dizzy. It also may be that during dancing, for example, the pounding in the head one might experience from anoxia could enhance a user's appreciation of the situation. More research is needed on this point.

Nitrous Oxide. Nitrous oxide is somewhat distinct in that it is a gas at room temperature and pressure. It is popular to divert anesthetic nitrous oxide for illegitimate use. The tanks can be used to fill balloons for ready sale at concerts, "raves," or parties. The acute pharmacologic and behavioral effects of subanesthetic concentrations of nitrous oxide are poorly understood. Certainly, it can produce euphoria ("laughing gas") and feelings of intoxication (Zacny, Coalson et al., 1994; Zacny, Klafta et al., 1995), but the qualitative nature of this intoxication appears to be different from that produced by anesthetic vapors such as isoflurane and sevoflurane or by other drugs of abuse (Zacny, Coalson et al. 1994; Zacny, Janiszewski et al., 1999). It should be remembered that nitrous oxide is very impotent as an anesthetic, requiring concentrations of about 15% to 20% to produce intoxication. In fact, many users breathe almost 100% nitrous oxide (for example, from a balloon). This action, of course, can lead to some anoxia and, as with nitrite-produced syncope, has acute psychological effects as well.

Another interesting aspect to nitrous oxide pharmacology is that, unlike vaporous anesthetics, it can produce good analgesia, as seen in animal models (Gillman & Lichtigfeld, 1994). Further, there is some evidence for opiate receptor involvement in the analgesic effects (Quock, Curtis et al., 1993), although opiate antagonists do not appear to reverse either anesthesia or subanesthetic intoxication with nitrous oxide (Zacny, Coalson et al., 1994).

Volatile Solvents, Fuels, and Anesthetics. This category includes a large collection of chemicals, which further research probably will reveal to have different profiles of acute effects as well, but the state of the science is insufficient at this point to propose a further subclassification. Among the prototypic chemicals for this class are 1,1,1-trichloroethane (TCE) and other halogenated hydrocarbons; toluene and other alkyl benzenes; butane and other alkanes; and various ketones, alcohols, and ethers (Table 1). It has been hypothesized that many of these commercial chemicals share profiles of acute effects with subanesthetic concentrations of volatile anesthetics such as halothane, sevoflurane, and isoflurane (Evans & Balster, 1991). Of course, ether has a long history of use as an abused anesthetic (Nagle, 1968). These anesthetics offer a safer alternative to the study of toluene and similar chemicals in humans, and they have been directly compared in many animal studies (Rees, Knisely et al., 1987). As a point of comparison, it is useful to recall that beverage alcohol (ethanol) also is a solvent and produces a type of anesthesia at very high blood levels. Ethanol actually is much less potent than the other solvents for acute central nervous system (CNS) effects, discouraging use by inhalation. Alcohol shares pharmacologic and behavioral effects with depressant drugs such as the barbiturates, nonbarbiturate sedatives, and benzodiazepines, and perhaps abuse of these solvents and anesthetics could be viewed clinically as special instances of abuse of depressant drugs. To be sure, the acute depressant-like intoxication and presentation of overdose can be the same among all these compounds.

History. The abuse of inhalants has a long history. Perhaps the best known instances are the use of anesthetics for purposes of intoxication that began with their discovery more than 200 years ago (Nagle, 1968). The euphoriant effects of nitrous oxide were noted by Sir Humphrey Davy, who synthesized the substance in 1798 and began calling it "laughing gas." Laughing gas subsequently was used as part of comedic traveling shows at the beginning of the 19th century. The early vapor anesthetics, including ether and chloroform, were used recreationally and as "nerve tonics," both by inhalation and drinking. It may seem odd to drink an anesthetic, but one must remember that alcohol is a highly volatile liquid with irritant properties, yet its oral consumption surprises no one.

Today, abused inhalants differ widely in their availability. Some, such as nitrous oxide and amyl nitrite, are under control of the FDA as prescription medications, although forms of nitrous oxide are available commercially (for example, as "whippets" and racing fuel). Commercial sales of volatile alkyl nitrites are regulated in the United States by the Consumer Product Safety Commission, a step that has greatly reduced the availability of most of these substances. However, cyclohexyl nitrite, which technically may not be an alkyl nitrite covered by the regulations, remains available in sex paraphernalia shops and through Internet sites. Many other types of abused inhalants can be found in homes or workplaces or are readily purchased at retail establishments. Gasoline, a very complex mixture of volatile compounds, is available everywhere, and butane lighter fluid is not very difficult to obtain. There have been discussions of strategies to prevent access to abused inhalants, to change their labeling, or to reformulate products to limit their abuse potential. Each of these strategies needs to be viewed on a case-by-case basis to be certain that it will achieve the desired effect and not result in abusers seeking potentially more toxic products that almost certainly cannot be restricted (for example, gasoline). Harwood (1995) has undertaken a policy analysis of the inhalant abuse problem in the United States, including the roles of treatment and prevention.

Epidemiology. Results of national surveys suggest that the prevalence of inhalant use in young adolescents exceeds that even of marijuana use (Edwards & Oetting, 1995). Data from the 1999 National Household Survey on Drug Abuse form the basis for estimating that more than two million youth aged 12 to 17 use inhalants, and 56,000 use them regularly. Among older youth and adults, the prevalence of inhalant use falls below that of marijuana, cocaine, and heroin, but current users remain a significant minority of substance abusers. Neumark and colleagues (1998) reviewed age, gender, ethnicity, and trends in the use of inhalants in the United States and found that such use is common among both sexes but disproportionately involves non-Hispanic white youths compared with other age and ethnic groups. Although many inhalant users quit as they reach young adulthood, it is incorrect to characterize this problem as a passing fad in youth. For about half of current users, duration of use exceeds one to two years, with about 10% using inhalants for six years or more (Neumark, Delva et al., 1998).

Abuse of inhalants is an even more significant problem in other parts of the world, particularly in the developing countries (Kozel, Sloboda et al., 1995).

Recent research points to the association of inhalant abuse with many other substance abuse, mental health, and social problems (Dinwiddie, 1998). Several studies have shown a clear progression from early inhalant use to later use of drugs such as cocaine and heroin. In one such study, researchers found that youth who had used inhalants by age 16 had more than a nine-fold greater likelihood of us-

ing heroin by age 32 than did youth who had not used inhalants, even when controlling for other risk factors associated with inhalant abuse (Johnson, Schütz et al., 1995). In another study, a history of inhalant use independently increased the odds of becoming an injection drug user by more than five-fold (Schütz, Chilcoat et al., 1994). In the latter study, the magnitude of the increased risk associated with inhalant use exceeded that for marijuana use.

ABSORPTION AND METABOLISM

The abused inhalants include compounds that are self-administered as gases, vapors, and aerosols. These three forms of inhalants have somewhat different absorption characteristics and require different methods of use (for example, balloons for gases and aerosol cans for aerosols). In the case of abused aerosol products such as spray paint, the likely "active ingredient" for abusers is the propellent (for example, butane) that exists in the aerosol can under pressure; however, the other materials in the cans (for example, pigments) also can be absorbed.

Probably the most useful way to think about the bioavailability of abused inhalants is to apply a knowledge of inhalation anesthesia. As has been mentioned, there is considerable overlap in some of the chemicals involved. Although individual inhalants differ somewhat, all are very lipophilic and have blood-brain partition coefficients of 1 to 5. It is important to know that most of these vapors are quite potent, probably requiring alveolar concentrations no greater than 10% for grossly intoxicating effects.

Gases and vapors rapidly penetrate deep into the lung and, because of their high lipophilicity, are rapidly absorbed and distributed into arterial blood. What distinguishes inhalant abuse from anesthetic use is that the partial pressure of the inhalant vapor inhaled generally is very high and quite variable over time, as users intermittently sniff from balloons or from rags or bags saturated with liquid. With these high concentrations in the inspired air, effects on the brain are almost immediate. As with anesthetics, key factors that would be expected to affect brain concentrations of inhalants are concentration in the inspired air, pulmonary ventilation rate, pulmonary blood flow, and the amount of body fat; however, the practical significance of these variables outside of a well-controlled anesthesia situation is uncertain. Because physical activity increases cardiac output, it is likely that inhalant distribution to the brain will be

TABLE 1. Pharmacologic Classification of Abused Inhalants

Class	Examples	Sources
Volatile alkyl nitrites	Amyl nitrite	Antianginal medication ampules
	Butyl nitrite	Room Odorizers
Nitrous oxide		Whipped creme chargers, cylinders for anesthesia, racing fuels, dairy industry foaming agent
Solvents, fuels, and anesthetics	Toluene	Adhesives, paint removers and thinners (toluol), inks, nail polish and remover, industrial solvents and degreasers
	Xylene	Adhesives and printing inks, paints and varnishes, pesticides
	Trichloroethane	A solvent in water repellants, automotive cleaners, paints, adhesives and silicone lubricants, correction fluids, spray paints and paint removers, spot removers and other cleaning products
	Trichloroethylene	Correction fluids, stains and varnishes, paint removers
	Methylene chloride	A solvent in water repellants, automotive cleaners, primers and paints, adhesives and silicone lubricants, correction fluids, spray paints and paint removers, rust and spot removers and other cleaning products
	Tetrachloroethylene	A solvent in water repellants, brake and carburetor cleaners, paints, adhesives and silicone lubricants, correction fluids, paint removers
	Butane, isopropane	Cigarette lighter fuel, aerosol propellent, bottled gas
	Ether, isoflurane	Anesthetics
	Ketones (MBK, MEK)	Solvents, adhesives.

markedly greater than when users are at rest. Inhalants easily cross the placenta and expose the fetus, with consequences that will be discussed later.

The situation with aerosols is somewhat different. Aerosol propellents typically are gases or vapors. Some of the constituents of aerosol products actually are droplets (that is, aerosols) when inhaled and, for these, the rapidity and efficiency of absorption are determined by particle size (median aerodynamic diameter). For all practical purposes, even aerosols have an almost immediate onset of action. Thus, it

is common for inhalant users to breathe the gas or vapor and instantly stumble or fall down, posing a risk to themselves and others.

It is likely that, for many use situations with inhalants, the concentrations in inspired air exceed concentrations that would be lethal if the user were to be exposed continuously. Lethal concentrations could occur, for example, if a user became unconscious while still exposed to the inhalant. This situation is probably the most common form of acute overdose. It happens when someone using a rag or a bag laden with solvent falls in such a way as to maintain contact with the solvent. Also, some users have devised methods for exposing themselves to inhalants without having to use their hands, such as for use in sexual situations, and become vulnerable to overdose while using the devices.

Elimination of inhalants is very rapid once the source is removed from the inspired air. For most of these chemicals, expired air is the major route of elimination. Those that are relatively insoluble in blood and brain (for example, TCE) are eliminated more quickly than those with greater solubility in these reservoirs (for example, toluene).

Most abused inhalants are metabolized to some extent, but this metabolism probably plays a greater role in determining their hepatic toxicity than their CNS effects. Another important factor affecting recovery is the duration of the use episode. Someone who has been inhaling for a few hours might achieve considerable accumulation in muscle, skin, and fat. For obese individuals, recovery can be a bit more prolonged, as the chemicals are more slowly relocated.

The nature of post-intoxication effects after an episode of inhalant abuse is poorly understood. It is reasonable to assume that they might produce a "hangover" and headaches sometimes are reported. Whether the aversiveness of post-intoxication motivates continued use is completely unknown. Nevertheless, intoxication with inhalants is of shorter duration than with other drugs of abuse, with the result that many health care providers, as well as friends and family of users, rarely see an inhalant abuser who is grossly intoxicated. Unless comatose, such users typically are not brought to emergency departments because they will have recovered before they get there. Law enforcement personnel occasionally encounter intoxicated users if they come upon them during a use episode, but there is little they can do, even in cases of driving under the influence, because of the rapid recovery time. Perhaps it is this lack of direct experience with intoxicated inhalant users and the difficulty of obtaining confirming clinical chemistry (to be discussed later) that has contributed to an under appreciation of the adverse public health effects of this form of substance abuse.

MECHANISMS OF ACTION

The neuropharmacologic mechanisms by which inhalant intoxication occurs are poorly understood. Once inhaled, solvents rapidly enter the brain and distribute to lipid-containing membranes within the CNS, placing them in proximity to key functional components. Although it is pre-sumed that the inhalants disrupt normal neural function, it is not clear which systems are most affected and the mechanism by which such disruption occurs. Even the question of whether specific receptors are affected by these agents remains unresolved.

Because of the properties that solvents share with alcohol, it is logical to turn to new discoveries about the mechanisms for the abuse-related effects of ethanol for hypotheses about how abused solvents might act in the brain. Currently, evidence is accumulating that ethanol and solvents can have effects at certain ligand-gated ion channel receptors, including those for gamma-aminobutyric acid (GABA), glutamate, and acetylcholine (Cruz, Balster et al., 2000; Cruz, Mirshahi et al., 1998; Mihic, Ye et al., 1997). Of particular interest is the discovery that these effects can be very selective for different structural subtypes of these heteromeric proteins, with different chemicals having somewhat different profiles of selectivity. Of particular importance is the finding that vaporous chemicals that do not have depressant-like acute behavioral effects (for example, flurothyl, a convulsant vapor) do not act like the abused chemicals in these in vitro procedures (Bowen, Wiley et al., 1996; Cruz, Balster et al., 2000). Nevertheless, definitive knowledge about the cellular mechanisms for the abuse of inhalants lags far behind our knowledge of most other classes of abused drugs.

Although most scientific evidence would support the view that most of the chemicals in this class of inhalants produces alcohol- and depressant drug-like effects, published descriptions include a much wider array of potential subjective and pharmacologic effects, including hallucinations, tremor, and seizures. Certainly vapors can have excitatory effects in animals (such as flurothyl); and animal studies provide some evidence that even aromatic hydrocarbons like benzene or the isoparaffins can produce a different profile of acute effects than the prototypic depressant solvents such as toluene (Tegeris & Balster, 1994; Balster, Bowen et al., 1997). Considering how many commercial products containing very complex mixtures are inhaled, it should not be surprising that users experience a diverse array of acute effects, depending on the product used.

ADDICTION LIABILITY

Many abused inhalants have behavioral and neurochemical effects similar to those seen with other depressant drugs of abuse (Balster, 1998). All of the vapors that have been tested produce clear, reversible, drug-like behavioral effects in animal studies (Evans & Balster, 1991). In addition, self-administration studies in primates (Wood, 1982) and humans (Zacny, Janiszewski et al., 1999) have shown toluene, chloroform, and nitrous oxide to have reinforcing properties. When given repeatedly to animals, many drugs of abuse produce sensitization to their locomotor stimulant effects, a phenomenon thought to reflect engagement of addictive processes in the brain. Trichloroethane has been shown to produce locomotor sensitization in mice (Bowen, Jones et al., 1997), and repeated toluene exposure in rats produces cross-sensitization to cocaine and increased cocaine-produced dopamine release (Beyer, Stafford et al., 2001). Indeed, toluene itself has been shown to enhance dopaminergic function in various portions of the brain reward system (reviewed in Balster, 1998), suggesting that there may be a common neural basis for abuse of inhalants and other well-studied drugs of abuse.

Tolerance and Dependence. Little is known about the development of tolerance to and dependence on inhalants, but in general they do not appear to be prominent features. It may be useful first to describe what has been learned from carefully controlled animal studies of tolerance and dependence, in which exposure conditions are easily manipulated. Under conditions in which many drugs of abuse show considerable tolerance development when given repeatedly, abused inhalants do not readily produce a significant degree of tolerance to their behavioral effects (Moser, Scimeca et al., 1985). It has also not been easy to demonstrate cross-tolerance with other depressant drugs of abuse. This fact is somewhat surprising because animal models for tolerance to ethanol are readily established. However, with continuous exposure (such as that achieved with mice in inhalation exposure chambers), a mild withdrawal syndrome can be observed with TCE (Evans & Balster, 1993); other vapors have not been systematically studied. The withdrawal effects appear within hours after discontinuation of exposure and can be considered excitatory in nature. Ethanol and barbiturates can suppress these withdrawal signs, suggesting a cross-dependence within the depressant class.

Inhalant abuse typically is episodic in nature and thus generally would not occur with sufficient frequency and intensity to maintain a constant exposure throughout a day, much less the weeks or months it might take for physical dependence to develop. Thus, it is not surprising that physical dependence on inhalants is not seen often, if at all. Signs and symptoms occurring a day or so after discontinuation of use (Evans & Raistrick, 1987) obviously would not correspond to the elimination of these chemicals from the body and may not represent a true abstinence syndrome so much as a manifestation of toxicity. There is little evidence of use of inhalants to avoid a withdrawal syndrome. Because of these factors, the *DSM-IV* of the American Psychiatric Association (1994) does not provide for a physiologic dependence subclassification of inhalation abuse or dependence. However, regular users of inhalants clearly can develop a pattern of uncontrolled use, marked by a devotion of considerable time and efforts to obtaining and using inhalants that is characteristic of all the substance abuse problems.

Clinical Chemistry. Although few, if any, clinical facilities will routinely conduct tests for the presence of abused inhalants, such tests can be ordered through special services provided by commercial laboratories. Typically, these tests are performed on blood and appear to be available mainly for the abused solvents such as toluene, TCE, and methyl ethyl ketone. Because inhalants are eliminated so rapidly after acute exposure, such tests would be expected to have a high probability of producing false negatives. The tests are being promoted for use in drug-free workplace or school programs, but do not appear to have the speed and accuracy needed for routine diagnosis. Nevertheless, technologic advances can be expected in this area. For example, new developments include the availability of a form of breath analyzer (ToxTrap®) that could be used to detect acute solvent use in the workplace or in drivers under the influence. Urine tests, such as those for the toluene metabolite hippuric acid, also are available.

TOXICITY/ADVERSE EFFECTS

It is difficult to summarize what is known and not known about the adverse consequences of inhalant abuse. The discussion that follows focuses almost exclusively on the subclass of inhaled solvents, fuels, and anesthetics. Their toxicity differs depending on which of this broad array of chemicals and chemical mixtures is being abused. The toxicology of commonly used solvents is reviewed in reference texts (Snyder, 1987), which can be consulted for specific information on compounds of interest. A brief overview of the information is provided here.

Nitrous oxide will be mentioned when appropriate, but the situation with alkyl nitrites probably is very different, involving different types of users and different use patterns. Clearly, the known side effects of organic nitrites used for smooth muscle relaxation would be relevant to abuse of these compounds, but a systematic study of the health consequences in nitrite abusers has not been done. Early in the AIDS epidemic, it was thought that nitrite use might be a cause of the immune dysfunction and Kaposi's sarcoma seen in gay men, but with the discovery of HIV and the lack of clear evidence for immunologic toxicity of nitrites under typical use conditions, this hypothesis now is rarely mentioned. For those interested in a fuller discussion of the health effects of nitrite abuse, other reviews may be helpful (Haverkos & Dougherty, 1988).

Acute Effects. Deaths related to the acute effects of inhalants are well documented (Bass, 1970; Garriott & Petty, 1980; Bowen, Daniel et al., 1999). There are two primary sources: behavioral toxicity and overdose. Because the solvent class of inhalants can produce profound intoxication and even anesthetic-like effects at high concentrations, it would not be surprising for accidents and injuries related to behavioral toxicity to occur. Vulnerability to these events probably is enhanced by the rapid onset of intoxication. Additive effects would be expected when these inhalants are used in combination with alcohol or other CNS depressant drugs. Overdose occurs when (as described earlier) users lose consciousness while being continually exposed, allowing lethal concentrations to accumulate in the brain. As with anesthetic vapors, the concentration-effect curves for inhalants are very steep, with toxic exposures achieved easily under the poorly regulated exposure conditions of actual use.

It appears that the proximate cause of most overdose deaths is CNS depression, leading to respiratory problems or suffocation. As mentioned earlier, treatment of overdose rarely occurs in emergency departments because overdose victims usually are either dead or recovered by the time they arrive. In addition to these overdose situations, at least some of the inhalants appear capable of producing acute cardiotoxicity, even in otherwise healthy young users. The mechanism may be increased sensitivity of the myocardium to circulating catecholamines, which may occur when an intoxicated individual engages in some strenuous activity. This phenomenon has been termed "sudden sniffing death" (Bass, 1970) and has been associated particularly with the abuse of aerosols containing chlorofluorocarbon and butane propellants and refrigerants such as Freon™ that contain them. The contribution of hypoxia to the acute toxicity of inhalants should be considered, es-

pecially with the use of nitrous oxide, in which even 100% concentrations are not lethal except for the loss of oxygen.

Chronic Toxicity. Because of the diverse array of chemicals subject to inhalant abuse, it is difficult to summarize their chronic toxicity. The situation is made even more complicated by the fact that few chronic users confine themselves to a single product or a single chemical agent. Add to this the fact that many abused commercial products are complex mixtures, and it is clear that the situation makes it difficult for a toxicologist to ascertain the specific etiology of any adverse health effects seen in inhalant users. Indeed, some adverse effects may be secondary to inhalant abuse and reflect lifestyle covariants seen in solvent abusers. These covariants may include such known predictors of poor health as homelessness, inadequate diet, and other substance abuse. Thus, data from case reports in inhalant abusers always should be viewed cautiously. Careful epidemiologic work that controls for key covariants in this population has yet to be done.

In animal studies, it is easier to study individual chemicals, but research in this area typically has been done to simulate the long duration and low concentration exposures that might be experienced in the home or workplace. Few studies attempt to model the repeated high concentration and intermittent exposure most typical of inhalant abusers. Having said this, many chronic inhalant abusers manifest adverse health effects, some of which can be used in diagnosing the problem. Common target organs are the nose and mouth area, lungs, brain, liver, and kidney. There also are physical dangers in using highly inflammable and explosive chemicals.

Neurotoxicity. Many, if not all, abused inhalants can be neurotoxic. Some components of abused products are well-characterized neurotoxicants. Among these are hexane and methyl-*n*-butyl-ketone, which produce axonopathies. The lead in leaded gasoline (still used in many countries throughout the world) produces classic demyelination. Other commonly abused chemicals (such as toluene, TCE, and propane) have less well described chronic effects on the brain and behavior. Animal studies and clinical observations suggest that they too can produce neurotoxic effects at high exposures, and brain scanning or autopsy reports of these and other solvents show many types of neuropathologies, including loss of white matter, brain atrophy, and damage to specific neural pathways. Imaging studies, neurologic assessments, and neuropsychological testing in chronic abusers also reveal myriad nervous system and behavioral abnormalities.

In Scandinavia, a pattern of behavioral abnormalities termed the "solvent syndrome" or "painter's syndrome" has been described, primarily in persons exposed to high concentrations in workplace settings. Whether this pattern applies to inhalant abusers is not known. When one considers that alcoholics can develop significant neurologic dysfunction with heavy use, it should not be surprising if at least some of the solvents caused the same dysfunction. Nitrous oxide abuse has been associated with a myeloneuropathy, possibly because of inactivation of vitamin B_{12}-dependent enzymes (Butzkueven & King, 2000).

Psychopathology. The association of early inhalant abuse with increased risk of cocaine and heroin addiction already has been mentioned. A similar association is seen with alcoholism. As reviewed by Dinwiddie (1998), increased risk of substance abuse problems also is accompanied by associations with delinquency and antisocial personality disorder. Less is known about the potential risk of other major psychiatric disorders.

Effects on Major Organ Systems. Many chronic solvent users develop irritation of the eyes, nose, and mouth and exhibit rhinitis, nose bleeding, conjunctivitis, and a localized skin rash. When these signs are accompanied by the odor of solvents on the breath or in clothing; by paint, adhesive, or other similar stains on clothing; or by possession of abusable products in unusual circumstances or amounts, inhalant abuse should be considered. With chronic use, inflammation of the lungs can result in coughing and may compromise respiration.

The liver is an important target in chronic exposure to many solvents, particularly those that undergo some metabolism. Of particular concern are some of the halogenated hydrocarbons, such as carbon tetrachloride. It could be speculated that persons with other types of liver disease, such as hepatitis or alcoholism, would be particularly vulnerable. Kidney damage also has been reported, in the form of glomerulonephritis, kidney stones, and renal tubular acidosis. Benzene and vinyl chloride are known carcinogens. Nitrites and methylene chloride can produce methemoglobinemia.

Fetal Solvent Syndrome. It has been estimated that as many as 12,000 women use inhalants while pregnant in the United States alone. The research on inhalant abuse and pregnancy (Jones & Balster, 1998) suggests that decreased fertility and spontaneous abortions in some women may be related to inhalant abuse. Clinical reports of adverse effects in the offspring of solvent abusers include low birth weight, facial and other physical abnormalities, microcephaly, and delayed neurologic and physical maturation. Followup studies have provided some evidence of residual deficits in cognitive, speech, and motor skills. Because certain features seen in these children resemble the fetal alcohol syndrome, a "fetal solvent syndrome" has been proposed. Whether these features result from direct teratologic effects of the abused chemicals or some lifestyle covariants associated with solvent abuse is unknown at this time. Nevertheless, confirmation of adverse effects of prenatal solvent exposure has been obtained in animal studies. Thus, clinicians should be alert to this possibility in patients who abuse inhalants during pregnancy.

FUTURE RESEARCH DIRECTIONS

Inhalant abuse almost certainly is the least understood substance abuse problem. This is primarily related to the fact that there has been little research in this area (Balster, 1997), generally because of mistaken beliefs about inhalant abuse that even exist within the scientific community. These beliefs include the ideas that (1) inhalant abuse is a transient phenomenon of adolescence that has relatively little associated morbidity and mortality, (2) abused inhalants have "nonspecific effects" on the brain and behavior that do not lend themselves to study with modern technologies in behavioral and molecular neurobiology, (3) laboratory studies of vapors and gases are very difficult to perform, and (4) there are too many chemicals to successfully sort out the similarities and differences in terms of their abuse potential and toxicity.

It is to be hoped that additional addiction scientists will be attracted to this important area of research. However, some unique problems inherent in the study of inhalant abuse should be mentioned. Perhaps the most significant is that it will be difficult to conduct laboratory-based human exposure studies of many of these compounds at behaviorally active concentrations. Such studies have been very important with other drugs of abuse. One approach to overcoming this problem may be to draw lessons about the effects of chemicals of this type by studying the medical use of general anesthetics. This approach has been used successfully by Zacny and colleagues (1994, 1995, 1999) and should be considered by others. It is particularly useful in studying nitrous oxide.

Animal studies of abused inhalants will be especially important because there are fewer limitations on the exposure conditions. Epidemiologic studies are made difficult by the numerous types of products and chemicals subject to inhalant abuse and by the fact that subclassifications have differed from study to study. There has been an increased appreciation that alkyl nitrite abuse differs from the rest, and this difference is reflected in separate analyses of prevalence data in many reports. The National Household Survey on Drug Abuse now contains a breakdown of specific subtypes of abused inhalant products, which should be useful for analyses. Thus, progress is being made in this area of research. Hopefully, such progress will lead to a better understanding of inhalant abuse and improved treatment and prevention strategies.

ACKNOWLEDGMENTS: The preparation of this chapter was supported by NIDA grant DA-03112. Dr. Ronald Wood has provided very useful instruction over the years on many aspects of inhalant abuse and provided some assistance with sections of this chapter as well.

REFERENCES

American Psychiatric Association (APA) (1994). *Diagnostic and Statistical Manual of Mental Disorders, 4th Edition (DSM-IV)*. Washington, DC: American Psychiatric Press.

Balster RL (1987). Abuse potential evaluation of inhalants. *Drug and Alcohol Dependence* 19(1):7-15.

Balster RL (1997). Inhalant abuse: A forgotten drug abuse problem. In LS Harris (ed.) *Problems of Drug Dependence 1996: Proceedings of the 58th Annual Scientific Meeting (NIDA Research Monograph 174)*. Rockville, MD: National Institute on Drug Abuse, 3-8.

Balster RL (1998). Neural basis of inhalant abuse. *Drug and Alcohol Dependence* 51:207-214.

Balster RL, Bowen SE, Evans EB et al. (1997). Evaluation of the acute behavioral effects and abuse potential of a C8-C9 isoparaffin solvent. *Drug and Alcohol Dependence* 46:125-135.

Bass M (1970). Sudden sniffing death. *Journal of the American Medical Association* 212:2075-2079.

Beyer SE, Stafford D, LeSage MG et al. (2001). Repeated exposure to inhaled toluene induces behavioral and neurochemical cross-sensitization to cocaine in rats. *Psychopharmacology* 154:198-204.

Bowen SE, Daniel J & Balster RL (1999). Deaths associated with inhalant abuse in Virginia from 1987 to 1996. *Drug and Alcohol Dependence* 53:239-245.

Bowen SE, Jones HE & Balster RL (1997) Repeated exposure to 1,1,1-trichloroethane produces both tolerance and sensitization to effects on mouse behavior. *Fundamental and Applied Toxicologist Supplement – The Toxicologist* 36: 62.

Bowen SE, Wiley JL, Evans EB et al. (1996). Functional observational battery comparing the effects of ethanol, 1,1,1-trichloroethane, ether and flurothyl. *Neurotoxicology and Teratology* 18:557-585.

Butzkueven H & King JO (2000). Nitrous oxide myelopathy in an abuser of whipped cream bulbs. *Journal of Clinical Neuroscience* 7:73-75.

Cruz SL, Balster RL & Woodward JJ (2000). Effects of volatile solvents on recombinant N-methyl-D-aspartate receptors expressed in Xenopus oocytes. *British Journal of Pharmacology* 131:1303-1308.

Cruz SL, Mirshahi T, Thomas B et al. (1998). Effects of the abused solvent toluene on recombinant NMDA and non-NMDA receptors expressed in *Xenopus* oocytes. *Journal of Pharmacology and Experimental Therapeutics* 286:334-340.

Dinwiddie SH (1998). In RE Tarter, RT Ammerman & PJ Ott (eds.) *Handbook of Substance Abuse: Neurobehavioral Pharmacology*. New York, NY: Plenum Press, 269-279.

Edwards RW & Oetting ER (1995). Inhalant abuse in the United States. In N Kozel, Z Sloboda & M De La Rosa (eds.) *Epidemiology of Inhalant Abuse: An International Perspective (NIDA Research Monograph 148)*. Rockville, MD: National Institute on Drug Abuse, 8-28.

Environmental Protection Agency (1987). *Household Solvent Products: A "Shelf" Survey with Laboratory Analysis* (EPA-OTS 560/5-87-006). Washington, DC: Office of Pesticides and Toxic Substances.

Evans AC & Raistrick D (1987). Phenomenology of intoxication with toluene-based adhesives and butane gas. *British Journal of Psychiatry* 150:769-773.

Evans EB & Balster RL (1991). CNS depressant effects of volatile organic solvents. *Neuroscience and Biobehavioral Reviews* 15:233-241.

Evans EB & Balster RL (1993). Inhaled 1,1,1-trichloroethane produced physical dependence in mice: Effects of drugs and vapors on withdrawal. *Journal of Pharmacology & Experimental Therapeutics* 264:726-733.

Garriott J & Petty CS (1980). Death from inhalant abuse: Toxicological and pathological evaluation. *Clinical Toxicology* 16:305-315.

Gillman MA & Lichtigfeld FJ (1994). Pharmacology of psychotropic analgesic nitrous oxide as a multipotent opioid agonist. *International Journal of Neuroscience* 76:5-12.

Harwood HJ (1995). Inhalants: A policy analysis of the problem in the United States. In N Kozel, Z Sloboda & M De La Rosa (eds.) *Epidemiology of Inhalant Abuse: An International Perspective (NIDA Research Monograph 148)*. Rockville, MD: National Institute on Drug Abuse, 274-303.

Haverkos HW & Dougherty JA, eds. (1988). *Health Hazards of Nitrite Inhalants (NIDA Research Monograph 83)*. Rockville, MD: National Institute on Drug Abuse.

Johnson EO, Schütz CG, Anthony JC et al. (1995). Inhalants to heroin: A prospective analysis from adolescence to adulthood. *Drug and Alcohol Dependence* 40:159-164.

Jones HE & Balster RL (1998). Inhalant abuse in pregnancy. *Obstetrics and Gynecology Clinics of North America* 25:153-167.

Kozel N, Sloboda Z & De La Rosa M, eds. (1995). *Epidemiology of Inhalant Abuse: An International Perspective (NIDA Research Monograph 148)*. Rockville, MD: National Institute on Drug Abuse.

Mihic SJ, Ye Q, Wock MJ et al. (1997). Sites of alcohol and volatile anaesthetic action on GABA$_a$ and glycine receptors. *Nature* 389:385-389.

Moser VC, Scimeca JA & Balster RL (1985). Minimal tolerance to the effects of 1,1,1-trichloroethane on fixed-ratio responding in mice. *Neurotoxicology* 6:35-42.

Nagle DR (1968). Anesthetic addiction and drunkenness. *International Journal of the Addictions* 3:26-30.

Neumark YD, Delva J & Anthony JC (1998). The epidemiology of adolescent inhalant drug involvement. *Archives of Pediatrics and Adolescent Medicine* 152:781-786.

Quock RM, Curtis BA, Reynolds BJ et al. (1993). Dose-dependent antagonism and potentiation of nitrous oxide antinociception by naloxone in mice. *Journal of Pharmacology & Experimental Therapeutics* 267:117-122.

Rees DC, Knisely JS, Balster RL et al. (1987). Pentobarbital-like discriminative stimulus properties of halothane, 1,1,1-trichloroethane, isoamyl nitrite, flurothyl and oxazepam in mice. *Journal of Pharmacology and Experimental Therapeutics* 241:507-515.

Schütz CG, Chilcoat HD & Anthony JC (1994). The association between sniffing inhalants and injecting drugs. *Comprehensive Psychiatry* 35:99-105.

Snyder R (1987). *Ethel Browning's Toxicity and Metabolism of Industrial Solvents, 2nd Edition, Vol. 1: Hydrocarbons.* Amsterdam, The Netherlands: Elsevier.

Tegeris JS & Balster RL (1994). A comparison of the acute behavioral effects of alkylbenzenes using a functional observational battery in mice. *Fundamental and Applied Toxicology* 22:240-250.

Wood RW (1982). Stimulus properties of inhaled substances. An update. In CD Mitchell (ed.) *Nervous System Toxicology.* New York, NY: Raven Press, 199-212.

Zacny JP, Coalson DW, Lichtor JL et al. (1994). Effects of naloxone on the subjective and psychomotor effects of nitrous oxide in humans. *Pharmacology and Biochemical Behavior* 49:573-578.

Zacny JP, Janiszewski D, Sadeghi P et al. (1999). Reinforcing, subjective, and psychomotor effects of sevoflurane and nitrous oxide in moderate-drinking health volunteers. *Addiction* 94:1817-1828.

Zacny JP, Klafta JM, Coalson DW et al. (1995). The reinforcing effects of brief exposures to nitrous oxide in healthy volunteers. *Drug and Alcohol Dependence* 42:197-200.

Chapter 12 | The Pharmacology of Steroids

Scott E. Lukas, Ph.D.

Drugs in the Class
Absorption and Metabolism
Pharmacologic Actions
Addiction Liability
Toxicity/Adverse Effects
Future Research Directions

The introduction of anabolic-androgenic steroids to the United States has been traced to the 1954 World Weightlifting Championships in Vienna, Austria, when the Soviet Union's coach informed the U.S. coach that Soviet team members were taking testosterone (Todd, 1987). In the ensuing years, use of anabolic-androgenic steroids by elite weight lifters, power lifters, and bodybuilders has increased. Over the years, use of these agents has spread to many professional sports, particularly those in which strength and body weight are important to success (as in football).

Testosterone was the drug of choice in the 1950s. In subsequent decades, it was replaced by more elegant synthetic compounds, primarily because of their slightly higher percent of anabolic versus androgenic effects and their relative resistance to detection by current laboratory tests. Use spread to collegiate and amateur athletes, as evidenced by the 50% positive tests obtained by the International Olympic Committee during unannounced urine screens in 1984 and 1985 (Yesalis, Anderson et al., 1990).

The 1990s saw a return to the use of testosterone, which is thought to be due to improved gas chromatographic methods of detecting the synthetic compounds and the continued difficulty of accurately detecting exogenously administered testosterone (Lukas, 1993). In the wake of anabolic-androgenic steroid abuse, athletes are using other types of performance-enhancing aids. Many of these are unregulated and are used primarily to enhance or boost the effects of steroids, but some have their own pharmacologic profiles that make them appealing. One recent example (February, 2002) is kynoselen, which has been used to treat AIDS patients in France. It is classified as a vitamin/mineral supplement composed of potassium, magnesium, selenium, B-12, and adenosine monophosphate (AMP), which, when combined, is advertised to act as an anabolic/anti-catabolic agent that reduces body fat. There are no scientific studies to support any of these contentions, but anecdotal reports and word of mouth advertising have made this one of the most sought after supplements. This pattern is not new, and it is safe to predict that within six months, at least a dozen variants of this product will be available.

DRUGS IN THE CLASS

Within the addiction field, the term "steroids" has come to define a group of compounds that have anabolic or tissue-building effects. However, because most also have some androgenic effects, they are more appropriately called anabolic-androgenic steroids. This profile of effects distinguishes them from the corticosteroids and the female gonadotrophic hormones, neither of which are subject to abuse. A rather large number of anabolic-androgenic steroids have been produced for human or veterinary use. The major source of abused steroids is diversion from licit manufacture and distribution, as clandestine laboratory synthesis of these products is very rare. The major distinction between use and abuse is that abusers employ supraphysiologic doses in order to increase muscle growth and enhance performance. It is the consequence of these extremely high doses that results in rather dangerous, but often reversible, organ toxicity.

The prototypic hormone, testosterone, is the standard to which all of the synthetic products are compared. It is one of four structurally distinct groups of anabolic-androgenic steroids. The other three groups are 17α-alkylated derivatives of testosterone, 17β-esterified derivatives of testosterone, and modified ring structure analogues (Wilson, 1988). The history of how testosterone and its effects on male sexual development and tissue building were discovered is well detailed by Kochakian (1990). Although hormonal involvement in male sexual development was known in 1849, it was not until 1930 that androsterone (a metabolite of testosterone) was isolated from human urine. In the 1940s, after chemists had succeeded in synthesizing testosterone, their efforts were directed toward separating its anabolic from its androgenic effects and developing a formulation that could be taken orally. The androgenic components of these synthetics have never been completely separated from the anabolic effects; only the relative proportions of the two have been manipulated. Commercially prepared products were used briefly during World War II to promote wound healing. In 1939, Boje postulated that anabolic-androgenic steroids might not only increase muscle mass, but improve physical performance as well.

Only a handful of anabolic-androgenic steroids are available in the United States and all have been placed in Schedule III of the federal Controlled Substances Act; many more products are available in foreign countries. A number of veterinary products are available in the United States; athletes frequently use preparations that are not labeled for human use when they cannot obtain the desired products. It is an interesting paradox that some young bodybuilders profess to be on strict diets and use only the purest of vitamin and dietary supplements, yet they take drugs for which use in humans has not been approved. Products that are not approved for use in the United States typically are obtained by mail order from abroad. Because the testing of these products in some other countries is not as stringent as that in the United States, individuals should be cautioned about using such products. Finally, there is an extensive black market of anabolic-androgenic steroids that supports a rather large percentage of inactive products that are falsely advertised as containing anabolic steroids.

Therapeutic Use. Although one might think that the therapeutic uses of anabolic-androgenic steroids is of less concern to the addiction medicine specialist, in reality, most physicians are asked to provide prescriptions for these drugs far more often than they are asked to help treat someone who is dependent on the drugs. Thus, knowledge of these medical situations may be useful in discussions with potential abusers because such individuals are likely to be aware of the medical reasons for their prescription and may use such information in their initial attempts to obtain legal medications to support their training or alter their appearance.

Misuse. Anabolic-androgenic steroids are abused by three distinct populations: (1) athletes who use them to improve performance, (2) aesthetes who use them solely to improve appearance and perhaps to gain some weight, and (3) the "fighting elite" who use them to enhance aggression and fighting skills (Brower, 1989). Identifying the specific population to which a patient belongs is the first step in understanding the pattern of use and determining the best treatment plan to follow.

Athletes: Athletes use anabolic-androgenic steroids for only one reason: to improve their performance. Perhaps one of the greatest mistakes clinicians make in dealing with athletes is attempting to dissuade their use on the grounds that the drugs cannot improve performance. In fact, this is not true. The older research studies that purported to show that the effects of anabolic-androgenic steroids were no different than placebo suffered from a number of methodological problems, did not control for motivation, and failed to document the amount of physical training. In addition, ethical considerations prevented the investigators from administering extremely high doses, which are considered necessary to achieve the muscle-building effect. Negative findings also have been attributed to the use of only one drug at a time in the research studies, whereas athletes in training typically use multiple drugs in combination.

The continued use of these drugs is based on the belief that they increase muscle capacity, reduce body fat, increase strength and endurance, and hasten recovery from injury (Haupt & Rovere, 1984). Many athletes also believe that anabolic-androgenic steroid-assisted training allows the user to increase both the frequency and the intensity of workouts—factors that contribute to any direct benefits of the drugs (Anderson & McKeag, 1985).

In the world of professional weightlifting and bodybuilding, anabolic-androgenic steroids are used in three basic patterns: "stacking," "pyramiding," and "cycling." *Stacking* is the practice of using multiple products at the same time. Users believe that the beneficial effects of one drug will complement those of another and that they will achieve real benefits only through the use of a specific combination. A *pyramid* plan involves starting with a low dose and then gradually increasing the dose until peak levels are achieved a number of weeks before competition. The individual then slowly reduces the drug dose. Because the beneficial effects of anabolic-androgenic steroids persist long after their use has been discontinued, athletes believe they will be "primed" for the competitive event. *Cycling* refers to the practice of using different combinations over a period of time in order to avoid the development of tolerance or loss of effectiveness. Thus, different combinations of drugs are used over a 6- to 12-week period, after which another drug or combination is substituted.

Aesthetes: Another group of users is composed of adolescent males who use these drugs primarily to increase their weight or to improve their physical appearance (Buckley, Yesalis et al., 1988; Yesalis, Streit et al., 1989; Wang, Fitzhugh et al., 1994; Tanner, Miller et al., 1995). The desire for weight gain among a group of adolescents who are not yet taking anabolic-androgenic steroids may place them at risk for initiating use (Wang, Fitzhugh et al., 1994). The trend is disturbing because many adolescents are unaware of the most serious risks associated with anabolic-androgenic steroid use. A study of the prevalence of anabolic-androgenic steroid use among 6th to 12th grade Canadian students found that 2.8% of respondents had used the drugs in the preceding year (Melia, Pipe et al., 1996). A third of the users had injected the drugs, and 29.2% of the injecting users reported that they had shared needles with friends. Young anabolic-androgenic steroid users also are likely to use other drugs, such as marijuana, smokeless tobacco, and cocaine (Durant, Rickert et al., 1993).

In general, the doses used by adolescents and others who want to improve their appearance are substantially lower than those used by adult athletes (Rogol & Yesalis, 1992). Further, the pattern of lower doses and intermittent cycles of use is likely to obviate the development of major side effects. However, because adolescent males are in transition due to hormonal changes associated with puberty, the drugs can have other significant effects. For example, the epiphyseal plate of the femur may close prematurely and actually stunt a boy's growth (Moore, 1988), which is contrary to what a significant number of adolescents believe. More importantly, these young users may be particularly sensitive to the increased aggressive effects resulting from their use (Rogol & Yesalis, 1992).

Apparently, a substantial proportion of adolescents are unaware of the side effects of anabolic-androgenic steroids. Although drug education programs have been slow to incorporate steroids into their lesson plans, the real reason the public is so unaware of the risks is that these drugs are probably not a severe health hazard when taken intermittently and in low to moderate doses (Rogol & Yesalis, 1992). Because programs that simply emphasize the negative aspects of drugs of abuse are ineffectual at curtailing use (Goldberg, Bents et al., 1991), the health professional should balance any discussion of anabolic-androgenic steroid abuse with factual information, rather than overstating the degree of potential harm. Such actions only serve to alienate the patient and instill a level of distrust. Young people know that only a small percentage of users actually experience very serious and deadly outcomes and believe that it will not happen to them. For the others, the side effects (except for some effects in women) are largely reversible.

Fighting Elite: Very little is known about this population of anabolic-androgenic steroid users. This profile was originally described by Brower (1989) and includes individuals who seek to increase their strength in order to perform a job. Another desired effect is the increase in aggressiveness that may help them with their jobs. Thus, bouncers at bars, security personnel, and even law enforcement officers have been reported to take these drugs (Dart, 1991; Swanson, Gaines et al., 1991).

Perhaps the most important concept to understand about anabolic-androgenic steroid abuse is that it does not follow typical patterns observed with traditional drugs of abuse such as cocaine, heroin, alcohol, nicotine, and marijuana. In this regard, along with most hallucinogens such as LSD, anabolic-androgenic steroids are not self-administered by laboratory animals, although a study in male rats demonstrated that the drugs may alter the sensitivity of brain reward systems (Clark, Lindenfeld et al., 1996). In that study, a two-week treatment with methandrostenolone alone had no effect on brain reward systems, but a 15-week treatment with a cocktail of three different anabolic-androgenic steroids resulted in a shift in the response patterns to brain electrical reward and amphetamine.

Self-Administration: The absence of a well-defined pattern of self-administration in animals is confirmed by the finding that humans cannot tell whether they have been given an active anabolic-androgenic steroid or placebo (Ariel & Saville, 1972). Marginal discriminations were made in two studies, but only after a period of extended testing had been employed (Freed, Banks et al., 1975; Crist, Stackpole et al., 1983). However, it is likely that it was the side effects of these drugs that were detected, rather than any positive reinforcing effects. As the latter are thought to regulate drug-taking behavior in both humans and animals, the question that remains is "why do humans use and abuse anabolic-androgenic steroids?"

It is well known that if the subjective effects of a psychoactive drug are sufficiently delayed after self-administration, then the drug's reinforcing efficacy decreases and drug-seeking behavior is reduced (Balster & Schuster, 1973). Although there are a few scattered anecdotal reports that high doses of anabolic-androgenic steroids can elevate mood, no controlled studies have demonstrated that these drugs produce immediate positive mood effects or euphoria. However, the lack of mood elevating effects in so-called "normal" volunteers is contrasted with the clear and significant improvement in mood when testosterone is given as replacement therapy in hypogonadal men (Su, Pagliaro et al., 1993). Both subjective and objective measures reflected an increase in energy level, sexual drive, and vitality in these men, suggesting that the hormonal status of an individual may very well dictate the psychoactive response to acute testosterone administration.

Anabolic-androgenic steroids can act within minutes to hours on cell membrane receptor sites, but the real beneficial effects of such action (such as protein synthesis) are not evident so quickly.

ABSORPTION AND METABOLISM
Anabolic-androgenic steroids are either taken orally or injected deep into the muscle; there is no intravenous formulation, nor is there a product that can be smoked. By far the greatest influence on subsequent development of toxic side effects is the route of administration. About half of an oral dose of testosterone is metabolized via the first-pass effect, so very large doses are needed. Some 17α analogues of testosterone like methyltestosterone resist such metabolism and so can be given orally in smaller doses. The oral route gives rise to a number of 17α-alkylated metabolites, which are formed in the liver. This overload, not only of the metabolizing enzymes, but because the doses taken are so high, causes significant stress on this organ.

Testosterone is metabolized to 5α-dihydrotestosterone (DHT) in certain tissues, such as the prostate gland, seminal vesicles, and pubic skin. Because DHT has two to three times the affinity for the androgen receptor as the parent hormone, the effects of testosterone are enhanced in these tissues. One of the more interesting aspects of testosterone's metabolic pathway is that it is converted to estradiol in tissues that contain an aromatase enzyme (Martini, 1982). The biological significance of circulating estrogens in males is unknown, but they may be involved with sex-hormone-binding globulin (SHBG) and lipoproteins. Further, the estrogen that results from this metabolic process may interact with estrogen receptors to produce an anabolic effect (Bardin, Catterall et al., 1990; Svare, 1990). The 17α-alkylated analogs discussed earlier are not metabolized to either DHT or estrogen. Instead, they interact with the androgen receptor (Wilson, 1988; Winters, 1990).

Thus, the overall profile of relative anabolic to androgenic effects is not due only to the parent compound, but also to the profile of metabolites that result. With the advent of widespread use of these drugs during athletic competition, a number of analytical laboratories have been set up to detect either the parent drug or its metabolites (Schanzer, 1996; Catlin, 1987). In addition to providing quantitative analyses of the various synthetic analogues, most labs attempt to measure the testosterone/epitestosterone ratio as a metric of exogenous testosterone administration.

PHARMACOLOGIC ACTIONS
About 95% of the testosterone in males is synthesized in the testes, while the remaining 5% comes from the adrenals. The cholesterol used in the synthetic pathway comes from acetate that is stored in the testes and not from circulating blood levels. Anabolic-androgenic steroids long have been thought to exert their effects in the periphery, primarily by increasing the rate of RNA transcription (see Lukas, 1993,

MOA

1996). About half of the circulating testosterone is tightly bound to SHBG, while the other half is lightly bound to albumin, from which it freely dissociates and from whence it can diffuse passively into target cells. After attaching to a steroid receptor in the cytoplasm, the hormone-receptor complex moves into the nucleus, where it binds to sites on the chromatin, resulting in new mRNA. If the target tissue is skeletal muscle, then new myofilaments are formed, which cause myofibrils to divide (Wilson, 1988; Rogivkin, 1976).

As it is not completely understood whether this activity occurs at the supraphysiologic doses typically taken by ana-bolic-androgenic steroid abusers, another mechanism was sought. It has been suggested that high doses of anabolic-androgenic steroids cross-react with glucocorticoid receptors, which control the catabolic rates of protein (Wilson, 1988; Mayer & Rosen, 1977; Raaka, Finnerty et al., 1989). The significance of the anticatabolic effect of these drugs often is ignored in lieu of the more direct effect of these steroids on protein synthesis. It also is possible that the stress of strenuous workouts is not felt by athletes taking these compounds, because the stress-induced increase in cortisol is somehow blocked. This action also would permit the workouts to be longer and more vigorous, further improving performance.

It is possible that the physical changes attributed to a direct effect of anabolic-androgenic steroids on protein synthesis actually may be mediated via a direct effect on the central nervous system. Such effects might result in increased motivation and intensity of training to a degree that performance is improved. Increased aggressive behavior also may play a role in the training process. It is likely that the use of supraphysiologic doses of these drugs can have both a direct effect on muscle tissue and an indirect effect on emotions by altering motivation and drive so that training periods are longer and more productive, resulting in improved performance.

The psychoactive effects of testosterone and related hormones long have been recognized and may reflect either organizational changes when a subject is exposed during a critical developmental period or activation effects that are observed during exposure to adults (Rubinow & Schmidt, 1996). The former are thought to be permanent, while the latter are transient and abate when exposure is terminated. Both males and females have a widely distributed array of testosterone receptors in the brain, and it appears that testosterone and related steroids activate different systems to stimulate the desirable physiologic effects as well as the undesirable psychiatric effects (Yates, 2000).

There is provocative evidence that anabolic-androgenic steroids interact directly with peripheral benzodiazepine receptors in the rat brain (Masonis & McCarthy, 1996). These receptors are mitochondrial proteins that are involved with regulating steroid synthesis and transport, so it seems plausible that their activation via exogenous anabolic-androgenic steroids could have an effect on behavior that is mediated by the receptors.

The increase in body weight, especially during the first weeks of use, almost certainly is attributable to the stimulation of mineral-corticoid receptors, resulting in sodium and, ultimately, water retention, as well as increasing amounts of circulating estrogen that has been aromatized from testosterone. This effect gives the muscles, particularly the deltoid, a "puffy" appearance.

The increase in red blood cell production is probably the major reason that long distance runners use these drugs: Endurance, rather than bulk muscle mass, is an asset in their sport. Blood volume probably increases as a result of erythropoietin synthesis. This effect is the result of direct action on bone marrow and easily leads to a rise in hematocrit (Narducci, Wagner et al., 1990).

ADDICTION LIABIILTY

Anabolic-androgenic steroid abuse includes a variety of social and psychological components that are not easy to imitate in either animal models or in currently validated methods of assessing abuse liability in human volunteers. The concepts of perception, motivation, and expectation play a more pivotal role in the initial use and subsequent abuse of these compounds.

It is difficult to determine whether the attraction of steroids is related to any beneficial effect on an individual's performance, as the drugs rarely are taken in the absence of a training program that includes exercise and sound nutrition (Bahrke & Yesalis, 1994). This concept punctuates the second aspect of anabolic-androgenic steroid abuse among athletes: It usually occurs during training periods, which typically can begin weeks and even months before a competitive event or season. The need for these drugs by most athletes decreases during actual competition, and so the active use can decline. However, with the advent of mandatory urine testing at major athletic events, the risk of being caught may curtail use, but because the urine tests are announced before the event, competitors have ample warning to stop using and allow the steroids to clear from the system. Thus, positive urine screens that are collected during actual competitive events usually are the result of high sensitivity of the analytical methods to detect minute amounts of metabolites that persist after use of anabolic-androgenic steroids is stopped. The competitor may be unaware that the drug remains in tissue for so long.

Surveys over the past decade have found that athletes are not the only individuals to use and abuse anabolic-androgenic steroids. Abuse now is seen in adult non-athletes and even in adolescents who may be using the drugs to improve their appearance (Yesalis, Kennedy et al., 1993). Women also use steroids, but all estimates indicate that the prevalence is much lower than in males.

These factors pushed the U.S. Congress to enact the Anabolic Steroids Control Act, which effectively placed all steroid compounds, including testosterone and its many analogues, in Schedule III of the federal Controlled Substances Act (states, of course, have the option of scheduling these drugs even more restrictively under state law). Schedule III contains opioids such as nalorphine, stimulants such as benzphetamine, and depressants such as butabarbital and thiopental.

Unfortunately, steroids no longer are tracked by the National Household Survey on Drug Abuse; however, the results of the 1994 survey (SAMHSA, 1996) indicate that overall lifetime use of anabolic-androgenic steroids among all individuals 12 years of age or older is about 0.52%. Except for heroin (0.9%), lifetime use of other drugs such as inhalants (5.8%), cocaine (10.4%), smokeless tobacco (17.2%) marijuana/hashish (31.2%), tobacco (73.3%), and alcohol (84.2%) was substantially higher than anabolic-androgenic steroids at that time.

Distribution of the anabolic-androgenic steroid problem is age-related, as lifetime use was highest in 18- to 25-year-olds (1.1%), followed by 26- to 34-year-olds (1.0%), 12- to 17-year-olds (0.7%), and 35+ year olds (0.2%). Use by males exceeded that by females (0.9% versus 0.2%), and use was equally distributed among Caucasian, African American and Hispanic ethnic groups (about 0.5%). The most recent Monitoring the Future Study for College Students and Young Adults, 1975-2000 (Johnston, O'Malley et al., 2001b) indicates that use within the preceding year dropped by 0.2% for young adults (ages 19 to 28), from 0.6% to 0.4%, and the distribution was nearly 3:1 for males to females. The Monitoring the Future Study for Second-

ary School Students, 1975-2000 (Johnston, O'Malley et al., 2001a) found that more than a half million 8th and 10th graders are using these drugs. An even larger percentage of high school seniors say they do not believe that the drugs are harmful. Specific findings indicate that use in the preceding year by 10th grade boys increased from 2.8% in 1999 to 3.6% in 2000, while use among 8th and 12th grade boys actually dropped by 0.3% and 0.6%, respectively. However, use among 8th, 10th, and 12th grade girls increased by 0.1%, 0.1%, and 0.3%, respectively, from 1999 to 2000. Lifetime prevalence rates for all 8th and 10th graders increased by 0.3% and 0.8% from 1999 to 2000, while 12th graders' rates decreased by 0.4%.

Two other indicators of potential abuse lie in the answers to questions regarding perceived harmfulness and ease of obtaining steroids. The long-term trends of perceived harmfulness by 12th graders was 63.8% in 1989 and peaked at 70.7% in 1992. This trend has slowly declined over the years, to 57.9% in 2000. It is noteworthy that, in 1992, the professional football player Lyle Alzado publicly claimed that steroids caused his brain cancer and so may have had an important effect on young people's beliefs at the time.

Long-term trends in perceived availability among 12th graders peaked in 1992, with 44.8% reporting that steroids were "very easy" to obtain. This belief declined to 40.3% in 1996, but rose to 44.8% of respondents in 2000.

While these values may seem small, the perceived increase in availability of anabolic-androgenic steroids was ranked behind only alcohol, marijuana, MDMA, cocaine, and LSD in the National Household Survey data. The use of all of these drugs (except marijuana) increased from 1999 to 2000. Thus, it is apparent that anabolic-androgenic steroids remain fairly easy to obtain in high schools and that fewer young people perceive them as harmful. These factors are reasons to remain concerned over the use of anabolic-androgenic steroids by youth.

Tolerance. Evidence supporting the development of tolerance is not strong, although there is a belief among users that cycling is a necessary practice to avoid its development. In various studies, 20% of weight lifters believed that tolerance develops, while more than 80% believed that dependence develops. Nevertheless, such concerns appear to be without hard empirical evidence. Thus, it must be assumed that the escalating doses that elite athletes use are not taken because of tolerance to drug effects, but to increase the magnitude of the desired effects. The doses are increased slowly in order to minimize the side effects or to allow time to acclimate to them. When presented with this fact, some users are likely to confuse their behavior with tolerance.

Dependence. Although there is little evidence of physical dependence on anabolic-androgenic steroids, there are a few detailed reports of clear signs of withdrawal when use of the drugs was stopped abruptly (Brower, Eliopulos et al., 1990; Brower, 1992; Brower, Blow et al., 1991). In a study of 49 male weight lifters (Brower, Blow et al., 1991), 84% reported experiencing withdrawal effects. The most frequently reported symptoms were craving for more steroids (52%), fatigue (43%), depressed mood state (41%), restlessness (29%), anorexia (24%), insomnia (20%), decreased libido (20%), and headaches (20%). Interestingly, 42% of these subjects were dissatisfied with their body image during withdrawal as well. Those who reported being dependent on anabolic-androgenic steroids generally took higher doses, completed more cycles of use, and reported more aggressive symptoms than those who did not report being dependent. However, the extent of dependence on anabolic-androgenic steroids in the larger population of users may be considerably smaller, as there have been no reported cases of withdrawal effects in female athletes or among patients who have been prescribed high doses for legitimate medical purposes.

Anabolic-androgenic steroids can, in fact, increase muscle mass and body weight, especially when used as part of a regular training program. However, many of the "black market" anabolic-androgenic steroid preparations sold during the late 1980s actually were devoid of any active ingredients, including anabolic-androgenic steroids. In spite of the spread of these counterfeit drugs, users claimed to have experienced improvements in performance. Herein lies the real difficulty in assessing the abuse liability of these compounds: Because they are not expected to have immediate beneficial effects, the delay in any improvement does not raise suspicion that the preparation may be inert. Nevertheless, whether the drugs actually increase muscle mass, improve performance, or increase endurance is not really the question that confronts the addiction medicine specialist. The fact that anabolic-androgenic steroid-seeking behavior exists and that extremely high doses are used over relatively long periods of time suggests that there is a problem and should trigger further inquiry and subsequent treatment.

Thus, while physical dependence on anabolic-androgenic steroids may be more rare than dependence on other drugs of abuse, the prudent clinician will be vigilant to identify the constellation of signs and symptoms that may signify dependence. Attempts to label the withdrawal signs and symptoms as opiate-like or ethanol-like may complicate the issue only because such an effort may conceal a real dependence on those drugs. Consequently, when obvious signs of distress are observed during periods of forced abstinence, it is worthwhile to consider the possibility that the individual may, in fact, be dependent on other drugs. There have been a few reports of opioid dependence in bodybuilders (Evans, Bowen et al., 1985; McBride, Williamson et al., 1996), and these individuals clearly met criteria for dependence on both drug classes. Thus, the possibility of polydrug abuse always should be considered when dealing with anabolic-androgenic steroid abusers.

TOXICITY/ADVERSE EFFECTS

Psychopathology. Controversy remains over the severity of anabolic-androgenic steroid-induced psychiatric effects, particularly those known as "roid rage." While case studies document a link between psychiatric effects and steroid use (Annitto & Layman, 1980; Freinhar & Alvarez, 1985; Conacher & Workman, 1989; Pope & Katz, 1987; Wilson, Prange et al., 1974), the eruption of frenzied violent behavior during a cycle of high-dose anabolic-androgenic steroids has been described in only a few case reports and a laboratory study. Pope and colleagues (2000) administered placebo or 600 mg/week of testosterone cypionate for six weeks each to 20- to 50-year-old males who did not have a history of psychiatric illness or steroid use. The order of exposure was randomized, and a six-week washout period was scheduled between treatments. Testosterone treatment resulted in 6% of the men becoming mildly hypomanic and 4% becoming markedly hypomanic, with increased aggressive responding in a simulated procedure. Responders and nonresponders did not differ on any demographic measure. The reasons for the highly variable individual responses is not known, but these data suggest that even modest doses of testosterone can induce psychiatric symptoms in certain "susceptible" individuals.

The constellation of symptoms appears to closely resemble those of hypomania or mania. The energized user of anabolic-androgenic steroids talks faster, has more energy, sleeps less and is more impulsive, even engaging in behaviors such as purchasing expensive automobiles (Pope & Katz, 1987). At the far end of the spectrum, mania may lead to delusions and even hallucinations. Interestingly, many individuals with body dysmorphic disorder present with delusions as well (Phillips, McElroy et al., 1994). Two studies (Perry, Yates et al., 1990; Pope & Katz, 1988) attempted to standardize the collection of these data and found that, using structured interviews, the incidence of a full affective syndrome was present in 22% of a population of 41 bodybuilders (Pope & Katz, 1988). Another 12% displayed psychotic symptoms that clearly emerged during anabolic-androgenic steroid use. The cohort of 20 weight lifters who used anabolic-androgenic steroids experienced more somatic, depressive, anxious, hostile, and paranoid complaints than those who did not use these drugs (Perry, Yates et al., 1990).

Empirical evidence of the effects of steroids in producing aggressive behavior has been obtained using the Karolinska Scale of Personality (Galligani, Renck et al., 1996) and a human laboratory model of aggression, the Point Subtraction Aggression Paradigm or PSAP (Cherek, 1981). Results from the personality scale indicated that a cohort of anabolic-androgenic steroid users exhibited significantly more verbal aggression, impulsiveness, and indirect aggression. Yates and colleagues (1992) reported that three measures of the Buss-Durkee Hostility Inventory (Buss & Durkee, 1957)—assault, indirect aggression, and verbal aggression—were elevated in a group of current or recent anabolic-androgenic steroid users. The PSAP paradigm directly measures the amount of provoked aggressive behavior in the laboratory by ostensibly taking away points (that are worth money) from an individual who believes he is playing against another person. In reality, the subject plays against a computer program, and the rate of provocation is controlled by the experimenter. Both aggressive and non-aggressive behavior is recorded, so the effects of various drugs on responding *per se* can be viewed independently of aggressive responding. Using this model, moderately high doses of testosterone cypionate (600 mg, intramuscularly, once a week) can be shown to increase aggressive responding in individuals who had not used steroids before (Kouri, Lukas et al., 1995).

Animal models confirm that anabolic-androgenic steroid administration increases aggressive behavior (Svare, 1990). As weight lifters and bodybuilders are reported to have used weekly doses three times those used in research studies, it is reasonable to suspect that aggressive behavior can result from such training programs.

Collectively, it appears that anabolic-androgenic steroid use can result in hypomania and even psychotic symptoms, while depression may emerge during withdrawal. The lack of well-controlled prospective studies has prevented a more definitive association between anabolic-androgenic steroid use and psychiatric disorders. It is unlikely that such data will become available in the near future as ethical constraints will preclude the conduct of any double-blind assessments of supraphysiological doses of these drugs.

Studies of the personalities of anabolic-androgenic steroid abusers by Cooper and colleagues (1996) identified a high rate of abnormal personality traits in a sample of 12 bodybuilders who used anabolic-androgenic steroids compared to a matched group who did not. In addition to being heavier than the controls, the users were more likely to score higher on measures of paranoia, schizoid, antisocial, borderline, histrionic, narcissistic, and passive-aggressive personality profiles. The incidence of abnormal personality traits before anabolic-androgenic steroid use began was not different in the study subjects than in the control group, suggesting that such disturbances are secondary to steroid use. Users also reported that they believe that anabolic-androgenic steroids not only enhance physical strength and athletic ability, but increase confidence, assertiveness, feelings of sexuality, and optimism (Schwerin & Corcoran, 1996).

In a study of 108 bodybuilders, Pope and colleagues (1993) noted a rather high percentage of anorexia nervosa and uncovered a body image disorder which they labeled *reverse anorexia*. This condition shares many signs and symptoms with body dysmorphic syndrome (Phillips, 1996). Sufferers view themselves as too small and weak, when in fact they are quite large and strong. The incidence of this disorder was 8% among anabolic-androgenic steroid users and was not observed in any of the non-users. The authors postulate that such body image disorders may have some influence on an individual's decision to use anabolic-androgen steroids. This condition has been called "muscle dysmorphia," as the persons affected become pathologically preoccupied with the degree of their muscularity (Pope, Gruber et al., 1997). Because the perceived size, shape, and attractiveness of one's body is related to self-esteem (Lombardo, 1992) and, in general, men want to be taller, three pounds heavier, and have wider shoulders (Wroblewski, 1997), anabolic-androgenic steroid use may be viewed as a way of attaining physical attractiveness. The similarity in profiles between body image disorders and drug use might suggest that anabolic-androgenic steroid abusers who present with a profile of body image disturbance may respond to the same treatments that have been used for body dysmorphic syndrome, for which serotonin reuptake inhibitors have been marginally successful (Hollander, Liebowitz et al., 1989). While there have been no published studies with anabolic-androgenic steroid users, fluoxetine has been marginally successful in a small sample of bodybuilders who presented with depression during withdrawal from anabolic-androgenic steroid use (Malone & Dimeff, 1992).

Collectively, these studies suggest that there is a growing number of individuals who are sufficiently dissatisfied with their appearance that they will seek out a variety of methods to improve their looks (Kanayama, Pope et al., 2001). Anabolic-androgenic steroids are the most prevalent way of pharmacologically altering body shape, but there are many other drugs that either enhance the effects of the steroids or exert their own effects to change appearance (Table 1). Thus, another clue that a person is using anabolic-androgenic steroids is the profile of other drugs that he or she is taking.

Effects on Major Organ Systems. A great deal is known about the side effects and toxic profile of anabolic-androgenic steroids. Side effects, which generally are reversible with cessation of drug use, are depicted in Figure 1. For practical purposes, the addiction medicine specialist should be able to recognize these signs, particularly when they emerge rather rapidly. More serious medical consequences and even toxic reactions appear to involve primarily blood chemistry, endocrine function, liver, the cardiovascular system, and the central nervous system. Reports that high-dose steroid use leads to certain malignancies have not been substantiated.

Blood: Administration of the 17α-alkylated androgens can cause a dramatic reduction in high-density lipoprotein (HDL) cholesterol, but because there is a nearly equal increase in low-density lipoprotein (LDL) cholesterol, there is no net change in total cholesterol levels (Friedl, 1990). Other agents such as nandrolone and testosterone esters fail to produce this profile (Friedl, 1990; Thompson, Curinane et al., 1989). Although the long-term detrimental effects of altered HDL/LDL ratios are known to predispose humans to atherosclerosis, studies linking anabolic-androgenic steroid use to increased rates of cardiac morbidity and mortality are few (McNutt, Ferenchick et al., 1988; Bowman, 1990). The lack of direct correlation may be attributable to the fact that different steroids have varied

effects on lipid dynamics (Thompson, Curinane et al., 1989). Thus, while users "stack" various drugs in order to improve the beneficial effects, this practice may actually afford some protection against certain side effects. Further, the relative paucity of coronary vascular disease in athletes who use the drugs may be due to a reduction in other risk factors (through diet, exercise, and reduction in body fat), which compensates for any negative contribution afforded by the HDL/LDL profile. Such protection, however, may not be present in individuals who use anabolic-androgenic steroids only to improve their appearance and do not engage in athletic activity. Platelet aggregation (Ferenchick, 1990) along with increased red blood cell production and slight increases in systolic blood pressure have been identified as important factors that increase an individual's risk for thromboembolic disorders (Wilson, 1988; Lenders, Demacker et al., 1988).

Endocrine: Because testosterone exerts an inhibitory action on the hypothalamic-pituitary axis, administration of natural or synthetic analogs of testosterone decrease testicular size and sperm count (Palacios, McClure et al., 1981; Allen & Suominen, 1984). Residual amounts of active metabolites may keep the levels of FSH and LH low, and—coupled with the relatively long cycle to produce sperm—the recovery is likely to be slow, but often is complete. Aromatization is the process by which steroid hormones are interconverted. For example, testosterone is converted to estradiol and estrone, so that high-dose male anabolic-androgenic steroid users can have circulating estrogen levels of normally cycling women (Wilson, 1988). These circulating estrogens exert the usual feminizing effects, such as gynecomastia. Compounds that resist aromatization (such as fluoxymesterolone, mesterolone, and stanozolol) may not produce these feminizing effects (Kashkin, 1992).

Reproductive: Males may receive anabolic-androgenic steroids for replacement therapy when the testicles fail to function, due to either congenital or traumatic factors, or when puberty is delayed and short stature would result. The doses that are prescribed, however, are much lower than those used by bodybuilders. The equivalent of 75 to 100 mg per week of testosterone suffices as replacement, but weight lifters and bodybuilders reportedly use weekly doses of 1,000 to 2,100 mg of metandienone (Yesalis, Herrick et al., 1988; Freed, Banks et al., 1975). Women occasionally are treated with androgens when metastatic breast cancer has spread to bone. Methyltestosterone is combined with

TABLE 1. Anabolic-Androgenic Steroids and Related Products

Popular/Trade Name	Chemical Name	Description of Uses/Actions
Anabolic-Androgenic Steroids (Human)		
Anabolicum vister®	quinbolone	Well tolerated but very weak androgen with a low side-effect profile.
Anadrol-50®	oxymetholone	One of the most powerful anabolic and androgenic steroids available.
Anavar®	oxandrolone	Now discontinued, but formerly popular.
Androderm®	testosterone patch	Slow-release formulation of testosterone, generally used for replacement therapy.
Androgel®	testosterone topical gel	Topical ointment formulation of testosterone.
Danocrine®	danazol	No anabolic, but mild androgenic effect; used to treat gynecomastia.
Deca-Durabolin®, Durabolin®	nandrolone decanoate, phenpropionate	Very popular injectable with high anabolic and low androgenic profile.
Delatestryl®	testosterone enanthate	Moderately powerful androgen in an injectable oil preparation; its effects are short lived.
Depo-Testosterone®	testosterone cypionate	Moderately powerful anabolic and androgen in an injectable oil preparation; its effects are relatively short-lived. Water retention is a problem.
Dianabol®	methandrostenolone	Popular oral preparation that has a rapid onset; moderate androgenic effects limits its use.
Halotestin®	fluoxymesterolone	A powerful androgen with little anabolic effect; increases strength with little weight gain.
Masterid®	drostanolone	A derivative of dihydrotestosterone (DHT), with a strong androgenic effect and little water retention; often used just before competition, as it is quickly metabolized.
Maxibolan®	ethylestrenol	A weak androgen that is favored by women; it is moderately effective, with little water retention, but is potentially toxic to the liver.
Metandren®, Testred®	methyltestosterone	An oral testosterone that is not very popular today, but still is taken because of its prominent android androgenic effects (aggression) and mild anabolic effects.
Oxandrin®	oxandrolone	Mild anabolic agent that increases strength without concomitant increase in mass; believed to be relatively safe, although liver toxicity is possible.
Permastril®	dromostanolone	Similar to Masterid.
Primobolan®	methenolone	Mild, but relatively safe anabolic agent with little androgenic effects; available in oral, buccal, and injectable depot formulations.
Proviron®	mesterolone	Less effective anabolic, as it is quickly metabolized to the diol metabolite and so may not reach receptors.
Stenox®	halotestin	Strong oral androgen and mild anabolic but rather toxic; weight gain is minimal.
Sustanon®	testosterone	Oil-based injectable preparation of four salts of testosterone (propionate, phenylpropionate, isocaproate, and decanoate) that are timed to release active testosterone from 1 to 30 days; pronounced anabolic and androgenic effects and less water retention.
Winstrol®	stanozolol	Oral preparation that has modest anabolic effects and weak androgenic effects; often "stacked" with other steroids; many counterfeits are available.

TABLE 1.   Anabolic-Androgenic Steroids and Related Products (continued)

Popular/Trade Name	Chemical Name	Description of Uses/Actions
Anabolic-Androgenic Steroids/Growth Promotants (Veterinary)		
Cheque Drops®	mibolerone	No longer popular; among the most toxic androgenic steroids; increases mass and aggression.
Drive®		Moderately strong androgen with mild androgenic activity and low liver toxicity.
Equipose®	boldenone	Strong anabolic with milder androgenic effects; often "stacked" with other steroids.
Finiject®	bolasterone	Popular injectable but no longer available; strong anabolic and androgenic effects.
Finaplix-H®	trenbolone	Implantable potent androgen; no longer available.
Implus®		Implantable combination of testosterone and estradiol; gynecomastia is a major side effect.
Nadrabolin®	nandrolone	Injectable long-acting version of Deca-Durabolin®; inexpensive and relatively easy to obtain.
Ralgrow®	zeranol	Implantable agent that increases weight in cattle, but is ineffective in humans.
Revalor®	trenbolone/estradiol	Implantable combination product of trenbolone and estradiol that will increase strength but little water retention; often used with dimethyl sulfoxide (DMSO) to promote skin absorption; renal toxicity is a common side effect.
Synovex-H®	testosterone/estradiol	Implantable combination of testosterone and estradiol, with a profile like Revalor®.
Winstrol-V®	stanozolol	Both oral and injectable preparation that has modest anabolic effects and weak androgenic effects and so often is "stacked" with other steroids; many counterfeits exist.
Supplements, Minerals, and Other Products		
Aldactazide®	aldactone/thiazide	Combination of the diuretics aldactone and thiazide; used to shed excess water.
Catapres®	clonidine	Antihypertensive taken to reduce steroid-induced elevated blood pressure.
Clomid®	clomiphene	Increases follicle-stimulating hormone, which in turn increases testosterone; typically used to avoid a "crash" after stopping steroids.
Cynomel® & others	cytomel	Synthetic thyroid hormone (T_3); used to increase basal metabolic rate by increasing synthesis of protein, carbohydrates, and fats; may work synergistically with steroids.
Cytadren®	aminogluthethimide	Used to treat Cushing's syndrome; inhibits production of androgens, estrogens, and cortisone.
EPO®	erythropoietin	Injectable protein hormone that stimulates red blood cell production in bone marrow; dangerous elevations in hematocrit has caused some deaths.
GHB®	gamma-hydroxybutyrate	General anesthetic; increases growth hormone secretion; contains a protein sparing effect; improves sleep quality; dangerous when combined with other CNS system depressants.
Glucophage®, Mellitron®	metformin	Oral hypoglycemic that mimics insulin; less toxic than phenformin.
Humulin R®	insulin	Natural pancreatic hormone; regulates glucose and helps glycogen and other nutrients enter muscles; typically used after a workout; very dangerous.

TABLE 1.   Anabolic-Androgenic Steroids and Related Products (continued)

Popular/Trade Name	Chemical Name	Description of Uses/Actions
Fenformin®	phenformin	Oral hypoglycemic agent; can produce lactic acidosis; not used as often as Glucophage.
IGF-1®	____	Insulin-like growth factor that is a structural analog of insulin; very short-acting and so combined with IGFBP-3 to extend its half-life.
Kyno-H®	kynoselen	A mixture of potassium, selenium, magnesium, vitamin B_{12}, and AMP that is promoted to inhibit protein breakdown; the claims have not been substantiated.
Lasix®	furosemide	Strong diuretic used before competitions to remove excess subcutaneous water; can induce electrolyte imbalance if used improperly.
Levothroid®	L-thyroxine	Synthetic thyroid hormone (T_4) used to increase the metabolism of carbohydrates, proteins, and fats; less popular than Cynomel®.
Naprosyn®, Naxen®	naproxen	Potent oral nonsteroidal agent that reduces inflammation, stiffness, and pain; can result in stomach ulcers.
Nubain®	nalbuphine	Opiate mixed agonist/antagonist pain killer; can be addictive.
Pregnyl®	human chorionic gonadotropin (HCG)	Natural protein hormone that mimics luteinizing hormone's effects to stimulate production of testosterone; used to counter negative feedback effects of exogenous steroids.
Protropin®	growth hormone (GH)	Synthetic version of human growth hormone; widely popular but may not be meeting expectations of protein buildup and breakdown of fat as an energy source; increases IGF-1 levels; cannot be detected by current testing procedures.
Pump N Pose®	synthol	A fatty acid that is injected into specific muscles to increase their size via encapsulation within the muscle fibers; gains are reported to be permanent, but this is unlikely, as it probably breaks down after a few years.
Slow-K®	potassium chloride	Slow-release formulation; used to prevent potassium depletion secondary to the use of strong diuretics.
Spiropent®	clenbuterol	Bronchodilator used to treat asthma; as a beta$_2$ agonist it burns fat, but its anabolic effects are limited to livestock, not humans.
Stadol®	butorphanol	Opioid analgesic; mixed agonist-antagonist; can be addictive.
Thiomucase®	____	A dispersing agent that is included with the injectable steroid to help it enter the system more quickly; also used alone to reduce fatty spots on the body.
Trisoralen®	trioxsalen	An oral medication that enhances pigmentation and thus promotes tanning to improve looks just before competition; not widely available.

estrogen (Premarin®) to help alleviate some of the signs and symptoms of menopause.

Both males and females might receive agents with more anabolic effects during treatment of a rare form of hereditary angioedema. Acquired aplastic anemia and myelofibrosis both result in deficiencies of red blood cell production, which is combated with drugs that have equal amounts of anabolic and androgenic effects. These drugs also can be useful in treating the trauma associated with burns and AIDS. Finally, steroids with more anabolic activity are useful in treating muscle wasting that is secondary to starvation.

Hepatic: Although a wide variety of medical disorders (and even exercise) can increase the amount of liver enzymes in the blood, this response is primarily limited to the use of oral, 17-alkylated anabolic-androgenic steroids. The relationship between these drugs and elevated enzyme levels exists because: (1) these orally effective drugs are metabolized by the liver, (2) the first pass effect delivers an exceptionally large percentage of the dose to the liver, and (3) abusers typically take excessive doses that further stress liver function. This profile often results in cholecystatic jaundice (Pecking, Lejolly et al., 1980) but, because inflammation and necrosis are not present, the symptoms are limited to an accumulation of bile that spills over into the blood. Interestingly, many bodybuilders use this side effect as a metric of their dosing regimen and titrate themselves to levels that just precipitate jaundice (Lukas, 1994).

Peliosis hepatitis is a disorder characterized by blood-filled cysts scattered throughout the liver; the history of this disorder and its relationship to anabolic-androgenic steroid abuse has been described in detail (Karch, 1993). It has been associated with the 17α-alkylated androgens, rarely results in symptoms, and probably resolves with discontinuation of steroid use (Westaby, Ogle et al., 1977).

The evidence linking 17α-alkylated androgens with hepatic tumors is well established. Except for the fact that the androgen-related adenomas are typically larger, the profile resembles that of women who take birth control pills. The risk of developing hepatocellular adenomas ranges from 1% to 3% of users (Friedl, 1990). As with peliosis hepatitis, these adenomas rarely result in symptoms and often are not documented except at autopsy.

Cardiovascular: Anabolic-androgenic steroids affect the cardiovascular system through their effects on HDL/LDL ratios and other blood products. However, there are reports that the drugs also directly affect myocardial tissue. The bulk of the evidence comes from animal studies in which high doses of methandrostenolone result in myocyte necrosis, cellular edema, and mitochondrial swelling (Appell, Heller-Umpfenbach et al., 1983; Behrendt & Boffin, 1977). As these changes cannot be produced by exercise alone, it is likely that they explain reports of anabolic-androgenic steroid users who suddenly die of cardiac arrest (Luke, Farb et al., 1991).

Other: A potential, but not well-documented, direct adverse effect of anabolic-androgenic steroid use during high-intensity training periods is an elevated incidence of traumatic injury, as typified by a case of bilateral quadriceps rupture (David, Green et al., 1995). While such injuries could be attributed to the fact that steroid users can train with the drugs to a level beyond what they could tolerate without the drugs, it also is possible that the growth of muscle mass is not paralleled by an increase in ligament support.

Women. Until recently, little was known about the psychiatric and medical effects of anabolic-androgenic steroid use by women. In a recent study of 75 dedicated female athletes, 33% reported current or past steroid use (Gruber & Pope, 2000). Not surprisingly, the users were more muscular than nonusers and reported using many other performance-enhancing drugs. Fifty-six percent of the users reported hypomanic symptoms during steroid use, while 40% reported depressive symptoms during withdrawal. This suggests that female users of steroids may be at risk for the same psychiatric symptoms as males (Honour, 1997). However, even the more serious side effects disappeared within three months of discontinuing steroid use, while benefits such as increases in lean body mass and increased diameter of muscle fibers remain (Hartgens, Kuipers et al., 1996).

FUTURE RESEARCH DIRECTIONS

With the advent of more sophisticated urine testing procedures, the likelihood that an athlete who uses anabolic-androgenic steroids can evade detection is decreasing. This situation has prompted the increased popularity of an entirely new generation of performance-enhancing drugs that can be taken without detection. Such drugs include human growth hormone (somatotropin), dihydroepiandrosterone (DHEA), erythropoietin, and thyroxine. Other drugs that may enhance performance include the mixed agonist/antagonist opioids such as butorphanol and nalbuphine (Wines, Gruber et al., 1999), the beta adrenergic agonist clenbuterol, "hormone helpers" such as gamma-hydroxybutyrate (GHB), clonidine and human chorionic gonadotropin (hCG), and testosterone stimulants such as clomiphene and human chorionic gonadotropin.

In addition, a variety of diuretics (including acetazolamide, furosemide, spironolactone, and triamterene) are used to help clear the anabolic-androgenic steroids and their metabolites from the urine in advance of drug testing. Knowledge of these drugs, where to obtain them, the doses to use, and even recipes for adding them to training programs can be found in a number of "underground" guides, as well as on a variety of Web sites frequented by athletes and others.

Because adolescents' use of anabolic-androgenic steroids has increased slightly in recent years, there is considerable concern that current drug abuse prevention programs are

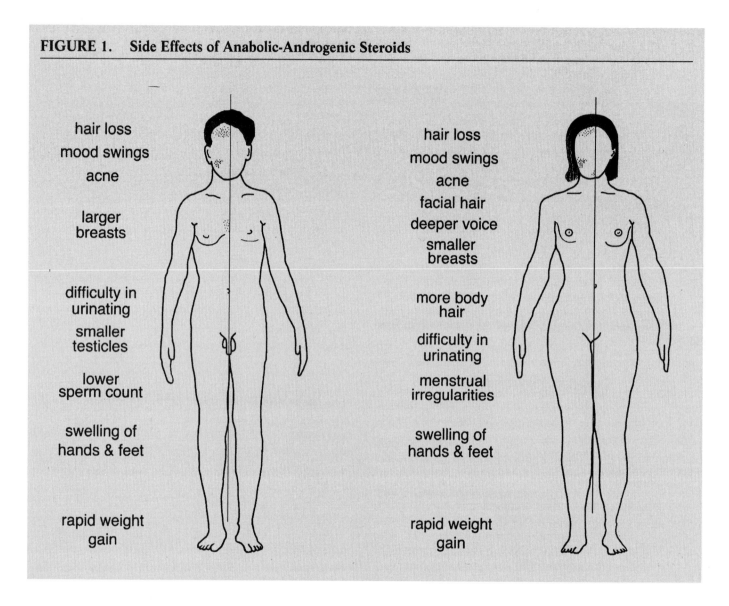

FIGURE 1.   Side Effects of Anabolic-Androgenic Steroids

failing to address steroid use. To this end, a recent program called Adolescents Training and Learning to Avoid Steroids (ATLAS) has been developed, and an initial efficacy study has been completed (Goldberg, MacKinnon et al., 2000). ATLAS is a team-oriented, gender-specific educational program that focuses on reducing intentions to use steroids, alcohol, and other drugs. The preliminary report is encouraging, depicting significant reductions in intention to use steroids and other drugs. This suggests that drug use among athletes (a historically difficult population) can be altered.

CONCLUSIONS

While the overall rate of abuse of anabolic-androgenic steroids remains lower than that of many other drugs, the potential organ damage from the typically large doses of steroids renders these drugs potentially dangerous. Recent trends toward increased use among adolescents, coupled with adolescents' reduced perceptions of harm associated with steroids, also is cause for concern.

As the anabolic-androgens have been placed in restrictive schedules under the federal Controlled Substances Act, a group of non-scheduled steroid alternatives or steroid "helpers" has emerged, and these could present an entirely different spectrum of health-related problems.

Finally, the clinician must remain vigilant in order to detect the early signs of anabolic-androgenic steroid use and be prepared to refer such patients to an appropriate treatment program.

ACKNOWLEDGMENT: This manuscript was supported by Research Scientist Award KO5 DA00343 from the National Institute on Drug Abuse. The author gratefully acknowledges the technical assistance of Carol Buchanan in its preparation.

REFERENCES

Allen M & Suominen J (1984). Effect of androgenic and anabolic steroids on spermatogenesis in power athletes. *International Journal of Sports Medicine* 5(Suppl):189.

Anderson W & McKeag B (1985). *The Substance Use and Abuse Habits of College Student Athletes. Research Paper No. 2.* Mission, KS: National Collegiate Athletic Association.

Annitto WR & Layman WA (1980). Anabolic steroids and acute schizophrenic episode. *Journal of Clinical Psychiatry* 41:143-144.

Appell H, Heller-Umpfenbach B, Feraudi M et al. (1983). Ultra-structural and morphometric investigations on the effects of training and administration of anabolic steroids on the myocardium of guinea pigs. *International Journal of Sports Medicine* 4:268-274.

Ariel G & Saville W (1972). The physiological effects of placebos. *Medicine and Science in Sports* 4:124.

Bahrke MS & Yesalis III CE (1994). Weight training: A potential confounding factor in examining the psychological and behavioural effects of anabolic-androgenic steroids. *Sports Medicine* 18(5):309-318.

Balster RL & Schuster CR (1973). Fixed-interval schedule of cocaine reinforcement: Effect of dose and infusion duration. *Journal of the Experimental Analysis of Behavior* 20(1):119-129.

Bardin CW, Catterall JF & Janne OA (1990). The androgen-induced phenotype. In GC Lin & L Erinoff (eds.) *Anabolic Steroid Abuse (NIDA Research Monograph 102).* Rockville, MD: National Institute on Drug Abuse, 131-141.

Behrendt H & Boffin H (1977). Myocardial cell lesions caused by an anabolic hormone. *Cell and Tissue Research* 181:423-426.

Boje O (1939). Doping. *Bulletin of Health Organization League of Nations* 8:439-469.

Bowman S (1990). Anabolic steroids and infarction. *British Medical Journal* 300:750.

Brower KJ (1989). Rehabilitation for anabolic-androgenic steroid dependence. *Clinics in Sports Medicine* 1:171-181.

Brower KJ (1992). Anabolic steroids: Addictive, psychiatric, and medical consequences. *American Journal on Addictions* 1(2):100-114.

Brower KJ, Blow FC, Young JP et al. (1991). Symptoms and correlates of anabolic-androgenic steroid dependence. *British Journal of Addiction* 86:759-768.

Brower KJ, Eliopulos GA, Blow FC et al. (1990). Evidence for physical and psychological dependence on anabolic-androgenic steroids in eight weightlifters. *American Journal of Psychiatry* 147:510-512.

Buckley WE, Yesalis CE, Friedl KE et al. (1988). Estimated prevalence of anabolic steroid use among male high school seniors. *Journal of the American Medical Association* 260:3441-3445.

Buss AH & Durkee A (1957). An inventory for assessing different kinds of hostility. *Journal of Consulting Psychology* 21:343-349.

Catlin DH (1987). Detection of drug use by athletes. In RH Strauss (ed.) *Drugs and Performance in Sports.* Philadelphia, PA: W.B. Saunders, 103-120.

Cherek DR (1981). Effects of smoking different doses of nicotine on human aggressive behavior. *Psychopharmacology* 75:339-345.

Clark AS, Lindenfeld RC & Gibbons CH (1996). Anabolic-androgenic steroids and brain reward. *Pharmacology, Biochemistry and Behavior* 53(3):741-745.

Conacher GN & Workman DG (1989). Violent crime possibly associated with anabolic steroid use. *American Journal of Psychiatry* 146:679.

Cooper CJ, Noakes TD, Dunne T et al. (1996). A high prevalence of abnormal personality traits in chronic users of anabolic-androgenic steroids. *British Journal of Sports Medicine* 30(3):246-250.

Crist DM, Stackpole PJ & Peake GT (1983). Effects of androgenic-anabolic steroids on neuromuscular power and body composition. *Journal of Applied Physiology* 54:366-370.

Dart R (1991). Drugs in the workplace: Anabolic steroid abuse among law enforcement officers. *Police Chief* 58(7):18.

David HG, Green JT, Grant AJ et al. (1995). Simultaneous bilateral quadriceps rupture: A complication of anabolic steroid abuse. *Journal of Bone and Joint Surgery (British edition)* 77(1):159-160.

Durant RH, Rickert VI, Ashworth CS et al. (1993). Use of multiple drugs among adolescents who use anabolic steroids. *New England Journal of Medicine* 328:922-926.

Evans WS, Bowen JN, Giordano FL et al. (1985). A case of stadol dependence [letter]. *Journal of the American Medical Association* 253(15):2191-2192.

Ferenchick BS (1990). Are androgenic steroids thrombogenic? *New England Journal of Medicine* 322:476.

Freed DLJ, Banks AJ, Longson D et al. (1975). Anabolic steroids in athletics: Crossover double-blind trial on weightlifters. *British Medical Journal* 2:471-473.

Freinhar JP & Alvarez W (1985). Androgen-induced hypomania. *Journal of Clinical Psychiatry* 46:354-355.

Friedl KE (1990). Reappraisal of the health risks associated with high doses of oral and injectable androgenic steroids. In GC Lin & L Erinoff (eds.) *Anabolic Steroid Abuse (NIDA Research Monograph 102).* Rockville, MD: National Institute on Drug Abuse, 142-177.

Galligani N, Renck A & Hansen S (1996). Personality profile of men using anabolic androgenic steroids. *Hormones and Behavior* 30(2):170-175.

Goldberg L, Bents R, Bosworth E et al. (1991). Anabolic steroid education and adolescents: Do scare tactics work? *Pediatrics* 87:283-286.

Goldberg L, MacKinnon DP, Elliot DL et al. (2000). The adolescents training and learning to avoid steroids program: Preventing drug use and promoting health behaviors. *Archives of Pediatrics and Adolescent Medicine* 154:332-338.

Gruber AJ & Pope HG Jr. (2000). Psychiatric and medical effects of anabolic-androgenic steriod use in women. *Psycotherapy and Psychosomatics* 69(1):19-26.

Hartgens F, Kuipers H, Wijnen JAG et al. (1996). Body composition, cardiovascular risk factors and liver function in long term androgenic-anabolic steroids using body builders three months after drug withdrawal. *International Journal of Sports Medicine* 17:429-433.

Haupt HA & Rovere GB (1984). Anabolic steroids: A review of the literature. *American Journal of Sports Medicine* 12:469-484.

Hollander E, Liebowitz MR, Winchel R et al. (1989). Treatment of body-dysmorphic disorder with serotonin reuptake blockers. *American Journal of Psychiatry* 146(6):768-770.

Honour JW (1997). Steroid abuse in female athletes. *Current Opinion in Obstetrics and Gynecology* 9:181-186.

Johnston LD, O'Malley PM & Bachman JG (2001a). *Monitoring the Future National Survey Results on Drug Abuse, 1975-2000. Volume I: Secondary School Students* (NIH Publication No. 01-4924). Bethesda, MD: National Institute on Drug Abuse.

Johnston LD, O'Malley PM & Bachman JG (2001b). *Monitoring the Future National Survey Results on Drug Abuse, 1975-2000. Volume II: College Students and Adults Ages 19-40* (NIH Publication No. 01-4925). Bethesda, MD: National Institute on Drug Abuse.

Kanayama G, Pope HG Jr. & Judson JI (2001). "Body image" drugs: A growing psychosomatic problem. *Psychotherapy and Psychosomatics* 70:61-65.

Karch SB (1993). Anabolic steroids. *The Pathology of Drug Abuse*. Boca Raton, FL: CRC Press, 355-373.

Kashkin KB (1992). Anabolic steroids. In JH Lowinson, P Ruiz, RB Millman & JG Langrod (eds.) *Substance Abuse: A Comprehensive Textbook, 2nd Edition*. Baltimore, MD: Williams & Wilkins, 380-395.

Kashkin KB & Kleber HD (1989). Hooked on hormones? An anabolic steroid addiction hypothesis. *Journal of the American Medical Association* 262(22):3166-3170.

Kochakian CD (1990). History of anabolic-androgenic steroids. In GC Lin & L Erinoff (eds.) *Anabolic Steroid Abuse (NIDA Research Monograph 102)*. Rockville, MD: National Institute on Drug Abuse, 29-59.

Kouri EM, Lukas SE, Pope HG Jr. et al. (1995). Increased aggressive responding in male volunteers following the administration of gradually increasing doses of testosterone cypionate. *Drug and Alcohol Dependence* 40:73-79.

Lenders JWM, Demacker PN, Vos JA et al. (1988). Deleterious effects of anabolic steroids on serum lipoproteins, blood pressure and liver function in amateur bodybuilders. *International Journal of Sports Medicine* 9:19-23.

Lombardo JA (1992). Anabolic-androgenic steroids. In GC Lin & L Erinoff (eds.) *Anabolic Steroid Abuse (NIDA Research Monograph 102)*. Rockville, MD: National Institute on Drug Abuse, 60-73.

Lukas SE (1993). Current perspectives on anabolic-androgenic steroid abuse. *Trends in Pharmacological Sciences* 14:61-68

Lukas SE (1994). *Steroids*. Hillside, NJ: Enslow Publishers.

Lukas SE (1996). CNS effects and abuse liability of anabolic-androgenic steroids. *Annual Review of Pharmacology and Toxicology* 36:333-357.

Luke J, Farb A, Virmani R et al. (1991). Sudden cardiac death during exercise in a weight lifter using anabolic androgenic steroids: Pathological and toxicological findings. *Journal of Forensic Sciences* 35(6):1441-1447.

Malone DA Jr. & Dimeff RJ (1992). The use of fluoxetine in depression associated with anabolic steroid withdrawal: A case series. *Journal of Clinical Psychiatry* 53(4):130-132.

Martini L (1982). The 5-alpha-reduction of testosterone in the neuroendocrine structures: Biochemical and physiological implications. *Endocrine Reviews* 3:1-25.

Masonis AE & McCarthy MP (1996). Direct interactions of androgenic/anabolic steroids with the peripheral benzodiazepine receptor in rat brain: Implications for the psychological and physiological manifestations of androgenic/anabolic steroid abuse. *Journal of Steroid Biochemistry and Molecular Biology* 58(56):551-555.

Mayer M & Rosen F (1977). Interaction of glucocorticoids and androgens with skeletal muscle. *Metabolism* 27:937-962.

McBride AJ, Williamson K & Petersen T (1996). Three cases of nalbuphine hydrochloride dependence associated with anabolic steroid use. *British Journal of Sports Medicine* 30(1):69-70.

McNutt RA, Ferenchick GF, Kirlin PC et al. (1988). Acute myocardial infarction in a 22 year old, world-class weightlifter using anabolic steroids. *American Journal of Cardiology* 62:164.

Melia P, Pipe A & Greenberg L (1996). The use of anabolic-androgenic steroids by Canadian students. *Clinical Journal of Sports Medicine* 6(1):9-14.

Moore WB (1988). Anabolic steroid use in adolescents. *Journal of the American Medical Association* 260:3484-3486.

Narducci WA, Wagner JC, Hendrickson TP et al. (1990). Anabolic steroids—A review of the clinical toxicology and diagnostic screening. *Clinical Toxicology* 28(3):287-310.

Palacios A, McClure RB, Campfield A et al. (1981). Effect of testosterone enanthate on testis size. *Journal of Urology* 26:46-48.

Pecking A, Lejolly JM & Najean Y (1980). Hepatic toxicity of androgen therapy in aplastic anemia. *Nouvelle Revue Francaise D'Hematologie* 22:257-265.

Perry PJ, Yates WR & Anderson KH (1990). Psychiatric effects of anabolic steroids: A controlled retrospective study. *Annals of Clinical Psychiatry* 2:11-17.

Phillips KA (1996). Body dysmorphic disorder: Diagnosis and treatment of imagined ugliness. *Journal of Clinical Psychiatry* 57(Suppl 8):61-4; discussion 65.

Phillips KA, McElroy SL, Keck PE Jr. et al. (1994). A comparison of delusional and nondelusional body dysmorphic disorder in 100 cases. *Psychopharmacology Bulletin* 30(2):179-186.

Pope HG Jr., Gruber AJ, Choi P et al. (1997). Muscle dysmorpnia. An underrecognized form of body dysmorphic disorder. *Psychosomatics* 38(6): 548-557.

Pope HG Jr. & Katz DL (1987). Body-builder's psychosis. *Lancet* 1:863.

Pope HG Jr. & Katz DL (1988). Affective and psychotic symptoms associated with anabolic steroid use. *American Journal of Psychiatry* 145(4):487-490.

Pope HG Jr., Katz DL & Hudson JI (1993). Anorexia nervosa and "reverse anorexia" among 108 male bodybuilders. *Comprehensive Psychiatry* 34(6):406-409.

Pope HG Jr., Kouri EM & Hudson JI (2000). Effects of supraphysiologic doses of testosterone on mood and aggression in normal men: A randomized controlled trial. *Archives of General Psychiatry* 57(2): 133-140.

Raaka BM, Finnerty M & Samuels HH (1989). The glucocorticoid antagonist 17 alpha-methyltestosterone binds to the 10S glucocorticoid receptor and blocks agonist-mediated disassociation of the 10S oligomer to the 4S deoxyribonucleic acid-binding subunit. *Molecular Endocrinology* 3:322-341.

Rogivkin BA (1976). The role of low molecular weight compounds in the regulation of skeletal muscle genome activity during exercise. *Medicine and Science in Sports* 8:104.

Rogol AD & Yesalis CE III (1992). Anabolic-androgenic steroids and the adolescent. *Pediatric Annals* 21(3):175, 179, 180-181, 183, 186-188.

Rubinow DR & Schmidt PJ (1996). Androgens, brain and behavior. *American Journal of Psychiatry* 153:974-984.

Schanzer W (1996). Metabolism of anabolic androgenic steroids. *Clinical Chemistry* 42(7):1001-1020.

Schwerin MJ & Corcoran KJ (1996). Beliefs about steroids: User vs. non-user comparisons. *Drug and Alcohol Dependence* 40(3):221-225.

Su TP, Pagliaro M, Schmidt PJ et al. (1993). Neuropsychiatric effects of anabolic steroids in male normal volunteers. *Journal of the American Medical Association* 269:2760-2764.

Substance Abuse and Mental Health Services Administration (SAMHSA) (1996). *National Household Survey on Drug Abuse: Main Findings 1994*. Washington, DC: U.S. Government Printing Office.

Svare BB (1990). Anabolic steroids and behavior: A preclinical research prospectus. In GC Lin & L Erinoff (eds.) *Anabolic Steroid Abuse (NIDA Research Monograph 102)*. Rockville, MD: National Institute on Drug Abuse, 224-241.

Swanson C, Gaines L & Gore B (1991). Abuse of anabolic steroids. *FBI Law Enforcement Bulletin* 60(8):19-23.

Tanner SM, Miller DW & Alongi C (1995). Anabolic steroid use by adolescents: Prevalence, motives, and knowledge of risks. *Clinical Journal of Sports Medicine* 5:108-115.

Thompson PB, Curinane AN, Sady SP et al. (1989). Contrasting effects of testosterone and stanozolol on serum lipoprotein levels. *Journal of the American Medical Association* 261:1165-1168.

Todd T (1987). Anabolic steroids: The gremlins of sport. *Journal of Sports History* 14:87-107.

Wang MQ, Fitzhugh EC, Yesalis CE et al. (1994). Desire for weight gain and potential risk of adolescent males using anabolic steroids. *Perceptual and Motor Skills* 78:267-274.

Westaby B, Ogle SJ, Paridians FJ et al. (1977). Liver damage from long-term methyltestosterone. *Lancet* 1(8032):261-263.

Wilson JD (1988). Androgen abuse by athletes. *Endocrine Review* 9:181-199.

Wilson IC, Prange AJ Jr. & Lara PP (1974). Methyltestosterone with imipramine in men: Conversion of depression to paranoid reaction. *American Journal of Psychiatry* 131:21-24.

Wines JD Jr., Gruber AJ, Pope HG Jr. et al. (1999). Nalbuphine hydrochloride dependence in anabolic steroid user. *American Journal on Addictions* 8(2):161-164.

Winters SJ (1990). Androgens: Endocrine physiology and pharmacology. In GC Lin & L Erinoff (eds.) *Anabolic Steroid Abuse (NIDA Research Monograph 102)*. Rockville, MD: National Institute on Drug Abuse, 113-130.

Wroblewski AM (1997). Androgenic-anabolic steroids and body dysmorphia in young men. *Journal of Psychosomatic Research* 42(3):225-234.

Yates WR (2000). Testosterone in psychiatry: Risks and benefits. *Archives of General Psychiatry* 57:155-156.

Yates WR, Perry P & Murray S (1992). Aggression and hostility in anabolic steroid users. *Biological Psychiatry* 31:1232-1234.

Yesalis C, Anderson W, Buckley W et al. (1990). Incidence of the non-medical use of anabolic-androgenic steroids. In GC Lin & L Erinoff (eds.) *Anabolic Steroid Abuse (NIDA Research Monograph 102)*. Rockville, MD: National Institute on Drug Abuse.

Yesalis CE, Herrick RT, Buckley WE et al. (1988). Self-reported use of anabolic androgenic steroids by elite powerlifters. *Physiology of Sports Medicine* 16:91-100.

Yesalis CE, Kennedy NJ, Kopstein AN et al. (1993). Anabolic-androgenic steroid use in the United States. *Journal of the American Medical Association* 270(10):1217-1221.

Yesalis CE, Streit AL, Vicary JR et al. (1989). Anabolic steroid use: Indications of habituation among adolescents. *Journal of Drug Education* 19:103-116.

SECTION 3 | Diagnosis, Assessment, and Early Intervention

Section Coordinator

Theodore V. Parran, Jr., M.D., FACP

Contributors

Sharon L. Baker, Ph.D.
Clinical Research Associate
Massachusetts General Hospital, and
Instructor in Psychology
Harvard Medical School
Boston, Massachusetts

Richard D. Blondell, M.D.
Professor of Family Medicine
Department of Family and Community Medicine
University of Louisville
Louisville, Kentucky

Joseph Conigliaro, M.D., M.P.H.
Associate Professor of Medicine and Epidemiology
University of Pittsburgh, and
VA Pittsburgh Healthcare System
Center for Health Equity Research and Promotion
Pittsburgh, Pennsylvania

Christine Delos Reyes, M.D.
Case-Western Reserve University
School of Medicine
Cleveland, Ohio

Kathleen Farkas, Ph.D., LISW, ACSW
Associate Professor
Mandel School of Applied Social Sciences
Case-Western Reserve University
School of Medicine
Cleveland, Ohio

Michael S. Fleming, M.D., M.P.H.
Professor, Family Medicine
Department of Family Medicine
University of Wisconsin
Madison, Wisconsin

David R. Gastfriend, M.D.
Chief, Addiction Research Program
Massachusetts General Hospital, and
Assistant Professor of Psychiatry
Harvard Medical School
Boston, Massachusetts

Allan W. Graham, M.D., FACP, FASAM
Medical Director
Chemical Dependency Treatment Services
Kaiser Permanente
Denver, Colorado

Paul J. Gruenewald, Ph.D.
Scientific Director
Prevention Research Center
Berkeley, California

Harold D. Holder, Ph.D.
Director
Prevention Research Center
Berkeley, California

Michael R. Liepman, M.D., FASAM
Kalamazoo Center for Medicine
Michigan State University
Kalamazoo, Michigan

Lisa M. Najavits, Ph.D.
Clinical Research Associate
Massachusetts General Hospital, and
Instructor in Psychology
Harvard Medical School
Boston, Massachusetts

Theodore V. Parran, Jr., M.D., FACP
Associate Clinical Professor of Medicine
Case-Western Reserve University
School of Medicine
Cleveland, Ohio

Sharon Reif, Ph.D.
Research Assistant
Massachusetts General Hospital
Boston, Massachusetts

Jerome E. Schulz, M.D., FASAM
Clinical Associate Professor
Department of Family Medicine
Eastern Carolina University
School of Medicine
Greenville, North Carolina

Andrew J. Treno, Ph.D.
Senior Research Scientist
Prevention Research Center
Berkeley, California

Elizabeth A. Warner, M.D.
Associate Professor of Medicine
Department of Internal Medicine
University of South Florida
Tampa, Florida

Chapter 1

Principles of Screening and Early Intervention

Joseph Conigliaro, M.D., M.P.H.
Christine Delos Reyes, M.D.
Theodore V. Parran, Jr., M.D., FACP
Jerome E. Schulz, M.D., FASAM

Screening
Assessment
Intervention
Followup Monitoring

Physicians are in a unique position to identify and help patients suffering from alcohol, tobacco, and other drug problems. In fact, up to 20% of visits to primary care physicians are related to such problems (Bradley, 1994). Patients with alcohol and other drug problems are twice as likely to consult a primary care physician as are patients without such problems (Rush, 1989). Moreover, a recent review of brief interventions for alcohol and drug problems concluded that primary care physicians can be effective in changing the course of patients' harmful drinking (Bien, Miller et al., 1993; Fleming, Barry et al., 1997).

Sadly, although physicians are the professionals most often cited by patients and families as the "most appropriate" source of advice and guidance about issues related to the use of alcohol, tobacco, and other drugs, they also are reported to be the "least helpful" in actually addressing these issues. Most diagnoses of abuse and addiction are missed by physicians and, even where a diagnosis is made, many physicians do not know how to develop an organized treatment plan. Clearly the basic clinical skills of screening, assessment, presenting the diagnosis, negotiating a treatment plan, and longitudinal monitoring—all skills that are used by physicians to manage other chronic illnesses—need

attention when it comes to issues of substance abuse and addiction.

SCREENING

Many standardized screening techniques are available to determine whether a patient has an alcohol or drug use disorder. However, before any attempt is made to assess a patient's alcohol and other drug use, the clinician must establish a relationship of rapport and trust with the patient. The best way to introduce screening questions is to give the patient a general idea of the content of the questions, their purpose, and the need for accurate answers. Questions about alcohol and other drug use are most appropriately asked as part of the history of personal habits such as smoking and coffee drinking. Questions should be asked forthrightly and in a non-judgmental manner to avoid engendering defensiveness on the part of the patient. (Assessing adolescents for alcohol and other drug problems is particularly challenging, and is discussed in detail in Section 13 of this text.)

For screening to be effective and accepted by patients, the following guidelines should be observed:

TABLE 1.   Presenting Complaints That Are "Red Flags" for Alcohol and Other Drug Problems

- Frequent absences from work or school
- History of frequent trauma/accidental injuries
- Depression
- Anxiety
- Labile hypertension
- Gastrointestinal symptoms
- Sexual dysfunction
- Sleep disorders.

- The patient should be alcohol-free at the time of the screening. Patients who have alcohol on their breath or who appear to be intoxicated often give unreliable responses, so consideration should be given to deferring the interview to a later time. If this is not possible, the patient's condition at interview should be noted in the medical record.

- The caregiver needs to be empathetic and non-threatening, to relate the purpose of the questions to the patient's health status, and to assure the patient that the information discussed will be treated as confidential.

- In some settings (such as waiting rooms), screening instruments can be given as self-report questionnaires, with instructions for patients to discuss the results with their health care provider.

- With patients who present for emergency treatment or who are temporarily impaired, it is best to wait until their condition has stabilized and they have become accustomed to the health care setting where the interview will take place.

The goal of screening determines the instrument to be used. If the goal is to identify existing disease, such as alcohol abuse or dependence, use of a formal screening instrument is appropriate. If, on the other hand, the goal is to prevent or identify at-risk drinking, then simple questions to assess quantity and frequency may be sufficient. Many experienced clinicians recommend a combined approach.

In the past, questions about quantity and frequency of alcohol or drug use were regarded as useless. This belief came from evaluating patients who already were alcoholic or drug-dependent and thus in considerable denial about their drug or alcohol use. Such patients tended to minimize and rationalize their drug and alcohol use. On the other hand, patients who are misusing alcohol and other drugs, but who are not yet alcohol- or drug-dependent, have not developed denial and thus usually are willing to tell physicians how often they use alcohol and other drugs, and how much they use (Williams, Aitken et al., 1985).

If patients do not drink, it is important to ask why they do not; there may be a personal or family history of alcohol problems. That should be documented as part of the patient's history. Such an exchange also presents an opportunity for the clinician to do primary prevention by supporting the patient in his or her choice not to use drugs or alcohol. Where there is a history of alcohol or drug problems, the patient chart should be labeled clearly to prevent prescribing any mood-altering drugs that may jeopardize his or her continued recovery. When the family history is positive, the patient should be educated about his or her increased risk of developing drug/alcohol problems.

If a patient does drink alcohol, the CAGE questions should be asked before quantity/frequency questions. One study (not in a primary care setting) showed that the CAGE was significantly less sensitive when administered after quantity/frequency questions had been asked (Steinweg, 1993). After the CAGE questions, patients should be asked how many days a week they drink alcohol; then, how many drinks they consume in an "average" day and what is the maximum number of drinks they have consumed on any given occasion during the preceding month.

The Alcohol Use Disorders Identification Test (AUDIT) is a longer, 10-item questionnaire that can identify at-risk or problem drinking as well as dependence (Babor, de la Fuente et al., 1992). Problem drinkers may not exhibit obvious consequences of their alcohol use, but still consume enough alcohol to increase the risk of associated medical and psychological problems. The length of the AUDIT, compared to the CAGE, may limit its ease of implementation; fortunately, however, the first three items have been found to be helpful in identifying early drinkers, who may be good candidates for brief interventions in primary care settings (Gordon, Maisto et al., 2001; Bush, Kivlahan et al., 1998).

The National Institute on Alcohol Abuse and Alcoholism (NIAAA) has developed "Healthy or Low Risk Drinking Guidelines." For men, the guidelines define low-risk drinking as no more than two drinks a day and no more than four

---

TABLE 2.   Physical Findings Suggestive of Alcohol and Other Drug Problems

- Mild tremor
- Odor of alcohol on breath
- Enlarged, tender liver
- Nasal irritation (suggestive of cocaine insufflation)
- Conjunctival irritation (suggestive of exposure to marijuana smoke)
- Labile blood pressure (suggestive of alcohol withdrawal)
- Tachycardia and/or cardiac arrhythmia
- "After Shave/Mouthwash" syndrome (to mask the odor of alcohol)
- Odor of marijuana on clothing.

drinks on a single occasion (at a rate less than one drink per hour). For women and patients over 65, the guidelines define low-risk drinking as no more than one drink a day and no more than three drinks on a single occasion. Women reach higher blood levels of alcohol than men after consuming equivalent amounts of alcohol because they are smaller and have less gastric alcohol dehydrogenase to metabolize alcohol. Pregnant patients and those with medical problems complicated by alcohol should abstain completely (NIAAA, 1995). These recommendations are derived by expert consensus and need further validation, although the limits recommended for older adults are consistent with data regarding the relationship between consumption and alcohol-related problems in this age group. The recommendations also are consistent with current evidence on the beneficial effects of moderate alcohol consumption.

If a patient is drinking more than the recommended amount of alcohol, is using any illicit drugs, or has one positive answer to the CAGE questions, he or she should be further assessed for alcohol or drug problems.

Two simple questions can increase the likelihood that screening will detect patients with alcohol problems. The first asks patients if they have ever had drinking problems. The second asks if they have had any alcohol to drink in the preceding 24 hours. If the answers to both questions are positive, the sensitivity for alcohol problems is 92% (Cyr & Wartman, 1988).

"Red Flags" for Alcohol and Other Drug Problems. Several common "chief complaints" cause patients with alcohol and other drug problems to seek medical care (Table 1). Some patients develop recurring "Monday flu" from weekend binge drinking or drug use, which requires them to obtain return-to-work slips because of frequent absenteeism. Others have labile blood pressure readings caused by alcohol withdrawal; in fact, withdrawal symptoms and poor medication compliance make treating hypertension a challenge in patients with alcohol and other drug problems.

Family members may present with the same symptoms as the drinking/drug-using patient. Trauma secondary to spousal abuse is common. Children may be seen for abdominal pain, headaches, or school problems.

Patients who abuse drugs other than alcohol may present with a variety of medical problems, each with specific signs and symptoms. Patients who abuse cocaine develop chest pain caused by vasoconstriction of the coronary arteries. Any young patient (<35 years old) with chest pain should be screened for cocaine abuse by urine toxicology screen for benzoylecgonine. Intranasal (snorting) of cocaine causes rhinorrhea, sinus, and dental problems. In severe cases, patients may perforate the nasal septum. Cocaine abuse causes seizures and (rarely) intraventricular hemorrhages. A chronic cough (especially if it produces *black* sputum) may result from crack cocaine abuse. Marijuana use should be considered in adolescents experiencing school difficulties, a chronic cough, or worsening of asthmatic conditions.

ASSESSMENT

Several strategies can be employed to assess patients who screen positive for alcohol or drug problems.

History. The first step is to take an expanded drug and alcohol history. Questions should focus on the consequences of the patient's alcohol and other drug use. One strategy is to ask simple followup questions to each positive response that the patient made to the CAGE questionnaire. These include questions about when, how, and why the patient cut down on drinking/drug use, and why it didn't last; who made comments about the patient's drinking, what happened to precipitate the comments, what the comments were, how many have been made by how many different people, and why they were annoying; what actions were embarrassing, in what way they were out of character, and over what period of time the guilt-producing actions persisted.

Further general assessment questions should focus on the consequences of the patient's alcohol or drug use in the spheres of life affected by addiction: self-respect, family, friends, finances, legal, school/occupation, and health.

TABLE 3.   Assessing Levels of Disease Severity

Domains ▶ ◀ Levels	Physiologic Dependence	Organ System Damage	Psychosocial Morbidity
Mild	One or more of the following: ■ Inability to stop ■ Insomnia ■ Irritability ■ Anxiety AUDIT (Questions 1–3)* combined score >5: ■ Frequency (1) ■ Average # of drinks (2) ■ Six or more drinks (3)	One of the following: ■ High normal GGT ■ Memory loss ■ Physical injury ■ Bloodshot eyes ■ Depression ■ Sexual dysfunction ■ High blood pressure ■ Gastritis/ulcers ■ Headaches ■ Osteoporosis	One of the following: CAGE: ■ Cut down (C) ■ Annoyed (A) ■ Guilty (G) AUDIT*: ■ Failed expectations (5) ■ Remorse (7) ■ Memory loss (8) ■ Injured self or others (9) ■ Concern expressed by others (10)
Moderate	Any of the above mild symptoms with one or more of the following: ■ Hand tremor ■ "Eye opener" ■ Diaphoresis ■ BAL ≥100 ■ Positive urine toxicology	Two or three of the following: ■ Elevated GGT ■ Memory loss ■ Injury/broken bones ■ Elevated MCV ■ Elevated liver function profile ■ Depression ■ Sexual dysfunction ■ High blood pressure ■ Gastritis/ulcers ■ Headaches ■ Osteoporosis	Two of the following: CAGE: ■ Cut down (C) ■ Annoyed (A) ■ Guilty (G) AUDIT*: ■ Failed expectations (5) ■ Remorse (7) ■ Memory loss (8) ■ Injured self or others (9) ■ Concern expressed by others (10)
Severe	Any of the above mild or moderate symptoms with one or more of the following: ■ Hallucinations ■ Seizures ■ DTs ■ BAL >200 ■ Prolonged positive toxicology	Four or more of the following: ■ Elevated GGT ■ Memory loss ■ Injury/broken bones ■ Elevated MCV ■ Elevated liver function profile ■ Depression ■ Sexual dysfunction ■ High blood pressure ■ Gastritis/ulcers ■ Headaches ■ Osteoporosis ■ Hepatomegaly ■ Elevated prothrombin time	Positive on three or more of the following: CAGE: ■ Cut down (C) ■ Annoyed (A) ■ Guilty (G) AUDIT*: ■ Failed expectations (5) ■ Remorse (7) ■ Memory loss (8) ■ Injured self or others (9) ■ Concern expressed by others (10)

*Alcohol Use Disorders Identification Test (numbers in parentheses denote specific item number).

SOURCE: National Institute on Alcohol Abuse and Alcoholism (NIAAA) (1995). *The Physician's Guide to Helping Patients with Alcohol Problems.* Rockville, MD: National Institutes of Health.

Specific questions should be asked about blackouts (loss of memory of events while intoxicated), changes and tolerance, and withdrawal symptoms. Medical problems that may be caused or exacerbated by alcohol or drug use (Table 2) should be identified (also see Section 10 of this text). For example, a history of pancreatitis, liver disease, or chronic gastrointestinal problems may signify chronic alcohol abuse. The patient should be asked about social or family problems commonly associated with alcohol and other drug misuse, such as a previous history of arrests for driving under the influence, job loss, financial problems, or family conflicts. *Repeated unsuccessful attempts to quit drinking alcohol or using drugs signifies alcohol or drug dependence rather than "problem use."* Such patients usually need a formal rehabilitation program to help them abstain from drugs and alcohol.

Physical Examination. Many "classic" physical findings of alcohol and other drug problems only become evident later in the course of the disease. More subtle early physical findings are listed in Table 3. For example, mild withdrawal can cause elevated blood pressure, tachycardia, and mild tremor. When patients binge drink, fatty deposits cause the liver to swell and be painful on palpation. Men may try to mask their alcohol use by using too much aftershave lotion or mouthwash. Women may use too much perfume or makeup to cover obvious signs of alcohol misuse. The smell of alcohol on a patient's breath should raise suspicion of alcohol problems. Hypertensive patients who drink alcohol often have wide fluctuations in their blood pressure readings. Alcohol withdrawal elevates the blood pressure, while intoxication may cause falsely low readings.

Laboratory Evaluation. There are no specific laboratory tests that confirm the diagnosis of alcohol or other drug problems. However, there are a number of laboratory tests that can help the clinician evaluate patients for potential alcohol or other drug problems; these are discussed in detail in Chapter 4 of this section.

Blood alcohol levels (BALs) and urine drug screens can be used to assess patients for possible alcohol and other drug problems; for example, a drug screen may be useful in evaluating an adolescent with school problems. However, these tests are controversial, so it is advisable to obtain the patient's (and/or parent's) permission before initiating such screens; in fact, failure to do so can cause irreparable damage to the physician-patient relationship. Blood and saliva alcohol tests and urine drug screens are critical components of many employee recovery programs (see the detailed discussion of these in Section 9 of this text).

Staging the Severity of the Disorder. Before formulating any treatment plan, physicians routinely assess the severity of the individual patient's disease state. "Staging the disease" is used in managing hypertension, diabetes, colon cancer, and certainly is necessary in drug/alcohol dependence. When effective screening tools are used (as outlined above), patients can be identified while their alcohol or other drug problem is marked by moderate to severe psychosocial morbidity and mild to nonexistent physiologic dependence and organ damage.

Clinically, it is helpful to assess the extent of the patient's alcohol or drug dependence within the general domains of physiologic dependence, organ system damage, and psychosocial morbidity (Table 3). This approach provides for a mild, moderate, or severe categorization of disease in each of the aforementioned domains. Stratifying alcohol or other drug problems in this way becomes useful when negotiating a treatment plan with patients across the continuum of readiness for behavior change and severity of disease.

A variety of instruments are available to guide such assessments; refer to Chapter 2 of this section for a complete discussion.

INTERVENTION

Once the assessment is complete, the patient should be given specific advice. Many physicians feel that presenting the diagnosis of alcohol or other drug problems or dependence is one of their most uncomfortable and difficult clinical tasks. Such discomfort often is caused by lack of knowledge, previous negative experiences, and a lack of appropriate skills. The following guidelines are offered to help physicians overcome these obstacles.

Non-Problem Use: If the patient does not drink or is within the range of low-risk consumption, the physician should provide prevention messages that support the patient's continued positive lifestyle choices. Patients with a positive family history of alcohol or other drug problems should be counseled about their increased risk of developing problems and their need for continued diligence. Patients who are not at risk can be given information about safe limits for alcohol use. In subsequent office visits, they should be screened periodically to verify that they have not developed problems with alcohol or drugs, especially if they have a positive family history.

TABLE 4. Pitfalls To Avoid When Presenting the Diagnosis: The DEATH Glossary

D: Drinking or drug use details are not relevant; talking with a drunk is not useful. When the diagnosis is presented, patients often launch into long explanations of why their dysfunctional drinking or drug use actually is not dysfunctional. It is important to redirect these discussions and move on. When patients have been actively drinking, they are not able to process much information and are emotionally labile. Therefore, the physician's message should be very brief and simple, such as "I am concerned about your drinking and/or drug use; let's schedule a time to talk about it. Please do not drink before that visit, because our time together is too important to have to talk through any alcohol."

E: Etiology. Patients often insist on an explanation for their addiction (such as stress, upbringing, depression, socioeconomic, or cultural causes). However, just as in presenting a diagnosis of hypertension, it is important to make the diagnosis and treat the condition, rather than speculating about the cause of the disease.

A: Arguments. Neither the physician nor the patient can hear anything when arguing, which also weakens the therapeutic relationship. It is much better to diffuse arguments with sympathy, respect, and support.

T: Threats, guilt, and shame do not promote recovery. If they did, the disease would provide its own cure! It is clear that threats, guilt, and shame are toxic to the physician-patient relationship.

H: Hedging hurts your credibility. Be clear, concise, and to the point. "Agreeing to disagree" with a patient who is in the precontemplative stage is much more therapeutic than appearing to be uncertain about and uncomfortable with making and presenting the diagnosis.

Problem Drinking/Drug Use: The patient who is not alcohol- or drug-dependent but who is a problem drinker should be encouraged to abstain from, or at least to reduce, his or her alcohol use. Such a patient should be strongly encouraged to abstain from all illicit drugs. The physician should articulate the medical concerns, being specific about the patient's alcohol use and the related medical issues. Such patients should be encouraged to verbalize their concerns about their alcohol or other drug use. The goal is for the patient to assume responsibility for deciding on a personal plan, while pursuing abstinence as a goal. If a patient does not wish to abstain, he or she should be asked to agree to a specific limit for alcohol use that is within the "safe" drinking guidelines. The physician should provide such a patient with educational information about low-risk drinking (NIAAA publishes an excellent patient handout that helps patients cut down on their drinking and suggests that they keep a diary of their progress).

When the physician recommends limits on alcohol consumption, it is critical that the patient be reassessed frequently to monitor his or her ability to comply with the recommended limits. For patients who are in the "at risk" range but do not meet the criteria for dependence, the physician should consider making a problem statement of "at-risk drinking/drug use" in the chart so as to identify the issue for future reference.

Alcohol or Other Drug Dependence: When the physician suspects that a patient is dependent on alcohol or other drugs, the diagnosis must be presented to the patient (brief intervention). A brief intervention is a physician/patient interaction, where the diagnosis of alcohol or drug dependence is clearly and concisely presented. This should be accompanied by a recommendation for abstinence and an offer to provide ongoing support. For a detailed discussion of brief interventions, consult Chapter 3 in this section.

Presenting the Diagnosis. In the past, much of the emphasis in presenting the diagnosis of alcohol or drug use disorder centered on the theory that health care professionals must confront patients, overcome denial, and motivate the patients toward treatment. This approach often led to arguments, harsh words, and—at times—the abrupt end of an otherwise therapeutic relationship. Although crisis interventions certainly can work to force previously unwilling patients into treatment, such interventions are difficult to do in many clinical settings. Using shame, guilt, threats, confrontation, arguments, and arbitrary treatment plans to motivate patients does not work and should be avoided.

In presenting the diagnosis, the physician should use the SOAPE mnemonic (Support, Optimism, Absolution, Plan, and Explanation; Clark, 1981). By demonstrating support for the patient and optimism about the patient's chances of resolving the problems caused by their disease (they do not need to feel guilty about a disease), the physician increases the likelihood that the patient will cooperate in deciding on an appropriate treatment plan. It may be helpful to copy the SOAPE and DEATH mnemonics (Tables 4 and 5) on a small card and refer to them during discussions with patients.

Another approach is to use the "Eight Basic Actions" outlined by Whitfield (1995). In one or two sentences the physician can: (1) state the specific diagnosis, (2) explain that it is a disease, (3) affirm that it is not the patient's fault, (4) state that it is the patient's responsibility, (5) encourage abstinence, (6) suggest a treatment plan, (7) offer to meet with a family member or supportive friend, and (8) suggest a return visit. Although perhaps not optimal, merely making these statements in a matter-of-fact, non-judgmental way is of significant therapeutic value.

Presenting the diagnosis is a discrete therapeutic intervention, separate from screening, diagnosis, and forming a treatment plan. Thus, it deserves a discrete office visit and negotiated followup to develop an individualized treatment plan. Only by maintaining a continuing dialogue about the issue of addiction can a practitioner accurately assess the patient's progress.

Assessing the Patient's Readiness To Change. The optimal approach to patients with any chronic disease, and especially to the patient with an addictive disorder, is to continue the dialogue over time to assess the patient's stage of readiness for behavior change. Patients typically move from precontemplation to contemplation, and then to action. At times, they regress through relapse back to precontemplation.

This model was first articulated and studied by Prochaska and DiClemente (1983) while they were studying smoking cessation. It places initial and often primary emphasis on the patient's willingness to begin change in his or her life, rather than emphasizing the physician's ability to design the optimal treatment plan. In addition to the diagnostic criteria and the severity of the disease, it introduces the patient's perceptions into the process of forming a treatment plan. The model hypothesizes that most people are at one of five stages of readiness for change regarding any problematic behavior in their lives. The stages are precontemplation, contemplation, action, maintenance, and relapse.

Patients who are in the *precontemplation* phase generally do not realize that a problem exists and thus are not

| TABLE 5. | Guidelines for Presenting the Diagnosis: The SOAPE Glossary |

S: **Support.** Use phrases such as, "we need to work together on this," "I am concerned about you and will follow up closely with you," and "as with all medical illnesses, the more people you work with, the better you will feel." These words reinforce the therapeutic relationship and strengthen the collaborative model of management.

O: **Optimism.** Most patients have "cut back" on their drinking or drug use several times, quit at times, and perhaps participated in some treatment. They have begun to expect failure and relapse, and to fear that they never will improve. By voicing a strong, ultimately optimistic message, the physician can help to re-motivate such patients. Use phrases such as, "you will get better," "no one deserves the pain and humiliation of this disease," "treatment works," "you can expect noticeable improvements in most areas of your life," and "with help, you will do well."

A: **Absolution.** Patients with addictive disorders usually blame themselves for their addiction. This pervasive sense of guilt, shame, and personal weakness tends to paralyze patients, impairing their ability to consider making life changes, and thus perpetuates the addiction cycle. One of the most important things a physician can do is to convince the patient that addiction is a disease, it is no one's fault, it is the physician's and patient's responsibility to work together toward recovery, and that recovery is likely.

P: **Plan.** Development of a treatment plan depends on the patient's readiness to make behavioral changes and the availability of resources. Use phrases such as, "there are many things we can pursue to help you recover," "I want you to seriously consider abstinence as an important aspect of your improvement," "building on what you have tried before is a good place to start," and "what do you think you can do at this point?"

E: **Explanatory Model.** As in all areas of medical practice, it is important to know what the patient believes about his or her illness. Beginning with the patient's beliefs and then helping him or her to consider a more therapeutic model is important when presenting any diagnosis. Use phrases such as "what is your idea of a person with alcohol or drug problems?," "your illness is not nearly that advanced," "this is an illness that responds to medical intervention and treatment, not a moral weakness," "you have been trying to use will power by itself to treat a disease; how about adding some treatment to your considerable will power?"

ready to take steps toward resolution. Expecting such a patient to accept a referral to Alcoholics Anonymous (AA) after one office visit is unrealistic and can set up both the patient and the physician for disappointment. "Agreeing to disagree" about the presence of a drinking problem and following up at future visits is a reasonable course of action.

Patients who are in the *contemplation* phase generally are aware of the problems in their lives. Often they are willing to entertain the possibility that some of their problems are related to—and at times caused by—substance abuse. Such patient usually are willing to discuss treatment options. They are more likely to keep followup appointments or to accept referrals. They often are willing to discuss the dysfunction caused by their substance use.

Patients who are in the *action* phase are very open to abstinence messages, and are likely to follow through with treatment recommendations, especially if those recommendations are the result of a negotiation between the physician and patient.

The *maintenance* phase is the so-called "relapse prevention" or "maintenance of behavior change" phase. Patients still require intermittent office monitoring, toxicology testing, pharmacotherapy, and ongoing assessment of their recovery program while in the maintenance phase.

When patients *relapse*, they often fail to keep appointments and refuse toxicology testing. Internal feelings of disappointment and shame can present as anger, sarcasm, or even suicidal ideation. Identifying relapse early and actively reaching out to the patient is extremely important. This is in direct contrast to the traditional clinical practice, in which patients who missed appointments were routinely dropped from the treatment program.

Assessing the patient's readiness to change allows the physician to negotiate appropriate patient-centered treatment plans. It also increases compliance, maintains the physician/patient relationship, and reduces staff frustration.

Negotiating a Treatment Plan. In older approaches to patient care, the role of the physician was overemphasized (that is, the physician formulated the treatment plan, prescribed medication, and recommended behavior change, while the patient merely complied with the physician's directives and directions). This physician-centered model of practice was characterized by relative noncompliance on the part of most patients, with the treatment of alcohol and drug problems no exception.

By contrast, the "negotiated model" for developing a treatment plan shifts the emphasis to include patient participation in the process, leading to much higher levels of patient compliance and satisfaction. The negotiated treatment plan model is applicable to many chronic illnesses in primary care and is essential when formulating treatment plans with alcohol and drug dependent patients. When used appropriately, this patient-centered approach results in treatment plans that are less time-consuming, simpler, more manageable, and productive of greater patient compliance.

Prognostic Factors That Influence Patient Outcomes: Several general prognostic indicators are worth evaluating to guide treatment planning and help establish realistic expectations. Positive prognostic factors often indicate either a less severe form or a less advanced stage of addiction. Such positive factors include lack of physiologic dependence, intact family/job, presence of prior treatment (prognosis for sobriety improves if patients have had one to three prior treatment experiences), absence of other psychiatric disease, presence of a long-term monitoring arrangement (as through a state medical society's Physician Effectiveness Program or an Employee Assistance Program). Negative prognostic factors indicate more severe, advanced, or complicated disease states. They include the presence of intoxication at office visits; loss of job, home, or family; multiple unsuccessful treatment attempts; severe physiologic dependence (as marked by a history of convulsions or *delirium tremens*); co-occurring psychiatric disorders (such schizophrenia, severe posttraumatic stress disorder (PTSD), or severe depression); and absence of long-term monitoring.

Applying Readiness for Change: When negotiating a treatment plan in the ambulatory setting, the severity of the disease and the patient's current stage of readiness for change are of primary importance.

If the patient is *precontemplative* and the severity of the disease is fairly mild, the urgency to intervene beyond an intermittent brief intervention is quite low. Pushing such a patient to accept treatment when he or she is not ready to do so threatens the physician-patient relationship and probably is not indicated. If possible, the patient's family members should be encouraged to learn more about alcohol and other drug dependence (either through various readings, family counseling, or participation in Al-Anon). If the disease is moderate in severity, there is more urgency to assess the disease and the patient's readiness. Additionally, the patient might be referred to an addiction specialist, presented with medical reasons for not drinking, and, if possible, referred for family counseling. If the patient is precontemplative and the disease is severe, a brief intervention should be performed at each visit. Such a patient should be referred to an addiction specialist and given strongly emphasized medical reasons not to drink. A crisis intervention should be considered (see below).

If the patient is *contemplative* and the disease is mild, the disease severity should be assessed frequently (every three to six months), and evidence of dysfunction and disability presented at least yearly. The patient should be encouraged to limit his or her drinking (move to the action stage) or to abstain. Consideration should be given to referring the family for more education about addiction. If the disease is moderate, evidence of dysfunction and medical reasons not to drink should be reemphasized at least twice a year. The physician should attempt to negotiate an agreement for referral to an addiction specialist and refer the family for more education. If the patient is contemplative and the disease is severe, evidence of dysfunction and medical complications should be presented at every visit. A primary care physician should insist on a referral to an addiction specialist and refer the family for more education and crisis intervention, if possible.

Even when patients affirm their willingness to undertake abstinence, it is critical to determine whether they are capable of achieving abstinence. To do so, the physician might negotiate a small change in activities and behaviors, then see the patient to assess his or her readiness and ability to make changes. Pharmacotherapy is an excellent test of "true" readiness.

The following questions are useful in negotiating a treatment plan with a patient who is ready for action. Answers should be corroborated whenever possible by interviews with other persons.

- Is the patient a danger to himself or others? (Suicide and vehicular homicide are serious consequences of alcohol and other drug disorders. Questions about suicidal ideation, impaired judgment while intoxicated, and *delirium tremens* thus are mandatory when assessing a patient.)

- Has the patient ever been able to stay sober for 3 or more days? (This question assesses the patient's ability to "self-detox.")

- What happened when the patient stopped drinking or using in the past? How serious was the withdrawal syndrome?

- Has the patient ever been able to stay completely abstinent for a long period of time? (Learning what has proved useful in the past and what the patient thinks can be added now is one of the most efficient and effective initial approaches to treatment planning.)

- Why did previous attempts fail to produce sobriety? (Factors that contributed to treatment failures should be identified and addressed.)

Evaluating Treatment Options. Selecting an appropriate treatment program can be difficult. The keys to identifying high-quality treatment programs are similar to the ways that generalists find specialists for referrals. Treatment programs need to be available and affordable to the patient and family. Good treatment programs communicate with the referring physician, coordinate on issues of toxicology testing and lab work, are open minded on issues of adjunctive pharmacotherapy, include family members in treatment, and insist on abstinence (Rogers & McMillin, 1992).

If inpatient or outpatient treatment are not options for the patient, Twelve Step groups can be recommended as sources of support to help the patient maintain abstinence (see Section 8). It also may be necessary to detoxify the patient on an outpatient basis (refer to Section 5). Guidance in evaluating treatment options is found in the *ASAM Patient Placement Criteria, Second Edition-Revised (2001)* (see the Appendix of this text for a summary).

Family Referral Resources. Family members frequently have misconceptions about alcohol and drug dependence. It is critically important to assess the family's belief systems and to educate family members toward a more therapeutic approach to this disease (also see Chapter 7 of this section). Resources available include an excellent book entitled "Freeing Someone You Love from Alcohol" (Rogers & McMillin, 1992). After family members have read this or similar books, they are more likely to agree to referral for individual counseling or family therapy. Finally, self-help organizations available to family members include Al-Anon, Alateen, Tough Love, and Families Anonymous. Family members will be much more likely to accept referral to self-help meetings if they have read about the programs and have had the chronic illness model presented by their physician.

In summary, negotiating a treatment plan can be simple and straightforward if several principles are observed and there is an accurate assessment of the severity of the disease and the patient's readiness for behavior change. For patients who are willing to consider making changes, the important issues to assess are what treatment options exist, which treatment options are most appropriate for the particular patient, and what treatment options are acceptable to the patient. Answering those questions can result in the development of a surprisingly comprehensive treatment plan. Of equal importance, the plan can be efficiently implemented and managed over time.

Negotiating a treatment plan is a discrete, independent clinical activity that deserves a separate visit or visits and should not be appended onto a visit in which the diagnosis is presented. If the patient is not ready to acknowledge a problem, then "agreeing to disagree" is an acceptable option. Frequent followup visits, during which the physician expresses ongoing concern about the patient's alcohol or other drug problem, is an acceptable "treatment plan" when working with a precontemplative patient.

Crisis Intervention. Crisis intervention is a major invasive procedure that is used to initiate treatment, particularly when the patient has a severe problem and is in the precontemplation stage. A crisis intervention is a group confrontation with the addicted individual. It must be carefully organized, rehearsed, and choreographed by a trained "intervention counselor." Each member of the group should be a "significant" person in the patient's life, and be prepared to state several experiences in which the patient's drinking or drug use adversely affected him or her. Given the weight of this objective evidence, the "wall of denial" breaks down sufficiently for most patients to enter a treatment program. Phrases and techniques that are coached by the intervention counselor include: "It's not you, it's the drinking." "It hurts me too much to see you continue in this painful disease." "You did not develop this on purpose, but you've got it." "We care about you, but hate your drinking." "I will not argue; this is what you did, this is when you did it, and this is how it made me feel." The common themes in these phrases include: (1) exhibiting positive regard toward the individual and negative regard toward the drinking, (2) obtaining specific data about specific events in order to confront patients adequately, and (3) validating the disease approach via statements about the obvious pain of this progressive illness. This approach allows the patient to relieve his or her guilt, become less defensive, and become more open to obtaining help with his or her disease. When organized and supervised by a well-trained intervention counselor, a crisis intervention can motivate patients who are contemplative or even precontemplative to enter a treatment program.

FOLLOWUP MONITORING
Patients should be monitored carefully to be sure that they are able to follow the physician's recommendations. Initially, such monitoring may require weekly followup visits. Seeing the patient regularly conveys that the physician is concerned about the patient's alcohol or other drug problem and cares about his or her progress.

At each visit, the physician should review the patient's progress and give positive reinforcement if the patient has been able to maintain the suggested limits. If there is concern that the patient is not following recommendations, a family member might be asked to verify the patient's history. Biochemical markers (such as GGT, CDT, blood or saliva alcohol levels, or urine drug screens) also might be used to assess patient compliance.

If a patient is not able to follow the recommended limits, the physician should consider referring him or her to an addiction medicine specialist or a formal rehabilitation program. Patients are more willing to follow recommendations if they have proved to themselves that they cannot control their alcohol or other drug use.

It is equally important for the physician to support and monitor patients who are abstaining from alcohol or drug use. Alcohol- or drug-dependent patients who have been involved in a treatment program should be asked to sign a medical release so that their physician can participate in their aftercare plan.

In addition to seeing the patient regularly, the physician should list alcohol or other drug dependence on the problem list in the patient's chart; the patient's "clean and sober" date also might be noted in the chart to remind the physician to provide positive reinforcement and support on recovery anniversaries (usually at 1, 3, 6, and 9 months, and then yearly thereafter). This reminder is another way to let patients know that the physician cares about their well-being and supports their continued commitment to recovery.

Problems in Recovery. A number of problems are commonly encountered by patients early in the recovery process. Depression is common and usually clears without treatment in the first few months. Severe depression or a history of past depression may indicate the need for an antidepressant to help reduce the risk of relapse.

Many patients experience sexual dysfunction early in recovery. The physician can reassure the patient that this is a common problem that will resolve with time.

Certain prescription medications can jeopardize a recovering patient's ability to abstain from alcohol and other illicit drugs. Specifically, benzodiazepines and narcotics should be avoided if at all possible, since both drug classes can significantly increase the likelihood of a relapse. Nonpharmacologic treatments should be used whenever possible.

Medications such as naltrexone and disulfiram may be helpful in early recovery (see Section 6). If the patient is attending AA meetings, the physician may need to give advice not to let AA members discourage the use of necessary medications; this is particularly important for patients with co-occurring psychiatric disorders. Although AA's official position is that groups should not interfere with members' medications, some AA members, acting on their own, may urge that all medications be discontinued.

Patients should be monitored for signs of potential relapse. It is possible to anticipate a relapse based on the patient's behavior and then to counsel him or her so as to minimize the risk of relapse and/or facilitate reentry into treatment.

Physicians often become frustrated when patients do not want to address their alcohol and other drug problems. It is important to remember that addiction is a chronic disorder, which presents an opportunity to work with the patient over time. The physician can continue to reaffirm concern and willingness to help.

Two common dangers are ignoring the problem and "preaching" to patients, as both techniques limit the physician's ability to help. An attitude of caring concern eventually will prevail. Even if a patient is unwilling to consider help with his or her alcohol or other drug problem, the physician still can help family members by recommending programs such as Al-Anon and Alateen.

REFERENCES

Babor TF, de la Fuente JR, Saunders J et al. (1992). *AUDIT—The Alcohol Use Disorders Identification Test: Guidelines for Use in Primary Health Care*. Geneva, Switzerland: World Health Organization.

Beresford TP, Blow FC, Hill E et al. (1990). Comparison of CAGE questionnaire and computer-assisted laboratory profiles in screening for covert alcoholism. *Lancet* 336:482-485.

Bien TH, Miller WR & Tonigan JS (1993). Brief intervention for alcohol problems: A review. *Addiction* 88:315-336.

Bradley KA (1994). The primary care practitioner's role in the prevention and management of alcohol problems. *Alcohol Health & Research World* 18:97-104.

Buchsbaum D (1994). Effectiveness of treatment in general medicine patients with drinking problems. *Alcohol Health & Research World* 18(2):140-145.

Bush K, Kivlahan DR, McDonnell MB et al. (1998). The AUDIT alcohol consumption questions (AUDIT-C): An effective brief screening test for problem drinking. *Archives of Internal Medicine* 158:1789-1795.

Clark WD (1981). Alcoholism: Blocks to diagnosis and treatment. *American Journal of Medicine* 71:285-286.

Cyr MG & Wartman SA (1988). The effectiveness of routine screening questions in the detection of alcoholism. *Journal of the American Medical Association* 259:51-54.

Fleming MF, Barry KL, Manwell LB et al. (1997). Brief physician advice for problem alcohol drinkers. *Journal of the American Medical Association* 277(13): 1039-1045.

Gordon AJ, Maisto SA, McNeil M et al. (2001). Three questions can detect hazardous drinkers. *Journal of Family Practice* 4:313-320.

Mayfield I, McLend G & Hall P (1971). The CAGE questionnaire: Validation of a new alcoholism screening instrument. *American Journal of Psychiatry* 127:1121-1123.

National Institute on Alcohol Abuse and Alcoholism (NIAAA) (1996). *How to Cut Down on Your Drinking*. Rockville, MD: NIAAA, National Institutes of Health.

National Institute on Alcohol Abuse and Alcoholism (NIAAA) (1995). *The Physicians' Guide to Helping Patients with Alcohol Problems*. Rockville, MD: NIAAA, National Institutes of Health.

Prochaska JO & DiClemente CC (1983). Stages and processes of self-change in smoking: Toward an integrative model of change. *Journal of Consulting and Clinical Psychology* 5:390-95.

Rogers RL & McMillin CS (1992). Choosing a treatment program. In *Freeing Someone You Love From Alcohol*. New York, NY: The Body Press.

Rush BR (1989). The use of family medical practices by patients with drinking problems. *Canadian Medical Association Journal* 140(1):35-38.

Steinweg DL & Worth H (1993). Alcoholism: The key to the CAGE. *American Journal of Medicine* 94:520-523.

Whitfield CL & Barker LR (1995). Alcoholism. In LR Barker, JR Burton & PD Zieve (eds.) *Principles of Ambulatory Medicine*. Baltimore, MD: Williams & Wilkins, 204-231.

Williams GD, Aitken SS & Malin H (1985). Reliability of self-reported alcohol consumption in a general population survey. *Journal of Studies on Alcohol* 46(3):223-227.

Chapter 2	# Laboratory Diagnosis

Elizabeth A. Warner, M.D.

Interpretation of Test Results
Body Fluids for Testing
Collection Procedures
Laboratory Methods
Drug-Specific Tests
Ethical Considerations

In evaluating a patient with a known or suspected substance use disorder, the clinician may use the laboratory to confirm findings obtained from the history and physical examination. Testing may include direct identification and measurement of suspected drugs of abuse in body fluids or tissues, or can indirectly measure the consequences of such use. The accurate interpretation of laboratory findings requires knowledge of the type of test performed, the limits of detection, and the recognition of the possibility of false positive and false negative tests (Wolff, Farell et al., 1999). Clinicians need to understand that the types of laboratory tests ordered to screen for substance use are intended for clinical care, rather than for legal proceedings. (For a discussion of drug testing in the workplace, refer to Section 9.)

Testing for substances of abuse often is performed in clinical settings (Lowinson, Ruiz et al., 1997). When suggested by clinical findings, laboratory tests can assist in the initial diagnosis of a substance use disorder, and can identify substances associated with overdose or trauma. Laboratory tests also are used both to monitor abstinence in patients in drug treatment programs and to monitor compliance with treatment, as in methadone treatment programs.

INTERPRETATION OF TEST RESULTS

Although tests for drugs of abuse are widely available and reasonably simple to perform, skill is required in the interpretation of the resulting data. Laboratory results must be interpreted in the clinical context (Osterloh, 1998). The clinician should know which drugs are detected by the tests ordered and how long the drug is detectable after use. Knowledge of which substances can give either false positive or false negative results also is important. Many laboratories use commercially available kits for drug testing. The manufacturers of these tests publish package inserts, which often report the concentration at which drugs are detected. The inserts also list drugs that cross-react with the assay and thus cause false positive tests.

Communication between the clinician and the laboratory is helpful, both in deciding which tests to order and in interpreting the test results.

BODY FLUIDS FOR TESTING

Virtually any body fluid or tissue can be assayed for drugs of abuse, but for practical purposes, such testing is limited to specimens that can be obtained in a reasonably non-invasive manner. Sources commonly used for drug testing

TABLE 1. Compounds That Can Cause False Positive Results in Urine Immunoassays

Amphetamines/	LSD
Methamphetamine	Amitriptyline
Bupropion	Chlorpromazine
Chloroquine	Doxepin
Chlorpromazine	Fluoxetine
Ephedrine	Haloperidol
Fenfluramine	Metoclopramide
Labetolol	Risperidone
Mexiletine	Sertraline
N-acetyl	Thioridazine
procainamide	Verapamil
Phentermine	
Phenylephrine	**Opiates**
Phenylpropanolamine	Ofloxacin
(PPA)	Papaverine
Propranolol	Rifampicin
Pseudoephedrine	
Quinacrine	**Phencyclidine (PCP)**
Ranitidine	Dextromethorphan
Selegiline	Diphenhydramine
(Eldepryl®)	Thioridazine
Trazodone	
Tyramine	**Propoxyphene**
	Cyclobenzaprine
Barbiturates	Diphenylhydramine
Phenytoin	Doxylamine
	Imipramine
Benzodiazepines	Methadone.
Oxaprozin	
Sertraline	

include urine and blood. Tests also are being developed for sweat, hair, and saliva.

Urine. Urine is the primary substance used to test for drugs of abuse because it is collected easily and non-invasively. A large quantity is available and drugs often are present in high concentrations. However, urine specimens are easily adulterated or substituted, so that an estimation of the authenticity of the urine may be needed (SAMHSA, 1999).

The temperature of recently collected urine specimens should approximate body temperature. An acceptable temperature range is 90° to 100° F. within four minutes of collection. A laboratory may refuse a urine specimen that is not within this temperature range.

Laboratories also may measure specific gravity, creatinine concentration, and pH to insure that specimens are within the range of normal human urine. A dilute urine has a creatinine concentration <20 mg/dL *and* a specific gravity <1.003. A substituted urine, which is not consistent with normal or dilute human urine, is defined as having a creatinine <5 mg/dL *and* a specific gravity ≤1.001 or >.020. In order for a urine specimen to be recorded as substitute, both creatinine and specific gravity must fall within the abnormal range.

In addition to diluting or substituting urine, donors may adulterate urine specimens. A specimen is considered adulterated if the nitrate concentration is >500 g/ml, if the pH is ≤3 or ≥11, if an exogenous substance is present in the urine, or if there is a higher concentration of an endogenous substance than should be found under normal physiologic concentration in the urine.

Multiple *in vivo* adulterants are available. They involve ingesting pills, capsules or "tea" to interfere with the laboratory test. Many of these products require increased fluid intake; in order not to dilute the urine excessively, they also may contain creatine or creatinine (Winecker & Goldberger, 1998).

In vitro adulterants include common household products, such as bleach, vinegar, liquid detergent, table salt, and baking soda, as well as commercially available kits, such as "Urine Luck," which can be added to urine to interfere with test results (Wu, Bristol et al., 1999).

Blood. Blood testing probably is more helpful than urine testing for quantitating recent ingestion. In addition, blood is less likely to be adulterated or substituted than urine. However, alcohol and other drugs generally are present in the blood for much shorter periods than in the urine. Also, venipuncture requires special training, is invasive, and poses a higher risk of infection to the personnel obtaining the specimen. Many injection drug users have poor venous access as the result of prior venous thrombosis, so obtaining specimens may be difficult.

Saliva. Saliva also has been used to screen for drugs of abuse. Saliva collection is non-invasive, and protection of privacy is not a concern with directly observed collection. Adulteration during sample collection is less likely with saliva than with urine. Measurement of drug concentrations in saliva can closely estimate circulating concentrations in plasma and can be used to assess for acute intoxication. On the other hand, drugs are measurable in the saliva for a shorter period of time, and the concentrations are lower than is the case with urine (Kidwell, Holland et al., 1998).

Hair. Hair has been used to test for drugs of abuse (McPhillips, Strang et al., 1998). It is assumed that the substances are deposited in the hair during keratonization and remain in the hair shaft in a fixed position indefinitely. Hair can be collected easily and non-invasively, and adulteration and substitution are less likely than with urine.

When testing hair, the immunoassay should target the parent drug or metabolite that is found in highest concentration in the hair. For example, after cocaine use, the metabolite benzoylecgonine is found in high concentrations in urine, while very little cocaine itself is found. The converse is true for hair. After use, the primary analyte found in hair is cocaine itself, with minimal amounts of benzoylecgonine (Spiehler, 2000).

Concentrations of drugs in hair are low, requiring sensitive assays. If hair is assumed to grow approximately 1 cm/month, the hair can give a qualitative account of the history of ingestion. However, hair testing is not helpful in assessing acute intoxication, because significant amounts of drug are not found in hair until one to two weeks after use (Spiehler, 2000).

Hair specimens require a more labor-intensive preparation than urine specimens, and there is some concern about passive accumulation of substances in hair. Theoretically, hair analysis can provide a history of the pattern of substance use over a longer time span than other studies, complementing the information obtained from short-term measures such as urine testing.

Sweat. Drugs also are secreted into sweat, which can be used to monitor substance use. Patches can be applied to the skin to absorb sweat. Such tests can identify drugs excreted over an extended period of time. However, sweat can be collected only in relatively small amounts, and quantitation of drug levels in sweat is difficult because it usually is not possible to measure the total amount of sweat secreted (Kidwell, Holland et al., 1998).

COLLECTION PROCEDURES

Proper collection and processing of specimens are essential to accurate results. Universal handling precautions are recommended for all specimens. The timing of the collection should be noted, so that results can be interpreted in the context of the time of ingestion. The identity of the person supplying the specimen needs to be confirmed and the specimen needs to be properly labeled. Chain of custody regulations in forensic or workplace testing have been developed to prevent laboratory misidentification, especially when the testing has legal implications (refer to Section 9). However, when testing is done for clinical purposes, chain of custody regulations are not routinely followed.

LABORATORY METHODS

The initial procedure for drug testing usually is a screening urine immunoassay (Wolff, Farell et al., 1999). Immunoassays are inexpensive, easily automated, and yield rapid results. In these tests, an antibody reacts to a portion of the drug or its metabolite. A major limitation of immunoassays is cross-reactivity: that is, the antibody interacts with antigens other than the one used to produce the antibody, yielding a false positive result (Colbert, 1994) (see Table 1).

Commercial immunoassays from different manufacturers use various antibodies, and not all assays share the same cross-reactivities. With the development of more specific antibodies, many currently available immunoassays no longer have cross-reactivities with substances previously reported to give false positive results. The package insert for an immunoassay should make it clear which compounds have been determined to cross-react with the assay. Such cross-reactivity information usually is listed for the parent drug, and does not include cross-reactivity information on endogenous metabolites (Colbert, 1994). Therefore, this information should be interpreted with caution, recognizing that metabolites of a compound may have cross-reactivity, even though the parent compound does not.

Because of the serious consequences that may ensue from a positive urine screen, positive tests on immunoassay often are confirmed with a second analytic procedure to verify the presence of a specific drug or metabolite. The second procedure should be independent of the initial test and should use a different technique and chemical principle from that of the initial test in order to ensure reliability and accuracy.

Chromatography is most commonly used as a confirmatory test. Gas chromatography with mass spectroscopy (GC/MS) couples the powerful separation potential of gas chromatography with the precise detection and identification capability of mass spectroscopy. This technique can

TABLE 2. Cutoff Values for Drug Screening Tests

Drug	SAMHSA Cutoff*	SAMHSA Confirmation*	Clinical Laboratories
Amphetamines	1,000 ng/mL	Amphetamine 500 ng/mL Methamphetamine 500 ng/mL (must also have presence of amphetamine 200 ng/mL)	1,000 ng/mL
Cannabinoids (THC-COOH)	50 ng/mL	15 ng/mL	50 or 100 ng/mL
Cocaine (benzoylecgonine)	300 ng/mL	150 ng/mL	300 ng/mL
Opiates	2,000 ng/mL	Morphine 2,000 ng/mL Codeine 2,000 ng/mL 6-Acetylmorphine 10 ng/ml (must be tested if morphine >2000 ng/mL)	300 ng/mL
Phencyclidine (PCP)	25 ng/mL	25 ng/mL	25 ng/mL
Barbiturates**	—	—	200 or 300 ng/mL
Benzodiazepines**	—	—	200 or 300 ng/mL
LSD**	—	—	0.5 ng/mL
Methadone**	—	—	150 or 300 ng/mL

*U.S. Department of Health and Human Services, 1994, 1997.
**Not included in federal workplace drug testing programs.

identify and quantify extremely small amounts of drugs or metabolites, rendering GC/MS the "gold standard" for confirming positive immunoassays. For workplace or forensic testing, confirming a positive immunoassay by GC/MS is required before reporting the test as positive (similar to performing a Western blot test to confirm a positive ELISA test when testing for HIV). However, in clinical practice, the laboratory may confirm a positive immunoassay when requested, but is not required to do so before reporting it as a positive test.

Cutoff. A cutoff is a defined concentration of an analyte in a specimen, at or above which the test is reported as positive and below which it is reported as negative. The cutoff concentration usually is significantly greater than the sensitivity of the assay and is chosen to minimize false positive and false negative results. If a drug is detected in a specimen in concentrations lower than the defined cutoff, the test will be reported as negative even though the drug was in fact detected. For screening tests, if a test is reported as negative, no further testing generally is done. If a specimen is reported as positive, a confirmatory test may be ordered.

Knowledge of the cutoff level for a particular test is helpful in estimating the length of time after drug ingestion that a test will be positive (Table 2). Lower cutoff levels are associated with longer detection times. Table 3 lists approximate duration of detection from the time of last use.

On-Site Testing. Point of care or on-site testing refers to tests that are performed outside of the laboratory. Commercially available immunoassay kits are available to test for commonly abused drugs. These tests are performed at the time of specimen collection. The assays are rapid and easy to perform and require little training. However, the interpretation of these tests is somewhat subjective. The tests lack adequate quality controls and are more expensive than tests performed in large numbers by laboratories. Such tests clearly are designed for use as screening tests. Moreover, recent studies show variable sensitivity and specificity compared to GC/MS (Division of Workplace Programs, 1999).

The manufacturers recommend that any positive results be confirmed by more specific laboratory methods. Nevertheless, many of these tests have been accepted for use in traffic testing and for workplace testing.

Federal Regulations. The U.S. Department of Health and Human Services (DHHS) and the Substance Abuse and Mental Health Services Administration (SAMHSA) have published guidelines for drug testing of federal workers (DHHS, 1994, 1997; SAMHSA, 1999), including the proper collection of specimens. Chain of custody procedures are defined to help ensure the validity of specimens. Initial screening tests are performed by immunoassay, followed by confirmation of all positive screening tests by gas chromatography/mass spectroscopy (GC/MS). The federal guidelines establish cutoff values for the five substances (amphetamines, cannabinoids, cocaine, opiates, and PCP) that are mandated in federal workplace drug testing (see Table 2). Although these cutoff values were developed for workplace testing for federal workers, many clinical laboratories have adopted them as well. Specimens obtained for clinical use, however, are not subject to these collection and testing requirements.

DRUG-SPECIFIC TESTS

Alcohol. Tests that are widely used to monitor recent alcohol ingestion include the GGT (gamma-glutamyl-peptidase), the AST (aspartate amino transferase), and the MCV (erythrocyte mean cell volume). Of these, the GGT is the most sensitive marker of alcohol abuse (Conigrave, Saunders et al., 1995). GGT levels are elevated in approximately 75% of persons diagnosed with alcohol dependence,

approximately 50% of patients hospitalized for alcohol-related problems, and approximately 30% of problem drinkers. It is important to note that the GGT is not specific for alcohol abuse and also is elevated in patients with fatty liver and those using certain medications, including anticonvulsants. GGT levels generally are reduced by half with two weeks of abstinence and can return to normal over six to eight weeks.

With abstinence, the MCV will fall, but because the lifespan of the RBC is 120 days, it may take approximately three months to see improvement in the MCV after abstinence. Non-alcohol related conditions that increase the MCV include chronic liver disease, hypothyroidism, folate deficiency, and megaloblastic disorders. Because the MCV takes longer to decline than the GGT, it is less helpful in following patients in the weeks after they enter alcohol treatment (Sillanaukee, 1996).

A less frequently used marker for alcohol abuse is the carbohydrate-deficient transferrin (CDT). In the setting of heavy alcohol ingestion, the glycosylation process of transferrin is impaired, rendering the transferrin missing some carbohydrate terminal chains, termed carbohydrate-deficient transferrin (CDT) (Litten, Allen et al., 1995). Drinking four to seven standard drinks per day (or about 50 to 80 grams of alcohol) for a week or more is required to elevate CDT levels. The half-life of CDT is approximately 15 days. Other etiologies of elevated CDT include advanced liver disease and genetic variations of transferrin. Since the CDT is not sufficiently sensitive or specific to detect alcohol abuse, it is not considered an acceptable test for screening, but may be used to monitor for abstinence or increased alcohol consumption (Laposata, 1999).

In one study (Yersin, Nicolet et al., 1995) that examined simultaneous measurements of CDT, GGT, and MCV in patients seen in an emergency department or primary care center, the sensitivity and specificity of the tests for a marker of alcohol consumption of >60 grams/day were 0.58 and 0.82 for the CDT, 0.69 and 0.65 for the GGT, and 0.27 and 0.91 for the MCV, respectively. The CDT was found to be the most sensitive and specific in a subgroup of men age less than 40 years (Yersin, Nicolet et al., 1995).

Serum transaminases, particularly aspartate amino transferase (AST) and alanine amino transferase (ALT), may be elevated in patients with alcohol abuse. However, these tests are not as sensitive a marker for alcohol abuse as the GGT. The AST usually is more elevated than the ALT in patients with alcohol-related liver disease. When the

TABLE 3. Approximate Duration of Detectability of Commonly Used Substances and Some of Their Metabolites in Urine (Based on Common Laboratory Cutoff Values)

Substance	Duration of Detectability
Barbiturates	
Short-acting	24 hours
Intermediate-acting (pentobarbital)	48 to 72 hours
Long-acting (phenobarbital)	16 days or more
Benzodiazepines	
Short-acting (triazolam)	24 hours
Intermediate-acting (temazepam, chlordiazepoxide)	40 to 80 hours
Long-acting (diazepam, nitrazepam)	7 days or more
Cannabinoids (marijuana): tetrahydrocannabinol	
Single use	3 days
Moderate use	4 days
Heavy use (daily)	10 days
Chronic heavy use	up to 36 days
Opioids	
Methadone (maintenance dosing)	7-9 days
Codeine/morphine	24 hours
6-Monoacetyl morphine	2 to 4 hours
Morphine glucuronides	48 hours
Codeine glucuronides	3 days
Propoxyphene/norpropoxyphene	6 to 48 hours
Dihydrocodeine	24 hours
Buprenorphine	48 to 56 hours
Buprenorphine conjugates	7 days
Stimulants	
Amphetamine	2 to 3 days
MDMA (Ecstasy)	30 to 48 hours
Methamphetamine	48 hours
Cocaine	6 to 8 hours
Cocaine metabolite/benzoylecgonine	2 to 3 days
Other	
Methaqualone	7 days or more
Phencyclidine (PCP)	8 days
LSD	24 hours
Nicotine	12 hours
Cotinine	2 to 3 days

SOURCE: Adapted with permission from Wolff K, Farrell M, Marsden J et al. (1999). A review of biological indicators of illicit drug use, practical considerations and clinical usefulness. *Addiction* 94(9):1279-1298.

transaminases are elevated and the ALT is more elevated than the AST, alcohol abuse is less likely to be the cause of the liver disease. While elevations of the transaminases may suggest alcohol-related liver disease, none of the abnormal liver enzymes can predict alcohol dependence or intoxication.

In summary, none of the currently available laboratory tests is sufficiently sensitive and specific to be used as routine screening tests for alcohol abuse.

Acute Alcohol Intoxication: Laboratory testing to confirm alcohol ingestion relies on measurement of ethanol from body fluids. These measurements can confirm recent alcohol intake, but do not necessarily determine degree of impairment, because some individuals develop tolerance to the effects of alcohol. Both blood and breath tests can estimate alcohol ingestion.

Blood alcohol concentration (BAC) detects alcohol use within the preceding few hours. Testing for alcohol levels in blood can be done through enzymatic analysis or gas chromatography of the headspace. Specimens for venipuncture should be drawn using an alcohol-free antiseptic. The enzymatic analysis measures the amount of NADH formed during oxidation of ethanol; this may produce falsely elevated readings in the presence of isopropanol, methanol, and ethylene glycol. High levels of acetone, similar to those found in DKA or starvation, can be metabolized to isopropanol, giving falsely elevated ethanol levels by the enzymatic analysis (Jones & Pounder, 1998).

In the headspace analysis, a specimen is obtained in a vacutainer tube that is not completely filled. Ethanol equilibrates between the blood and the air space (headspace) above the liquid. A portion of the vapor from the tube is injected onto a chromatographic column and then quantitated (Porter, 1999). Although gas chromatography is considered the gold standard for measuring ethanol in forensic laboratories, many clinical laboratories use enzymatic methods.

Most states define intoxication on the basis of whole blood alcohol levels; the most commonly used are 80 or 100 mg/dL. Clinical laboratories, however, measure ethanol in serum or plasma. Because the water content of serum is higher than that of whole blood, the same specimen will show a higher level of ethanol in serum than in whole blood (Frajola, 1993). An estimate of the ratio of serum to whole blood is 1.14/1.00. If a clinical specimen of serum or plasma is used to estimate whole blood levels, the appropriate correction needs to be calculated (Jones & Pounder, 1998).

Less invasive means of detecting the blood alcohol concentration include analysis of alcohol in the exhaled air. Breath alcohol testing generally is used in traffic law enforcement and workplace testing. The ratio of blood to breath concentration of alcohol is approximately 2100:1, although this probably underestimates venous levels by about 10%. (Jones & Pounder, 1998). In the United States, breath alcohol concentration usually is reported in grams/210 liters, so that a breath level of 0.1 gm/210 liters is equivalent to a whole blood alcohol level of 0.10 gm/dL.

In order to allow clearance of any ethanol that may be in the mouth, a 15-minute waiting period is required before a breath test is performed. The alveolar concentration of ethanol is most accurately measured when the subject takes a deep breath, with the measurement taken in the last third of the breath. Failure to obtain a deep breath specimen can lead to an underestimate of the blood alcohol level (Mason, Dubowski et al., 1976). In a study of patients with documented gastroesophageal reflux, breath alcohol analysis was not affected by the presence of such reflux (Kechagias, Jonsson et al., 1999).

Saliva also can be used to estimate serum ethanol concentration. The concentration of alcohol in saliva theoretically is similar to that in serum, although salivary alcohol levels do not correlate as well with breath tests in measuring blood alcohol levels (Bendtsen, Hultberg et al., 1999). Patients with chronic alcohol ingestion may have difficulty producing adequate salivary samples. This may be explained by some degree of parotid dysfunction related to chronic alcohol use. The U.S. Department of Transportation has approved on-site salivary tests that use swabs or cards for ethanol screening.

Alcohol also can be measured in the urine, which provides a qualitative marker of recent alcohol ingestion. The presence of alcohol in the urine suggests alcohol intake within about the preceding eight hours. However, urine concentrations are variable compared to blood levels and are related to the length of time the urine has been in the bladder, so quantitative measures of alcohol levels in the urine are difficult to interpret.

Amphetamines. Most screening tests for amphetamines are designed to detect *d*-amphetamine and *d*-methamphetamine, the most commonly abused amphetamines. However, there are a number of sympathomimetic amines with structures similar to amphetamines that may have cross-reactivity with the immunoassays, causing false positive results (Kraemer, Maurer et al., 1998).

Tests for amphetamines probably produce more false positives than any other frequently used tests for drugs of abuse. Examples of compounds that have been reported to cause positive results include the decongestants phenylpropanolamine, pseudoephedrine, and *l*-methamphetamine (a nasal decongestant used in Vick's® nasal inhaler) and appetite suppressants containing ephedrine or phentermine. (GC/MS tests can separate the stereoisomers of amphetamine and methamphetamine and identify other stimulants that lead to false positives.) Other prescription drugs, such as selegilene, are metabolized either to amphetamine or methamphetamine and also can cause false positive results.

Modifications of the immunoassay can detect 3,4-methylene-dioxymethamphetamine (MDMA, or "Ecstasy"), 3,4-methylenedioxyamphetamine (MDA), and 3,4-methylenedioxyethampehtamine (MDEA, or "Eve")—all illegal amphetamines with hallucinogenic activity. However, current immunoassays may require high concentrations of MDMA to show cross-reactivity. Therefore, one should not routinely assume that MDMA will be detected on an immunoassay. Instead, it is wise to review the package insert for the assay to determine the concentration of MDMA required to produce a positive result.

Since a significant amount of amphetamine and methamphetamine are excreted unchanged in the urine, most urinary detection methods are targeted for these compounds rather than their metabolites. Urine pH influences the excretion of amphetamines (Braithwaite, Jarvie et al., 1995). At high pH levels, there is a marked reduction in amphetamine and methamphetamine excretion (Porter, 1999). Individuals have been known to ingest large quantities of bicarbonate to reduce the amount of amphetamines excreted in the urine. The duration of detection of amphetamines in the urine by immunoassay is variable, but generally they can be detected for 24 hours after use (Simpson, Braithwaite et al., 1997).

Barbiturates. Barbiturates, which are central nervous system depressants, are divided into three categories, depending on their duration of action. Thiopental is an ultra short-acting barbiturate used in anesthesia. The short-acting barbiturates, which include pentobarbital (Nembutal®), secobarbital (Seconal®), and amobarbital (Amytal®), are the most widely abused. The long-acting barbiturates, such as phenobarbital, are used therapeutically as anticonvulsants and have low abuse potential. With the exception of phenobarbital, only a small portion of the parent drug is found in the urine. However, most urine immunoassays are directed toward the parent compound of secobarbital, using a cutoff concentration of either 200 or 300 ng/mL. The amount of cross-reactivity with other compounds varies with each assay.

The duration of detection following barbiturate use is variable and depends on dose. In general, short-acting barbiturates such as butalbital, pentobarbital, and secobarbital can be detected from one to four days after use, while long-acting barbiturates such as phenobarbital can be detected for several weeks after use (Porter, 1999). Testing for therapeutic levels of phenobarbital involves a separate assay; it is not an appropriate use of urine drug screens.

Benzodiazepines. The interpretation of urine immunoassays for benzodiazepines is complicated by the multiple drugs available, their variable potencies (allowing a large dose range), and their diverse metabolites, which may show poor cross-reactivity with commonly used immunoassays. Chlorazepate, chlordiazepoxide, diazepam, and temazepam typically are metabolized to oxazepam, which in turn is conjugated into an inactive glucuronide metabolite. The nitrobenzodiazepines, which include clonazepam, are metabolized to the 7-amino benzodiazepine (Drummer, 1998). Alprazolam, lorazepam, and triazolam are excreted as glucuronide conjugates, distinct from oxazepam glucuronide. Urine specimens usually contain little of the parent benzodiazepine (Fitzgerald, Rexin et al., 1994).

The most widely used screening tests for benzodiazepines employ the immunoassays. Many of the immunoassay kits are designed to detect unconjugated oxazepam, although some kits detect the glucuronide conjugates of benzodiazepines. Because the immunoassay is directed toward a specific benzodiazepine or its metabolites, false negatives can occur (Nishikawa, Ohtani et al., 1997). For example, an immunoassay that is targeted to detect oxazepam is less likely to detect clonazepam, lorazepam, or triazolam, unless they are present in high doses (Fitzgerald, Rexin et al., 1994).

The sensitivity of some immunoassays is increased by pretreating the urine with B-glucuronidase before performing the test. By cleaving the conjugate from the parent benzodiazepine, the immunoreactivity of the specimen is increased (Ropero-Miller, Garside et al., 1997), because the metabolites have a longer elimination half-life and are present in greater concentrations than the parent drug.

The cutoff for benzodiazepine immunoassays usually is either 200 or 300 ng/mL, which can detect high doses but may not detect a therapeutic dose. The high-potency benzodiazepines such as triazolam, which are prescribed in low doses, are more difficult to detect in immunoassays (Becker, Correll et al., 1993). The benzodiazepine antagonist, flumazenil, is not detected by immunoassay.

Urine can be adulterated with sodium chloride, peroxide, or detergents to obtain false negative results. Substances reported to give false positive results on immunoassay include oxaprozin and sertraline (Camara, Audette et al., 1995). At high concentrations, the nonsteroidal tolmetin has been found to give false negative results (Joseph, Dickerson et al., 1995). Because there is considerable variation in the half-life of benzodiazepines, it is difficult to estimate the time of use based on screening tests. In one study, a dose of diazepam 10 mg/day for five days produced positive urine immunoassays beginning one to three days after ingestion and continuing for up to a week after the medication was stopped (Verebey, Jukofsky et al., 1982).

Cocaine. Cocaine hydrochloride is the powdered form of cocaine. It is water-soluble and can be snorted or mixed with water and injected. The alkaloid form of cocaine, "crack" or freebase, is not water soluble, but vaporizes when heated, and can be smoked (Warner, 1993). Screening urine immunoassays measure benzoylecgonine, the major urinary cocaine metabolite, using a cutoff of 300 ng/mL. The detection of cocaine in the urine is variable and depends on the amount of drug ingested. The usual detection time after cocaine use is two to three days, although there are reports of positive urine assays up to 22 days after high-dose binges (Weiss & Gawin, 1988).

When combined with alcohol, cocaine can be transesterified to form cocaethylene. This substance has a longer elimination time than cocaine and often is present in the urine in similar or greater concentrations than cocaine. Immunoassays for benzoylecgonine are quite specific, and do not share the same difficulties with multiple false positives as the other drug screens. Immunoassays do not differentiate cocaine hydrochloride from crack cocaine, although specialized testing can detect a product of smoked cocaine (anhydroecgonine methyl ester) in the urine of individuals who smoke crack (Cone, Hillsgrove et al., 1994).

LSD. The hallucinogen LSD (lysergic acid diethylamide) is synthesized from lysergic acid and is structurally similar to the ergot alkaloids. LSD is extensively metabolized, so that less than 1% appears unchanged in the urine. The major human metabolite is nor-LSD (N-desmethyl-LSD). At a cutoff of 0.5 ng/mL, urine immunoassays detect LSD for two to five days after use (Schneider, Kuffer et al., 1998). Confirmatory testing can be done by chromatography.

One study found a 4% false-positive rate on immunoassay in patients and *in vitro* false positives with multiple drugs, including amitriptyline, chlorpromazine, doxepin, fluoxetine, haloperidol, metoclopramide, risperidone, sertraline, thioridazine, and verapamil (Ritter, Cortese et al., 1997). Because of the high number of false positives, caution must be exercised in interpreting these tests (Wu, Feng et al., 1997).

Marijuana. The most potent cannabinoid in the marijuana plant is tetrahydrocannabinol (THC), which composes about 1% to 2% of the leaves, stems, and seeds. When smoked, THC is absorbed quickly into the circulation, with an elimination half-life estimated to be between 20 and 30 hours. THC has a highly lipophilic nature and is stored in fat tissues, where it is slowly released back into the circulation. Most laboratories measure the active metabolite 11-nor-Δ^9-THC-9-carboxylic acid (THC-COOH).

Tests can be obtained with cutoff values of 20, 50, or 100 ng/mL. The current federally mandated cutoff for workplace testing is 50 ng/mL. Assays using 50 ng/mL can detect 23% to 53% more specimens than assays using 100 ng/mL (Huestis, Mitchell et al., 1994). A single marijuana cigarette can be detected for one to two days with a 50 ng/mL cutoff immunoassay (Huestis, Mitchell et al., 1995). At a cutoff of 20 ng/mL, heavy smokers had positive tests for as many as 46 consecutive days, and can take as many as 77 days to test negative for 10 consecutive days (Ellis, Mann et al., 1985).

A positive test is helpful in identifying past marijuana use, but it does not correlate with level of impairment. In the past, immunoassays gave false positive results with nonsteroidal anti-inflammatory drugs such as ibuprofen and naproxyn sodium. Current assays have been modified to eliminate this cross-reactivity. A host of adulterants, including bleach or detergent, can be added to urine samples to give false negative results. Confirmation of a positive screening immunoassay by GC/MS is done whenever there are legal implications.

There has been some debate about the degree to which passive exposure to marijuana smoke influences drug screens. In experimental studies using extreme conditions, urine specimens of individuals passively exposed to high concentrations of marijuana smoke did test positive on immunoassays (Cone, Johnson et al., 1987). However, on quantitative GC/MS, the concentrations of THC-COOH during more realistic exposures generally are less than 10 ng/mL (Mule & Casella, 1988).

Opioids. Because the primary purpose of opiate screens has been to detect heroin use, most urine immunoassays are targeted to morphine. The detection of other opioids, such as methadone and propoxyphene, requires specific tests. Both heroin and codeine are metabolized to morphine. In the process of heroin metabolism, 6-acetylmorphine (6-AM) is produced, which then is hydrolyzed to morphine. Poppy seeds contain small quantities of codeine and morphine, and ingestion of them can result in positive urine screens for 48 hours at a cutoff of 300 ng/mL (Hayes, Krasselt et al., 1987).

The presence of morphine in the urine can be produced by ingestion of heroin, codeine, morphine, or poppy seeds. The only finding that unequivocally proves heroin use is the detection of 6-acetylmorphine in the urine, as it is not a metabolite of morphine, codeine, or poppy seeds (Mule & Casella, 1988). However, 6-acetylmorpine is rapidly eliminated, and usually is detectable in the urine for less than eight hours after heroin use (Cone, Dickerson et al., 1993). Although federal regulations for workplace programs require testing for 6-AM when opiate immunoassays are positive, most clinical laboratories do not routinely check for 6-AM. Nonspecific positive opiate immunoassays can be confirmed through use of the GC/MS, which can identify individual opiates. In 1997, the federal government raised the cutoff for opioid testing in workplace programs from 300 ng/mL to 2000 ng/mL to reduce the number of false positive results, although many clinical laboratories still use a cutoff value of 300 ng/mL.

Little information is available about the detection of oxycodone and hydrocodone, but it appears that the currently available opiate immunoassays are less sensitive to these substances (Smith, Hughes et al., 1995). Dextromethorphan and the opioid antagonists nalmefene and naloxone do not cross-react with immunoassays for opiates (Storrow, Wians et al., 1994; Storrow, Magoon et al., 1995; Storrow, Hernandez et al., 1998). The opioids meperidine, fentanyl, and pentazocine generally are not detected in routine urine drug screens.

Methadone. Most drug testing for methadone is done to assess compliance with methadone therapy. Methadone is not detected in the standard drug screens. Screening immunoassays for methadone have little cross-reactivity with other opioids. At a cutoff value of 300 ng/mL, screening immunoassays detect methadone in the urine for two or three days after use. If there is concern that an individual may be spiking a urine specimen with methadone, further testing can be done to detect the presence of the major metabolite, 2-ethylidene-1,5-dimethyl-3,3-diphenylpyrrolidine (EDDP) (Simpson, Braithwaite et al., 1997).

Phencyclidine (PCP). PCP in powdered form ("angel dust") can be snorted or smoked, or the drug ingested in tablet form. The federal government requires PCP testing as part of drug screening programs for federal employees. Laboratories that are not federally regulated may include PCP in the drug screen, depending on the prevalence of PCP use in a given community.

At a cutoff value of 25 ng/dL, urine immunoassays are positive for approximately seven days after a single dose and for up to 21 days after chronic use. False positive tests for PCP can occur with thioridazine.

Saliva tests are promising because saliva levels of PCP are higher than blood levels and PCP may be more stable in saliva than in urine (Schneider, Kuffer et al., 1998).

Club Drugs. Standard urine drug screens do not detect many of the new "designer" drugs. At one time, MDMA and MDA were not detected by amphetamine immunoassays; however, newer generation tests have improved cross-reactivity to these compounds. The drugs ketamine and gamma-hydroxybutyrate (GHB) are not detected by routine urine drug tests.

ETHICAL CONSIDERATIONS

Although there are extensive guidelines for drug testing in the workplace, very few guidelines on the use of such tests for clinical purposes have been developed. In clinical practice, drug testing often is ordered, without informed consent, as a diagnostic test to guide treatment. The American Medical Association (AMA) and the U.S. Preventive Services Task Force (USPSTF) recommend asking about both drug and alcohol abuse when obtaining a patient history, but neither recommend routine laboratory screening for alcohol or drugs in asymptomatic adults. The AMA does encourage the use of blood alcohol tests and urine drug screens in hospitalized trauma patients, but it does not comment on the issue of informed consent in such circumstances (AMA, 1991). The USPSTF endorses drug testing in clinical situations in which "there is reasonable suspicion of substance abuse" and recommends obtaining informed consent prior to performing such tests (USPSTF, 1996). The American Academy of Pediatrics (AAP) recommends that physicians approach drug testing in the same manner as other diagnostic tests: as an aid in diagnosis and in formulating treatment recommendations. The AAP recommends that informed consent be obtained from competent adolescents, unless the adolescent lacks medical decisionmaking capacity or there are strong medical indications or legal requirements to test (AAP, 1996).

CONCLUSIONS

Laboratory testing in the evaluation of patients with known or suspected substance use disorders, when performed in an appropriate clinical setting, can assist in making an accurate diagnosis. However, the physician must understand the limitations of any test used. For alcohol, breath and blood testing can quantitate recent ingestion, but none of the markers for chronic alcohol abuse are ideal screening tests. For other drugs, urine testing can identify drug use, usually within the preceding few days, but does not confirm drug dependence.

An important distinction is that clinical testing that is intended to guide diagnosis and treatment planning does not follow the stringent requirements for workplace or forensic testing.

REFERENCES

American Academy of Pediatrics (AAP), Committee on Substance Abuse (1996). Testing for drugs of abuse in children and adolescents. *Pediatrics* 98(2 Pt. 1):305-307.

American Medical Association (AMA) (1991). Screening for alcohol and other drug use in trauma patients. Chicago, IL: The Association.

Becker J, Correll A, Koepf W et al. (1993). Comparative studies on the detection of benzodiazepines in serum by means of immunoassays (FPIA). *Journal of Analytical Toxicology* 17(2):103-108.

Bendtsen P, Hultberg J, Carlsson M et al. (1999). Monitoring ethanol exposure in a clinical setting by analysis of blood, breath, saliva, and urine. *Alcoholism: Clinical & Experimental Research* 23(9):1446-1451.

Braithwaite RA, Jarvie DR, Minty PS et al. (1995). Screening for drugs of abuse. I: Opiates, amphetamines and cocaine. *Annals of Clinical Biochemistry* 32(Pt 2):123-153.

Camara PD, Audette L, Velletri K et al. (1995). False-positive immunoassay results for urine benzodiazepine in patients receiving oxaprozin (Daypro®). *Clinical Chemistry* 41(1):115-116.

Colbert DL (1994). Drug abuse screening with immunoassays: Unexpected cross-reactivities and other pitfalls. *British Journal of Biomedical Science* 51(2):136-146.

Cone EJ, Dickerson S, Paul BD et al. (1993). Forensic drug testing for opiates. V. Urine testing for heroin, morphine, and codeine with commercial opiate immunoassays. *Journal of Analytical Toxicology* 17(3):156-164.

Cone EJ, Hillsgrove M & Darwin WD (1994). Simultaneous measurement of cocaine, cocaethylene, their metabolites, and "crack" pyrolysis products by gas chromatography-mass spectrometry. *Clinical Chemistry* 40(7):1299-1305.

Cone EJ, Johnson RE, Darwin WD et al. (1987). Passive inhalation of marijuana smoke: Urinalysis and room air levels of delta-9-tetrahydrocannabinol. *Journal of Analytical Toxicology* 11(3):89-96.

Conigrave KM, Saunders JB & Whitfield JB (1995). Diagnostic tests for alcohol consumption. *Alcohol & Alcoholism* 30(1):13-26.

Division of Workplace Testing Programs (1999). *An Evaluation of Non-Instrumental Drug Devices.* Rockville, MD: Substance Abuse and Mental Health Services Administration.

Drummer OH (1998). Methods for the measurement of benzodiazepines in biological samples. *Journal of Chromatography (B: Biomedical Sciences & Applications)* 713(1):201-225.

Ellis GMJ, Mann MA, Judson BA et al. (1985). Excretion patterns of cannabinoid metabolites after last use in a group of chronic users. *Clinical Pharmacology and Therapeutics* 38(5):572-578.

Fitzgerald RL, Rexin DA & Herold DA (1994). Detecting benzodiazepines: Immunoassays compared with negative chemical ionization gas chromatography/mass spectrometry. *Clinical Chemistry* 40(3):373-380.

Frajola WJ (1993). Blood alcohol testing in the laboratory: Problems and suggested remedies. *Clinical Chemistry* 39(3):377-379.

Hayes LW, Krasselt WG & Mueggler PA (1987). Concentrations of morphine and codeine in serum and urine after ingestion of poppy seeds. *Clinical Chemistry* 33(6):806-808.

Huestis MA, Mitchell JM & Cone EJ (1994). Lowering the federally mandated cannabinoid immunoassay cutoff increases true-positive results. *Clinical Chemistry* 40(5):729-733.

Huestis MA, Mitchell JM & Cone EJ (1995). Detection times of marijuana metabolites in urine by immunoassay and GC-MS. *Journal of Analytical Toxicology* 19(6):443-449.

Jenkins AJ & Cone EJ (1998). Pharmacokinetics: Drug absorption, distribution, and elimination. In SB Karch (ed.) *Handbook of Drug Abuse.* Boca Raton, FL: CRC Press, 151-202.

Jones AW & Pounder DJ (1998). Measuring blood-alcohol concentration for clinical and forensic purposes. In SB Karch (ed.) *Drug Abuse Handbook.* Boca Raton, FL: CRC Press, 327-355.

Joseph R, Dickerson S, Willis R et al. (1995). Interference by nonsteroidal anti-inflammatory drugs in EMIT and TDx assays for drugs of abuse. *Journal of Analytical Toxicology* 19(1): 13-17.

Kechagias S, Jonsson KA, Franzen T et al. (1999). Reliability of breath-alcohol analysis in individuals with gastroesophageal reflux disease. *Journal of Forensic Sciences* 44(4): 814-818.

Kidwell DA, Holland JC & Athanaselis S (1998). Testing for drugs of abuse in saliva and sweat. *Journal of Chromatography (B: Biomedical Sciences & Applications).* 713(1):111-135.

Kraemer T & Maurer HH (1998). Determination of amphetamine, methamphetamine and amphetamine-derived designer drugs or medicaments in blood and urine. *Journal of Chromatography (B: Biomedical Sciences & Applications)* 713(1):163-187.

Laposata M (1999). Assessment of ethanol intake. Current tests and new assays on the horizon. *American Journal of Clinical Pathology* 112(4):443-450.

LeBeau M, Andollo W, Hearn WL et al. (1999). Recommendations for toxicological investigations of drug-facilitated sexual assaults. *Journal of Forensic Sciences* 44(1):227-230.

Litten RZ, Allen JP & Fertig JB (1995). Gamma-glutamyltranspeptidase and carbohydrate deficient transferrin: Alternative measures of excessive alcohol consumption. *Alcoholism: Clinical & Experimental Research* 19(6):1541-1546.

Lowinson JH, Ruiz P, Millman RB et al., eds. (1997). *Substance Abuse: A Comprehensive Textbook, 3rd Edition.* Baltimore, MD: Williams & Wilkins.

Mason MF & Dubowski KM (1976). Breath-alcohol analysis: Uses, methods, and some forensic problems—Review and opinion. *Journal of Forensic Sciences* 21(1):9-41.

McPhillips MA, Strang J & Barnes TR (1998). Hair analysis. New laboratory ability to test for substance abuse. *British Journal of Psychiatry* 173(10):287-290.

Mule SJ & Casella GA (1988). Rendering the "poppy-seed defense" defenseless: Identification of 6-monoacetylmorphine in urine by gas chromatography/mass spectroscopy. *Clinical Chemistry* 34(7):1427-1430.

Nishikawa T, Ohtani H, Herold DA et al. (1997). Comparison of assay methods for benzodiazepines in urine. A receptor assay, 2 immunoassays, and gas chromatography-mass spectrometry. *American Journal of Clinical Pathology* 107(3):345-352.

Osterloh J (1998). Laboratory diagnoses and drug screening. In L Haddad, M Shannon & J Winchester (eds.) *Clinical Management of Poisoning and Drug Overdose*. Philadelphia, PA: W.B. Saunders.

Porter W (1999). Clinical toxicology. In C Burtis & E Ashwood (eds.) *Tietz Textbook of Clinical Chemistry*. Philadelphia, PA: W.B. Saunders, 906-981.

Ritter D, Cortese CM, Edwards LC et al. (1997). Interference with testing for lysergic acid diethylamide. *Clinical Chemistry* 43(4):635-637.

Ropero-Miller JD, Garside D & Goldberger BA (1997). Automated on-line hydrolysis of benzodiazepines improves sensitivity of urine screening by a homogeneous enzyme immunoassay. *Clinical Chemistry* 43(9):1659-1660.

Schneider S, Kuffer P & Wennig R (1998). Determination of lysergide (LSD) and phencyclidine in biosamples. *Journal of Chromatography (B: Biomedical Sciences & Applications)* 713(1):189-200.

Sillanaukee P (1996). Laboratory markers of alcohol abuse. *Alcohol & Alcoholism* 31(6):613-616.

Simpson D, Braithwaite RA, Jarvie DR et al. (1997). Screening for drugs of abuse (II): Cannabinoids, lysergic acid diethylamide, buprenorphine, methadone, barbiturates, benzodiazepines and other drugs. *Annals of Clinical Biochemistry* 34(Pt 5):460-510.

Smith ML, Hughes RO, Levine B et al. (1995). Forensic drug testing for opiates. VI. Urine testing for hydromorphone, hydrocodone, oxymorphone, and oxycodone with commercial opiate immunoassays and gas chromatography-mass spectrometry. *Journal of Analytical Toxicology* 19(1):18-26.

Spiehler V (2000). Hair analysis by immunological methods from the beginning to 2000. *Forensic Science International* 107(1-3):249-259.

Storrow AB, Hernandez AV & Norton JA (1998). Nalmefene and the urine opiate screen. *Clinical Chemistry* 44(2):346-348.

Storrow AB, Magoon MR & Norton J (1995). The dextromethorphan defense: Dextromethorphan and the opioid screen. *Academic Emergency Medicine* 2(9):791-794.

Storrow AB, Wians FH Jr., Mikkelsen SL et al. (1994). Does naloxone cause a positive urine opiate screen? *Annals of Emergency Medicine* 24(6):1151-1153.

Substance Abuse and Mental Health Services Administration (SAMHSA) (1999). *Guidance/Criteria for Specimen Validity Testing. Program Document 37.* Rockville, MD: U.S. Department of Health and Human Services.

U.S. Department of Health and Human Services (DHHS) (1994). Mandatory guidelines for federal workplace drug testing programs. *Federal Register* 59:29908.

U.S. Department of Health and Human Services (DHHS) (1997). Mandatory guidelines for federal workplace drug testing programs. *Federal Register* 62:5118.

U.S. Preventive Services Task Force (USPSTF) (1996). Screening for drug abuse. *Guide to Clinical Preventive Services*. Baltimore, MD: Williams & Wilkins, 583-594.

Verebey K, Jukofsky D & Mule SJ (1982). Confirmation of EMIT benzodiazepine assay with GLC/NPD. *Journal of Analytical Toxicology* 6:305-308.

Warner EA (1993). Cocaine abuse. *Annals of Internal Medicine* 119(3):226-235.

Weiss RD & Gawin FH (1988). Protracted elimination of cocaine metabolites in long-term, high-dose cocaine abusers. *American Journal of Medicine* 85(6):879-880.

Winecker RE & Goldberger BA (1998). Urine specimen suitability for drug testing. In SB Karch (ed.) *Drug Abuse Handbook*. Boca Raton, FL: CRC Press, 764-767.

Wolff K, Farrell M, Marsden J et al. (1999). A review of biological indicators of illicit drug use, practical considerations and clinical usefulness. *Addiction* 94(9):1279-1298.

Wu AH, Bristol B, Sexton K et al. (1999). Adulteration of urine by "Urine Luck." *Clinical Chemistry* 45(7):1051-1057.

Wu AH, Feng YJ, Pajor A et al. (1997). Detection and interpretation of lysergic acid diethylamide results by immunoassay screening of urine in various testing groups. *Journal of Analytical Toxicology* 21(3):181-184.

Yersin B, Nicolet J, DeCrey H et al. (1995). Screening for excessive alcohol drinking. *Archives of Internal Medicine* 155(17):1907-1911.

Chapter 3

Trauma Case Finding

Richard D. Blondell, M.D.

Importance of Prevention
Case Finding Among Trauma Patients
Initial Management
Diagnostic Assessment
Intervention

Traumatic injury is a leading cause of morbidity and mortality in the United States. It ranks first in years of life lost, first in utilization of hospital days, second in disability-adjusted life-years, and fourth in overall mortality (Gross, Anderson et al., 1999). There is a clear relationship between trauma and substance use disorders (Anda, Williamson et al., 1988). In fact, trauma may be but one of the many symptoms of problems related to alcohol and other drugs (Clark, McCarthy et al., 1985).

Alcohol is the major risk factor for virtually all categories of injury, including traffic crashes, burns and fires, drowning, air traffic injuries, occupational injuries, homicides, suicides, and domestic violence (NIAAA, 1997). Alcohol also causes physiologic effects that exacerbate the traumatic injury and complicate the medical and surgical management of the injured patient (Freeland, McMichen et al., 1993). Many intoxicated trauma patients who present to the hospital emergency department have a chronic alcohol use problem (Rivara, Jurkovich et al., 1993a).

Driving under the influence of alcohol clearly is related to driver injury and motor vehicle trauma (Cherpitel, 1992). Passengers, pedestrians, and bicyclists also are at risk for injuries from the intoxicated driver (Margolis, Foss et al., 2000). Alcohol is a factor in injuries resulting from interpersonal violence (Cesare, Morgan et al., 1990; Cherpitel, 1996). The quantity of alcohol consumed before a violent injury may be more predictive of injuries than the frequency of drinking (Borges, Cherpitel et al., 1998). Alcohol intoxication also reduces a person's ability to escape from a fatal fire (Marshall, Runyan et al., 1998).

The association of acute drug intoxication and traumatic injuries has not been as well studied. Although toxicology testing for alcohol is easily performed and can reflect the level of intoxication at the time of injury, urine screening tests may remain positive for several days after the acute intoxicating effects of the drugs have resolved. This makes it difficult to determine whether traumatic injuries are drug-related.

The vast majority of patients with minor injuries either do not seek medical attention or receive care in outpatient settings. In most areas of the United States, seriously injured patients are triaged to a network of trauma centers (Bazzoli & MacKenzie, 1995). Depending on the resources available and the services offered, trauma centers are classified as Level I, II, III, or IV.

TABLE 1.   Screening Instruments for Harmful and Dependent Drinkers

Screening	Harmful		Dependent	
	Sensitivity	Specificity	Sensitivity	Specificity
CAGE	75%	88%	76%	90%
TWEAK	87%	86%	84%	86%
AUDIT	85%	88%	83%	90%
Brief MAST	31%	98%	30%	99%
Breath alcohol analysis	20%	94%	20%	94%
Self-report	31%	89%	29%	89%

SOURCE: Reproduced with permission from Cherpitel CJ (1995). Screening for alcohol problems in the emergency department. *Annals of Emergency Medicine* 26:163-164.

Level I and II trauma centers provide a comprehensive level of care and usually are located in major tertiary care hospitals. Level I trauma centers have a major teaching mission as part of their care and typically are located in university hospitals or other major teaching hospitals.

Level III and IV trauma centers provide a limited range of services and often are located in community hospitals. Patients admitted to Level III and IV trauma centers with critical injuries usually are transferred to a Level I or II trauma center after initial assessment, resuscitation, and stabilization.

IMPORTANCE OF PREVENTION

Deaths from major trauma have a trimodal distribution and are characterized as immediate, early, and late (Trunkey, 1984). The pathophysiology of traumatic death is different for each mortality peak. Immediate deaths occur at the scene. These account for about half of the deaths from trauma and usually are due to a major disruption of the patient's anatomy (as in major brain injury, severe pulmonary contusion, or a laceration to the heart or a major blood vessel). Early deaths account for approximately 30% of trauma mortality and occur within the first few hours after the injury (for example, from shock due to blood loss from trauma to the lungs, abdominal contents or multiple fractures; injuries to the brain, spinal cord or lungs). Late deaths account for the remaining 20% of trauma mortality and occur within the first one to three weeks following injury. These deaths often are due to sepsis, respiratory failure, or multisystem organ failure.

Whereas improvements in the medical and surgical care rendered to trauma victims may produce incremental improvements in trauma's burden on morbidity and mortality, prevention has the potential to produce a quantum leap improvement. Prevention is the only way to prevent the majority of trauma deaths due to immediate causes and represents a method to prevent re-injury.

Trauma as a Chronic Disorder. Traditionally, traumatic injuries have been viewed as solitary, isolated events. However, the current view is that trauma is a chronic disorder with multiple risk factors (Waller, 1989). These may include physical, environmental, socioeconomic, and personality or psychological factors, all of which contribute to an increased risk of traumatic injury. For example, persons with certain physical disabilities (such as poor vision, unsteady gait, or osteoporosis) may be at increased risk for falls that result in fractures. Individuals who work in hazardous environments (such as coal mining or construction) may be at increased risk for injuries. Individuals who exhibit risk-taking behaviors are at increased risk for traumatic injury (Spain, Boaz et al., 1997).

Alcohol use is an important risk factor for traumatic injuries, and this risk appears to be dose-dependent (Anda, Williamson et al., 1988). Illicit drug use also appears to be a risk factor (Soderstrom, Smith et al., 1997). Re-injury is common among patients with alcohol-related injuries. Sims and colleagues (1989) found that violent trauma had a recurrence rate of 44% and a five-year mortality of 20%. In that study, 62% of the study patients had abused alcohol or drugs. Rivara and associates (1993b) found that trauma victims who were intoxicated at the time they presented to the trauma center were 2.5 times more likely to be readmitted for another injury than those who were not intoxicated; moreover, those with evidence of a chronic alcohol problem were 3.5 times more likely to be readmitted.

Prevention Efforts in Trauma Centers. Patients with acute illnesses in the later stages of an alcohol use disorder may have multiple hospital admissions related to cirrhosis, chronic pancreatitis, or esophageal varices. They frequently receive their care on the medical wards of the hospital. However, trauma may be the first obvious sign of an alcohol use disorder that brings the patient to the attention of the health care system. Moreover, trauma frequently captures the attention of the patient and creates a "teachable moment," in which the patient is receptive to information about his or her alcohol-related problem (Mitka, 1998). This creates a window of opportunity for the trauma center physician to intervene with the patient who has an alcohol use disorder, so as to prevent future injuries.

Phillips and associates (1999) have observed that the number of deaths due to substance abuse and an external cause (suicides, accidents, and homicides) in the first week of the month (when government benefit checks are mailed) is about 14% higher than in the last week of the preceding month. These data provide some insight into the magnitude of the reductions in mortality that may be possible if injuries related to substance use could be prevented. Early recognition, intervention, and appropriate referral of patients with alcohol and drug problems have the potential to reduce the morbidity and mortality associated with traumatic injuries (D'Onofrio, Bernstein et al., 1998). Although there is a unique opportunity to initiate treatment for patients with substance use disorders when they are hospitalized for a traumatic injury, this opportunity too often is missed (Lowenstein, Weissberg et al., 1990).

CASE FINDING AMONG TRAUMA PATIENTS

Physicians who provide care to injured patients can identify those who have alcohol- or drug-related problems through routine clinical assessments, the use of formal screening instruments, or routine laboratory testing (CSAT, 1995).

Clinical Assessment. Some patients who present to the hospital with trauma have injuries that obviously are related to chronic substance abuse (for example, an intoxicated driver involved in a motor vehicle crash who has lost his driver's license following two previous alcohol-related traffic crashes). Other patients who present with an alcohol-related injury may admit to a drinking problem if specifically asked, or they may have a history, documented in the medical record, of an alcohol or drug use disorder and have completed a course of treatment. Such patients do not require additional screening for substance use disorders. On the other hand, clinical assessment alone is not always reliable in detecting all patients whose injuries are alcohol-related. Gentilello and colleagues (1999b) assessed the accuracy of the clinical evaluation of 462 patients admitted to a trauma center. Overall, 23% of acutely intoxicated patients were not identified by their physicians. The percentage of patients who were not identified was higher in patients who had severe injuries, who were intubated, or who had been chemically paralyzed. Patients who had a negative blood alcohol concentration and who were falsely suspected of being intoxicated were more likely to be young, male, or perceived as being disheveled, uninsured, or having a low income.

Especially in patients who do not have an obvious substance use disorder, the routine use of screening instruments can enhance the physician's ability to determine which patients' injuries are related to alcohol or drug use.

Screening Instruments. Several instruments are available for the screening of alcohol problems in patients with trauma, including the CAGE questions (Ewing, 1984), the TWEAK questions (Russell, Martier et al., 1994), the AUDIT (Alcohol Use Disorders Identification Test; Babor & Grant, 1989), and the Brief MAST (Brief Michigan Alcoholism Screening Test; Pokorny, Miller et al., 1972) (see the Appendix of this text).

The aforementioned screening instruments have been extensively evaluated in emergency department settings by Cherpitel (1995a, 1995b, 1997, 1998), who compared

TABLE 2. Sensitivity, Specificity, and Positive Predictive Values for Different CAGE Scores at Varying Prevalences of Alcohol Abuse and Dependence

			Positive Predictive Value		
CAGE Score	Sensitivity	Specificity	10% Prevalence	20% Prevalence	30% Prevalence
≥ 1	86-90%	52-93%	15-20%	25-25%	40-50%
≥ 2	74-78%	76-96%	30-60%	55-75%	65-80%
≥ 3	44-54%	92-99%	60-75%	75-80%	80-95%
≥ 4	24-26%	100%	90-99%	95-99%	≥ 99%

SOURCE: Reproduced with permission from Schorling JB & Buchsbaum DG (1997). Screening for alcohol and drug problems. *Medical Clinics of North America* 81:845-865.

screening tests with patient self-reports and breath alcohol analyses (see Table 1). She found that the TWEAK appears to be the most sensitive of the screening instruments for the detection of harmful and dependent drinking in trauma patients. At the cutoff point of three positive answers, the sensitivity for the TWEAK questions was 87% for the detection of harmful drinking and 84% for the detection of dependent drinking. The AUDIT produced similar results using a cutoff score of 8. When a cutoff of two positive answers was used, the CAGE questions were almost as good as the TWEAK and the AUDIT screens.

However, these tests did not perform equally well in all racial, ethnic, or gender groups. The presence of injury also affected the specificity and sensitivity of the tests. Schorling and Buchsbaum (1997) evaluated the specificity, sensitivity, and positive predictive values for different cutoff levels for the CAGE questions (see Table 2).

Cherpitel (1997) concluded that more investigation is warranted before recommendations can be made with confidence about the use of particular screening instruments in an emergency setting. She observed that patient responses to structured questions were influenced by the skill level of the interviewing physician. Patients tended to reveal less when the CAGE was preceded by direct, close-ended questions about quantity and frequency of drinking. In such circumstances, the ability of the instrument to detect alcoholism was reduced.

There is no ideal screening instrument for use in emergency settings or for hospitalized trauma patients. The CAGE questions are familiar, easy to administer, and readily incorporated into the routine questions that are asked by nurses on initial patient assessment. They generally perform well when asked in a face-to-face interview that is not preceded by a series of quantity and frequency questions. Therefore, for most busy emergency rooms and inpatient hospital settings, the CAGE questions, followed by a few questions about quantity and frequency, may be the best current screening option for routine use.

Biochemical Markers. A number of laboratory tests have been used to screen for alcohol abuse in various patient groups (Hoeksema & de Boch, 1993). Because the liver is affected by excessive alcohol consumption, liver enzymes frequently are used as markers of excessive alcohol consumption. The most widely used are the gamma-glutamyltransferase (GGT), alanine aminotransferase (ALT), aspartate aminotransferase (AST), and the AST/ALT ratio. However, among trauma victims, injuries to the liver are common and limit the value of liver enzymes as screening tests for alcohol abuse.

The mean corpuscular volume (MCV) also has been used as a marker of excessive alcohol consumption. Although an elevated MCV may be a marker for heavy alcohol consumption, it lacks the sensitivity to be useful as a screening test among trauma patients (Spies, Emadi et al., 1995).

The carbohydrate deficient transferrin (CDT) is a promising new marker of heavy alcohol consumption (Litten, Allen et al., 1995). To date, the CDT has been used only in research settings; it is not available commercially for use in hospital laboratories. However, it may represent a useful test that can be incorporated into the evaluation of trauma victims in the future.

Because there is no single biological marker that appears to be effective in screening patients for alcohol or other substance use disorders in the trauma setting, investigators have evaluated a combination of markers (Nilssen, Ries et al., 1996). The values from three tests (GGT, MCV, and blood alcohol) have been used to develop a differentially "weighted alcohol markers" (WAM) score. In male patients, the WAM score was found to have a 75% sensitivity and an 83% specificity. For female patients, the values were 85% and 85%, respectively, using a different cutoff. Whether the WAM score (or a combination of other tests) are of practical value to trauma surgeons remains to be determined.

Toxicology Testing. In many trauma centers, toxicology testing is the screen that is used first to detect substance use disorders among injured patients. Samples of urine and blood are obtained routinely from trauma victims for other diagnostic purposes. It is simple to include toxicology testing of these specimens, and they are easily incorporated into the routine trauma medical orders. Such tests provide valuable information to trauma surgeons about the presence of a possible substance use disorder. More than 90% of patients who sustain a major injury while under the influence of alcohol or drugs, as evidenced by a toxicology screen, have an alcohol use disorder (Parran, Weber et al., 1995). The sensitivity of a positive blood alcohol concentration in detecting alcohol dependence ranges from 40% to 65%, while the specificity is approximately 85% (Soderstrom, Kufera et al., 1997; Soderstrom, Smith et al., 1997).

Urine toxicology tests are more difficult to interpret. Opioids and benzodiazepines often are given to patients early in the course of the management of their injuries, sometimes en route to the hospital. Although blood specimens usually are obtained early in the care of trauma patients, there may be a delay in obtaining a urine specimen. Therefore, any opiates or benzodiazepines detected may be from the therapeutic use of these drugs early in trauma care or due to legitimate therapeutic use rather than abuse.

The sensitivity, specificity, and predictive value of urine toxicology as a marker for substance use disorders among trauma victims has not been well studied. Nevertheless, those patients who have positive toxicology tests should be evaluated for a substance use disorder. The presence of cocaine or cannabinoids (marijuana) in the urine may indicate such a disorder. These substances have few therapeutic indications and are unlikely to be given to trauma victims early in the course of treatment. However, a positive toxicology screen does not mean that the patient was intoxicated at the time of injury, because the urine toxicology may be positive for a few days after the last use of cocaine and for a few weeks after the last use of marijuana.

Sometimes tobacco is mixed with marijuana and a small amount of crack cocaine and rolled into cigarette-like devices or packed into hollowed-out cigars. These are known as "blunts." These items may be used by even casual users of drugs and may result in a positive urine toxicology screen.

Limitations of Screening. Clinicians in trauma centers can use toxicology testing or any one of several available screening instruments to identify patients who have a substance use disorder. However, if lack of screening was the obstacle that prevented trauma centers from identifying alcoholics and drug addicts, then the solution would be straightforward. The health care objectives that are difficult to achieve in most trauma centers are adequate patient assessment for the severity of a substance use disorder, prompt medical detoxification to prevent withdrawal syndromes, effective and practical patient interventions, and efficient patient referral to a drug and alcohol rehabilitation program as needed.

INITIAL MANAGEMENT

Patients who present to the hospital with injuries sustained while under the influence of alcohol and/or drugs present a number of challenges to their physicians, including initial management and the need for prophylactic treatment to prevent the emergence of an alcohol or drug withdrawal syndrome. Acute alcohol intoxication appears to alter the initial assessment of the severity of an injury, resulting in an increased use of invasive diagnostic and therapeutic procedures (Jurkovich, Rivara et al., 1992). Ultimately, patients who are intoxicated with alcohol have similar outcomes to those who are not intoxicated (Thal, Bost et al., 1985). However, those who initially test positive for psychoactive drugs have been found to have a higher severity of injury, incidence of shock, and mortality.

Severity of the Disorder. It is difficult to assess the severity of an alcohol or drug problem in a patient with a major injury. Respiratory problems may interfere with the patient's ability to speak. Acute pain from a fracture may cause the patient to be unwilling to answer detailed questions about alcohol or drug use. A traumatic brain injury may impair the patient's cognitive ability and memory. The symptoms and signs of intoxication with alcohol or certain drugs may overlap with those of a traumatic brain injury, and the clinical course of a traumatic brain injury may be confused with the development of an alcohol withdrawal syndrome and vice versa.

Given the limitations of the initial patient evaluation in the face of major injury, the trauma surgeon often must rely on the patient's medical history, limited information from the patient or family members, and toxicology testing to predict which patients are at risk for the development of an alcohol or other drug withdrawal syndrome.

Management of Alcohol Intoxication and Withdrawal. Patients with more severe alcohol problems are at the greatest risk for the development of an alcohol withdrawal syndrome and *delirium tremens* (Spies & Rommelspacher, 1999). Patients with a high blood alcohol concentration (BAC) at admission or an acute illness may be at particularly high risk (Vinson, 1991; Ferguson, Suelzer et al., 1996). Clinical experience suggests that patients with a chronic alcohol use disorder who are more than 40 years old, who have a history of heavy or daily drinking for more than 10 years, who have an admission BAC greater than 250 mg/dl, who have a history of prior alcohol withdrawal or *delirium tremens*, or who report the signs and symptoms of alcohol withdrawal when not drinking, are at risk for developing alcohol withdrawal and *delirium tremens* (Fleming, 1992). Patients who have a toxicology screen positive for benzodiazepines or other sedatives may be at risk for a concurrent sedative withdrawal.

Prevention of Alcohol Withdrawal: The prevention and treatment of alcohol or drug withdrawal syndromes in trauma patients has not been well studied. Patients with concurrent medical problems usually are excluded from randomized clinical trials that evaluate the effectiveness of agents used for detoxification (Hayashida, Alterman et al., 1989). Randomized clinical trials of alcohol detoxification generally are conducted with patients presenting to inpatient or outpatient settings for alcohol rehabilitation. Based on a review of available data, Mayo-Smith (1997), writing for the ASAM Working Group on Pharmacologic Management of Alcohol Withdrawal, has recommended benzodiazepines as the treatment of choice to prevent the alcohol withdrawal syndrome.

Long-acting benzodiazepines such as diazepam often are avoided in trauma patients because of the risk of over-sedation, which can interfere with the serial neurological evaluation of patients with a closed head injury or lead to respiratory compromise of patients with chest injuries. For this reason, many surgeons prefer short-acting benzodiazepines such as lorazepam for routine prophylaxis of alcohol withdrawal in trauma patients. Lorazepam may be given on a scheduled basis or on a "symptom-triggered" basis to prevent alcohol withdrawal.

Scheduled benzodiazepines often are given to patients at high risk for the development of alcohol withdrawal. A typical order might be for 1 to 2 mg of lorazepam to be given every four to six hours on a scheduled basis, but not to be given if the patient is over-sedated. Additional doses may be given as needed for breakthrough symptoms. When given on a scheduled basis, lorazepam often is administered for two to three days and then, if the patient is stable, the dose is decreased gradually over three to five days.

Benzodiazepines may be given as needed to patients who are at low to moderate risk of alcohol withdrawal. Medications are given only if the patient develops the signs and symptoms of alcohol withdrawal. Frequently, objective scales, such as the Clinical Institute Withdrawal Assessment-Alcohol, Revised (CIWA-Ar) score, are used as the basis to administer these medications (Sullivan, Sykora et al., 1989). However, the signs and symptoms of traumatic injuries may compromise the validity of the CIWA-Ar or similar scales.

Thiamine should be given to any trauma patient suspected of having an alcohol use disorder to prevent the development of Wernicke's encephalopathy. Other medications (such as beta-antagonists, clonidine, and certain neuroleptics) are important adjuvants in the management of alcohol withdrawal.

Intravenous alcohol has been advocated for alcohol detoxification in trauma patients (Craft, Foil et al., 1994). Others oppose giving alcohol for detoxification (Murphy, Harwood et al., 1998). The clinical research data to support either view are limited. There is one prospective clinical trial involving 200 patients who were randomized into four treatment groups and admitted to an intensive care unit following the surgical resection of an abdominal tumor (Spies, Dublez et al., 1995). This limited study suggested that intravenous alcohol is as effective as benzodiazepines in the prophylaxis of alcohol withdrawal syndrome.

Management of the Withdrawal Syndrome: Trauma patients should be evaluated for concurrent problems before treatment for alcohol withdrawal is initiated. The development of alcohol withdrawal in such patients can be confusing because injuries may produce signs and symptoms that overlap or mimic the signs and symptoms of alcohol withdrawal. For example, in the two or three days following admission, patients with traumatic brain injuries can develop a constellation of signs and symptoms that closely resemble those of alcohol withdrawal.

Scheduled doses of sedatives frequently are used to treat alcohol withdrawal in trauma victims. Patients who fail to respond to intermittent doses may require a continuous infusion of lorazepam or midazolam, which can be titrated to treat the alcohol withdrawal syndrome while avoiding the risk of over-sedation. If the withdrawal syndrome is severe, a continuous infusion of propofol may be required, but patients usually require mechanical ventilation with this medication. Sedation can be continued until the patient is stable, at which time the dose is gradually reduced over several days. Patients weaned off sedatives too quickly may show rebound symptoms, demonstrating increased agitation that would require advancing the dose of sedatives.

Clonidine can be used to treat the hypertension and tachycardia associated with alcohol withdrawal. Pain can exacerbate the agitation associated with withdrawal. In such cases, intermittent doses of narcotics may be used, but continuous infusions of morphine or fentanyl sometimes are required and can be titrated to the desired effect by critical care nurses.

Management of Withdrawal Delirium: Patients who develop delirium may benefit from neuroleptics. Although haloperidol often is used for the delirium of alcohol withdrawal, there is evidence suggesting that this medication should be avoided in patients who have a closed head injury (Cardenas & McLean, 1992). Supportive care from a bedside "sitter" is the treatment of choice for many patients with delirium from a closed head injury.

Before detoxification treatment is initiated, trauma patients with alcohol dependence who develop delirium should be evaluated for causes other than alcohol withdrawal. There are many causes of delirium in alcohol-dependent trauma patients. For example, drugs that are given for therapeutic purposes (such as cimetidine to prevent peptic ulcers or corticosteroids for spinal cord injuries) may cause confusion in the trauma patient. Dehydration or volume loss may be associated with tachycardia and mental status changes. Abnormalities of the serum electrolytes (for example, hyponatremia) or endocrine abnormalities (such as hypothyroidism) may produce an altered brain function. Respiratory compromise may produce hypoxia or hypercapnia and cognitive dysfunction.

Alcoholics are at risk for the development of hepatic encephalopathy. Trauma patients are at risk for a number of infections, including pneumonia, intra-abdominal abscesses, and urinary tract infections, which may produce sepsis and mental confusion. Cardiac or cerebral ischemia may be confused with drug intoxication or alcohol withdrawal. Renal failure is not uncommon in trauma patients. Occasionally, urinary or fecal retention (bowel obstruction) can cause delirium, particularly in elderly patients.

Trauma patients frequently have closed head injuries and are at risk for intracranial pathology (such as subdural hematoma, intracerebral or subarachnoid hemorrhage), which typically are associated with an altered mental status. Sometimes trauma victims are visited by friends who bring to the hospital intoxicating substances, such as cocaine, that can cause confusion in a patient who is convalescing from traumatic injuries. Certain metabolic abnormalities (such as acidosis or hypoglycemia) also may produce delirium. The milieu of the intensive care unit (ICU) often causes sleep deprivation, which may progress to an "ICU psychosis" or a "sun-downing" syndrome that can mimic alcohol or drug withdrawal.

There are a number of unusual causes of altered mental status in trauma patients. Some patients may develop lead toxicity from drinking "moonshine" made in stills in which copper tubing is joined with lead-based solder. Other patients may have ingested hallucinogens that are undetected on routine toxicology screens. Some patients develop delirium, and no cause is ever diagnosed.

Management of Drug Intoxication and Withdrawal. Patients may be suspected of being at risk for withdrawal from sedatives, narcotics, or other drugs based on their clinical history and results of initial toxicology testing. Prophylactic treatment may be required to prevent withdrawal from these drugs of abuse.

Benzodiazepines: Withdrawal from short-acting benzodiazepines, such as alprazolam, may begin within the first 24 hours following hospital admission. Withdrawal from long-acting benzodiazepines, such as diazepam, may be delayed several days. Benzodiazepines can be given on a scheduled basis to replace the usual doses of these sedatives prior to admission and adjusted as needed, depending on clinical response. After the patient is clinically stable, doses may be reduced gradually over 7 to 14 days.

Opioids: Although opioid withdrawal is not necessarily life-threatening, it can complicate the clinical care of the trauma patient. Opioids often are given to trauma victims to relieve the pain of their injuries. However, patients who are dependent on opioids may require large doses for pain control and for the prevention of withdrawal. Adequate doses can be given, based on clinical response; when the patient is stable, these medications can be tapered gradually.

Cocaine and Amphetamines: Patients who binge on cocaine or amphetamines over several days experience insomnia. If they have a traumatic injury during the binge, they may present to the hospital in a confused and agitated state. If they sustain an injury following the binge, a toxicology screen may be positive, but the patient may appear to be sedated due to lack of sleep. Such sedation can mimic a closed head injury or intoxication from sedative drugs, but the patient may appear to have fairly normal cognitive function once aroused. Following a day or two of excessive sleep, the patient may awaken, become agitated, experience cravings for illicit drugs, and ask to leave the hospital. This restlessness and agitation can be controlled with benzodiazepines. Visitors who come to the hospital to visit such a patient may bring cocaine or amphetamines. Most hospital laboratories can perform a quantitative assessment of the level of the drug metabolites in the urine. Rising levels of cocaine or amphetamine metabolites following admission to the hospital suggest illicit use of these drugs while in the hospital.

DIAGNOSTIC ASSESSMENT

It often is difficult to obtain detailed information about the trauma victim's alcohol or drug use during the early stages of care because the surgeon's attention is appropriately focused on the patient's acute life-threatening problems. Information about the patient's alcohol or drug use can be obtained once the patient's condition has stabilized.

Trauma victims can be surprisingly open and honest about their alcohol and drug problems. The pain of traumatic injury and a positive toxicology screen can diminish the denial of an alcohol or drug problem. Many will answer affirmatively to simple, direct questions about their alcohol or drug problems (for example "Do you think you have a problem with alcohol?"). The diagnostic evaluation for the patient's severity of illness and willingness to change are best performed after the patient's acute medical and surgical problems have been stabilized, but before the patient

has an opportunity to re-deploy the defense of denial prior to discharge from the emergency department or hospital.

Severity of the Disorder. It is useful to classify the severity of the substance use disorder in the victim of alcohol or drug-related trauma as either "problem use," "abuse," or "dependence." The type of intervention that is performed depends of the severity of the disorder. For example, brief advice may be appropriate for patients who have problem use or minimal substance-related problems. On the other hand, referral to a treatment center is appropriate for patients who have serious alcohol or drug abuse problems or dependence.

Diagnostic instruments used in treatment centers or research settings, such as the AUDIT, SMAST, or the Diagnostic Interview Schedule-IV (Robins, Helzer et al., 2000) can be too time-consuming for most emergency departments and inpatient trauma services. A practical way to estimate the severity of disease in busy clinical settings is to use existing medical information, information from the patient's family, and the CAGE questions, followed by one or two simple questions about the quantity and frequency of alcohol or drug use.

Patients with severe substance use disorder often have a medical history of problems related to alcohol or drug abuse, such as pancreatitis, recurrent trauma, or skin abscesses from self-injections. They also may have lost jobs or spouses because of their use of drugs or alcohol or have prior arrests for driving while intoxicated or public intoxication. Patients who abuse drugs may have a history of drug-related criminal activity, being in jail or having served a prison sentence. Many trauma patients who are dependent have been to an alcohol or drug rehabilitation program, either voluntarily or as the result of a court order. Many have attended meetings of mutual help groups such as Alcoholics Anonymous.

Useful information to support a diagnosis of a severe alcohol or drug problem may be available from family members, but not always. Sometimes family members simply do not know the extent of the patient's abuse of drugs or alcohol. At other times, family members may not give accurate information because they also abuse drugs or alcohol or are trying to protect the patient. Parents may simply wish to assume that their son's or daughter's drinking or drug patterns are "normal" for the child's peer group.

Patients with severe disease may respond to direct questions. They may answer affirmatively to one or more of the CAGE questions, or readily admit to heavy daily drinking.

The patient's answer to a single question ("Have you ever had a drinking problem?" [Cyr & Wartman, 1988]) may produce information about the patient's severity of disease and willingness to change.

Willingness To Change. Before any intervention designed to change the patient's pattern of alcohol or drug use is attempted, it is useful to know something about the patient's willingness to change. The six-stage "readiness-to-change" model of Prochaska & DiClemente (1983) is a useful concept. For clinical purposes in emergency departments or on busy trauma services, their six-stage model can be collapsed into three stages: "not ready to change," "ambivalent," and "ready to change." Clinicians may have an intuitive sense of how much a given patient is willing to change after asking the patient questions to determine the severity of disease. If this is not the case, one direct question ("Do you think you need to change the way you drink?") can provide useful clinical information.

Patients with severe disease who are willing to change may be referred to an addiction medicine specialist for further evaluation and treatment. Patients who appear unwilling to change or who are ambivalent about change may respond to a brief intervention designed to increase their willingness to change and motivate them to seek help for their alcohol or drug problem.

INTERVENTION

The structured intervention for patients with alcohol problems developed by Johnson (1986) is one approach to intervening with victims of alcohol-related trauma. However, because the approach organizes the efforts of friends and family members during hours of rehearsing, it is difficult to coordinate during a hospitalization. Gentilello and associates (1988) performed a structured intervention according to the technique of Social Network Intervention with 17 alcoholic patients and found that all of them agreed to enter a 28-day alcohol treatment program. These methods are complicated, time-consuming, and require skilled coordinators.

Less demanding interventions of graduated intensity that are proportional to the patient's severity of disease may be effective (Gentilello, Donovan et al., 1995). Incorporating these graduated interventions into the routine of a busy trauma service is problematic. As is often the case in modern curative medicine, the immediate urgent problems often overshadow the importance of preventing long-term prob-

lems. "Brief interventions" also have been found to be effective. When trauma victims who were found to have an alcohol use disorder were given a single motivational interview by a psychologist trained in the use of brief interventions, the patients consumed fewer drinks per week over the 12 months following their hospital discharge than did the members of a control group who did not receive the intervention (Gentilello, Rivara et al., 1999a). However, this effect held primarily for patients who were considered to be problem drinkers and was less pronounced in alcohol-dependent patients.

A trend toward reduced rates of re-injury in the experimental group also was observed when compared to the control group at one to three years following hospital discharge, but this was not statistically significant.

In some hospitals, addiction medicine consultants or specialized teams are available to coordinate interventions during hospitalization and to refer patients to treatment at the time of discharge (Fuller, Diamond et al. 1995; McDuff, Solounias et al., 1996). These approaches appear to be effective (Fleming, Wilk et al., 1995; Barker, Knisely et al., 1999). Some addiction treatment programs will send a staff member to the hospital to evaluate a patient for rehabilitation prior to discharge.

Barriers to Intervention. Not all physicians have the skills to perform brief interventions, and it seems unlikely they will acquire them. In a recent survey of trauma surgeons, 76% were not familiar with the common alcohol and drug abuse screening instruments (Danielsson, Rivara et al., 1999). Reasons cited for not using them included "lack of time" and "not what I was trained to do." Although 88% responded that they were willing to devote time to these activities, it is not known if they actually would do so.

In large medical centers, it is not difficult for physicians or surgeons to refer their hospitalized patients to an addiction medicine consultant or substance abuse consult team or an inpatient substance abuse program. However, most community hospitals and small teaching hospitals do not offer these services. It can be difficult to refer patients to treatment, even when they are willing to enter an addiction treatment program. Many patients lack the resources to pay for such services. Waiting lists at publicly funded addiction treatment programs can be long, and patients can return to alcohol and drug use while waiting for an available bed. The effect of managed care on access to treatment is not clear. Some studies suggest that it poses a barrier to

TABLE 3. An Example of a FRAMES Intervention for Trauma Victims

Intervention Step	Example of Possible Dialogue
Feedback	"I am concerned that you had alcohol [and/or drugs] in your system when you had your injury."
Responsibility	"Only you can change your drinking habits [and/or use of drugs] to prevent this from happening again."
Action	"I want you to read this information and consider quitting drinking" (*for patients not ready to change*). "I want to have somebody come and talk with you about this" (*for patients ambivalent about changing*). "I want to set up an appointment for you to see someone for evaluation at a treatment center" (*for patients willing to change*).
Menu	"This (printed information/person) will review your options for the future so you don't get hurt again."
Empathy	"I know it's not easy to talk about this, but you don't deserve another injury."
Support	"If you reach out to others you can get a better life. It's not easy, but I think you can do it."

SOURCE: Adapted with permission from Miller & Rollnick (1991). *Motivational Interviewing: Preparing People to Change Addictive Behavior.* New York, NY: Guilford Press.

care (Rivara, Tollefson et al., 2000), while others suggest that managed care actually may improve access to addiction treatment (Deck, McFarland et al., 2000).

Simple and Practical Interventions. Nurses have a long tradition of commitment to patient education. Hospital nurses, particularly those who are nurse specialists, can be trained to deliver valuable information to patients with substance use disorders (Sommers, 1994; Dyehouse & Sommers, 1998).

Individuals who are involved with Alcoholics Anonymous (AA) are expected to do "Twelfth Step Work" and carry the message of AA to alcoholics. In the general hospital setting, they can be helpful in improving the outcomes of alcohol-related trauma victims (Collins & Barth, 1979; Blondell, Looney et al., 2001). By calling the local AA office, physicians sometimes can arrange for a layperson to visit a patient in the hospital. This visitor can share with the patient his or her own "experience, strength, and hope." This may be a practical and low-cost option in situations where specialized services are not available.

CONCLUSIONS

Trauma can be viewed as a recurrent illness, with risk factors that predict future injuries. Alcohol and drug abuse may be a significant risk factor. Patients who present to hospitals and emergency rooms with injuries should be screened for drug or alcohol problems. Those who are found to have such problems can be assessed for severity and willingness to change. Interventions directed at changing the course of a patient's alcohol or drug problems may be effective in guiding such patients into changing their behavior, obtaining appropriate treatment, and reducing the chance of future injuries.

Further research is needed to identify methods to accomplish these tasks that are simple, practical, and readily incorporated into the operations of the average emergency department, inpatient hospital service, or trauma center.

REFERENCES

Anda RF, Williamson DF & Remington PL (1988). Alcohol and fatal injuries among U.S. adults: Findings from the NHANES I epidemiologic follow-up study. *Journal of the American Medical Association* 260:2529-2532.

Babor TF & Grant M (1989). From clinical research to secondary prevention: International collaboration in the development of the Alcohol Use Disorders Identification Test (AUDIT). *Alcohol Health & Research World* 13:371-374.

Barker SB, Knisely JS & Dawson KS (1999). The evaluation of a consultation service for delivery of substance abuse services in a hospital setting. *Journal of Addictive Diseases* 18:73-82.

Bazzoli GJ & MacKenzie EJ (1995). Trauma centers in the United States: Identification and examination of key characteristics. *Journal of Trauma* 38:103-110.

Blondell RD, Looney SW, Northington AP et al. (2001). Can recovering alcoholics help hospitalized patients with alcohol problems? *Journal of Family Practice* 50:447.

Borges G, Cherpitel CJ & Rosovsky H (1998). Male drinking and violence-related injury in the emergency room. *Addiction* 93:103-112.

Cardenas DD & McLean Jr A (1992). Psychopharmacologic management of traumatic brain injury. *Physical Medicine and Rehabilitation Clinics of North America* 3:273-290.

Center for Substance Abuse Treatment (CSAT) (1995). *Alcohol and Other Drug Screening of Hospitalized Trauma Patients.* Rockville, MD: CSAT, Substance Abuse and Mental Health Services Administration.

Cesare J, Morgan AS, Felice PR et al. (1990). Characteristics of blunt and personal violent injuries. *Journal of Trauma* 30:176-182.

Cherpitel CJ (1992). Epidemiology of alcohol-related trauma. *Alcohol Health & Research World* 16:191-196.

Cherpitel CJ (1995a). Analysis of cut-points for screening instrument for alcohol problems in the emergency room. *Journal of Studies on Alcohol* 56:695-700.

Cherpitel CJ (1995b). Screening for alcohol problems in the emergency department. *Annals of Emergency Medicine* 26:158-166.

Cherpitel CJ (1996). Drinking patterns and problems and drinking in the event: An analysis of injury by cause among casualty patients. *Alcoholism: Clinical & Experimental Research* 20:1130-1137.

Cherpitel CJ (1997). Comparison of screening instruments for alcohol problems between black and white emergency room patients from 2 regions of the country. *Alcoholism: Clinical & Experimental Research* 21:1391-1397.

Cherpitel CJ (1998). Differences in performance of screening instruments for problem drinking among blacks, whites, and Hispanics in an emergency room population. *Journal of Studies on Alcohol* 50:420-426.

Clark DE, McCarthy E & Robinson E (1985). Trauma as a symptom of alcoholism [editorial]. *Annals of Emergency Medicine* 14:274.

Collins GB & Barth J (1979). Using the resources of AA in treating alcoholics in a general hospital. *Hospital & Community Psychiatry* 30:480-482.

Craft PP, Foil MB, Cunningham PRG et al. (1994). Intravenous ethanol for alcohol detoxification in trauma patients. *Southern Medical Journal* 87:47-54.

Cyr MG & Wartman SA (1988). The effectiveness of routine screening questions in the detection of alcoholism. *Journal of the American Medical Association* 259:51-54.

Danielsson PE, Rivara FP, Gentilello LM et al. (1999). Reasons why trauma surgeons fail to screen for alcohol problems. *Archives of Surgery* 134:564-568.

Deck DD, MacFarland BH, Titus JM et al. (2000). Access to substance abuse treatment services under the Oregon health plan. *Journal of the American Medical Association* 284:2093-2099.

D'Onofrio G, Bernstein E, Bernstein J et al. (1998). Patients with alcohol problems in the emergency department, part 1: Improving detection. *Academic Emergency Medicine* 5:1200-1209.

Dyehouse JM & Sommers MS (1998). Brief interventions after alcohol-related injuries. *Nursing Clinics of North America* 33:93-104.

Ewing JA (1984). Detecting alcoholism: The CAGE questionnaire. *Journal of the American Medical Association* 252:1905-1907.

Ferguson JA, Suelzer CJ, Eckert GJ et al. (1996). Risk factors of delirium tremens development. *Journal of General Internal Medicine* 11:410-414.

Fleming M (1992). Pharmacologic management of the nicotine, alcohol and other drug dependence. In M Fleming & K Barry (eds.) *Addictive Disorders.* St. Louis, MO: Mosby Yearbook, 44-74.

Fleming MF, Wilk A, Kruger J et al. (1995). Hospital-based alcohol and drug specialty consultation service: Does it work? *Southern Medical Journal* 88:275-282.

Freeland ES, McMicken DB & D'Onofrio G (1993). Alcohol and trauma. *Emergency Medicine Clinics of North America* 3:225-330.

Fuller MG, Diamond DL, Jordan ML et al. (1995). The role of a substance abuse consultation team in a trauma center. *Journal of Studies on Alcohol* 56:267-271.

Gentilello LM, Donovan DM, Dunn CW et al. (1995). Alcohol interventions in trauma centers: Current practice and future directions. *Journal of the American Medical Association* 274:1043-1048.

Gentilello LM, Duggan P, Drummond D et al. (1988). Major injury as a unique opportunity to initiate treatment in the alcoholic. *American Journal of Surgery* 56:558-561.

Gentilello LM, Rivara FP, Donovan DM et al. (1999a). Alcohol interventions in a trauma center as a means of reducing the risk of injury recurrence. *Annals of Surgery* 230:473-483.

Gentilello LM, Villaveces A, Ries RR et al. (1999b). Detection of acute alcohol intoxication and chronic alcohol dependence by trauma center staff. *Journal of Trauma* 47:1131-1139.

Gross CP, Anderson GF & Powe NR (1999). The relationship between funding by the National Institutes of Health and the burden of disease. *New England Journal of Medicine* 340:1881-1887.

Hayashida M, Alterman AI, McLellan T et al. (1989). Comparison effectiveness and costs of inpatient and outpatient detoxification of patients with mild-to-moderate alcohol withdrawal syndrome. *New England Journal of Medicine* 320:358-365.

Hoeksema HL & de Bock GH (1993). The value of laboratory tests for the screening and recognition of alcohol abuse in primary care patients. *Journal of Family Practice* 37:268-276.

Johnson VE (1986). *Intervention: How to Help Someone Who Doesn't Want Help*. Minneapolis, MN: Johnson Institute Books.

Jurkovich GJ, Rivara FP, Gurney JG et al. (1992). Effects of alcohol intoxication on the initial assessment of trauma patients. *Annals of Emergency Medicine* 21:704-708.

Litten RZ, Allen JP & Fertig JB (1995). Gamma-glutamyltranspeptidase and carbohydrate deficient transferrin: Alternative measures of excessive alcohol consumption. *Alcoholism: Clinical & Experimental Research* 19:1541-1546.

Lowenstein SR, Weissberg MP & Terry D (1990). Alcohol intoxication, injuries, and dangerous behaviors—and the revolving emergency department door. *Journal of Trauma* 30:1252-1257.

Margolis LH, Foss RD & Tolbert WG (2000). Alcohol and motor vehicle-related deaths of children as passengers, pedestrians, and bicyclists. *Journal of the American Medical Association* 283:2245-2248.

Marshall SW, Runyan CW, Bangdiwala SI et al. (1998). Fatal residential fires: Who dies and who survives. *Journal of the American Medical Association* 279:1633-1637.

Mayo-Smith MF et al. (1997). Pharmacological management of alcohol withdrawal. *Journal of the American Medical Association* 278:144-151.

McDuff DR, Solounias BL, Beuger M et al. (1996). A substance abuse consultation service. *American Journal on Addictions* 6:256-265.

Mitka M (1998). "Teachable moments" provide a means for physicians to lower alcohol abuse. *Journal of the American Medical Association* 279:1767-1768.

Murphy JT, Harwood A, Gotz M et al. (1998). Prescribing alcohol in a general hospital. *Journal of the Royal College of Physicians of London* 32:358-359.

National Institute on Alcohol Abuse and Alcoholism (NIAAA) (1997). Effects of alcohol on behavior and safety. In *Ninth Special Report to the U.S. Congress on Alcohol and Health* (NIH Publication No. 97-4017). Rockville, MD: NIAAA, National Institutes of Health, 247-274.

Nilssen O, Ries R, Rivara FP et al. (1996). The "WAM" score: Sensitivity and specificity of a user friendly biological screening test for alcohol problems in trauma patients. *Addiction* 91:255-262.

Parran Jr TV, Weber E, Tasse J et al. (1995). Mandatory toxicology testing and chemical dependence consultation follow up in a level-one trauma center. *Journal of Trauma* 38:278-280.

Phillips DP, Christenfeld N & Ryan NM (1999). An increase in the number of deaths in the United States in the first week of the month. *New England Journal of Medicine* 341:93-98.

Pokorny A, Miller B & Kaplan H (1972). The brief MAST: A shortened version of the Michigan Alcoholism Screening Test. *American Journal of Psychiatry* 129:342-345.

Prochaska JO & DiClemente CC (1983). Stages and processes of self-change in smoking: Toward an integrative model of change. *Journal of Consulting and Clinical Psychology* 5:390-395.

Rivara FP, Jurkovich GJ, Gurney JG et al. (1993a). The magnitude of acute and chronic alcohol abuse in trauma patients. *Archives of Surgery* 128:907-913.

Rivara FP, Koespell TD, Jurkovich GJ et al. (1993b). The effects of alcohol abuse on readmission for trauma. *Journal of the American Medical Association* 270:1962-1964.

Rivara FP, Tollefson S, Tesh E et al. (2000). Screening trauma patients for alcohol problems: Are insurance companies barriers? *Journal of Trauma* 48:115-118.

Robins LN, Helzer JE, Croughan J et al. (2000). Diagnostic Interview Schedule (DIS); Diagnostic Interview Schedule-IV (DIS-IV); Composite International Diagnostic Interview (CIDI) In *Handbook of Psychiatric Measures*. Washington, DC: American Psychiatric Press, 61-63.

Russell M, Martier SS, Sokol RJ et al. (1994). Screening for pregnancy risk-drinking. *Alcoholism: Clinical & Experimental Research* 18:1156-1161.

Schorlin JB & Buchsbaum DG (1997). Screening for alcohol and drug problems. *Medical Clinics of North America* 81:845-865.

Sims DW, Bivins BA, Obeid FN et al. (1989). Urban trauma: A chronic recurrent disease. *Journal of Trauma* 29:940-946.

Soderstrom CA, Kufera JA, Dischinger PC et al. (1997). A predictive model to detect trauma patients with BACs ≥50mg/dl. *Journal of Trauma* 42:67-73.

Soderstrom CA, Smith GS, Dischinger PC et al. (1997). Psychoactive substance use disorders among seriously injured trauma center patients. *Journal of the American Medical Association* 277:1769-1774.

Sommers MS (1994). Alcohol and trauma: The critical link. *Critical Care Nurse* April:82-93.

Spain DA, Boaz PW, Davidson DJ et al. (1997). Risk-taking behaviors among adolescent trauma patients. *Journal of Trauma* 43:423-426.

Spies CD, Dublez N, Funk W et al. (1995). Prophylaxis of alcohol withdrawal syndrome in alcohol-dependent patients admitted to the intensive care unit after tumour resection. *British Journal of Anesthesia* 75:734-737.

Spies CD, Emadi A, Neumann T et al. (1995). Relevance of carbohydrate-deficient transferrin as a predictor of alcoholism in intensive care patients following trauma. *Journal of Trauma* 39:742-748.

Spies CD & Rommelspacher H (1999). Alcohol withdrawal in the surgical patient: Prevention and treatment. *Anesthesia Analogue* 88:946-954.

Sullivan JT, Sykora K, Schneiclerman J et al. (1989). Assessment of alcohol withdrawal: The Revised Clinical Institute Withdrawal Assessment for Alcohol Scale (CIWA-Ar). *British Journal of Addiction* 84:1353-1357.

Thal ER, Bost & Anderson RJ (1985). Effects of alcohol and other drugs on traumatized patients. *Archives of Surgery* 120:708-712.

Trunkey DD (1984). Shock trauma. *Canadian Journal of Surgery* 27:479–486.

Vinson DC (1991). Admission alcohol level: A predictor of the course of alcohol withdrawal. *Journal of Family Practice* 33:161-167.

Waller JA (1989). Injury as disease. *Accident Analysis and Prevention* 19:13-20.

Chapter 4 | Brief Interventions

Allan W. Graham, M.D., FACP, FASAM
Michael F. Fleming, M.D., M.P.H.

Changing Perspectives on Outcomes
Defining Brief Interventions
Implementing Brief Interventions
Results of Brief Intervention

B rief intervention techniques, which have wide application in primary care, need to be extended more fully to include interventions for alcohol and drug use problems. Physicians and other health care professionals already use these counseling strategies to help patients change their dietary habits, lose weight, stop smoking, lower cholesterol, regulate blood pressure, and develop compliance with medication regimens. This chapter explores how the principles of brief intervention can be applied systematically to the delivery of health care to patients experiencing, or at risk for, addictive disorders.

CHANGING PERSPECTIVES ON OUTCOMES

Historically, treatment of alcohol-related disorders has focused on abstinence-based programs and outcomes. However, there is today an increasing public health emphasis on harm reduction as well. The goal of harm reduction is to reduce alcohol use to low-risk levels in the broad segment of drinkers who are not alcohol-dependent but who are statistically at increased risk for adverse consequences from their drinking. The ratio of problem drinkers to those severely affected by alcohol is estimated at about 4:1. Most people who experience alcohol-related injuries, health problems, or family difficulties do not meet the criteria for alcoholism; they just drink too much, often in high-risk situations (Fuchs, Stampfer et al., 1995; Gentilello, Cobean et al., 1993; Sobell, Cunningham et al., 1996). It also is becoming apparent that most problem drinkers who quit or reduce their alcohol use do so without specialized treatment (Sobell, Cunningham et al., 1996; Cunningham, Sobell et al., 1995, 1996; Sobell, Sobell et al., 1992; Sobell & Sobell, 1993). Studies suggest that just asking a problem drinker about alcohol consumption can reduce his or her alcohol use (Fleming, Manwell et al., 1999; Skinner, Allen et al., 1985). These findings parallel a large body of research showing that 80% to 90% of smokers who quit do so on their own with minimal professional intervention (Fiore, Novotny et al., 1990).

Traditional treatment for alcohol problems has relied predominantly on abstinence-based Twelve Step treatment models. In recent years, however, the alcohol field has shifted to include a broader range of treatment methods (NIAAA, 1994). A number of studies have demonstrated the efficacy of cognitive-behavioral therapies and guided self-change (Sobell & Sobell, 1993; Allen, Mattson et al., 1997). The harm reduction perspective acknowledges the need to address the spectrum of alcohol use disorders and to offer patients a broad range of prevention and treatment methods.

The shift to this broader view has important implications for the U.S. health care system. In the past, the physician's role was to identify persons with alcoholism and refer them for specialized treatment. However, research conducted over the past 10 years has demonstrated that the role of physicians has changed (Murray & Fleming, 1996; NIAAA, 1995b). A number of alcohol screening tests are available that are sensitive and specific. Clinical trials have shown the effectiveness of brief physician advice in reducing alcohol use and associated difficulties in problem drinkers (Wilk, Jensen et al., 1997; Fleming, Barry et al., 1997). The ability to follow patients and family members over a long period of time places physicians in a unique position to intervene and support the behavioral changes necessary to reduce the consequences of problem drinking. New pharmacologic agents also are expected to add significantly to the treatment options available to physicians; already several such drugs have demonstrated their efficacy: naltrexone (an opioid blocking agent), acamprosate (mechanism of action unclear), and ondansetron (selective serotonin 5-HT$_3$ receptor antagonist for early onset alcoholics).

Given the available data, reducing the adverse outcomes related to excessive drinking would seem to be a straightforward problem that is readily amenable to a variety of solutions. Identification of alcohol use problems in health care settings is relatively easy (Weaver, Jarvis et al., 1999; Saitz, 1999). Brief intervention techniques have been shown to reduce significantly the amount of hazardous drinking by medical patients (Wilk, Jensen et al., 1997; Fleming, Barry et al., 1997). Improvements in associated medical problems follow rather quickly once the patient ceases alcohol use. Potential financial rewards are plentiful, as measured by improved work performance and job attendance after excessive alcohol use is curtailed. Logically, then, it should be easy for health care systems to decrease the expense, morbidity, and mortality of alcohol abuse on the part of their members, but this has not necessarily been the case.

The first problem confronting any health delivery system is balancing competing demands for resources against anticipated beneficial outcomes (Ubel, 1999; Delamothe, 1994). Careful analysis of conflicting and complementary goals is essential in developing the best strategies for screening and brief interventions for alcohol use. Managed care, health maintenance organizations, and other health insurers are particularly mindful of the need to balance outcomes against costs as part of their capacity to survive in very competitive markets.

In general, the health care outcomes that are most likely to be promoted by insurers are those showing (1) dramatic changes in function (such as hip replacement), (2) large financial benefits over short periods of time (for example, preventing asthma-related hospitalizations with aggressive preventive therapies), and (3) wide popular support (such as breast cancer screening). Outcomes that seem to be less attractive to insurers and the public are those that require longer periods of time to show improvement (for example, pharmacotherapies for asymptomatic osteoporosis), have smaller immediate financial rewards to the health system (such as management of patients with chronic mental illness), or serve the politically disenfranchised (such as homeless persons). Because a particular outcome is achievable and even medically laudable does not mean that it can compete successfully against other laudable but perhaps more popular outcomes.

DEFINING BRIEF INTERVENTIONS

To be useful in primary care settings, intervention methods must be widely available, reliably applied, simple, and economical. These requirements make a compelling case for the widespread use of brief interventions, which are time-limited, patient-centered counseling strategies that focus on changing behavior and increasing medication compliance. Such strategies are widely used by physicians and other health care professionals in treating chronic diseases and effecting lifestyle changes. For example, these methods are used routinely to help patients change dietary habits, reduce weight, stop smoking, reduce cholesterol, and take medications correctly.

While definitions of brief intervention and brief counseling varies across trials and clinical programs, a number of common elements can be identified (Tables 1 and 2):

■ *Assessment*: "Tell me about your drinking?" "What does your family or partner think about your drinking?" "Have you had any problems related to your alcohol use?" "What do you think about your drinking?" "Have you ever been concerned about how much you drink?"

■ *Direct Feedback*: "As your doctor/therapist, I am concerned about how much you drink and how it is affecting your health." "The car crash is a direct result of your

TABLE 1.   Steps for Screening and Brief Intervention

STEP 1:   Ask about alcohol use:
   a. Inquire about the patient's alcohol consumption;
   b. Use the CAGE questionnaire.

STEP 2:   Assess for alcohol problems:
   a. Alcohol-related medical problems;
   b. Alcohol-related behavioral problems;
   c. Alcohol dependence.

STEP 3:   Advise appropriate action:
   a. If alcohol dependence is suspected;
      (1) advise him or her to abstain;
      (2) refer the patient to a specialist;
   b. If the patient is at risk for or evidences alcohol problems:
      (1) advise him or her to cut down;
      (2) set a drinking goal.

STEP 4:   Monitor the patient's progress.

alcohol use." "Your unborn child could develop a birth defect if you continue to drink."

- *Contracting, Negotiating, and Goal Setting*: "You need to reduce your drinking. What do you think about cutting down to three drinks two to three times per week?" "I would like you to use these diary cards to keep track of your drinking over the next two weeks. We will review these at your next visit."

- *Behavioral Modification Techniques*: "Here is a list of situations when people drink and sometimes lose control of their drinking. Let's talk about ways you can avoid these situations."

- *Self-help Directed Bibliotherapy*: "I would like you to review this booklet and bring it with you at your next visit. It would be very helpful if you would complete some of the exercises in this guide."

- *Followup and Reinforcement* (establishing a plan for supportive phone calls and followup visits): "I would like you to schedule a followup appointment in one month

to review your diary cards and answer any questions you might have. I also will ask one of the nurses to call you in a couple of weeks to see how things are going."

The number and duration of sessions have varied by trial and setting. The classic brief intervention performed by a physician or nurse usually requires 5 to 10 minutes and is repeated one to three times over a six- to eight-week period. Other trials that used therapists or psychologists as interventionists usually employed 30- to 60-minute counseling sessions over one to six visits. Some trials developed manuals or scripted workbooks; others allowed the professional to decide how to conduct the intervention, based on a training program. Some studies used the FRAMES mnemonic developed by Miller as a guide for the intervention (provide Feedback, Responsibility is the patient's, Advise about health matters, provide a Menu of options, express Empathy, and support Self-efficacy; Miller & Rollnick, 1991; Miller & Sanchez, 1994; see Chapter 3, Table 3).

Timing and Techniques of Brief Intervention. Timing and context are important: a patient's motivation to change alcohol use behaviors may be heightened during an alcohol-related illness, for example (Table 3). Studies show that patients are most likely to make behavior changes when they perceive that they have a problem (DiClemente, Fairhurst et al., 1991; DiClemente & Hughes, 1990; Prochaska & DiClemente, 1983), feel that they can be effective in making a change (Bandura, 1977), and are engaged as active participants in setting the goals to be achieved through the new behaviors (Miller & Rollnick, 1991; Ockene, Quirk et al., 1988).

Motivation may be enhanced through the use of patient-centered interviewing, which should incorporate the following elements (Delbanco, 1992a; Miller & Rollnick, 1991; Ockene, Quirk et al., 1988; Rollnick, Heather et al., 1992):

- Empathic, objective feedback of data;
- Meeting patient expectations;
- Working with ambivalence;
- Assessing the patient's readiness for change;
- Assessing barriers and strengths;
- Reinterpreting past experiences in light of current medical consequences;
- Negotiating a followup plan; and
- Providing hope.

TABLE 2.   A Lifestyle Risk Assessment Protocol

Date:

Name:

Age:

Why have you come today? What's wrong?

Injuries
Since your 18th birthday:
   Have you had a fracture or dislocation?
   Have you been injured in a traffic accident?
   Have you injured your head?
   Have you been injured in a fight?
   Have you been injured after drinking?

Exercise
Do you exercise regularly?
   Time per week for 20 minutes or more? ____

Stress and Social Network
Do you feel under stress?
   (Constantly, Often, Occasionally, Infrequently)
With whom do you live?
   (Alone, Spouse, Other relative, Group, Other)

Smoking
Have you ever smoked?
How many cigarettes daily do you smoke? ____

Diet
Do you regulate your diet for:
   Cholesterol
   Salt (sodium)
   Total calories or fat

Alcohol Use
Have you ever had a drinking problem?
Has anyone in the family had a drinking problem?
Have you ever felt you should cut down on your
   drinking?
Have people annoyed you by criticizing your drinking?
Have you ever felt bad or guilty about your drinking?
Have you ever had a drink first thing in the morning to
   steady your nerves or get rid of a hangover?
How many drinks do you have on a typical drinking
   day? ____
   (1 drink = 12 oz beer = 5 oz wine = 1.25 oz liquor)
How many days a week do you generally drink? ____

Health care professionals who address lifestyle issues within the context of medical consequences increase the effectiveness of their messages. Building a cooperative alliance is more effective in changing behavior than an authoritarian stance (Roche, Guray et al., 1991; Delbanco, 1992a, 1992b; Miller & Rollnick, 1991; Ockene, Quirk et al., 1988). The physician's words can have a major effect on future abstinence, frequency of drinking episodes, and behavioral impairment (Walsh, Hingson et al., 1992). Negotiating appropriate goals for cessation of drinking and other negative behaviors is a key to success (Sanchez-Craig & Lei, 1986). Providing a menu of options helps to tailor the treatment to the patient's learning style, motivational level, and the services available. Assuring a plan for followup, with objective, measurable, nonjudgmental goals, appears to enhance outcome (Kristenson, Ohlin et al., 1983).

Telephone contacts also can be important in improving compliance (Scivoletto, DeAndrade et al., 1992; Wasson, Gaudette et al., 1992).

Assessing the Patient's Readiness To Change: Research over the past decade has shown that individuals who succeed in changing their behavior move through a series of stages, involving precontemplation, contemplation, action, and maintenance (DiClemente, Fairhurst et al., 1991; DiClemente & Hughes, 1990; Prochaska & DiClemente, 1983). Such individuals typically shift back and forth among these stages as their level of motivation changes. Using these principles, Rollnick and colleagues (1992) created a 12-item "readiness to change" questionnaire for use in matching intervention techniques with a given patient's stage of readiness to change. The patient's stage does appear to be a significant predictor of future changes in alcohol consumption

---

(Heather, Rollnick et al., 1993). Matching stage of change with treatment choices is important in planning treatment, allocating resources, and developing referral plans.

Conceptualizing the Continuum of Risk: Early identification of alcohol or drug use problems is facilitated if clinicians begin to view such use as a point on a continuum, rather than as a dichotomy between problem use and no use at all (Fiellin, Reid et al., 2000). Conceptualizing such a continuum requires that the caregiver's focus be broadened to include persons whose drinking patterns have just begun to cause problems and those with an increased risk of future problems, injury, or harm. A simple categorization by levels of use (abstinent, light use, hazardous use, harmful use, and dependent) predicts the increasing probability of adverse consequences (Babor & Grant, 1992).

- "Hazardous use" can be defined as a level of alcohol consumption that is associated with a measurably increased risk of adverse consequences, such as trauma or accidents.

- "Harmful use" is a consumption pattern that contributes to a current problem or problems, such as esophagitis, gastritis, hypertension, insomnia, depression, or difficulties with interpersonal relationships.

- "Dependent use" is characterized by physical withdrawal symptoms (including tremor, diaphoresis, nausea, vomiting, and diarrhea) and the continued, compulsive use of alcohol despite adverse consequences.

IMPLEMENTING BRIEF INTERVENTIONS

Provider Issues. Screening and brief intervention clinical protocols should be incorporated into routine clinical care. Strategies might include the use of self-administered screening tests, nurses asking alcohol questions as part of routine vital signs, or reminder systems for clinicians to screen for alcohol problems. Self-help booklets, alcohol diary cards, lists of meetings of self-help groups such as Alcoholics Anonymous (AA), and referral information with phone numbers and names of alcohol specialists can help physicians and patients establish followup plans and strategies.

Maximizing provider effectiveness, assessing patient outcomes, and providing feedback to the staff are important steps that enhance provider participation, morale, and enthusiasm about screening and brief intervention. Efficient data collection, management, and analysis are needed to facilitate feedback and to promote meaningful outcome evaluation. For systematic interventions to work, providers need to have "buy-in" to the process and to feel they are effective clinically.

Systems Issues. Implementing screening and brief intervention is best approached as a systems issue, because any intervention program must be made to fit smoothly into the existing delivery system. There are many demands on the existing care team: Providers already are asked to perform a wide range of clinical tasks and prevention activities. These include performing routine physicals (sports, well woman, insurance), treating acute medical problems (trauma, infections, anxiety, headaches), managing chronic conditions (depression, hypertension, diabetes), and conducting prevention programs (breast cancer screening, nutrition and diet counseling, immunizations).

Strategies for implementing brief intervention in such a system include convincing purchasers (such as employers and governmental agencies) and payers (that is, insurance companies and health care maintenance organizations) to provide financial support and leadership. Purchasers of health insurance and providers will need to be convinced that the prevention and treatment of alcohol and drug problems will improve the health of their populations and reduce health care and social costs. Professional organizations need to take a more active role in encouraging payers and providers to allocate a level of resources that matches the magnitude of the problem. Establishing national standards for periodic alcohol screening, similar to those for mammographic screening, would set measurable goals for health plans and physician groups.

Another important consideration is the integration of specialized treatment with the general medical care system. Addiction treatment historically has occurred outside the traditional medical care system. Many treatment programs are freestanding community-based programs. In contrast to referral to other specialty referral systems (such as medical and surgical specialty clinics), addiction treatment programs do not routinely send copies of the patient assessment, treatment plan, or discharge summary to the referring physician or other provider. Nor do addiction medicine specialists routinely call the patient's physician or therapist to coordinate care and develop long-term treatment plans. Yet lack of communication between specialized treatment programs and the primary care team can have a serious adverse effect on the patient's long-term health outcomes.

One way to facilitate an integrated treatment process and to increase communication is to locate addiction treat-

TABLE 3.   Treatment Efficacy Affected by Comorbid Medical Problems

Motivation for making a behavior change is greatly increased when a patient becomes aware that the behavior is causally related to a current medical illness. Examples of increased intervention efficacy are listed below. It is important that health care providers make the most of these moments when patients are receptive to change.

TOBACCO
Differential smoking cessation rates measured one year after intervention demonstrate the effects of motivation and concurrent medical illness on successfully quitting.

Intervention	Quit Rate	Reference
Baseline yearly quit rate	2.5%	Fiscella, 1996
Hospital based stop-smoking consult service, no physician quit message	2.5%	Orleans, 1990
Physician counsel to quit	4.0%	Fiscella, 1996
With pregnant women	8%	Law, 1995
Community volunteers for quit studies	8–22%	Silagy, 1994
With nicotine replacement	15–25%	Silagy, 1994
Smoking clinic patients	10–22%	Silagy, 1994
With nicotine replacement	21–36%	Silagy, 1994
Victims of myocardial infarction	32%	Taylor, 1990
With nurse-managed intervention	61%	Taylor, 1990
Surgical oncology patients "usual care"	43%	Stanislaw, 1994
With nurse intervention	75%	Stanislaw, 1994

ALCOHOL
Effectiveness of alcohol use interventions is similarly subject to the differential effects of motivational state and of previously experienced alcohol-related life problems.

Intervention	Use after 6–24 months	Reference
At-risk drinkers, attending medical clinic	15% reduction	Wallace, 1988
Physician counsel to quit	30% reduction	Wallace, 1988
Health provider quit counsel	40% reduction	WHO, 1996
GGT feedback several times yearly	26% fewer sick days	Kristenson, 1983
	55% fewer hospital days	Kristenson, 1983
Alcoholics requesting treatment	90% reduction	Graham, 1995
	80% reduction	Project MATCH, 1997
Alcoholics receiving liver transplantation	80% abstinence	Knechle, 1992.

ment programs in close physical proximity to primary care settings and to carve in addiction treatment services, rather than using carved-out systems of behavioral care. Physicians are more likely to refer patients to a trusted colleague whose office is down the hall than to a stranger located many miles away in a different system of care. It also is easier for patients to accept and follow through with an in-house referral. Primary care providers and addiction medicine specialists need to be part of the same medical staff and care team. Patients benefit when their caregivers communicate and work together to provide coordinated, comprehensive care.

A Brief Intervention Action Plan. A brief intervention action plan should incorporate protocols and skills training that reflect the lessons learned from the research literature:

- Primary care physicians should be encouraged to establish routine alcohol screening procedures for all adult patients. Medical and surgical subspecialists should be encouraged to screen patients whose undetected alcohol use could affect treatment outcomes (for example, a patient at risk of postoperative *delirium tremens*). Quantity/frequency questions, used in combination with the CAGE, are the recommended screening method.

- Routine screening should be a standard part of preventive health care services as well. A reasonable goal is to screen 75% of all patients over age 14 for alcohol use disorders at least once every five years.

- Primary care physicians need to adapt the brief intervention skills they routinely use for other conditions to their work with at-risk drinkers. Tools such as NIAAA's *Training Physicians in Techniques for Alcohol Screening and Brief Intervention* (1997) can facilitate such adaptation.

- Clinics and physicians should establish working relationships with alcohol treatment programs, providers, and the self-help community.

- Specialized alcohol and drug treatment programs should be seamlessly integrated with primary care as part of the routine clinical practice of medicine. These programs should be located in close physical proximity to medical centers and outpatient clinics.

RESULTS OF BRIEF INTERVENTION

Studies of brief intervention in general hospitals, physicians' offices, and public health centers show that a surprisingly large percentage of heavy drinkers and alcoholics can reduce their intake by 20% to 50% after very brief counseling, even while others seem unresponsive to months of care.

Most of the trials discussed in this review specifically excluded persons who met the diagnostic criteria for alcohol dependence. While a number of trials included very heavy drinkers who probably were alcohol-dependent (Wallace, Cutler et al., 1988; WHO, 1996), a stratified analysis of this group was not reported.

Following the identification of a potential alcohol use problem, a brief intervention consisting of as little as a single visit has been associated with a 20% to 50% decrease in alcohol consumption (Chick, Lloyd et al., 1985; Wallace, Cutler et al., 1988; Babor & Grant, 1992; Fleming, Barry et al., 1997). However, changing addictive behaviors requires more than education: Specific strategies for brief intervention need to be implemented.

To present a clearer picture of the strengths and limitations of these outcome studies, seven examples are reviewed below. These studies illustrate the complexity of brief intervention trials and the challenges associated with community-based interventions. Two of the trials had negative results, while five had positive findings.

Trial 1. Kristenson and colleagues (1983) provided early evidence for the efficacy of brief interventions when they published a report of 585 male heavy drinkers who were followed for two to six years. Study data showed that 54% of these men drank more than 40 grams of ethanol per day (>3.5 drinks), 22% consumed 20 to 40 grams per day (2 to 3.5 drinks), and 24% drank less than 20 grams a day (<2 drinks). A substantial number of study participants had symptoms consistent with alcoholism: 30% experienced physical withdrawal, and 20% were early morning "relief" drinkers.

Patients were randomly assigned to control or intervention groups. Intervention patients received GGT tests monthly, physician visits every three months to discuss the GGT values, and a treatment goal of moderation of drinking. Patients in the control group were sent a letter informing them of their impaired liver tests, encouraged to live as usual but to restrict their alcohol consumption, and invited back two years later for new liver tests.

Followup measurements found identical decreases in GGT values for both groups: 28 I.U. at two years and 40 I.U. at four years. However, subjects in the intervention group had significantly fewer sick days (29 versus 52 days per year), hospital days (4.1 versus 9.1 days per year), and mortality rates (1.5% versus 3.3%) than those in the control group.

Trial 2. Wallace and colleagues (1988) studied the effect of physicians' advice to reduce drinking on patients who engaged in excessive alcohol consumption (defined as more than 20 drinks per week). The patients were part of a larger study evaluating the effects of physician intervention on heart disease. Of the study group, 909 subjects had drinking patterns that were deemed excessive.

Every patient received advice on smoking, exercise, and diet, as well as an educational booklet. Subjects in the control group received no specific advice about drinking, while those in the experimental group received advice from their physicians about the potentially harmful effects of their drinking. Patients in the experimental group also were shown a histogram comparing their weekly intake with national norms, given an informational booklet about sensible drinking, and scheduled for a followup appointment one month later. On return visits, physicians reviewed their drinking diaries and blood tests.

Twelve months later (with 82% followup), individuals in both the control and intervention groups showed statistically significant reductions in alcohol consumption. Those in the intervention group showed a twofold greater reduction than the controls (p<0.001 men, p<0.05 women). No substantial changes in cigarette consumption, exercise frequency, or weight reduction occurred in either group.

Trial 3. Israel and colleagues (1996) described a systematic, office-based, screening/intervention program involving 15,686 patients who attended private practices of 42 Canadian physicians. The patients were asked five questions related to their history of traumatic injury (Skinner, Holt et al., 1984). This technique identified 62% to 85% of the expected number of problem drinkers.

A sample of problem drinkers was randomized and prospectively assigned to receive either simple advice or cognitive-behavioral counseling for three hours, delivered over a period of one year. At 12 months (with 70% available at followup), subjects in the simple advice group reported a 46% reduction in their alcohol use, but showed no significant decrease in GGT levels, physician visits, or psychosocial problems. In contrast, the counseled patients reported larger reductions in alcohol use (70%) and showed significant decreases in GGT (32%), physician visits (34%), and psychosocial problems (85%).

A notably larger effect of treatment was seen in this study than in Wallace's study. The cost per patient in this study was $90 per at-risk drinker for the intervention, based on the use of 15 minutes of physician's time and three hours of nurse's time over one year. The counseling intervention is estimated to have saved three office visits over the ensuing two years for each patient who received the intervention.

Trial 4. Project TrEAT (Trial for Early Alcohol Treatment; Fleming, Barry et al., 1997) was designed to replicate the Medical Research Council trial (Wallace, Cutler et al., 1988) conducted in Great Britain. Physicians were recruited through the Wisconsin Research Network, local community hospitals, managed care organizations, and personal

contacts. For the study, 64 physicians were recruited from 17 clinics; they had a mean age of 46 years and a mean tenure of 13 years in practice. Study subjects were 774 men and women, age 18 to 65 years, who were randomized to a control group or a physician-delivered brief intervention group. Major inclusion criteria were number of drinks per week (15 to 50 drinks per week for men and 12 to 50 drinks per week for women), no evidence of alcohol dependence, and no alcohol treatment in the preceding 12 months. At 12-month followup, 723 subjects completed the interview, for a 93.4% followup rate.

Large decreases were found in average number of drinks per week, binge drinking, and excessive drinking in all groups at 6 and 12 months. The number of drinks consumed in the preceding week decreased from 19.1 at baseline to 11.5 at 12 months for the brief intervention group (40% decrease) and from 18.9 at baseline to 15.5 at 12 months for the controls (18% decrease) (p<.001). Men in the experimental group reduced their consumption slightly less than their female counterparts. The number of binge drinking episodes during the preceding 30 days decreased from 5.7 at baseline to 3.1 at 12 months for the experimental group (46% decrease) and from 5.3 at baseline to 4.2 at 12 months for the controls (21% decrease) (p<.001).

The investigators also found a difference in the number of hospital days used at 6 and 12 months for both men (p<.01) and women (p<.05), favoring intervention.

Trial 5. One of the first community-based U.S. trials, conducted at a family medicine teaching clinic in Texas, enlisted a sample of Mexican American subjects (Burge, Amodie et al., 1997). The trial screened 4,014 patients who came to the clinic for primary care. Of these, 279 were randomized into one of four groups: no treatment, patient education only, physician intervention only, and combined patient education and physician intervention. At 12-month followup, 78% of the subjects were assessed for alcohol use, health status, and GGT levels. No significant differences were found between the four groups; subjects in all groups demonstrated significant reductions in alcohol consumption, Addiction Severity Index variables, and GGT levels. This was a negative trial.

Trial 6. Discouraging results have been reported by investigators at Kaiser Permanente in Oregon, who conducted a brief intervention trial with at-risk drinkers in primary care settings (Senft, Polen et al., 1997). The investigators used the AUDIT (see the Rapid Reference section of this text for the 10 questions of the AUDIT instrument) to identify the study sujects. They defined a positive score as either in the range of 8 to 21, or as a score of ≥5 on question 1 (frequency) plus question 2 (quantity). The patient outcomes at 6 and 12 months were compared with patients who had been randomized to one of three control conditions: 30 seconds of advice about safe drinking levels, 15 minutes of motivational counseling, or a packet of printed materials. The 516 hazardous drinkers identified by the AUDIT (70% of whom were male) had a mean intake score of 10.5 and an average age of 42. At 12-month followup, 80% of the subjects completed a telephone interview. No differences between control conditions were found in the reported number of drinks per drinking day or number of drinks per week, nor were there differences in the use of medical care during the year following the interventions (the mean number of outpatient visits was 10.7 for the intervention group and 10.3 for the control group). Hospitalization rates also were similar: 15% for the intervention group and 14% for the control group.

Trial 7. Gentilello and colleagues (1999) studied the efficacy of providing brief alcohol interventions as a routine component of trauma care to reduce alcohol consumption and decrease trauma recidivism. For the study, 2,524 patients admitted to a Level 1 trauma center for treatment of an injury were screened for an alcohol problem through use of BAC, GGT, and the SMAST. Those with positive results were randomized to a brief intervention (n=366) or a control group (n=396). The intervention, conducted on or near the day of hospital discharge, consisted of a single motivational interview with a trained psychologist. Subjects were re-interviewed at 6 and 12 months to assess changes in their alcohol use. Trauma registries and Washington State databases were used to assess rates of hospital readmission and legal events. The investigators reported a significant reduction in alcohol use at 12 months post-intervention in the intervention group (decrease of 21.8 ±3.7 drinks per week) as compared to the control group (decrease of 6.7 ± 5.8) (p = 0.03). While there was a reduction in trauma events and readmission, these differences were not statistically significant.

CONCLUSIONS

A systematic strategy for intervention in and treatment of alcohol problems is needed in the American health care system. Such a strategy must address at least five domains:

- Identification of at-risk drinkers;

- Intervention with at-risk drinkers;

- Cost analysis of identification and intervention;

- Evaluation of outcomes in terms of morbidity, mortality, and health service utilization; and

- Integration of medical and behavioral health services (including addiction and mental health services) within the existing delivery system.

The research shows that routine use of brief interventions can effectively address these domains. However, such interventions must be able to compete successfully for resource dollars and staff time. Programs need to demonstrate cost-effectiveness to their financially focused constituencies, inside and outside of their respective health care organizations. Financial benefits accruing to employers (through decreased absenteeism and increased productivity) must be documented to demonstrate the cost-effectiveness of the intervention. Savings to businesses, judicial and prison systems, and community social service agencies need to be used to demonstrate the effectiveness of the alcohol intervention programs. In short, health care systems need to see tangible benefits for doing "the right thing" for the community (for example, lowering alcohol-related costs to society). Otherwise, the health system may not be able to continue to support the program. For example, the health care system could be offered tax incentives for decreased crime related to substance abuse treatment. It could be encouraged if companies continue to offer the particular system as one of the company's available health options. Health systems could be encouraged even more by employers who purchase health insurance to select systems featuring programs that have been shown to enhance workers' attendance and productivity.

Providers also need incentives to make the necessary changes in their practice routines. Quality improvement programs can provide opportunities to support changes in clinician practice behaviors. The establishment of monitoring systems to examine rates of alcohol use in persons being treated for hypertension, depression, or anxiety disorders can significantly change practice patterns. Clinician incentives can include financial reimbursement for this clinical activity, paid education time to attend training workshops, and quality improvement peer review programs. In the current system, it often is difficult for clinicians to receive compensation for alcohol and drug screening and brief intervention.

REFERENCES

Adams WL, Barry KL & Fleming MF (1996). Screening for problem drinking in older primary care patients. *Journal of the American Medical Association* 276(24):1964-1967.

Adams WL, Magruder-Habib K, Trued S et al. (1992). Alcohol abuse in elderly emergency department patients. *Journal of the American Geriatrics Society* 40(12):1236-1240.

Allen JP & Litten RZ (1998). Screening instruments and biochemical screening tests. In AW Graham & TK Schultz (eds.) *Principles of Addiction Medicine, Second Edition.* Chevy Chase, MD: American Society of Addiction Medicine, 263-271.

Allen JP, Litten RZ, Fertig JB et al. (1997). A review of research on the Alcohol Use Disorders Identification Test (AUDIT). Review. *Alcoholism: Clinical & Experimental Research* 21(4):613-619.

Allen JP, Mattson ME & Miller WR (1997). Matching alcoholism treatment to client heterogeneity: Project MATCH post treatment drinking outcomes. *Journal Studies on Alcohol* 58:7-29.

Anderson P & Scott E (1992). The effect of general practitioners' advice to heavy drinking men. *British Journal of Addiction* 87:1498-1508.

Armstrong MA, Midanik LT & Klatsky AL (1998). Alcohol consumption and utilization of health services in a health maintenance organization. *Medical Care* 36(11):1599-1605.

Babor T & Grant M (1992). *Project on Identification and Management of Alcohol Related Problems. Report on Phase II: A Randomized Clinical Trial of Brief Interventions in Primary Health Care.* Geneva, Switzerland: World Health Organization.

Bandura A (1977). *Social Learning Theory.* Englewood Cliffs, NJ: Prentice-Hall.

Bien TH, Miller WR & Tonigan JS (1993). Brief interventions for alcohol problems: A review. *Addiction* 88:315-335.

Borges G, Cherpitel CJ, Medina-Mora ME et al. (1998). Alcohol consumption in emergency room patients and the general population: A population-based study. *Alcoholism: Clinical & Experimental Research* 22(9):1986-1991.

Bradley KA, Boyd-Wickizer J, Powell SH et al. (1998). Alcohol screening questionnaires in women: A critical review. *Journal of the American Medical Association* 280(2):166-171.

Bradley KA, Bush KR, McDonell MB et al. (1998). Screening for problem drinking: Comparison of CAGE and AUDIT. Ambulatory Care Quality Improvement Project (ACQUIP). Alcohol Use Disorders Identification Test. *Journal of General Internal Medicine* 13(6):379-388.

Burge SK, Amodei N, Elkin B et al. (1997). An evaluation of two primary care interventions for alcohol abuse among Mexican-American patients. *Addiction* 92:1705-1716.

Bush B, Shaw S, Cleary P et al. (1987). Screening for alcohol abuse using the CAGE questionnaire. *American Journal of Medicine* 82:231-235.

Bush K, Kivlahan DR, McDonell MB et al. (1998). The AUDIT alcohol consumption questions (AUDIT-C): An effective brief screening test for problem drinking. Ambulatory Care Quality Improvement Project (ACQUIP). Alcohol Use Disorders Identification Test. *Archives of Internal Medicine* 158(16):1789-1795.

Caetano R, Tam T, Greenfield T et al. (1997). DSM-IV alcohol dependence and drinking in the U.S. population: A risk analysis. *Annals of Epidemiology* 7(8):542-549.

Chan AW, Pristach EA & Welte JW (1994). Detection by the CAGE of alcoholism or heavy drinking in primary care outpatients and the general population. *Journal of Substance Abuse* 6(2):123-135.

Chan AW, Pristach EA, Welte JW et al. (1993). Use of the TWEAK test in screening for alcoholism/heavy drinking in three populations. *Alcoholism: Clinical & Experimental Research* 17(6):1188-1192.

Chang G, Wilkins-Haug L, Berman S et al. (1999). Brief intervention for alcohol use in pregnancy: A randomized trial. *Addiction* 94(10):1499-1508.

Cherpitel CJ (1998). Differences in performance of screening instruments for problem drinking among blacks, whites and Hispanics in an emergency room population. *Journal of Studies on Alcohol* 59(4):420-426.

Chick J, Lloyd G & Crombie E (1985). Counseling problem drinkers in medical wards: A controlled study. *British Medical Journal* 290:965-967.

Cleary P, Miller M, Bush B et al. (1988). Prevalence and recognition of alcohol abuse in a primary care population. *American Journal of Medicine* 85:466-471.

Conigliaro J, Lofgren RP & Hanusa BH (1998). Screening for problem drinking: Impact on physician behavior and patient drinking habits. *Journal of General Internal Medicine* 13(4):251-256.

Cunningham JA, Sobell LS & Sobell MB (1996). Are disease and conceptions of alcohol abuse related to beliefs about outcome and recovery? *Journal of Applied Social Psychology* 26:773-780.

Cunningham JA, Sobell LS & Sobell MB (1995). Resolution from alcohol problems with and without treatment. *Journal of Substance Abuse* 7(3):365-372.

Cushman P (1992). Blood and liver markers in the estimation of alcohol consumption. In RZ Litten & JP Allen (eds.) *Measuring Alcohol Consumption: Psychosocial and Biochemical Methods.* Totowa, NJ: The Humana Press, Inc., 135-147.

Cyr M & Wartman S (1988). The effectiveness of routine screening questions in the detection of alcoholism. *Journal of the American Medical Association* 259(1):51-54.

Delamothe T (1994). Using outcomes research in clinical practice. *British Medical Journal* 308(6944):1583-1584.

Delbanco TL (1992a). Enriching the doctor-patient relationship by inviting the patient's perspective. *Annals of Internal Medicine* 116(5):414-418.

Delbanco TL (1992b). Patients who drink too much: Where are their doctors? *Journal of the American Medical Association* 267(5):702-703.

DiClemente C, Fairhurst S, Velasquez M et al. (1991). The process of smoking cessation: An analysis of pre-contemplation, contemplation, and preparation stages of change. *Journal of Consulting and Clinical Psychology* 59(2):295-304.

DiClemente C & Hughes S (1990). Stages of change profiles in outpatient alcoholism treatment. *Journal of Substance Abuse* 2:217-235.

Elvy G, Wells J & Baird K (1988). Attempted referral as intervention for problem drinking in the general hospital. *British Journal of Addiction* 83:83-89.

Ewing J (1984). Detecting alcoholism. *Journal of the American Medical Association* 252:1905-1907.

Fiore MC, Novotny TE, Pierce JP et al. (1990). Methods used to quit smoking in the United States. *Journal of the American Medical Association* 263(20):2760-2765.

Fiscella K & Franks P (1996). Cost-effectiveness of the transdermal nicotine patch as an adjunct to physicians' smoking cessation counseling. *Journal of the American Medical Association* 275(16):1247-1251.

Fleming MF, Barry KL, Manwell LB et al. (1998). At-risk drinking in a HMO primary care sample: Prevalence and health policy implications. *American Journal of Public Health* 88(1):90-93.

Fleming MF, Barry KL, Manwell LB et al. (1997). Brief physician advice for problem alcohol drinkers: A randomized controlled trial in community-based primary care practices. *Journal of the American Medical Association* 277:1039-1045.

Fleming MF, Manwell LB, Barry KL et al. (1999). Brief physician advice for alcohol problems in older adults: A randomized community-based trial. *Journal of Family Practice* 48:378-384.

Fleming MF, Mundt MP, French MT et al. (2000). Benefit-cost analysis of brief physician advice with problem drinkers in primary care settings. *Medical Care* 38(1):7-18.

Fleming MF, Mundt MP, French MT et al. (unpublished). Project TrEAT, a Trial for Early Alcohol Treatment: Four-year follow-up.

Friedman PD, Saitz R & Samet JH (1998). Management of adults recovering from alcohol or other drug problems: Relapse prevention in primary care. *Journal of the American Medical Association* 279: 1227-1231.

Fuchs CS, Stampfer MJ, Colditz GA et al. (1995). Alcohol consumption and mortality among women. *New England Journal of Medicine* 332(19):1245-1250.

Gentilello LM, Cobean RA, Walker AP et al. (1993). Acute ethanol intoxication increases the risk of infection following penetrating abdominal trauma. *Journal of Trauma* 34(5):669-674.

Gentilello LM, Rivara FP, Donovan DM et al. (1999). Alcohol interventions in a trauma center as a means of reducing the risk of injury recurrence. *Annals of Surgery* 230(4):473-480.

Girela E, Villanueva E, Hernandez-Cueto C et al. (1999). Comparison of the CAGE questionnaire versus some biochemical markers in the diagnosis of alcoholism. Depression among high utilizers of medical care. *Journal of General Internal Medicine* 14(8):461-468.

Goldberg HI, Ries RK et al. (1991). Alcohol counseling in a general medicine clinic: A randomized controlled trial of strategies to improve referral and show rates. *Medical Care* 29(7Suppl):JS49-JS57.

Graham AW (1991). Screening for alcoholism by life-style risk assessment in a community hospital. *Archives of Internal Medicine* 151(5):958-964.

Graham AW (1995). Positive outcomes after brief hospital interventions in patients seeking treatment for alcoholism (abstract). *Journal of Addictive Diseases* 14(1):139.

Hankin J, McCaul MD & Heussner J (2000). Pregnant, alcohol-abusing women. *Alcoholism: Clinical & Experimental Research* 24(8):1276-86.

Heather N, Rollnick S & Bell A (1993). Predictive validity of the readiness to change questionnaire. *Addiction* 88:1667-1677.

Israel Y, Hollander O et al. (1996). Screening for problem drinking & counseling by the primary care physician-nurse team. *Alcoholism: Clinical & Experimental Research* 20(8):1443-1450.

Kahan M, Wilson L & Becker L (1995). Effectiveness of physician-based interventions with problem drinkers: A review. *Canadian Medical Association Journal* 152:851-859.

Kristenson H, Ohlin H, Hulten-Nosslin M et al. (1983). Identification and intervention of heavy drinking in middle-aged men. Results and follow-up of 24-60 months of long-term study with randomized controls. *Alcoholism: Clinical & Experimental Research* 7(2):203-209.

Law M & Tang JL (1995). An analysis of the effectiveness of interventions intended to help people stop smoking. *Archives of Internal Medicine* 155(18):1933-1941.

Marlatt GA, Baer JS, Kivlahan DR et al. (1998). Screening and brief intervention for high-risk college student drinkers: Results from a 2-year follow-up assessment. *Journal of Consulting and Clinical Psychology* 66:604-615.

Mayfield D, McLeod G & Hall P (1974). The CAGE questionnaire: Validation of a new alcoholism screening instrument. *American Journal of Psychiatry* 131:1121-1123.

Miller W & Rollnick S (1991). *Motivational interviewing: Preparing People to Change Addictive Behavior.* New York, NY: Guilford Press.

Miller WR & Sanchez VC (1994). Motivating young adults for treatment and lifestyle change. In GS Howard & PE Nathan (eds.) *Alcohol Use and Misuse by Young Adults.* Notre Dame, IN: University of Notre Dame Press.

Monti PM, Colby SM, Barnett NP et al. (1999). Brief intervention for harm reduction with alcohol-positive older adolescents in a hospital emergency department. *Journal of Consulting and Clinical Psychology* 67(6):989-994.

Murray M & Fleming M (1996). Prevention and treatment of alcohol-related problems: An international medical education model. *Academic Medicine* 71(11):1204-1210.

National Institute on Alcohol Abuse and Alcoholism (NIAAA) (1994). *Eighth Special Report to the U.S. Congress on Alcohol and Health.* Alexandria, VA: NIAAA, National Institutes of Health.

National Institute on Alcohol Abuse and Alcoholism (NIAAA) (1995a). *Project MATCH Series, Vols. 1-3.* Rockville, MD: NIAAA, National Institutes of Health.

National Institute on Alcohol Abuse and Alcoholism (NIAAA) (1995b). *The Physicians' Guide to Helping Patients with Alcohol Problems.* Rockville, MD: NIAAA, National Institutes of Health.

National Institute on Alcohol Abuse and Alcoholism (NIAAA) (1997). *Training Physicians in Techniques for Alcohol Screening and Brief Intervention.* Training manual for *The Physicians' Guide to Helping Patients with Alcohol Problems.* Rockville, MD: NIAAA, National Institutes of Health.

O'Connor PG, Farren CK, Rounsaville BJ et al. (1997). A preliminary investigation of the management of alcohol dependence with naltrexone by primary care providers. *American Journal of Medicine* 103:477-482.

Ockene JK, Adams A, Hurley TG et al. (1999). Brief physician- and nurse practitioner-delivered counseling for high risk drinkers: Does it work? *Archives of Internal Medicine* 159(18):2198-2205.

Ockene J, Quirk M, Goldberg R et al. (1988). A residents' training program for the development of smoking intervention skills. *Archives of Internal Medicine* 148:1039-1045.

Orleans CT, Rotberg HL, Quade D et al. (1990). A hospital quit-smoking consult service: Clinical report and intervention guidelines. *Preventive Medicine* 19(2):198-212.

Prochaska J & DiClemente C (1983). Stages and processes of self-change of smoking: Toward an integrative model of change. *Journal of Consulting and Clinical Psychology* 51:390-395.

Roche A, Guray C & Saunders J (1991). General practitioners' experiences of patients with drug and alcohol problems. *British Journal of Addiction* 86:263-275.

Rollnick S, Heather N, Gold R et al. (1992). Development of a short 'readiness to change' questionnaire for use in brief, opportunistic interventions among excessive drinkers. *British Journal of Addiction* 87:743-754.

Rosman AS & Lieber CS (1992). Overview of current and emerging markers of alcoholism. In RZ Litten & JP Allen (eds.) *Measuring Alcohol Consumption: Psychosocial and Biochemical Methods.* Totowa, NJ: The Humana Press, Inc., 99-134.

Saitz R (1999). Screening tests for alcohol use disorders. *Annals of Internal Medicine* 130(9):779 (discussion 779-780).

Saitz R, Lepore MF, Sullivan LM et al. (1999). Alcohol abuse and dependence in Latinos living in the United States: Validation of the CAGE (4M) questions. *Archives of Internal Medicine* 159(7):718-724.

Saitz R, Mulvey KP, Plough A et al. (1997). Physician unawareness of serious substance abuse. *American Journal of Drug and Alcohol Abuse* 23:343-354.

Sanchez-Craig M (1980). Random assignment to abstinence or controlled drinking in a cognitive-behavioral program: Short-term effects on drinking behavior. *Addictive Behaviors* 5:35-39.

Sanchez-Craig M & Lei H (1986). Disadvantages to imposing the goal of abstinence on problem drinkers: An empirical study. *British Journal of Addiction* 81:505-512.

Sanchez-Craig M, Wilkinson DA & Davila R (1995). Empirically based guidelines for moderate drinking: 1-year results from three studies with problem drinkers. *American Journal of Public Health* 85(6):823-828.

Saunders J, Aasland O, Babor T et al. (1993). Development of the alcohol use disorders identification test (AUDIT): WHO collaborative project on early detection of persons with harmful alcohol consumption—II. *Addiction* 88:791-804.

Scivoletto S, DeAndrade A & Castel S (1992). The effect of a 'recall system' in the treatment of alcoholic patients. *British Journal of Addiction* 87:1185-1188.

Selzer M, Vinokur A & Van Rooijen I (1975). A self-administered Short Michigan Alcoholism Screening Test (SMAST). *Journal of Studies on Alcohol* 36:117-126.

Senft RA, Polen MR, Freeborn DK et al. (1997). Brief intervention in a primary care setting for hazardous drinkers. *American Journal of Preventive Medicine* 13:464-470.

Seppa K, Lepisto J & Sillanaukee P (1998). Five-shot questionnaire on heavy drinking. *Alcoholism: Clinical & Experimental Research* 22(8):1788-1791.

Seppa K, Makela R & Sillanaukee P (1995). Effectiveness of the alcohol use disorders identification test in occupational health screenings. *Alcoholism: Clinical & Experimental Research* 19(4):999-1003.

Skinner H, Allen B, McIntosh M et al. (1985). Lifestyle assessment: Just asking makes a difference. *British Medical Journal* 290:214-216.

Skinner H, Holt S, Schuller R et al. (1984). Identification of alcohol abuse using laboratory tests and a history of trauma. *Annals of Internal Medicine* 101:847-851.

Skinner H, Holt S, Sheu W et al. (1986). Clinical versus laboratory detection of alcohol abuse: The alcohol clinical index. *British Medical Journal* 292:1703-1708.

Sobell L, Cunningham J & Sobell M (1996). Recovery from alcohol problems with and without treatment: Prevalence in two populations surveys. *American Journal of Public Health* 86(7)966-972.

Sobell LC, Sobell MB & Toneatto T (1992). Recovery from alcohol problems without treatment. In N Heather, WR Miller & J Greeley (eds.) *Self-Control and the Addictive Behaviors.* New York, NY: Maxwell MacMillan, 198-242.

Sobell MB & Sobell LC (1993). *Problem Drinkers Guided Self-Change Treatment.* New York, NY: Guilford Press.

Steinbauer JR, Cantor SB, Holzer CE 3rd et al. (1998). Ethnic and sex bias in primary care screening tests for alcohol use disorders. *Annals of Internal Medicine* 129(5):353-362.

Taj N, Devera-Sales A & Vinson DC (1998). Screening for problem drinking: Does a single question work? *Journal of Family Practice* 46(4):328-335.

Taylor CB, Houston-Miller N, Killen JD et al. (1990). Smoking cessation after acute myocardial infarction: Effects of a nurse-managed intervention. *Annals of Internal Medicine* 113:118-123.

Ubel PA (1999). Physicians' duties in an era of cost containment: Advocacy or betrayal? *Journal of the American Medical Association* 282(17):1675.

Volk RJ, Steinbauer JR, Cantor SB et al. (1997). The Alcohol Use Disorders Identification Test (AUDIT) as a screen for at-risk drinking in primary care patients of different racial/ethnic backgrounds. *Addiction* 92(2):197-206.

Wallace P, Cutler S & Haines A (1988). Randomised controlled trial of general practitioner intervention in patients with excessive alcohol consumption. *British Medical Journal* 297:663-668.

Walsh DC, Hingson RW, Merrigan DM et al. (1992). The impact of a physician's warning on recovery after alcoholism treatment. *Journal of the American Medical Association* 267(5):663-667.

Wasson J, Gaudette C, Whaley F et al. (1992). Telephone care as a substitute for routine clinic follow-up. *Journal of the American Medical Association* 267(13):1788-1793.

Weaver MF, Jarvis MA & Schnoll SH (1999). Role of the primary care physician in problems of substance abuse. Review. *Archives of Internal Medicine* 159(9):913-924.

Wilk AI, Jensen NM & Havighurst TC (1997). Meta-analysis of randomized control trials addressing brief interventions in heavy alcohol drinkers. *Journal of General Internal Medicine* 12(5):274-283.

World Health Organization (WHO), Brief Intervention Group (1996). A cross-national trial of brief interventions with heavy drinkers. *American Journal of Public Health* 86(7):948-955.

Chapter 5 | Assessment

David R. Gastfriend, M.D.
Sharon Reif, Ph.D.
Sharon L. Baker, Ph.D.
Lisa M. Najavits, Ph.D.

Using Assessment Instruments in Treatment Planning
Characteristics of Valid Assessment Instruments
Instruments for Standardized Assessments
Introducing Assessment Instruments Into Practice

At its best, the clinical practice of addiction medicine offers treatments that, because they are tailored to the patient's needs, are effective and efficient. The rapid rise in health care costs has alarmed many employers and payers of care, including the federal government. Concern over costs, coupled with the perception that much care is unnecessary or provided inefficiently, has given rise to increasingly widespread techniques to manage health benefits and hold clinicians more accountable for the services provided (Institute of Medicine, 1990). Clinicians must continually advocate for their patients' access to quality care while remaining mindful of the demands for cost containment.

Over the past decade, the field of addiction medicine has been challenged to examine the status of patient evaluation after coming under particular scrutiny by the United States Congress, which asked the Institute of Medicine (IOM) to study treatment services for persons with alcohol problems. The IOM study noted that society is struggling with two cost-versus-quality questions that challenge clinicians to rethink our system of care: "First, how do we ensure that people get needed medical care without spending so much that other social objectives are compromised? Sec-

ond, how do we discourage unnecessary and inappropriate medical services without jeopardizing necessary, high-quality care?" The committee's report "Broadening the Base of Treatment for Alcohol Problems," defined a need for improvements in pretreatment assessment of alcohol problems so as to facilitate appropriate treatment decisions (IOM, 1990).

This thinking represented a departure from the 1980s, when the standard for treatment was to refer patients to the most intensive services they would accept. Current standards look to optimize the match between patient and treatment without relying on the assumption that the most promising treatment for a given patient is the most intensive treatment available. There is growing empirical support for matching strategies, although there is not yet uniformity in the variables used or the methods of implementation (Gastfriend & McLellan, 1997).

Any successful matching strategy must rely initially on the identification of key matching variables. Mattson and colleagues (1994) reviewed 31 empirical studies of treatment matching and identified at least four categories of clinical variables important to the matching process: (1) demographics, (2) addiction-specific characteristics such as severity, (3) intrapersonal characteristics such as psychopathology and motivation, and (4) interpersonal function, including environmental factors and social support.

Formal assessment instruments may provide the standardization and credibility necessary for effective treatment matching, which ideally becomes a critical step in overall treatment planning. Reviewers frequently require providers to assess patients in at least the following areas in order to justify their participation in a particular treatment: (1) diagnosis, (2) severity of addiction, and (3) motivation and rehabilitation potential. These areas roughly correspond to the matching variables identified by Mattson and colleagues (1994) and can be assessed using available instruments with known reliability and validity.

USING ASSESSMENT INSTRUMENTS IN TREATMENT PLANNING

The considerations cited above demand new approaches to clinical assessment and documentation. Whereas traditionally the patient record served only to communicate clinical data among providers, today it is crucial in determining what type of care the patient will receive and, indeed, whether the patient will receive care at all. Interest in assessment instruments no longer is limited to research domains, now that managed care entities require clinicians to justify and document decisions about treatment. As third-party payers demand increased communication between providers and managed care monitors, uniform assessment becomes a necessity. Patient evaluations that document the assessment process in an objective way offer the distinct advantage of providing justification for any treatment recommendations derived from them.

Formal assessment instruments for treatment planning generally offer several advantages over the conventional clinical interview for both treatment matching and treatment planning. A valid instrument offers a uniform inquiry, comprehensive coverage of essential areas, quantification of data, and standardization of the interpretations of the data. Assessments without instruments cannot provide these features, because interviewers may vary widely in style (for example, use of open- versus closed-ended questions), areas of inquiry (severity of substance dependence versus psychopathology), depth of inquiry (screening superficially in some areas versus detailed probing in others), units of measure (severity of drug use may be measured in terms of quantity, frequency, recency, and/or expenditures), and—most importantly—interviewers may vary widely in the assumptions they use in interpreting assessment results.

While a plethora of measures exists (Allen, 1995), the instruments presented in this chapter have been selected for their utility in treatment matching and treatment planning, their strong psychometric properties (reliability and validity), and the availability of data on their use. The instruments described provide information in the areas of clinical diagnosis, severity of substance abuse and dependence, and motivation and treatment readiness. Instruments may be combined to create a comprehensive battery that yields data for matching patients to levels of care, which presents exciting new possibilities for patient evaluation.

Clinical Diagnosis. Clinical diagnosis is perhaps the most fully developed assessment area because of the general acceptance of the criteria of the *Diagnostic and Statistical Manual of Mental Disorders* of the American Psychiatric Association (*DSM-IV;* 1994).

Several clinical interview instruments exist for establishing *DSM-IV* diagnoses of psychoactive substance use disorders. Of these, the Structured Clinical Interview for *DSM-IV* (SCID; First, Spitzer et al., 2001) is the most readily incorporated into a battery aimed at use in both research and clinical evaluation. Other measures are available, but the requirements for their administration may be less than ideal in most circumstances. The Schedule for Affective Disorders and Schizophrenia (SADS; Endicott & Spitzer, 1978), for example, requires interviewers with graduate degrees and fairly extensive clinical experience and can take up to 4 hours to administer. The Diagnostic Interview Schedule (DIS; Robins, Helzer et al., 1981) was designed for administration by non-clinicians and proceeds on a symptom-by-symptom basis, with the requirement that each question be read verbatim from a booklet (Hasin, 1991). The DIS also is available in a self-administered, computerized format.

The SCID thus provides a middle ground in terms of structure, level of expertise required for administration, and duration of the interview.

Substance Abuse and Dependence Severity. The term "severity" is used in relation to addiction to refer both to the severity of the addictive behavior itself (that is, the level of dependence and associated risks of withdrawal), and to functional impairments related to the addictive behavior (that is, the severity of the consequences of that behavior for other areas of life functioning). Assessment of severity for purposes of treatment matching and treatment planning must take into account both uses of the term.

Severity of the addictive behavior is a multidimensional construct. To illustrate this problem, consider two examples: One patient has severe dependence and uses infrequently but in binges of large amounts. These activities are self-destructive in terms of legal violations and physical injury to self and others. Another patient with severe dependence uses regularly without intoxication but with multiple medical, career, and family disruptions and losses.

An effective instrument must characterize these differing patterns and yield some absolute level of severity that renders a similar score for both patients. To accomplish this, the instrument must measure severity across multiple dimensions. Of the instruments available for assessing severity, one of the earliest and most widely used is the Addiction Severity Index (ASI; McLellan, Luborsky et al., 1980), which was the first to provide a multidimensional assessment of substance abuse severity. A more recently developed instrument is the Drinker Inventory of Consequences (DrInC; Miller, Tonigan et al., 1995), which provides a comprehensive assessment of the extent of alcohol problems other than consumption and dependence.

Motivation and Treatment Readiness. Patient treatment readiness is a fundamental consideration in addiction treatment planning, yet it often is evaluated on an intuitive basis. Clinicians routinely report motivation as a global quality, which they believe may predict the patient's likelihood of treatment success. For example, a 1990 pilot study of patients newly admitted for addiction treatment found that demographic factors and comorbidity collectively accounted for only one-third of the variance in outcomes, while nurses' global ratings of patients' motivation significantly added to the prediction of outcome (Marc A. Schuckit, personal communication).

Because treatment readiness is a more recent area of investigation, the repertoire of available instruments is less well studied than in the case of diagnosis or severity assessment. However, several instruments are available that assess various aspects of motivation and readiness for treatment. The RAATE-CE (Mee-Lee & Hoffman, 1992; Mee-Lee, 1985, 1988), assesses treatment readiness as a multidimensional construct that combines patient awareness of problems, behavioral intent to change, capacity to anticipate future treatment needs, and medical, psychiatric, or environmental impediments. The University of Rhode Island Change Assessment Scale (URICA; DiClemente &

Hughes, 1992) assesses Prochaska and DiClemente's (1992) stages of change model. The Stages of Change Readiness and Treatment Eagerness Scale (SOCRATES; Miller & Tonigan, 1996) assesses the three factors of Recognition, Ambivalence, and Taking Steps. The Circumstances, Motivation, Readiness, and Suitability Scale (CMRS; DeLeon, Melnick et al., 1994) measures patients' perceptions across the four related domains.

CHARACTERISTICS OF VALID ASSESSMENT INSTRUMENTS

An assessment instrument should demonstrate certain psychometric properties if it is to be accepted for clinical research or routine clinical use. The items that make up the instrument should have clear meanings, should be distinct and parsimonious (that is, non-redundant), and should relate to one another in a coherent way (for example, items that are logically connected should be grouped with one another in subscales). Different raters should be able to use the instrument and obtain similar ratings (*inter-rater reliability*) and the same patient should obtain similar results on two different, yet closely spaced administrations (*test-retest reliability*).

In addition to reliability, an instrument must have demonstrated validity. The instrument and its items should be based on an underlying logical framework, or construct. The instrument should make sense as an effort to assess the intended area: that is, it should demonstrate *face validity*. If an accepted "gold standard" measure exists, a comparative trial between the two instruments should yield similar results, demonstrating *convergent validity*. Different scores should distinguish different outcomes, demonstrating *predictive validity*. Finally, the instrument should obtain different results from those of another instrument designed for a different purpose (*discriminant validity*).

Issues in Patient Self-Report. One of the greatest challenges of clinical assessment in addiction treatment is the reliability of patient self-report. Effective interviewing depends on helping patients to understand the meaning of each question, to organize their recollections, and to avoid defensiveness about their behaviors. In general, the reliability of patient self-report can be improved by using a consistent sequence of questions, which progress from general to specific information, and an interview style that moves from an open-ended to a closed-ended question format.

What follows is the description of a set of instruments that incorporates these principles and that provides a comprehensive assessment capable of yielding sufficient information for treatment matching and/or treatment planning. The battery includes the SCID for *DSM-IV* (First, Spitzer et al., 2001), the Clinical Institute Withdrawal Assessment-Alcohol, Revised (CIWA-Ar; Sullivan, Sykora et al., 1989), the ASI (McLellan, Luborsky et al., 1980; McLellan, Kushner et al., 1992), and the RAATE-CE (Mee-Lee, 1985, 1988).

INSTRUMENTS FOR STANDARDIZED ASSESSMENTS

Structured Clinical Interview for DSM-IV (SCID).

The Structured Clinical Interview for *DSM-IV* (SCID) is a widely used, semistructured interview that obtains Axis I and II diagnoses using *DSM-IV* criteria. The SCID is designed for use with psychiatric, medical, or community-based normal adults (Spitzer, Williams et al., 1989). Its reliability and validity have been demonstrated in numerous studies. It is composed of one module for each major syndrome group in the *DSM-IV*: anxiety disorders, affective disorders, psychotic disorders, and substance use disorders. Each module may stand on its own for assessment of that particular diagnostic syndrome. Each question on the SCID corresponds to a specific *DSM-IV* criterion. The questions are sequenced to carefully obey the decision rule process and to yield a diagnosis only if the patient meets all requisite *DSM-IV* criteria.

The SCID is designed for use by a clinical evaluator trained at the master's or doctoral level, although in research settings it has been used by bachelor's level technicians with extensive training. Administration of Axis I and Axis II batteries may require more than two hours each for patients with multiple diagnoses. The Psychoactive Substance Use Disorders module may be administered by itself in 30 to 60 minutes, depending on the extent of the patient's substance use history and current involvement.

For the Psychoactive Substance Use Disorders module, the SCID poses a query for each *DSM-IV* criterion for abuse/dependence, first for alcohol and then for each non-alcohol psychoactive substance. The information is collected in such a way that it is possible to establish lifetime diagnoses, age of onset of first abuse or dependence, and current severity.

In a recent study, Kranzler and colleagues (1996) reported on the validity of SCID substance abuse diagnoses, using the SCID for *DSM-IIIR*. The researchers were able to demonstrate both concurrent and discriminant validity for both alcohol and drug abuse/dependence diagnoses with a number of related measures, including the ASI, with significance for the most part in the range of p<.001. For comorbid major depression and antisocial personality disorders, validity was established with a smaller number of concurrent measures in the significance range of p<.05 to p<.01. Concurrent validity was not demonstrated for comorbid anxiety. Predictive validity using measures of substance use at six-month followup generally was good and significant, with some variability across measures for abuse and dependence, but not for comorbid disorders.

One reason for the poorer showing of the SCID in diagnosing comorbid disorders may be that the *DSM-IIIR* version did not assess specifically for substance-induced disorders. Anxiety symptoms, in particular, tend to be high in early abstinence and can be difficult to differentially diagnose. The *DSM-IV* incorporates substance-induced mood disorders and substance-induced anxiety disorders as distinct categories with specific diagnostic criteria. The SCID for *DSM-IV* includes separate modules for obtaining substance-induced diagnoses, which are linked to the mood and anxiety modules by specific skip-out instructions. Improved validity for comorbid diagnoses might be expected with the presence of the substance-induced disorder modules.

Because the SCID is constructed around the *DSM-IV*, it uses symptom criteria based on the loss of behavioral control model for the spectrum of dependence-producing substances. Although it does measure criterion-based symptomatology, the SCID is too limited for a comprehensive treatment evaluation and should be supplemented with an instrument that has been designed for severity assessment, such as the ASI or the DrInC.

Clinical Institute Withdrawal Assessment-Alcohol, Revised (CIWA-Ar).

Often the first step in conducting an addiction assessment is to establish degree of risk associated with the current level of acute intoxication. The CIWA-Ar is a brief scale of 10 items (requiring less than two minutes to administer), which provides a clinical quantification of the severity of the alcohol withdrawal syndrome. The instrument was developed and reliability and validity data obtained on patients in alcohol withdrawal, although it has been shown to be useful in assessing withdrawal from other benzodiazepine drugs as well.

An observer rates the intensity of 10 common withdrawal symptoms and a total score is obtained by summing the ratings from the 10 items. It can be administered by trained non-medical personnel, such as detoxification unit workers or research assistants.

Addiction Severity Index (ASI). The ASI is a widely used semistructured interview that is designed to elicit information about areas of the patient's life that may contribute to and/or be affected by his or her substance use problem. The ASI assesses seven dimensions that typically are of foremost concern to patients with substance dependence. These are: Medical Status, Employment/Support Status, Drug/Alcohol Use, Legal Status, Family History, Family/Social Relationships (including family history), and Psychiatric Status. The ASI asks factual questions about the amount of alcohol and drug use within the preceding 30 days as well as lifetime use, about living arrangements and disruptions in relationships, and about the number of legal charges resulting in convictions.

The ASI has been used for both clinical and research purposes and has been incorporated into some large-scale intake and referral programs, such as the U.S. Target Cities Program demonstration project for city-wide drug treatment improvement and the Drug Evaluation Network System, which tracks trends in addiction treatment (Carise, McLellan et al., 1999). It is designed to be administered by a trained technician in approximately 40 to 60 minutes. It also is available in a self-administered, computerized format. A subset of items is used in followup interviews to assess the patient's progress over time. The ASI can be administered as frequently as once a month to assess serial change.

A potentially useful feature of the ASI is that it first establishes with the patient a detailed list of adverse behaviors and consequences of addiction. Then, having acknowledged these consequences, the patient is asked to assess the severity of his or her problems in each area. A Severity Rating Scale asks "How important to you now is treatment for these alcohol problems?" on a five-point scale, with potential responses ranging from "not at all important" to "extremely important."

The fact that the ASI, like most clinical interviews, relies heavily on historical data obtained from the patient, without access to external corroboration, presents a potential limitation to the validity of the data obtained. As a check on the subjective quality of the patient's self-report, the ASI incorporates the judgment of the rater about the patient's apparent comprehension or misrepresentation. In addition, there is an interviewer severity rating in which the interviewer is asked to estimate severity on each ASI dimension, using a 10-point scale. These ratings have been shown to produce reliable and valid estimates of patient status (McLellan, Luborsky et al., 1985; Hodgins & el-Guebaly, 1992).

The ASI provides a composite score for each dimension. Composite scoring increases standardization because, being mathematically derived, it obviates the need to use the rater's judgment to gauge the quantitative severity (McGahan, Griffith et al., 1986). Composite scores were constructed by selecting and combining items from each problem area that had the capacity to demonstrate change in patient status. The items included in each composite were shown to have fairly high internal consistency (alphas of .70 or higher on each of the composites). Comparison by the instrument's authors with other well-validated measures for each ASI dimension has shown significant convergent validity for all composite scores (McLellan, Luborsky et al., 1985).

The ASI was developed and initially validated in methadone maintenance populations, but since has been validated in other substance-dependent populations (Alterman, McDermott et al., 2000). It has shown excellent capabilities for characterizing severe dependence with multiple areas of dysfunction, such as homeless substance abusers (Argeriou, McCarty et al., 1994) and those with psychiatric impairment (Hodgins & el-Guebaly, 1992). However, because it was developed for use in more severely dependent heroin addicts, it primarily measures gross impairments associated with substance use. For example, it provides data on loss of income or employment, degree of legal involvement, and number of previous detoxifications. While in certain settings this may be a strength, in others it may represent a limitation. By itself, the ASI may lack sufficient resolution to adequately characterize problems in less severe patients such as alcoholic outpatients.

The ASI recently has been supplemented by an Expanded Female Version (ASI-F; Brown, Frank et al., 1995). The ASI-F was designed to be used in the same manner and for the same purposes as the ASI. Some of the new items refer to problems and situations unique to women, such as how many times the subject has been pregnant or given birth. Other items, while possibly more relevant to women, actually may apply to men as well. These include information on the gender and age of children, a history of sexually transmitted diseases, and a recent history of homelessness. The name "Female" thus is somewhat misleading, as the instrument can be used with male patients. This version of the ASI has established reliability and validity.

Severity-of-illness data based on past and recent history of drug use and consequences establish a baseline assessment of severity, but not an ongoing short-term measurement of improvement. To plan efficient individualized treatment, assessment of severity requires instruments that provide a comprehensive severity assessment at the time of admission, and also are sensitive and flexible enough to measure short-term treatment response (for example, within a five- to seven-day inpatient detoxification). The ASI was developed for re-administration, but at a minimum of 30-day intervals. It measures gross functional impairments that are not likely to change in brief time frames or in restrictive treatment settings.

Finally, the ASI and most severity-oriented evaluation tools lack items for assessing patient attitudes, cognitive understanding of chemical dependence, treatment expectations, and commitment to treatment. Yet these are areas of great significance in treatment and are widely regarded as concurrent indicators of progress. This is the basis for supplementing severity assessment with a measure of motivation and treatment readiness.

Recovery Attitude and Treatment Evaluator (RAATE-CE). The Recovery Attitude and Treatment Evaluator (RAATE-CE) was designed to quantify patient resistance and impediments to addiction treatment. The RAATE-CE is a clinician-rated structured interview that assesses five areas relevant to substance abuse treatment planning decisions: (1) degree of resistance to treatment, (2) degree of resistance to continuing care, (3) acuity of biomedical problems, (4) acuity of psychiatric problems, and (5) extent of social, family and/or environmental systems that are not supportive of recovery (Mee-Lee, Hoffman et al., 1992; Mee-Lee, 1985, 1988). It is designed to be administered by a trained counselor and requires approximately 35 minutes to complete.

The RAATE-CE consists of 35 items, rated on a one- to four-point fixed interval scale, on which higher scores represent greater resistance or impediments to recovery. A typical item asks, "Is the patient aware of an addiction problem?" The RAATE also permits serial assessment of treatment progress (Mee-Lee, 1988).

In a study of 139 public sector, high severity patients, inter-rater reliability on the five RAATE dimensions was reported to range from .59 to .77. Internal consistency coefficients ranged from .65 to .87 (Smith, Hoffman et al., 1992). Inter-rater reliability was higher with raters who had higher levels of clinical expertise. The validity of the RAATE-CE has been studied in 220 consecutive admissions to an inpatient addictions unit (Gastfriend, Filstead et al., 1995). Patients were assessed on the RAATE-CE by counselors shortly after admission, and the results were compared to patients' discharge dispositions. All five RAATE dimensions yielded one or more associations with subsequent treatment outcomes in the expected directions, thus providing initial evidence of predictive validity of the instrument. In particular, on the RAATE-B, C, D and E dimensions, significant mean group differences occurred between subjects who required extended hospital rehabilitation versus those discharged to less restrictive settings (p=.046 to .001). RAATE-B, D, and E significantly differentiated between the groups who would accept intensive treatments versus those who left against medical advice (p=.071 to <.001).

The RAATE-CE subsequently has been revised for use in clinical research (RAATE-CE/R). The RAATE-CE/R provides probe questions in preparation for each scored item and provides descriptive anchors to explain quantitative ratings. Preliminary reliability data indicate high inter-rater reliability, high internal consistency, independence of subscales, and a factor structure that partially supports the scale's original design (Najavits, Gastfriend et al., 1996).

INTRODUCING ASSESSMENT INSTRUMENTS INTO PRACTICE

In the authors' experience, most patients view these assessment instruments positively as a means to further understand themselves and as a thought-provoking inquiry. However, for a smaller subset, resistance to a structured interview format initially is strong, so that implementing the protocol requires attention to both clinical and interpersonal skills. Particularly if the data are to be used for research as well as clinical purposes, it is not uncommon for the patient to feel like a "research guinea pig." It often is helpful to explore such feelings at the outset of the interview. Feeling that the interviewer is concerned and interested in him or her as a person usually can dispel subjects' negative reactions to the interview. In situations in which research subjects subsequently will be receiving treatment, it also is helpful to emphasize that the results will enhance the staff's ability to help them. A supportive and nonjudgmental style, a conversational approach (rather than a checklist), and the opportunity to take a break if necessary are essential to developing an atmosphere of comfort and respect.

It is essential to provide thorough training in each instrument, regardless of the level of education and expertise of the clinician rater. Manuals for each of the instruments provide a basis for standardized training; training tapes also are available. Training can be tailored to meet site-specific as well as individual needs. It is important that training be treated as an iterative process. Ideally, raters need to receive feedback not only throughout the training process but intermittently thereafter in order to prevent slippage from the standardized administration. In addition to receiving feedback on their performance, it is important to elicit feedback from raters on an ongoing basis about their experiences in using the battery and to provide them with updates about the usefulness of the data they have collected.

Using Assessments To Individualize Treatment Planning. Studies on spontaneous smoking cessation have conceptualized motivation in terms of stages of behavioral change. This literature, subsequently generalized to all substance dependence, contradicts the view of low motivation as a trait characteristic, but rather describes a dynamic forward spiraling pattern (Prochaska & DiClemente, 1992) through which change efforts may successfully progress as a result of the interaction between patient and clinician (Miller & Rollnick, 1991). These findings suggest that the clinician needs to go beyond conventional data-gathering to measure and then influence the patient's motivational state (Prochaska & DiClemente, 1992).

The data-gathering processes involved in a clinical assessment can promote behavioral change by providing detailed objective feedback to the patient about his or her behaviors, symptoms, and consequences. Sometimes, the objective interview process itself may help the patient to move from the precontemplation stage to the contemplation stage (during which he or she becomes aware of a need to change). When further strategies are necessary to enhance this transition, comprehensive patient history data gathered with these instruments can be helpful in confronting denial about the degree to which substance use has been a causal factor in losses.

While the structured clinical interview may be a more powerful way of confronting the patient with his or her problems, alternatives do exist. These are paper and pencil questionnaires that can be completed by the patient in a relatively short period of time. The obvious advantage of such questionnaires is the time saved for the clinician interviewer. The obvious disadvantage is that the clinician interviewer does not have an opportunity to interact with the patient and thus loses a chance to obtain a better sense of the validity and reliability of what the patient is reporting. However, the results of such self-administered instruments can be used as a guide for the clinician or interviewer in future interactions with the patient.

Questionnaires with known reliability and validity for assessing severity and motivation/readiness to change can, however, be an invaluable adjunct to treatment matching and/or planning where a structured clinical interview is either not possible or not desirable. They may be used in conjunction with the full structured clinical interview described earlier, or as substitutes for some or all of the instruments. The instruments described below focus on the problem areas that are important not only in planning treatment, but in offering feedback to the patient regarding problems and accompanying attitudes.

Drinker Inventory of Consequences (DrInC). The Drinker Inventory of Consequences (DrInC) was developed to provide a comprehensive assessment of drinking problems and consequences, separate from consumption and dependence (Miller, 1995). Unlike the ASI, which assesses functional impairment across dimensions without reference to a specific causal connection to drinking, the DrInC asks the respondent to make a connection between drinking and his or her problems.

The DrInC is a paper and pencil questionnaire that can be completed in about 10 minutes. It asks about physical consequences ranging from hangovers to impact on sexual functioning; intrapersonal consequences such as guilt, shame, loss of interest, and loss of spirituality; social responsibility consequences relating to failure to meet obligations; interpersonal consequences regarding family and friends; and impulse control consequences, including motor vehicle crashes, fights, and arrests. It also contains a number of reverse-scored items as a validity check against blanket denial of all problems.

The pretreatment assessment version of the DrInC consists of two scales containing the same items. One set of items asks for yes/no responses to questions related to "Lifetime Consequences." The other set provides a Likert scale, which allows for an intensity measure of "Recent Consequences." There are other forms of the DrInC, including a short form, a version to be completed by the significant other, and an "Inventory of Drug Use Consequences" (InDUC).

The DrInC has demonstrated both internal consistency within subscales (generally in the .70 to .80 range) and independence between subscales. It has adequate test-retest reliability. It can be hand-scored and the raw scores easily transferred to a profile sheet. Separate profiles sheets for men and women reflect gender differences in the pattern of scores.

The advantage of the DrInC is that is quick and simple to administer. The disadvantage is that, because it is a paper and pencil questionnaire, there is no opportunity for a clinician or interviewer to probe responses.

University of Rhode Island Change Assessment Scale (URICA). The URICA measures the four theoretical stages of change proposed by Prochaska and DiClemente (1992): precontemplation, contemplation, action, and maintenance. It is designed to measure change across a variety of problem areas; specific versions have been adapted for alcohol- and drug-abusing populations. Items are in the form of a statement and are endorsed on a five-point scale from "strongly disagree" to "strongly agree." For example, a typical item is the statement, "As far as I'm concerned, I don't have any problems that need changing." The URICA is a paper-and-pencil questionnaire that requires about 10 minutes to complete

Both internal consistency and test-retest reliability have been established. The scale offers a single readiness score. It also has been used to profile patients in terms of their stage of change with mixed success (Abellanas & McLellan, 1993; DiClemente & Hughes, 1990).

Stages of Change Readiness and Treatment-Eagerness Scale (SOCRATES). The SOCRATES was designed to assess motivation for change in problem drinkers. It is a paper and pencil questionnaire with both a short (19-item) and a longer (39-item) version. The scale identifies three subgroups. The first group has been variously described as either "Uninvolved" or "Recognition," the second group as "Ambivalent," and the third group as either "Active" or "Taking Steps" (Isenhart, 1994; Miller & Tonigan, 1996). Reliability has been established.

Circumstances, Motivation, Readiness Scale (CMRS). The CMRS was designed to measure patient perceptions within the specific context of the therapeutic community. Patients endorse statements on each of four subscales, using a five-point scale ranging from "strongly disagree" to "strongly agree." There are 58 items. The scale yields a total score as well as four subscale scores. An example of an item on the Circumstances Subscale is, "I am sure that I would have come to treatment without the pressure of my legal involvement." The scale has been used to predict treatment retention in a therapeutic community (DeLeon,

Melnick et al., 1994). In the same study, discriminant and factor analyses confirmed the face validity of the four subscales. Internal consistency has been demonstrated.

CONCLUSIONS

The instruments described here provide clear benefits for initiating treatment planning. The SCID diagnostic assessment comprehensively assesses use of all addictive substances and yields definitive data on the need for psychiatric evaluation. The CIWA-Ar provides an objective assessment of the risk of alcohol withdrawal at the initiation of treatment. The ASI delineates case management needs and is ideal for outlining a comprehensive treatment plan. The RAATE determines the patient's acceptance and willingness to engage in active treatment and targets specific treatment impediments for intervention. There are as yet no standards for discrete scores or thresholds for categorizing patients for targeted treatments. Further research is needed to validate the use of these instruments for predicting individual treatment outcomes and for optimizing treatment plans.

All of the measures discussed, particularly when incorporated into treatment planning in some combination, can be expected to improve the uniformity, comprehensiveness, and inter-agency or inter-provider reliability of clinical assessment. Despite the costs of training, staff adaptation, and additional time for the duration of administration, these gains can be expected to yield improvements in time and, hopefully, cost efficiency in the long run.

ACKNOWLEDGMENT: Preparation of this chapter was supported by grant No. DA07693-02 from the National Institute on Drug Abuse, the Center for Substance Abuse Treatment, and the Parkside Medical Services Corporation, Parkside, IL.

REFERENCES

Abellanas L & McLellan AT (1993). "Stage of change" by drug problem in concurrent opioid, cocaine, and cigarette users. *Journal of Psychoactive Drugs* 25:307-313.

Allen JP (1995). *Assessing Alcohol Problems: A Guide for Clinicians and Researchers (NIAAA Treatment Handbook, Series 4).* Rockville, MD: National Institute on Alcohol Abuse and Alcoholism.

Alterman AI, McDermott PA, Cook TG et al. (2000). Generalizability of the clinical dimensions of the Addiction Severity Index to nonopioid-dependent patients. *Psychology of Addictive Behaviors* 14:287-294.

American Psychiatric Association (APA) (1994). *Diagnostic and Statistical Manual of Mental Disorders, 4th Edition (DSM-IV)*. Washington, DC: American Psychiatric Press.

Argeriou M, McCarty D, Mulvey K et al. (1994). Use of the Addiction Severity Index with homeless substance abusers. *Journal of Substance Abuse Treatment* 11:359-365.

Brown E, Frank D & Friedman A (1995). *Supplementary Administration Manual for the Expanded Female Version of the Addiction Severity Index (ASI) Instrument, The ASI-F*. Herndon, VA: Head & Co., Inc.

Carise D, McLellan AT, Gifford LS et al. (1999). Developing a national addiction treatment information system. An introduction to the Drug Evaluation Network System. *Journal of Substance Abuse Treatment* 17:62-77.

DeLeon, G, Melnick G, Kressler D et al. (1994). Circumstances, motivation, readiness, and suitability (the CMRS scales): Predicting retention in therapeutic community treatment. *American Journal of Drug and Alcohol Abuse* 20(4):495-515.

DiClemente CC & Hughes SO (1990). Stages of change profiles in outpatient alcoholism treatment. *Journal of Substance Abuse* 2:2172-2175.

Endicott J & Spitzer RL (1978). A diagnostic interview: The Schedule for Affective Disorders and Schizophrenia. *Archives of General Psychiatry* 35(7):837-844.

First MB, Spitzer RL, Gibbon ML et al. (2001). *Structured Clinical Interview for DSM-IV-TR Axis I Disorders, Research Version, Patient Version (SCID I/P)*. New York, NY: Biometrics Research Department, New York State Psychiatric Institute.

Gastfriend DR, Filstead WJ, Reif S et al. (1995). Validity of assessing treatment readiness in patients with substance use disorders. *American Journal on Addictions* 4(5):254-260.

Gastfriend DR & McLellan AT (1997). Treatment matching: Theoretic and practical implications. *Medical Clinics of North America* 81(4):1-22.

Hasin D (1991). Diagnostic interviews for assessment: Background, reliability, validity. *Alcohol Health & Research World* 15:293-302.

Hodgins D & el-Guebaly N (1992). More data on the Addiction Severity Index: Reliability and validity with the mentally ill substance abuser. *Journal of Nervous and Mental Disease* 180:197-201.

Institute of Medicine (1990). *Broadening the Base of Treatment for Alcohol Problems: A Report of a Study by a Committee of the Institute of Medicine, Division of Mental Health and Behavioral Medicine*. Washington, DC: National Academy Press.

Isenhart C (1994). Motivational subtypes in an inpatient sample of substance abusers. *Addictive Behaviors* 19:463-475.

Kranzler H, Kadden R, Babor T et al. (1996). Validity of the SCID in substance abuse patients. *Addiction* 91:859-868.

LaJeunesse C & Thorenson R (1988). Generalizing a predictor of male alcoholic treatment outcomes. *International Journal of Addiction* 23:183-205.

Letteri D, Nelson J & Sayers M (1985). *Alcoholism Treatment Assessment Research Instruments*. Rockville, MD: National Institute on Alcohol Abuse and Alcoholism.

Mattson ME, Allen JP, Longabaugh R et al. (1994). A chronological review of empirical studies matching alcoholic clients to treatment. *Journal of Studies on Alcohol* 12(Suppl):16-29.

McGahan P, Griffith J, Parente R et al. (1986). Composite scores from the Addiction Severity Index. Pittsburgh, PA: Penn-VA Center for Studies of Addiction (unpublished manuscript).

McLellan AT, Kushner H, Metzger D et al. (1992). The fifth edition of the Addiction Severity Index. *Journal of Substance Abuse Treatment* 9:199-213.

McLellan AT, Luborsky L, Cacciola J et al. (1985). New data from the addiction severity index—Reliability and validity in three centers. *Journal of Nervous and Mental Disease* 173:412-423.

McLellan AT, Luborsky L & Woody GE (1980). An improved diagnostic evaluation instrument for substance abuse patients: The Addiction Severity Index. *Journal of Nervous and Mental Diseases* 168:26-33.

Mee-Lee D (1985). The Recovery Attitude and Treatment Evaluator (RAATE) an instrument for patient progress and treatment assignment. *Proceedings of the 34th International Congress on Alcoholism and Drug Dependence* 424-426.

Mee-Lee D (1988). An instrument for treatment progress and matching: The Recovery Attitude and Treatment Evaluator (RAATE). *Journal of Substance Abuse Treatment* 5:183-186.

Mee-Lee D, Hoffmann NG & Smith MB (1992). *The Recovery Attitude and Treatment Evaluator Manual*. St. Paul, MN: New Standards, Inc.

Mee-Lee D, Shulman G, Fishman M et al. (2001). *ASAM Patient Placement Criteria for the Treatment of Substance-Related Disorders, Second Edition-Revised (PPC-2R)*. Chevy Chase, MD: American Society of Addiction Medicine.

Mee-Lee D, Shulman G & Gartner L (1996). *Patient Placement Criteria for the Treatment of Substance-Related Disorders, Second Edition (PPC-2)*. Chevy Chase, MD: American Society of Addiction Medicine.

Miller W & Rollnick S (1991). *Motivational Interviewing; Preparing People to Change Addictive Behavior*. New York, Guilford Press.

Miller W & Tonigan JS (1996). Assessing drinker's motivations for change: The Stages of Change Readiness and Treatment Eagerness Scale (SOCRATES). *Psychology of Addictive Behaviors* 10(2):81-89.

Miller W, Tonigan JS & Longabaugh R (1995). *The Drinker Inventory of Consequences (DrInC): An Instrument for Assessing Adverse Consequences of Alcohol Abuse. Test Manual (NIAAA Project MATCH Monograph Series, Volume 4)*. Rockville, MD: National Institute on Alcohol Abuse and Alcoholism.

Najavits LM, Gastfriend DR, Nakayama EY et al. (1996). A measure of readiness for substance abuse treatment: Psychometric properties of the RAATE research interview. *American Journal on Addictions*.

Prochaska JO & DiClemente CC (1992). Stages of change in the modification of problem behaviors. *Progress in Behavior Modification* 28:183-218.

Robins LN, Helzer JE, Croughan J et al. (1981). National Institute of Mental Health Diagnostic Interview Schedule. *Archives of General Psychiatry* 38(4):381-389.

Skre I, Onstad S, Torgersen S et al. (1991). High interrater reliability for the Structured Clinical Interview for DSM-IIIR Axis I. *Acta Psychiatrica Scandinavica* 84:167-173.

Smith B, Hoffman N & Nederhoed R (1992). The development and reliability of the RAATE-CE. *Journal of Substance Abuse* 4:355-363.

Spitzer RL, Williams JB, Gibbon M et al. (1992). The Structured Clinical Interview for DSM-IIIR (SCID) I: History, rationale and description. *Archives of General Psychiatry* 49:624-629.

Spitzer RL, Williams JB, Mirian G et al. (1989). *Instruction Manual for the Structured Interview for DSM-IIIR*. New York, NY: Biometrics Research Dept., New York State Psychiatric Institute, May 1.

Sullivan JT, Sykora K, Schneiderman J et al. (1989). Assessment of alcohol withdrawal: The revised Clinical Institute Withdrawal Assessment for Alcohol Scale (CIWA-Ar). *British Journal of the Addictions* 84:1353-1357.

Williams JB, Gibbon M, First MB et al. (1992). The Structured Clinical Interview for DSM-IIIR (SCID), II. Multisite test-retest reliability. *Archives of General Psychiatry* 49:630-636.

| Chapter 6 | # Environmental Approaches to Prevention |

Paul J. Gruenewald, Ph.D.
Harold D. Holder, Ph.D.
Andrew J. Treno, Ph.D.

The purposes of this chapter are threefold. First, it presents the conceptual underpinnings of the "environmental" approach to preventing alcohol, tobacco, and other drug problems, as developed from the public health model, and it compares and contrasts traditional individual approaches with environmental strategies. Second, it presents the primary research findings that have emerged in support of environmental approaches. Third, it discusses three multicomponent multisite projects that have developed out of these approaches to test the efficacy of various environmental strategies.

CONCEPTUAL UNDERPINNINGS

Environmental strategies for the reduction of alcohol and drug abuse have developed over the past three decades from scientific pre-intervention research to efficacy trials and, most recently, to effectiveness trials that attempt to assess the relative advantages of different prevention strategies (Holder, Flay et al., 1999). These advances have been supported by the accumulation of scientific knowledge about the causes and correlates of substance abuse behaviors at multiple levels, including the individual, the family, the peer group, the neighborhood environment, the enforcement communities, and the policy environment of communities, states, and nations. Innovative environmental prevention efforts have demonstrated the degree to which environmental change can effectively reduce problem outcomes. Within the foreseeable future, new prevention research will reveal the ways in which the combined forces of individual and environmental prevention can be focused to reduce alcohol- and drug-related harm.

Prior to the past three decades, most programs that have been developed to prevent alcohol- and other drug-related problems have been restricted to approaches that relied heavily upon various methods to persuade individuals to avoid use. Of particular note here are school-based drug programs that have focused either on conveying the dangers of use to youth or instilling "protective factors" such as resistance skills, family strengthening programs, and media-based campaigns focused on encouraging supportive health behaviors of different sorts (Botvin, Schinke et al., 1989; Hansen, 1994; Perry & Kelder, 1992; Flay & Sobel, 1983; Kumpfer, 1989). Such approaches attempt to alter the behavior of individuals by providing them with messages or strategies to prevent initiation, encourage desistance, or reduce use. Generally applied, such programs also may change the peer and family environments of young people by altering the behaviors of friends, parents, and siblings.

As a complement to these approaches, and in response to the observation that substance abuse involves more than the behaviors of individual substance abusers, environmental strategies have been developed and shaped into programs that communities can implement to reduce alcohol and drug problems (Howard, 1996; Holder, Grube et al., 1995; Pentz, 2000; Wagenaar & Perry, 1994). Although the environmental prevention strategies that were developed during this time differ somewhat from one another in terms of details, they share a number of common characteristics and a single common heritage.

The common heritage of these programs is the long history of policy, regulatory, and enforcement interventions that have attempted to restrain or reduce problems related to substance abuse, all of them changing in one way or another the environments of alcohol and drug users (Caulkins, 2000; Hingson & Howland, 1989; Holder, Flay et al., 1999). Thus, the social history of alcohol and drug abuse is replete with efforts by communities, states, and nations to reduce use, abuse, and problems through legal action, enforcement, and other forms of control, all in the realms of the economic, physical, and social environments of users. States and nations make alcohol and other drugs more expensive, ban their use, police their roadways for drunken drivers, and prohibit the provision of alcohol to minors. As a lesson learned from these efforts, prevention researchers have recognized that these types of interventions may be brought directly to bear upon problems in towns and cities that wish to intervene for the good of the community.

TRADITIONAL VERSUS ENVIRONMENTAL APPROACHES

Environmental approaches to the reduction of alcohol and other drug problems differ from traditional approaches in several important ways. First, and most obviously, traditional approaches seek to reduce problem levels by changing individual behaviors. Whether the problem behavior is drinking by youth, drunken driving, or injection drug use, the focus of traditional prevention is to alter the individual's proclivities to use, to encourage the individual to stop such use, or to change the individual's behavior so that problems related to use occur less frequently. In contrast, environmental approaches seek to change "community systems" that

are related to substance use and the occurrence of related problems.

Community systems are those functional groups of human social behaviors that make communities run: firefighters work collectively to prevent and put out fires, police to enforce laws, bar and restaurant owners to distribute alcohol and food, drug sellers to distribute illegal drugs (sometimes in public markets but often through social networks), and drinking networks to distribute alcohol to underage drinkers (Holder, 1998). The goal of environmental prevention is to alter the relationships of community systems to the individuals who use them. Such efforts often include changing formal institutions (as by reducing hours and days of sale of alcohol), but also may include attempts to change informal systems (for example, by breaking up markets for illegal drugs).

The second way in which the two approaches differ is in their use of the media. While traditional approaches use media messages to influence individuals, environmental approaches use the media to target policymakers. Changes in community systems cannot be accomplished without the support of relevant gatekeepers to systems that enable prevention efforts. Thus, media efforts in environmental prevention programs often are intended to motivate gatekeepers to pursue activities that are extensions of their normal efforts; for example, persuading the police chief to increase enforcement of laws against drinking and drug impaired driving, or against retail sale of alcohol to minors, or working with retailers to better manage service policies and practices, or securing support for community zoning restrictions to reduce the density of alcohol outlets, and so on.

A third distinction between environmental and traditional approaches to prevention is their orientation toward persons at risk. The individual-oriented approach typically targets individuals at risk, while the environmental approach targets the broader alcohol and drug environment. In the general parlance of prevention studies, environmental prevention programs are, in an important sense, universal prevention programs; they affect everyone in a community, including those not at-risk for alcohol problems. Environmental programs are rarely directed at specific subgroups (and then usually at geographically defined groups) and most often cannot be so directed. For example, a workplace based environmental preventive intervention may be aimed at altering workplace policies toward alcohol, but these policies will affect everyone at the workplace, not just those who abuse alcohol (Ames, 2000).

The primary consequences of this broad focus are the secondary effects of environmental prevention on persons not at risk. These individuals may have to accept greater regulation (as through reduced access to alcohol) or greater investments in enforcement efforts (for example, in the form of greater taxes for policing) in order to reduce alcohol or drug related risks for others. Thus, recent research that shows the degree to which non-abusers suffer collateral damage from alcohol and drug abuse (Wechsler, Moeykens et al., 1995; Gruenewald, Millar et al., 1996) may lead them to support the implementation of environmental prevention programs. The community thereby plays a key role in environmental prevention efforts.

In contrast to traditional approaches in which the broader community is conceptualized in terms of information disseminators and receivers, the environmental approach views the community as a resource to mobilize for structural and system change. This fourth distinction between environmental and individual prevention explains why environmental prevention often takes the form of policy interventions.

A final distinction is that traditional approaches seek to reduce demand for drugs, whereas environmental approaches generally seek either to reduce supply or risk associated with their use. Examples of efforts targeting supply include enforcement actions to reduce youth purchases of alcohol (Grube, 1997) and efforts at drug interdiction (Reuter, 1988). Examples of efforts targeting risks related to the supply of alcohol include responsible beverage service programs (Saltz & Stanghetta, 1997), safe needle programs (Caulkins, 2000), and efforts to change the distribution rather than the level of supply so as to ameliorate problem "hot spots" (Gruenewald & Treno, 2000).

CHRONIC VERSUS ACUTE PROBLEMS

Alcohol and drug use can be said to be related to both "acute" and "chronic" problem outcomes. Acute problems result from specific drinking or drug use events, such as drinking and driving or drug overdoses. Chronic problems occur as a consequence of the regular, and often excessive, use of alcohol or other drugs. Such persistent substance abuse leads to alcohol- and other drug-related disorders such as liver cirrhosis, hepatitis C, or addiction—all health conditions that are caused or made worse by regular use of these substances. Important examples of acute problems related to alcohol and drug use include drug overdoses and violence related to the crack cocaine epidemic (White &

Gorman, 2000), drinking and driving (Grube & Voas, 1996), and the host of problems attributed to binge drinking on college campuses (Wechsler, Moeykens et al., 1995).

Alcohol prevention programs that employ an environmental approach generally have targeted acute problems such as motor vehicle crashes, general injuries, and assaultive violence, rather than chronic medical conditions such as alcohol use disorder, alcohol dependence, alcoholism, or cirrhotic liver damage. In the case of illegal drugs, environmental efforts generally have targeted reductions in drug-related crime (White & Gorman, 2000).

While it is clear that environmental approaches to prevention may lead to reductions in alcohol or drug use, it is not the case that reductions in such use are a requisite for reductions in alcohol- or drug-related harm. In fact, the outcomes of environmental prevention efforts may not focus on reduced use *per se*, but rather on reduced harm resulting from use. Thus, prevention programs that are oriented toward regulating problem outcomes related to alcohol use, such as responsible beverage service (Saltz & Stanghetta, 1997), may reduce one harmful outcome related to alcohol use (motor vehicle crashes) without affecting the number of drinks or average consumption. It follows that environmental prevention programs may reduce proximal acute harms related to alcohol and drug abuse (such as motor vehicle crashes and needle-sharing among injection drug users) without changing the chronic problems that may result from prolonged use.

The importance of the focus on acute problems is illustrated by the social costs of alcohol and drug abuse in terms of years of life lost due to acute harm (Single, Robson et al., 1996). For example, the total economic costs of the tens of thousands of individuals killed and injured each year in alcohol-related motor vehicle crashes, violence, and premature death ($218 billion) accounts for a very substantial portion of the $246 billion total costs of alcohol abuse (1992 data; Harwood, Fountain et al., 1998).

When all acute harms related to drug and alcohol use are considered (including all injuries and violent crimes related to illegal drug use), the costs are estimated at $305 billion per year. The immediate short-term burden that acute alcohol and drug problems place on the health care and enforcement systems thus renders them more costly to society than many other major health problems.

Acute problems are so costly because they are distributed so widely in the population of drinkers and drug users. Thus, one often hears reference to the "prevention paradox" (Kreitman, 1986), which is the observation that while high-risk individuals produce more problems on an individual basis, lower-risk individuals produce more problems on an aggregate basis. So, if 100 high-risk drinkers produce problems 10% of the time (a higher individual risk), they will produce 10 problems in the aggregate. If 5,000 lower risk individuals produce problems 1% of the time (a lower individual risk), they will produce 100 problems in the aggregate. From a public health perspective of reducing aggregate alcohol and drug problems in the community, a focus on high- *and* low-risk individuals makes sense. Environmental strategies have the advantage of affecting all drinkers and drug users, regardless of their levels of use, and, importantly, affect all individuals at risk.

DOMAINS OF ENVIRONMENTAL PREVENTION

Environmental prevention programs act in three domains: the physical, the social, and the economic. Prevention programs may alter physical access by affecting proximity to sources of alcohol, drugs, and tobacco. College dormitories may prohibit alcohol in dorm rooms, college administrators may eliminate the sale of tobacco through vending machines, and public markets for illegal drugs may be disrupted by matrix enforcement programs (Caulkins, 2000). Environmental prevention programs may alter social access by affecting the social networks that encourage and enable distribution of these substances. They may alter social access to alcohol by restricting social activities at which alcohol is freely served (as during on-campus celebrations), reduce social access to tobacco through increased counter-advertising, and moderate social access to illegal drugs by establishing and enforcing drug-free zones in a community. Prevention programs may alter economic access by increasing the real costs of alcohol, drugs, and tobacco and changing the economic geography of availability.

The three domains of environmental influence interact in producing alcohol and drug problems. For example, physical, social, and economic availability of alcohol (represented by outlets, use by others, and beverage prices) intersect at places where alcohol problems occur. The presence of other drinkers at outlets exposes the patron of a bar both to social influences for drinking and much greater risks of violence (Homel, 1997). Prices for alcoholic beverages at bars are much greater than at off-premise establishments, changing both the nature of drinking at bars and its relationship to problem outcomes, such as driving while intoxicated and alcohol-related crashes (Gruenewald, Johnson et al., 2000).

The purchasing patterns of others at these establishments naturally influence the behaviors of drinking groups, as by encouraging much greater levels of intoxication (Hennessy & Saltz, 1993). Naturally, parallel arguments can be constructed for illegal drugs. Concentrated use of illegal drugs (for example, in and around crack houses) is associated with substantial degrees of crime and elevated rates of disease (Caulkins, 2000; White & Gorman, 2000). Prices of illegal drugs may be influenced by drug interdiction efforts (modestly), but certainly affect the distribution of drug purchases (Reuter & Caulkins, 1995). Favored drugs for abuse change as social access is restructured by enforcement efforts or other changes in informal social systems that support drug distribution.

The substantial costs of alcohol and drug use to society and the effectiveness of environmental prevention programs that target such synergistic interactions provide support for such strategies. Environmental prevention strategies often seek to disrupt the link between availability, use, and problems related to alcohol and drug use. Acting through community, county, state, and national systems, environmental prevention strategies attempt to affect relationships between system components and alcohol and drug problems for the population of alcohol and drug consumers.

THE STRUCTURE OF
ENVIRONMENTAL PREVENTION

Environmental prevention programs are part of the natural ecology of local communities—the psychological, social, and economic geographies of people, places, and things with which everyone interacts in daily life. Nothing in environmental prevention takes place in a vacuum, and everything is contingent on something else. Thus, in environmental prevention, the relationships between physical, social, and economic contexts of human behavior become very important. These relations are not naively additive, contributing to the balance sheet of risk and protective factors (Hawkins, Catalano et al., 1992), but represent ecological contexts that interact with the relationships between individual predispositions to problem outcomes and their realization in different settings (Gruenewald, Millar et al., 1993; Gruenewald & Treno, 2000; Stockwell & Gruenewald, 2001).

Individual use of drugs and alcohol produces problems. Drinking may lead to drinking and driving, or illegal drug use may lead to crime. The alcohol environment is not simply producing problems or influencing personal activities.

Instead, the environment creates a stage on which human activities play themselves out to produce problems. With this in mind, there are four ways in which the alcohol environment can affect problems related to drinking and drug use:

1. The alcohol environment may directly affect use (as when reduced availability leads to reduced use).

2. The alcohol environment may indirectly affect problems through its effect on use (as when reduced availability leads to reduced use and, hence, fewer problems related to use).

3. The alcohol environment may directly affect outcomes (as when increased safety belt use leads to reductions in alcohol-involved fatal crashes, independent of rates of alcohol use).

4. The alcohol environment may moderate the relationship between substance use and problem outcomes (as when densities of bars and restaurants moderate the relationship between traffic flow patterns and automobile crashes).

It is in the third and fourth arenas that the effects of the environment are most compelling, as environmental changes can accelerate or decelerate the rates of alcohol and drug problems (Gruenewald & Treno, 2000).

Direct Effects on Substance Use. The most obvious way in which environmental prevention activities reduce problems related to alcohol and drugs is to alter the behaviors of drinkers and drug users. Behavioral change was, in fact, the primary goal of prevention studies through much of the latter half of the 20th century. Environmental prevention research has demonstrated that demographic, economic, and physical restrictions on availability can reduce use and problems. For example, increasing the minimum legal drinking age to 21 has been linked to a 13% reduction in the number of high school seniors reporting drinking, as well as lower drinking levels across demographic groups (O'Malley & Wagenaar, 1991).

Price increases demonstrably are associated with declines in alcohol consumption (Kenkel & Manning, 1996), with heavy drinkers and youthful drinkers particularly sensitive to price changes (Coate & Grossman, 1988). Estimates from these studies suggest that if beer prices had been indexed to inflation over the past decades, youth drinking could be reduced by 9% and youth heavy drinking by 20% (Laixuthai & Chaloupka, 1993). Increases and decreases in the physical availability of alcohol have been linked to increases and decreases in alcohol sales (Gruenewald, Ponicki et al., 1993), suggesting that a 10% reduction in outlet densities would be associated with a 3% reduction in alcohol sales. Thus, in large aggregate studies across the United States, reductions in the demographic, economic, and physical availability of alcohol appear to be related to reductions in use.

Additional mechanisms also have been found through which the environment may directly affect drinking behaviors. For example, reductions have been achieved through the introduction of responsible beverage service programs, which are linked to lower levels of intoxication (Hennessy & Saltz, 1990), or local enforcement of underage sales laws, which can reduce underage alcohol sales in off-premise establishments by half (Grube, 1997). On the other hand, increases in alcohol use have been related to the privatization of alcohol monopolies, which yield lower prices, greater numbers of outlets, and increased sales (Wagenaar & Holder, 1996).

Environmental efforts to reduce underage access to alcohol have proved particularly effective. The implementation of community-based alcohol policies to reduce youth access have led to reduced sales to youth in on-premise outlets by 24% and off-premise outlets by 8%, with a concomitant 7% reduction in past 30-day drinking (Wagenaar, Murray et al., 2000).

Indirect Effects on Problems. Empirical studies have clearly demonstrated the potential impact of environmental change on problem outcomes such as traffic crashes. For example, raising the legal drinking age to 21 has been linked to a 20% reduction in single vehicle nighttime crashes (the commonly used surrogate for alcohol-involved crashes) among youthful drivers (O'Malley & Wagenaar, 1991; Wagenaar, Murray et al., 2000). Similarly, reflecting the potential impact of changes in the economic availability of alcohol, higher alcohol prices have been linked to lower rates of traffic deaths and cirrhosis mortality (Cook & Tauchen, 1982). Mandated server-training policies have been linked to reductions in alcohol-involved crashes (Holder & Wagenaar, 1994). Conversely, increased availability of spirits at bars and restaurants has been linked to substantial increases in alcohol-involved crashes (Holder & Blose, 1987). More recently, at the local level of neighborhoods within communities, lower densities of alcohol outlets have been linked to decreases in alcohol-involved crashes (Scribner, MacKinnon et al., 1994; Gruenewald, Millar et al., 1996;

Jewel & Brown, 1995), pedestrian injury collisions (LaScala, Gerber et al., 2000; LaScala, Johnson et al., 2001), and violence (Roncek & Maier, 1991; Scribner, MacKinnon et al., 1995; Stevenson, Lind et al., 1999; Gorman, Speer et al., 2001).

Direct Effects on Problems. As suggested in the previous section, environmental conditions that support drinking or drug use can indirectly affect problems. Changes in one can produce reductions in the other through a simple causal chain. Environmental prevention efforts also can directly affect problem outcomes and provide alternative paths to prevention.

Aspects of the psychological, social, economic, and physical environments apparently unrelated to alcohol and drug use can confound research efforts to evaluate any prevention activity, but they also can become an important part of environmental prevention as well. As a confound or "nuisance," these aspects of the environment disrupt simple cause-and-effect relationships between environmental prevention activities (such as reduced availability) and prevention outcomes (for example, reduced motor vehicle crashes). Any attempt to evaluate the effects of reduced alcohol availability on drinking and driving traffic crashes must isolate the unique effects of this policy from such factors as vehicle miles traveled by drivers, characteristics of urban and rural traffic flow, other safety measures on roadway systems (such as stoplights) and within automobiles (such as safety belts), and sources of distraction (like cell phones). Thus, differences in traffic flow rates and patterns can be shown to be substantive predictors of traffic crashes and pedestrian collisions in general, and alcohol-related motor vehicle crashes and pedestrian collisions in particular (Gruenewald, Millar et al., 1996; LaScala, Johnson et al., 2001). Sociodemographic characteristics of resident populations around retail centers (such as poverty) are related to violence independent of the number of alcohol outlets (Gorman, Speer et al., 2001). The availability of alcohol in different venues (such as taverns and grocery stores) may mitigate the effects of a price increase (Gruenewald & Treno, 2000; Osterberg, 2001).

However, the same "nuisance" factors also can become part of environmental prevention efforts. Thus, low rates of driving after drinking in urban settings where public transportation is widely available points to a natural environmental strategy for the reduction of alcohol-related crashes: safe ride programs. The former confounding variable now becomes a potential intervention. Greater or lesser rates of safety belt use may confound an evaluation of the direct effects of a liquor tax increase on alcohol-related fatal crashes, but become part of an effective strategy to reduce this particular alcohol-related harm. Thus, most environmental prevention studies recognize that the multiple environmental supports for problem outcomes are to be recognized and used in prevention efforts. As an example, Hingson and colleagues (1996) showed that a combination of media campaigns, enforcement of speed and DUI limits, and community awareness reduced fatal motor vehicle crashes by as much as 25%. Holder and colleagues (2000) demonstrated that environmental prevention programs oriented toward alcohol-related problems (such as alcohol-related crashes, violence, drownings, burns, and falls), rather than alcohol use, can be effective in reducing problems and changing patterns of use.

Effects on Relationships Between Substance Use and Problem Outcomes. Substance use and abuse are related to a variety of physiological conditions specific to the substance user, but when the locus of the problem is outside the person and in the environment, the environment becomes the moderator of all problem outcomes. The social, economic, and physical environments determine the nature of problems experienced by individuals. No violence occurs in the absence of social interaction, no motor vehicle crashes without cars or trucks, no falls occur without the opportunity for falling. Thus, participation in the routine activities of daily life condition the occurrences of problem outcomes (Felson, 1987). The environment may encourage or discourage alcohol and drug use (above), and it certainly moderates the relationship between use and problems related to specific drinking events, which are so productive of alcohol- and drug-related harm.

The moderating effects of environmental variables on the relationship between substance use and problem outcomes have been investigated in only a few studies to date. In each case, however, researchers found strong indications that environmental contexts focus problems in ways that can be taken advantage of in future preventive intervention programs. In the case of alcohol-related traffic crashes, as shown by Gruenewald and Treno (2000), local patterns of traffic flow are directly related to rates of motor vehicle crashes, but this relationship is significantly moderated by the presence of on-premise alcohol outlets (bars and restaurants). The location of alcohol outlets along different types of roadways affects drinking, driving, and crashing. Within low traffic flow areas of communities, greater numbers of alcohol outlets do not lead to significantly greater numbers of alcohol-related crashes. Within high traffic flow areas of communities, on the other hand, greater numbers of alcohol outlets lead to substantively greater numbers of alcohol-related crashes.

The differences in these contexts suggest that 10% greater densities of alcohol outlets will be related, systematically, to no change in crash rates within downtown areas with low traffic flow, to 20% greater crash rates within areas with greater traffic flow (particularly along highway systems). Clearly, regulations governing outlet densities and locations within community areas should be developed to be sensitive to these local characteristics.

Similar observations are beginning to emerge in studies of violence related to alcohol outlets and problems related to illegal drug markets. The frequently observed relationship between densities of alcohol outlets (particularly bars) and rates of violence (Roncek & Maier, 1991; Scribner, MacKinnon et al., 1995) must be supplemented with two other pieces of contextual information. First, rates of violence are not simply a function of the number of outlets and populations characteristics of a local area, but also are a function of population characteristics of people living in nearby areas (Gorman, Speer et al., 2001). Second, densities of alcohol outlets do not appear to be a direct source of violence in geographic areas, but rather a moderator of the rates at which populations produce violence (Gruenewald & Treno, 2000). Rates of assault are greater in neighborhoods with specific population characteristics (for example, more poverty, disorganization, immigration, and residential mobility). They are accelerated in neighborhoods with more taverns and off-premises alcohol establishments. A similar pattern is found with regard to illegal drug markets: Disrupting the geographic link between location of sales and location of users leads to reduced drug sales and problems (Moore, 1990).

EFFICACY TRIALS

Communities have an opportunity to act in important ways to reduce harm related to alcohol and other drugs. In the last decade of the 20th century, several important community-based environmental preventive intervention studies were undertaken. Each involved at least one aspect of the alcohol environment, and each employed a clearly environmental approach to prevention. These projects went beyond the scientific evidence to test whether environmental prevention efforts could be effective at the community level in preventing three harmful outcomes related to alcohol: drinking and driving, underage access and use, and violence related to alcohol.

The Saving Lives Project. The Saving Lives Project, conducted in six communities in Massachusetts, was designed to reduce alcohol-impaired driving and related problems such as speeding (Hingson, McGovern et al., 1996). In each participating community, a full-time coordinator from within city government organized a task force representing various city departments. Each project was funded at a rate of $1 per inhabitant per year, with half the funds paying the costs of a coordinator, police enforcement, program activities, and educational materials. Programs were designed locally and involved a host of activities, including media campaigns, business information programs, speeding and drunk driving awareness days, speed watch telephone hotlines, police training, high school peer-led education, Students Against Drunk Driving chapters, and college prevention programs.

The program evaluation involved a quasi-experimental design and five communities as controls. While the control communities were slightly more affluent than the experimental sites, they had similar demographic characteristics, rates of traffic citations, and fatal crashes. The outcome evaluation of the project included measures of fatal and injury crashes, safety belt use, telephone surveys, and traffic citations.

The study found that over the five years of the program, Saving Lives cities experienced a 25% decline in fatal crashes when compared to the rest of Massachusetts (that is, from 178 crashes to 120), a 42% reduction in fatal motor vehicle crashes within the experimental communities, a 47% reduction in the number of fatally injured drivers who tested positive for alcohol, and an 8% decline in crash injuries among 15- to 25-year-olds.

In addition, there was a decline in self-reported driving after drinking (specifically among youth). The greatest fatal and injury crash reductions occurred in the 15- to 25-year-old age group.

The CMCA Project. The Communities Mobilizing for Change on Alcohol (CMCA) project was designed to reduce access to alcohol among youth under the legal drinking age of 21 (Wagenaar, Murray et al., 2000). The project was composed of five core components intended to influence (1) community policies, (2) community practices, (3) youth alcohol access, (4) youth alcohol consumption, and subsequently (5) youth alcohol problems. Although the project clearly was communitywide in terms of the institutions involved, it was focused on youth under 21 years old.

The CMCA project recruited 15 communities (defined by school districts with at least 200 students in the ninth grade and that drew students from no more than three municipalities) in Minnesota and western Wisconsin before using randomization to determine which would be the intervention communities and which would be the control group. Seven pairs of communities were created by matching on their size, state, proximity to a college or university, and baseline data from an alcohol purchase survey. One member community of each pair then was selected randomly to be the intervention site when the time came to begin the community organizing. This yielded seven intervention sites and eight control sites, ranging in population from approximately 8,000 to 65,000, with an average of about 20,000. In this respect, the CMCA project is unique for its group randomized design (Murray, 1998).

The CMCA project hired a part-time local organizer from within each community who was trained and supervised by project staff. The part-time organizer was responsible for community organizing activities that activated the community members, who would, in turn, select interventions designed to influence underage access to alcohol. The interventions that could be selected included a broad array of programs that affect youth access: decoy operations with alcohol outlets (in which police typically have underage buyers purchase alcohol at selected outlets), citizen monitoring of outlets selling to youth, keg registration (which requires that purchasers of kegs of alcohol provide identifying information, thus establishing liability for resulting problems at parties where minors are drinking), sponsorship of alcohol-free events for youth, policy action to shorten hours of sale for alcohol, implementation of responsible beverage service training programs, and development of educational programs for youth and adults. The experimental sites were free to shape these interventions to their own ends.

Evaluation data were collected at baseline and at about 30 months after the interventions began. Results showed that merchants increased the frequency of checks for age identification, reduced sales to minors, and reported more care in controlling sales to youth (Wagenaar, Toomey et al., 1996). A telephone survey of 18- to 20-year-olds showed reductions in attempts to purchase alcohol, reduced levels of alcohol use, and reduced propensity to provide alcohol to other teens (Wagenaar, Murray et al., 2000). In addition, the project found a statistically significant net decline in drinking and driving arrests among 18- to 20-year-olds and disorderly conduct violations among 15- to 17-year-olds in the CMCA cities compared to the controls (Wagenaar, Murray et al., 2000).

The Community Trials Project. The Community Trials Project (Holder, Saltz et al., 1997) was a five-component, community-level intervention conducted in three experimental communities matched to three controls. The goals of the project were to reduce alcohol-related harm among all persons in the three experimental communities. The outcomes of the project reflected the primary sources of acute injury and harm related to alcohol: injuries and fatalities related to drinking and driving or to violence, drownings, burns, and falls (Holder & Howard, 1992). Each environmental prevention component was based on prior scientific evidence (Holder, Grube et al., 1995), but this mix of components had not been tested for mutually supportive or synergistic effects (Holder, Saltz et al., 1997). The project design recognized the complex systems environment in which environmental preventive interventions take place (Holder, 1998).

Population growth leads, in general, to corresponding growth in retail services that meet the demands of community residents, one of which is for alcohol. The numbers of outlets thus increases to meet the growing demand for alcohol from ever larger communities, which leads to increases in alcohol sales, and increased sales correspond to general increases in drinking levels and the use of multiple drinking contexts for the use of alcohol (such as bars, restaurants, friends' homes, and the like). Individuals may not be drinking more, but more individuals are drinking and in more different places, exposing themselves to different risks. Thus, alcohol-related injuries and deaths, the sequelae of the natural increase in drinking experienced by growing communities, may increase in community settings without corresponding increases in average drinking levels *per se*. Instead, shifts in routine drinking activities among different segments of the population (for example, more drinking at taverns and restaurants among young males as the number of these establishments increases) is related to greater levels of harm (such as alcohol-related motor vehicle crashes) at the population level.

Some likely consequences of the continued growth in supply of alcohol at the community level are greater access to alcohol among youth, increases in drinking and driving and alcohol-related motor vehicle crashes, increases in alcohol-related violence (particularly prevalent in bars and taverns), and other injuries related to alcohol use. At the population level, these problems can be prevented through the use of environmental preventive interventions that target specific links. For this purpose, Community Trials fielded five intervention components: (1) a "Media and Mobilization" component to develop community organization and support for the goals and strategies of the project; (2) a "Responsible Beverage Service" component to reduce service to intoxicated patrons at bars and restaurants; (3) a "Sales to Youth" component to reduce underage access; (4) a "Drinking and Driving" component to increase enforcement activities related to driving while intoxicated (DWI) offenses; and (5) an "Access" component to reduce the availability of alcohol. Each of these interventions were shown to have specific effects:

- The Media and Mobilization component led to a significant increase in coverage of alcohol issues in local newspapers and on local TV in the experimental communities, as compared with the matched control communities. Increased media coverage was important to gain leaders' support of specific alcohol policies and to increase public awareness of drinking and driving enforcement (Holder & Treno, 1997).

- The Responsible Beverage Services component yielded an increase in adoption of responsible alcohol serving policies in the experimental communities as compared with the control communities (Saltz & Stanghetta, 1997).

- The Sales to Youth component produced a significant reduction in alcohol sales to minors. Overall, off-premise outlets in experimental communities were half as likely to sell alcohol to minors as in the comparison sites. This outcome was the result of special training of clerks and managers to conduct age identification checks, the development of effective off-premise outlet policies and, especially, the threat of enforcement of lawsuits against sales to minors (Grube, 1997).

- The Drinking and Driving component produced increased enforcement of drinking and driving laws and a significant reduction in alcohol-involved traffic crashes overall (Voas, Holder et al., 1997).

- The Alcohol Access component achieved some of its goals, as all communities adopted some aspects of local

policies to reduce alcohol access, particularly concerning high-density, on-premises outlets. For example, one community introduced a ban on new outlets (Reynolds, Holder et al., 1997).

The final evaluation of the project covered the key problem areas through data collected in a large population survey and from archival sources (Gruenewald, 1997). Comparison of the effects of the interventions on relative risks of injury outcomes between matched communities found significant reductions in nighttime injury crashes (10% in experimental relative to comparison communities) and in crashes in which the driver was found by police to "have been drinking" (6%). Assault injuries observed in emergency departments declined by 43% in the intervention communities versus the comparison communities, and all hospitalized assault injuries declined by 2%. Examining the survey data, the evaluation reported a 49% decline in episodes of driving after "having had too much to drink" and 51% in self-reports of driving when "over the legal limit." Surprisingly, although the drinking population increased slightly in the experimental sites over the course of the study, there was a significant reduction in problematic alcohol use: The average number of drinks per occasion declined by 6%, and the variance in drinking patterns (an indirect measure of heavy drinking) declined by 21% (Holder, Gruenewald et al., 2000).

ENVIRONMENTAL STRATEGIES AND ALCOHOL POLICY

"Policy" usually refers to structural change, as through a regulation, law, or enforcement priority to reduce alcohol problems. As suggested by this review, communities have begun to go beyond policy to affect the drinking environment itself as an approach to reducing alcohol-involved problems. Local policymakers can establish the priorities for community action to reduce risky behavior involving drinking, which, in turn, can reduce the number of alcohol-involved problems. For example, local alcohol policies can make it a priority to enforce laws against drinking and driving, violence, or sales of alcohol to youth; mandate server training for bars, pubs, and restaurants; set written policies for responsible alcoholic beverage service by licensed retail establishments; or allocate enforcement resources to prevent alcohol sales to underage persons.

Local communities can have a say in the location of outlets, their number, and serving and enforcement practices. Existing national and state or provincial laws provide the legal basis for many local policies and can enable local communities to prioritize uses of existing resources within legal frameworks to achieve specific objectives. In short, national as well as state, regional, or provincial laws often establish the base for local policies, including legal drinking ages, regulation of alcohol outlets, the legal blood alcohol level for drinking and driving, advertising restrictions, and service to obviously intoxicated persons and underage persons. Local policies often address the implementation and enforcement of these existing laws.

In sum, environmental prevention strategies appear to have a critical role in reducing alcohol problems. Such strategies have demonstrated effectiveness in terms of population-level outcome measures (for example, reductions in alcohol-involved motor vehicle crashes) and drinking among both heavy and moderate users, and have been characterized by maintained effects extending beyond the initial implementation periods. They are politically feasible because they do not target specific subgroups in a discriminatory manner. In general, they are cost-effective because they do not require case finding, service provision, or cost maintenance. Moreover, environmental prevention strategies provide a number of levers for change, including tax codes, alcohol beverage control laws, laws regulating drinking and driving and minimum drinking ages, administrative regulation of outlets, planning and zoning regulations and conditional use permits, and law enforcement policies.

A number of issues do, however, remain unresolved. The first concerns the appropriate geographic level of implementation. In general, it may be argued that neighborhood problems such as drinking in public parks are best addressed through local initiatives, while broader community problems such as drinking and driving likely require community-wide strategies. A second issue concerns which administrative agencies provide the most appropriate levels for environmental intervention. Here it is important to adopt a community systems approach that views communities and neighborhoods as providing both challenges to and resources for the implementation of desired environmental change. Finally, the unique problems characterizing at-risk or underserved neighborhoods and populations should be addressed. Specifically, such populations and geographic units face unique circumstances in the development of environmental strategies and subsequently pose a substantial challenge to researchers and public policymakers.

ENVIRONMENTAL STRATEGIES AND DRUG POLICY

Environmental strategies for the reduction of harm related to the use of illicit drugs are in their infancy when compared to alcohol prevention program. As Caulkins (2000) points out, much of what is conceived as "environmental" is instead only "enforcement" when considering illegal substances. That the enforcement activities of police take place in the drug selling and drug using environment does make this sort of activity a form of environmental intervention, but whether it is prevention or selective incapacitation (the removal of drug users and sellers from activity on the streets) is another question. Ideally, the equivalent action with regard to alcohol (arrests for drunken driving) are intended to reduce this illegal activity by deterring driving after drinking, as described in specific and general deterrence theories (Voas, Holder et al., 1997). Arrests make enforcement an environmental prevention activity (that is, an action that may, in the future, discourage an apprehended, drunk driver from driving after drinking). In the arena of illegal drug sales, it is difficult to ascribe such preventive benefits to enforcement outside of the greater costs incurred by users through the disruption of drug supply networks (Moore, 1990), and the effects of enforcement in this domain remain largely uninvestigated. In a similar manner, greater costs for drugs may arise through the "War on Drugs" and other interdiction activities. However, the effectiveness of such strategies has been shown to be very limited (Reuter & Caulkins, 1995).

Other prevention strategies with regard to illegal drug use are oriented at individuals or families, not the environment of drug use. The majority of these efforts are programs to educate young people to resist use, to help moderate the dire consequences of disrupted families on youth use, and more general media campaigns to encourage users to stop and discourage non-users from beginning to use drugs (Advisory Council on the Misuse of Drugs, 1998). Strikingly, although there is extensive research literature discussing the many environments in which drug use and related crime take place, there is little literature on environmental prevention *per se* (Harrison & Backenheimer, 1998; Caulkins, 2000). Were one to modify community environments, what would be the consequences to illegal drug sales and use? What aspects of the community environment are most likely to enable reductions of sales and use? These questions remain largely unanswered.

CONCLUSIONS

Environmental prevention strategies can provide the necessary levers to alter the environment and to prevent alcohol- and drug-related problems. Environmental strategies are not limited to laws and regulations and thus provide extra-governmental means to achieve healthy communities. For example, responsible alcohol beverage service policies to reduce public intoxication, changes in the social environment of use through alterations in advertising, the establishment of enforcement priorities with respect to drinking and driving and retail sale of alcohol to youth, and changes in local planning and zoning reviews all are activities that go beyond law to environmentally shape behaviors in public and private settings. Similar prevention activities conducted with respect to drug and alcohol use hold promise for prevention efforts in the 21st century.

ACKNOWLEDGMENTS: The authors acknowledge the assistance of Drs. Robert Saltz, Marcia Russell, and Genevieve Ames in the preparation and editing of this manuscript. Research and preparation of this manuscript was supported by National Institute on Alcohol Abuse and Alcoholism Research Center grant No. P50-AA06282 and NIAAA grant No. R01-AA11968.

REFERENCES

Advisory Council on the Misuse of Drugs (1998). *Drug Use and the Environment.* London, England: Her Majesty's Stationery Office.

Ames GM (2000). Revisiting environmental approaches to prevention of workplace alcohol problems: Where do we go from here? In *Research in the Sociology of Organizations.* JAI Press.

Botvin GJ, Schinke SP & Orlandi MA (1989). Psychosocial approaches to substance abuse prevention: Theoretical foundations and empirical findings. *Crisis: The Journal of Crisis Intervention and Suicide Prevention* 10(1):62-77.

Caulkins JP (2000). Measurement and analysis of drug problems and drug control efforts. In D Duffee (ed.) *Measurement and Analysis of Crime and Justice, Vol. 4, Criminal Justice 2000.* Washington, DC: National Institute of Justice (NIJ 182411), 391-449.

Coate D & Grossman M (1988). Effects of alcoholic beverage prices and legal drinking ages on youth alcohol use. *Journal of Law & Economics* 31:145-171.

Cook PJ & Tauchen G (1982). Effect of liquor taxes on heavy drinking. *Bell Journal of Economics* 13:379-390.

Felson M (1987). Routine activities and crime prevention in the developing metropolis. *Criminology* 25:911-931.

Flay BR & Sobel JL (1983). The role of mass media in preventing adolescent substance abuse. In TJ Glynn, CG Leukefeld & JP Ludford (eds.) *Preventing Adolescent Drug Abuse: Intervention Strategies.* Rockville, MD: National Institute on Drug Abuse, 5-35.

Gorman D, Speer PW, Gruenewald PJ et al. (2001). Spatial dynamics of alcohol availability, neighborhood structure and violent crime. *Journal of Studies on Alcohol* 62:628-636.

Grube JW (1997). Preventing sales of alcohol to minors: Results from a community trial. *Addiction* 92:S251-S260.

Grube JW & Voas RB (1996). Predicting underage drinking and driving behaviors. *Addiction* 91:1843-1857.

Gruenewald PJ (1997). Analysis approaches to community evaluation. *Evaluation Review* 21:209-230.

Gruenewald PJ, Johnson FW, Millar A et al. (2000). Drinking and driving: Explaining beverage specific risks. *Journal of Studies on Alcohol* 61:515-523.

Gruenewald PJ, Millar AB & Treno AJ (1993). Alcohol availability and the ecology of drinking behavior. *Alcohol Health & Research World* 17:39-45.

Gruenewald PJ, Millar AB, Treno AJ et al. (1996). The geography of availability and driving after drinking. *Addiction* 91:967-983.

Gruenewald PJ, Ponicki WR & Holder HD (1993). The relationship of outlet densities to alcohol consumption: A time series cross-sectional analysis. *Alcoholism: Clinical & Experimental Research* 17:38-47.

Gruenewald PJ & Treno AJ (2000). Local and global alcohol supply: Economic and geographic models of community systems. *Addiction* 95:S537-S545.

Hansen WB (1994). Prevention of alcohol use and abuse. *Preventive Medicine* 23(5):683-687.

Harrison LD & Backenheimer M (1998). Research careers in unraveling the drug-crime nexus in the United States. *Substance Use and Misuse* 33:1763-2003.

Harwood H, Fountain D & Livermore G (1998). *The Economic Costs of Alcohol and Drug Abuse in the United States, 1992* (National Institute on Drug Abuse and National Institute on Alcohol Abuse and Alcoholism). Washington, DC: U.S. Government Printing Office.

Hawkins JD, Catalano RF & Miller JY (1992). Risk and protective factors for alcohol and other drug problems in adolescence and early adulthood: Implications for substance abuse prevention. *Psychological Bulletin* 112(1):64-105.

Hennessy M & Saltz RF (1993). Modeling social influences on public drinking. *Journal of Studies on Alcohol* 54:139-145.

Hennessy M & Saltz RF (1990). The situational riskiness of alcoholic beverages. *Journal of Studies on Alcohol* 51:422-427.

Hingson R & Howland J (1989). Alcohol, injury, and legal controls: Some complex interactions. *Law, Medicine & Health Care* 17:58-68.

Hingson R, McGovern T, Howland J et al. (1996). Reducing alcohol-impaired driving in Massachusetts: The Saving Lives program. *American Journal of Public Health* 86:791-797.

Holder HD (1998). *Alcohol and the Community: A Systems Approach to Prevention.* New York, NY: Cambridge University Press.

Holder HD & Blose JO (1987). Impact of changes in distilled spirits availability on apparent consumption: A time series analysis of liquor-by-the-drink. *British Journal of Addiction* 82:623-631.

Holder HD, Flay B, Howard J et al. (1999). Phases of alcohol problem prevention research. *Alcoholism: Clinical & Experimental Research* 23:183-194.

Holder HD, Grube JW, Gruenewald PJ et al. (1995). Community approaches to prevention of alcohol-related accidents. In RR Watson (ed.) *Drug and Alcohol Abuse Reviews, Vol. 7: Alcohol, Cocaine, and Accidents.* Totowa, NJ: Humana Press, Inc., 175-194.

Holder HD, Gruenewald PJ, Ponicki W et al. (2000). Effect of community-based interventions on high risk drinking and alcohol-related injuries. *Journal of the American Medical Association* 284:2341-2347.

Holder HD & Howard J, eds. (1992). *Community Prevention Trials for Alcohol Problems: Methodological Issues*. Westport, CT: Praeger Publishers.

Holder HD, Saltz RF, Grube JW et al. (1997). A community prevention trial to reduce alcohol-involved accidental injury and death: Overview. *Addiction* 92:S155-S171.

Holder HD & Treno AJ (1997). Media advocacy in community prevention: News as a means to advance policy change. *Addiction* 92:S189-S199.

Holder HD & Wagenaar AC (1994). Mandated server training and reduced alcohol-involved traffic crashes: A time series analysis of the Oregon experience. *Accident Analysis and Prevention* 26, 89-97.

Homel R (1997). *Policing for Prevention: Reducing Crime, Public Intoxication and Injury*. New York, NY: Criminal Justice Press.

Howard J (1996). Community organizing, public policy and the prevention of alcohol problems. *Alcoholism: Clinical & Experimental Research* 20(8 Suppl):265A-269A.

Jewell RT & Brown RW (1995). Alcohol availability and alcohol-related motor vehicle accidents. *Applied Economics* 27:759-765.

Kenkel D & Manning W (1996). Perspectives on alcohol taxation. *Alcohol Health & Research World* 20:230-238.

Kreitman N (1986). Alcohol consumption and the preventive paradox. *British Journal of Addiction* 81:353-363.

Kumpfer KI (1989). Prevention of alcohol and drug abuse: A critical review of risk factors and prevention strategies. In D Shaffler, I Philips & N Enzer (eds.) *Prevention of Mental Disorders, Alcohol, and Other Drug Use in Children and Adolescents*. Rockville, MD: Office of Substance Abuse Prevention, 309-371.

Laixuthai AF & Chaloupka FJ (1993). Youth alcohol use and public policy. *Contemporary Policy Issues* 11:70-81.

LaScala EA, Gerber D & Gruenewald PJ (2000). Demographic and environmental correlates of pedestrian injury collisions: A spatial analysis. *Accident Analysis and Prevention* 32:651-658.

LaScala EA, Johnson F & Gruenewald PJ (2001). Neighborhood characteristics of alcohol-related pedestrian injury collisions: A geostatistical analysis. *Prevention Science* 2:123-134.

Moore MH (1990). Supply reduction and drug law enforcement. In M Tonry & JQ Wilson (eds.) *Drugs and Crime, Vol. 13 of Crime and Justice: A Review of Research*. Chicago, IL: University of Chicago Press.

Murray D (1998). *Design and Analysis of Group-Randomized Trials*. New York, NY: Oxford University Press.

O'Malley PM & Wagenaar AC (1991). Effects of minimum drinking age laws on alcohol use, related behaviors and traffic crash involvement among American youth: 1976-1987. *Journal of Studies on Alcohol* 52:478-491.

Osterberg E (2001). Economic Availability. Chapter in review for *Alcohol Policy and the Public Good*.

Pentz MA (2000). Institutionalizing community-based prevention through policy change. *Journal of Community Psychology* 28(3).

Perry CL & Kelder SH (1992). Models for effective prevention. *Journal of Adolescent Health* 13(5):355-363.

Reuter P (1988). Quantity illusions and paradoxes of drug interdiction: Federal intervention into vice policy. *Law and Contemporary Problems* 51:233-252.

Reuter P & Caulkins JP (1995). Redefining the goals of drug policy: Report of a working group. *American Journal of Public Health* 85:1059-1063.

Reynolds R, Holder HD & Gruenewald PJ (1997). Community prevention and alcohol retail access. *Addiction* 92:S261-S272.

Roncek DW & Maier PA (1991). Bars, blocks, and crimes revisited: Linking the theory of routine activities to the empiricism of "hot spots." *Criminology* 29:725-753.

Saltz RF & Stanghetta P (1997). A community-wide responsible beverage service program in three communities: Early findings. *Addiction* 92:S237-S249.

Scribner RA, MacKinnon DP & Dwyer JH (1994). Alcohol outlet density and motor vehicle crashes in Los Angeles County cities. *Journal of Studies on Alcohol* 5:447-453.

Scribner RA, MacKinnon DP & Dwyer JH (1995). The risk of assaultive violence and alcohol availability in Los Angeles County. *American Journal of Public Health* 85:335-340.

Single E, Robson L, Xie X et al. (1996). *The Costs of Substance Abuse in Canada*. Ottawa, Canada: CCSA.

Stevenson RJ, Lind B & Weatherburn D (1999). The relationship between alcohol sales and assault in New South Wales, Australia. *Addiction* 94:397-410.

Stockwell T & Gruenewald PJ (2001). Controls on the physical availability of alcohol. In N Heather, TJ Peters & T Stockwell (eds.) *Handbook on Alcohol Dependence and Alcohol Related Problems*. New York, NY: John Wiley & Sons.

Voas RB, Holder HD & Gruenewald PJ (1997). The effect of drinking and driving interventions on alcohol-involved traffic crashes within a comprehensive community trial. *Addiction* 92:S221-S236.

Wagenaar AC & Holder HD (1996). The scientific process works: Seven replications now show significant wine sales increases after privatization. *Journal of Studies on Alcohol* 57:575-576.

Wagenaar AC, Murray DM, Gehan JP et al. (2000). Communities mobilizing for change on alcohol: Outcomes from a randomized community trial. *Journal of Studies on Alcohol* 61:85-94.

Wagenaar AC & Perry CL (1994). Community strategies for the reduction of youth drinking: Theory and application. *Journal of Research on Adolescence* 4:319-345.

Wagenaar AC, Toomey TL, Murray DM et al. (1996). Sources of alcohol for underage drinkers. *Journal of Studies on Alcohol* 57:325-333.

Wechsler H, Moeykens B, Davenport A et al. (1995). The adverse impact of heavy episodic drinkers on other college students. *Journal of Studies on Alcohol* 56:628-634.

White HR & Gorman DM (2000). Dynamics of the drug-crime relationship. In *Criminal Justice 2000, Vol. 1: The Nature of Crime: Continuity and Change*, 151-218.

| Chapter 7 | # The Family in Addiction |

Theodore V. Parran, Jr., M.D., FACP
Michael R. Liepman, M.D., FASAM
Kathleen Farkas, Ph.D., LISW, ACSW

The Importance of Family in Addiction
Family Consequences of Addiction
Family Adjustment to Addiction
The Physician's Role With Addicted Families
Models of Family Therapy

Many physicians do not consider it of great clinical importance to be aware of and attend to family issues in their patients. This is a grave error in caring for patients with chronic illness in general and addictive disorders in particular. In fact, it is vital to address family issues with the patient who has an alcohol or drug use disorder for the following reasons:

- Addictive disorders have a very high prevalence rate, produce a significant amount of morbidity (and, not uncommonly, mortality) in family members, and often are overlooked by physicians and other treatment providers.

- Addiction can be seen as a prototype for chronic illnesses that affect families.

- Addictive disorders overwhelmingly are familial in origin, genetically and environmentally, and heavily cluster in certain families.

- Family members can have a significant effect on the processes of addiction and recovery.

- Family education and therapy have been shown to have therapeutic value as part of addiction treatment.

- A number of simple, straightforward interventions are available to help family members of addicted patients.

For all of these reasons, learning about and addressing the family aspects of addiction are important to physicians and other caregivers.

The term "family of procreation" is used to indicate the nuclear family, including the individual's spouse and children, while the term "family of origin" describes the individual's parents and siblings. "Extended family" refers to all the known living relatives. "Family with addiction" or "addicted family" describes a family in which at least one (and, not infrequently, more than one) member suffers from an addictive disorder.

THE IMPORTANCE OF FAMILY IN ADDICTION
Given that the lifetime prevalence of addictive disorders is in the range of 10% to 13%, and the tendency of addictive disorders to manifest initially in late adolescence and early adulthood, addiction has a proportionately larger effect on family systems than most other chronic illnesses. At least a fourth of the population is part of a family that is affected by an addictive disorder in a first-degree relative. The data

also suggest that up to 90% of actively addicted individuals live at home with a family or significant other.

If physicians tend to overlook addiction in their patients, they are even more likely to miss the diagnosis of addiction in family members (Frank, Graham et al., 1992). As a result, the attendant dysfunction, morbidity, and risk of mortality are unrecognized, and the underlying cause of many somatic complaints is not identified and addressed (Graham, 1996; McGann, 1990).

Family attitudes can directly or indirectly encourage or permit the early experimentation with or use of mood-altering substances. For example, one of the most important predictors of childhood experimentation with tobacco is a parent who smokes. Families also can play an important role in discouraging substance abuse by family members and moving an individual toward recovery or, conversely, sheltering the family member from the adverse consequences of his or her substance use and thus enabling his or her continuing addiction. (Family enabling is a natural outgrowth of the normal phenomenon of caring and support that takes place to a greater or lesser extent in all families, but it can become distorted by an addictive disorder into impressively pathologic forms.)

Families often play a role in the progression and perpetuation of addictive behaviors, and family problems are widely recognized as an important risk factor for relapse.

Finally, continued use of mood-altering drugs by family members, or continued interpersonal strife within the family system, can precipitate relapse, especially during the early phases of abstinence or recovery.

FAMILY CONSEQUENCES OF ADDICTION

Addictions are among the most familial of diseases, with strong genetic components and significant environmental contributions. Living in a family affected by addiction can lead to induction of alcohol or other drug abuse in additional family members. It has been observed that heterosexual women who are married to or who live with addicted men are more likely to become addicted themselves (Klassen, Wilsnack et al., 1991; Lex, 1990; Wilsnack & Wilsnack, 1990, 1993); conversely, many drinking women who separate from or divorce addicted partners subsequently reduce their drinking or drug use.

Children who grow up in a home where alcohol or other drugs are abused, whether in the open or "under wraps," generally are at increased risk of developing addiction problems themselves. This may be related to genetic pre-

disposition (Heath, Cates et al., 1993; Swan, Carmelli et al., 1990; Goodwin, 1979; Reich, Cloninger et al., 1988; Cadoret, Troughton et al., 1986). Substance abuse prevention research suggests that smoking and drinking alcohol are two early steps in an adolescent's progression into illicit drug use (Kandel & Faust, 1975). Exposure to drinking and smoking in the home provides behavioral role models, tacit approval, and ease of access to the drugs, all of which encourage early experimentation.

Families can be harmed by the consequences of addiction in ways that include realignment of priorities and changing values, emergence of illness and disability, violence and exposure to other dangers, experience of early losses, and enabling others to become affected by alcohol or other drugs. Family rituals are one way that youngsters learn the values of their ancestors. Some families are more tolerant of deviance than others. Watching parents and relatives while they vacation, celebrate, or dine together permits children to observe and copy attitudes and behaviors, including those related to drug and alcohol intake, intoxication, coping with consequences, and reacting to those behaviors (Wolin, Bennett et al., 1979, 1980).

Alcohol and drug addiction are classified as behavioral disorders. Judgment and moral values are key determinants that govern behavior, but addiction repetitively and unpredictability impairs judgment and dissolves moral values, resulting in erratic and atypical behaviors. As the addicted person becomes progressively more enmeshed in obtaining and using alcohol or other drugs, his or her values are compromised. Dishonesty may surface first as "white lies" to cover up indiscretions, then as stealing, drug dealing, or involvement in other illicit behavior to obtain drugs—sometimes progressing even to more serious criminal activities. Sharing alcohol and other drugs in social situations may lead to early sexual activity, poor choices in sexual partners, sexual exploitation or traumatization, trading sex for drugs, promiscuity, and prostitution. Sporadic failures to honor religious, civic, and family responsibilities because of intoxication or withdrawal may accumulate to such an extent that the individual appears to shirk responsibility altogether.

Individuals in the recovery community often refer to their addiction as having been a major love relationship with a jealous "significant other," which just happened to be an inanimate mood-altering drug. As their relationship with the drug gradually hypertrophied, it crowded out and severely stressed all other major relationships in their lives—particularly their family relationships. Because psychoactive drugs often remain in the body for long periods of time, an episode of alcohol or other drug use may have spilled over into times that should have been, or were intended to be, devoted to other activities. As the addiction progressed through development of toxicity, tolerance, dependence, and obsession over acquisition and ingestion, the amount of time spent impaired increased, and the amount of time spent drug-free diminished.

An individual who abuses alcohol or other drugs has a substantially increased risk of illness or disability. Dangers such as traumatic injury and morbidity associated with the psychological and/or physiological effects of alcohol and other drugs increase the risk of hospitalization, permanent disability, and death (Burant, Liepman et al., 1992; Liepman, Nirenberg et al., 1987; Wartenberg & Liepman, 1987, 1990). The burden on the family increases during times when the alcohol- or drug-abusing member is ill or disabled.

Interpersonal verbal, physical, and sexual violence often erupts within addicted families, to the extent that addiction is clearly associated with an increased risk of domestic violence. When alcohol or sedative-hypnotics are involved, the anxiolytic effect may numb the perception or fear of harming loved ones. The amnestic effect of these drugs also may lead to memory blackouts that prevent recall of prior hurtful acts that were committed under the influence. Stimulants cause irritability, intensify aggression and expressions of anger, and enhance paranoia. If both the victim and the perpetrator of violence are intoxicated, they may be unable to de-escalate the conflict before it becomes dangerous. Sexual violence long has been associated with substance abuse and addiction, and particularly with the use of alcohol and stimulants. The ability of an intoxicated person to remain sensitive to the subtle cues of a sexual partner and to heed warnings may be diminished, leading to partner or date rape or to sexual insensitivity (Nirenberg, Liepman et al., 1990).

Active addiction carries with it a sevenfold increase in risk of mortality, so death of an addicted family member is all too common. While some may consider this a welcome opportunity for the family to rid itself of continuing exposure to danger and unhappiness, it tragically deprives children of parents or siblings and causes grief and loss of a valued family member. Family roles need to shift to adjust to such a loss. Some members may blame themselves or others in the family for the untimely death of the addicted parent or spouse. Loss of a role model may affect children,

and loss of a spouse and sexual partner may lead to more instability, sometimes accompanied by introduction of a new (all too often addicted) spouse/partner, whose presence as stepparent may be resented and resisted by the children. Loss of a parent or sibling may occur in other ways, as through institutionalization (in prison, a mental hospital, a foster or group home, or a nursing home) as the result of trauma or emotional problems, or through running away from home (Casey, 1991), adolescent pregnancy, and premature marriage, divorce or separation. Family addiction may lead to other family structural changes as various members remove themselves from an increasingly dysfunctional family (Liepman, White et al., 1986).

FAMILY ADJUSTMENT TO ADDICTION

Addictive disorders provide a model for understanding the effects and minimizing the impact of any chronic disease on families and individual family members. Such disorders often occur during periods of peak family involvement in the life cycle, are of gradual and insidious onset, involve aberrant behaviors as their earliest symptoms, and feature periods of relapse and remission. As such, addictive disorders alter family "rules, roles, and customs/rituals," and often cause family members to overlook the very existence of the disorder.

The early onset, gradual progression, and intermitten chronic nature of addictive disorders, coupled with the addict's resistance to the constructive influences exerted by family members, often lead other family members to resigned acceptance of the disordered member's addiction as an unchangeable trait of family life. This is particularly true in families where the addiction has persisted for a long time (decades or generations). Such families adjust to the chronic condition of addiction so completely that adjusting to recovery may become stressful; they do so by evolving various bizarre or at least self-defeating defensive routines. Knowledge of the stereotypical defense mechanisms that families develop in response to addiction can be helpful to physicians and addiction treatment professionals.

Typical defense mechanisms adopted by families include *classic denial* that there is a problem, *minimization* of the magnitude of the problem, *projection* of the problem or blame for the problem onto others, and *rationalization* or excusing the problem away (Barker, Whitfield et al., 1995). Through use of these mechanisms, family members attempt to protect themselves or to reinforce the normalcy and worth of their family system. Addicted families tend to employ

---

more and more *isolation* as a defense, minimizing the amount of potential embarrassment to which they are exposed, while at the same time limiting the exposure of their own members to other, healthier family systems (Graham 1996; Graham & Berolzheimer, 1993). In fact, families affected by addiction often are not even aware that addictive disease is present. If families do not identify addiction as a problem for an individual family member, then they are not able to recognize that addiction also is adversely affecting the family as a system.

All family systems develop typical patterns of interrelating with one another; these patterns have been termed family rules and family roles (Baird, 1992). The rules have been summarized as (1) "don't talk": discussing dysfunctional and painful drinking events by the family often is energetically suppressed; (2) "don't feel": suppressing feelings is common in addictive families, much as it is in addictive individuals; and (3) "don't trust": the disease of addiction almost inevitably results in repeated episodes of irresponsible and erratic behavior. This sort of behavior causes frequent disappointments to others and diminishes their ability to trust in others. The emphasis on the following rules may well provide some protective effect for individual family members, but it does not encourage the development of healthy, intimate, nurturing relationships.

Stereotypical family roles, first described by Wegscheider-Cruse (1989), now are widely accepted in popular culture. Wegscheider-Cruse postulated that children in families with alcoholism internalize limited and rigid family roles that can stay with them throughout their lives. Her descriptions of those roles (enabler, hero, scapegoat, lost child, mascot) are taught in virtually every program in the country today. It is important for physicians to be familiar with the roles in order to understand patients' actions within their family systems (Graham, 1996). Individuals may move from one role to another over time, but it is striking how often individuals adapt their behaviors to fit the assigned roles. For example, spouses and other family members may become enablers by acting as though the family's most important priority is helping the active alcoholic or addict to flourish over the short term, even at a substantial long-term cost (Kaufman, 1985; Liepman, 1993; Liepman, Wolper et al., 1982). Enablers typically become overinvolved with the addicted family member and align themselves with the addiction, sometimes assisting in defensive activities against others who would apply constructive influences against the addiction (Prochaska & DiClemente,

1986). Such alignments contribute to the prolongation or chronicity of the addictive disorder.

Cultural factors influence these interactions. In an elegant ethnographic study that compared Italian American and Irish American Roman Catholic cultures, Ames and colleagues (1985) examined the connection between alcohol abuse by the male alcoholic and domestic violence. The Irish American couples reported that the male did his drinking in a pub and any violent behavior seemed limited to those surroundings. Husbands and wives agreed that episodes of domestic violence would not be tolerated in their marital relationship, despite the rules of the Church concerning divorce. In contrast, the Italian American couples described the male's drinking as limited to the home, where his violence also erupted; both husbands and wives agreed that their marriages would continue despite the violence, "until death do us part." In the United States, where there are myriad cultures of origin and where marriages often bring together couples from different cultures, families may represent an interactive mixture of cultural rules and beliefs. In families of mixed cultural backgrounds, it is possible for the "rules" about use of alcohol and drugs, or behaviors associated with such use, to have critical protective elements deleted. This finding extends the notion advanced by Wolin and colleagues (1979, 1980) that family rituals are influenced by and promote transmission of family cultural beliefs to future generations.

Families have been observed to develop stereotyped repetitive oscillations between behavioral sequences that occur in association with ingestion of alcohol or other drugs and those associated with abstinence (called "family behavioral loops"; Liepman, Silvia et al., 1989; Silvia & Liepman, 1991). The results, like the story of Dr. Jekyll and Mr. Hyde, feature transformations under certain circumstances involving drinking or drug use. What is remarkable about such transformations is that, while the addicted person changes the character of his or her behavior, so do the other members of the family (Steinglass, Davis et al., 1977). The behavioral changes of family members are triggered by conditioned cues that indicate that the addicted person is currently sober or has relapsed.

THE PHYSICIAN'S ROLE WITH ADDICTED FAMILIES

Physicians have a unique opportunity to help families deal effectively with an addictive disorder in a family member. The clinical skills that any concerned physician should employ in dealing with family issues around addictive disorders include:

- Screening for addictive disease in the family and educating the family so that they can identify addiction in their family member.

- Helping family members to identify codependency issues and to make a "family diagnosis of addiction" (that is, morbidity, pain, and suffering in their own lives as a consequence of the addiction).

- Referring the family members for the help they need.

- Helping family members to identify and address their enabling behaviors.

Screening. Most families affected by addiction are missed by the health care team. This is due in part to family denial, and in part to families not having recognized the problem themselves. Sometimes, it is not recognized because the right questions never were asked. Given their high prevalence rate and significant effect on all family members, addictive disorders should become part of the routine family history. Simply asking all patients if they have a family history of alcohol or drug problems would improve detection considerably. However, the optimal approach to the family history of addiction is through the use of the family CAGE or f-CAGE (Frank, Graham et al. 1992). The f-CAGE is a clinical tool that permits screening for the symptoms of addiction without requiring that the individuals actually have made the diagnosis themselves. The f-CAGE markedly improves sensitivity and specificity of screening for family addictions.

An added value of adding the f-CAGE to the family interview is that it provides evidence of dysfunction and disability, or pain and suffering on the part of a loved one around his or her use of alcohol or drugs. This can be especially powerful data when it is time to present the diagnosis of a family member's addiction to the person being interviewed. It also is useful in the second task in dealing with addiction in families: helping the family make a diagnosis of addiction in the affected individual.

Another tool that can help in this effort is the use of a questionnaire such as the "Family Drinking Survey" (FDS) (Barker, Whitfield et al., 1995). The FDS incorporates 32 questions related to the family effects of alcohol or other drugs. The questions are divided into three clinical areas of inquiry: diagnosis of addiction, diagnosis of family addic-

tion (codependency resulting from the significant other's addiction), and enabling traits on the part of the family. The questions that help make the diagnosis of addiction in a family member, when combined with the results of the f-CAGE, can be extremely useful in convincing the family that they do in fact have an addicted member.

The Risk Inventory for Substance Abuse Affected Families is a tool to help physicians and other health professionals who work with children and family services (Olsen, Allen et al., 1996). The tool takes about 15 minutes to administer by a trained interviewer. It assesses the dimensions and consequences of substance abuse that make it difficult for parents to care safely and adequately for children. The scales include the areas of commitment to recovery, patterns of substance abuse, ability to meet children's needs, parental well-being, and neighborhood safety.

Addressing Codependency Issues. Questions that identify pain and suffering in the family as a result of addiction should be asked to identify codependence or family illness resulting from the addicted person's disease. The FDS identifies issues of family morbidity including self-pity, ruined occasions, arguments, anger or depression, worry, fear for safety, insomnia, and other somatic symptoms. Positive responses to the questions permit the physician to make and present the diagnosis of family illness. Counseling the family members about family addiction is more effective when it incorporates their own responses on the FDS, because it can identify ways in which the family's quality of life has been diminished by a family member's addiction.

Referrals for Care. The full range of treatment that individuals or families may need to address the family consequences of addiction is beyond the scope of this chapter. It is important for the physician to be aware of the broad range of treatment resources and to be able to help patients engage in the process. "Bibliotherapy," or recommending that individuals begin to read materials related to families and addiction, often is a good place to start. Materials from Al-Anon are quite useful, as are a number of self-help books. For individuals or families who are willing, referral to individual or family counseling can be extraordinarily helpful. In making such a referral, the physician needs to communicate with the therapist regarding the family illness and consequences that led to the referral. Otherwise individuals and even whole families can participate in counseling for long periods of time without ever disclosing the presence of the underlying addictive disorder. Finally, self-help groups for family members—including Al-Anon, Alateen,

Ala-Tot, Tough Love, and Families Anonymous—are available in every part of the country (contact information generally is found in the telephone book). Most such groups are organized on the principles and steps of Alcoholics Anonymous (AA), but focus on the recovery tasks of the individual family member who is experiencing pain from another's addictive disorder.

Addressing Enabling Behaviors. The final task for physicians to master is that of helping families identify and ultimately alter behaviors that enable the disease of addiction (Graham, 1996). Several question on the FDS assess family enabling, covering areas such as making excuses for the individual, avoiding situations that may prove embarrassing, trying to limit the family member's drinking or drug use, joining in the drinking or drug use, and altering schedules or habits to accommodate the family member's addictive behavior. Presenting information to help them understand how their actions may actually be sheltering the addicted person from appropriate consequences can be very helpful for families. However, it is important to remember that the identification of enabling behaviors is a late step in family treatment, and is useful only after families have progressed through the core steps discussed earlier.

No discussion of the tools available to help families deal with enabling behaviors would be complete without mention of the family crisis intervention. The crisis intervention essentially is a group confrontation with the addicted individual—one that is carefully organized, rehearsed, and choreographed by a trained "intervention counselor." Each member of the group is a "significant other" of the patient, and is prepared to describe several experiences in which the patient's drinking or drug use adversely affected him or her. With the weight of all of this objective evidence, presented by friends and family members, the "wall of denial" for many patients breaks down sufficiently to encourage the patient to enter a treatment program (Liepman, 1993; Liepman, Nirenberg et al., 1987; Liepman, Wolper et al., 1982).

Phrases and techniques that are coached by the intervention counselor include the following: "It's not you, it's the drinking," "It hurts me too much to see you continue in this painful disease," "You did not develop this on purpose, but you've got it," "We care about you, but hate your drinking," "I will not argue; this is what you did, this is when you did it, and this is how it made me feel." There are several common threads in these phrases: (1) exhibiting positive regard toward the individual but negative attitudes toward the drinking or drug use; (2) providing data about specific events; (3) validating the disease through statements about the obvious pain of this progressive illness—which destroys families, jobs, finances, legal standing, spirituality, and physical health—thus giving the patient permission to become less defensive; and (4) relieving guilt and reducing defensiveness by acknowledging that patients with addictive disorders did not intend to "catch it," but insisting that they need treatment nonetheless.

When organized and supervised by a well-trained intervention counselor, a crisis intervention motivates 8 of 10 patients who are at the contemplative or even precontemplative stage of change to agree to enter a treatment program. Even if it is not successful in engaging the index patient in treatment, a family crisis intervention usually alters the family system surrounding the index patient in a positive way by helping family members free themselves from their family member's addiction.

MODELS OF FAMILY THERAPY

Most physicians are not involved directly with family interventions and family treatment of addiction, but it is important to understand the models available. Often it is a non-using family member who seeks advice from the physician on how to engage the addicted individual in treatment.

Typically, families have tried and failed to influence the family member's drinking or drug use behavior before they seek professional help. There have been a number of recent advances in motivational techniques for family members. Community Reinforcement and Family Training (CRAFT) is an intervention that employs reinforcement principles (Meyers, Miller et al., 1999). Using cognitive-behavioral techniques, CRAFT teaches family members to use behavioral principles and to reduce their own stress levels. CRAFT has been studied for use with treatment-resistant alcoholics (Meyers & Smith, 1997).

Families with adolescents who require substance abuse treatment present special problems, given the complex issues of adolescent development, substance abuse, and family dynamics. Toumbourou and colleagues (2001) conducted an evaluation of the Behavioral Exchange Sytems Training (BEST) program, which is an eight-week parent group that supports and assists parents in coping with their adolescent's substance use. Parents participating in the BEST program showed reductions in mental health symptoms and increases in satisfaction and assertive parenting behaviors.

McGillicuddy and colleagues (2001) developed a coping skills training program for parents of substance-abusing adolescents. Skills training was associated with improved parental coping, family communication, and parental reports of their own functioning. Prosocial family therapy (PFT) is based on theories of risk and protective factors and integrates specific parent training with nonspecific family therapy (Blechman & Vryan, 2000). PFT is designed as a preventive intervention for juvenile offenders and their families.

The National Institute on Drug Abuse has funded the Youth Support Project (YSP), which also targets juvenile offenders. Many physicians who treat high-risk families struggle with ways to engage them in treatment interventions. YSP was developed especially for high-risk families—those who are difficult to enroll and to retain in addiction treatment (Dembo, Cervenka et al., 1999).

One of the most widely used family treatment approaches is behavioral couples therapy. In an extensive review of the literature, Epstein and McCrady (1998) found empirical support for the effectiveness of behavioral couples therapy; however, Fals-Stewart and Birchler (2001) have shown that fewer than 30% of the addiction treatment programs surveyed use behavioral couples therapy. Couples therapy has been shown to be effective in a variety of formats. Based on their extensive review of the literature, Thomas and Corcoran (2001) report that overall, all treatment conditions showed reduced substance use for up to two years after treatment had ended, although drinking tended to increase as time elapsed. (There is limited research on drug-using couples, minority groups, and low-income couples.)

As physicians watch patients and their families move through the transition points in the family life cycle, it is important to use anticipatory guidance in dealing with the stresses of such times in order to prevent relapses of recovering persons and initiation of new addictions in family members.

REFERENCES

Baird MA (1992). Care of family members and other affected persons. In MF Fleming & KL Barry (eds.) *Addictive Disorders*. St. Louis, MO: Mosby Year Book, 195-210.

Barker RL, Whitfield C & Davis J (1995). Alcoholism. In LR Barker, JR Burton & PD Zieve (eds.) *Principles of Ambulatory Medicine*. Baltimore, MD: Williams & Wilkins.

Bennett LA & Ames GM (1985). *The American Experience with Alcohol: Contrasting Cultural Perspectives*. New York, NY: Plenum Publishing Co.

Blechman E & Vryan K (2000). Prosocial family therapy: A manualized preventive intervention for juvenile offenders. *Aggression and Violent Behavior* 5:343-378.

Burant D, Liepman MR & Miller MM (1992). Mental health disorders and their impact on treatment of addictions. In MD Fleming & KL Barry (eds.) *Addictive Disorders*. St. Louis, MO: Mosby/Year Book Publishers, 315-337.

Cadoret RJ, Troughton E, O'Gorman TW et al. (1986). An adoption study of genetic and environmental factors in drug abuse. *Archives of General Psychiatry* 43:1131-1136.

Casey K (1991). *Children of Eve: The Shocking Story of America's Homeless Kids*. Hollywood, CA: Covenant House.

Dembo R, Cervenka K, Hunter B et al. (1999). Engaging high risk families in community based intervention services. *Aggression and Violent Behavior* 4:41-58.

Epstein E & McCrady B (1998). Behavioral couples treatment of alcohol and drug use disorders: Current status and innovations. *Clinical Psychology Review* 18:689-711.

Fals-Stewart W & Birchler GR (2001). A national survey of the use of couples therapy in substance abuse treatment. *Journal of Substance Abuse Treatment* 20:277-283.

Frank SH, Graham AV, Zyzanski SJ et al. (1992). Use of the Family CAGE in screening for alcohol problems in primary care. *Archives of Family Medicine* 1:209-216.

Garrett J, Landau J, Shea R et al. (1998). The ARISE Intervention: Using family and network links to engage addicted persons in treatment. *Journal of Substance Abuse Treatment* 15:333-343.

Garrett J, Landau-Stanton J, Stanton M et al. (1997). ARISE: A method for engaging reluctant alcohol- and drug-dependent individuals in treatment. *Journal of Substance Abuse Treatment* 14:235-248.

Goodwin DW (1979). Alcoholism and heredity: A review and hypothesis. *Archives of General Psychiatry* 36:57-61.

Graham AV (1996). Family Issues in Substance Abuse. *Faculty Development Program in Substance Abuse*. Rockville, MD: Center for Substance Abuse Prevention.

Graham AV & Berlozheimer N (1993). Alcohol abuse—A family disease. *Primary Care: Clinics in Office Practice* 20(1):121-130.

Graham AV, Zyzanski SJ & Reeb KG (1993). Family alcohol problems—A comparison of residents' recordings and patient telephone interviews. *Substance Abuse* 6:95-103.

Griner ME & Griner PF (1987). Alcoholism and the family. In HL Barnes, MD Aronson MD & TL Delbanco (eds.) *Alcoholism: A Guide for the Primary Care Physician*. New York, NY: Springer Verlag, 159-166.

Heath AC, Cates R, Martin NG et al. (1993). Genetic contribution to risk of smoking initiation: Comparisons across birth cohorts and across cultures. *Journal of Substance Abuse* 5:221-246.

Johnson VE (1986). *Intervention: How to Help Those Who Don't Want Help*. Minneapolis, MN: Johnson Institute.

Kandel D & Faust R (1975). Sequence and stages in patterns of adolescent drug use. *Archives of General Psychiatry* 32:923-932.

Kaufman E (1985). *Substance Abuse and Family Therapy*. New York, NY: Harcourt Brace Jovanovich, 221.

Klassen AD, Wilsnack SC, Harris TR et al. (1991). Partnership dissolution and remission of problem drinking in women: Findings from a US longitudinal survey. Presented at the Symposium on Alcohol, Family and Significant Others, Social Research Institute of Alcohol Studies and Nordic Council for Alcohol and Drug Research; Helsinki, Finland; March.

Lex BW (1990). Male heroin addicts and their female mates: Impact on disorder and recovery. *Journal of Substance Abuse* 2:147-175.

Liepman MR (1993). Using family influence to motivate alcoholics to enter treatment: The Johnson Institute Intervention Approach. In TJ O'Farrell (ed.) *Marital and Family Therapy in Alcoholism Treatment*. New York, NY: Guilford Press, 54-77.

Liepman MR, Nirenberg TD, Porges R et al. (1987). Depression associated with substance abuse. In OG Cameron (ed.) *Presentations of Depression: Depression in Medical and Other Psychiatric Disorders*. New York, NY: John Wiley & Sons, 131-167.

Liepman MR, Silvia LY & Nirenberg TD (1989). The use of Family Behavior Loop Mapping for substance abuse. *Family Relations* 38:282-287.

Liepman MR, White WT & Nirenberg TD (1986). Children in alcoholic families. In DC Lewis & CN Williams (eds.) *Providing Care for Children of Alcoholics: Clinical and Research Perspectives*. Pompano Beach, FL: Health Communications, Inc., 39-64.

Liepman MR, Wolper B & Vazquez J (1982). An ecological approach for motivating women to accept treatment for chemical dependency. In BG Reed, J Mondanaro & GM Beschner (eds.) *Treatment Services for Drug Dependent Women, Vol. II*. Rockville, MD: National Institute on Drug Abuse, 1-61.

McGann KP (1990). Self-reported illnesses in family members of alcoholics. *Family Medicine* 22(2):103-106.

McGillicuddy N, Rychtarik R, Duquette J et al. (2001). Development of a skill training program for parents of substance-abusing adolescents. *Journal of Substance Abuse Treatment* 20:59-68.

Meyers R, Miller W, Hill D et al. (1999). Community Reinforcement and Family Training (CRAFT): Engaging unmotivated drug users in treatment. *Journal of Substance Abuse* 10:291-308.

Meyers R & Smith JE (1997). Getting off the fence: Procedures to engage treatment-resistant drinkers. *Journal of Substance Abuse Treatment* 14:467-472.

Nirenberg TD, Liepman MR, Begin AM et al. (1990). The sexual relationship of male alcoholics and their female partners during periods of drinking and abstinence. *Journal of Studies on Alcohol* 51:565-568.

Olsen L, Allen D & Azzi-Lessing L (1996). Assessing risk in families affected by substance abuse. *Child Abuse and Neglect* 20(9):833-842.

Prochaska JO & DiClemente CC (1986). Towards a comprehensive model of change. In WR Miller & N Heather (eds.) *Treating Addictive Behaviors: Processes of Change*. New York, NY: Plenum Publishing Co., 3-27.

Reich T, Cloninger CR, Van Eerdewegh et al. (1988). Secular trends in the familial transmission of alcoholism. *Alcoholism: Clinical & Experimental Research* 12:458-464.

Silvia LY & Liepman MR (1991). Family behavior loop mapping enhances treatment of alcoholism. *Family & Community Health* 13:72-83.

Steinglass P, Davis DI & Berenson D (1977). Observations of conjointly hospitalized "alcoholic couples" during sobriety and intoxication: Implications for theory and therapy. *Family Process* 16:1-16.

Swan GE, Carmelli D et al. (1990). Smoking and alcohol consumption in adult male twins: Genetic heritability and shared environmental influences. *Journal of Substance Abuse* 2:39-50.

Thomas C & Corcoran J (2001). Empirically based marital and family interventions for alcohol abuse: A review. *Research on Social Work Practice* 11:549-575.

Toumbourou J, Blyth A, Bamberg J et al. (2001). Early impact of the BEST intervention for parents stressed by adolescent substance abuse. *Journal of Community and Applied Social Psychology* 11:291-304.

Wartenberg AA & Liepman MR (1987). Medical consequences of addictive behaviors. In TD Nirenberg & SA Maisto (eds.) *Developments in the Assessment and Treatment of Addictive Behaviors*. Norwood, NJ: Ablex, 49-85.

Wartenberg AA & Liepman MR (1990). Medical complications of substance abuse. In WD Lerner & MA Barr (eds.) *Handbook of Hospital-Based Substance Abuse Treatment*. New York, NY: Pergamon, 45-65.

Wilsnack SC & Wilsnack RW (1990). Epidemiology of women's drinking. *Journal of Substance Abuse* 3:133-157.

Wilsnack SC & Wilsnack RW (1993). Epidemiological research on women's drinking: Recent progress and directions for the 1990s. In ESL Gomberg & TD Nirenberg (eds.) *Women and Substance Abuse*. Norwood, NJ: Ablex, 62-99.

Wolin SJ, Bennett LA & Noonan DL (1979). Family rituals and the recurrence of alcoholism over generations. *American Journal of Psychiatry* 136(4B):589-593.

Wolin SJ, Bennett LA, Noonan DL et al. (1980). Disrupted family rituals: A factor in the intergenerational transmission of alcoholism. *Journal of Studies on Alcohol* 41:199-214.

SECTION
4

Overview of Addiction Treatment

Section Coordinators

Allan W. Graham, M.D., FACP, FASAM
Anne Geller, M.D., FASAM
Alexander F. DeLuca, M.D., FASAM

Contributors

Martin Adler, M.D.
Temple University School of Medicine
Philadelphia, Pennsylvania

Andrea G. Barthwell, M.D., FASAM
Deputy Director for Demand Reduction
Office of National Drug Control Policy
Executive Office of the President
The White House
Washington, DC

Frederic C. Blow, Ph.D.
University of Michigan
Ann Arbor, Michigan

Tacey A. Boucher, Ph.D.
Research Manager
Center for Addiction and Alternative Medicine Research
Minneapolis Medical Research Foundation
Minneapolis, Minnesota

Margaret K. Brooks, J.D.
Consultant on Legal Issues
Montclair, New Jersey

Lawrence S. Brown, Jr., M.D., M.P.H., FASAM
Clinical Associate Professor of Public Health
Weill Medical College of Cornell University, and
Senior Vice President
Addiction Research & Treatment Corporation
Brooklyn, New York

H. Blair Carlson, M.D., FACP, FASAM
Clinical Professor of Medicine
University of Colorado School of Medicine
Denver, Colorado

John N. Chappel, M.D., M.P.H., FASAM
Professor Emeritus of Psychiatry
University of Nevada School of Medicine, and
Medical Director
West Hills Hospital
Reno, Nevada

H. Westley Clark, M.D., J.D., M.P.H., FASAM
Director, Center for Substance Abuse Treatment
Substance Abuse and Mental Health Services Administration
Bethesda, Maryland

Dennis C. Daley, Ph.D.
Associate Professor of Psychiatry, and
Chief of Addiction Medicine Services
Western Psychiatric Institute and Clinic
Pittsburgh, Pennsylvania

Peter J. Delany, D.S.W.
Deputy Director
Division of Epidemiology, Services and Prevention Research
National Institute on Drug Abuse
National Institutes of Health
Bethesda, Maryland

Alexander F. DeLuca, M.D., FASAM
Private Practice of Medicine
New York, New York

John W. Finney, Ph.D.
Director, HSR&D
Center for Health Care Evaluation
VA Palo Alto Health Care System, and
Stanford University Medical Center
Palo Alto, California

Bennett W. Fletcher, Ph.D.
Senior Research Scientist
Division of Epidemiology, Services and Prevention Research
National Institute on Drug Abuse
National Institutes of Health
Bethesda, Maryland

Peter D. Friedmann, M.D., M.P.H.
Associate Professor of Medicine and Community Health
Division of General Internal Medicine
Brown University School of Medicine
Providence, Rhode Island

Richard K. Fuller, M.D.
Director, Division of Clinical and Prevention Research
National Institute on Alcohol Abuse and Alcoholism
National Institutes of Health
Bethesda, Maryland

Anne Geller, M.D., FASAM
Associate Professor of Clinical Medicine
Columbia College of Physicians and Surgeons
New York, New York

Allan W. Graham, M.D., FACP, FASAM
Medical Director
Chemical Dependency Treatment Services
Kaiser Permanente
Denver, Colorado

Susanne Hiller-Sturmhöfel, Ph.D.
Science Editor, Alcohol Research & Health
National Institute on Alcohol Abuse and Alcoholism
National Institutes of Health
Bethesda, Maryland

The Hon. Peggy Fulton Hora
Superior Court Judge
Alameda County, California

Thomas J. Kiresuk, Ph.D.
Chief Clinical Psychologist
Hennepin County Medical Center, and
Director, Program Evaluation Research Center, and
Director, Center for Addiction
   and Alternative Medicine Research
Minneapolis Medical Research Foundation
Minneapolis, Minnesota

G. Alan Marlatt, Ph.D.
Professor of Psychology, and
Director, Addictive Behaviors Research Center
University of Washington
Seattle, Washington

James R. McKay, Ph.D.
Treatment Research Institute
Penn-VA Center for Studies of Addiction
University of Pennsylvania
Philadelphia, Pennsylvania

A. Thomas McLellan, Ph.D.
Treatment Research Institute
Penn-VA Center for Studies of Addiction
University of Pennsylvania
Philadelphia, Pennsylvania

David Mee-Lee, M.D.
Chair, ASAM Criteria Committee and
   Coalition for National Clinical Criteria, and
Chief Editor, ASAM Patient Placement Criteria
Davis, California

Rudolf H. Moos, Ph.D.
Director Emeritus, HSR&D
Center for Health Care Evaluation
VA Palo Alto Health Care System, and
Stanford University Medical Center
Palo Alto, California

Patrick G. O'Connor, M.D., M.P.H.
Professor of Medicine
Yale University School of Medicine, and
Chief, Section of General Internal Medicine
Yale New Haven Hospital
New Haven, Connecticut

Richard Saitz, M.D., M.P.H., FACP
Associate Professor of Medicine and Epidemiology
Section of General Internal Medicine, and
Director, Clinical Addiction Research
   and Education (CARE) Unit
Boston University School of Medicine
Boston, Massachusetts

Jeffrey H. Samet, M.D., M.A., M.P.H.
Professor of Medicine and Public Health
Section of General Internal Medicine, and
Clinical Addiction Research and Education (CARE) Unit
Boston University School of Medicine
Boston, Massachusetts

The Hon. William G. Schma
Circuit Judge
Kalamazoo, Michigan

Joseph J. Shields, Ph.D.
Associate Professor of Social Work
Catholic University of America
Washington, DC, and
Social Science Analyst
Division of Epidemiology, Services and Prevention Research
National Institute on Drug Abuse
National Institutes of Health
Bethesda, Maryland

Gerald D. Shulman, M.A., M.A.C., FACATA
Training & Consulting Services in Behavioral Health
Jacksonville, Florida

Crystal E. Spotts, M.Ed.
Research Coordinator
Western Psychiatric Institute and Clinic
Pittsburgh, Pennsylvania

Alan I. Trachtenberg, M.D., Ph.D.
U.S. Public Health Service Medical Officer
Center for Substance Abuse Treatment
Substance Abuse and Mental Health Services Administration
Bethesda, Maryland

David B. Wexler
Lyons Professor of Law and Professor of Psychology
University of Arizona, and
Director, International Network on Therapeutic Jurisprudence
University of Puerto Rico
Ponce, Puerto Rico

Bruce J. Winick
Professor of Law
University of Miami School of Law
Coral Gables, Florida

Alex Wodak, M.D., FRACP
Director, Alcohol and Drug Service
St. Vincent's Hospital
Darlinghurst, New South Wales
Australia

Douglas Ziedonis, M.D., M.P.H.
Director, Division of Addiction Medicine
Department of Psychiatry
Robert Wood Johnson Medical School
Piscataway, New Jersey

Joan E. Zweben, Ph.D.
Clinical Professor of Psychiatry
University of California, San Francisco, and
Executive Director, 14th Street Clinic
    and East Bay Community Recovery Project
Oakland, California

Chapter 1

The Treatment of Alcoholism: A Review

Richard K. Fuller, M.D.
Susanne Hiller-Sturmhöfel, Ph.D.

Treatment Settings
Detoxification
Behavioral Treatment Approaches
Pharmacotherapies
Brief Interventions

According to the 1992 National Longitudinal Alcohol Epidemiologic Survey, a national household survey, approximately 7.5% of the U.S. population (about 14 million Americans) abuse and/or are dependent on alcohol (Grant, Harford et al., 1994). Further, according to the 1993 National Drug and Alcoholism Treatment Unit Survey, more than 700,000 persons receive alcoholism treatment on any given day (NIAAA, 1997). Of those persons, 13.5% receive inpatient treatment in either a residential setting or a hospital, and 86.5% are treated on an outpatient basis. Approaches currently used in the treatment of alcohol problems generally have been developed on the basis of three sources of information: (1) the experiences of recovering alcoholics and the professional staff who treat them, (2) research into human behavior, and (3) studies of potential medications (that is, pharmacological research).

Most treatment programs encourage patients to attend regular meetings of Alcoholics Anonymous (AA) or similar self-help groups that are based on a Twelve Step philosophy. Many treatment programs also use relapse prevention techniques to help patients acquire the skills necessary to prevent a relapse after they achieve initial abstinence. This approach is derived from therapeutic methods developed by behavioral psychologists. Cognitive-behavioral therapy (CBT) is based on learning theory, which posits that human behavior is largely learned and that learning processes can be used to change problem behaviors.

In addition to Twelve Step programs and behavioral therapies, one pharmacological agent, disulfiram (Antabuse®), has been available and used in alcoholism treatment since the late 1940s. In 1994, the U.S. Food and Drug Administration (FDA) also approved the medication naltrexone (ReVia™) for alcoholism treatment on the basis of randomized clinical trials. To date, however, naltrexone is not widely used, although such pharmacotherapy has shown promising results in improving treatment outcomes.

This chapter summarizes some of the characteristics and findings of recent alcoholism treatment research. It introduces the two general treatment settings (inpatient and outpatient) and reviews research into currently used alcoholism treatment approaches. These approaches include detoxification to manage alcohol withdrawal, nonpharmacologic treatment methods, pharmacotherapies, and brief interventions that are designed to be delivered by primary care physicians rather than alcoholism treatment specialists. For more in-depth information on these topics, the reader is referred to the chapters in Sections 5, 6, 7, and 8.

Alcoholism Treatment Research. Until recently, few controlled clinical studies had evaluated and compared the efficacy of various treatment approaches, particularly of AA and other Twelve Step programs that currently are the cornerstone of alcoholism treatment in the United States. Several factors may contribute to the paucity of controlled research on the efficacy of AA. First, AA became a central component of most treatment programs before stringent study designs and criteria for assessing treatment outcomes were introduced as standard procedures for determining the efficacy of alcoholism treatment. Second, researchers in the past have been deterred from studying AA for several reasons: AA programs can vary tremendously from group to group in the type and number of attendees, as well as in the meeting style; moreover, no standard definition of an AA member exists, and studying AA without perturbing its characteristics, such as the anonymity of its members, is difficult. Third, practitioners may be reluctant to enroll their patients in clinical studies of alcoholism treatments if the practitioners believe that the treatment to be evaluated is inferior to the traditional approaches already used.

TREATMENT SETTINGS

Various alcoholism treatments differ not only in the methods they use but also in the setting in which they are delivered. Thus, alcoholism treatment can be performed either in residential and hospital (inpatient) settings or in outpatient settings. Inpatient rehabilitation programs traditionally last 28 days and provide highly structured treatment services, including group therapy, individual therapy, and alcoholism education. In these settings, professional staff members are available around the clock to help manage the patient's acute medical and psychological problems during the initial treatment period (detoxification). Alternatively, the patient may receive only short-term inpatient detoxification services before being transferred to an outpatient setting for further rehabilitation.

Currently, the vast majority of alcoholic patients are treated in outpatient facilities. Those programs offer alcoholism treatment services of varying intensity and duration. Day hospital programs (for example, intensive outpatient programs) involve the patient for several hours a day, several days a week and were developed as alternatives to inpatient programs. Day hospital programs allow patients to maintain their family roles while simultaneously receiving treatment. Less intensive outpatient services generally offer counseling sessions (such as group sessions, individual sessions, and—if necessary—family or couples therapy) once or twice a week. For many patients, those services are intended as maintenance therapy after patients have received initial inpatient or intensive outpatient treatment.

Because of escalating health care costs, the focus in recent years has shifted away from inpatient treatment and toward outpatient treatment for all stages of recovery. This shift has resulted in an emphasis on outpatient detoxification and intensive outpatient services for initial treatment—approaches that are less expensive than inpatient treatment. In addition, the typical length of stay in inpatient programs has decreased substantially.

The effectiveness of inpatient treatment versus outpatient treatment is controversial. Finney and colleagues (Finney, Hahn et al., 1996) analyzed several studies and concluded that outpatient treatment is appropriate for most individuals who have sufficient social resources and who do not have serious co-occurring medical and/or psychiatric impairments. Conversely, inpatient treatment should be employed for clients who have serious co-occurring medical and/or psychiatric conditions, as well as for clients with few social resources and/or environments that are not supportive of recovery.

DETOXIFICATION

Sudden cessation of alcohol consumption in persons who have consumed alcohol regularly can lead to a variety of clinical symptoms that collectively are called "alcohol withdrawal syndrome." The manifestations of alcohol withdrawal can range from mild irritability, insomnia, and tremors to potentially life-threatening medical complications, such as seizures, hallucinations, and *delirium tremens*. Consequently, before beginning long-term alcoholism treatment, many patients require a detoxification period during which they become alcohol-free under controlled conditions. Depending on the severity of the withdrawal symptoms, such services can be delivered in either an inpatient or an outpatient setting.

Medically supervised detoxification frequently involves treatment with medications, particularly for patients with moderate to severe withdrawal symptoms. For most patients, benzodiazepines are the treatment of choice. An early randomized clinical trial demonstrated that benzodiazepines effectively prevented the development of *delirium tremens*

(Kaim, Klett et al., 1969). Since that study was conducted, benzodiazepine use has revolutionized the treatment of alcohol withdrawal syndrome. Initially, benzodiazepines were administered on a predetermined dosing schedule for several days, often in gradually tapering doses. Recent studies have shown, however, that lower overall benzodiazepine doses can be used if the dose is continually adjusted to the severity of the symptoms (Saitz, 1998). Because benzodiazepines have an abuse potential of their own, therapists should not prescribe them after the acute withdrawal period.

Current state-of-the-art alcohol detoxification begins with an assessment of the severity of the patient's withdrawal symptoms, using assessment tools such as the revised Clinical Institute Withdrawal Assessment for Alcohol (CIWA-Ar) (Sullivan, Sykora et al., 1989; Foy, March et al., 1988). This questionnaire evaluates the presence and severity of various withdrawal symptoms, such as nausea and vomiting; tremors; sweating; anxiety; agitation; tactile, auditory, and visual disturbances; headaches; and disorientation. The higher the patient's score on the CIWA-Ar, the greater his or her risk of experiencing serious withdrawal symptoms, such as seizures and confusion.

Patients who experience only mild withdrawal symptoms (a score below 8 points on the CIWA-Ar) do not require pharmacotherapy; however, they should be monitored for potential complications. Conversely, patients who experience withdrawal symptoms that either are moderate (a score of 8 to 15 points) or severe (a score of more than 15 points) should be treated with medications, such as benzodiazepines. Hayashida and colleagues (1989) demonstrated that patients with moderate withdrawal symptoms can be treated safely on an outpatient basis.

Recent work by Hayashida (1998) indicates that outpatient detoxification offers several advantages. For example, the patient may be able to use the same facility for both detoxification and subsequent long-term outpatient treatment. In addition, the patient may be able to more easily maintain family and social relationships and thus experience greater social support. Finally, the costs are lower for outpatient than for inpatient detoxification.

Outpatient detoxification is not appropriate, however, for patients who are at risk for life-threatening withdrawal symptoms, have other serious medical conditions, are suicidal or homicidal, have disruptive family or job situations, or cannot travel daily to the treatment facility. Moreover, outpatient detoxification is associated with significantly lower completion rates than inpatient detoxification

(Hayashida, Alterman et al., 1989). Finally, patients undergoing outpatient detoxification are at an increased risk of relapse during or shortly after detoxification because they have more access to alcoholic beverages. However, long-term outcomes (more than 6 months) do not appear to differ between patients who receive inpatient or outpatient detoxification (Hayashida, 1998).

BEHAVIORAL TREATMENT APPROACHES

The term "behavioral treatment" is used broadly here to include various nonpharmacologic therapies whose objective is to change behavior around alcohol consumption. These approaches include behavioral therapy, cognitive therapy, various types of psychotherapy, counseling, and other rehabilitative strategies.

Cognitive-Behavioral Therapy. One of the greatest challenges in the treatment of alcoholism and other addictions is the prevention of relapse. Patients have reported numerous factors that can trigger relapse. Some of those factors are internal to the patient, such as craving for alcohol, depression, and anxiety. Other factors are external, such as social pressure to drink; environmental cues associated with drinking (for example, visits to bars or restaurants or the smell of alcohol); problems in relationships with other people; and negative life events, such as the death or illness of a family member or loss of a job. To prevent relapses resulting from those factors, cognitive-behavioral therapy (CBT) is designed to help the patient identify high-risk situations for relapse, learn and rehearse strategies for coping with those situations, and recognize and cope with craving. Variations of CBT are widely used in alcoholism treatment under the label of "relapse prevention." In formal CBT, patients practice behavioral or cognitive skills to cope with high-risk situations through rehearsal, role playing, and homework.

Various studies have evaluated the efficacy of CBT (Longabaugh & Morgenstern, 1999). In the Project MATCH study, which compared the efficacy of three different treatment approaches, CBT achieved outcomes comparable to those of the other two therapies studied (Project MATCH Research Group, 1997a). This result may be surprising because CBT and other approaches, such as Twelve Step programs, appear to differ substantially. A recent review, however, identified elements common to Twelve Step programs and CBT-based approaches that may help explain their comparable results. For example, both approaches encourage the patient to pursue activities incompatible with drinking and to identify and cope with negative thinking (McCrady, 1994).

Motivational Enhancement Therapy. Another psychological-behavioral approach to alcoholism treatment that is receiving increasing attention is motivational enhancement therapy (MET). This method, which is based on the principles of motivational psychology, does not guide the patient step-by-step through recovery but strives to motivate the individual to use his or her own resources to change behavior. To that end, the therapist first assesses the type and severity of the patient's drinking-associated problems. On the basis of this initial assessment, the therapist provides structured feedback to stimulate the patient's motivation to change. The therapist also encourages the patient to make future plans and, during subsequent counseling sessions, attempts to maintain or increase the patient's motivation to initiate or to continue implementing change. (For more information on MET, see DiClemente, Bellino et al., 1999.)

AA and Twelve Step Facilitation Therapy. AA and similar self-help groups outline 12 consecutive activities, or steps, that alcoholics should achieve during the recovery process. For example, these steps specify that drinkers must admit that they are powerless over alcohol, make a moral inventory of themselves, admit the nature of their wrongs, make a list of everyone they have harmed, and make amends to those people. Alcoholics can become involved with AA before entering professional treatment, as part of their professional treatment, as aftercare following professional treatment, or instead of professional treatment. In addition, AA members can differ in the degree of their AA involvement (for example, how often they attend AA meetings, whether they become involved with a sponsor, or whether they actively participate in meetings).

Twelve Step Facilitation (TSF) is a formal treatment approach that has been developed to introduce clients to and involve them in AA and similar Twelve Step programs. Thus, TSF guides clients through the first five steps of the AA program and promotes AA affiliation and involvement. For example, therapists who use TSF actively encourage their patients to attend AA meetings, maintain a journal of their AA attendance and participation, obtain a sponsor, and work on completing the first five steps. In addition, participants receive reading assignments from the AA literature.

Although AA is the most popular self-help group for persons with drinking problems, its efficacy rarely has been assessed in randomized clinical trials. Most research on AA efficacy has compared the outcomes of persons who did or did not become involved in AA. Those studies have reported a consistent association between voluntary AA participation and abstinence. Because the studies are not randomized, however, some factor other than AA involvement may account for the results. (For example, it may be that persons who choose to attend AA have a greater motivation to become abstinent.)

To eliminate the possibility that another factor is responsible for the observed outcome and to demonstrate a cause and effect relationship between AA participation and outcome, researchers must conduct studies in which alcoholic patients are randomly assigned to AA and to one or more other treatments. To date, Walsh and colleagues (1991) and the Project MATCH Research Group (1997a) have conducted two major studies of AA, using random patient assignment. The findings of the both studies are summarized in the following section.

The study by Walsh and colleagues (Walsh, Hingson et al., 1991) included 227 alcohol-abusing participants whose employers had referred them to an employee assistance program. Participants were randomly assigned to one of three treatment options: (1) compulsory three-week inpatient treatment, followed by one year of attendance at AA meetings (hospital group), (2) compulsory attendance at AA meetings only (AA group), or (3) participants' choice of treatment. Participants were followed for two years (choice group). During that time, the investigators examined various drinking measures (such as abstinence rates), relapse rates (as measured by the need for hospitalization for additional treatment), and work-related outcomes (for example, proportion of participants who remained employed). The study results can be summarized as follows:

- On drinking measures, both the AA-only group and the choice group fared worse than the hospital group. For example, whereas 37% of the hospital group remained abstinent throughout the entire two-year study period, only 17% of the choice group and 16% of the AA-only group were continuously abstinent. Similarly, the percentage of patients who did not become intoxicated during the study period was significantly higher in the hospital group than in either the choice or the AA-only group.

- Participants in the AA-only group relapsed more often than did participants in the other two groups. Thus, 63% of the AA-only group required hospitalization for a relapse during the two-year study period, compared

TABLE 1.   Overall Outcomes of Clients in the Aftercare and Outpatient* Groups of the Project MATCH Study

Outcome Variable	Percentage of Clients According to Treatment Group**	
	Aftercare	Outpatient
Continuously abstinent for 1 year following treatment	35	20
Abstinent between 9 and 12 months after treatment	46	30
Drinking moderately without any problems between 9 and 12 months after treatment	7	12

* Aftercare clients were recruited into the study after receiving either inpatient or intensive outpatient treatment. Participants in the outpatient group received no intensive treatment before entering the study (Project MATCH Research Group, 1997a).

** The numbers represent the proportion of clients in the aftercare and outpatient samples who fulfilled the outcome variable indicated. For example, 35% of all aftercare clients and 20% of all outpatient clients remained continuously abstinent for 1 year following treatment.

with 23% of the hospital group and 38% of the choice group. As a result of the additional treatment required by the AA-only group, the estimated total costs incurred by the hospital group were about 10% higher than the costs incurred by the AA-only group.

■ Work-related outcome variables, such as the proportion of patients who remained employed over the study period, did not differ significantly among the three groups.

This study is important for several reasons. First, the counselors involved in the study allowed their clients to be randomly assigned to a treatment. Second, the study methodology was scientifically sound, because it compared the outcomes of three treatment approaches to which the participants had been randomly assigned. Third, the results suggest that an approach that integrates AA with professional treatment generally will achieve better outcomes than referral to AA alone. However, the study did not address whether inpatient and outpatient professional treatments can be equally effective in combination with AA participation.

Project MATCH. Project MATCH, a multisite study, primarily focused on identifying patient characteristics that would predict which patients would benefit most from a particular treatment approach. The study included two groups of participants. One group (the aftercare sample) was recruited at four facilities that provided aftercare services to patients who had received inpatient or day-hospital treatment and therefore had received some kind of intensive treatment. The other group (the outpatient sample) was recruited at five outpatient facilities and was composed of patients who had not received prior intensive inpatient or day-hospital treatment. As a result of their varied treatment histories, the two groups differed in certain patient characteristics. For example, the aftercare patients were more severely alcohol dependent when entering the study than were the outpatients.

Within both the aftercare samples and the outpatient samples, participants were randomly assigned to receive CBT, MET, or TSF. All interventions were delivered over a 12-week period in individual outpatient counseling sessions and were based on treatment manuals. To determine treatment efficacy, the study assessed several drinking-related variables. The primary variables, which were analyzed for the 90 days preceding treatment, the year following treatment, and the 90 days preceding the three-year followup, were the percentage of days on which the participants were abstinent and the number of drinks consumed per drinking day.

The study found that the aftercare sample generally achieved better treatment results than did the outpatient sample. For example, at one-year followup, 35% of the aftercare patients had remained continuously abstinent, compared with 20% of the outpatient sample. Similarly, a higher percentage of the aftercare sample than of the outpatient sample was abstinent between 9 and 12 months after treatment or was drinking moderately without problems during that period (see Table 1). Because the patients were not randomly assigned to either the aftercare sample or the outpatient sample, however, one cannot conclude that aftercare is superior to outpatient treatment. Instead, a variety of factors may help explain why the aftercare patients more commonly achieved continuous abstinence. For example, the total amount of care received may contribute to treatment outcome, because the aftercare patients had received previous care in addition to the treatment approaches included in the study. Alternatively, the period of enforced abstinence that the aftercare patients experienced during their inpatient treatment may have had a beneficial effect.

Although Project MATCH was not primarily concerned with comparing the three treatments for differential efficacy, the study's design allowed such analyses. In the aftercare sample, no differences were found in the efficacy of CBT, MET, and TSF during the year following treatment. Similarly, no differences or only small ones existed among the outpatients in the efficacy of the three treatments. Those differences that did exist usually indicated that TSF was most efficacious. For example, significantly more TSF-treated outpatients (24%) than either MET- or CBT-treated outpatients (14% and 15%, respectively) were continuously abstinent for one year after treatment (Project MATCH Research Group, 1997a). Similarly, the abstinence rate during the preceding 90 days at both the one- and three-year followups were slightly higher among the TSF-treated outpatients than among the MET-treated and CBT-treated outpatients (Project MATCH Research Group, 1998a).

Some differences existed in the time course over which the three treatments improved the outpatients' drinking patterns; no such differences existed, however, among aftercare patients. Thus, during the three months of therapy, only 28% of MET-treated outpatients, compared with 41% of the CBT- and TSF-treated outpatients, were continuously abstinent or drank moderately without problems (Project MATCH Research Group 1998b). During the three years following treatment, however, the percentage of abstinent days and number of drinks per drinking day reported by the MET-treated outpatients were comparable with those of the CBT- and TSF-treated outpatients. These findings suggest that patients may achieve control over their drinking problems more slowly with the less directive MET approach than with the CBT or TSF approaches; nevertheless, they experience long-term outcomes comparable with those of the two other therapies.

Patient Characteristics Predicting Treatment Outcome. The primary goal of the Project MATCH study was to determine patient characteristics that could predict which treatment approach would be most effective for a given patient. The study identified four patient-treatment matches—one in the aftercare sample and three in the outpatient sample.

First, when the aftercare patients were classified according to the severity of their dependence, those patients who had been more severely dependent achieved better results (that is, had more abstinent days and fewer drinks per drinking day) with TSF than with CBT (Project MATCH Research Group, 1997b). For example, among the TSF-treated patients, the most severely dependent were abstinent on 94% of the days after treatment compared with abstinence on 84% of the days in the most severely dependent CBT-treated patients. Conversely, the least severely dependent CBT-treated patients averaged 94% of abstinent days after treatment, compared with 89% of abstinent days in the least severely dependent TSF-treated patients. These findings suggest that among patients who have already received inpatient treatment, TSF may be more appropriate for highly dependent patients, whereas CBT may be more appropriate for less severely dependent patients.

Second, in the outpatient sample, MET was the most effective approach in the treatment of patients with high levels of anger (as determined by the Spielberger Anger Scale). MET-treated outpatients with greater levels of anger had a greater percentage of abstinent days and fewer drinks per drinking day than did outpatients with similar anger levels who were treated with CBT. For example, MET patients with high anger levels were abstinent on 85% of the days, compared with 75% of abstinent days for CBT patients with high anger levels (Project MATCH Research Group, 1998b). This match between anger level and treatment approach was observed at the one-year followup and persisted at the three-year followup (Project MATCH Research Group, 1998a).

Third, the Project MATCH results indicated that TSF and the resulting AA involvement were particularly effective for outpatients whose social networks (family members and friends) supported drinking. At the three-year followup, those patients had better outcomes with TSF than with MET (Longabaugh, Wirtz et al., 1998). Thus, outpatients in the upper median for a supportive drinking network who received TSF had 83% of abstinent days, compared with 66% of abstinent days among similar patients receiving MET. AA involvement was an important mediator of this effect: TSF-treated patients whose social network supported drinking and who became involved in AA had 91% abstinent days, compared with 60% abstinent days for similar patients who did not become involved in AA. AA involvement also enhanced treatment outcomes in patients whose social networks were supportive of drinking and who received either MET or CBT; however, this beneficial effect of AA involvement was smaller than among patients receiving TSF.

Researchers also observed the relationship among a drinker's social network, AA involvement, and treatment outcome in a recent long-term study of patients at 15 Department of Veterans Affairs hospitals (Humphreys, Mankowski et al., in press). The study found that replacing patients' social networks of drinking friends with the AA fellowship was at least partially responsible for the better outcomes observed in those who became involved with AA. Thus, treatment approaches that facilitate involvement in Twelve Step programs may be beneficial, particularly for persons whose social networks support drinking. For such individuals, a new social network of friends who support abstinence appears to be a key element in recovery.

Fourth, the Project MATCH findings indicated that for the first nine months following treatment, outpatients who were low in psychiatric severity as assessed by the Addiction Severity Index psychiatric subscale experienced more abstinent days and fewer drinks per drinking day when treated with TSF than with CBT. At the one-year followup, however, this difference between the treatment groups no longer existed.

Overall, the results of Project MATCH provide only limited support for the hypothesis that patients can be matched with optimal treatments on the basis of patient characteristics, because only 4 of a possible 21 matches (based on the number of treatments and patient characteristics evaluated) were detected. Moreover, one of the four matches had dissipated within one year after treatment. The findings do suggest, however, that some incremental improvement in outcome occurs if aftercare patients are screened for severity of dependence and outpatients are screened prior to treatment for anger and type of social network.

PHARMACOTHERAPIES

At present, therapists use primarily two types of medications in alcoholism treatment: (1) aversive medications, which deter the patient from drinking, and (2) anticraving medications, which reduce the patient's desire to drink.

Aversive Medications. The most commonly used aversive medication in alcoholism treatment is disulfiram, which has been available since the late 1940s. The medication causes an unpleasant reaction (involving nausea, vomiting, flushing, and increased blood pressure and heart rate) when the patient ingests alcohol. Early clinical studies of disulfiram therapy reported favorable outcomes among recovering alcoholics; however, most of those studies were not conducted according to the current standards of controlled clinical trials (Fuller & Roth, 1979).

Conversely, according to one large, well-designed study, disulfiram did not increase the rate of sustained abstinence or time to relapse among the patients (Fuller, Branchey et al., 1986). In addition, only a subgroup of study participants (patients who showed evidence of greater social stability) drank less frequently when taking disulfiram than did patients with similar characteristics who received placebo or no medication. Moreover, abstinence was related to the patients' compliance with the medication regimen. Because poor compliance can nullify disulfiram's effectiveness, some programs require staff members or relatives to observe the patient ingesting the medication. A randomized study (Chick, Gough et al., 1992) found that supervised disulfiram administration was more beneficial than supervised vitamin administration.

Anticraving Medications. Various brain chemicals have been implicated in mediating alcohol's pleasant effects and in contributing to the development of tolerance to and craving for alcohol. Accordingly, researchers have attempted to prevent alcohol's pleasant effects and craving for alcohol by developing medications that interfere with the actions of those brain chemicals. Two of those medications are naltrexone and acamprosate.

Naltrexone was the first agent in nearly 50 years to be approved by the FDA for alcoholism treatment. The approval was based on two randomized clinical trials reporting that naltrexone combined with psychosocial treatment reduced three-month relapse rates from 50% among patients who received a placebo to 25% among patients who received naltrexone (O'Malley, Jaffe et al., 1992; Volpicelli, Alterman et al., 1992). As with disulfiram, one study found that compliance with naltrexone was critical to obtaining favorable outcomes (Volpicelli, Rhines et al., 1997). Naltrexone acts by interfering with the actions of key brain chemicals called endogenous opioids. In response to alcohol, endogenous opioids activate certain brain cells and induce some of alcohol's pleasant effects (such as euphoria and reduced anxiety). By blocking the actions of endogenous opioids, naltrexone prevents alcohol from exerting its pleasant effects and may reduce the patient's desire to drink.

Acamprosate is another medication aimed at reducing alcohol craving. Researchers in Europe have studied the drug extensively; however, it is not yet commercially available in the United States. Scientists still do not know acamprosate's precise mechanism of action. However, the drug appears to interact with a certain type of receptor (the N-methyl-D-aspartate [NMDA] receptor) that is located on the surface of certain brain cells and which mediates the effects of another important brain chemical, glutamate. Controlled European studies have found that acamprosate treatment can almost double the abstinence rate among recovering alcoholics (Sass, Soyka et al., 1996). Researchers in the U.S. currently are conducting a multisite randomized clinical trial of acamprosate.

Future Directions in Pharmacotherapy. In addition to the medications described here, scientists are evaluating other pharmacotherapeutic approaches to alcoholism treatment (for more information on recent advances and future trends in pharmacotherapy, see Jonson & Ait-Daoud, 1999). For example, some researchers are testing medications targeting other brain chemicals (such as serotonin) that have been implicated in mediating alcohol's effects. To date, however, clinical trials of serotonin-targeting agents have not demonstrated efficacy in alcohol-dependent patients (Kranzler, Burleson et al., 1995; Johnson, Jasinski et al., 1996).

Some alcoholics suffer from co-occurring psychiatric conditions, such as depression and anxiety. In certain patients, these psychiatric conditions precede, and possibly even precipitate, alcohol abuse and dependence. In other patients, the psychiatric condition results from long-term alcohol abuse. It is plausible that at least in the former group of patients, treatment of the psychiatric illness may

decrease alcohol consumption because the patients no longer need to resort to alcohol to alleviate anxiety or depression. Three clinical trials of antidepressant medication therapy for alcoholism found that this treatment improved the patients' depression (Mason, Kocsis et al., 1996; McGrath, Nunes et al., 1996; Cornelius, Salloum et al., 1997). However, only one of the studies found that antidepressant therapy caused a major change in drinking levels (Cornelius, Salloum et al., 1997). Studies of the anti-anxiety medication buspirone in alcoholic patients have yielded conflicting results (Kranzler, Burleson et al., 1994; Malcolm, Anton et al., 1992).

Finally, other clinical trials are evaluating whether treatment efficacy can be increased by combining medications, because combination therapy is effective for the treatment of many other conditions, such as high blood pressure. It may be that these approaches will yield effective therapies to help alcoholics achieve long-term abstinence.

BRIEF INTERVENTIONS

Many persons with alcohol-related problems do not seek the help of an alcoholism treatment specialist, but rather receive care from a primary care provider. Brief intervention therapies are ideally suited to such settings. Such treatments can be completed in four or five office visits. In general, brief intervention begins with an assessment of the extent of the patient's alcohol-related problems (for example, impaired liver function or alcohol-related problems at work) and a discussion of the potential health consequences of continued drinking. The health care professional then offers advice on strategies to cut down on drinking (for nonalcohol-dependent patients only) or to abstain from drinking (for both dependent and nondependent patients). Such strategies can include setting specific goals for reducing the number of drinks consumed per day or per week and agreeing to written contracts that specify measures of progress toward changes in drinking behavior (for more information on such contracts, see Higgins & Petry, 1999).

Two controlled studies conducted in the United States and Canada have investigated the efficacy of brief interventions. Those studies demonstrated that brief interventions reduced drinking (Fleming, Barry et al., 1997; Israel, Hollander et al., 1996), alcohol-related problems (Israel, Hollander et al., 1996), and the patient's use of health care services (Fleming, Barry et al., 1997). The current challenge is to educate health care professionals about brief interventions and motivate them to employ this option (for more information on brief interventions, see Fleming & Manwell, 1999).

CONCLUSIONS

The past decade has seen remarkable advances in alcoholism treatment research. Researchers and treatment providers now have a better understanding of the effectiveness of nonpharmacologic treatments and of key elements in Twelve Step programs. In addition, research on effective pharmacotherapies for alcoholism is entering a new era. Finally, brief interventions delivered in primary care settings have been shown to be effective in reducing drinking among persons who have alcohol-related problems or who are at risk for such problems.

Substantial challenges remain, however, before the results of this research can be translated into improved treatment outcomes. For example, many treatment programs do not use pharmacotherapies, primarily for philosophical reasons—some treatment providers are reluctant to substitute one drug (the treatment medication) for another (the alcohol). Similarly, many primary care providers may not be aware of the usefulness and correct use of brief interventions. Consequently, all health care professionals working with persons who abuse or are dependent on alcohol—particularly addiction professionals—must be aware of improvements in alcoholism treatment and novel treatment options. Otherwise, patients with alcohol-related problems who could benefit from new approaches, such as pharmacotherapies, might be deprived of an opportunity for achieving long-term recovery.

ACKNOWLEDGMENT: Adapted with permission of the authors and publisher from Fuller RK & Hiller-Sturmhöfel S (1999). Alcoholism treatment in the United States: An overview. Alcohol Research & Health *23(2):78-85.*

REFERENCES

Chick J, Gough K, Faldowski W et al. (1992). Disulfiram treatment of alcoholism. *British Journal of Psychiatry* 161:84-89.

Cornelius JR, Salloum IM, Ehler JG et al. (1997). Fluoxetine in depressed alcoholics: A double-blind, placebo-controlled trial. *Archives of General Psychiatry* 54:700-705.

DiClemente C, Bellino L & Neavins T (1999). Motivation for change and alcoholism treatment. *Alcohol Research & Health* 23(2):78-85.

Finney JW, Hahn AC & Moos RH (1996). The effectiveness of inpatient and outpatient treatment for alcohol abuse: The need to focus on mediators and moderators of setting effects. *Addiction* 91:1773-1796.

Fleming ME, Barry KL, Manwell LB et al. (1997). Brief physician advice for problem alcohol drinkers: A randomized controlled trial in community-based primary care practices. *Journal of the American Medical Association* 277(13):1039-1045.

Fleming M & Manwell L (1999). Brief intervention in primary care settings. *Alcohol Research & Health* 23(2):128-137.

Foy A, March S & Drinkwater V (1988). Use of an objective clinical scale in the assessment and management of alcohol withdrawal in a large general hospital. *Alcoholism: Clinical & Experimental Research* 12:360-364.

Fuller RK & Roth HP (1979). Disulfiram for the treatment of alcoholism: An evaluation in 128 men. *Annals of Internal Medicine* 90:901-904.

Fuller RK, Branchey L, Brightwell DR et al. (1986). Disulfiram treatment of alcoholism: A Veterans Administration Cooperative Study. *Journal of the American Medical Association* 256:1449-1489,

Grant BF, Harford TC, Dawson DA et al. (1994). Prevalence of DSM-IV alcohol abuse and dependence: United States, 1992. *Alcohol Health and Research World* 18(3):243-248.

Hayashida M (1998). An overview of outpatient and inpatient detoxification. *Alcohol Health and Research World* 22(1):44-46.

Hayashida M, Alterman AI, McLellan AT et al. (1989). Comparative effectiveness and costs of inpatient and outpatient detoxification of patients with mild-to-moderate alcohol withdrawal syndrome. *New England Journal of Medicine* 320(6):358-364.

Higgins S & Petry N (1999). Contingency management. *Alcohol Research & Health* 23(2):122-127.

Humphreys K, Mankowski ES, Moss RH et al. (in press). Do enhanced friendship networks and active coping mediate the effect of self-help groups on substance abuse? *Annals of Behavioral Medicine.*

Israel Y, Hollander O, Sanchez-Craig M et al. (1996). Screening for problem drinking and counseling by the primary care physician-nurse team. *Alcoholism: Clinical & Experimental Research* 20:1443-1450.

Jonson B & Ait-Daoud N (1999). Medications to treat alcoholism. *Alcohol Research & Health* 23(2):99-106.

Johnson BA, Jasinski DR, Galloway GP et al. (1996). Ritanserin in the treatment of alcohol dependence—A multicenter clinical trial. *Psychopharmacology* 128:206-215.

Kaim SC, Klett CJ & Pothfeld B (1969). Treatment of the acute alcohol withdrawal state: A comparison of four drugs. *American Journal of Psychiatry* 125:1640-1646.

Kranzler HR, Burleson JA, Del Boca FK et al. (1994). Buspirone treatment of anxious alcoholics: A placebo-controlled trial. *Archives of General Psychiatry* 51:720-731.

Kranzler HR, Burleson JA, Korner P et al. (1995). Placebo-controlled trial of fluoxetine as an adjunct to relapse prevention in alcoholics. *American Journal of Psychiatry* 152:391-397.

Longabaugh R & Morgenstern J (1999). Cognitive-behavioral coping-skills therapy for alcohol dependence. *Alcohol Research & Health* 23(2):78-85.

Longabaugh R, Wirtz PW, Zweben A et al. (1998). Network support for drinking: Alcoholics Anonymous and long term matching effects. *Addiction* 93:1313-1333.

Malcolm R, Anton RF, Randall CL et al. (1992). A placebo-controlled trial of buspirone in anxious inpatient alcoholics. *Alcoholism: Clinical & Experimental Research* 16:1007-1013.

Mason BJ, Kocsis JH, Ritvo EC et al. (1996). A double-blind placebo-controlled trial of desipramine for primary alcohol dependence stratified on the presence or absence of major depression. *Journal of the American Medical Association* 275:761-767.

McCrady BS (1994). Alcoholics Anonymous and behavior therapy: Can habits be treated as diseases? Can diseases be treated as habits? *Journal of Consulting and Clinical Psychology* 62:1159-1166.

McGrath PJ, Nunes EV, Stewart JW et al. (1996). Imipramine treatment of alcoholics with major depression: A placebo-controlled clinical trial. *Archives of General Psychiatry* 53:232-240.

National Institute on Alcohol Abuse and Alcoholism (NIAAA) (1997). *Ninth Special Report to the U.S. Congress on Alcohol and Health.* Washington, DC: U.S. Department of Health and Human Services.

O'Malley SS, Jaffe AJ, Chang G et al. (1992). Naltrexone and coping skills therapy for alcohol dependence: A controlled study. *Archives of General Psychiatry* 49(11):881-887.

Project MATCH Research Group (1997a). Matching alcoholism treatments to client heterogeneity: Project MATCH posttreatment drinking outcomes. *Journal of Studies on Alcohol* 58:7-29.

Project MATCH Research Group (1997b). Project MATCH secondary a priori hypotheses. *Addiction* 92:1671-1698.

Project MATCH Research Group (1998a). Matching alcoholism treatments to client heterogeneity: Project MATCH three-year drinking outcomes. *Alcoholism: Clinical & Experimental Research* 22:1300-1311.

Project MATCH Research Group (1998b). Matching alcoholism treatments to client heterogeneity: Treatment main effects and matching effects on drinking during treatment. *Journal of Studies on Alcohol* 59:631-639.

Saitz R (1998). Introduction to alcohol withdrawal. *Alcohol Health and Research World* 22(1):5-12.

Sass H, Soyka M, Mann K et al. (1996). Relapse prevention by acamprosate. Results from a placebo-controlled study on alcohol dependence. *Archives of General Psychiatry* 53:673-680.

Sullivan JT, Sykora K, Schneiderman J et al. (1989). Assessment of alcohol withdrawal: The Revised Clinical Institute Withdrawal Assessment for Alcohol Scale (CIWA-Ar). *British Journal of Addiction* 84:1353-1357.

Volpicelli JR, Alterman AI, Hayashida M et al. (1992). Naltrexone in the treatment of alcohol dependence. *Archives of General Psychiatry* 49(11):876-880.

Volpicelli JR, Rhines KC, Rhines JS et al. (1997). Naltrexone and alcohol dependence. Role of subject compliance. *Archives of General Psychiatry* 54:737-742.

Walsh DC, Hingson RW, Merrigan DM et al. (1991). A randomized trial of treatment options for alcohol-abusing workers. *New England Journal of Medicine* 325(11):775-782.

Chapter 2	# The Treatment of Drug Addiction: A Review

Martin Adler, M.D.
Andrea G. Barthwell, M.D., FASAM
Lawrence S. Brown, Jr., M.D., M.P.H., FASAM, et al.

Goals of Drug Addiction Treatment
Treatment Approaches
Components of Addiction Treatment
Treatment in the Criminal Justice System
Treatment of Adolescents

Drug addiction is a complex illness. It is characterized by compulsive—at times uncontrollable—drug craving, seeking, and use, which persist even in the face of extremely negative consequences. For many people, drug addiction becomes chronic, with relapses possible even after long periods of abstinence.

Because addiction has so many dimensions and disrupts so many aspects of an individual's life, treatment for this illness never is simple. Drug treatment must help the individual stop using drugs and maintain a drug-free lifestyle, while achieving productive functioning in the family, at work, and in society. Effective treatment programs typically incorporate many components, each directed to a particular aspect of the illness and its consequences.

Three decades of scientific research and clinical practice have yielded a variety of effective approaches to addiction treatment. Extensive data show that such treatment is as effective as treatments for most other similarly chronic medical conditions.

Of course, not all drug treatment is equally effective. Research also has revealed a set of overarching principles that characterize the most effective drug addiction treatments and their implementation (Table 1).

GOALS OF DRUG ADDICTION TREATMENT

Drug addiction is a complex disorder that can involve virtually every aspect of an individual's functioning—in the family, at work, and in the community. Because of addiction's complexity and pervasive consequences, addiction treatment typically must involve many components. Some of those components focus directly on the individual's drug use. Others, like employment training, focus on restoring the addicted individual to productive membership in the family and society (Table 2).

Treatment of drug abuse and addiction is delivered in many different settings, using a variety of behavioral and pharmacological approaches. In the United States, more than 11,000 specialized drug treatment facilities provide rehabilitation, counseling, behavioral therapy, medication, case management, and other types of services to persons with drug use disorders.

TREATMENT APPROACHES

Research studies on drug addiction treatment typically have classified treatment into several general approaches or modalities. Treatment approaches and individual programs continue to evolve, and many programs in existence today

TABLE 1. Principles of Effective Treatment

1. **No single treatment is appropriate for all individuals.** Matching treatment settings, interventions, and services to each individual's particular problems and needs is critical to his or her ultimate success in returning to productive functioning in the family, workplace, and society.

2. **Treatment needs to be readily available.** Because individuals who are addicted to drugs may be uncertain about entering treatment, taking advantage of opportunities when they are ready for treatment is crucial. Potential treatment applicants can be lost if treatment is not immediately available or is not readily accessible.

3. **Effective treatment attends to multiple needs of the individual.** To be effective, treatment must address the individual's drug use and any associated medical, psychological, social, vocational, and legal problems.

4. **An individual's treatment and services plan must be assessed continually and modified as necessary to ensure that the plan meets the person's changing needs.** A patient may require varying combinations of services and treatment components during the course of treatment and recovery. In addition to counseling or psychotherapy, a patient at times may require medication, other medical services, family therapy, parenting instruction, vocational rehabilitation, and social and legal services. It is critical that the treatment approach be appropriate to the individual's age, gender, race/ethnicity, and culture.

5. **Remaining in treatment for an adequate period of time is critical for treatment effectiveness.** The appropriate duration for an individual depends on his or her problems and needs. Research indicates that, for most patients, the threshold of significant improvement is reached at about three months in treatment. After this threshold is reached, additional treatment can produce further progress toward recovery. Because people often leave treatment prematurely, programs should include strategies to engage and keep patients in treatment.

6. **Counseling (individual and group) and other behavioral therapies are critical components of effective treatment.** In therapy, patients address issues of motivation, build skills to resist drug use, replace drug-using activities with constructive and rewarding nondrug-using activities, and improve their problem-solving abilities. Behavioral therapy also facilitates interpersonal relationships and the individual's ability to function in the family and community.

7. **Medications are an important element of treatment for many patients, especially when combined with counseling and other behavioral therapies.** Methadone and levo-alpha-acetylmethadol (LAAM) are very effective in helping individuals addicted to heroin and other opiates stabilize their lives and reduce their illicit drug use. Naltrexone is an effective medication for some opiate addicts and some patients with co-occurring alcohol dependence. For persons addicted to nicotine, a nicotine replacement product (such as patches or gum) or an oral medication (such as bupropion) can be an effective component of treatment. For patients with co-occurring mental disorders, both behavioral treatments and medications can be critically important.

8. **Addicted or drug-abusing individuals with co-occurring mental disorders should have both disorders treated in an integrated way.** Because addictive disorders and mental disorders often occur in the same individual, patients presenting for either condition should be assessed and treated for the co-occurrence of the other type of disorder.

9. **Medical detoxification is only the first stage of addiction treatment and by itself does little to change long-term drug use.** Medical detoxification safely manages the acute physical symptoms of withdrawal associated with stopping drug use. While detoxification alone is rarely sufficient to help addicts achieve long-term abstinence, for some individuals it is a strongly indicated precursor to effective addiction treatment.

10. **Treatment does not need to be voluntary to be effective.** Strong motivation can facilitate the treatment process. Sanctions or enticements in the family, employment setting, or criminal justice system can increase significantly both entry into treatment and retention in treatment, as well as the success of treatment interventions.

11. **Possible drug use during treatment must be monitored continuously.** Lapses to drug use can occur during treatment. The objective monitoring of a patient's drug and alcohol use during treatment, as through urinalysis or other tests, can help the patient withstand urges to use drugs. Such monitoring also can provide early evidence of drug use so that the individual's treatment plan can be adjusted. Feedback to patients who test positive for illicit drug use is an important element of monitoring.

12. **Treatment programs should provide assessment for HIV/AIDS, hepatitis B and C, tuberculosis, and other infectious diseases, and counseling to help patients modify or change behaviors that place themselves or others at risk for infection.** Counseling can help patients avoid high-risk behaviors. Counseling also can help those who are already infected manage their illnesses.

13. **Recovery from drug addiction can be a long-term process and frequently requires multiple episodes of treatment.** As with other chronic illnesses, relapses to drug use can occur during or after successful treatment episodes. Addicted individuals may require prolonged treatment and multiple episodes of treatment to achieve long-term abstinence and fully restore functioning. Participation in self-help support programs during and following treatment often is helpful in maintaining abstinence.

SOURCE: *National Institute on Drug Abuse (1999).* Principles of Drug Addiction Treatment: A Research-Based Guide *(1999). Rockville, MD: NIDA (NIH Publication No. 99-4180), 1-3.*

do not fit neatly into traditional addiction treatment classifications.

Opioid Agonist Treatment. Also referred to as "opioid substitution therapy," agonist or maintenance treatment for opiate addicts usually is conducted in outpatient settings such as methadone treatment programs. These programs use a long-acting synthetic opiate medication, usually methadone or levo-alpha-acetylmethadol (LAAM), administered orally for a sustained period at a dose sufficient to prevent opiate withdrawal, block the effects of illicit opiate use, and decrease opiate craving. Patients stabilized on adequate, sustained doses of methadone or LAAM can function normally. They can hold jobs, avoid the crime and violence of the drug culture, and reduce their exposure to HIV by stopping or decreasing injection drug use and drug-related high-risk sexual behaviors.

Patients stabilized on opiate agonists can engage more readily in counseling and other behavioral interventions that are essential to recovery and rehabilitation. The best, most effective opiate agonist maintenance programs include individual and/or group counseling, as well as provision of, or referral to, other needed medical, psychological, and social services (Ball & Ross, 1991; Cooper, 1992; Dole, Nyswander et al., 1996; Lowinson, Payte et al., 1996; McLellan, Arndt et al., 1993; Novick, Joseph et al., 1990; Simpson, Joe et al., 1982; Simpson, 1981).

Narcotic Antagonist Treatment Using Naltrexone. Treatment of opiate addicts with naltrexone usually is conducted in outpatient settings, although initiation of the medication often begins following medical detoxification in a residential setting. Naltrexone is a long-acting synthetic opiate antagonist with few side effects that is taken orally, either daily or three times a week, for a sustained period of time. Candidates for therapy with naltrexone must be medically detoxified and opiate-free for several days before the drug can be given, to avoid precipitating an opiate abstinence syndrome. When naltrexone is used in this fashion, it completely blocks all the effects of self-administered opiates, including euphoria.

The theory behind this treatment is that the repeated lack of the desired opiate effects, as well as the perceived futility of using the opiate, will gradually result in breaking the habit of opiate addiction. Naltrexone itself has no subjective effects or potential for abuse and is not addicting. Patient noncompliance is a common problem. Therefore, a favorable treatment outcome requires that there also be a positive therapeutic relationship, effective counseling or therapy, and careful monitoring of medication compliance.

Many experienced clinicians have found naltrexone most useful for highly motivated, recently detoxified patients who desire total abstinence because of external circumstances, including impaired professionals, parolees, probationers, and prisoners in work-release status. Patients stabilized on naltrexone can function normally. They can hold jobs, avoid the crime and violence of the street culture, and reduce their exposure to HIV by stopping injection drug use and drug-related high-risk sexual behaviors (Cornish, Metzger et al., 1997; Greenstein, Arndt et al., 1984; Resnick, Schuyten-Resnick, 1979; Resnick & Washton, 1978).

TABLE 2. Components of Comprehensive Addiction Treatment

The best treatment programs provide a combination of therapies and other services to meet the needs of the individual patient.

Core components of addiction treatment:
Intake processing/assessment
Treatment planning
Clinical and case management
Substance use monitoring
Behavioral therapy and counseling
Pharmacotherapies
Self-help/peer support groups
Continuing care.

Ancillary services include:
Mental health services
Medical services
HIV/AIDS services
Educational services
Vocational services
Legal services
Financial services
Housing/transportation services
Family services
Child care services.

SOURCE: National Institute on Drug Abuse (1999). *Principles of Drug Addiction Treatment: A Research-Based Guide (1999).* Rockville, MD: NIDA (NIH Publication No. 99-4180), 14.

Outpatient Drug-Free Treatment. This treatment varies in the types and intensity of services offered. It costs less than residential or inpatient treatment and often is more suitable for individuals who are employed or who have extensive social supports. Low-intensity programs may offer little more than drug education and admonition. Other outpatient models, such as intensive day treatment, can be comparable to residential programs in services and effectiveness, depending on the individual patient's characteristics and needs. In many outpatient programs, group counseling is emphasized. Some outpatient programs are designed to treat patients who have medical or mental health problems in addition to their drug disorder (Higgins, Budney et al., 1994; Hubbard, Craddock et al., 1998; IOM, 1990; McLellan, Grisson et al., 1993; Simpson & Brown, 1998).

Long-Term Residential Treatment. Residential programs provide care 24 hours a day, generally in nonhospital settings. The best-known residential treatment model is the therapeutic community (TC), but residential treatment programs also employ other models, such as cognitive-behavioral therapy.

TCs are residential programs with planned lengths of stay of 6 to 12 months. TCs focus on the "resocialization" of the individual and use the program's entire "community"—including other residents, staff, and the social context—as active components of treatment. Addiction is viewed in the context of an individual's social and psychological deficits, so treatment focuses on developing personal accountability and responsibility and socially productive lives. Treatment is highly structured and can at times be confrontational, with activities designed to help residents examine damaging beliefs, self-concepts, and patterns of behavior and to adopt new, more harmonious and constructive ways to interact with others. Many TCs are quite comprehensive and include employment training and other support services on site.

Compared with patients in other forms of drug treatment, the typical TC resident has more severe problems, with more co-occurring mental health problems and more criminal involvement. Research shows that TCs can be modified to treat individuals with special needs, including adolescents, women, those with severe mental disorders, and individuals in the criminal justice system (Leukefeld, Pickens et al., 1991; Lewis, McCusker et al., 1993; Sacks, Sacks et al., 1998; Stevens & Glider, 1994; Stevens, Arbiter et al., 1989).

Short-Term Residential Programs. Short-term programs provide intensive but relatively brief residential treatment based on a modified Twelve Step approach. These programs originally were designed to treat alcohol problems, but during the cocaine epidemic of the mid-1980s, many began to treat illicit drug abuse and addiction. The original residential treatment model consisted of a three- to six-week hospital-based inpatient treatment phase, followed by extended outpatient therapy and participation in a self-help group such as Alcoholics Anonymous. Reduced health care coverage for addiction treatment has resulted in a diminished number of these programs, and the average length of stay under managed care review is much shorter than in early programs (Hubbard, Craddock et al., 1998; Miller, 1998).

Medical Detoxification. Detoxification is not, in itself, a treatment, but rather is a process whereby individuals are systematically withdrawn from addicting drugs in an inpatient or outpatient setting, typically under the care of a physician. Detoxification is most appropriately considered a precursor to treatment, because it is designed to address the acute physiological effects of stopping drug use. Medications are available for detoxification from opiates, nicotine, benzodiazepines, alcohol, barbiturates, and other sedatives. In some cases, particularly for the last three types of drugs, detoxification may be a medical necessity, and untreated withdrawal may be medically dangerous or even fatal.

Detoxification is not designed to address the psychological, social, and behavioral problems associated with addiction and therefore does not typically produce the type of lasting behavior changes necessary for recovery. Detoxification is most useful when it incorporates formal processes of assessment and referral to subsequent addiction treatment (Kleber, 1996).

COMPONENTS OF ADDICTION TREATMENT

This section presents several examples of treatment approaches and components that have been developed and tested for efficacy through research supported by the National Institute on Drug Abuse (NIDA). Each approach is designed to address certain aspects of drug addiction and its consequences for the individual, family, and society. The approaches are to be used to supplement or enhance—not replace—existing treatment programs.

This section is not a complete list of efficacious, scientifically based treatment approaches. Additional approaches are under development as part of NIDA's continuing support of treatment research and are reviewed in this section, as well as in Sections 6, 7, and 8.

Relapse Prevention. A form of cognitive-behavioral therapy, relapse prevention was developed for the treatment of problem drinking and adapted later for cocaine addicts. Cognitive-behavioral strategies are based on the theory that learning processes play a critical role in the development of maladaptive patterns of behavior. The goal of relapse prevention is to help addicted individuals learn to identify and correct their problematic behaviors. Relapse prevention encompasses several cognitive-behavioral strategies that facilitate abstinence as well as provide help for persons who experience relapse.

The relapse prevention approach to the treatment of cocaine addiction consists of a collection of strategies intended to enhance self-control. Specific techniques include exploring the positive and negative consequences of continued use, self-monitoring to recognize drug cravings early on and to identify situations that pose high risk of use, and developing strategies for coping with and avoiding high-risk situations and the desire to use. A central element of this treatment is anticipating the problems patients are likely to meet and helping them develop effective coping strategies.

Research indicates that the skills individuals learn through relapse prevention therapy remain after the completion of treatment. In one study, most persons receiving this cognitive-behavioral approach maintained the gains they made in treatment throughout the year following discharge (Carroll, Rounsaville et al., 1991, 1994; Marlatt & Gordon, 1985).

Supportive-Expressive Psychotherapy. Supportive-expressive psychotherapy is a time-limited, focused psychotherapy that has been adapted for heroin- and cocaine-addicted individuals. The therapy has two main components:

- *Supportive techniques* to help patients feel comfortable in discussing their personal experiences.

- *Expressive techniques* to help patients identify and work through interpersonal relationship issues.

Special attention is paid to the role of drugs in relation to problem feelings and behaviors and how problems may be solved without recourse to drugs.

The efficacy of individual supportive-expressive psychotherapy has been tested with patients in methadone maintenance treatment who had co-occurring psychiatric disorders. In a comparison with patients receiving only drug counseling, both groups fared similarly with regard to opiate use, but the supportive-expressive psychotherapy group had lower cocaine use and required less methadone. Also, the patients who received supportive-expressive psychotherapy maintained many of the gains they had made. In an earlier study, supportive-expressive psychotherapy, when added to drug counseling, improved outcomes for opiate addicts in methadone treatment with moderately severe psychiatric problems (Luborsky, 1984; Woody, McLellan et al., 1995, 1987).

Individualized Counseling. Individualized counseling focuses directly on reducing or stopping the addict's illicit drug use. It also addresses related areas of impaired functioning—such as employment status, illegal activity, family/social relations—as well as the content and structure of the patient's recovery program. Through its emphasis on short-term behavioral goals, individualized drug counseling helps the patient develop coping strategies and tools for abstaining from drug use and then maintaining abstinence. The addiction counselor encourages Twelve Step participation and makes referrals for needed supplemental medical, psychiatric, employment, and other services. Individuals are encouraged to attend sessions one or two times a week.

In a study that compared opiate addicts receiving methadone alone to those receiving methadone coupled with counseling, individuals who received methadone alone showed minimal improvement in reducing opiate use. The addition of counseling produced significantly more improvement. The addition of onsite medical, psychiatric, employment, and family services further improved outcomes.

In another study with cocaine addicts, individualized drug counseling, together with group counseling, was quite effective in reducing cocaine use. Thus, it appears that this approach has great utility with both heroin and cocaine addicts in outpatient treatment (McLellan, Arndt et al., 1993; McLellan, Woody et al., 1988; Woody, Luborsky et al., 1983; Crits-Cristoph, Siqueland et al., 2000).

Motivational Enhancement Therapy. Motivational enhancement therapy (MET) is a client-centered counseling approach that attempts to initiate behavior change by helping clients resolve their ambivalence about engaging in treatment and stopping drug use. This approach employs strategies to evoke rapid and internally motivated change in the client, rather than guiding the client stepwise through the recovery process. This therapy consists of an initial assessment battery session, followed by two to four individual treatment sessions with a therapist. The first treatment session focuses on providing feedback generated from the initial assessment battery to stimulate discussion regarding personal substance use and to elicit self-motivational statements. Motivational interviewing principles are used to strengthen motivation and build a plan for change. Coping strategies for high-risk situations are suggested and discussed with the client. In subsequent sessions, the therapist monitors change, reviews cessation strategies being used, and continues to encourage commitment to change or to sustained abstinence. Clients sometimes are encouraged to bring a significant other to sessions. This approach has been used successfully with alcoholics and with marijuana-dependent individuals (Budney, Kandel et al., 1997; Miller, 1996; Stephens, Roffman et al., 1994).

Combined Behavioral and Nicotine Replacement Therapy for Nicotine Addiction. This approach has two main components:

- The *transdermal nicotine patch or nicotine gum*, which is used to reduce the symptoms of withdrawal, producing better initial abstinence.

- A *behavioral component* to provide concurrent support and reinforcement of coping skills, yielding better long-term outcomes.

Behavioral skills training helps patients learn to avoid high-risk situations for smoking relapse and to plan strategies to cope with such situations. Patients practice their skills in treatment, social, and work settings. They learn coping techniques, such as cigarette refusal skills, assertiveness, and time management. The combined treatment is based on the rationale that behavioral and pharmacological treatments operate by different yet complementary mechanisms that produce potentially additive effects (Fiore, Kenford et al., 1994; Hughes, 1991; APA, 1996).

Community Reinforcement Approach (CRA) Plus Vouchers. CRA is an intensive 24-week outpatient therapy for the treatment of cocaine addiction. The treatment has dual goals:

- To achieve cocaine abstinence long enough for patients to learn new life skills that will help sustain abstinence.

- To reduce alcohol consumption for patients whose drinking is associated with cocaine use.

Patients attend one or two individual counseling sessions per week, where they focus on improving family relations, learn a variety of skills to minimize drug use, receive vocational counseling, and develop new recreational activities and social networks. Those who also abuse alcohol receive clinic-monitored disulfiram (Antabuse®) therapy. Patients submit urine samples two or three times a week and receive vouchers for cocaine-negative samples. The value of the vouchers increases with consecutive clean samples. Patients may exchange their vouchers for retail goods that are consistent with a cocaine-free lifestyle.

This approach facilitates patients' engagement in treatment and systematically aids them in gaining substantial periods of cocaine abstinence. The approach has been tested in urban and rural areas and used successfully in outpatient detoxification of opiate-addicted adults and with inner-city methadone maintenance patients who have high rates of intravenous cocaine abuse (Higgins, Budney et al., 1995, 1994; Silverman, Higgins et al., 1996).

Voucher-Based Reinforcement Therapy in Methadone Maintenance Treatment. Voucher-based reinforcement therapy helps patients achieve and maintain abstinence from illegal drugs by providing them with a voucher each time they provide a drug-free urine sample. The voucher has monetary value and can be exchanged for goods and services consistent with the goals of treatment. Initially, the voucher values are low, but their value increases with the number of consecutive drug-free urine specimens the individual provides. Cocaine- or heroin-positive urine specimens reset the value of the vouchers to the initial low value. The contingency of escalating incentives is designed specifically to reinforce periods of sustained drug abstinence.

Studies show that patients receiving vouchers for drug-free urine samples achieved significantly more weeks of abstinence and significantly more weeks of sustained abstinence than patients who were given vouchers independent of urinalysis results. In another study, urinalyses positive for heroin decreased significantly when the voucher program was started and increased significantly when the program was stopped (Silverman, Higgins et al., 1996; Silverman, Wong et al., 1996).

Day Treatment With Abstinence Contingencies and Vouchers. This approach was developed to treat homeless crack addicts. For the first two months, participants were required to spend 5.5 hours daily in the program, which provided lunch and transportation to and from shelters. Interventions included individual assessment and goal setting, individual and group counseling, multiple psychoeducational groups (for example, didactic groups on community resources, housing, cocaine, and HIV/AIDS prevention; establishing and reviewing personal rehabilitation goals; relapse prevention; and weekend planning), and patient-governed community meetings, in which patients reviewed contract goals and provided support and encouragement to each other. Individual counseling occurs once a week, and group therapy sessions are held three times a week. After two months of day treatment and at least two weeks of abstinence, participants graduated to a four-month work component that pays wages, which can be used to rent inexpensive, drug-free housing. A voucher system also rewards drug-free social and recreational activities.

This innovative day treatment was compared with treatment consisting of twice-weekly individual counseling and Twelve Step groups, medical examinations and treatment, and referral to community resources for housing and vocational services. Innovative day treatment followed by work and housing (dependent on drug abstinence) had a more positive effect on alcohol use, cocaine use, and days of homelessness (Milby, Schumacher et al., 1996).

The Matrix Model. The Matrix Model provides a framework for engaging stimulant abusers in treatment and helping them achieve abstinence. Patients learn about issues critical to addiction and relapse, receive direction and support from a trained therapist, become familiar with self-help programs, and are monitored for drug use by urine testing. The program includes education for family members affected by the addiction.

The therapist functions simultaneously as teacher and coach, fostering a positive, encouraging relationship with the patient and using that relationship to reinforce positive behavior change. The interaction between the therapist and the patient is realistic and direct but not confrontational or parental. Therapists are trained to conduct treatment sessions in a way that promotes the patient's self-esteem, dignity, and self-worth. A positive relationship between patient and therapist is a critical element for patient retention.

Treatment materials draw heavily on other tested treatment approaches. Thus, this approach includes elements pertaining to the areas of relapse prevention, family and group therapies, drug education, and self-help participation. Detailed treatment manuals contain work sheets for individual sessions; other components include family educational groups, early recovery skills groups, relapse prevention

groups, conjoint sessions, urine tests, Twelve Step programs, relapse analysis, and social support groups.

A number of projects have shown that participants treated with the Matrix Model demonstrate statistically significant reductions in drug and alcohol use, improvements in psychological indicators, and reductions in risky sexual behaviors associated with HIV transmission. These reports, along with evidence suggesting comparable treatment responses for methamphetamine users and cocaine users and demonstrated efficacy in enhancing naltrexone treatment of opiate addicts, provide a body of empirical support for the use of the model (Huber, Ling et al., 1997; Rawson, Shoptaw et al., 1995).

TREATMENT IN THE CRIMINAL JUSTICE SYSTEM

Research has shown that combining criminal justice sanctions with drug treatment can be effective in decreasing drug use and related crime. Individuals under legal coercion tend to stay in treatment for a longer period of time and do as well as or better than others not under legal pressure. Often, drug addicts come into contact with the criminal justice system earlier than other health or social systems, and intervention by the criminal justice system to engage the individual in treatment may help to interrupt and shorten a career of drug use. Treatment for the criminal justice-involved addict may be delivered prior to, during, after, or in lieu of incarceration.

Prison-Based Treatment Programs. Offenders with drug disorders may encounter a number of treatment options while incarcerated, including didactic drug education classes, self-help programs, and treatment based on therapeutic community (TC) or residential milieu therapy models. The TC model has been studied extensively and found to be quite effective in reducing drug use and recidivism to criminal behavior. Those in treatment should be segregated from the general prison population, so that the "prison culture" does not overwhelm progress toward recovery. As might be expected, treatment gains can be lost if inmates are returned to the general prison population after treatment. Research shows that relapse to drug use and recidivism to crime are significantly lower if the drug offender continues treatment after returning to the community.

Community-Based Treatment for Criminal Justice Populations. A number of criminal justice alternatives to incarceration have been tried with offenders who have drug disorders, including limited diversion programs, pretrial release conditional on entry into treatment, and conditional probation with sanctions. The drug court is a promising approach. Drug courts mandate and arrange for drug addiction treatment, actively monitor progress in treatment, and arrange other services for drug-involved offenders. Federal support for planning, implementation, and enhancement of drug courts is provided under the U.S. Department of Justice Drug Courts Program Office.

As a well-studied example, the Treatment Accountability and Safer Communities (TASC) program provides an alternative to incarceration by addressing the multiple needs of drug-addicted offenders in a community-based setting. TASC programs typically include counseling, medical care, parenting instruction, family counseling, school and job training, and legal and employment services. The key features of TASC include (1) coordination of criminal justice and drug treatment, (2) early identification, assessment, and referral of drug-involved offenders, (3) monitoring offenders through drug testing, and (4) use of legal sanctions as inducements to remain in treatment (Anglin & Hser, 1990; Hiller, Knight et al., 1996; Hubbard, Collins et al., 1998; Inciardi, Martin et al., 1997; Wexler, 1997a, 1997b; Wexler, Falkin et al., 1990).

TREATMENT OF ADOLESCENTS

Behavioral Therapy. As used in the treatment of adolescents, behavioral therapy incorporates the principle that unwanted behavior can be changed by clear demonstration of the desired behavior and consistent reward of incremental steps toward achieving it. Therapeutic activities include fulfilling specific assignments, rehearsing desired behaviors, and recording and reviewing progress, with praise and privileges given for meeting assigned goals. Urine samples are collected regularly to monitor drug use. The therapy aims to equip the patient to gain three types of control:

- *Stimulus control* helps patients to avoid situations associated with drug use and learn to spend more time in activities incompatible with drug use.

- *Urge control* helps patients to recognize and change thoughts, feelings, and plans that lead to drug use.

- *Social control* involves family members and other persons important in helping patients avoid drugs. A parent or significant other attends treatment sessions when possible and assists with therapy assignments and reinforcing desired behavior.

According to research studies, this therapy helps adolescents become drug free and increases their ability to remain drug free after treatment ends. Adolescents also show improvement in several other areas—employment/school attendance, family relationships, depression, institutionalization, and alcohol use. Such favorable results are attributed largely to including family members in therapy and rewarding drug abstinence verified by urinalysis (Azrin, Acierno et al., 1996; Azrin, McMahon et al., 1994; Azrin, Donohue et al., 1994).

Multidimensional Family Therapy (MDFT). MDFT is an outpatient family-based drug treatment approach for adolescents. It approaches adolescent drug use in terms of a network of influences (individual, family, peer, and community) and suggests that reducing unwanted behavior and increasing desirable behavior occur in multiple ways in different settings. Treatment includes individual and family sessions held in the clinic, in the home, or with family members at the family court, school, or other community locations.

During individual sessions, the therapist and adolescent work on important developmental tasks, such as decisionmaking, negotiation, and problem-solving skills. Teens acquire skills in communicating their thoughts and feelings to deal better with life stressors and vocational skills. Parallel sessions are held with family members. Parents examine their particular parenting styles, learn to distinguish influence from control, and learn how to have a positive and developmentally appropriate influence on their child (Diamond & Liddle, 1996; Schmidt, Liddle et al., 1996).

Multisystemic Therapy (MST). MST addresses the factors associated with serious antisocial behavior in children and adolescents who use drugs. These factors include characteristics of the adolescent (for example, favorable attitudes toward drug use), the family (poor discipline, family conflict, or parental drug abuse), peers (positive attitudes toward drug use), school (dropout, poor performance), and neighborhood (criminal subculture). By participating in intense treatment in natural environments (homes, schools, and neighborhood settings) most youths and families complete a full course of treatment. MST significantly reduces adolescent drug use during treatment and for at least six months following treatment. Reduced numbers of incarcerations and out-of-home placements of juveniles offset the cost of providing this intensive service and maintaining the clinicians' low caseloads (Henggeler, Pickrel et al., 1996;

Henggeler, Schoenwald et al., 1998; Schoenwald, Ward et al., 1996). (For more information on treatment of adolescents, see Section 13 of this text.)

ACKNOWLEDGMENT: Adapted by permission of the publisher from Principles of Drug Addiction Treatment: A Research-Based Guide *(1999). Rockville, MD: National Institute on Drug Abuse (NIH Publication No. 99-4180). Members of the expert panel for this publication were Martin W. Adler, Ph.D.; Andrea G. Barthwell, M.D., FASAM; Lawrence S. Brown, Jr., M.D., M.P.H., FASAM; James F. Callahan, D.P.A.; H. Westley Clark, M.D., J.D., M.P.H., FASAM; Richard R. Clayton, Ph.D.; Linda B. Cottler, Ph.D.; David P. Friedman, Ph.D.; Reese T. Jones, M.D.; Linda R. Wolf-Jones, D.S.W.; Linda Kaplan, CAE; A. Thomas McLellan, Ph.D.; Nancy K. Mello, Ph.D.; Charles P. O'Brien, M.D., Ph.D.; Eric J. Simon, Ph.D.; and George Woody, M.D.*

REFERENCES

American Psychiatric Association (APA) (1996). *Practice Guideline for the Treatment of Patients with Nicotine Dependence.* Washington, DC: American Psychiatric Press.

Anglin MD & Hser Y (1990). Treatment of drug abuse. In M Tonry & JQ Wilson (eds.) *Drugs and Crime.* Chicago, IL: University of Chicago Press, 393-460.

Azrin NH, Acierno R, Kogan E et al. (1996). Follow-up results of supportive versus behavioral therapy for illicit drug abuse. *Behavioral Research and Therapy* 34(1):41-46.

Azrin NH, Donohue B, Besalel VA et al. (1994). Youth drug abuse treatment: A controlled outcome study. *Journal of Child and Adolescent Substance Abuse* 3(3):1-16.

Azrin NH, McMahon PT, Donahue B et al. (1994). Behavioral therapy for drug abuse: A controlled treatment outcome study. *Behavioral Research and Therapy* 32(8):857-866.

Ball JC & Ross A (1991). *The Effectiveness of Methadone Treatment.* New York, NY: Springer-Verlag.

Budney AJ, Kandel DB, Cherek DR et al. (1997). College on problems of drug dependence meeting, Puerto Rico (June 1996). Marijuana use and dependence. *Drug and Alcohol Dependence* 45:1-11.

Carroll K, Rounsaville B & Keller D (1991). Relapse prevention strategies for the treatment of cocaine abuse. *American Journal of Drug and Alcohol Abuse* 17(3):249-265.

Carroll K, Rounsaville B, Nich C et al. (1994). One-year follow-up of psychotherapy and pharmacotherapy for cocaine dependence: Delayed emergence of psychotherapy effects. *Archives of General Psychiatry* 51:989-997.

Cooper JR (1992). Ineffective use of psychoactive drugs; methadone treatment is no exception. *Journal of the American Medical Association* 267(2):281-282.

Cornish JW, Metzger D, Woody GE et al. (1997). Naltrexone pharmacotherapy for opioid dependent federal probationers. *Journal of Substance Abuse Treatment* 14(6):529-534.

Crits-Cristoph P, Siqueland L, Blaine J et al. (2000). Psychosocial treatments for cocaine dependence: Results of the NIDA Cocaine Collaborative Study. *Archives of General Psychiatry.*

Diamond GS & Liddle HA (1996). Resolving a therapeutic impasse between parents and adolescents in Multidimensional Family Therapy. *Journal of Consulting and Clinical Psychology* 64(3):481-488.

Dole VP, Nyswander M & Kreek MJ (1996). Narcotic blockade. *Archives of Internal Medicine* 118: 304-309.

Fiore MC, Kenford SL, Jorenby DE et al. (1994). Two studies of the clinical effectiveness of the nicotine patch with different counseling treatments. *Chest* 105:524-533.

Greenstein RA, Arndt IC, McLellan AT et al. (1984). Naltrexone: A clinical perspective. *Journal of Clinical Psychiatry* 45(9 Part 2):25-28.

Henggeler SW, Pickrel SG, Brondino MJ et al. (1996). Eliminating (almost) treatment dropout of substance abusing or dependent delinquents through home-based multisystemic therapy. *American Journal of Psychiatry* 153:427-428.

Henggeler SW, Schoenwald SK, Borduin CM et al. (1998). *Multisystemic Treatment of Antisocial Behavior in Children and Adolescents.* New York, NY: Guilford Press.

Higgins ST, Budney AJ, Bickel WK et al. (1994). Incentives improve outcome in outpatient behavioral treatment of cocaine dependence. *Archives of General Psychiatry* 51:568-576.

Higgins ST, Budney AJ, Bickel WK et al. (1995). Outpatient behavioral treatment for cocaine dependence: One-year outcome. *Experimental & Clinical Psychopharmacology* 3(2):205-212.

Hiller ML, Knight K, Broome KM et al. (1996). Compulsory community-based substance abuse treatment and the mentally ill criminal offender. *Prison Journal* 76(2):180-191.

Hubbard RL, Collins JJ, Rachal JV et al. (1998). The criminal justice client in drug abuse treatment. In CG Leukefeld & FM Tims (eds.) *Compulsory Treatment of Drug Abuse: Research and Clinical Practice (NIDA Research Monograph 86).* Rockville, MD: National Institute on Drug Abuse.

Hubbard RL, Craddock SG, Flynn PM et al. (1998). Overview of 1-year follow-up outcomes in the Drug Abuse Treatment Outcome Study (DATOS). *Psychology of Addictive Behaviors* 11(4):291-298.

Huber A, Ling W, Shoptaw S et al. (1997). Integrating treatments for methamphetamine abuse: A psychosocial perspective. *Journal of Addictive Diseases* 16:41-50.

Hughes JR (1991). Combined psychological and nicotine gum treatment for smoking: A critical review. *Journal of Substance Abuse* 3:337-350.

Inciardi JA, Martin SS, Butzin CA et al. (1997). An effective model of prison-based treatment for drug-involved offenders. *Journal of Drug Issues* 27(2):261-278.

Institute of Medicine (IOM) (1990). *Treating Drug Problems.* Washington, DC: National Academy Press.

Kleber HD (1996). Outpatient detoxification from opiates. *Primary Psychiatry* 1:42-52.

Leukefeld C, Pickens R & Schuster CR (1991). Improving drug abuse treatment: Recommendations for research and practice. In RW Pickens, CG Luekefeld & CR Schuster (eds.) *Improving Drug Abuse Treatment (NIDA Research Monograph Series).* Rockville, MD: National Institute on Drug Abuse.

Lewis BF, McCusker J, Hindin R et al. (1993). Four residential drug treatment programs: Project IMPACT. In JA Inciardi, FM Tims & BM Fletcher (eds.) *Innovative Approaches in the Treatment of Drug Abuse*. Westport, CT: Greenwood Press, 45-60.

Lowinson JH, Payte JT, Joseph H et al. (1996). Methadone maintenance. In JH Lowinson, P Ruiz, RB Millman et al. (eds.) *Substance Abuse: A Comprehensive Textbook*. Baltimore, MD: Lippincott, Williams & Wilkins, 405-414.

Luborsky L (1984). *Principles of Psychoanalytic Psychotherapy: A Manual for Supportive-Expressive (SE) Treatment*. New York, NY: Basic Books.

Marlatt G & Gordon JR, eds. (1985). *Relapse Prevention: Maintenance Strategies in the Treatment of Addictive Behaviors*. New York, NY: Guilford Press.

McLellan AT, Arndt I, Metzger DS et al. (1993). The effects of psychosocial services in substance abuse treatment. *Journal of the American Medical Association* 269(15):1953-1959.

McLellan AT, Grisson G, Durell J et al. (1993). Substance abuse treatment in the private setting: Are some programs more effective than others? *Journal of Substance Abuse Treatment* 10:243-254.

McLellan AT, Woody GE, Luborsky L et al. (1988). Is the counselor an "active ingredient" in substance abuse treatment? *Journal of Nervous and Mental Disease* 176:423-430.

Milby JB, Schumacher JE, McNamara C et al. (1996a). Abstinence contingent housing enhances day treatment for homeless cocaine abusers. *NIDA Research Monograph Series 174*. Rockville, MD: National Institute on Drug Abuse.

Milby JB, Schumacher JE, Raczynski JM et al. (1996b). Sufficient conditions for effective treatment of substance abusing homeless. *Drug and Alcohol Dependence* 43:39-47.

Miller WR (1996). Motivational interviewing: Research, practice and puzzles. *Addictive Behaviors* 61(6):835-842.

Miller MM (1998). Traditional approaches to the treatment of addiction. In AW Graham & TK Schultz (eds.) *Principles of Addiction Medicine, Second Edition*. Washington, DC: American Society of Addiction Medicine.

Novick DM, Joseph J, Croxson TS et al. (1990). Absence of antibody to human immunodeficiency virus in long-term, socially rehabilitated methadone maintenance patients. *Archives of Internal Medicine* 150(1):97-99.

Rawson R, Shoptaw S, Obert JL et al. (1995). An intensive outpatient approach for cocaine abuse: The Matrix model. *Journal of Substance Abuse Treatment* 12(2):117-127.

Resnick RB, Schuyten-Resnick E & Washton AM (1979). Narcotic antagonists in the treatment of opioid dependence: Review and commentary. *Comprehensive Psychiatry* 20(2):116-125.

Resnick RB & Washton AM (1978). Clinical outcome with naltrexone: Predictor variables and followup status in detoxified heroin addicts. *Annals of the New York Academy of Sciences* 311:241-246.

Sacks S, Sacks J, DeLeon G et al. (1998). Modified therapeutic community for mentally ill chemical abusers: Background; influences; program description; preliminary findings. *Substance Use and Misuse* 32(9):1217-1259.

Schmidt SE, Liddle HA & Dakof GA (1996). Effects of multidimensional family therapy: Relationship of changes in parenting practices to symptom reduction in adolescent substance abuse. *Journal of Family Psychology* 10(1):1-16.

Schoenwald SK, Ward DM, Henggeler SW et al. (1996). MST treatment of substance abusing or dependent adolescent offenders: Costs of reducing incarceration, inpatient, and residential placement. *Journal of Child and Family Studies* 5:431-444.

Silverman K, Higgins ST, Brooner RK et al. (1996). Sustained cocaine abstinence in methadone maintenance patients through voucher-based reinforcement therapy. *Archives of General Psychiatry* 53:409-415.

Silverman K, Wong C, Higgins S et al. (1996). Increasing opiate abstinence through voucher-based reinforcement therapy. *Drug and Alcohol Dependence* 41:157-165.

Simpson DD (1981). Treatment for drug abuse: Follow-up outcomes and length of time spent. *Archives of General Psychiatry* 38(8):875-880.

Simpson DD & Brown BS (1998). Treatment retention and follow-up outcomes in the Drug Abuse Treatment Outcome Study (DATOS). *Psychology of Addictive Behaviors* 11(4):294-307.

Simpson DD, Joe GW & Bracy SA (1982). Six-year follow-up of opioid addicts after admission to treatment. *Archives of General Psychiatry* 39(11):1318-1323.

Stephens RS, Roffman RA & Simpson EE (1994). Treating adult marijuana dependence: A test of the relapse prevention model. *Journal of Consulting and Clinical Psychology* 62:92-99.

Stevens S, Arbiter N & Glider P (1989). Women residents: Expanding their role to increase treatment effectiveness in substance abuse programs. *International Journal of the Addictions* 24(5):425-434.

Stevens SJ & Glider PJ (1994). Therapeutic communities: Substance abuse treatment for women. In FM Tims, G De Leon & N Jainchill (eds.) *Therapeutic Community: Advances in Research and Application (NIDA Research Monograph 144)*. Rockville, MD: National Institute on Drug Abuse, 162-180.

Wexler HK (1997a). The success of therapeutic communities for substance abusers in American prisons. *Journal of Psychoactive Drugs* 27(1):57-66.

Wexler HK (1997b). Therapeutic communities in American prisons. In E Cullen, L Jones & R Woodward (eds.) *Therapeutic Communities in American Prisons*. New York, NY: Wiley & Sons.

Wexler HK, Falkin GP & Lipton DS (1990). Outcome evaluation of a prison therapeutic community for substance abuse treatment. *Criminal Justice and Behavior* 17(1):71-92.

Woody GE, Luborsky L, McLellan AT et al. (1983). Psychotherapy for opiate addicts: Does it help? *Archives of General Psychiatry* 40:639-645.

Woody GE, McLellan AT, Luborsky L et al. (1987). Twelve month follow-up of psychotherapy for opiate dependence. *American Journal of Psychiatry* 144:590-596.

Woody GE, McLellan AT, Luborsky L et al. (1995). Psychotherapy in community methadone programs: A validation study. *American Journal of Psychiatry* 152(9):1302-1308.

| Chapter 3 | # Components of Successful Addiction Treatment |

A. Thomas McLellan, Ph.D.
James R. McKay, Ph.D.

Rehabilitation Treatments in Addiction
Research on Factors Related to Treatment Outcomes

Addictive disorders result in dramatic costs to society in terms of lost productivity, social disorder, and health care utilization (IOM, 1995a, 1997; Harwood, Fountain et al., 1998). Over the past 20 years, many of the traditional forms of addiction treatment (such as methadone maintenance, therapeutic communities, outpatient drug-free, and others) have been evaluated multiple times and shown to be effective (McLellan, Woody et al., 1996; McLellan, O'Brien et al., 2000; Simpson, Joe et al., 1997; Ball & Ross, 1991). Importantly, this research has shown that the benefits obtained from addiction treatment typically extend beyond the reduction of substance use to areas that are important to society, such as reduced crime, reduced risk of infectious diseases, and improved social function. Finally, the research indicates that the funds spent on addiction treatment yield three- to seven-fold returns to the employer, to health insurers, and to society within the three years following treatment (Holder, Longabaugh et al., 1991).

How do these results translate into recommendations for providing successful addiction treatment? While the conclusions from this line of research are important and gratifying, they are not adequate to inform important clinical questions regarding the delivery of addiction treatment

services. Simply knowing that those who stay in treatment longer have better outcomes does not help when the funding and duration of treatment in "real world" settings are regularly reduced (McLellan, Grissom et al., 1997). Further, research demonstrating that highly specialized and resource-intensive treatments work with highly selected samples of patients may not be helpful to "real world" treatment professionals who have no prospects of accessing those treatments and very few of the patients on whom the treatment was tested. This is particularly true at the level of community-based public-sector treatment programs, which have been forced to operate under limited budgets and with little access to sophisticated services.

How can research in the treatment setting inform the decisions made by these parties? How can treatment professionals use information from research studies to upgrade or expand their treatment efforts within the practical constraints of available budgets and personnel? In seeking answers to these questions, the authors have reviewed the existing treatment outcome literature to summarize the available knowledge regarding the important patient and treatment factors that have been shown to influence the outcomes of addiction treatments. This was an important first step in recognizing and recommending proven, practical, and cost-effective treatment strategies that can be implemented by community-based addiction treatment programs. In this regard, the authors elected not to review literature on detoxification methods, on adolescent treatment, or on smoking cessation treatment, in order to better focus on standard treatments for drug and alcohol dependence, typically following detoxification.

From a methodological perspective, the review included only those clinical trials, treatment matching, or health services studies in which the patients were alcohol- or drug-dependent by contemporary criteria; in which the treatment provided was a conventional form of rehabilitation (any setting or modality); and in which either treatment processes or patient change was measured during as well as after treatment. Finally, methadone maintenance (as well as treatment with the long-acting drug levo-alpha-acetylmethadol [LAAM]) was included in the general category of outpatient rehabilitation treatments, rather than as a special category.

In the review that follows, the authors first discuss some of the basic assumptions underlying various forms of addiction treatment (for example, that patients are eligible for rehabilitation, that rehabilitation has realistic goals, and the like), because they set the stage for the clinical methods currently in use and for the types of studies that are found in the research literature.

Next, the authors discuss some considerations regarding definitions of "outcomes," the types of treatments that were included in the review, and the methodological standards that were set for articles to be included. With these assumptions and considerations in mind, they then review the treatment processes that contribute most significantly to the outcomes of addiction treatment.

REHABILITATION TREATMENTS IN ADDICTION

Patients For Whom Rehabilitation Is Designed. Detoxification is a relatively brief, usually medical procedure designed to stabilize the physical and emotional effects of recent termination of heavy alcohol and/or drug use. In contrast, rehabilitation is a much longer process, which usually involves multidisciplinary staff. It is designed for substance-dependent patients who have gotten past the initial detoxification/stabilization part of addiction treatment but who still have problems controlling their use of alcohol and/or other drugs and who are in need of behavioral change to regain control of their urges to use substances.

Purposes of Addiction Rehabilitation. The major purposes of rehabilitation treatments for alcohol and drug addiction are:

■ To prevent return to active substance use that would require detoxification/stabilization;

■ To assist the patient in developing control over urges to use alcohol or other drugs (usually through attaining and sustaining total abstinence from all drugs and alcohol); and

■ To assist the patient in regaining (or attaining for the first time) improved personal health and social function—both as a secondary part of the rehabilitation function and because these improvements in lifestyle are important for maintaining sustained control over substance use.

Rehabilitation Methods. Professional opinions regarding the underlying reasons for the loss of control over alcohol and drug use vary widely. Suggested causes include genetic predispositions, acquired metabolic abnormalities, learned negative behavioral patterns, self-medication of underlying psychiatric or physical medical problems, character flaws, lack of family and community support for positive function, and the like. For this reason, there is an equally wide range of treatment methods that have been applied to correct or ameliorate these underlying problems and to provide continuing support for the targeted changes in behavior. Methods have included such diverse elements as psychotropic medications to relieve underlying psychiatric problems; anti-craving medications to relieve alcohol and drug craving; acupuncture to correct acquired metabolic imbalances; educational seminars, films, and group sessions to correct false impressions about alcohol and drug use; group and individual counseling and therapy sessions to provide insight, guidance, and support for behavioral change; and peer help groups (such as Alcoholics Anonymous [AA], Narcotics Anonymous [NA], and Cocaine Anonymous [CA]) to provide continued support for the behavioral changes thought to be important in sustaining improvement.

At this writing, inpatient rehabilitation programs can be divided into three general categories (Simpson, 1997):

- Inpatient hospital-based treatment (now very rare): from 7 to 11 days;

- Non-hospital "residential rehabilitation": from 30 to 90 days; and

- Therapeutic communities: from six months to two years.

Outpatient forms of treatment (at least abstinence-oriented outpatient treatment) typically range from 30 to 120 days (Simpson, Joe et al., 1997). Many of the more intensive forms of outpatient treatment (such as intensive outpatient or day hospital) begin with full-day or half-day sessions, five or more times per week, for approximately one month. As the patient's rehabilitation progresses, the intensity of treatment is reduced to sessions of shorter duration (one to two hours), delivered twice a week to twice a month.

The final part of outpatient rehabilitation typically is called "continuing care" or "aftercare." It is characterized by biweekly to monthly support group meetings, which continue (in association with parallel activity in self-help groups) for as long as two years (McKay, Alterman et al., 1998). Maintenance forms of treatment (involving methadone or LAAM, for example) are designed to be of indeterminate length and may continue throughout the life of the patient.

Outcomes to Be Expected From Addiction Treatment. In earlier works (McLellan, Alterman et al., 1995; McLellan & Weisner, 1996), the authors have argued that outcome expectations for addiction treatment should not be confined simply to reduction of alcohol and drug use because the public, the payers of treatment, and even the patients themselves are interested in a broader definition of "rehabilitation." The authors also have argued that for addiction treatments to be seen as "worth it" to these stakeholders, the positive effects of addiction treatment should be sustained beyond the end of the treatment period and continue for at least 6 to 12 months. Most of the experienced researchers in the addiction field have adopted a similarly broad view of outcome expectations (see Simpson, 1997; Simpson, Joe et al., 1997; Holder, Longabaugh et al., 1991; IOM, 1995a, 1997).

In the review that follows, the authors have attempted to characterize outcomes broadly in terms of improved health, social function, and reductions in public health and safety concerns, rather than only in terms of reduced substance use, and to present findings from posttreatment evaluations. The review thus gives greater attention to studies in which multiple outcomes were measured 6 to 12 months following inpatient discharge or at the same points during the course of outpatient care.

RESEARCH ON FACTORS RELATED TO TREATMENT OUTCOMES

Patient factors have been much more widely studied than treatment setting, modality, process, and service factors as predictors of treatment outcome. Perhaps the major reason is that, while there have been many reliable and valid measures of various patient characteristics, there still are very few measures of treatment setting (Moos, Finney et al., 1990) or treatment services (McLellan, Cacciola et al., 1992; Barber, Mercer et al., 1996). Recent developments in the psychotherapy field have led to the creation of manual-based treatments and, with them, appropriate measures of treatment fidelity and integrity. More recently, the multisite NIAAA study of patient-treatment matching (Project MATCH Research Group, 1997) has resulted in several new manuals for the three treatments that were studied as part of that project, as well as additional manuals for measuring patient and treatment characteristics. Below, the authors review several dimensions or characteristics of treatment that have been studied and shown to have some relationship to treatment outcomes.

Treatment Setting. A large number of studies have investigated potential differences in outcome among various forms of inpatient and outpatient treatment. In the field of rehabilitation from alcohol dependence, there have been several important studies of the role of treatment setting. For example, studies by Alterman and colleagues (Alterman, Droba et al., 1992; Alterman, McLellan et al., 1994) randomly assigned alcohol-dependent patients to an equal term (28 to 30 days) in either inpatient or day-hospital treatment. Comparisons of many outcome measures in both studies showed essentially no significant differences between the groups, suggesting that the setting of care might not be an important contributor to outcome.

Reviews of the literature on inpatient and outpatient alcohol rehabilitation by Miller and Hester (1986) and Holder and colleagues (1991) also concluded that, across a range of study designs and patient populations, there was no significant advantage provided by inpatient care over outpatient care in the rehabilitation of alcohol dependence, despite the substantial difference in costs (but also see Chapter 4 of this section). It is important to note that a widely cited study by Walsh and colleagues (1991) did find a significant difference in outcome favoring an inpatient program. This difference was shown among employed alcohol-dependent patients who were assigned to either an inpatient program or to a very non-intensive form of outpatient treatment (largely AA meetings).

In the field of cocaine dependence treatment, there also have been several studies examining the role of treatment setting. Again, while there is evidence for high attrition rates (for example, Kang, Kleinman et al., 1991), there also is evidence that outpatient treatments for cocaine dependence can be effective, even for patients with relatively limited social resources. Alterman and colleagues (1994) compared the effectiveness of four weeks of intensive, highly structured day-hospital (DH) treatment (27 hours weekly) with inpatient (INP) treatment (48 hours weekly) for cocaine dependence. The subjects were primarily inner-city, African American males who were treated at a Veterans Administration Medical Center. The INP treatment completion rate of 89% was significantly higher than the DH completion rate of 54%. However, at seven months after treatment entry, self-reported outcomes indicated considerable improvements for both groups in drug and alcohol use, as well as family, social, legal, employment, and psychiatric problems. The finding of reduced self-reported cocaine use was supported by the results of urine screens. Both self-report and urine data indicated abstinence rates of 50% to 60% for both groups at followup assessment.

Similar findings have been shown in field studies of private addiction treatment programs that treat primarily cocaine and cocaine-plus-alcohol dependent patients (Pettinati, Belden et al., 1997; McLellan, Cacciola et al., 1992; Havassy, Hall et al., 1997). In all of these studies, patients who were assigned to one of several outpatient treatment programs were less likely to complete treatment than those assigned to inpatient programs. However, those who did complete treatment showed equal levels of improvement and outcome in the two settings. It is important to note that virtually all studies of this type have shown greater engagement and retention of patients in inpatient settings. This is particularly significant because the majority of this research was conducted among patients who were willing to accept random assignment to either treatment.

There have been at least two attempts to formalize clinical decision processes as to who should and should not be assigned to inpatient and outpatient settings of care (the Cleveland Criteria and the American Society of Addiction Medicine's Patient Placement Criteria). McKay and col-

leagues (1992) failed to show evidence for the predictive validity of the Cleveland placement criteria, at least when those criteria were applied to the assignment of alcohol- and drug-dependent patients to inpatient and day-hospital programs. That is, there were no significant differences in the six-month outcomes of those who met the Cleveland criteria for inpatient treatment and who had been randomly assigned to either inpatient or day-hospital treatment. In a similar study evaluating the psychosocial predictors of the American Society of Addiction Medicine's criteria, McKay and colleagues (1997) did find at least partial support for the predictive validity of these placement variables, although a full evaluation was not possible.

The most recent versions of the ASAM criteria have attempted to make very fine-grained decisions regarding placement in levels of care, as determined by the amount and quality of medical supervision and monitoring. Research is needed to determine the predictive validity of these finer distinctions and whether patients placed in settings and modalities with "more medical supervision" actually receive more medical contact or services than patients placed in settings where such services are not expected. Current work (Mee-Lee, Shulman et al., 2001; Gastfriend & McLellan, 1997) is in progress to inform our understanding about these clinical decision criteria.

Length of Treatment/Compliance With Treatment. Virtually all studies of rehabilitation have shown that patients who stay in treatment longer and/or who attend the most treatment sessions have the best posttreatment outcomes. Specifically, the multisite DATOS study has suggested that outpatient treatments of less than 90 days are more likely to result in early return to drug use and generally poorer response than treatments of longer duration (Simpson, Joe et al., 1997).

Although length of stay is a very robust positive predictor of treatment outcome, the nature of this relationship remains ambiguous. Clearly, one possibility is that patients who enter treatment gradually acquire new motivation, skills, attitudes, knowledge, and supports over the course of their stay in treatment; that those who stay longer acquire more of these favorable attributes and qualities; and that the gradual acquisition of these qualities or services is the reason for the favorable outcomes. A less attractive but equally plausible possibility is that better-motivated and better-adjusted patients come into treatment ready and able to change; that the decisions they made to change their lives were made in advance of their admission to treatment; and that, because of their greater motivation and "treatment readiness," they are likely to stay longer in treatment and to do more of what is recommended.

These two interpretations of the same facts have very different implications for treatment practice. If treatment gradually produces positive changes over time, it is clinically sound practice to retain patients longer to provide them with more benefits. Alternatively, if well-motivated, high-functioning, compliant patients enter treatment already in possession of the skills and supports they need to do well, then length of stay in treatment could be irrelevant to outcome. More research is needed on this important point.

Participation in AA/NA/CA. AA is, of course, recognized as a social organization and not a formal treatment. For this reason, and because of the anonymous quality of the group, not much research has been done to evaluate this important part of rehabilitation until recently (McCrady & Miller, 1993; Project MATCH Research Group, 1997). While there always has been consensual validation for the value of AA and other peer support forms of treatment, the past few years have witnessed the emergence of evidence showing that patients who have participated in AA, NA, and other peer support groups, who have a sponsor, or who have participated in fellowship activities have much better abstinence records than patients who have received rehabilitation treatments but who have not continued in AA. McKay and colleagues (1994, 1997) found that participation in posttreatment self-help groups predicted better outcomes among a group of cocaine- or alcohol-dependent veterans in a day-hospital rehabilitation program. Timko, Moos et al. (1994) found that more AA attendance was associated with better one-year outcomes among previously untreated problem drinkers, regardless of whether they received inpatient, outpatient, or no other treatment.

There has been less research on the use of self-help organizations among cocaine- and/or opiate-dependent patients. However, a recent study of cocaine-dependent patients participating in outpatient counseling and psychotherapy showed that, while only 34% attended a CA meeting, 55% of those who did so became abstinent, compared with only 38% of those who did not attend CA meetings. Interestingly, there were very few background characteristics that differentiated those who attended CA meetings from those who did not (Weiss, Griffin et al., 1996).

It is important to note that, in contemporary addiction treatment, AA has become synonymous with the last part of rehabilitation: aftercare. Virtually all alcohol treatment programs and most cocaine treatment programs refer patients to AA with instructions to get a sponsor, to "share and chair" at meetings, and to attend 90 meetings in 90 days as a continued commitment to sobriety. Thus, while the research studies to date generally have suggested that the peer-support component of rehabilitation is valuable, it also is difficult to sort out the extent to which AA attendance constitutes an active ingredient of successful treatment rather than simply being a marker of treatment compliance. In this regard, citing a relative paucity of well-controlled studies of the effect of AA participation on drinking among alcoholics, Vaillant (1996) concluded, "The jury is still out" (p. 269).

The Therapist or Counselor Who Provides Treatment. A growing body of research suggests that the counselor or therapist can make an important contribution to patient engagement and participation in treatment and to the posttreatment outcome. Perhaps the clearest example of the role of the counselor and the counseling process is found in a study of methadone-maintained patients, all of whom were within the same treatment program and receiving the same methadone dose, who were randomly assigned to receive counseling or no counseling in addition to the methadone (McLellan, Arndt et al., 1993). Results were unequivocal: 68% of patients assigned to the no counseling condition failed to reduce their drug use (confirmed by urinalysis) and 34% of those patients required at least one episode of emergency medical care. In contrast, no patient in the counseling group required emergency medical care, 63% showed sustained elimination of opiate use, and 41% showed sustained elimination of cocaine use over the six months of the trial.

A study by Fiorentine and Anglin (1996) as part of a larger "Target Cities" evaluation also demonstrated the contribution of counseling to drug rehabilitation. In that study, group counseling was the most common modality (averaging 9.5 sessions per month), followed by Twelve Step meetings (7.5 times per month), and individual counseling (4.7 times per month). Greater frequency of both group and individual counseling sessions was shown to reduce the likelihood of relapse over the subsequent month and the subsequent six months.

One important contribution of the study, given the cautions (cited previously) regarding the role of simple length of stay in determining treatment outcome, is that the relationships shown between more counseling and lower likelihood of relapse to cocaine use were seen even among patients who completed treatment—that is, among those who had approximately the same length of stay in the programs. Thus, it may be that, beyond the simple effects of attending a program, greater involvement in counseling activities is important to improved outcomes.

Many important questions remain. While patients who meet with a counselor during treatment appear to have better outcomes than do those who have no counselor, there are significant differences in outcome for patients treated by different counselors. There is little to indicate which qualities (personal, educational, philosophical, and the like) are important in determining who should and should not be a counselor and whether a given patient is likely to have good or poor outcomes when assigned to a particular counselor. It is important to note that these relationships have been examined primarily for individual therapy and counseling; it is not known whether the same effect would be seen in group therapy settings.

McLellan and colleagues (1988) found that assignment to one of five methadone maintenance counselors resulted in significant differences in treatment progress over the following six months. Specifically, patients transferred to one counselor achieved significant reductions in illicit drug use, unemployment, and number of arrests, while concurrently reducing their average methadone dose. By contrast, patients transferred to another counselor evidenced increased unemployment and illicit drug use, while their average methadone dose went up.

Although it is relatively clear that therapists and counselors differ considerably in the extent to which they are able to help their patients achieve positive outcomes, it is less clear what distinguishes more effective from less effective therapists. In an experimental study of two different therapist styles, Miller and colleagues (1993) found that a client-centered approach that employed reflective listening was more effective for problem drinkers than a directive, confrontational approach. In a review of the literature on therapist differences in addiction treatment, Najavits and Weiss (1994) concluded, "The only consistent finding has been that therapists' in-session interpersonal functioning is positively associated with greater effectiveness" (p. 683).

It should be noted that there are a variety of certification programs for counselors (including those of the Committee on Addiction Rehabilitation [CARF] and the Certified Addictions Counselor [CAC]), as well as physicians and other professionals who are certified to treat substance-dependent patients (including those certified by the American Society of Addiction Medicine, the American Academy of Addiction Psychiatry, and the American Psychological Association). These added qualification certificates are offered throughout the country, usually by professional organizations. While the efforts of these professional organizations to bring needed training and proficiency to the treatment of addicted persons are commendable, we were unable to find any published studies validating whether patients treated by "certified" addiction counselors, physicians, or psychologists have better outcomes than patients treated by non-certified individuals. This is an important gap in the existing literature. The results of such studies would be quite important for the licensing and certification efforts and health policy decisions of many states and health care organizations.

Medications. Over the past decade, the National Institute on Alcoholism and Alcohol Abuse (NIAAA) and the National Institute on Drug Abuse (NIDA) have sponsored a great deal of research aimed at developing useful medications for the treatment of addictive disorders. Great progress has been made in the development of new medications and in the application of existing medications for the treatment of particular conditions associated with substance dependence and for particular types of substance dependent patients. A review of the more than 200 randomly controlled trials of various types of addiction treatments is beyond the scope of this chapter. However, the latest scientific efforts to develop new medication for the treatment of addiction have been reviewed elsewhere (IOM, 1995b; O'Brien, 1997; Anton, 1995). What follows here is a brief overview of available medications (also see Section 6 of this text).

Medications for Opioid Addiction: Opiate receptor agonists, partial agonists, and antagonists are the three primary types of medications available for the treatment of opioid dependence. Agonist medications are prescribed either acutely, as part of an opioid detoxification protocol, or chronically in a "maintenance" regimen (to reduce drug craving, maximize the patient's tolerance, and eliminate the effects of lower potency "street" opiates). Methadone and LAAM have been used effectively as maintenance medications because of their slow onset of action and long half-life. Studies validated by a panel of impartial physicians and scientists in a National Institutes of Health (NIH) consensus conference confirmed major reductions in opiate use, crime, and the spread of infectious diseases in patients on methadone maintenance (NIH, 1997).

A partial agonist, buprenorphine, is newly approved by the U. S. Food and Drug Administration (FDA) for the treatment of opioid dependence in general practice settings. Buprenorphine, which is administered sublingually, is effective in reducing opiate craving for 24 to 36 hours (Bickel & Amass, 1995). The partial agonist actions of buprenorphine may have some advantages over methadone, such as few or no withdrawal symptoms on discontinuation and lower risk of overdose even if combined with other opiates (Bickel & Amass, 1995).

Among the most robust findings in the treatment literature is the relationship between dose of methadone and general outcome in methadone treatment (Ball & Ross, 1991; D'Aunno & Vaughn, 1992; IOM, 1995b): higher doses are more effective than lower doses. In a well-controlled double-blind multisite VA study, Ling and colleagues (1976) found that 100 mg per day of methadone was superior to 50 mg, as indicated by staff ratings of global improvement and by a drug use index composed of weighted results of opiate urine tests. In a more recent randomized double-blind study, Strain and colleagues (1993) compared 50 mg and 20 mg of methadone with a 0 mg placebo-only group. They found orderly dose-response effects on treatment retention, and they found that 50 mg was more effective than 20 mg or 0 mg at reducing opiate and cocaine use, as measured by urinalysis results.

In a randomized double-blind comparison of moderate (40 to 50 mg) and high (80 to 100 mg) dose methadone, Strain and colleagues (1996) found a significantly lower rate of opiate positive urine specimens among patients receiving the high dose of methadone (53% vs. 62%). They concluded that, although the higher dose was more effective, substantial opiate use can persist even among patients treated with 80 to 100 mg per day of methadone.

There are many other studies of opiate agonist medications, but space limitations do not permit more detail here (for additional information, see the IOM Report, 1995b, as well as Section 6 of this text).

Opioid receptor antagonists such as naltrexone produce neither euphoria nor dysphoria when prescribed to abstinent opiate addicts and have been on the market since 1984 (Kleber, 1987). Naltrexone is an orally administered opiate antagonist that blocks the actions of externally administered opiates (such as heroin) through competitive binding to opiate receptors for 48 to 72 hours (IOM, 1995b; O'Brien, 1997). Like methadone, naltrexone (marketed under the trade name ReVia®) is a maintenance medication, but compliance generally has been poor, with most field studies showing retention rates of less than 20%. It may be most useful in selected populations, when combined with social, employment, or criminal justice sanctions to increase compliance. For example, naltrexone has been used in the monitored treatment of physicians, attorneys, nurses, and other professionals (Ling & Wesson, 1984), where maintaining a license to practice is contingent on maintaining abstinence. In a recent controlled trial with opiate-dependent federal probationers, Cornish and colleagues (1998) showed that naltrexone combined with standard probation produced 70% less opiate use and 50% less reincarceration than probation alone.

Medications for Alcohol Dependence: Disulfiram (Antabuse®) has been used in the treatment of alcohol dependence for 30 years. It produces vomiting, facial flushing, and headaches if a patient drinks alcohol. Because of the severity of these effects, disulfiram has been used only with a relatively select group of well-supervised patients (Fuller, Branchey et al., 1986). More recently, the opiate antagonist naltrexone has been approved by the FDA for reducing drinking among alcohol-dependent patients. It blocks alcohol-mediated stimulation of endogenous opioids, thus blunting some of alcohol's euphoric effects (Volpicelli, Alterman et al., 1992; O'Malley, Jaffe et al., 1992). Naltrexone also has some side effects (nausea, headaches) in a minority of patients, but does not produce unpleasant physiological effects if the patient consumes alcohol (Volpicelli, Alterman et al., 1992; O'Malley, Jaffe et al., 1992).

More recently, European researchers have found encouraging results using acamprosate to block craving and the return to alcohol abuse. While acamprosate acts primarily on glutamate receptors rather than opiate receptors, as with naltrexone, the clinical results are remarkably similar (Sass, Soyka et al., 1996). Alcohol-dependent patients who take either medication have shown significantly lower relapse rates than those randomly assigned to placebo (Anton, 1995; O'Brien, 1997).

Medications for Stimulant Dependence: Over the past 10 years, many medications have been tried for the treatment of cocaine and/or other stimulant dependence, but there is not yet a safe and effective agent (IOM, 1995b; O'Brien, 1997). Research continues in this important area—and there have been indications of a potentially successful "vaccine" that may be able to rapidly bind to or cleave cocaine molecules, thereby inactivating them (see Fox, 1998).

This promising work currently is being tested in animal models, with clinical trials planned.

While the use of opiate and alcohol antagonists or blocking agents is increasing as addiction medicine physicians become more comfortable in prescribing adjunctive medications and as more addicted patients are treated by primary care physicians in office settings (Fleming, Barry et al., 1997), there still are relatively few patients who receive—or physicians who prescribe—such medications. The available literature in this area does not yet provide unambiguous conclusions about the parameters that are most effective when using medications. For example, a cautionary article by Miotto and colleagues (1997) warned about an unusually high rate of deaths (particularly suicides) among opiate-dependent individuals who were transferred to naltrexone therapy.

The responsible and appropriate use of antagonist or blocking medications in the treatment of addictive disorders may be among the most important topics for future research in the treatment field. The past 10 years have seen innovation and discovery in this area, but some physicians still are reluctant to prescribe these medications (IOM, 1995a). At this time, there is a need for long-term studies of patients who have been prescribed these medications, as well as of the most appropriate and efficient mix of psychosocial and pharmacological services to maximize the effects on the rehabilitation of various types of alcohol- and drug-dependent patients.

Provision of Specialized Services. The majority of patients admitted to addiction treatment have significant problems in one or more life areas, such as medical status, employment and self-support, family relations and/or psychiatric function (see, for example, McLellan & Weisner, 1996). The severity of such problems generally is predictive of their response to treatment and posttreatment outcome. Studies have documented that strategies designed to direct and focus specialized services to these addiction-related problems can be applied in standard clinical settings and can be effective in improving the results of addiction treatment. Again, this conclusion follows more than a decade of research showing that the addition of professional marital counseling (O'Farrell, 1995; O'Farrell, Choquette et al., 1987), psychotherapy (Carroll, Rounsaville et al., 1994; Woody, McLellan et al., 1995), and medical care (Fleming & Barry, 1992) produces clinically and significantly better outcomes than does addiction treatment alone.

It should be noted that the majority of these adjunctive forms of therapy and services have been most clearly associated with improved personal health and social function following treatment and are less related to reductions in alcohol and drug use. In addition, and not surprisingly, these treatments have been shown to be effective only in patients who have more severe problems in the target area (matching effect); that is, if there has been no indication of a relatively severe problem in the target area, typically there has been no evidence that providing the target therapy is effective or worthwhile.

A study by Milby and colleagues (1996) illustrates the importance of providing supplemental social support services to homeless, substance (typically cocaine and alcohol) dependent individuals who sought health care services (not explicitly drug abuse treatment) from the Birmingham Health Care for the Homeless Coalition. In that study, 176 subjects were recruited and randomized into one of two conditions, conducted in separate facilities:

- *Usual Care*: Twice weekly Twelve Step-oriented individual and group counseling, medical evaluation, and referral were offered for diagnosed conditions. Counselors referred patients to other agencies for housing and vocational services.

- *Enhanced Care*: Day treatment was offered five days a week for 5.5 hours a day. Transportation and lunch were provided. Day treatment was group-oriented around a community model. Multiple educational and psychologically oriented groups were provided on various topics and themes. Each client had an individual counselor and an individual treatment plan, with regularly supervised review of progress.

After two months, Enhanced Care subjects graduated to a four-month work/therapy phase in which day treatment was reduced to two afternoons per week and the remaining time was spent in supervised rehabilitation of dilapidated housing that ultimately would be used by the program for drug-free housing (including housing for the subjects themselves). Minimum wages were paid and subsidized housing was available for the participants during the work therapy phase. Importantly, participation in this second phase was contingent on drug-free urines (monitored weekly on randomly selected days) and continued participation in the day-treatment program.

Outcomes were measured at several points following admission and included multiple domains that were considered important to the "value" of the treatment program to the supporting agencies. With regard to treatment retention, 131 of the 176 individuals entered one of the two programs. Usual care (UC) patients attended an average of 0.6 days per week, or 29% of expected attendance. In contrast, Enhanced Care (EC) patients attended an average of 2.5 days per week, or 48% of expected attendance. At six-month followup, the EC patients showed significantly lower rates of use of cocaine, alcohol, and opiates than did the UC patients. In addition, the EC patients were twice as likely to be employed and four times less likely to be homeless than the UC patients. Some of these significant group differences disappeared at 12 months.

Although there were problems with the very low number of subjects recruited (approximately 10% of the total homeless population), the results of this study are important in that the differences were substantial and important from a health policy perspective and because these individuals were *not* applying for addiction treatment. The treatment was available from the project and was offered to individuals who requested only health screening services. Despite the lack of initial motivation for these services, the supplemental services included as part of addiction treatment were associated with significant and broad improvements.

These data are reminiscent of findings in the criminal justice system, where addiction treatments added to standard probation or parole typically improve the effects of those interventions (Cornish, Metzger et al., 1998; Inciardi, Martin et al., 1997).

Milby has suggested that the reasons his study was able to show significant differences is that the interventions were aimed at severely affected individuals, the components of the care provided were both necessary to and desired by the subjects, and the enhanced intervention was potent and well implemented. Milby believes that both addiction-focused interventions (such as drug counseling, aftercare, and AA) and survival services (drug-free housing, employment, or self-support skills) are necessary for effective treatment, but that neither is sufficient on its own.

Similar findings have emerged from studies of "Target Cities" projects in Los Angeles and Philadelphia (McLellan, Hagan et al., 1998), which showed that supplemental social services (such as drug-free housing, medical screening and referral, parenting classes, and employment counsel-

ing) were integrated effectively into standard outpatient drug treatment through the use of clinical case managers, and that patients who were assigned to "enhanced" service programs showed 20% to 40% improvements over patients assigned to standard outpatient programs.

Matching Patients With Treatments. The past two decades have witnessed substantial research that attempts to match patients with particular problems to the specific types, modalities, or settings of treatment thought to be best suited to their needs. The approach to patient-treatment matching that has received the greatest attention from treatment researchers involves attempts to identify the characteristics of individual patients that predict the best response to different forms of treatment (Mattson, Allen et al., 1994; Project MATCH Research Group, 1997). Another approach to matching is to assess patients' problem severity across a range of areas at intake and then to add specific treatment services according to the problems assessed (Gastfriend & McLellan, 1997). This approach has the potential to be particularly helpful for the patient who has multiple problems, as most substance-focused interventions are not designed to address serious co-occurring medical, psychiatric, family, or legal problems.

Substance users who have comorbid psychiatric problems may be particularly good candidates for the addition of focused, specialized services, in the form of professionally delivered psychotherapy, psychotropic medications, greater treatment intensity or structure, or a combination of all three. For example, recent studies suggest that tricyclic antidepressants may reduce both drinking and depression levels in alcoholics with major depression (Mason, Kocsis et al., 1996). Similarly, the anxiolytic buspirone may reduce drinking in alcoholics with a comorbid anxiety disorder (Kranzler & McLellan, 1995). Highly structured relapse prevention interventions also may be more effective than less structured interventions in decreasing cocaine use in subjects with comorbid depression (Carroll, Nich et al., 1995).

The impact of adding professionally delivered treatment services to a basic methadone program also was investigated by McLellan and colleagues (1993). In that study, patients were randomly assigned to receive (1) methadone only, (2) methadone plus standard counseling, or (3) methadone and counseling plus on-site medical, psychiatric, employment, and family therapy services (the "enhanced" condition). Although these additional services were not "matched" to patients on an individual basis, most of the patients in the study were polydrug abusers with relatively high problem levels in other areas. On most outcome measures, the best results were obtained in the enhanced condition, followed by methadone plus counseling, and then by methadone alone. Improvements in the enhanced condition were significantly better than those in the methadone plus counseling condition in the areas of employment, alcohol use, criminal activity, and psychiatric status. These results demonstrate the value of providing additional professional treatment services to polyproblem substance abusers, even when such services are not "matched" to specific problems at the level of the individual patient.

Another type of patient who can pose problems is the cocaine-dependent patient who is unable to achieve remission from cocaine dependence early in outpatient treatment. Several randomized studies suggest that highly structured cognitive-behavioral treatment is particularly efficacious with such individuals. In two outpatient studies with cocaine abusers, those who had more severe cocaine problems at intake had significantly better outcomes if they received structured relapse prevention rather than interpersonal or clinical management treatments (Carroll, Rounsaville et al., 1991, 1994).

In a third study, cocaine-dependent patients who continued to use cocaine during a four-week intensive outpatient treatment program had much better cocaine use outcomes if they subsequently received aftercare that included a combination of group therapy and a structured relapse prevention protocol delivered through individual sessions, rather than aftercare that consisted of group therapy alone (McKay, Alterman et al., 1997).

McLellan and colleagues recently attempted a different type of matching research in two inpatient and two outpatient private treatment programs (McLellan, Grissom et al., 1997). Patients in the study (n=130) were assessed with the Assessment Severity Index (ASI) at intake and placed in a program that was acceptable to both the EAP referral source and the patient. At intake, patients were randomized to either the standard or "matched" services condition. In the standard condition, the treatment program received information from the intake ASI and personnel were instructed to treat the patient in the standard manner, as though no evaluation study was ongoing. The programs were instructed not to withhold any services from patients in the standard condition. Patients who were randomly assigned to the matched services condition also were placed in one of the four treatment programs and their ASI infor-

mation was forwarded to that program. However, the programs agreed to provide at least three individual sessions in the areas of employment, family/social relations, or psychiatric health, delivered by a professionally trained staff person, when a patient evidenced a significant degree of impairment in one or more areas at intake. (For example, a patient whose intake ASI showed significant impairments in the areas of social and psychiatric functioning would receive at least six individual sessions, three by a psychiatrist and three by a social worker.)

The standard and matched patients were compared on a number of measures, including number of services received while in treatment, treatment completion rates, intake to 6-month improvements in the seven problem areas assessed by the ASI, and other key outcomes at six months. The following results were obtained. First, matched patients received significantly more psychiatric and employment services than standard patients, but not more family/social services or addiction services. Second, matched patients were more likely to complete treatment (93% vs. 81%), and showed more improvement in the areas of employment and psychiatric functioning than the standard patients. Third, while matched and standard patients had sizable and equivalent improvements on most measures of alcohol and drug use, matched patients were less likely to be re-treated for substance abuse problems during the six-month followup period. These findings suggest that matching treatment services to adjunctive problems can improve outcomes in key areas and also may be cost-effective, because it appears to reduce the need for subsequent treatment as the result of relapse.

Limitations of the Matching Approach: It is difficult to argue against the face validity of a treatment approach that stresses the importance of providing additional services to address co-occurring medical, economic, psychiatric, family, and legal problems. After all, standard addiction-focused interventions are not designed to address serious problems in other areas. If left untreated, co-occurring problems can increase the risk of poor treatment response and poor posttreatment outcomes. And, in some cases, it may be impossible even to initiate treatment for an addictive disorder until a severe co-occurring problem has been treated. In addition to benefits for the patients, the matching approach can reduce stress levels in clinicians who treat polyproblem individuals, provided that a team approach to treatment is taken and regular lines of communication are established among clinicians involved with a case.

The primary limitation of this approach concerns the potential lack of resources in a time of health care cost containment. Funding may not be available for adjunctive services in areas such as medical and psychiatric care, unless the problems are so severe that these co-occurring disorders can be considered "primary" or at least as critical as the substance use problem. Recent research has shown that addiction treatment programs vary widely in the number and frequency of adjunctive services they provide (McLellan, Grissom et al., 1993; D'Aunno & Vaughn, 1992), which may reflect differences among programs in the funding available for such services.

Obviously, it is impossible to match services to problems if the appropriate services are not available. The scarcity of resources underlies the need for accurate assessment and diagnosis of co-occurring problems, so as to ensure that patients who are in need of such services will stand a better chance of receiving them. Also, not all services may be potent enough to make a significant difference in the target problem area. For example, despite the importance of employment-related problems in predicting treatment outcomes and despite the range of interventions that have been developed to improve employment and self-support among substance-dependent patients (see French, Rachal et al., 1991), there is little evidence (Hall, Loeb et al., 1981, is an exception) that this type of specialized service is effective in improving the employment of the patients or in improving their abstinence from drugs.

A *caveat* also is in order concerning the addition of family or couples therapy (conjoint therapy) to addiction treatment. In studies in which couples behavioral marital therapy has been compared to other forms of outpatient treatment for alcoholics, such therapy frequently has been associated with superior outcomes (Holder, Longabaugh et al., 1991). However, there is less evidence that conjoint therapy is effective with polyproblem individuals or drug abusers, and there is some indication that it can produce worse outcomes with some patients under certain conditions. Longabaugh and colleagues (1995) randomized patients to three 20-session outpatient social learning-based conditions that varied in the amount of conjoint therapy included (0, 4, or 8 sessions). Analyses indicated that the 8-conjoint-session condition was least effective for patients who had either the worst or best relationship situations, as indicated by the patient's degree of investment in the relationship and the degree of support for abstinence from significant others.

Additional analyses with the same sample indicated that, according to the perceptions of both the patient and significant other, family functioning showed equal improvement from pre- to posttreatment in the individually focused (0 conjoint sessions) and relationally focused (4 or 8 conjoint sessions) conditions. However, the individually focused condition actually produced greater improvement in family functioning for patients characterized by a high degree of dependence on others (McKay, Longabaugh, et al., 1993).

The results of this study raise the possibility that, for patients with serious family or social problems, a limited number of conjoint treatment sessions may do more harm than good, especially if the sessions are substituted for standard alcohol or drug sessions. In such cases, providing a limited number of conjoint sessions may in a sense "open a can of worms" by encouraging both patient and significant other to air feelings of anger, hurt, or disappointment and then not providing enough time to work through the problems that have been identified.

CONCLUSIONS

This review has attempted to identify patient variables and treatment process variables that have been shown to be important in determining the outcome of addiction rehabilitation efforts. The research reviewed here suggests the following three points:

First, research has effectively established that treatment can be effective, but there are only preliminary indications as to *why* treatment is effective or *what it is* within treatment that makes it effective. Treatment researchers are only now beginning to develop the measures and models that will be necessary for the exploration of questions regarding why treatment works. If the outcomes research field really is to inform contemporary community-based treatment, then it will be necessary to move beyond the question of *whether* treatment works to the question of *how* treatment works. In turn, this will require a shift in methodology from the simple evaluation or comparison of treatment outcomes to the parametric study of the various types of treatment services and therapeutic processes delivered within those treatments, and their relationship to the target outcomes.

The suggested methodology will require measurement of more than just the target outcomes at a posttreatment followup point. Careful recording of the treatment services and processes provided during treatment will be necessary, as will the concurrent monitoring of during-treatment changes in patient attitude, cognition, motivation, affect, and behavior that are the interim goals of these processes. These types of "dose response" or "dose ranging" designs ultimately will permit the discovery of the important therapeutic milestones that patients must achieve along their route to recovery and the "active ingredients" within a treatment that are responsible for their achieving the milestones and, ultimately, for lasting outcomes following treatment. This is a line of inquiry that has been called for by several researchers within the field (see Simpson, 1997), but the present review has uncovered very few studies that have pursued such research. Thus, an important message of this chapter is a call to the treatment research field for more systematic work on this line of investigation.

Second, some patients have better prognoses at the start of treatment than others. The variables that suggest better prognosis include: (1) low severity of dependence and psychiatric symptoms at admission; (2) motivation beyond the precontemplation stage of change; (3) being employed or self-supporting; and (4) having family and social supports for sobriety.

Third, some treatment variables have reliably been shown to produce better and more enduring outcomes. The treatment variables associated with better outcomes include: (1) staying in treatment (at least outpatient treatment) longer and/or being more compliant with treatment; (2) having an individual counselor or therapist and more counseling sessions during treatment; (3) receiving proper medications (both anti-craving medications and medications for adjunctive psychiatric conditions); (4) participating in voucher-based, behavioral reinforcement interventions; (5) participating in AA, CA, or NA following treatment; and (6) having supplemental social services provided for adjunctive medical, psychiatric, and/or family problems.

It is important to note that none of these patient or treatment variables showed a completely unambiguous record of prediction, although all have shown replicated evidence across more than one type of primary drug problem (alcohol, cocaine, or opiates) and in more than one research evaluation. An important point raised by Holder and colleagues in their review of the alcohol rehabilitation literature (1991) is that many of the currently applied treatment practices and processes have not been shown to have an important association with treatment outcomes, and that many have not been studied at all. In fact, there are a number of therapeutic practices and procedures that remain prevalent in the field that have not shown indications of success, so more research clearly is needed to identify the "active ingredients" of treatment and the minimal effective doses of those ingredients.

ACKNOWLEDGMENTS: Preparation of this chapter was supported by grants from the Center for Substance Abuse Treatment, the National Institute on Drug Abuse, and The Robert Wood Johnson Foundation. A version of this paper was submitted as part of the Institute of Medicine's Committee on Community Based Addiction Treatments.

REFERENCES

Alterman AI, Droba M & McLellan AT (1992). Response to day hospital treatment by patients with cocaine and alcohol dependence. *Hospital & Community Psychiatry* 43(9):930-932.

Alterman AI, McLellan AT, O'Brien CP et al. (1994). Effectiveness and costs of inpatient versus day hospital cocaine rehabilitation. *Journal of Nervous & Mental Disease* 182:157-163.

Anton RF (1995). New directions in the pharmacotherapy of alcoholism. *Psychiatric Annals* 25: 353-362.

Ball JC & Ross A (1991). *The Effectiveness of Methadone Maintenance Treatment.* New York, NY: Springer-Verlag.

Barber JP, Mercer D, Krakauer I et al. (1996). Development of an adherence/competence rating scale for individual drug counseling. *Drug and Alcohol Dependence* 43:125-132.

Bickel WK & Amass L (1995). Buprenorphine treatment of opioid dependence: A review. *Experimental and Clinical Psychopharmacology* 3:477-489.

Carroll KM, Nich C & Rounsaville BJ (1995). Differential symptom reduction in depressed cocaine abusers treated with psychotherapy and pharmacotherapy. *Journal of Nervous & Mental Disease* 183(4):251-259.

Carroll KM, Rounsaville BJ, Nich C et al. (1994). One-year follow-up of psychotherapy and pharmacotherapy for cocaine dependence: Delayed emergence of psychotherapy effects. *Archives of General Psychiatry* 51(12):989-997.

Carroll KM, Rounsaville BJ & Gawin FH (1991). A comparative trial of psychotherapies for ambulatory cocaine abusers: Relapse prevention and interpersonal psychotherapy. *American Journal of Drug and Alcohol Abuse* 17:229-247.

Carroll KM, Rounsaville BJ, Gordon LT et al. (1994). Psychotherapy and pharmacotherapy for ambulatory cocaine abusers. *Archives of General Psychiatry* 51:177-187.

Cornish J, Metzger D, Woody G et al. (1998). Naltrexone pharmacotherapy for opioid dependent federal probationers. *Journal of Substance Abuse Treatment* 15(2):134-141.

D'Aunno T & Vaughn TE (1992). Variations in methadone treatment practices: Results from a national study. *Journal of the American Medical Association* 267:253-258.

Fiorentine R & Anglin DM (1996). More is better: Counseling participation and the effectiveness of outpatient drug treatment. *Journal of Substance Abuse Treatment* 13(4):232-240.

Fleming MF & Barry KL, eds. (1992). *Addictive Disorders.* St. Louis, MO: Mosby Yearbook Primary Care Series.

Fleming MF, Barry KL, Manwell LB et al. (1997). Brief physician advice for problem alcohol drinkers: A randomized controlled trial in community-based primary care practices. *Journal of the American Medical Association* 277:1039-1045.

Fox BS (1997). Development of a therapeutic vaccine for the treatment of cocaine addiction. *Drug and Alcohol Dependence* 48:153-158.

French MT, Rachal JV & Hubbard RL (1991). Conceptual framework for estimating the social cost of drug abuse. *Journal of Health & Social Policy* 2:1-22.

Fuller RK, Branchey L, Brightwell DR et al. (1986). Disulfiram treatment of alcoholism: A Veterans Administration cooperative study. *Journal of the American Medical Association* 256:1449-1489.

Gastfriend D & McLellan AT (1997). Treatment matching: Theoretical basis and practical implications. In J Samet & M Stein (eds.) *Medical Clinics of North America*. New York, NY: W.B. Saunders.

Hall SM, Loeb P, LeVois P et al. (1981). Increasing employment in ex-heroin addicts II: Methadone maintenance sample. *Behavioral Medicine* 12:453-460.

Harwood HJ, Fountain D & Livermore G (1998). *The Economic Costs of Alcohol and Drug Abuse in the United States*. Rockville, MD: National Institute on Drug Abuse.

Havassy BE, Hall SM & Wasserman DA (1997). Social support and relapse: Commonalities among alcoholics, opiate users, and cigarette smokers. *Addictive Behaviors* 16(5):235-246.

Holder HD, Longabaugh R, Miller WR et al. (1991). The cost effectiveness of treatment for alcohol problems: A first approximation. *Journal of Studies on Alcohol* 52:517-540.

Inciardi JA, Martin SS, Butzin CA et al. (1997). An effective model of prison-based treatment for drug-involved offenders. *Journal of Drug Issues* 27(2):261-278.

Institute of Medicine (IOM) (1995a). *Dispelling the Myths About Addiction*. Washington, DC: National Academy Press.

Institute of Medicine (IOM) (1995b). *Development of Medications for the Treatment of Opiate and Cocaine Addictions: Issues for the Government and Private Sector*. Washington, DC: National Academy Press.

Institute of Medicine (IOM) (1997). *Managing Managed Care: Quality Improvement in Behavioral Health*. Washington, DC: National Academy Press.

Kang SY, Kleinman PH, Woody GE et al. (1991). Outcomes for cocaine abusers after once-a-week psychosocial therapy. *American Journal of Psychiatry* 148:630-635.

Kleber HD (1987). Clonidine and naltrexone in the outpatient treatment of heroin withdrawal. *American Journal of Drug and Alcohol Abuse* 13:1-17.

Kranzler HR & McLellan AT (1995). Pharmacotherapies for alcoholism: Evolving theoretical and methodological perspectives. In H Kranzler (ed.) *Substance Abuse Treatment*. Baltimore, MD: Williams & Wilkins.

Ling W, Charuvastra VC, Kaim SC et al. (1976). Methadyl acetate and methadone as maintenance treatments for heroin addicts. *Archives of General Psychiatry* 33:709-720.

Ling W & Wesson DR (1984). Naltrexone treatment for addicted health care professionals: A collaborative private practice experience. *Journal of Clinical Psychiatry* 45(9):46-48.

Longabaugh R, Wirtz PW, Beattie MC et al. (1995). Matching treatment focus to patient social investment and support: 18 month follow-up results. *Journal of Consulting and Clinical Psychology* 63:296-307.

Mason BJ, Kocsis JH, Ritvo EC et al. (1996). A double-blind, placebo-controlled trial of desipramine for primary alcohol dependence stratified on the presence or absence of major depression. *Journal of the American Medical Association* 275:761-767.

Mattson ME, Allen JP, Longabaugh R et al. (1994). A chronological review of empirical studies matching alcoholics to treatment. *Journal of Studies on Alcohol* 12(Suppl):16-29.

McCrady BS & Miller WR (1993). *Research on Alcoholics Anonymous: Opportunities and Alternatives*. New Brunswick, NJ: Rutgers Center of Alcohol Studies.

McKay J, McLellan AT, Alterman A et al. (1998). Predictors of participation in aftercare sessions and self-help groups following completion of intensive outpatient treatment for substance abuse. *Journal of Studies in Alcohol*.

McKay JR, Alterman AI, McLellan AT et al. (1994). Treatment goals, continuity of care, and outcome in a day hospital substance abuse rehabilitation program. *American Journal of Psychiatry* 151:254-259.

McKay JR, Alterman AI, Cacciola JS et al. (1997). Group counseling vs. individualized relapse prevention aftercare following intensive outpatient treatment for cocaine dependence: Initial results. *Journal of Consulting and Clinical Psychology* 65:778-788.

McKay JR, Cacciola J, McLellan AT et al. (1997). An initial evaluation of the psychosocial dimensions of the ASAM criteria for inpatient and day hospital substance abuse rehabilitation. *Journal of Studies on Alcohol* 58:239-252.

McKay JR, Longabaugh R, Beattie MC et al. (1993). Does adding conjoint therapy to individually-focused alcoholism treatment lead to better family functioning? *Journal of Substance Abuse* 5:45-60.

McKay JR, McLellan AT & Alterman AI (1992). An evaluation of the Cleveland Criteria for Inpatient Treatment of Substance Abuse. *American Journal of Psychiatry* 149:1212-1218.

McLellan AT, Alterman AI, Woody GE et al. (1994). Great expectations: A review of the concepts and empirical findings regarding substance abuse treatment. In *Alcohol and Substance Dependence*. London, England: Royal Task Force on Substance Dependence.

McLellan AT, Arndt IO, Woody GE et al. (1993). Psychosocial services in substance abuse treatment? A dose-ranging study of psychosocial services. *Journal of the American Medical Association* 269(15):1953-1959.

McLellan AT, Cacciola J, Kushner H et al. (1992). The Fifth Edition of the Addiction Severity Index: Cautions, additions and normative data. *Journal of Substance Abuse Treatment* 9(5):461-480.

McLellan AT, Grissom G & Brill P (1997). Improved outcomes from treatment service "matching" in substance abuse patients: A controlled study. *Archives of General Psychiatry* 54:730-735.

McLellan AT, Grissom G, Durell J et al. (1993). Substance abuse treatment in the private setting: Are some programs more effective than others? *Journal of Substance Abuse Treatment* 10:243-254.

McLellan AT, Hagan TA, Meyers K et al. (1998). Supplemental social services improve outcomes in public addiction treatment. *Addiction* 93(10):1489-1499.

McLellan AT, Luborsky L, Cacciola J et al. (1995). New data from the Addiction Severity Index: Reliability and validity in three centers. *Journal of Nervous and Mental Disease* 173:412-423.

McLellan AT, O'Brien CP, Lewis D et al. (2000). Drug addiction as a chronic medical illness: Implications for treatment, insurance and evaluation. *Journal of the American Medical Association* 284:1689–1695.

McLellan AT & Weisner C (1996). Achieving the public health potential of substance abuse treatment: Implications for patient referral, treatment "matching" and outcome evaluation. In W Bickel & R DeGrandpre (eds.) *Drug Policy and Human Nature*. Philadelphia, PA: Williams & Wilkins.

McLellan AT, Woody GE, Luborsky L et al. (1988). Is the counselor an "active ingredient" in substance abuse rehabilitation? *Journal of Nervous and Mental Disease* 176:423-430.

McLellan AT, Woody GE, Metzger D et al. (1996). Evaluating the effectiveness of treatments for substance use disorders: Reasonable expectations, appropriate comparisons. *Milbank Quarterly* 74(1):51-85.

Mee-Lee D, Shulman J, Gartner L et al. (1996). *Patient Placement Criteria for the Treatment of Substance-Related Disorders, Second Edition (ASAM PPC-2)*. Chevy Chase, MD: American Society of Addiction Medicine.

Mee-Lee D, Shulman J, Fishman M et al. (2001). *ASAM Patient Placement Criteria for the Treatment of Substance-Related Disorders, Second Edition-Revised (ASAM PPC-2R)*. Chevy Chase, MD: American Society of Addiction Medicine.

Milby JB, Schumacher JE, Raczynski JM et al. (1996). Sufficient conditions for effective treatment of substance abusing homeless persons. *Drug and Alcohol Dependence* 43:39-47.

Miller WR & Hester RK (1986). Inpatient alcoholism treatment: Who benefits? *American Psychologist* 41:794-805.

Miller WR, Benefield RG & Tonigan JS (1993). Enhancing motivation for change in problem drinking: A controlled comparison of two therapist styles. *Journal of Consulting and Clinical Psychology* 61:455-461.

Miotto K, McCann MJ, Rawson RA et al. (1997). Overdose, suicide attempts and death among a cohort of naltrexone-treated opioid addicts. *Drug and Alcohol Dependence* 45:131-134.

Moos RH, Finney JW & Cronkite RC (1990). *Alcoholism Treatment: Context, Process and Outcome*. New York, NY: Oxford University Press.

Najavits LM & Weiss RD (1994). Variations in therapist effectiveness in the treatment of patients with substance use disorders: An empirical review. *Addiction* 89(6):679–688.

National Institutes of Health (NIH) (1997). Presentation at the Consensus Conference on the Treatment of Opiate Addiction, Bethesda, MD.

Nunes E, Quitkin F, Brady R et al. (1994). Antidepressant treatment in methadone maintenance patients. *Journal of Addictive Diseases* 13(3):13–24.

O'Brien CP (1997). A range of research-based pharmacotherapies for addiction. *Science* 278:66-70.

O'Farrell TJ (1995). Marital and family therapy. In RK Hester & WR Miller (eds.) *Handbook of Alcoholism Treatment Approaches (2nd Ed.)*. Needham Heights, MA: Allyn & Bacon.

O'Farrell TJ, Choquette KA & Cutter HSG (1987). Couples relapse prevention sessions after behavioral marital therapy for male alcoholics: Outcomes during the three years after starting treatment. *Journal of Studies on Alcohol*.

O'Malley SS, Jaffe AJ, Chang G et al. (1992). Naltrexone and coping skills therapy for alcohol dependence. *Archives of General Psychiatry* 49:881-887.

Pettinati HM, Belden PP, Evans BD et al. (1997). The natural history of outpatient alcohol and drug abuse treatment in a private health care setting. *Alcoholism: Clinical & Experimental Research* 45:345-349.

Project MATCH Research Group (1997). Matching alcoholism treatments to client heterogeneity: Project MATCH post treatment drinking outcomes. *Journal of Studies on Alcohol* 58:7–29.

Sass H, Soyka M, Mann K et al. (1996). Relapse prevention by acamprosate: Results from a placebo-controlled study on alcohol dependence. *Archives of General Psychiatry* 53:673-680.

Simpson DD (1997). Effectiveness of drug abuse treatment: Review of research from field settings. In JA Egertson, DM Fox & AI Leshner (eds.) *Treating Drug Abusers Effectively*. Cambridge, MA: Blackwell.

Simpson DD, Joe GW & Brown BS (1997). Treatment retention and follow-up outcomes in the Drug Abuse Treatment Outcome Study (DATOS). *Psychology of Addictive Behaviors* 11(4):294-301.

Strain EC, Bigelow GE, Liebson IA et al. (1996). Moderate versus high dose methadone in the treatment of opioid dependence. Poster session presented at the annual meeting of the College on Problems of Drug Dependence, San Juan, Puerto Rico; June.

Strain EC, Stitzer IA, Liebson IA et al. (1993). Dose-response effects of methadone in the treatment of opioid dependence. *Annals of Internal Medicine* 119:23-27.

Timko C, Moos RH, Finney JW et al. (1994). Outcome of treatment for alcohol abuse and involvement in Alcoholics Anonymous among previously untreated problem drinkers. *Journal of Mental Health Administration* 21:145–160.

Vaillant GE (1996). *The Natural History of Alcoholism*. Cambridge, MA: Harvard University Press.

Volpicelli JR, Alterman AI, Hayashida M et al. (1992). Naltrexone in the treatment of alcohol dependence. *Archives of General Psychiatry* 49:876-880

Walsh DC, Hingson R, Merrigan D et al. (1991). A randomized trial of treatment options for alcohol-abusing workers. *New England Journal of Medicine* 325:775–782.

Weiss RD, Griffin ML, Najavits LM et al. (1996). Self help activities in cocaine dependent patients entering treatment: Results from the NIDA Collaborative Cocaine Treatment Study. *Drug and Alcohol Dependence* 43(1-2):79-86.

Woody GE, McLellan AT, Luborsky L et al. (1995). Psychotherapy in community methadone programs: A validation study. *American Journal of Psychiatry* 152(9):1302–1308.

Effects of Setting, Duration, and Amount on Treatment Outcomes

Chapter 4

John W. Finney, Ph.D.
Rudolf H. Moos, Ph.D.

**Effect of Treatment Setting
Effect of Treatment Duration and Amount
Implications for Policymakers and Service Providers**

Addiction treatment researchers sometimes feel that their work is overlooked by policymakers and treatment providers. This has not been the case for researchers studying the effects of various treatment settings and different durations and amounts of treatment, because variations in these treatment dimensions have readily apparent, immediate cost implications. Several research reviews have examined the relative effectiveness of alcohol treatment in inpatient and outpatient settings (Annis, 1986; Mattick & Jarvis, 1994; Miller & Hester, 1986; Saxe, Dougherty et al., 1983) and of variations in treatment duration and amount (Babor, 1994; Bien, Miller et al., 1993; Mattick & Jarvis, 1994; Miller & Hester, 1986). Focusing on controlled studies employing random assignment or matching on patient pretreatment variables, each of these reviews concluded there was no evidence for the superiority of inpatient over outpatient treatment (a similar conclusion has been reached in reviews of drug abuse treatment research by Anglin & Hser, 1990, and Crits-Christoph & Siqueland, 1996, but also see Budde, Rounsaville et al., 1992), or for longer or more intensive treatment over briefer or less intensive treatment.

In this chapter, the authors re-examine the research evidence on the effects of treatment settings, duration, and amount, drawing heavily on more recent reviews of these topics (Finney, Hahn et al., 1996; Finney & Moos, 1996, 1998; Monahan & Finney, 1996; Moos & Finney, 1996a, 1996b; Moyer, Finney et al., 2002). The primary focus is research on the treatment of alcohol use disorders, although research on treatment of drug use disorders also is considered. The authors argue that research findings have been extrapolated to populations beyond those involved in the studies and that key issues remain to be addressed. Those issues include determining whether certain types of patients benefit more from treatment in inpatient and residential settings, whether certain types of patients benefit from longer or more intensive treatment, and whether—perhaps for many patients—treatment should be less intensive but spread out over longer periods.

EFFECT OF TREATMENT SETTING
Rationales for Inpatient and Outpatient Treatment. Four main rationales have been put forward for the superiority of inpatient and residential treatment settings. One is that

such settings provide a respite for patients, removing them from environments that are perpetuating their addiction, and allowing their efforts toward abstinence to be consolidated. Second, it has been argued that inpatient and residential settings allow patients to receive more treatment because they are less likely to drop out of treatment, treatment is more intensive, and patients are linked more effectively with aftercare. A third rationale is that inpatient and residential settings provide medical and psychiatric care (inpatient settings) and/or tangible and emotional support (inpatient and residential settings) to patients who otherwise would not have access to such care or support. Finally, some proponents argue that inpatient treatment suggests to patients that their problems are more severe than would be the case if treatment were offered in an outpatient setting.

Arguments in favor of outpatient treatment also have focused on the patient's usual life situation, but have emphasized the advantages of leaving the patient in, rather than removing him or her from, that context. Proponents have suggested that outpatient treatment provides an opportunity for more accurate assessments of the antecedents of substance use and for testing coping skills in real-life situations while the patient remains in a supportive therapeutic relationship. Thus, the theory goes, greater generalization of learning should take place than would be the case in the atypical environment of an inpatient treatment program (see Annis, 1986). In addition, it has been suggested that outpatient treatment mobilizes help in the patient's natural environment—as from a family physician or self-help groups—to a greater extent than does inpatient or residential treatment. Finally, proponents have argued that outpatient treatment results in a more successful transition to aftercare when, for example, a patient begins to attend self-help group meetings near his or her home while still in treatment.

Relevant Research. In a review of research on inpatient versus outpatient treatment for alcohol abuse, Finney and colleagues (1996) considered 14 relevant studies, including several studies not included in prior reviews. In those studies, inpatient treatment took various forms but usually was provided in an acute inpatient setting. In one study, the planned alterative to inpatient treatment was inpatient detoxification; in another, it was a wait-list control. In the remaining studies, the planned outpatient treatment ranged from day-hospital programs to individual and group outpatient treatment (including brief advice), to participation in self-help groups such as Alcoholics Anonymous.

Overall, the studies varied substantially in the content and amount of index treatment and aftercare.

The investigators initially summarized the studies' findings through use of a "box score" approach—that is, tallying whether inpatient and residential treatment was found to be significantly superior or inferior to, or not different from, the comparison condition in each study. Of the 14 studies, seven yielded significant setting effects on one or more drinking-related outcome variables at one or more followup points. In five studies, the outcome difference favored inpatient over outpatient treatment; in the other two, the outcome difference favored day-hospital over inpatient treatment. Patients in the "superior" setting usually received more treatment. When patients treated in outpatient settings did not first receive inpatient detoxification, they tended to show poorer outcomes than did patients treated in inpatient settings.

The box score approach to synthesizing the research literature has serious limitations. Nonsignificant differences between groups may simply reflect lack of statistical power; significant findings may emerge by chance when multiple tests for treatment effects are conducted and not adjusted for "experimentwise" error. Indeed, Finney, Hahn, and Moos (1996) found that the seven studies yielding significant setting effects had greater statistical power and conducted more treatment contrasts, on average, than the studies with no difference in outcome.

The shortcomings of box score reviews prompted the development of meta-analytic techniques that used between-group "effect sizes" (Cooper & Hedges, 1994). A between-group effect size is the difference in the average posttreatment functioning of two groups, divided by the pooled standard deviation of outcome scores within the two groups. An effect size (ES) allows one to determine by how many standard deviation units, or by what proportion of standard deviation unit, the functioning of one group is superior to that of another.

Initially, the authors had not conducted an ES analysis because the number of studies was small and it was felt that following the conventions of assigning a zero ES to findings simply reported as "nonsignificant," and of assigning the smallest possible ES consistent with $p < .05$ for findings simply reported as "statistically significant," could yield distorted results. However, after submitting the manuscript reporting the box score review, the authors were able to obtain additional data from several investigators. When the average cross-study ESs were calculated, only the three-month followup ES was significantly different from zero (for more details, see Finney & Moos, 1996). In addition, it should be noted that (1) Rychtarik and colleagues (2000) found no differences on primary outcome variables during an 18-month followup for alcohol patients randomly assigned to inpatient, intensive outpatient, and standard outpatient treatment, (2) a randomized trial of inpatient versus day-hospital treatment for cocaine abuse found no setting effects (Alterman, O'Brien et al., 1994; Budde, Rounsaville et al., 1992), and (3) reviews of the relevant research (by Anglin & Hser, 1990; Crits-Christoph & Siqueland, 1996) on outpatient methadone maintenance and outpatient drug-free treatment reported few differences in outcomes in comparison with residential therapeutic community programs.

How representative of patients typically receiving inpatient treatment are the participants in the existing studies of inpatient and outpatient alcohol treatment? The reports for eight of the 14 studies reviewed by Finney and colleagues (1996) did not indicate the percentage of patients in treatment who participated in the research. In the other six studies, the percentage of patients who participated was 14% (McLachlan & Stein, 1982), 22% (McKay, Alterman et al., 1995; two studies), 25% (Pittman & Tate, 1972), 54% (Chapman & Huygens, 1988), and 61% (Walsh, Hingson et al., 1991). In general, existing studies have examined a restricted set of patients and often have excluded patients with major medical or psychiatric disorders and/or an inability to commute to treatment. Three studies focused specifically on patients who presented for treatment at private hospitals, two focused on first admission patients, and one focused on workers in an Employee Assistance Program (EAP). Thus, the findings may not generalize well to populations of more impaired individuals and/or those with fewer social resources.

Is there evidence that such impaired patients would benefit more from inpatient or residential treatment? A diagnosis of a serious psychiatric disorder often has been an exclusion criterion in studies of inpatient versus outpatient alcohol treatment (see Finney, Hahn et al., 1996), precluding its examination as a matching variable. However, Ritson (1968) found that patients in outpatient treatment who had personality disorders tended to have poor outcomes; no relationship was found between personality disorders and outcome among inpatients.

With respect to social resources, Kissin and colleagues (1970) reported that more socially competent alcoholic patients experienced better outcomes in outpatient treatment, whereas socially unstable patients had better outcomes following inpatient treatment. Among both alcoholic and drug abusing patients with middle-level psychiatric severity in a study by McLellan, Luborsky et al. (1983), those who had more serious family, legal, and/or employment problems experienced poorer outcomes after receiving outpatient versus inpatient treatment.

Focusing on a different matching variable, Rychtarik and colleagues (2000) found that inpatients who were high in alcohol involvement had better outcomes than outpatients with high alcohol involvement; patients who had low alcohol involvement fared better following outpatient treatment than inpatient treatment. Similarly, patients with more cognitive impairment had better outcomes following inpatient than outpatient treatment. However, the study by Rychtarik et al. (2000) yielded no supporting evidence for the hypothesis that persons from environments promoting heavy drinking benefit more from a residential stay that provides a respite from that environment.

Scattered research findings such as these formed part of the basis for the *Patient Placement Criteria* of the American Society of Addiction Medicine (ASAM) (Mee-Lee, Shulman et al., 2001). The criteria attempt to match patients to five levels of care: (1) early intervention; (2) outpatient treatment; (3) intensive outpatient/partial hospitalization treatment; (4) residential/inpatient treatment; and (5) medically managed intensive inpatient treatment. Placement decisions are based on a patient's standing on six dimensions: (1) acute intoxication and/or withdrawal potential; (2) biomedical conditions and complications; (3) emotional/behavioral conditions or complications; (4) treatment acceptance/resistance; (5) relapse/continued use potential; and (6) recovery/living environment. More research is needed to determine the validity of these criteria and other patient-setting matching systems (Gastfriend, Lu et al., 2000; McKay, Cacciola et al., 1997).

As a concluding comment, the authors point out that research on treatment settings has focused on the relative *effectiveness* of inpatient and outpatient treatment. Not typically addressed in such studies is the relative ability of different settings to *retain* patients in treatment. The few studies that have examined this issue (Alterman, O'Brien et al., 1994; Bell, Williams et al., 1994; McKay, Alterman et al., 1995; Pettinati, Meyers et al., 1993; Stecher, Andrews et al., 1994) have found that a higher proportion of inpatients complete treatment, although with no difference in outcome when followups were conducted. Whether the enhanced treatment retention afforded by inpatient and residential settings would lead to better outcomes for certain types of patients (for example, those with few social resources) remains to be determined.

A more fundamental issue not addressed in existing studies is the relative *attractiveness* of treatment in each of the two types of settings: that is, their ability to induce potential patients to seek treatment. Patients involved in clinical trials already have opted for treatment. Under normal conditions of treatment delivery, inpatient and residential programs may be more effective than outpatient programs in attracting persons to treatment who are homeless or who lack access to transportation. If inpatient and residential programs are not available, administrators of such facilities may be able to point to "reduced demand" as evidence to support cutbacks in addiction treatment services.

EFFECT OF TREATMENT DURATION AND AMOUNT

This section reviews evidence for the effectiveness of brief interventions, longer versus shorter stays in inpatient and residential treatment, and the effects of participation in outpatient continuing care.

Brief Interventions. Five reviews have reported considerable support for the effectiveness of brief interventions for alcohol use disorders. Babor (1994), Bien and colleagues (1993), and Moyer and colleagues (2002) concluded that brief interventions were more effective than control conditions (typically "treatment as usual") for samples usually recruited in medical settings; in many cases, they were as effective as more intensive interventions for individuals presenting for alcohol treatment. Also, among multiple treatment approaches considered in two reviews by Miller and colleagues (Miller, Brown et al., 1995; Miller, Andrews et al., 1998), brief interventions had the highest score on the authors' effectiveness criterion. Finally, Project MATCH (Project MATCH Research Group, 1997), a large, multisite treatment trial, found that four planned sessions of motivational enhancement treatment were as effective as cognitive-behavioral and Twelve Step Facilitation treatments that were offered in 12 planned sessions.

Several points should be kept in mind when considering this evidence, however. First, Bien and colleagues (1993) reported that the average study effect size favoring brief interventions over a control condition was .38. Moyer and colleagues (2002) calculated average effect sizes for either aggregated drinking-related outcomes or for alcohol consumption at each of four followup intervals. Although all eight effect sizes indicated the superiority of brief interventions over control conditions for predominantly medical patients, seven were .26 or under (the effect size for alcohol consumption at followups of three months or less was .67), and the two effect sizes for followups at more than 12 months were not statistically significant. Thus, effect sizes for treating excessive drinking among patients in medical settings tend to fall between what Cohen (1988) termed a "small" and a "medium" effect and do not appear to endure for more than one year.

Second, Jonson and colleagues (1995) noted that the brief interventions in some of the studies reviewed by Bien, Miller, and Tonigan (1993) were considered to be more extended interventions in other studies. Moyer and colleagues (2002) suggested that, in studies comparing brief interventions versus more extended treatments for alcohol patients, the brief interventions are more intensive/extensive than in studies of brief interventions versus control conditions among medical patients. As an example, Monahan and Finney (1996) calculated that the average patient in the single-session "advice" condition in the well-known study by Edwards and colleagues (1977) actually received more than 30 hours of assessment and treatment during the year in which other participants were receiving extended treatment. However, 30 hours typically would be classified as extended treatment.

Third, Moyer and colleagues (2002) found that in studies of brief interventions versus treatment-as-usual control conditions, brief interventions were more effective only in those studies in which individuals with severe drinking problems had been excluded at the only followup point (>3 to 6 months) at which there was significant heterogeneity in effect across studies.

Fourth, aspects of the reviews by Miller and colleagues (Miller, Brown et al., 1995; Miller, Andrews et al., 1998) seem to favor finding positive effects for brief interventions. Brief interventions found to be superior to treatment-as-usual control conditions received a +2, whereas treatments found to be superior to another treatment approach received only a +1. Because of the typically lower severity of participants, studies of brief interventions in medical settings are more likely to have no-treatment control conditions (see Wilk, Jenson et al., 1997; Swearingen, Moyer et al., in press) than studies of more intensive/extensive treatment modalities. Also, Miller and colleagues (Miller, Brown et al., 1995; Miller, Andrews et al., 1998) classified a brief intervention that was found not significantly inferior to a more extensive intervention as "effective" (it received an effectiveness score of +1), whereas the more extensive comparison intervention received a score of –2. Thus, studies that found no difference in treatment outcome constituted "positive evidence" for the effectiveness of brief interventions. This aspect of Miller's box scoring system combines cost and effectiveness, two dimensions that should be considered separately so that their relationship can be determined from independent data.

Finally, in Project MATCH (Project MATCH Research Group, 1997), patients attended proportionately more of the four planned sessions of motivational enhancement therapy, on average, than they did of the 12 planned sessions of Twelve Step Facilitation and cognitive-behavioral treatment. In addition, all patients received eight hours of assessment prior to treatment and five followup contacts at three-month intervals, all of which may have had a therapeutic effect. Overall, the difference in treatment intensity between the motivational enhancement and the other two conditions was not as large as it first appeared.

Studies of brief interventions most often have been conducted with patients of low to moderate severity in terms of their alcohol use disorders (Babor, 1994). Research is needed to examine the effectiveness of brief interventions among patient populations that vary more substantially in severity. At present, however, patients with low to moderate alcohol severity, positive life contexts, and without severe skills deficits appear to be the best candidates for brief interventions. In this vein, Edwards and colleagues (1977) noted the social stability of the patients in their classic study of brief advice versus treatment and suggested that "patients with a lesser degree of social support might . . . be less able to respond to the advice regimen—extrapolation to a population of homeless men would be risky" (p. 1021).

Even with these *caveats*, the evidence supporting the effectiveness of low-cost brief interventions is impressive. A brief intervention might well be the first option even among alcohol-dependent persons presenting for treatment. Patients who do not respond could be offered more intensive/extensive treatment in a "stepped care" approach (Breslin, Sobell et al., 1998). Miller and Sanchez (1993) offered the acronym "FRAMES" to identify the six "active ingredients" of brief interventions they believe contribute to change in drinking behavior: **F**eedback on personal risk or impairment, emphasis on personal **R**esponsibility for change, clear **A**dvice to change, a **M**enu of alternative change

options, therapeutic **E**mpathy, and enhancement of patients' **S**elf-efficacy or optimism. Bien and colleagues (1993) also note that many brief interventions have included ongoing follow-through contacts with patients. Overall, the FRAMES elements may help patients enhance their motivation to change their drinking behavior, while ongoing contacts may supply the support needed by some individuals to maintain such change.

Length of Stay in Inpatient/Residential Treatment. Miller and Hester (1986) and Mattick and Jarvis (1994) reviewed several randomized trials that compared different lengths of inpatient or residential treatment for alcohol abuse. The studies consistently found no difference in outcome. Several more recent randomized trials also found no or only isolated (that is, only a few outcomes) beneficial effects for longer addiction treatment (Guydish, Werdegard et al., 1998; Guydish, Sorensen et al., 1999; Kamara & Van der Hyde, 1997, 1998a, 1998b; Nemes, Wish et al., 1999; Trent, 1998). In contrast, many naturalistic studies of addiction treatment have found that longer stays in treatment are associated with better outcomes, and even a reduction in premature mortality (Bunn, Booth et al., 1994). For example, longer stays in inpatient care (Peterson, Swindle et al., 1994; Timko, Finney et al., 1995), extended care (Moos, King et al., 1996), community residential care (Moos, Pettit et al., 1995; Rosenheck, Frisman et al., 1995; Simpson, 1981), and therapeutic communities (Condelli & Hubbard, 1994) have been associated with better treatment outcomes and psychosocial functioning, as well as lower readmission rates for subsequent inpatient care.

In addition, Monahan and Finney (1996) found that amount of treatment for alcoholism, indexed by treatment in inpatient, residential, and day-hospital settings, was related to treatment group abstinence rates across 150 treatment groups in 100 studies. On average, patients in the high-intensity treatment groups received 148 hours of treatment, as compared with 14 hours for patients in the low-intensity groups. After patient social stability, program ownership (private for-profit versus other), and several study design features were taken into account, the more intensively treated patients had a 15% better abstinence rate than did the less intensively treated patients.

It may be that beneficial effects of longer stays in inpatient and residential treatment apply only to more impaired patients who have fewer social resources. For example, Welte and colleagues (1981) found no relationship between length of stay (LOS) and outcomes for patients in alcoholism treatment who had more social stability; in contrast, among patients with less social stability, those who had longer stays also had better outcomes (but see Gottheil, McLellan et al., 1992; Messina, Wish et al., 1999).

Outpatient Care Following Inpatient Treatment. Most clinicians recommend additional outpatient treatment to maintain or enhance the therapeutic gains achieved during inpatient, residential, or intensive outpatient (such as day-hospital) treatment. Continuing outpatient treatment attempts to provide the ongoing support needed to continue a course of sobriety or to limit the course of a relapse. Ito and Donovan's (1986) review suggested a correlation between participation in aftercare and positive outcomes for alcohol patients. Hawkins and Catalano (1985) arrived at a similar conclusion with respect to patients with drug problems.

Two randomized controlled studies provide mixed support for continuing care for alcohol patients. O'Farrell and colleagues (1993) reported that continuing behavioral marital therapy and relapse prevention offered over the course of a full year yielded better outcomes than no continuing care. In contrast, no difference in outcome was found by Connors and colleagues (1992), who compared the effects of eight group aftercare sessions or eight telephone calls provided over a shorter (six-month) period with no aftercare.

Taken together, these reviews of treatment intensity, length of stay, and aftercare suggest that an effective strategy may be to provide lower intensity addiction treatment for a longer duration—that is, treatment spread out at a lower rate over a longer period (Moos, Finney et al., 1999; Stout, Rubin et al., 1999). As O'Brien and McLellan (1996) note: "The persistent changes produced by addiction . . . require continued maintenance treatment . . ." (p. 237). They point out that there are many chronic diseases—such as diabetes, hypertension, and asthma—that are "generally accepted as requiring life-long treatment" (p. 237).

The effectiveness of spreading addiction treatment over a longer period of time is suggested by the positive findings for outpatient care following inpatient treatment (Moos, Finney et al., 1999) and for brief interventions that incorporate extended contacts with patients. More extended treatment may improve patient outcomes because it provides patients with ongoing support and the potential to discuss and resolve problems prior to the occurrence of a full-blown relapse. In this vein, brief interventions may be most effective for relatively healthy patients who have intact community support systems. Patients who have severe

alcohol or drug dependence, concomitant psychiatric disorders, and/or deficient social resources appear to be appropriate candidates for longer and more intensive treatment to address their multiple disorders (see Higgins, Budney et al., 1993; Crits-Christoph & Siqueland, 1996).

IMPLICATIONS FOR POLICYMAKERS AND SERVICE PROVIDERS

Past research on addiction treatment settings, amount, and duration, along with reviews of this research, have had a positive effect on health care policy by calling into question the blanket application of expensive forms of treatment. For example, in the early 1980s, insurance coverage for alcoholism treatment often was available only for inpatient care. If a socially stable individual wanted treatment that was covered by his health plan, inpatient treatment was the only option.

At this point, however, the pendulum may have swung too far in the other direction. Insurers and benefit managers have used findings for selected samples to justify denying inpatient and residential treatment to persons who need such treatment. An important agenda over the next decade will be to determine whether certain types of patients derive greater benefit from inpatient and residential treatment or longer-term/more intensive treatment.

With respect to treatment setting, the authors believe that the best approach today is the one recommended in previous reviews: (1) provide outpatient treatment for those individuals who have sufficient social resources and no serious medical or psychiatric impairment; (2) use less costly intensive outpatient treatment for patients who have failed with brief interventions or for whom a more intensive intervention seems warranted, but who do not need the structured environment of a residential setting; (3) retain residential options for those with few social resources and/or a living environment that is a serious impediment to recovery; and (4) reserve inpatient treatment options for individuals with serious medical and psychiatric conditions.

With respect to treatment duration and amount, existing research indicates that uncomplicated patients should be provided less intensive treatment, while patients with more complex disorders should receive more intensive treatment. For many patients, outpatient treatment (in some cases, following an initial episode of residential care) should be provided over an extended period.

Overall, it should be borne in mind that, although they are very important from a cost perspective, the setting in which addiction treatment takes place and, to a lesser extent, the duration and amount of treatment given, are distal variables in determining patients' posttreatment functioning. Other treatment variables, such as the treatment modality employed (Finney & Monahan, 1996; Miller, Brown et al., 1995; Miller, Andrews et al., 1998), the combination of treatment services offered (McLellan, Arndt et al., 1993; McLellan, Grissom et al., 1993), and the characteristics of the therapist (Hser, 1995; Najavits & Weiss, 1994; Najavits, Crits-Christoph et al., 2000), have a more direct effect on posttreatment functioning.

REFERENCES

Alterman AI, O'Brien CP, McLellan AT et al. (1994). Effectiveness and costs of inpatient versus day hospital cocaine rehabilitation. *Journal of Nervous and Mental Disease* 182:157-163.

Anglin MD & Hser Y-I (1990). Treatment of drug abuse. In M Tonry & JQ Wilson (eds.) *Drugs and Crime (Vol. 13)*. Chicago, IL: University of Chicago Press.

Annis HM (1986). Is inpatient rehabilitation cost effective? Con position. *Advances in Alcohol and Substance Abuse* 5:175-190.

Babor TF (1994). Avoiding the horrid and beastly sin of drunkenness: Does dissuasion make a difference? *Journal of Consulting and Clinical Psychology* 62:1127-1140.

Bell DC, Williams ML, Nelson R et al. (1994). An experimental test of retention in residential and outpatient programs. *American Journal of Drug and Alcohol Abuse* 20:331-340.

Bien TH, Miller WR & Tonigan JS (1993). Brief interventions for alcohol problems: A review. *Addiction* 88:315-336.

Breslin F, Sobell MB, Sobell LC et al. (1998). Problem drinkers: Evaluation of stepped-care approach. *Journal of Substance Abuse* 10:217-232.

Budde D, Rounsaville F & Bryant K (1992). Inpatient and outpatient cocaine abusers: Clinical comparisons at intake and one-year follow-up. *Journal of Substance Abuse Treatment* 9:337-343.

Bunn JY, Booth BM, Loveland-Cook CA et al. (1994). The relationship between mortality and intensity of inpatient alcoholism treatment. *American Journal of Public Health* 84: 211-214.

Chapman PLH & Huygens I (1988). An evaluation of three treatment programmes for alcoholism: An experimental study with 6- and 18-month follow-ups. *British Journal of Addiction* 83:67-81.

Cohen J (1988). *Statistical Power Analysis for the Behavioral Sciences (2nd Ed.)*. Hillsdale, NJ: Lawrence Erlbaum.

Condelli WS & Hubbard RL (1994). Relationship between time spent in treatment and client outcomes from therapeutic communities. *Journal of Substance Abuse Treatment* 11:25-33.

Connors GJ, Tarbox AR & Faillace LA (1992). Achieving and maintaining gains among problem drinkers: Process and outcome results. *Behavior Therapy* 23:449-474.

Cooper H & Hedges LV, eds. (1994). *The Handbook of Research Synthesis*. New York, NY: Russell Sage Foundation.

Crits-Christoph P & Siqueland L (1996). Psychosocial treatment for drug abuse: Selected review and recommendations for national health care. *Archives of General Psychiatry* 53:749-756.

Edwards G, Orford J, Egert S et al. (1977). Alcoholism: A controlled trial of "treatment" and "advice." *Journal of Studies on Alcohol* 38:1004-1031.

Finney JW, Hahn AC & Moos RH (1996). The effectiveness of inpatient and outpatient treatment for alcohol abuse: The need to focus on mediators and moderators of setting effects. *Addiction* 91:1773-1796.

Finney JW & Monahan SC (1996). The cost effectiveness of treatment for alcoholism: A second approximation. *Journal of Studies on Alcohol* 57:229-243.

Finney JW & Moos RH (1996). Effectiveness of inpatient and outpatient treatment for alcohol abuse: Effect sizes, research design issues, and explanatory mechanisms (Response to Commentaries). *Addiction* 91:1813-1820.

Finney JW & Moos RH (1998). Psychosocial treatment for alcohol use disorders. In PE Nathan & JM Gorman (eds.) *Treatments That Work*. New York, NY: Oxford University Press, 156-166.

Gastfriend DR, Lu S-H & Sharon E (2000). Placement matching: Challenges and technical progress. *Substance Use & Misuse* 35: 2191-2213.

Gottheil E, McLellan AT & Druley KA (1992). Length of stay, patient severity and treatment outcome: Sample data from the field of alcoholism. *Journal of Studies on Alcoholism* 53:69-75.

Guydish J, Sorensen JL, Chan M et al. (1999). A randomized trial comparing day and residential drug abuse treatment: 18-month outcomes. *Journal of Consulting and Clinical Psychology* 67:428-434.

Guydish J, Werdegard D, Sorensen JL et al. (1998). Drug abuse day treatment: A randomized clinical trial comparing day and residential treatment programs. *Journal of Consulting and Clinical Psychology* 66:280-289.

Hawkins JD & Catalano RF (1985). Aftercare in drug abuse treatment. *International Journal of the Addictions* 20:917-945.

Higgins ST, Budney AJ, Bickel WK et al. (1993). Achieving cocaine abstinence with a behavioral approach. *American Journal of Psychiatry* 150:763-769.

Hser Y-I (1995). Drug treatment counselor practices and effectiveness. *Evaluation Review* 19:389-408.

Ito J & Donovan DM (1986). Aftercare in alcoholism treatment: A review. In WR Miller & N Heather (eds.) *Treating Addictive Behaviors: Processes of Change*. New York, NY: Plenum, 435-452.

Jonson H, Hermansson U, Ronnberg S et al. (1995). Comments on brief intervention of alcohol problems: A review of a review. *Addiction* 90:1118-1120.

Kamara SG & Van der Hyde VA (1997). Outcomes of regular vs. extended alcohol/drug outpatient treatment. I. Relapse, aftercare, and treatment re-entry. *Medicine and Law* 16: 607-620.

Kamara SG & Van der Hyde VA (1998a). Employment outcomes of regular versus extended outpatient alcohol and drug treatment. *Medicine and Law* 17:625-632.

Kamara SG & Van der Hyde VA (1998b). Outcomes of regular versus extended outpatient alcohol/drug treatment. Part II. Medical, psychiatric, legal and social problems. *Medicine and Law* 17:131-142.

Kissin B, Platz A & Su WH (1970). Social and psychological factors in the treatment of chronic alcoholism. *Journal of Psychiatric Research* 8:13-27.

Mattick RP & Jarvis T (1994). In-patient setting and long duration for the treatment of alcohol dependence? Out-patient care is as good. *Drug and Alcohol Review* 13:127-135.

McKay JR, Alterman AI, McLellan AT et al. (1995). The effect of random versus nonrandom assignment in a comparison of inpatient and day hospital rehabilitation for male alcoholics. *Journal of Consulting and Clinical Psychology* 63:70-78.

McKay JR, Cacciola JS, McLellan AT et al. (1997). An initial evaluation of the psychosocial dimensions of the American Society of Addiction Medicine criteria for inpatient versus intensive outpatient substance abuse rehabilitation. *Journal of Studies on Alcohol* 58:239-252.

McLachlan JFC & Stein RL (1982). Evaluation of a day clinic for alcoholics. *Journal of Studies on Alcohol* 43:261-272.

McLellan AT, Arndt IO, Metzger DS et al. (1993). The effects of psychosocial services in substance abuse treatment. *Journal of the American Medical Association* 269:1953-1959.

McLellan AT, Grissom GR, Brill P et al. (1993). Private substance abuse treatments: Are some programs more effective than others? *Journal of Substance Abuse Treatment* 10:243-254.

McLellan AT, Luborsky L, Woody GE et al. (1983). Predicting response to alcohol and drug abuse treatments: Role of psychiatric severity. *Archives of General Psychiatry* 40:620-625.

Mee-Lee D, Shulman G, Fishman M et al. (2001). *Patient Placement Criteria for the Treatment of Substance-Related Disorders, Second Edition-Revised (ASAM PPC-2R).* Chevy Chase, MD: American Society of Addiction Medicine.

Messina NP, Wish ED & Nemes S (1999). Therapeutic community treatment for substance abusers with antisocial personality disorder. *Journal of Substance Abuse Treatment* 17:121-128.

Miller WR, Andrews NR, Wilbourne P et al. (1998). A wealth of alternatives: Effective treatments for alcohol problems. In WR Miller & N Heather (eds.) *Treating Addictive Behaviors (2nd Ed.).* New York, NY: Plenum Press, 203-216.

Miller WR, Brown JM, Simpson TL et al. (1995). What works? A methodological analysis of the alcohol treatment outcome literature. In RK Hester & WR Miller (eds.) *Handbook of Alcoholism Treatment Approaches: Effective Alternatives.* Boston, MA: Allyn and Bacon, 12-44.

Miller MR & Hester RK (1986). Inpatient alcoholism treatment: Who benefits? *American Psychologist* 41:794-805.

Miller WR & Sanchez VC (1993). Motivating young adults for treatment and lifestyle change. In G Howard (ed.) *Issues in Alcohol Use and Misuse by Young Adults.* Notre Dame, IN: University of Notre Dame Press.

Monahan SC & Finney JW (1996). Explaining abstinence rates following treatment for alcohol abuse: A quantitative synthesis of patient, research design, and treatment effects. *Addiction* 91:787-805.

Moos RH & Finney JW (1996a). Inpatient and outpatient treatment for substance abuse: Implications for VA services. *VA Health Services Research & Development Forum* June:4-5.

Moos RH & Finney JW (1996b). *Inpatient and Outpatient Treatment for Substance Abuse: Current Findings and Implications for VA Services.* Palo Alto, CA: Department of Veterans Affairs Health Care System, Psychiatry Services and Center for Health Care Evaluation: HSR&D Field Program.

Moos RH, Finney JW, Ouimette PC et al. (1999). A comparative evaluation of substance abuse treatment: I. Treatment orientation, amount of care, and 1-year outcomes. *Alcoholism: Clinical & Experimental Research* 23:529-536.

Moos RH, King M & Patterson M (1996). Outcomes of residential treatment of substance abuse in hospital- versus community-based programs. *Psychiatric Services* 47:68-74.

Moos RH, Pettit E & Gruber V (1995). Longer episodes of community residential care reduce substance abuse patients' readmission rates. *Journal of Studies on Alcohol* 56:433-443.

Moyer A, Finney JW, Swearingen CE et al. (2001). Brief interventions for alcohol problems: A meta-analytic review of controlled investigations in treatment-seeking and non-treatment-seeking populations. *Addiction* 97:279-292.

Najavits LM, Crits-Christoph P & Dierberger A (2000). Clinicians' impact on the quality of substance use disorder treatment. *Substance Use & Misuse* 35:2161-2190.

Najavits LM & Weiss RD (1994). Variation in therapist effectiveness in the treatment of patients with substance use disorders: An empirical review. *Addiction* 89:679-688.

Nemes S, Wish E & Messina N (1999). Comparing the impact of standard and abbreviated treatment in a therapeutic community: Findings from the District of Columbia Treatment Initiative Experiment. *Journal of Substance Abuse Treatment* 17:339-347.

O'Brien CP & McLellan AT (1996). Myths about the treatment of addiction. *Lancet* 347:237-240.

O'Farrell TJ, Choquette KA, Cutter HSG et al. (1993). Behavioral Marital Therapy with and without additional couples relapse prevention sessions for alcoholics and their wives. *Journal of Studies on Alcohol* 54:652-666.

Peterson K, Swindle R, Phibbs C et al. (1994). Determinants of readmission following inpatient substance abuse treatment: A national study of VA programs. *Medical Care* 32: 535-550.

Pettinati HM, Meyers K, Jensen JM et al. (1993). Inpatient vs outpatient treatment for substance abuse revisited. *Psychiatric Quarterly* 64:173-182.

Pittman DJ & Tate RL (1972). A comparison of two treatment programs for alcoholics. *Journal of Social Psychiatry* 18:183-193.

Project MATCH Research Group (1997). Matching alcoholism treatment to client heterogeneity: Project MATCH posttreatment drinking outcomes. *Journal of Studies on Alcohol* 58:7-29.

Ritson B (1968). The prognosis of alcohol addicts treated by a specialised unit. *British Journal of Psychiatry* 114:1019-1029.

Rosenheck R, Frisman L & Gallup P (1995). Effectiveness and cost of specific treatment elements in a program for homeless mentally ill veterans. *Psychiatric Services* 46:1131-1139.

Rychtarik RG, Connors GJ, Wirtz PW et al. (2000). Treatment settings for persons with alcoholism: Evidence for matching clients to inpatient versus outpatient care. *Journal of Consulting and Clinical Psychology* 68:277-289.

Saxe L, Dougherty D, Esty K et al. (1983). *The Effectiveness and Costs of Alcoholism Treatment (Health Technology Case Study 22).* Washington, DC: Office of Technology Assessment.

Simpson DD (1981). Treatment for drug abuse: Follow-up outcomes and length of time spent. *Archives of General Psychiatry* 38:875-880.

Stecher BM, Andrews CA, McDonald L et al. (1994). Implementation of residential and nonresidential treatment for the dually diagnosed homeless. *Evaluation Review* 18:689-717.

Stout RL, Rubin A, Zwick W et al. (1999). Optimizing the cost-effectiveness of alcohol treatment: A rationale for extended case monitoring. *Addictive Behaviors* 24:17-35.

Swearingen CE, Moyer A & Finney JW (in press). Alcoholism treatment outcome studies, 1970-1998: An expanded look at the nature of the research. *Addictive Behaviors.*

Timko C, Finney JW & Moos RH (1995). Short-term treatment careers and outcomes of previously untreated alcoholics. *Journal of Substance Abuse* 7:43-59.

Trent LK (1998). Evaluation of a four- versus six-week length of stay in the Navy's alcohol treatment program. *Journal of Studies on Alcohol* 59:270-279.

Walsh DC, Hingson RW, Merrigan DM et al. (1991). A randomized trial of treatment options for alcohol-abusing workers. *New England Journal of Medicine* 325(11):775-782.

Welte J, Hynes G, Sokolow L et al. (1981). Effect of length of stay in inpatient alcoholism treatment on outcome. *Journal of Studies on Alcohol* 42:483-491.

Wilk AI, Jenson NM & Havighurst TC (1997). Meta-analysis of randomized control trials addressing brief interventions in heavy alcohol drinkers. *Journal of General Internal Medicine* 12:274-283.

| Chapter 5 | # The ASAM Placement Criteria and Matching Patients to Treatment |

David Mee-Lee, M.D.
Gerald D. Shulman, M.A., M.A.C., FACATA

When considering treatment matching, treatment planning, and the use of patient placement criteria, certain distinctions and definitions must be clarified, particularly the distinction between "placement matching" and "modality matching." In placement matching, a patient is referred to a particular setting, such as intensive outpatient or residential care, while modality matching attempts to match a patient's needs to a specific treatment approach (such as motivational enhancement therapy), regardless of setting. When placement matching is disconnected from modality matching, treatment is likely to be less effective because it fails to respond to the individual needs of the patient. (Gastfriend, Lu et al., 2000).

Good treatment planning thus combines modality matching (for all pertinent problems and priorities identified in the assessment) with placement matching (which identifies the least intensive level of care that can safely and effectively provide the resources that will meet the patient's needs (Mee-Lee, 1998).

SELECTING AN APPROPRIATE TREATMENT
Evolving Approaches to Treatment Matching. The process of matching patients to treatment services has evolved through at least four approaches, each with a fundamentally different philosophy (Mee-Lee, 2001).

Complications-driven treatment gives only cursory attention to the diagnosis of substance use disorder. In this approach, rather than actively treating the primary alcohol or other drug disorder that is causing the patient's symptoms, only the secondary complications or sequelae are addressed. The gastritis or bleeding esophageal varices are controlled, the depression is medicated, fractures are splinted or pinned, but care for the addictive disorder is superficial or non-existent.

In contrast, *diagnosis, program-driven treatment* recognizes the primacy of the substance use disorder, but the diagnosis alone drives the treatment plan, rather than the specific assessed needs of the patient. Patients are assigned to fixed lengths of stay in programs with static approaches, often in response to available funding or benefit structures.

Individualized, assessment-driven treatment emphasizes multidimensional assessment. Problems are identified and prioritized in the context of the patient's severity of illness and level of function. Treatment services are matched to the patient's needs over a continuum of care (Shulman, 1994). Ongoing assessment of progress and treatment

FIGURE 1. A Model of Individualized, Assessment-Driven Treatment

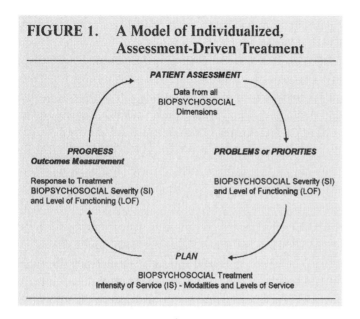

PATIENT ASSESSMENT
Data from all
BIOPSYCHOSOCIAL
Dimensions

PROGRESS
Outcomes Measurement

Response to Treatment
BIOPSYCHOSOCIAL Severity (SI)
and Level of Functioning (LOF)

PROBLEMS or PRIORITIES

BIOPSYCHOSOCIAL Severity (SI)
and Level of Functioning (LOF)

PLAN
BIOPSYCHOSOCIAL Treatment
Intensity of Service (IS) - Modalities and Levels of Service

response influences future treatment recommendations. This continuous quality improvement cycle—assessment, treatment matching, level of care placement, and progress evaluation through assessment (see Figure 1)—represents an approach to care that much of the addiction treatment field still struggles to implement (Mee-Lee, 1998).

In *outcomes-driven treatment*, which is the newest approach, the promise of matching patients to treatment has yet to be fully realized. For all the current rhetoric about outcomes, performance measures, accountability, and evidence-based treatment, this approach to addiction treatment is only just beginning to be articulated and actualized.

Uses of Placement Criteria. Placement criteria are irrelevant to the first two approaches to patient placement (complications-driven and program-driven treatment). In the latter two approaches (assessment-driven treatment and outcomes-driven treatment), however, placement criteria play an integral role by providing a structure for assessment that focuses on the patient's assessed needs. Criteria also provide a nomenclature to describe an expanded set of treatment options and guidelines to promote the use of a broader continuum of services. Overall, the placement criteria are intended to enhance the efficient use of limited resources, increase patient retention in treatment, prevent dropout and relapse, and thus improve patient outcomes.

The Concept of "Unbundling." At present, most addiction treatment services are "bundled," meaning that a

number of different services are packaged together and paid for as a unit. Similarly, the first edition of the ASAM criteria "bundled" clinical services with environmental supports in fixed levels of care. Today, however, there is increasing recognition that clinical services can be and often are provided separately from environmental supports. Indeed, many managed care companies and public treatment systems are suggesting that treatment modality and intensity be "unbundled" from the treatment setting.

Unbundling is a practice that allows any type of clinical service (such as psychiatric consultation) to be delivered in any setting (such as a therapeutic community). With unbundling, the type and intensity of treatment are based on the patient's needs and not on limitations imposed by the treatment setting. The unbundling concept thus is designed to maximize individualized care and to encourage the delivery of necessary treatment in any clinically feasible setting.

A transition to unbundled treatment would require a paradigm shift in state program licensure and reimbursement. In terms of treatment, there would no longer be "programs" but rather a constellation of services to meet the needs of each patient. The systems currently in use for billing, reimbursement, and funding would not support unbundled treatment. All of these obstacles are reasons for delaying an abrupt change to the new paradigm, but the ASAM criteria encourage exploration of unbundling by suggesting ways to match risk and severity of needs with specific services and intensity of treatment.

UNDERSTANDING THE ASAM PATIENT PLACEMENT CRITERIA

Four features characterize the ASAM Patient Placement Criteria: (1) individualized treatment planning, (2) ready access to services, (3) attention to multiple treatment needs, and (4) ongoing reassessment and modification of the plan.

Functionally, the criteria are used to match treatment settings, interventions, and services to each individual's particular problems and (often-changing) treatment needs. The ASAM criteria advocate for individualized, assessment-driven treatment and the flexible use of services across a broad continuum of care.

The criteria also advocate for a system in which treatment is readily available, because patients are lost when the treatment they need is not immediately available and readily accessible. By expanding the criteria to incorporate outpatient care, especially for those in early stages of readiness to change, the ASAM criteria have helped to reduce waiting

FIGURE 2.   A Decision Tree to Match Assessment with Treatment Planning and Placement

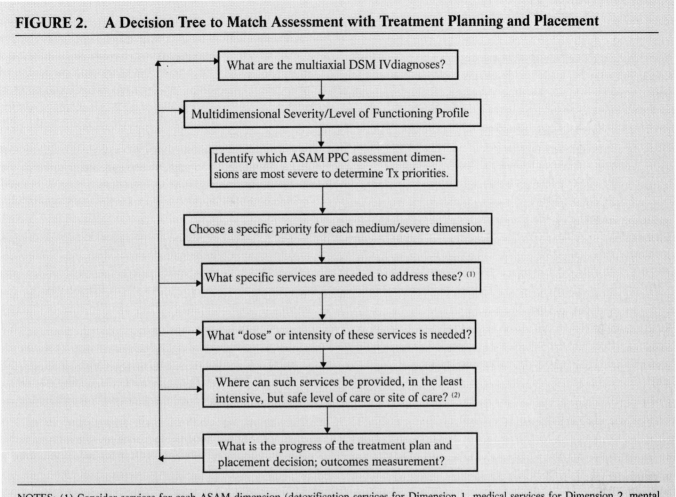

NOTES: (1) Consider services for each ASAM dimension (detoxification services for Dimension 1, medical services for Dimension 2, mental health services for Dimension 3, motivational interviewing/counseling/intervention for Dimension 4). (2) If medically managed treatment is necessary, a Level IV setting is used. If medically monitored treatment is appropriate, a Level III setting, "23-hour bed" or hospital-based partial hospitalization program may be appropriate.

lists for residential treatment and thus have improved access to care.

The criteria are based on a philosophy that effective treatment attends to multiple needs of each individual, not just his or her alcohol or drug use. To be effective, treatment must address any associated medical, psychological, social, vocational, and legal problems. Through its six assessment dimensions, the ASAM criteria underscore the importance of multidimensional assessment and treatment (Figure 2).

Objectivity. The criteria are as objective, measurable, and quantifiable as possible. Certain aspects of the criteria require subjective interpretation. In this regard, the assessment and treatment of substance-related disorders are no different from biomedical or psychiatric conditions in which diagnosis or assessment and treatment are a mix of objectively measured criteria and experientially based professional judgments.

Principles Guiding the Criteria. Several important principles have guided development of the ASAM criteria.

Goals of Treatment: The goals of intervention and treatment (including safe and comfortable detoxification, motivational enhancement to accept the need for recovery, the attainment of skills to maintain abstinence, and the like) determine the methods, intensity, frequency, and types of services provided. The health care professional's decision to prescribe a type of service, and subsequent discharge of a patient from a level of care, are based on how that treatment and its duration will influence the resolution of the dysfunction and positively alter the prognosis for the patient's long-term outcome.

Thus, in addiction treatment, the treatment may extend beyond simple resolution of observable biomedical distress to the achievement of overall healthier functioning. The patient demonstrates a response to treatment through new insights, attitudes, and behaviors. Addiction treatment programs have as their goal not simply stabilizing the patient's condition but altering the course of the patient's disease.

Individualized Treatment Plan: Treatment should be tailored to the needs of the individual and guided by an individualized treatment plan that is developed in consultation with the patient. Such a plan should be based on a comprehensive biopsychosocial assessment of the patient and, when possible, a comprehensive evaluation of the family as well.

The plan should list problems (such as obstacles to recovery, knowledge or skill deficits, dysfunction, or loss), strengths (such as readiness to change, a positive social support system, and a strong connection to a source of spiritual support) and priorities (such as obstacles to treatment and risks, identified within the list of problems and arranged according to severity), goals (a statement to guide realistic, achievable, short-term resolution or reduction of the problems), methods or strategies (the treatment services to be provided, the site of those services, the staff responsible for delivering treatment), and a timetable for follow-through with the treatment plan that promotes accountability.

The plan should be written to facilitate measurement of progress. As with other disease processes, length of service should be linked directly to the patient's response to treatment (for example, attainment of the treatment goals and degree of resolution of the identified clinical problems).

Choice of Treatment Levels: Referral to a specific level of care must be based on a careful assessment of the patient. The goal that underlies the criteria is the placement of the patient in the most appropriate level of care. For both clinical and financial reasons, the preferred level of care is the least intensive level that meets treatment objectives, while providing safety and security for the patient. Moreover, while the levels of care are presented as discrete levels, in reality they represent benchmarks or points along a continuum of treatment services that could be used in a variety of ways, depending on a patient's needs and response. A patient could begin at a more intensive level and move to a more or less intensive level of care, depending on his or her individual needs.

Continuum of Care: In order to provide the most clinically appropriate and cost-effective treatment system, a continuum of care must be available. Such a continuum may be offered by a single provider or multiple providers. For the continuum to work most effectively, it is best distinguished by three characteristics: (1) seamless transfer between levels of care, (2) philosophical congruence among the various providers of care, and (3) timely arrival of the patient's clinical record at the next provider. It is most helpful if providers envision admitting the patient into the continuum *through* their program rather than admitting the patient *to* their program.

Many providers of treatment services offer only one of the many levels of care described. In such situations, movement between levels might mean referring the patient out of the provider's own network of care. While lack of reimbursement for some levels of care, or lack of availability of other levels of care may render this impossible at present, the goal of these criteria is to stimulate the development of efficient and effective services that can be made available to all patients.

Progress Through the Levels of Care: As a patient moves through treatment in any level of care, his or her progress in all six dimensions should be continually assessed. Such multidimensional assessment ensures comprehensive treatment. In the process of patient assessment, certain problems and priorities are identified as justifying admission to a particular level of care. The resolution of those problems and priorities determines when a patient can be treated at a different level of care or discharged from treatment. The appearance of new problems may require services that can be effectively provided at the same level of care, or that require a more or less intensive level of care.

Each time the patient's response to treatment is assessed, new priorities for recovery are identified. The intensity of the strategies incorporated in the treatment plan helps to determine the most efficient and effective level of care that can safely provide the care articulated in the individualized

---

treatment plan. Patients may, however, worsen or fail to improve in a given level of care or with a given type of program. When this happens, changes in the level of care or program should be based on a reassessment of the treatment plan, with modifications to achieve a better therapeutic response.

Length of Stay: The length of stay or service is determined by the patient's progress toward achieving his or her treatment plan goals and objectives. Fixed length of stay or program-driven treatment is not individualized and does not respond to the particular problems of a given patient. While fixed length of stay programs are more convenient and predictable for the provider, they may be less effective for individuals.

Clinical Versus Reimbursement Considerations: The ASAM criteria describe a wide range of levels and types of care. Not all of these services are available in all locations, nor are they covered by all payers. Clinicians who make placement decisions are expected to supplement the criteria with their own clinical judgment, their knowledge of the patient, and their knowledge of the available resources. The ASAM criteria are not intended as a reimbursement guideline, but rather as a clinical guideline for making the most appropriate placement recommendation for an individual patient with a specific set of symptoms and behaviors. If the criteria only covered the levels of care commonly reimbursable by private insurance carriers, they would not address many of the resources of the public sector and, thus, would tacitly endorse limitations on a complete continuum of care.

Treatment Failure: Two incorrect assumptions are associated with the concept of "treatment failure." The first is that the disorder is acute rather than chronic, so that the only criterion for success is total and complete amelioration of the problem. Such expectations are recognized as inappropriate in the treatment of other chronic disorders, such as diabetes or hypertension. No one expects that simply because a patient has been treated on one occasion for his or her hypertension, there will never be another episode. The same recognition of chronicity should be applied to the treatment of addictive disorders, for which appropriate criteria would involve reductions in the intensity or severity of symptoms, the duration of symptoms, and the frequency of symptoms.

The second assumption is that responsibility for treatment "failure" always rests with the patient (as in, "The patient was not ready"). However, poor treatment outcomes also may be related to a provider's failure to provide services tailored to the patient's needs.

Finally, there is a concern that some benefit managers require that a patient "fail" at one level of care as a prerequisite for approving admission to a more intensive level of care (for example, "failure" in outpatient treatment as a prerequisite for admission to inpatient treatment). In fact, such a requirement is no more rational than treating every patient in an inpatient program or using a fixed length of stay for all. Such a strategy potentially puts the patient at risk because it delays care at a more appropriate level of treatment, and potentially increases health care costs if restricting the appropriate level of treatment allows the addictive disorder to progress.

The ASAM Criteria and State Licensure or Certification. The ASAM criteria contain descriptions of treatment programs at each level of care, including the setting, staffing, support systems, therapies, assessments, documentation, and treatment plan reviews typically found at that level. This information should be useful to providers who are preparing to serve a particular group of patients, as well as to clinicians who are making placement decisions. Nevertheless, the descriptions are not requirements and are not intended to replace or supersede the relevant statutes, licensure, or certification requirements of any state.

ASSESSMENT DIMENSIONS
The ASAM criteria identify the following problem areas (dimensions) as the most important in formulating an individualized treatment plan and in making subsequent patient placement decisions. (Note that the information given here is for the adult criteria only. A detailed discussion of the adolescent criteria is found in Section 13 of this text.)

Dimension 1: Acute Intoxication and/or Withdrawal Potential. What risk is associated with the patient's current level of acute intoxication? Is there significant risk of severe withdrawal symptoms or seizures, based on the patient's previous withdrawal history, amount, frequency, and recency of discontinuation or significant reduction of alcohol or other drug use? Are there current signs of withdrawal? Does the patient have supports to assist in ambulatory detoxification, if medically safe? Has the patient been using multiple substances in the same drug class? Is there a withdrawal scale score available?

In the adult ASAM Placement Criteria, detoxification services can be provided at any of five levels of care. Specific criteria, organized by drug class (alcohol, sedative-hypnotics, opioids, and the like) guide the decision as to which detoxification level is safe and efficient for a patient in withdrawal.

Dimension 2: Biomedical Conditions and Complications. Are there current physical illnesses, other than withdrawal, that need to be addressed because they are exacerbated by withdrawal, create risk, or may complicate treatment? Are there chronic conditions that affect treatment? Is there need for medical services that might interfere with treatment?

Dimension 3: Emotional, Behavioral, or Cognitive Conditions and Complications (diagnosable mental disorders or mental health problems that do not present sufficient signs and symptoms to reach the diagnostic threshold). Are there current psychiatric illnesses or psychological, behavioral, emotional, or cognitive problems that need to be addressed because they create or complicate treatment? Are there chronic conditions that affect treatment? Do any emotional, behavioral, or cognitive problems appear to be an expected part of the addictive disorder, or do they appear to be autonomous? Even if connected to the addiction, are they severe enough to warrant specific mental health treatment? Is the patient suicidal, and if so, what is the lethality? Is the patient able to manage the activities of daily living? Can he or she cope with any emotional, behavioral, or cognitive problems? If the patient has been prescribed psychotropic medications, is he or she compliant?

Dimension 4: Readiness to Change. Is the patient actively resisting treatment? Does the patient feel coerced into treatment? How ready is the patient to change? If he or she is willing to accept treatment, how strongly does the patient disagree with others' perception that she or he has an addictive or mental disorder? Does the patient appear to be compliant only to avoid a negative consequence, or does he or she appear to be internally distressed in a self-motivated way about his or her alcohol or other drug use or mental health problem? At what point is the patient in the stages of change? Is leverage for change available?

Dimension 5: Relapse, Continued Use, or Continued Problem Potential. Is the patient in immediate danger of continued severe mental health distress and/or alcohol or drug use? Does the patient have any recognition or understanding of, or skills in, coping with his or her addictive or mental disorder in order to prevent relapse, continued use, or continued problems such as suicidal behavior? How severe are the problems and further distress that may continue or reappear if the patient is not successfully engaged in treat-

ment at this time? How aware is the patient of relapse triggers, ways to cope with cravings to use, and skills to control impulses to use or impulses to harm self or others? What is the patient's ability to remain abstinent or psychiatrically stable, based on history? What is the patient's current level of craving and how successfully can he or she resist using? If on psychotropic medications, is the patient compliant? If the patient has another chronic disorder (such as diabetes), what is the history of compliance with treatment for that disorder?

Dimension 6: Recovery Environment. Do any family members, significant others, living situations, or school or work situations pose a threat to the patient's safety or engagement in treatment? Does the patient have supportive friendships, financial resources, or educational or vocational resources that can increase the likelihood of successful treatment? Are there legal, vocational, or social service agency or criminal justice mandates that may enhance the patient's motivation for engagement in treatment? Are there transportation, child care, housing, or employment issues that need to be clarified and addressed?

The prognosis for resolution of problems in the various dimensions depends on the clinician's knowledge of problem severity and the level of difficulty in resolving these problems. This knowledge then forms the basis for the clinician and patient participating together in establishing a mutually agreeable treatment plan. The goals for each problem may need to be reviewed from the standpoint of resolution of the acute crisis and/or alteration of the course of the chronic illness.

Interactions Across Dimensions in Assessing for Level of Care. The ASAM criteria function best when individuals are assessed in each dimension independently and also in terms of the interaction across dimensions. For example, when assessing an individual for severity, a history of moderate or severe withdrawal *without* any current intoxication or withdrawal, or current intoxication without a history of significant withdrawal problems should generate a lesser level of concern than a combination of a history of moderate or severe withdrawal *with* current symptoms of intoxication or withdrawal.

In reality, there is considerable interaction across dimensions. For example, significant problems with readiness to change (Dimension 4), coupled with a poor recovery environment (Dimension 6) or moderate problems with relapse or continued use (Dimension 5), may increase the risk of relapse. Another commonly seen combination involves problems in Dimension 2 (such as chronic pain that distracts the patient from the recovery process) coupled with problems in Dimensions 4, 5, or 6.

The converse also is true. For example, problems with relapse potential (Dimension 5) may be offset by a high degree of readiness to change (Dimension 4) or a very supportive recovery environment (Dimension 6). The interaction of these factors may result in a lower level of severity than is seen in any dimension alone.

The lesson here is that assessments are most accurate when they take into account all of the factors (dimensions) that affect each individual's receptivity and ability to engage in treatment at a particular point in time.

Continued Service and Discharge Criteria. In a departure from earlier editions, the current edition of the criteria (*ASAM Patient Placement Criteria for the Treatment of Substance-Related Disorders, Second Edition-Revised [ASAM PPC-2R]*; Mee-Lee, Shulman et al., 2001) contains only admission criteria, leaving the decisions about continued service, transfer, or discharge to general guidelines and the judgment of the treatment professional. This change was made in recognition of the fact that, in the process of patient assessment, certain problems and priorities are identified as justifying admission to a particular level of care. It is the resolution of those problems and priorities that determines when a patient can be treated at a different level of care or discharged. The appearance of new problems may require services that can be provided effectively at the same level of care, or transfer of the patient to a more or less intensive level of care.

The assessment process for continued service or discharge/transfer is the same as for admission, with the reassessment of multidimensional severity determining the treatment priorities, intensity of needed services, and the decision about ongoing level of care. Decisions concerning continued service, transfer, or discharge involve review of the treatment plan and assessment of the patient's progress. That is, they involve the same type of multidimensional assessment process that led to admission to the current level of care.

LEVELS OF CARE

The ASAM criteria conceptualize treatment as a continuum marked by five basic levels of care, which are numbered in Roman numerals from Levels 0.5 through Level IV. Thus, the ASAM criteria provide the addiction field with a nomenclature for describing the continuum of addiction services, as follows:

Level 0.5:   Early Intervention
Level I: Outpatient Services
Level II: Intensive Outpatient/Partial Hospitalization Services
Level III: Residential/Inpatient Services
Level IV: Medically Managed Intensive Inpatient Services

Within each level, a decimal number (ranging from **.1 to .9**) expresses gradations of intensity within the existing levels of care. This structure allows improved precision of description and better "inter-rater" reliability by focusing on five broad levels of care. Thus the ASAM criteria describe gradations within each level of care. For example, a **II.1** level of care provides a benchmark for intensity at the minimum description of Level II care (also see the Rapid Reference section of this text for a summary crosswalk of the levels of care).

Level 0.5: Early Intervention. Professional services for early intervention constitute a service for specific individuals who, for a known reason, are at risk of developing substance-related problems or for those for whom there is not yet sufficient information to document a substance use disorder.

Level I: Outpatient Treatment. Level I encompasses organized, non-residential services, which may be delivered in a wide variety of settings. Addiction or mental health treatment personnel provide professionally directed evaluation, treatment, and recovery service. Such services are provided in regularly scheduled sessions and follow a defined set of policies and procedures or medical protocols.

Level I outpatient services are designed to treat the individual's level of clinical severity and to help the individual achieve permanent changes in his or her alcohol- and drug-using behavior and mental functioning. To accomplish this, services must address major lifestyle, attitudinal, and behavioral issues that have the potential to undermine the goals of treatment or inhibit the individual's ability to cope with major life tasks without the non-medical use of alcohol or other drugs.

In the current edition (*ASAM PPC-2R*), Level I has been expanded to promote greater access to care for dual diagnosis patients, unmotivated patients who are mandated into treatment, and others who previously only had access to care if they agreed to intensive periods of primary treatment. The expansion reflects recent knowledge of and experience with cognitive behavioral therapies such as motivational interviewing, motivational enhancement, solution-focused therapy, and stages of change work, all of which may be appropriate for patients who previously would have been turned away as not ready for treatment, or in denial and thus in need of coerced intensive treatment. The expansion thus can enhance access to care and facilitate earlier engagement of patients in treatment, thereby allowing better utilization of resources and improving the effectiveness of recovery efforts.

Level II: Intensive Outpatient Treatment/Partial Hospitalization. Level II is an organized outpatient service that delivers treatment services during the day, before or after work or school, in the evening, or on weekends. For appropriately selected patients, such programs provide essential education and treatment components while allowing patients to apply their newly acquired skills within "real world" environments. Programs have the capacity to arrange for medical and psychiatric consultation, psychopharmacological consultation, medication management, and 24-hour crisis services.

Level II programs can provide comprehensive biopsychosocial assessments and individualized treatment plans, including formulation of problem statements, treatment goals, and measurable objectives—all developed in consultation with the patient. Such programs typically have active affiliations with other levels of care, and their staff can help patients access support services such as child care, vocational training, and transportation.

Level III: Residential/Inpatient Treatment. Level III encompasses organized services staffed by designated addiction treatment and mental health personnel who provide a planned regimen of care in a 24-hour live-in setting. Such services adhere to defined sets of policies and procedures. They are housed in, or affiliated with, permanent facilities where patients can reside safely. They are staffed 24 hours a day. Mutual and self-help group meetings generally are available on-site.

Level III encompasses four types of programs: Level III.1: Clinically Managed Low-Intensity Residential Treatment; Level III.3: Clinically Managed Medium-Intensity Residential Treatment; Level III.5: Clinically Managed High-Intensity Residential Treatment; and Level III.7: Medically Monitored Inpatient Treatment.

The defining characteristic of all Level III programs is that they serve individuals who need safe and stable living environments in order to develop their recovery skills. Such living environments may be housed in the same facility where treatment services are provided or they may be in a separate facility affiliated with the treatment provider.

Level IV: Medically Managed Intensive Inpatient Treatment. Level IV programs provide a planned regimen of 24-hour medically directed evaluation, care, and treatment of mental and substance-related disorders in an acute care inpatient setting. They are staffed by designated addiction-credentialed physicians, including psychiatrists, as well as other mental health- and addiction-credentialed clinicians. Such services are delivered under a defined set of policies and procedures and have permanent facilities that include inpatient beds.

Level IV programs provide care to patients whose mental and substance-related problems are so severe that they require primary biomedical, psychiatric, and nursing care. Treatment is provided 24 hours a day, and the full resources of a general acute care hospital or psychiatric hospital are available. The treatment is specific to mental and substance-related disorders; however, the skills of the interdisciplinary team and the availability of support services allow the conjoint treatment of any co-occurring biomedical conditions that need to be addressed.

PLACEMENT DILEMMAS

Even those using the ASAM criteria regularly encounter "real world" dilemmas surrounding access, reimbursement, funding, resource allocation, and availability of services, particularly for patients with co-occurring medical or psychiatric disorders.

Co-Occurring Disorders. When the first edition of the ASAM criteria was published in 1991, the criteria were designed for programs that offered only addiction treatment services. However, even that early edition also acknowledged that some patients come to treatment with medical (Dimension 2) and psychiatric (Dimension 3) disorders that coexist with their substance-related problems. Clinical reality suggests that programs and practitioners who are committed to meeting the total needs of the patients they serve must be able to meet the needs of such dual diagnosis patients. This concept is particularly relevant today, as the range of patient needs and clinical variability continues to broaden.

Factors contributing to this clinical reality include the expansion of substance use and substance-related disorders in younger populations; greater sensitivity to substance use

TABLE 1.   Matching Patients Who Have Co-Occurring Disorders to Services

Patients	Services
Addiction-Only Patients: Individuals who exhibit substance abuse or dependence problems without co-occuring mental health problems or diagnosable Axis I or II disorders.	**Addiction Only Services (AOS):** Services are directed toward the amelioration of substance-related disorders. No services are available for the treatment of co-occurring mental health problems or diagnosable disorders. (Such a program is clincially inappropriate for dually diagnosed individuals.)
Patients With Co-Occurring Mental Health Problems of Mild to Moderate Severity: Individuals who exhibit (1) sub-threshold diagnostic (traits, symptoms) Axis I or II disorders or (2) diagnosable but stable Axis I or II disorders (for example, bipolar disorder but compliant with and stable on medication).	**Dual Diagnosis Capable (DDC):** The primary focus is on substance use disorders, but the program is capable of treating patients with sub-threshold or diagnosable but stable Axis I or II disorders. Psychiatric services are available on-site or by consultation; at least some staff are competent to understand and identify signs and symptoms of acute psychiatric conditions.
Patients With Co-Occurring Mental Health Problems of Moderate to High Severity: Individuals who exhibit moderate to severe diagnosable Axis I or II disorders, who are not stable and require mental health as well as addication treatment.	**Dual Diagnosis Enhanced (DDE):** Psychiatric services are available on-site or are closely coordinated; all staff are crosstrained in addiction and mental health disorders and are competent to understand and identify signs and symptoms of acute psychiatric conditions and to treat mental health problems along with the substance use disorders. Treatment for the mental and substance use disorders is integrated (similar to a traditional "dual diagnosis" program).

SOURCE: Mee-Lee D, Shulman GD, Fishman M et al. (2001). *ASAM Patient Placement Criteria for the Treatment of Substance Related Disorders, Second Edition-Revised (ASAM PPC-2R).* Chevy Chase, MD: American Society of Addiction Medicine.

problems in the mental health, welfare, and criminal justice systems; and increased commitment to earlier intervention in substance use disorders in preference to fragmented services and incarceration. A major factor has been the growing body of scientific evidence pointing to addictive disorders as diseases of the brain; another is the development of pharmacotherapies for addiction. Greater understanding of the uses and effects of psychosocial and cognitive-behavioral strategies also has heightened awareness of a broadened range of modalities to meet individual needs.

The *ASAM PPC-2R* thus incorporates criteria that address the large subset of individuals who present for treatment with co-occurring Axis I substance-related disorders and Axis I/Axis II mental disorders. Individuals with such co-occurring disorders (often referred to as "dual diagnoses") can be conceptualized as belonging to one of two general categories:

- *Moderate Severity Disorders*: Patients present with stable mood or anxiety disorders of moderate severity (including resolving bipolar disorder), or with personality disorders of moderate severity (although some persons with severe levels of antisocial personality disorder may be appropriately placed in this group), or with signs and symptoms of a mental health disorder that are not so severe as to meet the diagnostic threshold.

TABLE 2. Application of the ASAM Criteria to Clinical Presentations

Use of the *ASAM Patient Placement Criteria* in treatment planning involves much more than simply a decision about level of care. The assessment dimensions and the broad continuum of care surveyed by the ASAM dimensions provide an opportunity to focus treatment, consistent with a disease management approach. The following vignettes, which represent segments of comprehensive assessments, are designed to illustrate some of the more common problems encountered in determining severity of illness, developing treatment plans, and making placement decisions. Each vignette illustrates an initial response, a discussion, and a revised response.

CASE 1: Mr. G

Mr. G is a 29-year-old Mexican-American male who has been in the U.S. for five years. He has 2 DUI convictions involving driving under the influence of alcohol, and faces assault charges arising from a bar fight while intoxicated. He is at a very early stage of readiness to change and is not prepared to acknowledge that he has a drinking problem (ASAM Dimension 4). He recently was evicted from his housing because of disturbances he caused while intoxicated; as a result, he has no place to live (ASAM Dimension 6).

Initial Response. Because of his low readiness to change (Dimension 4) and homelessness (Dimension 6), Mr. G is referred to an ASAM Level III.5 residential treatment program.

Discussion. Placing Mr. G at a level of care as intensive as Level III.5 (because of his low readiness to change) is likely to harden his resistance. While his homelessness unquestionably is a problem, the appropriate response is to help him find housing in other than a treatment setting.

Revised Response. Assuming that he has no severe problems in other Dimensions, a better choice would be to place Mr. G in a Level I outpatient treatment program, using motivational enhancement therapies to engage him in treatment, and to help him find housing separate from the treatment program.

CASE 2: Ms. P

A 16-year-old woman is brought to the emergency department of an acute care hospital with a report that, in the course of an argument with her parents, she has thrown a chair. Her parents suspect drug intoxication is the cause and report that she has been staying out unusually late at night and mixing with "the wrong crowd." They report a great deal of family discord, anger, and frustration, particularly directed by the young woman toward her father. Ms. P has no history of psychiatric or addiction treatment.

The parents both are present in the emergency department, although Ms. P was brought in by the police after her mother called for help. An emergency physician and a nurse from the psychiatric unit jointly evaluate Ms. P; they agree that she needs to be hospitalized in view of the animosity at home, her violent behavior, and the possibility that she is using an unknown drug. Following the ASAM assessment dimensions, they organize the clinical information as follows:

Dimension 1: Acute Intoxication and/or Withdrawal Potential: Although she was intoxicated at the time of the chair-throwing incident, Ms. P no longer is intoxicated and has not been using alcohol or other drugs in sufficient quantities or for a long enough period of time to suggest the possibility of a withdrawal syndrome.

Dimension 2: Biomedical Conditions and Complications: Ms. P is not taking any medications, is physically healthy, and has no current complaints.

Dimension 3: Emotional, Behavioral, or Cognitive Conditions and Complications: Ms. P has complex problems with anger management, as evidenced by the chair-throwing incident, but is not impulsive at present if separated from her parents, especially her father.

Dimension 4: Readiness to Change: Ms. P is willing to talk to a therapist, blames her parents for being overbearing and not trusting her, and agrees to come into treatment, but does not want to be at home with her father.

Dimension 5: Relapse, Continued Use, or Continued Problem Potential: The team concludes that Ms. P is likely to engage in drug use if released. They believe that, if she returns home immediately, there may be a reoccurrence of the fighting and, possibly, violence.

Dimension 6: Recovery Environment: Ms. P's parents are frustrated and angry as well. They are mistrustful of their daughter and want her hospitalized to provide a break in the family fighting.

Initial Response. Based on Ms. P's recent history of violent acting out, the emergency physician and the psychiatric nurse recommend that she be admitted to the hospital's psychiatric unit, at least for the night.

Discussion. Ms. P's acting out occurred when she was intoxicated, which she no longer is. The major conflict appears to be a family issue, particularly between Ms. P and her father. There is no indication of a severe or imminently dangerous biomedical, emotional, behavioral, or cognitive problem that requires the resources of a medically managed intensive inpatient setting.

Revised Response. The initial goal is to separate Ms. P from her father, which might be done by arranging for Ms. P to stay with a relative or family friend overnight, or by having Ms. P and her mother stay at a motel for the night. Based on the available information, Ms. P's behavior and conflict with her parents may reflect normal adolescent struggles rather than psychopathology. To address this, outpatient family counseling should be considered.

In crisis or mandated treatment situations, clinicians often come under pressure from family or referral agencies to provide a certain level of care. However, when the essential information is organized according to the ASAM dimensions, the patient's real severity and needs are more easily identified. This leads to a more appropriate clinical plan and avoids wasteful use of resources by focusing on the services needed to meet the patient's individual needs.

■ *High Severity Disorders*: Patients present with schizophrenia-spectrum disorders, severe mood disorders with psychotic features, severe anxiety disorders, or severe personality disorders (such as fragile borderline conditions).

Individuals whose co-occurring mental disorders best fit within the category of moderate severity disorders are appropriately treated in programs designed to treat primary substance use disorders. Those with concurrent high severity mental disorders, however, generally are best managed in dual diagnosis specialty programs that can offer integrated mental health and addiction treatment approaches. Some patients may require immediate stabilization of their psychiatric symptoms before they can be engaged in ongoing addiction treatment and recovery. Depending on the severity of their symptoms, such patients may require referral to medical and/or psychiatric services outside the *ASAM PPC-2R* levels of care (see Table 1).

Once stabilization has been achieved, the initial placement for recovery services should reflect an assessment of the patient's status in all six dimensions. The principle here is that the highest severity problem (particularly those in Dimensions 1, 2, or 3) should determine the patient's initial placement. Subsequent resolution of this problem creates an opportunity to transfer the patient to a less intensive level of care. Addressing the individual's recovery needs thus may involve a sequence of services across several levels of care (involving a "step-down" or "step-up" process). For example, a patient who is assessed in Dimension 2 as dangerously hypertensive should be placed in a Level III.7 or Level IV program to stabilize his or her medical condition before being transferred to a Level I program for treatment of the addictive disorder.

What should be avoided is the notion of "averaging" severity across dimensions to arrive at a placement determination.

Patients whose biomedical or psychiatric disorders are so severe that stabilizing them is the highest priority are most appropriately treated in a medical or psychiatric facility or unit before addiction treatment is initiated.

Assessment of Imminent Danger. If a patient has problems in Dimensions 4 and 5 that require 24-hour supervision and treatment interventions (such as boundary setting), without which treatment services cannot be effectively delivered, and/or the individual is in imminent danger, then the mere addition of room and board would be inadequate to meet the individual's needs. Such a patient needs placement in a residential program that offers clinical staff and services 24 hours a day in order to respond to the patient's issues that pose the imminent danger. Assessment of risk should guide the decision.

Mandated Level of Care or Length of Service. In some cases, an individual is referred for treatment at a specific level of care and/or for a specific length of service (for example, an offender in the criminal justice system may be given a choice of a prison term or a fixed length of stay in a treatment center). Such mandated or court-ordered referrals may not be based on clinical considerations and thus may be inconsistent with a placement decision arrived at through the ASAM criteria. In such a case, the provider should make reasonable attempts to have the order amended to reflect the assessed clinical level or length of service.

If the court order or other mandate cannot be amended, the individual may be continuing treatment at a level of care or for a length of stay greater than is clinically indicated. The resident's readiness for discharge or transfer and the staff's attempts to implement a clinically appropriate placement should be noted in the clinical record, and the treatment plan should be updated in a manner that provides the resident with the opportunity to continue the recovery process at the same level of care even though it could be continued at a less intensive level of care.

Logistical Impediments. Logistical problems can arise anywhere but are found most frequently in rural and underserved inner-city areas. When logistical considerations are an impediment to the indicated services (for example, lack of available transportation is a barrier to a patient's access to an indicated outpatient program), an outpatient service combined with unsupervised/minimally supervised housing may be an appropriate treatment intervention. In cities or towns, such a domiciliary option might be found in a group living situation (such as a Salvation Army program, motel accommodations, YMCA/YWCA, or mission). In rural and other underserved areas, options could include (1) the creation of a supervised housing situation by using unused treatment beds, (2) assertive community treatment models in which the treatment is brought to rural areas (such as Native American settlements) and provided in weekend intensive models at sites such as community centers and churches, (3) vans that are sent out to pick up patients and bring them to a treatment site, and (4) using a van or motor home as an office or group therapy room.

Need for a Safe Environment. When a patient lives in a recovery environment that is so toxic as to preclude recovery efforts (as through victimization or exposure to an active addict) and a Level I or II outpatient service is indicated, the patient may need referral to a safe place to live while in treatment, as well as to treatment itself.

Assuring Individualized Treatment. Many programs claim to provide individualized care, but how is the referring clinician to know that such care actually is provided? There are at least three efficient ways to determine whether a program is providing truly individualized treatment:

1. Take 10 closed clinical case records and compare the treatment plans. If the reviewer cannot clearly distinguish patients by their treatment plans, the treatment is not individualized.

2. Review the progress notes and determine whether they relate back to the objectives or strategies in the treatment plan.

3. For programs that receive reimbursement from multiple payers, compare lengths of service with sources of payment. If the lengths of stay correspond to payer type, then the program is payment-driven rather than offering individualized treatment.

Exceptions to the Patient Placement Criteria. In making treatment placement decisions, three important factors override the patient-treatment match with regard to levels of care:

1. Lack of availability of appropriate, criteria-selected care;

2. Failure of a patient to progress at a given level of care, so as to warrant a reassessment of the treatment plan with a view to modifying the treatment approach. Such situations may require transfer to a specialized program at the same level of care or to a more intensive or less intensive level of care to achieve a better therapeutic response; and

3. State laws regulating the practice of medicine or licensure of a facility that require the use of different criteria.

Unique clinical presentations or extenuating circumstances require some flexibility in application of the criteria to ensure the safety and welfare of the patient.

RESEARCH ON THE ASAM CRITERIA

Since the publication of the first edition, there has been over a decade of experience with the ASAM criteria. Use of the second edition (*ASAM PPC-2*; Mee-Lee, Shulman et al., 1996) has been mandated or recommended to publicly funded treatment programs in nearly 30 states by the U.S. Department of Defense and by two large health maintenance organizations. While this does not constitute universal acceptance, there clearly is movement toward the common language they provide to the providers and managers of care, as well as a strong focus on multidimensional assessment and individualized care.

Formal research into the criteria also is encouraged. In the earliest such study (Plough, Shirley et al., 1996), counselors used a simple, one-page summary of the criteria. The results suggested that use of even a primitive version of the ASAM criteria is associated with improved treatment retention.

In 1994, the National Institute on Drug Abuse (NIDA) funded the first randomized controlled trial using the ASAM criteria, and it is hoped that clinical outcomes research will drive future revisions of the criteria. There also have been two retrospective studies: one applied an abbreviated *PPC-1* algorithm to telephone survey data (Morey, 1996), while the other implemented only the psychosocial dimensions (McKay, Cacciola et al., 1997). A solution has been developed to address the problem of interviewer ease of use of criteria, and this solution has been tested in three prospective studies. It consists of a comprehensive implementation designed by Gastfriend and his associates that offers the counselor a sequence of questions and scoring options on the screen of a microcomputer (Turner, Turner et al., 1999).

There have been two naturalistic studies and one randomized controlled trial of placement criteria (the results of which are not yet published). Overall, the early studies have shown adequate reliability, good concurrent validity, and some degree of predictive validity (Gastfriend, Lu et al., 2000).

CONCLUSIONS

Four important missions underlie the ASAM criteria: (1) to enable patients to receive the most appropriate and highest quality treatment services, (2) to encourage the development of a broad continuum of care, (3) to promote the effective, efficient use of care resources, and (4) to help protect access to and funding for care. The use of placement criteria in treatment planning thus represents far more than a narrow utilization review or case management process. Correctly applied and implemented, the ASAM criteria can assist in improving the "placement match" by redesigning the place of treatment and the level of care.

Effective implementation of the newest version of the ASAM criteria (*ASAM PPC-2R*) will require a shift in thinking toward outcomes-driven case management. A variety of treatment agencies will need to make this shift, including regulatory agencies, clinical and medical staff, and referral sources (such as courts, probation officers, child protective services, employers, and employee assistance professionals [Heatherton, 2000]).

The ASAM criteria offer a system for improving the "modality match" through the use of multidimensional assessment and treatment planning that permits more objective evaluation of patient outcomes. With improved outcome analysis driving treatment decisions, the problem of access to care and funding of treatment can be championed more effectively.

REFERENCES

American Psychiatric Association (APA) (1994). *Diagnostic and Statistical Manual of Mental Disorders, 4th Edition (DSM-IV)*. Washington, DC: American Psychiatric Press.

Gartner L & Mee-Lee D, eds. (1995). *The Role and Current Status of Patient Placement Criteria in the Treatment of Substance Use Disorders* (Treatment Improvement Protocol No. 13). Rockville, MD: Center for Substance Abuse Treatment.

Gastfriend DR, Lu S & Sharon E (2000). Placement matching: Challenges and technical progress. *Substance Use & Misuse* 35(12-14):2191-2213.

Gastfriend DR & McLellan AT (1997). Treatment matching: Theoretic basis and practical implications. *Medical Clinics of North America* 81(4):945-966.

Gregoire TK (2000). Factors associated with level of care assignment in substance abuse treatment. *Journal of Substance Abuse Treatment* 18:241-248.

Heatherton B (2000). Implementing the ASAM criteria in community treatment centers in Illinois: Opportunities and challenges. *Journal of Addictive Diseases* 19(2):109-116.

Hoffmann NG, Halikas JA, Mee-Lee D et al. (1991). *Patient Placement Criteria for the Treatment of Psychoactive Substance Use Disorders (PPC-1)*. Washington, DC: American Society of Addiction Medicine.

McKay JR, Cacciola JS, McLellan AT et al. (1997). An initial evaluation of the psychosocial dimensions of the American Society of Addiction Medicine criteria for inpatient vs. intensive outpatient substance abuse rehabilitation. *Journal of Studies on Alcohol* 58(5):239-252.

Mee-Lee D (2001a). Persons with addictive disorders, system failures, and managed care. In EC Ross (ed.) *Managed Behavioral Health Care Handbook*. Gaithersburg, MD: Aspen Publishers, Inc., 225-266.

Mee-Lee D (2001b). Treatment planning for dual disorders. *Psychiatric Rehabilitation Skills* 5(1):52-79.

Mee-Lee D (1998). Use of patient placement criteria in the selection of treatment. In AW Graham & TK Schultz (eds.) *Principles of Addiction Medicine, Second Edition*. Chevy Chase, MD: American Society of Addiction Medicine.

Mee-Lee D, Shulman GD, Fishman M et al. (2001). *ASAM Patient Placement Criteria for the Treatment of Substance-Related Disorders, Second Edition-Revised (ASAM PPC-2R)*. Chevy Chase, MD: American Society of Addiction Medicine.

Mee-Lee D, Shulman GD & Gartner L (1996). *ASAM Patient Placement Criteria for the Treatment of Substance-Related Disorders, Second Edition (ASAM PPC-2)*. Chevy Chase, MD: American Society of Addiction Medicine.

Miller WR & Rollnick S (2002). *Motivational Interviewing: Preparing People for Change*. New York, NY: Guilford Press.

Morey LC (1996). Patient placement criteria: Linking typologies to managed care. *Alcohol Health & Research World* 20(1):36-44.

National Institute on Drug Abuse (NIDA) (1994). *Mental Health Assessment and Diagnosis of Substance Abusers* (Clinical Report Series). Rockville, MD: NIDA, National Institutes of Health.

National Institute on Drug Abuse (NIDA) (1999). *Principles of Drug Addiction Treatment: A Research-Based Guide*. Rockville, MD: NIDA, National Institutes of Health.

National Institute on Drug Abuse (NIDA) (1997). *Treatment of Drug-Dependent Individuals With Comorbid Mental Disorders* (Research Monograph 172). Rockville, MD: NIDA, National Institutes of Health.

Plough A, Shirley L, Zaremba N et al. (1996). *CSAT Target Cities Demonstration Final Evaluation Report*. Boston, MA: Office for Treatment Improvement.

Prochaska JO, DiClemente CC & Norcross JC (1992). In search of how people change: Applications to addictive behaviors. *American Psychologist* 47:1102-1114.

Project MATCH Research Group (1997). Matching alcoholism treatments to client heterogeneity: Project MATCH posttreatment drinking outcomes. *Journal of Studies on Alcohol* 58:7-29.

Shulman GD (1994). Continued treatment for substance abuse: An effective system for referral. *Continuing Care* 13:27-33.

Turner WM, Turner KH, Reif S et al. (1999). Feasibility of multidimensional substance abuse treatment matching: Automating the ASAM Patient Placement Criteria. *Drug and Alcohol Dependence* 55:35-43.

| Chapter 6 | # Relapse Prevention: Clinical Models and Intervention Strategies |

Dennis C. Daley, Ph.D.
G. Alan Marlatt, Ph.D.
Crystal E. Spotts, M.Ed.

Recovery, Lapse, and Relapse
Treatment Outcomes and Relapse Rates
Relapse Precipitants
Models of Relapse Prevention
Studies of Relapse Prevention Approaches
Clinical Interventions

Individuals with substance use disorders (SUDs) face the possibility of relapse once they stop using alcohol or other drugs even if they have a successful treatment episode (NIDA, 1999; NIAAA, 2000). In response to this fact, increasing emphasis has been placed on the maintenance stage of the change process for individuals with all types and combinations of SUDs. A number of relapse prevention (RP) approaches and clinical strategies have been developed to help clinicians address relapse issues. The principles and concepts of RP are used with SUDs (Marlatt & Gordon, 1985; Dimeff & Marlatt, 1998; Tims & Leukefeld, 1987; Daley & Marlatt, 1997a; Marlatt, Barrett & Daley, 1999) as well as other addictive disorders and problems of impulse control, including smoking, compulsive overeating, sexual offenses, and sexual addiction (Daley & Ross, 2000), violence and criminal offenses (Gondolf, 2001; Gorski & Kelley, 1996; Peters & Steinberg, 2000), marital problems, psychiatric disorders, and comorbid addictive disorder and psychiatric illness (Wilson, 1992; Daley & Lis, 1995; Weiss, Najavits et al., 1998; Daley & Roth, 2001).

This chapter summarizes clinical strategies used to reduce relapse risk. Definitions of recovery, lapse, and relapse are provided; treatment outcomes studies are summarized;

common relapse precipitants are delineated; and models of RP are reviewed briefly. The clinical interventions discussed represent the most common issues or themes espoused in the various RP models. The chapter is based on a review of the empirical and clinical literature and the authors' clinical experience.

RECOVERY, LAPSE, AND RELAPSE

Recovery refers to the process of initiating abstinence from alcohol or other drug use, as well as making intrapersonal and interpersonal changes to maintain abstinence over time. A process often initiated by involvement in professional treatment, recovery is best viewed as a long-term and ongoing process rather than an endpoint (Dimeff & Marlatt, 1995; NIDA, 1999). Specific changes can occur in any of the following areas: physical, psychological, behavioral, interpersonal, family, social, spiritual, and financial (Daley & Marlatt, 1997a, 1997b; Daley, 2001). Recovery tasks and areas of clinical focus are contingent on the stage or phase of recovery the individual is in (Brown, 1995; Washton, 2001, 2002). Recovery and relapse are mediated by the severity and degree of damage caused by the SUD, the presence of a comorbid psychiatric or medical illness, and the individual's coping skills, motivation, and support system. Although some individuals achieve full recovery, others achieve only partial recovery (Gorski, 1986). The latter group is at risk for multiple relapses over time, yet still can benefit from the cumulative effects of multiple treatments.

Recovering from an SUD involves gaining information, increasing self-awareness, developing skills for sober living, and following a program of change. The program of change may involve therapy or counseling, adjunctive pharmacotherapy, participation in self-help programs, and self-management approaches. A publication from the National Institute on Drug Abuse (NIDA; 1999) delineating the principles of treatment for drug addiction emphasized that, in addition to professional treatment, case management, and self-help groups, the addicted patient often needs help with family, vocational, mental health, medical, educational, legal, financial, and social issues and problems.

In the early phases of recovery, the patient relies more on external supports and help from professionals, sponsors, or other members of support groups. As recovery progresses, the patient places more reliance on himself or herself to handle problems and the challenges of living a sober life. The information and skills learned as part of RP offer an excellent mechanism to prepare patients for this "maintenance" phase of recovery.

The term *lapse* refers to the initial episode of alcohol or other drug use after a period of abstinence (Marlatt & Gordon, 1985). A lapse can end quickly or lead to a relapse of varying proportions. The effects of the initial lapse are mediated by the person's affective and cognitive reactions. A full-blown relapse is more likely in the individual who has a strong perception of violating the abstinence rule (Marlatt, 1985a). Although some individuals experience a full-blown relapse and return to pretreatment levels of substance abuse, others use alcohol and drugs problematically but do not return to previous levels of abuse, and thus suffer fewer harmful effects as a result. Patients in relapse vary in the quantity and frequency of their substance use, as well as the medical and psychosocial sequelae that accompany a relapse.

Marlatt (1985a) defines *relapse* as "a breakdown or setback in a person's attempt to change or modify any target behavior" (p. 3). NIDA's Cue Extinction (CE) model of RP defines relapse as "an unfolding process in which the resumption of substance abuse is the last event in a long series of maladaptive responses to internal or external stressors or stimuli" (NIDA, 1993, p. 39). Thus, relapse can be understood not only as the event of resuming substance use after a period of improvement, but also as a process in which indicators are observable before actual substance use resumes (Gorski, 1986; Daley & Marlatt, 1997b).

TREATMENT OUTCOMES AND RELAPSE RATES

Early studies and reviews of the outcome literature reported rates of relapse of more than 70% among alcohol- and drug-abusing patients participating in treatment (Hunt, Barnett et al., 1971; Emrick, 1974; Miller & Hester, 1980; Catalano, Howard et al., 1988). Most relapses occur within the first year of treatment, with two-thirds occurring within the first 90 days. Patients who remain in treatment the longest generally have the best outcomes (NIDA, 1997a, 1997b).

More recent studies and reports in the outcomes literature demonstrate that treatment of addictive disorders is effective in reducing relapse rates and improving the functioning of persons with substance use disorders. McLellan and colleagues (2000) reviewed more than 100 clinical trials of drug addiction treatment and reported that most studies showed significant reductions in substance use, improved personal health, and reduced social pathology. Patients treated for addiction had favorable outcomes during treatment, and at 6- and 12-month followup (for example, at 12-month followup, 40% to 60% of patients had been continuously abstinent and 15% to 30% had not used substances addictively). These positive outcomes are similar to those seen with other chronic medical conditions such as diabetes, hypertension, and asthma. Also, as with other chronic disorders, persons with SUDs have difficulties in adhering to treatment, sometimes drop out early, and may relapse to substance use.

A report by NIDA (1997b) of a study of 10,010 drug users in nearly 100 treatment programs in 11 cities showed that all four treatment approaches studied were effective in reducing drug use, reducing illegal acts, improving employment rates, and reducing suicidal thoughts and behaviors. Another NIDA publication (1999) summarized the positive effects of 12 different scientifically based treatment approaches, including RP.

Several publications by the Center for Substance Abuse Treatment (CSAT; 1999, 2000a, 2000b) and the most recent report to Congress by the National Institute on Alcohol Abuse and Alcoholism (NIAAA) on alcohol and health (2000) describe positive outcomes for substance abusers who have received professional treatment, including (1) reduced rates of substance use; (2) reduced medical costs for patients and families a year after treatment; (3) reduced rates of criminal behaviors, re-arrests, and re-incarcerations; (4) improved psychological functioning; and (5) improved family productivity, more mothers reunited with their children, and reduced dependence on welfare.

The results of Project MATCH (1998), a large-scale study of 1,726 alcohol-dependent patients who were randomly assigned to one of three manual-driven treatment approaches (Twelve Step Facilitation, cognitive-behavioral therapy, or motivational enhancement therapy) (NIAAA 1995a, 1995b), show that significant reductions in alcohol use (in terms of total days used as well as number of drinks per day) observed in the first year after treatment were sustained over the three-year followup period. Thirty percent were totally abstinent in months 37 to 39 and those who did drink were abstinent about two-thirds of the time. In an earlier analysis of the alcohol treatment outcome literature, Miller and colleagues (1995) reported that there was a "significant treatment effect on at least one alcohol measure for at least one followup point" (p. 17) for 146 of 211 studies (69%).

Simpson and colleagues (1986) followed a group of 405 opioid addicts for 12 years after their admission to drug abuse treatment. At year 12, 26% were using opioids on a daily basis, 39% were using some opioids, 61% were using marijuana, 47% were using other drugs, and 27% were drinking more than 4 oz. of alcohol per day. However, there was a significant reduction in daily opioid use, from 47% at year 1 to 26% at year 12.

Hoffmann and Harrison (1986, 1989) followed 1,957 adults with SUDs who were treated in five different treatment centers. They reported that approximately half of the patients were abstinent for the entire two-year period. These results, however, come from a naturalistic study that lacked randomized design and a control group. The Comprehensive Assessment and Treatment Outcome Research group followed 8,087 patients from 38 inpatient programs and 1,663 patients from 19 outpatient programs for a year (Hoffman & Miller, 1992). Abstinence rates at 12 months were 60% for the 4,635 inpatients contacted (57.3% of the inpatient cohort) and 68% for the outpatient subjects contacted (62.5% of the total outpatient cohort) at 12 months. Even when these rates are adjusted, and assuming a 70% relapse rate for missing cases, abstinence rates at one year would be 44% for the inpatient cohort and 52% for the outpatient cohort. The researchers also reported that, at the one-year followup, patients who received professional treatment evidenced the following significant changes: (1) a reduction in medical care for expensive hospital services from 21% to 10% (n=4,541); (2) a decrease in work problems, including absenteeism, from 41% to 7% (n=2,719); and (3) a decrease in traffic violations from 16% to 7% (n=5,567).

RELAPSE PRECIPITANTS

Relapse rarely is caused by any single factor and often is the result of an interaction of individual, situational, physiologic, and sociocultural factors (Dimeff & Marlatt, 1995; Marlatt, 1996a). Relapse is best viewed as a "dynamic" process in which the person's readiness to change interacts with other external and internal factors (Marlatt, 1996b). Specific precipitants of relapse vary substantially from one experience to the next even within the same individual.

Catalano and colleagues (1988) reviewed the literature on relapse in alcoholism, heroin addiction, and smoking and classified relapse precipitants in three categories: (1) pretreatment factors, such as the degree of substance dependence or psychiatric impairment, (2) treatment factors, such as the type and length of addictive disorder treatment, and (3) post-treatment factors, such as family and social supports or social skills. Daley (1989a) reviewed the literature on recovery and relapse across all addictions and classified relapse precipitants into eight categories: (1) affective variables such as depression or anxiety; (2) behavioral variables such as inadequate coping skills or leisure management skills; (3) cognitive variables such as attitudes and beliefs about recovery or relapse or low self-efficacy; (4) environmental and relationship variables such as social pressures to use substances, lack of productive roles, and poor levels of social support; (5) physiologic variables such as post-acute withdrawal, cravings caused by conditioned responses to substance stimuli, physical pain, or medication use for medical problems; (6) psychological or psychiatric variables such as level of motivation to change or the presence of a comorbid psychiatric disorder; (7) spiritual variables such as excessive guilt or shame, feeling empty, or a lack of meaning in life; and (8) treatment system variables such as the clinician's knowledge and skills and effect on the patient, as well as access to the services needed.

The most widely cited taxonomy for relapse precipitants is that developed by Marlatt, who classified the determinants for alcoholics, smokers, heroin addicts, gamblers, and overeaters into two broad categories: intrapersonal and interpersonal (Marlatt, 1985a, 1996a; Marlatt, Barrett et al.,

1999). This classification scheme has been found useful in other countries (Sandahl, 1984; Annis, 1986) and is supported by prospective studies (Miller, Westerberg et al., 1996; Hodgins, el-Guebaly et al., 1995). It also has been used as the basis of research protocols (Carroll, Rounsaville et al., 1991), treatment protocols (George, 1989; Daley, 1989b), and patient recovery guides (Daley, 1987, 2000).

Intrapersonal determinants of relapse include negative emotional states, negative physical states, positive emotional states, testing of personal control, and urges and temptations. Marlatt's research found that the determinant most often involved in relapse of alcoholics, smokers, and heroin addicts was negative emotional states: 38% of alcoholics, 37% of smokers, and 19% of heroin addicts relapsed in response to a negative affective state (Marlatt, 1985a). Shiffman (1982) reported that negative affect or stress was a factor in 52% of relapses of smokers. LaBounty and colleagues (1992) found that significantly more anxious patients reported relapsing to cope with depression, anxiety, and anger compared with matched control subjects without anxiety problems.

Interpersonal factors in relapse include relationship conflict, social pressure to use substances, and positive emotional states associated with some type of interaction with others (Saunders & Allsop, 1991; Tucker, Vuchinich et al., 1991). Social pressure to use drugs was identified by 36% of heroin addicts, 32% of smokers, and 18% of alcoholics as contributing to their relapses (Marlatt, 1985a). Havassy and colleagues (1991) reported that greater social support and spousal support predicted a lower risk of relapse among alcoholics, opiate users, and cigarette smokers completing treatment.

Miller and colleagues (1996) found lack of coping skills to be most predictive of relapse. Also, recent antecedents were more predictive of relapse than ones in the distant past. Allsop and colleagues (2000) categorized the process of relapse and found that treatment self-efficacy and cognitive functioning both were predictors of treatment outcome and time to lapse and relapse. McKay (1999) examined the relationship between cocaine use and alcohol use in a study with cocaine users and concluded that alcohol is a potential relapse precipitant for cocaine users. This finding also was supported by the work of Rawson and colleagues, who reported that alcohol use among cocaine addicts increases the risk of relapse by eight times and marijuana use increases it by five times (Rawson, Huber et al., in press). In a quality improvement survey of more than 100 outpatients with comorbid SUDs and psychiatric disorders, Daley, Salloum et al. (1996) asked patients to identify factors contributing to relapse, as well as factors that aided their recovery. The five factors identified most often as contributing to relapse were inability to manage stress or negative emotional states (69%), interpersonal conflicts with family or others (29%), poor adherence to professional treatment (25%), negative thinking (11%), and low motivation to change (10%).

MODELS OF RELAPSE PREVENTION

RP generally refers to two types of clinical interventions: (1) any individual or group psychosocial treatment aimed at reducing substance use relapse rates and improving clinical outcome (for example, community reinforcement, contingency management, cognitive-behavioral therapies, individual or group drug counseling approaches, and the like) and (2) specific RP models that focus primarily on the issues and skills seen as most relevant to enhancing the patient's ability to maintain abstinence and make broader lifestyle changes to reduce the need for substances (Dimeff & Marlatt, 1995; Washton, 2001, 2002). In addition, pharmacotherapeutic strategies combined with psychosocial treatments also are used as part of an overall treatment strategy to reduce relapse risk and improve abstinence rates (NIDA, 1997a, 1997b; McLellan, Lewis et al., 2000; NIAAA, 2000).

Treatment Approaches Incorporating RP Principles. Addiction rehabilitation programs include lectures and groups on RP as part of their overall treatment protocol, so as to expose patients to major issues and principles of RP that they can use in their ongoing recovery. Many clinical models of care focus on RP as one component of the overall treatment. The cognitive-behavioral coping skills therapy approach developed by Kadden and colleagues (NIAAA, 1995a), as adapted for use in the Project MATCH study, aimed to help patients develop coping skills to manage cravings and thoughts of drinking alcohol, refuse offers to drink, cope with a lapse to prevent it from leading to a relapse, and understand "seemingly irrelevant decisions" that may lead to relapse. Twelve Step facilitation therapy, another treatment provided in Project MATCH (NIAAA, 1995b), aimed to reduce relapse risk by helping patients understand and use the AA program (that is, attend meetings, become active in various aspects of the Twelve Step program, and get and use an AA sponsor). The individual drug counseling (IDC) (NIDA, 2000) and group drug counseling (GDC) (NIDA, 2001) models used in a large multisite outpatient treatment study of cocaine dependence placed considerable attention on issues of relapse and its prevention. Both IDC and GDC provided specific treatment sessions on relapse, as well as the opportunity for patients to discuss lapses and relapses and strategies to reestablish abstinence if relapse occurred. The MATRIX model of structured outpatient treatment developed by Rawson and colleagues for the treatment of cocaine and methamphetamine dependence includes an extensive module on RP (Matrix Center, 1989; Obert, McCann et al., 2000).

Similarly, the Washton model of outpatient addiction treatment (2001, 2002) incorporates RP as a major focus of treatment. A unique feature of the Washton approach is the use of three different types of groups, depending on the patient's stage of change: a self-evaluation group for patients in the precontemplation, contemplation, or decision stage of change; an initial abstinence group (IAG) for patients in the action stage who are ready to make the behavior changes needed to stop using substances; and a relapse prevention group (RPG) for patients who have graduated from the IAG. The RPG is based on the cognitive-behavioral model of Marlatt and Gordon (1985) and incorporates skills training, cognitive reframing, and lifestyle interventions. An "extended" RPG is available for patients who have established sobriety and who wish to explore in detail the issues pertinent to their inner emotional life as well as interpersonal relationship patterns that lead to desires to use substances to alleviate painful affects (Washton, 2002).

Specific Models of RP. Various models of RP are described in the literature, and many of these have been adapted for use in clinical trials (for summaries of various RP models, see Connors, Maisto et al., 1996; Marlatt, 1996a; and Daley, 1988). RP models include the following:

■ Marlatt and Gordon's cognitive-behavioral approach (1985; Marlatt, Barrett et al., 1999).

■ Annis's cognitive-behavioral approach (1991), which incorporates concepts of Marlatt's model with Bandura's self-efficacy theory.

■ Daley's psychoeducational approach (Daley & Marlatt, 1997a; Daley, 2000), which adapted Marlatt's classification of relapse precipitants to a treatment protocol that can be used in individual or group sessions.

■ Gorski's neurologic impairment model, which incorporates elements from the disease model of addiction and relapse, as well as Marlatt's model (2000).

■ Zackon, McAuliffe and Chien's recovery training and self-help model (NIDA, 1994).

■ The MATRIX neurobehavioral model of treatment of Rawson and colleagues, which includes RP as a central component of treatment (Matrix Center, 1989; Rawson, Obert et al., 1993a; Rawson, Shoptaw et al., 1995; Shoptaw, Reback et al., 1998; Obert, McCann et al., 2000).

■ Washton's intensive outpatient model (2001, 2002), which includes significant attention to RP during the third phase of treatment.

■ The coping/social skills training (CSST) model of Monti and colleagues (1989, 1993).

■ The CE model developed by Childress and colleagues (NIDA, 1993).

Despite any differences in theoretical underpinnings, clinical philosophy of treatment, or intervention strategies, these RP approaches have many components in common. They focus on the need for patients with SUDs to (1) have a broad repertoire of cognitive and behavioral coping strategies to draw on for handling high-risk situations and warning signs of relapse; (2) make lifestyle changes so as to decrease the need for alcohol, drugs, or tobacco; (3) increase healthy activities; (4) prepare for interrupting lapses so that they do not develop into full-blown relapse; and (5) prepare for interrupting relapses so that adverse consequences can be minimized. Most RP models incorporate strategies from Marlatt's original conceptualization of relapse.

STUDIES OF RELAPSE PREVENTION APPROACHES

Many reports and studies show that RP does help improve recovery and reduce relapse rates. Carroll (1996) reviewed randomized controlled trials on the effectiveness of RP among smokers (12 studies), alcohol abusers (6 studies), marijuana abusers (1 study), cocaine abusers (3 studies), opiate addicts (1 study), and other drug abusers (1 study). She found that the strongest evidence for the efficacy of RP is seen in smokers and concluded that "there is good evidence for relapse prevention approaches compared with no-treatment controls, . . . and added that "outcomes where relapse prevention may hold greater promise include reducing severity of relapses when they occur, durability of effects after cessation, and patient-treatment matching" (p. 53). Patients with higher levels of impairment along dimensions such as psychiatric severity and addiction severity appear to benefit most from RP, compared with those with less severe levels of impairment. Thus, RP can be especially helpful for patients with co-occurring mental disorders.

Irvin and colleagues (1999) conducted a meta-analysis of 26 published and unpublished clinical trials on RP conducted between 1978 and 1995, involving a total sample of 9,504 participants. These studies assessed the efficacy of RP as a cognitive-behavioral intervention and were consistent with Marlatt and Gordon's approach to RP. Outcomes assessed included substance use and overall psychosocial adjustment. The strongest treatment effects for RP were found for alcohol and polysubstance use. Effects were weaker for smoking and cocaine. It appeared that individual, group, and marital modalities were equally effective, but the research cautioned that the sample sizes were wide in range. Another finding was that medication is very helpful in reducing relapse rates, particularly in the treatment of alcohol problems.

In a randomized clinical trial, Carroll and colleagues (1991) compared 21 outpatient cocaine abusers receiving RP with 21 receiving interpersonal psychotherapy (IPT). RP was more effective than IPT for patients with more severe cocaine problems ($p < .01$) and to some extent for those with greater psychiatric severity ($p < .05$). In another randomized clinical trial of treatment involving 97 outpatient cocaine abusers, Carroll and colleagues (1994) compared RP with an operationalized clinical management condition and pharmacotherapy condition (desipramine hydrochloride or placebo). At one-year followup, they found a significant psychotherapy-by-time effect, indicating a delayed response to treatment among patients who received RP. This response was determined by random regression analyses using the Addiction Severity Index cocaine composite scores (estimate, 0.061; SE=0.02; z=2.11; p=.03). Goldstein and colleagues (1989) also found a significant delayed effect for an experimental RP condition (n=49), as compared with an educational support control condition (n=40) at six months for smokers treated in a 10-week group program. The abstinence rate for RP at six months was 36.7%, compared with 17.5% for the control condition (χ^2=4.16, df=1, $p < .05$; G^2=1.87; df=4, p=.759). Rawson and colleagues (in press) found a similar "sleeper effect" for RP with cocaine addicts. These findings of delayed effects of RP are consistent with

the notion that learning new ways to cope with high-risk situations takes time.

In a study of 60 men with alcoholism, Saunders and Allsop (1991) found that subjects receiving RP returned to heavy alcohol use at a rate of four to seven times less rapidly than subjects in a discussion control group at the 6-month followup period (z=1.9, $p < .03$). Heavy drinking was defined as consumption of 30 or more standard drinks in a week or more than eight drinks consumed on any one day of drinking. Chaney and O'Leary (1978) compared subjects receiving an RP skills training intervention (n=14) with those in a discussion control group (n=24) at 12-month followup. Subjects who received RP drank less, had fewer episodes of intoxication, experienced less severe lapses for shorter periods of time, and stopped drinking significantly sooner after a relapse, as compared with patients in the discussion group control condition. The mean number of "days drunk" in the RP condition was 11.1 (SD=14.3), compared with 64 (SD=88.3) in the control condition (df=37, t=2.21, $p < .05$). The mean "total number of drinks" was 399.8 for RP, compared with 1,592 for the control condition ($p < .05$).

Koski-Jannes (1992) found greater treatment adherence and satisfaction, reduced lengths of inpatient treatment, and fewer alcohol-related arrests among patients who received RP compared with patients who received other treatment modalities. A study of hospitalized male alcoholics found that patients who received RP (n=20) compared with IPT (n=19) drank on fewer days, drank less alcohol, were more likely to complete a course of aftercare treatment (80% versus 57.9%), and had a slightly higher rate of continuous abstinence at 6-month followup (50% versus 42.1%) (Ito, Donovan et al., 1988).

Stephens and colleagues (1994) randomly assigned 161 men and 51 women seeking help for marijuana dependence to either RP or a social support (SSP) discussion intervention. Twelve-month outcomes of 167 subjects contacted (79% of sample) showed substantial reductions in the frequency of marijuana use (RP, x=14.78, SD=11.96, compared with SSP, x=14.30, SD=12.2) and associated problems, but no substantial differences between the two interventions on days of use, related problems, or abstinence rates. A study by Wells and colleagues (1994) of outpatient cocaine abusers, comparing RP with Twelve Step counseling (TSC), found that subjects in both treatment conditions reduced their use of cocaine, marijuana, and alcohol use at the 12-week post-treatment period. However, RP subjects were more likely to maintain a reduced drinking level at 12 weeks (p <.04). Mean drinking in TSC at baseline was 7.67 (SD=8.89) days in the preceding 30 days, compared with 9.85 (SD=8.97) days in the RP condition. This decreased to 5.00 (SD=7.90) and 7.16 (SD=9.45) for TSC and 7.90 (SD=8.36) and 8.40 (SD=9.43) for RP at posttreatment and six-month followup, respectively.

Kranzler and colleagues (1995) assessed the effects of fluoxetine (Prozac®) as an adjunct to RP in 101 alcoholics and found that subjects in both the fluoxetine and placebo groups reduced their number of drinking days and the number of drinks per drinking day at six-month followup. Mean drinking days were 45.3 (SD=12.6) and mean drinks per drinking day were 9.8 (SD=4.0) in the fluoxetine group, compared with 43.4 (SD=12.4) mean drinking days and 9.8 (SD=6.2) mean drinks per drinking day in the placebo group. Because there were no notable differences between the fluoxetine and placebo groups, the investigators concluded that RP was a factor in improved drinking outcomes.

A study by O'Malley and colleagues (1992) of naltrexone (ReVia®) and coping skills in an alcohol-dependent population (n=97) documented naltrexone's efficacy over placebo, but also found a therapy-by-medication effect, indicating that the patients who received RP/coping skills and naltrexone were less likely to relapse to heavy drinking after a lapse than were patients in the other group. Data analysis using a proportional hazards model found that those receiving RP had one-fourth the risk of relapse of those in the placebo plus coping skills condition (p <.05). Stevens and colleagues (1993) compared 666 control subjects receiving usual care to 453 hospitalized smokers who received a single RP session. RP subjects had better total abstinence rates at 3 months (20.5% versus 13.7%) and 12 months (21% versus 16.7%) and were more likely to have consecutive abstinence during the followup period (p=.0002).

Several studies found that RP administered in groups is as efficacious as RP delivered in individual sessions (Graham, Annis et al., 1996; Schmitz, Oswald et al., 1997). McKay and colleagues (1997) randomized 98 cocaine users to standard group or RP individual sessions and determined that those who endorsed a goal of total abstinence when entering treatment had better outcomes in RP than those in standard group counseling. The RP condition was more effective in limiting the use of cocaine among those patients that did use the drug in months 1 to 3. Investigators also found better outcomes at months 13 to 24 among patients who received RP than in those who received

standard group counseling or other treatment modalities. Results showed that, although 45.5% of patients in standard group treatment used cocaine on more than 15% of the study days, only 4.6% of those in the RP condition used cocaine (t=8.25, df=1, p.01).

Several studies included spouses in the RP intervention. A study of the first relapse episodes and reasons for terminating relapses of men with alcoholism who were treated with their spouses found that the relapses of patients receiving RP in addition to behavioral marital therapy were shorter than those of patients not receiving RP (Maisto, McKay et al., 1995). Relapses of subjects in the RP condition lasted 6.5 days, compared with 21.8 days in the non-RP condition (t=1.96, df=22, p=.05). In a study of 59 married alcoholics, O'Farrell (1993) found that in couples assessed to be "high distress," abstinence rates at 12 months were highest for those who received behavioral marital therapy (BMT) in combination with RP. Alcoholics who received RP after completing BMT had more days of abstinence, fewer days of drinking and, for those with the poorest functioning at baseline, improved marriages compared with those who received only BMT (F=5.07, 1/57df, p=.028) (O'Farrell, Choquette et al., 1993).

There are several limitations to studies on RP (Carroll, 1996; Marlatt, 1996b; Daley & Marlatt, 1997c). First, there is no consensus as to how to define or measure relapse. Second, some studies have used RP as the single treatment intervention for cessation of substance use rather than for maintenance of change once substance use was stopped. Third, studies usually do not differentiate between subjects who are motivated to change their substance use behavior and those who have little or no motivation to change. Fourth, in some studies, sample sizes are small and there is not enough power to detect statistical differences between experimental and control conditions. Fifth, studies do not always use random assignment or operationalize the therapy being compared against RP, making it difficult to determine what factors contribute to treatment effects. Finally, the followup period often is short-term. Despite these limitations, the literature generally favors the efficacy of RP and shows that RP strategies enhance the recovery of individuals with SUDs.

CLINICAL INTERVENTIONS

This section describes practical RP clinical interventions that reflect the approaches of numerous clinicians and researchers who have developed specific models of RP and/or written patient-oriented RP recovery materials. The literature emphasizes individualizing RP strategies, taking into account the patient's level of motivation, severity of substance use, ego functioning, and sociocultural environment. These RP interventions can be provided in individual or group sessions (many RP programs were designed for small groups of participants) (Monti, Adams et al., 1989; Washton, 2002; Daley, 2001; Rawson, Huber et al., in press; NIDA, 1993).

The use of experiential learning or action techniques such as role playing or behavioral rehearsal, metaphors, monodramas, psychodrama, bibliotherapy, use of workbooks, a daily inventory, interactive videos, and homework assignments makes learning an active experience for the patient. Such techniques enhance self-awareness, decrease defensiveness, and encourage behavioral change (Matrix Center, 1989; Daley, 1988, 2000; Gorski, 1986; NIDA, 1993, 1994; Dimeff & Marlatt, 1995).

In RP groups, action techniques provide numerous opportunities for the clinician to elicit feedback and support for individual patients from their peers, to identify common themes and issues related to RP, and to practice specific cognitive or interpersonal skills. For example, the leader of a treatment group set up a role play in which a male cocaine addict in recovery was offered cocaine by another addict who was not in recovery. Other group members were instructed to imagine that they also were in this situation and asked to pay close attention to their thoughts and feelings as they observed the role play. Although the patient refused the substance offered during the actual role play, the post-role play discussion revealed several interesting facts.

First, the patient's body language and affect during the role play were viewed by observers as giving mixed messages to the addict who was offering the drug, thus opening the door for the person to continue to pressure the addict to use the drugs. Group members felt that ambivalence about sobriety often is perceived by other addicts offering substances. Second, although the patient said to the person offering cocaine that he did not want to use the drug, his internal dialogue was much more ambivalent, and strong thoughts of getting high on cocaine emerged. This observation took the patient somewhat by surprise because he reported to the group that he did feel his commitment to abstinence was strong. Finally, when other group members shared their reactions about what it was like for them to imagine being in this situation, it became apparent that most felt that such interpersonal encounters tap the "addicted part" of them that still wants to use substances. Although

some patients were not surprised by this feeling, others were. Such experiential learning often leads patients to look beneath the surface and examine internal thoughts, feelings, and desires. Once patients are aware of their internal struggles, the clinician can help them to explore, develop, and practice strategies to manage the social pressures they expect to face.

The following strategies are taken from the various models of RP and other treatment models that incorporate relapse issues. Several clinical examples are provided.

Help patients anticipate their high-risk relapse factors and develop coping skills or strategies to manage them. The need to recognize and manage high-risk factors is an essential component of RP. High-risk factors involve intrapersonal and interpersonal situations in which the patient feels vulnerable to substance use (Marlatt & Gordon, 1985; Daley & Marlatt, 1997b). Relapse is more likely to occur as the result of lack of coping skills than the high-risk situation itself, so the clinician should assess the client's coping style to identify targets for clinical intervention (Marlatt, 1985b; Miller, Westerberg et al., 1996). Findings from the Relapse Replication and Extension Project (RREP) indicate that the availability of coping skills is a protective factor that reduces relapse risk, whereas ineffective coping skills are a consistent predictor of relapse (Connors, Longabaugh et al., 1996).

The meaning of specific high-risk factors also varies among patients. RP strategies and interventions therefore need to take into account the nuances of each patient's high-risk factors. For example, two patients identified depression as a serious relapse risk. In the first case, depression was described as the rather common and normal feeling experienced when the patient realized that his drug addiction caused serious problems in his relationships with his wife and children. Getting his family involved in his treatment, facilitating their attendance at self-help meetings, helping him make amends to them and spend time with them led to improvement in his mood. In the second case, the patient's depression worsened significantly the longer she was sober from alcohol. Although she felt that some of the behavioral and cognitive strategies explored in therapy were helpful in improving her mood, it was not until she took an antidepressant that she experienced the full benefits of treatment. Both of these patients reported that an improved mood was a significant factor in their ability to prevent a subsequent relapse to addiction.

For some patients, identifying high-risk factors and developing new coping strategies for each is inadequate because they can identify many risk factors. Such patients need help in taking a more global approach to recovery and may need to learn specific problem-solving skills. Marlatt (1985c), for example, suggested that in addition to teaching patients "specific" RP skills to deal with high-risk factors, the clinician also should use "global" approaches such as problem-solving or skills-training strategies (such as behavioral rehearsal, covert modeling, and assertiveness training), cognitive reframing (such as coping imagery, reframing reactions to lapse/relapse), and lifestyle interventions (such as meditation, exercise, and relaxation).

Help patients identify and manage relapse warning signs, which are part of the process of relapse. Patients are better prepared for the challenges of recovery if they understand that relapse occurs in a context and that clues or warning signs often precede an actual lapse or relapse. Although a relapse can result from an impulsive act, it also is possible that attitudinal, emotional, cognitive, and/or behavioral changes are evident days, weeks, or even longer before the actual ingestion of substances (Daley, 2000; Marlatt, 1985d). An individual's clues or warning signs can be conceptualized as links in a relapse chain (Brownell & Rodin, 1990; Daley & Marlatt, 1997b). Warning signs may be overt and obvious, such as stopping or reducing treatment sessions or self-help meetings without discussing this decision with a therapist or sponsor, or experiencing a significant increase in strong cravings for substances. Warning signs also may be overt and idiosyncratic or unique to the patient. For example, a drug-dependent patient reported that one of his principal warning signs was the return of dishonest behaviors. His review of several past relapses helped him to discover that even before obvious signs of relapse were present, he would start to exhibit dishonest behaviors such as lying, scamming others, and stealing money from his employer. Shortly thereafter, the more obvious relapse warning signs emerged, such as thoughts of needing some action, contacting old friends who still were using drugs, dropping out of treatment, and reducing contact with Narcotics Anonymous (NA) friends and sponsor.

Patients in treatment for the first time can benefit from reviewing common relapse warning signs identified by others in recovery. The clinician can ask the patient to review the relapse experience in detail to learn the connections between thoughts, feelings, events, or situations and relapse to substance use. A survey (n=511) of an RP model developed by one of the authors, as well as a workbook used in conjunction with that program, found that "Understanding the Relapse Process" was the topic rated most useful by patients participating in a residential addiction treatment program (Daley, 1989a).

Help patients identify feelings and manage negative emotional states. Negative affective states such as depression and anxiety are factors in a substantial number of relapses (Hatsukami, Pickins et al., 1981; LaBounty, Hatsukami et al., 1992; Pickens, Hatsukami et al., 1985; Hodgins, El-Guebaly et al., 1995). Zackon (1989) believed that addicts frequently relapse as a result of joylessness in their lives. Shiffman and colleagues (1985) found that coping responses for high-risk situations were less effective for smokers who were depressed. Other negative affective states associated with relapse include anger and boredom (Rosellini & Worden, 1985, 1989; Daley, 1998). The acronym HALT, frequently cited by members of Alcoholics Anonymous (AA) and NA, speaks to this important issue of negative affect when it warns not to become too **H**ungry, too **A**ngry, too **L**onely, or too **T**ired.

Interventions that help patients develop appropriate coping skills for managing negative emotional states depend on the issues and needs of the individual. For example, strategies for dealing with the depression that accompanies the realization that addiction has caused havoc in one's life may differ from those for dealing with the more severe form of depression seen in bipolar or major depressive illness. Interventions to help the patient who occasionally gets angry and seeks solace in substances can differ from those needed to help the patient who is chronically angry. The former may need help in expressing anger appropriately rather than suppressing it, whereas the chronically angry patient may need to learn how to contain angry feelings, because such feelings often are expressed impulsively and inappropriately. The latter patient can benefit from cognitive techniques that help challenge and change angry thoughts. The chronically angry person also may benefit from seeing his or her angry disposition as a "character defect." Psychotherapy and/or use of the Twelve Step program of AA and NA are appropriate interventions to help modify such an ingrained character trait.

Interventions for patients who report feelings of chronic boredom, emptiness, or joylessness similarly depend on the specific nature of the emotional state. One patient may need help in learning how to use free time or how to have fun without substances. Another may need help in developing new relationships or finding new activities that provide a sense of meaning in life and an emotional connection to others. The patient also may need to alter beliefs about fun, excitement, and what is important in life. The authors have encountered many addicts who report that being drug-free was boring compared with the "high" provided by the drug or the behaviors associated with obtaining the drug or "living on the edge." In such a case, the patient needs to change not only behaviors, but also beliefs and attitudes.

Help patients identify and prepare to handle direct and indirect social pressures to engage in substance use. Direct and indirect social pressures often lead to increased thoughts and desires to use substances, as well as anxiety about one's ability to refuse offers to drink alcohol or use other drugs. In some instances, the patient can be taken by surprise at the strength of such pressure, especially when it is unexpected. For example, a heroin-addicted woman who had been drug-free for several months received an unplanned visit from an old friend with whom she used to get high. After the patient invited the friend to her home, the friend casually asked if she wanted to get high on crack. The patient said she did not want to do so. The friend then asked the patient if she could smoke crack in her house. The patient reluctantly agreed and, later in the evening, smoked crack herself. The next day she reflected on this experience and felt guilty for using drugs. However, she told herself that, if she was going to relapse, it might as well be on her drug of choice, so she called her dealer and bought heroin. In reviewing this experience with her clinician, the patient realized that she was not fully prepared to refuse social pressures to use drugs and thus had made two "apparently irrelevant decisions" that affected her relapse (that is, allowing her drug-using friend to enter her home and then allowing her friend to smoke crack cocaine in front of her), and that those decisions affected her relapse.

The clinician can help the patient to identify high-risk relationships (for example, living or socializing with or dating an active substance abuser) and social situations or events in which the patient may be exposed to or offered substances. The next step is to assess the effects of these social pressures on the patient's thoughts, feelings, and behaviors. Planning, practicing, and implementing coping strategies is the next step. Coping strategies include avoidance of high-risk people, situations, and events when appropriate and the use of verbal, cognitive, and behavioral skills. Rehearsing ways to refuse offers of drugs or alcohol is one practical and easy-to-use intervention. The final step of this process involves teaching the patient to evaluate the results of a given coping strategy and to modify it as needed.

Although some social situations cannot be avoided, it is not unusual for a patient to sabotage recovery by making what Marlatt refers to as "apparently irrelevant decisions" that are a "set-up" for relapse. For example, a recovering cocaine-dependent patient accepted a date with a man she knew was still using drugs and put herself in a very risky situation. An alcoholic who had been sober for several months went on a weekend golfing trip with several friends with whom he used to drink. Because the weekend trips commonly involved excessive drinking, simply accepting the invitation put himself at higher risk of relapse. Although both of these individuals successfully resisted pressures to use substances, they reported feeling extremely awkward, anxious, and "close" to using.

In some cases, pressure to use alcohol or other drugs results from relationships with active substance abusers or being part of a high-risk social network in which substance use plays a significant role. Therefore, the patient needs to assess his or her social network and, if needed, learn ways to limit or end relationships that pose a high risk of relapse (Zackon, McAuliffe et al., 1994).

Help patients improve their interpersonal communications and relationships and develop a recovery support system. Many researchers and clinicians address RP from a broader perspective that includes a focus on interpersonal relationships and support systems (Barber & Crisp, 1995; Johnson & Herringer, 1993; Havassy, Hall et al., 1991; Daley, 1996). The model of Monti and colleagues (1989) includes considerable focus on interpersonal skills such as giving and receiving criticism, refusing offers of alcohol, refusing requests, developing close and intimate relationships, and enhancing social support networks. McGrady (1989) has modified Marlatt's cognitive-behavioral model of RP and applied it to couples in recovery. O'Farrell and colleagues (1993) developed an RP protocol for use in combination with BMT. Maisto and colleagues (1995) found that alcoholics and their spouses who were treated with RP in addition to marital therapy had shorter and less severe relapses than patients not receiving RP. Daley (1989a) and Gorski and Miller (1988) emphasized the need to involve family or significant others in developing RP plans or intervening in the process of a lapse or relapse.

Positive family and social supports generally enhance recovery for the substance-dependent member. Families are more likely to support the recovery of the addicted member if they are engaged in treatment and have an opportunity to ask questions, share their concerns and experiences, learn practical coping strategies, and learn behaviors to avoid (Daley & Raskin, 1991). This opportunity is more likely to occur if the member with the SUD understands the effect of an addictive disorder on the family and makes amends for some of its adverse effects.

Patients can be encouraged to become involved in self-help support groups. Sponsors, other recovering members of self-help groups, personal friends, and employers can become part of an individual's RP network. Following are some suggested steps for helping patients develop a RP network. First, the patient needs to identify who to include in or exclude from this network. Others who abuse substances, harbor strong negative feelings toward the recovering person, or who generally are not supportive of recovery usually should be excluded. The patient then can determine how and when to ask for support or help. Behavioral rehearsal can help the patient practice ways to make specific requests for support. Rehearsal also helps to increase confidence and clarify thoughts and feelings about reaching out for help. Some patients feel guilty or ashamed and question whether they deserve the support of others. Other patients have such strong pride that asking for support is very difficult. Rehearsal can help to clarify the patient's ambivalence about asking for help or support from others. This process helps the patient better understand how the person being asked for support can respond, thus preparing the patient for potentially negative responses from others.

Some patients find it helpful to put their action plan into writing. The action plan can address the following issues: how to communicate about and deal with relapse warning signs and high-risk situations, how to interrupt a lapse, how to intervene if a relapse occurs, and the importance of exploring all the details of a lapse/relapse after the patient is stable so that it can be used as a learning experience. A plan can make both the recovering person and family feel more in control, even when faced with the possibility of an actual relapse. The plan helps everyone involved take a proactive approach to recovery, rather than waiting passively for the problem to worsen.

Assess patients for psychiatric comorbidities and facilitate treatment for any coexisting disorders. Numerous studies and clinical reports have noted the high rates of co-occurring psychiatric disorders among patients with SUDs (Robins & Regier, 1991; Kessler, McGonagle et al., 1994; Daley & Moss, 2002; O'Connell & Beyer, 2002). Patients with dual diagnosis are at higher risk of relapse to substance use than those with only a substance use diagnosis because of the effect of psychiatric symptoms on motivation, judgment, and functioning. In addition, patients with dual diagnosis who resume substance use frequently fail to adhere to psychiatric treatment and comply poorly with pharmacotherapy, psychotherapy, and/or self-help program attendance. RP strategies can be adapted to the problems and symptoms of the patient's psychiatric disorder. Monitoring moods or behaviors, enhancing social support systems, participating in pleasant activities, developing routine and structure in daily life, learning to cope with persistent psychiatric symptoms associated with chronic or recurrent forms of psychiatric illness, and identifying early warning signs of psychiatric relapse and developing appropriate coping strategies are helpful interventions for patients with dual diagnosis (Daley & Lis, 1995; Daley, 1994; Daley & Roth, 2001).

Negative mood states that are part of a major mood or anxiety disorder may require pharmacotherapy in addition to psychotherapy and involvement in self-help programs. Patients on medications for these or other psychiatric disorders also benefit from developing strategies for dealing with well-meaning members of self-help programs who pressure them to stop their medication use because it is perceived as detrimental to recovery from their SUD.

Help patients understand and manage their cravings to use substances as well as "cues" that trigger cravings. A strong desire or craving for a substance can be triggered by exposure to environmental or internal cues associated with prior use. Cues such as the sight or smell of the substance can trigger cravings that are evidenced in increased thoughts of using and physiologic changes (for example, anxiety). Research has not been able to establish craving as predictive of relapse. One reason for this could be that the concept of craving is not clearly defined across autonomic, behavioral, or subjective domains. Further, trials looking at craving and relapse may be measuring different aspects of the phenomenon (Drummond, Litten et al., 2000). What is clear is that craving has clinical meaning, and medications are being developed and used in conjunction with therapy or counseling to reduce craving (Li, 2000; Meyer, 2000).

Volkow and Fowler (2000) have presented a theory of addiction and relapse that derives from positron emission tomography studies. They hypothesize that the dopamine stimulation that occurs with long-term drug use leads to disruption of brain circuitry involved in regulating drives. This disruption, in turn, leads to a conditioned response (that is, craving) when exposed to stimuli, which leads to compulsive drug-taking (Stuss & Benson, 1986; Volkow, Ding et al., 1996; Volkow & Fowler, 2000; O'Brien, Childress et al., 1998; McKay, 1999).

CE treatment (NIDA, 1993) is one method used to help patients identify drug-use triggers and master or learn to control the conditioned response to those triggers. This treatment differs from the traditional focus on "avoiding people, places, and things" and instead involves exposing the patient to specific cues associated with substance use. CE aims to enhance behavioral and cognitive coping skills as well as the patient's confidence in his or her ability to resist the desire to use. Systematic relaxation, behavioral alternatives, visual imagery, and cognitive interventions are used in CE. Several studies have validated CE (McCusker & Brown, 1995; Monti, Rohsenow et al., 1993; Drummond & Glautier, 1994; O'Brien, Childress et al., 1990; Staiger, Greeley et al., 1999).

The clinician can provide information about cues and how they trigger cravings for alcohol or other drugs. Monitoring and recording cravings, associated thoughts, and outcomes in a daily log or journal can help patients become more vigilant and prepare them to cope when they occur. Cognitive interventions include changing thoughts about the craving or desire to use, challenging euphoric recall, talking oneself through the craving, thinking beyond the high by identifying negative consequences of using (immediate and delayed) and positive benefits of not using, using AA/NA/ Cocaine Anonymous recovery slogans, and delaying the decision to use. Behavioral interventions include avoiding, leaving, or changing situations that trigger or worsen a craving; redirecting activities or becoming involved in pleasant activities; obtaining help or support from others by admitting and talking about cravings and hearing how others have survived them; attending self-help support group meetings; or taking medications such as disulfiram (Antabuse®) or naltrexone (ReVia®) that reduce craving and increase confidence in the ability to cope.

Marlatt (1985a) described an interesting experiential strategy for managing craving. The patient is instructed to "detach" from his or her craving by externalizing and labeling it. Similar to a surfer who must learn to ride the waves so as not to get wiped out, the addicted patient imagines "riding the crest" of an urge or craving, maintaining balance until the crest has finally broken and the wave of feeling

subsides. The CE model includes a similar strategy, in which the patient uses "mastery imagery" to view himself or herself defeating the craving, for example, by driving a large tank and crushing the craving (NIDA, 1993).

Help patients identify and manage patterns of thinking that increase relapse risk. Cognitive distortions or errors in thinking are associated with mental health disorders (Beck, 1976) and SUDs (Beck, Wright et al., 1994; Ellis, McInerney et al., 1988) and have been implicated in relapse (Marlatt, 1985c, 1985d). Marlatt (1985b) observed that "the patient's cognitive errors and distortions may increase the probability that an initial slip will develop into a total relapse" (p. 250). Twelve Step programs refer to these patterns as "stinking thinking" and suggest that recovering persons need to alter their thinking if they are to remain alcohol- and drug-free.

Teaching patients to identify their negative thinking patterns or cognitive errors (for example, black-and-white thinking, overgeneralizing, catastrophizing, jumping to conclusions, and so forth) and to evaluate how these affect recovery and relapse is one strategy. Patients then can be taught to use counter-thoughts to challenge their thinking errors or specific negative thoughts. One way to achieve this is to have the patient discuss or write down (1) specific relapse-related thoughts (for example, "relapse can't happen to me"; "I'll never use alcohol or drugs again"; "I can control my use of alcohol or other drugs"; "a few drinks, tokes, pills, lines won't hurt"; "recovery isn't happening fast enough"; "I need alcohol or other drugs to have fun"; and "my problem is cured"); (2) what is wrong with such thinking in terms of potential effect on relapse; and (3) new self-statements or thoughts that counteract negative thinking (Daley & Marlatt, 1997c).

Many of the AA and NA slogans were devised to help alcoholics and drug addicts alter their thinking and survive desires to use substances. Slogans such as "this too will pass," "let go and let God," and "one day at a time" have helped many patients manage thoughts of using.

Help patients work toward a more balanced lifestyle. In addition to identifying and managing intrapersonal and interpersonal high-risk relapse factors, patients can benefit from global changes to restore or achieve balance in their lives (Marlatt, 1985e; Wanigaratne, 1990). Development of a healthy lifestyle is seen as important in reducing stress that makes the patient more vulnerable to relapse. Lifestyle can be assessed by evaluating patterns of daily activities, sources of stress, stressful life events, daily hassles and uplifts, the balance between wants (activities engaged in for pleasure or self-fulfillment) and shoulds (external demands), health, exercise and relaxation patterns, interpersonal activities, and religious beliefs (Marlatt, 1985e). Helping patients to develop positive habits or substitute indulgences (such as jogging, meditation, relaxation, exercise, hobbies, or creative tasks) for an addictive disorder can help to balance their lifestyles (O'Connell & Alexander, 1994). Patients with a need for greater adventure or action may become involved in more challenging activities (Daley, 1987; George, 1989).

Combine pharmacologic adjuncts with psychosocial treatments. Some patients benefit from pharmacologic interventions to attenuate or reduce cravings for alcohol or other drugs, enhance motivation to stay sober, and increase confidence in their ability to resist relapse or reduce the severity of an actual relapse (Volpicelli, Alterman et al., 1992; NIDA, 1999; NIAAA, 2000). A review of 375 articles, including 41 studies by Garbutt and colleagues (1999), found that naltrexone and acamprosate are the most helpful pharmacologic adjuncts for use with alcoholics. Patients who were given naltrexone were much less likely to continue drinking than were control subjects. In a study of naltrexone combined with coping skills/RP training (N+RP) or supportive therapy (N+ST), O'Malley and colleagues (1992) found that subjects in the N+RP arm who returned to drinking were less likely to experience a relapse to heavy drinking than were those who received N+ST.

Medications for opiates include agonist or substitution therapy with methadone or levo-alpha-acetylmethadol (LAAM) (APA, 1995). These medications are designed to reduce drug craving and decrease illicit substance use. LAAM dosing can be as infrequent as three times a week, compared with daily dosing with methadone (Tennant, Rawson et al., 1986). The opiate antagonist naltrexone can be used to block the euphoric effects of opiate drugs, which can lead to an extinction of drug craving (Wikler, 1973; Wikler & Pesco, 1967). Adherence to oral naltrexone regimens sometimes is a problem, and an injectable form of this medication is under development. Buprenorphine (Buprenex®), a mixed agonist-antagonist with less abuse potential, has been found to reduce relapse risk among opiate addicts (Ling, Wesson et al., 1996; Pani, Maremmani et al., 2000).

A survey of AA members' attitudes about taking a medication to help prevent relapse yielded an interesting finding. Only 17% of the 277 AA members surveyed believed they should *not* take a medication; more than 50% of the sample thought medication that helped reduce drinking was a good idea (Rychtarik, Connors et al., 2000).

Treatment of psychiatric symptoms with appropriate medications has important implications for recovery and reducing relapse risk. Kranzler and colleagues (1994) conducted a randomized, 12-week, placebo-controlled trial of buspirone in 61 anxious alcoholics who also received weekly RP. Patients receiving buspirone showed greater retention in treatment at 12 weeks, as well as reduced anxiety, a slower return to heavy alcohol use, and fewer drinking days than those who received placebo. In a randomized, controlled, double-blind clinical trial of 100 alcoholic patients, Gottlieb and colleagues (1994) found that, among the 57 high-risk patients who reported cravings for alcohol at baseline, relapse rates were 90% for patients receiving placebo compared with 65% for those receiving atenolol, a beta-adrenergic blocker. This study also found that poor treatment adherence was strongly associated with adverse outcomes. A series of pilot studies and clinical trials of patients with dual diagnosis conducted by the authors' research group at the University of Pittsburgh Medical Center found that fluoxetine was effective in decreasing both depressive symptoms and alcohol use among severely depressed alcoholics (Cornelius, Salloum et al., 1993). The authors also found that patients with dual diagnoses who had only a partial response to a selective serotonin reuptake inhibitor benefitted from the addition of naltrexone to their treatment (Salloum, Cornelius et al., 1998). The authors currently are conducting two double-blind, placebo-controlled studies, one with selective serotonin reuptake inhibitors plus naltrexone for depressed alcoholics and another with lithium with or without valproate for bipolar alcoholics.

Prepare patients to interrupt lapses and relapses as early as possible in the process to minimize damage caused by setbacks. Patients should have an emergency plan to follow if they lapse so that a full-blown relapse can be avoided. However, if a full-blown relapse occurs, the patient needs to have strategies to interrupt it. The specific intervention strategies should be based on the severity of the patient's lapse or relapse, coping mechanisms, and prior history of relapse. Helpful interventions include using self-talk or behavioral procedures to stop a lapse or relapse; asking family, AA or NA sponsors, friends, or professionals for help; carrying an emergency card with names and phone numbers of others who can be called on for support; or carrying a reminder card that gives specific instructions as to what to do if a lapse or relapse occurs (Daley, 2000; Marlatt, 1985d). Marlatt recommends developing a relapse contract with patients that outlines specific steps to take in the event of a future relapse. The aim of this contract is to formalize or reinforce the patient's commitment to change.

Once a relapsed patient is stable, analyzing lapses or relapses is a valuable process that can aid in ongoing recovery. The patient can identify warning signs that preceded actual substance use, as well as the high-risk factors that could have played a role in the relapse. This process can help the patient reframe a "failure" as a "learning" experience and prepare for future high-risk situations. It also can help the patient determine if any irrelevant decisions were made that affected relapse.

Facilitate the transition between levels of care for patients completing residential or hospital-based IPT programs, or structured partial hospital (PH) or intensive outpatient programs (IOP). Patients can make significant gains in residential or day treatment programs only to have the gains negated because of failure to adhere to ongoing outpatient or aftercare treatment. Interventions used to enhance treatment entry and adherence that also lower the risk of relapse include providing a single session of motivational therapy before discharge from IPT, using telephone or mail reminders of initial treatment appointments, and providing reinforcers for appropriate participation in treatment activities or for providing drug-free urine tests (Kadden & Mauriello, 1991; Miller & Rollnick, 1991; Higgins & Silverman, 1999). In a quality improvement survey, the authors found that a single motivational therapy session provided to hospitalized psychiatric patients with comorbid SUDs led to a nearly twofold increase in the show rate for the initial outpatient appointment (Daley & Zuckoff, 1999). Patients who complied with their initial appointment had a reduced risk of treatment dropout and subsequent psychiatric and/or substance use relapse.

Incorporate strategies to improve adherence to treatment. Numerous studies and reports show that patients who are retained in treatment show better outcomes, including lower relapse rates, than those who drop out early (NIDA, 1997a, 1997b). Many clinical and systems strategies have been shown to improve adherence to treatment among patients with SUDs and dual disorders (Daley & Zuckoff, 1999; NIAAA, 1998).

CONCLUSIONS

A variety of clinical treatment models and specialized RP approaches have been developed for patients with SUDs, both to reduce relapse risk and to improve psychosocial functioning. Many of the cognitive and behavioral interventions described in these RP approaches can be adapted for use with patients who have additional problems, such as other compulsive disorders, impulse control disorders, or comorbid psychiatric illnesses. RP interventions aim to help patients maintain change over time and address the most common issues and problems raising vulnerability to relapse. RP also aims to help patients make broader lifestyle changes that reduce stress and facilitate personal growth and satisfaction.

Studies indicate that RP has efficacy in reducing both relapse rates and the severity of lapses or relapses. Clinical RP strategies can be used throughout the continuum of care in primary rehabilitation programs, halfway houses, or therapeutic community programs, as well as in outpatient and aftercare programs. In addition, family members can be included in educational and therapy sessions and involved in the development of RP plans for members with SUDs. Pharmacotherapy added to RP is also helpful to some patients.

Many of the RP approaches described in the literature are short-term or brief treatments and can be provided in individual or group sessions, making them attractive and cost-effective. Most clinical models of RP are supported by user-friendly, interactive recovery materials such as books, workbooks, videos, and audiotapes. These supplemental materials provide additional information and support to patients, who can learn to use self-management techniques of RP on their own, after completion of formal treatment.

ACKNOWLEDGMENTS: The authors gratefully acknowledge Cindy Hurney, administrative manager at the Center for Psychiatric and Chemical Dependency Services, for her help in preparing this manuscript, and Dr. Allan Graham and Bonnie Wilford for their editorial suggestions.

Preparation of this chapter was supported in part by grant DA09421-04 from the National Institute on Drug Abuse and grant AA11929 from the National Institute on Alcohol Abuse and Alcoholism.

REFERENCES

American Psychiatric Association (APA) (1995). Practice guidelines for the treatment of patients with substance use disorders: Alcohol, cocaine, opioids. *Supplement to American Journal of Psychiatry* 152(11).

Allsop S, Sanders B & Phillips M (2000). The process of relapse in severely dependent male problem drinkers. *Addiction* 95(1):95-106.

Annis H (1986). A relapse prevention model for treatment of alcoholics. In W Miller & N Heather (eds.) *Treating Addictive Behaviors: Process of Change.* New York, NY: Plenum Books.

Annis H (1991). A cognitive-social learning approach to relapse: Pharmacotherapy and relapse prevention counseling. *Alcohol and Alcoholism* 1(Suppl):527-530.

Barber JG & Crisp BR (1995). Social support and prevention of relapse following treatment for alcohol abuse. *Research on Social Work Practice* 5(3):283-296.

Beck A (1976). *Cognitive Therapy and the Emotional Disorders.* New York, NY: New American Library.

Beck A, Wright F & Liese B (1994). *Cognitive Therapy of Substance Abuse.* New York, NY: Guilford Press.

Brown S (1995). *Treating the Alcoholic: A Developmental Model of Recovery, 2nd Edition.* New York, NY: John Wiley & Sons.

Brownell K & Rodin J (1990). *The Weight Maintenance Survival Guide.* Dallas, TX: The LEARN Education Center.

Carroll KM (1996). Relapse prevention as a psychosocial treatment: A review of controlled clinical trials. *Experimental and Clinical Psychopharmacology* 4(1):46-54.

Carroll KM, Rounsaville BJ & Gawin FH (1991). A comparative trial of psychotherapies for ambulatory cocaine abusers: Relapse prevention and interpersonal psychotherapy. *American Journal of Drug and Alcohol Abuse* 17(3):229-247.

Carroll KM, Rounsaville BJ, Nich C et al. (1994). One-year follow-up of psychotherapy and pharmacotherapy for cocaine dependence. Delayed emergence of psychotherapy effects. *Archives of General Psychiatry* 51(12):989-997.

Catalano R, Howard M, Hawkins J et al. (1988). Relapse in the addictions: Rates, determinants, and promising prevention strategies. *1988 Surgeon General's Report On Health Consequences Of Smoking.* Washington, DC: Office of Smoking and Health, Department of Health and Human Services.

Center for Substance Abuse Treatment (CSAT) (1999). Treatment succeeds in fighting crime. In *Substance Abuse in Brief.* Rockville, MD: CSAT, Substance Abuse and Mental Health Services Administration (December).

Center for Substance Abuse Treatment (CSAT) (2000a). Substance abuse treatment reduces family dysfunction, improves productivity. In *Substance Abuse in Brief.* Rockville, MD: CSAT, Substance Abuse and Mental Health Services Administration (April).

Center for Substance Abuse Treatment (CSAT) (2000b). Treatment cuts medical costs. In *Substance Abuse in Brief.* Rockville, MD: CSAT, Substance Abuse and Mental Health Services Administration (May).

Chaney E & O'Leary M (1978). Skill training with alcoholics. *Journal of Consulting and Clinical Psychology* 46(5):1092-1104.

Connors GJ, Longabaugh R & Miller WR (1996). Looking forward and back to relapse: Implications for research and practice. *Addiction* 91(Suppl):191-196.

Connors GJ, Maisto SA & Donovan DM (1996). Conceptualizations of relapse: A summary of psychological and psychobiological models. *Addiction* 91(Suppl):S5-S13.

Cornelius JR, Salloum IM, Cornelius MD et al. (1993). Fluoxetine trial in suicidal depressed alcoholics. *Psychopharmacology Bulletin* 29:195-199.

Cornelius JR, Salloum IM, Day NL et al. (1996). Patterns of suicidality and alcohol use in alcoholics with major depression. *Alcoholism: Clinical & Experimental Research* 20:1451-1455.

Cornelius JR, Perkins KA, Salloum IM et al. (1999). Fluoxetine vs. Placebo for the smoking of depressed alcoholics. *Journal of Clinical Psychopharmacology* 19:183-184.

Daley DC (1987). *Relapse: A Guide for Successful Recovery.* Bradenton, FL: Human Services Institute.

Daley DC (1988). *Relapse Prevention: Treatment Alternatives and Counseling Aids.* Bradenton, FL: Human Services Institute.

Daley DC (1989a). Five perspectives on relapse in chemical dependency. *Journal of Chemical Dependency Treatment* 2(2):3-26.

Daley DC, ed. (1989b). *Relapse: Conceptual, Research and Clinical Perspectives.* New York, NY: Haworth Medical Publishing.

Daley DC (1994). *Preventing Relapse.* Center City, MN: Hazelden.

Daley DC (1996). *Improving Communication and Relationships.* Holmes Beach, FL: Learning Publications.

Daley DC (1998). *Coping With Feelings Workbook, Revised Edition.* Holmes Beach, FL: Learning Publications.

Daley DC (2000). *Relapse Prevention Workbook for Recovering Alcoholics and Drug Dependent Persons, 3rd Edition.* Holmes Beach, FL: Learning Publications.

Daley DC (2001). Substance use disorders. In DC Daley & IM Salloum (eds.) *A Clinician's Guide to Mental Illness.* New York, NY: McGraw Hill/Hazelden.

Daley DC & Lis J (1995). Relapse prevention: Intervention strategies for mental health clients with comorbid addictive disorders. In A Washton (ed.) *Psychotherapy and Substance Abuse: A Practitioner's Handbook.* New York, NY: Guilford Press, 243-263.

Daley DC & Marlatt GA (1997a). Relapse prevention: Cognitive and behavioral interventions. In J Lowinson, P Ruiz, RB Millman et al. (eds.) *Substance Abuse: A Comprehensive Textbook, 3rd Edition.* Baltimore, MD: Williams & Wilkins, 458-466.

Daley DC & Marlatt GA (1997b). *Therapist's Guide for Managing Your Alcohol or Drug Problem.* San Antonio, TX: Psychological Corporation.

Daley DC & Marlatt GA (1997c). *Managing Your Alcohol or Drug Problem.* San Antonio, TX: Psychological Corporation.

Daley DC & Miller J (2001). *Addiction in Your Family: Helping Yourself and Your Loved Ones.* Holmes Beach, FL: Learning Publications.

Daley DC & Moss HB (2002). *Dual Disorders: Counseling Clients with Chemical Dependency and Mental Illness, 3rd Edition.* Center City, MN: Hazelden.

Daley DC & Raskin MS (1991). *Treating the Chemically Dependent and Their Families.* Newbury Park, CA: Sage Publications.

Daley DC & Ross JR (2000). *Relapse Prevention Workbook for Sexually Compulsive Behavior.* Holmes Beach, FL: Learning Publications.

Daley DC & Roth L (2001). *When Symptoms Return: A Guide to Relapse in Psychiatric Illness, 2nd Edition.* Holmes Beach, FL: Learning Publications.

Daley DC & Zuckoff A (1999). *Improving Treatment Compliance: Counseling and System Strategies for Substance Use and Dual Disorders.* Center City, MN: Hazelden.

Daley DC, Salloum IM & Spotts CE (1996). Survey of relapse factors among dual diagnosis outpatients (unpublished data). Quality Improvement Study.

Daley DC, Salloum IM, Zuckoff A et al. (1998). Increasing treatment compliance among outpatients with depression and cocaine dependence: Results of a pilot study. *American Journal of Psychiatry* 155:1611-1613.

DeLeon G (1990-91). Aftercare in therapeutic communities. Special issue: Relapse prevention in substance misuse. *International Journal of the Addictions* 25(9A-10A):1225-1237.

Dimeff LA & Marlatt GA (1995). Relapse prevention. In R Hester & W Miller (eds.) *Handbook of Alcoholism Treatment Approaches, 2nd Edition.* Boston, MA: Allyn & Bacon, 176-194.

Dimeff LA & Marlatt GA (1998). Preventing relapse and maintaining change in addictive behaviors. *Clinical Psychology: Science and Practice* 5(4):513-525.

Drummond DC & Glautier S (1994). A controlled trial of cue-exposure treatment in alcohol dependence. *Journal of Consulting and Clinical Psychology* 62(4):809-817.

Drummond DC, Litten RZ, Lowman C et al. (2000). Craving research: Future directions. *Addiction* 95(Suppl 2):S247-255.

Ellis A, McInerney J, DiGiuseppe R et al. (1988). *Rational-Emotive Therapy with Alcoholics and Substance Abusers.* New York, NY: Pergamon.

Emrick C (1974). A review of psychologically oriented treatment of alcoholism. *Journal of Studies on Alcohol* 35:523-549.

Garbutt JC, West SL, Carey TS et al. (1999). Pharmacological treatment of alcohol dependence: A review of the evidence. *Journal of the American Medical Association* 281(14):1318-1325.

George W (1989). Marlatt and Gordon's relapse prevention model. *Journal of Chemical Dependency Treatment* 3(2):125-152.

Goldstein MG, Niaura R, Follick MJ et al. (1989). Effects of behavioral skills training and schedule of nicotine gum administration on smoking cessation. *American Journal of Psychiatry* 146(1):56-60.

Gondolf EW (2001). *Relapse, Reuniting, and Progress.* Holmes Beach, FL: Learning Publications.

Gorski T (1986). Relapse prevention planning: A new recovery tool. *Alcohol Health and Research World* 1:6-11.

Gorski T (2000). The CENAPS model of relapse prevention therapy (CMRPT). *Approaches to Drug Abuse Counseling.* Rockville, MD: National Institute on Drug Abuse.

Gorski TT & Kelly JM (1996) *Counselor's Manual for Relapse Prevention with Chemically Dependent Criminal Offenders.* Rockville, MD: Substance Abuse and Mental Health Services Administration.

Gorski T & Miller M (1988). *Staying Sober Workbook.* Independence, MO: Independence Press.

Gottlieb LD, Horwitz RI, Kraus ML et al. (1994). Randomized controlled trial in alcohol relapse prevention: Role of atenolol, alcohol craving, and treatment adherence. *Journal of Substance Abuse Treatment* 11(3):253-258.

Graham K, Annis H, Brett P et al. (1996). A controlled field trial of group versus individual cognitive-behavioural training for relapse prevention. *Addiction* 91(8):1127-1139.

Hatsukami D, Pickins R & Svikis D (1981). Post-treatment depressive symptoms and relapse to drug use in different age groups of an alcohol and other drug abuse population. *Drug and Alcohol Dependence* 8(4):271-277.

Havassy BE, Hall SM & Wasserman DA (1991). Social support and relapse: Commonalities among alcoholics, opiate users, and cigarette smokers. *Addictive Behaviors* 16(5):235-246.

Higgins ST & Silverman K, eds. (1999). *Motivating Behavior Change Among Illicit Drug Abusers: Research on Contingency Management.* Washington, DC: American Psychological Association.

Hodgins DC, El-Guebaly N & Armstrong S (1995). Prospective and retrospective reports of mood states before relapse to substance use. *Journal of Consulting and Clinical Psychology* 63:400-407.

Hoffmann N & Harrison P (1986). *CATOR 1986 Report: Findings Two Years After Treatment.* St. Paul, MN: CATOR.

Hoffmann N & Harrison P (1989). Relapse: Conceptual and methodological issues. *Journal of Chemical Dependency Treatment* 2(2):27-52.

Hoffmann NG & Miller NS (1992). Treatment outcomes for abstinence-based programs. *Psychiatric Annals* 22(8):402-408.

Hunt W, Barnett L & Branch L (1971). Relapse rates in addiction programs. *Journal of Clinical Psychology* 27:455-456.

Irvin JE, Bowers CA, Dunn ME et al. (1999). Efficacy of relapse prevention: A meta-analytic review. *Journal of Consulting and Clinical Psychology* 67(4):563-570.

Ito JR, Donovan DM & Hall JJ (1988). Relapse prevention and alcohol aftercare: Effects on drinking outcome, change process, and aftercare attendance. *British Journal of Addiction* 83:171-181.

Johnson E & Herringer LG (1993). A note on the utilization of common support activities and relapse following substance abuse treatment. *Journal of Psychology* 127(1):73-77.

Kadden RM & Mauriello IJ (1991). Enhancing participation in substance abuse treatment using an incentive system. *Journal of Substance Abuse Treatment* 8:133-144.

Kessler RC, McGonagle KA, Zhao S et al. (1994). Lifetime and 12-month prevalence of DSM-IIIR psychiatric disorders in the United States. Results from the National Comorbidity Survey. *Archives of General Psychiatry* 51:8-19.

Koski-Jannes A (1992). *Alcohol Addiction and Self-Regulation: A Controlled Trial of Relapse Prevention Program for Finnish Inpatient Alcoholics.* Helsinki, Finland: The Finnish Foundation for Alcohol Studies.

Kranzler HR, Burleson JA, Del Boca FK et al. (1994). Buspirone treatment of anxious alcoholics. A placebo-controlled trial. *Archives of General Psychiatry* 51(9):720-731.

Kranzler HR, Burleson JA, Korner P et al. (1995). Placebo-controlled trial of fluoxetine as an adjunct to relapse prevention in alcoholics. *American Journal of Psychiatry* 152(3):391-397.

LaBounty LP, Hatsukami D, Morgan SF et al. (1992). Relapse among alcoholics with phobic and panic symptoms. *Addictive Behaviors* 17(1):9-15.

Laws DR, Hudson SM & Ward T, eds. (2000). *Remaking Relapse Prevention with Sex Offenders.* Thousand Oaks, CA: Sage Publications.

Li TK (2000). Clinical perspectives for the study of craving and relapse in animal models. *Addiction* 95(Suppl 2):S55-S60.

Ling W, Wesson DR, Charuvastra C et al. (1996). A controlled trial comparing buprenorphine and methadone maintenance in opioid dependence. *Archives of General Psychiatry* 53:401-407.

Maisto SA, McKay JR & O'Farrell TJ (1995). Relapse precipitants and behavioral marital therapy. *Addictive Behaviors* 20(3):383-393.

Marlatt GA (1985a). Relapse prevention: Theoretical rationale and overview of the model. In GA Marlatt & J Gordon (eds.) *Relapse Prevention: A Self-Control Strategy for the Maintenance of Behavior Change*. New York, NY: Guilford, 3-70.

Marlatt GA (1985b). Situational determinants of relapse and skill-training interventions. In GA Marlatt & J Gordon (eds.) *Relapse Prevention: A Self-Control Strategy for the Maintenance of Behavior Change*. New York, NY: Guilford, 71-127.

Marlatt GA (1985c). Cognitive factors in the relapse process. In GA Marlatt & J Gordon (eds.) *Relapse Prevention: A Self-Control Strategy for the Maintenance of Behavior Change*. New York, NY: Guilford, 128-200.

Marlatt GA (1985d). Cognitive assessment and intervention procedures for relapse prevention. In GA Marlatt & J Gordon (eds.) *Relapse Prevention: A Self-Control Strategy for the Maintenance of Behavior Change*. New York, NY: Guilford, 201-279.

Marlatt GA (1985e). Lifestyle modification. In GA Marlatt & J Gordon (eds.) *Relapse Prevention: A Self-Control Strategy for the Maintenance of Behavior Change*. New York, NY: Guilford, 280-350.

Marlatt GA (1996a). Taxonomy of high-risk situations for alcohol relapse: Evolution and development of a cognitive-behavioral model. *Addiction* 91(Suppl 1):S37-S49.

Marlatt GA (1996b). Lest taxonomy become taxidermy: A comment on the relapse replication and extension project. *Addiction* 91(Suppl 1):147-154.

Marlatt GA & Gordon J, eds. (1985). *Relapse Prevention: A Self-control Strategy for the Maintenance of Behavior Change*. New York, NY: Guilford Press.

Marlatt GA, Barrett K & Daley DC (1999). Relapse prevention. In M Galanter & HD Kleber (eds.) *Textbook of Substance Abuse, 2nd Edition*. Washington, DC: American Psychiatric Press, 353-365.

The Matrix Center (1989). *The Neurobehavioral Treatment Model Volume II: Group Sessions*. Beverly Hills, CA: Matrix Center.

McCusker CG & Brown K (1995). Cue-exposure to alcohol-associated stimuli reduces autonomic reactivity, but not craving and anxiety, in dependent drinkers. *Alcohol and Alcoholism* 30(3):319-327.

McGrady B (1989). Extending relapse prevention to couples. *Addictive Behaviors* 14:69-74.

McKay JR (1999). Studies of factors of relapse to alcohol, drug, and nicotine use: A critical review of methodologies and findings. *Journal of Studies on Alcohol* 60:566-576.

McKay JR, Alterman AI, Cacciola JS et al. (1997). Group counseling versus individualized relapse prevention aftercare following intensive outpatient treatment for cocaine dependence: Initial results. *Journal of Consulting and Clinical Psychology* 65(5):778-788.

McKay JR, Alterman AI, Cacciola JS et al. (1999a). Continuing care for cocaine dependence: Comprehensive 2-year outcomes. *Journal of Consulting and Clinical Psychology* 67(3):420-427.

McKay JR, Alterman AI, Rutherford MJ et al. (1999b). The relationship of alcohol use to cocaine relapse in cocaine dependent patients in an aftercare study. *Journal of Studies on Alcohol* 60(2):176-180.

McKay JR, Rutherford MJ, Alterman AI et al. (1995). An examination of the cocaine relapse process. *Drug and Alcohol Dependence* 38(1):35-43.

McLellan AT, Lewis DC, O'Brien CP et al. (2000). Drug dependence, a chronic medical illness: Implications for treatment, insurance, and outcomes evaluation. *Journal of the American Medical Association* 284(13):1689-1695.

Meyer RE (2000). Craving: What can be done to bring the insights of neuroscience, behavioral science and clinical science into synchrony. *Addiction* 95(Suppl 2):S219-S227.

Miller W & Hester R (1980). Treating the problem drinker: Modern approaches. *The Addictive Behaviors: Treatment of Alcoholism, Drug Abuse, Smoking and Obesity*. New York, NY: Pergamon Press.

Miller WR & Rollnick S (1991). *Motivational Interviewing: Preparing People to Change Addictive Behavior*. New York, NY: Guilford Press.

Miller WR, Brown JM, Simpson TL et al. (1995). What works? A methodological analysis of the alcohol treatment outcome literature. In R Hester & W Miller (eds.) *Handbook of Alcoholism Treatment Approaches, 2nd Edition*. Boston, MA: Allyn & Bacon, 12-44.

Miller WT, Westerberg VS, Harris RJ et al. (1996). What predicts relapse? Prospective testing of antecedent models. *Addiction* 91(Suppl):S155-S171.

Monti P, Adams D, Kadden R et al. (1989). *Treating Alcohol Dependence*. New York, NY: Guilford Press.

Monti PM, Rohsenow DJ, Rubonis AV et al. (1993). Cue exposure with coping skills treatment for male alcoholics: A preliminary investigation. *Journal of Clinical and Consulting Psychology* 61(6):1011-1019.

National Institute on Alcohol Abuse and Alcoholism (NIAAA) (1995a). *Cognitive-Behavioral Coping Skills Therapy Manual: A Clinical Research Guide for Therapists Treating Individuals with Alcohol Abuse and Dependence*. Rockville, MD: NIAAA, National Institutes of Health.

National Institute on Alcohol Abuse and Alcoholism (NIAAA) (1995b). *Twelve Step Facilitation Therapy Manual: A Clinical Research Guide for Therapists Treating Individuals with Alcohol Abuse and Dependence*. Rockville, MD: NIAAA, National Institutes of Health.

National Institute on Alcohol Abuse and Alcoholism (NIAAA) (1998). *Strategies for Facilitating Protocol Compliance in Alcoholism Treatment Research*. Rockville, MD: NIAAA, National Institutes of Health.

National Institute on Alcohol Abuse and Alcoholism (NIAAA) (2000). Highlights from the 10th Special Report to Congress. *Alcohol Research & Health* 24(1).

National Institute on Drug Abuse (NIDA) (1993). *Cue Extinction Techniques: NIDA Technology Transfer Package*. Rockville, MD: NIDA, National Institutes of Health.

National Institute on Drug Abuse (NIDA) (1994). *Recovery Training and Self-Help, 2nd Edition*. Rockville, MD: NIDA, National Institutes of Health.

National Institute on Drug Abuse (NIDA) (1997a). Beyond the therapeutic alliance: Keeping the drug-dependent individual in treatment. In L Simon Onken, JD Blaine & JJ Boren (eds.) *NIDA Research Monograph 165*. Rockville, MD: NIDA, National Institutes of Health.

National Institute on Drug Abuse (NIDA) (1997b). Study sheds new light on the state of drug abuse treatment nationwide. *NIDA Notes* 12(5):1-8.

National Institute on Drug Abuse (NIDA) (1999). *Principles of Drug Addiction Treatment: A Research-Based Guide*. Rockville, MD: NIDA, National Institutes of Health.

National Institute on Drug Abuse (NIDA) (2000). *Individual Drug Counseling for Cocaine Addiction: The Cocaine Collaborative Model*. Rockville, MD: NIDA, National Institutes of Health.

National Institute on Drug Abuse (NIDA) (2001). *Group Drug Counseling for Cocaine Dependence: The Cocaine Collaborative Model*. Rockville, MD: NIDA, National Institutes of Health.

Nigam R, Schottenfeld R & Kosten TR (1992). Treatment of dual diagnosis patients: A relapse prevention group approach. *Journal of Substance Abuse Treatment* 9(4):305-309.

Obert JL, McCann MJ, Marinelli-Casey P et al. (2000). The matrix model of outpatient stimulant abuse treatment: History and description. *Journal of Psychoactive Drugs* 32(2):157-164.

O'Brien CP, Childress AR, Ehrman R et al. (1998). Conditioning factors in drug abuse: Can they explain compulsion? *Psychopharmacology* 12:15-22.

O'Brien CP, Childress AR, McLellan T et al. (1990). Integrating systematic cue exposure with standard treatment in recovering drug dependent patients. *Addictive Behaviors* 15(4):355-365.

O'Connell D & Beyer E, eds. (2002). *Managing the Dually Diagnosed Patient, 2nd Edition*. New York, NY: Haworth Medical Publishing.

O'Connell DF & Alexander CN (1994). *Self Recovery Treating Addictions Using Transcendental Meditation and Maharishi Ayur-Veda*. New York, NY: Haworth Press.

O'Farrell TJ (1993). Couples relapse prevention sessions after a behavioral marital therapy couples group program. In TJ O'Farrell (ed.) *Treating Alcohol Problems: Marital and Family Interventions*. New York, NY: Guilford Press, 305-326.

O'Farrell TJ, Choquette KA, Cutter HS et al. (1993). Behavioral marital therapy with and without additional couples relapse prevention sessions for alcoholics and their wives. *Journal of Studies on Alcohol* 54(6):652-666.

O'Malley SS, Jaffe AJ, Chang G et al. (1992). Naltrexone and coping skills therapy for alcohol dependence. *Archives of General Psychiatry* 49:881-887.

Pani PP, Maremmani I, Pirastu R et al. (2000). Buprenorphine: A controlled clinical trial in the treatment of opioid dependence. *Drug and Alcohol Dependence* 60:39-50.

Peters RH & Steinberg ML (2000). Substance abuse treatment services in U.S. prisons. In D Shewan & J Davies (eds.) *Drugs and Prisons*. London, England: Harwood Academic Publishers, 89-116.

Pickens R, Hatsukami D, Spicer J et al. (1985). Relapse by alcohol abusers. *Alcoholism: Clinical & Experimental Research* 9(3):244-247.

Project MATCH (1998). Matching alcoholism treatments to client heterogeneity: Project MATCH three-year drinking outcomes. *Alcoholism: Clinical & Experimental Research* 22(6):1300-1311.

Rawson RA, Huber A, McCann M et al. (in press). A comparison of contingency management and cognitive-behavioral approaches for cocaine dependent methadone maintained individuals.

Rawson RA, Obert JL, McCann MJ et al. (1993a). Relapse prevention models for substance abuse treatment. Special issue: Psychotherapy for the addictions. *Psychotherapy* 30(2):284-298.

Rawson RA, Obert JL, McCann MJ et al. (1993b). Relapse prevention strategies in outpatient substance abuse treatment. Special series: Psychosocial treatment of the addictions. *Psychology of Addictive Behaviors* 7(2):85-95.

Rawson RA, Shoptaw SJ, Obert JL et al. (1995). An intensive outpatient approach for cocaine abuse treatment. *Journal of Substance Abuse Treatment* 12(2):117-127.

Robins LN & Regier DA (1991). *Psychiatric Disorders in America: The Epidemiologic Catchment Area Study*. New York, NY: Free Press.

Rosellini G & Worden M (1985). *Of Course You're Angry*. Center City, MN: Hazelden.

Rosellini G & Worden M (1989). *Of Course You're Anxious*. Center City, MN: Hazelden.

Rychtarik RG, Connors GJ, Dermen KH et al. (2000). Alcoholics Anonymous and the use of medications to prevent relapse: An anonymous survey of member attitudes. *Journal of Studies on Alcohol* 61:134-138.

Salloum IM, Cornelius JR, Thase ME et al. (1998). Naltrexone utility in depressed alcoholics. *Psychopharmacology Bulletin* 34(1):111-115.

Sandahl C (1984). Determinants of relapse among alcoholics: A cross-cultural replication study. *International Journal of the Addictions* 19(8):833-848.

Saunders B & Allsop S (1991). Alcohol problems and relapse: Can the clinic combat the community? *Journal of Community and Applied Social Psychology* 1(3):213-221.

Schmitz JM, Oswald LM, Jacks SD et al. (1997). Relapse prevention treatment for cocaine dependence: Group vs. individual format. *Addictive Behaviors* 22(3):405-418.

Shiffmann S (1982). Relapse following smoking cessation: A situational analysis. *Journal of Consulting and Clinical Psychology* 50:71-86.

Shiffman S, Read L, Maltese J et al. (1985). Preventing relapse in ex-smokers: A self-management approach. In GA Marlatt & J Gordon (eds.) *Relapse Prevention: A Self-Control Strategy for the Maintenance of Behavior Change*. New York, NY: Guilford Press, 472-520.

Shoptaw S, Reback CJ, Frosch DL et al. (1998). Stimulant abuse treatment as HIV prevention. *Journal of Addictive Diseases* 17(4):19-32.

Simpson DD, Joe GW, Lehman WE et al. (1986). Addiction careers: Etiology, treatment and 12-year follow-up outcomes. *Journal of Drug Issues* 12:107-123.

Staiger PK, Greeley JD & Wallace SD (1999). Alcohol exposure therapy: Generalization and changes in responsivity. *Drug and Alcohol Dependence* 57(1):29-40.

Stephens RS, Roffman RA & Simpson EE (1994). Treatment adult marijuana dependence: A test of the relapse prevention model. *Journal of Consulting and Clinical Psychology* 62(1):92-99.

Stevens VJ, Glasgow RE, Hollis JF et al. (1993). A smoking-cessation intervention for hospital patients. *Medical Care* 31:65-72.

Stuss DT & Benson DF (1986). *The Frontal Lobes*. New York, NY: Raven Press.

Tennant FS Jr., Rawson RA, Pumphrey E et al. (1986). Clinical experiences with 959 opined-dependent patients treated with levo-alpha-acetylmethadol (LAAM). *Journal of Substance Abuse Treatment* 3:195-202.

Tims F & Leukefeld C, eds. (1987). *Relapse and Recovery in Drug Abuse (NIDA Research Monograph 72)*. Rockville, MD: NIDA, National Institutes of Health.

Tucker JA, Vuchinich RE & Gladsjo JA (1990-1991). Environmental influences on relapse in substance use disorders. Special issues: Environmental factors in substance misuse and its treatment. *International Journal of the Addictions* 25(7A-8A):1017-1050.

Volkow ND, Ding Y-S, Fowler JS et al. (1996). Cocaine addiction: Hypothesis derived from imaging studies with PET. *Journal of Addictive Disorders* 15:55-71.

Volkow ND & Fowler JS (2000). Addiction, a disease of compulsion and drive: Involvement of the orbitofrontal cortex. *Cerebral Cortex* (10):318-325.

Volpicelli JR, Alterman AI, Hayashida M et al. (1992). Naltrexone in the treatment of alcohol dependence. *Archives of General Psychiatry* 49:876-880.

Wanigaratne S (1990). *Relapse Prevention for Addictive Behaviors*. London, England: Blackwell Scientific Publications.

Washton AM (2001). Group therapy: A clinician's guide to doing what works. In R Coombs (ed.) *Addiction Recovery Tools: A Practical Headbook*. Newbury Park, CA: Sage Publications.

Washton AM (2002). Outpatient groups at different stages of substance abuse treatment: preparation, initial abstinence, and relapse prevention. In DW Brook & HI Spitz (eds.) *The Group Therapy of Substance Abuse*. New York, NY: Haworth Medical Publishing.

Weiss RD, Najavits LM & Greenfield SF (1998). A relapse prevention group for patients with bipolar and substance use disorders. *Journal of Substance Abuse Treatment* 16(1):47-54.

Wells EA, Peterson PL, Gainey RR et al. (1994). Outpatient treatment for cocaine abuse: A controlled comparison of relapse prevention and Twelve-Step approaches. *American Journal of Drug and Alcohol Abuse* 20(1):1-17.

Wikler A (1973). Dynamics of drug dependence: Implications of a conditioning theory for research and treatment. *Archives of General Psychiatry* 28:611-616.

Wikler A & Pesco FT (1967). Classical conditioning of a morphine abstinence phenomenon, reinforcement of opioid-drinking behavior and "relapse" in morphine addicted rats. *Psychopharmacologia* 10:255-284.

Wilson PH (1992). *Principles and Practices of Relapse Prevention*. New York, NY: Guilford Press.

Zackon F (1989). Relapse and "re-joyment": Observations and reflections. *Journal of Chemical Dependency Treatment* 2(2):67-80.

Zackon F, McAuliffe W & Chien J (1994). *Addict Aftercare: Recovery Training and Self-Help*. Rockville, MD: NIDA, National Institutes of Health.

Chapter 7

Ethical Issues in Addiction Treatment

H. Westley Clark, M.D., J.D., M.P.H., FASAM
Margaret K. Brooks, Esq.

Patient Autonomy
Informed Consent
Privacy
Establishing an Ethical Stance

A number of ethical principles are central to medical practice. Foremost among these is the physician's obligation to put the patient's health first. Close behind is respect for the patient's autonomy (which includes the patient's right to make his or her own medical decisions, as well as the right to be left alone), and the patient's privacy or confidentiality. The physician also has a general duty to protect society when the patient's condition poses a threat to others.

Most of the time, these ethical principles are congruent. However, physicians who screen, assess, or treat patients for addictive disorders sometimes find themselves in situations where ethical principles conflict. For example, a physician who suspects a patient has an addictive disorder may face a conflict between an obligation to put the patient's health first and respect for the patient's autonomy. Should the physician press the patient about his or her substance use and order medical tests, out of concern for the patient's health? Or should the physician drop the subject if the patient indicates that he or she does not wish to discuss it, out of respect for the patient's autonomy? What should a physician do if the patient's health plan will not pay for the kind of treatment that is needed? Which ethical principles should guide the physician who believes that a patient's addictive disorder poses a danger to the patient's safety: the duty to the patient's health or the duty to protect the patient's privacy? Is coerced treatment ethical?

These questions and others are explored in this chapter. The first section begins with a discussion of the relationship between patient autonomy and the physician's obligation to counsel patients about the health risks of substance use. It then turns to the concept of informed consent and examines the questions raised when a patient is not competent to make his or her own decisions or is not willing to enter treatment voluntarily.

The next section concerns privacy of information about a patient's addictive disorders. It begins with a brief discussion of confidentiality of medical information and why it is important. It then turns to an overview of the legal guidelines that govern privacy of medical information. Finally, it examines three situations in which the physician can be called on to resolve an ethical dilemma between the obligation to maintain confidentiality and the duty to protect the patient and/or society.

PATIENT AUTONOMY

Americans attach extraordinary importance to their right to be left alone. We pride ourselves on having perfected a social and political system that limits how far the government—and others—can intrude on our "space" or control what we do. The principle of autonomy is enshrined in the Constitution, and the courts repeatedly have affirmed the right of citizens to make their own decisions on fundamental issues.

Medicine places a high value on patient autonomy. Patients consult physicians on their own initiative when they decide they have reached a level of discomfort with a particular problem. The physician who is consulted by a patient about a condition, such as back pain, is expected to outline the causes and suggest possible preventive measures and available treatments. The physician certainly can make a recommendation, but must recognize that the patient has the right to choose among the recommended treatments or to refuse them altogether. Rarely will a physician consider forcing advice on a patient, even if convinced that the patient is making a wrong choice.

When a patient is in denial about his or her abuse of alcohol or drugs, however, deference to patient autonomy can shift. The principles of autonomy and privacy, so critical to honest communication between physician and patient, can sometimes, in the context of drug and alcohol abuse, seem to work against what the physician sees as the patient's best interests.

Dealing With Denial. Traditionally, respect for the patient's autonomy has made physicians reluctant to ask questions about areas not directly related to the presenting condition, particularly if those areas are sensitive. Until recent years, patients' annual physicals rarely included questions about alcohol consumption, and physicians were even more reluctant to question patients about drug use. However, a physician who screens or assesses patients for addictive disorders (whether by observing the patient, performing laboratory tests, or administering behavioral questionnaires) is seeking information about lifestyle and personal habits that carry a good deal of stigma. Both patient and physician may view such inquiries as intrusions on the patient's autonomy (as well as his or her privacy).

Nevertheless, when a physician suspects that a patient, who arrives at the office with another presenting complaint, also is abusing drugs or alcohol, he or she must take the initiative if the patient does not raise the issue. In such a case, the physician has an ethical duty to act if there is reason to believe that the patient's use of alcohol or drugs is affecting his or her health.

The difficulty is that raising the issue sometimes is not enough. Denial is an integral part of addictive disorders. Individuals in denial fail to recognize or are reluctant to acknowledge their problem, or they find ways to deny or minimize the extent of their alcohol or drug use because they are ambivalent about giving up such use. What is the proper balance between respect for the principle of autonomy and the physician's responsibility for the patient's health when dealing with a patient in denial? Should the physician raise the issue and then drop it at the slightest hint of resistance on the part of the patient? Or should he or she intervene more forcefully—by talking with the patient, conducting medical tests, or involving the family?

Talking With the Patient. To fulfill the ethical responsibility to the patient, the physician should do more than simply raise the issue. He or she should provide relevant information, engage the patient in discussion and, if the patient shows resistance, follow up in future visits. How far the physician can intrude on the patient's autonomy will depend a great deal on the strength of the physician-patient relationship. Unless a firm foundation of trust and understanding has been established, persistent questions or a forceful confrontation can backfire and ultimately strengthen the patient's resistance.

In most cases, it is only the individual with the addictive disorder who can take action to change his or her behavior. Although the physician can supply information and encouragement, it is the patient who must make the decision to change.

Ordering Laboratory Tests. Must, or should, a physician obtain the patient's consent before ordering a drug screen? It is most likely that the law does not require the patient's consent. Ordinarily, a physician does not ask a patient to sign a consent form before sending blood or urine for other testing. However, ordering laboratory tests to screen patients for addictive disorders is different. And failing to consult the patient can undermine the physician's efforts to induce the patient to acknowledge the problem.

Screening urine or blood for drugs is not the routine practice in primary care settings. Patients expect to be screened for blood sugar and cholesterol, but they do not expect their physician to screen them for drug use. A patient confronted with the results of a test he or she did not know about and for which he or she did not give consent may feel betrayed by the physician, which is a shorthand

---

way of saying that he or she will be angry that the physician did not show respect for the patient's autonomy. The physician runs the risk that such a situation will damage the relationship with the patient. The patient may refuse to participate in any further discussions about alcohol or drug use. Tactically, therefore, the better practice is to obtain the patient's permission for blood or urine tests for alcohol or drugs.

A second reason the physician should obtain the patient's permission before employing laboratory drug screens has to do with the patient's right to privacy. If the physician orders a test, the patient's third-party payer will know about it and perhaps the result as well. The physician's decision to order a drug screen tells the third-party payer a good deal, even if the result is negative. Therefore, it is the patient, not the physician, who should decide whether it is appropriate and necessary for the health insurer to have this information.

A third reason is financial. The patient's third-party payer may not cover drug screens as a matter of course. The advent of managed care has narrowed the range of tests a physician can order on a routine basis. If the patient's insurance carrier or health maintenance organization (HMO) will not cover the test, the patient should have the opportunity to decide whether he or she is willing to pay for the test out of pocket, a decision that should be made before the test is ordered.

Unfortunately, there is a good chance that if the physician consults the patient and asks permission to perform a drug screen, the patient will refuse to agree to the test. However, this result leaves the door open to further discussion with the patient about possible drug problems. The patient likely will appreciate the physician's concern for his or her autonomy and privacy, and thus may be more open than would be the case if the physician was perceived as acting "behind the patient's back" and therefore could not be trusted. The physician might begin such a discussion by asking, in a neutral way, why the patient does not want to have a drug screen.

The physician is likely to encounter fewer problems if the order is for a test of liver function. Patients are less likely to be surprised that such a test has been ordered, and the test results still provide an opening for a conversation about the health effects of alcohol or drug use.

When the Patient Is an Older Adult. The physician who suspects an older adult patient is abusing alcohol or drugs must be especially sensitive. As we age, most of us become more sensitive to perceived threats to our autonomy. Because of the stigma surrounding addictive disorders, a patient whose physician suggests that he or she may be drinking too much or abusing drugs (legal or illegal) might conclude that the physician is suggesting that whatever brought him or her for a medical visit has an emotional basis or that the patient's functioning or capacity is diminished. If an older adult thinks that his or her autonomy is being threatened, the patient may be more likely to point to the "normal" infirmities of old age as the source of the difficulty, rather than acknowledging a problem with alcohol or other drugs.

Most older adults are unaware that the way their bodies metabolize alcohol and drugs (including prescription medications) changes as they age and that the amount of alcohol or drugs they consumed without obvious adverse consequences when they were younger can harm their health and even incapacitate them. Moreover, many older adult patients take multiple prescription drugs to control their cholesterol, blood pressure, diabetes, depression, or anxiety. They may not be aware that their prescription medications can interact with each other and with any alcohol or nonprescription drugs they consume, interfering with the therapeutic effects of their medications. An approach that emphasizes these issues provides a better opportunity to engage an older adult patient in a discussion about addictive disorders without posing a threat to his or her autonomy.

INFORMED CONSENT

Autonomy also is at the root of our belief that a patient has the right to decide what treatment he or she will accept, and even whether he or she will accept treatment at all. When a physician asks a patient to sign an "informed consent" agreement, he or she is affirming that the patient has the right to make decisions about his or her medical care.[1]

---

[1] Of course, physicians do not ask patients to sign informed consent forms each time medical decisions are made. When we go for routine blood tests or an electrocardiogram, or when we get a flu shot or start an antibiotic for bronchitis, no one asks us to sign a form consenting to treatment. Generally, informed consent forms are used when the patient will undergo an invasive procedure that poses a risk of adverse physical consequences, when the patient chooses a treatment that the physician has warned him or her may be ineffective, or when the law requires the physician to get informed consent because the test can result in serious adverse *legal* or *psychological* consequences and asking the patient to sign the form impresses on him or her the importance of the decision to be made. (For example, in some states, a patient must sign an informed consent form when an HIV test is performed.)

"Informed consent" has two components. First, the patient's decision to undergo a course of treatment must be based on knowledge and competency. The physician must give the patient the kind and amount of information the patient needs to make an intelligent ("informed") choice, and the patient must be capable of understanding the information and making a decision. Second, the patient's decision must be voluntary—that is, a product of his or her free will. What happens when one of these conditions cannot be met—when the patient is not fully informed or competent to make a decision for himself or herself or when he or she is coerced into treatment?

Informed = Knowledge Plus Competency. *Information*: The physician is obligated to give the patient all the information he or she needs to make a decision. This information should include the physician's opinion of the patient's diagnosis, an outline of the available treatment alternatives, a description of what each alternative involves (including its benefits and risks), an explanation of the consequences should the patient decline treatment altogether, and responses to the patient's questions. Often, the physician also helps the patient evaluate the treatment alternatives in accordance with the patient's values, hopes, and fears.

With the growth of managed care, physician and patient no longer have an exclusive relationship. The managed care organization has intruded itself into the relationship. Many managed care contracts shift some financial risk from the managed care company to the physician. In some plans, the contract gives physicians whose patients do not use expensive (or extensive) services a financial bonus. In other plans, the contract limits the services for which the physician will be reimbursed. (Note that such contracts do not limit the services the physician can provide—only those for which he or she will be compensated.) In this way, many managed care plans create incentives that can impinge on medical judgment.

If a physician allows financial incentives or disincentives to influence treatment recommendations, or to discharge a patient who has exhausted benefits under the contract, that physician has placed financial interests before his or her obligation to the patient's health—a clear ethical violation.

Because managed care places (often hidden) limits on certain forms of treatment, ethicists have begun to suggest that the physician should inform the patient about any economic issues that could influence either the physician's recommendation or the patient's decision. Providing "economic informed consent" ensures that the patient knows about any limitations the managed care plan or insurer imposes on treatment before making a decision.

Competence (Decision-Making Capacity): The concept of informed consent is based on the assumption that the patient has "decisional capacity." Decisional capacity means that the patient is able to understand the physician's explanation of the diagnosis, prognosis, treatment alternatives, and likely outcome if treatment is refused, and is able to go through the complex process of assessing that information in accordance with his or her personal system of values. Most patients have decisional capacity. However, the physician may encounter questions about decisional capacity in dealing with two groups: adolescents and older adults.

Adolescents. Adolescents do not have the same legal status as full-fledged adults, and there are certain decisions that society does not allow them to make. Below a certain age (which varies from state to state), adolescents must attend school and cannot drive, marry, or sign binding contracts. In some states, the adolescent's right to consent to medical treatment—or to refuse treatment—also differs from an adult's right.

In more than half the states, adolescents have the right to consent on their own to addictive disorder screening, assessment, or treatment, while in other states, a parent must be notified and/or consent.[2] In states that deem adolescents competent to consent to addictive disorder treatment (and which therefore do not require parental consent), the physician has no ethical dilemma; he or she can provide whatever treatment is appropriate (and to which the adolescent patient consents).

It is in those states that require parental consent or notification that the physician sometimes encounters a complex ethical quandary. The difficulty arises when an adolescent who seeks assessment or treatment refuses to permit communication with a parent. If the physician believes that the adolescent does need treatment, he or she has three choices:

CHOICE 1: The physician can treat the adolescent without consulting a parent.

---

[2]Presumably, a parent whose child seeks treatment will consent. A parent or guardian who refuses to consent to treatment that a physician believes is necessary to an adolescent's well-being could face charges of child neglect.

The Dilemma: The physician who treats an adolescent without parental consent or notification is acting in accordance with the ethical principles of putting the patient's health first and respecting the patient's autonomy (and privacy), but may be violating the law. Although violation of the parental consent/notification law most likely is not a criminal offense, it could put the physician's professional license at risk or expose him or her to a lawsuit by the adolescent's parents. It is unlikely, however, that a physician treating an adolescent would be faced with either eventuality if the treatment provided is not controversial or intrusive, does not put the adolescent at risk, and is carried out in a responsible, non-negligent manner. In such circumstances, it would be difficult for a parent (or licensing authority) to show that any harm was done. This is particularly true if the physician made a reasoned decision and acted in good faith and out of concern for the adolescent. Contrary to popular belief, most lawyers do not chase after cases that are complex, time-consuming, expensive, and difficult to win. Convincing an attorney to take on such a case would not be easy.

Factors to Consider: The physician who is considering whether to offer treatment without parental consent or notification in a state that requires it should consider the following factors:

- The adolescent's age. Society accords adolescents more autonomy as they get older. A physician who might decline to treat a 14-year-old without parental consent in a state that requires it might have fewer qualms about treating a 17-year-old in similar circumstances.

- The adolescent's maturity. Chronological age clearly is not the only measure. There are 14-year-olds who have maturity beyond their years and emotionally immature 17-year-olds with poor social skills and reasoning ability.

- The adolescent's family situation. Adolescents in need of addictive disorder treatment may be estranged from their families. Those who refuse to permit parental notification may have good reason to do so. Forcing them to involve parents who have failed them is neither ethical nor good clinical practice. Reconciliation with the family may be vital to an adolescent's recovery, but circumstances may dictate that it be abandoned or postponed to a later stage of treatment.

- The severity of the adolescent's addictive disorder and the danger it poses to his or her life or health.

- The kind of treatment to be provided. The more intrusive and intensive the proposed treatment, the more risk the physician assumes in treating an adolescent without parental consent. For example, a physician offering an outpatient course of treatment is on firmer ground than one proposing intensive outpatient or residential treatment.

- The physician's possible liability for refusing to treat the patient. State law may impose a duty to treat patients in need.

- The financial consequences. If the physician treats an adolescent without parental consent, he or she may not be paid.

CHOICE 2: The physician can refuse to treat the adolescent.

The Dilemma: Refusing to treat the adolescent adheres to the letter of state laws that consider adolescents incompetent to make medical decisions and it shows respect for the patient's privacy, but it may violate the ethical principle that requires the physician to put the patient's health first. In some states, it also violates a law requiring physicians to treat patients in medical need.

CHOICE 3: The physician can call the adolescent's parent to try to obtain consent to treat the adolescent.

The Dilemma: Calling the parent and treating the adolescent complies with the letter of state law and is in accordance with the ethical principle that puts the patient's health first. However, it clearly violates the adolescent's right to privacy. Moreover, the federal confidentiality rules complicate this choice. If the physician is subject to the federal confidentiality rules (discussed later), he or she is prohibited from contacting a parent unless the adolescent consents. The sole exception allows a treatment program director to contact a parent when the life or physical wellbeing of an adolescent is threatened.[3]

---

[3]Federal confidentiality regulations prohibit physicians and others who provide alcohol and drug screening, assessment, and treatment from communicating with anyone, including a parent, unless the adolescent consents. The sole exception allows the director of an addiction treatment program to communicate "facts relevant to reducing a threat to the life or physical

Older Adults. Most older adults are fully capable of understanding medical information, weighing the treatment alternatives, and making and articulating decisions. A small percentage of older patients clearly are incapable of participating in a decisionmaking process. In such cases, the older adult may have signed a health care proxy or may have a court-appointed guardian to make such decisions.

The real difficulty arises when a physician is screening or assessing an older adult whose mental capacity lies between those two extremes. The patient may have fluctuating capacity, with "good days" and "bad days," or periods of greater or lesser alertness depending on the time of day. The patient's condition can be transient or deteriorating. Diminished capacity may affect some parts of his or her ability to comprehend information and make complex decisions, but not others.

In caring for an older adult patient whose decisional capacity is less than optimal, how can the physician help the patient to understand the information presented, appreciate the implications of each alternative treatment, and make a "rational" decision, based on the patient's best interests? And what can the physician do if the patient appears to be not competent to make his or her own health care decision? Although there are no easy answers to these questions, there are several possible approaches.

Present information carefully. The physician can help the patient who appears to have diminished capacity through a gradual information-gathering and decisionmaking process. Information should be presented in a way that allows the patient to absorb it gradually, clarify and restate information as necessary, and summarize the issues already covered at regular intervals. Each alternative and its consequences should be laid out and examined separately. Finally, the physician can help the patient identify his or her values and link those values to the alternatives. By helping the patient narrow his or her focus and proceeding step-by-step, the physician may gain assurance that the patient has understood the choices and acted in his or her own best interests.

Enlist the help of a health or mental health professional. If helping the patient through a process of gradual information-gathering and decisionmaking is not working, the physician can suggest that physician and patient jointly consult a mental health professional or a health professional who is familiar with the patient's history and has a better understanding of the obstacles to decisionmaking. Or, the physician could suggest a specialist who can help determine why the patient is having difficulty and whether he or she has the capacity to give informed consent.

Enlist the help of family or close friends. Another approach is for the physician to suggest that the patient call in a family member or close friend who can help them organize the information and sort through the alternatives. Asking the patient who would be helpful could gain endorsement of this approach.

Consult a family member or friend. If the patient cannot grasp the information or come to a decision, the physician might ask the patient to allow him or her to consult a family member or close friend. If the patient consents, the physician should lay out the concerns to the family member or friend. It may be that the patient already has planned for the possibility of incapacity and has signed a durable power of attorney or health care proxy.

Guardianship. A guardian is a person appointed by a court to manage some or all aspects of another person's life. Anyone seeking appointment of a guardian must show the court that the individual is disabled in some way by disease, illness, or senility and that the disability prevents that individual from performing the tasks necessary to manage one or more areas of his or her life.

Each state handles guardianship proceedings differently, but some principles apply across the board: Guardianship is not an all-or-nothing state. Courts generally require that the person seeking appointment of a guardian prove the individual's incapacity in a variety of tasks or areas. Courts can apply different standards to different life tasks—managing money, managing a household, making health care decisions, and entering contracts. A person can be found incompetent to make contracts and manage money but competent to make his or her own health care decisions (or vice versa), and the guardianship will be limited accordingly. Guardianship limits the older adult's autonomy and is an expensive process. It should be considered only as a last resort.

Voluntariness Versus Coercion. A growing proportion of patients in addictive disorder treatment has been forced

---

wellbeing of the [adolescent seeking services] or any other individual to the minor's parent, guardian, or other person authorized under state law to act in the minor's behalf, when the program director believes that the adolescent, because of extreme youth or mental or physical condition, lacks the capacity to decide rationally whether to consent to the notification of a parent or guardian," and (2) "The program director believes the disclosure to a parent or guardian is necessary to cope with a substantial threat to the life or physical well-being of the adolescent or someone else" (42 CFR §§2.14[c] and [d]).

into treatment by family, an employer, or the criminal justice system. A spouse can give his or her partner an ultimatum—enter treatment "or else;" an employer can require treatment as a condition of retaining a job; or a criminal justice agency can require a defendant to enter treatment as a condition of probation, parole, or suspension of charges.

Critics of coerced treatment contend that it is unethical because it violates the principle of autonomy. Some critics are particularly concerned when it is the criminal justice system that is mandating treatment and holding out the possibility that a criminal defendant will avoid incarceration. Some critics charge that the power imbalance in such circumstances is especially annihilative to autonomy.

Proponents counter that, although coerced treatment unquestionably impinges on a patient's autonomy, it does not violate it altogether, even in the criminal context. The patient may not want to enter treatment, but always has a choice and retains the right to refuse. He or she may not like the consequences (losing a spouse, losing a job, or being incarcerated on criminal charges), but still retains the autonomy to make the decision. Proponents also point out that patients who stay in treatment for at least 90 days have better outcomes than those who leave earlier. To the extent that coercion raises retention rates, they argue, it works to improve the odds that the patient will have a positive outcome.

PRIVACY

Patients expect their physicians to treat information about them confidentially. Medicine values patients' privacy because it relies on patients to provide physicians with accurate information. By giving privacy protections to medical information, society assures patients that they can discuss things with their physicians without worrying about what others will hear or think.

Confidentiality is especially important when a patient has an addictive disorder, because of the widespread perception that such persons are weak and/or morally impaired. A patient considering treatment might be concerned that, if an insurer or HMO learns that his or her traumatic injuries were related to alcoholism, it will be difficult or impossible to obtain coverage for hospitalization costs or that his or her insurance will be canceled. Similarly, a patient may fear that his or her relationships with a spouse, parents, children, an employer, or friends would suffer if they learned about his or her problems with alcohol or drugs. If a patient has marital problems, information about an addictive disorder could have an effect on divorce or custody proceedings. A patient whose problem becomes known to his employer could lose an expected promotion—or a job. Adverse consequences such as these can deter patients from admitting to problems with alcohol or drugs and from obtaining treatment for those problems.

This section begins with a description of the statutory and regulatory sources of guidance on confidentiality of information about patients' addictive disorder screening, assessment, or treatment. It then turns to the questions raised when the principle of maintaining patients' confidentiality conflicts with other ethical principles.

Sources of Guidance. *Federal Law*: In the early 1970s, Congress passed legislation to protect information about patients in addictive disorder treatment and directed the Department of Health and Human Services (DHHS) to issue regulations protecting patients' confidentiality. The law is codified at 42 U.S.C. §290dd-2. The implementing federal regulations, titled "Confidentiality of Alcohol and Drug Abuse Patient Records," are contained in 42 CFR Part 2 (Volume 42 of the Code of Federal Regulations, Part 2).

Federal confidentiality rules apply to almost all addictive disorder treatment programs in the United States. They prohibit programs and their counselors from disclosing any information (written or oral) about any applicant, patient, or former patient unless (1) the patient has consented in writing (on the form required by the regulations), or (2) another very limited exception specified in the regulations applies. The rules apply whether or not the person seeking information already has the information, has other ways of obtaining it, has official status, is authorized by state law, or has a subpoena or search warrant.

The federal rules permit disclosures in only nine limited circumstances:

1. When a patient signs a consent form that complies with the regulations' requirements.

2. When a disclosure does not identify the patient as a substance abuser.

3. When program staff members consult among themselves.

4. When the disclosure is to a "qualified service organization" that provides services to the program.

5. When there is a medical emergency.

6. When the program must report child abuse or neglect.

7. When a patient commits a crime at the program or against staff members.

8. When the information is for research, audit, or evaluation purposes.

9. When a court issues a special order authorizing disclosure.

The federal law and regulations restrict communications more tightly in many instances than either the physician-patient or the attorney-client privilege. Violating the regulations is punishable by a fine of up to $500 for a first offense and up to $5,000 for each subsequent offense (42 CFR §2.4).

Physicians who practice primary care probably are not subject to the federal confidentiality law and regulations.[4] However, when a general care practice includes someone whose primary function is to provide addictive disorder assessment or treatment and the practice benefits from "federal assistance,"[5] it must comply with the federal rules for handling information about patients who may have alcohol or drug problems.

Although most primary care physicians are not subject to the federal rules, they should handle information about patients' addictive disorders with great care. The best prac-

tice for those not subject to the federal confidentiality rules is voluntary compliance.

In 1996, the Congress passed another law—the Health Insurance Portability and Accountability Act, Public Law 104-191 (HIPAA)—part of which mandated the establishment of standards for the privacy of "individually identifiable health information." To carry out that mandate, DHHS issued a set of regulations governing patients' privacy that apply to a wide range of "health care providers." These HIPAA regulations appear in Volume 45 of the Code of Federal Regulations, Parts 160 and 164. Health care providers who are covered by HIPAA must comply with the regulations by April 14, 2003.

HIPAA regulations are not as restrictive as the federal confidentiality rules. Practitioners who are subject to both sets of rules must follow the more restrictive standard.

State Law: State laws also offer some protection to medical information. Most clinicians—and patients—think of these laws as the "physician-patient privilege." Strictly speaking, the physician-patient privilege is a rule of evidence that governs whether a physician can be compelled to testify in a court case about a patient. In many states, however, the laws offer wider protection, and some states have special confidentiality laws that explicitly prohibit practitioners from divulging information about patients without their consent. States often include such prohibitions in professional licensing laws; such laws generally prohibit licensed professionals from divulging information about patients and make unauthorized disclosures grounds for disciplinary action, including license revocation.

Each state has its own set of rules, which means that the scope of protection offered by state law varies widely. Whether a communication (or laboratory test result) is "privileged" or "protected" depends on a number of factors:

The type of professional holding the information and whether he or she is licensed or certified by the state: Most state laws do cover licensed physicians.

The context in which the information was communicated: Some states limit protection to information a patient communicates to a physician in private, in the course of the medical consultation, and do not protect information disclosed to a physician in the presence of a third party, such as a spouse. Other states protect information the patient tells the physician when others are present as well as information the physician gains during examination.

---

[4]For many years, there was confusion as to whether general medical care settings such as primary care clinics or hospital emergency departments were subject to the federal law and regulations because they provided addictive disorder diagnosis, referral, and treatment as part of their services. In 1995, DHHS revised the definition of the kinds of "programs" subject to the regulations so as to make it clear that *the regulations do not generally apply to a general medical care facility* unless that facility (or person) "holds itself out as providing, and provides, alcohol or drug abuse diagnosis, treatment or referral for treatment. . . ." (42 CFR §2.11).

[5]"Federally assisted" programs include the following: (1) programs run directly by or under contract for the federal government; (2) programs carried out under a federal license, certification, registration, or other authorization, including certification under the Medicare program, authorization to conduct a methadone maintenance treatment program, or registration to dispense a drug that is regulated by the Controlled Substances Act to treat alcohol or drug abuse; (3) programs supported by any federal department or agency of the United States, even when the federal support does not directly pay for the alcohol or drug abuse diagnosis, treatment, or referral activities; (4) programs conducted by state or local governments unit that are supported by federal funding that could be (but is not necessarily) spent for the treatment program; and (5) tax-exempt programs.

The circumstances in which "confidential" information will be or was disclosed: Some states protect medical information only when that information is sought in a court proceeding. If a physician divulges information about a patient in any other setting, the law does not recognize that there has been a violation of the patient's right to privacy. Other states protect medical information in many different contexts.

How the right to privacy is enforced: State legal protection of medical information is useful only when it is backed by enforcement of the law. Although enforcement remains relatively rare, states can discipline professionals who violate their patients' privacy, allow patients to sue physicians for damages, or criminalize behavior that violates patients' privacy.

Exceptions to any general rule protecting the privacy of information:

■ *Consent*: All states permit physicians to disclose information if the patient consents, although states have different requirements about consent. In some states, it must be written; in others, it can be oral. Some states require different consent forms for disclosures about different diseases.

■ *Reporting Infectious Diseases*: All states require physicians to report certain infectious diseases to public health authorities, although states' definitions of reportable diseases vary.

■ *Reporting Child Abuse and Neglect*: All states require physicians to report child abuse and neglect to child protective services, although states' definitions of child abuse vary.

■ *Duty to Warn*: Most states also require physicians to report credible threats a patient makes to harm others.

When Confidentiality Conflicts With Other Ethical Principles. When the principle of confidentiality conflicts with a physician's ethical responsibility to others, which principle takes precedence?

Employer or Employee: To whom does a physician owe loyalty when treating a patient who has been referred by an employer as a condition of retaining a job? Is it to the employer, who is relying on the physician to help the employee recover and remain (or return) to work? Or is it to the patient (the employee)? The employer likely will require reports from the physician on the patient's progress in treatment. What should the physician do if the employee is not attending or complying with treatment? This question appears most starkly when the employee is in a safety-sensitive position and the physician is concerned that his or her behavior poses an immediate risk to other employees or to the public. To which ethical principle should the physician adhere: the obligation to safeguard the patient's privacy or the obligation to protect those who might be harmed by the patient's actions?

The best way to avoid having to grapple with this problem in an emergency (always a difficult and unpleasant experience) is to create agreed-upon ground rules before treatment begins. If an employer requires reports, the physician must have the patient sign a consent form authorizing communications with the employer. Physician and patient must agree on what kinds of information will be reported, and that agreement should be made part of the consent form. (Unfortunately, the patient can revoke his consent at any time.) Of course, the employer also must be willing to accept whatever limitations the agreement places on the kinds of information it will receive.

Reports to employers usually include information about attendance and progress in treatment. In most cases, it would be inappropriate for the physician to include detailed clinical information in such reports. However, employers can require more information when safety-sensitive employees are in treatment. Employers may want to hear about positive results from a drug screen test, and the physician may want to be able to report continued drug use by an employee in a safety-sensitive position. The physician can discharge his or her duty to the public at large (and to the employer) without violating the patient's right to privacy if the patient signs a consent form that documents his or her understanding that certain types of behavior would be reported to the employer.

Parent and Society or Adolescent: Adolescence is a time of testing limits. Even adolescents who are not involved in substance use or abuse engage in behavior that alarms adults. Adolescents in addictive disorder treatment may engage in hazardous activities such as renewed drug-taking, criminal activity, risky sexual conduct, or other self-destructive behaviors. If an adolescent patient's conduct poses a serious threat to his or her life or health, and if counseling seems not to be productive in reducing that behavior, what should the physician do? Should he or she notify the adolescent's parents?

The physician's primary duty is to preserve the adolescent's health or life. If events have reached a life-or-death stage, and notifying the adolescent's parents without consent is the only way to save that life, the physician would have to do so.

There are steps the physician can take to reduce the conflict between the obligation to maintain a patient's privacy and the obligation to safeguard the adolescent's health. Before beginning to treat an adolescent who has a history of risk-taking behavior, the physician could ask the adolescent to sign a consent form that authorizes the physician to disclose, to an adult the adolescent trusts, any behavior that takes a dangerous turn. (The adolescent can revoke such a consent at any time.) The adult named could be a parent or other relative, a minister or youth counselor, or anyone else with whom the adolescent has a good rapport. An adolescent entering treatment might consent to this arrangement because he or she may believe, as do many people entering treatment, that he or she will not suffer a relapse. An added benefit of this kind of request is that it demonstrates to the adolescent that the physician takes the patient's privacy very seriously and will not disclose information to others without the patient's consent.[6]

---

[6]Physicians who are subject to the federal confidentiality rules cannot call an adolescent's parents without the adolescent's consent. Notifying another adult the adolescent trusts permits the physician to alert someone who then can disclose the information to others (including the adolescent's parents) if he or she does so without revealing the fact that the adolescent is in treatment for an addictive disorder. (The federal rules have this requirement even if the adolescent's parents already know he or she is in treatment.)

Even if the physician's conduct is not circumscribed by the federal rules, however, calling the parents may not be the best or wisest option, as the patient (or other patients) may become reluctant to trust a physician who has notified parents over an adolescent's objections.

There are other options for the physician who is subject to the federal rules. For more information, see Winters (1999a, 199b).

Society or Patient: When a patient presents a danger to others, is the physician's obligation to the patient or to society? Most physicians know that, in most states, legislators and the courts have determined that their duty to warn supersedes their duty to protect a patient's privacy. The law requires a warning to the potential victim or someone in a position to protect the potential victim. The duty to warn, however, does not completely nullify the patient's right to privacy. The physician can warn others of potential danger without disclosing extraneous information about the patient, including information about his or her use of drugs and alcohol. Physicians who are subject to federal confidentiality rules are required to issue the warning in a way that minimizes harm to the patient's privacy.

ESTABLISHING AN ETHICAL STANCE

The chapter has examined some of the ethical principles at the core of medical practice and considered the ways in which screening, assessing, or treating a patient for addictive disorders can challenge those principles. Physicians can avoid or minimize potential ethical dilemmas if they remain aware of the sources of potential conflict, keep the purposes of the ethical principles in mind, discuss potential conflicts with patients at the beginning of treatment, and take prophylactic steps to reduce conflicts to a few relatively rare situations.

NOTE: The views and opinions expressed herein are those of the authors and do not necessarily reflect the views, opinions, or policies of the Substance Abuse and Mental Health Services Administration or the U.S. Department of Health and Human Services.

REFERENCES

Winters KC, ed. (1999a). *Screening and Assessment for Adolescent Substance Use (Treatment Improvement Protocol 31).* Rockville, MD: Center for Substance Abuse Treatment.

Winters KC, ed. (1999b). *Treatment of Adolescent Substance Use (Treatment Improvement Protocol 32).* Rockville, MD: Center for Substance Abuse Treatment.

| Chapter 8 | # Linking Addiction Treatment With Other Medical and Psychiatric Treatment Systems |

Peter D. Friedmann, M.D., M.P.H.
Richard Saitz, M.D., M.P.H., FACP
Jeffrey H. Samet, M.D., M.A., M.P.H.

Barriers to Optimal Linkage
Benefits of Linked Services
Models of Linked Services
Prospects for Improved Linkage

Persons with substance use problems are at substantial risk for coexisting medical and mental health problems (see Sections 10 and 11), so it comes as little surprise that they present in substantial numbers in medical and mental health settings. Similarly, patients in addictive disorder treatment commonly experience medical and psychiatric problems, which can distract from recovery work and increase relapse risk. In both medical and addictive disorder treatment settings, the provision of comprehensive care for individuals with alcohol and other drug use disorders presents challenges to clinicians, who traditionally have been concerned only with issues reflecting their own training and perspectives. For example, medical practitioners typically address the toxic effects of a particular substance, such as seizures or cirrhosis, or the health consequences of a high-risk lifestyle, such as viral hepatitis or HIV. Psychiatrists and other mental health professionals focus on the mental health issues so prevalent among substance-abusing patients. Meanwhile, addiction medicine specialists typically focus on the individual's destructive preoccupation with obtaining and consuming a psychoactive chemical substance and the negative consequences of such actions. For the patient, these problems are insepa-

rable, yet the providers operate in separate systems of care, each with its own—often exclusive—focus. For example, the medical literature contains multiple instances of medical practitioners not attending to the addictive disorders of their patients by failing to screen, intervene, or refer (Moore, Bone et al., 1989; Saitz, Mulvey et al., 1997a). Similarly, many patients in addictive disorder treatment programs report unmet psychological and medical needs (Etheridge, Craddock et al., 1995). Substance-abusing patients with psychiatric or medical illnesses sometimes are bounced between systems—told that they must be abstinent before they can get treatment for their psychiatric and medical problems, or that they are too sick (medically or psychiatrically) to get into an addiction treatment program—resulting in a clinical "Catch-22."

Patients who present with complex, interrelated, comorbid problems make apparent the gaps between these parallel yet separate systems of care. The growth of addiction medicine will help to close these gaps. However, for most systems that lack access to a certified addiction medicine physician (Laine, Newschaffer et al., 2000), linkages across the separate medical, mental health, and addictive disorder disciplines will be needed to improve the quality of care delivered to patients with addictive disorders. This chapter briefly reviews the barriers to linkages between primary medical care, mental health, and addictive disorder services; outlines the potential benefits of such linkages; and describes published linkage models.

BARRIERS TO OPTIMAL LINKAGE

Many barriers impede better linkage of services. One well-documented problem has been the perspective of many medical practitioners that addressing alcohol and drug abuse issues is not providing medical care and thus is beyond his or her purview (Chappel & Schnoll, 1977). This point of view is slowly changing within the profession. Medical education about these issues was sorely deficient in past years (Lewis, Niven et al., 1987). In the mid-1980s, medical students' suboptimal knowledge, perceived responsibility for caring for patients with alcoholism, and confidence in clinical skills was related to reported screening and referral practices; resident physicians perceived even less of a responsibility for care, had less confidence in their skills, and had more negative attitudes (Geller, Levine et al., 1989). These reports suggested that curricula needed improvement and that education, although necessary, may not be sufficient to maintain appropriate attitudes and practices on the part of physicians. Efforts to rectify that situation have been under way, most notably in the past decade, with development of appropriate standards, curricula, and effective addictive disorder educators within many disciplines, including most recently an effort by the Health Resources and Services Administration (HRSA) and the Center for Substance Abuse Treatment (CSAT) to have addiction educators in place in every health professional school in the United States (Adger, Macdonald et al., 1999; Brown, Marcus et al., 2001; Isaacson, Fleming et al., 2000; Sirica, 1995; Haack, Adger et al., 2002). Nevertheless, progress requires time, dedicated resources, attention to continuing medical education, and maintenance of high quality care.

Similarly, addiction medicine specialists often have viewed the medical and mental health issues of recovering individuals as secondary to their substance use problems. This perspective does not lend itself to effective collaborative efforts.

Medical clinicians in practice generally report having received minimal training in substance use disorders, and they screen inadequately for preclinical cases (Friedmann, McCullough et al., 2000; Isaacson, Fleming et al., 2000). Because they neither find patients with less severe addictive

disorders nor follow up those who have had success in treatment, most physicians have experienced few successes. This latter product of poor linkages biases the spectrum of medical providers' clinical experience and further discourages physician involvement. In effect, only patients who do poorly and develop severe medical and psychosocial problems are "visible" (Cohen & Cohen, 1984). In such an environment, it is difficult to convince even well-meaning providers that the diagnosis and management of these disorders are worthwhile; however, training can help overcome these barriers (Adams, Ockene et al., 1998; Saitz, Sullivan et al., 2000; D'Onofrio, Nadel et al., 2002)

Payment and Service Linkage. In our current health care system, payment for addictions and mental health care has been limited, compared with payments for other medical services (Goldman, McCulloch et al., 1998; Schoenbaum, Zhang et al., 1998). Although there have been efforts to achieve parity for health care benefits, parity is not the norm. Moreover, many managed behavioral health plans have "carved out" addictive disorder benefits, separating the financing of care for mental and addictive disorders from that for the rest of the patient's ailments (Larson, Samet et al., 1997; Stein, Reardon et al., 1999; Sturm, 1999; Sturm & McCulloch, 1998). Although such plans have reduced the utilization of services for addictive disorders, the effect they have had on outcomes, quality of care, integration of care, and physician attitudes remains unclear. Such separate systems can foster the continuation of episodic, poorly coordinated care for substance-abusing patients.

Current systems of payment also do not cover addictive disorder services provided by primary care physicians. Financial reimbursements to medical and behavioral health clinicians generally are taken from separate budgets, and the financial benefits occur late. Consequently, the cost of treatment for an addictive disorder that prevents subsequent HIV infection may be appreciated as a treatment expense, rather than as a savings of future medical care costs. Another financial disincentive to linked services is the perception that costs of such care may be limitless. The fear of the cost of appropriate addictive disorder services persists, despite analyses that document the limited effect even a worst case scenario would have on health care expenditures (Sturm, Zhang et al., 1999).

Confidentiality Concerns. Well-meaning concerns about patient confidentiality also can be barriers to effectively linked medical, mental health, and addictions care. Practical difficulties can interfere with obtaining timely two-way written releases of information. Addictive disorder information must be specified in information releases so it can be shared. This history often is kept separate from the standard medical record, a phenomenon that can occur in the case of HIV infection as well. Although these approaches serve a noble purpose, to protect patient confidentiality, they can impede integrated care.

Stigma remains a fundamental barrier to progress in the treatment of any patient with alcohol or drug abuse. In addition to effects on patient behavior, such as limiting recognition of needs and readiness to accept services, stigma can manifest as medical clinicians not wanting to spend time dealing with drug and alcohol issues, or it can lead to a perception of diminished stature of providers who work in this field. Both outgrowths of stigma prevent overall progress.

Medical and mental health providers can inadequately appreciate the efficacy of treatment for addictive disorders. The overwhelmingly supportive body of research appears infrequently in the medical literature. For example, physicians do not appreciate the comparable therapeutic value of treatment for alcohol or heroin dependence relative to standard treatment for other chronic disorders, such as diabetes mellitus or asthma (McLellan, Woody et al., 1996; McLellan, Lewis et al., 2000; O'Brien & McLellan, 1996).

In summary, the barriers to an integrated system of care for patients with substance use disorders are manifold. Barriers include issues of professional responsibility, education among providers, financial disincentives, concerns about confidentiality, and stigma, among others. Although the barriers can appear to be extensive, they are not insurmountable. On the "macro" level, addressing linkage at the systems level would go a long way toward improving integrated care. Examples of systems approaches include implementation of the following: linkage models of care, payment systems that encourage linkage, and quality measures that value coordinated care. Parity of health care benefits for mental health, addictive disorders, and medical problems (as in Connecticut and Minnesota) would help to reduce stigma and improve care coordination, but impediments to the care of addictive disorders in primary care settings exist even in states where parity legislation has been enacted. These impediments include the arbitrary health insurance practice of discounting or denying primary care reimbursement for visits in which the provider indicates a mental or addictive disorder as the primary diagnosis (Bosl, 2001).

Confidentiality issues also can be addressed at a systems level (that is, by having all care occur under the umbrella of one health system, thereby facilitating records availability), and at an individual patient-physician level, by having office systems that prompt clinicians and office staff to advise patients to sign appropriate releases to allow all of their health care providers to communicate. Recently published and future studies demonstrating the feasibility and effectiveness of these models should help to convince payers and practitioners of the need to move in this direction.

The advent of office-based opioid substitution therapy is expected to enhance communication between some primary medical care providers and methadone treatment staff members. At the clinician level, various approaches can be taken simultaneously to help overcome barriers. Physician attitudes, skills, and practices can be changed by active-learning educational programs (Adams, Ockene et al., 1998; Saitz, Sullivan et al., 2000). Convincing theoretical and empirically proven benefits of linked services also will lead clinicians to favor better-integrated care.

BENEFITS OF LINKED SERVICES

Effective linkage may benefit individuals with substance use problems in the following common scenarios: when issues related to addictive disorders are not addressed in primary care and mental health settings, when medical and mental health issues are not addressed in addictive disorder treatment, and when the patient is seen in two or more of these settings but no effective communication between the systems occurs.

From a patient's perspective, the potential for improved overall care is the motivating force for linkage of systems (Table 1). One example is a patient on methadone maintenance who receives a pharmacotherapy, such as rifampin (Rifadin®) or nevirapine (Viramune®), which can decrease methadone blood levels. Without coordination of care, changes in methadone levels on initiation of pharmacotherapy might lead to withdrawal symptoms or toxicity, concern about methadone diversion, or potential relapse. Other examples of improved quality of care from such linkages include better pain control in addicted patients, proper attribution of side effects of medications (versus substance use), and better access to detoxification and treatment for patients in the medical system. A profound benefit of linked systems would be the improved wellbeing of individual patients, in terms of addictive disorder severity, medical and

---

TABLE 1. Benefits of Linking Addiction Treatment With Other Medical and Psychiatric Services

From the Patient's Perspective

- Improves overall quality of care.

- Facilitates access to addictive disorder treatment for patients in medical care settings.

- Enhances access to primary medical care for patients receiving addictive disorder treatment.

- Improves patient wellbeing in terms of addictive disorder severity and medical problems.

- Provides care that may be easier to access.

- Increases the patient's satisfaction with his or her health care.

From the Primary Care Provider's Perspective

- Promotes screening of all patients for alcohol problems.

- Facilitates inclusion of alcohol and drug causes when considering a differential diagnosis.

- Allows more achievable access to the addictive disorder treatment system.

- Supports the prevention of relapse to alcohol and drug abuse.

- Encourages other mental health services for primary care patients.

- Enhances adherence with appointments and medical regimens.

- Provides addictive disorder training opportunities for personnel.

From the Addiction Treatment Provider's Perspective

- Improves addictive disorder treatment outcomes.

- Reduces stigma about addictive disorder issues among medical providers.

- Provides training opportunities about addictive disorder-related medical problems.

- Promotes healthier behaviors.

- Enhances medical providers' appreciation of the value of addictive disorder treatment.

- Creates support for reimbursement parity for addictive disorder services.

- Develops ongoing quality improvement efforts within addictive disorder programs.

From a Societal Perspective

- Reduces costs related to health care, criminal justice, and loss of productivity.

- Reduces duplication of services and administrative costs.

- Improves health outcomes of specific populations.

---

psychiatric problems, and overall quality of life (D'Aunno, 1997). A pragmatic patient benefit is the provision of a convenient service; this positive development would require careful assessment of the appropriateness of likely increased service utilization. Finally, linking services also may decrease stigma.

From the perspective of the primary care provider and the mental health clinician, possible benefits of linkage include early identification of and relapse prevention for substance use disorders (Friedmann, Saitz et al., 1998), more consideration given to alcohol and drug problems in the formulation of differential diagnoses, better access to addictive disorder treatment services, enhanced patient adherence to appointments and medications, and addictive disorder training opportunities for personnel.

From an addiction treatment provider's perspective, stronger linkages could yield improved outcomes of addictive disorder treatment, similar to that demonstrated with the addition of needed psychosocial services (McLellan, Arndt et al., 1993; McLellan, Hagan et al., 1998). Ready availability of needed medical and mental health services also would allow addictive disorder professionals to do what they do best: focus on the core substance use issues. Exposure to examples of successful treatment could reduce stigma on the part of medical and mental health professionals toward addictive disorders and enhance their appreciation of the value of addictive disorder treatment. Bringing addictive disorder treatment closer to mainstream medical care and exposing its similarities to the care of other chronic illnesses could support the effort to achieve reimbursement parity for addictive disorders. Addictive disorder providers could learn about the medical and mental health complications of addictions and enhance their appreciation of clients' conditions, health care needs, and prevention approaches. Conceivably, the linkage of services could provide an opportunity to affect other behavior-related issues, such as sexually transmitted diseases (including HIV) and smoking. Finally, linkage of services could enhance quality improvement efforts within addictive disorder treatment systems—a relatively recent requirement for accreditation by the Joint Commission on Accreditation of Healthcare Organizations—by taking lessons from medical settings that have grappled with these issues as part of the restructuring of medical care systems.

From a societal perspective, stronger linkages can reduce long-term costs, including savings from HIV infections and other health-related sequelae of substance use averted, reduced incarceration and other criminal justice expenditures, and increased productivity. Other benefits include reduced duplication of services across these systems. Finally, a potential public health achievement would be improved health outcomes for specific populations burdened with the substantial morbidity associated with alcohol or drug use disorders.

MODELS OF LINKED SERVICES

Alcohol and drug-abusing patients use services in "inefficient" ways (for example, emergency department presentations rather than outpatient clinic visits), and they do not receive care in the continuous, longitudinal, and comprehensive manner essential for the high-quality management of any chronic disease (Bodenheimer, 2000; Kimball & Young, 1994; Saitz, Mulvey et al., 1997b). Two basic models have been proposed to bring the system of care for patients with substance use disorders closer to a primary care or chronic disease management model (Table 2). One model uses a centralized approach in which treatment of addictive disorders, primary medical care, and mental health services are co-located at a single site. A different model uses a distributive approach to facilitate effective patient referrals to services at different sites. This section describes these models of linked primary medical, mental health, and addictive disorder services and reviews the available evidence of their success in facilitating the multidisciplinary care of addicted patients.

Centralized Models. Centralized or on-site models bring primary care, mental health, and/or addictive disorder services together at a single site. This fully integrated, "one-stop shopping" model has been best described in primary care medical clinics and in addictive disorder treatment programs. In addition to overcoming the substantial political, bureaucratic, attitudinal, and financial barriers that separate addicted persons from needed services (CSAT, 1993; Umbricht-Schneiter, Ginn et al., 1994), centralized delivery overcomes the problems of geographic separation, patient disorganization, and poor motivation that inhibit patients with addictive disorders from keeping outside appointments (Teitelbaum, Walker et al., 1992; Umbricht-Schneiter, Ginn et al., 1994).

Willenbring and Olson (1999) have reported favorable results for a model of integrated alcohol treatment in a primary care clinic for poorly motivated, medically ill alcoholics. Their model included (1) at least monthly visits, (2) outreach to patients who missed appointments, (3) clinic notes that cued the primary care physician or nurse practitioner to monitor alcohol intake at each visit, (4) physician- or nurse practitioner-delivered brief advice that emphasized reducing the harm from alcohol use and cutting down rather than strict abstinence, (5) verbal and graphic feedback of improvement and deterioration in biological markers such as gamma-glutamyl transferase (GGT), and (6) on-site mental health services as needed (Willenbring, Olson et al., 1995). In a randomized design, medically ill alcoholic patients in the integrated clinic were compared with similar patients referred to traditional alcoholism treatment and ambulatory medical care. During two years of followup, patients in the integrated clinic had improved drinking outcomes (including greater abstinence), returned twice as often for outpatient visits, and experienced lower mortality. Although this model may prove too elaborate for many primary care settings, it serves as a starting point for a disease management system for substance use disorders similar to those

---

TABLE 2.   Features of Centralized and Distributive Integrated Service Models

---

Centralized Models

- Addiction treatment delivered at primary medical care and mental health services sites.

- Addiction providers located in group health maintenance organizations, private practices, or clinics.

- Behavioral medicine and primary medical provider offices co-located in shared space.

- Addiction treatment delivered at public health clinics (for example, sexually transmitted infections, HIV, or tuberculosis care).

- Addiction treatment delivered in a general hospital with proximate medical and mental health clinics.

- Addiction treatment and primary care services co-located in a community mental health setting.

- Addiction-trained nurse practitioner or physician available in a primary care practice to prescribe and monitor naltrexone, to prescribe and monitor buprenorphine, and to initiate and manage detoxification.

- Addiction and mental health specialty teams present in medical care sites (for example, consult teams in emergency departments or hospitals).

- Smoking cessation counseling and pharmacotherapy delivered as part of primary care (brief intervention in doctor's offices, emergency departments, and hospitals).

- Primary medical care and mental health services delivered at addiction treatment sites.

- Medical and mental health providers or clinic located at a methadone treatment program.

- Co-located primary care and addiction care.

- An integrated alcohol and medical clinic.

- An addiction medicine physician with medical and psychiatric skills.

- A multiservice community agency with a central location.

Distributive Models

- Health maintenance organizations or preferred provider organizations with defined, yet decentralized referral networks.

- Addiction triage and referral or central intake and assessment centers that perform medical and mental health assessments and referral for multiple addiction treatment programs.

- Community-based case management.

- Evaluation at addiction treatment sites, with external referral for ongoing medical and mental health care.

- Defined networks of providers with facilitated communication and financial/contractual links and systems.

- Informal links between clinicians or agencies, facilitated by releases of information, transportation, and case management.

- A multiservice community agency with a single owner but several locations.

---

used for asthma, diabetes mellitus, and congestive heart failure (Bodenheimer, 2000; Finney, Willenbring et al., 2000). With further study, this model may prove cost-effective for recalcitrant alcohol-dependent patients or for other poorly motivated or complicated substance-abusing patients.

Less resource-intensive intervention models developed for problem drinkers in primary care also have proved feasible. The cost analysis of Project TrEAT, a randomized study of physician-delivered brief interventions, showed substantial improvements in drinking outcomes and substantial savings for society and health systems (Fleming, Mundt et al., 2000). A primary care study from the University of Massachusetts reported that 2.5 hours of primary care provider training in patient-centered alcohol brief intervention was feasible (Adams, Ockene et al., 1998) and reduced alcohol consumption among problem drinkers

(Ockene, Adams et al., 1999). An early study suggested that simple feedback about changes in biological markers, such as GGT in alcoholic patients, can itself reduce sick days, hospital days, and mortality (Kristenson, Ohlin et al., 1983). Saitz and colleagues demonstrated that a systems intervention (physician prompting with suggested courses of action) can improve counseling for alcohol problems and reduce drinking (Saitz, Horton et al., in press). In another model of alcohol treatment in primary care, O'Connor reported the successful treatment of a series of alcohol-dependent patients with naltrexone (ReVia®) (O'Connor, Farren et al., 1997). Other models have successfully incorporated behavioral health personnel into primary care practices (Bray & Rogers, 1997; Kunnes, Niven et al., 1993). However, if these efforts are to be generalized to primary care settings as they exist today, substantial training of clinicians will be required.

Few American studies have integrated treatment of illicit drug dependence into primary care, although general practitioners frequently participate in the management of these disorders elsewhere in the world. Under the terms of the Drug Addiction Treatment Act of 2000, qualifying American physicians are able to provide office-based treatment of opioid dependence with Schedule III, IV, or V pharmacologic agents approved by the U.S. Food and Drug Administration (FDA). Sublingual buprenorphine (Subutex®) and a combination of buprenorphine and naloxone (Suboxone®) recently were approved for this purpose. Several studies have found that buprenorphine works as well as methadone for patients with opiate addiction of mild to moderate severity. In a 12-week randomized trial of 46 opiate-dependent patients treated with buprenorphine maintenance, there was higher retention in the primary care setting than in a drug treatment program (78% versus 52%, $p = 0.06$), and lower rates of opioid use based on urine toxicology (63% versus 85%, $p < 0.01$) (O'Connor, Oliveto et al., 1998). With the development and dissemination of new pharmacologic therapies for alcohol and other drug use disorders, the impetus for addictive disorder services in the primary care setting will only increase.

Centralized models of primary medical and mental health care in addiction treatment settings also improve addicted patients' access to these services (Friedmann, Alexander et al., 1999). For example, Umbricht-Schneiter and colleagues (1994) found that 92% of patients randomly assigned to a centralized model in a methadone treatment program received medical services, compared with only 35%

of patients referred to a local clinic (Umbricht-Schneiter, Ginn et al., 1994). Such integrated models also have been found to promote delivery of HIV-related care, medication adherence, and outpatient medical services (Friedmann, Lemon et al., 2001; Newschaffer, Laine et al., 1998; Samet, Stein et al., 1995; Selwyn, Budner et al., 1993). An analysis of data gathered from New York State Medicaid claims found that regular drug abuse and medical care reduced hospitalizations by approximately 25% among HIV-positive and HIV-negative patients with drug abuse diagnoses (Laine, Hauck et al., 2001). A recent randomized trial of integrated primary care in an addiction treatment program concluded that integrated care is cost-effective for patients with addictive disorder-related medical conditions (Weisner, Mertens et al., 2001).

Integration of addictive disorder treatment and community mental health services similarly reduces relapse and improves social stability for patients dually diagnosed with addictive disorders and mental illness (Bach-Beisel, Scott et al., 1999; Baker, 1991; Crits-Christoph & Siqueland, 1996).

In general, patients with nicotine dependence, at-risk drinking, and low-severity illicit drug use can be managed in primary care settings without subspecialty addiction medicine consultation. On the other hand, patients with addictive disorders or dependence generally should be cared for in collaboration with addiction specialists (whether integrated in a primary care office or located elsewhere). All patients should have primary and preventive health care—again, where this care is delivered will depend on the system of care. An ideal centralized model of care can provide the addiction, mental health, and medical care at a single site. Whether specialty addiction medicine or addiction psychiatry services are delivered at an addiction specialty treatment site or within the primary care setting, the key is that systems be integrated to deliver the most appropriate and efficient care.

Distributive Models. In light of the lack of parity for the treatment of substance use disorders and the absence of unified budgets for medical and behavioral health services (Mechanic, 1999), most providers lack resources to provide comprehensive, centralized services for addicted patients (Friedmann, Alexander et al., 1999). Moreover, patients (especially those in long-term recovery) may object to long-term primary care in settings primarily identified as addiction treatment programs. Therefore, the development and dissemination of effective decentralized or distributive models is an important step toward service integration in the current health care environment.

Successful referral is the central task of the distributive model. Anecdote and limited data suggest that simple referral alone cannot integrate the care of addicted patients in primary care settings. For example, among 1,440 patients in addiction treatment with a primary care physician, 45% reported that the physician who cared for them was unaware of their addictive disorder (Saitz, Mulvey et al., 1997a). A study of one community in California similarly noted that 45% of drug users had contact with the mainstream health care system in a given year, but medical or mental health providers were major client referral sources or destinations for fewer than 10% of addictive disorder programs (Weisner & Schmidt, 1995). Thus, the substantial interorganizational distance between addiction treatment programs and mainstream health care presents great barriers to successful referral. Because substance-abusing populations can have disorganized lifestyles and poor motivation, contemporary distributive models typically use case management to facilitate referrals. Community-based case management can effectively link substance-dependent patients to needed services (Ashery, 1992; Brindis, Pfeffer et al., 1995).

In addiction disorder treatment programs, distributive arrangements are commonly used to link patients to medical and mental health services (Friedmann, D'Aunno et al., 2000; Samet, Saitz et al., 1996; Peter D. Hart Research Associates, 1999). Distributive arrangements range, for example, from an addictive disorder treatment unit that contracts with a local group practice to provide physical examinations and routine medical care to its patients, to one that makes *ad hoc* referrals to a local community mental health center. The advantage of this model is that it makes use of existing health care systems. For example, in an ongoing study, patients in an inpatient detoxification unit receive a facilitated referral to primary care in the local community from a multidisciplinary team (physician, nurse, and social worker) (Samet, Larson et al., in press). This model requires no rearrangement of existing health care delivery systems. It does require efforts (and therefore costs) to assure that linkage is facilitated.

Case management or transportation assistance can facilitate these referrals (Friedmann, D'Aunno et al., 2000; Friedmann, Lemon et al., 2001; Schwartz, Baker et al., 1997). A study of public addiction treatment programs found that contracted referral with case management increased medi-cal services utilization twofold to threefold over *ad hoc* referrals (McLellan, Hagan et al., 1999). More recent work has emphasized the importance of transportation assistance to increase the delivery of needed services (Friedmann, D'Aunno et al., 2000b; Friedmann, Lemon et al., 2001).

In summary, several effective models of centralized and distributive linkage in primary care and specialty addiction treatment settings have been developed. Addiction interventions in medical settings are appropriate for at-risk drinkers and substance use disorders of mild-to-moderate severity, medically ill substance-dependent patients who refuse formal treatment referral, and substance-dependent patients who receive rehabilitative counseling elsewhere yet would benefit from substance-related pharmacotherapy and management of their medical problems. With adequate support, primary care physicians also can have a productive role in outpatient detoxification (O'Connor, Waugh et al., 1995). Minimally motivated patients who will accept only harm reduction interventions can benefit from management in the primary care setting as well. For patients in formal addiction treatment, linkage to needed medical and psychological services can improve access to health care, improve physical and mental health, and reduce relapse.

Both centralized and distributive models show promise for integrating care across these systems. The distributive model predominates in the United States (Friedmann, D'Aunno et al., 2000). Although it can be less effective than the centralized model in linking substance-abusing patients to needed services (Friedmann, Lemon et al., 2001; Umbricht-Schneiter, Ginn et al., 1994), its relatively low cost, flexibility, and adaptability (especially to integration of secondary and tertiary care services), suggest that the distributive model, with further refinements, is likely to remain the shape of integrated services in the near future.

PROSPECTS FOR IMPROVED LINKAGE

Despite the enormity of the challenge, the time is right for a transformation in the configuration of addictive disorder treatment and health care services. A number of signs suggest that a window of opportunity exists for innovation. The staggering burden of medical and mental health problems affecting substance-abusing patients is now well documented, from HIV, hepatitis C, and drug overdose, to depression, anxiety, and victimization (Liebschutz, Mulvey et al., 1997; O'Connor, Selwyn et al., 1994; Schiff, 1997; Sporer, 1999). The enormous economic burden that substance use problems place on our society, through costs related to health care, criminality/incarceration, and loss of productivity, increasingly is recognized and forces policymakers to consider alternative approaches to the management and care of this population (NIDA & NIAAA, 1998). Moreover, advances in the diagnosis and treatment of substance-related disorders, including pharmacologic and behavioral approaches applicable in the primary care setting, promise to change the approach to clinical management of these prevalent disorders.

Primary care and disease management systems are not restricted to physicians, but rather require a multidisciplinary team. Thus, the reported sense of overburdening of physicians should not preclude the development of linkage systems but rather influence its development so that its implementation does not solely rely on physicians' functions (St. Peter, Reed et al., 1999). The ability to treat addictive disorders in less intensive settings will promote cost savings and cost-effectiveness. Increased attention to the improvement of quality in health care systems also presents opportunities to address linkage to addictive disorder treatment as a quality issue. Finally, the current era has seen rapid reorganization of health care services. Despite the difficulties associated with such periods, they challenge policymakers to rethink inadequate systems and can create a climate of innovation toward the delivery of high-quality, comprehensive, and integrated care for patients with substance use disorders.

REFERENCES

Adams A, Ockene JK, Wheeler EV et al. (1998). Alcohol counseling: Physicians will do it. *Journal of General Internal Medicine* 13:692-698.

Adger H Jr, Macdonald DI & Wenger S (1999). Core competencies for involvement of health care providers in the care of children and adolescents in families affected by substance abuse. *Pediatrics* 103:1083-1084.

Ashery RS, ed. (1992). *Progress and Issues in Case Management* (NIH publication no. ADM 92-1946). Rockville, MD: National Institute on Drug Abuse.

Bach-Beisel J, Scott J & Dixon L (1999). Co-occurring severe mental illness and substance use disorders: A review of recent research. *Psychiatric Services* 50:1427-1434.

Baker F (1991). *Coordination of Alcohol, Drug Abuse, and Mental Health Services* (Publication no. SMA 00-3360, Technical Assistance Publication Series, No. 4). Rockville, MD: Center for Substance Abuse Treatment.

Bodenheimer T (2000). Disease management in the American market. *British Medical Journal* 320:563-566.

Bosl RH (2001). The illusion of parity [letter]. *Internal Medicine News* 2001:8, May 15.

Bray JH & Rogers JC (1997). The linkages project: Training behavioral health professionals for collaborative practice with primary care physicians. *Families, Systems & Health* 15:55-61.

Brindis CD, Pfeffer R & Wolfe A (1995). A case management program for chemically dependent clients with multiple needs. *Journal of Case Management* 4:22-28.

Brown RL, Marcus M, Amodeo M et al. (2001). The HRSA-AMERSA interdisciplinary faculty development fellowship program in substance abuse [abstract]. *Substance Abuse* 22:127.

Center for Substance Abuse Treatment (CSAT) (1993). *State Methadone Maintenance Treatment Guidelines* (DHHS Publication No. SMA 93-1991). Rockville, MD: CSAT, Substance Abuse and Mental Health Services Administration.

Chappel JN & Schnoll SH (1977). Physician attitudes: Effect on the treatment of chemically dependent patients. *Journal of the American Medical Association* 237:2318-2319.

Cohen P & Cohen J (1984). The clinician's illusion. *Archives of General Psychiatry* 41:1178-1182.

Crits-Christoph P & Siqueland L (1996). Psychosocial treatment for drug abuse: Selected review and recommendations for national health care. *Archives of General Psychiatry* 53:749-756.

D'Aunno TA (1997). Linking substance abuse treatment and primary health care. In JA Egertson, DM Fox & AI Leshner (eds.) *Treating Drug Abusers Effectively.* Malden, MA: Blackwell Publishers, 311-351.

D'Onofrio G, Nadel ES, Degutis LC et al. (2002). Improving emergency medicine residents' approach to patients with alcohol problems: A controlled educational trial. *Annals of Emergency Medicine* 40:50-62.

Etheridge RM, Craddock SG, Dunteman GH et al. (1995). Client services in two national studies of community-based drug abuse treatment programs. *Journal of Substance Abuse* 7:9-26.

Finney JW, Willenbring ML & Moos RH (2000). Improving the quality of VA care for patients with substance-use disorders: The Quality Enhancement Research Initiative (QUERI) substance abuse module. *Medical Care* 38:I105-I113.

Fleming MF, Mundt MP, French MT et al. (2000). Benefit-cost analysis of brief physician advice with problem drinkers in primary care settings. *Medical Care* 38:7-18.

Friedmann PD, Alexander JA, Jin L et al. (1999). On-site primary care and mental health services in outpatient drug abuse treatment units. *Journal of Behavioral Health Services & Research* 26:80-94.

Friedmann PD, D'Aunno TA, Jin L et al. (2000). Medical and psychosocial services in drug abuse treatment: Do stronger linkages promote client utilization? *Health Services Research* 35:443-465.

Friedmann PD, Lemon SC, Stein MD et al. (2001). Linkage to medical services in the Drug Abuse Treatment Outcome Study. *Medical Care* 39:284-295.

Friedmann PD, McCullough D, Chin MH et al. (2000). Screening and intervention for alcohol problems. A national survey of primary care physicians and psychiatrists. *Journal of General Internal Medicine* 15:84-91.

Friedmann PD, Saitz R & Samet JH (1998). Management of adults recovering from alcohol or other drug problems: Relapse prevention in primary care. *Journal of the American Medical Association* 279:1227-1231.

Geller G, Levine DM, Mamon JA et al. (1989). Knowledge, attitudes, and reported practices of medical students and house staff regarding the diagnosis and treatment of alcoholism. *Journal of the American Medical Association* 261:3115-3120.

Goldman W, McCulloch J & Sturm R (1998). Costs and use of mental health services before and after managed care. *Health Affairs* 17:40-52.

Haack MR & Adger H Jr., eds. (2002). Strategic plan for interdisciplinary faculty development. Arming the nation's health professional workforce for a new approach to substance use disorders. *Substance Abuse* 23(3 Suppl).

Isaacson JH, Fleming M, Kraus M et al. (2000). A national survey of training in substance use disorders in residency programs. *Journal of Studies on Alcohol* 61:912-915.

Kimball HR & Young PR (1994). Statement on the generalist physician from the American Boards of Family Practice and Internal Medicine. *Journal of the American Medical Association* 271:315-316.

Kristenson H, Ohlin H, Hulten-Nosslin MB et al. (1983). Identification and intervention of heavy drinking in middle-aged men: Results and follow-up of 24-60 months of long-term study with randomized controls. *Alcoholism: Clinical & Experimental Research*, 7:203-209.

Kunnes R, Niven R, Gustafson T et al. (1993). Financing and payment reform for primary health care and substance abuse treatment. *Journal of Addictive Diseases* 12:23-42.

Laine C, Hauck WW, Gourevitch MN et al. (2001). Regular outpatient medical and drug abuse care and subsequent hospitalization of persons who use illicit drugs. *Journal of the American Medical Association* 285:2355-2362.

Laine C, Newschaffer C, Zhang D et al. (2000). Models of care in New York State Medicaid substance abuse clinics. Range of services and linkages to medical care. *Journal of Substance Abuse Treatment* 12:271-285.

Larson MJ, Samet JH & McCarty D (1997). Managed care of substance abuse disorders. Implications for generalist physicians. *Medical Clinics of North America* 81:1053-1069.

Lewis DC, Niven RG, Czechowicz D et al. (1987). A review of medical education in alcohol and other drug abuse. *Journal of the American Medical Association* 257:2945-2948.

Liebschutz JM, Mulvey KP & Samet JH (1997). Victimization among substance-abusing women. Worse health outcomes. *Archives of Internal Medicine* 157:1093-1097.

McLellan AT, Arndt IO, Metzger DS et al. (1993). The effects of psychosocial services in substance abuse treatment. *Journal of the American Medical Association* 269:1953-1959.

McLellan AT, Hagan TA, Levine M et al. (1998). Supplemental social services improve outcomes in public addiction treatment. *Addiction* 93:1489-1499.

McLellan AT, Hagan TA, Levine M et al. (1999). Does clinical case management improve outpatient addiction treatment. *Drug and Alcohol Dependence* 55:91-103.

McLellan AT, Lewis DC, O'Brien CP et al. (2000). Drug dependence, a chronic medical illness: Implications for treatment, insurance, and outcomes evaluation. *Journal of the American Medical Association* 284:1689-1695.

McLellan AT, Woody GE, Metzger D et al. (1996). Evaluating the effectiveness of addiction treatments: Reasonable expectations, appropriate comparisons. *Milbank Quarterly* 74:51-85.

Mechanic D (1999). Integrating mental health into a general health care system. *Hospital and Community Psychiatry* 45:893-897.

Moore RD, Bone LR, Geller G et al. (1989). Prevalence, detection, and treatment of alcoholism in hospitalized patients. *Journal of the American Medical Association* 261:403-407.

National Institute on Drug Abuse & National Institute on Alcohol Abuse and Alcoholism (NIDA & NIAAA) (1998). In HJ Harwood, D Fountain & D Livermore (eds.) *The Economic Costs of Alcohol and Drug Abuse in the United States—1992.* Accessed at: HTTP://WWW.NIDA.NIH.GOV/ECONOMICCOSTS/INDEX.HTML. Accessed June 25, 2001.

Newschaffer CJ, Laine C, Hauck WW et al. (1998). Clinic characteristics associated with reduced hospitalization of drug users with AIDS. *Journal of Urban Health* 75:153-169.

O'Brien CP & McLellan AT (1996). Myths about the treatment of addiction. *Lancet* 347:237-240.

O'Connor PG, Farren CK, Rounsaville BJ et al. (1997). A preliminary investigation of the management of alcohol dependence with naltrexone by primary care providers. *American Journal of Medicine* 103:477-482.

O'Connor PG, Oliveto AH, Shi JM et al. (1998). A randomized trial of buprenorphine maintenance for heroin dependence in a primary care clinic for substance users versus a methadone clinic. *American Journal of Medicine* 105:100-105.

O'Connor PG, Selwyn PA & Schottenfeld RS (1994). Medical care for injection-drug users with human immunodeficiency virus infection. *New England Journal of Medicine* 331:450-459.

O'Connor PG, Waugh ME, Carroll K et al. (1995). Primary care-based ambulatory opioid detoxification: The results of a clinical trial. *Journal of General Internal Medicine* 10:255-260.

Ockene JK, Adams A, Hurley TG et al. (1999). Brief physician and nurse practitioner-delivered counseling for high-risk drinkers: Does it work? *Archives of Internal Medicine* 159:2198-2205.

Peter D. Hart Research Associates (1999). *The Road to Recovery. A Landmark National Study on Public Perceptions of Alcoholism and Barriers to Treatment.* New York, NY: The Recovery Institute.

Saitz R, Horton NJ, Sullivan LM et al. (in press). Addressing alcohol problems in primary care: A cluster randomized, controlled trial of a systems intervention (the Screening and Intervention in Primary Care (SIP) Study). *Annals of Internal Medicine.*

Saitz R, Mulvey KP, Plough A et al. (1997a). Physician unawareness of serious substance abuse. *American Journal of Drug and Alcohol Abuse* 23:343-354.

Saitz R, Mulvey KP & Samet JH (1997b). The substance abusing patient and primary care: Linkage via the addiction treatment system? *Substance Abuse* 18:187-195.

Saitz R, Sullivan LM & Samet JH (2000). Training community-based clinicians in screening and brief intervention for substance abuse problems: Translating evidence into practice. *Substance Abuse* 21:21-32.

Samet JA, Stein MD & O'Connor PG (1995). Models of medical care for HIV-infected drug users. *Substance Abuse* 16:131-139.

Samet JH, Larson MJ, Horton NJ et al. (in press). Linking alcohol and drug dependent adults to primary medical care: A randomized controlled trial of a multidisciplinary health evaluation in a detoxification unit (the Health Evaluation and Linkage to Primary Care [HELP] Study). *Addiction.*

Samet JH, Saitz R & Larson MJ (1996). A case for enhanced linkage of substance abusers to primary medical care. *Substance Abuse* 17:181-199.

Schiff ER (1997). Hepatitis C and alcohol. *Hepatology* 26:39S-42S.

Schoenbaum M, Zhang W & Sturm R (1998). Costs and utilization of substance abuse care in a privately insured population under managed care. *Psychiatric Services* 49:1573-1578.

Schwartz M, Baker G, Mulvey KP et al. (1997). Improving publicly funded substance abuse treatment: The value of case management. *American Journal of Public Health* 87:1659-1664.

Selwyn PA, Budner NW, Wasserman WC et al. (1993). Utilization of on-site primary care services by HIV-seropositive and seronegative drug users in a methadone maintenance program. *Public Health Reports* 108:492-500.

Sirica C, ed. (1995). *Training About Alcohol and Substance Abuse for All Primary Care Physicians* (conference proceedings, October 2-5, 1994). New York, NY: Josiah Macy Jr. Foundation.

Sporer KA (1999). Acute heroin overdose. *Annals of Internal Medicine* 130:584-590.

St. Peter RF, Reed MC, Kemper P et al. (1999). Changes in the scope of care provided by primary care physicians. *New England Journal of Medicine* 341:1980-1985.

Stein B, Reardon E & Sturm R (1999). Substance abuse service utilization under managed care: HMOs versus carve-out plans. *Journal of Behavioral Health Services & Research* 26:451-456.

Sturm R (1999). Tracking changes in behavioral health services: How have carve-outs changed care? *Journal of Behavioral Health Services & Research* 26:360-371.

Sturm R & McCulloch J (1998). Mental health and substance abuse benefits in carve-out plans and the Mental Health Parity Act of 1996. *Journal of Health Care Finance* 24:82-92.

Sturm R, Zhang W & Schoenbaum M (1999). How expensive are unlimited substance abuse benefits under managed care? *Journal of Behavioral Health Services & Research* 26:203-210.

Teitelbaum M, Walker A, Gabay M et al. (1992). *Analysis of Barriers to the Delivery of Integrated Primary Care Services and Substance Abuse Treatment: Case Studies of Nine Linkage Program Projects.* Rockville, MD: Health Resources and Services Administration and Abt Associates, Inc.

Umbricht-Schneiter A, Ginn DH, Pabst KM et al. (1994). Providing medical care to methadone clinic patients: Referral vs. on-site. *American Journal of Public Health* 84:207-210.

Weisner C & Schmidt LA (1995). Expanding the frame of health services research in the drug abuse field. *Health Services Research* 30:707-726.

Weisner C, Mertens J, Parthasarathy S et al. (2001). Improved effectiveness from integrating primary medical care with addiction treatment. Presented at American Society of Addiction Medicine 32nd Annual Medical-Scientific Conference, Los Angeles, CA; April 20.

Willenbring ML & Olson DH (1999). A randomized trial of integrated outpatient treatment for medically ill alcoholic men. *Archives of Internal Medicine* 159:1946-1952.

Willenbring ML, Olson DH, Bielinski J et al. (1995). Treatment of medically ill alcoholics in the primary-care setting. In T Beresford & E Gomberg (eds.) *Alcohol and Aging.* New York, NY: Oxford University Press, 249-259.

Chapter 9 | Complementary and Alternative Therapies

Tacey A. Boucher, Ph.D.
Thomas J. Kiresuk, Ph.D.
Alan I. Trachtenberg, M.D., M.P.H.

Many therapies and practices in addiction treatment in the United States can be labeled "complementary" or "alternative" therapies (CAT). Alternative health practices, in general, have been gaining in popularity and prevalence in the U.S. for at least the last half century (Kessler, Davis et al., 2001). Over the past decade, scientific publications and the popular press have raised awareness of these therapies and their widespread use by the public. Surveys suggest that a large percentage of physicians are willing to consider the possibility that at least some alternative therapies hold promise for the treatment of various symptoms of disease (Boucher & Lenz, 1998). In addition, the National Institutes of Health has been supporting the scientific evaluation of alternative therapies through the National Center for Complementary and Alternative Medicine (NCCAM), formerly the Office of Alternative Medicine, since 1992. While definitive outcome data may not yet be available for many of these therapies, preliminary findings suggest that some may have efficacy. Moreover, some alternative therapies may offer symptomatic relief, comfort, or other benefits when the treatments are supported by the health beliefs of the patient. For example, traditional treatments (based on cultural health traditions of the community), if safe and inexpensive, can form a useful component of culturally competent, community-oriented comprehensive care, especially for rural, remote, and culturally distinct populations.

The goal of this chapter is to provide basic information to researchers and practitioners unfamiliar with complementary and alternative therapies for the treatment of addiction, so they can answer the questions of patients who are using or considering such therapies for their mental or physical health problems, as well as to provide useful information to clinicians who are willing to consider or use alternative therapies for patients who have special needs and for whom traditional therapies have been ineffective or unacceptable.

To this end, the chapter reviews several of the most frequently used or promising therapies, such as acupuncture, biofeedback, and nutrition. For each modality, a brief description is provided, followed by a summary of the current state of the science. Some of the primary debates and questions facing both researchers and practitioners are discussed as well.

OVERVIEW OF COMPLEMENTARY AND ALTERNATIVE THERAPIES

The use of CAT extends around the world and, in many countries, constitutes the major form of treatment. Therapies seem to gain a designation of "alternative" in U.S. medicine if they come from the medical traditions of other cultures or originate outside the hospital-based, research-oriented biomedical culture of the West. If so, they are subjected (sometimes properly so) to greater skepticism and more demands for evidence than if they came from a surgical research center or other regular medical setting. Unfortunately, this skepticism has made it difficult for either proponents or curious researchers to accumulate acceptable data to support or refute their efficacy.

American consumers, however, have demonstrated less skepticism than their physicians. Consumers spent an estimated $27 billion out of pocket on CAT in 1997, and research suggests that they used CAT for a variety of conditions, visiting CAT providers more frequently than they did primary care physicians (Eisenberg, Davis et al., 1998). Use of CAT does not appear restricted by social class, educational levels, or gender (Wolsko, Ware et al., 2000; Eisenberg, Davis et al., 1998).

Patient and physician surveys are not the only indication of CAT's increasing use. For instance, CAT courses now are offered in more than half of U.S. medical schools and in growing numbers of public health programs. The University of Minnesota School of Medicine now offers a minor in CAT. Some health plans have started to reimburse for CAT services such as chiropractic and acupuncture, and others are expected to follow suit (Stoneham, 1998). Eight states mandate insurance coverage for at least one form of CAT, while seven states mandate insurance coverage specifically of acupuncture (Sturm & Unutzer, 2000-2001). Changes in terminology from "unconventional" or "alternative" to "complementary" and "integrative" speak to the increasing cooperation between conventional and alternative health disciplines.

Three recent studies have found that CAT is widely used by individuals with self-reported mental conditions, including substance use disorders, depression, and anxiety (Druss & Rosenheck, 2000; Kessler, Soukap et al., 2000; Unutzer, Klap et al., 2000). The lack of a "magic bullet" to treat most substance use disorders and the high rates of relapse may help to explain the interest in CAT among practitioners of addiction medicine. Physicians may be more willing to refer patients to CAT practitioners for complaints that conventional medicine has been unable to address. For example, the appearance of crack cocaine in the 1980s probably contributed to the popularity of acupuncture in treatment centers and drug courts throughout the U.S.

CAT and Addiction Medicine. Some of the landmarks in the history of addiction medicine demonstrate the recurrent interaction of standard practice with modalities and practices considered by many to be "alternative." In the late 1800s, for example, sanitaria for persons with alcohol and opiate disorders offered, among other things, saline and electric baths. At the turn of the century, street vendors sold remedies for every complaint imaginable, including alcoholism and "soldier's sickness" (morphine addiction). The remedies themselves were not regulated and often contained a variety of addictive ingredients, including morphine and cocaine (Morgan, 1981). In the mid-1900s, treatment took a spiritual path, as individuals participating in Alcoholics Anonymous (AA) and other self-help groups were instructed to turn their lives over to a Higher Power (Miller, 1990; Chappel, 1993). Today, Twelve Step programs and other programs based on the AA model are the most popular forms of intervention in the U.S. (Vaillant, Clark et al., 1993; Peteet, 1993). This utilization occurs even though the Twelve Step approach came from outside the biomedical establishment and still suffers from a paucity of randomized clinical trial data.

Although many significant findings have been reported over the past two decades regarding the physiological, neurochemical, and pharmacological basis of addiction, many scientists and physicians no longer seek a "magic bullet," but a combination of therapies to prevent or treat addictive disease. Efforts to broaden the practitioner's treatment arsenal have run parallel with the growing popular acceptance of CAT. Addiction treatment programs increasingly use a combination of conventional and alternative methods, as in the use of acupuncture in conjunction with counseling and methadone. Within the past three decades, researchers have begun to take an active role in exploring the potential of CAT therapies for the treatment of addictive disorders. The fluid nature of CAT's boundaries and the changing nature of addiction medicine provide a rich and varied field for research.

Defining CAT. CAT represents a wide range of interventions that are not currently considered an integral part of the conventional medical system in the U.S. Attempts to create an operational definition have been limited in part by changing attitudes, as well as a growing body of clinical experience and scientific data. Such definitions are culturally relative and specific to the jurisdictions in which they occur.

Such variation is demonstrated by the acceptance of acupuncture in conventional medicine in France as merely another specialty, like surgery or psychiatry. Similarly, German medicine incorporates a well-regulated and accepted role for phytomedical (herbal) and even homeopathic remedies. In the United States, the National Institutes of Health's NCCAM groups CAT into five domains: (1) mind/body interventions, (2) biologically based treatments, (3) manipulative and body-based methods, (4) energy therapies, and (5) alternative medical systems.

The label "CAT" may be applied to entire systems of medicine (such as Ayurvedic Medicine), a specific modality or therapy (such as massage or ear acupuncture), a profession or practice (such as naturopathy), or an explanation of efficacy (such as spiritual rather than behavioral or neurochemical). The particular use of a modality also may be considered CAT, such as the use of dietary restrictions and recommendations for the prevention of relapse to drugs and alcohol, in contrast to heart disease or diabetes, for which dietary treatments are conventional. Similarly, spirituality has become a standard of care in addiction medicine through Twelve Step programs, but not for the treatment of cancer. Definitions of CAT also have been unable to distinguish between certain lifestyle choices and therapeutic regimes, such as a vegetarian diet, prayer, art therapy, or meditation. This chapter will not resolve these problems of definition but will attend to those practices commonly understood to be representative of CAT.

Researching CAT. Although the application of "Western" research methodology to the realm of CAT research is relatively recent, it would be shortsighted to assume that the difference between CAT and conventional therapies is that the former are unproved and the latter are proven. While there is scant knowledge about the efficacy of CAT modalities, it generally is accepted that many treatments currently recommended by U.S. physicians also lack adequate evidence of efficacy (Goldstein, 1989). Nevertheless, the relative absence of scientific validation is particularly detrimental to physician acceptance of CAT (Schachter, Weingarten et al., 1993; Himmel, Schulte et al., 1993; Visser & Peters, 1990; Wharton & Lewith, 1986; Hadley, 1988; Marshall, 1992; Berman, Singh et al., 1995). At present, case studies, clinical data, and pilot studies with inadequate power, randomization, and/or controls constitute the majority of CAT research.

Controlled clinical trials have become the "gold standard" in the process of confirming or refuting the effectiveness of medical interventions. Skepticism of new treatments is justified because numerous treatments throughout history initially have been applied with enthusiasm, only later to be found ineffective or even detrimental (Shapiro & Morris, 1978). Neither conventional nor CAT modalities should be excluded from this process simply on the basis of their origin. However, it is important for researchers studying CAT to have an understanding of the special methodological problems inherent in researching some of these treatments. It also is important to strive for clarity in the interpretation and communication of research results. For example, there is an important and often overlooked difference between a study that fails to find effectiveness and one that finds ineffectiveness (including the need for the latter study sample to be much larger than that for the former study). Additionally, improvements in laboratory measurements do not always translate into improvements in the health outcomes associated with those measurements. Rigorous application of clinical epidemiology is essential, and neither conventional nor CAT modalities should be excluded from the evidence-based decision process simply on the basis of their origin.

In particular, difficulties arise around the issue of standardization. Other obstacles, such as blindedness, also need to be considered. Acupuncture has become the most thoroughly researched and used CAT modality for the treatment of addiction in the U.S. The methodological challenges inherent to CAT and addiction research may be illustrated by the acupuncture experience (see McLellan for a review; McLellan, Grossman et al., 1993).

Standardization: Many CAT therapies are rooted in philosophies and theories that focus on the entire person (or even the entire community) rather than on a disease entity. For example, in traditional Chinese medicine, individuals addicted to alcohol may be "diagnosed" with a number of different patterns of disharmony, such as "damp heat condition of the liver" or "kidney yin heart deficiency." Traditional treatment methods would vary, based on this alternative system of assessment.

In the interests of clinical expediency and research efficiency, however, treatment protocols for addictive disorders (among others) often are standardized, rather than individualized. The CAT protocol most commonly studied in the U.S. for addiction treatment was derived from the clinical practice at Lincoln Hospital in New York and was adopted by the National Acupuncture Detoxification Association (NADA). The acupuncture method consists of three to five needles placed in each ear, and is referred to as bilateral auricular acupuncture (Smith & Khan, 1988; Culliton & Kiresuk, 1996; Brumbaugh, 1993), or "Acudetox."

However, in clinical practice, the issue of standardization is controversial. The number of needles and the placement may vary from one practitioner to the next, as may the use of unilateral or bilateral auricular placement or the use of other body points. The needles may or may not be moved or twirled. The skin may or may not be penetrated. Electrical current and moxibustion (which are standard in general acupuncture but not in the NADA protocol) may or may not be used. The number of sessions attended over a given period of time also varies widely. As a result of this variation, it is difficult to compare results across studies, and the relevance of research protocols to clinical practice has been questioned.

Other Methodological Issues: These issues remain complex. If standardized points are to be used, how should these points reliably be identified? Some practitioners locate points by experience or by the responses of individual patients, while others use a galvanometer that measures skin impedance or conductivity. This relates to the level of practitioner experience. While double-blind studies of acupuncture would be ideal, only an untrained practitioner could be blinded to whether they were delivering a "true" or "control" treatment. However, untrained acupuncturists might lack the skills to know by site or patient reaction whether they are needling the appropriate location, thereby calling into question treatment reliability. To date, reliability has taken priority over blindedness, and a double-blind trial of acupuncture has not been conducted.

Regarding appropriate control groups, the identification of "placebo" or "sham" needling points also has been controversial. This is due, in part, to the inability of the majority of studies to find significant variation between "true" and "sham" treatment groups (Avants, Margolin et al., 1995; Lipton, Brewington et al., 1994). Other studies, however, have demonstrated such differences (Washburn, Fullilove et al., 1993; Avants, Margolin et al., 2000).

There are other important debates. For example, electroacupuncture has been shown to release endorphins, which has been hypothesized to be the primary mechanism of action in the relief of opiate withdrawal symptoms. However, unstimulated needles have not been shown to have the same effect (Ulett, Han et al., 1998; McLellan, Grossman et al., 1993). If the endorphin system is an important mechanism for the efficacy of acupuncture in treating addiction (Ulett, Han et al., 1998; McLellan, Grossman et al., 1993; Brewington, Smith et al., 1994; Kosten, Kreck et al., 1986; Pomeranz, 1987), further investigation of electroacupuncture is warranted.

Finally, researchers have failed to design a fair or standard set of expectations for acupuncture. Trials of acupuncture may deal with several stages of addiction, from detoxification (the majority of animal studies) to relapse prevention (U.S. human trials). Whether acupuncture is effective for any particular stage of treatment is a question yet to be addressed.

Many practitioners and researchers question whether CAT can be accurately evaluated using conventional standards for research. Due to variations in philosophy, the individualization of treatments, and the difficulties in assigning appropriate placebos, some researchers and practitioners claim that Western science is not capable of assessing the efficacy of many alternative therapies. However, before CAT is further integrated into the health care system by physicians, clinics, and managed care organizations, it must be subjected to evaluation using methodologically sound research strategies (Lewith, Kenyon et al., 1996). In the interim, it seems wise to maintain a reasonable skepticism while not arbitrarily discounting any approach that may improve treatment outcomes or reduce somatic complaints associated with addictive disorders.

Placebo and Nonspecific Effects: Particular attention has been paid to the relationship of CAT to placebo effects. At this time, the extent to which the effects of modalities like acupuncture are the result of placebo effects, rather than neurophysiologically induced treatment effects, remains unclear. Classically defined, a placebo effect is an effect that occurs after the administration of a therapeutically inactive substance. An example of a placebo treatment would be the substitution of a sugar pill for an active medication. If the patient's physiological response to the sugar pill is similar to the effects that normally would result from active treatment, a placebo effect is said to have occurred. Nonspecific effects are effects that occur after treatments that do not use medication or procedures that have known or presumed mechanisms of action. In conventionally treated alcoholics, for example, nonspecific treatments (as defined by Frank [1973]) such as information, evaluation only, advice, encouragement, and exhortation, have been shown to have salutary effects (Miller & Hester, 1980; Miller & Baca, 1983; Powell, Penick et al., 1985; McLellan, Lubrosky et al., 1985).

This is of more than academic interest, since variously defined placebo and nonspecific treatments have been reported to be as effective as certain forms of surgery, to influence the effectiveness and action of medications and hypnosis analgesia in dentistry, to enhance tolerance of pain, to increase survival rates in the elderly, to reduce postsurgical lengths of stay and requests for pain medication and, in certain individuals and cultures, to cause death (Adler & Cohen, 1975; Justice, 1987; Lefcourt, 1973; Mumford, Schlesinger et al., 1982; Richter, 1957). Jerome Frank's work (1973) on the role of persuasion in healing has been followed by many reviews of the topic, indicating its importance to any form of treatment delivery (Kiresuk, 1988; Bowers & Clum, 1988; Shapiro, Struening et al., 1980).

Early accusations that the therapeutic effects of alternative therapies such as acupuncture were attributable to suggestibility stimulated experimentation on animals and an investigation of the inhibitory effects of naloxone on hypnotic analgesia in humans. Both lines of inquiry indicated that the effects of acupuncture were not explained by suggestion alone. The role of nonspecific effects in acupuncture, as in many approaches to addiction treatment, has not been studied adequately.

However, it should be noted that the placebo and its effects are not simple concepts. For example, Shapiro recounts conflicting finds in placebo research (Kiresuk, 1988). Efforts to replicate research findings have failed, even when identical procedures were used on highly similar populations and when the same subjects were given identical placebo stimuli in different environments. The placebo effect has not been consistently identified with particular patient characteristics that would label certain individuals as "placebo reactors," nor has it been found to be consis-

tently related to the attributes of suggestibility, acquiescence, social desirability, dependency, external locus of control, and particular psychopathology.

In a major review and critique of the placebo literature, Kienle and Kiene (1996) challenged the commonly accepted 35% placebo effect concept popularized by Beecher. They found that Beecher had been misquoted in 10 of the 15 studies referring to his work.

In their review of oft-cited placebo studies, Kienle and Kiene pointed out that the possibility of a specific effect being produced by a procedure never can be entirely ruled out:

> If our analyses erase doubts about the existence of the placebo effect in its narrow sense (i.e., true therapeutic effects achieved by mere imitation of a therapy), it does not rule out the possibility that the patient's self-healing powers may be influenced by a wide variety of non-pharmacological approaches (p.51).

Self-healing powers also may be influenced by a variety of nontherapeutic distortions, such as conditions of administration in clinical versus research settings. Kaptchuk (2001) has argued that these distortions have strong implications for research, but they also may have clinical repercussions. Moreover, practitioner attitudes and behaviors, as well as styles of health care, have been shown to produce measurable differences in outcomes. These findings could have significance for CAT research and practice (Kaptchuk, 2001). A recent study even has reopened questions about the clinical significance of the placebo effect. Its authors conclude that "the use of placebo outside the aegis of a controlled, properly designed clinical trial cannot be recommended" (Hrobjartsson & Gotzsche, 2001).

ACUPUNCTURE AND ELECTROACUPUNCTURE

In 1973, Wen and Cheung noted that opium addicts being treated with postsurgical analgesic electroacupuncture reported relief from withdrawal symptoms. Wen conducted a series of studies using electroacupuncture on opiate-dependent rodents and humans; his preliminary results suggested that opiate withdrawal symptoms could be mitigated through use of electroacupuncture (Brewington, Smith et al., 1994). Research on humans combined naloxone with electroacupuncture, yielding a drug-free rate of 51% at one-year followup. Wen's distinctions between craving and abstinence and between detoxification and subsequent psychosocial rehabilitation give power to his research (Wen & Cheung, 1973; Wen & Teo, 1975; Wen, 1979).

Five animal studies of electroacupuncture have been conducted using opiate-addicted rats and mice, each demonstrating a significant decrease in morphine withdrawal symptoms in the electroacupuncture group compared to controls (Brewington, Smith et al., 1994). Findings suggest that electroacupuncture may alleviate symptoms associated with addiction to various substances and may be responsible for various neurophysiologic changes observed. However, there have been no systematic controlled studies of electroacupuncture for the treatment of addiction in humans. Further, the majority of studies have been criticized for faulty methodology, such as inadequate controls or, in the animal studies, excessive electrical current. To date no significant negative side effects have been reported.

Research in the U.S. has focused on daily auricular acupuncture therapy without electrical stimulation, based on a three- to five-point auricular acupuncture protocol established by Smith and colleagues at Lincoln Hospital in New York (Smith & Khan, 1988). Smith began treating detoxifying drug addicts with acupuncture in the mid-1970s, and his early clinical research showed promising results. Smith's protocol was used in the first two placebo-controlled studies conducted by Bullock and colleagues (1987, 1989), and the method subsequently was adopted as the standard treatment by the 4,000-member NADA.

Both electroacupuncture and acupuncture are based on the belief that health is determined by a balanced flow of qi, the vital life energy present in all living organisms. Practitioners identify 12 major energy pathways, called meridians, each linked to a specific internal organ or system. Acupoints exist along the meridians; in a traditional treatment setting, the practitioner places approximately 10 to 12 small stainless steel needles into the skin at points consistent with the diagnosis. This placement is said to help correct and rebalance the flow of qi and consequently to restore health. During electroacupuncture, the needle is linked to a small device that delivers mild electricity to the acupuncture site.

A proposed hypothesis of addiction states that when naturally occurring endogenous opioids (such as enkephalins and endorphins) occupy specific receptor sites in the brain, individuals experience wellbeing and the absence of craving. Drugs such as ethanol may displace endogenous opioids by acting at agonist binding sites, over time inhibiting the production of the natural endorphins. Craving may be linked to the deficiency of enkephalins and endorphins, as well as other genetic or ethanol-related neurochemical deficits (McLellan, Grossman et al., 1993; Brewington, Smith et al., 1994; Kosten, Kreck et al., 1986; Culliton & Kiresuk, 1996).

The work of Pomeranz and colleagues (1987) provides support for the use of acupuncture to treat addictive disorders. The work of Pomeranz suggests that acupuncture stimulates peripheral nerves, which send messages to the brain to release endorphins. Ulett agrees that endorphins are involved, based on work showing that naloxone can prevent electroacupuncture-induced analgesia (Ulett, Han et al., 1998). Like Wen, Ulett emphasizes the importance of electrical stimulation of needles during treatment and suggests that manual acupuncture for addictions may be little more than a placebo. Steiner reported that acupuncture had been shown to alter levels of other central neurotransmitters, including serotonin and norepinephrine, and also to affect regulation of hormones such as prolactin, oxytocin, thyroid hormone, corticosteroid, and insulin (Steiner, May et al., 1982). These findings suggest a preliminary model for the efficacy of acupuncture for the treatment of pain, as well as opiate and alcohol addiction.

Acupuncture has been studied in the treatment of heroin, alcohol, cocaine, and nicotine addiction. It is not considered effective in reducing the symptoms of nicotine withdrawal (White, Resch et al., 1999). Several reviews of the literature have outlined study findings to date (see Table 1).

Two controlled studies of alcoholic populations conducted by Bullock and colleagues (Bullock, Umen et al., 1987; Bullock, Culliton et al., 1989) resulted in significantly improved program attendance and less self-reported need for alcohol among the acupuncture group. The second study also found that placebo subjects self-reported over two times the number of drinking episodes and had twice the number of admissions to a hospital detoxification unit than did the subjects treated with acupuncture. Other studies have shown mixed results (Toteva & Malinov, 1996; Worner, Zeller et al., 1992; Sapir-Weiss et al., 1999). In the first large-scale randomized placebo-controlled trial (Bullock, Kiresuk et al., 2002), subjects (n=503) were randomized to one of four treatment groups: (1) no acupuncture, (2) four-point ear acupuncture, (3) non-specific (sham) acupuncture, or (4) individualized acupuncture. The

TABLE 1. Review Articles: Acupuncture in Addiction Treatment

Author(s)	Year	Focus	Drug(s)
Culliton & Kiresuk	1996	General review	multiple
Brewington, Smith et al.	1994	Review of efficacy	multiple
Brumbaugh	1994	Summary of practice	multiple
Brumbaugh	1993	History and protocol	multiple
McLellan, Grossman et al.	1993	Research methodology	multiple
Ter Riet, Kleijnen et al.	1990	Meta-analysis	multiple
Smith & Kahn	1988	General review	multiple
Whitehead	1978	Review of efficacy	multiple
Blum, Newmeyer et al.	1978	Review of neurochemical mechanisms	opiates

investigators found no significant differences between treatment groups in alcohol consumption or desire for alcohol (Bullock, Kiresuk et al., 2002).

Preliminary trials of acupuncture for the treatment of cocaine addiction have had mixed outcomes (Smith, 1988; Otto, Quinn et al., 1998; Avants, Margolin et al., 2000). However, the results of the first randomized placebo-controlled study, conducted by Bullock and colleagues (n=438) found that cocaine use did not differ significantly in the acupuncture and control groups (Bullock, Kiresuk et al., 1999). Moreover, the results of a multisite randomized controlled trial by Margolin and colleagues (n=620) showed no differences by treatment condition on any outcome measure. The use of acupuncture for the treatment of cocaine addiction is not supported by these studies.

TRANSCUTANEOUS CRANIAL ELECTRICAL STIMULATION

Transcutaneous cranial electrical stimulation (TCES), also known as TENS or CES, was a Russian invention, originally called "electrosleep," and was used in the 1950s for the treatment of insomnia (Brewington, Smith et al., 1994). Sometimes known as "Limoges current," this treatment consists of high-frequency, low-intensity electrical stimulation that has, among other things, been shown to decrease patient requirements for anesthesia and analgesia during abdominal surgery (Mignon, Lauderbach et al., 1996). Treatment effect is thought to be mediated by the release of central endogenous opioids. In a typical TCES session, surface electrodes are placed in the mastoid region (behind the ear) and, as in electroacupuncture, stimulated through use of a low amperage alternating current.

Several studies have examined the role of TCES in the treatment of addictive disorders, particularly with opiates; however, evidence in support of the therapy is weak. In a review of the literature by Brewington and colleagues (1994), three studies were identified as having somewhat positive results for the treatment of opiates. However, serious methodological flaws and a fourth study reporting that TCES is less effective than methadone reduce confidence in these findings (Gossop, Bradley et al., 1984). A fifth study, by Gariti and colleagues (1992), was a randomized, double-blind study of hospitalized opiate and cocaine users who were detoxified by use of TCES. The rate of completion for the 12-day study was 88%. However, other than a comfortable detoxification, there were no significant differences between the active and placebo groups.

Fewer studies of TCES have been conducted in alcohol-addicted populations, and available studies have focused primarily on the reduction of anxiety and depression rather than consumption. These studies either have had serious methodological difficulties or yielded findings that failed to provide adequate support (Patterson, Patterson et al., 1993; Patterson, Krupitsky et al., 1994; Brewington, Smith et al., 1994). More recently, Taub and colleagues (1994) conducted a study using TCES for the treatment of alcoholism. Even when it was administered in conjunction with AA and counseling, the investigators failed to find support for TCES as an effective treatment for alcoholism.

BIOFEEDBACK

Biofeedback did not develop out of any single healing tradition or discipline, but evolved in the 1950s and 1960s from several disciplines, including electronics and psychophysiology. Researchers envisioned a wide range of possible applications for the new modality (Winer, 1977). The 1960s were especially active periods of research into biofeedback. While the concept of controlling physiological functions was not new in the West, the outstanding finding of early work was that highly specific responses could be learned (Winer, 1977).

Research on the effectiveness of biofeedback for addiction treatment has been varied and the outcomes have been questionable. Some confusion has arisen as a result of the variety of biofeedback methods used. In the early 1970s, EEG alpha biofeedback was discounted as largely ineffective, particularly for the treatment of addictive disorders. The addition of theta brainwave training to the alpha protocol has resulted in more positive clinical reports (Fahrion, 1995; Peniston & Kulkosky, 1990). Other researchers have turned to EMG or thermal biofeedback techniques, and preliminary studies have shown some efficacy (Denney, Baugh et al., 1991; Taub, Steiner et al., 1994).

Despite investigator and clinician preferences, research has suggested that these three conditions have much the same effect on brainwaves. In one study, adults in treatment for addictive disorders were given one of three types of EEG biofeedback: EMG, standard alpha-theta feedback, or alpha feedback alone. The authors reported no significant differences, using quantitative EEG, between groups in the percentage of time in theta-alpha crossover or in the ratio of theta amplitude to alpha amplitude, averaged over a session. These findings suggest that all three conditions can be effective in achieving positive therapeutic outcomes (Trudeau, 2000). However, due to a paucity of rigorous research, the specific mechanism of biofeedback in the treatment of addictive disorders is unknown, as is the extent of its efficacy.

In the 1970s and 1980s, the Menninger Center for Applied Psychophysiology began using alpha-theta brainwave training to treat patients suffering from addictive disorders, with generally positive results. This work was modified by Peniston in the late 1980s, sparking a wave of research and

criticism (Graap & Freides, 1998). Studies to date have shown similar responses regardless of the patient's drug of choice, although biofeedback has not yet been applied to methamphetamine addiction (Fahrion, 1995). Previous studies of alpha-theta feedback have suggested effects on various measures of mood and personality associated with clinical outcomes (Fahrion, Walters et al., 1992; Peniston & Kulkosky, 1990). The studies have not yet controlled for the placebo and nonspecific effects inherent in increments of any therapy.

EMG biofeedback teaches the subject to reduce muscle tension rather than attempting to affect brainwaves. Research linking EMG biofeedback to the treatment of addictions has been scarce. The findings of case studies have been mixed, and only one randomized controlled trial has been conducted (Taub, Steiner et al., 1994), with EMG biofeedback as one of the four treatment arms (n=125). The study found support for the use of EMG biofeedback for use in the prevention of relapse in alcoholics, and the EMG group did significantly better than the control group at the end of treatment and at followup.

Research has demonstrated that the use of alcohol or nicotine results in poor performance during biofeedback sessions. The ability of smokers to modulate blood pressure is restricted when compared to nonsmokers and the ability to manipulate skin temperature appears to be greatest in nonsmokers and impossible for those who smoke just prior to the biofeedback session (DeGood & Valle, 1978; Birnbaumer, Elbert et al., 1992; Grimsley, 1990; Schneider, Elbert et al., 1993).

HYPNOSIS

Hypnotic suggestion in one form or another has been used in healing throughout the world since ancient times, and was a focal point of treatment in early Greek healing temples (Alternative Medicine, 1994). However, the roots of modern hypnosis can be traced to the 18th century work of Franz Anton Mesmer. Mesmer used what he called "magnetic healing" to treat a variety of psychological and psychophysiological disorders (Alternative Medicine, 1994). Hypnotic methods have varied widely across time and still vary among practitioners (Katz, 1980). Despite controversy over the validity of hypnosis, historically it has been one of the most important techniques of psychotherapy (Katz, 1980).

In 1958, the American Medical Association (AMA) formally sanctioned the use of hypnosis as a valid medical treatment, and over the past 50 years, the clinical application of hypnosis by physicians, dentists, psychologists, and other health professionals for numerous ailments, including addictive disorders, has increased (Alternative Medicine, 1994). Hypnosis attempts to place patients in a state of attentive and focused concentration. Practitioners typically either lead patients through relaxation and mental imagery exercises, often using suggestion, or teach clients a form of self-hypnosis that can be practiced at home. Contrary to popular folklore, patients must be willing to undergo hypnosis, and despite being relatively unaware of their external environment, are capable of responding to stimuli (Alternative Medicine, 1994).

Research and clinical reports repeatedly have demonstrated that hypnotic methods are capable of generating notable changes in memory, cognition, perception, and physiology in susceptible subjects (Katz, 1980). Studies have shown that hypnosis may result in decreased sympathetic nervous system activity, oxygen consumption and carbon dioxide elimination, lowered blood pressure and heart rate, and increased activity in certain kinds of brain waves (Spiegel, Bloom et al., 1989). However, the difficulties in defining hypnosis, the inability to externally measure the presence of hypnotic states, and the lack of standardized methods in research have hampered efforts at systematic evaluation (Stoil, 1989). Moreover, the mechanism of action of hypnosis is unknown.

To say that "hypnosis" has been used as a treatment for an addictive disorder means that the patient could have been exposed to any of 20 or more strategies, including suggestions to reduce urges, symptom substitution, ego strengthening, or cue sensitization (Katz, 1980). Therefore, it is difficult to compare the few controlled studies that have been conducted. However, practitioner claims of cure rates as high as 95% have never been verified through controlled research (Haxby, 1995). Several case studies using either hypnotherapy or self-hypnosis for the treatment of substance abuse have reported successful outcomes (Page & Handley, 1993; Orman, 1991), and some clinical data has demonstrated high rates of abstinence (Johnson & Karkut, 1994; Schwartz, 1992).

Overall, however, the results of controlled trials have not supported these preliminary findings. A review of four studies conducted prior to 1975 evaluated hypnosis negatively (Miller, Brown et al., 1995), while more recent studies have demonstrated some short-term benefits that were not maintained through followup (Rabkin, Boyko et al., 1984; Hyman, Stanley et al., 1986; Lambe, Osier et al., 1986).

Moreover, hypnosis research has been criticized for lack of proper controls, insufficient followup, and poor reporting of data (Johnston & Donoghue, 1971; Katz, 1980; Holroyd, 1980). Most researchers and modern practitioners believe that hypnosis alone is not an effective therapy, although it may enhance the effects of other therapies (Haxby, 1995; Stoil, 1989).

TRANSCENDENTAL MEDITATION

Transcendental Meditation (TM) was introduced to the U.S. in the 1960s by the Maharishi Mahesh Yogi as a simplified form of yoga (Alternative Medicine, 1994). Derived from the ancient Vedic tradition of India, TM is a significant component of the modern version of Ayurvedic medicine (O'Connell & Alexander, 1995). Proponents claim that TM is a truly holistic modality that addresses physiological, psychological, spiritual, and environmental/social factors. However, the Maharishi Mahesh Yogi and TM have been accused of deceptive practices and fraud. Some critics even cite evidence of considerable harm they claim can result from the practice of TM (Singer, 1992; Alexander, 1992; Chopra, 1992; Tompkins, 1992; Skolnick, 1992). Since its introduction, TM has been used for stress management and health maintenance, as well as a cure for conditions such as high blood pressure, chronic pain, and addiction.

TM philosophy holds that repetitive or perpetual stressors (chronic stress) may result in an ineffective or destructive stress response, producing homeostatic imbalance or disease in the body. TM proponents contend that substance abuse arises in an attempt to achieve homeostasis: "substance abuse is an attempt to optimize one's psychophysiological state [using] exogenous chemicals" (Walton & Levitsky, 1995). They add that substance abuse results in increased imbalance, distress, and eventually more drug use. Therefore, the objective of TM is to optimize psychophysiological function and balance, simply and naturally, thus interrupting the cycle of drug use and need for addiction. Proponents clearly state that this view does not exclude the possibility that genetic factors predispose some individuals to addiction. Mechanisms involved in the maintenance of homeostasis may be affected by genetic differences, inclining these individuals toward substance misuse and addiction (Walton & Levitsky, 1995).

Studies indicate that during TM, physiological arousal is significantly decreased compared to simply resting with the eyes closed, as indicated by lowered respiration rate, skin conductance level, and plasma lactate level. Studies also have shown that in as few as four months, TM significantly increases serotonin and reduces cortisol, and that TM results in a more rapid mobilization, habituation, and stability of autonomic response to stressful stimuli than various control conditions (O'Connell & Alexander, 1995b). The implications of these findings for addiction medicine have been reviewed in several publications (O'Connell & Alexander, 1995a).

More than 30 studies have been conducted on the efficacy of TM for the treatment of addiction. While rates of success have ranged from 65% in a controlled study of recidivist alcoholics (with two-year followup) to 98% in a retrospective analysis of drug use among TM program participants, most of the studies have lacked rigorous methods and appropriate controls. Methodological difficulties have included a failure to control for the type of drug(s) used, the subject's history of use, or the severity of misuse. Moreover, studies often are retrospective, lack appropriate randomization and controls, rarely are blinded, and usually are conducted by researchers affiliated with the Maharishi University.

Gelderloos and colleagues (1991) reviewed 24 studies and positively evaluated all of them, despite often serious methodological flaws. Success in these studies was measured by "discontinued or reduced use"; however, reduced use was not quantified and abstinence not reported separately. Moreover, for 10 of the 24 studies, the authors simply cited a percentage of subjects who "succeeded," without adequately defining the criteria by which success was assessed.

More recently, TM, biofeedback, and electroneurotherapy were compared in a randomized controlled trial conducted by Taub and colleagues (1994). At two-year followup, the TM and biofeedback groups significantly increased their non-drinking days compared to the electric neurotherapy and AA/counseling controls. However, because non-drinking days were used as the primary indicator, rather than rates of abstinence, these findings are difficult to interpret and compare.

RELAXATION TRAINING

Relaxation training can take a number of forms, and sometimes is considered to be either a form of or a component of meditation. "Relaxation" groups sometimes are used as controls in meditation research. Because of the variety of definitions and methods in use, studies of relaxation training are difficult to compare. For the purposes of this chapter, relaxation does not include the practice of TM (see above).

In general, the intent of relaxation training in treating addictive disorders has been to provide a substitute for the sedative effects of drugs such as alcohol and tobacco. However, the validity of this philosophy has been questioned, as many drugs are consumed for their euphoric, rather than tranquilizing, effects (Klajner, Hartman et al., 1984; Surawy & Cox, 1986). Further, relaxation training for the treatment of addiction has not fared well in evaluations of past research (Holder, Longabaugh et al., 1991; Miller, Brown et al., 1995). While one study did show a reduction in measures of anxiety through the use of relaxation training, the reduction in anxiety was not linked to a reduction in drug consumption (Ormrod & Budd, 1991). Finally, biofeedback (Taub, Steiner et al., 1994) has been shown to be more effective than relaxation for treating substance use disorders, as measured by abstinence rates.

RESTRICTED ENVIRONMENTAL STIMULATION (REST)

The late 1950s and 1960s marked the beginning of academic interest in research on sensory deprivation and restricted environments' effects on the mind and body (Lilly, 1956; Suedfeld, 1964; Lawes, 1963). By the 1970s, interest had expanded to include research on the effects of restricted environmental stimulation therapies (REST) on smoking and drinking behaviors (Suedfeld, Landon et al., 1972; Suedfeld & Ikard, 1974; Jacobson, 1971; Suedfeld & Best, 1977; Rank & Suedfeld, 1978).

Chamber REST and flotation REST are two methods used to produce a sensory-deprivation environment. In chamber REST, the individual is placed in a light- and sound-proof room for 12 to 24 hours, or longer, with only a comfortable bed, a toilet, and access to food. Flotation REST also takes place in an enclosed room or capsule, where the individual lies in a pool of water heated to skin temperature and supersaturated with Epsom salts to a specific gravity of 1.26 to 1.28. There the individual floats effortlessly for 30 to 150 minutes (Borrie, 1990-1991).

Researchers and practitioners have suggested a number of potential psychological and psychotherapeutic uses for REST in both adolescent and adult populations. By isolating the individual from the majority of sensory stimuli (visual, auditory, tactile, gustatory, and olfactory), REST attempts to reduce stress and increase introspection, allowing the body to rebalance and heal (Borrie, 1990-1991).

Various studies have shown that REST may result in a number of significant biochemical changes, including reduced plasma and urinary cortisol levels, plasma renin, ACTH, and aldosterone levels, lowered blood pressure, and enhanced EEG alpha activity following treatment (Turner & Fine, 1983; Barabasz, Barabasz et al., 1983; McGrady, Turner et al., 1987; Borrie, 1990-1991). It also has been hypothesized that REST may stimulate the release of beta-endorphins and thus stimulate the brain's reward mechanism. REST has been offered by advocates as an alternative method to stimulate pleasure centers, in place of alcohol or drugs.

The majority of clinical research involving REST and addictive disorders has focused on smoking behavior. In preliminary quasi-experimental and clinical designs, chamber REST has shown better results in smoking cessation than flotation REST. Some evidence indicates that chamber REST may result in significant reductions in smoking behavior, which may be sustained through a two-year followup (Suedfeld, 1990; Suedfeld & Ikard, 1974; Suedfeld, Landon et al., 1972). There also is some evidence to suggest that REST is more effective when combined with other treatment modalities. A six-month followup of a multimodal program using REST, self-management, and social support found an 88% rate of abstinence. Another study combined REST with hypnosis and reported abstinence rates of 47% at four months posttreatment (Barabasz, Baer et al., 1986). While flotation REST has been considered unsuccessful for promoting smoking cessation (Borrie, 1990-1991), there is some evidence that the psychotic-like symptoms of persons intoxicated with PCP and LSD may be reduced through use of this therapy, and that flotation REST may be useful for the treatment of drug withdrawal symptoms (Borrie, 1990-1991).

Less research has been conducted on REST for the treatment of alcohol dependence, although preliminary studies of both flotation and chamber REST have shown positive results (Rank & Suedfeld, 1978; Borrie, 1990-1991).

NUTRITION AND VITAMINS

Food and nutrition long have played an important role in various healing traditions. For example, in traditional Chinese medicine, food is categorized by its energetic qualities. Prevention-oriented prescriptions are emphasized, but in the case of illness, dietary interventions are tailored according to the physical characteristics of the patient and the illness disturbance (Alternative Medicine, 1994). Western medical traditions also have recognized the importance of nutrition, using foods and vitamins for the prevention and treatment of disease. Moreover, Western science has demonstrated links between basic vitamin-mineral deficiencies and some severe, chronic, and even terminal diseases, such as iron and anemia, vitamin C and scurvy, and vitamin D and rickets. Conventional medicine also has begun to incorporate nutritional substances in the prevention, reduction, and elimination of various disease states, such as the use of lithium for the treatment of bipolar disorders (Schou, 1997).

An increasing number of clinical settings have begun to incorporate nutritional therapies. In 1990, the American Dietetic Association took the position that improved nutritional status can improve the efficacy of addiction treatment through the effects of supplements, modified diets, and nutrition education (Beckley-Barrett & Mutch, 1990); to date, this statement has not been revised. Some advocates of nutritional therapy attribute depression and other ailments commonly found in drug users to nutritional deficits, undiagnosed hypoglycemia, and unidentified food allergies, and claim that these ailments can be treated through special diets, exercise, and vitamin and mineral supplements.

While scientists seem to agree that excessive intake of alcohol and other drugs may cause a number of nutritional deficiencies, including malnutrition and thiamine deficiency (Werbach, 1991; Mohs, Watson et al., 1990; Watson & Mohs, 1990), the link between nutritional disorders and addiction has not been fully accepted. Further, the belief that special diets or nutritional supplements may be viable adjunctive or stand-alone treatments for addictive disorders has not been adequately researched.

Preliminary human studies have shown positive results for nutritional programs or supplements used in the treatment of alcoholism, including increased abstinence, reduced craving, and decreased depression (Biery, Williford et al., 1991; Mathews-Larson & Parker, 1987; Brown, Blum et al., 1990; Blum, Trachtenberg et al., 1988). In the early 1980s, one study of alcoholics conducted in a VA medical center compared a standard treatment group (which employed counseling and Twelve Step meetings) to a standard treatment group with the addition of a whole foods diet, nutritional supplements, and nutritional education. After six months, 81% of the nutrition group had maintained abstinence, compared to 38% of the control group (Guenther,

1983). A clinical study followed patients through a 28-day treatment program that involved both counseling and nutrition. At one year posttreatment, 74% of those treated for alcoholism remained abstinent (Beasley, Grimson et al., 1991). A third study conducted a six-month followup of 100 patients who had received six weeks of outpatient counseling and nutritional therapy; the researchers reported that 81% were abstinent from alcohol (Mathews-Larson & Parker, 1987). Des Maisons (1996) conducted a preliminary trial of 29 subjects, each of whom had two DUI offenses, and 29 self-selected controls. Following use of a dietary protocol, alcohol consumption and recidivism were significantly reduced in the treatment group.

Preliminary studies of amino acid supplementation (with neurotransmitter precursors) also have shown promising results for the treatment of alcohol and cocaine addiction; however, no large-scale controlled trials have been conducted. Amino acid supplements were tested in an open trial on 30 alcoholic patients and 30 patients addicted to cocaine. Rates of relapse were 13% for the alcohol active treatment group and 20% for the cocaine active treatment group, as compared with 53% and 87%, respectively, for the placebo-treated controls (Blum, Trachtenberg et al., 1988).

However, detailed experimental or clinical studies are limited, and published studies frequently are outdated, lack methodological rigor, or lack adequate sample size (Mohs, Watson et al., 1990). Preliminary animal studies of the effects of various nutrients on withdrawal and free-choice ethanol consumption also have shown promise (Werbach, 1991; Collipp, Kris et al., 1984; Eriksson, Pekkanen et al., 1980; Pekkanen, 1980; Forander, Kohonen et al., 1958; Register, Marsh et al., 1972; Rogers, Pelton et al., 1956). The majority of human and animal studies have been restricted to alcoholism, neglecting the effects of nutritional therapies on other addictive disorders. Research on nutrition has been slow because of the lack of resources to follow up on promising preliminary results (Alternative Medicine, 1994).

HERBAL REMEDIES

The use of herbal remedies to treat illness dates from prehistoric times. The earliest written records detailing the use of medicinal herbs are found in Mesopotamian clay tablets, dated earlier than 2,000 BC. Numerous cultures have produced descriptions and systems of herbal medicine.

Between 2,000 BC and 1 AD, the Chinese, Greek, and East Indian peoples all created materia medica that involved reviews of up to 1,000 substances. The current version of the Chinese materia medica contains over 5,500 entries (Alternative Medicine, 1994). While less than 10% of plants today have been extensively studied for medicinal applications, about 25% of Western medicines contain plant material (Alternative Medicine, 1994; McKenna, 1996). Further, the modern use of nearly 75% of plant-derived pharmaceutical products directly correlates with their traditional uses (Mack, 1997).

Critics argue that synthetic compound screening and combinatorial chemistry are more efficient and legitimate methods for determining pharmaceutical leads than pursuing ancient nostrums based on anecdotal evidence (Mack, 1997). Proponents point to the prevalence of plant materials in modern medicines and speak of the advantages of acknowledging thousands of years of experimentation and folk knowledge. For example, the Chinese ethnopharmacopoeia is written, taught in medical schools, and has been used and revised over thousands of years.

Difficulties in herbal research include: (1) the lack of a methodology capable of studying the herb as a whole, rather than its component parts or derivatives, (2) difficulties in securing a standardized preparation of herbs and herbal compounds, so that the results of trials will be reliable and valid, and (3) the cost of meeting U.S. Food and Drug Administration guidelines for the introduction of new pharmaceuticals. Because botanicals are not patentable (although they can be patented for use) producers of herbal remedies may not recover their expenses, and pharmaceutical companies will not risk the loss (Mack, 1997; Alternative Medicine, 1994). While many herbal remedies have few or no side effects, others can be toxic if improperly administered.

Despite the barriers, some research on herbal medicines for the treatment of addictive disorders has been conducted. The majority of this research has been conducted on traditional Chinese herbs. For example, Leguminosae Pueraria lobata (kudzu) is a perennial vine native to eastern Asia, which also is widely available in the southern United States (Keung & Vallee, 1993; Althoff, 1994). An extract from the root, radix pueraria, has been used in traditional Chinese medicine for thousands of years as an antipyretic, antidiarrhetic, diaphoretic, antiemetic, amethystic, as well as an anti-inebriation agent (Keung & Vallee, 1993; Xie,

Lin et al., 1994). An "anti-drunkenness" effect first was reported in 600 AD, and radix pueraria was described as a treatment for alcoholism circa 1580 AD (Keung & Vallee, 1993).

The mechanism of radix pueraria for the treatment of alcohol abuse is as yet elusive, although it seems unlikely that the herb works through either the ADH or the ALDH enzyme systems (Keung, 1993; Keung, Lazo et al., 1995). It has been hypothesized that kudzu may work through the serotonergic systems of the brain or through the calcium channels regulator (Lee, 1996).

One of the primary animal models used in the research of kudzu and its isoflavones, diadzin and diadzein, for the treatment of alcoholism (Keung & Vallee, 1993; Keung, Lazo et al., 1995) has been soundly criticized (McMillen & Williams, 1995; Piercy & Myers, 1995; Lankford, Roscoe et al., 1991; Lankford & Myers, 1994). However, four studies using Wistar (P) rats reported similar findings, including decreased peak blood alcohol levels, shortened sleep time induced by ethanol intoxication, and reduced free-choice ethanol intake (Xie, Lin et al., 1994; Lee, 1996). Research currently is underway at Harvard Medical School on the use of kudzu for the treatment of alcoholism in humans (Overstreet, Lee et al., 1998, 1996).

Other herbs and herbal compounds have been identified by practitioners as effective in the reduction of craving and as adjuncts to the process of detoxification (Petri & Takach, 1990; Shanmugasundaram, Subramaniam et al., 1986), but virtually no work has been done to assess their efficacy.

HALLUCINOGENS

The hallucinogenic properties of lysergic acid diethylamide (LSD) were discovered by Hofmann in 1943 (Abbott, Aldridge et al., 1996). At the time of their introduction in the U.S. and Europe in the late 1940s and 1950s, LSD and other potent agents became available to large populations for religious, recreational, and scientific purposes. By the mid-1960s, it appeared that medicine had found a new tool for generating insights into the mechanisms of nerve cell transmission or the phenomenology of schizophrenia, as well as a potential treatment for a number of psychiatric disorders (Riedlinger & Riedlinger, 1994).

However, beginning in 1968, a series of papers were published on the potential dangers of hallucinogens and, by the mid-1970s, the majority of investigations of therapeutic uses of hallucinogens had ceased (Halpern, 1996; Abbott,

Aldridge et al., 1996). It is difficult to know which came first, political and societal pressure to abandon research, or the belief that models of therapy were lacking validity (McKenna, 1996; Abbott, Aldridge et al., 1996; Halpern, 1996). Only recently, with the introduction of new agents such as ibogaine, has there been a resurgence of interest in the potential utility of hallucinogens.

It is hypothesized that craving may be attenuated through the use of agonists/antagonists of the neurotransmitter serotonin (5-HT) (Halpern, 1996). Like DMT, mescaline, and psilocybin, LSD is characterized by a serotonergic pharmacology (McKenna, 1996) and is an agonist/antagonist at the discrete serotonin receptors 5-HT[1] and 5-HT[2]. If serotonin mediates reward-related behavior, then LSD and other hallucinogens may exhibit anticraving features (Halpern, 1996). Ibogaine also has an effect on serotonergic pharmacology and is an NMDA antagonist. Preclinical data suggest that these compounds are effective in attenuating the development of tolerance and in decreasing the symptoms of dependence on all abused substances examined to date (Popik, Layer et al., 1995).

During the 1960s and 1970s, the use of LSD to treat alcoholism was examined more thoroughly than any other therapeutic application of hallucinogenic agents. Reviews of these studies are mixed (Halpern, 1996; Abbott, Aldridge et al., 1996; Ludwig, Levine et al., 1970). Studies of hallucinogens conducted in the 1960s and 1970s have been criticized on the basis of their varied methodology, dosing, and criteria for improvement, as well as their failure to adhere to the now-accepted double-blind, placebo-controlled standards. It now appears that, while case studies and data from open trials resulted in encouraging findings, controlled studies failed to replicate these results (Halpern, 1996). A review of the controlled studies conducted during that era suggests that, in the majority of studies, there were no differences between treatment and control groups and that LSD may even possess some antitherapeutic effects (Ludwig, Levine et al., 1970).

Based on a review of single dose studies, it has been suggested that the anti-addictive properties offered by hallucinogens may be of limited duration. Peak theories recommend dosing at intervals that would provide the addict a continuous or steady-state benefit, perhaps every one or two months (Halpern, 1996). However, before considering further testing involving dosing, the clinical difficulties of administering hallucinogenic agents to patients must be addressed. In addition to their current status as Schedule I controlled substances, these include: (1) the need to monitor patients for hours or even days after the agent is administered to minimize adverse effects, (2) the need for therapists to be extensively trained as guides for the sessions, and (3) the degree of adjustment and accommodation that would be required by psychotherapists who wish to incorporate these drugs into their practices (Riedlinger & Riedlinger, 1994).

Ibogaine: The root bark of a West African shrub, *Tabernanthe iboga*, yields the psychoactive indole alkaloid known as ibogaine (Rezvani, Overstreet et al., 1995). Ibogaine is a stimulant, but at high doses has hallucinogenic properties. Historically, ibogaine has been used in ritual ways by various indigenous populations, and has been used by hunters and warriors to remain awake for long periods. Like the classic hallucinogens, ibogaine is classified as a Schedule I controlled substance by the U.S. Drug Enforcement Administration (Popik, Layer et al., 1995). However, ibogaine is available throughout much of the European community, and in some locations is available as a treatment for addiction (Sheppard, 1994). Extremely high doses of ibogaine may be fatal (Popik, Layer et al., 1995).

Studies have been conducted to document the effects of ibogaine on a variety of animal populations. It has been shown to attenuate alcohol intake and reduce cocaine preference (Rezvani, Overstreet et al., 1995; Sershen, Hashim et al., 1994). Other research has focused on the effects of ibogaine on dopaminergic systems, opioid systems, serotonergic systems, intracellular calcium regulation, cholinergic systems, gamma-aminobutyric acidergic systems, voltage-dependent sodium channels, glutamatergic systems, *s* receptors, and adrenergic systems (see Popik, Layer et al., 1995, for a review). Because ibogaine appears to be dose-, setting-, gender-, and species-specific, further testing is needed.

Anecdotal reports regarding the efficacy of ibogaine as a treatment for addiction have been impressive, and preliminary human case studies using single doses of 700 to 1,800 mg of ibogaine for the treatment of heroin addiction have been encouraging but inconclusive (Sheppard, 1994). Despite its use with clinical populations in Europe, no controlled clinical data are available on the use of ibogaine for the treatment of addiction.

OTHER ALTERNATIVE THERAPIES

Several other alternative therapies have been used to treat addictive disorders. At this time, clinical and controlled data on efficacy is lacking. A brief description of each follows.

Light Therapy. Light therapy probably is best known for its use as a treatment for seasonal affective disorder (SAD), a depressive disorder characterized by seasonal onset. While a specific mechanism of action for the efficacy of light therapy has not been identified, SAD may be linked to serotonin deficits. A connection between SAD and some addictive disorders has been proposed on the basis of preliminary case studies (Satel & Gawin, 1989; McGrath & Yahia, 1993) and basic science research (Dilsaver & Majchrzak, 1988). However, studies looking for seasonal patterns of alcoholism have produced contradictory findings (Eastwood & Stiasny, 1978; Poikolainen, 1982; APA, 1988). Currently, proponents suggest the use of light therapy as an adjunct to standard treatment modalities for patients with seasonal patterns of dependence.

Yoga and Tai-chi. Yoga is a discipline that has been practiced in India for thousands of years as part of a lifestyle based on Vedic scriptures. In modern times, the practice of yoga has adopted various components of this traditional lifestyle and involves postures, flowing movements, breathing, and meditation. Over 70 years of scientific research have shown that, through the practice of yoga, an individual can learn to control certain physiological parameters, including blood pressure, cardiac and respiratory function, and brain waves (Alternative Medicine, 1994). It has been suggested that there may be some potential in the use of yoga for the treatment of addictive disorders and their related consequences. The rationale for using yoga is similar to that of biofeedback, although no scientific evidence exists regarding the mechanism of action. One pilot study (N=59) has been conducted on the use of yoga for the treatment of opiate misuse (Shaffer & LaSalvia, 1997). All subjects received daily doses of methadone and the treatment group was taught hatha yoga, while the controls participated in traditional psychodynamic group therapy. The investigators found no significant differences in outcomes between the treatment group and the controls.

Tai-chi is a form of mid-range boxing that has been practiced in China for centuries. The philosophy and practice of Tai-chi applies the principles of Yin and Yang and other elements of traditional Chinese medicine. As the popularity of Tai-chi increases in North America, it has been suggested that Tai-chi may assist individuals in the process of withdrawal and relapse prevention. No studies have been published on the efficacy of Tai-chi for the treatment of addictive disorders, although it has been shown to improve balance function and reduce the number of dangerous falls in the elderly (Li, Hong et al., 2001; Hartman, Manos et al., 2000).

Eye Movement Desensitization and Reprocessing. Eye movement desensitization and reprocessing (EMDR) is a relatively new psychological method based on the belief that eye movement, such as the rapid eye movement experienced during sleep, can stimulate the brain's self-healing capacities (Coates, 1996). Research to date has focused on patients dealing with the psychological consequences of traumatic events such as sexual assault, combat, or grief (Shapiro, Vogelmann-Sine et al., 1994; Montgomery & Ayllon, 1994; Silver, Brooks et al., 1995). EMDR has been recommended for the treatment of addicts who have a history of mental trauma and who have progressed through the initial stage of withdrawal. Proponents believe that EMDR may aid recovery by helping addicts to confront their denial and distortions (Shapiro, Vogelmann-Sine et al., 1994). Research on the efficacy of EMDR for the treatment of substance abuse is ongoing.

Homeopathy. The theory of homeopathy first was described 200 years ago by Samuel Hahnemann (Abbott & Stiegler, 1996). In the early part of the 19th century, homeopathy was introduced in the U.S., where its apparent success in treating cholera won it many allies. By 1900, there were 22 medical schools, more than 100 hospitals, and around 15,000 practitioners in the U.S. dedicated to the practice of homeopathy. However, with the introduction of effective pharmacotherapies in the 1920s and the standardization of conventional physician training programs, homeopathic hospitals and schools all but disappeared from the U.S. (Starr, 1982). Almost all women's medical colleges, which had been primarily homeopathic, were lost as well. While homeopathy remained part of the "medical landscape" in places like Germany, England, and India, interest in homeopathy was almost totally absent from American medicine until a resurgence began in the 1970s.

Homeopathy is based on the "Law of Similars," derived in part from observations made by Hippocrates. The law states that certain pharmacologically active substances are able to cure symptoms similar to those which they cause: "like cures like" (Anonymous, 1995). Hahnemann began testing this hypothesis by administering small doses of various substances to healthy volunteers to determine the agents' symptom profiles. He then administered the substances to patients by giving them substances that evoked symptoms

similar to the patient's symptom profile (Mirman, 1994). Classical homeopathy asserts that each patient should receive one remedy tailored to his or her particular needs, while pluralist practitioners often prescribe several tinctures to a single patient.

The aspect of homeopathic theory that most disturbs critics is that many of the remedies are "potentized" by dilution with a water-alcohol solution. The final concentration may be diluted to a concentration as low as 10:20,000—far below the point at which any molecules of the medicine can be detected in the solution (Alternative Medicine, 1994). To date, no one has been able to provide an adequate explanation for the possible mechanism of homeopathy. Moreover, meta-analyses and reviews of homeopathic research have come to different conclusions regarding the efficacy of the modality (Reilly, Taylor et al., 1994; Kleijnen, Knipschild et al., 1991; Hill & Doyon, 1990; Bellavite, 1990; Walach & Righetti, 1996; Kurz, 1992). In some cases, skeptics have been forced to admit some evidence of efficacy (Kleijnen, Knipschild et al., 1991), while proponents of homeopathy have re-reviewed those analyses, saying that no such conclusion is possible (Linde, Scholz et al., 1999).

Homeopathy is being used to treat addiction in parts of Europe, in the United Kingdom and—to a lesser extent—in the United States. To date, no research on the treatment of substance abuse has been published in biomedical journals.

Aromatherapy. Aromatherapy is a branch of herbal medicine in which fragrant essential oils, extracted from various plants, are inhaled or applied to the skin, primarily for the sake of their odor. Many essential oils are highly toxic if ingested orally, and aromatherapy materials should be kept out of the reach of children. Advocates believe that specific olfactory sensations, evoked by the oils, promote health and can be useful in the prevention and treatment of disease. The odor of each oil is said to have specific physiologic and/or psychologic properties.

Clinical reports suggest that this modality can be used for the treatment of addiction. However, no data are available on the efficacy of aromatherapy for this purpose.

CULTURALLY SPECIFIC HEALING THERAPIES

Cultural differences exist regarding the use and meaning of psychoactive drugs. For example, psychoactive substances have been used in religious ceremonies or rituals across cultures and time, from the use of alcohol in Jewish and Christian ceremonies to the use of peyote by Native Americans, or opium in certain Hindu marriage ceremonies

(Westermeyer, Lyfoung et al., 1991). Cultural differences in treatment philosophies and modalities also exist. There follows a case discussion involving Native American treatment of alcoholism. Many of the issues raised in this case are applicable to the debates regarding other culturally distinct communities and peoples.

It long has been recognized that alcohol is a major drug of abuse among Native Americans, who have a mortality rate from alcoholism three to four times that of the U.S. population (Seale & Muramoto, 1993). Further, Native Americans tend to do poorly in standard addiction treatment programs, as measured by reported rates of relapse (Kivlahan, Walker et al., 1985; Query, 1985; Hanson, 1985). Inhalant abuse is a particularly prevalent and dangerous problem among Native American youth. American Indian tribes are recognized as having unique cultures, heritage, and needs. Thus it has been suggested that treatment services for this and other minority populations need to be more sensitive to the cultural perspectives and issues of importance to the populations served (Hanson, 1985).

The range of Native American practices used for the treatment of drug and alcohol abuse is quite diverse, including sweat lodges, herbs, cultural reeducation, peyote rituals, and sun dances (Hall, 1986; Beauvais & LaBoueff, 1985). Although cultural supports are given attention by some treatment centers, the availability of culturally specific programs is limited, and funding is scarce (Seale & Muramoto, 1993).

The lack of agreement among treatment professionals and the literature regarding the meaning of "culturally specific" or "culturally appropriate" treatments have made replication and research difficult. The terms imply that the programs are in some way designed for, adapted to, or responsive to the needs of the individual, based on his or her cultural heritage. However, the essential differences between culturally specific and non-specific programs have not been defined. Moreover, there are no standards for defining the cultural competence of counselors, or formal policies in place for regulating referrals of clients to culturally specific treatment programs.

Despite the argument that cultural identification may influence the patient's response to treatment (Babor & Mendelson, 1986; Iber, 1986; Flores, 1985-1986; Hall, 1986), research results have been contradictory (Beauvais, 1992; Brady, 1995; Flores, 1985-1986; Hanson, 1985; Parker, Jamous et al., 1991; Rhodes, Mason et al., 1988; Beauvais & LaBoueff, 1985; Westermeyer & Peake, 1983; Westermeyer & Neider,

1986; Gutierres, Russo et al., 1994). Some evidence suggests that Native Americans who withdraw temporarily from their cultural communities may have better rates of recovery (Westermeyer & Peake, 1983). Conclusions and recommendations have been drawn from epidemiologic data, as controlled research has not been conducted.

At this point, research on treatment outcomes has failed to separate the cultural influences from the demographic differences among ethnic groups, using the appropriate statistical controls (Babor & Mendelson, 1986). Not all tribes or individuals are going to respond identically to any given situation (Beauvais & La Boueff, 1985), and ethnicity is not the only factor to be considered, as addictive disorders also vary with age, gender, education, and socioeconomic status (Seale & Muramoto, 1993; Westermeyer & Peake, 1983). Further, researchers have failed to consider the possibility that culturally specific programs also may be used to treat non-native peoples (Babor & Mendelson, 1986), a point which, if verified, could contribute to future support and funding.

SPIRITUALITY AND PRAYER

Although spirituality and religion frequently are used in the prevention and treatment of addiction, drugs and alcohol also have been used during religious rituals and in the quest for transcendence. From the use of alcohol in Jewish and Christian ceremonies to the use of opium at certain Hindu marriage ceremonies, psychoactive drugs in ritual are common, transcending culture and time (Westermeyer, Lyfoung et al., 1991). Further, drugs or mixtures with hallucinogenic properties may be used to bring about religious visions. The use of psychoactive herbal drugs in the quest for transcendence predates history and spans the globe (Miller, 1997).

There is evidence to suggest that, for some individuals, participation in new religions actually may relieve psychiatric symptoms and psychological distress, including substance abuse and dependence. By providing community, the New Religious Movements may serve a "halfway house" function, helping participants recover and reintegrate into the mainstream (Muffler, Langrod et al., 1997).

Indigenous therapies for the treatment of addictions often have incorporated aspects of the spiritual. Spirit dancing, peyote ceremonies, and Shakerism have been used by Native Americans; spiritual churches, "voodoo," and black Hebrew divine healing by African Americans. Hispanic traditions have used Curanderismo, Pentecostalism, and Espiritismo for the treatment of addictive disorders (Singer & Borrero, 1984). For example, in Espiritismo it is believed that people may be made ill or cured by spirits. The treatment of spiritists, then, involves mediums who perform spiritual consultations and conduct cleansing rituals (Singer & Borrero, 1984; Muffler, Langrod et al., 1997). Healing that addresses a patient's faith and culture may be an effective method of treatment (Muffler, Langrod et al., 1997; Miller, 1997).

Evangelical and Pentecostal churches teach individuals seeking treatment to pray and to depend on God. This belief teaches that by accepting Jesus Christ as savior, an individual may be "born again," free himself or herself from the mistakes of the "former" life, and thus recover. Programs like Teen Challenge developed with the belief that religious conversion is the only reality capable of combating addictions (Muffler, Langrod et al., 1997).

Mainline Protestant denominations and Roman Catholicism are more frequently associated with addiction treatment than other religious or spiritual forms in the U.S. Historically, many programs emphasized religious values, but have been transformed into more secular approaches. The majority of efforts sponsored by Protestant and Catholic churches have been institutionalized and are housed in hospitals or community centers rather than church facilities. The influence of earlier Protestant treatment efforts, and the emphasis on religious values, still is seen in popular Twelve Step programs such as Alcoholics Anonymous and Narcotics Anonymous. Successful completion of the steps in these programs requires that members turn their lives over to God or some Higher Power.

Religious involvement seems to be a major source of help for individuals trying to change involuntary habits. In a large number of studies, epidemiological research has demonstrated a negative correlation between personal "religiousness" and substance use (Benson, 1992). However, there has been no direct research into spirituality/prayer as a treatment for substance abuse. A body of research does provide evidence that spiritual healing can occur even when psychological factors have been controlled, as in plant or animal research (Hodges & Scofield, 1995). However, whether prayer is a nonspecific treatment or whether it is efficacious has yet to be determined. Studies on the efficacy of prayer and spirituality are necessary to further its potential use in the treatment of substance abuse, primarily in relapse prevention.

EFFICACY AND EFFECTIVENESS OF CAT

There may be confusion regarding the benefits to be obtained from CAT, as with any current treatment of addictive disorders. In the treatment of medical conditions, benefits may consist of alleviation or cure of the underlying illness or disease. In this sense, antibiotic treatment of certain forms of respiratory illness may be considered efficacious. On the other hand, many treatments can be shown to be effective in dealing with symptoms related to cancer, even though the underlying condition does not improve. In addiction treatment, even if proper controls cannot be put together to adequately show efficacy, treatments that lack efficacy may still have "effectiveness" for some populations. If the treatment procedure helps the patient to access treatment, if dropout rates are reduced, if employment rates improve or other side effects are alleviated, then that treatment has effectiveness and may be worthwhile. At this time, probably all forms of addiction treatment—conventional and CAT—can be considered potentially effective but not efficacious.

Spontaneous Remission. The addiction literature is full of evidence that some individuals "mature out" of their addictive disorders (Klingemann, 1991; Stall & Biernacki, 1986; Klingemann, 1992; Tuchfield, 1981; Prugh, 1986). The most familiar example of addicts maturing out or spontaneously remitting can be seen in the many recovered nicotine addicts. Of all those who stop smoking, 80% to 90% will do so on their own (Sobell, Elingstad et al., 2000). Another well-known example of addicts who spontaneously stopped using is the American servicemen who stopped using heroin on their return from Vietnam. In addition, we know that the majority of humans who use psychoactive drugs (including nicotine, caffeine, and alcohol), never misuse substances (Kalant, 1989).

If there are interventions that can interrupt addiction or increase the probability of spontaneous remission or maturing out, then these would be valuable tools in the clinical armamentarium. Many of the CAT treatments described in this chapter may serve this purpose.

Dropouts and Relapse. Conventional treatment approaches to addiction have been criticized on a number of levels. Dropout rates from most treatment programs are extremely high; rates of 50% or more are common for alcohol misuse and 75% to 85% for cocaine or crack cocaine addiction (Hoffman, Caudill et al., 1994; Vaillant, Clark et al., 1993; Chappel, 1993; Mammo & Weinbaum, 1991). Some facilities do not include dropout rates in their outcome data thus significantly inflating their success rates and misrepresenting their capabilities. A 25% overall success rate (success measured as abstinence) is typical in conventional treatment facilities. Further, despite the substantial amounts of time, energy, and money expended by conventional treatment facilities, there has been scant assessment of the effect of their programs on costs to society or reduction in arrest rates.

Critics also have pointed out that treatment facilities often are not available or accessible to special populations and that the high rate of dropout and relapse of these special populations suggests that their needs are not being met. Further, critics question whether current programs are unable to handle the full scope of physiological, sociological, and psychological problems of clients, all of which must be addressed during recovery.

One way to improve the outcomes of existing programs would be to increase the frequency, intensity, and/or types of treatment services offered. Many studies have indicated that increasing the number of modalities provided increased rates of treatment success (Hoffman, Caudill et al., 1994). In this context, alternative therapies promise to expand and enrich the treatment continuum.

CONCLUSIONS

There are several reasons to consider the use of CAT. Some treatments show promise in preliminary clinical reports and early research efforts (as described above), and early research suggests that at least some effectiveness or utility may be expected. In addition, however, many of the treatments described in this chapter have the capacity to elicit salubrious changes in personal and interpersonal status. One of the lessons of biofeedback, yoga, Tai-chi, relaxation, and transcendental meditation is that the individual can learn to control his or her own mental and physical processes. In this way, the gateway to the concept of self-efficacy may be opened. A common concept underlying many alternative therapies is the elicitation and strengthening of natural healing processes. This concept of self-healing may be one of the learning experiences of the patients.

These aspects may help account for the current excitement and curiosity about use of CAT. It has been demonstrated that patients are finding their way through conventional and CAT systems, even in the absence of secure information regarding efficacy. It is the responsibility of therapists to help these individuals by providing information regarding the potential benefits and dangers of CAT, and to be open to the possibility that there may be avenues

for personal and interpersonal growth in addition to narrowly defined symptom reduction and management, leading patients to a community of supportive people and strengthened capacity to interact with the larger world around them.

NOTE: The views and opinions expressed herein are those of the authors and do not necessarily reflect the views, opinions, or policies of the Substance Abuse and Mental Health Services Administration or the U.S. Department of Health and Human Services.

REFERENCES

Abbott A, Stead LF, White AR et al. (2002). Hypnotherapy for smoking cessation. In *The Cochrane Library, Issue 1*. Oxford, England: Update Software.

Abbott A & Stiegler G (1996). Support for scientific evaluation of homeopathy stirs controversy. *Nature* 383.

Abraham HD, Aldridge AM & Gogia P (1996). The psychopharmacology of hallucinogens. *Neuropsychopharmacology* 14:285-298.

Ades J & Lejoyeaux M (1993). Clinical evaluation of acamprosate to reduce alcohol intake. *Alcohol and Alcoholism* (Suppl 2):275.

Adler R & Cohen N (1975). Behaviorally conditioned immunosuppression. *Psychosomatic Medicine* 33:333-340.

Alexander CN (1992). Closing the chapter on Maharishi Ayur-Veda (Letter). *Journal of the American Medical Association* 267(10):1337.

Allen J (1989). Overview of alcoholism treatment: Settings and approaches. *Journal of Mental Health Administration* 16(2):55-62.

Alling FA, Johnson BD & Elmoghazy E (1990). Cranial electrostimulation (CES) use in the detoxification of opiate-dependent patients. *Journal of Substance Abuse Treatment* 7:173.

Althoff S (1994). Weed for alcoholics. *Natural Health* 24(2):18.

Amaro H (1999). An expensive policy: The impact of inadequate funding for substance abuse treatment. *American Journal of Public Health* 89(5):657-659.

Anderson E & Anderson P (1987). General practitioners and alternative medicine. *Journal of the Royal College of General Practitioners* 37:52-55.

Annis HM (1985). Is inpatient rehabilitation of the alcoholic cost-effective? *Advances in Alcoholism and Substance Abuse* 1-2:175.

Anonymous (1994a). *Alternative Medicine: Expanding Medical Horizons: A Report to the National Institutes of Health on Alternative Medical Systems and Practices in the United States* (NIH Publication No. 94-066). Rockville, MD: National Institute on Drug Abuse.

Anonymous (1994b). Much ado about nothing? *Consumer Reports* 59(3):201-206.

Anonymous (1995). What is Homeopathy: BOIRON Reference Guide. France: BOIRON.

Avants SK, Margolin A, Chang P et al. (1995). Acupuncture for the treatment of cocaine addiction. *Journal of Substance Abuse Treatment* 12(3):195-205.

Avants SK, Margolin A, Holford TR et al. (2000). A randomized controlled trial of auricular acupuncture for cocaine dependence. *Archives of Internal Medicine* 160(15):2305-2312.

Babor RF & Mendelson JH (1986). Ethnic/religious differences in the manifestation and treatment of alcoholism. *Annals of the New York Academy of Sciences* 472:46-59.

Barabasz AF, Baer L, Sheehan DV et al. (1986). A three-year follow-up of hypnosis and restricted environmental stimulation therapy for smoking. *International Journal of Clinical & Experimental Hypnosis* 34(3):169-181.

Barabasz M, Barabasz AF & Mullin CS (1983). Effects of brief Antarctic isolation on absorption and hypnotic susceptibility—preliminary results and recommendations: A brief communication. *International Journal of Clinical and Experimental Hypnosis* 31(4):235-238.

Beasley JD, Grimson RC, Bicker AA et al. (1991). Follow-up of a cohort of alcoholic patients through 12 months of comprehensive biobehavioral treatment. *Journal of Substance Abuse Treatment* 8(3):133-142.

Beauvais F (1992). An integrated model for prevention and treatment of drug abuse among American Indian youth. *Journal of Addictive Diseases* 11(3):63-81.

Beauvais F & LaBoueff S (1985). Drug and Alcohol abuse intervention in American Indian communities. *International Journal of the Addictions* 20(1):139-171.

Beckley-Barrett LM & Mutch PB (1990). Position of the American Dietetic Association: Nutrition intervention in treatment and recovery from chemical dependency. *Journal of the American Dietetic Association* 90(9):1274-1277.

Bellavite P (1990). Research in homeopathy: Data, problems and prospects (Review) (Italian). *Annali dell Istituto Superiore di Sanita* 26(2):179-187.

Benson PL (1992). Religion and substance use. In JF Schumaker (ed.) *Religion and Mental Health.* New York, NY: Oxford University Press, 211-220.

Berman BM, Singh BK, Lao L et al. (1995). Physicians' attitudes toward complementary or alternative medicine: A regional survey. *Journal of the American Board of Family Practice* 8(5):361-366.

Biery JR, Williford JH & McMullen EA (1991). Alcohol craving in rehabilitation: Assessment of nutrition therapy. *Journal of the American Dietetic Association* 91(4):463-466.

Birnbaumer N, Elbert T, Rockstroh B et al. (1992). Effects of inhaled nicotine on instrumental learning of blood pressure responses. *Biofeedback and Self Regulation* 17(2):107-123.

Blum K, Newmeyer JA & Whitehead C (1978). Acupuncture as a common mode of treatment for drug dependence: Possible neurochemical mechanisms. *Journal of Psychedelic Drugs* 10(2):105-115.

Blum K, Trachtenberg MC, Elliott CE et al. (1988). Enkephalinase inhibition and precursor amino acid loading improves inpatient treatment of alcohol and polydrug abusers: Double-blind placebo-controlled study of the nutritional adjunct SAAVE. *Alcohol* 5(6):481-493.

Borrie RA (1990-1991). The use of restricted environmental stimulation therapy in treating addictive behaviors (Review). *International Journal of the Addictions* 25(7A-8A):995-1015.

Bowers TG & Clum GA (1988). Relative contribution of specific and nonspecific treatment effects: Meta-Analysis of placebo-controlled behavior therapy research. *Psychological Bulletin* 103(3):315-323.

Brady K (1995). Prevalence, consequences and costs of tobacco, drug, and alcohol use in the United States. In CM Circa (ed.) *Training About Alcohol and Substance Abuse for All Primary Care Physicians.* Proceedings of a conference sponsored by the Josiah Macy, Jr. Foundation, October 2-5, 1994, Phoenix, AZ.

Brewington V, Smith M & Lipton D (1994). Acupuncture as a detoxification treatment: An analysis of controlled research. *Journal of Substance Abuse Treatment* 11(4):289-307.

Brown RJ, Blum K & Trachtenberg MC (1990). Neurodynamics of relapse prevention: A neuronutrient approach to outpatient DUI offenders. *Journal of Psychoactive Drugs* 22(2):173-87.

Brumbaugh AG (1993). Acupuncture: New perspectives in chemical dependency treatment. *Journal of Substance Abuse Treatment* 10(1):35-43.

Brumbaugh AG (1994). Acupuncture. In NS Miller (ed.) *Principles of Addiction Medicine.* Chevy Chase, MD: American Society of Addiction Medicine.

Bullock ML, Culliton PD & Olander RT (1989). Controlled trial of acupuncture for severe recidivist alcoholism. *Lancet* 1(8652):1435-1439.

Bullock ML, Kiresuk TJ, Sherman RM et al. (2002). A large randomized placebo controlled study of auricular acupuncture for alcohol dependence. *Journal of Substance Abuse Treatment* 22(2):71-77.

Bullock ML, Pheley AM, Kiresuk TJ et al. (1997). Characteristics and complaints of patients seeking therapy at a hospital-based alternative medicine clinic. *Journal of Alternative and Complementary Medicine* 3(1):31-37.

Bullock ML, Umen AJ, Culliton PD et al. (1987). Acupuncture treatment of alcoholic recidivism: A pilot study. *Alcoholism, Clinical & Experimental Research* 11(3):292-295.

Chappel J (1993). Long-term recovery from alcoholism. *Recent Advances in Addictive Disorders* 16(1):177-187.

Chiauzzi E & Liljegren S (1993). Taboo topics in addiction treatment. An empirical review of clinical folklore. *Journal of Substance Abuse Treatment* 10(3):303-316.

Chopra D (1992). Closing the chapter on Maharishi Ayur-Veda (Letter). *Journal of the American Medical Association* 267(10):1338.

Coates C (1996). Sympathetic threads. *Common Boundary* 40-45.

Collipp PJ, Kris VK, Castro-Magana M et al. (1984). The effects of dietary zinc deficiency on voluntary alcohol drinking in rats. *Alcoholism* 8(6):556-559.

Cowan JD (1993). Alpha-theta brainwave biofeedback: The many possible theoretical reasons for its success. *Biofeedback* 21(2):11-16.

Cronan TA, Kaplan RM, Posner L et al. (1989). Prevalence of the use of unconventional remedies for arthritis in a metropolitan community. *Arthritis & Rheumatism* 32(12):1604-1607.

Culliton P & Kiresuk T (1996). Overview of substance abuse acupuncture treatment research. *Journal of Alternative and Complementary Medicine* 2(1):149-159.

DeGood DE & Valle RS (1978). Self-reported alcohol and nicotine use and the ability to control occipital EEG in a biofeedback situation. *Addictive Behaviors* 3:13-18.

Denney MR, Baugh JL & Hardt HD (1991). Sobriety outcome after alcoholism treatment with biofeedback participation: A pilot inpatient study. *International Journal of the Addictions* 26(3):335-341.

Des Maisons KB (1996). Addictive nutrition as a treatment intervention for multiple offense drunk drivers (Dissertation). The Union Institute.

Dilsaver SC & Majchrzak MJ (1988). Bright artificial light produces subsensitivity to nicotine. *Life Sciences* 42:225-230.

Eastwood MR & Stiasny LS (1978). Psychiatric disorder, hospital admission, and season. *Archives of General Psychiatry* 35:769-771.

Eisenberg DM, Kessler RC, Foster C et al. (1993). Unconventional medicine in the United States. Prevalence, costs, and patterns of use. *New England Journal of Medicine* 328(4):246-52.

Eriksson K, Pekkanen L & Russi M (1980). The effects of dietary thiamin on voluntary ethanol drinking and ethanol metabolism in the rat. *British Journal of Nutrition* 43(1):1-13.

Fahrion SL (1995). Human potential and personal transformation. *Subtle Energies* 6(1):55-88.

Fahrion SL, Walters ED, Coyne L et al. (1992). Alterations in EEG amplitude, personality factors, and brain electrical mapping after alpha-theta brainwave training: A controlled case study of an alcoholic in recovery. *Alcoholism: Clinical & Experimental Research* 16(3):547-552.

Fink M, Gutenbrunner C, Rollnik J et al. (2001). Credibility of a newly designed placebo needle for clinical trials in acupuncture research. *Forschende Komplementarmedizin und Klassiche Naturheikunde* 8(6):368-372.

Flores PJ (1985-1986). Alcoholism treatment and the relationship of Native American cultural values to recovery. *International Journal of the Addictions* 20(11-12):1707-1726.

Forander O, Kohonen J & Suomalainen H (1958). *Quarterly Journal of Studies on Alcohol* 19:379-387.

Frank J (1973). *Persuasion and Healing.* Baltimore, MD: Johns Hopkins University Press.

Garbutt JC, West SL, Carey TS et al. (1999). Pharmacological treatment of alcohol dependence: A review of the evidence. *Journal of the American Medical Association* 281(14):1318-1325.

Gariti P, Auriacombe M, Incmikoski R et al. (1992). A randomized double-blind study of neuroelectric therapy in opiate and cocaine detoxification. *Journal of Substance Abuse* 4(3):299-308.

Garrity JF (2000). Jesus, peyote, and the holy people: Alcohol abuse and the ethos of power Navajo healing. *Medical Anthropology Quarterly* 14(4):521-542.

Gelderloos P, Walton KG, Orme-Johnson D et al. (1991). Effectiveness of the Transcendental Meditation program in preventing and treating substance misuse: A review. *International Journal of the Addictions* 26(3):293-325.

Goldstein A (1989). Introduction. In A Goldstein (ed.) *Molecular and Cellular Aspects of the Drug Addictions.* New York, NY: Springer-Verlag, xiii-xviii.

Gossop M, Bradley B, Strang J et al. (1984). The clinical effectiveness of electrostimulation vs. oral methadone in managing opiate withdrawal. *British Journal of Psychiatry* 144:203-208.

Grimsley D (1990). Nicotine effects on biofeedback training. *Journal of Behavioral Medicine* 13(3):321-326.

Guenther RM (1983). Nutrition and alcoholism. *Journal of Applied Nutrition* 35(1):44-46.

Gutierres SE, Russo NF & Urbanski L (1994). Sociocultural and psychological factors in American Indian drug use: Implications for treatment. *International Journal of the Addictions* 29(14):1761-1786.

Hadley C (1988). Complementary medicine and the general practitioner: A survey of general practitioners in the Wellington area. *New Zealand Medical Journal* 101:766-768.

Hall RL (1986). Alcohol treatment in American Indian populations: An indigenous treatment modality compared with traditional approaches. *Annals of the New York Academy of Sciences* 472:168-178.

Halpern JH (1996). The use of hallucinogens in the treatment of addiction. *Addiction Research* 4(2):177-189.

Hanson B (1985). Drug treatment effectiveness: The case of racial and ethnic minorities in America—Some research questions and proposals. *International Journal of the Addictions* 20(1):99-137.

Haxby D (1995). Treatment of nicotine dependence (Review). *American Journal of Health-System Pharmacy* 52(3):265-281.

Hester R (1994). Outcome research: Alcoholism. In M Galanter & H Kleber (eds.) *The American Psychiatric Press Textbook of Substance Abuse Treatment.* Washington, DC: American Psychiatric Press, 35-43.

Hill C & Doyon F (1990). Review of randomized trials of homeopathy. *Revue and Epidemiologie et de Sante Publique* 38(2):139-147.

Himmel W, Schulte M & Kochen MM (1993). Complementary medicine: Are patients' expectations being met by their general practitioners? *British Journal of General Practice* 43(371):232-235.

Hodges RD & Scofield AM (1995). Is spiritual healing a valid and effective therapy? *Journal of the Royal Society of Medicine* 88:203-207.

Hoffman JA, Caudill BD, Koman JJ et al. (1994). Comparative cocaine abuse treatment strategies: Enhancing client retention and treatment exposure. *Journal of Addictive Diseases* 13(4):115-128.

Holder H, Longabaugh R, Miller W et al. (1991). The cost effectiveness of treatment for alcoholism: A first approximation. *Journal of Studies on Alcohol* 52(6):517-540.

Holroyd J (1980). Hypnosis treatment for smoking: An evaluative review. *International Journal of Clinical and Experimental Hypnosis* 28(4):341-357.

Hyman G, Stanley R, Burrows G et al. (1986). Treatment effectiveness of hypnosis and behavior therapy in smoking cessation: A methodological refinement. *Addictive Behaviors* 11(4):355-365.

Iber FL (1986). Treatment and recovery in alcoholism: Contrast between results in white men and those in special populations. *Annals of the New York Academy of Sciences* 472:189-194.

Jacobson GR (1971). Sensory deprivation and field dependence in alcoholics. (Unpublished doctoral dissertation). Illinois Institute of Technology.

Johnson D & Karkut R (1994). Performance by gender in a stop-smoking program combining hypnosis and aversion. *Psychological Reports* 75(2):851-857.

Johnston EJ & Donoghue JR (1971). Hypnosis and smoking: A review of the literature. *American Journal of Clinical Hypnosis* 13(4):265-272.

Jou TH (1991). *The Tao of Tai-Chi Chuan: Way to Rejuvenation.* Warwick, NY: Tai-Chi Foundation.

Justice B (1987). *Who Gets Sick: Thinking and Health.* Houston, TX: Peak Press.

Kalant H (1989). The nature of addiction: An analysis of the problem. *Molecular and Cellular Aspects of the Drug Addictions.* New York, NY: Springer-Verlag, 1-28.

Katz N (1980). Hypnosis and the addictions: A critical review. *Addictive Behaviors* 5:41-47.

Keung WM (1993). Biochemical studies of a new class of alcohol dehydrogenase inhibitors from Radix puerariae. *Alcoholism: Clinical & Experimental Research* 17(6):1254-1260.

Keung WM, Lazo O, Kunze L et al. (1995). Daidzin suppresses ethanol consumption by Syrian golden hamsters without blocking acetaldehyde metabolism. *Proceedings of the National Academy of Sciences* 92(19):8990-8993.

Keung WM & Vallee BL (1993). Daidzin and daidzein suppress free-choice ethanol intake by Syrian golden hamsters. *Proceedings of the National Academy of Sciences* 90(21):10008-10012.

Kienle GS & Kiene H (1996). Placebo effect and placebo concept: A critical methodological and conceptual analysis of reports on the magnitude of the placebo effect. *Alternative Therapies* 2(6):39-54.

Kiresuk TJ (1988). The placebo effect: Public policy and knowledge transfer. *Knowledge: Creation, Diffusion, Utilization* 9(4):435-475.

Kivlahan DR, Walker D, Donovan DM et al. (1985). Detoxification recidivism among urban American Indian alcoholics. *American Journal of Psychiatry* 142(12):1467-1470.

Klajner F, Hartman L & Sobell M (1984). Treatment of substance abuse by relaxation training: A review of its rationale, efficacy and mechanisms. *Addictive Behaviors* 9(1):41-55.

Kleijnen J, Knipschild P & Ter Riet G (1991). Clinical trials of homeopathy. *British Medical Journal* 302(6772):316-323.

Klingemann HK (1992). Coping and maintenance strategies of spontaneous remitters from problem use of alcohol and heroin Switzerland. *International Journal of the Addictions* 27(12):1359-1388.

Klingemann HK (1991). The motivation for change from problem alcohol and heroin use. *British Journal of Addiction* 86(6):727-744.

Kosten TR, Kreck MJ, Ragunath J et al. (1986). A preliminary study of beta endorphin during chronic naltrexone maintenance treatment in ex-opiate addicts. *Life Sciences* 31(1):5559.

Kurz R (1992). Clinical medicine vs. Homeopathy. *Paditrie und Padologie* 27(2):37-41.

Lambe R, Osier C & Franks P (1986). A randomized controlled trial of hypnotherapy for smoking cessation. *Journal of Family Practice* 22(1):61-65.

Lankford MF & Myers RD (1994). Genetics of Alcoholism: Simultaneous presentation of a chocolate drink diminishes alcohol preference in high drinking HAD rats. *Pharmacology, Biochemistry and Behavior* 49(2):417-225.

Lankford MF, Roscoe AK, Pennington SN et al. (1991). Drinking of high concentrations of ethanol versus palatable fluids in alcohol-preferring (P) rats: Valid animal model of alcoholism. *Alcohol* 8:293-299.

Lawes TGG (1963). Schizophrenia, "Sernyl", and sensory deprivation. *British Journal of Psychiatry* 109:243-250.

Lee DY (1996). Animal Studies of NPI-028 for Addiction (herbal compound). Unpublished data.

Lefcourt H (1973). The functions of illusions of control and freedom. *American Psychologist* 28(3):417-425.

Lewith GT, Kenyon JN & Lewis PJ (1996). *Complementary Medicine: An Integrated Approach*. Oxford, England: Oxford University Press.

Lilly JC (1956). *Mental Effects of Reduction of Ordinary Levels of Physical Stimuli on Intact, Healthy Persons* (Psychiatric Research Reports, No. 5). Washington, DC: American Psychiatric Association.

Lipton DS, Brewington V & Smith M (1994). Acupuncture for crack-cocaine detoxification: Experimental evaluation of efficacy. *Journal of Substance Abuse Treatment* 11(3):205-215.

Ludwig A, Levine J & Stark L (1970). *LSD and Alcoholism: A Clinical Study of Treatment Efficacy*. Springfield, IL: Charles C Thomas.

Mack A (1997). Biotechnology turns to ancient remedies in quest for sources of new therapies. *The Scientist* 11(1):8-9.

Mammo A & Weinbaum D (1991). Some factors that influence dropping out from outpatient alcoholism treatment facilities. *Journal of Studies on Alcohol* 54(1):92-101.

Margolin A, Kleber HD, Avants SK et al. (2002). Acupuncture for the treatment of cocaine addiction: A randomized controlled trial. *Journal of the American Medical Association* 287(1):55-63.

Marshall R (1992). Integration of alternative and orthodox practices among general practitioners in Auckland, New Zealand. In W Andritzky (ed.) *Yearbook of Cross-Cultural Medicine and Psychotherapy*. Berlin, Germany: VWB - Verlag fur Wissonschaft und Bildung, 133–143.

Mathews-Larson J & Parker RA (1987). Alcoholism treatment with biochemical restoration as a major component. *International Journal of Biosocial Research* 9(1):92-104.

McGrady A, Turner JW, Fine TH et al. (1987). Effects of biobehaviorally-assisted relaxation training on blood pressure, plasma renin, cortisol, and aldosterone levels in borderline essential hypertension. *Clinical Biofeedback and Health: An International Journal* 10(1):16-25.

McGrath RE & Yahia M (1993). Preliminary data on seasonally related alcohol dependence. *Journal of Clinical Psychiatry* 54(7):260-262.

McKenna DJ (1996). Plant hallucinogens: Springboards for psychotherapeutic drug discovery. *Behavioural Brain Research* 73:109-115.

McLellan AT, Grossman DS, Blaine JD et al. (1993). Acupuncture treatment for drug abuse: A technical review. *Journal of Substance Abuse Treatment* 10(6):569-576.

McLellan A, Lubrosky L, Cacciola J et al. (1985). New data from the Addiction Severity Index. Reliability and validity in three centers. *Journal of Nervous and Mental Diseases* 172:412-423.

McMillen BA & Williams HL (1995). Volitional consumption of ethanol by fawn-hooded rats: Effects of alternative solutions and drug treatments. *Alcohol* 12(4):345-350.

Miller WR (1990). Spirituality: The silent dimension in addiction research. The 1990 Leonard Ball Oration. *Drug and Alcohol Review* 9:259-266.

Miller WR (1997). Spiritual aspects of addictions treatment and research. *Mind/Body Medicine* 2(1):37-43.

Miller W & Baca L (1983). Two-year follow-up of bibliotherapy and therapist-directed controlled drinking training for problem drinkers. *Behavioral Therapy* 14:441-450.

Miller WR, Brown JM, Simpson TL et al. (1995). What works? A methodological analysis of the alcohol treatment outcome literature. In RK Hester & WR Miller (eds.) *Handbook of Alcoholism Treatment Approaches: Effective Alternatives, 2nd Edition*. Boston, MA: Allyn & Bacon, 12-44.

Miller W & Hester R (1980). The addictive behaviors: Treatment of alcoholism, drug abuse, smoking and obesity. *Treating the Problem Drinker: Modern Approaches*. Oxford, England: Pergamon Press.

Mirman JI (1994). *What the Hell Is Homeopathy?* New Hope, MN: New Hope Publishers.

Mohs ME, Watson RR & Leonard-Green T (1990). Nutritional effects of marijuana, heroin, cocaine, and nicotine. *Journal of the American Dietetic Association* 90(9):1261-1267.

Montgomery R & Ayllon T (1994). Eye movement desensitization across subjects: Subjective and physiological measures of treatment efficacy. *Journal of Behavior Therapy and Experimental Psychiatry* 25(3):217-230.

Morgan HW, ed. (1981). *Drugs in America: A Social History, 1800-1980.* Syracuse, NY: Syracuse University Press.

Morrison H (1995). Nature's Prozac. *Natural Health* 25(3):80-88.

Muffler J, Langrod JG, Richardson JT et al. (1997). Religion. In JH Lowinson, P Ruiz, RB Millman et al. (eds.) *Substance Abuse: A Comprehensive Textbook, 3rd Edition.* Baltimore, MD: Williams and Wilkins, 492-499.

Mumford E, Schlesinger H & Glass G (1982). The effects of psychological intervention on recovery from surgery and heart attacks: An analysis of the literature. *American Journal of Public Health* 7 2(2):141-151.

O'Connell DF (1995). Possessing the self: Maharishi Ayur-Veda and the process of recovery from addictive diseases. In DF O'Connell & CN Alexander (eds.) *Self Recovery: Treating Addictions Using Transcendental Meditation and Maharishi Ayur-Veda.* New York, NY: Harrington Park Press, 459-496.

O'Connell DF & Alexander CN (1995). Introduction: Recovery from addictions using Transcendental Meditation and Maharishi Ayur-Veda. In DF O'Connell & CN Alexander (eds.) *Self Recovery: Treating Addictions Using Transcendental Meditation and Maharishi Ayur-Veda.* New York, NY: Harrington Park Press, 1-12.

Orman D (1991). Reframing of an addiction via hypnotherapy: A case presentation. *American Journal of Clinical Hypnosis* 33(4):263-271.

Ormrod J & Budd R (1991). A comparison of two treatment interventions aimed at lowering anxiety levels and alcohol consumption amongst alcohol abusers. *Drug and Alcohol Dependence* 27(3):233-243.

Page R & Handley G (1993). The use of hypnosis in cocaine addiction. *American Journal of Clinical Hypnosis* 36(2):120-123.

Parker L, Jamous M, Marek R et al. (1991). Traditions and innovations: A community-based approach to substance abuse prevention. *Rhode Island Medical Journal* 74:281-286.

Patterson M, Krupitsky E, Flood N et al. (1994). Amelioration of stress in chemical dependency detoxification by transcranial electrostimulation. *Stress Medicine* 10:115-126.

Patterson MA, Patterson L, Winston JR et al. (1993). Electrostimulation in drug and alcohol detoxification: Significance of stimulation criteria in clinical success. *Addiction Research* 1:130-144.

Pekkanen L (1980). Effects of thiamin deprivation and antagonism on voluntary ethanol intake in rats. *Journal of Nutrition* 110:937-944.

Peniston EG & Kulkosky PJ (1990). Alcoholic personality and alpha-theta brainwave training. *Medical Psychotherapy* 3:37-55.

Peniston EG & Kulkosky PJ (1989). Alpha-theta brainwave training and beta-endorphin levels in alcoholics. *Alcoholism: Clinical & Experimental Research* 13(2):271-279.

Peteet JR (1993). A closer look at the role of a spiritual approach in addictions treatment. *Journal of Substance Abuse Treatment* 10(3):263-267.

Petri G & Takach G (1990). Application of herbal mixtures in rehabilitation after alcoholism. *Planta Medica* 56(6):692-693.

Piercy KT & Myers RD (1995). Tomato juice, chocolate drink, and other fluids suppress volitional drinking of alcohol in the female Syrian golden hamster. *Physiology and Behavior* 57(6):1155-1161.

Poikolainen K (1982). Seasonality of alcohol-related hospital admissions has implications for prevention. *Drug and Alcohol Dependence* 10:65-69.

Pomeranz B (1987). Scientific basis of acupuncture. *Acupuncture: Textbook and Atlas.* Berlin, Germany: Springer-Verlag.

Popik P, Layer RT & Skolnick P (1995). 100 years of ibogaine: Neurochemical and pharmacological actions of a putative anti-addictive drug. *Pharmacological Reviews* 47(2):235-253.

Powell B, Penick E, Read M et al. (1985). Comparison of three outpatient treatment interventions: A twelve-month follow-up of men alcoholics. *Journal of Studies on Alcohol* 46(4):309-312.

Prugh T (1986). Recovery without treatment. *Alcohol Health and Research World* 11(1)(24):71-72.

Query JMN (1985). Comparative admission and follow-up study of American Indians and whites in a youth chemical dependency unit on the North Central Plains. *International Journal of the Addictions* 20(3):489-502.

Rabkin SW, Boyko E, Shane F et al. (1984). A randomized trial comparing smoking cessation programs utilizing behaviour modification, health education, or hypnosis. *Addictive Behaviors* 9:157-173.

Rank D & Suedfeld P (1978). Positive reactions of alcoholic men to sensory deprivation. *International Journal of the Addictions* 13(5):807-815.

Register UD, Marsh SR, Thurston DT et al. (1972). Influence of nutrients on intake of alcohol. *Journal of the American Dietetic Association* 61:159-162

Reilly D, Taylor M, Beattie N et al. (1994). Is evidence for homeopathy reproducible? *Lancet* 344(8937):1601-1606.

Rezvani AH, Overstreet DH & Lee Y (1995). Attenuation of alcohol intake by ibogaine in three strains of alcohol-preferring rats. *Pharmacology, Biochemistry and Behavior* 52(3):615-620.

Rhodes ER, Mason RD, Eddy P et al. (1988). The Indian Health Service approach to alcoholism among American Indian and Alaska Natives. *Public Health Reports* 103(6):621-627.

Richter C (1957). On the phenomenon of sudden death in animals and man. *Psychosomatic Medicine* 72(3):191-198.

Riedlinger TJ & Riedlinger JE (1994). Psychedelic and entactogenic drugs in the treatment of depression. *Journal of Psychoactive Drugs* 26(1):41-55.

Rogers LL, Pelton RB & Williams RJ (1956). Amino acid supplementation and voluntary alcohol consumption by rats. *Journal of Biological Chemistry* 220(1):321-323.

Satel SL & Gawin FH (1989). Seasonal cocaine abuse. *American Journal of Psychiatry* 146:534-535.

Schachter L, Weingarten MA & Kahan EE (1993). Attitudes of family physicians to nonconventional therapies. *Archives of Family Medicine* 2:1268-1270.

Schneider F, Elbert T, Heimann H et al. (1993). Self-regulation of slow cortical potentials in psychiatric patients: Alcohol dependency. *Biofeedback and Self Regulation* 18(1):23-32.

Schou M (1997). Forty years of lithium treatment (Review). *Archives of General Psychiatry* 54(1):21-23.

Schwartz J (1992). Methods of smoking cessation (Review). *Medical Clinics of North America* 76(2):451-476.

Seale JP & Muramoto ML (1993). Substance abuse among minority populations. *Primary Care Clinics in Office Practice* 20(1):167-180.

Sershen H, Hashim A & Lajtha A (1994). Ibogaine reduces preference for cocaine consumption in C57BL/6 by mice. *Pharmacology, Biochemistry and Behavior* 47:13-19.

Shaffer HJ & LaSalvia TA (1997). Comparing Hatha Yoga with dynamic group psychotherapy for enhancing methadone maintenance treatment: A randomized clinical trial. *Alternative Therapies in Health and Medicine* 3(4):57-66.

Shanmugasundaram E, Subramaniam U, Santhini R et al. (1986). Studies on brain structure and neurological function in alcoholic rats controlled by an Indian medicinal formula (SKV). *Journal of Ethnopharmacology* 17:225-245.

Shapiro A & Morris L (1978). *Placebo Effects in Medical and Psychological Therapies: Handbook of Psychotherapy and Behavior Change.* New York, NY: John Wiley & Sons.

Shapiro A, Struening E & Shapiro E (1980). The reliability and validity of a placebo test. *Journal of Psychiatric Research* 55:253-290.

Shapiro F, Vogelmann-Sine S & Sine LF (1994). Eye movement desensitization and reprocessing: Treating trauma and substance abuse. *Journal of Psychoactive Drugs* 26(4):379-391.

Sheppard SG (1994). A preliminary investigation of ibogaine: Case reports and recommendations for further study. *Journal of Substance Abuse Treatment* 11(4):379-385.

Silver S, Brooks A & Obenchain J (1995). Treatment of Vietnam War veterans with PTSD: A comparison of eye movement desensitization and reprocessing, biofeedback, and relaxation training. *Journal of Traumatic Stress* 8(2):337-342.

Singer MT (1992). Closing the chapter on Maharishi Ayur-Veda (Letter). *Journal of the American Medical Association* 267(10):1337.

Singer M & Borrero MG (1984). Indigenous treatment of alcoholism: The case of Puerto Rican spiritism. *Medical Anthropology* 8(4):246-73.

Skolnick AA (1992). Closing the chapter on Maharishi Ayur-Veda (Letter). *Journal of the American Medical Association* 267(10):1339-1340.

Smith MO (1988). Acupuncture treatment for crack: Clinical survey of 1500 patients treated. *American Journal of Acupuncture* 16(3):241-247.

Smith MO & Khan I (1988). An acupuncture programme for the treatment of drug-addicted persons. *Bulletin on Narcotics* 40(1):35-41.

Spiegel D, Bloom JR, Kraemer HC et al. (1989). Effect of psychosocial treatment on survival of patients with metastatic breast cancer. *Lancet* 2(8668):888-891.

Stall R & Biernacki P (1986). Spontaneous remission from the problematic use of substances: An inductive model derived from a comparative analysis of the alcohol, opiate, tobacco, and food/obesity literatures. *International Journal of the Addictions* 21(1):1-23.

Steiner RP, May DL & Davis AW (1982). Acupuncture therapy for the treatment of tobacco smoking addiction. *American Journal of Chinese Medicine* 10(1-4):107-121.

Stoil M (1989). Problems in the evaluation of hypnosis in the treatment of alcoholism. *Journal of Substance Abuse Treatment* 6:31-35.

Suedfeld P (1964). Attitude manipulation in restricted environments: I. Conceptual structure and response to propaganda. *Journal of Abnormal and Social Psychology* 68:242-247.

Suedfeld P (1990). Restricted environmental stimulation and smoking cessation: A fifteen-year progress report. *International Journal of the Addictions* 25:861-888.

Suedfeld P & Best JA (1977). Satiation and sensory deprivation combined in smoking therapy: Some case studies and unexpected side-effects. *International Journal of the Addictions* 12(2-3):337-359.

Suedfeld P & Ikard F (1974). The use of sensory deprivation in facilitating the reduction of cigarette smoking. *Journal of Consulting and Clinical Psychology* 42:888-895.

Suedfeld P, Landon PB, Pargament R et al. (1972). An experimental attack on smoking: Attitude manipulation in restricted environments, III. *International Journal of the Addictions* 7:721-733.

Surawy C & Cox T (1986). Smoking behaviour under conditions of relaxation: A comparison between types of smokers. *Addictive Behaviors* 11(2):187-191.

Taub E, Steiner SS, Weingarten E et al. (1994). Effectiveness of broad spectrum approaches to relapse prevention in severe alcoholism: A long-term, randomized, controlled trial of transcendental mediation, EMG biofeedback and electronic neurotherapy. *Alcoholism Treatment Quarterly* 11(1/2):187-220.

Ter Riet G, Kleijnen J & Knipschild P (1990). A meta-analysis of studies into the effect of acupuncture on addiction. *British Journal of General Practice* 40(338):379-382.

Tompkins VD (1992). Closing the chapter on Maharishi Ayur-Veda (Letter). *Journal of the American Medical Association* 267(10):133139.

Tuchfield BS (1981). Spontaneous remission in alcoholics: Empirical observations and theoretical implications. *Journal of Studies on Alcohol* 42(7):626-641.

Turner JW & Fine TH (1983). Effects of relaxation associated with brief restricted environmental stimulation therapy (REST) on plasma cortisol, ACTH and LH. *Biofeedback and Self-Regulation* 8(1):115-126.

U.S. Department of Health and Human Services (USDHHS) (2000). *Treating Tobacco Use and Dependence: A Clinical Practice Guideline.* Washington, DC: USDHHS.

Vaillant G, Clark W, Cyrus C et al. (1993). Prospective study of alcoholism treatment: Eight year follow-up. *American Journal of Medicine* 75:455-463.

Visser GJ & Peters L (1990). Alternative medicine and general practitioners in The Netherlands: Towards acceptance and integration. *Family Practice* 7(3):227-232.

Walach H & Righetti M (1996). Homeopathy: Principles, status of research, research design. *Wiener Klinische Wochenschrift* 108(20):654-63.

Walton KG & Levitsky D (1995). A neuroendocrine mechanism for the reduction of drug use and addiction by transcendental meditation. In DF O'Connell & CN Alexander (eds.) *Self Recovery: Treating Addictions Using Transcendental Meditation and Maharishi Ayur-Veda.* New York, NY: Harrington Park Press, 89-118.

Washburn AM, Fullilove RE, Fullilove MT et al. (1993). Acupuncture heroin detoxification: A single-blind clinical trial. *Journal of Substance Abuse Treatment* 10(4):345-351.

Watson RR & Mohs ME (1990). Effects of morphine, cocaine, and heroin on nutrition. *Alcohol, Immunomodulation, and AIDS* 325:413-418.

Wen HL (1979). Acupuncture and electrical stimulations (AES) outpatient detoxification. *Modern Medicine in Asia* 15:39-43.

Wen HL & Cheung SYC (1973). Treatment of drug addiction by acupuncture and electrical stimulation. *Asian Journal of Medicine* 9:138-141.

Wen HL & Teo SW (1975). Experience in the treatment of drug addiction by electro-acupuncture. *Modern Medicine in Asia* 11:23-24.

Werbach MR (1991). Alcoholism. *Nutritional Influences on Mental Illness: A Sourcebook of Clinical Research.* Tarzana, CA: Third Line Press, 18-47.

Westermeyer J, Lyfoung T, Westermeyer M et al. (1991). Opium addiction among Indochinese refugees in the U.S.: Characteristics of addictions and their opium use. *American Journal of Drug and Alcohol Abuse* 17(3):267-277.

Westermeyer J & Neider J (1986). Cultural affiliation among American Indian alcoholics: Correlations and change over a ten-year period. *Annals of the New York Academy of Sciences* 472:179-188.

Westermeyer J & Peake E (1983). A ten-year follow-up of alcoholic Native Americans in Minnesota. *American Journal of Psychiatry* 140(2):189-194.

Wharton R & Lewith G (1986). Complementary medicine and the general practitioner. *British Medical Journal* 292(6534):1498-1500.

Whitehead PC (1978). Acupuncture in the treatment of addiction: A review and analysis. *International Journal of the Addictions* 13(1):1-16.

Winer LR (1977). Biofeedback: A Guide to the clinical literature. *American Journal of Orthopsychiatry* 47(4):626-638.

Worner TM, Zeller B, Schwarz H et al. (1992). Acupuncture fails to improve treatment outcome in alcoholics. *Drug and Alcohol Dependence* 30(2):169-173.

Xie CI, Lin RC, Antony V et al. (1994). Daidzin, an antioxidant isoflavonoid, decreases blood alcohol levels and shortens sleep time induced by ethanol intoxication. *Alcoholism: Clinical & Experimental Research* 18(6):1443-1447.

Chapter 10

Harm Reduction as an Approach to Treatment

Alex Wodak, M.D., FRACP

Harm reduction policies and programs, which span prevention and treatment, aim to decrease the adverse health, social, and economic consequences of drug use without necessarily diminishing drug consumption (Wodak & Saunders, 1995). This approach has gained increasing support over the past decade, while more conventional approaches increasingly have appeared ineffective, expensive, and counterproductive (Nadelmann, 1989; Riley, 1996).

WHAT IS HARM REDUCTION?

Defining Harm Reduction. The term "harm reduction," sometimes known as "harm minimization," has not been defined by an official body and consequently has been used with a bewildering variety of interpretations (Strang, 1993). The ambiguity of the term adds to the confusion of an area already complicated by lack of terminological clarity and excessive emotional fervor. The alcohol and drug field also is characterized by attempts to force dichotomous categorizations, even though most phenomena in the discipline are distributed on a continuum. Harm reduction is better considered as a difference in emphasis rather than a radical departure from conventional responses.

Although harm reduction approaches are not intended primarily to reduce consumption of drugs, this often is an unintended long-term result. For example, random breath testing was introduced to reduce the incidence of alcohol-related road crash deaths and serious injuries by deterring intoxicated citizens from driving. This has had the unanticipated benefit of encouraging many car drivers, who form the majority of the adult population, to consume less alcohol. Similarly, many drug users who have attended needle exchange programs for some time canvass the idea of achieving abstinence and request referral to drug treatment (Lurie, Reingold et al., 1993).

History of Harm Reduction. Although harm reduction often is misrepresented as a recent development in the alcohol and drug field, it has a long history. Like Moliere's character M. Jourdain, who discovered after more than 40 years that he had been speaking prose without knowing it, some clinicians and policymakers have discovered that they have long been practicing harm reduction. In ancient China, authorities attempted unsuccessfully to limit alcohol consumption as a means of preventing inebriated citizens falling into wintery canals and freezing to death. Although it was not possible to eliminate public intoxication, the simple installation of barriers around the canals was found to effectively prevent such deaths. Compulsory safety belt legislation was introduced from the 1960s in a number of countries when authorities became alarmed by increasing numbers of alcohol-related road crash deaths. Efforts at that time to reduce per capita alcohol consumption were singularly unsuccessful. Ensuring that almost all car drivers wore safety belts while driving had no effect on alcohol consumption or drunk driving but did dramatically reduce alcohol-related road crash deaths and serious injuries. Support for harm reduction policies and programs increased in the mid-1980s following the recognition of the central role of injecting drug users in the HIV pandemic in many countries and the realization that uncontrolled epidemics involving injecting drug users had immense health, social, and economic costs.

Misconceptions About Harm Reduction. To some, harm reduction means the employment of any measures likely to reduce an adverse consequence of illicit drug use. A more expanded view of harm reduction emphasizes maximizing the potential benefits of mood-altering substances as well. For example, inadequate doses of opioids too often are prescribed in the management of cancer pain, where they result in considerable distress from inadequate pain relief. Such subtherapeutic doses usually are prescribed in response to excessive fears of inducing drug dependence, even among patients who have a very limited life expectancy. Similarly, current restrictions on medicinal use of cannabis to ameliorate distressing symptoms of cancer or AIDS are of concern to many advocates of harm reduction, who favor the same kind of rigorous evaluation of costs and benefits for this approach as in other medical attempts to prolong life or alleviate suffering (Kassirer, 1997).

Harm reduction often is misconstrued as dismissing any role for law enforcement. On the contrary, harm reduction usually involves a far closer partnership between law enforcement and health professionals than generally occurs in conventional approaches to drug treatment. In many countries, police have been persuaded of the importance of not interfering with the functioning of needle exchange and methadone programs, in order to ensure that significant community benefits are not jeopardized. Also, health workers have come to appreciate the considerable difficulties of enforcing drug laws and the importance of collaborative work in certain areas, such as reducing alcohol-related violence. In many countries where harm reduction has been well accepted for some years, police have begun to reverse their earlier opposition to methadone programs and have supported expansion of drug treatment. They also have been influenced by impressive evidence of crime reduction following enrollment of addicts in methadone treatment (Maddux & Desmond, 1979), as well as increasing concern that excessive reliance on use reduction often leads to serious corruption among police officers.

A concern often expressed about harm reduction strategies is their potential for communicating a message that condones drug use. Such concerns have been expressed, for instance, about mass media programs that encourage drinking groups to nominate a nondrinking "designated driver," since this message might seem to condone drunkenness in other group members. Similarly, concerns have been expressed about educational campaigns that provide information about methods for solvent inhalation that reduce the risk of fatalities and other harm. Many of these concerns could be alleviated by more carefully targeting the educational message to those already involved in hazardous drug use. In considering such strategies, it should be kept in mind that the public health sector always has been in favor of reducing the immediate drug-related harm, even if this involves some risk of a more distant hazard or can be seen as condoning drug use.

For some, harm reduction always will be simply the thin edge of the ugly wedge of drug legalization. For others in more hostile environments, or where the paramount immediate objective is preventing or controlling an epidemic of HIV infection among injecting drug users, achieving even minimal harm reduction is a major accomplishment, while talk of substantial drug policy reform is a luxurious distraction. A third group are convinced that the major benefits achieved in many communities from harm reduction justifies taking reform further, including rigorously evaluating some form of controlled availability of currently illicit drugs.

It is difficult to deny that harm reduction has in some countries appeared to open up drug policy as an issue, but this is not, in itself, reason enough to permanently suppress all consideration of harm reduction policies and programs.

Examples of Harm Reduction Approaches. Needle exchange and methadone maintenance programs are the most commonly cited exemplars of harm reduction. The rationale for needle exchange is to increase the supply of sterile injecting equipment while decreasing the availability of contaminated injecting equipment in order to reduce the spread of HIV among injecting drug users. At the time of their introduction in many countries in the late 1980s, there was a fear that the benefits of reducing HIV spread might be at the cost of inadvertently increasing drug consumption. No evidence has emerged over the past decade to support this fear (Lurie, Reingold et al., 1993). In many parts of the world, increased demand for treatment followed the introduction of needle exchange programs (Lurie, Reingold et al., 1993).

Methadone maintenance programs provide an oral, legal, and long half-life drug as a replacement for an intravenous, illegal, and short half-life drug. Enrollment in methadone programs is associated with multiple benefits (Ward, Mattick et al., 1992), including decreased mortality, morbidity, HIV infection (Caplehorn & Ross, 1995), and crime. Social functioning also improves (Ward, Mattick et al., 1992). Supporters of harm reduction welcome these benefits, while accepting that all patients continue to consume a mood-altering substance (methadone) and a small proportion continue to inject (considerably reduced quantities of) heroin. Better, they argue, to have a patient taking methadone who is well, employed, not committing crime, HIV-negative, and who occasionally injects heroin, than someone who intermittently engages in drug-free treatment but has become HIV-positive, commits crime, is unemployed, injects heroin frequently, but does not take methadone.

Official Responses to Harm Reduction. Reduction of drug-related harm is a logical target of national and international drug policy. In fact, harm reduction has been explicitly accepted as national drug policy in a number of developed countries, including Australia, Canada, and France. Although the United Nations International Drug Control Programs (UNDCP) is responsible for coordinating international illicit drug law enforcement and global supply control initiatives, even this organization has offered muted endorsement of harm reduction (Executive Director, 1994): "in recent years the increased attention on drug abuse has led to an intense debate on how best to reduce the damage inflicted on the individual and society. Insofar as UNDCP is involved in this debate its position can be only the following: there is no fixed formula, no panacea to remedy the global ill of drug abuse. Entrenched confrontation at the national and international levels must be tempered with pragmatism. While ridding the world of drug abuse remains a central objective, it is a long-term goal. Therefore, the most useful short-term outlook should aim to contain the immediate threat to society."

A document drawn up by an Expert Committee of the World Health Organization (WHO) used the term "harm reduction" in the sense of preventing adverse consequences of drug use without setting out primarily to reduce drug consumption (WHO, 1993). This interpretation of harm reduction has existed comfortably and apparently without controversy in an organization that carefully positions itself in the middle ground of the family of nations. Examples of harm reduction referred to in the document included needle exchange to control the spread of HIV among injecting drug users, nicotine patches for tobacco users, and attempts to reduce physical injuries associated with alcohol intoxication by making environments in which people drink less dangerous. The committee commented that "in the harm minimization approach, attention is directed to the careful scrutiny of all prevention and treatment strategies in terms of their intended and unintended effects on levels of drug-related harm" (WHO, 1993).

A series of international conferences on the reduction of drug-related harm have been held annually following an initial conference in Liverpool, England, in 1990. In 1996, an International Harm Reduction Association and an Asian Harm Reduction Network were established. Other regional harm reduction networks have been established in Central and Eastern Europe, South America, Africa, and Oceania. The first National Harm Reduction Conference in the United States was held in Oakland, CA, in 1996, organized by the National Harm Reduction Coalition.

Almost all developed countries that have a significant problem with injecting drug use have established needle exchange programs. As federal funding is still prohibited for these programs in the U.S., the scale of implementation of needle exchange is limited to areas that choose to mount local initiatives, through which 55 needle exchange programs provide almost eight million syringes (Wodak & Lurie, 1997). Programs in some other developed countries, such as Sweden, also are quite restricted. In 1994, needle programs exchanged over 10 million syringes from over 4,000 outlets in Australia. A few developing countries have established needle exchange programs, and such programs have established in Russia.

Methadone programs now operate in all countries belonging to the European Union and are growing very rapidly in Austria, Belgium, France, Germany, and Spain. Methadone programs exist in a number of Asian countries, including Nepal, Thailand, and Hong Kong. A number of developing countries are likely to establish methadone programs in the next few years.

The growing international acceptance of methadone was confirmed in a recent survey carried out by the Health Department of Canada (Ruel, 1996). Long-term methadone maintenance was accepted in 16 countries by 1995, including Australia, Canada, Denmark, Finland, France, Germany, Hong Kong, Hungary, Israel, Italy, Mexico, The Netherlands, New Zealand, Spain, Switzerland, and the U.S. Three countries (Belgium, England, and Sweden) regarded methadone with eventual withdrawal as the only acceptable form of treatment. Controls and regulations differ considerably. Switzerland had the highest number of patients/million (2,000) followed by Hong Kong (1,818), Belgium (1,000), Australia (964), Netherlands (732), Denmark (542), New Zealand (495), Spain (459) and the U.S. (441).

Methadone programs for inmates now operate in correctional systems in five countries, pilot needle exchange for inmates is being evaluated in prisons in Switzerland and Germany, and bleach to decontaminate needles and syringes is provided to prisoners in 13 countries (Dolan, Wodak et al., 1995).

Public Support for Harm Reduction. Strong community support for needle exchange has been demonstrated in two community opinion surveys in Australia, where 90% of respondents supported needle exchange in a survey in New South Wales (Schwartzkopf, Spooner et al., 1990), while the proportion of Western Australian respondents supporting needle exchange increased from 76% to 87% after participants heard a brief tape explaining the rationale for the program (Lenton, 1994). Although anticipated public opposition to needle exchange programs often is used by opponents to justify maintenance of the ban on such programs in the U.S., a national public opinion poll found that 66% of respondents supported such programs (Henry J. Kaiser Family Foundation, 1996).

While these opinion surveys are encouraging, authorities in several countries have encountered local opposition to the establishment of needle exchange and methadone treatment programs. Opposition is not unique to these services, as local communities often oppose other drug treatment services and even fire stations or other public utilities that are well accepted if located elsewhere.

HARM REDUCTION AND ADDICTION TREATMENT

Harm reduction has had a significant effect on drug treatment, changing the focus from the rapid achievement of a drug-free state to acceptance of incremental improvements that represent the best that particular individuals can manage at certain times. Clinicians working in a harm reduction framework usually are very conscious of the considerable difficulties experienced by many drug-dependent persons, particularly those who also are disadvantaged by poverty, poor housing, racial discrimination, unemployment, limited educational opportunities, and squalid neighborhoods with high crime rates. The objectives of harm reduction treatment are negotiated by the clinician and the patient, with the latter free to set specific goals and targets.

Harm reduction also encourages clinicians to take a broader view of alcohol and drug problems and their amelioration. Treatment and prevention are regarded as indivisible parts of the same whole. For example, harm reduction approaches broaden treatment from an exclusive preoccupation with intensive therapies for persons with alcohol dependence to the much earlier brief interventions with persons engaged in problem drinking. This shift in emphasis is justified by the epidemiological observation that it is the very large number of persons with moderately heavy aggregate consumption who account for the majority of alcohol-related problems in society (Kreitman, 1986).

Harm reduction also has influenced smoking cessation programs. Many smokers who reduce their consumption frequently resume previous levels of tobacco use (or compensate by subconsciously adjusting their inhalation to maintain blood nicotine and tar levels). As a result, the efficacy of using harm reduction approaches with cigarette smokers has been questioned. The use of nicotine substitution (as chewing gum, skin patches, and nasal sprays) has many parallels with methadone maintenance programs for heroin users (Russell, 1993). In both cases, a less damaging variant of the addictive substance is provided for a period of time, during which the powerful reinforcing cues that support continuation of drug-seeking behavior are allowed to dissipate gradually. It is accepted in both cases that some persons may continue their use of less damaging addictive substance for a lengthy period and that a small number may continue indefinitely.

Outcomes of Harm Reduction Approaches. *Methadone Treatment*: There is compelling evidence for the effectiveness of methadone treatment against a range of important outcomes drawn from a large literature, including some randomized controlled studies and a large number of observational studies (Ward, Mattick et al., 1992). For example, methadone treatment has been demonstrated to reduce deaths from drug overdose, total mortality, morbidity, HIV risk behavior, HIV seroprevalence, HIV seroincidence, unemployment rates, and crime. The plausibility and consistency of these findings is extremely impressive. Improved outcomes are seen with higher doses of methadone, strengthening the confidence in these findings. Methadone programs also are far more successful than other treatment modalities in attracting and retaining large numbers of drug users. In general, retention in drug treatment is closely linked to satisfactory outcomes.

Needle Exchange: Six studies of needle exchange funded by the U.S. government concluded that these programs reduce HIV transmission and do not lead to increased drug use (National Commission on Acquired Immune Deficiency Syndrome, 1991; United States General Accounting Office, 1993b; Lurie, Reingold et al., 1993; Satcher, 1995; National Research Council and Institute of Medicine, 1995; Office of Technology Assessment, 1995).

As more data has become available over time, confidence in the findings of these major studies has increased (Wodak & Lurie, 1997). Comparisons of needle exchange participants with nonparticipants generally have shown a reduction in high-risk behaviors among the former. A reduction of at least one-third in the incidence of HIV among injecting drug users who participated in needle exchange programs was estimated using a mathematical model. A single study (Hagan, Des Jarlais et al., 1995), as yet unreplicated, demonstrated that non-participants in exchange programs had a seven- to eight-fold increase in risk of infection with hepatitis B or hepatitis C, as compared to injecting drug users who attended a needle exchange program.

A recent ecological study of needle exchange programs and HIV seroprevalence among injecting drug users involved 29 cities in many countries where serial data on HIV seroprevalence was available (Hurley, Jolley et al., 1996). Mean initial seroprevalence was approximately 3% in cities that introduced needle exchange programs and those that did not. At the conclusion of the study, mean seroprevalence rates were considerably lower in locations with a needle exchange program (6%) than in those without (21%).

The mean annual increase in seroprevalence, weighted according to the number of subjects sampled, was 3.6% in cities without and 0.2% in cities with needle exchange programs. Although a standard methodology for measurement of HIV seroprevalence between and within cities was not used, it is difficult to envisage any systematic design flaw capable of producing these results.

Using conservative assumptions drawn from published studies, it has been estimated that between 4,000 and 10,000 HIV infections could have been prevented in the U.S. if needle exchange programs had been implemented at the same rate they have been in Australia. These infections ultimately will cost up to half a billion U.S. dollars in HIV/AIDS treatment costs (Lurie & Drucker, 1996).

ALTERNATIVES TO HARM REDUCTION
Societal responses to illicit drug use once were sharply divided into law enforcement, education, and treatment approaches. A more contemporary division has been into categories labeled "supply reduction," "demand reduction," and "harm reduction."

Demand Reduction. "Demand reduction" typically involves a range of educational measures, including mass campaigns, school campaigns, and programs directed at established drug users and high-risk groups. Treatment of drug users is classified as a form of demand reduction.

Some measures clearly intended to reduce demand also reduce supply and *vice versa*. For example, methadone treatment might be regarded as simply reducing demand for drugs in a small number of heroin dependent individuals; however, those seeking entry to methadone maintenance programs usually are severely dependent and probably include many of the heaviest consumers in the community. Removing these individuals from the heroin market has an effect on demand as well. Because many of these users also are likely to traffick in drugs, their entry into treatment may temporarily disrupt the heroin supply system to some degree.

Supply Reduction. "Supply reduction," also sometimes referred to as "use reduction," forms the core of traditional international drug policy. The paramount aim of use reduction is to decrease consumption of mood-altering substances. Any reduction in harm is regarded as a bonus.

In terms of strategies, supply reduction usually involves attempts to reduce crop production, drug production, drug transport from countries of origin to countries of destination (interdiction), drug entry to the country of destination (customs), drug distribution (police) and financial surveillance.

Supply reduction is based on the implicit premise that adverse consequences of drug use are closely correlated with consumption. This relationship is valid in the case of legal drugs like alcohol and tobacco. Both drugs have significant intrinsic toxicity and adverse health consequences, which correlate closely with individual or societal levels of consumption. Consumption of alcohol and tobacco correlates closely with changes in price or availability. Decreases in price or increases in availability of alcohol and tobacco almost invariably result in increased consumption and worse health outcomes. The converse also is true. Above a certain threshold, alcohol toxicity increases: linearly for some conditions, exponentially for others, and in a J curve relationship for yet other conditions (Edwards, Anderson et al., 1994). Tobacco toxicity generally is linear, but there seems to be no threshold below which smokers can consume with impunity.

Among developed countries, one of the strongest supporters of supply reduction is the United States. The Anti-Drug Abuse Act passed by Congress in 1988 stated in §5252-B that "it is the declared policy of the United States to create a Drug-Free America by 1995."

Contrasts Between Harm Reduction and Alternative Approaches. One of the most fundamental differences between the harm reduction and supply reduction approaches is the judgment implicit in harm reduction that it is more effective to establish and reach achievable but suboptimal goals than to nominate but fail to reach unachievable and utopian goals. The public health tradition accepts that incremental improvements often are all that can be achieved in areas of great complexity and difficulty. Aggregate results from the combination of multiple interventions often are very rewarding, even if each intervention produces relatively minor benefits.

An elderly and somewhat decrepit Groucho Marx responded to the question, "What do you think of old age?" by noting that it was better than the alternative. This remark encapsulates the spirit of harm reduction. Harm reduction programs do not pretend to be a panacea, but they do have a strong case to be regarded as more effective than alternative approaches that rely almost exclusively on supply reduction.

Outcomes of Alternative Approaches. A review of the global illicit drug situation by a body charged with responsibility for international supply reduction concluded that "countries that are not suffering from the harmful consequences of drug abuse are the exception rather than the rule" (International Narcotics Control Board, 1993). This deterioration in the global illicit drug situation occurred despite progressive strengthening of illicit drug law enforcement over several decades.

Illicit drug use was a problem in only a few developed countries a generation ago. During the 1960s, illicit drug use spread to a number of developed countries. During the 1980s, illicit drug use began to spread to most developing countries. By the early 1990s, it was estimated that there were over 5 million drug injectors (Mann, Tarantola et al., 1992) spread over more than 120 countries (Stimson & Choopanya, in press). These changes reflected a steady growth in global cultivation and production of illicit drugs. Technological changes in transport, communications, and computers made movement of contraband substances and profits around the globe much easier for drug traffickers, while control of illicit drug trafficking became much more difficult for law enforcement authorities.

This inexorable deterioration of the global illicit drug situation was accompanied by increasingly serious consequences of illicit drug use. Soon after the AIDS epidemic first was identified in the early 1980s, it was recognized that HIV had spread alarmingly in populations of injecting drug users in several developed countries, including the United States. HIV has irrevocably changed the nature of injecting drug use and has had an equally dramatic influence on the way injecting drug users are perceived. Hepatitis C is recognized to be globally more prevalent among injecting drug users than HIV, even in those countries where HIV prevalence has reached alarming levels (Garfein, Vlahov et al., 1996). Although there is some uncertainty about the natural history of hepatitis C, it is apparent that this infection results in considerable mortality and morbidity, albeit in a smaller proportion and after a longer interval than HIV infection. Multidrug resistant tuberculosis has appeared as a significant health problem in some countries and is thought to be closely associated with uncontrolled HIV epidemics in injecting drug users.

Outcomes of Demand Reduction Approaches: There is a large literature evaluating the effectiveness of efforts to reduce demand for illicit substances through the use of educational programs. However, there is little evidence of significant and sustained reduction in demand from mass, school-based, or specially targeted educational campaigns (Cohen, 1993). Some educational programs have demonstrated improvements in knowledge, others in attitudes, some in both. But evidence of reduced consumption or more significantly, a reduction in drug-related problems, is scant.

Demand for illicit substances appears to be greater in populations with high levels of youth unemployment, poor housing, limited educational opportunities, poor health services, and neglected, crime-ridden neighborhoods. It is difficult to assess the role of these factors in stimulating demand for drugs. However, lack of data for the influence of these factors on demand should not be taken as evidence that they are unimportant.

Outcomes of Supply Reduction Approaches: A substantial literature, including empirical (Riley, 1996; Commission on Narcotic Drugs, 1995) and theoretical (Riley, 1996; Wisotsky, 1986; Thornton, 1991; Center for Strategic and International Studies, 1993) studies, document the relative ineffectiveness of supply reduction and predict continuing failure. An impressive study, commissioned by the U.S. Army and carried out by the RAND Corporation, evaluated the return on a one dollar investment in a variety of measures designed to reduce the societal cost of cocaine. The return was 17 cents for crop reduction and eradication in South America, 32 cents for interdicting transport of cocaine between South America and the U.S., 52 cents for U.S. customs and police, and $7.48 for treatment of cocaine users (Rydell & Everingham, 1994).

The ineffectiveness of supply reduction and the likelihood of continuing failure prompted a review body to despair that "over the past two decades in Australia, we have devoted increased resources to drug law enforcement, we have increased the penalties of drug trafficking, and we have accepted increasing inroads on our civil liberties as part of the battle to curb the drug trade. All the evidence shows, however, not only that our law enforcement agencies have not succeeded in preventing the supply of illicit drugs to Australian markets, but that it is unrealistic to expect them to do so. If the present policy of prohibition is not working, then it is time to give serious consideration to the alternatives, however radical they may seem" (Parliamentary Joint Committee on the National Crime Authority, 1989).

Consideration of alternatives (Nadelmann, 1992) is now beginning in a number of countries and has even been undertaken by the research arm of the U.S. Congress (U.S. General Accounting Office, 1993a).

The experience of most countries has been that global drug production for decades increased almost every year, apart from occasional reductions in production caused by bad weather in growing areas. Illicit drug use is spreading to more and more countries around the world. The range of drugs used has increased. Many countries have experienced an exponential growth in drug-related crime and other adverse outcomes. The response to this national and global deterioration of the illicit drug situation has been an ever-increasing emphasis on attempts to restrict the supply of illicit drugs. International collaboration has increased. More funds have been allocated to attempts to reduce drug cultivation and production. Penalties for drug trafficking or drug use have been increased. Drug squads have been expanded. The number of prison inmates serving sentences for drug-related offenses has increased. Financial surveillance has been intensified.

A comparison of the effectiveness of harm reduction and supply reduction suggests that attempted harm elimination rarely has been successful, while attempted harm reduction rarely has failed. To many, harm reduction has been a way of curbing the excesses of a drug policy that has unrealistically emphasized supply reduction.

The alarming possibility exists that supply reduction may have inadvertently exacerbated health problems. Emphasis on supply reduction and public health goals may be inimical. Anti-opium policies adopted in Hong Kong (1945), Thailand (1959), and Laos (1972) were followed by the disappearance of opium smoking, which was replaced by heroin injecting (Westermeyer, 1976), setting the scene for a later epidemic of HIV infection among injecting drug users in Thailand in 1988, which then seeded uncontrolled epidemics involving the general populations of Thailand, Burma, Malaysia, Vietnam, China, and India.

CONCLUSIONS

It is likely that harm reduction will be increasingly accepted as a legitimate component of a modern response to mood-altering drugs, along with efforts to decrease demand and restrict supplies. A more effective response to the problems of illicit drugs requires a better balance of these elements rather than an almost exclusive reliance on supply reduction. If, as expected, harm reduction is accepted increasingly around the world, including the U.S. (in spirit if not name), treatment for drug users will change considerably, with more satisfactory outcomes for drug users, clinicians, and communities.

REFERENCES

Caplehorn JRM & Ross MW (1995). Methadone maintenance and the like-lihood of risky needle sharing. *International Journal of Addiction* 30(6):685–698.

Center for Strategic and International Studies (1993). *The Transnational Drug Challenge and the New World Order: New Threats and Opportunities.* Washington, DC: The Center.

Cohen J (1993). Achieving a reduction in drug-related harm through education. In N Heather, A Wodak, E Nadelmann et al. (eds.) *Psychoactive Drugs and Harm-reduction: From Faith to Science.* London, England: Whurr Publishers, 65–76.

Commission on Narcotic Drugs (1995). *Economic and Social Consequences of Drug Abuse and Illicit Trafficking: An Interim Report.* Vienna, Austria: United Nations Economic and Social Council.

D'Aunno T & Vaughn TE (1992). Variations in methadone treatment practices: Results from a national study. *Journal of the American Medical Association* 267:253–258.

Department of Health (1985). *National Campaign Against Drug Abuse.* Canberra, Australia: Australian Government Publishing Service, 2.

Des Jarlais DC, Hagan H, Friedman SR et al. (1995). Maintaining low HIV seroprevalence in populations of injecting drug users. *Journal of the American Medical Association* 274:1226–1231.

Dolan K, Wodak A & Penny R (1995). AIDS behind bars: Preventing HIV spread among incarcerated drug injectors (Editorial). *AIDS* 9:825–832.

Edwards G, Anderson P, Babor TF et al. (1994). *Alcohol Policy and the Public Good.* Oxford, England: Oxford University Press, 41–74.

Executive Director, United Nations International Drug Control Program (1994). 37th Session of the Commission on Narcotic Drugs. Vienna, 13th April.

Garfein RS, Vlahov D, Galai N et al. (1996). Viral infections in short-term injection drug users: The prevalence of the hepatitis C, B, human immunodeficiency and human T-lymphotropic viruses. *American Journal of Public Health* 86:655–661.

Glantz LH & Mariner WK (1996). Annotation: Needle exchange programs and the law-time for a change (Editorial). *American Journal of Public Health* 86:1077–1078.

Hagan H, Des Jarlais DC, Friedman SR et al. (1995). Reduced risk of hepatitis B and hepatitis C among injection drug users in the Tacoma syringe exchange program. *American Journal of Public Health* 85:1531–1537.

Hartnoll R, Mitcheson M, Battersby A et al. (1980). Evaluation of heroin maintenance in controlled trial. *Archives of General Psychiatry* 37:877–884.

Henry J. Kaiser Family Foundation (1996). *The Kaiser Survey on Americans and AIDS/HIV.* Menlo Park, CA: The Foundation.

Holmberg SD (1996). The estimated prevalence and incidence of HIV in 96 large US metropolitan areas. *American Journal of Public Health* 86:642–654.

Hurley S, Jolley D & Kaldor J (1996). In S Hurley & JRG Butler (eds.) *An Economic Evaluation of Aspects of the Australian HIV/AIDS Strategies.* Canberra, Australia: Australian Government Publishing Service, 56–60.

Institute of Medicine (1990). *Broadening the Base of Treatment For Alcohol Problems.* Washington DC: National Academy Press.

International Narcotics Control Board (INCB) (1993). *Report of the International Narcotics Control Board for 1993.* Vienna, Austria: INCB.

Kahn JG (1993). Are NEPs cost-effective in preventing HIV infection? In P Lurie, AL Reingold, B Bowser et al. (eds.) *The Public Health Impact of Needle Exchange Programs in the United States and Abroad (Volume I).* San Francisco, CA: University of California.

Kaldor J, Elford J, Wodak A et al. (1993). HIV prevalence among IDUs in Australia: A methodological review. *Drug and Alcohol Review* 12:175–184.

Kassirer JP (1997). Federal foolishness and marijuana (editorial). *The New England Journal of Medicine* 336:366–367.

Kreitman N (1986). Alcohol consumption and the prevention paradox. *British Journal of Addiction* 81:353–363.

Lenton S (1994). *Illicit Drug Use, Harm Reduction and the Community: Attitudes to Cannabis Law and Needle and Syringe Provision in Western Australia* (Technical Report). Perth, Australia: National Centre for Research into the Prevention of Drug Abuse.

Lurie P & Drucker E (1996). *An Opportunity Lost: Estimating the Number of HIV Associated with the U.S. Government Opposition to Needle Exchange Programs.* Presented at XI International Conference on AIDS; Vancouver, British Columbia; July 7–12.

Lurie P, Reingold AL, Bowser B et al. (1993). *The Public Health Impact of Needle Exchange Programs in the United States and Abroad* (Vol. I). San Francisco, CA: University of California.

MacDonald M, Wodak A, Ali R et al. (1997). HIV prevalence and risk behaviour in needle exchange attenders: A national study. The Collaboration of Australian Needle Exchanges. *Medical Journal of Australia* 166(5):237–240.

Maddux JF & Desmond DP (1979). Crime and drug abuse: An area analysis. *Criminology* 19:281–302.

Mann JM, Tarantola DJM & Netter TW (1992). *AIDS in the World. The Global AIDS Policy Coalition.* Cambridge, MA: Harvard University Press, 406–411.

Nadelmann E (1989). Drug prohibition in the United States: Costs, consequences and alternatives. *Science* 245(4921):939–947.

Nadelmann E (1992). Thinking seriously about alternatives to drug prohibition. *Daedalus* 121:85–132.

National Commission on Acquired Immune Deficiency Syndrome (1991). *The Twin Epidemics of Substance Use and HIV.* Washington, DC: The Commission.

National Research Council and Institute of Medicine (1995). *Preventing HIV Transmission. The Role of Sterile Needles and Bleach.* Washington, DC: National Academy Press.

Office of Technology Assessment (OTA) (1995). *The Effectiveness of AIDS Prevention Efforts.* Washington, DC: The Office.

Parliamentary Joint Committee on the National Crime Service (1989). Canberra, Australia: Publications Office.

Riley KJ (1996). *Snow Job?: The War Against International Cocaine Trafficking.* New Brunswick, NJ: Transaction Publishers.

Ruel J-M (1996). *International Survey of the Use of Methadone in the Treatment of Narcotic Addiction.* Ottawa, Canada: Health Canada.

Russell MAH (1993) Reduction of smoking-related harm: The scope for nicotine replacement. In N Heather, A Wodak, E Nadelmann et al. (eds.) *Psychoactive Drugs and Harm-reduction: From Faith to Science.* London, England: Whurr Publishers, 153–167.

Rydell CP & Everingham SS (1994). *Controlling Cocaine. Supply Versus Demand Programs.* Santa Monica, CA: RAND Drug Policy Research Center.

Satcher D (1995). *Note to Jo Ivey Boufford.* Available from the Drug Policy Foundation, 4455 Connecticut Avenue, NW, Suite B500, Washington, DC, 20008.

Schwartzkopf J, Spooner S, Flaherty B et al. (1990). *Community Attitudes to Needle & Syringe Exchange and to Methadone Programs* (A 90/6). Sydney, Australia: New South Wales Department of Health.

Stimson GV (1996). Has the United Kingdom averted an epidemic of HIV-1 infection amongst drug injectors? (Editorial). *Addiction* 91(8):1085–1088.

Stimson GV & Choopanya K (in press). Global perspectives on drug injecting. In GV Stimson, DC des Jarlais & A Ball (eds.) *Drug Injecting and HIV Infection: Global Dimensions and Local Responses.*

Strang J (1993). Drug use and harm reduction: Responding to the challenge. In N Heather, A Wodak, E Nadelmann et al. (eds.) *Psychoactive Drugs and Harm-reduction: From Faith to Science.* London, England: Whurr Publishers, 3–20.

Strang J & Gossop M (1996). Heroin Prescribing in the British System: Historical Review. *European Addiction Research* 2:185–193.

Thornton M (1991). *The Economics of Prohibition.* Salt Lake City, UT: University of Utah Press.

Uchtenhagen A, Dobler-Mikola A & Gutzwiller F (1996). Medical prescription of narcotics. Background and intermediate results of a Swiss national project. *European Addiction Research* 2:201–207.

Uchtenhagen A, Gutzwiller F, Dobler-Mikola A et al. (1996). *Program for A Medical Prescription of Narcotics. Interim Report of the Research Representatives.* Zurich, Switzerland: University of Zurich, Institute for Social and Preventive Medicine.

U.S. General Accounting Office (1993a). *Confronting the Drug Problem: Debate Persists on Enforcement And Alternative Approaches* (Report No. GAO/GGD-93-82). Washington, DC: U.S. Government Printing Office.

U.S. General Accounting Office (1993b). *Needle Exchange Programs: Research Suggests Promise as an AIDS Prevention Strategy* (Report No. GAO/HRD-93-60). Washington, DC: U.S. Government Printing Office.

Ward J, Mattick R & Hall W (1992). *Key Issues in Methadone Maintenance Treatment.* Kensington, Australia: New South Wales University Press.

Westermeyer J (1976). The pro-heroin effects of anti-opium laws in Asia. *Archives of General Psychiatry* 33:1135–1139.

White House (The) (1989). *Drug Control Strategy.* Washington, DC: Government Printing Office, 11.

Wiley J & Samuel M (1989). Prevalence of HIV infection in the USA. *AIDS* 3(Suppl 1):71–78.

Wisotsky S (1986). *Breaking the Impasse in the War on Drugs.* Westport, CT: Greenwood Press.

Wodak A (1992). HIV infection and injecting drug use in Australia: Responding to a crisis. *Journal of Drug Issues* 22(3):549–562.

Wodak A & Lurie P (1997). A tale of two countries: Attempts to control HIV among injecting drug users in Australia and the United States. *Journal of Drug Issues* 27(1):117–134.

Wodak A & Saunders W (1995). Harm reduction means what I choose it to mean (editorial). *Drug and Alcohol Review* 14:269–271.

World Health Organization (WHO), Expert Committee on Drug Dependence (1993). *WHO Technical Report Series (28th Report).* Geneva, Switzerland: World Health Organization.

Chapter 11

Special Issues in Treatment: Drug Courts

H. Blair Carlson, M.D., FACP, FASAM
The Hon. Peggy Fulton Hora
The Hon. William G. Schma

Definitions
A New Approach to an Old Problem
Why Drug Treatment Courts Work
The Courts and Physicians Working Together

The number of drug offenders sentenced to state prisons each year has increased nearly 12-fold, from 9,000 in 1980 to 107,000 in 1998. Most of this growth is a direct result of the "War on Drugs" and the resulting escalation in penalties for drug possession, trafficking, and use. Communities first attempted to "build out" of the problem, spending hundreds of millions of dollars on new prisons, only to find that they could not afford to operate or maintain them (U.S. Department of Justice, 1993). In the year 2000, the United States reached an unhappy benchmark: two million of its citizens were behind bars. With 5% of the world's population, the U.S. has 25% of the world's prisoners (*Newsweek*, 2000).

Over the past 10 years, it has become abundantly clear that incarceration alone is totally ineffective in addressing alcohol and drug abuse and addiction, let alone recidivism to criminal behavior. Society also has come to realize that prison is a scarce resource best employed to isolate violent offenders from the community. These realizations, coupled with an increased knowledge of the neurobiology of addiction and its treatment, have led to an understanding by the community and the criminal justice system that collabora-tive projects such as drug treatment courts are the most intelligent way to address this problem.

A drug treatment court (DTC) is a collaborative pro-gram of judicially supervised treatment and recovery within the criminal justice system. This specialized system of courts was created to address spiraling numbers of drug-related offenses and offenders, which have swelled court dockets over the past decade. DTCs represent a major retooling of the criminal justice system, as well as a new court role in society as an interdisciplinary, problem-solving community institution with therapeutic implications—in short, a part-ner in public health (Hora, Schma et al., 1999).

From fewer than a dozen in 1991, the number of DTCs has increased to almost 700 today, in communities as di-verse as New York City and Las Cruces, NM. DTCs are found in all but one state, Vermont, where there is a court in the planning stage. There are DTCs in Puerto Rico, one federal DTC, tribal DTCs (which are called Healing to Wellness Courts), and international DTCs.

This chapter will examine the therapeutic underpinnings of drug treatment courts and explain how they differ from traditional criminal courts. Treatment opportunities in the

TABLE 1.   Recommended Assessment Procedures

Keep assessments brief. DTCs frequently use the Addiction Severity Index (ASI), which can be completed very quickly.

Identify clients' expectations. DTCs fully outline the program in participants' handbooks. Treatment providers also explain the DTC to the participant.

Provide clear orientation. The referral to a DTC is made at the time of the defendant's first appearance, the arraignment. He or she is referred to the court coordinator before the next court appearance. After viewing the DTC session, the judge reviews the written behavioral contract with each participant. If the defendant wants to proceed, a full orientation with the court coordinator/case manager is scheduled. Each defendant, on request, also is referred to legal counsel to discuss the legal options.

Offer clients options. DTC participation always is voluntary. The participant may opt out at any time and proceed with regular criminal case adjudication.

Keep it simple. The client handbook has clear, understandable information for each participant. Written reminders are given out at every court session. There are written attendance records of meetings and other appointments. Everyone tries to use clear and simple language. Participants who cannot read are helped by other participants who can.

Involve significant others. Family participation is encouraged. Couples counseling and family days are options at the treatment programs. Children and partners always are welcome in court and are identified by name by the judge. "Toxic families" that are detrimental to the participants' recovery are prohibited. Restraining orders may be ordered to protect the participant from a spouse, partner, parent, or sibling.

criminal justice system will be explored, as will the key components of effective DTCs. The chapter will focus on the role of these courts within the treatment community and describe opportunities for collaboration between the court system and the health care community, particularly addiction specialists.

DEFINITIONS

A DTC is a judicially supervised, treatment-driven program for non-violent substance-abusing criminal offenders. It is a collaborative effort that involves judges, prosecutors, defense attorneys, probation officers, treatment providers, and other persons or agencies that interact with addicts whose behavior has brought them into the criminal justice system. Participation by the offender is voluntary.

In this universe, the court serves as a convener and coordinator of related services in a continuum of care for substance-abusing individuals.

DTCs are as varied in form and format as the diverse legal and treatment cultures from which they spring. Some

courts divert offenders from the criminal justice system entirely; some accept only misdemeanants, others only felons. There are DTCs solely for alcoholics, or only cocaine or heroin users, while others accept anyone whose criminal involvement is related to substance use. There are gender-specific courts and courts that enroll only juveniles. Re-entry DTCs recently have emerged to serve adjudicated substance-abusing offenders who are returning to society on parole or probation.

DTCs rely on the principle that the coercive powers of the court system can contribute to recovery from addiction to alcohol and other drugs. Contradicting the popular notion that drug-dependent offenders are best dealt with by adjudication and sanctions, DTCs embrace the scientific premise that alcohol and other drug dependence is a chronic, relapsing medical condition (McLellan, Lewis et al., 2000). The authoritative and supervisory power of the judge is critical to this approach to treatment. However, the participation of a judge in the rehabilitation process represents a dramatic shift in legal thought and judicial behavior.

A NEW APPROACH TO AN OLD PROBLEM

Through the collaborative efforts of defense attorneys and prosecutors, treatment providers, the court coordinator or case manager, community policing agencies, and probation officials, a criminal defendant in a DTC is given an opportunity to engage in an alternative to the criminal "business as usual" and, in its place, to pursue a program of addiction treatment and recovery.

DTCs employ a series of "carrots and sticks" to induce treatment compliance and lifestyle changes in a criminal defendant. The ultimate payoff for the participant is dismissal of the charges, having a sentence set aside, or imposition of a lesser penalty. By choosing to participate in a DTC, a criminal defendant avoids serving a substantial period of incarceration and gains sobriety and a crime-free lifestyle. "A [DTC] establishes an environment that the participant can understand: a system in which clear choices are presented and individuals are encouraged to take control of their own recovery" (U.S. Department of Justice, 1997).

The operations of drug courts are defined by 10 key components:

1. Drug courts integrate alcohol and other drug treatment services with justice system case processing.

2. Using a nonadversarial approach, prosecution and defense counsel promote public safety while protecting participants' due process rights.

3. Eligible participants are identified early and promptly placed in the drug court program.

4. DTCs provide access to a continuum of alcohol, drug, and related treatment and rehabilitation services.

5. Abstinence is monitored through frequent alcohol and other drug testing.

6. A coordinated strategy governs DTC responses to participants' compliance.

7. Ongoing judicial interaction with each DTC participant is essential.

8. Monitoring and evaluation measure the achievement of program goals and gauge its effectiveness.

9. Continuing interdisciplinary education promotes effective DTC planning, implementation, and operations.

10. Forging partnerships among DTCs, public agencies, and community-based organizations generates local support and enhances the DTC's effectiveness.

When these components are employed, the courtroom is transformed into an arena in which a judge is the central figure of a team that is focused on the participants' recovery. The prosecutor screens each candidate for eligibility and makes sure each candidate is appropriate for participation in the DTC. The defense counsel verifies that clients know of the voluntary nature of DTC participation, are aware of all their legal options, and make a knowing and intelligent waiver of their rights, including their confidentiality rights. Opposing counsel thus focuses on the participant's progress, rather than on the merits of the pending case. A close, interpersonal, and therapeutic relationship develops between the judge and the participant, who is encouraged to develop the tools he or she needs to maintain sobriety and recovery. Participants often enter into written contracts, agreeing to certain behaviors (data show that such contracts are more likely to induce compliance, whether it is taking medication or engaging in addiction treatment) (Winick, 1991). A typical contract includes attending treatment, court dates, self-help meetings, and other appointments on time; complying with all rules; waiving confidentiality; paying fees and fines; taking presumptive urine tests without waterloading, adulteration, or counterfeiting; agreeing to refrain from drinking alcohol or taking other drugs or associating with people who do; abstaining from use of poppy seeds, over-the-counter or prescription medications without prior approval, or other things that could yield a false result on a urine test; and making a 12- to 18-month commitment to treatment.

Although the judge remains the final arbiter of all issues, he or she receives input from the entire team, including the participant. If a problem arises, such as a use episode, it is not unusual for a participant to arrive in court having already discussed the problem with the treatment provider and a probation officer and/or court coordinator, who will present a recommendation to the judge (which might involve jail time, increased meetings, and/or increased urine tests). When participants themselves propose the sanctions, they are more likely to comply with them and not to feel coerced by the "system" or the judge. A person who proposes his or her own "punishment" is more likely to think it fair.

Confidentiality waivers are mandatory, as are waivers of judicial ethical issues such as the prohibition on *ex parte*

TABLE 2. Recommended Strategies for Initiating Treatment

Initiate treatment goals. Treatment goals for DTCs are sobriety, program retention, and maintenance of a crime-free lifestyle. Goals are explained in the participants' handbook and the written behavioral contract, as well as by the judge, case coordinator, attorneys, and treatment providers.

Establish treatment attendance. Participants must bring written proof of attendance to each court date. Unverifiable meetings are not allowed except in unusual circumstances. For instance, a participant may be going out of town for a business trip and be allowed to attend Twelve Step meetings in the area he or she will be visiting. If away for an extended stay, urine testing may be arranged, often with the help of another DTC.

Schedule frequent contacts. Frequent court appearances are a hallmark of DTCs. Daily contact with the case coordinator or treatment provider may be required in volatile relapse situations. At a minimum, weekly contacts are maintained throughout the life of the program in some DTCs.

Use positive incentives to reinforce treatment participation. In the Hayward, CA, DTC, the local Deputy Sheriffs' Association provides the DTC with tickets for Oakland A's games to use as rewards for good performance. There may be a drawing for theater or county fair tickets, a Halloween pumpkin, or a tote bag, or tee shirt from the latest conference attended by the judge. To be eligible for the drawing, a participant must have a negative urine test and have attended all meetings. Drawings are held on a random basis, and participants who have missed a meeting are quite upset when they are not eligible to participate. One treatment provider awards food vouchers and bus tickets to participants who meet their goals.

Call no shows. The court coordinator calls all participants who have failed to appear in court. If there is no response, the bailiff immediately asks the community policing liaison to serve a bench warrant. Through this approach, participants are taught that it is better to appear and test positive than to fail to appear. Program retention and participation lead to negative urine tests; the opposite is not true.

Create a positive environment. Because court appearances are so personalized by the judge, participants develop a positive attitude toward coming to court. Most treatment providers have court meetings so that participants can develop friendships. Participants help each other find jobs and transportation and even cook Thanksgiving dinner together before marathon holiday meetings. Everyone feels good because of the positive atmosphere in the courtroom.

Discontinue use of psychoactive substances. While there was some initial resistance to uniform "no alcohol" clauses for DTC participants, such requirements now are standard (U.S. Department of Justice, 2000). DTC contracts also include a prohibition on the use of prescription drugs prescribed for others and, of course, prohibit the use of illicit substances.

Establish a daily schedule. Treatment meetings, self-help groups, employment, job training or job seeking, education, volunteer work, and court appointments keep a DTC participant on a tight schedule. Some participants have had to change work shifts and find new employment because working late-night shifts triggered a craving for stimulants to stay awake. Daytime employment and an early bedtime seem to help reduce stimulant craving.

Initiate a urinalysis schedule. Most DTCs require frequent, random, observed urine tests. Night and weekend testing, long-distance testing, and daily testing as a sanction all are employed.

Assess psychiatric comorbidity. Posttraumatic stress disorder (PTSD) and clinical depression are the most commonly observed psychiatric problems among DTC participants. Many DTCs have mutual help groups for co-occurring disorders such a bipolar and schizophrenia. A mental health assessment is ordered for those who are not being program-compliant, rather than assuming that the participant is "treatment resistant." The incidence of comorbidity for this population is very high.

Assess associated compulsive sexual behaviors. Treatment providers who work with stimulant abusers in DTCs have special sex addiction groups. DTCs also offer confidential and anonymous HIV testing and education, as well as testing and education for hepatitis B and C and other sexually transmitted diseases (STDs). Many participants have worked as prostitutes, which raises not only STD issues but also PTSD issues that must be addressed in treatment.

Provide crisis resolution. The court, the case manager, and treatment providers all need to be aware of the need for suicide and homicide assessment, psychiatric referrals, and necessary medical referrals. Participants may need extra support in times of personal crisis and stepped-up relapse prevention services at these times. The court may order an emergency psychiatric assessment or additional services.

communications, simply because the treatment providers, mental health professionals, and physicians must be able to communicate with the court coordinator/case manager and the team. Written waivers that comply with federal statutes are mandatory. Judges must be able to talk to team members individually without inhibition. Participants must understand their rights to confidentiality and the judges' prohibition on *ex parte* communication and be willing to provide a written waiver as a condition of entering DTC. This team concept of drug treatment courts uniquely facilitates an individual's treatment progress. It is not unusual for a participant to ask that the arresting officer be present at his or her graduation. Police officers, including the bailiff in the courtroom, become supporters and benefactors rather than enemies. Similarly, supporting actors such as community-based treatment providers, community policing officers, housing authority personnel, mental health professionals, and physicians have a unique new relationship with the courts and a voice not previously heard.

Most DTCs have three phases: an initiation of abstinence phase, in which the participant comes to court weekly; a treatment phase, in which the participant meets with the judge twice a month; and a relapse prevention phase, with monthly court dates. Frequent contact with and monitoring by the judge is essential to the success of the DTC participant. The court monitors the participant's treatment program, attendance, and drug test results. As the ultimate authority figure in this system, the judge also is important in motivating and encouraging participants. The judge praises, cajoles, kids, threatens, harangues, and does whatever it takes to keep the participant in treatment and recovery. As Dr. John Chappel, Professor of Medicine at the University of Nevada, Reno, sees it, "The role of the judge is to coerce treatment until sobriety becomes tolerable." Treatment may be delivered in a variety of settings: a community-based program, a day treatment model, outpatient, inpatient, residential, or in-custody. Using graduated sanctions, the court usually begins with the least restrictive model, as indicated by an assessment tool such as the Addiction Severity Index (ASI). The participant is moved to more restrictive placements as needed. Placing a participant in a more restrictive environment is not phrased in terms of punishment; rather, participants are encouraged to see the change as necessary to their recovery. At intake, a social needs assessment is completed, along with an alcohol and drug use assessment. Mental health, housing, physical health, employment, education, and other legal entangle-

ments are addressed. Periods of abstinence, confirmed by weekly, random urine tests, are required for each phase—typically at 30, 90, and 180 days.

There is aftercare planning, and participants petition the court to "graduate," typically at the end of 12 to 18 months and with at least 180 days of sobriety. To receive such approval, the participant must demonstrate a knowledge of addiction and have a plan for relapse prevention. The participant also is invited to become involved in a DTC alumni group. In order to graduate, the participant must have a clean and sober living environment, as well as full-time employment or full-time student status; all fees and fines must be paid or substantial amounts of volunteer work completed. Graduating participants also must have a drivers' license, insurance and proof of registration of all vehicles, and be able to show that there are no outstanding tickets or warrants. They must have a high school diploma or GED and either take literacy classes, if they are English-speaking, or enroll in a class for students learning English as a Second Language (ESL). The whole person is transformed by the DTC; abstinence alone is not enough.

When a participant submits a positive urine test, misses meetings or appointments, fails to participate, or otherwise breaks program rules, sanctions are imposed immediately. Such sanctions may include payment for the urine test, increased meeting attendance (30 meetings in 30 days, for example), demotion to an earlier phase, requirement to perform volunteer work or short stints of jail time (usually one day to no more than one week at a time) or, the ultimate sanction, removal from the program and (in a pre-plea model) reentry into the criminal system or (post-adjudication) sentencing, including incarceration. Consistent non-compliance may trigger a mental health assessment, as many DTC participants have undiagnosed comorbid mental health problems such as clinical depression, posttraumatic stress disorder, bipolar disorder, or schizophrenia. Program dismissal is reserved for the most serious offenses, such as attempts to falsify or adulterate a urine sample, leaving without permission, or being arrested for a violent offense.

The focus of the DTC team is not on punishment, but on treatment compliance and program retention. Rewards may include an earn-down of program fees, a reduction in the number of court appearances, and awarding of certificates (with much cheering and applause from the audience) to mark the completion of each phase.

In a DTC, it is not unusual to hear a public defender recommend jail time, while a prosecutor argues that only increased meetings are required. The adversarial system is put on hold in DTC; defense counsel and the prosecution are equal team members whose interest is in treatment and recovery, not convictions or acquittals. At any point in the process, the participant may opt out of the DTC and into the traditional criminal justice case processing system, with all the attendant rights and remedies.

WHY DRUG TREATMENT COURTS WORK

There is support for DTCs on many fronts and from all factions of the political spectrum. First, it is clear that coerced treatment works. "Research indicates that a person coerced to enter treatment by the criminal justice system is likely to do as well as one who volunteers" (Hubbard, Marsden et al., 1989; Maugh & Anglin, 1994; Anglin & Hser, 1990). In fact, there is debate about the "voluntariness" of any addiction treatment, since most addicts come to treatment because of legal problems, concerns in their personal lives, problems with job performance, or for health reasons (Hora & Schma, 1998). Second, addiction treatment is as successful as treatment for other chronic diseases and saves $7 for every treatment dollar spent (California Department of Alcohol and Drugs, 1992). It costs more than $22,000 per year to incarcerate a prisoner, while effective out-patient treatment with random drug screens may be had for about $2,500. Roughly 60% of untreated drug offenders are re-arrested within the first year, whereas 80% to 98% of DTC graduates are arrest-free after one year (OJP, 2000). Moreover, because of the requirement for interdisciplinary training, DTC judges and other team members are aware of the likelihood of relapse and know how to respond appropriately. DTCs are in a unique position to recognize these temporary setbacks as learning experiences for the participant and the treatment team.

Courts have come to accept their changing role from neutral, uninvolved arbiter to becoming problem-solvers who look at cases holistically. There also is support for the proposition that judicial job satisfaction is increased if judges work therapeutically (Chase & Hora, 2000). The Bureau of Justice Assistance, an arm of the U.S. Department of Justice, recently promulgated trial court performance standards. Standard 4.5 says, "The trial court anticipates new conditions and emergent events and adjusts its operations as necessary" (BJA, 1997). Clearly, DTCs address "new conditions and emergent events."

In 2001, the U.S. Conference of Chief Justices and the Conference of State Court Administrators adopted a joint resolution endorsing DTCs and problem-solving courts based on the drug court model, the first resolution of its kind. The resolution commits all 50 Chief Justices and State Court Administrators "to take steps nationally and locally to expand the principles and methods of well functioning drug courts into ongoing court operations." It also pledges to "encourage the broad integration, over the next decade, of the principles and methods employed in problem solving courts into the administration of justice."

Law enforcement support for DTCs is strong because officers see that recovery presents a long-term solution to a community's and an individual's problems with alcohol or other drugs. Formal liaisons between community police and DTCs are encouraged through the Community Policing Mentor Court Network of the National Association of Drug Court Professionals.

THE COURTS AND PHYSICIANS WORKING TOGETHER

"Given what is known about the many social, medical, and legal consequences of drug abuse, effective drug abuse treatment should, at a minimum, be integrated with criminal justice, social, and medical services" (Executive Office of the President, The White House, 2000). DTCs and the criminal justice system can be powerful allies for addiction medicine specialists. Through DTCs, physicians and judges have initiated a whole new dialogue about alcohol and other drug problems. The group Physicians' Leadership on National Drug Policy, based at Brown University's Center for Alcohol & Addiction Studies, has partnered with the American Judges Association to develop a curriculum for the joint training of judges and physicians. The resulting program was piloted in Fort Worth, TX, in 1999, and replicated in Philadelphia. In each session, 16 local physicians and psychologists met with almost 50 criminal and family law judges for a day of joint training.

The partnership has extended to other venues, as well: judges have participated in Congressional and U.S. Mayoral briefings. For the first time, judges presented a panel at the 2000 annual meeting of the American Society of Addiction Medicine (ASAM). Addiction medicine specialists teach courses on alcohol and other drug problems at the National Judicial College and in many of the states, as well. The time is ripe for local coalitions of judges and other players in the criminal justice system to team up with addiction medicine specialists to educate one another in how to be more effective in working with their mutual clients/patients.

Judges in the criminal justice system may have more to say about a patient's treatment that the physician does. Questions relating to involvement with the justice system should be added to patient histories as a case-finding tool for alcohol and other drug problems.

Physicians should acquaint themselves with their local drug treatment courts and, if there isn't one currently in operation, lead a community coalition to ask that one be established. Most courts have long-range strategic, operational, and action plans developed with community input; DTCs should be part of those plans. Local grand juries, with the help of addiction medicine specialists, should study DTCs and make recommendations for appropriate use of those courts in their own communities. At the very least, state chapters of ASAM should provide assistance to judges who have questions about alcohol and other drug issues. Judges have the power to appoint such physicians as expert advisors to the court. We are at a unique place in history in our ability to foster these new and exciting collaborations. Let this chapter, co-authored by two judges, be the first step.

REFERENCES

Anglin MD & Hser Y (1990). Legal coercion and drug abuse treatment: Research findings and social policy implications. In JA Inciardi (ed.) *Handbook of Drug Control in the United States.*

Barthwell AG (1995). Interventions/Wilmer: A continuum of care for substance abusers in the criminal justice system. *Journal of Psychoactive Drugs* 27-39.

Bureau of Justice Assistance (BJA) (1997). *Trial Court Performance Standards With Commentary.* Washington, DC: U.S. Department of Justice, Bureau of Justice Assistance.

California Department of Alcohol and Drugs (1992). CALDATA. Sacramento, CA: The Department.

Carlson B (1995). Prison-Based Treatment. *Alcoholism and Drug Abuse Weekly.*

Center for Substance Abuse Treatment (1995a). *Treatment Improvement Protocol Series, No. 17.* Rockville, MD: Substance Abuse and Mental Health Services Administration, U.S. Department of Health and Human Services.

Center for Substance Abuse Treatment (1995b). *Treatment Improvement Protocol Series, No. 21.* Rockville, MD: Substance Abuse and Mental Health Services Administration, U.S. Department of Health and Human Services.

Center for Substance Abuse Treatment (1999). *Treatment Improvement Protocol Series, No. 23.* Rockville, MD: Substance Abuse and Mental Health Services Administration, U.S. Department of Health and Human Services.

Chase DJ & Hora PF (2000). The implications of therapeutic jurisprudence for judicial satisfaction. *Court Review* 37:12.

Drug Courts Program Office (1997). *Defining Drug Courts: The Key Components.* Washington, DC: Office of Justice Programs, U.S. Department of Justice.

Drug Courts Program Office (2000). *The Interrelationship Between the Use of Alcohol and Other Drugs: Summary Overview for Drug Court Practitioners.* Washington, DC: Office of Justice Programs, U.S. Department of Justice and the Drug Court Clearinghouse and Technical Assistance Project, American University (NCJ178940).

Drug Strategies Institute (1996). *Keeping Score 1996: What Are We Getting for Our Federal Drug Control Dollars?* Washington, DC: The Institute, 9-10.

Hora PF, Schma WG & Rosenthal JTA (1999). Therapeutic jurisprudence and the drug treatment court movement: Revolutionizing the criminal justice system's response to drug abuse and crime in America. *Notre Dame Law Review* 74:439.

Hora PF & Schma WG (1998). Legal intervention. In White & Wright (eds.) *Addiction Intervention: Strategies To Motivate Treatment-Seeking Behavior.* New York, NY: Hayworth Press.

Hubbard R, Marsden M, Rachal J et al. (1989). *Drug Abuse Treatment: A National Study of Effectiveness.* Chapel Hill, NC: University of North Carolina Press.

Inciardi JA (1996). *A Corrections-Based Continuum of Effective Drug Abuse Treatment.* Washington, DC: U.S. Department of Justice, National Institute of Justice.

Lipton DS (1996). Prison-based therapeutic communities: Their success with drug-abusing offenders. *National Institute of Justice Journal.*

Maugh TH II & Anglin MD (1994). Court-ordered drug treatment does work. *The Judges' Journal.*

McLellan AT, Lewis DC, O'Brien CP et al. (2000). Drug dependence, a chronic medical illness: Implications for treatment, insurance, and outcomes. *Journal of the American Medical Association.*

Office of Justice Programs (1993). *National Directory of Corrections Construction, 1993 Supplement.* Washington, DC: National Institute of Justice and Bureau of Justice Assistance, U.S. Department of Justice.

OJP Drug Court Clearinghouse and Technical Assistance Project (2000). *Drug Court Update.* Washington, DC: American University.

Warren RK (1998). Re-engineering the Court Process. Presentation at the Great Lakes Court Summit, Madison, WI.

Winick B (1991). Harnessing the power of the bet: Wagering with the government as a mechanism for social and individual change. *University of Miami Law Review* 45:737-814.

Therapeutic Jurisprudence

Bruce J. Winick
David B. Wexler

Therapeutic jurisprudence is the study of the law's healing potential (Wexler & Winick, 1996, 1991; Winick, 1997b). An interdisciplinary approach to legal scholarship that has a reform agenda, therapeutic jurisprudence seeks to assess the therapeutic and counter-therapeutic consequences of the law and how it is applied, as well as to increase the former and diminish the latter. It is an approach to the law that uses the tools of the behavioral sciences to assess the law's therapeutic effects and, when consistent with other important legal values, to reshape law and legal processes in ways that can improve the psychological functioning and emotional wellbeing of the individuals affected.

PHILOSOPHIC ROOTS OF THERAPEUTIC JURISPRUDENCE

Daicoff (2000) has noted that therapeutic jurisprudence is one of the major vectors of a growing movement in the law "towards a common goal of a more comprehensive, humane, and psychologically optimal way of handling legal matters." In addition to therapeutic jurisprudence, these vectors include (among others) preventive law, restorative justice, facilitative mediation, holistic law, collaborative divorce, and specialized treatment courts. Such specialized courts—"problem-solving courts," as they are becoming known—include drug treatment courts (Hora, Schma et al., 1999), domestic violence courts (Fritzler & Simon, 2000; Winick, 2000), and mental health courts (Rottman & Casey, 1999; Casey & Rottman, 2000).

Specialized treatment courts such as drug treatment courts are related to therapeutic jurisprudence (Hora, Schma et al., 1999) but are not synonymous with that concept. Instead, specialized treatment courts often employ the principles of therapeutic jurisprudence to enhance their functioning (Conference of Chief Justices & Conference of State Court Administrators, 2000). Such principles include ongoing judicial intervention, close monitoring of and immediate response to behavior, integration of treatment services with judicial case processing, multidisciplinary involvement, and collaboration with community-based and government organizations.

THERAPEUTIC JURISPRUDENCE AND DRUG COURTS

Therapeutic jurisprudence was developed in the late 1980s as an interdisciplinary approach to legal scholarship and law reform. Although drug treatment courts developed independently of therapeutic jurisprudence, they can be seen as taking a complementary approach to the processing of drug cases, inasmuch as their goal is the rehabilitation of the offender. Drug courts use the legal process, and particularly the role of the judge, to accomplish this goal.

Therapeutic jurisprudence already has produced a large body of interdisciplinary scholarship that analyzes principles of psychology and the behavioral sciences and attempts to understand how those principles can be used in the legal system to improve mental health outcomes (Wexler & Winick, 1996). Recent scholarship has focused on how judges in specialized problem-solving courts can employ the principles of therapeutic jurisprudence in their work (Casey & Rottman, 2000; Fritzler & Simon, 2000; Winick, 2000). Indeed, a recent symposium issue of *Court Review*, a publication of the American Judges Association, was devoted entirely to therapeutic jurisprudence and its application by the courts (Court Review, 2000).

An important insight of therapeutic jurisprudence is that the way in which judges and other legal officers fulfill their roles has inevitable consequences for the mental health and psychological wellbeing of the persons with whom they interact. Because drug treatment court judges consciously view themselves as therapeutic agents in dealing with offenders, they can be seen as playing a therapeutic jurisprudence role. In fact, an understanding of the approach of therapeutic jurisprudence and of the psychological and social work principles it employs can improve the functioning of drug treatment court judges.

Judge-defendant interactions are central to the functioning of drug treatment courts. Judges therefore need to understand how to convey empathy, how to recognize and deal with denial, and how to apply principles of behavioral psychology and motivation theory. They need to understand the psychology of procedural justice, which teaches that persons appearing in court experience greater satisfaction and comply more willingly with court orders when they are given a sense of voice and validation and treated with dignity and respect (Winick, 1999).

Judges need to know how to structure court practices in ways that maximize their therapeutic potential; for example, even such mundane matters as the ordering of cases in the courtroom can maximize the chance that defendants awaiting their turn before the judge can experience vicarious learning. Offenders who accept diversion to drug treatment court are, in effect, entering into a type of behavioral contract with the court, and judges therefore should understand the psychology of such behavioral contracting and how it can be used to increase motivation, compliance, and effective performance (Wexler, 1991; Winick, 1991).

Drug treatment court judges also need to understand how to deal with feelings of coercion on the part of offenders (Winick, 1997a). A degree of legal coercion is undeniably present when a drug offender is arrested and must decide whether to face the consequences of trial and potential punishment in the criminal court or instead accept diversion and a course of treatment supervised by the drug treatment court. However, a body of literature on the psychology of choice suggests that if the defendant experiences this choice as coerced, his or her attitude, motivation, and chances for success in the treatment program may be undermined. On the other hand, experiencing the choice as voluntarily made and non-coerced is more conducive to success. Judges therefore should not attempt to pressure offenders to accept diversion to drug treatment court, but should remind them that the choice is entirely theirs. A body of psychological work on what makes individuals feel coerced suggests that judges should strive to treat offenders with dignity and respect, to inspire their trust and confidence that the judge has their best interests at heart, to provide them a full opportunity to participate, and to listen attentively to what they have to say. Judges who treat drug court offenders in this fashion increase the likelihood that the offender will experience treatment as a voluntary choice, will internalize the goals of treatment, and will act in ways that help to achieve those goals.

Although therapeutic jurisprudence can help drug court judges to more effectively fulfill their roles in the drug treatment process, it is important to recognize that therapeutic jurisprudence does not necessarily support all actions that may be regarded as pro-treatment. Nor does therapeutic jurisprudence take a position as to whether increased or decreased criminalization or penalties for possession of drugs are warranted. Indeed, unless there are independent justifications for criminalization, therapeutic jurisprudence would not support continued criminalization solely to provide a stick-and-carrot approach to inducing criminal defendants to accept treatment in a drug court diversion program.

CONCLUSIONS

In summary, then, therapeutic jurisprudence can contribute much to the functioning of drug treatment courts, and such courts can provide rich laboratories from which to generate and refine approaches to therapeutic jurisprudence. But the two perspectives are merely vectors moving in a common direction; they are not identical concepts.

Therapeutic jurisprudence and drug treatment courts share a common cause as they strive to understand how legal rules and court practices can be designed to facilitate the rehabilitative process. Each has much to offer the other.

REFERENCES

Casey P & Rottman DB (2000). Therapeutic jurisprudence in the courts. *Behavioral Sciences & the Law* 18:445-457.

Conference of Chief Justices & Conference of State Court Administrators (2000). CCJ Resolution 22 & COSCA Resolution 4. *In Support of Problem-Solving Courts.*

Court Review (2000). Special Issue on Therapeutic Jurisprudence. *Court Review* 37:1-68.

Daicoff S (2000). The role of therapeutic jurisprudence within the comprehensive law movement. In DP Stolle, DB Wexler & BJ Winick (eds.) *Practicing Therapeutic Jurisprudence: Law as a Helping Profession.* Durham, NC: Carolina Academic Press, 465-492.

Fritzler RB & Simon LMJ (2000). The development of a specialized domestic violence court in Vancouver, Washington utilizing innovative judicial paradigms. *University of Missouri-Kansas City Law Review* 69:139-177.

Hora PF, Schma WG & Rosenthal JTA (1999). Therapeutic jurisprudence and the drug treatment court movement: Revolutionizing the criminal justice system's response to drug abuse and crime in America. *Notre Dame Law Review* 74:439-537.

Rottman DB & Casey P (1999). Therapeutic jurisprudence and the emergence of problem-solving courts. *National Institute of Justice Journal* (Summer) 12-19.

Wexler DB (1991). Inducing therapeutic compliance through the criminal law. In DB Wexler & BJ Winick (eds.) *Essays in Therapeutic Jurisprudence.* Durham, NC: Carolina Academic Press, 187-198.

Wexler DB & Winick BJ (1991). *Essays in Therapeutic Jurisprudence.* Durham, NC: Carolina Academic Press.

Wexler DB & Winick BJ (1996). *Law in a Therapeutic Key: Developments in Therapeutic Jurisprudence.* Durham, NC: Carolina Academic Press.

Winick BJ (2000). Applying the law therapeutically in domestic violence cases. *University of Missouri-Kansas City Law Review* 69:33-91.

Winick BJ (1997a). Coercion and mental health treatment. *Denver University Law Review* 74:1145-1168.

Winick BJ (1991). Harnessing the power of the bet: Wagering with the government as a mechanism of social and individual change. In DB Wexler & BJ Winick (eds.), *Essays in Therapeutic Jurisprudence.* Durham, NC: Carolina Academic Press, 219-290.

Winick BJ (1997b). The jurisprudence of therapeutic jurisprudence. *Psychology, Public Policy, and Law* 3:184-206.

Chapter 12

Special Issues in Treatment: Incarcerated Populations

Peter J. Delany, D.S.W.
Joseph J. Shields, Ph.D.
Bennett W. Fletcher, Ph.D.

Characteristics of the Inmate Population
Health and Social Needs of Inmates
Models of Treatment for the Offender
Assessment and Placement

Over the past three decades it has been public policy to treat drug use and addiction primarily as a public safety issue requiring a criminal justice intervention. Martinson's (1974) influential article "What Works? Questions and Answers about Prison Reform" and his conclusion that "nothing works" provided the basis for a shift from the rehabilitation of addicts in prison toward one of "just desserts" and incapacitation (Hollin, 1999; Taxman, 2000). This shift led to the initiation of tough mandatory sentencing guidelines for drug possession and trafficking by federal and state legislatures, the elimination of parole options, and changes in law enforcement practices leading to an increased focus on street crime and efforts to target street-level users and sellers. These changes, combined with high rates of criminal and drug use recidivism among released inmates, have led to an alarming increase in the number of persons incarcerated in jails and prisons (Falkin, Wexler et al., 1992; Leukefeld & Tims, 1993; U.S. Department of Justice, 1995; Belenko & Peugh, 1999; Belenko, 2000; Peters & Steinberg, 2000).

As the prison population has increased, the percentage of inmates receiving needed treatment has declined. In 1998, more than 1.8 million persons were incarcerated: 1,178,978

in state prisons, 123,041 in federal prisons, and another 592,462 in local jails (Beck & Mumola, 1999)—at a total cost of more than $30 billion. This population is more than three times the number incarcerated in 1980 (Belenko & Peugh, 1999; Belenko, 2000). Much of the increase in the prison population is directly attributable to an increased number of persons arrested for drug possession, drug dealing, and other drug-related offenses remanded into custodial care. Of those incarcerated in 1998, approximately 65% had serious involvement with drugs (regular use at least once a week for more than a month). This percentage represents 1.2 million individuals, with the number growing to almost 1.4 million when persons with alcohol-related problems are included (Beck & Mumola, 1999; Belenko & Peugh, 1999; Mumola, 1999). By comparing these estimates with the number of inmates who actually received treatment in the period 1990 through 1999, Belenko and Peugh (1999) calculated that, in the early 1990s, approximately 16% of inmates who needed treatment actually received treatment. By 1999, this percentage had declined to only 13% who were receiving some form of addiction treatment (anything from drug education programs, group counseling, or self-help groups to intensive therapeutic community-type treatment programs). Of the remaining 87% of inmates who are identified as in need of treatment, there is a question as to whether they were in a position to participate in treatment. For instance, because treatment effects diminish over time (which is particularly likely in the case of an inmate who is returned to the general prison population), there is a question as to when treatment is most effective in the incarceration period. Some of the more traditional models would enroll the inmate into the treatment program 9 to 18 months before release (Knight, Simpson et al., 1999; Martin, Butzin et al., 1999; Wexler, Melnick et al., 1999). However, inmates facing long prison sentences may not benefit from traditional treatment models. Research is needed to develop effective treatment that can be offered to the long-term prisoner. Without intervention, it is likely that most of prisoners will return to drug use and/or crime within a year after being released (Belenko & Peugh 1999; Martin, Butzin et al., 1999).

A more pressing and broadly relevant issue revolves around how the correctional system and the health system can work together to develop and implement a continuum of care that breaks the cycle of drug use and crime for the thousands of inmates being released back into the community.

The effect of illicit drug use on public safety has been established by a number of researchers, who have documented previous drug-related offenses of criminal justice populations. These include offenses such as simple possession of drugs, possession with intent to distribute, or distribution and manufacturing; predatory crimes such as assault, theft, burglary, and robbery; prostitution; and crimes of deceit such as fraud and confidence games (Hunt, 1990; Speckart & Anglin, 1986). Statistical and anecdotal evidence also documents a relationship between drug use and various forms of domestic violence, such as spouse abuse, child abuse and maltreatment, and sexual abuse (ONDCP, 2000). These behaviors have noteworthy implications for the wellbeing of individuals as well as the communities to which they return.

Drug abuse in itself is a threat to the public health and thus is subject to public health intervention. Poverty and poor health often are part of the drug-using lifestyle. The combination of crime, drug use, and poverty create particular vulnerabilities to infectious diseases such as HIV/AIDS, tuberculosis, and hepatitis, as well as physical and sexual trauma. Many addicts suffer from dysfunctional and splintered family relationships, inadequate schooling, and

unstable, impoverished, and violent environments. Most do not have the social or work skills needed to obtain or maintain gainful employment, which limits their ability to access necessary social and health services in the community (Anno, 1991; Belenko & Peugh, 1999; McDonald, 1995; Wexler, Lipton et al., 1988).

In the early 1970s, when Martinson (1974) concluded that "nothing works," the addiction treatment field was in its relative infancy, and few treatment strategies or models were capable of demonstrating consistent effectiveness. Over the past 20 years, however, we have seen the development of structured behavioral and multimodal treatment approaches, which have been shown in careful studies to reduce drug use and recidivism and improve post-incarceration outcomes, especially when paired with post-incarceration treatment and support services (Andrews, Zinger et al., 1990; Falkin, Wexler et al., 1992; Hiller, Knight et al., 1999, 1996; Inciardi, Martin et al., 1997; Gendreau, 1996; Lipton, 1995; Pelissier & McCarthy, 1993; Peters & Steinberg, 2000; Sherman, Gottfredson et al, 1997). This research has moved the field away from the notion that "nothing works" toward a focus on "what works." The research provides a framework on which to construct new therapeutic and rehabilitative interventions and programs for offenders. The challenge is to successfully translate the research findings into effective practice (Hollin, 1999).

Every year thousands of inmates who have had little or no treatment will be released back into the community. These men and women will return to their communities and face a high probability of returning to a drug-using lifestyle and, eventually, reincarceration. The question is how to reconcile public safety and public health concerns while providing an integrated model of care that understands addiction as a chronic health condition that requires both behavioral and health interventions within a system that is primarily focused on criminal justice. In short: How do we incorporate the latest science-based findings on treatment effectiveness while respecting the safety mission of the criminal justice system?

The purpose of this chapter is to raise issues that must be addressed in developing prison-based treatment alternatives. First, the chapter reviews the demographic characteristics of the prison population, as well as the common health, behavioral, and social problems that they encounter. Second, it describes the types of strategies that currently exist in correctional settings. Finally, it discusses a treatment process model that has demonstrated empirical validity and its application in prison settings and continuing-care programs.

CHARACTERISTICS OF
THE INMATE POPULATION

The inmate population in American prisons and jails is not a homogenous group, nor does it mirror the overall U.S. population. It is critically important that custodial and treatment providers working in correctional settings be aware of these differences when developing and implementing effective addiction services.

The overall demographic profile of the inmate population is of a group that is primarily male, young, a member of a racial or ethnic minority group, and possessed of few educational and vocational resources. Although current numbers are small, the percentage of female and older inmates is expected to increase in the near future.

In fact, most inmates in federal and state prisons and local jails are younger than age 40 (approximately 70%), with an average age of 31.9 for state prisoners, 37.0 for federal prisoners, and 29.2 for jail inmates. Belenko and Peugh (1999) noted that, although the number of inmates older than age 50 is quite small compared with the overall inmate population (approximately 5% and 2% of regular drug users in federal and state prisons, respectively), the number is rising at a rapid pace. This is primarily the result of longer sentences mandated by "truth in sentencing" requirements as well as "three strike" legislation. As might be expected, older inmates often have more and more serious medical needs than younger inmates, which has implications for the development of specialized medical services and the recruitment and hiring of specially trained staff members. Studies suggest that the average cost of caring for an inmate older than 50 years is almost three times the cost of care for an average 30-year-old inmate (Belenko & Paugh, 1999).

Overall, the percentage of regular drug users older than age 40 represents a small but significant subpopulation of inmates (13% of state prisoners, 29% of federal prisoners, and 11% of jail inmates). These inmates are likely to have been hard-core drug users for long periods of time and are susceptible to the many physical and mental health problems that are associated with such long-term use. They also are likely to have been through various treatment programs, and to be multiple and repeat offenders. If this trend toward an aging and ailing prison population continues, as it is expected to do, it will have serious implications for the development and delivery of all services, including addiction and medical care within prisons and jails.

Although only 8% of the incarcerated population are women, the number of women inmates has increased dramatically in recent years, primarily because of the larger number of women being arrested for drug-related behaviors such as theft, driving under the influence, prostitution, passing bad checks, and other forms of fraud (Immarigen & Chesney-Lind, 1992). Henderson (1998) found that most of these women also have drug-related problems. Findings from a number of studies indicate that women differ significantly from men in the types of crimes they commit. For example, women are less likely to commit violent crimes and are more likely to be under the influence of drugs or alcohol at the time of their arrest (Belenko & Peugh, 1999).

Research also indicates that female drug-abusing inmates have higher rates of physical health problems (for example, HIV/AIDS and other sexually transmitted diseases), mental health problems (such as depression and anxiety), and histories of physical and sexual abuse than their male counterparts. They also tend to be from lower socioeconomic backgrounds; to have limited educational backgrounds, few vocational skills, and poor work histories; and to have responsibility for the care of at least one minor child (Henderson, 1998). These findings have led many treatment providers to call for the establishment of special programs for women that focus more clearly on issues related to family reunification and enhancing support structures that change the status of the children of these women.

Although, in general, the racial and ethnic characteristics of the drug-using inmate population mirror the general inmate population, they do not reflect the racial and ethnic characteristics of the adult population at large. Although whites make up 76% of the general population, they compose only 39% of the inmate population. In contrast, African Americans make up 11% of the general population but approximately 41% of the inmate population. Hispanics represent 9% of the general population and approximately 18% of the inmate population (Belenko & Peugh, 1999). These data raise some important questions for corrections, treatment, and medical practitioners in terms of cultural competence and treatment planning.

Other demographic characteristics of the inmate population indicate that they are less likely to be married, more likely to have low educational attainment and poor employment histories, and more likely to be below the poverty level than the general population (Belenko & Peugh, 1999).

HEALTH AND SOCIAL NEEDS OF INMATES

The demographic characteristics of the inmate population form the context for understanding their health and social needs. The documented relationship between crime, poverty, and poor physical and mental health, coupled with the high-risk lifestyles of drug users, render the inmate population in need of comprehensive services (Anno, 1991; Belenko & Peugh, 1999). Many drug-abusing inmates enter prison with dental problems, nutritional deficiencies, liver problems, general infections, and injuries as the result of street violence (shootings, stabbings, and so forth), all of which are in need of medical attention. Of particular concern is the increasing incidence of HIV among inmates. Injection drug use (IDU) is the second most common means of exposure to HIV in the U.S., accounting for approximately a third of all cases among adults (Belenko & Peugh, 1999). Among inmates, IDU is the most common source of HIV infection (Hammett & Widom, 1996). It is estimated that 25% of the inmates in state prisons, or between 250,000 and 300,000 persons, are IDUs and that approximately half have a history of needle sharing (Belenko & Peugh, 1999). Noninjecting drug users also are at risk of HIV through associated behaviors, such as prostitution and exchanging sex for drugs, particularly given the prevalence of multiple sex partners (Hammett, 2000).

In addition to high rates of HIV infection, the incidence of confirmed AIDS cases among inmates has increased dramatically in recent years (from 179 cases in 1985 to 5,009 in 1995, or more than six times the rate among the U.S. population at large. Currently, AIDS is the second leading cause of death among prison inmates, increasing by 94% between 1991 and 1995 (Belenko & Peugh, 1999). As the incidence of HIV continues to grow, prisons and jails will face enormous challenges and costs in providing services to this population.

Given the relationship between drug use and the medical conditions discussed earlier, it is important that the medical response to these conditions not be isolated and separated from services for the treatment of addictive disorders.

In addition to physical health problems, inmates face a number of issues related to mental health. For example, the co-occurrence of addictive disorder and mental disorders among correctional populations is receiving increased

attention. Ditton (1999) reported that, by the middle of 1998, approximately 7% of federal prisoners, 16% of state prisoners, and 16% of jail inmates (a total of 238,000 persons) had a diagnosable mental illness. The most common of these are schizophrenia, personality disorders, major depression, and anxiety. A study conducted in California state prisons found that the rate of schizophrenia was two to three times greater than in a matched sample from the general population (Belenko & Peugh, 1999). The National Coalition for the Mentally Ill has estimated that there are one-third more mentally ill persons in jails then there are patients in mental hospitals (Dimascio, 1995). Despite the number of inmates in need of mental health services, few are receiving any form of treatment: in 1996, only 3% of state and federal inmates were being treated in mental health programs (Camp & Camp, 1996).

Closely associated with mental health status is the issue of sexual and physical abuse, which often are viewed as a causal factor in the onset of mental illness. Belenko and Peugh (1999) reported that among inmates who are regular drug users, a substantial proportion have histories of such abuse: for example, 45% of women and 13% of men in state prisons; 33% of women and 7% of men in federal prisons; and 31% of women and 6% of men in jail have been physically abused. The data make clear that the issue of abuse is especially important to understanding the situation of women inmates and needs to be considered when developing treatment services for that population.

In addition to the multiple medical and mental health issues that require increased integration of care between the prison setting and the community, the reality of poverty, low education, and poor employment skills create particular risks for the substance-using inmate on release. Belenko and Peugh (1999) reported that almost 40% of drug users lived below the poverty level, as compared with the slightly more than 12% of the general population. Most of these individuals have less than a high school education and poor work histories, with only 64% reporting that they had either full- or part-time work before arrest, whereas approximately 30% acquired income through illegal means.

It is clear that substance-using inmates present a diverse and complex clinical picture for the medical, treatment, and correctional staff. Although there remains some lack of agreement about the importance of treatment programming, this appears to be more an issue of differing priorities than a disagreement as to whether treatment can be effective. However, all can agree that prison provides a unique opportunity to engage this high-risk, hard-to-reach population, often earlier in their addiction career than might have occurred had there been no legal involvement (Anglin & Hser, 1989).

Continued supervision after release can increase participation in community-based drug treatment services and the likelihood that the individual's long-term health and social needs will be addressed and positive outcomes achieved (Anglin & Hser, 1990; Tims, Fletcher et al., 1991; Hubbard, Marsden et al., 1989; Simpson & Sells, 1982). The challenge for the correctional system and the professionals who work in those systems is to find ways to better define roles, areas of expertise, and the integration of service components to address the gaps in service delivery that affect the quality of care offered in the correctional setting. If not, the health and social needs of these individuals will continue to impede their recovery, and the cycle of crime, poverty, and drug use will continue.

MODELS OF TREATMENT FOR THE OFFENDER

As mentioned earlier, prisons and jails vary significantly in the types of treatment services and programs that are available to inmates. Brown (1993) examined the types of services available in correctional settings and who provided those services. He identified the following five models.

Incarceration Without Specialized Services: This model is probably the most common and, depending on institutional resources, can provide educational programming, vocational counseling, casework, discharge planning, and individual and/or group counseling. In this model, services typically are provided by institutional and some contract personnel. Although the model addresses some deficits, it may not specifically address drug and criminal lifestyle issues.

Incarceration With Drug Education and/or Counseling: This model is the second most commonly found program. It often includes drug education and targeted counseling, including HIV and AIDS education, counseling, and testing. Services often are provided by institutional staff members, and group counseling techniques are favored. Brown (1993) noted, however, that although there may be support for treatment, issues of security become dominant, especially in maximum security facilities.

Incarceration in Dedicated Residential Units: There has been significant growth in this model since 1992. Many, if not most, of these programs are modeled on therapeutic communities. Some of the most heavily researched programs include Stay'N Out in New York, Cornerstone in Oregon, Key in Delaware, and the Amity at Donovan Prison in California. These programs focus on the group process and reward growth with increased responsibility. Residents are expected not only to attend educational groups and counseling, but also must help maintain the behavior and environment of the program. Staff typically are drawn from both inside and outside the institution, and include recovering addicts. Although recovering persons who have felony records have been excluded in the past, they increasingly are recognized as valuable assets to prison-based treatment programs.

Incarceration With Client-Initiated and/or Client-Maintained Services: In this model, inmates take responsibility for initiating programs, although interested corrections staff members or outside groups such as prison ministries may assist. Most often, these are Twelve Step recovery programs, such as Narcotics Anonymous (NA) and Alcoholics Anonymous (AA), which seek to help inmates change behavior and maintain a drug-free lifestyle. Brown (1993) also reports that Muslim faith groups operating in prisons target the elimination of drug use, leading to a sober life. Not as much is known about client-driven programs, but they make few demands on staff members and resources, other than the coordination of space.

Incarceration With Specialized Services for Problems Other Than Drug Abuse: This model includes specialized services such as college-level study in a degree program, or other educational and vocational training. Services often are provided by outside organizations, such as local colleges or vocational training institutes.

Treatment Goals and Approaches. As noted, drug abuse treatment in correctional settings has expanded over the past decade, primarily in response to the rapid increase in the number of drug offenders entering the prison system (Leukefeld & Tims, 1993). A growing body of empirical research linking positive outcomes among drug-abusing offenders with treatment, both in prison and in the community, has helped to fuel this expansion (Martin, Butzin et al., 1999; Wexler, Melnick et al., 1999; Knight, Simpson et al., 1999).

More recently, movements by Arizona, California, Massachusetts, Florida, and other states are aimed at redirecting nonviolent offenders who have serious drug problems into the community-based treatment system rather than into prison. How well these efforts will succeed remains an open question, as the criminal justice, drug treatment, mental health, social service, and social welfare systems grapple with issues related to screening and assessment, capacity, linking systems, and information needs. However, programs such as those mandated by California's Proposition 36 do not diminish the need to address the limitations of drug treatment within prisons for those offenders who will continue to be incarcerated and to have serious drug problems (Hollin, 1999; Leukefeld & Tims, 1990).

Taxman (2000) argues that the lack of infrastructure continues to undermine most efforts to treat drug users across the criminal justice system. A structure needs to be in place that allows treatment providers to design, develop, and implement protocols that do not as yet universally exist across the criminal justice system. In addition, many addiction treatment programs are added onto an existing system without adequate attention to how the treatment services will be integrated into the correctional program. The result, Taxman (2000) suggests, is that treatment goals are viewed as secondary to correctional goals, rather than as a core component of efforts toward behavioral change on the part of the drug-using offender. Too often, treatment is perceived as a "luxury" rather than as a necessary part of corrections programming. This perception is, in part, due to a focus by researchers and practitioners on outcomes of individual offenders and the application of those outcomes as indicators of the effectiveness of the system. Work by Simpson (1997) and colleagues (Simpson, Joe et al., 1997b) has focused more attention on the treatment system, taking up the more complex question of what types of interventions work with which offenders and under what conditions. This type of approach is much more challenging for both researchers and practitioners, but it offers an opportunity to highlight gaps in the infrastructure of correctional institutions that offer treatment. It also provides a framework for asking questions that can lead to a better integration of the public safety and public health systems.

Stages of Treatment and Opportunities for Systems Integration. The stage-based treatment model, which draws on the work of Simpson and colleagues (Simpson, 1997; Simpson, Joe et al., 1997b; Joe, Simpson et al., 1999), incorporates multiple components to enhance the engagement of the drug user in the treatment process and to help that individual make the transition to early recovery. Additional work has identified some very specific interventions that can be used to augment these processes (Blankenship, Dansereau et al., 1999; Czuchry & Dansereau, 2000; Dees & Dansereau, 1997; DeLeon, 2000; Joe, Simpson et al., 1999; Simpson, 1997). An underlying theme of this research is the notion that effective treatment does not end at the prison door (Inciardi, Martin et al., 1997; Wexler, Melnick et al., 1999). Quite the opposite, prison-based treatment should be just the beginning of a series of interventions aimed at developing a strong recovery program that includes new prosocial skill sets that reduce the likelihood of relapse, recidivism, and return to custody.

The stage-based model is intended as a framework to help treatment and custodial staff define their roles and consider how services might be integrated to create a system of care that incorporates the principles of effective treatment for the offender (NIDA, 1999). The model outlines the goals of each stage and suggests specific questions that the leadership might ask to better integrate services across their unique system. Additionally, the model points to where duplication of effort occurs and focuses on empirically supported components.

ASSESSMENT AND PLACEMENT

One of the most important steps in the treatment process is the assessment and placement of the offender within the correctional system. Taxman (2000) noted that it is very typical for the addiction treatment system, the medical system, and the custodial system to carry out separate assessments of inmates' needs, with little or no exchange of information across the systems. Not only is this inefficient in terms of resource allocation, but it also interferes with good treatment planning and can lead to inappropriate placement of the offender and a missed opportunity to engage the offender in the treatment process.

To form an integrated assessment and placement process that enhances information-sharing and leads to better planning and allocation of resources, several questions must be addressed:

- What is the best mix of validated instruments to assess the offender's:

  □ motivation and readiness for treatment;

  □ problem severity (including his or her history and current status across the dimensions of criminal justice, addictive disorder, mental health, physical health, family and social relationships, and employment and vocation);

  □ safety risk;

  □ special needs (developmental, neurologic, health, including HIV status and risk); and

  □ length of sentence as it relates to treatment need?

- Who will be responsible for conducting the assessments?

- Where in the process will the information be gathered?

- What protocols will be used to share information with the offender and other systems? What information should not be shared?

- Will one person or multiple people be charged with coordinating information?

- Will the offender, public safety, and public health personnel agree to one integrated treatment plan, or will there be multiple plans that are shared to reduce replication and increase mutual support?

- How will risk and health needs be used in determining placement, taking into account the offender's needs and system realities?

The goal here is to integrate the assessment and placement phases across multiple systems so as to adequately address both the public health and public safety needs of the offender and the systems involved. Integrating the assessment also allows corrections and treatment staff members to begin to determine the extent to which the offender's criminality is dominated by his or her drug use (Farabee & Leukefeld, 2001). In this model, placement becomes a multidimensional process that can be categorized according to safety level, type and availability of treatment services, and duration of services necessary to respond to both problem severity and risk (Simpson, 1997; Hiller, Knight et al., 1999).

Induction. Although there is ample evidence that treatment does not need to be voluntary to be effective (NIDA, 1999), a mandate for prison-based treatment by the court or by corrections and prison health care personnel does not always translate into readiness to enter treatment or, for that matter, to change behaviors that support drug use and criminality (Taxman, 2000). In correctional programming, this can be a significant problem, as there often is a significant lag time between prison entry and treatment entry. For many, this period may be several years, and it cannot be assumed that offender motivation to enter treatment and make lifestyle changes has remained stable over time. As a result, correctional, treatment, and health care personnel must pay particular attention to the fit between the offender's motivation and the services provided. Failure to address the fit can have a considerable effect on entry into treatment, retention, compliance during treatment, and post-release outcomes, including the decision to continue treatment post-release (Battjes, Onken et al., 1999; Farabee, Simpson et al., 1995; Joe, Simpson et al., 1999; Simpson, 1997; Taxman, 2000).

Research into the development of induction interventions shows promise in this area. Induction interventions seek to enhance treatment readiness "by helping individuals examine consequences of different levels of treatment engagement and by helping them identify resources (both internal and external) that can be used in maximizing outcomes (Blankenship, Dansereau et al., 1999, p. 432)." One model, *The Treatment Readiness Program,* was developed at Texas Christian University (TCU) as a complement to correctional programming. This model is aimed at building motivation to achieve outcomes such as being drug-free. It also attempts to enhance the inmates' confidence in the value and contribution of the treatment process to achieving those outcomes. An important aspect of this model for correctional programs is that it was designed to address limitations in education and cognitive functioning of the type often encountered in the offender population (Blankenship, Dansereau et al., 1999).

In considering the use of induction techniques to address offender motivation and readiness to enter prison-based treatment, corrections professionals need to examine several issues. For example, when and where will induction techniques have the greatest effect on the offender's motivation and readiness to enter treatment? Who will deliver the interventions? Of the evidence-based induction models, which one best aids the system in terms of offender and correctional programming needs, as well as resource availability (staff skills and funding for training and maintenance)? Can the model be adapted to current programming? How will induction interventions enhance or inhibit the offender's ability to engage in the treatment process?

Engagement. Induction interventions are important in that they help offenders better understand what treatment is and is not and what outcomes can be achieved at different levels of effort. Shifting the balance of cost and benefits of actively engaging in treatment requires motivating both the drug-abusing offender and the program to engage in a recovery process in which the offender and the correctional institution are active partners in the offender's recovery. This approach focuses more on strategies that increase internal motivation and lessen the reliance on external, more coercive factors. Early engagement, as defined by Simpson and colleagues (Joe, Simpson et al, 1999; Simpson, 1997, 2001;

Simpson, Joe et al., 1997b), includes two major components: program participation and the therapeutic relationship, both of which must be addressed to engage the client in the treatment process. Court mandates and coercive factors within the correctional system initially can facilitate attendance and compliance with treatment activities, but they rarely are sufficient to maintain progress. Behavioral strategies, such as contingency management procedures that offer social recognition and tokens or coupons that can be used to purchase supportive items (for example, phone cards or personal hygiene items), can help to increase participation and other positive behaviors early in treatment (Hiller, Rowan-Szal et al., 1996; Simpson, 2000).

Building an active therapeutic relationship requires attention to the inmate's cognitive involvement and satisfaction with the process. It also requires an immediate focus on the perceived needs of the offender, which may have more to do with feeling safe in the prison environment and receiving medical care than with changing behaviors that lead to abstinence and prosocial behaviors (Battjes, Onken et al., 1999). Cognitive counseling techniques, such as those developed by Dansereau and colleagues (Blankenship, Dansereau et al., 1999; Dansereau, Dees et al., 1995; Pitre, Dansereau et al., 1998), have been used successfully with correctional populations to improve offender and staff engagement in the treatment process. This intervention, "node-link mapping," is based on a visual representation system to help illustrate the drug user's problems and issues that surface during treatment, with the goal of improving communication and developing solution-oriented thinking and action planning. In general, the researchers have found that the techniques contribute to a greater sense of motivation and confidence and higher levels of satisfaction and participation among both offenders and staff members.

The integration of enhanced counseling techniques aimed at fostering the therapeutic relationship and increasing offender participation in the treatment process requires some research and consultation, similar to the process of integrating induction strategies into prison programming. Perhaps the most important issues that staff members need to address revolve around identification of the best evidence-based approach that will meet the system's needs, as well as determining whether resources will be sufficient to train for and maintain this intervention.

Early Recovery. Taxman (2000) noted that the conceptual framework for recovery requires the offender to pass through several stages of recovery and to make lasting behavioral and social changes. During the early recovery phase, programming should focus on helping the offender develop problem recognition skills, as well as self-management and relapse prevention skills. In addition to cognitive mapping (Dansereau, Dees et al., 1995; Pitre, Dansereau et al., 1998), TCU has developed a number of specialized cognitive and social skill interventions that can be integrated into existing programs to help the offender recognize and self-diagnose problems and acquire skills to improve his or her functioning. These interventions include materials focusing on communication skills and sexual health for men and women (Bartholomew, Hiller et al., 2000; Bartholomew, Rowan-Szal et al., 1994; Hiller, Rowan-Szal et al., 1996), on HIV/AIDS prevention (Boatler, Knight et al., 1994), on improving relationships with peers and family, and on replacing dysfunctional relationships (Knight & Simpson, 1996). The protocols are based on a significant body of research and are easily accessed by program staff members. The major issue for personnel to consider is how to use the interventions most effectively within the existing program structure.

Monitoring. Another important role for treatment, corrections, and medical personnel is that of monitoring service utilization and the progress made in treatment and feeding this information back to the service system to facilitate continuous treatment planning. As the offender moves through the treatment process, needs for various services and interventions will arise. For example, the offender may need additional specialized counseling, medication for a previously undiagnosed psychiatric disorder, or family therapy and parenting training as he or she moves toward transition into the community (NIDA, 1999). Because of the multiple systems and cultures that the offender must operate within while involved in prison-based treatment, it is incumbent on personnel from the various systems to find ways to share and coordinate information, so as to deliver high-quality treatment and increase the likelihood that the offender will complete the primary phase of treatment.

Transition to Community Support. In general, a body of research shows reductions in drug use and criminal behavior after prison-based treatment (Simpson, Wexler et al., 1999; Pearson & Lipton, 1999). An important and consistent observation is that better results are obtained if offenders enter community-based treatment during their transition into the community. The most favorable results are obtained by those who complete community-based treatment and continue in aftercare (Martin, Butzin et al., 1999; Wexler, Melnick et al., 1999; Knight, Simpson et al., 1999).

This research suggests that prison-based treatment can effectively engage the inmate in a process of recovery, but that process needs to continue as the individual transitions back into the community. The prison treatment environment naturally limits the inmate's exposure to situations that increase the risk of relapse. For example, in prison-based treatment there is little opportunity to learn how to handle social situations with peers who are using drugs or alcohol, or of encountering situations that produce a conditioned craving response through a prior association with drug use. The addicted offender can learn to avoid relapse or to cope with these situations if treatment continues in the community. There is a higher risk of relapse and recidivism if community-based treatment is unavailable or refused, with re-arrest and re-incarceration as the likely consequences. The challenge for corrections and criminal justice personnel, prison-based treatment providers, and community-based treatment programs is to capitalize on the progress made in prison treatment settings to improve retention of the patient who is returning to the community.

The primary goal of this stage, then, is to help the offender gain greater mastery over the cognitive, behavioral, and social skills necessary for problem recognition and self-management and to develop relapse prevention skills. The primary goal for the correctional treatment program is to optimize relationships with community-based treatment and correctional programs to initiate linkages to new support networks that will maintain progress as the offender leaves the institutional setting.

An issue about which little is known is the congruence between prison-based approaches to treatment and the approaches found in community-based programs, and how that affects decisions by the offender to remain in treatment on release. For example, a prison program may employ a therapeutic community-based approach, with a heavy emphasis on using peer influence to support social behavior characterized as "right living," whereas a community-based program may emphasize a medical model in which addiction is addressed as a neurologic or behavioral disorder without regard for social or environmental factors. The lack of apparent congruence in the approaches used by various drug abuse treatment programs may create difficulties in transitioning from one program to another. (Lack of congruence may be confusing to the new "patient" who must "relearn" how to cope with the addiction.) There is a risk that the patient will drop out of treatment rather than re-engage in a new recovery process. Obviously, more research

is needed to better determine how to facilitate transitions between programs. In developing linkages, correctional programming staff members may want to look closely at their partners in the community, including treatment staff members, criminal justice staff members, and family and friends of the offender, who again will become part of the support network. Some questions that should be addressed include:

- How can key community treatment staff members be introduced to the offender and identify his or her individual needs before release to community treatment?

- When there is a lack of congruence in treatment approaches between prison-based treatment and community-based treatment, what orientation and induction strategies are necessary to help the offender transition to a community-based program while maintaining gains made during prison treatment?

- Can community-based programs integrate better with prison programs to provide a more congruent treatment approach that furthers the progress already made in prison?

- How will criminal justice staff members be informed of therapeutic progress? What is needed to facilitate a partnership to achieve successful treatment outcomes?

- How can criminal justice staff members participate in the treatment process?

- Is there a partnership between the individual, the treatment provider, and the criminal justice staff members?

Maintenance. Much of what was effective during prison-based treatment and the transition to community-based care continues to be helpful during the maintenance stage, although the focus shifts to relapse prevention and the development of positive social networks, including self-help programs, that support an abstinent and legitimate lifestyle. At this stage, the patient and the treatment and criminal justice staff members can be expected to struggle with how much and what kind of treatment is needed.

Research into the neuroscience of addiction shows that chronic drug use produces persistent changes in the structure and biochemical function of the brain (NIDA, 1999). Given this long-lasting damage, it is perhaps not surprising that the behavioral attributes of addiction, including criminality, resemble a chronic disorder that, for many addicts, has an effective treatment but no cure. The concept of addiction as a chronic long-term disorder suggests that treatment should be expected to continue over a long period—perhaps over the life of the patient—so that the harm resulting from episodes of lapse or relapse can be minimized.

A number of questions must be addressed at this stage: What are the implications of chronic, long-term care models on the public health and public safety systems? What are the criteria that indicate enough progress to release the individual from supervision in the public health and public safety systems? Does the system tolerate the individual returning to treatment when there are problems, without re-entry into the legal system?

FUTURE DIRECTIONS
IN PRISON-BASED TREATMENT

The fundamental assumption in this chapter is that there are social benefits to both the public health and public safety to be derived from providing addiction treatment to criminal offenders. These benefits are measured in reduced drug use, reduced criminal behavior, and avoidance of many drug-related adverse medical and social problems. The benefits of treatment can vary, however, depending on the type of treatment, how it is delivered, and how the individual responds to it. The pressing issues for the public health and public safety communities are to improve both the quality and performance of treatment and to incorporate evidence-based interventions into everyday practice.

An organizing principle of this chapter is the view that addiction produces changes in the structure and biochemical functioning of the brain. These changes often are accompanied by behavioral attributes and social consequences that do not necessarily diminish once drug use has ceased. More recent research suggests that the brain does not recover over time, once abstinence is achieved, although we have yet to understand how fully such recovery occurs or how much time it requires.

What should be the future direction of addiction treatment in the criminal justice system? Recent trends in criminal justice, such as drug courts and other forms of therapeutic jurisprudence are attempts to take advantage of the potential benefits of blending public health and public safety concerns in dealing with the national problem of drug abuse and addiction. The criminal justice setting can provide strong external motivation for the offender to change his or her behavior. Especially when deciding whether to seek treatment and during the period of engagement, the offender can benefit from close monitoring and supervision, which criminal justice systems provide. Although the criminal jus-

tice system can provide sanctions for incorrigibly bad behavior, it is less clear how well it can reinforce positive behaviors.

Dealing with offenders can be frustrating, as can treating drug addiction. The question for both criminal justice professionals and clinical providers is how to provide criminal justice oversight in a way that maximizes its therapeutic value. A decision to punish behavior never should be reflexive, but rather should be a considered decision that attempts to address the twin goals of public health and safety. More research is needed to determine the effectiveness of various criminal justice sanctions, both positive and negative, under what circumstances they work best, and when they do not work.

Likewise, it is important to understand how to improve the ability of the criminal justice system to work with drug abuse treatment providers as well as other health and social services systems in the community. Not only are the problems of drug addiction long lasting, but they are also multiple and complex. A "seamless" system of care that provides continuity of services from incarceration to re-integration into the community may provide the best opportunity to realize the potential for blending public health and safety.

ACKNOWLEDGMENT: The authors express their appreciation for the editorial assistance of Keri-Lyn Coleman in the preparation of this chapter.

REFERENCES

Andrews DA, Zinger I, Hoge RD et al. (1990). Does treatment work? A clinically relevant and psychologically informed meta-analysis. *Criminology* 28:369-404.

Anglin MD & Hser Y (1989). Legal coercion and drug abuse treatment: Research findings and policy implications. In JA Inciardi (ed.) *Handbook of Drug Control in the United States.* Westport, CT: Greenwood Press.

Anglin MD & Hser Y (1990). Treatment of drug abuse. In M Tonry & JQ Wilson (eds.) *Drugs and Crime.* Chicago, IL: University of Chicago Press.

Anno J (1991). *Prison Health Care: Guidelines for the Management of an Adequate Delivery System.* Washington, DC: U.S. Department of Justice, National Institute of Corrections, National Commission on Correctional Health Care.

Bartholomew NG, Hiller ML, Knight K et al. (2000). Effectiveness of communication and relationship skills training for men in substance abuse treatment. *Journal of Substance Abuse Treatment* 18(3):217-225.

Bartholomew NG, Rowan-Szal GA, Chatham LR et al. (1994). Effectiveness of a specialized intervention for women in a methadone program. *Journal of Psychoactive Drugs* 26(3):249-255.

Battjes RJ, Onken LS & Delany PJ (1999). Drug abuse treatment entry and engagement: A report of a meeting on treatment readiness. *Journal of Consulting and Clinical Psychology* 55(5):643-657.

Beck AJ & Mumola CJ (1999). Prisoners in 1998. *Bureau of Justice Statistics Bulletin*. Washington, DC: U.S. Department of Justice, Office of Justice Programs, Bureau of Justice Statistics.

Belenko S (2000). The challenges of integrating drug treatment into the CJ process. *Albany Law Review* 63(3):833-876.

Belenko S & Peugh J (1999). *Behind Bars: Substance Abuse and America's Prison Population* (Technical report). New York, NY: National Center on Addiction and Substance Abuse.

Blankenship J, Dansereau DF & Simpson DD (1999). Cognitive enhancements of readiness for corrections-based treatment for drug abuse. *Prison Journal* 79(4):431-445.

Boatler JF, Knight K & Simpson DD (1994). Assessment of an AIDS intervention program during drug abuse treatment. *Journal of Substance Abuse Treatment* 11(4):367-372.

Brown BS (1993). In CG Leukefeld & FM Tims (eds.) *Drug Abuse Treatment in Prisons and Jails (NIDA Research Monograph 118)*. Rockville, MD: National Institute on Drug Abuse.

Camp GM & Camp CG (1996). *The Corrections Yearbook: 1996*. South Salem, NY: Criminal Justice Institute.

Czuchry M & Dansereau DF (2000). Drug abuse treatment in criminal justice settings: Enhancing community engagement and helpfulness. *American Journal of Drug and Alcohol Issues* 26(4):537-552.

Dansereau DF, Dees SM, Greener JM et al. (1995). Node-link mapping and the evaluation of drug abuse counseling sessions. *Psychology of Addictive Behaviors* 9(3):125-203.

Dees SM & Dansereau DF (1997). *A Jumpstart for Substance Abuse Treatment: Readiness Activities* (TCU/CETOP Manual for Counselors). Fort Worth, TX: Institute for Behavioral Research, Texas Christian University.

DeLeon G (2000). *The Therapeutic Community*. New York, NY: Springer Publishing Company.

Ditton PM (1999). *Mental Health and Treatment of Inmates and Probationers: Bureau of Justice Statistics Special Report*. Washington, DC: U.S. Department of Justice, Office of Justice Programs.

Falkin GP, Wexler HK & Lipton DS (1992). Drug treatment in state prisons. In *Extent and Adequacy of Insurance Coverage for Substance Abuse Services, Institute of Medicine Report: Treating Drug Problems Vol. II (NIDA Services Research Series No. 3)*. Rockville, MD: National Institute on Drug Abuse.

Farabee D & Leukefeld CG (2001). Recovery and the criminal justice system. In FM Tims, CG Leukefeld & JJ Platt (eds.) *Relapse and Recovery in Addictions*. New Haven, CT: Yale University Press, 40-59.

Farabee D, Simpson DD, Dansereau DF et al. (1995). Cognitive inductions into treatment among drug users on probation. *Journal of Drug Issues* 25:669-682.

Gendreau P (1996). The principles of effective intervention with offenders. In A Harland (ed.) *Choosing Correctional Options that Work*. Newbury Park, CA: Sage Publications.

Hammett TM (2000). HIV/AIDS and other infectious diseases in correctional populations. Paper Presented at the Drug Abuse Treatment in the Correctional System: The 2nd Annual NIDA/NDRI Research to Practice Conference, Bethesda, MD.

Hiller ML, Knight K, Broome KM et al. (1996). Legal pressures and treatment retention in a national sample of long-term residential programs. *Criminal Justice and Behavior* 25(4):463-481.

Hiller ML, Knight K & Simpson DD (1999). Prison-based substance abuse treatment, residential aftercare and recidivism. *Addiction* 94:833-842.

Hiller ML, Rowan-Szal GA, Bartholomew NG et al. (1996). Effectiveness of a specialized women's intervention in a residential treatment program. *Substance Abuse & Misuse* 31(6):771-783.

Hollin CR (1999). Treatment programs for offenders: Meta-analysis, "what works," and beyond. *International Journal of Law and Psychiatry* 22(3-4):361-372.

Hubbard RL, Marsden ME, Rachal JV et al. (1989). *Drug Abuse Treatment: A National Study of Effectiveness*. Chapel Hill, NC: University of North Carolina Press.

Inciardi BW, Fletcher & Horton AM Jr., eds. (n.d.) *The Effectiveness of Innovative Strategies in the Treatment of Drug Abuse*. Westport, CT: Greenwood Press, 182-203.

Inciardi JA, Martin SS, Butzin CA et al. (1997). An effective model of prison-based treatment for drug-involved offenders. *Journal of Drug Issues* 27(2): 261-278.

Joe GW, Simpson DD & Broome KM (1999). Patient and program attributes related to treatment process indicators in DATOS. *Drug and Alcohol Dependence* 57(2):127-136.

Knight K & Simpson DD (1996). Influences of family and friends on client progress during drug abuse treatment. *Journal of Drug Abuse Treatment* 8(4):417-429.

Knight K, Simpson DD, Chatham LR et al. (1997). An assessment of prison-based drug treatment: Texas in-prison therapeutic community program. *Journal of Offender Rehabilitation* 24(3/4):75-100.

Knight K, Simpson DD & Hiller ML (1996). Evaluation of prison-based treatment and aftercare: process and outcomes. Presented at the Annual Meeting of the American Psychological Association, Toronto, Canada; August.

Knight K, Simpson DD & Hiller M (1999). Three year reincarceration outcomes for in-prison therapeutic community treatment in Texas. *Prison Journal* 79(3):337-351.

Leukefeld CG & Tims FM (1990). Compulsory treatment for drug abuse. *Journal of Substance Abuse Treatment* 10:77-84.

Leukefeld CG & Tims FM (1993). Directions for research and practice. In C Leukefeld & F Tims (eds.) *Drug Abuse Treatment in Prisons and Jails (NIDA Research Monograph 118)*. Rockville, MD: National Institute on Drug Abuse.

Leukefeld CG, Tims FM & Platt JJ (2001). Future directions in relapse. In FM Tims, CG Leukefeld, & JJ Platt (eds.) *Relapse and Recovery in Addictions*. New Haven, CT: Yale University Press, 402-413.

Lipton D, Martinson R & Wilks J (1975). *The Effectiveness of Correctional Treatment*. New York, NY: Praeger Publishers.

Lipton DS (1995). *The Effectiveness of Treatment for Drug Abusers under Criminal Justice Supervision* (Research Report). Washington, DC: U.S. Department of Justice, National Institute of Justice.

Martin SS, Butzin CA, Saum CA et al. (1999). Three-year outcomes of therapeutic community treatment for drug-involved offenders in Delaware: From prison to work release to aftercare. *Prison Journal* 79(3):294-320.

Martinson R (1974). What works? Questions and answers about prison reform. *Public Interest* 35:22-45.

McDonald DC (1995). *Managing Prison Health Care and Costs (Research Report)*. Washington, DC: U.S. Department of Justice, National Institute of Justice.

McDonald DC (2000). Health care coordination. Paper presented at Drug Abuse Treatment in the Correctional System: The 2nd Annual NIDA/NDRI Research to Practice Conference, Bethesda, MD.

Mumola CJ (1999). *Substance Abuse and Treatment, State and Federal Prisoners in 1997. Bureau of Justice Statistics Special Report*. Washington, DC: U.S. Department of Justice, Office of Justice Programs, Bureau of Justice Statistics.

Mumola CJ & Beck AJ (1997). Prisoners in 1996. *Bureau of Justice Statistics Bulletin*. Washington, DC: U.S. Department of Justice, Office of Justice Programs, Bureau of Justice Statistics.

National Institute on Drug Abuse (NIDA) (1999). *Principles of Drug Addiction Treatment: A Research-Based Guide*. Washington, DC: U.S. Government Printing Office.

Office of National Drug Control Policy (ONDCP) (2000). *National Drug Control Strategy*. Washington, DC: U.S. Government Printing Office.

Pearson FS & Lipton DS (1999). A meta-analytic review of the effectiveness of corrections-based treatments for drug abuse. *Prison Journal* 79(4):384-410.

Pelissier B & McCarthy D (1993). Evaluation of the Federal Bureau of Prisons Drug Treatment Programs. In CG Leukefeld & FM Tims (eds.) *Drug Abuse Treatment in Prisons and Jails (NIDA Research Monograph 118)*. Rockville, MD: National Institute on Drug Abuse, 261-278.

Peters RH & Steinberg ML (2000). Substance abuse treatment services in U.S. prisons. In D Shewan & J Deavies (eds.) *Drugs and Prisons*. London, England: Harwood Academic Publishers, 89-116.

Pitre U, Dansereau DF, Newbern D et al. (1998). Residential drug abuse treatment for probationers: Use of node-link mapping to enhance participation and progress. *Journal of Substance Abuse Treatment* 15(6):535-543.

Sherman LW, Gottfredson D, MacKenzie D et al. (1997). *Preventing Crime: What Works, What Doesn't, What's Promising: Report to Congress*. Washington. DC: Office of Justice Programs.

Simpson DD (1997). Effectiveness of drug abuse treatment: A review of research from field settings. In JA Egertson, DM Fox & AI Leshner (eds.) *Treating Drug Abusers Effectively*. Cambridge, MA: Blackwell Publishers of North America.

Simpson DD (2000). Research Summary: Focus on Treatment Process and Outcomes. Fort Worth, TX: Institute for Behavioral Research, Texas Christian University.

Simpson DD (2001). Modeling treatment process and outcomes (editorial). *Addiction* 96(2):207-211.

Simpson DD & Sells S (1982). Effectiveness of treatment for drug abuse: An overview of the DARP research program. *Advances in Alcohol and Substance Abuse Treatment* 2:7-29.

Simpson DD, Joe GW, Dansereau DF et al. (1997a). Strategies for improving methadone treatment process and outcomes. *Journal of Drug Issues* 27(2):239-260.

Simpson DD, Joe GW, Rowan-Szal GA & Greener JM (1997b). Drug abuse treatment process components that improve retention. *Journal of Substance Abuse Treatment* 14(6):565-572.

Simpson DD, Wexler HK & Inciardi JA (1999). Introduction. *Prison Journal* 79(3):291-293.

Speckart G & Anglin MD (1986). Narcotics and crime: A causal modeling approach. *Journal of Quantitative Criminology* 2(1):3-28.

Taxman F (1999). Unraveling "What Works" for offenders in substance abuse services. *National Drug Court Institute Review* II(2)Winter: 93-133.

Taxman F (2000). Effective practices for protecting public safety through substance abuse treatment (unpublished manuscript). Rockville, MD: National Institute on Drug Abuse.

Tims FM, Fletcher BW & Hubbard RL (1991). Treatment outcomes for drug abuse clients. In RW Pickens, CG Leukefeld & CR Schuster (eds.) *Improving Drug Abuse Treatment (NIDA Research Monograph 106)*. Rockville, MD: National Institute on Drug Abuse.

U.S. Department of Justice (1995). *Prisoners in 1994*. Washington DC: Bureau of Justice Statistics.

Weisner C & Schmidt LA (1995). Expanding the frame of health services research in the drug abuse field. *Health Services Research* 30(5):707-726.

Wexler HK, Lipton DS & Johnson BD (1988). *A Criminal Justice System Strategy for Treating Cocaine-Heroin Abusing Offenders in Custody*. Washington, DC: National Institute of Justice.

Wexler HK, Melnick G, Lowe L et al. (1999). Three-year reincarceration outcomes for Amity in-prison therapeutic community and aftercare in California. *Prison Journal* 79(3):321-336.

Primary Medical Care in Correctional Settings

H. BLAIR CARLSON, M.D., FACP, FASAM

Programs that treat addicted inmates in prisons and jails often do not incorporate physicians, nurses, physician assistants, and other health care workers, or they significantly limit their roles. Nevertheless, health care personnel who have contact with inmate-addicts in correctional dispensaries and infirmaries do have several important roles:

1. They are responsible for the recognition, assessment, and appropriate treatment of inmates who are intoxicated, at risk of major withdrawal, or in the throes of an abstinence syndrome. These situations often constitute medical emergencies and require the attention of trained medical professionals.

2. They must recognize, accurately diagnose, and treat the consequences of alcohol and drug abuse. This includes infections resulting from intravenous drug use, such as HIV, hepatitis, and endocarditis. Organ disorders as the result of alcohol abuse are common among inmate populations and must be addressed as well.

3. They must learn how to prescribe appropriately for drug-addicted inmates. This often involves the proper treatment of pain in opiate-dependent individuals. The judicious use of other psychoactive medications in addicts who have mental disorders should not be avoided, but rather addressed carefully and intelligently.

4. Nurses, physician assistants, and physicians are part of a complex system in any jail or prison. Their professional advice and counsel is needed. They should work to engender a trusting relationship with custodial and administrative staff, so that their opinions and recommendations are heard and acted upon when appropriate.

5. Finally, a most important role involves providing credible counseling. The term "brief intervention" has come to describe an interaction between a health professional and a patient in which the professional is able to help move the patient toward a change in his or her risky behaviors—no matter how miniscule the movement may seem to be (Miller & Rollnick, 1991). Health professionals who work with inmates must, in a compassionate and credible manner, counsel their patients about addiction. There is an abundant literature about such interactions between caregiver and patient demonstrating that brief interventions can be effective in motivating persons to want to change their behaviors. Suggestions as to how to make a change and where to get help are more likely to be accepted from a credible, compassionate, and savvy caregiver.

The FRAMES mnemonic is useful in approaching these interactions. As adapted for work with incarcerated populations, FRAMES helps the caregiver to remember the following points:

- **F**eedback usually is provided following an assessment, in which the information gained from history, physical, or laboratory results serves as a catalyst for feedback about risk and the need to change a risky behavior. A caregiver who listens reflectively often helps a patient to think about his or her pattern of behaviors and the consequences of those behaviors.

- **R**esponsibility for change lies with the patient. This should be made clear, implicitly and explicitly.

- **A**dvice to change or to think about change or to recognize the difficulties caused by a behavior are not easily ignored when given by a health care professional and may have surprisingly positive results.

- **M**enus or options for where to get help give an inmate some choice in the matter. Options are limited in correctional settings, but health care staff should know what is available in the institution and be savvy about schedules, what happens in a treatment program, and how to make it possible for an inmate to get into treatment within the system. Counseling sessions, Twelve Step programs, facilitated groups, and even a therapeutic community may be available.

- **E**mpathic counsel is critical. Inviting the patient to come back and report how things are going is a good idea.

- **S**elf-efficacy often is a forgotten part of effective counseling in addiction medicine. The health care professional must help the patient believe that he or she *can* succeed. Such encouragement must be reinforced over and over. Optimism about the patient's recovery is the cornerstone of a successful therapeutic relationship.

At the time of any encounter, the clinician and patient together can view the problem sheet in the medical record, which should clearly indicate the patient's alcohol or other drug problem. The simple presence of this information in the patient's chart sends a strong message that can help keep the patient focused on a significant problem in her or his life. Addressing the problem as it appears in the medical record should be a frequent event.

In addition to clinic visits for medical complaints, there are other times when a discussion of the items on the problem list become suitable. For example, the standards of the National Commission on Correctional Health Care call for health reviews that are oppotunities to identify alcohol and other drug problems during the mental health evaluation, health promotion and disease prevention encounters, periodic screening, special needs treatment planning, and the periodic health assessment. In practice, this means looking at the problem sheet with the patient and pausing at the addiction problem long enough to encourage the patient to talk about what this means to him or her at the moment and what kinds of help the patient wants and needs.

The clinician then listens carefully to the patient's response and decides what the most appropriate next comment should be. And so it goes: correctional health care becomes more interesting.

REFERENCE

Miller W & Rollnick S (1991). *Motivational Interviewing: Preparing People to Change Addictive Behavior.* New York, NY: Guilford Press.

Twelve Step Programs in Correctional Settings

JOHN N. CHAPPEL, M.D., M.P.H., FASAM

Alcoholism and other drug addictions pose a major problem for physicians and other health care workers in correctional settings, because inmates' continued drinking and drug use threaten both individual and institutional health. Fortunately, both Alcoholics Anonymous (AA) and Narcotics Anonymous (NA) can bring their meetings and accompanying Twelve Step programs into institutional settings.

THE BENEFITS
Any inmate who decides to work a Twelve Step program of recovery in AA or NA will become more responsible in his or her behavior, more honest, more open to change, and less obsessed or absorbed by his or her own selfish needs. Correctional staff, from the warden on down, need to be educated as to these benefits. The physician can play an important role in this essential educational process.

GETTING STARTED
In 1942, AA members from San Francisco brought the first AA meeting into San Quentin prison at the request of Warden Duffy. That historic event taught all the lessons required to bring the benefits of Twelve Step programs to any correctional institution today.

First, the prison superintendent or warden must set the rules and regulations under which Twelve Step groups are to function inside the prison. AA and NA members who enter a correctional facility are guided by AA policy, which calls for them to "obey the rules of the facility you are visiting. . . . The only thing we take in is our message. Take nothing out: no letters, messages or notes. Don't promise anything but sobriety."

Next, a member of the prison staff should be appointed the AA or NA group sponsor. (The physician might suggest this role to a health care professional who works in the prison.) The staff sponsor inside the prison works with an AA or NA sponsor outside the facility to plan and conduct the first meeting.

The importance of inviting AA or NA to bring the Twelve Step message into the prison cannot be overemphasized. Many AA and NA members are reluctant to enter correctional facilities. Those who have been incarcerated in the past are not certain they will be welcome, or even allowed to enter. Those who have not been in prison or jail are not certain they want to enter. Yet, despite their reluctance and anxiety, most AA and NA members respond positively to requests for help. They take seriously the AA motto: "When anyone, anywhere reaches out for help, I want the hand of AA always to be there—for that I am responsible."

Contact with local AA groups can be made by calling the number listed in the local telephone book and asking for someone on the Correctional Facilities Committee or the Hospitals and Institutions Committee. If the local AA group does not have either of these committees, the request for help will prompt the formation of one. Also, help always can be obtained from AA World Services, at the number listed below.

HOW IT WORKS
Working a Twelve Step program of recovery in AA or NA does something for an individual that modern medicine cannot do. The process not only makes sobriety tolerable—and long-term sobriety possible—it also helps to change or improve personality disorders or traits. These beneficial changes require work on the part of the individual. Time and energy are put into being honest, open, and willing to change. This is not easy in the prison setting, where survival appears to depend on just the opposite traits. The physician or other health care professional can facilitate the effectiveness of the Twelve Step program by being knowledgeable about and supportive of the following essential elements:

1. *Meetings*: These are the gatherings where AA and NA members share their experiences, strength, and hope. In meetings, they are protected by the tradition of anonymity, where nothing that is seen or heard in the meeting is taken out. As an inmate practices sharing in meetings, he or she develops better self-observation, respect for the experiences of others, and a sense of his or her own story, which helps to develop integrity.

2. *Home Groups*: When an inmate makes an AA or NA group his or her "home group," the members of that group become like an extended family. Having a home group helps an inmate develop acceptance and tolerance of self and others.

3. *Sponsorship*: Each member of AA or NA is expected to choose a sponsor, who will mentor him or her through the Twelve Step program of recovery. This mentoring system helps the member and the sponsor as well, as there is evidence that the process of being a sponsor and passing along what one has learned to another strengthens sobriety and reduces the risk of relapse.

4. *Step Work*: The Twelve Steps combine thought, attitude, and action. Working the steps is not easy, especially when the inmate reaches Steps 4 and 5. The steps put the inmate on the path of personal growth and development. Chapters 5 and 6 of *Alcoholics Anonymous* (the Big Book) provide a good introduction to the steps, while the Twelve Steps and Twelve Traditions (see Section 8 of this text), written 15 years later, provide more depth and experience for each step.

5. *Spirituality*: Inmates who work a Twelve Step program of recovery are likely to have spiritual experiences. These usually involve something good happening for which there is no explanation. A common spiritual experience is a reduction in craving for alcohol or other drugs, often associated with working Steps 2 and 3.

Correctional health staff often must deal with inmates' mistaken belief that Twelve Step programs are "religions." This is not true. The only requirement for membership is a desire to stop drinking or using drugs (Tradition 3). There is no creed, no theology, no doctrine to be learned or followed. Atheists and agnostics are welcome and do well in the programs. The home group can serve as a functional Higher Power for the individual who is unwilling or unable to accept the concept of God unattached to any religion.

There is much more that physicians and other correctional health professionals can learn about Twelve Step programs and their value in correctional settings. Twelve Step programs such as AA, NA, or Alanon not only benefit inmates, they also provide value to the correctional institution and the community to which the inmate eventually returns.

RECOMMENDED READING

The following publications can be obtained from AA World Services, PO Box 459, Grand Central Station, New York, NY 10163, or by phone at 212/870-3312.

AA in Correctional Facilities: A pamphlet describing the steps in starting an AA program in a correctional facility.

AA in Prison: Inmate to Inmate: A booklet containing the stories of 32 inmates.

It Sure Beats Sitting in a Cell: A pamphlet introducing AA in prison and afterwards.

| Chapter 13 | # Special Issues in Treatment: Women |

Joan E. Zweben, Ph.D.

Within the past decade, treatment providers have devoted increasing attention to defining and addressing the unique needs of women. Gender disparities were largely ignored until the 1970s, when interest grew in the biomedical and psychosocial aspects of women's use of alcohol and other drugs. Prompted by the women's movement, the federal government initiated efforts to focus scientific and public attention on women's issues (Blume, 1992, 1998). This focus has generated new research, services specifically tailored to women's needs, new materials for clinicians in the field, and reconsideration of public policy issues. However, there still are many ways in which the needs of women in alcohol and drug treatment remain unmet.

This chapter presents information on the epidemiology of alcohol and drug use among women and on circumstances that increase women's problems with addictive disorders and affect their recovery. It discusses treatment issues specific to women, including the relationship of drug and alcohol use problems to psychiatric and medical conditions.

EPIDEMIOLOGY

Gender Differences in Alcohol and Other Drug Use. Several large-scale epidemiologic studies document gender differences in the use of alcohol and almost all other drugs, with higher rates found in men (Kessler, McGonagle et al., 1994; Regier, Farmer et al., 1990). The Epidemiological Catchment Area study, with data collected in the 1980s, reported that men had five times greater one-month prevalence rates for alcohol and three times greater one-month prevalence for other drugs (Regier, Farmer et al., 1990). The more recent National Comorbidity Study (Kessler, McGonagle et al., 1994) documented similar differences, but the gap appears to be diminishing. The most recent National Household Survey on Drug Abuse (Greene, Marsden et al., 2000), conducted in 1998, showed smaller gender differences for all age groups except adolescents aged 12 to 17 years. For this group, the gap virtually disappeared for alcohol, marijuana, cocaine, and cigarettes. Thus, gender patterns are evolving according to changing social conditions, with reported rates of use becoming more similar for men and women.

Common Psychiatric Disorders in Women With Addictive Disorders. Most women in treatment for addictive disorders have at least one coexisting mental disorder. The higher the level of care, the greater the likelihood of one or more disorders. Both the Epidemiologic Catchment Area Study (Regier, Farmer et al., 1990) and the National

---

Comorbidity Study (Kessler, McGonagle et al., 1994) found that women were more likely to have any affective disorders than men (with the exception of mania, for which rates were the same). Women were significantly more likely than men to have experienced a major depressive episode, with data from the National Comorbidity Study showing a lifetime prevalence of 21.3% and a 12-month prevalence of 12.9% for women, compared with 12.7% and 7.7% for men. Dysthymia also was more common in women, with a lifetime prevalence of 8% and a 12-month prevalence of 3% compared with 4.8% and 2.1% for men (Kessler, McGonagle et al., 1994).

Women also had a higher lifetime and 12-month prevalence of three or more disorders (Kessler, McGonagle et al., 1994). In addition, women who have experienced childhood sexual abuse are at greatly increased risk of developing a wide range of psychopathology, particularly bulimia and alcohol and other drug dependence (Kendler, Bulik et al., 2000). In this carefully done twin study, the researchers concluded that their results could not be explained by background familial factors.

MEDICAL CONSIDERATIONS

Alcohol. The influence of alcohol on women's health has been much more carefully studied than have other drugs. Although women are less likely than men to drink heavily or even moderately (Dawson & Archer, 1992), when they do so, they are more vulnerable to alcohol-related liver damage, cardiovascular disease, and brain damage (NIAAA, 2000). Negative consequences occur at lower levels of consumption and after much shorter periods of drinking. A recent large prospective study that followed 13,000 adults for 12 years found that women developed alcohol-related liver disease at approximately half the consumption levels of men (Becker, Deis et al., 1996). For women, the risk of alcohol-induced liver disease and alcohol-related cirrhosis rose once consumption levels exceeded 7 to 13 drinks (84 to 156 g of alcohol) per week, half the quantity found for men. Alcohol increased women's susceptibility to myopathy and cardiomyopathy, and studies suggest that female alcoholics suffer from a generalized skeletal fragility that goes beyond the risk of falls (NIAAA, 2000). A review of studies of alcohol absorption, distribution, elimination, and impairment explored the mechanisms by which women achieve higher blood alcohol concentrations than men after drinking equivalent amounts of alcohol, even when doses are adjusted for body weight (Mumenthaler, Taylor et al.,

1999). The review also noted women's relatively greater susceptibility to alcohol's effects on cognitive functions, such as divided attention and memory. Their review concluded that the menstrual cycle is not likely to affect alcohol pharmacokinetics and is not a significant influence on alcohol's effects on performance.

The relationship between drinking and breast cancer risk has been studied since the 1980s. The effect appears to be modest and dose-related, and the form of alcohol appears to be irrelevant. Alcohol consumption raises breast cancer risk even after adjustment for age, family history, and other known dietary and reproductive risk factors (NIAAA, 2000).

Prenatal Alcohol Exposure. Drinking during pregnancy remains a serious concern, with physicians in a key position to reinforce social norms that encourage the elimination of drinking during this time. Fetal alcohol syndrome (FAS) is a set of birth defects considered the single leading nonhereditary cause of mental retardation. The growth deficiency and characteristic set of facial traits tend to become more normal over time, but the alcohol-induced damage to the developing brain is enduring. These mental impairments include deficits in general intellectual functioning and specific difficulties with learning, memory, attention, and problem solving, in addition to manifestations in psychosocial arenas. The impairments are dose-related and may be evident in children without the distinguishing physical features of FAS (NIAAA, 2000).

Several terms have been developed to describe alcohol-related conditions. The term "alcohol-related birth defects" refers to alcohol-related physical abnormalities of the skeleton and certain organ systems (for example, heart and kidney) that occur in the absence of the characteristic growth deficiency and facial characteristics of FAS.

The term "alcohol-related neurodevelopmental disorder" refers to the mental impairments in the absence of FAS. The introduction of a new diagnostic system for categorizing fetal alcohol effects has facilitated more systematic research. Neuroimaging studies provide insight into the structural damage to the brain, and specific patterns of behavioral impairment have been more carefully delineated. Heavy prenatal exposure to alcohol leads to neurobehavioral impairment, but the effects of lower levels of exposure are less clear, although documented in some studies (NIAAA, 2000). Compounding these defects are the caregiving deficits in the child's immediate family when one or both parents are drinking heavily. These deficits include inconsistent nurturance; lack of parental support, monitoring, and communication; high levels of conflict; and physical and sexual abuse (Young, 1997). Comprehensive treatment of the substance-abusing woman needs to address these wide-ranging needs, as described later in this chapter and in Section 10.

Other Drugs. Although evidence on gender differences in the effects of drug use is not extensive at this time, there are indications that gender may be a factor for understanding the pharmacokinetic effects of other drugs. A study of treatment-seeking female cocaine users concluded that some women may have greater vulnerability to the effects of cocaine relative to men, resulting in more rapid progression of pathology (McCance-Katz, Carroll et al., 1999). Biomedical research also suggests that women may be more sensitive to some behavioral effects of cocaine. Mechanisms suggested include female steroid hormones (Woolfolk, McCreary et al., 1999), estrogen (Sell, Scalzitti et al., 1999), and differences in receptor function (Carmona, Tella et al., 1999). Current investigations of the influence of menstrual cycle phase have yielded contradictory results (Mendelson, Sholar et al., 1999; Sholar, Mendelson et al., 1999; Sofuoglu, Dudish-Poulsen et al., 1999).

Unfortunately, little evidence exists in the literature to explain the possible differences between men and women resulting from the use of other drugs such as heroin. The limited evidence available indicates the need for vigorous early education and intervention efforts, as well as more prevention efforts specifically targeted to women.

A woman's substance use is heavily influenced by her male partner (Amaro, Zuckerman et al., 1989; Anglin, Hser et al., 1987; Hser, Anglin et al., 1987), and she can underestimate her level of harm if her main reference point is her partner's behavior.

Domestic Violence. A Bureau of Justice report indicated that, in 1994, more than half a million women were treated in hospital emergency departments for violence-related injuries, usually inflicted by an intimate partner (Rand & Strom, 1997). At least 4.4 million women in the United States each year suffer from related health problems.

Women who have been battered report that their general health is fair or poor, that they have had sexually transmitted diseases and other gynecologic problems, and that they have needed medical care and not received it. Chronic headaches, as well as hearing, vision, and concentration problems, can reflect neurologic damage. A variety of stress-related symptoms, such as irritable bowel syndrome,

also can manifest (Campbell & Lewandowski, 1997). For these reasons, psychosocial treatment efforts must integrate good medical care to be fully comprehensive. It is especially important that residential and outpatient programs without such care on site develop effective case management. Addiction medicine specialists can help such programs develop protocols and procedures to ensure that the counseling staff members are aware of the woman's medical status and its implications for participation in treatment and are clear in their role to facilitate adherence to treatment recommendations. Larger programs have found that a "medical coordinator" who functions as a medical case manager can provide more systematic attention to medical concerns.

HIV/AIDS and Hepatitis C. Women account for a steadily increasing proportion of AIDS cases. More than 90,000 women have been diagnosed and reported with AIDS attributed to injection drug use and sexual relations with an HIV-infected partner. The preponderance of women reported with AIDS in 1999 were African American, with high rates in Hispanic women as well. Similar patterns of increase, particularly among women of color, also are beginning to be apparent in the distribution of hepatitis C cases reported.

Socially sanctioned imbalance of power plays a major role in influencing risk reduction behavior in women. Inasmuch as the condom remains the major method to reduce sexual transmission of HIV, women are at a disadvantage for determining their exposure. Women must either gain the cooperation of their male partners in using a condom or must decide not to have sexual relations if the man refuses (Amaro, 1995; Amaro & Hardy-Fanta, 1995). Many women lack the self-esteem and communication skills to negotiate condom use. Young women in particular often lack the fortitude to insist if their partner balks at the prospect of using a condom. Addicted women are at an additional disadvantage in attempting to practice safer sex. Many women fear emotional or physical abuse if they do so. Indeed, a woman's greatest risk of assault is from her male partner (Koss, Goodman et al., 1994). The development of an effective protective method that is under the woman's control and can be used without the knowledge of her sexual partner is a key element in reducing women's risk.

For the HIV-infected woman, managing her caretaking responsibilities often is an issue added to the physical and psychiatric burdens of the disease. They can worry about transmission of the virus to family members and must be

---

both well informed and reassured. They struggle with how to address their health issues and possible death with their children. Women who have given birth to HIV-positive children have an added layer of anxiety and guilt. Those who become pregnant must choose whether to carry the child to term. Women in these circumstances often are socially isolated and welcome the opportunity to share with other women in the group format, as this sharing can enable them to bypass their shame and express their feelings more openly, with less fear of rejection (Chung & Magraw, 1992).

PSYCHIATRIC DISORDERS

The need for treatment interventions that are sensitive to gender differences has brought increasing attention to co-occurring disorders and their effect on substance-abusing women. It is preferable to address other coexisting mental disorders in an integrated approach. Although the addiction treatment field has made great progress in addressing dual disorders in the past decade, advances in understanding and practice vary greatly in their degree of dissemination. Physicians can expect wide variation in sophistication and responsiveness among community providers and should attempt to refer or place the patient according to specific conditions and behaviors that indicate the need for particular services or levels of care. These conditions and behaviors are described in the recent revision of ASAM's *Patient Placement Criteria* (*ASAM PPC-2R*; Mee-Lee, Shulman et al., 2001), in which community service levels are described in terms of "addiction treatment only (AOS)," programs that focus primarily if not exclusively on addiction; programs that are "dual diagnosis capable (DDC)," for those whose psychiatric disorders have been stabilized; and those that are "dual diagnosis enhanced (DDE)," for those who are unstable or disabled to the extent of needing specific psychiatric support, monitoring, and accommodation. Many community providers describe themselves as offering treatment for co-occurring psychiatric disorders without having the resources to handle the full range of problems. A clear picture of the strengths and limits of programs available in the community can lead to more appropriate referrals, as well as help in guiding the development of services needed to fill the gaps.

It has become more widely accepted in the addiction treatment community that psychotropic medications are compatible with recovery, especially when prescribed by physicians knowledgeable about addiction. Indeed, appro-

priately prescribed medications enhance the effects of psychosocial interventions. Effective pharmacotherapy requires careful education and a clear treatment contract (Gastfriend & Lillard, 1998). "The essential principles are that pharmacotherapy targets specific symptoms, is time limited, is modified only one change at a time, is monitored for compliance, and is provided only in the context of a comprehensive psychosocial treatment plan" (p. 1002). The physician's role as a member of a multidisciplinary team is crucial to achieving these objectives. Counseling staff members typically are responsible for implementing major elements of the plan, and good communication and a structure for coordination improve patient cooperation with physician recommendations.

Anxiety Disorders. As a group, these disorders constitute the most common psychiatric disorders among women, with a total lifetime prevalence of 30.5% and a 12-month prevalence of 22.6% (Kessler, McGonagle et al., 1994). The experience of anxiety is characterized by sensations of nervousness, tension, apprehension, and fear that arise from the anticipation of internal or external danger. It can be easy to underestimate her level of distress when a woman's description is viewed as "dramatic"; in earlier eras, women reporting the same symptoms as men often were labeled "hysterics." Both depression and anxiety can occur in the context of a wide variety of other disorders, and it may be difficult to disentangle the interacting elements and identify the predominant disorders. When anxiety symptoms do not resolve with abstinence, a variety of psychosocial interventions can be used, selected to address the tasks specific to the woman's stage of recovery.

In early recovery, calming reassurance, reality-oriented support, exercise, meditation, breathing management, and other relaxation techniques can be helpful when added to group activities designed to encourage exchange of experiences and transmission of skills. In the later stages of treatment, a variety of supportive, cognitive, and psychodynamic therapies can be used, but anxiety-arousing explorations should be avoided in early recovery. Insight-oriented therapy should be used in the context of a firm recovery support system (including regular self-help group attendance) by a therapist familiar with recovery issues. Familiarity with relapse hazards, warning signs, and prevention strategies is important.

Severe or chronic anxiety can be a significant relapse hazard, so it is important to develop a medication stance that does not make a virtue out of excessive suffering. However, the patient must develop new ways of coping with distress, and it is undesirable to seek to eliminate most of the unpleasant feeling states that are inevitable in recovery. Benzodiazepines, commonly prescribed for anxiety disorders, are problematic for those with a personal or family history of alcoholism or other drug dependence. They are best avoided when possible or used in circumscribed situations (Gastfriend & Lillard, 1998). Non-reinforcing alternatives, such as sedating antidepressants or buspirone (BuSpar®) for anxiety or trazodone (Desyrel®) for insomnia, are recommended.

Of all the anxiety disorders, posttraumatic stress disorder (PTSD) is viewed as a key obstacle to improving treatment outcome. In the National Comorbidity Study, the estimated lifetime prevalence of PTSD was 7.8%, with a striking gender difference—a prevalence of 10.4% in women as compared with 5.0% in men—even when researchers controlled for gender differences in the types of most upsetting trauma (Kessler, Sonnega et al., 1995). This finding is consistent with several studies by Breslau and colleagues (1991, 1997a, 1997b). Wasserman and colleagues (1997) concluded that the relationship between gender and PTSD is robust across patient populations. Rape and sexual molestation were the most frequently reported "most upsetting event(s)," with childhood parental neglect and childhood physical abuse reported more frequently by women. Female victims were more than twice as likely as male victims to develop PTSD (20% compared with 8.2%). A lifetime history of at least one other disorder was present in 79% of women with PTSD, and more than a third of the women with PTSD failed to recover, even after many years and even if they received professional treatment.

Participants in addiction treatment have much higher rates of traumatic experiences and PTSD than the general population. Studies of both residential and outpatient treatment programs that serve both middle-class insured and indigent populations show high levels of childhood abuse and adult trauma (Boyd, Blow et al., 1993; Dansky, Brady et al., 1996; Gil-Rivas, Fiorentine et al., 1997; Janikowski & Glover, 1994; Teets, 1997; Wasserman, Havassy et al., 1997; Yandow, 1989). These findings require treatment providers to equip themselves to meet complex needs. Many programs are ill-equipped to handle them. As Brown and colleagues (Brown, Huba et al., 1995) demonstrated, such a high "level of burden" promotes early dropout, increases the difficulty of treatment in a variety of ways, and makes it more difficult to obtain a positive outcome.

Childhood experiences set the stage for later manifestation of a wide range of disorders and enhance the likelihood of dysfunctional coping responses in adulthood (Zweben, Clark et al., 1994). Studies differ in terms of the types of trauma they consider and how they measure it, making it difficult to compare across studies. Using a conservative definition of childhood sexual abuse (that is, excluding non-physical contact), Russell and Wilsnack reported that more than one third of female children experienced sexual abuse by the age of 18 years. Addictive disorder is only one of many sequelae. Other sequelae include low self-esteem, depression, suicide, anxiety, difficulties in interpersonal relationships, sexual dysfunction, and a tendency toward revictimization (Wasserman, Havassy et al., 1997). These girls are at nearly a fourfold-increased risk of any psychiatric disorder and a threefold risk of addictive disorder (Finkelhor & Dziuba-Leatherman, 1994).

It appears that among adult stressors, rape is the most consistently severe in its effect (Breslau, Davis et al., 1991). Koss and Burkart (1989) noted that almost half of the victims of rape seek some type of professional psychotherapy, often years after the assault. One study indicated that nearly 20% of the women who reported rapes in 1984 had attempted suicide and as many as 80% to 97% developed symptoms of PTSD (Green, 1994).

Mood Disorders. In assessing for depression, it is important to rule out the direct effects of alcohol, illicit drugs, or medications, as well as general medical conditions common in women, such as hypothyroidism, that can lower mood. For diagnostic purposes, negative mood states that are the direct effect of alcohol or illicit drugs generally clear within two to three weeks, with symptoms of longer duration suggesting an independent mood disorder (Brown & Schuckit, 1988; Brown, Inaba et al., 1995). Distress, which is not the same as depression, can persist for a long period of time. It is important to inquire carefully, because women in recovery often use the term "depressed" to describe brooding anxiety, misery, obsessive guilt, apprehension, and other forms of wretchedness that are not synonymous with clinical depression.

It also is important to remember that a sad or depressed mood is only one of many signs and symptoms of a clinically significant depression and may not be the most prominent feature. Other indications include disturbances in emotional, cognitive, behavioral, or somatic regulation. The mood disturbance itself can include apathy, anxiety, or irritability along with, or instead of, sadness. Not all clinically depressed patients feel sad, and many who feel sad are not clinically depressed. Clinicians need to have good skills for drawing patients out and helping them describe their feelings. Women in subcultures that place a high value on functioning can mask depressive symptoms. Those in leadership or caregiver roles can initially manifest depression in more disguised forms, especially if they have a high investment in performance or in continuing to function despite distress. Some depressed women do not describe a low mood, but their interest in or capacity for pleasure or enjoyment may be markedly reduced, making it difficult for them to experience rewards in recovery or to invest in new social relationships with others who do not drink or use drugs.

Eating Disorders. Despite the recognition that eating disorders are relatively common in substance-abusing women, careful assessment is not routine in most programs and integrated treatment is rare. An eating disorder is a severe disturbance in eating behavior that is consistently associated with a psychological or behavioral syndrome. Eating disorders are more prevalent among substance-abusing women than in the general population, and substance-abusing women report more disordered eating behavior than women in the general population. A review of the comorbidity of eating disorders and addictive disorder (Holderness, Brooks-Gunn et al., 1994) indicated that bulimia is more common than anorexia. Krahn and colleagues (Krahn, Kurth et al., 1992; Krahn, 1991) studied eating abnormalities and substance use (including alcoholism) and suggested that levels of symptoms below the threshold required to meet criteria for eating disorders are important for the clinician to address. They caution that dieting-related attitudes and behaviors in young women may be related to increased susceptibility to alcohol and other drug use.

Among alcohol- and drug-using women, there are many possible relationships between substance use and eating disorders. The eating disorder may be present before the onset of alcohol and drug problems. Eating disorders can coexist with substance use in a variety of ways. For example, heroin may be appealing because it facilitates vomiting. Drinking alcohol can provide the feeling of release also gained from vomiting. Stimulants are attractive because they make women feel powerful and suppress the appetite. Alcohol can be used to suppress the panic associated with bingeing and vomiting or to quash the shame that follows an episode. Eating disorders also can be part of a pattern of symptom substitution in abstinent substance us-

ers. For example, women concerned about weight gain once abstinent from stimulants may begin to vomit or purge to cope with their anxiety about attractiveness.

It is important for programs serving women to develop proficiency in addressing eating disorders, especially given the demise of many specialized eating disorder programs. As secrecy is a feature of both disorders, careful inquiry is important during the initial assessment, and observation by staff members is necessary throughout treatment. A woman in treatment may gain 20 to 30 pounds without a disorder being addressed by her individual counselor or in her groups. Eating disorder specialists agree that treatment of this condition requires specialized training. A thorough medical evaluation should assess possible problems and be part of a plan for nutritional stabilization, including strategies to stop aberrant eating behaviors, as well as medication planning and discharge planning that actively address both disorders (Marcus & Katz, 1990). Addiction specialists should avoid the temptation to apply an adapted Twelve Step model as the sole treatment for eating disorders and should be selective about which elements are applied. Cognitive-behavioral approaches to eating disorders, which are well-supported by empirical evidence, are designed to reduce dietary restraint (in contrast with promoting abstinence from particular foods), address abnormal attitudes about body weight and shape, and alter thinking about eating and personal control. Psychotherapy to address related personal issues is encouraged much earlier in the recovery process (Wilson, 1997) than is the case with addictive disorders.

Borderline Personality Disorder. When receiving a patient with a borderline diagnosis, it is important to review the diagnosis for accuracy. Misdiagnosis of borderline personality disorder unfortunately is quite common, because of confusion of borderline characteristics with the behaviors exhibited during active alcohol and drug use and early recovery. Although the *DSM-IV* (APA, 1994) introduced clear criteria for differential diagnosis, patients diagnosed before that time or from settings in which diagnostic rigor is not the norm may be improperly classified. Thus, it is advisable to reconsider the diagnosis. This reconsideration is especially important because borderline patients are viewed in many settings as difficult and unrewarding to treat. Clinicians treating addictive disorder are accustomed to seeing women present with behaviors consistent with borderline personality disorder, who settle down markedly and look far less pathologic with a year or so of sobriety and a good recovery program.

Enduring characteristics of borderline personality disorder include unstable mood and self image; unstable, intense, interpersonal relationships; extremes of overidealization and devaluation; and marked shifts from baseline to impulsive outbursts, anxiety states, or other extreme moods. Prevalence of borderline personality disorder is estimated to be about 2% of the general population, 10% of those seen in outpatient mental health clinics, and 20% of psychiatric inpatients. Women constitute about 75% of those with the diagnosis (APA, 2000).

Initial formulations and discussion of borderline personality disorder emerged from the psychoanalytic tradition and predated the empirical literature that established a relationship between borderline pathology and childhood physical and sexual abuse. This tradition downplayed the possibility that abuse experiences were real, in favor of the view that fantasy distortion, strong impulses in a weak ego structure, maternal conflicts, and separation and loss experiences were decisive. The possibility that fearfulness, anger, and suspicion of the borderline patient might have its roots in real childhood trauma was minimized (van der Kolk, 1994). Cultural denial of childhood abuse was pervasive until the attention to PTSD created a knowledge base that revised earlier notions about abuse as mere fantasy (Herman, 1992a, 1992b). Herman, van der Kolk, and others have explored the possibility that actual traumatic experiences play a key role in the etiology of borderline pathology.

SPECIAL POPULATIONS

Variations in cultural subgroups and sexual orientation also play an important role in treatment. Gender roles vary greatly, especially among immigrant groups, in which the degree of acculturation determines many of the constraints on the woman's role. Use of alcohol and other drugs may be taboo for women, so recognition of their use, or seeking treatment for problems related to use, may be impossible. Those from patriarchal cultures can face strong taboos about disclosing family secrets, especially around interpersonal violence. Women can fear abandonment if they violate cultural norms. Those disclosing sexual violations can risk severe devaluation within or expulsion from their community, and they can lack the hope for improvement that could propel them past this barrier. Institutional racism causes many to fear the police, social services, and mental health agencies that might provide alternative resources (Brainin-Rodriguez, 1998; Comas-Dias & Greene, 1994). Culturally sensitive and specific education and prevention messages

have begun to be developed for some women in some subgroups, but much more work in this area remains to be done.

Another subgroup of women is at particular risk because of the extensive use of alcohol and drugs as part of the culture. The subculture of lesbian women influences the risk factors and treatment-seeking behavior of this group. Socializing patterns built around bars and drug-sharing increase the risk of addiction but do not necessarily lead to recognition of the attendant problems. These women generally are more dependent on lesbian friendship networks than on families of origin or marital bonds, and their adaptive system of mutual reliance may be inappropriately pathologized as codependence. Historically, lesbian bars were seen as gathering places and safe arenas for self-expression and, in many areas, they still are the only place where such behavior can occur. Even when problems are recognized, they can avoid treatment agencies if they fear discrimination or lack of understanding about their specific needs (Hall, 1993).

ADDITIONAL TREATMENT ISSUES

Management and Retention Issues. New work on readiness to change shows promise for improving women's treatment. Brown and colleagues (Brown, Melchior et al., 2000) noted that candidates for addiction treatment can vary in their commitment to make changes in a variety of areas that will affect their prospects. They have developed a Steps of Change Model that covers four areas in which changes may be relevant: (1) domestic violence, (2) risky sexual behaviors, (3) addictive disorder behaviors, and (4) emotional problems. Their work supports the hypothesis that the most immediate or threatening problems will be what a woman focuses on first, and she selects her treatment modality accordingly. Women with addictive disorders who are in domestic violence situations are relatively resistant to addressing their alcohol and drug use. They are preoccupied with achieving greater safety and see their alcohol and other drug problems as secondary. By contrast, women with other mental health problems are more receptive to treatment for their addictive disorders. Treatment providers need to be willing to start by addressing those problems the woman is most ready to change while cultivating readiness in other areas identified by the clinician as important for long-term success.

The epidemiologic finding that women have high rates of three or more disorders has consequences for treatment.

The number and severity of problems experienced by women clients, as well as related problems experienced by staff and community members, can be translated into a measure of level of burden. In studies of high burden clients, such women tend to be at greatest risk of early termination and poor outcomes even when they do remain in treatment for longer periods of time (Brown, Huba et al., 1995). Integrated treatment for multiple disorders thus is especially important in designing or selecting a treatment program to meet women's needs.

It generally is agreed by providers that women-only programs or activities are an important aspect of effective treatment, although research on this question has not been systematic and findings are inconclusive. An examination of the services offered in women-only programs compared with mixed-gender programs in southern California found that the most consistent difference was the provision of services specific to women's needs, particularly those associated with pregnancy and parenting (Grella, Polinsky et al., 1999). These services included parenting classes; children's activities; and pediatric, prenatal, and postpartum services. Women-only programs also were more likely to assist with housing, transportation, job training, and practical skills training. Thus, even though programs can present themselves as doing individualized treatment planning, women-only programs appear to be better equipped to meet women's needs. These programs also were more likely to be funded through the Medicaid system instead of fees or private insurance, reflecting the lower socioeconomic status of their client population.

Physical and Sexual Abuse and Domestic Violence. Although more than a third of women with PTSD fail to recover after many years, even with professional treatment, the average duration of symptoms was shorter among women in treatment (Kessler, Sonnega et al., 1995), suggesting that existing treatments did confer some benefit. Co-occurring psychopathology typically is associated with less-favorable treatment outcomes. However, in a study by Gil-Rivas, Fiorentine et al. (1997), abused clients were more likely than their non-abused counterparts to participate in counseling and just as likely to complete treatment and remain drug-free during and up to 6 months after treatment.

It has been noted that children with battered mothers experience posttraumatic stress reactions themselves. These children often are subjected to ongoing marital conflict, family dysfunction, dislocations and relocations of home, lack of parental care, economic and social disadvantage, and in-teractions with the police and court. Preschool children are more vulnerable to the effects of domestic violence (Campbell & Lewandowski, 1997) than older children.

Children develop a variety of other problems in response to traumatic events, including thought suppression, sleep problems, exaggerated startle responses, developmental regressions, deliberate avoidances, panic, irritability, psychophysiologic disturbances, hypervigilance, and fear of recurrence. Children can engage in repetitive play in which the trauma is reenacted, cope by psychic numbing and withdrawal, show uncharacteristic behavior patterns, and/or become fearful of mundane things (Campbell & Lewandowski, 1997). Cognitive and emotional problems include a preoccupation with physical aggression, withdrawal and suicidal ideation, anxiety, depression, and social withdrawal. Behavioral problems include conduct problems, hyperactivity, diminished social competence, school problems, bullying, truancy, clinging behaviors, and speech disorders. Physical symptoms include bed-wetting, sleep disturbances, headaches, gastrointestinal problems, and failure to thrive (Campbell & Lewandowski, 1997). The extensive variety and complexity of children's reactions to domestic violence argue for routine assessment and case management for these families.

Treatment Culture. Women clients and treatment providers have noted that the male-dominated treatment culture characteristic of some programs (particularly many therapeutic communities) is not conducive to meeting women's needs (Brown, Sanchez et al., 1996). They stress the importance of a more supportive and less confrontational approach to treatment. In addition to the gender imbalance in the client population, reliance on aggressive confrontation contributed to premature dropout and a treatment environment that did not seem safe enough to explore vulnerable issues. An emphasis on harsh confrontation is particularly problematic in populations with a high frequency of traumatic experiences. Treatment methods that exacerbate a woman's sense of powerlessness discourage her from revealing and exploring key issues. In addition, women with severe psychiatric disorders can decompensate and leave treatment if confrontation is too intense. Reducing the emphasis on confrontation and broadening the skill base of clinicians has proved a difficult task in some treatment modalities, particularly those that rely primarily on staff members without advanced professional training. Although these practitioners may have extensive training and many have acquired addiction credentials, the style of intervention they learned first is difficult to change, particularly if it involves role models who were important in personal recovery.

Both the National Institute on Drug Abuse (NIDA) and the Center for Substance Abuse Treatment (CSAT) have funded specialized research and treatment demonstration programs focused on women, and these programs have enhanced the development of provider groups committed to improving women's treatment. Additional resources made available through CSAT's Addiction Technology Transfer Centers, launched in the mid-1990s, made it easier to broaden the skill base of front-line practitioners working with an indigent population. There appears to be less coordinated activity focused on women in treatment facilities that serve the insured population.

Provider groups serving women also emphasize the importance of female leadership at all levels of the organization to serve as role models and to avoid perpetuating the view that major decisionmaking influence is reserved for men. Some programs hire only female staff members to simplify the task of dealing with sensitive issues such as incest, rape, and battering. Male staff members in a residential program are in a difficult situation and must have clear boundaries and a supervision structure that protects them and the patients from potential boundary violations. This situation also is an issue for female staff members, particularly in areas with a large lesbian population, as boundary violations among women usually are more taboo to discuss.

Women and the Criminal Justice System. Women constitute the fastest growing segment of the criminal justice population nationally and yet have the fewest appropriate social services available to them (Wellisch, Anglin et al., 1993). Women today are more likely than men to serve time in prison for drug offenses (Bureau of Justice Statistics, 1994). Between 1982 and 1991, the number of women arrested for drug offenses increased 89% (Wellisch, Anglin et al., 1993). Since 1991, increasing numbers of women have been incarcerated for crimes committed in the service of drug use. Half the women reported committing their crimes while under the influence of drugs or alcohol, and about 40% reported using drugs daily before arrest. Fifty-three percent of the women in federal prison were unemployed at the time of arrest (Bureau of Justice Statistics, 1994).

Typically, incarcerated women report that they started using drugs at an early age. These women commonly were confronted with obstacles such as absent parents, educa-tional setbacks, parenthood, poverty, drug accessibility (Department of Justice Statistics, 1994), and minimal social resources (Wellisch, Anglin et al., 1993). Most came from communities in which crime was rampant. Additionally, most were victims of childhood sexual and/or physical abuse, as well as traumatic experiences as adults. Consequently, they had high rates of depressive and other psychiatric disorders (Jordan, Schlenger et al., 1996). They often suffered from low self-esteem, depression, addiction, and shame, and frequently attempted to self-medicate their struggle with illicit drugs.

Insufficient job skills as a result of poor education undermine self-esteem in incarcerated women. Low income or poverty results in desperation, thus making illegal activities more acceptable, especially in the service of drug use. Major child-rearing responsibilities with inadequate social support systems contribute to the development of psychiatric disorders in mothers and behavior problems in children (Jordan, Schlenger et al., 1996). Thirty-four percent of the women in U.S. prisons report being sexually abused, and another 34% report being physically abused (Bureau of Justice Statistics, 1994). Women's social status and gender roles affect sexual risk behaviors and the ability to take steps to reduce the risk of HIV infection (Amaro, 1995), contributing to the high incidence of HIV in drug-using and incarcerated women.

Intergenerational and familial transmission of drug use and associated criminality makes the obstacles confronting these women more debilitating. National data on women in prison show that 40% of the women reported that an immediate family member also was in jail (Bureau of Justice Statistics, 1994). In California, 59% of inmate women reported that family members were currently incarcerated (Arnaudy, Lee et al., 1996). One-third of the inmates reported that a parent or guardian had abused drugs or alcohol. For these and other complex and interwoven factors, it is necessary to intervene decisively in prison pre-release programs to break the cycle of drug use and criminality and to include family members in the treatment experience whenever possible.

Prison-based treatment is growing rapidly, and specialized programs for women are included in this development. Both research and clinical experience indicate that community-based services after treatment in prison significantly increases the percentage of offenders who remain drug-free 18 months after release. Thus, programs in large states such as California emphasize the importance of a seamless transition to services in the community and provide substantial funding to accomplish these goals.

CONCLUSIONS

Although gender differences have been well-studied in specific areas, there are many gaps in our understanding. Biomedical effects are far better understood for alcohol than for the illicit drugs. Research and treatment funding incentives over the past 20 years have provided a much better understanding of women's treatment needs and preferences. Removing obvious barriers, such as transportation and child care, increases women's participation in treatment. Treatment for women must be comprehensive, including their spouses, partners, and children. Research is needed to determine how best to intervene with children to reduce the negative effects of their parents' addictive disorders.

Programs need to be capable of addressing co-occurring mood and anxiety disorders, particularly PTSD and eating disorders. When queried, women report that women-only groups and other activities and role models at all levels of decisionmaking in the organization are important to them. It is to be hoped that controlled research will clarify which gender-specific components are most influential in improving outcomes.

REFERENCES

Amaro H (1995). Love, sex and power. Considering women's realities in HIV prevention. *American Psychologist* 50(6):437-447.

Amaro H & Hardy-Fanta C (1995). Gender relations in addiction and recovery. *Journal of Psychoactive Drugs* 27(4):325-356.

Amaro H, Zuckerman B & Cabral H (1989). Drug use among adolescent mothers: A profile of risk. *Pediatrics* 84:144-151.

American Psychiatric Association (APA) (1994). *Diagnostic and Statistical Manual of Mental Disorders, 4th Edition (DSM-IV)*. Washington DC: American Psychiatric Press.

American Psychiatric Association (APA) (2000). *Diagnostic and Statistical Manual of Mental Disorders, 4th Edition (DSM-IV-TR)*. Washington DC: American Psychiatric Press.

Anglin MD, Hser YI & McGothlin W (1987). Sex differences in addict careers II: Becoming addicted. *American Journal of Drug and Alcohol Abuse* 13(1-2):59-71.

Arnaudy M, Lee S & Relojo E (1996). *Report on the Health Care Status of Incarcerated Women*. San Francisco, CA: Department of Public Health.

Becker U, Deis A, Sorensen TI et al. (1996). Prediction of risk of liver disease by alcohol intake, sex and age: A prospective population study. *Hepatology* 23(5):1025-1029.

Blume S (1992). Alcohol and other drug problems in women. In JH Lowinson, P Ruiz, RB Millman et al. (eds.) *Substance Abuse: A Comprehensive Textbook*. Baltimore, MD: Williams and Wilkins, 794-807.

Blume SB (1998). Understanding addictive disorders in women. In AW Graham & TK Schultz (eds.) *Principles of Addiction Medicine, Second Edition*. Chevy Chase, MD: American Society of Addiction Medicine.

Boyd CJ, Blow F & Orgain LS (1993). Gender differences among African-Americans. *Journal of Psychoactive Drugs* 25(4):301-305.

Brainin-Rodriguez J-E (1998). Traumatic experiences in substance abusing women. Paper presented at the Traumatic Experiences in Substance Abusing Women: Implications for Recovery, San Francisco, CA; January 29.

Breslau N, Davis GC, Andreski P et al. (1991). Traumatic events and posttraumatic stress disorder in an urban population of young adults. *Archives of General Psychiatry* 48:216-222.

Breslau N, Davis GC, Andreski P et al. (1997a). Sex differences in post-traumatic stress disorder. *Archives of General Psychiatry* 54(11):1044-1048.

Breslau N, Davis GC, Peterson EL et al. (1997b). Psychiatric sequelae of posttraumatic stress disorder in women. *Archives of General Psychiatry* 54(1):81-87.

Brown S & Schuckit M (1988). Changes in depression among abstinent alcoholics. *Journal of Studies on Alcohol* 49(5):412-417.

Brown SS, Inaba RK, Gillin JC et al. (1995). Alcoholism and affective disorder; clinical course of depressive symptoms. *American Journal of Psychiatry* 152(1):45-51.

Brown V, Sanchez S, Zweben JE et al. (1996). Challenges in moving from a traditional therapeutic community to a women and children's TC model. *Journal of Psychoactive Drugs* 28(1):39-46.

Brown VB, Huba GJ & Melchior LA (1995). Level of burden: Women with more than one co-occurring disorder. *Journal of Psychoactive Drugs* 27(4):321-325.

Brown VB, Melchior LA, Panter AT et al. (2000). Women's steps of change and entry into drug abuse treatment. A multidimensional stages of change model. *Journal of Substance Abuse Treatment* 18(3):231-240.

Bureau of Justice Statistics (1994). *Women in Prison*. Washington, DC: U.S. Department of Justice.

Campbell JC & Lewandowski LA (1997). Mental and physical health effects of intimate partner violence on women and children. *Psychiatry Clinics of North America* 20(2):353-374.

Carmona GN, Tella SR, Greig NH et al. (1999). The gender-specified psychomotor stimulatory effects of cocaine may not be due to hepatic mechanisms. In LS Harris (ed.) *Problems of Drug Dependence, 1998 (NIDA Research Monograph 179)*. Bethesda, MD: National Institute on Drug Abuse, 149.

Chung JY & Magraw MM (1992). A group approach to psychosocial issues faced by HIV-positive women. *Hospital & Community Psychiatry* 43(9):981-894.

Comas-Dias L & Greene B, eds. (1994). *Women of Color: Integrating Ethnic and Gender Identities in Psychotherapy*. New York, NY: Guilford Press.

Dansky BS, Brady KT, Saladin ME et al. (1996). Victimization and PTSD in individuals with substance use disorders: Gender and racial differences. *American Journal of Drug Alcohol Abuse* 22(1):75-93.

Dawson D & Archer L (1992). Gender differences in alcohol consumption: Effects of measurement. *British Journal of Addiction* 87(1):119-123.

Finkelhor D & Dziuba-Leatherman D (1994). Victimization of children. *American Psychologist* 49(3):173-183.

Gastfriend DR & Lillard P (1998). Anxiety disorders. In AW Graham & TK Schultz (eds.) *Principles of Addiction Medicine, Second Edition*. Chevy Chase, MD: American Society of Addiction Medicine, 993-1006.

Gil-Rivas V, Fiorentine R, Anglin MD et al. (1997). Sexual and physical abuse: Do they compromise drug treatment outcomes? *Journal of Substance Abuse Treatment* 14(4):351-358.

Green BL (1994). Psychosocial research in traumatic stress: An update. *Journal of Traumatic Stress* 7:341-362.

Greene JM, Marsden ME, Sanchez RP et al. (2000). *National Household Survey on Drug Abuse: Main Findings 1998*. Rockville, MD: Department of Health and Human Services, Office of Applied Studies.

Grella CE, Polinsky ML, Hser YI et al. (1999). Characteristics of women-only and mixed-gender drug abuse treatment programs. *Journal of Substance Abuse Treatment* 17(1-2):37-44.

Hall JM (1993). Lesbians and alcohol: Patterns and paradoxes in medical notions and lesbians' beliefs. *Journal of Psychoactive Drugs* 25(2):109-119.

Herman J (1992a). Complex PTSD: A syndrome in survivors of prolonged and repeated trauma. *Journal of Traumatic Stress* 5:377-391.

Herman J (1992b). *Trauma and Recovery*. New York, NY: Basic Books.

Holderness CC, Brooks-Gunn J & Warren MP (1994). Co-morbidity of eating disorders and substance abuse review of the literature. *International Journal of Eating Disorders* 16(1):1-34.

Hser YI, Anglin MD & McGlothlin W (1987). Sex differences in addict career, I: Initiation of use. *American Journal of Drug and Alcohol Abuse* 13(1-2):33-57.

Janikowski TP & Glover NM (1994). Incest and substance abuse: Implications for treatment professionals. *Journal of Substance Abuse Treatment* 11(3):177-183.

Jordan KB, Schlenger WE, Fairbank JA et al. (1996). Prevalence of psychiatric disorders in incarcerated women. II. Convicted felons entering prison. *Archives of General Psychiatry* 53:513-519.

Kendler KS, Bulik CM, Silberg J et al. (2000). Childhood sexual abuse and adult psychiatric and substance use disorders in women. *Archives of General Psychiatry* 57:953-959.

Kessler RC, McGonagle KA, Zhao S et al. (1994). Lifetime and 12 month prevalence of DSM-IIIR psychiatric disorders in the United States. *Archives of General Psychiatry* 51:8-19.

Kessler RC, Sonnega A, Bromet E et al. (1995). Posttraumatic stress disorder in the National Comorbidity Survey. *Archives of General Psychiatry* 52(12):1048-1060.

Koss MP & Burkhart BR (1989). A conceptual analysis of rape victimization. *Psychology of Women Quarterly* 13:27-40.

Koss MP, Goodman LA, Browne A et al. (1994). *No Safe Heaven: Male Violence Against Women at Home, at Work, and in the Community*. Washington DC: American Psychological Association.

Krahn D, Kurth C, Demitrack M et al. (1992). The relationship of dieting severity and bulimic behaviors to alcohol and other drug use in young women. *Journal of Substance Abuse* 4(4):341-353.

Krahn DD (1991). The relationship of eating disorders and substance abuse. *Journal of Substance Abuse* 3(2):239-253.

Marcus RN & Katz JL (1990). Inpatient care of the substance-abusing patient with a concomitant eating disorder. *Hospital & Community Psychiatry* 41(1):59-63.

McCance-Katz EF, Carroll KM & Rounsaville BJ (1999). Gender differences in treatment-seeking cocaine abusers—Implications for treatment and prognosis. *American Journal on Addictions* 8:300-311.

Mee-Lee D, Shulman G, Fishman M et al. (2001). *ASAM Patient Placement Criteria for the Treatment of Substance-Related Disorders, Second Edition-Revised (ASAM PPC-2R)*. Chevy Chase, MD: American Society of Addiction Medicine.

Mendelson JH, Sholar MB, Mello NK et al. (1999). Cocaine pharmacokinetics in men and in women during two phases of the menstrual cycle. In LS Harris (ed.) *Problems of Drug Dependence, 1998 (NIDA Research Monograph 179)*. Rockville, MD: National Institute on Drug Abuse, 149.

Mumenthaler MS, Taylor JL, O'Hara R et al. (1999). Gender differences in moderate drinking effects. *Alcohol Research & Health* 23(1):55-64.

National Institute on Alcohol Abuse and Alcoholism (NIAAA) (2000). *10th Special Report to the U.S. Congress on Alcohol and Health*. Rockville, MD: U.S. Department of Health and Human Services.

Rand MR & Strom K (1997). *Violence-Related Injuries Treated in Hospital Emergency Departments (Bureau of Justice Statistics Special Report NCJ-156921)*. Washington, DC: Bureau of Justice.

Regier DA, Farmer ME, Rae DS et al. (1990). Comorbidity of mental disorders with alcohol and other drug abuse. *Journal of the American Medical Association* 264(19):2511-2518.

Root MP (1989). Treatment failures: The role of sexual victimization in women's addictive behavior. *American Journal of Orthopsychiatry* 59(4):542-549.

Russell SA & Wilsnack S (1991). Adults survivors of childhood sexual abuse: Substance abuse and other consequences. In P Roth (ed.) *Alcohol and Drugs Are Women's Issues, Vol. I*. Netuchen, NJ: Women's Action Alliance and The Scarecrow Press.

Sell SL, Scalzitti JM, Thomas ML et al. (1999). The influence of ovarian hormones on the acute locomotor response to cocaine in female rats. In LS Harris (ed.) *Problems of Drug Dependence, 1998 (NIDA Monograph 179)*. Rockville, MD: National Institute on Drug Abuse, 148.

Sholar MB, Mendelson JH, Mello NK et al. (1999). Gender differences in ACTH and cortisol response to I.V. cocaine administration. In LS Harris (ed.) *Problems of Drug Dependence, 1998 (NIDA Research Monograph 179)*. Rockville, MD: National Institute on Drug Abuse, 150.

Sofuoglu M, Dudish-Poulsen S, Nelson D et al. (1999). Subjective effects of cocaine are altered by gender and menstrual phase in humans. In LM Harris (ed.) *Problems of Drug Dependence, 1998 (NIDA Research Monograph 179)*. Rockville, MD: National Institute on Drug Abuse, 150.

Teets JM (1997). The incidence and experience of rape among chemically dependent women. *Journal of Psychoactive Drugs* 29(4):331-336.

van der Kolk B (1994). The body keeps score: Memory and the evolving psychobiology of posttraumatic stress. *Harvard Review of Psychiatry* 1(5):253-265.

Wasserman DA, Havassy BE & Boles SM (1997). Traumatic events and post-traumatic stress disorder in cocaine users entering private treatment. *Drug and Alcohol Dependence* 46(1-2):1-8.

Wellisch J, Anglin MD & Prendergast ML (1993). Numbers and characteristics of drug-using women in the criminal justice system: Implications for treatment. *Journal of Drug Issues* 23:7-30.

Wilson GT (1997). Eating disorders and addictive disorders. In KD Brownell & CG Fairburn (eds.) *Eating Disorders and Obesity: A Comprehensive Handbook*. New York, NY: Guilford Press.

Woolfolk DR, McCreary AC & Cunningham KA (1999). An electrophysiologic study of ventral tegmental area dopamine neurons in male vs. female rats. In LS Harris (ed.) *Problems in Drug Dependence, 1998 (NIDA Research Monograph 179)*. Rockville, MD: National Institute on Drug Abuse, 148.

Yandow V (1989). Alcoholism in women. *Psychiatric Annals* 19:243-247.

Young NK (1997). Effects of alcohol and other drugs on children. *Journal of Psychoactive Drugs* 29(1):23-42.

Zweben JE, Clark HW & Smith DE (1994). Traumatic experiences and substance abuse: Mapping the territory. *Journal of Psychoactive Drugs* 26(4):327-345.

| Chapter 14 | # Special Issues in Treatment: Older Adults |

Frederic C. Blow, Ph.D.

An Invisible Epidemic
Drinking Practices and Problems Among Older Adults
Problems With Prescription and OTC Medications
Screening and Assessment
Approaches to Treatment

Substance abuse, particularly of alcohol and prescription drugs, among adults 60 years and older is one of the fastest growing health problems facing the country. Yet, even as the number of older adults suffering from these disorders climbs, the situation remains underestimated, underidentified, underdiagnosed, and undertreated. Until relatively recently, alcohol and prescription drug misuse, which affect up to 17% of older adults, was not discussed in either the addiction or gerontology literature (D'Archangelo, 1993; NIAAA, 1988; Minnis, 1988; Atkinson, 1984, 1990).

AN INVISIBLE EPIDEMIC

Because of insufficient knowledge, limited research data, and hurried office visits, health care providers often overlook alcohol and drug misuse and abuse among older adults. Diagnosis can be difficult because symptoms of addictive disorders in older individuals sometimes mimic symptoms of other medical and behavioral disorders often seen in this population, such as diabetes, dementia, and depression. Drug trials of new medications often do not include older subjects, so a clinician has no way of predicting or recognizing an adverse reaction or unexpected psychoactive effect.

Other factors responsible for the lack of attention to addictive disorders in older adults include fears of cohort disapproval of and shame about use and misuse of substances, along with a reluctance to seek professional help for what many older adults consider a private matter. In the same vein, relatives of older individuals with substance use disorders, and particularly their adult children, often are ashamed of the problem and choose not to address it. "Ageism" also contributes to the problem and to the silence, in that younger adults often unconsciously assign different quality-of-life standards to older adults. Such attitudes are reflected in remarks like, "Grandmother's cocktails are the only thing that makes her happy," or "What difference does it make; he won't be around much longer anyway."

There is an unspoken but pervasive assumption that it is not worth treating older adults for substance use disorders. Behaviors that are considered a problem in younger adults do not inspire the same urgency when they occur in older adults. Along with the impression that alcohol or drug problems cannot be successfully treated in older adults, there is an assumption that treatment for this population is a waste of health care resources.

These attitudes not only are callous, they also rest on misperceptions. Most older adults can and do live independently: less than 5% of adults over age 65 live in nursing or personal care homes. Moreover, Grandmother's cocktails are not cheering her up: Older adults who "self-medicate" with alcohol or prescription drugs are more likely to characterize themselves as lonely and to report lower levels of life satisfaction (Hendricks, Johnson et al., 1991). Older women with alcohol problems are more likely to have had a problem-drinking spouse, to have lost their spouses to death, to have experienced depression, and to have been injured in falls (Wilsnack & Wilsnack, 1995).

The reality is that misuse and abuse of alcohol and other drugs take a greater toll on affected older adults than on younger adults. In addition to the psychosocial issues that are unique to older adults, aging also ushers in biomedical changes that influence the effects that alcohol and drugs have on the body. Alcohol abuse, for example, can accelerate the normal decline in physiologic functioning that occurs with age (Gambert & Katsoyannis, 1995). In addition, alcohol misuse can elevate older adults' already high risk of injury, illness, and socioeconomic decline (Tarter, 1995).

Alcohol Disorders. Problems stemming from alcohol consumption, including the interaction of alcohol with prescribed and over-the-counter (OTC) drugs, far outnumber any other addictive disorder among older adults. Community prevalence rates range from 3% to 25% for "heavy alcohol use" and from 2.2% to 9.6% for "alcohol abuse," depending on the population sampled (Liberto, Oslin et al., 1992). A study found that 15% of men and 12% of women aged 60 years and older who were treated in primary care clinics regularly drank in excess of limits recommended by the National Institute on Alcohol Abuse and Alcoholism (NIAAA; that is, no more than one drink per day) (Saunders, 1994; Adams, Barry et al., 1996; NIAAA, 1995).

The differences in the prevalence rates resulting from these studies illustrate the difficulty in identifying exactly how widespread the current problem is. One researcher has suggested that alcohol abuse among older adults is easily hidden, partly because of its similarities to other diseases common as one ages and partly because elders remind clinicians of a parent or grandparent (Beresford, 1995). Studies in Australia and similar data from the United States (Curtis, Geller et al., 1989) found that clinicians recognized alcoholism in only a third of older hospitalized patients who had the disorder. Moreover, many of the signs and symptoms of alcohol abuse among younger populations are not so easily detected in older adults, simply because most older adults no longer are in the work force, have smaller social networks, and drive less often.

Problems With Prescription Drugs. The abuse of illicit drugs is rare among older adults, except for those who abused them in their younger years (Jinks & Raschko, 1990; Myers, Weissman et al., 1984). Prescribed opioids are an infrequent problem as well: only 2% to 3% of noninstitutionalized older adults receive prescriptions for opioid analgesics (Ray, Thapa et al., 1993) and most of those do not develop problems with those drugs. One study, for example, found that only 4 of nearly 12,000 patients who were prescribed morphine for self-administration became addicted (Hill & Chapman, 1989).

Although little published information exists, a far greater concern for drug misuse or abuse is the large number of older adults using prescription sedative-hypnotics, particularly benzodiazepines, without proper physician supervision (Gomberg, 1992). Older patients are prescribed benzodiazepines more than any other age group, and North American studies demonstrate that 17% to 23% of drugs prescribed to older adults are benzodiazepines (D'Archangelo, 1993). The dangers associated with these prescription drugs include problematic effects because of age-related changes in drug metabolism, interactions among prescriptions, and interactions with alcohol.

Unfortunately, these agents, especially those with longer half-lives, often result in unwanted side effects that influence functional capacity and cognition, which place the older person at greater risk of falling and for institutionalization (Roy & Griffin, 1990). Older users of these drugs experience more adverse effects than do younger adults, including excessive daytime sedation, ataxia, and cognitive impairment. Attention, memory, physiologic arousal, and psychomotor abilities often are impaired as well, and drug-related delirium or dementia can be wrongly labeled as Alzheimer's disease.

DRINKING PRACTICES AND PROBLEMS AMONG OLDER ADULTS

Despite a certain heterogeneity in drinking practices, there are substantial differences between an older and a younger adult's response to alcohol, most of which stem from the physiologic changes wrought by the aging process.

Adults older than age 65 are more likely to be affected by at least one chronic illness, many of which can make them more vulnerable to the negative effects of alcohol consumption. In addition, three age-related changes significantly affect the way an older person responds to alcohol: (1) a decrease in body water, (2) an increase in sensitivity and a decrease in tolerance to alcohol, and (3) a decrease in the metabolism of alcohol in the gastrointestinal tract.

As lean body mass decreases with age, total body water also decreases, while fat increases. Because alcohol is water soluble and not fat soluble, this change in body water means that, for a given dose of alcohol, the concentration of alcohol in the bloodstream is greater in an older person than in a younger person. For this reason, the same amount of alcohol that has little effect in youth can cause intoxication in the older person (Smith, 1995; Vestal, McGuire et al., 1977). This effect explains the increased sensitivity and decreased tolerance to alcohol as individuals age. Researchers speculate that the change in relative alcohol content, combined with slower reaction times frequently observed in older adults, are responsible for some of the accidents and injuries that plague this age group (Salthouse, 1985; Ray, 1992).

The decrease in gastric alcohol dehydrogenase enzyme that occurs with age is another factor that exacerbates problems with alcohol. This enzyme plays a key role in the absorption of alcohol in the gastric mucosa. With decreased alcohol dehydrogenase, alcohol is metabolized more slowly, so the blood alcohol level remains elevated for a longer period of time. With the stomach less actively involved in metabolism, an increased strain is placed on the liver (Smith, 1995).

Comorbidities. Although alcohol can negatively affect a person of any age, the interaction of age-related physiologic changes and the consumption of alcohol can trigger or exacerbate other serious problems, including the following:

- Increased risk of hypertension, cardiac arrhythmia, myocardial infarction, and cardiomyopathy;

- Increased risk of hemorrhagic stroke;

- Impairments in the immune system;

- Cirrhosis and other liver diseases;

- Decreased bone density;

- Gastrointestinal bleeding;

- Depression, anxiety, and other mental health problems; and

- Malnutrition.

Other biomedical changes that occur with aging include cognitive impairments, which are both confused with and exacerbated by alcohol use. Chronic alcoholism can cause serious, irreversible changes in brain function, although this change is more likely to be seen in older adults who have a long history of alcoholism. Alcohol use also can have direct neurotoxic effects, leading to a characteristic syndrome called alcohol-related dementia (ARD) or can be associated with the development of other dementing illnesses such as Alzheimer's disease or Wernicke-Korsakoff's syndrome, an illness characterized by anterograde memory deficits, gait ataxia, and nystagmus. Indeed, several researchers have cast doubt on the existence of ARD as a neuropathologic disease and suggest that most cases of ARD are, in fact, Wernicke-Korsakoff's syndrome.

Sleep patterns typically change with increasing age (Haponik, 1992). Increased episodes of sleep with rapid eye movement (REM), decreased REM length, decreased stage III and IV sleep, and increased awakenings are common, all of which can be worsened by alcohol use. Moeller and colleagues (1993) demonstrated in younger subjects that alcohol and depression had additive effects on sleep disturbances when they occur together.

One study concluded that sleep disturbances, especially insomnia, can be a potential etiologic factor in the development of late-life alcohol problems or in precipitating relapse to alcohol use. This hypothesis is supported by a study demonstrating that abstinent alcoholics experienced insomnia, frequent awakenings, and REM fragmentation. However, when the subjects ingested alcohol, sleep periodicity normalized and REM sleep was temporarily suppressed, suggesting that alcohol may be used by some older adults to self-medicate for sleep disturbances.

Classifying Drinking Practices and Problems Among Older Adults. Physiologic changes, as well as changes in the kinds of responsibilities and activities pursued by older adults, make established criteria for classifying alcohol problems largely irrelevant to this population.

Two classic models for understanding alcohol problems—the medical diagnostic model and the at-risk, heavy, and problem drinking classification—include criteria that may not adequately apply to many older adults and may lead to underidentification of drinking problems (Atkinson, 1990).

TABLE 1.   Applying DSM-IV Diagnostic Criteria to Older Adults

Diagnostic criteria for alcohol dependence are subsumed within the DSM-IV's *general criteria for substance dependence. Dependence is defined as a "maladaptive pattern of substance use, leading to clinically significant impairment or distress, as manifested by three (or more) of the following, occurring at any time in the same 12-month period" (American Psychiatric Association, 1994, p. 181). There are special considerations when applying DSM-IV criteria to older adults with alcohol problems.*

Criteria	Special Considerations in Older Adults
1. Tolerance	May have problems with even low levels of intake because of increased sensitivity to alcohol and higher blood alcohol levels.
2. Withdrawal	Many late-onset alcoholics do not develop physiologic dependence.
3. Taking larger amounts or over a longer period than was intended.	Increased cognitive impairment can interfere with self-monitoring; drinking may exacerbate cognitive impairment.
4. Unsuccessful efforts to cut down or control use	Same issues across the lifespan.
5. Spending much time to obtain and use alcohol and to recover from its effects	Negative effects can occur at relatively low levels of use.
6. Giving up activities because of use	May engage in fewer activities, making detection of problems more difficult.
7. Continuing use despite physical or psychological problems caused by use	May not know or understand that problems are related to use, even after medical advice.

SOURCE: Modified from American Psychiatric Association (1994). *Diagnostic and Statistical Manual of Mental Disorders, 4th Edition (DSM-IV).* Washington, DC: American Psychiatric Press.

DSM-IV: Most clinicians rely on the conventional medical model defined in the American Psychiatric Association's *Diagnostic and Statistical Manual of Mental Disorders, Fourth Edition (DSM-IV*; 1994) for classifying the signs and symptoms of alcohol-related problems. The *DSM-IV* employs specific criteria to distinguish between those drinkers who abuse alcohol and those who are dependent on alcohol.

Although widely used, the *DSM-IV* criteria (Table 1) may not apply to many older adults who do not experience the specified legal, social, or psychological consequences of alcohol use. For example, the criterion that describes "a failure to fulfill major role obligations at work, school, or home" is less applicable to a retired person who has minimal familial responsibilities. Nor does the criterion "continued use of the substance(s) despite persistent or recurrent problems" always apply. Many older alcoholics do not realize that their persistent or recurrent problems are, in fact, related to their drinking, a view likely to be reinforced by health care professionals who often attribute such problems, in whole or in part, to the aging process or age-related comorbidities.

Although tolerance is one of the *DSM-IV* criteria for a diagnosis of substance dependence—and one weighted heavily by clinicians performing an assessment for substance dependence—the thresholds of consumption often considered by clinicians as indicative of tolerance may be set too high for older adults because of their altered sensitivity to and body distribution of alcohol (Atkinson, 1990). The lack of tolerance to alcohol does not necessarily mean that an older adult does not have a drinking problem or is not experiencing serious negative effects as a result of his or her drinking. Furthermore, many late onset alcoholics have not developed physiologic dependence, and they do not exhibit signs of withdrawal.

The drinking practices of many older adults who do not meet the diagnostic criteria for abuse or dependence nevertheless pose a risk of complicating an existing medical or psychiatric disorder. Consuming one or two drinks per day, for example, can lead to increased cognitive impairment in patients who already have Alzheimer's disease, can lead to worsening of sleep problems in patients with sleep apnea, or can interact with medications in a way that alters the therapeutic effect or causes adverse side effects. A barrier to good clinical management in such cases may be the lack of understanding of the risks of so-called "moderate drinking." Limiting access to treatment because symptoms do not meet the rigorous diagnostic criteria of the *DSM-IV* can preclude an older patient from making significant improvements in the quality of his or her life.

At-Risk, Heavy, and Problem Drinking: Some experts on aging issues use the model of at-risk, heavy, and problem drinking in place of the *DSM-IV* model of alcohol abuse and dependence because it allows for more flexibility in characterizing drinking patterns. In this classification scheme, an *at-risk drinker* is one whose patterns of alcohol use, although not yet causing problems, can bring about adverse consequences, either to the drinker or to others. Engaging in occasional moderate drinking at social gatherings and then driving home is an example of at-risk drinking. Although an accident may not occur, all the elements of a disaster are present.

As their names imply, the terms *heavy* and *problem* drinking signify more hazardous levels of consumption than at-risk drinking. Although the distinction between the terms heavy and problem is meaningful to alcohol treatment specialists interested in differentiating severity of problems among younger alcohol abusers, it may have less relevance for older adults (Atkinson & Ganzini, 1994), who may experience pervasive consequences at lower levels of consumption because of their heightened sensitivity to al-

cohol or the presence of such coexisting disorders as diabetes mellitus, hypertension, cirrhosis, or dementia.

In general, the threshold for at-risk alcohol use decreases with advancing age. Although an individual's health and functional status determine the degree of effect, the pharmacokinetic and pharmacodynamic effects of alcohol on aging organ systems result in higher peak blood alcohol levels and increased responsiveness to doses that caused little impairment at a younger age. For example, body sway increases and the capacity to think clearly decrease with age after a standard alcohol load, even when controlling for blood alcohol levels (Beresford & Lucey, 1995; Vogel-Sprott & Barrett, 1984; Vestal, McGuire et al., 1977).

Certain medical conditions, such as hypertension and diabetes mellitus, can be made worse by regular drinking of relatively small amounts of alcohol. In addition, the tendency "to take the edge off" with alcohol during times of stress and its subsequent effect on cognition and problem-solving skills can provoke inadequate or destructive responses, even in those older adults whose overall consumption is less than that of some younger, problem-free social drinkers. Moreover, older drinkers who do not meet the substance abuse criteria for "recurrent use" behavior or consequences nevertheless may pose potential risk to themselves or others.

For many adults, the phenomenon of aging, with its accompanying physical vulnerabilities and distinctive psychosocial demands, may be the key risk factor for alcohol problems. To differentiate older drinkers, a Consensus Panel convened by the Center for Substance Abuse Treatment (CSAT, 1998) recommended using the terms "at-risk" and "problem drinkers" to describe older adults. As discussed earlier, not only do the concepts of quantity/frequency implicit in the term heavy drinking have less application to older populations, but also the "distinction between heavy and problem drinking narrows with age" (Atkinson & Ganzini, 1994, p. 300). In the two-stage conceptualization recommended by the CSAT panel, the "problem drinker" category included those who otherwise would fall into the "heavy" and "problem" drinking classifications in the more traditional model, as well as those who would meet the *DSM-IV* criteria for abuse and dependence.

Age-Appropriate Levels of Consumption. In its *Physician's Guide to Helping Patients With Alcohol Problems*, NIAAA offers recommendations for low-risk drinking. For individuals over the age of 65, NIAAA recommends "no more than one drink per day" (NIAAA, 1995). The

TABLE 2.   Clinical Characteristics of Early and Late Onset Problem Drinkers

Variable	Early Onset	Late Onset
Age at onset	Various: < 25, 40, 45 years	Various: > 55, 60, 65 years
Socioeconomic status	Tends to be lower	Tends to be higher
Drinking in response to stressors	Common	Common
Family history of alcoholism	More prevalent	Less prevalent
Extent and severity of alcohol problems	More psychosocial, legal problems, greater severity	Fewer psychosocial, legal problems, lesser severity
Alcohol-related chronic illness (cirrhosis, pancreatitis, cancers)	More common	Less common
Psychiatric comorbidities	Cognitive loss is more severe, less reversible	Cognitive loss is less severe, more reversible
Age-associated medical problems aggravated by alcohol (hypertension, diabetes mellitus, drug-alcohol interactions)	Common	Common
Treatment compliance and outcome	Possible less compliant; relapse rates do not vary by age of onset (Atkinson et al., 1990; Blow, Walton et al., 1997; Schonfeld & Dupree, 1991).	Possibly more compliant; relapse rates do not vary by age of onset (Atkinson et al., 1990; Blow, Walton et al., 1997; Schonfeld & Dupree, 1991).

SOURCE: Blow FC, ed. (1999). *Substance Abuse Among Older Adults (Treatment Improvement Protocol No. 26).* Rockville, MD: Center for Substance Abuse Treatment.

following refinements of the recommendations also are offered:

- No more than one drink per day;
- A maximum of two drinks on any drinking occasion (New Year's Eve, weddings, and the like); and
- Somewhat lower limits for women.

A standard drink is one can (12 oz.) of beer or ale, a single shot (1.5 oz.) of hard liquor, a glass (5 oz.) of wine, or a small glass (4 oz.) of sherry, liqueur, or aperitif. Promoting these limits helps to establish a "safety zone" for healthy older adults who drink. Older men and women who do not have serious or unstable medical problems and who are not taking psychoactive medications are unlikely to incur problems with alcohol if they adhere to these guidelines. The goal is to foster sensible drinking that avoids health risks, while allowing older adults to obtain the beneficial effects that can accrue from careful use of alcohol.

Drinking Patterns Among Older Adults. Although more research on addictive disorders among older adults is needed, studies to date suggest three ways of categorizing older adults' problem drinking: early versus late onset drinking, continuous versus intermittent drinking, and binge drinking.

Early Onset Versus Late Onset Problem Drinking: One of the most striking and potentially useful findings in contemporary geriatric research is the new understanding about the age at which individuals begin experiencing alcohol-related problems. Although it appears that alcohol use declines with increasing age for most adults (Temple & Leino, 1989), some persons begin to experience alcohol-related problems at about ages 55 to 60 (Table 2).

Early onset drinkers tend to have longstanding alcohol-related problems that generally begin before age 40 (most often in their 20s and 30s). In contrast, late onset drinkers generally experience their first alcohol-related problem after age 40 or 50 (Atkinson, 1984, 1994).

Early Onset Drinkers: Early onset drinkers comprise the majority of older patients who receive treatment for alcohol abuse, and they tend to resemble younger alcohol abusers in their reasons for use. Throughout their lives, early onset drinkers have turned to alcohol to cope with a range of psychosocial or medical problems. Psychiatric comorbidity is common in this group, particularly the major affective disorders (major depression, bipolar disorder) and thought disorders. For the most part, they continue their established abusive drinking patterns as they age (Schonfeld & Dupree, 1991; Atkinson, 1984; Atkinson, Turner et al., 1985).

Late Onset Drinkers: In comparison, late onset drinkers appear to be psychologically and physically healthier. Some studies have found that late onset drinkers are more likely to have begun or to have increased drinking in response to recent losses, such as the death of a spouse or a divorce, a change in health status, or retirement (Hurt, Finlayson et al., 1988; Finlayson, Hurt et al., 1988). Because late onset drinkers have a shorter history of problem drinking and thus fewer health problems than early onset drinkers, health care providers tend to overlook their drinking. In addition, this group's psychological and social pathology, family relationships, past work history, and lack of involvement with the criminal justice system contradict the familiar "picture" of an alcoholic. Late onset drinkers frequently appear too healthy, too "normal" to raise suspicions about problem drinking.

The literature suggests that about a third of older adults with drinking problems are late onset drinkers. Late onset alcoholism often is milder and more amenable to treatment than early onset drinking (Atkinson & Ganzini, 1994), and

it sometimes resolves spontaneously. When appraising their situation, late onset drinkers often view themselves as affected by developmental stages and circumstances related to growing older. Early onset drinkers are more likely to have exacerbated their adverse circumstances through their history of problem alcohol use (Atkinson, 1994).

Data from the Epidemiologic Catchment Area (ECA) study, a large-scale, community-based survey of psychiatric disorders including alcohol abuse and dependence, provide relevant information on the occurrence of late onset alcoholism, which has been defined by various researchers as occurring after ages 40, 45, 50, or 60 years. From the ECA study, 3% of male alcoholics between 50 and 59 years reported first having a symptom of alcoholism after age 49, compared with 15% of those between 60 and 69 and 14% of those between 70 and 79. For women, 16% between 50 and 59 years reported a first symptom of alcoholism after the age of 50, with 24% of women between 60 and 69 and 28% of women between 70 and 79. These percentages suggest that late onset alcoholism is a significant problem, especially among women. (Gender differences are discussed later.)

Both early and late onset problem drinkers appear to use alcohol almost daily, outside social settings, and at home alone. Both are more likely to use alcohol as a palliative, self-medicating measure in response to hurts, losses, and affective changes, rather than as a socializing agent.

Although there is controversy over the issue of whether early and late onset distinctions influence treatment outcomes (Atkinson, 1994), problem onset affects the choice of intervention. For example, late onset problem drinkers usually respond better than early onset drinkers to brief interventions, because late onset problems tend to be milder and are more sensitive to informal social pressure (Atkinson, 1994; Moos, Mertens et al., 1993). The essential similarities and differences between early and late onset drinkers are outlined in Table 2. The most consistent findings concern medical and psychiatric comorbidity; demographic and psychosocial factors are less consistent. Little is known about the effect of early versus late onset on the complications and treatment outcomes of concomitant medication and alcohol use.

Continuous Versus Intermittent Drinking: Another way of understanding patterns of drinking over the lifespan is to look at the timeframes in which people drink and the frequency of their drinking. In contrast to ongoing, continuous drinking, *intermittent drinking* refers to regular, perhaps daily, heavy drinking that has resumed after a stable period of abstinence of three to five years or more (NIAAA, 1995).

Intermittent drinking problems are easy to overlook but crucial to identify. Even problem drinkers who have been sober for many years are at risk of relapse as they age. For this reason, during routine health screenings, it is important for clinicians to take a history that includes both current and lifetime use of alcohol, so as to identify evidence of past alcohol problems. Armed with this information, they can help their older patients anticipate situations that tend to provoke relapse and plan strategies to address them before they occur.

Binge Drinking: Binge drinking generally is defined as short periods of loss of control over drinking, alternating with periods of abstinence or much lighter alcohol use. A *binge* usually is defined as any drinking occasion in which an individual consumes five or more standard drinks. For older adults, a binge is defined as four or more drinks per occasion. Individuals who are alcohol-free throughout the work week, but engage in Friday night or holiday "benders" would be considered binge drinkers.

Identifying older binge drinkers can be difficult because many of the usual clues, including problems in the workplace or arrests for driving while intoxicated, occur less often among aging adults who no longer work or drive. Although research is needed on the natural history of binge drinkers as they age, anecdotal observations indicate that younger binge drinkers who survive to their later years often become continuous or near-daily drinkers.

Risk Factors for Alcohol Abuse. *Gender*: Studies indicate that older men are much more likely than older women to have alcohol-related problems (Myers, Weissman et al., 1984; Atkinson, 1990). Since the issue first was studied, most adults with alcohol problems in old age have been found to have a long history of problem drinking, and most of them have been men (D'Archangelo, 1993; Helzer, Burnam et al., 1991). About 10% of men report a history of heavy drinking at some point in their lives. Forty-three percent of veterans (who can be assumed to be mostly men and mostly alcohol- as opposed to drug-abusers) receiving long-term care were found to have a history of addictive disorders (Joseph, Ganzini et al., 1995; D'Archangelo, 1993).

Men who drink have been found to be two to six times more likely to have medical problems than women who drink (Adams, Yuan et al., 1993), even though women are more vulnerable to the development of cirrhosis.

Older women are less likely to drink and less likely to drink heavily than are older men. The ratio of male-to-female alcoholics, however, is an open question. One study found "a higher than expected number of females" (Beresford, 1995, p. 11), whereas another study of older patients in treatment facilities found a ratio of 2:1 (83 men to 42 women) (Gomberg, 1995).

Epidemiologic studies and clinical research reports consistently suggest a later onset of problem drinking among women (Gomberg, 1995; Hurt, Finlayson et al., 1988; Moos, Mertens et al., 1993). In one study by Gomberg (1995), for example, women reported a mean age at onset of 46.2 years, whereas men reported 27.0 years. Further, 38% of older female patients but only 4% of older male patients reported onset of alcohol problems within the preceding 10 years.

A number of other differences between older male and female alcoholics have been reported: In contrast to men, women are more likely to be widowed or divorced, to have had a problem-drinking spouse, and to have experienced depression (Gomberg, 1993). Women also report more negative effects of alcohol than men, greater use of prescribed psychoactive medications than men, and more drinking with their spouses (Gomberg, 1994).

Although research has not identified any definite risk factors for drinking among older women, Wilsnack and Wilsnack (1995) suggested that increased amounts of free time and lessening of role responsibilities can serve as an etiologic factor. It also should be noted that women generally are more vulnerable than men to social pressure, so their movement into retirement communities where drinking is common probably has an effect.

These differences between men and women have implications for treatment. Women of all ages are less likely than men to appear at treatment facilities. Among older women who may be socially isolated or homebound, outreach is particularly important. Families, physicians, staff of senior centers and senior housing, and the police all play important roles in helping to identify women who have problems with alcohol. To be effective, however, all of these potential outreach agents must be sensitive to women's feelings of stigma, shame, and social censure.

Loss of Spouse: Alcohol abuse is more prevalent among older adults who have been separated or divorced and among men who have been widowed. Some researchers have hypothesized that a significant triad of disorders may be triggered in older men when their wives die, including

---

depression, development of alcohol problems, and suicide. The highest rate of completed suicide among all population groups is in older white men who become depressed and drink heavily after the death of their spouses (NIAAA, 1988; Brennan & Moos, 1996).

Other Losses: As individuals age, they not only lose their spouses but also other family members and friends to death and separation. Retirement can mean loss of income as well as job-related social support systems and the structure and self-esteem that work provides. Other losses include diminished mobility (greater difficulty using public transportation where available, inability to drive or driving limited to the daylight hours, problems walking); impaired sensory capabilities, which may be isolating even when the elder is in physical proximity to others; and declining health because of chronic illnesses.

Health Care Settings: High rates of alcoholism are consistently reported in medical settings, indicating the need for screening and assessment of patients seen for problems other than addictive disorders (Douglass, 1984; Liberto, Oslin et al., 1992; Adams, Barry et al., 1996). Among community-dwelling older adults, investigators have found a prevalence rate of alcoholism in the range of 2% to 15% (Gomberg, 1992b; Adams, Barry et al., 1996), and a rate in the range of 18% to 44% among general medical and psychiatric inpatients (Colsher, Wallace et al., 1990; Saunders, Copeland et al., 1991).

Addictive Disorder Earlier in Life: A strong relationship exists between developing a substance use disorder earlier in life and experiencing a recurrence in later life. Some recovering alcoholics with long periods of sobriety undergo a recurrence of alcoholic drinking as a result of major losses or an excess of discretionary time (Atkinson & Ganzini, 1994). Among the 10% of older men who reported a history of heavy drinking at some point in their lives, widespread physical and social problems occurred in later life (Colsher, Wallace et al., 1990). Drinking problems early in life confer a greater than fivefold risk of late-life psychiatric illness, despite cessation of heavy drinking. Indeed, some research suggests that a previous drinking problem is the strongest predictor of a problem in later life (Welte & Mirand, 1992).

Comorbid Psychiatric Disorders: Estimates of primary mood disorder occurring in older alcoholics vary from 12% to 30% or more (Finlayson, Hurt et al., 1988; Koenig & Blazer, 1996). Although research does not support the notion that mood disorders precede alcoholism in older adults,

there is evidence that such disorders may be either precipitating or maintenance factors in late onset drinking. Depression, for example, appears to precipitate drinking, particularly among women. Some problem drinkers of both sexes who do not meet the clinical criteria for depression often report feeling depressed before the first drink on a drinking day (Dupree, Broskowski et al., 1984; Schonfeld & Dupree, 1991).

Patients with severe cognitive impairment generally drink less than non-impaired alcohol users. Among individuals who are only mildly impaired, however, alcohol use can increase as a reaction to lower self-esteem and perceived loss of memory. Axis II disorders are more likely to be associated with early onset interpersonal and alcohol-related problems and less likely to affect the individual for the first time at age 60 or older. Late onset alcohol abuse is less to be associated with psychological or psychiatric problems and more likely to be linked to age-associated losses. The exception might be the intermittent drinker who has been in control and whose alcohol or psychiatric problems surface again later in life.

Family History of Alcohol Problems: There is substantial cumulative evidence that genetic factors are important in alcohol-related behaviors. For example, researchers studying the genetic vulnerability of a group of male alcoholics contend that such men often have a history of early drinking that worsens over time (Schuckit, 1989).

Although most human genetic studies of alcohol use have been conducted on relatively young subjects, several studies using a twin registry of U.S. veterans have focused on significantly older individuals (Swan, Carmelli et al., 1990). The results of these studies provide strong evidence that drinking behaviors are greatly influenced by genetics throughout the lifespan (Heller & McClearn, 1995; Atkinson, 1984).

Concomitant Substance Use: The substances most commonly abused by older adults in addition to alcohol are nicotine and psychoactive prescription medications. Both nicotine and prescription drug abuse are far more prevalent among older adults who also abuse alcohol than among the general population in this age group (Goldberg, Burchfiel et al., 1994; Colsher, Wallace et al., 1990; Finlayson, Hurt et al., 1988). Concomitant use of prescribed benzodiazepines and alcohol also is common among older adults, especially older women. This concomitant use includes non-abusive use of both substances, which may be harmful even at modest doses: for example, consuming one or two drinks a day in combination with a small dose of a sedative at night. A similar concern is raised by the concomitant use of alcohol and opiates prescribed for pain relief. Although there is little empirical evidence in this area, clinical practice suggests that dual addiction decreases the effectiveness of specific interventions and increases the severity of symptoms.

Although there is little research on the abuse of other illicit substances (heroin, cocaine, marijuana) by older adults, therapists and health care personnel are seeing more older adults who present with symptoms of illicit drug abuse. Many of these older users of illicit drugs obtain their drugs from a younger relative or partner who uses or sells drugs.

Tobacco: Smoking is the major preventable cause of premature death in the U.S., accounting for an estimated 5 million years of potential life lost (U.S. Preventive Services Task Force, 1996). Every year, tobacco smoking is responsible for one of every five American deaths (U.S. Preventive Services Task Force, 1996). Despite these compelling statistics, however, 25.5% of U.S. adults (48 million adults) are current smokers.

Surveys show that cigarette smoking, although fairly widespread among older adults, declines sharply after age 65. In 1994, approximately 28% of men aged 45 to 64 reported current use of cigarettes; among those age 65 and older, however, this figure was only about 13%. In the younger age group (aged 45 to 64), women have lower smoking rates than men, but after age 65, the levels are similar. Approximately 23% of women aged 45 to 64 reported smoking cigarettes in 1994, whereas about 11% of those aged 65 and older currently smoked. Although the trend in use declines with age, the problem remains significant, with more than 4 million older adults smoking regularly.

Smoking is a "major risk factor for at least 6 of the 14 leading causes of death among individuals 60 years and older (that is, heart disease, cerebrovascular disease, chronic obstructive pulmonary disease, pneumonia/influenza, lung cancer, colorectal cancer) and a complicating factor of at least three others" (Cox, 1993, p. 424).

Current cigarette smoking also is "associated with an increased risk of losing mobility in both men and women" (LaCroix, Guralnik et al., 1993). Not surprisingly, older adult smokers have a "70% overall risk of dying prematurely" (Caruthers, 1992, p. 2257), and fewer smokers "make it to the ranks of older adults as compared with nonsmokers and quitters" (Cox, 1993, p. 423). In addition to increasing the risk of disease, smoking also can affect the performance of prescription drugs used to treat chronic disorders. For example, smokers tend to require higher doses of benzodiazepines to achieve efficacy than do nonsmokers (Ciraulo, Shader et al., 1995).

Smoking in older problem drinkers is far more prevalent than in the general older adult population, making tobacco use the most common substance use disorder among older adults. Some researchers estimate that 60% to 70% of older male alcohol users smoke a pack of cigarettes a day (Finlayson, Hurt et al., 1988), an assessment consistent with studies indicating that the prevalence of smoking among alcoholics generally is greater than 80%.

Although there have been few studies on interventions that are especially useful in helping older adults stop smoking, the advantages of quitting at any age are clear (Orleans, Jepson et al., 1994a; Rimer & Orleans, 1994). Two years after stopping, for example, the risk of stroke begins to decrease. Mortality rates for chronic obstructive pulmonary disease decline; bronchitis, pneumonia, and other infections decrease; and respiratory symptoms such as cough, wheezing, and sputum production lessen (U.S. Preventive Services Task Force, 1996). As another example, a 60-year-old male smoker who quits can expect to reduce his risk of smoking-related illness by about 10% over the next 15 years (Cox, 1993).

As with alcohol and drug abuse, studies suggest that many clinicians fail to counsel patients about the health effects of smoking, despite the fact that older smokers are more likely to quit than younger smokers. Tailoring smoking cessation strategies to older adults so that their unique concerns and barriers to quitting are addressed improves success rates. Brief interventions, for example, can more than double 1-year quit rates for older adults (Rimer & Orleans, 1994). In one study of older smokers who used transdermal nicotine patches, 29% of the subjects quit smoking for 6 months (Orleans et al., 1994a). Because there is little evidence that adults in recovery from alcohol problems relapse when they stop smoking, efforts to reduce substance abuse among older adults also should include tobacco smoking (Hurt, Eberman et al., 1993).

Psychoactive Drugs: Older adults' use of psychoactive drugs combined with alcohol is a growing concern. In a study of inpatients aged 65 and older in an addiction treatment program, 12% had combined dependence on alcohol and one or more prescription drugs (Finlayson, Hurt et al., 1988). In addition, an early report by Schuckit and Morrissey (1979) found that two-thirds of women in an alcohol treatment center had received prescriptions for abusable drugs, usually hypnotic and antianxiety drugs, and one-third reported abusing them. The drug-abusing women in this study reported more suicide attempts and early antisocial problems and had received more psychiatric care than the alcoholic women who did not abuse their prescriptions.

An additional concern is that psychoactive drugs can combine with alcohol to create adverse drug reactions. A study found that the combination of alcohol and OTC pain medications was the most common source of adverse drug reactions among older patients (Forster, Pollow et al., 1993). Such drug interactions result from a lack of understanding among physicians, pharmacists, and older adults themselves about the potential dangers of consuming alcohol when taking certain medications, even those sold without prescriptions.

PROBLEMS WITH PRESCRIPTION AND OTC MEDICATIONS

Adults aged 65 and older consume more prescribed and over-the-counter medications than any other age group in the U.S. Although older adults constituted less than 13% of the population in 1991, they received 25% to 30% of all prescriptions and experienced more than half of all reported adverse drug reactions leading to hospitalization (Woods & Winger, 1995; Ray, Thapa et al., 1993; Sheahan, Hendricks et al., 1989). Some 80% to 86% of adults older than age 65 reportedly suffer from one or more chronic diseases or conditions, and an estimated 83% of adults older than 65 take at least one prescription drug (Hazelden Foundation, 1991; Ray, Thapa et al., 1993). In fact, 30% of those older than 65 take eight or more prescription drugs daily (Sheahan, Hendricks et al., 1989).

A large share of prescriptions for older adults are for psychoactive drugs that carry the potential for misuse, abuse, or dependence. In 1983, one-fourth of community-dwelling older adults used psychotherapeutic drugs on a regular basis for sleep disorders or chronic pain, as well as for anxiety and mood regulation (Finlayson, 1995). Approximately 25% to 28% of older adults reported use of a psychoactive drug within the preceding year, and 20% used a tranquilizer daily. Indeed, 27% of all tranquilizer prescriptions and 38% of hypnotic prescriptions in 1991 were written for older adults. Moreover, older adults apparently are more likely to continue use of psychoactive drugs for longer periods than their younger counterparts (Sheahan, Hendricks et al., 1989; Woods & Winger, 1995).

Patterns of Use. The use patterns of psychoactive prescription drug users can be described as a continuum that ranges from appropriate use for medical or psychiatric indications through misuse by the patient or the prescribing health care practitioner to persistent abuse and dependence as defined by the *DSM-IV* (APA, 1994). Because older adults are less likely to use psychoactive medications nontherapeutically, problems with drugs generally fall into the misuse category and are unintentional. For example, older patients are more likely to misunderstand directions for appropriate use—a problem that is compounded by the multiple prescriptions they receive, often from multiple physicians, each of whom is unaware of a colleague's treatments. In these circumstances, overdose, additive effects, and adverse reactions from combining drugs are more likely to occur.

Unintentional misuse can progress into abuse if an older adult continues to use a medication nontherapeutically for the effects it provides, much as an abuser of any drug does.

Adults can become physiologically dependent on psychoactive medications without meeting the *DSM* criteria for dependence. Tolerance and physical dependence can develop when some psychoactive medications (benzodiazepines, opioids) are taken regularly at the therapeutically appropriate dose for relatively brief periods of time. An abstinence syndrome or withdrawal effects can occur if the drug is stopped precipitously. This type of iatrogenically induced physiologic dependence is not usually accompanied by any tendency on the part of the patient to escalate the dose during or after medically supervised withdrawal, to experience cravings after discontinuation, or subsequently to continue use (Woods & Winger, 1995; Portenoy, 1993). In other words, adults can become dependent on psychoactive medications without realizing it.

Risk Factors for Misuse and Abuse of Psychoactive Drugs. A variety of factors influence the use and potential for misuse or abuse of psychoactive prescription drugs and over-the-counter medications by older adults. The aging process, with its physiologic changes, accumulating physical health problems, and other psychosocial stressors, makes prescription drug use both more likely and more risky. The most consistently documented correlates of psychoactive prescription drug use are old age, poor physical health, and female gender (Cooperstock & Parnell, 1982; Sheahan, Hendricks et al., 1989; Finlayson, 1995).

Among older women, use of psychoactive drugs is correlated with middle- and late-life divorce, widowhood, less education, poorer health and chronic somatic problems, higher stress, lower income, and more depression and anxiety (Gomberg, 1995; Closser & Blow, 1993). Major losses of economic and social supports, factors related to the provider and health care system, and previous or coexisting drug, alcohol, or mental health problems also seem to increase vulnerability to misuse or abuse of prescribed medications.

Data from the 1984 ECA survey (Regier, Farmer et al., 1990) confirm that anxiety disorders are relatively prevalent in the general population of adults older than 65 years, with 7.3% of older respondents reporting an incident within the past month. Older women are nearly twice as likely as older men to develop a diagnosable anxiety disorder. Bereavement precipitates anxiety in nearly one-fourth of survivors during the first 6 months after the death of a loved one, and in nearly two-fifths of those left behind during the second six-month period. Anxiety also is common after a bereavement or other traumatic event (Salzman, 1993a).

System and Environmental Influences. A variety of health care system-related and environmental factors also place older adult users of psychoactive prescription drugs at risk of misuse of these substances. For example, potentially dangerous prescribing practices include ordering medications without adequate diagnoses or other documented indicators of symptoms, prescribing them for too long a time without appropriate medical monitoring of drug reactions and patient compliance with the prescribed regimen, selecting drugs known to have a high potential for side effects in older adults at the doses given, ordering drugs without knowing or reviewing whether they interact adversely with other medications the patient is taking, and failing to provide adequate and comprehensible instructions for patients about how and when to take medications and what side effects to expect and report. Problems also occur when the prescriber fails to consider the influence of aging on the effects of drugs in the body.

Adverse Effects. The chronic administration of psychoactive substances to older adults, even at therapeutic doses, has been associated with a variety of adverse central nervous system effects, including diminished psychomotor performance, impaired reaction time, loss of coordination, ataxia, falls, excessive daytime drowsiness, confusion, aggravation of emotional state, rage, and amnesia, as well as the development of physiologic dependence manifested by withdrawal effects when the drugs are suddenly discontinued (Fouts & Rachow, 1994). Psychoactive medications have been implicated in 23% of adverse drug reactions among nursing home residents (Joseph, 1995). Side effects from these drugs range from constipation, dry mouth, or urinary difficulty to such severe reactions as hip fractures from falls, withdrawal seizures or delirium, and worsened depression leading to suicide attempts (APA, 1994). However, all undesirable reactions may be more serious in frail older adults and in those with multiple chronic diseases, and thus cannot be ignored (Solomon, Manepalli et al., 1993).

Anxiolytics: An estimated 95% of benzodiazepine prescriptions for older adults in this country are ordered for anxiety and insomnia, with only 5% used as adjuncts for general anesthesia, as muscle relaxants, or as anticonvulsants (Ray, Thapa et al., 1993). Numerous studies, including the 1990 American Psychiatric Association Task Force report, have concluded that most use of these agents is appropriate, with only occasional overprescribing by physicians for some patient subgroups or misuse by patients (Salzman, 1990, 1993b; Winger, 1993; Woods & Winger, 1995). Even among the small group of respondents to household surveys who have acknowledged taking benzodiazepines that were not prescribed for them (less than 6%), most borrowed pills from significant others and used them for symptom relief rather than for recreational purposes. Moreover, worldwide experience with the short-term use of benzodiazepines to relieve acute anxiety, situational stress, and transient insomnia indicates that these medications are unusually safe and efficacious, with very little liability for dose increases, prolonged use, or addiction (Salzman, 1993b).

Benzodiazepine use for longer than four months is of particular concern among older adults. The aging process decreases the body's ability to absorb and metabolize drugs, allowing the drug to accumulate more rapidly than in younger persons and increasing the likelihood of toxicity and adverse effects. Benzodiazepines have variable rates of absorption, with metabolism occurring primarily in the liver. Because the longer-acting benzodiazepines have active metabolites, some of which have very long half-lives—up to 200 hours in the case of flurazepam (Dalmane®)—the duration of action often is longer than expected. These drugs also are more likely to produce residual sedation and other adverse effects, such as decreased attention, memory, cognitive function, and motor coordination, as well as increased injuries related to falls or motor vehicle crashes (Solomon, Manepalli et al., 1993; Fouts & Rachow, 1994; Ray, Thapa et al., 1993; Winger, 1993).

By contrast, some shorter-acting benzodiazepines are not as likely to produce toxic or dependence-inducing effects with chronic dosing. One reason is that these drugs have no active metabolites. Moreover, because the oxidative pathway often is impaired in older adults and in those with liver disease, it is best to choose drugs that are not metabolized by this pathway. Such drugs include oxazepam (Serax®) and lorazepam (Ativan®).

Unfortunately, both long- and short-acting benzodiazepines can produce physiologic dependence, even when taken at therapeutic doses and for as short a period as two months (Woods & Winger, 1995). Many of the most unpleasant withdrawal effects can be alleviated by gradually tapering the dose rather than stopping it abruptly. Even if the dose is tapered, however, withdrawal symptoms are experienced by 40% to 80% of patients who discontinue benzodiazepines after four to six months of regular use (Miller, Whitcup et al., 1985; Speirs, Navey et al., 1986). Symptoms such as anxiety, agitation, lethargy, nausea, loss of appetite, insomnia, dizziness, tremor, poor coordination, difficulty concentrating, depersonalization, or confusion can occur after stopping either long or short half-life benzodiazepines. Symptoms usually peak toward the end of the tapered discontinuation and disappear altogether within three to five weeks (Winger, 1993). However, in a few psychiatric patients, the withdrawal syndrome has been known to persist for several months (Solomon, Manepalli et al., 1993).

Salzman (1993b) makes a compelling case that chronic benzodiazepine use may be appropriate for patients he characterizes as older (but not necessarily elderly), with a number of chronic illnesses and compromised physical and/or psychosocial functioning. This group includes patients who often are in pain, dysphoric, or depressed, as well as those who are anxious, suffering from insomnia, or unwilling to visit their physicians. Chronic users of this type can experience side effects from benzodiazepines or incur mild interactions with other drugs they are taking, but they are not purposefully abusing psychoactive drugs or mixing them with alcohol. Benzodiazepine prescriptions seem to be clearly indicated for patients with overwhelming stress or anxiety that compromises functioning for short periods of time and for chronically medically ill, usually older, patients (Salzman, 1993b).

Sedative-Hypnotics: Sleep disturbances are a common complaint among older adults, occurring in approximately half of Americans older than age 65 who live at home and in two-thirds of those in long-term care facilities. Complaints about insomnia, which increase with advancing age, occur in conjunction with a variety of psychiatric, medical, or pharmacologic problems, as well as the changing circadian rhythms that accompany the aging process (NIH, 1990; Fouts & Rachow, 1994).

Benzodiazepines have replaced older and more toxic hypnotics (secobarbital, ethchlorvynol, glutethimide), which have a high addiction liability and difficult-to-treat overdose potential and which also tend to accumulate in older adults with chronic dosing as their capabilities for drug absorption and elimination diminish (Solomon, Manepalli et al., 1993; Bezchlibnyk-Butler & Jeffries, 1995). Nearly two of five prescriptions for benzodiazepines (38%) in 1991 were written for older patients (NIH, 1990; Fouts & Rachow, 1994). As with anxiolytics, the shorter-acting hypnotic benzodiazepines generally are favored over the longer acting ones that tend to accumulate in older adults and produce undesirable effects in the central nervous system. Currently, the most commonly prescribed hypnotic benzodiazepines are oxazepam (Serex®), temazepam (Restoril®), triazolam (Halcion®), and lorazepam (Ativan®) (Fouts & Rachow, 1994).

Unfortunately, like the anxiolytics, hypnotics also tend to be prescribed for longer than needed for efficacy, a situation that leads to the well-known drawbacks of withdrawal and rebound insomnia (Fouts & Rachow, 1994). In 1990, for example, 23% of adults who used benzodiazepine hypnotics (mostly the short-acting triazolam) had used them nightly for at least four months (Woods & Winger, 1995).

Sleep: Although aging changes sleep architecture, decreasing the amount of time spent in the deeper levels of sleep (stages 3 and 4) and increasing the number and duration of awakenings during the night, these new sleep patterns do not appear to bother most medically healthy older adults who recognize and accept that their sleep will not be as sound or as regular as when they were younger (NIH, 1990). Rather, insomnia complaints among older adults usually are associated with a secondary medical or psychiatric disorder, psychosocial changes and stressors, or the use of medications that interfere with sleep (NIH, 1990).

Among the drugs causing poor sleep patterns are the antidepressant monoamine oxidase inhibitors and selective serotonin reuptake inhibitors; antiParkinson medications; appetite suppressors; the beta-blocker for hypertension, propranolol (Inderal®); and alcohol. Sleep apnea, in particular, may be aggravated by the use of a benzodiazepine (Culebras, 1992). Insomnia also has been related to depression and anxiety, Alzheimer's disease, Parkinson's disease, cardiovascular disease, arthritis, pain, urinary problems, prostate disease, pulmonary disease, hyperthyroidism, and endocrinopathies. Sleep disruption as well as anxiety commonly accompany other psychosocial adjustments, such as retirement, bereavement, dislocation, or traumatic situations (NIH, 1990). Sleep complaints also are associated with female gender, living alone or in a nursing facility, activity limitations, and sleep habits, such as excessive daytime napping.

With respect to treatment of insomnia, a 1990 National Institutes of Health consensus development conference statement on sleep disorders in older adults specifically cautioned against relying on benzodiazepines as the mainstay for managing insomnia (NIH, 1990). Although these medications can be useful for short-term amelioration of temporary sleep problems, no studies demonstrate their long-term effectiveness beyond 30 continuous nights, and tolerance and dependence develop rapidly (NIH, 1990; Salzman, 1993b). In fact, symptomatic treatment of insomnia with medications should be limited to 7 to 10 days, with frequent monitoring and reevaluation if the prescribed drug will be used for more than two to three weeks. Intermittent dosing at the smallest possible dose is preferred, and no more than a 30-day supply of hypnotics should be prescribed. Given the changes associated with drug metabolism among older patients, all hypnotic medications should be used with caution, especially those with long half-lives (NIH, 1990; Fouts & Rachow, 1994). As with the anxiolytic benzodiazepines, withdrawal effects signifying physiologic dependence are common concomitants of precipitous medication discontinuation, especially of the short-acting compounds. The REM sleep rebound effects from abruptly stopping a chronically administered benzodiazepine can last one to three weeks or longer (Fouts & Rachow, 1994).

Furthermore, benzodiazepines and other sedative-hypnotics, used for sleep induction can cause confusion and equilibrium problems in older users who get up frequently during the night (to go to the bathroom). When treating older adults, situations likely to increase the incidence of falls with subsequent injury should be avoided at all costs. In addition, drugs taken at night for sleep induction will be potentiated by any alcohol the individual has used during the evening.

Instead of relying on drugs as a first line of approach, treatment initially should be directed toward any underlying disorder (depression, alcoholism, panic states, anxiety). Having the patient keep a sleep diary may be useful in obtaining a more objective clarification of sleep patterns, because insomnia is notoriously subjective. Also, the importance of good sleep hygiene cannot be underestimated (NIH, 1990; Fouts & Rachow, 1994). Patients may need to be educated about regularizing bedtime, restricting daytime naps, using the bedroom only for sleep and sexual activity, avoiding alcohol and caffeine, reducing evening fluid intake and heavy meals, taking some medications in the morning, limiting exercise immediately before retiring, and substituting behavioral relaxation techniques (NIH, 1990; Fouts & Rachow, 1994).

Withdrawal from sedative-hypnotic medications should be carefully monitored. Withdrawal is characterized by increased pulse rate, hand tremor, insomnia, nausea or vomiting, and anxiety. Seizures can occur. Hallucinations similar to those associated with alcoholic *delirium tremens* also may be present.

Several precautions about particular drugs should be noted. Specifically, triazolam (Halcion®) rapidly achieved notoriety and was banned in the United Kingdom and other European countries shortly after its 1979 introduction, when reports emerged of bizarre, idiosyncratic panic and delusional reactions, as well as adverse side effects of confusion, agitation, and anxiety (Woods & Winger, 1995; Winger, 1993). More serious side effects still are more consistently and more frequently reported with triazolam than with temazepam, a similar short-acting benzodiazepine (Woods & Winger, 1995). It appears that older patients are more likely than younger ones to experience increased sedation and psychomotor impairment with this medication and to report an increased incidence of adverse behavioral reactions at doses greater than 0.125 mg (Fouts & Rachow, 1994).

Another recently introduced but popular hypnotic, zolpidem (Ambien®), does not have the anxiolytic, muscle relaxant, or anticonvulsant properties of benzodiazepines. It has been marketed as a safer sleep medication because it does not disrupt physiologic sleep patterns at low doses and appears to have relatively mild dose-related adverse effects. However, zolpidem is much more costly than the benzodiazepines, an important consideration for low-income older patients. Also, lower doses (beginning at 5 mg) must be used in older patients to avoid hazardous confusion and falls (Winger, 1993; Fouts & Rachow, 1994; Ray, Thapa et al., 1993; Bezchlibnyk-Butler & Jeffries, 1995). Because of its relatively recent introduction, there is as yet only limited information on the possible undesirable effects of zolpidem for the older patient.

Several antihistamines, which generally are used for the relief of allergies and are available as over-the-counter medications, also are taken as sleeping aids because of their sedating properties (for example, Benadryl®). Antihistamines also are combined with over-the-counter analgesics and marketed as nighttime pain medications (such as Tylenol PM®). However, older adults appear to be more susceptible to adverse anticholinergic effects from these substances and are at increased risk of orthostatic hypotension and central nervous system depression or confusion. In addition, antihistamines and alcohol potentiate one another, further exacerbating the above conditions as well as any problems with balance. Because tolerance develops within days or weeks, these antihistamines have questionable efficacy and are not recommended for older adults who are living alone (Ray, Thapa et al., 1993; Fouts & Rachow, 1994; NIH, 1990; Bezchlibnyk-Butler & Jeffries, 1995).

Opioid Analgesics: An estimated 2% to 3% of noninstitutionalized older adults receive prescriptions for opioid analgesics (Ray, Thapa et al., 1993). Opioids are undeniably effective in the management of severe pain, such as that occurring after surgery and serious trauma, and periodically in some medical illnesses (such as gout or inflammatory bowel disease). This acute pain usually is short-lived and resolves within days to weeks. Opioid analgesics also are used to treat cancer-related pain, which is experienced by nearly all patients with advanced disease and by a third to half of patients in earlier stages. The use of opioid medications for these purposes is widely acceptable in medical practice (Portenoy, 1993).

In addition to the rapid development of tolerance and physiologic dependence, other problems are associated with opioid prescriptions for older patients. Opioid dose requirements decrease with age: The onset of action is slowed by the decreased rate of gastrointestinal absorption of orally ingested narcotics, and the duration of action is longer because of older patients' decreased metabolism and liver functioning. Older adults also have more adverse side effects because of changes in receptor sensitivity with age. The less potent opioids, codeine and propoxyphene (Darvon®), cause sedation and mild, dose-related impairment of psychomotor performance, whereas the more potent opioids, such as oxycodone (Percodan®) and intramuscular meperidine (Demerol®), induce substantial impairment of vision, attention, and motor coordination. No apparent relation between age and sedation is observed in patients treated with morphine and pentazocine (Talwin®) (Solomon, Manepalli et al., 1993; Ray, Thapa et al., 1993).

The prescribing of opioid analgesics for chronic nonmalignant pain is a controversial issue. Although long-term treatment of chronic pain with opiates or opioids has not traditionally been accepted by either patients or physicians, a growing body of evidence suggests that prolonged opioid therapy may be both effective and feasible (see Section 12 of this text). Convincing and persuasive testimony also has been given by a number of clinicians as to the successful management of lengthy opioid treatment in patients with chronic nonmalignant pain (Portenoy, 1993).

Opioid withdrawal is accompanied by restlessness, dysphoric mood, nausea or vomiting, muscle aches, tearing and yawning, diarrhea, fever, and insomnia. Although opioid withdrawal is uncomfortable, it is not life-threatening or particularly dangerous compared with untreated withdrawal from benzodiazepines.

SCREENING AND ASSESSMENT

Although the vast majority (87%) of older adults see physicians regularly, it has been estimated that 40% of those who are at risk do not self-identify or seek services for addictive disorders. Moreover, they are unlikely to be identified by their physicians, despite the frequency of contact. Because most older adults live in the community and fewer than 5% of those older than age 65 live in nursing or personal care homes, training supervisors in such residences does not offer a reasonable strategy for increasing problem identification. To ensure that older adults receive needed screening, assessment, and intervention services, stepped-up identification efforts by health care providers and multitiered, nontraditional case-finding methods within the community will be needed (DeHart & Hoffmann, 1995).

Most older adults see a medical practitioner several times a year, often for conditions that lend themselves to collateral discussion of the patients' drinking habits. Thus, the primary care setting provides an opportunity for screening that is currently underused, as is the hospital. Home health care providers have unparalleled opportunities to observe isolated, homebound seniors for possible problems and, if addictive disorder is suspected, to administer a nonthreatening screening instrument.

Identification of addictive disorders among older adults should not be the purview of health care workers alone. Friends and family of older adults and staff members of senior centers, including drivers and volunteers who see older adults on a regular basis, are intimately acquainted with their habits and daily routines. Frequently, they are in the best position to detect those behavioral changes that signal a possible problem. Leisure clubs, health fairs, congregate meal sites, Meals-on-Wheels®, and senior day care programs also provide venues in which older adults can be encouraged to self-identify. The National Council on Aging, for example, sponsors a depression awareness program that features a computerized, self-administered depression test. The computer offers anonymity and immediate results. It also avoids confidentiality problems and seems to offer a feasible model for mass screening for drinking problems.

In contrast to younger persons, whose problems with alcohol and other drugs often are identified as a result of an action initiated by a family member, spouse, employer, school, police, or the courts, a substantial proportion of older adults' addictive disorders go undetected. Unless health, social service, and community service providers understand that alcohol and prescription drugs can pose serious problems for older adults, and take the initiative in getting them the help they need, their quality of life will be diminished, independence compromised, and physical deterioration accelerated.

Asking Screening Questions. Screening questions should be asked in a confidential setting and in a nonthreatening, nonjudgmental manner. Many older adults are acutely sensitive to the stigma associated with alcohol and other drug use and are far more willing to accept a "medical" as opposed to a "psychological" or "mental health" diagnosis as an explanation for their problems. Prefacing questions with a link to a medical condition can make them more palatable. For example, "I'm wondering if alcohol may be the reason why your diabetes isn't responding as well as it should?" or "Sometimes one prescription drug can affect how well another medication is working. Let's go over the drugs you're taking and see if we can figure this problem out."

It is vitally important to avoid using stigmatizing terms like "alcoholic" or "drug abuser" during these encounters.

Cognition and Collateral Reporting. Impaired cognition interferes with screening, making it difficult to obtain complete and accurate answers. Although it is important to respect the older adult's autonomy, collateral participation from family members or friends may be necessary in situations in which a coherent response is unlikely. In this case, the screener should first ask for the older adult's permission to question others on his or her behalf. If possible, the screen should be administered to collaterals in private, using a nonconfrontational approach, such as: "I'm concerned about your father's deteriorating condition and wonder if his use of alcohol may be having a negative effect. Have you or anyone else in the family had any concerns about his drinking?" Because circumstances differ within families, family members may not know or may be unwilling to respond honestly to such an inquiry. Another question that skilled clinicians find useful in collateral screening is, "Has anyone in your family ever had a problem with drinking?" A positive response suggests that a problem may exist and that more in-depth questioning should follow.

Sometimes collateral screening unleashes a family member's simmering anger toward the older adult for both past and current alcohol-related behaviors. It is important to be alert to this possibility and to be prepared to work with the family member to discourage a confrontation with the older adult when the screen concludes.

Screening Instruments. The CAGE questionnaire (Ewing, 1984) and the Michigan Alcoholism Screening Test-Geriatric Version (MAST-G; Blow, Brower et al., 1992a) are two well-known alcohol screening instruments that have been validated for use with older adults. One of the most widely used alcohol screens, the CAGE consists of four questions, can be self-administered even by those with low literacy, and can be modified to screen for use of other drugs. Positive responses on the CAGE are for lifetime problems, not current ones. Before administering the CAGE, the MAST-G, or any other screen, it is important to ascertain that the person does currently drink alcohol and that the questions that are endorsed are for problems that they have experienced recently, usually within the past year.

Although two or more positive responses are considered indicative of an alcohol problem, a positive response to any CAGE question by an older adult should prompt further exploration. The CAGE is most effective in identifying more serious problem drinkers, and is less effective for women problem drinkers than their male counterparts.

TABLE 3.   Physical Symptom Screening Triggers

- Sleep complaints; observable changes in sleeping patterns; unusual fatigue, malaise, or daytime drowsiness; apparent sedation (a formerly punctual older adult begins to oversleep and is not ready when the senior center van arrives);

- Cognitive impairment, memory or concentration disturbances, disorientation or confusion (family members have difficulty following an older adult's conversation, the older adult no longer is able to participate in a usual weekly bridge game or to track the plot on daily soap operas);

- Seizures, malnutrition, muscle wasting;

- Liver function abnormalities;

- Persistent irritability (without obvious cause) and altered mood, depression, or anxiety;

- Unexplained complaints about chronic pain or other somatic complaints;

- Incontinence, urinary retention, difficulty urinating;

- Poor hygiene and self-neglect;

- Unusual restlessness and agitation;

- Complaints of blurred vision or dry mouth;

- Unexplained nausea and vomiting or gastrointestinal distress;

- Changes in eating habits;

- Slurred speech;

- Tremor, motor uncoordination, shuffling gait;

- Frequent falls and unexplained bruising.

SOURCE: Blow FC, ed. (1999). *Substance Abuse Among Older Adults (Treatment Improvement Protocol No. 26).* Rockville, MD: Center for Substance Abuse Treatment.

The MAST-G was developed specifically for older adults and has high sensitivity and specificity in this population in a wide range of settings, including primary care clinics, nursing homes, and older adult congregate housing locations. Triggers for physical symptom screening are listed in Table 3.

With some older adults, it may be impossible to understand the true effect of their alcohol and drug use or to recommend appropriate treatment services without a full assessment of their physical, mental, and functional health.

Assessing Functional Abilities. Functional health refers to a person's capacity to perform two types of everyday tasks: activities of daily living (ADLs), which include ambulating, bathing, dressing, feeding, and using the toilet, and instrumental activities of daily living (IADLs), which include managing finances, preparing meals, shopping, taking medications, and using the phone. Limitations in these domains, sometimes referred to as "disabilities," can result in an inadequate diet, mismanagement of medications or finances, or other serious problems. These disabilities are major risk factors for institutionalization and are more likely than physical illness or mental health problems to prompt older adults to seek treatment.

Impairments in functional abilities are common in older adults who have medical and psychiatric disorders. For instance, 90% of adults older than age 65 require the use of corrective lenses and 50% of adults older than 65 have some degree of hearing loss (Plomp, 1978). Sensory impairments affect older adults in subtle ways that are not always immediately obvious to health practitioners, but which need to be anticipated, identified, and incorporated into treatment practices. For example, clinicians should ensure that older patients can read their prescriptions or hear what is said in a group therapy session. When not considered and compensated for, functional impairments can obstruct treatment. For example, it would be futile to enroll an older patient who is obese and has limited mobility in a program housed in a facility with steep flights of stairs and no elevator. Likewise, it makes little sense to recommend an evening program to an older adult who cannot drive at night and who does not have someone else to drive him or her.

Alcohol use can diminish IADLs and ADLs. Although alcohol-related functional impairments potentially are reversible, they should be considered when planning a treatment regimen. There are known complications of and differences between alcohol use in men and women related to compromised functional abilities and ADLs. In a study of older adults with a history of past alcohol abuse, impairment in ADLs was twice as common in women as in men (Ensrud, Nevitt et al., 1994). In addition, alcohol use was more strongly correlated with functional impairment than were smoking, age, use of anxiolytics, stroke, or diminished grip strength.

Cognitive Impairment. The presence of cognitive impairment or dementia significantly alters treatment decisions.

TABLE 4.   Life Changes Associated With Substance Abuse in Older Adults

Emotional and Social Problems	
■ Bereavement and sadness ■ Loss of 　□ Friends 　□ Family members 　□ Social status 　□ Occupation and sense of professional identity 　□ Hopes for the future 　□ Ability to function.	■ Sense of being a "nonperson" ■ Social isolation and loneliness ■ Reduced self-regard or self-esteem ■ Family conflict and estrangement ■ Problems in managing leisure time/boredom ■ Loss of physical attractiveness (especially important for women).
Medical Problems	
■ Physical distress ■ Chronic pain ■ Physical disabilities and handicapping conditions ■ Insomnia.	■ Sensory deficits 　□ Hearing 　□ Sight ■ Reduced mobility ■ Cognitive impairment and change.
Practical Problems	
■ Impaired self-care ■ Reduced coping skills ■ Decreased economic security or new poverty status because of 　□ Loss of income 　□ Increased health care costs.	■ Dislocation 　□ Move to new housing or family moves away 　□ Homelessness 　□ Inadequate housing.

SOURCE: Blow FC, ed. (1999). *Substance Abuse Among Older Adults (Treatment Improvement Protocol No. 26)*. Rockville, MD: Center for Substance Abuse Treatment.

It is particularly important to distinguish between dementia and delirium, which often are mistaken for each other in older patients.

Dementia: Dementia is a chronic, progressive, and generally irreversible cognitive impairment that is sufficient to interfere with an individual's daily living. Dementia also limits an individual's ability to interact in traditional group settings. Common causes of dementia include Alzheimer's disease, vascular disorders (multi-infarct dementia), and alcohol-related dementia. Dementia also makes it more difficult to monitor outcomes of drinking (patients can forget they drank), to get into treatment, and to benefit from treatment.

Changes in cognition are not unusual as people age, and they increase in frequency with each decade. Such changes, which are experienced in varying degrees, include minor short-term memory loss and difficulty with certain mathematical functions. However, significant memory loss, impaired abstract thinking, confusion, difficulty communicating, extreme emotional reactions and outbursts, and disorientation to time, place, and person are signs of cognitive impairment and are not part of the normal aging process.

Dementia can range from a mild level of cognitive impairment that is easily managed to a severe stage that can require intensive treatment and nursing home care. Symptoms may not be equally present in all older adults.

Screening for significant cognitive dysfunction can be accomplished easily by any of a number of screening instruments. Patients who have been medically detoxified should not be screened for several weeks after detoxification because, until fully recovered, they can exhibit some reversible cognitive impairment. Either of two screens should be used: the Orientation/Memory/Concentration Test, which is simple and can be completed in the office, or the Folstein Mini-Mental Status Exam (MMSE), which is an acceptable alternative. It should be noted that in the assessment of older problem drinkers who recently (in the preceding 30 to 60 days) attained sobriety in an outpatient setting, the MMSE can be insensitive to subtle cognitive impairments. Moreover, because the MMSE is weak on visual-spatial testing, which is likely to show some abnormality in many recent heavy drinkers and does not include screening tests of abstract thinking and visual memory, use of the "draw-a-clock task" (Watson, Arfken et al., 1993) and the Neurobehavioral Cognitive Status Examination (NCSE) should be used as supplements.

Delirium: Also known as "acute confusional state" and "acute brain syndrome," delirium is an alteration of mental status that usually can be reversed with medical treatment. Symptoms can occur in any combination and may be intermittent.

Delirium is a potentially life-threatening illness that requires acute intervention, usually hospitalization. The cognitive losses experienced with delirium, unlike the effects of dementia, often can be reversed with proper medical treatment.

Benzodiazepine use before hospitalization has been demonstrated to be a significant risk factor for the development of delirium among hospitalized older adults. This finding suggests that these individuals had classical withdrawal delirium from the benzodiazepines or that mild withdrawal, in addition to other risk factors, greatly increases the incidence of delirium. The Confusion Assessment Method (CAM) is widely used as a brief, sensitive, and reliable screening measure for detecting delirium. A positive delirium screen should be followed by careful clinical diagnostics based on *DSM-IV* criteria and any associated cognitive impairment be followed clinically using the MMSE.

Life changes associated with alcohol and other drug use in older adults are listed in Table 4.

APPROACHES TO TREATMENT

Moving the Older Adult Into Treatment. After determining that an older adult can benefit from a reduction in or complete abstinence from alcohol use, the clinician must assess the patient's understanding of this benefit. Many older adults may not know that their alcohol use is affecting their

health. Because patient understanding and cooperation are essential both in eliciting accurate information and following through on the treatment plan prescribed, clinicians should use the assessment process as an opportunity to educate the older adult and to motivate him or her to accept treatment.

Interacting With Older Adults: Many health care professionals rarely interact with older adults. To facilitate the assessment process with this population, clinicians should adhere to the following guiding principles:

- Areas of concern most likely to motivate older patients are physical health, the loss of independence and function, financial security, and maintenance of independence.

- Assessment and treatment decisions must include the patient to be successful. This is particularly relevant to older adults, who may be very uncomfortable in formalized addiction treatment programs that do not include their peers or address their specific developmental and health needs.

- Depending on an individual's particular situation, it may be important to include family members in treatment or intervention discussions (understanding that children can vacillate between a desire to help and denial, and that the patient's right to confidentiality always must be respected).

- Addiction is a chronic disorder that ebbs and flows. Thus, patients' needs will change over time and will require different types and intensities of treatment.

- Because many older adults have several health care providers (including visiting nurses, social workers, adult day care staff, religious personnel), it is important to include this network as a resource in assessment and in providing treatment.

- Given the complex health needs of older adults, health care providers may need assistance from experienced nonmedical personnel to adequately assess the totality of treatment issues and choices. Providers should be aware of their limitations, both in providing addiction treatment and in assessing and treating mental or physical health needs.

- All treatment strategies must be culturally competent and, to the extent possible, incorporate appropriate ethnic considerations (rituals).

■ Overarching continuity of care issues and considerations should be identified and addressed, especially in rural and minority communities where emergency room staff members often function as primary care providers.

Selecting a Treatment Modality. The least intensive treatment options should be explored first: *brief intervention* and *motivational counseling*. Although these approaches may be sufficient to address the problem for some older patients, for others they will function as pre-treatment strategies. These less intensive options will not resolve the latter patient's alcohol or other drug problems, but can help to move him or her into specialized treatment by helping to overcome resistance to and ambivalence about changing alcohol or drug use behavior.

Like treatment itself, pretreatment activities in some cases may be conducted best in the patient's home, perhaps coupled with other personal or social services or with home-based detoxification services. This approach is ideal for the large number of at-risk older adults who are homebound. Such pretreatment can be conducted by visiting nurses, housing authority staff, and social workers. Community health agencies often have staff members designated to make visits to older adults in their homes, and some in-home treatment programs have a visiting nurse who identifies and treats addictive disorder in the home.

Brief Intervention for At-Risk Drinkers. Research has shown that 10% to 30% of nondependent problem drinkers reduce their drinking to moderate levels after a brief intervention by a physician or other clinician (also see Section 3). A brief intervention is one or more counseling sessions, which can include strategies to enhance motivation for change, patient education, assessment and direct feedback, contracting and goal-setting, behavior modification, and the use of written materials such as self-help manuals (Fleming, Barry et al., 1997b). Brief intervention techniques have been used to reduce alcohol use in adolescents, in adults younger than age 65 who are nondependent problem drinkers and, most recently, in older adults (Blow, in press; Fleming, Barry et al., 1997a). All of these activities can be conducted by trained clinicians, home health care workers, psychologists, social workers, and professional counselors (physicians, nurses, physicians' assistants).

Conducting Brief Interventions: Older adults present unique challenges to those applying brief intervention strategies for reducing alcohol consumption. Because many older at-risk and problem drinkers are ashamed of their drinking, intervention strategies need to be especially non-confrontational and supportive. Thus, a brief intervention with an older adult should include the following steps:

1. Customized feedback on the patient's responses to screening questions about drinking patterns and other health habits, such as smoking and nutrition.

2. Discussion of the types of drinkers in the U.S. and how the patient's drinking patterns fit into the population norms for his or her age group.

3. The patient's reasons for drinking. This step is particularly important because the practitioner needs to understand the role of alcohol in the context of the older patient's life, including coping with loss and loneliness.

4. Consequences of heavier drinking. Some older patients can experience problems in physical, psychological, or social functioning even though their alcohol consumption is below cutoff levels.

5. Reasons to cut down or quit drinking. Maintaining independence, physical health, financial security, and mental capacity can be key motivators in this age group.

6. Sensible drinking limits and strategies for cutting down or quitting. Strategies that are useful in this age group include developing social opportunities that do not involve alcohol, getting reacquainted with hobbies and interests from earlier in life, and pursuing volunteer activities, if possible.

7. A drinking agreement in the form of a written agreement. Agreed-upon drinking limits that are signed by the patient and the practitioner are particularly effective in changing drinking patterns.

8. Help in coping with risky situations. Social isolation, boredom, and negative family interactions can present special problems in this age group.

9. Summary of the session.

When older adults are motivated to take action on their own behalf, the prognosis for positive change is extremely favorable. The key to inspiring motivation is the clinician's caring style, willingness to view the older adult as a full partner in his or her recovery, and capacity to provide hope and encouragement as the older adult progresses through the referral, treatment, and recovery processes.

Motivational Counseling: As a result of the work pioneered by Prochaska and DiClemente, clinicians now understand that people can respond quite differently to recommendations to alter or give up longstanding or previously pleasurable behaviors. Their reactions depend, to a great extent, on their individual readiness to change (Prochaska, DiClemente et al., 1992). For example, the screening or assessment findings can confirm one individual's suspicions about the negative effects of alcohol on personal health, and lead to an immediate commitment to abstain or begin tapering off. For another patient, the assessment may be a revelation that must be processed over time before any changes can be made. Still others may be unconvinced by the findings and unpersuaded of the need to make any changes at all.

Motivational counseling acknowledges differences in readiness and offers an approach for "meeting people where they are" that has proved effective with older adults (Miller & Rollnick, 1991). In this approach, an understanding and supportive counselor listens respectfully and accepts the older adult's perspective on the situation as a starting point, then helps the individual identify the negative consequences of drinking or drug use, helps the patient shift perceptions about the effects of his or her drinking or drug-taking habits, empowers the individual to generate insights about and solutions for his or her problem, and expresses belief in and support for the older adult's capacity for change. Motivational counseling is an intensive process that enlists patients in their own recovery by avoiding labels, avoiding confrontation (which usually results in greater defensiveness), accepting ambivalence about the need to change, inviting patients to consider alternative ways of solving problems, and placing the responsibility for change on the patient. This process also can help offset the denial, resentment, and shame invoked during an intervention and can serve as a prelude to cognitive-behavioral therapy (Miller & Rollnick, 1991).

Specialized Treatment: For some older adults, especially those who are late-onset drinkers or drug users with strong social supports and no mental health comorbidities, pretreatment approaches can prove quite effective, and followup brief interventions and empathic support for positive change may be sufficient for continued recovery. There is, however, a subpopulation of older adults who will need more intensive treatment.

Despite the resistance seen in some older problem drinkers or drug users, treatment is worth pursuing. Studies show that older adults are more compliant with treatment and have treatment outcomes as good as or better than those of younger patients (Oslin, Pettinati et al., 1997; Atkinson, 1995).

Program Philosophy and Basic Principles. The alcohol treatment literature on older adults suggests incorporating the following six features into treatment of the older alcoholic (Schonfeld & Dupree, 1995):

1. Age-specific group treatment that is supportive and nonconfrontational and that aims to build or rebuild the patient's self-esteem.

2. A focus on coping with depression, loneliness, and loss (such as death of a spouse or retirement).

3. A focus on rebuilding the client's social support network.

4. A pace and content of treatment appropriate for the older person.

5. Staff members who are interested and experienced in working with older adults.

6. Linkages with medical services, services for the aging, and institutional settings for referral into and out of treatment, as well as case management.

Building from these six features, treatment programs for older adults should adhere to the following principles:

- Treat older adults in age-specific settings wherever feasible.

- Create a culture of respect for older patients.

- Adopt a broad, holistic approach to treatment that emphasizes age-specific psychological, social, and health problems.

- Keep the treatment program flexible.

- Adapt treatment as needed in response to the patient's gender.

Holistic Treatment Based on Age-Specific Problems. In treating older adults, treatment programs need to focus on more than just the patient's alcohol or drug use disorder. As people age, the likelihood of multiple antecedent conditions for problem behaviors increases. In other words, the individual's psychological and health problems tend to become more complex, multiply determined, and interactive. Research suggests that older adults with alcohol problems often drink in response to loneliness, depression, and poor social support networks (Schonfeld & Dupree, 1995). Researchers also have identified chronic pain as a high-risk condition for addictive disorders.

A number of interrelated emotional, social, medical, spiritual, and practical problems or changes characterize the older adult's experiences. Some of these problems can precipitate the abuse of alcohol or other drugs. Those that initiate, sustain, or interact with the addictive disorder provide a focus for a holistic treatment approach that is tailored to the needs of the individual.

Discussing life changes with patients can help them develop insight into the causes of their addictive disorders. For example, while discussing salient nondrinking problems with an older adult, the drinking problem often emerges naturally as a topic of conversation. Although the problems associated with aging can be overwhelming, patients need not accept them passively. They can develop a self-care skill or positive attitude and can obtain appropriate help, such as the pharmacologic alleviation of pain, management of grief, or skills for improving relationships.

Program Flexibility. The goals, setting, and duration of treatment may well be different for each patient. For example, the first step toward ending problem drinking may involve finding safe, affordable housing for one patient, resolving depression for a second, or improving relationships with a caregiving daughter for a third. Every element of treatment, from work assignments to exercise programs, should be tailored to the needs and abilities of each individual patient.

It may be necessary to stop treatment when illnesses or hospitalization intervene. Schedule adjustments may be needed in recognition of the fatigue levels of older individuals. The treatment setting may need to shift from clinic to home during a period of convalescence from a hip fracture or an illness. One patient may need twice as many treatment sessions to master steps toward self-sufficiency as another client. One individual may need to continue treatment for two years to achieve his or her goals, while another patient attains his goals within six months.

Treatment Approaches. The following general approaches have been found effective in the treatment of older adults:

- Cognitive-behavioral approaches;
- Group-based approaches;
- Individual counseling;
- Medical and psychiatric approaches;
- Marital and family involvement or family therapy; and
- Case management/community-linked services and outreach.

Not every approach will be needed by every patient. Instead, the clinician can individualize the treatment plan by selecting the specific services a particular patient needs. Information to guide the plan comes from interviews; mental status examinations; physical examinations; laboratory, radiologic, and psychometric tests; and social network assessments, among others.

Discharge Plans and Continuing Care. Effective discharge planning is essential to case management for older adults because their social networks may have shrunk as a result of their addictive disorders, physical limitations, or the loss of family members and friends. In this context, it is vitally important for counselors or case managers to help patients tap into available community resources by assisting them in identifying ongoing needs (income maintenance, housing), scheduling services (homemakers, eye care, hearing tests, financial planning), and obtaining equipment (large-number telephones, large-screen computers, walkers, and other devices).

As part of the discharge process, a counselor or case manager should develop an aftercare plan in consultation with the patient. For older adults, such a program may entail arranging transportation to followup appointments and reminders to note dates and times on the calendar, as well as fulfilling more traditional functions, such as monitoring progress to prevent or reduce the risk of relapse. Standard features of most discharge plans for older adults include the following:

- Participation in age-appropriate Alcoholics Anonymous, Pills Anonymous, Rational Recovery, women's, or other support groups.

- Ancillary services needed to maintain independence in the community.

- Ongoing medical monitoring.

- Involvement of an appropriate case manager as needed to advocate for the patient and to ensure that needed services are provided.

Aftercare and recovery services for older persons differ in some respects from those typically offered by addiction treatment programs, in which fraternization is discouraged. Programs oriented to older adults often sponsor socialization groups or weekly treatment alumnae meetings, which are run by peer counselors in long-term recovery. Others allow patients to return to the program to participate in group therapy. Still others initiate a network of contacts for older adults and teach them how to expand it.

Special Treatment Issues for Prescription Drugs. Because so many problems with prescription drugs stem from unintentional misuse, approaches to patients with a prescription drug problem differ in some important respects from treatment for alcohol problems. Issues that need to be addressed as part of treatment include educating and assisting patients who misuse prescribed medications to comply consistently with dosing instructions, providing informal or brief counseling for patients who are abusing a prescribed substance with deleterious consequences, and engaging drug-dependent patients in the formal treatment system at an appropriate level of care. In addition, it is important for providers to understand how other practitioners' prescribing behavior contributes to the problem, so that they can address the problem, both with the patient and with the uninformed health care professional.

Medication Noncompliance: Experts estimate that as many as 70% of depressed older patients fail to take a fourth to a half of their medications, leading to wide fluctuations in blood levels and jeopardizing the efficacy of therapy (NIH, 1991). Such widespread problems with compliance requires intensive efforts to determine the reasons for the problems and to educate patients about medication management.

Medication noncompliance can take the following forms:

- Omitting doses or changing the frequency or timing of doses;

- Doubling up doses after forgetting to take the previous dose;

- Taking the entire day's medications in the morning to alleviate the fear of forgetting to take a later dose;

- Increasing doses or dosing frequency;

- Taking the wrong drugs;

- Borrowing or sharing drugs;

- Supplementing prescribed drugs with over-the-counter medications or "leftover" medications from an earlier illness;

- Continuing to use alcohol or other contraindicated drugs or foods while taking the prescribed medications;

- Engaging in contraindicated activities while taking the medications (driving motor vehicles, spending time in the sun);

- Failing to tell the prescribing physician about all other medications (prescribed and over-the-counter) being used or to report significant or unexpected side effects or adverse reactions; and

- Storing medications improperly (not refrigerating those that require a continued cold temperature) or using prescriptions with expired expiration dates.

In general, the causes of noncompliance with a prescribed medication regimen can be categorized as follows:

- Misunderstanding or a lack of knowledge about the drug.

- An inability to manage the medication regimen, either because it is too complex or because the patient has persistent memory problems and needs regular supervision.

- Insufficient resources for purchasing or storing the medications.

- Intentional misuse to obtain results other than those for which the drug was prescribed (for example, using pain medication to sleep, relax, or soften negative affect).

Unless interventions address the real reasons for noncompliance, they are not likely to be effective. If initial observations and questions about prescription drug use suggest misuse, more information will be needed so that remedies can be appropriately targeted. For example, if a 73-year-old woman is skipping doses of her blood pressure medication, the provider needs to learn whether this happens because (1) the patient only takes the medicine when she feels ill rather than on the prescribed schedule, (2) the medicine sometimes makes her feel unpleasantly dizzy, (3) the patient frequently forgets whether she took the medicine, or (4) the patient cannot afford the drug, either regularly or sporadically.

If the patient's noncompliance is the result of economic considerations, teaching her how to manage her medications by separating them into container compartments for each day of the week (or hour of the day) will not be helpful. That strategy might be appropriate, however, for another patient who has suffered a stroke and has real difficulty with short-term memory.

The patient and the health care practitioner share a responsibility for ensuring that the patient understands all dosing instructions, the purposes of the medications prescribed, and the unpleasant side effects or adverse reactions that should be reported to the doctor. However, providers also can instruct patients to take advantage of pharmacists' services in providing personal advice and computer-generated instructions about specific drugs, side effects of varying intensity and seriousness, contraindications for use, and when beneficial effects can be anticipated. Many materials are available that have been developed specifically for older adults to enhance medication compliance. These materials can be obtained from numerous sources, including home health care agencies, state and local offices on aging, the Substance Abuse and Mental Health Services Administration (through the National Clearinghouse for Alcohol and Drug Information), the National Council on Aging, and the American Association of Retired Persons.

Treatment providers can help empower older adults to ask more questions and optimize the benefits of their contacts with medical professionals. Older patients with some cognitive or sensory impairments may not be able to adhere to complicated medication regimens. In such cases, treatment providers can identify and educate family members or other professional or volunteer advocates and caregivers about the need to assist the older adult with this task.

When the clinician identifies a medication compliance problem, arrangements should be made for an initial but intensive monitoring of the patient's use of the problematic drug. Monitoring may be undertaken by visiting or public health nurses or other designated medical staff members. The objective is to determine whether the problems with use continue despite all attempts to correct the underlying reasons for noncompliance. If the patient appears to be intentionally noncompliant, the behavior is characteristic of abuse.

The intervention for such behavior would depend on an accurate and indepth assessment of the social, medical, and psychological problems that may be driving the addictive disorder (such as depression, bereavement, a medical condition, social isolation, physical pain, insomnia). Assessment results then provide the basis for an individualized treatment plan that includes and ranks mechanisms for addressing each issue. Unless the abuse has resulted in a serious crisis, it usually is appropriate to try psychosocial approaches first, including grief therapy, sleep management training, relaxation techniques, socialization (day care) programs, psychotherapy, and acupuncture.

Once treatment begins to resolve the underlying issues, a decision needs to be made as to whether the older adult should remain on the problematic drug at a reduced dose, discontinue use altogether, or switch to an alternative prescription with less addictive potential. The choice will depend on what options are available and the severity of the problems experienced as a result of the addictive disorder. An open discussion of these issues with the patient, an addiction medicine specialist, and the patient's primary care physician is recommended.

ACKNOWLEDGMENT: Adapted by permission of the publisher from Blow FC, ed. (1999). Substance Abuse Among Older Adults (Treatment Improvement Protocol No. 26). Rockville, MD: Center for Substance Abuse Treatment.

REFERENCES

Adams WL, Barry KL & Fleming MF (1996). Screening for problem drinking in older primary care patients. *Journal of the American Medical Association* 276(24):1964-1967.

Adams WL, Yuan Z, Barboriak JJ et al. (1993). Alcohol-related hospitalizations of elderly people: Prevalence and geographic location in the United States. *Journal of the American Medical Association* 270(10):1222-1225.

Administration on Aging (n.d.). A Profile of Older Americans. Accessed at: HTTP://WWW.AOA.DHHS.GOV/AOA/PAGES/PROFIL95.HTML.

American Psychiatric Association (APA) (1994). *Diagnostic and Statistical Manual of Mental Disorders, 4th Edition (DSM-IV)*. Washington, DC: American Psychiatric Press.

Atkinson R (1985). Persuading alcoholic patients to seek treatment. *Comprehensive Therapy* 11(11):16-24.

Atkinson RM (1984). Substance use and abuse in late life. In RM Atkinson (ed.) *Alcohol and Drug Abuse in Old Age*. Washington, DC: American Psychiatric Press, 1-21.

Atkinson RM (1990). Aging and alcohol use disorders: Diagnostic issues in the elderly. *International Psychogeriatrics* 2:55-72.

Atkinson RM (1994). Late onset problem drinking in older adults. *International Journal of Geriatric Psychiatry* 9:321-326.

Atkinson RM (1995). Treatment programs for aging alcoholics. In T Beresford & E Gomberg (eds.) *Alcohol and Aging*. New York, NY: Oxford University Press, 186-210.

Atkinson RM & Ganzini L (1994). Substance abuse. In CE Coffey & JL Cummings (eds.) *Textbook of Geriatric Neuropsychiatry*. Washington, DC: American Psychiatric Press, 297-321.

Atkinson RM, Turner JA, Kofoed LL et al. (1985). Early versus late onset alcoholism in older persons: Preliminary findings. *Alcoholism: Clinical & Experimental Research*, 9:513-515.

Beresford TP (1995). Alcoholic elderly: Prevalence, screening, diagnosis, and prognosis. In TP Beresford & E Gomberg (eds.) *Alcohol and Aging*. New York, NY: Oxford University Press, 3-18.

Beresford TP & Lucey MR (1995). Ethanol metabolism and intoxication in the elderly. In TP Beresford & ES Gomberg (eds.) *Alcohol and Aging.* New York, NY: Oxford University Press, 117-127.

Bezchlibnyk-Butler KZ & Jeffries JJ (eds.) (1995). *Clinical Handbook of Psychotropic Drugs, 5th Edition.* Toronto, Canada: Hogrefe & Huber.

Blow FC, ed. (1998). *Substance Abuse Among Older Adults (Treatment Improvement Protocol No. 26).* Rockville, MD: Center for Substance Abuse Treatment.

Blow FC (in press). The spectrum of alcohol interventions for older adults. In ESL Gomberg, AM Hegedus & RA Zucker (eds.) *Alcohol Problems and Aging.* Rockville, MD: National Institute on Alcohol Abuse and Alcoholism.

Blow FC, Brower KJ, Schulenberg JE et al. (1992a). The Michigan Alcoholism Screening Test—Geriatric Version (MAST-G): A new elderly-specific screening instrument. *Alcoholism: Clinical & Experimental Research* 16:372.

Brennan PL & Moos RH (1996). Late-life problem drinking: Personal and environmental risk factors for 4-year functioning outcomes and treatment seeking. *Journal of Substance Abuse* 8:167-180.

Caruthers M (1992). Health promotion in the elderly. *American Family Physician* 45:2253-2259.

Chermack ST, Blow FC, Hill EM et al. (1996). The relationship between alcohol symptoms and consumption among older drinkers. *Alcoholism: Clinical & Experimental Research* 20(7):1153-1158.

Ciraulo DA, Shader RI, Greenblatt DJ et al. (1995). *Drug Interactions in Psychiatry, 2nd Edition.* Baltimore, MD: Williams & Wilkins.

Closser MH & Blow FC (1993). Special populations: Women, ethnic minorities, and the elderly. *Psychiatric Clinics of North America* 16(1):199-209.

Colsher PL, Wallace RB, Pomrehn PR et al. (1990). Demographic and health characteristics of elderly smokers: Results from established populations for epidemiologic studies of the elderly. *American Journal of Preventative Medicine* 6:61-70.

Cooperstock R & Parnell P (1982). Research on psychotropic drug use: A review of findings and methods. *Social Science and Medicine* 16:1179-1196.

Cox JL (1993). Smoking cessation in the elderly patient. *Clinics in Chest Medicine* 14(3):423-428.

Culebras A (1992). Update on disorders of sleep and the sleep-wake cycle. *Psychiatric Clinics of North America* 15:467-489.

Curtis JR, Geller G, Stokes EJ et al. (1989). Characteristics, diagnosis, and treatment of alcoholism in elderly patients. *Journal of the American Geriatrics Society* 37:310-316.

D'Archangelo E (1993). Substance abuse in later life. *Canadian Family Physician* 39:1986-1993.

DeHart SS & Hoffmann HG (1995). Screening and diagnosis of "alcohol abuse and dependence" in older adults. *International Journal of the Addictions* 30:1717-1747.

Douglass RL (1984). Aging and alcohol problems: Opportunities for socioepidemiologic research. In M Galanter (ed.) *Recent Developments in Alcoholism.* New York, NY: Plenum Press, 251-266.

Dupree LW, Broskowski H & Schonfeld L (1984). The Gerontology Alcohol Project: A behavioral treatment program for elderly alcohol abusers. *Gerontologist* 24:510-516.

Ensrud KE, Nevitt MC, Yunis C et al. (1994). Correlates of impaired function in older women. *Journal of the American Geriatrics Society* 42:481-489.

Finlayson R, Hurt R, Davis L et al. (1988). Alcoholism in elderly persons: A study of the psychiatric and psychosocial features of 216 inpatients. *Mayo Clinic Proceedings* 63:761-768.

Finlayson RE (1995). Misuse of prescription drugs. *International Journal of the Addictions* 30(13&14):1871-1901.

Fleming M, Barry KL, Adams W et al. (1997a). Guiding Older Adult Lifestyles (Project GOAL): The effectiveness of brief physician advice for alcohol problems in older adults. Manuscript submitted for publication.

Fleming MF, Barry KL, Manwell LB et al. (1997b). Brief physician advice for problem alcohol drinkers: A randomized controlled trial in community-based primary care practices. *Journal of the American Medical Association* 277:1039-1045.

Forster LE, Pollow R & Stoller EP (1993). Alcohol use and potential risk for alcohol-related adverse drug reactions among community-based elderly. *Journal of Community Health* 18:225-239.

Fouts M & Rachow J (1994). Choice of hypnotics in the elderly. *P&T News* 14(8):1-4.

Gambert SR & Katsoyannis KK (1995). Alcohol-related medical disorders of older heavy drinkers. In TP Beresford & E Gomberg (eds.) *Alcohol and Aging.* New York, NY: Oxford University Press, 70-81.

Goldberg RJ, Burchfiel CM, Reed DM et al. (1994). A prospective study of the health effects of alcohol consumption in middle-aged and elderly men: The Honolulu Heart Program. *Circulation* 89:651-659.

Gomberg ESL (1992). Medication problems and drug abuse. In FJ Turner (ed.) *Mental Health and the Elderly.* New York, NY: Free Press, 355-374.

Gomberg ESL (1993). Recent developments in alcoholism: Gender issues. In M Galanter (ed.) *Recent Developments in Alcoholism: Volume. 11.* New York, NY: Plenum Press, 95-107.

Gomberg ESL (1994). Risk factors for drinking over a woman's life span. *Alcohol Health and Research World* 18:220-227.

Gomberg ESL (1995). Older women and alcohol use and abuse. In M Galanter (ed.) *Recent Developments in Alcoholism: Volume 12. Alcoholism and Women.* New York, NY: Plenum Press, 61-79.

Graham K, Clarke D, Bois C et al. (1996). Addictive behavior of older adults. *Addictive Behaviors* 21(3):331-348.

Haponik EF (1992). Sleep disturbances of older persons: Physicians' attitudes. *Sleep* 15(2):168-172.

Hazelden Foundation (1991). *How to Talk to an Older Person Who Has a Problem With Alcohol or Medications.* Center City, MN: Hazelden Foundation.

Heller DA & McClearn GE (1995). Alcohol, aging, and genetics. In TP Beresford & E Gomberg (eds.) *Alcohol and Aging.* New York, NY: Oxford University Press, 99-114.

Helzer JE, Burnam A & McEvoy LT (1991). Alcohol abuse and dependence. In LN Robins & DA Reigier (eds.) *Psychiatric Disorders in America: The Epidemiologic Catchment Area Study.* New York, NY: Free Press, 81-115.

Hendricks J, Johnson TP, Sheahan SL et al. (1991). Medication use among older persons in congregate living facilities. *Journal of Geriatric Drug Therapy* 6(1):47-61.

Hill HF & Chapman CR (1989). *Clinical Effectiveness of Analgesics in Chronic Pain States* (NIDA Research Monograph Series, No. 95). Rockville, MD: National Institute on Drug Abuse, 102-109.

Hurt RD, Eberman KA, Slade J et al. (1993). Treating nicotine addiction in patients with other addictive disorders. In CT Orleans & J Slade (eds.) *Nicotine Addiction: Principles and Management*. New York, NY: Oxford University Press, 310-326.

Hurt RD, Finlayson RE, Morse RM et al. (1988). Alcoholism in elderly persons: Medical aspects and prognosis of 216 patients. *Mayo Clinic Proceedings* 63:753-760.

Institute of Medicine (IOM) (1990). *Broadening the Base of Treatment for Alcohol Problems*. Washington, DC: National Academy Press.

Jinks MJ & Raschko RR (1990). A profile of alcohol and prescription drug abuse in a high-risk community-based elderly population. *Drug Intelligence and Clinical Pharmacy* 24:971-975.

Joseph CL (1995). Alcohol and drug misuse in the nursing home. *International Journal of the Addictions* 30(13&14):1953-1983.

Joseph CL, Ganzini L & Atkinson R (1995). Screening for alcohol use disorders in the nursing home. *Journal of the American Geriatrics Society* 43:368-373.

Koenig HG & Blazer DG (1996). II. Depression. In JE Birren (ed.) *Encyclopedia of Gerontology: Age, Aging, and the Aged. Vol. I.* San Diego, CA: Academic Press, 415-428.

LaCroix AZ, Guralnik JM, Berkman LF et al. (1993). Maintaining mobility in late life: Smoking, alcohol consumption, physical activity, and body mass index. *American Journal of Epidemiology* 137:858-869.

Liberto JG, Oslin DW & Ruskin PE (1992). Alcoholism in older persons: A review of the literature. *Hospital and Community Psychiatry* 43(10):975-984.

Miller F, Whitcup S, Sacks M et al. (1985). Unrecognized drug dependence and withdrawal in the elderly. *Drug and Alcohol Dependence* 15:177.

Miller WR & Rollnick S (1991). *Motivational Interviewing*. New York, NY: Guilford Press.

Minnis J (1988). Toward an understanding of alcohol abuse among the elderly: A sociological perspective. *Journal of Alcohol and Drug Education* 33(3):32-40.

Moeller FG, Gillin JC, Irwin M et al. (1993). A comparison of sleep EEGs in patients with primary major depression and major depression secondary to alcoholism. *Journal of Affective Disorders* 27:39-42.

Moos RH, Mertens JR & Brennan PL (1993). Patterns of diagnosis and treatment among late-middle-aged and older substance abuse patients. *Journal of Studies on Alcohol* 54:479-488.

Myers JK, Weissman MM, Tischler GL et al. (1984). Six-month prevalence of psychiatric disorders in three communities: 1980-1982. *Archives of General Psychiatry* 41:959.

National Institute on Alcohol Abuse and Alcoholism (NIAAA) (1988). Alcohol and aging. *Alcohol Alert* 2:1-5.

National Institute on Alcohol Abuse and Alcoholism (NIAAA) (1995). *The Physicians' Guide to Helping Patients With Alcohol Problems*. Rockville, MD: NIAAA, National Institutes of Health.

National Institutes of Health (NIH) (1990). The treatment of sleep disorders in older people. *Consensus Development Conference Statement* 8(3):1-22.

National Institutes of Health (NIH) (1991). Diagnosis and treatment of depression in late life. *Consensus Development Conference Statement* 9(3):1-27.

Orleans CT, Jepson C, Resch N et al. (1994a). Quitting motives and barriers among older smokers. *Cancer* 74:2055-2061.

Oslin D, Liberto JG, O'Brien J et al. (1997). Naltrexone as an adjunctive treatment for older patients with alcohol dependence. *American Journal of Geriatric Psychiatry* 5:324-332.

Oslin DW, Pettinati H, Volpicelli JR et al. (1997). Enhancing treatment compliance in elderly alcoholics: A new psychosocial intervention model. Paper presented at the annual meeting of the Gerontologic Society of America, Washington, DC.

Plomp R (1978). Auditory handicap of hearing impairment and the limited benefit of hearing aids. *Journal of the Acoustic Society of America* 63:533-549.

Portenoy RK (1993). Therapeutic use of opioids: Prescribing and control issues. In JR Cooper, DJ Czechowicz, SP Molinari et al. (eds.) *Impact of Prescription Drug Diversion Control Systems on Medical Practice and Patient Care (NIDA Research Monograph 131)*. Rockville, MD: National Institute on Drug Abuse, 35-50.

Prochaska JO, DiClemente CC & Norcross JC (1992). In search of how people change: Applications to addictive behaviors. *American Psychologist* 47(9):1102-1114.

Ray WA (1992). Psychotropic drugs and injuries among the elderly: A review. *Journal of Clinical Psychopharmacology* 12:386-396.

Ray WA, Thapa PB & Shorr RI (1993). Medications and the older driver. *Clinics in Geriatric Medicine* 9(2):413-438.

Regier DA, Farmer ME, Rae DS et al. (1990). Comorbidity of mental disorders with alcohol and other drug abuse. *Journal of the American Medical Association* 264(19):2511-2518.

Rimer BK & Orleans CT (1994). Tailoring smoking cessation for older adults. *Cancer* 74:2051-2054.

Roy W & Griffin M (1990). Prescribed medications and the risk of falling. *Topics in Geriatric Rehabilitation* 5(20):12-20.

Salthouse TA (1985). Speed of behavior and its implications for cognition. In JE Birren & KW Schaie (eds.) *Handbook of the Psychology of Aging*. New York, NY: Van Nostrand & Reinhold, 400-426.

Salzman C (1990). *Benzodiazepine Dependence, Toxicity, and Abuse: A Task Force Report of the American Psychiatric Association*. Washington, DC: American Psychiatric Press.

Salzman C (1993a). Benzodiazepine treatment of panic and agoraphobic symptoms: Use, dependence, toxicity, abuse. *Journal of Psychiatric Research* 27:97-110.

Salzman C (1993b). Issues and controversies regarding benzodiazepine use. In JR Cooper, DJ Czechowicz, SP Molinari et al. (eds.) *Impact of Prescription Drug Diversion Control Systems on Medical Practice and Patient Care (NIDA Research Monograph 131)*. Rockville, MD: National Institute on Drug Abuse, 68-88.

Saunders PA (1994). Epidemiology of alcohol problems and drinking patterns. In RM John, MT Copeland, MT Aboou-Saleh et al. (eds.) *Principles and Practice of Geriatric Psychiatry*. New York, NY: John Wiley & Sons, 801-805.

Saunders PA, Copeland JR, Dewey ME et al. (1991). Heavy drinking as a risk factor for depression and dementia in elderly men: Findings from the Liverpool Longitudinal Community Study. *British Journal of Psychiatry* 159:213-216.

Schonfeld L & Dupree LW (1991). Antecedents of drinking for early- and late-onset elderly alcohol abusers. *Journal of Studies on Alcohol* 52:587-592.

Schonfeld L & Dupree LW (1995). Treatment approaches for older problem drinkers. *International Journal of the Addictions* 30(13&14):1819-1842.

Schuckit MA (1989). *Drug and Alcohol Abuse, 3rd Edition.* New York, NY: Plenum Press.

Schuckit MA & Morrissey ER (1979). Drug abuse among alcoholic women. *American Journal of Psychiatry* 136:607-611.

Sheahan SL, Hendricks J & Coons SJ (1989). Drug misuse among the elderly: A covert problem. *Health Values* 13(3):22-29.

Smith JW (1995). Medical manifestations of alcoholism in the elderly. *International Journal of the Addictions* 30(13&14):1749-1798.

Solomon K, Manepalli J, Ireland GA et al. (1993). Alcoholism and prescription drug abuse in the elderly: St. Louis University grand rounds. *Journal of the American Geriatric Society* 41(1):57-69.

Speirs CJ, Navey FL, Broods DJ et al. (1986). Opisthotonos and benzodiazepine withdrawal in the elderly. *Lancet* 2:1101.

Swan GE, Carmelli D, Rosenman RH et al. (1990). Smoking and alcohol consumption in adult male twins: Genetic heritability and shared environmental influences. *Journal of Substance Abuse* 2:39-50.

Tarter RE (1995). Cognition, aging, and alcohol. In TP Beresford & E Gomberg (eds.) *Alcohol and Aging.* New York, NY: Oxford University Press, 82-97.

Temple MT & Leino EV (1989). Long-term outcomes of drinking: A 20 year longitudinal study of men. *British Journal of Addiction* 84:889-899.

U.S. Preventive Services Task Force (1996). *Guide to Clinical Preventive Services.* Baltimore, MD: Williams & Wilkins.

Vestal RE, McGuire EA, Tobin JD et al. (1977). Aging and ethanol metabolism. *Clinical Pharmacology and Therapeutics* 21:343-354.

Vogel-Sprott M & Barrett P (1984). Age, drinking habits, and the effects of alcohol. *Journal of Studies on Alcohol* 45:517-521.

Watson YI, Arfken CL & Birge SJ (1993). Clock completion: An objective screening test for dementia. *Journal of the American Geriatrics Society* 41:1235-1240.

Welte & Mirand (1992).

Wilsnack SC & Wilsnack RW (1995). I. Drinking and problem drinking in U.S. women: Patterns and recent trends. *Recent Developments in Alcoholism* 12:29-60.

Winger G (1993). Other abused drugs: Benzodiazepines and sedatives. In *Fourth Triennial Report to Congress on Drug Abuse and Drug Abuse Research From the Secretary, Department of Health and Human Services.* Rockville, MD: National Institute on Drug Abuse.

Woods JH & Winger G (1995). Current benzodiazepine issues. *Psychopharmacology* 118:107-115.

SECTION 5 | Management of Intoxication and Withdrawal

Section Coordinator
Michael F. Mayo-Smith, M.D., M.P.H.

Contributors

Raymond Anton, M.D.
Alcohol Research Center
Center for Drug and Alcohol Programs
Medical University of South Carolina
Charleston, South Carolina

William E. Dickinson, D.O., FASAM, FAAFP
Medical Director
Providence Behavioral Health Services
Everett, Washington

Steven J. Eickelberg, M.D., FASAM
President, PerforMax
Private Practice of Sport Psychiatry,
Addiction Medicine and Psychiatry,
Occupational and Organizational Psychiatry
Scottsdale, Arizona

David A. Gorelick, M.D., Ph.D.
Chief, Clinical Pharmacology Section
Intramural Research Program
National Institute on Drug Abuse
National Institutes of Health, and
Adjunct Professor of Psychiatry
University of Maryland School of Medicine
Baltimore, Maryland

Mark K. Greenwald, Ph.D.
Addiction Research Institute
Department of Psychiatry and Behavioral Neurosciences
Wayne State University School of Medicine
Detroit, Michigan

Christine L. Kasser, M.D.
Private Practice of Medicine
Germantown, Tennessee

Thomas R. Kosten, M.D.
Deputy Chief, Psychiatry Service
VA Connecticut Healthcare System, and
Professor of Psychiatry
Yale University School of Medicine
New Haven, Connecticut

Romana Markvitsa, M.D.
Department of Psychiatry
Cedars-Sinai Medical Center
Los Angeles, California

Michael F. Mayo-Smith, M.D., M.P.H.
Director, Primary Care Service Line
VA New England Healthcare System, and
Assistant Professor of Medicine
Harvard Medical School
Boston, Massachusetts

Katherine G. Mellott, M.D.
Department of Psychiatry
Cedars-Sinai Medical Center
Los Angeles, California

Hugh Myrick, M.D.
Alcohol Research Center
Center for Drug and Alcohol Programs
Medical University of South Carolina
Charleston, South Carolina

Patrick G. O'Connor, M.D., M.P.H.
Professor of Medicine
Yale University School of Medicine, and
Chief, Section of General Internal Medicine
Yale New Haven Hospital
New Haven, Connecticut

Susan M. Stine, M.D., Ph.D.
Associate Professor
Addiction Research Institute
Substance Abuse Research Division
Department of Psychiatry and Behavioral Neurosciences
Wayne State University School of Medicine
Detroit, Michigan

Jeffery N. Wilkins, M.D.
Director, Addiction Medicine Services
Cedars-Sinai Medical Center, and
Adjunct Professor of Psychiatry
UCLA School of Medicine
Los Angeles, California

Chapter 1

Management of Intoxication and Withdrawal: General Principles

Hugh Myrick, M.D.
Raymond Anton, M.D.
Christine L. Kasser, M.D.

Intoxication States
Withdrawal States
Special Populations

The first stage of treating individuals with substance use disorders is the recognition of intoxication and withdrawal states. The treatment of patients who are under the influence of, or experiencing withdrawal from, alcohol and other drugs of abuse requires an understanding of many variables. These variables include an appreciation of the natural history and variants of such syndromes, a complete assessment of the patient's individual medical, psychiatric, and social issues, and a knowledge of the uses and limitations of a variety of behavioral and pharmacologic interventions. All therapies must be individualized to each patient's needs and adjusted to reflect the patient's response to treatment.

This chapter will serve as an introduction to the identification and management of intoxication and withdrawal states, with the management of specific substances to be reviewed in subsequent chapters in this section.

INTOXICATION STATES

Intoxication is the mood-altering state produced when alcohol or another drug of abuse is taken. The recognition of intoxication states is of paramount importance to clinicians. Intoxication states can range from euphoria or sedation to life-threatening emergencies when overdose occurs. Typically, each substance of abuse has a set of signs and symptoms that are seen during intoxication.

Identification and treatment of intoxication can lead to prevention of withdrawal phenomenon and provide an avenue for entry into treatment. The challenge to the clinician, however, is diagnosis, because intoxication can mimic many psychiatric and medical conditions.

Identification and Management of Intoxication. The identification of intoxication begins with the collection of patient data through a patient history, physical examination, and laboratory screening. Of immediate concern is life-threatening intoxication or overdose. Thus, the first priority is general supportive care and resuscitative actions, as needed. It is important to determine not only the severity of the substance ingestion, but also the patient's level of consciousness, the substances involved, and any complicating medical disorders.

Historical information regarding substance use usually can be obtained from the patient. Questions regarding the quantity and frequency of substance use provide valuable information to the clinician. Discovering chronic patterns of substance use may aid in subsequent referral to addiction treatment. However, some individuals may be unable, or unwilling, to provide such information. In such cases, the patient's companions or family may be able to provide important information.

Standardized questionnaires for self-administration by the patient or for use by the physician are designed to elicit answers related to alcohol use (see the discussion of screening and assessment instruments in Section 3).

Toxicology screens provide valuable information regarding the type, or types, of substances used. Of toxicology screens, urine is the most widely used specimen because of the ease with which a sample is obtained, the relatively high concentrations of drugs and metabolites present in urine, and the stability of metabolites when frozen (Council on Scientific Affairs, 1987). Drug screens can aid in the differential diagnosis when atypical symptoms are present. Such screening can be particularly helpful in cases where little clinical history is available.

Screening for alcohol is accomplished primarily by Breathalyzer®, blood alcohol, or urine alcohol levels. Laboratory assays that measure increases in liver enzymes—such as gamma-glutamyl transpeptidase (GGT), aspartate aminotransferase (AST), and alanine aminotransferase (ALT)—can be helpful in identifying alcohol use. Although alcohol is not the only cause of an increase in GGT, and does not increase in younger drinkers, this assay is a reliable predictor of drinking behavior. A biologic assay to monitor alcohol intake involves carbohydrate-deficient transferrin (CDT). CDT may be a more sensitive and specific indicator of heavy alcohol consumption (Litten, Allen et al., 1995).

WITHDRAWAL STATES

Withdrawal syndrome is the predictable constellation of signs and symptoms following abrupt discontinuation of, or rapid decrease in, intake of a substance that has been used consistently for a period of time. The signs and symptoms of withdrawal usually are the opposite of a substance's direct pharmacologic effects. Substances in a given pharmacologic class produce similar withdrawal syndromes; however, the onset, duration, and intensity are variable, depending on the particular agent used, the duration of use, and the degree of neuroadaptation.

Evidence for the cessation of or reduction in use of a substance may be obtained by history or toxicology. Additionally, the clinical picture should not correspond to any of the organic mental syndromes, such as organic hallucinosis (APA, 1994). Withdrawal may, however, be superimposed on any organic mental syndrome. Therefore, a thorough physical examination is necessary, including appropriate laboratory analysis of basic organ functions.

The term "detoxification" implies a clearing of toxins. However, for individuals with physiologic substance dependence, detoxification is defined as the management of the withdrawal syndrome.

Goals of Detoxification. Detoxification is the process by which a substance on which an individual is physically dependent is gradually eliminated from the body. The three immediate goals of detoxification are (1) to provide a safe withdrawal from alcohol or other drug(s) of dependence and enable the patient to become free of nonprescribed medications, (2) to provide a withdrawal that is humane and that protects the patient's dignity, and (3) to prepare the patient for ongoing treatment of his or her dependence (CSAT, 1995a).

Many risks are associated with withdrawal, some of which are influenced by the setting in which detoxification occurs. For example, in persons who are severely dependent on alcohol, abrupt, untreated cessation of drinking may result in marked hyperautonomic signs, seizures (which may be recurrent), withdrawal delirium, or even death. Other sedative-hypnotics also can produce life-threatening withdrawal syndromes. Withdrawal from opiates and stimulants produces severe discomfort, but generally is not life-threatening. It may, however, present a danger to those who are debilitated by advanced HIV disease, medical sequelae of addiction, advanced age, coronary artery disease, and other medical problems. Moreover, risks to the patient and society are not limited to the severity of the patient's physical disturbance, particularly when the detoxification is conducted in an outpatient setting. Outpatients experiencing withdrawal symptoms may self-medicate with alcohol or other drugs that can interact with withdrawal medications in an additive fashion or precipitate overdose.

A caring staff, a supportive environment, sensitivity to cultural issues, confidentiality, and the selection of appropriate detoxification medications (as needed) are important components of a humane withdrawal. However, staff must be firm as well as sympathetic and have experience in dealing with difficult behaviors that often accompany detoxification. Supportive others (family members, friends, or employers) should be enlisted whenever possible to assist in the care of the patient during outpatient detoxification.

During detoxification, patients may form therapeutic relationships with treatment staff or other patients and may become aware of alternatives to an alcohol- or drug-using lifestyle. Detoxification is an opportunity to offer patients information and to motivate them for longer-term treatment. Unfortunately, managed care organizations and other third-party payers often regard detoxification as separate from other phases of alcohol and other drug treatment, as though detoxification occurs in isolation from such treatment. In clinical practice, this separation cannot exist: Detoxification is but one component of a comprehensive treatment strategy.

General Principles of Management. Some detoxification procedures are specific to particular drugs, while others are based on general principles of treatment and are not drug-specific. The general principles are presented here, while subsequent chapters address specific treatment protocols for each class of drugs.

There is a risk of serious adverse consequences for some patients who undergo withdrawal. As such, an initial medical assessment is important to determine the need for medication and medical management. Such an assessment should include evaluation of predicted withdrawal severity and medical or psychiatric comorbidity.

While the severity of a given patient's withdrawal cannot always be predicted with accuracy, helpful information includes the amount and duration of alcohol or other drug use, the severity of the patient's prior withdrawal experiences (if any), and the patient's medical and psychiatric history. A widely used instrument in clinical and research settings for the initial assessment and ongoing monitoring of alcohol withdrawal is the Clinical Institute Withdrawal Assessment of Alcohol-Revised (CIWA-Ar). The CIWA-Ar is a short test that rates the severity of withdrawal, as observed by the clinician. In general, low scores (9 or less) suggest that pharmacotherapy may not be required, whereas high scores (10 or more) indicate a greater risk of seizures and *delirium tremens.*

Every means possible should be used to ameliorate the patient's withdrawal signs and symptoms. Medication should not be the only component of treatment, as psychological support is extremely important in reducing the patient's distress during detoxification.

The duration of detoxification is not a clearly defined, discrete period of time. Because detoxification often requires a greater intensity of services than other types of treatment, there is a practical value in defining a period during which a person is "in detoxification." The detoxification period usually is defined as the time during which the patient receives detoxification medications, even though some signs and symptoms may persist for a much longer period. Another way of defining the detoxification period is by measuring the duration of withdrawal signs or symptoms. However, the duration of these symptoms may be difficult to determine in a correctly medicated patient, because symptoms of withdrawal are largely suppressed by the medication.

Another problem in defining the duration of detoxification is the fact that many patients may have prolonged withdrawal signs or symptoms, or "protracted abstinence syndrome." Symptoms of the syndrome include disturbances of sleep, anxiety, irritability, and mood instability. The very existence of the protracted abstinence syndrome has been the subject of considerable controversy (Geller, 1994). Physicians often find it difficult to distinguish symptoms caused by drug withdrawal from those caused by a patient's underlying mental disorder, if one is present. The signs and symptoms of protracted withdrawal thus are not as predictable as those of acute withdrawal, which produces measurable signs that researchers can study in animals under controlled laboratory conditions; protracted withdrawal, on the other hand, often is confined to distress symptoms for which there are no animal models.

The plan of care for detoxification should be individualized to account for the considerable variation among patients in terms of signs and symptoms of withdrawal. The best outcomes are obtained by tailoring the detoxification regimen to meet the needs of individual patients. The initial plan of care for detoxification should be adjusted to reflect the patient's response to the treatment provided.

Pharmacologic Management: There are two general strategies for pharmacologic management of withdrawal: suppressing withdrawal through use of a cross-tolerant medication, and reducing signs and symptoms of withdrawal through alteration of another neuropharmacological process. Either, or both, may be used to manage withdrawal syndromes effectively. In order to suppress withdrawal with cross-tolerant medication, a longer acting medication typically is used to provide a milder, controlled withdrawal. Examples include use of methadone for opiate detoxification and diazepam for alcohol detoxification. Medications that are not cross-tolerant are used to treat specific signs and symptoms of withdrawal. Examples include use of clonidine for opiate or alcohol withdrawal.

Detoxification alone rarely constitutes adequate treatment. The provision of detoxification services without continuing treatment at an appropriate level of care constitutes less than optimal use of limited resources. The appropriate level of care and content of treatment following detoxification must be clinically determined, based on the patient's individual needs. Biopsychosocial factors to be considered in determining the continuing treatment plan include medical and psychiatric conditions, motivation, relapse potential, and available support systems. These factors correspond to the dimensions of illness described in the *ASAM Patient Placement Criteria for the Treatment of Substance-Related Disorders, Second Edition-Revised (ASAM PPC-2R*; Mee-Lee, Shulman et al., 2001).

Detoxification Settings. The initial assessment should facilitate the selection of the appropriate level of care for detoxification. Detoxification may take place in a variety of inpatient and outpatient settings. Multiple instruments have been designed to facilitate selection of an appropriate level of care. The *ASAM PPC-2R* contains detailed guidelines for matching patients to an appropriate intensity of services for detoxification.

Detoxification is conducted in both inpatient and outpatient settings. Both types of settings initiate recovery programs that may include referrals for problems such as medical, legal, psychiatric, and family issues.

Inpatient Detoxification: Inpatient detoxification is offered in medical hospitals, psychiatric hospitals, and medically managed residential treatment programs. As described by Alling (1992), inpatient detoxification has several advantages to outpatient detoxification. First, the inpatient detoxification restricts the patient's access to substances of abuse. Second, inpatient detoxification allows the clinician to closely monitor the patient for serious withdrawal symptoms and adjust medications as indicated. Such monitoring is especially important if the patient is dependent on high doses of alcohol or other sedative-hypnotic drugs. Finally, detoxification in an inpatient facility can be accomplished more rapidly than in an outpatient setting.

In the case of detoxification from alcohol, about 20% of those undergoing treatment for alcohol withdrawal must be treated as inpatients. Relative indications for inpatient treatment include a history of alcohol withdrawal seizures or delirium, pregnancy, medical or psychiatric illness, or lack of a reliable support system (Saitz & O'Malley, 1997; Myrick & Anton, 2000). Inpatient care of alcohol withdrawal can be 10 to 20 times as expensive as outpatient care. Generally, therefore, it is reserved for those expected to have severe withdrawal symptoms and to require a more intensive level of care (such as patients with a history of severe withdrawal symptoms).

Outpatient Detoxification: Outpatient detoxification usually is offered in community mental health centers, methadone maintenance programs, addiction treatment programs, and private clinics. Alling (1992) cites several advantages of outpatient detoxification. First, it is much less expensive than inpatient treatment. Second, the patient's life is not disrupted to the degree that it is during inpatient treatment. Finally, the patient does not undergo the abrupt transition from a protected inpatient setting to the everyday home and work settings.

Emergency departments are important components of outpatient detoxification, as they often serve as a gateway to detoxification services. Detoxification programs may rely on emergency department staff to assess and initiate treatment for patients with medical conditions or medical complications that occur during detoxification. For social model programs, emergency departments often serve as a safety net for patients who need medical treatment. For the addict who has overdosed or who is experiencing a medical complication of abuse, the emergency department may be the initial point of contact with the health care system and serve as a source of case identification and referral to detoxification. Many patients experiencing alcohol withdrawal seizures present initially to an emergency department where they are taken after a seminal episode.

Considerations in Selecting a Setting: The best detoxification setting for a given patient may be defined as the least restrictive, least expensive setting in which the goals of detoxification can be met. The ability to meet this standard assumes that treatment choices always are based primarily on a patient's clinical needs. A comprehensive evaluation of the patient often indicates what therapeutic goals might be achieved realistically during the time allotted for the detoxification process.

Treatment providers should consider detoxification settings and patient matching within the context of two fundamental principles of high-quality patient care. The first is that the patient's needs should drive the selection of the most appropriate setting. The severity of the patient's withdrawal symptoms and the intensity of care required to ensure appropriate management of these symptoms are of primary importance.

Pressures to achieve cost savings are having a significant effect on the selection of treatment settings for detoxification. Many insurance companies, managed care organizations, and other payers have adopted stringent policies concerning reimbursement for alcohol and other drug detoxification services. These policies govern not only the setting in which the services are provided, but also the maximum number and duration of detoxification episodes that are covered benefits.

Such policies give insufficient weight to the variety of factors that affect the selection of a setting in which the patient has the greatest likelihood of achieving satisfactory detoxification. Some persons in need of detoxification, for example, may not be appropriate candidates for outpatient detoxification because of environmental impediments such as a spouse who is using alcohol or other drugs. Such a patient may be more appropriately detoxified in a residential setting such as a recovery house or other residential environment that is free of alcohol and other drug use.

Panelists convened by the federal Center for Substance Abuse Treatment expressed concern that important clinical decisions often are driven by economic rather than clinical considerations (CSAT, 1995a). They affirmed that the dominant principle in patient placement is that detoxification is cost-effective only if it is appropriate to the needs of the individual patient.

Use of the ASAM Patient Placement Criteria: The *ASAM PPC-2R* is intended for use as a clinical tool for matching patients to appropriate levels of care. The criteria reflect a clinical consensus of adult and adolescent treatment specialists and incorporate the results of a comprehensive peer review by professionals in addiction treatment. The ASAM criteria describe levels of treatment that are differentiated by the following characteristics: (1) degree of direct medical management provided, (2) degree of structure, safety, and security provided, and (3) degree of treatment intensity provided.

The ASAM criteria offer a variety of options, on the premise that each patient should be placed in a level of care that has the appropriate resources (staff, facilities, and services) to assess and treat that patient's substance use disorder.

Relapse. Many individuals undergo detoxification more than once, and some do so many times. When recently de-pendent persons return for repeat detoxification, it generally is with a more realistic expectation of what is needed to remain free from alcohol and other drugs. O'Brien and colleagues (1991) point out that compliance and relapse in addictive disease are comparable to rates of relapse in other illnesses, such as diabetes and hypertension. Therefore, they recommend comparable long-term treatment. While addicted persons are at increased risk of relapse at certain points in their recovery, relapse can occur at any time. The relapsed patient is an appropriate candidate for detoxification and continuing treatment, including relapse prevention education.

SPECIAL POPULATIONS

While researchers have not yet thoroughly evaluated withdrawal strategies for certain populations, patients in several groups clearly require special consideration.

Pregnant and Nursing Women. Special concerns attend detoxification during pregnancy. For example, withdrawal from opiates can result in fetal distress, which can lead to premature labor or miscarriage (Miller, 1998; Mitchell, 1994). On the other hand, opioid substitution therapy, coupled with good prenatal care, generally is associated with good maternal and fetal outcomes (Miller, 1998; Mitchell, 1994; Kreek, 1979). Although offspring of women on opioid maintenance therapy tend to have a lower birth weight and smaller head circumference than drug-free newborns, no developmental differences at six months of age have been documented. Use of clonidine in pregnant women should be considered investigational and done only in the setting of a research protocol.

Federal panels recommend that all pregnant and nursing women be advised of the potential risks of drugs that are excreted in breast milk (CSAT, 1993a; CSAT, 1995a). Nevertheless, they advise that detoxification protocols should not be modified for nursing women unless there is specific evidence that the detoxification medication enters the breast milk in amounts that could be harmful to the nursing infant (CSAT, 1995a; CSAT, 1993a). Women who are using benzodiazepines, antidepressants, or antipsychotic medications should not breastfeed (CSAT, 1995a). (Also see the chapter on perinatal addiction in Section 10.)

Persons Who Are HIV-Positive. A diagnosis of HIV infection does not change the indications for detoxification medications, which can be used in HIV-positive persons in the same way they are used in uninfected patients. A federal panel advises that the detoxification process need not be altered by the presence of HIV infection (CSAT, 1993c; 1993e; 1995a).

Patients With Other Medical Conditions. Brain-injured patients are at risk for seizures (CSAT, 1995a). If an alcohol- or other drug-abusing patient who has sustained trauma to the head becomes delirious, the exact cause of the delirium must be determined. Slower medication tapers should be used in patients with seizure disorders (CSAT, 1995a). Doses of anticonvulsant medications should be stabilized before sedative-hypnotic withdrawal begins. The treatment of individuals with past alcohol or sedative-hypnotic withdrawal seizures is controversial. In such a situation, the use of anticonvulsant agents (carbamazepine, valproate) should be considered, either alone or in combination with benzodiazepines.

Patients with cardiac disease require continued clinical assessment (Chiang & Goldfrank, 1990). Because a withdrawal seizure—or even the physiologic stress of withdrawal—may complicate the patient's cardiac condition, it may be necessary to withdraw the drug at a slower-than-normal rate. Treatment providers also should be alert to the possibility of interactions between cardiac medications and the agents used to manage detoxification.

Severe liver or renal disease can slow the metabolism of both the drug of abuse and the detoxification medication. Use of shorter acting detoxification drugs and a slower taper are appropriate for such patients, but require precautions against drug accumulation and oversedation (Chiang & Goldfrank, 1990).

Pain patients may not require detoxification from prescribed medications unless they meet the *DSM-IV* criteria for opiate abuse or dependence (CSAT, 1995a). However, treatment providers should exercise caution when prescribing medications for chronic pain patients who have a history of addictive disorders. Also, any patient who has taken opiates or sedative-hypnotics for a prolonged period of time should be weaned from them gradually.

Patients With Psychiatric Comorbidities. It is difficult to assess accurately underlying psychopathology in a patient who is undergoing detoxification (CSAT, 1995a). Drug toxicity or organic psychiatric symptoms (particularly with amphetamines and cocaine, hallucinogens, or phencyclidine) can mimic psychiatric disorders. For this reason, a thorough psychiatric evaluation should be conducted after two to three weeks of abstinence.

At the time they are evaluated for detoxification, some patients with underlying psychiatric disorders already are using antidepressants, neuroleptics, anxiolytics, or lithium. Although staff may believe that such patients should discontinue all psychoactive drugs immediately, a federal panel advises that this course of action may not be in the best interest of the patient (CSAT, 1995a). Abrupt cessation of psychotherapeutic medications may cause withdrawal symptoms or reemergence of symptoms of the underlying psychopathology. Thus decisions about discontinuing the medication should be deferred temporarily. If, however, the patient has been abusing the prescribed medication or the psychiatric condition clearly was caused by the patient's alcohol or other drug abuse, the rationale for discontinuing the medication is more compelling. Individuals who use both sedative-hypnotics and alcohol pose a real challenge for detoxification, which generally should be conducted in an inpatient setting and over a prolonged period of time.

During detoxification, some patients decompensate into psychosis, depression, or severe anxiety. In such cases, careful evaluation of the withdrawal medication regimen is of paramount importance. Anxiety symptoms can cause an overestimation of withdrawal severity on the CIWA-Ar and therefore overmedication of withdrawal. If the decompensation is the result of inadequate dosing with the withdrawal medication, the appropriate response is to increase that medication. If the dose of the withdrawal medication appears to be adequate, other medications may need to be added. Before selecting that alternative, however, it is important to consider the potential side effects of the additional medication and the possibility of interaction with the withdrawal medication. If withdrawal medications are adequate and appropriate but the patient continues to decompensate, nonaddicting psychotropic medications (such as antipsychotics, anticonvulsants, or antidepressants) may be indicated for the treatment of psychoses, depression, or anxiety emerging during withdrawal. After detoxification is completed, the patient's need for medications should be reassessed. A trial period with no medications may be indicated.

Adolescents. Adolescents in detoxification pose somewhat different clinical issues than do adults. Chief among these is that physical dependence generally is not as severe and the adolescent patient's response to detoxification usually is more rapid than that of the adult (CSAT, 1995a; 1993d). Behavioral problems may be more indirect, and the potential for suicide needs to be evaluated carefully.

Adolescents who are undergoing detoxification need a structured environment that is nurturing and supportive. This is especially important because adolescents are notorious for leaving treatment against medical advice. Also, adolescents should be housed separately from adults. Decisions about involving the family in treatment should be made on a case-by-case basis and should reflect an assessment of family functioning.

Note: Federal regulations allow methadone detoxification of adolescents, but state regulations vary. Methadone detoxification is rare in this age group.

Older Adults. Because of the increased likelihood of medical comorbidities, it is essential to conduct a complete assessment and careful monitoring of the patient for comorbid conditions, such as respiratory or cardiac disease, or diabetes (Wartenberg & Nirenberg, 1995). In addition, aging patients may be taking a number of prescription and over-the-counter drugs, so the possibility of drug interactions cannot be ignored. For these reasons, detoxification in a medically monitored or medically managed setting often is required (CSAT, 1995a).

The cumulative effects of years of drinking may lead to more severe withdrawal symptoms in elderly persons (Anton & Becker, 1995), so the shorter-acting benzodiazepines may be of more clinical utility in this population given their lower risk of oversedation. It may be necessary to reduce the doses of detoxification medications because of older patients' slowed metabolism or coexisting medical disorders.

Persons in Criminal Justice Settings. Persons who are incarcerated or in detention in holding cells or elsewhere should be assessed for dependence on alcohol or other drugs, because untreated withdrawal from alcohol and sedative-hypnotics can be life threatening (CSAT, 1995a; 1994b). While heroin withdrawal is not life threatening to a healthy individual, it can be very difficult for the patient and should be treated appropriately.

Patients who have been on maintenance therapy before being incarcerated should continue to receive their usual dose of medication if the expected period of incarceration is less than two weeks. If it is to be longer, the maintenance therapy should be discontinued gradually. Individuals who are on methadone maintenance may experience severe withdrawal symptoms if the medication is stopped abruptly. Indeed, methadone abstinence symptoms may persist for weeks or months and include severe vomiting and diarrhea, which can lead to complications. Pain may be severe and intractable.

Detoxification protocols need not be modified for incarcerated persons, except to the extent that state laws restrict the use of methadone or LAAM in criminal justice settings. In such cases, linkages with local methadone detoxification programs are advised.

In dealing with incarcerated patients, the physician needs to be aware that, in most prisons, there is an underground market for psychoactive medications. Patients may try to deceive caregivers about their dependence in order to obtain drugs for sale to others. For this reason, prison medical staff need special training in patient assessment and detoxification (CSAT, 1994b).

CONCLUSIONS

The recognition and treatment of intoxication and withdrawal states represent important initial steps in the treatment of alcohol or other drug addiction. The primary goal of managing intoxication and withdrawal states is the prevention of morbidity and mortality. Whereas the treatment of intoxication often takes place in a medical setting, the treatment of withdrawal can occur in either an inpatient or an outpatient setting. Many variables must be taken into consideration in providing optimum care to patients who are undergoing treatment of withdrawal states. The *ASAM PPC-2R* can aid the clinician in matching patients to the appropriate levels of care for ongoing treatment of their addictive disorders.

ACKNOWLEDGMENT: This work was supported in part by an NIH NIAAA Center grant, an NIH NIAAA K Award, and a VA Merit Review.

REFERENCES

Alling FA (1992). Detoxification and treatment of acute sequelae. In JH Lowinson, P Ruiz & RB Millman (eds.) *Substance Abuse: A Comprehensive Textbook.* Baltimore, MD: Williams & Wilkins, 402-415.

American Psychiatric Association (APA) (1994). *Diagnostic and Statistical Manual of Mental Disorders, 4th Edition.* Washington, DC: American Psychiatric Press.

Anton RF & Becker HC (1995). Pharmacology and pathophysiology of alcohol withdrawal. In HR Kranzler (ed.) *Handbook of Experimental Pharmacology, Volume 114: The Pharmacology of Alcohol Abuse.* New York, NY: Springer-verlag, 315-367.

Center for Substance Abuse Treatment (CSAT) (1995a). *Detoxification from Alcohol and Other Drugs (Treatment Improvement Protocol Series, Number 19).* Rockville, MD: Substance Abuse and Mental Health Services Administration.

Center for Substance Abuse Treatment (CSAT) (1993d). *Guidelines for Improving the Treatment of Alcohol and Other Drug-Abusing Adolescents (Treatment Improvement Protocol Series, Number 4).* Rockville, MD: Substance Abuse and Mental Health Services Administration.

Center for Substance Abuse Treatment (CSAT) (1994a). *Intensive Outpatient Treatment for Alcohol and Other Drug Abuse (Treatment Improvement Protocol Series, Number 8).* Rockville, MD: Substance Abuse and Mental Health Services Administration.

Center for Substance Abuse Treatment (CSAT) (1995b). *LAAM in the Treatment of Opioid Addiction (Treatment Improvement Protocol Series, Number 22).* Rockville, MD: Substance Abuse and Mental Health Services Administration.

Center for Substance Abuse Treatment (CSAT) (1995c). *Matching Treatment to Patient Needs in Opioid Substitution Therapy (Treatment Improvement Protocol Series, Number 20).* Rockville, MD: Substance Abuse and Mental Health Services Administration.

Center for Substance Abuse Treatment (CSAT) (1994b). *Planning for Alcohol and Other Drug Abuse Treatment for Adults in the Criminal Justice System (Treatment Improvement Protocol Series, Number 17).* Rockville, MD: Substance Abuse and Mental Health Services Administration.

Center for Substance Abuse Treatment (CSAT) (1993a). *Pregnant, Substance-Using Women (Treatment Improvement Protocol Series, Number 2).* Rockville, MD: Substance Abuse and Mental Health Services Administration.

Center for Substance Abuse Treatment (CSAT) (1993e). *Screening for Infectious Diseases Among Substance Abusers (Treatment Improvement Protocol Series, Number 6).* Rockville, MD: Substance Abuse and Mental Health Services Administration.

Center for Substance Abuse Treatment (CSAT) (1993b). *State Methadone Treatment Guidelines (Treatment Improvement Protocol Series, Number 1).* Rockville, MD: Substance Abuse and Mental Health Services Administration.

Center for Substance Abuse Treatment (CSAT) (1993c). *Treatment for HIV-Infected Alcohol and Other Drug Abusers (Treatment Improvement Protocol Series, Number 15).* Rockville, MD: Substance Abuse and Mental Health Services Administration.

Chiang W & Goldfrank L (1990). The medical complications of drug abuse. *Medical Journal of Australia* 152:83-88, January.

Cochin J & Kornetsky C (1964). Development and loss of tolerance to morphine in the rat after single and multiple injections. *Journal of Pharmacological and Experimental Therapeutics* 145:1-10.

Council on Scientific Affairs (1987).

Geller A (1998). Management of protracted withdrawal. In AW Graham & TK Schultz (eds.) *Principles of Addiction Medicine, Second Edition.* Chevy Chase, MD: American Society of Addiction Medicine.

Kreek MJ (1979). Methadone disposition during the perinatal period in humans. *Pharmacology, Biochemistry and Behavior* 11:7-13.

Litten RZ, Allen JP & Fertig JB (1995). Gamma-glutamyltranspeptidase and carbohydrate-deficient transferrin-alternative measures of excessive alcohol consumption. *Alcoholism: Clinical & Experimental Research* 19:1541-1546.

Mee-Lee D, Shulman G, Fishman M et al. (2001). *Patient Placement Criteria for the Treatment of Substance-Related Disorders, 2nd Edition-Revised (ASAM PPC-2R).* Chevy Chase, MD: American Society of Addiction Medicine.

Miller LJ (1998). Detoxification of the addicted woman in pregnancy. In AW Graham & TK Schultz (eds.) *Principles of Addiction Medicine, Second Edition.* Chevy Chase, MD: American Society of Addiction Medicine.

Mitchell JL (1994). Treatment of the addicted woman in pregnancy. In NS Miller (ed.) *Principles of Addiction Medicine, First Edition.* Chevy Chase, MD: American Society of Addiction Medicine.

Myrick H & Anton R (2000). Clinical management of alcohol withdrawal. *CNS Spectrums* 5(2): 22-32.

O'Brien CP, Childress AR & McLellan AT (1991). *Conditioning Factors May Help to Understand and Prevent Relapse in Patients Who Are Recovering from Drug Dependence (NIDA Research Monograph Number 106).* Rockville, MD: National Institute on Drug Abuse.

Saitz R & O'Malley SS (1997). Pharmacotherapies of alcohol abuse. Withdrawal and treatment. *Medical Clinics of North America* 81(4):881-907.

Wartenberg AA & Nirenberg TD (1995). Alcohol and drug abuse in the older patient. In W Reichel (ed.) *Care of the Elderly: Clinical Aspects of Aging, Edition 4.* Baltimore, MD: Williams & Wilkins, 133-141.

Summary of the ASAM Patient Placement Criteria for Adult Patients in Need of Detoxification Services

Dimension 1, Acute Intoxication and/or Withdrawal Potential, is the first of the six primary assessment areas to be evaluated in making treatment and placement decisions. The range of clinical severity seen in this dimension has given rise to multiple levels of intensity in the management of detoxification.

In this context, detoxification refers not only to the attenuation of the physiological and psychological features of withdrawal syndromes, but also to the process of interrupting the momentum of compulsive use in persons diagnosed with substance *dependence*. Because of the force of this momentum and the inherent difficulties in overcoming it even when there is no clear withdrawal syndrome, this phase of treatment frequently requires a greater intensity of services initially in order to establish treatment engagement and patient role induction. This is, of course, critical to the course of treatment because of the impossibility of engaging a patient in treatment while that patient is caught up in the cycle of frequent intoxication and withdrawal.

TREATMENT LEVELS WITHIN DIMENSION 1

Level I-D: Ambulatory Detoxification Without Extended On-Site Monitoring. Level I-D detoxification is an organized outpatient service, which may be delivered in an office setting, health care or addiction treatment facility, or in a patient's home by trained clinicians who provide medically supervised evaluation, detoxification and referral services according to a predetermined schedule. Such services are provided in regularly scheduled sessions. Level I-D services should be delivered under a defined set of policies and procedures or medical protocols.

Outpatient detoxification services should be designed to treat the patient's level of clinical severity and to achieve safe and comfortable withdrawal from mood-altering drugs (including alcohol) and to effectively facilitate the patient's transition into ongoing treatment and recovery.

Level II-D: Ambulatory Detoxification With Extended On-Site Monitoring. Level II-D detoxification is an organized outpatient service, which may be delivered in an office setting, health care or addiction treatment facility by trained clinicians who provide medically supervised evaluation, detoxification and referral services. Level II-D services are provided in regularly scheduled sessions. They are deliv-

ered under a defined set of policies and procedures or medical protocols. Outpatient services are designed to treat the patient's level of clinical severity and to achieve safe and comfortable withdrawal from mood-altering drugs (including alcohol) and to effectively facilitate the patient's entry into ongoing treatment and recovery.

Essential to this level of care is the availability of appropriately credentialed and licensed nurses (such as registered nurses or licensed practical nurses), who monitor patients over a period of several hours each day of service.

Level III-D: Residential/Inpatient Detoxification. Criteria are provided for two types of Level III detoxification programs: Level III.1-D and III.5-D (Clinically Managed Residential Detoxification) and Level III.7-D (Medically Monitored Inpatient Detoxification). The "residential" level of care has, in the past, been synonymous with rehabilitation services, whereas detoxification services and the "inpatient" level of care have been synonymous with acute inpatient hospital care. With the increased availability and utilization of Medically Monitored Inpatient Detoxification Services, the terms "residential" and "inpatient" are being used more broadly to contrast ambulatory ("outpatient") detoxification with non-ambulatory ("residential" or "inpatient") detoxification services. The difference between these two levels of detoxification is the intensity of clinical services, particularly as demonstrated by the degree of involvement of medical and nursing professionals.

Level III.1-D and III.5-D: Clinically Managed Residential Detoxification (sometimes referred to as "social setting detoxification") is an organized service that may be delivered by appropriately trained staff, who provide 24-hour supervision, observation and support for patients who are intoxicated or experiencing withdrawal. Clinically managed residential detoxification is characterized by its emphasis on peer and social support.

This level provides care for patients whose intoxication/withdrawal signs and symptoms are sufficiently severe to require 24-hour structure and support. However, the full resources of a Level III.7-D, medically monitored inpatient detoxification service, are not necessary.

Some clinically managed residential detoxification programs are staffed to supervise self-administered medications for the management of withdrawal. All programs at this level rely on established clinical protocols to identify patients who are in need of medical services beyond the capacity of the facility and to transfer such patients to more appropriate levels of care.

Level III.7-D: Medically Monitored Inpatient Detoxification is an organized service delivered by medical and nursing professionals, which provides for 24-hour medically supervised evaluation and withdrawal management in a permanent facility with inpatient beds. Services are delivered under a defined set of physician-approved policies and physician-monitored procedures or clinical protocols.

This level provides care to patients whose withdrawal signs and symptoms are sufficiently severe to require 24-hour inpatient care. It sometimes is provided by overlapping with Level IV-D services (as a "step-down" service) in a specialty unit of an acute care general or psychiatric hospital. Twenty-four hour observation, monitoring and treatment are available. However, the full resources of an acute care general hospital or a medically managed intensive inpatient treatment program are not necessary.

Level III.7-D detoxification also can be provided by overlapping with Level IV-D detoxification as a step-down service in a specialty unit of a general or psychiatric hospital.

Level IV-D: Medically Managed Intensive Inpatient Detoxification. Level IV-D detoxification is an organized service delivered by medical and nursing professionals that provides for 24-hour medically directed evaluation and withdrawal management in an acute care inpatient setting. Services are delivered under a defined set of physician-approved policies and physician-managed procedures or medical protocols.

Level IV-D provides care to patients whose withdrawal signs and symptoms are sufficiently severe to require primary medical and nursing care services. Twenty-four hour observation, monitoring and treatment are available. Although Level IV-D is specifically designed for acute medical detoxification, it also is important to assess the patient and develop a care plan for any treatment priorities identified in Dimensions 2 through 6.

SOURCE: Mee-Lee D, Shulman G, Fishman M et al. (2001). *ASAM Patient Placement Criteria for the Treatment of Substance-Related Disorders, Second Edition-Revised (ASAM PPC-2R).* Chevy Chase, MD: American Society of Addiction Medicine. Reprinted by permission of the publisher.

Chapter 2

Management of Alcohol Intoxication and Withdrawal

Michael F. Mayo-Smith, M.D., M.P.H.

Alcohol Intoxication
Alcohol Withdrawal
Pharmacologic Management
Common Treatment Issues

Management of alcohol intoxication and withdrawal is one of the clinical issues most frequently encountered by specialists in addiction medicine. Effective approaches, with a strong scientific basis, have been developed to reduce the incidence of serious complications.

ALCOHOL INTOXICATION

Clinical Picture. As blood alcohol concentration rises, so too does the clinical effect on the individual (Herrington, 1987). At a blood alcohol concentration between 20 mg% and 99 mg%, loss of muscular coordination begins. Changes in mood, personality, and behavior accompany these blood alcohol levels. As the blood alcohol level rises to the range of 100 mg% to 199 mg%, neurologic impairment occurs, accompanied by prolonged reaction time, ataxia, incoordination, and mental impairment.

At a blood alcohol level of 200 mg% to 299 mg%, very obvious intoxication is present, except in those with marked tolerance. Nausea and vomiting, as well as marked ataxia, may occur. As the level rises to 300 mg% to 399 mg%, hypothermia may occur, along with severe dysarthria and amnesia, with Stage I anesthesia.

At blood alcohol levels between 400 mg% and 799 mg%, the onset of alcoholic coma occurs. The precise level at which this occurs depends on tolerance: Some persons experience coma at levels of 400 mg%, while others do not experience it until the level approaches 600 mg%.

Serum levels of alcohol between 600 mg% and 800 mg% often are fatal. Progressive obtundation develops, accompanied by decreases in respiration, blood pressure, and body temperature. The patient may develop urinary incontinence or retention, while reflexes are markedly decreased or absent. Death may occur from the loss of airway protective reflexes (with subsequent airway obstruction by the flaccid tongue), from pulmonary aspiration of gastric contents, or from respiratory arrest arising from profound central nervous system (CNS) depression.

Management. Management of alcohol intoxication and overdose remains supportive. The most important goal is to prevent severe respiratory depression and to protect the airway to prevent aspiration. Even with very high blood alcohol levels, survival is probable as long as the respiratory and cardiovascular systems can be supported. As with all patients with impaired consciousness, intravenous glucose and thiamine should be given; however, these are of particular importance in alcohol intoxication. Ethanol can impair gluconeogenesis, with an increased risk of hypoglycemia, and chronic alcoholism places the individual at increased risk of thiamine deficiency. It also is important to assess whether the patient has ingested other drugs in addition to alcohol, as these may further suppress the central nervous system and alter the approach to treatment.

Alcohol is rapidly absorbed, so induction of emesis or gastric lavage usually is not indicated unless a substantial ingestion has occurred within the preceding 30 to 60 minutes, or unless other drug ingestion is suspected. Ipecac-induced emesis may be useful at the scene (for example, with children at home), if it can be given within a few minutes of exposure. Similarly, gastric lavage is indicated only if the patient presents in the emergency department soon after ingestion. Activated charcoal does not efficiently absorb ethanol, but may be given if other toxins have been ingested.

Enhancement of elimination has a very limited role to play. Over 90% of alcohol is oxidized in the liver and, at the levels seen clinically, the rate of oxidation follows zero-order kinetics; that is, it is independent of time and concentration of the drug. Elimination thus occurs at a fixed rate, with the level falling at a rate of about 20 mg/dl/hour. In extreme cases, hemodialysis can be used, as it efficiently removes alcohol, but it is needed only rarely because supportive care usually is sufficient.

Hemoperfusion and forced diuresis are not effective. High doses of oral or intravenous fructose will moderately increase alcohol metabolism. Large fructose doses, however, cause gastrointestinal upset, lactic acidosis, hyperuricemia, and osmotic diuresis, which make this approach of little clinical value.

At present there is no known agent that is effective as an alcohol antagonist, reversing the effects of alcohol in the same manner that naloxone reverses opiate intoxication. While human laboratory studies have shown that CNS stimulants such as amphetamines and caffeine can overcome some of the sedation and psychomotor impairment produced by acute alcohol intoxication, they are not useful clinically. Such stimulants have significant toxicities, which limit their use at higher doses. In patients with clinically significant alcohol ingestions, they would pose the risk of producing a mixed CNS depressant/stimulant intoxication (Gorelick, 1993). Benzodiazepine antagonists such as flumazenil do not block or reverse alcohol intoxication (Broaden & Goa, 1991).

The acutely intoxicated patient may exhibit some agitation as part of the intoxication syndrome. This is best managed non-pharmacologically. Support and reassurance can go a long way in dealing with agitation in an acutely intoxicated patient. On rare occasions, if pharmacologic intervention is needed to manage a mildly or moderately intoxicated individual's behavior in a medical setting, intramuscular administration of a rapid onset, short-acting benzodiazepine (such as lorazepam), alone or in combination with a neuroleptic agent such as haloperidol, can be useful. Caution must be exercised in regard to a potential synergistic response between the alcohol already in the patient's system and an exogenously administered sedative-hypnotic, so this approach should be used only as a last resort and not in individuals with high blood alcohol levels.

ALCOHOL WITHDRAWAL

Clinical Picture. The clinical manifestations of alcohol withdrawal begin 6 to 24 hours after the last drink, sometimes arising before the blood alcohol level has returned to zero.

Early withdrawal signs and symptoms include anxiety, sleep disturbances, vivid dreams, anorexia, nausea, and headache. Physical signs include tachycardia, elevation of blood pressure, hyperactive reflexes, sweating, and hyperthermia. A tremor, best brought out by extension of the hands or tongue, may appear; this tremor has a rate of 6 to 8 cycles per second and appears on electromyography to be an exaggeration of normal physiologic tremor.

Alcohol withdrawal seizures can occur at various times, but most occur within 48 hours of cessation. Alcohol withdrawal delirium, or *delirium tremens*, typically begins 48 to 72 hours after the last drink and is preceded by the typical signs and symptoms of early withdrawal, although these may be masked or delayed by other illnesses or medications. Signs of sympathetic hyperactivity (such as tachycardia, hypertension, fever, and diaphoresis) often are profound and are hallmarks of alcohol withdrawal delirium. The mortality rate is thought to be 1% to 5% and increases with delayed diagnosis, inadequate treatment, and concurrent medical conditions.

Pathophysiology. Goldstein and Goldstein proposed in 1961 that dependency develops as a cell or organism makes homeostatic adjustments to compensate for the primary effect of a drug (Goldstein & Goldstein, 1961). As described in Section 2, the primary effect of alcohol on the brain is depressant. With chronic exposure, there are compensatory adjustments to this chronic depressant effect, with down-regulation of inhibitory systems and up-regulation of excitatory systems. With abrupt abstinence from alcohol, these relative deficiencies in inhibitory influences and relative excesses in excitatory influences suddenly are unmasked, leading to the appearance of withdrawal phenomena. The withdrawal symptoms last until the body readjusts to the absence of the alcohol and establishes a new equilibrium.

Two neurotransmitter systems appear to play a central role in the development of alcohol withdrawal. Alcohol exerts its effects in part by directly or indirectly enhancing the effect of GABA, a major inhibitory neurotransmitter. GABA mediates typical sedative-hypnotic effects such as sedation, muscle relaxation, and a raised seizure threshold. Chronic alcohol intake leads to an adaptive suppression of GABA activity. A sudden relative deficiency in GABA neurotransmitter activity is produced with alcohol abstinence, and is believed to contribute to the anxiety, increased psychomotor activity, and predisposition to seizures seen in withdrawal.

While alcohol enhances the effect of GABA, it inhibits the sensitivity of autonomic adrenergic systems, with a resulting upregulation concurrent with chronic alcohol intake. The discontinuation of alcohol leads to rebound overactivity of the brain and peripheral noradrenergic systems. Increased sympathetic autonomic activity, arising from increased neuronal activity in the locus ceruleus area of the brain stem, contributes to such acute manifestations as tachycardia, hypertension, tremor, diaphoresis, and anxiety. Norepinephrine and its metabolites are elevated in plasma, urine, and cerebral spinal fluid during withdrawal; levels of metabolites correlate significantly with the sympathetic nervous system signs of withdrawal (Hawley, Major et al., 1985).

Research is beginning to identify a large number of other neural effects of chronic alcohol intake, including effects on neuronal calcium channels, on glutamate receptors, on cyclic AMP systems, and on the hypothalamic-pituitary-adrenal neuroendocrine axis. However, the importance of these in producing the clinical manifestations of alcohol withdrawal and their implications for treatment are uncertain at this time.

Clinical Presentation. "If the patient be in the prime of life and if from drinking he has trembling hands, it may be well to announce beforehand either delirium or convulsions" (Hippocrates, circa 400 BC). As the quotation reveals, the relationship of heavy alcohol intake to certain syndromes has been recognized since ancient times. However, it was not until the 18th century that the clinical manifestations of alcohol withdrawal were clearly delineated. As is evident in the writings of Sutton, the vivid descriptions of severe withdrawal written at that time remain relevant today:

> It is preceded by tremors of the hands, restlessness, irregularity of thought, deficiency of memory, anxiety to be company, dreadful nocturnal dreams when the quantity of liquor through the day has been insufficient: much diminution of appetite, especially an aversion to animal food; violent vomiting in the morning and excessive perspiration from trivial causes. Confusion of thought arises to such height that objects are seen of the most hideous forms, and in positions that it is physically impossible they can be so situated; the patients generally sees flies or other insects; or pieces of money which he anxiously desires to possess. . . .

For the most part, clinicians believed that these symptoms were a consequence of alcohol itself, and it was not until the second half of the 20th century that their relationship to the cessation of chronic alcohol intake—a relationship taken for granted today—was established. In 1953, Victor and Adams reported their careful observations of 286 consecutive alcoholic patients admitted to an inner-city hospital, revealing the consistent relationship of the cessation of alcohol to the emergence of clinical symptoms (Victor & Adams, 1953). Their findings were supported in 1955 by a study by Isbell and colleagues, in which 10 former morphine addicts were given large quantities of alcohol for 7 to 87 days and then withdrawn abruptly without sedation (Isbell, Fraser et al., 1955).

Over the next two decades, the concept of an alcohol withdrawal syndrome was firmly established by further animal and human studies, and diagnostic criteria based on empirical observation were developed.

The current understanding of the alcohol withdrawal syndrome is reflected in the diagnostic criteria of the *Diagnostic and Statistical Manual of Mental Disorders, 4th Edition* (APA, 1994).

Hallucinations: In mild alcohol withdrawal, patients may experience perceptual distortions of a visual, auditory, and tactile nature. Lights may seem too bright or sounds too loud and startling. A sensation of "pins and needles" may be experienced. In more severe cases of withdrawal, these misperceptions may develop into frank hallucinations. Visual hallucinations are most common and frequently involve some type of animal life, such as seeing a dog or rodent in the room. Auditory hallucinations may begin as unformed sounds (such as clicks or buzzing) and progress to formed voices. In contrast to the auditory hallucinations of schizophrenia, which may be of religious or political significance, these voices often are of friends or relatives and frequently are accusatory in nature. Tactile hallucinations may involve a sensation of bugs or insects crawling on the skin.

In milder cases of withdrawal, the patient's sensorium is otherwise clear and the patient retains insight that the hallucinations are not real. In more severe withdrawal, this insight may be lost. In the past, it was thought that the hallucinations could become chronic, developing into a state labeled "chronic alcoholic hallucinosis." However, with improved psychiatric nosology and more careful clinical observation, the existence of this entity has not been confirmed and it is not contained in current diagnostic classifications.

Withdrawal Seizures: Grand mal seizures are another manifestation of alcohol withdrawal. Withdrawal seizures occurred in 23% of the patients studied by Victor and Adams, in 33% of the patients in Isbell's study who drank for 48 to 87 days, and in 11% of placebo-treated patients who were enrolled in prospective controlled studies examining the effectiveness of benzodiazepines in symptomatic withdrawal (Mayo-Smith, Cushman et al., 1997). Withdrawal seizures usually begin within 8 to 24 hours after the patient's last drink and may occur before the blood alcohol level has returned to zero. Most are generalized major motor seizures, occurring singly or in a burst of several seizures over a period of one to six hours.

Although fewer than 3% of withdrawal seizures evolve into status epilepticus, alcohol withdrawal has been found to be a contributing cause in up to 15% of status epilepticus patients (Alldredge, Lowenstein et al., 1993). Seizures peak 24 hours after the last drink, corresponding to the peak of withdrawal-induced EEG abnormalities, which include increased amplitude, a photomyoclonic response, and spontaneous paroxysmal activity. These EEG abnormalities are transient, in keeping with the brevity of the convulsive attacks. Except for this brief period following withdrawal, the incidence of EEG abnormalities in patients with withdrawal seizures is not greater than in the normal population. The risk of withdrawal seizures appears to be in part genetically determined, and is increased in patients with a history of prior withdrawal seizures or in those who are undergoing concurrent withdrawal from benzodiazepines or other sedative-hypnotic drugs.

There also is evidence that the risk of seizures increases as an individual undergoes repeated withdrawals (Booth & Blow, 1993). This association has been described as a "kindling effect," which refers to animal studies demonstrating that repeated subcortical electrical stimulation is associated with increases in seizure susceptibility (Ballenger & Post, 1978). Animal studies have supported this kindling hypothesis in alcohol withdrawal, demonstrating that submitting animals to repeated alcohol withdrawal episodes increases their risk of withdrawal seizures.

Alcohol Withdrawal Delirium: Withdrawal is highly individualized in both severity and duration. For up to 90% of patients, withdrawal does not progress beyond the relatively mild symptoms described above, peaking between 24 and 36 hours and gradually subsiding. In other patients, however, the manifestations steadily worsen and can progress into a severe life-threatening delirium accompanied by an autonomic storm: hence the term *delirium tremens* (DTs). DTs generally appear 72 to 96 hours after the last drink.

In their classic presentation, DTs are marked by all the signs and symptoms of mild withdrawal but in a much more pronounced form, with the development of marked tachycardia, tremor, diaphoresis, and fever. The patient develops global confusion and disorientation to place and time. The patient may become absorbed in a separate psychic reality, often believing himself or herself to be in a location other than the hospital, and misindentifies staff as personal acquaintances. Hallucinations are frequent, and the patient may have no insight into them. Without this insight, they can be extremely frightening to the patient, who may react in a way that poses a threat to his own or the staff's safety. Marked psychomotor activity may develop, with severe agitation in some cases or continuous low level motor activity in others, so that activities such as efforts to get out of bed can last for hours. Severe disruption of the normal sleep-wake cycle also is common, and may be marked by the absence of clear sleep for several days.

The duration of the delirium is variable, but averages two to three days in most studies. In some cases, the delirium is relatively brief, lasting only a few hours before the patient regains orientation. In other cases, the patient remains delirious for several days, with reports of periods as long as 50 days before the confusion clears (Wolf, 1993).

As noted, severe withdrawal develops in only a minority of individuals. While accurate knowledge of characteristics that place patients at risk for severe withdrawal would

---

be of great use clinically, well-done research on this question has been very limited. Surprisingly, the amount of daily intake and duration of heavy drinking have not been correlated consistently with the severity of withdrawal, although a certain amount is required to induce dependence. There is evidence, however, that individuals with a high alcohol level at the time of presentation (greater than 300 mg/dl) or who present after having a withdrawal seizure appear to be at higher risk for progressing to severe withdrawal or DTs.

Older individuals appear at higher risk for developing confusion and delirium when undergoing withdrawal (Kraemer, Mayo-Smith et al., 1997). This confusion in older patients may not involve the severe autonomic manifestations of classic DTs and may be a manifestation of the increased susceptibility of older persons to development of delirium with any significant medical illness or hospitalization.

Management. The first step in managing the patient with alcohol withdrawal is to perform an assessment for the presence of medical and psychiatric problems. Chronic alcohol intake is associated with the development of many acute and chronic medical problems. The clinician needs to determine whether these are acute conditions that require hospital treatment or chronic conditions that may alter the approach to management of withdrawal because they could be exacerbated significantly by the development of withdrawal or its treatment.

Pertinent laboratory tests generally include complete blood count, electrolytes, magnesium, calcium, phosphate, liver enzymes, urine drug screen, pregnancy test (when appropriate), and Breathalyzer® or blood alcohol level. Others, depending on suspected co-occurring conditions, may include skin test for tuberculosis, chest x-ray, electrocardiogram, and tests for viral hepatitis, other infections, or sexually transmitted diseases.

General management also involves maintaining adequate fluid balance, correction of electrolyte deficiencies, and attendance to the patient's nutritional needs. Patients in early withdrawal often are overhydrated, so that aggressive hydration usually is not necessary unless there have been significant fluid losses from vomiting or diarrhea (Beard & Knott, 1968). Supportive care and reassurance from nursing personnel are important elements of comfortable detoxification and help to facilitate continuing treatment.

Supportive non-pharmacologic care is an important and useful element in the management of all patients undergoing withdrawal. Simple interventions such as reassurance, reality orientation, monitoring of signs and symptoms of withdrawal, and general nursing care are effective. It is important to note that these measures do not prevent the development of major complications such as seizures and are not adequate by themselves to manage the patient with severe withdrawal or delirium, in which case pharmacologic intervention is required.

Alcohol Withdrawal Severity Scales. Because alcohol withdrawal involves a constellation of nonspecific findings, efforts have been made to develop structured withdrawal severity assessment scales to objectively quantify the severity of withdrawal. A number of such scales have been published in the literature. The most extensively studied and best known is the Clinical Institute Withdrawal Assessment-Alcohol, or CIWA, and a shortened version known as the CIWA-A Revised, or CIWA-Ar. The CIWA-Ar has well-documented reliability, reproducibility, and validity based on comparisons to ratings of withdrawal severity by experienced clinicians. The CIWA-Ar and similar scales require two to five minutes to complete and have proved useful in a variety of settings, including detoxification units, psychiatric units, and general medical/surgical wards. Such scales allow rapid documentation of the patient's signs and symptoms and provide a simple summary score that facilitates accurate and objective communication among staff.

In the case of the CIWA-Ar, a score of 9 or less indicates mild withdrawal, a score of 10 to 18 indicates moderate withdrawal, and a score above 18, suggests severe withdrawal. Moreover, it has been shown that high scores are predictive of the development of seizures and delirium; thus, use of the CIWA-Ar can contribute to appropriate triage of patients to levels of treatment.

PHARMACOLOGIC MANAGEMENT

The medical literature on the pharmacologic management of alcohol withdrawal has been comprehensively reviewed as part of the American Society of Addiction Medicine's efforts to develop evidence-based Clinical Practice Guidelines (Mayo-Smith, Cushman et al., 1997). This review of the evidence indicated that the cornerstone of pharmacologic management of withdrawal is the use of benzodiazepines.

Benzodiazepines. Benzodiazepines are pharmacologically cross-tolerant with alcohol and have the similar effect of enhancing the effect of GABA-induced sedation. A specific benzodiazepine receptor site has been identified on the GABA receptor complex. It is believed that the provision of benzodiazepines alleviates the acute deficiency of GABA neurotransmitter activity that occurs with sudden cessation of alcohol intake.

Well-designed studies consistently have shown that benzodiazepines are more effective than placebo in reducing the signs and symptoms of withdrawal. In addition, meta-analysis of prospective placebo-controlled trials of patients admitted with symptomatic withdrawal have shown a highly significant reduction in seizures, with a risk reduction of 7.7 seizures per 100 patients treated, as well as in delirium, with a risk reduction of 4.9 cases of delirium per 100 patients treated.

Trials comparing different benzodiazepines indicate that all are similarly efficacious in reducing signs and symptoms of withdrawal. However, longer-acting agents such as diazepam and chlordiazepoxide may be more effective in preventing seizures. Longer-acting agents also may contribute to an overall smoother withdrawal course, with a reduction in breakthrough or rebound symptoms. On the other hand, pharmacologic data and clinical experience suggest that longer-acting agents can pose a risk of excess sedation in some patients, including elderly persons and patients with significant liver disease. In such patients, shorter-acting agents such as lorazepam or oxazepam may be preferable.

Another consideration in the choice of benzodiazepine is the rapidity of onset. Certain agents with rapid onset of action (such as diazepam, alprazolam, and lorazepam) demonstrate greater abuse potential than do agents with a slower onset of action (such as chlordiazepoxide and oxazepam). This consideration may be of relevance in an outpatient setting or for patients with a history of benzodiazepine or other substance abuse. However, when rapid control of symptoms is needed, medications with faster onset offer an advantage.

A final consideration in the choice of benzodiazepine is cost, as these agents vary considerably in price. Given the evidence of equal efficacy, if a particular agent is available to a practitioner or program at a lower cost, that is a legitimate factor to consider.

Studies have indicated that non-benzodiazepine sedative-hypnotics also are effective in reducing the signs and symptoms of withdrawal, but non-benzodiazepine agents have not been as extensively studied, and the size of studies with them is not adequate to draw conclusions as to their degree of effectiveness in reducing seizures and de-

lirium. Benzodiazepines have a greater margin of safety, with a lower risk of respiratory depression, as well as overall lower abuse potential than do the non-benzodiazepine agents. Phenobarbital, a long-acting barbiturate, still is used by some programs, as it is long-acting, has well-documented anticonvulsant activity, is inexpensive, and has low abuse liability

Determining the Dose: In the majority of studies examining the effectiveness of various medications for withdrawal, the medications were given in fixed amounts at scheduled times (such as chlordiazepoxide 50 mg every six hours) and were given for periods of five to seven days. However, it has been shown that many patients can go through withdrawal with only minor symptoms even though they receive little or no medication. An alternative to giving medication on a fixed schedule is known as symptom-triggered therapy. In this approach, the patient is monitored through use of a structured assessment scale and given medication only when symptoms cross a threshold of severity. Well-designed studies have demonstrated that this approach is as effective as fixed-dose therapy, but leads to the administration of significantly less medication and a significantly shorter duration of treatment (Saitz, 1994). Symptom-triggered therapy also facilitates the delivery of large amounts of medication quickly to patients who evidence rapidly escalating withdrawal and thus reduces the risk of undertreatment that may arise with the use of fixed doses.

For programs specializing in the management of addiction, use of a symptom-triggered approach with the utilization of a severity scale offers significant advantages. However, there may be situations in which the provision of fixed doses remains appropriate. For example, with patients admitted to general medical or surgical wards, the nursing staff may not have the training or experience to implement the regular use of scales to monitor patients. In certain patients, such as those with severe coronary artery disease, the clinician may wish to prevent the development of even minor symptoms of withdrawal. Finally, because a history of past withdrawal seizures is a risk factor for seizures during a withdrawal episode, and because withdrawal seizures usually occur early in the course of withdrawal, some practitioners administer fixed doses to patients with a history of withdrawal seizures.

Whenever fixed doses are given, it is very important that allowances be made to provide additional medication if the fixed dose should prove inadequate to control symptoms. Treatment should allow for a degree of individualization so that patients can receive large amounts of medication rapidly if needed.

In all cases, medications should be administered by a route that has been shown to have reliable absorption. Therefore, the benzodiazepines should be administered orally or, when necessary, intravenously. An exception is lorazepam, which has good intramuscular and sublingual absorption. In the past, intramuscular (IM) administration was commonly used. However, for most agents IM absorption is extremely variable, leading to problems when rapid control of symptoms is necessary and also with delayed appearance of oversedation when large amounts are administered.

Examples of some treatment regimens consistent with current recommendations are shown in Table 1.

Other Agents. Beta adrenergic blocking agents, such as atenolol and propanolol, as well as centrally acting alpha adrenergic agonists, such as clonidine, also are effective in ameliorating symptoms in patients with mild to moderate withdrawal, primarily by reducing the autonomic nervous system manifestations of withdrawal. However, these agents do not have known anticonvulsant activity, and the studies to date have not been large enough to determine their effectiveness in reducing seizures or delirium. Beta blockers pose a particular problem in this regard because delirium is a known, albeit rare, side effect of these drugs. In addition, there is concern that selective reduction in certain manifestations of withdrawal may mask the development of other significant withdrawal symptoms and make it difficult to utilize withdrawal scales to guide therapy.

Carbamazepine has been widely used in Europe for alcohol withdrawal, and it has been shown to be equal in efficacy to benzodiazepines for patients with mild to moderate withdrawal. It is without significant toxicity when used in 7-day protocols for alcohol withdrawal and is associated with less psychiatric distress and a faster return to work. Carbamazepine does not potentiate the CNS and respiratory depression caused by alcohol, does not inhibit learning (an important side effect of larger doses of benzodiazepines), and has no abuse potential. It has well-documented anticonvulsant activity and prevents alcohol withdrawal seizures in animal studies. However, studies of adequate size to assess its efficacy in preventing withdrawal seizures or delirium are not yet available.

Carbamazepine currently is available only in oral form, making it difficult to titrate doses rapidly for the more symptomatic or rapidly worsening patient. For these reasons, and because of their proven efficacy, the benzodiazepines remain the recommended agents.

Carbamazepine sometimes is used as an adjunctive agent, as in patients who have a history of recurrent withdrawal seizures, with prominent mood lability during withdrawal or with concurrent benzodiazepine withdrawal.

Neuroleptic agents, including the phenothiazines and the butryphenone haloperidol, demonstrate some effectiveness in reducing the signs and symptoms of withdrawal, and for a period of time were used extensively for that purpose. However, these agents are less effective than benzodiazepines in preventing delirium and actually lead to an increase in the rate of seizures. Neuroleptic agents are widely used to calm agitated patients and are useful for this purpose in the setting of alcohol withdrawal as well. They should not be used alone, but always in conjunction with a benzodiazepine; moreover, neuroleptic agents with less effect on the seizure threshold, such as haloperidol, should be selected.

It long has been recognized that magnesium levels often are low during alcohol withdrawal. Closer study has found that magnesium levels usually are normal at admission, but then drop during the course of withdrawal, before spontaneously returning to normal as symptoms subside. Only one randomized trial of magnesium during withdrawal has been performed, and that study found no difference in severity of withdrawal or rate of seizures, even after adjustment for magnesium levels. Providing supplemental oral magnesium to patients with a documented low magnesium level is without significant risk, but routine administration of magnesium, either oral or intramuscular, for withdrawal no longer is recommended.

One agent whose use for the management of alcohol withdrawal still is encountered occasionally is alcohol itself. Case series describing oral or intravenous alcohol for the prevention or treatment of withdrawal symptoms have been published, but no controlled trials evaluating the safety or relative efficacy of this approach—either compared to placebo or to benzodiazepines—have been performed. Intravenous alcohol infusions require close monitoring because of the potential toxicity of alcohol. As a pharmacologic agent, ethyl alcohol has numerous adverse effects, including its well known hepatic, gastrointestinal, and neurologic toxicities, as well as its effects on mental status and judgment. Given the proven efficacy and safety of benzodiazepines, the use of alcohol for detoxification is discouraged by addiction specialists.

TABLE 1.   Examples of Specific Pharmacologic Treatment Regimens

Monitoring

Monitor the patient every 4 to 8 hours using the CIWA-Ar until the score has been below 8-10 for 24 hours; use additional assessments as needed.

Symptom-Triggered Medication Regimens

Administer one of the following medications every hour when the CIWA-Ar is $\geq$ 8-10:

- Chlordiazepoxide 50-100 mg
- Diazepam 10-20 mg
- Oxazepam 30-60 mg
- Lorazepam 2-4 mg

(Other benzodiazepines may be used at equivalent substitutions.)

Repeat the CIWA-Ar one hour after every dose to assess need for further medication.

Structured Medication Regimens

The physician may feel that the development of even mild to moderate withdrawal should be prevented in certain patients (for example, in a patient experiencing a myocardial infarction) and thus may order medications to be given on a predetermined schedule. One of the following regimens could be used in such a situation:

- Chlordiazepoxide 50 mg every 6 hours for four doses, then 25 mg every 6 hours for eight doses.
- Diazepam 10 mg every 6 hours for four doses, then 5 mg every 6 hours for eight doses.
- Lorazepam 2 mg every 6 hours for four doses, then 1 mg every 6 hours for eight doses.

(Other benzodiazepines may be substituted at equivalent doses.)

It is very important that patients receiving medication on a predetermined schedule be monitored closely and that additional medication be provided should the doses given prove inadequate.

Agitation

For the patient who displays increasing agitation or hallucinations that have not responded to oral benzodiazepines alone, one of the following medications may be used:

- Haloperidol 2 to 5 mg IM alone or in combination with 2 to 4 mg of lorazepam.
- Intravenous diazepam given slowly every 5 minutes until the patient is lightly sedated. Begin with 5 mg for two doses. If needed, increase to 10 mg for two doses, then 20 mg every 5 minutes.

Given the risk of respiratory depression, the patient on this regimen should be closely monitored, with equipment for respiratory support immediately available.

(Other phenothiazines and benzodiazepines may be substituted at equivalent doses.)

Phenytoin: The routine use of phenytoin has been advocated as a method to prevent the occurrence of withdrawal seizures, and there is some evidence from early trials that it may be effective for this purpose. However, more recent and more methodologically sound trials have failed to show evidence that phenytoin is effective in preventing recurrent withdrawal seizures. Moreover, studies have shown that appropriately used benzodiazepines are extremely effective in preventing withdrawal seizures and that the addition of phenytoin does not lead to improved outcomes (Kasser,

1994). For these reasons, the routine use of phenytoin has been largely abandoned.

Thiamine: A final agent with an important role in the management of patients withdrawing from alcohol is thiamine. Alcoholics are at risk for thiamine deficiency, which may lead to Wernicke's disease and the Wernicke-Korsakoff syndrome. Wernicke's disease is an illness of acute onset characterized by the triad of mental disturbance, paralysis of eye movements, and ataxia. The ocular abnormality usually is weakness or paralysis of abduction (sixth nerve palsy), which invariably is bilateral, although rarely symmetric. It is accompanied by diploplia, strabismus, and nystagmus. The ataxia primarily affects gait and stance. Mental status changes typically involve a global confusional-apathetic state but, in some patients, a disproportionate disorder of retentive memory is apparent.

Wernicke's disease is a neurologic emergency that should be treated by the immediate parenteral administration of thiamine, with a dose of 50 mg intravenously and 50 mg intramuscularly. Delay in provision of thiamine increases the risk of permanent memory damage. The provision of intravenous glucose solutions may exhaust a patient's reserve of B vitamins, acutely precipitating Wernicke's disease. Therefore, intravenous glucose always should be accompanied by the administration of thiamine in the alcoholic patient. Ocular palsies may respond within hours, while the gait and cognitive problems of Wernicke's improve more slowly.

As the apathy, drowsiness, and confusion recede, the patient may be left with a sometimes permanent defect in retentive memory and learning known as Korsakoff's psychosis. To reduce the risk of these sequelae, all patients presenting with alcohol withdrawal should receive 50 to 100 mg of thiamine at the time of presentation, followed by oral supplementation for several weeks. Patients with symptoms of Wernicke's disease, those who are to receive glucose-containing IV solutions, and those at high risk of malnutrition should receive their initial dose parenterally.

COMMON TREATMENT ISSUES

Locating Treatment Services. As both research and clinical experience demonstrated that pharmacologic therapy can significantly reduce the incidence of major complications associated with alcohol withdrawal, it became common practice to admit patients to the hospital to provide three to seven days of medication. However, such intensive therapy is not necessary for many patients, and increasing interest has been shown in managing withdrawal on an outpatient basis. Such therapy clearly is less expensive than the inpatient alternative, but currently is the source of some controversy because the factors that may be used to identify patients for whom this therapy is appropriate have not been delineated clearly. Nevertheless, for patients with only mild withdrawal, no history of seizures or DTs, and no concurrent significant medical or psychiatric problems, such an approach seems reasonable.

Such patients should have a responsible individual to monitor them, they should be seen on a daily basis until they have stabilized, and transportation to emergency medical services should be available. In addition, many programs are concentrating on sharply reducing the length of stay for patients undergoing withdrawal. Patients may be treated in an observation unit or admitted for a one-day stay. If significant withdrawal symptoms do not develop, and the withdrawal is easily controlled with little or no medication, patients can be discharged or transferred to an intensive outpatient rehabilitation program. Patients who experience severe withdrawal symptoms, however, need the close monitoring and nursing support of an inpatient unit (see the Appendix to Chapter 1 of this section.)

Management of the Patient Following a Withdrawal Seizure. The patient who presents after experiencing a withdrawal seizure raises a number of management issues. It is important to recognize that not all seizures in alcohol-dependent patients are the result of withdrawal. In epidemiologic studies, it is clear that the rate of epilepsy and seizures rises in parallel with the amount of an individual's alcohol intake. Alcoholics are at higher risk for seizures unrelated to withdrawal. A careful history of the temporal relationship of alcohol intake to the seizure should be obtained, and the diagnosis of withdrawal seizure should be made only if there is a clear history of a marked decrease or cessation of drinking in the 24 to 48 hours preceding the seizure.

All patients who present with their first seizure warrant hospital admission for observation and evaluation. At a minimum, this should involve a thorough neurologic examination and brain imaging, with lumbar puncture and EEG also appropriate in many cases. Patients who are known to have a history of withdrawal seizures and who present with a seizure that can be attributed clearly to withdrawal may not require a full repeat evaluation. If the seizure was generalized and without focal elements, and if a careful neurologic examination reveals no evidence of focal deficits, there is no suspicion of meningitis and there is no history of recent major head trauma, additional testing has an extremely low yield and may be safely omitted.

There is a 6- to 12-hour period during which there is an increased risk of seizures. Withdrawal seizures often are multiple, with a second seizure occurring in one case out of four. For the patient who presents with a withdrawal seizure, rapid treatment is indicated to prevent further episodes. The parenteral administration of a rapid-acting benzodiazepine such as diazepam or lorazepam may be effective (D'Onofrio, Rathlev et al., 1999). Several studies have shown that phenytoin is no more effective than placebo in preventing recurrent seizures (Rathlev, D'Onofrio et al., 1994). Initial treatment should be followed by oral doses of long-acting benzodiazepines over the ensuing 24 to 48 hours.

Early studies indicated that a withdrawal seizure placed the patient at increased risk for progression to DTs. Admission of patients after a withdrawal seizure for monitoring and treatment with benzodiazepines therefore is a reasonable and safe approach.

Management of the Patient With Delirium. The patient who progresses to delirium raises a number of special management issues. Older studies showed a mortality rate of up to 30% in DTs but, with modern care, mortality has been reduced to less than 1%. The principles of successful treatment involve adequate sedation and meticulous supportive medical care. Such patients require close nursing observation and supportive care, which frequently necessitates admission to an intensive care unit. Careful management of fluids and electrolytes is important, given the patient's inability to manage his own intake and the presence of marked autonomic hyperactivity. Delirium often is encountered in patients admitted for acute medical problems whose alcohol dependence was not recognized and whose withdrawal was not adequately treated. A high index of suspicion for the development of infection—whose presenting signs may be masked by the fever, tachycardia, and confusion of the underlying delirium—is essential, as is careful management of coexisting medical conditions.

The use of cross-tolerant sedative-hypnotics has been shown to reduce mortality in DTs and is recommended (Kasser, 1997). However, such medications have not been shown to reverse the delirium or reduce its duration. The goal is to sedate the patient to a point of light sleep. This will control the patient's agitation, preventing behavior posing a risk to him- or herself and to staff, and allow staff to provide necessary supportive medical care. The use of intravenous benzodiazepines with rapid onset, such as diazepam, has been shown to provide more rapid control of the patient's symptoms. An example of a widely used regimen is given in Table 2.

The main complication of therapy with diazepam is respiratory depression. Whenever this approach is used, providers should have equipment and personnel immediately available to provide respiratory support if needed. One advantage of diazepam is that its peak onset occurs within five minutes of intravenous administration. This allows the provider to deliver repeat boluses and titrate sedation quickly without fear of a delayed appearance of oversedation. Once established, delirium can be expected to last for a number of hours, so diazepam offers another advantage in that its longer half-life helps maintain sedation with less chance of breakthrough agitation. Massive doses of benzodiazepines may be needed to control the agitation of patients in DTs, with hundreds and even thousands of milligrams of diazepam or its equivalent used over the course of treatment. The practitioner should not hesitate to use whatever amounts are needed to control the agitation.

There have been reports of the use of continuous intravenous drips of short-acting agents such as lorazepam or triazolam. Existing evidence suggests that this approach is no more effective than the use of boluses of longer acting agents and is extremely expensive.

In the agitated patient, benzodiazepines can be supplemented with the addition of neuroleptic agents such as haloperidol. As has been discussed, such agents should not be used alone. Also, neuroleptic agents with less effect on seizure threshold, such as haloperidol, should be used.

In patients whose withdrawal is not readily controlled with oral benzodiazepines and who are beginning to demonstrate signs of agitation, intramuscular administration of a combination of lorazepam and a neuroleptic such as haloperidol often is effective in calming the patient, thus avoiding the need to use intravenous administration.

CONCLUSIONS

It is important to remember that successful management of withdrawal is only the first—and sometimes the most easily achieved—step toward the primary goal of treating the patient's underlying addiction to alcohol. Development of a plan to engage the patient in treatment is a critical component of withdrawal and must not be overlooked.

REFERENCES

Alldredge BK & Lowenstein DH (1993). Status epilepticus related to alcohol abuse. *Epilepticus* 34:1033-1037.

American Psychiatric Association (1994). *Diagnostic and Statistical Manual of Mental Disorders, 4th Edition (DSM-IV).* Washington, DC: American Psychiatric Press.

Ballenger JC & Post RM (1978). Kindling as a model for alcohol withdrawal syndromes. *British Journal of Psychiatry* 133:1-14.

Booth BM & Blow FC (1993). The kindling hypothesis: Further evidence from a U.S. national study of alcoholic men. *Alcohol and Alcoholism* 28:593-598.

Broaden RN & Goa KL (1991). Flumazenil: A reappraisal of its pharmacological properties and therapeutic efficacy as a benzodiazepine antagonist. *Drugs* 42(6):1061-1089.

D'Onofrio G, Rathlev NK, Ulrich AS et al. (1999). Lorazepam for the prevention of recurrent seizures related to alcohol. *New England Journal of Medicine* 340:915-919.

Goldstein DB & Goldstein A (1961). Possible role of enzyme inhibition and repression in drug tolerance and addiction. *Biochemistry and Pharmacology* 8:48.

Gorelick DA (1993). Overview of pharmacologic treatment of alcohol and other drug addictions: Intoxication, withdrawal and relapse prevention. *Psychiatric Clinics of North America* 16(1):141-156.

Hawley RJ, Major LF, Schulman EA et al. (1985). Cerebrospinal fluid 3-methoxy-4-hydroxyphenylglycol and norepinephrine levels in alcohol withdrawal: Correlations with clinical signs. *Archives of General Psychiatry* 42(11):1056-1062.

Isbell H, Fraser HF, Wikler A et al. (1955). An experimental study of the etiology of "rum fits" and delirium tremens. *Quarterly Journal of Studies of Alcohol* 16:1-33.

Kasser C, Mayo-Smith M et al. (1998). *Management of Alcohol Withdrawal Delirium (Clinical Practice Guideline).* Chevy Chase, MD: American Society of Addiction Medicine.

Kraemer KL, Mayo-Smith MF & Calkins DR (1997). Impact of age on severity, course and complications of alcohol withdrawal. *Archives of Internal Medicine* 157:2234-2241.

Mayo-Smith MF, Cushman P, Hill AJ et al. (1997). Pharmacological management of alcohol withdrawal: A meta-analysis and evidence-based practice guideline. *Journal of the American Medical Association.*

Rathlev NK, D'Onofrio G, Fish SS et al. The lack of efficacy of phenytoin in prevention of recurrent alcohol related seizures. *Annals of Emergency Medicine* 23:513-518.

Victor M & Adams RD (1953). Effect of alcohol on the nervous system. *Research Publication of the Association for Research in Nervous and Mental Diseases* 32:526-523

Wolf KM, Shaughnessy AF & Middleton DB (1993). Prolonged delirium tremens requiring massive doses of medication. *Journal of the American Board of Family Practice* 6:502-504.

Chapter 3

Management of Sedative-Hypnotic Intoxication and Withdrawal

William E. Dickinson, D.O., FASAM, FAAFP
Michael F. Mayo-Smith, M.D., M.P.H.
Steven J. Eickelberg, M.D., FASAM

Sedative-Hypnotic Intoxication and Overdose
Sedative-Hypnotic Withdrawal
Patient Evaluation and Management
Common Treatment Issues

Sedative-hypnotic medications decrease activity, moderate excitement, exert a calming effect, produce drowsiness, and facilitate sleep. They are among the most widely used prescription drugs in the United States. Misuse of and dependence on these drugs have occurred since their introduction.

Sedative-hypnotics stimulate the inhibitory neurotransmitters in the GABA receptors. While all sedatives and hypnotics have mild stimulant properties at low doses, their primary effect is to decrease central nervous system (CNS) function.

Drugs in this class that are commonly associated with severe withdrawal states (in addition to alcohol) include methaqualone, glutethimide, phenobarbital, and short-acting benzodiazepines such as alprazolam and triazolam. Sedative drugs associated with less severe clinical withdrawal states include meprobamate, diazepam, chlordiazepoxide, and lorazepam.

SEDATIVE-HYPNOTIC
INTOXICATION AND OVERDOSE

Clinical Picture. The signs and symptoms of sedative-hypnotic intoxication and overdose are similar for the various drugs in the class. The patient with mild to moderate toxicity presents with slurred speech, ataxia, and uncoordination similar to that seen with alcohol intoxication. On occasion, particularly in the older adults, a paradoxical agitated confusion and even delirium may be produced. At more severe stages of intoxication, stupor and coma develop. With the older non-benzodiazepine agents, toxicity may progress, ultimately leading to fatal respiratory arrest or cardiovascular collapse. Overdose with these older agents also may be associated with a variety of agent-specific clinical manifestations, such as bullous skin lesions with barbiturates ("barb blisters"), details of which can be found in textbooks on toxicologic emergencies (Osborn & Goldfrank, 1994).

An additional problem with several of the older sedative-hypnotics is that, with regular use, tolerance may develop to the drugs' therapeutic effects but not to their lethal effects. The maintenance dose then may approach the lethal dose and the therapeutic index decreases. Toxicity and overdose thus can occur with only small increases over the individual's regular intake.

On the other hand, benzodiazepines virtually never lead to death when ingested by themselves. A lethal dose has

TABLE 1. Diagnosis of Sedative-Hypnotic Overdose

History
- Sedative-hypnotic use (ask about drug, amount, time of last use);
- Polydrug abuse;
- Use multiple sources of information (family, hospital records, etc.).

Physical Examination
- Central nervous system depression;
- Respiratory depression.

Laboratory Tests
- Rule out hypoglycemia, acidemia, fluid and electrolyte abnormalities;
- Toxicology screens for sedative-hypnotics and other drugs.

not been established for any of the benzodiazepines and there are very few well-documented cases of death due to ingestion of benzodiazepines alone. The few deaths that have occurred all involved short-acting high potency benzodiazepines such as alprazolam and triazolam (Litovitz, 1987) or administration of benzodiazepines by an intravenous route. However, inappropriate intramuscular use of chlordiazepoxide can lead to erratic absorption, producing respiratory compromise. The benzodiazepines are free of toxic effects on peripheral (non-CNS) organ systems in either long-term use or acute overdose.

Despite their safety, benzodiazepines continue to be a major cause of overdose and continue to pose a significant problem because, while safe by themselves, they act synergistically with other agents when ingested in combination. Mixed overdoses—such as those involving benzodiazepines in combination with alcohol, major tranquilizers, antidepressants, or opiates—can be fatal. This result is true for the non-benzodiazepine agents as well.

Management. Assessment and maintenance of the airway and, when necessary, ventilatory support, form the cornerstone in managing sedative-hypnotic overdose. Many of the benzodiazepine agents slow gut motility and some—

such as phenobarbital, meprobamate, glutethimide, and ethchlorvinyl—can form concretions in the stomach. Therefore, evacuation of the gastrointestinal tract with a large bore orogastric tube is the next step, provided an active gag reflex is elicited or the airway is protected by intubation. A slurry of 1.0g/kg activated charcoal, together with a dose of cathartic, should be given. Repeated doses of activated charcoal, at 0.5 to 1.0g/kg every two to four hours (or a similar amount delivered by slow continuous nasogastric infusion) may be helpful, particularly for barbiturate or other non-benzodiazepine ingestions. Some of these agents have an extensive entero-hepatic circulation, and repeated doses of charcoal have been shown to speed their elimination.

Alkalization of the urine also may be helpful in eliminating phenobarbital, but forced diuresis has not been shown to be helpful for any drugs in the class. In extreme cases, hemoperfusion may have a role.

Measurement of serum levels can be helpful in documenting the identity and amounts of agents ingested, as well as in tracking levels over time. However, immediate clinical management is based on the patient's condition rather than serum levels.

Flumazenil is a competitive antagonist with very weak agonist properties at the benzodiazepine receptor (Howland, 1994). It can reverse the sedative effects of benzodiazepines, but not of the other agents or alcohol. Overall, it has found a role in reversing the effects of short-acting benzodiazepines, such as midazolam after medical procedures. It also may be used when benzodiazepines have been ingested alone as an overdose. In such settings, slow IV titration in amounts not exceeding 1 mg is recommended, with monitoring for the recurrence of sedation. The effects of flumazenil are short-lived, and symptoms may return in 30 to 60 minutes. Moreover, its use has been associated with seizures and cardiac arrhythmias. These adverse effects are more likely to occur when it is administered rapidly in large amounts and in patients who have ingested a sedative-hypnotic in combination with a substance capable of causing seizures, such as a tricyclic antidepressant (Spivey, 1992). Persons who are physiologically dependent on benzodiazepines are at high risk of seizures when they are given flumazenil. Flumazenil thus has not found a role as part of the standard "coma cocktail" (containing thiamine, glucose, and naloxone) because it produces a rapid benzodiazepine withdrawal. Its use in mixed overdoses or in patients who have used benzodiazepines chronically is limited due to the risk of adverse effects.

SEDATIVE-HYPNOTIC WITHDRAWAL

Clinical Picture. The use of most sedative, hypnotic, and/or anxiolytic agents can result in the development of psychological dependence, physical dependence, or addiction. (In this chapter, "dependence" is used to refer to the host's neurophysiological adaptation to regular or chronic sedative-hypnotic use. The definition of dependence includes adaptation to substance use that leads to an abstinence syndrome with the abrupt and, at times, tapered cessation of use.) Withdrawal is tantamount to, and is defined by, the signs and symptoms contained within the abstinence syndrome. This syndrome can occur with both high- and low-dose use—even use at therapeutic levels monitored by a physician. The evolutionary development of dependence to sedative-hypnotic compounds is similar across the classes of the benzodiazepines, the barbiturates, and the nonbarbiturate/nonbenzodiazepine agents.

All of the sedative-hypnotic agents covered in this chapter are substances that currently, or in the recent past, have enjoyed widespread use. All possess well-documented, clinically important dependence and withdrawal characteristics. Marked similarities exist between the withdrawal syndromes seen with the benzodiazepines, the barbiturates, and the non-barbiturate/non-benzodiazepine agents, all of which resemble the acute alcohol withdrawal syndrome in many ways. This resemblance is related to the properties of the binding site in the brain (the GABA receptor). Differences in withdrawal syndrome characteristics among sedative-hypnotic compounds primarily reflect differences in the rate at which dependence is induced, the rapidity with which symptoms occur on discontinuation of the drug, and the severity of those symptoms.

A clinically significant withdrawal syndrome is most apt to occur following discontinuation of daily therapeutic dose (low dose) use of a sedative-hypnotic for at least four to six months or, at doses that exceed two to three times the upper limit of recommended therapeutic use (high dose), for more than two to three months. The time course and severity of the sedative-hypnotic withdrawal syndrome reflects the influences of three pharmacologic factors: (1) dose, (2) duration of use, and (3) duration of drug action (also see Figure 1). (For the purposes of this discussion, duration of drug action is directly related to the elimination half-life at steady-state conditions.) Withdrawal severity has been related to dose and duration of treatment. Latency to onset of withdrawal is related to the elimination half-life (Woods, Katz et al., 1992). Clinical research with benzodi-

TABLE 2. Clinical Manifestations of Sedative-Hypnotic Withdrawal	
Vital Signs ■ Tachycardia ■ Hypertension ■ Fever	**Ears** ■ Tinnitus
	Gastrointestinal ■ Anorexia ■ Diarrhea ■ Nausea
Central Nervous System ■ Agitation ■ Anxiety ■ Delirium ■ Hallucinations ■ Insomnia ■ Irritability ■ Nightmares ■ Sensory disturbances ■ Tremor	**High-Dose (Severe) Withdrawal** ■ Seizures ■ Delirium ■ Death.

azepines has identified additional drug and host factors that influence the onset and severity of the withdrawal syndrome; these factors are elaborated upon in the following sections.

The spectrum of signs and symptoms that are experienced most often during the course of withdrawal are summarized in Table 2. Considerable variation exists among patients in terms of the signs and symptoms of the abstinence syndrome. Although Figure 1 appears to indicate that withdrawal follows a smooth and predictable course, most patients experience significant moment-to-moment quantitative and qualitative variations in their signs and symptoms. Salzman (1997) reviewed the frequency of various symptoms of benzodiazepine withdrawal. Anxiety, insomnia, restlessness, agitation, irritability, and muscle tension were very frequent. Less frequent were nausea, diaphoresis, lethargy, aches and pains, coryza, hyperacusis, blurred vision, nightmares, depression, hyperreflexia, and ataxia. Psychosis, seizures, confusion, paranoid delusions, hallucinations, and persistent tinnitus were uncommon. The areas under the curves in Figure 1 outline the potential time course and withdrawal severity characteristics. The multitude of signs and symptoms outlined in Table 2 illustrates that, in the absence of the knowledge that a patient is withdrawing from a sedative-hypnotic, a number of

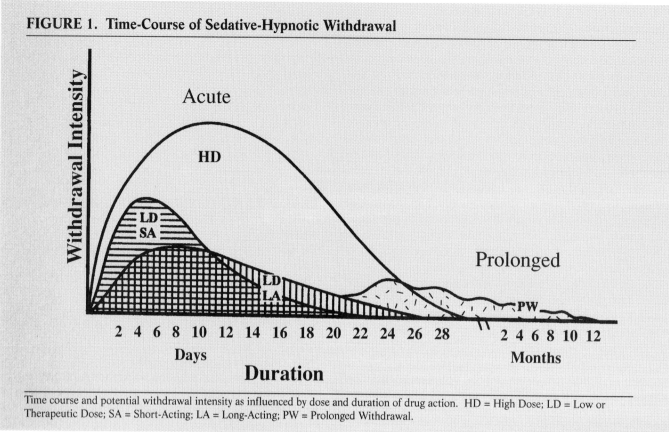

FIGURE 1. Time-Course of Sedative-Hypnotic Withdrawal

Time course and potential withdrawal intensity as influenced by dose and duration of drug action. HD = High Dose; LD = Low or Therapeutic Dose; SA = Short-Acting; LA = Long-Acting; PW = Prolonged Withdrawal.

medical and/or psychiatric differential diagnoses would be entertained to explain the patient's condition.

Benzodiazepines: Benzodiazepine use, dependence, and withdrawal are much more thoroughly researched than other classes of sedative-hypnotic compounds. Soon after chlordiazepoxide (Librium®, 1960) and diazepam (Valium®, 1961) became available commercially, clinical reports were published documenting a high-dose discontinuation withdrawal syndrome with severe characteristics (seizures, depression, delirium, psychosis) (Hollister, Motzenbecker et al., 1961; Essig, 1966). Reports of a withdrawal syndrome following discontinuation of long-term use of benzodiazepines at therapeutic doses were published within the following decade (Covi, Park et al., 1973). It now is well established that benzodiazepine dependence, withdrawal, and difficulties in discontinuing chronic benzodiazepine use are influenced by multiple pharmacological and host factors (as discussed later in this chapter).

Barbiturates: Reports in the medical literature evidenced an emerging awareness of barbiturate dependence and an abstinence syndrome as early as the 1940s. The first American paper (Isbell, 1950) directly addressing the barbiturate withdrawal syndrome was followed by a clinical study that chronicled the signs and symptoms of the barbiturate abstinence syndrome (Isbell, Altschul et al., 1950). Further studies quantified, with high-dose use, the duration of barbiturate ingestion necessary for the appearance of mild, moderate, and severe withdrawal symptoms (Fraser, Wikler et al., 1958; Isbell & White, 1953). The first evidence that an abstinence syndrome could occur following long-term therapeutic (low-dose) barbiturate use was published nearly two decades later (Covi, Lipman et al., 1973; Epstein, 1980).

Treatment of barbiturate withdrawal with barbiturate substitution was reported as early as 1953 (Isbell & White, 1953). In 1970 and 1971, Smith and Wesson reported on a protocol that employs phenobarbital substitution, stabilization, and tapering to treat barbiturate dependence. Their technique remains the "gold standard" for the management of all sedative-hypnotic classes or mixed sedative-hypnotic withdrawal.

Nonbarbiturate/Nonbenzodiazepine Agents: The medical literature contains case reports documenting the full spectrum of sedative-hypnotic withdrawal signs and symptoms from this group of compounds. Of greatest concern are the multitude of reports documenting severe withdrawal syndromes, marked by delirium, psychosis, hallucinations, hyperthermia, cardiac arrests, and death (Essig, 1964; Sadwin & Glen, 1958; Lloyd & Clark, 1959; Phillips, Judy et al., 1957; Swanson & Okada, 1963; Flemenbaum & Gumby, 1971; Swartzburg, Lieb et al., 1973, Vestal & Rumack, 1974).

Signs and Symptoms of Discontinuation. The signs and symptoms experienced following the discontinuation of benzodiazepine use have been categorized and attributed to at least four different etiologies: (1) symptom recurrence or relapse, (2) rebound, (3) pseudowithdrawal, and (4) true withdrawal.

Symptom recurrence or relapse is characterized by the recurrence of symptoms (such as insomnia or anxiety) for which the benzodiazepine initially was taken. The symptoms are similar in character to the condition that existed prior to drug treatment. Relapse may occur following discontinuation, with or without the prior existence of benzodiazepine dependence. Reemergence of symptoms is quite common, exceeding 60% to 80% for anxiety and insomnia disorders (Rickels, Case et al., 1986a; Greenblatt, Miller et al., 1990). Symptom recurrence can present rapidly or slowly over days to months following drug discontinuation.

This pattern can have important implications for routine reassessment of the need for continued benzodiazepine use. The need for the benzodiazepine is reevaluated, with attention given to dose and duration. When the need is diminished or eliminated, so should be the benzodiazepine.

Rebound is marked by the development of symptoms, within hours to days of drug discontinuation, that are qualitatively similar to the disorder for which the benzodiazepine initially was prescribed. However, the symptoms are transiently more intense than they were prior to drug treatment. Insomnia and anxiety disorders are the best studied examples (Rickels, Fox et al., 1988). Rebound symptoms are of short duration and are self-limited (Greenblatt, Miller et al., 1990), which distinguishes this syndrome from recurrence.

Pseudowithdrawal and over-interpretation of symptoms may occur when expectations of withdrawal lead to the experiencing of abstinence symptoms. This effect has been observed in study patients who discontinued placebo medication or continued benzodiazepine use but believed that the benzodiazepine had been discontinued (Winokur & Rickels, 1981). In addition, expectations of symptoms often are negatively influenced by concerns registered in the media or by friends and/or physician(s).

True withdrawal is marked by the emergence of psychological and somatic signs and symptoms following the discontinuation of benzodiazepines in an individual who is physically dependent on the drug. The withdrawal syndrome can be suppressed by the reinstitution of the discontinued benzodiazepine or another cross-tolerant sedative-hypnotic. Withdrawal from benzodiazepines results from a reversal of the neuroadaptive changes in the central nervous system that were induced by chronic benzodiazepine use. Withdrawal reflects a relative temporal and temporary diminution of central nervous system GABA-ergic neuronal inhibition.

Considerable individual variations and variability over time exist among patients who discontinue benzodiazepine use. The benzodiazepine withdrawal syndrome has been documented to include any of the spectrum of signs and symptoms listed in Table 2. Any combination of signs and symptoms may be experienced with varying severity throughout the initial one to four weeks of abstinence. None of the signs or symptoms of the abstinence syndrome are pathognomonic of benzodiazepine withdrawal. Many signs and symptoms are identical to those of anxiety or depressive disorder. Common symptoms include tremor, muscle twitching, nausea and vomiting, impaired concentration, restlessness, anxiety, anorexia, blurred vision, irritability, insomnia, sweating, and weakness. Common clinical signs include tachycardia, hypertension, hyperreflexia, mydriasis, and diaphoresis. The presence of neuropsychiatric symptoms— including perceptual distortions and hypersensitivity to light, sound, and touch—are common. Many believe these "sensory-perceptual symptoms" are most indicative of neurophysiological withdrawal, but they rarely occur in the absence of some of the aforementioned adrenergic or anxiety symptoms. Lack of clinical signs should not be considered tantamount to the absence of a withdrawal syndrome.

The clinical withdrawal picture can consist primarily of subjective symptoms, accompanied by few or no concurrently observable hyper-adrenergic signs or vital sign fluctuations (as seen with acute alcohol withdrawal).

These discontinuation syndromes often occur in combination. For example, considerable overlap exists between the symptoms of recurrence in anxiety and insomnia disorders and the signs and symptoms of rebound and withdrawal. Clinical techniques that treat, minimize, and attenuate benzodiazepine abstinence symptoms also effectively alleviate rebound. As a result, attention to sorting out rebound from withdrawal is unnecessary (if not impossible). However, symptom recurrence or relapse is common. Clinicians must be attuned to the emergence or persistence of clinically important symptoms of relapse during and after the period of acute withdrawal.

Prolonged Withdrawal: Some physicians (Smith & Wesson, 1983; Smith & Seymour, 1991; Landry, Smith et al., 1992) report, and clinical experience confirms, that a small proportion of patients, following long-term benzodiazepine use, experience a prolonged syndrome of withdrawal. The signs and symptoms may persist for weeks to months following discontinuation. The syndrome is notable for its irregular and unpredictable day-to-day course and qualitative and quantitative differences in symptoms from both the pre-benzodiazepine use state and the acute withdrawal period. Patients with prolonged withdrawal often experience slowly abating—albeit characteristic waxing and waning—symptoms of insomnia, perceptual disturbances, tremor, sensory hypersensitivity(ies), and anxiety.

Role of the GABA-Benzodiazepine Receptor Complex. Benzodiazepine action in the central nervous system is mediated by the Gamma-aminobutyric-acid-Benzodiazepine-Receptor-Complex [GABA-BDZ-R-Complex] (Haefly, 1975; Costa, Guidotti et al., 1975). Work by numerous investigators has shown that GABA is the primary central nervous system inhibitory neurotransmitter. Activation of the GABA receptor induces the opening of a neuronal, membrane-bound chloride ion channel, located within the GABA-BDZ-R-Complex. Neuronal inhibition results from neuronal membrane hyperpolarization secondary to the flow of chloride ions down the electrochemical gradient into the neuron. Benzodiazepines bind allosterically to a "benzodiazepine receptor" (called the "omega receptor"), located on the GABA-BDZ-R-Complex. Benzodiazepines positively modulate and influence the GABA-Chloride channel relationship.

A series of studies by Miller and colleagues (1988a, 1988b, 1989; Miller, 1991) illustrated that, in mice, behavioral tolerance and discontinuation syndromes are temporally associated with molecular/receptor level adaptations. The investigators reported that, as tolerance to the ataxia-inducing effects of lorazepam developed behaviorally, benzodiazepine and GABA receptors were down-regulated (through decreased receptor number, decreased GABA-receptor function, and diminished protein synthesis for GABA receptors). After lorazepam was administered for four weeks, it was abruptly discontinued. Concurrent with signs of withdrawal, GABA-receptors were up-regulated, and GABA-receptor complex function was enhanced (as evidenced by greater affinity for GABA, increased affinity of the benzodiazepine receptor for benzodiazepines, increased benzodiazepine receptor number).

The rate of onset of behavioral tolerance to alprazolam and clonazepam followed by an abstinence syndrome upon abrupt discontinuation was similarly computed and then compared with lorazepam in a subsequent report (Miller, 1991). Tolerance and withdrawal developed more rapidly with alprazolam (four days for tolerance; two days for withdrawal) than with lorazepam and clonazepam, which were similar (seven days for tolerance; four days for withdrawal) (Miller, Greenblatt et al., 1988a, 1988b; Miller, 1991). These studies also demonstrated that tolerance is primarily a pharmacodynamic, neuroadaptive phenomena (brain and plasma levels remained constant throughout the period of chronic administration).

File (1993) comments that it is premature to link our current observations of neurochemical changes to behavior etiologically, since multiple potential explanations exist. Events may (1) be independent yet occur simultaneously, (2) reflect neuroadaptive changes resulting from compensatory mechanisms, or (3) be causally linked. Despite numerous unanswered questions, it is apparent that the primary neuroadaptive response occurs at the GABA-BDZ-R-Complex. This system then influences changes in other neurotransmitter systems, depending on the neuroanatomical location of the GABA-BDZ-R-Complex. The benzodiazepine discontinuation syndrome subsequently is influenced, if not mediated, by numerous neurotransmitter systems.

Pharmacologic Characteristics Affecting Withdrawal. Pharmacologic factors are primarily responsible for the relationship between various benzodiazepines and the differing clinical manifestations of benzodiazepine withdrawal syndrome.

Pharmacokinetics: Benzodiazepine pharmacokinetics determine the onset of discontinuation symptoms following chronic use. Cessation of use is followed by declining blood levels of drug at receptor sites, brain, blood, and peripheral tissues, with the rate of decline determined primarily by the elimination half-life. The onset, duration, and severity of the withdrawal syndrome correlate with declining serum levels of drug (Hollister, Motzenbecker et al., 1961; Tyrer, Rutherford et al., 1981; Schweizer & Rickels, 1998; Miller, Greenblatt et al., 1988a, 1988b, 1989).

Onset of withdrawal from short-acting benzodiazepines (such as lorazepam, oxazepam, triazolam, alprazolam, and temazepam) occurs within 24 hours of cessation (Rickels, 1986b), with peak severity of withdrawal occurring within one to five days following cessation (Rickels, Case et al., 1986b; Schweizer & Rickels, 1990). With long-acting benzodiazepines (such as diazepam, chlordiazepoxide, and clonaz- epam), onset of withdrawal occurs within five days of cessation (Rickels, 1986) and withdrawal severity peaks at one to nine days (Schweizer & Rickels, 1990).

Duration of acute withdrawal, from the temporal onset to the resolution of symptoms, can be as long as 7 to 21 days for short-acting and 10 to 28 days for long-acting benzodiazepines. While there is a difference in the type or number of withdrawal symptoms following discontinuation of short- or long-acting benzodiazepines (Rickels, Case et al., 1986b; Schweizer & Rickels 1990), withdrawal symptoms from short-acting benzodiazepines are experienced as being more intense than those associated with long-acting drugs, and are of more rapid onset following abrupt discontinuation (Tyrer, Rutherford et al., 1981; Rickels, 1986b; Schweizer & Rickels, 1990).

Dose and Duration of Use: Higher doses and longer use place patients at greater risk for increased withdrawal severity. Daily benzodiazepine use for 10 days or less can lead to transient insomnia when the medications are stopped. A withdrawal syndrome can follow discontinuation of short-term (<2 to 3 months') low dose therapeutic use, but most symptoms, if present at all, are rated as mild (such as insomnia) and are easily managed. On discontinuation of long-term (>1 year) therapeutic (low-dose) use, withdrawal is common and is accompanied by moderate to severe symptoms in 20% to 100% of patients (Rickels, Case, et al., 1986b; Schweizer & Rickels, 1990). Discontinuation of high-dose (>4 to 5 times the high end of the therapeutic range for more than 6 to 12 weeks) benzodiazepine use leads to moderate withdrawal in all patients, and severe withdrawal signs and symptoms in most patients (Hollister, Motzenbecker et al., 1961).

Beyond one year of continuous benzodiazepine therapy, the duration of use becomes a less important factor in the severity of withdrawal (Rickels, Schweizer et al., 1990). Use beyond one year may, however, predispose patients to prolonged withdrawal sequelae.

Potency: Tolerance to the sedative and hypnotic effects develops most rapidly to shorter acting, higher potency benzodiazepines (such as triazolam and alprazolam). Withdrawal from these agents may be more intense and require more aggressive attention and longer periods of medical monitoring than is the case with other benzodiazepines (Dickinson, Rush et al., 1990; Malcolm, Brady et al., 1993).

Host Factors Affecting Withdrawal. In addition to the aforementioned pharmacologic influences, host factors are implicated in patients' susceptibility to dependence and in the difficulty they encounter in discontinuing benzodiazepines once they become dependent. Clinically important patient factors include:

Psychiatric Comorbidity: The primary clinical indication for benzodiazepine use involves treatment of the highly prevalent conditions of insomnia, anxiety, thought, and mood disorders. It follows that patients with chronic psychiatric disorders who are maintained on benzodiazepines for more than three to six months will, in addition to their psychiatric condition (adequately treated or not), also be physically dependent on the benzodiazepine. Numerous benzodiazepine discontinuation studies highlight the high (40% to 100%) prevalence of active concurrent psychiatric disorders seen at intake of study participants (Rickels, Case et al., 1986b; Schweizer & Rickels, 1990; Rickels, Schweizer et al., 1990; Malcolm, Brady et al., 1996; Romach, Busto et al., 1995). Most of these studies demonstrate a correlation between the patients' degree of psychopathology and their withdrawal symptom severity and difficulty in discontinuing use.

Rickels and colleagues (1986b) reported on 119 patients discontinuing long-term, therapeutic-dose use. They noted a 90% prevalence of initial, active psychopathology with diagnoses that included generalized anxiety disorder (44%), panic disorder (27%), depression (14%), and other (7%). Patients with greater psychopathology required more support and assurance. The intensity of the withdrawal syndrome was seen as partially a function of the degree of psychopathology and other premorbid personality variables.

Rickels and colleagues (1990) studied abrupt and tapered discontinuation of long-term, therapeutic-dose benzodiazepine use. They found that 79% to 84% of patients had clinically significant, active symptoms of anxiety and or depression at intake (primary psychiatric diagnoses included generalized anxiety disorder, panic disorder, and major depression). They reported significantly greater withdrawal severity in patients diagnosed with more initial psychopathology, dependent personality disorder, or neuroticism. Increased withdrawal symptoms also have been associated with high initial anxiety or depression and decreased educational level (Woods, Katz et al., 1992).

Clinicians conducting benzodiazepine discontinuation thus must obtain psychiatric histories while remaining vigilantly watchful for, and prepared to manage, the emergence or reemergence of psychiatric disorders. Clinicians also must be aware that patients with psychiatric symptoms or disorders often experience more severe withdrawal symptoms and have greater difficulty discontinuing use.

Concurrent Use of Other Substances: Concurrent regular use of other dependence-producing substances increases the complexity of the benzodiazepine abstinence syndrome and the clinical situation as a whole. Additional sedative-hypnotic substance use contributes to a withdrawal syndrome of increased severity and less predictable course. For example, opioid substance withdrawal contributes an additional cluster of signs and symptoms. Anxiety, agitation, irritation, hyper-arousal, and the adrenergic components of opioid and benzodiazepine withdrawal are additive, often overlap, and lead to an exacerbation of symptoms. Psychomotor stimulant withdrawal symptoms contribute factors from the opposite end of the withdrawal spectrum (for example, apathy, hypersomnia, and lethargy). When stimulant withdrawal is combined with sedative-hypnotic withdrawal, the clinical picture is variable, with hypersomnolence and lethargy mixed with symptoms of severe agitation, depression, irritability, and somatosensory hypersensitivity. Initial hypersomnolence and lethargy can mask symptoms of benzodiazepine withdrawal, particularly involving benzodiazepines with a longer half-life.

Several factors underscore the need for clinicians to be aware of the high co-occurrence of alcoholism, anxiety disorders, and/or benzodiazepine dependence and their potential influence on the benzodiazepine withdrawal syndrome:

- A high percentage of alcoholics use benzodiazepines regularly, ranging from 29% (Busto & Sellers, 1991), to 33% (Busto, Simpkins et al., 1983) to 76% (Ciraulo, Barnhill et al., 1988).

- The rate of comorbid alcohol abuse and anxiety disorders is reported to be 18% to 19% (Regier, Farmer et al., 1990).

- Alcoholics have a high propensity for dependence on benzodiazepines (Ciraulo, Barnhill et al., 1988; Sellers, Ciraulo et al., 1993).

Moderate alcohol use (exceeding one beer or drink per day) is a more significant predictor of benzodiazepine withdrawal severity than dose or half-life of the drug (Rickels, Schweizer et al., 1990). Patients with high-dose benzodiazepine use who present for inpatient addiction treatment exhibit a high rate (70% to 96%) of concurrent dependence on other substances (Romach, Busto et al., 1995; Malcolm, Brady et al., 1993). Almost all of these patients reported histories of dependence on other substances. DuPont (1988) reported that >20% of patients newly admitted to inpatient addiction treatment reported using benzodiazepines at least weekly, 73% of heroin users reported greater than weekly use, and >15% of heroin users used benzodiazepines daily (Griffiths & Wolf, 1990).

It is uncommon for drug addicts to use a benzodiazepine as an initial or primary drug of use (Smith & Landry, 1990). Instead, benzodiazepines are used in combination with other psychoactive drugs. In addition, a high rate of benzodiazepine use in methadone maintenance clinics is supported by numerous clinical surveys.

Consequently, clinicians must be aware of, and suspect, benzodiazepine use in patients with any substance use disorders. Conversely, in high-dose benzodiazepine users, other substance use must be assumed until ruled out.

Family History of Alcohol Dependence: Mood changes associated with lability or benzodiazepine abuse (and increased propensity to develop dependence) have been reported following controlled clinical administration of diazepam and alprazolam in adult sons of severe alcoholics (Ciraulo, Barnhill et al., 1988; Cowley, Roy-Byrne et al., 1991, 1992). Similar findings with alprazolam were reported recently in adult daughters of alcoholics (Ciraulo, Sarid-Segal et al., 1996). This predisposition to abuse benzodiazepines is important, because at least one study implicates a linkage of paternal history of alcoholism with increased withdrawal severity in patients discontinuing alprazolam use (Dickinson, Rush et al., 1990).

Concurrent Medical Conditions: Benzodiazepine withdrawal should be avoided during acute medical or surgical conditions because the physiologic stress of withdrawal can adversely and unnecessarily affect the course of the medical condition. On the other hand, continued benzodiazepine use rarely has a negative effect on acute medical conditions. In an acute medical situation, the goal of therapy for a patient dependent on benzodiazepines is to provide adequate stabilization of the benzodiazepine dose so as to prevent withdrawal.

Clinicians need to be secure in their understanding of the indications for discontinuing long-term benzodiazepine use in patients with chronic medical conditions. This understanding is particularly critical when evaluating the discontinuation of sedative-hypnotics in patients with conditions that are significantly influenced by adrenergic and psychologic stress factors (such as cardiac arrhythmia, asthma, systemic lupus erythematosus, and inflammatory bowel disease). The risks of exacerbating the medical condition through acute withdrawal or a protracted withdrawal course may outweigh the longer term benefits of benzodiazepine discontinuation.

In general, patients with chronic medical conditions experience benzodiazepine withdrawal more severely than others. Clinicians and patients must be aware that, during withdrawal, difficulties in managing the medical condition (diabetes, cardiovascular disease, thyroid disease, and arthritis) may emerge. The rate of discontinuation is an important factor. Slower rates can improve the success of detoxification. Achieving lower doses of benzodiazepine use is an acceptable intermediate (and, in some patients, final) goal. It is important to stabilize both the patient's physical and psychologic health at reduced benzodiazepine levels before proceeding with further reductions.

Age: The use of anxiolytics peaks between the ages of 50 and 65, while the use of hypnotics is most frequent in the oldest age range (Woods, Katz et al., 1992). Hepatic microsomal enzyme oxidase system (MEOS) efficiency decreases with age. Elderly patients may have elimination half-lives that are two to five times slower than the rate in younger adults for benzodiazepines eliminated through the MEOS (all benzodiazepines except for lorazepam, temazepam, and oxazepam). The withdrawal syndrome for elderly persons who are discontinuing oxidatively metabolized benzodiazepines may be quite prolonged and/or approach the severity of high-dose withdrawal secondary to the pharmacokinetic factors of aging. The withdrawal course can become especially pernicious following discontinuation of long-acting benzodiazepines that are metabolized to sedative-hypnotic compounds with longer elimination half-lives (such as diazepam, chlordiazepoxide, and flurazepam).

Gender: Worldwide, women are prescribed benzodiazepines twice as often as men; hence, twice as many women as men are likely to become dependent (Gabe, 1993). Possibly compounding this trend are reports that female gender is a significant predictor of increased withdrawal severity in patients undergoing tapered cessation of long-term, therapeutic benzodiazepine use (Rickels, Schweizer et al, 1990). However, gender has not been implicated as an influential factor in abrupt cessation of long-term, therapeutic-dose use (Schweizer, Rickels et al., 1990).

PATIENT EVALUATION AND MANAGEMENT
Evaluation and Assessment. Evaluating patients for benzodiazepine cessation and detoxification requires a combination of clinical, diagnostic, consultation and liaison, counseling, and pharmacologic management skills. To be effective, the clinician must be flexible and able to tolerate ambiguities and variations in the course of withdrawal, while supporting the patient (who generally experiences significant apprehension and anxiety). Clinical evaluation and assessment of the patient typically include the following steps:

Step 1: Determine the reason(s) the patient or referral source is seeking evaluation of sedative-hypnotic use and/or discontinuation. Determine the indication(s) for the patient's drug use. A discussion with the referring physician should be standard practice. Discussion with any other referring person(s) or close family members often is helpful. Seek evidence to answer the question as to whether the patient's use is improving his or her quality of life or causing significant disability and/or exacerbating the original condition. Discuss the patient's expectations.

Step 2: Take a sedative-hypnotic use history, including, at a minimum, the dose, duration of use, substance(s) used, and the patient's clinical response to sedative-hypnotic use at present and over time. The history should include attempts at abstinence (including previous detoxification[s]), symptoms experienced with changing the dose, and reasons for increasing or decreasing the dose. The history should include behavioral responses to sedative-hypnotic use and adverse or toxic side effects. For long-term users, a determination of the current pharmacologic efficacy and clinical efficacy should be sought.

Step 3: Elicit a detailed accounting of other alcohol or psychoactive drug use, including medical and non-medical, prescribed and over-the-counter drugs, current and past, as well as the sequelae of such use. In addition to prior withdrawal experiences, the history also should include prior periods of abstinence and abstinence attempts.

Step 4: Take a psychiatric history, including current and past psychiatric diagnoses, hospitalizations, suicide attempts, treatment, psychotherapy, and therapists (names and locations). Ask if alcohol and/or other drugs were used during or near the time any psychiatric diagnoses were made. Ask if the evaluator was aware of the patient's alcohol and/or drug use.

Step 5: Take a family history of substance use, psychiatric, and medical disorders.

Step 6: Take a current and past medical history of the patient, including illnesses, trauma, surgery, medications, allergies, and history of loss of consciousness, seizure(s), or seizure disorder.

Step 7: Take a psychosocial history, including current social status and support system.

Step 8: Perform a physical and mental status examination.

Step 9: Conduct a laboratory urine drug screen for substances of abuse. An alcohol Breathalyzer® test (if available) often is helpful in providing immediate evidence of alcohol use that was not disclosed in the history. Remember that these are therapeutic tools. Trust the patient, but check the urine. Depending on the patient's profile, a complete blood count, blood chemistry panel, liver enzymes, viral hepatitis panel, HIV test, TB test, pregnancy test, and/or ECG test may be indicated.

Step 10: Complete an individualized assessment, taking into account all aspects of the patient's presentation and history and, in particular, focusing on factors that would significantly influence the presence, severity, and time course of withdrawal.

Step 11: Arrive at a differential diagnosis, including a comprehensive list of diagnoses that have been considered. This greatly aids clinical management decisions as the patient's symptoms diminish, emerge, or change in character during and after drug cessation.

Step 12: Determine the appropriate setting for detoxification.

Step 13: Determine the most efficacious detoxification method. In addition to proven clinical and pharmacologic efficacy, the method selected should be one that the physi-

cian and clinical staff in the detoxification setting are comfortable with and experienced in administering.

Step 14: Obtain the patient's informed consent.

Step 15: Initiate detoxification. Ongoing physician involvement is central to appropriate management of detoxification. Subsequent to the patient assessment, development of the treatment plan, and obtaining patient consent, the individualized discontinuation program should be initiated. The physician closely monitors and flexibly manages (adjusting as necessary) the dosing or detoxification strategy to provide the safest, most comfortable and efficacious course of detoxification. To achieve optimal results,

TABLE 3. Sedative-Hypnotic Withdrawal Substitution Dose Conversions

Drug	Dose Equal to 30 mg of Phenobarbital (mg)
Benzodiazepines	
Alprazolam (Xanax®)	0.5–1
Chlordiazepoxide (Librium®)	25
Clonazepam (Klonopin®)	1–2
Clorazepate (Tranxene®)	7.5
Diazepam (Valium®)	10
Estazolam (ProSom®)	1
Flurazepam (Dalmane®)	15
Lorazepam (Ativan®)	2
Oxazepam (Serax®)	10–15
Quazepam (Doral®)	15
Temazepam (Restoril®)	15
Triazolam (Halcion®)	0.25
Barbiturates	
Pentobarbital (Nembutal®)	100
Secobarbital (Seconal®)	100
Butalbital (Fiorinal®)	100
Amobarbital (Amytal®)	100
Phenobarbital	30
Nonbarbiturates-Nonbenzodiazepines	
Ethchlorvynol (Placidyl®)	500
Glutethimide (Doriden®)	250
Methyprylon (Noludar®)	200
Methaqualone (Quaalude®)	300
Meprobamate (Miltown®)	1,200
Carisoprodol (Soma®)	700
Chloral Hydrate (Noctec®)	500

the physician and patient will need to establish a close working relationship. A withdrawal contract is a useful tool.

Management. For patients who are dependent on sedative-hypnotics, there are two primary options for the detoxification process: tapering or substitution and tapering.

Gradual dose reduction (tapering) is the most widely used and most logical method of benzodiazepine discontinuation. The taper method is indicated for use in (1) an outpatient ambulatory setting, (2) patients with therapeutic-dose benzodiazepine dependence, (3) patients who are dependent only on benzodiazepines, and (4) patients who can reliably present for regular clinical followup during and after detoxification (Rickels, DeMartinis et al., 1996; Smith & Landry, 1990; Ashton, 1991; Alexander & Perry, 1991; Schweizer & Rickels, 1998; Busto & Sellers, 1991).

Tapering: With the taper method, the patient is slowly and gradually weaned from the benzodiazepine on which he or she is dependent, using a fixed-dose taper schedule. The dose is decreased on a weekly to every-other-week basis. The rate of discontinuation for long-term users (>1 year) should not exceed 5 mg diazepam equivalents per week (12.5 mg chlordiazepoxide or 15 mg phenobarbital equivalents) or 10% of the current (starting) dose per week, whichever is smaller. The first 50% of the taper is usually smoother, quicker, and less symptomatic than the last 50% (Rickels, DeMartinis et al., 1996; Schweizer, Rickels et al., 1990). For the final 25% to 35% of the taper, the rate and/or dose reduction schedule should be slowed to half the previous dose reduction per week and the reduction accomplished at twice the original tapering interval. If symptoms of withdrawal occur, the dose should be increased slightly until the symptoms resolve and the subsequent taper schedule commenced at a slower rate.

Some patients may want to accelerate the reduction. This acceleration is better tolerated and can be encouraged early in the reduction. As a general rule, patients tolerate more dose reduction and with shorter intervals early in the tapering process and then require decreased dose reduction over longer intervals as the taper progresses and the dose is reduced. A common error is trying to push the taper process too quickly.

Brief office visits should be conducted at least weekly to facilitate regular assessment of the patient for withdrawal symptoms, general health, taper compliance, and use of supportive therapy. Taper medications should be closely controlled by prescribing an amount sufficient only for the time period until the next visit. The prescriber should give a clear message to the patient that lost, misplaced, or stolen medication will not be replaced. A withdrawal contract between the clinician and the patient is advisable. A copy of the written schedule of daily doses, covering multiple weeks to months, helps the patient adhere to the reduction plan.

Patients who are unable to complete a simple taper program should be reevaluated and, if indicated, an alternative detoxification method chosen. Some patients may require a substitution and taper program or a period of hospitalization to receive more intensive monitoring and support in order to complete drug discontinuation.

Substitution and Taper: Substitution and taper methods employ cross-tolerant long-acting benzodiazepines (such as chlordiazepoxide or clonazepam) or phenobarbital to substitute, at equipotent doses, for the sedative-hypnotic(s) on which the patient is dependent (Table 3). Chlordiazepoxide, clonazepam, and phenobarbital are the most widely used substitution agents for a number of important reasons:

- At steady state, there is negligible inter-dose serum level variation with these drugs;

- With tapering, a more gradual reduction in serum levels, reducing the risk of that withdrawal symptoms will emerge; and

- Each of the drugs has a low abuse potential (phenobarbital is lowest, followed by clonazepam and then chlordiazepoxide).

Phenobarbital offers the added advantage of rarely inducing behavioral disinhibition and possesses broad clinical efficacy in the management of withdrawal from all classes of sedative-hypnotic agents. Clinical experience shows that phenobarbital is most useful and effective in patients with polysubstance dependence, high-dose dependence, and in patients with unknown dose or erratic "polypharmacy" drug use.

If hepatomegally or elevated liver tests are a problem, then oxazepam may be a good substitute (Smith & Landry, 1990). Lorazepam could be considered, but its abuse liability is much higher than that of oxazepam (Griffiths & Wolf, 1990).

Uncomplicated Substitution and Taper: This method is used in outpatient settings for patients who are discontinuing use of short half-life benzodiazepines or for those who are unable to tolerate gradual tapering.

1. Calculate the equivalent dose of chlordiazepoxide, clonazepam, or phenobarbital using the Substitution Dose Conversion Table (Table 3). Individual variation in clinical responses to "equivalent" doses can vary, so close clinical monitoring of patient response to substitution is necessary. Adjustments to the initially calculated dose schedule are to be expected.

2. Provide the substituted drug in a divided dose. For chlordiazepoxide, oxazepam, or phenobarbital, give three to four doses per day. For clonazepam, two to three doses per day usually are sufficient.

3. While the substituted agent is achieving steady state levels on a fixed dose schedule, provide the patient with PRN doses of the benzodiazepine he or she has been using. This will help to suppress breakthrough symptoms of withdrawal. Do this for the first week only, then discontinue PRN drug dosing.

4. Stabilize the patient on an adequate substitution dose (same dose on consecutive days without the need for regular PRN doses). This usually is accomplished within 1 week.

5. Gradually reduce the dose. The dose is decreased on a weekly to every-other-week basis, as in the simple taper model. The rate of discontinuation is 5 mg diazepam equivalents per week (or 12.5 mg chlordiazepoxide equivalents or 15 mg phenobarbital equivalents), as shown in Table 3; or 10% of the current (starting) dose per week. The first half of the taper usually is smoother, quicker, and less symptomatic than the latter half.

6. For the final 25% to 35% of the taper, the rate and/or dose reduction should be slowed. If symptoms of withdrawal occur, hold the taper for three to four days to stabilize the patient, then resume the process. Some patients may wish to accelerate the reduction. This is better tolerated early in the taper. Care should be taken not to push the taper too quickly.

7. Support the patient with short but frequent visits, as described above. Taper medication should be closely controlled by prescribing only enough medication for the time period until the next visit.

Sedative-Hypnotic Tolerance Testing: This method is employed when the degree of dependence is difficult to determine. Such a situation is common in high-dose, erratic-dose, illicit source, polysubstance, or alcohol plus sedative-hypnotic use. Testing is best done in a setting that offers 24-hour medical monitoring. Pentobarbital is used because of its rapid onset of action, short half-life, ease with which signs of toxicity can be monitored, and ease with which it can be replaced by phenobarbital once the patient has been stabilized.

1. 200 mg pentobarbital is given orally every two hours for up to 24 to 48 hours.

2. Doses are held for signs of toxicity (intoxication), which develop in the following progression at increasing serum levels: fine lateral sustained nystagmus, coarse nystagmus, slurred speech, ataxia, and somnolence. Doses are held with the development of coarse nystagmus and slurred speech and subsequently resumed with the resolution of the signs of toxicity.

3. After 24 to 48 hours, the total amount of administered pentobarbital is divided by the number of days it was administered. This amount is the 24-hour stabilizing dose.

4. The stabilizing dose is administered in divided doses over the next 24 hours to ensure adequate substitution. The patient's response determines the indications for upward or downward adjustments in the dose.

5. Once the patient is stable on a consistent dose for 24 hours, phenobarbital is substituted for pentobarbital (Table 3).

6. A gradual dose reduction of phenobarbital is conducted, as described under substitution and tapering.

Withdrawal Emergence PRN Phenobarbital Substitution: This procedure is best used in a 24-hour medically monitored setting. It provides the smoothest and most effective treatment for sedative-hypnotic withdrawal for patients who are unable to complete outpatient tapering regimens, or who are high-dose users, polysubstance-dependent, and experiencing considerable comorbid psychopathology.

1. Signs and symptoms of withdrawal are treated as needed (PRN) with 30 to 60 mg of phenobarbital every one to four hours. The period of PRN dosing is determined by the elimination of most withdrawal signs and symptoms and is influenced by the duration of action of the substances(s) the patient is discontinuing.

---

2. The patient is monitored hourly to ensure adequate dosing and to prevent oversedation. Ideally, a balance is achieved between the signs and symptoms of withdrawal and those of phenobarbital intoxication.

3. When the patient has received similar 24-hour phenobarbital dose totals for two consecutive days, the total dose for those two days is divided by 2 to arrive at the stabilizing dose.

4. The stabilizing dose is given in divided-dose increments over the next 24 hours, which may require medication administration every three to four hours for patients with high tolerance.

5. Once the patient is stabilized, a gradual taper is initiated, as described above.

Patients often can be transferred from an inpatient setting to an intensive (medically monitored) outpatient program once they are stabilized and well established on the tapering portion of the protocol.

Appropriate Clinical Setting. Patients who have polysubstance dependence (including sedatives and hypnotics), mixed alcohol with other sedative-hypnotic use, high-dose hypnotic sedative use, erratic behavior, incompatible use histories, involvement with illicit sources, and extensive mental health issues are best served in an inpatient facility that offers 24-hour medical monitoring.

Adjunctive Withdrawal Management Measures. *Carbamazepine*: Adjunctive carbamazepine therapy is not widely used, although clinical protocols and patient selection for this method are being studied. Initial reports on small clinical trials using carbamazepine showed encouraging but mixed effectiveness and utility (Klein, Uhde et al., 1986; Klein, Colvin et al., 1994; Ries, Roy-Byrne et al., 1989; Garcia-Borresuerro, 1990; Schweizer, Rickels et al., 1991). Pages and Ries (1998) reviewed further use of carbamazepine and found it to be an effective adjunct. Schweizer and colleagues (1991) studied 40 patients with a history of difficulty discontinuing long-term therapeutic benzodiazepines. Significantly more patients treated with carbamazepines were benzodiazepine-free at five weeks. Patients receiving carbamazepine (but not the clinicians evaluating them) reported a larger reduction in withdrawal severity compared with patients taking placebo. Ries and colleagues (1989) and Pages and Ries (1998) reported protocols for the use of carbamazepine: 600 mg per day (usually 200 mg

TID) is used alone or in combination with a three-day benzodiazepine taper.

Chlordiazepoxide is useful because of its longer half-life and low abuse potential. Phenobarbital can be added PRN to this protocol for breakthrough withdrawal symptoms.

Carbamazepine is continued for a minimum of two to three weeks after the three-day benzodiazepine taper is completed and can be tapered to monitor for return of withdrawal symptoms. Elderly patients who are discontinuing benzodiazepines have been treated successfully with carbamazepine at doses of 400 to 500 mg per day.

Adverse consequences of carbamazepine use can include GI upset, neutropenia, thrombocytopenia, and hyponatremia, necessitating initial and ongoing laboratory evaluation and monitoring.

Sodium Valproate: Reports indicate that sodium valproate is effective in attenuating the benzodiazepine withdrawal syndrome. Valproate possesses GABA-ergic actions and anticonvulsant effects (Harris, Roache et al., 2000; Apelt & Emerich, 1990). Valproate also may suppress N-methyl-D-aspartate (NMDA) and reduce L-glutamate responses (Harris, Roach et al., 2000; Zeise, Kasparon et al., 1991). Rickels, Schweizer et al. (1999) found that valproate-treated patients were 2.5 times more likely to be benzodiazepine-free at five weeks post-taper, compared with a placebo group.

Valproate doses of 250 mg TID (250 mg BID if over age 60) can be used in combination with a three-day benzodiazepine taper. Chlordiazepoxide is a useful choice because of its long half-life and low abuse potential. Calculate the equivalent chlordiazepoxide dose for the amount of current benzodiazepine being discontinued. Give one-half to two-thirds of this dose spaced equally over the first day (24 hours); one-third spaced equally over the second day (second 24 hours); and 10% to 20% spaced equally over the third day (third 24 hours). Phenobarbital can be used for breakthrough withdrawal symptoms. Valproate is continued for a minimum of two to three weeks after the three-day benzodiazepine taper is completed. Longer treatment may improve the proportion of patients who remain benzodiazepine-free. Valproate can be tapered to monitor for return of withdrawal symptoms.

Valproate has been used to treat anxiety. It has fewer side effects than carbamazepine. It can be used both inpatient and outpatient. For these reasons, further studies may strengthen the role of valproate in the treatment of benzodiazepine withdrawal. Side effects (including elevated liver function tests, thrombocytopenia, bone marrow suppression, and pancreatitis), drug reactions (including rash and erythema multiforme), gastric upset, and behavioral changes require close monitoring.

Propranolol: Tyrer and colleagues (1981) clearly demonstrated that propranolol alone does not affect the rate of successful benzodiazepine discontinuation or the incidence of withdrawal symptoms for discontinuation of chronic benzodiazepine use. However, propranolol treatment did diminish the severity of adrenergic signs and symptoms of withdrawal. Propranolol is not cross-tolerant with sedative-hypnotic drugs and should not be used as the sole therapeutic agent in managing sedative-hypnotic withdrawal. Propranolol can be used, in doses of 60 to 120 mg per day, divided TID or QID, as an adjunct to one of the aforementioned withdrawal methods. However, clinicians need to be mindful that propranolol treatment will diminish some of the very symptoms and signs that are monitored to determine substitution doses.

Clonidine: Clonidine has been shown to be ineffective in treating benzodiazepine withdrawal. Doses sufficient to decrease serum levels of norepinephrine metabolites had minimal attenuating effect on the benzodiazepine withdrawal syndrome. One significant result of this study was the demonstration that increased norepinephrine activity plays a small role in the overall benzodiazepine withdrawal syndrome.

Buspirone: Buspirone is a non-benzodiazepine anxiolytic drug that is not cross-tolerant with benzodiazepines or other sedative-hypnotic drugs. Schweizer and colleagues (1986) demonstrated that buspirone substitution in patients undergoing abrupt or gradual benzodiazepine discontinuation failed to protect against the symptoms of withdrawal.

Trazodone: Trazodone is useful in the management of benzodiazepine withdrawal. Trazodone decreased anxiety in benzodiazepine-tapered patients (Ansseau & Roeck, 1993). Trazodone improved patients' ability to remain benzodiazepine-free after a four-week taper of the benzodiazepine. In one study, two-thirds of the patients treated with trazodone, compared with 31% of patients treated with placebo, were benzodiazepine-free at five weeks post-taper (Rickels, Schweizer et al., 1999). Trazodone can be used to improve sleep during benzodiazepine tapering and when

benzodiazepine-free. Side effects may include dry mouth, morning hangover, drowsiness, dizziness, and priapism.

Cognitive-Behavioral Therapy: Two studies (Spiegel, Bruce et al., 1994; Otto, Pollack et al., 1993) demonstrate that, in patients with panic disorder, adding cognitive-behavioral therapy to alprazolam discontinuation improved the rate of successful alprazolam discontinuation. Spiegel and colleagues (1994) reported that patients in the combined taper and cognitive-behavioral therapy groups had greater rates of abstinence from alprazolam at six months than did those who underwent taper alone.

Prolonged Benzodiazepine Withdrawal. Some physicians (Smith & Wesson, 1983; Smith & Seymour, 1991; Landry, Smith et al., 1992) report, and clinical experience confirms, that a small proportion of patients, following long-term benzodiazepine use, experience a prolonged syndrome in which withdrawal signs and symptoms persist for weeks to months following discontinuation. This prolonged withdrawal syndrome is noted for its irregular and unpredictable day-to-day course and qualitative and quantitative differences in symptoms from both the pre-benzodiazepine use state and the acute withdrawal period. Patients with prolonged withdrawal often experience slowly abating, albeit characteristic, waxing and waning symptoms of insomnia, perceptual disturbances, tremor, sensory hypersensitivity(ies), and anxiety.

Smith and Wesson (1983) propose that protracted symptoms reflect long-term receptor site adaptations. Higgitt and Fonagy (1983) propose that a comprehensive etiologic model of the prolonged syndrome must include a psychological component that can be explained through cognitive and behavioral models. They observe that many patients with persistent withdrawal symptoms resemble patients with somatization disorders. The patients often experience acute withdrawal more severely and may be "sensitized to anxiety." In addition to a potential lack of effective coping mechanisms away from benzodiazepines, such patients often possess a perceptual and/or cognitive style that leads to apprehensiveness, body sensation amplification and mislabeling, and misinterpretation.

Management: Before entertaining the existence of a prolonged withdrawal syndrome, physicians must rule out psychiatric conditions. A distinguishing characteristic of protracted withdrawal from anxiety disorders is the gradual diminution and eventual resolution of symptoms with benzodiazepine withdrawal.

Propranolol in doses of 10 to 20 mg four times a day often is helpful in attenuating anxiety or tremors. Lower doses of sedating antidepressant medications—such as trazodone, amitriptyline, imipramine, or doxepin—are helpful in treating insomnia. Frequent clinical followup for education, supportive psychotherapy, and regular reassurance are strongly advised. Frequent reassessment of the working diagnosis is recommended.

COMMON TREATMENT ISSUES

Formal treatment is indicated for nearly all patients with substance use and addictive disorders. Among sedative-hypnotic users, treatment most often is indicated for polysubstance users, high-dose users, and/or patients in whom addiction is diagnosed. The support, education, and recovery training available in most treatment programs are valuable to many patients who are dependent on sedative-hypnotics. On the other hand, patients with long-term, therapeutic use problems should not be coerced to participate in programs designed to treat addictive disorders, as they often feel out of place and unable to relate to their peers.

Participation in specific components of treatment, tailored to each patient's individual needs, can be helpful and non-threatening. Patients who choose to participate in treatment often discover an immense source of support and encouragement, in addition to learning and practicing coping skills that facilitate drug discontinuation and abstinence.

REFERENCES

Alexander B & Perry P (1991). Detoxification from benzodiazepines: Schedules and strategies. *Journal of Substance Abuse Treatment* 8:9-17.

American Psychiatric Association (APA) (1994). *Diagnostic and Statistical Manual of Mental Disorders, 4th Edition*. Washington, DC: American Psychiatric Press.

Annsseau M & DeRoeck J (1993). Trazodone in benzodiazepine dependence. *Journal of Clinical Psychiatry* May:189-191.

Apelt S & Emrich H (1990). Letter. *American Journal of Psychiatry* 147(7):950-951.

Ashton H (1987). Benzodiazepine withdrawal: Outcome in 50 patients. *British Journal of Addiction* 665-671.

Ashton H (1991). Protracted withdrawal syndromes from benzodiazepines. *Journal of Substance Abuse Treatment* 8:19-28.

Barter G & Cormack M (1996). The long-term use of benzodiazepines; Patients' views, accounts and experiences. *Family Practice* 13 (6):491.

Busto U & Sellers E (1991). Anxiolytics and sedative/hypnotics dependence. *British Journal of Addiction* 86:1647-1652.

Busto U, Simpkins J & Sellers EM (1983). Objective determination of benzodiazepine use and abuse in alcoholics. *British Journal of Addiction* 78:429-435.

Ciraulo DA, Barnhill JG, Greenblatt DJ et al. (1988). Abuse liability and clinical pharmacokinetics of alprazolam in alcoholic men. *Journal of Clinical Psychiatry* 49:333-337.

Ciraulo DA, Sarid-Segal O, Knapp C et al. (1996). Liability to alprazolam abuse in daughters of alcoholics. *American Journal of Psychiatry* 153:956-958.

Costa E, Guidotti A et al. (1975). Evidence for the involvement of GABA in the actions of benzodiazepines. In E Costa & P Greengard (eds.) *Mechanisms and Actions of Benzodiazepines*. New York, NY: Raven Press, 141-161.

Covi L, Lipman RS, Pattison JH et al. (1973). Length of treatment with anxiolytic sedatives and response to their sudden withdrawal. *Acta Psychiatrica Scandinavica* 49:51-64.

Covi L, Park LC & Lipman RS (1973). Factors affecting withdrawal response to certain minor tranquilizers. In JO Cole & JR Wittenborn (eds.) *Drug Abuse: Social and Pharmacological Aspects*. Springfield, IL: Charles C Thomas, 93-108.

Cowley DS, Roy-Byrne PP, Gordon C et al. (1992). Response to diazepam in sons of alcoholics. *Alcoholism: Clinical & Experimental Research* 16:1057-1063.

Cowley DS, Roy-Byrne PP, Hommer DW et al. (1991). Sensitivity to benzodiazepines in sons of alcoholics. *Biological Psychiatry* 29:104-112.

Dickinson W, Rush PA & Radcliffe AB (1990). Alprazolam use and dependence: A retrospective analysis of 30 cases of withdrawal. *Western Journal of Medicine* 152(5):604-608.

DuPont RL (1988). Abuse of benzodiazepines: The problems and solutions. *American Journal of Alcohol and Drug Abuse* 14S:1-69.

Epstein RS (1980). Withdrawal symptoms from chronic use of low-dose barbiturates. *American Journal of Psychiatry* 137(1):107-108.

Essig CF (1964). Addiction to nonbarbiturate sedative and tranquilizing drugs. *Clinical Pharmacology and Therapeutics* 5(3):334-343.

Essig CF (1966). Newer sedative drugs that can cause states of intoxication and dependence of barbiturate type. *Journal of the American Medical Association* 196(8):126-129.

File SE (1993). The biology of benzodiazepine dependence. In C Hallstrom (ed.) *Benzodiazepine Dependence*. New York, NY: Oxford University Press, 95-118.

Flemenbaum A & Gumby B (1971). Ethchlorvynol (Placidyl®) abuse and withdrawal. *Diseases of the Nervous System* 32:188-191.

Fraser HF, Wikler A, Essig CF et al. (1958). Degree of physical dependence induced by secobarbital or phenobarbital. *Journal of the American Medical Association* 166:126-129.

Gabe J (1993). Women and tranquilizer use: A case study in the social politics of health and health care. In C Hallstrom (ed.) *Benzodiazepine Dependence*. New York, NY: Oxford University Press, 350-363.

Garcia-Borresuerro D (1990). Treatment of benzodiazepine withdrawal symptoms with carbamazepine. *Psychiatry and Clinical Neuroscience* 241:145-150.

Greenblatt DJ, Miller LG & Shader RI (1990). Benzodiazepine discontinuation syndromes. *Journal of Psychiatric Research* 24(Suppl):73-79.

Griffiths R (1995). [Commentary on a review by Woods and Winger] Benzodiazepines: Long-term use among patients is a concern and abuse among polydrug abusers is not trivial. *Psychopharmacology* 118:116-117.

Griffiths R & Wolf B (1990). Relative abuse liability of different benzodiazepines in drug abusers. *Journal of Clinical Psychopharmacology* 10(4):237.

Haefly W (1975). Possible involvement of GABA in the central actions of benzodiazepines. In E Costa & P Greengard (eds.) *Mechanisms of Action of Benzodiazepines*. New York, NY: Raven Press, 162-202.

Harris J, Roache J & Thornton J (2000). A role for valproate in the treatment of sedative-hypnotic withdrawal and for relapse prevention. *Alcohol & Alcoholism* 35(4):319-323.

Higgitt A & Fonagy P (1983). Benzodiazepine dependence syndromes and syndromes of withdrawal. In C Hallstrom (ed.) *Benzodiazepine Dependence*. New York, NY: Oxford University Press, 58-70.

Hollister LE, Bennett LL, Kimbell I et al. (1961). Diazepam in newly admitted schizophrenics. *Diseases of the Nervous System* 24:746-750.

Hollister LE, Motzenbecker FP & Degan RO (1961). Withdrawal reactions for chlordiazepoxide (Librium®). *Psychopharmacologia* 2:63-68.

Howland MA (1994). Flumazenil. In LR Goldfrank, NE Flemenbaum, NA Lewin et al. (eds.) *Toxicologic Emergencies*. Norfolk, CT: Appleton & Lange, 805-810.

Isbell H (1950). Addiction to barbiturates and the barbiturate abstinence syndrome. *Annals of Internal Medicine* 33:108-121.

Isbell H, Altschul S et al. (1950). Chronic barbiturate intoxication: An experimental study. *Archives of Neurology and Psychiatry* 64:1-28.

Isbell H & White WM (1953). Clinical characteristics of addictions. *American Journal of Medicine* 14:558-565.

King M, Gabe J, Williams P et al. (1990). Long term use of benzodiazepines: The views of patients. *British Journal of General Practice* 194-196.

Klein RL, Colvin V et al. (1994). Alprazolam withdrawal in patients with panic disorder and generalized anxiety disorder: Vulnerability and effect of carbamazepine. *American Journal of Psychiatry* 151:1760-1766.

Klein RL, Uhde TW et al. (1986). Preliminary evidence for the utility of carbamazepine in alprazolam withdrawal. *American Journal of Psychiatry* 143:326-336.

Lader R (1993). Guidelines for the prevention and treatment of benzodiazepine dependence: Summary of a report from the Mental Health Foundation. *Addiction* 88:1707-1708.

Landry MJ, Smith DE, McDuff DR et al. (1992). Benzodiazepine dependence and withdrawal: Identification and medical management. *Journal of the American Board of Family Practice* 5:167-176.

Litovitz T (1987). Fatal benzodiazepine toxicity. *American Journal of Emergency Medicine* 5:472-473.

Lloyd EA & Clark LD (1959). Convulsions and delirium incident to glutethimide (Doriden®). *Diseases of the Nervous System* 20:1-3.

Malcolm R, Brady TK et al. (1993). Types of benzodiazepines abused by chemically dependent inpatients. *Journal of Psychoactive Drugs* 25(4):315-319.

Miller L (1991). Chronic benzodiazepine administration: From patient to gene. *Journal of Clinical Pharmacology* 31:492-495.

Miller L, Greenblatt DJ et al. (1988a). Chronic benzodiazepine administration I: Tolerance is associated with benzodiazepine receptor down regulation and decreased GABA$_A$ receptor function. *Journal of Pharmacology and Experimental Therapy* 246:170-176.

Miller L, Greenblatt DJ et al. (1988b). Chronic benzodiazepine administration II: Discontinuation syndrome is associated with up regulation of GABA$_A$ receptor complex binding and function. *Journal of Pharmacology and Experimental Therapy* 146:177-281.

Miller L, Greenblatt DJ et al. (1989). Chronic benzodiazepine administration III: Up regulation of GABA$_A$ receptor complex binding and function associated with chronic benzodiazepine agonist administration. *Journal of Pharmacology and Experimental Therapy* 248:1096-1101.

Miller L, Greenblatt DJ et al. (1990). Chronic benzodiazepine administration IV: A partial agonist produces behavioral effects without tolerance or receptor alternations. *Journal of Pharmacology and Experimental Therapy* 254:33-38.

Osborn H & Goldfrank LR (1994). Sedative-hypnotic agents. In LR Goldfrank, NE Flemenbaum, NA Lewin et al. (eds.) *Toxicologic Emergencies*. Norfolk, CT: Appleton & Lange, 787-804.

Otto MN, Pollack MH, Sachs GS et al. (1993). Discontinuation of benzodiazepine treatment: Efficacy of cognitive behavioral therapy for patients with panic disorder. *American Journal of Psychiatry* 150:1485-1490.

Pages K & Ries R (1998). Use of anticonvulsants in benzodiazepine withdrawal. *American Journal on Addictions* 7(3):198.

Phillips RM, Judy FR & Judy HE (1957). Meprobamate addiction. *Northwest Medicine* 56:453-454.

Regier DA, Farmer ME et al. (1990). Comorbidity of mental disorders with alcohol and other drug abuse. Results from the epidemiologic catchment area (ECA) study. *Journal of the American Medical Association* 264(19):2511-2518.

Rickels K, Case WG, Downing RW et al. (1986a). One-year follow-up of anxious patients treated with diazepam. *Journal of Clinical Psychopharmacology* 6:32-36.

Rickels K, Case WG, Schweizer E et al. (1986b). Low-dose dependence on chronic benzodiazepine users: A preliminary report. *Psychopharmacology Bulletin* 22:407-415.

Rickels K, DeMartinis N, Rynn M et al. (1996). Pharmacologic strategies for discontinuing benzodiazepine treatment. *Journal of Clinical Psychopharmacology* 19(6 Suppl.2):128.

Rickels K, Fox IL & Greenblatt DJ (1988). Clorazepate and lorazepam: Clinical improvement and rebound anxiety. *American Journal of Psychiatry* 145:312-317.

Rickels K, Schweizer E et al. (1990). Long-term therapeutic use of benzodiazepines. I. Effects of abrupt discontinuation. *Archives of General Psychiatry* 47:899-907.

Rickels K, Schweizer E, Garcia-Espana F et al. (1999). Trazodone and valproate in patients discontinuing long-term benzodiazepine therapy; Effects on withdrawal symptoms and taper outcome. *Psychopharmacology* 141:1-5.

Ries RK (1991). Benzodiazepine withdrawal: Clinicians' ratings of carbamazepine treatment versus traditional taper methods. *Journal of Psychoactive Drugs* 23(1):73-76.

Ries RK, Roy-Byrne PP et al. (1989). Carbamazepine treatment for benzodiazepine withdrawal. *American Journal of Psychiatry* 146(4):536-537.

Romach M, Busto U, Somer GR et al. (1995). Clinical aspects of chronic use of alprazolam and lorazepam. *American Journal of Psychiatry* 152:1161-1167.

Roy-Byrne P, Ward N & Donnelly P (1989). Valproate in anxiety and withdrawal syndromes. *Journal of Clinical Psychiatry* 50 (Suppl):44.

Sadwin A & Glen RS (1958). Addiction to glutethimide (Doriden®). *American Journal of Psychiatry* 115:469-470.

Salzman C (1997). The benzodiazepine controversy: Therapeutic effects versus dependence, withdrawal and toxicity. *Psychopharmacology* 4:279-282.

Schweizer E & Rickels K (1998). Benzodiazepine dependence and withdrawal: A review of the syndrome and its clinical management. *Acta Psychiatrica Scandinavica* 393(Suppl):95-101.

Schweizer E, Rickels K, Case G et al. (1990). Long-term therapeutic use of benzodiazepines: Effects of gradual taper. *Archives of General Psychiatry* 47:908.

Schweizer E, Rickels K, Case G et al. (1991). Carbamazepine treatment in patients discontinuing long-term benzodiazepine therapy. *Archives of General Psychiatry* 48:448.

Sellers E, Ciraulo DA, DuPont RL et al. (1993). Alprazolam and benzodiazepine dependence. *Journal of Clinical Psychiatry* 54(Suppl 10):64-75.

Smith DE & Landry M (1990). Benzodiazepine dependency discontinuation: Focus on the chemical dependency detoxification setting and benzodiazepine-polydrug abuse. *Journal of Psychiatric Research* 24 (Suppl 2):145-156.

Smith DE & Seymour RB (1991). Benzodiazepines. In NS Miller (ed.) *Comprehensive Handbook of Drug and Alcohol Addiction*. New York, NY: Marcel Dekker, 405-426.

Smith DE & Wesson DR (1983). Benzodiazepine dependency syndromes. *Journal of Psychoactive Drugs* 15:85-95.

Spiegel DA, Bruce TJ, Gregg SF et al. (1994). Does cognitive behavioral therapy assist slow-taper alprazolam discontinuation in panic disorder? *American Journal of Psychiatry* 151:876-881.

Spivey WH (1992). Flumazenil and seizures: Analysis of 43 cases. *Clinical Therapeutics* 14:292-305.

Swanson LA & Okada T (1963). Death after withdrawal of meprobamate. *Journal of the American Medical Association* 184:780-781.

Swartzburg M, Lieb J & Schwartz AH et al. (1973). Methaqualone withdrawal. *Archives of General Psychiatry* 29:46-47.

Tyrer P, Rutherford D & Huggett (1981). Benzodiazepine withdrawal symptoms and propanolol. *Lancet* 1:520-522.

Vestal R & Rumack B (1974). Glutethimide dependence: Phenobarbital treatment. *Annals of Internal Medicine* 80:670-673.

Winokur A & Rickels K (1981). Withdrawal and pseudowithdrawal reactions from diazepam therapy. *Archives of Clinical Psychiatry* 42:442-444.

Woods J, Katz J & Winger G (1992). Benzodiazepines: Use, abuse and consequences. *Pharmacological Reviews* 44(2):151.

Woods J & Winger G (1995). Current benzodiazepine issues. *Psychopharmacology* 118:107-115.

Zeise M, Kasparow S & Zieglgansberger W (1991). Valproate suppresses N-methyl-D-aspartate-evoked, transient depolarizations in the rat neocortex in vitro. *Brain Research* 544:345-348.

Chapter 4 | Management of Opioid Intoxication and Withdrawal

Patrick G. O'Connor, M.D., M.P.H.
Thomas R. Kosten, M.D.
Susan M. Stine, M.D., Ph.D.

Opioid Intoxication and Overdose
Opioid Withdrawal

Opioids include substances that are derived directly from the opium poppy (such as morphine and codeine), the semisynthetic opioids (such as heroin), and the purely synthetic opioids (such as methadone and fentanyl).

These compounds share several pharmacologic effects, including sedation, respiratory depression, and analgesia, and common clinical features of intoxication and withdrawal. This chapter reviews the clinical features of opioid intoxication and withdrawal.

While all drugs in the class are associated with clinical withdrawal syndromes, those associated with the most severe withdrawal include heroin, methadone, morphine, oxycodone, oxymorphone, and meperidine.

OPIOID INTOXICATION AND OVERDOSE

Clinical Picture. Opioid intoxication and overdose may present in a variety of settings. While mild to moderate intoxication (as evidenced by euphoria or sedation) usually is not life-threatening, severe intoxication or overdose is a medical emergency that causes many preventable deaths and thus requires immediate attention (Sporer, 1999). In a retrospective analysis of consecutive cases of presumed opioid overdose in patients initially managed by emergency medical services (EMS) personnel in an urban setting, 16% either were dead or in full cardiopulmonary arrest at the time of the initial EMS evaluation (Sporer, Firestone et al., 1996). As the prevalence of heroin use has increased in the United States, the incidence of opioid overdose has increased as well. For example, one population-based study performed in King County, WA, demonstrated a 134% increase in the number of opioid overdose deaths between 1990 and 1999 (MMWR, 2000).

Increases in opioid overdose deaths have been seen outside the U.S. as well (Hall & Darke, 1998). Despite these increases, opioid overdose can be treated successfully, if patients present in a timely manner and general principles of overdose management (as well as specific therapies for opioid overdose) are employed.

The pharmacologic actions responsible for opioid intoxication and overdose involve a specific set of opioid receptors, particularly those in the central nervous system (CNS) (Martin, 1983; Jaffe & Martin, 1990). These opioid receptors include the mu, kappa, and delta types, which also interact with endogenous substances, including the endorphins (Bozarth & Wise, 1984). Of primary concern in the management of overdose are interactions with mu receptors in the CNS, which can lead to sedation and respiratory depression. The mechanism of respiratory depression with opioids presumably is direct suppression of respiratory centers in the brain stem and medulla (Martin, 1983).

The level of tolerance to opioids can have a significant effect on an individual's risk of opioid overdose. In addition, tolerance to respiratory depression may be slower than tolerance to euphoric effects, thus explaining why overdose occurs so often, even among "experienced" opioid users (White & Irvine, 1999). Recently detoxified patients or those who have experienced intentional or unintentional abstinence from opioids for any reason may be particularly susceptible to death from heroin overdose (Tagliaro, De Battisti et al., 1998). While injecting opioids may be the route of administration associated with the highest risk of overdose, increasingly popular non-injection routes are associated with significant risk as well (Darke & Ross, 2000).

Myosis ("pinpoint pupils") is an important pharmacologic effect that can be used as a sign to identify possible opioid intoxication. Other pharmacologic effects of the opioids, including gastrointestinal hyposecretion and dysmotility, are less important in the consideration of opioid intoxication.

Diagnosis. As with most clinical challenges, evaluation of opioid intoxication begins with the collection of patient data through a detailed history and physical examination (Table 1). An important issue in the patient with moderate to severe respiratory depression is the immediate institution of pharmacologic and supportive therapies to ameliorate morbidity and prevent mortality.

When available historical information can be obtained concerning opioid use (including the specific drug, amount, and time of last use), either directly from the patient or from friends and family members, this information can supplement available hospital records. In addition to opioid abuse, it is important to ask about use of other drugs or alcohol because of the likelihood of polydrug abuse (Gould & Kleber, 1974; Kosten, Gawin et al., 1986). Identification of polydrug use has important implications for patient management; for example, identification of the frequent co-occurrence of heroin and benzodiazepine overdose may indicate the need for additional therapy directed at reversing the benzodiazepine component of the overdose with flumazenil (Dunton, Schwam et al., 1988). This also is true in cases of suspected opioid overdose in children who are at high risk of co-occurring opioid and benzodiazepine toxic-

---

TABLE 1. Diagnosis of Opioid Overdose

History
- Opioid use (ask about drug, amount, time of last use)
- Polydrug abuse
- Use multiple sources of information (family, hospital records, etc.)

Physical Examination
- Central nervous system depression
- Respiratory depression
- Myosis
- Needle tracks

Laboratory Tests
- Rule out hypoglycemia, acidemia, fluid and electrolyte abnormalities
- Toxicology screens for opioids and other drugs.

---

ity and who thus may require management of both upon presentation for medical care (Perry & Shannon, 1996).

Physical examination of the intoxicated patient may find CNS and respiratory depression, as well as pinpoint pupils and direct evidence of drug use, such as needle tracks or soft tissue infection.

The laboratory can provide important supportive information in the evaluation of opioid intoxication (see Section 3).

In addition, acute mental status changes from HIV-related opportunistic infections may mimic those of opioid intoxication (O'Connor, Selwyn et al., 1994). Patients who present with symptoms of such intoxication also may have other important causes of depressed mental status, such as hypoglycemia, acidemia, or other fluid and electrolyte disorders. Thus, toxicology screening should be performed immediately in emergency settings (Council on Scientific Affairs, 1987). Urine toxicology is preferred, because urine contains higher concentrations of drugs and their metabolites than serum. Results usually are qualitative, indicating only the presence or absence of specific substances. Even when the results of toxicologic screening are not available until after acute management has been initiated, drug screening may support the diagnosis of drug intoxication, and also may reveal the presence of other drugs not suspected on initial evaluation. Benzodiazepine abuse is common among

---

patients with opioid dependence, and some benzodiazepines (such as alprazolam) may not be readily detectable by standard urine techniques. Newer approaches involving the examination of serum may be useful in documenting previously unsuspected benzodiazepine abuse (Rogers, Hall et al., 1997).

Kellerman and colleagues (1987) examined the effects of drug screening on suspected overdose in a study of 405 adult patients who presented to an emergency department. While initial clinical management did not change significantly on the basis of the toxicology results, implications for treatment beyond the acute event were noted. Poor followup of drug screening also was demonstrated in a study of alcohol intoxication in patients injured in motor vehicle crashes. In that study, none of 47 patients who had alcohol levels between 200 and 500 milligrams per deciliter were referred for a substance abuse followup visit (Chang & Astrachan, 1988). Thus toxicology screening is useful not only for acute management, but also for planning care after discharge from the acute setting (O'Connor, Samet et al., 1994).

Opioid use and overdose also may be complicated by the effects of substances employed to "cut" drugs purchased on the street. Along with inert substances present to add bulk, active substances—including dextromethorphan, lidocaine, and scopolamine—may be present. One report of overdoses that contained significant amounts of scopolamine documented the potential clinical importance of this problem (MMWR, 1996).

Although the classic "triad" of respiratory depression, coma, and pinpoint pupils usually alerts clinicians to the possibility of opioid overdose, atypical presentations may cause some initial confusion. In a study of 43 hospitalized patients who received naloxone for a clinically suspected narcotic overdose, only two overdose patients had the classic triad, suggesting that a high index of suspicion should be maintained in certain patients who may have atypical presentations (Whipple, Quebbeman et al., 1994).

Management. In a case of suspected opioid intoxication, general supportive management must be instituted simultaneously with the specific antidote, naloxone (Table 2) (Sporer, 1999). Adult basic life support and adult advanced cardiac life support need to be available (AHA, 1992a, 1992b). The physician needs to assure that an adequate airway is established and that respiratory and cardiac function are appropriately assessed and managed. Adequate intravenous access is essential so that fluids and pharmacologic agents can be administered as needed. Finally, frequent

---

TABLE 2. Management of Opioid Overdose

General Supportive Management
- Assess and clear airway
- Support ventilation (if needed)
- Assess and support cardiac function
- Intravenous access and fluids.

Specific Pharmacologic Therapy
- Naloxone hydrochloride: 0.4 to 0.8 mg initially, repeated as necessary.

---

monitoring of vital signs and cardiorespiratory status is required until it is clearly established that the opioid and any other intoxicating substances have been cleared from the patient's system.

In the course of managing patients with suspected opioid overdose, clinicians need to be aware of the co-occurrence of acute medical problems and the exacerbation of chronic medical problems often seen in this population (O'Connor, Selwyn et al., 1994; Cherubin & Sapira, 1993). For example, prolonged hypoxia in overdose survivors can result in rhabdomyolysis and myocardial infarction (Melandri, Re et al., 1996). Other issues, such as acute infections, trauma, and chronic liver disease, may have major implications for management of the overdose patient (Cherubin & Sapira, 1993).

Pharmacologic Therapies. When a patient presents to an emergency department with pinpoint pupils and respiratory depression, pharmacologic therapy for opioid dependence should be instituted immediately (Sporer, 1999). Naloxone hydrochloride, a pure opioid antagonist, can effectively reverse the CNS effects of opioid intoxication and overdose. An initial intravenous dose of 0.4 to 0.8 mg will quickly reverse neurologic and cardiorespiratory depression. The onset of action of intravenously administered naloxone, as manifested by antagonism of opioid overdose, is approximately two minutes. Although intravenous naloxone should work more rapidly than subcutaneous naloxone, one study demonstrated that the subcutaneous route may be just as effective for managing patients before they arrive in the emergency department (Wanger, Brough et al., 1998). In that study, the authors speculated that "The slower rate of absorption via the s.q. route was offset by the delay in establishing an IV" (Wanger, Brough et al., 1998).

Overdose with opioids that are more potent (such as fentanyl) or longer acting (such as methadone) may require higher doses of naloxone given over longer periods of time, as by ongoing naloxone infusion.

In patients who do not respond to multiple doses of naloxone, alternative causes of the failure to respond must be considered. Along with the need to monitor patients for continued naloxone requirements, another important consideration to anticipate in administering naloxone is the possibility of initiating a significant withdrawal syndrome.

Followup Care. Pharmacologic management of opioid overdose is relatively straightforward in comparison to the challenge of engaging opioid dependent patients into medical care and addiction treatment once the overdose event has resolved. In one study of 77 persons admitted to hospital for management of opioid overdose, 64% left the hospital against medical advice after an average stay of less than six hours, while only half the subjects seemed interested in counseling (Seidler, Stuhlinger et al., 1996). Despite these and similar findings, clinicians who manage overdose patients should establish the need for ongoing addiction treatment as the major goal of patient management while caring for overdose-related complications.

For medical personnel, two common questions concern which patients seen in the emergency department can be discharged and when they can be discharged. Clearly, patients with major acute medical or psychiatric comorbidities, including suicidal ideation, should be hospitalized for further treatment. In the absence of these issues, resolution of the symptoms of intoxication and establishment of followup referrals for addiction, medical, and psychiatric care are necessary before a patient can be discharged safely. In a study of 573 emergency department patients, a group of investigators developed a clinical prediction rule to identify patients with opioid overdose who could be safely discharged 1 hour after naloxone administration. The authors reported that patients who can be safely discharged are those who (1) can mobilize as usual, (2) have oxygen saturation on room air of >92%, (3) have a respiratory rate >10 breaths/min and <20 breaths/min, (4) have a temperature of >35.0° C. and <37.5° C. (5) have a heart rate >50 beats/min and <100 beats/min, and (6) have a Glasgow Coma Scale score of 15. Such patients are at lower risk of adverse events (Christenson, Etherington et al., 2000).

Recent evidence suggests that naloxone also may have a role in the prevention and treatment of opioid overdose when used in the community by drug users themselves. This concept is based on the fact that most users of illicit opiates have witnessed overdoses and many (up to a third in one study) have witnessed overdose-related deaths (Strang, Powis et al., 1999). In the population studied, 89% of the subjects who had witnessed an overdose death said they would have given naloxone to the overdose victim had they know of its availability and use (Strang, Powis et al., 1999). Clearly, this concept is complicated by a number of logistical, medico-legal, ethical, and other problems that would need to be addressed. However, the approach may warrant further research, possibly including controlled clinical trials (Darke & Hall, 1997).

OPIOID WITHDRAWAL

The opioid abstinence syndrome is characterized by two phases (Himmelsbach, 1942; Martin & Jasinski, 1969). In the initial phase, opioid-dependent patients experience acute withdrawal. This was followed by the more chronic signs of a protracted abstinence syndrome. Current pharmacotherapeutic strategies are based on this duality.

Acute Withdrawal. In the initial opioid withdrawal phase, the patient typically experiences a range of symptoms for various lengths of time. Such symptoms include gastrointestinal (GI) distress (such as diarrhea and vomiting), thermoregulation disturbances, insomnia, muscle and joint pain, and marked anxiety and dysphoria. Although these symptoms generally include no life-threatening complications, the acute withdrawal syndrome causes marked discomfort, often prompting continuation of opioid use even in the absence of any opioid-associated euphoria.

Chronic Dependence and Protracted Abstinence. In patients with a chronic history of opiate dependence, acute withdrawal, and detoxification are only the beginning of treatment. Himmelsbach (1942), reporting on 21 prisoners addicted to morphine, observed that "physical recovery requires not less than six months of total abstinence." Factors he measured included temperature, sleep, respiration, weight, basal metabolic rate, blood pressure, and hematocrit. The times required for return to baseline ranged from one week to about six months. Martin and Jasinski (1969) reported in a subsequent study that this phase persisted for six months or more after withdrawal and that it was associated with "altered physiological function." They found decreased blood pressure, decreased heart rate and body temperature, myosis, and a decreased sensitivity of the respiratory center to carbon dioxide, beginning about six weeks after withdrawal and persisting for 26 or more weeks. They

---

TABLE 3. Clinical Manifestations of Opioid Withdrawal

Vital Signs	**Central Nervous System**	**Eyes**	**Skin**
■ Tachycardia	■ Restlessness	■ Pupillary dilation	■ Piloerection
■ Hypertension	■ Irritability	■ Lacrimation	**Gastrointestinal**
■ Fever	■ Insomnia	**Nose**	■ Nausea
	■ Craving	■ Rhinorrhea	■ Vomiting
	■ Yawning		■ Diarrhea

---

also found increased sedimentation rates (which persisted for months) and questionable EEG changes.

Martin and Jasinski also postulated a relationship between the protracted abstinence syndrome and relapse. Based on similar observations, Dole (1972) concluded that "human addicts almost always return to use narcotics" after hospital detoxification. In his paper, he reviewed the relative importance of metabolic and conditioned factors in relapse and concluded that the underlying drive is metabolic, arguing that "psychological factors are only triggers for relapse."

The concept of protracted abstinence has been controversial (Satel, Kosten et al., 1993), but remains a useful model for scientific hypothesis testing and development of new therapeutic approaches (Stine & Kosten, 1994). Accordingly, Dole recommended methadone maintenance treatment, even though "it does establish physical dependence." Since, as Dole pointed out, methadone continues physical dependence, protracted abstinence may continue to be a problem whenever detoxification from methadone is undertaken. However, the recent development of new pharmacologic agents may prove to ameliorate this problem.

In addition to biological considerations, psychosocial concomitants of opioid dependence also necessitate longer, more specialized adjunct treatments for these additional problems.

Clinical Picture. Withdrawal from opioids results in a specific constellation of symptoms. Although some opioid withdrawal symptoms overlap withdrawal from sedative-hypnotics, opioid withdrawal generally is considered less likely to produce severe morbidity or mortality. Clinical phenomena associated with opioid withdrawal include neurophysiologic rebound in the organ systems on which opioids have their primary actions (Jaffe, 1990). Thus, the generalized CNS suppression that occurs with opioid use is replaced by increased CNS activity.

The severity of opioid withdrawal varies with the dose and duration of drug use. In addition, route of administration appears to be important as well. Data from one study suggests that injection drug use is associated with significantly higher withdrawal symptom scores than was inhaled opioid use (Smolka & Schmidt, 1999). The time to onset of opioid withdrawal symptoms depends on the half-life of the drug being used. For example, withdrawal may begin four to six hours after the last use of heroin, but up to 36 hours after the last use of methadone (Jaffe, 1990).

Neuropharmacologic studies of opioid withdrawal have supported the clinical picture of increased CNS noradrenergic hyperactivity (Jaffe, 1990; Gunne, 1959). Therapies to alter the course of opioid withdrawal (such as clonidine) are designed to decrease this hyperactivity, which occurs primarily at the locus ceruleus. Evidence for the role of noradrenergic hyperactivity in opioid withdrawal has been provided by studies showing elevated norepinephrine metabolite levels (Crawley, Laberty et al., 1979).

Diagnosis. Opioid withdrawal involves a constellation of clinical manifestations (Table 3). Early findings may include abnormalities in vital signs, including tachycardia and hypertension. Bothersome CNS system symptoms include restlessness, irritability, and insomnia. Opioid craving also occurs in proportion to the severity of physiologic withdrawal symptoms. Pupillary dilation can be marked. A variety of cutaneous and mucocutaneous symptoms (including lacrimation, rhinorrhea, and piloerection—also known as "gooseflesh") can occur as well. Patients frequently report yawning and sneezing. Gastrointestinal symptoms, which initially may be mild (anorexia), can progress in moderate to severe withdrawal to include nausea,

---

vomiting, and diarrhea. This combination of symptomatology and intense craving frequently leads to relapse to drug use.

As with the onset of withdrawal, the duration also varies with the drug used. For example, the meperidine abstinence syndrome may peak within 8 to 12 hours and last only four to five days (Jaffe, 1990), whereas heroin withdrawal symptoms generally peak within 36 to 72 hours and may last for 7 to 14 days (Dole, 1972).

A protracted abstinence syndrome has been described, in which a variety of symptoms may last beyond the typical acute withdrawal period (Schuckit, 1989). Findings in prolonged and protracted abstinence may include mild abnormalities in vital signs and continued craving (Wen, Ho et al., 1984). Despite the extensive literature on protracted withdrawal, a universal definition and diagnostic criteria are lacking, making diagnosis difficult in individual patients (Satel, Kosten et al., 1993).

Management. As in the management of opioid intoxication and overdose, management of opioid withdrawal involves a combination of general supportive measures and specific pharmacologic therapies. It is very important for the physician to do a thorough evaluation to rule out other medical problems that may be complicating the opioid withdrawal. In patients hospitalized for other medical disorders, the severity of their underlying clinical conditions may affect the selection of withdrawal therapy (O'Connor, Samet et al., 1994).

In addition to assessment of general health problems, it is important to obtain objective information to help guide the management of patients undergoing opioid withdrawal. Thus, a physical examination should be performed to detect specific findings consistent with withdrawal in order to establish the diagnosis.

General supportive measures for managing withdrawal include providing a safe environment and adequate nutrition, as well as reassuring patients that their symptoms will be taken seriously. The decision as to whether to perform opioid detoxification on an outpatient or inpatient basis depends on the presence of comorbid medical and psychiatric problems, the availability of social supports (such as family members to provide monitoring and transportation), and the presence of polydrug abuse. The preferred method of detoxification also may affect this decision; for example, methadone detoxification has been restricted by federal legislation to inpatient settings or specialized licensed outpatient drug treatment programs (Federal Register, 1989), although

more recent federal initiatives may allow some opioid-based treatments to be used under less restricted circumstances (O'Connor, 2000).

In the course of managing opioid withdrawal, clinicians also need to be able to address medical problems seen in this population (O'Connor, Selwyn et al., 1994; Cherubin & Sapira, 1993). Issues such as acute bacterial infections and HIV-related problems may complicate withdrawal presentation and management.

Pharmacologic Therapies. A variety of pharmacologic therapies have been developed to assist patients through a safer, more comfortable opioid withdrawal. These therapies involve the use of opioid agonists (such as methadone), an alpha-2 adrenergic agonist (such as clonidine), and an opioid antagonist (such as naltrexone or naloxone) in combination with clonidine, with sedation, or with general anesthesia, and a mixed opioid agonist/antagonist (buprenorphine) (O'Connor & Fiellin, 2000). While some of these therapies are used widely in clinical practice (for example, clonidine and methadone), others are considered more experimental.

Slow Methadone Detoxification: Clinically, it is important to distinguish between withdrawal from short-acting opioids such as heroin (plasma half-life of morphine, the main metabolite: three to four hours) and long-acting opioids such as methadone (plasma half-life: 13 to 47 hours). For short-acting opioids, the natural course of withdrawal generally is relatively brief, but more intense and associated with a higher degree of discomfort than with equivalent doses of long-acting opioids. However, there is considerable individual variation, so that strong early withdrawal symptoms from methadone are possible, as are delayed severe heroin withdrawal symptoms.

One treatment strategy that employs this general principle is to stabilize heroin addicts on methadone, then slowly decrease the methadone dose. Initially, methadone may be given in 5 mg increments as the physical signs of abstinence begin to appear (Jackson & Shader, 1973), up to a total of 10 to 20 mg over the first 24 hours. Larger methadone doses are required to treat patients who use heroin of greater purity and who have larger opioid habits; for such patients, a routine starting dose might be 20 mg rather than 5 mg.

Once a stabilizing dose has been reached, methadone is tapered by 20% a day for inpatients, leading to a one- to two-week procedure. Alternatively, the dose is tapered by 5% per day for outpatients, in a gradual cessation phase lasting as long as six months (Margolin & Kosten, 1991).

Senay and colleagues (1977) studied the effects of rapid (reductions of 10% of initial dose per week) and gradual (3% per week) outpatient cessation under double-blind conditions. They found that the 10% weekly decrements were associated with higher drop-out rates, increased illicit opioid use, and elevated levels of subjective distress. The authors recommended a dose-tapering rate of about 3% per week from methadone maintenance.

On such a regimen, successful detoxification can be achieved by as many as 80% of inpatients and 40% of outpatients, when success is measured in terms of completion of detoxification and a withdrawal-free naloxone challenge test. The longer duration of the procedure and the greater discomfort make the outpatient detoxification with methadone especially vulnerable to patient drop-out and continuing illicit opioid use.

Clonidine Detoxification: Gold and colleagues (1978) reported amelioration of opioid withdrawal symptoms by use of clonidine and postulated that both morphine and clonidine blocked activation of the locus ceruleus, a major noradrenergic nucleus that shows increased activity during opioid withdrawal. While opioids exert their effect through opiate receptors, clonidine activates alpha-2 adrenergic receptors. Consequently, clonidine does not possess the potential for physical dependence and abuse seen with opioids.

In a subsequent outpatient study (Washton & Resnick, 1980), clonidine was reported to "reduce or eliminate most of the commonly reported withdrawal symptoms," including lacrimation, rhinorrhea, restlessness, muscle pain, joint pain, and gastrointestinal symptoms. However, symptoms such as lethargy and insomnia persisted. Sedation and dizziness due to orthostatic hypotension were reported as the most significant side effects of clonidine.

The protocol involved administering 0.1 mg of clonidine every four to six hours as needed for withdrawal discomfort on the first day, followed by an increase in clonidine by 0.1 or 0.2 mg per day, to a maximum of 1.2 mg, according to each patient's blood pressure and withdrawal symptoms. The average maximum dose used in the study was 0.8 mg. Toward the end of the detoxification period (days 5 to 7 in heroin detoxification), the clonidine dose was tapered by 0.1 to 0.2 mg daily to avoid rebound hypertension, headaches, and the reemergence of withdrawal symptoms. Success was defined as becoming opiate-free in 10 days and undergoing a naloxone challenge without opioid withdrawal. In this study (Washton & Resnick, 1980), 80% of methadone-maintained patients (taking 5 to 40 mg per day), but only 36% of heroin-dependent patients were successfully detoxified.

Another study (Charney, Sternburg et al., 1981) confirmed the 80% completion rate for clonidine-assisted methadone detoxification, but found that withdrawal symptoms of anxiety, restlessness, insomnia, and muscle aches were the most resistant to clonidine treatment. In an outpatient study comparing a slow methadone taper (at 1 mg decrements, beginning with a 20 mg daily methadone dose) with a clonidine detoxification over 10 to 13 days, Kleber and colleagues (1985) demonstrated equal effectiveness, with 40% of subjects successfully completing detoxification. In a six-month followup, about a third of the subjects in each group had maintained abstinence. However, the authors noted that clonidine offered some advantages for outpatient detoxification, in that it poses minimal risk of diversion to illicit use, is not a controlled substance and therefore is more widely available to general physicians, and shortens the detoxification period from 20 days (for the methadone taper) to 10 to 13 days.

Some reports suggest that clonidine does not induce euphoria (Gold, Redmond et al., 1978), while other reports suggest reinforcing properties associated with this drug in animals (Asin & Wirtshafter, 1985). The reinforcing properties are relatively weak (Davis & Smith, 1977) and are not morphine-like in animals. Although there have been case reports of street abuse (Lauzon, 1992), this has not become a widespread problem.

Recently lofexidine, an analogue of clonidine that also is an agonist at the alpha-2 noradrenergic receptor, has shown promise as a detoxification agent. It generally is reported to be as effective as clonidine (Lin, Strang et al., 1997; Carnwath & Hardman, 1998; Bearn, Gossop et al., 1998), but more economical and with fewer side effects. This medication is not available for use in the U.S., but is undergoing clinical trials as an opiate detoxification agent.

Combined Clonidine and Naltrexone Treatment: Although clonidine alone "ameliorates signs and symptoms, it does not alter the time course of opiate withdrawal" (Kleber, Topazian et al., 1987). The authors found that addition of the opioid antagonist naltrexone to clonidine shortened the duration of withdrawal without increasing patient discomfort. However, the small naltrexone doses used in this study were clinically impractical, because they were not commercially available. Vining and colleagues (1988) compared two rapid outpatient opioid detoxifications (over four and five days), using clonidine and naltrexone. In that study, the smallest naltrexone dose was 12.5 mg, or one-quarter of a scored 50 mg naltrexone tablet (Trexan®). In the four-day protocol, subjects underwent a naloxone challenge test, followed by clonidine therapy administered three times a day. The first naltrexone dose (12.5 mg) was given the afternoon of the first day, after preloading with clonidine at 0.2 to 0.3 mg. Naltrexone was increased to 25 mg on the second day, 50 mg on the third day, and 100 mg on the fourth day. Clonidine was given at 0.1 to 0.3 mg three times per day, as needed, for the first three days, and three times at 0.1 mg on the fourth day.

The authors reported that 75% of patients successfully completed detoxification and were discharged on maintenance doses of naltrexone. There was no difference in withdrawal symptoms or severity between the four- and five-day protocols. Most patients reported that withdrawal was "relatively comfortable." Persistent symptoms included anxiety, restlessness, insomnia, joint pain, and muscle aches. Diazepam 10 mg twice a day on days 1 and 2 was found to be very effective for persistent restlessness and muscle aches. In addition, clonidine lowered blood pressure significantly, but resulted in no clinical problems. In summary, the authors found that combined clonidine and naltrexone therapy had the advantage of "being more rapid and probably more successful in the outpatient setting." The completion rate of 75% (compared to 40% for methadone or clonidine alone) is another significant advantage. Finally, the initiation of naltrexone during withdrawal eased the patients' transition into naltrexone maintenance treatment. A review of clonidine detoxification compared with clonidine and naltrexone detoxification is available in the Cochrane Database (Gowing, Ali et al., 2000b).

Buprenorphine Detoxification: Buprenorphine is a high-affinity, partial mu opioid agonist that has been approved by the U.S. Food and Drug Administration (FDA) as a pharmacotherapy for opioid dependence (Bickel & Amass, 1995; Ling, Rawson et al., 1994). The introduction of buprenorphine into the drug treatment marketplace (perhaps as a controlled substance) is of intense scientific interest and great public health significance. Despite its higher unit-dose cost compared to methadone, bupre-norphine may expand access to narcotic treatment. This could reduce the disparity between the number of opioid-addicted individuals and the number of treatment slots available to them, and facilitate general medical care of addicted individuals (Lewis, 1999; NIH Consensus Panel, 1999; Rounsaville & Kosten, 2000).

Most Phase 1 and 2 medication development studies with buprenorphine have been conducted using parenteral and sublingual (s.l.) liquid formulations, and the s.l. liquid has been extensively studied in Phase 3 clinical trials. The buprenorphine s.l. tablet is available in two forms. One formulation contains only buprenorphine ("mono" tablet). The second formulation ("combination" tablet) contains buprenorphine and the opioid antagonist naloxone in a 4:1 ratio, which is designed to discourage illicit diversion and intravenous use. The "mono" form would be employed in the clinical setting, while the "combo" form would be suitable for take-home use. Pharmacokinetic studies have found that the buprenorphine s.l. liquid formulation differs in bioavailability from the s.l. tablet. In volunteers who are not maintained on buprenorphine (Mendelson, Upton et al., 1997; Nath, Upton et al., 1999) and volunteers who are maintained on daily buprenorphine (Schuh & Johanson, 1999), the tablet has been shown to produce blood levels that are about 50% to 60% those achieved with the liquid. Thus, tablet doses used in clinical practice probably will exceed those shown to be effective in past controlled studies with the sublingual solution.

Clinical research over the past 10 years has established that buprenorphine (as well as buprenorphine with naloxone) is a safe and effective alternative to methadone (Bickel, Stitzer et al., 1988a; Johnson, Jaffe et al., 1992; Strain, Stitzer et al., 1994; Ling, Wesson et al., 1996; Ling, Charuvastra et al., 1998; Uehlinger, Deglon et al., 1998; Liu, Cai et al., 1997; Bouchez, Beauverie et al., 1998; Amass, Kamien et al., in press 2001) and levomethadyl acetate hydrochloride (LAAM) (Chutuape, Johnson et al., 1999) for opioid agonist maintenance treatment. Treatment with buprenorphine also produces significant and substantial improvements in psychosocial functioning over time (Strain, Stitzer et al., 1996). Buprenorphine also has unique features that permit novel uses, which may alter current strategies for maintenance and detoxification (Bickel & Amass, 1995; Amass, Washington et al., in press 2001). In particular, buprenorphine's ceiling on agonist activity reduces the danger of overdose, may limit its abuse liability (Walsh, Preston et al., 1994, 1995), and has low toxicity even at high intravenous doses (Lange, Fudala et al., 1990; Huestis, Umbricht et al., 1999), thereby increasing the dose range over which it may be administered safely. Buprenorphine also can produce sufficient tolerance to block the effects of exogenously administered opioids (Bickel, Stitzer et al., 1988b; Rosen,

Wallace et al., 1994; Walsh, Preston et al., 1995), suggesting that it may help to reduce illicit opioid use.

Buprenorphine's slow dissociation from mu opioid receptors results in a long duration of action (ideal for a maintenance medication) and also diminishes withdrawal signs and symptoms on discontinuation (Amass, Bickel et al., 1994; Bickel, Amass et al., 1997; Cheskin, Fudala et al., 1994; Fudala, Jaffe et al., 1990; Jasinski, Johnson et al., 1985; Seow, Quigley et al., 1986), making it particularly useful for opioid detoxification. Such qualities may make buprenorphine an advance in detoxification treatment by permitting accelerated buprenorphine detoxification without significant withdrawal distress. It has been investigated in clinical pilot studies as a treatment for opioid withdrawal. One study randomly assigned 45 heroin-dependent patients to buprenorphine (2 mg) or methadone (30 mg) for three weeks, followed by a taper over a four-week period, and found that the two approaches produced equivalent results (Bickel, Stitzer et al., 1988a). Another study compared a gradual (36-day) to a more rapid (12-day) buprenorphine taper (initially 8 mg) and found that the gradual approach was superior (Amass, Bickel et al. 1994). A study that compared a three-day course of buprenorphine (3 mg) to a five-day course of clonidine found that those approaches were equivalent (Cheskin, Fudala et al., 1994), although another study found that a longer course of buprenorphine (10 days) was superior to clonidine (Nigam, Ray et al., 1993). A larger study (O'Connor, Carroll et al., 1997) compared 162 heroin dependent patients detoxified in a primary care setting who were randomized to three 8-day treatment protocols: clonidine, combined clonidine and naltrexone, and buprenorphine. Participants in the combined clonidine and naltrexone group and the buprenorphine group were more likely to complete detoxification than the clonidine group, while the buprenorphine group experienced less severe withdrawal symptoms than the other two groups.

Another study provided further evidence that step-down buprenorphine detoxification minimizes withdrawal symptoms, thus reducing the need for concurrent medication (Vignau, 1998).

A review (Gowing, Ali et al., 2000a) with stringent criteria, selecting only studies with randomized or quasi-randomized prospective designs comparing buprenorphine with another form of treatment, found only five studies that met selection criteria. It concluded that buprenorphine has the potential to relieve heroin withdrawal and possibly methadone withdrawal, but many aspects of treatment pro-tocols and the influence of variables such as the opioid used, dose of methadone, and route of administration require further investigation. In conclusion, although buprenorphine is promising, data on the clinical effectiveness of shorter and longer detoxifications with buprenorphine remain limited (Amass, Bickel et al., 1994; Bickel, Amass et al., 1997). More research is needed to compare the effectiveness of different detoxification regimens to optimize buprenorphine dose-tapering schedules.

Methadone-to-Buprenorphine Transfer: It is anticipated that some patients will need to be transferred from methadone to buprenorphine for maintenance or detoxification. This demand will be driven by several factors. First, there is the unique pharmacology of buprenorphine, leading to its more favorable safety profile and longer duration of action (thus permitting less frequent dosing) relative to methadone (Amass, Washington et al., in press 2001; Bickel, Amass et al., 1999; Fudala, Jaffe et al., 1990; Schottenfeld, Pakes et al., 2000).

Second, given its status as a novel treatment option (which may differentially attract or retain novelty-seeking individuals [Helmus, Downey et al., in press 2001]), buprenorphine may engender less fear of stigma than methadone.

Third, because of its enhanced safety, buprenorphine may be used effectively in office-based primary care (that is, outside the domain of standard narcotic treatment programs) (O'Connor, Carroll et al., 1997; O'Connor & Kosten, 1998). It also may be appropriate as an early intervention strategy for those with short addiction histories (for example, adolescents), or with less physical dependence. Buprenorphine can produce withdrawal discomfort among opioid-dependent volunteers under certain conditions, which may be due to more than one mechanism (Bickel & Amass, 1995; Johnson, Cone et al., 1989). Low buprenorphine doses may provide too-little agonist effect (that is, insufficient substitution) relative to the maintenance opioid (such as heroin). In this case, raising the buprenorphine dose may or may not surmount this problem. Put another way, the partial agonist profile of buprenorphine may limit its ability to suppress opioid abstinence signs and symptoms. Alternatively, buprenorphine may directly precipitate withdrawal discomfort, in which case higher doses would be expected to aggravate the problem. Among individuals maintained on the long-acting, full mu opioid agonist methadone, the high-affinity partial mu agonist buprenorphine is capable of abruptly reducing the extent of mu opioid receptor stimulation. This would be expected to reduce opioid agonist symptoms and/or increase withdrawal symptoms.

This principle has been amply demonstrated in humans: Partial mu opioid agonists such as nalorphine and butorphanol (Preston, Bigelow et al., 1988a, 1989) can, in methadone-maintained individuals, abruptly precipitate opioid withdrawal signs and symptoms that are functionally similar to those produced by the antagonist naloxone. Obviously, it would be ideal to avoid (or at least minimize) this problem because this discomfort may translate into attrition and relapse. It is important to note that, among individuals maintained on shorter-acting mu opioid agonists like morphine (relative to the longer-acting agonist methadone), buprenorphine administered alone did not precipitate a significant opioid withdrawal syndrome (Fudala, Bridge et al., 1998; Mendelson, Jones et al., 1996, 1999; Schuh, Walsh et al., 1996). Bickel and Amass (1995) proposed tentative guidelines for inducting heroin abusers onto buprenorphine, which involve considering the amount of heroin used and maintaining a sufficient interval (at least 12 hours) between the last heroin use and the first buprenorphine dose. They recommended that the induction dose of buprenorphine be administered when patients are beginning to experience opioid withdrawal, so that buprenorphine can suppress those symptoms.

Clinical experience with administering initial doses of buprenorphine to heroin abusers suggests that an interval of six hours probably is sufficient to minimize the risk of precipitated withdrawal. However, transferring patients from a longer-acting agonist such as methadone to buprenorphine without producing significant withdrawal discomfort, attrition, or relapse to drug use, has been shown to be more challenging, as discussed next.

Inpatient Challenge Studies of Buprenorphine's Effects in Methadone-Maintained Research Volunteers: Several clinical studies have investigated the possibility of switching methadone-maintained research volunteers to buprenorphine. Four programmatic studies examined the effect of time interval between the last methadone maintenance dose and the initial buprenorphine dose (Preston, Bigelow et al., 1988b; Strain, Preston et al., 1992, 1995; Walsh, June et al., 1995). Most subjects in the four studies were maintained on methadone 30 mg/day. When buprenorphine was administered to the volunteers, buprenorphine significantly increased opioid withdrawal effects at two hours post-methadone (Strain, Preston et al., 1992), but not at 20 to 22 hours (Preston, Bigelow et al., 1988b; Strain, Preston et al., 1992),

nor at 40 hours (Walsh, June et al., 1995). Results of another study in which buprenorphine was administered intravenously at about a 20-hour interval (Mendelson, Upton et al., 1997) also are consistent with these data. The time interval of about 24 hours is relevant, because this is the customary methadone dosing interval employed in clinical practice and these studies therefore provide encouraging evidence that an outpatient transfer could succeed.

Only Walsh and colleagues (1995) have systematically addressed whether methadone maintenance dose influences the response to buprenorphine. One group of volunteers in that study was maintained on 30 mg/day and a second group of volunteers was maintained on 60 mg/day. The first group of volunteers received 60 mg and, in these individuals, buprenorphine precipitated a dose-dependent increase in opioid withdrawal symptoms. In contrast, buprenorphine did not precipitate significant increases in opioid withdrawal in the second group of volunteers, who received 30 mg. This study was limited by lack of either random assignment to different groups (between-subject design) or, alternatively, a within-subject controlled design.

Three studies (Strain, Preston et al., 1992, 1995; Walsh, June et al., 1995) have directly addressed whether buprenorphine dose-dependently precipitates opioid withdrawal in methadone-maintained volunteers. This variable can be interpreted as reflecting the degree of antagonist (or partial agonist) capacity of the challenge drug. In the studies by Strain and colleagues (1992, 1995), buprenorphine (five active doses from 0.5 to 8 mg IM) precipitated mild withdrawal at the two-hour interval. However, withdrawal severity was not dose-related.

Attempts at a Full Methadone-to-Buprenorphine Transfer (Inpatient and Outpatient): Five studies have directly examined, or are now examining, a full medication transfer. Kosten and Kleber (1988) reported the first outpatient trial of the methadone-to-buprenorphine (s.l. liquid) transition. In this open-label study, there were 16 volunteers. However, only half were methadone-maintained (25 mg/day), while the other half were using heroin. The eight methadone patients were assigned to receive 2 mg (n=4), 4 mg (n=2), or 8 mg (n=2) per day. Patients were inducted onto buprenorphine within 24 hours after their last methadone dose. Therefore, the dosing parameters of this study are comparable to the inpatient challenge studies of Preston and colleagues (1988a) and Strain and colleagues (1995). The investigators reported that most patients completed the protocol. However, one patient exhibited persistent withdrawal symptoms and four patients reported headaches during the initial transfer period. Overall, heroin use was relatively low, with 78% of all samples testing drug-free. Across the entire sample (n=16), withdrawal symptoms were highest on the first two test days. Withdrawal symptom ratings varied by buprenorphine dose, but were not dose-dependent. Limitations of this study include the open-label design, small group, and attendant problems of data interpretation (for example, lack of dose-dependent changes in the dependent measures).

In an open-label study, Banys and colleagues (1994) examined the ability of s.l. liquid buprenorphine to suppress opioid withdrawal 26 to 31 hours after discontinuing methadone. Fifteen participants were allowed to take three low doses of buprenorphine over several hours (0.15 mg at baseline, then 0.15 mg 1 hour later, and 0.3 mg 2 hours later) in an effort to relieve withdrawal signs and symptoms. There were substantial individual differences reported in the ability of buprenor-phine to suppress opioid withdrawal. Six subjects reported relief with buprenorphine, four subjects reported partial relief, and five subjects reported no relief at all. In short, these buprenorphine doses provided inadequate agonist effect to offset methadone abstinence symptoms. These data suggest that individual differences may affect the efficacy of the medication transfer.

Lukas and colleagues (1984) conducted the first double-blind, double-dummy pilot study of three males—maintained on three different methadone doses (25, 58, and 60 mg/day)—who were switched abruptly to buprenorphine 2 mg subcutaneously. Physiologic (including EEG), behavioral, and subjective ratings were collected during methadone stabilization, the abrupt transfer, buprenorphine stabilization, then detoxification. They found that buprenorphine did not fully substitute for methadone during the transfer: Withdrawal signs and symptoms peaked within the first several days of buprenorphine (depending on the measure) and abated during buprenorphine stabilization. The authors did not report any differences between subjects during substitution of buprenorphine for methadone (that is, no effect of moderate [n=2] versus low [n=1] methadone dose), which could have been due to the very small sample size.

At present, the only other published study of the methadone-to-buprenorphine (s.l. liquid) full transfer is a within-subject, double-blind, double-dummy procedure with inpatient volunteers (Levin, Fischman et al., 1997). A moderate methadone maintenance dose (60 mg) was tapered over a few days (40 mg, 30 mg, 30 mg, then 0 mg) before initiating buprenorphine (4 mg on day 1, followed by 8 mg). Like Kosten and Kleber (1988), the protocol of Levin and colleagues (1997) demonstrated some qualified success, in that 79% (15 of 19) of participants who began the dose-taper completed the transfer. In the Levin study, the one-day methadone placebo—which produced a 48-hour interval between the last active methadone dose and the first active buprenorphine dose—significantly increased opioid withdrawal symptoms to a "moderate" level. Peak withdrawal symptom scores occurred just prior to the first buprenorphine dose. Opioid withdrawal symptoms remained elevated, but were not significantly worsened, by the first two buprenorphine daily doses (4 mg, then 8 mg). Withdrawal symptoms gradually were suppressed by subsequent daily doses of buprenorphine (8 mg) and returned to baseline during buprenorphine stabilization (8 mg/day). Thus, the initial buprenorphine doses might have been too low, since they did not rapidly suppress methadone abstinence withdrawal symptoms (see Banys, Clark et al., 1994, above).

Levin and colleagues (1997) reported that the participants who dropped out cited an "inability to tolerate the withdrawal symptoms." A second limitation is that there was no control group against which to evaluate the methadone dose-taper. (However, the within-subject design did permit analysis of symptom changes over time). In addition, individuals were given access to, and used, significant amounts of ancillary medications (mean oxazepam dose of 45 mg/day and mean clonidine dose of 0.3 mg/day) to alleviate withdrawal discomfort during the transfer period. For this reason, the study by Levin and colleagues (1997) cannot be compared directly with previous studies, which did not permit use of these medications. It also is difficult to extrapolate this study to outpatient conditions.

In a recent small double-blind, double-dummy pilot study (Greenwald, Schuh et al., manuscript submitted), five male heroin-dependent outpatient volunteers were transferred from methadone 60 mg (with one intervening 45 mg dose) to the buprenorphine s.l. tablet. Subjective effects and vital signs were collected before the transfer (methadone 60 mg and 45 mg), and on buprenorphine days 1 and 2 (8 mg/day), and days 7 and 8 (16 mg/day).

The one-day methadone dose-taper did not significantly alter opioid withdrawal or agonist symptoms. On transfer day 1, buprenorphine significantly increased withdrawal symptoms (which peaked later that evening), and decreased agonist symptoms and dose preference, as compared to methadone stabilization. On buprenorphine transfer day 2, withdrawal symptoms and blood pressure were elevated, but agonist symptoms and dose preference did not significantly differ from methadone stabilization levels. The amount of self-reported heroin use decreased from before methadone stabilization and did not increase during the transfer. One week later, buprenorphine 16 mg doses increased agonist effects. Therefore, a one-day methadone dose-taper to 45 mg was well tolerated relative to 60 mg/day stabilization and the transition from methadone 45 mg to buprenorphine 8 mg tablet resulted in a time-related (throughout the same day) increase in opioid withdrawal symptoms, which peaked during the evening (about 6 to 18 hours) after the first buprenorphine 8 mg dose. This suggests that, in practice, peak symptoms might occur outside the clinical setting, thereby increasing the probability of heroin use. Importantly, the protocol used in this pilot study was able to shorten the duration of withdrawal discomfort to about one day, relative to the results of Levin and colleagues (1997).

These preliminary results suggest that it is feasible to transfer outpatients on methadone 60 mg/day to the buprenorphine 8 mg/day s.l. tablet, although refinements are needed to improve the tolerability and clinical efficacy of this protocol. In contrast, the dose-taper used by Levin and colleagues (1997) probably was too extreme, leading to methadone abstinence withdrawal, and the initial buprenorphine doses did not rapidly suppress this withdrawal. It would seem reasonable to propose that, in future studies, the magnitude and duration of the methadone dose-taper (from a starting level of 60 mg) should strike a compromise between the protocols used in the two studies, as from an intermediate 30 mg dose of methadone to 8 mg of buprenorphine. However, the increased opioid withdrawal symptoms experienced by the outpatients in the Greenwald study did not lead to increased attrition, even though they were associated with decreased ratings of dose adequacy and dose preference (relative to their pre-study methadone dose). In addition, if the first daily transfer dose of buprenorphine does precipitate withdrawal, it may be useful to consider increased subsequent buprenorphine doses (to provide additional agonist) to suppress this withdrawal. Moreover, buprenorphine 16 mg can decrease residual opioid withdrawal after brief stabilization on buprenorphine 8 mg/day, and was preferred by participants to 60 mg/day methadone stabilization. These data imply that higher buprenorphine doses may be useful in suppress-ing residual withdrawal symptoms and initiating heroin abstinence in some individuals immediately after the transfer, and also may be preferred.

Buprenorphine in Agonist-to-Antagonist Treatment: Buprenorphine has been used in several experimental studies (Kosten & Kleber, 1988; Bickel, Stitzer et al., 1988a; Kosten, Morgan et al., 1989) as a transitional agent between agonists (such as methadone or heroin) and antagonists (such as naloxone or naltrexone). In one study, Kosten and Kleber (1988) substituted buprenorphine at 2, 4, and 8 mg for 20 mg to 30 mg of methadone or heroin for one month without precipitating substantial withdrawal symptoms, although buprenorphine may act as an opioid antagonist at doses as low as 8 mg. After chronic administration, buprenorphine produces less physical dependence than do pure agonists, as suggested by the minimal withdrawal symptoms that occur when buprenorphine is stopped, and by the use of relatively higher antagonist doses that are needed to precipitate withdrawal in buprenorphine-maintained volunteers (Eissenberg, Greenwald et al., 1996). After one month of buprenorphine stabilization, the drug was abruptly discontinued and a small dose of naltrexone given 24 hours later.

The investigators observed that the transition to buprenorphine generally was well-tolerated. The subsequent abrupt discontinuation of buprenorphine was associated with "minimal withdrawal" in the 2 mg and 4 mg buprenorphine groups, and a low dose of naltrexone (1 mg) did not precipitate withdrawal. However, subjects in the 8 mg group reported a more substantial increase in withdrawal symptoms when buprenorphine was stopped.

Because of these properties, Kosten examined whether buprenorphine might facilitate the transition from opioid agonists to antagonists in a three-step process: (1) buprenorphine substitution for agonists such as methadone, (2) buprenorphine induced reduction in physical dependency, and (3) discontinuation of buprenorphine with rapid introduction of naltrexone.

In a study testing that hypothesis, Kosten and colleagues (1989) used intravenous naloxone to challenge five opioid-addicted patients who were maintained on 3 mg sublingual buprenorphine. Induction onto naltrexone was attempted in all of those patients who completed 30 days on buprenorphine. The buprenorphine discontinuation and induction onto naltrexone included blinded discontinuation of the buprenorphine, followed by double-blind, placebo-controlled challenges with high-dose naloxone. Five male opioid-addicted patients maintained on buprenorphine 3 mg sublingually for one month as outpatients were abruptly discontinued from buprenorphine by blinded, placebo substitution and enlisted in a placebo-controlled, double-blind challenge with intravenous naloxone at 0.5 mg/kg. The naloxone was given over a 20-minute period using a 10 mg/ml solution. Significant withdrawal symptoms were precipitated. However, the severity of withdrawal was about two-thirds the severity for methadone patients (Abstinence Rating Scale = 22; SD = 9.3) and less than a third of the full Abstinence Rating Scale score of 45. Moreover, five hours after this naloxone challenge, withdrawal symptoms were at baseline levels, and oral naltrexone was given at either 12.5 mg or 25 mg without precipitating further withdrawal symptoms. The authors felt that the withdrawal syndrome was milder for buprenorphine than for pure opioid agonists, "suggesting a partial resetting of the opioid receptors by the antagonist activity of buprenorphine."

In some situations, combination drug treatment may facilitate greater patient acceptance of agonist-antagonist switching. Thus, Gerra and colleagues (2000) have shown that the early use of naltrexone during detoxification in combination with benzodiazepines and clonidine facilitated naltrexone acceptance by patients. Umbricht and colleagues (1999), in a study comparing buprenorphine taper alone and buprenorphine with naltrexone, suggested that the combination treatment may reduce the severity of withdrawal symptoms.

The use of buprenorphine stabilization of opioid addicts before switching to naltrexone has the advantage of psychosocial stabilization prior to detoxification. This approach thus may represent a compromise approach between acute detoxification and long-term treatment of chronic dependence.

The foregoing techniques (clonidine/naltrexone and buprenorphine/naltrexone) may be combined in a clinical protocol that places methadone patients or heroin addicts on buprenorphine for several weeks to stabilize and engage them in the psychosocial aspects of treatment. This could be followed by rapid transition to naltrexone, using clonidine to relieve any withdrawal symptoms caused by stopping the buprenorphine. Such combination approaches are reviewed in Stine and Kosten (1992). These generally have been small pilot studies. Larger clinical trials of buprenorphine-to-naltrexone transitions, with and without clonidine, are needed and have potential to lead to shorter, more cost-effective treatment alternatives (to long-term maintenance) for patients who need more treatment than brief detoxification.

Followup Care. As with the management of opioid overdose, medical detoxification is an important first step in the treatment of opioid addiction. It must be made clear that detoxification alone, without plans for ongoing drug treatment, is not adequate to manage patients (O'Connor, Samet et al., 1994). Thus, at the initiation of detoxification, arrangements for ongoing treatment need to be assured.

CONCLUSIONS

The management of opioid intoxication and withdrawal requires that physicians be familiar with the basic pharmacologic properties of opioids and the clinical manifestations of opioid overdose and withdrawal. Patients experiencing intoxication and withdrawal require careful evaluation and supportive management. In addition, specific pharmacologic therapies such as naloxone and clonidine may play a major role in the management of these conditions.

ACKNOWLEDGMENTS: This work was supported by the National Institute on Drug Abuse grants R01-DA05626 (TRK), K05-DA0454 (TRK), P50-DA09250, and the Veterans Administration Mental Illness Research, Education and Clinical Center (MIRECC).

REFERENCES

Albanese AP, Gevirtz C, Oppenheim B et al. (2000). Outcome and six-month follow up of patients after ultra rapid opiate detoxification (UROD). *Journal of Addictive Diseases* 19(2):11-28.

Amass L, Bickel WK, Higgins ST et al. (1994). A preliminary investigation of outcome following gradual or rapid buprenorphine detoxification. *Journal of Addictive Diseases* 13(3):33-45.

Amass L, Kamien JB, Branstetter SA et al. (in press 2001). A controlled comparison of the buprenorphine-naloxone tablet and methadone for opioid maintenance treatment: Interim results. In LS Harris (ed.). *Problems of Drug Dependence 1999 (NIDA Research Monograph).* Rockville, MD: National Institute on Drug Abuse.

Amass L, Washington DCL, Kamien JB et al. (in press 2001). Thrice-weekly supervised dosing with the combination buprenorphine-naloxone table is preferred to daily supervised dosing by opioid-dependent humans. *Drug and Alcohol Dependence.*

American Heart Association (AHA), Emergency Cardiac Care Committee and Subcommittees (1992a). Adult advanced cardiac life support. *Journal of the American Medical Association* 268:2199-2241.

American Heart Association (AHA), Emergency Cardiac Care Committee and Subcommittees (1992b). Adult basic life support. *Journal of the American Medical Association* 268:2184-2198.

Asin K & Wirtshafter D (1985). Clonidine produces a conditioned place preference in rats. *Psychopharmacology* (Berl) 85(3):383-385.

Banys P, Clark HW, Tusel DJ et al. (1994). An open trial of low dose buprenorphine in treating methadone withdrawal. *Journal of Substance Abuse Treatment* 11:9-15.

Bearn J, Gossop M & Strang J (1998). Accelerated lofexidine treatment regimen compared with conventional lofexidine and methadone treatment for inpatient opiate detoxification. *Drug and Alcohol Dependence* 50(3):227-232.

Bickel W, Amass L, Crean JP et al. (1999). Buprenorphine dosing every 1, 2, or 3 days in opioid-dependent patients. *Psychopharmacology (Berl)* 146(2):111-118.

Bickel WK & Amass L (1995). Buprenorphine treatment of opioid dependence: A review. *Experimental and Clinical Psychopharmacology* 3:477-489.

Bickel WK, Amass L, Higgins ST et al. (1997). Effects of adding behavioral treatment to opioid detoxification with buprenorphine. *Journal of Consulting and Clinical Psychology* 65(5):1-81.

Bickel WK, Stitzer MI, Bigelow GE et al. (1988a). A clinical trial of buprenorphine: Comparison with methadone in the detoxification of heroin addicts. *Clinical Pharmacology and Therapeutics* 43:72-78.

Bickel WK, Stitzer MI, Bigelow GE et al. (1988b). Buprenorphine: Dose-related blockade of opioid challenge effects in opioid dependent humans. *Journal of Pharmacology and Experimental Therapeutics* 247:47-53.

Bouchez J, Beauverie P & Touzeau D (1998). Substitution with buprenorphine in methadone- and morphine sulfate-dependent patients. Preliminary results. *European Addiction Research* (4 Suppl) 1:8-12.

Bozarth MA & Wise RA (1984). Anatomically distinct opiate receptor fields mediate reward and physical dependence. *Science* 224:514-517.

Carnwath T & Hardman J (1998). Randomized double-blind comparison of lofexidine and clonidine in the outpatient treatment of opiate withdrawal. *Drug and Alcohol Dependence* 50(3):251-254.

Chang G & Astrachan BN (1988). The emergency department surveillance of alcohol intoxication after motor vehicle accidents. *Journal of the American Medical Association* 260:2533-2536.

Charney DS, Heninger GR, Kleber HD et al. (1986). The combined use of clonidine and naltrexone as a rapid, safe, effective treatment for abrupt withdrawal from methadone. *American Journal of Psychiatry* 143:831-837.

Charney DS, Sternburg DE, Kleber HD et al. (1981). The clinical use of clonidine in abrupt withdrawal from methadone. *Archives of General Psychiatry* 38:1273-1277.

Cherubin CE & Sapira JD (1993). The medical complications of drug addiction and the medical assessment of the intravenous drug user: 25 years later. *Annals of Internal Medicine* 119(10):1017-28.

Cheskin LJ, Fudala PJ & Johnson RE (1994). A controlled comparison of buprenorphine and clonidine for acute detoxification from opioids. *Drug and Alcohol Dependence* 36(2):115-21.

Christenson J, Etherington J, Grafstein E et al. (2000). Early discharge of patients with presumed opioid overdose: Development of a clinical prediction rule. *Academic Emergency Medicine* 7(10):1110-1118.

Chutuape MA, Johnson RE, Strain EC et al. (1999). Controlled clinical trial comparing maintenance treatment efficacy of buprenorphine (buprenorphine), levomethadoneadoneadyl acetate (LAAM) and methadone (m). In LS Harris (ed.) *Problems of Drug Dependence 1998 (NIDA Research Monograph No. 179)*. Rockville, MD: National Institute on Drug Abuse, 74.

Council on Scientific Affairs (CSA) (1987). Scientific issues in drug testing. *Journal of the American Medical Association* 257:3110-3114.

Crawley JN, Laberty RN & Roth RH (1979). Clonidine reversal of increased norepinephrine metabolite levels during morphine withdrawal. *European Journal of Pharmacology* 57:247-255.

Cucchia AT, Monnat M, Spagnoli J et al. (1998). Ultra-rapid opiate detoxification using deep sedation with oral midazolam: Short and long-term results. *Drug and Alcohol Dependence* 52(3):243-250.

Darke S & Hall W (1997). The distribution of naloxone to heroin users. *Addiction* 92(9):1195-1199.

Darke S & Ross J (2000). Fatal heroin overdoses resulting from non-injecting routes of administration, NSW, Australia, 1992-1996. *Addiction* 95(4):569-573.

Davis WM & Smith SG (1977). Catecholaminergic mechanisms of reinforcement: Mechanismns of reinforcement: Direct assessment by drug self-administration. *Life Sciences* 20:483-492.

Dawe S & Gray JA (1995). Craving and Drug reward: A comparison of methadone and clonidine in detoxifying opiate addicts. *Drug and Alcohol Dependence* 39(3):207-12.

Dole VP (1972). Narcotic addiction, physical dependence and relapse. *New England Journal of Medicine* 286:988-992.

Dunton AW, Schwam E, Pittman V et al. (1988). Flumazenil. U.S. Clinical Pharmacology Studies. *European Journal of Anaesthesiology* 581-595.

Eissenberg T, Greenwald MK, Johnson RE et al. (1996). Buprenorphine's physical dependence potential: antagonist-precipitated withdrawal in humans. *Journal of Pharmacology and Experimental Therapeutics* 276(2):449-59.

Federal Register (1989). Methadone: Rules and Regulations. *Federal Register* 54:8954.

Fudala PJ, Bridge TP, Herbert S et al. and the Buprenorphine+Naloxone Collaborative Study Group (1998). A multisite efficacy evaluation of a buprenorphine+naloxone product for opiate dependence treatment. *Problems of Drug Dependence 1998 (NIDA Research Monograph 179)*. Rockville, MD: National Institute on Drug Abuse, 105.

Fudala PJ, Jaffe JH, Dax EM et al. (1990). Use of buprenorphine in the treatment of opioid addiction. II. Physiologic and behavioral effects of daily and alternate-day administration and abrupt withdrawal. *Clinical Pharmacology and Therapeutics* 47:525-534.

Fultz JM & Senay EC (1975). Guidelines for the hospitalized narcotic addicts. *Annals of Internal Medicine* 82:815-818.

Gerra G, Zaimovic A, Rustichelli P et al. (2000). Rapid opiate detoxification in outpatient treatment: Relationship with naltrexone compliance. *Journal of Substance Abuse Treatment* 18(2):185-191.

Gold MS, Pottash AC, Sweeney DR et al. (1980). Opiate withdrawal using clonidine. *Journal of the American Medical Association* 243:343-346.

Gold M, Redmond DE & Kleber HD (1978). Clonidine blocks acute opiate withdrawal symptoms. *Lancet* 2:599-600.

Gould LC & Kleber HD (1974). Changing patterns of multiple drug use among applicants. *Archives of General Psychiatry* 31:408-415.

Gowing L, Ali R & White J (2000a). Buprenorphine for the management of opioid withdrawal. In The Cochrane Database of Systematic Reviews. *Cochrane Library* Issue 3.

Gowing L, Ali R & White J (2000b). Opioid antagonists and adrenergic agonists for the management of opioid withdrawal. *Cochrane Database Systematic Reviews* (2):CD002021.

Greenwald MK, Schuh KJ & Stine SM (in submission). Transferring heroin-dependent outpatients stabilized on moderate-dose meet: A preliminary study. *Drug and Alcohol Dependence.*

Gunne LN (1959). Noradrenaline and adrenaline in the rat brain during acute and chronic morphine administration and during withdrawal. *Nature* 184:150-151.

Hall W & Darke S (1998). Trends in opiate overdose deaths in Australia, 1979-1995. *Drug and Alcohol Dependence* 52(1):71-77.

Helmus T, Downey KK, Arfken C et al. (in press 2001). Novelty seeking among heroin dependent poly-drug abusers entering buprenorphine treatment. *Drug and Alcohol Dependence.*

Himmelsbach CK (1942). Clinical studies of drug addiction: Physical dependence, withdrawal and recovery. *Archives of Internal Medicine* 69:766-772.

Huestis MA, Umbricht A, Preston KL et al. (1999). Safety of buprenorphine: No clinically relevant cardio-respiratory depression at high IV doses. In LS Harris (ed.) *Problems of Drug Dependence (NIDA Research Monograph No. 179)*. Rockville, MD: National Institute on Drug Abuse.

Jackson AH & Shader RI (1973). Guidelines for the withdrawal of narcotic and general depressant drugs. *Diseases of the Nervous System* 34:162-166.

Jaffe JH (1990). Drug addiction and drug abuse. In AG Gilman, TW Rall, AS Nies & P Taylor (eds.) *Goodman and Gilman's The Pharmacological Basis of Therapeutics, 8th Ed.* New York, NY: Pergamon Press, 522-573.

Jaffe JH & Martin WR (1990). Opioid analgesics and antagonists. In AG Gilman, TW Rall, AS Nies & Taylor P (eds.) *Goodman and Gilman's The Pharmacological Basis of Therapeutics, 8th Ed.* New York, NY: Pergamon Press, 485-521.

Janiri L, Mannelli P, Persico AM et al. (1994). Opiate detoxification of methadone maintenance patients using lefetamine, clonidine and buprenorphine. *Drug and Alcohol Dependence* 36(2):139-145.

Jasinski DR, Johnson DR & Kocher TR (1985). Clonidine and morphine withdrawal: Differential effects on signs and symptoms. *Archives of General Psychiatry* 42:1063-1066.

Jasinski DR, Pevnick JS & Griffith JD (1978). Human pharmacology and abuse potential of the analgesic buprenorphine. *Archives of General Psychiatry* 35:510-516.

Johnson RE, Cone EJ, Henningfield JE et al. (1989). A controlled trial of buprenorphine in the treatment of heroin addiction. I. Physiological and behavioral effects during a rapid dose induction. *Clinical Pharmacology and Therapeutics* 46:335-343.

Johnson RE, Jaffe JH & Fudala PJ (1992). A controlled trial of buprenorphine treatment for opioid dependence. *Journal of the American Medical Association* 267:2750-2755.

Kahn A, Mumford JP, Rogers GA et al. (1997). Double-blind study of lofexidine and clonidine in the detoxification of opiate addicts in hospital. *Drug and Alcohol Dependence* 44(1):57-61.

Kellerman AL, Fikn SD, Logerfo JP et al. (1987). Impact of drug screening and suspected overdose. *Annals of Emergency Medicine* 16:1206-1216.

Kleber HD, Riordan CE, Rounsaville B et al. (1985). Clonidine in outpatient detoxification from methadone maintenance. *Archives of General Psychiatry* 42:391-394.

Kleber HD, Topazian M, Gaspari J et al. (1987). Clonidine and naltrexone in the outpatient treatment of heroin withdrawal. *American Journal of Drug and Alcohol Abuse* 13:1.

Kosten TR, Gawin FH, Rounsaville BJ et al. (1986). Cocaine use among opioid addicts: Demographic and diagnostic factors in treatment. *American Journal of Drug and Alcohol Abuse* 12:1-16.

Kosten TR & Kleber HD (1988). Buprenorphine detoxification from opioid dependence: A pilot study. *Life Science* 42:635-641.

Kosten TR & Kleber HD (1984). Strategies to improve compliance with narcotic antagonists. *American Journal of Alcohol and Drug Abuse* 10:249-266.

Kosten TR, Morgan C & Kleber HD (1992). Phase II clinical trials of buprenorphine: Detoxification and induction onto naltrexone. *NIDA Research Monograph 121.* Rockville, MD: *National Institute on Drug Abuse*, 101-119.

Kosten TR, Morgan CH, Krystal JH et al. (1989). Rapid detoxification procedure using buprenorphine and naloxone. *American Journal of Psychiatry* 147:1349.

Laberty R & Roth RH (1980). Clonidine reverses the increased norepinephrine increase during morphine withdrawal in rats. *Brain Research* 182:482-485.

Lange WR, Fudala PJ, Dax EM et al. (1990). Safety and side effects of buprenorphine in the clinical management of heroin addiction. *Drug and Alcohol Dependence* 26:19-28.

Lauzon P (1992). Two cases of clonidine abuse/dependence in methadone-maintained patients. *Journal of Substance Abuse Treatment* 9(2):125-127.

Lawental E (2000). Ultra rapid opiate detoxification as compared to 30-day inpatient detoxification program—A retrospective follow-up study. *Journal of Substance Abuse* 11(2):173-181.

Levin FR, Fischman MW, Connerney I et al. (1997). A protocol to switch high-dose, methadone-maintained subjects to buprenorphine. *American Journal of Addictions* 6:105-116.

Lewis DC (1999). Access to narcotic addiction treatment and medical care: prospects for the expansion of methadone maintenance treatment. *Journal of Addictive Diseases* 18:5-21.

Lin SK, Strang J, Su LW et al. (1997). Double blind randomized controlled trial of lofexidine versus clonidine in the treatment of heroin withdrawal. *Drug and Alcohol Dependence* 48(2):127-33.

Ling W, Charuvastra C, Collins JF et al. (1998). Buprenorphine maintenance treatment of opiate dependence: A multicenter, randomized clinical trial. *Addiction* 93(4):475-86.

Ling W, Rawson RA & Compton MA (1994). Substitution pharmacotherapies for opioid addiction: From methadone to LAAM and buprenorphine. *Journal of Psychoactive Drugs* 26(2):119-128.

Ling W, Wesson DR, Charuvastra C et al. (1996). A controlled trial comparing buprenorphine and methadone maintenance in opioid dependence. *Archives of General Psychiatry* 53:401-407.

Liu Z, Cai Z, Wang XP et al. (1997). Rapid detoxification of heroin dependence by buprenorphine. *Chung Kuo Yao Li Hsueh Pao* 18(2):112-114.

Loimer N, Hofmann P & Chaudhry H (1993). Ultrashort noninvasive opiate detoxification [letter]. *American Journal of Psychiatry* 150(5):839.

Loimer N, Lenz K, Schmid R et al. (1991). Technique for greatly shortening the transition from methadone to naltrexone maintenance of patients addicted to opiates. *American Journal of Psychiatry* 148(7):933-935.

Loimer N, Schmid R, Lenz K et al. (1990). Acute blocking of naloxone-precipitated opiate withdrawal symptoms by methohexitone. *British Journal of Psychiatry* 157:748-752.

Loimer N, Schmid R, Presslich O et al. (1988). Naloxone treatment for opiate withdrawal syndrome [letter]. *British Journal of Psychiatry* 153:851-852.

Lukas SE, Jasinski DR & Johnson RE (1984). Electroencephalographic and behavioral correlates of buprenorphine administration. *Clinical Pharmacology and Therapeutics* 36:127-132.

Margolin A & Kosten TR (1991). Opioid detoxification and maintenance with blocking agents. In NS Miller (ed.) *Comprehensive Handbook of Drug and Alcohol Addiction.* New York, NY: Marcel Dekker, 1127-1141.

Martin WR (1983). Pharmacology of opioids. *Pharmacology Reviews* 35:283-323.

Martin WR & Jasinski DR (1969). Physiological parameters of morphine dependence in man: Tolerance, early abstinence, protracted abstinence. *Journal of Psychiatric Research* 7:9-17.

Melandri R, Re G, Lanzarini C et al. (1996). Myocardial damage and rhabdomyolysis associated with prolonged hypoxic coma following opiate overdose. *Journal of Toxicology and Clinical Toxicology* 34(2):199-203.

Mello MK & Mendelson JH (1980). Buprenorphine suppresses heroin use by heroin addicts. *Science* 207:657-659.

Mendelson J, Jones RT, Fernandez I et al. (1996). Buprenorphine and naloxone interactions in opiate-dependent volunteers. *Clinical Pharmacology and Therapeutics* 60:105-114.

Mendelson J, Jones RT, Welm S et al. (1999). Buprenorphine and naloxone combinations: The effects of three dose ratios in morphine-stabilized, opiate-dependent volunteers. *Psychopharmacology (Berl)* 141:37-46.

Mendelson J, Upton RA, Everhart ET et al. (1997). Bioavailability of sublingual buprenorphine. *Journal of Clinical Pharmacology* 37(1):31-37.

Morbidity and Mortality Weekly Reports (1996). Scopolamine poisoning among heroin users—New York City, Newark, Philadelphia, and Baltimore, 1995 and 1996. *Morbidity and Mortality Weekly Reports* 45(22):457-460.

Morbidity & Mortality Weekly Reports (2000). 49(28):636-640.

Nath RP, Upton RA, Everhart ET et al. (1999). Buprenorphine pharmacokinetics: Relative bioavailability of sublingual tablet and liquid formulations. *Journal of Clinical Pharmacology* 39(6):619-623.

Nigam AK, Ray R & Tripathi BM (1993). Buprenorphine in opiate withdrawal: A comparison with clonidine. *Journal of Substance Abuse Treatment* 10(4):391-394.

NIH Consensus Panel (1999). NIH Consensus Panel recommends expanding access to and improving methadone treatment programs for heroin addiction. *European Addiction Research* 5:50-51.

O'Connor PG (2000). Treatment of opioid dependence—New data and new opportunities. *New England Journal of Medicine* 343:1332-1335.

O'Connor PG, Carroll KM, Shi JM et al. (1995). A randomized trial of three methods of primary care-based outpatient opioid detoxification. *Journal of General and Internal Medicine* 10(s):47.

O'Connor PG, Carroll KM, Shi JM et al. (1997). Three methods of opioid detoxification in a primary care setting. A randomized trial. *Annals of Internal Medicine* 127(7):526-530.

O'Connor PG & Fiellin DA (2000). Pharmacologic treatment of heroin-dependent patients. *Annals of Internal Medicine* 133(1):40-54.

O'Connor PG & Kosten TR (1998). Rapid and ultrarapid opioid detoxification techniques. *Journal of the American Medical Association* 279(3):229-134.

O'Connor PG, Samet JH & Stein MD (1994). Management of hospitalized intravenous drug users. Role of the internist. *American Journal of Medicine* 96:551-558.

O'Connor PG, Selwyn PA & Schottenfeld RS (1994). Medical management of injection-drug users with HIV infection. *New England Journal of Medicine* 331:450-459.

O'Connor PG, Waugh ME, Carroll KM et al. (1995). Primary care-based ambulatory opioid detoxification: The results of a clinical trial. *Journal of General and Internal Medicine* 10:255-260.

Perry HE & Shannon MW (1996). Diagnosis and management of opioid- and benzodiazepine-induced comatose overdose in children. *Current Opinions in Pediatrics* 8(3):243-247.

Petry NM, Bickel WK & Badger GJ (1999). A comparison of four buprenorphine dosing regimens in the treatment of opioid dependence. *Clinical Pharmacology and Therapeutics* 66:306-314.

Pfab R, Hirtl C & Zilker T (1999). Opiate detoxification under anesthesia: No apparent benefit, but suppression of thyroid hormones and risk of pulmonary and renal failure. *Journal of Toxicology & Clinical Toxicology* 37(1):43-50.

Presslich O, Loimer N, Lenz K et al. (1989). Opiate detoxification under general anesthesia by large doses of naloxone. *Journal of Toxicology & Clinical Toxicology* 27(4-5):263-270.

Preston KL, Bigelow GE & Liebson IA (1988a). Butorphanol-precipitated withdrawal in opioid-dependent human volunteers. *Journal of Pharmacological and Experimental Therapeutics* 246:441-448.

Preston KL, Bigelow GE & Liebson IA (1988b). Buprenorphine and naloxone alone and in combination in opioid-dependent humans. *Psychopharmacology* 94:484-490.

Preston KL, Bigelow GE & Liebson IA (1989). Antagonist effects of nalorphine in opioid-dependent human volunteers. *Journal of Pharmacology and Experimental Therapeutics* 248:929-937.

Rabinowitz J, Cohen H, Tarrasch R et al. (1997). Compliance to naltrexone treatment after ultra-rapid opiate detoxification: An open label naturalistic study. *Drug and Alcohol Dependence* 47(2):77-86.

Riordan CE & Kleber HD (1980). Rapid opiate detoxification with clonidine and naloxone. *Lancet* 1:1039-1080.

Rogers WO, Hall MA, Brissie RM et al. (1997). Detection of alprazolam in three cases of methadone/benzodiazepine overdose. *Journal of Forensic Sciences* 42(1):155-156.

Rosen MI, Wallace EA, McMahon TJ et al. (1994). Buprenorphine: duration of blockade of effects of intramuscular hydromorphone. *Drug and Alcohol Dependence* 35:569-580.

Rounsaville BJ & Kosten TR (2000). Treatment for opioid dependence: Quality and access. *Journal of the American Medical Association* 283:1337-1339.

San L, Puig M, Bulbena A et al. (1995). High risk of ultrashort noninvasive opiate detoxification [letter]. *American Journal of Psychiatry* 152(6):956.

Satel SL, Kosten TR, Schuckit MA et al. (1993). Should protracted withdrawal from drugs be included in DSM-IV? *American Journal of Psychiatry* 150(5):695-704.

Scherbaum N, Klein S, Kaube H et al. (1998). Alternative strategies of opiate detoxification: Evaluation of the so-called ultra-rapid detoxification. *Pharmacopsychiatry* 31(6):205-209.

Schottenfeld RS, Pakes J, O'Connor P et al. (2000). Thrice weekly versus daily buprenorphine maintenance. *Biological Psychiatry* 47:1072-1079.

Schuckit MA (1989). Opiates and other analgesics. *In Drug and Alcohol Abuse: A Clinical Guide to Diagnosis and Treatment, 3rd Ed.* New York, NY: Plenum Publishing Co., 118-142.

Schuckit N (1988). Clonidine and the treatment of withdrawal. *Drug Abuse and Alcoholism Newsletter* 17:1-4.

Schuh KJ & Johanson CE (1999). Pharmacokinetic comparison of the buprenorphine sublingual liquid and tablet. *Drug and Alcohol Dependence* 56:55-60.

Schuh KJ, Walsh SL, Bigelow GE et al. (1996). Buprenorphine, morphine and naloxone effects during ascending morphine maintenance in humans. *Journal of Pharmacological and Experimental Therapeutics* 278:836-846.

Seidler D, Stuhlinger GH, Fischer G et al. (1996). After antagonization of acute opiate overdose: A survey at hospitals in Vienna. *Addiction* 91(10):1479-1487.

Senay EC, Dorus W, Goldberg F et al. (1977). Withdrawal from methadone maintenance. *Archives of General Psychiatry* 34:361-367.

Seow SS, Quigley AJ, Ilett KF et al. (1986). Buprenorphine: A new maintenance opiate? *Medical Journal of Austria* 144(8):407-411.

Smolka M & Schmidt LG (1999). The influence of heroin dose and route of administration on the severity of the opiate withdrawal syndrome. *Addiction* 94(8):1191-1198.

Sporer KA (1999). Acute heroin overdose. *Annals of Internal Medicine* 130(7):584-590.

Sporer KA, Firestone J & Isaacs SM (1996). Out-of-hospital treatment of opioid overdoses in an urban setting. *Academy of Emergency Medicine* 3(7):660-667.

Stephenson J (1997). Experts debate merits of 1-day opiate detoxification under anesthesia. *Journal of the American Medical Association* 277(5):363-364.

Stine S & Kosten T (1994). Reduction of opiate withdrawal-like symptoms by cocaine abuse during methadone and buprenorphine maintenance. *American Journal of Drug and Alcohol Abuse* 20(4):445-458.

Stine SM & Kosten TR (1992). Use of drug combinations in treatment of opioid withdrawal. *Journal of Clinical Psychopharmacology* 12:203-209.

Strain EC, Preston KL, Liebson IA et al. (1992). Acute effects of buprenorphine, hydromorphone and naloxone in methadone-maintained volunteers. *Journal of Pharmacology and Experimental Therapeutics* 261:985-993.

Strain EC, Preston KL, Liebson IA et al. (1995). Buprenorphine effects in methadone-maintained volunteers: Effects at two hours after methadone. *Journal of Pharmacological and Experimental Therapeutics* 272:628-638.

Strain EC, Stitzer ML, Liebson IA et al. (1994). Comparison of buprenorphine and methadone in the treatment of opioid dependence. *American Journal of Psychiatry* 151(7):1025-1030.

Strain EC, Stitzer ML, Liebson IA et al. (1996). Buprenorphine versus methadone in the treatment of opioid dependence: Self-reports, urinalysis, and Addiction Severity Index. *Journal of Clinical Psychopharmacology* 16:58-67.

Strang J, Bearn J & Gossop M (1997). Opiate detoxification under anaesthesia [editorial] [see comments]. *British Medical Journal* 315(7118):1249-1250.

Strang J, Powis B, Best D et al. (1999). Preventing opiate overdose fatalities with take-home naloxone: Pre-launch study of possible impact and acceptability. *Addiction* 94(2):199-204.

Tagliaro F, De Battisti Z, Smith FP et al. (1998). Death from heroin overdose: Findings from hair analysis. *Lancet* 351(9120):1923-1925.

Uehlinger C, Deglon J, Livoti S et al. (1998). Comparison of buprenorphine and methadone in treatment of opioid dependence. Swiss multicenter study. *European Addiction Research* 4 Suppl 1:13-18.

Umbricht A, Montoya I, Hoover DR et al. (1999). Naltrexone shortened opioid detoxification with buprenorphine. *Drug and Alcohol Dependence* 56(3):181-190.

Vignau J (1998). Preliminary assessment of a 10-day rapid detoxification programme using high dosage buprenorphine. *European Addiction Research* (4 Suppl) 1:29-31.

Vining E, Kosten TR & Kleber HD (1988). Clinical utility of rapid clonidine-naltrexone detoxification for opioid abusers. *British Journal of Addiction* 83:567-575.

Walsh SL, June HL, Schuh KJ et al. (1995). Effects of buprenorphine and methadone in methadone-maintained subjects. *Psychopharmacology (Berl)* 119:268-276

Walsh SL, Preston KL, Bigelow GE et al. (1995). Acute administration of buprenorphine in humans: Partial agonist and blockade effects. *Journal of Pharmacological and Experimental Therapeutics* 274:361-372.

Walsh SL, Preston KL, Stitzer ML et al. (1994). Clinical pharmacology of buprenorphine: Ceiling effects at high doses. *Clinical Pharmacology and Therapeutics* 55:569-580.

Washton AM & Resnick RB (1980). Clonidine for opiate detoxification: Outpatient clinical trials. *American Journal of Psychiatry* 137:1121-1122.

Wanger K, Brough L, Macmillan I et al. (1998). *Academic Emergency Medicine* 5(4):293-299.

Wen HL, Ho WK & Wen PY (1984). Comparison of the effectiveness of different opioid peptides in depressing heroin withdrawal. *European Journal of Pharmacology* 100:155-162.

Whipple JK, Quebbeman EJ, Lewis KS et al. (1994). Difficulties in diagnosing narcotic overdoses in hospitalized patients. *Annals of Pharmacotherapy* 28(4):446-450.

White JM & Irvine RJ (1999). Mechanisms of fatal opioid overdose. *Addiction* 94(7):961-972.

Zielbauer P (1999). State knew of risky heroin treatment before patient deaths. *New York Times*. October 31, 41.

Ultra Rapid Opiate Detoxification

Susan M. Stine, M.D., Ph.D.
Mark K. Greenwald, Ph.D.
Thomas R. Kosten, M.D.

A recent and controversial development, which has arisen from use of the clonidine-naltrexone combination, is ultra rapid inpatient detoxification from opiates, using sedatives and anesthetics in combination with opiate antagonists.

Ultra rapid opiate detoxification (UROD) first was described in a study of 12 opiate-dependent patients who were given naloxone while under general anesthesia (Loimer, Schmid et al., 1988). Loimer and associates (1990) also reported a protocol involving barbiturate anesthesia with methohexitone (100 mg intravenous pretreatment, followed by 400 mg intravenously) and naltrexone (10 mg intravenously). This protocol allowed the successful detoxification of patients from opiates in 48 hours, but required intensive medical treatment (involving intubation and artificial ventilation), as well as the risks of anesthesia; therefore, it is controversial.

RESEARCH INTO
ULTRA RAPID DETOXIFICATION.

Subsequent studies of this technique (O'Connor & Kosten, 1998; Scherbaum, Klein et al., 1998) have used various approaches to both the detoxification and the sedation or general anesthesia. These studies generally have been small and methodologically limited, have not compared ultra rapid detoxification to other methods, and have provided little long-term followup, as reviewed by O'Connor and Kosten (1998). This has led many clinicians to raise serious questions about the widespread use of this procedure. For example, in one study in which detoxified patients were followed up by telephone interview, only 10% continued naltrexone maintenance therapy for seven months (Rabinowitz, Cohen et al., 1997). As reviewed by O'Connor and Fiellin (2000), two studies have demonstrated that substantial withdrawal symptoms persist well beyond the detoxification period (Scherbaum, Klein et al., 1998; Cucchia, Monnat et al., 1998). In addition, the expense of this procedure (up to $7,500), the additional risk associated with general anesthesia, and safety concerns (San, Puig et al., 1995; Pfab, Hirtl et al., 1999) limit its usefulness in clinical practice (O'Connor & Kosten, 1998). General

anesthesia with intubation, however, avoids the significant the risk of vomiting and aspiration, which may occur with sedation. In at least one instance, safety concerns led to the termination of a clinical program that provided ultra rapid detoxification (Zielbauer, 1999).

Although many investigators have suggested that the procedure should be limited to clinical trials until its safety and efficacy can be established (Strang, Bearn et al., 1997), interest in this procedure and consumer demand for it remain intense, and some recent studies are relatively encouraging. Albanese and colleagues (2000) evaluated six-month outcome data for 93 men and 27 women treated with ultra rapid detoxification, followed by naltrexone maintenance and an aftercare program. Outcome was assessed through urine drug screens, report from a significant other, or report from a therapist. All of the study group were reported to be relapse-free. However, this study is limited by lack of a prospective randomized controlled design.

Another recent study, by Hensel and Kox (2000), reported followup data from 72 opioid-dependent patients (whose drugs of abuse had included morphine, codeine, heroin, and methadone), who were detoxified with propofol general anesthesia using the ultra rapid method and subsequently treated with long-term naltrexone maintenance and a supportive psychotherapy program. At 12 months, 49 patients (68%) were abstinent from opiates, 17 had relapsed, and 6 were lost to followup. The investigators reported that methadone patients had more withdrawal symptoms than did the other addicts. This study also had design limitations (related to the absence of an open trial and lack of random assignment to a comparison group).

A third study (Lawental, 2000), which compared ultra rapid detoxification with 30-day inpatient detoxification, concluded that ultra rapid detoxification was less effective. In this study, 81 of 87 patients who were detoxified in 30 days and 82 of 139 patients who were detoxified by ultra rapid detoxification were interviewed by telephone 12 to 18 months after their participation in the program. Interview results suggested that ultra rapid detoxification was more expensive and less effective than traditional treatment. While this study was limited by its retrospective design and lack of randomized assignment, it does support longer-term biopsychosocial treatment alternatives over rapid detoxification.

Conclusions. Ultra rapid opiate detoxification remains a controversial but possibly promising and certainly intensely investigated new approach. It may be the only treatment acceptable to certain otherwise healthy patients who are unwilling to interrupt their work or personal schedules for longer term detoxification. It also may facilitate rapid induction to and maintenance on naltrexone. Nevertheless, the risks remain considerable and much research remains to be done on long-term outcomes.

REFERENCES

Albanese AP, Gevirtz C, Oppenheim B et al. (2000). Outcome and six-month follow up of patients after ultra rapid opiate detoxification (UROD). *Journal of Addictive Diseases* 19(2):11-28.

Cucchia AT, Monnat M, Spagnoli J et al. (1998). Ultra-rapid opiate detoxification using deep sedation with oral midazolam: Short and long-term results. *Drug and Alcohol Dependence* 52(3):243-250.

Hensel M, Wolter S & Kox WJ (2000). EEG controlled rapid opioid withdrawal under general anaesthesia. *British Journal of Anaesthesia* 84(2):236-238.

Lawental E (2000). Ultra rapid opiate detoxification as compared to 30-day inpatient detoxification program—A retrospective follow-up study. *Journal of Substance Abuse* 11(2):173-181.

Loimer N, Schmid R, Lenz K et al. (1990). Acute blocking of naloxone-precipitated opiate withdrawal symptoms by methohexitone. *British Journal of Psychiatry* 157:748-52.

Loimer N, Schmid R, Presslich O et al. (1988). Naloxone treatment for opiate withdrawal syndrome [letter]. *British Journal of Psychiatry* 153:851-852.

O'Connor PG & Fiellin DA (2000). Pharmacologic treatment of heroin-dependent patients. *Annals of Internal Medicine* 133(1):40-54.

O'Connor PG & Kosten TR (1998). Rapid and ultrarapid opioid detoxification techniques. *Journal of the American Medical Association* 279(3):229-134.

Pfab R, Hirtl C & Zilker T (1999). Opiate detoxification under anesthesia: No apparent benefit, but suppression of thyroid hormones and risk of pulmonary and renal failure. *Journal of Toxicology & Clinical Toxicology* 37(1):43-50.

Rabinowitz J, Cohen H, Tarrasch R et al. (1997). Compliance to naltrexone treatment after ultra-rapid opiate detoxification: An open label naturalistic study. *Drug and Alcohol Dependence* 47(2):77-86.

San L, Puig M, Bulbena A et al. (1995). High risk of ultrashort noninvasive opiate detoxification [letter]. *American Journal of Psychiatry* 152(6):956.

Scherbaum N, Klein S, Kaube H et al. (1998). Alternative strategies of opiate detoxification: Evaluation of the so-called ultra-rapid detoxification. *Pharmacopsychiatry* 31(6):205-209.

Strang J, Bearn J & Gossop M (1997). Opiate detoxification under anaesthesia [editorial] [see comments]. *British Medical Journal* 315(7118):1249-1250.

Zielbauer P (1999). State knew of risky heroin treatment before patient deaths. *New York Times.* October 31, 41.

Management of Stimulant, Hallucinogen, Marijuana, Phencyclidine, and Club Drug Intoxication and Withdrawal

Chapter 5

Jeffery N. Wilkins, M.D.
Katherine G. Mellott, M.D.
Romana Markvitsa, M.D.
David A. Gorelick, M.D., Ph.D.

Stimulants
Hallucinogens
Marijuana
Phencyclidine (PCP)
MDMA ("Ecstasy")
Gamma-Hydroxybutyrate (GHB)
Flunitrazepam (Rohypnol®)
Serotonin Syndrome
Multiple Drug Withdrawal
Population-Specific Considerations

This chapter reviews the treatment of acute intoxication and withdrawal states associated with the use of stimulants such as cocaine and methamphetamine (including their smokable forms "crack" and "ice"); hallucinogens such as lysergic acid diethylamide (LSD); marijuana; dissociative anesthetics such as phencyclidine (PCP) and ketamine; and "club drugs" such as 3,4-methylenedioxymethamphetamine (MDMA or "Ecstasy") and gamma-hydroxybutyrate (GHB). It also reviews the treatment of the serotonin syndrome and withdrawal from multiple drugs. Psychiatric and medical complications are considered separately because they often are treated with different modalities and in different settings (for example, in psychiatric versus medical emergency departments). Not all of the substances reviewed here have clinically distinct intoxication or withdrawal syndromes, nor are there pharmacologic treatments for all such syndromes (see Table 1).

Successful treatment of acute intoxication, overdose, or withdrawal can facilitate entry into addiction treatment by reducing uncomfortable withdrawal symptomatology that negatively reinforces drug-taking. Even when successful, these early stages of treatment often are followed by relapse to substance use, with patients reentering a "revolving door" of repeated detoxification programs. For drugs without a physiologically prominent withdrawal syndrome, such as marijuana, LSD, PCP, and MDMA, there may be little benefit to short-term treatment focused on alleviating acute withdrawal. Short-term treatment of acute intoxication or withdrawal does not obviate the need for long-term treatment of addiction.

Pharmacologic treatment of drug intoxication and overdose generally follows one of three approaches (Gorelick, 1993): (1) increased clearance of drug from the body, either by increasing catabolism, increasing excretion, or both;

TABLE 1.   Presence of Clinically Distinct Substance Intoxication or Withdrawal Syndromes, According to DSM-IV Criteria

Substance	Intoxication Delirium	Intoxication Psychosis	Intoxication	Withdrawal
Stimulants	Yes	Yes	Yes	Yes
Marijuana	Yes	Yes	Yes	No
Hallucinogens	Yes	Yes	Yes	No
Phencyclidine	Yes	Yes	Yes	No

(2) blockade of the neuronal site to which the drug binds to exert its effect (as through the use of naloxone to block the opiate receptor in the treatment of opiate overdose); and (3) counteracting effects of the drug through alternative neuropharmacologic action.

Pharmacologic treatment of any drug withdrawal syndrome generally follows one of two approaches (Gorelick, 1993): (1) suppression by a cross-tolerant medication from the same pharmacologic class—usually a longer-acting one to provide a milder, controlled withdrawal (as in the use of the opioid methadone for opiate detoxification)—and (2) reducing the signs and symptoms of withdrawal by targeting the neurochemical or receptor systems that mediate withdrawal (as in the use of the non-opiate clonidine to treat opiate withdrawal).

The application of these pharmacologic treatment approaches to the drugs reviewed in this chapter is limited. There may be no practical method for altering drug clearance (as with hallucinogens and marijuana), or no specific drug receptor site(s) has been identified. Even when a receptor site has been identified, there may not yet exist a clinically useful antagonist. Finally, current understanding of the neuropharmacological processes that mediate intoxication or withdrawal may be too limited to suggest appropriate pharmacologic interventions. Thus, clinical stabilization, supportive management, and palliation of symptoms often remain the mainstays of treatment.

STIMULANTS
Stimulant Intoxication. The acute psychological and medical effects of cocaine, amphetamines, and other stimulants are attributable principally to increases in catecholamine neurotransmitter activity. Enhanced catecholamine activity occurs through blockade of the presynaptic neurotransmit-

ter reuptake pumps (as by cocaine) and by presynaptic release of catecholamines (as by amphetamines) (King & Ellinwood, 1997; Johanson & Fischman, 1989). The resulting stimulation of brain reward circuits (the corticomesolimbic dopamine circuit) is thought to mediate the desired (and addicting) psychological effects of stimulants. The resulting stimulation of the sympathetic nervous system leads to peripheral vasoconstriction (with organ ischemia), increased heart rate, and lowered seizure threshold, among other adverse effects. Table 2 lists medical complications of stimulant intoxication.

Blockade of catecholamine presynaptic binding sites or postsynaptic receptors should, in principle, be an effective treatment for stimulant intoxication. However, with limited exceptions (such as haloperidol for stimulant-induced psychosis or phentolamine for hypertension), no such medication has yet proved broadly effective, especially in attenuating the desirable or reinforcing effects of stimulant intoxication (Gorelick, 1995).

Another method of attenuating the effects of cocaine intoxication might be to decrease cocaine availability in the central nervous system (CNS) by binding it peripherally with anticocaine antibodies or by increasing its catabolism (Gorelick, 1997). The latter approach could be implemented with catalytic antibodies (Mets, Winger et al., 1998) or the endogenous cocaine-metabolizing enzyme butyrylcholinesterase (BChE, E.C. 3.1.1.8) (Hoffman, Morasco et al., 1996; Mattes, Belendiuk et al., 1998).

Table 3 gives an overview of treatment for the psychiatric and medical complications of stimulant intoxication.

Psychological and Behavioral Effects of Stimulant Intoxication: The initial desired effects of stimulant intoxication include increased energy, alertness, and sociability; elation; euphoria; and decreased fatigue, need for sleep, and appetite (Hurlbut, 1991). At this stage, users do not seek or need treatment. With high-dose or repeated use, however, stimulant intoxication usually progresses to unwanted effects such as anxiety, irritability, interpersonal sensitivity, hypervigilance, suspiciousness, grandiosity, impaired judgment, stereotyped behavior, and psychotic symptoms such as paranoia and hallucinations. In some case series, more than half of chronic cocaine and amphetamine users reported psychotic symptoms (Cubells, Kranzler et al., 2000; Hall, Hando et al., 1996; Satel, Southwick et al., 1991c; Serper, Chou et al., 1999). However, these results may reflect selection bias among users who come to medical or research attention. Stimulant users typically remain alert and oriented, but the delusional state may impair judgment, cognition, and attention.

Patients with stimulant-induced psychoses may closely resemble those with acute schizophrenia and may be misdiagnosed as such (Harris & Batki, 2000; Rosse, Collins et al., 1994; Serper, Chou et al., 1999; Shaner, Roberts et al., 1998). Cocaine-induced psychosis may differ from acute schizophrenic psychosis in having less thought disorder and bizarre delusions and fewer negative symptoms such as alogia and inattention (Serper, Chou et al., 1999). Stimulant-induced hallucinations may be auditory, visual, or somatosensory (Cubells, Kranzler et al., 2000). Tactile hallucinations are especially typical of stimulant psychosis, such as the sensation of something crawling under the skin (formication). Panic reactions are common, and may evolve into a panic disorder (Schuckit, 2000). This may be exacerbated by anxiety elicited by the physiological symptoms commonly associated with stimulant use, such as palpitations and hyperventilation.

Very severe stimulant intoxication may produce an excited delirium or organic brain syndrome that can be fatal (Karch & Stephens, 1999; Ruttenber, McAnally et al., 1999). Patients should be evaluated promptly for an acute neurological lesion (for example, intracranial bleeding) or a preexisting neuropsychiatric condition and treated aggressively.

Management of Psychological and Behavioral Effects of Stimulant Intoxication: The initial clinical evaluation should include a drug use history and drug toxicology to confirm stimulant intoxication. As the patient's condition permits, further evaluation should rule out other potential medical (hyperthyroidism, hypoglycemia) or neuropsychiatric (panic or bipolar affective disorder) conditions (Brady

& Duncan, 1999). The initial treatment approach is non-pharmacologic (Khantzian & McKenna, 1979; Roth, Benowitz et al., 1998). The patient should be observed in a quiet environment with minimal sensory stimulation to avoid exacerbating symptoms. Treatment staff should interact in a calm and confident manner, using the "ART" approach developed at the Haight Ashbury Free Clinic in San Francisco: **A**cceptance of the patient's immediate needs (such as pain relief or use of the bathroom), **R**eassurance that the condition is due to the drug and likely will dissipate within a few hours, and **T**alkdown, to provide reality orientation and avoid hostility. All procedures should be explained to the patient before initiation.

Most experts prefer benzodiazepines (such as diazepam [10 to 30 mg PO or 2 to 10 mg IM or IV] or lorazepam [2 to 7 mg PO, IM, or IV]) over neuroleptics to control severe agitation, anxiety, or psychotic symptoms (Goldfrank & Hoffman, 1991; Roth, Benowitz et al., 1998; Schuckit, 2000). The former protect against the CNS and cardiovascular toxicities of cocaine, while the latter may worsen the sympathomimetic and cardiovascular effects, lower the seizure threshold, and increase the risk of hyperthermia. Parenteral benzodiazepine dosing may be repeated every 5 to 10 minutes until sedation is achieved. If a neuroleptic is needed to control psychosis, a high-potency agent such as haloperidol (5 to 10 mg PO, IM, or IV) or droperidol (2.5 to 5 mg IV) is preferred because of its minimal anticholinergic activity. Medications with anticholinergic activity should be avoided because they may contribute to delirium and hyperthermia (by impairing heat dissipation from sweating). One recent controlled trial found IV droperidol as effective as IV lorazepam in controlling stimulant-induced agitation, with droperidol causing less sedation and requiring fewer repeat doses (Richards, Derlet et al., 1998). There is little published experience with the newer atypical neuroleptics (such as clozapine, risperidal, quetiapine, and olanzapine). Less potent neuroleptics, such as chlorpromazine, have been associated with anticholinergic or hypotensive episodes (Smart & Anglin, 1987) and may inhibit the metabolism of amphetamine (Weiss, Greenfield et al., 1994). Chlorpromazine has been used safely in treating children with severe amphetamine poisoning (Callaway & Clark, 1994).

Physical restraints to control agitation or violent behavior should be avoided unless absolutely necessary. The use

TABLE 2. Acute Medical Complications of Stimulant Intoxication

Organ System	Medical Effects
HEENT	Pupil dilation; headache; bruxism
Pulmonary*	Hyperventilation, dyspnea; cough; chest pain; wheezing; hemoptysis; acute exacerbation of asthma; barotrauma (pneumothorax, penumomediastinum, pulmonary edema)
Cardiovascular	Tachycardia; palpitations; increased blood pressure; arrhythmia; chest pain; myocardial ischemia or infarction; ruptured aneurysm; cardiogenic shock
Neurologic	Headache; agitation; psychosis; tremor, hyperreflexia; small muscle twitching; tics; stereotyped movements; myoclonus; seizures; cerebral hemorrhage or infarct (stroke); cerebral edema
Gastrointestinal	Nausea, vomiting; mesenteric ischemia; bowel infarction or perforation
Renal	Diuresis; myoglobinuria; acute renal failure
Body Temperature	Mild fever; malignant hyperthermia
Other	Rhabdomyolysis.

*All pulmonary complications except hyperventilation and pulmonary edema come primarily from the smoked route of administration.

SOURCES: Ghuran & Nolan, 2000; Neiman, 2000; Schuckit, 2000; Tashkin, 2001.

of restraints can increase risk of hyperthermia and rhabdomyolysis, with resulting severe medical complications (Hurlbut, 1991; Roth, Benowitz et al., 1998).

A psychotic or agitated patient who has not responded to initial treatment should be hospitalized until the episode has resolved. This usually occurs within a few days if no more stimulants are ingested (Schuckit, 2000). Psychiatric symptoms that persist beyond a few days suggest an etiology other than stimulant use (Hurlbut, 1991; Satel, Seibyl et al., 1991b).

Medical Effects of Stimulant Intoxication: Mild stimulant intoxication (the state desired by users) is accompanied by one or more self-limiting physiological effects such as restlessness, tachycardia, hyperventilation, mydriasis, bruxism, headache, diaphoresis, or tremor. These do not usually bring the individual to medical attention or require treatment. Higher doses or repeated use are associated with

more serious medical events, including myocardial ischemia or infarction (usually reflected in chest pain), cardiac arrhythmia, hypertension, seizures, stroke, hyperthermia, or rhabdomyolysis (Ghuran & Nolan, 2000; Neiman, Haapaniemi et al., 2000; Nzerue, Hewan-Lowe et al., 2000; Richards, Johnson et al., 1999). Medical complications associated with stimulant intoxication are summarized in Table 2.

Stimulant use should be high on the list of possible diagnoses for any younger patient presenting with one of these events, especially in the absence of other risk factors. Urine and/or blood samples for toxicological analysis always should be obtained to determine what drugs, if any, the patient has ingested recently. Even if an apparently adequate history has been obtained, the patient or collateral informants may not know the true content of any street drugs that have been used. A history of stimulant use within the preceding 96 hours or a positive toxicology test is highly suggestive. The actual blood cocaine concentration has little prognostic significance (Blaho, Logan et al., 2000).

Non-traumatic chest pain is a common presenting complaint among stimulant users who seek acute medical care. The differential diagnosis includes myocardial ischemia or infarction, aortic dissection, pneumothorax or pneumomediastinum (especially among drug smokers), endocarditis or pneumonia (especially among injection drug users), pulmonary embolus, myocarditis or cardiomyopathy, or musculoskeletal pain after a seizure (Hahn & Hoffman, 2001). The ECG is not always helpful because of its low sensitivity and positive predictive value (36% and 18%, respectively, in one study) and the high frequency of early repolarization among the young, male patients most likely to present with cocaine-associated chest pain (Hahn & Hoffman, 2001; Lange & Hillis, 2001). The best diagnostic tool for acute myocardial infarction is serial levels of blood CPK-MB fraction. (Total CPK may be elevated because of trauma or rhabdomyolysis.) Serum troponin levels are being used with increasing frequency because of their greater sensitivity and specificity.

Patients who present with non-traumatic stimulant-associated chest pain usually should be observed for 12 to 24 hours while undergoing evaluation (Hahn & Hoffman, 2001). The vast majority of such patients (> 90%) will not have acute myocardial infarction (Weber, Chudnofsky et al., 2000). Resolution of symptoms with a negative evaluation warrants discharge to home with followup outpatient evaluation (for example, a cardiac stress test). Patients who have persistent chest pain despite standard treatment, hypotension, congestive heart failure, or cardiac arrhythmia require hospitalization for further evaluation and treatment. Even patients with confirmed acute myocardial infarction have a favorable prognosis, possibly because of their relatively young age and good underlying health (Ghuran & Nolan, 2000).

Rhabdomyolysis may be due to a direct effect of the drug, hyperthermia, excessive muscle activity, or trauma (Roth, Benowitz et al., 1998). The usual symptoms of myalgia and muscle tenderness and swelling often are absent in rhabdomyolysis associated with stimulants. The diagnosis is suggested by a plasma CK level greater than five times normal (with other tissue sources ruled out) and a urine dipstick positive for heme but without red blood cells (indicating free myoglobin [or hemoglobin] in the urine).

Management of Medical Effects of Stimulant Intoxication: The first priority in the management of severe acute stimulant intoxication is maintenance of basic life-support functions. Vital signs and neurologic status should be monitored closely. Activated charcoal and/or gastric lavage with isotonic saline may be helpful if a large amount of stimulant has been taken orally within the preceding hour, as by a "bodypacker" (Roth, Benowitz et al., 1998; Schuckit, 2000). This can be done by oral intake or via nasogastric tube in the awake, cooperative patient. A nasogastric tube may be used after endotracheal intubation in the unconscious patient. Activated charcoal (50 to 100 g orally) may be just as effective as gastric lavage and minimizes the risk of aspiration. Severe hypertension (for example, diastolic BP >120) that lasts more than 15 minutes should be treated promptly to avoid CNS hemorrhage (Schuckit, 2000). Rhabdomyolysis should be treated vigorously with intravenous fluid to maintain a urine output of >2 ml/kg/hour so as to avoid myoglobinuric renal failure (Roth, Benowitz et al., 1998; Schuckit, 2000). Maintenance of urine pH above 5.6 with sodium bicarbonate (1 mmol/kg IV) helps to prevent the dissociation and precipitation of myoglobin.

Benzodiazepines in sedative doses are the initial treatment of choice for both acute cardiovascular and CNS toxicity from stimulants (Baumann, Perrone et al., 2000; Ghuran & Nolan, 2000; Roth, Benowitz et al., 1998). Hypertension or tachycardia that does not respond to sedation alone may be treated with an alpha-adrenergic blocker such as phentolamine (2 to 10 mg IV over 10 minutes). Beta-adrenergic blockers such as propranolol or esmolol are contraindicated because of the risk of unopposed alpha-adrenergic stimulation by the stimulant, resulting in vasoconstriction and worsening hypertension (Ramoska & Sacchetti, 1985). The combined alpha- and beta-adrenergic blocker labetalol actually shows little alpha-adrenergic antagonism in clinical practice and also should be avoided (Ghuran & Nolan, 2000). If alpha-adrenergic blockade is ineffective, direct vasodilation with sodium nitroprusside infusion (0.25 to 10 μg/kg/min) or nitroglycerin (5 to 100 μg IV) can be used. There is no evidence that rapid lowering of blood pressure compromises peripheral (including cerebral) circulation in an otherwise intact patient. Calcium channel blockers may reduce vasospasm, but their role remains unclear (Hahn & Hoffman, 2001). They enhance CNS toxicity in animal studies, have shown inconsistent effects in case series, and may accelerate gas-

TABLE 3. Treatment of Acute Stimulant Intoxication

Clinical Problem	Moderate Syndrome	Severe Syndrome
Anxiety; agitation	Provide reassurance; place in a quiet, non-threatening environment.	Give diazepam (10-30 mg PO, 2-10 mg IM, IV); or lorazepam (2-4 mg PO, IM, IV); may repeat every 1 to 3 hours.
Paranoia; psychosis	Place in a quiet, non-threatening environment; give benzodiazepines for sedation.	Give a high-potency neuroleptic (e.g., haloperidol) or an atypical neuroleptic.
Hyperthermia	Monitor body temperature; place patient in a cool room.	If >102° F (oral), use external cooling with cold water, ice packs, hypothermic blanket; if >106° F, use internal cooling; epigastric lavage with iced saline.
Seizures	Diazepam (2-20 mg IV, <5 mg/min); or lorazepam (2-8 mg).	For status epilepticus: IV diazepam or phenytoin (15-20 mg/kg IV, <150 mg/min; or phenobarbital (25-50 mg IV).
Hypertension	Monitor blood pressure closely; give benzodiazepines.	If diastolic >120 for 15 minutes, give phentolamine (2-10 mg IV over 10 minutes).
Cardiac arrhythmia	Monitor ECG, vital signs; give benzodiazepines for sedation.	As appropriate for specific rhythm, based on ACLS criteria.
Myocardial infarction	Give benzodiazepines for sedation; supplemental oxygen; sublingual nitroglycerin for vasodilation; aspirin for anti-clotting; morphine for pain.	Give nitrates IV for coronary artery dilation; phentolamine (2-10 mg IV) to control BP; thrombolysis, angioplasty (if clot confirmed, no hemorrhage).
Rhabdomyolysis	Use IV hydration to maintain urine output >2 ml/kg/hour.	Force diuresis with aggressive intravenous hydration.
Increased urinary drug excretion	Give 8 oz of cranberry juice TID or ammonium chloride (500 mg PO every 3-4 hours) until urine pH <6.6 (if renal and hepatic function are normal)	Same as for moderate intoxication.
Recent (few hours) oral drug ingestion	Administer activated charcoal orally or gastric lavage via nasogastric tube (if patient is awake and cooperative).	Use gastric lavage via nasogastric tube after endotracheal intubation (if patient is unconscious).

trointestinal drug absorption (for example, after rupture of cocaine packets ingested by "bodypackers") (Ghuran & Nolan, 2000).

Treatment of cocaine-induced cardiac arrhythmias begins with correction of any exacerbating conditions such as myocardial ischemia, hypoxia, electrolyte abnormalities, or acid-base disturbance (Ghuran & Nolan, 2000; Hahn & Hoffman, 2001; Lange & Hillis, 2001). Many arrhythmias will resolve without specific treatment as the drug is eliminated from the body and sympathetic hyperactivity subsides. Cocaine, as a sodium channel blocker, itself acts as a class I antiarrhythmic agent. Therefore, class IA antiarrhythmic medications (such as quinidine, procainamide, or disopyramide) should be avoided because of their potential additive effect on QRS and QT interval prolongation and interference with cocaine metabolism. Wide-complex supraventricular tachycardias may respond to alkalinization with sodium bicarbonate. Ventricular tachycardia can be treated with lidocaine. If the arrhythmia is associated with symptomatic hypotension, an intravenous bolus of hypertonic sodium bicarbonate followed by cardioversion may be helpful. Treatment of specific arrhythmias should follow ACLS guidelines, published by the American Heart Association.

The treatment of stimulant-associated myocardial ischemia or infarction largely resembles that for non-drug-associated ischemia, with the exception of avoiding use of beta-adrenergic blockers and labetolol (Ghuran & Nolan, 2000; Hahn & Hoffman, 2001; Lange & Hillis, 2001). Initial treatment includes oxygen, benzodiazepine for sedation, morphine for pain, sublingual nitroglycerin for vasodilation, and aspirin for antiplatelet action, while evaluation is continuing. Further treatment can include phentolamine and/or intravenous nitrates (10 μg/kg/min) to lower blood pressure and reverse coronary artery vasoconstriction. The calcium channel blocker verapamil (10 mg) can be used to reduce coronary artery vasospasm.

The role of thrombolysis or percutaneous transluminal coronary angioplasty in confirmed myocardial infarction remains uncertain (Hahn & Hoffman, 2001). Many cocaine-associated infarctions may be due to vasospasm rather than clot formation, making thrombolysis irrelevant. In addition, cocaine users are at increased risk of intracranial hemorrhage. Both thrombolysis and angioplasty have been safely and effectively used in non-hemorrhagic patients with focal lesions confirmed by coronary angiography in whom blood pressure was well controlled (Shah, Dy et al., 2000).

Elevated body temperature (>102° F. orally) should be managed aggressively to avert hyperthermic crisis (as by cold-water sponging, cooling blankets, ice packs, ice-water gastric lavage, or cold peritoneal lavage) (Roth, Benowitz et al., 1998; Schuckit, 2000). Untreated hyperthermia may result in rhabdomyolysis and renal failure.

Intravenous benzodiazepines (diazepam 5 to 10 mg or lorazepam 2 to 10 mg over two minutes, repeated as needed) are recommended to control seizures stemming from stimulant intoxication (Roth, Benowitz et al., 1998). Because diazepam may cause apnea or laryngospasm, intubation trays should be available (Schuckit, 2000). Fosphenytoin (15 to 20 mg/kg at 100 to 150 mg/min) or phenobarbital (15 to 20 mg/kg over 20 minutes) also can be used. However, the latter may cause hypotension or prolonged sedation.

Excretion of amphetamine can be increased by acidifying the urine to pH < 6.6 (as with 500 mg of oral ammonium chloride every 3 to 4 hours), which inhibits renal reabsorption of amphetamine (Jenkins & Cone, 1998). The actual clinical usefulness of this maneuver is uncertain (Callaway & Clark, 1994; Weiss, Greenfield et al., 1994). Acidification is contraindicated if renal or hepatic function are abnormal (Weiss, Greenfield et al., 1994) or in overdose situations, when plasma acidification may compromise cardiovascular function (Hurlbut, 1991).

Stimulant Withdrawal. Abrupt cessation of stimulant use is associated with depression, anxiety, fatigue, difficulty concentrating, anergia, anhedonia, increased drug craving, increased appetite, hypersomnolence, and increased dreaming (due to increased REM sleep) (Coffey, Dansky et al., 2000; Cottler, Shillington et al., 1993; Lago & Kosten, 1994). The initial period of intense symptoms is commonly termed the "crash," but most symptoms are mild and selflimited, resolving within one to two weeks without treatment. One early study of cocaine addicts in outpatient treatment described a triphasic withdrawal syndrome lasting several weeks, but this pattern has not been found in subsequent inpatient or outpatient studies of cocaine withdrawal (Coffey, Dansky et al., 2000; Lago & Kosten, 1994; Satel, Price et al., 1991a).

Hospitalization for stimulant withdrawal rarely is indicated on medical grounds and has not been shown to improve the short-term outcome for stimulant addiction (Mulvaney, Alterman et al., 1999; Rosenblum, Foote et al., 1996). Pharmacologic treatment has focused more on long-

TABLE 4. Acute Psychological and Behavioral Effects of Intoxication with LSD, Marijuana, Phencyclidine (PCP), and MDMA

Effects	LSD	Marijuana	Phencyclidine	MDMA
"Abnormal" overall behavior and appearance	x x	x	x x x	x
Disoriented to person, place, time, or situation	x x	none	x x	none
Impaired memory	x	x x	x x	x
Inappropriate affect	x x x	x	x x x	x x
Depressed mood	x x	x	x x	x
Overly elated mood	x x x	x x	x x	x x x
Confused, disorganized thinking	x x	x x	x x x	x
Hallucinations	x x x	x	x x x	x
Delusions	x/x x x	x x x	x x	?
Bizarre behavior	x x x	x	x x x	?
Suicidal or danger to self	x x	x x	x x	?
Homicidal or danger to others	x x	x	x x x	x
Poor judgment	x/x x x	x x x	x x x	x x

Relative weighting: x = mild; x x = moderate; x x x = marked;
/ = common/rare; ? = insufficient research.
MDMA = 3,4-methylenedioxymethamphetamine

term treatment of addiction than on short-term treatment of acute withdrawal. Most clinical trials that used medication during the early withdrawal period have continued to use such medication for at least several weeks, with the additional goal of treating the addiction itself (Gorelick, 1995) (also see Section 6).

Medical Effects of Stimulant Withdrawal: The first week of stimulant withdrawal has been associated with myocardial ischemia (Nademanee, Gorelick et al., 1989), possibly due to coronary vasospasm. Other medical effects of stimulant withdrawal are relatively minor, including nonspecific musculoskeletal pain, tremors, chills, and involuntary motor movement (Khantzian & McKenna, 1979). These rarely require specific medical treatment.

Management of Stimulant Withdrawal: The stimulant withdrawal syndrome has been hypothesized to be the result of decreased levels of brain dopamine activity resulting from chronic stimulant exposure. This so-called "dopamine deficiency" hypothesis of withdrawal has not been consistently supported by clinical studies (Gill, Gillespie et al., 1991; Satel, Price et al., 1991a; Volkow, Fowler et al., 1992), but has generated use of dopamine agonists to treat cocaine withdrawal. Most commonly used are bromocriptine and amantadine, two medications already marketed for the treatment of parkinsonism, which also is a dopamine deficiency disease.

Clinical trials have yielded inconsistent results (Gorelick, 1995; Teller & Devenyi, 1988). The dopamine amino acid precursor L-dopa, which also is used to treat parkinsonism, was effective in reducing cocaine withdrawal symptoms in one small inpatient case series (Wolfsohn & Angrist, 1990). No controlled clinical trial has directly compared the benefits of medication versus a supportive milieu.

Symptoms of stimulant withdrawal are best treated supportively by allowing the patient to sleep and eat as much as necessary (Schuckit, 2000). Short-acting benzodiazepines such as lorazepam may be helpful in selected patients who develop agitation or sleep disturbance. Severe (suicidal ideation) or persistent (>2 to 3 weeks) depression may require antidepressant treatment (Schuckit, 2000; Weiss, Greenfield et al., 1994) and psychiatric admission. The risk of relapse is high during the early withdrawal period, in part because drug craving is easily triggered by encounters with drug-associated stimuli. This issue is better addressed by psychosocial treatment, such as cognitive-behavioral therapy and relapse prevention, than by medication.

Administration of a cross-tolerant or similarly acting stimulant has not been systematically evaluated as a short-term treatment for stimulant withdrawal. Antidepressants have been used because, like cocaine, they inhibit presynaptic neurotransmitter reuptake, and because depression is a common symptom of stimulant withdrawal. No controlled clinical trials have evaluated the effectiveness of antidepressants for this purpose.

HALLUCINOGENS

Hallucinogen Intoxication. Hallucinogens fall into two different chemical groups: serotonin- or tryptamine-related (including lysergic acid diethylamide [LSD], psilocybin, or N,N-dimethyltryptamine [DMT]) and the phenylethylamine- or amphetamine-related (including 3,4,5-trimethoxyphenyl-ethylamine [mescaline], 3,5-dimethoxy-4-methylamphetamine [DOM, STP], or 3,4,5-trimethoxyamphetamine [TMA]). All share enough clinical similarities with LSD to be classified as LSD-like hallucinogens (Abraham, Aldridge et al., 1996). 3,4-methylenedioxymethamphetamine (MDMA, "Ecstasy") has characteristics of both a hallucinogen and a stimulant and is considered below. Phencyclidine (PCP) and its close analogue ketamine can be abused for their hallucinogenic effects, but differ substantially in their range of effects and mechanisms of action. They are considered in their own section, below.

Psychological and Behavioral Effects of Hallucinogen Intoxication: The psychological effects of hallucinogen intoxication are summarized in Table 4 (Abraham, Aldridge et al., 1996; Brust, 1998) (also see Section 2). The subjective experience is influenced greatly by set and setting; that is, the expectations and personality of the user, coupled with the environmental and social conditions of use. Mood can vary from euphoria and feelings of spiritual insight to depression, anxiety, and terror. Perception usually is intensified and distorted, with alterations in the sense of time, space, and body boundaries. Hallucinations (especially visual and auditory) are common. Cognitive function may range from

clarity to confusion and disorientation, although reality testing usually remains intact.

A "bad trip" usually takes the form of an anxiety attack or panic reaction, with the user feeling out of control (Kulig, 1990; Strassman, 1984; Weiss, Greenfield et al., 1994). An experience of depersonalization may precipitate the fear of losing one's mind permanently. Panic reactions are more common in those who have limited experience with hallucinogens, but previous "positive" experiences provide no protection against an adverse reaction (Pechnick & Ungerleider, 1997). Hallucinogens may trigger a transient psychosis even in psychologically normal users; however, a true psychotic episode is rare. Hallucinogen-induced psychosis may resemble acute paranoid schizophrenia (Pechnick & Ungerleider, 1997). The two usually can be distinguished because patients with schizophrenia tend to have auditory (rather than visual) hallucinations and a history of prior mental illness. Hallucinogen users, unlike patients with schizophrenia, usually retain at least partial insight that their psychosis is drug-related.

Hallucinogen ingestion may result in an acute toxic delirium that is characterized by delusions, hallucinations, agitation, confusion, paranoia, and inadvertent suicide attempts (as through attempts to fly or perform other impossible activities) (Weiss, Greenfield et al., 1994).

Medical Effects of Hallucinogen Intoxication: Acute medical complications of hallucinogen intoxication that require treatment are rare (Table 5) (Brust, 1998). Dizziness, paresthesias, or tremor may occur. Body temperature should be monitored and any elevation treated promptly. Dry skin, increased muscle tone, agitation, and seizures are warning signs of a potential hyperthermic crisis. Patients may not respond to anticonvulsant medication until body temperature is lowered.

Oral LSD is rapidly absorbed, so that ipecac-induced vomiting or gastric lavage usually are not helpful and may exacerbate the patient's psychological distress. There is no evidence that LSD binds to charcoal. Gastric lavage may be useful in psilocybin ingestion, or when there is doubt as to the identity of the ingested mushrooms (Schwartz & Smith, 1988).

Management of Hallucinogen Intoxication: Initial treatment is non-pharmacologic. The patient should be placed in a quiet environment with minimal sensory stimulation, but should be observed because of the risk of unintended self-injury (as the result of delusions or hallucinations) or

TABLE 5. Acute Medical Complications of Intoxication With LSD, MDMA, Marijuana, or Phencyclidine (PCP)

Organ System	LSD	MDMA	Marijuana	PCP (Stage I)	PCP (Stage II)	PCP (Stage III)
HEENT	Pupil dilation	Bruxism; headache; trismus; dry mouth	Pupil constriction; conjunctival injection; headache	Horizontal nystagmus; lid reflex lost; variable pupil size; laryngeal/pharyngeal reflexes hyperactive; ↑ tearing; ↑ saliva	Corneal reflex lost; disconjugate gaze; pupils mid-position and reactive; laryngeal/pharyngeal reflexes diminished; ↑ tearing; ↑ saliva	"Eyes open" coma; pupil dilation; laryngeal/pharyngeal reflexes absent; ↑ tearing; ↑ saliva
Skin	Piloerection; diaphoresis	Diaphoresis; flushing		Diaphoresis; flushing	Diaphoresis; flushing	Diaphoresis; flushing
Pulmonary			Mild tachypnea	Moderate tachypnea	Periodic breathing, apnea, pneumonia, pulmonary edema	
Cardiovascular	↑ HR; ↑ BP	↑ HR ↑ BP (rarely, ↓ BP)	↑ HR, ↓ BP orthostatic hypotension	Mildly ↑ HR, BP	Moderately ↑ HR, BP	Greatly ↑ HR, BP; high-output cardiac failure
Neurologic	Hyperreflexia; tremors; seizures	Tremor; trismus; ↑ muscle tone	Tremor; ↓coordination; ataxia	Conscious; muscle rigidity; repetitive movements; hyperreflexia	Stupor to mild coma; tonic-clonic seizures; deep pain response intact; muscle rigidity, muscle twitching	Deep coma; tonic-clonic seizures; stroke; deep pain response absent; generalized myoclonus, opisthotonus, or decerebrate posturing; deep tendon reflexes absent
Gastrointestinal	Nausea, vomiting	Nausea; ↓ appetite	↑ appetite	Nausea; vomiting	Protracted vomiting	
Renal	Urinary retention	Acute renal failure	Urinary retention	Acute renal failure		
Body Temperature	↑ or ↓	↑ (possible malignant hyperthermia)		Mild ↑	Moderate ↑	Possible malignant hyperthermia
Other		Rhabdomyolysis		Rhabdomyolysis		

MDMA = 3,4-methylenedioxymethamphetamine; HR = heart rate; BP = blood pressure

SOURCES: Carroll, 1990; Ghuran & Nolan, 2000; Kalant, 2000; Leikin, Krantz et al., 1989; Milhorn, 1991; Schuckit, 2000; Selden, Clark et al., 1990.

of suicide (as the result of depression). The presence of a familiar person usually is comforting. Unless the patient presents in an acutely agitated or threatening state, physical restraints are contraindicated because they may exacerbate anxiety and increase the risk of rhabdomyolysis associated with muscle rigidity or spasms. The use of "gentle restraints" in combination with muscle massage and individualized counseling may be helpful (Miller, Gay et al., 1992).

The "talk-down" or reassurance technique may be helpful. The clinician, in a concerned and nonjudgmental manner, discusses the patient's anxiety reaction, stressing that the drug's effects are temporary and that the patient will recover completely.

For patients who do not respond to reassurance alone, oral benzodiazepines such as lorazepam (1 to 2 mg) or diazepam (10 to 30 mg) are the drugs of choice (Strassman, 1984). When oral medication is too slow, or the patient will not take oral medication, intramuscular lorazepam (2 mg, repeated hourly as needed) may be effective. If benzodiazepines are insufficient, a high-potency neuroleptic such as haloperidol (5 to 10 mg orally or 2 mg intramuscularly) is recommended. The role of the atypical antipsychotics in this situation remains unclear. Anti-parkinson medication should be available to treat acute dystonic reactions or other possible acute neuroleptic side effects (Strassman, 1984). Phenothiazines should be avoided because they have been associated with poor outcomes (Leikin, Krantz et al., 1989) and may exacerbate an unsuspected anticholinergic poisoning.

Patients usually recover sufficiently after several hours and may be released into the care of a responsible relative or friend. If psychosis does not resolve within one or two days, ingestion of a longer-acting drug such as PCP or DOM should be suspected (Schuckit, 2000). Symptoms that persist beyond a few days raise the strong likelihood of a preexisting or concurrent psychiatric or neurological condition. Psychiatric problems that last more than a month probably are related to preexisting psychopathology.

Treatment for hallucinogen-induced delirium generally follows the guidelines for simple intoxication: Isolate the patient and minimize sensory input until effects of the drug have worn off. Reassurance that the delirium will abate as the drug is metabolized also may be helpful. Pharmacologic treatment is not necessary in most cases and may confuse the clinical picture. If medication is needed, a drug with few anticholinergic properties is preferred for the reasons listed above; for example, diazepam may be given 15 to 30 mg orally, repeating 5 to 20 mg every three to four hours as needed (Weiss, Greenfield et al., 1994).

Hallucinogen Withdrawal. Withdrawal symptoms, including fatigue, irritability, and anhedonia, are reported by about 10% of hallucinogen users (Cottler, Schuckit et al., 1995), but there is no evidence to suggest a clinically significant hallucinogen withdrawal syndrome (Khantzian & McKenna, 1979; Pechnick & Ungerleider, 1997). The rapid development of tolerance (within three to four days) may explain in part why use of LSD-like drugs generally is intermittent. There currently is no role for medication in the treatment of hallucinogen withdrawal.

MARIJUANA

Marijuana Intoxication. The major psychological and physiological effects of marijuana are mediated by the interaction of delta-9-tetrahydrocannabinol (THC) with specific cannabinoid (CB1) receptors on nerve cells (Ameri, 1999), the regional distribution of which in the human brain is consistent with the known effects of marijuana (Glass, Dragunow et al., 1997). In animal studies, THC effects are reduced or blocked by CB1 receptor antagonists (Huestis, Gorelick et al., 2001).

Psychological and Behavioral Effects of Marijuana Intoxication: The initial—usually desired—psychological effects of marijuana intoxication include relaxation, euphoria, slowed time perception, altered (often intensified) sensory perception, increased awareness of the environment, and increased appetite. As with hallucinogens, psychological set and social setting can substantially influence the quality of the experience. Higher doses, repeated use, or a stressful setting are associated with adverse effects such as hypervigilance, anxiety, paranoia, derealization and depersonalization (commonly associated with altered time sense) (Mathew, Wilson et al., 1993), acute panic (associated with anxiety), illusions or hallucinations (usually auditory or visual), psychosis, or delirium (Brust, 1998). Preexisting psychopathology increases the risk of adverse events such as panic attack or psychosis (Szuster, Pontius et al., 1988). Table 4 summarizes the adverse psychological effects of marijuana intoxication.

Psychotic states resulting from marijuana intoxication are rare (Hurlbut, 1991), except in individuals with a preexisting or underlying psychotic condition. Some cases may be the result of adulterants such as PCP or LSD. Delirium is even rarer, but may occur with very large doses. Oral ingestion of marijuana may produce a higher incidence of adverse reactions than does smoking. The latter route of administration provides an immediate, titratable effect (by varying depth and duration of inhalation), while the former produces no immediate effect. This may provoke the user into taking repeated doses while awaiting the (delayed) effect, resulting in a larger than intended cumulative dose.

Medical Effects of Marijuana Intoxication: The acute physiological effects of oral or smoked marijuana intoxication include conjunctival injection ("red eye"), tachycardia, orthostatic hypotension and dry mouth (Table 5). These generally are mild, self-limiting, and do not require medical treatment (Selden, Clark et al., 1990). There are no established cases of human fatalities from pure marijuana overdose. Intravenous use of marijuana, while extremely rare, is associated with a serious syndrome of tachycardia, hypotension, fever, vomiting, diarrhea, and rhabdomyolysis, which may progress to renal failure (Brandenburg & Wernick, 1986).

Management of Marijuana Intoxication: Adverse effects of marijuana intoxication tend to be self-limited and

TABLE 6. Procedures for Managing Acute Phencyclidine (PCP) Intoxication

Procedure	Stage I	Stage II	Stage III
Monitor level of consciousness	Yes	Yes	Yes
Monitor vital signs	Yes	Yes	Yes
Collect blood and urine samples for toxicology	Yes	Yes	Yes
Lower body temperature	Loosen clothing	Sponging, ice packs	Sponging, ice packs
Catheterize urinary bladder	No	Yes	Yes
Gastric lavage	No	Sometimes	Yes
Oral suctioning	Rarely	Gently, as needed	Yes
Tracheal suctioning	No	Sometimes	Yes
Insert nasogastric tube	No	Sometimes	Yes
Neuromuscular blockade and mechanical ventilation	No	Sometimes	Sometimes

SOURCE: Milhorn, 1991.

often can be managed without medication. The patient should be kept in a quiet environment and offered supportive reassurance. If immediate pharmacologic intervention is needed to control severe agitation or anxiety, benzodiazepines are preferred to neuroleptics, although there are no controlled studies to confirm this. Psychosis usually responds promptly to low doses of antipsychotic medication (Schnoll & Daghestani, 1986).

A synthetic, selective CB1 receptor antagonist currently is undergoing human trials (Huestis, Gorelick et al., 2001). Should this or a similar compound prove safe and effective, it could be used to treat marijuana intoxication in the same way that naloxone acts on opiate intoxication.

Marijuana Withdrawal. Acute marijuana withdrawal, although not a recognized syndrome in the *DSM-IV* (APA, 1994), is reported by 16% to 25% of heavy marijuana users (Cottler, Schuckit et al., 1995; Wiesbeck, Schuckit et al., 1996) and about half of those seeking treatment for

marijuana dependence (Budney, Novy et al., 1999). Symptoms include irritability, anxiety, anger, restlessness, anorexia, insomnia, diaphoresis, nausea, diarrhea, muscle twitches, and flu-like symptoms. The syndrome almost always is mild and self-limited.

Management of Marijuana Withdrawal: Marijuana withdrawal rarely requires medical treatment. The antidepressant bupropion (300 mg/day) exacerbated marijuana withdrawal symptoms in a small case series (Haney, Ward et al., 2001). The serotonergic antidepressant trazodone has been reported helpful in relieving severe withdrawal insomnia (Duffy & Milin, 1996).

PHENCYCLIDINE (PCP)
Phencyclidine Intoxication. PCP and its analogue ketamine are dissociative anesthetics that produce a range of intoxicated states, which can be grouped into three stages (Gorelick & Balster, 1995; Rappolt, Gay et al., 1980):

Stage I—conscious, with psychological effects but (at most) mild physiological effects; Stage II—stuporous or in a light coma, yet responsive to pain; and Stage III—comatose and unresponsive to pain. The main effects of PCP and ketamine appear to be mediated by their action as noncompetitive antagonists of the NMDA-glutamate excitatory amino acid neurotransmitter receptor, although direct effects on other neurotransmitter systems (such as dopamine) may occur at high doses (Gorelick & Balster, 1995; Jentsch & Roth, 1999).

Treatment of PCP intoxication is largely supportive and aimed at controlling or reversing specific signs and symptoms (Baldridge & Bessen, 1990). No clinically useful PCP antagonist is yet available. The anticonvulsant lamotrigine (300 mg daily), which inhibits glutamate release, was found to reduce the psychological and cognitive effects of ketamine in a small experimental trial (Anand, Charney et al., 2000).

Ketamine is a PCP analogue, legally marketed as an anesthetic, which has pharmacologic effects similar to those of PCP, although shorter acting and somewhat less potent. In recent years, ketamine has enjoyed increasing popularity as a substance of abuse and "club drug" (Dotson, Ackerman et al., 1995; Rome, 2001). The spectrum of psychiatric complications from ketamine intoxication appears similar to that from PCP, but there is very little published data on the treatment of ketamine intoxication.

Psychological and Behavioral Effects of PCP Intoxication: Table 4 summarizes the psychological and behavioral effects of PCP intoxication and overdose. The time course of psychological effects is highly variable and unpredictable, so that even a recovering patient should be kept under observation until all symptoms have resolved (typically at least 12 hours) (Baldridge & Bessen, 1990; Woolf, Vourakis et al., 1980). Patients may "emerge" from one stage of intoxication to the next; that is, a stuporous or comatose patient in Stage II or III may enter Stage I and become agitated and delirious (Milhorn, 1991; Rappolt, Gay et al., 1980). Similarly, a conscious patient in Stage I may suddenly become comatose (Baldridge & Bessen, 1990). The entire clinical episode may require up to six weeks to resolve (Schuckit, 2000).

The psychiatric manifestations of Stage I intoxication can resemble a variety of psychiatric syndromes, making differential diagnosis difficult in the absence of toxicology results or a history of recent PCP intake. Common syndromes seen in treatment settings include delirium, psychosis without delirium, catatonia, hypomania with euphoria, and depression with lethargy. Agitated or bizarre behavior, with increased risk of violence, can occur with any psychiatric presentation (Gorelick & Balster, 1995; Hurlbut, 1991). Because of the analgesic effect of PCP, patients may not report the existence of even serious injuries (which may be self-inflicted) (Brust, 1998).

Medical Effects of PCP Intoxication: PCP intoxication at the mild Stage I desired by users is associated with few serious medical complications (see Table 5) (Gorelick & Balster, 1995). Common medical effects at this stage include nystagmus (especially horizontal), tachycardia, increased blood pressure, ataxia, dysarthria, numbness, increased salivation, and hyperreflexia (Brust, 1998; Weiss, Greenfield et al., 1994). Higher stages are associated with severe medical effects (Table 5), including hypertension, stroke, cardiac failure, seizures, rhabdomyolysis, acute renal failure, coma, and death.

Management of Psychological and Behavioral Effects of PCP Intoxication: Mild Stage I PCP intoxication is best treated without medication. The patient should be isolated in a quiet room with unobtrusive observation, and external stimuli eliminated as much as possible. Frequent or intrusive contact or aggressive medical intervention may worsen the situation and should be avoided. Reassuring, reality-oriented communication ("talking down") rarely works with such patients (Brust, 1998). Urine acidification may increase renal clearance of PCP, but is of doubtful clinical utility at this level of intoxication (Gorelick, Wilkins et al., 1986). Cranberry juice, commonly used as a urine acidifier in the non-medical setting, never has been clearly shown to decrease urine pH (Soloway & Smith, 1988). Benzodiazepines should be used if medication is needed to control severe anxiety, agitation, or psychotic behavior (Gorelick & Balster, 1995), although they may delay renal clearance of PCP at high doses (Milhorn, 1991).

If benzodiazepines are insufficient to control psychosis, high-potency neuroleptics such as haloperidol (5 mg IM) or droperidol should be used (Giannini, Underwood et al., 2000). They are less likely than other neuroleptics to produce anticholinergic or cardiovascular side effects that may exacerbate PCP's own anticholinergic and cardiovascular effects. Because neuroleptics may lower the seizure threshold, they should be avoided if seizures are a concern. No controlled trials have compared the efficacy and safety of benzodiazepines directly with the neuroleptics (Gorelick & Balster, 1995).

Management of Medical Effects of PCP Intoxication: The mild medical effects commonly associated with Stage I

TABLE 7. Medications for Treating Acute Phencyclidine (PCP) Intoxication

Medication	STAGE I Conscious	STAGE II Stuporous to Unconscious; Deep Pain Response Intact	STAGE III Unconscious, Unresponsive to Deep Pain
Syrup of ipecac	Not indicated	Not indicated	Not indicated
Activated charcoal	Not indicated	If needed	50-150 g initially, then 30-40 g every 6-8 hours
Diazepam	For agitation: 10-30 mg orally or 2.5 IV, up to 25 mg total	For muscle rigidity: same dosage, IM or IV, as for agitation in Stage I	For muscle rigidity: same as for Stage II. For status epilepticus: 5-10 mg IV, to 30 mg total
Lorazepam	For agitation: 2-4 mg IM as needed	Not indicated	Not indicated
Haloperidol	For psychosis: 5-10 mg	Not indicated	Not indicated
Ascorbic Acid	Not indicated	For urine pH < 5.5: 0.5-1.5 g every 4-6 hours as needed	As for Stage II
Hydralazine	Not indicated	For hypertension: 5-10 mg IV	For hypertension: 10-20 mg IV
Propranolol	Not indicated	For hypertension: 1 mg IV every 30 mins as needed up to 8 mg total	As for Stage II
Furosemide	Not indicated	For increased urinary output: 20-40 mg IV every 6 hours.	As for Stage II
Aminophylline	Not indicated	For bronchospasm: 250 mg IV	As for Stage II

IV = intravenous; IM = intramuscular.
SOURCE: Milhorn, 1991.

intoxication usually do not need specific medical treatment. Tachycardia and hypertension can be treated with beta-blockers such as propranolol, or calcium channel blockers such as verapamil, although there are no controlled trials to substantiate their efficacy.

Stage II and III intoxication are medical emergencies that require treatment in a comprehensive medical setting to maintain life-support functions until the drug has been eliminated from the body (Gorelick & Balster, 1995). Tables 6 and 7 summarize medical treatments for acute PCP intoxication. In this context, increasing the renal clearance of PCP with forced diuresis and urine acidification (pH <5) may be helpful (Brust, 1998). This can be done by administering ammonium chloride—2.75 mEq/kg in 60 ml of saline every six hours through a nasogastric tube and 2 gm of IV ascorbic acid in 500 ml of IV fluid every six hours (Weiss, Greenfield et al., 1994). IM ascorbic acid also has been used successfully (Giannini, Loiselle et al., 1987). Caution should be exercised to avoid causing metabolic acidosis, especially in the presence of drugs such as barbiturates and salicylates, whose renal clearance is delayed by acidification.

Another pharmacokinetic approach currently undergoing animal testing is administration of anti-PCP monoclonal antibody binding fragments (Hardin, Wessinger et al., 1998). These antibody fragments bind to PCP molecules in the body and prevent them from entering the brain, thereby reducing the acute effects of a PCP dose. Further research is needed to establish the safety and efficacy of this antibody approach in humans.

Phencyclidine Withdrawal. Although a PCP withdrawal syndrome is not recognized in the *DSM-IV*, about one-quarter of heavy PCP users report withdrawal symptoms (Cottler, Schuckit et al., 1995), including depression, anxiety, irritability, hypersomnolence, diaphoresis, and tremor (Brust, 1998; Tennant, Rawson et al., 1981), although it is not clear to what extent these represent a true withdrawal syndrome. Tricyclic antidepressants such as desipramine may reduce the psychological symptoms associated with discontinuation of PCP use, but there is no evidence that such treatment improves the outcome of PCP addiction (Giannini, Loiselle et al., 1993; Tennant, Rawson et al., 1981).

Prolonged Psychiatric Sequelae (Flashbacks): All hallucinogens and PCP have the potential to trigger long-lasting (days to weeks) psychiatric sequelae, ranging from prolonged states of anxiety or depression to both mild and pronounced psychotic states. A patient's risk of a prolonged psychiatric reaction appears to depend on several factors: the patient's premorbid psychopathology, the number of prior exposures to the drug, and the patient's history of polydrug use (Strassman, 1984). Prolonged reactions occasionally are reported in apparently well-adjusted individuals who have no obvious risk factors. Some users, while maintaining otherwise normal functioning, suffer from perceptual disorders that may last for years, including auditory and visual hallucinations such as after images seen from moving objects. Prolonged psychotic reactions to PCP are almost always associated with premorbid psychopathology (Erard, Luisada et al., 1980; Gwirtsman, Winkop et al., 1984).

Treatment of prolonged anxiety or depression usually is psychosocial, but may involve medication if symptoms become sufficiently severe. Treatment of prolonged psychosis essentially follows guidelines for treatment of chronic functional psychosis. Patients may present with wide-ranging symptomatology: apathy, insomnia, hypomania, dissociative states, formal thought disorder, hallucinations, delusions, and paranoia. An observation period of at least several days with no or minimal medication (such as sedatives) is helpful to ensure an accurate diagnosis.

The term "flashback" has been given to brief episodes (usually lasting a few seconds) in which aspects of a previous hallucinogenic drug experience are unexpectedly re-experienced. Flashbacks are associated principally with the LSD-like hallucinogens, although they can occur following use of MDMA, PCP, and, occasionally, marijuana (Abraham, Aldridge et al., 1996; Strassman, 1984; Weiss, Greenfield et al., 1994). Flashbacks can precipitate considerable anxiety, particularly if the original drug experience had negative overtones. Re-experience of perceptual effects is most common, but somatic and emotional components of the original experience also may reoccur. Flashbacks may occur spontaneously or be triggered by stress, exercise, another drug (such as marijuana), or a situation reminiscent of the original drug experience.

Flashbacks almost always are brief and self-limiting. Treatment usually involves no more than alleviating anxiety with supportive reassurance. Over time, flashbacks tend to decrease in frequency, duration, and intensity, as long as no further hallucinogens are taken (Strassman, 1984). Benzodiazepines may be helpful in treating secondary anxiety. Neuroleptics are not indicated, as haloperidol has been reported to transiently worsen flashbacks (Moskowitz, 1971; Strassman, 1984). Recent case reports suggest that selective serotonin reuptake inhibitor antidepressants or naltrexone may help reduce flashbacks (Lerner, Oyffe et al.,

1997; Young, 1997). Flashbacks that occur more than a year after the original drug experience suggest another etiology, such as a functional psychosis.

CLUB DRUGS

"Club drugs" are a pharmacologically heterogeneous group of drugs associated with a youth subculture that revolves around late-night dance parties known as "raves" or "trances" (Doyon, 2001; Rome, 2001). The illicit use of these substances was popularized in this setting because of their perceived ability to enhance the sensory experience and allow for long periods of dancing to repetitive music. Common club drugs include MDMA ("Ecstasy"), an amphetamine analogue with stimulant and hallucinogenic properties, as well as gamma-hydroxybutyrate (GHB) and flunitrazepam (Rohypnol®), both of which are CNS depressants.

MDMA ("Ecstasy")

"Ecstasy" is the common street name for 3,4-methylenedioxymethamphetamine (MDMA). Related amphetamine analogues such as 3,4-methylenedioxyethylamphetamine (MDEA, "Eve"), 3,4-methylenedioxyamphetamine (MDA), and N-methyl-1-(3,4- methylene-dioxyphenyl)-2-butanamine (MBDB) also may be present in street preparations. The effects of MDMA are those of a stimulant combined with a mild hallucinogen. "Herbal Ecstasy" often refers to preparations containing the stimulant ephedrine. "Liquid Ecstasy" is a street name for gamma-hydroxybutyrate (GHB) (see the discussion below).

MDMA was introduced in 1914 as an appetite suppressant, but was not approved for medical use and is not currently manufactured by any pharmaceutical company (Burgess, O'Donohoe et al., 2000; Doyon, 2001; Kalant, 2001; Murray, 2001). It was used experimentally as a psychotherapy enhancer in the 1960s and 1970s and became popular as a "recreational" drug, especially on college campuses and dance clubs. Following increasing reports of toxicity, it was restricted in 1977 under the Misuse of Drugs Act in the United Kingdom and placed in Schedule I of the U.S. Controlled Substances Act in 1985.

MDMA usually is taken orally as a pill or tablet, at doses of 50 to 250 mg per tablet. Less commonly, it may be held under the tongue, added to beverages as a powder, or taken intranasally (Rome, 2001). MDMA often is taken concurrently with other drugs, such as LSD (in a combination called "candyflipping"), for enhanced effect. Dextromethorphan (available in over-the-counter cough medicines) also is a frequent concomitant drug, and may be substituted for MDMA in street preparations (Baggott, Heifets et al., 2000). "Stacking" refers to the practice of taking multiple MDMA doses over a short period of time, often alternating with other drugs to enhance the experience. For example, amphetamine or cocaine may be used initially to augment the experience, followed later by a CNS depressant such as alcohol, marijuana, or GHB to temper the "coming down" (Rome, 2001). Menthol, camphor, or ephedrine may be applied to the nasal mucosa or chest wall to enhance the drug experience (Doyon, 2001).

MDMA has good oral bioavailability and readily crosses the blood-brain barrier (Doyon, 2001; Kalant, 2001). The onset of action is within 30 minutes and peak plasma concentrations are achieved in one to three hours (Doyon, 2001). The elimination half-life is seven to eight hours. Because MDMA is a weak acid, this is delayed to 16 to 31 hours with alkaline urine. MDMA is metabolized by several hepatic microsomal enzymes, chiefly CYP2D6. Individuals who are genetically deficient in CYP2D6 (up to 10% of Caucasians) are theoretically at increased risk of developing MDMA toxicity (de la Torre, Farre et al., 2000).

MDMA appears to have non-linear kinetics because the higher-affinity enzymes become saturated at relatively low drug concentrations (Kalant, 2001). This results in disproportionately large increases in drug concentrations in response to small increases in dose (de la Torre, Farre et al., 2000) and may account for the poor correlation between plasma concentration and toxicity (Henry, Jeffreys et al., 1992). A major MDMA metabolite is methylenedioxyamphetamine (MDA), which also is pharmacologically active and has a longer elimination half-life of 16 to 38 hours.

MDMA acts at presynaptic nerve endings to release monoamine neurotransmitters by interfering with the monoamine transporters (reuptake pumps) (Burgess, O'Donohoe et al., 2000; Doyon, 2001; Kalant, 2001). The predominant effect is on serotonin, but catecholamine neurotransmitters also are affected. In animal studies, MDMA causes a dose-dependent depletion of serotonin and a reduction in functional serotonin transporters. Chronic MDMA exposure causes a reduction in serotonergic neurons and degeneration of serotonergic axons. The relevance of these animal findings to MDMA serotonin neurotoxicity in human users is controversial, in part because most animal studies use MDMA doses far higher than those used by humans (Vollenweider, Gamma et al., 1999). Chronic

MDMA users do have lower serotonin and serotonin metabolite concentrations in cerebrospinal fluid, lower density of serotonin transporters in brain (demonstrated by PET scanning), and reduced hormone response to stimulation of the serotonin system (Curran, 2000; Kalant, 2001; McCann, Eligulashvili et al., 2000; Vollenweider, Gamma et al., 1999). Many of these changes show a significant correlation with degree of MDMA exposure, consistent with a direct causal relationship. However, several methodologic limitations weaken the conclusiveness of most human studies. These limitations include lack of knowledge of subjects' baseline function prior to MDMA use and inability to control for use of other drugs and lifestyle factors that also could influence brain function.

MDMA Intoxication. The diagnosis of MDMA intoxication is made by history of drug intake and/or analysis of unused drug. Most signs and symptoms are not specific to MDMA, but resemble those of stimulants or hallucinogens. MDMA is not detected by routine urine or blood drug screens, which may be positive for amphetamines (products of MDMA metabolism) (Doyon, 2001).

Gastric lavage with activated charcoal may be helpful within the first hour after ingestion, especially if other drugs also have been taken. Induced emesis is not recommended because of the risk of CNS depression (Doyon, 2001). Acidification of urine would quicken MDMA elimination, but usually is contraindicated because it would increase the risk of metabolic acidosis and exacerbate renal toxicity from rhabdomyolysis (Doyon, 2001).

Psychological and Behavioral Effects of MDMA Intoxication: Low to moderate oral doses of MDMA (50 to 150 mg) typically produce an intense initial effect (known as "coming on" or "rush"), especially if taken on an empty stomach, that may last 30 to 45 minutes (Rome, 2001). These desired effects include increased wakefulness and energy, euphoria, heightened sensory perception, sociability, and increased empathy and sense of closeness to others (Burgess, O'Donohoe et al., 2000; Doyon, 2001; Kalant, 2001). The latter effects led to experimental use of MDMA as an aid to psychotherapy (Murray, 2001). The initial phase is followed by several hours of less intense experience ("plateau"), during which repetitive dancing is common. Users start to "come down" three to six hours after ingestion (Rome, 2001).

Undesired effects may occur with repeated use or at higher doses. These include hyperactivity, insomnia, anxiety, agitation, flight of ideas, hallucinations, depersonali-zation, and bizarre or reckless behavior. Some users develop panic attacks, brief psychotic episodes, or delirium, which usually resolve rapidly as the drug effect wears off. Initial treatment should be the same as for hallucinogen intoxication: placement in a quiet, reassuring environment, with observation to reduce the risk of unintended self-injury. Physical restraints are contraindicated because they may exacerbate anxiety and increase the risk of rhabdomyolysis. If severe or persisting symptoms require medication, benzodiazepines are preferred. Neuroleptics should be avoided as much as possible because they may increase the risk of hyperthermia and seizures. A high-potency neuroleptic such as haloperidol should be used if necessary. The role of the atypical antipsychotics in this situation remains unclear. A recent human study found that a single dose of citalopram (40 mg IV) significantly reduced the mood and perceptual effects of experimental MDMA intoxication (Liechti, Baumann et al., 2000), suggesting that selective serotonin uptake inhibitors might have a future role in treating MDMA intoxication.

A few users may develop persisting depression or recurrent psychotic symptoms or panic attacks, which require psychiatric treatment.

Medical Effects of MDMA Intoxication: The acute physical effects of MDMA at low to moderate doses resemble those of a stimulant: increased muscle tension, jaw clenching, tooth grinding (bruxism), restlessness, ataxia, headache, nausea, decreased appetite, dry mouth, dilated pupils, and increased heart rate and blood pressure (Burgess, O'Donohoe et al., 2000; Doyon, 2001; Kalant, 2001). Doses >200 mg are associated with life-threatening toxicities that can be grouped into four major syndromes. Most dangerous is hyperthermia, which results from a combination of increased physical activity (as through vigorous dancing), warm environment (as in a crowded, poorly ventilated dance club), and disruption of thermoregulation by the drug, often exacerbated by dehydration (Doyon, 2001; Kalant, 2001). The syndrome may resemble that of severe heatstroke. The high body temperature causes rhabdomyolysis (with resulting myoglobinuria and renal failure), liver damage, and/or disseminated intravascular coagulation (resulting in hemorrhage). Treatment is based on early recognition, close monitoring of serum creatinine kinase levels (to detect rhabdomyolysis), and reversal of the hyperthermia. Core body temperatures >102° F. call for urgent measures such as ice-water sponging, gastric or bladder lavage with cool liquids, and intravenous infusion of chilled saline. Muscle paralysis with intubation may be required for refractory, ongoing rhabdomyolysis. Rhabdomyolysis treatment includes vigorous hydration and alkalinization of the urine to minimize myoglobin precipitation in the renal tubules.

Benzodiazepines help control both the hyperthermia and agitation. Neuroleptics should be avoided because they interfere with heat dissipation and lower the seizure threshold. Recent case series suggest that dantrolene (1 mg/kg IV) also may be very helpful. Because of similarities between MDMA toxicity and the serotonin syndrome (see the discussion below), serotonin antagonists such as methysergide and cyproheptadine have been used successfully.

Acute hepatic toxicity from MDMA may be related to metabolism into reactive intermediaries that deplete hepatic glutathione, resulting in cell death (Kalant, 2001). The clinical picture can vary from a mild hepatitis (marked by enlarged, tender liver and elevated serum liver enzymes) that resolves spontaneously over several weeks to fulminant liver failure requiring transplantation. Liver toxicity may be exacerbated by hyperthermia.

Acute cardiovascular toxicity from MDMA is the result of increased catecholamine activity (Kalant, 2001). This may cause hypertension, with risk of blood vessel rupture and hemorrhage, or tachycardia and cardiac arrhythmia. The preferred treatment is an adrenergic antagonist with both alpha and beta blocking activity, combined with a vasodilator such as nitroglycerin or nitroprusside if needed to control blood pressure. A pure beta-adrenergic blocker should be avoided because of the remaining unopposed alpha-adrenergic stimulation, resulting in vasoconstriction and worsening hypertension. Hypertensive crisis unresponsive to mixed adrenergic blockers and vaso-dilators should be treated with an alpha-adrenergic antagonist such as phentolamine (Ghuran & Nolan, 2000). Cardiac ischemia or arrhythmia should be treated by standard clinical protocols such as the American Heart Association's Advanced Cardiac Life Support (ACLS) guidelines. Agitation should be controlled with a short-acting benzodiazepine such as lorazepam.

Acute neurologic toxicity from MDMA often is the result of hyponatremia ("water intoxication"), which may cause seizures and intracranial fluid shifts that compress the brain stem into the foramen magnum (Kalant, 2001). The hyponatremia is caused by loss of sodium in sweat (as during vigorous dancing in a warm environment) and hemodilution from drinking large amounts of water and the antidiuretic effect of MDMA. The conservative initial treatment is fluid restriction. Profound hyponatremia has been treated with hypertonic saline solution (Halachanova, Sansone et al., 2001). Intravenous benzodiazepines should be used to control seizures.

MDMA Withdrawal. Symptoms during the first few days after MDMA use may resemble a mild form of stimulant withdrawal or "crash," with depression, anxiety, fatigue, and difficulty concentrating (Kalant, 2001; Rome, 2001). These usually resolve without treatment.

Medical Effects of MDMA Withdrawal: There is no evidence of a physically prominent or distinctive withdrawal syndrome associated with MDMA that would require specific pharmacologic treatment. Users may complain of muscle pain and stiffness in the jaw, neck, lower back, and limbs for the first two to three days after use (Kalant, 2001), which may be the result of MDMA-induced muscle tension and the vigorous dancing often associated with MDMA use. There is some evidence of increased variability of heart rate and blood pressure for several days after MDMA use.

GAMMA-HYDROXYBUTYRATE (GHB)

Gamma-hydroxybutyrate (GHB or "liquid Ecstasy") is a naturally occurring metabolite of the neurotransmitter gamma-aminobutyric acid (GABA). It was synthesized in 1960 as an anesthetic agent, but currently is used medically only as a treatment for narcolepsy (approved in Europe; experimental in the U.S.) (Doyon, 2001; Shannon & Quang, 2000). GHB became popular in the late 1980s as a dietary supplement, sleep aid, and bodybuilding agent. Recreational use was promoted by its reputed aphrodisiac, disinhibitory, and amnestic effects, short duration of action, absence of "hangover," and nondetectability by standard drug screens. Reports of adverse effects led the U.S. Food and Drug Administration (FDA) to ban over-the-counter sales in 1990. Further federal regulation was hindered by the Dietary Supplement Health and Education Act of 1994, until GHB was placed in CSA Schedule I by Congressional action in the Hillary J. Farias and Samantha Reid Date-Rape Drug Prohibition Act of 2000 (O'Connell, Kaye et al., 2000). In response to these restrictions, users turned to the legal precursors gammabutyrolactone (GBL, an industrial solvent found in floor strippers and some household products) and 1,4-butanediol (1,4-BD), which are readily metabolized to GBH in the body. In 1999, the FDA asked manufacturers to voluntarily recall GBL and issued a public health alert on 1,4-BD. All three drugs still can be obtained in the U.S., either as stock imported from Europe, sold legally as dietary supplements, or manufactured in clandestine laboratories.

GHB is taken orally as a liquid or in a powder mixed into drinks. A typical dose is one to three teaspoons or capfuls. GHB is rapidly absorbed from the gastrointestinal tract and readily crosses the blood-brain barrier. Effects begin within 15 minutes of ingestion and last 2 to 4 hours. The blood elimination half-life is about 30 minutes, largely due to rapid redistribution into other tissues. GHB is metabolized to succinic semialdehyde, which eventually enters the Krebs cycle. Less than 5% of parent drug appears in the urine.

The mechanism of action of GHB is not completely understood. Because of its structural similarity to gamma-aminobutyric acid (GABA), it is thought to interact with central GABA receptors (Doyon, 2001). Specific GHB receptors also have been identified in mammalian brain.

GHB Intoxication. The diagnosis of GHB intoxication is based on clinical suspicion, a history of drug intake, and/or analysis of unused drug. The signs and symptoms are not specific for GHB, but resemble those of any CSN depressant. GHB is not detected by routine drug toxicology assays.

There is no proven antidote for GHB intoxication. Physostigmine, naloxone, and flumazenil have reversed some GHB effects in small case series or animal studies (Caldicott & Kuhn, 2001; Shannon & Quang, 2000), but should be considered experimental. Gastric lavage usually is not helpful because of rapid GHB absorption, but activated charcoal may be.

Psychological and Behavioral Effects of GHB Intoxication: The desired acute effects of GHB at low oral doses (<20 mg/kg) include relaxation, euphoria, sedation, disinhibition, sociability, and anterograde amnesia (Doyon, 2001; Shannon & Quang, 2000). Higher doses produce somnolence, confusion, and hallucinations. Unintended overdose may occur because of GHB's very steep dose-response curve and the great variability in potency of street preparations. First-time users often underestimate the potency of GHB. The effects are prolonged and intensified when taken with other CNS depressants, such as alcohol. Patients recovering from acute GHB intoxication may wake up abruptly with a clear sensorium, or may go through a brief period of agitation and combativeness.

Medical Effects of GHB Intoxication: Low to moderate oral doses of GHB may cause headache, dizziness, ataxia,

hypotonia, and vomiting (Doyon, 2001; Shannon & Quang, 2000). Higher doses (≥ 30 mg/kg) may cause incontinence, myoclonic movements, bradycardia, hypotension, hypothermia, generalized tonic-clonic seizures, and coma. Most patients recover completely within several hours with supportive care and do not require intubation. However, death may result from respiratory depression, so that intubation and mechanical ventilation may be indicated in severe cases. Seizures should be controlled with benzodiazepines, symptomatic bradycardia with atropine, and symptomatic hypotension with intravenous saline. Similar adverse effects occur with GBL and 1,4-BD (Zvosec, Smith et al., 2001).

GHB Withdrawal. Cessation of chronic GHB or GBL use leads to a discrete withdrawal syndrome resembling that of sedative-hypnotic withdrawal: Anxiety, restlessness, insomnia, tremor, nystagmus, tachycardia, and hypertension usually appear within six hours of last drug use (Chin, 2001; Dyer, Roth et al., 2001). Left untreated, mild symptoms usually resolve gradually over one to two weeks (Dyer, Roth et al., 2001). More severe withdrawal may cause delirium with hallucinations, psychosis, agitation, and autonomic instability (Sivilotti, Burns et al., 2001). GHB withdrawal seizures have not been reported.

Most cases of GHB withdrawal can be effectively managed through use of a long-acting benzodiazepine, tapering the dose after the symptoms have been controlled (as for sedative-hypnotic withdrawal) (Dyer, Roth et al., 2001; Chin, 2001). Severe cases may require high doses (several hundred mg) or parenteral administration. Patients unresponsive to benzodiazepines may benefit from pentobarbital, propofol (Sivilotti, Burns et al., 2001), or chloral hydrate (Dyer, Roth et al., 2001).

FLUNITRAZEPAM (Rohypnol®)

Flunitrazepam (Rohypnol®, also known as "roofies," or the "date rape pill") is a potent, fast-acting benzodiazepine that frequently causes anterograde amnesia (Rome, 2001; Schwartz, Milteer et al., 2000). It is legally manufactured and marketed in Europe and Latin America, but is illegal in the U.S. because of its association with "date rape." It comes in 1 mg and 2 mg tablets. Flunitrazepam is difficult to detect with routine toxicology screens because of its low concentration and short half-life.

Flunitrazepam Intoxication. Flunitrazepam intoxication resembles intoxication with other benzodiazepines, and features sedation, disinhibition, anterograde amnesia, confusion, ataxia, bradycardia, hypotension, and respiratory depression. Overdose rarely is life-threatening unless the drug is combined with another CNS depressant, such as alcohol. Treatment is supportive; activated charcoal and gastric lavage may be helpful. When respiratory depression or circulatory compromise are severe, the benzodiazepine antagonist flumazenil (Romazicon®) may be used, albeit cautiously. Flumazenil precipitates acute withdrawal in patients who are physically dependent on benzodiazepines and lowers the seizure threshold, thus increasing the risk of withdrawal seizures. Flumazenil is effective for about 20 minutes, so that repeated dosing is necessary to avoid resedation by flunitrazepam, which has a half-life of at least nine hours.

Flunitrazepam Withdrawal. A typical sedative-hypnotic withdrawal syndrome can develop after cessation of chronic flunitrazepam use, as is the case with any benzodiazepine (Woods & Winger, 1997). Withdrawal symptoms can develop up to 36 hours after the last dose and include anxiety, tremors, insomnia, and agitation. Treatment of withdrawal involves supportive measures and substitution with cross-tolerant medications such as lorazepam or clonazepam, followed by gradual tapering.

SEROTONIN SYNDROME

The serotonin syndrome may account for some of the severe complications associated with intoxication and overdose on amphetamines or MDMA, especially when used in combination with other drugs or medications that increase serotonergic activity (Demirkiran, Jankovic et al., 1996; Henry, Jeffreys et al., 1992). The syndrome is a triad of signs and symptoms, consisting of cognitive and behavioral changes (confusion, agitation, lethargy, delirium, or coma), autonomic instability (low-grade fever, tachycardia, diaphoresis, nausea, vomiting, diarrhea, dilated pupils, abdominal pain, hypertension, tachypnea), and neuromuscular changes (myoclonus, nystagmus, hyperreflexia, rigidity, trismus, tremor) (Carbone, 2000; Mason, Morris et al., 2000). Each component of the triad appears in about half of patients, sometimes making diagnosis difficult (Carbone, 2000).

The differential diagnosis includes neuroleptic malignant syndrome (with which it is most commonly confused), sepsis, heat stroke, *delirium tremens*, and sympathomimetic or anticholinergic poisoning (Carbone, 2000; Mason, Mor-

ris et al., 2000). Patients with neuroleptic malignant syndrome differ from those with serotonin syndrome in that they are more likely to present with extrapyramidal signs and autonomic instability and rarely present with the neuromuscular changes common in serotonin syndrome (Carbone, 2000; Gillman, 1999).

The serotonin syndrome is the result of excessive stimulation of 5-HT1A receptors in the nervous system (Carbone, 2000; Mason, Morris et al., 2000). This can occur through several different pathways: activation of serotonin receptors by agonists, enhanced release of serotonin (by MDMA or amphetamines), decreased presynaptic serotonin reuptake (by cocaine or SSRI antidepressants), decreased serotonin metabolism (by amphetamines or monoamine oxidase inhibitors), and increased serotonin synthesis. The serotonin syndrome is most commonly seen after ingestion of two or more drugs with such actions, but also may occur with a single drug. The true incidence is unknown (Mason, Morris et al., 2000).

The onset of the serotonin syndrome generally is within 24 hours of medication initiation, increase in dose, or overdose (Mason, Morris et al., 2000). Laboratory abnormalities are nonspecific, but elevated CPK, liver transaminases, WBC, serum bicarbonate, and evidence of disseminated intravascular coagulation (DIC) may occur in severe cases (Carbone, 2000; Mason, Morris et al., 2000). In severe cases, or in the absence of appropriate diagnosis and treatment, there may be progression to rhabdomyolysis, hyperthermia, renal failure, DIC, and death (Carbone, 2000; Mason, Morris et al., 2000).

Effective treatment of the serotonin syndrome requires early identification, immediate discontinuation of all serotonergic medications, close monitoring, and supportive care, usually including intravenous hydration (Carbone, 2000; Gillman, 1999; Mason, Morris et al., 2000). Such treatment usually results in a benign, self-limited course. Seventy percent of patients recover with no complications within 24 hours (Mason, Morris et al., 2000). Muscle rigidity and spasm should be controlled with benzodiazepines to prevent rhabdomyolysis. Severe forms of the syndrome may require more aggressive measures, including neuromuscular blocking agents, mechanical ventilation, and external cooling. Nonselective serotonin receptor blockers, such as cyproheptadine or methysergide, have decreased the syndrome's intensity and duration in case series, but they have not yet been evaluated in controlled clinical trials and are not FDA-approved for this indication (Carbone, 2000; Gillman, 1999; Mason, Morris et al., 2000).

WITHDRAWAL FROM MULTIPLE DRUGS

Multiple Sedative-Hypnotics. Withdrawal from dependence on multiple sedative-hypnotic agents, including alcohol, is best managed in the same way as withdrawal from a single such drug: by using tapering dosages of a single, longer-acting sedative-hypnotic (Gorelick & Wilkins, 1986; Schuckit, 2000). It usually is safest to focus on managing withdrawal of the longer-acting drug. The time course of withdrawal from multiple sedative-hypnotics is more unpredictable than from single drugs; for example, there may be a bimodal time course of symptomatology if one drug is short-acting and the other is longer-acting. The rate at which the dose is tapered usually should not exceed 10% per day. Safe withdrawal may be facilitated by use of an anticonvulsant such as carbamazepine or valproate, even in the absence of epilepsy or withdrawal seizures. Both medications have been used successfully to treat withdrawal from single sedative-hypnotics (Harris, Roache et al., 2000), but have not been studied in multiple drug withdrawal.

Sedative-Hypnotics With Other Drugs. In the pharmacologic management of patients withdrawing from both sedative-hypnotics and CNS stimulants, it is preferable to treat the sedative-hypnotic withdrawal first, since this poses the greatest difficulty and medical risk. For concurrent addiction to sedative-hypnotics and opiates, concurrent pharmacologic treatment is recommended (Gorelick & Wilkins, 1986; Schuckit, 2000). The patient may be stabilized on an opiate (preferably oral methadone, although codeine can be used if methadone is not available) at the same time that the sedative-hypnotic dose is tapered by 10% per day. Once the sedative-hypnotic withdrawal is completed, opiate withdrawal can begin. Clonidine has been suggested as adjunctive treatment for such mixed sedative-hypnotic and opiate withdrawal, because it can alleviate withdrawal symptoms from both drug classes, but this has not been evaluated systematically.

POPULATION-SPECIFIC CONSIDERATIONS

Neonates. Neonatal drug exposure is a substantial public health problem. Many drugs of abuse are readily transferred from the maternal circulation across the placenta to the fetus. Thus, perinatal drug use by the mother raises the possibility of drug intoxication and/or withdrawal in the newborn (Wagner, Katkaneni et al., 1998). National surveys in the U.S. suggest that up to a quarter-million newborns each year have been exposed to illegal drugs (Kandall, 1999; Smeriglio & Wilcox, 1999). Obtaining an accurate maternal drug use history for the several days preceding delivery is essential and should include information from collateral sources when available. Meconium is a more sensitive substrate for neonatal toxicology than is urine (Lester, El Sohly et al., 2001; Moore, Negursz et al., 1998; Smeriglio & Wilcox, 1999; Wagner, Katkaneni et al., 1998), in part because it reflects exposure over a longer period of time (several weeks).

Neonatal signs and symptoms of drug intoxication or withdrawal often are nonspecific, including sedation, irritability, restlessness, hypertonia, hyperreflexia, tremors, poor feeding, abnormal sleep patterns, respiratory difficulty, and seizures (Kandall, 1999; Wagner, Katkaneni et al., 1998). Stimulants (such as cocaine), marijuana, LSD, and PCP all have been associated with a neonatal withdrawal syndrome, although one that usually is less intense than the opiate withdrawal syndrome.

Perinatal use of stimulants by the mother can be associated with either bradycardia or tachycardia in the newborn (Plessinger, 1998). The additive cardiovascular effects of the stimulant and the normal catecholamine surge during labor may cause fetal distress and retard delivery (Wagner, Katkaneni et al., 1998). These cardiac effects usually resolve as the drug is eliminated from the body. Neonatal stimulant intoxication may be associated with irritability, tremors, hyperactivity, abnormal movements, excessive sucking, and high-pitched and excessive crying for 1 to 2 days, followed by a period of lethargy and hyporeactivity (Kandall, 1999; Wagner, Katkaneni et al., 1998).

Treatment of drug-exposed newborns is largely supportive, with avoidance of overstimulation (Wagner, Katkaneni et al., 1998). Pharmacologic treatment should be used cautiously because it has its own potential for morbidity. Phenobarbital is the preferred medication for newborns with non-opiate drug withdrawal who do require pharmacologic treatment, as when seizures are a factor (Kandall, 1999; Wagner, Katkaneni et al., 1998). A loading dose of 10 to 20 mg/kg/day (in two divided doses, given one to two hours apart) is given until withdrawal is controlled, followed by a maintenance dose of 5 mg/kg/day. After stabilization, doses are tapered by 20%/day for five days, then 20% every 12 hours. Phenobarbital has a long half-life, so plasma concentrations should be checked periodically to avoid drug accumulation and overtreatment.

Older Adults. Little information is available regarding pharmacologic treatment of intoxication, overdose, and withdrawal in elderly patients and how it might differ from treatment in younger individuals. Benzodiazepines should be used with caution in elderly patients because of an increased risk of development of overdose, dependence, and withdrawal (Shorr & Robin, 1994). Older adults are more susceptible to medication-induced delirium, so any medication must be used cautiously in this population (Sumner & Simons, 1994). The recommended dosing approach is "start low and go slow"; that is, start the medication at a lower dose and increase the dose in smaller increments than would be used in younger individuals. Because delirium may present with diverse clinical features, it should be considered in any elderly patient who evidences a change in mental status, personality, or behavior.

Adolescents. There has been little systematic study of drug intoxication or withdrawal in adolescents. Recent research suggests that symptoms of drug dependence and withdrawal similar to those in adults are present in adolescent substance users (Stewart & Brown, 1995), suggesting that adolescents may respond to the same treatment methods that are used in adults. Future clinical research is needed to determine optimal treatment approaches for adolescents.

Women. There has been little systematic study of possible gender differences in the treatment of intoxication, overdose, and withdrawal. Limited anecdotal evidence suggests that pharmacologic treatment for women is similar to that for men, taking into account possible gender differences in medication pharmacokinetics. One area requiring special attention is the effects of intoxication, overdose, and withdrawal and their treatment in pregnancy and the fetus. For example, the benefit to mother and fetus of successful withdrawal treatment must be weighed against the possible ill effects on the fetus of medications such as benzodiazepines and anticonvulsants (Briggs, Freeman et al., 1990), and the risks of inadequately treated withdrawal. Another area in need of further research is the influence of the menstrual cycle on intoxication and withdrawal and their treatment.

REFERENCES

Abraham HD, Aldridge AM & Gogia P (1996). The psychopharmacology of hallucinogens. *Neuropsychopharmacology* 14:285-298.

Ameri A (1999). The effects of cannabinoids on the brain. *Progress in Neurobiology* 58:315-348.

American Psychiatric Association (APA) (1994). *Diagnostic and Statistical Manual of Mental Disorders, 4th Edition*. Washington, DC: American Psychiatric Press.

Anand A, Charney DS, Oren DA et al. (2000). Attenuation of the neuropsychiatric effects of ketamine with lamotrigine. *Archives of General Psychiatry* 57:270-276.

Baggott M, Heifets B, Jones R et al. (2000). Chemical analysis of ecstasy pills. *Journal of the American Medical Association* 284(17):2190.

Baldridge EB & Bessen HA (1990). Phencyclidine. *Emergency Medicine Clinics of North America* 8(3):541-550.

Baumann BM, Perrone J, Hornig SE et al. (2000). Randomized, double-blind, placebo-controlled trial of diazepam, nitroglycerin, or both for treatment of patients with potential cocaine-associated acute coronary syndromes. *Academic Emergency Medicine* 7:878-885.

Blaho K, Logan B, Winbery S et al. (2000). Blood cocaine and metabolite concentrations, clinical findings, and outcome of patients presenting to an ED. *American Journal of Emergency Medicine* 18(5):593-598.

Brady WJ Jr & Duncan CW (1999). Hypoglycemia masquerading as acute psychosis and acute cocaine intoxication. *American Journal of Emergency Medicine* 17(3):318-319.

Brandenburg D & Wernick R (1986). Intravenous marijuana syndrome. *Western Journal of Medicine* 145:94-96.

Briggs GG, Freeman RK & Yaffe SJ (1990). *Reference Guide to Fetal and Neonatal Risk: Drugs in Pregnancy and Lactation, 3rd Edition*. Baltimore, MD: Williams & Wilkins.

Brust JCM (1998). Acute neurologic complications of drug and alcohol abuse. *Neurologic Clinics of North America* 16(2):503-519.

Budney AJ, Novy PL & Hughes JR (1999). Marijuana withdrawal among adults seeking treatment for marijuana dependence. *Addiction* 94(9):1311-1321.

Burgess C, O'Donohoe A & Gill M (2000). Agony and ecstasy: A review of MDMA effects and toxicity. *European Psychiatry* 15: 287-294.

Caldicott D & Kuhn M (2001). Gamma-hydroxybutyrate overdose and physostigmine: Teaching new tricks to an old drug. *Annals of Emergency Medicine* 37(1):99-102.

Callaway CW & Clark RF (1994). Hyperthermia in psychostimulant overdose. *Annals of Emergency Medicine* 24:68-75.

Carbone JR (2000). The neuroleptic malignant and serotonin syndromes. *Emergency Medicine Clinics of North America* 18(2): 317-325.

Carroll ME (1990). PCP and hallucinogens. *Advances in Alcohol & Substance Abuse* 9(1-2):167-190.

Chin RL (2001). A case of severe withdrawal from gamma-hydroxybutyrate. *Annals of Emergency Medicine* 37(5):551-552.

Coffey SF, Dansky BS, Carrigan MH et al. (2000). Acute and protracted cocaine abstinence in an outpatient population: A prospective study of mood, sleep and withdrawal symptoms. *Drug and Alcohol Dependence* 59:277-286.

Cottler LB, Schuckit MA, Helzer JE et al. (1995). The DSM-IV field trial for substance use disorders: Major results. *Drug and Alcohol Dependence* 38:59-69.

Cottler LB, Shillington AM, Compton III WM et al. (1993). Subjective reports of withdrawal among cocaine users: Recommendations for DSM-IV. *Drug and Alcohol Dependence* 33:97-104.

Cubells JF, Kranzler HR, McCance-Katz E et al. (2000). A haplotype at the DBH locus, associated with low plasma dopamine beta-hydroxylase activity, also associates with cocaine-induced paranoia. *Molecular Psychiatry* 5(1):56-63.

Curran HV (2000). Is MDMA ("Ecstasy") neurotoxic in humans? An overview of evidence and of methodological problems in research. *Neuropsychobiology* 42:34-41.

de la Torre R, Farre M, Ortuno J et al. (2000). Non-linear pharmacokinetics of MDMA ('Ecstasy') in humans. *British Journal of Clinical Pharmacology* 49:104-109.

Demirkiran M, Jankovic J & Dean JM (1996). Ecstasy intoxication: An overlap between serotonin syndrome and neuroleptic malignant syndrome. *Clinical Neuropharmacology* 19:157-164.

Dotson JW, Ackerman DL & West JL (1995). Ketamine abuse. *Journal of Drug Issues* 25(4):751-757.

Doyon S (2001). The many faces of ecstasy. *Current Opinion in Pediatrics* 13:170-178.

Duffy A & Milin R (1996). Case study: Withdrawal syndrome in adolescent chronic cannabis users. *Journal of American Academy of Child and Adolescent Psychiatry* 35:1618-1621.

Dyer JE, Roth B & Hyma BA (2001). Gamma-hydroxybutyrate withdrawal syndrome. *Annals of Emergency Medicine* 37(2):147-153.

Erard R, Luisada PV & Peele R (1980). The PCP psychosis: Prolonged intoxication or drug precipitated functional illness? *Journal of Psychedelic Drugs* 12(3-4):235-250.

Ghuran A & Nolan J (2000). Recreational drug misuse: Issues for the cardiologist. *Heart* 83:627-633.

Giannini AJ, Loiselle RH, DiMarzio LR et al. (1987). Augmentation of haloperidol by ascorbic acid in phencyclidine intoxication. *American Journal of Psychiatry* 144:1207-1209.

Giannini AJ, Loiselle RH & Graham BH (1993). Behavioral response to buspirone in cocaine and phencyclidine withdrawal. *Journal of Substance Abuse Treatment* 10:523-527.

Giannini AJ, Underwood NA & Condon M (2000). Acute ketamine intoxication treated by haloperidol: A preliminary study. *American Journal of Therapeutics* 7:389-391.

Gill K, Gillespie HK & Hollister LE (1991). Dopamine depletion hypothesis of cocaine dependence: A test. *Human Psychopharmacology* 6:25-29.

Gillman PK (1999). The serotonin syndrome and its treatment. *Journal of Psychopharmacology* 13(1):100-109.

Glass M, Dragunow M & Faull RLM (1997). Cannabinoid receptors in the human brain: A detailed anatomical and quantitative autoradiographic study in the fetal, neonatal and adult human brain. *Neuroscience* 77(2):299-318.

Goldfrank LR & Hoffman RS (1991). The cardiovascular effects of cocaine. *Annals of Emergency Medicine* 20:165-175.

Gorelick DA (1997). Enhancing cocaine metabolism with butyrylcholinesterase as a treatment strategy. *Drug and Alcohol Dependence* 48:159-165.

Gorelick DA (1993). Overview of pharmacological treatment approaches for alcohol and other drug addiction: Intoxication, withdrawal, and relapse prevention. *Psychiatric Clinics of North America* 16(1):141-156.

Gorelick DA (1995). Pharmacologic therapies for cocaine addiction. In NS Miller & MS Gold (eds.) *Pharmacologic Therapies for Drug and Alcohol Addiction.* New York, NY: Marcel Dekker, 143-157.

Gorelick DA & Balster RL (1995). Phencyclidine (PCP). In FE Bloom & DJ Kupfer (eds.) *Psychopharmacology: The Fourth Generation of Progress.* New York, NY: Raven Press, 1767-1776.

Gorelick DA & Wilkins JN (1986). Special aspects of human alcohol withdrawal. In M Galanter (ed.) *Recent Developments in Alcoholism, 4th Edition.* New York: Plenum Press, 283-305.

Gorelick D, Wilkins J & Wong C (1986). Diagnosis and treatment of chronic phencyclidine abuse. *NIDA Research Monograph 64.* Rockville, MD: *National Institute on Drug Abuse*, 218-228.

Gwirtsman HE, Winkop W, Gorelick DA et al. (1984). Phencyclidine intoxication: Incidence, clinical patterns, and course of treatment. *Research Communications in Psychology, Psychiatry, and Behavior* 9:405-410.

Hahn I-H & Hoffman RS (2001). Cocaine use and acute myocardial infarction. *Emergency Medicine Clinics of North America* 19(2):493-510.

Halachanova V, Sansone RA & McDonald S (2001). Delayed rhabdomyolysis after ecstasy use. *Mayo Clinic Proceedings* 76(1):112-113.

Hall W, Hando J, Darke S et al. (1996). Psychological morbidity and route of administration among amphetamine users in Sydney, Australia. *Addiction* 91(1):81-87.

Haney M, Ward AS, Comer SD et al. (2001). Bupropion SR worsens mood during marijuana withdrawal in humans. *Psychopharmacology* 155:171-179.

Hardin JS, Wessinger WD, Proksch JW et al. (1998). Pharmacodynamics of a monoclonal antiphencyclidine Fab with broad selectivity for phencyclidine-like drugs. *Journal of Pharmacology and Experimental Therapeutics* 285:1113-1122.

Harris D & Batki SL (2000). Stimulant psychosis: Symptom profile and acute clinical course. *American Journal on Addictions* 9(1):28-37.

Harris JT, Roache JD & Thornton JE (2000). A role for valproate in the treatment of sedative-hypnotic withdrawal and for relapse prevention. *Alcohol & Alcoholism* 35(4):319-323.

Henry JA, Jeffreys CJ & Dawling S (1992). Toxicity and deaths from 3,4-methylenedioxymethamphetamine ("Ecstasy"). *Lancet* 340:384-387.

Hoffman RS, Morasco MS & Goldfrank LR (1996). Administration of purified human plasma cholinesterase protects against cocaine toxicity in mice. *Clinical Toxicology* 34:259-266.

Huestis MA, Gorelick DA, Heishman SJ et al. (2001). Blockade of effects of smoked marijuana by the CB1-selective cannabinoid receptor antagonist SR141716. *Archives of General Psychiatry* 58:322-328.

Hurlbut KM (1991). Drug-induced psychoses. *Emergency Medicine Clinics of North America* 9(1):31-52.

Jenkins AJ & Cone EJ (1998). Pharmacokinetics: Drug absorption, distribution, and elimination. In SB Karch (ed.) *Drug Abuse Handbook.* Boca Raton, FL: CRC Press, 151-201.

Jentsch JD & Roth RH (1999). The neuropsychopharmacology of phencyclidine: From NMDA receptor hypofunction to the dopamine hypothesis of schizophrenia. *Neuropsychopharmacology* 20:201-225.

Johanson CE & Fischman MW (1989). The pharmacology of cocaine related to its abuse. *Pharmacological Review* 41:3-52.

Kalant H (2001). The pharmacology and toxicology of "ecstasy" (MDMA) and related drugs. *Canadian Medical Association Journal* 165(7):917-928.

Kandall SR (1999). Treatment strategies for drug-exposed neonates. *Clinics in Perinatology* 26(1):231-243.

Karch SB & Stephens BG (1999). Drug abusers who die during arrest or in custody. *Journal of the Royal Society of Medicine* 92:110-113.

Khantzian EJ & McKenna GJ (1979). Acute toxic and withdrawal reactions associated with drug use and abuse. *Annals of Internal Medicine* 90:361-372.

King GR & Ellinwood Jr EH (1997). Amphetamines and other stimulants. In JH Lowinson, P Ruiz, RB Millman & JF Langrod (eds.) *Substance Abuse: A Comprehensive Textbook, 3rd Edition*. Baltimore, MD: Williams & Wilkins, 207-223.

Kulig K (1990). LSD. *Emergency Medicine Clinics of North America* 8(3):551-558.

Lago JA & Kosten TR (1994). Stimulant withdrawal. *Addiction* 89:1477-1481.

Lange RA & Hillis LD (2001). Cardiovascular complications of cocaine use. *New England Journal of Medicine* 345(5):351-358.

Leikin JB, Krantz AJ, Zell-Kanter M et al. (1989). Clinical features and management of intoxication due to hallucinogenic drugs. *Medical Toxicology and Adverse Drug Experiences* 4(5):324-350.

Lerner AG, Oyffe I, Isaacs G et al. (1997). Naltrexone treatment of hallucinogen persisting perception disorder. *American Journal of Psychiatry* 154:437.

Lester BM, El Sohly M, Wright LL et al. (2001). The maternal lifestyle study: Drug use by meconium toxicology and maternal self-report. *Pediatrics* 107(2):309-317.

Liechti ME, Baumann C, Gamma A et al. (2000). Acute psychological effects of 3,4-methylenedioxymethamphetamine (MDMA, "ecstasy") are attenuated by the serotonin uptake inhibitor citalopram. *Neuropsychopharmacology* 22(5):513-521.

Mason PJ, Morris VA & Balcezak TJ (2000). Serotonin syndrome. Presentation of 2 cases and review of the literature. *Medicine* 79(4):201-209.

Mathew RJ, Wilson WH, Humphreys D et al. (1993). Depersonalization after marijuana smoking. *Biological Psychiatry* 33:431-441.

Mattes CE, Belendiuk GW, Lynch TJ et al. (1998). Butyrylcholinesterase: An enzyme antidote for cocaine intoxication. *Addiction Biology* 3:171-188.

McCann UD, Eligulashvili V & Ricaurte GA (2000). (±)3,4-Methylenedioxymethamphetamine ("Ecstasy")-induced serotonin neurotoxicity: Clinical studies. *Neuropsychobiology* 42:11-16.

Mets B, Winger G, Cabrera C et al. (1998). A catalytic antibody against cocaine prevents cocaine's reinforcing and toxic effects in rats. *Proceedings of the National Academy of Sciences* 95:10176-10181.

Milhorn TH (1991). Diagnosis and management of phencyclidine intoxication. *American Family Physician* 43(4):1293-1302.

Miller PL, Gay GR, Ferris KC et al. (1992). Treatment of acute adverse psychedelic reactions: "I've tripped and I can't get down." *Journal of Psychoactive Drugs* 24(3):277-279.

Moore C, Negursz A & Lewis D (1998). Determination of drugs of abuse in meconium. *Journal of Chromatography* B713:137-146.

Moskowitz D (1971). Use of haloperidol to reduce LSD flashbacks. *Military Medicine* 136:754-757.

Mulvaney FD, Alterman AI, Boardman CR et al. (1999). Cocaine abstinence symptomatology and treatment attrition. *Journal of Substance Abuse Treatment* 16(2):129-135.

Murray JB (2001). Ecstasy is a dangerous drug. *Psychological Reports* 88:895-902.

Nademanee K, Gorelick DA, Josephson MA et al. (1989). Myocardial ischemia during cocaine withdrawal. *Annals of Internal Medicine* 111:376-380.

Neiman J, Haapaniemi HM & Hillblom M (2000). Neurological complications of drug abuse: Pathophysiological mechanisms. *European Journal of Neurology* 7:595-606.

Nzerue CM, Hewan-Lowe K & Riley Jr LJ (2000). Cocaine and the kidney: A synthesis of pathophysiologic and clinical perspectives. *American Journal of Kidney Diseases* 35(5):783-795.

O'Connell T, Kaye L & Plosay III JJ (2000). Gamma-hydroxybutyrate (GHB): A newer drug of abuse. *American Family Physician* 62:2478-2482.

Pechnick RN & Ungerleider JT (1997). Hallucinogens. In JH Lowinson, P Ruiz, RB Millman & JF Langrod (eds.) *Substance Abuse: A Comprehensive Textbook, 3rd Edition*. Baltimore, MD: Williams & Wilkins, 230-238.

Plessinger MA (1998). Prenatal exposure to amphetamines: Risks and adverse outcomes in pregnancy. *Obstetrics & Gynecology Clinics of North America* 25(1):119-138.

Ramoska ER & Sacchetti AD (1985). Propanolol-induced hypertension in treatment of cocaine intoxication. *Annals of Emergency Medicine* 14(11):1112-1113.

Rappolt RT, Gay GR & Farris RD (1980). Phencyclidine (PCP) intoxication: Diagnosis in stages and algorithms of treatment. *Clinical Toxicology* 16:509-529.

Richards JR, Derlet RW & Duncan DR (1998). Chemical restraint for the agitated patient in the emergency department: Lorazepam versus droperidol. *Journal of Emergency Medicine* 16(4):567-573.

Richards JR, Johnson EB, Stark RW et al. (1999). Methamphetamine abuse and rhabdomyolysis in the ED: A 5-year study. *American Journal of Emergency Medicine* 17:681-685.

Rome ES (2001). It's a rave new world: Rave culture and illicit drug use in the young. *Cleveland Clinic Journal of Medicine* 68(6):541-550.

Rosenblum A, Foote J, Magura S et al. (1996). Follow-up of inpatient cocaine withdrawal for cocaine-using methadone patients. *Journal of Substance Abuse Treatment* 13(6):467-470.

Rosse RB, Collins JP Jr, Fay-McCarthy M et al. (1994). Phenomenologic comparison of the idiopathic psychosis of schizophrenia and drug-induced cocaine and phencyclidine psychoses: A retrospective study. *Clinical Neuropharmacology* 17(4):359-369.

Roth BA, Benowitz NL & Olson KR (1998). Emergency management of drug abuse-related disorders. In SB Karch (ed.) *Drug Abuse Handbook*. Boca Raton, FL: CRC Press, 567-639.

Ruttenber AJ, McAnally HB & Wetli CV (1999). Cocaine-associated rhabdomyolysis and excited delirium: Different stages of the same syndrome. *American Journal of Forensic Medicine & Pathology* 20(2):120-127.

Satel SL, Price LH, Palumbo JM et al. (1991a). Clinical phenomenology and neurobiology of cocaine abstinence: A prospective inpatient study. *American Journal of Psychiatry* 148:1712-1716.

Satel SL, Seibyl JP & Charney DS (1991b). Prolonged cocaine psychosis implies underlying major psychopathology. *Journal of Clinical Psychiatry* 52(8):349-350.

Satel SL, Southwick SM & Gawin FH (1991c). Clinical features of cocaine-induced paranoia. *American Journal of Psychiatry* 148(4):495-498.

Schnoll SH & Daghestani AN (1986). Treatment of marijuana abuse. *Psychiatric Annals* 16:249-254.

Schuckit MA (2000). *Drug and Alcohol Abuse. A Clinical Guide to Diagnosis and Treatment, 5th Edition*. New York, NY: Kluwer Academic/Plenum.

Schwartz RH, Milteer R & LeBeau MA (2000). Drug-facilitated sexual assault ("date rape"). *Southern Medical Journal* 93(6):558-561.

Schwartz RH & Smith DE (1988). Hallucinogenic mushrooms. *Clinical Pediatrics* 27(2):7073.

Selden BS, Clark RF & Curry SC (1990). Marijuana. *Emergency Medicine Clinics of North America* 8(3):527-539.

Serper MR, Chou JC, Allen MH et al. (1999). Symptomatic overlap of cocaine intoxication and acute schizophrenia at emergency presentation. *Schizophrenia Bulletin* 25(2):387-394.

Shah DM, Dy TC, Szto GY et al. (2000). Percutaneous transluminal coronary angioplasty and stenting for cocaine-induced acute myocardial infarction: A case report and review. *Catheterization & Cardiovascular Interventions* 49:447-451.

Shaner A, Roberts LJ, Eckman TA et al. (1998). Sources of diagnostic uncertainty for chronically psychotic cocaine abusers. *Psychiatry Research* 49(5):684-690.

Shannon M & Quang LS (2000). Gamma-hydroxybutyrate, gamma-butyrolactone, and 1,4-butanediol: A case report and review of the literature. *Pediatric Emergency Care* 16(6):435-440.

Shorr RI & Robin DW (1994). Rational use of benzodiazepines in the elderly. *Drugs and Aging* 4:9-20.

Sivilotti ML, Burns MJ, Aaron CK et al. (2001). Pentobarbital for severe gamma-butyrolactone withdrawal. *Annals of Emergency Medicine* 38(6):660-665.

Smart RG & Anglin L (1987). Do we know the lethal dose of cocaine? *Journal of Forensic Sciences* 32:303-312.

Smeriglio VL & Wilcox HC (1999). Prenatal drug exposure and child outcome. *Clinics in Perinatology* 26(1):1-16.

Soloway MS & Smith RA (1988). Cranberry juice as a urine acidifier. *Journal of the American Medical Association* 260:1465.

Stein MD (1999). Medical consequences of substance abuse. *Psychiatric Clinics of North America* 22(2):351-370.

Stewart DG & Brown SA (1995). Withdrawal and dependency symptoms among adolescent alcohol and drug abusers. *Addiction* 90:627-635.

Strassman RJ (1984). Adverse reactions of psychedelic drugs: A review of the literature. *Journal of Nervous and Mental Disease* 172(10):577-595.

Sumner AD & Simons RJ (1994). Delirium in the hospitalized elderly. *Cleveland Clinic Journal of Medicine* 61:258-262.

Szuster RR, Pontius EB & Campos PE (1988). Marijuana sensitivity and panic anxiety. *Journal of Clinical Psychiatry* 49:427-429.

Tashkin DP (2001). Airway effects of marijuana, cocaine, and other inhaled illicit agents. *Current Opinion in Pulmonary Medicine* 7:43-61.

Teller DW & Devenyi P (1988). Bromocriptine in cocaine withdrawal-Does it work? *International Journal of the Addictions* 23:1197-1205.

Tennant FS, Rawson RA & McCann M (1981). Withdrawal from chronic phencyclidine dependence with desipramine. *American Journal of Psychiatry* 138:845-847.

Volkow ND, Fowler JS & Wolf AP (1992). Effects of chronic cocaine abuse on postsynaptic dopamine receptors. *American Journal of Psychiatry* 147:719-724.

Vollenweider FX, Gamma A, Liechti M et al. (1999). Is a single dose of MDMA harmless? *Neuropsychopharmacology* 21(4):598-600.

Wagner CL, Katkaneni LD, Cox TH et al. (1998). The impact of prenatal drug exposure on the neonate. *Obstetrics & Gynecology Clinics of North America* 25(1):169-194.

Weber JE, Chudnofsky CR, Boczar M et al. (2000). Cocaine-associated chest pain: How common is myocardial infarction? *Academic Emergency Medicine* 7(8):873-877.

Weiss RD, Greenfield SF & Mirin SM (1994). Intoxication and withdrawal syndromes. In SE Hyman (ed.) *Manual of Psychiatric Emergencies*. Boston, MA: Little, Brown & Co, 279-293.

Wiesbeck GA, Schuckit MA, Kalmijn JA et al. (1996). An evaluation of the history of a marijuana withdrawal syndrome in a large population. *Addiction* 91(10):1469-1478.

Wolfsohn R & Angrist B (1990). A pilot trial of levodopa/carbidopa in early cocaine abstinence. *Journal of Clinical Psychopharmacology* 10:440-442.

Woods JH & Winger G (1997). Abuse liability of flunitrazepam. *Journal of Clinical Psychopharmacology* 17(3 Suppl 2):1S-57S.

Woolf DS, Vourakis C & Bennett G (1980). Guidelines for management of acute phencyclidine intoxication. *Critical Care Update* 7(6):16-24.

Young CR (1997). Sertraline treatment of hallucinogen persisting perception disorder. *Journal of Clinical Psychiatry* 58:85.

Zvosec D, Smith S, McCutcheon JR et al. (2001). Adverse events, including death, associated with the use of 1,4-butanediol. *New England Journal of Medicine* 344(2):87-94.

SECTION 6 | Pharmacologic Interventions

Section Coordinators
David A. Gorelick, M.D., Ph.D.
Raye Z. Litten, Ph.D.

Contributors

Lowell C. Dale, M.D.
Associate Professor of Medicine, and
Associate Director, Mayo Clinic
   Nicotine Dependence Center
Rochester, Minnesota

Jon O. Ebbert, M.D.
Assistant Professor of Medicine
Mayo Clinic Nicotine Dependence Center
Rochester, Minnesota

David A. Gorelick, M.D., Ph.D.
Chief, Clinical Pharmacology Section
Intramural Research Program
National Institute on Drug Abuse
National Institutes of Health, and
Adjunct Professor of Psychiatry
University of Maryland School of Medicine
Baltimore, Maryland

Mark K. Greenwald, Ph.D.
Addiction Research Institute
Department of Psychiatry
   and Behavioral Neurosciences
Wayne State University School of Medicine
Detroit, Michigan

J. Taylor Hays, M.D.
Assistant Professor of Medicine, and
Associate Director, Mayo Clinic
   Nicotine Dependence Center
Rochester, Minnesota

Richard D. Hurt, M.D., FASAM
Professor of Medicine, and
Director, Mayo Clinic
   Nicotine Dependence Center
Rochester, Minnesota

Jerome H. Jaffe, M.D.
Adjunct Clinical Professor of Psychiatry
University of Maryland
School of Medicine
Baltimore, Maryland

Thomas R. Kosten, M.D.
Chief, Psychiatry Service
VA Connecticut Healthcare System, and
Associate Professor of Psychiatry
Yale University School of Medicine
New Haven, Connecticut

Henry R. Kranzler, M.D.
Professor of Psychiatry, and
Associate Scientific Director
Alcohol Research Center
University of Connecticut School of Medicine
Farmington, Connecticut

Walter Ling, M.D.
Director of Research
Los Angeles Addiction Treatment Research Center, and
Associate Clinical Professor of Psychiatry
University of California, Los Angeles
Los Angeles, California

Raye Z. Litten, Ph.D.
Treatment Research Branch
National Institute on Alcohol Abuse
   and Alcoholism
Bethesda, Maryland

Judith Martin, M.D.
Medical Director, 14th Street Clinic
   and East Bay Community Recovery Project
Oakland, California

J. Thomas Payte, M.D.
Founder and Medical Director
Drug Dependence Associates
San Antonio, Texas

Andrew J. Saxon, M.D.
Professor, Department of Psychiatry
   and Behavioral Sciences
University of Washington, and
Center of Excellence in Substance Abuse
   Treatment and Education
Puget Sound Health Care System
Seattle, Washington

David E. Smith, M.D.
Founder, Medical Director and President
Haight Ashbury Free Clinics, and
Associate Clinical Professor of
   Occupational Health and Clinical Toxicology
University of California, San Francisco
San Francisco, California

Susan M. Stine, M.D., Ph.D.
Associate Professor
Addiction Research Institute
Substance Abuse Research Division
Department of Psychiatry and Behavioral Neurosciences
Wayne State University School of Medicine
Detroit, Michigan

Donald R. Wesson, M.D.
Chair, ASAM Medications Development Committee, and
Consultant, CNS Medications Development
Oakland, California

Jeffery N. Wilkins, M.D.
Director, Addiction Medicine
Cedars-Sinai Medical Center, and
Adjunct Professor of Psychiatry
UCLA School of Medicine
Los Angeles, California

Joan E. Zweben, Ph.D.
Clinical Professor of Psychiatry
University of California, San Francisco, and
Executive Director, 14th Street Clinic
   and East Bay Community Recovery Project
Oakland, California

Chapter 1 | Pharmacologic Interventions for Alcoholism

Henry R. Kranzler, M.D.
Jerome H. Jaffe, M.D.

Drugs Used to Deter Alcohol Consumption
Pharmacotherapies for Postwithdrawal
Affective Disturbances

This chapter reviews the literature on the use of medications to prevent relapse in alcoholics. Rather than reviewing the literature exhaustively, the focus of the chapter is on those developments that are of current interest to the clinician or that are likely to yield important clinical advances in the future. The reader is referred to a number of other reviews published recently that augment the topics covered here (Garbutt, West et al., 1999; Swift, 1999; Kranzler, 2000; Myrick, Brady et al., 2001).

DRUGS USED TO DETER ALCOHOL CONSUMPTION

Among the major challenges in the months after cessation of drinking in alcoholics are the prevention of relapse to drinking and the management of persistent emotional and physiologic disturbances. Pharmacologic agents can be used to deter alcohol consumption in several ways. Alcohol-sensitizing drugs make the ingestion of alcohol aversive or hazardous. Some drugs appear to reduce alcohol intake by reducing the reinforcing effects of alcohol or by reducing the urge or craving to ingest it. The treatment of persistent psychiatric symptoms is postulated to reduce the risk of relapse by removing motivation to use alcohol as "self-medication" to control such symptoms. Each of these approaches to pharmacotherapy is discussed in detail below.

Alcohol-Sensitizing Agents. Sensitizing agents alter the body's response to alcohol, making its ingestion unpleasant or toxic. Disulfiram (Antabuse®) and carbimide are two drugs of this type that have been used to treat alcoholism. Both inhibit aldehyde dehydrogenase (ALDH), the enzyme that catalyzes the oxidation of acetaldehyde to acetic acid. If alcohol is ingested after this enzyme is inhibited, blood acetaldehyde levels rise. As a result, in the case of disulfiram, the disulfiram-ethanol reaction (DER) develops. The DER generally varies in intensity both with the dose of disulfiram and with the volume of alcohol ingested. In its mild form, the syndrome includes warmness and flushing of the skin, especially that of the upper chest and face; increased heart rate; palpitations; and decreased blood pressure. Nausea, vomiting, shortness of breath, sweating, dizziness, blurred vision, and confusion also can occur. Most reactions last about 30 minutes and are self-limited. Occasionally, the DER can be severe and include marked tachycardia, hypotension, bradycardia, or even cardiac arrest secondary to vagal stimulation associated with retching or vomiting. Cardiovascular collapse, congestive heart failure, and convulsions have been reported. Although severe reactions usually are associated with high doses of disulfiram (more than 500 mg/day), combined with more than 2 ounces of alcohol, deaths have occurred at lower doses and after a single drink (Lindros, Stowell et al., 1981; Peachey, Brien et al., 1981; Peachey, Maglana et al., 1981; Sellers, Naranjo et al., 1981).

A variety of agents, such as oral hypoglycemics and trichomonacides, also can produce unpleasant effects when combined with ethanol, as a consequence of their inhibition of ALDH. However, given their other actions, these drugs generally are unsuitable for use as sensitizing agents in the treatment of alcoholism.

The use of alcohol-sensitizing agents has intuitive appeal. Consequently, these drugs long have been used in the rehabilitation of alcoholic patients (Favazza & Martin, 1974), despite the absence of methodologically sound evaluations demonstrating their clinical efficacy. Most studies undertaken before the last decade failed to include measures of compliance or adequate controls, both of which now generally are considered essential elements in the evaluation of the efficacy of a medication for treatment of alcohol dependence (Kranzler, Mason et al., 1997). Except for the Veterans Affairs Cooperative Study (see below), only a few studies of disulfiram have incorporated these elements, and such studies generally have had small samples or used ill-defined outcome measures.

The efficacy of alcohol-sensitizing agents in the prevention or limitation of relapse in alcoholics remains to be demonstrated. However, in selected samples of alcoholics with whom special efforts are made to ensure compliance, these drugs can be of utility. Unfortunately, at the present time, no guidelines can be offered either to identify those patients for whom disulfiram is most likely to have a beneficial effect or for specific psychosocial interventions to enhance compliance with particular patients. The following discussion is limited to disulfiram, which is the only aversive agent that is widely used in clinical practice.

Disulfiram is absorbed almost completely after oral administration. It is metabolized rapidly to diethyldithiocarbamate (DDC), which in turn is degraded to diethylamine and several other substances, including carbon disulfide. The detection of carbon disulfide in breath provides a measure of compliance. Because disulfiram inhibits ALDH by binding to it irreversibly, renewed enzyme activity requires the synthesis of new protein. This effect is the basis for the admonition to avoid alcohol consumption for at least two weeks from the time disulfiram last was ingested, because it can produce the DER.

Adverse effects from disulfiram are common. In addition to its effects on ALDH, disulfiram inhibits a variety of other enzymes, including dopamine beta-hydroxylase (DBH). Although disulfiram reduces clearance rates of chlordiazepoxide (Librium®) and diazepam (Valium®), benzodiazepines that do not require hydroxylation before excretion (such as lorazepam [Ativan®] and oxazepam [Serax®]) are not altered. Disulfiram also can reduce the clearance, increase the elimination half-life, and lead to higher peak plasma levels of desipramine (Norpramin®) and imipramine (Tofranil®) (Ciraulo, Barnhill et al., 1985). Clearance of phenytoin (Dilantin®) and warfarin (Coumadin®) is reduced, and dose adjustments are required to avoid adverse effects (Hoyumpa & Schenker, 1982; Sellers, Naranjo et al., 1981).

Chick (1999) reviewed safety issues in the use of disulfiram for the treatment of alcohol dependence and found that common side effects include drowsiness, lethargy, and fatigue. Other more serious adverse effects, such as optic neuritis, peripheral neuropathy, and hepatotoxicity, are rare. The inhibition of DBH by disulfiram and its metabolite DDC results in increased dopamine levels. The exacerbation of psychotic symptoms in schizophrenics and occasionally their appearance in nonschizophrenics, as well as the development of depression, may be linked to this action. As with the neuropathic effects, the psychiatric effects are uncommon and may depend for their appearance on higher doses of disulfiram. Alcoholics with low cerebrospinal fluid DBH activity are more likely to develop dysphoric or psychotic symptoms in response to disulfiram (Major, Lerner et al., 1979; Sellers, Naranjo et al., 1981). Thus, in addition to the toxicity of the DER caused by the accumulation of acetaldehyde, adverse effects of disulfiram or its metabolites can occur as a result of multiple drug interactions, alterations in levels of normal body constituents and neurotransmitters, and other toxic effects.

Although disulfiram has been used in the treatment of alcoholism for many years, problems in designing adequate experiments have made it difficult to assess its efficacy. Its approval by the U.S. Food and Drug Administration (FDA) preceded the implementation of rigorous requirements for efficacy that now must be satisfied for a drug to be marketed in the United States. In the few controlled studies that have been conducted, the difference in outcome between subjects taking disulfiram and those given placebo is minimal. One problem is that patients easily determine what they are taking, making it impossible to implement a true double-blind study. Another problem has been poor verification of compliance.

In a large, multicenter study conducted by the Veterans Affairs Cooperative Studies Group, more than 600 male alcoholics were assigned randomly to groups receiving either 1 mg/day of disulfiram or a therapeutic dose of 250 mg/day, or to a control group that was told they were not receiving disulfiram. Patients assigned to the disulfiram groups were told they were being given the drug, but neither patients nor staff knew the dose. The capsules provided to patients in the different groups were indistinguishable, and all contained riboflavin, which permitted the monitoring of compliance. Among the significant findings were the following: There was a direct relationship between compliance with drug therapy (in all three groups) and complete abstinence. Among patients who resumed drinking, those taking a therapeutic dose of disulfiram had significantly fewer drinking days than did patients in the other two groups. However, in terms of a variety of outcome measures, including length of time to first drink, unemployment, social stability, or number of men totally abstinent, there was no significant difference among the three groups. The researchers concluded that disulfiram can be helpful in reducing the frequency of drinking in men who cannot remain abstinent (Fuller, Branchey et al., 1986), although they conceded that such a finding may have arisen by chance (given the large number of statistical analyses).

Disulfiram usually is given orally. Because the risk of side effects and of toxic hazards increases with the dose, the daily dose prescribed in the U.S. has been limited to 250 to 500 mg/day. However, efforts to titrate the dose of disulfiram in relation to a challenge dose of ethanol indicate that some patients require in excess of 1 g/day of disulfiram to reach blood levels sufficient to produce the DER (Brewer, 1984). Moreover, the clinical use of a challenge dose of ethanol to demonstrate to the patient the potential for adverse effects of disulfiram in combination with alcohol is not generally used in the U.S., although it is thought to enhance the efficacy of the medication (Brewer, 1984).

The requirement that disulfiram undergo bioactivation before it can inhibit ALDH (Yourick & Faiman, 1991) may explain the need for a higher dose in some patients. At the dose that is used clinically, faulty bioactivation in some individuals can yield too low a concentration of the active metabolite to inhibit ALDH. The clinical use of the sulfoxide metabolite of disulfiram that directly antagonizes the activity of ALDH can eliminate much of the variability in response observed with disulfiram. Because that metabolite is potent and has favorable pharmaceutical characteristics, its use as a transdermal or sustained-release formulation may be feasible, thereby offering the prospect of improved compliance.

Disulfiram has been given by subcutaneous implantation of 100 mg tablets (Esperal®) in the abdominal wall (Wilson, Davidson et al., 1980). In most cases, blood levels of disulfiram and DDC after implantation probably are too low to exert alcohol-sensitizing effects for a period long enough to justify the implant, and benefits seen after implantation appear to be primarily the result of psychological factors (Bergstrom, Ohlin et al., 1982; Sellers, Naranjo et al., 1981). Such psychological factors may interact or overlap with factors related to compliance; this was shown by Fuller and colleagues (1986) to be a potent predictor of treatment outcome.

Careful efforts to enhance compliance with disulfiram can serve to augment the deterrent effects of the medication. Behavioral efforts that may be of value include providing the patient with incentives, contracting with the patient and a significant other to work together to ensure compliance, providing regular reminders and other information to the patient, and using behavioral training and social support (Allen & Litten, 1992). Azrin and colleagues (1982) found that a trial program of stimulus control training, role playing, communication skills training, and recreational and vocational counseling improved outcome in disulfiram-treated patients compared with those receiving placebo. Chick and colleagues (1992) assessed the efficacy of supervised disulfiram treatment as an adjunct to outpatient treatment of alcoholism. During a six-month treatment period, patients received disulfiram 200 mg/day or placebo under the supervision of an individual nominated by the patient. Under those circumstances, disulfiram significantly increased abstinent days and decreased total drinks consumed; these effects were confirmed by parallel changes in gamma-glutamyltranspeptidase (GGTP) levels. Supervision of the use of disulfiram may be an essential element (Brewer, Meyers et al., 2000). However, because the enhancement of compliance with disulfiram therapy generally requires substantial efforts (Azrin, Sisson et al., 1982), use of the drug outside of a well-organized treatment program probably is not warranted.

TABLE 1.   Placebo-Controlled Trials of Naltrexone for Alcohol Dependence[1]

Reference[2]	N	Study Duration[3]	Comment[4]
Volpicelli et al., 1992	70	12	NTX 50 mg/day orally delayed time to first drink and reduced risk of heavy drinking.
O'Malley et al., 1992	101	12	NTX 50 mg/day orally resulted in fewer drinking days and heavy drinking days. NTX and ST particularly efficacious in preventing initiation of drinking; NTX and CBT particularly efficacious in preventing relapse to heavy drinking.
Oslin et al., 1997	44	12	NTX 50 mg/day orally reduced risk of relapse to heavy drinking.
Volpicelli et al., 1997	97	12	In ITT, NTX 50 mg/day orally = PLA on self-reported drinking, but NTX superior on transaminase levels. In highly compliant subjects, NTX superior on self-report measures.
Hersh et al., 1998	64	8	NTX 50 mg/day orally = PLA on alcohol and cocaine use in subjects with comorbid alcohol and cocaine use disorders.
Kranzler et al., 1998	20	8	Sustained release NTX injection reduced frequency of heavy drinking.
Anton et al., 1999	131	12	NTX 50 mg/day orally reduced drinking frequency and drinks/drinking day and delayed relapse to heavy drinking.
Kranzler et al., 2000	183	12	NTX 50 mg/day orally associated with more adverse effects, poorer medication compliance, and greater attrition from treatment than PLA. NTX = NEF = PLA on drinking outcomes.
Chick et al., 2000	175	12	In ITT, NTX 50 mg/day orally = PLA on all outcomes. In compliant subjects, NTX produced greater reductions in GGTP level, in overall alcohol consumption, and on a measure of alcohol craving.
Heinala et al., 2001	121	12	NTX 50 mg/day orally reduced risk of relapse to heavy drinking, but only in group that received coping skills therapy. Targeted treatment sustained this difference.

[1]Reprinted from Kranzler (2000), by permission of the Medical Council on Alcoholism
[2]All studies, except that of Chick, Anton et al. (2000); Chick, Howlett et al. (2000) and Heinala, Alho et al. (2001, Finland), were conducted in the United States and were single-site studies
[3]Treatment period only (weeks)
[4]Only statistically significant differences reported

CBT = cognitive-behavioral therapy	ITT = intention-to-treat analysis	NTX = naltrexone
PLA = placebo	ST = supportive therapy	

Patients should be warned carefully about the hazards of disulfiram, including the need to avoid over-the-counter preparations containing alcohol or drugs that interact adversely with disulfiram. A warning also should be provided

TABLE 2.   Placebo-Controlled Trials of Fluoxetine[1]

Reference	Country	N	Study Duration[2]	Comment[3]
Naranjo et al., 1990	Canada	29	4 wk	FLX 60mg/day (but not 40mg/day) reduced drinks/day
Gerra et al., 1992	Italy	28	1 mo	FLX 40mg/day reduced drinks/day in FHP patients only
Gorelick & Paredes, 1992	U.S.	20	4 wk	FLX to a maximum of 80mg/day transiently reduced drinks/day
Kranzler et al., 1995	U.S.	101	12 wk	FLX 60mg/day was comparable to placebo on all drinking outcomes
Janiri et al., 1996	Italy	50	2 mo	FLX 20mg/day increased proportion abstinent
Kabel & Petty, 1996	U.S.	28	12 wk	FLX 60mg/day was comparable to placebo on all drinking outcomes

[1]Reprinted from Kranzler (2000), by permission of the Medical Council on Alcoholism.
[2]Treatment period only [for the study by Gerra et al. (1992), this is the duration of each treatment received].
[3]Only statistically significant differences reported.

wk = weeks   FLX = fluoxetine   mo = month(s)   FHP = family-history-positive

are needed. Moreover, the number of patients treated in double-blind studies of these medications has been comparatively small, and longer-term outcome studies are lacking. A number of studies currently are under way to evaluate these effects further, including the range of patient groups for which the medications are efficacious, their optimal duration of use, and the most appropriate psychosocial and pharmacologic treatments to be used in combination with them.

Serotonergic Agents: LeMarquand and colleagues (1994a,b) have reviewed the extensive experimental literature that links 5-HT neurotransmission to alcohol consumption. In rodents, 5-HT precursors and selective serotonin reuptake inhibitors (SSRIs) consistently decrease ethanol consumption (LeMarquand, Pihl et al., 1994a).

A variety of SSRIs have been tested in humans to determine their effects on alcohol consumption. They include zimelidine (Amit, Brown et al., 1985; Naranjo, Sellers et al., 1984), fluvoxamine (Kranzler, Del Boca et al., 1993; Angelone, Bellini et al., 1998), viqualine (Naranjo, Sullivan et al., 1989), sertraline (Pettinati, Volpicelli et al., 2000), citalopram (Naranjo, Sellers et al., 1987; Naranjo, Poulos et al., 1992; Naranjo, Bremner et al., 1995; Balldin, Berggren et al., 1994; Tiihonen, Ryynanen et al., 1996), and fluoxetine (Naranjo, Kadlec et al., 1990; Gerra, Caccavari et al., 1992; Gorelick & Paredes, 1992; Kranzler, Burleson et al., 1995; Kabel & Petty, 1996). In the paragraphs that follow, the focus is on the two most intensively studied SSRIs, fluoxetine (Table 2) and citalopram (Table 3).

Naranjo and colleagues (1990) first reported that fluoxetine (Prozac®) reduced alcohol consumption. These investigators found that 60 mg/day of fluoxetine reduced average daily alcohol consumption by approximately 17% from baseline levels, whereas treatment with fluoxetine 40 mg/day or placebo had no effect. When alcoholics on an inpatient unit were given access to alcohol, fluoxetine pretreatment initially reduced alcohol consumption, but the effect did not persist (Gorelick & Paredes, 1992). By using a crossover design, Gerra and colleagues (1992) compared the effects of fluoxetine, acamprosate (discussed in detail later), and placebo on alcoholics who had a positive family history with volunteers who had a negative family history.

TABLE 3.   Placebo-Controlled Trials of Citalopram[1]

Reference	Country	N	Study Duration[2]	Comment[3]
Naranjo et al., 1987	Canada	39	4 wk	CIT 40mg/day increased abstinent days and decreased drinks/day
Naranjo et al., 1992	Canada	16	1 wk	CIT 40mg/day increased abstinent days and decreased drinks/day
Balldin et al., 1994	Sweden	30	5 wk	CIT 40mg/day decreased drinks/day for lighter drinkers only
Naranjo et al., 1995	Canada	62	12 wk	CIT 40mg/day decreased drinks/day for first week only
Tiihonen et al., 1996	Finland	62	4 mo	CIT 40mg/day increased study retention and improved drinking outcomes (by informant report)

[1]Reprinted from Kranzler (2000), by permission of the Medical Council on Alcoholism.
[2]Treatment period [for crossover studies (Naranjo et al. 1987, 1992), this is the duration of each treatment received].
[3]Only statistically significant differences reported.

CIT = citalopram   wk = week(s)   mo = months

Although they found both active medications to be superior to placebo in reducing the number of drinks consumed, the effect of fluoxetine was significant only in the patients with a positive family history, whereas acamprosate produced a significant reduction only in the patients with a negative family history. Kabel and Petty (1996) showed no advantage for fluoxetine over placebo among severe alcoholics recruited from an alcoholism treatment program at a Veterans Affairs Medical Center. A 12-week, placebo-controlled trial of fluoxetine in combination with coping skills psychotherapy in 101 alcohol-dependent subjects showed no overall advantage to the active drug on drinking outcomes (Kranzler, Burleson et al., 1995). A further analysis of the data showed a paradoxical effect among the subgroup of patients with high levels of both premorbid vulnerability and alcohol-related problems; in that subgroup, fluoxetine appeared to reduce the beneficial effects of coping skills training (Kranzler, Burleson et al., 1996).

Citalopram (Celexa®) is the other SSRI whose effects on alcohol consumption have been studied reasonably extensively. Naranjo and colleagues (1987) first reported that citalopram 40 mg/day (but not 20 mg/day) reduced the number of drinks per day and increased the number of abstinent days relative to baseline drinking in nondepressed, early-stage problem drinkers. Subsequently, citalopram 40 mg/day was shown to reduce alcoholic drinks significantly and to increase the number of abstinent days in non-depressed, alcohol-dependent subjects (Naranjo, Poulos et al., 1992). However, when citalopram 40 mg/day was combined with a brief psychosocial intervention in a 12-week treatment trial, the active drug was superior to placebo in reducing the number of daily alcoholic drinks only during the first week of treatment (Naranjo, Bremner et al., 1995). In a five-week, placebo-controlled study of citalopram 40 mg/day in a sample of heavy drinkers, Balldin and colleagues (1994) found no overall difference between treatment groups. However, when the data were reanalyzed on the basis of a median split on the pretreatment level of alcohol consumption, subjects in the lighter drinking subgroup had lower daily alcohol intake with citalopram compared with placebo.

In a three-month, placebo-controlled study of citalopram 40 mg/day in alcohol-dependent subjects, Tiihonen and colleagues (1996) found a significant advantage of the active medication on study retention and on collateral informants' reports of the patients' condition. In this study, there also was a trend toward reduced alcohol consumption and GGTP levels in the citalopram group.

One possible explanation for the variable findings in studies of the effects of SSRIs on drinking behavior lies in the diversity of subjects in the various study groups. Many of the studies were conducted with heavy drinkers who were not seeking to reduce or stop their drinking. Some, but not all, studies examined medication effects in the context of psychotherapeutic treatment. Overall, these studies suggest that SSRIs are efficacious only in heavy drinkers or in certain subgroups of alcoholics. For example, Gerra and colleagues (1992) found an effect of fluoxetine only in alcoholics who had a positive family history of alcoholism. Balldin and colleagues (1994) found an effect of citalopram only among the heavier drinkers in their patient sample.

By using a different approach to subtyping alcoholism, Kranzler and colleagues (1996) found that high-risk/severity (Type B) alcoholism (one characteristic of which is an earlier age of alcoholism onset) showed a poorer response to fluoxetine than to placebo. Pettinati and colleagues (2000) examined the interaction of alcoholic subtype with medication effects in a placebo-controlled trial of sertraline (Zoloft®). In that study, low-risk/severity (Type A) alcoholics (those with later age of alcoholism onset) drank on fewer days and were more likely to be abstinent in the 12-week treatment trial when treated with sertraline compared with placebo. In contrast, Type B alcoholics showed better outcomes on these measures with placebo treatment; however, the effects did not reach statistical significance. In a similar vein, although not an SSRI, ondansetron (Zofran®, a 5-HT$_3$ antagonist) was shown by Johnson and colleagues (2000) to produce a selective beneficial effect in early-onset alcoholics (those with onset of problem drinking before age 25). Specifically, at a dose substantially lower than that used to exert the antiemetic effects for which the medication is approved, ondansetron was superior to placebo in the proportion of abstinent days and the intensity of alcohol intake. Among late-onset alcoholics, the effects of ondansetron on drinking behavior were, in nearly all respects, comparable to those of placebo. Prospective studies that aim to match SSRI treatment with alcoholic subtypes (based either on age of onset or on a more complex subtyping procedure) can define a clearer role for such medications in the treatment of heavy drinking or alcohol dependence.

Agents Affecting Other Neurotransmitter Systems. *Acamprosate* (calcium acetylhomotaurinate), an amino acid derivative, affects both gamma-aminobutyric acid and excitatory amino acid (glutamate) neurotransmission (the latter effect most likely being the one that is important for its therapeutic effects in alcoholism). The medication is approved for use throughout Europe, based on a series of studies there (Table 4). A camprosate was approved for use in the U.S. in 2004, and a large, multicenter clinical trial recently has been completed here.

In an initial single-center trial in France, acamprosate was found to be twice as effective as placebo in reducing the rate at which alcoholics returned to drinking (Lhuintre, Moore et al., 1985). Subsequently, a multicenter study in France (Lhuintre, Moore et al., 1990) showed that acamprosate treatment produced a greater reduction in GGTP levels than did placebo treatment; however, data on drinking behavior *per se* were not reported. In another large, multicenter study in France (Paille, Guelfi et al., 1995), acamprosate was associated with significantly better rates of clinic attendance and more abstinent days, with the high-dose acamprosate showing the best outcomes, the placebo group the poorest outcomes, and the low-dose acamprosate group intermediate outcomes on these measures.

Three placebo-controlled studies of acamprosate for alcohol dependence have been conducted in Belgium. Roussaux and colleagues (1996) found no difference in drinking outcomes or biochemical measures among alcoholics recruited from an inpatient setting. However, acamprosate was shown to enhance treatment retention and the maintenance of abstinence among alcoholics in a study by Pelc and colleagues (1996). In a second study, Pelc and colleagues (1997) compared two doses of acamprosate to placebo in a multicenter study. Both acamprosate-treated groups had significantly better outcomes than placebo-treated patients on abstinent days, the proportion of patients achieving abstinence for the entire trial, the time to first alcoholic drink, and liver enzyme levels. Although there were some trends suggesting that the higher dose of acamprosate was superior to the lower dose of that medication, such trends did not reach statistical significance.

Subsequent multicenter studies have been conducted in Belgium, the Netherlands, and Luxembourg (Geerlings, Ansoms et al., 1997), Austria (Whitworth, Fischer et al., 1996), Germany (Sass, Soyka et al., 1996), and Italy (Poldrugo, 1997; Tempesta, Janiri et al., 2000). In all of

TABLE 4.   Acamprosate Treatment of Alcohol Dependence: Placebo-Controlled Trials[1]

Reference	Country	N	Study Duration[2]	Comment[3]
Lhuintre et al., 1985	France	85	3/0	ACA (25mg/kg/day) more likely to remain abstinent than PLA
Lhuintre et al., 1990	France	569	3/0	ACA (1.3 g/day) had lower GGTP level than PLA
Gerra et al., 1992	Italy	28	1/0	ACA (1.3 g/day) that was negative for family history of alcoholism had lower mean quantity of alcoholic drinks
Pelc et al., 1996	Belgium	102	6/0	ACA[4] had greater treatment retention, fewer days drinking, was more likely to remain abstinent, and had greater reduction in GGTP level than PLA.
Paille et al., 1995	France	538	12/6	ACA (1.3 or 2 g/day) had greater treatment retention, fewer days drinking, and greater likelihood of normal GGTP than PLA. Effects on study retention and abstinence persisted during F/U.
Roussaux et al., 1996	Belgium	127	3/0	ACA[4] had drinking and related outcomes comparable to those of PLA.
Sass et al., 1996	Germany	272	12/12	ACA[4] had greater treatment retention and fewer days drinking and was more likely to remain abstinent than PLA. Effects on drinking persisted during F/U.
Whitworth et al., 1996	Austria	448	12/12	ACA[4] had fewer days drinking and was more likely to remain abstinent than PLA. Effects on drinking persisted during F/U.
Geerlings et al. 1997	Benelux	262	6/6	ACA[4] had greater treatment retention, fewer days drinking and greater likelihood of remaining abstinent than PLA.
Poldrugo, 1997	Italy	246	6/6	ACA[4] had greater treatment retention, fewer days drinking, greater likelihood of remaining abstinent, and lower rate of abnormal GGTP than PLA. Difference in likelihood of abstinence persisted during F/U.
Pelc et al., 1997	Belgium	188	3/0	ACA (1.3 or 2 g/day) had greater treatment retention, fewer days drinking, was more likely to remain abstinent, and had greater reduction in GGTP and ASAT levels than PLA.
Besson et al., 1998	Switzerland	110	12/12	ACA[4] had fewer days drinking and was more likely to remain abstinent during treatment. Patients receiving disulfiram and ACA had best outcomes; those receiving neither drug had poorest outcomes. Patients receiving either ACA or DSF had intermediate outcomes.
Chick et al., 2000	United Kingdom	581	6/1	ACA (2 g/day) had drinking outcomes comparable to those of PLA. Transient beneficial effects were seen on desire to drink and on anxiety symptoms in ACA.
Tempesta et al., 2000	Italy	330	6/3	ACA (2 g/day) had delayed relapse to drinking, fewer days drinking, and greater likelihood of remaining abstinent than PLA. Among patients who drank during treatment, ACA had fewer drinking episodes and lower mean quantity of alcohol consumption than PLA. Lower drinking frequency persisted during F/U.

[1]Reprinted from Kranzler (2000), by permission of the Medical Council on Alcoholism.
[2]Treatment period/followup period (months).
[3]Only statistically significant differences reported.
[4]Dosage was dependent on body weight (1.3 g/day for subjects weighing <60 kg; 2 g/day for subjects weighing ≥60 kg).

ACA = acamprosate group   DSF = disulfiram   F/U = followup period   GGTP = gamma-glutamyltransferase   PLA = placebo group the studies, there were significant advantages for acamprosate over placebo. However, in a study conducted in England, Chick and colleagues (2000) failed to find any beneficial effects of the active drug on drinking behavior. Transient beneficial effects of acamprosate were observed on desire to drink and on anxiety symptom ratings. Unlike other multicenter studies of acamprosate, nearly a third of the patients had relapsed to drinking by the time of randomization, which may help to explain the absence of a medication effect.

One study of acamprosate has implications for the use of that medication in combination with disulfiram (Besson, Aeby et al., 1998). In that study, patients were randomly assigned to receive acamprosate or placebo, with randomization separate for patients who were taking disulfiram. Acamprosate was shown to be superior to placebo on measures of total abstinence and on cumulative abstinent days. Interestingly, the group receiving both acamprosate and disulfiram showed a significantly greater percentage of abstinent days than any of the other three groups. One explanation offered by the investigators for the marked effect of combination therapy was that acamprosate reduced the need to drink, whereas disulfiram enhanced the cognitive effects of self-control over drinking. Given that the design was not fully randomized, additional studies of this combination therapy are needed to evaluate it appropriately.

Together, studies in more than 4,000 patients (a substantially greater number than have been studied with naltrexone) provide consistent evidence of the efficacy of acamprosate in alcoholism rehabilitation. On the basis of these findings and the benign side-effect profile of acamprosate, it appears to be of considerable value for the treatment of alcohol dependence. Results of the U.S. trial, which have not yet been published, are positive and, although modest, appear to be of a magnitude comparable to the effect observed in many of the studies described earlier (Mason & Goodman, 2000).

Summary. To the present, the most promising agents that directly reduce alcohol consumption are the opiate antagonists and acamprosate. Further research is required with these agents to identify the conditions under which they are most efficacious. Specifically, it remains to be determined which patient groups, dose schedules, duration of therapy, and concomitant psychosocial treatments are optimal for the use of these medications. Moreover, trials that compare and/or combine medications that show initial promise for relapse prevention (including SSRIs) are needed to determine the best strategies for relapse prevention in alcoholics.

PHARMACOTHERAPIES FOR POSTWITHDRAWAL AFFECTIVE DISTURBANCES

Although many alcoholics feel considerably better after their acute withdrawal symptoms abate, for many others the anxiety, insomnia, and general distress of the acute withdrawal syndrome merge imperceptibly into a postwithdrawal state that can last for weeks or months. Some aspects of this postacute withdrawal (such as irritability or insomnia) are referred to as "protracted withdrawal." Other symptoms can represent the emergence of diagnosable psychiatric disorders. Whether the treatment of either the persistent withdrawal symptoms or the comorbid disorders will result in a generally better outcome remains uncertain.

Multiple factors can play a causal role in the production of mood disturbances in the postwithdrawal period, including (1) heavy alcohol intake, (2) acute and protracted withdrawal, (3) alcohol-induced damage to the central nervous system, (4) damage to the central nervous system from indirect effects of alcohol (for example, head trauma or thiamine deficiency), (5) social, economic, and interpersonal losses, (6) antecedent psychiatric disorders, and (7) a cluster of signs and symptoms that may be referred to as the "defeat/depression/hypophoria cluster."

Many of the early studies of pharmacotherapy for mood disturbances were carried out before the full extent of this diagnostic heterogeneity was recognized (Ciraulo & Jaffe, 1981). Consequently, treatment usually was directed at target symptoms of depression and anxiety in unselected groups of detoxified alcoholics. Under these circumstances, unless the patient samples are unusually homogeneous by chance or the drug in question works powerfully across diagnostic and etiologic categories, consistent positive findings are unlikely.

Today, there is renewed interest in the incidence and prevalence of comorbid psychiatric disturbances among individuals with alcohol abuse/dependence. Epidemiologic studies have shown high rates of comorbidity of drug dependence and psychiatric disorders in alcohol-dependent individuals in the community (Regier, Farmer et al., 1990; Kessler, McGonagle et al., 1994; Kessler, Crum et al., 1997; Grant & Harford, 1995). It also is evident that most alcoholics who seek treatment meet lifetime criteria for psychiatric disorders in addition to alcoholism. Among the more common of these disorders are major depression, bipolar disorder, antisocial personality disorder, drug dependence, borderline personality disorder, phobias, and attention deficit disorder—residual type (hyperactivity syndrome) (Behar & Winokur, 1979; Hesselbrock, Meyer et al., 1985; Mullaney & Trippett, 1979; Nace, Saxon et al., 1983; Wood, Wender et al., 1983; Ross, Frederick et al., 1988).

Among the drugs that have been used or proposed to treat anxiety and depression in the postwithdrawal state are tricyclic antidepressants, SSRI antidepressants, benzodiazepines and other anxiolytics, phenothiazines and other dopaminergic blockers, and lithium. The use of these drugs in alcoholics requires careful consideration of the potential for adverse effects in this patient population, which may be attributable to co-occurring medical disorders (often present among alcoholics) and the pharmacokinetic effects of acute and chronic alcohol consumption. For example, it has been shown that chronic ethanol administration increases clearance of imipramine and desipramine, thereby reducing the therapeutic potential of these medications (Ciraulo, Alderson et al., 1982; Ciraulo, Barnhill et al., 1988). Further, disulfiram can interact with these and other medications used to treat comorbid psychiatric disorders in alcoholics (Ciraulo, Barnhill et al., 1985; Gorelick, 1993). Although indications for the use of these medications in alcoholics are similar to those for nonalcoholic populations and can be arrived at only through careful psychiatric diagnosis, the choice of medications should take into account the increased potential for drug interactions among alcoholics.

Tricyclic Antidepressants (TCAs). TCAs once were widely used in the treatment of alcoholic patients. However, because alcoholics routinely had been excluded from antidepressant trials, firm evidence of the efficacy of TCAs in such patients began to be available only as the routine use of these agents was declining in favor of the SSRIs. In most studies of TCAs, a therapeutically inadequate dose was used and no effort was made to compensate for the fact that both cigarette smoking and heavy drinking can stimulate liver enzymes that metabolize drugs (Ciraulo & Jaffe, 1981). Ciraulo and colleagues (1982) have shown that the intrinsic clearance of imipramine in alcoholics is 2.5 times that of control subjects. After a standard 150 mg dose of imipramine, alcoholics have steady-state concentrations of imipramine and its metabolites that are subtherapeutic. The effect on imipramine clearance is greater than that on desipramine clearance (Ciraulo, Barnhill et al., 1988).

Nunes and colleagues (1993) conducted an open-label study in which alcoholics with primary major depression or dysthymic disorder who responded to imipramine treatment were randomly assigned to continue on imipramine or switch to placebo. Despite a small sample size, there was a trend for the active drug to prevent a relapse to depression and heavy drinking. In a study of outpatient alcoholics with primary depression that was conducted by McGrath and colleagues (1996), imipramine treatment was found to result in a modest improvement in depressive symptoms, but no overall effect on drinking measures.

In a study of secondary depression in alcoholics, in which desipramine or placebo treatment was initiated after a median of 8 days of abstinence, the active drug was found to be superior in reducing both depressive symptoms and heavy drinking (Mason, Kocsis et al., 1996). The antidepressant response that was observed suggests that the common practice of requiring a period of two to four weeks before initiating antidepressant therapy may be excessive.

Selective Serotonin Reuptake Inhibitors. There are a limited number of studies with SSRIs, such as fluoxetine, in the treatment of major depression in alcoholics. A small, open-label study of inpatient alcoholics who were depressed and suicidal showed that fluoxetine reduced depressive symptoms and alcohol consumption (Cornelius, Salloum et al., 1993). Subsequently, a 12-week, placebo-controlled, double-blind study by the same investigators showed fluoxetine to be superior in reducing both depressive symptoms and total alcohol consumption in 51 patients diagnosed with major depression and alcohol dependence (Cornelius, Salloum et al., 1997). Similarly, in a placebo-controlled trial of fluoxetine for relapse prevention in alcoholics (Kranzler, Burleson et al., 1995), the subgroup with current major depression showed a greater reduction in depressive symptoms in response to the active drug. However, the size of the subsample was too small in that study to permit a meaningful evaluation of the effect of reduced depression on alcohol consumption.

Although it has only modest inhibitory effects on serotonin reuptake, the antidepressant nefazodone has predominant serotonergic effects. Roy-Byrne and colleagues (2000) found this medication to be beneficial in decreasing depressive symptoms in depressed alcoholics. However, after controlling for changes in depressive symptoms, investigators found that nefazodone showed no effect on drinking behavior.

Even if one accepts the view that most instances of postwithdrawal depression and "blues" will remit spontaneously within a few days to several weeks (Schuckit, 1983; Brown & Schuckit, 1988), there are some patients whose severe and persistent depression requires treatment. In such cases, antidepressants may be used. However, because alcoholics may be less compliant with the recommended dose than are nonalcoholic patients, and because heavy drinking and smoking can increase clearance of TCAs (Ciraulo, Alderson et al., 1982; Ciraulo, Barnhill et al., 1988; reviewed in Sands, Knapp et al., 1995), the monitoring of TCA plasma levels is recommended or the use of an SSRI should be considered. The choice of an SSRI over a TCA probably is warranted by the greater safety profile of the newer medications, particularly in relation to the risk of suicide by medication overdose.

Benzodiazepines and Other Anxiolytics. Benzodiazepines are widely used in the treatment of acute alcohol withdrawal. However, anxiety, depression, and sleep disturbances can persist for months after withdrawal. Consequently, it is unclear where withdrawal ends and other causes of anxiety and disturbed sleep begin. Nevertheless, most nonmedical personnel involved in the treatment of alcoholism are opposed to the use of medication that can induce any variety of dependence. The pros and cons of the use of benzodiazepines in alcoholics and other patients with addictive disorders during the postwithdrawal period for the management of anxiety or insomnia was the topic of a recent debate (Ciraulo & Nace, 2000), which augments the discussion that follows.

The increased risk of dependence notwithstanding, there may be an important role for the judicious use of benzodiazepines in alcoholics. The dropout rate from alcoholism rehabilitation often is very high, frequently because of a relapse to drinking. To the extent that early relapse is a result of continued withdrawal-related symptoms (such as anxiety, depression, and insomnia) that can be suppressed by low doses of benzodiazepines, retention in treatment may be enhanced (Kissin, 1977). Moreover, for some patients, benzodiazepine dependence, if it does occur, may be more benign than alcoholism.

These important potential benefits must be weighed against the dual risks of benzodiazepine overdose and of physical dependence on benzodiazepines. While benzodiazepines alone are comparatively safe, even in overdose, their combination with other brain depressants (including alcohol) can be lethal. Although there is little doubt that alcoholics are vulnerable to the development of dependence on the benzodiazepines, the probability of abuse and dependence may be lower than is generally believed (Bliding, 1978; Marks, 1978; Ciraulo, Barnhill et al., 1990). However, dependence on both alcohol and benzodiazepines can increase depressive symptoms (Schuckit, 1983), and the combination of alcohol and benzodiazepine dependence may be more difficult to treat than the alcoholism alone (Sokolow, Welte et al., 1981).

The benzodiazepines currently available for clinical use differ substantially in terms of pharmacokinetics, acute euphoriant effects, and frequency of reported dependence. It is likely, therefore, that not all benzodiazepines have the same potential for abuse. Kissin (1977) believed that chlordiazepoxide was the benzodiazepine of choice for use in alcoholics. Wolf and colleagues (1990) offered evidence that diazepam, lorazepam, and alprazolam have greater abuse potential than chlordiazepoxide and clorazepate. Bliding (1978) reported low levels of abuse with oxazepam. Jaffe and colleagues (1983) found that, in recently detoxified alcoholics, halazepam produces minimal euphoria even at supratherapeutic doses. A number of partial agonist and mixed agonist/antagonist compounds currently in development may offer an advantage over approved benzodiazepines for use in alcoholics.

Buspirone (BuSpar®), a nonbenzodiazepine anxiolytic, appears to exert its effects largely through its agonist activity at serotonergic autoreceptors. It is equal to diazepam in the relief of anxiety and associated depression in outpatients with moderate to severe anxiety (Goldberg & Finnerty, 1979; Jacobson, Dominguez et al., 1985). Buspirone may, however, have several advantages: It is less sedating than diazepam or clorazepate, does not interact with alcohol to impair psychomotor skills, and does not appear to have abuse liability (Mattila, Aranko et al., 1982; Seppala, Aranko et al., 1982; Griffith, Jasinski et al., 1986). In contrast to benzodiazepines, however, buspirone does not have acute anxiolytic effects, nor is it useful in the treatment of alcohol withdrawal.

A double-blind, placebo-controlled trial of buspirone in alcoholics (Bruno, 1989) showed significantly greater retention in treatment and greater decreases in alcohol craving, anxiety, and depression scores in buspirone-treated patients. Although both groups showed significant declines in alcohol consumption during the study, buspirone treatment did not differentially reduce alcohol consumption. Tollefson and colleagues (1992), using a double-blind study design, also reported an advantage for buspirone over placebo in abstinent alcoholics with comorbid generalized anxiety disorder. Those investigators found that buspirone-treated subjects were less likely to discontinue treatment prematurely and had greater reductions in anxiety than did placebo-treated subjects. Although a subjective, global measure of improvement in drinking was observed for the active drug group, measures of alcohol consumption were not reported. Kranzler and colleagues (1994), using a double-blind, placebo-controlled design, also found that buspirone was superior to placebo in terms of retention in treatment among a group of anxious alcoholics. The active drug also delayed relapse to heavy drinking and, during a six-month posttreatment followup period, it reduced the number of drinking days. The beneficial effects of buspirone on both anxiety and drinking were most evident among the patients with the highest baseline anxiety scores.

In contrast to these three reports, a placebo-controlled study by Malcolm and colleagues (1992) showed the drug to have no advantage over placebo on anxiety or drinking measures in an anxious, severely alcohol-dependent patient sample. Although there appears to be a role for buspirone in the treatment of generalized anxiety in alcoholics, further research is needed to identify the most appropriate patient group in which to use the drug.

Phenothiazines and Other Dopaminergic Blockers. These drugs are of obvious importance in the treatment of alcoholics with comorbid psychotic disorders (such as schizophrenia). Several studies have compared the effects of dopaminergic blockers with those of placebo on symptoms of anxiety, tension, or depression during the postwithdrawal phase (Behar & Winokur, 1979; Rada & Kellner, 1979; Smith, 1978). As with most studies of TCAs, patients on placebo showed substantial improvement, and differences in favor of the active drugs were not great. In one study, a low dose of thioridazine (Mellaril®) was superior to placebo in the reduction of tension and insomnia, but the placebo group did better in terms of work and activity (Hague, Wilson et al., 1976).

The selective dopaminergic receptor blocker tiapride also was studied in depressed and anxious alcoholics (Shaw, Majumdar et al., 1987). Although the study's findings are limited by a high dropout rate, subjects treated with the active drug drank less and had longer periods of abstinence than did patients treated with placebo. Patients treated with tiapride evidenced less neuroticism, anxiety, and depression; expressed greater satisfaction with their social situations and

physical health; and exhibited fewer physical complications of alcoholism (Shaw, Majumdar et al., 1987). In a subsequent study (Shaw, Waller et al., 1994), tiapride-treated patients were more likely than placebo-treated patients to abstain from alcohol and to report greater subjective feelings of wellbeing, and they were less likely to use health services.

At present, given the equivocal results of trials of antipsychotic drugs in alcoholics and the potential for adverse effects such as tardive dyskinesia, long-term use of these medications in alcoholics who do not have coexisting psychotic disorders probably is not warranted. However, additional research on the role of tiapride in alcoholism treatment does appear to be warranted.

Lithium. Studies of lithium conducted in the 1970s, including some that used placebo controls (Kline, Wren et al., 1974; Merry, Reynolds et al., 1976), showed that lithium-treated patients experienced fewer days of pathologic drinking. However, the rates of attrition from treatment in these studies were high. Subsequently, Fawcett and colleagues (1987) found that compliance with either lithium or placebo was associated with abstinence in alcoholics who were not selected for coexisting depression. Moreover, compliant patients taking active medication who had therapeutic serum levels (0.4 mEq/L or greater) were abstinent more often than were compliant subjects with subtherapeutic lithium levels. After the first six months, however, even the subjects who were compliant early in the study tended to stop taking their medication. Nevertheless, the association between early compliance and sobriety persisted, suggesting that the beneficial effects of lithium are greatest in the early months after detoxification. The beneficial effect of lithium did not appear to be mediated by an antidepressant effect, because it did not affect mood in patients who were depressed.

Dorus and colleagues (1989) conducted a multicenter, double-blind, placebo-controlled trial in depressed and nondepressed alcoholic veterans. A total of 457 male alcoholics, of whom approximately a third were depressed, were assigned randomly to receive either 600 or 1,200 mg/day of lithium or a comparable number of placebo capsules. No significant differences between lithium-treated and placebo-treated patients were found on any of a variety of outcome measures, including number of drinking days, alcohol-related hospitalizations, and severity of depression. The lack of efficacy was observed for both the depressed and the nondepressed subjects. This large, carefully conducted trial suggests that lithium should be reserved for the treatment of alcoholics who have comorbid bipolar disorder. A study by Fawcett and colleagues (2000), in which there was no advantage to lithium over placebo in alcoholics who were not selected for a comorbid psychiatric disorder, is consistent with this conclusion.

CONCLUSIONS

In general, with the exception of the central role that benzodiazepines play in the treatment of alcohol withdrawal, pharmacotherapy has not yet had a demonstrably large effect on alcoholism treatment. However, recent developments, including approval of naltrexone for relapse prevention in the U.S. and Europe, and of acamprosate in Europe, suggest that the use of medications eventually can contribute substantially to the treatment of alcoholism. Nevertheless, there remain a considerable number of questions that must be examined before medications can be used widely in the treatment of alcohol dependence. In addition to the issues discussed earlier in regard to specific agents (concerning the optimal duration of use of naltrexone), the safety and efficacy of medications for treatment of alcohol dependence must be examined in women, in various ethnic and racial groups, and in adolescent and geriatric populations.

Unfortunately, little has changed since Gorelick (1993) observed that data on pharmacotherapy for relapse prevention in these groups are virtually nonexistent. Also virtually nonexistent are cost-effectiveness and cost-benefit data that would support the routine coverage of pharmacologic treatments for alcoholism under standard medical insurance plans.

Increasingly, however, psychiatric comorbidity is being recognized as an important determinant of the effectiveness of alcoholism rehabilitation. Persistent psychiatric disturbances interfere with psychosocial treatments. Thus, pharmacologic agents that are effective in treating psychiatric symptomatology may provide important benefits in relapse prevention. Anxiolytics that appear to have little abuse potential, such as buspirone, and antidepressants that also can influence ethanol intake warrant careful evaluation in the treatment of anxious and depressed alcoholics.

However, the relationship between substance use and psychiatric symptomatology is complex (Myers, Borg et al., 1986; Kranzler & Rounsaville, 1998). Drugs that ameliorate persistent mood and anxiety symptoms will not necessarily produce changes in alcohol consumption once a significant degree of alcohol dependence develops. This lack of change can occur even if pathologic mood states are important in the initiation of heavy drinking. Once the neuroadaptive changes and the complex learning that constitute the dependence syndrome occur, alcohol dependence becomes autonomous (Edwards & Gross, 1976; Wikler, 1980). It does not resolve simply because one major contributing factor is brought under control. Efforts to change pathologic alcohol use patterns must accompany any treatment, including pharmacotherapy, that is aimed at control of pathologic mood states. The challenge for those who treat alcoholics is to combine medication effectively with psychotherapy and self-help group participation (Meza & Kranzler, 1996).

Drugs that directly affect alcohol consumption may be most useful as adjuncts to cognitive-behavioral relapse prevention treatment (O'Malley, Jaffe et al., 1992). In this regard, the drugs that appear most promising are naltrexone and acamprosate. A number of studies of these medications, administered in conjunction with psychotherapy, are under way. As the research literature on the use of these drugs grows, it will be possible to assess their utility in conjunction with a variety of psychotherapies or as one element in a multimodal program for the treatment of alcoholism. Efforts to match medications with specific subgroups of alcoholics also is a promising strategy.

As with the use of medications to treat comorbid psychopathology, the use of medications to reduce drinking must be integrated with psychosocial treatment. Although medications have not become a mainstream therapy in alcoholism treatment programs, combining medications with self-help group participation can represent a particular challenge. Abstinence-oriented groups such as Alcoholics Anonymous see the alcohol-sensitizing agents as supportive of their goal of total abstinence and are willing to work with physicians around the issues of proper dose, compliance, and early detection of side effects. However, such groups historically have been less supportive of other pharmacotherapies for alcoholism. Thus, it may be necessary to communicate to the groups the view that effective pharmacotherapy of associated anxiety and mood disturbances is complementary, rather than competitive, with abstinence-oriented change and support systems. Similarly, the use of medications to reduce the risk of relapse through direct effects on craving or drinking behavior should be seen as potentially additive or synergistic to self-help efforts.

It does not seem unduly optimistic to predict that within the next few years, a number of medications will have been shown convincingly to be efficacious for the treatment of comorbid psychopathology and/or the prevention of relapse in alcoholics. In anticipation of these developments, attention also must be directed to enhancing the acceptability of these medications to the alcoholism treatment community as a standard ingredient in alcoholism rehabilitation.

REFERENCES

Allen JP & Litten RZ (1992). Techniques to enhance compliance with disulfiram. *Alcoholism: Clinical & Experimental Research* 16:1035-1041.

Amit Z, Brown Z, Sutherland A et al. (1985). Reduction in alcohol intake in humans as a function of treatment with zimelidine: Implications for treatment. In CA Naranjo & EM Sellers (eds.) *Research Advances in New Psychopharmacological Treatments for Alcoholism.* Amsterdam, The Netherlands: Elsevier.

Amit Z, Smith BR, Brown ZW et al. (1982). An examination of the role of TIQ alkaloids in alcohol intake: Reinforcers, satiety agents or artifacts. In F Bloom, J Barchas, M Sandler et al. (eds.) *Beta-Carbolines and Tetrahydroisoquinolines.* New York, NY: Alan R. Liss.

Angelone SM, Bellini L, Di Bella D et al. (1998). Effects of fluvoxamine and citalopram in maintaining abstinence in a sample of Italian detoxified alcoholics. *Alcohol and Alcoholism* 33:151-156.

Anton RF, Moak DH, Latham PK et al. (2000). Posttreatment results of combining naltrexone and cognitive-behavior therapy for the treatment of alcoholism. *Journal of Clinical Psychopharmacology* 21:72-77.

Anton RF, Moak DH, Waid R et al. (1999). Naltrexone and cognitive behavioral therapy for the treatment of outpatient alcoholics: Results of a placebo-controlled trial. *American Journal of Psychiatry* 156:1758-1764.

Azrin NH, Sisson RW, Meyers R et al. (1982). Alcoholism treatment by disulfiram and community reinforcement therapy. *Journal of Behavior Therapy and Experimental Psychiatry* 13:105-112.

Balldin J, Berggren U, Engel J et al. (1994). Effect of citalopram on alcohol intake in heavy drinkers. *Alcoholism: Clinical & Experimental Research* 18:1133-1136.

Behar D & Winokur G (1979). Research in alcoholism and depression: A two-way street under construction. In RW Pickens & LL Heston (eds.) *Psychiatric Factors in Drug Abuse.* New York, NY: Grune & Stratton, 125-152.

Bergstrom B, Ohlin H, Lindblom PE et al. (1982). Is disulfiram implantation effective? *Lancet* 1:49-50.

Besson J, Aeby F, Kasas A et al. (1998). Combined efficacy of acamprosate and disulfiram in the treatment of alcoholism: A controlled study. *Alcoholism: Clinical & Experimental Research* 22:573-579.

Bliding A (1978). The abuse potential of benzodiazepines with special reference to oxazepam. *Acta Psychiatrica Scandinavica* (Suppl 24):111-116.

Brewer C (1984). How effective is the standard dose of disulfiram? A review of the alcohol-disulfiram reaction in practice. *British Journal of Psychiatry* 144:200-202.

Brewer C, Meyers RJ & Johnsen J (2000). Does disulfiram help to prevent relapse in alcohol abuse? *CNS Drugs* 14:329-341.

Brown SA & Schuckit MA (1988). Changes in depression among abstinent alcoholics. *Journal of Studies on Alcohol* 49:412-417.

Bruno F (1989). Buspirone in the treatment of alcoholic patients. *Psychopathology* 22(Suppl 1):49-59.

Chick J (1999). Safety issues concerning the use of disulfiram in treating alcohol dependence. *Drug Safety* 20:427-435.

Chick J, Anton R, Checinski K et al. (2000). A multicentre, randomized, double-blind, placebo-controlled trial of naltrexone in the treatment of alcohol dependence or abuse. *Alcohol and Alcoholism* 35:587-593.

Chick J, Gough K, Falkowski W et al. (1992). Disulfiram treatment of alcoholism. *British Journal of Psychiatry* 161: 84-89.

Chick J, Howlett H, Morgan MY et al. (2000). United Kingdom multicentre acamprosate study (UKMAS): A six-month prospective study of acamprosate versus placebo in preventing relapse after withdrawal from alcohol. *Alcohol and Alcoholism* 35:176-187.

Ciraulo DA & Jaffe JH (1981). Tricyclic antidepressants in the treatment of depression associated with alcoholism. *Journal of Clinical Psychopharmacology* 1:146-150.

Ciraulo DA & Nace E (2000). Benzodiazepine treatment of anxiety or insomnia in substance abuse patients. *American Journal of Addictions* 9:276-284.

Ciraulo DA, Alderson LM, Chapron DJ et al. (1982). Imipramine disposition in alcoholics. *Journal of Clinical Psychopharmacology* 2:2-7.

Ciraulo DA, Barnhill J & Boxenbaum HG (1985). Pharmacokinetic interaction of disulfiram and antidepressants. *American Journal of Psychiatry* 142:1373-1374.

Ciraulo DA, Barnhill JG & Jaffe JH (1988). Clinical pharmacokinetics of imipramine and desipramine in alcoholics and normal volunteers. *Clinical Pharmacology and Therapeutics* 43:509-518.

Ciraulo DA, Barnhill JG, Jaffe JH et al. (1990). Intravenous pharmacokinetics of 2-hydroxyimipramine in alcoholics and normal controls. *Journal of Studies on Alcohol* 51:366-372.

Cohen G & Collins MS (1970). Alkaloids from catecholamines in adrenal tissues: Possible role in alcoholism. *Science* 167:1749-1751.

Cornelius JR, Salloum IM, Cornelius MD et al. (1993). Fluoxetine trial in suicidal depressed alcoholics. *Psychopharmacology Bulletin* 29:195-199.

Cornelius JR, Salloum IM, Ehler JG et al. (1997). Fluoxetine in depressed alcoholics: A double-blind, placebo-controlled trial. *Archives of General Psychiatry* 54:700-705.

Dorus W, Ostrow DG, Anton R et al. (1989). Lithium treatment of depressed and nondepressed alcoholics. *Journal of the American Medical Association* 262:1646-1652.

Edwards G & Gross MM (1976). Alcohol dependence: Provisional description of a clinical syndrome. *British Medical Journal* 1:1058-1061.

Favazza AR & Martin P (1974). Chemotherapy of delirium tremens: A survey of physicians' preferences. *American Journal of Psychiatry* 131:1031-1033.

Fawcett J, Clark DC, Aagesen CA et al. (1987). A double-blind, placebo-controlled trial of lithium carbonate therapy for alcoholism. *Archives of General Psychiatry* 44:248-256.

Fawcett J, Kravitz HM, McGuire M et al. (2000). Pharmacological treatments for alcoholism: Revisiting lithium and considering buspirone. *Alcoholism: Clinical & Experimental Research* 24:666-674

Fuller RK, Branchey L, Brightwell DR et al. (1986). Disulfiram treatment of alcoholism: A Veteran's Administration Cooperative Study. *Journal of the American Medical Association* 256:1449-1455.

Garbutt JC, West SL, Carey TS et al. (1999). Pharmacological treatment of alcohol dependence: A review of the evidence. *Journal of the American Medical Association* 281:1318-1325.

Geerlings PJ, Ansoms C & van den Brink W (1997). Acamprosate and prevention of relapse in alcoholics. *European Addiction Research* 3:129-137.

Gerra G, Caccavari R, Delsignore R et al. (1992). Effects of fluoxetine and Ca-acetyl-homotaurinate on alcohol intake in familial and nonfamilial alcohol patients. *Current Therapeutic Research* 52:291-295.

Goldberg HL & Finnerty RJ (1979). The comparative efficacy of buspirone and diazepam in the treatment of anxiety. *American Journal of Psychiatry* 136:1184-1187.

Gorelick DA (1993). Recent developments in pharmacological treatment of alcoholism. In Galanter M (ed.) *Recent Developments in Alcoholism, Vol. 11.* New York, NY: Plenum Press, 413-427.

Gorelick DA & Paredes A (1992). Effect of fluoxetine on alcohol consumption in male alcoholics. *Alcoholism: Clinical & Experimental Research* 16:261-265.

Grant BF & Harford TC (1995). Comorbidity between DSM-IV alcohol use disorders and major depression: Results of a national survey. *Drug and Alcohol Dependence* 39:197-206.

Griffith JD, Jasinski DR, Casten GP et al. (1986). Investigation of the abuse liability of buspirone in alcohol-dependent patients. *American Journal of Medicine* 80(Suppl 3B):30-35.

Hague WH, Wilson LG, Dudley DL et al. (1976). Post-detoxification drug treatment of anxiety and depression in alcoholic addicts. *Journal of Nervous and Mental Diseases* 162:354-359.

Heinala P, Alho H, Kiianmaa K et al. (2001). Targeted use of naltrexone without prior detoxification in the treatment of alcohol dependence: A factorial double-blind, placebo-controlled trial. *Journal of Clinical Psychopharmacology* 21:287-292.

Hersh D, Van Kirk JR & Kranzler HR (1998). Naltrexone treatment of comorbid alcohol and cocaine use disorders. *Psychopharmacology* 139:44-52.

Hesselbrock MN, Meyer RE & Keener JJ (1985). Psychopathology in hospitalized alcoholics. *Archives of General Psychiatry* 42:1050-1055.

Hiller JM, Aangel LM & Simon EJ (1981). Multiple opiate receptors: Alcohol selectively inhibits binding to delta receptors. *Science* 214:468-469.

Hoyumpa AM & Schenker S (1982). Major drug interactions: Effect of liver disease, alcohol and malnutrition. *Annual Review of Medicine* 33:113-149.

Jacobson AF, Dominguez RA, Goldstein BJ et al. (1985). Comparison of buspirone and diazepam in generalized anxiety disorder. *Pharmacotherapy* 5:290-296.

Jaffe JH, Ciraulo DA, Nies A et al. (1983). Abuse potential of halazepam and diazepam in patients recently treated for acute alcohol withdrawal. *Clinical Pharmacology and Therapeutics* 34:623-630.

Jaffe AJ, Rounsaville B, Chang G et al. (1996). Naltrexone, relapse prevention and supportive therapy with alcoholics: An analysis of patient treatment matching. *Journal of Consulting and Clinical Psychology* 64:1044-1053.

Janiri L, Gobbi G, Mannelli P et al. (1996). Effects of fluoxetine at antidepressant doses on short-term outcome of detoxified alcoholics. *International Clinical Psychopharmacology* 11:109-117.

Johnson BA, Roache JD, Javors MA et al. (2000). Ondansetron for reduction of drinking among biologically predisposed alcoholic patients: A randomized controlled trial. *Journal of the American Medical Association* 284:963-971.

Kabel DI & Petty F (1996). A double blind study of fluoxetine in severe alcohol dependence: Adjunctive therapy during and after inpatient treatment. *Alcoholism: Clinical & Experimental Research* 20:780-784.

Kessler RC, Crum RM, Warner LA et al. (1997). Lifetime co-occurrence of DSM-IIIR alcohol abuse and dependence with other psychiatric disorders in the National Comorbidity Study. *Archives of General Psychiatry* 54:313-321.

Kessler RC, McGonagle KA, Zhao S et al. (1994). Lifetime and 12-month prevalence of DSM-IIIR psychiatric disorders in the United States. *Archives of General Psychiatry* 51:8-19.

Kissin B (1977). Medical management of the alcoholic patient. In B Kissin & H Begleiter (eds.) *The Biology of Alcoholism, Vol. 5. Treatment and Rehabilitation of the Chronic Alcoholic.* New York, NY: Plenum Press, 55-103.

Kline NS, Wren JC, Cooper TB et al. (1974). Evaluation of lithium therapy in chronic and periodic alcoholism. *American Journal of Medical Sciences* 268:15-22.

Kranzler HR, ed. (1995). *The Pharmacology of Alcohol Abuse.* New York, NY: Springer Publishing.

Kranzler HR (2000). Pharmacotherapy of alcoholism: Gaps in knowledge and opportunities for research. *Alcohol and Alcoholism* 35:537-547.

Kranzler HR & Rounsaville BJ, eds. (1998). *Dual Diagnosis: Substance Abuse and Comorbid Medical and Psychiatric Disorders.* New York, NY: Marcel Dekker.

Kranzler HR, Burleson JA, Del Boca FK et al. (1994). Buspirone treatment of anxious alcoholics: A placebo-controlled trial. *Archives of General Psychiatry* 51:720-731.

Kranzler HR, Burleson JA, Korner P et al. (1995). Placebo-controlled trial of fluoxetine as an adjunct to relapse prevention in alcoholics. *American Journal of Psychiatry* 152:391-397.

Kranzler HR, Burleson JA, Brown J et al. (1996). Fluoxetine treatment seems to reduce the beneficial effects of cognitive-behavioral therapy in Type B alcoholics. *Alcoholism: Clinical & Experimental Research* 20:1534-1541.

Kranzler HR, Del Boca F, Korner P et al. (1993). Adverse effects limit the usefulness of fluvoxamine for the treatment of alcoholism. *Journal of Substance Abuse Treatment* 10:283-287.

Kranzler HR, Mason BJ, Pettinati HM et al. (1997). Methodological issues in pharmacotherapy trials with alcoholics. In M Hertzman & D Feltner (eds.) *The Handbook of Psychopharmacology Trials.* New York, NY: New York University Press, 213-245.

Kranzler HR, Modesto-Lowe V & Nuwayser ES (1998). A sustained-release naltrexone preparation for treatment of alcohol dependence. *Alcoholism: Clinical & Experimental Research* 22:1074-1079.

Kranzler HR, Modesto-Lowe V & Van Kirk J (2000). Naltrexone vs. nefazodone for treatment of alcohol dependence: A placebo-controlled trial. *Neuropsychopharmacology* 22:493-503.

Kranzler HR, Tennen H, Penta C et al. (1997). Targeted naltrexone treatment in early problem drinkers. *Addictive Behaviors* 22:431-436.

LeMarquand D, Pihl RO & Benkelfat C (1994a). Serotonin and alcohol intake, abuse, and dependence: Findings of animal studies. *Biological Psychiatry* 36:395-421.

LeMarquand D, Pihl RO & Benkelfat C (1994b). Serotonin and alcohol intake, abuse, and dependence: Clinical evidence. *Biological Psychiatry* 36:326-337.

Lhuintre JP, Moore ND, Saligaut C et al. (1985). Ability of calcium bis acetyl homotaurinate, a GABA agonist, to prevent relapse in weaned alcoholics. *Lancet* 1:1014-1016.

Lhuintre JP, Moore N, Tran G et al. (1990). Acamprosate appears to decrease alcohol intake in weaned alcoholics. *Alcohol & Alcoholism* 25:613-622.

Lindros KO, Stowell A, Pikkarainen P et al. (1981). The disulfiram (Antabuse)-alcohol reaction in male alcoholics: Its efficient management by 4-methylpyrazole. *Alcoholism: Clinical & Experimental Research* 5:528-530.

Major LF, Lerner P, Ballenger JK et al. (1979). Dopamine beta-hydroxylase in the cerebrospinal fluid: Relationship to disulfiram induced psychosis. *Biological Psychiatry* 14:337-344.

Malcolm R, Anton RF, Randall CL et al. (1992). A placebo-controlled trial of buspirone in anxious inpatient alcoholics. *Alcoholism: Clinical & Experimental Research* 16:1007-1013.

Marks J (1978). *The Benzodiazepines: Use, Misuse, Abuse.* Lancaster, England: MTP Press, Ltd.

Mason B & Goodman A (2000). Acamprosate: New preclinical and clinical research. Presented at the 23rd Annual Scientific Meeting of the Research Society on Alcoholism; June 24-29, Denver, CO.

Mason BJ, Kocsis JH, Ritvo EC et al. (1996). A double-blind, placebo-controlled trial of desipramine for primary alcohol dependence stratified on the presence or absence of major depression. *Journal of the American Medical Association* 275:761-767.

Mason BJ, Ritvo EC, Morgan RO et al. (1994). A double-blind, placebo-controlled pilot study to evaluate the efficacy and safety of oral nalmefene HCl for alcohol dependence. *Alcoholism: Clinical & Experimental Research* 18:1162-1167.

Mason BJ, Salvato FR, Williams LD et al. (1999). A double-blind, placebo-controlled study of oral nalmefene for alcohol dependence. *Archives of General Psychiatry* 56:719-724.

Mattila MJ, Aranko K & Seppala T (1982). Acute effects of buspirone and alcohol on psychomotor skills. *Journal of Clinical Psychiatry* 43:56-60.

McCaul ME, Wand GS, Rohde C et al. (2000). Serum 6-beta-naltrexol levels are related to alcohol responses in heavy drinkers. *Alcoholism: Clinical & Experimental Research* 24:1385-1391.

McGrath PJ, Nunes EV, Stewart JW et al. (1996). Imipramine treatment of alcoholics with primary depression. *Archives of General Psychiatry* 53:232-240.

Merry J, Reynolds CM, Bailey J et al. (1976). Prophylactic treatment of alcoholism by lithium carbonate. *Lancet* 2:481-482.

Meyer RE (1986). How to understand the relationship between psychopathology and addictive disorders: Another example of the chicken and the egg. In RE Meyer (ed.) *Psychopathology and Addictive Disorders.* New York, NY: Guilford Press.

Meza E & Kranzler HR (1996). Closing the gap between alcoholism research and practice: The case for pharmacotherapy. *Psychiatric Services* 47:917-920.

Mullaney JA & Trippett CJ (1979). Alcohol dependence and phobias: Clinical description and relevance. *Psychiatry* 135:565-573.

Myers RD, Borg S & Mossberg R (1986). Antagonism by naltrexone of voluntary alcohol selection in the chronically drinking macaque monkey. *Alcohol* 3:383-388.

Myrick H, Brady KT & Malcolm R (2001). New developments in the pharmacotherapy of alcohol dependence. *American Journal on Addictions* 10(Suppl):3-15.

Nace CP, Saxon JJ & Shore N (1983). A comparison of borderline and nonborderline alcoholic patients. *Archives of General Psychiatry* 40:54-56.

Naranjo CA, Bremner KE & Lanctot KL (1995). Effects of citalopram and a brief psycho-social intervention on alcohol intake, dependence, and problems. *Addiction* 90:87-99.

Naranjo CA, Kadlec KE, Sanhueza P et al. (1990). Fluoxetine differentially alters alcohol intake and other consummatory behaviors in problem drinkers. *Clinical Pharmacology and Therapeutics* 47:490-498.

Naranjo CA, Poulos CX, Bremner KE et al. (1992). Citalopram decreases desirability, liking, and consumption of alcohol in alcohol-dependent drinkers. *Clinical Pharmacology and Therapeutics* 51:729-739.

Naranjo CA, Sellers EM, Roach CA et al. (1984). Zimelidine-induced variations in alcohol intake by nondepressed heavy drinkers. *Clinical Pharmacology and Therapeutics* 35:374-381.

Naranjo CA, Sellers EM, Sullivan JT et al. (1987). The serotonin uptake inhibitor citalopram attenuates ethanol intake. *Clinical Pharmacology and Therapeutics* 41:266-274.

Naranjo CA, Sullivan JT, Kadlec KE et al. (1989). Differential effects of viqualine on alcohol intake and other consummatory behaviors. *Clinical Pharmacology and Therapeutics* 46:301-309.

Nunes EV, McGrath PJ, Quitkin FM et al. (1993). Imipramine treatment of alcoholism with comorbid depression. *American Journal of Psychiatry* 150:963-965.

O'Malley SS, Jaffe AJ, Chang G et al. (1992). Naltrexone and coping skills therapy for alcohol dependence: A controlled study. *Archives of General Psychiatry* 49:894-898.

O'Malley SS, Jaffe AJ, Rode S et al. (1996a). Experience of a "slip" among alcoholics treated with naltrexone or placebo. *American Journal of Psychiatry* 153:281-283.

O'Malley SS, Jaffe AJ, Chang G et al. (1996b). Six-month follow-up of naltrexone and psychotherapy for alcohol dependence. *Archives of General Psychiatry* 53:217-224.

Oslin D, Liberto JG, O'Brien J et al. (1997). Naltrexone as an adjunctive treatment for older patients with alcohol dependence. *American Journal of Geriatric Psychiatry* 5:324-332.

Paille FM, Guelfi JD, Perkins AC et al. (1995). Double-blind randomized multicentre trial of acamprosate in maintaining abstinence from alcohol. *Alcohol & Alcoholism* 30:239-247.

Peachey JE, Brien JF, Roach CA et al. (1981). A comparative review of the pharmacological and toxicological properties of disulfiram and calcium carbimide. *Journal of Clinical Psychopharmacology* 1:21-26.

Peachey JE, Maglana S, Robinson GM et al. (1981). Cardiovascular changes during the calcium carbimide-ethanol interaction. *Clinical Pharmacology and Therapeutics* 29:40-46.

Pelc I, Le Bon O, Lebert P et al. (1996). Acamprosate in the treatment of alcohol dependence: A 6-month postdetoxification study. In M Soyka (ed.) *Acamprosate in Relapse Prevention of Alcoholism.* Berlin, Germany: Springer-Verlag, 133-142.

Pelc I, Verbanck P, Le Bon O et al. (1997). Efficacy and safety of acamprosate in the treatment of detoxified alcohol-dependent patients. A 90-day placebo-controlled dose-finding study. *British Journal of Psychiatry* 171:73-77.

Pettinati HM, Volpicelli JR, Kranzler HR et al. (2000). Sertraline treatment for alcohol dependence: Interactive effects of medication and subtype. *Alcoholism: Clinical & Experimental Research* 24:1041-1049.

Poldrugo F (1997). Acamprosate treatment in a long-term community-based alcohol rehabilitation programme. *Addiction* 92:1537-1546.

Rada RR & Kellner R (1979). Drug treatment in alcoholism. In JM Davis & D Greenblatt (eds.) *Psychopharmacology Update: New and Neglected Areas.* New York, NY: Grune & Stratton, 105-144.

Regier DA, Farmer ME, Rae DS et al. (1990). Comorbidity of mental disorders with alcohol and other drug abuse. Results from the Epidemiologic Catchment Area (ECA) Study. *Journal of the American Medical Association* 264:2511-2518.

Ross HE, Frederick B, Glaser MD et al. (1988). The prevalence of psychiatric disorders in patients with alcohol and other drug problems. *Archives of General Psychiatry* 45:1023-1031.

Roussaux JP, Hers D & Ferauge M (1996). Does acamprosate diminish the appetite for alcohol in weaned alcoholics? [in French]. *Journal de Pharmacie de Belgique* 51:65-68.

Roy-Byrne PP, Pages KP, Russo JE et al. (2000). Nefazodone treatment of major depression in alcohol-dependent patients: A double-blind, placebo-controlled trial. *Journal of Clinical Psychopharmacology* 20:129-136.

Sands BF, Knapp CM & Ciraulo DA (1995). Interaction of alcohol with therapeutic drugs and drugs of abuse. In HR Kranzler (ed.) *The Pharmacology of Alcohol Abuse.* New York, NY: Springer-Verlag, 475-512.

Sass H, Soyka M, Mann K et al. (1996). Relapse prevention by acamprosate: Results from a placebo controlled study on alcohol dependence. *Archives of General Psychiatry* 53:673-680.

Schuckit M (1983). Alcoholic patients with secondary depression. *American Journal of Psychiatry* 140:711-714.

Sellers EM, Naranjo CA & Peachey JE (1981). Drugs to decrease alcohol consumption. *New England Journal of Medicine* 305:1255-1262.

Seppala T, Aranko K, Mattila MJ et al. (1982). Effects of alcohol on buspirone and lorazepam actions. *Clinical Pharmacology and Therapeutics* 32:201-207.

Shaw GK, Majumdar SK, Waller S et al. (1987). Tiapride in the long-term management of alcoholics of anxious or depressive temperament. *British Journal of Psychiatry* 150:164-168.

Shaw GK, Waller S, Majumdar SK et al. (1994). Tiapride in the prevention of relapse in recently detoxified alcoholics. *British Journal of Psychiatry* 165:515-523.

Smith CM (1978). *Alcoholism: Treatment.* Montreal, Ontario, Canada: Eden Press.

Sokolow L, Welte J, Hynes G et al. (1981). Multiple substance use by alcoholics. *British Journal of Addiction* 76:147-158.

Swift RM (1999). Drug therapy for alcohol dependence. *New England Journal of Medicine* 340:1482-1490.

Swift RM, Whelihan W, Kuznetsov O et al. (1994). Naltrexone-induced alterations in human ethanol intoxication. *American Journal of Psychiatry* 151:1463-1467.

Tempesta E, Janiri L, Bignamini A et al. (2000). Acamprosate and relapse prevention in the treatment of alcohol dependence: A placebo-controlled study. *Alcohol and Alcoholism* 35:202-209.

Tiihonen J, Ryynanen O-P, Kauhanen J et al. (1996). Citalopram in the treatment of alcoholism: A double-blind placebo-controlled study. *Pharmacopsychiatry* 29: 27-29.

Tollefson GD, Montague-Clouse J & Tollefson SL (1992). Treatment of comorbid generalized anxiety in a recently detoxified alcohol population with a selective serotonergic drug (Buspirone). *Journal of Clinical Psychopharmacology* 12:19-26.

Volpicelli J, O'Brien C, Alterman A et al. (1992). Naltrexone in the treatment of alcohol dependence. *Archives of General Psychiatry* 49:867-880.

Volpicelli J, Rhines KC, Rhines JS et al. (1997). Naltrexone and alcohol dependence: Role of subject compliance. *Archives of General Psychiatry* 54:737-742.

Volpicelli JR, Watson NT, King AC et al. (1995). Effect of naltrexone on alcohol "high" in alcoholics. *American Journal of Psychiatry* 152:613-615.

Whitworth AB, Fischer F, Lesch OM et al. (1996). Comparison of acamprosate and placebo in long-term treatment of alcohol dependence. *Lancet* 347:1438-1442.

Wikler A (1980). *Opioid Dependence.* New York, NY: Plenum Press.

Wilson A, Davidson WJ & Blanchard R (1980). Disulfiram implantation: A trial using placebo implants and two types of controls. *Journal of Studies on Alcohol* 41:429-436.

Wolf B, Iguchi MY & Griffiths RR (1990). Sedative/tranquilizer use and abuse in alcoholics currently in outpatient treatment: Incidence, pattern and preference. In LS Harris (ed.) *Problems of Drug Dependence 1989 (NIDA Research Monograph 95).* Rockville, MD: National Institute on Drug Abuse, 376-377.

Wood D, Wender PH & Reimherr FW (1983). The prevalence of attention deficit disorder, residual type, or minimal brain dysfunction, in a population of male alcoholic patients. *American Journal of Psychiatry* 140:95-98.

Yourick JJ & Faiman MD (1991). Disulfiram metabolism as a requirement for the inhibition of rat liver mitochondrial low Km aldehyde dehydrogenase. *Biochemical Pharmacology* 42:1361-1366.

Pharmacologic Interventions for Benzodiazepine and Other Sedative-Hypnotic Addiction

Chapter 2

Donald R. Wesson, M.D.
David E. Smith, M.D., FASAM
Walter Ling, M.D.

Issues in Diagnosing Dependence
Indications for Initiating Withdrawal
Benzodiazepine Withdrawal Syndromes
Pharmacologic Management of Withdrawal
Postwithdrawal Treatment

This chapter focuses on pharmacotherapies for physical dependence on benzodiazepines and other prescription sedative-hypnotics. In the final section, the chapter discusses treatment of patients who ingest sedative-hypnotics in addition to other psychoactive drugs.

The pharmacologic classification of sedative-hypnotics draws attention to the therapeutic applications of these drugs. Sedative-hypnotics generally are prescribed to treat anxiety and insomnia. They are known as "depressants" because, in high doses, they obtund consciousness and reduce respiration. In overdose, they can produce coma and death.

The term "depressants" should be used with caution in referring to the sedative-hypnotics because of the potential for confusion with depression as a mood disorder. This potential for confusion is compounded by the observation that clinical depression often is present in individuals who are dependent on sedative-hypnotics; in such individuals, chronic use of sedative-hypnotics appears to cause or exacerbate clinical depression.

While the usual effect of sedative-hypnotics is sedation or sleep induction, under some conditions, sedative-hypnotics may produce euphoria, stimulation, and behavioral disinhibition. Elevation of mood often is fragile and may change quickly from euphoria to agitation, sadness, or rage. The combination of stimulation and impaired judgment may result in aggressive, violent or criminal behavior.

Alcohol has a pharmacologic profile that qualifies it as a sedative-hypnotic. By convention, however, alcohol generally is considered in a class by itself.

Benzodiazepine agonists usually are included in the category of sedative-hypnotics. In contrast to the generic term "sedative-hypnotic," which by convention may refer to barbiturates and medications of several different chemical classes, "benzodiazepines" refers to a class of medications that are variations on a common chemical structure.

In medical therapeutics, the benzodiazepines largely have replaced the short-acting barbiturates and other non-barbiturate sedative-hypnotics that were available before 1960. More recently, imidazopyridine derivatives (such as alpidem, zolpidem [Ambien®, Stilnox®, Myslee®], and zaleplon [Sonata®]) have been introduced. Although chemically distinct from benzodiazepines, these medications bind selectively to the brain omega-1 receptor, a subunit of the GABA-BZ receptor. Subjects with a history of drug abuse experience effects similar to zaleplon and triazolam (Rush, Frey et al., 1999) or zolpidem and triazolam (Rush & Griffiths, 1996). Trazodone, an antidepressant often used for its hypnotic effects in patients with a history of substance abuse, appears to have fewer subjective effects that would lead to its abuse (Rush, Baker et al., 1999).

The pharmacology of benzodiazepines and other sedative-hypnotics is described in detail in Section 2.

ISSUES IN DIAGNOSING DEPENDENCE

Most patients who develop sedative-hypnotic dependence do so while being treated for an anxiety disorder or insomnia. The majority of such patients have an underlying disorder that must be addressed either before or after detoxification. Clinical trials with patients treated for panic disorder with benzodiazepines provide useful insights into therapeutic dose benzodiazepine tolerance and the issues to be considered when initiating benzodiazepine discontinuation.

With the exception of alcohol, sedative-hypnotics are not often primary drugs of abuse; that is, they are not taken daily to produce intoxication. Even among drug addicts, sedative-hypnotic abuse usually is intermittent and only rarely results in physical dependence. Some individuals become dependent on sedative-hypnotics while using drugs purchased on illicit markets for self-medication of symptoms caused by stimulant or opiate abuse.

Neuroadaptation versus Physiologic Dependence. Chronic exposure to sedative-hypnotics induces alterations in brain function at the neuroreceptor level; these changes are termed "neuroadaptation." An understanding of physical dependence is best achieved through an understanding of how benzodiazepines and other sedative-hypnotics interact with the brain receptors.

Benzodiazepines exert their physiologic effects by attaching to a subunit of gamma-aminobutyric acid (GABA) receptors. The GABA receptor is made up of an ion channel and several subunits that bind to different drugs: one subunit binds GABA, another benzodiazepines, and another barbiturates. The receptor subunits that are separate from, but functionally coupled to, the GABA receptor are said to be allosterically bound to the GABA receptor. The subunit that binds benzodiazepines has been designated the benzodiazepine receptor (Squires & Braestrup, 1977; Braestrup, Albrechtsen et al., 1977; Möhler & Okada, 1977).

Benzodiazepines that enhance the effect of GABA are called "agonists." Although receptors typically are named

for the endogenous ligand that is an agonist at the receptor, the natural ligand for the benzodiazepine receptor has not yet been identified. Several endogenous nonbenzodiazepine compounds that attach to the receptor have been identified; however, it has not been established that these compounds attach to the receptor during normal physiologic function.

GABA is the major inhibitory neurotransmitter in the brain and GABA synapses, distributed throughout the brain and spinal cord, comprise as many as 40% of all synapses. The physiologic function of GABA synapses is to modulate the polarization of neurons. The GABA receptor does this by opening or closing chloride ion channels (ionophores). Opening chloride channels allows more chloride ions to enter neurons. The influx of negatively charged chloride ions increases the electrical gradient across the cell membrane and makes the neuron less excitable. Closing the channels decreases electrical polarization and makes the cell more excitable. Attachment of an agonist at the benzodiazepine receptor facilitates the effect of GABA (that is, it opens the chloride channel). The clinical effects are anxiety reduction, sedation, and increased seizure threshold.

Substances that attach to the benzodiazepine receptor and close the channel produce an opposite effect: they are anxiogenic and lower the seizure threshold. Compounds such as betacarboline that produce an effect that is the opposite of the benzodiazepine agonists are termed "inverse agonists." Some compounds attach with high affinity to the benzodiazepine receptor but neither increase nor decrease the effect of GABA. In the absence of a benzodiazepine agonist or inverse agonist, these compounds are neutral ligands (they attach to the receptor and block the effects of both agonists and inverse agonists but activate no effects in the receptor). Consequently, neutral ligands are called "antagonists." If the receptor is occupied by an agonist or inverse agonist, an antagonist will displace the agonist or inverse agonist. (Displacement of a benzodiazepine agonist has clinical utility. For example, the benzodiazepine antagonist flumazenil [Romazicon®] was marketed in the United States in 1992 to reverse the sedation produced by a benzodiazepine following a surgical procedure or overdose.)

The interaction of benzodiazepine receptors with their ligand is extremely complex. Attachment of the ligands can alter the pharmacology of the receptor (as by altering the number of receptors or changing the affinity of the ligand for the receptor). With chronic exposure to benzodiazepines, there is neurochemical evidence that the functional coupling of the benzodiazepine receptor with the GABA receptor is decreased (Friedman, Gibbs et al., 1996).

Distinguishing Physical Dependence From Substance Use Disorder. Patients may be physically dependent on a benzodiazepine but not have a substance abuse disorder. In the minds of many patients and physicians, physical dependence is synonymous with addiction or a substance abuse disorder. An unfortunate choice of terms in the *Diagnostic and Statistical Manual of Mental Disorders, 4th Edition* (*DSM-IV*; APA, 1994) adds to the confusion. The *DSM-IV* diagnostic criteria for substance abuse were developed primarily for drugs not used in a medical context. In the *DSM-IV* nomenclature, "drug dependence" refers to a disorder more severe than "drug abuse." "Physical dependence" and "characteristic withdrawal syndrome" are diagnostic criteria included in "drug dependence," but physical dependence alone is not sufficient to establish a diagnosis of a benzodiazepine-related substance abuse disorder. (This seemingly arcane distinction often is lost.) Some patients conclude that they are addicted if they stop a medication and withdrawal symptoms emerge.

The diagnostic criteria are sufficiently broad that they can reasonably accommodate abuse of and dependence on prescription drugs used in a medical context. *DSM-IV* diagnosis of "substance dependence" requires a maladaptive pattern of substance use leading to clinically significant impairment or distress (American Psychiatric Association, 1994). Seven criteria are listed; three or more criteria are required for a diagnosis of substance dependence. The first two criteria are tolerance and drug withdrawal; a diagnosis of substance abuse disorder requires at least one other of the five remaining criteria.

Sensible use of the diagnostic criteria requires some interpolation and judgment, taking into consideration the medical context and the nature of the patient's underlying problem. For example, Criteria 3 and 4 relate to a patient's loss of control over drug-taking behavior; that is, "the drug often is used in larger amounts or over a longer period than intended," or "there is persistent use, or unsuccessful efforts to cut down or control substance use." In a medical context, a patient would fulfill these criteria if he or she frequently took more of the medication than was prescribed, stealthily obtained the medication from multiple physicians, or insisted on using it beyond the duration intended by the prescribing physician.

Criterion 5 involves the patient spending a great deal of time in activities necessary to obtain the substance or to recover from its effects (this would include seeing multiple physicians to obtain additional prescriptions). Criterion 6 involves the patient giving up important social, occupational, or recreational activities because of substance use. Criterion 7 involves continued use of the medication even though the patient is experiencing a physical or psychological problem that is caused or exacerbated by continued use of the substance.

Biological Vulnerabilities. In the addiction literature, it is common to read that benzodiazepines are likely to be abused by individuals who have a history of sedative-hypnotic abuse or "polydrug" abuse. This statement is true, but the underlying reasoning is circuitous. After sedative-hypnotic dependence has occurred, it is fairly certain that the individual is at risk for sedative abuse, dependence, or both if he or she resumes use of a sedative-hypnotic drug. However, predicting in advance who will abuse or become dependent on a sedative-hypnotic is a much less certain enterprise.

Studies of the reinforcing properties of benzodiazepines show that these drugs are not effective reinforcers for most individuals (Chutuape & de Wit, 1994; de Wit, Johanson et al., 1984). A growing body of evidence suggests that benzodiazepines are euphorogenic for some individuals. In one study, for example, the mood-elevating effects of alprazolam were experienced more intensely by daughters of alcoholics than by subjects with no history of parental alcohol dependence (Ciraulo, Sarid-Segal et al., 1996). Similar results were seen in sons of alcoholics (Cowley, Roy-Byrne et al., 1992, 1994). Animal studies suggest that concurrent administration of nonpsychoactive medications can selectively affect the development of physical dependence. For example, in the rat, concurrent administration of nifedipine, a calcium channel blocker, was found to facilitate development of physical dependence on barbital but not on diazepam (Suzuki, Mizoguchi et al., 1995).

A hotly debated issue is the vulnerability of alcohol abusers to benzodiazepine abuse and dependence. Both alcohol and benzodiazepines enhance the effects of GABA at the $GABA_A$ receptor complex. One concern is that the combination of alcohol and benzodiazepines may result in increased neurocognitive and behavioral toxicity (Hollister, 1990). Another is that alcohol, through its effect on receptor function, may increase the likelihood of uncoupling of the benzodiazepine receptor. *In vitro* data suggest that alcohol can produce alterations of $GABA_A$ receptor binding and function (Klein, Mascia et al., 1995).

INDICATIONS FOR INITIATING WITHDRAWAL

Presence of a Substance Use Disorder. From the point of view of an addiction medicine specialist, a primary reason for discontinuing use of a sedative-hypnotic drug is the presence of a coexisting substance use disorder involving a second (or multiple) drug(s). It is impossible to adequately assess the therapeutic benefits or risks of treatment of an underlying disorder with sedative-hypnotic drugs while a patient is concurrently abusing alcohol, cocaine, or other substances.

Development of Physical Dependence. Physical dependence on sedative-hypnotics (principally benzodiazepines) is a cause for concern, but it may be an acceptable state if (1) the medication is medically indicated; (2) the medication continues to be effective in ameliorating the patient's symptoms and it is not producing significant behavioral or organ toxicity; and (3) the patient has not been diagnosed with a substance use disorder.

Other Indications. Beyond a substance use disorder, there are other reasons for initiating withdrawal of a sedative-hypnotic drug; for example, if the treatment is inducing difficulties with memory or producing adverse behavioral reactions such as irritability, anger, rage, or hostility.

Benzodiazepines and Memory: Knowledge about the amnestic effects of benzodiazepines derives from many sources, including animal studies (Dickinson-Anson, Mesches et al., 1993); clinical case reports of patients' experiences; experiments with nonpatient volunteers (Ott, Rohloff et al., 1988; Fleishaker, Sisson et al., 1993; Ingum, Beylich et al., 1993); studies of recall in patients undergoing medical procedures; and studies of neurocognitive function in patients receiving long-term treatment with benzodiazepines and after benzodiazepine discontinuation (Tonne, Hiltunen et al., 1991). Some studies suggest that the amnestic effects produced by benzodiazepines and alcohol are mediated through the benzodiazepine receptor linked to $GABA_A$ (Dickinson-Anson, Mesches et al., 1993). Other studies have found that the benzodiazepine antagonist, flumazenil, blocks the sedative but not the amnesic effects of midazolam (Curran & Birch, 1991).

Experimental studies often use memory tasks that are unique to the laboratory situation. This has led some to question the generalizability of the laboratory data (Moussaoui, 1986).

Memory is a complex process requiring integration of many aspects of neurocognitive function. At some dose, all benzodiazepines can produce impairment of memory. Considerable evidence suggests that benzodiazepine-induced memory defects are produced because the drug impairs the transfer of newly acquired information to long-term storage (Barbee, 1993):

> The memory impairment is for events following the ingestion of the benzodiazepine. This type of memory impairment, often referred to as "anterograde amnesia," is similar to an alcohol "blackout." Amnesia may be partial or complete for an interval of time. The memory impairment is dose dependent and more profound as the dose of the benzodiazepine is increased. Unlike the memory impairment produced by anticholinergic medications such as scopolamine, recall of information acquired before the ingestion of the benzodiazepine is not impaired (Barbee, 1993).

The term "retrograde amnesia" can be a source of confusion because it is used to refer to different timeframes in the medical and pharmacology literature, and in the legal and lay literature. In the medical and pharmacology literature, the term "anterograde amnesia" refers to the inability to remember events *following* the ingestion of a drug, while "retrograde amnesia" refers to the inability to remember events that *preceded* drug ingestion. The literature on benzodiazepines contains mentions of retrograde amnesia (Ott, Rohloff et al., 1988), but the references are to contrast retrograde amnesia with anterograde amnesia. No studies have shown that benzodiazepines produce retrograde amnesia. In fact, some studies suggest that small to moderate doses of a benzodiazepine may produce enhanced recall of events that occurred prior to drug ingestion (Ott, Rohloff et al., 1988).

Benzodiazepine-induced memory impairment is not merely a function of sedation. In an experimental study of healthy volunteers, midazolam-induced sedation was reversed by the benzodiazepine antagonist flumazenil, whereas the memory impairment was not (Curran & Birch, 1991). In contrast, acute effects (neuropsychological impairment in humans) of diazepam were observed in memory measures at all times. Tolerance to the effects of benzodiazepines on memory appears never to fully develop (Gorenstein, Bernik et al., 1994).

The amnestic effects of benzodiazepines are useful properties in anesthetic practice (Deppe, Sipperly et al., 1994; Berggren, Eriksson et al., 1983), but in other therapeutic uses, memory impairment is an undesirable side effect.

Paradoxical Reactions: Although the benzodiazepines generally have the effect of reducing anxiety and anger, some patients respond to these drugs with an increase in anger, rage, or hostility. Because the effect is contrary to the expected effect, it often is referred to as a "paradoxical reaction." This effect has been mentioned episodically in the medical literature (Lader & Petursson, 1981; Lader & Morton, 1991; Freedman, 1990; Goldney, 1977; Hall & Zisook, 1981; Feldman, 1986). The reasons that some individuals respond paradoxically are not well understood. Set and setting are factors, as demonstrated by the fact that paradoxical reactions are said to occur frequently in prison populations (Brown, 1978) and in patients with borderline personality disorders (Cole & Kando, 1993).

BENZODIAZEPINE WITHDRAWAL SYNDROMES

Withdrawal from high doses of sedative-hypnotics can be severe and even life-threatening. Therapeutic doses of benzodiazepines taken for months to years produce physiologic dependence and a significant discontinuation syndrome in about 50% of patients (Tyrer, 1993). Management of these withdrawal syndromes is described in detail in Section 5.

Symptom Rebound. After cessation of a benzodiazepine, an intensified return of the symptoms (such as insomnia or anxiety) for which the benzodiazepine was prescribed is called "symptom rebound." The term comes from sleep research in which rebound insomnia frequently is observed following sedative-hypnotic use. Symptom rebound lasts a few days to a few weeks following drug discontinuation (APA, 1990). Symptom rebound is the most common withdrawal syndrome following prolonged benzodiazepine use.

Symptom Reemergence (or Recrudescence). Patients' symptoms of anxiety, insomnia, or muscle tension may have abated during benzodiazepine treatment. When the benzodiazepine is stopped, symptoms may return to the same level as before the benzodiazepine therapy was initiated. The reason for distinguishing between symptom rebound and symptom reoccurrence is that symptom reoccurrence suggests that the original symptoms have not been adequately treated, whereas symptom rebound suggests a form of withdrawal syndrome (APA, 1990).

Some patients can ingest therapeutic doses of benzodiazepines for many months or years and then abruptly stop them without developing symptoms other than those that were present before benzodiazepine treatment. Other patients taking the same doses of benzodiazepines over long periods develop new symptoms after the benzodiazepine is stopped. Such symptoms can be disabling and may persist for many months.

Protracted Withdrawal. Some clinicians have described a more prolonged benzodiazepine withdrawal syndrome that is severe and disabling (Ashton, 1991).

Waxing and waning intensity of symptoms is characteristic of the low-dose protracted benzodiazepine withdrawal syndrome. Patients sometimes are asymptomatic for several days, then, without apparent reason, they become acutely anxious. Often, there are concomitant physiologic signs (such as dilated pupils, increased resting heart rate, and elevated blood pressure). The intense waxing and waning is important in distinguishing symptoms of low-dose withdrawal from symptom reemergence.

Protracted benzodiazepine withdrawal has no pathognomonic signs or symptoms. The differential diagnosis includes agitated depression, generalized anxiety disorder, panic disorder, partial complex seizures, and schizophrenia. Other symptoms that have been attributed to protracted benzodiazepine withdrawal include anxiety; increased sensitivity to sound, light, and touch (Lader, 1990); tinnitus (Busto, Fornazzari et al., 1988); and psychotic depression. The time course of symptom resolution is the primary feature differentiating symptoms generated by withdrawal from symptom reemergence. Symptoms from protracted benzodiazepine withdrawal wax and wane but gradually subside with continued abstinence, whereas symptom reemergence and symptom sensitization do not.

In the early 1980s, clinicians hypothesized that low-dose benzodiazepine withdrawal is mediated by neuroadaptation of the GABA receptor (Wesson & Smith, 1982); however, neurochemical evidence was lacking. The pathophysiology of a protracted withdrawal syndrome from benzodiazepines remains incompletely understood. Some drugs or medications may facilitate neuroadaptation by increasing the affinity of benzodiazepines for their receptors. Phenobarbital, for example, increases the affinity of diazepam for benzodiazepine receptors (Skolnick, Concada et al., 1981; Olsen & Loeb-Lundberg, 1981). Prior treatment with a barbiturate has been found to increase the intensity of withdrawal symptoms (Covi, Lipman et al., 1973). Patients at increased risk for development of the low-dose withdrawal syndrome are those with a family or personal history of alcoholism, those who use alcohol daily, or those who use other sedatives concurrently with benzodiazepines. Case control studies suggest that patients with a history of addiction, particularly to other sedative-hypnotics, are at high risk for low-dose benzodiazepine dependence (Ciraulo, Barnhill et al., 1988). The short-acting, high-milligram potency benzodiazepines appear to produce a more intense low-dose withdrawal syndrome.

A protracted withdrawal syndrome has been described for most drugs that induce physical dependence, including alcohol (Geller, 1991). The signs and symptoms generally attributed to protracted withdrawal syndromes consist of irritability, anxiety, insomnia, and mood instability.

The Dependence/Withdrawal Cycle. When dependence arises during therapeutic use of benzodiazepines, it often occurs in a predictable sequence of phases. The clinical course described here most often occurs during long-term treatment of a generalized anxiety disorder, panic disorder, or severe insomnia.

Stages in the development of benzodiazepine dependence include:

Pretreatment Phase: Even before treatment, the distressing symptoms of anxiety or insomnia vary in intensity from day to day, depending on life stresses and the waxing and waning of the patient's underlying disorder.

Therapeutic Response Phase: When treatment with a benzodiazepine is started, patients often have initial side effects, such as drowsiness. Tolerance to unwanted sedation usually develops within a few days. The therapeutic phase, in which the patient's symptoms are ameliorated or reduced by benzodiazepine treatment, may last for months to years.

Symptom Escape and Dose Escalation Phase: During long-term treatment, benzodiazepines may lose their effectiveness in controlling symptoms. For some patients, this "symptom escape" coincides with a period of increased life stress; for others, no unusual psychological stressor is apparent. Patients often are aware that the medication "no longer works" or that its effect is qualitatively different.

As the usual dose of benzodiazepines loses effectiveness, the patient may increase his or her benzodiazepine consumption in the hope that symptoms again will be controlled. As the daily dose increases, the patient may develop

subtle benzodiazepine toxicity that is difficult to diagnose without psychometric assessment. This is a common clinical problem that generally goes unrecognized. It has not received sufficient research attention, and evidence at this time is scanty and indirect. Although many studies have demonstrated that acute doses of benzodiazepines impair cognitive function, there has been little study of the effect of benzodiazepines over prolonged periods of use. One psychometric study, which compared long-term benzodiazepine users with subjects who were benzodiazepine-abstinent, found that the long-term benzodiazepine users performed poorly on tasks involving visual-spatial ability and sustained attention (Golombok, Moodley et al., 1988). Clinically, the patient may not be aware that his or her impairment is benzodiazepine induced. Coping skills that previously were bolstered by the benzodiazepine become compromised. Some patients make suicide attempts or exhibit self-defeating behavior that otherwise would be out of character.

The symptom escape phase does not appear to be an invariable consequence of long-term treatment with benzodiazepines. Some patients are vulnerable to developing withdrawal symptoms; others are not. Patients who have experienced symptom escape and dose escalation appear most likely to have a protracted withdrawal syndrome.

Withdrawal Phase: A patient who stops taking a benzodiazepine or whose daily dose falls below 25% of the peak maintenance dose may become increasingly symptomatic. Such symptoms may be the result of symptom rebound, symptom reemergence, or the beginning of a withdrawal syndrome. The symptoms that occur during this phase may represent a mixture of new symptoms with symptoms that were present during the "pretreatment phase." During the first few weeks, it is not possible to know exactly what is producing such symptoms or to accurately predict their duration.

Symptoms of the same type that occurred during the pretreatment phase suggest symptom rebound or symptom reemergence. New symptoms, particularly alterations in sensory perception, suggest the beginning of a withdrawal syndrome. Increasing the benzodiazepine dose may diminish the symptoms if they are due to benzodiazepine withdrawal.

Resolution Phase: The duration of the resolution phase is highly variable. Most patients experience symptom rebound lasting only a few weeks, while others have a severe, protracted abstinence syndrome that lasts months to a year

TABLE 1. Characteristics of Syndromes Related to Benzodiazepine Withdrawal

Syndrome	Signs/Symptoms	Time Course	Response to Reinstitution of Benzodiazepine
High-dose withdrawal	Anxiety, insomnia, nightmares, major motor seizures, psychosis, hyperpyrexia, death.	Begins 1 or 2 days after a short-acting benzodiazepine is stopped; 3 to 8 days after a long-acting benzodiazepine is stopped.	Signs and symptoms reverse 2 to 6 hours following a hypnotic dose of a benzodiazepine.
Symptom rebound	Same symptoms that were present before treatment.	Begins 1 to 2 days after a short-acting benzodiazepine is stopped; 3 to 8 days after a long-acting benzodiazepine is stopped. Lasts 7 to 14 days.	Signs and symptoms reverse 2 to 6 hours following a hypnotic dose of a benzodiazepine.
Protracted, low-dose withdrawal	Anxiety, agitation, tachycardia, palpitations, anorexia, blurred vision, muscle cramps, insomnia, nightmares, confusion, muscle spasms, psychosis, increased sensitivity to sounds and light, and paresthesias.	Signs and symptoms emerge 1 to 7 days following discontinuation of the benzodiazepine to below the usual therapeutic dose.	Signs and symptoms reverse 2 to 6 hours following a sedative dose of a high-potency benzodiazepine.
Symptom reemergence	Recurrence of the same symptoms that were present before taking a benzodiazepine (e.g., anxiety, insomnia).	Symptoms emerge when the benzodiazepine is stopped and continue unabated with time.	Signs and symptoms reverse 2 to 6 hours following a usual therapeutic dose of a benzodiazepine.

or more. During early abstinence, the patient's symptoms generally vary in intensity from day to day. If abstinence from benzodiazepines is maintained, symptoms gradually return to their baseline level. An encouraging finding of one discontinuation study was that "patients who were able to remain free of benzodiazepines for at least five weeks obtained lower levels of anxiety than before benzodiazepine discontinuation" (Rickels, Schweizer et al., 1990).

The physician's response during the withdrawal phase is critical to achieving a resolution. Some physicians interpret a patient's escalating symptoms as evidence of the patient's "need" for benzodiazepine treatment and reinstate therapy at higher doses or switch the patient to another benzodiazepine. Reinstitution of a benzodiazepine usually does not achieve satisfactory symptom control and may prolong the recovery process. Benzodiazepine withdrawal, using one of the strategies described below, generally achieves the best long-term outcome.

PHARMACOLOGIC MANAGEMENT OF WITHDRAWAL

Benzodiazepine withdrawal strategies must be tailored to suit three possible dependence situations: (1) high-dose withdrawal (following use of doses greater than the recommended therapeutic dose for more than one month), (2) low-dose withdrawal (following use of doses below those in the upper range of Table 2), and (3) a combined high-dose and low-dose withdrawal (following daily high doses

TABLE 2. Benzodiazepines and Sedative-Hypnotics and Their Phenobarbital Withdrawal Equivalents

Generic Name	Trade Name	Common Therapeutic Indication(s)	Therapeutic Dose Range (mg/day)	Dose Equal to 30 mg of Phenobarbital Withdrawal (mg)[b]
Benzodiazepines				
alprazolam	Xanax®	sedative, anti-panic	0.75-6	1
chlordiazepoxide	Librium®	sedative	15-100	25
clonazepam	Klonopin®	anti-convulsant	0.5-4	2
clorazepate	Tranxene®	sedative	15-60	7.5
diazepam	Valium®	sedative	4-40	10
estazolam	ProSom®	hypnotic	1-2	1
flumazenil	Mazicon®	benzodiazepine antagonist	NA	NA
flurazepam	Dalmane®	hypnotic	15-30	15
halazepam	Paxipam®	sedative	60-160	40
lorazepam	Ativan®	sedative	1-16	2
midazolam	Versed®	IV sedative	NA	NA
oxazepam	Serax®	sedative	10-120	10
prazepam	Centrax®	sedative	20-60	10
quazepam	Doral®	hypnotic	15[a]	15
temazepam	Restoril®	hypnotic	15-30[a]	15
triazolam	Halcion®	hypnotic	0.125-0.50	0.25
Barbiturates				
amobarbital	Amytal®	sedative	50-100	100
butabarbital	Butisol®	sedative	45-120	100
butalbital	Fiorinal®, Sedapap®	sedative/analgesic[c]	100-300	100
pentobarbital	Nembutal®	hypnotic	50-100[c]	100
secobarbital	Seconal®	hypnotic	50-100[c]	100
Others				
buspirone	BuSpar®	anti-anxiety	15-60	—[d]
chloral hydrate	Noctec®, Somnos®	hypnotic	250-1,000	500
ethchlorvynol	Placidyl®	hypnotic	500-1,000	500
glutethimide	Doriden®	hypnotic	250-500	250
meprobamate	Miltown®, Equanil®, Equagesic®	sedative	1,200-1,600	1,200
methylprylon	Noludar®	hypnotic	200-400	200
zaleplon	Sonata®	hypnotic	5-20	10
zolpidem	Ambien®, Stillnox®	hypnotic	5-10	5

NA = Not applicable

[a]Usual hypnotic dose

[b]Phenobarbital withdrawal conversion equivalence is not the same as therapeutic dose equivalency. Withdrawal equivalence is the amount of the drug that 30 mg of phenobarbital will substitute for and prevent serious high-dose withdrawal signs and symptoms.

[c]Butalbital is usually available in combination with opiate or non-opiate analgesics.

[d]Not cross-tolerant with barbiturates.

for more than six months), in which both a high-dose sedative-hypnotic withdrawal syndrome and a low-dose benzodiazepine withdrawal syndrome occur concurrently.

High-Dose Benzodiazepine Withdrawal. Abrupt discontinuation of a sedative-hypnotic in a patient who is severely dependent on the drug can result in serious medical complications and even death. There are three general strategies for safely withdrawing patients from sedative-hypnotics, including benzodiazepines.

The first method is to use decreasing doses of the drug of dependence. Gradual reduction of the benzodiazepine of dependence is used primarily in medical settings to treat dependence arising from treatment of an underlying condition. The patient must be cooperative, able to adhere to dosing regimens, and not concurrently abusing alcohol or other drugs.

The second method is to substitute phenobarbital for the addicting agent and then gradually to withdraw the substitute medication (Smith & Wesson, 1970, 1971). The pharmacologic rationale for phenobarbital substitution is that phenobarbital is long-acting, so that little change in blood levels of phenobarbital occurs between doses. This allows the safe use of progressively smaller daily doses. Phenobarbital is safer than the shorter-acting barbiturates because the lethal dose of phenobarbital is many times higher than the toxic dose, and the signs of toxicity (such as sustained nystagmus, slurred speech, and ataxia) are easy to observe. Finally, phenobarbital intoxication usually does not produce disinhibition, so most patients view it as a medication rather than as a drug of abuse.

Phenobarbital substitution also can be used to withdraw patients who have lost control of their benzodiazepine use or who are polydrug dependent.

The third method, used for patients who are dependent on both alcohol and a benzodiazepine, is to substitute a long-acting benzodiazepine, such as chlordiazepoxide, and then taper it over one to two weeks.

The method selected depends on the particular benzodiazepine, the involvement of other drugs of dependence, and the clinical setting in which detoxification is to take place.

Stabilization Phase: The patient's history of drug use during the month preceding treatment is used to compute the stabilization dose of phenobarbital. Although many addicts exaggerate the number of pills they are taking, the patient history remains the best guide to initiating pharmacotherapy for withdrawal. Patients who have overstated the amount of drug they are taking will become intoxicated during the first day or two of treatment. Such intoxication is easily managed by omitting one or more doses of phenobarbital and recalculating the daily dose.

The patient's average daily sedative-hypnotic dose is converted to phenobarbital equivalents, and the daily amount is divided into three doses. (The conversion equivalents for various benzodiazepines and for other sedative-hypnotics are given in Table 2.)

The computed phenobarbital equivalent is given in three or four doses daily. If the patient is using significant amounts of other sedative-hypnotics (including alcohol), the amounts of all the drugs are converted to phenobarbital equivalents and added together (for example, 30 cc of 100 proof alcohol is equivalent to 30 mg of phenobarbital for withdrawal purposes). The maximum starting phenobarbital dose is 500 mg per day.

Before each dose of phenobarbital is given, the patient is checked for signs of phenobarbital toxicity; these include sustained nystagmus, slurred speech, or ataxia. Of these, sustained nystagmus is the most reliable. If nystagmus is present, the scheduled dose of phenobarbital is withheld. If all three signs are present, the next two doses of phenobarbital are withheld and the daily dose of phenobarbital for the following day is halved.

If the patient is in acute withdrawal and has had or is in danger of having withdrawal seizures, the initial dose of phenobarbital is administered by intramuscular injection. If nystagmus and other signs of intoxication develop one to two hours after the intramuscular dose, the patient is in no immediate danger of barbiturate withdrawal.

Patients are maintained on the initial dosing schedule of phenobarbital for two days. If the patient has no signs of withdrawal or phenobarbital toxicity (slurred speech, nystagmus, unsteady gait), then phenobarbital withdrawal is initiated.

Withdrawal Phase: Unless the patient develops signs and symptoms of phenobarbital toxicity or sedative-hypnotic withdrawal, the phenobarbital dose is decreased by 30 mg per day. Should signs of phenobarbital toxicity develop during withdrawal, the daily phenobarbital dose is decreased by 50% and the 30 mg per day withdrawal continued from the reduced phenobarbital dose. If the patient has objective signs of sedative-hypnotic withdrawal, the daily dose is increased by 50% and the patient restabilized before the withdrawal is continued.

Low-Dose Benzodiazepine Withdrawal. Most patients experience only mild to moderate symptom rebound, which disappears after a few days to a week. In such cases, no special treatment is needed. However, the patient may need reassurance that rebound symptoms are common and will subside.

Some patients have severe symptoms that are quite unlike anything they have experienced previously. The phenobarbital regimen described above will not be adequate to suppress these symptoms to tolerable levels. For such patients, there are several pharmacologic options.

One strategy is to increase the phenobarbital dose to 200 mg per day and then to slowly taper the phenobarbital over several months.

Another approach is to block somatic symptoms, such as tachycardia, with propranolol. A dose of 20 mg every six hours can be used, alone or in combination with phenobarbital, to reduce the intensity of withdrawal symptoms (Tyrer, Rutherford et al., 1981). This schedule is continued for two weeks and then stopped. Even after phenobarbital withdrawal is complete, propranolol can be used episodically as needed to control tachycardia, increased blood pressure, and anxiety. However, continuous propranolol therapy for more than two weeks is not recommended, because propranolol itself may result in symptom rebound when discontinued after prolonged use (Glaubiger & Lefkowitz, 1977).

POSTWITHDRAWAL TREATMENT

Withdrawal usually is successful when the patient cooperates, but many patients do not remain abstinent. For patients with an underlying anxiety disorder, relapse may mean that the patient is unable or unwilling to tolerate the symptoms that reemerge following detoxification. For patients with a dual diagnosis, outcomes other than drug abstinence must be considered. Fortunately, there now are pharmacologic alternatives to benzodiazepines and the older sedative-hypnotics for the treatment of anxiety. In addition, cognitive-behavioral therapies and other psychotherapeutic and behavioral treatments for anxiety have shown efficacy.

Detoxification alone is not adequate treatment of sedative-hypnotic dependence, but rather should be seen as the first step in the recovery process. Adjunctive use of medications such as carbamazepine, imipramine, and buspirone has been found to result in significantly higher discontinua-

tion rates—carbamazepine (91%), buspirone (85%), and imipramine (79%)—compared to placebo (58%) (Rickels, Case et al., 1990).

Because of its low abuse potential and benign side effects, buspirone would seem a likely candidate for the treatment of anxiety following benzodiazepine discontinuation. Buspirone appears to act as a serotonin HT1A partial agonist (Taylor & Moon, 1991). However, in a crossover study, buspirone did not appear to lessen the intensity of benzodiazepine withdrawal (Schweizer & Rickels, 1986). There is some suggestion that patients with a history of benzodiazepine abuse may be unusually resistant to the anxiolytic effects of buspirone (Schweizer, Rickels et al., 1986). Buspirone does not appear to be efficacious in managing panic disorders (Sheehan, Raj et al., 1993) or social phobias. On the other hand, some success has been reported with the use of buspirone in postdetoxification treatment of generalized anxiety in alcoholics may have utility (Tollefson, Montague-Clouse et al., 1992).

Because benzodiazepines may cause or exacerbate cognitive impairment in older adults, buspirone may be a particularly useful alternative to the benzodiazepines for managing anxiety in this population (Steinberg, 1994).

Supportive individual psychotherapy or self-help recovery group support virtually always is needed as part of the recovery plan for patients who have a sedative-hypnotic substance abuse disorder.

Treatment Placement. Treatment strategies for sedative-hypnotic dependence cannot be separated from the realities of evolving health care delivery. Physicians often are in the position of devising not the optimal treatment plan, but one that can be negotiated with the patient and the payer. The realities of today's fractured health care dictate rethinking pharmacologic treatment strategies for sedative-hypnotic dependence. Health care payers and the agents of managed care often have simplistic and unrealistic criteria for assigning patients to level of care. (By contrast, the *ASAM Patient Placement Criteria* [Mee-Lee, Shulman et al., 2001] are clinically derived and should be followed whenever possible.)

Some—if not most—of the assessment and treatment of sedative-hypnotic dependence thus must be accomplished on an outpatient basis. The assessment and treatment of physical dependence is more complex for the physician and carries more risk for the patient on an outpatient than on an inpatient basis. For example, in an inpatient setting, the patient's access to medications can be controlled more completely, the patient's response to medications can be observed more closely, and the patient is not tempted to drive an automobile while experiencing toxicity or withdrawal symptoms.

Risks associated with outpatient management of withdrawal can be reduced by establishing clear goals, employing a systematic assessment procedure, and devising a clearly defined treatment protocol. Assessment and treatment protocols help the physician to systematically accumulate the information needed to initiate treatment and monitor treatment progress. Well-structured assessment and treatment protocols also are useful in negotiating with treatment payers and managed care entities for payment of the treatment the patient needs. Detailed medical records can be important in documenting the patient's clinical course and adverse events, and can buttress the physician's argument for a more intensive level of care, when needed.

CONCLUSIONS

Benzodiazepines have many therapeutic uses. In the treatment of some conditions, such as panic disorders, long-term use of benzodiazepines is an appropriate strategy. Physical dependence is not always an avoidable complication. Before initiating a course of prolonged therapy, the physician should discuss with the patient the possibility that the patient will develop new or intensified symptoms when use of the benzodiazepine is discontinued.

For patients whose benzodiazepine dependence develops during pharmacotherapy, such dependence does not necessarily amount to a substance use disorder. To label it as substance abuse unnecessarily stigmatizes the patient and the prescribing physician.

REFERENCES

American Psychiatric Association (APA) (1994). *Diagnostic and Statistical Manual of Mental Disorders, 4th Edition (DSM-IV).* Washington, DC: American Psychiatric Association, 886.

American Psychiatric Association (APA), Task Force on Benzodiazepine Dependency (1990). *Benzodiazepine Dependency, Toxicity, and Abuse.* Washington, DC: American Psychiatric Press.

Apelt S & Emrich HM (1990). Sodium valproate in benzodiazepine withdrawal [letter]. *American Journal of Psychiatry* 147:950-951.

Ashton H (1991). Protracted withdrawal syndromes from benzodiazepines. *Journal of Substance Abuse Treatment* 8:19-28.

Barbee JG (1993). Memory, benzodiazepines, and anxiety: integration of theoretical and clinical perspectives. *Journal of Clinical Psychiatry* 54(Suppl):86-97; discussion 98-101.

Berggren L, Eriksson I, Mollenholt P et al. (1983). Sedation for fibreoptic gastroscopy: A comparative study of midazolam and diazepam. *British Journal of Anaesthesia* 55:289-296.

Braestrup C, Albrechtsen R & Squires R (1977). High densities of benzodiazepine receptors in human cortical areas. *Nature* 269:702-704.

Brown CR (1978). The use of benzodiazepines in prison populations. *Journal of Clinical Psychiatry* 39:219-222.

Busto U, Fornazzari L & Naranjo CA (1988). Protracted tinnitus after discontinuation of long-term therapeutic use of benzodiazepines. *Journal of Clinical Psychopharmacology* 8:359-362.

Chutuape MA & de Wit H (1994). Relationship between subjective effects and drug preferences: Ethanol and diazepam. *Drug and Alcohol Dependence* 34:243-251.

Ciraulo DA, Barnhill JG, Greenblatt DJ et al. (1988). Abuse liability and clinical pharmacokinetics of alprazolam in alcoholic men. *Journal of Clinical Psychiatry* 49:333-337.

Ciraulo DA, Sarid-Segal O, Knapp C et al. (1996). Liability to alprazolam abuse in daughters of alcoholics. *American Journal of Psychiatry* 153:956-958.

Cole JO & Kando JC (1993). Adverse behavioral events reported in patients taking alprazolam and other benzodiazepines. *Journal of Clinical Psychiatry* 54(Suppl):49-61; discussion 62-63.

Covi L, Lipman RS, Pattison JH et al. (1973). Length of treatment with anxiolytic sedatives and response to their sudden withdrawal. *Acta Psychiatrica Scandinavica* 49:51-64.

Cowley DS, Roy-Byrne PP, Godon C et al. (1992) Response to diazepam in sons of alcoholics. *Alcoholism: Clinical & Experimental Research* 16:1057-1063.

Cowley DS, Roy-Byrne PP, Radant A et al. (1994). Eye movement effects of diazepam in sons of alcoholic fathers and male control subjects. *Alcoholism: Clinical & Experimental Research* 18:324-332.

Curran HV & Birch B (1991). Differentiating the sedative, psychomotor and amnesic effects of benzodiazepines: A study with midazolam and the benzodiazepine antagonist, flumazenil. *Psychopharmacology* 103:519-523.

Deppe SA, Sipperly ME, Sargent AI et al. (1994). Intravenous lorazepam as an amnestic and anxiolytic agent in the intensive care unit: A prospective study. *Critical Care Medicine* 22:1248-1252.

de Wit H, Johanson CE & Uhlenhuth EH (1984). Reinforcing properties of lorazepam in normal volunteers. *Drug and Alcohol Dependence* 13:31-41.

Dickinson-Anson H, Mesches MH, Coleman K et al. (1993). Bicuculline administered into the amygdala blocks benzodiazepine-induced amnesia. *Behavioral and Neural Biology* 60:1-4.

Farre M, de la Torre R, Gonzalez ML et al. (1997). Cocaine and alcohol interactions in humans: neuroendocrine effects and cocaethylene metabolism. *Journal of Pharmacology and Experimental Therapeutics* 283:164-176.

Feldman MD (1986). Paradoxical effects of benzodiazepines. *North Carolina Medical Journal* 47:311-312.

Fleishaker JC, Sisson TA, Sramek JJ et al. (1993). Psychomotor and memory effects of two adinazolam formulations assessed by a computerized neuropsychological test battery. *Journal of Clinical Pharmacology* 33:463-469.

Freedman DX (1990). Benzodiazepines: Therapeutic, biological and psychosocial issues. Symposium summary. *Journal of Psychiatric Research* 24(Suppl 2):169-174.

Friedman LK, Gibbs TT & Farb DH (1996). Gamma-aminobutyric acid A receptor regulation: Heterologous uncoupling of modulatory site interactions induced by chronic steroid, barbiturate, benzodiazepine or GABA treatment in culture. *Brain Research* 707(1):100-109.

Geller A (1991). Protracted abstinence. In NS Miller (ed.) *Comprehensive Handbook of Drug and Alcohol Addiction*. New York, NY: Marcel Dekker, 905-913.

Glaubiger G & Lefkowitz R (1977). Elevated beta-adrenergic receptor number after chronic propranolol treatment. *Biochemical and Biophysical Research Community* 78:720-725.

Goldney RD (1977). Paradoxical reaction to a new minor tranquilizer. *Medical Journal of Australia* 1:139-140.

Golombok S, Moodley P & Lader M (1988). Cognitive impairment in long-term benzodiazepine users. *Psychological Medicine* 18:365-374.

Gorenstein C, Bernik MA & Pompeia S (1994). Differential acute psychomotor and cognitive effects of diazepam on long-term benzodiazepine users. *International Clinical Psychopharmacology* 9:145-153.

Griffiths R & Roache J (1985). Abuse liability of benzodiazepines. A review of human studies evaluating subjective and/or reinforcing effects. In D Smith & D Wesson (eds.) *The Benzodiazepines: Current Standards for Medical Practice*. Hingham, MA: MTP Press, 209-225.

Hall RC & Zisook S (1981). Paradoxical reactions to benzodiazepines. *British Journal of Clinical Pharmacology* 11(Suppl 1):99S-104S.

Harrison M, Busto U, Naranjo CA et al. (1984). Diazepam tapering in detoxification for high-dose benzodiazepine abuse. *Clinical Pharmacology and Therapeutics* 36:527-533.

Henning RJ & Wilson LD (1996). Cocaethylene is as cardiotoxic as cocaine but is less toxic than cocaine plus ethanol. *Life Sciences* 59:615-627.

Hollister LE (1990). Interactions between alcohol and benzodiazepines. *Recent Developments in Alcoholism* 8:233-239.

Hollister LE, Bennett LL, Kimbell I et al. (1963). Diazepam in newly admitted schizophrenics. *Diseases of the Nervous System* 24:746-750.

Ingum J, Beylich KM & Moriand J (1993). Amnesic effects and subjective ratings during repeated dosing of flunitrazepam to healthy volunteers. *European Journal of Clinical Pharmacology* 45:235-240.

Jatlow P, Elsworth JD, Bradberry CW et al. (1991) Cocaethylene: A neuropharmacologically active metabolite associated with concurrent cocaine-ethanol ingestion. *Life Sciences* 48:1787-1794.

Klein RL, Mascia MP, Whiting PJ et al. (1995). GABA_A receptor function and binding in stably transfected cells: Chronic ethanol treatment. *Alcoholism: Clinical & Experimental Research* 19:1338-1344.

Lader M (1990). Drug development optimization—Benzodiazepines. *Agents and Actions Supplements* 29:59-69.

Lader M & Morton S (1991). Benzodiazepine problems. *British Journal of Addictions* 86:823-828.

Lader M & Petursson H (1981). Benzodiazepine derivatives—Side effects and dangers. *Biological Psychiatry* 16:1195-1201.

Lecrubier Y & Judge R (1997). Long-term evaluation of paroxetine, clomipramine and placebo in panic disorder. Collaborative Paroxetine Panic Study Investigators. *Acta Psychiatrica Scandinavica* 95:153-160.

Lecrubier Y, Bakker A, Dunbar G et al. (1997). A comparison of paroxetine, clomipramine and placebo in the treatment of panic disorder. Collaborative Paroxetine Panic Study Investigators. *Acta Psychiatrica Scandinavica* 95:145-152.

Lydiard RB, Lesser IM, Ballenger JC et al. (1992). A fixed-dose study of alprazolam 2 mg, alprazolam 6 mg, and placebo in panic disorder. *Journal of Clinical Psychopharmacology* 12:96-103.

McElroy SL, Keck PE Jr & Lawrence JM (1991). Treatment of panic disorder and benzodiazepine withdrawal with valproate [letter]. *Journal of Neuropsychiatry and Clinical Neuroscience* 3:232-233.

Mee-Lee D, Shulman G, Gastfriend D et al. (2001). *ASAM Patient Placement Criteria for the Treatment of Substance-Related Disorders, Second Edition-Revised*. Chevy Chase, MD: American Society of Addiction Medicine.

Modell JG (1997). Protracted benzodiazepine withdrawal syndrome mimicking psychotic depression [letter]. *Psychosomatics* 38:160-161.

Möhler H & Okada T (1977). Benzodiazepine receptors: Demonstration in the central nervous system. *Science* 198:849-851.

Moussaoui D (1986). Benzodiazepines and memory. *Encephale* 12:315-319.

Nabeshima T, Tohyama K & Kameyama T (1988). Reversal of alcohol-induced amnesia by the benzodiazepine inverse agonist Ro 15-4513. *European Journal of Pharmacology* 155:211-217.

Noyes R Jr, Burrows GD, Reich JH et al. (1996). Diazepam versus alprazolam for the treatment of panic disorder. *Journal of Clinical Psychiatry* 57:349-355.

O'Connor R (1993). Benzodiazepine dependence—A treatment perspective and an advocacy for control. *NIDA Research Monograph Series*. Rockville, MD: National Institute on Drug Abuse, 266-269.

Oehrberg S, Christiansen PE, Behnke K et al. (1995). Paroxetine in the treatment of panic disorder. A randomised, double-blind, placebo-controlled study. *British Journal of Psychiatry* 167:374-379.

Olsen R & Loeb-Lundberg F (1981). Convulsant and anti-convulsant drug binding sites related to GABA-regulated chloride ion channels. In E Costa, G DiChiari & G Gessa (eds.) *GABA and Benzodiazepine Receptors*. New York, NY: The Raven Press.

Ott H, Rohloff A, Aufdembrinke B et al. (1988). Anterograde and retrograde amnesia after lormetazepam and flunitrazepam. *Psychopharmacology Series* 6:180-193.

Ozdemir V, Bremner KE & Naranjo CA (1994). Treatment of alcohol withdrawal syndrome. *Annals of Medicine* 26:101-105.

Pevnick JS, Jasinski DR & Haertzen CA (1978). Abrupt withdrawal from therapeutically administered diazepam. *Archives of General Psychiatry* 35:995-998.

Randall T (1992). Cocaine, alcohol mix in body to form even longer lasting, more lethal drug. *Journal of the American Medical Association* 267:1043-1044.

Richens A, Davidson DL, Cartlidge NE et al. (1994). A multicentre comparative trial of sodium valproate and carbamazepine in adult onset epilepsy. *Journal of Neurology, Neurosurgery, and Psychiatry* 57:682-687.

Rickels K, Case WG, Schweizer E et al. (1990). Benzodiazepine dependence: management of discontinuation. *Psychopharmacology Bulletin* 26:63-68.

Rickels K, Schweizer E, Case WG et al. (1990). Long-term therapeutic use of benzodiazepines. 1. Effects of abrupt discontinuation [published erratum appears in *Archives of General Psychiatry* 1991 Jan;48(1):51]. *Archives of General Psychiatry* 47:899-907.

Robinson GM, Sellers EM & Janecek B (1981). Barbiturate and hypnosedative withdrawal by a multiple oral phenobarbital loading technique. *Clinical Pharmacology and Therapeutics* 30:71-76.

Rosenbaum JF, Moroz G & Bowden CL (1997). Clonazepam in the treatment of panic disorder with or without agoraphobia: A dose-response study of efficacy, safety, and discontinuance. Clonazepam Panic Disorder Dose-Response Study Group. *Journal of Clinical Psychopharmacology* 17:390-400.

Roy-Byrne PP, Ward NG & Donnelly P (1989). Valproate in anxiety and withdrawal syndromes. *Journal of Clinical Psychiatry* 50:44-48.

Rush CR, Baker RW & Wright K (1999). Acute behavioral effects and abuse potential of trazodone, zolpidem and triazolam in humans. *Psychopharmacology (Berlin)* 144(3):220-233.

Rush CR, Frey JM & Griffiths RR (1999). Zaleplon and triazolam in humans: Acute behavioral effects and abuse potential. *Psychopharmacology (Berlin)* 145(1):39-51.

Rush CR & Griffiths RR (1996). Zolpidem, triazolam, and temazepam: Behavioral and subject-rated effects in normal volunteers. *Journal of Clinical Psychopharmacology* 16(2):146-157.

Salloum IM, Cornelius JR, Daley DC et al. (1995). The utility of diazepam loading in the treatment of alcohol withdrawal among psychiatric inpatients. *Psychopharmacology Bulletin* 31:305-310.

Schechter MD (1997). Discrimination of cocaethylene in rats trained to discriminate between its components. *European Journal of Pharmacology* 320:1-7.

Schweizer E & Rickels K (1986). Failure of buspirone to manage benzodiazepine withdrawal. *American Journal of Psychiatry* 143:1590-1592.

Schweizer E, Rickels K, Case WG et al. (1991). Carbamazepine treatment in patients discontinuing long-term benzodiazepine therapy. Effects on withdrawal severity and outcome. *Archives of General Psychiatry* 48:448-452.

Schweizer E, Rickels K & Lucki I (1986). Resistance to the anti-anxiety effect of buspirone in patients with a history of benzodiazepine use [letter]. *The New England Journal of Medicine* 314:719-720.

Sellers EM, Naranjo CA, Harrison M et al. (1983). Oral diazepam loading: Simplified treatment of alcohol withdrawal. *Clinical Pharmacology and Therapeutics* 34:822-826.

Sheehan DV & Harnett-Sheehan K (1996). The role of SSRIs in panic disorder. *Journal of Clinical Psychiatry* 57(Suppl 10):51-58.

Sheehan DV, Raj AB, Harnett-Sheehan K et al. (1993). The relative efficacy of high-dose buspirone and alprazolam in the treatment of panic disorder: A double-blind, placebo-controlled study. *Acta Psychiatrica Scandinavica* 88:1-11.

Skolnick P, Concada V, Barker J et al. (1981). Pentobarbital: dual action to increase brain benzodiazepine receptor affinity. *Science* 211:1448-1450.

Smith D & Wesson D (1970). A new method for treatment of barbiturate dependence. *Journal of the American Medical Association* 213:294-295.

Smith D & Wesson D (1971). A phenobarbital technique for withdrawal of barbiturate abuse. *Archives of General Psychiatry* 24:56-60.

Squires RF & Braestrup C (1977). Benzodiazepine receptors in rat brain. *Nature* 266:732-734.

Steinberg JR (1994). Anxiety in elderly patients. A comparison of azapirones and benzodiazepines. *Drugs and Aging* 5:335-345.

Suzuki T, Mizoguchi H, Motegi H et al. (1995). Effects of nifedipine on physical dependence on barbital or diazepam in rats. *Journal of Toxicological Sciences* 20:415-425.

Taylor DP & Moon SL (1991). Buspirone and related compounds as alternative anxiolytics. *Neuropeptides* 19(Suppl):15-19.

Tollefson GD, Montague-Clouse J & Tollefson SL (1992). Treatment of comorbid generalized anxiety in a recently detoxified alcoholic population with a selective serotonergic drug (buspirone). *Journal of Clinical Psychopharmacology* 12:19-26.

Tonne U, Hiltunen AJ, Vikander B et al. (1991). Neuropsychological changes during steady-state drug use, withdrawal and abstinence in primary benzodiazepine-dependent patients. *Acta Psychiatrica Scandinavica* 91:299-304.

Tyrer P (1993). Benzodiazepine dependence: A shadowy diagnosis. *Biochemical Society Symposium* 59:107-119.

Tyrer P, Rutherford D & Huggett (1981). Benzodiazepine withdrawal symptoms and propranolol. *Lancet* 1:520-527.

Wesson DR & Smith DE (1982). Low dose benzodiazepine withdrawal syndrome: Receptor site medicated. *California Society for the Treatment of Alcoholism and Other Drug Dependencies News* 9:1-5.

Winokur A, Rickels K, Greenblatt DJ et al. (1980). Withdrawal reaction from long-term, low-dosage administration of diazepam. A double-blind, placebo-controlled case study. *Archives of General Psychiatry* 37:101-105.

Woods SW, Nagy LM, Koleszar AS et al. (1992). Controlled trial of alprazolam supplementation during imipramine treatment of panic disorder. *Journal of Clinical Psychopharmacology* 12:32-38.

| Chapter 3 | # Pharmacologic Interventions for Opioid Addiction |

Susan M. Stine, M.D., Ph.D.
Mark K. Greenwald, Ph.D.
Thomas R. Kosten, M.D.

Naltrexone
Methadone
LAAM
Buprenorphine

Studies on the nature of opioid addiction have described an abstinence syndrome characterized by two phases (Himmelsbach, 1942; Martin & Jasinski, 1969): a relatively brief initial phase in which opioid-dependent patients experience acute withdrawal, followed by a protracted abstinence syndrome. Current pharmacotherapeutic strategies are based on this distinction.

Acute Withdrawal. The acute withdrawal syndrome is precipitated by abstinence from opioids. It consists of a wide range of symptoms that persist for various lengths of time. Symptoms include gastrointestinal (GI) distress (such as diarrhea and vomiting), thermal regulation disturbances, insomnia, muscle pain, joint pain, marked anxiety, and dysphoria. Although these symptoms generally include no life-threatening complications, the acute withdrawal syndrome causes marked discomfort, often prompting continuation of opioid use, even in the absence of any opioid-associated euphoria (see Section 5 for a detailed discussion of the management of opioid withdrawal).

Dependence and Protracted Abstinence. In patients with a history of opiate dependence, acute withdrawal and detoxification are only the beginning of treatment. Himmelsbach (1942), reporting on 21 prisoners addicted to morphine, observed that "physical recovery requires not less than six months of total abstinence." Factors he measured included temperature, sleep, respiration, weight, basal metabolic rate, blood pressure, and hematocrit. The times required for return to baseline ranged from one week to about six months. Martin and Jasinski (1969) reported in a subsequent study that the period of protracted abstinence persisted for six months or more following withdrawal and that it was associated with "altered physiological function." They found decreased blood pressure, decreased heart rate and body temperature, miosis, and a decreased sensitivity of the respiratory center to carbon dioxide, beginning about six weeks after withdrawal and persisting for 26 to 30 or more weeks. They also found increased sedimentation rates (which persisted for months) and questionable EEG changes.

Martin and Jasinski also postulated a relationship between the protracted abstinence syndrome and relapse. Based on similar observations, Dole (1972) concluded that "human addicts almost always return to use narcotics" after hospital detoxification. In his paper, Dole reviewed the relative importance of metabolic and conditioned factors in relapse and concluded that the underlying drive is metabolic, arguing that "psychological factors are only triggers for relapse." The concept of protracted abstinence has been controversial (Satel, Kosten et al., 1993), but remains a useful model for scientific hypothesis testing and development of new therapeutic approaches (Stine & Kosten, 1994). Accordingly, Dole recommended methadone maintenance treatment, even though "it does establish physical dependence." Since, as Dole pointed out, methadone continues physical dependence, protracted abstinence may remain a problem at a later time when detoxification from methadone is undertaken.

In addition to biological considerations, psychosocial concomitants of opioid dependence also necessitate longer, more specialized adjunct treatments for these and additional problems. Fortunately, the recent development of new pharmacologic agents may help to address these problems.

NALTREXONE

Naltrexone is a long-acting opioid antagonist that provides complete blockade of opioid receptors when taken at least three times a week for a total weekly dose of about 350 mg (Kosten & Kleber, 1984). Because the reinforcing properties of opioids are completely blocked, naltrexone is theoretically an ideal maintenance agent in the rehabilitation of opioid addicts. However, this optimistic theoretical perspective is contradicted by clinical reality, as reflected in treatment retention rates of only 20% to 30% over six months.

Multiple factors appear to account for such poor retention (Kleber, 1987). Opioid antagonists, unlike methadone, do not provide any narcotic effect. Therefore, if antagonists are stopped, there is no immediate reminder in the form of withdrawal. In addition, craving for narcotics may continue during naltrexone treatment. Nevertheless, for some patients (such as health care professionals, business executives, or probation referrals), for whom there is an external incentive to comply with naltrexone therapy and to remain drug-free, naltrexone has been very effective.

A pharmacologic approach to patient noncompliance may be the development of an injectable, long-acting depot preparation of naltrexone, which would eliminate the need for daily intake. Other supportive measures to increase compliance include family therapy and several behavior modification approaches (Kosten & Kleber, 1984).

Clinically, naltrexone is initiated following acute withdrawal from opioids. There should be at least a five- to seven-day opioid-free period for the short-acting narcotics and a 7- to 10-day period for the long-acting agents. This, of course, does not apply to withdrawal medicated with the

---

TABLE 1. Methadone-Drug Interactions

Drugs That Induce CYP450 Enzyme Activity
Rifampin
Phenytoin
Ethyl alcohol
Barbiturates
Carbamazepine

Drugs That Inhibit CYP450 Enzyme Activity
Cimetidine
Ketoconazole
Erythromycin

---

naltrexone-clonidine combination (see Section 5). The initial dose of naltrexone used generally is 25 mg on the first day, followed by 50 mg daily or an equivalent of 350 mg weekly, divided into three doses (100, 100, and 150 mg). The principal reason for the reduced dose on day 1 is the potential for gastrointestinal side effects, such as nausea and vomiting. This occurs in about 10% of patients taking naltrexone. In most cases, GI upset is relatively mild and transient, but in some cases it may be so severe as to cause discontinuation of the naltrexone. The most serious (but far less frequent) potential side effect of naltrexone is liver toxicity; however, 50 mg daily has been given safely to opioid addicts (Brahen, Capone et al., 1988).

In summary, although naltrexone has not lived up to expectations, for selected patients who are opioid-dependent, it may represent the best form of maintenance pharmacotherapy.

METHADONE

The initial pharmacologic rationale for long-term methadone maintenance was its ability to relieve the protracted abstinence syndrome and to block heroin euphoria (Dole, 1972; Kosten, 1990). However, an equally important benefit of longer-term maintenance has proved to be the opportunity it affords for psychosocial stabilization in the context of symptom relief. Good treatment retention, improved psychosocial adjustment, and reduced criminal activity are among the benefits reported (Cooper, Altman et al., 1983; Dole, 1972). No serious side effects are associated with continued methadone use (Kleber, 1987). Minor side effects, such as constipation, excess sweating, drowsiness, and decreased sexual interest and performance, have been noted. In addition, neuroendocrine studies have shown normalization of stress hormone responses and reproductive functioning (both of which are significantly disrupted in heroin users) after several months of stabilization on methadone (Kreek, 1981). Women stabilized on methadone generally have uneventful pregnancies. Newborns of methadone-maintained women may experience opioid withdrawal symptoms, but these are readily treated. Long-term followup of 27 children who had been exposed to methadone *in utero* found no cognitive impairment in the preschool years (Kaltenbach & Finnegan, 1988). (For a detailed discussion of methadone maintenance, see Chapter 4 of this section.)

A series of large-scale studies has demonstrated that patients maintained on doses of 60 mg or more of methadone a day had better treatment outcomes than those maintained on lower doses and that doses below 60 mg appear to be inadequate for most patients (Hartel, Selwyn et al., 1988; Hartel, Schoenbaum et al., 1989; Hartel, 1989-1990; Ball & Ross, 1991; Caplehorn & Bell, 1991). These studies also confirm that medical decisions should not be based on public biases but on scientific knowledge and clinical evaluation. In particular, the study by Ball and Ross (1991) showed that opiate use was directly related to methadone dose levels and that the effectiveness of methadone was even greater for patients on a 70 mg dose and was still more pronounced for patients on 80 mg a day or more.

A recent factor mandating higher doses is the current purity of street heroin: opioid cross-tolerance implies that the amount of heroin needed to produce euphoria would be prohibitively expensive for someone maintained on a sufficiently high dose of methadone. However, today's high-purity street heroin has required even higher methadone doses to achieve cross-tolerance.

High doses and pure street drugs also may increase the risk of toxicity if patients try to override the cross-tolerance with illicit heroin, since tolerance to respiratory depression may not be as complete as that to euphoria. The functional biological distinction between these pharmacologic effects in animal and binding studies resulted in the proposal of two subclasses of mu receptors (Pasternak & Wood, 1986; Pasternak, 1993; Reisine & Pasternak, 1996), although receptor cloning experiments have not yet confirmed the existence of these mu subclasses (Chen, Mestek et al., 1993; Reisine & Bell, 1993).

Many diverse factors may, in theory, significantly modify the pharmacologic effectiveness of methadone. Three types of factors that have been shown to significantly modify the metabolic breakdown of methadone in the body, and thus potentially its pharmacologic effectiveness, are: (1) chronic diseases, including chronic liver disease, chronic renal disease, and possibly other diseases; (2) drug interactions, including interactions of methadone with rifampin and phenytoin in man, possibly with ethanol and disulfiram and, also, by inference from animal studies, interactions of methadone with phenobarbital, diazepam, desipramine, and other drugs, as well as with estrogen steroids, cimetidine, and antiviral agents used in treatment of HIV (Friedland, Schwartz et al., 1992); and (3) altered physiologic states, especially pregnancy.

The liver in particular may play a central role in several aspects of methadone disposition, involving not only methadone metabolism and clearance but also storage and subsequent release of unchanged methadone. In a study by Kreek and colleagues (1978), unchanged methadone persisted in the liver for up to six weeks and methadone disposition was significantly altered only in a patient subgroup with moderately severe but compensated cirrhosis. These factors have been reviewed in detail by Kreek (1986) and Stine (1997).

Of the multiple medical problems that result from direct and/or indirect effects of opioid use, chronic liver disease is the most common. For example, 50% to 60% of all heroin addicts entering methadone maintenance have biochemical evidence of chronic liver disease, either secondary to infection (hepatitis B and C) or alcohol-induced liver disease. Chronic liver disease in all its forms has major implications for medication use. For example, opioid medications for treatment of dependence (such as methadone, LAAM, and buprenorphine); medications (such as Isoniazid® and Rifampin®) that are prescribed for other diseases that are prevalent in drug users, such as tuberculosis; as well as drugs used to treat or prevent opportunistic infections (such as trimethoprim-sulfamethoxazole) and some antiretroviral agents (such as Didanosine®) may have hepatotoxic effects (O'Connor, Selwyn et al., 1994; Kreek, Garfield et al., 1976; Sawyer, Brown et al., 1993; Schwartz, Brechbuhl et al., 1990). Other diseases commonly coexisting with chronic opioid dependence that can affect maintenance pharmacotherapy are bacterial infections and tuberculosis, particularly "extrapulmonary" manifestations of tuberculosis in

HIV-infected individuals (Braun, Byers et al., 1990; Barnes, Bloch et al., 1991), and drug-resistant forms of tuberculosis (Small, Shafer et al., 1993; CDC, 1991).

With the increasing number of HIV-infected patients in methadone maintenance programs, it is important to define potential interactions between methadone and antiviral agents used in the treatment of HIV. A study of possible interactions between methadone and zidovudine (Azidothymidine® or AZT) has shown that serum levels of methadone are not affected by this drug, but that some patients who receive methadone maintenance treatment may show a potentially toxic increase in serum levels of AZT (Friedland, Schwartz et al., 1992). However, the authors caution against making changes in the dose of AZT; instead, they suggest careful clinical monitoring for signs of dose-related AZT toxicity.

The assessment of new antiretroviral drug efficacy, as well as the determination of patients' prognosis and rate of disease progression, were revolutionized in 1996 with the introduction of commercial assays that quantitate the amount of HIV RNA in plasma. The introduction of new antiretroviral agents has raised justifiable hope of a new therapeutic era for HIV-infected patients, but also has introduced new complexities related to potential drug toxicities and interactions. This also is an issue for current research.

In response to concerns about HIV and drug injection as a mode of transmission, methadone maintenance has been accorded renewed attention. Given that there are more than a million chronic intravenous heroin users in the United States, the magnitude of this problem becomes clear. Prevalence studies in New York City from 1984 to 1985 found that less than 10% of methadone-maintained patients who entered treatment before 1978 were HIV-positive, compared to more than half of heroin addicts who were not in treatment (Des Jarlais, Friedman et al., 1992). Similarly, a prospective study in Philadelphia found an HIV seroconversion rate four times higher in active intravenous heroin users than in methadone-maintained patients (Metzger, Woody et al., 1993). Other studies documented a dramatically reduced HIV seroprevalence rate for patients who were successfully maintained on methadone, as compared to active injecting drug users (Barthwell, Senay et al., 1989; Novick, Joseph et al., 1990; Tidone, Sileo et al., 1987). Methadone maintenance thus appears to be extremely effective in reducing injection-related risk factors for HIV.

The importance of psychosocial treatment as an adjunct to methadone pharmacotherapy also was emphasized by the Ball and Ross study (1991). Recent refinements of this component, as well as treatment-matching studies of the appropriate treatment intensity for patients with varying disability, are an active focus of clinical research (Avants, Ohlins et al., 1996). In general, for successful rehabilitation, length of treatment with methadone is best seen in terms of years rather than months. For many patients, 5 to 10 years—or even a lifetime—of methadone maintenance may be required. However, most programs attempt to withdraw their patients after about a year of treatment (Kleber, 1987). At that time, the pharmacologic component of protracted withdrawal may still present a problem, but the slow decrease in methadone dose plus ongoing therapeutic support in a context of psychosocial stability often renders this problem more manageable.

From an organizational and public health perspective, early treatment termination, illicit use of non-narcotic substances (such as cocaine or alcohol), and diversion of the take-home dose of methadone to the illicit market remain significant issues for most methadone maintenance programs. While concurrent substance use also is a problem (initially, 20% to 50% of methadone patients use cocaine and 25% to 40% abuse alcohol), several effective treatment interventions have been developed, including behavioral approaches and pharmacologic interventions. Diversion of take-home doses is of concern to every methadone maintenance program, although its impact on illicit opioid use remains small (methadone accounts for about 4% of opioids used on the street). Diversion could be eliminated through the use of LAAM, a methadone alternative, which has a duration of action of up to three days and thus obviates the need for take-home doses (Ling, Charuvastra et al., 1976; Kleber, 1987), as well as by use of the buprenorphine+naloxone combination medication approved late in 2002 (Suboxone®).

LAAM

Levo-alpha-acetylmethadol (LAAM) is a derivative of methadone. Its duration of action is up to three days, which makes a three-times-a-week dosing schedule possible. The principal disadvantage of such a long duration of action is the time necessary to reach a steady state and to stabilize the patient at an appropriate comfort level. However, with increased recognition of the shortcomings of methadone maintenance (which involve incomplete suppression of abstinence due to rapid metabolism in some patients, the need for daily dosing, and the potential for diversion of take-home doses), LAAM offers a distinct advantage for some patients.

In spite of these advantages, LAAM at high doses recently has been shown to increase the risk of sudden cardiac death because of prolongation of the QT interval (Schwetz, 2001; Deamer, Wilson et al., 2001). As a result, LAAM has been removed from the market in Europe and has become a relatively contraindicated agent for treatment in the U.S. Thus, for most patients, LAAM is unlikely to be the treatment of choice.

BUPRENORPHINE

Buprenorphine is a high-affinity partial mu opioid agonist that, in October 2002, was approved by the U.S. Food and Drug Administration (FDA) as a pharmacotherapy for opioid dependence (Bickel & Amass, 1995; Ling, Rawson et al., 1994). The introduction of buprenorphine as an agent for the treatment of opioid dependence is of intense scientific interest and great public health significance. Despite its higher unit-dose cost compared to methadone, buprenorphine may expand access to narcotic treatment. This could reduce the disparity between the number of opioid-addicted individuals and the number of treatment slots available to them, and facilitate general medical care of addicted individuals (Lewis, 1999; NIH Consensus Panel, 1999; Rounsaville & Kosten, 2000).

Most Phase 1 and 2 medication development studies with buprenorphine have been conducted using parenteral and sublingual (s.l.) liquid formulations, and the s.l. liquid has been extensively studied in Phase 3 clinical trials. The buprenorphine s.l. tablet is available in two forms. One formulation (Subutex®) contains only buprenorphine ("mono" tablet). The second formulation (Suboxone®) contains buprenorphine and the opioid antagonist naloxone in a 4:1 ratio, which is designed to discourage illicit diversion and intravenous use. The "mono" form would be employed in the clinical setting, while the "combo" form would be suitable for take-home use. Pharmacokinetic studies have found that the buprenorphine s.l. liquid formulation differs in bioavailability from the s.l. tablet. In volunteers who are not maintained on buprenorphine (Mendelson, Upton et al., 1997; Nath, Upton et al., 1999) and volunteers who are maintained on daily buprenorphine (Schuh & Johanson, 1999), the tablet has been shown to produce blood levels

that are about 50% to 60% those achieved with the liquid. Thus, tablet doses used in clinical practice probably will exceed those shown to be effective in past controlled studies with the sublingual solution.

Clinical research over the past 10 years has established that buprenorphine (and buprenorphine with naloxone) is a safe and effective alternative to methadone (Bickel, Stitzer et al., 1988a; Johnson, Jaffe et al., 1992; Strain, Stitzer et al., 1994; Ling, Wesson et al., 1996; Ling, Charuvastra et al., 1998; Uehlinger, Deglon et al., 1998; Liu, Cai et al., 1997; Bouchez, Beauverie et al., 1998; Amass, Kamien et al., in press 2001) and LAAM (Chutuape, Johnson et al., 1999) for opioid agonist maintenance treatment. Treatment with buprenorphine produces significant and substantial improvements over time in psychosocial functioning (Strain, Stitzer et al., 1996). Buprenorphine also has unique features that permit novel uses, which may alter current strategies for maintenance and detoxification (Bickel & Amass, 1995; Amass, Washington et al., in press 2001). In particular, buprenorphine's ceiling on agonist activity reduces the danger of overdose, may limit its abuse liability (Walsh, Preston et al., 1994, 1995), and has low toxicity even at high intravenous doses (Lange, Fudala et al., 1990; Huestis, Umbricht et al., 1999), thereby increasing the dose range over which it may be administered safely. Buprenorphine also can produce sufficient tolerance to block the effects of exogenously administered opioids (Bickel, Stitzer et al., 1988b; Rosen, Wallace et al., 1994; Walsh, Preston et al., 1995), suggesting that it may help to reduce illicit opioid use.

Buprenorphine's slow dissociation from mu opioid receptors results in a long duration of action (ideal for a maintenance medication) and also diminishes withdrawal signs and symptoms on discontinuation (Amass, Bickel et al., 1994; Bickel, Amass et al., 1997; Cheskin, Fudala et al., 1994; Fudala, Jaffe et al., 1990; Jasinski, Pevnick et al., 1978; Seow, Quigley et al., 1986), making it particularly useful for opioid detoxification. Such qualities may make buprenorphine an advance in detoxification treatment by permitting accelerated buprenorphine detoxification without significant withdrawal distress. It has been investigated in clinical pilot studies as a treatment for opioid withdrawal. One study randomly assigned 45 heroin-dependent patients to buprenorphine (2 mg) or methadone (30 mg) for three weeks, followed by a taper over a four-week period, and found that the two approaches produced equivalent results (Bickel, Stitzer et al., 1988a). Another study compared a gradual (36-day) to a more rapid (12-day) buprenorphine taper (initially 8 mg) and found that the gradual approach was superior (Amass, Bickel et al. 1994). A study that compared a three-day course of buprenorphine (3 mg) to a five-day course of clonidine found that those approaches were equivalent (Cheskin, Fudala et al., 1994), although another study found that a longer course of buprenorphine (10 days) was superior to clonidine (Nigam, Ray et al., 1993). A larger study (O'Connor, Carroll et al., 1997) compared 162 heroin- dependent patients detoxified in a primary care setting who were randomized to three 8-day treatment protocols: clonidine, combined clonidine and naltrexone, and buprenorphine. Participants in the combined clonidine and naltrexone group and the buprenorphine group were more likely to complete detoxification than the clonidine group, while the buprenorphine group experienced less severe withdrawal symptoms than the other two groups.

Another study provided further evidence that step-down buprenorphine detoxification minimizes withdrawal symptoms, thus reducing the need for concurrent medication (Vignau, 1998).

A review (Gowing, Ali et al., 2000a) with stringent criteria, selecting only studies with randomized or quasi-randomized prospective designs comparing buprenorphine with another form of treatment, found only five studies that met selection criteria. It concluded that buprenorphine has the potential to relieve heroin withdrawal and possibly methadone withdrawal, but many aspects of treatment protocols and the influence of variables such as the opioid used, dose of methadone, and route of administration require further investigation. In conclusion, although buprenorphine is promising, data on the clinical effectiveness of shorter and longer detoxifications with buprenorphine remain limited (Amass, Bickel et al., 1994; Bickel, Amass et al., 1997). More research is needed to compare the effectiveness of different detoxification regimens so as to optimize buprenorphine dose-tapering schedules.

Methadone-to-Buprenorphine Transfer. It is anticipated that some patients will be transferred from methadone to buprenorphine for maintenance or detoxification. This decision will be driven by several factors. First, there is the unique pharmacology of buprenorphine, leading to its more favorable safety profile and longer duration of action (thus permitting less-frequent dosing) relative to methadone (Amass, Washington et al., in press 2001; Bickel, Amass et al., 1999; Fudala, Jaffe et al., 1990; Petry, Bickel et al., 1999; Schottenfeld, Pakes et al., 2000).

Second, given its status as a novel treatment option (which may differentially attract or retain novelty-seeking individuals [Helmus, Downey et al., in press 2001]), buprenorphine may engender less fear of stigma than methadone.

Third, due to its enhanced safety, buprenorphine may be used effectively in office-based primary care (that is, outside the domain of standard narcotic treatment programs) (O'Connor, Carroll et al., 1997; O'Connor & Kosten, 1998). It also may be appropriate as an early intervention strategy for those with short addiction histories (for example, adolescents), or with less physical dependence. Buprenorphine can produce withdrawal discomfort among opioid-dependent volunteers under certain conditions, which may be due to more than one mechanism (Bickel & Amass, 1995; Johnson, Cone et al., 1989). Low buprenorphine doses may provide too-little agonist effect (that is, insufficient substitution) relative to the maintenance opioid (such as heroin). In this case, raising the buprenorphine dose may or may not surmount this problem. Put another way, the partial agonist profile of buprenorphine may limit its ability to suppress opioid abstinence signs and symptoms. Alternatively, buprenorphine may directly precipitate withdrawal discomfort, in which case higher doses would be expected to aggravate the problem. Since among individuals maintained on the long-acting, full mu opioid agonist methadone, the high-affinity partial mu-agonist buprenorphine is capable of abruptly reducing the extent of mu opioid receptor stimulation. This would be expected to reduce opioid agonist symptoms and/or increase withdrawal symptoms.

This principle has been amply demonstrated in humans: Partial mu opioid agonists such as nalorphine and butorphanol (Preston, Bigelow et al., 1988b, 1989) can, in methadone maintained individuals, abruptly precipitate opioid withdrawal signs and symptoms that are functionally similar to those produced by the antagonist naloxone. Obviously, it would be ideal to avoid (or at least minimize) this problem because this discomfort may translate into attrition and relapse. It is important to note that, among individuals maintained on shorter-acting mu opioid agonists like morphine (relative to the longer-acting agonist methadone), buprenorphine administered alone did not precipitate a significant opioid withdrawal syndrome (Fudala, Bridge et al., 1998; Mendelson, Jones et al., 1996, 1999; Schuh, Walsh et al., 1996). Bickel and Amass (1995) proposed tentative guidelines for inducting heroin abusers onto buprenorphine, which involve considering the amount of heroin used and maintaining a sufficient interval (at least 12 hours) between the last heroin use and the first buprenorphine dose. They recommended that the induction dose of buprenorphine be administered when patients are beginning to experience opioid withdrawal, so that buprenorphine can suppress those symptoms.

Clinical experience with administering initial doses of buprenorphine to heroin abusers suggests that an interval of six hours probably is sufficient to minimize the risk of precipitated withdrawal. However, transferring patients from a longer-acting agonist such as methadone to buprenorphine without producing significant withdrawal discomfort, attrition, or relapse to drug use, has been shown to be more challenging.

Inpatient Challenge Studies of Buprenorphine's Effects in Methadone-Maintained Research Volunteers. Several clinical studies have investigated the possibility of switching methadone-maintained research volunteers to buprenorphine. Four programmatic studies examined the effect of time interval between the last methadone maintenance dose and the initial buprenorphine dose (Preston, Bigelow et al., 1988; Strain, Preston et al., 1992, 1995; Walsh, June et al., 1995). Most subjects in the four studies were maintained on methadone 30 mg/day. When buprenorphine was administered to the volunteers, buprenorphine significantly increased opioid withdrawal effects at two hours post-methadone (Strain, Preston et al., 1992), but not at 20 to 22 hours (Preston, Bigelow et al., 1988b; Strain, Preston et al., 1992), nor at 40 hours (Walsh, June et al., 1995). Results from another study in which buprenorphine was administered intravenously at about a 20-hour interval (Mendelson, Upton et al., 1997) also are consistent with these data. The time interval of about 24 hours is relevant, because this is the customary methadone dosing interval employed in clinical practice and these studies therefore provide encouraging evidence that an outpatient transfer could succeed.

Only Walsh and colleagues (1995) have systematically addressed whether methadone maintenance dose influences the response to buprenorphine. One group of volunteers in that study was maintained on 30 mg/day, and a second group of volunteers was maintained on 60 mg/day. The first group of volunteers received 60 mg and, in these individuals, buprenorphine precipitated a dose-dependent increase in opioid withdrawal symptoms. In contrast, buprenorphine did not precipitate significant increases in opioid withdrawal in the second group of volunteers, who received 30 mg.

This study was limited by lack of either random assignment to different groups (between-subject design) or, alternatively, a within-subject controlled design.

Three studies (Strain, Preston et al., 1992, 1995; Walsh, June et al., 1995) have directly addressed whether buprenorphine dose-dependently precipitates opioid withdrawal in methadone-maintained volunteers. This variable can be interpreted as reflecting the degree of antagonist (or partial agonist) capacity of the challenge drug. In the studies by Strain and colleagues (1992, 1995), buprenorphine (five active doses from 0.5 to 8 mg IM) precipitated mild withdrawal at the two-hour interval. However, withdrawal severity was not dose-related.

Attempts at a Full Methadone-to-Buprenorphine Transfer (Inpatient and Outpatient). Five studies have directly examined, or are now examining, a full medication transfer. Kosten and Kleber (1988) reported the first outpatient trial of the methadone-to-buprenorphine (s.l. liquid) transition. In this open-label study, there were 16 volunteers. However, only half of these were methadone-maintained (25 mg/day), while the other half were using heroin. The eight methadone patients were assigned to receive 2 mg (n=4), 4 mg (n=2), or 8 mg (n=2) per day. Patients were inducted onto buprenorphine within 24 hours after their last methadone dose. Therefore, the dosing parameters of this study are comparable to the inpatient challenge studies of Preston and colleagues (1988a) and Strain and colleagues (1995). The investigators reported that most patients completed the protocol. However, one patient exhibited persistent withdrawal symptoms and four patients reported headaches during the initial transfer period. Overall, heroin use was relatively low, with 78% of all samples testing drug-free. Across the entire sample (n=16), withdrawal symptoms were highest on the first two test days. Withdrawal symptom ratings varied by buprenorphine dose, but were not dose-dependent. Limitations of this study include the open-label design, small group, and attendant problems of data interpretation (for example, lack of dose-dependent changes in the dependent measures).

In an open-label study, Banys and colleagues (1994) examined the ability of s.l. liquid buprenorphine to suppress opioid withdrawal 26 to 31 hours after discontinuing methadone. Fifteen participants could take three low doses of buprenorphine over several hours (0.15 mg, 0.15 mg one hour later, then 0.3 mg two hours later), in an effort to relieve withdrawal signs and symptoms. There were substantial individual differences reported in the ability of buprenorphine to suppress opioid withdrawal. Six subjects reported relief with buprenorphine, four subjects reported partial relief, and five subjects reported no relief at all. In short, these buprenorphine doses provided inadequate agonist effect to offset methadone abstinence symptoms. These data suggest that individual differences may affect the efficacy of the medication transfer.

Lukas and colleagues (1984) conducted the first double-blind, double-dummy pilot study of three males—maintained on three different methadone doses (25, 58 and 60 mg/day)—who were switched abruptly to buprenorphine 2 mg/day, subcutaneously. Physiologic (including EEG), behavioral, and subjective ratings were collected during methadone stabilization, the abrupt transfer, buprenorphine stabilization, and detoxification. They found that buprenorphine did not fully substitute for methadone during the transfer: Withdrawal signs and symptoms peaked within the first several days of buprenorphine (depending on the measure), and abated during buprenorphine stabilization. The authors did not report any differences between subjects during substitution of buprenorphine for methadone (that is, no effect of moderate [n=2] versus low [n=1] methadone dose), which could have been due to the very small sample size.

At present, the only other published study of the methadone to buprenorphine (s.l. liquid) full transfer is a within-subject, double-blind, double-dummy procedure with inpatient volunteers (Levin, Fischman et al., 1997). A moderate methadone maintenance dose (60 mg) was tapered over a few days (40 mg, 30 mg, 30 mg, then 0 mg) before initiating buprenorphine (4 mg on day 1, followed by 8 mg). Like Kosten and Kleber (1988), the protocol of Levin and colleagues (1997) demonstrated some qualified success, in that 79% (15 of 19) of participants who began the dose-taper completed the transfer. In the Levin study, the one-day methadone placebo—which produced a 48-hour interval between the last active methadone dose and the first active buprenorphine dose—significantly increased opioid withdrawal symptoms to a "moderate" level. Peak withdrawal symptom scores occurred just prior to the first buprenorphine dose. Opioid withdrawal symptoms remained elevated, but were not significantly worsened, by the first two buprenorphine daily doses (4 mg, then 8 mg). Withdrawal symptoms gradually were suppressed by subsequent daily doses of buprenorphine (8 mg) and returned to baseline during buprenorphine stabilization (8 mg/day). Thus, the initial buprenorphine doses might have been too low, since

they did not rapidly suppress methadone abstinence withdrawal symptoms (see Banys, Clark et al., 1994, above).

Levin and colleagues (1997) reported that the participants who dropped out cited an "inability to tolerate the withdrawal symptoms." A second limitation is that there was no control group against which to evaluate the methadone dose-taper. (However, the within-subject design did permit analysis of symptom changes over time.) In addition, individuals were given access to, and used, significant amounts of ancillary medications (mean oxazepam dose of 45 mg/day and mean clonidine dose of 0.3 mg/day) to alleviate withdrawal discomfort, even though concurrent use of buprenorphine and benzodiazepines is not advised. For this reason, the study by Levin and colleagues (1997) cannot be compared directly with previous studies, which did not permit use of these medications. It also is difficult to extrapolate this study to outpatient conditions.

In a recent small double-blind, double-dummy pilot study (Greenwald, Schuh et al., manuscript submitted), five male heroin-dependent outpatient volunteers were transferred from methadone 60 mg (with one intervening 45 mg dose) to the buprenorphine s.l. tablet. Subjective effects and vital signs were collected before the transfer (methadone 60 mg and 45 mg), on buprenorphine days 1 and 2 (8 mg/day), and on days 7 and 8 (16 mg/day).

The one-day methadone dose-taper did not significantly alter opioid withdrawal or agonist symptoms. On transfer day 1, buprenorphine significantly increased withdrawal symptoms (which peaked later that evening), and decreased agonist symptoms and dose preference, as compared to methadone stabilization. On buprenorphine transfer day 2, withdrawal symptoms and blood pressure were elevated, but agonist symptoms and dose preference did not significantly differ from methadone stabilization levels. Amount of self-reported heroin use decreased from before methadone stabilization and did not increase during the transfer. One week later, buprenorphine 16 mg doses increased agonist effects. Therefore, a one-day methadone dose-taper to 45 mg was well tolerated relative to 60 mg/day stabilization, and the transition from methadone 45 mg to buprenorphine 8 mg tablet resulted in a time-related (throughout the same day) increase in opioid withdrawal symptoms, which peaked during the evening (about 6 to 18 hours) after the first buprenorphine 8 mg dose. This suggests that, in practice, peak symptoms might occur outside the clinical setting, thereby increasing the probability of heroin use. Importantly, the protocol used in this pilot study was able to shorten the duration of withdrawal discomfort to about one day, relative to the results of Levin and colleagues (1997).

These preliminary results suggest that it is feasible to transfer outpatients on methadone 60 mg/day to the buprenorphine 8 mg/day s.l. tablet, although refinements are needed to improve the tolerability and clinical efficacy of this protocol. In contrast, the dose-taper used by Levin and colleagues (1997) probably was too extreme, leading to methadone abstinence withdrawal, and the initial buprenorphine doses did not rapidly suppress this withdrawal. It would seem reasonable to propose that, in future studies, the magnitude and duration of the methadone dose-taper (from a starting level of 60 mg) should strike a compromise between the protocols used in the two studies, as from an intermediate 30 mg dose of methadone to 8 mg of buprenorphine. However, the increased opioid withdrawal symptoms experienced by the outpatients in the Greenwald study did not lead to increased attrition, even though they were associated with decreased ratings of dose adequacy and dose preference (relative to their pre-study methadone dose). In addition, if the first daily transfer dose of buprenorphine does precipitate withdrawal, it may be useful to consider increased subsequent buprenorphine doses (to provide additional agonist) to suppress this withdrawal. Moreover, buprenorphine 16 mg can decrease residual opioid withdrawal after brief stabilization on buprenorphine 8 mg/day, and was preferred by participants to 60 mg/day methadone stabilization. These data imply that higher buprenorphine doses may be useful in suppressing residual withdrawal symptoms and initiating heroin abstinence in some individuals immediately after the transfer, and also may be preferred.

Buprenorphine in Agonist-to-Antagonist Treatment. Buprenorphine has been used in several experimental studies (Kosten & Kleber, 1988; Bickel, Stitzer et al., 1988a; Kosten, Krystal et al., 1989) as a transitional agent between agonists (such as methadone or heroin) and antagonists (such as naloxone or naltrexone). In one study, Kosten and Kleber (1988) substituted buprenorphine at 2, 4 and 8 mg for 20 to 30 mg of methadone or heroin for one month without precipitating substantial withdrawal symptoms, although buprenorphine may act as an opioid antagonist at doses as low as 8 mg. After chronic administration, buprenorphine produces less physical dependence than do pure agonists, as suggested by the minimal withdrawal symptoms that occur when buprenorphine is stopped, and by the use of relatively higher antagonist doses that are needed to precipitate withdrawal in buprenorphine-maintained volunteers (Eissenberg, Greenwald et al., 1996). After one month of buprenorphine stabilization, the drug was abruptly discontinued and a small dose of naltrexone given 24 hours later.

The investigators observed that the transition to buprenorphine generally was well-tolerated. The subsequent abrupt discontinuation of buprenorphine was associated with "minimal withdrawal" in the 2- and 4-mg buprenorphine groups, and a low dose of naltrexone (1 mg) did not precipitate withdrawal. However, subjects in the 8 mg group reported a more substantial increase in withdrawal symptoms when buprenorphine was stopped.

Because of these properties, Kosten and Kleber (1988) examined whether buprenorphine might facilitate the transition from opioid agonists to antagonists in a three-step process: (1) buprenorphine substitution for agonists such as methadone, (2) buprenorphine-induced reduction in physical dependence, and (3) discontinuation of buprenorphine with rapid introduction of naltrexone.

In a study testing that hypothesis, Kosten and colleagues (1989) used intravenous naloxone to challenge five opioid-addicted patients who were maintained on 3 mg s.l. buprenorphine. Induction onto naltrexone was attempted in all of those patients who completed 30 days on buprenorphine. The buprenorphine discontinuation and induction onto naltrexone included blinded discontinuation of the buprenorphine, followed by double-blind, placebo-controlled challenges with high-dose naloxone. Five male opioid-addicted patients maintained on buprenorphine 3 mg sublingually for one month as outpatients were abruptly discontinued from buprenorphine by blinded, placebo substitution and enlisted in a placebo-controlled, double-blind challenge with intravenous naloxone at 0.5 mg/kg. The naloxone was given over a 20-minute period using a 10 mg/ml solution. Significant withdrawal symptoms were precipitated. However, the severity of withdrawal was about two-thirds the severity for methadone patients (Abstinence Rating Scale = 22; SD = 9.3) and less than a third of the full Abstinence Rating Scale score of 45. Moreover, five hours after this naloxone challenge, withdrawal symptoms were at baseline levels and oral naltrexone was given at either 12.5 mg or 25 mg without precipitating further withdrawal symptoms. The authors felt that the withdrawal syndrome was milder for buprenorphine than for pure opioid agonists, "suggesting a partial resetting of the opioid receptors by the antagonist activity of buprenorphine."

In some situations, combination drug treatment may facilitate greater patient acceptance of agonist-antagonist switching. Thus, Gerra and colleagues (2000) have shown that the early use of naltrexone during detoxification in combination with benzodiazepines and clonidine facilitated naltrexone acceptance by patients. Umbricht and colleagues (1999), in a study comparing buprenorphine taper alone and buprenorphine with naltrexone, suggested that the combination treatment may reduce the severity of withdrawal symptoms.

The use of buprenorphine to stabilize opioid addicts before switching them to naltrexone has the advantage of psychosocial stabilization prior to detoxification. This approach thus may represent a compromise between acute detoxification and long-term treatment of chronic dependence.

The foregoing techniques (clonidine/naltrexone and buprenorphine/naltrexone) may be combined in a clinical protocol that places methadone patients or heroin addicts on buprenorphine for several weeks to stabilize and engage them in the psychosocial aspects of treatment. This could be followed by rapid transition to naltrexone, using clonidine to relieve any withdrawal symptoms caused by stopping the buprenorphine. Such combination approaches are reviewed in Stine and Kosten (1992). These generally have been small pilot studies. Larger clinical trials of buprenorphine-to-naltrexone transitions, with and without clonidine, are needed and have potential to lead to shorter, more cost-effective treatment alternatives (to long-term maintenance) for patients who need more treatment than brief detoxification.

ACKNOWLEDGMENTS: This work was supported by National Institute on Drug Abuse grants R01-DA05626 (TRK), K05-DA0454 (TRK), and P50-DA09250, and the Veterans Affairs Mental Illness Research, Education and Clinical Center (MIRECC).

REFERENCES

Albanese AP, Gevirtz C, Oppenheim B et al. (2000). Outcome and six-month follow up of patients after ultra rapid opiate detoxification (UROD). *Journal of Addictive Diseases* 19(2):11-28.

Amass L, Bickel WK, Higgins ST et al. (1994). A preliminary investigation of outcome following gradual or rapid buprenorphine detoxification. *Journal of Addictive Diseases* 13(3):33-45.

Amass L, Kamien JB, Branstetter SA et al. (In press 2001). A controlled comparison of the buprenorphine-naloxone tablet and methadone for opioid maintenance treatment: Interim results. In LS Harris (ed.) *Problems of Drug Dependence 1999 (NIDA Research Monograph Series)*. Bethesda, MD: National Institute on Drug Abuse.

Amass L, Washington DCL, Kamien JB et al. (In press 2001). Thrice-weekly supervised dosing with the combination buprenorphine-naloxone table is preferred to daily supervised dosing by opioid-dependent humans. *Drug and Alcohol Dependence.*

Asin K & Wirtshafter D (1985). Clonidine produces a conditioned place preference in rats. *Psychopharmacology (Berlin)* 85(3):383-385.

Avants SK, Ohlin R & Margolin A (1996). Matching methadone-maintained patients to psychosocial treatments. In SM Stine & TR Kosten (eds.) *New Treatments for Opiate Dependence*. New York, NY: Guilford Press, 3:149-170.

Ball JC & Ross A (1991). *The Effectiveness of Methadone Maintenance Treatment*. New York, NY: Springer-Verlag.

Banys P, Clark HW, Tusel DJ et al. (1994). An open trial of low dose buprenorphine in treating methadone withdrawal. *Journal of Substance Abuse Treatment* 11:9-15.

Barnes PF, Bloch AB, Davidson PT et al. (1991). Tuberculosis in patients with human immunodeficiency virus infection. *New England Journal of Medicine* 1644-1650.

Barthwell A, Senay E, Marks R et al. (1989). Patients successfully maintained with methadone escaped human immunodeficiency virus infection. *Archives of General Psychiatry* 46:957-958.

Bearn J, Gossop M & Strang J (1998). Accelerated lofexidine treatment regimen compared with conventional lofexidine and methadone treatment for in-patient opiate detoxification. *Drug and Alcohol Dependence* 50(3):227-232.

Bickel WK & Amass L (1995). Buprenorphine treatment of opioid dependence: A review. *Experimental and Clinical Psychopharmacology* 3:477-489.

Bickel W, Amass L, Crean JP et al. (1999). Buprenorphine dosing every 1, 2, or 3 days in opioid-dependent patients. *Psychopharmacology (Berlin)* 146(2):111-118.

Bickel WK, Amass L, Higgins ST et al. (1997). Effects of adding behavioral treatment to opioid detoxification with buprenorphine. *Journal of Consulting and Clinical Psychology* 65(5):1-81.

Bickel WK, Stitzer MI, Bigelow GE et al. (1988a). A clinical trial of buprenorphine: Comparison with methadone in the detoxification of heroin addicts. *Clinical Pharmacology and Therapeutics* 43:72-78.

Bickel WK, Stitzer MI, Bigelow GE et al. (1988b). Buprenorphine: Dose-related blockade of opioid challenge effects in opioid dependent humans. *Journal of Pharmacology and Experimental Therapeutics* 247:47-53.

Bouchez J, Beauverie P & Touzeau D (1998). Substitution with buprenorphine in methadone- and morphine sulfate-dependent patients. Preliminary results. *European Addiction Research* 4(Suppl)1:8-12.

Brahen LS, Capone TJ & Capone DM (1988). Naltrexone: Lack of effect on hepatic enzymes. *Journal of Clinical Pharmacology* 28:64-70.

Braun MM, Byers RH, Heyward WL et al. (1990). Acquired immunodeficiency syndrome and extrapulmonary tuberculosis in the United States. *Archives of Internal Medicine* 150:1913-1916.

Caplehorn JRM & Bell J (1991). Methadone dosage and retention of patients in maintenance treatment. *Medical Journal of Australia* 154:195-199.

Carnwath T & Hardman J (1998). Randomized double-blind comparison of lofexidine and clonidine in the outpatient treatment of opiate withdrawal. *Drug and Alcohol Dependence* 50(3):251-254.

Carroll ME, Carmona GN, May SA et al. (1992). Buprenorphine effects on self-administration of smoked cocaine base and orally delivered phencyclidine, ethanol and saccharin in rhesus monkeys. *Journal of Pharmacology and Experimental Therapeutics* 261:26-37.

Centers for Disease Control and Prevention (CDC) (1991). Nosocomial transmissions of multidrug-resistant tuberculosis among HIV-infected persons—Florida and New York, 1988-1991. *Morbidity and Mortality Weekly Reports* 40:585-602.

Charney DS, Sternberg DE, Kleber HD et al. (1981). The clinical use of clonidine in abrupt withdrawal from methadone. *Archives of General Psychiatry* 38:1273-1277.

Chen Y, Mestek A, Liu J et al. (1993). Molecular cloning and functional expression of a mu-opioid receptor from rat brain. *Molecular Pharmacology* 44:8-12.

Cheskin LJ, Fudala PJ & Johnson RE (1994). A controlled comparison of buprenorphine and clonidine for acute detoxification from opioids. *Drug and Alcohol Dependence* 36(2):115-121.

Chutuape MA, Johnson RE, Strain EC et al. (1999). Controlled clinical trial comparing maintenance treatment efficacy of buprenorphine (buprenorphine), levomethadoneadoneadyl acetate (LAAM) and methadone (m). In LS Harris (ed.) *Problems of Drug Dependence 1998 (NIDA Research Monograph 179)*. Rockville, MD: National Institute on Drug Abuse, 74.

Cooper JR, Altman F, Brown B et al. (1983). *Research on the Treatment of Narcotic Addiction: State of the Art*. Rockville, MD: National Institute on Drug Abuse.

Davis WM & Smith SG (1977). Catecholaminergic mechanisms of reinforcement. Mechanisms of reinforcement: Direct assessment by drug self-administration. *Life Sciences* 20:483-492.

Deamer RL, Wilson DR, Clark DS et al. (2001). Torsades de pointes associated with high dose levomethadyl acetate (ORLAAM). *Journal of Addictive Diseases* 20(4):7-14.

Des Jarlais DC, Friedman SR, Woods J et al. (1992). HIV infection among intravenous drug users: Epidemiology and emerging public health perspectives. In JH Lowinson, P Ruiz & RB Millman (eds.) *Substance Abuse: A Comprehensive Textbook*. Baltimore, MD: Williams & Wilkins, 734-743.

Dole VP (1972). Narcotic addiction, physical dependence and relapse. *New England Journal of Medicine* 286:988-992.

Dole VP & Nyswander ME (1965). A medical treatment for diacetylmorphine (heroin) addiction. *Journal of the American Medical Association* 193:646-650.

Doxey JC, Everitt JE, Frank LW et al. (1977). A comparison of the effects of buprenorphine and morphine on the blood gases of conscious rats. *British Journal of Pharmacology* 60:118P.

Eissenberg T, Greenwald MK, Johnson RE et al. (1996). Buprenorphine's physical dependence potential: antagonist-precipitated withdrawal in humans. *Journal of Pharmacology and Experimental Therapeutics* 276(2):449-459.

Foldes BS, Shivaku Y, Matsuo S et al. (1979). The influence of methadone derivatives on the isolated myenteric plexus-longitudinal muscle preparation of the guinea pig ileum. *Advances in Pharmacological Research and Practice: Proceedings of the Congress of the Hungarian Pharmacological Society* 5:165-170, 201.

Friedland A, Schwartz E, Brechbuhl AB et al. (1992). Pharmacokinetic interactions of zidovudine and methadone in intravenous drug using patients with HIV infection. *Journal of the Acquired Immune Deficiency Syndrome* 5:619-626.

Fudala PJ, Bridge TP, Herbert S et al. (1998). A multisite efficacy evaluation of a buprenorphine/naloxone product for opiate dependence treatment. *NIDA Research Monograph 179*. Rockville, MD: National Institute on Drug Abuse, 105.

Fudala PJ, Jaffe JH, Dax EM et al. (1990). Use of buprenorphine in the treatment of opioid addiction. II. Physiologic and behavioral effects of daily and alternate-day administration and abrupt withdrawal. *Clinical Pharmacology and Therapeutics* 47:525-534.

Gerra G, Zaimovic A, Rustichelli P et al. (2000). Rapid opiate detoxification in outpatient treatment: Relationship with naltrexone compliance. *Journal of Substance Abuse Treatment* 18(2):185-191.

Gold MS, Redmond DE & Kleber HD (1978). Clonidine in opiate withdrawal. *Lancet* 11:929-930.

Gold ME, Redmond DC & Kleber HD (1978). Clonidine blocks acute opiate-withdrawal symptoms. *Lancet* 2:599-602.

Gowing L, Ali R & White J (2000a). Buprenorphine for the management of opioid withdrawal. *The Cochrane Database of Systematic Reviews*, Issue 3.

Gowing L, Ali R & White J (2000b). Opioid antagonists and adrenergic agonists for the management of opioid withdrawal. *The Cochrane Database Systematic Reviews* (2):CD002021.

Greenwald MK, Schuh KJ & Stine SM (In submission 2001). Transferring heroin-dependent outpatients stabilized on moderate-dose methadone to the buprenorphine sublingual tablet: A preliminary study. *Drug and Alcohol Dependence*.

Hartel D (1989-1990). Cocaine use, inadequate methadone dose increase risk of AIDS for IV drug users in treatment. *NIDA Notes* 5(1).

Hartel D, Schoenbaum EE, Selwyn PA et al. (1989). Temporal patterns of cocaine use and AIDS in intravenous drug users in methadone maintenance [Abstract]. *5th International Conference on AIDS*, Stockholm, Sweden, June.

Hartel D, Selwyn PA, Schoenbaum EE et al. (1988). Methadone maintenance treatment and reduced risk of AIDS and AIDS-specific mortality in intravenous drug users [Abstract 8526]. *4th International Conference on AIDS*, Stockholm, Sweden, June.

Helmus T, Downey KK, Arfken C et al. (in press 2001). Novelty seeking among heroin dependent poly-drug abusers entering buprenorphine treatment. *Drug and Alcohol Dependence*.

Hensel M, Wolter S & Kox WJ (2000). EEG controlled rapid opioid withdrawal under general anaesthesia. *British Journal of Anaesthesia* 84(2):236-238.

Himmelsbach CK (1942). Clinical studies of drug addiction; Physical dependence, withdrawal and recovery. *Archives of Internal Medicine* 69:766-772.

Huestis MA, Umbricht A, Preston KL et al. (1999). Safety of buprenorphine: No clinically relevant cardio-respiratory depression at high IV doses. In LS Harris (ed.) *Problems of Drug Dependence 1998 (NIDA Research Monograph 179).* Rockville, MD: National Institute on Drug Abuse, 62.

Jackson AH & Shader RI (1973). Guidelines for the withdrawal of narcotic and general depressant drugs. *Diseases of the Nervous System* 34:162-166.

Jasinski DR, Pevnick JS & Griffith JD (1978). Human pharmacology and abuse potential of the analgesic buprenorphine. *Archives of General Psychiatry* 35:501-516.

Johnson RE, Cone EJ, Henningfield JE et al. (1989). A controlled trial of buprenorphine in the treatment of heroin addiction. I. Physiological and behavioral effects during a rapid dose induction. *Clinical Pharmacology and Therapeutics* 46:335-343.

Johnson RE, Fudala PJ & Jaffe JH (1992). A controlled trial of buprenorphine for opioid dependence. *Journal of the American Medical Association* 267:2750-2755.

Johnson RE, Jaffe JH & Fudala PJ (1992). A controlled trial of buprenorphine treatment for opioid dependence. *Journal of the American Medical Association* 267:2750-2755.

Kaltenbach K & Finnegan L (1988). Children exposed to methadone in-utero: Cognitive ability in preschool years. *NIDA Research Monograph 81.* Rockville, MD: National Institute on Drug Abuse.

Kleber H, Topazian M, Gaspari J et al. (1987). Clonidine and naltrexone in the outpatient treatment of heroin withdrawal. *American Journal of Drug and Alcohol Abuse* 13(1-2):1-17.

Kleber HD (1987). Treatment of narcotic addicts. *Psychiatric Medicine* 3:389-418.

Kleber HD, Riordan CE, Rounsaville B et al. (1985). Clonidine in outpatient detoxification from methadone maintenance. *Archives of General Psychiatry* 42:391-394.

Kosten TR (1990). Current pharmacotherapies for opioid dependence. *Psychopharmacology Bulletin* 26:69-74.

Kosten TR & Kleber HD (1988). Buprenorphine detoxification from opioid dependence: A pilot study. *Life Sciences* 42:611-635.

Kosten TR & Kleber HD (1984). Strategies to improve compliance with narcotic antagonists. *American Journal of Drug and Alcohol Abuse* 10:249-266.

Kosten TR, Krystal JH, Charney DS et al. (1989). Rapid detoxification from opioid dependence. *American Journal of Psychiatry* 146:1349.

Kosten TR, Schottenfeld R, Ziedonis D et al. (1993). Buprenorphine versus methadone maintenance for opioid dependence. *Journal of Nervous and Mental Disease.*

Kreek MJ (1986). Factors modifying the pharmacological effectiveness of methadone. *NIDA Monograph Series.* Rockville, MD: National Institute on Drug Abuse.

Kreek MJ (1981). Medical management of methadone-maintained patients. In JH Lowinson & P Ruiz (eds.) *Substance Abuse: Clinical Problems and Perspectives.* Baltimore, MD: Williams & Wilkins, 660-673.

Kreek MJ, Garfield JW, Gutjahr CL et al. (1976). Rifampin-induced methadone withdrawal. *New England Journal of Medicine* 294:1104-1106.

Kreek MJ, Oratz M & Rothschild MA (1978). Hepatic extraction of long- and short-acting narcotics in the isolated perfused rabbit liver. *Gastroenterology* 75:88-94.

Lange WR, Fudala PJ, Dax EM et al. (1990). Safety and side effects of buprenorphine in the clinical management of heroin addiction. *Drug and Alcohol Dependence* 26:19-28.

Lauzon P (1992). Two cases of clonidine abuse/dependence in methadone-maintained patients. *Journal of Substance Abuse Treatment* 9(2):125-127.

Lawental E (2000). Ultra rapid opiate detoxification as compared to 30-day inpatient detoxification program—A retrospective follow-up study. *Journal of Substance Abuse Treatment* 11(2):173-181.

Levin FR, Fischman MW, Connerney I et al. (1997). A protocol to switch high-dose, methadone-maintained subjects to buprenorphine. *American Journal of Addiction* 6:105-116.

Lewis DC (1999). Access to narcotic addiction treatment and medical care: Prospects for the expansion of methadone maintenance treatment. *Journal of Addictive Diseases* 18:5-21.

Lin SK, Strang J, Su LW et al. (1997). Double blind randomized controlled trial of lofexidine versus clonidine in the treatment of heroin withdrawal. *Drug and Alcohol Dependence* 48(2):127-133.

Ling W, Charuvastra C, Collins JF et al. (1998). Buprenorphine maintenance treatment of opiate dependence: A multicenter, randomized clinical trial. *Addiction* 93(4):475-486.

Ling W, Charuvastra VC, Kaim SC et al. (1976). Methadyl acetate and methadone as maintenance treatments for heroin addicts. *Archives of General Psychiatry* 33:709-720.

Ling W, Rawson RA & Compton MA (1994). Substitution pharmacotherapies for opioid addiction: From methadone to LAAM and buprenorphine. *Journal of Psychoactive Drugs* 26(2):119-128.

Ling W, Wesson DR, Charuvastra C et al. (1996). A controlled trial comparing buprenorphine and methadone maintenance in opioid dependence. *Archives of General Psychiatry* 53:401-407.

Liu Z, Cai Z, Wang XP et al. (1997). Rapid detoxification of heroin dependence by buprenorphine. *Chung Kuo Yao Li Hsueh Pao* 18(2):112-114.

Loimer N, Schmid R, Lenz K et al. (1990). Acute blocking of naloxone-precipitated opiate withdrawal symptoms by methohexitone. *British Journal of Psychiatry* 157:748-752.

Loimer N, Schmid R, Presslich O et al. (1988). Naloxone treatment for opiate withdrawal syndrome [letter]. *British Journal of Psychiatry* 153:851-852.

Lukas SE, Jasinski DR & Johnson RE (1984). Electroencephalographic and behavioral correlates of buprenorphine administration. *Clinical Pharmacology and Therapeutics* 36:127-132.

Margolin A & Kosten TR (1991). Opioid detoxification and maintenance with blocking agents. In NS Miller (ed.) *Comprehensive Handbook of Drug and Alcohol Addiction.* New York, NY: Marcel Dekker, 1127-1141.

Martin WR, Eades CG, Thompson JA et al. (1976). The effects of morphine- and nalorphine-like drugs in the nondependent and morphine-dependent chronic spinal dog. *Journal of Pharmacology and Experimental Therapy* 197:517-532.

Martin WR & Jasinski DR (1969). Physiological parameters of morphine dependence in man: Tolerance, early abstinence, protracted abstinence. *Journal of Psychiatric Research* 7:9-17.

Mello NK, Mendelson JH, Bree MP et al. (1989). Buprenorphine suppresses cocaine self-administration by Rhesus monkeys. *Science* 245:859-862.

Mendelson J, Jones RT, Fernandez I et al. (1996). Buprenorphine and naloxone interactions in opiate-dependent volunteers. *Clinical Pharmacology and Therapeutics* 60:105-114.

Mendelson J, Jones RT, Welm S et al. (1999). Buprenorphine and naloxone combinations: The effects of three dose ratios in morphine-stabilized, opiate-dependent volunteers. *Psychopharmacology (Berlin)* 141:37-46.

Mendelson J, Upton RA, Everhart ET et al. (1997). Bioavailability of sublingual buprenorphine. *Journal of Clinical Pharmacology* 37(1):31-37.

Metzger DS, Woody GE, McLellan AT et al. (1993). Human immunodeficiency virus seroconversion among intravenous drug users in- and out-of-treatment: An 18 month prospective follow-up. *Journal of Acquired Immune Deficiency Syndrome* 6:1049-1056.

Nath RP, Upton RA, Everhart ET et al. (1999). Buprenorphine pharmacokinetics: Relative bioavailability of sublingual tablet and liquid formulations. *Journal of Clinical Pharmacology* 39(6):619-623.

National Institutes of Health (NIH) Consensus Panel (1999). NIH Consensus Panel recommends expanding access to and improving methadone treatment programs for heroin addiction. *European Addiction Research* 5:50-51.

Nickander R, Booher R & Miles H (1974). L-a-acetylmethadol and its N-demethylated metabolites have potent opiate actions in guinea pig isolated ileum. *Life Sciences* 41:2011-2017.

Nigam A, Ray R & Tripathi BM (1993). Buprenorphine in opiate withdrawal: A comparison with clonidine. *Journal of Substance Abuse Treatment* 10(4):391-394.

Novick DM, Joseph H, Croxson TS et al. (1990). Absence of antibody to human immunodeficiency virus in long-term, socially rehabilitated methadone maintenance patients. *Archives of Internal Medicine* 150:97-99.

O'Connor P & Kosten TR (1998). Rapid and ultrarapid opioid detoxification techniques [see comments]. *Journal of the American Medical Association* 279(3):229-234.

O'Connor P, Carroll K, Shi JM et al. (1997). Three methods of opioid detoxification in a primary care setting. A randomized trial. *Annals of Internal Medicine* 127(7):526-530.

O'Connor PG & Fiellin DA (2000). Pharmacologic treatment of heroin-dependent patients. *Annals of Internal Medicine* 133(1):40-54. Review.

O'Connor PG, Selwyn PA & Schottenfeld RS (1994). Medical care for injection drug users with human immunodeficiency virus infection. 331(7):450-459.

Pasternak GW (1993). *Neuropharmacology* 16:1-18.

Pasternak GW & Wood PJ (1986). *Life Sciences* 38:1889-1898.

Petry NM, Bickel WK & Badger GJ (1999). A comparison of four buprenorphine dosing regimens in the treatment of opioid dependence. *Clinical Pharmacology and Therapeutics* 66:306-314.

Pfab R, Hirtl C & Zilker T (1999). Opiate detoxification under anesthesia: No apparent benefit but suppression of thyroid hormones and risk of pulmonary and renal failure. *Journal of Toxicology—Clinical Toxicology* 37(1):43-50.

Pickworth WB, Johnson RE, Holicky BA et al. (1993). Subjective and physiologic effects of intravenous buprenorphine in humans. *Clinical Pharmacology and Therapeutics* 53:570-576.

Preston KL, Bigelow GE & Liebson IA (1988a). Butorphanol-precipitated withdrawal in opioid-dependent human volunteers. *Journal of Pharmacological and Experimental Therapeutics* 246:441-448.

Preston KL, Bigelow GE & Liebson IA (1988b). Buprenorphine and naloxone alone and in combination in opioid-dependent humans. *Psychopharmacology* 94:484-490.

Preston KL, Bigelow GE & Liebson IA (1989). Antagonist effects of nalorphine in opioid-dependent human volunteers. *Journal of Pharmacology and Experimental Therapeutics* 248:929-937.

Rabinowitz J, Cohen H, Tarrasch R et al. (1997). Compliance to naltrexone treatment after ultra-rapid opiate detoxification: An open label naturalistic study. *Drug and Alcohol Dependence* 47(2):77-86.

Reisine T & Bell GI (1993). Molecular biology of opioid receptors. *Trends in Neuroscience* 16:506-510.

Reisine T & Pasternak G (1996). Opioid analgesics and antagonists. In JG Hardman & LE Limbird (eds.) *Goodman and Gilman's Pharmacological Basis of Therapeutics, 9th Edition.* New York, NY: McGraw-Hill, 521-557.

Research Triangle Institute (RTI) (1984). Bioavailability and pharmacokinetics/pharmacodynamics of l-a-acetylmethadol and its metabolites: Metabolism and pharmacokinetics of drugs. *Final Report for Contract #771-80-3705, Task #2*, September.

Resnick RB, Galanter M, Pycha C et al. (1992). Buprenorphine: An alternative to methadone for heroin dependence treatment. *Psychopharmacology Bulletin* 28(1):109-113.

Resnick RB, Resnick E & Galanter M (1991). Buprenorphine responders: A diagnostic subgroup of heroin addicts? *Progress in Neuro-Psychopharmacology and Biological Psychiatry* 15:531-538.

Rosen MI, Wallace EA, McMahon TJ et al. (1994). Buprenorphine: Duration of blockade of effects of intramuscular hydromorphone. *Drug and Alcohol Dependence* 35:569-580.

Rounsaville BJ & Kosten TR (2000). Treatment for opioid dependence: Quality and access. *Journal of the American Medical Association* 283:1337-1339.

San L, Puig M, Bulbena A et al. (1995). High risk of ultrashort noninvasive opiate detoxification [letter]. *American Journal of Psychiatry* 152(6):956.

Satel S, Kosten T, Bulbena A et al. (1993). Should protracted withdrawal from drugs be included in DSM-IV? [see comments]. *American Journal of Psychiatry* 150(5):695-704.

Sawyer RC, Brown LS, Narong PG et al. (1993). Evaluation of a possible pharmacological interaction between rifampin and methadone in HIV seropositive injecting drug users. In *Abstracts of the Ninth International Conference on AIDS/Fourth STD World Congress, Berlin, Germany, June 6-11.* London, England: Wellcome Foundation, 501 Abstract.

Schottenfeld RS, Pakes J, O'Connor P et al. (2000). Thrice weekly versus daily buprenorphine maintenance. *Biological Psychiatry* 47:1072-1079.

Schottenfeld RS, Pakes J, Ziedonis D et al. (1993). Buprenorphine: Dose-related effects on cocaine-abusing opioid dependent humans. *Biological Psychiatry*.

Schuh KJ & Johanson CE (1999). Pharmacokinetic comparison of the buprenorphine sublingual liquid and tablet. *Drug and Alcohol Dependence* 56:55-60.

Schuh KJ, Walsh SL, Bigelow GE et al. (1996). Buprenorphine, morphine and naloxone effects during ascending morphine maintenance in humans. *Journal of Pharmacological and Experimental Therapeutics* 278:836-846.

Schwartz EL, Brechbuhl AB, Kahl P et al. (1990). Altered pharmacokinetics of zidovudine in former IV drug-using patients receiving methadone. In *Abstracts of the Sixth International Conference on AIDS, San Francisco, June 20-24, Vol 3.* San Francisco, CA: University of California, 194. Abstract.

Schwetz BA (2001). From the Food and Drug Administration. *Journal of the American Medical Association* 285(21):2705.

Senay EC, Dorus W, Goldberg F et al. (1977). Withdrawal from methadone maintenance. *Archives of General Psychiatry* 34:361-367.

Seow SS, Quigley AJ, Ilett KF et al. (1986). Buprenorphine: A new maintenance opiate? *Medical Journal of Austria* 144(8):407-411.

Small PM, Shafer RW, Hopewell PC et al. (1993). Exogenous reinfection with multidrug-resistant Mycobacterium tuberculosis in patients with advanced HIV infection. *New England Journal of Medicine* 328:1137-1144.

Smits SE (1974). The analgesic activity of l-a-acetylmethadol and two of its metabolites in mice. *Research in Commun. Chemistry, Pathology and Pharmacology* 8:575-578.

Smits SE & Booher R (1973). Analgesic activity of some of the metabolites of methadone and alpha-acetylmethadol in mice and rats. *Federation Proceedings* 32:764.

Stine SM (1997). New developments in methadone treatment and matching treatments to patient. In SM Stine & TR Kosten (eds.) *New Treatments for Opiate Dependence.* New York, NY: Guilford Press, 3:121-172.

Stine S & Kosten T (1994). Reduction of opiate withdrawal-like symptoms by cocaine abuse during methadone and buprenorphine maintenance. *American Journal of Drug and Alcohol Abuse* 20(4):445-458.

Stine SM & Kosten TR (1992). Use of drug combinations in treatment of opioid withdrawal. *Journal of Clinical Psychopharmacology* 12:203-209.

Strain EC, Preston KL, Liebson IA et al. (1992). Acute effects of buprenorphine, hydromorphone and naloxone in methadone-maintained volunteers. *Journal of Pharmacological and Experimental Therapeutics* 261:985-993.

Strain EC, Preston KL, Liebson IA et al. (1995). Buprenorphine effects in methadone-maintained volunteers: Effects at two hours after methadone. *Journal of Pharmacological and Experimental Therapeutics* 272:628-638.

Strain EC, Stitzer ML, Liebson IA et al. (1994). Comparison of buprenorphine and methadone in the treatment of opioid dependence. *American Journal of Psychiatry* 151(7):1025-1030.

Strain EC, Stitzer ML, Liebson IA et al. (1996). Buprenorphine versus methadone in the treatment of opioid dependence: Self-reports, urinalysis, and Addiction Severity Index. *Journal of Clinical Psychopharmacology* 16:58-67.

Strang J (1985). Abuse of buprenorphine. *Lancet* 725.

Strang J, Bearn J & Gossop M (1997). Opiate detoxification under anaesthesia [editorial] [see comments]. *British Medical Journal* 315(7118):1249-1250.

Tidone L, Sileo F, Goglio A et al. (1987). AIDS in Italy. *American Journal of Drug and Alcohol Abuse* 13(4):485-486.

Uehlinger C, Deglon J, Livoti S et al. (1998). Comparison of buprenorphine and methadone in treatment of opioid dependence. Swiss multicenter study. *European Addiction Research* 4(Suppl)1:13-18.

Umbricht A, Montoya I, Hoover DR et al. (1999). Naltrexone shortened opioid detoxification with buprenorphine. *Drug and Alcohol Dependence* 56(3):181-190.

Vignau J (1998). Preliminary assessment of a 10-day rapid detoxification programme using high dosage buprenorphine. *European Addiction Research* 4(Suppl)1:29-31.

Vining E, Kosten TR & Kleber HD (1988). Clinical utility of rapid clonidine-naltrexone detoxification for opioid abusers. *British Journal of Addiction* 83:567-575.

Walsh SL, June HL, Schuh KJ et al. (1995). Effects of buprenorphine and methadone in methadone-maintained subjects. *Psychopharmacology (Berlin)* 119:268-276.

Walsh SL, Preston KL, Bigelow GE et al. (1995). Acute administration of buprenorphine in humans: Partial agonist and blockade effects. *Journal of Pharmacological and Experimental Therapeutics* 274:361-372.

Walsh SL, Preston KL, Stitzer ML et al. (1994). Clinical pharmacology of buprenorphine: Ceiling effects at high doses. *Clinical Pharmacology and Therapeutics* 55:569-580.

Washton AM & Resnick RB (1980). Clonidine for opiate detoxification: Outpatient clinical trials. *American Journal of Psychiatry* 137:1121-1122.

Winger G, Skjoldager P & Woods JH (1992). Effects of buprenorphine and other opioid agonists and antagonists on alfentanil and cocaine reinforced responding in rhesus monkeys. *Journal of Pharmacology and Experimental Therapeutics* 261:311-317.

Zielbauer P (1999). State knew of risky heroin treatment before patient deaths. *New York Times* October 31, 41.

Prescribing Buprenorphine for the Treatment of Opioid Addiction

DONALD R. WESSON, M.D.

On October 8, 2002, the U.S. Food and Drug Administration (FDA) approved buprenorphine sublingual tablets for use in the treatment of addiction. Concurrently, the Drug Enforcement Administration (DEA) designated all formulations of buprenorphine approved for use in the United States—Buprenex®, Suboxone®, and Subutex®—as Schedule III *narcotics*. (The class designation of narcotic has important regulatory and clinical ramifications independent of the Schedule II designation.)

In issuing its approval, FDA asked the drugs' manufacturer to develop a comprehensive risk management program that involves close monitoring of drug distribution channels and adverse event reports.

PRESCRIBING QUALIFICATIONS

Physicians who wish to prescribe Suboxone or Subutex for the treatment of opiate dependence must be specially qualified, either through certification in addiction medicine by the American Society of Addiction Medicine or the American Osteopathic Academy of Addiction Medicine, or through completion of a Certificate of Added Qualifications (CAQ) of the American Psychiatric Association. Physicians who do not hold any of these certifications may qualify by completing an approved training course.

Qualified physicians must submit a notice of intent to prescribe buprenorphine to the federal Center for Substance Abuse Treatment (CSAT) and obtain a unique identifying number from the U.S. Drug Enforcement Administration (DEA). (An application form can be downloaded from the federal web site WWW.BUPRENORPHINE.SAMHSA.GOV.) Other restrictions include limits on the number of patients an individual physician or physician group may treat in an office setting.

Although buprenorphine may not be prescribed for the treatment of addiction except under the conditions established by the Drug Addiction Treatment Act of 2000, the package insert does not alert physicians to this fact, and it is likely that practitioners outside the addiction treatment community will not know of the special requirements for prescribing Suboxone and Subutex.

CAUTIONS IN USING THE DRUG

While Buprenex, an injectable formulation of buprenorphine, is marketed for the treatment of moderate to severe pain, it should not be used in the treatment of addiction. Only formulations of buprenorphine that are FDA-approved for the treatment of opiate dependence (that is, Suboxone and Subutex) may be legally prescribed for this purpose.

Also, a widely misunderstood provision of the Code of Federal Regulations (21 U.S.C. 1307.07) allows physicians to administer a narcotic medication to an opioid addict to alleviate withdrawal symptoms while arrangements are being made to admit such a patient to an addiction treatment program. Many physicians have assumed that this provides a three-day window in which they can administer narcotic drugs such as buprenorphine for the purpose of detoxification. However, the DEA's web site contains an explicit prohibition against use of buprenorphine under the so-called "three day rule."

BUPRENORPHINE AND PAIN MANAGEMENT

The analgesic effects of full opioids will be attenuated in patients who are maintained on buprenorphine, which attaches to the mu opioid receptor with high affinity. In effect, buprenorphine blocks access of the full opioid to the receptor, which is why it attenuates the effects of heroin. In addition, the patient may have developed tolerance to opioids. Trauma, surgery, or an acute illness requiring treatment with full opioid agonists thus may require larger doses of opioid analgesics, but the patient must be carefully monitored while being treated with short-acting opioids. As the buprenorphine leaves the receptor and is metabolized, the patient's opioid requirements may decrease. Unfortunately, there are not yet any well-controlled clinical studies to guide practice in such situations.

CONCLUSIONS

The approval of buprenorphine signifies more than the availability of a new medication. The conjunction of the Drug Abuse Treatment Act of 2000 and the launch of Suboxone and Subutex reverses more than 40 years of prohibition against physician use of agonist therapy to treat opiate dependence outside of specially licensed clinics. If office-based opiate agonist treatment ever is to become accepted clinical practice, physicians will have to demonstrate to the FDA and DEA that they can prescribe opioid agonists to opioid-dependent patients responsibly and without creating any public health problems. This is an opportunity all addiction specialists should cherish and protect.

ACKNOWLEDGMENTS: Gail Jara, Walter Ling, M.D., and Monika Koch reviewed drafts of this manuscript and provided many useful suggestions.

Chapter 4

Opioid Maintenance Treatment

J. Thomas Payte, M.D.
Joan E. Zweben, Ph.D.
Judith Martin, M.D.

Unique Aspects of Opioid Addiction
Clinical Issues in Maintenance Pharmacotherapy
Maintenance Treatment Using Methadone
Maintenance Treatment Using LAAM
Maintenance Treatment Using Buprenorphine
Psychosocial Interventions
Growth, Controversy, and Future Challenges

Of an estimated 810,000 opiate addicts in the United States, approximately 179,000 are involved in opioid maintenance treatment (OMT) using methadone and levo-alpha-acetylmethadol (LAAM), making it the largest single treatment intervention for this population (NIH-CDC, 1997). Thirty-five years of extensive research and clinical experience have quieted somewhat the passions aroused by this approach, while public health concerns—combined with an extensive educational effort—have made OMT somewhat more available to those who need it. However, it is apparent that, for each patient in an existing treatment slot, there are approximately five persons addicted to opiates for whom OMT is not available (Payte, 1997b).

During the 1990s, several major scientific bodies examined the evidence regarding treatment benefits and access barriers; they concluded that OMT is effective and that barriers to obtaining it need to be reduced (National Consensus Development Panel, 1998; Rettig & Yarmolinsky, 1995). Physicians often are startled by the discrepancy between the benefits of OMT documented by scientific research and the public's perceptions of such treatment; for this reason, it is necessary to begin with a description of the context in which OMT takes place.

The use of opioids as a maintenance pharmacotherapy began with the use of methadone by Dole and Nyswander in the 1960s (Dole & Nyswander, 1965). Negative attitudes toward OMT have been common since that time among physicians, other treatment staff, patients, and the general public. These attitudes often stem from the perception that methadone treatment is "just substituting one addicting drug for another." Rather than a simple substitution or replacement for illicit opioids, OMT involves a stabilization or correction of a possible lesion or defect in the endogenous opioid system (Dole, 1988; Goldstein, 1991). The neurobiological mechanism remains poorly understood even among physicians and will be elaborated later in this chapter.

This simple intervention, by reducing craving and preventing withdrawal, virtually eliminates the hazards of needles, frees the patient from preoccupation with obtaining illicit opioids, and enhances overall function, thus enabling the patient to make use of available psychosocial interventions. Nevertheless, a set of regulatory requirements unmatched by anything in medicine continues to contribute to the stigmatization of OMT as a treatment modality and creates many barriers to providing treatment to those who

---

need it. Despite reviews of regulatory barriers and inadequate capacity, negative attitudes continue to influence daily practice (Rettig & Yarmolinsky, 1995).

Negative attitudes affect medical practice in a variety of ways (Zweben & Payte, 1990). Physicians in other medical settings sometimes refuse to treat a patient who discloses that he or she is receiving maintenance pharmacotherapy. Occasionally, patients are told that they must withdraw from maintenance pharmacotherapy to receive treatment for other medical conditions. A physician may withhold medication needed for symptomatic relief, thus causing unnecessary discomfort and pain. Patients are keenly sensitive to disgust, distrust, and a begrudging manner and often forego needed medical treatment because they cannot tolerate an adversarial relationship with the health care provider. Although long-standing educational efforts have modified negative attitudes in many quarters, they remain common enough to constitute a hazard to high-quality patient care.

As with any chronic illness, there can be denial and hesitation on the part of the patient who needs long-term treatment. Contrary to common beliefs, many heroin addicts enter OMT with great ambivalence and want to discontinue maintenance therapy as soon as possible. Indeed, the initial hope of many practitioners, policymakers, and regulators was that methadone could be used to transition patients to a drug-free lifestyle and then be withdrawn. This has not proved to be the case. Repeated studies suggest that only 10% to 20% of patients who discontinue methadone are able to remain abstinent (McLellan, 1983), a range consistent with clinical impressions and the findings of subsequent studies (Ball & Ross, 1991). This range is similar to that seen with many chronic medical conditions for which control requires the use of medication.

The known risks of discontinuing OMT, with predictable relapse to intravenous heroin use, become increasingly critical when viewed in the context of the HIV epidemic. These risks, when compared to the proven safety and efficacy of long-term methadone treatment, suggest that long-term—even indefinite—OMT is appropriate and even essential for a significant proportion of eligible patients.

OMT currently is viewed as treatment of a chronic medical disorder, with the goal of achieving control of the heroin addiction and avoiding the ravages of the untreated disease (Hser, Hoffman et al., 2001).

Treatment should
patient continues to be

to remain in treatment, remains at risk of relapse to heroin or other substance use, suffers no significant adverse effects from continued methadone maintenance treatment, and as long as continued treatment is indicated in the professional judgment of the physician (Payte & Khuri, 1993b).

Patients do seek to discontinue maintenance for nonmedical but very real and practical reasons (for example, transportation or scheduling difficulties) and to escape continued disruption of their lives associated with the burdensome restrictions, regulations, and structure of the treatment delivery system. For patients who attempt withdrawal, it is important for practitioners to provide encouragement along with the best medical and supportive treatment available, without fostering unrealistic expectations or unnecessary guilt, and to provide a means for rapid readmission in the event of relapse or impending relapse to the use of illicit opiates (ASAM, 1991).

UNIQUE ASPECTS OF OPIOID ADDICTION

Although this chapter focuses on medical aspects of OMT, it is commonly accepted that addictive disorders are complex phenomena that involve the interaction of biological, psychosocial, and cultural variables, all of which need to be addressed if treatment is to be effective. As a medical modality based on proper use of opioid agonist medication, it should be clear that the medication itself is central to and the foundation of OMT as a treatment modality. However, favorable treatment outcomes require that the medical intervention be integrated with a host of other therapies and supportive and rehabilitative services. Much of the destructive behavior of treatment professionals results from inappropriate expectations, particularly the belief that heroin addicts could avoid drug use if they were sufficiently motivated.

Dole always has held the view that there is something unique about opioid addiction that makes it difficult for patients to remain free of illicit heroin use for extended periods of time. In their early work, Dole and Nyswander (1967) postulated the existence of a "metabolic disease," a view supported and refined by subsequent biomedical research. Dole won the Albert Lasker Clinical Medicine ~~Research Award~~ in 1988 for his work in this area. He sum- ~~Journal of the American~~ ~~in~~ which he wrote:

If pancakes for lunch are wrong, we don't want to be right.

It is postulated that the high rate of relapse of addicts after detoxification from heroin use is due to persistent derangement of the endogenous ligand-narcotic receptor system and that methadone in an adequate daily dose compensates for this defect. Some patients with long histories of heroin use and subsequent rehabilitation on a maintenance program do well when the treatment is terminated. The majority, unfortunately, experience a return of symptoms after maintenance is stopped. The treatment, therefore, is corrective but not curative for severely addicted persons. A major challenge for future research is to identify the specific defect in receptor function and to repair it. Meanwhile, methadone maintenance provides a safe and effective way to normalize the function of otherwise intractable narcotic addicts.

In Dole's view, the persistent receptor disorder is the result of chronic opiate use, leading to down-regulation of the modulating system and possibly also to suppression of the endogenous ligands. Goldstein (1991) supported the concept of a metabolic disease as well as a genetic predisposition to that disease. Goldstein suggested that genetic influence carries an exceptional vulnerability to the disease in the presence of certain environmental influences. Kreek (1992) suggested that multiple genes may account for different degrees of vulnerability to developing addiction. Other research also supports the view that heroin addiction has a genetic component (Pickens, 1997; Merikangas, Stolar et al., 1998; Tsuang, Lyons et al., 1998). Further research is needed to define the metabolic disease process and the respective roles of genetic predisposition and environmental exposure.

Positron emission tomography scans that look at cerebral metabolism in opiate-addicted patients suggest that methadone maintenance at least partly normalizes cerebral glucose metabolism, compared with patients withdrawn from methadone and in sustained remission (Galynker, Watras-Ganz et al., 2000). A key question for future research is whether it is possible to restore normal functioning without maintenance therapy and, if so, how to accomplish this function.

CLINICAL ISSUES IN MAINTENANCE PHARMACOTHERAPY

Maintenance pharmacotherapy is based on the use of a medication to maintain chronic opioid users in a normal state for 24 hours or more, avoiding any impairment in the form of sedating, obtunding, or euphoric effects and preventing the onset of the opioid withdrawal syndrome. For opioid agonist (maintenance) treatment *per se*, the sole criterion for success is a reduction in or cessation of illicit opioid use, thus allowing the patient to achieve the broader goals of restoration of function and improved quality of life (Goldstein, 1991). Cessation of OMT *never* should be a criterion for success. Instead, practitioners are encouraged to focus on improved social integration and quality-of-life issues for persons with chronic opioid addiction, rather than the relentless pursuit of eliminating all medication as the primary goal of treatment.

Goals of Pharmacotherapy. Kreek (1992) outlined the goals of treatment and the properties of desirable opioid agonist medications as follows:

1. Prevention or reduction of withdrawal symptoms.
2. Prevention or reduction of drug craving.
3. Prevention of relapse to use of addictive drugs.
4. Restoration to or toward normalcy of any physiologic function disrupted by chronic drug use.

Profile of Potential Psychotherapeutic Agents. Characteristics of potential psychotherapeutic agents can be defined as follows:

1. Such medications are effective after oral administration.
2. They have a long biological half-life (>24 hours).
3. They have minimal side effects during chronic administration.
4. They are safe (that is, they lack true toxic or serious adverse effects).
5. They are efficacious for a substantial proportion of persons with the disorder.

Initial Dose. In most cases, patients being evaluated for admission to OMT have developed significant tolerance to opioids and demonstrate objective signs of withdrawal as a sign of current opioid physical dependence. The response to the initial dose of agonist medication provides valuable information about tolerance levels and the target "therapeutic window." Significant relief during peak (four to eight) hours is evidence that the dose is in the range of the established level of tolerance and may not require further escalation. The absence of relief suggests that the dose is well short of the therapeutic window. The initial dose of methadone is no more than 30 mg in most cases and, under federal regulations, is limited to no more than a 30 mg first dose or 40 mg on the first day.

Induction. After the initial dose, the induction phase allows for subsequent careful adjustments of the dose to achieve elimination of drug craving and prevention of withdrawal, while avoiding the risk of intoxication or overdose associated with accumulation of methadone (Kaufman, Payte et al., 1995; Payte & Khuri, 1993a). The induction phase can be considered to last until the patient has been on a stable dose for 4 to 5 days (half-lives). An understanding of steady-state pharmacokinetics is essential.

Maintenance. Once a stable dose is established, based on the presence of desired clinical effects, elimination of craving, and prevention of withdrawal, the maintenance phase begins. Maintenance continues until such a time that there is a reason to alter the treatment. Most methadone-maintained patients do well on a dose range of 60 to 120 mg a day, although some patients require less and some require more.

As the patient who is on maintenance surfaces from his or her addiction and begins to work on major life changes, the need for daily visits to the dispensing window and for regular counseling can change as well. Patients who do well and who improve according to specified criteria set out in federal regulations can earn take-home medications for unsupervised dosing. As of May 2001, these guidelines allow patients to take home up to six doses a week after nine months, two weeks of medication after the first year, and 30-day doses after the second year of treatment. (However, many states may have more restrictive regulations.)

Medical Maintenance: Medical maintenance, designed for "stable, recovered" patients on methadone, is an effort to release the patient from burdensome attendance in an opioid treatment program (OTP) by allowing a physician who is affiliated with the clinic, but in office practice, to prescribe or administer the maintenance medication. In April 2000, the Center for Substance Abuse Treatment (CSAT) circulated draft guidelines describing medical maintenance. These guidelines were developed after more than 10 years of pilot projects showed that this approach to care works and that it improves the quality of life for patients (Salsitz, Joseph et al., 2000).

"Medical maintenance" generally refers to attendance that is reduced to one or two visits per month, with a minimum number of supportive services, and is offered to selected stable patients. Two models have emerged. The first was designed by Des Jarlais and colleagues (1985) as a feasibility study and subsequently was reported by Novick. According to the model, medical maintenance is defined as the treatment of rehabilitated methadone maintenance patients in a general medical setting rather than a licensed clinic. Selection criteria called for a minimum of five years in treatment, with essentially perfect compliance for a period of three years. Results are excellent in terms of enhanced retention and reduced rates of addictive disorder or lost medication (Novick & Joseph, 1991; Novick, Joseph et al., 1994; Novick, Pascarelli et al., 1988).

The other model, developed by Senay, differs in several ways. Admission to the study was based on performance rather than time in treatment, with only six months of excellent performance required. The reduced attendance and services were provided in a methadone program, with continued periodic counseling and urine drug screens. The Senay model also demonstrated an excellent treatment outcome (Senay, Barthwell et al., 1993, 1994).

An obvious advantage to both models is a reduced level or intensity of care and cost of treatment, thus freeing resources for patients just entering treatment, while stable rehabilitated patients benefit from ongoing OMT with a minimum of cost and disruption of their lives. As mentioned earlier, many patients risk their abstinence and, in an AIDS epidemic, their lives, in an effort to withdraw from methadone for nonmedical reasons. For those who are attempting to free themselves from clinic constraints, rather than from the effects of daily medication, medical maintenance could be an acceptable solution. Current regulations require a federal waiver for medical maintenance.

Pain Management. The undertreatment of pain in methadone- and LAAM-maintained patients remains a serious problem. In cases of acute pain associated with surgery, trauma, or dental work, the physicians or dentists involved often, and incorrectly, assume that the maintenance dose of methadone also will relieve any pain. Some may fear that a methadone-maintained addict might become dangerous if given opioid analgesia. The minimum essentials of management of acute pain in OMT patients were summarized as follows in the *Journal of Maintenance in the Addictions* (Payte, 1997a):

> Patients being maintained with methadone or LAAM require special considerations for acute pain management in surgical or trauma situations. OMT patients are often denied any analgesia and serious under-treatment of pain is common. Maintenance

patients develop full tolerance to the analgesic effects of the maintenance dose of methadone. During OMT a cross-tolerance develops to all opioid agonist drugs, accounting for the "blockade" effect. Early research demonstrated that stable OMT patients could not distinguish 20 mg IV morphine from IV saline. Hence: *The usual maintenance dose does not provide any analgesia, and adequate analgesia will require higher doses of opioid agonists given more frequently than in the non-tolerant patient.*

Methadone has a half-life of 24 to 36 hours, but its analgesic effects range from four to six hours, which is similar to morphine in both potency and duration (Reisine & Pasternak, 1996). Morphine, Dilaudid®, codeine, and other agonist drugs are appropriate for OMT patients. Mixed agonist-antagonists (pentazocine, butorphanol, nalbuphine) and partial agonists (buprenorphine) *must not be used*, as they will precipitate an opioid withdrawal syndrome. Meperidine and propoxyphene should be avoided because of the risk of seizures at the higher doses required to produce analgesia in OMT patients.

In summary: (1) Continue maintenance treatment without interruption. (2) Provide adequate individualized doses of opioid agonists, which must be titrated to the desired analgesic effect. The proper dose is enough! (3) Doses should be given more frequently and on a fixed schedule rather than "as needed for pain."

Pregnancy and Opioid Agonist Treatment. Of the various topics covered in this chapter, issues relating to opioid agonist treatment during pregnancy remain the most controversial and emotionally charged. This is largely attributable to the neonatal opioid withdrawal syndrome, which is the most visible and dramatic sequela of passive addiction in the neonate. Efforts to treat, prevent, and minimize neonatal opioid withdrawal have predominated since the results of the first 13 pregnancies were reported in 1969 (Wallach, Jerez et al., 1969). Maternal withdrawal can result in potentially dangerous fetal distress, and methadone maintenance is considered the treatment of choice for opioid-addicted pregnant women.

This issue is addressed in detail in Section 10.

Hepatitis C. The hepatitis C virus (HCV) was isolated in 1988, with the first serologic test for HCV antibody available in 1990. It is estimated that 1.8% of the U.S. population is infected and that the overall mortality rate is 2% (result-

---

TABLE 1. Symptoms of Acute Hepatitis C

- Flu-like illness
- Fatigue, malaise, fever, chills
- Anorexia, loss of appetite
- Nausea and occasional vomiting
- Dark urine (the color of cola drinks)
- Vague abdominal discomfort, especially in right quadrant
- Jaundice, with yellow eyes, skin, and mucous membranes.

SOURCE: Adapted from Barthwell & Gibert, 1993.

---

ing in 8,000 to 10,000 deaths per year) (Alter, 1997). Studies suggest that the prevalence in intravenous drug users ranges from 50% to 90% (Barthwell & Gibert, 1993; Novick, Reagan et al., 1997), with some providers reporting even higher rates when they are able to test all their clinic patients.

Novick and colleagues (1997) concluded that, from 1978 to 1983, HCV had become well-established in the addict population. High rates are found even in those with short histories of addictive disorders. In a later publication, Novick (2000) reported HCV positivity rates of 66% to 88% of all injection drug users, with 77% in persons using for one year or less, and 94% in persons who had injected drugs for at least 10 years. HCV becomes chronic in 85% of infected persons but progresses slowly. Cirrhosis is seen in 20% to 30% and also develops slowly—in most cases, over 10 to 20 years.

HCV is a blood-borne pathogen transmitted by direct contact with blood or blood products—in the addict population, usually contaminated needles. Injection drug use is considered the risk factor for acquisition in about 35% of reported cases. HCV also can be spread by sexual contact, but the risks are considered lower (Barthwell & Gibert, 1993). Inasmuch as the risk factors are similar, it is not surprising that co-infection rates are high (CDC, 2001; Herrero Martinez, 2001). For example, in some sample populations, more than 90% of injection drug users who are HIV-positive also are infected with hepatitis C (Cahoon-Young, 1997). HCV infection appears to cause increased morbidity and mortality in those with HIV infection (Monga, Rodriguez-Barradas et al., 2001).

Approximately 50% to 75% of acute HCV infections in adults are asymptomatic. If symptoms are present, they include those listed in Table 1.

Tong and el-Farra (1996) described the course of HCV infection in 125 patients with a history of injection drug use. The mean age at which drug use was initiated was 23.1 years, with presentation to a tertiary care center in California occurring approximately 20 years later (Liver Center, Pasadena, CA, unpublished observation). The most common presenting symptoms were fatigue, abdominal pain, anorexia, and weight loss. The initial workup indicated 26% had chronic hepatitis, 37% had chronic active hepatitis, 36% had cirrhosis, and 0.8% had hepatocellular carcinoma. Alcohol use increases the severity of the disease (Novick, 2000).

Since 1998, the standard treatment for HCV has been a combination of interferon injection and oral ribavirin (Virazole®). For the patient this means three shots a week and two pills a day for 6 to 12 months. Viral titers are obtainable but do not have a clear relationship to symptoms or stage of illness; however, they can be used to monitor antiviral treatment and to diagnose remission, defined as undetectable viral load. Response to treatment depends partly on the viral type. Most needle-users are infected with the more resistant type 1, which requires a full year of treatment. With treatment, long-term remission rates are about 40% (Novick, 2000).

Studies are under way to determine whether these remission rates apply to patients in methadone maintenance treatment. Sylvestre (2002) treated 50 eligible methadone-maintained patients with active HCV and concomitant liver fibrosis with interferon-ribavirin combination therapy and reported a 64% virologic response rate in patients who completed treatment and 54% on an intent-to-treat basis. This finding is comparable to patients without a history of injection drug use.

Much debate exists about patient selection. The difficulty of treating patients who have chaotic lives and the interaction of interferon with drugs of abuse and with alcohol are cited as reasons to restrict treatment to stable patients who have at least six months of abstinence. However, treatment may be the "only chance" for patients, who almost certainly will be denied access to liver transplantation, should they need it (Koch & Banys, 2001).

Well-established treatment programs are seeing an increasing number of patients who become ill and die. It is important that programs develop educational interventions to encourage health practices (such as complete elimination of alcohol) that are likely to prolong the period of good health. Advocacy will be needed to ensure that patients have access to emerging treatments.

Patients With Psychiatric Comorbidities. The high rate of comorbidity of psychiatric and addictive disorders (Regier, Farmer et al., 1990; Kessler, McGonagle et al., 1994) obligates treatment providers to equip themselves to address both problems. In addition, psychiatric severity (as measured by the Addiction Severity Index) strongly predicts clinical outcome (O'Brien, Woody et al., 1984). Woody and colleagues (1986) examined the efficacy of two kinds of professional psychotherapy and drug abuse counseling typically provided in methadone programs as a function of global psychiatric status ratings of the patients. They found that low-severity patients benefited from both drug abuse counseling (focused on current life problems) and psychotherapy (employing supportive-expressive and cognitive-behavioral approaches). Patients with high levels of psychiatric symptoms were lower in all areas of pretreatment functioning and did not improve as much as patients with less severe problems. However, the addition of psychotherapy did maximize their improvement in many areas. Professionally trained therapists, integrated into the ongoing program, improved outcome for these difficult patients.

Depression and dysthymia are common co-occuring disorders in the opiate addiction treatment population. Rounsaville and Kleber (1985) compared opiate addicts with similar severity and duration of use and found those who sought treatment had higher lifetime rates of dysphoric disorders and current major depression. Life crises and depressive symptoms posed a substantial risk of relapse, which lessened for those who remained in treatment (Kosten, Rounsaville et al., 1986). Antidepressant medications can be prescribed in conjunction with opioid agonist treatment without ill effects, although lower doses of tricyclics may be desirable in some patients (Maany, Dhopesh et al., 1989). For patients at high risk or those known to have poor compliance, antidepressants may be dispensed along with opioid agonist medication.

Anxiety disorders also are common, with symptoms abating with a combination of an adequate methadone dose and the provision of counseling or psychotherapy over a period of time (Musselman & Kell, 1995).

Schizophrenia is relatively uncommon in opioid treatment patients (O'Brien, Woody et al., 1984; Rounsaville, Weissman et al., 1982), although most programs have some

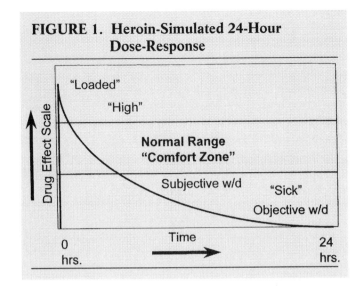

FIGURE 1. Heroin-Simulated 24-Hour Dose-Response

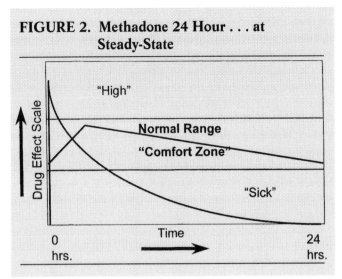

FIGURE 2. Methadone 24 Hour . . . at Steady-State

patients with the disorder. Based on historical references and clinical observations, some clinicians have proposed that opioids have antipsychotic properties (Comfort, 1977; Verebey, 1982). Clinicians have described a subgroup of patients, such as the one who referred to methadone as his "sanity syrup," who appear calmed and stabilized by the medication; when their doses drop, they become disorganized. It also is likely that the high degree of structure characteristic of many treatment programs has a beneficial effect on these patients by providing a sense of safety and security.

It is common to find reports of personality disorders, particularly antisocial personality disorder, in the heroin-using population, but it is important to view these findings with caution. Criteria in editions of the *Diagnostic and Statistical Manual of Mental Disorders* before the *DSM-IV* (APA, 1994) failed to distinguish behaviors characteristic of alcohol and drug users from personality traits that were more enduring. The self-preoccupation of the opioid agonist treatment patient in the stabilization phase (comparable to other patients who are newly abstinent or in early recovery) was too readily interpreted as narcissistic preoccupation characteristic of personality disorder. In addition, symptoms of posttraumatic stress disorder can be mistaken for personality disorder. As clinicians come to uderstand the high prevalence of emotional trauma in addicted persons, they will note that apparent lack of feelings and/or interpersonal connection may represent numbing symptoms (for example, feelings of detachment or estrangement, restricted

range of emotions) seen in posttraumatic stress disorder. It is important to be attentive to these potential confusions because personality disorder—and especially antisocial personality disorder—carries a poor prognosis and often evokes negative staff attitudes. It is advisable to be wary of psychiatric disorders diagnosed at or shortly after admission, because many patients look more pathologic than they will after their medication has been stabilized and they have begun to make use of psychosocial services.

MAINTENANCE TREATMENT USING METHADONE

Heroin Versus Methadone. The active opioid addict typically experiences rapid and wide swings from a brief "high," fading into a period of normalcy, which can be described as the "comfort zone." This period is followed by the beginnings of subjective withdrawal, which soon develops into the full objective withdrawal syndrome typical of opioid addiction. This cycle is particularly evident in the patient who engages in intravenous injection or snorting of potent short-acting opioids such as heroin. A full cycle from "sick" to "high" to "normal" to "sick" can occur in 24 hours or less (Figure 1). The sensation of the "rush" is associated with a very rapid increase in blood levels, to a point somewhat above the therapeutic window. The "high" is experienced during the time that drug levels remain above the therapeutic window (Figure 2).

Steady State. Methadone, regularly administered at steady state, is present at levels sufficient to maintain normalcy (comfort zone or therapeutic window) throughout

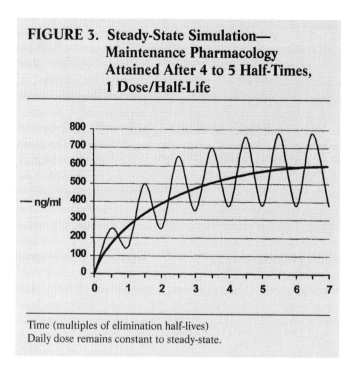

**FIGURE 3. Steady-State Simulation—
Maintenance Pharmacology
Attained After 4 to 5 Half-Times,
1 Dose/Half-Life**

Time (multiples of elimination half-lives)
Daily dose remains constant to steady-state.

the dosing interval—usually 24 hours. With the next maintenance dose, there is a gradual rise in blood level, reaching a peak at three to four hours. Typically, the peak level is less than two times the trough level. There is a gradual decline over the rest of the 24-hour period, back to the trough level. At no time does the rate or extent of change in blood levels cause a sensation of being high or result in withdrawal symptoms.

Induction. This is the most critical phase of treatment: At this state, patients are 6.7 times more likely to die than untreated heroin addicts (Caplehorn & Drummer, 1999). About 42% of drug-related deaths occurred during the first week of OMT (Zador & Sunjic, 2000). In a 1992 study, 10 OMT deaths were reported; all 10 patients had been in treatment less than seven days (Drummer, Opeskin et al., 1992). Such deaths still occur in the U.S.

The safe and effective introduction of methadone requires an understanding of steady-state pharmacologic principles (Benet, Kroetz et al., 1996). In general, steady-state levels are reached after a drug is administered for four to five half-lives (methadone has a half-life of 24 to 36 hours). The clinical significance is that, with daily dosing, a significant portion of the previous dose remains in the bloodstream, resulting in increased peak and trough methadone levels

after the second and subsequent doses. Thus, the levels of methadone increase daily, even without an increase in dose. The rate of increase levels off as steady state is achieved at four to five half-lives (five to eight days; see Figure 3). Patients who are uncomfortable at 24 hours but were comfortable during the first 4 to 12 hours probably need more time, not more medication. Methadone dose can be increased by up to 10 mg/day until significant relief is realized during the peak methadone levels, three to eight hours after dose. At that point, the dose should be held constant for three to five days to allow the patient to reach a steady state at that dose. Further dose adjustments may be needed to find the optimal dose.

During the induction phase, it is helpful to observe patients three to four hours after they are given a dose of methadone. Additional methadone can be provided when significant objective withdrawal persists during peak methadone levels.

Duration and Dose. As part of the "regulatory counterattack" (Courtwright, Joseph et al., 1989) of the early 1970s, regulators responded to a self-imposed question: How long should treatment last, and how much methadone should be given? Efforts to limit the duration of treatment occurred initially at the federal level and later were initiated by some individual state methadone authorities. Based on an extensive review of the research literature on the prognosis of patients who have been withdrawn from methadone, as well as the safety of continued maintenance treatment, the American Society of Addiction Medicine supports the principle that methadone maintenance treatment is most effective as a long-term modality (ASAM, 1991).

Dose: Until recently, clinical practice in relation to methadone dose has been guided by regulation and treatment philosophy, rather than by clinical judgment. Documentation of the need for adequate dose to achieve positive outcome has improved treatment practices in many settings (Ball & Ross, 1991). Efforts to establish dose should be focused on achieving and maintaining the desired clinical response, rather than on adherence to arbitrary dose practices set by policy or regulation. There is no scientific or clinical basis for an arbitrary dose ceiling on methadone or other agonist medication (Kaufman, Payte et al., 1995). However, despite the presence of abundant evidence in the research literature, inadequate dosing remains common. When a patient continues to use heroin, the first response should be to ensure the adequacy of the maintenance drug dose. Once dose has been determined to be adequate, appropriate behavioral and psychosocial interventions can be effective.

Techniques to Assure Adequacy of Dose: The proper dose of methadone is "enough." How much is enough? "The amount required to produce the desired response for the desired duration of time, with an allowance for a margin of effectiveness and safety" (Payte & Khuri, 1993a). In most cases, clinical observation and patient reporting are adequate to make appropriate dose determinations.

Blood Levels in Dose Determination: Mean, random, or trough levels of methadone do not define an adequate dose. The clinical utility of blood levels is based on peak and trough values to define a rate of change, or a peak-to-trough ratio.

In the methadone clinic setting, patients occasionally experience problems in maintaining stability on a given dose of methadone. Statements such as "My dose isn't holding me," "I wake up sick every morning," "My dose only lasts a few hours," "I have drug hunger every night," or "I get sleepy at work but start getting sick by bedtime" are not uncommon in OMT programs. These clinical problems may not respond to simple dose adjustments and may suggest wide fluctuations over the dosing interval (rapid metabolism).

As early as 1978, it was suggested that serial methadone levels could result in dramatic clinical improvement, with a "flattening of the curve" associated with a divided-dose regimen in those methadone maintenance patients who were experiencing problems on a single daily dose (Walton, Thornton et al., 1978). Researchers in the early 1980s compared 24-hour methadone levels in two groups of patients, all of whom received 80 mg a day. One of the groups was composed of patients who were doing very well in treatment, while the patients in the other group were doing poorly in terms of drug use, compliance, and the like. The results showed the stable group to have a mean of 410 ng/mL at 24 hours, whereas the poor performers had a mean of 101 ng/mL (Tennant, Rawson et al., 1984). It has become clear that the same dose may vary in efficacy among individuals and that patients may be doing poorly as a result of inadequate dosing rather than because they are "bad patients."

Several researchers support blood levels greater than 150 to 200 ng/mL at all times for optimum results (Dole, 1988; Holmstrand, Anggard et al., 1978; Loimer & Schmid, 1992). There is growing consensus that levels above 400 ng/mL can represent an optimum level in providing adequate cross-tolerance to make ordinary doses of intravenous heroin ineffective (nonreinforcing) during OMT (Loimer, Schmid et al., 1991).

Methadone peak, trough, and mean levels, and the rate of elimination (half-life) can be influenced by several factors. Individual differences in the metabolism of methadone, poor absorption, changes in urinary pH, effects of concomitant medications, diet, and even vitamins are among the possible factors that can influence the 24-hour dose-response curve of methadone. Pregnancy, particularly during the third trimester, is associated with significant decrease in trough methadone levels, suggesting increased rates of metabolism of methadone (Pond, Kreek et al., 1985).

Blood levels can be very useful in evaluating suspected drug interactions (discussed later in this chapter). Blood levels can identify patients who may benefit from a divided-dose regimen or demonstrate the effectiveness of a divided-dose regimen.

Procedure for Obtaining Blood Levels: Ideally, peak blood levels should be drawn at three (two to four) hours after a dose and trough levels at 24 hours. Patients already on a divided dose, such as every 12 hours, should have two- to three-hour and 12-hour specimens. A trough level alone is of little clinical value unless it is extremely low or very high.

Interpretation: Blood levels are interpreted in the context of a clinical presentation for which the laboratory values can supplement clinical judgment. The peak level at two to four hours should be no more than twice the trough level. A peak/trough ratio of 2 or less is ideal (peak/trough = ratio). Ratios greater than 2 suggest rapid metabolism. The rate of change is of greater clinical significance than the actual levels. For example, a patient with a 24-hour level of 350 ng/mL after a peak of 1,225 ng/mL (1,225/350 = 3.5, indicating rapid metabolism) may be experiencing early opioid withdrawal, whereas a patient with a trough of 150 ng/mL and a peak of 250 ng/mL (250/150 = 1.7, indicating a normal metabolism) may be quite comfortable. These clinical examples are best illustrated with two brief case histories.

> At the time he was admitted, Patient A was using $150 of heroin a day. He was disabled and under treatment for a severe seizure disorder, using carbamazepine (Tegretolt). On the basis of his clinical presentation, the daily dose of carbamazepine was gradually adjusted to 180 mg. At that time, he was symptomatic in less than 24

hours. Initial methadone levels were 118 ng/mL at three hours and less than 25 ng/mL at 24 hours. The dose was gradually increased, and the dosing interval was decreased, until the patient was receiving 100 mg of methadone every six hours. The result was a modest improvement in peak/trough ratio from 9.8 to 5.8, but levels remained well below therapeutic levels. Cimetidine (Tagamett) was added to inhibit metabolism, and the patient was stabilized clinically at methadone 100 mg and cimetidine 300 mg every six hours. Mean levels at two and six hours were 219 and 136 ng/mL, with a ratio of 1.6. Despite the low levels, the marked flattening of the curve provided excellent stability over the dosing interval.

Patient B, a 39-year-old woman, is an insulin-dependent diabetic with a severe seizure disorder, alcoholism in remission, chronic opioid addiction, bulimia, anxiety, and depression. Phenytoin (Dilantin®) 400 mg daily provided adequate control of the seizure activity. On the basis of persistent craving and withdrawal, methadone levels were performed the day after admission. They showed a peak of 38 ng/mL and 0 ng/mL at 24 hours while on methadone 100 mg once daily. Methadone was gradually increased to 100 mg every six hours, resulting in dramatic clinical improvement, with three- and six-hour levels of 224 and 101 (ratio of 2.2). The final stabilizing dose was 120 mg every six hours (254/155 = 1.6), providing an excellent clinical response (Grudzinskas, Woosley et al., 1996).

The preceding examples are not common in clinical practice but do illustrate the need for flexibility in pursuit of the goals of providing effective treatment, comfort, and relief for the patient by making sound decisions based on clinical presentation, supported by appropriate laboratory procedures. It also should be apparent that any effort to set a specific ceiling or maximum dose of methadone, LAAM, or other opioid agonist by policy or regulation is not based on scientific, clinical, or laboratory evidence. Such efforts are destined to be counterproductive. When arbitrary dose ceilings are applied, the patient is denied adequate care, and the physician is limited in the exercise of his or her clinical judgment.

One additional use of methadone blood levels may be in the nursing mother. Research shows that breastfeeding is safe for mothers on methadone and suggests that the amount of methadone in breastmilk correlates to maternal blood levels, not dose. Blood levels in the therapeutic range were found to be safe for breastfeeding infants (Geraghty, Graham et al., 1997; McCarthy, 2000; Wojnar-Horton, Kristensen et al., 1997).

Methadone-Drug Interactions. Clinical experience suggests that concomitant medications can either induce or inhibit CYP450 activity on methadone metabolism (Grudzinskas, Woosley et al., 1996). Considerable flexibility in dosing may be required to stabilize some patients whose metabolism has been altered by drug interactions or naturally occurring altered rates of metabolism. Metabolism of methadone is largely a function of enzyme activity in the liver. The group of enzymes is known as CYP450 enzymes (see the Table on page 736). Drugs that stimulate or induce CYP450 activity can precipitate opioid withdrawal by accelerating metabolism, thus shortening duration and diminishing intensity of the effect of methadone. Other drugs tend to inhibit this enzyme activity, slowing the metabolism and extending the duration of the drug effect.

A review of interactions with HIV medications confirmed that interactions have been documented and are at present poorly understood and unpredictable (Gourevitch & Friedland, 2000). Clinicians who treat patients with AIDS and hepatitis C should be alert to possible medication interactions and the need to adjust methadone dose accordingly.

MAINTENANCE TREATMENT USING LAAM
LAAM was developed in 1948. By 1952, it had been observed to suppress opioid withdrawal for more than 72 hours (Fraser & Isbell, 1952). LAAM was evaluated in opioid addiction in the late 1960s and 1970s, ignored in the 1980s, and resurrected in 1990 by the Medications Development Division of the National Institute on Drug Abuse (Fudala, Vocci et al., 1997). LAAM was approved for use in the treatment of opioid addiction by the U.S. Food and Drug Administration (FDA) in 1993 (Marion, 1995).

A derivative of methadone, LAAM is similar to methadone in its safety profile, side effects, drug interactions, and efficacy. LAAM differs from methadone in its slow onset and long duration of action, and thus is given every other day or three times a week. The extended action is due to sequential metabolism to nor-LAAM and dinor-LAAM, both of which are more potent and longer acting than the parent drug. Because LAAM has slow onset of action, the patient may find it hard to wait for the agonist effects and be tempted to use illicit opiates during the induction phase. This action poses a risk of overdose when the full activity of LAAM asserts itself several hours later. For this reason, some practitioners stabilize the patient on methadone for weeks or months and then transfer the patient to LAAM, once the therapeutic dose of methadone is determined. If LAAM is the induction medication, it is helpful to observe the patient four to eight hours after ingestion of the first dose, which usually is no more than 30 mg. With LAAM, the onset of action generally begins around four hours after ingestion and peaks at about 10 hours. Steady-state may not be achieved for 7 to 10 days after a dose change.

Conversion from methadone to LAAM is simple, with the LAAM dose being 1.2 to 1.3 times the methadone dose, given every 48 hours, with a 0% to 40% increase in LAAM dose for a 72-hour interval.

LAAM has not been studied in pregnancy, so patients who become pregnant are converted to methadone. For women of childbearing age, monthly pregnancy tests are required.

LAAM is not recommended for nursing mothers and persons younger than 18 years (Marion, 1995).

New labeling applied to LAAM in May 2001 changes the clinical approach to care. On the basis of studies showing an increased risk of sudden cardiac death in patients given high doses of LAAM, the drug has been removed from the market in Europe. In the U.S., the new label warns about prolonged QT interval and gives guidelines for acceptable corrected QT interval before LAAM dosing. In addition, the label specifically states that there should be an advantage over other treatment, such as methadone, before a patient is transferred to LAAM. Federal regulations require that medications used in opioid treatment programs must follow FDA labeling and that sound clinical reasons for any deviation from label advice must be documented in the patient chart (42 CFR, 8.12, h.4.). Aside from the greater comfort enjoyed by some patients, the principal advantages of LAAM are evident early in treatment in the form of reduced travel, disruption of routine, and clinic attendance, without the need for take-home doses. Patients in work settings in which drug testing occurs are greatly relieved by the absence of toxicology screens to detect LAAM. The new label for LAAM, and the federal regulations published in May 2001, allow for LAAM take-home use, although many state regulations still prohibit this option.

MAINTENANCE TREATMENT USING BUPRENORPHINE

Buprenorphine is a partial opioid agonist. Pharmacologic studies show that buprenorphine combines a strong affinity for the opioid receptors with a low intrinsic activity. A significant advantage is that, as a partial agonist with antagonist properties, buprenorphine has a considerable margin of safety with little chance for a lethal overdose. However, patients with a high tolerance may find that buprenorphine's agonist activity is not sufficient to control their symptoms. Since the mid-1970s, when the potential benefits of buprenorphine in treating opioid addiction first were noted, extensive clinical investigations of the drug have been completed.

Buprenorphine has been used widely as an injectable analgesic. Intravenous buprenorphine has been reported as a significant drug of abuse in Europe, New Zealand, and Australia. In October 2002, the FDA approved two sublingual tablet forms. One is a single product, and the other is a combination of naloxone (Narcan®) with buprenorphine. It is expected that the combination product will reduce the potential for diversion to intravenous use.

Numerous studies have confirmed the safety and efficacy of buprenorphine in maintenance treatment. Studies have found that an 8 mg dose of buprenorphine is equivalent in efficiency to methadone doses of 35 to 60 mg in terms of patient retention and avoidance of opioid-positive urine samples. High-dose methadone is uniformly superior to low-dose methadone and lower doses of buprenorphine (Johnson & Fudala, 1992; Kosten, Schottenfeld et al., 1993; Ling, Rawson et al., 1994). A subsequent study found that 8 mg buprenorphine did not compare favorably with methadone doses of 80 mg/day (Ling, Wesson et al., 1996). This finding suggests that doses in the range of 16 mg/day or more might be required in some patients. However, buprenorphine's agonist activity shows a ceiling effect, with little added benefit above 32 mg.

PSYCHOSOCIAL INTERVENTIONS

Physicians who work in clinics focused on opioid maintenance pharmacotherapy typically find that counseling and case management vary widely in quality and comprehensiveness. In many states, the introduction of methadone was permitted only if accompanied by a serious rehabilitative effort, but recent changes in funding have undermined efforts to maintain comprehensive services. Inasmuch as medication makes other changes possible, but does not in itself produce them, it is important to preserve the capacity of programs to provide a broad spectrum of care.

In many programs, psychosocial interventions are provided by counselors, who range widely in educational level and professional training. The counselor's task is to identify and address specific problems in the areas of drug use, physical health, interpersonal relationships (including family interaction), psychological problems, and educational or vocational goals (Zweben, 1991). Short- and long-term treatment plans provide structure for the counseling sessions and a tool by which to monitor the patient's progress and quality of care. The counselor often serves as a case manager as well, initiating screening for medication and other program services; attending to issues concerning program rules, privileges, and policies; and providing links to other agencies.

Clinics that have access to professionally trained staff may offer psychotherapy to selected patients. Typically, this access is found in programs involved in research or professional training. Motivational enhancement strategies (Miller & Rollnick, 1991; Miller, Zweben et al., 1994) have been introduced to address patient resistance to giving up alcohol, cocaine, and continuing (even if reduced) heroin use. This approach offers an alternative to harsh confrontation and encourages counselors to meet patients wherever they are prepared to begin and to move forward from there. Other psychological issues and interventions are reviewed by Zweben (1991).

The philosophy of providing comprehensive services is supported by recent research. McLellan and colleagues (McLellan, 1983; McLellan, Alterman et al., 1994; McLellan, Arndt et al., 1993; McLellan, Grissom et al., 1997) have demonstrated that the addition of enhanced onsite professional services led to better results than basic counseling alone. Quality, quantity, and the match between the patient's specific problem areas (for example, vocational, family, or psychiatric) and the services offered all led to demonstrably better outcomes in a variety of populations (McLellan, Grissom et al., 1997; McLellan, Hagan et al., 1998). A quality assurance process that monitors and encourages a close fit between the patient's needs and the services delivered is likely to produce the best outcome, in contrast to a "cookie cutter" approach in which most patients receive a similar mix of services.

Phased programs allow treatment to be individualized within a highly structured, systematic process that allows the patient to move forward, achieving tangible markers of progress. Hoffman and Moolchan (1994) described one such model, divided into three phases: intensive stabilization, commitment, and rehabilitation. Staff/patient ratios can be adjusted according to the levels of support and assistance required by the patient at each stage, and specific activities can be tailored to the individual's needs. Services can be provided onsite or through a network of referral sources in the community. In the later stages, the patient can be tracked into a tapering phase or a medical maintenance phase, with a reinforcement phase used as followup.

GROWTH, CONTROVERSY, AND FUTURE CHALLENGES

Any physician who becomes involved in the treatment of an OMT patient has an important task beyond that of medical practitioner: education and advocacy. A few minutes spent educating family members, clinical providers, employers, and others can have a major effect in reducing stigma and improving the way the patient is treated in a variety of systems of care. The patient who feels that his or her physician is knowledgeable and concerned will make a far greater effort to comply with that physician's treatment recommendations.

An issue that merits attention, although there is little literature on the subject, involves middle-class individuals who use illicit opiates but who would not consider seeking treatment in the system that currently delivers OMT. A study of Empire Blue Cross and Blue Shield subscribers in the New York metropolitan area found that approximately 141,000 opiate users were insured between 1982 and 1992 and that, at the end of the study, 85,000 still were insured by that plan (Eisenhandler & Drucker, 1993). This research suggests that there is a large population of mainstream, working, insured opiate users who are not well described because they are not reached by government agencies, which historically have been the source of data on opiate addiction. Clinicians observe that many of these patients are referred to more "middle-class" treatment facilities, in which staff members who are not knowledgeable about opiate addiction may harbor negative attitudes toward those who use these drugs. Some of these patients substitute alcohol or benzodiazepines as a more socially acceptable remedy. Many of the longer-term opiate users clearly would be candidates for OMT, if the treatment system were comparable to that for other medical conditions. In the interim, they make themselves known by presenting for assessment and treatment for HIV disease and, more recently, HCV.

Oversight and Regulatory Challenges. Since the early 1970s, methadone maintenance and withdrawal treatment have been influenced by regulations promulgated by the FDA, in consultation with the National Institute on Drug Abuse (NIDA) and the U.S. Drug Enforcement Administration (DEA). In addition, some states have adopted their own regulations, most of which are based on federal regulations but may be more restrictive in their provisions. There is little question that these regulations, in their current form, have failed to ensure the quality of patient care and have had some unintended consequences (Dole, 1992, 1995; Rettig & Yarmolinsky, 1995). A 1995 report by the Institute of Medicine estimated that only 18% to 36% of heroin users were enrolled in methadone treatment in that year (Rettig & Yarmolinsky, 1995). A consensus statement issued in 1998 by the National Institutes of Health supported the chronic disease model of opiate addiction and pointed to methadone maintenance as the best available treatment (NIH-CDC, 1997). Since then, efforts to improve access to treatment have taken several forms.

The most significant is a transition of primary federal oversight responsibilities from FDA to CSAT. Major revisions of regulations, guidelines, and standards are part of this transition, which implements revised federal regulations published in May 2001. CSAT sponsored a study on the feasibility and effect of an accreditation system for OTPs, using existing accrediting bodies for outpatient mental health facilities, as well as the Joint Commission on Accreditation of Healthcare Organizations and the Commission on Accreditation of Rehabilitation Facilities. The revised federal regulations call for OTPs to become accredited by the year 2003. CSAT also has published Guidelines for the Accreditation of Opioid Treatment Programs.

Changes involving more flexibility in take-home unsupervised dosing and the elimination of artificial barriers to admission to methadone maintenance programs have the potential to make medical decisions part of everyday life in treatment programs. In addition, some previously regulated areas are to be incorporated into clinic-specific policies and procedures. For example, each clinic must have policies to reduce diversion of medication. In the past, regulations that attempted to thwart diversion might have dictated use of liquid medications, locked boxes, and inspection of returned bottles, leaving none of the decisions to clinic policy. Another area is the requirement for continued performance evaluation. Each clinic is to designate the outcome measures to be followed, reflecting the clinic's own philosophy of care and based on current research about opiate addiction. This task has the potential to put decisions about delivery of care into the hands of clinic administrators rather than regulatory bodies.

Although these changes have been made at the federal level, many states still have not changed their regulations to come into conformance with them, so it remains to be seen when and how much clinical ground actually is won.

An urgent need to increase access to treatment while improving and ensuring the quality of that treatment drives the need for restructuring. In this context, two other changes deserve mention. One is the Drug Addiction Treatment Act of 2000, signed by President Clinton in October 2000, which allows office-based prescription of narcotics for the treatment of addiction, with certain restrictions.

Because the act contains specific requirements for training, courses in the use of buprenorphine have been offered to physicians around the country, pending FDA approval of buprenorphine, which is expected to be classified in Schedule IV or V of the federal Controlled Substance Act. Clinical trials of buprenorphine have shown it to be effective and safe in office-based practice as a maintenance medication.

Also, work is under way on office-based use of methadone (office-based opioid treatment, or OBOT) to expand treatment capacity. CSAT is evaluating several such projects around the country. OBOT currently is available and successful in several nations outside the U.S., including Canada. (See the following chapter for a complete discussion of OBOT.)

REFERENCES

Alter MJ (1997). Epidemiology of hepatitis C. *NIH Consensus Development Conference on Management of Hepatitis C.* Bethesda, MD: National Institutes of Health, 67-70.

American Psychiatric Association (APA) (1994). *Diagnostic and Statistical Manual of Mental Disorders, 4th Edition (DSM-IV).* Washington, DC: American Psychiatric Press.

American Society of Addiction Medicine (ASAM) (1991). *American Society of Addiction Medicine Policy Statement on Methadone Treatment.* Washington, DC: American Society of Addiction Medicine.

Ball JC & Ross A (1991). *The Effectiveness of Methadone Maintenance Treatment.* New York, NY: Springer-Verlag, 283.

Barthwell AG & Gibert CL (1993). *Screening for Infectious Diseases Among Substance Users (Treatment Improvement Protocol Series, No. 6)*. Rockville, MD: Center for Substance Abuse Treatment.

Benet LZ, Kroetz DL & Sheiner LB (1996). Pharmacokinetics: The dynamics of drug absorption, distribution, and elimination. In JG Hardman, LE Limbird, PB Molinoff et al. (eds.) *Goodman & Gilman's The Pharmacological Basis of Therapeutics*. New York, NY: McGraw-Hill, 23.

Cahoon-Young B (1997). Prevalence of hepatitis C virus in women: Who's getting it, why and co-infection with HIV. *Perspective on the Epidemiology, Treatment and Interventions for the Hepatitis C Virus*. Presented at: Haight Ashbury Free Clinics, Inc., Diagnostic Support Services, 14th Street Clinic and Medical Group; March 20, 1997; San Francisco, CA.

Caplehorn JR & Drummer OH (1999). Mortality associated with New South Wales methadone programs in 1994: Lives lost and saved. *Medical Journal of Australia* 170(3):104-109.

Centers for Disease Control and Prevention (CDC) (2001). Prevalence of hepatitis C virus infection among clients of HIV counseling and testing sites—Connecticut, 1999. *Morbidity and Mortality Weekly Reports* 5(27):577-581.

Comfort A (1977). Morphine as an antipsychotic. Relevance of a 19th-century therapeutic fashion. *Lancet* 2(8035):448-449.

Courtwright D, Joseph H & Des Jarlais D (1989). Methadone maintenance—Interview with Vincent Dole. *Addicts Who Survived: An Oral History of Narcotic Use in America, 1923-1965*. Knoxville, TN: University of Tennessee Press, 331-343.

Des Jarlais DC, Joseph H, Dole VP et al. (1985). Medical maintenance feasibility study. *NIDA Research Monograph 58*. Rockville, MD: National Institute on Drug Abuse, 101-110.

Dole VP (1988). Implications of methadone maintenance for theories of narcotic addiction. *Journal of the American Medical Association* 260(20):3025-3029.

Dole VP (1992). Hazards of process regulations. The example of methadone maintenance. *Journal of the American Medical Association* 267(16):2234-2235.

Dole VP (1995). On federal regulation of methadone treatment. *Journal of the American Medical Association* 274(16):1307.

Dole VP & Nyswander M (1965). A medical treatment for diacetylmorphine (heroin) addiction—A clinical trial with methadone hydrochloride. *Journal of the American Medical Association* 193(8):646-650.

Dole VP & Nyswander ME (1967). Heroin addiction—A metabolic disease. *Archives of Internal Medicine* 120(1):19-24.

Drummer OH, Opeskin K, Syrjanen M et al. (1992). Methadone toxicity causing death in ten subjects starting on a methadone maintenance program. *American Journal of Forensic Medicine and Pathology* 13(4):346-350.

Eisenhandler J & Drucker E (1993). Opiate dependency among the subscribers of a New York area private insurance plan. *Journal of the American Medical Association* 269(22):2890-2891.

Fraser HF & Isbell H (1952). Actions and addiction liabilities of alpha-acetylmethadol in man. *Journal of Pharmacology and Experimental Therapy* 105:458-465.

Fudala PJ, Vocci F, Montgomery A et al. (1997). Levomethadyl acetate (LAAM) for the treatment of opioid dependence: A multisite, open-label study of LAAM safety and an evaluation of the product labeling and treatment regulations. *Journal of Maintenance in the Addictions* 1(2):9-39.

Galynker II, Watras-Ganz S, Miner C et al. (2000). Cerebral metabolism in opiate-dependent subjects: Effects of methadone maintenance. *Mount Sinai Journal of Medicine* 67(5 & 6):381-387.

Geraghty B, Graham EA, Logan B et al. (1997). Methadone levels in breast milk. *Journal of Human Lactation* 13(3):227-230.

Goldstein A (1991). Heroin addiction: Neurobiology, pharmacology, and policy. *Journal of Psychoactive Drugs* 23(2):123-133.

Gourevitch MN & Friedland GH (2000). Interactions between methadone and medications used to treat HIV infection: A review. *Mount Sinai Journal of Medicine* 67(5 & 6):429-436.

Grudzinskas CV, Woosley RL, Payte JT et al. (1996). The documented role of pharmacogenetics in the identification and administration of new medications for treating drug abuse. *Problems of Drug Dependence, 1995 (NIDA Research Monograph 58)*. Rockville, MD: National Institute on Drug Abuse, 60-63.

Harper RG, Solish GI, Purow HM et al. (1974). The effect of a methadone treatment program upon pregnant heroin addicts and their newborn infants—Short-term, ambulatory detoxification of opiate addicts using methadone. *Pediatrics* 54(3):300-305.

Herrero Martinez E (2001). Hepatitis B and hepatitis C co-infection in patients with HIV. *Reviews in Medical Virology* 11(4):253-270.

Hoegerman G & Schnoll S (1991). Narcotic use in pregnancy. *Clinical Perinatology* 18(1):51-76

Hoffman JA & Moolchan ET (1994). The phases-of-treatment model for methadone maintenance: Implementation and evaluation. *Journal of Psychoactive Drugs* 26(2):181-197.

Holmstrand J, Anggard E & Gunne LM (1978). Methadone maintenance: Plasma levels and therapeutic outcome. *Clinical Pharmacology and Therapeutics* 23(2):175-180.

Hser Y-I, Hoffman V, Grella C et al. (2001). A 33-year follow-up of narcotics addicts. *Archives of General Psychiatry* 58:503-508.

Jarvis M, Knisely J & Schnoll S (1996). Changes in metabolism of methadone during pregnancy. *NIDA Research Monograph Series*. Rockville, MD: National Institute on Drug Abuse, 129.

Jarvis MA & Schnoll SH (1994). Methadone treatment during pregnancy. *Journal of Psychoactive Drugs* 26(2):155-161.

Johnson RE & Fudala PJ (1992). Background and design of a controlled clinical trial (ARC 090) for the treatment of opioid dependence. *Statistical Issues in Clinical Trials for the Treatment of Opiate Dependence (NIDA Research Monograph Series)*. Rockville, MD: National Institute on Drug Abuse, 14-24.

Kaltenbach KA (1994). Effects of in-utero opiate exposure: New paradigms for old questions. *Drug and Alcohol Dependence* 36(2):83-87.

Kaltenbach K & Finnegan LP (1984). Developmental outcome of children born to methadone maintained women: A review of longitudinal studies. *Neurotoxicology and Teratology* 6(4):271-275.

Kaltenbach K & Finnegan LP (1987). Perinatal and developmental outcome of infants exposed to methadone in-utero. *Neurotoxicology and Teratology* 9(4):311-313.

Kaltenbach K, Comfort M, Rajagopal D & Kumaraswamy G (1996). Methadone maintenance of > 80 mg during pregnancy. *NIDA Research Monograph 174.* Rockville, MD: National Institute on Drug Abuse, 128.

Kaltenbach K, Silverman N & Wapner R (1993). Methadone maintenance during pregnancy. In MW Parrino (ed.) *State Methadone Treatment Guidelines (Treatment Improvement Protocol Series, No. 1).* Rockville, MD: Center for Substance Abuse Treatment, 85-93.

Kaufman J, Payte JT & McLellan AT (1995). Treatment standards and optimal treatment. In RA Rettig & A Yarmolinski (eds.) *Institute of Medicine—Federal Regulation of Methadone Treatment.* Washington, DC: National Academy Press, 185-216.

Kessler RC, McGonagle KA, Zhao S et al. (1994). Lifetime and 12-month prevalence of *DSM-IIIR* psychiatric disorders in the United States. Results from the National Comorbidity Survey. *Archives of General Psychiatry* 51(l):8-19.

Koch M & Banys P (2001). Liver transplantation and opioid dependence. *Journal of the American Medical Association* 285(8):1056-1058.

Kosten TR, Rounsaville BJ & Kleber HD (1986). A 2.5-year follow-up of depression, life crises, and treatment effects on abstinence among opioid addicts. *Archives of General Psychiatry* 43(8):733-738.

Kosten TR, Schottenfeld R, Ziedonis D et al. (1993). Buprenorphine versus methadone maintenance for opioid dependence. *Journal of Nervous and Mental Disease* 181(6):358-364.

Kreek MJ (1979). Methadone disposition during the perinatal period in humans. *Pharmacology, Biochemistry and Behavior* 11(Suppl):7-13.

Kreek MJ (1992). Rationale for maintenance pharmacotherapy of opiate dependence. In CP O'Brien & JH Jaffe (eds.) *Addictive States* (Research Publications: Association for Research in Nervous and Mental Disease). New York, NY: Raven Press, 205-230.

Ling W, Rawson RA & Compton MA (1994). Substitution pharmacotherapies for opioid addiction: From methadone to LAAM and buprenorphine. *Journal of Psychoactive Drugs* 26(2):119-128.

Ling W, Wesson DR, Charuvastra C et al. (1996). A controlled trial comparing buprenorphine and methadone maintenance in opioid dependence. *Archives of General Psychiatry* 53(5):401-407.

Loimer N & Schmid R (1992). The use of plasma levels to optimize methadone maintenance treatment. *Drug and Alcohol Dependence* 30(3):241-246.

Loimer N, Schmid R, Grunberger J et al. (1991). Psychophysiological reactions in methadone maintenance patients do not correlate with methadone plasma levels. *Psychopharmacology (Berlin)* 103(4):538-540.

Maany I, Dhopesh V, Arndt IO et al. (1989). Increase in desipramine serum levels associated with methadone treatment. *American Journal of Psychiatry* 146(12):1611-1613.

Marion IJ, ed. (1995). *LAAM in the Treatment of Opiate Addiction (Treatment Improvement Protocol, No. 22).* Rockville, MD: Center for Substance Abuse Treatment.

McCarthy JJ & Posey BL (2000). Methadone levels in human milk. *Journal of Human Lactation* 16(2):115-120.

McLellan AT (1983). Patient characteristics associated with outcome. In JR Cooper, F Altman, BS Brown et al. (eds.) *Research on the Treatment of Narcotic Addiction: State of the Art (NIDA Monograph Series).* Rockville, MD: National Institute on Drug Abuse, 500-529.

McLellan AT, Alterman AI, Metzger DS et al. (1994). Similarity of outcome predictors across opiate, cocaine, and alcohol treatments: Role of treatment services. *Journal of Consulting and Clinical Psychiatry* 62(6):1141-1158.

McLellan AT, Arndt IO, Metzger DS et al. (1993). The effects of psychosocial services in substance abuse treatment. *Journal of the American Medical Association* 269(15):1953-1959.

McLellan AT, Grissom GR, Zanis D et al. (1997). Problem-service "matching" in addiction treatment. A prospective study in 4 programs. *Archives of General Psychiatry* 54(8):730-735.

McLellan AT, Hagan TA, Levine M et al. (1998). Supplemental social services improve outcomes in public addiction treatment. *Addiction* 93(10):1489-1499.

Merikangas KR, Stolar M, Stevens DE et al. (1998). Familial transmission of substance use disorders. *Archives of General Psychiatry* 55:973-979.

Miller WR & Rollnick S (1991). *Motivational Interviewing: Preparing People to Change Addictive Behavior.* New York, NY: Guilford Press.

Miller WR, Zweben A, DiClemente CC et al. (1994). *Motivational Enhancement Therapy Manual (Project Match Series, No. 2).* Rockville, MD: National Institute on Drug Abuse.

Monga HK, Rodriguez-Barradas MC, Breaux K et al. (2001). Hepatitis C virus infection-related morbidity and mortality among patients with human immunodeficiency virus infection. *Clinical Infectious Diseases* 33(2):240-247.

Musselman DL & Kell MJ (1995). Prevalence and improvement in psychopathology in opioid dependent patients participating in methadone maintenance. *Journal of Addictive Diseases* 14(3):67-82.

National Consensus Development Panel on Effective Medical Treatment of Opiate Addiction (1998). Effective medical treatment of opiate addiction. *Journal of the American Medical Association* 280(22):1936-1943.

National Institutes of Health-Centers for Disease Control and Prevention (NIH-CDC) (1997). *Effective Medical Treatment of Heroin Addiction (NIH Consensus Statement).* Bethesda, MD: National Institutes of Health.

Novick DM (2000). The impact of hepatitis C virus infection on methadone maintenance treatment. *Mount Sinai Journal of Medicine* 67(5 & 6):437-443.

Novick DM & Joseph H (1991). Medical maintenance: The treatment of chronic opiate dependence in general medical practice. *Journal of Substance Abuse Treatment* 8(4):233-239.

Novick DM, Joseph H, Salsitz EA et al. (1994). Outcomes of treatment of socially rehabilitated methadone maintenance patients in physicians' offices (medical maintenance): Follow-up at three and a half to nine and a fourth years. *Journal of General Internal Medicine* 9(3):127-130.

Novick DM, Pascarelli EF, Joseph H et al. (1988). Methadone maintenance patients in general medical practice. A preliminary report. *Journal of the American Medical Association* 259(22):3299-3302.

Novick DM, Reagan KJ, Croxson TS et al. (1997). Hepatitis C virus serology in parenteral drug users with chronic liver disease. *Addiction* 92(2):167-171.

O'Brien CP, Woody GE & McLellan AT (1984). Psychiatric disorders in opioid-dependent patients. *Journal of Clinical Psychiatry* 45(12 Pt 2):9-13.

Payte JT (1997a). Clinical take-homes [column]. *Journal of Maintenance in the Addictions* 1(2):103-104.

Payte JT (1997b). Methadone maintenance treatment: The first thirty years. *Journal of Psychoactive Drugs* 29(2):149-153.

Payte JT & Khuri ET (1993a). Principles of methadone dose determination. In M Parrino (ed.) *CSAT State Methadone Treatment Guidelines (Treatment Improvement Protocol Series, No. 1).* Rockville, MD: Center for Substance Abuse Treatment, 47-58.

Payte JT & Khuri ET (1993b). Treatment duration and patient retention. In MW Parrino (ed.) *State Methadone Treatment Guidelines (Treatment Improvement Protocol Series, No. 1).* Rockville, MD: Center for Substance Abuse Treatment, 119-124.

Pickens RW (1997). Genetic and other risk factors in opiate addiction. *NIH Consensus Development Conference on Effective Medical Treatment of Heroin Addiction.* Bethesda, MD: National Institutes of Health, 33-36.

Pond SM, Kreek MJ, Tong TG et al. (1985). Altered methadone pharmacokinetics in methadone-maintained pregnant women. *Journal of Pharmacology and Experimental Therapeutics* 233(1):1-6.

Regier DA, Farmer ME, Rae DS et al. (1990). Comorbidity of mental disorders with alcohol and other drug abuse. Results from the Epidemiologic Catchment Area (ECA) Study. *Journal of the American Medical Association* 264(19):2511-2518.

Reisine T & Pasternak G (1996). Opioid analgesics and antagonists. In JG Hardman, LE Limbird, PB Molinoff et al. (eds.) *Goodman & Gilman's The Pharmacological Basis of Therapeutics.* New York, NY: McGraw-Hill.

Rettig R & Yarmolinsky A, eds. (1995). *Institute of Medicine—Federal Regulation of Methadone Treatment.* Washington, DC: National Academy Press.

Rounsaville BJ & Kleber HD (1985). Untreated opiate addicts. How do they differ from those seeking treatment? *Archives of General Psychiatry* 42(11):1072-1077.

Rounsaville BJ, Weissman MM, Wilber CH et al. (1982). The heterogeneity of psychiatric diagnosis in treated opiate addicts. *Archives of General Psychiatry* 39:161-169.

Salsitz EA, Joseph H, Frank B et al. (2000). Methadone medical maintenance (MMM): Treating chronic opioid dependence in private medical practice—A summary report (1983-1998). *Mount Sinai Journal of Medicine* 67(5 & 6):388-397.

Senay EC, Barthwell A, Marks R et al. (1994). Medical maintenance: An interim report. *Journal of Addictive Diseases* 13(3):65-69.

Senay EC, Barthwell AG, Marks R et al. (1993). Medical maintenance: A pilot study. *Journal of Addictive Diseases* 12(4):59-76.

Soepatmi S (1994). Developmental outcomes of children of mothers dependent on heroin or heroin/methadone during pregnancy. *Acta Paediatrica Supplement* 404(9):36-39.

Swift RM, Dudley M, DePetrillo P et al. (1989). Altered methadone pharmacokinetics in pregnancy: Implications for dosing. *Journal of Substance Abuse* 1(4):453-460.

Sylvestre D (2002). Treating hepatitis C in methadone maintenance patients: A preliminary report. *Drug and Alcohol Dependence* 66(3).

Tennant FS Jr, Rawson RA, Cohen A et al. (1984). Methadone plasma levels and persistent drug abuse in high dose maintenance patients. *Problems of Drug Dependence, 1983 (NIDA Research Monograph 49).* Rockville, MD: National Institute on Drug Abuse, 262-268.

Tong MJ & el-Farra NS (1996). Clinical sequelae of hepatitis C acquired from injection drug use. *Western Journal of Medicine* 164(5):399-404.

Tsuang MT, Lyons MJ, Meyer JM et al. (1998). Co-occurrence of abuse of different drugs in men. *Archives of General Psychiatry* 55:967-972.

Verebey K, ed. (1982). Opioids in mental illness: Theories, clinical observations and treatment possibilities. *Annals of the New York Academy of Sciences* 398:1-512.

Wallach RC, Jerez E & Blinick G (1969). Pregnancy and menstrual function in narcotics addicts treated with methadone. The Methadone Maintenance Treatment Program. *American Journal of Obstetrics and Gynecology* 105(8):1226-1229.

Walton RG, Thornton TL & Wahl GF (1978). Serum methadone as an aid in managing methadone maintenance patients. *International Journal of Addiction* 13(5):689-694.

Wittmann BK & Segal S (1991). A comparison of the effects of single- and split-dose methadone administration on the fetus: Ultrasound evaluation. *International Journal of Addiction* 26(2):213-218.

Wojnar-Horton RE, Kristensen JH, Yapp P et al. (1997). Methadone distribution and excretion into breast milk of clients in a methadone maintenance programme. *British Journal of Clinical Pharmacology* 44(6):543-547.

Woody GE, McLellan AT, Luborsky L et al. (1986). Psychotherapy for substance abuse [published erratum appears in *Psychiatric Clinics of North America* 1990 Mar; 13(l): xiii]. *Psychiatric Clinics of North America* 9(3):547-562.

Zador D & Sunjic S (2000). Deaths in methadone maintenance treatment in New South Wales, Australia 1990-1995. *Addiction* 95(1):77-84.

Zweben JE (1991). Counseling issues in methadone maintenance treatment. *Journal of Psychoactive Drugs* 23(2):177-190.

Zweben JE & Payte JT (1990). Methadone maintenance in the treatment of opioid dependence. A current perspective. *Western Journal of Medicine* 152(5):588-599.

Special Issues in Office-Based Opioid Treatment

Chapter 5

Andrew J. Saxon, M.D.

Epidemiologic and Regulatory Issues
Research Issues
Clinical Issues

Current interest in office-based approaches to the treatment of opioid addiction springs from a recognition that the numbers and needs of opioid-dependent individuals are overwhelming the capacity of the existing treatment system. Most such individuals cannot gain access to opioid agonist therapy, which is the most effective intervention yet devised for this disorder (National Consensus Development Panel, 1998). Meanwhile, indicators of opioid-related health care costs and criminal justice contacts continue to surge (NIJ, 1999; Sporer, 1999), as do the number of opioid-related deaths (Sporer, 1999). Many opioid-dependent individuals also have unique and serious medical and psychiatric problems that the existing treatment system cannot always address and that contribute to morbidity and mortality (National Consensus Development Panel, 1998). Office-based opioid therapy (OBOT) offers one potential avenue in the drive to ameliorate this unsatisfactory situation.

This chapter reviews some of the historical and regulatory events that shaped our current treatment system and account for some of the ongoing gaps in services for opioid-dependent individuals. Office-based treatment can effectively fill some of these gaps, in part because office-based treatment can encompass two distinct treatment paradigms. First, OBOT offers a less structured, more flexible, and more personalized form of intervention for opioid-dependent patients who have succeeded in the traditional treatment system of opioid agonist clinics licensed by the U.S. Food and Drug Administration (FDA), but who need to continue in pharmacotherapy. Second, OBOT offers a potential alternative route of entry into treatment for opioid-dependent individuals who, for a variety of reasons, have not had access to adequate treatment, or to reengagement in treatment for individuals who have not achieved their goals in the traditional treatment system.

A summary of the rapidly accruing evidence for the benefits of transferring selected, stable methadone-treated patients into office-based settings precedes a synopsis of more preliminary efforts to apply and evaluate the office-based approach for less stable patients newly entering treatment. Results of these investigations of office-based treatment then guide a discussion of clinical issues pertinent to conducting office-based treatment with opioid-dependent patients.

EPIDEMIOLOGIC AND REGULATORY ISSUES

Over the past decade, the purity of heroin sold in the U.S. has increased, while the price has decreased (Bach & Lantos, 1999). Heroin-related emergency department visits have increased from 33,900 in 1990 to 97,287 in 2000 (SAMHSA 2002; Greenblatt, 1997). Heroin-related overdose deaths reported to the Drug Abuse Warning Network increased from 2,300 in 1991 to 4,330 in 1998 (SAMHSA, 1999, 2000). Overdose accounts for only half the overall observed mortality in heroin users, who exhibit mortality rates 6 to 20 times those of age-matched populations (Barnett, 1999; Darke & Zador, 1996).

A subset of the heroin-using population engages in repeated criminal activity (Hanlon, Nurco et al., 1990). The Arrestee Drug Abuse Monitoring Program (NIJ, 2000) provides urine toxicology results for the year 1999 for 30,000 male arrestees in 34 sites around the country and 10,000 female arrestees in 32 sites. These data show that, in 1999, adult male arrestees tested positive for recent opiate use at a median site rate of 6.0%, up from 5.5% in 1997. Female arrestees tested positive for recent opiate use at a rate of 8.0%, slightly down from 8.2% in 1997.

Despite these trends, most opioid-dependent individuals cannot access adequate treatment services. Estimates of the number of heroin users in the U.S. range from 500,000 to 1 million (SAMHSA, 1999; Hamid, Curtis et al., 1997), but, for a variety of reasons—historical, geographic, social, medical, and legal—only 138,000 to 170,000 of these individuals receive opioid agonist treatment. Although apparently portraying a deteriorating situation, the data also reflect a circumstance that has been prevalent throughout the past 100 years.

The mobilization of office-based treatment as a response to this problem does not represent a true innovation but rather a return to a once commonly used strategy. Thousands of untreated opioid-dependent individuals also worried society in the early part of the 20th century. Before the Harrison Narcotic Act was enacted in 1914, no legal restrictions limited the right of physicians to prescribe opioid medications for the care of patients considered addicted. Although controversy raged then, as it does now, about how best to handle opioid-dependent individuals, many experts of that generation already had recognized the high likelihood that opioid-dependent patients would resume opioid use after enforced detoxification. Physicians in many areas of the country thus viewed opioid addiction as a medical disorder; they advocated and practiced the ongoing prescribing of opioids from their offices as a reasonable and apparently useful way to manage the problem.

Most of these physicians conducted this part of their work in a responsible way. A minority may have allowed their practices to become conduits for controlled substances out of a profit motive without always providing adequate medical care. On the basis of a small number of reports of this type of inappropriate prescribing, concern about the safety and wisdom of prescribing opioids to addicts increased in the medical profession itself as well as among regulators and the general public. In 1919, the United States Supreme Court ruled that the Harrison Act disallowed such prescribing to addicts for "maintenance" purposes (Musto, 1987). This decision effectively ended the first era of office-based treatment for opioid addiction.

Such a wholesale shift in policy left patients without access to the opioids on which they depended. Many municipalities responded by creating publicly funded and administered opioid maintenance clinics (Musto, 1987). For example, when New York City experienced one of its waves of heroin addiction after World War I, a clinic under the auspices of the city health department treated 8,000 heroin-dependent patients with prescribed heroin (Wren, 1998). These pioneer efforts at agonist pharmacotherapy ended within a few years when the Narcotic Division of the Federal Prohibition Unit shut down these maintenance clinics as violators of the Harrison Act (Musto, 1987). Thus, from the 1920s onward, physicians were actively discouraged from treating heroin-dependent individuals and, indeed, medical school curricula provided no training to physicians in this regard. In essence, opioid addiction was reconceptualized as a criminal justice rather than a medical problem. Convicted violators of federal narcotics laws caused an overload in the federal penal system, so Congress established federal narcotics hospitals at Lexington, KY, and Forth Worth, TX, in the 1930s. Despite high recidivism rates, these isolated facilities remained the only treatment option for opioid-dependent individuals until the advent of methadone maintenance 30 years later (Musto, 1987).

In some respects, the severance of opioid addiction treatment from the general practice of medicine actually was exaggerated in the 1970s when opioid agonist therapy, in the form of methadone maintenance, once again was permitted and, to some extent, promulgated. Federal methadone regulations (21 CFR Part 291) promulgated in 1972 and the Narcotic Addict Treatment Act of 1974 mandated a closed distribution system for methadone, with special licensing by both federal and state authorities. These regulations effectively made it illegal for physicians not associated with a licensed program to treat opioid-dependent patients with agonist pharmacotherapy in an office setting. Until very recently, a private physician would have to obtain an additional registration from the U.S. Drug Enforcement Administration, annual certification by the U.S. Department of Health and Human Services, and approval by state drug authorities to provide opioid agonist therapy (Cooper, 1995). Less than a handful of physicians around the country have been willing to negotiate this bureaucratic maze. As a result, the only option for patients who desired opioid agonist pharmacotherapy was to enroll in a specialized, licensed methadone treatment program. Once again, most practicing physicians were deprived of exposure to and experience in treating opioid-dependent patients.

The divergence between mainstream medicine and opioid addiction treatment has had some unfortunate consequences. Opioid addiction causes considerable medical morbidity as a consequence of drug effects and intravenous route of administration (Cushman, 1980). Medical problems common in users of illicit opiates include infectious diseases such as pneumonia, tuberculosis, endocarditis, as well as sexually transmitted diseases (Haverkos & Lange, 1990); soft tissue infections (Makower, Pennycock et al., 1992); bone and joint infections (Chandrasekar & Narula, 1986); central nervous system infections (Rubin, 1987); and viral hepatitis (Chamot, de Saussure et al., 1992), particularly hepatitis C (Dieperink, Willenbring et al., 2000). In addition, HIV infection and AIDS pose a massive problem among intravenous drug users (Chamot, de Saussure et al, 1992; Selwyn, Alcabes et al, 1992). Noninfectious problems also typically occur in the lungs (O'Donnell & Pappas, 1988), the central and peripheral nervous systems (Rubin, 1987), the vascular system (Makower, Pennycock et al., 1992), and the musculoskeletal system (Makower, Pennycock et al., 1992). Licensed opioid agonist treatment programs often lack the resources to provide comprehensive medical care (Cooper, 1995), with the result that comorbid medical disorders may be unattended, delaying care and driving up its ultimate cost. Total health care costs related to heroin addiction have reached $1.2 billion annually (SAMHSA, 1999).

Similarly, a high prevalence of Axis I psychiatric comorbidity, particularly mood and anxiety disorders, is seen among patients who are addicted to opioids (Brooner, King et al., 1997; Mason, Kocsis et al., 1998), and licensed programs typically cannot provide the treatment these conditions require (Cooper, 1995).

Were the divide between general medical practice and opioid agonist treatment to be bridged, patients would have improved access to simultaneous care for these serious comorbid medical and psychiatric conditions.

Many potential patients who need and desire opioid agonist treatment and are willing to enroll in licensed programs cannot overcome the barriers to entry. Geography creates an impossible hurdle for some. Seven states (Idaho, Mississippi, Montana, North Dakota, South Dakota, Vermont, and Wyoming) do not offer licensed opioid agonist treatment. New Hampshire instituted its first program in 2000. West Virginia instituted its first program in 2001. In states that do offer such programs, the licensed clinics, by virtue of economic necessity and neighborhood acceptance, tend to be sited primarily in urban locations (Cooper, 1995; Wren, 1997). Even within larger metropolitan areas, specific neighborhoods or communities can bar licensed clinics (Cooper, 1995; Roane, 1997). A few patients who reside in states or communities without opioid agonist clinics or in rural areas invest considerable effort in traveling to other states or cities to obtain treatment; most, who cannot afford the time or cost, simply must forgo it (Wren, 1997).

Inadequate treatment capacity creates another barrier for potential patients who do live in reasonable proximity to a licensed clinic (Schwartz, Brooner et al., 1999). Many clinics have waiting lists that discourage potential patients from even attempting entry (Modie, 1999). Many more potential patients lack the financial resources to pay for their treatment (Modie, 1999). Although OBOT would not necessarily cost less than treatment in a licensed clinic, insurance companies and managed care organizations might be more likely to reimburse at least some of the expense of physician office visits, particularly if comorbid conditions were addressed (Schwartz, Brooner et al., 1999).

Finally, the very nature of licensed opioid agonist treatment clinics, with the potential to be recognized and stigmatized by passersby, waiting lines for medication administration, rigid attendance policies, and lack of privacy, deters some potential patients (Hunt, Lipton et al., 1985).

Many of the latter concerns pertain most directly to long-term, stable patients who have achieved a measure of rehabilitation in opioid agonist treatment. Such patients have ceased illicit drug use and, in most cases, have employment and family responsibilities (Salsitz, Joseph et al., 2000; Schwartz, Brooner et al., 1999). To make their sched-

TABLE 1.   Studies of Stable Methadone-Treated Patients Transferred to Office-Based Opioid Therapy

Author	Year	Method	Requirements for Entry	N	Methadone Dose (take-home)	Protocol Retention	Use of Illicit Opiates	Use of Other Illicit Substances
Salsitz et al.	2000	Naturalistic program evaluation	Employment; 4-5 years on methadone; 3 years no illicit use	158	Mean=60 mg (30-day supply)	83.5%; median retention =13.8 years	None	15/158 excessive cocaine use
Schwartz et al.	1999	Naturalistic program evaluation	Employment; 5 years on methadone; 5 years no illicit use	21	Mean=71.4 mg (28-day supply)	71.4% over 12 years	None	2/21-1 cocaine positive UA; 1/21-1 positive barb UA
Merrill	2001	Naturalistic program evaluation	1 year on methadone; 1 year no illicit use; responsible with take-home medications	31	Not yet reported (30-day supply)	Not yet reported	Not yet reported	Not yet reported
Senay et al.	1993	Randomized clinical trial: medical maintenance vs. control	Employment; 1 year on methadone; 6 months no illicit use	130	N/A (14-day supply)	73% reached 1 year for both conditions	2 experimental; 1 control	14 experimental; 8 control
Fiellin et al.	2001	Randomized clinical trial: office-based vs. clinic treatment	Stable income, >1 year on methadone; 1 year free of illicit opioid use; no dependence on other substances	22 office; 24 standard	Mean=69 mg office (7-day supply); mean=70 mg standard (2-7 day supply)	82% office; 79% standard over 6 months	55% office; 42% standard	Cocaine use: 27% office; 25% standard
King et al.	2000	Randomized clinical trial: office-based vs. monthly clinic pick-up vs. clinic	Employment; 1 year on methadone; 1 year free of illicit substance use; 2 years of no problems	26 office; 27 monthly pick-up; 21 routine clinic care	Mean=63 mg (28-day supply vs. 3-7 day supply)	89% office; 89% monthly clinic; 90% routine clinic over 6 months	0% office; 7% monthly clinic; 0% routine clinic	0% office; 0% monthly clinic; 5% routine clinic

ules accommodate frequent clinic visits with waits for medication, to hold up their travel plans to obtain regulatory approval, and to bring them to a locale where unstable patients with residual drug use congregate may undermine rather than support their rehabilitation (Salsitz, Joseph et al., 2000; Schwartz, Brooner et al., 1999). In addition, many of these rehabilitated patients already have derived maximum benefit from counseling and other services available at licensed clinics. Moving stable patients out of the restrictive clinic setting while continuing their agonist phar-

macotherapy would permit reallocation of clinic resources to patients who most need them.

Three important developments have now altered the landscape. Since March 2000, the FDA has allowed licensed opioid agonist treatment programs to apply for exceptions so that stable, long-term patients can enter methadone medical maintenance and have visits to obtain medication less frequently than once per week. The Children's Health Act of 2000, signed into law in October 2000, included a provision waiving the requirements of the Narcotic Addict

Treatment Act to permit qualified physicians to dispense or prescribe Schedule III, IV, or V narcotic drugs or combinations of such drugs that are approved by the FDA for the treatment of heroin addiction. This change allows qualified physicians to prescribe certain opioid agonist medications in an office-based setting. In October 2002, the FDA approved buprenorphine and buprenorphine+naloxone for the treatment of opioid dependence. These medications were placed in Schedule III, and so are available for use in OBOT.

Clearly, our current treatment system cannot accommodate all the opioid-dependent individuals who want or need treatment. A century ago, office-based treatment met with some success in the United States. A resurrection of office-based treatment now would remove geographic, social, and regulatory barriers for both new and rehabilitated patients and thus make opioid agonist treatment more widely available. New legislation and a loosening of earlier regulations will permit implementation of this idea. Because of the divide between opioid agonist treatment and general medical practice, some physician education and training in management of opioid-dependent patients with pharmacotherapy no doubt will be necessary. Considerable data, described in detail below, offer instruction to physicians.

RESEARCH ISSUES

Research Related to Stable, Long-Term Patients in Office-Based Practice. Several investigations have demonstrated the general safety and utility of transferring patients who have achieved specified degrees of stability through initial treatment in a licensed methadone clinic into an office-based setting (Table 1). The concept of transferring stable methadone patients to office-based practice originated with Novick and colleagues of New York City, who have used this procedure since 1983 and have documented their findings in several reports over the years (Novick, Pascarelli et al., 1988; Novick & Joseph, 1991; Novick, Joseph et al., 1994).

A recent summary of their work describes outcomes for 158 total patients (Salsitz, Joseph et al., 2000). Stringent standards were set for patients to participate in the program. Until 1996, patients were required to have completed five years of methadone treatment; this subsequently was reduced to four years, although all patients actually accepted had at least six years of methadone treatment. At the time of entry, all participants had to have at least three years without illicit drug use, excessive alcohol use, or criminal activity. All had to verify employment or other productive

activity. Additional criteria addressed the need for financial, emotional, and social stability. Patients who met the criteria were transferred from their methadone programs to the care of internists or family physicians in a hospital-based practice. The physicians, most of whom had little familiarity with treating opioid addiction, received specific training from physicians with experience in methadone agonist treatment. The average methadone dose at entry was 60 mg/day. Patients attended two office visits in the first month and then advanced to a monthly reporting and dosing schedule. At each office visit, they provided a specimen for urine toxicology screening and took a dose of methadone under observation to confirm tolerance. They received annual physical examinations from their office-based provider along with routine medical care as needed.

To remain in compliance with the office-based program, patients had to avoid methadone misuse or loss, avoid illicit drug use, attend all appointments, pay fees, and maintain acceptable office comportment. Only 26 patients (16.5%) ever failed to meet these standards, 15 for uncontrollable use of cocaine and 11 for other violations. Eighteen of the "failed patients" returned to their clinics of origin. Patients had a projected median retention time of 13.8 years in office-based treatment. During the years of this investigation, 12 subjects voluntarily and successfully tapered off methadone. Of 99 active patients, 27 required dose increases, while 10 achieved dose reductions.

A retrospective analysis detected several differences between successful and unsuccessful office-based patients. Successful patients were more likely to be married or in stable relationships, were more likely to have had multiple prior treatment episodes in traditional methadone programs, and had more total years of treatment in traditional methadone programs before entering office-based treatment.

A similar, although smaller, uncontrolled trial was conducted in Baltimore by Schwartz, Brooner and colleagues (1999). The sample consisted of 21 patients enrolled during a four-month period in 1985 and 1986. This program required that patients have at least five years' documented abstinence from illicit drug use in a traditional methadone program, as well as no alcohol abuse. Patients also were required to have self-supporting employment and emotional and social stability. Those who used psychotropic medications for psychiatric disorders were excluded. All patients transferred to the private office practice were under the care of a single physician. For the first six months, patients visited the office every two weeks, at which time they gave a urine specimen, had a brief interview with the physician, and received a 14-day supply of methadone. They subsequently advanced to visits every 28 days and a 28-day supply of medication. Only minor medical problems were addressed by the primary practitioner, with most health care services delivered by outside referral. Average methadone dose over the course of the project was 71.4 mg/day. To remain in compliance with the office-based program, patients had to avoid methadone misuse or loss, have accurate return of outstanding medication doses during a "call-back" procedure, avoid illicit drug or alcohol use, attend all appointments, and avoid legal problems leading to arrest.

During 12 years of followup, six patients (28.6%) failed to comply and were transferred back to their original methadone program: two for legal problems, three for positive urine tests, and one for a combination of problems. Of all urine specimens collected, only 0.5% showed any positive results. Not a single patient failed any of the 65 random medication call-backs conducted.

A third uncontrolled trial of the transfer of stable clinic-treated patients to an office-based setting has been initiated in Seattle (Merrill, Jackson et al., 2002). The two programs described above gained permission to provide methadone treatment outside the established guidelines by obtaining an Investigational New Drug approval by the FDA to conduct research. The Seattle program was the first to obtain extensive FDA waivers to establish a clinical program allowing stabilized patients to receive methadone in a medical setting, with extended take-home privileges. Thirty-one patients who attended the licensed methadone clinic no more often than three times a week and who had 12 months of clinical stability (demonstrating responsibility with take-home medication, no urine drug tests positive for illicit drugs, consistent clinic attendance, and psychiatric stability) were transferred to an internal medicine clinic in a public hospital for primary medical care and methadone treatment. General internal medicine specialists cared for the patients after attending several training sessions on opioid addiction and agonist therapy. Ongoing counseling beyond physician visits was not required, but was available through the licensed clinic. Trained pharmacists dispensed the medication through a satellite hospital pharmacy in the medical clinic.

Patients who demonstrated stability in office-based care could be advanced to monthly medication pick-ups. Subjects supplied monthly urine toxicology specimens and had to comply with periodic medication call-backs. Patients who required intensive monitoring or treatment could be returned immediately to the licensed methadone clinic. Preliminary 12-month results showed 28 of 31 patients still in office-based treatment, with two patients choosing to leave the program voluntarily, and one found to be in relapse at entry and returned to licensed clinic care.

Although the three investigations described certainly suggest that most highly stable methadone patients can safely transfer to office-based care, the lack of control groups in these open trials precludes conclusions about whether fewer subjects would deteriorate if they remained in traditional methadone clinics. A few controlled investigations of stable methadone patients in office-based practice have been completed. The largest of these controlled trials, although a very worthwhile study that addressed many of the concerns pertinent to office-based practice, did not represent, in the strictest sense, a trial of office-based practice because of the methodology employed. In the study, Senay and colleagues (Senay, Barthwell et al., 1993) worked with a group of 130 patients who had received at least one year of methadone treatment, who had six months of negative urine toxicologies, steady employment or productive activity, no arrests, general program compliance, and who had no current legal involvement. Patients were assigned randomly to either an experimental (two of three subjects) or a control condition (one of three subjects). The experimental condition consisted of a monthly visit with a physician; observed ingestion of methadone every 14 days, with 13 take-home doses for use between visits; three random urine toxicology screens per year; and random medication call-backs. Patients were required to attend at least one counseling session and leave one nonrandom urine specimen per month in their clinic of origin. Thus, the experimental subjects did continue ongoing contact with their traditional methadone programs, a situation not typical of most office-based paradigms. The control subjects remained in their clinics of origin for six months and then entered the experimental program. The report of this study did not provide methadone dose levels. Subjects continued in either the experimental or control conditions if they provided negative urine specimens, paid their fees, and refrained from criminal activity or lateness. During the first six months, 89% of experimental and 85% of control subjects remained in the program. At one year, 73% of both groups remained. Of the patients removed from the program, 70% were for positive urine specimens, while 30% were for other causes. Removal rates did not differ by condition. The report of this study does not mention the results of the medication call-backs. The advantages of this study derive from its randomized, controlled methodology and from its enrollment of subjects who had far less time in traditional methadone programs and less stable time than did the subjects in the studies described earlier by Salsitz and colleagues (2000) or Schwartz and colleagues (1999). Obviously, subjects of the type in the Senay (1993) study comprise a much larger proportion of typical methadone clinic populations than do the exceedingly stable patients in the other studies. The disadvantage of the Senay study resides in the fact that all subjects continued some attendance and counseling at their clinics of origin. Hence, the study really only demonstrates that most moderately stable methadone patients can manage adequately with observed ingestion of medication only once every 14 days and monthly contact with a physician, but it conveys little about office-based practice independent of a traditional methadone program.

Two small controlled studies have, however, assessed office-based practice for stable methadone patients without confounds from ongoing clinic involvement. In one study (Fiellin, O'Connor et al., 2001), 46 patients already receiving methadone agonist therapy at a licensed treatment program were randomly assigned to be transferred to office-based treatment with an internal medicine physician (n=22) or to remain in standard clinic treatment (n=24). Eligibility requirements for participants included more than a year of methadone treatment; one year's abstinence from use of illicit opiates, as reflected by negative monthly random urine specimens; no current evidence of dependence on other substances; no significant medical or psychiatric conditions that could be compromised by the transfer; a source of legal income; and stable housing. Of note is the fact that only slightly more than 10% of the clinic's total population met these criteria, which clearly are less stringent than those employed in the studies by Salsitz and colleagues (2000) and Schwartz and colleagues (1999). The average methadone dose for the subjects assigned to the office-based treatment condition was 69 mg. Average dose for those assigned to remain in standard clinic treatment was 70 mg. The six physicians who provided the office-based treatment and their staff members received training in management of patients on opioid agonist therapy.

Subjects assigned to office-based treatment received a weekly supply of methadone from the physician's office. They had an initial one-hour office visit in which a history and physical were performed. They subsequently met with their physician monthly. Subjects assigned to remain in standard clinic treatment came to the clinic one to three times a week to pick up their methadone. All subjects provided monthly urine specimens and quarterly hair specimens for toxicologic analysis. If a patient's urine was positive for opiates or cocaine or negative for methadone, a repeat urine specimen was obtained within one week. If this repeat specimen also tested positive for opiates or cocaine or negative for methadone, patients were considered out of compliance with the protocol, removed from the study, and transferred back to routine care. During a six-month followup interval, 18% of the office-based subjects and 21% of the standard clinic subjects violated the study criteria and were transferred back to routine care. By either urinalysis, hair toxicology, or self-report, 55% of office-based and 42% of standard clinic subjects had evidence of illicit opiate use, while 27% and 25%, respectively, had evidence of cocaine use.

Hair toxicology testing at baseline in this study allowed for some valuable observations. Although all subjects had submitted 12 consecutive negative monthly urine specimens before entering the study, hair testing found evidence of illicit drug use in the preceding 90 days by 44% of the subjects. While the failure of monthly urine testing to detect all substance use does not come as a surprise (Saxon, Calsyn et al., 1990), positive hair testing at baseline did act as a predictor of substance use during followup. Among those with positive hair toxicology at baseline, 90% had evidence of illicit use during followup. In contrast, only 20% of those with negative baseline hair toxicology had such evidence at followup.

In another controlled study (King, Stoller et al., 2002), 73 subjects who were receiving methadone treatment were randomly assigned to one of three conditions: (1) medication pick-up every 28 days in a physician's office away from the licensed treatment program, (2) medication pick-up every 28 days, with a monthly physician visit at the licensed treatment clinic, or (3) continued routine clinic care, with medication pick-up once or twice a week at the clinic. Eligibility requirements for participants included continuous methadone treatment and absence of any positive monthly urine specimens over the preceding 12 months, full-time employment, and no failed medication recalls or problems handling medication over the preceding 24 months. About 25% of patients from two different clinics met these criteria. The average methadone dose was 63 mg/day. The four physicians who provided the office-based treatment had

TABLE 2. Studies of Patients Admitted Directly to Office-Based Opioid Treatment

Author	Year	Method	Requirements for Entry	N	Methadone Dose (take-home)	Protocol Retention	Use of Illicit Opiates	Use of Other Illicit Substances
Hutchinson et al.	2000	Naturalistic program evaluation	Opioid dependence	204	Methadone; mean initial dose=43 mg	42.4% of 119 followed up at 12 months	2% daily heroin for subjects in continuous treatment	0% daily benzodiazepine for subjects in continuous treatment
Gossop et al.	1999	Non-randomized comparison: GP office vs. clinic	Opioid dependence	155-GP; 297 clinic	Methadone; mean initial dose =51 mg (GP) or 48 mg (clinic)	6 months: 66% GP; 60% clinic	< 10 days heroin use per month, both groups	Reduced significantly and equally for both groups
Vignau & Brunelle	1998	Non-randomized comparison: GP office vs. clinic	Opioid dependence	32-GP; 37 clinic	Buprenorphine; mean=5.9 mg/d (GP) or 6.6mg/d (clinic)	6 months: 70% GP; 60% clinic	N/A	N/A
O'Connor et al.	1998	Randomized clinical trial: Primary care clinic vs. drug clinic treatment	Opioid dependence	23 in each condition	Buprenorphine: 22 mg Mon/Wed; 40 mg Fri	12 weeks: 78% primary care; 52% drug clinic	63% positive UAs primary care; 85% drug clinic	33% cocaine positive UAs both conditions
Fudala et al.	2001	Randomized clinical trial: Buprenorphine vs. buprenorphine +naloxone vs. placebo	Opioid dependence	326 total subjects	Buprenorphine 16 mg/d vs. Buprenorphine +naloxone 16/4 mg /d vs. placebo	Not yet reported	Placebo > than 2 other conditions	Not yet reported
Ling	2002	Naturalistic study	Opioid dependence	582	Buprenorphine +naloxone 2/0.5 mg/d to 24/6 mg /d	Estimated 66% at 16 weeks (study still in progress)	Estimated 27% UAs positive at 16 weeks	Not yet reported

previous experience treating patients with methadone agonist therapy. All subjects received a single 20-minute counseling session per month. The 28-day pick-up subjects received counseling from their physicians. The routine care subjects received counseling from clinic counselors. All subjects submitted to a monthly random medication recall procedure. All subjects gave two urine specimens per month. The 28-day pick-up subjects provided a routine, nonrandom specimen at the time of their scheduled physician visits and also produced a random urine specimen at the time of the medication recall. The routine care patients gave a routine random urine specimen once a month, just as did the other clinic patients, and provided a second random speci-

men at the time of their medication recall. An innovative stepped-care counseling intensification procedure was used so that subjects who exhibited problems such as a positive urine specimen or failed medication recall could be transferred back to the clinic for five weekly medication visits until they again attained stability. They would then resume treatment in their assigned research condition. About 90% of subjects in each research condition completed six months of randomized care. Only four patients submitted positive specimens over six months (one by missing a specimen, which counted as positive; one for repeated evidence of cocaine and benzodiazepines; and two for a single specimen that was positive for morphine), while 19 failed a medication recall. These problems resulted in 21 subjects (29%) entering intensified counseling. No subjects in office-based care gave a positive urine specimen. The three groups did not differ significantly in the likelihood that patients would experience a negative outcome.

Consideration of the overall data obtained from patients who have achieved some measure of stability on methadone therapy delivered in a clinic setting show fairly convincingly that most can transfer successfully to office-based care. In addition, in virtually all cases, patients who fail in office-based treatment because of substance relapse or rule violations can be returned to routine clinic care to receive intensified counseling and monitoring without undue harm. The controlled studies also suggest that relapse or other problems in previously stable patients in office-based practice occur at rates no greater than those of similarly stable patients who remain in routine clinic care.

Research Related to Patients Entering Directly Into Office-Based Practice. Although policies and attitudes in the U.S. have, until relatively recently, steered practitioners away from the idea of bringing unstable street addicts directly into office-based treatment, other countries have, out of necessity and an innovative spirit, embraced this concept more quickly (Table 2).

For example, in Scotland, most patients who receive methadone have it prescribed in general practitioners' offices and ingest it in community pharmacies (Gruer, Wilson et al., 1997; Hutchinson, Taylor et al., 2000; Peters & Reid, 1998; Weinrich & Stuart, 2000; Wilson, Watson et al., 1994). These general practitioners receive training specific to this endeavor (Hutchinson, Taylor et al., 2000). A one-year followup of 204 opioid-dependent patients who entered such a paradigm in 1996 has been reported by Hutchinson and colleagues (2000). A total of 58 general practitioners provided treatment to these patients. The study report does not specify the frequency or content of office visits, so practitioners presumably arranged their interventions on an individualized basis. The report also does not explicitly mention the frequency with which methadone doses were taken under observation, but it implies that this occurred on a daily or near-daily basis. Methadone dose levels are reported only for the 50 subjects who remained in continuous treatment for 12 months and who completed followup interviews. These subjects began at an average dose of 43 mg and increased to an average dose of 65 mg at 12 months. Followup interviews at 12 months were com-

pleted with 119 subjects (58.3%). Predictors of failure at followup included prostitution, unstable living arrangements, higher proportion of drug-using associates, higher daily drug expenditures, a higher level of benzodiazepine use, and a higher proportion of income from illegal sources. Among the 119 subjects followed, 50 (42.4%) remained continuously on methadone for 12 months, 34 (28.8%) interrupted and then resumed methadone treatment, and 35 stopped methadone treatment. In the group who stopped treatment, 39% did so because of imprisonment, 33% did so because they were taking other drugs or misbehaving in the pharmacy, and 27% left voluntarily because they disliked the program. In one analysis, the researchers imputed missing data for followup failures by carrying forward their baseline values. In this analysis, daily opiate injecting for the entire cohort declined from 80% at baseline to 43% at 12 months, the mean daily amount spent on drugs from £63 to £38, and the mean number of acquisitive crimes in the preceding month declined from 18 to 11. Another analysis that examined subjects followed up at 12 months compared 50 subjects who remained continuously on methadone with 57 subjects who interrupted methadone treatment during the first 6 months. Only 2% of those who remained continuously on methadone reported daily opiate injecting at 12 months compared with 21% of those with interrupted treatment. Continuous treatment subjects were spending a daily mean of £4 on drugs at 12 months, compared with £16 for those with interrupted treatment. Continuous treatment subjects committed a mean of three acquisitive crimes in the preceding month, compared with five for those with interrupted treatment.

England also has had a policy since the 1980s of encouraging opioid-dependent individuals to get methadone treatment through office-based treatment by general practitioners (Gossop, Marsden et al., 1999). A nonrandomized comparison study evaluated subjects who began methadone in 1995, either in a specialist drug clinic (n=297) or with a general practitioner (n=155). Training required for general practitioners was not specifically mentioned. At baseline, the two groups were similar in illicit drug use except that the specialist clinic group had greater use of amphetamines. The mean initial methadone dose was 51 mg (SD=18.7) for the general practitioner group and 48 mg (SD=19.1) for the specialist clinic group. General practitioners prescribed less than daily dispensing for 43% of their patients, while specialist clinics allowed less than daily dispensing for only

25% of their patients. Only 14% of general practitioners required that methadone administration (at retail pharmacies) be supervised. Frequency of office visits with general practitioners was not specified. Followup at six months was achieved with 76% of the original sample.

At six months, 66% of general practitioner patients and 60% of specialized clinic patients remained in treatment. In both groups, heroin use was reduced, on average, from more than 19 days per month at baseline to less than 10 days per month at followup; there was no significant difference between groups. All other substance use was reduced significantly and similarly for both groups. Drug injecting decreased among the general practitioner group from 53% to 41% and among the specialist clinic group from 66% to 53%. Non-drug-related crime fell among both groups, but significantly more so among the general practitioner group.

France did not offer agonist pharmacotherapy to opioid-dependent individuals until the introduction of methadone at specialist addiction centers in 1995 (Vignau & Brunelle, 1998). Shortly thereafter, buprenorphine became available in France for the treatment of opioid addiction, and general practitioners, regardless of their training, gained permission to prescribe it for this indication (Moatti et al., 1998; Vignau & Brunelle, 1998). Today, general practitioners in France can prescribe up to 28 days' supply of take-home medications and a maximum daily buprenorphine dose of 16 mg. More than 50,000 patients have received buprenorphine in this office-based paradigm. A nonrandomized comparison study examined outcomes for opioid-dependent patients in France who were treated with buprenorphine by general practitioners (n=32), compared with patients treated with buprenorphine at specialized addiction centers (n=37) (Vignau & Brunelle, 1998). The general practitioners had a fixed frequency of consultations, although the report does not specify the frequency. General practitioners performed urine testing weekly, required cannabis abstinence, and could arrange psychosocial services but did not necessarily have such services available. The addiction centers had a variable frequency of consultations, had no systematic frequency of urine testing, did not require cannabis abstinence, but had psychosocial services directly available. Apparently, subjects self-selected their own treatment venues.

The two groups differed at baseline on important variables. The patients treated in the addiction centers were older, less likely to be employed, had more polydrug use, experienced many more episodes of overdose, and were more likely to be injecting heroin. Doses of buprenorphine (5.9 mg/day for the general practitioner group versus 6.6 mg/day in the addiction center group) were relatively low in both groups. Treatment retention at 180 days was approximately 70% in the general practitioner group and about 60% in the addiction center group. Addiction Severity Index scores improved similarly for both groups from baseline to 90 days.

The first U.S. study to evaluate a quasi-office-based approach to opioid-dependent individuals just entering treatment also used buprenorphine as an agonist pharmacotherapeutic agent (O'Connor, Oliveto et al., 1998). Potential subjects with other drug or alcohol addiction, recent cocaine use, or complex medical or psychiatric comorbidities were excluded. Subjects were assigned randomly to receive 12 weeks of buprenorphine pharmacotherapy, either in a primary care setting or in a drug treatment setting that typically provided methadone treatment. The primary care setting was housed in a clinic designed to handle the primary care needs of substance users and psychiatric patients. Physicians in the primary care setting relied on a manual-guided clinical management protocol. Subjects assigned to the primary care setting (n=23) received an initial one-hour visit with a primary care provider, who took a substance use and medical history, created a treatment plan, made a referral to group psychotherapy, and prescribed buprenorphine. The subjects then saw their primary care provider in weekly 20-minute sessions. Group therapy conducted by a primary care nurse practitioner occurred weekly for 50 minutes, with a self-help focus on promoting abstinence.

Subjects assigned to the drug treatment setting (n=23) received a standard set of services, including individualized substance abuse counseling and weekly relapse prevention group therapy. In both settings, subjects attended five days during week 1, with a buprenorphine dose escalation beginning at 2 mg and doubling daily until the dose reached 32 mg on day 5. From weeks 2 through 12, subjects attended clinic three times a week and received observed buprenorphine doses of 22 mg on Mondays and Wednesdays and 40 mg on Fridays. Thus, this study totally avoided prescribing of take-home medications. Subjects in both settings also gave urine specimens three times a week. Patients were terminated from the study for missing three consecutive medication doses or for failure to attend group therapy. Successful completion of 12 weeks of treatment was observed for 78% of the subjects in primary care, compared with 52% of the subjects in drug treatment. Urine specimens were positive for opiates in 63% of urine specimens provided by primary care subjects, compared with 85% of drug treatment subjects. Primary care subjects showed a decreasing trend of opiate-positive specimens over time, whereas drug treatment subjects did not. Roughly a third of urine specimens in both groups tested positive for cocaine (O'Connor, Oliveto et al., 1998).

This study lends some support to the notion that treatment-seeking opioid-dependent patients can derive as much benefit from treatment in an office-based setting as from a drug treatment setting. Nevertheless, the researchers themselves properly note several aspects of the study design that limit its applicability to a true office-based setting. The primary care setting in this study required many more visits and more observed medication administration than would be practical in a typical office-based practice. The clinic used for the primary care setting had much more familiarity and expertise with substance-using patients than would most office-based settings. The study excluded patients with the medical and psychiatric complications commonly seen in opioid-dependent treatment seekers.

Another, much larger study in the U.S. also examined a quasi-office-based approach for opioid-dependent patients just entering treatment (Paul Fudala, Ph.D, personal communication, 2001). This study differed from the others in that it did not compare an office-based with a clinic approach, but rather compared different medication strategies within a quasi-office-based setting. In this randomized, double-blind, placebo-controlled, multicenter trial, 326 subjects were randomly assigned to receive either (1) buprenorphine 16 mg/day, (2) buprenorphine 16 mg+naloxone 4 mg/day, or (3) placebo. Medication was administered in office-based settings affiliated with Veterans Affairs Medical Centers. Subjects received their doses five days a week, with take-home medications given for weekends and holidays. The trial was terminated early because of the demonstrated efficacy of buprenorphine+naloxone compared with placebo. Subjects treated with either buprenorphine alone or buprenorphine+naloxone had a greater proportion of urine specimens that were negative for opiates than did the subjects given placebo. The rate of adverse events was manageable and comparable between the two active treatments.

The largest study yet conducted of office-based treatment, A Multicenter Safety Trial of Buprenorphine+Naloxone for the Treatment of Opiate Dependence, has been completed and data are being analyzed (Walter Ling, M.D., personnel communication, 2002). This uncontrolled, natu-ralistic investigation will examine outcomes for 582 opiate-dependent individuals newly entering office-based treatment. Patients were not excluded for psychiatric or medical problems (other than pregnancy, because buprenorphine+ naloxone is not approved for use in pregnant patients), so long as the treating physician could manage the problems on her or his own or by appropriate referral. Patients were treated by 38 physicians in six states with buprenorphine+ naloxone, in doses ranging from 2 mg/0.5 mg to 24 mg/6 mg per day. Medications were dispensed by institutional and community pharmacies. Physicians and pharmacists involved in the study received at least 8 hours of training in the pharmacology of buprenorphine+naloxone and issues pertinent to office-based treatment of opioid addiction. Treatment lasted up to a year. Patients were seen by the physicians at least twice in the first week of treatment, at least weekly during weeks 2 through 12 of treatment, at least biweekly from weeks 13 to 26, and monthly thereafter until week 52. For stable patients, medication dispensing followed a pattern similar to the office visits, so that in the final six months of treatment, patients could have monthly medication pick-ups. Urine toxicology screens were obtained onsite at each office visit. Relapse prevention counseling were available and encouraged, but not required. Patients who became stable early in treatment had the option to taper the dose of buprenorphine+naloxone between weeks 7 and 9 and to complete treatment at that time.

An interim analysis involving 344 subjects who had been enrolled for at least 16 weeks found an overall treatment retention rate of 66%. Among 157 subjects who completed four months of treatment, the rate of opiate-positive urine screens in month 4 was 27.5%. When the results of this study are published, they will greatly inform the field about the feasibility, safety, and practice patterns of office-based treatment for opioid addiction using buprenorphine+ naloxone.

All of these early evaluations of direct entry to office-based treatment for opioid addiction support its viability as a treatment option and show its acceptance by patients, physicians, and pharmacists. Treatment retention in these office-based investigations did not fall markedly below— nor did illicit opiate use rise strikingly above—rates reported in recent clinic-based investigations of opioid agonist treatment, even though the European studies discussed here used doses of agonist medications that currently would be considered less than optimal.

CLINICAL ISSUES

Although the totality of clinical experience with office-based treatment remains somewhat limited, the body of evidence reviewed above does encourage some synthesis of relevant ideas and recommendations related to clinical practice in an office setting. Again, it makes sense to divide this discussion into two segments: one most pertinent to care of long-term, stable patients who are transferred from a licensed program to office-based care, and one focused on management of patients who are admitted directly to an office-based setting.

Patient assessment and appropriate selection of patients for transfer from clinic-based to office-based care obviously are key elements of this paradigm. A comparison of the various studies discussed earlier gives rise to the expected impression that more stringent selection criteria with more required time and stability in clinic-based treatment lead to better success after transfer to office-based treatment. When several years of treatment and stability are required (Salsitz, Joseph et al., 2000; Schwartz, Brooner et al., 1999), patients exhibit no illicit opioid use and minimal other substance use and most remain in the protocol for many years. Within the group of subjects in the study by Salsitz and colleagues (2000), more episodes of methadone treatment and longer time in treatment were associated with a greater likelihood of a good outcome after transfer to office-based care. When less stringent selection criteria are used (Fiellin, O'Connor et al., 2001; Senay, Barthwell et al., 1993), illicit drug use is more likely to manifest in the office-based setting. The hair toxicology performed in the Connecticut study (Fiellin, O'Connor et al., 2001) also provides insights into this issue. Hair testing detected illicit substance use for some subjects who were believed by their program to be substance-free on the basis of monthly urine screens. Positive hair testing at baseline in that study clearly predicted substance use during the experimental paradigm for subjects in either office-based or standard clinic care. Because hair testing remains unavailable in most clinical settings, an alternative might be to obtain weekly or more frequent urine screens for some period of time before the anticipated transfer of any apparently stable patient from a licensed clinic to office-based care.

How thoroughly to assess and how stringently to screen patients for potential transfer to office-based care also depends on how much illicit substance use would be tolerated in the office-based setting. The programs thus far reported in the literature and reviewed here tolerated very little use

before initiating protective transfer of the patient back to standard clinic care. In view of the fact that patients in office-based methadone treatment may have substantial quantities of take-home methadone doses in their possession, this conservative approach toward illicit drug use makes sense. Safety concerns would dictate that patients who are using illicit drugs should not have any (or have only a negligible supply of) take-home methadone to minimize the potential for overdose. Also, patients who use illicit drugs may pose a greater risk of diverting methadone to raise cash to buy drugs. Nevertheless, the controlled studies indicate that substance use did not differ on the basis of treatment in office-based versus standard clinic care (Fiellin, O'Connor et al., 2001).

What remains unknown is whether patients transferred to office-based care who experience more than a few brief episodes of substance use will continue to deteriorate in office-based care and need protective transfer back to standard clinic care, or whether such relapses could be contained as effectively within the office-based setting, presuming a practical mechanism exists to limit the number of take-home doses of methadone provided until stability is regained. The report of Salsitz and colleagues (2000) described the need for termination of 15 patients with serious abuse of cocaine that could not be treated within private practice, but it does not specify what measures might be taken within an office-based setting to address this type of problem. The stepped care intensification procedure used in the study by King and colleagues (2002) offered one model for handling instability in the office-based setting that does not preclude rapid return to office-based care. Future studies could help to answer this question through controlled trials that randomly assign office-based patients undergoing a substance use relapse either to stay in office-based care or to receive protective transfer back to standard clinic care.

Further, office-based practitioners no doubt vary in their ability to tolerate and manage relapse. Some may feel very uncomfortable and immediately wish to transfer the patient back to standard clinic care, while others may prefer to intensify services in other ways, as through an increased number of office visits, a referral to counseling or self-help groups, or an increase in the methadone dose.

Concerns about relapse lead directly to a consideration of techniques for monitoring stable patients in office-based practice. All the studies described used urine testing, which would be common practice in licensed agonist treatment clinics. With the exception of the study by Senay and colleagues (1993), these studies typically tested urine specimens at least monthly, often in a nonrandom fashion. In the study by Fiellin and colleagues (2001), subjects who provided a specimen that was positive for drugs were required to give another specimen within the following week. The study by King and colleagues (2002) used a monthly, random medication call-back schedule that also required subjects to give a random urine specimen. Rates of illicit drug use were lower in this study than in the study by Fiellin and colleagues (2001), even though the subject populations appear to be relatively similar. Despite the dangers of comparing results across different studies, these observations lead to speculation that the random nature of the call-back procedures in the King (2002) study may have deterred some illicit drug use. Although the regular and frequent call-back procedure used in that study might prove somewhat cumbersome in a purely clinical setting, the data argue for physicians who provide opioid agonist treatment in an office-based setting to institute some type of call-back procedure. The office-based subjects in the King (2002) study were highly satisfied with their treatment, even though the call-back procedures meant that they had to visit their physician's office twice rather than once a month. A call-back procedure obviously also helps to minimize the risk of inappropriate or excessive medication use or diversion.

A monitoring plan that would be practical in an office-based setting would involve monthly nonrandom urine specimens at the time of scheduled office visits; a few unscheduled call-backs per year, with medication checks and provision of random urine specimens; and a very quick call-back after any positive urine specimen to obtain a repeat specimen within a few days. The latter part of the plan dictates that the physician must use a toxicology laboratory with a rapid turnaround time and must remain vigilant and act on positive test results as soon as they are received from the lab. Alternatively, with the technology to conduct onsite urine testing now readily available, an office setting with that capacity could detect illicit drug use at the time of the office visit. A more frequent medication pick-up schedule could be instituted immediately, along with plans to return for repeat urine monitoring.

The clinical management of methadone pharmacotherapy clearly encompasses another major component of office-based treatment for transferred patients. A substantial number of subjects in the investigation by Salsitz and

colleagues (2000) required methadone dose changes. Physicians who treat patients with methadone in office-based practice need to remain alert to the need for alterations in medication dose. Methadone stereoisomer plasma concentrations can change over time in response to a variety of somewhat unpredictable environmental factors, and such changes could lead to variations in clinical medication effects (Eap, Bertschy et al., 1998; Rostami-Hodjegan, Wolff et al., 1999). Thus, physicians should frequently inquire about symptoms such as rhinorrhea, lacrimation, chills, nausea, diarrhea, muscle aches, and insomnia, and assess whether these symptoms could be related to opioid withdrawal. They should query patients about thoughts of drug use or cravings. If such symptoms are occurring, an increase in the methadone dose should be given serious consideration. Similarly, physicians should ask about possible methadone side effects (such as constipation, excess sedation, or lowered libido) that may suggest the need for a reduction in methadone dose. In the absence of serious side effects or serious risk of relapse to drug use, the patient's wishes about dose changes often serve as the best guide to clinical decisionmaking (Maddux, Desmond et al., 1995).

Psychosocial interventions form another potentially valuable element of office-based treatment for transferred patients. It would be expected, in general, that such interventions would be brief and might be minimal or unnecessary for the highly stable, long-term patients seen in the studies by Salsitz and colleagues (2000) and Schwartz and colleagues (1999). In the context of an office visit, it would be desirable for the physician to ask about the patient's drug and alcohol use and cravings; how the patient is doing at work and/or with family or child care responsibilities, financial and housing circumstances; about psychiatric and medical status; and about use of leisure time. In most cases, long-term patients will indicate in a few words that they have maintained stability in these areas of their lives. In the event that a patient acknowledges some problem or added stress, a few moments to delineate the scope of the difficulty, express concern and empathy, and provide support, advice, and encouragement may suffice to assist the patient in coping with mild or moderate distress. If the problem seems more severe, the office-based physician must either arrange more frequent sessions with the patient or have ready access to referral to counseling resources. Some of the office-based paradigms described earlier (King, Stoller et al., 2002; Merrill, Jackson et al., 2002) had ongoing arrangements for temporary intensification of counseling services at the original licensed treatment program.

The clinical management of unstable, opioid-dependent patients newly entering office-based treatment poses some challenges that overlap those of already stabilized clinic patients, but also some that are distinct. Patients who enter directly into office-based care exhibit marked reductions in substance use, risk behavior, and criminality; also, they have much higher rates of drop-out and drug use than do stable patients. Even in the study by O'Connor and colleagues (1998), which excluded subjects with recent cocaine use or serious psychiatric or medical problems, rates of drop-out and substance use were substantial. With the exception of that study, most investigations of direct entry into office-based treatment have applied no exclusions to admission, so little direct scientific information exists to guide patient selection. To a great extent, then, patient selection for direct entry into office-based treatment must rely on the specific areas of expertise and clinical skills of the treating physician. Through thorough assessment, including a complete history and physical examination, the physician should ascertain whether he or she can comfortably manage—either by direct care and/or by adequate referral networks—the combination of substance use problems, general medical problems, psychiatric problems, and life crises likely to arise in the treatment of each patient. Physicians should exercise caution and refer patients who are not good candidates for their practice settings to licensed treatment programs. Although the early evidence suggests that some patients who enter directly into office-based opioid agonist therapy have a smooth treatment course, many certainly remain unstable for some time. Physicians who accept patients directly into office-based treatment will have to be able to tolerate and deal with some serious and unexpected clinical events.

As with stable, transferred patients, appropriate monitoring strategies will help the physician to stabilize patients newly entering office-based treatment. Again, no solid scientific data are available to guide precise techniques or monitoring schedules. Urine toxicology testing and periodic medication call-backs, coupled with regular clinical evaluation, likely will continue to serve as the mainstays of monitoring.

Medication dispensing schedules allow another method of managing instability. For transferred, stable patients, weekly or more frequent dispensing schedules make no sense because such patients could obtain equivalent schedules at licensed clinics. For newly entering patients, on the other hand, tight control of medication dispensing, when practical, likely enhances the patient's progress toward stability. Buprenorphine and buprenorphine+naloxone are the only agonist medications approved for the treatment of patients directly entering office-based care in the U.S. Although daily observation of medication ingestion would not be practical in most office-based settings, buprenorphine can be administered effectively three times a week (O'Connor, Oliveto et al., 1998), a schedule that probably is feasible in some office-based settings and/or their affiliated community pharmacies.

Monitoring and dispensing schedules will vary much more for newly entering patients, with more intensity of services expected initially, later decreasing as indicators of stability appear. Such indicators would include generally compliant behavior; regular, timely attendance at scheduled office visits; successful compliance with medication callbacks; negative urine toxicology tests; productive use of time; supportive interpersonal relationships; and the absence of criminal justice involvement. As such signs of stability appear, medication dispensing can be liberalized from three times a week to once a week, biweekly, or monthly, with an appropriate number of take-home doses. The frequency of scheduled office visits, urine testing, and medication callbacks can be adjusted in a similar fashion. If signs of instability reappear, any or all of these monitoring techniques can be readjusted for greater frequency.

As in the treatment of stable, transferred patients, careful pharmacotherapy of newly entering patients can contribute to their stability. The physician needs considerable skill to prescribe buprenorphine, particularly in view of its potential to precipitate opioid withdrawal during induction of patients with high levels of physical dependence (Jacobs & Bickel, 1999; Strain, Preston et al., 1995; Walsh, Preston et al., 1995). This characteristic of buprenorphine generally dictates initiation of pharmacotherapy at low doses, followed by dose escalation as soon as the patient demonstrates medication tolerance. Throughout the course of treatment, as in the care of transferred patients, the physician will need to be alert to the signs and symptoms described earlier and be ready to adjust the dose.

Psychosocial treatments may be even more important to patients who are newly entering office-based treatment than to stable patients who already have received regular counseling at a licensed program. Scant scientific data are available to provide reliable instruction as to the optimal modality or frequency of psychosocial treatments for these patients. The uncontrolled studies conducted in Britain did not evaluate the variety of psychosocial treatments prescribed by physicians. The study by O'Connor and colleagues (1998) used weekly physician visits and weekly group therapy—an intensity of psychosocial services that might not be available or reimbursable in most clinical settings. Studies of various intensities of psychosocial services in licensed methadone programs (Avants, Margolin et al., 1999; Calsyn, Wells et al., 1994; McLellan, Arndt et al., 1993) do offer some illumination on this point: patients who receive minimal psychosocial services do not fare as well as those who receive moderate or high levels of services (however, the lower cost-effectiveness of more intensive services may nullify any slight advantage they hold over moderate services [Avants, Margolin et al., 1999; Kraft, Rothbard et al., 1997]). In the absence of any more definitive information, these findings would argue for the value of at least monthly counseling for a patient newly entering office-based treatment. If the physician does not wish to provide this service, ancillary office staff or an outside counselor to whom patients are referred could do so. The intensity of psychosocial services then could be titrated to the response of each individual patient.

Many of the studies summarized here used some form of brief physician training before the physician engaged in office-based care of opioid-dependent patients. As with many aspects of office-based opioid treatment, little empirical evidence exists to specify the optimal training method. Practicing physicians have limited amounts of time in their schedules for training, so a brief course makes sense. At present, physicians are eligible to practice office-based treatment of opioid addiction on completion of eight hours of formal training.

CONCLUSIONS

Patients who are addicted to opioids have posed a perennial challenge to the health care system. In recent decades, the system has tried to meet the challenge by providing opioid agonist pharmacotherapy at licensed treatment programs. This approach has greatly improved the outcomes and lives of many patients, but has failed to accommodate many others because of inadequate capacity and because, for some individuals, attendance at such a program creates undue hardships. Good scientific data now show that transfer of patients who have one or two years of demonstrated stabil-

ity in a licensed methadone program to office-based care leads to outcomes comparable to those obtained if the patients had continued at a licensed clinic. If such patients become unstable in office-based care, they can be transferred safely back to clinic care.

Many such patients prefer office-based care and have more time for productive activities when receiving treatment in an office setting. Moreover, transferring such patients to office-based care opens treatment slots in methadone clinics to previously untreated patients. Now that several hundred patients have been treated in office settings, the appropriate management techniques (including patient selection, monitoring, and pharmacotherapy) have been reasonably well established.

Early evidence from studies of office-based care of opioid-dependent patients newly entering treatment likewise suggests that such care is reasonable for many such patients and that their short-term outcomes appear nearly equivalent to those achieved with similar patients in traditional licensed programs. Although this approach holds a great deal of promise, implementation of optimal management techniques awaits completion of additional rigorous research.

As more knowledge accrues about office-based treatment of opioid addiction, and as it becomes a more widespread practice, a number of positive "ripple effects" likely will ensue. The "treatment gap" should narrow as more patients who live in a variety of locations and have varying needs gain access to opioid agonist treatment. The medical and addiction treatment systems will reintegrate. Not only will medical and psychiatric comorbidities be attended to more fully, but physicians may become more willing to address substance use problems other than opioid addiction. Society in general will benefit from reductions in crime and its associated costs, as well as an increased engagement in the workforce by previously unemployable individuals, and possibly an overall decline in health care expenditures.

REFERENCES

Avants SK, Margolin A, Sindelar JL et al. (1999). Day treatment versus enhanced standard methadone services for opioid-dependent patients: A comparison of clinical efficacy and cost. *American Journal of Psychiatry* 156(1):27-33.

Bach PB & Lantos J (1999). Methadone dosing, heroin affordability, and the severity of addiction. *American Journal of Public Health* 89(5):662-665.

Barnett PG (1999). The cost-effectiveness of methadone maintenance as a health care intervention. *Addiction* 94(4):479-488.

Brooner RK, King VL, Kidorf M et al. (1997). Psychiatric and substance use comorbidity among treatment-seeking opioid abusers. *Archives of General Psychiatry* 54(1):71-80.

Calsyn DA, Wells EA, Saxon AJ et al. (1994). Contingency management of urinalysis results and intensity of counseling services have an interactive impact on methadone maintenance treatment outcome. *Journal of Addictive Diseases* 13(3):47-63.

Chamot E, de Saussure PH, Hirschel B et al. (1992). Incidence of hepatitis C, hepatitis B and HIV infections among drug users in a methadone maintenance programme [letter]. *AIDS* 6:430-431.

Chandrasekar PH & Narula AP (1986). Bone and joint infections in intravenous drug abusers. *Reviews of Infectious Diseases* 6:904-911.

Cooper JR (1995). Including narcotic addiction treatment in an office-based practice. *Journal of the American Medical Association* 273(20):1619-1620.

Cushman P (1980). The major medical sequelae of opioid addiction. *Drug and Alcohol Dependence* 5:239-254.

Darke S & Zador D (1996). Fatal heroin "overdose": A review. *Addiction* 91(12):1765-1772.

Dieperink E, Willenbring M & Ho SB (2000). Neuropsychiatric symptoms associated with hepatitis C and interferon alpha: A review. *American Journal of Psychiatry* 157:867-876.

Eap CB, Bertschy G, Baumann P et al. (1998). High interindividual variability of methadone enantiomer blood levels to dose ratios [letter]. *Archives of General Psychiatry* 55(1):89-90.

Fiellin DA, O'Connor PG, Chawarski M et al. (2001). Methadone maintenance in primary care: A randomized controlled trial. *Journal of the American Medical Association* 286:1724-1731.

Gossop M, Marsden J, Stewart D et al. (1999). Methadone treatment practices and outcome for opiate addicts treated in drug clinics and in general practice: Results from the National Treatment Outcome Research Study. *British Journal of General Practice* 49(438):31-34.

Greenblatt J (1997). *Year-End Preliminary Estimates from the 1996 Drug Abuse Warning Network*. Rockville, MD: Office of Applied Studies, U.S. Department of Health and Human Services.

Gruer L, Wilson P, Scott R et al. (1997). General practitioner centred scheme for treatment of opiate dependent drug injectors in Glasgow. *British Medical Journal* 314(7096):1730-1735.

Hamid A, Curtis R, McCoy K et al. (1997). The heroin epidemic in New York City: Current status and prognoses. *Journal of Psychoactive Drugs* 29(4):375-391.

Hanlon TE, Nurco DN, Kinlock TW et al. (1990). Trends in criminal activity and drug use over an addiction career. *American Journal of Drug & Alcohol Abuse* 16(3-4):223-238.

Haverkos HW & Lange WR (1990). Serious infections other than human immunodeficiency virus among intravenous drug abusers. *Journal of Infectious Diseases* 161:894-902.

Hunt DE, Lipton DS, Goldsmith DS et al. (1985). "It takes your heart": The image of methadone maintenance in the addict world and its effect on recruitment into treatment. *International Journal of the Addictions* 20(11-12):1751-1771.

Hutchinson SJ, Taylor A, Gruer L et al. (2000). One-year follow-up of opiate injectors treated with oral methadone in a GP-centred programme. *Addiction* 95(7):1055-1068.

Jacobs EA & Bickel WK (1999). Precipitated withdrawal in an opioid-dependent outpatient receiving alternate-day buprenorphine dosing [letter]. *Addiction* 94(1):140-141.

King VL, Stoller KB, Hayes M et al. (2002). A multicenter randomized evaluation of methadone medical maintenance. *Drug and Alcohol Dependence* 65(2):137-148.

Kraft MK, Rothbard AB, Hadley TR et al. (1997). Are supplementary services provided during methadone maintenance really cost-effective? *American Journal of Psychiatry* 154(9):1214-1219.

Maddux JF, Desmond DP & Vogtsberger KN (1995). Patient-regulated methadone dose and optional counseling in methadone maintenance. *American Journal on Addictions* 4(1):18-32.

Makower RM, Pennycook AG & Moulton C (1992). Intravenous drug abusers attending an inner city accident and emergency department. *Archives of Emergency Medicine* 9:32-39.

Mason BJ, Kocsis JH, Melia D et al. (1998). Psychiatric comorbidity in methadone maintained patients. *Journal of Addictive Diseases* 17(3):75-89.

McLellan AT, Arndt IO, Metzger DS et al. (1993). The effects of psychosocial services in substance abuse treatment. *Journal of the American Medical Association* 269(15):1953-1959.

Merrill JO, Jackson TR, Schulman BA et al. (2002). Methadone maintenance in primary care. *Journal of General Internal Medicine*.

Moatti JP, Souville M, Escaffre N et al. (1998). French general practitioners' attitudes toward maintenance drug abuse treatment with buprenorphine. *Addiction* 93(10):1567-1575.

Modie N (1999). More heroin addicts may be offered treatment. *Seattle Post-Intelligencer* December 8.

Musto DF (1987). *The American Disease*. New York, NY: Oxford University Press.

National Consensus Development Panel on Effective Medical Treatment of Opiate Addiction (Consensus Development Panel) (1998). Effective medical treatment of opiate addiction. *Journal of the American Medical Association* 280(22):136-143.

National Institute of Justice (NIJ), U.S. Department of Justice (2000). *Arrestee Drug Abuse Monitoring Annual Report, 1999 Adult Program Findings*. Available at: WWW.NCJRS.ORG/PDFFILES1/NIJ/99ADLTFIND.PDF.

Novick DM & Joseph H (1991). Medical maintenance: The treatment of chronic opiate dependence in general medical practice. *Journal of Substance Abuse Treatment* 8(4):233-239.

Novick DM, Joseph H, Salsitz EA et al. (1994). Outcomes of treatment of socially rehabilitated methadone maintenance patients in physicians' offices (medical maintenance): Follow-up at three and a half to nine and a fourth years. *Journal of General Internal Medicine* 9(3):127-130.

Novick DM, Pascarelli EF, Joseph H et al. (1988). Methadone maintenance patients in general medical practice. A preliminary report. *Journal of the American Medical Association* 259(22):3299-3302.

O'Connor PG, Oliveto AH, Shi JM et al. (1998). A randomized trial of buprenorphine maintenance for heroin dependence in a primary care clinic for substance users versus a methadone clinic. *American Journal of Medicine* 105(2):100-105.

O'Donnell AE & Pappas LS (1988). Pulmonary complications of intravenous drug abuse, experience at an inner city hospital. *Chest* 94:251-253.

Peters AD & Reid MM (1998). Methadone treatment in the Scottish context: Outcomes of a community-based service for drug users in Lothian. *Drug & Alcohol Dependence* 50(1):47-55.

Roane KR (1997). Legislation for those with a methadone clinic next door. *New York Times*, April 6.

Rostami-Hodjegan A, Wolff K, Hay AW et al. (1999). Population pharmacokinetics of methadone in opiate users: Characterization of time-dependent changes. *British Journal of Clinical Pharmacology* 48(1):43-52.

Rubin AM (1987). Neurologic complications of intravenous drug abuse. *Hospital Practice* 22:279-288.

Salsitz EA, Joseph H, Fran B et al. (2000). Methadone medical maintenance (MMM): Treating chronic opioid dependence in private medical practice—A summary report (1983-1998). *Mount Sinai Journal of Medicine* 67(5-6):388-397.

Saxon AJ, Calsyn DA, Haver VM et al. (1990). A nationwide survey of urinalysis practices of methadone maintenance clinics. Utilization of laboratory services. *Archives of Pathology & Laboratory Medicine* 114(1):94-100.

Schwartz RP, Brooner RK, Montoya ID et al. (1999). A 12-year follow-up of a methadone medical maintenance program. *American Journal on Addictions* 8(4):293-299.

Selwyn PA, Alcabes P & Hartel D (1992). Clinical manifestations and predictors of disease progression in drug users with human immunodeficiency virus infection. *New England Journal of Medicine* 327:1697-1703.

Senay EC, Barthwell AG, Marks R et al. (1993). Medical maintenance: A pilot study. *Journal of Addictive Diseases* 12(4):59-76.

Sporer KA (1999). Acute heroin overdose. *Annals of Internal Medicine*, 130(7):584-590.

Strain EC, Preston KL, Liebson IA et al. (1995). Buprenorphine effects in methadone-maintained volunteers: Effects at two hours after methadone. *Journal of Pharmacology & Experimental Therapeutics* 272(2):628-638.

Substance Abuse and Mental Health Services Administration (SAMHSA) (1999). Press Release, July 22, 1999. Available at: HTTP://WWW.SAMHSA.GOV/PRESS/99/990722NR.HTM.

Substance Abuse and Mental Health Services Administration (SAMHSA) (2000). *Mortality Data from the Drug Abuse Warning Network, 1998.* Available at WWW.SAMHSA.GOV/OAS/DAWN.HTM#MECOMP.

Substance Abuse and Mental Health Services Administration (SAMHSA) (2002). *Year-End 2000 Emergency Department Data from the Drug Abuse Warning Network.* Available at WWW.SAMHSA.GOV/OAS/DAWN.HTM#EDCOMP.

Vignau J & Brunelle E (1998). Differences between general practitioner- and addiction-centre-prescribed buprenorphine substitution therapy in France. *European Addiction Research* 4(Suppl 1):24-28.

Walsh SL, Preston KL, Bigelow GE et al. (1995). Acute administration of buprenorphine in humans: Partial agonist and blockade effects. *Journal of Pharmacology & Experimental Therapeutics* 274(1):361-372.

Weinrich M & Stuart M (2000). Provision of methadone treatment in primary care medical practices: Review of the Scottish experience and implications for U.S. policy. *Journal of the American Medical Association* 283(10):1343-1348.

Wilson P, Watson R & Ralston GE (1994). Methadone maintenance in general practice: Patients, workload, and outcomes. *British Medical Journal* 309(6955):641-644.

Wren CS (1997). Ex-addicts find methadone more elusive than heroin. *New York Times*, February 2.

Wren CS (1998). Holding an uneasy line in the long war on heroin; Methadone emerged in city now debating it. *New York Times*, October 3.

| Chapter 6

Pharmacologic Interventions for Cocaine, Crack, and Other Stimulant Addiction

David A. Gorelick, M.D., Ph.D.

Cocaine Addiction
Choice of Medication
Amphetamine Addiction
Special Treatment Situations

Pharmacologic treatment of cocaine addiction is widely practiced in the United States. An anonymous mail survey of physicians practicing addiction medicine found that 59% of respondents used medication to help prevent relapse to cocaine use after initial abstinence. Fifteen different medications were reported used, despite the physicians' own doubts about their effectiveness (Gorelick, Halikas et al., 1994). This finding reflects the lack of agreement on effective pharmacotherapy for cocaine addiction (including the absence of any medication approved by the U.S. Food and Drug Administration [FDA] for this indication) and the paucity of replicated, scientifically rigorous studies to support the efficacy of any particular medication (Gorelick, 1999; O'Leary & Weiss, 2000). Despite this state of knowledge, both clinical and scientific interest in pharmacologic treatment continues to be stimulated by the often disappointing success rate of current psychosocial treatment approaches (Carroll, 2000; Carroll & Schottenfeld, 1997).

This chapter reviews the current state of pharmacologic treatment of cocaine addiction, including choice of medication and medications for use in special treatment situations, such as patients with mixed addictions or psychiatric comorbidities. Emphasis is given to the use of medications in clinical practice, rather than to laboratory studies or preclinical pharmacology. (For more detailed coverage of pharmacology, see Section 2.)

Most of the clinical and clinical research literature deals with cocaine, rather than other stimulants such as the amphetamines or methylphenidate; therefore, little mention is made of the latter in this chapter. The extent to which findings related to cocaine addiction can be extrapolated to other stimulant addictions remains unclear.

COCAINE ADDICTION

Goals of Treatment. The goals of pharmacologic treatment of cocaine addiction are the same as for any other treatment modality; that is, to help patients abstain from cocaine use and regain control of their lives. The behavioral mechanisms by which medication achieves these goals are poorly understood and can vary across patients and medications. In theory, medication could shift the balance of reinforcement away from cocaine-taking in favor of other behaviors through several mechanisms: (1) by reducing or eliminating the positive reinforcement from taking a cocaine dose (for example, by reducing the euphoria or "high"), (2) by reducing or eliminating a subjective state (such as "craving") that predisposes to taking cocaine, (3) by reducing or eliminating negative reinforcement from taking a cocaine dose (as by reducing withdrawal-associated dysphoria), (4) by making cocaine-taking aversive, or (5) by increasing the positive reinforcement obtained from non-cocaine-taking behaviors. Currently available medications are considered to act by one or more of the first three mechanisms, and these mechanisms are the focus of research in medications development. No research addresses the fourth mechanism (which would be analogous to use of disulfiram [Antabuse®] in treating alcoholism). The fifth mechanism is crucial to successful treatment because it ensures that other behaviors are reinforced to replace cocaine-taking as the latter is extinguished, but such medications do not exist. In current practice, this mechanism is engaged by psychosocial interventions that address issues such as vocational rehabilitation, the patient's social network, and use of leisure time.

Because of the importance of this mechanism, as well as other factors, medication almost never is used without some psychosocial treatment component. Few controlled clinical trials explicitly compare the efficacy of medication use with and without psychosocial treatment (Carroll, Rounsaville et al., 1994; Henningfield & Singleton, 1994), so the relative contributions of pharmacologic and psychosocial treatments are unknown. The type, intensity, and duration of psychosocial treatment that should accompany pharmacologic treatment are questions with little data to guide clinical decisionmaking (Carroll, 1997). At a minimum, one would expect that addressing psychosocial factors that influence medication compliance would improve treatment outcome.

Pharmacologic Mechanisms. At least four pharmacologic approaches are potentially useful in the treatment of cocaine addiction (Gorelick, 1999). These approaches are (1) substitution treatment with a cross-tolerant stimulant (analogous to methadone maintenance treatment of opiate addiction), (2) treatment with an antagonist medication that blocks the binding of cocaine at its site of action (true pharmacologic antagonism, analogous to naltrexone [ReVia®] treatment of opiate addiction), (3) treatment with a medication that functionally antagonizes the effects of cocaine (as by reducing the reinforcing effects of or craving for cocaine), and (4) alteration of cocaine pharmacokinetics so that less drug reaches or remains at its site(s) of action in the brain.

No medication currently is approved by the FDA for the treatment of cocaine addiction, chiefly because no medication has met the scientifically rigorous standard of consistent, statistically significant efficacy in replicated, controlled clinical trials. Most current clinical and research attention has focused on the second and third approaches mentioned above: reducing or blocking cocaine's actions, either directly at its neuronal binding site (true pharmacologic antagonism) or indirectly by otherwise reducing its reinforcing effects. The first approach has been evaluated in a small number of clinical trials, with mixed results. The fourth approach has not yet been used clinically, but has shown promise in some animal studies and a Phase I clinical trial.

Cocaine has two major neuropharmacologic actions: blockade of presynaptic neurotransmitter reuptake pumps, resulting in psychomotor stimulant effects, and blockade of sodium ion channels in nerve membranes, resulting in local anesthetic effects (Gorelick, 1999; Newman, 2000). Cocaine's positively reinforcing effects are believed to derive from its blockade of the dopamine reuptake pump, causing presynaptically released dopamine to remain in the synapse and enhancing dopaminergic neurotransmission (Gorelick, 1999; Wise, 1998). Cocaine's local anesthetic effects are believed to contribute to cocaine-induced kindling, the phenomenon by which previous exposure to cocaine sensitizes the individual so that later exposure to low doses produces an enhanced response.

CHOICE OF MEDICATION

Antidepressants. *Heterocyclic Antidepressants*: Tricyclic and other heterocyclic antidepressants are the most widely used and best studied class of medications for the treatment of cocaine addiction. Their use is based both on the clinical observation of frequent depressive symptoms among cocaine addicts seeking treatment and on their pharmacologic mechanism of increasing biogenic amine neurotransmitter activity in synapses. Such increase is achieved by inhibiting presynaptic neurotransmitter reuptake pumps, thus ameliorating a hypothesized neurotransmitter deficiency, especially of dopamine, caused by chronic cocaine use.

Desipramine (Norpramin®) was the first medication found effective in an outpatient, double-blind, controlled clinical trial—a finding that received wide publicity even before the complete study was published in a peer-reviewed journal. As a result, desipramine is the best studied of the tricyclic antidepressants, with more than a half dozen controlled clinical trials in the published literature. Typical doses are 150 to 300 mg/day (about 2.5 mg/kg), similar to those used in the treatment of depression. Although an early meta-analysis found desipramine significantly effective in reducing relapse to cocaine use, although not in initiating abstinence (Levin & Lehman, 1991; Delucchi, 1992), later and larger controlled trials have not confirmed desipramine's efficacy (Arndt, Dorozynsky et al., 1992; Campbell, Thomas et al., 1994; Carroll, Nich et al., 1995) or have found it effective only for short periods (4 or 6 but not 8 or 12 weeks) and in less severely addicted patients (Carroll, Rounsaville et al., 1994; Kosten, Morgan et al., 1992).

Retrospective data analyses suggest that patient characteristics can account for some of the differential efficacy of desipramine in various studies; for example, patients with depression (Ziedonis & Kosten, 1991) and without antisocial personality disorder (Arndt, McLellan et al., 1994) may respond best to desipramine.

One factor that can influence efficacy is plasma level of medication. Preliminary evidence from some clinical trials suggests that desipramine can have a therapeutic "ceiling" in terms of plasma level, with steady-state plasma levels above 200 ng/mL associated with poorer outcomes than lower levels (Khalsa, Gawin et al., 1993). This ceiling effect can be related, in part, to anecdotal reports that, at higher desipramine doses (and presumably higher plasma levels), some patients have subjective effects that they experience as somewhat similar to those produced by cocaine itself, with consequent stimulation of cocaine craving (Weiss & Mirin, 1989). These findings would support keeping desipramine at moderate dose levels, rather than pushing for the maximum tolerated dose, and adjusting the dose downward if the patient is taking concomitant medication (such as methadone) that inhibits desipramine metabolism.

There is no convincing pharmacologic rationale for preferring desipramine over other heterocyclic antidepressants. Limited experience with imipramine (Tofranil®) and maprotiline (Ludiomil®) at antidepressant doses found equivocal evidence of efficacy (Brotman, Witkie et al., 1988; Nunes, McGrath et al., 1995).

No unexpected or medically serious side effects have been reported to date from clinical trials of tricyclic antidepressants. However, patients who relapse to cocaine use while still on antidepressant medications could, in theory, be at increased risk of cardiovascular side effects. Both cocaine and the tricyclics have quinidine-like membrane effects that, when superimposed, could lead to cardiac arrhythmias or sudden death. The concurrent administration of cocaine and desipramine (blood levels above 100 ng/mL) to research volunteers has produced additive increases in heart rate and blood pressure (Fischman, Foltin et al., 1990). This potential cardiotoxicity, although not yet actually observed in any clinical trial, should be considered when prescribing tricyclics for patients with other cardiovascular risk factors, such as a history of coronary artery disease, arrhythmia, or recent myocardial infarction.

Selective Serotonin Reuptake Inhibitors (SSRIs): Antidepressants that specifically block the presynaptic serotonin reuptake pump have attracted interest because of the role of serotonin in inhibiting appetitive behaviors (Sellers, Higgins et al., 1991). Four double-blind, controlled clinical trials have not found any advantage for fluoxetine (Prozac®; 20, 40, or 60 mg/day) over placebo (Batki, Washburn et al., 1996; Covi, Hess et al., 1995; Grabowski, Rhoades et al., 1995), although treatment retention was improved in two of the studies.

Monoamine Oxidase Inhibitors: The rationale for use of monoamine oxidase (MAO) inhibitors lies in their effect of increasing brain levels of biogenic amine neurotransmitters by inhibiting a major catabolic enzyme. Limited open-label experience with phenelzine, at antidepressant doses of 30 to 90 mg/day, suggests that this medication can reduce cocaine and other stimulant use (Brewer, 1993; Maletzky, 1977). However, its clinical usefulness may be limited by the need for dietary and concomitant medication restrictions to avoid precipitating a hypertensive crisis, as well as by the theoretical possibility of potentiating cocaine-induced effects should the patient relapse to cocaine use while still taking the medication. Some researchers have argued that fear of such an aversive, potentially life-threatening reaction is what motivates abstinence while taking an MAO inhibitor (Brewer, 1993), making the mechanism of action analogous to that of disulfiram for alcoholism.

Current research is focusing on selective MAO inhibitors that act only on MAO type B, the predominant type in the brain, while sparing MAO type A, the predominant type in the gastrointestinal tract. It is inhibition of MAO in the gastrointestinal tract that produces a hypertensive crisis ("cheese reaction") after ingestion of tyramine-containing foods or certain catecholaminergic medications. Selegiline (Eldepryl®), marketed for the treatment of parkinsonism, is fairly selective for MAO type B at recommended doses (10 mg/day) and is being studied as a treatment for cocaine addiction. However, one small, open-label outpatient study found it ineffective (Tennant, Tarver et al., 1993), and a recently completed multisite controlled clinical trial reportedly found little evidence for efficacy.

Other Antidepressants: The "second generation" antidepressant bupropion (Wellbutrin®) has attracted interest because it increases brain dopamine activity by binding to the same presynaptic dopamine reuptake site as does cocaine. Although well tolerated by cocaine addicts at antidepressant doses (100 mg three times a day), a double-blind, placebo-controlled trial among inpatients found no significant effect on cocaine craving (Hollister, Krajewski et al., 1992), and a multisite outpatient-controlled clinical trial in methadone-maintained cocaine addicts found no significant effect on cocaine use (Margolin, Kosten et al., 1995).

Nefazodone (Serzone®), another second generation antidepressant, had no significant effect on cocaine use in a controlled clinical trial among cocaine-abusing women (Specker, Crosby et al., 2000).

Ritanserin, a 5-HT$_2$ receptor antagonist developed as an antidepressant, attracted interest because of animal studies showing that it reduced cocaine self-administration (although this effect was not replicated in all studies). However, two recent controlled clinical trials found ritanserin no better than placebo in reducing cocaine use (Cornish, Maany et al., 2001; Johnson, Chen et al., 1997).

Dopamine Agonists (Anti-Parkinson agents). A variety of dopamine agonist medications have been tried for the treatment of cocaine addiction, based on the dopamine depletion hypothesis (Dackis & Gold, 1985), although the data supporting the hypothesis in human subjects are equivocal (Gorelick, 1999). Dopamine agonists, by stimulating synaptic dopamine activity, would ameliorate the effects of decreased dopamine activity caused by cessation of cocaine use; these include anhedonia, anergia, depression, and cocaine craving. In rats, dopamine receptor agonists such as bromocriptine (Parlodel®) and lisuride reduce cocaine self-administration and reverse the reduced metabolic rate and elevated intracranial self-stimulation threshold produced in dopaminergic mesocorticolimbic brain areas after cessation of chronic cocaine administration (Clow & Hammer, 1991; Markou & Koob, 1992; Pulvirenti & Koob, 1994).

Bromocriptine, pergolide (Permax®), and amantadine (Symmetrel®), all marketed for the treatment of parkinsonism (another dopamine deficiency condition), are the most commonly used dopamine agonist medications. Studies of cocaine craving among hospitalized cocaine addicts have yielded mixed results (Eiler, Schaefer et al., 1995; Wang, Kalbfleisch et al., 1994). Results of outpatient

double-blind clinical trials with bromocriptine are inconclusive. Several such trials from one research group have consistently found bromocriptine (2.5 to 10 mg/day) better than placebo, but they used psychological symptoms rather than actual cocaine use as the outcome measure, making the relevance of the results to addiction treatment unclear (Giannini, Folts et al., 1989). Of two small (7 and 29 patients, respectively), short-term (10 and 15 days, respectively) outpatient trials using urine toxicology results as the outcome measure, the first found an increase in cocaine-negative urine tests but had no placebo comparison group (Tennant & Sagherian, 1987), while the second found no significant decrease in cocaine-positive urine tests (Moscovitz, Brookoff et al., 1993). A third, larger (69 patients) placebo-controlled trial found no significant effect on cocaine use (Hill, Wilkins et al., 1996). Two controlled clinical trials of pergolide found it worse than placebo (Levin, McDowell et al., 1999; Malcolm, Herron et al., 2001).

The use of bromocriptine is limited by side effects such as headache, nausea, and abdominal cramps. These side effects tend to be related to high individual doses (2.5 mg or more) and rapid dose escalation. They can be avoided by use of low starting doses, divided daily doses (three or four times a day), and limiting dose increases to no more often than every three days. Bromocriptine should be used very cautiously in postpartum women because of an increased risk of vasospastic complications and seizures (Bakht, Kirshon et al., 1990).

Results of clinical trials of amantadine also have been disappointing. Only one of six well-designed double-blind, placebo-controlled studies found that amantadine (200 to 400 mg/day) reduced cocaine use more than did placebo (Alterman, Droba et al., 1992; Arndt, Dorozynsky et al., 1992; Kampman, Volpicelli et al., 2000; Kolar, Brown et al., 1992; Kosten, Morgan et al., 1992; Weddington, Brown et al., 1991). However, a recent re-analysis of one of the negative studies found a significant benefit from amantadine (100 mg 3 times a day) among patients with more severe cocaine withdrawal symptoms (Kampman, Volpicelli et al., 2000).

Pramipexole (Mirapex®), a potent dopamine receptor agonist marketed for Parkinson's disease, was found in a single case report to abolish cocaine craving and use at 1.5 mg/day (Rosenbaum & Fredman, 1999).

The amino acid L-DOPA, a precursor for the synthesis of catecholamines, has been used to increase brain dopamine levels in the treatment of cocaine addiction, both alone and in combination with carbidopa (Sinemet®), a peripheral amino acid decarboxylase inhibitor that prevents systemic side effects by blocking the conversion of L-DOPA to dopamine outside the brain. This approach is successful in the treatment of parkinsonism, but it has had only mixed success in short-term, open-label studies of cocaine addiction at doses in the low range of those used to treat parkinsonism (Rosen, Flemenbaum et al., 1986; Tennant, Tarver et al., 1993). L-tyrosine, the amino acid precursor of L-DOPA, reduced cocaine craving in a small (12 patients) double-blind study of inpatients (Cold, 1996), but was not effective in reducing cocaine use in two outpatient clinical trials at 2 g every eight hours (open-label) or 800 or 1,600 mg twice a day (double-blind) (Galloway, Frederick et al., 1996; Thomas, Campbell et al., 1996).

Disulfiram. Disulfiram (Antabuse®) can be considered a functional dopamine agonist because it blocks the conversion of dopamine to norepinephrine by the enzyme dopamine-alpha-hydroxylase, thereby increasing dopamine concentrations. Interest in disulfiram as a treatment for cocaine addiction initially was generated by suggestions of its efficacy in patients with both cocaine addiction and alcoholism, a common comorbidity. Two recent controlled clinical trials in cocaine addicts with concurrent opiate dependence (being treated with methadone or buprenorphine), but without alcoholism, found disulfiram (250 mg/day) significantly better than placebo in promoting cocaine abstinence (George, Chawarski et al., 2000; Petrakis, Carroll et al., 2000). A human laboratory study found that pretreatment with disulfiram (250 mg daily for three days) significantly prolonged cocaine's plasma half-life, increased plasma cocaine concentrations, and potentiated the tachycardic and hypertensive effects of intranasal cocaine (1 or 2 mg/kg) (McCance-Katz, Kosten et al., 1998). These findings suggest that disulfiram may be a promising new treatment for cocaine addiction, although raising a caution about potential adverse drug interactions should patients use cocaine while on the medication.

Stimulants. By analogy with methadone maintenance treatment of opiate addiction (see Chapters 3, 4, and 5 of this section) or nicotine replacement treatment of tobacco dependence (see Chapter 7 of this section), maintenance treatment of cocaine addicts with stimulant medication might be clinically beneficial in reducing cocaine craving and use. As with methadone, advantages might include use of the less medically risky oral route of administration (ver-

sus injected or smoked cocaine), use of pure medication of known potency (thus avoiding contaminant effects or inadvertent overdose), and use of a medication with slower onset and longer duration of action (thus avoiding "rush"/"crash" cycling) (Gorelick, 1998).

Several orally active psychomotor stimulants marketed for the treatment of attention deficit/hyperactivity disorder (ADHD) and narcolepsy or as appetite suppressants (anorexiants) have been used to test the substitution approach, with only limited success. An early case series of five patients (without ADHD) who received methylphenidate (Ritalin®, up to 100 mg/day; recommended doses for ADHD or narcolepsy are 10 to 60 mg/day) for two to five weeks found it detrimental (Gawin, Riordan et al., 1985). Cocaine craving and use increased in four patients, and there was concern about the abuse potential of methylphenidate (which is classified in Schedule II of the federal Controlled Substances Act). More recent experience with sustained-release methylphenidate (20 mg twice a day) suggests it may have less abuse potential, although its efficacy remains uncertain (Grabowski, Roache et al., 1997; Roache, Grabowski et al., 2000). A recent controlled clinical trial found sustained-release d-amphetamine (30 or 60 mg/day) better than placebo in reducing the proportion of cocaine-positive urine samples over 12 weeks (Grabowski, Rhoades et al., 2000b). Another Schedule II anorexiant, phenmetrazine (Preludin®), increased cocaine use in a small, open-label outpatient study when used at or slightly above the recommended dose of 50 to 75 mg/day (Tennant, Tarver et al., 1993).

Several marketed stimulants with less abuse potential (Schedule IV) have yielded disappointing results. Pemoline (Cylert®, 75 to 225 mg/day for several weeks) did not reduce cocaine use in a case series of outpatients without ADHD (Margolin, Avants et al., 1996), although it does seem effective in patients with comorbid ADHD. Diethylpropion (up to 75 mg/day for two weeks) did not reduce cocaine craving (both spontaneous and cocaine-cue elicited) among inpatients in a double-blind trial (Alim, Rosse et al., 1995). Mazindol was ineffective in three double-blind outpatient studies (at 1, 2, or 2 to 4 mg/day) (Kosten, Steinberg et al., 1993; Margolin, Avants et al., 1995; Stine, Krystal et al., 1995).

In principle, cocaine itself, in a slow-onset formulation or route of administration, might be used for agonist maintenance treatment (Gorelick, 1998; Walsh, Haberny et al., 2000), in the same way that slow-onset transdermal or transbuccal nicotine is used to treat addiction to rapid-onset smoked nicotine (cigarettes). Oral cocaine (100 mg four times a day) significantly attenuates the response to an intravenous cocaine challenge (25 mg) (Walsh, Haberny et al., 2000) and, in the form of coca tea, has been used successfully to reduce cocaine smoking in an open-label case series in Lima, Peru (where oral cocaine products are legal) (Llosa, 1994).

Neuroleptics. The older (so-called "typical") neuroleptics marketed in the U.S. for treatment of psychosis, which are potent dopamine receptor antagonists (chiefly D_2 [postsynaptic] subtype), do not appear to significantly alter cocaine craving or use, as evidenced by clinical experience with cocaine-abusing schizophrenics who receive chronic neuroleptic treatment (Brady, Anton et al., 1990; Farren, Hameedi et al., 2000; Ohuoha, Maxwell et al., 1997). The neuroleptic flupenthixol, which is not marketed in the U.S. but is available in Canada and Europe, markedly decreased cocaine craving and use in a case series of 10 Bahamian "crack" cocaine addicts, but results of a double-blind, outpatient trial in the U.S. have not yet been published (Soyka & De Vry, 2000).

Greater efficacy was expected from the newer "atypical" neuroleptics, in part because of their different spectrum of receptor binding (that is, to dopamine D_1 and serotonin). However, recent controlled clinical trials did not find olanzapine (Zyprexa®, 10 mg/day) (Reid, Leiderman et al., 2000) or risperidone (Risperdal®, 1 to 6 mg/day) (Grabowski, Rhoades et al., 2000a; Levin, McDowell et al., 1999) any better than placebo in reducing cocaine use.

Caution should be exercised when prescribing any neuroleptic to cocaine users because of their potential vulnerability to the neuroleptic malignant syndrome, based on their presumed cocaine-induced dopamine depletion (Akpaffiong & Ruiz, 1991). Cocaine or amphetamine users also can be at elevated risk of neuroleptic-induced movement disorders (Decker & Ries, 1993; van Harten, van Trier et al., 1998) and for cardiovascular side effects from clozapine (Clozaril®) (Farren, Hameedi et al., 2000).

Anticonvulsants. Anticonvulsants have been tried in the treatment of cocaine addiction because they block the development of cocaine-induced kindling in animals. Kindling (increased neuronal sensitivity to a drug because of prior intermittent exposure) has been hypothesized as a neurophysiologic mediator of cocaine craving in humans (Halikas & Kuhn, 1990). Carbamazepine (Tegretol®) has been the most studied, but the promise of early open-label studies has not been confirmed in controlled trials. Four of five double-blind outpatient trials found no significant effect on cocaine craving or use (Lima, Lima et al., 2000; Montoya, Levin et al., 1995).

Other anticonvulsants have shown inconsistent effects in small-scale studies. Gabapentin (Neurontin®, 800 to 2,400 mg/day) and lamotrigine (Lamictal®, 300 mg/day), which are considered to influence glutamatergic kindling mechanisms, were found to reduce cocaine use in some (Margolin, Avants et al., 1998; Myrick, Henderson et al., 2001; Raby, 2000) but not all (Berger, Leiderman et al., 2000) open-label trials and case series. Valproic acid (Depakene®) was ineffective in both a small, open-label study (500 to 1,000 mg/day) (Tennant, Tarver et al., 1993) and a recent controlled clinical trial (1,500 mg/day) (Reid, Leiderman et al., 2000). Phenytoin (Dilantin®, 300 mg/day) significantly reduced cocaine use in a double-blind outpatient trial, especially at serum concentrations above 6.0 µg/mL (Crosby, Pearson et al., 1996), but did not alter self-administration of smoked cocaine or the drug's psychological effects in a human laboratory study at concentrations of 8 to 20 µg/mL (Sofuoglu, Pentel et al., 1999).

Nutritional Supplements and Herbal Products. *Nutritional Supplements*: The use of amino acid mixtures, either alone or with other nutritional supplements (vitamins and minerals), has been widely publicized in the drug abuse treatment field, encouraged by their freedom from the regulations imposed on prescription medications and their perceived safety and absence of side effects. Proprietary mixtures, including tyrosine and L-tryptophan (the amino acid precursor of serotonin), have been marketed with claims of efficacy (Blum, Allison et al., 1988), but a double-blind, 28-day cross-over study found no significant effect of tyrosine and tryptophan (1 g of each daily) on cocaine craving or withdrawal symptoms (Chadwick & Gregory, 1990). L-carnitine (500 mg/day) plus coenzyme Q10 (200 mg/day) was no better than placebo in an eight-week controlled clinical trial (Reid, Leiderman et al., 2000).

Herbal Products: Various herbal and plant-derived products have been touted as treatments for drug abuse, but few have undergone controlled clinical evaluation. One that has received substantial publicity, but not yet clinical evaluation, is ibogaine, an indole alkaloid found in the root bark of the West African shrub *Tabernanthe iboga*. This compound has been claimed to suppress cocaine (and opiate and alcohol) withdrawal and craving for several months after a single oral dose (Szumlinski, Maisonneuve et al., 2001). Ginkgo biloba (120 mg/day for 8 weeks) was no better than placebo in a controlled clinical trial (Kampman, Majewska et al., 2000).

Lithium. Both double-blind and open-label studies have found lithium, at doses and plasma levels used in the treatment of bipolar disorder, ineffective for the treatment of cocaine addiction (Nunes, McGrath et al., 1990).

Calcium Channel Blockers. Calcium channel blockers have been suggested as treatment for cocaine addiction because of their effects on neurotransmitter release and inhibition of cocaine's psychological effects in some, but not all, studies of human research volunteers (Kosten, Woods et al., 1999). However, amlodipine (Norvasc®), diltiazem (Cardizem®), and nifedipine (Procardia®) showed little or no efficacy in two open-label outpatient case series (Malcolm, Brady et al., 1999; Tennant, Tarver et al., 1993), nor did nimodipine (Nimotop®) reduce cocaine craving in a double-blind inpatient study (Rosse, Alim et al., 1994).

Other Medications. Fenfluramine, a serotonin-releasing agent formerly marketed as an appetite suppressant, was not effective in reducing cocaine use in a double-blind trial among methadone-maintained cocaine addicts (Batki, Bradley et al., 1996). It was withdrawn from the market in 1997. A controlled clinical trial of the beta-adrenergic blocker propanolol (up to 80 mg/day) found it no better than placebo, except in outpatients with more severe cocaine withdrawal (Kampman, Volpicelli et al., 2001). Naltrexone, a mu-opiate receptor antagonist marketed for the treatment of alcoholism and opiate dependence, showed some efficacy at 50 mg/day in cocaine-dependent outpatients without alcohol or opiate dependence, but only when combined with relapse prevention therapy (Schmitz, Stotts et al., 2001). Baclofen (Lioresal®, 20 mg three times a day), a gamma-aminobutyric acid B (GABA$_B$) receptor agonist marketed as a muscle relaxant, reduced cocaine craving and use in a small case series (Ling, Shoptaw et al., 1998). GABA is an inhibitory neurotransmitter that inhibits dopamine release and attenuates the reinforcing effects of cocaine in rats (Roberts & Brebner, 2000).

Medication Combinations. Concurrent use of two different medications is being studied in the hope that such combinations will enhance efficacy while minimizing side effects, either by acting on a single neurotransmitter system by two different mechanisms or by acting on two different neurotransmitter systems. Concurrent open-label use of the dopaminergic agents bupropion and bromocriptine (Parlodel®) in outpatient cocaine addicts has been found safe, albeit with little suggestion of efficacy (Montoya, Preston et al., 2002). Concurrent use of pergolide (a dopamine D$_1$/D$_2$ receptor agonist) and haloperidol (Haldol®, a dopamine D$_2$ receptor antagonist), designed to produce relatively pure D$_1$ agonist action, also found little evidence of efficacy (Malcolm, Moore et al., 1999).

The combined use of the dopamine releaser phentermine and the serotonin releaser fenfluramine, each marketed as an appetite suppressant, received substantial publicity as the so-called "phen-fen" treatment for obesity and addictive disorder. This medication combination had mixed results in the outpatient treatment of cocaine addiction (Kampman, Rukstalis et al., 2000). The combination no longer is available since the withdrawal of fenfluramine because of its association with primary pulmonary hypertension and valvular heart disease (Connolly & McGoon, 1999). Combinations that replace fenfluramine with an SSRI such as fluoxetine have not been systematically evaluated.

Other Physical Treatments. Acupuncture is an ancient Chinese treatment that involves mechanical (with needles), thermal (moxibustion), or electrical (electroacupuncture) stimulation of specific points on the body surface (Brewington, Smith et al., 1994). The mechanism of action is unknown; speculation has included stimulation of endogenous opiate systems. Acupuncture of the ear has enjoyed growing popularity as a treatment for drug withdrawal (Brewington, Smith et al., 1994; Lipton, Brewington et al., 1994), but there have been few controlled trials of efficacy. Three single-blind trials in cocaine-dependent patients (two inpatient, one outpatient) found no benefit over standard treatment (Bullock, Kiresuk et al., 1999; Otto, Quinn et al., 1998). A larger controlled outpatient trial found significantly less cocaine use over eight weeks in patients receiving auricular acupuncture than in those receiving sham acupuncture (needle insertion at presumed inactive sites) or relaxation counseling (Avants, Margolin et al., 2000).

Transcranial magnetic stimulation (TMS) involves activation of brain cells by magnetic fields generated by electromagnetic coils placed on the scalp. Repetitive TMS is being evaluated as a treatment for depression and other neuropsychiatric disorders (Wassermann & Lisanby, 2001). The recent finding that TMS of the prefrontal cortex induces dopamine release in subcortical structures (Strafella, Paus et al., 2001) suggests that TMS is worth evaluating as a potential treatment for drug addiction.

AMPHETAMINE ADDICTION

Relatively few clinical trials have evaluated pharmacologic treatment of addiction to amphetamines. The antidepressant imipramine (150 mg/day) was not effective in reducing methamphetamine use in a 180-day controlled clinical trial, although it did improve treatment retention (Galloway, Newmeyer et al., 1996). Fluoxetine (20 mg/day) was reported effective in reducing or eliminating drug use for two weeks to several months in amphetamine abusers participating in an outpatient open-label case series (Polson, Fleming et al., 1993). However, a more recent controlled clinical trial found fluoxetine ineffective in reducing methamphetamine use (Batki, Moon et al., 2000). Calcium channel blockers also have generated inconsistent results. Isradipine (DynaCirc®) reduced the psychological effects (including craving) of a methamphetamine challenge in a human laboratory study (Johnson, Roache et al., 1999), whereas amlodipine (5 or 10 mg/day) was ineffective in reducing methamphetamine use in a controlled clinical trial (Batki, Moon et al., 2001). Anecdotal clinical evidence from Great Britain (where prescribing amphetamine for addiction treatment is legal) suggests that substitution treatment with dexamphetamine elixir (10 to 90 mg/day) can be safe and effective for some amphetamine addicts (Charnaud & Griffiths, 1998; White, 2000), although this approach remains to be validated by controlled clinical trials.

SPECIAL TREATMENT SITUATIONS

Mixed Addictions. *Opiate Addiction*: Concurrent opiate use, including addiction, is a common clinical problem among cocaine addicts. Some addicts use cocaine and opiates simultaneously (as in the so-called "speedball") to enhance the drugs' subjective effects. Up to 20% or more of opiate addicts in methadone maintenance treatment also use cocaine for a variety of reasons, including continuation of prior polydrug abuse, replacement for the "high" no longer obtained from opiates, self-medication for the sedative effects of high methadone doses, or attenuation of opiate withdrawal symptoms (Schottenfeld, Pakes et al., 1993). Three different pharmacologic approaches have been used for the treatment of such dual cocaine and opiate addiction: (1) adjustment of methadone dose, (2) maintenance with another opiate medication, and (3) addition of a medication targeting the cocaine addiction.

Higher methadone doses (usually 60 mg or more daily) generally are associated with less opiate use by patients in methadone maintenance. This relationship also holds in general for cocaine use among patients in methadone maintenance (Tennant & Shannon, 1995), although exceptions have been reported (Grabowski, Rhoades et al., 1993). Increasing the methadone dose as a contingency in response to cocaine use can be effective in reducing such use (and more so than decreasing the methadone dose in response to a cocaine-positive urine sample) (Stine, Freeman et al., 1992; Tennant & Shannon, 1995). Some evidence is available that cocaine use can lower serum methadone concentrations (Tennant & Shannon, 1995).

Buprenorphine (Buprenex®) is a partial opiate agonist (mu-receptor agonist/kappa-receptor antagonist) that is newly approved in the U.S. for the treatment of addiction. it is marketed worldwide as an opiate analgesic and in Europe as a treatment for opiate dependence (see Chapters 3, 4 and 5, this section). With sublingual administration, buprenorphine can be as effective as high-dose methadone as a maintenance treatment for opiate dependence. Its advantages over methadone (a pure mu-receptor agonist) reside in buprenorphine's milder withdrawal syndrome and higher therapeutic index (that is, safety in overdose). Some open-label studies in opiate addicts who used cocaine (but who were not necessarily cocaine-dependent) found that cocaine use was reduced along with opiate use, but later controlled clinical trials found no significant effect of buprenorphine on cocaine use, even when opiate use was substantially reduced (Compton, Ling et al., 1995). More recent studies in patients who were dependent on both opiates and cocaine suggest that cocaine use is reduced at higher buprenorphine doses (12 to 16 mg/day) (Montoya, Gorelick et al., 1996; Schottenfeld, Pakes et al., 1993).

Non-opiate medications for the treatment of cocaine addiction frequently are evaluated in methadone-maintained, opiate-dependent outpatients because the methadone maintenance component ensures good treatment retention and compliance, making medication trials easier to conduct and complete. A variety of the medications discussed earlier, including desipramine, amantadine, bromocriptine, and fluoxetine, have been studied in methadone-maintained cocaine addicts, with inconsistent results. A recent controlled clinical trial found that desipramine (150 mg/day) significantly facilitated both opiate and cocaine abstinence in opiate-dependent cocaine abusers receiving either methadone (65 mg/day) or buprenorphine (12 mg/day) (Oliveto, Feingold et al., 1999). No studies have explicitly and directly compared medication efficacy in methadone-maintained versus opiate-free cocaine addicts.

Pharmacodynamic and pharmacokinetic interactions between methadone and the other treatment medication could account for some of the variability in results, although these interactions have not been well studied. Methadone maintenance has been found to increase desipramine plasma levels by inhibiting desipramine metabolism (Kosten, Gawin et al., 1990; Maany, Dhopesh et al., 1989).

Alcoholism: Alcoholism is a common problem among cocaine addicts, both in the community and in treatment settings, with rates of comorbidity as high as 90% (Gorelick, 1992). Alcohol use by cocaine addicts is associated with poorer treatment outcome (Gorelick, 1992; Carroll, Nich et al., 1998), which can be related to a variety of factors, including production of the toxic psychoactive metabolite cocaethylene (Gorelick, 1992), stimulation of cocaine craving by alcohol (Gorelick, 1992), and alteration of medication metabolism by the hepatic effects of alcohol (which has not been directly studied in cocaine addicts).

Two medications used in the treatment of alcoholism have been studied in the treatment of outpatients dually dependent on cocaine and alcohol. Disulfiram (Antabuse®), at the dose commonly used to treat alcoholism (250 mg/day), substantially decreased both cocaine and alcohol use (Carroll, Nich et al., 1998; Higgins, Budney et al., 1993). Naltrexone (ReVia®), a mu-opiate receptor antagonist marketed for the treatment of alcoholism (see Chapter 1, this section) and opiate dependence (see Chapter 3, this section), also substantially decreased both cocaine and alcohol use at 150 mg/day (Oslin, Pettinati et al., 1999), but not at 50 mg/day (Carroll, Ziedonis et al., 1993; Hersh, Van Kirk et al., 1998), the dose typically used in treatment of alcohol or opiate dependence.

Psychiatric Comorbidities. Treatment-seeking cocaine addicts have high rates of psychiatric comorbidity (that is, psychiatric diagnoses other than another substance use disorder), with rates as high as 65% for lifetime disorders and 50% for current disorders (Rounsaville, Anton et al., 1991; Thevos, Brady et al., 1993). The commonest comorbid disorders tend to be major depression, bipolar spectrum, phobias, and posttraumatic stress disorder. Personality disorders are common among treatment-seeking cocaine addicts, with rates in this population as high as 69% (Weiss, Mirin et al., 1993). The most common of these is antisocial personality disorder, which is associated with poor response to treatment (Arndt, McLellan et al., 1994).

Depression: Antidepressants appear to vary in their efficacy for reducing cocaine use among patients with comorbid major depression, although there have been few direct comparisons or controlled clinical trials. Desipramine, imipramine, and bupropion have shown some efficacy (Nunes, McDowell et al., 2000; Ziedonis & Kosten, 1991), whereas fluoxetine (20 or 40 mg a day) has not (Cornelius, Salloum et al., 1998; Schmitz, Averill et al., 2001). Venlafaxine (Effexor®, 150 mg/day) showed some efficacy in a recent open trial (McDowell, Levin et al., 2000).

Bipolar Disorder: Case series suggest that anticonvulsant mood stabilizers such as valproate and carbamazepine (Tegretol®) (Brown, Suppes et al., 2001; Goldberg, Garno et al., 1999) are more effective than lithium (Nunes, McGrath et al., 1990) in reducing cocaine use among cocaine addicts with bipolar or cyclothymic disorder. Combining lithium with an anticonvulsant can be helpful in treatment-resistant patients (Goldberg, Garno et al., 1999).

Attention Deficit/Hyperactivity Disorder: Up to 10% of adult cocaine addicts seeking treatment have either adult ADHD or a history of childhood ADHD (Levin, Evans et al., 1998b). Stimulant and dopaminergic medications are the mainstay of treatment for ADHD, suggesting that some of these patients may be self-medicating their ADHD with cocaine. Several case series and clinical trials show that such medications successfully treat ADHD symptoms and reduce cocaine use in adults: methylphenidate (up to 120 mg/day), dextroamphetamine (up to 60 mg/day), methamphetamine (15 mg/day), pemoline (up to 75 mg three times a day), and bupropion (up to 100 mg three times a day) (Castaneda, Levy et al., 2000; Downey, Schubiner et al., 1999; Levin, Evans et al., 1998c. An open-label case series found bupropion (100 mg three times a day) similarly effective in adolescents with co-occurring ADHD and stimulant abuse (Riggs, Leon et al., 1998).

Schizophrenia: Although schizophrenia is not a common comorbid psychiatric disorder among cocaine addicts, cocaine use and abuse are common among treatment-seeking schizophrenic patients (Farren, Hameedi et al., 2000; Krystal, D'Souza et al., 1999). Clinical experience indicates that typical neuroleptics, at doses that are effective in the treatment of schizophrenia, do not significantly alter cocaine craving or use (Brady, Anton et al., 1990; Farren, Hameedi et al., 2000; Ohuoha, Maxwell et al., 1997). One exception may be flupenthixol, a mixed dopamine D_1/D_2 receptor and $5\text{-}HT_{2A}$ receptor antagonist that is not marketed in the U.S. (Soyka & De Vry, 2000). Depot flupenthixol (40 mg of decanoate intramuscularly every two weeks) reduced cocaine use and improved psychopathology in a small case series of cocaine-using schizophrenic patients (Levin, Evans et al., 1998a). Several case series suggest that newer "atypical" neuroleptics, such as clozapine, can significantly reduce cocaine and other drug use among schizophrenic patients (Buckley, McCarthy et al., 2000; Volavka, 1999; Zimmet, Strous et al., 2000).

Use of cocaine or amphetamines can exacerbate or provoke neuroleptic-induced movement disorders (Decker & Ries, 1993; van Harten, van Trier et al., 1998) and increase vulnerability to the neuroleptic malignant syndrome (Akpaffiong & Ruiz, 1991).

Scattered case reports suggest that at least some medications used in cocaine addicts, such as mazindol (Seibyl, Brenner et al., 1992) and tricyclic antidepressants (Krystal, D'Souza et al., 1999), can be effective in cocaine-abusing schizophrenics. Imipramine (150 to 200 mg/day) has been reported effective in reducing cocaine abuse when used to treat postpsychotic depression in schizophrenic patients (Siris, Bermanzohn et al., 1991), although attention must be paid to potential pharmacokinetic interactions with neuroleptics and anticholinergic interactions with anti-Parkinson medications.

Medical Comorbidities. Few data have been systematically or prospectively collected to guide the pharmacotherapy of cocaine addiction in medically ill patients, making this an important issue for future clinical research. Prudent clinical practice would require a careful medical evaluation of any patient before starting medication, with special attention to medical conditions common in cocaine addicts. Such conditions would include viral hepatitis and alcoholic liver disease, which might alter the metabolism of prescribed medications, and HIV infection. The presence of the latter necessitates caution in prescribing medications with a known potential for inhibiting immune function. Clinical experience suggests that buprenorphine and bupropion can be used safely in HIV-positive patients (Avants, Margolin et al., 1998).

Gender-Specific Issues. Women tend to be excluded from or underrepresented in many clinical trials of cocaine abuse pharmacotherapy (Gorelick, Montoya et al., 1998), in part because of concern, embodied in former FDA regulations, over risk to the fetus and neonate should a female subject become pregnant. Thus, there is a substantial lack of information about gender-specific issues of pharmacotherapy in general (Yonkers, Kando et al., 1992) and the pharmacotherapy of cocaine addiction in particular. This situation should improve in the future because FDA and

National Institutes of Health regulations now require appropriate representation of women in clinical trials. Meanwhile, clinicians must deal on an *ad hoc* basis with the treatment implications of possible gender differences in medication pharmacokinetics (such as those resulting from differences in body mass and composition) and in pharmacodynamics (such as those related to the menstrual cycle or exogenous hormones such as oral contraceptives) (Yonkers, Kando et al., 1992).

In the absence of directly relevant and systematically collected data, caution should be used when prescribing medications to pregnant addicts and those with pregnancy potential, keeping in mind both the risks of medication and the risks of continued cocaine use. Most medications proposed for the treatment of cocaine addiction (such as tricyclic antidepressants, fluoxetine, bupropion, and bromocriptine) appear to have little potential for morphologic teratogenicity or disruption of pregnancy, although there is little or no data on behavioral teratogenicity (Miller, 1994). Some exceptions are amantadine (associated with pregnancy complications), lithium (associated with cardiac malformations and neonatal toxicity [Moore, 1995]), anticonvulsants (associated with increased risk of congenital malformations [Yerby, 1994]), and neuroleptics (which can be associated with nonspecific congenital anomalies and neonatal withdrawal). Bromocriptine should be used cautiously in the postpartum period because of the risk of vasospastic complications and seizures (Bakht, Kirshon et al., 1990).

Age. Although adolescents make up a substantial minority of heavy cocaine users, they have been excluded from clinical trials of cocaine pharmacotherapies because of legal and informed consent considerations. On the basis of the scarcity of published case reports, it appears that medication is not often used in the treatment of adolescent cocaine addiction (Center for Substance Abuse Treatment, 1993).

CONCLUSIONS AND FUTURE PROSPECTS

The absence of any medication that meets FDA standards for efficacy and safety leaves physicians with little clear-cut guidance for pharmacologic treatment of stimulant addiction. Among existing medications marketed for other indications, none has yet been proved broadly effective in replicated controlled clinical trials. Disulfiram appears the most promising, especially for patients with comorbid alcohol abuse. Tricyclic antidepressants such as desipramine and imipramine (but not SSRIs such as fluoxetine) can be of some use in patients with milder dependence or comorbid depression, whereas dopaminergic agents such as amantadine and bromocriptine can be of use in patients who are experiencing a prominent withdrawal syndrome. Anticonvulsants such as gabapentin, lamotrigine, and phenytoin (but not carbamazepine) have shown promise in small-scale studies and warrant further evaluation. The stimulant maintenance approach also warrants further evaluation using medications with less abuse potential (for example, pemoline, or sustained-release methylphenidate or amphetamine), or perhaps even a slow onset (for example, oral or transdermal) form of cocaine itself.

More sophisticated patient-treatment matching can enhance the efficacy of current medications by taking into account both patient characteristics that can influence treatment response (for example, severity of addiction, psychiatric comorbidity, or concomitant medications) and characteristics of the psychosocial treatment accompanying the medication (Carroll, Rounsaville et al., 1994). For example, some medications can be effective in patients who are experiencing severe cocaine withdrawal, even when they are not effective in cocaine addicts as a group (Kampman, Volpicelli et al., 2000, 2001).

Future progress in pharmacologic treatment for cocaine addiction is likely to come from development of new medications with novel mechanisms of action. New medications should evolve from an improved understanding of the neuropharmacology of cocaine addiction and animal studies of the interactions of cocaine with novel compounds (Carroll, Howell et al., 1999; Gorelick, 1999; Newman, 2000). Preclinical studies with compounds that bind tightly and long-lastingly to the same presynaptic dopamine transporter site as does cocaine (thereby keeping cocaine from acting), but which do not themselves produce robust reinforcing effects (such as the experimental compound GBR-12909), suggest that these compounds may be useful as functional cocaine "antagonists" (Froimowitz, Wu et al., 2000; Howell & Wilcox, 2001). Manipulation of brain dopamine activity with selective dopamine receptor ligands has attenuated the rewarding effects of cocaine in several animal studies but has not always been effective in human studies (Carroll, Howell et al., 1999; Childress & O'Brien, 2000; Haney, Collins et al., 1999). Other neuropharmacologic approaches being studied for possible therapeutic use include manipulation of neurotransmitter/hormone systems that interact with the mesolimbic dopamine reward circuit (Wise, 1998), stimulation of kappa opioid receptors (Shippenberg, Chefer et al., 2001), blockade of excitatory amino acid receptors

(Pulvirenti, Balducci et al., 1997), stimulation of GABA activity (either by activation of $GABA_B$ receptors [Ling, Shoptaw et al., 1998; Roberts & Brebner, 2000] or by inhibition of GABA metabolism [Gerasimov, Schiffer et al., 2001]), and inhibition of the hypothalamic-pituitary-adrenal system (Sarnyai, Shaham et al., 2001).

The failure of existing medications to show consistent efficacy in the treatment of cocaine addiction has prompted growing interest in pharmacokinetic approaches: that is, preventing ingested cocaine from entering the brain and/or enhancing its elimination from the body (Gorelick, 1997). The former approach could be implemented by active or passive immunization to produce binding antibodies that keep cocaine from crossing the blood-brain barrier. The latter approach could be implemented by administration of an enzyme (butyrylcholinesterase) that catalyzes cocaine hydrolysis or by immunization with a catalytic antibody. These pharmacokinetic approaches already have shown promise in attenuating cocaine's behavioral effects in animals (Baird, Landry et al., 2000; Carmona, Schindler et al., 1998; Carrera, Ashley et al., 2001). A recent phase I study of a cocaine vaccine (that is, active immunization against cocaine) in healthy volunteers yielded promising results: the vaccine was well tolerated, and detectable anti-cocaine antibody levels persisted for up to nine months (Kosten, Roberts et al., 2000).

Regardless of which medications show promise in the future, their adoption into clinical practice should be guided by acceptable scientific proof of efficacy and safety, based on data from replicated, well-designed, controlled clinical trials.

REFERENCES

Akpaffiong MJ & Ruiz P (1991). Neuroleptic malignant syndrome: A complication of neuroleptics and cocaine abuse. *Psychiatric Quarterly* 62:299-309.

Alim TN, Rosse RB, Vocci FJ Jr et al. (1995). Diethylpropion pharmacotherapeutic adjuvant therapy for inpatient treatment of cocaine dependence: A test of the cocaine-agonist hypothesis. *Clinical Neuropharmacology* 18:183-195.

Alterman AI, Droba M, Antelo R et al. (1992). Amantadine may facilitate detoxification of cocaine addicts. *Drug and Alcohol Dependence* 31:19-29.

Arndt IO, Dorozynsky L, Woody GE et al. (1992). Desipramine treatment of cocaine dependence in methadone-maintained patients. *Archives of General Psychiatry* 49:888-893.

Arndt IO, McLellan AT, Dorozynsky L et al. (1994). Desipramine treatment for cocaine dependence. *Journal of Nervous and Mental Disease* 182:(3)151-156.

Avants SK, Margolin A, DePhilippis D et al. (1998). A comprehensive pharmacologic-psychosocial treatment program for HIV-seropositive cocaine- and opioid-dependent patients. *Journal of Substance Abuse Treatment* 15:261-265.

Avants SK, Margolin A, Holford TR et al. (2000). A randomized controlled trial of auricular acupuncture for cocaine dependence. *Archives of General Psychiatry* 160:2305-2312.

Baird TJ, Landry DW, Winger G et al. (2000). A novel anti-cocaine antibody (mAb 15A10) and butyryl-cholinesterase (BChE) alter cocaine self-administration in rats. *Drug and Alcohol Dependence* 60(Suppl 1):S10.

Bakht FR, Kirshon B, Baker T et al. (1990). Postpartum cardiovascular complications after bromocriptine and cocaine use. *American Journal of Obstetrics and Gynecology* 162:1065-1066.

Batki SL, Bradley M, Herbst M et al. (1996). A controlled trial of fenfluramine in cocaine dependence. *Problems of Drug Dependence, 1995 (NIDA Research Monograph 162).* Rockville, MD: National Institute on Drug Abuse, 148.

Batki SL, Moon J, Bradley M et al. (2000). Fluoxetine in methamphetamine dependence—A controlled trial: Preliminary analysis. *Problems of Drug Dependence, 1999 (NIDA Research Monograph 180).* Bethesda, MD: National Institute on Drug Abuse, 235.

Batki SL, Moon J, Delucchi K et al. (2001). Amlodipine treatment of methamphetamine dependence, a controlled outpatient trial: Preliminary analysis. *Drug and Alcohol Dependence* 63(Suppl 1):S12.

Batki SL, Washburn AM, Delucchi K et al. (1996). A controlled trial of fluoxetine in crack cocaine dependence. *Drug and Alcohol Dependence* 41:137-142.

Berger SP, Leiderman D, Majewska M et al. (2000). A NIDA-sponsored cocaine rapid efficacy screening trial of gabapentin, lamotrigine and reserpine. *Drug and Alcohol Dependence* 60(Suppl 1):S16.

Blum K, Allison D, Trachtenberg MC et al. (1988). Reduction of both drug hunger and withdrawal against advice rate of cocaine abusers in a 30-day inpatient treatment program by the neuronutrient tropamine. *Current Therapeutic Research* 43:1204-1214.

Brady K, Anton R, Ballenger JC et al. (1990). Cocaine abuse among schizophrenic patients. *American Journal of Psychiatry* 147:1164-1167.

Brewer C (1993). Treatment of cocaine abuse with monoamine oxidase inhibitors. *British Journal of Psychiatry* 163:815-816.

Brewington V, Smith M & Lipton D (1994). Acupuncture as a detoxication treatment: An analysis of controlled research. *Journal of Substance Abuse Treatment* 11:289-307.

Brotman AW, Witkie SM, Gelenberg AJ et al. (1988). An open trial of maprotiline for the treatment of cocaine abuse. *Journal of Clinical Psychopharmacology* 8:125-127.

Brown ES, Suppes T, Adinoff B et al. (2001). Drug abuse and bipolar disorder: Comorbidity or misdiagnosis? *Journal of Affective Disorder* 65:105-115.

Buckley PF, McCarthy M, Chapman P et al. (2000). Craving reduction and clozapine response in patients with comorbid substance abuse and schizophrenia. *Biological Psychiatry* 47(Suppl):18S-19S.

Bullock ML, Kiresuk TJ, Pheley AM et al. (1999). Auricular acupuncture in the treatment of cocaine abuse: A study of efficacy and dosing. *Journal of Substance Abuse Treatment* 16:31-38.

Campbell JL, Thomas HM, Gabrielli W et al. (1994). Impact of desipramine or carbamazepine on patient retention in outpatient cocaine treatment: Preliminary findings. *Journal of Addictive Diseases* 13:191-199.

Carmona GN, Schindler CW, Shoaib M et al. (1998). Attenuation of cocaine-induced locomotor activity by butyrylcholinesterase. *Experimental and Clinical Psychopharmacology* 6:274-279.

Carrera MRA, Ashley JA, Wirsching P et al. (2001). A second-generation vaccine protects against the psychoactive effects of cocaine. *Proceedings of the National Academy of Sciences* 98:1988-1992.

Carroll FI, Howell LL & Kuhar MJ (1999). Pharmacotherapies for treatment of cocaine abuse: Preclinical aspects. *Journal of Medicinal Chemistry* 42:2721-2736.

Carroll KM (1997). Integrating psychotherapy and pharmacotherapy to improve drug abuse outcomes. *Addictive Behavior* 22:233-245.

Carroll KM (2000). Implications of recent research for program quality in cocaine dependence treatment. *Substance Use and Misuse* 35:2011-2030.

Carroll KM & Schottenfeld R (1997). Nonpharmacologic approaches to substance abuse treatment. *Medical Clinics of North America* 81:927-944.

Carroll KM, Nich C & Rounsaville BJ (1995). Differential symptom reduction in depressed cocaine abusers treated with psychotherapy and pharmacotherapy. *Journal of Nervous and Mental Disease* 183:251-259.

Carroll KM, Nich C, Ball SA et al. (1998). Treatment of cocaine and alcohol dependence with psychotherapy and disulfiram. *Addiction* 93:713-728.

Carroll KM, Rounsaville BJ, Gordon LT et al. (1994). Psychotherapy and pharmacotherapy for ambulatory cocaine abusers. *Archives of General Psychiatry* 51:177-187.

Carroll KM, Ziedonis D, O'Malley S et al. (1993). Pharmacologic interventions for alcohol- and cocaine-abusing individuals. *American Journal on Addictions* 2(1):77-79.

Castaneda R, Levy R, Hardy M et al. (2000). Long-acting stimulants for the treatment of attention-deficit disorder in cocaine-dependent adults. *Psychiatric Services* 51:169-171.

Center for Substance Abuse Treatment (1993). *Guidelines for the Treatment of Alcohol- and Other Drug-Abusing Adolescents (Treatment Improvement Protocol Series, No. 4).* Rockville, MD: Center for Substance Abuse Treatment.

Chadwick MJ & Gregory DL (1990). A double-blind amino acids, L-tryptophan and L-tyrosine, and placebo study with cocaine-dependent subjects in an inpatient chemical dependency treatment center. *American Journal of Drug and Alcohol Abuse* 16:275-286.

Charnaud B & Griffiths V (1998). Levels of intravenous drug misuse among clients prescribed oral dexamphetamine or oral methadone: A comparison. *Drug and Alcohol Dependence* 52:79-84.

Childress AR & O'Brien CP (2000). Dopamine receptor partial agonists could address the duality of cocaine craving. *Trends in Pharmacological Science* 21:6-9.

Clow DW & Hammer RP (1991). Cocaine abstinence following chronic treatment alters cerebral metabolism in dopaminergic reward regions. *Neuropsychopharmacology* 4(1):71-75.

Cold JA (1996). NeuRecover-SA® in the treatment of cocaine withdrawal and craving, a pilot study. *Clinical Drug Investigation* 12:1-7.

Compton PA, Ling W, Charuvastra VC et al. (1995). Buprenorphine as a pharmacotherapy for cocaine abuse: A review of the evidence. *Journal of Addictive Diseases* 14(3):97-114.

Connolly HM & McGoon MD (1999). Obesity drugs and the heart. *Current Problems in Cardiology* 24:745-792.

Cornelius JR, Salloum IM, Thase ME et al. (1998). Fluoxetine versus placebo in depressed alcoholic cocaine abusers. *Psychopharmacology Bulletin* 34:117-121.

Cornish JW, Maany I, Fudala PJ et al. (2001). A randomized, double-blind, placebo-controlled study of ritanserin pharmacotherapy for cocaine dependence. *Drug and Alcohol Dependence* 61:183-189.

Covi L, Hess JM, Kreiter NA et al. (1995). Effects of combined fluoxetine and counseling in the outpatient treatment of cocaine abusers. *American Journal of Drug and Alcohol Abuse* 21:327-344.

Crosby RD, Pearson VL, Eller C et al. (1996). Phenytoin in the treatment of cocaine abuse: A double-blind study. *Clinical Pharmacology and Therapeutics* 59:458-468.

Dackis CA & Gold MS (1985). Pharmacological approaches to cocaine addiction. *Journal of Substance Abuse Treatment* 2:139-145.

Decker KP & Ries RK (1993). Differential diagnosis and psychopharmacology of dual disorders. *Psychiatric Clinics of North America* 16:(4)703-718.

Delucchi KL (1992). Research on desipramine in the treatment of cocaine abuse: A critique of Levin and Lehman's meta-analysis. *Journal of Clinical Psychopharmacology* 12(5):367-369.

Downey KK, Schubiner H & Schuster CR (1999). Double-blind placebo controlled stimulant trial for cocaine-dependent ADHD adults. *Problems of Drug Dependence, 1999 (NIDA Research Monograph 180).* Rockville, MD: National Institute on Drug Abuse, 116.

Eiler K, Schaefer MR, Salstrom D et al. (1995). Double-blind comparison of bromocriptine and placebo in cocaine withdrawal. *American Journal of Drug and Alcohol Abuse* 21:65-79.

Farren CK, Hameedi FA, Rosen MA et al. (2000). Significant interaction between clozapine and cocaine in cocaine addicts. *Drug and Alcohol Dependence* 59:153-163.

Fischman MW, Foltin RW, Nestadt G et al. (1990). Effects of desipramine maintenance on cocaine self-administration by humans. *Journal of Pharmacology and Experimental Therapeutics* 253(2):760-770.

Froimowitz M, Wu K-M, Moussa A et al. (2000). Slow-onset, long-duration 3-(3',4'-dichlorophenyl-)-1-indanamine monoamine reuptake blockers as potential medications to treat cocaine abuse. *Journal of Medicinal Chemistry* 43:4981-4992.

Galloway GP, Frederick SL, Thomas S et al. (1996). A historically controlled trial of tyrosine for cocaine dependence. *Journal of Psychoactive Drugs* 28:305-309.

Galloway GP, Newmeyer J, Knapp T et al. (1996). A controlled trial of imipramine for the treatment of methamphetamine dependence. *Journal of Substance Abuse Treatment* 13:493-497.

Gawin FH, Riordan CA & Kleber HD (1985). Methylphenidate use in non-ADD cocaine abusers—A negative study. *American Journal of Drug and Alcohol Abuse* 11:193-197.

George TP, Chawarski MC, Pakes J et al. (2000). Disulfiram versus placebo for cocaine dependence in buprenorphine-maintained subjects: A preliminary trial. *Biological Psychiatry* 47:1080-1086.

Gerasimov MR, Schiffer WK, Gardner EL et al. (2001). GABAergic blockade of cocaine-associated cue-induced increases in nucleus accumbens dopamine. *European Journal of Pharmacology* 414:205-209.

Giannini AJ, Folts DJ, Feather JN et al. (1989). Bromocriptine and amantadine in cocaine detoxification. *Psychiatry Research* 29:11-16.

Goldberg JF, Garno JL, Leon AC et al. (1999). A history of substance abuse complicates remission from acute mania in bipolar disorder. *Journal of Clinical Psychiatry* 60:733-740.

Gorelick DA (1992). Alcohol and cocaine: Clinical and pharmacological interactions. *Recent Developments in Alcoholism* 11:37-56.

Gorelick DA (1997). Enhancing cocaine metabolism with butyrylcholinesterase as a treatment strategy. *Drug and Alcohol Dependence* 48:159-165.

Gorelick DA (1998). The rate hypothesis and agonist substitution approaches to cocaine abuse treatment. *Advances in Pharmacology* 42:995-997.

Gorelick DA (1999). Pharmacological treatment of cocaine addiction. *Einstein Quarterly Journal of Biology and Medicine* 16:61-69.

Gorelick DA, Halikas JA & Crosby RD (1994). Pharmacotherapy of cocaine dependence in the United States: Comparing scientific evidence and clinical practice. *Substance Abuse* 15:209-213.

Gorelick DA, Montoya ID & Johnson EO (1998). Sociodemographic representation in published studies of cocaine abuse pharmacotherapy. *Drug and Alcohol Dependence* 49:89-93.

Grabowski J, Rhoades H, Elk R et al. (1993). Methadone dosage, cocaine and opiate abuse. *American Journal of Psychiatry* 150(4):675.

Grabowski J, Rhoades H, Elk R et al. (1995). Fluoxetine is ineffective for treatment of cocaine dependence or concurrent opiate and cocaine dependence: Two placebo-controlled, double-blind trials. *Journal of Clinical Psychopharmacology* 15:163-174.

Grabowski J, Rhoades H, Silverman P et al. (2000a). Risperidone for the treatment of cocaine dependence: Randomized, double-blind trial. *Journal of Clinical Psychopharmacology* 20:305-310.

Grabowski J, Rhoades H, Stotts A et al. (2000b). d-Amphetamine for treatment of cocaine dependence: Randomized double-blind, placebo-controlled trials. *Drug and Alcohol Dependence* 60(Suppl 1):S77.

Grabowski J, Roache JD, Schmitz JM et al. (1997). Replacement medication for cocaine dependence: Methylphenidate. *Journal of Clinical Psychopharmacology* 17:485-488.

Halikas JA & Kuhn KL (1990). A possible neurophysiological basis of cocaine craving. *Annals of Clinical Psychiatry* 2:79-83.

Haney M, Collins ED, Ward AS et al. (1999). Effect of a selective dopamine D_1 agonist (ABT-431) on smoked cocaine self-administration in humans. *Psychopharmacology* 143:102-110.

Henningfield JE & Singleton EG (1994). Managing drug dependence: Psychotherapy or pharmacotherapy? *CNS Drugs* 1(5):317-322.

Hersh D, Van Kirk JR & Kranzler HR (1998). Naltrexone treatment of comorbid alcohol and cocaine use disorders. *Psychopharmacology* 139:44-52.

Higgins ST, Budney AJ, Bickel WK et al. (1993). Disulfiram therapy in patients abusing cocaine and alcohol. *American Journal of Psychiatry* 150(4):675-676.

Hill JL, Wilkins JN & Gorelick DA (1996). Double-blind outpatient trial of bromocriptine for treatment of cocaine abuse. *Problems of Drug Dependence, 1995 (NIDA Research Monograph 162).* Rockville, MD: National Institute on Drug Abuse, 145.

Hollister LE, Krajewski K, Rustin T et al. (1992). Drugs for cocaine dependence: Not easy. *Archives of General Psychiatry* 49:905.

Howell LL & Wilcox KM (2001). The dopamine transporter and cocaine medication development: Drug self-administration in nonhuman primates. *Journal of Pharmacology and Experimental Therapeutics* 298:1-6.

Johnson BA, Chen YR, Swann AC et al. (1997). Ritanserin in the treatment of cocaine dependence. *Biological Psychiatry* 42:932-940.

Johnson BA, Roache JD, Bordnick PS et al. (1999). Isradipine, a dihydropyridine-class calcium channel antagonist, attenuates some of d-methamphetamine's positive subjective effects: a preliminary study. *Psychopharmacology* 144:295-300.

Kampman KM, Majewska MD, Tourian K et al. (2000). A pilot trial of piracetam and ginkgo biloba for the treatment of cocaine dependence. *Drug and Alcohol Dependence* 60(Suppl 1):S106.

Kampman KM, Rukstalis M, Pettinati H et al. (2000). The combination of phentermine and fenfluramine reduced cocaine withdrawal symptoms in an open trial. *Journal of Substance Abuse Treatment* 19:77-79.

Kampman KM, Volpicelli JR, Alterman AI et al. (2000). Amantadine in the treatment of cocaine-dependent patients with severe withdrawal symptoms. *American Journal of Psychiatry* 157:2052-2054.

Kampman KM, Volpicelli JR, Mulvaney F et al. (2001). Effectiveness of propranolol for cocaine dependence treatment may depend on cocaine withdrawal symptom severity. *Drug and Alcohol Dependence* 63:69-78.

Khalsa ME, Gawin FH, Rawson R et al. (1993). A desipramine ceiling in cocaine abusers. *Problems of Drug Dependence, 1992 (NIDA Research Monograph 132)*. Rockville, MD: National Institute on Drug Abuse, 18.

Kolar A, Brown B, Weddington W et al. (1992). Treatment of cocaine dependence in methadone maintenance clients: A pilot study comparing the efficacy of desipramine and amantadine. *International Journal of the Addictions* 27:849-868.

Kosten TR, Gawin FH, Morgan C et al. (1990). Evidence for altered desipramine disposition in methadone-maintained patients treated for cocaine abuse. *American Journal of Alcohol and Drug Abuse* 16:329-336.

Kosten TR, Morgan CM, Falcione J et al. (1992). Pharmacotherapy for cocaine-abusing methadone-maintained patients using amantadine or desipramine. *Archives of General Psychiatry* 49:894-898.

Kosten TR, Roberts JSC, Bond J et al. (2000). Longitudinal safety and immunogenicity of a therapeutic cocaine vaccine. *Drug and Alcohol Dependence* 60(Suppl 1):S250.

Kosten TR, Steinberg M & Diakogiannis IA (1993). Crossover trial of mazindol for cocaine dependence. *American Journal on Addictions* 2:161.

Kosten TR, Woods SW, Rosen MI et al. (1999). Interactions of cocaine with nimodipine: A brief report. *American Journal on Addictions* 8:77-81.

Krystal JH, D'Souza DC, Madonick S et al. (1999). Toward a rational pharmacotherapy of comorbid substance abuse in schizophrenic patients. *Schizophrenia Research* 35(Suppl):S35-S49.

Levin FR & Lehman AF (1991). Meta analysis of desipramine as an adjunct in the treatment of cocaine addiction. *Journal of Clinical Psychopharmacology* 11:374-378.

Levin FR, Evans SM, Coomaraswammy S et al. (1998a). Flupenthixol treatment for cocaine abusers with schizophrenia: A pilot study. *American Journal of Drug and Alcohol Abuse* 24:343-360.

Levin FR, Evans SM & Kleber HD (1998b). Prevalence of adult attention-deficit hyperactivity disorder among cocaine abusers seeking treatment. *Drug and Alcohol Dependence* 52:15-25.

Levin FR, Evans SM, McDowell DM et al. (1998c). Methylphenidate treatment for cocaine abusers with adult attention-deficit/hyperactivity disorder: A pilot study. *Journal of Clinical Psychiatry* 59:300-305.

Levin FR, McDowell D, Evans SM et al. (1999). Pergolide mesylate for cocaine abuse: A controlled preliminary trial. *American Journal on Addictions* 8:120-127.

Lima AR, Lima MS, Soares BGO et al. (2000). Carbamazepine for cocaine dependence (CD002023). *Cochrane Library: Cochrane Database of Systematic Reviews*, 3; Oxford, England: Update Software.

Ling W, Shoptaw S & Majewska D (1998). Baclofen as a cocaine anti-craving medication: A preliminary clinical study. *Neuropsychopharmacology* 18:403-404.

Lipton DS, Brewington V & Smith M (1994). Acupuncture for crack-cocaine detoxification: Experimental evaluation of efficacy. *Journal of Substance Abuse Treatment* 11:205-215.

Llosa T (1994). The standard low dose of oral cocaine used for treatment of cocaine dependence. *Substance Abuse* 15:215-220.

Maany I, Dhopesh V, Arndt IO et al. (1989). Increase in desipramine serum levels associated with methadone treatment. *American Journal of Psychiatry* 146:1611-1613.

Malcolm R, Brady KT, Moore J et al. (1999). Amlodipine treatment of cocaine dependence. *Journal of Psychoactive Drugs* 31:117-120.

Malcolm R, Herron J, Sutherland SE et al. (2001). Adverse outcomes in a controlled trial of pergolide for cocaine dependence. *Journal of Addictive Diseases* 20:81-92.

Malcolm R, Moore JA, Brady KT et al. (1999). Pergolide/haloperidol for the treatment of cocaine dependence. *Problems of Drug Dependence, 1999 (NIDA Research Monograph 180)*. Rockville, MD: National Institute on Drug Abuse, 165.

Maletzky BM (1977). Phenelzine as a stimulant drug antagonist. *International Journal of the Addictions* 12(5):661-665.

Margolin A, Avants SK & Kosten TR (1995). Mazindol for relapse prevention to cocaine abuse in methadone-maintained patients. *American Journal of Drug and Alcohol Abuse* 21:469-481.

Margolin A, Avants SK & Kosten TR (1996). Pemoline for the treatment of cocaine dependence in methadone-maintained patients. *Journal of Psychoactive Drugs* 28:301-304.

Margolin A, Avants SK, DePhilippis D et al. (1998). A preliminary investigation of lamotrigine for cocaine abuse in HIV-seropositive patients. *American Journal of Drug and Alcohol Abuse* 24:85-101.

Margolin A, Kosten TR, Avants SK et al. (1995). A multicenter trial of bupropion for cocaine dependence in methadone maintained patients. *Drug and Alcohol Dependence* 40:125-131.

Markou A & Koob GF (1992). Bromocriptine reverses the elevation in intracranial self-stimulation thresholds observed in a rat model of cocaine withdrawal. *Neuropsychopharmacology* 7(3):213-224.

McCance-Katz EF, Kosten TR & Jatlow P (1998). Chronic disulfiram treatment effects on intranasal cocaine administration: Initial results. *Biological Psychiatry* 43:540-543.

McDowell DM, Levin FR, Seracini AM et al. (2000). Venlafaxine treatment of cocaine abusers with depressive disorders. *American Journal of Drug and Alcohol Abuse* 26:25-31.

Miller LJ (1994). Psychiatric medication during pregnancy: Understanding and minimizing risks. *Psychiatric Annals* 24:69-75.

Montoya I, Gorelick D, Preston K et al. (1996). Buprenorphine for treatment of dually-dependent (opiate and cocaine) individuals. *Problems of Drug Dependence, 1995 (NIDA Research Monograph 162).* Rockville, MD: National Institute on Drug Abuse, 178.

Montoya ID, Levin FR, Fudala P et al. (1995). Double-blind comparison of carbamazepine and placebo for treatment of cocaine dependence. *Drug and Alcohol Dependence* 38:213-219.

Montoya ID, Preston K, Rothman R et al. (2002). Open-label pilot study of bupropion plus bromocriptine for treatment of cocaine dependence. *American Journal of Drug and Alcohol Abuse* 28:1-8.

Moore JA (1995). An assessment of lithium using the IEHR evaluative process for assessing human developmental and reproductive toxicity of agents. *Reproductive Toxicology* 9:175-210.

Moscovitz H, Brookoff D & Nelson L (1993). A randomized trial of bromocriptine for cocaine users presenting to the emergency department. *Journal of General Internal Medicine* 8:1-4.

Myrick H, Henderson S, Brady KT et al. (2001). Gabapentin in the treatment of cocaine dependence: A case series. *Journal of Clinical Psychiatry* 62:19-23.

Newman AH (2000). Novel pharmacotherapies for cocaine abuse 1997-2000. *Expert Opinion in Therapeutic Patents* 10:1095-1122.

Nunes EV, McDowell D, Rothenberg J et al. (2000). Desipramine treatment for cocaine-dependent patients with depression. *Drug and Alcohol Dependence* 60(Suppl 1):S160.

Nunes EV, McGrath PJ, Wager S et al. (1990). Lithium treatment for cocaine abusers with bipolar spectrum disorders. *American Journal of Psychiatry* 147(5):655-657.

Nunes EV, McGrath PJ, Quitkin FM et al. (1995). Imipramine treatment of cocaine abuse: Possible boundaries of efficacy. *Drug and Alcohol Dependence* 39:185-195.

Ohuoha DC, Maxwell JA, Thomson LE 3rd et al. (1997). Effect of dopamine receptor antagonists on cocaine subjective effects: A naturalistic case study. *Journal of Substance Abuse Treatment* 14:249-258.

O'Leary G & Weiss RD (2000). Pharmacotherapies for cocaine dependence. *Current Psychiatry Reports* 2:508-513.

Oliveto AH, Feingold A, Schottenfeld R et al. (1999). Desipramine in opioid-dependent cocaine abusers maintained on buprenorphine vs. methadone. *Archives of General Psychiatry* 56:812-820.

Oslin DW, Pettinati HM, Volpicelli JR et al. (1999). The effects of naltrexone on alcohol and cocaine use in dually addicted patients. *Journal of Substance Abuse Treatment* 16:163-167.

Otto KC, Quinn C & Sung Y-F (1998). Auricular acupuncture as an adjunctive treatment for cocaine addiction: A pilot study. *American Journal on Addictions* 7:164-170.

Petrakis IL, Carroll KM, Nich C et al. (2000). Disulfiram treatment for cocaine dependence in methadone-maintained opioid addicts. *Addiction* 95:219-228.

Polson RG, Fleming PM & O'Shea JK (1993). Fluoxetine in the treatment of amphetamine dependence. *Human Psychopharmacology* 8:55-58.

Pulvirenti L & Koob GF (1994). Lisuride reduces intravenous cocaine self-administration in rats. *Pharmacology Biochemistry and Behavior* 47:(4)819-822.

Pulvirenti L, Balducci C & Koob GF (1997). Dextromethorphan reduces intravenous cocaine self-administration in the rat. *European Journal of Pharmacology* 321:279-283.

Raby WN (2000). Gabapentin therapy for cocaine cravings. *American Journal of Psychiatry* 157:2058-2059.

Reid MS, Leiderman D, Casadonte P et al. (2000). A controlled trial of olanzapine, valproate or coenzyme Q10/L-carnitine versus placebo for the treatment of cocaine dependence. *Drug and Alcohol Dependence* 60(Suppl 1):S179.

Riggs PD, Leon SL, Mikulich SK et al. (1998). An open trial of bupropion for ADHD in adolescents with substance use disorders and conduct disorder. *Journal of American Academy of Child and Adolescent Psychiatry* 37:1271-1278.

Roache JD, Grabowski J, Schmitz JM et al. (2000). Laboratory measures of methylphenidate effects in cocaine-dependent patients receiving treatment. *Journal of Clinical Psychopharmacology* 20:61-68.

Roberts DC & Brebner K (2000). GABA modulation of cocaine self-administration. *Annals of the New York Academy of Sciences* 909:145-158.

Rosen H, Flemenbaum A & Slater V (1986). Clinical trial of carbidopa-l-dopa combination for cocaine. *American Journal of Psychiatry* 143:1493.

Rosenbaum JF & Fredman SJ (1999). Pramipexole treatment for cocaine cravings. *American Journal of Psychiatry* 156:1834.

Rosse RB, Alim TN, Fay-McCarthy M et al. (1994). Nimodipine pharmacotherapeutic adjuvant therapy for inpatient treatment of cocaine dependence. *Clinical Neuropharmacology* 17:348-358.

Rounsaville BJ, Anton SF, Carroll K et al. (1991). Psychiatric diagnoses of treatment-seeking cocaine abusers. *Archives of General Psychiatry* 48:43-51.

Sarnyai Z, Shaham Y & Heinrichs SC (2001). The role of corticotropin-releasing factor in drug addiction. *Pharmacological Reviews* 53:209-243.

Schmitz JM, Averill P, Stotts AL et al. (2001). Fluoxetine treatment of cocaine-dependent patients with major depressive disorder. *Drug and Alcohol Dependence* 63:207-214.

Schmitz JM, Stotts AL, Rhoades HM et al. (2001). Naltrexone and relapse prevention treatment for cocaine-dependent patients. *Addictive Behaviors* 26:167-180.

Schottenfeld R, Pakes J, Ziedonis D et al. (1993). Buprenorphine: Dose-related effects on cocaine and opioid use in cocaine-abusing opioid-dependent humans. *Biological Psychiatry* 34:66-74.

Seibyl JP, Brenner L, Krystal JH et al. (1992). Mazindol and cocaine addiction in schizophrenia. *Biological Psychiatry* 31:1172-1183.

Sellers EM, Higgins GA, Tomkins DM et al. (1991). Opportunities for treatment of psychoactive substance use disorders with serotonergic medications. *Journal of Clinical Psychiatry* 52(Suppl 12):49-54.

Shippenberg TS, Chefer VI, Zapata A et al. (2001). Modulation of the behavioral and neurochemical effects of psychostimulants by κ-opioid receptor systems. *Annals of the New York Academy of Sciences* 937:50-73.

Siris SG, Bermanzohn PC, Mason SE et al. (1991). Antidepressant for substance-abusing schizophrenic patients: A minireview. *Progress in Neuropsychopharmacology and Biological Psychiatry* 15:1-13.

Sofuoglu M, Pentel PR, Bliss RL et al. (1999). Effects of phenytoin on cocaine self-administration in humans. *Drug and Alcohol Dependence* 53:273-275.

Soyka M & De Vry J (2000). Flupenthixol as a potential pharmacotreatment of alcohol and cocaine abuse/dependence. *European Neuropsychopharmacology* 10:325-332.

Specker S, Crosby R, Borden J et al. (2000). Nefazodone in the treatment of females with cocaine abuse. *Drug and Alcohol Dependence* 60(Suppl 1):S179.

Stine SM, Freeman M, Burns B. Effect of methadone dose on cocaine abuse in a methadone program. *American Journal on Addictions* 1(4):294-303.

Stine SM, Krystal JH, Kosten TR et al. (1995). Mazindol treatment for cocaine dependence. *Drug and Alcohol Dependence* 39:245-252.

Strafella AP, Paus T, Barrett J et al. (2001). Repetitive transcranial magnetic stimulation of the human prefrontal cortex induces dopamine release in the caudate nucleus. *Journal of Neuroscience* 21:RC157:1-4.

Szumlinski KK, Maisonneuve IM & Glick SD (2001). Iboga interactions with psychomotor stimulants: Panacea in the paradox? *Toxicon* 39:75-86.

Tennant F & Shannon J (1995). Cocaine abuse in methadone maintenance patients is associated with low serum methadone concentrations. *Journal of Addictive Diseases* 14:67-74.

Tennant F, Tarver A, Sagherian A et al. (1993). A placebo-controlled elimination study to identify potential treatment agents for cocaine detoxification. *American Journal on Addictions* 2:299-308.

Tennant FS & Sagherian AA (1987). Double-blind comparison of amantadine and bromocriptine for ambulatory withdrawal from cocaine dependence. *Archives of Internal Medicine* 147:109-112.

Thevos AK, Brady KT, Grice D et al. (1993). A comparison of psychopathy in cocaine and alcohol dependence. *American Journal on Addictions* 2:279-286.

Thomas HM, Campbell J, Laster L et al. (1996). Efficacy of two doses of tyrosine in retaining crack cocaine abusers in outpatient treatment. *Problems on Drug Dependence, 1995 (NIDA Research Monograph 162)*. Rockville, MD: National Institute on Drug Abuse, 148.

van Harten PN, van Trier JCAM, Horwitz EH et al. (1998). Cocaine as a risk factor for neuroleptic-induced acute dystonia. *Journal of Clinical Psychiatry* 59:128-130.

Volavka J (1999). The effects of clozapine on aggression and substance abuse in schizophrenic patients. *Journal of Clinical Psychiatry* 60(Suppl 12):43-46.

Walsh SL, Haberny KA & Bigelow GE (2000). Modulation of intravenous cocaine effects by chronic oral cocaine in humans. *Psychopharmacology* 150:361-373.

Wang RIH, Kalbfleisch J, Cho JK et al. (1994). Bromocriptine, desipramine, and trazodone alone and in combination to cocaine dependent patients. *Problems on Drug Dependence, 1993 (NIDA Research Monograph 141)*. Rockville, MD: National Institute on Drug Abuse, 437.

Wassermann EM & Lisanby SH (2001). Therapeutic application of repetitive transcranial magnetic stimulation: A review. *Clinical Neurophysiology* 112:1367-1377.

Weddington WW, Brown BS, Haertzen CA et al. (1991). Comparison of amantidine and desipramine combined with psychotherapy for treatment of alcoholism and drug abuse. *American Journal of Alcohol and Drug Abuse* 17(2):137-152.

Weiss RD & Mirin SM (1989). Tricyclic antidepressants in the treatment of alcoholism and drug abuse. *Journal of Clinical Psychiatry* 50(Suppl 7):4-9.

Weiss RD, Mirin SM, Griffin ML et al. (1993). Personality disorders in cocaine dependence. *Comprehensive Psychiatry* 34:145-149.

White R (2000). Dexamphetamine substitution in the treatment of amphetamine abuse: An initial investigation. *Addiction* 95:229-238.

Wise RA (1998). Drug-activation of brain reward pathways. *Drug and Alcohol Dependence* 51:13-22.

Yerby MS (1994). Pregnancy, teratogenesis, and epilepsy. *Neurology Clinics* 12:749-771.

Yonkers KA, Kando JC, Cole JO et al. (1992). Gender differences in pharmacokinetics and pharmacodynamics of psychotropic medication. *American Journal of Psychiatry* 149:587-595.

Ziedonis DM & Kosten TR (1991). Pharmacotherapy improves treatment outcome in depressed cocaine addicts. *Journal of Psychoactive Drugs* 23(4):417-425.

Zimmet SV, Strous RD, Burgess ES et al. (2000). Effects of clozapine on substance use in patients with schizophrenia and schizoaffective disorder: A retrospective survey. *Journal of Clinical Psychopharmacology* 20:94-98.

| Chapter 7 | # Pharmacologic Interventions for Tobacco Dependence |

Richard D. Hurt, M.D.
Jon O. Ebbert, M.D.
J. Taylor Hays, M.D.
Lowell C. Dale, M.D.

Pathophysiology of Tobacco Dependence
Measuring Nicotine Exposure
Nicotine Replacement Therapy
Non-Nicotine Products
Combination Pharmacotherapies
Unproven Pharmacotherapies
Tobacco Dependence in Alcoholics

Tobacco has been used since the earliest recorded history of the western hemisphere, but cigarettes are a product of the latter part of the 19th century. It was not until the early part of the 20th century that cigarettes were mass-produced and marketed in an effective way, with the result that annual consumption increased from less than 4 billion cigarettes in 1905 to more than 100 billion just 20 years later (McNally, 1932). The epidemic of tobacco-caused diseases emerged in the mid-20th century and now has spread throughout the world. An estimated 10 million tobacco-caused deaths per year are expected to occur by the year 2030 (Peto, Lopey et al., 1994).

The tobacco industry responded to these staggering figures first by denying the relationship of cigarettes to disease and then by mounting a public relations campaign to deceive the public (Hurt & Robertson, 1998). The first major product change came in the 1950s, when filters were added to cigarettes for "health reassurance."

The first Surgeon General's report on the health consequences of smoking was published in 1964, but the first Surgeon General's report on nicotine addiction did not appear until 1988. It is well known now that the tobacco industry knew about and exploited nicotine addiction dec-

ades before this report was issued. As concerns about the health effects of smoking continued to rise, the tobacco industry responded once again with deception by promoting its low tar/low nicotine cigarettes as a safer alternative. The pattern continues today, with one tobacco manufacturer promoting a new nicotine delivery system (Eclipse®) as a safer alternative for cigarette smokers (Fagerström, Hughes et al., 2000), while other companies announce work on a tobacco with lower levels of carcinogens.

The common thread woven through the history of the major tobacco companies is their pursuit of the most efficient instrument for the delivery of nicotine, which they perfected in the modern cigarette: a highly sophisticated and refined nicotine delivery device. It is important for those who treat patients for tobacco dependence to understand that the nicotine replacement products used in treatment are relatively inefficient in delivering nicotine compared with cigarettes. It is to be hoped that newer pharmacotherapies will be more efficacious than the treatments now available.

Great strides have been made in the development of safe and effective pharmacotherapies for smoking cessation (Hughes, Goldstein et al., 1999). The U.S. Food and Drug Administration (FDA) has approved five products for the treatment of tobacco dependence in the United States, with two additional second-line medications included in the recent U.S. Public Health Service Guideline (Fiore, Bailey et al., 2000). Additional products have been approved for use in the United Kingdom, and many others are undergoing testing or are under development. Because pharmacotherapy has been established as a cornerstone of treatment of the tobacco-dependent patient, research and development of newer medications are likely to continue.

Given the insidious way in which the tobacco industry promotes its deadly product, health care providers will need novel approaches to treat tobacco dependence effectively, so as to help individual patients and promote the public health. Unlike other medical conditions, such as infectious diseases for which prevention and treatment efforts can decrease disease incidence, tobacco dependence has an eager, well-funded industry to promote continuation of the problem.

It is encouraging that the wider availability of pharmacotherapy has resulted in an eightfold increase in the number of quit attempts. There were approximately 1 million quit attempts using pharmacotherapy in the early 1990s, compared with more than 8 million in 1998 (Burton, Gitchell et al., 2000).

PATHOPHYSIOLOGY OF TOBACCO DEPENDENCE

Nicotine has complex and wide-ranging effects on the central nervous system (CNS). Nicotine activates native nicotinic acetylcholine receptors in the mesolimbic system of the brain. Many of these neurons project to the mesolimbic dopamine system, where dopamine release is stimulated (Watkins, Koob et al., 2000). Repeated exposure to high concentrations of nicotine causes up-regulation of the nicotinic acetylcholine receptors, leading to an absolute increase in the number of these receptors in smokers compared with nonsmokers (Balfour, 1991). Although not completely understood, it generally is assumed that nicotinic acetylcholine receptor up-regulation is critical to the development of tolerance to and dependence on nicotine.

Nicotinic acetylcholine receptors are located in all areas of the human brain. Nicotine causes the release of norepinephrine, glutamate, vasopressin, serotonin, gamma-aminobutyric acid (GABA), beta-endorphins, and other neurotransmitters. There are high concentrations of nicotinic acetylcholine receptors in the mesolimbic system and locus ceruleus. The former is important in the pleasure and reward phenomenon, whereas the latter is important in cognitive function.

In the mesolimbic system (and specifically in the nucleus accumbens), nicotine causes the release of dopamine, believed to be associated with nicotine's reinforcing effects; this area also is involved with the reinforcing effects of amphetamines, cocaine, and opiates (Clarke, 1993; DiChiara & Imperato, 1988; Pontieri, Tanda et al., 1996). Dopamine appears to mediate these reinforcing properties, which are critical to the addictive process (DiChiara, 2000). Because dopaminergic transmission within the nucleus accumbens is modulated by GABA, it has been postulated that GABA antagonists might inhibit nicotine-induced increases in dopamine (Dewey, Brodie et al., 1999). It has been demonstrated that nicotine-induced dose-dependent increases in feelings of pleasure occur simultaneously with increases in the functional magnetic resonance imaging of neuronal activity that occurs in the nucleus accumbens, amygdala, cingulate, and frontal lobes (Stein, Pankiewicz et al., 1998).

Tobacco dependence in smokers has been hypothesized to have a genetic component as well (Carmelli, Swan et al., 1992). Twin studies have confirmed an inherited component for tobacco use and dependence and, recently, familial transmission of smoking has been observed across three generations of families (Cheng, Swan et al., 2000). It has been hypothesized that multiple genetic polymorphisms relating to dopamine release, dopamine transmission, dopamine receptors, and nicotine metabolism are important inherited factors that influence the initiation and perpetuation of tobacco use (Lerman, Caporaso et al., 1999; Sabol, Nelson et al., 1999). However, substance dependence is complex and involves multiple genetic and environmental risk factors (Kendler, Neale et al., 1999). Further work is needed to study the spectrum of inheritable traits that influence genetic susceptibility to tobacco dependence.

MEASURING NICOTINE EXPOSURE

One approach to the therapeutic use of nicotine replacement products for the treatment of tobacco dependence is to determine the level of nicotine exposure of an individual. Once this exposure is determined, a nicotine replacement dose that approximates the dose the individual receives from smoking can be prescribed. However, there are several factors that make this task difficult. Smokers exposed to the same nicotine by inhaling tobacco smoke have marked interindividual differences in the venous nicotine concentrations achieved (Dale, Hurt et al., 1995; Gourlay & Benowitz, 1997). Cigarette smoking produces initial arterial nicotine concentrations that are several-fold higher than concomitant venous nicotine levels (Henningfield, Stapleton et al., 1993). In addition, nicotine has a short half-life of 120 minutes and, with smoking, tends to have peaks and troughs in both the venous and the arterial circulation.

For these reasons, a non-nicotine biologic measure is needed to estimate nicotine exposure. Cotinine, the major metabolic product of nicotine, has a half-life of 18 to 20 hours and can be used to quantify an individual's exposure to nicotine. The use of blood nicotine and cotinine concentrations is similar to the manner in which clinicians use fasting plasma glucose and glycosylated hemoglobin to determine glycemic control in patients with diabetes. Plasma glucose is used to determine the "real-time" glucose levels, whereas glycosylated hemoglobin provides an estimate of longer-term glycemic control. Venous nicotine concentrations give an assessment (albeit less than arterial levels) of acute nicotine exposure, whereas cotinine integrates nicotine exposure over a period of two to three days.

Minor tobacco alkaloids such as nornicotine, trans-3-hydroxycotinine, and anabasine can be measured in body fluids (Jacob, Yu et al., 1999). Anabasine is a tobacco alkaloid that is not a metabolic product of nicotine. Anabasine is present in the urine of tobacco users but not in the urine of patients using nicotine replacement therapy. Anabasine thus can be especially useful in distinguishing abstinent tobacco users who are using nicotine replacement therapy from those who are continuing to use tobacco.

NICOTINE REPLACEMENT THERAPY

According to the practice guideline published by the U.S. Public Health Service, every patient who attempts to stop smoking should be treated with pharmacotherapy (Fiore, Bailey et al., 2000). Clinical trials have shown that, in general, adding pharmacotherapy to a behavioral intervention doubles the success rate. Because of its demonstrated efficacy in multiple clinical trials, nicotine replacement therapy remains a mainstay of pharmacotherapy for the treatment of tobacco dependence.

To date, the FDA has approved several nicotine replacement products, including nicotine gum, nicotine patches, a nicotine nasal spray and, most recently, a nicotine vapor inhaler. The first two now are available over the counter, while the latter two are available by prescription only.

Physicians who prescribe nicotine replacement therapy for tobacco dependence should individualize the dose and duration of treatment and schedule followup office visits or telephone calls to monitor the patient's response. The dose and duration of therapy should be based on the patient's subjective need for relief of withdrawal symptoms and support of abstinence.

Nicotine Gum. Nicotine gum has been available for many years, and both the 2 mg and 4 mg doses are available as over-the-counter products. Venous nicotine concentrations achieved through the proper use of nicotine gum are relatively low compared with those produced by smoking cigarettes (Russell, Raw et al., 1980). Nevertheless, nicotine gum is effective in the treatment of tobacco dependence. The 4 mg dose seems to be more effective in smokers who are more dependent (Glover, Sachs et al., 1996; Sachs, 1995) and is recommended for those who smoke 25 or more cigarettes per day.

Patients should be instructed to bite into a piece of the nicotine gum a few times until a mild tingling or peppery taste indicates nicotine release. The patient then should "park" the gum between the cheek and gum for several minutes before chewing it again. This cycle allows for buccal absorption and should be repeated for about 30 minutes per piece of gum. Because the rapidity of absorption of nicotine is lowered by a more acidic pH, patients should be instructed not to drink beverages or eat while using the gum. When nicotine gum is used as a single agent, most patients should chew a minimum of 10 to 15 pieces per day to achieve initial abstinence. The most common adverse effects of nicotine gum are nausea and indigestion, which can be minimized with the proper chewing technique. Other adverse effects reported include gingival soreness and mouth ulcerations.

Nicotine Patch. Nicotine patch therapy, which was introduced in 1991, delivers a steady dose of nicotine for 16 to 24 hours. The once-daily dosing requires little effort on the part of the patient, resulting in high compliance. Nicotine patches are available without a prescription in doses of 7, 11, 14, 21, and 22 mg, which deliver nicotine over 24 hours, and a 15-mg patch that delivers nicotine over 16 hours. In almost every randomized clinical trial performed to date, the nicotine patch has been shown to be effective compared with placebo, usually with a doubling of the stop rate. Standard-dose nicotine patch therapy begins with a dose of 21 or 22 mg/24 hours or 15 mg/16 hours. Most regimens continue this dose for several weeks before tapering over a period of a few weeks. However, single-patch

TABLE 1. Initial Nicotine Patch Dose, Based on Baseline Serum Cotinine Concentration (While Smoking)

Cotinine (ng/mL)	Nicotine Patch Dose
<200	14-22 mg/day
200-300	22-44 mg/day
>300	>44 mg/day

dosing is not effective in all smokers. In fact, it has been shown that a standard dose (21 or 22 mg/24 hours) of nicotine patch therapy achieves a median serum cotinine level of only 54% of the cotinine concentrations achieved through smoking (Dale, Hurt et al., 1995; Hurt, Dale et al., 1993). Lighter smokers with lower baseline cotinine concentrations have higher stop rates, suggesting that their nicotine replacement needs are more adequately met than those of heavier smokers (Hurt, Dale et al., 1994).

Because of the observation that many patients are underdosed at standard nicotine patch doses, efforts have been made to study increases in dosing to improve the efficacy of this treatment. The limited number of reported studies have yielded mixed results. However, use of higher doses of nicotine patch therapy (that is, more than one patch at a time) can be appropriate for smokers who previously failed single-dose patch therapy or for those whose nicotine withdrawal symptoms were not relieved sufficiently with standard therapy (Hughes, 1995). This approach can be especially important for heavy smokers because they will be significantly underdosed with single-dose patch therapy (Dale, Hurt et al., 1995).

High-dose nicotine patch therapy has been shown to be safe and well tolerated in patients who smoke more than 20 cigarettes per day (Dale, Hurt et al., 1995; Fredrickson, Hurt et al., 1995). By employing the concept of therapeutic drug monitoring, the clinician can use serum cotinine concentrations to tailor the nicotine replacement dose so that it is close to 100% replacement. A baseline cotinine concentration is obtained while the smoker is smoking his or her usual number of cigarettes. An initial nicotine patch dose based on the cotinine level (or cigarettes per day) is prescribed. After the patient reaches steady state (>3 days of nicotine patch therapy and not smoking), the serum cotinine level is rechecked. The replacement dose then can be adjusted according to the steady-state cotinine level. Percentage replacement for a given dose of nicotine patch therapy can be expressed as follows:

$$\text{Percentage replacement} = \frac{\text{Baseline serum cotinine}}{\text{Steady-state serum cotinine}} \times 100$$

Table 1 shows the recommended initial dosing of nicotine patch therapy based on serum cotinine levels. Higher percentage replacement has been shown to reduce nicotine withdrawal symptoms (Dale, Hurt et al., 1995), but the efficacy for long-term abstinence of such an approach has not been completely established (Dale, Hurt et al., 1995; Hughes, Lesmes et al., 1999; Jorenby, Smith et al., 1995; Sachs, Benowitz et al., 1995; Tonnesen, Paoletti et al., 1999). Nevertheless, this concept can be used to titrate more precisely the dose to reach higher levels of nicotine replacement in the more severely addicted patient.

In special populations, such as pregnant women, in which there is a need to use the lowest possible effective dose, monitoring serum cotinine can be used to keep the replacement levels close to baseline.

Individualizing the nicotine patch dose is warranted because of the interindividual variability of baseline nicotine and cotinine concentrations among smokers who smoke a similar number of cigarettes per day. There also is interindividual variability in steady-state serum cotinine while receiving nicotine patch therapy during abstinence from smoking (Dale, Hurt et al., 1995; Hurt, Dale et al., 1992). Serum cotinine is the test of choice for calculating the percentage replacement, even though urine nicotine or cotinine can be used (Lawson, Hurt et al., 1998a,b). Blood can be drawn at any time of the day for this assessment (Lawson, Hurt et al., 1998a).

If serum cotinine testing is not available, the replacement dose can be estimated based on the number of cigarettes smoked per day. Table 2 shows the recommended initial dosing of nicotine patch therapy based on the number of cigarettes smoked per day, which has been shown to correlate with the cotinine concentrations shown in Table 1 (Dale, Hurt et al., 1995).

After initiation of nicotine patch therapy on the stop date, the patient should have a followup visit or a telephone counseling session within the first two weeks and periodically thereafter. Abstinence from smoking during the first two weeks of patch therapy has been shown to be highly predictive of long-term abstinence (Hurt, Dale et al., 1994; Kenford, Fiore et al., 1994). Thus, the first two weeks of nicotine patch therapy are critical. Alterations in therapy at followup depend on how well the patient is maintaining abstinence from smoking and the relief of withdrawal symptoms. If the patient continues to smoke at all during the first two weeks, the treatment must be changed, either by adding additional pharmacotherapy (using the concept of percentage replacement, as described earlier) or intensifying the behavioral counseling. Nicotine patch doses should be increased for patients who experience pronounced withdrawal symptoms such as irritability, anxiety, loss of concentration, or craving, or for patients who do not achieve 100% replacement based on the second serum cotinine level.

Although the various nicotine patches have quite comparable pharmacokinetic profiles, there are differences between brands that could lead to higher percentage replacement (Gariti, Alterman et al., 1999). Thus, measuring cotinine is a more accurate method of assessing the adequacy of nicotine replacement and avoiding "over replacement."

Most patients use the nicotine patch for four to eight weeks, but it is safe to use it longer if needed to maintain abstinence. Optimal length of treatment has not been determined.

Side effects of nicotine patch therapy are relatively mild and include localized skin reactions at the patch site. Such reactions generally begin to occur about four weeks after initiation of patch therapy. Lesions vary from erythema to erythema plus vesicles. Topical corticosteroid therapy sometimes is helpful in controlling these local symptoms. Rotation of the patches to different sites of the skin helps to reduce the frequency of this side effect. In rare instances, a generalized skin eruption can occur, requiring that nicotine patch therapy be discontinued. Although sleep disturbance is another side effect that has been attributed to nicotine patch therapy, it often is difficult to ascertain whether this is attributable to nicotine withdrawal or to the administration of nicotine during the evening hours. In a sleep study of smokers who were trying to stop, the best quality of sleep was observed in those receiving a 22 mg/24 hours nicotine patch dose compared with placebo (Wetter, Fiore et al., 1995). If there is a concern that nicotine patch therapy is causing sleep disturbance, the patch can be removed at night to see if the sleep disturbance resolves.

Shortly after nicotine patches reached the market, some concern was expressed in the lay press that smokers might be at increased risk of myocardial infarction if they contin-

TABLE 2. Initial Nicotine Patch Dose, Based on Number of Cigarettes Smoked Daily

Cigarettes per Day	Patch Dose* (mg/day)
<10	7-14
10-20	14-22
21-40	22-44
>40	44+

* Nicotine patches are available in the following doses: 7, 11, 14, 15, 21, and 22 mg.

ued to smoke while using the patch (Hwang & Waldholz, 1992). This exposure in the press led to hearings at the FDA, which concluded that there is no cause for concern. Subsequent studies have shown no adverse effects in smokers with a history of coronary disease who are receiving the 14- or 21-mg patch doses (Joseph, Norman et al., 1996; Working Group, 1994), nor were there adverse effects on lipids or markers of homeostasis in nonsmokers who received nicotine patch therapy (Thomas, Davies et al., 1995). Nicotine patch doses up to 63 mg/day were not associated with short-term adverse cardiovascular effects in smokers (Zevin, Jacob et al., 1998). Standard nicotine patch doses have been shown to reduce exercise-induced myocardial ischemia (assessed by exercise thallium studies) in smokers who were trying to stop smoking (Mahmarian, Moye et al., 1997). Experimentally, nicotine patch doses of up to 44 mg/day for four weeks have not adversely affected the early patency of coronary artery bypass grafts in dogs (Clouse, Yamaguchi et al., 2000). However, transdermal nicotine can increase the production of and response to nitric oxide in the bypass grafts, which usually would produce vasodilatation (Clouse, Yamaguchi et al., 2000).

In summary, the risks of nicotine patch therapy in smokers with cardiovascular disease are small and are substantially outweighed by the potential benefits of stopping smoking (Benowitz & Gourlay, 1997).

Nicotine Nasal Spray. Nicotine nasal spray delivers nicotine directly to the nasal mucosa. It has been found to be effective in randomized clinical trials (Schneider, Olmstead et al., 1995). This device delivers nicotine more rapidly than other therapeutic nicotine replacement delivery systems and reduces withdrawal symptoms more quickly than nicotine gum (Hurt, Offord et al., 1998; Schneider, Lunell et al., 1996). The reduction in withdrawal symptoms may be partially attributable to the rapidity with which nicotine is absorbed from the nasal mucosa and the resulting arterial venous differences in the plasma concentration of nicotine (Gourlay & Benowitz, 1997). Each spray contains 0.5 mg of nicotine, and one dose is one spray in each nostril (a total of 1 mg). Recommended dosing is one to two doses per hour, not to exceed five doses per hour or 40 doses per day. When using the nicotine nasal spray as a single agent, most patients initially use 12 to 16 doses per day. The recommended length of treatment is up to 12 weeks of ad lib use, followed by a tapering schedule. The nicotine nasal spray can be used in combination with other nicotine replacement products or with bupropion (Zyban®). Patients should be instructed to spray against the lower nasal mucosa and not to sniff spray into the upper nasal passages or to attempt to inhale it. The most common adverse side effects are rhinorrhea, nasal and throat irritation, watery eyes, and sneezing. These irritant side effects decrease significantly within the first week of use, independent of dose (Hurt, Dale et al., 1998).

Because the nicotine nasal spray is a more rapid delivery device than other nicotine replacement products, there was early concern that the spray could have long-term abuse liability (Sutherland, Stapleton et al., 1992). More recent information indicates that the potential for abuse is low (Schuh, Schuh et al., 1997).

Nicotine Inhaler. The nicotine vapor inhaler has been shown to be effective in placebo-controlled trials (Leischow, Nilsson et al., 1996). This device is a plastic holder into which a cartridge containing a cotton plug impregnated with 10 mg of nicotine is inserted. The device delivers a nicotine vapor that is absorbed through the oral mucosa in much the same way as nicotine gum. Although the device is called an inhaler, this is something of a misnomer because little of the nicotine vapor reaches the pulmonary alveoli, even with deep inhalations. Positron emission tomography studies show that only a small amount of radiolabeled nicotine reaches the lungs, and that most of it is absorbed through the oral pharynx, so the inhaler does not provide high arterial levels of nicotine in the manner of cigarettes (Bergström, Nordberg et al., 1995; Lunell, Bergström et al., 1996; Lunell, Molander et al., 2000). When the nicotine inhaler is used as a single therapy, efficacy is increased when more than six cartridges per day are used. Nicotine replacement levels

based on serum cotinine concentrations vary from 43% to more than 60%, depending on the number of nicotine cartridges used per day, with six cartridges associated with higher levels of replacement and improved abstinence rates (Hjalmarson, Nilsson et al., 1997; Leischow, Nilsson et al., 1996). The recommended initial dose of the nicotine inhaler when used alone is 6 to 16 cartridges per day. The recommended length of treatment is approximately 12 weeks, followed by a tapering schedule, although the inhaler could be used longer. Although this device requires frequent puffing to deliver substantial amounts of nicotine, the puffing mimics some of the behavior of smoking.

Because it is a unique delivery device, the nicotine inhaler lends itself to being used in combination with other nicotine replacement products and/or bupropion. Adverse effects generally are mild and most often involve mouth or throat irritation, with occasional coughing.

Sublingual Nicotine Tablet and Nicotine Lozenge. A new nicotine replacement product, a sublingual tablet, has been tested in double-blind, placebo-controlled trials and is available in the United Kingdom and parts of Europe (Glover, Glover et al., in press; Wallström, 2000; Molander, 2000). The nicotine sublingual tablet, which delivers 2 mg of nicotine, has been well accepted by smokers in clinical trials. Although the method of delivery (transbuccal) is similar to that of nicotine gum, the sublingual tablet is simpler to use and can improve patient compliance. Side effects appear to be mild and transient (Wallström, Sand et al., 1999).

A 1 mg nicotine lozenge also is being marketed in some parts of the world. Similar to the nicotine sublingual tablet, the lozenge delivers nicotine across the buccal mucosa. There are no published reports about efficacy of this delivery device.

Summary. With the exception of the nicotine lozenge, all of the approved nicotine replacement products discussed here have been found to be effective in randomized, placebo-controlled trials, usually with a doubling of the stop rate in the active treatment group. These products have proved to be remarkably safe. As the number and availability of such products have increased, the number of attempts to stop smoking by American smokers has increased dramatically (Burton, Gitchell et al., 2000). Although all of the nicotine replacement products seem to be equally effective, there are differences in compliance with the recommended dose. There are, however, no notable differences between the products when used at standard doses, nor their effects on withdrawal symptom discomfort, perceived helpfulness, and general efficacy (Hajek, West et al., 1999).

NON-NICOTINE PRODUCTS

Bupropion (Zyban®). The relationship between smoking and depression has been well documented. Smokers are more likely than nonsmokers to have a history of major depression (Anda, Williamson et al., 1990; Glassman, Helzer et al., 1990; Hall, Munoz et al., 1991). During the course of an attempt to stop smoking, many smokers develop a depressed affect, and some become overtly depressed (Borrelli, Niaura et al., 1996; Covey, Glassman et al., 1990; Glass, 1990; Tsoh, Humfleet et al., 2000). The development of a depressed affect during an attempt to stop smoking is associated with relapse to smoking (Hall, Munoz et al., 1994; Shiffman, 1982). This association has raised the question of the role antidepressants might play in treating tobacco dependence and has led to the study of the efficacy of antidepressants in treating smokers. Of the antidepressants tested, bupropion is the first non-nicotine pharmacologic treatment approved for the treatment of tobacco dependence.

Bupropion is a monocyclic antidepressant that inhibits the reuptake of both norepinephrine and dopamine (Ascher, Cole et al., 1995). Dopamine release in the mesolimbic system and the nucleus accumbens is thought to be the basis for the reinforcing properties of nicotine and other drugs of addiction (Clarke, 1993; DiChiara & Imperato, 1988; Pontieri, Tanda et al., 1996). It does not appear that bupropion works through its antidepressant activity. Rather, it is hypothesized that the efficacy of bupropion in smoking cessation stems from its dopaminergic activity on the pleasure and reward pathways in the mesolimbic system and nucleus accumbens. Recently, bupropion also has been shown to have an antagonist effect on nicotinic acetylcholine receptors (Fryer & Lukas, 1999; Slemmer, Martin et al., 2000). Thus, its mechanism of action likely is multifactorial.

Sustained-release bupropion has been shown to be effective in a dose-response study (Hurt, Sachs et al., 1997) and in a study combining bupropion with nicotine patch therapy (Jorenby, Leischow et al., 1999). In the former study, smokers were randomly assigned to receive bupropion at 100, 150, or 300 mg/day or placebo. A significant dose-response effect was detected at all time points, and the smoking abstinence rates for the 150- and 300-mg treatment groups were significantly higher than placebo at the end of treatment and at one year. In addition, there was an attenuation of weight gain during the treatment period for those who were continuously abstinent while receiving the 300 mg/day dose (however, the attenuation of weight gain did not persist at one-year followup). Treatment with bupropion alone or in combination with the nicotine patch resulted in a significantly higher long-term rate of abstinence from smoking than did use of either the nicotine patch alone or placebo (Jorenby, Leischow et al., 1999). Smoking abstinence rates were higher with combination therapy than with bupropion alone, but the differences were not statistically significant.

Treatment with bupropion should be initiated about one week before the patient's stop date, at an initial dose of 150 mg/day for three days, then 150 mg twice a day. The usual length of treatment is 6 to 12 weeks, but bupropion can be used safely for much longer. As with other antidepressants, a small risk (0.1%) of seizures is associated with this medication. Therefore, bupropion is contraindicated in patients who have a history of seizures, serious head trauma (such as a skull fracture or a prolonged loss of consciousness), an eating disorder (anorexia nervosa or bulimia), or concomitant use of medications that lower the seizure threshold. The most common adverse side effects are insomnia and dry mouth. Cardiovascular and sexual adverse effects are uncommon. Recent reports from the FDA suggest that treatment-emergent hypertension can occur during treatment with bupropion, especially when it is used in combination with nicotine patch therapy. Therefore, periodic blood pressure measurements during treatment are advised.

In an assessment of the predictors of successful outcome, bupropion was found to be effective in treating cigarette smokers, independent of all other characteristics studied. However, lower smoking rate, prior abstinence from smoking for brief periods (<24 hours) or long periods (>4 weeks), and male gender all were predictors of better outcome, independent of the bupropion dose (Dale, Glover et al., 2001). Further, bupropion appears to be equally effective in smokers with or without a history of depression or in recovering alcoholics and nonalcoholics alike (Hayford, Patten et al., 1999).

Bupropion also has been tested as an agent for relapse prevention. In a large study, more than 700 smokers received open-label bupropion (300 mg/day) treatment for seven weeks. Those who were abstinent from smoking at the end of the open-label period were assigned randomly to

TABLE 3. Items and Scoring for the Fagertröm Test for Nicotine Dependence

Questions	Answers	Points
1. How soon after you wake up do you smoke your first cigarette?	Within 5 minutes	3
	6-30 minutes	2
	31-60 minutes	1
	After 60 minutes	0
2. Do you find it difficult to refrain from smoking in places where it is forbidden (in church, at the library, in cinema, etc.)?	Yes	1
	No	0
3. Which cigarette would you hate most to give up?	The first one in the morning	1
	All others	0
4. How many cigarettes per day do you smoke?	10 or less	0
	11-20	1
	21-30	2
	31 or more	3
5. Do you smoke more frequently during the first hours after waking than during the rest of the day?	Yes	1
	No	0
6. Do you smoke if you are so ill that you are in bed most of the day?	Yes	1
	No	0

SOURCE: Fagerström KO (1978). Measuring degree of physical dependence to tobacco smoking with reference to individualization of treatment. *Addictive Behavior* 3:235-241.

active or placebo bupropion for the remainder of the year, then followed for a subsequent year (Hays, Hurt et al., 2001). Smoking abstinence rates were significantly higher in the bupropion group compared with placebo at the end of medication therapy (week 52) and at week 78, but not at 104 weeks. The median time to relapse was significantly longer for subjects who received bupropion compared with placebo, and there was significantly less weight gain in the bupropion group compared with placebo at weeks 52 and 104. As with the dose-response study, the best overall predictor of successful relapse prevention was assignment to active bupropion (Hurt, Wolter et al., 2001). There was a medication effect that was independent of any predictor except older age and no or minimal weight gain during the open-label phase.

Predictors of successful relapse prevention included lower baseline smoking rates, a Fagerström Tolerance Ques-

tionnaire score lower than 6 (Table 3), and initiation of smoking at an older age. As with the dose-response study, the extended use of bupropion for relapse prevention is effective for smokers with or without a history of depression (Cox, Patten et al., in press).

Because of the high prevalence of a history of depression in smokers, clinicians often encounter smokers who want to stop smoking but already are being treated with an antidepressant. The question arises as whether to discontinue the current antidepressant before starting bupropion or to simply add bupropion to that regimen. There is no drug-drug interaction to preclude the use of bupropion with either selective serotonin reuptake inhibitors or tricyclic antidepressants. Thus, adding bupropion to a selective serotonin reuptake inhibitor is preferable to discontinuing that medication and using bupropion only. Although one study showed no serious adverse effects (Chengappa,

Kambhampati et al., in press), patients receiving two antidepressants should be monitored carefully. The use of monoamine oxidase inhibitors is a contraindication for use of bupropion. In summary, bupropion has utility in the general smoking population, seems to attenuate the weight gain associated with stopping smoking, and can be used to prevent relapse to smoking.

Nortriptyline (Aventyl®). Nortriptyline is a tricyclic antidepressant that is recommended as a second-line drug for smoking cessation (Fiore, Bailey et al., 2000). Two randomized clinical trials have shown a significant effect with active nortriptyline compared with placebo (Hall, Reus et al., 1998; Prochazka, Weaver et al., 1998). In these studies, the maximal dose range was 75 to 100 mg/day, and the length of treatment was 8 to 12 weeks. The most common adverse effects were sedation and dry mouth. As with bupropion, nortriptyline produced higher smoking abstinence rates than placebo, independent of a history of depression. However, increases in negative affect after quitting smoking were attenuated by nortriptyline (Hall, Reus et al., 1998).

Clonidine (Catapres®). Clonidine is a centrally acting alpha-agonist that can be used as a second-line drug (Fiore, Bailey et al., 2000). It is available in both oral or transdermal forms. The transdermal form is easier to use, with a recommended dose of 0.2 mg/day for 3 to 10 weeks. The clonidine patch should be initiated a week before the patient's stop date and changed weekly thereafter. Common side effects include dry mouth and drowsiness.

COMBINATION PHARMACOTHERAPIES

A few studies have examined nicotine replacement products used in combination. One study used the combination of nicotine patch therapy and bupropion. The U.S. Public Health Service Guideline recommends that combining the nicotine patch with a self-administered form of nicotine replacement therapy, either nicotine gum or nicotine nasal spray, is more effective than a single form of nicotine replacement. This approach should be encouraged if a patient is unable to stop smoking by using a single first-line pharmacotherapy.

It is not clear whether the superiority of combination therapy is due to the use of two types of delivery systems or to the fact that two delivery systems tend to produce higher blood nicotine levels. The former seems to be the main reason for improved success with combination therapy, but more research is needed. Nicotine patch therapy combined with nicotine gum has been shown to reduce nicotine withdrawal symptoms (Fagerström, Schneider et al., 1993) and to improve abstinence outcomes when compared with placebo gum and nicotine patch therapy alone (Kornitzer, Boutsen et al., 1995). Nicotine patch therapy for five months, combined with nicotine nasal spray for one year, produced higher rates of abstinence from smoking than did nicotine patch therapy with placebo nasal spray (Blondal, Gudmundsson et al., 1999a). Treatment with the nicotine vapor inhaler plus nicotine patch seems to significantly increase smoking abstinence rates beyond that seen with the inhaler plus placebo patch (Bohadana, Nilsson et al., 2000).

UNPROVEN PHARMACOTHERAPIES

Anxiolytics have not been shown to be effective in helping patients stop smoking (Hughes, Stead et al., 1999). Specifically, buspirone has not been shown to have efficacy in a placebo-controlled trial (Schneider, Olmstead et al., 1996). Antidepressants other than bupropion and nortriptyline have been tested and generally have been found to be ineffective in producing long-term abstinence from smoking. Doxepin (Adapin®) was reported to be effective in one small clinical trial, which has not been replicated (Edwards, Murphy et al., 1989). Fluoxetine (Prozac®) has been tested in a large randomized clinical trial, but the main results have not been reported, presumably because there was no main effect in the active versus placebo arms. Fluoxetine was not found to enhance nicotine inhaler therapy (Blondal, Gudmundsson et al., 1999b). Paroxetine (Paxil®) has been tested in combination with nicotine patch therapy and showed no added value in improving abstinence rates (Killen, Fortmann et al., 2000).

The antihypertensive mecamylamine was shown to have efficacy in a small trial of smokers (Rose, Behm et al., 1994). A much larger, unpublished study combining mecamylamine and nicotine in a single patch versus placebo showed no main effect on smoking abstinence rates. Despite the theoretical role that dopamine plays as a critical mediator of the reinforcing effects of nicotine, administration of carbidopa/levodopa (Sinemet®, a dopamine agonist) in doses used to treat Parkinson's disease showed no efficacy compared with placebo (Hurt, Ahlskog et al., 2000). Finally, naltrexone (ReVia®) did not show efficacy compared with placebo in a randomized, clinical trial using naltrexone and the nicotine patch (Wong, Wolter et al., 1999); however, other studies suggest that it may have some short-term effects (Brauer, Behm et al., 1999; Covey, Glassman et al., 1999).

TOBACCO DEPENDENCE IN ALCOHOLICS

Tobacco-caused diseases account for 19% of all deaths in the U.S., while alcoholism and other non-nicotine drug dependence account for another 6% (McGinnis & Foege, 1993). The prevalence of smoking among alcoholics and those dependent on other drugs is two to three times that of the general population (Bobo, 1989; Kozlowski, Henningfield et al., 1993; Kozlowski, Jelinek et al., 1986). Thus, it is estimated that alcoholics may constitute as much as 26% of all smokers (DiFranza & Guerrera, 1989).

The importance of treating tobacco dependence in alcoholic and non-nicotine substance abusers is highlighted by the fact that tobacco-caused diseases account for more than 50% of all deaths, whereas alcohol-related conditions account for more than 30% of deaths in patients previously treated in an inpatient addiction treatment program (Hurt, Offord et al., 1996). The fact that tobacco-caused diseases were the leading cause of death in patients treated for alcoholism and other non-nicotine drug dependence provides compelling evidence that the treatment of tobacco dependence is imperative in these high-risk patients. Not only are mortality rates higher, but there is a marked decrease in the general and mental health status of current tobacco users who have a history of an alcohol problem, compared with nontobacco users with no history of an alcohol problem (Patten, Schneekloth et al., 2001).

Efforts have been made to treat nicotine as a drug of dependence in addiction treatment programs (Hurt, Eberman et al., 1994; Joseph, Nichol et al., 1990). Specific smoking interventions have been developed for individuals who also are alcohol dependent (Martin, Calfas et al., 1997). For alcoholic patients who have a history of a major depressive disorder, effective interventions have focused on managing negative mood (Patten, Martin et al., 1998). A variety of cognitive strategies should be considered in treating tobacco dependence in persons in recovery, and more is to be learned about facilitating tobacco dependence treatment among those early in recovery (Sussman, in press).

Data on pharmacotherapies for tobacco dependence in alcoholics are very limited. In general, alcoholic smokers have more severe nicotine dependence than do nonalcoholics with higher smoking rates, higher baseline blood cotinine levels, and higher Fagerström Tolerance Questionnaire scores (Hughes, 1993; Hurt, Dale et al., 1995). In a *post hoc* analysis of smokers receiving standard nicotine patch therapy, recovering alcoholics achieved an initial smoking abstinence rate of 46% at the end of treatment, but this rate dropped to 0 at one-year followup (Hurt, Dale et al., 1995). Only one placebo-controlled, nicotine patch trial has focused on recovering alcoholic smokers, and end-of-treatment smoking abstinence rates were 37% and 26%, respectively, for those assigned to a 21 mg nicotine patch or placebo (Novy, Hughes et al., 1998).

Surprisingly, among smokers receiving nicotine patch therapy, recovering alcoholics have been shown to have more difficulty stopping smoking than current alcoholics or nonalcoholics (Hays, Schroeder et al., 1999). Because alcoholics are likely to be heavier smokers than nonalcoholics, high-dose nicotine patch therapy seems justified for these patients, who have a high risk of mortality from tobacco-caused diseases. Further, combinations of nicotine replacement therapies or combinations of nicotine replacement and non-nicotine products, such as bupropion or nortriptyline, seem indicated as well. As mentioned earlier, bupropion seems to be effective in smokers, irrespective of their history of depression or alcoholism (Hayford, Patten et al., 1999). Finally, for recovering alcoholic smokers, more intense behavioral treatments (such as residential treatment) may be indicated (Hays, Wolter et al., 2001).

CONCLUSIONS

Much progress has been made in recent years in treating tobacco dependence. There are now five FDA-approved medications, two of which are readily available as over-the-counter products. An evidence-based guideline published by the U.S. Public Health Service extends our understanding of effective treatments and encourage clinicians to be more persistent in recognizing tobacco users and more aggressive in treating them. The guideline clearly outlines the potential use of the five approved medications as first-line drugs and two additional medications as second-line drugs. It encourages the use of combinations of these medications when appropriate.

Clearly, for a medical problem of the magnitude of smoking, more—and more effective—pharmacotherapies are needed.

REFERENCES

Anda RF, Williamson DF, Escobedo LG et al. (1990). Depression and the dynamics of smoking: A national perspective. *Journal of the American Medical Association* 264:1541-1545.

Ascher JA, Cole JO, Colin JN et al. (1995). Bupropion: A review of its mechanism of antidepressant activity. *Journal of Clinical Psychiatry* 56(9):395-401.

Balfour DJK (1991). The neurochemical mechanisms underlying nicotine tolerance and dependence. In JA Pratt (ed.) *The Biological Basis of Drug Tolerance and Dependence.* London, England: Academic Press, 121-151.

Benowitz NL & Gourlay SG (1997). Cardiovascular toxicity of nicotine: Implications for nicotine replacement therapy. *Journal of the American College of Cardiology* 29:1422-1431.

Bergström M, Nordberg A, Lunell E et al. (1995). Regional deposition of inhaled 11C-nicotine vapor in the human airway as visualized by positron emission tomography. *Clinical Pharmacology and Therapeutics* 57(3):309-317.

Blondal T, Gudmundsson LJ, Olafsdottir I et al. (1999a). Nicotine nasal spray with nicotine patch for smoking cessation: Randomized trial with six year follow up. *British Medical Journal* 318:285-288.

Blondal T, Gudmundsson LJ, Tomasson K et al. (1999b). The effects of fluoxetine combined with nicotine inhalers in smoking cessation—A randomized trial. *Addiction* 94(7):1007-1015.

Bobo JK (1989). Nicotine dependence and alcoholism epidemiology and treatment. *Journal of Psychoactive Drugs* 21:323-329.

Bohadana A, Nilsson F, Rasmussen T et al. (2000). Nicotine inhaler and nicotine patch as a combination therapy for smoking cessation. A randomized, double-blind, placebo-controlled trial. *Archives of Internal Medicine* 160:1-7.

Borrelli B, Niaura R, Keuthen NJ et al. (1996). Development of major depressive disorder during smoking cessation treatment. *Journal of Clinical Psychiatry* 57:534-538.

Brauer LH, Behm FM, Westman EC et al. (1999). Naltrexone blockade of nicotine effects in cigarette smokers. *Psychopharmacology* 143(4):339-346.

Burton SL, Gitchell JG & Shiffman S (2000). Use of FDA-approved pharmacologic treatments for tobacco dependence—United States, 1984-1998. *Morbidity and Mortality Weekly Report* 49(29):665-668.

Carmelli D, Swan GE, Robinette D et al. (1992). Genetic influence on smoking. A study of male twins. *New England Journal of Medicine* 327:829-833.

Cheng LS, Swan GE & Carmelli D (2000). A genetic analysis of smoking behavior in family members of older adult males. *Addiction* 95(3):427-435.

Chengappa KNR, Kambhampati RK, Perkins KA et al. (2001). Bupropion sustained release as a smoking cessation treatment in remitted depressed patients maintained on treatment with selective serotonin reuptake inhibitor antidepressants. *Journal of Clinical Psychiatry* 62(7):503-508.

Clarke PB (1993). Nicotine dependence—Mechanisms and therapeutic strategies. *Biochemical Society Symposia* 59:83-95.

Clouse WD, Yamaguchi H, Phillips MR et al. (2000). Effects of transdermal nicotine treatment on structure and function of coronary artery bypass grafts. *Journal of Applied Physiology* 89:1213-1223.

Covey LS, Glassman AH & Stetner F (1990). Depression and depressive symptoms in smoking cessation. *Comprehensive Psychiatry* 31:350-354.

Covey LS, Glassman AH & Stetner F (1999). Naltrexone effects on short-term and long-term smoking cessation. *Journal of Addictive Diseases* 18(1):31-40.

Cox LS, Patten CA, Niaura RS et al. (In press). Efficacy of bupropion for relapse prevention in smokers with a past history of major depression or alcoholism. *Journal of Clinical Psychiatry.*

Dale LC, Glover ED, Sachs DPL et al. (2001). Bupropion for smoking cessation: Predictors of successful outcome. *Chest* 119:1357-1364.

Dale LC, Hurt RD, Offord KP et al. (1995). High-dose nicotine patch therapy: Percentage of replacement and smoking cessation. *Journal of the American Medical Association* 274(17):1353-1358.

Dewey SL, Brodie JD, Gerasimov M et al. (1999). A pharmacologic strategy for the treatment of nicotine addiction. *Synapse* 31(1):76-86.

DiChiara G (2000). Role of dopamine in the behavioral actions of nicotine related to addiction. *European Journal of Pharmacology* 393(1-3):295-314.

DiChiara G & Imperato A (1988). Drugs abused by humans preferentially increase synaptic dopamine concentrations in the mesolimbic system of freely moving rats. *Proceedings of the National Academy of Sciences* 85(14):5274-5278.

DiFranza JR & Guerrera MP (1989). Hardcore smokers [letter]. *Journal of the American Medical Association* 261(18):2634-2635.

Edwards NB, Murphy JK, Downs AD et al. (1989). Doxepin as an adjunct to smoking cessation: A double-blind pilot study. *American Journal of Psychiatry* 146(3):373-376.

Fagerström KO, Hughes JR, Rasmussen T et al. (2000). Randomised trial investigating effect of a novel nicotine delivery device (Eclipse) and a nicotine oral inhaler on smoking behaviour, nicotine and carbon monoxide exposure, and motivation to quit. *Tobacco Control* 9:327-333.

Fagerström KO, Schneider NG & Lunell E (1993). Effectiveness of nicotine patch and nicotine gum as individual versus combined treatments for tobacco withdrawal symptoms. *Psychopharmacology* 111:271-277.

Fiore MC, Bailey WC, Cohen SJ et al. (2000). *Treating Tobacco Use and Dependence (Clinical Practice Guideline).* Rockville, MD: U.S. Department of Health and Human Services, Public Health Service.

Fredrickson PA, Hurt RD, Lee GM et al. (1995). High dose transdermal nicotine therapy for heavy smokers: Safety, tolerability and measurement of nicotine and cotinine levels. *Psychopharmacology* 122:215-222.

Fryer JD & Lukas RJ (1999). Noncompetitive functional inhibition at diverse, human nicotinic acetylcholine receptor subtypes by bupropion, phencyclidine and ibogaine. *Journal of Pharmacology and Experimental Therapeutics* 288(1):88-92.

Gariti P, Alterman AI, Barber W et al. (1999). Cotinine replacement levels for a 21 mg/day transdermal nicotine patch in an outpatient treatment setting. *Drug and Alcohol Dependence* 54(2):111-116.

Glass RM (1990). Blue mood, blackened lungs: Depression and smoking [editorial]. *Journal of the American Medical Association* 264:1583-1584.

Glassman AH, Helzer JE, Covey LS et al. (1990). Smoking, smoking cessation, and major depression. *Journal of the American Medical Association* 264:1546-1549.

Glover ED, Glover PN, Franzon M et al. (In press). A comparison of a nicotine sublingual tablet and placebo for smoking cessation. *Nicotine and Tobacco Research.*

Glover ED, Sachs DPL, Stitzer ML et al. (1996). Smoking cessation in highly dependent smokers with 4 mg nicotine polacrilex. *American Journal of Health Behavior* 20(5):319-332.

Gourlay SG & Benowitz NL (1997). Arteriovenous differences in plasma concentration of nicotine and catecholamines and related cardiovascular effects after smoking, nicotine nasal spray, and intravenous nicotine. *Clinical Pharmacology and Therapeutics* 62(4):453-463.

Hajek P, West R, Foulds J et al. (1999). Randomized comparative trial of nicotine polacrilex, a transdermal patch, nasal spray, and an inhaler. *Archives of Internal Medicine* 159:2033-2038.

Hall SM, Munoz R & Reus V (1991). Smoking cessation, depression and dysphoria. *Problems of Drug Dependence, 1990 (NIDA Research Monograph 105)*. Rockville, MD: National Institute on Drug Abuse, 312-313.

Hall SM, Munoz RF & Reus VI (1994). Cognitive-behavioral intervention increases abstinence rates for depressive-history smokers. *Journal of Consulting and Clinical Psychology* 62(1):141-146.

Hall SM, Reus V, Munoz R et al. (1998). Nortriptyline and cognitive-behavioral therapy in the treatment of cigarette smoking. *Archives of General Psychiatry* 55:683-690.

Hayford KE, Patten CA, Rummans TA et al. (1999). Efficacy of bupropion for smoking cessation in smokers with a former history of major depression or alcoholism. *British Journal of Psychiatry* 174:173-178.

Hays JT, Hurt RD, Rigotti N et al. (2001). A randomized controlled trial of sustained-release bupropion for pharmacologic relapse prevention following smoking cessation. *Annals of Internal Medicine.* 135:423-433.

Hays JT, Schroeder DR, Offord KP et al. (1999). Response to nicotine dependence treatment in smokers with current and past alcohol problems. *Annals of Behavioral Medicine* 21(3):244-250.

Hays JT, Wolter TD, Eberman KM et al. (2001). Residential (inpatient) treatment compared with outpatient treatment for nicotine dependence. *Mayo Clinic Proceedings* 76(2):124-133.

Henningfield JE, Stapleton JM, Benowitz NL et al. (1993). Higher levels of nicotine in arterial than in venous blood after cigarette smoking. *Drug and Alcohol Dependence* 33(1):23-29.

Hjalmarson A, Nilsson F, Sjöström L et al. (1997). The nicotine inhaler in smoking cessation. *Archives of Internal Medicine* 157:1721-1728.

Hughes JR (1993). Treatment of smoking cessation in smokers with past alcohol/drug problems. *Journal of Substance Abuse Treatment* 10:181-187.

Hughes JR (1995). Treatment of nicotine dependence. Is more better? [editorial]. *Journal of the American Medical Association* 274(17):1390-1391.

Hughes JR, Goldstein MG, Hurt RD et al. (1999). Recent advances in the pharmacotherapy of smoking. *Journal of the American Medical Association* 281(1):72-76.

Hughes JR, Lesmes GR, Hatsukami DK et al. (1999). Are higher doses of nicotine replacement more effective for smoking cessation? *Nicotine and Tobacco Research* 1:169-174.

Hughes JR, Stead LF & Lancaster T (1999). Anxiolytics and antidepressants for smoking cessation (Cochrane Review). *The Cochrane Library, Issue 4.* Oxford, England: Update Software.

Hurt RD & Robertson CR (1998). Prying open the door to the tobacco industry's secrets about nicotine: The Minnesota Tobacco Trial. *Journal of the American Medical Association* 280:1173-1181.

Hurt RD, Ahlskog E, Croghan GA et al. (2000). Carbidopa/levodopa for smoking cessation: A pilot study with negative results. *Nicotine and Tobacco Research* 2:71-78.

Hurt RD, Dale LC, Croghan GA et al. (1998). Nicotine nasal spray for smoking cessation: Pattern of use, side effects, relief of withdrawal symptoms, and cotinine levels. *Mayo Clinic Proceedings* 73:118-125.

Hurt RD, Dale LC, Fredrickson PA et al. (1994). Nicotine patch therapy for smoking cessation combined with physician advice and nurse follow-up—One-year outcome and percentage nicotine replacement. *Journal of the American Medical Association* 271(8):595-600.

Hurt RD, Dale LC, Offord KP et al. (1992). Inpatient treatment of severe nicotine dependence. *Mayo Clinic Proceedings* 67:823-828.

Hurt RD, Dale LC, Offord KP et al. (1993). Serum nicotine and cotinine levels during nicotine patch therapy. *Clinical Pharmacology and Therapeutics* 54(1):98-106.

Hurt RD, Dale LC, Offord KP et al. (1995). Nicotine patch therapy for smoking cessation in recovering alcoholics. *Addiction* 90:1541-1546.

Hurt RD, Eberman KM, Croghan IT et al. (1994). Nicotine dependence treatment during inpatient treatment for other addictions: A prospective intervention trial. *Alcoholism: Clinical & Experimental Research* 18(4):867-872.

Hurt RD, Offord KP, Croghan GA et al. (1998). Temporal effects of nicotine nasal spray and gum on nicotine withdrawal symptoms. *Psychopharmacology* 140:98-104.

Hurt RD, Offord KP, Croghan IT et al. (1996). Mortality following inpatient addictions treatment: Role of tobacco use in a community-based cohort. *Journal of the American Medical Association* 275(14):1097-1103.

Hurt RD, Sachs DPL, Glover ED et al. (1997). A comparison of sustained-release bupropion and placebo for smoking cessation. *New England Journal of Medicine* 337:1195-1202.

Hurt RD, Wolter TD, Rigotti N et al. (2001). Bupropion for pharmacologic relapse prevention to smoking: Predictors of outcome. *Addictive Behaviors* 26:1-15.

Hwang SL & Waldholz M (1992). Heart attacks reported in patch users still smoking. *The Wall Street Journal*, June, B1.

Jacob PI, Yu L, Shulgin AT et al. (1999). Minor tobacco alkaloids as biomarkers for tobacco use: Comparison of users of cigarettes, smokeless tobacco, cigars, and pipes. *American Journal of Public Health* 89(5):731-736.

Jorenby DE, Leischow SJ, Nides M et al. (1999). A controlled trial of sustained-release bupropion, a nicotine patch, or both for smoking cessation. *New England Journal of Medicine* 340(9):685-691.

Jorenby DE, Smith SS, Fiore MC et al. (1995). Varying nicotine patch dose and type of smoking cessation counseling. *Journal of the American Medical Association* 274(17):1347-1352.

Joseph AM, Nichol KL, Willenbring ML et al. (1990). Beneficial effects of treatment of nicotine dependence during an inpatient substance abuse treatment program. *Journal of the American Medical Association* 263:3043-3046.

Joseph AM, Norman SM, Ferry LH et al. (1996). The safety of transdermal nicotine as an aid to smoking cessation in patients with cardiac disease. *New England Journal of Medicine* 335(24):1792-1798.

Kendler KS, Neale MC, Sullivan P et al. (1999). A population-based twin study in women of smoking initiation and nicotine dependence. *Psychological Medicine* 29(2):299-308.

Kenford SL, Fiore MC, Jorenby DE et al. (1994). Predicting smoking cessation. Who will quit with and without the nicotine patch. *Journal of the American Medical Association* 271(8):589-594.

Killen JD, Fortmann SP, Schatzberg AF et al. (2000). Nicotine patch and paroxetine for smoking cessation. *Journal of Consulting and Clinical Psychology* 68(5):883-889.

Kornitzer M, Boutsen M, Dramaix M et al. (1995). Combined use of nicotine patch and gum in smoking cessation: A placebo-controlled clinical trial. *Preventive Medicine* 24(1):41-47.

Kozlowski LT, Henningfield JE, Keenan RM et al. (1993). Patterns of alcohol, cigarette, and caffeine and other drug use in two drug abusing populations. *Journal of Substance Abuse Treatment* 10:171-179.

Kozlowski LT, Jelinek LC & Pope MA (1986). Cigarette smoking among alcohol abusers: A continuing and neglected problem. *Canadian Journal of Public Health* 77:205-207.

Lawson GM, Hurt RD, Dale LC et al. (1998a). Application of serum nicotine and plasma cotinine concentrations to assess nicotine replacement in light, moderate, and heavy smokers undergoing transdermal therapy. *Journal of Clinical Pharmacology* 38(6):502-509.

Lawson GM, Hurt RD, Dale LC et al. (1998b). Application of urine nicotine and cotinine excretion rates to assess nicotine replacement in light, moderate and heavy smokers undergoing transdermal therapy. *Journal of Clinical Pharmacology* 38(6):510-516.

Leischow SJ, Nilsson F, Franzon M et al. (1996). Efficacy of the nicotine inhaler as an adjunct to smoking cessation. *American Journal of Health and Behavior* 20(5):364-371.

Lerman C, Caporaso NE, Audrain J et al. (1999). Evidence suggesting the role of specific genetic factors in cigarette smoking. *Health Psychology* 18(1):14-20.

Lunell E, Bergström M, Antoni G et al. (1996). Nicotine deposition and body distribution from a nicotine inhaler and a cigarette studied with positron emission tomography [letter]. *Clinical Pharmacology and Therapeutics* 59(5):593-594.

Lunell E, Molander L, Ekberg K et al. (2000). Site of nicotine absorption from a vapour inhaler—Comparison with cigarette smoking. *European Journal of Clinical Pharmacology* 55(10):737-741.

Mahmarian JJ, Moye LA, Nasser GA et al. (1997). Nicotine patch therapy in smoking cessation reduces the extent of exercise-induced myocardial ischemia. *American College of Cardiology* 30(1):125-130.

Martin JE, Calfas KJ, Patten CA et al. (1997). Prospective evaluation of three smoking interventions in 205 recovering alcoholics: One-year results of Project SCRAP-Tobacco. *Journal of Consulting and Clinical Psychology* 65(1):190-194.

McGinnis JM, Foege WH (1993). Actual causes of death in the United States. *Journal of the American Medical Association* 270:2207-2212.

McNally WD (1932). The tar in cigarette smoke and its possible effects. *American Journal on Cancer* 162:1502-1514.

Molander L, Lunell E, Fagerström KO (2000). Reduction of tobacco withdrawal symptoms with a sublingual nicotine tablet: A placebo controlled study. *Nicotine and Tobacco Research* 2:187-191.

Novy PL, Hughes JR, Jensen JA et al. (1998). The efficacy of the nicotine patch in recovering alcoholic smokers [abstract]. *College for Problems of Drug Dependence: Proceedings of the 60th Annual Scientific Meeting (NIDA Monograph Series, No. 179)*. Rockville, MD: National Institute on Drug Abuse, 91.

Patten CA, Martin JE, Myers MG et al. (1998). Effectiveness of cognitive-behavioral therapy for smokers with histories of alcohol dependence and depression. *Journal of Studies on Alcohol* 59:327-335.

Patten CA, Schneekloth TD, Morse RM et al. (2001). Effect of current tobacco use and history of an alcohol problem on health status in hospitalized patients. *Addictive Behaviors* 26:129-136.

Peto R, Lopey AD, Boreham J et al. (1994). Mortality from smoking in developed countries 1950-2000. *Indirect Estimate from National Vital Statistics*. Oxford, England: Oxford University Press.

Pontieri FE, Tanda G, Orzi F et al. (1996). Effects of nicotine on the nucleus accumbens and similarity to those of addictive drugs. *Nature* 382:255-257.

Prochazka AV, Weaver MJ, Keller RT et al. (1998). A randomized trial of nortriptyline for smoking cessation. *Archives of Internal Medicine* 158:2035-2039.

Rose JE, Behm FM, Westman EC et al. (1994). Mecamylamine combined with nicotine skin patch facilitates smoking cessation beyond nicotine patch treatment alone. *Clinical Pharmacology and Therapeutics* 56(1):86-99.

Russell MAH, Raw M & Jarvis MJ (1980). Clinical use of nicotine chewing gum. *British Medical Journal* 280:1599-1602.

Sabol SZ, Nelson ML, Fisher C et al. (1999). A genetic association for cigarette smoking behavior. *Health Psychology* 18(1):7-13.

Sachs DPL (1995). Effectiveness of the 4-mg dose of nicotine polacrilex for the initial treatment of high-dependent smokers. *Archives of Internal Medicine* 155:1973-1980.

Sachs DPL, Benowitz NL, Bostrom AG et al. (1995). Percent serum replacement and success of nicotine patch therapy. *American Journal of Respiratory and Critical Care Medicine* 151:A688.

Schneider NG, Lunell E, Olmstead RE et al. (1996). Clinical pharmacokinetics of nasal nicotine delivery: A review and comparison to other nicotine systems. *Clinical Pharmacokinetics* 31(1):65-80.

Schneider NG, Olmstead R, Mody FV et al. (1995). Efficacy of a nicotine nasal spray in smoking cessation: A placebo-controlled, double-blind trial. *Addiction* 90(12):1671-1682.

Schneider NG, Olmstead RE, Steinberg C et al. (1996). Efficacy of buspirone in smoking cessation: A placebo-controlled trial. *Clinical Pharmacology and Therapeutics* 60:568-575.

Schuh KJ, Schuh LM, Henningfield JE et al. (1997). Nicotine nasal spray and vapor inhaler: Abuse liability assessment. *Psychopharmacology* 130(4):352-361.

Shiffman S (1982). Relapse following smoking cessation: A situational analysis. *Journal of Consulting and Clinical Psychology* 50:71-86.

Slemmer JE, Martin BR & Damaj MI (2000). Bupropion is a nicotinic antagonist. *Journal of Pharmacology and Experimental Therapeutics* 295(1):321-327.

Stein EA, Pankiewicz J, Harsch HH et al. (1998). Nicotine-induced limbic cortical activation in the human brain: A functional MRI study. *American Journal of Psychiatry* 155(8):1009-1015.

Sussman S (in press). Smoking cessation among persons in recovery. *Substance Use and Misuse*.

Sutherland G, Stapleton JA, Russell MAH et al. (1992). Randomized controlled trial of nasal nicotine spray in smoking cessation. *Lancet* 340:324-329.

Thomas GAO, Davies SV, Rhodes J et al. (1995). Is transdermal nicotine associated with cardiovascular risk? *Journal of the Royal College of Physicians of London* 29(5):392-396.

Tonnesen P, Paoletti P, Gustavsson G et al. (1999). Higher dosage nicotine patches increase one-year smoking cessation rates: Results from the European CEASE trial. *European Respiratory Journal* 13:238-246.

Tsoh JY, Humfleet GL, Munoz RF et al. (2000). Development of major depression after treatment for smoking cessation. *American Journal of Psychiatry* 157:368-374.

Wallström M, Nillson F, Hirsch JM (2000). A randomized, double-blind placebo-controlled clinical evaluation of a nicotine sublingual tablet in smoking cessation. *Addiction* 95:1161-1171.

Wallström M, Sand L, Nilsson F et al. (1999). The long-term effect of nicotine on the oral mucosa. *Addiction* 94(3):417-423.

Watkins SS, Koob GF & Markou A (2000). Neural mechanisms underlying nicotine addiction: Acute positive reinforcement and withdrawal. *Nicotine and Tobacco Research* 2(1):19-37.

Wetter DW, Fiore MC, Baker TB et al. (1995). Tobacco withdrawal and nicotine replacement influence objective measures of sleep. *Journal of Consulting and Clinical Psychology* 63(4):658-667.

Wong GY, Wolter TD, Croghan GA et al. (1999). A randomized trial of naltrexone for smoking cessation. *Addiction* 94(8):1227-1237.

Working Group for the Study of Transdermal Nicotine in Patients with Coronary Artery Disease (Working Group) (1994). Nicotine replacement therapy for patients with coronary artery disease. *Archives of Internal Medicine* 154:989-995.

Zevin S, Jacob P & Benowitz NL (1998). Dose-related cardiovascular and endocrine effects of transdermal nicotine. *Clinical Pharmacology and Therapeutics* 64:87-95.

Chapter 8

Pharmacologic Interventions for Other Drug and Multiple Drug Addictions

Jeffery N. Wilkins, M.D.
David A. Gorelick, M.D., Ph.D.

Marijuana
Anabolic Steroids
Phencyclidine
Hallucinogens
Inhalants
Nicotine With Other Drugs
Opiates With Other Drugs

Pharmacologic treatment of individuals with addiction can follow at least five different strategies (Gorelick, 1993). Patients can be given medications with pharmacologic actions similar to those of the target drug (for example, cross-tolerant agonists), with the goal of substitution (as when methadone is employed for opioid dependence or nicotine for tobacco dependence). A second approach is to use antagonists or receptor blockers, with the goal of preventing or blunting the action of the target drug (as when the opiate receptor antagonist naltrexone [ReVia®] is used in the treatment of opioid dependence). A third approach uses medications that alter neural mechanisms mediating reinforcement or drug craving (other than by acting at the same drug receptor). A fourth approach is to increase drug metabolism or clearance from the body, with the goal of reducing the intensity and/or duration of drug effects. A final approach is to use medication to produce a conditioned aversion to the drug, with the goal of reducing or reversing the reinforcing qualities of the target drug (such as disulfiram [Antabuse®] in the treatment of alcoholism).

This chapter focuses on pharmacologic therapies for the following single substances: marijuana, anabolic steroids, phencyclidine (PCP), hallucinogens (such as lysergic acid diethylamide [LSD], 3,4-methylenedioxymethamphetamine [MDMA, "Ecstasy"], N,N-dimethyltryptamine [DMT], and mescaline), and inhalants (volatile substances, including solvents), as well as the following mixed addictions: nicotine with other drugs, opiates with other drugs (alcohol, cocaine), and cocaine with PCP. Few of the potential treatment strategies listed above have been tried with these drugs. In almost all cases, the pharmacologic treatments described must be considered experimental or unproven, in that they lack any rigorous clinical data (as from controlled clinical trials) to support their use. Therefore, in most cases the mainstay of treatment is psychosocial modalities (see Section 7).

This chapter includes a discussion of the potential use of hallucinogenic drugs as pharmacologic agents in the treatment of addiction. This use of hallucinogens received considerable attention in the 1950s and 1960s, then waned for a variety of social, legal, and ethical reasons. It has recently gained renewed attention.

MARIJUANA

At present, there is no recognized or proven role for pharmacotherapy in the short- or long-term treatment of marijuana abuse or dependence. No medication has any substantial body of clinical experience to support its use. Thus, the mainstay of treatment remains psychosocial. L-tryptophan, the amino acid precursor of serotonin, has been used in some patients, but it is unclear to what extent its effects went beyond its ability to induce sedation and sleep (Zweben & O'Connell, 1992). Trazodone (Desyrel®), an antidepressant that tends to induce sleep by increasing ser-otonin activity, has been used to treat cases of severe insomnia associated with marijuana withdrawal (Duffy & Milin, 1996).

Future research in psychopharmacology may well open new opportunities for pharmacologic treatment. A specific marijuana (cannabinoid) receptor has been identified on nerve cell membranes (Ameri, 1999), with a regional distribution in human brain consistent with the known effects of marijuana (Glass, Dragunow et al., 1997). In principle, the development of specific cannabinoid receptor agonists or antagonists could lead to a pharmacologic treatment for marijuana abuse, using the strategy either of cross-tolerant agonist substitution or of receptor blockade. A newly developed synthetic, highly specific cannabinoid receptor antagonist blocks the physiologic and psychological effects of marijuana in animals and humans (Huestis, Gorelick et al., 2001). This compound (SR141716) is undergoing phase III trials in humans.

ANABOLIC STEROIDS

There is no established medication for the treatment of anabolic steroid abuse (Brower, 1997; Lukas, 1996). Two pharmacologic treatment approaches have been suggested: hormonal treatments to restore hypothalamic-pituitary-gonadal dysfunction caused by use of steroids, and medications to relieve specific symptoms associated with steroid withdrawal. Neither approach has been systematically evaluated for efficacy or safety.

The first approach could be implemented with tapering doses of a long-acting steroid such as testosterone enanthate (for example, 200 to 400 mg intramuscularly initially, tapering by 50 to 100 mg every one to two weeks). This approach could be considered analogous to treating heroin withdrawal with a long-acting opiate such as methadone. Other possible treatments include human chorionic gonadotropin or synthetic forms of luteinizing hormone-releasing hormone to stimulate testosterone production, or anti-estrogenic agents such as clomiphene (for example, 50 mg

twice a day for 10 to 14 days) to reduce the elevated estradiol levels associated with anabolic steroid use.

The second approach uses standard psychotropic medications to target the depression, irritability, and aggression often associated with anabolic steroid use, although these symptoms often resolve without medication. The selective serotonin reuptake inhibitor (SSRI) antidepressant fluoxetine (Prozac®) was reported helpful in one case series (Malone & Dimeff, 1992). The use of tricyclic antidepressants has been discouraged by some on theoretical grounds because their cardiovascular and anticholinergic effects might exacerbate the cardiotoxicity and urinary retention (because of prostatic hypertrophy) associated with anabolic steroid use. There also is a case report of exacerbation of steroid-induced psychological symptoms by the tricyclic antidepressant imipramine (Tofranil®) (Wilson, Prange et al., 1974). Low-dose neuroleptics (such as phenothiazine-equivalent doses of about 200 mg daily) have been reported effective for managing steroid induced psychosis, hostility, and agitation (Weiss, Greenfield et al., 1994).

PHENCYCLIDINE

PCP is a synthetic dissociative anesthetic that gained popularity as an abused drug in the 1960s and no longer is legally available in the United States (Gorelick & Balster, 1995). A synthetic analogue, ketamine, still is used clinically and marketed legally in the U.S., although it also is subject to abuse (Dotson, Ackerman et al., 1995). There is little systematic experience with pharmacologic treatment of PCP addiction. Almost all published studies involve psychosocial treatment approaches, which usually have poor long-term success rates (Daghestani & Schnoll, 1989; Gorelick & Wilkins, 1989; Gorelick, Wilkins et al., 1989). Both the tricyclic antidepressant desipramine (Norpramin®) and the anxiolytic buspirone (BuSpar®) have significantly improved psychological symptoms such as depression in small outpatient-controlled clinical trials, but neither medication significantly reduced PCP use when compared with a double-blind placebo (Giannini, Loiselle et al., 1993; Giannini, Malone et al., 1986). There is no published experience with pharmacologic treatment of ketamine abuse (Dotson, Ackerman et al., 1995).

PCP in Combination With Cocaine or Marijuana. PCP often is smoked with cocaine ("space basing") or marijuana ("primos"). There is very little literature on the treatment of these dual addictions, and no clinical trial has shown any medication to be effective. The antidepressant desipramine has been used because of its possible effectiveness in the treatment of separate PCP or cocaine addiction. In a double-blind study of 20 chronic PCP/cocaine users, desipramine (200 mg/day) significantly reduced symptoms associated with withdrawal but had less effect on actual drug use (Giannini, Loiselle et al., 1987).

HALLUCINOGENS

Hallucinogens are a varied group of plant-derived alkaloids and synthetic compounds that have in common the ability to produce sensory, perceptual, and cognitive changes without impairing attention or level of consciousness (that is, with a clear sensorium) (Abraham, Aldridge et al., 1996). They include compounds that influence serotonergic neurotransmission, such as LSD, psilocybin, and DMT, and those that influence catecholaminergic neurotransmission (such as mescaline and amphetamine analogues like MDMA).

At present, no pharmacologic treatment is available for the treatment of hallucinogen abuse (Abraham, Aldridge et al., 1996; Smith & Seymour, 1994). Several retrospective case reports suggest that long-term treatment with monoamine oxidase inhibitors (such as phenelzine) or SSRI antidepressants (fluoxetine, sertraline [Zoloft®]) can reduce the acute psychological effects of LSD, whereas treatment with tricyclic antidepressants (imipramine, desipramine) or lithium may enhance LSD effects (Bonson & Murphy, 1996). Single doses of the SSRI antidepressant citalopram (Celexa®) or the $5-HT_{2A/C}$ receptor antagonist ketanserin attenuated many of the acute psychological effects of MDMA in human experimental studies (Liechti, Baumann et al., 2000; Liechti, Saur et al., 2000), whereas a dose of the dopamine D_2 receptor antagonist haloperidol (Haldol®) attenuated only the mania-like mood effect (Liechti & Vollenweider, 2000). These findings suggest that medications affecting serotonergic neurotransmission are a promising area for development of pharmacologic treatments for hallucinogen abuse.

The mainstay of treatment remains psychosocial intervention, which can require residential treatment in patients with severe personality disorganization. Prolonged psychotic reactions appear to occur chiefly in individuals who have preexisting psychiatric disorders; these can be difficult to distinguish from hallucinogen-induced precipitation or exacerbation of a preexisting psychotic disorder such as schizophrenia (Boutros & Bowers, 1996). Regardless of etiology, such psychotic reactions can require treatment with antipsychotic medication (Boutros & Bowers, 1996; Smith & Seymour, 1994). Low doses of a high potency neuroleptic have been recommended (such as 2 to 5 mg haloperidol) (Giannini, 1994).

LSD use has been associated with perceptual abnormalities, such as illusions, distortions, and hallucinations, persisting or recurring intermittently for long periods (up to years) after the last LSD use (hallucinogen persisting perception disorder in *DSM-IV*) (Abraham, Aldridge et al., 1996; Smith & Seymour, 1994). When these abnormalities occur after a period of normal perceptual functioning, they are termed "flashbacks." Case reports suggest that sertraline, naltrexone, or clonidine (Catapres®) can be helpful in the treatment of both persisting perceptual abnormalities and flashbacks (Young, 1997; Lerner, Oyffe et al., 1997; Lerner, Gelkopf et al., 2000). Some anecdotal experience suggests that neuroleptics such as haloperidol can transiently worsen flashbacks (Moskowitz, 1971; Strassman, 1984). These perceptual disorders can be associated with secondary depression or anxiety disorders such as panic and agoraphobia. In such cases, treatment with benzodiazepines or SSRI antidepressants has been reported to be helpful (Smith & Seymour, 1994).

Experimental Treatment Using Hallucinogens. Within four years of its discovery, LSD (Delysid®) was marketed as an adjunct to psychotherapy (Ulrich & Patten, 1991). Over the following decades, it was used clinically as pharmacologic treatment for a variety of psychiatric disorders, including depression, anxiety, alcoholism, and drug abuse (Abraham, Aldridge et al., 1996; Savage & McCabe, 1973; Strassman, 1995). Other hallucinogens such as mescaline, psilocybin, and DMT also were used, but to a much lesser extent. Because hallucinogens were considered to induce a temporary "model" psychosis, it was hoped that study of their effects might unlock some of the neurochemical mysteries of psychiatric disorders (Vollenweider, 1998). The literature accompanying Delysid® recommended that psychiatrists take it themselves in order to better understand the subjective experiences of their schizophrenic patients.

LSD was given orally as a psychiatric treatment in two ways: (1) one or two high doses (usually 200 to 800 μg), with or without formal psychotherapy, to generate a cathartic or transforming emotional experience (this so-called psychedelic approach was popular in North America), or (2) multiple low doses (usually 25 to 200 μg) as an adjunct to psychotherapy to break down therapeutic resistance and enhance access to unconscious material (the so-called psycholytic approach, popular in Europe) (Strassman, 1995).

LSD is one of the most frequently studied pharmacologic treatments for alcohol dependence, albeit with no published studies since the early 1970s (Abraham, Aldridge et al., 1996; Mangini, 1998). Most existing studies have serious methodologic flaws, such as no control or comparison groups, poorly characterized patient samples, and vaguely defined or unspecified outcome measures. At least nine published randomized controlled trials have been reported, all of which used the psychedelic approach. Only three trials (two double-blind) found significantly more improvement in the LSD group than in the comparison group at followup intervals of 2 to 12 months. In two of the three studies, the advantage of LSD treatment no longer was present after 6 or 12 months. No controlled trials have evaluated the psycholytic approach, so its efficacy remains undetermined.

LSD administration in medical and research settings was considered safe, with low rates of psychosis and suicidality and little or no potential for addiction or overdose (Mangini, 1998; Strassman, 1995). As use spread outside the medical setting in the mid-1960s, reports of adverse reactions, behavioral toxicity, and misuse or abuse increased sharply. Research with hallucinogens was criticized for inadequate controls and followup. These concerns led policymakers in many countries to place LSD and other hallucinogenic drugs under strict regulatory controls (for example, they were reclassified as Schedule I drugs in the U.S.). This action stopped virtually all clinical research with hallucinogens (Gouzoulis-Mayfrank, Hermle et al., 1998; Pechnick & Ungerleider, 1997).

Interest in clinical research with hallucinogens has revived over the past decade. The U.S. Food and Drug Administration has approved several studies of hallucinogenic drugs in humans. In addition to LSD, other hallucinogenic drugs being studied in the U.S. and Europe include MDMA, ibogaine, DMT (Strassman, 1996), psilocybin (Gouzoulis-Mayfrank, Thelen et al., 1999), mescaline (Hermle, Gouzoulis-Mayfrank et al., 1998), and ketamine (Krupitsky & Grinenko, 1997). MDMA has attracted interest as an alternative to LSD because of its shorter duration of action and reportedly milder hallucinogenic properties (Strassman, 1995).

Ibogaine, derived from the West African plant *Tabernanthe iboga*, recently attracted interest because of anecdotal reports that a single high-dose (>1 g) treatment alleviated withdrawal symptoms and produced long-term abstinence (>3 months) in heroin and polydrug addicts (Mash, Kovera et al., 1998). To date, no controlled clinical trials have been conducted. Concern about possible ibogaine toxicity has limited its use. Several deaths have been associated with the administration of ibogaine, and neurotoxicity, especially in the cerebellum, has been reported in animal studies. Ibogaine's mechanism of action remains unclear; it influences several different neurotransmitter systems (Szumlinski, Maisonneuve et al., 2001). In many, but not all, rodent studies, ibogaine pretreatment reduced cocaine and heroin self-administration and blunted the locomotor stimulation produced by cocaine.

The use of hallucinogens also is being investigated in the treatment of depression, obsessive-compulsive disorder, and posttraumatic stress disorder (Moreno & Delgado, 1997; Riedlinger & Riedlinger, 1994). The presumed benefits to psychotherapy include a lessening of patients' "fear responses," which often inhibit patients' ability to deal with traumatic situations, facilitation of interpersonal dyadic relationships with therapists, spouses, and others in their social support network, and accelerating formation of the therapist/patient relationship.

INHALANTS

Inhalants are a heterogeneous group of volatile abused substances that include adhesives, aerosols, solvents, anesthetics, gasoline, cleaning agents, and nitrites (Brouette & Anton, 2001; Dinwiddie, 1994). Because these agents usually are marketed legally for commercial purposes, they generally are inexpensive and readily available. Many inhalant abusers entering treatment have co-occurring psychiatric and addictive disorders, typically involving alcohol and marijuana, that can complicate treatment.

There is no clear role for pharmacologic treatment in inhalant addiction; the mainstay of treatment is psychosocial (Brouette & Anton, 2001; Dinwiddie, 1994). Limited case reports suggest that those rare patients who experience withdrawal symptoms may benefit from benzodiazepines.

NICOTINE WITH OTHER DRUGS

Nicotine and Alcohol. More than half of alcohol-dependent individuals also are dependent on nicotine, whereas about one quarter of nicotine-dependent individuals also are dependent on alcohol (Kandel, Huang et al., 2001). Nicotine and alcohol appear to reciprocally facilitate each other's use (Hughes, 1993). Tobacco-related diseases are a substantial cause of morbidity and mortality in alcoholic patients. In view of these facts, it makes good clinical sense to address both alcohol and nicotine dependence whenever they coexist. There is no evidence that such a concurrent focus hinders treatment of alcohol dependence or increases the risk of relapse (Bien & Burge, 1991; Hughes, 1993; Hurt, Eberman et al., 1994).

Medications used for the separate treatment of alcoholism (such as disulfiram [Antabuse®] or naltrexone) or nicotine dependence (such as nicotine gum) have not yet been evaluated systematically for their use in the treatment of co-occurring nicotine and alcohol dependence. A controlled clinical trial found no benefit from naltrexone in the treatment of nicotine dependence, either alone or in combination with a nicotine skin patch (Wong, Wolter et al., 1999).

Nicotine and Other Drugs. More than half of individuals who are dependent on illicit drugs also are dependent on nicotine (Kandel, Huang et al., 2001). Up to 98% of opiate-dependent individuals, including patients in methadone maintenance treatment, smoke cigarettes (Richter & Ahluwalia, 2000; Richter, Gibson et al., 2001). Treatment for nicotine dependence often is neglected in the context of other addictions, largely because of the belief that smoking cessation might have an adverse effect on abstinence from other drugs. This belief is not supported by the limited research done to date. Addicted patients often express a strong interest in quitting smoking and doing so does not adversely affect their future course (Hurt, Eberman et al., 1994; Burling, Marshall et al., 1991; Richter, Gibson et al., 2001; Sees & Clark, 1993). No clinical trials have yet addressed the issue of concurrent pharmacologic treatment for nicotine dependence (as with nicotine replacement therapy) and other drug dependence (for example, methadone maintenance therapy for heroin addiction).

OPIOIDS WITH OTHER DRUGS

Opioids and Alcohol. Alcoholism is a common problem among opiate-dependent individuals, including those in methadone maintenance treatment (Chatham, Rowan-Szal et al., 1995; Shaffer & LaSalvia, 1992). Concurrent treatment with disulfiram, at the same doses used to treat alcoholism alone, can be effective in reducing alcohol intake among patients in methadone maintenance (Liebson, Bigelow et al., 1973). The careful medication monitoring and incentives for compliance that are possible in a metha-done maintenance program can make disulfiram treatment more effective than it is in other treatment settings.

Opioids and Cocaine. Cocaine use is common among opiate addicts (Grella et al., 1997) and is associated with greater opiate use even among those in methadone maintenance treatment (DeMaria, Sterling et al., 2000). A popular pattern involves simultaneous use of the two drugs ("speed balling"), which is said to provide a qualitatively better subjective experience ("high") than either drug alone (Walsh, Sullivan et al., 1996). For patients already in methadone maintenance, increasing the methadone dose (usually to >60 mg/day) can reduce both opiate and cocaine use (Stine, Burns et al., 1991; Tennant & Shannon, 1995). The opiate antagonist naltrexone, marketed for the treatment of opiate dependence (and alcoholism), has shown modest success in reducing cocaine use in patients without opiate dependence (Schmitz, Stotts et al., 2001), but it has not been evaluated in patients addicted to both opiates and cocaine.

Buprenorphine (Buprenex®), a partial opioid agonist (kappa-receptor agonist, mu-receptor antagonist), is marketed worldwide as a parenteral analgesic. It is as effective (given sublingually) as methadone for substitution treatment of opiate dependence. Some animal drug self-administration studies have suggested that it also might be effective in reducing cocaine use (Rodefer, Mattox et al., 1997). Several clinical trials found no influence of buprenorphine on cocaine use among opiate addicts at doses that significantly decreased opiate use (Compton, Ling et al., 1995). A few trials using higher doses (12 to 16 mg/day sublingually) have found significant reductions in both cocaine and opiate use (Montoya, Gorelick et al., 1996; Schottenfeld, Pakes et al., 1993).

CONCLUSIONS

This chapter reviewed approaches to pharmacologic treatment of addiction to several individual drugs of abuse, including marijuana, anabolic steroids, PCP, and inhalants, as well as to some common mixed addictions, including nicotine or opiates with alcohol and other drugs, and cocaine with PCP. In most cases, there is little or no published literature to guide the choice of pharmacologic treatment and no clinical trials to support the efficacy of any treatment. Thus, the mainstay of treatment for marijuana, anabolic steroid, PCP, hallucinogen, or inhalant abuse is psychosocial interventions. The use of pharmacologic treatments remains a question for which the physician must rely almost exclusively on his or her own experience and judgment, with very little help from the medical or scientific literature. Future research may alter this situation and spur the development of effective new pharmacologic treatments. Two intriguing areas now gaining attention are compounds that interact with cannabinoid receptors in the brain (such as specific "marijuana antagonists") and the use of hallucinogenic drugs in the treatment of addiction.

REFERENCES

Abraham HD, Aldridge AM & Gogia P (1996). The psychopharmacology of hallucinogens. *Neuropsychopharmacology* 14:285-298.

Ameri A (1999). The effects of cannabinoids on the brain. *Progress in Neurobiology* 58:315-348.

American Psychiatric Association (1994). *Diagnostic and Statistical Manual of Mental Disorders, 4th Edition (DSM-IV)*. Washington, DC: American Psychiatric Association.

Bien TH & Burge R (1991). Smoking and drinking, a review of the literature. *International Journal of the Addictions* 25(12):1429-1454.

Bonson KR & Murphy DL (1996). Alterations in responses to LSD in humans associated with chronic administration of tricyclic antidepressants, monoamine oxidase inhibitors or lithium. *Behavioural Brain Research* 73:229-233.

Boutros NN & Bowers MB Jr (1996). Chronic substance-induced psychotic disorders: State of the literature. *Journal of Neuropsychiatry & Clinical Neurosciences* 8:262-269.

Brouette T & Anton R (2001). Clinical review of inhalants. *American Journal on Addictions* 10:79-94.

Brower KJ (1997). Withdrawal from anabolic steroids. *Current Therapy in Endocrinology & Metabolism* 6:338-343.

Burling TA, Marshall GD & Seidner AL (1991). Smoking cessation for substance abuse inpatients. *Journal of Substance Abuse* 3(3):269-276.

Chatham LR, Rowan-Szal GA, Joe GW et al. (1995). Heavy drinking in a population of methadone-maintained clients. *Journal of Studies on Alcohol* 56:417-422.

Compton PA, Ling W, Charuvastra VC et al. (1995). Buprenorphine as a pharmacotherapy for cocaine abuse: A review of the evidence. *Journal of Addictive Diseases* 14(3):97-114.

Daghestani AN & Schnoll SH (1989). Phencyclidine abuse and dependence. In American Psychiatric Association Task Force on Treatment of Psychiatric Disorders (ed.) *Treatments of Psychiatric Disorders, Vol. 2*. Washington, DC: American Psychiatric Press, 1209-1218.

DeMaria PA Jr, Sterling R & Weinstein SP (2000). The effect of stimulant and sedative use on treatment outcome of patients admitted to methadone maintenance treatment. *American Journal on Addictions* 9:145-153.

Dinwiddie SH (1994). Abuse of inhalants: A review. *Addiction* 89:925-939.

Dotson JW, Ackerman DL & West JL (1995). Ketamine abuse. *Journal of Drug Issues* 25(4):751-757.

Duffy A & Milin R (1996). Case study: Withdrawal syndrome in adolescent chronic cannabis users. *Journal of the American Academy of Child & Adolescent Psychiatry* 35:1618-1621.

Giannini AJ (1994). Inward the mind's I: Description, diagnosis, and treatment of acute and delayed LSD hallucinations. *Psychiatric Annals* 24(3):134-136.

Giannini AJ, Loiselle RH & Giannini MC (1987). Space-based abstinence: Alleviation of withdrawal symptoms in combinative cocaine-phencyclidine abuse. *Clinical Toxicology* 25(6):493-500.

Giannini AJ, Loiselle RH & Graham BH (1993). Behavioral response to buspirone in cocaine and phencyclidine withdrawal. *Journal of Substance Abuse Treatment* 10:523-527.

Giannini AJ, Malone DA, Giannini MC et al. (1986). Treatment of depression in chronic cocaine and phencyclidine abuse with desipramine. *Journal of Clinical Pharmacology* 26(3):211-214.

Glass M, Dragunow M & Faull RLM (1997). Cannabinoid receptors in the human brain: A detailed anatomical and quantitative autoradiographic study in the fetal, neonatal and adult human brain. *Neuroscience* 77(2):299-318.

Gorelick DA (1993). Overview of pharmacological treatment approaches for alcohol and other drug addiction: Intoxication, withdrawal, and relapse prevention. *Psychiatric Clinics of North America* 16(1):141-156.

Gorelick DA & Balster RL (1995). Phencyclidine (PCP). In FE Bloom & DJ Kupfer (eds.) *Psychopharmacology: The Fourth Generation of Progress*. New York, NY: Raven Press, 1767-1776.

Gorelick DA & Wilkins JN (1989). Inpatient treatment of PCP abusers and users. *American Journal of Drug and Alcohol Abuse* 15:1-12.

Gorelick DA, Wilkins JN & Wong C (1989). Outpatient treatment of PCP abusers. *American Journal of Drug and Alcohol Abuse* 15:367-374.

Gouzoulis-Mayfrank E, Hermle L, Thelen B et al. (1998). History, rationale and potential of human experimental hallucinogenic drug research in psychiatry. *Pharmacopsychiatry* 31(Suppl 2):63-68.

Gouzoulis-Mayfrank E, Thelen B, Habermeyer E et al. (1999). Psychopathological, neuroendocrine and autonomic effects of 3,4-methylenedioxyethylamphetamine (MDE), psilocybin and d-methamphetamine in healthy volunteers. Results of an experimental double-blind placebo-controlled study. *Psychopharmacology* 142(1):41-50.

Grella CE, Anglin MD & Wugalter SE (1997). Patterns and predictors of cocaine and crack use by clients in standard and enhanced methadone maintenance treatment. *American Journal of Drug and Alcohol Abuse* 23:15-42.

Hermle L, Gouzoulis-Mayfrank E & Spitzer M (1998). Blood flow and cerebral laterality in the mescaline model of psychosis. *Pharmacopsychiatry* 31(Suppl 2):85-91.

Huestis MA, Gorelick DA, Heishman SJ et al. (2001). Blockade of effects of smoked marijuana by the CB1-selective cannabinoid receptor antagonist SR141716. *Archives of General Psychiatry* 58:322-328.

Hughes JR (1993). Treatment of smoking cessation in smokers with past alcohol/drug problems. *Journal of Substance Abuse Treatment* 10:181-187.

Hurt RD, Eberman KM, Croghan IT et al. (1994). Nicotine dependence treatment during inpatient treatment for other addictions: A prospective intervention trial. *Alcoholism: Clinical & Experimental Research* 18:867-872.

Kandel DB, Huang FY & Davies M (2001). Comorbidity between patterns of substance use dependence and psychiatric syndromes. *Drug and Alcohol Dependence* 64(2):233-241.

Krupitsky EM & Grinenko AY (1997). Ketamine psychedelic therapy (KPT): A review of the results of ten years of research. *Journal of Psychoactive Drugs* 29(2):165-183.

Lerner AG, Gelkopf M, Oyffe I et al. (2000). LSD-induced hallucinogen persisting perception disorder treatment with clonidine: An open pilot study. *International Clinical Psychopharmacology* 15(1):35-37.

Lerner AG, Oyffe I, Isaacs G et al. (1997). Naltrexone treatment of hallucinogen persisting perception disorder. *American Journal of Psychiatry* 154:437.

Liebson I, Bigelow G & Flamer R (1973). Alcoholism among methadone patients: A specific treatment method. *American Journal of Psychiatry* 130:483-485.

Liechti M & Vollenweider FX (2000). Acute psychological and physiological effects of MDMA ("Ecstasy") after haloperidol pretreatment in healthy humans. *European Neuropsychopharmacology* 10(4):289-295.

Liechti ME, Baumann C, Gamma A et al. (2000). Acute psychological effects of 3,4-methylenedioxymethamphetamine (MDMA, "ecstasy") are attenuated by the serotonin uptake inhibitor citalopram. *Neuropsychopharmacology* 22(5):513-521.

Liechti M, Saur MR, Gamma A et al. (2000). Psychological and physiological effects of MDMA ("Ecstasy") after pretreatment with the 5-HT(2) antagonist ketanserin in healthy humans. *Neuropsychopharmacology* 23(4):396-404.

Lukas SE (1996). CNS effects and abuse liability of anabolic-androgenic steroids. *Annual Review of Pharmacology & Toxicology* 36:333-357.

Malone DA Jr & Dimeff RJ (1992). The use of fluoxetine in depression associated with anabolic steroid withdrawal: A case series. *Journal of Clinical Psychiatry* 53:130-132.

Mangini M (1998). Treatment of alcoholism using psychedelic drugs: A review of the program of research. *Journal of Psychoactive Drugs* 30(4):381-418.

Mash DC, Kovera CA, Buck BE et al. (1998). Medication development of ibogaine as a pharmacotherapy for drug dependence. *Annals of the New York Academy of Sciences* 844:274-292.

Montoya I, Gorelick D, Preston K et al. (1996). Buprenorphine for treatment of dually-dependent (opiate and cocaine) individuals. Problems of Drug Dependence, 1995 (*NIDA Research Monograph 162*). Rockville, MD: National Institute on Drug Abuse, 178.

Moreno FA & Delgado PL (1997). Hallucinogen-induced relief of obsessions and compulsions. *American Journal of Psychiatry* 154(7):1037-1038.

Moskowitz D (1971). Use of haloperidol to reduce LSD flashbacks. *Military Medicine* 136:754-757.

Pechnick RN & Ungerleider JT (1997). Hallucinogens. In JH Lowinson, P Ruiz, P Millman et al. (eds.) *Substance Abuse: A Comprehensive Textbook, 3rd Edition*. Baltimore, MD: Williams & Wilkins, 230-238.

Richter KP & Ahluwalia JS (2000). A case for addressing cigarette use in methadone and other opiate treatment programs. *Journal of Addictive Diseases* 19(4):35-52.

Richter KP, Gibson CA, Ahluwalia JS et al. (2001). Tobacco use and quit attempts among methadone maintenance clients. *American Journal of Public Health* 91(2):296-299.

Riedlinger TJ & Riedlinger JE (1994). Psychedelic and entactogenic drugs in the treatment of depression. *Journal of Psychoactive Drugs* 26(1):41-55.

Rodefer JS, Mattox AJ, Thompson SS et al. (1997). Effects of buprenorphine and an alternative nondrug reinforcer, alone and in combination on smoked cocaine self-administration in monkeys. *Drug and Alcohol Dependence* 45:21-29.

Savage C & McCabe L (1973). Residential psychedelic (LSD) therapy for the narcotic addict: A pilot study. *Archives of General Psychiatry* 28(6):808-814.

Schmitz JM, Stotts AL, Rhoades HM et al. (2001). Naltrexone and relapse prevention treatment for cocaine-dependent patients. *Addictive Behavior* 26(2):167-180.

Schottenfeld RS, Pakes J, Ziedonis D et al. (1993). Buprenorphine: Dose-related effects on cocaine and opioid use in cocaine-abusing opioid-dependent humans. *Biological Psychiatry* 34:66-74.

Sees KL & Clark HW (1993). When to begin smoking cessation in substance abusers. *Journal of Substance Abuse Treatment* 10(2):189-195.

Shaffer HJ & LaSalvia TA (1992). Patterns of substance use among methadone maintenance patients. *Journal of Substance Abuse Treatment* 9:143-147.

Smith DE & Seymour RB (1994). LSD: History and toxicity. *Psychiatric Annals* 24(3):145-147.

Stine SM, Burns B & Kosten T (1991). Methadone dose for cocaine abuse. *American Journal of Psychiatry* 148(9):1268.

Strassman RJ (1984). Adverse reactions of psychedelic drugs: A review of the literature. *Journal of Nervous and Mental Disease* 172(10):577-595.

Strassman RJ (1995). Hallucinogenic drugs in psychiatric research and treatment. *Journal of Nervous and Mental Disease* 183:127-138.

Strassman RJ (1996). Human psychopharmacology of N,N-dimethyltryptamine. *Behavioral Brain Research* 73(1-2):121-124.

Szumlinski KK, Maisonneuve IM & Glick SK (2001). Iboga interactions with psychomotor stimulants: Panacea in the paradox? *Toxicon* 39(1):75-86.

Tennant F & Shannon J (1995). Cocaine abuse in methadone maintenance patients is associated with low serum methadone concentrations. *Journal of Addictive Diseases* 14(1):67-74.

Ulrich RF & Patten BM (1991). The rise, decline, and fall of LSD. *Perspectives in Biology & Medicine* 34(4):561-578.

Vollenweider FX (1998). Advances and pathophysiological models of hallucinogenic drug actions in humans: A preamble to schizophrenia research. *Pharmacopsychiatry* 31(Suppl):92-103.

Walsh SL, Sullivan JT, Preston KL et al. (1996). Effects of naltrexone on response to intravenous cocaine, hydromorphone and their combination in humans. *Journal of Pharmacology and Experimental Therapeutics* 279:524-538.

Weiss RD, Greenfield SF & Mirin SM (1994). Intoxication and withdrawal syndromes. In SE Hyman (ed.) *Manual of Psychiatric Emergencies*. Boston, MA: Little, Brown & Co, 279-293.

Wilson IC, Prange AJ & Lapp PP (1974). Methyltestosterone and imipramine in men: Conversion of depression to paranoid reaction. *American Journal of Psychiatry* 131:21-24.

Wong GY, Wolter TD, Croghan IT et al. (1999). A randomized trial of naltrexone for smoking cessation. *Addiction* 94:1227-1237.

Young CR (1997). Sertraline treatment of hallucinogen persisting perceptual disorder. *Journal of Clinical Psychiatry* 58:85.

Zweben JE & O'Connell K (1992). Strategies for breaking marijuana dependence. *Journal of Psychoactive Drugs* 24(2):165-171.

SECTION

7

Behavioral Interventions

Section Coordinator
Allan W. Graham, M.D., FACP, FASAM

Contributors

Richard A. Brown, Ph.D.
Butler Hospital
Brown University School of Medicine
Providence, Rhode Island

Kathleen M. Carroll, Ph.D.
Professor of Psychiatry
Yale University School of Medicine
VA Connecticut Healthcare Center
New Haven, Connecticut

Dennis C. Daley, Ph.D.
Associate Professor of Psychiatry, and
Chief of Addiction Medicine Services
Western Psychiatric Institute and Clinic
Pittsburgh, Pennsylvania

George DeLeon, Ph.D.
Center for Therapeutic Community Research
National Development
    and Research Institutes, Inc.
New York, New York

P. Joseph Frawley, M.D.
Private Practice of Medicine
Santa Barbara, California

Marc Galanter, M.D., FASAM
Professor of Psychiatry and
Director, Division of
    Alcoholism and Drug Abuse
New York University School of Medicine
New York, New York

Michael G. Goldstein, M.D.
Bayer Institute of Health Care Communication
West Haven, Connecticut

Allan W. Graham, M.D., FACP, FASAM
Associate Medical Director
Chemical Dependency Treatment Services
Kaiser Permanente
Denver, Colorado

Stephen T. Higgins, Ph.D.
Human Behavioral Pharmacology Laboratory
Department of Psychiatry
University of Vermont
Burlington, Vermont

Christopher W. Kahler, Ph.D.
Center for Alcohol and Addiction Studies
Department of Psychiatry and Human Behavior
Brown University
Providence, Rhode Island

Donald J. Kurth, M.D., FASAM
Chief of Addiction Medicine
Loma Linda University Behavioral
    Medicine Center, and
Associate Professor of Psychiatry
Loma Linda University
Loma Linda, California

Delinda E. Mercer, Ph.D.
Instructor, Department of Psychiatry
Center for the Study of Addictions
University of Pennsylvania
Philadelphia, Pennsylvania

James O. Prochaska, Ph.D.
Director and Professor
Cancer Prevention Research Center
University of Rhode Island
Kingston, Rhode Island

Bruce J. Rounsaville, M.D.
Professor of Psychiatry
Yale University School of Medicine
VA Connecticut Healthcare Center
New Haven, Connecticut

Crystal E. Spotts, M.Ed.
Research Coordinator
Western Psychiatric Institute and Clinic
Pittsburgh, Pennsylvania

Jennifer W. Tidey, Ph.D.
Center for Alcohol and Addiction Studies
Department of Psychiatry and Human Behavior
Brown University
Providence, Rhode Island

Michael J. Zvolensky, Ph.D.
Department of Psychology
University of Vermont
Burlington, Vermont

| Chapter 1 | # Enhancing Motivation To Change |

James O. Prochaska, Ph.D.

The Stages of Change
Using the Stages of Change Model to Motivate Patients

What motivates people to take action? The answer to this key question depends on what type of action is to be taken. What moves people to start therapy? What motivates them to continue therapy? What moves people to progress in therapy, or to continue to progress after therapy? Answers to these questions can provide better alternatives to one of the field's most pressing concerns: What types of therapeutic interventions would have the greatest effect on the entire population at risk for or experiencing addictive disorders?

What motivates people to change? The answer to this question depends in part on where they start. What motivates people to begin thinking about change can be different from what motivates them to begin preparing to take action. Once prepared, different forces can move people to take action.

Once action is taken, what motivates people to maintain that action? Conversely, what causes people to regress or relapse to their addictive behaviors?

Fortunately, the answers to this complex set of questions may be simpler, or at least more systematic, than the questions themselves. To appreciate the answers, it is helpful to begin with the author's model of change (Prochaska

& DiClemente, 1983; Prochaska, DiClemente et al., 1992; Prochaska, Norcross et al., 1994).

THE STAGES OF CHANGE

Change is a process that unfolds over time through a series of stages: precontemplation, contemplation, preparation, action, maintenance, and termination.

Precontemplation is a stage in which the individual does not intend to take action in the foreseeable future (usually measured as the next six months). The individual may be at this stage because he or she is uninformed or underinformed about the consequences of a given behavior. Or he or she may have tried to change a number of times and become demoralized about his or her ability to do so. Individuals in both categories tend to avoid reading, talking, or thinking about their high-risk behaviors. In other theories, such individuals are characterized as "resistant" or "unmotivated" or "not ready" for therapy or health promotion programs. In fact, traditional treatment programs were not ready for such individuals and were not motivated to match their needs.

Individuals who are in the precontemplation stage typically underestimate the benefits of change and overestimate its costs, but are unaware that they are making such mistakes. If they are not conscious of making such mistakes, it is difficult for them to change. As a result, many remain "stuck" in the precontemplation stage for years, with considerable resulting harm to their bodies, themselves, and others.

There appears to be no inherent motivation for people to progress from one stage to the next. The stages are not like stages of human development, in which children have inherent motivation to progress from crawling to walking, even though crawling works very well and even though learning to walk can be painful and embarrassing.

Instead, two major forces can move people to progress. The first is *developmental events*. In the author's research, the mean age of smokers who reach long-term maintenance is 39 years. Those who have passed 39 recognize it as an age to reevaluate how one has been living and whether one wants to die from that lifestyle or whether one wants to enhance the quality and quantity of the second half of life.

The other naturally occurring force is *environmental events*. A favorite example is a couple who were both heavy smokers. Their dog of many years died of lung cancer. This death eventually moved the wife to quit smoking. The husband bought a new dog. So even the same events can be processed differently by different people.

A common belief is that people with addictive disorders must "hit bottom" before they are motivated to change. So family, friends, and physicians wait helplessly for a crisis to occur. But how often do people turn 39 or have a dog die? When individuals show the first signs of a serious physical illness, such as cancer or cardiovascular disease, the persons around them usually become mobilized to help them seek early intervention. Evidence shows that early interventions often are lifesaving, and so it would not be acceptable to wait for such a patient to "hit bottom."

In opposition to such a passive stance, a third force that has been created to help patients with addictions progress beyond the precontemplation stage is called *planned interventions*.

Contemplation is a stage in which an individual intends to take action within the ensuing six months. Such a person is more aware of the benefits of changing, but also is acutely aware of the costs. When an addicted person begins to seriously contemplate giving up a favorite substance, his or her awareness of the costs of changing can increase. There is no free change. This balance between the costs and benefits of change can produce profound ambivalence,

which may reflect a type of love-hate relationship with an addictive substance, and thus can keep an individual stuck at the contemplation stage for long periods of time. This phenomenon often is characterized as "chronic contemplation" or "behavioral procrastination." Such individuals are not ready for traditional action-oriented programs.

Preparation is a stage in which an individual intends to take action in the immediate future (usually measured as the ensuing month). Such a person typically has taken some significant action within the preceding year. He or she generally has a plan of action, such as participating in a recovery group, consulting a counselor, talking to a physician, buying a self-help book, or relying on a self-change approach. It is these individuals who should be recruited for action-oriented treatment programs.

Action is a stage in which the individual has made specific, overt modifications in his or her lifestyle within the preceding six months. Because action is observable, behavior change often has been equated with action. But in the Transtheoretical Model, action is only one of six stages. In this model, not all modifications of behavior count as action. An individual must attain a criterion that scientists and professionals agree is sufficient to reduce the risk of disease. In smoking, for example, only total abstinence counts. With alcoholism and alcohol abuse, many believe that only total abstinence can be effective, whereas others accept controlled drinking as an effective action.

Maintenance is a stage in which the individual is working to prevent relapse, but does not need to apply change processes as frequently as one would in the action stage. Such a person is less tempted to relapse and is increasingly confident that he or she can sustain the changes made. Temptation and self-efficacy data suggest that maintenance lasts from six months to about five years.

One of the common reasons for early relapse is that the individual is not well prepared for the prolonged effort needed to progress to maintenance. Many persons think the worst will be over in a few weeks or a few months. If, as a result, they ease up on their efforts too early, they are at great risk of relapse.

To prepare such individuals for what is to come, they should be encouraged to think of overcoming an addiction as running a marathon rather than a sprint. They may have wanted to enter the 100th running of the Boston Marathon. But they know they would not succeed without preparation and so would not enter the race. With some preparation, they might compete for several miles but still would fail to finish the race. Only those who are well prepared could maintain their efforts mile after mile.

Using the Boston Marathon metaphor, people know they have to be well prepared if they are to survive Heartbreak Hill, which runners encounter at about mile 20. What is the behavioral equivalent of Heartbreak Hill? The best evidence available suggests that most relapses occur at times of emotional distress. It is in the presence of depression, anxiety, anger, boredom, loneliness, stress, and distress that humans are at their emotional and psychological weak point.

How does the average person cope with troubling times? He or she drinks more, eats more, smokes more, and takes more drugs to cope with distress (Mellinger, Balter et al., 1978). It is not surprising, therefore, that persons struggling to overcome addictive disorders will be at greatest risk of relapse when they face distress without their substance of choice. While emotional distress cannot be prevented, relapse can be prevented if patients have been prepared to cope with distress without falling back on addictive substances.

If so many Americans rely on oral consumptive behavior as a way to manage their emotions, what is the healthiest oral behavior they could use? Talking with others about one's distress is a means of seeking support that can help prevent relapse. Another healthy alternative is exercise. Physical activity helps manage moods, stress, and distress. Also, 60 minutes a week of exercise can provide a recovering person with more than 50 health and mental health benefits. Exercise thus should be prescribed to all sedentary patients with addictions. A third healthy alternative is some form of deep relaxation, such as meditation, yoga, prayer, massage, or deep muscle relaxation. Letting the stress and distress drift away from one's muscles and one's mind helps the patient move forward at the most tempting of times.

Termination is a stage at which an individual has zero temptation and 100% self-efficacy. No matter whether they are depressed, anxious, bored, lonely, angry, or stressed, such persons are certain they will not return to their old unhealthy habits as a method of coping. It is as if they never acquired the habit in the first place. In a study of former smokers and alcoholics, fewer than 20% of each group had reached the stage of no temptation and total self-efficacy (Snow, Prochaska et al., 1992). Although the ideal is to be cured or totally recovered, it is important to recognize that, for many patients, a more realistic expectation is a lifetime of maintenance.

USING THE STAGES OF CHANGE MODEL TO MOTIVATE PATIENTS

The stages of change model can be applied to identify ways to motivate more patients at each phase of planned interventions for the addictions. The five phases are (1) recruitment, (2) retention, (3) progress, (4) process, and (5) outcomes.

Recruitment. Too few studies have paid attention to the fact that professional treatment programs recruit or reach too few persons with addictions. Across all diagnoses in the *Diagnostic and Statistical Manual of Mental Disorders, 4th Edition* (American Psychiatric Association, 1994), fewer than 25% of persons with addictive disorders enter professional treatment in their lifetimes (Veroff, Douvon et al., 1981a, 1981b). With smoking, the deadliest of addictions, fewer than 10% ever participate in a professional treatment program (USDHHS, 1990).

Given that addictive disorders are among the costliest of contemporary conditions, it is crucial to motivate many more persons to participate in appropriate treatment. These conditions are costly to the addicted individuals, their families and friends, their employers, their communities, and their health care systems. Health professionals no longer can treat addictive disorders just on a case basis; instead, they must develop programs that can reach addicted persons on a population basis.

Governments and health care systems are seeking to treat addictive disorders on a population basis. But when they turn to the largest and best clinical trials of addiction therapies, they find less than completely positive outcomes (Luepker, Murray et al., 1994; COMMIT, 1995; Glasgow, Terborg et al., 1995; Ennett, Tabler et al., 1994). Whether the trials were conducted in work sites, schools, or entire communities, the results are remarkably similar: No significant effects compared with the control conditions.

If we examine more closely one of these trials, the Minnesota Heart Health Study, we can find hints of what went wrong (Lando, Pechacek et al., 1995). With smoking as one of the targeted behaviors, nearly 90% of the smokers in treated communities reported seeing media stories about smoking, but the same was true with smokers in the control communities.

Only about 12% of smokers in the treatment and control conditions said their physicians talked to them about smoking in the preceding year. If one looks at what percentage participated in the most powerful behavior change

FIGURE 1. **Pre-Therapy Stage Profiles for Premature Terminators, Appropriate Terminators, and Continuers**

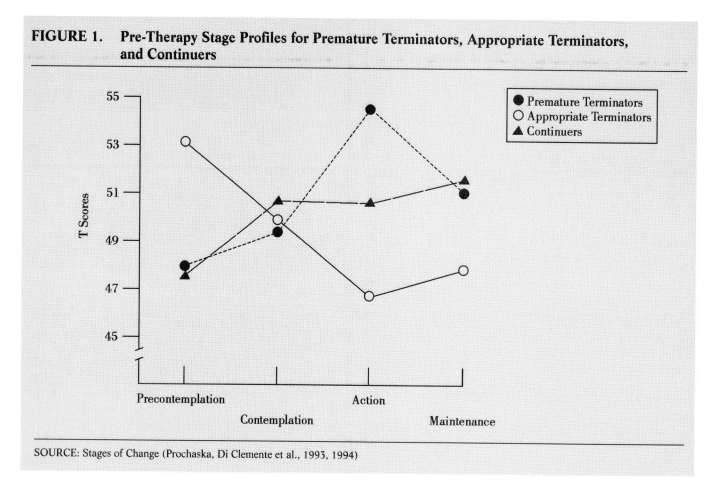

SOURCE: Stages of Change (Prochaska, Di Clemente et al., 1993, 1994)

programs (clinics, classes, and counselors), it is apparent that only 4% of smokers participated in the past five years of planned interventions. Even when state-of-the-science smoking cessation clinics are offered at no charge, only 1% of smokers are recruited (Lichtenstein & Hollis, 1992).

There simply will be little effect on the health of the nation if our best treatment programs reach so few persons with the deadliest of addictions.

How can more people with addictive disorders be motivated to seek the appropriate help? By changing both paradigms and practices. There are two paradigms that need to be changed. The first is an action-oriented paradigm that construes behavior change as an event that can occur quickly, immediately, discretely, and dramatically. Treatment programs that are designed to have patients immediately quit abusing substances are implicitly or explicitly designed for the portion of the population in the preparation stage.

The problem is that, with most unhealthy behaviors, fewer than 20% of the affected population are prepared to take action. Among smokers in the U.S., for example, about 40% are in the precontemplation stage, 40% in the contemplation stage, and 20% in the preparation stage (Velicer, Fava et al., 1995). Among college students who abuse alcohol, about 85% are in the pre-contemplation stage, 10% in the contemplation stage, and 5% in the preparation stage. When only action-oriented interventions are offered, fewer than 20% of the at-risk population is being recruited. In order to meet the needs of the entire addicted population, interventions must meet the needs of the 40% in the precontemplation and the 40% in the contemplation stages.

By offering stage-matched interventions and applying proactive or outreach recruitment methods in three large-scale clinical trials, the author and colleagues have been able to motivate 80% to 90% of smokers to enter a treatment program (Prochaska, Velicer et al., 2000, 2001). Comparable participation rates were generated with college students who abuse alcohol, even though 75% were in the precontemplation stage (Laforge, 2001). These results represent a quantum increase in our ability to move many more people to take the action of starting therapy.

The second paradigm change that is required is movement from a passive-reactive approach to a proactive approach. Most professionals have been trained to be passive-reactive: to passively wait for patients to seek their services and then to react. The problem with this approach is that most persons with addictive disorders never seek such services.

The passive-reactive paradigm is designed to serve populations with acute conditions. The pain, distress, or discomfort of such conditions can motivate patients to seek the services of health professionals. But the major killers today are chronic lifestyle disorders such as the addictions. To treat the addictions seriously, professionals must learn how to reach out to entire populations and offer them stage-matched therapies.

Regions of the National Health Service in Great Britain are training health professionals in these new paradigms. More than 6,000 physicians, nurses, counselors, and health educators have been trained to interact proactively at each stage of change with their entire patient populations who smoke or abuse alcohol, drugs, or food.

What happens if professionals change only one paradigm and proactively recruit entire populations to action-oriented interventions? This experiment has been tried in one of the largest U.S. managed care organizations (Lichtenstein & Hollis, 1992). Physicians spent time with every smoker in an effort to persuade him or her to enroll in a state-of-the-art action-oriented clinic. If that did not work, nurses spent up to 10 minutes encouraging the smoker to enroll, followed by 12 minutes with a health educator and a counselor call to the home. The base rate was 1% participation.

This most intensive recruitment protocol motivated 35% of smokers in precontemplation to enroll. However, only 3% actually entered the program, 2% completed it, and none showed improved outcomes. From a combined contemplation and preparation group, 65% enrolled, 15% entered the program, 11% completed it, and some had an improved outcome.

In the face of this evidence, there may be several answers to the question: What can move a majority of people to enter a professional treatment program for an addictive disorder? One is the availability of professionals who are motivated and prepared to proactively reach out to entire populations and offer them interventions that match whatever stage of change they are in.

Retention. What motivates patients to continue in therapy? Or conversely, what moves clients to terminate counseling quickly and prematurely, as judged by their counselors? A meta-analysis of 125 studies found that nearly 50% of clients drop out of treatment (Wierzbicki & Pekarik, 1993). Across studies, there were few consistent predictors of premature termination. Although addictive disorder, minority status, and lower education predicted a higher percentage of dropouts, these variables did not account for much of the variance.

At least five studies are available on dropouts from a stage model perspective on addictive disorder, smoking, obesity, and a broad spectrum of psychiatric disorders. These studies found that stage-related variables were more reliable predictors than demographics, type of problem, severity of problem, and other problem-related variables. Figure 1 presents the stage profiles of three groups of patients with a broad spectrum of psychiatric disorders (Brogan, Prochaska et al., 1999; Prochaska, DiClemente et al., 1992). In that study, the investigators were able to predict 93% of the three groups: premature terminators, early but appropriate terminators, and those who continued in therapy (Brogan, Prochaska et al., 1999).

Figure 1 shows that the before-therapy profile of the entire group who dropped out quickly and prematurely (40%) was a profile of persons in the precontemplation stage. The 20% who finished quickly but appropriately had a profile of patients who were in the action stage at the time they entered therapy. Those who continued in long-term treatment were a mixed group, with most in the contemplation stage.

The lesson is clear: Persons in the precontemplation stage cannot be treated as if they are starting in the same place as those in the action stage. If they are pressured to take action when they are not prepared, they simply will leave therapy.

For patients in the action stage who enter therapy, what would be an appropriate approach? One alternative would be to provide relapse prevention strategies like those described by Dr. Alan Marlatt. But would relapse prevention strategies make any sense with the 40% of patients who enter in the precontemplation stage? What might be a good

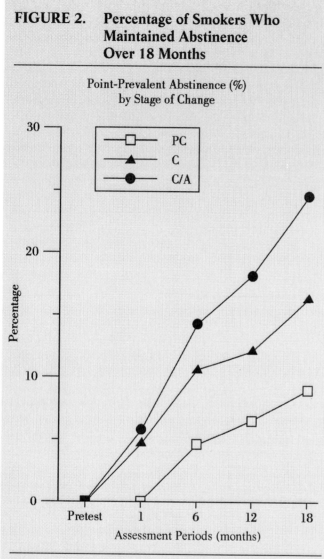

FIGURE 2. Percentage of Smokers Who Maintained Abstinence Over 18 Months

Point-Prevalent Abstinence (%) by Stage of Change

□ PC
▲ C
● C/A

Percentage

Pretest 1 6 12 18

Assessment Periods (months)

NOTE: Groups were in the following stages at the time of entry into treatment: Precontemplation (PC), Contemplation (C), and Preparation (C/A) (N=570).

tempted to leave early." The therapist then can explore whether the patient has been pressured to enter therapy. How do such patients react when someone tries to pressure or coerce them into quitting an addiction when they are not ready? Can they tell the therapist if they feel pressured or coerced? It is only feasible to encourage them to take steps when they are most ready to succeed.

The author and colleagues have conducted four studies with stage-matched interventions in which retention rates of persons entering interventions in the precontemplation stage can be examined. What is clear is that, when treatment is matched to stage, persons in the precontemplation stage will remain in treatment at the same rates as those who start in the preparation stage. This result was consistent in clinical trials in which patients were recruited proactively (the therapist reached out with an offer of help), as well as in trials in which patients were recruited reactively (they asked for help).

What motivates people to continue in therapy? Receiving treatments that match their stage of readiness to change.

Progress. What moves people to progress in therapy and to continue to progress after therapy? Figure 2 presents an example of what is called the *stage effect*. The stage effect predicts that the amount of successful action taken during and after treatment is directly related to the stage at which the person entered treatment (Prochaska, DiClemente et al., 1992). In the study cited, interventions with smokers ended at six months. The group of smokers who started in the precontemplation stage showed the least amount of effective action, as measured by abstinence at each assessment point. Those who started in the contemplation stage made significantly more progress, while those who entered treatment already prepared to take action were most successful at every assessment.

The stage effect has been found across a variety of problems and populations, including rehabilitative success for brain injury and recovery from anxiety and panic disorders after random assignment to placebo or effective medication (Beitman, Beck et al., 1994; Lam et al., 1988). In the latter clinical trial, the psychiatrist leading the trial concluded that patients need to be assessed for their stage of readiness to benefit from medication and to be helped through the stages so that they are well prepared before being placed on the medication.

One strategy for applying the stage effect clinically involves setting realistic goals for brief encounters with match for them? Experience suggests a dropout prevention approach, because such patients are likely to leave early if they are not helped to continue.

With patients who begin therapy in the pre-contemplation stage, it is useful for the therapist to share key concerns: "I'm concerned that therapy may not have a chance to make a significant difference in your life, because you may be patients at each stage of change. A realistic goal is to help patients progress one stage in brief therapy. If a patient moves relatively quickly, he or she may be able to progress two stages. The results to date indicate that, if a patient progresses one stage in one month, the likelihood of his or her taking effective action by six months is doubled. If the patient progresses two stages, the likelihood that he or she will take effective action increases three to four times (Prochaska, Velicer et al., 2000). Setting realistic goals thus can enable many more people to enter therapy, continue in therapy, progress in therapy, and continue to progress after therapy.

The first result reported from England with the 6,000 health professionals trained in this approach to the addictions is a dramatic increase in the morale of the health professionals involved. They can see progress with most of their patients, where they once saw failure when immediate action was the only criterion for success. They are much more confident that they have treatments that can match the stages of all of their patients rather than the small number who are prepared to take immediate action.

A lesson here is that the models of therapy selected should be good for the mental health of the therapist as well as the patient. After all, the professional is engaged in therapy for a lifetime, while most patients are involved for only a brief time.

As managed care organizations move to briefer and briefer therapies for the addictions and other disorders, there is a danger that most health professionals will feel pressured to produce immediate action. If this pressure is transferred to patients who are not prepared for such action, most patients will not be reached or not retained in treatment. A majority of patients can be helped to progress in treatment through relatively brief encounters, but only if realistic goals are set for both patient and therapist. Otherwise, there is a risk of demoralizing and demotivating both patient and therapist.

Process. In order to help motivate patients to progress from one stage to the next, it is necessary to know the principles and processes of change that can produce such progress.

Principle 1: The rewards for changing must increase if patients are to progress beyond precontemplation. In a review of 12 studies, all showed that the perceived benefits were higher in the contemplation than in the precontemplation stage (Prochaska, Velicer et al., 1994). This pattern held true across 12 problem behaviors: use of cocaine, smok-

ing, delinquency, obesity, inconsistent condom use, unsafe sex, sedentary lifestyles, high-fat diets, sun exposure, radon testing, mammography screening, and physicians practicing behavioral medicine.

A technique that can be used in population-based programs involves asking a patient in the pre-contemplation stage to describe all the benefits of a change such as quitting smoking or starting to exercise. Most persons can list four or five. The therapist can let the patient know that there are 8 to 10 times that number, and challenge the patient to double or triple the list for the next meeting. If the patient's list of benefits of exercise begins to indicate many more motives, such as a healthier heart, healthier lungs, more energy, healthier immune system, better moods, less stress, better sex life, and enhanced self-esteem, he or she will be more motivated to begin to seriously contemplate such a change.

Principle 2: The "cons" of changing must decrease if patients are to progress from contemplation to action. In 12 of 12 studies, the author and colleagues found that the perceived costs of changing were lower in the action than in the contemplation stage (Prochaska, Velicer et al., 1994).

Principle 3: The relative weight assigned to benefits and costs must cross over before a patient will be prepared to take action. In 12 of 12 studies, the costs of changing were assessed as higher than the rewards in the precontemplation stage, but in 11 of 12 the rewards were assessed as higher than the costs in the action stage. The sole exception involved quitting cocaine. In that study, a large percentage of treatment was delivered to inpatients. We interpret this exception to mean that the actions of these patients may have been more under the social control of residential care than under their self-control. At a minimum, their pattern would not bode well for immediate discharge.

It should be noted that, if raw scores are used to assess these patterns, it would appear that the rewards for changing are seen as greater than the costs, even by persons in the precontemplation stage. It is only when standardized scores are used that clear patterns emerge, with the costs of changing always perceived as greater than the rewards. This suggests that, compared with their peers at other stages of change, persons in the precontemplation stage underestimate the rewards and overestimate the costs of change.

Principle 4: The strong principle of progress holds that, to progress from precontemplation to effective action, the rewards for changing must increase by one standard deviation (Prochaska, 1994).

Principle 5: The weak principle of progress holds that, to progress from contemplation to effective action, the perceived costs of changing must decrease by one-half standard deviation.

Because the perceived rewards for changing must increase twice as much as the perceived costs decrease, twice as much emphasis must be placed on the rewards than the costs of changing. What is striking here is that the author and colleagues believe they have discovered mathematical principles for the degree to which positive motivations must increase and negative motivations must decrease. Such principles can produce much more sensitive assessments to guide interventions, giving therapists and patients feedback for when therapeutic efforts are producing progress and when they are failing. Together, they can modify methods if movement is needed for the patient to become adequately prepared for action.

Principle 6: It is important to match particular processes of change with specific stages of change. Table 1 presents the empirical integration found between processes and stages of change. Guided by this integration, the following processes would be applied to patients in the precontemplation stage:

1. *Consciousness raising* involves increased awareness of the causes, consequences, and responses to a particular problem. Interventions that can increase awareness include observations, confrontations, interpretations, feedback, and education. Some techniques, such as confrontation, pose considerable risk in terms of retention and are not recommended as highly as motivational enhancement methods such as personal feedback about the current and long-term consequences of continuing the addictive behavior. Increasing the costs of not changing is the corollary of raising the rewards for changing. So consciousness-raising should be designed to increase the perceived rewards for changing.

2. *Dramatic relief* involves emotional arousal about one's current behavior and the relief that can come from changing. Fear, inspiration, guilt, and hope are some of the emotions that can move persons to contemplate changing. Psychodrama, role-playing, grieving, and personal testimonies are examples of techniques that can move people emotionally.

   It should be noted that earlier literature on behavior change concluded that interventions such as education and fear arousal did not motivate behavior

change. Unfortunately, many interventions were evaluated in terms of their ability to move people to immediate action. However, processes such as consciousness raising and dramatic relief are intended to move people to the contemplation rather than the action stage. Therefore, their effectiveness should be assessed according to whether they lead to the expected progress.

3. *Environmental reevaluation* combines both affective and cognitive assessments of how an addiction affects one's social environment and how changing would affect that environment. Empathy training, values clarification, and family or network interventions can facilitate such reevaluation.

   For example, a brief media intervention aimed at a smoker in precontemplation might involve an image of a man clearly in grief saying, "I always feared that my smoking would lead to an early death. I always worried that my smoking would cause lung cancer. But I never imagined it would happen to my wife." Beneath his grieving face appears this statistic: "50,000 deaths per year are caused by passive smoking" (California Department of Health). In 30 seconds, this message achieves consciousness raising, dramatic relief, and environmental reevaluation.

4. *Self-reevaluation* combines both cognitive and affective assessments of an image of one's self free from addiction. Imagery, healthier role models, and values clarification are techniques that can move individuals in this type of intervention. Clinically, patients first look back and reevaluate how they have lived as addicted individuals. As they progress into the preparation stage, they begin to develop a focus on the future as they imagine how life could be if they were free of addiction.

5. *Self-liberation* involves both the belief that one can change and the commitment and re-commitment to act on that belief. Techniques that can enhance such willpower include public rather than private commitments. Motivational research also suggests that individuals who have only one choice are not as motivated as if they have two choices (Miller, 1977). Three choices are even better, but four choices do not seem to enhance motivation. Wherever possible, then, patients should be given three of the best choices for applying each process. With smoking cessation, for example, there are at least three good choices: (1) quitting "cold turkey," (2) using

TABLE 1.   Stages of Change in Which Change Processes Are Emphasized

	Stages of Change				
	Precontemplation	Contemplation	Preparation	Action	Maintenance
Processes	Consciousness raising				
	Dramatic Relief				
	Environmental reevaluation				
		Self-reevaluation			
			Self-liberation		
				Contingency management	
				Helping relationships	
				Counterconditioning	
					Stimulus control

nicotine replacement therapy, and (3) using nicotine fading. Asking clients to choose which alternative they believe would be most effective for them and which they would be most committed to can enhance their motivation and their self-liberation.

6. *Counterconditioning* requires the learning of healthier behaviors that can substitute for addictive behaviors. Counterconditioning techniques tend to be quite specific to a particular behavior. They include desensitization, assertion, and cognitive counters to irrational self-statements that can elicit distress.

7. *Contingency management* involves the systematic use of reinforcements and punishments for taking steps in a particular direction. Because successful self-changers rely much more on reinforcement than punishment, it is useful to emphasize reinforcements for progressing rather than punishments for regressing. Contingency contracts, overt and covert reinforcements, and group recognition are methods of increasing reinforcement and incentives that increase the probability that healthier responses will be repeated.

To prepare patients for the longer term, they should be taught to rely more on self-reinforcements than social reinforcements. Clinical studies show that many patients expect much more reinforcement and recognition from others than they actually receive. Relatives and friends may take action for granted. Average acquaintances typically generate only a few positive consequences early in the action stage. Self-reinforcements obviously are much more under self-control and can be given more quickly and consistently when temptations to lapse or relapse are resisted.

8. *Stimulus control* involves modifying the environment to increase cues that prompt healthy responses and decrease cues that lead to relapse. Avoidance, environmental re-engineering (such as removing addictive substances and paraphernalia), and attending self-help groups can provide stimuli that elicit healthy responses and reduce the risk of relapse.

9. *Helping relationships* combine caring, openness, trust, and acceptance, as well as support for changing. Rapport building, a therapeutic alliance, counselor calls, buddy systems, sponsors, and self-help groups can be excellent resources for social support. If patients become dependent on such support to maintain change, the support will need to be carefully faded, lest termination of therapy becomes a condition for relapse.

FIGURE 3.   Point-Prevalence Abstinence (%) for Four Treatment Groups at Pre-Test and at 6, 12, and 18 Months

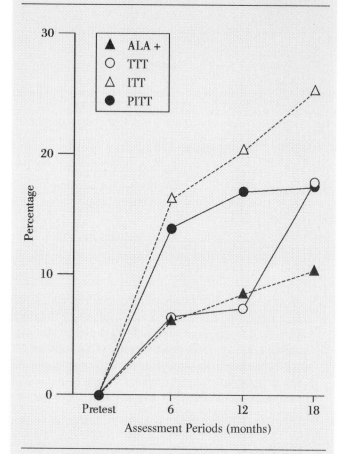

NOTE: ALA+ = standardized manuals; TTT = individualized stage-matched manuals; ITT = interactive computer reports; PITT = personalized counselor calls.

Competing theories of therapy have implicitly or explicitly advocated alternative processes of enhancing motivation for change. Is it ideas or emotions that move people? Is it values, decisions, or dedication? Do contingencies incentivize humans, or is behavior determined by environmental conditions or habits? Or is it the therapeutic relationship that is the common healer across all therapeutic modalities?

The answer to each of these questions is "yes." Therapeutic processes originating from competing theories can be compatible when they are combined in a stage-matched paradigm. With patients in earlier stages of change, motivation can be enhanced through more experiential processes that produce healthier cognitions, emotions, evaluations, decisions, and commitments. In later stages, it is possible to build on such solid preparation and motivation by emphasizing more behavioral processes that can help condition healthier habits, reinforce these habits, and provide physical and social environments that support healthier lifestyles freer from addictions.

Outcomes. What is the result when all of these principles and processes of change are combined to help patients and entire populations move toward action on their addictions? A series of clinical trials applying stage-matched interventions offers lessons about the future of behavioral health care generally and treatment of the addictions specifically.

In a large-scale clinical trial, the author and colleagues compared four treatments: (1) a home-based action-oriented cessation program (standardized), (2) stage-matched manuals (individualized), (3) a computerized expert system plus manuals (interactive), and (4) counselors plus an expert system and manuals (personalized). Patients (739 smokers) were randomly assigned by stage to one of the four treatments (Prochaska, DiClemente et al., 1993).

In the expert system condition, participants completed 40 questions by mail or telephone. Their responses were entered into a central computer, from which feedback reports were generated. These reports informed participants about their stage of change, the benefits and costs of changing, and change processes appropriate to their stages of change. At baseline, participants were given positive feedback on what they were doing correctly and guidance on which principles and processes they needed to apply to progress. In two progress reports delivered over the following six months, participants also received positive feedback on any improvement in any of the variables relevant to progress.

Thus, demoralized and defensive smokers could begin to progress without having to quit and without having to work too hard. Smokers in the contemplation stage could begin to take small steps, such as delaying their first cigarette in the morning for an additional 30 minutes. They could choose small steps that would increase their self-efficacy and help them become better prepared for quitting.

In the personalized condition, smokers received four proactive counselor calls over the six-month intervention period. Three of the calls were based on the expert system's reports. Counselors reported much more difficulty in interacting with participants without any progress data. Without scientific assessments, it was more difficult for both patients and counselors to know whether any significant progress had occurred since their last interaction.

Figure 3 presents point-prevalence abstinence rates for each of the four treatment groups over 18 months, with treatment ending at six months. Results with the two self-help manual conditions were parallel for 12 months, but the stage-matched manuals achieved better results at 18 months. This is an example of a *delayed action effect*, which often is observed with stage-matched programs and which others have observed with self-help programs. It takes time for participants in early stages to progress all the way to action. Therefore, some treatment effects as measured by action will be observed only after considerable time has elapsed. But it is encouraging to find treatments producing therapeutic effects months and even years after active treatment has ended.

The expert system alone and expert system-plus-counselor conditions produced comparable results for 12 months. Then, the effects of the counselor condition flattened out, whereas the expert system condition effects continued to increase. Potential reasons for the delayed differences between these conditions include the possibility that participants in the personalized condition may have become somewhat dependent on the social support and social control of the counselor calling. The last call occurred after the six-month assessment, and benefits would be observed at 12 months. Termination of the counselor calls could result in no further progress because of the loss of social support and control. The classic pattern in smoking cessation clinics is rapid relapse that begins as soon as treatment is terminated. Some of this rapid relapse could well be due to the sudden loss of social support or social control provided by the counselors and other participants when active treatment ends.

The next test was to demonstrate the efficacy of the expert system when applied to an entire population recruited proactively. With more than 80% of 5,170 smokers participating and less than 20% in the preparation stage, this study demonstrated significant benefits of the expert system at each six-month followup (Prochaska, Velicer et al., 2001). Moreover, the advantages over proactive assessment alone increased at each followup for the full two years as-

sessed. The implications here are that expert system interventions in a population can continue to demonstrate benefits long after the intervention has ended.

The efficacy of the expert system intervention was demonstrated again in a health maintenance organization (HMO) population of 4,000 smokers, with 85% participation (Prochaska, Velicer et al., 2000). In the first population-based study, the expert system was 34% more effective than assessment alone; in the second, it was 31% more effective. These differences were clinically significant as well. Although working on a population basis, the investigators were able to show a level of success normally found only in intensive clinic-based programs with low participation rates of more carefully selected samples of smokers. The implication is that, once expert systems are developed and show effectiveness with one population, they can be transferred to, and show replicable results in, other populations.

Enhancing Interactive Interventions: In recent benchmarking research, the author and colleagues have been attempting to create enhancements to the expert system to produce even better outcomes. In the first enhancement, which involved a study of an HMO population, a personal digital assistant (PDA) designed to bring the behavior under stimulus control was added (Prochaska, Velicer et al., 2000). However, this action-oriented intervention did not enhance the study outcomes on a population basis. In fact, the original expert system alone was twice as effective as the system plus the PDA enhancement. This result suggests that (1) more is not necessarily better, and (2) providing interventions that are mismatched to stage can make outcomes markedly worse.

Counselor Enhancements: In the HMO population, counselors plus expert system computer-based interventions were outperforming expert systems alone at 12 months. But at 18 months, results for the counselor enhancement had declined, whereas those for the expert systems alone had increased. Both interventions were producing identical outcomes of 23.2% abstinence, which are excellent for an entire population. Why did the effect of the counselor condition drop after the intervention? A leading hypothesis is that patients can become dependent on counselors for social support and social monitoring. Withdrawing those social influences may place such patients at increased risk of relapse. The expert system, in contrast, tends to maximize self-reliance. In a current clinical trial, the author and colleagues are "fading out" the counselor intervention over time in an effort to minimize dependence on the counselor. If fading is effective, it will have implications for how counseling should be terminated: gradually over time rather than suddenly.

It seems clear that the most powerful change programs will combine the personalized benefits of counselors and consultants with the individualized, interactive, and data-based benefits of expert system computer-based interventions. However, studies to date have not demonstrated that the more costly counselors, who have been the most powerful change agents, actually add value over expert system interventions alone. These findings have clear implications for the cost-effectiveness of expert systems for entire populations in need of health promotion programs.

Interactive Versus Non-Interactive Interventions: Another important goal of the HMO study was to assess whether an interactive intervention (specifically, a computer-based expert system) is more effective than non-interactive communications (such as self-help manuals) when the results are adjusted to control for the number of intervention contacts (Velicer, Prochaska et al., 1999). At 6, 12, and 18 months for groups of smokers receiving a series of one, two, three, or six interactive versus non-interactive contacts, the interactive interventions (expert system) outperformed the non-interactive manuals. The difference at 18 months was at least 5%—a difference between treatment conditions assumed to be clinically significant. These results clearly support the hypothesis that interactive interventions will outperform the same number of non-interactive interventions.

These results support the assumption that the most powerful health promotion programs for entire populations will be interactive. Reports in the clinical literature support the hypothesis that interactive interventions such as behavioral counseling produce better long-term abstinence rates (20% to 30%) than do non-interactive interventions such as self-help manuals (10% to 20%). In assessing these results, it should be kept in mind that traditional action-oriented programs were implicitly or explicitly recruiting for populations of individuals in the preparation stage, whereas the studies cited here involved proactively recruited smokers, of whom fewer than 20% were in the preparation stage. Even so, long-term abstinence rates were in the 20% to 30% range for the interactive interventions and in the 10% to 20% range for non-interactive interventions. The implications are clear. Providing interactive interventions through the use of computer-based expert systems is likely to produce better outcomes than relying on non-interactive communications such as newsletters, media, or self-help manuals.

CONCLUSIONS

It seems clear that the future of health promotion programs lies in stage-matched, proactive, interactive inter-ventions. Much greater effects can be generated through the use of proactive programs because participation rates are increased, even if efficacy rates are lower. But proactive programs also can produce outcomes comparable to those of traditional reactive programs. While it is counterintuitive to suggest that outcomes for groups that are proactively recruited can match those of individuals who reach out for help, that is what informal comparisons strongly suggest. For example, in a comparison of results at 18-month followup for all subjects who received three expert system interventions in a study of reactive intervention and a study of proactive intervention, the abstinence curves were remarkably similar (Prochaska, DiClemente et al., 1993; Prochaska, Velicer et al., 2001).

The results with the counseling plus expert system conditions were even more impressive. Proactively recruited smokers, working with both counselors and the expert system, achieved higher rates of abstinence at each followup than did the smokers who had called for help. These results are partially attributable to the fact that the proactive counseling protocol has been revised and, it is to be hoped, improved on the basis of previous data and experience. But the point is that if it is possible to reach out and offer people improved behavior-change programs that are appropriate for their stage of readiness to change, it ought to be possible to produce efficacy or abstinence rates at least equal to those seen with individuals who reach out for help. Unfortunately, there is no experimental design that would make it possible to assign study subjects randomly to proactive versus reactive recruitment programs. Thus, one is left with informal but provocative comparisons.

If these results continue to be replicated, therapeutic programs will be able to produce unprecedented effects on entire populations. To do so will require scientific and professional shifts: (1) from an action paradigm to a stage paradigm, (2) from reactive to proactive recruitment, (3) from expecting participants to match the needs of programs to having programs match the needs of patients, and (4) from clinic-based to population-based programs that apply individualized and interactive intervention strategies.

REFERENCES

American Psychiatric Association (APA) (1994). *Diagnostic and Statistical Manual of Mental Disorders, 4th Edition (DSM-IV)*. Washington, DC: American Psychiatric Press.

Beitman BD, Beck NC, Deuser W et al. (1994). Patient stages of change predicts outcome in a panic disorder medication trial. *Anxiety* 1:64-69.

Brogan ME, Prochaska JO & Prochaska JM (1999). Predicting termination and continuation status in psychotherapy using the Transtheoretical Model. *Psychotherapy* 36:105-113.

COMMIT Research Group (1995). COMMunity Intervention Trial for Smoking Cessation (COMMIT): I. Cohort results from a four-year community intervention. *American Journal of Public Health* 85:183-192.

Ennett ST, Tabler NS, Ringwolt CL et al. (1994). How effective is drug abuse resistance education? A meta-analysis of Project DARE outcome evaluations. *American Journal of Public Health* 84:1394-1401.

Glasgow RE, Terborg JR, Hollis JF et al. (1995). Take Heart: Results from the initial phase of a work-site wellness program. *American Journal of Public Health* 85:209-216.

Laforge RE (2001). A Proactive Individualized Program for College Drinkers (NIAAA grant proposal).

Lam CS, McMahon BT, Priddy DA et al. (1988). Deficit awareness and treatment performance among traumatic head injury adults. *Brain Injury* 2:235-242.

Lando HA, Pechacek TF, Pirie PL et al. (1995). Changes in adult cigarette smoking in the Minnesota Heart Health Program. *American Journal of Public Health* 85:201-208.

Lichtenstein E & Hollis J (1992). Patient referral to smoking cessation programs: Who follows through? *Journal of Family Practice* 34:739-744.

Luepker RV, Murray DM, Jacobs DR et al. (1994). Community education for cardiovascular disease prevention: Risk factor changes in the Minnesota Heart Health Program. *American Journal of Public Health* 84:1383-1393.

Mellinger GD, Balter MB, Uhlenhuth EH et al. (1978). Psychic distress, life crisis, and use of psychotherapeutic medications: National Household Survey Data. *Archives of General Psychiatry* 35:1045-1052.

Miller WR (1985). Motivation for treatment: a review with special emphasis on alcoholism. *Psychological Bulletin* 98:84-107.

Prochaska JO (1994). Strong and weak principles for progressing from Precontemplation to Action based on twelve problem behaviors. *Health Psychology* 13:47-51.

Prochaska JO & DiClemente CC (1983). Stages and processes of self-change of smoking: Toward an integrative model of change. *Journal of Consulting and Clinical Psychology* 51:390-395.

Prochaska JO, DiClemente CC & Norcross JC (1992). In search of how people change: Applications to the addictive behaviors. *American Psychologist* 47:1102-1114.

Prochaska JO, DiClemente CC, Velicer WF et al. (1993). Standardized, individualized, interactive and personalized self-help programs for smoking cessation. *Health Psychology* 12:399-405.

Prochaska JO, Norcross JC & DiClemente CC (1994). *Changing for Good*. New York, NY: William Morrow.

Prochaska JO, Velicer WF, Fava JL et al. (2001). Evaluating a population-based recruitment approach and a stage-based expert system intervention for smoking cessation. *Addictive Behaviors* 26:583-602.

Prochaska JO, Velicer WF, Fava JL et al. (2000). Counselor and stimulus control enhancements of a stage-matched expert system for smokers in a managed care setting. *Preventive Medicine* 32:39-46.

Prochaska JO, Velicer WF, Rossi JS et al. (1994). Stages of change and decisional balance for twelve problem behaviors. *Health Psychology* 13:39-46.

Snow MG, Prochaska JO & Rossi JS (1992). Stages of change for smoking cessation among former problem drinkers: A cross-sectional analysis. *Journal of Substance Abuse* 4:107-116.

U.S. Department of Health and Human Services (DHHS) (1990). *The Health Benefits of Smoking Cessation: A Report of the Surgeon General*. Washington, DC: U.S. Government Printing Office.

Velicer WF, Fava JL, Prochaska JO et al. (1995). Distribution of smokers by stage in three representative samples. *Preventive Medicine* 24:401-411.

Velicer WF, Prochaska JO, Fava JL et al. (1999). Interactive versus non-interactive and dose response relationships for stage matched smoking cessation programs in a managed care setting. *Health Psychology* 18:1-8.

Veroff J, Douvan E & Kulka RA (1981a). *The Inner America*. New York, NY: Basic Books.

Veroff J, Douvan E & Kulka RA (1981b). *Mental Health in America*. New York, NY: Basic Books.

Wierzbicki M & Pekarik G (1993). A meta-analysis of psychotherapy dropout. *Professional Psychology: Research and Practice* 29:190-195.

Chapter 2 | Group Therapies

Dennis C. Daley, Ph.D.
Delinda E. Mercer, Ph.D.
Crystal E. Spotts, M.Ed.

Group therapies are used widely in the treatment of substance use disorders in short-term residential rehabilitation, long-term therapeutic community, partial hospital, intensive outpatient, drug-free outpatient, and aftercare programs. In these contexts, groups are used to address early recovery issues such as initiating abstinence and engaging the patient in a recovery process (Matrix, 1989; McAuliffe & Albert, 1992; Washton, in press, a), relapse prevention Daley & Marlatt, 1997a; Schmitz, Oswald et al., 1997; Washton, in press, b), anger management (Reilly & Shropshire, 2000), and co-occurring psychiatric disorders (Daley & Thase, 2000; Daley & Moss, 2002; Najavits, Weiss et al., 1995; Khantzian, Golden et al., 1999). Group therapies also are widely used in the treatment of specific clinical populations, particularly women (Covington, 1999); alcoholics (Monti, Abrams et al., 1989; Yalom, Bloch et al., 1978); persons in the criminal justice system (Peters & Hills, 1999; Gorski & Kelly, 1996); those dependent on marijuana (Roffman, Stephens et al., 1988), cocaine (Gottheil, Weinstein et al., 1998; McAuliffe & Albert, 1992; Malik, Washton et al., 1995), methamphetamine (Obert, McCann et al., 2000), or opiates (NIDA, 1994); and families of substance users (Vannicelli, 1995).

For structured treatment programs such as residential, therapeutic community, partial hospital, or intensive outpatient programs, group therapies often are the principal modality of clinical intervention.

This chapter provides an overview of group therapies. It reviews the goals, types, and limitations of group therapies as they are used to treat substance use disorders. Training and supervision issues are discussed. The chapter reflects the authors' review of the empirical and clinical literature on group therapies, as well as their direct experience, including experience with clinical trials.

GOALS OF GROUP THERAPIES

The goal of addiction treatment is to help the patient initiate and maintain abstinence and to make the personal or lifestyle changes needed to support abstinence. Group therapies help patients achieve these goals by creating a milieu in which members of a group can bond with each other, thus reducing the stigma associated with addiction and the humiliation of having lost control of one's own behavior (Washton, in press, a). The specific ways in which groups can help achieve this include (1) providing education on addiction, recovery, and relapse, (2) resolving ambivalence by overcoming denial and enhancing motivation to change, (3) instilling hope and optimism for change, (4) providing an opportunity to give and receive feedback from peers, (5) teaching recovery skills to manage the addictive disorder over the long term, (6) understanding and resolving problems contributing to or resulting from the addictive disorder, rather than avoiding such problems, (7) providing a context in which the patient can identify with others and give and receive support, (8) creating an experience of positive membership in a recovery-oriented group in which feelings, thoughts, and conflicts can be freely expressed, (9) preparing the patient for involvement in long-term treatment, and (10) facilitating the patient's interest in participating in self-help programs in addition to treatment groups (Yalom, 1985; Flores, 1988; Daley, Mercer et al., 1998a; Washton, 1997; McAuliffe & Albert, 1992).

Treatment groups provide a context in which addicted persons can gain support, encouragement, feedback, and confrontation from peers who understand from personal experience how addicted individuals think, feel, and act, including the manipulations, schemes, and diversions they sometimes use to rationalize their substance use and other maladaptive behaviors (Washton, in press, a & b).

ORGANIZATION OF GROUP THERAPIES

Group therapies vary in their theoretical underpinnings, structure, format, rules, number and duration of sessions, clinical focus, size, types of patients accepted, requirements for abstinence, approach to the group model, relative focus on content or process, and role of the group leader. For example, psychoeducational groups are more structured and content focused, depend on the leader to facilitate discussion of educational material, and can accommodate larger numbers of patients than do therapy groups. Therapy groups usually are limited to 8 to 12 persons, with the content of discussions determined by the participants. Leaders are less verbally active in these groups and serve more as facilitators of members' exploration of problems and sharing of support and feedback.

Although some groups incorporate principles and information from self-help groups such as Alcoholics Anonymous (AA), Narcotics Anonymous (NA), or Cocaine Anonymous (CA), therapy groups differ from self-help groups in their focus on in-depth exploration of psychological, interpersonal, and personal issues.

Structured inpatient, residential, partial hospital, and intensive outpatient treatment programs can last from several weeks to a year, thus exposing patients to a considerable number of group sessions. For example, a large, multisite study of outpatient treatment for cocaine addiction (Crits-Cristoph, Siqueland et al., 1997) offered 39 individual sessions to patients in three of the four treatment conditions, in addition to 24 group counseling sessions, over a period of six months of active treatment and three additional monthly individual booster sessions.

Types of Group Therapies. Although many different types and structures of group treatments are available for the treatment of addictive disorders, many of the problems or issues addressed are similar (Table 1).

Group therapists or counselors employ a variety of techniques, such as providing education, eliciting support and feedback from members, confronting problematic behaviors, clarifying problems and feelings, helping the group remain focused, facilitating participant self-disclosure, teaching coping skills, and integrating experiential strategies relevant to the problems or issues being discussed (for example, using role-play to address interpersonal issues or conflicts, monodramas to address internal conflicts, and so forth).

Group therapies for substance use disorders generally fall into one of the following categories:

Milieu Groups: Milieu groups are offered in residential programs and usually involve a group meeting to start and/or end the day. A community group may review the upcoming day's schedule, discuss issues pertinent to the community of patients, ask each patient to state a goal for the day, or have patients listen to and reflect on the reading of the day (for example, an inspirational reading from a recovery book such as *24 Hours a Day*). A wrap-up group may review the day's activities and provide participants a chance to reflect on experiences and insights from the day's treatment activities.

Psychoeducational Groups: Psychoeducational groups provide information about specific topics related to addiction and recovery, and help patients begin to learn how to cope with the challenges of recovery (for example, how to resist social pressure to use substances or how to reduce boredom). These groups use a combination of lectures, discussions, educational videos, behavioral rehearsals, and completion of written assignments such as a recovery workbook or personal journal.

Skill Groups: Skill groups are aimed at helping patients develop and/or improve their intrapersonal and interpersonal skills. For example, these groups teach problem-

TABLE 1.   Issues and Problems Commonly Addressed in Recovery Groups

Physical/Lifestyle Issues

Tolerance, physical withdrawal, and the need for detoxification

Craving Management

Medication for the addiction

Medical problems and the addition

Sexuality issues, HIV/AIDS, and other sexually transmitted diseases

Importance of exercise, rest, relaxation, and nutrition in recovery

Types and purposes of treatment

Defining personal goals

Structuring time

Engaging in non-substance-using activities

Achieving balance in life

Regular use of recovery tools in daily life.

Psychological/Behavioral/Spiritual Issues

Understanding and identifying emotions and feelings and their effect on relapse

Managing anxiety

Managing depression

Managing feelings of emptiness

Managing boredom

Reducing shame and guilt

Grief and loss issues

Self-esteem

Self-defeating and therapy-sabotaging behaviors

Psychiatric comorbidities

Relapse and personal growth

High risk factors or dangerous situations for relapse

Relapse warning signs

Relapse set-ups

Lapse/relapse interruption

Spirituality

Meditation.

Understanding Addiction and Recovery

Understanding addiction (etiology, symptoms, effects)

Effects of specific substances (alcohol, cocaine, marijuana, et al.)

Acceptance of addiction

Motivation to change and motivational struggles

Tips for quitting alcohol or drug use

Pros and cons of change

Pros and cons of abstinence

Denial and other defenses

Stages of change

Phases of recovery and domains of recovery (physical, psychological, family, social, spiritual)

Addictive thinking

Other addictions.

Family/Interpersonal/Social Domains

Effects of addiction on family and interpersonal relationships

Role of the family in treatment/recovery

Resolving marital or family conflicts

Making amends to family or others

Managing high-risk people, places, and events

Engaging in healthy leisure interests

Addressing social life and relationship problems or deficits

Resisting social pressures to drink alcohol or use other drugs

Presenting a history of addictive disorders to the employer

Facing versus avoiding interpersonal conflicts

Learning to ask for help and support

Love and intimacy

Self-help programs in recovery

The Twelve Steps

Seeking and using an AA or NA sponsor

Recovery clubs.

---

solving methods, stress management, cognitive strategies, and relapse prevention strategies.

Therapy or Counseling Groups: These groups are unstructured and give the participants an opportunity to create their own agenda. Any of the issues presented in Table 1 can be discussed. These groups focus more on insight and raising self-awareness than on education or skill development. Some clinics provide gender-specific therapy or counseling groups so that women and men can work separately on their concerns and problems.

More extensive discussions of various group approaches for addiction, such as interactional group therapy (Yalom, 1985; Flores, 1988), modified dynamic group therapy (Khantzian, Halliday et al., 1990; Khantzian, Golden et al., 1999), cognitive-behavioral (McAuliffe & Albert, 1992), psychoeducational and problem-solving (Daley, Mercer et al., 1998a), skills training (Monti, Abrams et al., 1989), and recovery stage-specific groups (Washton, in press, a & b) can be found in texts cited in the references.

Format of Group Therapy Sessions. Group sessions usually last from 60 to 90 minutes. Groups can be limited to a specific number of sessions or be open-ended, so that the patient can attend for as long as needed. Programs vary in the frequency of sessions as well. For example, the Matrix model of addiction treatment, developed by Rawson and colleagues (Rawson, Shoptaw et al., 1995), offered 20 individual sessions during the first six months of an intensive outpatient program that included many group sessions. In a variation of this model, three individual sessions are provided to patients during the course of a 16-week treatment episode (Obert, McCann et al., 2000). The Washton structured outpatient model involves group therapy two to four times each week in combination with weekly individual counseling sessions (Malik, Washton et al., 1995). Interestingly, the last model explicitly acknowledges that, "although group therapy is the core treatment modality for most patients, some are not able to tolerate group as a result of psychiatric and/or interpersonal impairment. Treatment for these patients can consist of individual therapy two to three times a week" (p. 286).

Phase 1 Therapy Sessions: In a study conducted by the authors (Daley, Mercer et al., 1998b), patients participated in 90-minute sessions each week for 12 weeks. Each session focused on a specific topic relevant to early or middle recovery. At every session, patients were encouraged to abstain from all substances, seek and use a sponsor, participate in self-help groups, and use the "tools" of recovery (for example, talking about versus acting on strong cravings, reaching out for support, and the like). Patients were encouraged to socialize with each other before the start of the session while the group leader administered a Breathalyzer® test.

Each group session began with a check-in period (10 to 20 minutes in duration), during which time patients briefly reported any substance use, strong cravings, or "close calls." This was followed by a review of the topic for the session, lasting 40 to 60 minutes. Although the group leader had a specific curriculum for each meeting, the session was conducted in a way that encouraged patients to relate to the material in a personal way. Each session provided materials from a workbook that contained information about the topic and several questions for the patients to complete to relate the material to their own lives. During these discus-

sions, patients were encouraged to ask questions, share personal experiences related to the psychoeducational material, give each other feedback, and identify strategies to manage their problems in recovery.

Each session ended with a brief review of patients' plans for the coming week (10 to 15 minutes). Patients could discuss self-help meetings and other steps they could take toward recovery. Just before the session closed, patients recited the Serenity Prayer of AA.

Topics of Phase 1 therapy sessions included the following:

- *Session 1—Understanding Addiction:* Addiction was defined as a biopsychosocial disorder in which multiple factors contributed to its development and maintenance. Symptoms of addiction were reviewed in terms of the *Diagnostic and Statistical Manual of Mental Disorders, 4th Edition* (American Psychiatric Association, 1994), with a focus on obsession, compulsion, tolerance changes, physiologic dependence, and psychosocial impairment.

- *Sessions 2 and 3—The Process of Recovery:* Effects of addiction on all areas of functioning and the concept of denial were reviewed. Recovery was defined as a long-term process of abstinence and change involving multiple domains: physical, psychological, family, social, and spiritual. Each patient identified and discussed one area of change and a plan to achieve such change. Feedback was elicited from peers about the plan.

- *Sessions 4 and 5—Social and Interpersonal Issues in Recovery:* The group discussed cravings, internal and external triggers, and enabling behaviors on the part of other people in the patient's life. Major emphasis was given to identifying and learning to manage direct and indirect social pressures to engage in substance use (people, places, events, and things). The effects of addiction on family and social relationships and activities were described, and patients discussed strategies to address interpersonal problems in early recovery. Finally, components of healthy relationships were discussed.

- *Sessions 6 and 7—Self-Help Groups and Support Systems:* The importance of participating in Twelve Step programs of AA, NA, and CA was emphasized in all group sessions; these two sessions provided specific information on types of meetings, sponsorship, the Twelve Steps, and other tools of recovery. Barriers and negative perceptions or experiences with self-help programs were discussed, as were the benefits of self-help programs. Discussions also addressed sources of support outside AA, NA, and CA (for example, family, friends, recovery clubs, and organizations); barriers to asking for help; and ways to actually ask others for help.

- *Sessions 8 and 9—Managing Feelings in Recovery:* These sessions focused on understanding the connection between feelings and substance use and becoming aware of "high risk" emotional states associated with relapse. Strategies to manage feelings were reviewed, and patients were asked to develop a plan to address one emotional state they felt was a problem for them (such as anger, anxiety, boredom, depression, or loneliness). An entire session focused on understanding and dealing with guilt and shame, as these feelings are so common among patients in early recovery.

- *Sessions 10, 11, and 12—Relapse Prevention and Maintenance:* Relapse was defined as both a process and an event, with both obvious and covert warning signs. These sessions focused on helping patients identify and manage warnings of relapse, as well as individual high-risk situations. Common risk factors identified in research studies were reviewed to help patients learn to anticipate and prepare to address them. Strategies for maintaining recovery over time and using the tools of recovery on a daily basis also were discussed.

Phase 2 Problem-Solving Groups: Phase 2 groups met for 90 minutes weekly for 12 sessions. The goals were to help patients identify, rank, and discuss their problems in recovery and identify strategies to manage these problems to reduce relapse risk. Sessions provided an opportunity for patients to give and receive support and feedback from peers. After the check-in period—in which patients reported on any episodes of use, strong cravings, or close calls—they were asked to identify a problem or recovery issue for discussion in the group. Often, more than one member would identify a similar problem or issue for discussion. The issues and problems reviewed in the psychoeducational groups were revisited frequently.

Issues discussed often involved struggles with motivation to change or remain abstinent; persistent obsessions; compulsions and close calls to use cocaine or other substances; actual lapses or relapses; boredom with sobriety; upsetting emotional states (for example, anxiety, anger, depression); concerns or experiences with self-help programs; the Twelve Steps or a sponsor; interpersonal problems and pressures to use substances; financial, job, and lifestyle problems; other addictions; and spirituality.

At the end of each session, patients were asked to state their plans for the coming week in terms of attendance at self-help meetings or other steps they could take to aid their recovery or resolve a problem.

Group Process Issues: In both Phase 1 and Phase 2, group counselors had to attend to the group process to keep the group focused and productive. This attention required counselors to engage quiet members in discussions and facilitate their self-disclosure and to limit or redirect members who talked too much and tried to dominate group discussions, listened poorly to fellow group members, or tried to use the group to obtain individual therapy from the leader. Counselors kept the group from going off on unrelated tangents or talking in generalities, balanced the discussions between problems and coping strategies, facilitated group members' sharing of support and feedback, and addressed impasses or problems in the group. In Phase 1 groups, the counselor had to ensure that the curriculum for each session was covered, because this was viewed as an important part of treatment.

Obstacles to Group Therapies: Other researchers who have written about group treatments identify problems with group participants that create obstacles to treatment. Washton (in press, a) reports the following problems among members of therapy groups: lateness and absenteeism, intoxication, hostility and chronic complaining, silence and lack of participation, terse and superficial presentations, factual reporting and focusing on externals, proselytizing and hiding behind AA, and playing co-therapist. In his classic text on group psychotherapy, Yalom identified a number of "recurring behavioral constellations" (1985, p. 375) that occur in the treatment group. He identified these constellations as monopolist, schizoid, silent, boring, help-rejecting complainer, self-righteous moralist, psychotic, narcissistic, and borderline. Because the problems affect the group as a whole, the leader must have strategies to address any that arise in the course of a group session.

Family Psychoeducational Workshops: Family psychoeducational workshops (FPWs) and other family programs often are used to educate the family, provide support, help reduce the family's burden, increase helpful behaviors, and

---

decrease unhelpful behaviors (Anderson, Reiss et al., 1986; Daley, Bowler et al., 1992; McAuliffe & Albert, 1992; Washton, 1995; Obert, McCann et al., 2000).

FPWs are semi-structured sessions in which specific information is provided to patients and families in the context of a group of families. Support is provided, and families are encouraged to share their questions, concerns, and feelings. Strong affect always is present in these workshops, and some sharing of emotion is necessary. However, opening up families too much can be counterproductive, so education and support are the main areas of focus. Thus, the group leader must be careful not to allow the group to become a venue for sharing deep-seated emotions. Interactive discussion is encouraged because it increases participants' understanding of addiction and recovery.

The specific material covered in FPWs depends on the amount of time available. Possibilities include:

■ *An Overview of Substance Abuse and Dependence:* Prevalence, symptoms, causes, and basic concepts (such as various degrees of substance use problems, denial, obsession, compulsion, tolerance, psychiatric comorbidity, and the like).

■ *Effects of Substance Use Disorders:* The effects on the individual, the family system, and specific family members, including children.

■ *An Overview of Recovery:* Recovery issues for the affected person (physical, psychological or emotional, social, family, spiritual, other) and how to measure outcomes.

■ *An Overview of Treatment Resources:* Treatment resources and approaches for the affected individual.

■ *How the Family Can Help:* Enabling behaviors for the family to avoid and behaviors that are helpful in supporting the addicted family member's recovery.

■ *Family Recovery Issues:* How the family member can recover from the adverse effects of addiction and involvement in a close relationship with an addicted member.

■ *Self-Help Programs:* Programs available for addicted individuals and their family members, how such programs can help the family, and how to access them.

■ *Relapse:* Warning signs of relapse, the importance of relapse prevention planning, how the family can be involved, and how to deal with an actual lapse or relapse of an addicted family member.

In the cocaine collaborative study (Daley, Mercer et al., 1998b), the authors offered a single FPW during the first month of treatment. The purpose of the session was to educate families about the study, to seek their help in supporting the patients' compliance with treatment, and to provide education about addiction, recovery, their effect on the family, and community resources available to the family.

Anecdotal reports across a range of addictive disorders suggest an association between relapse and the absence or availability of social supports. This underscores the value of involving family members in supporting the patient's recovery efforts through their participation in FPW sessions.

EMPIRICAL VALIDATION OF GROUP THERAPIES

Recent years have witnessed a number of studies that have compared different models of psychotherapy and/or counseling for addictive disorders (NIAAA, 2000; NIDA, 1999). Most studies funded by the National Institute on Drug Abuse (NIDA) and the National Institute on Alcohol Abuse and Alcoholism (NIAAA) involve individual and/or pharmacotherapeutic interventions. Despite the widespread use of group therapies in addiction treatment, controlled trials of group interventions have been somewhat limited, and many studies report results from "programs" that involve multiple components (that is, individual plus group, multiple types of group treatments, or group plus other services). However, researchers and clinicians agree on the importance of group therapies, and groups remain one of the principal modalities of treatment in most residential, therapeutic community, partial hospital, intensive outpatient, and aftercare programs.

The interest in researching various models of psychotherapy has led to the development of treatment manuals that describe the various psychotherapeutic approaches. Psychotherapy outcomes studies have found that such manuals have an important, positive effect on the quality of both research and clinical practice. In fact, the use of treatment manuals has become a standard practice in research studies because they help ensure that therapists or counselors are providing treatment in a defined, measurable way. This practice also appears to reduce the variance among therapists providing what is nominally the same treatment.

Adherence to Group Sessions and Treatment Dropout. Most randomized clinical trials show significant reductions in drug use, improved health, and reduced social pathology (McLellan, Lewis et al., 2000). Patients who comply with sessions and attend a sufficient number of sessions show better outcomes than those who drop out prematurely. However, two of the major problems in the treatment of addictive disorders and co-occurring psychiatric disorders are poor adherence with session attendance or medications and early termination (Daley & Zuckoff, 1999).

Reasons for Dropping Out of Group Treatment: In the cocaine collaborative study by the authors, patients were assessed to learn the reasons for early termination of treatment. The reasons most commonly cited were time problems (42.7%), the relapse to use or the desire to use (30.7%), not finding group sessions helpful (29.3%), wanting a different treatment, such as individual therapy (30.7%), improvement in the problem (18.7%), other unspecified reasons (18.7%), unwillingness to participate in treatment (16%), and need for hospitalization (13.3%).

Limitations of Research. Although evidence suggests that group treatments are effective for substance use disorders, limitations to the research conducted on group treatments arise from two sources: variations in content and differences in process. A level of interaction and complexity must be taken into consideration, over and above the content of the intervention and the counselor's skill in conducting it. Very often, group programs are studied rather than a single group intervention. For example, studies of intensive outpatient programs (IOPs) often evaluate a comprehensive program that involves several different types of groups that together make up the IOP. Therefore, it is unclear how much each type of group actually contributes to the treatment outcome. In addition, studies sometimes involve a combination of group and individual treatments, making it difficult to determine how much each intervention contributes to the outcome.

GROUP THERAPIES FOR CO-OCCURRING DISORDERS

Community surveys and clinical studies document high rates of co-occurring psychiatric and substance use disorders (Robins & Regier, 1991; Kessler, McGonagle et al., 1994; O'Connell, in press). Group therapy appears to be helpful to patients with such co-occurring disorders. Considerable clinical research supports the use of various group treatments for so-called "dual diagnosis" patients, including those with chronic and persistent mental disorders (Minkoff & Drake, 1991; Montrose & Daley, 1995; Daley & Moss, 2002).

Several investigators have developed and are testing in clinical trials the effects of manual-driven group treatments. Najavits and colleagues (Najavits, Weiss et al., 1995; Najavits & Weiss, 1998) developed a cognitive-behavioral therapy model for women with posttraumatic stress disorder (PTSD). Their cognitive-behavioral therapy protocol involves 24 weekly group sessions, which are divided into "units" dealing with problems that are frequently encountered. An introductory unit of two sessions provides education on PTSD and substance use disorders (SUDs) and introduces the women to community resources and self-help programs. A behavioral unit of seven sessions teaches skills to manage the SUD and PTSD, addressing issues such as setting a daily schedule, structuring time, nurturing the self, learning to ask for help and support from others, identifying and managing triggers for both disorders, managing ambivalence about change, and learning to deal with life stressors. A unit of six sessions teaches cognitive strategies, such as changing maladaptive thoughts or cognitive distortions associated with SUD or PTSD. A unit of six sessions focuses on improving communication skills and interpersonal relationships. (This unit also addresses issues such as self-protection in relationships, rebuilding trust, and healthy relationship thinking.) The final unit of three sessions reviews the experience of group and termination issues with a focus on ongoing supports, knowing how to judge progress or deterioration, and the importance of a continuing care plan. At the time the group treatment contract is signed an interview is conducted with each patient before he or she enters the group, and ways to benefit from this treatment are reviewed. An individual HIV counseling session is provided to each patient within the first three weeks of treatment, at which time an HIV risk assessment is completed and education and counseling on HIV issues are provided. Homework assignments and action techniques such as role-play are used throughout this protocol.

A study of 17 women enrolled in this treatment program found major improvements in substance use, trauma-related symptoms, suicide cognitions about substance use, and didactic knowledge of topics covered in treatment sessions (Najavits, Weiss et al., 1998). Although this finding suggests that group treatment can be helpful to substance-abusing women with PTSD, the results are tentative because of the lack of a control group.

Weiss and colleagues (2000) compared an integrated model of group treatment (IGT) for bipolar patients with substance use disorders to group drug counseling (GDC) combined with standard psychiatric treatment. Both IGT and GDC are manual-driven treatments that involve 20 weekly group sessions lasting one hour each. IGT focuses on issues pertinent both to substance use and bipolar illness, whereas GDC focuses solely on addictive disorder issues. GDC patients address psychiatric issues in separate sessions with a mental health professional. GDC is an adaptation of the model used in the cocaine collaborative study (Crits-Cristoph, Siqueland et al., 1997; Daley, Mercer et al., 2002). The primary aim of GDC is to help patients manage their substance use disorder, whereas the goal of IGT is to help patients manage both disorders. In an uncontrolled quality improvement study of 117 patients who participated in the authors' integrated dual diagnosis intensive outpatient program (Daley & Those, 2000), there was a steady weekly decrease in mean scores for the Beck Anxiety Inventory (BAI), Beck Depression Inventory (BDI), and Addiction Severity Index (ASI) from baseline to week 4. The mean rating of both BAI and BDI scores declined from "moderate" to "mild" by week 4, and the mean ASI scored was 58% lower at week 4 than at baseline.

THE NEED FOR PHYSICIAN SUPPORT

Physicians and other addiction professionals who do not provide group therapies can play a significant role in supporting and facilitating patients' participation in groups. First, they can educate, encourage, and persuade patients to participate in groups as part of their overall treatment program. It is helpful for all clinical staff members to give patients a consistent message about the value of groups. The physician can use his or her status as a healer to help the patient make a decision to participate.

Second, the physician can monitor and discuss the patient's group participation. This task allows the physician to identify and resolve any barriers related to the patient's continued participation, to understand the reasons for poor adherence or early dropout, and to help the patient re-engage in group.

Third, the physician can collaborate with group therapists about patients' clinical status or problems with adherence. A physician may see a patient for management of withdrawal, for management of a co-occurring psychiat-

ric disorder, or to provide medications (such as naltrexone or disulfiram). If, during such a visit, the physician learns that the patient is not adhering to the plan to attend or participate actively in group therapy, the physician can facilitate a discussion with the group leader or even hold a joint meeting with the patient and group therapist to try to resolve the problem. Again, the message the patient receives from this collaboration is that the group is an important part of the overall treatment plan and is valued by the physician.

COUNSELOR TRAINING AND SUPERVISION

Counselor Training. To provide effective group treatment, it is necessary for counselors or therapists to be familiar with and skillful in addiction treatment and group therapy. It goes without saying that training in these areas is necessary when one is beginning in the field and that ongoing training and supervision help to keep counselors abreast of current developments in the field and enthusiastic about their work.

The knowledge base that one should have to provide competent addiction treatment involves knowledge of the effects of the various drugs of abuse and which drugs are commonly used in combination and their interactions, as well as the medical, psychological, social, family, and spiritual consequences of addiction. It also is necessary to understand the processes of recovery and relapse and the strategies or tools that can help the recovering person to manage the recovery process. The clinician should be familiar with the Twelve Step self-help approach of AA or NA for addiction recovery and with alternative self-help resources for patients who are not comfortable with Twelve Step programs.

In terms of group counseling or therapy, counselors should have an understanding of counseling theory and experience in counseling individual patients. Such understanding and experience are necessary because situations can arise in any group that require the group counselor to intervene in a therapeutic way with an individual while continuing to conduct the group. Conducting groups thus involves an additional level of complexity compared to working with individuals, in that the group leader must be able to understand and respond to individual as well as group dynamics or group process issues simultaneously. This ability involves understanding the ongoing process that is a key part of the group experience. "Group process" refers to the attitudes and interaction of the group members and leaders (Daley, Mercer et al., 1998a; NIDA, 2002).

It also is important for the counselor to be familiar with the stages of groups: the beginning, the middle or working stage, and the ending or closing stage. The group leader should be familiar with the kinds of interventions he or she will use most often and how to deal with problem situations that occur most commonly in groups. Basic intervention skills include active listening, clarification and questioning, information giving, summarization, encouraging and supporting, modeling, eliciting feedback, and addressing problems that commonly arise (for example, a member who dominates the group, resistant members who are reluctant to participate, a member who tries to assume the role of the leader, mutually hostile members, insensitive or destructive feedback, and members who try to challenge the leader).

Counselor Supervision. Supervision is a very important, meaningful part of the practice of group treatment, yet it often is overlooked or provided in a less than optimal manner. Generally speaking, it is always a good idea to provide the group counselor with access to someone who has more experience and expertise in the field, to whom the counselor can bring any problems as they emerge. It also is important to communicate that supervision is not primarily about evaluation of the counselor's work, but rather an opportunity for the counselor to air problems, hone his or her skills, and continue to learn.

Counselors in the cocaine collaborative study protocol received ongoing supervision that involved weekly meetings or telephone conversations with their supervisor. The goals of supervision were to ensure that the group sessions conformed to the research protocol and that the best possible clinical treatment was being delivered. Because this study was for comparative research, adherence to the counseling approach was of utmost importance. For this reason, an adherence scale was developed in conjunction with the group drug counseling manual and was used by the supervisors to rate videotaped group sessions.

An adherence scale provides specific operational definitions of desired interventions. These definitions make it clear to counselors what interventions should be incorporated into their work and make it easy for supervisors to point out strengths and deficiencies when giving feedback. Adherence scales associated with a treatment manual can be a useful tool for both research and clinical purposes, in that they allow researchers to assess whether therapists are following the specified treatment manual. They are helpful in showing that treatments can be differentiated from one another and in assessing the extent to which counselors incorporate techniques from other treatments. They are useful clinically in training and supervision of a particular model of treatment.

Counselor Satisfaction. It is important that counselors feel satisfied with the group approach they are providing and with the clinical environment in which they work. When counselors are dissatisfied, burnout, indifferent treatment, and departures from appropriate counseling behavior often result. Dissatisfied counselors also tend to feel less positive about their work and to express less confidence in their patients' ability to achieve recovery; such feelings can undermine the patients' own perception of their ability to recover.

LIMITATIONS OF GROUP THERAPIES

Although group therapies offer many benefits, they also have some limitations with which the clinician should be familiar. One of the most common is an overemphasis on group treatment at the expense of individual treatment. As part of an ongoing quality improvement effort, one of the authors (D.D.) has met with small focus groups of patients (totaling more than 1,000 over a period of several years) in a broad range of addiction and dual diagnosis inpatient, partial hospital, and outpatient treatment programs to inquire about what they liked and disliked about treatment. Although most patients participating in group treatment were able to articulate benefits of the group, a consistent criticism heard over many years has been a concern that they did not receive any or enough individual therapy. Patients often reported that there were certain types of problems or issues that they would not discuss in group sessions and that they preferred the privacy and confidentiality afforded by an individual counseling or therapy session. (Examples that patients reported of the personal problems difficult to disclose in group sessions included experiences as a victim and/or perpetrator of violence, sexual abuse, child abuse, some types of deviant behaviors, the presence of certain psychiatric symptoms, and conflicts related to sexual identity or behaviors.)

Confidentiality issues were cited as another reason for reluctance to disclose personal information in some group sessions. This was particularly true of patients who participated in a group session in which another member was from the same neighborhood or shared mutual friends.

Patients who had difficulty with assertiveness or disclosing personal problems reported that it was easy for them to blend into the background in a group. Although this felt "safe," the patients recognized that this feeling led to less than optimal gain from group therapy. Some patients described attending group sessions in which the leader did not control participants who talked too much or who listened poorly to others, or leaders who did not engage quiet members in group discussions.

Social anxiety or phobias are common among patients with substance use disorders (Myrick & Brady, 1997). Daley and Salloum (1996) administered the Davidson Brief Social Phobia questionnaire to 128 outpatients and found that more than a third reported high levels of social anxiety and avoidance behavior. Specifically, patients reported high levels of anxiety about speaking at AA or NA meetings or in a group therapy session. As a result of social anxiety, patients may choose to limit participation in therapy or self-help group discussions, miss group sessions, or drop out prematurely. They often do so without discussing their reasons with a therapist, counselor, or sponsor.

CONCLUSIONS

The research literature and clinical experience suggest a number of points that are important to an understanding of group therapies for substance use disorders.

First, group therapies play a critical role in addiction treatment and should be supported by all clinicians, regardless of whether they actually provide group sessions themselves.

Second, different group therapies can be used, depending on a given patient's progress in relation to the stages of change and the treatment context.

Third, a combination of group and individual treatment probably is optimal. (This issue is important because group therapy is the primary and often sole modality offered by many addiction treatment programs.)

Fourth, careful staff training and ongoing supervision appear to enhance the effectiveness of group therapies. Traditional addiction counseling may be very effective, but only when it is supported by good clinical supervision and opportunities for ongoing training.

Fifth, patients who participate in group therapies often benefit from pharmacotherapies as well. Considerable research indicates that a combination of behavioral treatments and medications improve treatment outcomes (NIDA, 1997 & 1999; McLellan, Lewis et al., 2000; NIAAA, 2000).

Sixth, self-help programs and group therapies are different in their purpose and structure. Group therapies can encourage self-help attendance, provide education, and explore experiences and resistances. Therapy groups are different from self-help programs in that they are designed to explore psychological, personal, and interpersonal issues in a safe environment in which self-disclosure, self-awareness, and self-change are encouraged and valued.

Seventh, treatment personnel must be sensitive to the fact that substance use disorders are debilitating, chronic, and relapsing in nature and cause many problems for the individual, the family and society. As with other chronic disorders, they require ongoing management.

Professional group therapy is one approach to initiating and continuing this process to the maintenance phase of recovery.

ACKNOWLEDGMENTS: The authors gratefully acknowledge the help of Cindy Hurney, administrative coordinator at the Center for Psychiatric and Chemical Dependency Services, for her help in preparing this manuscript, and of Dr. Allan Graham for his critique and editorial suggestions.

Preparation of this chapter was supported in part by grant DA09421-04 from the National Institute on Drug Abuse and grant AA11929 from the National Institute on Alcohol Abuse and Alcoholism.

REFERENCES

American Psychiatric Association (1994). *Diagnostic and Statistical Manual of Mental Disorders, 4th Edition (DSM-IV)*. Washington, DC: American Psychiatric Press.

Anderson CM, Reiss DJ & Hogarty GE (1986). *Schizophrenia and the Family*. New York, NY: Guilford Press.

Covington SS (1999). *A Woman's Journal*. San Francisco, CA: Jossey-Bass Publishers.

Crits-Christoph P, Siqueland L, Blaine J et al. (1997). The National Institute on Drug Abuse collaborative cocaine treatment study: Rationale and methods. *Archives of General Psychiatry* 54: 721-726.

Daley DC & Marlatt GA (1997a). *Managing Your Drug or Alcohol Problem: Therapist Guide*. San Antonio, TX: The Psychological Corporation.

Daley DC & Salloum IM (1996). *Social Anxiety Among Dual Diagnosis Outpatients*. Unpublished data.

Daley DC & Thase ME (2000). *Dual Disorders Recovery Counseling: Integrated Treatment for Substance Use and Mental Health Disorders*. Independence, MO: Herald House/Independence Press.

Daley DC & Zuckoff A (1999). *Improving Treatment Compliance: Counseling and System Strategies for Substance Use and Dual Disorders*. Center City, MN: Hazelden.

Daley DC, Bowler K & Cahalane H (1992). Approaches to patient and family education with affective disorders. *Patient Education and Counseling* 19:163-174.

Daley DC, Mercer D & Carpenter G (2002). *Group Drug Counselinig for Cocaine Dependence. Therapy Manuals for Addiction, Manual 4.* Bethesda, MD: National Institute on Drug Abuse.

Daley DC, Mercer D & Carpenter G (1998a). *Group Drug Counseling Manual.* Holmes Beach, FL: Learning Publications, Inc.

Daley DC, Mercer D & Carpenter G (1998b). *Group Drug Counseling Participant Recovery Workbook.* Holmes Beach, FL: Learning Publications, Inc.

Daley DC & Moss HB (2002). *Dual Disorders: Counseling Clients with Chemical Dependency and Mental Illness, 3rd Edition.* Center City, MN: Hazelden.

Flores PJ (1988). *Group Psychotherapy with Addicted Populations.* New York, NY: Haworth Press.

Gorski TT & Kelly JM (1996). *Counselor's Manual for Relapse Prevention with Chemically Dependent Criminal Offenders.* Rockville, MD: Substance Abuse and Mental Health Services Administration.

Gottheil E, Weinstein SP, Sterling RC et al. (1998). A randomized controlled study of the effectiveness of intensive outpatient treatment for cocaine dependence. *Psychiatric Services* 49(6):782-787.

Kazdin (1986). (Delinda).

Kessler RC, McGonagle KA, Zhao S et al. (1994). Lifetime and 12-month prevalence of DSM-IIIR psychiatric disorders in the United States. Results from the National Comorbidity Survey. *Archives of General Psychiatry* 41:8-19.

Khantzian EJ, Golden SJ & McAuliffe WE (1999). Group therapy. In M Galanter & HD Kleber (eds.) *Textbook of Substance Abuse Treatment.* Washington, DC: American Psychiatric Press, 367-378.

Khantzian EJ, Halliday KS & McAuliffe WE (1990). *Addiction and the Vulnerable Self: Modified Dynamic Group Therapy for Substance Abusers.* New York, NY: Guilford Press.

Malik R, Washton AM & Stone-Washton N (1995). Structured outpatient treatment. In AM Washton (ed.) *Psychotherapy and Substance Abuse: A Practitioner's Handbook.* New York, NY: Guilford Press, 285-294.

The Matrix Center (1989). *The Neurobehavioral Treatment Model Volume II: Group Sessions.* Beverly Hills, CA: Matrix Center.

McAuliffe WE & Albert J (1992). *Clean Start: An Outpatient Program for Initiating Cocaine Recovery.* New York, NY: Guilford Press.

McLellan AT, Lewis DC, O'Brien CP et al. (2000). Drug dependence, a chronic medical illness: Implications for treatment, insurance, and outcomes evaluation. *Journal of the American Medical Association* 284(13):1689-1695.

Minkoff K & Drake RE (1991). *Dual Diagnosis of Major Mental Illness and Substance Disorder.* San Francisco, CA: Jossey-Bass.

Monti PM, Abrams DB, Kadden RM et al. (1989). *Treating Alcohol Dependence.* New York, NY: Guilford Press.

Montrose K & Daley D (1995). *Celebrating Small Victories: A Primer of Approaches and Attitudes for Helping Clients with Dual Disorders.* Center City, MN: Hazelden.

Myrick H & Brady KT (1997). Social phobia in cocaine-dependent individuals. *American Journal on Addictions* 6(2):99-104.

Najavits LM & Weiss RD (1998). "Seeking safety" outcome of a new cognitive-behavioral psychotherapy for women with posttraumatic stress disorder and substance dependence. *Journal of Traumatic Stress* 11:437-456.

Najavits LM, Weiss RD & Liese BS (1995). Group cognitive-behavioral therapy for women with PTSD and substance use disorder. *Journal of Substance Abuse Treatment* 13(1):13-22.

Najavits LM, Weiss RD, Shaw SR et al. (1998). A clinical profile of women with posttraumatic stress disorder and substance dependence. *Psychology of Addictive Behaviors* 13(2):98-104.

National Institute on Alcohol Abuse and Alcoholism (NIAAA) (2000). Highlights from the 10th Special Report to Congress. *Alcohol Research & Health* 24(1).

National Institute on Drug Abuse (NIDA) (1994). *Addict Aftercare: Recovery Training and Self-Help, 2nd Edition.* Rockville, MD: NIDA.

National Institute on Drug Abuse (NIDA) (1997). Study sheds new light on the state of drug abuse treatment nationwide. *NIDA Notes* 12(5):1-8.

National Institute on Drug Abuse (NIDA) (1999). *Principles of Drug Addiction Treatment: A Research-Based Guide.* Rockville, MD: NIDA.

Obert JL, McCann MJ, Marinelli-Casey P et al. (2000). The matrix model of outpatient stimulant abuse treatment: History and description. *Journal of Psychoactive Drugs* 32(2):157-164.

O'Connell D, ed. (in press). *Managing the Dually Diagnosed Patient, 2nd Edition.* New York, NY: Haworth Press.

Peters RH & Hills HA (1999). Community treatment and supervision strategies for offenders with co-occurring disorders: What works? In E Latessa (ed.) *Strategic Solutions: The International Community Corrections Association Examines Substance Abuse.* Lanham, MD: American Correctional Association, 81-137.

Rawson RA, Shoptaw SJ, Obert JL et al. (1995). An intensive outpatient approach for cocaine abuse treatment. *Journal of Substance Abuse Treatment* 12(2):117-127.

Reilly PM & Shropshire MS (2000). Anger management group treatment for cocaine dependence: Preliminary outcomes. *American Journal of Drug and Alcohol Abuse* 26(2):161-177.

Robins LN & Regier DA (1991). *Psychiatric Disorders in America.* New York, NY: Free Press.

Roffman RA, Stephens RS & Simpson EE (1988). Relapse prevention with adult chronic marijuana smokers. In DC Daley (ed.) *Relapse: Conceptual, Research and Clinical Perspectives.* Binghamton, NY: Haworth Press, 241-257.

Schmitz JM, Oswald LM, Jacks SD et al. (1997). Relapse prevention treatment for cocaine dependence: Group vs. individual format. *Addictive Behaviors* 22(3):405-418.

Vannicelli M (1995). Group psychotherapy with substance abusers and family members. In AM Washton (ed.) *Psychotherapy and Substance Abuse: A Practitioner's Handbook.* New York, NY: Guilford Press, 337-356.

Washton AM (1997). Structured outpatient group treatment. In JH Lowinson, P Ruiz, RB Millman & JG Langrod (eds.) *Substance Abuse: A Comprehensive Textbook, 3rd Edition.* Baltimore, MD: Williams & Wilkins, 440-447.

Washton AM, ed. (1995). *Psychotherapy and Substance Abuse: A Practitioner's Handbook.* New York, NY: Guilford Press.

Washton AM (in press, a). Outpatient groups at different stages of substance abuse treatment: Preparation, initial abstinence, and relapse prevention. In DW Brook & HI Spitz (eds.) *The Group Psychotherapy of Substance Abuse.* Washington, DC: American Psychiatric Press.

Washton AM (in press, b). Group therapy: A clinician's guide to doing what works. In R Coombs (ed.) *Addiction Recovery Tools: A Clinician's Headbook.* Newbury Park, CA: Sage Publications.

Weiss RD, Griffin ML, Greenfield SF et al. (2000). Group therapy for patients with bipolar disorder and substance dependence: Results of a pilot study. *Journal of Clinical Psychiatry* 61(5):361-367.

Yalom ID (1985). *The Theory and Practice of Group Psychotherapy.* New York, NY: Basic Books.

Yalom ID, Bloch S, Bond G et al. (1978). Alcoholics in interactional group therapy: An outcome study. *Archives of General Psychiatry* 35:419-425.

Chapter 3 | Individual Psychotherapy

Bruce J. Rounsaville, M.D.
Kathleen M. Carroll, Ph.D.

When Is Psychotherapy Indicated?
Specialized Knowledge Necessary for Therapy With Addicts
Common Issues and Strategies
Efficacy Research
Empirically Validated Treatments

This chapter focuses on aspects of individual therapy that are unique to the one-to-one format of treatment delivery. The chapter presents guidelines on individual therapy that are applicable to those persons who are dependent on alcohol as well as other drugs. The chapter emphasizes a review of research findings relative to illicit drugs because the extensive literature on psychosocial treatments for alcoholics has been reviewed elsewhere (Miller & Heather, 1998; Institute of Medicine, 1990; Babor, 1994).

The history of individual psychotherapy for addictive disorders has been one of importation of methods first developed to treat other conditions. Thus, when psychoanalytic and psychodynamic therapies were the predominant modality for treating most mental disorders, published descriptions of the dynamics of substance abuse or of therapeutic strategies arose from using this established general modality to treat the special population of individuals with addictive disorders (Blatt, McDonald et al., 1984). Similarly, with the development of behavioral techniques, client-centered therapies, and cognitive behavioral treatments, earlier descriptions based on other types of patients were followed by discussions of the special modifications needed to treat addictive disorders.

Psychosocial treatment approaches that have originated with treating addictive disorders, such as Alcoholics Anonymous (AA) and therapeutic communities, have emphasized large and small group treatment settings. Although always present as a treatment option, individual psychotherapy has not been the predominant treatment modality for drug abusers since the 1960s, when inpatient Twelve Step-informed milieu therapy, group treatments, methadone maintenance, and therapeutic community approaches came to be the fixtures of addictive disorder treatment programs.

In fact, these newer modalities derived their popularity from the failures of dynamically informed ambulatory individual psychotherapy when it was used as the sole treatment for addictive disorders. There are several reasons why this approach was poorly suited to the needs of addicts when it was offered as the sole ambulatory treatment.

First, the lack of emphasis on symptom control and the lack of structure in the therapist's typical stance allowed the patient's continued drug or alcohol use to undermine the treatment. Therapists did not develop methods for addressing the patient's needs for coping skills because this removal of symptoms was seen as palliative and likely to result in symptom substitution. As a result, substance use often continued unabated while the treatment focused on underlying dynamics. The major strategy that is now common to all currently practiced psychotherapies for addictive disorders is to place primary emphasis on controlling or reducing drug use, while pursuing other goals only after such use has been at least partly controlled. This means that either (1) the individual therapist uses techniques designed to help the patient stop alcohol or drug use as a central part of the treatment, or (2) the therapy is practiced in the context of a comprehensive treatment program in which other aspects of the treatment curtail the patient's use of alcohol or other drugs (for example, pharmacotherapy or residential treatment).

A second major misfit between individual dynamic therapy and addictive disorders is the anxiety-arousing nature of such therapy, coupled with the lack of structure provided by the neutral therapist. Because addicts frequently react to increased anxiety or other dysphoric affects by resuming substance use, it is important to introduce anxiety-arousing aspects of treatment only after a strong therapeutic alliance has been developed or within the context of other supportive structures (for example, an inpatient unit, a strong social support network, or methadone maintenance). Such supports guard against relapse to substance use when the patient experiences heightened anxiety and dysphoria in the context of therapeutic exploration.

Individual psychotherapy has become a resurgent approach since the 1980s, as the limitations of other modalities have become apparent (for example, methadone maintenance without ancillary services) (Dole, Nyswander et al., 1976; Ball & Ross, 1991), and necessary modifications in technique have been made to address the factors underlying earlier failures. A major development in recent years is the growing list of individual psychotherapies for addictive disorders that have demonstrated efficacy in rigorously conducted randomized clinical trials (DeRubeis & Crits-Christoph, 1998; Leshner, 1999; McLellan & McKay, 1998).

Two key research developments have encouraged renewed interest in individual psychotherapies. The first development was the publication of results of Project MATCH, a landmark multisite clinical trial in which three months of treatment with one of three individual psychotherapies—motivational enhancement treatment (MET)

(Miller, Zweben et al., 1992), Twelve Step facilitation (TSF) (Nowinski, Baker et al., 1992), and cognitive-behavioral therapy (CBT) (Kadden, Carroll et al., 1992)—were followed by marked and sustained reductions in alcohol consumption (Project MATCH Research Group, 1997, 1998). To illustrate, in all three conditions, patients, on average, entered treatment drinking more than 80% of days, rapidly reduced their consumption to less than 15% of days, and kept those levels down at followup visits over three years.

The second development was the growing evidence for the efficacy of brief psychotherapies (Babor, 1994; Bien, Miller et al., 1993; MTP Research Group, 2001; Wilk, Jensen et al., 1997). This approach includes brief advice to nondependent, heavy substance users in medical settings (Babor, Grant et al., 1994; WHO Brief Intervention Study Group, 1996). There also was mounting evidence for the efficacy of four or fewer sessions of MET, one of the three treatments included in Project MATCH.

To encourage more widespread use of efficacious treatments, the National Institute on Drug Abuse (NIDA), the National Institute on Alcohol Abuse and Alcoholism, and the Center for Substance Abuse Treatment disseminated training manuals for many of these treatments, either through the Internet from their web sites (WWW.NIDA.NIH.GOV or WWW.NIAAA.NIH.GOV) or in a printed format that can be ordered through the National Clearinghouse on Alcohol and Drug Abuse Information (P.O. Box 2345, Rockville, MD 20847).

WHEN IS PSYCHOTHERAPY INDICATED?

Some form of behavioral therapy should be considered as a treatment option for all patients who seek help for a substance use disorder. Treatment seekers represent only about 20% of community members who meet the criteria for current substance use disorders (Norquist & Regier, 1996), and they are likely to represent the more severe end of the spectrum, as most of those who seek treatment do so only after numerous unsuccessful attempts to stop or reduce drug use on their own (Robins, 1979). The alternatives to psychotherapy are either pharmacologic or structural (as through sequestration from access to drugs and alcohol in a residential setting), and both treatments have limited effectiveness if not combined with psychotherapy or counseling. Removal from the substance-using setting is a useful and sometimes necessary part of treatment, but it seldom is sufficient in itself, as demonstrated by the high relapse rates typically seen from residential detoxification programs or incarceration during the year after the patient's return to his or her community (Hubbard, Rachal et al., 1984; O'Donnell, 1969; Simpson, Joe et al., 1982; Vaillant, 1966).

Psychotherapy and Pharmacotherapy. The most powerful and commonly used pharmacologic approaches to drug abuse are maintenance on an agonist that has an action similar to that of the abused drug (for example, methadone for opioid addicts or nicotine gum for cigarette smokers), use of an antagonist that blocks the effect of the abused drug (for example, naltrexone for opioid addicts), the use of an aversive agent that provides a powerful negative reinforcement if the drug is used (for example, disulfiram for alcoholics), or the use of agents that reduce the desire to use the substance (for example, naltrexone and acamprosate for alcoholics). Although all of these agents are widely used, they seldom are employed without adjunctive psychotherapy, because, for example, naltrexone maintenance alone for opioid dependence is plagued by high rates of premature dropout (Kleber & Kosten, 1984; Rounsaville, 1995), and disulfiram use without adjunctive psychotherapy has not been shown to be superior to placebo (Fuller, Branchey et al., 1986; Allen & Litten, 1992).

In particular, the large body of literature on the effectiveness of methadone maintenance points to the success of methadone maintenance in retaining opioid addicts in treatment and reducing their illicit opioid use and illegal activity (Ball & Ross, 1991). However, there is a great deal of variability in success rates across different methadone maintenance programs, which is at least partially due to wide variations in the provision and quality of psychosocial services (Ball & Ross, 1991; Corty & Ball, 1987).

The shortcomings of even powerful pharmaco-therapies delivered without psychotherapy were convincingly demonstrated by McLellan and colleagues at the Philadelphia Veterans Affairs Medical Center (McLellan, Arndt et al., 1993). In a 24-week trial, 92 opioid addicts were randomly assigned to receive either (1) methadone maintenance alone, without psychosocial services; (2) methadone maintenance with standard psychosocial services, which included regular individual meetings with a counselor; or (3) enhanced methadone maintenance, which included regular counseling plus access to on-site psychiatric, medical, employment, and family therapy. In terms of drug use and psychosocial outcomes, the best outcomes were seen in the enhanced methadone maintenance condition, with intermediate outcomes for the standard methadone services condition, and

poorest outcomes for the methadone alone condition. Although a few patients did reasonably well in the methadone alone condition, 69% had to be transferred out of that condition within three months of the study inception because their substance use did not improve or even worsened or because they experienced significant medical or psychiatric problems that required a more intensive level of care. The results of this study suggest that, although methadone maintenance alone can be sufficient for a small subgroup of patients, the majority will not benefit from a purely pharmacologic approach, and the best outcomes are associated with higher levels of psychosocial treatments. Even when the principal treatment is seen as pharmacologic, psychotherapeutic interventions are needed to complement the pharmacotherapy by (1) enhancing the motivation to stop substance use by taking the prescribed medications, (2) providing guidance for the use of prescribed medications and management of side effects, (3) maintaining motivation to continue taking the prescribed medications after the patient achieves an initial period of abstinence, (4) providing relationship elements to prevent premature termination, and (5) helping the patient develop the skills to adjust to a life without drug and alcohol use.

The elements that psychotherapy can offer to complement pharmacologic approaches are likely to be needed even if "perfect" pharmacotherapies become available. This is because the effectiveness of even the most powerful pharmacotherapies is limited by patients' willingness to comply with them, and the strategies found to enhance compliance with pharmacotherapies (monitoring, support, encouragement, education) are inherently psychosocial. Moreover, the provision of a clearly articulated and consistently delivered psychosocial treatment in the context of a primarily pharmacologic treatment is an important strategy for reducing noncompliance and attrition, thereby enhancing outcomes in clinical research and clinical treatment (Carroll, 1997).

Moreover, the importance of psychotherapy and psychosocial treatments is reinforced by recognition that the repertoire of pharmacotherapies available for treatment of drug addicts is limited to a handful, with the most effective agents limited in their utility to treatment of opioid dependence (Senay, 1989; Jaffe & Kleber, 1989; O'Brien & Woody, 1989; O'Brien, 1997) and alcohol dependence (Fuller, Branchey et al., 1986; Volpicelli, Alterman et al., 1992; O'Malley, Jaffe et al., 1992; Whitworth, Fischer et al., 1996; Sass, Soyka et al., 1996). Effective pharmacotherapies for dependence on cocaine, marijuana, hallucinogens, sedative-hypnotics, and stimulants have not yet been developed, and talking therapies remain the principal approaches for the treatment of these classes of drugs (Kosten & McCance-Katz, 1995; Meyer, 1992; Kleber, 1989; Kosten, 1989).

Although the foregoing has emphasized the need for psychotherapy to enhance the effectiveness of pharmacotherapy, this section would not be complete without considering the role of pharmacotherapy to enhance the efficacy of psychotherapy. These two treatments have different mechanisms of action and targeted effects that can counteract the weaknesses of either treatment alone. Psychotherapies effect change by psychological means in psychosocial aspects of drug abuse, such as motivation, coping skills, dysfunctional thoughts, or social relationships. Their weaknesses include limited effects on the physiologic aspects of drug use or withdrawal. Also, the effects of behavioral treatments tend to be delayed, requiring practice, repeated sessions, and a "working through" process.

In contrast, the strengths of pharmacologic treatments are their rapid actions in reducing immediate or protracted withdrawal symptoms, drug craving, and/or the rewarding effects of continued drug use. In effect, pharmacotherapies for drug dependence reduce the patients' immediate access to and preoccupation with drugs, freeing the patient to address other concerns such as long-term goals or interpersonal relationships.

Dropout from psychotherapy is reduced because drug urges and relapse are mitigated by the effects of the medication. Greater duration of abstinence can further enhance the effects of psychotherapy because substance-related effects on attention and mental acuity are prevented, maximizing new learning that therapy can induce. Because of the complementary actions of psychotherapies and pharmacotherapies, combined treatment has a number of potential advantages. As reviewed later, research evidence on combined treatment is sparse but generally supportive of this approach. Although factors such as cost and patient acceptance can limit use of combined approaches, it is important to note that no studies have shown that combined treatments are less than effective with either psychotherapy or pharmacotherapy alone.

Individual Versus Group Therapy. If psychotherapy is necessary for at least a substantial number of treatment-seeking drug addicts, when is individual therapy a better choice than other modalities such as family therapy or group

therapy? Because group therapy has become the modal format for psychotherapy of drug addicts, evaluation of the role of individual therapy should take the strengths and weaknesses of group therapy as its starting point.

A central advantage of group over individual psychotherapy is economy, which is a major consideration in an era of generally skyrocketing health care costs and increasingly curtailed third-party payments for the treatment of addictive disorders. Groups typically have a minimum of six members and a maximum of two therapists, yielding at least a threefold increase in the number of patients treated per therapist hour. Although the efficacy of group versus individual therapy has not been systematically studied with drug addicts, no evidence is available from other populations that individual psychotherapy yields superior benefits (Smith, Glass et al., 1980). Moreover, nearly all major schools of individual psychotherapy have been adapted to a group format.

In addition to the general concept that group therapy can be just as effective as but less expensive than individual therapy, there are aspects of group therapy that can be argued to make this modality more effective than individual treatment of drug addicts. For example, given the social stigma attached to having lost control of substance use, the presence of other group members who acknowledge having similar problems can provide comfort. Related to this aspect, other group members who are farther along in their recovery from addiction can act as models to illustrate that attempting to stop drug and alcohol use is not a futile effort. These more experienced group members can offer a wide variety of coping strategies that go beyond the repertoire known even by the most skilled individual therapist. Moreover, group members frequently can act as "buddies" who offer continued support outside of the group sessions in a way that most professional therapists do not.

Finally, the "public" nature of group therapy, with its attendant aspects of confession and forgiveness, coupled with the pressure to publicly confess future slips and transgressions, provides a powerful incentive to avoid relapse. The ability to publicly declare the number of days sober, coupled with the fear of having to publicly admit to "falling off the wagon," are strong forces that push an individual toward recovery. This public affirmation or shaming can be all the more crucial in combating a disorder that is characterized by a failure of internalized mechanisms of control. Addicted persons have been characterized as having poorly functioning internal self-control mechanisms (Khantzian,

1978, 1985; Khantzian & Schneider, 1986; Wurmser, 1979), and the group process—with many eyes watching—provides a robust source of external control.

Moreover, because the group is composed of recovering addicts, members may be better able to detect each other's attempts to conceal relapse or early warning signals for relapse than would an individual therapist who may not have personal experience with an addictive disorder.

Given these strengths of group therapy, what are the advantages of individual therapy that can justify its greater expense? First, a key advantage of individual therapy is that it provides privacy. Although self-help groups such as AA attempt to protect the confidentiality of group members by asking for first names only, and routine group therapy procedures involve instructions to members to keep identities of individuals and the contents of sessions confidential, participation in group therapy always risks a breach in confidentiality, especially in small communities. Although publicly admitting to one's need for help can be a key element of the recovery process, it is a step that is very difficult to take, particularly when the problems associated with substance use have not yet become severe. Public knowledge of drug and alcohol use still can ruin careers and reputations.

Second, the individualized pace of individual therapy allows the therapist more flexibility to address the patient's problems as they arise, whereas group therapy can be "out of sync" with some members while suiting the needs of the majority. This situation is particularly an issue for open groups that add new members throughout the life of the group, necessitating repetition of many therapeutic elements so as to acquaint new members with the group's history and to address the needs of individuals who have just begun treatment.

Third, from the patient's point of view, individual therapy allows a much higher percentage of therapy time to concentrate on issues that are uniquely relevant to that individual. Members of therapy groups usually have the experience of spending many hours discussing issues that are not problems for them, and the individual tailoring of therapy sessions to fit particular needs ultimately can be more efficient.

Fourth, logistical issues make individual therapy more practical in many settings. Given the decentralization of much mental health service delivery, individual therapy is most feasible for many mental health professionals or medical practitioners who do not have a caseload of addicts large enough to conduct group treatment. If group therapy is to be started with a new group, it can be many weeks before enough members are screened to be entered into a new group, resulting in patients' discouragement and high dropout rates while awaiting the onset of treatment. If group therapy involves addition to an ongoing group, this situation can present formidable obstacles to joining. Also, unless group therapy is offered in the context of a large clinic or practice with many ongoing groups, scheduling can be very difficult for those patients whose employer is not apprised of the need for treatment.

Fifth, the process and structure of individual therapy can confer unique advantages in dealing with some kinds of problems presented by patients. For example, individual therapy can be more conducive to the development of a deepening relationship between the patient and therapist over time, which can allow exploration of relationship elements not possible in group therapy. Alternatively, patients with particular personality disorders, such as borderline or schizoid patients, may be unable to get involved with other group members, as also is the case with patients who are so shy that they cannot bring themselves to attend group sessions.

SPECIALIZED KNOWLEDGE NECESSARY FOR THERAPY WITH ADDICTS

This section bases its recommendations on the supposition that most individual psychotherapists who attempt to work with addicts obtained their first psychotherapy experience and training with other groups of patients, such as those typically seen at inpatient or outpatient general psychiatric clinics. This supposition is based on the status of addiction treatment as a subspecialty placement within training programs for the major professions that practice psychotherapy, including psychologists, psychiatrists, and social workers. Thus, to treat addicts, the task for the typical psychotherapist is to acquire necessary new knowledge and modify already learned skills.

Pharmacology, Use Patterns, Consequences, and Course of Addiction. The principal areas of knowledge to be mastered by the beginning therapist are pharmacology, use patterns, consequences, and course of addiction for the major types of abused substances. For therapy to be effective, it is useful not only to obtain the textbook knowledge about frequently abused drugs but also to become familiar with street knowledge about drugs (for example, slang names, favored routes of administration, prices, and availability) and the clinical presentation of individuals when they are intoxicated or experiencing withdrawal from the various abused drugs. This knowledge has many important uses in the course of individual therapy.

First, it fosters a therapeutic alliance by allowing the therapist to convey an understanding of the addict's problems and the world in which the addict lives. This issue is especially important when the therapist is from a different racial or social background from the patient. In engaging the patient in treatment, it is important to emphasize that the patient's primary presenting complaint is likely to be substance abuse, even if many other issues also are amenable to psychotherapeutic interventions. Hence, if the therapist is not comfortable and familiar with the nuances of problematic drug and alcohol use, it can be difficult to forge an initial working alliance. Moreover, by knowing the natural history of addiction and the course of drug and alcohol effects, the clinician can be guided in helping the patient anticipate problems that will arise in the course of initiating abstinence. For example, knowing the typical type and duration of withdrawal symptoms can help the addict recognize their transient nature and develop a plan for successfully completing an ambulatory detoxification.

Second, knowledge of drug actions and withdrawal states is crucial for diagnosing comorbid psycho-pathology and for helping the patient to understand and manage dysphoric affects. It has been observed in clinical situations and demonstrated in laboratory conditions (Mendelson & Mello, 1966; Mirin, Meyer et al., 1980; Nathan & O'Brien, 1971; Gawin & Ellinwood, 1988) that most abused drugs, such as opioids or cocaine, are capable of producing constellations of symptoms that mimic psychiatric syndromes, such as depression, mania, anxiety disorders, or paranoia. Many of these symptomatic states are completely substance-induced and resolve spontaneously when such use is stopped. It often is the therapist's job to determine whether or not presenting symptoms are part of an enduring, underlying psychiatric condition or a transient, drug-induced state. If the former, simultaneous treatment of the psychiatric disorder is appropriate; if the latter, reassurance and encouragement to maintain abstinence usually are the better course.

This need to distinguish transient substance-induced affects from enduring attitudes and traits also is an important psychotherapy task. Affective states have been shown to be linked closely with cognitive distortions, as Beck and colleagues (Beck, 1967; Beck, Rush et al., 1979) have dem-

onstrated in their delineation of the cognitive distortions associated with depression. While experiencing depressive symptoms, a patient is likely to have a profoundly different view of himself or herself, the future, the satisfactions available in life, and his or her important interpersonal relationships. These views are likely to change radically with remission of depressive symptoms, even if the remission of symptoms is induced by pharmacotherapy and not by psychotherapy or actual improvement in life circumstances (Simons, Garfield et al., 1984). Because of this tendency for substance-related affective states to greatly color the patient's view of self and world, it is important for the therapist to be able to recognize these states so that the associated distorted thoughts can be recognized as such rather than being taken at face value. Moreover, it is important that the patient also be taught to distinguish between sober and substance-affected conditions and to recognize when, in the colloquial phrase, it is "the alcohol talking" and not the person's more enduring sentiments.

Third, learning about drug and alcohol effects is important in detecting when patients have relapsed or come to sessions intoxicated. It is seldom useful to conduct psychotherapy sessions when the patient is intoxicated and, when this happens, the session should be rescheduled for a time when the patient can participate while sober. For alcoholics, noticing the smell of alcohol or using a Breathalyzer® is a useful technique for detecting intoxication. A number of inexpensive and rapid urine tests are commercially available that can be used in the office to detect recent drug use. Samples also can be sent to commercial laboratories for verification. The clinician then must rely on his or her own clinical skills to determine whether or not the patient is drug free and able to participate fully in the psychotherapy.

Other Treatment and Self-Help Group Philosophies and Techniques. A second area of knowledge to be mastered by the psychotherapist is an overview of treatment philosophies and techniques for the range of treatments and self-help groups that are available to substance-using patients. As noted above, the early experience of attempting individual psychotherapy as the sole treatment of the more severe types of drug addiction was marked by failure and early dropout. Hence, for many addicts, individual psychotherapy is best conceived as a component of a multifaceted program of treatment to help the patient overcome a chronic, relapsing condition. In fact, one function of individual psychotherapy can be to help the patient choose which additional therapies to employ in his or her attempt to stop using alcohol or other drugs. Thus, even when the therapist is a solo practitioner, he or she should know when detoxification is necessary, when inpatient treatment is appropriate, and what pharmacotherapies are available.

Another major function of knowing about the major alternative treatment modalities for addicts is to be alert to the possibility that different treatments can provide contradictory recommendations that may confuse the patient or foster the patient's attempts to sabotage treatment. Unlike a practitioner whose treatment is likely to be sufficient in itself, the individual psychotherapist does not have the option of simply instructing the patient to curtail other treatments or participation in self-help groups while individual treatment is taking place. Rather, it is vital that the therapist attempt to adjust his or her own work to bring the psychotherapy into accord with other treatments.

A commonly occurring set of conflicts arises between the treatment goals and methods employed by professional therapists and those of Twelve Step self-help movements such as AA, Cocaine Anonymous (CA), and Narcotics Anonymous (NA). For example, the recovery goal for many who use a Twelve Step approach is a life of complete abstinence from psychotropic medications. This approach may conflict with professional advice when the therapist recommends use of psychopharmacologic treatments for co-occurring psychiatric disorders such as depression, mania, or anxiety. Although the Twelve Step literature supports use of appropriately prescribed medications of all kinds, many individual members draw the line at prescribed psychotropic medications. In the face of disapproval from fellow members, patients may prematurely discontinue psychotropic medications and experience relapse of psychological symptoms, with consequent return to substance use.

To avoid this situation, it is important for the therapist who recommends or prescribes psychotropic medications to warn the patient about the apparent contradiction between the Twelve Step admonition to lead a drug-free life and the clinician's use of prescribed psychotropic medications. One way to approach this issue is to describe the psychiatric condition for which the medications are prescribed as a disease separate from the addictive disorder and to impress on the patient that medications are as necessary for the treatment of this separate condition as insulin would be for diabetes. The fact that the medications are intended to affect brain functioning and attendant mental symptoms, while insulin affects other parts of the body, is less important than the concept that two diseases are present and not one.

A second common area of conflict between some forms of psychotherapy and the Twelve Step philosophy is the role played by family members. The Al-Anon approach tends to suggest that family members get out of the business of attempting to control the addict's use of drugs and alcohol. Separate meetings are held for family members and addicts. In contrast, many therapists encourage involvement of family members in dealing with family dynamics that can foster substance use and/or in acting as adjunctive therapists (Anton, Hogan et al., 1981; Stanton & Todd, 1982). As with the use of psychotropic medications, the major way to prevent a patient's confusion is to anticipate the areas of contradictory advice and to provide a convincing rationale for the therapist's recommendations. In doing so, it is advisable to acknowledge that different strategies appear to work for different individuals and that alternative approaches may be employed sequentially if the initial plan fails.

COMMON ISSUES AND STRATEGIES

This section reviews issues that must be addressed, if not emphasized, in order for individual psychotherapy to be effective. As noted in reviewing the difficulties encountered by early psychodynamic practitioners, the central modification that is required of psychotherapists is to be aware that the patient being treated is an addict. Hence, even when attempting to explore other issues in depth, the therapist should (1) devote at least a small part of every session to monitoring the patient's most recent successes and failures in controlling or curtailing substance use and (2) be willing to interrupt other work to address slips and relapses as they occur.

Implicit in the need to remain focused on the patient's substance use is the recognition that psychotherapy with these patients entails a more active therapist stance than does treatment of patients with other psychiatric disorders, such as depression or anxiety. This need is related to the fact that the principal symptom of substance abuse—compulsive use—is at least initially gratifying, whereas it is the long-term consequences of substance use that induce pain and the desire to stop. In contrast, the principal symptoms of depression or anxiety disorders are inherently painful and alien. Because of this key difference, psychotherapy with addicts typically requires both empathy and structured limit-setting, whereas the need for limit-setting is less marked in psychotherapy with depressed or anxious patients.

Beyond these key elements, this section also elaborates on the following set of psychotherapy tasks: enhancing motivation to stop drug use, teaching coping skills, changing reinforcement contingencies, fostering management of painful affects, improving interpersonal functioning, and enhancing social supports. Although different schools of thought about therapeutic action and behavior change can vary in the degree to which emphasis is placed on the various tasks, some attention to each area is likely to be part of any successful treatment.

Enhancing Motivation. Cummings (1979) has noted that addicted persons most often enter treatment not with the goal to stop, but rather to return to the days when drug and alcohol use was enjoyable. The natural history of substance abuse (Robins, 1979) typically is characterized by an initial period of episodic use lasting months to years in which substance-related consequences are minimal and use is perceived as beneficial. Even at the time of treatment-seeking, which usually occurs only after substance-related problems have become severe, patients usually can identify many ways in which they want or feel the need for drugs or alcohol and have difficulty developing a clear picture of what life without these substances might be like. To be able to achieve and maintain abstinence or controlled use, such patients need a clear conception of their treatment goals. Several investigators (DiClemente, Prochaska et al., 1985; Prochaska & DiClemente, 1986) have postulated stages in the development of addicts' thinking about stopping use, beginning with precontemplation, moving through contemplation, and culminating with determination as the ideal cognitive set with which to derive the greatest benefit from treatment.

Regardless of the treatment type, an early task for psychotherapists is to gauge the patient's level of motivation to stop his or her substance use by exploring the patient's treatment goals. In this task, it is important to challenge overly quick or glib assertions that the patient's goal is to stop using substance altogether. One way to approach the patient's likely ambivalence is to attempt an exploration of the patient's perceived benefits from use of alcohol or drugs, or his or her perceived need for them. To obtain a clear report of the patient's positive attitudes toward substance use, it may be necessary to elicit details of the patient's early involvement with drugs and alcohol. After the therapist has obtained a clear picture of the patient's perceived needs and desires, it is important to counter these perceptions by exploring the advantages of a drug-free life.

As noted earlier, although virtually all types of psychotherapy for addiction address the issue of motivation and goal-setting to some extent, motivational therapy or interviewing (Miller & Rollnick, 1991; Miller, Zweben et al., 1992) makes this the sole initial focus of treatment. Motivational approaches, which usually are quite brief (for example, two to four sessions) are based on principles of motivational psychology and are designed to produce rapid, internally motivated change by seeking to maximize patients' motivational resources and commitment to abstinence. Active ingredients of these approaches are hypothesized to include objective feedback of personal risk or impairment, emphasis on personal responsibility for change, clear advice to change, a menu of alternative change options, therapist empathy, and facilitation of patient self-efficacy (Miller, Zweben et al., 1992). Motivational approaches have substantial empirical evidence supporting their effectiveness with alcoholics (Babor, 1994; Holder, Longabaugh et al., 1991), but have not yet been widely applied or evaluated for drug-abusing populations.

One major controversy in this area is whether controlled use can be an acceptable alternative treatment goal to abstinence from all psychoactive drugs (Douglas, 1986; Cook, 1988). Many, if not most, patients enter treatment with a goal of controlled use, especially of alcohol (Sanchez-Craig & Wilkinson, 1986/1987), and failure to address the patient's presenting goal may result in failure to engage the patient. At the heart of the issue is whether or not drug abuse is seen as a categorical disease, for which the only treatment is abstinence, or as a set of habitual dysfunctional behaviors that are aligned along a continuum of severity (Edwards & Gross, 1976). For illicit drugs of abuse (such as cocaine or heroin), it is unwise for a professional therapist to take a position that advocates any continued use, because such a stance allies the therapist with illegal and antisocial behavior. Even advocates of controlled use as an acceptable treatment goal usually acknowledge that patients with more severe dependence should seek an abstinence goal. In practice, the therapist cannot force the patient to seek any goal that the patient does not choose. The process of arriving at an appropriate treatment goal frequently involves allowing the patient to make several failed attempts to achieve a goal of controlled use. This initial process may be necessary to convince the patient that a goal of abstinence is more appropriate.

Teaching Coping Skills. The most enduring challenge in treating addicts is to help the patient avoid relapse after achieving an initial period of abstinence (Marlatt & Gordon, 1985). A general tactic for avoiding relapse is to identify specific circumstances that increase an individual's likelihood of resuming substance use and to help the patient anticipate and practice strategies (for example, refusal skills, recognizing and avoiding cues for craving) for coping with these high-risk situations. Approaches that emphasize the development of coping skills include CBT (Martlatt & Gordon, 1985; Kadden, Carroll et al., 1992), in which a systematic effort is made to identify high-risk situations and master alternative behaviors, as well as coping skills intended to help the patient avoid drug use when these situations arise. A postulate of this approach is that proficiency in coping skills that are generalizable to a variety of problem areas will help foster durable change. Evidence is emerging that points to the durability and, in some cases, the delayed emergence of effects of coping skills treatments (Carroll, Rounsaville et al., 1994a; O'Malley, Jaffe et al., 1996). For other approaches, enumeration of risky situations and development of coping skills are less structured (Luborsky, 1984; Rounsaville, Gawin et al., 1985) and embedded in a more general exploration of patients' wishes and fears.

Changing Reinforcement Contingencies. Edwards and colleagues (Edwards & Gross, 1976; Edwards, 1986; Edwards, Arif et al., 1981) have noted that a key element of deepening dependence on alcohol or other drugs is the rise of substance-related behavior to the top of an individual's list of priorities. As dependence deepens, it can take precedence over concerns about work, family, friends, possessions, and health. As compulsive use becomes a part of every day, previously valued relationships or activities may be given up, so that the rewards available in daily life are narrowed progressively to those derived from use of the substance. When such use is ended, its absence may leave the patient with a need to fill the time that had been spent using drugs or alcohol and to find rewards to substitute for those derived from their use.

The ease with which the patient can rearrange priorities is related to the level of achievement before he or she became involved with alcohol or drugs and the degree to which substance use destroyed or replaced valued relationships, jobs, or hobbies. Because the typical course of illicit drug use entails initiation of compulsive use between the ages of 12 and 25 years (Kandel & Faust, 1975), many patients come to treatment without having achieved satisfactory adult relationships or vocational skills. In such cases, achieving a drug- and alcohol-free life may require a lengthy process of vocational rehabilitation and development of meaningful relationships.

Individual psychotherapy can contribute importantly to this process by helping maintain the patient's motivation throughout the recovery process and by helping the patient to explore factors that have interfered with achievement of rewarding ties to others.

An example of an approach that actively changes reinforcement contingencies is the one developed by Higgins and colleagues (Budney & Higgins, 1998; Higgins, Delaney et al., 1991; Higgins, Budney et al., 1993, 1994a), which incorporates positive incentives for abstinence into a community reinforcement approach (Sisson & Azrin, 1989).

Fostering Management of Painful Affects. Marlatt and Gordon (1980) demonstrated that dysphoric affects are the most commonly cited precipitant for relapse, and many psychodynamic clinicians (Khantzian, 1985; Wurmser, 1979) have suggested that failure of affect regulation is a central dynamic underlying the development of compulsive alcohol or drug use. Moreover, surveys of psychiatric disorders in treatment-seeking populations concur in demonstrating high rates of depressive disorders (Hesselbrock, Meyer et al., 1985; Khantzian & Treece, 1985; Rounsaville, Weissman et al., 1982).

A key element in developing ways to handle powerful dysphoric affects is learning to recognize and identify the probable cause of such feelings. The difficulty in differentiating among negative emotional states has been identified as a common characteristic among addicts (Khantzian, 1985; Wurmser, 1979). To foster the development of mastery over dysphoric affects, most psychotherapies include techniques for eliciting strong affects within a protected therapeutic setting and then enhancing the patient's ability to identify, tolerate, and respond appropriately to them. Given the demonstrated efficacy of pharmacologic treatments for affective and anxiety disorders (Beckman & Leber, 1985) and the high rates of these disorders seen in treatment-seeking populations, the individual psychotherapist should be alert to the possibility that a patient may benefit from combined treatment with psychotherapy and medications.

Moreover, as evidence points to the difficulty many patients face in articulating strong affect (Keller, Carroll et al., 1995), which can have an effect of treatment response

(Taylor, Parker et al., 1990), clinicians should be alert to the need to assess and address difficulties in expression of affect and cognition when working with addicts in psychotherapy.

Improving Interpersonal Functioning and Enhancing Social Supports. A consistent finding in the literature on relapse is the protective influence of an adequate network of social supports (Marlatt & Gordon, 1985; Tims & Leukefeld, 1986). Gratifying friendships and intimate relationships provide a powerful source of rewards to replace those obtained from drug and alcohol use, and the threat of losing those relationships can furnish a strong incentive to maintain abstinence. Typical issues presented by addicts are the loss of or damage to valued relationships that occurred when alcohol or drug use became the individual's principal priority, failure to have achieved satisfactory relationships even before having initiated substance use, and inability to identify friends or intimates who are not, themselves, engaged in substance abuse. For some types of psychotherapy (such as interpersonal therapy and supportive-expressive treatment), working on relationship issues is the central focus of the work, while for others this aspect is implied in other therapeutic activities such as identifying risky and protective situations (Marlatt & Gordon, 1985).

A major potential limitation of individual psychotherapy as the sole treatment for alcohol or drug dependence is its failure to provide adequate social supports to patients who lack a supportive social network of friends who are not engaged in substance abuse. Individual psychotherapy can fill only one to several hours per week of a patient's time.

Again, although most approaches address these issues to some degree in the course of treatment, approaches that emphasize the development of a strong relationship with persons who are not substance users are traditional counseling, TSF (Nowinski, Baker et al., 1992), and other approaches that underline the importance of involvement in self-help groups. Self-help groups offer a fully developed social network of welcoming individuals who are understanding and committed to leading a substance-free life. Moreover, in most urban and suburban settings, self-help meetings are held daily or several times a week, and a sponsor system is available to provide the recovering person with individual guidance and support on a 24-hour basis, if needed. For psychotherapists who are working with addicts, encouraging patients to become involved in self-help groups can provide a powerful source of social support that protects the patient from relapse while the work of therapy progresses.

EFFICACY RESEARCH

As noted above, early efforts to engage and treat drug users with dynamically oriented individual psycho-therapy as the sole treatment were marked by failure. These failures led researchers to focus increasingly on the evaluation of psychotherapy as a treatment for addiction in terms of the context in which individual psychotherapy is delivered most effectively as well as the types of patients most likely to benefit from individual psychotherapy. Hence, the following section reviews empiric evidence for the effectiveness of individual psychotherapy by substance of abuse and treatment setting. The section reviews findings from the growing number of studies that have used rigorous methodologies associated with the Technology Model of psychotherapy research (Waskow, 1984; Carroll & Rounsaville, 1991). Akin to specification of the formulation and dosage of medications in pharmacotherapy trials, this approach has generated methods for specifying the techniques to be evaluated, for training therapists to use these techniques consistently, and for monitoring the dose and delivery of these techniques over the course of clinical trials. These methodologic features include random assignment to treatment conditions, specification of treatments in manuals, selection of well-trained therapists committed to the type of approach they conduct in the trial, extensive training of therapists, ongoing monitoring of therapy implementation, multidimensional ratings of outcome by independent evaluators blind to the study treatment received by the patient, and adequate sample sizes.

In this review, the authors have focused on studies of opiate and cocaine addicts because the more extensive literature on psychosocial treatments of alcohol has received detailed review elsewhere (Miller & Heather, 1986; Institute of Medicine, 1990; Babor, 1994).

Individual Psychotherapy for Opioid Dependence. *Opioid Maintenance Therapy:* Only a few studies have evaluated the efficacy of formal psychotherapy to enhance outcomes with opioid maintenance therapies. The landmark study in this area was done by Woody and colleagues (1983) and recently was replicated in community settings (Woody, McLellan et al., 1995). Although the original study is now more than 15 years old, it is reviewed here because it remains an impressive demonstration of the benefits and role of psychotherapy in the context of methadone maintenance. In the study, a total of 110 opiate addicts entering a methadone maintenance program were randomly assigned to one of three treatments: drug counseling alone; drug counseling plus supportive-expressive psychotherapy (SE), which is a short-term dynamic approach; or drug counseling plus cognitive psychotherapy, a structured cognitive approach. After a six-month course of treatment, although the SE and cognitive psychotherapy groups did not differ significantly from each other on most measures of outcome, subjects who received either form of professional psychotherapy evidenced greater improvement in more outcome domains than the subjects who received drug counseling alone (Woody, Luborsky et al., 1983). Moreover, gains made by the subjects who received professional psychotherapy were sustained over a 12-month followup period, whereas subjects who received drug counseling alone evidenced some attrition of gains (Woody, McLellan et al., 1987).

The study also demonstrated differential responses to psychotherapy as a function of patient characteristics, which can point to the best use of psychotherapy (relative to drug counseling) when resources are scarce. Although methadone-maintained opiate addicts with lower levels of psychopathology tended to improve regardless of whether they received professional psychotherapy or drug counseling, those with higher levels of psychopathology tended to improve only if they received psychotherapy.

Contingency Management: Several studies have evaluated the use of contingency management to reduce the use of illicit drugs in addicts who are maintained on methadone. In these studies, a reinforcer (reward) is provided to patients who demonstrate specified target behaviors such as providing drug-free urine specimens, accomplishing specific treatment goals, or attending treatment sessions. For example, offering methadone take-home privileges contingent on reduced drug use is an approach that capitalizes on an inexpensive reinforcer that is potentially available in all methadone maintenance programs. Stitzer and colleagues (Stitzer & Bigelow, 1978; Stitzer, Bickel et al., 1986) did extensive work in evaluating methadone take-home privileges as a reward for decreased illicit drug use. In a series of well-controlled trials, these researchers demonstrated (1) the relative benefits of positive (for example, rewarding desired behaviors such as abstinence) compared with negative (for example, punishing undesired behaviors such as continued drug use through discharges or dose reductions) contingencies (Stitzer, Bickel et al., 1986), (2) the attrac-

tiveness of take-home privileges over other incentives available within methadone maintenance clinics (Stitzer & Bigelow, 1978), and (3) the relative effectiveness of rewarding drug-free urine specimens compared with other target behaviors (Iguchi, Lamb et al., 1996).

Silverman and colleagues (1996), drawing on the compelling work of Higgins and colleagues (described later), evaluated a voucher-based contingency management system to address concurrent illicit drug use (typically cocaine) among methadone-maintained opioid addicts. In this approach, urine specimens are required three times a week to systematically detect all episodes of drug use. Abstinence, verified through drug-free urine screens, is reinforced through a voucher system in which patients receive points redeemable for items consistent with a drug-free lifestyle that are intended to help the patient develop alternate reinforcers to drug use (for example, movie tickets and sporting goods).

In a very elegant series of studies, Silverman and colleagues (1996a, 1996b, 1998) have demonstrated the efficacy of this approach in reducing illicit opioid and cocaine use and producing a number of treatment benefits in this very difficult population.

Behavioral Therapies: Opioid antagonist treatment (naltrexone) offers many advantages over methadone maintenance, including the fact that it is nonaddicting and can be prescribed without concerns about diversion, has a benign side effect profile, and can be less costly in terms of demands on professional time and of patient time than the daily or near-daily clinic visits required for methadone maintenance (Rounsaville, 1995). Most important are the behavioral aspects of treatment, as unreinforced opiate use allows extinction of relationships between cues and drug use. Although naltrexone treatment is likely to be attractive only to a minority of opioid addicts (Greenstein, Arndt et al., 1984), naltrexone's unique properties make it an important alternative to methadone maintenance.

However, naltrexone has not, despite its many advantages, fulfilled its promise. Naltrexone treatment programs remain comparatively rare and underutilized as compared to methadone maintenance programs (Rounsaville, 1995). This situation is largely due to problems with retention, particularly during the induction phase, when an average of 40% of patients drop out during the first month of treatment and 60% drop out by three months (Greenstein, Fudala et al., 1992). In the 1970s, several preliminary evaluations of behavioral interventions used to address naltrexone's weaknesses, including providing incentives for compliance with naltrexone (Grabowski, O'Brien et al., 1979; Meyer, Mirin et al., 1976) and the addition of family therapy to naltrexone treatment (Anton, Hogan et al., 1981), suggested the promise of these strategies. However, the interventions were not widely adopted, compliance remained a major problem, and naltrexone treatment and research dropped off considerably until the past few years, when the need for alternatives to methadone maintenance stimulated a modest revival of interest in naltrexone.

Some of the most recent promising data about strategies to enhance retention and outcome in naltrexone treatment have come from investigations of contingency management approaches. Preston and colleagues (1999) found improved retention and naltrexone compliance with an approach that provided vouchers for naltrexone compliance, as compared with standard naltrexone treatment that did not provide vouchers. Carroll (2001) found that reinforcement of naltrexone compliance and drug-free urine specimens, alone or in combination with family involvement in treatment, improved retention and reduced drug use among recently detoxified opioid-dependent individuals.

Individual Psychotherapy for Cocaine Dependence. Compared with the results of trials evaluating pharmacologic treatment of cocaine dependence, evaluations of behavioral therapies—particularly contingency management, CBT, and manualized disease-model approaches—have been much more promising (DeRubeis & Crits-Christoph, 1998; Van Horn & Frank, 1998). Because of the lack of an effective pharmacologic platform for cocaine dependence (analogous to methadone maintenance for the treatment of opioid dependence), behavioral therapies for cocaine-dependent individuals have had to focus on key outcomes such as retention and the inception and maintenance of abstinence, rather than placing initial emphasis on secondary psychosocial problems (for example, family, psychological, legal problems). Major findings from randomized controlled trials evaluating each of these treatments for adult cocaine dependent groups are summarized here.

Contingency Management; Perhaps the most exciting findings pertaining to the effectiveness of behavioral treatments for cocaine dependence have been the reports by Higgins and colleagues (1991, 1993, 1994) on the use of behavioral incentives for abstinence, as described earlier. The strategy of Higgins has four organizing features that are grounded in principles of behavioral pharmacology: (1) drug use and abstinence must be swiftly and accurately detected, (2) abstinence is posi-

tively reinforced, (3) drug use results in loss of reinforcement, and (4) emphasis is placed on the development of reinforcers to compete with drug use (Budney & Higgins, 1998). In this approach, urine specimens are required three times weekly to systematically detect all episodes of drug use. Abstinence, verified through drug-free urine screens, is reinforced through a voucher system in which patients receive points redeemable for items consistent with a drug-free lifestyle (such as movie tickets and sporting goods).

In a series of well-controlled clinical trials, Higgins has demonstrated high acceptance, retention, and rates of abstinence for patients receiving this approach, as compared with standard counseling oriented toward Twelve Step programs (Higgins, Delaney et al., 1991; Higgins, Budney et al., 1993). Rates of abstinence do not decline substantially when less valuable incentives are substituted for the voucher system (Higgins, Budney et al., 1993). The value of the voucher system itself, as opposed to other program elements, in producing good outcomes was demonstrated by comparing the behavioral system with and without the vouchers (Higgins, Budney et al., 1994a). Although the strong effects of this treatment declined somewhat after the contingencies were terminated, the voucher system has been shown to have durable effects (Higgins, Wong et al., 2000). Moreover, the efficacy of a variety of contingency management procedures (including vouchers, direct payments, and free housing) has been replicated in other settings and samples, including cocaine-dependent individuals within methadone maintenance (Silverman, Wong et al., 1998), homeless addicts (Milby, Schumacher et al., 1996), and freebase cocaine users (Kirby, Marlowe et al., 1998).

These findings are of great importance because contingency management procedures are potentially applicable to a wide range of target behaviors and problems, including treatment retention and compliance with pharmacotherapy (such as retroviral therapies for individuals with HIV). For example, Iguchi, Lamb et al. (1996) showed that contingency management can be used effectively to reinforce desired treatment goals (for example, looking for a job) in addition to abstinence.

Nevertheless, despite the very compelling evidence of the effectiveness of these procedures in promoting retention in treatment and reducing cocaine use, the procedures rarely are used in clinical treatment programs. One major impediment to broader use is the expense associated with the voucher program; average earnings for patients are about $600 (Higgins, Budney et al., 1994a; Silverman, Higgins et al., 1996; Silverman, Wong et al., 1996). Recently developed low-cost contingency management (CM) procedures may be a way to bring these effective approaches into general clinical use. In a recently completed study, Petry and colleagues (2000) demonstrated that a variable ratio schedule of reinforcement that provides access to large reinforcers (but at low probabilities) is effective in retaining subjects in treatment and reducing substance use. Rather than earning vouchers, subjects earn the chance to draw from a bowl and win prizes of varying magnitudes. The prizes range from small $1 prizes (bus tokens, McDonald's coupons) to large $20 prizes (portable radios, watches, and phone cards), to jumbo $100 prizes (for example, small televisions).

This system is far less expensive than the standard voucher system, because only a proportion of behaviors are reinforced with a prize. In a study of 42 alcohol-dependent veterans who were randomly assigned to standard treatment or standard treatment plus CM, 84% of the CM subjects were retained in treatment throughout an 8-week period, compared with 22% of standard treatment subjects. By the end of the treatment period, 69% of those receiving CM had not experienced a relapse to alcohol use, but only 39% of those receiving standard treatment were abstinent (Petry, Martin et al., 2000). A controlled evaluation of this promising approach for the treatment of cocaine dependence is ongoing.

Cognitive-Behavioral Therapies; Another behavioral approach that was shown to be effective in treating cocaine abusers is CBT. This approach is based on social learning theories on the acquisition and maintenance of substance use disorders (Carroll, 1999b). Its goal is to foster abstinence by helping the patient master an individualized set of coping strategies as an effective alternative to substance use. Typical skills include fostering the patient's resolve to stop using cocaine and other substances by exploring positive and negative consequences of continued use, functional analysis of substance use (that is, understanding substance use in relationship to its antecedents and consequences), development of strategies for coping with cocaine craving, identification of seemingly irrelevant decisions that could culminate in high-risk situations, preparation for emergencies and coping with a relapse to substance use, and identifying and confronting thoughts about substance use.

A number of randomized clinical trials among several diverse cocaine-dependent populations have demonstrated that (1) compared with other commonly used psychotherapies for cocaine dependence, CBT appears to be particularly more effective with more severe cocaine users or those with comorbid disorders (Carroll, Rounsaville et al., 1991, 1994a; McKay, Alterman et al., 1997; Maude-Griffin, Hohenstein et al., 1998); (2) CBT is significantly more effective than less intensive approaches that have been evaluated as control conditions (Carroll, Nich et al., 1998; Monti, Rohsenow et al., 1997); and (3) CBT is as or more effective than manualized disease-model approaches (Carroll, Nich et al., 1998; Maude-Griffin, Hohenstein et al., 1998). Moreover, CBT appears to be a particularly durable approach, with patients continuing to reduce their cocaine use even after they leave treatment (Carroll, Rounsaville et al., 1994b; Carroll, Nich et al., 2000).

Manualized Disease-Model Approaches: Until very recently, treatment approaches based on disease models were widely practiced in the U.S., but virtually no well-controlled randomized clinical trials had evaluated their efficacy alone or in comparison with other treatments. Thus, another important finding emerging from randomized clinical trials that has great significance for the treatment community is the effectiveness of manualized disease-model approaches. One such approach is TSF (Nowinski, Baker et al., 1992), a manual-guided, individual approach that is intended to be similar to widely used approaches that emphasize principles associated with disease models of addiction and that has been adapted for use with cocaine-dependent individuals. Although this treatment has no official relationship with AA or CA, its content is intended to be consistent with the Twelve Steps of AA, with primary emphasis given to Steps 1 through 5 and the concepts of acceptance (for example, to help the patient accept that he or she has the illness, or disease, of addiction) and surrender (for example, to help the patient acknowledge that there is hope for sobriety through accepting the need for help from others and a "Higher Power"). In addition to abstinence from all psychoactive substances, a major goal of the treatment is to foster active participation in self-help groups. Patients are actively encouraged to attend AA or CA meetings, become involved in traditional fellowship activities, and maintain journals of their self-help group attendance and participation.

In a comparison of TSF, CBT, and clinical management (a supportive approach in which patients received comparable empathy, support, and other "common elements" of psychotherapy but none of the unique "active ingredients" of TSF or CBT) for alcoholic cocaine-dependent individuals, TSF was found to be significantly more effective than clinical management and was comparable to CBT in reducing cocaine use (Carroll, Nich et al., 1998). In addition, a one-year followup suggested that gains from treatment were maintained for subjects who received TSF or CBT, who reported continuing to reduce their cocaine use throughout the followup period, compared with subjects who received clinical management. Moreover, there was a strong relationship between the attainment of significant periods of abstinence during treatment and abstinence during followup, which emphasizes that the inception of abstinence, even for comparatively brief periods, is an important goal of treatment (Carroll, Nich et al., 2000; Higgins, Wong et al., 2000).

More recently, the NIDA Collaborative Cocaine Treatment Study, a multisite randomized trial of psychotherapeutic treatments for cocaine dependence (Crits-Christoph, Siqueland et al., 1999), also offered strong evidence of the effectiveness of a similar approach: individual drug counseling. In that study, 487 cocaine-dependent subjects in four sites were randomly assigned to one of four manual-guided treatment conditions: (1) cognitive therapy (Beck, Wright et al., 1993) plus group drug counseling; (2) SE therapy, a short-term psychodynamically oriented approach, plus group drug counseling; (3) individual drug counseling plus group drug counseling; or (4) group drug counseling alone. The treatments offered were intensive (36 individual and 24 group sessions over 24 weeks, for a total of 60 sessions) and were met with comparatively poor retention. On average, patients completed less than half the sessions offered, with higher rates of retention for subjects assigned to cognitive therapy or SE therapy. On the whole, outcomes were good, with all groups significantly reducing their cocaine use from baseline; however, the best cocaine outcomes were seen for subjects who received individual drug counseling (a related point is that this study suggests that psychodynamic and cognitive approaches, which rarely have been studied with this population, may not be optimal initial approaches for general populations of cocaine users) (Carroll, 1999a).

Considered together with the findings of Project MATCH (Project MATCH Research Group, 1997), TSF was found to be comparable to CBT and MET (Miller, Zweben et al., 1992) in reducing alcohol use among 1,726 alcohol-dependent individuals. The findings from these studies offer compelling support for the efficacy of manual-guided disease-model approaches. This finding has important clinical implications because these approaches are similar to the dominant model applied in most community treatment programs (Horgan & Levine, 1998) and thus can be more easily mastered by "real-world" clinicians than approaches such as CM or CBT—treatments whose theoretical underpinnings may not be seen as highly compatible with disease-model approaches (although such incompatibility has yet to be demonstrated).

Moreover, it is critical to recognize that the evidence supporting disease-model approaches has emerged from well-conducted clinical trials in which therapists were selected on the basis of their expertise in this approach and were trained and closely supervised so as to foster high levels of adherence and competence in delivering the treatments, and it remains to be seen whether these approaches will be as effective when applied under less-than-ideal conditions. Likewise, these professional, individual approaches should be distinguished from merely referring patients to self-help meetings. It is of note that a large randomized trial that directly compared referral to self-help with professional treatments found poorer outcomes with high rates of treatment utilization for the patients referred to self-help compared with inpatient treatment (Walsh, Hingson et al., 1991).

Individual Psychotherapy for Marijuana Dependence. Although marijuana is the most commonly used illicit substance, treatment of marijuana abuse and dependence is a comparatively understudied area to date, in part because comparatively few individuals present for treatment with a primary complaint of marijuana abuse or dependence. Currently, no effective pharmacotherapies for marijuana dependence exist, and only a few controlled trials of psychosocial approaches have been completed. Stephens and colleagues (2000) compared a delayed-treatment control group with a two-session motivational approach and with an intensive (14-session) relapse prevention approach. They found better marijuana outcomes for the two active treatments compared with the delayed-treatment control group but found no significant differences between the brief and the more intensive treatment. More recently, a replication and extension of that study, involving a multisite trial of 450 marijuana-dependent patients, compared three approaches: (1) a delayed treatment control, (2) a two-session motivational approach, and (3) a nine-session combined motivational/coping skills approach. Results suggested that both active treatments were associated with significantly greater reductions in marijuana use than the delayed treatment control through a nine-month followup period (MTP Research Group, 2001). Moreover, the nine-session intervention was significantly more effective than the two-session intervention, and this effect also was sustained through the nine-month followup period.

EMPIRICALLY VALIDATED TREATMENTS

The empirical evidence reviewed here and the literature on behavioral treatments of alcoholism reviewed elsewhere (Babor, 1994; Miller & Heather, 1998) suggest the following:

■ To date, most studies suggest that individual psychotherapy is superior to control conditions as a treatment for patients with substance use disorders. This finding is consistent with the bulk of findings from psychotherapy efficacy research in areas other than substance use, which suggests that the effects of many psychotherapies are clinically and statistically significant and are superior to no treatment and placebo conditions (Lambert & Bergin, 1994).

■ No particular type of individual psychotherapy was found to be consistently superior as a treatment for substance use disorders.

■ The effects of even comparatively brief psychotherapies appear to be durable among patients with substance use disorders.

Ongoing Development of Innovative Behavioral Therapies. Our review of rigorously conducted efficacy research on psychotherapies for substance use disorders provides support for the use of a number of innovative approaches: SE treatment for opioid addicts, CBT for cocaine dependence, community reinforcement treatment with contingency management for cocaine dependence, and contingency management for a wide range of substance use disorders.

The growing list of empirically validated treatments is attributable, in part, to the behavioral therapies initiative begun in the early 1990s by NIDA (Onken, Blaine et al., 1997). That initiative was begun to encourage development and testing of new and improved psychotherapies for drug addicts. Although strong evidence suggests that addiction treatment works, the field needs better methods, as too few addicts enter treatment, complete treatment, and achieve lasting improvement. Better treatment ideas can come from any source, but widespread adoption of new methods should be reserved for those treatments with proven efficacy.

The behavioral therapies initiative was instituted to promote the process of moving new treatments from the stage in which they represent "good ideas" to one in which they are shown to be effective, are fully specified in training manuals, and are ready for use in community programs. This process is guided by a new stage model of behavioral therapies research (Rounsaville, Carroll et al., 2001; Onken, Blaine et al., 1997), demarcating three divisions in a rigorous scientific process that leads from initial innovation through efficacy research to effectiveness research. Stage I consists of pilot/feasibility testing, manual writing, training program development, and adherence/competence measure development for new and untested treatments. Stage II initially consists of randomized clinical trials (RCTs) to evaluate efficacy of manualized and pilot-tested treatments that have shown promise or efficacy in earlier studies. Stage II research also can address mechanisms of action or effective components of treatment for approaches with evidence of efficacy derived from RCTs. Stage III consists of studies to evaluate transportability of treatments whose efficacy has been demonstrated in at least two RCTs. Key Stage III research issues revolve around (1) generalizability (that is, will this treatment maintain effectiveness with different practitioners, patients, and settings?), (2) implementation issues (that is, what kinds of training by what kinds of trainers are necessary to train what kinds of clinicians to learn a new technique?), (3) cost-effectiveness issues (that is, compared with the costs of learning and implementing this treatment, what are the savings, particularly in comparison to existing methods?), and (4) consumer/marketing issues (that is, how acceptable is a new treatment to clinicians, patients, and payers outside of research settings?).

The stage model was developed in an attempt to bridge the gap (Institute of Medicine, 1998) between research and practice in the treatment of addiction. Although psychotherapies are widely practiced, the types of treatments most widely used have not been shown to be effective in RCTs. Conversely, comparatively few practitioners use the empirically validated treatments listed above. This gap is attributable to bottlenecks at Stage I and Stage III.

At the front end, creative clinicians have proffered many new treatments, but few of the originators have had an opportunity to prove the efficacy of their treatments in clinical trials. As a result, many promising, potentially effective treatments have been ignored. By following guidelines for Stage I research (Rounsaville, Carroll et al., 2001; Onken,

Blaine et al., 1997), clinicians can move their treatments to a stage at which efficacy testing can take place.

Another bottleneck occurs after a treatment is shown to be efficacious in rigorous clinical trials, but before community programs are ready to adopt the new treatments. The role of Stage III research is to answer important questions about a new treatment's effectiveness and cost-effectiveness in real-world settings.

In addition to articulating the stage model, NIDA has taken a major role in Stage III research by developing the National Drug Abuse Treatment Clinical Trials Network (CTN). The CTN is a network of academically based regional research and training centers that are linked in partnership with clinical treatment programs to provide the infrastructure for large-scale trials to evaluate the effectiveness of promising pharmacologic and/or behavioral treatments in representative community settings. NIDA's CTN plays a unique role for behavioral treatments. Unlike medication treatments that are distributed for profit by commercial pharmaceutical manufacturers, behavioral treatments have no organizational resources or advocates to promote their dissemination into community practice.

From the preceding summary, it is clear that the empirical literature offers only the most general sort of guidance about the choice of which individual psychotherapy is likely to be useful for a particular patient and when in the course of treatment it should be offered. Hence, the following recommendations are made on the basis of clinical experience rather than research evidence. With this *caveat*, it is suggested that individual psychotherapy may have the following uses: (1) to serve as an initial treatment or an introduction into treatment, (2) to treat patients with low levels of substance dependence, (3) to treat patients who failed in other modalities, (4) to complement other ongoing treatment modalities for selected patients, and (5) to help the patient solidify gains after achievement of stable abstinence.

Psychotherapy as Initial Treatment. As noted previously, a key advantage of individual therapy is the privacy and confidentiality it affords. This aspect can make individual therapy or counseling an ideal setting in which to clarify the treatment needs of patients who are in early stages (that is, contemplation or precontemplation) of thinking about changing their patterns of substance use (Prochaska & DiClemente, 1986). Notably, the growing evidence for the efficacy of brief (two to four sessions) MET suggests that this can be sufficient for certain patients. For individuals with severe dependence who deny the seriousness of their

involvement, a course of individual therapy in which the patient is guided to a clear recognition of the problem can be an essential first step toward more intensive approaches such as residential treatment or methadone maintenance. An important part of this process may involve allowing the patient to fail one or more times at strategies that have a low probability of success, such as attempting to cut down on substance use without stopping or attempting outpatient detoxification.

A general principle underlying this process is the successive use of treatments that involve greater expense and/or patient involvement only after less intensive approaches have been shown to fail. Hence, brief individual treatment may be sufficient alone or may serve a cost-effective triage function.

Psychotherapy for Patients With Mild to Moderately Severe Substance Dependence. Although less studied with nonalcoholic drug abusers, the drug dependence syndrome concept (Edwards, Arif et al., 1981) has received considerable attention in the study of alcoholism. This concept, first described by Edwards and Gross (1976), suggests that drug dependence is best understood as a constellation of cognitions, behaviors, and physical symptoms that underlie a pattern of progressively diminished control over drug use. This dependence syndrome is conceived to be aligned along a continuum of severity, with higher levels of severity associated with poorer prognosis and the need for more intensive treatment, and lower levels of severity requiring less intensive interventions. The dependence syndrome construct has generated a large empiric literature, suggesting its validity with alcoholics (Edwards, 1986). Moreover, several scales have been developed for gauging the severity of alcohol dependence (Skinner, 1981; Stockwell, Hodgson et al., 1979; Chick, 1980). Generally, measures of quantity and frequency of alcohol use show a high correlation with dependence severity, and similar quantity/frequency indices for other drugs of abuse can be an adequate gauge of dependence severity. Evidence from studies of individuals who are mildly to moderately dependent on alcohol has indicated that a brief course of psychotherapy is sufficient for many to achieve substantial reductions in or abstinence from drinking (Miller & Heather, 1998; Babor, 1994; Sanchez-Craig & Wilkinson, 1986/1987; Edwards, 1986; Wallace, Cutler et al., 1988; WHO Brief Intervention Study Group, 1996). Although these findings have yet to be replicated with other types of substance use disorders, they are likely to be generalizable.

Psychotherapy for Patients Who Failed in Other Therapies. Although numerous predictors of outcomes for addiction treatment have been identified (Luborsky & McLellan, 1978; McLellan, Alterman et al., 1994; Carroll, Powers et al., 1993), few are robust, and still fewer have been evaluated in terms of the issue of matching patients to treatments (McLellan, O'Brien et al., 1980). As a result, the choice of treatment often involves a degree of trial and error. Each type of treatment has its strengths and weaknesses, which can result in a better or worse "fit" for a particular patient. For example, individual therapy is more expensive but more private than group therapy, more enduring and less disruptive to normal routine than residential treatment, and less troubled by side effects and medical contraindications than pharmacotherapies. Each of these advantages may be crucial to a patient who has responded poorly to other therapeutic approaches.

Psychotherapy as Ancillary Treatment. In considering psychotherapy as part of an ongoing comprehensive program of treatment, it is useful to distinguish between treatment of opioid addicts and alcoholics, for which powerful pharmacologic approaches are available, and treatment of other drugs of abuse, for which strong alternatives to psychosocial treatments are not yet available (Kosten & McCance-Katz, 1995). For alcoholics, naltrexone, acamprosate, and disulfiram have strong potential for reducing relapse rates. However, the effectiveness of disulfiram in the absence of a strong psychosocial treatment was no greater than placebo (Fuller, Branchey et al. 1986), and studies demonstrating the efficacy of naltrexone and acamprosate were done only in the context of a comparatively intense psychosocial intervention (Volpicelli, Alterman et al., 1992; O'Malley, Jaffe et al., 1992; Sass, Soyka et al., 1996; Whitworth, Fischer et al., 1996). For opioid-dependent patients, the modal approach is methadone maintenance, which is used with the majority of those in treatment, whereas an alternative pharmacotherapy, naltrexone, can be highly potent for the minority who choose this approach. Because of their powerful and specific pharmacologic effects, either to satisfy the need for opioids or to prevent illicit opioids from yielding their desired effect, these agents—provided that they are delivered with at least minimal counseling—can be sufficient for many opioid addicts (McLellan, Alterman et al., 1994). The choice of those who might benefit from additional individual psychotherapy may be guided by the unique but robust empiric findings of Woody and colleagues (1984, 1985) and McLellan and colleagues (1980), which suggest that psychotherapy is most likely to be of benefit to those opioid addicts with high levels of psychiatric symptoms as measured by the Addiction Severity Index (ASI) (McLellan, Luborsky et al., 1980) or with a diagnosis of major depression as defined in the *Diagnostic and Statistical Manual of Mental Disorders, 4th Edition* (APA, 1994). Because the benefits of psychotherapy can be maximized when instituted relatively soon after the patient enters treatment, screening instruments such as the ASI (McLellan, Luborsky et al., 1980) or the Beck Depression Inventory (Beck, Ward et al., 1970) could be used to quickly identify those with psychopathology or depression, alerting staff to the need to refer the client for psychotherapy.

For non-opioid drugs of abuse, an active search for effective pharmacotherapies currently is under way. In the interim, the mainstay of treatment for such patients remains some form of psychosocial treatment offered in a group, family, residential, or individual setting. For cocaine use, forms of treatment that currently have empirical support include behavioral therapy and CBT (Carroll, Rounsaville et al., 1994b; Higgins, Budney et al., 1994b). Some evidence suggests that these forms of treatment can be of particular benefit to patients who are rated higher in severity of cocaine dependence (Carroll, Rounsaville et al., 1994b), have substantial depressive symptoms (Carroll, Nich et al., 1995), or have substantial family support (Higgins, Budney et al., 1994b). However, there is as yet no strong empirical evidence as to the optimal duration of treatment, nor are there clear guidelines for matching patients to treatment.

For other types of drug abuse, in the absence of empirically validated guidelines, the choice of individual psychotherapy can be based on such factors as expense, logistical considerations, patient preference, or the clinical fit between the patient's presenting picture and the treatment modality (for example, family therapy is ruled out for those without families).

Psychotherapy After Achievement of Sustained Abstinence. As noted earlier, an individual who experiences frequent relapses or who is only tenuously holding onto abstinence can be a poor candidate for certain types of psychotherapy, particularly those that involve bringing into focus painful and anxiety-provoking clinical material as an inevitable part of helping the patient master his or her dysphoric affects or avoid recurrent failures in establishing enduring intimate relationships. In fact, some arousal of anxiety or frustration may occur with most types of psychotherapy, even those that are conceived as being primarily supportive. Because of this situation, individual psychotherapy may be effective for many individuals only after they have achieved abstinence through some other treatment approach, such as residential treatment, methadone maintenance, or group therapy. Given the vulnerability of these patients to relapse (which can extend over a lifetime), and the frequency with which dysphoric affects or interpersonal conflict are noted as precipitants of relapse (Marlatt & Gordon, 1980), individual psychotherapy may be particularly indicated for those whose psychopathology or disturbed interpersonal functioning is found to endure after the achievement of abstinence. Given findings pointing to the delayed emergence of effects of individual psychotherapy for both cocaine (Carroll, Rounsaville et al., 1994b; Carroll, Nich et al., 2000) and opioid (Woody, McLellan et al., 1995) addicts, psychotherapy aimed at these enduring issues can be helpful not only for such problems independent of their relationship to drug use, but also as a form of insurance against the likelihood that these continuing problems eventually will lead to relapse.

REFERENCES

Alexander F & French T (1946). *Psychoanalytic Therapy: Principles and Applications.* New York, NY: Ronald Press.

Allen JP & Litten RZ (1992). Techniques to enhance compliance with disul-firam. *Alcoholism: Clinical & Experimental Research* 16:1035-1041.

American Psychiatric Association (APA) (1994). *Diagnostic and Statistical Manual of Mental Disorders, 4th Edition (DSM-IV).* Washington, DC: American Psychiatric Press.

Anton RF, Hogan I, Jalali B et al. (1981). Multiple family therapy and naltrexone in the treatment of opioid dependence. *Drug and Alcohol Dependence* 8:157-168.

Babor TF (1994). Avoiding the horrid and beastly sin of drunkenness: Does dissuasion make a difference? *Journal of Consulting and Clinical Psychology* 62:1127-1140.

Babor TF, Grant M, Acuda W et al. (1994). A randomized clinical trial of brief interventions in primary care: Summary of an WHO project. *Addiction* 89:657-660.

Ball JC & Ross A (1991). *The Effectiveness of Methadone Maintenance Treatment.* New York, NY: Springer-Verlag.

Beck AT (1967). *Depression: Clinical, Experimental and Theoretical Aspects.* New York, NY: Hoeber.

Beck AT, Rush AJ, Shaw BF et al. (1979). *Cognitive Therapy of Depression.* New York, NY: Guilford Press.

Beck AT, Ward CH & Mendelson M (1970). An inventory for measuring depression. *Archives of General Psychiatry* 4:461-471.

Beck AT, Wright FD, Newman CF et al. (1993). *Cognitive Therapy of Substance Abuse.* New York, NY: Guilford Press.

Beckman EE & Leber WR (1985). *Handbook of Depression: Treatment, Assessment and Research.* Homewood, IL: Dorsey Press.

Bibring E (1954). Psychoanalysis and the dynamic psychotherapies. *Journal of American Psychoanalysis Association* 2:745-770.

Bien TH, Miller WR & Tonigan JS (1993). Brief interventions for alcohol problems: A review. *Addiction* 88:315-335.

Blatt S, McDonald C, Sugarman A et al. (1984). Psychodynamic theories of opiate addiction: New directions for research. *Clinical Psychology Review* 4:159-189.

Brunswick AF (1979). Black youth and drug use behavior. In GM Beschner & AS Friedman (eds.) *Youth Drug Abuse.* Lexington, MA: Lexington Books, 52-66.

Budney AJ & Higgins ST (1998). *A Community Reinforcement Plus Vouchers Approach: Treating Cocaine Addiction.* Rockville, MD: NIDA.

Carroll KM (1999a). Old psychotherapies for cocaine dependence . . . revisited. *Archives of General Psychiatry* 56:505-506.

Carroll KM (1999b). Behavioral and cognitive behavioral treatments. In BS McCrady & EE Epstein (eds.) *Addictions: A Comprehensive Guidebook.* New York, NY: Oxford University Press, 250-267.

Carroll KM (1997). Manual-guided psychosocial treatment: A new virtual requirement for pharmacotherapy trials? *Archives of General Psychiatry* 54:923-928.

Carroll KM & Rounsaville BJ (1991). Can a technology model be applied to psychotherapy research in cocaine abuse treatment? In LS Onken & JD Blaine (eds.) *Psychotherapy and Counseling in the Treatment of Drug Abuse (NIDA Research Monograph 104).* Rockville, MD: National Institute on Drug Abuse, 91-104.

Carroll KM, Ball SA, Nich C et al. (2001). Targeting behavioral therapies to enhance naltrexone treatment of opioid dependence: Efficacy of contingency management and significant other involvement. *Archives of General Psychiatry* 58:755-761.

Carroll KM, Nich C & Rounsaville BJ (1995). Differential symptom reduction in depressed cocaine abusers treated with psychotherapy and pharmacotherapy. *Journal of Nervous and Mental Disease* 183:251-259.

Carroll KM, Nich C, Ball SA et al. (1998). Treatment of cocaine and alcohol dependence with psychotherapy and disulfiram. *Addiction* 93:713-728.

Carroll KM, Nich C, Ball SA et al. (2000). One year follow-up of disulfiram and psychotherapy for cocaine-alcohol abusers: Sustained effects of treatment. *Addiction* 95:1335-1349.

Carroll KM, Powers MD, Bryant KJ et al. (1993). One-year follow-up status of treatment-seeking cocaine abusers: Psychopathology and dependence severity as predictors of outcome. *Journal of Nervous and Mental Disease* 181:71-79.

Carroll KM, Rounsaville BJ & Gawin FH (1991). A comparative trial of psychotherapies for ambulatory cocaine abusers: Relapse prevention and interpersonal psychotherapy. *American Journal of Drug and Alcohol Abuse* 17:229-247.

Carroll KM, Rounsaville BJ, Gordon LT et al. (1994a). Psychotherapy and pharmacotherapy for ambulatory cocaine abusers. *Archives of General Psychiatry* 51:177-187.

Carroll KM, Rounsaville BJ, Nich C et al. (1994b). One year follow-up of psychotherapy and pharmacotherapy for cocaine dependence: Delayed emergence of psychotherapy effects. *Archives of General Psychiatry* 51:989-997.

Chick J (1980). Alcohol dependence: Methodological issues in its measurement: Reliability of the criteria. *British Journal of Addiction* 75:175-186.

Cook CH (1988). The Minnesota model in the management of drug and alcohol dependency: Miracle, method or myth? Part I. The philosophy and the program. *British Journal of Addiction* 83:625-634.

Corty E & Ball JC (1987). Admissions to methadone maintenance: Comparisons between programs and implications for treatment. *Journal of Substance Abuse Treatment* 4:181-187.

Crits-Christoph P, Siqueland L, Blaine J et al. (1999). Psychosocial treatments for cocaine dependence: Results of the National Institute on Drug Abuse Collaborative Cocaine Study. *Archives of General Psychiatry* 56: 495-502.

Cummings N (1979). Turning bread into stones: Our modern anti-miracle. *American Psychology* 34:1119-1129.

DeRubeis RJ & Crits-Christoph P (1998). Empirically supported individual and group psychological treatments for adult mental disorders. *Journal of Consulting and Clinical Psychology* 66:37-52.

DiClemente CC, Prochaska JO & Gibertini M (1985). Self-efficacy and the stages of self-change of smoking. *Cognitive Therapy and Research* 9(2):181-200.

Dole VP, Nyswander ME & Warner A (1976). Methadone maintenance treatment: A ten-year perspective. *Journal of the American Medical Association* 235:2117-2119.

Douglas DB (1986). Alcoholism as an addiction: The disease concept reconsidered. *Journal of Substance Abuse Treatment* 3:115-120.

Edwards G (1986). The alcohol dependence syndrome: A concept as stimulus to enquiry. *British Journal of Addiction* 81:171-183.

Edwards G & Gross MM (1976). Alcohol dependence: Provisional description of a clinical syndrome. *British Medical Journal* 1:1058-1061.

Edwards G, Arif A & Hodgson R (1981). Nomenclature and classification of drug and alcohol related problems. *Bulletin of the World Health Organization* 59:225-242.

Fuller R, Branchey L, Brightwell D et al. (1986). Disulfiram treatment of alcoholism: A Veteran's Administration cooperative study. *Journal of the American Medical Association* 256:1449-1455.

Gawin FH & Ellinwood EH (1988). Stimulants: Actions, abuse, and treatment. *New England Journal of Medicine* 318:1173-1183.

Grabowski J, O'Brien CP, Greenstein R et al. (1979). Effects of contingent payments on compliance with a naltrexone regimen. *American Journal of Drug and Alcohol Abuse* 6:355-365.

Greenstein RA, Arndt IC, McLellan AT et al. (1984). Naltrexone: A clinical perspective. *Journal of Clinical Psychiatry* 45:25-28.

Greenstein RA, Fudala PJ & O'Brien CP (1992). Alternative pharmacotherapies for opiate addiction. In JH Lowinson, P Ruiz & RB Millman (eds.) *Comprehensive Textbook of Substance Abuse, 2nd Edition.* New York, NY: Williams & Wilkins, 562-573.

Hall SM, Havassy BE & Wasserman DA (1991). Effects of commitment to abstinence, positive moods, stress, and coping on relapse to cocaine use. *Journal of Consulting and Clinical Psychology* 59:526-532.

Hesselbrock MN, Meyer RE & Keener JJ (1985). Psychopathology in hospitalized alcoholics. *Archives of General Psychiatry* 42:1050-1055.

Higgins ST, Budney AJ, Bickel WK et al. (1993). Achieving cocaine abstinence with a behavioral approach. *American Journal of Psychiatry* 150:763-769.

Higgins ST, Budney AJ, Bickel WK et al. (1994a). Participation of significant others in outpatient behavioral treatment predicts greater cocaine abstinence. *American Journal of Drug and Alcohol Abuse* 20:47-56.

Higgins ST, Budney AJ, Bickel WK et al. (1994b). Incentives improve outcome in outpatient behavioral treatment of cocaine dependence. *Archives of General Psychiatry* 51:568-576.

Higgins ST, Delaney DD, Budney AJ et al. (1991). A behavioral approach to achieving initial cocaine abstinence. *American Journal of Psychiatry* 148:1218-1224.

Higgins ST, Wong CJ, Badger GJ et al. (2000). Contingent reinforcement increases cocaine abstinence during outpatient treatment and one year follow-up. *Journal of Consulting and Clinical Psychology* 68:64-72.

Holder HD, Longabaugh R, Miller WR et al. (1991). The cost effectiveness of treatment for alcohol problems: A first approximation. *Journal of Studies on Alcohol* 52:517-540.

Horgan CM & Levine HJ (1998). The substance abuse treatment system: What does it look like and whom does it serve? Preliminary findings from the Alcohol and Drug Services Study. In S Lamb, MR Greenlick & D McCarty (eds.) *Bridging the Gap Between Practice and Research: Forging Partnerships with Community-Based Drug and Alcohol Treatment.* Washington, DC: National Academy Press, 186-197.

Hubbard RL, Marsden ME, Rachal JV et al. (1989). *Drug Abuse Treatment: A National Study of Effectiveness.* Chapel Hill, NC: University of North Carolina Press.

Hubbard RL, Rachal JV, Craddock SG et al. (1984). Treatment Outcome Prospective Study (TOPS): Client characteristics and behaviors before, during, and after treatment. In FM Tims & JP Ludford (eds.) *Drug Abuse Treatment Evaluation: Strategies, Progress, and Prospects (NIDA Research Monograph 51).* Rockville, MD: National Institute on Drug Abuse, 42-68.

Iguchi MY, Lamb RJ, Belding MA et al. (1996). Contingent reinforcement of group participation versus abstinence in a methadone maintenance program. *Experimental and Clinical Psychopharmacology* 4:1-7.

Institute of Medicine (1990). *Broadening the Base of Treatment for Alcohol Problems.* Washington, DC: National Academy Press.

Institute of Medicine (1998). *Bridging the Gap Between Practice and Research: Forging Partnerships with Community-based Drug and Alcohol Treatment.* Washington, DC: National Academy Press.

Jaffe JH & Kleber HD (1989). Opioids: General issues and detoxification. In TB Karasu (ed.) *Treatment of Psychiatric Disorders.* Washington, DC: American Psychiatric Press, 1309-1331.

Kadden R, Carroll KM, Donovan D et al. (1992). *Cognitive-behavioral Coping Skills Therapy Manual: A Clinical Research Guide for Therapists Treating Individuals with Alcohol Abuse and Dependence (NIAAA Project MATCH Monograph 3).* Rockville, MD: National Institute on Alcohol Abuse and Alcoholism.

Kandel D & Faust R (1975). Sequence and stages in patterns of adolescent drug use. *Archives of General Psychiatry* 32:923-932.

Keller DS, Carroll KM, Nich C et al. (1995). Differential treatment response in alexithymic cocaine abusers: Findings from a randomized clinical trial of psychotherapy and pharmacotherapy. *American Journal on Addictions* 4:234-244.

Khantzian EJ (1978). The ego, the self and opiate addiction: Theoretical and treatment considerations. *International Review of Psychoanalysis* 5:189-198.

Khantzian EJ (1985). The self-medication hypothesis of addictive disorders: Focus on heroin and cocaine dependence. *American Journal of Psychiatry* 142:1259-1264.

Khantzian EJ & Schneider RJ (1986). Treatment implications of a psychodynamic understanding of opioid addicts. In RE Meyer (ed.) *Psychopathology and Addictive Disorders.* New York, NY: Guilford Press.

Khantzian EJ & Treece C (1985). DSM-III psychiatric diagnosis of nar- cotic addicts. *Archives of General Psychiatry* 42:1067-1071.

Kirby KC, Marlowe DB, Festinger DS et al. (1998). Schedule of voucher delivery influences initiation of cocaine abstinence. *Journal of Con- sulting and Clinical Psychology* 66:761-767.

Kleber HD, ed. (1989). Psychoactive substance use disorders (not alco- hol). In TB Karasu (ed.) *Treatments of Psychiatric Disorders*. Washington, DC: American Psychiatric Press, 1183-1484.

Kleber HD & Kosten TR (1984). Naltrexone induction: Psychologic and pharmacologic strategies. *Journal of Clinical Psychiatry* 45:29.

Kosten TR (1989). Pharmacotherapeutic interventions for cocaine abuse: Matching patients to treatments. *Journal of Nervous and Mental Diseases* 177:379-389.

Kosten TR & Kleber HD (1984). Strategies to improve compliance with narcotic antagonists. *American Journal on Drug and Alcohol Abuse* 10:249-266.

Kosten TR & McCance-Katz E (1995). New pharmacotherapies. In JM Oldham & MB Riba (eds.) *American Psychiatric Press Review of Psy- chiatry*, Vol. 14. Washington, DC: American Psychiatric Press, 105-126.

Kosten TR, Rounsaville BJ & Kleber HD (1987). A 2.5 year follow-up of cocaine use among treated opioid addicts: Have our treatments helped? *Archives of General Psychiatry* 44:281-284.

Lambert MJ & Bergin AE (1994). The effectiveness of psychotherapy. In AE Bergin & SL Garfield (eds.) *Handbook of Psychotherapy and Behavior Change, 4th Edition*. New York, NY: John Wiley & Sons, 143-189.

Leshner AI (1999). Science-based views of drug addiction and its treat- ment. *Journal of the American Medical Association* 282:1314-1316.

Liebson IA, Tommasello A & Bigelow GE (1978). A behavioral treatment of alcoholic methadone patients. *Annals of Internal Medicine* 89:342-344.

Luborsky L (1984). Principles of psychoanalytic psychotherapy: A manual for supportive-expressive (SE) treatment. New York, NY: Basic Books.

Luborsky L & McLellan AT (1978). Our surprising inability to predict the outcomes of psychological treatments with special reference to treat- ments for drug abuse. *American Journal of Drug and Alcohol Abuse* 5:387-398.

Marlatt GA & Gordon GR (1980). Determinants of relapse: Implications for the maintenance of behavior change. In PO Davidson & SM Davidson (eds.) *Behavioral Medicine: Changing Health Lifestyles*. New York, NY: Brunner/Mazel, 410-452.

Marlatt GA & Gordon J (eds.) (1985). *Relapse Prevention*. New York: Guilford Press.

Maude-Griffin PM, Hohenstein JM, Humfleet GL et al. (1998). Superior efficacy of cognitive-behavioral therapy for crack cocaine abusers: Main and matching effects. *Journal of Consulting and Clinical Psy- chology* 66:832-837.

McCance-Katz E & Kosten TR (in press). Overview of potential treat- ment medications for cocaine dependence. In P Bridge, N Chiang & B Tai (eds.) *Medication Development for the Treatment of Cocaine Dependence: Issues in Clinical Efficacy Trials (NIDA Research Mono- graph Series)*. Rockville, MD: National Institute on Drug Abuse.

McKay JR, Alterman AI, Cacciola JS et al. (1997). Group counseling ver- sus individualized relapse prevention aftercare following intensive outpatient treatment for cocaine dependence. *Journal of Consulting and Clinical Psychology* 65:778-788.

McLellan AT & McKay JR (1998). The treatment of addiction: What can research offer practice? In S Lamb, MR Greenlick & D McCarty (eds.) *Bridging the Gap Between Practice and Research: Forging Partner- ships with Community Based Drug and Alcohol Treatment*. Washington, DC: National Academy Press, 147-185.

McLellan AT, Alterman AI, Metzger DS et al. (1994). Similarity of out- come predictors across opiate, cocaine, and alcohol treatments: Role of treatment services. *Journal of Consulting and Clinical Psychology* 62:1141-1158.

McLellan AT, Arndt IO, Metzger DS et al. (1993). The effects of psycho- social services in substance abuse treatment. *Journal of the American Medical Association* 269:1953-1959.

McLellan AT, Luborsky L, O'Brien CP et al. (1980). An improved diag- nostic evaluation instrument for substance abuse patients: The Addiction Severity Index. *Journal of Nervous and Mental Diseases* 168:26-33.

McLellan AT, O'Brien CP, Kron R et al. (1980). Matching substance abuse patients to appropriate treatments. *Drug and Alcohol Dependence* 5:189-195.

Mendelson JH & Mello NK (1966). Experimental analysis of drinking behavior in chronic alcoholics. *Annals of the New York Academy of Science* 133:828-845.

Meyer RE (1992). New pharmacotherapies for cocaine dependence . . . revisited. *Archives of General Psychiatry* 49:900-904.

Meyer RE, Mirin SM, Altman JL et al. (1976). A behavioral paradigm for the evaluation of narcotic antagonists. *Archives of General Psychia- try* 33:371-377.

Milby JB, Schumacher JE, Raczynski JM et al. (1996). Sufficient condi- tions for effective treatment of substance abusing homeless persons. *Drug and Alcohol Dependence* 43:23-28.

Miller WE & Heather N, eds. (1986). *Treating Addictive Behaviors, 2nd Edition*. New York, NY: Plenum Press.

Miller WR & Rollnick S (1991). *Motivational Interviewing: Preparing People to Change Addictive Behavior*. New York, NY: Guilford Press.

Miller WR, Zweben A, DiClemente CC et al. (1992). *Motivational En- hancement Therapy Manual: A Clinical Research Guide for Therapists Treating Individuals With Alcohol Abuse and Dependence (NIAAA Project MATCH Monograph 2)*. Rockville, MD: National Institute on Alcohol Abuse and Alcoholism.

Mirin SR, Meyer RE & McNamme B (1980). Psychopathology and mood duration in heroin use: Acute and chronic effects. *Archives of Gen- eral Psychiatry* 33:1503-1508.

Monti PM, Rohsenow DJ, Michalec E et al. (1997). Brief coping skills treatment for cocaine abuse: Substance abuse outcomes at three months. *Addiction* 92:1717-1728.

MTP Research Group (2001). Treating cannabis dependence: Findings from a multisite study. Under review.

Nathan PE & O'Brien JS (1971). An experimental analysis of the behavior of alcoholics and nonalcoholics during prolonged experimental drink- ing: A necessary procure of behavior therapy? *Behavioral Therapy* 2:455-476.

Norquist GS & Regier DA (1996). The epidemiology of psychiatric disorders and the *de facto* mental health care system. *Annual Review of Medicine* 47:473-479.

Nowinski J, Baker S & Carroll KM (1992). *Twelve-Step Facilitation Therapy Manual: A Clinical Research Guide for Therapists Treating Individuals With Alcohol Abuse and Dependence (NIAAA Project MATCH Monograph 1)*. Rockville, MD: National Institute on Alcohol Abuse and Alcoholism.

O'Brien CP (1997). A range of research-based pharmacotherapies for addiction. *Science* 278:66-70.

O'Brien CP & Woody GE (1989). Antagonist treatment: Naltrexone. In TB Karasu (ed.) *Treatments of Psychiatric Disorders*. Washington, DC: American Psychiatric Press, 1332-1340.

O'Donnell JA (1969). *Narcotic Addicts in Kentucky. Public Health Service Publication 1981*. Washington, DC: Government Printing Office.

O'Donnell JA, Voss HL, Clayton RR et al. (1976). *Young Men and Drugs: A Nationwide Survey (NIDA Research Monograph 5)*. Washington, DC: National Institute on Drug Abuse.

O'Malley SS, Jaffe AJ, Chang G et al. (1992). Naltrexone and coping skills therapy for alcohol dependence. *Archives of General Psychiatry* 49:881-887.

O'Malley SS, Jaffe AJ, Chang G et al. (1996). Six month follow-up of naltrexone and psychotherapy for alcohol dependence. *Archives of General Psychiatry* 53:217-224.

Onken LS, Blaine JD & Battjes R (1997). Behavioral therapy research: A conceptualization of a process. In SW Henngler & R Amentos (eds.) *Innovative Approaches For Difficult to Treat Populations*. Washington, DC: American Psychiatric Press, 477-485.

Petry NM, Martin B, Cooney JL et al. (2000). Give them prizes and they will come: Contingency management treatment of alcohol dependence. *Journal of Consulting and Clinical Psychology* 68:250-257.

Preston KL, Silverman K, Umbricht A et al. (1999). Improvement in naltrexone treatment compliance with contingency management. *Drug and Alcohol Dependence* 54:127-135.

Prochaska JO & DiClemente C (1986). Toward a comprehensive model of change. In WR Miller & N Heather (eds.) *Treating Addictive Behaviors: Processes of Change*. New York, NY: Plenum Press, 3-27.

Project MATCH Research Group (1997). Matching Alcohol Treatments to Client Heterogeneity: Project MATCH posttreatment drinking outcomes. *Journal of Studies on Alcohol* 58:7-29.

Project MATCH Research Group (1998). Matching Alcoholism Treatments to Client Heterogeneity: Project MATCH three-year drinking outcomes. *Alcoholism: Clinical & Experimental Research* 22:1300-1311.

Robins LN (1979). Addicts' careers. In RI DuPont, A Goldstein, J O'Donnell & B Brown (eds.) *Handbook on Drug Abuse*. Rockville, MD: National Institute on Drug Abuse.

Rounsaville BJ (1995). Can psychotherapy rescue naltrexone treatment of opioid addiction? In L Onken & J Blaine (eds.) *Potentiating the Efficacy of Medications: Integrating Psychosocial Therapies With Pharmacotherapies in the Treatment of Drug Dependence (NIDA Research Monograph 105)*. Rockville, MD: National Institute on Drug Abuse, 37-52.

Rounsaville BJ & Kleber HD (1985). Psychotherapy/counseling for opiate addicts: Strategies for use in different treatment settings. *International Journal of Addiction* 20:869-896.

Rounsaville BJ, Carroll KM & Onken LS (2001). NIDA's stage model of behavioral therapies research: Getting started and moving on from Stage I. *Clinical Psychology: Science and Practice* 8:133-142.

Rounsaville BJ, Gawin FH & Kleber HD (1985). Interpersonal psychotherapy (IPT) adapted for ambulatory cocaine abusers. *American Journal of Drug and Alcohol Abuse* 11:171-191.

Rounsaville BJ, Glazer W, Wilber CH et al. (1983). Short-term interpersonal psychotherapy in methadone-maintained opiate addicts. *Archives of General Psychiatry* 40:629-636.

Rounsaville BJ, Weissman M, Kleber HD et al. (1982). Heterogeneity of psychiatric diagnosis in treated opiate addicts. *Archives of General Psychiatry* 39:161-166.

Sampson DD, Savage LJ & Lloyd MR (1979). Follow-up evaluation of treatment of drug abuse during 1969 to 1972. *Archives of General Psychiatry* 36:772-780.

Sanchez-Craig M & Wilkinson DA (1986/1987). Treating problem drinkers who are not severely dependent on alcohol. *Drugs and Society* 1(2/3):39-67.

Sass H, Soyka M, Mann K et al. (1996). Relapse prevention by acamprosate. *Archives of General Psychiatry* 53:673-680.

Schmitz JM, Oswald LM, Jacks SD et al. (1997). Relapse prevention treatment for cocaine dependence: Group vs. individual format. *Addictive Behaviors* 22:405-418.

Senay E (1989). Methadone maintenance. In TB Karasu (ed.) *Treatments of Psychiatric Disorders*. Washington, DC: American Psychiatric Press, 1341-1358.

Silverman K, Higgins ST, Brooner RK et al. (1996). Sustained cocaine abstinence in methadone maintenance patients through voucher-based reinforcement therapy. *Archives of General Psychiatry* 53:409-415.

Silverman K, Wong CJ, Higgins ST et al. (1996). Increasing opiate abstinence through voucher-based reinforcement therapy. *Drug and Alcohol Dependence* 41:157-165.

Silverman K, Wong CJ, Umbricht-Schneiter A et al. (1998). Broad beneficial effects of cocaine abstinence reinforcement among methadone patients. *Journal of Consulting and Clinical Psychology* 66:811-824.

Simons AD, Garfield SL & Murphy GE (1984). The process of change in cognitive therapy and pharmacotherapy for depression. *Archives of General Psychiatry* 41:45-51.

Simpson DD, Joe GW & Bracy SA (1982). Six-year follow-up of opioid addicts after admission to treatment. *Archives of General Psychiatry* 39:1318-1326.

Sisson RW & Azrin NH (1989). The community reinforcement approach. In RK Hester & WR Miller (eds.) *Handbook of Alcoholism Treatment Approaches*. New York, NY: Pergamon, 242-258.

Skinner HA (1981). Primary syndromes of alcohol abuse: Their management and correlates. *British Journal of Addiction* 76:63-76.

Smith M, Glass C & Miller T (1980). *The Benefits of Psychotherapy*. Baltimore, MD: Johns Hopkins Press.

Stanton MD & Todd TC, eds. (1982). *The Family Therapy of Drug Abuse and Addiction*. New York, NY: Guilford Press.

Stephens RS, Roffman RA & Curtin L (2000). Comparison of extended versus brief treatments for marijuana use. *Journal of Consulting and Clinical Psychology* 68:898-908.

Stitzer ML & Bigelow GE (1978). Contingency management in a methadone maintenance program: Availability of reinforcers. *International Journal on Addiction* 13:737-746.

Stitzer ML, Bickel WK, Bigelow GE et al. (1986). Effect of methadone dose contingencies on urinalysis test results of polydrug-abusing methadone maintenance patients. *Drug and Alcohol Dependence* 18:341-348.

Stockwell T, Hodgson R, Edwards G et al. (1979). The development of a questionnaire to measure severity of alcohol dependence. *British Journal of Addiction* 74:79-87.

Taylor GJ, Parker JD & Bagby RM (1990). A preliminary investigation of alexithymia in men with psychoactive substance dependence. *American Journal of Psychiatry* 147:1228-1230.

Tims F & Leukefeld C, eds. (1986). *RAUS—Relapse and Recovery in Drug Abuse (NIDA Research Monograph)*. Rockville, MD: National Institute on Drug Abuse.

Vaillant GE (1966). Twelve-year follow-up of New York addicts. *American Journal of Psychiatry* 122:727-737.

Van Horn DH & Frank AF (1998). Psychotherapy for cocaine addiction. *Psychology of Addictive Behaviors* 12:47-61.

Volpicelli JR, Alterman AI, Hayashida M et al. (1992). Naltrexone in the treatment of alcohol dependence. *Archives of General Psychiatry* 49:876-880.

Wallace P, Cutler S & Haines A (1988). Randomised controlled trial of general practitioner intervention in patients with excessive alcohol consumption. *British Medical Journal* 297:663-668.

Walsh DC, Hingson RW, Merrigan DM et al. (1991). A randomized trial of treatment options for alcohol-abusing workers. *New England Journal of Medicine* 325:775-782.

Waskow IE (1984). Specification of the technique variable in the NIMH Treatment of Depression Collaborative Research Program. In JBW Williams & RL Spitzer (eds.) *Psychotherapy Research: Where Are We and Where Should We Go?* New York, NY: Guilford Press.

Whitworth AB, Fischer F, Lesch OM et al. (1996). Comparison of acamprosate and placebo in long-term treatment of alcohol dependence. *Lancet* 347:1438-1442.

WHO Brief Intervention Study Group (1996). A cross-national trial of brief interventions with heavy drinkers. *American Journal of Public Health* 86:948-955.

Wikler A (1980). *Opioid Dependence: Mechanisms and Treatment*. New York, NY: Plenum Press.

Wilk AI, Jensen NM & Havighurst TC (1997). Meta-analysis of randomized controlled trials addressing brief interventions in heavy alcohol drinkers. *Journal of General Internal Medicine* 12:274-283.

Woody GE, Luborsky L, McLellan AT et al. (1983). Psychotherapy for opiate addicts: Does it help? *Archives of General Psychiatry* 40:639-645.

Woody GE, McLellan AT, Luborsky L et al. (1984). Severity of psychiatric symptoms as a prediction of benefits from psychotherapy: The Veterans Administration-Penn study. *American Journal of Psychiatry* 141:1172-1177.

Woody GE, McLellan AT, Luborsky L et al. (1985). Sociopathy and psychotherapy outcome. *Archives of General Psychiatry* 42:1081-1086.

Woody GE, McLellan AT, Luborsky L et al. (1987). Twelve-month follow-up of psychotherapy for opiate dependence. *American Journal of Psychiatry* 144:590-596.

Woody GE, McLellan AT, Luborsky L et al. (1995). Psychotherapy in community methadone programs: A validation study. *American Journal of Psychiatry* 152:1302-1308.

Wurmser L (1979). *The Hidden Dimension: Psychopathology of Compulsive Drug Use*. New York, NY: Jason Aronson.

Chapter 4

Community Reinforcement and Contingency Management

Stephen T. Higgins, Ph.D.
Jennifer W. Tidey, Ph.D.

Conceptual Framework
Treatment of Alcohol Abuse and Dependence
Treatment of Cocaine Abuse and Dependence
Treatment of Opioid Abuse and Dependence
Treatment of Other Abuse and Dependence

This chapter reviews the research supporting the efficacy of the community reinforcement approach (CRA) and contingency management (CM) procedures for treating alcohol or other drug abuse and dependence. CRA and CM are based in the theoretical framework of operant conditioning, which is the study of how reinforcing and punishing environmental consequences alter the form and frequency of voluntary behavior. The chapter describes how alcohol and drug use and abuse are conceptualized within an operant framework and reviews controlled studies on the efficacy of CRA and CM in the treatment of abuse and dependence.

These interventions have been researched most extensively with regard to treating alcohol, cocaine, and opioid dependence, which are the main foci of this chapter. More recently, they have been extended to other forms of substance abuse and dependence and to special populations. Those advances are reviewed as well. The review is restricted to controlled studies published in peer-reviewed journals. (The only exceptions occur when an uncontrolled study is mentioned as the first in a series of studies that included a controlled trial.)

CONCEPTUAL FRAMEWORK

Alcohol and drug use can be considered a form of operant behavior that is maintained, in part, by the reinforcing effects of the substances involved (Goldberg & Stolerman, 1986). The reliable observation that abused substances function as reinforcers with humans and laboratory animals supports that position (Griffiths, Bigelow et al., 1980). Most substances that are abused by humans are voluntarily consumed by a variety of species (Young & Herling, 1986). Neither a prior history of exposure nor physical dependence is necessary for these substances to support voluntary consumption in normal laboratory animals. These commonalities across species and substances support the position that reinforcement is a fundamental determinant of substance use, abuse, and dependence.

Within this framework, all physically intact humans are considered to possess the necessary neurobiologic systems to experience alcohol- and drug-induced reinforcement and hence to develop use, abuse, and dependence. Genetic or acquired characteristics (for example, a family history of alcoholism or psychiatric disorder) are recognized as factors that affect the probability of developing abuse and

Figure 1.   Comparison of the CRA and Control Groups on Key Dependent Measures

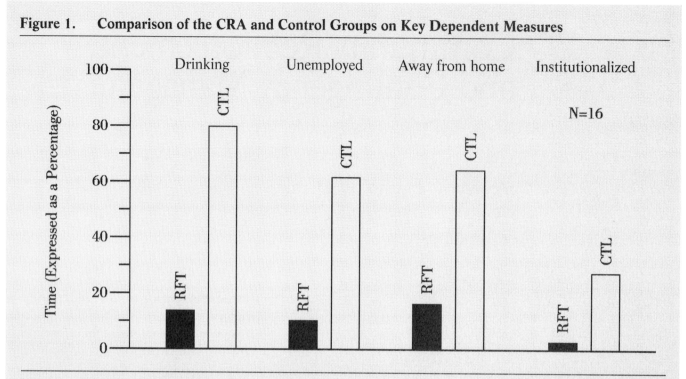

Comparison of the CRA and control groups on key dependent measures during the 6 months of followup hospital discharge: mean percentage of time spent drinking, unemployed, away from home, and institutionalized. From Hunt GM & Azrin NH (1973).   A community-reinforcement approach to alcoholism. *Behavior Research and Therapy* 11:91-104. Reprinted by permission of the publisher.

dependence, but are not deemed to be necessary for the problem to emerge. Instead, substance use is considered a normal, learned behavior that falls along a continuum, ranging from little use with few problems to excessive use with many untoward effects. The same principles of learning are assumed to operate across this continuum.

Treatments developed within this framework are designed to reorganize the environment of the user to systematically weaken the influence of reinforcement obtained through alcohol or drug use. Primary emphasis is on decreasing such use by increasing the availability and frequency of alternative reinforcing activities, especially those that are incompatible with a substance-abusing lifestyle.

Alcohol or drug use can be decreased by arranging the environment so that aversive events or the loss of reinforcing events occur as a consequence of such use. The following discussion illustrates how this general strategy is implemented in CRA and CM interventions.

TREATMENT OF ALCOHOL ABUSE AND DEPENDENCE

Community Reinforcement Approach. The seminal CRA study was conducted with 16 patients admitted to a state hospital in rural southern Illinois for treatment of alcoholism (Hunt & Azrin, 1973). These men were divided into eight matched pairs. Pair members were randomly assigned to receive CRA plus standard hospital care or standard care alone. Standard hospital care consisted of 25 didactic sessions of one hour each, involving lectures on Alcoholics Anonymous, alcoholism, and related medical problems.

CRA was designed to rearrange and improve the quality of the reinforcers obtained by patients through their vocational, family, social, and recreational activities. The goal was for these reinforcers to be available and of high quality when the patient was sober, and unavailable when drinking resumed. Plans for rearranging these reinforcers were individualized to conform to each patient's unique situation.

First, immediate barriers to participation in treatment were addressed, such as pending legal matters or other crises. For pressing legal matters, for example, staff members would help the patient find an appropriate lawyer. Second, vocational counseling was provided (Azrin & Besalel, 1980). Third, marital and family therapy was initiated during hospitalization and continued after discharge. Couples and other family members received training in positive communication skills to facilitate negotiation of contracts for reciprocally reinforcing changes in the patient's and family members' behavior, including alcohol abstinence on the part of the patient (Azrin, Naster et al., 1973). For those without family, attempts were made to identify someone in the community who was willing to serve as a surrogate family member. Fourth, social counseling was implemented to promote interactions with other friends and relatives who had low tolerance for drinking and to discourage interactions with drinkers. To further this process, staff members renovated a former tavern to serve as an alcohol-free social club that patients and their wives could attend for social activities. Finally, patients were taught to solve problems that previously had resulted in drinking, and they participated in behavioral rehearsals with the therapist to acquire new and more effective skills for resolving such situations without drinking.

On discharge from the hospital, CRA patients received a tapered schedule of counseling sessions: once or twice a week during the first month and then once a month across the next several months.

In the six months after hospital discharge, time spent drinking was 14% for participants in CRA versus 79% for those in standard treatment. Those treated with CRA had superior outcomes on a number of other outcome measures as well (Figure 1).

Improving CRA: CRA subsequently was expanded to include disulfiram therapy, with monitoring by a significant other (SO) to ensure medication compliance. Additionally, counseling directed at healthy methods of crisis resolution was added, as was a "buddy" system in which individuals in the alcoholic's neighborhood volunteered to be available to give assistance with practical issues such as auto repair. Finally, a switch from individual to group counseling was made to reduce costs (Azrin, 1976).

Twenty matched pairs of hospitalized men were randomly assigned to either the "improved" version of CRA or standard hospital care (which included advice to take disulfiram but no steps to ensure medication compliance).

During the six months after hospital discharge, outcomes achieved with CRA were superior to standard care in terms of time spent drinking (2% versus 55%), time unemployed (20% versus 56%), time away from family (7% versus 67%), and time spent institutionalized (0% versus 45%). The CRA group spent 90% or more time abstinent during a two-year followup period; comparable data were not reported for the standard treatment group.

Investigators at the University of New Mexico extended CRA to the treatment of homeless alcoholics (Smith, Meyers et al., 1998). A total of 106 adults were randomly assigned to receive CRA or standard care. Drinking levels declined more in the CRA condition than standard care through one year from intake, although both groups showed marked and undifferentiated improvements in employment and housing stability.

Social Club: One study completed as part of the original CRA series examined the effects of adding the social club described earlier to a standard regimen of outpatient counseling (Mallams, Godley et al., 1982). The club was designed to have the social atmosphere of a tavern but without alcohol. Individuals had to be abstinent to attend. Forty male and female alcoholic patients were randomly assigned to a group that was encouraged to attend the social club or to a control group that was not. At three-month followup, drinking in the social club group decreased from a baseline average of 4.67 oz. of alcohol consumed daily to 0.85 oz., whereas in the control group values were 3.56 and 3.32 oz., respectively. Greater improvements in the social club than control group were observed in ratings of behavioral impairment and time spent in heavy drinking situations.

Disulfiram Therapy: Another trial by Azrin and colleagues (1982) dissociated the effects of monitored disulfiram therapy from the other aspects of CRA. In a parallel-groups design, 43 male and female outpatients were randomized to receive usual care plus disulfiram therapy without compliance support, usual care plus disulfiram therapy involving SOs to support compliance, or CRA in combination with disulfiram therapy and support from SOs. CRA in combination with disulfiram and compliance procedures produced the greatest reductions in drinking, disulfiram in combination with compliance procedures but without CRA produced intermediate results, and the usual care plus disulfiram therapy without compliance support produced the poorest outcome. Interestingly, married patients did equally well with the full CRA treatment or disulfiram plus compliance procedures alone. Only unmarried patients appeared to need CRA treatment plus monitored disulfiram to achieve abstinence.

This study was the first full report on the efficacy of CRA with less-impaired outpatients. With these less-impaired individuals, treatment group differences were noted on measures of drinking only, whereas in the prior studies with more severe hospitalized alcoholics, differences were discerned on measures of time institutionalized and employed.

Helping SOs: Sisson and Azrin (1986) adapted CRA for use with the SOs of treatment-resistant alcoholics. Twelve SOs were randomly assigned to receive the CRA intervention (n=7) or a standard program (n=5) involving group instruction about alcohol and the disease model of alcoholism. The CRA intervention included education about alcohol problems, information and discussion of the positive consequences of not drinking, assistance in involving the alcoholic in healthy activities, increasing the involvement of the SO in social and recreational activities, and training in how to respond to drinking episodes (including dangerous situations) and how to recommend treatment entry to the alcoholic family member. In the control group, none of the alcoholics entered treatment during the three-month followup and their drinking remained unchanged. In the CRA group, by contrast, six of seven alcoholics entered treatment and average drinking decreased from 25 days per month at pretreatment to fewer than five days per month posttreatment. A more recent study conducted at the University of New Mexico replicated those findings, demonstrating greater efficacy of CRA than either a Johnson Institute confrontational intervention or Al-Anon facilitation therapy in helping SOs get unmotivated alcoholics into treatment (Miller, Meyers et al., 1999).

Conclusions: The evidence is strong in support of CRA's efficacy in treating alcohol-dependent patients, even when the clinical situation is complicated by homelessness. The evidence also supports the efficacy of CRA in helping SOs facilitate treatment entry among individuals who are unmotivated for treatment. CRA seems to have unrealized potential for the treatment of other special populations whose problems involve alcohol abuse or dependence, including patients with serious mental illness or other medical disorders such as HIV or other infectious disease. (Uses of CRA with adolescent substance users and adults with cocaine and opiate dependence are reviewed later in this chapter.) A therapist's manual on the use of CRA to treat alcohol abuse and dependence is available (Meyers & Smith, 1995).

Contingency Management. The goal of CM is to systematically weaken substance use and strengthen abstinence (Higgins & Silverman, 1999). Contingencies are arranged so that reinforcing or punishing events are contingent on the use of alcohol or other drugs or other behaviors deemed important to the treatment process, such as medication compliance or regular attendance at counseling sessions. Often, but not always, CM procedures are implemented as a component of a more comprehensive treatment intervention.

In the treatment of alcohol abuse and dependence, CM procedures have been used to reduce drinking and to increase compliance in taking medications and with other components of treatment (Higgins & Petry, 1999).

Reducing Drinking: The first randomized trial to examine the efficacy of CM in the treatment of alcohol dependence was conducted with chronic offenders under public inebriation statutes (Miller, 1975). Twenty arrestees were randomly assigned to a CM or control group. By reducing their drinking, those in the CM group earned housing, employment, medical care, and meals through several cooperating social service agencies. Sobriety was assessed through direct staff observation of gross intoxication and randomly administered blood alcohol concentrations (BACs). BACs of less than 0.01% maintained services, whereas BACs of 0.01% or more, or gross intoxication, resulted in termination of services for five days. Subjects in the control group received the same goods and services, independent of BACs or intoxication.

Subjects in the CM and control groups were arrested an average of 1.7 ± 1.2 and 1.4 ± 1.1 times during a two-month baseline period. During the two-month intervention period, arrests decreased to a mean of 0.3 ± 0.5 in the CM group and remained relatively unchanged at 1.3 ± 0.8 in the control group. (See Miller, Hersen et al. [1974] for an early controlled case study of the use of CM to treat alcohol dependence.)

After a relatively long period without research on the use of CM in the treatment of alcohol abuse and dependence, a clinical trial was reported recently in which 42 alcohol-dependent clients entering an intensive outpatient treatment program were randomly assigned to standard treatment plus CM or standard treatment alone (Petry, Martin et al., 2000). Standard treatment consisted of five hours per day of group sessions focused on relapse prevention, in addition to social and recreational training and participation in Twelve Step-oriented groups. This intensive treatment was provided for four weeks and was followed by aftercare consisting of similar group sessions one to three days per week. In both groups, patients met with a research assistant daily during intensive treatment and weekly during aftercare to provide a breath sample. In the CM group, patients earned the chance to compete for a prize for each negative BAC they submitted and for each of three preset activities they completed each week. Prizes ranged in value from $1 to $100. Of the patients assigned to the CM condition, 84% remained in treatment for the eight-week treatment period, compared with only 22% of those assigned to the standard treatment condition. By the end of the treatment period, 69% of the patients in the CM group had not experienced a relapse to alcohol use, compared with 39% of those in the standard treatment condition.

Use With Special Populations: The authors are not aware of any reports of clinical trials involving the use of CM to treat alcohol abuse and dependence in special populations, but successful controlled case studies involving the use of CM to reduce drinking among schizophrenic veterans (Peniston, 1988) and adolescent alcohol abusers (Brigham, Rekers et al., 1981) have been reported.

Increasing Treatment Compliance: CM can be used to increase treatment compliance. For example, alcohol abuse and dependence are a frequent cause of discharge from methadone treatment for opiate dependence (Bickel, Marion et al., 1987). At least three experimental reports support the efficacy of CM for increasing disulfiram compliance in this population (Bickel, Rizzuto et al., 1989; Liebson, Bigelow et al., 1973; Liebson, Tommasello et al., 1978). A preliminary report indicated that requiring alcoholic methadone-maintenance patients to ingest disulfiram as a condition for obtaining their daily methadone dose significantly reduced their alcohol use (Liebson, Bigelow et al., 1973). That report was followed by a well-controlled study (Liebson, Tommasello et al., 1978) in which 23 alcoholic methadone patients were randomly assigned to one of two groups: 13 patients received methadone treatment contingent on compliance with disulfiram therapy, while 10 control subjects also received a recommendation of disulfiram therapy, but noncompliance had no effect on their methadone treatment. During the 180-day study period, subjects in the methadone-contingent group spent 2% of study days drinking, as compared with 21% for the control group. Similar results

were reported by Bickel and colleagues (1989) using a controlled case-study design.

Robichaud and colleagues (1979) used a within-subject reversal design to evaluate the efficacy of mandated disulfiram therapy in a study conducted with 21 industrial employees referred for job-related problems with alcohol. Treatment consisted exclusively of mandatory supervised disulfiram ingestion. The main dependent variable was absenteeism. Median absenteeism rates, which had been 9.8% during a 24-month baseline period, decreased to 1.7% during almost one year of treatment.

Gallant and colleagues (Gallant, Bishop et al., 1968, 1973; Gallant, Faulkner et al., 1968) conducted a series of experimental studies that examined the efficacy of mandated treatment in criminal justice populations. In the initial study (Gallant, Bishop et al., 1968), 84 repeat offenders under public inebriation statutes were randomized to (1) six months of mandated weekly group therapy, (2) six months of mandated group therapy plus observed disulfiram ingestion three times a week, (3) observed disulfiram therapy three times a week with no other intervention, and (4) usual sentencing, with an informal suggestion by the judge to attend the alcoholism clinic. For participants in groups 1, 2, and 3, noncompliance was to result in individuals being incarcerated for a minimum of 60 days, but that contingency was not systematically enforced. Less than 10% of the assigned subjects were available for the six-month followup evaluation, which precluded drawing any meaningful conclusions from the study.

Results were no better in a followup study by the same group that included an inpatient treatment component (Gallant, Bishop et al., 1973). Finally, Ditman and colleagues (1967) reported similarly poor results in the ability of mandated treatment to significantly affect outcome with chronic offenders.

In contrast, Gallant and colleagues (1968) reported good success with compulsory treatment of alcoholics with more serious criminal offenses. Nineteen criminal alcoholics were randomly assigned to either a group for which attendance in outpatient alcoholism treatment was a requirement for parole, or to a control group for which attendance after the first appointment was urged but not required. (Criminal alcoholics were defined as persons who recently served a sentence of a year or more in a state penitentiary for a major offense that was directly or indirectly associated with alcohol use.) Subjects in the compulsory group were instructed that failure to attend a scheduled clinic visit was a violation of parole, for which they would be returned to prison to serve out their time (typically several years).

Ninety percent (9 of 10) of treatment-compulsory subjects attended treatment regularly for at least six months, compared with only 11% (1 of 9) of treatment-voluntary subjects. At 12 months, 70% (7 of 10) of contingent subjects were abstinent and working during their parole, whereas 78% (7 of 9) of treatment-voluntary subjects were either in prison or had violated parole and were at large.

The reasons for the different outcomes in the studies conducted with the chronic offenders and the more serious criminals are unclear, but law enforcement officials appeared more willing to enforce the contingencies with the latter group and the more serious offenders faced lengthier sentences for noncompliance.

Ersner-Hershfield and colleagues (1981) reported that compliance improved when offenders found guilty of driving under the influence (DUI) offenses were required to submit a $50 deposit at the first treatment session and then permitted to earn back a $5 check by attending treatment and turning in self-reports of recent drinking. (Readers interested in the efficacy of compulsory treatment for DUI offenders may want to examine a report by Ries [1982], which was not published in a peer-reviewed journal but provides evidence that one year of compulsory treatment can reduce DUI recidivism.)

Conclusions: CM has been used less extensively in the treatment of alcohol abuse and dependence than with other substances, partially because of the difficulty of objectively monitoring alcohol intake. Unlike most illicit drugs, in which urinalysis provides an objective marker of drug use during the several days preceding the test, the only practical objective measure of alcohol use is the BAC. Unfortunately, BAC provides evidence of use only during the few hours preceding the test. Considering that alcohol often is abused in an episodic or binge manner, this absence of a biological marker with an appropriate detection duration makes it difficult to reinforce or punish alcohol use. Nevertheless, the reports by Miller (1975) and Brigham and colleagues (1981) suggest that this difficulty can be overcome by relying on a combination of observations by others in the subject's natural environment and by randomly scheduled BAC tests. An alternative strategy is to target behaviors that are more readily monitored and incompatible with alcohol use, which is the rationale behind the use of monitored disulfiram therapy and compulsory treatment. The study by Azrin and

colleagues (1982) on the use of monitored disulfiram therapy as part of CRA and the studies described earlier with alcoholic patients in methadone maintenance illustrate ways in which disulfiram compliance can be reinforced effectively when the contingencies are managed systematically.

The criminal justice system would seem to be an ideal setting for making greater use of compulsory disulfiram therapy as a less expensive alternative to incarceration, but the controlled studies needed to evaluate the efficacy of that strategy are not available. As the studies by Gallant and colleagues (1968) on compulsory treatment illustrate, getting consequences implemented by the criminal justice system in a systematic and timely manner is no small challenge. Yet another alternative is to reinforce both negative BAC tests and compliance with other treatment goals deemed to be incompatible with drinking. The study by Petry and colleagues (2000) demonstrated the efficacy of this combined approach. Overall, CM appears to have more to offer alcohol treatment in general and treatment of alcoholic offenders in particular than currently is being realized.

TREATMENT OF COCAINE ABUSE AND DEPENDENCE

Community Reinforcement Approach. Several controlled trials completed at the University of Vermont demonstrate the efficacy of an intervention that combines CRA and CM for outpatient treatment of cocaine dependence. The seminal studies were two trials that compared CRA in combination with contingent voucher-based reinforcement with standard drug abuse counseling (Higgins, Delaney et al., 1991; Higgins, Budney et al., 1993a). The first trial, of 12 weeks' duration, assigned consecutively admitted clinic patients to the respective treatment groups, whereas the second trial, of 24 weeks' duration, used random patient assignment. In both trials, CRA plus vouchers retained patients in treatment longer and resulted in greater cocaine abstinence than did standard counseling. For example, in the randomized trial, 58% of patients assigned to the CRA-plus-vouchers treatment completed 24 weeks of treatment, compared with 11% of patients assigned to standard counseling. Further, 68% and 42% of patients in the CRA-plus-vouchers group achieved 8 and 16 weeks of continuous cocaine abstinence, compared with 11% and 5% of those in the counseling group.

Significantly greater cocaine abstinence was documented by urinalysis at 9- and 12-month followup in the CRA-plus-vouchers group than in the standard counseling

Figure 2.   Mean Duration of Continuous Cocaine Abstinence

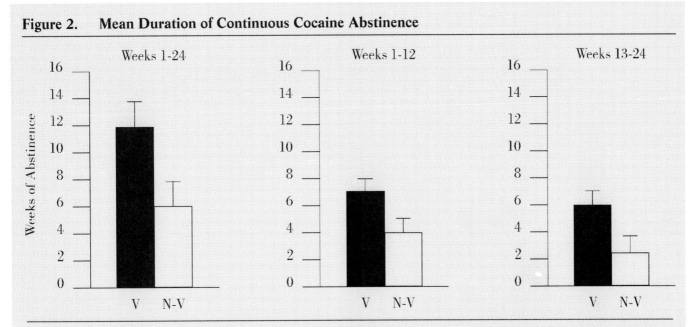

Mean duration of continuous cocaine abstinence, as documented by urinalysis testing in each treatment group during weeks 1-24, 1-12, and 13-24 of treatment. Solid and shaded bars indicate the voucher (V) and no-voucher (N-V) groups. Error bars represent + S.E.M. From Higgins ST, Budney AJ, Bickel WK et al. (1994). Incentives improve treatment retention and cocaine abstinence in ambulatory cocaine-dependent patients. *Archives of General Psychiatry* 51:568-576. Reprinted by permission of the publisher.

group, whereas the groups showed comparable and significant improvements on the Addiction Severity Index (ASI) (Higgins, Budney et al., 1995).

Disulfiram Therapy: Approximately 60% of the cocaine-dependent patients in these trials also were alcohol dependent. As described above, monitored disulfiram therapy is a core component of CRA and thus was offered to all individuals who reported evidence of concurrent alcohol dependence and abuse. An uncontrolled chart review identified a significant association between disulfiram therapy and reductions in both alcohol and cocaine use (Higgins, Budney et al., 1993b). Results from that uncontrolled study were supported by two randomized trials. In a pilot study, 18 outpatients being treated for alcohol and cocaine addiction were randomized to receive disulfiram or naltrexone therapy (Carroll, Ziedonis et al. 1993). Disulfiram therapy resulted in greater reductions in drinking and cocaine use than naltrexone therapy. In a larger randomized trial involving 117 outpatients who used both alcohol and cocaine (Carroll, Nich et al., 1998), abstinence from alcohol and cocaine use increased twofold to threefold among those engaged in Twelve Step programs or treated with cognitive-behavioral therapies in combination with disulfiram, compared with those engaged in Twelve Step programs or treated with psychosocial therapies alone.

Helping SOs: A trial with SOs of drug abusers demonstrated the efficacy of CRA in helping SOs facilitate entry into treatment among alcoholic family members (Kirby, Marlowe et al., 1999). In the trial, 32 concerned SOs were randomly assigned to receive CRA or to participate in a Twelve Step program. At 10 weeks after clinic contact, CRA was significantly better than a Twelve Step approach in facilitating treatment entry by the family member. Similarly positive results were observed in a recent trial involving 90 subjects, in which CRA proved superior to Al-Anon and Nar-Anon in promoting treatment entry among family members with cocaine and other drug dependence. (Meyers, Miller et al., 2002).

Conclusions: CRA combined with CM is an efficacious treatment for cocaine dependence. Importantly, studies of that approach provided some of the earliest evidence that cocaine dependence could be managed effectively in outpatient settings. In the course of assessing the efficacy of this combined treatment, it was learned that most patients also

Figure 3.   Abstinence Post-Treatment (Point Prevalence)

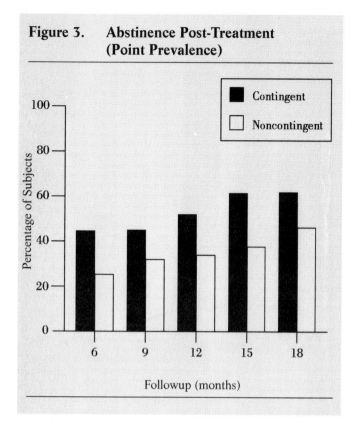

were alcohol dependent. That observation provided an opportunity to apply monitored disulfiram therapy to this population. Subsequent controlled trials demonstrated the efficacy of monitored disulfiram therapy for decreasing cocaine and alcohol use in those who used both substances. Consistent with what has been demonstrated with alcoholics, CRA is efficacious in assisting SOs in motivating family members in need of addiction treatment to access those services. Finally, the voucher component of such combined interventions has been shown to be efficacious in reducing cocaine use in several controlled trials. (A therapists' manual on CRA plus voucher treatment for cocaine dependence is available at no cost from the National Institute on Drug Abuse [Budney & Higgins, 1998].)

Contingency Management. In the CM procedure used in combination with CRA in studies conducted at the University of Vermont, patients' continued abstinence from cocaine was reinforced with vouchers that could be exchanged for retail items. The voucher system was in effect for weeks 1 through 12 of a 24-week intervention. The value of the vouchers increased with each consecutive cocaine-

negative specimen delivered, while cocaine-positive specimens reset the value of vouchers back to their initial level. Those who were continuously abstinent (as evidenced by cocaine-negative urine tests) earned the equivalent of $997.50 during weeks 1 through 12.

In a randomized trial, 40 patients were assigned to receive CRA with or without vouchers (Higgins, Budney et al., 1994). Seventy-five percent of patients in the group with vouchers completed 24 weeks of treatment, compared with 40% in the group without vouchers. Average duration of continuous cocaine abstinence in the two groups was 11.7 ± 2.0 weeks in the voucher group versus 6.0 ± 1.5 in the no-voucher group (Figure 2). At the end of the 24-week treatment period and during followup, significant decreases from pretreatment scores were observed in both treatment groups on the ASI family/social and alcohol scales, with no differences found between the groups (Higgins, Budney et al., 1995). Both groups decreased on the ASI drug scale, but the magnitude of change was significantly greater in the voucher than the no-voucher group, and only the voucher group showed a significant improvement on the ASI psychiatric scale. In a more recent randomized trial that examined the efficacy of contingent vouchers in combination with CRA (Higgins, Wong et al., 2000), positive effects on cocaine abstinence remained discernible through 12 months posttreatment and 15 months after discontinuation of the voucher program (Figure 3).

The seminal study demonstrating the generalizability of this approach to inner-city alcohol and drug users examined the efficacy of the voucher program with cocaine-using methadone maintenance patients (Silverman, Higgins et al., 1996). During a 12-week study, subjects in the experimental group (n=19) received vouchers that could be exchanged for retail items, contingent on cocaine-negative urine tests. A matched control group (n=18) received the vouchers independent of urinalysis results. Both groups received a standard form of outpatient drug abuse counseling. Cocaine use was substantially reduced in the experimental group but remained relatively unchanged in the control group (Figure 4). Use of opiates also decreased in the contingent group during the voucher period, even though the contingency was associated exclusively with cocaine use. Subsequent randomized trials in the same group (Silverman, Wong et al., 1998; Silverman, Chutuape et al., 1999) and others (Kirby, Marlowe et al., 1998) further demonstrated the efficacy of this approach in decreasing cocaine use among inner-city drug users.

Figure 4.   Longest Duration of Sustained Cocaine Abstinence

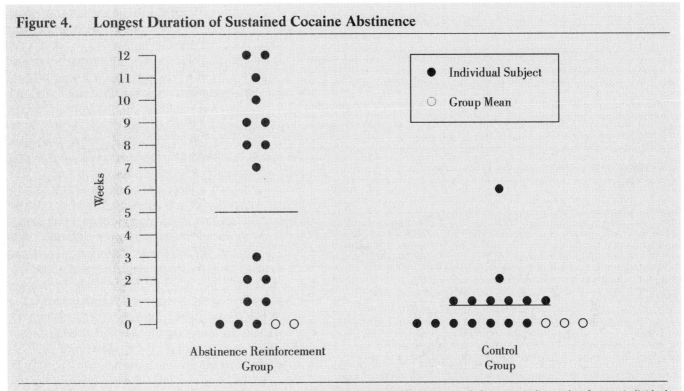

Longest duration of sustained cocaine abstinence achieved during the 12-week voucher condition. Each data point indicates data from an individual subject and the lines represent group means. Subjects in the reinforcement and control conditions are displayed in the left and right columns, respectively. Open circles represent early study dropouts. From Silverman K, Higgins ST, Brooner RK et al. (1996). Sustained cocaine abstinence in methadone maintenance patients through voucher-based reinforcement therapy. *Archives of General Psychiatry* 53:409-415. Reprinted by permission of the publisher.

Use With Special Populations: A recently completed study supported the efficacy of vouchers in promoting abstinence from cocaine and heroin and encouraging participation in vocational training among pregnant and recently postpartum women (Silverman, Svikis et al., 2001). The study involved 40 women who continued to use cocaine and heroin despite receiving methadone and intensive psychosocial treatment. Half of the women were randomly assigned to a therapeutic workplace (TW) intervention, whereas the other half were assigned to a control group. Women in the TW condition earned vouchers for cocaine and heroin abstinence and for participating in vocational training. Across a 24-week assessment, 40% of the women assigned to the TW group were abstinent on 75% or more of the testing occasions, compared with 10% of the women in the control group. This study was an initial report. Future reports on longer-term abstinence and the acquisition of vocational skills are planned.

An approach that combined day treatment with access to work therapy and a housing contingency demonstrated the efficacy of CM with homeless persons who used cocaine and other substances (Milby, Schumacher et al., 1996). In the study, 176 homeless persons who used cocaine and other substances were randomly assigned to receive enhanced or usual care. Enhanced care involved two months of intensive clinic attendance five days a week. During the final four months of the six-month treatment period, the intensity of day treatment was reduced, and subjects could participate in a work therapy program that involved refurbishing houses. They could also reside in the refurbished housing for a modest rental fee. Participation in the work program and housing were contingent on abstinence. Usual

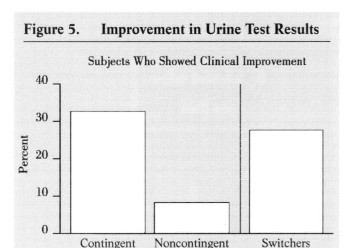

Figure 5.   Improvement in Urine Test Results

Subjects Who Showed Clinical Improvement

Percentages of subjects whose urine test results improved 10% or more from baseline to intervention periods and submitted at least 12 consecutive drug-free tests during the intervention period are shown for the original contingent and noncontingent take-home groups and also for the group of noncontingent subjects who received delayed exposure to the contingent protocol later in treatment. From Stitzer ML, Iguchi MY & Felch LJ (1992). Contingent take-home incentive: Effects on drug use of methadone maintenance patients. *Journal of Consulting and Clinical Psychology* 60(6):927-934. Reprinted by permission of the publisher.

care consisted of twice-weekly drug abuse counseling and referral to community agencies for housing and vocational services.

At the two-month assessment, the percentage of patients whose urine tests were positive for cocaine had decreased from a baseline of approximately 60% to 30% in the enhanced group. In the usual-care group, positive tests increased from 55% at baseline to 65%. The percentage of negative test results also was higher in the enhanced than in the usual-care group at the 6- and 12-month followup assessments, although the differences no longer were statistically significant. Enhanced care also produced greater reductions in alcohol use and fewer days of homelessness at the 6- and 12-month assessments. A followup study by the same investigators systematically replicated those findings (Milby, Schumacher et al., 2000).

A preliminary investigation of the use of CM in persons with co-occurring cocaine use and serious mental illness also was promising (Shaner, Roberts et al., 1997). A within-subject reversal design was used with two male veterans whose cocaine abuse had been refractory to various prior treatment efforts. Both spent their monthly Social Security benefit

checks on cocaine and other substances, were homeless, and required frequent hospitalizations. Over a period of several weeks, these two individuals were given an opportunity to earn $25 a day for cocaine abstinence. Compared to before and after intervention levels, cocaine use decreased significantly in both patients during the period when the CM intervention was in place. These results are being pursued in clinical trials in which mental health clinics will use Social Security benefits to reinforce abstinence among patients with co-occurring mental and substance use disorders (Ries & Comtois, 1997).

Conclusions: Little doubt remains that cocaine use can be reduced with CM. Nevertheless, important practical issues remain to be resolved. These include how such interventions might be deployed in community clinics, where resources to support material incentives are limited and regular urine testing may not be possible. In such situations, goods and services for use as incentives might be obtained through donations from community businesses. Other incentives might be accessed through existing community resources (such as swimming pools and basketball courts) (Higgins, Budney et al., 1994; Kirby, Amass et al., 1999). The reliable efficacy of CM demands that it be incorporated into community clinics, but exactly how that can be done remains unclear.

TREATMENT OF OPIOID ABUSE AND DEPENDENCE

Methadone and other opioid substitution therapies represent an important modality for the treatment of opioid dependence (NIH-CDC, 1997). These treatments are efficacious in suppressing heroin use and associated criminal activity (Ball & Ross, 1991) but do not decrease other forms of drug use and related problems common in this population (Silverman, Preston et al., 1998).

Community Reinforcement Approach. There are two controlled studies of CRA treatment of opioid dependence. In one, 181 methadone maintenance patients were randomly assigned to CRA (n=52), CRA combined with relapse prevention therapy (n=62), or standard drug abuse counseling (n=67) (Abbott, Weller et al., 1998). In this study, CRA did not involve the use of vouchers. Results were restricted to the treatment period. The two CRA groups were combined for data analysis purposes as the relapse prevention sessions were to be delivered after the main treatment period. Somewhat more patients in the CRA groups (89%) than the standard group (78%) achieved at least three weeks of continuous opioid abstinence, and the CRA groups exhibited greater before and after treatment reductions in self-reported drug use.

In the other study, CRA in combination with vouchers was compared with drug abuse counseling in 39 opioid-dependent patients who were undergoing buprenorphine detoxification (Bickel, Amass et al., 1997). The voucher program was modified so that half of the available vouchers could be earned by opiate-free urine tests and the other half by participating in activities identified as part of the CRA therapy. More subjects assigned to the CRA-plus-vouchers group completed the 24-week detoxification protocol (53% versus 20%) and more achieved at least eight weeks of continuous abstinence from illicit opiates (47% versus 15%).

Conclusions: These two trials suggest that CRA is efficacious in reducing illicit drug use among patients receiving opioid substitution therapy. The efficacy of vouchers and other CM procedures with this population is well established (see below). Studies further evaluating the efficacy of CRA with and without contingent vouchers in this population would be helpful in more fully elucidating how this treatment approach can be used to optimize outcomes during opioid substitution therapy.

Contingency Management. The methadone take-home privilege, in which an extra daily dose of methadone is dispensed to the patient for ingestion on the following day, offers a convenient and effective incentive for CM protocols (Stitzer & Bigelow, 1978). Studies by Stitzer and colleagues (1982) and Iguchi and colleagues (1988) examined take-home incentives in methadone patients who abused benzodiazepines. When take-home privileges could be earned by providing drug-free urine toxicology results, temporary abstinence (12 to 20 weeks) was observed in about 50% of study patients during the contingent take-home intervention. Magura and colleagues (1988) found that one month of contracting for contingent take-home privileges resulted in 34% of their polydrug-dependent subjects achieving abstinence, while Milby and colleagues (1978) reported that a similar percentage of clients responded to a take-home incentive program.

Most of these studies focused on selected groups of patients identified with polydrug problems and used within-subject designs to evaluate the efficacy of contingent take-home programs. In a randomized clinical trial (Stitzer, Iguchi et al., 1992), take-home incentives were examined in 54 newly admitted methadone maintenance patients. Half

the group received take-home privileges contingent on abstinence from illicit drug use, while the other half received the take-home doses noncontingently. Overall, 32% of the contingent patients achieved sustained periods of abstinence during the intervention (mean, 9.4 weeks; range, 5 to 15 weeks), compared with approximately 10% in the control group (Figure 5). The beneficial effect of contingent take-home delivery was replicated within the group of noncontingent patients, who switched to the contingent intervention after their six-month evaluation in the main study (partial crossover design).

Take-home deliveries can be used in combination with other programmed consequences as an "incentive package." A study by McCaul and colleagues (1984) examined the effects of an incentive package on relapse to opiate drug use during a 90-day ambulatory methadone detoxification. Patients were randomly assigned to a control or contingent intervention condition. In the contingent group, opiate abstinence resulted in a take-home day and $10 cash, whereas opiate use resulted in increased counseling contact, urine sample collection, and data questionnaire requirements. The contingent procedure was effective in delaying relapse.

Another effective consequence for reducing supplemental drug use is a methadone dose change. Suppression of opiate use during outpatient methadone detoxification was achieved in a study in which the contingent incentive for opiate abstinence was an increase in the methadone dose of up to 20 mg (Higgins, Stitzer et al., 1986). Non-contingent dose increases failed to produce the same degree of abstinence. Another study extended the evaluation of dose-change incentives by showing that decreases in polydrug abuse could be demonstrated during methadone maintenance when the methadone dose was increased above original maintenance levels as a result of drug-free urine toxicology results, and when the dose was decreased below original maintenance levels as a consequence of drug-positive urine toxicology results (Stitzer, Bickel et al., 1986).

Evaluating still other reinforcers, the study by Silverman and colleagues (1996) demonstrated the efficacy of contingent voucher-based reinforcement for reducing cocaine abuse among methadone-maintenance patients. Reductions in drug use during ambulatory detoxification also were reported in a controlled trial by Hall and colleagues (1979), which used small amounts of money ($4 to $10 per sample) to reinforce drug-free urine specimens. Similarly, positive results were achieved by using vouchers in an extended detoxification (Piotrowski, Tusel et al.,1999). Chutuape and colleagues (1999) provided preliminary evidence that combining a seven-day inpatient detoxification with subsequent outpatient CM (in which the patient could choose between contingent vouchers or medication take-home doses) reduced sedative use among methadone maintenance patients.

Carroll and colleagues (1995) were unsuccessful in an attempt to use a small amount of contingent monetary reinforcement (subjects could earn $15 weekly for three consecutive negative urine screens, in conjunction with weekly prenatal care and relapse prevention groups) to increase drug abstinence in pregnant methadone-maintained patients (n=7). Compared with a randomized control group in which patients received standard methadone treatment (n=7), no increases in drug abstinence were observed in the intervention group. Requiring an entire week of abstinence to earn a reinforcer may have been too large a response requirement, considering the relatively small amounts of the monetary reinforcer.

The possible negative influence of reinforcer delay and response requirement is supported by the results of a study by Rowan-Szal and colleagues (1994), who examined the influence of these factors in decreasing supplemental drug use and increasing counseling participation among methadone maintenance patients. Subjects could earn stars exchangeable for low-cost retail items by attending individual and group counseling sessions. Stars earned also were displayed on bulletin boards in counselors' offices. Subjects were randomly assigned to high reward (four stars required per back-up reinforcer), low reward (eight stars required per reinforcer), and delayed reward (stars could not be redeemed until the end of the three-month intervention) treatment conditions. Only the high reward condition reduced drug use and increased counseling attendance.

Treatment-Termination Contracting. Another commonly used intervention is the contingent availability of further methadone treatment. The studies of mandated disulfiram therapy described earlier demonstrated that treatment outcomes could be improved for alcoholic methadone patients by using the threat of treatment termination. McCarthy and Borders (1985) showed that structured treatment involving the threat of methadone termination for failure to meet specified standards of drug-free urine submissions reduced illicit opiate use.

Medication Compliance: Naltrexone is an opioid antagonist that is effective in reducing illicit opioid abuse, but it is not used widely because of difficulties in maintaining medication compliance. Preston and colleagues (1999) demonstrated the efficacy of contingent vouchers for that purpose. A total of 58 opioid-dependent patients were randomly assigned to one of three groups: contingent vouchers for compliance with a three-times-a-week naltrexone regimen, vouchers provided independent of naltrexone compliance, and a no-voucher group. The contingent group was retained in treatment longer and ingested more medication than either comparison group. The positive effect on naltrexone compliance was replicated in a subsequent randomized clinical trial (Carroll, Ball et al., 2001).

Conclusions: Structured CM programs have considerable efficacy in reducing drug abuse by patients enrolled in opioid substitution therapy. That conclusion is consistent with the results of a meta-analysis examining the efficacy of CM in this population (Griffith, Rowan-Szal et al., 2000). The studies reviewed earlier demonstrate that contingent use of positive incentives can delay relapse during detoxification and reduce supplemental drug use during maintenance treatment. Further research is needed to focus on ways to optimize the utility and cost-effectiveness of incentives that are readily available in the context of methadone clinic operations. Also needed is research to further characterize treatment nonresponders and to identify more efficacious CM and other interventions for use with them. Combining brief hospitalizations with subsequent outpatient incentive programs may be effective with more severe patients. Finally, the use of vouchers or other CM interventions to enhance naltrexone compliance merits investigation.

Contingent negative incentives can decrease supplemental drug use among opioid replacement patients. However, positive incentives have the advantage of keeping patients in treatment, whereas negative incentives (particularly those involving methadone dose decreases or threat of treatment termination) may result in treatment dropout. Treatment dropout or termination among severely dependent individuals can have serious, life-threatening consequences and should be avoided if possible. Whether positive and negative incentives can be used together to increase the potency of CM for improving outcomes during opioid substitution therapy merits investigation.

TREATMENT OF OTHER ABUSE AND DEPENDENCE

Community Reinforcement Approach. Azrin and colleagues (1994) adapted CRA for use with adolescent users of alcohol and other drugs. The intervention had three components:

stimulus control, urge control, and social control/contracting. The stimulus control component involved assisting the young people in identifying situations that were "safe" or "risky" for substance use, in combination with therapist-assisted problem-solving about how to increase the amount of time spent in safe situations and decrease the time spent in risky situations. Urge control involved teaching youth to recognize the early internal events that were precursors to alcohol or drug use and how to interrupt those internal events with alternative activities that are incompatible with substance use. Social control/contracting focused on involving parents in providing youth with opportunities to engage in safe activities, contingent with their compliance with activities that are incompatible with substance use.

Twenty-six youth were randomly assigned to receive individualized CRA therapy or a group-delivered alternative treatment involving supportive-expressive therapy. Over a six-month treatment period, the youth assigned to CRA engaged in significantly less drug use than did those assigned to supportive-expressive therapy. Such differences remained evident in posttreatment followup assessments conducted on average of nine months after treatment discontinuation (Azrin, Acierno et al., 1996).

Contingency Management. A controlled case study completed with two adults dependent on cocaine and marijuana demonstrated the sensitivity of chronic marijuana use to voucher-based reinforcement of abstinence (Budney, Higgins et al., 1991). Those findings were replicated in a recent randomized trial completed with marijuana-dependent adult outpatients (Budney, Higgins et al., 2000). A total of 60 men and women were assigned to one of three 14-week treatments: motivational enhancement (M), M plus behavioral coping-skills therapy (MBT), or M and BT plus voucher-based reinforcement of abstinence (MBTV). M involved four therapy sessions of 60 to 90 minutes focused on enhancing participants' motivation to abstain from marijuana use. MBT included an additional eight one-hour sessions focused on coping skills (for example, dealing with urges, drug refusal training, and the like). MBTV included all of the above, in addition to vouchers delivered contingent on marijuana-negative results in twice-weekly urine tests over weeks 3 to 14 of treatment. The voucher program generally operated the same way as those described earlier in the sections on cocaine abuse and dependence, but at about half the voucher value. No differences between the treatment groups were found in retention, but patients assigned to MBTV achieved significantly greater marijuana abstinence

during the intervention period than those assigned to the two other treatments. For example, 50% and 40% of those assigned to MBTV achieved four and seven weeks of continuous abstinence, compared with 30% and 5% of those assigned to MBT and 10% and 5% of those assigned to M. A greater percentage of participants assigned to MBTV were found to be abstinent at the end-of-treatment assessment, compared with those assigned to MBT or M (35%, 10%, 5%, respectively). Followup status was not assessed in this trial.

A recently completed feasibility study demonstrated the sensitivity of marijuana use by schizophrenic outpatients to monetary incentives for abstinence (Sigmon, Steingard et al., in press). A total of 18 regular marijuana users with serious mental illness participated in the study. They were not seeking substance abuse treatment, but were willing to attempt abstinence as part of the study. During two baseline conditions, participants received monetary rewards independent of their urinalysis results. During three incentive conditions, participants received varying amounts of money only if urine toxicology results indicated marijuana abstinence. Instructions issued before the incentive condition informed participants about when abstinence would need to be initiated to allow sufficient clearance time before the incentive conditions began. The amount of money that could be earned ranged from $25 to $100 per negative specimen in twice-weekly testing.

Abstinence increased in the contingent compared with the baseline conditions, thus demonstrating the sensitivity of marijuana use to the reinforcement contingencies. With several individuals, smoking was not sensitive to the contingencies, even when the monetary amount was increased to the $100 per test value.

An important practical question not answered in this initial feasibility study was how much the incentives could have been reduced in value without losing efficacy among those who were sensitive to the incentives. That question merits investigation.

Voucher-based reinforcement of abstinence was successfully extended to the treatment of pregnant smokers in a recent clinical trial (Donatelle, Prows et al., 2000). A total of 220 pregnant smokers were randomly assigned to a treatment group involving contingent vouchers for abstinence or to a control group. Women in both groups received smoking cessation self-help kits. Those in the treatment group were asked to include an SO in treatment. All participants were telephoned monthly and asked to self-report smoking status. Those in the treatment condition who reported abstinence were invited to the clinic to provide a saliva specimen. If the specimen confirmed abstinence, the participant earned a $50 voucher and the SO received a voucher as well. A greater percentage of smokers in the treatment condition (32%) than in the control condition (9%) were abstinent at eight months' gestation, and that difference was maintained at the two-month postpartum assessment (21% versus 6%).

Two feasibility studies support the potential for extending CM to the treatment of smoking among adolescents (Corby, Roll et al., 2000) and schizophrenics (Roll, Higgins et al., 1998). A similar procedure was used in both studies. Smokers who were not trying to quit but who were willing to try to stop smoking as part of a study were offered the challenge of not smoking for five consecutive days—a difficult challenge for most regular cigarette smokers. Under baseline conditions, subjects were encouraged to abstain but received no monetary incentive when they did so. Under the intervention condition, participants earned money by submitting breath carbon monoxide readings indicative of recent abstinence three times a day. In both populations, participants achieved higher abstinence rates in the incentive than the baseline conditions.

The results with the schizophrenic smokers have been systematically replicated, although the addition of nicotine replacement therapy did not enhance the efficacy of the monetary incentives (Tidey, O'Neill et al., in press). Results from several rigorous laboratory-based studies also support the sensitivity of smoking among schizophrenics to reinforcement contingencies and other environmental manipulations (Tidey, Higgins et al., 1999; Tidey, O'Neill et al., 1999).

Conclusions: The extension of CRA to adolescents is quite promising, considering how few controlled trials have been conducted of treatments for that population. It is to be hoped that the promising findings with CRA in adolescents will be followed up with additional trials. The extensions of CM to marijuana dependence are encouraging as well. Concerns had been expressed that the relatively long elimination half-life of marijuana might represent an insurmountable obstacle to effective CM interventions because users would have to abstain for so long before collecting the first reward. The research described earlier leaves little doubt that such issues can be surmounted even

among individuals with serious mental illness. Logical next steps in this area of investigation are to examine the effects of contingent incentives on longer-term abstinence among marijuana-dependent outpatients who are without serious mental illness and to move the studies with schizophrenics from initial feasibility assessments to formal treatment interventions.

The successful extension of vouchers to the treatment of pregnant smokers could represent an important breakthrough. The 32% abstinence rates at the end-of-pregnancy assessment observed by Donatelle and colleagues exceeded the usual 20% or lower levels commonly observed among pregnant smokers. Indeed, those results were sufficiently encouraging to help foster a national initiative by The Robert Wood Johnson Foundation to support research on the use of incentives and other motivational interventions to increase smoking abstinence in pregnant women (Orleans, Barker et al., 2000).

Finally, the feasibility studies of the use of CM with adolescent and schizophrenic cigarette smokers provide a strong rationale for conducting randomized clinical trials to examine whether CM increases quit rates among adolescent and schizophrenic smokers—two populations for whom effective smoking-cessation treatments are sorely needed.

CONCLUSIONS

Within an operant framework, alcohol and other drug use is considered a normal, learned behavior that can be fruitfully conceptualized to fall along a continuum, ranging from light use with no problems to heavy use with many untoward effects. The same basic learning processes are assumed to operate across the substance-use continuum. Treatment strategies based on this conceptual framework attempt to weaken the reinforcement obtained from substance use and related activities and to enhance the material and social reinforcement obtained from other sources, particularly from participation in activities deemed to be incompatible with a substance-abusing lifestyle. CRA and CM procedures are based on this general strategy and are efficacious in treating patients whose dependence involves alcohol, cocaine, opioids, polydrugs, and certain other substances. CRA and CM offer no "magic bullets" for the treatment of these disorders and, as discussed earlier, much more remains to be learned about each of them. Those limitations notwithstanding, CRA and CM offer a range of empirically based and effective strategies for treating some of the most challenging populations and daunting aspects of substance abuse and dependence.

ACKNOWLEDGMENT: Preparation of this chapter was supported by grants RO1 DA09378, and RO1 DA14002 RO1 DA08076, from the National Institute on Drug Abuse.

REFERENCES

Abbott PJ, Weller SB, Delaney HD et al. (1998). Community reinforcement approach in the treatment of opiate addicts. *American Journal of Drug and Alcohol Abuse* 24:17-30.

Azrin NH (1976). Improvements in the community-reinforcement approach to alcoholism. *Behaviour Research and Therapy* 14:339-348.

Azrin NH & Besalel VA (1980). *Job Club Counselor's Manual.* Baltimore, MD: University Park Press.

Azrin NH, Acierno R, Kogan ES et al. (1996). Follow-up results of supportive versus behavioral therapy for illicit drug use. *Behaviour Research and Therapy* 34:41-46.

Azrin NH, Donohue B, Besalel VA et al. (1994). Youth drug abuse treatment: A controlled outcome study. *Journal of Child and Adolescent Substance Abuse* 3:1-16.

Azrin NH, Naster BJ & Jones R (1973). Reciprocity counseling: A rapid learning based procedure for marriage counseling. *Behaviour Research and Therapy* 11:364–382.

Azrin NH, Sisson RW, Meyers R et al. (1982). Alcoholism treatment by disulfiram and community reinforcement therapy. *Journal of Behavior Therapy and Experimental Psychiatry* 13:105-112.

Ball JC & Ross A (1991). *The Effectiveness of Methadone Maintenance Treatment.* New York, NY: Springer-Verlag.

Bickel WK & Amass L (1995). Buprenorphine treatment of opioid dependence: A review. *Experimental and Clinical Psychopharmacology* 3:477-489.

Bickel WK, Amass L, Higgins ST et al. (1997). Effects of adding behavioral treatment to opioid detoxification with buprenorphine. *Journal of Consulting and Clinical Psychology* 65:803-810.

Bickel WK, Marion I & Lowinson JH (1987). The treatment of alcoholic methadone patients: A review. *Journal of Substance Abuse Treatment* 4:15-19.

Bickel WK, Rizzuto P, Zielony RD et al. (1989). Combined behavioral and pharmacological treatment of alcoholic methadone patients. *Journal of Substance Abuse* 1:161-171.

Brigham SL, Rekers GA, Rosen AC et al. (1981). Contingency management in the treatment of adolescent alcohol drinking problems. *Journal of Psychology* 109:73-85.

Budney AJ & Higgins ST (1998). *The Community Reinforcement Plus Vouchers Approach: Manual 2: National Institute on Drug Abuse Therapy Manuals for Drug Addiction* (NIH Publication No. 98-4308). Rockville, MD: National Institute on Drug Abuse.

Budney AJ, Higgins ST, Delaney DD et al. (1991). Contingent reinforcement of abstinence with individuals abusing cocaine and marijuana. *Journal of Applied Behavior Analysis* 24:657-665.

Budney AJ, Higgins ST, Radonovich KJ et al. (2000). Adding voucher-based incentives to coping-skills and motivational enhancement improves outcomes during treatment for marijuana dependence. *Journal of Consulting and Clinical Psychology* 68:1051-1061

Carroll KM, Ball SA, Nich C et al. (2001). Targeting behavioral therapies to enhance naltrexone treatment of opioid dependence: Efficacy of contingency management and significant other involvement. *Archives of General Psychiatry* 58:755-761.

Carroll KM, Chang G, Behr H et al. (1995). Improving treatment outcome in pregnant, methadone-maintained women. *American Journal on Addictions* 4:56-59.

Carroll KM, Nich C, Ball SA et al. (1998). Treatment of cocaine and alcohol dependence with psychotherapy and disulfiram. *Addiction* 93:713-728.

Carroll KM, Ziedonis D, O'Malley S et al. (1993). Pharmacologic interventions for alcohol- and cocaine-abusing individuals: A pilot study of disulfiram vs. naltrexone. *American Journal on Addictions* 2:77–79.

Chutuape MA, Silverman K & Stitzer ML (1999). Contingent reinforcement sustains post-detoxification abstinence from multiple drugs: A preliminary study with methadone patients. *Drug and Alcohol Dependence* 54:69-81.

Corby EA, Roll JM, Ledgerwood DM et al. (2000). Contingency management interventions for treating the substance abuse of adolescents: A feasibility study. *Experimental and Clinical Psychopharmacology* 8:371-376.

Ditman KS, Crawford GG, Forgy EW et al. (1967). A controlled experiment on the use of court probation for drunk arrests. *American Journal of Psychiatry* 124:64-67.

Donatelle RJ, Prows SL, Champeau D et al. (2000). Randomized controlled trial using social support and financial incentives for high risk pregnant smokers: Significant other supporter (SOS) program. *Tobacco Control* 9 (Suppl III):iii67-iii69.

Ersner-Hershfield SM, Connors GJ & Maisto SA (1981). Clinical and experimental utility of refundable deposits. *Behavioral Research and Therapy* 19:455-457.

Gallant DM, Bishop MP, Faulkner MA et al. (1968). A comparative evaluation of compulsory (group therapy and/or Antabuse) and voluntary treatment of the chronic alcoholic municipal court offender. *Psychosomatics* 9:306-310.

Gallant DM, Bishop MP, Mouledoux A et al. (1973). The revolving-door alcoholic. *Archives of General Psychiatry* 28:633-635.

Gallant DM, Faulkner M, Stoy B et al. (1968). Enforced clinic treatment of paroled criminal alcoholics. *Quarterly Journal of Studies on Alcohol* 29:77-83.

Goldberg SR & Stolerman IP, eds. (1986). *Behavioral Analysis of Drug Dependence.* Orlando, FL: Academic Press.

Griffith JD, Rowan-Szal GA, Roark RR et al. (2000). Contingency management in outpatient methadone treatment: A meta-analysis. *Drug and Alcohol Dependence* 58:55-66.

Griffiths RR, Bigelow GE & Henningfield JE (1980). Similarities in animal and human drug taking behavior. In NK Mello (ed.) *Advances in Substance Abuse: Behavioral and Biological Research, Vol 1.* Greenwich, CT: JAI Press, 1-90.

Hall SM, Bass A, Hargreaves WA & Loeb P (1979). Contingency management and information feedback in outpatient heroin detoxification. *Behavioral Therapy* 10:443-451.

Higgins ST & Petry NM (1999). Contingency management: Incentives for sobriety. *Alcohol Research & Health* 23:122-127.

Higgins ST & Silverman K (1999). *Motivating Behavior Change Among Illicit Drug Abusers: Research on Contingency Management Interventions*. Washington, DC: American Psychological Association.

Higgins ST, Budney AJ, Bickel WK et al. (1993a). Achieving cocaine abstinence with a behavioral approach. *American Journal of Psychiatry* 150:763-769.

Higgins ST, Budney AJ, Bickel WK et al. (1993b). Disulfiram therapy in patients abusing cocaine and alcohol. *American Journal of Psychiatry* 150:675-676.

Higgins ST, Budney AJ, Bickel WK et al. (1994). Incentives improve treatment retention and cocaine abstinence in ambulatory cocaine-dependent patients. *Archives of General Psychiatry* 51:568-576.

Higgins ST, Budney AJ, Bickel WK et al. (1995). Outpatient behavioral treatment for cocaine dependence: One-year outcome. *Experimental and Clinical Psychopharmacology* 3:205-212.

Higgins ST, Delaney DD, Budney AJ et al. (1991). A behavioral approach to achieving initial cocaine abstinence. *American Journal of Psychiatry* 148:1218-1224.

Higgins ST, Stitzer ML, Bigelow GE et al. (1986). Contingent methadone delivery: Effects on illicit-opiate use. *Drug and Alcohol Dependence* 17:311-322.

Higgins ST, Wong CJ, Badger GJ et al. (2000). Contingent reinforcement increases cocaine abstinence during outpatient treatment and 1-year of follow-up. *Journal of Consulting and Clinical Psychology* 68:64-72.

Hunt GM & Azrin NH (1973). A community-reinforcement approach to alcoholism. *Behaviour Research and Therapy* 11:91-104.

Iguchi MY, Stitzer ML, Bigelow GE et al. (1988). Contingency management in methadone maintenance: Effects of reinforcing and aversive consequences on illicit polydrug use. *Drug and Alcohol Dependence* 22:1-7.

Kirby KC, Amass L & McLellan AT (1999). Research on contingency management treatment of drug dependence: Clinical implications and future directions. In ST Higgins & K Silverman (eds.) *Motivating Behavior Change Among Illicit Drug Abusers: Research on Contingency Management Interventions*. Washington, DC: American Psychological Association, 327-344.

Kirby KC, Marlowe DB, Festinger DS et al. (1998). Schedule of voucher delivery influences initiation of cocaine abstinence. *Journal of Consulting and Clinical Psychology* 66:761-767.

Kirby KC, Marlowe DB, Festinger DS et al. (1999). Community reinforcement training for family and significant others of drug abusers: A unilateral intervention to increase treatment entry of drug users. *Drug and Alcohol Dependence* 56:85-96.

Liebson IA, Bigelow GE & Flamer R (1973). Alcoholism among methadone patients: A specific treatment model. *American Journal of Psychiatry* 130(4):483-485.

Liebson IA, Tommasello A & Bigelow GE (1978). A behavioral treatment of alcoholic methadone patients. *Annals of Internal Medicine* 89:342-344.

Magura S, Casriel C, Goldsmith DS et al. (1988). Contingency contracting with polydrug-abusing methadone patients. *Addictive Behaviors* 13(1):113-118.

Mallams JH, Godley MD, Hall GM et al. (1982). A social-systems approach to resocializing alcoholics in the community. *Journal of Studies on Alcohol* 43:1115-1123.

McCarthy JJ & Borders OT (1985). Limit setting on drug abuse in methadone maintenance patients. *American Journal of Psychiatry* 142(12):1419-1423.

McCaul ME, Stitzer ML, Bigelow GE et al. (1984). Contingency management interventions: Effects on treatment outcome during methadone detoxification. *Journal of Applied Behavior Analysis* 17(1):35-43.

Meyers RJ, Miller WR, Smith JE et al. (2002). A randomized trial of two methods for engaging treatment refusing drug users through concerned significant others. *Journal of Consulting and Clinical Psychology* 70:1182-1185.

Meyers RJ & Smith JE (1995). *Clinical Guide to Alcohol Treatment: The Community Reinforcement Approach*. New York, NY: Guilford Press.

Milby JB, Garrett C, English C et al. (1978). Take-home methadone: Contingency effects on drug-seeking and productivity of narcotic addicts. *Addictive Behaviors* 3(3-4):215-220.

Milby JB, Schumacher JE, Raczynski JM et al. (1996). Sufficient conditions for effective treatment of substance abusing homeless persons. *Drug and Alcohol Dependence* 43(1-2):39-47.

Milby JB, Schumacher JE, McNamara C et al. (2000). Initiating abstinence in cocaine abusing dually diagnosed homeless persons. *Drug and Alcohol Dependence* 60:55-67.

Miller PM (1975). A behavioral intervention program for chronic public drunkenness offenders. *Archives of General Psychiatry* 32:915-918.

Miller PM, Hersen M & Eisler RM (1974). Relative effectiveness of instructions, agreements, and reinforcement in behavioral contracts with alcoholics. *Journal of Abnormal Psychology* 83(5):548-553.

Miller WR, Meyers RJ & Tonigan JS (1999). Engaging the unmotivated in treatment for alcohol problems: A comparison of three strategies for intervention through family members. *Journal of Consulting and Clinical Psychology* 67:688-697.

NIH-CDC (1997). *Effective Medical Treatment of Heroin Addiction*. NIH Consensus Statement. Bethesda, MD: National Institutes of Health.

Orleans CT, Barker DC, Kaufman NJ et al. (2000). Helping pregnant smokers quit: Meeting the challenge in the next decade. *Tobacco Control* 9 (Suppl III): iii6-iii11.

Peniston EG (1988). Evaluation of long-term therapeutic efficacy of behavior modification program with chronic male schizophrenic patients. *Journal of Behavior Therapy and Experimental Psychiatry* 19:95-101.

Petry NM, Martin B, Cooney JL et al. (2000). Give them prizes, and they will come: Contingency management for treatment of alcohol dependence. *Journal of Consulting and Clinical Psychology* 68:250-257.

Piotrowski NA, Tusel DJ, Sees KL et al. (1999). Contingency contracting with monetary reinforcers for abstinence from multiple drugs in a methadone program. *Experimental and Clinical Psychopharmacology* 7:399-411.

Preston KL, Silverman K, Umbricht A et al. (1999). Improvement in naltrexone treatment compliance with contingency management. *Drug and Alcohol Dependence* 54:127-135.

Ries RE (1982). *The Traffic Safety Effectiveness of Educational Counseling Programs for Multiple Offense Drunk Drivers*. Washington, DC: Department of Transportation, National Highway Traffic Safety Administration.

Ries RK & Comtois KA (1997). Managing disability benefits as part of treatment for persons with mental illness and comorbid drug/alcohol disorders: A comparative study of payees and non-payee participants. *American Journal on Addictions* 6:330-338.

Robichaud C, Strickler D, Bigelow G et al. (1979). Disulfiram maintenance employee alcoholism treatment: A three-phase evaluation. *Behavior Research & Therapy* 17:618-621.

Roll JM, Higgins ST, Steingard S et al. (1998). Investigating the use of monetary reinforcement to reduce the cigarette smoking of schizophrenics: A feasibility study. *Experimental and Clinical Psychopharmacology* 6:157-161.

Rowan-Szal G, Joe GW, Chatham LR et al. (1994). A simple reinforcement system for methadone clients in a community-based treatment program. *Journal of Substance Abuse Treatment* 11:217-223.

Shaner, A, Roberts LJ, Eckman TA et al. (1997). Monetary reinforcement of abstinence from cocaine among mentally ill patients with cocaine dependence. *Psychiatric Services* 48:807-810.

Sigmon SC, Steingard S, Badger GJ et al. (in press). Contingent reinforcement of marijuana abstinence among individuals with serious mental illness: A feasibility study. *Experimental and Clinical Psychopharmacology* 8:509-517.

Silverman K, Chutuape MA, Bigelow GE et al. (1999). Voucher-based reinforcement of cocaine abstinence in treatment-resistant methadone patients: Effects of reinforcer magnitude. *Psychopharmacology* 146:128-138.

Silverman K, Higgins ST, Brooner RK et al. (1996). Sustained cocaine abstinence in methadone maintenance patients through voucher-based reinforcement therapy. *Archives of General Psychiatry* 53:409-415.

Silverman K, Preston KL, Stitzer ML et al. (1998). Treatment of cocaine abuse in methadone maintenance patients. In ST Higgins & JL Katz (eds.) *Cocaine Abuse Research: Pharmacology, Behavior, and Clinical Application*. San Diego, CA: Academic Press, 363-388.

Silverman K, Svikis D, Robles E et al. (2001). A reinforcement-based therapeutic workplace for the treatment of drug abuse: Six-month abstinence outcomes. *Experimental and Clinical Psycho-pharmacology* 9:14-23.

Silverman K, Wong CH, Umbricht-Schneiter A et al. (1998). Broad beneficial effects of reinforcement for cocaine abstinence in methadone patients. *Journal of Consulting and Clinical Psychology* 66:811-824.

Sisson RW & Azrin AH (1986). Family-member involvement to initiate and promote treatment of problem drinkers. *Journal of Behaviour Research and Therapy* 17:15-21.

Smith JE, Meyers RJ & Delaney HD (1998). The community reinforcement approach with homeless alcohol-dependent individuals. *Journal of Consulting and Clinical Psychology* 66:541-548.

Stitzer ML & Bigelow GE (1978). Contingency management in a methadone maintenance program: Availability of reinforcers. *International Journal of the Addictions* 13:737-746.

Stitzer ML, Bickel WK, Bigelow GE et al. (1986). Effect of methadone dose contingencies on urinalysis test results of polydrug-abusing methadone-maintenance patients. *Drug and Alcohol Dependence* 18(4):341–348.

Stitzer ML, Bigelow GE, Liebson IA et al. (1982). Contingent reinforcement for benzodiazepine-free urines: Evaluation of a drug abuse treatment intervention. *Journal of Applied Behavior Analysis* 15(4):493-503.

Stitzer ML, Iguchi MY & Felch LJ (1992). Contingent take-home incentive: Effects on drug use of methadone maintenance patients. *Journal of Consulting and Clinical Psychology* 60(6):927-934.

Tidey JW, Higgins ST, Bickel WK et al. (1999). Effects of response requirement and the availability of an alternative reinforcer on cigarette smoking by schizophrenics. *Psychopharmacology* 145: 52-60.

Tidey JW, O'Neill SC & Higgins ST (1999). Effects of abstinence on cigarette smoking among outpatients with schizophrenia. *Experimental and Clinical Psychopharmacology* 7:347-353.

Tidey JW, O'Neill SC & Higgins ST (in press). Effects of contingent monetary reinforcement and transdermal nicotine on cigarette smoking in schizophrenics. *Experimental and Clinical Psychopharmacology*.

Young AM & Herling S (1986). Drugs as reinforcers: Studies in laboratory animals. In SR Goldberg & IP Stolerman (eds.) *Behavioral Analysis of Drug Dependence*. Orlando FL: Academic Press, 9-67.

Chapter 5

Behavioral Interventions in Smoking Cessation

Christopher W. Kahler, Ph.D.
Michael J. Zvolensky, Ph.D.
Michael G. Goldstein, M.D.
Richard A. Brown, Ph.D.

Social Learning Theory
Multicomponent Treatment Programs
Preparation Stage
Cessation Stage
Maintenance Stage
Behavioral Approaches and Comorbid Mood Problems
Smoking Cessation in Addiction Treatment Programs
Smoking Cessation in Primary Care

Of approximately 1 billion cigarette smokers world wide (Wald & Hackshaw, 1996), about 48 million live in the United States (CDC, 1999a). About 27.6% of men and 22.1% of women in the U.S. are current smokers (CDC, 1999a); just under 82% of these individuals are daily smokers. Rates of cigarette smoking in the U.S. have declined from a peak of 42.4% in 1965 to 24.7% in 1997, but have remained relatively constant since 1990 (CDC, 1999b). In contrast, smoking rates among adolescents actually have increased, from 27.5% in 1991 to 36.4% in 1997 (CDC, 1998a). Smoking is especially prevalent among persons with 9 to 11 years of education and those living below the poverty level. About 5% of the U.S. population have smoked cigars in the past month (CDC, 1999c), and rates of smokeless tobacco use are only slightly lower (CDC, 1998b).

The consequences of tobacco use for the public health are enormous. Tobacco use has been linked to increased risk of cancer, heart disease, stroke, complications of pregnancy (such as low birth weight), and chronic obstructive pulmonary disease (DHHS, 1988) and is the leading cause of preventable death in the United States (McGinnis & Foege, 1993), resulting in more than 430,000 deaths each

year (CDC, 1997). Costs of medical care, lost productivity, and forfeited earnings because of smoking-related disability are estimated at more than $100 billion per year (CDC, 1994a; Miller, Zhang et al., 1993).

Tobacco users are well aware of the possible benefits of quitting (CDC, 1990). Just more than 40% of smokers have stopped smoking for at least one day in the past year (CDC, 1999a), and 70% would like to quit smoking altogether (CDC, 1994b). Unfortunately, only about 4% of those attempting to quit smoking on their own remain abstinent for a full year (Cohen, Lichtenstein et al., 1989). Abstinence rates in trials of intensive behavioral and/or pharmacologic treatments are considerably higher, but still are in the 20% to 30% range (Brown & Emmons, 1991; Fiore, Bailey et al., 2000). It has become increasingly apparent that multiple quit attempts often are required before stable long-term abstinence is achieved (Cohen, Lichtenstein et al., 1989; Fiore, Bailey et al., 2000). This chapter describes a variety of behavioral interventions that can improve smokers' odds of quitting. It begins by outlining social learning theory and the principal elements of multicomponent behavioral interventions in freestanding smoking cessation programs. It then addresses smoking among substance-using populations.

Finally, it covers procedures for intervening effectively with smokers in primary care settings.

In discussing behavioral interventions, the chapter focuses primarily on cigarette smoking among adults, for which research and clinical applications have been most well developed. However, smoking among adolescents and the use of other tobacco products are serious public health concerns. There are few theoretical reasons to expect that behavioral principles tested in adults do not apply equally to adolescents, although there is scant research on treating adolescents. Recommendations for treating cigarette smoking in adults generally can be applied to other tobacco products (Fiore, Bailey et al., 2000).

SOCIAL LEARNING THEORY

Cognitive social learning theory provides a useful framework for conceptualizing behavioral treatment of tobacco dependence (Bandura, 1997). This theory has been extended to treatment of other substances, such as alcohol, in which similar processes may operate (Abrams & Niaura, 1987). In this model, smoking and other tobacco use are viewed as a learned behavior that is acquired through classical and operant conditioning, modeling, and other cognitive processes (Bandura, 1986). Through pairing over time, various external and interoceptive stimuli (for example, drinking coffee, feeling stressed, celebrating at a party [Niaura, Rohsenow et al., 1988]) come to be associated with smoking behavior. These stimuli or *antecedents* then can trigger an urge to smoke. Once the smoker smokes a cigarette (the *behavior*), he or she experiences the rewarding *consequences* (for example, relaxation), thereby increasing the likelihood of future smoking. Smokers develop certain expectations about the effects of smoking that, in turn, influence their smoking behavior. Positive outcome expectancies (for example, "smoking will relax me") increase the likelihood of continued smoking, whereas negative outcome expectancies (such as "smoking increases my risk of heart disease") increase the likelihood of quitting.

The general rationale for behavioral treatment is that, with practice and skills training, the automatic chain of events (antecedent behavior consequences) leading to smoking can be disrupted, and smoking behavior can be replaced with alternative behaviors. The learning of nonsmoking skills occurs through a series of success experiences. These skills are practiced in both group and individual sessions and outside of treatment. As smokers become more proficient in the skills, their self-efficacy for quitting increases, thus increasing the likelihood that they can successfully stop smoking.

MULTICOMPONENT TREATMENT PROGRAMS

Whereas the earliest behavioral treatments tended to focus on the application of a single technique, multicomponent programs have become dominant over the past 20 to 25 years (Shiffman, 1993). Multicomponent treatments have success rates that generally are greater than programs using only one or two behavioral and psychosocial strategies (American Psychiatric Association, 1996; Schwartz, 1992). Multicomponent group treatments typically yield six-month quit rates of about 20% to 25% (APA, 1996; Schwartz, 1992), although rates of 50% or better have been reported (Schwartz, 1987; USDHHS, 1988).

Multicomponent packages are likely to be effective because they address multiple factors that precipitate or maintain smoking (Brown & Emmons, 1991; Brown, Goldstein et al., 1993). The combination of multimodal behavioral and pharmacologic interventions appears to have increased efficacy relative to either treatment alone (APA, 1996; Hughes, 1995). Current recommendations are that all smokers be offered some pharmacologic aid to cessation, except when contraindications exist (Fiore, Bailey et al., 2000). Although pharmacologic approaches are beyond the scope of this chapter, the authors do address "nicotine fading," which can serve as an alternative for smokers who desire a nonpharmacologic approach or for whom pharmacotherapy is otherwise inappropriate.

Multicomponent treatments traditionally have been delivered in a group format. This approach takes advantage of the social support of group treatment, reduces financial costs, and facilitates involvement of multiple therapists who may have overlapping but distinct therapeutic skills. The intensity of multicomponent treatments, both in terms of the number of sessions and the length of sessions, can vary according to setting. It has been shown, however, that intensity of treatment is associated positively with abstinence. Thus, it is recommended that interventions include a minimum of four sessions of at least 10 minutes' duration (Fiore, Bailey et al., 2000). The type of clinician providing treatment (for example, physician, psychologist, or nurse) does not appear to affect intervention efficacy (Fiore, Bailey et al., 2000).

Possible components of a behavioral cessation program are outlined below. It is useful to think of multicomponent cessation programs as comprising three interrelated phases:

preparation, quitting, and maintenance. These phases can overlap in time, and some principles and methods are useful in more than one phase.

PREPARATION STAGE

A "preparation" period before quitting smoking, the length of which can vary according to program needs, is beneficial. It has three key objectives. First, it allows the patient's motivation to quit and commitment to the program to be clarified and reinforced. Second, it allows a target quit day to be clearly established, thus allowing the patient time to prepare mentally and develop coping strategies for quitting smoking. Third, it affords time for the patient to self-monitor daily smoking behavior and analyze smoking triggers (that is, antecedents).

Reinforce Motivation and Commitment to Quit. Even smokers who enroll in cessation programs may be ambivalent about the prospect of quitting. Although acknowledging rational reasons for quitting, they may dread the prospect, lack confidence, feel hopelessly addicted, and secretly question whether the health risks could ever really affect them. This feeling can be especially true of smokers who have tried to quit and failed. The preparation phase offers an opportunity to help smokers resolve their ambivalence and strengthen their commitment to quitting. However, throughout treatment, motivation needs to be monitored for potential setbacks.

For many smokers, the expected short-term benefits of smoking (for example, "smoking calms my nerves") override the more distant negative consequences (such as potentially life-threatening illnesses). The challenge is to move smokers from general acceptance of potential negative consequences ("smoking is dangerous to health") to personalized acceptance ("smoking is dangerous to *my own* health") (Fishbein, 1977). Encouraging smokers to consider their smoker's cough and other current physical symptoms is one way to make negative consequences more personally salient. When appropriate, exploring the consequences of the illness or premature death of a loved one or what they will miss if they themselves die prematurely also can be a powerful motivator. A concurrent focus on the health benefits of quitting can be especially effective in motivating and sustaining efforts to quit smoking (Brown & Emmons, 1991).

A useful approach to enhance motivation involves having patients write down their specific, self-relevant reasons for wanting to stop smoking and for wanting to continue smoking. Listing reasons to continue smoking may seem unhelpful, but doing so can help patients identify likely barriers to quitting.

Designate a Target Quit Day. The patient should designate a target quit day at the beginning of the cessation program. This task gives the patient a specific date to work toward and should be chosen to allow sufficient time for acquisition of skills for maintaining cessation and preventing relapse.

Self-Monitor Smoking Behavior. Having the patient keep a written record of cigarettes smoked can help increase knowledge about the factors that cue and maintain smoking behavior. Self-monitoring also interrupts the automatic smoking habit by encouraging the patient to think about every cigarette smoked and why it was smoked. This procedure often reduces the number of cigarettes smoked per day (Abrams & Wilson, 1979).

Patients can be given preprinted cards or "wrap sheets" to use in recording the time of day and the situation in which each cigarette is smoked (for example, talking on the phone). Recording mood at the time of each cigarette also can be useful. Situational notations allow the patient to identify antecedents that trigger smoking.

Patients typically find self-monitoring of smoking behavior inconvenient. It thus is important for the clinician to present the rationale for self-monitoring clearly and to follow through at every session by reviewing the patient's wrap sheets so as to highlight the relevance of the information to the cessation effort. For example, it is useful to ask the patient what he or she learned about smoking behavior and its patterns over the course of a typical week; specifically, what moods commonly were triggers of smoking, during which times of the day he or she smoked most often, and which people or events typically triggered smoking.

CESSATION STAGE

Self-Management. Sometimes termed "self-control" or "stimulus control," self-management procedures are a critical component of behavioral interventions for smoking. They refer to strategies intended to rearrange environmental cues that trigger smoking or to alter the consequences of smoking. By using wrap sheets, patients develop a list of trigger situations. They then begin to intervene in these situations to break up the smoking behavior chain (situation/urge/smoke) by using one of three general strategies: (1) avoid the trigger situation, (2) alter or change the trigger situation, and (3) use an alternative or substitute in place of the cigarette to respond to the trigger situation.

Examples of avoiding trigger situations include forgoing a coffee break at work with other smokers, leaving the table after dinner, and avoiding social situations involving alcohol.

Altering a trigger situation might involve drinking tea or juice in the morning instead of coffee, watching television in the bedroom (a nonsmoking room) rather than in the living room, and placing cigarettes in the trunk of the car before driving.

Alternative or substitute responses can be used in conjunction with avoiding or altering trigger situations or in situations that cannot be avoided or altered. Alternatives may include sugarless candy or gum, chewing on cut-up vegetables such as carrot or celery sticks or on toothpicks, employing relaxation techniques in stressful situations, or using activities such as needlework that keep the hands occupied. Patients should choose strategies they think will work for them and then try out different approaches, rejecting those that are not useful, until they have successfully managed all or most trigger situations without smoking.

Several other stimulus control techniques can be useful in disrupting associations between smoking and trigger situations. In hierarchical reduction, smokers reduce or eliminate smoking in progressive fashion from the easiest to the most difficult situations. Increasing the time interval between cigarettes is a strategy that allows smoking only at designated times (Levinson, Shapiro et al., 1971; Cinciripini, Lapitsky et al., 1995). This procedure gradually reduces smoking while simultaneously severing associations between trigger situations and smoking. Finally, smoking only in "deprived situations" (for example, in the basement or garage) encourages smokers to narrow their range of smoking situations while breaking pleasurable associations with smoking.

Relaxation Training. Relaxation techniques provide smokers with methods for coping more effectively with stress, which is a common trigger of relapse (Marlatt & Gordon, 1985; Shiffman, 1982). The Benson relaxation response is a meditative, breathing-based technique that is easily taught to patients and readily mastered with moderate amounts of practice (Benson, 1975). Progressive muscle relaxation and imagery-based relaxation approaches are viable alternatives (Jacobson, 1983). It should be noted that, although relaxation training has been incorporated into many successful multicomponent programs, its use has failed to demonstrate incremental treatment effects when combined with other procedures (Brown & Emmons, 1991).

Social Support. Positive social support both within (for example, from the clinician) and outside of treatment has been shown to increase cessation rates (Fiore, Bailey et al., 2000; Mermelstein, Cohen et al., 1986). Social support can be a source of motivation for quitting and of positive reinforcement for maintaining abstinence. Social support can provide a buffer against stressful life events that might precipitate a relapse. Clinicians should encourage patients' efforts at cessation, communicate care and concern for their well-being, and encourage open discussion about their experiences during quitting. Encouraging patients to access social supports outside of treatment may be helpful; such social supports might include making specific requests to friends and family members to take steps to support patients' abstinence efforts.

Nicotine Fading. Nicotine fading is a procedure in which patients work toward a target quit day by switching to progressively lower nicotine content cigarettes over a period of several weeks. The rationale is that reducing nicotine intake gradually reduces physical dependence. Fading can reduce the intensity of withdrawal symptoms on the quit day and make quitting less difficult. (Information on the nicotine yields of current cigarette brands is available from the Federal Trade Commission [1997].) Patients frequently report mild withdrawal symptoms throughout the brand-switching phase, suggesting a diffusion of the withdrawal effects that ordinarily would be experienced all at once if they had not used the fading procedure.

The best multicomponent programs involving nicotine fading produced quit rates of 40% or better at long-term followup (Etringer, Gregory et al., 1984; Foxx & Brown, 1979; Lando & McGovern, 1985). Those rates are among the highest for behavioral, nonaversive procedures (Glasgow & Lichtenstein, 1987).

Nicotine fading may not be appropriate for smokers who already use low nicotine content cigarettes (currently, 0.05 mg nicotine). Such smokers can change to another brand with equal nicotine yield to disrupt the taste and comfort associated with smoking their regular brand.

It should be noted that actual reductions in nicotine intake may be less than those suggested by the published nicotine yield of the cigarette, because smokers often compensate by smoking more cigarettes or changing the topography of their smoking behavior. Patients should be cautioned about this possibility and advised to minimize such changes.

MAINTENANCE STAGE

Because most smokers who initially quit resume smoking within several months of treatment (Hunt & Bespalec, 1974), maintenance is a critical issue for smoking cessation programs. The most commonly used behavioral maintenance strategies are based on the relapse prevention model (Marlatt & Gordon, 1985), the main components of which are described below. Research on the effectiveness of relapse prevention components has been mixed, with relapse prevention treatments generally outperforming no-treatment controls but rarely outperforming credible alternative treatments (Carroll, 1996; Ockene, Emmons et al., 2000). A notable exception is a study by Stevens and Hollis (1989), in which relapse prevention booster sessions produced higher abstinence rates than both social support and no treatment.

Identifying and Coping With Situations That Pose High Risk of Relapse. Relapse prevention theory (Marlatt & Gordon, 1980, 1985) proposes that the ability to cope with "high-risk" situations for relapse determines an individual's likelihood of maintaining abstinence. High-risk situations often involve at least one of the following elements: negative moods, positive moods, social situations involving alcohol, and being in the presence of smokers. To help patients identify high-risk situations, a clinician can ask, "If you were to slip and smoke a cigarette after quit day, in what situation would it be?" For each high-risk situation identified, the patient can develop a set of strategies for managing the situation without smoking. He or she should be reminded that high-risk situations are functionally similar to the trigger situations addressed in the cessation stage and can be handled by applying similar self-management strategies (that is, avoid, alter, or use a substitute), as well as other problem-solving skills.

Abstinence Violation Effect. A common response to a "slip" or episode of smoking after cessation is one of self-defeating attributions and negative emotional reactions. This response has been termed the "abstinence violation effect" and has been postulated to increase the risk of continued smoking after an initial slip (Marlatt & Gordon, 1985). The main task that a patient faces if a slip does occur is to prevent the slip from becoming a relapse. Patients can be informed in advance that the abstinence violation effect is a natural reaction to having a slip. They can be instructed in cognitive and behavioral procedures to "fight off" this negative emotional reaction so as not to continue to smoke if a slip does occur.

Lifestyle Change. Marlatt and Gordon (1985) discuss the concept of replacing a negative addiction (such as smoking) with a "positive addiction" such as increasing participation in activities that are incompatible with smoking and are a source of pleasure. Patients are encouraged to set aside time as often as possible (ideally, on a daily basis) for this purpose. It is in this context that patients are strongly encouraged to engage in some type of regular physical exercise. Vigorous exercise has been shown to enhance smoking cessation in women (Marcus, Albrecht et al., 1999). Exercise can be a good alternative to dieting for individuals who are concerned about postcessation weight gain and can moderate increases in negative mood, which often are associated with nicotine withdrawal (Abrams, Monti et al., 1987; Shiffman, 1982, 1984).

BEHAVIORAL APPROACHES AND COMORBID MOOD PROBLEMS

Smokers typically exhibit higher rates of major depressive disorder (MDD) (Breslau, Kilbey et al., 1991; Glassman, Helzer et al., 1990; Kendler, Neale et al., 1993) and depressive symptoms (Anda, Williamson et al., 1990) than nonsmokers, although exceptions have been noted (Covey, Hughes et al., 1994). Lifetime prevalence rates of MDD are particularly high among smokers entering smoking cessation programs, with observed rates ranging from 22% to 61% (Hall, Muñoz et al., 1996; Hall, Reus et al., 1998; Hall, Muñoz et al., 1994; Glassman, Stetner et al., 1988). A number of studies have shown that affective distress at the beginning of treatment (Brown, Kahler et al., 2001; Kinnunen, Doherty et al., 1996) and after quitting (Ginsberg, Hall et al., 1995; Covey, Glassman et al., 1990; West, Hajek et al., 1989) predict poor outcome. Although an association between a history of MDD and smoking outcome has not been found in some studies (Hall, Muñoz et al., 1994; Ginsberg, Hall et al., 1995), MDD history has been associated with poorer smoking outcome at both 4 weeks (Glassman, Stetner et al., 1988) and 10 weeks after the quit date (Glassman, Covey et al., 1993), and particularly poor outcomes have been shown in smokers with recurrent MDD (Brown, Kahler et al., 2001; Glassman, Covey et al., 1993).

Given the negative association between mood problems and abstinence, cessation treatments that provide behavioral strategies for managing depressive symptoms and negative moods have generated substantial interest. Two studies have found significant effects of depression coping skills for smokers with an MDD history; however, in both of these studies, the experimental treatment had greater therapist contact time than the control (Hall, Muñoz et al., 1994; Hall, Reus et al., 1998). In a study equating for therapist contact, the effect was not replicated (Hall, Muñoz et al., 1996). Recently, Brown and colleagues (Brown, Kahler et al., 2001) found that cessation treatment incorporating cognitive-behavioral therapy for depression was particularly effective for smokers with recurrent MDD, even when equating for therapist contact time. Elements of this treatment approach are described later in this chapter. In none of the studies conducted to date have depression coping skills been found to improve negative mood during quitting or to reduce the effect of negative mood on outcome.

Cognitive-Behavioral Treatment for Depression. The Coping with Depression course (Brown & Lewinsohn, 1984a, 1984b; Lewinsohn, Antonuccio et al., 1984) can serve as a basis for treatment of comorbid mood problems in smoking cessation (Brown, Kahler et al., 2001). The major elements of the course include (1) daily monitoring of mood and factors influencing mood, (2) contracting for achievable, systematic increases in pleasant activities to maintain or improve mood and to prevent the onset of depressive symptoms after cessation, (3) cognitive self-management techniques for reducing negative thoughts and for increasing positive thoughts (Lewinsohn, Antonuccio et al., 1984), (4) the ABC Technique for identifying and challenging distorted, depressive thoughts (Ellis & Harper, 1961), and (5) assertiveness training using modeling, role-playing, and homework exercises, including situations that involve social pressure to smoke. These treatment elements are readily incorporated into behavioral cessation programs and can be helpful for smokers with a history of recurrent MDD (Brown, Kahler et al., 2001).

SMOKING CESSATION IN ADDICTION TREATMENT PROGRAMS

Comorbidity of Nicotine Dependence and Other Substance Use Disorders. An accumulation of evidence indicates a high co-occurrence of cigarette smoking and other addictive disorders. Approximately 85% of nonrecovering alcoholics smoke on a daily basis compared with approximately 25% of individuals in nonalcoholic populations (Bobo, 1989). Relative to those who are not dependent on alcohol, individuals with a history of alcohol dependence are nearly five times more likely to smoke regularly (Kozlowski & Ferrence, 1990), to smoke at a higher rate, and to have greater difficulty in quitting smoking (Burling & Ziff, 1988; Istvan & Matarazzo, 1984). The same pattern of findings is evident in those who seek treatment for alcohol problems. Across studies, approximately 70% to 90% of those who seek treatment for alcohol problems are smokers (Jarman & Kellett, 1979; Joseph, Nichol et al., 1990).

High rates of smoking also are found among individuals who use illicit drugs. For example, Rounsaville and colleagues (1985) found that 97% of opiate addicts in inpatient treatment were daily smokers. Sees and Clark (1993) found, in a large, heterogeneous sample of addictive disorder patients, that 77% of the cocaine addicts and 85% of the heroin addicts regularly smoked cigarettes. In the general population, smoking prevalence is high for persons who have heavy substance use histories. Chronic marijuana users are nearly four times as likely as those who do not use marijuana to be moderately to severely nicotine dependent (Henningfield, Clayton et al., 1990). Likewise, the prevalence of cocaine dependence is almost 10 times higher in persons with moderate nicotine dependence than in normal control participants (Breslau, Kilbey et al., 1991).

Smoking-Related Morbidity and Mortality Among Individuals With Substance Use Disorders. The health risks of combined smoking and addictive disorders exceed even those of the general population of smokers. In fact, a synergistic tobacco-alcohol effect appears to confer a greater risk of certain medical problems, such as cancer. Alcohol consumption combined with cigarette smoking greatly increases the risk of oral, pharyngeal, laryngeal, esophageal, and lung cancer relative to smoking alone, drinking alone, or neither smoking nor drinking (Sees & Clark, 1993). Blot and colleagues (1988) found a 35-fold increase in smoking-related cancer in men who were both heavy cigarette smokers and heavy alcohol drinkers compared with nonsmoking men who rarely drank. Although smoking and excessive alcohol consumption appear to have a synergistic effect on cancer risk, these effects appear to be additive for cardiovascular and respiratory diseases (NIAAA, 1984).

Attitudes Toward Smoking Cessation. *Interest and Success in Quitting*: Across studies, more than half of all patients surveyed while in treatment report that they want to quit smoking and maintain a "moderate" degree of interest in doing so (Bobo, Gilchrist et al., 1987; Hurt, Eberman et al., 1993; Kozlowski & Ferrence, 1990). This interest is not related to an erroneous belief that quitting smoking is "easier" than stopping other types of alcohol or drug use. In fact, approximately 50% of patients enrolled in drug or alcohol treatment report that giving up cigarettes would be "as hard" or "harder" than giving up their primary drug of abuse (Kozlowski, Ferrence et al., 1990).

The perceived difficulty of quitting smoking can explain why most patients would like to try to quit smoking only after they complete drug or alcohol treatment (Kozlowski, Ferrence et al., 1990). Despite their interest in doing so, it is rare for patients to quit smoking after treatment for another addiction. In studies in drug-abusing populations, nearly 90% of patients who were smokers during treatment were current smokers at followup (Hurt, Eberman et al., 1993; Rounsaville et al., 1985). Quit rates are low among those who desire to quit smoking yet remain "active" in their drug or alcohol use, with approximately 17% having stopped smoking at followup assessment (Hughes, 1993).

Staff and Program Support for Quitting: Despite interest in quitting among patients with addictive disorders, support for smoking cessation interventions within addiction treatment programs appears weak. Less than 50% of program personnel encourage patients to quit smoking, and 40% believe that smoking cessation should not be provided within the context of addiction treatment (Bobo & Gilchrist, 1983; Kozlowski, Skinner et al., 1989). Less than 15% of alcohol treatment programs encourage and/or provide smoking cessation treatment (Sees & Clark, 1993).

Concern about smoking cessation during treatment relates to issues concerning (1) whether cessation efforts will jeopardize abstinence from alcohol or drugs and/or (2) doubt that alcohol- and drug-addicted patients can mount a serious effort to quit smoking.

Perhaps the most compelling reason that treatment personnel's attitudes about smoking cessation during addiction treatment should change is that there is little, if any, evidence that smoking cessation impairs alcohol or drug treatment outcomes (Bobo, McIlvain et al., 1998). In fact, smoking cessation during alcohol and/or drug treatment actually can improve outcomes, albeit marginally. For example, slightly higher rates of abstinence from alcohol use were reported among those who successfully quit smoking, compared to those who did not (Bobo, Gilchrist et al., 1987; Bobo, McIlvain et al., 1998; Joseph, Nichol et al., 1990a).

There can be additive benefits when treatment involves targeting multiple behavior problems, particularly if they are functionally related to a common risk process (for example, deficits in drink-drug refusal skills). Moreover, applying coping skills to certain substances (such as alcohol) and not others (such as nicotine) can send a "psychologically conflicting" message to patients about their substance use. This inconsistent message can be most problematic for those addictive disorders that typically rely on inhalation-based methods of administration, such as marijuana dependence.

Outcomes of Behavioral Smoking Cessation Interventions With Addiction Treatment Patients. Finding ways to enhance motivation to quit smoking during drug and alcohol treatment is an important and timely endeavor, which is only beginning to garner serious scientific attention (Orleans & Hutchinson, 1993). In one of the earlier studies in this area, Burling and colleagues (1991) randomly assigned patients in a residential alcohol program to either behavioral smoking treatment or a wait-list control. Those offered smoking treatment were significantly more likely to continue in residential alcohol treatment, and approximately one-third actually quit smoking; however, smoking cessation was not maintained at followup.

In another investigation, behavioral smoking treatment was provided to volunteers on an inpatient addiction treatment unit and compared with smoking rates for patients who volunteered for a control group (Hurt, Eberman et al., 1993). At followup assessment, approximately 12% of the smokers in the treatment condition and 0% of the nontreated smokers were abstinent from smoking (see also, Bobo, McIlvain et al., 1998; Bobo, Slade et al., 1995; Burling, Marshall et al., 1991). In another investigation, smokers who were former problem drinkers (with at least three months' sobriety) were assigned to standard behavioral care, standard behavioral care plus exercise, or standard behavioral care plus nicotine replacement (Hurt, Eberman et al., 1993). At 12-month followup, 27% of the participants were not smoking, with no significant differences between conditions. Finally, Joseph and colleagues (Joseph, Nichol et al., 1990a, 1990b) reported similar findings for abstinence rates after a policy-related smoking ban in an inpatient alcohol treatment program for persons who had or had not received a brief, behavioral smoking cessation intervention.

Clinical Recommendations. The provision of smoking cessation treatment for individuals who seek treatment for alcohol and drug problems is in an early stage of development. Although voluntary smoking cessation efforts do not appear to have a negative effect on sobriety, quit rates are low (Bobo, McIlvain et al., 1998). Moreover, conclusions based on available studies are necessarily limited because of the selection bias for study participants. Randomized trials to evaluate the effects of brief motivational approaches and the differential efficacy of behavioral, pharmacologic, and combined interventions are needed. The authors recommend that addiction treatment programs draw on the findings of empirical work in primary care settings, which are described in the following section. In brief, addiction treatment personnel can follow primary care guidelines by identifying smokers, advising them to quit, providing motivational interventions for those who are not ready to quit, and offering assistance to those who are ready to quit.

SMOKING CESSATION IN PRIMARY CARE

Physicians are in a unique position to provide smoking cessation treatment because they have multiple opportunities over a period of years to intervene with patients who smoke. Even if a patient is asymptomatic, the clinician can link the patient's smoking to increased risk of future disease. The widespread adoption of smoke-free policies in hospitals and other health care institutions provides additional opportunities for intervention. Perhaps the most compelling reason to focus on physician-delivered smoking cessation interventions is that they increase abstinence rates (Ockene, 1987; Kottke, Battista et al., 1988; Fiore, Bailey et al., 2000) and are highly cost-effective, especially when compared with such medical practices as treatment of mild to moderate hypertension or hypercholesterolemia (Cummings, Rubin et al., 1989).

Although most primary care physicians recognize the importance of smoking cessation as a disease-preventive measure, few are confident in their ability to help patients stop smoking (Ockene, Aney et al., 1988; Orleans, 1985). Only 37% of smokers who saw a physician in the preceding year reported being advised to quit by a health care provider, and only 15% reported that a physician provided them specific assistance to quit smoking (Goldstein, Niaura et al., 1997). The following discussion provides guidelines and suggestions for implementing smoking cessation interventions in medical settings, both with patients who are willing to quit and with patients who are not ready to commit to quitting.

The Five As. In April 1996, after a comprehensive review and meta-analysis of the existing scientific literature, the Smoking Cessation Guideline Panel commissioned by the federal Agency for Health Care Policy and Research released *Smoking Cessation Clinical Practice Guideline No. 18* (Fiore, Bailey et al., 1996). These guidelines recently were updated by the Tobacco Use and Dependence Guideline Panel in a new publication by the U.S. Public Health Service (PHS), *Treating Tobacco Use and Dependence* (Fiore, Bailey et al., 2000). On the basis of the empirical literature, the PHS guidelines provide clinicians with a five-step strategy for cessation interventions in medical care settings, referred to as the "Five As." The five steps are (1) **A**sk—systematically identify all tobacco users at every visit; (2) **A**dvise—strongly advise all smokers to quit; (3) **A**ssess—identify smokers willing to make a quit attempt (and provide a motivational intervention if they are not willing to quit); (4) **A**ssist—aid the patient in quitting, including counseling and pharmacotherapy; and (5) **A**rrange—schedule followup contact. Each step is discussed in detail below.

Ask (identification): Although more than 70% of smokers see a physician each year, smoking status is identified in only about two-thirds of clinic visits (Thorndike, Riggotti et al., 1998). The enactment of procedures and systems that routinely identify and document smoking status in health care settings is critical, resulting in about three times higher rates of smoking cessation interventions by clinicians and almost two times higher quit rates among patients (Fiore, Bailey et al, 2000). Methods of documenting and identifying tobacco users include expanded vital sign sheets that incorporate tobacco use status along with blood pressure, pulse, and temperature, as well as reminder systems such as chart stickers or prompts on computer records.

Kottke and colleagues (Kottke, Battista et al., 1988; Kottke, Solberg et al., 1990) suggest additional organizational components and systems to aid in delivery of effective, consistent counseling in primary care settings. These components include establishing a specific smoking policy that clearly delineates roles and is endorsed by all staff members and enacting maintenance programs such as regular auditing of charts to provide feedback to staff members, spirit-building activities (for example, parties for achieving modest goals), and repeated skills-training sessions.

Advice: Smokers report that a physician's advice to quit smoking often is an important factor in their decision to make a quit attempt (Ockene, 1987; Pederson, Baskerville et al., 1982). This is supported by clinical trials, which found that brief advice (less than three minutes) by a clinician to quit smoking increases the odds of abstinence by about 30%, compared with the absence of such advice

(Fiore, Bailey et al., 2000). Thus, smokers should be provided at least a brief intervention at each office visit.

It also appears that brief motivational messages from a physician followed by more intensive interventions delivered by an allied health professional can reduce the time burden on physicians, make counseling more likely, and produce significantly increased cessation rates compared with brief physician advice alone (Hollis, Lichtenstein et al., 1993). The addition of nurse-delivered interventions to brief physician advice in a primary care setting produced quit rates of 7.1% at one year, compared with 3.9% for brief physician advice alone (Hollis, Lichtenstein et al., 1993).

Assessment: Patients present with differing levels of motivation for quitting smoking, and interventions should be based on the patient's readiness to change. The Stages of Change model identifies five discrete stages of readiness to change: precontemplation, contemplation, preparation, action, and maintenance (Prochaska & DiClemente, 1986; Prochaska & Goldstein, 1991). Individuals at the precontemplation stage, who constitute as many as 40% of current smokers seen in a typical medical practice (Velicer, Fava et al., 1995), are not considering stopping smoking in the foreseeable future. Individuals in the contemplation stage, who account for an additional 40% of smokers (Velicer, Fava et al., 1995), are considering making a quit attempt within the next 6 months, but have not yet made a firm commitment to change. For smokers in either the precontemplation or contemplation stages, intervention should be aimed at increasing motivation by using methods outlined later in this chapter.

About 20% of smokers who seek medical care are in the preparation stage and are intending to quit smoking in the next month (Velicer, Fava et al., 1995). Many of these patients have made a quit attempt in the past year or have taken small steps toward quitting, such as cutting down on the number of cigarettes they smoke (Prochaska & Goldstein, 1991). These smokers should be encouraged to set a specific quit day and be offered additional assistance, as described later.

Smokers in the action stage are actively trying to quit. In this stage, relapse is the rule rather than the exception, especially during the first few weeks after quitting. Finally, maintenance, defined as a stage beginning six months after quitting, is characterized by continued use of processes to prevent slips or relapse. It is important to note that smokers often transition in and out of stages of change. The

average smoker takes three or more cycles through the stages of change over several years before finally reaching a stable period of maintenance (Prochaska & Goldstein, 1991). Therefore, it is vital to arrange continued followup assessments for patients who are in the action and maintenance stages.

Assistance: All patients who are willing to attempt to quit smoking should be provided with assistance from physicians and other health care providers. Interventions delivered by many types of providers increase the likelihood of smoking cessation, suggesting that smoking cessation interventions should be delivered by as many clinicians and types of clinicians as feasible (Fiore, Bailey et al., 2000). A strong dose-response relationship is found between the intensity of person-to-person contact and smoking cessation outcomes (Fiore, Bailey et al., 2000). Although time is at a premium during office-based visits, the delivery of 10 or more minutes of counseling by other professional staff members can be feasible in some settings. Increasing the intensity of counseling from less than 3 minutes to 3 to 10 minutes increases quit rates by more than 20% (Fiore, Bailey et al., 2000).

Intervention can include many of the components of treatment outlined in this chapter, including setting a quit date, providing encouragement, anticipating challenges to quitting, identifying strategies to cope with triggers to smoke, and involving other sources of support, such as family and friends. Self-help manuals are important tools that enhance the capacity of the clinician to provide information and advice; materials are available through agencies such as the National Cancer Institute, U.S. Public Health Service, American Cancer Society, American Heart Association, American Lung Association, and CDC's Office on Smoking and Health. Finally, except when special circumstances exist, all smokers willing to quit should be offered pharmacotherapy along with an explanation that such medication can reduce withdrawal symptoms and increase success rates (Fiore, Bailey et al., 2000). First-line pharmacotherapies include nicotine replacement therapies (gum, inhaler, nasal spray, or patch) and bupropion SR (Zyban®).

Followup (Arrange): Advice to quit and other smoking interventions should be followed up by the clinician. Such followup contacts can be used to monitor readiness to change over time, so that obstacles to change can be addressed and support can be offered when a decision to quit is made. For smokers who are attempting to quit, the clinician should schedule a specific time to connect immediately after quit day to reinforce successes and troubleshoot difficulties in cessation efforts, including use and potential side effects of medication. Followup contacts provide an opportunity to work with patients who have lapsed to smoking. The clinician can empathize with the patient about difficulties in maintaining abstinence, help the patient view a lapse as a learning experience that is part of the normal process of quitting, and encourage the patient to continue his or her efforts to quit.

Motivating Smokers to Quit. By recognizing that most smokers who visit a physician's office are not ready to stop smoking, physicians can modify their own expectations, modulate their efforts to encourage all patients to quit smoking, and develop strategies to attain intermediate outcomes, such as moving a precontemplator to the contemplation stage or motivating a contemplator to take small steps toward quitting (Prochaska & Goldstein, 1991). Patients who are unwilling to attempt to quit may be uninformed or underinformed about smoking, demoralized about their ability to change, or defensive and resistant to change (Prochaska & Goldstein, 1991).

A useful and effective method for exploring readiness to change is to have patients rate on a numerical scale (for example, from 0 to 10) the importance they attach to quitting smoking and the confidence they have in their ability to quit (Rollnick, Mason et al., 1999). Once a patient has provided these ratings, the clinician can inquire further about factors that influence each rating. For example, the clinician might ask, "What made you give a rating of 4 to the importance of quitting rather than a 0?" In this way, the patient is prompted to generate reasons to quit smoking on his or her own. Self-generated motivational statements such as these may be especially likely to foster change and should be reinforced by the clinician.

Similarly, exploration of confidence ratings can reveal roadblocks that prevent more motivated patients from taking action and help identify potential strategies for overcoming such roadblocks. For example, the clinician might ask "What would help you to increase your confidence from a 6 to a 7 or an 8?"

For patients who have low importance ratings or are in the precontemplation stage, personalized information and feedback can raise awareness of the ways in which smoking is affecting their health. Such personalized feedback is more likely to be effective than mini-lectures about the general health effects of smoking (Miller & Rollnick, 1991). Feedback can take several forms, including evidence of the effects of smoking on a particular patient's laboratory findings (for example, carbon monoxide levels, pulmonary function tests, high-density lipoprotein), effects of smoking on disease states (for example, presence of angina, angiographic findings, asthma attacks), and the relationship between smoking and risk (for example, risk of sudden death or recurrent myocardial infarction). Feedback about the deleterious effects of continued smoking should be paired with feedback about smoking cessation's beneficial effects on health and reduction of morbidity.

After each piece of information, the clinician should elicit the patient's reactions and questions and then empathize with and validate the concerns before providing new information.

For patients who attach high levels of importance to quitting but are not taking action because of lack of confidence, the clinician can emphasize that it may take several quit attempts before the patient is finally successful. Empathic statements, such as "I recognize that it's difficult for many patients to quit," and statements of support, such as "When you are ready to quit, I'm willing to help," can help patients in the contemplation stage feel heard and understood (Prochaska & Goldstein, 1991). Statements such as "I'm glad that you're thinking about quitting" are especially useful because they reinforce the patient's interest in quitting. It is useful to explore contemplators' reasons for continued smoking as well as barriers to quitting so that potential solutions for overcoming barriers can be discussed (Prochaska & Goldstein, 1991). Contemplators who become chronically "stuck" in this stage can benefit from encouragement to take small steps toward action, such as cutting down the number of cigarettes they smoke, delaying their first cigarette of the day, or trying to quit for just 24 hours (Prochaska & Goldstein, 1991).

A commitment to change is unlikely to occur in one brief session. Instead, the goal of intervention with a patient who is not committed is to move him or her closer to change. Followup visits can allow for continued monitoring of readiness and repeated interventions to enhance motivation and facilitate quitting.

Intensive Case Management. In some settings, it can be feasible to develop more intensive smoking cessation programs than those typically available through a primary care physician. Such programs show substantial promise. DeBusk and colleagues (1994) evaluated a case management system that included the following components: (1) in-hospital counseling by a physician, lasting approximately two

---

minutes; (2) an in-hospital comprehensive assessment and counseling session conducted by a nurse trained in behavioral problem-solving skills; (3) provision of a self-help manual focusing on relapse prevention and a relaxation audiotape; and (4) telephone calls by the nurse 48 hours and one week after hospital discharge and monthly for six months. Patients who relapsed after discharge also were offered one additional visit with the nurse for further counseling, as well as nicotine gum or transdermal nicotine. This treatment was compared with a usual care condition that included physician counseling about smoking cessation, nutritionist counseling about dietary change during hospitalization, and physician-managed, lipid-lowering drug therapy after hospital discharge. Patients in the usual care group also had access to a group smoking cessation program and group exercise rehabilitation at a number of community facilities. The intensive case management system produced a one-year smoking cessation rate of 70%, compared with a rate of 53% for usual care for patients hospitalized with an acute myocardial infarction (p=0.03) (DeBusk, Miller et al., 1994). These findings highlight the utility of developing specialized intensive systems for use in intervening with smokers over extended periods of time.

CONCLUSIONS

Treating tobacco use is an important public health priority. Although efficacious behavioral and pharmacologic interventions have been identified, many clinicians may not apply these interventions routinely with smokers and other tobacco users. Increased awareness of the need to assess and intervene with tobacco users, as well as increased knowledge about available treatment options, is needed. Addiction treatment programs are a promising arena for intervening in tobacco use, but more research on interventions with this population is required. Primary care settings are another arena where physicians and medical staff can have a powerful effect on tobacco use and its associated health problems.

Although there are a number of promising behavioral interventions for tobacco users, it is clear that more work is needed. Knowledge about the most effective elements of motivational interventions is limited, and relapse remains the rule rather than the exception among smokers who attempt to quit. Further study of the behavioral as well as the biological and pharmacologic processes that lead to relapse is required to refine existing interventions and identify promising new approaches to treating tobacco use and dependence.

REFERENCES

Abrams DB & Niaura RS (1987). Social learning theory. In HT Leonard (ed.) *Psychological Theories of Drinking and Alcoholism*. New York, NY: Guilford Press, 131-178.

Abrams DB & Wilson GT (1979). Self-monitoring and reactivity in the modification of cigarette smoking. *Journal of Consulting and Clinical Psychology* 47:243-251.

Abrams DB, Monti PM, Pinto RP et al. (1987). Psychosocial stress and coping in smokers who relapse or quit. *Health Psychology* 6:289-303.

American Psychiatric Association (1996). Practice guideline for the treatment of patients with nicotine dependence. *American Journal of Psychiatry* 153(Suppl):1-31.

Anda RF, Williamson DF, Escobedo LG et al. (1990). Depression and the dynamics of smoking: A national perspective. *Journal of the American Medical Association* 264:1541-1545.

Bandura A (1986). *Social Foundations of Thought and Action: A Social Cognitive Theory*. Englewood Cliffs, NJ: Prentice-Hall.

Bandura A (1997). *Self-Efficacy: The Exercise of Control*. New York, NY: W. H. Freeman & Co.

Battjes RJ (1988). Smoking as an issue in alcohol and drug abuse treatment. *Addictive Behaviors* 13:225-230.

Benson H (1975). *The Relaxation Response*. New York, NY: Avon Books.

Blot WJ, McLaughlin JK, Winn DM et al. (1988). Smoking and drinking in relation to oral and pharyngeal cancer. *Cancer Research* 48:3282-3287.

Bobo JK (1989). Nicotine dependence and alcoholism epidemiology and treatment. *Journal of Psychoactive Drugs* 21:323-329.

Bobo JK & Davies CM (1993). Recovering staff and smoking in chemical dependency programs in rural Nebraska. *Journal of Substance Abuse Treatment* 10:221-227.

Bobo JK & Gilchrist LD (1983). Urging the alcoholic client to quit smoking cigarettes. *Addictive Behaviors* 8:297-305.

Bobo JK, Gilchrist LD, Schilling RF et al. (1987). Cigarette smoking cessation attempts by recovering alcoholics. *Addictive Behaviors* 12:209-215.

Bobo JK, McIlvain HE, Lando HA et al. (1998). Effect of smoking cessation counseling on recovery from alcoholism: Findings from a randomized community intervention trial. *Addiction* 93:877-887.

Bobo JK, Slade J & Hoffman AL (1995). Nicotine addiction counseling for chemically dependent patients. *Psychiatric Services* 46:945-947.

Breslau N, Kilbey M & Andresky P (1990). Nicotine dependence in an urban population of young adults: Prevalence and co-morbidity with depression, anxiety, and other substance dependencies. In L Harris (ed.) *Problems of Drug Dependence 1990: Proceedings of the 52nd Annual Scientific Meeting of the Committee on Problems of Drug Dependence (NIDA Research Monograph 105)*. Washington, DC: U.S. Department of Health and Human Services, 458-459.

Breslau N, Kilbey M & Andreski P (1991). Nicotine dependence, major depression, and anxiety in young adults. *Archives of General Psychiatry* 48:1069-1074.

Brown RA & Emmons KM (1991). Behavioral treatment of cigarette dependence. In JA Cocores (ed.) *The Clinical Management of Nicotine Dependence*. New York, NY: Springer-Verlag, 97-118.

Brown RA, Goldstein MG, Niaura R et al. (1993). Nicotine dependence: Assessment and management. In A Stoudemire & BS Fogel (eds.) *Psychiatric Care of the Medical Patient*. New York, NY: Oxford University Press.

Brown RA, Kahler CW, Niaura R et al. (2001). Cognitive-behavioral treatment for depression in smoking cessation. *Journal of Consulting and Clinical Psychology* 69:471-480.

Brown RA & Lewinsohn PM (1984a). *Coping With Depression: Course Workbook*. Eugene, OR: Castalia Press.

Brown RA & Lewinsohn PM (1984b). A psychoeducational approach to the treatment of depression: Comparison of group, individual, and minimal contact procedures. *Journal of Consulting and Clinical Psychology* 52(5):774-783.

Burling TA, Marshall GD & Seidner AL (1991). Smoking cessation for substance abuse inpatients. *Journal of Substance Abuse* 3:269-276.

Burling TA & Ziff DC (1988). Tobacco smoking: A comparison between alcohol and drug abuse inpatients. *Addictive Behaviors* 13:185-190.

Carroll KM (1996). Relapse prevention as a psychosocial treatment: A review of controlled clinical trials. *Experimental and Clinical Psychopharmacology* 4:46-54.

Centers for Disease Control and Prevention (CDC) (1990). Smokers' beliefs about the health benefits of smoking cessation—20 U.S. communities, 1989. *Morbidity and Mortality Weekly Report* 39: 653-656.

Centers for Disease Control and Prevention (CDC) (1993). Physician and other health-care professional counseling of smokers—United States, 1991. *Morbidity and Mortality Weekly Report* 42:854-857.

Centers for Disease Control and Prevention (CDC) (1994a). Medical-care expenditures attributable to cigarette smoking—United States, 1993. *Morbidity and Mortality Weekly Report* 43:469-472.

Centers for Disease Control and Prevention (CDC) (1994b). Cigarette smoking among adults—United States, 1993. *Morbidity and Mortality Weekly Report* 43:925-929.

Centers for Disease Control and Prevention (CDC) (1997). Smoking-attributable mortality and years of potential life lost—United States, 1984. *Morbidity and Mortality Weekly Report* 46:444-451.

Centers for Disease Control and Prevention (CDC) (1998a). Tobacco use among high school students—United States, 1997. *Morbidity and Mortality Weekly Report* 47:229-293.

Centers for Disease Control and Prevention (CDC) (1998b). State specific prevalence among adults of current cigarette smoking and smokeless tobacco use and per capita tax-paid sales of cigarettes—United States, 1997. *Morbidity and Mortality Weekly Report* 47:922-926.

Centers for Disease Control and Prevention (CDC) (1999a). Cigarette smoking among adults—United States, 1997. *Morbidity and Mortality Weekly Report* 48:993-996.

Centers for Disease Control and Prevention (CDC) (1999b). Tobacco use—United States, 1990-1999. *Morbidity and Mortality Weekly Report* 48:986-993.

Centers for Disease Control and Prevention (CDC) (1999c). State specific prevalence of current cigarette smoking among adults and cigar smoking among adults—United States, 1998. *Morbidity and Mortality Weekly Report* 48:1034-1039.

Cinciripini PM, Lapitsky L, Seay S et al. (1995). The effects of smoking schedules on cessation outcome: Can we improve on common methods of gradual and abrupt nicotine withdrawal? *Journal of Consulting and Clinical Psychology* 63:388-399.

Cohen S, Lichtenstein E, Prochaska JO et al. (1989). Debunking myths about self-quitting. *American Psychologist* 44:1355-1365.

Colletti G & Brownell K (1982). The physical and emotional benefits of social support: Applications to obesity, smoking and alcoholism. In M Hersen, R Eisler & P Miller (eds.) *Progress in Behavior Modification*, Vol. 13. New York, NY: Academic Press.

Covey LS, Glassman AH & Stetner F (1990). Depression and depressive symptoms in smoking cessation. *Comprehensive Psychiatry* 31:350-354.

Covey LS, Hughes DC, Glassman AH et al. (1994). Ever-smoking, quitting, and psychiatric disorders: Evidence from the Durham, North Carolina, epidemiologic catchment area. *Tobacco Control* 3:222-227.

Cumming SR, Rubin SM & Oster G (1989). The cost-effectiveness of counseling smokers to quit. *Journal of the American Medical Association* 261:75-79.

Curry S, Wagner EH & Grothaus LC (1990). Intrinsic and extrinsic motivation for smoking cessation. *Journal of Consulting and Clinical Psychology* 58:310-316.

DeBusk R, Miller N, Superko HR et al. (1994). A case-management system for coronary risk factor modification after acute myocardial infarction. *Annals of Internal Medicine* 120:721-729.

Ellis A & Harper RA (1961). *A Guide to Rational Living*. Hollywood, CA: Wilshire.

Etringer BD, Gregory VR & Lando HA (1984). Influence of group cohesion on the behavioral treatment of smoking. *Journal of Consulting and Clinical Psychology* 52:1080-1086.

Federal Trade Commission (1997). *Tar, Nicotine, and Carbon Monoxide of the Smoke of 1206 Varieties of Domestic Cigarettes*. Washington, DC: Federal Trade Commission.

Fiore MC, Bailey WC, Cohen SJ et al. (1996). *Smoking Cessation: Clinical Practice Guideline No. 18)*. Rockville, MD: U.S. Department of Health and Human Services, Public Health Service, Agency for Health Care Policy and Research, Centers for Disease Control and Prevention.

Fiore MC, Bailey WC, Cohen SJ et al. (2000). *Treating Tobacco Use and Dependence: Clinical Practice Guidelines*. Rockville, MD: U.S. Department of Health and Human Services, Public Health Service.

Fishbein M (1977). Consumer beliefs and behavior with respect to cigarette smoking: A critical analysis of the public literature. In Federal Trade Commission (ed.) *Report to Congress: Pursuant to the Public Health Cigarette Smoking Act, for the Year 1976*. Washington, DC: Federal Trade Commission.

Foxx RM & Brown RA (1979). Nicotine fading and self-monitoring for cigarette abstinence or controlled smoking. *Journal of Applied Behavior Analysis* 12:111-125.

Garvey AJ, Bliss RE, Hitchcock JL et al. (1992). Predictors of smoking relapse among self-quitters: A report from the normative aging study. *Addictive Behaviors* 17:367-377.

Ginsberg D, Hall SM, Reus VI et al. (1995). Mood and depression diagnosis in smoking cessation. *Experimental and Clinical Psychopharmacology* 3(4):389-395.

Ginsberg D, Hall S & Rosinski M (1992). Partner support, psychological treatment, and nicotine gum in smoking treatment: An incremental study. *International Journal of the Addictions* 27(5):503-514.

Glasgow RE & Lichtenstein E (1987). Long-term effects of behavioral smoking cessation interventions. *Behavior Therapy* 18:297-338.

Glasser W (1976). *Positive Addictions*. New York, NY: Harper & Row.

Glassman AH, Covey LS, Dalack GW et al. (1993). Smoking cessation, clonidine, and vulnerability to nicotine among dependent smokers. *Clinical Pharmacology and Therapeutics* 54:670-679.

Glassman AH, Helzer JE, Covey LS et al. (1990). Smoking, smoking cessation, and major depression. *Journal of the American Medical Association* 264(12):1546-1549.

Glassman AH, Stetner F, Walsh BT et al. (1988). Heavy smokers, smoking cessation, and clonidine. *Journal of the American Medical Association* 259(19):2863-2866.

Goldstein MG, Niaura R, Wiley-Lessne C et al. (1997). Physicians counseling smokers. A population-based survey of patients' perceptions of health care provider-delivered smoking cessation interventions. *Archives of Internal Medicine* 157:1313-1319.

Hall SM, Muñoz RF & Reus VI (1994). Cognitive-behavioral intervention increases abstinence rates for depressive-history smokers. *Journal of Consulting and Clinical Psychology* 62(1):141-146.

Hall SM, Muñoz RF, Reus VI et al. (1996). Mood management and nicotine gum in smoking treatment: A therapeutic contact and placebo-controlled study. *Journal of Consulting and Clinical Psychology* 64(5):1003-1009.

Hall SM, Reus VI, Muñoz RF et al. (1998). Nortriptyline and cognitive-behavioral therapy in the treatment of cigarette smoking. *Archives of General Psychiatry* 55:683-690.

Henningfield JE, Clayton R & Pollin W (1990). Involvement of tobacco in alcoholism and illicit drug use. *British Journal of Addiction* 85:279-292.

Hollis JF, Lichtenstein E, Vogt TM et al. (1993). Nurse-assisted counseling for smokers in primary care. *Annals of Internal Medicine* 118:521-559.

Hughes JR (1993). Treatment of smoking cessation in smokers with past alcohol/drug problems. *Journal of Substance Abuse Treatment* 10:181-187.

Hughes JR, ed. (1995). Combining behavioral therapy and pharmacotherapy for smoking cessation: An update. In LS Onken, JD Blaine & JJ Boren (eds.) *NIDA Research Monograph 150*. Washington, DC: U.S. Department of Health and Human Services.

Hunt WA & Bespalec DA (1974). An evaluation of current methods of modifying smoking behavior. *Journal of Clinical Psychology* 30:431-438.

Hurt RD, Eberman KM, Croghan IT et al. (1994). Nicotine dependence treatment during inpatient treatment for other addictions: A prospective intervention trial. *Alcoholism: Clinical & Experimental Research* 18:867-872.

Hurt RD, Eberman KM, Slade J et al. (1993). Treating nicotine addiction in patients with other addictive diseases. In CT Orleans & J Sade (ed.) *Nicotine Addiction: Principles and Management*. New York, NY: Oxford University Press, 310-326.

Istvan J & Matarazzo JD (1984). Tobacco, alcohol, and caffeine use: A review of their interrelationships. *Psychological Bulletin* 95:301-326.

Jacobson E (1983). *Progressive Relaxation, 2nd Edition*. Chicago, IL: University of Chicago Press.

Jarman CM & Kellett JM (1979). Alcoholism in the general hospital. *British Medical Journal* 132:469-472.

Joseph AM, Nichol KL & Anderson H (1990a). Effect of treatment for nicotine dependence on alcohol and drug treatment outcomes. *Addictive Behavior* 18:635-644.

Joseph AM, Nichol KL, Willenbring ML et al. (1990b). Beneficial effects of treatment of nicotine dependence during an inpatient substance abuse treatment program. *Journal of the American Medical Association* 263:3043-3046.

Kendler KS, Neale MC, MacLean CJ et al. (1993). Smoking and major depression: A causal analysis. *Archives of General Psychiatry* 50:36-43.

Kinnunen T, Doherty K, Militello FS et al. (1996). Depression and smoking cessation: Characteristics of depressed smokers and effects of nicotine dependence. *Journal of Consulting and Clinical Psychology* 64(4):791-798.

Kottke TE, Battista RN, DeFriese GH et al. (1988). Attributes of successful smoking cessation in medical practice: A meta-analysis of 39 controlled trials. *Journal of the American Medical Association* 259(19):2882-2889.

Kottke TE, Solberg LL & Brekke ML (1990). Beyond efficacy testing: Introducing preventive cardiology into primary care. *American Journal of Preventive Medicine* 6(Suppl):77-83.

Kozlowski LT & Ferrence RG (1990). Statistical control in research on alcohol and tobacco: An example from research on alcohol and mortality. *British Journal of Addiction* 85:271-278.

Kozlowski LT, Ferrence RG & Corbit T (1990). Tobacco use: A perspective for alcohol and drug researchers. *British Journal of Addiction* 85:245-300.

Kozlowski LT, Skinner W, Kent C et al. (1989). Prospects for smoking treatment in individuals seeking treatment for alcohol and other drug problems. *Addictive Behavior* 14:273-278.

Kozlowski LT, Wilkinson A, Skinner W et al. (1989). Comparing tobacco cigarette dependence with other drug dependencies: Greater or equal "difficulty quitting" and "urges to use," but less pleasure from cigarettes. *Journal of the American Medical Association* 261: 898-901.

Lando HA & McGovern PG (1985). Nicotine fading as a nonaversive alternative in a broad-spectrum treatment for eliminating smoking. *Addictive Behaviors* 52:1080-1086.

Lando HA, McGovern P & Stipfle C (1989). Public service application of an effective clinic approach to smoking cessation. *Health Education Research* 4:103-109.

Levinson BL, Shapiro D, Schwartz GE et al. (1971). Smoking elimination by gradual reduction. *Behavior Therapy* 2:477-487.

Lewinsohn PM, Antonuccio DO, Breckenridge JS et al. (1984). *The Coping With Depression Course: A Psychoeducational Intervention for Unipolar Depression*. Eugene, OR: Castalia Press.

Lichtenstein E, Antonuccio DO & Rainwater G (1977, April). *Unkicking the Habit: The Resumption of Cigarette Smoking*. Paper presented at the annual meeting of the Western Psychological Association, Seattle, WA.

Lichtenstein E, Glasgow RE & Abrams DB (1986). Social support in smoking cessation: In search of effective interventions. *Behavior Therapy* 17:607-619.

Marcus BH, Albrecht AE, Parisi AF et al. (1999). Efficacy of exercise as an aid for smoking cessation in women. *Archives of Internal Medicine* 159:1229-1234.

Marlatt GA & Gordon JR (1980). Determinants of relapse: Implications for the maintenance of behavior change. In PO Davidson & SM Davidson (eds.) *Behavioral Medicine: Changing Health Lifestyles.* New York, NY: Brunner/Mazel.

Marlatt GA & Gordon JR (1985). *Relapse Prevention.* New York, NY: Guilford Press.

McGinnis J & Foege W (1993). Actual causes of death in the United States. *Journal of the American Medical Association* 270:2207-2212.

Mermelstein R, Cohen S, Lichtenstein E et al. (1986). Social support and smoking cessation and maintenance. *Journal of Consulting and Clinical Psychology* 54:447-453.

Miller WR & Rollnick S (1991). *Motivational Interviewing: Preparing People to Change Addictive Behaviors.* New York, NY: Guilford Press.

Miller LS, Zhang X, Rice DP et al. (1993). State estimates of total medical care expenditures attributable to cigarette smoking. *Public Health Reports* 113:447-458.

National Institute on Alcohol Abuse and Addiction (NIAAA) (1984). *Fifth Special Report to the U. S. Congress on Alcohol and Health from the Secretary of Health and Human Services.* Washington, DC: U.S. Government Printing Office.

Niaura RS, Rohsenow DJ, Binkoff JA et al. (1988). Relevance of cue reactivity to understanding alcohol and smoking relapse. *Journal of Abnormal Psychology* 97(2): 133-152.

Ockene JK (1987). Smoking intervention: The expanding role of physicians. *American Journal of Public Health* 77:782-783.

Ockene JK, Aney J, Goldberg RJ et al. (1988). A survey of Massachusetts physicians' smoking intervention practices. *American Journal of Preventive Medicine* 4:14-20.

Ockene JK, Emmons KM, Mermelstein RJ et al. (2000). Relapse and maintenance issues for smoking cessation. *Health Psychology* 19 (Suppl):17-31.

Orleans CT (1985). Understanding and promoting smoking cessation: Overview and guidelines for physician intervention. *Annual Review of Medicine* 36:51-61.

Orleans CT & Hutchinson D (1993). Tailoring nicotine addiction treatments for chemical dependency patients. *Journal of Substance Abuse Treatment* 10:197-208.

Pederson LL, Baskerville JC & Wanklin JM (1982). Multivariate statistical models for predicting change in smoking behavior following physician advice to quit smoking. *Preventive Medicine* 11:536-549.

Prochaska JO & DiClemente CC (1986). Towards a comprehensive model of change. In WR Miller & N Heather (eds.) *Treating Addictive Disorders: Processes of Change.* New York, NY: Plenum Press.

Prochaska JO & Goldstein MG (1991). Process of smoking cessation: Implications for clinicians. *Clinics in Chest Medicine* 12(4):727-735.

Rollnick S, Mason P & Butler C (1999). *Health Behavior Change: A Guide for Practitioners.* London: Churchill Livingstone.

Rounsaville BJ, Kosten TR, Weissman MM et al. (1985). *Evaluating and Treating Depressive Disorders in Opiate Addicts.* Washington, DC: U.S. Government Printing Office.

Schachter S (1982). Recidivism and self-cure of smoking and obesity. *American Psychologist* 37(4):436-444.

Schwartz JL (1992). Methods of smoking cessation. *Medical Clinics of North America* 76:451-76.

Schwartz JL (1987). *Review and Evaluation of Smoking Cessation Methods: The United States and Canada, 1978-1985.* Bethesda, MD: U.S. Department of Health and Human Services, Public Health Service, National Institutes of Health, National Cancer Institute, Division of Cancer Prevention and Control.

Sees KL & Clark HW (1993). When to begin smoking cessation in substance abusers. *Journal of Substance Abuse Treatment* 10:189-195.

Shiffman S (1982). Relapse following smoking cessation: A situational analysis. *Journal of Consulting and Clinical Psychology* 50:71-86.

Shiffman S (1984). Coping with temptations to smoke. *Journal of Consulting and Clinical Psychology* 52:261-267.

Shiffman S (1985). Coping with temptations to smoke. In S Shiffman & T Wills (eds.) *Coping and Substance Abuse.* Orlando, FL: Academic Press.

Shiffman S (1993). Smoking cessation treatment: Any progress? *Journal of Consulting and Clinical Psychology* 61:718-722.

Stevens VJ & Hollis JF (1989). Preventing smoking relapse, using an individually tailored skills-training technique. *Journal of Consulting and Clinical Psychology* 57:420-424.

Thorndike AN, Rigotti NA, Stafford RS et al. (1998). National patterns in the treatment of smokers by physicians. *Journal of the American Medical Association* 279:604-608.

U.S. Department of Health and Human Services (DHHS) (1988). *The Health Consequences of Smoking: Nicotine Addiction. A Report of the Surgeon General.* Rockville, MD: U.S. Public Health Service, Office on Smoking and Health.

U.S. Department of Health and Human Services (DHHS) (1989). *Reducing the Health Consequences of Smoking: 25 Years of Progress. A Report of the Surgeon General.* Rockville, MD: U.S. Public Health Service, Office on Smoking and Health.

Velicer WF, Fava JL, Prochaska JO et al. (1995). Distribution of smokers by stage in three representative samples. *Preventive Medicine* 24: 401-411.

Wald NJ & Hackshaw AK (1996). Cigarette smoking: An epidemiological overview. *British Medical Bulletin* 52:3-11.

West RJ, Hajek P & Belcher M (1989). Severity of withdrawal symptoms as a predictor of outcome of an attempt to quit smoking. *Psychological Medicine* 19:981-985.

Chapter 6 | Network Therapy

Marc Galanter, M.D., FASAM

Conditioning and Conditioned Cues
Social Cohesiveness as a Vehicle for Reinforcing Abstinence
Network Therapy in Office Practice
Principles of Network Treatment

Recent years have seen considerable progress toward developing psychosocial modalities specific to the treatment of addiction. The situation today is quite different than it was when Alcoholics Anonymous (AA) emerged more than a half century ago in a climate of inadequate physician attention to the rehabilitation of alcoholics. Professionals in the addictions field now have access to a variety of therapeutic techniques, including variants of cognitive therapy, motivational enhancement, and family and group therapy modalities—all tailored to the needs of patients with alcohol or drug disorders.

The clinician in office practice, however, often is uncertain as to how to integrate these approaches to meet the needs of a given patient. On the face of it, there is no obvious relationship, for example, between the use of cognitively oriented approaches such as relapse prevention and the engagement of family support to secure improved motivation.

To address this dilemma, this chapter examines network therapy (Galanter, 1999), a comprehensive modality that has been disseminated to practitioners over the past two decades, and more recently standardized and studied in the clinical research setting. Network therapy is designed to provide clinicians with a method of integrating multiple approaches developed specifically for management of the addicted patient.

Support for addiction treatment itself has expanded over time, and recognition of the severity of the problem in the 1970s initially led to an increase in resources for inpatient care. The availability of beds in designated units increased by 62% from 1977 to 1984, with all of the net gain in the private sector (NIAAA, 1987). Also at that time, the "Minnesota Model" for inpatient management (Cook, 1988), incorporating a protracted inpatient stay, became a standard of treatment for many middle-class addicts. However, a subsequent wave of cost-containment initiatives reduced occupancy rates at nonpublic facilities to as low as 60% by 1990 (*Alcoholism and Drug Abuse Week*, 1990) and even lower more recently. This decline has been fueled by a lack of empirical support for the relative advantage of inpatient over ambulatory care (Institute of Medicine, 1990).

Managing addicted patients in office practice can in fact be less costly than inpatient care, but reports on its relative effectiveness in standard office practice have not been positive. In an early survey of psychiatrists in practice, Hayman (1956) found that very few professed an appreciable degree of success in treating alcoholics in an office setting.

No difference in outcome was found when outpatients were offered individual therapy as a treatment added to medical monitoring alone (Braunstein, Powell et al., 1983), nor was insight-oriented therapy found to enhance the effectiveness of outpatient milieu treatment for alcoholism (Olson, Ganley et al., 1981). Indeed, Vaillant (1981), commenting on alcoholism treatment, observed that "The greatest danger of this is wasteful, painful psychotherapy that bears analogy to someone trying to shoot a fish in a pool. No matter how carefully he aims, the refracted image always renders the shot wide of its mark." As conventionally practiced, individual therapy does not appear to be an effective tool for rehabilitation of the addicted patient.

A number of issues can be considered in formulating a new approach to office-based therapy. Recent years have witnessed both research-based and clinical support for the importance of securing abstinence as an initial step in addiction treatment, rather than awaiting results of an exploratory therapy (Nathan & McCrady, 1986/1987; Gitlow & Peyser, 1980; Gallant, 1987). This position has been strengthened by the widespread acceptance of AA, which is strongly oriented toward abstinence. To implement a regimen of abstinence, clinical researchers have developed a number of structured techniques, focusing on cognitive-behavioral change (Marlatt & Gordon, 1985; Annis, 1986) and interpersonal support from family and peers (Stanton & Thomas, 1982; Kaufman & Kaufman, 1979; Galanter, 1993b). Therefore, this chapter will consider how these approaches can be adapted to an office practice oriented toward individual therapy so as to promote abstinence and effective rehabilitation.

Such an integrated approach is referred to as "network therapy" because it draws on the support of a group of family and peers who are introduced into therapy sessions. The term derives from the work of Speck and Attneave (1974), who used a large support group drawn from the patient's family and social network as a tool for psychiatric management. Such networks were used for both psychological and practical aid in addressing acute psychiatric illness, so as to avert a hospitalization until the acute symptoms remitted. Once mobilized, the network became available to aid in ambulatory rehabilitation as well.

To define what this approach must accomplish, it is necessary to examine some unique characteristics of the substance dependence syndrome.

This chapter first considers the clinical implications of the conditioned abstinence syndrome in terms of its rel-evance to relapse prevention techniques directed at the conditioned cues that precipitate substance use. Next, it examines the role of social cohesiveness in stabilizing the substance-abusing patient in treatment and defines how family members and peers can be integrated into the patient's treatment in the office setting so as to make use of this potent vehicle for reinforcing abstinent behavior. Clinical examples and the particulars of the integrated technique are then given. Altogether then, network therapy is defined as integrating relapse prevention techniques into a therapeutic approach that brings family and peer members into the individual treatment setting.

CONDITIONING AND CONDITIONED CUES

For many clinicians, the problems of relapse and loss of control, embodied in the criteria for substance dependence in the *Diagnostic and Statistical Manual of Mental Disorders, 4th Edition* (American Psychiatric Association, 1994), epitomize the pitfalls inherent in addiction treatment. Because addicted patients typically experience pressure to relapse and ingest alcohol or drugs, they are seen as poor candidates for stable treatment. The concept of "loss of control" has been used to describe addicts' inability to limit consumption reliably once an initial dose is taken (Gallant, 1987).

Conditioned Abstinence. These clinical phenomena generally are described anecdotally but can be explained mechanistically as well, by recourse to the model of conditioned withdrawal, which relates the pharmacology of dependence-producing drugs to the behaviors they produce. Wikler (1973), an early investigator of addiction pharmacology, developed this model to explain the spontaneous appearance of drug craving and relapse. He pointed out that drugs of dependence typically produce compensatory responses in the central nervous system at the same time that their direct pharmacologic effects are felt, and these compensatory effects partly counter the drugs' direct action. Thus, when an opiate antagonist is administered to an addict maintained with morphine, latent withdrawal phenomena are unmasked. Similar compensatory effects are observed in alcoholics maintained with alcohol, who evidence evoked response patterns characteristic of withdrawal while still clinically intoxicated (Begleiter & Porjesz, 1979).

Wikler studied addicts who were maintained with morphine and then thrown into withdrawal with a narcotic antagonist. After several trials of precipitated withdrawal, he found that a full-blown withdrawal response could be elicited in his subjects when a placebo antagonist was administered. He concluded that the withdrawal had been conditioned and was later elicited by a conditioned cue—in this case, the syringe used to administer the placebo. This hypothesized mechanism was later confirmed by O'Brien and colleagues (1977), who elicited conditioned withdrawal by using sound tones as conditioned cues. This concept helps to explain addictive behavior outside the laboratory.

A potential addict who has begun to drink or use another drug heavily may be repeatedly exposed to an external stimulus (such as a certain mood state) while drinking. Subsequent exposure to these cues thus can produce conditioned withdrawal symptoms, which the individual subjectively experiences as craving. A dramatic example of this phenomenon is seen among heroin addicts, who may experience a severe withdrawal syndrome when they return to the neighborhoods where they previously had used heroin, even after years away from the drug. In such cases, the setting of the neighborhood itself serves as a cue that produces the signs and symptoms of withdrawal (McAuliffe, 1982; Galanter, 1983).

Implications for Treatment. The conditioned withdrawal model helps explain why relapse is such a frequent and unanticipated aspect of addiction treatment. Exposure to conditioned cues (ones that were repeatedly associated with drug use) can precipitate reflexive drug craving during the course of therapy, and such cue exposure also can initiate a sequence of unconditioned behaviors that lead addicts unwittingly to relapse to drug use.

Loss of control can be the product of conditioned withdrawal, described by Ludwig and colleagues (1978) and long recognized on a practical level by members of AA. The sensations associated with the ingestion of an addictive drug, such as the odor of alcohol or the euphoria produced by opiates, are temporally associated with the pharmacologic elicitation of a compensatory response to that drug and later can produce drug-seeking behavior. For this reason, the first drink can serve as a conditioned cue for further drinking. Patients thus have a very limited capacity to control consumption once a single dose of drug has been taken.

Case 1: A 30-year-old cocaine addict undergoing treatment was abstinent and well motivated for two months, but occasionally drank socially. One evening he sought out a cocaine dealer on an impulse, then purchased and insufflated 1 g of cocaine. After returning home, he bought more cocaine and continued to take the drug over the course of the entire night. Examination of this sequence of events in his next therapy session revealed that he had been sitting in a restaurant bar with a date whom he knew to use cocaine. After having two drinks, he had gone to the rest room—a place where he occasionally had used cocaine before entering treatment. It was after this event that he bought the cocaine.

The patient acknowledged that he had been exposed to a number of cues that had been associated with his previous cocaine consumption: a sexually charged situation with a cocaine user, consumption of alcohol, and a physical setting in which he had used cocaine in the past.

Changes in mood state also can become conditioned stimuli for drug-seeking behavior, and the addict can become vulnerable to relapse through reflexive response to a specific affective state. Such phenomena have been described clinically by Khantzian (1985) as self-medication. Such mood-related cues, however, are not necessarily mentioned spontaneously by the patient in conventional therapy. This situation is because the triggering feeling may not be associated with a memorable event and the drug use may avert emergence of memorable distress.

More dramatic is the phenomenon of affect regression, which Wurmser (1977) observed among addicted patients studied in a psychoanalytic context. He pointed out that when addicts suffer narcissistic injury, they are prone to a precipitous collapse of ego defenses and the consequent experience of intense and unmanageable affective flooding. In the face of such vulnerability, they handle stress poorly and can turn to drugs for relief. This vulnerability can be considered in light of the model of conditioned withdrawal, in which drug seeking can become an immediate reflexive response to stress, thereby undermining the stability and effectiveness of a patient's coping mechanisms.

The model of conditioned drug seeking has been applied to development of treatment techniques that attempt to train patients to recognize drug-related cues and thus to avoid relapse. Annis (1986), for example, has used a self-report schedule to assist patients in identifying the cues, situations, and moods that are most likely to lead them to alcohol craving. Marlatt and Gordon (1985) evolved an approach they described as "relapse prevention," whereby patients are taught strategies for avoiding the consequences of the alcohol-related cues they have identified. A similar concept has been used to extinguish cocaine craving through cue exposure in a clinical laboratory (Childress, McLellan et al., 1988).

These approaches can be introduced as part of a single-modality behavioral regimen, but they also can be used in expressive and family-oriented psychotherapy. For example, Ludwig and colleagues (1978) suggested the approach of cognitive labeling; namely, associating drinking cues with readily identified guideposts to aid the patient in consciously avoiding the consequences of prior conditioning. Similarly, the author (1983) has described a process of guided recall to explore the sequence of antecedents in given episodes of craving or drinking slips that was not clear to the patient. These approaches can be employed concurrently with an examination of general adaptive problems in an exploratory therapy.

The conditioning approach described here is useful in understanding the relationship between the pharmacology and behaviors associated with drugs of abuse. The test of an explanatory approach is whether it yields options that can be adapted to practice. This means that a stable ongoing treatment (one in which cues related to drug seeking can be addressed) must be secured.

In light of the need for practical applications, this chapter next considers the interpersonal modality necessary to secure an addicted patient's engagement in treatment and compliance. This approach has been termed "network therapy" because family members and friends are enlisted to provide an ongoing network of support for recovery.

SOCIAL COHESIVENESS AS A VEHICLE FOR REINFORCING ABSTINENCE

Social cohesiveness is defined as the sum of all forces that act on members of a group to keep them engaged (Cartwright & Zander, 1962). It can be an important factor in binding a patient to the therapeutic context, even when he or she is inclined to drop out. Dependency on a therapist, affinity for members of a therapy group, or bonds to spouse and children in family therapy all are examples of this phenomenon.

Cohesiveness is particularly important in addiction rehabilitation, as it often is the principal vehicle for retaining the addicted patient in therapy when relapse threatens.

Peer-Led Programs. In studies of the emergence of cohesiveness in AA and other mutual help groups, the author and colleagues have found that, when inductees become engaged, they experience an improvement in emotional well-being. This enhanced well-being stabilizes conformity with the group's norms because compliance is operantly reinforced by a positive affective response to involvement in the group (Galanter, Talbott et al., 1990; Galanter, 1990). Drug-free therapeutic communities promote intense relat-

edness among members as a vehicle for addiction rehabilitation (De Leon, 1989). Alcoholism has been treated by recourse to group practices in cohesive subcultures. This is seen in peyote rituals in Native American communities in the southwestern United States and in espiritismo practices among Puerto Rican Americans (Albaugh & Anderson, 1974; Singer & Borrero, 1984).

AA in particular provides an example of how group cohesiveness can be highly influential in addiction rehabilitation. At AA meetings, reinforcement for involvement is regularly provided as members are given effusive, ritualized approval by the group, both when they speak informally and when they recount their histories at anniversaries of their sobriety. An individual member develops close ties to a member who serves as a sponsor to supervise his or her recovery, and this relationship is a predictor of good outcome (Emrick, 1989). On an institutional level as well, the AA approach has been integrated into hospital-based programs, which encourage patients to sustain ties to fellow AA members after discharge (Cook, 1988). In a study of physicians who successfully completed an AA-oriented residential program, the author and colleagues found that, even two years after discharge, they attended more than five AA meetings each week and were in contact with their AA sponsors twice a week (Galanter, Talbott et al., 1990).

Importantly, AA illustrates the feasibility of combining strong, cohesive ties with cognitive-behavioral techniques. For example, members are inculcated to avoid the "persons, places, and things" that are cues to drinking. They learn mottos and phrases that serve as cognitive labels for avoidance of problematic attitudes and situations (Ludwig, Bendfeldt et al., 1978). These aspects of the Twelve Step approach illustrate how the labeling of cues for conditioned withdrawal can be wedded to a social therapy, thereby enhancing the addict's motivation to apply such labeling as a way to avoid relapse. AA members are reinforced when they discuss the avoidance of cues at AA meetings or with their sponsors in the organization.

Unfortunately, however, many addicted patients reject the option of involvement in AA, while others drop out after their initial meetings (Brandsma, Maultsby et al., 1980). Accordingly, there is a strategic advantage in a therapeutic approach that draws on preexisting cohesive ties—those of family and close friends—as a starting point in treatment. The latter approach also can protect against early dropping out, which might take place in a self-help group setting populated by relative strangers. It can help the therapist to encourage a reluctant patient to continue attendance at AA meetings.

Professionally Led Treatment. Professionals can draw on a network of cohesive relationships to enhance the outcome of treatment. For example, an evaluation of the outcome of Speck and Attneave's network therapy for psychotic patients (Schoenfeld, Halevey et al., 1986) demonstrated that considerable benefit derived from use of existing social ties to family and friends. Enhanced outcome was reported as well when the community reinforcement techniques developed by Hunt and Azrin (1973) were augmented by greater social relatedness in a club-like setting (Mallams, Godley et al., 1982). Similarly, the author and colleagues (Galanter, Castaneda et al., 1987) improved retention rates and increased social recovery by integrating a peer-led format into a professionally directed alcohol treatment program.

Not surprisingly, the cohesiveness and support offered by group and family therapy have been found effective in rehabilitating addicted patients. Yalom and colleagues (1978) reported on benefits derived when interactional group therapy was used as an adjunct to recovery techniques. Couples group therapy has been shown to benefit alcoholics and to diminish the likelihood of treatment dropout (Gallant, Rich et al., 1970; McCrady, Stout et al., 1991). Even counseling spouses of alcoholics in the absence of their alcoholic partners ultimately yields effective treatment (Dittrich & Trapold, 1984). Observations like these have led experienced clinicians to develop addiction rehabilitation techniques based on expertise in the practice of family therapy and have yielded a number of clinical monographs on the use of established family therapy techniques in addiction (Stanton & Thomas, 1982; Kaufman & Kaufman, 1979; Steinglass, Bennett et al., 1987).

NETWORK THERAPY IN OFFICE PRACTICE

Having examined the benefits of introducing behavioral techniques and social cohesion into ongoing treatment of the addicted patient, this chapter next considers the model of network therapy for addiction (Galanter, 1993a, 1987). It offers a pragmatic approach to augmenting conventional individual therapy that draws on recent advances to enhance the effectiveness of office management of the addicted patient.

Couples. Couples therapy for addiction has been described in both ambulatory and inpatient settings, and good marital adjustment has been found to be associated with a diminished likelihood of dropping out and a positive overall outcome (Stanton & Thomas, 1982; Kaufman & Kaufman, 1979; McCrady, Stout et al., 1991; Dittrich & Trapold, 1984; Galanter, 1987; Noel, McCrady et al., 1987; Moos & Moos, 1984).

It is recognized, however, that a spouse must be involved in an appropriate way. Constructive engagement should be distinguished from a codependent relationship (Cermak, 1986) or overly involved interaction, which is thought to be a problem in recovery. Indeed, couples managed with a behavioral orientation showed greater improvement in alcoholism than those treated with interactional therapy, in which attempts were made to engage them in relational change (O'Farrell, Cutter et al., 1985). Therefore, it is important for clinicians to accord each member of the couple an appropriate and differentiated role, so that the spouse is not placed in a position of pressing the patient to comply with treatment. Thus, we consider here a simple, behaviorally oriented device for making use of the marital relationship: namely, working with a couple to enhance the effectiveness of disulfiram therapy.

In controlled trials, the use of disulfiram has yielded relatively little benefit when patients are responsible for taking their doses on their own (Fuller & Williford, 1980). This situation occurs largely because disulfiram is effective only when used as instructed, typically on a daily basis. Alcoholics who forget to take required doses are likely to resume drinking. Indeed, such "forgetting" often reflects the initiation of a sequence of conditioned drug-seeking behaviors.

Although patient characteristics have not been shown to predict compliance with a disulfiram regimen (Schuckit, 1985), changes in the format of patient management have been found to have a beneficial effect on outcomes (Brubaker, Prue et al., 1987). For example, the involvement of a spouse in observing the patient's consumption of disulfiram yields a considerable improvement in outcome (Keane, Foy et al., 1984; Azrin, Sisson et al., 1982; Galanter, 1989). Patients alerted to take disulfiram each morning by this external reminder are less likely to experience conditioned drug seeking when exposed to addictive cues and are more likely to comply with the dosing regimen on subsequent days.

The technique (Galanter, 1993a) also helps to clearly define the roles in therapy of both the alcoholic and spouse (typically the wife) by avoiding the spouse's need to monitor drinking behaviors she cannot control. The spouse does not actively remind the alcoholic to take each disulfiram dose. She merely notifies the therapist if she does not observe the pill being ingested on a given day. Decisions about managing compliance then are shifted to the therapist, and the couple avoids becoming entangled in a dispute over the patient's attitude and the possibility of secret drinking. By means of this technique, most alcoholics in one clinical trial (Galanter, 1993b) experienced marked improvement and sustained abstinence over the period of treatment.

A variety of other behavioral devices shown to improve outcomes can be incorporated into a couples format. For example, one study found that scheduling a new patient's first appointment as soon as possible after an initial telephone contact improved outcomes by diminishing the possibility of an early loss of motivation (Stark, Campbell et al., 1990). Spouses also can be engaged in history-taking at the outset of treatment to minimize the introduction of denial into the patient's representation of the illness (Liepman, Nierenberg et al., 1989). The initiation of treatment with such a technique is illustrated in the following case report.

Case 2: A 39-year-old alcoholic man was referred for treatment. Both the patient and his wife were initially engaged by the psychiatrist in a telephone exchange so that all three could plan for the patient to remain abstinent on the day of the first session. They agreed that the wife would meet the patient at his office at the end of the work day and accompany him to the appointment. This action would ensure that cues presented by his friends going out for a drink after work would not lead him to drink.

In the session, an initial history was taken from the spouse as well as the patient, allowing her to expand on the negative consequences of the patient's drinking, thus heading off any effort to minimize the problem.

A review of the patient's medical status revealed no evidence of relevant organ damage, and the option of initiating his treatment with disulfiram was discussed. The patient, with the encouragement of his wife, agreed to take his first dose that day, continue under her observation, and then be evaluated by his internist within a few days. Subsequent sessions with the couple were dedicated to dealing with implementation of this plan. Concurrent individual therapy was initiated as well.

Patients who take disulfiram in this manner have acquired a cognitive label to help them avoid a sudden and unanticipated relapse. The potential efficacy of this approach is illustrated by the reaction of the patient described in Case 2, an attorney who experienced a precipitous collapse of psychological defenses on receiving an incorrect report about his share of the partnership's profits. If the patient had been taking disulfiram as described here, his knowledge of a potential disulfiram reaction could have alerted him to avoid going out to get a drink. Patients who are maintained with disulfiram, as described, for an initial year of recovery thus have the opportunity to deal in therapy with the issues that precipitate craving, without exposing themselves unduly to the threat of relapse. In the lawyer's case, adherence to the plan would have allowed him to address the psychodynamic underpinnings of his job-related anxieties in the therapy, rather than by reflexive drinking.

It is important to clarify certain aspects of engaging a collateral—particularly a spouse—in the treatment process. Long-standing conflicts between members of an alcoholic couple should not be allowed to interfere with the disulfiram monitoring. For example, the spouse should not be placed in a role in which he or she must demand compliance. This is why the patient is vested with the responsibility of ingesting the disulfiram in a way that is clearly visible to the spouse; the spouse's role is only to notify the therapist in a telephone message if the patient is not seen taking the pill on a given morning. Discussions of compliance thus are initiated by the therapist and not by the spouse. In this way, the role of the spouse as enforcer is eliminated. This is compatible with the approach suggested by Al-Anon, which encourages the spouse to avoid responsibility for managing the partner's drinking problem.

Larger Networks. In an evaluation of family treatment for alcohol problems reported by the Institute of Medicine (1990), McCrady and colleagues concluded that "research data support superior outcomes for family-involved treatment, enough so that the modal approach should involve family members and carefully planned interventions." Indeed, the idea of the therapist intervening with family and friends to initiate treatment was introduced by Johnson (1986) as one of the early ambulatory techniques in the addiction field (Gitlow & Peyser, 1980; Gallant, 1987). More broadly, the availability of greater social support to patients has been shown to be an important predictor of positive outcomes in addiction treatment (McLellan, Woody et al., 1983).

In light of this, it is important to consider what would serve as a useful paradigm for the involvement of family and social supports in office treatment. Such a paradigm also can be used to enhance the stability of the technique for disulfiram observation already described.

The demonstrated utility of directive and behaviorally oriented approaches for preventing relapse might protect against an unstructured exploration of the family as a system. There are, however, two options for stabilizing abstinence: ecologic and problem-solving family treatment. The ecologic approach, developed by Minuchin and colleagues (1967) and others, emphasizes the engagement of resources from the patient's family and social environment. It presumes that the patient's pathology is embedded in the broader social context and acknowledges that this context must be used to achieve recovery. Problem-solving family therapy, developed by Haley (1977) and others, relies on an initial assessment of the principal presenting symptom, and subsequent treatment is directed at the problem itself, rather than at restructuring family relationships. Through these approaches, the therapist can develop an option that parallels the community reinforcement behavioral approach used in multimodality clinics (Hunt & Azrin, 1973).

The author reported a positive outcome for this approach with a series of 60 patients treated in network therapy (Galanter, 1993b). These patients attended one network session a week in the first month and subsequent sessions less frequently—typically bimonthly after a year of ambulatory care. Individual therapy was carried out concomitantly once or twice a week. On average, the networks had 2.3 members, and the most frequent participants were mates, peers, parents, or siblings.

Case 3: Friends of a 46-year-old alcohol-dependent man sought help in securing his abstinence. At the psychiatrist's suggestion, they brought him to a conjoint session in which he vowed that he could stop drinking on his own. An agreement was made among the network members, the patient, and the psychiatrist that they would maintain contact so that they could act together in case the patient's suggested approach did not succeed. Two months later, after the patient had required brief hospitalization for detoxification after a relapse to drinking, members of the network prevailed on him to accept treatment. The patient and network members then agreed that he would participate in individual therapy and would meet with the network and psychiatrist at regular intervals. Six months later, the patient suffered a relapse; one of the network members consulted the psychiatrist and stayed with the patient in his home for a day to ensure that he would not drink. He and other network members then brought the patient to the psychiatrist's office to reestablish a plan for abstinence.

This case illustrates how members of a network can help counter a patient's inclination to deny his or her drinking problem in the initial stages of engagement, as well as during relapse. It also demonstrates the value of a network in providing the psychiatrist with the means of communicating with a relapsing patient and of assisting in reestablishing his or her abstinence.

However, the case also points to the quandary posed by a disorder in which a nonpsychotic patient is subject to uncontrolled, damaging behavior. To what extent should members of the network be encouraged to intervene in the patient's life? Is it proper for the clinician to support their pressing an intoxicated patient to let one of them stay in his or her home? To exercise proper caution, the therapist must carefully assess the motives and judgment of network members, as well as the patient's capacity to respond positively to their intervention. The therapist must anticipate as much as possible the patient's response to an intervention, both while intoxicated and later. Despite a clear need for caution, it should be noted that members of AA have for years assumed an active role in helping fellow members terminate relapses. This aspect of AA underlines the meaningful support that family and friends who are close to a recovering person can provide. Incidentally, their support can be instrumental in helping the therapist ensure that the addicted patient is motivated to attend meetings and become engaged in AA.

The network is most valuable during conjoint sessions with the patient when it supports the therapist's suggestions for helping the patient avoid relapse. For example, network involvement can be vital in countering the patient's denial of his or her own vulnerability to relapse. As illustrated in the following case vignette, an effective intervention need involve no more than the network members' providing advice in the therapy session. The patient's relationship with personally chosen network members and the patient's ability to respond to their efforts to help him or her are potent tools in securing compliance. In the following case, the network members were instrumental in ensuring that the patient would remove himself from conditioned environmental cues for substance use during the period of early abstinence.

Case 4: A 23-year-old man who had insufflated heroin for a year had recently begun using it intravenously. He abused alcohol and marijuana as well. In a psychiatric consultation that the patient solicited, he agreed to bring in his uncle, his cousin, and a friend for support and to take naltrexone each day under the observation of his uncle. In the ensuing session with this network, the patient expressed reluctance to move temporarily to his parents' home so as to avoid friends who would expose him to regular drinking and marijuana use.

After discussing the importance of this added security with his network members and the psychiatrist, the patient concurred with the consensus that he did need to make the move. The patient conceded, on the basis of advice of network members, that it was more important to avoid the drug cues of his peer group than to insist on independence from his parents.

Sustaining the Network. Yalom (1974) has described anxiety-reducing tactics used in therapy groups with alcoholics to avert disruptions and promote cohesiveness. These tactics include setting an agenda for the session and using didactic instruction. In the network format, a cognitive framework can be provided for each session by starting with the patient recounting events related to cue exposure or substance use since the last meeting. Network members then are expected to comment on this report to ensure that all are engaged in a mutual task with correct, shared information. Their reactions to the patient's report are addressed as well.

Case 5: An alcoholic began one of his early network sessions by reporting a minor lapse in abstinence. This report was disrupted by an outburst of anger from his older sister. She said that she had "had it up to here" with his frequent unfulfilled promises of sobriety. The psychiatrist addressed this source of conflict by explaining in a didactic manner how behavioral cues affect vulnerability to relapse. This didactic approach was adopted to defuse the assumption that relapse is easily controlled and to relieve consequent resentment. He then led members in planning concretely with the patient how he might avoid further drinking cues in the days until their next conjoint session.

This case illustrates the importance of maintaining an appropriate therapeutic milieu in the network sessions. In volunteering to participate, members agree to help the patient but not to subject their own motives to scrutiny. In this aspect, the network format differs materially from the systemic family therapy approach, because it avoids subjecting network members to the demands of addressing their own motives. The didactic or intellectualized approach employed in Case 5 thus can be helpful in neutralizing ex-

cessive anger toward the patient without scrutinizing the reasons for a network member's anger.

In addition, the patient is expected to help maintain amicable relations with network members to protect the supportive milieu. This protection is made explicit in both network and individual sessions. For example, if a network member is absent for a few sessions, the patient is expected to discuss the matter with that member and to resolve any outstanding issues to promote the member's return. Any difficulty the patient may experience in carrying out this role is viewed as an issue to be addressed in individual sessions.

The network thus is conceived as an active collaboration in which conflicts are minimized to ensure optimal function, as they would be on the work site or a sports team. When led effectively, members are inclined to be effective team members. They develop a positive transference toward the therapist and are willing to support the therapist's views.

Conditioned Withdrawal and Anxiety. Patients undergoing detoxification from chronic use of depressant medications often experience considerable anxiety, even when the dose is reduced gradually (APA, 1990). The expectation of distress (Monti, Rohsenow et al., 1988), coupled with conditioned withdrawal phenomena, can cause patients to balk at completing a detoxification regimen. In individual therapy, the psychiatrist would have little leverage in such a situation. When augmented with network therapy, however, the added support can be valuable in securing the patient's compliance.

Case 6: A patient elected to undertake detoxification from chronic use of diazepam (approximately 60 mg per day). In network meetings with the patient, her husband, and her friend, the psychiatrist discussed the need for added support toward the end of her detoxification. As her dose was brought to 2 mg three times a day, she became anxious, said that she had never intended to stop completely, and insisted on being maintained permanently at that low dose.

Network members supportively but explicitly pointed out that this had not been the plan. She then agreed to the original detoxification agreement, and her dose was reduced to zero over 6 weeks.

The Contingency Contract. Contingency contracting, as used in behavioral treatment (Hall, Cooper et al., 1977), stipulates that an unpalatable contingency will be applied if a patient engages in a prohibited behavior. Crowley (1984) successfully applied this technique to cocaine addicts by preparing a written contract with each patient, stating that a highly aversive consequence would be initiated for any use of the proscribed drug. As an example, at the time he or she enters treatment, an addicted physician would sign a letter to the state medical licensing board in which the physician admits his or her addiction. Any violation of the treatment protocol would result in the therapist mailing the letter to the board. This approach can be adapted to the network setting as well.

Case 7: A patient regularly attended network and individual therapy sessions and also attended Narcotics Anonymous (NA) meetings. Nonetheless, he frequently slipped into cocaine use. In a network session, the patient agreed to random weekly urine tests, with the samples to be collected by his friend, a member of the network. In discussions with network members, he further agreed to prepare a letter to his employer indicating that he was an addict and not suitable to remain on the job. The patient signed an agreement stating that the letter would be mailed by the psychiatrist if any of his weekly urinalyses revealed that he had ingested cocaine. He remained substance free with this regimen over the ensuing year, and his improved status was discussed in network sessions over that time. He continued to be substance free after the contingency was discontinued as well.

Complementing Individual Therapy. Psychotherapeutic approaches have been found to yield improved outcomes when combined with approaches such as AA (Emrick, 1989), methadone maintenance (Woody, Luborsky et al., 1983), and cocaine management techniques (Rounsaville, Gawin et al., 1985). In the context of network therapy, individual expressive sessions can complement the abstinence orientation of network meetings if the therapist closely attends to conditioned cues for substance use. Once abstinence is stabilized, network sessions can augment the psychotherapy with support for the patient's general social recovery.

Even after the patient's abstinence is apparently stable, it is important to examine in therapy the patient's thoughts about drinking, dreams related to substance use, and responses to environmental drinking cues. They alert the patient to the need to be aware of the long-term risk of relapse. They also provide revealing clues to ongoing conflicts, which may be apparent only in their expression in the symbolism of addiction.

Although network sessions can be terminated before long-term individual therapy comes to an end, it is essential that network members remain available if the patient should experience difficulties at a later date, as illustrated in the next case vignette.

Case 8: An alcoholic woman had been seen in network and individual sessions for 16 months and had been abstinent for a year. Because of the woman's stability, a final network session was scheduled with her husband and two friends. Discussion there initially focused on her successful recovery, as evidenced by her beginning a new job in the preceding month. Those present agreed that any of the network members could contact the therapist if the patient relapsed in the future. The patient indicated that she would discuss any lapse in abstinence with both the network members and the therapist.

Empirical Research. Two recent studies have been added to the body of empirical research on network therapy. In one, the technique was standardized relative to a structured treatment manual. In the second, an assessment was made of the feasibility of training clinicians in the technique.

Standardization: Contemporary research on psychosocial treatment modalities requires a structured manual that explains how the treatment should be carried out in a clinical setting. Only in this manner can reliability be achieved across clinicians in the application of therapeutic techniques. Such a manual, 122 pages in length, was developed for network therapy (Galanter & Keller, 1994). Using the manual, 17 clinicians were trained in the network technique and then tested for their ability to distinguish network procedures in a reliable manner from conventional family systems therapy. For both modalities, videotape segments of respective sessions were shown and scored by mental health professionals. The treatments were found to be differentiable with a high degree of reliability (Keller et al., 1996).

The Network Therapy Rating Scale used with the latter group of subjects was applied in a second study in which the efficacy of clinical training was assessed in terms of the results of addiction treatment in a clinical context.

Treatment Outcomes: In another study (Galanter, Castaneda et al., 1997), 19 third-year psychiatric residents without experience in addiction treatment or in outpatient therapy were given a 13-hour course in network therapy. They then undertook the treatment of cocaine addicts and were supervised by clinicians experienced in the network therapy technique. Altogether, 24 patients were treated over the course of 24 weeks. Of this group, 79% of the urine samples obtained each week were negative for cocaine, and 42% of the patients produced clean urine samples during the weeks immediately preceding completion of treatment.

Overall, this outcome, along with treatment retention rates, compared favorably with those reported in several studies of cocaine treatment in the medical literature in which experienced therapists were used. These results suggest that naive mental health trainees can be taught to apply network therapy for effective treatment management.

Two studies were done on the feasibility of technology transfer of network therapy out of the original training setting. The first involved community-based counselors (Keller & Galanter, 1999), while the second (Galanter, Keller et al., 1998) reached psychiatrists by means of the Internet. For the counselors, training methods included a didactic seminar, role-playing, use of videotaped illustrations, and clinical supervision. They applied the network approach to a sample of 10 cocaine-abusing patients who were being treated concurrently with the standard program (treatment as usual). The patients were compared with a cohort of 20 cocaine abusers who received only treatment as usual. Over the course of treatment, the network-augmented patients had significantly fewer positive urine tests than did members of the comparison group, although they were not significantly different in terms of treatment retention. This finding suggests the potential of enhancing treatment in a conventional community setting by applying network support in addition to conventional care.

Another technology transfer study (Galanter, Keller et al., 1998) included a course given for alcoholism treatment, conducted on the Internet. It combined network therapy with naltrexone treatment for alcoholism. The first 679 parties who accessed the course on the Internet included a group of 210 unique respondents, of whom 154 were psychiatrists. More than half of the psychiatrists completed the course and evaluated it. Most indicated that it helped them understand "a good deal" about the management of alcoholism and the use of network therapy and naltrexone. This result suggests the feasibility of using the Internet as a vehicle for teaching network therapy in addiction psychiatry, an area in which the need for advanced training often goes unmet.

PRINCIPLES OF NETWORK TREATMENT

The following is an abstract of the manual for applying network therapy. It can be adapted to the needs of a given patient and to the relative availability of potential network members.

Begin a Network as Soon as Possible

1. It is important to see the patient promptly, as the window of opportunity for openness to treatment generally is brief. A week's delay can result in loss of motivation or relapse to drinking.

2. If the patient is married, engage the spouse early on, preferably at the time of the first telephone call. Point out that addiction is a family problem. The spouse generally can be enlisted in assuring that the patient arrives at the office with a day's sobriety.

3. In the initial interview, frame the exchange so that a good case is built for the grave consequences of the patient's addiction. Do this before the patient can introduce his or her system of denial. This approach avoids putting the spouse or other network member in the awkward position of having to contradict the patient's statements.

4. Make clear that the patient needs to be abstinent, beginning immediately. (A tapered detoxification may be necessary with some drugs, such as the sedative-hypnotics.)

5. Start an alcoholic patient on disulfiram treatment as soon as possible—in the office at the time of the first visit, if possible. Instruct the patient to continue taking disulfiram under the observation of a network member.

6. Start to build a network for the patient at the first visit. Involve the patient's family members and close friends.

7. From the very first meeting, consider how to ensure the patient's sobriety until the next meeting and plan that with the network. Initially, the immediate companionship of network members, a plan for daily AA attendance, and planned activities all may be necessary.

Manage the Network With Care

1. Include persons who are close to the patient, who have a long-standing relationship with him or her, and who are trusted. Avoid members with substance use problems. Avoid superiors and subordinates at work, as they have an overriding relationship with the patient that is independent of friendship.

2. Recruit a balanced group. Avoid a network composed solely of the parental generation, or of younger people, or of persons of the opposite sex. Sometimes a nascent network selects itself for a consultation if the patient is reluctant to address his or her own problem. Such a group will go on to supportively engage the patient in the network, with careful guidance from the therapist.

3. Assure that the mood of meetings is trusting and free of recrimination. Do not allow the patient or the network members to be made to feel guilty or angry in meetings. Explain issues of conflict in terms of the problems presented by addiction, rather than engaging in discussions around personality conflicts.

4. Set a directive tone by giving explicit instructions to support and ensure abstinence. A feeling of teamwork should be promoted, and psychologizing or impugning of members' motives avoided.

5. Meet as frequently as necessary to ensure abstinence—perhaps once a week for a month, every second week for the next few months, and every month or two by the end of a year.

6. Assure that the network has no agenda other than to support the patient's abstinence. As that abstinence is stabilized, the network can help the patient plan for a new drug-free lifestyle. Do not allow the network to be distracted by issues of family relations or allow the focus to shift to other members' problems.

Keep the Network's Agenda Focused

1. *Maintain Abstinence*: At the beginning of each session, the patient and the network members should report any exposure of the patient to alcohol or drugs. The patient and network members should be instructed as to the nature of relapse and should work with the clinician to develop a plan to sustain abstinence. Cues to conditioned drug seeking should be examined.

2. *Support the Network's Integrity*: Everyone has a role in this step: The patient is expected to assure that network members keep their meeting appointments and stay involved with the treatment. The therapist sets meeting times and summons the network for any emergency, such as relapse. (The therapist does whatever is necessary to secure stability of the membership if the patient is having difficulty in doing so.) Members of the network are responsible for attending network sessions and engaging in other supportive activities with the patient.

3. *Secure Future Behavior*: The therapist should combine any and all treatment modalities necessary to ensure the patient's stability. This step might involve establishing a stable, drug-free residence; avoiding substance-abusing friends; attending Twelve Step meetings; using medications such as disulfiram or blocking agents; observing urinalyses; and obtaining ancillary psychiatric care. Written agreements can be useful. This step also may involve a mutually acceptable contingency contract, with penalties for violation of understandings.

Make Use of AA and Other Self-Help Groups

1. Patients should be expected to attend meetings of AA or related groups at least two to three times, with followup discussion in therapy.

2. If a patient has reservations about attending self-help group meetings, the therapist should try to help the patient understand how to deal with them. Issues such as social anxiety should be explored if they make a patient reluctant to participate. Generally, resistance to AA can be related to other areas of inhibition in a person's life, as well as to the denial of addiction.

3. As with other spiritual involvements, the therapist should not probe the patient's motivation or commitment to AA, once he or she has engaged. Rather, it is important to allow the patient to work out issues on his or her own, but be prepared to listen as needed.

CONCLUSIONS

The model of addictive behavior and office-based treatment presented here deals with the influence of pharmacologically conditioned drinking cues on relapse into substance dependence, and it employs a cognitive-behavioral approach to averting relapse. To engage addicted patients while treatment is applied and to motivate them to overcome the effect of addictive cues, a network of persons close to the patient can be brought into the therapy sessions and augment the individual treatment. Specific network techniques draw on the variety of relationships among the patient, the family, and peers.

ACKNOWLEDGMENT: This chapter was adapted in part from articles by the author in the Journal of Psychiatric Treatment and Evaluation *(1983;5:551),* Advances in Alcohol and Substance Abuse *(1987;6:159), and* Psychiatric Annals *(1989;19:226), and the manual* Network Therapy for Alcohol and Drug Abuse *(Galanter M, New York, NY, Basic Books, 1993).*

REFERENCES

Albaugh BJ & Anderson PO (1974). Peyote in the treatment of alcoholism among American Indians. *American Journal of Psychiatry* 131:1247-1250.

American Psychiatric Association (APA) (1990). *Benzodiazepine Dependence, Toxicity, and Abuse: A Task Force Report of the American Psychiatric Association.* Washington, DC: American Psychiatric Association.

American Psychiatric Association (APA) (1994). *Diagnostic and Statistical Manual of Mental Disorders, 4th Edition.* Washington, DC: American Psychiatric Association.

Annis HM (1986). A relapse prevention model for treatment of alcoholics. In WE Miller & N Heather (eds.) *Treating Addictive Behaviors: Processes of Change.* New York, NY: Plenum.

Azrin NH, Sisson RW, Meyers R et al. (1982). Alcoholism treatment by disulfiram and community reinforcement therapy. *Journal of Behavioral Therapy and Experimental Psychiatry* 13:105-112.

Begleiter H & Porjesz B (1979). Persistence of a subacute withdrawal syndrome following chronic ethanol intake. *Drug and Alcohol Dependence* 4:353-357.

Brandsma JM, Maultsby MC & Welsh RJ (1980). *Outpatient Treatment of Alcoholism: A Review and Comprehensive Study.* Baltimore, MD: University Park Press.

Braunstein WB, Powell BJ, McGowan JF et al. (1983). Employment factors in outpatient recovery of alcoholics: A multi-variate study. *Addictive Behavior* 8:345-551.

Brubaker RG, Prue DM & Rychtarik RG (1987). Determinants of disulfiram acceptance among alcohol patients: A test of the theory of reasoned action. *Addictive Behavior* 12:43-52.

Cartwright D & Zander A (1962). *Group Dynamics: Research and Theory.* Evanston, IL: Row, Peterson.

Cermak TL (1986). *Diagnosing and Treating Codependence.* Minneapolis, MN: Johnson Institute Books.

Childress AR, McLellan AT, Ehrman R et al. (1988). Classically conditioned responses in opioid and cocaine dependence: A role in relapse? In BA Ray (ed.) *Learning Factors in Substance Abuse (NIDA Research Monograph 84).* Rockville, MD: National Institute on Drug Abuse.

Cook CCH (1988). The Minnesota model in the management of drug and alcohol dependency: Miracle, method, or myth? *British Journal of Addiction* 83:625-634.

Crowley TJ (1984). Contingency contracting treatment of drug-abusing physicians, nurses, and dentists. In J Grabowski, ML Stitzer & JF Henningfeld (eds.) *Drug Abuse Treatment (NIDA Research Monograph 46).* Rockville, MD: National Institute on Drug Abuse.

De Leon G (1989). Therapeutic communities for substance abuse: Overview of approach and effectiveness. *Bulletin of the Society of Psychology of Addictive Behavior* 3:140-147.

Dittrich JE & Trapold MA (1984). A treatment program for wives of alcoholics: An evaluation. *Bulletin of the Society of Psychology of Addictive Behavior* 3:91-102.

Emrick CD (1989). Alcoholics Anonymous: Membership characteristics and effectiveness as treatment. In M Galanter (ed.) *Recent Developments in Alcoholism, Vol. 7.* New York, NY: Plenum.

Fuller RK & Williford WO (1980). Life-table analysis of abstinence in a study evaluating the efficacy of disulfiram. *Alcoholism: Clinical & Experimental Research* 4:298-301.

Galanter M (1983). Cognitive labelling: Psychotherapy for alcohol and drug abuse: An approach based on learning theory. *Journal of Psychiatric Treatment and Evaluation* 5:551.

Galanter M (1987). Social network therapy for cocaine dependence. *Advances in Alcohol and Substance Abuse* 6:159-175.

Galanter M (1989). Management of the alcoholic in psychiatric practice. *Psychiatric Annals* 19:266-270.

Galanter M (1990). Cults and zealous self-help movements: A psychiatric perspective. *American Journal of Psychiatry* 147:543-551.

Galanter M (1993a). Network therapy for addiction: A model for office practice. *American Journal of Psychiatry* 150:28-36.

Galanter M (1993b). Network therapy for substance abuse: A clinical trial. *Psychotherapy* 30:251-258.

Galanter M (1999). *Network Therapy for Alcohol and Drug Abuse, Expanded Edition.* New York, NY: Guilford Press.

Galanter M, Castaneda R & Salamon I (1987). Institutional self-help therapy for alcoholism: Clinical outcome. *Alcoholism: Clinical & Experimental Research* 11:424-429.

Galanter M & Keller D (1994). *Network Therapy for Substance Abuse: A Therapist's Manual.*

Galanter M, Keller D & Dermatis H (1997a). Network therapy for addiction: Assessment of the clinical outcome of training. *American Journal of Drug and Alcohol Abuse* 23:355-367.

Galanter M, Keller DS & Dermatis H (1997b). Using the internet for clinical training: A course on network therapy for substance abuse, MED.NYU.EDU/SUBSTANCEABUSE/COURSE. *Psychiatric Services* 48:999 ff.

Galanter M, Keller D, Dermatis H et al. (1998). Use of the Internet for addiction education. *American Journal on Addictions* 7:7-13.

Galanter M, Talbott D, Gallegos K et al. (1990). Combined Alcoholics Anonymous and professional care for addicted physicians. *American Journal of Psychiatry* 147: 64-68

Gallant M (1987). *A Guide to Diagnosis, Intervention, and Treatment.* New York, NY: W.W. Norton.

Gallant M, Rich A, Bey E et al. (1970). Group psychotherapy with married couples. *Journal of the Louisiana State Medical Society* 122:41-44.

Gitlow SE & Peyser HS (1980). *A Practical Treatment Guide.* New York, NY: Grune & Stratton.

Haley J (1977). *Problem Solving Therapy.* San Francisco, CA: Jossey-Bass.

Hall SM, Cooper JL, Burmaster S et al. (1977). Contingency contracting as a therapeutic tool with methadone maintenance clients. *Behavioral Research Therapy* 15:438-441.

Hayman M (1956). Current attitudes to alcoholism of psychiatrists in Southern California. *American Journal of Psychiatry* 112:485-493.

Hunt GM & Azrin NH (1973). A community-reinforcement approach to alcoholism. *Behavioral Research Therapy* 11:91-104.

Institute of Medicine (1990). *Broadening the Base of Treatment for Alcohol Problems*. Washington, DC: National Academy Press.

Johnson VE (1986). *How to Help Someone Who Doesn't Want Help*. Minneapolis, MN: Johnson Institute Books.

Kaufman E & Kaufman PN (eds.) (1979). *Family Therapy of Drug and Alcohol Abuse*. New York, NY: Gardner Press.

Keane TM, Foy DW, Nunn B et al. (1984). Spouse contracting to increase Antabuse compliance in alcoholic veterans. *Journal of Clinical Psychology* 40:340-344.

Keller DS & Galanter M (1999). Technology transfer of network therapy to community-based addictions counselors. *Journal of Substance Abuse Treatment* 16:183-189

Keller D, Galanter M & Weinberg S (1997). Validation of a scale for network therapy. *Journal of Drug and Alcohol Abuse* 23:115-127.

Khantzian EJ (1985). The self-medication hypothesis of addictive disorders: Focus on heroin and cocaine dependence. *American Journal of Psychiatry* 142:1259-1264.

Liepman MR, Nierenberg TD & Begin AM (1989). Evaluation of a program designed to help family and significant others to motivate resistant alcoholics to recover. *American Journal of Drug and Alcohol Abuse* 15:209-222.

Ludwig AM, Bendfeldt F, Wikler A et al. (1978). "Loss of control" in alcoholics. *Archives of General Psychiatry* 35:370-373.

Mallams JH, Godley MD, Hall GM et al. (1982). A social-systems approach to resocializing alcoholics in the community. *Journal of the Study of Alcoholism* 43:1115-1123.

Marlatt GA & Gordon J (1985). *Relapse Prevention: Maintenance Strategies in the Treatment of Addictive Behaviors*. New York, NY: Guilford Press.

McAuliffe WE (1982). A test of Wikler's theory of relapse: The frequency of relapse due to conditioned withdrawal sickness. *International Journal of Addiction* 17:19-33.

McCrady BS, Stout R, Noel N et al. (1991). Effectiveness of three types of spouse-involved behavioral alcoholism treatment. *British Journal of Addiction* 86:1415-1424.

McLellan AT, Woody GE, Luborsky L et al. (1983). Increased effectiveness of substance abuse treatment: A prospective study of patient-treatment "matching." *Journal of Nervous and Mental Diseases* 171:597-605.

Minuchin S, Montalvo B, Guerney BG et al. (1967). *Families of the Slums*. New York, NY: Basic Books.

Monti PM, Rohsenow DJ, Abrams DB et al. (1988). Social learning approaches to alcohol relapse: Selected illustrations and implications. In BA Ray (ed.) *Learning Factors in Substance Abuse (NIDA Research Monograph 84)*. Rockville, MD: National Institute on Drug Abuse.

Moos RH & Moos BS (1984). The process of recovery from alcoholism, III: Comparing functioning in families of alcoholics and matched control families. *Journal of the Study of Alcoholism* 45:111-118.

Nathan PE & McCrady BS (1986/1987). Bases for the use of abstinence as a goal in the treatment of alcohol abusers. *Drugs and Society* 1(2/3):109-131.

National Institute on Alcohol Abuse and Alcoholism (NIAAA) (1987). *Alcoholism and Health*. Washington, DC: U.S. Government Printing Office.

Nation's treatment providers forced to ration care (1990). *Alcoholism and Drug Abuse Week* February 28 (newsletter).

Noel NE, McCrady BS, Stout RL et al. (1987). Predictors of attrition from an outpatient alcoholism treatment program for couples. *Journal of Studies on Alcohol* 48:229-235.

O'Brien CP, Testa T, O'Brien TJ et al. (1977). Conditioned narcotic withdrawal in humans. *Science* 195:1000-1002.

O'Farrell TJ, Cutter HSG & Floyd FJ (1985). Evaluating behavioral marital therapy for male alcoholics: Effects on marital adjustment and communication before and after treatment. *Behavioral Therapy* 16:147-167.

Olson RP, Ganley R, Devine VT et al. (1981). Long-term effects of behavioral versus insight-oriented therapy with inpatient alcoholics. *Journal of Consulting and Clinical Psychology* 49:866-877.

Rounsaville BJ, Gawin FH & Kleber HD (1985). Interpersonal psychotherapy adapted for ambulatory cocaine users. *American Journal of Drug and Alcohol Abuse* 11:171-191.

Schoenfeld P, Halevey J & Hemley van der Velden E (1986). The long-term outcome of network therapy. *Hospital & Community Psychiatry* 37:373-376.

Schuckit MA (1985). A one-year follow-up of men alcoholics given disulfiram. *Journal of Studies on Alcohol* 46:191-195.

Singer M & Borrero MG (1984). Indigenous treatment for alcoholism: The case of Puerto Rican spiritualism. *Medical Anthropology* 8:246-273.

Speck R & Attneave C (1974). *Family Networks*. New York, NY: Vintage Books.

Stanton MD & Thomas TC, eds. (1982). *The Family Therapy of Drug Abuse and Addiction*. New York, NY: Guilford Press.

Stark MJ, Campbell BK & Brinkerhoff CV (1990). "Hello, may we help you?" A study of attrition prevention at the time of the first phone contact with substance-abusing clients. *American Journal of Drug and Alcohol Abuse* 15:209-222.

Steinglass P, Bennett LA, Wolin SJ et al. (1987). *The Alcoholic Family*. New York, NY: Basic Books.

Vaillant GE (1981). Dangers of psychotherapy in the treatment of alcoholism. In MH Bean & NE Zinberg (eds.) *Dynamic Approaches to the Understanding and Treatment of Alcoholism*. New York, NY: Free Press.

Wikler A (1973). Dynamics of drug dependence. *Archives of General Psychiatry* 28:611-616.

Woody GE, Luborsky L, McLellan AT et al. (1983). Psychotherapy for opiate addicts: Does it help? *Archives of General Psychiatry* 40:639-645.

Wurmser L (1977). Mrs. Pecksniff's horse? Psychodynamics of compulsive drug use. In JD Blaine & DS Julius (eds.) *Psychodynamics of Drug Dependence (NIDA Research Monograph 12)*. Rockville, MD: National Institute on Drug Abuse.

Yalom ID (1974). Group therapy and alcoholism. *Annals of the New York Academy of Science* 233:85-103.

Yalom ID, Bloch S, Bond G et al. (1978). Alcoholics in interactional group therapy. *Archives of General Psychiatry* 35:419-425.

| Chapter 7 | # Therapeutic Communities |

Donald J. Kurth, M.D., FASAM

History and Evolution
The Daytop Model
Features of the Modern TC
Referral Criteria
Criticisms of the TC Model

The modern addiction therapeutic community (TC) is a powerful therapeutic tool that, over the past several decades, has helped hundreds of thousands of addicts and alcoholics achieve abstinence-based recovery. Abstinence rates of more than 90% for many years after treatment are documented in well-established TCs.

Historically, the TC has been used to treat a variety of problems in living, but the modern addiction TC or "concept TC" is a hybrid of self-help and public support geared toward the treatment of addictive and co-occurring psychiatric disorders.

The philosophic foundation of the modern therapeutic community is personal responsibility for one's behavior and the belief that change is fully possible if the individual exerts the personal effort to follow the teachings of the program.

Evolving out of Alcoholics Anonymous (AA) in the 1960s, the modern addiction TC still retains many of the underpinnings of the Twelve Step approach to treatment. Drug addiction is viewed as a "whole person" disorder and therefore is treated with a holistic approach. Emotions and feelings are considered important and can be explored in depth, but change is based on action. That action is the responsibility of the individual. As in Twelve Step recovery, the individual is not expected to walk this road alone. The community is available to help the addict at every step of the way.

In the TC philosophy, drug or alcohol use is considered a symptom of a complex disorder involving the whole person. Self-destructive and defeating patterns of behavior and thought processes are thought to disrupt both the individual's lifestyle and society's functioning. Although genetic, environmental, and pharmacologic contributions to addiction are recognized, the individual is held fully responsible for his or her own disorder, behavior, and recovery. Addiction is regarded as the symptom, rather than the disorder. The problem is the behavior of the person, not the drug.

HISTORY AND EVOLUTION

The modern TC is a new application of an ancient concept. The Dead Sea Scrolls found at Qumron document the first TC. The communal practices of an ascetic religious sect, perhaps the Essenes, include the "Rules of Community." The Essene code denounces "the ways of the spirit of falsehood" and speaks of the problems of greed, lying, cruelty, brazen insolence, lust, and "walking the ways of darkness and guile."

Righteous and healthy living required strict adherence to the rules and teachings of the community.

Violation of the Rules of Community incurred sanctions resembling, although much harsher than, the sanctions used in the modern addiction TC. For violations such as lying, bearing a grudge, foolish speech or laughter, sleeping during a community meeting, or leaving a community meeting, sanctions could include periods of banishment from the community or limited rations or privileges.

At about the time Jesus walked the earth, a group of healers (therapeutrides) of the "incurable" diseases of the soul lived in Alexandria, Egypt. Philo Judaeus (25 BC to 45 AD) described the group as professing "an art of medicine for [excessive] pleasures and appetites . . . the immeasurable multitude of passions and vices" (Slater, 1984). As in the modern TC philosophy, diseases of the soul were seen as manifesting themselves through the whole person. Healing was regarded as occurring through some form of community involvement.

The Washingtonians (founded by a group of drinkers) later appeared in the United States as a 19th century precursor to AA. Although the Washingtonians did not survive as a group, several of their methods are still apparent in the modern addiction TC. These include the commitment to abstinence, proselytizing its message to others, and the practice of self-appraisal during group meetings.

The conceptual and organizational lineage of the modern addiction TC began about 1921 with the Oxford Group—also known as The Buchmanites, the First Century Christians Fellowship, and Moral Rearmament (Glaser, 1974). A branch of the Oxford Group in Akron, Ohio, evolved into AA in 1935 under the guidance of Bill Wilson and Doctor Bob Smith. A Santa Monica, California, AA group evolved into Synanon in 1958 under the guidance of AA members. From Synanon sprang Daytop Village in New York City, under the guidance of Monsignor William O'Brien. From Daytop, more than 100 other therapeutic communities have developed around the world.

The Oxford Group (or Oxford Movement) began in the second decade of the 20th century as the First Century Christian Fellowship. Founded by Lutheran evangelist minister Frank Buchman, the early Oxford Group preached a return to the purity and innocence of the early church. This spiritual rebirth was to be applied to all forms of human suffering. Although alcoholism and mental illness were not the primary focus of the Oxford Group, they were certainly seen as signs of spiritual deficit and thus were encompassed by the Oxford Group's principles.

The Reverend Buchman headquartered the Oxford Movement in New York City, where Dr. Samuel Shoemaker, pastor of Calvary Episcopal Church, became involved as well. During this period, the philosophies of the Quakers and Anabaptists (precursors to the Mennonites and Amish) began to influence the movement. These early influences carry through to the foundation of the modern addiction TC. Concepts and practices such as the work ethic, mutual concern, and sharing guidance are basic to the TC philosophy. Evangelical values such as honesty, purity, unselfishness, love, making amends for harm done, and working well with others all can be traced to this era (Ray, 1999; Wilson, 1957).

The thread continues even today. Although not directly related to the Oxford Group, "Oxford House" is the name of a self-run, self-supported sober living housing initiative that was begun in Silver Spring, Maryland, in 1975 and now includes more than 450 sober-living houses situated throughout the U.S.

The Twelve Steps of AA evolved directly from the Six Steps of the Oxford Group. Together with the Twelve Traditions and the Twelve Concepts, the Twelve Steps embody the principles that guide the individual in recovery. The concepts of confessing to others and making amends, and the belief that individual change requires conversion to belief in the group are principles derived directly from the Oxford Group. Other AA principles include admitting one's loss of control over alcohol and surrendering to one's "Higher Power," performing self-examination, seeking help from one's Higher Power in changing one's self, making amends to others, praying in the personal struggle, and helping others to engage in a similar process. Some striking differences are found, however. AA deviated from the Oxford requirement of a religious God by allowing each AA member to develop his or her own concept of a Higher Power. Although AA does not require a Christian god, its principles do stress that one's power to change is derived from a power greater than one's self. Nonsectarian AA, in fact, allows the Higher Power to be the AA group. This concept of the group as Higher Power is further developed in Synanon and later TCs, as it evolved into reliance on self and group process as the medium of individual behavioral change.

Fifteen years before Synanon appeared on the scene in the U.S., however, psychiatric hospital TCs began to develop in Great Britain. Pioneered by Maxwell Jones, the

---

TABLE 1. Characteristics of the Psychiatric (Jones) TC

1. The total organization is seen as affecting therapeutic outcomes.

2. The social organization is useful in creating a milieu that maximizes therapeutic effects and is not simply the background for treatment.

3. A core element is democratization: the social environment provides opportunities for patients to take an active part in the affairs of the institution.

4. All relationships are therapeutic.

5. The qualitative atmosphere of the social environment is therapeutic in that it is balanced between acceptance, control, and tolerance for disruptive activities.

6. Great value is placed on communication.

7. The orientation of the group is toward productive work and a quick return to society.

8. Educational techniques and group pressure are used for constructive purposes.

9. There is a diffusion of authority from staff to patients.

SOURCE: Adapted from DeLeon G (2000), after Kennard D (1983).

---

first of these appeared as a social rehabilitation unit at Belmont Hospital in England in the mid-1940s. The Jones TC embraced the therapeutic nature of the total environment as a treatment tool (Table 1). Although the Jones TC is used today as a viable treatment method in Great Britain, its application to the treatment of addictive disorders occurred only in the context of dual diagnoses patients. Some addictive disorder treatment adaptation of the Jones TC model has occurred in the U.S. in the Veterans Administration hospitals. There is little data about the efficacy of treatment in this application.

The evolution of Synanon from an AA group resulted in the concepts, program model, and basic practices that have become the essential elements of all modern addiction TCs. Synanon's charismatic founder, Chuck Dederich, integrated his AA experiences with other philosophical, pragmatic, and psychological influences to create the Synanon program. The unique encounter group process ("the game") evolved from weekly AA meetings. Distinct psychological changes were evident as a result of this process. The participants recognized this change as a new form of therapy and, within a year, the weekly meetings expanded into a residential community. In August 1959, the organization was officially founded to treat any addict, regardless of the chemical of choice. The name Synanon apparently was coined during the confused mumbling of a heroin addict who was having trouble pronouncing the word "seminar," fusing it with the word "symposium." Despite its role in the evolution of the modern TC, Synanon never considered itself a TC, but rather an alternative community for teaching and living.

Synanon evolved from AA and, as a result, the precepts of AA are fundamental to Synanon and to all modern addiction TCs. Still, the evolution did occur, and the differences are what created the TC as a distinct approach. Self-help recovery, a belief that the ability to change and heal lies within the individual, and a belief that healing occurs as a result of a therapeutic relationship with others who have a similar affliction all are philosophies common to both programs. The AA traditions and program activities lead directly to the TC's individual self-reliance, organizational self-reliance, and its schedule of regular groups and meetings.

The numbering system of AA's Twelve Steps did not carry through to Synanon, but the same stages of recovery are very much a part of the Synanon program and the other modern addiction TCs as well. Steps 1 to 3 are embodied in the TC's early phase recovery, which emphasizes breaking through denial and engaging in the change process. Steps 4 to 9 are seen in the mid-phase recovery period of intense self-examination and socialization. This period involves taking a personal inventory, sharing confession with another person, and making amends. Steps 10 to 12 are reflected in the maturational process and increased autonomy that develops in the re-entry phase of the TC. This phase requires continued personal honesty, humbly asking for help to sustain recovery, and actively helping others.

Critical differences, however, define the addiction TC as a new treatment modality. These include the residential setting, organizational structure, and profile of participants, goals, philosophy, and ideological orientation.

Initially, residents could graduate from Synanon. Soon, however, Synanon (like AA) abandoned the concepts of graduation or completion of the program. In AA, when participants are fully integrated in society, they continue to participate in the program of recovery and continue to attend group meetings. This participation is analogous, perhaps, to continuing to attend church. In the case of 24-hour-a-day residential Synanon, completion of the program signified quite a different situation. All activities of a person's life were to occur within the highly structured hierarchical organization, with no sort of re-entry or re-integration back into society as a whole. Synanon embraced AA's Seventh Tradition of fiscal independence with entrepreneurial spirit, developing profit-making businesses as well as pursuing both public and private funding. Although any member could rise within the hierarchy, the management was never democratic but rather oligarchical.

THE DAYTOP MODEL

Monsignor William O'Brien, a young priest, and Dr. Daniel Casriel, a Manhattan psychiatrist, first attempted to apply the concept of a TC specifically to the treatment of drug addiction. With the help of Joseph Shelly, chief probation officer of Brooklyn, New York, and Alexander Basson, a doctoral student who wrote the first grant, funds were obtained from the National Institute on Mental Health to develop an addiction TC.

The new program needed a director, and none of the initial applicants had been willing to take the job. So, Basson called the New York office of AA. A gentleman with no experience in treating drug addiction named Dean Colcord was sent to apply and was hired as the first director of Daytop Lodge (later to become Daytop Village).

Daytop Lodge opened with 25 beds on September 1, 1963, in Staten Island, NY. Dean Colcord had spent three weeks visiting the Westport Synanon to learn how it operated. Daytop applied the Synanon program with a strong dose of AA to the public sector treatment of addiction.

The founding of Daytop marked a milestone in the development of the modern TC (Table 2).

The modern TC rests on a foundation of secular ideology with certain existential assumptions, including the following:

- *Self-Determination*: A core value is self-determination. Each individual is seen as the captain of his or her own ship and the one who determines the path of his or her life.

- *Individual Responsibility*: The TC philosophy holds each individual fully responsible for his or her own behavior. No matter the genetic predisposition or environmental or family influences, each person is seen as fully and completely responsible for his or her own behavior.

- *Self-Change*: The concept of self change is regarded as possible through personal commitment and adherence to recovery teachings.

FEATURES OF THE MODERN TC

The addiction TC is a powerful tool for changing behavior, and its efficacy is well documented in the literature. It is less clear how and why this therapeutic modality is so effective in changing difficult behaviors for which so many other methods are not successful.

Components of a TC Program. Several features characterize TC programs that follow the Daytop Village model and other first-generation therapeutic communities (DeLeon, 2000).

Community Separateness: TC-oriented programs have their own identities and are housed in a space or locale that is separated from other agency or institutional programs or units or generally from the drug-related environment. In residential settings, clients remain away from outside influences 24 hours a day for several months before earning the privilege of a brief visit to the outside community. In nonresidential "day treatment" settings, the individual spends 4 to 8 hours a day in the TC environment and is monitored

---

TABLE 2. The Daytop Philosophy

I am here because there is no refuge, finally, from myself. Until I confront myself in the eyes and hearts of others, I am running. Until I suffer them to share my secrets, I have no safety from them. Afraid to be known, I can know neither myself nor any other, I will be alone. Where else but in our common ground, can I find such a mirror? Here, together, I can at last appear clearly to myself not as a giant of my dreams nor the dwarf of my fears, but as a person, part of a whole, with my share in its purpose. In this ground, I can take root and grow not alone any more as in death but alive to myself and to others. *Author: Richard Beauvais*

---

by peers and family while outside the TC. Even in the least restrictive outpatient settings, TC-oriented programs and components are in place. This is designed to help members gradually detach from old networks and relate to the drug-free peers in the program.

A Community Environment: The TC environment prominently features communal spaces and collective activities. Walls carry signs declaring the philosophy of the program, the messages of right living and recovery. Cork boards and blackboards are used to identify all participants by name, seniority level, and job function in the program. Daily schedules are posted as well. These visuals display an organizational picture of the program that the individual can relate to and comprehend, thus promoting program affiliation.

Community Activities: The TC philosophy holds that, to be effective, treatment and educational services must be provided within a context of the peer community. Thus, with the exception of individual counseling, all activities are programmed in collective formats. These activities include at least one daily meal prepared, served, and shared by all members; a daily schedule of groups, meetings, and seminars; jobs performed in teams; organized recreational/leisure time; and ceremonies and rituals (to mark birthdays, phase/progress graduations, and the like).

Staff Rules and Functions: Staff members are a mix of self-help professionals who are themselves in recovery and other helping professionals (medical, legal, mental health, and educational), who are integrated through cross-training grounded in the TC perspective and community approach. Professional skills define the function of staff members (for example, nurse, physician, lawyer, teacher, administrator, case worker, clinical counselor). Regardless of professional discipline or function, however, the generic *role* of all staff members is that of community members who, rather than providers and treaters, are viewed as rational authorities, facilitators, and guides in the self-help community method.

Peers as Role Models: Members who demonstrate the expected behaviors and reflect the values and teachings of the community are viewed as role models. Indeed, the strength of the community as a context for social learning relates to the number and quality of its role models. All members of the community are expected to be role models: roommates; older and younger residents; and junior, senior, and directorial staff. TCs require these multiple role models to maintain the integrity of the community and to ensure the spread of social learning effects.

A Structured Day: The structure of the program relates to the TC perspective, particularly the view of the client and recovery. Ordered activities conducted in a regular routine counter the characteristically disordered lives in which clients have lived and distract from negative thinking and boredom—factors that are thought to predispose individuals to drug use. Structured activities also are regarded as facilitating the acquisition of self-structure on the part of the individual, as expressed in time management; planning, setting, and meeting goals; and general accountability. Thus, regardless of its length, the day has a formal schedule of therapeutic and educational activities with prescribed formats, fixed times, and routine procedures.

Work as Therapy and Education: Consistent with the TC's self-help approach, all clients are responsible for the daily management of the facility (for example, cleaning, meal preparation and service, maintenance, purchasing, security, scheduling, preparation for group meetings, seminars, activities, and the like). In the TC, the various work roles mediate essential educational and therapeutic effects. Job functions strengthen affiliation with the program through participation, provide opportunities for skill development, and foster self-examination and personal growth through performance challenge and program responsibility. The scope and depth of clients' work depends on the program (for example, institutional versus free-standing facility) and client resources (levels of psychological function, social and life skills).

TABLE 3. Fundamental Changes in TCs After the Founding of Daytop Village

1. Marks the shift from being an alternative community for deviant addicts who presumably could not function in mainstream society to a human services agency preparing individuals for reintegration into a larger society.

2. Marks the shift from indefinite tenure in the same residential community to a planned duration of residential stay guided by a treatment plan and protocol.

3. Marks the shift from complete or partial private and entrepeneurial sources of support to virtually sole reliance on public funding for operational budgets, necessitating compliance with requirements for accountability and oversight by external boards of directors.

4. Marks a de-emphasis of charismatic leaders and increased importance of peer leadership, staff members as role models, and multiple decision makers.

5. Marks the inclusion of increasing proportions of nonrecovering staff in primary clinical and administrative roles from varied professional disciplines.

6. Develops aftercare programs for those who complete the residential phase of treatment.

7. Reintegrates AA Twelve Step principles and traditions into the treatment protocol of many residential TCs.

8. Includes gradual rapprochement between psychiatric and addiction TC models and methods.

9. Adapts the TC for special populations and in special settings such as mental health facilities and correctional institutions.

10. Marks the development of a research and evaluation knowledge base by independent and program-based investigative teams.

11. Codifies competency requirements for staff training, staff credentialing, and program accreditation.

12. Develops regional, national, and international TC organizations.

13. Promulgates and disseminates the TC for addictions worldwide through training, program development, technical assistance, and research.

SOURCE: Adapted from DeLeon G (2000). *The Therapeutic Community: Theory, Model, and Method.* New York, NY: Springer Publishing Company.

Phase Format: The treatment protocol, or plan of therapeutic and educational activities, is organized into phases that reflect a developmental view of the change process. Emphasis is placed on incremental learning at each phase, so as to move the individual to the next stage of recovery.

TC Concepts: Formal and informal curricula are focused on teaching the TC perspective, particularly its self-help recovery concepts and view of right living. The concepts, messages, and lessons are repeated in the various groups, meetings, seminars, and peer conversations, as well as in readings, signs, and personal writings.

Peer Encounter Groups: The principal community or therapeutic group is the encounter, although other forms of therapeutic, educational, and support groups are employed as needed. The minimal objective of the peer encounter is similar to TC-oriented programs—to heighten the individual's awareness of specific attitudes or behavior patterns that need to be modified. However, the encounter process can differ in degree of staff direction and intensity, depending on the client subgroups (for example, adolescents, prison inmates, and the dually diagnosed).

Awareness Training: All therapeutic and educational interventions involve raising the individual's awareness of the effects of his or her conduct and attitudes on himself or herself and the social environment and, conversely, the effect of the behaviors and attitudes of others on the individual and his or her environment.

Emotional Growth Training: Achieving the goals of personal growth and socialization involves teaching individuals how to identify feelings, express them appropriately, and manage them constructively through the interpersonal and social demands of communal life.

Planned Duration of Treatment. The optimal length of a full program involvement must be consistent with the TC goals of recovery and its developmental view of the change process. How long the individual must be involved in the program depends on his or her phase of recovery, although a minimum period of intensive involvement is required to assure internalization of the TC teachings. The duration of treatment of the traditional therapeutic community generally is 12 to 18 months.

Continuity of Care. Completion of primary treatment is a stage in the recovery process. It is followed by aftercare services, which are an essential component of the TC model. Whether implemented within the main program or separately (as in residential or nonresidential halfway houses or ambulatory settings), the perspective and approach guiding aftercare programming must be *continuous* with that primary treatment in the TC. Thus, the views of right living and self-help recovery and the use of a peer network are essential to enhance the appropriate use of vocational, educational, mental health, social, and other typical aftercare or re-entry services.

REFERRAL CRITERIA

For the physician in office-based practice, either as an addiction medicine specialist or simply as a perceptive, caring physician willing to address patients' addictive disorders, a question often arises as to which type of treatment is most appropriate for a particular patient. This question may not be easy to answer, but may well be the critical step that makes the difference between life and death for that particular human being.

Any one of four specific characteristics would qualify an addict and/or alcoholic for treatment in a TC (Table 4). But just what does such a person look like? Although a complete answer to this question could fill a volume or more, a few examples may serve to illustrate the broad outlines of the characteristics that might define a patient as a good candidate for treatment in a therapeutic community.

Case 1: The first example involves a patient who is abusing drugs or alcohol and who has begun to experience negative consequences of those behaviors but still is able to stop such use when the negative consequences are pointed out. For example, a young woman drinks only two or three times a year, but has three wine coolers at the office Christ-

mas party and perhaps even a joint offered by a co-worker. If stopped for driving under the influence, such an individual may seek help for the problem, either on her own initiative or through a referral from the courts. Such an individual may not in fact be addicted to alcohol or drugs, and probably can stop drinking and using on her own if she understands that negative consequences are directly and causally related to her substance use. She certainly does not need to participate in a long-term residential treatment program such as a TC.

Case 2: Another case involves a 44-year-old engineer who began drinking in college and has continued to drink heavily throughout his adult life. His family life may be stressed, but he still is married. His children are adolescents and not home very much. He may have had a DUI arrest 10 years earlier and, as a result, attended AA meetings briefly. But he found that he could not tolerate all the talk about God and Higher Power, so he drifted away from the meetings and continued to drink.

He was regarded as someone with high potential at the time he finished engineering school 20 years earlier, but he has not lived up to those expectations. He is resentful of his employer for not promoting him as he feels he deserves. His employer, on the other hand, is on the verge of firing him because he seems to have trouble making it to work on Mondays, especially after long weekends. He drinks 6 to 8 vodka martinis every day when he gets home from work. But he generally does not drink in the morning, except on the weekend. He does not consider himself an alcoholic.

Outpatient treatment probably will not be effective for this patient. He already has been to AA and found that it did not apply to his situation. If he is even slightly ready to change, he probably can do very well in hospital-based detoxification followed by inpatient rehabilitation for 30 days or so. This detoxification should be followed by outpatient treatment in either a partial hospitalization or intensive outpatient treatment program, with perhaps the additional support of a sober-living home. Finally, gradual transition back to his own home and work responsibilities over several weeks would give this fellow a good chance to build a strong foundation for a program of recovery that can well last him for the rest of his life.

Again, although his life is beginning to fall apart at the seams, this individual still has a lot going for him. He has a house, family, job, finances, and probably some social life left intact. The rest can be repaired or resurrected simply by adding some consistent sobriety to the equation.

TABLE 4. Indicators of the Presenting Disorder Among Typical TC Clients

A Life in Crisis

- Clients have a history of out-of-control behavior with respect to drug use, criminality, and often sexuality.

- Clients evidence suicidal potential through overdose.

- Clients are at risk of injury or death through other drug-related means.

- Clients exhibit a high degree of anxiety and fear concerning violence, jail, illness, or death.

- Clients have a history of profound personal losses (financial, relationships, employment).

Inability to Maintain Abstinence

- Clients are unable to maintain any significant period of drug abstinence or sobriety on their own; characterized by multiple substance use although oftne having a primary drug of choice.

- Clients have some previous treatment experiences, self-initiated attempts at abstinence, or cycles of short-term medical detoxification.

Social and Interperson Dysfunction

- Clients have a diminished capacity to function responsibly in any social or interpersonal setting.

- Clients are involved in the drug lifestyle (friends, places, activities), have a poor record of maintaining employment or school responsibilities, and have minimal or dysfunctional social relations with parents, spouses, and friends outside the drug lifestyle.

- Clients need a TC that focuses on the broad socialization or habilitation of the individual building these basic skills and fostering the individual's progress through developmental stages that previously were missed.

Antisocial Lifestyle

- Clients have criminal histories involving illegal activities, incarceration, and court proceedings: Some were involved with the criminal justice system as juveniles; a considerable number are legally referred to treatment.

- Clients have other characteristics that are highly correlated with drug use, including exploitation, abuse, and violence; attitudes of disaffiliation with mainstream society; and the rejection of absence of prosocial values.

SOURCE: Adapted from DeLeon G (1995). Therapeutic Communities for Addictions: A Theoretical Framework. *International Journal of the Addictions* 30(12):1603-1645.

Case 3: A third patient is a 34-year-old dentist who began drinking in high school and smoked a little marijuana as well. He did well in college without working very hard but found that it was easier to study if he used cocaine occasionally for those all-nighters at final exam time. After finishing dental school, he took over his father's dental practice and did well for a few years. After a skiing injury to his back, he began taking prescription Vicodin® and later OxyContin® for the pain. He has had three surgeries on his back, but still has pain.

The state physician diversion program interceded after he was investigated for writing excessive prescriptions for narcotics in the name of his office manager, and he currently is in the state's physician diversion program. He has completed three inpatient treatment programs. The first program was a one-week detoxification program with outpatient followup. That program proved to be barely a bump in the road of the progression of his disease. The second program consisted of inpatient detoxification followed by four weeks of inpatient rehabilitation in the standard Twelve Step format. Finally, after urinalysis showed continued opioid use, his license was suspended and he was referred to a 90-day modified TC program that specializes in treating professionals.

He completed the program and did well for six months posttreatment. Then he began to use heroin intravenously and again was found out through random urine testing. At this point, his wife and children have left him and he is in the throes of a divorce. He no longer has health insurance, and his car has been repossessed. He is living in an apartment that his father has been paying for from his retirement income. The diversion program is about to revoke his license and discharge him from the program for failure to derive benefit from treatment. This person is an excellent candidate for a residential modern addiction TC. He is at high risk of death. He probably has hepatitis B and C and can acquire AIDS if he continues in his current lifestyle. There is little or nothing left in his life to repair or resurrect. He is in need of a new lifestyle and renovation of his behavior patterns, which is exactly what a TC has to offer. He may be reaching a state of desperation necessary for him to make the commitment needed to succeed in the TC environment.

These examples illustrate the fact that treatment in a TC is not appropriate for every person with a drug or alcohol problem. The commitment of time, money, and surrender to the program is significant. What makes the dentist in Case 3 a good candidate for a TC is clear from that illustration. His life is in crisis, he is unable to maintain abstinence, his social and interpersonal dysfunction has permeated every aspect of his life, and he has begun to display the antisocial lifestyle typical of end-stage addicts.

If such a patient has the good fortune to cross paths with a physician who is perceptive and knowledgeable enough to refer him to an appropriate addiction TC, he may have a chance to survive. In fact, in some ways, he actually may have a better chance than someone like the engineer in Case 2.

Many patients seem to do better with a little external motivation. In the case of the dentist, the state diversion program may impose some requirements that will help him to remain focused on his recovery while going through the tough times of personal re-development in the TC process. Requirements imposed through probation or parole orders can be helpful as well. Such requirements may sound harsh, but are appropriate when balanced with the fact that the patients have a fatal illness and have failed at every other form of therapy. Admission to a TC may be the only defense between the addict and death in the street.

Application to Specific Population Groups. Those dealing with specific subpopulations have not overlooked the powerful rate of successful outcome of the therapeutic community. In particular, prison, adolescent, and dually diagnosed persons all have good recovery rates in TC programs. Broader applications are now being evaluated.

CRITICISMS OF THE TC MODEL

Critics of TCs generally fall into one of two groups: those who believe that TCs cost too much and those who believe that the treatment is too harsh.

Treatment in a 12- to 18-month residential TC program certainly costs more than attending AA or Narcotics Anonymous meetings. That is why this modality is reserved for those who have failed at lesser forms of treatment, usually on more that one occasion. However, TC treatment costs just a fraction of incarceration—usually about one third the price per resident per year. Even that cost is easily recouped by the lower rates of relapse or recidivism in TC programs.

The "rough edges" of TC life have been smoothed over the years in response to public opinion and payer oversight. Still, treatment in the modern addiction TC is the most difficult thing most residents will ever do. Generally, TC treatment is reserved for those who have had multiple treatment failures and who are at high risk of dying of the disease. The goal of the modern addiction TC is to rebuild human lives from the ground up. Some struggle and effort are required to achieve that change.

CONCLUSIONS

The modern addiction TC is a powerful therapeutic tool with broad application to changing human behavior. With roots in ancient times, the TC evolved out of AA into a highly structured, often publicly funded, highly successful therapeutic modality. The Daytop model has developed into a traditional TC agency and has been the progenitor of TC programs around the world. Despite its shortcomings, the TC has returned hundreds of thousands of "hopeless" addicts and alcoholics to useful, productive lives.

REFERENCES

Agnew R (1991). The interactive effect of peer variables on delinquency. *Criminology* 29:47-72.

Anglin MD & Hser Y (1990a). Legal coercion and drug abuse treatment: Research findings and social policy implications. In JA Inciardi & JR Biden Jr. (eds.) *Handbook of Drug Control in the United States.* New York, NY: Greenwood Publishing Group, 151-176.

Anglin MD & Hser Y (1990b). Treatment of drug abuse. In M Tonry & JQ Wilson (eds.) *Crime and Justice: An Annual Review of Research, Vol. 13.* Chicago, IL: University of Chicago Press, 393-460.

Anglin MD, Nugent JF & Ng LKY (1976). Synanon and Alcoholics Anonymous: Is there really a difference? *Addiction Therapist* 1(4):6-9.

Bandura A (1977). *Social Learning Theory*. Englewood Cliffs, NJ: Prentice-Hall.

Barr H (1986). Outcome of drug abuse treatment on two modalities. In G DeLeon & JI Ziegenfuss (eds.) *Therapeutic Communities for Addictions*. Springfield, IL: Charles C Thomas, 97-108.

Barton E (1994). The adaptation of the therapeutic community to HIV/AIDS. In *Proceedings of the Therapeutic Communities of America, 1992 Planning Conference: Paradigms—Past, Present and Future*. Chantilly, VA; December 6-9.

Bell DC (1994). Connection in Therapeutic Communities. *International Journal of the Addictions* 29:525-543.

Brown BS (1998). Towards the year 2000. Drug use—Chronic and relapsing or a treatable condition? *Substance Use and Misuse* 33(12):2515-2520.

Carroll JFX & McGinley I (1998). Managing MICA clients in a modified Therapeutic Community with enhanced staffing. *Journal of Substance Abuse Treatment* 15(6):565-577.

Condelli WS & Hubbard RL (1994). Client outcomes from therapeutic communities. In FM Tims, G DeLeon & N Jainchill (eds.) *Therapeutic Community: Advances in Research and Application (NIDA Research Monograph 144*. Rockville, MD: National Institute on Drug Abuse, 80-98.

DeLeon G (1995). Therapeutic communities for addictions: A theoretical framework. *International Journal of the Addictions* 30(12):1603-1645.

DeLeon G (1988). Legal pressure in therapeutic communities. In CG Leukefeld & FM Tims (eds.) *Compulsory Treatment of Drug Abuse: Research and Clinical Practice (NIDA Research Monograph 86)*. Rockville, MD: National Institute on Drug Abuse.

DeLeon G (2000). *The Therapeutic Community: Theory, Model, and Method*. New York, NY: Springer Publishing Company.

Glaser FB (1974). Some historical and theoretical background of a self-help addiction treatment program. *American Journal of Drug and Alcohol Abuse* 1:37-52.

Jainchill N (1994). Co-morbidity and therapeutic community treatment. In FM Tims, G DeLeon & N Jainchill (eds.) *Therapeutic Community: Advances in Research and Application (NIDA Research Monograph 144)*. Rockville, MD: National Institute on Drug Abuse, 209-231.

Jainchill N, Battacharya G & Yagelka J (1995). Therapeutic communities for adolescents. In E Rahdert & D Czechowicz (eds.) *Adolescent Drug Use: Clinical Assessment and Therapeutic Interventions (NIDA Research Monograph 156)*. Rockville, MD: National Institute on Drug Abuse, 190-217.

Kennard D (1983). *An Introduction to Therapeutic Communities*. London, England: Rutledge and Kegan Paul.

Kerr DH (1986). The therapeutic community: A codified concept for training and upgrading staff members working in a residential setting. In G DeLeon & JI Ziegenfuss (eds.) *Therapeutic Communities for Addictions*. Springfield, IL: Charles C Thomas, 55-63.

Kooyman M (1993). *The Therapeutic Community for Addicts: Intimacy, Parent Involvement and Treatment Outcome*. Amsterdam, The Netherlands: Swets and Zeitlinger.

Liberty HI, Johnson BD, Jainchill N et al. (1998). Dynamic recovery: Comparative study of therapeutic communities in homeless shelters for men. *Journal of Substance Abuse Treatment* 15(5):401-423.

Lipton DS (1999). Therapeutic community treatment programming in corrections. In CR Hollin (ed.) *Handbook of Offender Assessment and Treatment*. London, England: John Wiley & Sons, Ltd.

Messina NR, Wish ED & Nemes S (1999). Therapeutic community treatment for substance abusers with anti-social personality disorder. *Journal of Substance Abuse Treatment* 17(1-2):121-128.

Nielsen A & Scarpitti F (1997). Changing the behavior of substance abusers: Factors influencing the effectiveness of therapeutic communities. *Journal of Drug Issues* 27(2):279-298.

Nuttbrock LA, Rahav M, Rivera I et al. (1998). Outcomes of homeless mentally ill chemical abusers in community residences and a therapeutic community. *Psychiatric Services* 49:68-76.

Preston CA & Viney LL (1984). Self- and ideal self-perception of drug addicts in therapeutic communities. *International Journal of the Addictions* 19(7):805-818.

Ray R (1999). The Oxford Connection [online].

Sacks S, DeLeon G, Bernhardt AI et al. (1997). A modified therapeutic community for homeless mentally ill chemical abusers. In G DeLeon (ed.) *Community as Method: Therapeutic Communities for Special Populations and Special Settings*. Westport, CT: Greenwood Publishing Group, 19-37.

Silberstein CH, Metzger EI & Galanter M (1997). The Greenhouse: A modified therapeutic community for mentally ill homeless addicts at New York University. In G DeLeon (ed.) *Community as Method: Therapeutic Communities for Special Populations and Special Settings*. Westport, CT: Greenwood Publishing Group, 53-65.

Slater MR (1984). An Historical Perspective of Therapeutic Communities (thesis proposal to the MSS program, University of Colorado at Denver).

Stevens SJ, Arbiter N & McGrath R (1997). Women and children: Therapeutic community substance abuse treatment. In G DeLeon (ed.) *Community as Method: Therapeutic Communities for Special Populations and Special Settings*. Westport, CT: Greenwood Publishing Group, 129-142.

Talbot ES (1998). *Therapeutic Community Experiential Training: Facilitator's Guide*. Kansas City, MO: University of Missouri-Kansas City, Mid-America Technology Transfer Center.

Wilson B (1957). *Alcoholics Anonymous Comes of Age: A Brief History of AA*. New York, NY: Alcoholics Anonymous World Services.

Winick C & Evans JT (1997). A therapeutic community program for mothers and their children. In G DeLeon (ed.) *Community as Method: Therapeutic Communities for Special Populations and Special Settings*. Westport, CT: Greenwood Publishing Group, 143-160.

Yablonsky L (1989). *The Therapeutic Community*. New York, NY: Gardner Press.

Zweben JE & Smith DE (1986). Changing attitudes and policies toward alcohol use in the therapeutic community. *Journal of Psychoactive Drugs* 18(3):253-260.

Recent Research Into Therapeutic Communities

GEORGE DeLEON, PH.D.

Research into therapeutic communities (TCs) has focused on elaborating the theories and methods embodied in the TC approach to addiction treatment, on the development of instruments to assess client motivation and readiness for treatment, on measuring clinical progress, on defining and validating the essential elements of the TC model, on identifying elements in the TC environment that affect risk for clients dropping out of treatment, and on providing a conceptual framework of the treatment process. Such inquiries have been productive:

- *Theoretical Framework*: Research has contributed to the development of a comprehensive theoretical framework for the TC approach. Such a framework is useful in guiding clinical practice, program planning, treatment improvement, and empirical studies of the treatment process and client-treatment matching.

- *Program Diversity*: Empirical studies have identified the essential elements of the TC program model and have differentiated among TC programs to describe "standard" and "modified" programs. They also have identified factors that contribute to client dropout.

- *Motivation*: The role of motivation and readiness factors in entry into and retention in TC programs has been assessed, and initial studies have measured these factors in the TC treatment process.

- *Clinical Assessment*: Multiple instruments have been developed to measure client progress.

TC studies fall into two phases: the early (circa 1973-1989) and current (1990-present) studies. In each phase, studies focused on certain questions or areas of inquiry that are relevant to policy as well as science. The key questions, findings, and conclusions of the research in each phase are summarized here from a variety of literature reviews (such as Anglin & Hser, 1990; DeLeon, 1984, 1985, 2000; Hubbard, Marsden et al., 1989; Gerstein & Harwood, 1990; Simpson & Sells, 1982; Simpson, Joe et al., 1997; Tims, DeLeon et al., 1994; Tims & Ludford, 1984).

EARLY RESEARCH

The lines of inquiry in early studies focused on three key questions: (1) Who are the clients of TCs? (2) What are the success rates of TCs? and (3) What do we know about retention in TCs?

Clients Treated in TC Programs. TCs serve persons with severe substance use disorders, including those who are marked by social and psychological dysfunction and criminal deviancy, as well as persistent use of alcohol and illegal drugs. Approximately 70% of persons admitted to TC programs have co-occurring mental and addictive disorders. This psychosocial profile is fairly uniform across TC programs, cultures, and time frames. Moreover, there is an overall trend toward greater morbidity in more recent times, especially in terms of cognitive impairments, depression, and anxiety.

Effectiveness of TC Treatment. As measured in terms of improvements in functioning (such as reductions in drug use and criminal involvement and increased employment), more than half of all persons admitted to TCs have a positive outcome. These behavioral outcomes are positively associated with good psychological outcomes, as measured in terms of positive mental and emotional state, self-perception, and quality of life.

Across studies, length of stay in treatment is the most consistent predictor of positive outcomes.

Retention in Treatment. One-year retention rates differ across programs, but have steadily increased over the years. Dropout rates peak between 30 and 90 days following admission, declining thereafter. Predictors of dropout status include severe criminality, psychopathology, poor motivation, and lack of readiness for treatment.

Early studies confirmed that TCs were serving the most difficult-to-treat patient population. Their findings documented the TC perspective that substance abuse is a disorder of the whole person and underscored the need to maximize retention and treatment completion rates.

CURRENT RESEARCH

In recent years, TCs have modified their practices and adapted their approach to meet the needs of special populations, as well as adjust to various settings and changing funding patterns. In particular, the emergence of managed care and other pressures to reduce treatment costs has challenged the need for long-term residential treatment of the type offered by traditional TCs.

A second issue that has emerged, concurrent with these adaptations, is the fidelity of modern TC programs to the original concept. Thus areas of current inquiry include (1) the therapeutic and cost effectiveness of TC programs for special populations and special settings and (2) the boundaries of the TC treatment model and methods.

Standard TCs. The national multimodality survey studies uniformly showed that community-based standard TC residential programs still serve patients with the most severe substance use disorders, compared with other treatment modalities. Admission profiles suggest that contemporary TCs continue to serve a population that evidences considerable social and psychological dysfunction in addition to substance use disorders.

Long-term residential programs obtain positive outcomes in terms of reduced drug use and criminal activity and increased employment and psychological adjustment, which were comparable to outcomes for modalities that serve individuals with less severe substance use disorders.

While costs of long-term residential treatment exceeded those associated with other treatment modalities, these were offset by increased benefits, particularly those involving cost savings linked to reductions in criminal activities.

Current studies show that the planned duration of treatment in TCs is shorter than in earlier years. However, positive outcomes still are strongly associated with longer stays. The differential outcomes associated with relatively longer or shorter duration of treatment remain to be clarified in studies that match patients to appropriate planned durations of care.

Modified TCs. In modified TCs that specialize in the care of patients with co-occurring mental and substance use disorders, criminal justice populations, adolescents, and homeless persons, studies have found significant reductions in substance use and criminal activity, and improvements in employment and psychological functioning. Such improvements were positively correlated with longer duration of treatment. Associated reductions in expenditures related to criminal activity and mental health services tended to offset the higher treatment costs for residential care.

Aftercare or services beyond the period of active residential treatment were found to be a critical component of stable outcomes. From this, it can be concluded that, regardless of the duration of care in a TC, the presence of suitable aftercare is an important predictor of positive treatment outcome. Aftercare models should be integrated with the primary TC experience in terms of philosophy and treatment methods employed.

Based on these results, it is possible to state that TCs provide a cost-effective alternative to traditional institutional care in the mental health, acute hospital, and correctional systems.

CONCLUSIONS

The TC has evolved into a major treatment for substance use and related disorders. The efficacy of such treatment is supported by research documenting the effectiveness of the TC approach for a variety of clients and problems.

To a considerable extent, success of the current research agenda depends on scientific elaboration of the "black box" of treatment process in a TC. Thus the evolution of the scientific knowledge base through the early and current phases gradually has shifted the research question from *whether* TCs work to *how* they work.

REFERENCES

Anglin MD & Hser YI (1990). Treatment of drug abuse. In M Tonry & JQ Wilson (eds.) *Crime and Justice: An Annual Review of Research, Vol. 13.* Chicago, IL: University of Chicago Press, 393-460.

DeLeon G (1984). Program-based evaluation research in therapeutic communities. *Drug Abuse Treatment Evaluation: Strategies, Progress and Prospects; Research, Analysis and Utilization System (NIDA Research Monograph 51).* Rockville, MD: National Institute on Drug Abuse, 69-87.

DeLeon G (1985). The therapeutic community: Status and evolution. *International Journal of Addictions* 20(6-7):823-844.

DeLeon G, ed. (1997). *Community as Method: Therapeutic Communities for Special Populations and Special Settings.* Westport, CT: Greenwood Publishing Group, 12.

DeLeon G (2000). *The Therapeutic Community: Theory, Model and Method.* New York, NY: Springer Publishing Co.

Gerstein DR & Harwood JH, eds. (1990). *Treating Drug Problems, Vol. 1: A Study of the Evaluation, Effectiveness, and Financing of Public and Private Drug Treatment Systems (Report of the Institute of Medicine).* Washington, DC: National Academy Press.

Hubbard RL, Marsden ME, Rachal JV et al. (1989). *Drug Abuse Treatment: A National Study of Effectiveness.* Chapel Hill, NC: The University of North Carolina Press.

Simpson DD, Joe GW & Brown BS (1997). Treatment retention and follow-up outcomes in the Drug Abuse Treatment Outcome Study (DATOS). *Psychology of Addictive Behaviors* 11:294-307.

Simpson DD & Sells SB (1982). Effectiveness of treatment for drug abuse: An overview of the DARP research program. *Advances in Alcohol and Substance Abuse* 2:7-29.

Tims FM, DeLeon G & Jainchill N, eds. (1994). *Therapeutic Community: Advances in Research and Application (NIDA Research Monograph 144).* Rockville, MD: National Institute on Drug Abuse.

Tims FM & Ludford JP, eds. (1984). *Drug Abuse Treatment Evaluation: Strategies, Progress and Prospects (NIDA Research Monograph 51).* Rockville, MD: National Institute on Drug Abuse.

| Chapter 8 | # Aversion Therapies |

P. Joseph Frawley, M.D.

Principles of Conditioning
Uses of Aversion Therapy
Safety of Aversion Therapy
Acceptability of Aversion Therapy
Criticisms of Aversion Therapy
Aversion Therapy as Part of a Multimodality Treatment Program

Aversion therapy, or counter-conditioning, is a powerful tool in the treatment of alcohol and other drug addiction. Its goal is to reduce or eliminate the "hedonic memory" or craving for a drug and to simultaneously develop a distaste and avoidance response to the substance. Unlike punishments (jail, firings, fines, divorce, hangovers, cirrhosis, and the like), which often are delayed in time from the use episode, aversion therapy relies on the immediate association of the sight, smell, taste, and act of using the substance with an unpleasant or "aversive" experience.

This treatment is not designed to appeal to the logical part of the individual's brain, which often is all too aware of the negative consequences of alcohol and other drug use, but to the part of the brain where emotional attachments are made or broken through experienced associations of pleasure or discomfort. Aversion therapy provides a means of achieving control over injurious behavior for a period of time, during which alternative and more rewarding modes of response can be established and strengthened (Bandura, 1969).

People Need Care—Behavior Needs Modification. It is important not to confuse aversion with punishment. In punishment, it is the individual who receives the negative consequence, while in aversion therapy the negative consequence is *only* paired with the act of using a drug. This has a very important benefit to self-esteem. While the patient is engaging in positive recovery activities, he or she is receiving immediate positive support for a new way of behaving and thinking. It is only when the patient is engaging in an old behavior—alcohol or drug use—that he or she experiences immediate and consistent discomfort. Hence, self-esteem is rebuilt by separating the drug from the self (Smith, 1982).

In non-addicted populations, hangovers have been cited as a significant reason to cut down or stop drinking (Smith, Bookner et al., 1988). However, the hangover is delayed in time from the actual use of alcohol; thus, for the alcoholic, who drinks for the immediate euphorogenic effects of alcohol, a hangover often is ineffective in producing aversion because it is delayed in time from use of the substance whose immediate effect was experienced as pleasant or euphoric. Moreover, the discomfort of a hangover, while logically understood to be the result of drinking, is blamed on "drinking too much" (weakness) rather than drinking at all (disease). Even worse, alcohol may be used to cure the withdrawal ("hair of the dog"), which ensures that emotionally, the patient perceives the alcohol as a solution, not a problem.

Contrary to popular belief, disulfiram (Antabuse®) is not an aversion treatment. In aversion therapy for alcohol addiction, alcohol is not absorbed into the system (Smith, 1982). With disulfiram, alcohol must be absorbed and metabolism begun for it to produce its toxic effect (Ritchie, 1980). Aversion relies on safe but uncomfortable experiences that can be repeated, while disulfiram reactions can be life-threatening, even in healthy persons. For this reason, patients today are not given alcohol at the same time that they are prescribed disulfiram. As a result, they have not actually experienced a disulfiram reaction. Thus, disulfiram does not change the way the addict feels about alcohol. He or she may fear the consequence of drinking, just as he or she fears being arrested for drinking and driving; nevertheless, he or she still retains the euphoric recall of past episodes of drinking alcohol and hence the craving for the alcohol itself. Aversion works to eliminate or reduce euphoric recall by recording new negative experiences with the drug (Cannon, Baker et al., 1986).

In fact, spontaneous aversions are common, because the capacity to develop aversions is a biological defense mechanism. Silva and Rachman (1987) published a study of 125 students and hospital employees, 105 (84%) of whom had a history of natural aversions. There were an average of 3.5 aversions per person (females > males) and 70.1% had been present since childhood.

PRINCIPLES OF CONDITIONING

Ivan Pavlov noted that the repetitive pairing of a bell with food soon led to a "conditioned response" in dogs, who salivated at the sound of the bell alone, even with no food present. This type of pairing or training is called "classical conditioning."

B.F. Skinner expounded on the observation that the nervous system is so constructed that organisms will reduce or avoid behavior that is consistently paired with negative consequences, and increase behavior that is rewarded. This type of learning is called "operant conditioning." Both types of learning can be shown to occur in addiction (Hoeschen, 1991). Aversion therapy uses these principles in reversing the drug-rewarded learning and conditioned reflex to seek drugs.

The development of an aversion can be very specific. Inadequate treatment can occur when aversion is developed only to one type of alcoholic beverage (Lemere & Voegtlin,

1940; Quinn & Henbest, 1967). In professional alcohol addiction treatment, for example, 50% of trials may be with the addict's favorite brand or type of liquor, but the other trials include a range of alcoholic beverages (Lemere, Voegtlin et al., 1942; Smith, 1982).

Repetition is an essential part of training and conditioning (Schwartz, 1978). Adequate trials are needed to develop an aversion (Lemere, Voegtlin et al., 1942) and to maintain and reinforce it to prevent extinction (Voegtlin, Lemere et al, 1941; Smith, Frawley et al., 1991).

Addicts Already Have Been Conditioned by the Drug Prior to Entry Into Treatment. Studies have shown that alcoholics increase the number of swallows and amount of salivation in response to the sight of alcohol, as compared to non-alcoholics (Pomerleau, Fertig et al., 1983). Studies of smokers seeking to quit show that those who are least likely to quit have a much larger conditioned drop in pulse (presumably to compensate for the increase in pulse rate caused by smoking) when presented with a cigarette (Niaura, Abrams et al., 1989). Cocaine-dependent addicts experience progressively steeper drops in skin temperature and increased galvanic skin response (a sign of arousal) when viewing progressively more intense and explicit pictures of cocaine use. These responses can be shown to decay in strength as time away from the drug increases.

The presence of these phenomena suggests that one of the consequences of addiction is that the body becomes conditioned to drink or use drugs in the presence of certain stimuli. This may contribute to the sensation of physical craving experienced by addicts. The availability of drugs such as heroin or cocaine in the environment also influences craving (Sherman, Zinser et al., 1989; Weddington, Brown et al., 1990; Gawin & Kleber, 1986).

USES OF AVERSION THERAPY

Aversion Therapy in Smoking Cessation. It is estimated that more than 80% of smokers wish to quit but feel compelled to continue smoking because of the difficulty of stopping; indeed, the annual spontaneous recovery rate for smokers is less than 5% (Sachs, 1991). Sachs (1986, 1991) reviewed modern smoking cessation treatments and concluded that programs that use rapid smoking aversion had superior outcomes. Hall and Lando reported in separate studies that the best results were reported by programs in which aversion was combined with several other modalities, including relapse prevention, relaxation training, written exercises, contract management, booster sessions of aversion, and group support. In patients with cardiopulmonary disease, Hall has provided data both for and against the use of satiation aversion. In one study, patients treated with health motivation, self-management, film models and verbal commitment had better outcomes than those treated with satiation aversion, relaxation training, and role play. On the other hand, Hall reported that those on a waiting list had no abstinence compared with those treated with satiation aversion, 50% of whom achieved two-year abstinence. No myocardial ischemia or significant arrhythmia were found in a group of 18 treated patients. Five patients with ischemic changes on the treadmill did not experience the changes during the satiation treatment.

Much of the research on aversion therapy for smoking cessation has focused on improved outcomes with aversive smoking (puffing or inhaling smoke from the cigarette in a rapid manner to induce nicotine toxicity, often including nausea) (Erickson, Tiffany et al., 1983). While nicotine is taken into the system during this treatment, the aversion developed to smoking is adequate to prevent relapse despite the transient presence of nicotine in the bloodstream during treatment. Faradic aversion (mild electrical stimulus applied to the forearm) has been used commercially for smoking cessation since 1972 (Smith, 1988). With faradic aversion, the smoke is not inhaled, but merely puffed. Inhaling during faradic aversion may lead to early relapse because of maintenance of the nicotine dependence (Berecz, 1972). One advantage of this form of treatment is that less medically sophisticated staff can supervise the administration of the treatment. In both forms of treatment, patients personally administer the aversive agent (rapid smoking or electrical stimulus) to themselves, while the therapist serves as a coach. In the case of faradic aversion, each time a patient brings a cigarette toward his or her lips, a mild electrical stimulus is administered automatically by a 9-volt battery. The stimulus is activated by a string attached to the smoker's wrist. The therapist also instructs the patient in relapse prevention methods, and behavior and dietary changes that help maintain abstinence and achieve comfort during the initial period following smoking cessation. Smith (1988) contacted 59% of 556 patients treated with this method in a commercial program and found that 52% had achieved continuous abstinence at one year.

Aversion Therapy for Alcohol Addiction. The spontaneous recovery rate for alcoholism is influenced by a variety of factors, including severity of problems, age, and the presence of a co-occurring psychiatric disorder. Nevertheless,

the annual spontaneous recovery rate estimated by Vaillant in his study of the natural history of alcoholism was 2% to 3% (Vaillant, 1983). In 1949, Voegtlin and Broz published a 10.5-year followup of 3,125 patients treated with aversion therapy. One-year abstinence rates of 70% were reported using chemical aversion therapy with minimal counseling.

There are three well-conducted controlled trials of aversion therapy. Boland and colleagues (1978) evaluated the six-month abstinence rates for 50 lower socioeconomic alcoholics, using lithium as a chemical aversive agent. Twenty-five patients given emetic aversion with lithium had 36% total abstinence, as compared to 12% for the 25 patients given control treatment (p<0.05). Cannon and colleagues (1981) divided 20 Veterans Administration patients into three groups and found that there was little difference in outcome between seven patients given chemical aversion and those given control treatment (both groups, however, had extremely high abstinence rates: 170-180 days for the chemical aversion group versus 158-180 days for the control group). Both did better than seven patients receiving faradic aversion. However, the groups were small, there may have been some ceiling effect, and the subjects had to drink some alcohol during the actual testing sessions, which could counteract any aversion being developed.

In the private sector, Smith and Frawley (1991) compared 249 inpatients receiving aversion therapy as part of a multimodality treatment program with 249 inpatients from a large (>9,000 patient) treatment registry of patients receiving multimodality treatment, but without aversion therapy. All were matched on 17 baseline characteristics. Of the patients receiving aversion therapy, 84.7% had total abstinence from alcohol at six months, compared with 72.2% in the control group (p<0.01); at one year, 79% of those treated with aversion had maintained abstinence, versus 67% of those without such treatment (p<0.05). The group showing the greatest benefit from aversion therapy was the daily drinkers (84% versus 67%, p<0.001).

While the majority of patients in the study were treated with chemical aversion therapy, a subsample of 28 patients received faradic aversion instead. The decision to prescribe faradic aversion instead of chemical aversion within clinical practice usually is based on the patient's medical condition. If the patient has a medical contraindication to chemical aversion therapy, then faradic is prescribed. Jackson and Smith (1978) reported that patients selected in this way had nearly identical abstinence rates. In a more recent study, the same results were found (Smith, Frawley et al., 1997).

Nausea Aversion: As reported by Smith (1982), "The usual treatment session involves having the patient take nothing except clear liquids by mouth for six hours prior to treatment. This reduces the likelihood of aspiration of solid stomach contents during treatment. The patient, after receiving a full explanation of the treatment procedure, is taken to the treatment room, which is small in size and has shelves containing all types of alcoholic beverages along the walls. It also has cutouts of various liquor ads on the walls. The intent is to have the majority of the patient's visual stimuli associated with alcohol beverages and visual cues for drinking. The patient is then seated in a comfortable chair with an attached large emesis basin. The patient then receives an injection of pilocarpine and ephedrine to induce an autonomic arousal and an oral dose of emetine. The emetic effect begins in approximately five to eight minutes. Prior to that time, the patient is given two 10 oz. glasses of warm water with a small amount of added salt. The water provides a volume of easily vomited material, while the salt content tends to counteract the excessive loss of electrolytes during the procedure. Shortly before the expected onset of nausea, the nurse administering the treatment pours a drink of the patient's preferred alcoholic beverage and mixes it with an equal amount of warm water. The patient then is instructed to smell the beverage and to take a small mouthful, swish it around in the mouth to get the full flavor of it, and then to spit it out into the basin. This 'sniff, swish, and spit' phase is designed to insure that the patient has well-defined visual, olfactory, and gustatory sensations associated with the preferred beverage prior to the onset of the aversive stimulus of nausea. The nausea and vomiting ensue shortly thereafter and the procedure is altered to that of 'sniff, swish, and swallow.' The alcoholic beverage swallowed is shortly returned as emesis so that no significant amount of alcohol is retained to be absorbed, an event that would negate the treatment. After an intensive conditioning session in the treatment room, lasting 20 to 30 minutes, the patient is returned to the hospital room, where 30 minutes later, another drink of alcoholic beverage is given containing an oral dose of emetine and tartar emetic, which induces a slower-acting residual nausea lasting up to three hours. The average patient receives five treatment sessions, which are given every other day over a 10-day period of time."

Faradic Aversion Therapy for Alcohol: As reported by Smith (1982), "During each session, a pair of electrodes is attached to the forearm of the dominant hand and placed approximately two inches (0.05 dm) apart. The electrodes are attached to an electrostimulus machine capable of delivering 1 to 20 mA (DC, constant current). The faradic therapist runs an ascending series of test stimuli to determine the level of stimulus perceived as aversive by the patient on that particular day (there is a relatively wide variance between patients and within the same individual from day to day).

"The treatment paradigm consists of pairing an aversive level of electrostimulation with the sight, smell, and taste of alcoholic beverages. At the direction of the therapist (forced choice trial) the patient reaches for a bottle of alcoholic beverage, pours some of it in a glass and tastes it without swallowing. Electrostimulus onset occurs randomly throughout the entire behavior continuum, from reaching for the bottle through tasting the alcoholic beverage. The number of electrostimuli with each trial varies from 1 to 8. An additional 10 free choice trials are designed so that the patient is negatively reinforced, with removal of the aversive stimulus if he or she selects a nonalcoholic choice such as fruit juice. The patient is instructed not to swallow any alcohol at any time throughout the faradic session, and this behavior is closely monitored by the therapist."

Sessions last 20 to 45 minutes, depending on the individual patient. Following the aversion conditioning session in the treatment room, the patient returns to his or her room, listens to a relaxation tape, makes a list of positive changes with sobriety, and contrasts them with the negative consequences of continued use.

Aversion Therapy for Marijuana Dependence. The spontaneous recovery rate from marijuana dependence is not known and, like that for alcohol and nicotine, probably depends on multiple factors. Chemical aversion using emetine has been used for marijuana dependence. In clinical practice, aversion therapy for marijuana uses faradic aversion. The protocol for faradic aversion is similar to that of the treatment for alcohol, except that it uses a variety of bongs, drug paraphernalia, and visual imagery. An artificial marijuana substitute and marijuana aroma are used in treatment. A one-year abstinence rate of 84% was reported following five days of treatment, combined with three weekly group sessions on self-management techniques.

Aversion Therapy for Cocaine/Amphetamine Dependence. The spontaneous recovery rate from cocaine or amphetamine dependence is not known. Rawson and colleagues (1986) followed 30 patients who had requested information about stopping cocaine, but had not used treatment for an eight-month period; 47% were reported at the followup point to be using cocaine at least monthly. No total abstinence figures are available. Frawley and Smith (1990) reported the use of chemical aversion for the treatment of cocaine dependence. In this treatment, an artificial cocaine substitute called Articaine® was developed from tetracaine, mannitol, and quinine. Patients snorted this substance and paired it with nausea induced by emetine. Of those so treated, 56% were continuously abstinent and 78% currently abstinent (that is, for the prior 30 days) at six months following treatment; at 18 months, 38% were continuously abstinent and 75% currently abstinent. For those treated for both alcohol and cocaine, 70% were continuously and currently abstinent from cocaine at six months and 50% were continuously abstinent and 80% currently abstinent at 18 months following treatment.

Frawley and Smith (1992) reported a 53% one-year continuous abstinence rate in 156 cocaine and/or amphetamine dependent patients treated with aversion. This was based on a 73% followup rate. Outcomes for chemical and faradic aversion were not significantly different. The report also compared patients treated for alcohol and cocaine problems before the institution of cocaine aversion, when only aversion therapy for alcohol was available, with those who received aversion therapy for both alcohol and cocaine. The addition of the aversion for cocaine produced statistically significantly improved abstinence rates in this population. The increase in cocaine abstinence in the second group compared to the first (55% versus 88%) is greater than the decrease on followup from the first to the second group (84% versus 64%). Because of the lower followup rate in the second study, this research needs replication.

Aversion for Heroin Addiction. Copemann (1976) employed a unique approach to aversion therapy by pairing aversive stimuli to cognitive images of heroin use. Patients were asked to verbalize only after they had conjured up a strong mental image. A second part of the treatment asked addicts to conjure images of socially appropriate behavior, involving employment, education, or nondrug entertainment. Latency to verbalization was measured. Copemann found that, at baseline, addicts could rapidly conjure up positive thoughts about heroin use, but had significant delays in conjuring up thoughts about rewarding nondrug activities. Subjects were in a halfway house for heroin addicts and

received group therapy in conjunction with relaxation therapy in addition to the aversion treatment. A faradic stimulator was used. Once addicts had conjured up drug images, faradic aversion was applied. At other times, addicts were given 15 seconds to conjure images of nondrug socially appropriate behavior to prevent aversion from being applied. With this training over an average of 15 sessions (range 5 to 25), latency for drug-related images increased, while that for socially appropriate images decreased. Thirty of 50 patients completed the treatment and, at 24 months, 80% (24 of 30) were reported to be drug-free.

SAFETY OF AVERSION THERAPY

Faradic aversion has virtually no unwanted side effects and has been found to be safe for patients with pacemakers and pregnant women (because the current only travels between two electrodes on the arm).

To be eligible for chemical aversion therapy, patients must be free of medical contraindications such as esophageal varices, serious coronary artery disease, or active GI pathology. Emetine is given only orally, effectively eliminating the risk of cardiotoxic effects of IM emetine, since very little of the orally administered emetine is absorbed (Kattwinkel, 1949; Loomis, 1986). Emetine exerts its principal action by irritating the GI tract, hence stimulating the afferent vagus nerve to stimulate the vomiting center in the medulla. Oral emetine is effective in stimulating nausea in more than 95% of cases, while intramuscular emetine produces nausea only 30% to 40% of the time, probably through excretion in the bile (Klatskin & Friedman, 1948; Loomis, 1986). Pilocarpine and ephedrine are not used in patients with asthma or serious hypertension, while tartar emetic is held for patients with excessive diarrhea or prolonged nausea. Smith and colleagues (1991, unpublished data) found that there was no increased incidence of medical utilization or hospitalization in the six months after treatment in a group treated with aversion therapy, as compared to matched controls treated without aversion.

There are some contraindications to covert sensitization, similar to those for chemical aversion; however, with this therapy, emesis can be prevented in most cases. The drawback to covert aversion therapy is that the induction of nausea or other aversive state is not as predictable as with medication and requires more patient preparation (Elkins, 1985).

Satiation therapy with nicotine has been studied by Hall and colleagues in 18 patients (nine men and nine women;

average age 45.8 years) with pulmonary and cardiac disease. Nine had definite or probable cardiac ischemia, but none showed ischemic changes during rapid smoking. Premature ventricular contractions were not increased above baseline by rapid smoking.

ACCEPTABILITY OF AVERSION THERAPY

Selecting the appropriate treatment for a particular patient involves the patient having full informed consent. The practitioner needs to counsel the patient about the risks of continuing the addiction and the risks, benefits, and expected outcomes of various methods of treatment. Studies of patients who voluntarily received aversion therapy do not show higher rates of leaving against medical advice than is found in patients in Minnesota Model programs (Smith & Frawley, 1990; Gilmore, 1985; Patton, 1979).

Chemical aversion therapy has been reviewed and approved as a treatment for alcoholism by the National Center for Health Services Research and Health Care Technology Assessment (Carter, 1987), the body charged with determining which services should be reimbursable under Medicare. A 1987 OCHAMPUS demonstration project recommended coverage for chemical aversion therapy for alcoholism (Mendes, 1992). A California Medical Association Scientific Advisory Panel approved aversion therapy as appropriate treatment as part of a multimodality program (CMA, 1984). The American Society of Addiction Medicine includes aversion therapy as an appropriate part of treatment for alcoholism and other drug dependencies (ASAM, 1986). In a 1987 review, the American Medical Association's Council on Scientific Affairs found that the available research for the efficacy of faradic aversion for alcohol was weak, but that there was moderate support for the efficacy of chemical aversion. The Council found some support for both faradic and rapid smoking aversion techniques. However, the report emphasized that there have been few controlled trials. The Office of Technology Assessment of the U.S. Congress found that aversion therapy was effective for some patients under certain conditions (Saxe, Dovaterty et al., 1983).

CRITICISMS OF AVERSION THERAPY

Much of the criticism of aversion therapy is similar to criticisms of other forms of addiction treatment and stems from a lack of multiple well-designed controlled trials and the need to identify which treatment is appropriate for a given patient (IOM, 1990; Saxe, Dovaterty et al., 1983). Wilson (1987) has summarized a variety of such criticisms, including (1) greater medical expense than some other forms of treatment, (2) intrusiveness of aversion, and (3) the theoretical framework of aversive conditioning. While aversion therapy is more expensive than some other forms of treatment, the OCHAMPUS demonstration project did compare costs of OCHAMPUS beneficiaries admitted to the hospital with other forms of treatment and found the average cost to be slightly less for aversion therapy (which may be partially attributable to the shorter length of stay for aversion).

The principle that, when treatment outcomes are the same, the least intrusive treatment should be tried first has been raised by Wilson (1987) and echoed by Carter (1987). As further work is done on patient-treatment matching, patients for whom aversion clearly is more effective should be offered this treatment before less effective but less intrusive treatment. Smith, Frawley and Polissar (1991) found significantly better outcomes with aversion therapy in males and daily drinkers, and Boland, Mellor and Revusky (1978) found significantly better outcomes with aversion therapy in indigent male alcoholics. This work should be replicated.

The theoretical framework of aversion conditioning as a treatment does not exclude the need to develop alternative modes of behavior as part of a multimodality treatment program. Silva and Rachman (1987) demonstrated that aversions are common and can persist for a long time. Cannon and colleagues (1986) demonstrated a relationship between the strength of an aversion and the duration of abstinence following treatment.

AVERSION THERAPY AS PART OF A MULTIMODALITY TREATMENT PROGRAM

Relapse to alcohol and drug use is the result of a variety of factors. Patients who report that aversion therapy greatly reduced their urges have the best outcome (Frawley & Smith, 1992). In addition to craving, however, relapse may be related to reflex-conditioned responses to drink or use in response to either external cues such as being around others who drink or use drugs, or going to parties, or may be in response to internal cues such as negative or positive emotional states (Frawley & Smith, 1992; Marlatt & Gordon, 1980). The development of new, more appropriate responses to these emotional states and a change in the recovering person's associations remain important goals of treatment. Aversion therapy does not interfere with their development, but instead enhances the readiness of the patient to avoid the alcohol or drug and thus prepares him or her for new approaches and patterns that do not involve chemicals. Frawley and Smith (1992) found that the use of support groups was associated with improved abstinence in patients treated with aversion for cocaine and methamphetamine dependence.

CONCLUSIONS

Aversion therapy is an important tool to help patients achieve abstinence from alcohol and other drugs. The knowledgeable clinician should be aware of the risks, benefits, and expected outcomes for this approach to treatment.

ACKNOWLEDGMENT: The author wishes to acknowledge the assistance of James W. Smith, M.D., FASAM, who has reviewed the manuscript and conducted much of the research on aversion therapy.

REFERENCES

American Medical Association (AMA) (1987). Aversion therapy (Report of the Council on Scientific Affairs). *Journal of the American Medical Association* 258(18):2562-2566.

American Society of Addiction Medicine (ASAM) (1986). *Statement on Treatment for Alcoholism and Other Drug Dependencies.* Chevy Chase, MD: The Society.

Bandura A (1969). *Principles of Behavior Modification.* New York, NY: Holt, Rinehart and Winston, 509.

Berecz JM (1972). Reduction of cigarette smoking through self-administered aversion conditioning: A new treatment model with implications for public health. *Social Science and Medicine* 6:57-66.

Boland FJ, Mellor CS & Revusky S (1978). Chemical aversion treatment of alcoholism: Lithium as the aversive agent. *Behavior Research and Therapy* 16:401-409.

California Medical Association (CMA), Scientific Advisory Panels on General and Family Practice and Internal Medicine and the Committee on Alcoholism and Other Drug Dependence (1984). *Medical Practice Question: Is Aversion Therapy for the Treatment of Alcoholism Considered Accepted Medical Practice or Is It Investigational?* San Francisco, CA: California Medical Association.

Cannon DS, Baker TB, Gino A et al. (1986). Alcohol-aversion therapy: Relation between strength of aversion and abstinence. *Journal of Consulting and Clinical Psychology* 54(6):825-830.

Cannon DS, Baker TB & Wehl CK (1981). Emetic and electric shock alcohol aversion therapy: Six- and twelve-month follow-up. *Journal of Consulting and Clinical Psychology* 49(3):360-368.

Carter E (1987). Chemical aversion therapy for the treatment of alcoholism. *Health Technology Assessment Reports, 4.* Washington, DC: National Center for Health Care Services Research and Health Care Technology Assessment.

Copemann CD (1976). Drug addiction: II. An aversive countercontitioning technique for treatment. *Psychological Reports* 38:1271-1281.

Elkins RL (1985). Aversion therapy for alcoholism: Chemical, electrical, or verbal imagery? *International Journal of the Addictions* 10(2):157-209.

Erickson LM, Tiffany ST, Martin EM et al. (1983). Aversive smoking therapies: A conditioning analysis of therapeutic effectiveness. *Behavior Research and Therapy* 21(60):595-611.

Frawley PJ & Smith JW (1992). One-year follow-up after multimodal inpatient treatment for cocaine and methamphetamine dependence. *Journal of Substance Abuse Treatment* 9(4):271-286.

Frawley PJ & Smith JW (1990). Chemical aversion therapy in the treatment of cocaine dependence as part of a multimodal treatment program: Treatment outcome. *Journal of Substance Abuse Treatment* 7:21-29.

Gawin FH & Kleber HD (1986). Abstinence symptomatology and psychiatric diagnosis in cocaine abusers. *Archives of General Psychiatry* 43:107-113.

Gilmore K (1985). *Hazelden Primary Residential Treatment Program: 1983 Profile and Patient Outcome.* Center City, MN: Hazelden Foundation.

Hoeschen LE (1991). The pharmacokinetics and pharmacodynamics of alcohol and drugs of addiction. In NS Miller (ed.) *Comprehensive Handbook of Drug and Alcohol Addiction.* New York, NY: Marcel Dekker, 745-746.

Institute of Medicine (IOM) (1990). *Broadening the Base of Treatment for Alcohol Problems.* Washington, DC: National Academy Press.

Jackson TR & Smith JW (1978). A comparison of two aversion treatment methods for alcoholism. *Journal of Studies on Alcohol* 39(1):187-191.

Kattwinkel EE (1949). Death due to cardiac disease following the use of emetine hydrochloride in conditioned-reflex treatment of chronic alcoholism. *New England Journal of Medicine* 240(25):995-997.

Klatskin G & Friedman H (1948). Emetine toxicity in man: Studies on the nature of early toxic manifestations, their relation to the dose level, and their significance in determining safe dosage. *Annals of Internal Medicine* 28:892-915.

Lemere F & Voegtlin (1940). Conditioned reflex therapy of alcoholic addiction: Specificity of conditioning against chronic alcoholism. *California and Western Medicine* 53(6):1-4.

Lemere F, Voegtlin WL, Broz WR et al. (1942). Conditioned reflex treatment of chronic alcoholism: VII. *Diseases of the Nervous System* 3(8):59-62.

Loomis TA (1986). *Emetine Risk Analysis for the Shadel Hospital's Aversion Therapy Program.* Arlington, VA: Drill, Freiss, Hays, Loomis & Shaffer.

Marlatt GA & Gordon JR (1980). Determinants of relapse: Implications for the maintenance of behavior change. In PO Davidson & SM Davidson (eds.) *Behavioral Medicine: Changing Health Lifestyles.* New York, NY: Bruner/Mazel.

Mendes E (1992). Letter to Honorable Jamie L. Whitten, Chairman, Committee on Appropriations, House of Representatives, Washington, DC.

Niaura R, Abrams D, Demuth B et al. (1989). Responses to smoking-related stimuli and early relapse to smoking. *Addictive Behaviors* 14:419-428.

Patton M (1979). *The Outcomes of Treatment: A Study of Patients Admitted to Hazelden in 1976.* Center City, MN: Hazelden Foundation.

Pomerleau OF, Fertig J, Baker L et al. (1983). Reactivity to alcohol cue in alcoholics and non-alcoholics: Implications for a stimulus control analysis of drinking. *Addictive Behaviors* 8:1-10.

Quinn JT & Henbest R (1967). Partial failure of generalization in alcoholics following aversion therapy. *Quarterly Journal of Studies on Alcohol* 28:70-75.

Rawson RA, Obert JL, McCann MJ et al. (1986). In LS Harris (ed.) *Cocaine Treatment Outcome: Cocaine Use Following Inpatient, Outpatient and No Treatment (NIDA Research Monograph 67)*. Rockville, MD: National Institute on Drug Abuse, 271-277.

Ritchie JM (1980). The aliphatic alcohols. In AG Gilman, LS Goodman & A Gilman (eds.) *The Pharmacological Basis of Therapeutics, 6th Edition*. New York, NY: Macmillan.

Sachs DPL (1991). Advances in smoking cessation treatment. *Current Pulmonology* 12:139-198.

Sachs DPL (1986). Cigarette smoking: Health effects and cessation strategies. *Clinics in Geriatric Medicine* 2(2):337-363.

Saxe L, Dovaterty D, Esty K et al. (1983). Research on the effectiveness of alcoholism treatment. *Health Technology Case Study 22: The Effectiveness and Costs of Alcoholism Treatment*. Washington, DC: Office of Technology Assessment, U.S. Congress, 43-53.

Schwartz B (1978). *Psychology of Learning and Behavior, Chapter 4, Pavlovian Conditioning*. New York, NY: W.W. Norton & Co., 55.

Sherman JE, Zinser MC, Sideroff SI et al. (1989). Subjective dimensions of heroin urges: Influence of heroin-related and affectively related stimuli. *Addictive Behaviors* 14:611-623.

Silva P & Rachman S (1987). Human food aversions: Nature and acquisition. *Behavior Research and Therapy* 25(6):457-468.

Smith C, Bookner S & Dreher F (1988). Effects of alcohol intoxication and hangovers on subsequent drinking. *NIDA Research Monograph 90*. Rockville, MD: National Institute on Drug Abuse, 366.

Smith JW (1988). Long-term outcome of clients treated in a commercial stop smoking program. *Journal of Substance Abuse* 5:33-36.

Smith JW (1982). Treatment of alcoholism in aversion conditioning hospitals. In EM Pattison & E Kaufman (eds.) *Encyclopedic Handbook of Alcoholism*. New York, NY: Gardner Press, 874-884.

Smith JW & Frawley PJ (1990). Long-term abstinence from alcohol in patients receiving aversion therapy as part of a multimodal inpatient program. *Journal of Substance Abuse Treatment* 7:77-82.

Smith JW, Frawley PJ & Polissar L (1997). Six- and twelve-month abstinence rates in inpatient alcoholics treated with either faradic aversion or chemical aversion compared with matched inpatients from a treatment registry. *Journal of Addictive Diseases* 16(1):5-24.

Smith JW, Frawley PJ & Polissar L (1991). Six- and twelve-month abstinence rates in inpatient alcoholics treated with aversion therapy compared with matched inpatients from a treatment registry. *Alcoholism: Clinical & Experimental Research* 15(5):862-870.

Vaillant GE (1983). *The Natural History of Alcoholism: Causes, Patterns and Paths to Recovery*. Cambridge, MA: Harvard University Press, 128.

Voegtlin WL & Broz WR (1949). The conditioned reflex treatment of chronic alcoholism. X. An analysis of 3125 admissions over a period of ten and a half years. *Annals of Internal Medicine* 30:580-597.

Voegtlin WL, Lemere F, Broz WR et al. (1941). Conditioned reflex therapy of chronic alcoholism: IV. A preliminary report on the value of reinforcement. *Quarterly Journal of Studies on Alcohol* 2(3):505-511.

Weddington WW, Brown BS, Haertzen CA et al. (1990). Changes in mood, craving, and sleep during short-term abstinence reported by male cocaine addicts. *Archives of General Psychiatry* 47:861-868.

Wilson GT (1987). Chemical aversion conditioning as a treatment for alcoholism: A re-analysis. *Behavior Research and Therapy* 25(6):503-516.

SECTION
8

Twelve Step Programs and Other Recovery-Oriented Interventions

Section Coordinator
Jerome E. Schulz, M.D., FASAM

Contributors

John N. Chappel, M.D., M.P.H., FASAM
Professor Emeritus of Psychiatry
University of Nevada at Reno School of Medicine, and
Medical Director
West Hills Hospital
Reno, Nevada

Barbara S. McCrady, Ph.D.
Center of Alcohol Studies
Rutgers—The State University of New Jersey
Piscataway, New Jersey

Jerome E. Schulz, M.D., FASAM
Clinical Professor
ECU Family Medicine
Eastern Carolina University
Greenville, North Carolina

Deborah Share
Center of Alcohol Studies
Rutgers—The State University of New Jersey
Piscataway, New Jersey

Twelve Step Programs and Other Recovery-Oriented Interventions

Chapter 1

Jerome E. Schulz, M.D., FASAM

Alcoholics Anonymous
Narcotics Anonymous
Cocaine Anonymous
Other Twelve Step Support Groups
The Physician's Role

Today, millions of people worldwide are living fuller and more complete lives because of their involvement in Twelve Step recovery groups. This discussion of recovery groups will emphasize Alcoholics Anonymous (AA) and its basic philosophy. Other programs—including Al-Anon, Alateen, Narcotics Anonymous, Cocaine Anonymous, and Adult Children of Alcoholics—also will be described.

ALCOHOLICS ANONYMOUS

History. AA began in 1935 when a stockbroker (Bill W) met with a physician (Dr. Bob). Bill W was an alcoholic who had a spiritual experience during his fourth detoxification in December 1934, following a visit from a recovering alcoholic friend who was a member of a religious group called the Oxford Movement. A few months later when a business venture failed during a trip to Akron, Ohio, Bill W's thoughts turned to alcohol as a means to ease the pain. He decided to try to talk to another alcoholic who was also a member of the Oxford Movement. He arranged a meeting with Dr. Bob, an actively drinking alcoholic who was unenthusiastic about meeting with Bill. What was to be a brief meeting lasted several hours and marked the beginning of

Alcoholics Anonymous. Over the following months, Bill W and Dr. Bob began to formulate the basic philosophies of Alcoholics Anonymous, which included reaching out to other alcoholics to help themselves stay sober.

The principles that came to guide the organization were published in *Alcoholics Anonymous* (widely known as the "Big Book") (AA, 1976) in 1939. This publication represented the final break from the Oxford Movement and any apparent connection with a particular religious orientation. It established AA for all alcoholics, including atheists and agnostics.

Overview and Philosophy. The preamble of *Alcoholics Anonymous*, which frequently is read at the beginning of AA meetings, points out many important facts about how AA works: "Alcoholics Anonymous is a fellowship of men and women who share their experience, strength and hope with each other that they may solve their common problem and help others to recover from alcoholism. The only requirement for membership is a desire to stop drinking. There are no dues or fees for AA membership; we are self-supporting through our own contributions. AA is not allied with any sect, denomination, politics, organization or institution; does not wish to engage in any controversy; neither

---

TABLE 1.   The Twelve Steps of Alcoholics Anonymous

1. We admitted we were powerless over alcohol; that our lives had become unmanageable;

2. Came to believe that a Power greater than ourselves could restore us to sanity;

3. Made a decision to turn our will and our lives over to the care of God as we understood Him;

4. Made a searching and fearless moral inventory of ourselves;

5. Admitted to God, to ourselves, and to another human being the exact nature of our wrongs;

6. Were entirely ready to have God remove all these defects of character;

7. Humbly asked Him to remove our shortcomings;

8. Made a list of all persons we had harmed, and became willing to make amends to them all;

9. Made direct amends to such people wherever possible, except when to do so would injure them or others;

10. Continued to take personal inventory and when we were wrong promptly admitted it;

11. Sought through prayer and meditation to improve our conscious contact with God as we understood Him, praying only for knowledge of His will for us and the power to carry that out; and

12. Having had a spiritual experience (awakening) as the result of these steps, we tried to carry this message to alcoholics, and to practice these principles in all our affairs.

SOURCE: Reprinted by permission of Alcoholics Anonymous World Service, Inc. Permission to reprint this material does not mean that AA has reviewed or approved the contents of this publication, nor that AA agrees with the views expressed herein.

---

endorses nor opposes any causes. Our primary purpose is to stay sober and help other alcoholics to achieve sobriety."

The Twelve Steps of AA (Table 1) describe both the spiritual basis and the necessary actions, which form the backbone of recovery for AA members. AA is a spiritual, not a religious, program: As the AA preamble states, AA is not allied with any sect or denomination.

The Twelve Steps have been applied effectively to many other problems in life, such as narcotics, cocaine, gambling, sex, emotions, shopping, and eating disorders. They require a willingness to look at oneself and change to become a "healthier" human being who can live harmoniously with others.

The Twelve Traditions (Table 2), which were formulated in 1945, are the guidelines that help Alcoholics Anonymous groups survive and function smoothly. The traditions grew out of conflicts that threatened AA's early existence.

Membership and Structure. More than 100,000 AA groups with more than 2.1 million members exist in 146 countries worldwide (AA, 2001); all are guided by the Twelve Traditions, yet no individual or group is "in charge."

The General Service Office in New York City serves as a clearinghouse for AA information and publications, under the direction of the General Service Board, which is composed of both alcoholics and nonalcoholics. Neither the Office nor the Board has any authority over AA members or groups. Both are responsible to the AA groups and report annually at the General Service Conference attended by members selected by groups in the United States and Canada. This large, loosely structured, leaderless, democratic system works because AA closely follows the Twelve Traditions. AA has a web site for further information.

Each AA group is autonomous (as defined in the fourth tradition). This tradition allows AA groups to vary widely in how they apply the Twelve Steps and Twelve Traditions.

Membership in AA is simple to obtain: All that is required is to attend a meeting and, according to the third tradition, "have a desire to stop drinking." There is no formal application process or paperwork. Groups may have a phone list so individuals can support and help each other between meetings, but participation is strictly optional. Each member is encouraged to develop his or her personal phone list for use in times of need.

TABLE 2.   The Twelve Traditions of Alcoholics Anonymous

1. Our common welfare should come first; personal recovery depends on AA unity.

2. For our group purpose there is but one ultimate authority—a loving God as He may express Himself in our group conscience. Our leaders are but trusted servants; they do not govern.

3. The only requirement for AA membership is a desire to stop drinking.

4. Each group should be autonomous except in matters affecting other groups or AA as a whole.

5. Each group has but one primary purpose—to carry its message to the alcoholic who still suffers.

6. An AA group ought never endorse, finance, or lend the AA name to any related facility or outside enterprise, lest problems of money, property, and prestige divert us from our primary purpose.

7. Every AA group ought to be fully self-supporting, declining outside contributions.

8. Alcoholics Anonymous should remain forever nonprofessional, but our service centers may employ special workers.

9. AA, as such, ought never be organized; but we may create service boards or committees directly responsible to those they serve.

10. Alcoholics Anonymous has no opinion on outside issues; hence the AA name ought never be drawn into public controversy.

11. Our public relations policy is based on attraction rather than promotion; we need always maintain personal anonymity at the level of press, radio, and films.

12. Anonymity is the spiritual foundation of all our traditions, ever reminding us to place principles before personalities.

SOURCE: Reprinted by permission of Alcoholics Anonymous World Service, Inc. Permission to reprint this material does not mean that AA has reviewed or approved the contents of this publication, nor that AA agrees with the views expressed herein.

Meetings. AA holds both open and closed meetings. Anyone may attend an open meeting, whereas closed meetings are restricted to alcoholics and anyone with a desire to stop drinking. AA meetings usually open with the Serenity Prayer (Table 3), after which each participant may introduce himself or herself by saying, "My name is ____, and I'm an alcoholic." There may be several readings, including the Twelve Traditions, "How it Works," the "Promises" (described later), and a daily reflection. At many open meetings, a speaker gives the classic AA talk about "how it was, what happened, and how it is now." Speakers usually talk for an hour or less. They almost never use notes or scripts, because they believe that such spontaneity helps them "talk from the heart and not the head."

In closed meetings, group members may discuss one of the Twelve Steps, a specific topic (such as resentments, fear, or anger) or a reading from *Alcoholics Anonymous* (1976), which serves as the textbook for AA. The Big Book has sold over 20 million copies in over 40 languages. An important part of the Big Book, entitled "How it Works" (Chapter 5), often is read at the beginning of AA meetings. The Twelve

Steps are part of "How it Works" and also are discussed in the AA publication *Twelve Steps and Twelve Traditions* (1951)—the "12 by 12"—which describes the important aspects of each of the steps and traditions.

AA meetings usually last an hour, and most meetings close with the Lord's Prayer or the Serenity Prayer (described later in the chapter). Many newcomers initially are uncomfortable with the apparent Christian orientation expressed by the Lord's Prayer; however, in the context of AA, the prayer is viewed as a commonly remembered ritual that reminds group members of their need for something other than self in maintaining sobriety. In fact, each group can use any ritual it wishes to open or close the meeting.

Meetings often are followed by socializing over coffee to give members a chance to continue to talk about the meeting topic or just to interact without alcohol—a new experience for most alcoholics. It also gives the newcomer a chance to get to know the other group members.

Types of Groups. As AA has grown, many special groups have developed because of the autonomous nature of each AA group. When patients report that they feel uncomfortable at an AA meeting, referral to a special interest group may be helpful. Most large metropolitan areas have special meetings for women, young people, older adults, gays and lesbians, African Americans, and other racial/ethnic groups. Nonsmoking AA meetings are becoming very common. In many areas, there are special meetings for professionals such as nurses, physicians, attorneys, and clergy.

One special group for physicians, psychologists, dentists, veterinarians, educators, and anyone with a doctoral degree is International Doctors in AA (IDAA). IDAA was founded in upstate New York in 1947 by several physicians (three from Canada) and a psychologist. The program is based on the principles of Alcoholics Anonymous. There are more than 6,000 members internationally, many of whom attend the annual IDAA meeting, which is held in different parts of the country (and Canada).

Sponsorship. Sponsorship is a basic AA concept. A sponsor generally is someone of the same sex who has been in AA for at least a year. The sponsor becomes a mentor and role model for the newcomer and is an example of how the AA program works. Newcomers are asked to call their sponsors whenever they are thinking about drinking or are having problems (which is very common for newcomers). It also is common for a newcomer to talk with his or her sponsor on the telephone between meetings and to meet with the sponsor regularly to discuss progress. The sponsor helps and guides the newcomer to work the Twelve Steps.

Newcomers are urged to find a sponsor as soon as possible, and groups often appoint temporary sponsors. AA will provide temporary contacts through the local treatment facilities committee. These temporary contacts can introduce the newcomer to local meetings and members of the fellowship. Sponsorship frequently is a lifelong relationship. After some time in recovery, the AA member may be asked to sponsor a new member. In one 10-year followup, 91% of alcoholics who became sponsors were in stable sobriety (Cross, Morgan et al., 1990).

Anniversaries. Sobriety anniversaries are important milestones in AA. Many groups give a "white chip" (a poker chip) to the newcomer attending his or her first AA meeting or the person who has had a relapse and comes back to AA. The white chip signifies surrender and a willingness to try something new to overcome alcoholism. When the newcomer reaches into his or her pocket for drinking money, the chip is a reminder not to drink. Newcomers are given a new chip (different colors) at 1, 2, 3, 6, 9, and 12 months, signifying their continuing sobriety and commitment to re-

covery. Some groups give out medallions instead of chips. A medallion may have the Serenity Prayer on one side and something about AA on the other side, along with the number of months or years the member has been sober. Anniversaries are special times in AA and may be celebrated with a cake and party.

The "dry date," which is the first drug- or alcohol-free day, is an important date for physicians to acknowledge. This date can be put on the patient's problem list along with the diagnosis of alcoholism. Physicians can show support and interest in their patients' recovery by acknowledging anniversaries.

AA Slogans. Because many alcoholics suffer permanent cognitive deficits due to their chronic alcohol intake, AA has many simple slogans and sayings that are repeated frequently at meetings. When recovering alcoholics are having difficulty, these slogans can redirect their thinking and make them less likely to use alcohol or other mood-altering chemicals to overcome their frustration. The physician's commitment to the patient's recovery is obvious when the physician knows enough about AA to use the slogans.

"One day at a time" is one of the oldest slogans in AA. This slogan emphasizes a basic AA philosophy—that the alcoholic has to be concerned only with today. A lifetime of sobriety can overwhelm many alcoholics. This slogan helps relieve that pressure. Recovering alcoholics may go on a roaring drunk tomorrow, but they need to stay sober just today. Along with drinking problems, alcoholics have all kinds of fears and irrational concerns about what may happen tomorrow, next week, or in the next 100 years. This simple five-word slogan helps them live in the present and take care of just today's problems.

"Easy does it" is another frequently heard slogan. Alcoholics early in recovery tend to want to get everything resolved immediately. They expect years of problems to be resolved the minute they become sober. They frequently want to go on diets, start exercising, quit smoking, and resolve all their personal conflicts. This behavior usually fails and can result in a relapse. "Easy does it" helps recovering alcoholics realize they need to go slowly.

"Let go and let God" emphasizes the spiritual aspect of AA. For alcoholics, attempts to control their drinking can spill over into trying to exert excessive control over other areas of their lives. They overanalyze situations and can develop resentments, which can be fatal errors for the recovering alcoholic. The slogan helps the alcoholic realize that there is a Higher Power ("God, as we understand Him")

TABLE 3.   The Serenity Prayer of Alcoholics Anonymous

"God grant me the serenity to accept the things I cannot change, the courage to change the things that I can, and the wisdom to know the difference."

SOURCE: Reprinted by permission of Alcoholics Anonymous World Service, Inc.

to help them if they can just "let go." The Serenity Prayer (Table 3) has a similar philosophy.

"Keep it simple" is directed toward the alcoholic's knack for complicating things. In AA, members are told not to drink, to go to meetings, to read the Big Book, to work the steps, and to reach out to other suffering alcoholics (doing Twelfth Step work). In other words, they should stay focused and directed on what is important and let go of the rest.

HOW is an acronym frequently heard at AA meetings. It stands for **H**onesty, **O**penness, and **W**illingness. The steps of AA require members to be honest with themselves, with their Higher Power, and with the people around them. For many, this is the first time in their lives (or at least in many years) that they have been truly honest. For most alcoholics, the process of recovery is gradual and does not result in immediate change. Openness helps alcoholics overcome their narrow-minded attitudes. They need to be encouraged to share what they are feeling and to be open to new ideas. They need to be willing to listen, to share feelings, and to try sometimes uncomfortable, new behaviors.

HALT is an acronym that warns alcoholics not to allow themselves to become too **H**ungry, too **A**ngry, too **L**onely, or too **T**ired, because an excess of any of these can lead to relapse.

"First things first" emphasizes what alcoholics always must remember: Staying sober is the most important priority in their lives.

Serenity Prayer. The Serenity Prayer (Table 3) is basic to AA. It offers a simple solution to many frustrations that alcoholics (and, for that matter, everyone) experience in life. Almost all AA meetings either open or close with this prayer. Alcoholics use the Serenity Prayer during the day to help them deal with frustrating and stressful situations.

AA Promises. An essential aspect of AA recovery is the "Promises," which AA says will happen if a person works the AA program to the best of his or her ability. The promises are as follows:

"If we are painstaking about this phase of our development, we will be amazed before we are halfway through. We are going to know a new freedom and a new happiness. We will not regret the past nor wish to shut the door on it. We will comprehend the word 'serenity' and we will know peace.

"No matter how far down the scale we have gone, we will see how our experience can benefit others. That feeling of uselessness and self-pity will disappear.

"We will lose interest in selfish things and gain interest in our fellows. Self-seeking will slip away.

"Our whole attitude and outlook upon life will change. Fear of people and of economic insecurity will leave us. We will intuitively know how to handle situations which used to baffle us. We will suddenly realize that God is doing for us what we could not do for ourselves.

"Are these extravagant promises? We think not! They are being fulfilled among us—sometimes quickly, sometimes slowly. They will always materialize if we work for them" (Alcoholics Anonymous, 1976).

The promises frequently are read at the beginning or end of AA meetings. They help AA members realize that life without alcohol can be rich and rewarding.

Outcomes. In five membership surveys conducted by AA over the 15-year period from 1977 to 1989, analysis "strongly suggests that about half those who come to AA are gone within three months" (Alcoholics Anonymous, 1989). Possible explanations for this dropout rate include resistance to outside coercion to go to meetings, denial of the presence of the disease, and mistaken beliefs about AA. The number of members sober for more than five years increased to 47% in 1998, and the average length of sobriety of members increased to over seven years (Alcoholics Anonymous, 1998). Members attend an average of two meetings a week, and in the under 30 age group, the percentage of women attending meetings has increased to 38%.

Other outcome studies are discussed in Chapter 2.

NARCOTICS ANONYMOUS

History. "We cannot change the nature of the addict or addiction. We can help to change the old lie 'Once an addict, always an addict' by striving to make recovery more available. God help us to remember this difference" (Narcotics Anonymous, 1983)—this is the basic premise of Narcotics

Anonymous (NA). The concepts of NA began at the U.S. Public Health Service Hospital in Lexington, Kentucky, in 1947 (Peyrot, 1985). In 1953, a group of AA members, who also were addicts, started a group in Sun Valley, California, from which NA grew. This group emphasized the need for NA to follow the Twelve Steps and Twelve Traditions of AA. NA was formed because of the discomfort many narcotic and other drug addicts felt when attending AA meetings. At NA meetings, members are able to share problems related to drugs other than alcohol. The Twelve Steps are the same, except for Step 1, which in NA is changed from "alcohol" to "addiction," and the Twelfth Step, which in NA is changed from "alcoholic" to "addict." By refocusing from a specific substance (alcohol) to addiction, NA was able to include all drugs.

NA's philosophy is that drug addiction is a disease that is progressive and lifelong and involves more than the use of drugs. Recovery is based on abstinence from all mood-altering drugs, including alcohol. Through the Twelve Steps, the addict is encouraged to work toward freedom, good will, creative action, and personal growth.

Because the drugs they use are illegal, NA members characteristically are suspicious and manipulative early in recovery. Other group members can help identify these problems in themselves and provide suggestions as to how to overcome them. The goal of recovery is more than abstinence from mood-altering chemicals—it is to live life so that mood-altering chemicals are no longer needed to experience positive feelings. By associating with other people in recovery, the addict is able to see the benefits of being "straight and clean."

Structure and Meetings. The structure of NA is almost identical to that of AA. The basic unit is the "group." A World Service Office is NA's information center. There is a web site. NA meetings are similar to those of AA and generally can be classified as discussion, step, or speaker meetings. Sponsorship is an integral part of the NA program. All newcomers are urged to find a sponsor (Narcotics Anonymous, 1983). AA slogans and sayings also are used in NA, which estimates that there are approximately 27,000 meetings worldwide (in over 70 countries) and "hundreds of thousands" of members.

Literature. NA has its own "Big Book," entitled *Narcotics Anonymous* (1983), which outlines the principles of NA and contains the personal stories of early NA members. *Welcome to Narcotics Anonymous* is an excellent NA pam-

---

TABLE 4. The Al-Anon Preamble

The Al-Anon Family Groups are fellowships of relatives and friends of alcoholics who share their experience, strength, and hope in order to solve their common problems. We believe alcoholism is a family illness and that changed attitudes can aid recovery.

Reprinted from *This is Al-Anon*, by permission of Al-Anon Family Group Headquarters, Inc.

---

phlet that explains the principles of NA to the newcomer. A valuable resource for patients interested in NA, the pamphlet states: "Our message is simple: We have found a way to live without using drugs and we are happy to share it with anyone for whom drugs are a problem."

Staying Clean on the Outside is another resource to give to patients when they leave a treatment program. For people in communities without an NA group, the World Service Office provides an *NA Group Starter Kit* that describes how to start an NA group.

COCAINE ANONYMOUS

Cocaine Anonymous (CA) groups exist in many metropolitan areas of the country. CA was founded in Hollywood, California, in 1982 and has a World Service Office in Los Angeles, which hosts a Web site. CA is based on the Twelve Steps. Its groups are open to anyone who is suffering from addiction to cocaine. The first step of CA is "We admitted we were powerless over cocaine and *all other mind-altering substances*: that our lives had become unmanageable." Most cocaine addicts also attend either Narcotics Anonymous or Alcoholics Anonymous meetings. At NA and AA, they can find people with longer periods of being chemically free. Most cocaine addicts also are addicted to other drugs and alcohol.

OTHER TWELVE STEP SUPPORT GROUPS

Over the past 20 years, more than 100 support groups have started based on the Twelve Steps of AA. Additional information is available at HTTP://WWW.ONLINERECOVERY.ORG.

Family Support Groups. If there are 20 million alcoholics in the United States and the life of each alcoholic affects four other individuals, then approximately 80 million persons are affected by alcoholism in some way. This estimate is very close to the findings of a Gallup poll, which found that 24% of persons interviewed said that their life had been affected by an alcoholic in some way (Robertson, 1988).

As the field of alcohol and drug addiction has become more sophisticated, the concept of addiction being a family disease has emerged. Everyone in the family is affected—not just the identified alcoholic or addict. Based on this understanding, Twelve Step support groups for the family members of alcoholics have grown rapidly. These support groups all emphasize that even if the person who is addicted to drugs or alcohol continues to use, the family members can get help. The emphasis is on helping the family member, not the drug- or alcohol- addicted person.

Al-Anon. The oldest family program is Al-Anon, which was started by Lois Wilson (wife of Bill W). Early in the history of AA, wives frequently would accompany their husbands to AA meetings. While the men were having their meeting, the wives would get together to talk and support each other. Many members of these groups tried to follow the Twelve Steps and to apply them to their own lives. They began to see that they also were affected by alcoholism and that they needed help and support in their recovery. In 1950, Lois Wilson and several other spouses started their own Central Service Center and published the first Al-Anon literature—*Purposes and Suggestions for Al-Anon Family Groups*. Focusing on themselves, not the alcoholic, was the major theme of this work. This simple philosophy was revolutionary in its meaning and application to people who previously had spent most of their energy and time concentrating on the alcoholic.

Philosophy: Like AA, Al-Anon is a spiritual (not religious) program based on Twelve Steps. The steps are similar to AA's, with the exception of Step Twelve, which states: "Having had a spiritual awakening as the result of these steps, we tried to carry this message to others, and to practice these principles in all our affairs." Two main ideas are stressed by Al-Anon (Anthony, 1977): The first is that alcoholism is a disease. This principle is emphasized in the Al-Anon Preamble (Table 4), which is read at the opening of most Al-Anon meetings to help members learn to free themselves of feeling responsible for the alcoholic's disease.

The second major Al-Anon principle emphasizes that the program is for the relative or friend, not the alcoholic. This idea is emphasized in the Al-Anon welcome: "We welcome you to the (name of the group) and hope you will find in this fellowship the help and friendship we have been privileged to enjoy. We who live, or who have lived, with the problem of alcoholism understand as perhaps few others can. We, too, were lonely and frustrated, but in Al-Anon we discover that no situation is truly hopeless and that it is possible for us to find contentment, and even happiness, whether or not the alcoholic continues to drink. We urge you to try our program. It has helped many of us find solutions that lead to serenity. So much depends on our own attitudes, and as we learn to place our problem in its true perspective, we find it loses its power to dominate our thoughts and our lives" (Al-Anon, 1981).

The Al-Anon program teaches people to look at what they can do to feel better about themselves and to caringly "let go" of the alcoholics. This concept is called "tough love," which means stopping "enabling behaviors" and making the alcoholic responsible for the consequences of his or her drinking and alcoholism. Al-Anon describes this idea in a pamphlet called *Detachment* (1979). Members are encouraged to "let go of our obsession with another's behavior and begin to lead happier and more manageable lives." Al-Anon helps members learn:

- Not to suffer because of the action or reactions of other people.

- Not to allow ourselves to be used or abused in the interest of another's recovery.

- Not to do for others what they should do for themselves.

- Not to manipulate situations so others will eat, go to bed, get up, pay bills, etc.

- Not to cover up another's mistakes or misdeeds.

- Not to create a crisis.

- Not to prevent a crisis if it is in the natural course of events.

Newcomers often come into Al-Anon with resentments and anger that they have not previously acknowledged. Al-Anon helps them view the alcoholic as someone with a disease instead of someone who is "trying to get them." Step One points out that they are powerless over alcohol and that they have no control over the alcoholic. Steps Two and Three help the person reach outside herself or himself for help from a "Higher Power." "Letting go" of control and trusting a Higher Power are basic concepts of Al-Anon.

Membership and Meetings: The third tradition of Al-Anon states: "The only requirement for membership is that there be a problem of alcoholism in a relative or friend."

There are more than 27,000 Al-Anon groups worldwide. Al-Anon meetings usually start with the Serenity Prayer, the preamble, and the welcome and are followed by introductions. There are speaker, discussion, and step meetings. The meetings emphasize sharing, support, and encouragement to work on oneself.

Meetings usually last an hour and have a standard closing: "The opinions expressed here were strictly those of the persons who gave them. Take what you like and leave the rest. A few special words to those of you who haven't been with us long: Whatever your problems, there are those among us who have had them too. If you try to keep an open mind, you will find help. You will come to realize that there is no situation too difficult to be bettered and no unhappiness too great to be lessened. We aren't perfect. The welcome we give you may not show the warmth we have in our hearts for you. After a while, you'll discover that though you may not like all of us, you'll love us in a very special way—the same way we already love you" (Al-Anon, 1981).

The leader then emphasizes that everything said in the meeting is considered confidential. Frequently there is a social time after the meeting for further support and sharing.

Literature: In 1966 Al-Anon published *Al-Anon Family Groups* (1966), which is equivalent to the Big Book in AA. This book sets down the basic principles of Al-Anon and tells the stories of the founders. Al-Anon's *Twelve Steps and Twelve Traditions* (1981) discusses the steps and traditions from an Al-Anon perspective. *One Day at a Time in Al-Anon* (1973) is a daily meditation guide that many members read for inspiration and guidance. Al-Anon also publishes over 50 pamphlets on special topics such as men in Al-Anon, denial, alcoholism as a family disease, and adult children of alcoholics. (Pamphlets are available from Al-Anon Family Group Headquarters, Inc., P.O. Box 862, Midtown Station, New York, NY 10018-0862, or from a local Al-Anon office.)

Alateen. Alateen is a separate program of Al-Anon Family Groups. Started by a California teenager in 1957, Alateen is specifically for teenagers and follows the Al-Anon steps and traditions. Every Alateen group has an active Al-Anon member who serves as a sponsor for the group. The sponsor provides guidance and stability to the group and helps the group stay focused on the Twelve Steps and Twelve Traditions. A key to being a good sponsor is to guide without dominating. The group can hold a group inventory and decide to get a new sponsor if the relationship is unsatisfactory. Alateen meetings frequently are held at the same place as Al-Anon meetings, but in different rooms. Many schools host Alateen meetings. A referral to Alateen can be made through the local Al-Anon office.

Alateen has its own literature especially directed to teenagers. In *Hope for Children of Alcoholics—Alateen* (1973), there is a chapter devoted to explaining alcoholism in terms teenagers can understand. Alcoholics are described as anyone and not necessarily "skid row bums." The sources of the alcoholic's obsession, addiction, and compulsion are defined. The family disease concept is discussed, with an emphasis on denial, anger, and anxiety, as well as adolescents' feelings about being "caught in the middle." The alcoholic is described as sick and unable to control his or her alcohol intake or reactions. The slogans are explained, and one chapter contains personal stories to help teenagers feel that they are not alone. At the end of the book, there is a detailed discussion of how to start an Alateen group. A special page labeled "Remember" encourages group members to focus on the common problem of alcoholism and not to gossip, waste time, be impatient, or talk about what happens in the group outside of the group. As the members become older, they are encouraged to join Al-Anon to continue their recovery.

Adult Children of Alcoholics. Adult Children of Alcoholics (ACOA) is a relatively new movement, which has developed rapidly over the past 30 years. In the 1970s, researchers began trying to identify common characteristics of adults raised in alcoholic homes. In the late 1970s, a small group of previous Alateen members started an Alanon meeting called "Hope for Adult Children of Alcoholics". Several books were published on the topic (Black, 1982; Wegscheider, 1981; Woititz, 1981) and served as the impetus for other support groups for adult children of alcoholics (by some estimates, as many as 30 to 40 million people). Because the movement grew rapidly, it did not have the advantage of time to develop and mature, as did AA and Al-Anon, and many different groups developed. Al-Anon started having special meetings for adult children of alcoholics. Groups such as the National Association for Children of Alcoholics started. There was a lack of clarity about what the groups should and should not do. Many groups had no one who had any extended time in recovery to help provide guidance and direction. Some groups emphasized therapy over support, with heavy confrontation instead of relying on the Twelve Steps and Twelve Traditions. Although these problems still exist in some groups, most ACOA groups have matured and now offer excellent support for adult

---

TABLE 5.   Communicating With Addicted Patients About Recovery

1. If you think your patient is an alcoholic, tell him (her).

2. Tell him he is suffering from an illness, not a moral weakness.

3. Tell him alcoholism is progressive and can only get worse if he continues to drink.

4. Tell him his illness is treatable.

5. Try to get him to admit his troubles are caused by drinking not the other way around.

6. Tell him where help is available—clinics, detox units, therapy groups, etc.

7. Tell him about AA.

8. Go to an AA meeting yourself to see how it works.

9. Get a local AA meeting list.

10. Get to know some AA members for referral purposes.

---

children of alcoholics. The national center is Adult Children of Alcoholics World Service Organization (ACA WSO, P.O. Box 3216, Torrance, CA 90510). The center also hosts a Web site.

The "Problem" is read at the opening of meetings:

> Many of us found that we had several characteristics in common as a result of being brought up in alcoholic or other dysfunctional households. We had come to feel isolated and uneasy with other people, especially authority figures. To protect ourselves, we became people pleasers, even though we lost our own identities in the process. All the same we would mistake any personal criticism as a threat. We either became alcoholics ourselves, married them, or both. Failing that, we found other compulsive personalities, such as workaholic, to fulfill our sick need for abandonment. We lived life from the standpoint of victims. Having an overdeveloped sense of responsibility, we preferred to be concerned with others rather than ourselves. We got guilt feelings when we trusted ourselves, giving in to others. We became reactors rather than actors, letting others take the initiative. We were dependent personalities, terrified of abandonment, willing to do almost anything to hold on to a relationship in order not to be abandoned emotionally. We kept choosing insecure relationships because they matched our childhood relationship with alcoholic or dysfunctional parents. These symptoms of the family disease of alcoholism or other dysfunction

made us 'co-victims'—those who take on the characteristics of the disease without necessarily ever taking a drink. We learned to keep our feelings down as children and keep them buried as adults. As a result of this conditioning, we often confused love with pity, tending to love those we could rescue. Even more self-defeating, we became addicted to excitement in all our affairs, preferring constant upset to workable solutions. This is a description, not an indictment.

If physicians are aware of these common characteristics, they can identify patients who are adult children of alcoholics. Until they are identified, these individuals can be overusers of the medical system and frustrating for physicians to treat. By referring patients to ACOA, physicians can be instrumental in helping them start a program of recovery.

Meetings: Most ACOA meetings last 90 minutes. They usually start with the Serenity Prayer and a welcome. The Twelve Steps, the problem, and the solution (which describes what ACOA recommends for recovery) often are read. At some meetings, the characteristics are read. A member may talk about a step or characteristic and how it affects his or her life. Then each member of the group has the opportunity to share his or her feelings about the topic or talk about any other concerns he or she may have. The meeting usually closes with a prayer. Members are invited to socialize after meetings.

Newcomers are encouraged to attend six meetings to help them become comfortable with the group and develop

---

the trust that is essential to recovery. Sponsors are an important part of ACOA, and newcomers are encouraged to get a sponsor. Most groups have phone lists and encourage members to call each other for support. As with AA and Al-Anon, an important part of recovery in ACOA is reaching out to others. ACOA members are willing to take people to meetings and can be a helpful resource for physicians.

THE PHYSICIAN'S ROLE

To be able to help alcoholics and drug addicts, physicians need to be familiar with recovery support groups, especially the Twelve Step programs. The physician can work as a facilitator to help patients attend meetings. Project MATCH (1997) showed that trained professionals who support meeting attendance in a positive noncoercive way could improve their patient's acceptance of Twelve Step programs. There are several advantages to referring patients to Twelve Step programs:

- Meetings are free of cost. (AA's Preamble states "There are no dues or fees for AA membership.")

- Meetings are accessible even in the smallest of towns.

- No records are kept of attendance, and anonymity is assured.

- Participants do not have to be sober to attend a meeting. (The only requirement for membership is a desire to stop drinking.)

- Persons from all racial and ethnic backgrounds and socioeconomic groups are welcome. Being unemployed, African American, and unmarried does *not* predict an unfavorable outcome with Twelve Step meeting attendance (Miller, 1995).

- The newcomer develops a feeling of "self-value" as he or she becomes part of the group.

Twelve Step groups work supportively with other therapies. They provide the newcomer with many other new positive experiences (Bassin, 1975; Canavan, 1983).

- Attending group meetings helps overcome the patient's feelings of "terminal uniqueness" and isolation.

- Groups educate patients about the disease process of addiction and hold out the hope of recovery.

- Group members offer newcomers unconditional support as they struggle with early recovery, which the group characterizes as a positive, joyful experience.

- Groups help members learn basic social skills. Members become less self-obsessed and more aware of the feelings of others.

- Groups provide a "reality base" for addicts in recovery, overcoming the isolation and thinking disorders that prevent addicts from comprehending the potential consequences of their behavior and illuminating errors and dangers in the member's thinking.

- Groups help members with the inevitable setbacks experienced in recovery.

- Groups help members constructively use the time formerly occupied by alcohol and drug use.

Making Referrals to Twelve Step Programs. In the 1996 triennial AA member survey, only 8% of newcomers reported coming to meetings through a physician's referral. This finding is unfortunate because AA and other self-help programs can be a valuable resource for physicians in helping their addicted patients.

There are several ways to refer patients. AA has a listed phone number in most cities and will provide volunteers to contact the patient and explain AA. After obtaining the patient's permission, the physician should initiate contact with the self-help group in the patient's presence. Giving the patient the telephone number with a recommendation to call usually is not successful. Sisson and Mallams (1981) randomly assigned newly diagnosed alcoholics to two types of referral. The first group was told to call AA and go to a meeting. The second group was put in direct contact with an AA member while in the physician's office. None of the first group attended a meeting; the entire second group did. Most addiction treatment programs incorporate a strong self-help component and will encourage patients to attend Twelve Step meetings as a regular part of their aftercare program.

Alcoholics Anonymous: The physician may find it helpful to keep a list of AA members willing to do "Twelfth Step" work. Some physicians accompany patients to AA meetings (nonalcoholic physicians may be allowed to attend closed meetings if they are with patients, or physicians may select an open AA meeting). Although such attendance is time-consuming for the physician, it demonstrates to the patient the physician's sincere belief in the importance of AA to recovery. Physicians can obtain a current list of nearby AA meetings from the local AA office (frequently listed in directories as "Intergroup" or "Central Office"). Such lists usually include a brief description of the type of meeting, whether it is a special interest group, and if it is nonsmoking. A summary, published by AA, of how physicians can help alcoholic patients is included as Table 5.

Narcotics Anonymous: Referrals to NA are similar to those for AA. NA often has a listed phone number; many treatment programs also have lists of NA meetings. If neither of these resources is available, the Narcotics Anonymous World Service Office in Van Nuys, California can provide help and a wealth of information about NA.

Al-Anon: In most cities, Al-Anon has a listed phone number. If not, the AA office often will provide the location and times of Al-Anon meetings. Al-Anon has a Family Group Headquarters and a Web site. The more physicians know about Al-Anon, the more effectively they can make referrals. An excellent way to learn is to talk with Al-Anon members about their experiences with the program and to attend a meeting. It is also helpful for the physician to have a list of Al-Anon members who are willing to take new members to Al-Anon meetings and to encourage patients to attend at least six meetings.

Adult Children of Alcoholics: Because there is considerable variation in ACOA groups, physicians must be familiar with the group to which they refer patients. Good groups usually have members who have been involved in other Twelve Step programs and who provide stability and experience. A group can offer support and caring when the pain of being an adult child of an alcoholic begins to surface. The group should not allow "cross talk" (confrontation or interruptions), so that the meeting feels "safe" to the new member. The purpose of ACOA groups is "to shelter and support newcomers in confronting denial; to comfort those mourning their early loss of security, trust and love; and to teach the skills for reparenting themselves with gentleness, humor, love, and respect" (Jacobson, 1987).

Because alcoholism is an inherited disease, ACOA patients should be screened carefully and referred if there is any suggestion of an addictive disorder. Although ACOA patients may appear to be emotionally stable, they often are fragile under their carefully constructed external shell. They need to be treated with care, understanding, and gentleness by the physician.

Making the Referral Work. A knowledgeable, empathetic physician can "prepare" the patient to help overcome the initial fear and apprehension about attending a Twelve Step meeting. The physician should acknowledge the patient's ambivalence (which is not denial) about stopping drinking (Miller & Rollnick, 1991). The following suggestions will help the referral work:

1. Know the meetings in your area and refer each patient to a meeting that will meet his or her needs. Meetings have different "personalities" (Tonigan, Ashcroft et al., 1995). If they are unhappy with a meeting, help them find another.

2. Help patients make direct contact with members of the group.

3. Give patients a "prescription" to attend a meeting.

4. Tell them what is going to happen at the meeting and how meetings are structured.

5. Encourage them to socialize by arriving early and staying late after the meeting

6. Encourage patients to pick a *temporary* sponsor early to increase their chances of staying clean and sober. Tell them to pick someone of the same sex with at least one year of sobriety. Tell them it is okay to change sponsors if necessary.

7. Talk about their fears and apprehensions about attending a meeting and dispel any inaccurate myths or beliefs they may have about Twelve Step support groups.

8. Encourage them to attend frequent meetings but initially do not push or coerce them.

9. Schedule them for a followup visit to discuss their experience at meetings. If they have been attending regularly, encourage them to pick a "home" group and become more active. Being actively involved in the program is a better predictor of a successful outcome than the number of meetings attended (Montgomery, Miller et al., 1995).

Potential Problems With Referrals. Patient objections to AA and other mutual help groups typically are expressed in the following ways (Anonymous, 1982):

"I don't believe in God." AA is a spiritual program that is not allied with any particular religion and does not require the members to believe in anything except a Higher Power ("God, as we understand Him"). There are many atheists and agnostics in AA. *Alcoholics Anonymous* (the Big Book) contains an entire chapter for agnostics (Chapter 4), which the physician may recommend to patients who offer this objection.

"I don't like to talk in a group." There is no requirement to talk at an AA meeting. Members can say they "pass" if they do not wish to talk in front of the group.

"I can't stand all the smoke." Nonsmoking group meetings are available in most geographic areas. In others, large groups divide into smoking and nonsmoking sections.

"I don't have a way to get there." Transportation usually can be arranged for an interested newcomer by calling AA.

"I don't want anyone to know about my drinking." Anonymity is a basic concept of AA. Things said in a meeting stay there; no AA member has the right to break the anonymity of another member.

"I can't stay sober." The third tradition of AA clearly states, "The only requirement for AA membership is a desire to stop drinking." Many oldtimers spent a long time attending meetings before they were able to stay sober, and they understand the plight of the newcomer.

Group Problems: The patient may have difficulty identifying with the members of his or her self-help group. If the patient has attended a meeting several times and still has this feeling, he or she should be referred to a different group. In large metropolitan areas, there are many varieties of self-help groups (involving, for example, young people, senior citizens, gays/lesbians, nonsmokers, women, African Americans, and Hispanic Americans).

Twelve Step "Docs": Although AA as an organization encourages members to cooperate with their physicians, individual AA members may give patients inappropriate advice about stopping essential drugs, such as antidepressants, antipsychotics, naltrexone, disulfiram, or other medications. If patients are using these medications, physicians should caution them about this possibility. Frequently, communication between the physician and the patient's sponsor can overcome this problem. It may be wise to tell patients not to discuss their medication at meetings (Chappel & DuPont, 1999).

Gender Orientation: Women sometimes have a problem with AA because of the masculine perspective of most AA literature. However, AA groups now are very receptive to women, who do well in the program. There also are AA meetings exclusively for women.

Limitations of Twelve Step Groups. Physicians need to understand the limitations of AA and other Twelve Step approaches (Anonymous, 1972):

- AA does not solicit members; it will only reach out to those who ask for help.

- AA does not keep records of membership (although some AA groups will provide phone lists for group members).

- AA does not engage in research.

- There is no formal control or followup on members by AA.

- AA does not make any medical or psychiatric diagnoses. Each member needs to decide if he or she is an addict.

- AA as a whole does not provide housing, food, clothing, jobs, or money to newcomers (although individual members may do so).

- AA is self-supporting through its own members' contributions; it does not accept money from any outside sources.

Support in Recovery. The patient who participates in a mutual help group may show certain warning signs of an impending relapse. Early in sobriety, patients often experience excessive euphoria, which can lead to overconfidence and relapse.

The first sign of a potential relapse may be a patient's unwillingness to discuss the recovery program with his or her physician, a behavior that may indicate the patient has decreased the frequency of or stopped attending meetings. This behavior can lead to the "dry drunk syndrome," which is characterized by irritability and unwillingness to share feelings. The patient loses his or her reality base and reverts to distorted thinking. New resentments and a multitude of other negative feelings can lead to drinking to relieve the pain. At this point, patients may request mood-altering chemicals to relieve anxiety. Such a request is a "red flag" that a relapse may be imminent.

To assess a patient's recovery status, the physician can ask a few simple questions (Chappel, 1992).

- "What are you working on in your recovery program and with your sponsor?"

- "What step are you working on?"

- "What meetings are you attending?"

- "How are you using your phone list?"

Patients in a good recovery program will be very open to answering and discussing any of these questions. The questions stimulate patients' thinking about what working a program of recovery really means. Using the information elicited, physicians often can make suggestions about their patients' recovery and decrease the likelihood of a relapse.

Physicians also can show an interest in their patients' recovery by acknowledging anniversaries, using the slogans, and caringly asking at each visit about how a patient is doing in his or her recovery. Alcoholism and drug addiction should be included on patient problem lists to help prevent inadvertent prescribing of medications that may endanger recovery.

Physicians also can counsel patients during high-risk times, such as periods of extreme stress. Encouraging patients to attend more meetings and contact their sponsor during such periods can prevent relapse. Patients frequently complain to their physicians about AA. By listening attentively to patients' concerns and then encouraging them to continue attending meetings, physicians can allow patients to vent their frustration while maintaining attendance at meetings.

CONCLUSIONS

Twelve Step programs have over 66 years' experience in helping alcoholics, addicts, and family members recover from addiction and its consequences. Almost all patients afflicted with addictive disease will have a more rewarding recovery if they actively participate in a Twelve Step program. Physicians can play an important role by helping their patients understand these programs and encouraging them to participate in meetings.

Physicians need to know how to use Twelve Step and other support groups effectively to help alcoholics, addicts, and family members recover from the disease of drug and alcohol addiction.

REFERENCES

Alcoholics Anonymous (1982). *AA as a Resource for the Medical Profession.* New York, NY: Alcoholics Anonymous World Service, Inc.

Alcoholics Anonymous (1966). *Al-Anon Family Groups.* New York, NY: Al-Anon Family Group Headquarters, Inc.

Alcoholics Anonymous (1981). *Al-Anon's Twelve Steps & Twelve Traditions.* New York, NY: Al-Anon Family Group Headquarters, Inc.

Alcoholics Anonymous (1973). *Alateen—Hope for Children of Alcoholics.* New York, NY: Al-Anon Family Group Headquarters, Inc.

Alcoholics Anonymous (1976). *Alcoholics Anonymous.* New York, NY: Alcoholics Anonymous World Service, Inc.

Alcoholics Anonymous (1984). *Another Look.* Van Nuys, CA: Narcotics Anonymous World Service Office, Inc.

Alcoholics Anonymous (1972). *A Brief Guide to Alcoholics Anonymous.* New York, NY: Alcoholics Anonymous World Service, Inc.

Alcoholics Anonymous (1989). *Comments on AA's Triennial Surveys, 1989.* New York, NY: Alcoholics Anonymous World Service.

Alcoholics Anonymous (1979). *Detachment.* New York, NY: Al-Anon Family Group Headquarters, Inc.

Alcoholics Anonymous (1998). *Fact Sheet,* AA Website.

Alcoholics Anonymous (n.d.). *Grapevine.* New York, NY: Alcoholics World Service, Inc.

Alcoholics Anonymous (1983). *Narcotics Anonymous.* Van Nuys, CA: World Service Office, Inc.

Alcoholics Anonymous (1973). *One Day at a Time in Al-Anon.* New York, NY: Al-Anon Family Group Headquarters, Inc.

Alcoholics Anonymous (1983). *Sponsorship.* Van Nuys, CA: Narcotics Anonymous World Service Office, Inc.

Alcoholics Anonymous (1975). Ten tips from Alcoholics Anonymous for family doctors. *Medical Times* 103(6):74-76.

Alcoholics Anonymous (1983). *The Triangle of Self-Obsession.* Van Nuys, CA: World Service Office, Inc.

Alcoholics Anonymous (1952). *Twelve Steps and Twelve Traditions.* New York, NY: Alcoholics Anonymous World Service, Inc.

Anthony M (1977). Al-Anon. *Journal of the American Medical Association* 238(10):1062-1063.

Bassin A (1975). Psychology in action. *American Psychologist* 30(6): 695-696.

Black C (1982). *It Will Never Happen to Me!* Denver, CO: M.A.C. Printing and Publishing Division.

Canavan D (1983). Impaired physicians program-support groups. *Journal of the Medical Society of New Jersey* 80(11):953-954.

Chappel JN (1992). Effective use of AA and NA in treating patients. *Psychiatric Annals* 22:409-418.

Chappel JN & Dupont RL (1999). Twelve-step and mutual-help programs for addictive disorders. *Psychiatric Clinics of North America* 22(2): 425-445.

Cross GM, Morgan CW, Mooney AJ et al. (1990). Alcoholism treatment: A ten year follow up study. *Alcoholism: Clinical & Experimental Research* 14(2):169-173.

Jacobson S (1987). The 12-step program and group therapy for adult children of alcoholics. *Journal of Psychoactive Drugs* 19(3):253-255.

Miller NS & Verinis JS (1995). Treatment outcome for impoverished alcoholics in abstinence-based program. *International Journal of the Addictions* 30(6):753-763.

Miller WR & Rollnick (1991). *Motivational Interviewing: Preparing People to Change Addictive Behavior.* New York, NY: The Guilford Press.

Montgomery HA, Miller WR & Tonigan JS (1995). Does Alcoholics Anonymous involvement predict treatment outcome? *Journal of Substance Abuse Treatment* 12(4):241-246.

Peyrot M (1985). Narcotics Anonymous: Its history, structure and approach. *International Journal of the Addictions* 20(10):1509-1522.

Project MATCH Research Group (1997). Matching alcoholism treatment to client heterogeneity: Project MATCH post treatment drinking outcomes. *Journal of Studies on Alcohol* 58:7-28.

Robertson N (1988). *Getting Better Inside Alcoholics Anonymous.* New York, NY: Ballantine Books.

Sheeren M (1988). The relationship between relapse and involvement in Alcoholics Anonymous. *Journal of Studies on Alcohol* 49: 104-106.

Sisson RW & Mallams JH (1981). The use of systematic encouragement and community access procedures to increase attendance at Alcoholics Anonymous and Al-Anon meetings. *American Journal of Drug and Alcohol Abuse* 8(3):371-376.

Tonigan S, Ashcroft F & Miller W (1995). AA group dynamics and 12-step activity. *Journal of Studies on Alcohol* 56:616-621.

Vaillant GE (1983). *The Natural History of Alcoholism: Causes, Patterns, and Paths to Recovery.* Cambridge, MA: Harvard University Press.

Wegscheider S (1981). *Another Chance.* Palo Alto, CA: Science and Behavior Books.

Woititz J (1981). *Adult Children of Alcoholics.* Pompano Beach, FL: Health Communications, Inc.

| Chapter 2 | # Recent Research Into Twelve Step Programs |

Barbara S. McCrady, Ph.D.
Deborah Share

Utilization of AA
AA and Population Subgroups
The Effectiveness of AA
and Treatments Based on AA
Mechanisms of Change in AA
and Twelve Step Oriented Treatment
Future Directions

Alcoholics Anonymous (AA) is ubiquitous, both in the United States and around the world, with a growth rate of 11.5% internationally and 7.2% domestically in the decade from 1981 to 1990 (Mäkelä, Arminen, et al., 1993). The formal structure of AA is similar across nations, although there is some variability in emphasis on different parts of the AA program and differences in the demography of membership is apparent, depending on the cultural context in which AA occurs (Mäkelä et al., 1996).

Although most addiction professionals have some familiarity with AA and other self-help groups based on Twelve Step principles, those professionals' scientific knowledge about AA often is more limited. The past decade has witnessed an explosion of research on AA and on treatments designed to facilitate involvement in AA. Despite earlier skepticism about the possibility of conducting research on AA, researchers have used a range of methodologies, including ethnographic methods, epidemiologic studies, longitudinal studies of treatment-seeking and nontreatment-seeking populations, controlled clinical trials, and meta-analyses to develop a body of new research about AA that has some coherence, confirms some previous findings

and beliefs, and challenges others. McCrady and Miller (1993) reviewed AA research up to the early 1990s, and McCrady (1996) reviewed additional literature published through 1996.

This chapter provides a selective review of earlier research on AA and a more comprehensive review from 1995 through 2000. It addresses several major topics, including patterns of utilization of AA, the unique experiences and views of AA among specific population groups, the effectiveness of AA and treatments designed to facilitate AA involvement, and processes of change associated with involvement with AA and other Twelve Step programs. The chapter concludes with methodological comments and directions for future research. Research on other Twelve Step programs for substance use disorders is very limited, but will be included where relevant data exist.

UTILIZATION OF AA

AA members enter the program by a number of routes, including self-referral or referral by family or friends, referral from treatment centers, or through coercion from the legal system, employers, or the social welfare system.

Population Studies. Population surveys provide information on utilization of AA in the general and alcohol-problemed populations. Hasin and Grant (1995) examined data from the National Health Interview Survey of 43,809 adults in the United States. Among the survey population, 5.8% had attended AA at some point in their lives. Room and Greenfield's (1993) household survey of 2,058 adults revealed similar results: 10% of men and 8% of women had attended AA at some point. Room and Greenfield further distinguished between AA attendance for personal problems with drinking and AA attendance for other reasons, and found that 3.1% of respondents had attended AA for their own drinking problems. Weisner and colleagues (1995) reported that AA attendance among respondents with a history of alcohol dependence or social consequences from their drinking was even higher (22% and 15%, respectively). Their data also suggested that, over the period 1979 to 1990, the probability of attending AA increased among young men (from 1.4% in 1979 to 5.8% in 1990) and among those with more evidence of alcohol dependence (from 11% to 22%) and more social consequences of drinking (from 4% to 15%). Such increases may be due to increased treatment resources and more mandatory referrals to treatment.

Help-Seeking Populations. A different perspective on the utilization of AA is provided by studies of patterns of help-seeking among individuals seeking assistance for an alcohol problem. Narrow and colleagues (1993), using data from the Epidemiologic Catchment Area Survey, reported that among individuals with substance abuse disorders who sought help, 36% used AA and other voluntary support services, compared to 83% who used professional services. Timko and colleagues (1993) examined treatment utilization among individuals who first contacted an information and referral center, or who underwent alcohol detoxification. One year later, 75% had sought treatment: 18% had attended only AA or another self-help group (24% of help-seekers), 25% had sought only outpatient treatment (33% of help-seekers), and 32% had sought only inpatient/residential treatment (43% of help-seekers). AA involvement was high among treatment seekers, with 66% of outpatients and 68% of inpatients also attending AA.

By the time of an eight-year followup (Timko, Moos et al., 2000), 17% still had sought no treatment, and 14% had attended only AA. The majority (53%) participated in both formal treatment and AA. Study subjects who attended AA (either AA alone or in conjunction with treatment) showed a pattern of steady and consistent involvement over time: 71 to 108 meetings in the first year, 230 to 260 meetings in the subsequent two years, and 362 to 434 meetings in years 4 to 8.

Mandated Populations. Although there has been considerable controversy about the current criminal justice practice of mandating individuals to attend AA, little research has examined the actual process of criminal justice referral to AA. Speiglman (1994) selected four counties in California that varied in the degree to which they used presentencing screening strategies to deal with repeat offenders through the use of driving under the influence (DUI) statutes. Two of the four counties referred cases to AA, referring 37% to 40% of cases. Interestingly, offenders who were represented by private attorneys were more likely to be referred to AA than those who had public representation. However, among offenders also mandated to parole or to participation in probation-defined treatment, the vast majority (88% to 97%) were required to attend AA. Frequency of attendance also was specified and typically involved two to three required meetings per week.

Patterns of Utilization of AA. Both cross-sectional and longitudinal studies provide information about patterns of utilization of AA. Data from the Epidemiologic Catchment Area Study (Narrow, Regier et al., 1993) suggest that individuals who attend AA or other self-help groups make about twice as many visits to meetings as to professional treatment. Alcoholics who attend AA averaged 44.8 visits/person/year, or just under one meeting per week. Data from Timko and colleagues (1993) also suggest fairly substantial utilization rates among AA attenders, with subjects who attended AA—with or without outpatient treatment—remaining involved, on average, for about six months, with an average rate of attendance of two meetings per week. Subjects who received inpatient treatment were involved longer, but at the same frequency of attendance.

Several innovative methodologies have been used to study patterns of affiliation over time. McCrady and colleagues (1996) examined weekly records of AA attendance among outpatients and reported three distinct patterns of affiliation: (1) positive affiliation, characterized by either immediate, regular attendance, or gradually increasing attendance over the course of treatment, (2) negative affiliation, characterized by initially higher rates of attendance, which decreased over the course of treatment, and (3) nonaffiliation, characterized by little or no involvement. Morgenstern and colleagues (1996) identified three distinct patterns of posttreatment involvement with AA that were similar to McCrady and colleagues' within-treatment findings. Optimal responders attended meetings daily and often sought advice from AA members, partial responders attended meetings frequently but rarely sought advice from AA members, and nonresponders did not engage with AA. Caldwell and Cutter (1998) also examined characteristics of involvement among three groups of alcoholics 10 weeks after treatment. Those with low levels of attendance (less than 20 meetings) were least likely to see themselves as alcoholics, less likely to accept the concept of a Higher Power, and least likely to join an AA group. High AA attenders (at least 70 meetings in 10 weeks) saw their drinking problems as the most serious, accepted the concepts of powerlessness and a Higher Power, took advantage of the informal support and sharing associated with AA, and had worked the first five steps in AA. Humphreys and colleagues (1995), in studying patterns of change over time, noted that subjects who were able to attain stable abstinence over a three-year period initially were actively involved with AA, attending approximately two meetings per week for the first year. However, AA involvement decreased over the following two years so that, although remaining abstinent, subjects attended AA rarely, averaging about one meeting per month.

Mäkelä (1994) studied anniversary announcements published in a Finnish AA newsletter to track AA membership over time. Over three consecutive years, he found that the probability of remaining sober and involved with AA was about 67% for those with one year of sobriety, 85% for those with two to five years of sobriety, and 90% for those with more than five years of sobriety.

Finally, Smith (1993) conducted semistructured interviews with members of AA who had at least two years' sobriety to characterize patterns of social affiliation with AA. She described three patterns of affiliation: those who were affiliative from the beginning of involvement, those who were socially distant at first but later became more involved, and those who remained distant from interactions with other group members despite continued attendance at AA meetings. Those who affiliated gradually seem to have followed a common pattern: first forming a connection with one person in AA; then focusing on specific content of stories told at meetings and through the literature, working the steps with encouragement from the sponsor without much group affiliation; and, finally, performing some service work within the organization despite personal discomfort.

Factors Associated With Successful Affiliation With AA. Despite the diversity of the membership of AA, research shows that certain factors are associated with more successful affiliation with AA. Research to identify characteristics of those more likely to affiliate with AA is directed toward identifying factors that are most associated with successful affiliation and does not imply that individuals without those characteristics will not affiliate. A number of individual studies have reported characteristics predictive of affiliation with AA, including male gender (Room & Greenfield, 1993), more serious alcohol problems (Caetano, 1993; Hasin & Grant, 1995; Morgenstern, Labouvie et al., 1997; Timko, Finney et al., 1993), greater commitment to abstinence (Morgenstern, Labouvie et al.,1997), more social support to stop drinking (Hasin, Labouvie et al., 1995), less support from and more stress in marriage/intimate relationships (Humphreys, Finney et al., 1994), fewer psychological problems such as depression or poor self-esteem (Timko, Finney et al., 1993), use of a more avoidant style for coping with problems (Humphreys, Finney et al., 1994), and having a greater desire to find meaning in life (Project MATCH Research Group, 1997a). Most findings, however, are supported by only one recent study. Findings are contradictory for some variables, such as education, where affiliation is predicted by greater education among whites but less education among Hispanic Americans; or marital status, where unmarried status predicts affiliation among Hispanics (Caetano, 1993), but being married generally is predictive of affiliation in population surveys.

The more controversial personal characteristic of spirituality or religiosity has inspired some recent research. Professionals and the public alike believe that individuals who are more religious will be more successful in AA because of the intrinsically spiritual nature of the recovery program. A recent survey found that program directors in Department of Veterans Affairs (VA) facilities were less likely to refer a patient to AA if the individual was an atheist (Humphreys, 1997). Research by Winzelberg and Humphreys (1999) looked at the relationships among clinician referral to Twelve Step groups, client religiosity, group attendance, and client outcomes. They too found that professionals were less likely to refer patients to Twelve Step groups if the patients engaged in fewer religious behaviors. However, though more frequent religious behaviors predicted Twelve Step meeting attendance, clinician referral to such groups increased attendance regardless of religiosity. Finally, attendance at Twelve Step groups predicted better outcomes, again irrespective of religiousness. The authors concluded that success in Twelve Step groups is not predicated on religious behaviors and that clinicians ought to make equal efforts to advise Twelve Step group attendance to both religious and less religious patients. Similar research on NA found that spiritual beliefs could predict NA attendance. However, because only 6% of the variance in attendance was accounted for, the authors similarly concluded that religiosity should not be considered a crucial variable in client referral (Christo & Franey, 1995).

Psychiatric comorbidity is another patient characteristic whose relationship with AA participation is unclear. Higher levels of psychiatric severity in these individuals point to questions of the applicability as well as the benefit of Twelve Step participation for this group. Tomasson and Vaglum (1998) determined that the presence or absence of most comorbid disorders was unrelated to AA attendance in an aftercare sample of alcoholics, although the presence of comorbid disorders was associated with higher rates of professional help-seeking. Schizophrenia, however, was the one diagnosis associated with lower rates of attendance. In a study of substance abuse patients, Ouimette and colleagues (1999) found that during treatment, individuals with substance abuse only and those with both substance abuse and personality disorders attended Twelve Step meetings more frequently than did substance abusers with psychotic, anxiety, or depression diagnoses. However, in the continuing care phase, there were no significant differences among the groups in frequency of Twelve Step meeting attendance.

Another factor associated with AA attendance and success for individuals is the orientation of their treatment program. A large sample of inpatients in VA treatment programs of differing orientations (cognitive-behavioral, Twelve Step, or eclectic) was assessed for individuals' participation and involvement in Twelve Step groups, as well as for treatment outcome (Humphreys, Huebsch et al., 1999a). Humphreys and his colleagues found that not only were patients in the Twelve Step and eclectic programs more frequent participants in Twelve Step groups, but also that the positive relationship between self-help group involvement and positive substance use outcome was even stronger for those coming from Twelve Step- or eclectically oriented programs. The authors concluded that program orientation is thus a crucial moderating factor in enhancing self-help group attendance as well as received benefit.

AA AND POPULATION SUBGROUPS

Two contrasting views of AA lead to different predictions about AA and different population subgroups. One perspective suggests that AA is a program of recovery for alcoholics and that the common experience of alcoholism should supercede superficial individual differences. Because AA groups are autonomous, individual meetings may take on the character of the predominant population in attendance, allowing for meetings that are comfortable for persons of different backgrounds. In the United States, "special interest" groups for certain subpopulations (such as women, gays and lesbians, young people, and certain racial/ethnic groups) are very common (Mäkelä, Arminen et al., 1996).

An alternative perspective is that, because AA was developed by educated, middle-aged, white, Christian, heterosexual males, its relevance to less educated, young, or older persons, persons of color, non-Christians, gays and lesbians, or women is suspect. AA's own triennial surveys have found an increase in the proportion of women in AA, as well as a decrease in the age of AA members (cited in Mäkelä, Arminen et al., 1996), and observation of AA meetings clearly reveals broad diversity among the membership. Research data about the relevance of AA to various subgroups are limited though increasing.

Women. Four articles published in the past decade specifically have examined women and AA. Smith (1992) recruited a convenience sample of women attending AA and compared them with women in outpatient alcoholism treatment. The women in AA tended to be older, were more likely to be employed, and showed some evidence of having more severe drinking problems than the women in the comparison groups. Kaskutas (1994) studied women attending Women for Sobriety (WFS) meetings, approximately 25% of whom also attended AA. The women attended AA for reasons somewhat different than for attending WFS: AA was cited as the program most crucial to their staying sober, although the fellowship, support, sharing, and spirituality in AA all were cited as important as well. The women perceived WFS as most valuable for the nurturing atmosphere, involvement with an all-women's program, and exposure to positive female role models. The women in the sample also reported reasons they did not attend AA, including a feeling that they did not fit in, a perception that AA is too punitive and focused on shame and guilt, and disagreement with program principles related to powerlessness, surrender, and reliance on a Higher Power, and a perception that AA is male-dominated.

Beckman (1993), in a review of the literature on AA, Twelve Step-oriented treatment, and women, concluded that women were underrepresented in studies of AA, but that AA involvement seemed to be associated with more positive drinking outcomes.

Humphreys and colleagues (1994) compared substance abusers who were actively involved in either AA or NA following a treatment episode with those who did not attend self-help groups. They found that women and men were equally likely to be involved in a Twelve Step program. However, in comparing individuals who were actively involved in AA with those who had been active but then dropped out, the authors found that a greater proportion of women than men dropped out of their self-help groups.

Cultural, Racial, and Ethnic Subgroups. Research on involvement in AA by cultural, racial, and ethnic subgroups is limited. A recent study by Kaskutas and colleagues (1999) examined previous self-help group participation among African American and white treatment seekers. African Americans more frequently reported prior NA or Cocaine Anonymous exposure, with a trend toward more previous AA exposure. Of those who had been exposed to AA in the past, 76% of African Americans versus 55% of whites said they had gone to AA as a part of prior treatment, whereas more whites had gone to AA through other referrals or on their own. Active participation was equivalent for both groups, as measured by mean AA affiliation scale scores. However, analysis of the individual items from the affiliation scale revealed differential manners of participation. African Americans were more likely than whites to identify themselves as AA members (64% vs. 54%), to say they had a spiritual awakening through AA (38% vs. 27%), and to have done service at an AA meeting recently (48% vs. 37%). African Americans were less likely than whites to have a sponsor currently (14% vs. 23%) and less likely to have read AA literature recently (67% vs. 77%). These patterns held true after controlling for prior treatment and exposure to AA during treatment.

A study comparing Hispanics and non-Hispanic whites examined treatment utilization and outcome differences in a treatment-seeking sample (Arroyo, Westerberg et al., 1998). They found that, at six-month followup, Hispanics engaged in more formal treatment sessions but fewer AA meetings than the non-Hispanic whites. However, alcohol-related outcomes were similar at followup for both groups,

implying that ultimate outcomes are similar for Hispanics and non-Hispanic whites, despite the finding that they engage in different treatment paths. One possible explanation for the finding that Hispanics participated less in AA is that the Hispanics were more likely to be living with others at intake and thus may have been better able to turn to those persons for social support rather than a support group like AA. Another possible explanation is that Hispanics may not have viewed self-help groups as being as effective as formal approaches.

Tonigan and colleagues (1998) reported that in the outpatient arm of Project MATCH, similar proportions of whites, Hispanics, and African Americans attended AA at any followup period considered. However, the results from the aftercare arm of the study showed different results: While Hispanics and African Americans did not differ from Caucasians in AA attendance at the beginning of the followup period, the two groups differed significantly from whites in AA attendance later in the followup period. Tonigan and colleagues (1998) also reported on a subsample from Project MATCH participants from Albuquerque, NM. There they found that although Hispanics attended fewer AA meetings, they reported being more committed to AA than whites (as evidenced by working the steps, having or being a sponsor, and celebrating AA birthdays). AA predicted better drinking outcomes in both Hispanics and whites.

Humphreys and colleagues (1994) reported that among substance abusers who were followed up one year after treatment intake, there were no significant racial differences between those individuals who were actively involved in a Twelve Step program and those who were not. When dropouts from Twelve Step groups were compared with those who remained involved, no significant differences were attributable to race/ethnicity. They also found that African Americans who were involved in self-help groups improved more in the areas of drug, alcohol, and medical problems than did African Americans who were not participating. Thus the authors concluded that members of racial/ethnic groups, such as African Americans, attend and drop out of self-help groups at the same rates as whites; self-help group participation also was found to improve outcomes for African Americans.

Earlier data reported by Caetano (1993) from a national survey showed that, in general, Hispanics, African Americans, and whites tended to endorse equally the basic tenets of the disease model. All groups held fairly positive views of AA (meaning that they would be more likely to recommend it than any other treatment modality). Some variability was noted in support for AA, with 97% of Hispanics, 94% of whites, 87% of African Americans, and 76% of Asian Americans recommending AA as a resource. Caetano also reported that Hispanics in the sample were more likely to have had contact with AA (12%) than either whites or African Americans (5%).

Age-Specific Groups. Several studies have suggested a strong association between AA/NA involvement and abstinence in adolescents, similar to that found in adults (these studies are reviewed in the section on the effectiveness of AA). However, only one recent study has focused on the experience of an age-specific group in AA. Hohman and LeCroy (1996) examined a sample of adolescents who had completed inpatient treatment. About 44% of the study subjects had participated in AA. Adolescents who had attended AA were more likely to have experienced prior treatment, experienced more feelings of hopelessness, had family who had participated less in their treatment program, and currently were more likely to have friends who did not use alcohol or drugs. However, only 23% of the variance in affiliation with AA was explained by these four variables.

Dually Diagnosed Individuals. Research on substance abusers with comorbid psychiatric disorders has, until recently, been focused primarily on a comparison of the substance use, psychiatric, and other life outcomes of those with multiple diagnoses compared to those with substance use disorders alone. Recent research also supports understanding of those dually diagnosed individuals in AA. Pristach and Smith (1999) looked at attitudes and participation in AA in a sample of 60 psychiatric inpatients who had comorbid alcohol use disorders. The sample was divided by type of disorder, including affective disorders, personality or adjustment disorders, psychotic disorders, and other substance use disorders. Overall, 37% of the sample reported at least weekly attendance at AA. Pro-AA sentiments were common among those involved, and such attitudes were associated with regular past AA attendance. Those who had attended AA previously reported being more likely to attend AA after treatment than those who had never attended AA; they also reported feeling comfortable with AA. In contrast to Tomasson and Vaglum's (1998) finding that alcohol abusers with comorbid schizophrenia were less likely to attend AA, Pristach and Smith found no difference in past AA attendance for schizophrenic individuals compared with other dually diagnosed patients.

An important implication of the presence of comorbid disorders is the need for prescription medications. The subject of medication use by AA members is a particularly important one, given that medications play a larger role in mental health treatment today and that AA is commonly viewed as antimedication. In an anonymous survey, Rychtarik and colleagues (2000) assessed AA members' attitudes toward the use of medication, either to prevent relapse or to treat other disorders. (Medications included antidepressants, pain medications, anxiolytics, lithium, antipsychotics, naltrexone, and disulfiram.) Regarding medication to prevent relapse, 53% of the sample thought that use of medications was either a good idea or might be a good idea, 17% reported that they did not like the idea of medication and believed the individual should not take it, and 12% said they would recommend that another member discontinue medication use. About 29% said they had been encouraged to stop taking any type of medication, and an additional 20% had heard of others who had been encouraged to discontinue use. Of those who were encouraged to stop medication use, 31% actually stopped.

Gays and Lesbians. Research on the experience of gays and lesbians in relation to AA is limited. One ethnographic study (Hall, 1994) recruited lesbians who had been in recovery for at least one year. All respondents were familiar with AA; 74% were actively involved. Hall identified three sources of tension for the lesbians in AA. First, they reported a tension between a sense of assimilation and a sense of differentiation. The women said they felt that AA was a program in which people of very different backgrounds could relate because of their common concerns, but at times they viewed AA as a white, male, heterosexist organization. Second, they said they understood the value of the authority of AA as a prescription for sobriety, but at times viewed AA more as a program that provided a set of tools for recovery. The perceived sexist language in the AA literature and the lack of focus on lesbian issues made following the program prescriptively a difficult task. Finally, the women said they experienced tension between the strongly individual focus of AA and their perception of the importance of examining issues in a cultural context.

THE EFFECTIVENESS OF AA AND TREATMENTS BASED ON AA

Answering the apparently simple question, "Does AA work?" is a challenge. One approach is to look at the success of AA as an organization—the broad dissemination of the program around the world and the large membership suggest that AA has been enormously successful in attracting persons to AA as a program of recovery. The AA triennial surveys also point to the substantial proportion of abstaining, long-term members, as do Mäkelä's (1994) studies of stability of sobriety in AA. More difficult questions, however, have less clear-cut answers: "Is AA *the most effective* approach to alcohol dependence?" and "Is AA involvement *necessary* to successful resolution of alcohol problems?" Research to answer these questions has used several methodologies: (1) randomized clinical trials comparing AA to different forms of alcoholism treatment, (2) studies examining the unique contribution of AA to the prediction of success, (3) randomized clinical trials of treatments designed to involve individuals in the program and beliefs of AA, and (4) single group evaluation studies of treatments designed to involve individuals in the program and beliefs of AA. Review of these four lines of evidence provides some provocative answers to questions about the relative effectiveness of AA.

Therapeutic Effectiveness of AA. Randomized clinical trials (RCTs), in which persons are randomly assigned to different treatment conditions, are considered the most rigorous experimental tests of therapeutic effectiveness. Only three RCTs that compared AA to different forms of treatment have been reported in the research literature, and no RCT has been reported since 1991 (Walsh, Hingson et al., 1991). Each of the three RCTs has serious methodological problems, and all used populations mandated to treatment, so it is difficult to draw specific conclusions about the effectiveness of AA from these studies.

However, many studies have examined the contribution of AA attendance and involvement to the prediction of successful resolution of a drinking problem. One of the most consistent and robust findings is that there is a positive correlation between AA attendance and drinking outcomes. Studies of treatment populations in the early 1990s (Hoffmann & Miller, 1992; Johnson & Herringer, 1993), found that patients who attended AA were significantly more likely to be abstinent 1 year after treatment than those who did not attend AA. More recent research has supported these earlier findings. For example, an evaluation of VA patients diagnosed with alcohol dependence (Fortney, Booth et al., 1998) found that patients who were attending AA three months after treatment were 3.7 times more likely to be abstinent as patients who were not involved with AA. Stud-

ies of nontreatment populations (Schuckit, Tipp et al., 1997) found that AA involvement was one of a handful of significant predictors of long-term (greater than five years) abstinence. Long-term, eight-year followups of individuals who had either presented to an information and referral center or received detoxification (Timko, Moos et al., 2000, 1999), found that AA attendance was significantly, though weakly, correlated with less alcohol consumption, less intoxication, more abstinence, and fewer symptoms of alcohol dependence or alcohol-related problems. They also found that persons who had been involved with AA were more likely to have positive long-term outcomes than those who had received no treatment. Compared to those who received treatment without AA, those who attended AA alone were more likely to be abstinent up to three years after initial contact, but outcomes were equivalent at the eight-year followup. Outcomes were comparable for persons who attended treatment alone or who combined treatment with AA.

Controlled Trials of Treatments Based on Twelve Step Principles. AA and Twelve Step-oriented treatments have close conceptual links in their adherence to the classic disease concept of alcoholism, emphasis on abstinence, the importance of AA involvement, and working the Twelve Steps. Differences between AA and other Twelve Step treatment programs are substantial, however, and the two should not be equated. Unfortunately, the empirical literature often ignores this distinction and reports results of Twelve Step-oriented treatments as though they are studies of AA. Several important randomized clinical trials, nonrandomized clinical trials, and single group evaluation studies of treatments based on Twelve Step principles have been reported over the past several years.

The most prominent and visible randomized clinical trial, Project MATCH (Project MATCH Research Group, 1997a, 1997b, 1998a, 1998b), was designed to study the interactions between specific patient characteristics and one of three structured 12-week outpatient individual treatments: Twelve Step Facilitation (TSF), Motivational Enhancement Therapy (MET), or Cognitive-Behavior Therapy (CBT). Participants were 1,726 persons diagnosed with alcohol abuse or dependence (952 outpatients and 774 aftercare patients) who were recruited from among 4,481 patients screened at nine participating clinical research units. Participants were assessed thoroughly, then randomly assigned to one of the three treatments. Clinicians were nested within treatments, received extensive training prior to the study, and were carefully supervised throughout. Treatment was delivered over a three-month period. Individuals assigned to TSF or CBT could receive up to 12 manual-guided treatment sessions, while MET participants received up to four treatment sessions over the same 12-week period. All participants were followed for 15 months from baseline, with research contacts scheduled every three months. Participants in the outpatient arm of the study were contacted again 39 months after the initial baseline evaluation, and their functioning over the preceding three months was assessed.

Although Project MATCH was not designed specifically to study the main effects of the three study treatments, some treatment main effects did emerge. During treatment (Project MATCH Research Group, 1998a), patients in the outpatient arm of the study were more likely to maintain abstinence or moderate drinking if they received CBT or TSF rather than MET (41% vs. 28%). One year after treatment, patients in the three treatments had comparable outcomes in the percentage of days that they were abstinent, as well as the mean number of drinks consumed per day (Project MATCH Research Group, 1997a). Two variables favored the TSF treatment: Patients who had participated in TSF treatment were more likely to have maintained continuous abstinence and were less likely to have relapsed to heavy drinking after treatment. At the three-year followup of the outpatient arm of the study, few significant differences among the three treatment conditions were noted, but, as at the one-year followup, patients who had received the TSF treatment were more likely to have been abstinent during the three months prior to the three-year followup. Also, compared to patients who had participated in CBT, TSF subjects had a significantly greater percentage of abstinent days during the preceding three months (Project MATCH Research Group, 1998b).

Several significant client-treatment matching effects were found. During treatment, no client-treatment matches affected drinking (Project MATCH Research Group, 1998a). However, during the first year after treatment, patients who had low levels of psychiatric symptoms had more days of abstinence if they had received the TSF rather than the CBT treatment (Project MATCH Research Group, 1997a). Aftercare patients with higher levels of alcohol dependence also had better outcomes with TSF. In contrast, those patients who were low in alcohol dependence had better outcomes with CBT (Project MATCH Research Group, 1997b). One other matching hypothesis that did not involve the TSF treatment was significant: outpatients high in anger had better drinking outcomes with MET than with CBT (Project MATCH Research Group, 1997b). The positive match between angry clients and MET was maintained at the three-year followup (Project MATCH Research Group, 1998b).

A second important matching finding emerged at three years: Outpatients whose social networks were highly supportive of their drinking had better outcomes if they received TSF rather than MET treatment (Longabaugh, Wirtz et al., 1998).

Although the positive findings from Project MATCH are significant, most of the matching hypotheses tested were *not* supported, including primary and secondary matching hypotheses related to gender, sociopathy and Antisocial Personality Disorder, other DSM diagnoses, alcoholic subtypes, cognitive impairment or conceptual level, motivation and readiness to change, self-efficacy, assertion of autonomy, meaning seeking, and other aspects of social functioning.

Naturalistic Studies of Treatments Based on Twelve Step Principles. In contrast to randomized clinical trials, which typically include strict experimental controls to maximize internal validity, naturalistic study designs evaluate existing treatment programs and patient populations. Experimental controls are lacking, but the inclusion of a broader sample and the evaluation of extant treatments without attempting to influence the treatment itself provide information complementary to that obtained from RCTs.

In the largest comparative study of Twelve Step-based treatments, Moos and colleagues (1999) studied 3,698 male veterans being treated at 1 of 15 VA treatment units. The treatment units were classified as Twelve Step-oriented, Cognitive-Behavioral Therapy oriented, or Eclectic. No patients were excluded from the study, and 97% of the patients were followed successfully one year after treatment. Overall, patients improved significantly in drinking, symptoms of alcohol dependence, psychological problems, and social functioning. Patients who participated in Twelve Step-oriented treatment were about 1.5 times as likely to be abstinent as patients whose treatment was cognitive-behavioral in orientation (Ouimette, Finney et al., 1997). Patients from both types of programs, however, were more likely to be employed than patients whose treatment was more eclectic in focus.

Patient-treatment matching also was examined in the VA study (Ouimette, Finney et al., 1999), but there was no evidence that specific patient characteristics predicted differential response to either Twelve Step-oriented or Cognitive-Behavioral Therapy.

Single group evaluations of treatments based on Twelve Step principles typically have studied inpatient treatment programs. Most studies have focused on private treatment centers, whose populations typically are more socially stable than patients in public treatment programs. The largest study of this type (Hoffmann & Miller, 1992) reported that 67% to 75% of participants reported abstinence six months after treatment, and 60% to 68% abstinent rates at a 12-month followup. However, study attrition was substantial, and the investigators estimated that abstinence rates would have been 56% to 65% at six months, and 34% to 42% at 12 months, if patients lost to followup were considered to have relapsed.

An evaluation of 1,083 patients treated at the Hazelden treatment program (Stinchfield & Owen, 1998) reported, with better than 70% followup rates, that six months after discharge, 59% of patients said they had not used alcohol or drugs since discharge; at the 12-month followup, 53% said they had not used alcohol or drugs since discharge. If patients lost to followup are included as treatment failures, adjusted rates of continuous abstinence were 45% at six months and 37% at 12 months—results very comparable to those reported by Hoffmann and Miller (1992).

MECHANISMS OF CHANGE IN AA AND TWELVE STEP-ORIENTED TREATMENT

AA Involvement Among AA Members. No recent research has examined processes of involvement with AA outside of treatment. However, several studies from the early 1990s provide important information about the process of affiliation with AA. Brown and Peterson (1991) surveyed AA members' views of the relative importance of aspects of the AA program. Working the steps, having a sponsor, telling their story at a meeting, and daily meditations were seen as most important. In a second sample, members of AA, as well as other Twelve Step groups, were surveyed. Respondents believed in a Higher Power, that they would recover with the help of their Higher Power, and that they were powerless over alcohol or another problem for which they sought help. Additionally, respondents reported a number of behavioral changes that facilitated recovery, including attending group meetings, avoiding people, places, and things associated with their problem, making amends, working the Fourth and Fifth Steps, praying, telling their story at a meeting, and maintaining a regular pattern of sleep.

Snow and colleagues (1994) used a broader theoretical model to describe the types of cognitive and behavioral processes used by AA members to facilitate change. Half of their sample were current members of AA; another 35% had attended at some point. Current members of AA were more likely to use helping relationships, stimulus control ("people, places, and things"), and behavioral management strategies to maintain sobriety. Those who attended more frequently used more behavioral processes of change. Snow and colleagues also examined the processes of change used by those with the strongest affiliation to AA. They found that those with the greatest affiliation reported greater importance for helping relationships, stimulus control, behavior management, and consciousness-raising processes (Snow, Prochaska et al., 1994).

Morgenstern and colleagues (1996) reported that the processes used in AA depended on the degree of involvement with AA. Those subjects who attended daily meetings and turned to other AA members for advice also were more likely to have a sponsor, to work the steps, to be involved with AA service, to read AA literature, and to pray.

AA Involvement Among Patients in Twelve Step Programs. An alternative approach to studying affiliation with AA is to study the process of acceptance of Twelve Step beliefs during treatment. McCrady and colleagues (1996), reporting on an outpatient sample, found that among outpatients in treatment designed to facilitate AA involvement, 50% had a sponsor by the end of treatment, 57% reported working the initial steps in AA, and 36% reported being involved with AA activities and socializing with other AA members. Morgenstern and colleagues (1996) found that, during Twelve Step-oriented residential or outpatient treatment, participants became more accepting of several beliefs, including their own powerlessness over alcohol and the existence of a Higher Power.

Mediators of the Influence of AA on Outcomes. Research has gone beyond merely examining correlations between AA involvement and drinking outcomes to considering what aspects of AA involvement relate to drinking outcomes. Montgomery and colleagues (1995) distinguish AA *attendance* from AA *involvement*, which includes, in addition to attendance, the degree of involvement with various aspects of AA—such as participation during meetings, having a sponsor, leading meetings, working specific steps, or doing Twelfth Step work (Tonigan, Toscova et al., 1996). Montgomery and colleagues (1995) reported that AA involvement and attendance were moderately correlated (.45); however, involvement, not attendance, correlated with posttreatment alcohol consumption (r = –.44) in a sample of patients in an inpatient Twelve Step treatment program.

Using Project MATCH data, Tonigan and colleagues (2000) examined the nature of participants' experience with AA. As in other research, there was a positive correlation between AA-related actions and the degree to which patients were abstinent. Tonigan and colleagues anticipated that there would be two aspects of experience with AA—a subjective dimension and a behavioral dimension. Statistically, however, experiences with AA seemed to reflect one major dimension rather than two. Greater participation was reflected in a combination of factors: a spiritual awakening, God-consciousness, the perception that attending AA meetings was helpful, actually attending AA meetings, being involved with other AA-related practices, and completing more steps. They also found that participation in AA during treatment and in the first six months after treatment predicted better drinking outcomes in the second six months after treatment (Tonigan, Miller et al., 2000).

Three studies have examined mediators of the relationship between specific aspects of AA involvement and outcome. Christo and Franey (1995) found that, although neither spiritual beliefs nor believing in addiction as a disease predicted drug use outcomes, both predicted NA attendance, which was related to reduced drug use. Morgenstern and colleagues (1997) examined a complex set of mediational pathways to abstinence after Twelve Step-oriented treatment. They found that several variables predicted affiliation with AA after treatment, including perceived past and future harm from alcohol use, anticipated benefits from abstinence, degree of commitment to abstinence, and drinking problem severity (Morgenstern, Labouvie et al., 1997). In turn, affiliation with AA one month after treatment predicted that subjects would use behavioral coping strategies to stay abstinent and would have a greater commitment to abstinence six months after treatment. AA affiliation one month after treatment also was a strong predictor of drinking status at six months' posttreatment. Additional analyses suggested that AA led to a positive drinking outcome in part because it enhanced individuals' general use of strategies for dealing with alcohol.

Another study using Project MATCH data (Longabaugh, Wirtz et al., 1998) tested the pathway by which patients with extensive social supports for drinking did better if they receive TSF. The investigators found that patients who received TSF were more likely to become involved with AA than other patients and that this involvement with AA, in turn, predicted better drinking outcomes.

Social Support. Given the nature of self-help groups, it is easy to understand why consideration of social factors, such as social context, social network, and social support, is important when studying Twelve Step groups and their relation to substance use disorders. Surprisingly, few studies have looked directly at the complex relationships that exist in groups like AA and the social aspects of substance abusers' lives.

As described in the section on effectiveness, involvement with Twelve Step groups is related to improved substance use outcomes. Thus one way to look at the substance abuser in a social context is to look at what role social support plays in this established pathway from self-help group involvement to positive outcomes. Humphreys and colleagues (1999b) examined whether a social variable mediates this pathway. They assessed a group of male veterans with substance use disorders for participation in NA, CA, and AA, general friendship quality and friends' support for abstinence at followup, and substance use outcomes. Once the established relationship between Twelve Step participation and outcome was found, statistical analyses were used to find that both friendship variables partially mediated the relationship between Twelve Step participation and outcome. In other words, the investigators concluded that part of the reason that self-help groups are so effective is that they improve the quality of friendships and how much friends support abstinence. These improvements in friendship quality then predicted better drinking outcomes (Humphreys, Mankowski et al., 1999b).

Involvement in self-help groups may influence the nature of a substance abuser's social network. Humphreys and Noke (1997) followed male inpatient substance abusers after treatment and examined AA, NA, or CA participation and social network outcomes. They found that increased group participation predicted both better quality of general friendship and less support of substance use by friends at followup. Individuals involved significantly in Twelve Step groups (involved in at least two of three Twelve Step activities measured) actually increased the size of their friendship networks by an average of 16%; those *not* significantly involved in Twelve Step groups showed no change in the size of their friendship networks. The greater increase in social network size was attributable to the fact that those significantly more involved in Twelve Step groups increased their numbers of friends in Twelve Step programs, not because those less involved with Twelve Step groups lost friends. Finally, Humphreys and Noke (1997) found that those who had networks composed almost entirely of Twelve Step members experienced better friendship quality than did others who held social networks composed of almost no Twelve Step members.

Social variables also may function as moderators of the relationship between Twelve Step participation and outcome. Although the Project MATCH studies are reviewed elsewhere in this chapter, one study by Longabaugh, Wirtz et al. (1998) is of particular interest here. In examining the effects of matching patient characteristics with specific treatment modalities, Longabaugh and colleagues found that TSF treatment, which aimed to involve patients in AA, was more effective than MET for individuals who had social networks that were supportive of drinking. Those with low support for drinking had similar outcomes, regardless of treatment type. The investigators also found that AA participation mediated the interaction between treatment type and network support for drinking. In other words, TSF treatment emphasized AA involvement and thus helped to create improved social networks, which in turn predicted better drinking outcomes. This was especially true for those individuals who had networks that supported their drinking behavior.

FUTURE DIRECTIONS

Research on AA has become increasingly sophisticated over the past decade, and a body of accrued knowledge provides a richer and more articulated research-based picture of AA than was available previously. However, important gaps in the research remain.

Self-Selection Bias. Research on self-help groups is confounded by the existence of self-selection bias (Fortney, Booth et al., 1998) created by differences among treatment groups that have not been accounted for by researchers. Self-selection bias may affect factors that predict outcomes, but are not a component of the treatment under examination. These variables may be included inadvertently when treatment effects are calculated, when they should be controlled instead. Given that many studies of self-help groups tend to be observational or naturalistic, attempts to minimize self-selection bias should be considered in designing studies, and problems with self-selection bias should be considered when interpreting research results. Fortney, Booth et al. (1998) proposed a special statistical technique that could be used to control for such outcome bias.

Population Subgroups. The population of the United States is racially and ethnically diverse. That racial and ethnic diversity is not well represented in AA, but the membership of AA is diverse in age, socioeconomic status, and gender. The research literature, however, provides little information about the experience, utilization, and barriers to use of AA for different groups. Data are particularly scant for young people, older adults, gays and lesbians, and persons mandated to attend AA.

Data from AA's triennial surveys and studies of persons in Twelve Step-oriented treatment indicate that the majority of individuals who try AA do not continue or affiliate. Research to understand the lack of affiliation is needed. It is possible that some reasons for non-affiliation with AA are amenable to therapeutic intervention. Although Twelve Step-oriented treatment programs are designed to facilitate involvement, little is known about the active elements in these programs that stimulate involvement, and no research has focused specifically on this aspect of AA.

Other Twelve Step Programs. One of the most notable gaps in the research literature is the paucity of research on other Twelve Step recovery programs, such as Cocaine Anonymous or Narcotics Anonymous. There is virtually no systematic research on these organizations or the persons who affiliate with them. Given the prevalence of other drug dependence, a concerted effort to develop research on the other Twelve Step groups is needed.

Process Research. Although impressive and thoughtful research has been conducted in an effort to understand the linkages between personal and social network characteristics, dimensions of AA involvement over time, and outcome, there continue to be notable gaps in the process research literature. The nature of an individual's involvement with AA evolves over time, but research has yet to capture any aspect of that evolution. A current initiative of the National Institute on Alcohol Abuse and Alcoholism (NIAAA) to fund research into spirituality may provide some initial perspectives on the evolution of spirituality with recovery. AA involvement is rich and multitextured, and development of models to study multidimensional involvement over time is a challenge for future researchers.

CONCLUSIONS

This chapter has reviewed a substantial body of research on AA and other Twelve Step groups. AA is used widely in the United States: 6% to 10% of the population has attended an AA meeting, with that rate doubling or tripling among those with drinking problems. Use is growing most quickly among young men, who also are the most likely to be mandated to treatment. Increasingly, the legal system is referring individuals to AA. When individuals seek help voluntarily, a substantial proportion use AA, either as their sole source of assistance or in conjunction with formal treatment. Typically, individuals become actively involved in AA for several months, attending meetings about twice a week. There is, however, considerable variability in patterns of affiliation, with some individuals becoming increasingly committed over time, while others gradually slip away from the program. Longer-term involvement is less common, but those who stay with AA for more than a year are very likely to continue their involvement for many years.

AA is such a heterogeneous organization that it is difficult to draw generalizations about who is most or least likely to affiliate. There is little evidence of problems with affiliation among specific subpopulations, but concerns about aspects of the AA program have been documented, particularly among women. It may be that the presence of special interest groups within AA and modifications of the program at the local level can effectively address these concerns. Overall, data suggest that individuals who have more severe problems, more concern about their drinking, a greater commitment to staying abstinent, less support from a spouse, a social network supportive of drinking, a history of turning to others for support, and a greater desire to find meaning in their lives may be most likely to affiliate with AA.

Substantial research on the process of change and outcomes associated with AA involvement has been reported over the past five years. AA involvement clearly is correlated with positive outcomes in terms of reduced drinking, improved psychological functioning, and better social support. Research suggests that members actively use the core of the AA program: they attend meetings, work the steps, get a sponsor, and tell their story at meetings. Overall, the more active they are with AA, the better are their outcomes. The positive effect of AA seems at least partially attributable to the clear cognitive and behavioral changes that members make, as well as to improved social supports.

Other research has focused on treatment programs based in AA philosophy and procedures. Studies of formal treatments that draw from the core beliefs of AA have yielded mixed results, but evidence generally suggests that these programs yield outcomes comparable to or better than programs based in other treatment philosophies.

Finally, there is increased methodological sophistication and creativity in research on AA. Concepts of AA involvement capture more fully the core of the AA program, while several new measures that have good psychometric properties have been developed. A more varied population of problem drinkers is being examined, including subpopulations that differ in age, race/ethnicity, and the presence of comorbid psychiatric disorders. Diverse and complementary methodologies have contributed to a richer, data-based understanding of AA, which should continue to expand over the next decade.

ACKNOWLEDGMENT: Preparation of this chapter was supported in part by NIAAA grants R01 AA07070 and T32 AA 07569.

REFERENCES

Arroyo JA, Westerberg VS & Tonigan JS (1998). Comparison of treatment utilization and outcome for Hispanics and non-Hispanic whites. *Journal of Studies on Alcohol* 59:286-291.

Beckman LJ (1993). Alcoholics Anonymous and gender issues. In BS McCrady & WR Miller (eds.) *Research on Alcoholics Anonymous: Opportunities and Alternatives*. New Brunswick, NJ: Rutgers Center of Alcohol Studies, 233-248.

Brown HP & Peterson JH (1991). Assessing spirituality in addiction treatment. Development of the Brown-Peterson Recovery Progress Inventory (BPRPI). *Alcoholism Treatment Quarterly* 8:41-50.

Caetano R (1993). Ethnic minority groups and Alcoholics Anonymous: A review. In BS McCrady & WR Miller (eds.) *Research on Alcoholics Anonymous: Opportunities and Alternatives*. New Brunswick, NJ: Rutgers Center of Alcohol Studies, 209-232.

Caldwell PE & Cutter HSG (1998). Alcoholics Anonymous affiliation during early recovery. *Journal of Substance Abuse Treatment* 15:221-228.

Christo G & Franey C (1995). Drug users' spiritual beliefs, locus of control and the disease concept in relation to Narcotics Anonymous attendance and six-month outcomes. *Drug and Alcohol Dependence* 38:51-56.

Fortney J, Booth B, Zhang M et al. (1998). Controlling for selection bias in the evaluation of Alcoholics Anonymous as aftercare treatment. *Journal of Studies on Alcohol* 59:690-697.

Hall JM (1994). The experiences of lesbians in Alcoholics Anonymous. *Western Journal of Nursing Research* 16:556-576.

Hasin DS & Grant BF (1995). AA and other help seeking for alcohol problems: Former drinkers in the U.S. general population. *Journal of Substance Abuse* 7:281-292.

Hoffmann NG & Miller NS (1992). Treatment outcomes for abstinence-based programs. *Psychiatric Annals* 22:402-408.

Hohman M & LeCroy CW (1996). Predictors of adolescent AA affiliation. *Adolescence* 31:339-352.

Humphreys K (1997). Clinicians' referral and matching of substance abuse patients to self-help groups after treatment. *Psychiatric Services* 48:1445-1449.

Humphreys K, Finney JW & Moos RH (1994). Applying a stress and coping framework to research on mutual help organizations. *Journal of Community Psychology* 22:312-327.

Humphreys K, Huebsch PD, Finney JW et al. (1999a). A comparative evaluation of substance abuse treatment: V. Substance abuse treatment can enhance the effectiveness of self-help groups. *Alcoholism: Clinical & Experimental Research* 23:558-563.

Humphreys K, Mankowski ES, Moos RH et al. (1999b). Do enhanced friendship networks and active coping mediate the effect of self-help groups on substance abuse? *Annals of Behavioral Medicine* 21:54-60.

Humphreys K, Mavis BE & Stoffelmayer BE (1994). Are twelve step programs appropriate for disenfranchised groups? Evidence from a study of posttreatment mutual help involvement. *Prevention in Human Services* 11:165-179.

Humphreys K, Moos RH & Finney JW (1995). Two pathways out of drinking problems with professional treatment. *Addictive Behaviors* 20:427-441.

Humphreys K & Noke JM (1997). The influence of posttreatment mutual help group participation on the friendship networks of substance abuse patients. *American Journal of Community Psychology* 25:1-16.

Johnson E & Herringer LG (1993). A note on the utilization of common support activities and relapse following substance abuse treatment. *Journal of Psychology* 127:73-78.

Kaskutas LA (1994). What do women get out of self-help? Their reasons for attending Women for Sobriety and Alcoholics Anonymous. *Journal of Substance Abuse Treatment* 11:185-195.

Kaskutas LA, Weisner C, Lee M et al. (1999). Alcoholics Anonymous affiliation at treatment intake among white and black Americans. *Journal of Studies on Alcohol* 60:810-816.

Longabaugh R, Wirtz PW, Zweben A et al. (1998). Network support for drinking, Alcoholics Anonymous and long-term matching effects. *Addiction* 93:1313-1333.

Mäkelä K (1993). International comparisons of Alcoholics Anonymous. *Alcohol Health & Research World* 17:228-234.

Mäkelä K (1994). Rates of attrition among the membership of Alcoholics Anonymous in Finland. *Journal of Studies on Alcohol* 55:91-95.

Mäkelä K, Arminen I, Bloomfield K et al. (1996). *Alcoholics Anonymous as a Mutual-Help Movement.* Madison, WI: University of Wisconsin Press.

McCrady BS (1996). Recent research in Twelve Step programs. In AW Graham & TK Schultz (eds.) *Principles of Addiction Medicine, Second Edition.* Chevy Chase, MD: American Society of Addiction Medicine, 707-718.

McCrady BS, Epstein EE & Hirsch LS (1996). Issues in the implementation of a randomized clinical trial that includes Alcoholics Anonymous: Studying AA-related behaviors during treatment. *Journal of Studies on Alcohol* 57:604-612.

McCrady BS & Miller WR (1993). *Research on Alcoholics Anonymous: Opportunities and Alternatives.* New Brunswick, NJ: Rutgers Center of Alcohol Studies.

Montgomery HA, Miller WR & Tonigan JS (1995). Does Alcoholics Anonymous involvement predict treatment outcome? *Journal of Substance Abuse Treatment* 12:241-246.

Moos RH, Finney JW, Ouimette PC et al. (1999). A comparative evaluation of substance abuse treatment: I. Treatment orientation, amount of care, and 1-year outcomes. *Alcoholism: Clinical & Experimental Research* 23:529-536.

Morgenstern J, Kahler CW, Frey RM et al. (1996). Modeling therapeutic response to 12-step treatment: Optimal responders, nonresponders, and partial responders. *Journal of Substance Abuse* 8:45-59.

Morgenstern J, Labouvie E, McCrady BS et al. (1997). Affiliation with Alcoholics Anonymous after treatment: A study of its therapeutic effects and mechanisms of action. *Journal of Consulting and Clinical Psychology* 65:768-777.

Narrow WE, Regier DA, Rae DS et al. (1993). Use of services by persons with mental and addictive disorders. *Archives of General Psychiatry* 50:95-107.

Ouimette PC, Finney JW, Gima K et al. (1999). A comparative evaluation of substance abuse treatment: III. Examining mechanisms underlying patient-treatment matching hypotheses for 12-Step and Cognitive-Behavioral Treatments for substance abuse. *Alcoholism: Clinical & Experimental Research* 23:545-551.

Ouimette PC, Finney JW & Moos RH (1997). Twelve-Step and Cognitive-Behavioral Treatment for substance abuse: A comparison of treatment effectiveness. *Journal of Consulting and Clinical Psychology* 65:230-240.

Ouimette PC, Gima K, Moos RH et al. (1999). A comparative evaluation of substance abuse treatment: IV. The effect of comorbid psychiatric diagnoses on amount of treatment, continuing care, and 1-year outcomes. *Alcoholism: Clinical & Experimental Research* 23:552-557.

Pristach CA & Smith CM (1999). Attitudes towards Alcoholics Anonymous by dually diagnosed psychiatric outpatients. *Journal of Addictive Diseases* 18:69-76.

Project MATCH Research Group (1997a). Matching alcoholism treatments to client heterogeneity: Project MATCH posttreatment drinking outcomes. *Journal of Studies on Alcohol* 58:7-29.

Project MATCH Research Group (1998b). Matching alcoholism treatments to client heterogeneity: Project MATCH three-year drinking outcomes. *Alcoholism: Clinical & Experimental Research* 22:1300-1311.

Project MATCH Research Group (1998a). Matching alcoholism treatments to client heterogeneity: Treatment main effects and matching effects on drinking during treatment. *Journal of Studies on Alcohol* 59:631-639.

Project MATCH Research Group (1997b). Project MATCH secondary a priori hypotheses. *Addiction* 92:1671-1698.

Room R & Greenfield T (1993). Alcoholics Anonymous, other 12-step movements and psychotherapy in the US population, 1990. *Addiction* 88:555-562.

Rychtarik RG, Connors GJ, Dermen KH et al. (2000). Alcoholics Anonymous and the use of medications to prevent relapse: An anonymous survey of member attitudes. *Journal of Studies on Alcohol* 61:134-138.

Schuckit MA, Tipp JE, Smith TL et al. (1997). Periods of abstinence following the onset of alcohol dependence in 1,853 men and women. *Journal of Studies on Alcohol* 58:581-589.

Smith AR (1993). The social construction of group dependency in Alcoholics Anonymous. *Journal of Drug Issues* 23:689-704.

Smith LN (1992). A descriptive study of alcohol-dependent women attending Alcoholics Anonymous, a regional council on alcoholism and an alcohol treatment unit. *Alcohol & Alcoholism* 27:667-676.

Snow MG, Prochaska JO & Rossi JS (1994). Processes of change in Alcoholics Anonymous: Maintenance factors in long-term sobriety. *Journal of Studies on Alcohol* 55:362-371.

Speiglman R (1994). Mandated AA attendance for recidivist drinking drivers: Ideology, organization, and California criminal justice practices. *Addiction* 89:859-868.

Stinchfield R & Owen P (1998). Hazelden's model of treatment and its outcome. *Addictive Behaviors* 23:669-683.

Timko C, Finney JW, Moos RH et al. (1993). The process of treatment selection among previously untreated help-seeking problem drinkers. *Journal of Substance Abuse* 5:203-220.

Timko C, Moos RH, Finney JW et al. (2000). Long-term outcomes of alcohol use disorders: Comparing untreated individuals with those in Alcoholics Anonymous and formal treatment. *Journal of Studies on Alcohol* 61:529-540.

Timko C, Moos RH, Finney JW et al. (1999). Long-term treatment careers and outcomes of previously untreated alcoholics. *Journal of Studies on Alcohol* 60:437-447.

Tomasson K & Vaglum P (1998). Psychiatric co-morbidity and aftercare among alcoholics: A prospective study of a nationwide representative sample. *Addiction* 93:423-431.

Tonigan JS, Connors GJ & Miller WR (1998). Special populations in Alcoholics Anonymous. *Alcohol Health & Research World* 22:281-285.

Tonigan JS, Miller WR & Connors GJ (2000). Project MATCH client impressions about Alcoholics Anonymous: Measurement issues and relationship treatment outcome. *Alcoholism Treatment Quarterly* 18:25-41.

Tonigan JS, Toscova R & Miller WR (1996). Meta-analysis of the literature on Alcoholics Anonymous: Sample and study characteristics moderate findings. *Journal of Studies on Alcohol* 57:65-72.

Walsh DC, Hingson RW, Merrigan DM et al. (1991). A randomized trial of treatment options for alcohol-abusing workers. *New England Journal of Medicine* 325:775-782.

Weisner C, Greenfield T & Room R (1995). Trends in the treatment of alcohol problems in the U.S. general population, 1979-1990. *American Journal of Public Health* 85:55-60.

Winzelberg A & Humphreys K (1999). Should patients' religiosity influence clinicians' referral to 12-Step self-help groups? Evidence from a study of 3, 018 male substance abuse patients. *Journal of Consulting and Clinical Psychology* 67:790-794.

Chapter 3

Spirituality and the Recovery Process

John N. Chappel, M.D., M.P.H., FASAM

Spirituality and Medicine
Spirituality and Religion
Benefits of Spirituality
Attainment of Spiritual Health
Spirituality in Clinical Practice

The greatest revolution in our generation is the discovery that human beings, by changing the inner attitudes of their minds, can change the outer aspects of their lives (William James, 1842-1910).

SPIRITUALITY AND MEDICINE

The past decade has seen a remarkable interest in and acceptance of the role of spirituality in human medicine. Recent articles in many peer-reviewed specialty journals have addressed the subject of spirituality and primary care (Waldfogel, 1997), rheumatology (Nicassio, Schumann et al., 1997), dermatology (Thomsen, 1998), orthopedic surgery (White, 1999), family medicine (Ellis, Vinson et al., 1999; Daaleman & Frey, 1999), oncology (Rousseau, 2000), and end-of-life care (Daaleman & VendeCreek, 2000). A special article in the *American Journal of Medicine* reviewed the literature and concluded that:

Physicians need to learn to be open to discussing spiritual concerns with their patients; to address these issues in a respectful, careful, and professional way; and to know how and when to refer patients

to other members of the health care team for spiritual support (Astrow, Puchalski et al., 2001).

According to Lukoff and colleagues (1992), "Health professionals have not accorded religious and spiritual issues in clinical practice the attention warranted by their prominence in human experience." Medical undergraduate and specialty training virtually ignores religious and spiritual issues. Even psychiatry offers little or no instruction in this area, which so often can have a profound effect on patients' lives (Sansone, Khatain et al., 1990). The reasons for this omission are rooted in two important influences. The first, and perhaps more important, is that modern medical ethics demand that physicians provide equal care regardless of their patients' (or their own) religious beliefs (American Psychiatric Association, 1990). The second is the explosion in medical technology and the resulting emphasis on biomedical issues in medical education and practice.

In 1994 the National Institute for Healthcare Research was funded by the John Templeton Foundation to award grants to U.S. medical schools to support the development of curricula in spirituality and medicine. By 1998 nearly

100 medical schools had expressed interest in applying for the award. Among the key components of these curricula is "including a spiritual assessment as part of a routine history. Students learn clinical and ethical guidelines for discussing a patient's spiritual or religious beliefs and values in a respectful, nonjudgmental, and non-imposing fashion" (Puchalski & Larson, 1998).

These interests and activities have not gone unchallenged. A group of chaplains published an article in the *New England Journal of Medicine* that questioned the validity of the evidence linking religious activities to health, particularly if physicians are being encouraged to prescribe religious activities for their patients. They concluded:

> Most important, we are concerned that attempts to obtain scientific evidence of the health benefits of religious activity and to use such activity instrumentally in achieving beneficial outcomes not only are superficial but also suggest that the value of religion derives from its effects on health. Religion is more that a collection of views and practices, and its value cannot be determined instrumentally; it is a spiritual way of being in the world (Sloan & Bagiella, 2001).

SPIRITUALITY AND RELIGION

Such debate and discussion reflect the importance of separating religion from spirituality in medical practice. Religion, which is found wherever humans exist, is characterized by organization. Each religion has its own theology, doctrine, creeds, catechisms, and liturgical practices, all of which are intended to enhance each member's spirituality. The problem for physicians is the value judgments about people with different beliefs. These responses may range from tolerance through disapproval to rejection and even genocide. During the Renaissance, when scientific discoveries conflicted with religious doctrine, medicine began to be separated from religion as ethical guidelines for medical practice were developed (Americal Psychiatric Association, 1990).

The current discussions of spirituality and medicine strikingly omit reference to addiction medicine and the form of spirituality developed by Alcoholics Anonymous (AA). This spirituality is expressed operationally in the Twelve Steps of AA. As a Protestant minister's son and a psychiatrist, the author has had a long-term interest in spiritual health, but it was only with service as a nonalcoholic member of the General Service Board of AA that the difference between spirituality and religion became clear.

Those who practice addiction medicine have a distinct advantage over colleagues in other branches of medicine. The Twelve Steps offer a template that can be recommended to patients and used personally. The Steps were empirically derived over three years by a slowly growing group of chronic alcoholics who kept asking the question, "How can we stay sober?" (AA, 1976). The Twelve Steps therefore can be considered the product of field research, the effectiveness of which is being supported by recent clinical research (Emrich, 1999).

There is evidence that working a Twelve Step program is not participating in a religion:

1. All the modern religions that have examined the Twelve Steps have come to the conclusion that the Steps do not conflict with their beliefs.

2. AA has spread around the world and is working well in many non-Christian countries.

3. Joining AA does not require learning any theology, creed, or catechism. Tradition 3 of AA affirms that the only requirement for membership is a desire to stop drinking. Atheists are welcome and do well in the program. Bill W (1967) recommended to atheists and agnostics that they make the group their Higher Power, because "most of their AA group is sober, and they are drunk . . . I know how they feel because I was once that way myself."

4. In over 60 years, not one documented or reported fight or act of violence based on arguments over spirituality has occurred between AA members.

Spirituality can be defined as the relationship between an individual and a transcendent or higher being or force or mind of the universe (Peterson & Nelson, 1987). This relationship is personal to the individual and does not require affiliation with any religion; in fact, religion is not necessary for a person to have a spiritual experience or to develop his or her own spirituality. While spirituality does not require religion, it does require theology: that is, a theory of this higher being, mind, or power. AA wisely adds that "whatever this higher power is, it is not me."

Addiction medicine, however, cannot ignore spiritual issues. If former patients are asked about the factors that led to their long-term recovery from alcohol or other drug addictions, a large number mention spiritual experiences or motivation. The most important source of such spiritual experiences in recovery is participation in a Twelve Step program such as AA. The Twelve Step approach to spirituality thus is one that specialists in addiction medicine should understand, clinically support, and communicate to their colleagues who care for alcohol- and other drug-addicted patients.

BENEFITS OF SPIRITUALITY

The spiritual life is a journey, and each person's journey is different (Thomsen, 1998). Common questions as one moves along this journey are:

Why do people live?
Does life have meaning?
Is there a higher power?
Why do people suffer?
Why is this happening to me?
(Rousseau, 2000)

Why should an individual make any effort to develop spirituality or work on his or her spiritual health? The principal reason for making the effort concerns the benefits that result:

Humility. Khantzian and Mack (1989) state that "the power and awe engendered by an outside universe and our humble place in it instill a sense of a force or power greater than ourselves." They argue that this experience "may be a step in the direction of taming and transforming infantile omnipotence and serving in early childhood to establish a capacity for object love." "In this context God serves as a 'self-object' in transition from self-love to object love and provides much needed authority and structure within the self."

Humility can be a powerful stimulus for healing by engendering honesty and a willingness to accept help. In humility, one comes to know one's self as a fallible individual who makes mistakes. It thus is unnecessary to make excuses, to blame others, or to tell lies when a problem arises.

Inner Strength. The experience of a higher power within oneself leads to a sense of being able to deal with adversity. This makes it possible for the individual to face painful situations and to continue the struggles that so often are necessary in life. This internal experience requires active work, such as that involved in Step 11, through prayer and meditation.

A Sense of Meaning and Purpose. Spiritual experience often leads to a greater interest and intention in living. This may be as specific as promoting healing in medical practice or as general as working to improve or sustain the quality of life on earth. Such an experience is a major reason for associating service with spiritual health.

Robert Coles, a child analyst, spent years studying children from different cultures and various religious backgrounds. He concluded that most, if not all, children struggle with the concept of God and attempt to find meaning and purpose in their lives. His concluding comment is: "So it is that we connect with one another, move in and out of one another's lives, teach and heal and affirm one another, across space and time—yet how young we are when we start wondering about it all, the nature of the journey and of the final destination!" (Coles, 1990).

Acceptance and Tolerance. The internal experience of being accepted and cared for by a power greater than oneself leads to acceptance of one's self. This is the first step toward accepting others as they are. Acceptance and tolerance are facilitated by humility, with the individual recognizing the fact that living his or her own life is difficult enough without trying to direct, control, or destroy the lives of others. Acceptance also can be a powerful antidote for shame.

Harmony. Closely related to acceptance is the experience of being in harmony with the universe. This experience leads to an interest in preserving and protecting our environment. It also leads to a sense of connectedness to all other human beings and living things.

Other qualities could be described, including the sobriety that is so important in addiction medicine. However, more benefit is derived from focusing on a few specific issues rather than dwelling on complex theoretical issues.

Booth (1991) described spirituality as "an inner attitude that emphasizes energy, creative choice, and a powerful force for living." Four qualities reflect healthy spirituality: truth (honesty), energy (vitality), love, and acceptance. AA puts it more simply: "Spirituality is the ability to get our minds off ourselves" (Pittman, 1988).

ATTAINMENT OF SPIRITUAL HEALTH

The attainment of physical and mental health requires more than the belief that they can be experienced. Both require active effort and practice on the part of each individual. The roles of exercise, nutrition, and physiologic monitoring have been well established. Less is known about the relationship between body and mind, but most humans practice thinking, problem-solving, management and expression of feelings, and the maintenance of long-term relationships in a social support system.

What areas of practice and exercise are needed to attain and maintain a relationship with a higher power? Five activities could be postulated as useful:

Prayer. Attempts to communicate with a higher power have been effective for many persons. Books have been written on how to pray. One simple fact to remember is that communication with another includes listening as well as talking. Anyone can pray: at issue are the results. As one recovering alcoholic said, "I came into this program a drunken atheist. Today I pray. As an atheist, I faked prayer in the beginning. The results have altered my view of the cosmos. This change in a drunken, hardcore, cynical atheist is a miracle beyond human comprehension" (AA, 1985). Prayer can be as simple as "Help" in the morning and "Thank you" in the evening. AA's Serenity Prayer asks for serenity to accept "the things I cannot change," which includes others, and "the courage to change the things I can," which relates to one's self.

Maintaining an Open Mind. Clearing the mind through meditation may be a way of opening one's self to the experience of a higher power. Many persons experience new ideas and energy—in addition to mental and physical benefits—when they practice meditation. The best results appear to be obtained through disciplined practice. Working Steps 6 and 7 can be very useful in this process.

Discussion. Much can be learned from the experience of others. Unfortunately, social prohibitions make discussion of spiritual issues difficult; for example, military personnel are cautioned not to discuss religion because of the arguments that so often ensue. Anxiety at the prospect of ridicule or rejection is another barrier to discussion of spiritual issues. The Twelve Step programs, by valuing personal experience and refusing to evaluate or judge the experience of another, have created a forum in which it is comfortable for many persons to discuss their spiritual beliefs and experiences or lack thereof.

Reading. The recorded thoughts and experiences of others can be useful in developing one's own ideas and experiences. The classic literature of each of the world's great religions provides examples that often are stimulating and inspiring. Kurtz and Ketcham (1992) have gathered stories

from both religious and secular sources to illustrate the spirituality of imperfection.

As yet, no empirical data exist to support the relationship of these activities to healing. The amount of time and energy that should be devoted to the attainment of spiritual health is unknown. In this regard, it is useful to recall the example of aerobic exercise: although the aspects of such exercise are easily measurable, it took years for scientists to demonstrate its beneficial effect on physical health and longevity. However, many persons who experienced the benefits of aerobic exercise in their own lives did not wait for the controlled studies: they made the effort, noted how much better they felt, and modified their lifestyles accordingly.

The same is true of activities that contribute to mental and spiritual health. As potentially beneficial activities are identified and practiced on a regular basis, it will be possible to measure their effects on different areas of health.

SPIRITUALITY IN CLINICAL PRACTICE

The specialist in addiction medicine or addiction psychiatry must have a working knowledge of the potential role of spirituality in enhancing recovery from alcoholism and other drug addictions. Knowledge and skill in supporting a patient's spiritual experience and the work necessary to develop and maintain spiritual health do not require spiritual beliefs on the part of the health care professional. The atheist or agnostic physician is at no greater disadvantage than is the physician who smokes or is overweight in helping patients deal with those problems. In any case, the physician should refrain from any attempt to persuade the patient to adopt a particular set of religious beliefs. In this context, the physician may wish to consult the following guidelines, which are adapted from principles articulated by the American Psychiatric Association (1990):

- Maintain respect for each patient's beliefs.

- Obtain information about the religious or ideologic orientation and beliefs of the patient so that they can be attended to in the course of treatment.

- If conflict arises in relation to such beliefs, handle it with a concern for the patient's vulnerability to the physician's attitudes.

- Develop empathy for the patient's sensibilities and particular beliefs.

- Do not impose one's own religious, antireligious, or ideologic concepts in the course of therapeutic practice.

Some patients may wish to enter a religiously based treatment program, and there is no reason to discourage them. After studying several programs in New York and surveying the literature, Muffler and colleagues (1992) concluded that "religious programs have demonstrated successful outcomes comparable to those of secular treatment regimens. Religious commitment and treatment by religious practitioners are playing a vital role for many in addictive treatment care."

Know Alcoholics Anonymous. AA is recommended because it is a spiritual program that is not a religion. This fact is not always recognized in the professional literature. For example, Galanter (1990), although he recommends the clinical use of AA, refers to it as a zealous self-help group and compares it to a cult. After describing Bill W's initial spiritual experience, he states that "Bill went on from this experience to preach to other alcoholics and, as with the cultic groups described above, the forces of shared belief and group cohesiveness have become central in the engagement process of AA." The key fact missed in this description is that, after a few months of preaching in which he failed to sober up a single alcoholic, Bill W stopped preaching and began sharing his experience. It took less than three years for AA to discover that a religious approach did not work for many alcoholics. AA then separated from the Oxford Movement and included only a uniquely personal spiritual experience with a higher power, as each individual understood that concept.

Learn About the Benefits Associated With Spiritual Health. These include the humility, inner strength, sense of meaning and purpose, evidence of acceptance and tolerance, and sense of harmony with others and the world already described. Kurtz and Ketcham (1992) add gratitude and forgiveness as benefits of spiritual health; indeed, their finding in this area is that "the experience of being able to forgive was preceded by some experience of being forgiven."

CONCLUSIONS

Although powerful arguments can be made against including spiritual issues in addiction medicine, an even stronger case can be made for their inclusion. The experiences of so many recovering alcoholics and other drug addicts cannot be ignored. Thus it is useful for the physician to practice acceptance of the varied spiritual experiences of patients and to support those experiences as helpful in recovery.

Practitioners of addiction medicine and addiction psychiatry have an obligation to demonstrate knowledge and skill in supporting spiritual issues in the treatment of addictive disorders.

References

Alcoholics Anonymous (1976). *AA: Alcoholics Anonymous: The Story of How Many Thousands of Men and Women Have Recovered from Alcoholism, 3rd Edition.* New York, NY: Alcoholics Anonymous World Service, Inc.

Alcoholics Anonymous (1985). *AA: Best of the Grapevine.* New York, NY: AA Grapevine, Inc.

American Psychiatric Association (1990). Committee on Religion and Psychiatry: Guidelines regarding possible conflict between psychiatrists' religious commitments and psychiatric practice. *American Journal of Psychiatry* 47:542.

Anandarajah G & Hight E (2001). Spirituality and medical practice: Using the HOPE questions as a practical tool for spiritual assessment. *American Family Physician* 63(1):81-89.

Anonymous (1944). Bill W: Basic concepts of Alcoholics Anonymous. *New York State Medical Journal* 44:1805-1810.

Anonymous (1978). *Webster's New Twentieth Century Dictionary.* Ann Arbor, MI: Collins World Publishing.

Astin JA (1998). Why patients use alternative medicine: Results of a national study. *Journal of the American Medical Association* 279(19):1548-1553.

Astrow AB, Puchalski CM & Sulmasy DP (2001). Religion, spirituality, and health care: Social, ethical, and practical considerations. *American Journal of Medicine* 110:283-287.

Benson H & Friedman R (1996). Harnessing the power of the placebo effect and renaming it "Remembered wellness." *Annual Review of Medicine* 47:193-199.

Bill W (1967). *As Bill Sees It.* New York, NY: Alcoholics Anonymous World Service, Inc..

Booth L (1991). *When God Becomes a Drug: Breaking the Chains of Religious Addiction and Abuse.* New York, NY: Tarcher-Perigree Books.

Carroll S (1991). Spirituality and purpose in life in addiction recovery. *Journal of Studies on Alcohol* 54:297-301.

Chibnall JT & Duckro PN (2000). Does exposure to issues of spirituality predict medical students' attitudes toward spirituality in medicine? *Academic Medicine* 75(6):661.

Coles R (1990). *The Spiritual Life of Children.* Boston, MA: Houghton-Mifflin Co.

Craigie FC, Liu IY, Larson DB et al. (1988). A systematic analysis of religious variables in the Journal of Family Practice, 1976-1986. *Journal of Family Practice* 27:509-513.

Cross GM, Morgan CW, Mooney AJ, Martin CA & Rafter JA (1990). Alcoholism treatment: A ten year followup study. *Alcoholism: Clinical & Experimental Research* 14(2): 169-173.

Daaleman TP & Frey B (1999). Spiritual and religious beliefs and practices of family physicians: A national survey. *Journal of Family Practice* 48:98-104.

Daaleman TP & VandeCreek L (2000). Placing religion and spirituality in end-of-life care. *Journal of the American Medical Association* 284(19):2514-2517.

Dorr D, Bonner JW & Reid V (1983). Follow-up of sixty-one physicians after psychiatric treatment. *Journal of Clinical Psychology* 39(6):1038-1042.

Ellis MR, Vinson DC & Ewigman B (1999). Addressing spiritual concerns of patients: Family physicians' attitudes and practices. *Journal of Family Practice* 48(2):105-109.

Emrick CD (1999). Alcoholics Anonymous and other 12-step groups. In M Galanter & HD Kleber (eds.) *Textbook of Substance Abuse Treatment, 2nd Edition*. Washington, DC: American Psychiatric Press.

Galanter M (1990). Cults and zealous self-help movements: A psychiatric perspective. *American Journal of Psychiatry* 147(5): 543-551.

Goldfarb LM, Galanter M, McDowell D, Lifshutz H & Dermatis H (1996). Medical student and patient attitudes toward religion and spirituality in the recovery process. *American Journal of Drug and Alcohol Abuse* 22(4):549-561.

Hatch RL, Burg MA, Naberhaus DS et al. (1998). The Spiritual Involvement and Beliefs Scale: Development and testing of a new instrument. *Journal of Family Practice* 46(6):476-486.

Hiatt JF (1986). Spirituality, medicine and healing. *Southern Medical Journal* 79:736-743.

Khantzian EJ & Mack JE (1989). Alcoholics Anonymous and contemporary psychodynamic theory. In M Galanter (ed.) *Recent Developments in Alcoholism*. New York, NY: Plenum Press, 67-89.

Koenig HG (2001). Spiritual assessment in medical practice. *American Family Physician* 63(1):30-31.

Kuhn C (1988). A spiritual inventory of the medically ill patient. *Psychiatric Medicine* 6:87-89.

Kurtz E & Ketcham K (1992). *The Spirituality of Imperfection: Modern Wisdom From Classic Stories*. New York, NY: Bantam Books.

Levin JS, Larson DB & Puchalski CM (1997). Religion and spirituality in medicine: Research and education. *Journal of the American Medical Association* 278(9):792-793.

Lukoff D, Lu F & Turner R (1992). Toward a more culturally sensitive DSM-IV. *Journal of Nervous and Mental Disease* 180(11):673-682.

McLellan AT, Lewis DC, O'Brien CP et al. (2000). Drug dependence, a chronic medical illness. *Journal of the American Medical Association* 284(13):1689-1695.

Muffler J, Langrod JG & Larson D (1992). "There is a balm in Gilead": Religion and substance abuse treatment. In J Lowinson (ed.) *Substance Abuse: A Comprehensive Textbook*. Baltimore, MD: Williams & Wilkins, 584-595.

Nicassio PM, Schumann C, Kim J et al. (1997). Psychosocial factors associated with complementary treatment use in fibromyalgia. *Journal of Rheumatology* 24(10):2008-2013.

Peterson EA & Nelson K (1987). How to meet your client's spiritual needs. *Journal of Psychological Nursing* 25:34-39.

Pittman B (1988). *Stepping Stones to Recovery*. Seattle, WA: Glen Abbey Books, Inc.

Post SG, Puchalski CM & Larson DB (2000). Physicians and patient spirituality: Professional boundaries, competency, and ethics. *Annals of Internal Medicine* 132(7):578-583.

Puchalski CM & Larson DB (1998). Religion and spirituality in medicine: Research and education. *Journal of the American Medical Association* 278(9):792-793.

Rousseau P (2000). Spirituality and the dying patient. *Journal of Clinical Oncology* 18(9):2000-2002.

Sansone RA, Khatain K & Rodenhauser P (1990). The role of religion in psychiatric education: A national survey. *Academic Psychiatry* 14:34-38.

Sloan RP & Bagiella E (2001). Spirituality and medical practice: A look at the evidence. *American Family Physician* 63(1):33-34.

Sulmasy DP (1999). Is medicine a spiritual practice? *Academic Medicine* 74(9):1002-1005.

Thomsen RJ (1998). Spirituality in medical practice. *Archives of Dermatology* 134:1443-1446.

Veach TL & Chappel JN (1992). Measuring spiritual health: A preliminary study. *Substance Abuse* 13(3): 139-147.

Waldfogel S (1997). Spirituality in medicine. *Primary Care* 24(4):963-976.

White AA (1999). Compassionate patient care and personal survival in orthopedics: A 35-year perspective. *Clinical Orthopaedics and Related Research* 361:250-260.

SECTION 9

Alcohol and Drug Problems in the Workplace

Section Coordinator
Donald Ian Macdonald, M.D., FASAM

Contributors

Robert L. DuPont, M.D., FASAM
President, Institute for Behavior & Health, Inc.
Rockville, Maryland, and
Clinical Professor
Georgetown University School of Medicine
Washington, DC

Paul H. Earley, M.D., FASAM
President
Earley Corporation
Smyrna, Georgia

James L. Ferguson, D.O.
Chief Medical Review Officer
Employee Health Programs, Inc.
Bethesda, Maryland

Dale J. Kaplan, LCSW-C, MDWAC
Vice President for Clinical Services
Employee Health Programs, Inc.
Bethesda, Maryland

Donald Ian Macdonald, M.D., FASAM
Chairman and Medical Director
Employee Health Programs, Inc.
Bethesda, Maryland

Carl Selavka, Ph.D., D-ABC
Institute for Behavior & Health, Inc.
Rockville, Maryland

G. Douglas Talbott, M.D., FACP, FASAM
Founder and Medical Director
Talbott Recovery Campus
Atlanta, Georgia

Robert E. Willette, M.D.
President
Duo Research
Denver, Colorado

| Chapter 1

The Role of the Medical Review Officer

Donald Ian Macdonald, M.D., FASAM
Robert L. DuPont, M.D., FASAM
James L. Ferguson, D.O.

Medical review of workplace drug tests affords new challenges and opportunities to the field of addiction medicine. Thousands of physicians who act as medical review officers (MROs) are convinced that the expertise they offer makes drug-free workplace programs more effective and that such programs are deterrents to casual drug use and of benefit to those workers with alcohol or other drug problems who are detected and referred to treatment earlier in the course of their disease than they otherwise would be.

A 1986 Presidential Executive Order directed the U.S. Department of Health and Human Services (DHHS) to develop and publish scientific and technical guidelines for workplace drug testing of federal employees. These guidelines (DHHS, 1988) significantly increased public acceptance of drug testing by establishing rigid certification procedures for laboratories and placing final responsibility for the review of drug tests with a physician—designated, for the first time, an MRO. The medical review field grew dramatically when, late in 1989, the U.S. Department of Transportation (DOT) mandated widespread testing of transportation workers in safety-sensitive positions (DOT, 1989) and included the requirement for medical review. Further growth occurred as the courts and other government agencies and private employers acknowledged the protection offered by the expertise of a physician and as more and more employers added MROs to their testing programs, even when not required to do so.

On August 1, 2001, a new generation of the DOT regulations took effect. The regulations reflect the newest research data, over 10 years' experience with workplace testing, and more than 100 technical corrections to the existing rules. In addition, many of the Operating Administrations within DOT have aligned their programs. In non-mandated programs, however, there are significant variations from the DOT standard, reflecting other federal rules as well as any relevant state or municipal rules. In general, programs that are most closely modeled after the DOT guidelines are the most defensible legally because of their past success in withstanding court challenges.

In the regulations initially promulgated by DHHS (1988), the only qualifications specified for MROs were that such an official must be a "licensed physician with a knowledge of substance abuse disorders." However, it quickly became apparent that additional qualifications would be needed. In fact, the 2001 regulations require that MROs not only be licensed, but have "clinical experience in controlled substances abuse disorders." They also require attendance at a training course at least once every three years and certification by a nationally recognized certifying board. The American Society of Addiction Medicine and other organizations responded to this need by offering education and certification programs.

As the laws and regulations governing workplace drug testing change and as drug-using individuals devise ever more challenging ways to "beat" the testing system, the practicing MRO must find a way to keep his or her knowledge up to date.

INITIATING THE MEDICAL REVIEW PROCESS

The medical review process begins when the MRO receives a drug test result from a laboratory and ends when he or she reports the result. The specific duties, however, vary according to the test result.

Negative Results. For negative test results, the MRO's role is twofold. First, the MRO reviews the laboratory result to find conditions that may modify the result, such as a statement about specimen dilution. These conditions need to be reported by the MRO to the employer, and employers need to be advised as to appropriate actions in response. Second, MROs review the Chain of Custody and Control Form (CCF) to look for evidence of errors in the collection process. MROs are considered to be the gatekeepers of the drug testing process, and are responsible for verifying that correctable errors are, in fact, corrected if it is possible to do so.

Non-Negative Results (including positive, adulterated, substituted, and invalid test results). The review of non-negative drug test results is the principal MRO function. Before reporting a result as non-negative, the MRO should be satisfied that: (1) the correct specimen was tested (and not somehow mixed up with someone else's, for example); (2) the laboratory accurately performed the necessary analyses; and (3) there was no legitimate medical explanation for the non-negative test result. To resolve these questions, the MRO must understand forensic collection and chain-of-custody procedures, know what the toxicology laboratory does, and be familiar with the relevant laws and regulations. Each employee who has a laboratory-confirmed non-negative test must be interviewed and the relevant paperwork from the laboratory and collection sites reviewed. During this review, the MRO may find it necessary to speak with the Designated Employer Representative (DER), with the individual who collected the urine, with laboratory personnel, and/or with the employee's physician or pharmacy. On occasion, the MRO may wish to examine the worker. Additional laboratory testing may be required, possibly including reanalysis of the specimen.

Invalid Test: Some specimens cannot be tested because of an interfering substance, because they are too dilute or concentrated, or because their pH is out of range. Some medications interfere with the screening process and, occasionally, adulterating substances have been added. If the laboratory cannot completely identify an adulterant or other interfering substance, the results are reported to the MRO as "invalid." The MRO must review the results, interview the donor, and report the results to the employer as "test cancelled." In all DOT cases, an immediate observed recollection of the urine is ordered. However, if the problem is a legitimate prescription rather than an adulterant, a repeat of the test may not be necessary.

Adulterated/Substituted Test: If the laboratory can identify an adulterant, the result comes to the MRO as "adulterated." In cases of extreme dilution that is not consistent with human urine, the results are reported to the MRO as "substituted." Adulterated and substituted results also must be reviewed by the MRO, and are reported to the employer as "refusal to test," with the reason (for example, "refusal to test because of adulteration with glutaraldehyde).

Recordkeeping: When any laboratory report arrives that is not a negative, a chart should be prepared to track all of the relevant paperwork and notes of all MRO interactions with the worker and others. Because the information in such a chart may be subpoenaed, the MRO should treat it with at least as much care as is used in a clinical chart. Under federal testing programs, the MRO is required to keep records of all non-negative tests for five years. In practice, this is a good rule for unregulated programs as well. Many MROs retain such records even longer.

The MRO Interview: The MRO obtains the name of the worker from the CCF after the collector transmits it. The MRO then should make at least three attempts to contact the donor at the numbers on the CCF during the 24 hours after the document is received. If the MRO is unable to contact the donor during that time, he or she should ask the DER to contact the donor and inform the donor that he or she must call the MRO within 72 hours. The DER also should warn the donor that if he or she does not contact the MRO, the MRO will report the results to the employer after 72 hours.

If contact is made, the MRO should identify the donor by asking him or her to provide the identification number used during the drug test collection (usually the donor's Social Security number). Then the MRO should explain the review process and the role of the MRO in that process. Most importantly, the MRO must warn the employee that the MRO is required to provide to the employer and/or appropriate government agencies any information disclosed to the MRO during the review process if it might affect the performance of safety-sensitive duties. Some have called this a drug testing "Miranda" warning.

If the donor is willing to proceed with the interview, the MRO should relay the test result and make note of the individual's reaction (or lack of reaction) to the news.

CONTRACTUAL ISSUES

Before beginning the process of medical review, the MRO should have a written contract with the employer, spelling out in detail the services to be provided. Medical review is only one of many components of a drug-free workplace program and the successful MRO will either provide the other components or be able to direct the employer to them. Organizations called "consortia" or "third-party administrators" (C/TPAs) provide overall program management, policy review, educational materials, training programs, and random sampling of employees, and contract out for laboratory, MRO, and collection services. MROs may function as C/TPAs, but they must be careful to follow the regulations that prohibit them from having a financial relationship with laboratories whose tests they review (DOT, 2000).

SELECTING A LABORATORY

When dealing with urine testing for the so-called "HHS 5" drugs (that is, drugs specified by the Department of Health and Human Services for federally mandated workplace testing programs), it is strongly recommended that MROs work only with laboratories that have been certified under the DHHS rules requiring academic credentials, regular inspections, and satisfactory performance on the testing of regularly submitted blind proficiency specimens (DuPont, 1989, 1990). When testing materials other than urine (such as hair, oral fluids, or sweat), laboratory selection involves careful review of quality control procedures. Until DHHS publishes guidance on the use of alternative methods of testing, consultation with a forensic toxicologist may be desirable.

Before a test may be called positive, its designated analyte must test positive both by an approved immunoas-

say and by confirmation with gas chromatography/mass spectrometry (GC/MS). The GC/MS is so specific that some have called it a "chemical fingerprint." Screening tests are less specific than GC/MS and may be positive on the basis of compounds that are in some way chemically similar to the sought-after analytes. To discount the possibility of drug tests being read as positive in individuals who may have passively inhaled marijuana, DHHS has established testing cutoff levels, below which an analyte may be present but not reportable. The DHHS certification program includes only the HHS 5 drugs (cocaine, marijuana, phencyclidine [PCP], amphetamines, and opiates); it does not include certification for the testing of additional drugs, such as benzodiazepines and barbiturates, which often are included in non-federally mandated testing panels.

On-site testing kits, called "point of collection" kits by DHHS, are widely advertised and sold, but are not currently allowed under the DOT or DHHS rules, principally because they are screening tests only. When an individual who screens positive for amphetamines because of a non-prescription cold medicine is held under suspicion, even temporarily, harm is done. Unlike breath alcohol determinations, which have some direct correlation with impairment, positive urine drug tests—even when confirmed—do not. In recognition of this, the DHHS and DOT programs have been set up to deter drug use, but are not designed to determine fitness for duty on any given day. On the other hand, the Nuclear Regulatory Commission (NRC), which has higher safety requirements, does use on-site screening as a condition of work.

The Federal Drug Testing Advisory Board (DTAB) is in the process of evaluating point of collection testing kits and can be expected to recommend that DHHS approve their use, under rigid guidelines, as screening devices. However, positive screens from these kits will require confirmation, as do positive urine screens under the present system.

DTAB also is evaluating tests that use alternative specimens such as hair, sweat, and oral fluids. Standards for tests of this type can be expected in the near future, as can standards for other drugs of abuse, such as 3,4-methylenedioxymethamphetamine (MDMA) and methylenedioxymethampethamine (MDA).

COLLECTING THE SPECIMEN

Although federal guidelines minimize the MRO's responsibility in this area, the MRO is required to check each collection form for signature and collector remarks. In addition to this administrative function, the MRO should confirm that, in cases involving non-negative test results, the chain of custody was not broken. The MRO also should be prepared to deal with problems of "shy bladder" and with issues of dilution, substitution, and adulteration.

Choice of Specimen. Urine is the preferred specimen for determining drug use in workplace programs. Drugs and/or their metabolites are excreted into urine, where they tend to accumulate and concentrate, at least between voidings. Urine is an easier specimen to obtain and to analyze. It can be readily transported and stored for short periods of time at room temperature, for several days under refrigeration, and indefinitely when frozen. On the other hand, urine concentrations of drugs and their metabolites can be affected by time of day, degree of hydration (that is, how much liquid a person has consumed), exercise (loss of water through sweat), certain dietary habits, and drugs, so it is more difficult with urine than with blood to relate any single test result to the amount of drug taken or when it was taken.

Chain of Custody. The employee being tested should not lose sight of his or her specimen from the moment the cup is filled until the specimen is securely and forensically sealed. For each DOT collection, a DOT-approved printed form, the CCF, should be used to identify the sample, with an identifying number unique to that form.

The specimen bottle should be sealed with tamper-evident tape that is dated by the collector and that contains the unique number from the individual's collection site form; the tape should be initialed by the donor. In some testing programs, collection of a split specimen is required. A split specimen is a single-void specimen that has been divided into two bottles, each forensically identified and sealed, and sent together to the laboratory (DOT, Office of Drug Enforcement and Program Compliance, 1995; DOT, 2000). During the sample's progress through the laboratory, strict chain-of-custody procedures should be observed and be carefully documented.

Privacy Issues. Because drug users routinely seek ways to beat the drug testing system, observed collections are a part of testing programs for the military and in the criminal justice and treatment systems. To increase the acceptance of testing programs in the civilian workplace, collections are not routinely observed but, to provide the system with some protection, there have been "privacy trade-off" measures. Among these are turning off the water supply to the area of the collection, adding blueing to the water in the commode, and taking the temperature of the freshly voided urine specimen.

"Shy Bladder": The DOT rules state that an employee who does not produce an adequate volume of urine may be given fluids in an amount up to 40 ounces and be given up to three hours to complete the collection. For employees who are unable to provide an adequate specimen within three hours, a physical examination may be performed. The MRO may counsel the employer in this regard. The MRO is responsible for making the final determination, based on his or her own evaluation or a copy of the evaluation by another physician. The consequences of an unexplained "shy bladder" are the same as the consequences of a "refusal to test," which in most cases is the same as the consequences of a positive test result.

DOT rules limit acceptable medical explanations for failure to provide a specimen to (1) physiological causes (for example, urinary system dysfunction) and (2) pre-existing and documented psychological conditions (such as one designated in the most recent edition of the *Diagnostic and Statistical Manual of Mental Disorders* (APA, 1994). Assertions of "situational anxiety" and dehydration are considered unverifiable and thus are not acceptable explanations.

Dilution, Substitution, or Adulteration. The tabloid *High Times* and other drug-oriented publications keep users informed of ways to escape detection in drug tests. As solutions to one strategy emerge, new strategies appear and are marketed.

Dilution of the Specimen: One of the most commonly used ways to avoid detection involves diluting the urine so that the concentration of the analyte falls below the cutoff level. Because it is very difficult to maintain the temperature of a specimen that is substituted for the user's own urine or to maintain the temperature of a specimen to which water has been added, the temperature of each specimen should be measured within four minutes of the time of void. If the temperature falls outside the 90 to 100 degree range, a note should be made on the chain-of-custody form, and an observed collection should be obtained immediately. Both the first and second specimens should be sent to the laboratory for analysis.

The most often used method of diluting a specimen involves drinking a large quantity of fluids. Dilute specimens produced in this fashion are of normal temperature and thus are not detectable at the point of collection. They are reported by the laboratory as dilute if they have a specific gravity below 1.003 and a creatinine of less than 0.2 gm/dL. Although many dilute specimens represent attempts to beat the test, it is important to exercise judgement in their interpretation because most contain no measurable amount of drug. When a dilute negative report is received, the DOT rules (DOT, 2000) allow the employer to order a second unobserved collection if the employer wishes to do so and has a written policy in place that specifies a second collection. The policy must treat all employees the same, but may differ according to the reason for testing. For example, line workers must be treated the same as managers, but pre-employment tests may be repeated, while random tests need not be. In such cases, some combination of escorting an individual to the site and restricting fluids on the way to the site is recommended.

Adulteration of the Specimen: When attempts to adulterate are noted by the collector, an observed collection should be performed immediately. Some, but not all, adulterated specimens interfere with the laboratory's ability to conduct the usual screening immunoassays. When a laboratory reports that a specimen is "invalid," the MRO should call the laboratory director to obtain the director's advice as to how to proceed.

Urinaid®, a trade name for glutaraldehyde, was a popular additive that increased the light absorbency of the most commonly used screening test, the enzyme multiplied immunoassay (EMIT®), and made the test unreadable. Urinaid became less popular when it was discovered that alternate screening immunoassay tests could be used and that glutaraldehyde could be detected by GC/MS. It was quickly replaced by "MaryJane Superclean 13," which turned out to be clear detergent and was detected by its ability to make suds. The next adulterant to appear was "Klear," which is potassium nitrite and which interfered with the GC/MS. DOT rules require that an observed collection sample be obtained immediately from anyone who has a specimen that is invalid and who does not have a legitimate medical reason for that being so.

Substitution of the Specimen: Specimens in which the creatinine level is less than or equal to 5 mg/dl, and specific gravity is less than or equal to 1.001, are termed "substituted." Clinical studies compiled and published by DHHS have shown that specimens diluted to this extreme are not consistent with human urine, and therefore should not be tested by laboratories or verified by MROs as if they were human urine.

MRO Review of Adulterated/Substituted Specimens: The new DOT rules require MROs to follow essentially the same verification process for specimens reported as adulterated, substituted, or invalid as they do for laboratory positives. Donors must be contacted, identified, Mirandized, and given an opportunity to discuss the result and to offer a legitimate medical reason for it. In some cases, a physical examination may be required to verify their statements. Donors also must be given an opportunity to have split specimens reanalyzed.

Flaws in the Collection Process. When the MRO finds evidence of possible flaws in the collection process, he or she should report them to the employer. Flaws such as the absence of blue dye in the commode or requiring an individual to disrobe for collection are important, but do not affect the chain of custody or the validity of a positive test.

At the time of the first interview with the donor, the MRO should ask about the collection procedure to ascertain whether the donor handed his or her specimen to the collector and whether the collector sealed the package in the presence of the donor and had the donor initial the sealed package. Frequently, the donor will not recall all of these details. Grounds for cancellation may exist if the MRO is told that a donor's unsealed specimen was placed on a counter on which there were other unsealed specimens and that the donor was dismissed before the specimen was sealed. (DOT tests may be cancelled only if the collector agrees that an error occurred.) Other grounds for cancellation might include sending the donor home or to the waiting room while the collector sealed the specimen package, or the donor's inability to fill the specimen bottle on first effort and over the course of time adding urine to the original bottle. In each of these cases, the MRO should call the collector and check the story. If the collector denies the story and is able to convince the MRO of his or her competence and experience, the MRO would notify the client that the collection has been questioned, but sounds defensible. If, on the other hand, the MRO has a reasonable doubt as to whether the specimen could have been switched, he or she should discuss the problem with the employer. If there is an undisputed error that could work against the donor's right to a fair test, the MRO may cancel the test result.

Re-analysis of Results. In the course of interviewing a donor of a positive, adulterated, or substituted sample, the MRO must notify the individual that the specimen is being kept at the laboratory and may be shipped to another laboratory for re-analysis if the donor requests it within 72 hours. For DOT tests, the MRO must honor the request and make payment the employer's responsibility. For non-DOT tests, there is no standard as to who pays for re-analysis.

A split specimen sent to the second laboratory is sent directly to GC/MS. No screening test is performed and there is no cutoff level other than the laboratory's scientific limit of detection. Adulterated and substituted specimens are reanalyzed with the same cutoffs as in the initial confirmatory tests. If the initial result is confirmed, there is no action except notification of the donor and the employer. If it is not confirmed, the specimen is checked for adulterants. If none are found, both the original test result and the re-analysis are canceled. During the time that the re-analysis is being processed, the donor may not occupy a safety-sensitive position.

INTERPRETING TEST RESULTS

For four of the HHS 5 drugs (the exception being PCP), there may be a legitimate medical explanation for a non-negative test result (Hawks & Chiang, 1986). To properly assess this possibility, the MRO should develop, use, and document a standard checklist for non-negative test results with each class of drugs. When a possible explanation involving medical use is suggested, the MRO should secure documentation in the form of a conversation with the prescribing physician or pharmacy, and/or obtain appropriate written documentation for the record.

Alcohol. Breath testing for alcohol has been mandated by the Department of Transportation for most of the individuals who fall under the drug testing rules. DOT does not require medical review of these tests because there is no legitimate medical explanation for having a BAC level of 0.04 while on duty. DOT does not accept alcohol tolerance as a defense against actions under these rules.

Marijuana. Marinol®, a synthetic form of delta-9-tetrahydrocannabinol (THC), is legally prescribed for nausea related to chemotherapy and for appetite stimulation in AIDS. Either of these indications may be a legitimate medical explanation for a positive test. So too is marijuana use that has been court-approved for the treatment of glaucoma. The enactment of propositions in a number of states calling for legal use of marijuana for a much wider set of medical circumstances may complicate the MRO's decision in private industry. In federal testing programs, however, DOT and DHHS have advised MROs not to consider use under these propositions as legitimate medical use and there-

fore not to accept such use as a reason to reverse a test result that is positive for cannabinoids (Interagency Coordination Group, 1997).

Marijuana, because of its lipid solubility, may remain in the body for extended periods of time, but it will not remain at levels above the cutoff for very long. It has been shown that, at the DHHS-recommended screening cutoff level of 50 ng/mL, mean detection time after a single high-dose marijuana cigarette is less than two days (Interagency Coordination Group, 1997). In the chronic user, higher levels have been reported for as long as 70 days but, in most cases, allowing any more than a month for this possibility is generous. In any case, this explanation does not change the test result.

The employee may try to convince the MRO that the reason for the positive test was marijuana smoked years ago or exposure to marijuana smoked by a friend or co-worker. In establishing its guidelines, DHHS set its testing cutoff levels high enough to discount both of these possibilities. Subsequent studies showing that passive exposure accounts for only very low urine levels of cannabinoids allowed DHHS to lower the cutoff levels from those written into its initial guidelines. Although positive tests may result from eating marijuana brownies, such ingestion, even if proven, is not considered legitimate medical use or a reason to reverse a positive test report. (The same is true of hemp cookies and a confection called "seedie sweeties.")

Cocaine. Cocaine is never prescribed but may be used legally by emergency physicians as a topical anesthetic in a compound called TAC (tetracaine, adrenalin, and cocaine) or by ophthalmologists, dentists, and ENT physicians in a 1% to 4% solution. The MRO should ask the donor who tests positive for cocaine if he or she recently has consulted a physician or dentist, or been in an emergency room. If the answer is affirmative, the MRO should ask about procedures that might have required local anesthesia. If a history of possible use within two to three days of the drug test is obtained, the donor should be asked to have the treating physician call the MRO or to send a copy of the pertinent medical record. The names of many drugs with anesthetic properties incorporate the "-caine" suffix (such as lidocaine and procaine), but none of them test positive for benzoylecgonine, the metabolite of cocaine that is monitored in the urine.

Amphetamines. A number of widely used over-the-counter medications, such as pseudoephedrine, have chemical structures similar to the amphetamines and may

---

test positive on the screening test, but only amphetamine and methamphetamine and drugs that metabolize to them will be confirmed by the GC/MS test. The MRO should be aware of the long list of medications that do result in positive GC/MS confirmation, including those that contain amphetamine (such as Dexedrine®) and methamphetamine (Desoxyn®) and those that the body breaks down to methamphetamine (Benzphetamine® and Selegiline®) and amphetamine (Amphetaminil®). This list is only partial and does not include amphetamine-containing prescriptions from Mexico and other countries.

Among non-prescription medications, only the Vicks® nasal inhaler causes a GC/MS confirmed positive test. Further laboratory analysis can distinguish Vicks from the form of methamphetamine with high abuse potential. Amphetamines come in two forms, with those that refract light to the right—the most psychoactive forms—called "dextro" or "d-forms." The methamphetamine in Vicks refracts to the left and is called "levo" or "l-methamphetamine." Some MROs routinely request and some laboratories routinely perform d-l (chiral) separations on all tests that are positive for methamphetamine. If less than 80% l-methamphetamine is present, the MRO cannot accept that the Vicks inhaler caused the positive result and must call the test positive (DOT, 1997a).

Opiates. Interpretation of opiate positives can be confused by the ingestion of poppy seeds and poppy seed pastes, because they are products of the same plants that yield morphine and codeine. Because of this possibility, for all morphine or codeine levels below 15,000 ng/ml, there must either be a laboratory report confirming the presence of 6-monoacetylmorphine in the specimen or clinical evidence of unauthorized use. If the level of either opiate is 15,000 ng/ml or higher, the worker must present evidence of a legitimate medical explanation. At less than that level, the burden of proof rests on the MRO to show illegitimate use and, although documentation of legitimate prescriptions usually is sought and frequently obtained, the donor is not required to prove legitimate prescription use. For "clinical evidence," the MRO often must rely on the history given by the donor; this may, but rarely does, include an admission of heroin use. Physical examination of individuals who test positive for opiates largely have been abandoned by MROs because only rarely did such examinations yield evidence of current use.

Because federal programs test only for morphine and codeine, prescriptions for other opiates (such as hydrocodone and hydromorphone) that do not contain or metabolize to morphine or codeine cannot explain a positive test. Most often, the clinical evidence comes as an admission of taking a drug prescribed for another. Approximately half of MROs consider such an admission sufficient evidence of "inappropriate use," but some MROs disagree. Part of their concern involves the severity of the assessed penalty (for example, job loss) relative to the gravity of the offense, their concern that workers are not adequately warned against self-incrimination, and their belief that such use is not what the program was designed to deter. A compromise position (which usually requires a change in company policy) is to call the test result positive and expedite a speedy assessment and return to work.

Other Drugs. Although the federal laboratory certification program and testing are limited to the HHS 5 drugs, MROs often are asked to review drug tests that are positive for a variety of other compounds, the yield for which is low in terms of reportable abuse. Most often these panels include testing for the benzodiazepines or barbiturates. MROs who express concern about prescription drug abuse must recognize that most workplace testing programs were set up to deter the use of "street" drugs and accept the fact that such programs are not effective at dealing with the problem of prescription abuse.

If a legitimate medical explanation is found and documented, the test should be reported to the employer as a negative test.

Foreign Medications. The DOT policy on foreign medications (DOT, 2000) allows the reversal of a drug test result that is positive for medications that were imported for personal use consistent with an indicated medical condition, provided there is adequate documentation of foreign travel and verification of a legal prescription or evidence of non-prescription status in the country of issue and appropriate indications for use.

Safety Concerns. Even though there may be a legitimate medical explanation for a drug test result, the MRO may be concerned about use of the drug by an individual who works in a safety-sensitive position. To deal with this possibility, DOT regulations specify that, "As the MRO, you *must* report drug test results and medical information you learned as part of the verification process to third parties without the employee's consent if you determine, in your reasonable medical judgment, that (1) the information may result in the employee being found to be medically unqualified, or (2) the information indicates that continued performance by the employee of his or her safety-sensitive function is likely to pose a significant safety risk" (DOT, 2000). Under this provision, an MRO might reverse a positive test result when there is a legitimate prescription for amphetamine, but may contact the employer to express his or her concern about the narcolepsy for which the amphetamine was prescribed.

REPORTING THE RESULTS

At the conclusion of the review process, the MRO notifies the donor and employer of the findings. The findings may be:

- *Negative* (including reversals on the basis of legitimate medical explanations); and *Negative, dilute*;
  - □ A negative result may include shy bladder with a legitimate medical explanation in an individual who presents with no evidence of drug use.

- *Positive* (including positive results confirmed on reanalysis); and *Positive, dilute*.

- *Cancelled,* because of:
  - □ Fatal flaws or uncorrected correctable flaws;
  - □ Failure to reconfirm on reanalysis; and
  - □ Invalid specimens with or without medical justification;
  - □ Shy bladder in a current employee who has an acceptable medical explanation.

- *Refusal to test*, because of:
  - □ Specimen adulteration/substitution;
  - □ Insufficient amount of urine provided without a legitimate explanation;
  - □ Worker late for test or left the collection site before the test could be completed;
  - □ Worker refused to permit direct observation of the test as required;
  - □ Worker refused to cooperate with the testing process or refused to take a second test when asked to do so.

THE FUTURE OF MRO PRACTICE

The contemporary perspective on alcohol and drug abuse in the workplace is rooted in a new understanding of addiction as a biopsychosocial disorder, with a renewed emphasis on brain biology (Nahas & Burks, 1997; DuPont, 1997). As a consequence, MRO practice is challenging and constantly changing, providing physicians who specialize in addiction medicine with an additional arena in which to exercise their expertise and interest.

The major challenge for the future of addiction prevention and treatment in the workplace is to develop comprehensive programs that are compassionate as well as tough. Such programs must operate in the public interest in ways that respect not only the interests of all involved, but also the dignity of workers and their families, including the dignity of persons with addictive disorders.

In a free and open society, many hurdles faced by workplace alcohol and drug programs will not be dealt with easily, but they must be addressed if workplace programs are to achieve their full life-saving potential.

REFERENCES

American Correctional Association and Institute for Behavior and Health, Inc. (1991). *Monograph: Drug Testing of Juvenile Detainees.* Washington, DC: Office of Juvenile Justice and Delinquency Prevention, Office of Justice Programs, U.S. Department of Justice.

American Psychiatric Association (APA) (1994). *Diagnostic and Statistical Manual of Mental Disorders, 4th Edition (DSM-IV).* Washington, DC: American Psychiatric Press.

Anonymous (1998). Scientists combat effects of popular adulterant on workplace testing programs. *Workplace Substance Abuse Advisor* 12(7).

Anonymous (n.d.[a]). An evaluation of preemployment drug testing. *Journal of Applied Psychology* 75:629-639.

Anonymous (n.d. [b]). Medical Review Officer training. *MRO Alert.*

Anonymous (n.d. [c]). *MRO Update.* Arlington Heights, IL: American College of Occupational and Environmental Medicine.

Anonymous (n.d. [d]). *The Medical Review Officer Handbook, Sixth Edition.* Research Triangle Park, NC: Quadrangle Research LLC.

DuPont RL (1989). Drugs in the American workplace: Conflict and opportunity, part II: Controversies in workplace drug use prevention. *Social Pharmacology* 3:147-164.

DuPont RL (1990). Medicines and drug testing in the workplace. *Journal of Psychoactive Drugs* 22:451-459.

DuPont RL (1997). *The Selfish Brain: Learning from Addiction.* Washington, DC: American Psychiatric Press.

Hawks RL & Chiang CN (1986). *Urine Testing for Drugs of Abuse: Research Monograph 73.* Rockville, MD: National Institute on Drug Abuse.

Huestis MA, Mitchell J & Cone EJ (1995). Detection times of marijuana metabolites in urine by immunoassay and GC/MS. *Journal of Analytical Toxicology* October:19.

Interagency Coordination Group (1997). *Action Regarding California Proposition 215 and Arizona Proposition 22.* Washington, DC: White House Office of National Drug Control Policy, U.S. Department of Justice, Office of Personnel Management & U.S. Department of Health and Human Services.

Nahas GG & Burks TF (1997). *Drug Abuse in the Decade of the Brain.* Amsterdam, The Netherlands: IOS Press.

National Treasury Employees Union v. Von Raab, 489 U.S. 656 (1989).

Schwartz RH (1988). Urine testing in the detection of drugs of abuse. *Archives of Internal Medicine* 148:2407-2412.

Skinner v. Railway Labor Executives' Association, 489 U.S. 602 (1989).

U.S. Department of Health and Human Services (DHHS) (1988). Mandatory guidelines for federal workplace drug testing programs. *Federal Register* 1998:53:11970.

U.S. Department of Health and Human Services (DHHS) (1998). Substance Abuse and Mental Health Services Administration, Testing Split (Bottle B) Specimens for Adulterants, March 9.

U.S. Department of Transportation (DOT) (2000). 49 CFR Part 40 Procedures for Transportation Workplace Drug Testing Programs, Section 40.33,i.

U.S. Department of Transportation (DOT) (1997a). Guidance on Recent Drug Initiatives in California and Arizona, January.

U.S. Department of Transportation (DOT) (1994a). Limitation on alcohol use by transportation workers. *Federal Register* 1994:59:7302.

U.S. Department of Transportation (DOT) (1996). Procedures for transportation workplace drug and alcohol testing programs; Insufficient specimens and other issues. *Federal Register* 1996:61:37693

U.S. Department of Transportation (DOT) (1994b). *Urine Specimen Collection Procedures Guidelines for Transportation Workplace Drug Testing Programs.* Washington, DC: Government Printing Office.

U.S. Department of Transportation (DOT) (1997b). Procedures for Workplace Testing Programs, 49 CFR Part 40, Section 40.25 Procedures (E)(2)(B)(ii), January 10.

U.S. Department of Transportation (DOT) (1989). Procedures for transportation workplace drug testing programs. *Federal Register* 1989;54:11979.

U.S. Department of Transportation (DOT), Office of Drug Enforcement and Program Compliance (1995). 49 CFR Part 40 Interpretation, December 14.

The Role of the Substance Abuse Professional

Chapter 2

Donald Ian Macdonald, M.D., FASAM
Dale J. Kaplan, LCSW-C, MDWAC

SAP Qualifications
SAP Role and Responsibilities
Challenges in the SAP Process

The substance abuse professional (SAP) is an individual who assesses, refers, and evaluates compliance with treatment recommendations on the part of workers who have failed a workplace alcohol or drug test. The role of the SAP was created in law. Qualifications and responsibilities initially were defined in the Omnibus Transportation Employee Testing Act of 1991 (102nd Congress, 1991) and subsequently were clarified in regulations issued by the U.S. Department of Transportation (DOT; 1995). Subsequent revisions significantly strengthened the SAP's role and responsibilities (DOT, 2001).

The federal SAP model, expanded beyond the areas governed by DOT, increasingly is used by nonregulated employers to evaluate and retain workers who admit to alcohol or drug use or who test positive for alcohol or other drugs.

SAP QUALIFICATIONS

DOT Minimum Requirements. By statute, the SAP *must* have knowledge of and clinical experience in the diagnosis and treatment of alcohol- and drug-related disorders. He or she also must be knowledgeable about pertinent DOT rules and regulations. The *Substance Abuse Professional*

Procedures Guidelines for Transportation Drug and Alcohol Testing Programs (DOT, 2001) are a useful reference in this regard. The guidelines call for the SAP to be: (1) a licensed physician (M.D. or D.O.), (2) a licensed or certified psychologist, (3) a licensed or certified social worker, (4) a certified employee assistance professional (CEAP), (5) an alcohol and drug abuse counselor certified by the National Association of Alcoholism and Drug Abuse Counselors (NAADAC), or (6) an individual certified by the International Certification Reciprocity Consortium (ICRC).

SAP Training and Certification. Beginning in 2004, all SAPs must have passed an examination given by a nationally recognized professional or training organization. After initial certification, SAPs will be required to complete 12 hours of additional training that meets DOT standards in each three-year period (DOT, 2000). SAPs must be prepared to provide evidence of their credentials and qualifications to DOT, to the employer, and to the employee upon request.

Additional Requirements. The authors believe the SAP qualifications that have been encoded in federal regulations (and which, by definition, represent a series of legislative and regulatory compromises) are insufficient to allow SAPs to provide adequate assessment and management of many workers. Assessment of individuals who have failed an alcohol or drug test is, at best, a challenge. To rise to this challenge, SAPs also must be able to recognize co-occurring mental disorders, understand the reliability of various drug testing technologies, and have knowledge that encompasses a broad array of workplace safety concerns.

Conflict of Interest. In response to the practice of some professionals who provide "free" evaluations and then refer the evaluated personnel to their own treatment programs, the DOT rules specifically prohibit self-referral or referral to any person or organization in which the SAP has a financial interest. The only exceptions to this self-referral policy are (1) a public agency, such as a state or county, (2) a person under contract to supply services to the employer, (3) a sole source of therapeutically appropriate treatment, or (4) a provider who is covered under the worker's health insurance plan and who is reasonably accessible to the worker (DOT, 2000).

SAP ROLE AND RESPONSIBILITIES

The SAP has several roles. First, he or she must assess each individual who is referred and make a decision as to the extent of that person's alcohol or drug problem, if any. Second, the SAP must make a recommendation for the worker to participate in an appropriate treatment or education program. When the worker has completed such a program, the SAP must meet with the worker for a reassessment in order to evaluate the level of compliance with the initial recommendation for remediation. If the worker has complied with the recommendations and made adequate progress, the SAP must prepare a letter to the employer attesting to that determination (such a letter also should include recommendations for return-to-duty and followup drug and/or alcohol testing and for any aftercare deemed necessary). Throughout this process, the SAP has the final authority to make recommendations and determinations about treatment participation and compliance, but only the employer may decide to return a worker to duty.

Preparing for the SAP Interview. A prerequisite to the assessment must be the employee's willingness to sign a consent form allowing the SAP to communicate with the worker's employer, supervisor, significant other(s), treatment providers (past, present, and future), and others (such as a probation officer), as needed. Although it is possible for the SAP and the Medical Review Officer (MRO) to share

certain information without such a signed consent, it is good practice to obtain one (DOT, 2000). With the proper consents in place, the SAP can be assured of permission to disclose information to the MRO or to the employer that would, in most counseling situations, be considered confidential.

Conducting the SAP Interview. DOT rules require that the initial SAP assessment be conducted in person. Much of the information needed can be collected as part of a thorough biopsychosocial history. In this process, the assessor inquires about the worker's health history and explores any legal, financial, workplace, family, or other personal problems. The SAP should solicit a history of past treatment for substance abuse or mental disorders, as well as any family history of substance use or mental health problems. The SAP also should solicit information from significant others, workplace supervisors, and any treatment professionals who have been in contact with the worker. Beyond specific information about drinking or drug use, these individuals should be asked about the worker's overall functioning. Such information can be useful in breaking through denial and determining the availability and quality of environmental supports (or lack thereof) for the worker during and after treatment.

Because financial considerations limit the amount of time available for SAP assessments, the authors strongly recommend the use of structured assessment tools that can be self-administered and that are demonstrated to be valid and reliable. Indeed, such tools lend additional credibility to the assessment process. For example, the Brief Symptom Inventory (Anonymous, 1993) consists of 53 questions that screen for mental illness. It can be scored quickly, so that results can be reviewed with the worker at the time of administration. The Drug Abuse Screening Test (DAST; Skinner, 1982) is a 28-question instrument, while the Alcohol Use Disorders Identification Test (AUDIT; Allen, Litten et al., n.d.) contains 10 questions. Each of these instruments is well researched, easily scored, and very useful in the assessment process.

Finally, the SAP should assess the worker's ability to afford any recommended treatments, as well as the appropriateness of providers in the network covered by the worker's health plan. However, the SAP's recommendation for treatment should not be based on such financial considerations.

Formulating Treatment Recommendations. In most cases, the conservative position is to lean toward recommending treatment. In the authors' experience, most employees who test positive for alcohol or drug use already have progressed to dependence.

At a minimum, the SAP should recommend that the worker attend an educational program or support group meetings. However, in the authors' experience, most workers who are referred only for these interventions test positive on subsequent drug tests. With an increased understanding of denial, the experienced SAP usually recommends more than educational interventions. The SAP must have a consistent method of determining the types and intensity of treatment to recommend. In this regard, the *ASAM Patient Placement Criteria for the Treatment of Substance-Related Disorders, Second Edition-Revised* (*ASAM PPC-2R*; Mee-Lee, Shulman et al., 2001) is a useful tool. To use the *ASAM PPC-2R*, the assessor solicits information during the personal interview that addresses the worker's situation in each of six dimensions:

1. Potential for acute intoxication or withdrawal;

2. Biomedical conditions and complications;

3. Emotional, behavioral, or cognitive conditions and complications;

4. Readiness to change;

5. Potential for relapse, continued use, or continued problems; and

6. Recovery/living environment.

Basing the assessment on the six dimensions of the ASAM patient placement criteria (Mee-Lee, Shulman et al., 2001) allows the SAP to recommend one of the following levels of care (also see the Rapid Reference section of this text):

Level 0.5:	Early Intervention
Level I:	Outpatient Treatment
Level II:	Intensive Outpatient Treatment/Partial Hospitalization
Level III:	Residential/Inpatient Treatment
Level IV:	Medically Monitored Inpatient Treatment.

Reporting the Assessment Results. The SAP must inform the employer in writing of the assessment results and any treatment recommendations. Such a letter, on the SAP's letterhead, must contain at least the following information (DOT, 2000):

1. The employee's name and social security number.

2. The employer's name and address.

3. The reason for the initial assessment (that is, the specific violation of rules and the date on which it occurred).

4. The date of the initial SAP assessment.

5. The SAP's recommendation for educational or treatment intervention(s).

Reassessment and the Return-to-Work Process. The DOT rules require that, before an employee may return to work, he or she must meet in person with the SAP and provide documentation of his or her compliance with the recommendations made at the time of the initial assessment.

In preparation for such a reassessment, the SAP should have obtained a status report (written and oral) from the educational or treatment program to which the worker was referred, as well as a record of any alcohol or drug tests performed while the worker was in the program. In addition to attendance, the report should comment on the worker's behavior and level of effort. Treatment program staff typically will have discovered additional important information about the worker, which can be useful in the reassessment.

Any followup (aftercare) recommendations made by the treatment program should be taken into consideration. Possible relapse triggers should be addressed, with special attention to the severity of any substance abuse or dependence or coexisting mental disorder. In considering the risk of relapse, the SAP should evaluate the quality of the worker's support systems, both at home and in the workplace.

Testing Recommendations. For workers who have failed a mandated drug or alcohol test, the DOT rules require a negative test before returning to work and a minimum of six random unannounced tests in the first year after return to work. Followup random testing may be recommended for up to 60 months.

DOT rules allow the SAP to recommend testing for alcohol or other drugs in addition to the substance found in the initial test. If company policy allows it, the SAP may recommend testing for drugs (such as benzodiazepines) that are not part of the DOT drug panel, but such non-DOT tests must be performed with a different set of collection

TABLE 1.   Sample Minimum Testing Schedule

Reason for Failed Test	Months 1-2	Month 3	Months 4-6	Months 7-12	Years 2-5
Use of a drug prescribed to another person	1 test per month	1 test per month	1 test per month	1 test every other month	No further testing required
Use of cocaine or methamphetamine	1 test per month	2 tests per month	1 test per month	1 test per quarter	1 test per quarter
Use of marijuana, alcohol, or other drugs	2 tests per month	2 tests per month	1 test per month	1 test per month	1 test per quarter

forms and a separate void. Because cocaine is associated with a higher risk of relapse and has a shorter half-life than marijuana, for example, the authors usually recommend more frequent testing of those who abuse cocaine than of workers whose problem is with marijuana.

The use of observed collections is allowed under DOT rules and should be recommended for all return-to-work and follow-up testing. Unfortunately, the majority of collection sites will not perform an observed collection.

In formulating a recommendation for testing, the SAP should consider the substance used, the report of the treatment facility, the assessed degree of dependence, the risk of relapse, and the degree of stress reported at work and at home, as well as general safety issues.

The value of testing as a relapse prevention tool and as a safety warning system cannot be overestimated. The authors believe that the conservative stance is to test early and often. Specifically, it is the authors' advice that the SAP recommend random unannounced drug and/or alcohol testing for a period of 60 months, based on an understanding that substance abuse is a chronic, recurring disorder and a belief that testing can be an effective tool in relapse prevention. In consideration of these factors, a typical minimum testing schedule is shown in Table 1.

At any time after the employee's first year back on the job, the SAP may modify or eliminate the testing requirements. Any recommendations for followup alcohol or drug

testing and for other aftercare made by the SAP should follow the worker to subsequent employers.

For the employee, the consequences of failing a return-to-work test or any subsequent test can be severe. The most extreme example probably is that of pilots, who are not allowed to fly again if they have a second positive DOT test. In such a situation, the worker is apt to forget that he or she was less than honest with the SAP who recommended a return to work. In at least one such case, a worker filed suit against a SAP, charging that the SAP "should have known" that the worker was not being completely honest. The SAP needs to tell the worker that it is his or her personal responsibility to understand the possible consequences under federal rules and company policy of a second failed drug test. A statement signed by the worker that acknowledges such responsibility should be included in the return-to-work agreement.

Reporting the Reassessment and Return-to-Work Recommendation. Under DOT rules, the SAP is required to report the results of the reassessment to the employer in writing, describing whether the employee has complied with the recommendations made at the time of the initial assessment. This report should incorporate all of the information in the initial assessment letter, as well as the following:

1. The name of the practice or program that provided the treatment.

2. The dates during which the worker participated in treatment.

3. A clinical description of the treatment program.

4. A clinical assessment of the worker's degree of compliance with the treatment recommendation.

5. A followup testing plan.

6. A discussion of the worker's continuing care needs, including recommendations for ongoing treatment, aftercare, and/or support group services (DOT, 2000).

The Return-to-Work Decision. While the SAP offers information and a recommendation, DOT rules clearly state that the actual decision to reinstate a worker is the sole responsibility of the employer. The federal Americans with Disability Act (ADA) requires that employers make reasonable accommodations for the workers' disability, including alcoholism or drug dependence.

Monitoring Compliance. Once an employee has returned to work, compliance with the SAP's recommendations should be monitored (this monitoring is not required but is strongly recommended in the DOT rules). The monitoring function, which is the employer's responsibility, may be conducted directly by the employer or may be delegated to an MRO, the SAP, or to an Employee Assistance Program (EAP). A good compliance system would monitor:

■ Alcohol or drug use (through testing);

■ Attendance at self-help groups;

■ Participation in counseling, treatment sessions, and aftercare; and

■ Job performance.

In developing a monitoring system, clinicians need to remember that addiction is a chronic, recurring disorder and that relapse always is a possibility.

CHALLENGES IN THE SAP PROCESS

Financial Issues. Federal rules require the employer to identify the SAP, but they do not require the employer to pay for the SAP's services. Often the issue of payment is determined by existing management-labor agreements or company policy. The SAP should clarify payment issues with the worker before conducting the assessment.

Denial. Denial, which is a characteristic feature of substance abuse disorders, can greatly impede the assessment process. In a worker who is referred because of a failed alcohol or drug test, the potential for denial is greatly magnified. Such a worker presents for assessment only because DOT rules or company policies require him or her to do so in order to return to the job. The worker typically claims that the drug test results are an error and attempts to convince the assessor that he or she does not have a problem with alcohol or other drugs. Because such an individual may be early in the course of developing abuse or dependence, the initial assessment may find little evidence on which to base a diagnosis. The SAP, who may be more accustomed to dealing with individuals who undergo assessment voluntarily or under a court order, must be prepared for such denial. Otherwise, the naive SAP can be induced to spend the majority of the assessment time trying to understand how the failed test was wrong.

Delay. For financial and other reasons, workers may postpone their initial SAP assessment, or their entry into treatment, or their posttreatment assessment. Others may try to avoid the SAP assessment or recommendations altogether by changing employers without informing the new employer of the failed alcohol or drug test. Each delay makes the SAP's work more difficult. In fact, a long delay may compel the SAP to perform an extensive reassessment. To address this issue, the SAP should prepare a memorandum of understanding (MOU) for each worker to sign, outlining the contract between the SAP and the worker. A major part of this agreement should include the timeframes that the SAP determines appropriate for each step in the process, including how much time the worker is allowed to comply with the SAP's recommendations before a repeat initial assessment is required.

Federal Rules. For the SAP who has had little experience with regulated programs, the DOT rules may seem difficult to learn and hard to follow. The SAP needs to become comfortable in sharing information with employers that, in nonregulated roles, would be considered confidential (in fact, confidentiality issues are specifically addressed in the DOT rules).

In workplace programs, the SAP's role is unique. The individuals who are assessed are not the SAP's clients or patients, but employees referred for assessment of their ability to function in a critical and often safety-sensitive job.

Before initiating an assessment, the SAP should be knowledgeable about any applicable DOT rules and be aware that, in addition to the general rules, each of the DOT operating agencies (also called "modes") may have specific requirements. The latest revisions of the DOT rules bring increased consistency to the modes in describing the SAP's responsibilities, but significant modal differences remain. For example, the Coast Guard identifies the role of the SAP in the return-to-work process following a failed drug test, but requires an MRO to certify that the chance of relapse is low before allowing an employee to return to work. The Federal Aviation Administration (FAA) assigns much of this responsibility to the FAA flight surgeon, who makes a final return-to-work decision based on the recommendations of the MRO and the SAP as well as other information.

In addition to the DOT requirements, the SAP also should be familiar with the employer's company policies as they relate to requirements for return to work and willingness to pay for assessment and treatment.

CONCLUSIONS

Evaluation by a qualified SAP can be an effective avenue for providing much-needed assistance to workers and employers. With the help of a Substance Abuse Professional, an employer gains a productive employee and does not have to bear the costs involved in hiring and training a new person. The employee's family is profoundly affected when he or she is able to regain control over his or her life. And the employee is given an opportunity to succeed and prosper rather than becoming a potential financial or criminal problem in the greater community.

REFERENCES

Allen J, Litten R, Fertig J et al. (n.d.). Review of research on the Alcohol Use Disorders Identification Test (AUDIT). *Alcoholism: Clinical & Experimental Research* 21:613-619.

Anonymous (1993). *BSI®: Brief Symptom Inventory.* Minneapolis, MN: National Computer Systems, Inc.

Mee-Lee D, Shulman G, Fishman M et al. (2001). *ASAM Patient Placement Criteria for the Treatment of Substance-Related Disorders, Second Edition-Revised.* Chevy Chase, MD: American Society of Addiction Medicine.

Skinner H (1982). The Drug Abuse Screening Test (DAST). *Addictive Behaviors* 7:363-371.

U.S. Department of Transportation (DOT) (1995). Procedures for Transportation Workplace Drug and Alcohol Testing Programs; Final Rule. *Federal Register* 49 CFR Part 40, April 19.

U.S. Department of Transportation (DOT) (2000). Procedures for Transportation Workplace Drug and Alcohol Testing Programs; Final Rule. *Federal Register* 49 CFR Part 40, December.

U.S. Department of Transportation (DOT) (2001). Substance Abuse Professional Procedures Guidelines for Transportation Drug and Alcohol Testing Programs. Washington, DC: Office of the Secretary, Drug Enforcement and Program Compliance, DOT, August.

102nd Congress (1991). Omnibus Transportation Employee Testing Act of 1991 (P.L. 102-143), October 28.

Chapter 3

Drug Testing in the Workplace

Robert E. Willette, Ph.D.

Guidelines for Workplace Drug Testing
Types of Workplace Drug Testing
The Science of Workplace Drug Testing
Requirements for Reliable Laboratories

The courts consistently have held that employers have a duty to provide a safe workplace and a right to expect employees to perform their work in a safe and efficient manner. The U.S. Department of Transportation (DOT) has issued regulations that require the testing of some 7 million transportation workers in the private sector. In addition, the federal government enforces various laws designed to prevent, detect, and eliminate illegal drug use in the workplace. In response to such mandates, many government agencies and private employers have initiated drug testing programs to assure workforce reliability. Because these programs affect the livelihoods of individuals, it is important to understand how drug testing operates, or should operate, and how to select the appropriate drug testing procedures and a competent testing laboratory.

GUIDELINES FOR WORKPLACE DRUG TESTING

Contemporary programs for workplace drug testing must conform to federal regulations codified in the 1988 publication, *Mandatory Guidelines for Federal Workplace Drug Testing Programs* (DHHS). The guidelines address laboratory procedures, drugs to be tested, testing cutoff levels, and specific reporting requirements, including mandatory medical review. They also require the use of immunoassays approved by the U.S. Food and Drug Administration (FDA) for screening and gas chromatography/mass spectrometry (GC/MS) to confirm the presence of drugs.

Even though many companies had launched drug testing programs by the time the federal guidelines were issued 1988, the presence of specific federal regulations, coupled with a program for federal certification of drug testing laboratories and the government's successful defense of federal testing policies before the United States Supreme Court, created a climate hospitable to the implementation of drug testing programs in both the public and private sectors.

The 1990s were a period of maturation for drug testing. Arbitrators and courts further defined what employers could and could not do. Certified drug testing laboratories developed better procedures for processing and testing specimens. The federal government refined and expanded its regulations to include mandatory random alcohol testing for certain transportation workers. On the other side, however, a wide array of techniques and chemicals intended to defeat drug testing became available; these were designed to adulterate, dilute, and substitute specimens.

Notwithstanding such techniques, workplace drug testing programs have been extremely successful. For example, following implementation of its testing program, the U.S. Navy saw the rate of positive test results drop from 47% in 1981 to less than 1% by 2000. Other employers have seen similar reductions in detected drug use.

TYPES OF WORKPLACE DRUG TESTING

Workplace drug testing can be used for multiple purposes (Johnson & Quandar, 1998):

Pre-employment Testing. Pre-employment testing is considered preventive because it denies employment to persons who are identified as drug users before they begin work. Almost all companies that conduct any type of drug testing use pre-employment testing, which is the most frequently used form of situational testing.

Reasonable Cause Testing. "Reasonable cause" testing is used when an employee's unsafe or unacceptable job conduct clearly points to a problem that may involve drug use. This form of testing is conducted when an employer believes, based on objective evidence, that a particular employee is unable to perform his or her duties satisfactorily by virtue of impairment from drugs or alcohol. Such inability to perform may include, but is not limited to, a decrease in the quality or quantity of the employee's productivity, judgment, reasoning, concentration, and psychomotor control, as well as marked behavioral changes. Accidents, deviations from safe working practices, and erratic workplace conduct—indicative of impairment—are other examples of reasonable cause situations.

Random Testing. A random selection technique is one in which all persons in a defined population have an equal chance of being tested. Random testing sometimes is referred to as "unannounced testing" because the salient feature is the absence of advance notice. It also is called "no-cause testing" because the selection of employees for testing is unrelated to a specific performance problem. These two factors—no notice and no cause—are responsible for the unpopularity of this testing method. Overall, random testing is the most controversial drug testing option because it pits the employer's desires, which often mirror broad societal interests, against the employee's privacy interest.

Post-Accident Testing. Testing after an accident has occurred involves testing of an individual who is directly involved in a motor vehicle crash or other accident or near-accident. Post-accident testing resembles reasonable cause testing in that both are based on specific events. However,

in post-accident testing, indicators of employee impairment need not be present for testing to occur.

Periodic Testing. Periodic testing is a catch-all category that includes drug tests conducted at designated intervals. Such tests usually are conducted as an adjunct to routine checkups or recertification of occupational licenses. However, periodic testing has limited efficacy in deterring or detecting on-the-job alcohol or drug use because users may simply abstain for a period of time prior to the scheduled test. Also, the personnel who collect drug test specimens as part of a medical evaluation do not always adequately guard against specimen substitution.

Rehabilitation Testing. The frequency and manner of testing employees in rehabilitation programs before they return to work are determined by rehabilitation program professionals. The key person could be a medical review officer (MRO) or a substance abuse professional (SAP) who is employed by the company. Although the principal role of the MRO is the evaluation of positive test results, this role could be expanded to include rehabilitation functions (such as setting an unannounced testing schedule for the employee and deciding when an employee is fit to return to work).

The use of unannounced testing after an employee returns to work from a rehabilitation program is determined by management or senior supervisors close to the job and familiar with the employee's duties. When the job involves safety-sensitive duties, unannounced testing should occur more frequently and be more unpredictable; the period of aftercare monitoring also should be longer. These steps are taken to maximize assurance that an employee will remain drug-free. The frequency of unannounced testing following rehabilitation can vary from once every three months to once every three days, with the norm about once a month. The length of posttreatment monitoring usually ranges from one to five years.

THE SCIENCE OF WORKPLACE DRUG TESTING

Analytical Chemistry. The analytical chemist must identify and measure the amount of a specific chemical present in a given sample. When the sample is taken from a biological specimen, such as blood or urine, the chemist's task is complicated by the fact that thousands of other chemicals also are present in the sample. The chemist thus must separate the chemical or drug of interest from all other chemicals and characterize it in a manner that provides sufficient information to identify it with some degree of scientific certainty; in most circumstances, this identification must meet the legal or forensic standard of certainty "beyond a reasonable doubt." (Testing in counseling situations usually is conducted at a somewhat lower standard.)

The analytical chemist uses two methods to achieve the necessary separation and identification: immunoassays and chromatography. To achieve a forensic-quality result, it has become common practice to use both techniques in combination. Other combinations also may be acceptable, but the typical drug testing scenario employs an immunoassay as an initial test (often called a "screen"), followed by a chromatographic analysis as a confirmatory test.

Immunoassays: Immunoassays separate a specific chemical, or group of closely related chemicals, from everything else in the sample by attracting or binding the target chemical to an antibody designed to recognize it. This is similar to the principle underlying allergies and immunizations. Antibodies initially are obtained by injecting animals with a specifically designed "antigen" and collecting the antisera. Today, most antibodies are cloned from selected lines of antibodies.

The assay also requires a "marker" molecule that will indicate when the target drug is present. This is accomplished by adding the drug, attached to an enzyme or a radioactive or fluorescent molecule, to the assay mixture. When the target drug is present in the sample, it competes with the marker molecule for binding sites on the antibody, thus releasing the marker into the surrounding solution. The amount of marker displaced is proportional to the amount of drug present. The displacement can be measured by an appropriate instrument, such as a spectrophotometer or scintillation counter.

Immunoassays have the advantage of high sensitivity. This means that immunoassays can detect very low concentrations of the target drug. This often makes it possible to detect drug use for relatively long periods of time. The cutoff level (that is, the concentration above which the test response is said to be positive) can be adjusted to almost any level within certain limitations. Thus, detection periods can be adjusted to match program goals.

Immunoassays can be adapted to high-volume, rapid testing, which reduces the cost of simultaneous screening for more than one drug. With newer immunoassays and modern analyzers, testing can be fully automated, employing computer-driven panels and barcode readers.

One of the challenges in designing immunoassays is to make them quite specific for a given drug or closely related group of drugs. However, if many closely related drugs fall into the same class, as with amphetamines, the assay may cross-react with several drugs that have an amphetamine-like structure. For this reason, a separate test must be used to confirm the initial result.

Other immunoassays, such as that used to detect the cocaine metabolite, benzoylecgonine, are extremely specific and do not detect any other chemical, except for very high concentrations of cocaine itself.

Immunoassays for marijuana are designed to detect delta-9-tetrahydrocannabinol (THC), which is the major psychoactive ingredient in marijuana and other cannabis products. The metabolite, THC-9-acid, is used to produce the antibodies for these assays and as the standard for calibrating the analysis. However, the antibodies tend to attract or cross-react in varying degrees with several other THC metabolites. Thus, a response in this assay measures the total of cross-reacting metabolites that are present. Nevertheless, the total response does reflect the relative amount of THC present in the specimen.

Chromatography: As used in analytical chemistry, chromatography takes advantage of the different properties of chemicals and drugs that permit them to be separated from each other. This requires passing the mixture of chemicals over an absorbent material that allows some chemicals to "move" faster than others. A detector is used to detect each chemical as it emerges from the system. The separation system most commonly used is gas chromatography (GC) and the detector most widely used is a mass spectrometer (MS). In combination, this method is called "gas chromatography/mass spectrometry" (GC/MS).

GC/MS analysis begins with an extraction step. For example, a portion of a urine specimen is treated with certain specific chemicals that make the target drug less soluble in the urine. The drug and other similar molecules then are removed from the urine with a solvent in which the drug is more soluble. Alternatively, the urine sample can be passed through a solid that attracts the drug molecules. The drug is retrieved from the solvent or solid and concentrated to a very small residue. This extraction step helps remove the drug from the many other chemicals in the urine, simplifying the next stage of analysis.

The concentrated extract is dissolved in a small amount of solvent and injected into the inlet of a long, narrow tube, known as a chromatographic column. Sometimes, the extract must be treated with other reagents to produce a derivative that is more stable or volatile than the parent drug. The column is coiled up inside a heated oven and is arranged for a stream of gas to flow through the column. When the extract is injected into the stream of gas, it is swept through the column. Each of the chemicals present in the extract is attracted to the column packing or coating to varying degrees. Therefore, some pass through more rapidly than others, which are slowed by their attraction to the column. If the proper conditions are selected, the target drug will be separated away from all other components.

The next step in the assay is to detect each of the separated components as it emerges from the other end of the column. Several types of detectors are used for this purpose. A mass spectrometer records a spectrum of the molecules entering it, separated by their molecular weight or their mass. The drug molecules emerge from the column into the MS, which separates all components present according to their molecular weight. While more than one chemical can have the same molecular weight, each has a unique structure. It is the differences in structure that permit the various molecules to be separated in the extraction and the chromatography steps.

In order to characterize the chemical or mixture of chemicals that emerge from the GC column, most mass spectrometers cause the molecules to break into pieces or "fragment." Under the same operating conditions, each chemical gives rise to the same fragmentation pattern. It is this fragmentation information that makes the MS detector so powerful. Because the fragmentation pattern can vary from instrument to instrument or from day to day, it is necessary to run known standards along with any unknown samples in order to make the comparison. The extraction process, the chromatographic and mass separations, and the matching of fragmentation patterns all combine to provide unequivocal evidence that a drug or its metabolite is present in a sample.

Beyond the simple presence of the drug or its metabolite, the concentration of the drug also must be measured in order to prove that the signals measured in the mass spectrometer are due to the drug and not to any "background noise" caused by the sample or the instrument. A cutoff level is established on the basis of experiments using samples containing known amounts of the drug. During actual analyses, known standards must be included in the analysis in order to establish the appropriate calibration of signals produced by the sample. In order to make this extremely accurate, an "internal standard" is added to the sample before it is extracted. This produces a fixed relationship between the drug and the internal standard. By comparing the ratios for the standards against the ratio from a sample, the concentration can be calculated.

Other Assays: It should be noted that other chromatographic assays are in use and available for drug testing. The most common of these are thin layer chromatography (TLC) and high pressure liquid chromatography (HPLC). Since these two methods do not offer the same degree of accuracy as GC/MS or other MS methods, their use as confirmatory assays has been discouraged. However, new instruments using HPLC as the chromatographic system, coupled with a MS detector, have provided a valuable system for drugs that cannot survive GC conditions. Accordingly, it is anticipated that this and other forms of mass spectrometry will be allowed under the revised DHHS *Mandatory Guidelines*.

Validating the Sample. In addition to testing for the presence of specific drugs, it has become necessary for laboratories also to conduct tests to "validate" the specimen (that is, to determine whether the specimen actually is urine and is free from external contamination). This need arises from the development of numerous products and techniques for adulterating or substituting a specimen. Initially, such efforts employed common household products such as bleach or Drano®. More recently, commercial products specifically designed for this purpose have become available. They are advertised in drug culture magazines such as *High Times* and are readily available for purchase over the Internet. (In fact, a simple search on "drug test" will generate more than a thousand hits.)

Among the most common adulterants are "Urinaid" (glutaraldehyde), various salts of nitrous acid, an oxidizing agent ("Klear"), other oxidizing agents such as the chromates ("Urine Luck"), and enzymes ("Stealth"). The more sophisticated products actually destroy some drugs, such as the metabolite of THC and opiates, while others interfere with the screening or confirmatory assays. Because most workplace drug testing programs do not involve observed specimen collection, it is simple for donors to add such products to their specimens. To combat such efforts, laboratories conduct various tests to detect the adulterants, and these are incorporated in both the DHHS and DOT standards.

Other tactics commonly employed to foil the test involve substituting someone else's specimen or the individual's own "clean" specimen (collected during a period of non-use) and adding water or other liquids to the specimen in an effort to dilute it sufficiently to lower the drug concentration below the cutoff level of the assay

TABLE 1. Invalid Urine Specimens

A specimen is considered:

- **Dilute** if the creatinine is <20 mg/dl *and* the specific gravity is <1.003.

- **Substituted** (the specimen does not exhibit the clinical signs or characteristics associated with normal human urine) if the creatinine concentration is ≤5 mg/dL *and* the specific gravity is ≤1.001 or ≥1.020.

- **Adulterated** if the nitrite concentration is ≥500 ug/mL; or if an exogenous substance (a substance that is not ordinarily a constituent of urine) is present; of if an endogenous substance is present at a higher than normal concentration.

(Table 1). Such specimens usually are detected in the laboratory by measuring the creatinine concentration and specific gravity of the sample and comparing the results to established standards for what constitutes a specimen that is consistent with normal human urine.

In federally regulated programs and in most government agency and company programs, a report by the laboratory that the specimen is adulterated or "not consistent with normal human urine" is treated as a refusal to submit a specimen. Most custody forms signed by donors incorporate a statement certifying that the specimen is the donor's own and has not been adulterated or altered in any manner.

Establishing Cutoff Levels. Several factors determine whether a specimen will be reported as positive for the presence of a drug. The choice of cutoff or reporting level is somewhat arbitrary, and can be adjusted for different purposes. Generally, higher cutoff levels detect more recent use but permit more drug use to go undetected. In general, the cutoff levels dictated by the DHHS *Mandatory Guidelines* are moderately high because they are selected to serve as a deterrent to drug use rather than being designed to detect all drug users. This approach also minimizes analytical false positive results.

Factors Confounding Test Results. Most drug test results provide proof of illegal drug use. However, there are circumstances in which a plausible alternative explanation must be considered.

Cocaine: Cocaine is a Schedule II controlled drug that is used in certain surgical procedures. If a test is positive for cocaine (usually detected as its primary metabolite benzoylecgonine), such surgical procedures are readily verified.

In addition, there are two possible avenues for unintentional ingestion of cocaine. The first involves imported herbal teas containing real coca leaves. Although such teas are illegal, this fact may not be known to the user at the time. Because of the rarity with which such teas are seen, strong evidence would be required to determine that this is a plausible explanation for a positive cocaine result.

Alternatively, as little as 25 mg of cocaine could be placed in a drink, consumed without being detected, and produce a test result that is positive for cocaine for up to two days. Before such an explanation could be accepted, however, credible witnesses would have to be available to verify the events.

Marijuana: As described earlier, the psychoactive ingredient in marijuana, delta-9-tetrahydrocannabinol (THC), is quite fat soluble and is stored throughout the body. The accepted half-life of THC is about 24 hours. Normally, a positive result following the smoking or eating of a single "joint" (about 1/2 gram) can be obtained for no more than three days, while heavy or frequent use can produce a positive result for up to two weeks. Thus, if a test yields a positive result, the explanation that the subject had just one joint several days earlier is not plausible.

Passive inhalation is possible but highly improbable. At a 50 ng/mL immunoassay cutoff level, it would take several days of repeated exposure to the smoke of about 30 joints in an unventilated small space to produce a positive result. Even under these extreme conditions, quantitative levels of the primary THC metabolite generally do not exceed 35 ng/ml. Exposure to the smoke of eight joints over one hour under these conditions on six consecutive days does not exceed 75 ng/ml of total cross-reacting metabolites (as measured in an immunoassay). In test situations, only one of 400 specimens collected exceeded 10 ng/ml on the GC/MS confirmation, and it was 12 ng/ml.

It is possible that ingesting marijuana cooked into food will produce a positive result for several days. However, this is unlikely and a credible witness would have to testify to the nature of the food and the quantity of marijuana it contained.

Morphine and Codeine: A test that is positive for morphine may result from four possible sources. The least likely is pure morphine, which usually is administered only in a hospital. Codeine is metabolized to morphine, so both usually are present following codeine use. This can be verified through the existence of a valid prescription. Usually, the codeine level is very high, especially if the use was recent. Occasionally, the level of codeine is lower than that of morphine and may be too low to detect, since it is excreted faster than its metabolite morphine. However, the morphine level will be quite low as well.

Heroin is very rapidly metabolized to morphine, which would be found in high concentrations. Some codeine usually is present as well, because it is a natural constituent of opium and remains as a contaminant in the heroin. It usually is not possible to conclude that an individual used heroin in the absence of any other evidence of such use, such as needle marks or other physiological signs. If heroin use is suspected or there is no other plausible explanation, the laboratory should be asked to retest the specimen for the presence of 6-acetylmorphine (6-AM), an intermediate metabolite between heroin and morphine. Its presence is conclusive proof of heroin use. A detection level of at least 10 ng/ml is required. The DHHS *Mandatory Guidelines* require that all specimens positive for morphine at a 2,000 ng/mL cutoff level be analyzed for 6-AM.

Also, many poppy seeds that are used in baking are obtained from opium poppies. Depending on their source, some poppy seeds contain sufficient amounts of morphine to produce a positive test result after they are ingested. Codeine usually is present at about 10% of the morphine level.

Amphetamines: Amphetamine is a relatively small and simple molecule. Because of its close chemical relationship to natural neurotransmitters—the chemicals responsible for many of the body's functions—many drugs are available that are very similar in chemical structure to amphetamine. Some are available over-the-counter in cold and diet preparations, such as phenylpropanolamine (PPA) and ephedrine. Because of this close chemical similarity, many of these drugs may be detected in immunoassay screens, which are designed to detect amphetamine-like drugs. This does not pose any problem when appropriate confirmatory methods are used, with the following exception.

The most widely abused amphetamines are dextro- or *d*-amphetamine (Dexedrine®), racemic or *dl*-amphetamine (Benzedrine®), *d*-methamphetamine (Methedrine®), and dl-methamphetamine. The racemic or *dl*-forms of these drugs usually are a product of clandestine laboratories that use phenyl-2-propanone as a starting material. The optically active *d*-forms, which are the most potent isomers, can be diverted from legitimate medical sources or produced illicitly from drugs such as ephedrine or pseudoephedrine. Laboratories conducting GC/MS assays can readily identify these two drugs and have an assay available to distinguish between the *d*-, *l*- or *dl*-forms.

Overuse of Vicks® inhalers also can give rise to the positive identification of methamphetamine in the urine of the user, because Vicks Inhalers contain *l*-desoxyephedrine, another chemical name for *l*-methamphetamine, the weakly active isomer of *d*-methamphetamine. Concentrations approaching 2,000 ng/ml have been seen under experimental and natural conditions. Accordingly, it is necessary for laboratories adopt a new assay to confirm the presence of amphetamines. The most promising derivative reagent is (-)-(trifluoroacetyl)prolyl chloride (TFP). Interpretation of such results can reveal which isomer or isomers were consumed. It also must be recognized that extremely high concentrations of *l*-methamphetamine can result from abuse of the inhalers. It is known that users extract the drug from many inhalers and mainline the residue.

Another amphetamine-like drug, 3,4-methylenedioxy-methamphetamine (MDMA or "Ecstasy") can be detected by some of the commercial immunoassays and confirmed by GC/MS. These assays are routinely conducted by the military but have not become widely available in commercial laboratories. The proposed revision of the DHHS *Mandatory Guidelines* would require testing for MDMA and related drugs.

Alternative Specimens for Testing. The federal government, primarily through the Division of Workplace Programs within the U.S. Department of Health and Human Services (DHHS), has conducted an intensive evaluation of specimens other than urine. Based on information gathered through public conferences, workshops, working groups, and the like, the revised DHHS *Mandatory Guidelines* are expected to permit the use of oral fluids (mixed saliva), sweat, and hair. The guidelines also are expected to permit the testing of urine and oral fluids at the collection site (called "point of collection testing," or POCT) with instrumented or non-instrumented devices or at local instrumented screening laboratories (known as "instrumented initial testing facilities," or IITF). Several drafts of the revised guidelines have been circulated for public comment and DHHS plans formal publication as a Notice of Proposed Rule Making before the end of 2004. Once the revised guidelines are released, they will permit DOT to adopt many or all of these techniques.

In the interim, alternate testing methods are in use outside of federally regulated programs. Employers now can choose from a variety of testing approaches to find the most appropriate specimen for various purposes. For example, testing oral fluids helps to overcome current problems with adulteration in urine testing, as all collections are observed and the ability to dilute or adulterate the specimen is negligible. Hair testing permits a look back at drug use over time. Sweat testing is a facile means of monitoring drug use over time. All of these approaches can be used to create a complementary package to better deter illicit drug use and to help those involved in such use.

REQUIREMENTS FOR RELIABLE LABORATORIES

An obvious requirement for a reliable drug testing program is the use of a laboratory that meets the highest standards. Several factors determine the overall reliability of a laboratory. As noted earlier, there are laboratory accreditation and certification programs specifically designed for laboratories that perform urine drug testing for employment purposes. It is prudent to use only accredited or certified laboratories (see the discussion, following).

Whether certified or not, it is essential to understand what to look for in selecting the best laboratory available. First, the laboratory should be participating in at least one, and preferably all, of the proficiency testing (PT) programs that are available.

It is essential that the laboratory have a written manual of operating procedures, which should include a detailed description of every step in handling and analyzing specimens. Each page should be dated and signed to show that it is continually updated as the laboratory modifies its procedures. The manual must explain everything the laboratory is doing to ensure that test results are properly reviewed and recorded. In addition to the chain of custody procedures used for the collection of specimens, the laboratory must maintain the chain of custody of specimens and test samples during the entire testing process.

The laboratory must inspect each urine container. Each should be assigned a unique identifying number, or accession number, or the one on the label and custody form may be used. Some laboratories place several copies of the same preprinted number on the specimen bottle. These extra labels are used to identify test tubes containing the specimen or any other container. Bar coded labels are widely used to further ensure that accession numbers are not misread or entered incorrectly.

Integrity of the specimen is maintained by labeling specimen and aliquot containers. To maintain chain of custody, the original specimen container should not leave the secured or limited access part of the laboratory. A completely new aliquot must be obtained from the original container when performing a confirmatory or repeat test. Matching the numbers is essential in order to avoid confusing the specimens. Only one specimen container can be open at a time.

Positive specimens should be stored frozen in a secure place and there should be a way to identify everyone who has had access to them. The laboratory also should be able to track exactly where each specimen has been from the time it entered the lab until it was stored. All records associated with the testing should be filed in an easily retrievable yet secure manner.

The staff of the laboratory must, at the very least, meet state requirements. These vary from state to state. The laboratory should have an internal certification program for each staff position and be certified or licensed by the state and one of the appropriate boards or societies. The laboratory should be able to provide access to a well-informed staff capable of offering sound advice about drug testing, selection of appropriate cutoff levels, and interpretation of results.

An important consideration in laboratory selection pertains to the materials the lab will supply. Most will provide all the specimen containers, request forms, evidence tape or sealers for specimen bottles, packaging materials (such as plastic bags and boxes), and mailing or freight forms. Some laboratories also offer overnight courier delivery as part of their service.

Every laboratory should have a comprehensive quality assurance (QA) program that involves constant surveillance of all aspects of laboratory operations, such as staff training and certification, preparation of reagents, internal chain-of-custody procedures, quality control, equipment functions and maintenance, and the reporting of results. Quality control (QC) is a significant part of the QA program. QC is intended to ensure the accuracy of results by including samples with known concentrations with every batch of specimens that is analyzed. Some samples are "open," or known to the operators, allowing them to evaluate the performance of each batch, while other samples are "blind."

Laboratory Certification and Accreditation. An official registry of federally certified drug testing laboratories is compiled by DHHS and published in the *Federal Register*. These laboratories meet the federal standards for performance (proficiency) testing and certification created by the National Institute on Drug Abuse for laboratories engaged in drug testing for federal agencies and employers covered by drug testing regulations issued by DOT, the Nuclear Regulatory Commission, and the Departments of Defense and Energy. The certification program began in October 1987, with 65 laboratories certified through 2001. Even if a company is not required to use one of these certified laboratories, it is sound practice to do so.

REFERENCES

Cody JT & Valtier S (2001). Effects of Stealth® adulterant on immunoassay testing for drugs of abuse. *Journal of Forensic Toxicology* 25:466.

Cody JT, Valtier S & Kuhlman J (2001). Analysis of morphine and codeine in samples adulterated with Stealth®. *Journal of Forensic Toxicology* 25:572.

Cook JD, Caplan YH et al. (2000). The characterization of human urine for specimen validity determination in workplace drug testing: A review. *Journal of Forensic Toxicology* 24:579.

DuPont RL, Griffen DW, Siskin BR et al. (1995). Random drug tests at work: The probability of identifying frequent and infrequent users of illicit drugs. *Journal of Addictive Diseases* 14:1-17.

Johnson BL & Quandar JD (1998). Drug-free workplace programs. In AW Graham & TK Schultz (eds.) *Principles of Addiction Medicine, Second Edition*. Chevy Chase, MD: American Society of Addiction Medicine.

LeBeau MA, Miller ML & Levine B (2001). Effect of storage temperature on endogenous SHB levels in urine. *Forensic Science International* 46:688.

Moore KA, Slerov J et al. (2001). Urine concentration of ketamine and norketamine following illegal consumption. *Journal of Forensic Toxicology* 25:583.

Niedbala RS, Kardos KW et al. (2001a). Detection of marijuana use by oral fluid and urine analysis following single-dose administration of smoked and oral marijuana. *Journal of Forensic Toxicology* 25:289.

Poch GK, Klette KL & Anderson C (2000). The quantitation of 2-oxo-3-hydroxy lysergic acid diethylamide (O-H-LSD) in human urine specimens, a metabolite of LSD: Comparative analysis using liquid chromatography-selected ion monitoring mass spectrometry and liquid chromatography-ion trap mass spectrometry. *Journal of Forensic Toxicology* 24:170.

Sklerov JH, CoMagluilo J et al. (2001). Liquid chromatography-electrospray ionization mass spectrometry for the detection of lysergide and a major metabolite, 2-oxo-3-hydroxy-LSD, in urine and blood. *Journal of Forensic Toxicology* 24:543.

Tsai JSC, el-Sohly MA et al. (2000). Investigation of nitrite adulteration on the immunoassay and GC-MS analysis of cannabinoids in urine specimens. *Journal of Forensic Toxicology* 24:708.

U.S. Department of Health and Human Services (DHHS) (1988). Mandatory guidelines for federal workplace drug testing programs. *Federal Register* 11979-11989; April 11.

Chapter 4

Drug Testing in Addiction Treatment and Criminal Justice Settings

Robert L. DuPont, M.D., FASAM
Carl Selavka, Ph.D., D-ABC

Testing in Treatment and Correctional Settings
The Science of Non-Workplace Drug Testing
Who and When to Test
Selecting a Laboratory
Selecting a Test Specimen

This chapter examines the uses of drug testing in addiction treatment and criminal justice settings. It is designed to complement two related chapters in this volume: Chapter 3 of this section, on drug testing in the workplace, which highlights the complex and continuously evolving rules and regulations encountered in the interpretation of drug testing, and Chapter 3 of Section 3, which discusses the use of laboratory tests in the diagnosis and treatment of substance use disorders.

The chapter does retrace some ground covered in other chapters, particularly those on the MRO and on drug testing in the workplace, but it does so from the perspective of drug testing in addiction treatment and criminal justice settings, both of which are large environments of unique importance to addiction medicine.

TESTING IN TREATMENT AND CORRECTIONAL SETTINGS

Testing for drugs of abuse has a long history in the context of emergency medicine, where the diagnosis of severely impaired, often unconscious, patients is an urgent priority (DuPont, 1997). By the 1960s, medical examiners were routinely testing for drugs of abuse in unexplained deaths.

In the late 1960s, there was a rapid expansion of drug abuse treatment (White, 1998), which led to the routine use of drug testing to identify relapses to non-medical drug use and to validate the effectiveness of the drug abuse treatment process itself (DuPont & Greene, 1973). At the same time, agencies of the criminal justice system began to test for drugs of abuse in a variety of correctional settings (DuPont, 1971).

In the early 1980s, there was an interest in extending drug testing to non-clinical populations to reduce the overall demand for illegal drugs. The first large non-clinical population exposed to drug testing was the U.S. military, which instituted universal random urine drug testing in the wake of the 1981 crash on the aircraft carrier Nimitz. The Navy was alarmed when it found that large numbers of the sailors involved in the accident had been using illicit drugs and medications without prescriptions. Subsequent drug testing found that the other armed services had similarly high levels of non-medical drug use. After random testing was instituted for all members of the armed services, the rate of drug use in the military fell dramatically.

In 1986, when the devastating crack cocaine epidemic began, the national response included the first widespread use of drug testing in the civilian workplace. Based on the earlier success of military drug testing, the primary focus of drug testing in the civilian workforce was on pre-employment testing and on jobs that were safety or security sensitive. Workplace drug testing was codified into federal regulations covering federally regulated industries such as nuclear power and transportation (DHHS, 1988). The 1988 federal guidelines became the *de facto* standard for drug testing in the workplace, although they actually applied only to the narrow segments of the civilian workforce that were subject to federally mandated drug testing. One of the principal concerns of the DHHS *Guidelines* was to distinguish medical from non-medical use of drugs, so as not to put at risk employees who were using legitimately prescribed medications (Macdonald & DuPont, 1998). The development of the role of the Medical Review Officer (MRO) was a major innovation of this federal initiative.

The federal guidelines were a successful effort to capture the best practices in use at the time and to ensure that no employee was falsely accused of using illegal drugs, even at the expense of missing many drug abusers in the drug testing net that was cast in the civilian workforce. In the years since the regulations first were published, there have been only a few minor changes made in the drug testing aspects of the federal standards. This inertia has had the effect of freezing in place most workplace drug testing to the technology, and the political compromises, of the mid-1980s. For example, the federal guidelines address only urine drug tests and then only tests for five drugs: marijuana, cocaine, morphine/codeine, amphetamine/ methamphetamine, and phencyclidine. Because these five drugs were defined as the testing targets by the National Institute on Drug Abuse (NIDA), they often are referred to as the "NIDA 5" or "HHS 5" drugs. Not present on the federal list of drugs to be tested are synthetic opiates (such as methadone, oxycodone, hydrocodone, and meperidine), MDMA, LSD, GHB, barbiturates, benzodiazepines, and literally dozens of other widely abused drugs.

The cutoff levels used in the federally mandated urine drug tests are conservative, reflecting the relatively primitive drug testing technology available in the mid-1980s. While there is an argument for limiting workplace tests to the NIDA 5 drugs, this panel of drugs is far too restrictive for use in drug treatment, where the range of drugs used by patients is wider than the limited five-drug screen.

Because of concerns surrounding possible false identification of workers as drug abusers, federal guidelines for drug tests require a wide range of protections and hold laboratories to the highest levels of forensic practice. Requirements include formal chain-of-custody procedures, immunoassay screens, gas chromatography/mass spectrometry (GC/MS) confirmation, involvement of a Medical Review Officer to interpret positive results, routine laboratory proficiency testing and inspections, and retention of positive urine samples for a year to allow for retesting where the results are in dispute. Such requirements substantially increase the cost of drug testing and seldom are necessary in drug treatment settings.

There are several reasons that standards for drug testing in addiction treatment and criminal justice settings are different from those for workplace testing. In the workplace, a single positive drug test commonly leads to serious consequences, including suspension, mandatory treatment, and termination of employment. Such tests must withstand legal challenges, so employers want the most defensible testing protocols.

Drug testing in addiction treatment and criminal justice settings is different on all counts. First, a single positive drug test is unlikely to have drastic consequences; rather, a pattern of drug test results is more likely to be the reason for action. Second, there seldom is a legal challenge to drug tests in the addiction treatment and criminal justice settings. If a drug test conducted in a treatment setting is challenged, the standard in drug treatment is totally different from the standard in the workplace. Finally, the high costs of workplace protections can be borne by employers, but are unsustainable in resource-constrained treatment programs and criminal justice systems.

Although testing in addiction treatment and criminal justice settings is not governed by the 1988 DHHS guidelines for workplace drug testing, many laboratories focus their work on urine tests, and then only for the HHS 5 drugs. Similarly, many commercial laboratories limit their cutoff levels to those incorporated in the federal guidelines. The development of the entire drug testing field has been inhibited by these static and restrictive general guidelines. Following the federal guidelines does confer some protection on employers and others concerned about possible legal challenges to their drug testing programs. However, these modest legal protections are accompanied by the significant costs attendant on reduced detection of active users of illicit drugs and greatly increased testing costs.

There have been dramatic developments in drug testing technology over the past 15 years. Most early tests were time- and labor-intensive, relatively insensitive, and non-selective. The science of drug testing has progressed so that drugs of abuse (or, in the case of marijuana and cocaine, their metabolites) can be identified reliably at much lower concentrations. There also have been rapid developments in the ability to test for drugs of abuse in biological matrices other than blood and urine.

Drug testing once required large, highly sophisticated, and expensive equipment. Two decades ago, it took days for highly trained scientists to complete testing on a single sample. Such testing was a minor part of the work of clinical laboratories. However, the heightened interest in the identification of drugs of abuse, coupled with concern over the reliability of test results, has lifted the practice of clinical chemistry in general. More rigorous scientific processes and routine quality assurance testing have become commonplace.

Today reliable, low-cost, on-site testing is available. In modern laboratories, the drug testing process has been computerized and mechanized so that sensitivity and reliability have increased while costs have declined dramatically. All of these changes in the science and the practice of drug testing have important implications for the users of drug tests, including physicians who work in the addiction treatment and criminal justice systems. Specifically, improved drug testing technology—with lower costs, the ability to identify more drugs, and increased reliability—have solidified and expanded the roles of drug testing in addiction treatment and criminal justice settings.

THE SCIENCE OF NON-WORKPLACE DRUG TESTING

On any given day, about 1 million Americans are in addiction treatment, while another 4 million are under the supervision of an agency of the criminal justice system (ONDCP, 2000). All of the treatment population, and more than half of the criminal justice population, use illegal drugs to produce what is recognized today as brain reward (DuPont & Gold, 1995). Whether the drug is smoked, snorted, swallowed, injected, or taken in any other way, the reward-inducing chemicals enter the user's bloodstream, which rapidly transports the chemicals to the target organ: the mid-brain pleasure centers (DuPont, 2000). Once in the body, drugs of abuse are not limited to acting in the blood and the brain. Rather, they are distributed rapidly to all parts of the body. For this reason, they can be identified in every tissue, from vital organs like the liver and kidneys

to sweat, hair, and fingernails. Ethyl alcohol, because it is volatile, also is easily detected in the user's breath, while no other commonly used drug of abuse is found in breath samples.

In the 1980s, urine was the standard biological matrix for drug detection because the kidneys concentrate drugs and other substances removed from blood and because urine is easily obtained (compared to blood, which was the primary biological fluid used in emergency departments and by medical examiners in early drug detection efforts). To penetrate the blood-brain barrier, abused drugs generally are highly lipid-soluble. The lack of water solubility of drugs of abuse retards their removal from the blood by the kidneys.

Abused drugs are metabolized primarily in the liver to more water-soluble metabolites. These metabolites are rapidly removed by the kidneys from the blood into the urine. While most drugs of abuse are cleared from the blood to relatively low levels within a few hours of administration, metabolites of abused drugs typically are detected in the urine for up to one to three days after the last drug use. The urine of many drug users tests negative for drugs of abuse at standard cutoff levels less than 48 hours after their last drug use. This is true except when prior drug use has been heavy and chronic, in which case urine samples may test positive for somewhat longer periods of time. Even under the circumstance of heavy chronic use, however, urine tests usually are negative for abused drugs within a week of the last drug use. The exception to this general rule is marijuana, for which heavy chronic use can produce a positive urine test for up to a month in the most extreme cases. However, most individuals who occasionally use marijuana produce negative urine test results at standard cutoffs within one to three days of their last use of the drug.

The cells that generate hair, fingernails, and toenails incorporate drugs and drug metabolites that are in the blood at the time the tissues are produced. Therefore, the tissues represent the equivalent of an historical record of drug ingestion. Head hair grows at a rate of about half an inch per month, so a hair sample 1.5 inches long contains a record of drug use over approximately the preceding 90 days. Therefore, routine use of hair testing in the treatment setting can significantly increase the amount of information available to clinicians (Paterson, McLachlan-Troup et al., 2001).

Fingernails take several months to grow out from root to end, so scrapings from fingernails contain an even longer record of drug use (Lemos, Anderson et al., 2000; Ropero-Miller, Goldberger et al., 2000). Toenails grow even more slowly, so they contain a record of drug use over an even longer period of time.

Because drugs clear from the blood rapidly, testing of blood, serum and plasma offers the shortest window of detection for drug use—usually less than 24 hours. Urine has a detection window of one to three days, while hair and nails provide much longer windows. Testing of oral fluids (saliva mixed with other fluid found in the mouth) affords a detection window that approximates that of blood (Niedbala, Kardos et al., 2001a, 2001b), while sweat testing affords a detection window that is variable, depending on how long the sweat patch collection device is worn—generally, one to two weeks (Moody & Cheever, 2001; Huestis, Cone et al., 2001; O'Neal, Crouch et al., 2001). Sweat testing using a direct method (Crouch, Cook et al., 2001), even in an office setting (Kintz, Cirimele et al., 2000), also is possible for some drugs.

Immunoassays and Mass Spectrometry. Achieving the goal of forensic defensibility in drug testing requires the use of more than one analysis by different techniques in order to report a positive result. Use of an inexpensive preliminary screening test lowers the overall cost of analysis, since most tested individuals have negative initial results. To fulfill the requirements of high accuracy and low cost, samples first are tested using sensitive, relatively inexpensive immunoassay techniques. When immunoassay screening tests are positive, a more specific and more expensive confirmatory detection technique is used. The most widely used confirmatory method couples a separation technique—gas chromatography (GC)—with a highly selective identification technique—mass spectrometry (MS)—which are combined in the extremely powerful GC/MS technique.

Immunoassays employ antibodies that selectively bind to drugs and/or drug metabolites. Generally, drug test immunoassays set up competition between the target drug/metabolite and a roughly equivalent chemical that facilitates highly sensitive detection. This detection step following the drug/metabolite-antibody interaction may use enzymes, latex agglutination, fluorescence, chemilluminescence, radioactivity, or simple color reactions to determine the approximate concentration of the drug/metabolite in the tested sample. Such testing produces a semiquantitative result with the screening immunoassay test. Laboratories have many inexpensive, automated immunoassay options available to rapidly rule out or presumptively indicate the presence of drugs/metabolites. However, immunoassays respond to many substances that have similar chemical structures. Because of their high sensitivity and low specificity, negative results from immunoassay can be trusted, but a presumptively positive immunoassay result must be confirmed through use of a more specific method.

GC/MS is recognized as the "gold standard" for routine confirmation of positive drug test results. Confirmatory testing for drugs of abuse begins with chemical extraction of drugs/metabolites from urine, hair, a sweat patch, or an oral fluid collection device. This extraction pre-concentrates the target substances, increasing the already high sensitivity of this method. Then the extracted sample is introduced into the GC, where it is vaporized before undergoing chromatographic separation. Separated components are automatically introduced into the mass spectrometer, which creates unique identifiable fragments of each drug/metabolite. This step has extremely high specificity. When all GC/MS quality parameters are met, it is virtually impossible to generate false-positive results; that is, a positive result without the presence of a specific drug or drug metabolite. GC/MS drug test results are specific to the chemical identified, with virtually no possibility of cross-reactivity or a false positive identification of a single, specific drug or drug metabolite.

Confirmatory tests add significantly to the cost of drug testing and seldom are justified in addiction treatment and criminal justice settings (although they may be necessary when a single drug test result is likely to have serious consequences and/or be subject to legal challenge). In lieu of routine confirmatory testing or the use of Medical Review Officers, staff of the treatment program or correctional facility may inform test subjects not to use over-the-counter cold preparations containing stimulants because they can trigger an immunoassay test positive for amphetamines or methamphetamines. Similarly, they may advise subjects to refrain from eating poppy seeds, which can produce a test result that is positive for opiates. These are reasonable ways to manage the limitations of the immunoassay screen without resort to routine laboratory confirmation. Nevertheless, it is prudent to have in place a process for dealing with disputed drug test results that includes re-testing samples, testing new samples, and/or testing hair samples that cover the period in dispute.

On-site Versus Laboratory Tests. On-site drug tests are available for urine and oral fluids. On-site urine tests have been subject to significant scientific and regulatory review, which has detected wide variations in quality. Several manufacturers have emerged as providers of reasonably accurate devices for on-site applications. Careful review of the literature (Peace, Tarnai et al., 2000) or discussion with a toxicologist involved in clinical and workplace applications of on-site urine testing is useful before implementing such an approach. On-site testing of oral fluids is relatively new and significant hurdles to its widespread use remain. The biggest drawback to testing of oral fluids is that such tests are relatively insensitive to marijuana, although they reliably detect cocaine, methamphetamine, and heroin. On-site testing of hair and sweat patches are not yet available but are technically feasible and therefore likely to become commonplace during the next 5 to 10 years.

Most on-site test devices are regulated by the U.S. Food and Drug Administration (FDA), so they must meet certain standards for accuracy, precision, and linearity of response at specific cutoff levels for drugs/metabolites in urine or oral fluids. Because FDA-cleared devices are not subject to ongoing review by the FDA, manufacturing issues have arisen with some cleared devices in the past. Therefore, an important programmatic feature of all on-site drug testing applications in the workplace is the routine forwarding of all positive and selected negative samples to a laboratory, to confirm the on-site results and ensure that the overall testing program meets forensic standards. This expensive step is not necessary in most treatment and criminal justice contexts. However, even in treatment and criminal justice settings, it is desirable to send a group of both positive and negative samples off-site for confirmation to verify that the on-site drug testing device is producing acceptable results. If the validity of the on-site results is not supported, use of the specific on-site approach should be reconsidered.

On-site drug testing is used in workplace programs to rapidly cull out negative specimens and identify presumptively positive specimens for further confirmatory testing. This is effective because, in many workplace settings, more than 95% of samples are negative for drug use. Forensic toxicology laboratories repeat the initial screening test using immunoassays and then confirm presumptive positive results through the use of GC/MS or another competent molecular identification method. This is necessary because on-site devices do not provide forensically defensible results. On the other hand, for most substances, the on-site results are confirmed, so policies can be implemented to remove the subjects quickly from safety-sensitive positions, pending the results of laboratory confirmation tests.

Most drug abuse treatment programs and agencies of the criminal justice system find on-site tests useful and seldom need to confirm results except in special cases. On-site drug tests cover only a limited number of abusable drugs, with a single cutoff for each class of drug. The cost of such tests on a "per drug class" basis generally is higher than equivalent laboratory services when laboratories are used to confirm the initial test finding prior to reporting. Therefore, when flexibility is needed in a drug treatment program or in the criminal justice system, on-site drug tests may not meet the need. In general, on-site drug testing is helpful in post-accident testing and in other scenarios where results are needed immediately. Certain other situations in prisons, probation and parole settings, and in specific clinical applications also may use on-site tests to advantage.

It is important to recognize that on-site urine drug testing retains the shortcomings of laboratory-based urine testing, such as a short detection window, vulnerability to cheating (adulteration, substitution and interfering adulteration), inability to detect heroin use because of the poppy seed problem, absence of tests for drugs other than the HHS 5, and privacy concerns at collection. In addition, on-site testing introduces problems not present in laboratory testing, such as reduced accuracy and ambiguity of handling the immunoassay positive result pending laboratory confirmation. None of these problems is an absolute barrier to on-site testing in addiction treatment and criminal justice settings. Nevertheless, consultation with an attorney, a qualified third party administrator, and a toxicologist is helpful when implementing on-site testing.

WHO AND WHEN TO TEST

Because testing for abused drugs, even using unconfirmed urine tests, is expensive in the context of drug treatment and the criminal justice system, a cost-benefit strategy is needed to guide the testing process. The basic concept is that either a test with a long detection window is used (for example, a sweat patch covering several weeks or a hair test covering up to three months) or urine testing is performed on a frequent random basis so that the population is subject to drug testing at any time. Heavy drug users will be positive at nearly all times on all tests. Intermittent users present a more difficult challenge. One study (DuPont, Griffen et al., 1995) showed that random urine tests are highly effective in identifying regular users of any illegal drug, but that they must be repeated often to identify occasional users.

A test with a long detection window is most appropriate for subjects at low risk of drug use, while frequent random urine tests are appropriate for high-risk subjects, such as those early in the treatment process. Sweat patch and hair tests are more resistant to cheating, which can be a major advantage.

Before an individual enters addiction treatment, at the time of the initial evaluation, it often is desirable to conduct a hair test because tests of hair (and sweat patches) permit a rough estimation of the frequency of drug use, making it possible to distinguish between an individual who uses a drug only occasionally and an individual who uses a drug intensively and continuously. Moreover, the use of sequential segments of a hair sample from a given patient permits the determination of the relative drug use history for the tested individual month-by-month over several months. Such segmental analysis of a hair sample is not often necessary, but it is useful in some clinical settings.

There are several points in the criminal justice system at which early surveillance with an appropriate drug test can provide the information needed to plan appropriate interventions and ongoing evaluation. For example, testing drug offenders at the point of arrest or arraignment can provide judges in rapid resolution programs (including the popular "drug court" systems) with information that is useful in introducing a drug treatment component into the offender's sentence. Urine drug tests usually are employed, which can cause an issue for the court if the time from arrest to arraignment should include a weekend or other period greater than two or three days, because a negative urine test at the time of arraignment no longer reliably represents the drug use status at the time of arrest. A better strategy would be to use either urinalysis closer to the time of arrest, or to replace the urine test with a hair test. The cost of hair tests, although greater than that of urinalysis, is offset by the significantly greater reliability of this method of testing.

Testing of probationers and parolees has long use in improving the outcomes of these intermediate "conditional releases." When such testing includes random, frequent urinalysis for the appropriate classes of drugs, lower relapse rates are seen. On the other hand, it would be far more cost effective and easier to manage a program for probation and parole officers if sweat tests or hair tests were employed. The need for routine contact to collect samples is the greatest cost and liability of programs for parolees and probationers, and both hair and sweat tests require less frequent contact between probation officers and their assigned

populations. While the argument often is made that contact should be frequent enough to allow for routine urinalysis without additional burden, the reality—especially in times of straitened fiscal circumstances—is that parole officers' contacts with offenders occurs far less frequently than most program managers would prefer and that frequent urine drug test programs would require.

Drug testing among incarcerated individuals is widespread, often involves on-site urinalysis, and has demonstrated episodic success in reducing or eradicating drug use in prisons and jails. The reduced cost of on-site testing (compared to laboratory testing) is accompanied by the problem of testing by less qualified individuals and a lack of control over sample collection and integrity. More importantly, poor followup skills on the part of contract medical staff or administrators ill-prepared to deal with drug issues, or facing the reality that positive results indicate a continued problem of drug infiltration, can lead to questionable practices that undercut the effectiveness of the program. Examples include announced tests (which allow time to stop drug use prior to urine collection), non-random selection (so that tests can be anticipated or avoided), or the use of on-site devices made for emergency medical settings, which employ higher cutoff values than do tests more appropriately used in correctional settings.

SELECTING A LABORATORY

Several significant choices must be made when considering the laboratory or laboratories employed for drug testing services in addiction treatment and criminal justice settings. While cost is an important factor, it may be even more important to consider specific needs for materials provided, testing timeliness, scope of available drug testing, access to toxicology experts, and specific quality assurance and accreditation elements. Most commercial clinical laboratories can turn around reports for negatives in urine testing within 48 hours. However, positive drug test reports may take as long as five to seven days. This is one component of a drug testing service that must be carefully contracted. Larger laboratories tend to have shorter positive reporting times, but the availability of some other services (such as specialized reporting and different cutoff levels) and access to experts generally are more problematic with larger laboratories.

At present, no single laboratory offers drug testing of all matrices (hair, sweat, oral fluids, and urine). Therefore, to maintain flexibility and reduce costs, programs must use multiple laboratories and suppliers.

The federal government has an accreditation standard that must be met by laboratories that provide testing for federally mandated testing programs. While the number of federally mandated drug tests is a small fraction of the total number of workplace tests conducted each year, the National Laboratory Certification Program (NLCP), which is governed by DHHS-promulgated standards, may be used to differentiate the 60+ laboratories that have obtained NLCP certification from all others. It is important to stress that NLCP accreditation currently only covers urine drug testing for the HHS 5 drugs, although DHHS is in the process of promulgating similar accreditation standards for oral fluids, hair, sweat, and on-site urine drug tests. Many excellent laboratories are not NLCP-accredited, primarily because they do not seek out contracts for federally mandated testing or because they use matrices other than urine.

Most laboratories that perform hair testing are not NLCP accredited, yet many have instituted sophisticated quality assurance features similar to those of certified laboratories. Such laboratories can provide forensically defensible results. Since NLCP accreditation covers only urine testing for the HHS 5 drugs, clinicians who use drug testing for other drugs of abuse must seek out laboratories which, although potentially NLCP-accredited, cannot necessarily provide the same level of quality in testing for the non-NLCP drugs. Careful review of services for the other drugs is essential before contracting with such laboratories.

SELECTING A TEST SPECIMEN

In both the addiction treatment and criminal justice systems, urine is the standard matrix for drug tests for many reasons, including familiarity, cost, and the range of abused substances that can be identified. Two problems that are serious disadvantages of urine testing in the workplace are less of a problem in treatment or criminal justice settings. The first is the problem of cheating. This is a major issue in the workplace because observed collection is rarely used, while it is routinely used in treatment and criminal justice testing. Second, the poppy seed problem virtually eliminates the value of opiate testing in the workplace. This is not a problem in treatment or criminal justice settings because test subjects are advised not to eat poppy seeds.

In contrast, sweat, oral fluids, and hair offer unique advantages in some situations. Sweat patch testing is uniquely valuable in monitoring individuals 24 hours a day when patches are changed every week or two. Hair testing is particularly valuable in testing over longer periods of time

in low-risk settings (an entire year can be monitored with just four tests). Oral fluids are easy to collect, which is especially useful for on-site testing for cocaine or heroin. On the other hand, oral fluids rarely detect marijuana, because oral pH and other factors make the low concentration of THC metabolites difficult to detect. These alternative matrices have not been well-integrated into testing protocols, although they are expected to be more widely used in the future.

Few commercial drug testing laboratories today routinely test for MDMA (Caplan & Goldberger, 2001), ketamine (Logan, 2001), oxycodone, GHB (LeBeau, Miller et al., 2001; Kalasinsky, Dixon et al., 2001), and LSD (Poch, Klette et al., 2000; Sklerov, CoMagluilo et al., 2001), even though all of these drugs are widely abused and laboratory methods of testing for them have been validated.

CONCLUSIONS

The range of drug tests available to clinicians is expanding rapidly as the sensitivity of the tests increases and the cost of the tests declines. Drug testing will become even easier and less expensive in the future. This will place the responsibility for deciding who to test, when to test, and how to test where it belongs, on the addiction medicine physician, who then can determine how best to achieve the goals of the addiction treatment and criminal justice systems.

In the future, the limiting factors in drug testing are less likely to be scientific than political and regulatory. The political problem involves significant privacy concerns. Regulatory problems relate primarily to workplace testing. Neither is relevant to drug testing in addiction treatment or criminal justice settings.

The future of drug testing lies outside these boundaries, established more than a decade ago, in the domain of multiple matrices, an expanded scope of target drugs, and appropriate use of on-site testing applications.

REFERENCES

Caplan YH & Goldberger BA (2001). Alternative specimens for workplace drug testing. *Journal of Forensic Toxicology* 25:396. (Author's note: The information in this article already had been overtaken by events at the time of publication, but it represents the most recent peer-reviewed article available on federal standard-setting. For current information, refer to the DHHS web site [HTTP://WORKPLACE.SAMHSA.GOV] or a toxicologist familiar with alternate matrix specialties.)

Cody JT & Valtier S (2001). Effects of Stealth® adulterant on immunoassay testing for drugs of abuse. *Journal of Forensic Toxicology* 25:466.

Cody JT, Valtier S & Kuhlman J (2001). Analysis of morphine and codeine in samples adulterated with Stealth®. *Journal of Forensic Toxicology* 25:572.

Cook JD, Caplan YH et al. (2000). The characterization of human urine for specimen validity determination in workplace drug testing: A review. *Journal of Forensic Toxicology* 24:579.

Crouch DJ, Cook RF et al. (2001). The detection of drugs of abuse in liquid perspiration. *Journal of Forensic Toxicology* 25:625.

DuPont RL (1997). Drug testing. In NS Miller, MS Gold & DE Smith (eds.) *Manual of Therapeutics for Addictions.* New York, NY: Wiley-Liss, Inc.

DuPont RL (1971). Profile of a heroin-addiction epidemic. *New England Journal of Medicine* 285:320-324.

DuPont RL (2000). *The Selfish Brain—Learning from Addiction.* Rochester, MN: Hazelden.

DuPont RL & Gold MS (1995). Withdrawal and reward: Implications for detoxification and relapse prevention. *Psychiatric Annals* 25:663-668.

DuPont RL & Greene MH (1973). The dynamics of a heroin addiction epidemic. *Science* 181:716-722.

DuPont RL, Griffen DW, Siskin BR et al. (1995). Random drug tests at work: The probability of identifying frequent and infrequent users of illicit drugs. *Journal of Addictive Diseases* 14:1-17.

Huestis MA, Cone EJ et al. (2001). Monitoring opiate use in substance abuse treatment patients with sweat and urine drug testing. *Journal of Forensic Toxicology* 24:609.

Kalasinsky KS, Dixon MM et al. (2001). Blood, brain, and hair GHB concentrations following fatal overdose. *Journal of Forensic Science* 46:728.

Kintz P, Cirimele V, Ludes B et al. (2000). Detection of cannabis in oral fluid (saliva) and forehead wipes (sweat) from impaired drivers. *Journal of Forensic Toxicology* 25:144.

LeBeau MA, Miller ML & Levine B (2001). Effect of storage temperature on endogenous SHB levels in urine. *Forensic Science International* 46:688.

Lemos NP, Anderson RA & Robertson JR (2000). The analysis of methadone in nail clippings from patients in a methadone-maintenance program. *Journal of Forensic Toxicology* 24:656.

Logan BK (2001). Amphetamines: An update on forensic issues. *Journal of Forensic Toxicology* 25:583.

Macdonald DI & DuPont RL (1998). The role of the medical review officer. In AW Graham & TK Schultz (eds.) *Principles of Addiction Medicine, Second Edition.* Chevy Chase, MD: American Society of Addiction Medicine.

Massing M (1998). *The Fix: Under the Nixon Administration, America Had an Effective Drug Policy—We Should Restore It (Nixon Was Right).* New York, NY: Simon & Schuster.

Moody DE & Cheever ML (2001). Evaluation of immunoassays for semiquantitative detection of cocaine and metabolite or heroin and metabolites in extracts of sweat patches. *Journal of Forensic Toxicology* 25:190.

Moore KA, Slerov J et al. (2001). Urine concentration of ketamine and norketamine following illegal consumption. *Journal of Forensic Toxicology* 25:583.

Niedbala RS, Kardos KW et al. (2001a). Detection of marijuana use by oral fluid and urine analysis following single-dose administration of smoked and oral marijuana. *Journal of Forensic Toxicology* 25:289.

Niedbala RS, Kardos KW et al. (2001b). Immunoassay for detection of cocaine metabolites in oral fluids. *Journal of Forensic Toxicology* 25:62.

Office of National Drug Control Policy (ONDCP) (2000). *National Drug Control Strategy—2000 Annual Report.* Washington, DC: ONDCP, Executive Office of the President, The White House.

O'Neal CL, Crouch DJ et al. (2001). The effects of collection methods on oral fluid codeine concentrations. *Journal of Forensic Toxicology* 24:536.

Paterson S, McLachlan-Troup N et al. (2001). Qualitative screening of drugs of abuse in hair using GC-MS. *Journal of Forensic Toxicology* 25:203.

Peace MR, Tarnai LD & Poklis A (2000). Performance evaluation of four on-site drug-testing devices for detection of drugs of abuse in urine. *Journal of Forensic Toxicology* 24:589.

Poch GK, Klette KL & Anderson C (2000). The quantitation of 2-oxo-3-hydroxy lysergic acid diethylamide (O-H-LSD) in human urine specimens, a metabolite of LSD: Comparative analysis using liquid chromatography-selected ion monitoring mass spectrometry and liquid chromatography-ion trap mass spectrometry. *Journal of Forensic Toxicology* 24:170.

Ropero-Miller JD, Goldberger BA et al. (2000). The disposition of cocaine and opiate analytes in hair and fingernails of humans following cocaine and codeine administration. *Journal of Forensic Toxicology* 24:496.

Sklerov JH, CoMagluilo J et al. (2001). Liquid chromatography-electrospray ionization mass spectrometry for the detection of lysergide and a major metabolite, 2-oxo-3-hydroxy-LSD, in urine and blood. *Journal of Forensic Toxicology* 24:543.

Tsai JSC, el-Sohly MA et al. (2000). Investigation of nitrite adulteration on the immunoassay and GC-MS analysis of cannabinoids in urine specimens. *Journal of Forensic Toxicology* 24:708.

U.S. Department of Health and Human Services (DHHS) (1988). Mandatory guidelines for federal workplace drug testing programs. *Federal Register* 11979-11989; April 11.

White WL (1998). *Slaying the Dragon—The History of Addiction Treatment and Recovery in America.* Philadelphia, PA: Chestnut Health Systems—Lighthouse Institute.

Chapter 5

Physician Health Programs and the Addicted Physician

G. Douglas Talbott, M.D., FACP, FASAM
Paul H. Earley, M.D., FASAM

Substance Use Disorders
Relapse to Alcohol or Drug Use

In the general population in the United States, the lifetime prevalence of any substance abuse or dependence disorder has been estimated to be 26.6% (14.4% for alcohol dependence and 7.5% for drug dependence (Kessler, 1994). Experts suggest that the lifetime risk for physicians is somewhat higher. Some of this risk is related to access to drugs in the course of medical practice, particularly when those drugs are dispensed or administered directly by the physician. Thus, dependence on controlled drugs has been described as an "occupational hazard" for physicians.

Within medicine, subtler differences appear: for example, the literature indicates that the proportion of female physicians hospitalized for substance-related disorders has increased in recent years, while medical residents in anesthesiology and psychiatry experience higher rates of substance use than do residents in other specialties.

SUBSTANCE USE DISORDERS

Although the alcohol or drug addict may focus his or her attention on different substances with varied toxic effects, addiction specialists view substance dependence as a single disease with multiple and varying presentations. Substance dependence is a chronic disorder whose genetic, psycho-logical, social, family, and environmental factors influence both its inception and its course. It is characterized by:

- Continuous or periodic loss of control over drinking or drug use (compulsivity is a primary symptom of the disease).

- Preoccupation with the use of alcohol or other drugs despite adverse consequences.

- Distortions in thinking, most notably denial.

Substance dependence can occur alone, but also appears in combination with other medical or psychiatric illnesses and develops a complex interaction with these concomitant disorders. Left untreated, substance dependence is progressive and often fatal.

The affected physician rarely recognizes substance dependence as a problem in his or her life until secondary consequences occur in the realms of profession, family, legal status, or health. Even at that point, most impaired physicians view their substance use as a product of other difficulties, rather than as the cause.

Patterns of Substance Use and Addiction in Physicians. The relationship between substance use and addiction is not linear, but an increase in substance use in a physician population is likely to correlate with an increase in the incidence of addictive disease in that population. Access also plays a critical role in the type of drug(s) used and abused. For example, emergency physicians appear more likely to use illicit drugs, while psychiatrists use more benzodiazepines than do physicians in other specialties.

The specific drug(s) of abuse also influence the course of the disorder in terms of how it emerges and progresses. For example, anesthesiologists often appear in treatment addicted to the synthetic opioid agent fentanyl (Sublimaze®) or similar agents. A drug commonly used in anesthesiology, fentanyl is associated with the rapid development of substance dependence. Physicians addicted to it typically develop intense tolerance and drug-seeking behavior over a series of months rather than years. Nevertheless, relapse rates among anesthesiologists addicted to fentanyl are comparable to relapse rates for other physicians who participate in a well-designed Physician Health Program.

Protocol. The care of substance-abusing physicians has three components: (1) comprehensive assessment, (2) detoxification, medical stabilization, and primary treatment, and (3) long-term continuing care and monitoring.

Comprehensive Assessment: A comprehensive assessment by one or more professionals experienced in the evaluation of addiction and its concomitant problems in physicians, and approved by the state medical licensing board or the Physician Health Program, is necessary to determine if professional impairment or potential impairment is present.

The assessment should determine, with a reasonable degree of medical certainty, whether the physician is impaired or potentially impaired because of habitual or excessive use of controlled drugs, alcohol, or other substances. Any coexisting physical or mental problems also should be reported, including an opinion as to whether such problems may have contributed significantly to the events leading to the assessment. Mental disorders and substance use diagnoses should conform to *DSM-IV* criteria (American Psychiatric Association, 1994).

The assessment team also must determine whether issues involving public health and safety or violations of ethical standards require that the physician be reported to the medical board, if a report has not already been made.

If there is controversy or contention over the events leading to an intervention and professional impairment is suspected, assessment by a team approved by the board or

Physician Health Program should include evaluations by specialists in addiction medicine, psychology and neuropsychiatry, and psychiatry. Regardless of whether the referral was made by the Physician Health Program or the medical board, the physician must agree to provide a written authorization for full disclosure of information arising from the assessment to the board, the program, or both. Failure to comply with such a request should precipitate an immediate report to the medical board. Physicians who self-report for assessment or treatment are referred to the Physician Health Program during treatment. Depending on the severity of the addictive disease and concomitant morbidity, some physicians may need to report directly to the medical board as well as to the Physician Health Program.

At the time the initial assessment is completed, if all parties agree that substance dependence is present and the physician agrees to proceed with treatment, he or she may elect to begin treatment immediately at the assessment facility. However, the physician also should have the option of beginning treatment at a facility other than where the assessment was performed, so long as the other facility is approved by the medical board as appropriate for the care of physicians with addictive disorders.

If, on the other hand, the physician denies that substance use is present, but the assessor (or assessment team) believes that substance dependence is in fact present, the physician may proceed to a second independent assessment. If the case does not involve a complaint or report to the medical board, the medical director of the Physician Health Program generally is directly involved in determining where the second assessment will occur. If the case does involve a complaint or report to the medical board, the board will be involved as a concerned party in selecting the time and place for the second assessment.

Assessment results should be given to the medical board only with the physician's written consent.

Detoxification, Medical Stabilization, and Primary Treatment: When a physician is assessed as having impairment or potential impairment, he or she is required to satisfactorily complete primary treatment in a program approved by the medical board and the Physician Health Program.

Multidisciplinary addiction treatment is aimed at reducing denial; increasing self-care; treating the coexisting family, medical, and psychiatric problems; and helping the physician learn to protect himself or herself from the addictive disorder. Comprehensive treatment typically involves

TABLE 1. 16 Areas of Progress in Recovery

1. Meetings
2. Sponsor
3. Monitoring
4. Emotional traps (anger, guilt, depression, anxiety, insomnia)
5. Additions to/subtractions from the addiction history (secrets)
6. Compulsive behavior (sex, food, nicotine, gambling, theft, spending)
7. Current therapy/treatment/medications (prescribed and over-the-counter)
8. Relationships (family, spouse, parents, children, friends)
9. Physical health/exercise program
10. Leisure time/fun
11. Work (professional status, duties, attitudes)
12. Financial status
13. Legal/licensure status
14. Additional training and/or continuing medical education
15. Spiritual program
16. "Soft" part of the recovery program.

SOURCE: GD Talbott & LR Crosby, eds. (2001). *Problem Physicians: A National Perspective* (A Report to the Georgia Composite State Board of Medical Examiners).

individual and group therapy, Twelve Step or other spiritual programs, medication as needed, written assignments, psychoeducation, family education and therapy, and workplace/lifestyle restructuring.

Most treatment facilities use the patient placement criteria of the American Society of Addiction Medicine (*ASAM PPC-2R*; Mee-Lee, Shulman et al., 2001) to guide decisions about the intensity and duration of services required. It generally is accepted, however, that physicians require a longer duration of treatment, preferably in a treatment milieu with expertise in treating physicians and other health care professionals. The presence of comorbid medical or psychiatric conditions also may prolong the primary treatment. Other reasons for a longer duration of treatment include:

- Physicians must meet a higher standard for recovery because of concerns about public safety.

- The credibility of the physician community is endangered by a single physician's relapse.

- Addicted physicians are quite clever at concealing their illness and mimicking good recovery skills, so a somewhat prolonged treatment process may be necessary to help the physician to incorporate and internalize genuine recovery skills.

Of course, if the physician remains impaired or potentially impaired at the completion of primary treatment, extended treatment is required.

In any case, when the patient is discharged from treatment, he or she must sign a written authorization to provide full disclosure of the treatment records to the medical board or the Physician Health Program. Failure to comply with this request typically precipitates an immediate report to the medical board.

Continuing Care and Monitoring: On successful completion of primary treatment and, when necessary, extended residential care, the physician enters into continuing care. While tailored to each physician's needs, such care generally involves individual, group, and family therapy. (Group therapy, some of which involves physician peers, has been shown to be the most effective method of reducing denial and orienting the physician to a lifestyle that reduces the risk of relapse.)

Attendance at peer group meetings, analysis of bodily fluids, and participation in recovery-based therapy and support groups also are important. Most physician support groups are modeled after Twelve Step programs such as Alcoholics Anonymous (AA) and Narcotics Anonymous (NA), with additional spiritual support systems as needed.

Continuing care is performed under an agreement called a "continuing care contract" or "monitoring agreement" (samples of which are presented in Appendices 1 and 2, following). Such agreements cover, at a minimum:

- Continuing care therapy to be delivered;

- Attendance at mutual help group meetings;

- Bodily fluid analysis;

- Modifications in the physician's professional practice;

- Practice monitoring by peers/others;

- Additional continuing care assignments;

- Protocols to be followed if the physician should require mood-altering drugs for a medical problem;

- Contingencies that will occur should a patient relapse to substance use; and

- Names of individuals who will support the physician in his or her ongoing recovery.

If a physician has not been reported to the medical board, the contract is between the physician and the Physician Health Program. In all other cases, the contract is under the purview of the medical board. If a physician has a coexisting mental disorder, additional contractual provisions may be necessary.

Structured posttreatment monitoring should be provided to recovering physicians for at least five years. In this regard, ongoing review of recovery progress is helpful (Table 1).

Board Considerations. The medical board's first priority is to assure the safety of patients. In addition, the board may encourage a physician to seek professional help and rehabilitation. Physician health programs or other therapeutic programs geared to this type of problem manage many cases in which a physician seeks help with substance abuse, at least initially. When impairment rises to the level that a physician must cease practicing temporarily and seek either inpatient or intensive outpatient treatment, the impaired physician is obliged to report this treatment to the board.

If impairment is the only issue, and the physician self-reports, the physician may be asked to sign an agreement not to resume practice without the approval of the treatment team and the board. In such a case, the physician must appear before the Impairment Committee of the board and present evidence that he or she can practice with reasonable skill and safety. A private, nondisciplinary consent order may be entered into with the board before the physician is allowed to resume practice. Such an order generally involves 5 years of monitoring, as well as terms and conditions specific to the physician's case.

If there are complaints that the physician has violated the law or harmed patients in the course of his or her impairment, a full investigation should be initiated. If the evidence supports the allegations, appropriate public sanctions may be imposed.

RELAPSE TO ALCOHOL OR DRUG USE

An addicted physician who returns to practice does so under the presumption that he or she can practice with skill and safety. A relapse—while not unexpected in a chronic, relapsing disorder—entails consequences that are especially severe for recovering physicians, particularly in terms of legal and public safety concerns.

In fact, return to use of addicting substances is the final incident in a series of events that defines a relapse. Prior to the chemical relapse, the addicted physician commonly exhibits characteristic behaviors that signal an impending return to alcohol or drug use. Any use of addicting chemicals by a recovering physician probably indicates a significant reoccurrence of illness and demands careful scrutiny.

In diagnosing a relapse, the following facts should be considered:

- Abnormalities in emotional behavior often precede relapse (in the language of AA, this is "stinking thinking").

- Relapse may be partial (a slip) with limited consequences, or may be defined as sustained partial remission.

- The risk of relapse never ends. Relapse can occur at any time in an individual who has an addictive disorder.

- The more comprehensive the monitoring during the first 5 years after treatment, the less the chance of relapse.

Denial, shame, and fear of consequences following return to use of mood-altering substances prevent many relapsing physicians from seeking help. Nevertheless, it is imperative that a relapsing physician be detected and helped as soon as possible. Clinical experience across multiple treatment centers suggests that physicians who relapse often exhibit a very rapid downhill course. Swift intervention can prevent dire consequences, including risk of harm to self or others. Allowing a relapsing physician to continue in his or her medical practice not only puts patients and the public at risk, but also may lead to serious physical and emotional consequences to the relapsing physician, many of whom commit suicide or die of an accidental overdose.

The key to prevention and early detection of relapse in the physician lies in close monitoring (see the checklist, following). When conducted by a physician or therapist on a timely basis, such monitoring generally can detect impending relapse. As with other relapsing/remitting disorders such as diabetes and rheumatoid arthritis, proactive guidelines should be developed at the time of treatment. A relapse contract (see Appendix 3, following) should be completed by the patient, the family, and significant others in the physician's support system.

Protocol. Once relapse is detected, the physician should be evaluated by a multidisciplinary team composed of medical, psychiatric, and addiction medicine specialists, as well as a neuropsychiatrist and a family therapist. The team then makes a determination as to whether the physician is experiencing a partial or full relapse. The following protocol is recommended:

Investigating the Relapse: When members of the physician's support system suspect relapse, an immediate informal conference should occur between members of the Physician Health Program and the supervising physician (if appropriate). At this point, the group must decide:

- Whether immediate action should be taken to encourage (or, if necessary) insist that the physician leave his or her medical practice pending further assessment.

- Whether the physician should be admitted directly to an appropriate program for assessment or treatment to prevent untoward consequences, including the need for medical detoxification and observation for possible suicidal behavior.

- Whether immediate analysis of appropriate bodily fluids (blood, urine, breath, or hair) should be considered.

- Whether the medical board should be informed of the relapse, if the physician is not already known to the board. If the physician is under an active consent order with the board, other reporting issues may need to be resolved.

Evaluating the Course of Action: The evaluation group (or, when appropriate, the assessment team) should carefully consider:

- The relapsed physician's emotional state;

- The recovery program prior to the relapse;

- The length of the physician's sobriety and the extent of the relapse; and

- The psychological dynamics of the relapse (for example, was the relapse triggered by poor recovery skills, emerging unresolved emotional traumas, or character pathology?).

Once the evaluation criteria are considered, the relapsed physician should be presented with the group's findings and given several options for additional treatment. If the physician has "slipped" (defined as short-term chemical use with little or no psychological, legal, or physical damage), the treatment team may suggest adjustment of the physician's recovery plan in lieu of readmission to a treatment program. Significant relapse, on the other hand, warrants treatment in a relapse-specific treatment program.

The team also needs to consider the legal consequences or potential patient safety issues posed by the relapse.

Informing the Medical Board: The treatment team should provide recommendations to the medical board. Their report should include the following information:

- Whether the drug(s) used in the relapse is other than the initial drug(s) of choice.

- The longest length of time the physician has had in recovery prior to the relapse.

- The length of time the physician has been in relapse.

- The effect the relapse has had on others, including the physician's patients.

- The physician's response to the intervention (that is, his or her willingness to accept personal responsibility for the relapse).

- The drugs used in the relapse.

- Whether the physician practices in a high-risk position (for example, one that affords access to high potency synthetic narcotics such as fentanyl). Such a physician may need to be reassigned to another type of practice to reduce his or her risk of relapse.

- Any known professional boundary violations or improprieties that have occurred as part of or separate from the relapse to alcohol or drug use.

- Whether the physician has complied with his or her continuing care contract.

- Other factors relevant to the relapse, such as family, job, stress, and physical illness (particularly pain).

- Whether the physician's registration with the federal Drug Enforcement Administration (DEA) should be voluntarily surrendered or held in suspension.

Restoring the Physician to Practice: Once the physician successfully completes a specialized relapse treatment program, as recommended by the evaluation group or assessment team, and attends to the recovery activities outlined in the relapse contract, the recovering physician must petition the evaluation group and the Medical Board to lift any license suspension. Such a petition must include:

- A general description of the quality of the physician's recovery.

- Written reports by the physician's treatment program and evaluation team.

- Evidence of participation in physician-specific support groups (in compliance with the continuing care contract).

- Evidence of participation in a Twelve Step group.

- Results of randomly administered bodily fluid screens, as obtained under chain-of-custody provisions in conformance with the rules of the evaluation team and the medical board. (Testing must be performed by a laboratory certified by the National Institute on Drug Abuse.)

Board Considerations. Recurring relapses generally incur progressively severe sanctions, including public suspension. The physician, the monitor, or the treatment program must report a relapse to the medical board as soon as possible. Lifting of the suspension occurs only after a physician has entered and completed treatment and has advocacy to return to the practice of medicine, *and* the physician has appeared before the Impairment Committee and obtained the Medical Board's approval to resume practice under a consent order. Progressively longer suspensions generally follow multiple relapses.

In restoring a relapsed physician to practice, careful consideration should be given to whether to return the recovering physician's DEA registration.

CONCLUSIONS

Collaborative multicenter outcome studies on the treatment of physicians with substance use disorders have established that, with satisfactory completion of primary treatment and extended physician-specific comprehensive monitoring, the large majority of physicians are able to achieve and maintain recovery. Eventually, most such physicians are able to re-enter the practice of medicine, to practice with competence, and to maintain a high level of public safety. In fact, physicians who complete comprehensive treatment and enter an abstinence-based recovery process often report that their skills after treatment (especially those related to the art of medicine) are more acute than at any other time in their careers.

ACKNOWLEDGMENT: Adapted with the permission of the editors from GD Talbott & LR Crosby, eds. (2001). Problem Physicians: A National Perspective *(A Report to the Georgia Composite State Board of Medical Examiners).*

REFERENCES

American Psychiatric Association (APA) (1994). *Diagnostic and Statistical Manual of Mental Disorders, 4th Edition (DSM-IV).* Washington, DC: American Psychiatric Press.

Angres D, Talbott GD & Bettinardi-Angres K (1999). *Healing the Healer: The Addicted Physician.* Madison, CT: Psychosocial Press.

Argren B (1996). Should a physician always be a physician? *Tidsskr Nor Laegeforen* (Norwegian) 116(12):1504.

Bloom JD, Resnick M, Ulwelling JJ et al. (1991). Psychiatric consultation to a state board of medical examiners. *American Journal of Psychiatry* 148(10):1366-1370.

Breen KJ (1998). Doctors who self-administer drugs of dependence. *Medical Journal of Australia* 169(8):404-405.

Canavan DI (1993). Addiction disorders of New Jersey physicians. *New Jersey Medicine* (11):861-862.

Carlson HB, Dilts SL & Radcliffe S (1994). Physicians with substance abuse problems and their recovery environment: A survey. *Journal of Substance Abuse Treatment* 11(2):113-119.

Centrella M (1994). Physician addiction and impairment—Current thinking: A review. *Journal of Addictive Diseases* 12(1):91-105.

Femino J & Nirenberg TD (1994). Treatment outcome studies on physician impairment: A review of the literature. *Rhode Island Medicine* 77(10):345-350.

Flaherty JA & Richman JA (1993). Substance use and addiction among medical students, residents, and physicians. *Psychiatric Clinics of North America* 16(1):189-197.

Gallegos KV, Lubin B, Bowers C et al. (1992). Relapse and recovery: Five to ten year follow-up study of chemically dependent physicians—The Georgia experience. *Maryland Medical Journal* 41(4):315-319.

Goldman L, Myers M & Dickstein L, eds. (2000). *The Handbook of Physician Health.* Chicago, IL: American Medical Association.

Gross R (1992). When physicians treat their own families. *New England Journal of Medicine* 326(13):895 (discussion 895-896).

Kessler RC (1994). Lifetime and 12-month prevalence of DSM-IIIR psychiatric disorders in the United States. *Archives of General Psychiatry* 51:8-19.

Lang DA, Nye GS & Jara G (1993). Physician diversion program experience with successful graduates. *Journal of Psychoactive Drugs* 25(2):159-164.

Mee-Lee D, Shulman GD, Fishman M et al. (2001). *ASAM Patient Placement Criteria for the Treatment of Substance-Related Disorders, Second Edition, Revised (ASAM PPC-2R).* Chevy Chase, MD: American Society of Addiction Medicine.

Milkman H & Sunderwirth S (1987). *Craving for Ecstasy: The Consciousness and Chemistry of Escape.* Lexington, MA: Lexington Books.

Penn JE (1991). Physician behavior and the family. *Ohio Medicine* 87(9):439-440.

Pickens R (1985). Relapse by alcohol abusers. *Alcoholism: Clinical & Experimental Research* 9:244-247.

Rakatansky H & Moclair W (1994). The Physician's Health Committee of the Rhode Island Medical Society. *Rhode Island Medicine* 77(10):343-344.

Reading EG (1992). Nine years' experience with chemically dependent physicians: The New Jersey experience. *Maryland Medical Journal* 41(4):325-329.

Steindler EM (1984). Physician impairment: Past, present, and future. *Journal of the Medical Association of Georgia* 73(11):741-743.

Summer GL (1994). Physician impairment: Current concepts. *Alabama Medicine* 64(4):24-25.

Summer GL (1992). Self-medication in physicians. *Alabama Medicine* 61(8):19-21.

Summer GL (1993). The implications of relapse for the physician with chemical dependency. *Alabama Board of Medical Examiners Newsletter*, Spring.

Talbott GD (1992). Alcoholics anonymous and addicted health professionals: The Georgia experience. *Journal of the Medical Association of Georgia* 81(10):565-8.

Talbott GD (1983). The disease of chemical dependency—From concept to precept. *Counselor* 1(4):18-19.

Talbott GD, Angres D & Gallegos KV (1997). Physicians and other health professionals. In JH Lowinson et al. (ed.) *Substance Abuse: A Comprehensive Textbook, Third Edition*. Baltimore, MD: Williams & Wilkins.

Talbott GD & Gallegos KV (1998). Impairment and recovery in physicians and other health professionals. In AW Graham & TK Schultz (eds.) *Principles of Addiction Medicine, Second Edition*. Chevy Chase, MD: American Society of Addiction Medicine.

Talbott GD & Gander O (1975). Alcoholism, the disease a medical fact. *Journal of the Medical Association of Georgia* 64:331-333.

Udel MM (1984). Chemical abuse/dependence: Physicians' occupational hazard. *Journal of the Medical Association of Georgia* 73(11):775-778.

Uzvch L (1994). The promise and challenge of physician profiling. *Nebraska Medical Journal* 79(8):298-299.

Ziegler PP (1995). Monitoring impaired physicians: A tool for relapse prevention. *Pennsylvania Medicine* 10:38-40.

Ziegler PP (1994). Recognizing the chemically dependent physician. *Pennsylvania Medicine* 97(3)36-38.

APPENDIX 1. Sample Continuing Care Contract

Discharge Date: _____

Name: _____

Home Address: _____

Telephone: (H): _____ (W): _____

The following continuing care plan is a set of recommendations that have been developed by the clinical treatment team. It utilizes the expertise gained from years of treating chemically dependent individuals. Our experience is that patients who follow these guidelines significantly enhance their recovery. Where appropriate, impaired networks, boards, employers, families and referral sources have provided input regarding the recommendations presented in this plan. It is not meant to be a binding legal agreement, but a recommended recovery plan. We recommend adherence to this plan for a period of 5 years.

I agree to abstain completely from taking any mood-changing chemical except as cleared by my primary physician and monitoring physician (and when appropriate, in consultation with an addiction medicine specialist). I also agree to have my primary physician and monitor clear any and all medications (prescribed, over-the-counter, or herbal/nutritional) before using them. I agree not to self-prescribe. Listed below are any and all current medications prescribed/cleared by my attending physician:

I will ask my primary care physician and/or monitor to assist me with care or followup of the medical conditions listed below.

I agree to follow the terms of the family and the continuing care relapse plans.

If I change address, I agree to notify the Continuing Care Director at least 2 weeks before such a move in order to develop a new support network.

I agree to complete, submit for review to my monitoring professional, and mail to the treatment program completed Continuing Care Quarterly Monitoring Reports every 3 months for 5 years.

Discharge Date: _____

Listed below are any and all current legal/licensure issues: _____

_____

_____

Relapse prevention suggestions for return to work include: _____

I will be returning to work at the following location: _____

Company: _____

Address: _____

Telephone: _____

My return to work date is: _____

It is suggested that I work no more than 40 hours per week, unless agreed on and cleared by my monitor.

Discharge Date: _____

Until I return to work, I will be following a schedule that will include the following:

The following is my primary physician. I agree to execute a continuing care release to my primary physician including full address prior to my discharge.

Name: _____

Address: _____

Telephone: _____

I will utilize the following as my monitor/monitors. I agree to execute a continuing care release to each member of my monitoring team (including full address) prior to my discharge.

Monitor's Name: _____   Telephone: _____

Address: _____

Other Name: _____   Telephone: _____

Address: _____

I agree to contact my monitor/monitors the Monday following discharge and then as directed.

I agree to random/observed urine/blood monitoring drug screens to be set up by my monitor and agree to pay for these urine/blood drug screens.

Plan: _____

Frequency: _____

Drop Site: _____

I have asked the following person to be my sponsor. I agree to utilize my sponsor to continue to work a daily recovery program.

Name: _____   Telephone: _____

Address: _____

I agree to the following living recommendations: _____

I understand that the recommendation is that I attend daily meetings for 90 days and then 4 to 7 meetings per week for the duration of this continuing care plan. I understand that my aftercare/monitoring groups can count in that total if my monitor approves. I have obtained a home group and will develop a regular plan for meeting attendance.

Home Group: _____

Meeting Schedule:

    Monday: _____

    Tuesday: _____

    Wednesday: _____

    Thursday: _____

    Friday: _____

    Saturday: _____

    Sunday: _____

The day, time, and location of my Health Professionals group is:

    Day: _____

    Time: _____

    Location: _____

The day, time, and location of my Continuing Care group is:

    Day: _____

    Time: _____

    Location: _____

I agree to participate in recommended therapy as indicated below. I also agree to complete a continuing care release, including full address, for all therapeutic parties listed below:

Family Therapist: _____ Telephone: _____

Address: _____

Individual Therapist: _____ Telephone: _____

Address: _____

Medication: _____ Telephone: _____

Management: _____

Address: _____

Recommendations for return visits include:

    ☐ 3 Month Return Visit: _____ ☐ 6 Month Return Visit: _____

    ☐ Annually for 5 years thereafter. If I am unable to attend a scheduled return visit, I will contact the Continuing Care Director in writing with reason for absence.

In addition to this plan, I will be under contract with the following: _____

I have identified the following barriers to maintaining a drug-free lifestyle: _____

In addressing the preceding barriers, I would like to commit to the following recovery activities:

    Spiritual: _____

    Leisure/Social: _____

    Physical Health: _____

    Other: _____

I will comply with the treatment center Business Office agreement.

The above continuing care plan has been explained to my satisfaction, and I understand its contents.

_____
Patient Name (Printed)

_____
Patient Signature   Date

_____
Continuing Care Director's Signature   Date

APPENDIX 2.   Sample Quarterly Monitoring Agreement

Name _____ Occupation/Profession _____ Specialty _____

Street _____ City _____ State _____ Zip _____

Home telephone _____ Daytime/office telephone _____

Today's Date _____ Discharge Date _____ Sobriety Date _____

Part I.   Status Changes (Please circle YES or NO and write where needed.)

1. Has your sobriety date changed since you completed formal treatment?   YES   NO

    a.   If YES, did you seek help?   YES   NO

    b.   If YES, are you back in recovery?   YES   NO

    Your new sobriety date, if applicable

2. Your marital status is (circle):   Single   Married   Divorced   Separated   Widowed

    a.   Changed since discharge?   YES   NO

    b.   Have you ever been divorced?   YES   NO

3. Are you smoking now?   YES   NO

4. Is your life out of balance in any of these areas?   YES   NO

    a.   If YES (circle):   Sex   Food   Gambling   Spending   Work   Other _____

5. Are you taking any prescribed medications?   YES   NO

    a.   If YES, please list _____

6. Any trouble with your licensure status now?   YES   NO

    a.   If YES, please explain _____

7. Any legal status troubles now (such as traffic violations or civil actions)?   YES NO

    a.   If YES, please explain _____

8. Any employment status or job location change? YES NO

    a.   If YES, please explain _____

Part II.   Recovery Activities

Please indicate how many **times per month** you engage in the following activities. If the item does not apply, write "N/A" in the appropriate bracket. Please do not leave any blank spaces.

_____   9. Attend a Twelve Step group meeting

_____ 10. Contact a Twelve Step sponsor

_____ 11. Perform Twelve Step service work

_____ 12. Attend a professional group meeting

_____ 13. Contact a professional monitor

_____ 14. Attend a Continuing Care Group meeting

_____ 15. Attend individual therapy or counseling sessions

_____ 16. Exercise for 30- to 60-minute sessions

_____ 17. Take time for regular meditation/reflection

_____ 18. Contact your primary physician

_____ 19. Attend therapy/counseling sessions with family/spouse/other persons

_____ 20. Spend an hour or more in recreational or social activities

_____ 21. Attend continuing medical education or other professional training.

Other Activities (note any change in frequency)

_____ 22. Number of hours worked **per week**

_____ 23. Number of random urine/blood drug screens completed **this quarter**.

APPENDIX 3.   Sample Relapse Contract

I, _____, agree to perform the following within 24 hours should I use any alcohol or other mood altering drugs:

- ☐ Contact my sponsor
- ☐ Attend an AA/NA meeting and pick up a white chip when applicable
- ☐ Contact my monitoring professional in my area to inform him/her of my relapse
- ☐ Contact the Continuing Care Associate at my treatment center to inform him/her of my relapse.

I, _____, a member of the family or significant other, agree to encourage the patient to contact the monitoring professional to inform him/her of the relapse. I agree to contact my sponsor and home Al-Anon group for additional suggestions. I agree to contact the monitoring professional and Continuing Care associate at the treatment center as outlined above, if the patient is unwilling to do so.

I, _____, will complete and return this contract to my treatment provider within 30 days of my discharge.

SECTION 10

Medical Disorders and Complications of Addiction

Section Coordinator
Richard Saitz, M.D., M.P.H.

Contributors

Edward A. Alexander, M.D.
Section of Nephrology
Boston University School of Medicine
Boston, Massachusetts

Daniel P. Alford, M.D., M.P.H.
Section of General Internal Medicine
Department of Medicine
Boston University School of Medicine
Boston, Massachusetts

Sanford Auerbach, M.D.
Department of Neurology and Psychiatry
Boston University School of Medicine, and
Director, Sleep Disorders Center
Boston Medical Center
Boston, Massachusetts

John C.M. Brust, M.D.
Department of Neurology
Harlem Hospital Center and
Columbia College of Physicians & Surgeons
New York, New York

Jose Carlos T. DaSilva, M.D., M.P.H.
Section of Nephrology
Boston University School of Medicine
Boston, Massachusetts

Linda C. Degutis, Dr.P.H.
Associate Professor
Section of Emergency Medicine
Yale University School of Medicine
New Haven, Connecticut

Gail D'Onofrio, M.D., M.S.
Associate Professor
Section of Emergency Medicine
Yale University School of Medicine
New Haven, Connecticut

David A. Fiellin, M.D.
Department of Internal Medicine
Yale University School of Medicine
New Haven, Connecticut

Howard S. Friedman, M.D.
Clinical Professor
Division of Cardiology
Department of Medicine
New York University School of Medicine
New York, New York

Paul S. Haber, M.D., FRACP
Head of Drug Health Service
Royal Prince Alfred Hospital, and
Department of Medicine
University of Sydney
Sydney, Australia

Alan Ona Malabanan, M.D., FACE
Section of Endocrinology, Diabetes and Nutrition
Department of Medicine
Boston University School of Medicine
Boston, Massachusetts

Elizabeth Mirabile-Levin, M.D.
Pulmonary Center
Boston University School of Medicine
Boston, Massachusetts

Ann Marie Pagliaro, M.S.N., Ph.D. Candidate
Professor and Director
Substance Abusology Research Unit
University of Alberta
Edmonton, Alberta, Canada

Louis A. Pagliaro, M.S., Pharm.D., Ph.D.
Professor of Pharmacopsychology
University of Alberta
Edmonton, Alberta, Canada

Richard Saitz, M.D., M.P.H., FACP
Associate Professor of Medicine and Epidemiology
Clinical Addiction Research and Education Unit
Section of General Internal Medicine
Departments of Medicine and Epidemiology
Boston University School of Medicine
Boston, Massachusetts

Jussi J. Saukkonen, M.D.
Assistant Professor of Medicine
Pulmonary Center
Boston University School of Medicine
Boston, Massachusetts

Carol A. Sulis, M.D.
Associate Professor of Medicine
Section of Infectious Diseases
Department of Medicine
Boston University School of Medicine
Boston, Massachusetts

Michael F. Weaver, M.D.
Assistant Professor
  of Internal Medicine and Psychiatry
Medical College of Virginia
Virginia Commonwealth University
Richmond, Virginia

Kevin Wilson, M.D.
Pulmonary Center
Department of Medicine
Boston University School of Medicine
Boston, Massachusetts

Medical and Surgical Complications of Addiction

Richard Saitz, M.D., M.P.H., FACP

Persons with addictive disorders often do not receive regular health care (Saitz, Mulvey et al., 1997). As a result, their medical care for acute and chronic conditions can be fragmented and inefficient. Furthermore, they miss opportunities to receive preventive health care (Samet, Friedmann et al., 2001). In addition to the direct effects of intoxication, overdose, and withdrawal, abused substances can affect every body system. Substance abuse and dependence are associated with behaviors that place individuals at risk of health consequences that are not directly related to use of the substance. Regular health care can lead to improved health for persons with addictive disorders (Laine, Hauck et al., 2001; Samet, Friedmann et al., 2001; Samet, Saitz et al., 1996). Such care could be accessed at general medical or addiction treatment delivery sites.

This section will address the wide range of health consequences of alcohol and other drug use, focusing on the most common and most serious illnesses, mainly by organ system. This introductory chapter will review preventive care, addiction care during medical hospitalization, the medical consequences of substance abuse and dependence, the management of common medical problems in persons

with addictive disorders, and consequences in older adults. Preventive care for healthy adults, as well as issues specific to persons with addictive disorders, are presented herein because any health care contact is an opportunity for persons with addictive disorders or dependence to obtain such care. Subsequent chapters will address the epidemiology, diagnosis, and management of consequences of substance use in detail, focusing on HIV/AIDS, tuberculosis and other infectious diseases, renal and metabolic disorders, endocrine and reproductive consequences, hepatitis, cirrhosis and other liver diseases, gastrointestinal consequences, neurologic complications, cardiac consequences, respiratory and sleep disorders, injury, and management of addicted surgical patients.

ROUTINE AND PREVENTIVE CARE

In the early 20th century, preventive health care meant a thorough and detailed evaluation focused on examination and testing. The "executive physical," a "one-size-fits-all" approach in which more tests were better, evolved from this approach. Over the past several decades, however, preventive care expert panels have recommended targeted evaluations based on age and other risk factors (U.S.

Preventive Services Task Force, 1996). The rationale for these targeted evaluations is based on the notion that time and resources are limited and, perhaps more importantly, the recognition that preventive care can result not only in benefit, but also in harm (such as a perforated colon from a colonoscopy performed as a result of an occult blood test that turns out to be a false-positive test for colorectal cancer). In addition, some preventive testing predicted to offer health benefit has been shown to offer no benefit in terms of length and quality of life when evaluated in controlled clinical trials (for example, screening chest radiographs in smokers). The approach presented here follows a targeted strategy based on the known effectiveness of interventions. Although disagreements exist among professional and other organizations (and their guidelines) regarding some details, most recommendations are in agreement when it comes to which diseases should be identified during their preclinical stages. Ongoing updates of recommendations by the U.S. Preventive Services Task Force (3rd edition, 2000-2002) can be accessed at HTTP://WWW.AHRQ.GOV/CLINIC/PREVENIX. HTM.

Medical History. The medical history in an asymptomatic person with an addictive disorder (in addition to a thorough alcohol and drug use history) should include an assessment of sexual practices and behaviors, including condom use; dental care, including use of floss and brushing with fluoride toothpaste; diet (fat, cholesterol, fruit, grain, vegetable, and overall caloric intake); physical activity; calcium intake; use of lap and shoulder belts when in vehicles; use of helmets when riding a bicycle or motorcycle; presence of a firearm and smoke detector in the household; and cardiopulmonary resuscitation knowledge in the household. These assessments are recommended because they can lead to counseling interventions, depending on the answers.

For persons with addictive disorders, screening for depression and anxiety, assessment of sexual practices, intention to conceive a child, and behavior that might lead to injury are particularly important. Such patients should be asked specifically about substance use before operating a motor vehicle, riding with intoxicated drivers, heterosexual sex without contraception, and sex while intoxicated. In addition, a thorough history must include any medications used, allergies, and past immunizations or courses of chemoprophylaxis (as for tuberculosis, menopause, or to prevent folate deficiency). Alcoholics are at higher risk of folate deficiency, and this is of particular importance for women of childbearing age, whose fetuses are at risk of neural tube defects.

Additional history is needed to determine if the patient belongs to a high-risk group that would indicate additional preventive interventions. For example, patients should be asked about chronic medical illnesses, whether they live in an institutional setting, contact with active cases of tuberculosis, recency of immigration, cardiovascular risk factors (smoking, cholesterol elevation, family history of heart disease, and diabetes), history or family history of cancer, travel patterns, receipt of blood products, drug injection, and occupation.

Physical Examination. The physical examination may be complete and should certainly address body systems related to any reported symptoms. In asymptomatic persons, height, weight, blood pressure, and a cardiac examination listening for murmurs should be performed. The height and weight should be used to determine the body mass index and assess nutritional status. Most preventive recommendations include the breast physical examination for adult women, although the evidence for benefit is absent until age 40, when there is less risk from misidentification of benign lesions (Kerlikowske, 1997; Kerlikowske & Ernster, 2000; Kerlikowske, Grady et al., 1995; Sox, 1998). Most masses detected in young women will be benign, but may require investigation once detected to rule out malignancy. Testicular examination for young men as well as rectal and prostate examinations (all to screen for cancers) are recommended by some specialty organizations (American Cancer Society and American Urological Association) but not by generalist organizations (American College of Physicians-American Society of Internal Medicine and U.S. Preventive Services Task Force) because of the absence of evidence for benefit (U.S. Preventive Services Task Force, 1996). The risk of breast cancer is, and prostate and colorectal cancer may be, increased by even moderate alcohol consumption (Fuchs, Stampfer et al., 1995; Smith-Warner, Spiegelman et al., 1998; Bagnardi, Blangiardo et al., 2001), such cancers are not more common in addicted persons.

Persons with alcohol, tobacco, and other drug abuse should have the cervical, axillary, supraclavicular, and inguinal lymph node regions examined for lymphadenopathy. Tuberculosis, chancroid, syphilis, and HIV are more common in persons with addictive disorders who present with lymphadenopathy. Supraclavicular nodes can be the presenting sign of lung cancer in tobacco users. Smokers and alcohol users should have a thorough examination of the oral cavity to look for premalignant and malignant lesions to which they are particularly susceptible, synergistically. Tobacco-stained teeth can serve as a focus for discussion. Examination of the liver is advisable, if only to draw attention to the many possible complications of drug and alcohol use. Even asymptomatic persons can have the small hard liver of cirrhosis or the enlarged liver of chronic viral or alcohol-related hepatitis. Skin examination can reveal signs of injection drug use, the wrinkles associated with tobacco use, or the palmar erythema of alcoholism.

Tests. All adults should be screened for hypercholesterolemia with a fasting lipid profile (serum low-density lipoprotein, high-density lipoprotein, and total cholesterol and triglycerides) or a random (nonfasting) serum total cholesterol and high-density lipoprotein (National Cholesterol Education Program, 2001). Hypertriglyceridemia is associated with alcoholism and can be a cause of pancreatitis. Primary prevention—that is, identifying patients with hyperlipidemia who have no clinically evident coronary artery disease—can decrease the risk of heart disease and death. A serum hemoglobin, mean corpuscular volume (MCV), or a hemoglobin electrophoresis should be checked in men and women who might be contemplating parenting. The purpose of the screen is to detect the common thalassemia traits and to provide genetic counseling. An unsuspected anemia or pancytopenia can be found in persons with alcoholism or HIV.

All women who have had sexual intercourse should have a cervical cytology (Papanicolaou smears) performed every one to three years to detect the premalignant lesions of cervical cancer. Smokers are at higher risk of cervical cancer. Adolescents and young adults should have urine chlamydia testing performed. Although a pelvic examination without testing is not routinely indicated, addicted persons are at risk of sexually transmitted diseases, and genital warts, abnormal vaginal discharge, or herpetic lesions can be seen.

Yearly mammography should be offered to women, beginning at age 40 or 50. Randomized trials show minimal benefit below the age of 50, and almost half of the women screened will suffer a false positive and the consequences of further testing to clarify the diagnosis (Elmore, Barton et al., 1998). Breast self-examination is of no proven benefit (Thomas, Gao et al., 2002) and increases the risk of a benign breast biopsy. Mortality from breast cancer can be decreased by regular physical examination and screening mammography. A family history of breast cancer can indicate the need for earlier testing or referral to a specialist for genetic testing.

Prostate cancer screening remains controversial. The serum prostate specific antigen (PSA) test is recommended by specialty organizations, but many other groups (including all generalist physician organizations) stop short of such a recommendation. All men aged 50 years and older who have a life expectancy of at least 10 to 15 years should be counseled about the option of prostate cancer screening (Barry, 2001). The controversy is due to the current state of the science: Prostate cancer usually has a very long preclinical phase, it is not yet possible to predict accurately which cases will progress, the testing is neither sensitive nor specific, the evaluation for a positive test is invasive, the treatment results in significant complications (including erectile dysfunction and incontinence). Only one study (of senecal) has shown a decrease in cancer-related mortality (Holmberg, Bill-Axelson et al., 2002). In that study, only a small fraction of the tumors were PSA-detected. The Pivot study should help to resolve the controversy (Wilt & Brower, 1997). Patients who choose to be screened might do so because of the belief they will benefit (a belief shared by some physicians and scientists), but this benefit is by no means certain. Those who are at higher risk of prostate cancer, including African Americans and those with a family history of the disease, may use that information to help make decisions about screening, beginning at age 40.

Colorectal cancer screening, however, is not controversial. Colorectal cancer mortality can be decreased in adults aged 50 years and older (younger for those with risk factors or familial disease) by a variety of approaches. Currently recommended approaches include yearly fecal occult blood testing, flexible sigmoidoscopy every five years, and both procedures or colonoscopy every 10 years (Rex, Johnson et al., 2000). Positive occult blood testing or sigmoidoscopy should be followed by an examination of the complete colon. Older adults (aged 65 or older) should have thyroid function testing (serum thyroid-stimulating hormone) because abnormalities are common, difficult to recognize clinically, and easily treatable. Vision and hearing testing should be performed routinely in older adults. Bone mineral density (BMD) testing should be done for older menopausal women and younger menopausal women with risk factors if an intervention to prevent osteoporosis would be instituted as a result (U.S. Preventive Services Task Force, 2002). This testing is of particular importance for persons with inadequate calcium intake, excessive alcohol use, physical inactivity, smoking, and a family history of osteoporosis. Persons with addictive disorders can have poor diets, little sun exposure, and minimal intake of milk products; screening for vitamin D deficiency with a 25-hydroxyvitamin D should be considered.

Persons with addictive disorders who have been sexually active or who use injection drugs should be screened routinely for sexually transmitted diseases with a serologic test for syphilis, HIV, and chlamydia (using the ligase chain reaction in a urine or cervical specimen). Specific consent should be obtained for the HIV test, as should pre- and posttest counseling. Because of the implications and the potential to trigger relapse, the timing of HIV testing must be individualized, with input from the patient, preferably to a time when recovery is stable. The serologic test for syphilis (rapid plasma reagin [RPR] or Venereal Disease Research Laboratory [VDRL]) frequently is falsely positive in injection drug users (as is the serum rheumatoid factor and the partial thromboplastin time), reflecting a generalized activation of the immune system. As a result, the screening test should not be used as evidence of syphilis—instead, the result should be confirmed by a treponemal test such as the microhemagglutination test for *Treponema pallidum* (MHA-TP) or the fluorescent treponemal antibody (FTA) tests.

Users of injection drugs, those with alcohol abuse, and persons with multiple sexual partners or high-risk sexual activity should have the international normalized ratio (INR), the serum bilirubin, transaminases (aspartate aminotransferase [AST] and alanine aminotransferase [ALT]), and the serum albumin and alkaline phosphatase checked as screening tests for chronic hepatitis and cirrhosis (and the serum albumin for nutritional status as well). The serum pre-albumin will give a more stable view of long-term nutritional status, as it fluctuates less than the serum albumin. Abnormal liver enzymes, INR, or serum bilirubin tests should be followed by hepatitis B (surface antigen and core antibody) and C antibody testing. Previously vaccinated individuals should have the antisurface hepatitis B antibody determined to assess current immunoprotection. Injection drug users and those who practice anal intercourse and who are not from endemic areas should be tested for immunity to hepatitis A. Injection drug users and those with HIV risk factors should have a urinalysis and serum creatinine to assess the presence of silent renal disease.

Among other risk factors, persons with alcoholism and other drug abuse without past known tuberculosis should be screened for asymptomatic infection with *Mycobacterium tuberculosis*, using a 5 tuberculin unit intradermal injection read at 48 hours (provided a previous test is not known to have been positive). A positive test in such persons is 10 mm of induration (5 mm if immune deficiency is present); in such cases, a chest radiograph should be performed (ATS & CDC, 2000a). Provided the radiograph is not consistent with active tuberculosis, prophylactic pharmacotherapy should be considered regardless of age (ATS & CDC, 2000b).

Preventive Counseling. All patients should be counseled about healthy dietary habits (limiting saturated fat and favoring fruits, vegetables, legumes, fiber, and grains) and physical activity (at least 20 minutes of aerobic exercise three times a week). All alcohol and other drug abusers should be counseled about safer sexual practices (abstinence and condom use), and injection drug users should be educated about sterile injection practices. Women of childbearing age and their partners should be counseled about contraceptive options.

All persons should be counseled that, in addition to their addiction specialty care, they should engage in regular primary and preventive health care with a primary care physician. Linkage of patients to primary medical care has many potential benefits, including improved prevention, management of chronic conditions, coordination of the many health care services needed by patients with addictive disorders, and support in relapse prevention efforts (Friedmann, Saitz et al., 1998; Laine, Hauck et al., 2001; Samet, Friedmann et al., 2001). In addition, because psychiatric illness is so common in addicted patients, linkage to mental health care should be offered when appropriate. This linkage can be accomplished through a primary care physician.

Those persons who store or carry weapons should be reminded of gun safety. All patients should be advised about seat belt and helmet use. Referrals for both regular eye and dental care should be routine. Preventive advice about safe lifting is warranted to prevent low back injury.

Immunizations. Immunizations for adults include tetanus toxoid every 10 years (presuming an initial series has been given); this is particularly important for injection drug users, who can expose themselves to tetanus (Gardner & Peter, 2001; Gardner & Schaffner, 1993; Talan & Moran, 1998). Hepatitis B vaccination (a series of three injections) is indicated for injection drug users, health care workers, persons with hepatitis C, and those with high-risk sexual practices who lack immunity (core or surface antibody). Hepatitis A vaccination (two injections) is indicated for travelers, those with any chronic liver disease, those who practice anal intercourse, and injection drug users, when negative for immunity (immunoglobulin G to hepatitis A). Pneumococcal vaccination should be administered to all persons age 65 years and older and those with chronic cardiopulmonary disease (including heart disease, more common in smokers, and reactive airway diseases such as obstructive lung disease and asthma, which are more common in smokers and users of inhaled drugs). Alcoholism is a specific recognized indication for the vaccine, and many practitioners believe other drug addiction also is a reasonable indication. When childhood vaccinations are unknown, consideration should be given to a primary series for polio; measles, mumps, and rubella; and varicella vaccination. Many adults will have immunity to these diseases but, if unknown, testing is warranted, given that many persons with addictive disorders may be in group living situations, sometimes with children and young adults, in which measles and varicella infections can spread easily.

Influenza vaccination should be given yearly to all persons with addictive disorders. It is particularly indicated for those with cardiopulmonary disease and older adults, but is cost-effective for general populations too, and of particular utility for those living in group settings.

Chemoprophylaxis. Aspirin is reasonable as primary prevention for myocardial infarction in men, particularly men with risk factors (Gaziano, Skerrett et al., 2000). Smoking is a strong risk factor for coronary artery disease. Although randomized trials are not available, there is no reason to believe women would not benefit. However, the benefit of aspirin does not likely outweigh the risks of serious central nervous system or gastrointestinal bleeding in alcoholics without symptoms of coronary disease because they are at risk of gastritis, thrombocytopenia, coagulopathy, and trauma. Women of childbearing age should take folate 400 μg daily to prevent neural tube defects (CDC, 1992). Because of the risk of thiamine, vitamin D, pyridoxine, niacin, riboflavin, zinc, and folic acid deficiency in alcoholics and those with deficient diets, a daily multivitamin including 400 IU vitamin D, 100 mg thiamine, and 1 mg folic acid can be recommended. If serum 25-hydroxyvitamin D is low, repletion should begin with 50,000 IU vitamin D weekly for four weeks. Because magnesium deficiency is common in alcoholism, replacement by encouraging the use of foods with a high magnesium content (such as peanuts) or a magnesium supplement (magnesium oxide tablets or magnesium hydroxide-containing antacids) is recommended. If the INR is known to be elevated, a trial of vitamin K is warranted, although generally the INR elevation in addicted persons

will be due to liver disease and not to vitamin deficiency. Men and women, particularly those with deficient diets, should assure adequate calcium intake in their diets or should use supplements (1 g elemental calcium daily for all but postmenopausal women, who should receive 1.5 g).

Raloxifene [Evista®], alendronate [Fosamax®], and risedronate [Actonal®]) may be used for the prevention of osteoporosis in postmenopausal women (Delmas, Bjarnason et al., 1997; Hosking, Chilvers et al., 1998; McClung, Geusens et al., 2001), although the risks and benefits for addicted persons are difficult to predict. Risks for osteoporosis are higher in alcoholics and some other addicted persons, but the interaction between estrogen and alcohol on breast cancer is not clear, and the side effects of the drugs in alcoholics and those with liver disease are not known.

CARE DURING HOSPITALIZATION

Because of the burden of illness carried by persons with addictive disorders, they can require transfer from addiction treatment to a general hospital, or they can be admitted there directly. During a medical hospitalization, three areas deserve particular attention: (1) management of the drug withdrawal, (2) pain management, and (3) common comorbidities (O'Connor, Samet et al., 1994). Treatment (including brief interventions, which are well suited to medical hospital settings), is covered in Sections 4-8 of this text. Withdrawal is addressed in detail in Section 5 and pain management in Section 12, but several points are relevant to medical hospitalizations specifically.

Withdrawal. When a history of alcohol dependence and recent use is obtained, withdrawal should be anticipated. Symptoms should be treated as they appear. Persons not yet symptomatic with withdrawal but with past alcohol-related seizures or concomitant acute medical or surgical conditions (which increase the risk of withdrawal) should be treated with a benzodiazepine (that is, 10 to 20 mg diazepam [Valium®] or 1 to 2 mg lorazepam [Ativan®]) to prevent convulsions or delirium [Mayo-Smith, 1997]).

Because the symptoms of withdrawal may not be distinguishable from systemic symptoms of infection, heart disease, or neurologic conditions, treatment for withdrawal should proceed while investigations to identify other treatable medical disorders continue. Although the use of standardized withdrawal scales generally is encouraged, their lack of specificity requires that the information they provide be considered in the context of the coexisting medical illness. Nevertheless, patients hospitalized for withdrawal

TABLE 1.   Selected Medical Disorders Related to Alcohol and Other Drug Use

Cardiovascular	*Alcohol*: Cardiomyopathy, atrial fibrillation (holiday heart), hypertension, dysrhythmia, masks angina symptoms, coronary artery spasm, myocardial ischemia, high-output states, coronary artery disease, sudden death. *Cocaine*: Hypertension, myocardial infarction, angina, chest pain, supraventricular tachycardia, ventricular dysrhythmias, cardiomyopathy, cardiovascular collapse from bodypacking rupture, moyamoya vasculopathy, left ventricular hypertrophy, myocarditis, sudden death, aortic dissection. *Tobacco*: Atherosclerosis, stroke, myocardial infarction, peripheral vascular disease, cor pulmonale, erectile dysfunction, worse control of hypertension, angina, dysrhythmia. *Infection*: Endocarditis, septic thrombophlebitis.
Cancer	*Alcohol*: Aerodigestive (lip, oral cavity, tongue, pharynx, larynx, esophagus, stomach, colon), breast, hepatocellular and bile duct cancers. *Tobacco*: Oral cavity, larynx, lung, cervix, esophagus, pancreas, kidney, stomach, bladder. *Injection or high-risk sexual behavior*: Hepatocellular carcinoma related to hepatitis C.
Endocrine/Reproductive	*Alcohol*: Hypoglycemia and hyperglycemia, diabetes, ketoacidosis, hypertriglyceridemia, hyperuricemia and gout, testicular atrophy, gynecomastia, hypocalcemia and hypomagnesemia because of reversible hypoparathyroidism, hypercortisolemia, osteopenia, infertility, sexual dysfunction. *Opiates*: Osteopenia, alteration in gonadotropins, decreased sperm motility, menstrual irregularities. *Cocaine*: Diabetic ketoacidosis. *Tobacco*: Graves' disease, azoospermia, erectile dysfunction, osteopenia, osteoporosis, fractures, estrogen alterations, insulin resistance. *Any addiction*: Amenorrhea.
Hepatic	*Alcohol*: Steatosis (fatty liver), acute and chronic hepatitis (infectious [that is, B or C] or toxic [that is, acetaminophen]), alcoholic hepatitis, cirrhosis, portal hypertension and varices, spontaneous bacterial peritonitis. *Opiates*: Granulamatosis. *Cocaine*: Ischemic necrosis, hepatitis. *Injection or high-risk sexual behavior*: Infectious hepatitis B and C (acute and chronic) and delta.
Hematologic	*Alcohol*: Macrocytic anemia, pancytopenia because of marrow toxicity and/or splenic sequestration, leukopenia, thrombocytopenia, coagulopathy because of liver disease, iron deficiency, folate deficiency, spur cell anemia, burr cell anemia. *Tobacco*: Hypercoagulability. *Injection or high-risk sexual behavior*: Hematologic consequences of liver disease, hepatitis C-related cryoglobulinemia and purpura.
Infectious	*Alcohol*: Hepatitis C. pneumonia, tuberculosis (including meningitis), HIV, sexually transmitted diseases, spontaneous bacterial peritonitis, brain abscess, meningitis. *Opiates*: Aspiration pneumonia. *Tobacco*: Bronchitis, pneumonia, upper respiratory tract infections. *Injection*: Endocarditis, cellulitis, pneumonia, septic thrombophlebitis, septic arthritis (unusual joints, that is, sternoclavicular), osteopyelitis (including vertebral), epidural and brain abscess, mycotic aneurysm, abscesses and soft tissue infections, mediastinitis, malaria, tetanus. *Injection or high-risk sexual behavior*: Hepatitis B, C, and delta; HIV; sexually transmitted diseases.
Neurologic	*Alcohol*: Peripheral and autonomic neuropathy, seizure, hepatic encephalopathy, Korsakoff's dementia, Wernicke's syndrome, cerebellar dysfunction, Marchiafava-Bignami syndrome, central pontine myelinolysis, myopathy, amblyopia, stroke, withdrawal delirium, hallucinations, toxic leukoencephalopathy, subdural hematoma, intracranial hemorrhage. *Opiates*: Seizure (overdose and hypoxia), compression neuropathy. *Cocaine*: Stroke, seizure, status epilepticus, headache, delirium, depression, hypersomnia, cognitive deficits. *Tobacco*: Stroke, small vessel ischemia and cognitive deficits. *Any addiction*: Compression neuropathy.
Nutritional	*Alcohol*: Vitamin and mineral deficiencies (B_1, B_6, riboflavin, niacin, vitamin D, magnesium, calcium, folate, phosphate, zinc). *Any addiction*: Protein malnutrition.

Other Gastrointestinal	*Alcohol*: Gastritis, esophagitis, pancreatitis, diarrhea, malabsorption (because of pancreatic exocrine insufficiency, or folate or lactase deficiency), parotid enlargement, malignancy, colitis, Barrett esophagus, gastroesophageal reflux, Mallory-Weiss syndrome, gastrointestinal bleeding.
	Opiates: Constipation, ileus, intestinal pseudo-obstruction.
	Cocaine: Ischemic bowel and colitis.
	Tobacco: Peptic ulcers, gastroesophageal reflex, malignancy (pancreas, stomach).
	Any addiction: Overdose from bodypacking.
Prenatal and Perinatal	*Alcohol*: Fetal alcohol effects and syndrome.
	Opiates: Neonatal abstinence syndrome, including seizures.
	Cocaine: Placental abruption, teratogenesis, neonatal irritability.
	Tobacco: Teratogenesis, low birth weight, spontaneous abortion, abruptio placentae, placenta previa, perinatal mortality, sudden infant death syndrome, neurodevelopmental impairment.
Perioperative	*Alcohol*: Withdrawal, perioperative complications (delirium, infection, bleeding, pneumonia, delayed wound healing, dysrhythmia), hepatic decompensation, hepatorenal syndrome, death.
	Opiates: Withdrawal, inadequate analgesia.
	Cocaine: Hypersomnia and depression in withdrawal, mimicking of postoperative neurologic complications, complications from underlying drug-induced cardiopulmonary disease.
	Tobacco: Pulmonary infection, difficulty weaning, respiratory failure, reactive airways exacerbations.
Pulmonary	*Alcohol*: Aspiration, sleep apnea, respiratory depression, apnea, chemical or infectious pneumonitis.
	Opiates: Respiratory depression/failure, emphysema, bronchospasm, exacerbation of sleep apnea, pulmonary edema.
	Cocaine: Nasal septum perforation, gingival ulceration, perennial rhinitis, sinusitis, hemoptysis, upper airway obstruction, fibrosis, hypersensitivity pneumonitis, epiglottitis, pulmonary hemorrhage, pulmonary hypertension, pulmonary edema, emphysema, interstitial fibrosis, hypersensitivity pneumonia.
	Tobacco: Lung cancer, chronic obstructive pulmonary disease, reactive airways, pneumonia, bronchitis, pulmonary hypertension, interstitial lung disease, pneumothorax.
	Injection: Pulmonary hypertension, talc granulomatosis, septic pulmonary embolism, pneumothorax, emphysema, needle embolization.
	Inhalation: Pulmonary edema, bronchospasm, bronchitis, granulomatosis, airway burns.
Renal	*Alcohol*: Hepatorenal syndrome, rhabdomyolysis and acute renal failure, volume depletion and prerenal failure, acidosis, hypokalemia, hypophosphatemia.
	Opiates: Rhabdomyolysis, acute renal failure, factitious hematuria.
	Cocaine: Rhabdomyolysis and acute renal failure, vasculitis, necrotizing angiitis, accelerated hypertension, nephrosclerosis, ischemia.
	Tobacco: Renal failure, hypertension.
	Injection or high-risk sexual behavior: Focal glomerular sclerosis (HIV, heroin), glomerulonephritis from hepatitis or endocarditis, chronic renal failure, amyloidosis, nephrotic syndrome (hepatitis C).
Sleep	*Alcohol*: Apnea, periodic limb movements of sleep, insomnia, disrupted sleep, daytime fatigue.
	Opiates: Insomnia.
	Cocaine: Hypersomnia in withdrawal.
	Tobacco: Insomnia, increased sleep latency.
Trauma	*Alcohol*: Motor vehicle crash, fatal and nonfatal injury, physical and sexual abuse.
	Cocaine: Death during "Russian Roulette."
	Opiates: Motor vehicle crash, other violent injury.
	Tobacco: Burns, smoke inhalation.
	Any addiction: Sexual and physical abuse.
Musculoskeletal	*Alcohol*: Rhabdomyolysis, compartment syndromes, gout, saturnine gout, fracture, osteopenia, osteonecrosis.
	Opiates: Osteopenia.
	Cocaine: Rhabdomyolysis.
	Any addiction: Compartment syndromes, fractures.

as well as for other medical conditions have had favorable outcomes when treated with symptom-triggered therapy (Jaeger, Lohr et al., 2001; Saitz, Mayo-Smith et al., 1994; Daeppen, Gache et al., 2002).

Similarly, opiate and other drug withdrawal should be identified and managed pharmacologically, both for patient comfort as well as to prevent complications of the medical disorder for which the patient was hospitalized. Patients who already are in treatment for opiate or long-acting sedative dependence should have their treating clinician contacted when they are hospitalized, so that any prescribed ongoing treatment can be continued. Similarly, addiction treatment providers should communicate directly with hospital physicians to facilitate appropriate treatment, after obtaining permission from the patient. Doses for patients not on long-acting opiate treatment should be adequate to prevent withdrawal and should be administered to allow treatment of the underlying medical disorder (that is, 20 mg methadone, repeated in two hours, then given daily or in divided doses twice a day).

At hospital admission, when deciding on the best treatment for the patient, the patient's disposition at discharge should be anticipated. If the patient plans to abstain from the substance at hospital discharge, the substituted opioid can be tapered if symptoms allow. Alternatively, a dose sufficient to avoid withdrawal can be maintained during the hospitalization for those who intend to continue drug use or to enter a maintenance treatment program. Again, symptoms of withdrawal can mimic medical disorders. In addition to providing comfort and helping to prevent the more serious complications of withdrawal (such as convulsions from alcohol withdrawal), specific treatment of withdrawal controls the autonomic symptoms that can worsen a patient's medical condition (such as tachycardia during a myocardial infarction) and helps the patient cooperate with treatment for the medical condition that prompted hospitalization.

Another consideration for the management of withdrawal in hospitalized patients is the route of administration of the drug. Delirious patients should receive intravenous medications (such as diazepam or lorazepam), whereas others who cannot take medications by mouth should receive medications via a route associated with reliable absorption for the particular drug (that is, lorazepam intramuscularly for alcohol withdrawal or methadone [40% to 50% of the oral dose in three to four divided doses] intramuscularly for opiate dependence).

Pain. Pain management often becomes an issue during medical hospitalization of addicted patients. Physicians and nurses may fear providing pain control with opioids when a patient is addicted to them, because of the fear of causing or worsening addiction. This management style generally results in inadequate pain management and frustration for patient and provider alike. Clearly, patients with addictive disorders usually are very tolerant to the substance they use. In the case of opiate dependence, pain control can be achieved only with substantially higher doses of opioids, with careful reassessment of the dose effect and timing to make appropriate adjustments. Once a dose is determined, pain medications should be given on a regular schedule rather than as needed, to avoid making the patient demand medication to relieve uncontrolled symptoms.

Comorbidities. Finally, while patients are hospitalized, several comorbidities should be considered. First, because psychiatric comorbidity is common (in particular antisocial personality disorder, anxiety, and depression), attention to behavioral issues is important. Hospital staff members should take extra care to explain hospital procedures, while setting firm limits. Patients should be assured that their medical, psychiatric, and addiction-related symptoms and pain will be attended to. Discussing withdrawal and pain treatment regimens with the patient can help avoid later problems and disagreements and help allay the fears and preconceptions patients may have about providers.

Screening for coexisting medical disorders (such as HIV, hepatitis, and tuberculosis) during a medical hospitalization should be considered because the acute care setting may provide the only medical care received by the patient. Nevertheless, when such testing is done, consideration should be given to the patient's readiness to hear and handle the results and to arranging followup medical care for the condition. For HIV testing in particular, pretest (reasons for testing, past testing, assessment of risk behaviors, the implications of test results, and the risks and benefits) and posttest counseling must be provided. In a recent survey, most patients in detoxification centers thought HIV testing should be available during detoxification (Pugatch, Levesque et al., 2001). Treatment for coexisting medical and psychiatric conditions should be made available.

MEDICAL CONSEQUENCES OF ALCOHOL, TOBACCO, AND OTHER DRUG USE

Medical consequences of addiction may be due to drug-specific effects, methods of administration, contaminants in or vehicles for drugs used, behavioral habits associated with substance use, or common comorbidities (Table 1). In this portion of the chapter, the medical consequences of addiction are reviewed and organized by drug and then by organ system or clinical area. More details can be found in the chapters in this section. Although some lifestyle choices and risk behaviors span more than one substance, consequences are discussed once to avoid redundancy.

Alcohol. The medical consequences of alcohol use are seen in almost every organ system of the body. Women are more susceptible to many of the effects at lower doses because of less first-pass metabolism of alcohol and lower body weights on average (Bradley, Badrinath et al., 1998). Although moderate drinking can have some beneficial effects for selected individuals, two drinks per day for women and three drinks per day for men increases the risk of death (Doll, Peto et al., 1994; Holman, English et al., 1996).

Withdrawal, Seizures, and Delirium Tremens: Although the direct medical consequences of alcohol withdrawal (hyper-autonomic states, seizures, and delirium) are covered in detail in Section 5, mention is made here because they are common, often are managed in acute care general medical hospitals, and can lead to death. Many patients in withdrawal can be managed as outpatients with or without medication, provided symptoms are minimal and there is little comorbidity that would complicate outpatient management or place patients at higher risk of complications of withdrawal. Alcohol withdrawal symptoms, such as diaphoresis and tremor, begin 6 to 48 hours after the last drink (Saitz & O'Malley, 1997). Such withdrawal symptoms may resolve spontaneously or require treatment with benzodiazepines. Benzodiazepines are the only medications proven, compared with placebo, to ameliorate symptoms of withdrawal, to decrease the risk of seizures and delirium and, compared with paraldehyde (Thompson, Johnson et al., 1975), to speed achievement of a calm but awake state in patients experiencing delirium (Mayo-Smith, 1997; Saitz & O'Malley, 1997). Signs found on physical examination include tremor, moist warm skin, agitation, tachycardia, or hypertension, although these signs may be absent. The tachycardia can complicate underlying medical conditions such as coronary artery disease by precipitating angina or myocardial infarction.

Pharmacologic treatment is indicated for asymptomatic patients at higher risk of complications (acute medical, surgical, or psychiatric comorbidity; past seizures; and past delirium) and for those with significant symptoms (on the Clinical Institute Withdrawal Assessment for Alcohol, Revised, a score of >8-15) to prevent progression to seizures or delirium and for patient comfort (Mayo-Smith, 1997). Seizures, when they occur, almost always resolve spontaneously. They can recur and generally do so within six hours of the first seizure. Benzodiazepines prevent further seizures and progression to *delirium tremens* (DTs). Phenytoin (Dilantin®) and other anticonvulsants are not indicated unless there is another cause or suspected cause for the seizures in addition to alcohol. DTs (hyperautonomia and disorientation/confusion) should be managed in a setting where frequent and intensive monitoring is possible because of the risk of death from the condition and its treatment. Other medications besides the benzodiazepines can be used as adjunctive therapies, provided the patient receives benzodiazepines. These include beta-blockers for tachycardia determined to be the result of withdrawal, clonidine (Catapres®) for hypertension, and haloperidol (Haldol®) for psychosis or agitation, when these signs and symptoms fail to respond to benzodiazepines. Other drugs (such as gabapentin [Neurontin®] and carbamazepine [Tegretol®]), although they may alleviate symptoms, should not be used as monotherapy for withdrawal in patients for whom treatment is indicated to prevent complications. Barbiturates are reasonable alternatives to the benzodiazepines but have a lower margin of safety and no placebo-controlled evidence for efficacy.

Neurologic Consequences: Neurologic complications are perhaps some of the most well known. Alcohol intoxication can lead to head trauma. The signs and symptoms of intracranial hemorrhage—particularly subdural hematoma—can be confused with intoxication. Imaging of the brain is indicated when there are signs of significant head trauma and abnormal mental status, focal neurologic deficits are present, or when neurologic symptoms do not resolve with declining alcohol levels. Alcoholics are at higher risk of tuberculosis, which can manifest as tuberculous meningitis (Ogawa, Smith et al., 1987). DTs are the diagnosis of exclusion (by lumbar puncture) when fever and delirium are present in an alcoholic. In addition to withdrawal seizures, alcohol can lower the seizure threshold in epileptics, and seizures may be the presenting sign of an intracranial hemorrhage.

Ischemic stroke may be less common in moderate drinkers, but heavy drinkers are at higher risk of ischemic and hemorrhagic stroke, related to an interplay with smoking, trauma, hypertension, folic acid deficiency and hyperhomo-cystinemia, and cardiomyopathy (Renaud, 2001). For example, the overall risk of stroke in women is increased in those who consume just more than one standard drink per day (Bradley, Badrinath et al., 1998). Cognitive impairment may be caused acutely by Wernicke-Korsakoff disease because of thiamine deficiency, presenting with confusion, ataxia, or nystagmus. Parenteral thiamine, 100 mg administered before glucose, is the initial treatment. Chronically, Wernicke-Korsakoff disease can develop into Korsakoff's syndrome, a memory impairment classically characterized by confabulation.

More commonly, chronic alcoholism is associated with a nonspecific dementia and volume loss on head computed tomography. Toxic leukoencephalopathy, or damage of cerebral white matter, can contribute to the dementia seen with alcoholism (Filley & Kleinschmidt-DeMasters, 2001). Marchiafava-Bignami disease, caused by lesions in the corpus callosum, is rare. Also rare is central pontine myelinolysis, which is seen in conjunction with alcoholism and too rapid correction of hyponatremia. Alcoholic cerebellar dysfunction is not so rare; it results in ataxia and incoordination, and often is irreversible. Alcoholics can suffer from peripheral neuropathy, usually from vitamin deficiency, pressure on a nerve, or ethanol toxicity. The classic presentation of alcoholic polyneuropathy is of sensory disturbance, including burning, pain, and numbness in a stocking-glove distribution.

Gastrointestinal Consequences: Gastrointestinal problems are very common in the alcoholic patient. Alcohol is directly toxic to the gastric mucosa and can lead to gastritis. Gastritis can be asymptomatic or can present as epigastric burning, nausea, vomiting, anemia, or hematemesis (coffee grounds emesis). Vomiting can lead to a Mallory-Weiss tear and hematemesis. Alcohol can lead to stomatitis, esophagitis, duodenitis, esophageal cancer, and gastric cancer. Endoscopy is warranted for persistent reflux symptoms or epigastric pain, particularly if weight loss is present, or if patients are aged 40 years and older.

Liver and pancreatic consequences of alcohol use are among the most well known. Hepatitis ranges in severity from an asymptomatic elevation of the hepatic transaminases to critical illness with hepatic failure. In alcoholic hepatitis, AST usually is higher than ALT. A higher ALT concentration suggests another or a concomitant etiology, such as hepatitis C, for which alcohol abuse is a risk factor. Heavy alcohol use accelerates the progression to cirrhosis in hepatitis C and interferes with the success of treatment

(Ohnishi, Matsuo et al., 1996; Wiley, McCarthy et al., 1998). Hepatic steatosis can cause elevations in serum transaminases. Although steatohepatitis is best diagnosed by liver biopsy, clinically it often is diagnosed when serology for hepatitis B and C are negative, the abnormality persists with abstinence, and an ultrasound examination is consistent with the diagnosis.

Classic alcoholic hepatitis presents with fever, leukocytosis, right upper-quadrant pain and tenderness, and elevations of the AST concentration out of proportion to ALT elevations. Management consists of abstinence from alcohol as well as of supportive care, with attention to fluid and electrolyte balance, vitamin K for coagulopathy, clotting factor replacement when there is active bleeding and coagulopathy, and attention to volume and mental status. Patients with coagulopathy, hyperbilirubinemia, and hepatic encephalopathy are at high risk of death. Corticosteroids have been shown to decrease mortality in selected cases of alcoholic hepatitis, and propylthiouracil, colchicine, and pentoxifylline (Trental®) have shown promising results in some studies, although they are not yet standard treatments (Akriviadis, Botla et al., 2000; Akriviadis, Steindel et al., 1990; Christensen & Gluud, 1995; Imperiale & McCullough, 1990; Orrego, Blake et al., 1987; Trinchet, Beaugrand et al., 1989). Similarly, oxandrolone has been reported to decrease mortality in patients with alcoholic hepatitis and significant malnutrition (Mendenhall, Moritz et al., 1993).

Cirrhosis can develop in chronic alcohol users either as a consequence of hepatitis C, recurrent alcoholic hepatitis, or, simply, chronic heavy use. An increase in the incidence of cirrhosis can be detected in populations drinking two to three standard drinks per day compared with nondrinkers (Anderson, 1995; Holman, English et al., 1996; Thun, Peto et al., 1997), although heavier amounts are more commonly associated with the condition (that is, 40 to 60 g/day of ethanol for men and less [20 g] for women) (Batey, Burns et al., 1992; Lieber, 1995; Norton, Batey et al., 1987; Parrish, Dufour et al., 1993). Cirrhosis leads to hypoalbuminemia, coagulopathy, and hyperbilirubinemia. Hepatocellular carcinoma can occur, particularly when hepatitis C is present (Yamauchi, Nakahara et al., 1993). It can be cured surgically if detected early enough.

Complications of cirrhosis portend a poor prognosis. These complications include hepatic encephalopathy, esophageal or gastric variceal bleeding, ascites and spontaneous bacterial peritonitis, volume overload and edema, and hepatorenal syndrome. When cirrhosis and alcoholic hepatitis coexist, the prognosis is poor (35% to 50% four- to five-year survival), particularly when drinking continues (Chedid, Mendenhall et al., 1991; Powell & Klatskin, 1968). End-stage liver disease of many etiologies can be addressed with liver transplantation. Patients transplanted because of alcoholic liver disease have similar prognoses to those transplanted for other causes of liver failure (Bird, O'Grady et al., 1990). Many liver transplantation programs have required defined periods of abstinence (often six to 12 months) before patients will be evaluated for this extensive surgery and scarce resource, although assessing relapse risk without requiring an arbitrary period of abstinence is an alternative approach (Gish, Lee et al., 1993).

Chronic alcohol use increases the risk of acetaminophen toxicity, even at doses of 4 g daily, particularly when the patient has been fasting; cases of fulminant hepatic failure have been reported (Schiodt, Rochling et al., 1997).

Pancreatitis often presents as epigastric pain, sometimes radiating to the back, in chronic heavy alcohol users. The other common cause in the United States is gallstones. The serum amylase often is elevated unless there has been chronic pancreatic damage. The amylase is neither sensitive nor specific for pancreatitis (Salt & Schenker, 1976). In alcoholics, amylase often is elevated because of chronic parotitis. Abdominal computed tomography is the most sensitive and specific test, but it is not indicated unless the presentation is atypical, fever is present, or the patient does not improve as expected. Severity can range from mild epigastric pain after eating, with some nausea, to a mortal condition complicated by acidosis, adult respiratory distress syndrome, and hypovolemia. Predictors of death include hyperglycemia, anemia, hypoxemia, acidosis, older age, leukocytosis, elevated blood urea nitrogen, lactate dehydrogenase or AST, hypocalcemia, or hypovolemia (Ranson, Rifkind et al., 1976). The only treatment proven to decrease mortality is volume repletion, best accomplished with intravenous normal saline (Marshall, 1993). Standard therapy includes nothing by mouth, volume repletion, and pain control by using opiates parenterally. Antibiotics should be considered in the presence of unexplained fever. Surgical consultation should be obtained when other diagnoses are being considered and when consideration is given to necrotizing pancreatitis.

When acute episodes resolve, a return to drinking can lead to recurrent episodes and ultimately to constant pain and chronic pancreatitis, loss of pancreatic exocrine function with greasy stools and malabsorption, and even loss of pancreatic endocrine function manifested by hyperglycemia and diabetes (Steer, Waxman et al., 1995). The prognosis is markedly worse with any ongoing alcohol consumption (Lankisch, Imoto et al., 2001). Oral pancreatic enzyme supplementation with meals then is indicated, although pain management is difficult and often requires opiates. Serum amylase and lipase often are normal, although calcifications may be seen on abdominal radiographs.

Hematologic Consequences: In addition to the iron deficiency anemia that can result from gastrointestinal hemorrhage or chronic blood loss (from variceal bleeding, gastritis, Mallory-Weiss tears, coexisting ulcers, esophagitis, or gastrointestinal cancers), alcoholics can develop a pancytopenia (leukopenia, thrombocytopenia, and anemia) from alcohol's direct toxic effects on the bone marrow (Colman & Herbert, 1980; Larkin & Watson-Williams, 1984). The leukopenia can increase the risk of infections. Splenic sequestration as a result of the splenomegaly associated with cirrhosis and portal hypertension can cause a pancytopenia.

Alcoholics often have not only leukopenia but also an impaired quantitative and qualitative white blood cell response to infection (Larkin & Watson-Williams, 1984). The thrombocytopenia can lead to serious bleeding (as a result of trauma or varices, for example), when the platelet count is below 50,000. The anemia can be severe.

Alcoholics can be folate deficient, with a megaloblastic anemia. Thus, the MCV, often used to assist in the differential diagnosis of anemia, can be misleadingly normal, with iron deficiency lowering the MCV and hemolytic anemias related to liver disease with reticulocytosis or megaloblastic processes simultaneously increasing it. In these cases, the red cell distribution width should be elevated.

The treatment for bone marrow suppression is abstinence, for iron deficiency it is identification of the cause and iron replacement, and for folate deficiency it is folate (after testing for concomitant vitamin B_{12} deficiency and giving treatment, as needed). A reticulocytosis should be seen within one to two weeks of instituting appropriate treatment. A significant thrombocytosis often develops within days of abstinence. Coagulopathy (manifested as easy bleeding and ecchymoses), confirmed by elevation of the INR and prolongation of the partial thromboplastin time, usually is a result of chronic liver disease, although a trial of vitamin K replacement is warranted at least once. Anemias can be the result of abnormal red blood cell membranes in patients with cirrhosis (that is, spur and burr cell anemia).

Cardiovascular Consequences: In addition to the transient hypertension seen during withdrawal, heavy drinking (three or more standard drinks per day) is associated with chronic hypertension, which can lead to end-organ cardiac, retinal, renal, and vascular damage (Criqui, 1987; Gitlow, Dziedzic et al., 1986). Hypertension can be the result of even low levels of regular consumption. Although persons who in retrospect prove to be safe drinkers of moderate amounts appear to have a lower incidence of coronary heart disease events, chronic heavy drinking can lead to alcoholic cardiomyopathy and congestive heart failure (Urbano-Marquez, Estruch et al., 1989). Echocardiogram reveals diffuse hypokinesis and often four-chamber dilatation. If left ventricular thrombosis is seen, patients are at higher risk of embolic stroke. Treatment consists of alcohol abstinence (which can, in some cases, lead to an increase in the left ventricular ejection fraction), and standard treatments for congestive heart failure (which include angiotensin-converting-enzyme inhibitors or antagonists, furosemide [Lasix®] or other loop diuretics, nitrates, and sometimes digoxin).

Evaluation for sustained ventricular dysrhythmias in symptomatic patients is warranted and may lead to anti-arrhythmic therapy (with amiodarone [Cordarone®]) or implantation of an automatic implantable cardioverter defibrillator to decrease the risk of sudden death (Hohnloser, 1999). Anticoagulation with warfarin may be indicated when there is a ventricular clot, but the risk-benefit balance often is unclear, particularly when the patient is not abstinent. Atrial fibrillation ("holiday heart") can occur as a consequence of alcohol use or withdrawal, is not restricted to holidays, and usually resolves spontaneously (Ettinger, Wu et al., 1978; Klatsky, 1998; Kupari & Koskinen, 1991; Rich, Siebold et al., 1985). If the dysrhythmia persists after treatment for withdrawal (with benzodiazepines and, in this case, beta-blockers) and abstinence, other etiologies (for example, hyperthyroidism, hypertension, ischemic heart disease, and cardiomyopathy) should be evaluated, and additional treatment (electrical or chemical cardioversion and anticoagulation) should be considered.

Moderate drinking (<2 standard drinks per day) has been associated with fewer cardiovascular events and decreased mortality in men (but not in average-risk women) (Thun, Peto et al., 1997), although no randomized trials have been done of this pharmacologic agent with known side effects. And binge amounts have adverse cardiovascular consequences (Poikolainen, 1998). The epidemiologic findings of benefit for moderate drinking can be confounded by alternative explanations, such as differences in social characteristics that remain unaccounted for (Camacho, Kaplan et al., 1987; Kromhout, Bloemberg et al., 1996; Muntwyler, Hennekens et al., 1998). Recent studies have suggested that, if there is a benefit, it may be most pronounced in patients who have the same alcohol dehydrogenase genotype that may predispose them to alcoholism (Hines, Stampfer et al., 2001). Clearly, nondrinkers should not begin to drink for cardiovascular benefit.

Renal and Metabolic Consequences: Renal and metabolic consequences of alcohol use often are seen in acute care settings. Hepatitis C can lead to nephrotic syndrome and glomerulonephritis with or without cryoglobulinemia and purpura (Johnson, Gretch et al., 1993). Cirrhosis can be complicated by the almost always fatal renal ischemic disorder, hepatorenal syndrome. Chronic renal insufficiency may be seen in persons who ingest home-distilled alcohol made with lead equipment (Nolan & Shaikh, 1992). Acute renal failure from rhabdomyolysis can occur after alcohol intoxication.

Fluid and electrolyte abnormalities are very common and often are minimized and overlooked in alcoholics who present for medical care. Many patients with alcoholism who present for medical treatment will be volume-depleted from vomiting, diarrhea, and diuresis. Volume repletion is best accomplished orally, when possible, and with intravenous normal saline, at least until the patient no longer manifests postural changes in blood pressure and heart rate and excess losses are not continuing. Acidosis can be a medical emergency. The first step is to distinguish between a non-anion gap and an anion gap acidosis. If an anion gap is not present, diarrhea is the most common cause in alcoholics. If an anion gap is present, the differential diagnosis is broad but, in the alcoholic, lactic acidosis (from sepsis, injury, severe pancreatitis, or after convulsion), ketoacidosis, and ingestion should be considered first. To rule out ingestion, in addition to the history (which may be unreliable), the measured serum osmolality should be compared with the calculated osmolality (accounting for the serum ethanol in the calculation). If no osmolar gap is present, ethylene glycol and methanol ingestions are unlikely. These ingestions require prompt treatment with fomepizole, hemodialysis, or both to prevent blindness or death (Brent, 2001).

Alcoholic ketoacidosis is common (Fulop, 1993; Wrenn, Slovis et al., 1991). The glucose concentration can be high, normal, or low, and the urine ketones can be negative (although serum ketones should be positive). The treatment is volume expansion, and the substrate is given as 5% dextrose in normal saline (preceded by thiamine). In the absence of ketones or an osmolar gap, lactic acidosis is the next most serious diagnosis to consider, mainly because it can be the only clue to an unrecognized etiology (such as myocardial infarction or recent convulsion).

Alkalemia is not uncommon in alcoholics, either from respiratory alkalosis related to liver disease and hyperventilation or metabolic alkalosis from vomiting. Treatment for withdrawal (holding diuretics if the patient is on them, control of vomiting with antiemetics, and abstinence from alcohol, combined with volume repletion) can help speed the resolution of the alkalemia, which is important because alkalemia can be associated with hypokalemia and hypomagnesemia from secondary hyperaldosteronism.

When dextrose is given to malnourished alcoholics, severe hypophosphatemia can be unmasked and require treatment (Knochel, 1980). Hypomagnesemia is common in alcoholics, as a result of diuretic use, hypokalemia, and reversible hypoparathyroidism resulting from impaired parathyroid hormone release when the magnesium cofactor is deficient (Laitinen, Lamberg-Allardt et al., 1991). The latter condition also leads to hypocalcemia, which does not respond to calcium replacement; rather, it responds to magnesium repletion. The hypokalemia often seen in alcoholics with hyperaldosteronism from volume depletion and diuretic use will not correct until magnesium is replaced. Serum levels do not reflect total body magnesium stores, so empiric replacement is the best approach. Oral replacement of magnesium and phosphate is possible with magnesium-containing antacids and milk, but this approach often is limited by an inability to take food by mouth or by diarrhea (which worsens the deficiencies). Intravenous replacement, with cardiac monitoring in the case of severe hypophosphatemia, may be necessary. Hyperglycemia or hypoglycemia can be seen in alcoholism as a result of pancreatic insufficiency or, in the case of end-stage cirrhosis, as a result of depleted glycogen stores, which is a very poor prognostic sign.

Trauma: Injury is a common consequence of both alcohol and drug intoxication, but may be more likely in alcohol abusers (Rees, Horton et al., 2002). Trauma, including physical and sexual abuse, can lead to poorer addiction treatment outcomes (Liebschutz, Savetsky, et al., 2002). Alcohol can interfere with balance and coordination, thus predisposing to injury. It also interferes with judgment, and some heavy drinkers already have a predisposition to risk-taking. Binge drinking poses a particular risk of injury and accidents (Anda, Williamson et al., 1988). Patients who present to emergency departments and trauma centers with serious injuries are far more likely than others to have used alcohol recently (Cherpitel, 1993). The high frequency of injury in persons with heavy alcohol use suggests that facilities where such persons are seen for health care (that is, emergency departments and trauma centers) should routinely screen for alcohol problems and refer patients with alcohol-related disorders for treatment in order to prevent additional injury. Such strategies have proved successful in randomized trials (Gentilello, Rivara et al., 1999). Moreover, addiction specialists should be attuned to the high rates of injury (both past trauma and the risk of future injury) when counseling alcoholics. Injury can be a motivating factor for discontinuing alcohol use, or a focus of counseling to prevent future injuries.

Infectious Diseases: Alcohol can lead to infectious consequences by various mechanisms. Alcoholics can have impaired defenses because of undernutrition, splenic dysfunction, leukopenia and impaired granulocyte function, as well as suppression of the gag reflex during intoxication and overdose. Because of these risks, fever in an alcoholic must not be attributed to a minor viral syndrome or withdrawal unless other causes have been reasonably excluded. For example, although fever and confusion might be attributable to a postictal state or DTs, cerebrospinal fluid examination is warranted to exclude the possibility of meningitis. Although the treatment is the same as for nonaddicted persons, pneumonia is more common in alcoholics, alcoholism increases the risk of mortality, and hospital treatment is more costly because it takes longer (Saitz, Ghali et al., 1997). Concomitant smoking increases the risk by impairing the mucociliary elevator. Causes include aspiration (commonly of anaerobic organisms), *S. pneumoniae*, atypical organisms, viruses, *Haemophilus influenzae*, and *Klebsiella pneumoniae*.

Tuberculosis is a consideration, particularly when the symptoms are more chronic, weight loss is present, and upper lobe infiltrates appear on the chest x-ray in alcoholics who are homeless, have immigrated from a country where the disease is endemic, are known to have a previous positive tuberculin skin test, or have had contact with an active case. Because HIV is more common in alcoholics than in the general population, *Pneumocystis carinii* pneumonia and other opportunistic infections must be considered when pneumonia is diagnosed. Treatment for all of these conditions involves hospitalization in severe cases and antimicrobial therapy directed at the known or likely etiologies, along with observation and treatment for withdrawal symptoms.

Other infectious diseases seen in alcoholics include sexually transmitted diseases, spontaneous bacterial peritonitis, brain abscess, and meningitis. Meningitis in alcoholics has a broader differential diagnosis than in the general population. It can be due to *S. pneumoniae, Listeria monocytogenes*, gram-negative bacilli and, in younger persons, *Neisseria meningitidis*. Brain abscess can result from poor dentition, leading to transient bacteremia and local infection, for example, in a preexisting subdural hematoma. Spontaneous bacterial peritonitis occurs in patients with cirrhosis and ascites. Symptoms can include only fever or abdominal discomfort or encephalopathy, with any one of these symptoms absent. Abdominal tenderness may be minimal or absent. Diagnosis is made by paracentesis, which should be done when there is any clinical suspicion.

Spontaneous bacterial empyema can occur when pleural effusion is present (Kirchmair, Allerberger et al., 1998). Sexually transmitted diseases, including HIV, are more common in heavy alcohol users, in part because of sexual risk-taking behavior (CDC, 2000). Treatment for all of these conditions is guided by local epidemiology, frequently updated resources (for example, *The Medical Letter* or handbooks of antimicrobial therapy), and national treatment guidelines for targeted and empiric antimicrobial therapy (Niederman, Mandell et al., 2001; Workowski, 2000).

Musculoskeletal Consequences: Musculoskeletal consequences can occur from the chronic heavy use of alcohol. Intoxication to the point of overdose may result in the individual remaining in one position for prolonged periods of time. In addition to compression nerve palsies, rhabdomyolysis (with hyperphosphatemia, hyperkalemia, hypocalcemia, and acute renal failure) can develop and cause a compartment syndrome—a surgical emergency that requires release of the pressure by incision of the skin and fascia along with debridement of necrotic tissue. Diagnosis is made when there is a tense edematous limb, often with evidence of trauma, initially with severe pain and later with anesthesia. Because physical signs and symptoms are variable and unreliable, the diagnosis often is pursued with intracompartmental pressures; a newer method, near infrared spectroscopy, shows promise in avoiding delays in treatment

(Giannotti, Cohn et al., 2000). Surgical consultation is required.

Hyperuricemia and gout are more common in alcoholism. Gout classically presents as podagra, an edematous, exquisitely painful, erythematous great toe. Treatment is with colchicine, using caution in renal or hepatic insufficiency, or indomethacin (Indocin®), using caution in the presence of gastritis or renal insufficiency. The cyclooxygenase-2-specific nonsteroidal anti-inflammatory agents can be effective in gout and have the advantage that they are safer in patients who are at risk of gastrointestinal bleeding, although they have deleterious renal effects. A brief course of corticosteroids or a single injection of adrenocorticotropic hormone may be safer choices for the alcoholic. Chronic treatment in the setting of renal disease, tophaceous gout, or polyarticular gout should be with allopurinol (Lopurin®) or probenecid (Benemid®). Saturnine gout is diagnosed when the hyperuricemia is associated with past "moonshine" use (Ehrlich & Chokatos, 1966; Klinenberg, 1969). Hyperuricemia can lead to renal insufficiency.

Excessive alcohol use (more than one drink a day for women, two for men, and binge drinking) increases the risk of skeletal fracture. What component of this increased risk is due to a higher risk of trauma and what is attributable to alcohol-related osteopenia is unclear. Although moderate alcohol use can be associated with an increase in BMD (either because of alcohol's effect on estrogens or other hormones, or because of a lifestyle factor associated with increased BMD), excessive consumption leads to osteopenia. Heavy alcohol use can lead to osteonecrosis of bone, such as that at the femoral head.

Oncologic Risks: Alcohol is a risk factor for a number of cancers. These include malignancies of the lip, oral cavity, pharynx, larynx, esophagus, stomach, breast, liver, intrahepatic bile ducts, prostate, and colon (Bagnardi, Blangiardo et al., 2001). Although most of these cancers are associated with heavy alcohol use, often in association with smoking, the increased risk of the cancers often is detectable in large populations at more moderate levels (Anderson, 1995; Holman, English et al., 1996; Thun, Peto et al., 1997). For example, breast cancer risk increases with consumption of one to two standard drinks per day on average (Fuchs, Stampfer et al., 1995; Smith-Warner, Spiegelman et al., 1998).

Pulmonary Consequences: Alcohol intoxication can lead to respiratory depression and aspiration, leading to a chemical or infectious pneumonia. Tachypnea can be the result of pulmonary infection, respiratory alkalosis of liver disease, alcohol withdrawal, or compensation for a metabolic acidosis.

Endocrinologic Consequences: Alcohol causes sexual dysfunction and hypogonadism in men, both through direct effects on the testes and through secondary effects in chronic liver disease, in which gynecomastia may be seen. Alcohol delays menopause and is associated with menstrual disorders such as dysmenorrhea and metrorrhagia. Amounts as little as one drink per week have been associated with decreased fertility in women (Jensen, Hjollund et al., 1998). Alcohol increases the high-density lipoprotein fraction of cholesterol which, in part, explains observed decreases in coronary artery disease in moderate drinkers; however, it also increases serum triglycerides, which can lead to heart disease, hepatic steatosis, and pancreatitis.

Consequences in the Perioperative Patient: Heavy alcohol consumption is a risk factor for postoperative complications (Tonnesen & Kehlet, 1999). In the perioperative period, attention must be given to identifying a risk of withdrawal, managing the withdrawal, and managing the pain. Elective surgery can be an opportune time to try to achieve abstinence, both as treatment for alcohol dependence and to prevent perioperative morbidity. This approach can reduce morbidity, as has been demonstrated in at least one randomized trial (Tonnesen, Rosenberg et al., 1999).

Vitamin Deficiencies: Alcoholics are prone to vitamin deficiency because of malabsorption and poor dietary intake (Green, 1983; Hoyumpa, 1986; Lieber, 1984; Russell, 1980; Ryle & Thomson, 1984). Alcohol has been associated with deficiencies of fat-soluble vitamins when there is malabsorption because of pancreatic disease and also with deficiencies of thiamine, pyridoxine, niacin, riboflavin, vitamin D, and zinc. Symptoms commonly seen in alcoholics may not be due to intoxication or withdrawal. For example, thiamine deficiency can cause confusion and ataxia, whereas diarrhea, abdominal discomfort, amnesia, anxiety, insomnia, nausea, seizure, and ataxia may be the result of pellagra. A clue to this diagnosis is the coexistence of glossitis and rash in sun-exposed areas, but these more specific features may be absent (Kertesz, 2001). Vitamin replacement is safe and should be done empirically.

Sleep: Although alcohol can help nonalcoholics fall asleep, it also can be stimulating and lead to disrupted sleep and daytime fatigue. In the alcoholic, a drink may be required to sleep, but sleep is quite disrupted. This situation also is true of the alcoholic in recovery, who may relapse because of intolerable insomnia (Brower, Aldrich et al., 2001). Alcohol increases the risk of obstructive sleep apnea and worsens the disease because of its depressant effects on respiration and relaxation of the upper airway. Alcohol can increase the risk of periodic limb movements of sleep. Treatment of insomnia in the alcoholic involves attention to sleep hygiene as well as pharmacotherapy with drugs with a low or no risk of dependence, such as trazodone (Desyrel®).

Fetal, Neonatal, and Infant Consequences: Use of alcohol during pregnancy, even in amounts considered to be moderate in nonpregnant adults, can lead to mental retardation and neurobehavioral deficits in children. The fetal alcohol syndrome involves craniofacial abnormalities, neurologic abnormalities, and growth retardation (Anonymous, 2000). Affected individuals may have some or all of the manifestations of the syndrome. The neurologic disabilities persist into adulthood. Because no safe amount of alcohol during pregnancy has been identified and there is no treatment for the effects of alcohol on the fetus, abstinence is recommended during pregnancy.

Tobacco. Tobacco use increases the risk of death. In addition, it causes cosmetic effects such as stained teeth, stained fingers, wrinkles, and many medical illnesses.

Withdrawal: Although nicotine withdrawal is not life-threatening, the craving can complicate treatment for other medical illnesses. Nicotine replacement should be provided for medically ill patients who are hospitalized. Bupropion (Zyban®) is an alternative. Nicotine replacement can precipitate myocardial ischemia, but the alternative, smoking a cigarette, also can do so. Therefore, in general, even smokers with coronary artery disease can use nicotine replacement, unless they are experiencing unstable angina or myocardial infarction.

Neurologic Consequences: Tobacco use is associated with atherosclerosis, peripheral vascular disease and, therefore, cerebrovascular disease and ischemic and hemorrhagic stroke. Atherosclerotic disease can involve small vessels and result in cognitive deficits.

Gastrointestinal Consequences: Smoking is a cause of gastric and duodenal ulcers. Smoking can cause and exacerbate gastroesophageal reflux disease. Smoking interferes with ulcer healing. These diseases can require pharmacotherapy in addition to smoking cessation, as with histamine type 2 receptor antagonists, proton pump inhibitors, or antibiotics for *Helicobacter pylori.*

Hematologic Consequences: Although data are conflicting, smoking is known to have hypercoagulable effects, and it can be a risk factor for deep vein thrombosis (Goldhaber, Grodstein et al., 1997).

Cardiovascular Consequences: Smoking can lead to poorer control of hypertension (Buhler, Vesanen et al., 1988) and causes atherosclerosis. Smokers thus are at higher risk of myocardial infarction and sudden death. Moreover, smoking appears to potentiate the risks of heart attack conferred by hyperlipidemia and diabetes. Smoking can precipitate angina by causing vasospasm and hypercoagulability, and it can precipitate dysrhythmia. Smokers are at higher risk of cerebrovascular disease and stroke and peripheral vascular disease, which leads to intermittent claudication, pain, and loss of limb. Smoking lowers the beneficial serum high-density lipoprotein subfraction of cholesterol. The risk of heart disease (Kawachi, Colditz et al., 1994) and peripheral vascular disease and stroke morbidity and mortality decreases soon after smoking cessation.

Renal Consequences: The renal consequences of tobacco dependence are limited primarily to the effects of atherosclerosis of the renal arteries, which can lead to ischemic renal failure and hypertension from renal artery stenosis.

Injury: Although smoking does not increase the level of risk associated with risk-taking behavior, tobacco dependence can lead to house fires, smoke inhalation, and death, as well as other accidental death (Leistikow, Martin et al., 2000). Anecdotally, smoking in medically ill patients using oxygen has resulted in facial and airway burns and fires.

Infectious Consequences: Because of its pulmonary effects, smoking increases the risk of acute and chronic bronchitis and pneumonia. Smokers have more frequent upper respiratory infections. These risks decrease with cessation.

Oncologic Risks: Smoking has been associated with the following cancers: oral cavity, larynx, lung, esophagus, bladder, kidney, pancreas, stomach, and cervix. In addition, smokers with one smoking-related cancer are at higher risk for a second one. These risks decrease with cessation.

Pulmonary Consequences: Smoking leads to chronic bronchitis and emphysema, collectively referred to as "chronic obstructive pulmonary disease" (COPD). Smoking is the leading cause of both COPD and bronchogenic carcinoma. The risks of both of these mortal diagnoses can be lowered with smoking cessation. Smoking cessation can slow the steady decline in pulmonary function seen in COPD (Scanlon, Connett et al., 2000). Smoking leads to pulmonary hypertension, interstitial lung disease, and pneumo-

thorax. Although some lung cancers can be treated surgically if detected early, chemotherapeutic approaches have been disappointing. Treatment for COPD is somewhat disappointing, particularly when the patient continues to smoke. Effective treatments include bronchodilators, oxygen for hypoxemia and, less commonly, corticosteroids.

Endocrinologic Consequences: Cigarette use is known to increase the risk of Graves' disease (hyperthyroidism) and hypothyroidism (Winsa, Mandahl et al., 1993). Smoking and nicotine itself can increase insulin resistance (including detrimental effects on lipids and glucose) and risk of diabetes. Estrogen is decreased in male and female smokers, as is sperm number and function in men (Michnovicz, Hershcopf et al., 1989; Vine, Margolin et al., 1994). Smoking is one of the leading causes of erectile dysfunction, mainly because of atherosclerosis. Cigarette use is associated with decreased BMD, osteoporosis, and fractures.

Consequences in the Perioperative Patient: Smoking increases the risk of postoperative pulmonary complications, including pneumonia, atelectasis, reactive airways exacerbations, and respiratory failure. Smoking cessation before elective surgery is advisable, although it should be done at least two months before surgery (Bluman, Mosca et al., 1998; Tisi, 1987; Warner, Offord et al., 1989). Current smokers should pay particular attention to pulmonary toilet perioperatively. Incentive spirometry should be used, along with use of bronchodilators.

Sleep: Nicotine increases the time it takes to fall asleep (sleep latency). Abstinence in tobacco-dependent individuals (that is, withdrawal) increases daytime sleepiness.

Fetal, Neonatal, and Infant Consequences: Tobacco use during pregnancy causes low birth weight, spontaneous abortion, and perinatal mortality, among other consequences. The risks of sudden infant death syndrome and neurodevelopmental impairment are increased, although studies have had difficulty separating the effects of tobacco, alcohol, nutrition, and social situations.

Opiates, Cocaine, and Other Drugs. The complications of other drugs often are related to route of administration. Injection and inhalation of drugs have particular consequences. In addition to route of administration, drugs have unique organ systems complications.

Injection Drug Use: Injection of drugs leads to a break in the skin barrier that protects against infection. As a result, skin and soft tissue infections are common in injection drug users (Stein, 1990). Most commonly, cellulitis is caused by staphylococci and streptococci. Treatment should be with a semisynthetic penicillin or first-generation cephalosporin or vancomycin. Abscess usually is caused by *Staphylococcus aureus* and requires surgical drainage in addition to antibiotic treatment. However, one must be aware of local epidemiology and practices because there have been reports of unusual pathogens (that is, *Pseudomonas aeruginosa* and *Serratia* species) and polymicrobial infections from use of saliva to prepare the injection (Cherubin & Sapira, 1993; Levin, Weinstein et al., 1984). Furthermore, injection drug users sometimes use antibiotics obtained without prescription, which places them at risk of infection with resistant organisms. Soft tissue infections can progress to become serious and life-threatening if fasciitis develops or if there is significant local ischemia, as with cocaine injection (Murphy, DeVita et al., 2001). Intravenous injection can result in septic thrombophlebitis, as well as arterial injection with embolus and digital ischemia and infection. Injection can lead to venous valvular damage in the extremities, marked by leg ulcers, edema, and a propensity to develop deep vein thrombosis. Although rare, tetanus can develop as a result of nonsterile injection (Cherubin & Sapira, 1993; Talan & Moran, 1998).

Injection drug use spreads bloodborne pathogens when needles or other equipment are shared or when the drug user engages in risky behaviors. Regarding sexually transmitted infections, false-positive screening tests for syphilis often are found in injection drug users. Treponemal-specific tests are needed to determine the diagnosis (fluorescent treponemal antibody, or microhemagglutination test for *T. pallidum*). Bloodborne pathogens spread by injection or risky behaviors, including HIV, hepatitis B, hepatitis C, and malaria. Hepatitis B can develop into a chronic infection, and HIV and hepatitis C almost invariably are chronic illnesses that require long-term management strategies by clinicians familiar with the complexities of their care.

Hepatitis can lead to cirrhosis and its sequelae, including death, and HIV to opportunistic infections and death. Antiviral drugs for these infections exist (their use is beyond the scope of this introductory chapter). Altered mentation can result from HIV infection and liver disease. Similarly, opportunistic infections in AIDS can lead to stroke.

One of the most serious infectious consequences of injection drug use is bacterial endocarditis. In an injection drug user, as in an alcohol user, fever cannot be taken lightly. If there is an identifiable cause (such as pneumonia or cellulitis), it should be treated. Pneumonia is common in injection drug users, either because of aspiration, septic embolization, or exposure to pathogens such as *M. tuberculosis*. Injection drug users can have septic arthritis in unusual locations (sternoclavicular or sacroiliac joints), spinal epidural or vertebral infections, osteomyelitis, or meningitis. However, a significant proportion of patients with fever and no identifiable cause will have an unrecognized serious illness, most often endocarditis (Samet, Shevitz et al., 1990). Missing this diagnosis can be fatal. A cardiac murmur may not be present. The classic "textbook" signs of subacute bacterial endocarditis, most of which are immunologic phenomena, often are not present in drug users with acute bacterial, often right-sided (that is, tricuspid valve) endocarditis (Roberts & Slovis, 1990). Therefore, blood cultures should be taken, and close observation (often in the hospital) instituted; many authorities recommend empiric antibiotic treatment while awaiting culture results. If endocarditis is diagnosed, treatment is with bactericidal antibiotics for four to six weeks. Mycotic aneurysms; endophthalmitis; congestive heart failure; brain, spleen, or myocardial abscesses and emboli; renal failure from interstitial nephritis; pulmonary septic emboli with effusions; stroke; and heart block can complicate the course. Selected uncomplicated cases can be treated with shorter courses (DiNubile, 1994). Patients who have multiple emboli or hemodynamic decompensation may require surgical intervention and valve replacement.

In addition to infectious complications, injection of drugs can lead to pulmonary talc granulomatosis from injected crushed tablets containing talc, pulmonary hypertension from granulomatous disease or drug-related vasoconstriction, needle embolization, pneumothorax or hemothorax from injection into large central veins gone awry, and pulmonary emphysema related or unrelated to talc granulomatosis. Granulomatosis can occur in the liver from injection of talc. Nephropathy related to injection drug use, primarily because of HIV infection, is a common renal complication. Amyloidosis and nephrotic syndrome can occur because of chronic skin infections. Hepatitis C infection can lead to glomerulonephritis. The coagulopathy that results from liver and kidney disease in injection drug users can lead to neurologic complications—namely, hemorrhagic stroke. Cerebral infarction has resulted from injection of crushed tablets and even of a melted suppository (intravenously and via inadvertent intra-arterial injection) (Bitar & Gomez, 1993).

Inhalation of Drugs: Consequences of inhalation that are not related to the specific substance inhaled are primarily pulmonary. Inhalation of drugs has effects related to the size of the particles: larger particles affect the airways, while smaller ones reach the alveoli. Complications include granulomatous responses to fibrogenic substances such as talc, chronic bronchitis from inhaled smoke (regardless of whether the drug involved is marijuana, nicotine, cocaine, and so forth), bronchospasm (as from inhaled cocaine), barotrauma with resultant pneumothorax or pneumomediastinum from prolonged breath holding or stimulant use, hemoptysis from airway irritation, and emphysema from inhaled tobacco, marijuana, or opiates (Johnson, Smith et al., 2000; Pare, Cote et al., 1989). Freebasing can lead to upper airway and facial burns.

Withdrawal: Withdrawal from opiates often is seen in patients with medical illnesses who require hospitalization. Although the withdrawal is not fatal in an otherwise healthy person, it should be treated for symptomatic relief to prevent hyperadrenergic states that complicate treatment of the acute medical problems (for example, coronary syndromes) and to allow the patient to be sufficiently comfortable so that he or she can complete medical treatment and link to addiction treatment.

Neurologic Consequences: As with alcohol users, drug users may suffer from incoordination and exposure to risky situations that can lead to injury, including head injury or (in the case of involvement with illegal drugs or difficult social situations) injury from stabbings and gunshots. Seizures can occur as a result of sedative withdrawal (barbiturates and benzodiazepines), stimulant use (methamphetamines and cocaine), or proconvulsant metabolites (meperidine [Demerol®]). Similarly, hemorrhagic stroke can occur with use of methamphetamines, phenylpropanolamine, lysergic acid diethylamide, and phencyclidine from hypertension, vasculitis, or other vascular mechanisms. Cocaine use can lead to both hemorrhagic and ischemic strokes (Johnson, Devous et al., 2001; McEvoy, Kitchen et al., 2000). Anabolic steroids can cause stroke by promoting hypercoagulability. Although classic syndromes of dementia have not been described for users of drugs other than alcohol, chronic cognitive deficits can be seen in users of cocaine, sedatives (barbiturate), and toluene. Neuropathy (including plexopathies and Guillan-Barré syndrome) may be caused by heroin use, compression neuropathy in any drug user, quadriplegia in glue sniffers, and combined systems degeneration from vitamin B_{12} deficiency induced

by nitrous oxide use. Parkinsonism can develop from the use of a meperidine analogue, MPTP.

Gastrointestinal Consequences: In addition to viral hepatitis, which is almost universal in injection drug users, cocaine itself can cause hepatic necrosis, probably because of ischemia. Ecstasy and phencyclidine use has been reported to cause liver failure (Andreu, Mas et al., 1998; Armen, Kanel et al., 1984). Androgenic steroids can cause hepatic toxicity. Chronic diarrhea can be a result of laxative abuse, whereas anticholinergic and opiate abuse will cause constipation. "Bodypacking" (transporting cocaine, heroin, or other drugs in bags that are swallowed) can lead to mechanical obstruction of the intestines. Rupture can lead to overdose and death from respiratory arrest or cardiovascular collapse.

Hematologic Consequences: Amyl nitrate, isobutyl nitrate, and other "poppers" can cause methemoglobinemia. The arterial partial pressure of oxygen is normal, the saturation is low, and cyanosis is present. Methemoglobin can be measured. The treatment is with methylene blue (Wartenberg, 1990).

Cardiovascular Consequences: In addition to the infectious complications of drug abuse that are related to route of administration (endocarditis and myocardial abscess), drugs of abuse can directly affect the heart and blood vessels. Cocaine can cause severe hypertension, cardiac dysrhythmias, angina, myocardial infarction, sudden death, and stroke. As with treatment for hypertension in cocaine users, nitrates and benzodiazepines are first-line agents. For these acute coronary syndromes, oxygen and aspirin are first line as well, and calcium channel blockers (verapamil [Calan®]), phentolamine, thrombolysis, or angioplasty (with anticoagulants as indicated) are second-line treatments (Lange & Hillis, 2001). Sedation with a benzodiazepine can be helpful. Labetalol (Normodyne®) is, in theory, an alternative because of its alpha- and beta-blocking effects but, because its effects are predominantly beta-blocking, it should be avoided. Chest pain often occurs during or after cocaine use, but most persons evaluated in emergency departments with chest pain and cocaine use do not have myocardial infarction (Feldman, Fish et al., 2000). Nonetheless, heart attacks do occur and are thought to be related to coronary vasospasm, *in situ* thrombosis, or the accelerated development of atherosclerosis because of cocaine (or underlying atherosclerotic coronary artery disease, from smoking, for example). As with treatment for hypertension in cocaine users, calcium channel blockers, nitrates, and benzodiazepines are preferred. Cardiomyopathy can occur as a consequence of cocaine use (Nademanee, 1992). Other stimulants (for example, phenylpropanolamine and amphetamines) can produce cardiac complications. Anabolic steroids can lead to coronary artery disease as well as cardiomyopathy. Drugs with anticholinergic effects (muscle relaxants, antihistamines, and antidepressants) cause tachycardia and can cause dysrhythmias in intoxication or overdose. Inhalants (volatile fluorocarbons) can cause dysrhythmias, as can anesthetic gases.

Renal and Metabolic Consequences: Aside from the previously discussed infectious and injection-related renal complications of other drugs of abuse, any drug that leads to sedation with intoxication or overdose (such as, heroin and barbiturates) can lead to muscle compression and rhabdomylysis and to acute renal failure. Rhabdomyolysis can be seen with amphetamine, cocaine, and phencyclidine use. Persons who abuse prescription drugs (opiates) can present with factitious hematuria (red blood cells in the urine and flank pain, feigning nephrolithiasis) to obtain opiate prescriptions because no radiologic test or procedure is 100% sensitive for kidney stones and because nephrolithiasis is invariably (and appropriately) treated with opiates. Cocaine can lead to accelerated hypertension and renal failure, hypertensive nephrosclerosis, thrombotic microangiopathy, and renal infarction. Amphetamines can result in a drug-related polyarteritis nodosa. Ecstasy use can lead to hyponatremia when users drink excess water to prevent the hypovolemia associated with its use. Toluene inhalation can lead to metabolic acidosis.

Injury: Although much of the literature focuses on alcohol as a risk factor for injury, cocaine and other drugs also have been associated with an increased risk of motor vehicle crash and other violent injuries, including fatal shootings (Marzuk, Tardiff et al., 1992). Persons in a detoxification program for opiates or cocaine have a very high risk of injury (20% in each of five consecutive six-month periods) (Rees, Horton et al., 2001).

Infectious Consequences of Drug Use: Most of the infectious complications of drug use are related to injection or risky sexual practices, as discussed previously. As with alcohol users, users of other drugs engage in high-risk sexual behaviors that place them at risk of sexually transmitted diseases, including HIV. Diagnosis and treatment are the same as in nondrug users. Similarly, drug users are at risk of pneumonia from aspiration related to overdose and tuberculosis.

Oncologic Risks: Although the magnitude of risk remains unclear, marijuana, when smoked, can lead to squamous cell carcinoma of the oral cavity and to lung cancer (Tashkin, 2001).

Pulmonary Consequences: In addition to injection complications, the lungs are affected by many illicit drugs. Drugs that produce sedation with use or overdose can lead to respiratory depression and death. Naloxone (Narcan®) and flumazenil (Romazicon®) can reverse the effects in opiate and benzodiazepine users, respectively. Atelectasis can develop, as can aspiration and chemical pneumonitis; these do not require antibiotic treatment but are managed with airway management, incentive spirometry, chest physiotherapy, and oxygen. More specifically, marijuana use can lead to obstructive lung disease (Johnson, Smith et al., 2000) and fungal infection from contamination. Cocaine use can lead to nasal septal perforation, sinusitis, epiglottitis, upper airway obstruction, and hemoptysis, primarily from irritant and vasoconstrictive effects. Cocaine use can lead to pulmonary hemorrhage, edema, hypertension, emphysema, interstitial fibrosis, and hypersensitivity pneumonitis.

The treatment for most of these diseases is withdrawal of the cocaine and supportive care, although corticosteroids and bronchodilators are warranted in some cases. Pulmonary hypertension and edema can result from use of stimulants (specifically amphetamines). Opiate use can lead to bronchospasm, as a result of their stimulation of histamine release, and pulmonary edema in the setting of overdose. The pulmonary consequences of sedatives are limited primarily to respiratory depression and arrest from overdose, worsening of sleep-disordered breathing, as well as tachypnea, hyperventilation, and respiratory alkalosis from withdrawal syndromes. Inhalants can lead to methemoglobinemia (treated with methylene blue), tracheobronchitis, asphyxiation, and hypersensitivity pneumonitis. Nitrous oxide can cause respiratory depression and hypoxemia. Anabolic steroids can induce prothrombotic states and lead to pulmonary embolism.

Endocrinologic Consequences: Most drugs of abuse can affect hormone levels, particularly thyroid hormones, gonadotropins, antidiuretic hormone, sex steroids, and the hypothalamic-pituitary-adrenal axis, but the clinical implications often are unclear. Opiates can impair gonadotropin release. Clinically, men may have impaired sperm motility, and women may have menstrual and ovulatory irregularities. This mechanism may explain the reduced BMD seen in heroin addicts (Pedrazzoni, Vescovi et al., 1993).

Cocaine is a risk factor for the more frequent occurrence of diabetic ketoacidosis, in part because of adrenergic effects (Warner, Greene et al., 1998). Barbiturate use can lead to osteomalacia from vitamin D deficiency. The deficiency results from stimulation of the cytochrome hepatic metabolism of substances, including thyroid hormone and hydrocortisone, which are of note when treating patients with these drugs. Clinical metabolic consequences have been clearly linked to use of anabolic steroids. Women develop androgenization, and lipids are adversely affected.

Consequences in the Perioperative Patient: Several issues arise in the perioperative period with users of other drugs. First, it is essential to assess (through the history and toxicologic screens) what drugs have been used. Second, attention to and treatment of withdrawal symptoms can avert development of tachycardia and hypertension, which may complicate interpretation of assessments and operative and anesthetic treatments. Third, the anesthesiologist must be informed of any recent drug use because of potential interactions between beta-blockers and cocaine and because of the potentiation of sedative and anesthetic drugs. Finally, anesthesia and pain management generally require much higher doses than usual in the opiate-dependent patient. Nutritional issues often require attention in addicted persons undergoing surgery, as wound healing may be impaired.

Vitamin Deficiencies: Nitrous oxide abuse is a well-known cause of vitamin B_{12} deficiency.

Sleep: Clearly, stimulants, including caffeine, can suppress sleep, which often is an intended effect. Opioids and nicotine tend to reduce sleep. Benzodiazepines, often used to help with sleep, do reduce the time it takes to fall asleep. Many persons with addictive disorders also experience sleep disturbances, because of the drug used, lifestyles, or comorbid psychiatric conditions. Sleep problems can contribute to the desire to use drugs for self-medication. In fact, opioids are effective for the management of restless legs syndrome and periodic movements of sleep, a treatment an opioid-dependent person may have discovered accidentally. The management of sleep disorders, particularly insomnia, therefore is difficult but important in addicted persons. Attention to sleep hygiene (that is, a quiet location, using the bed only for sleep and sex, and elimination of napping) and judicious use of drugs less likely to lead to misuse, such as trazodone, are the best approaches.

Fetal, Neonatal, and Infant Consequences: No clear teratogenic effects of opiates are known. Although many studies of the issue have been conducted, studies that did find effects often did not control for the effects of important confounders such as nutrition, alcohol, and tobacco use. However, opiate exposure *in utero* can lead to the neonatal abstinence syndrome, including seizures. Detoxification, when agreeable to the patient, is best done during the second trimester to prevent this complication.

Benzodiazepines have been associated with cleft lip and palate, but the studies of benzodiazepines, like other studies of teratogenesis in drug users, may have been confounded by alcohol use. Toluene use appears to cause an embryopathy, and other inhalants have caused various nonspecific effects, including preterm labor and intrauterine growth retardation. The effects of caffeine in pregnancy are controversial. It probably is relatively safe, although some reports of increased fetal loss suggest minimizing its use during pregnancy.

Dextroamphetamine (Dexedrine®) does appear to be associated with teratogenesis. Cocaine can induce teratogenic effects and neonatal irritability, and also may cause behavioral and learning disorders. But again, many of these reports are difficult to interpret because other maternal factors (including other drug use, inadequate health care, and malnutrition) might account for the findings (Frank, Augustyn et al., 2001).

COMMON MEDICAL PROBLEMS IN PERSONS WITH ADDICTIVE DISORDERS

Persons with addictive disorders suffer from the same medical conditions as nonaddicted persons, but addiction can interfere with the disease or its management. A general medical textbook should be consulted about the diagnosis and management of these disorders; however, several points specific to addiction and common medical problems are discussed here.

Treatment adherence is a problem with addicted and nonaddicted persons alike, but it takes on particular importance with the management of chronic medical illnesses. Cardiovascular diseases are the most common cause of death in the U.S. Coronary artery disease is particularly common in persons with alcohol and other drug abuse because of concomitant tobacco dependence. The person with addiction and anginal chest pain (which lasts at least five minutes, is pressure-like, and often is accompanied by dyspnea, nausea, diaphoresis, and radiation to the jaw or arm) must be taken seriously, with consideration given to a cardiac etiology by examination of the electrocardiogram, cardiac enzymes, and exercise tolerance testing, when appropriate.

Angina can be complicated by alcohol, opiate, and sedative withdrawal, as well as cocaine and other stimulant use when the hyperadrenergic states precipitate anginal attacks. Beta blockers are drugs of choice for managing angina (and for preventing death in persons with coronary artery disease) and are helpful in decreasing sympathetic outflow associated with drug withdrawal. They should be administered to persons withdrawing from alcohol, opiates, and sedatives when underlying coronary artery disease is suspected or present, as well as during acute myocardial infarction or unstable angina. However, cocaine should be avoided when beta-blockers are used because of the unopposed vasoconstriction that can result.

Aspirin is a standard treatment to decrease mortality after myocardial infarction and during unstable angina. Aspirin and other treatments for acute coronary events (heparin, tissue plasminogen activator, and similar anticoagulants) can be problematic in persons who have a potential site for internal bleeding, such as alcoholics with gastritis or liver disease, or intracranial bleeding that is unrecognized. Nitrates and calcium channel blockers often are used in the management of coronary heart disease, and there are no particular considerations applicable to addicted patients with these drugs.

The diagnosis of hypertension can be problematic in persons with addictive disorders. A single elevated blood pressure should not be equated with the diagnosis of hypertension (Joint National Committee VI, 1997). Blood pressure elevation can be a product of pain, withdrawal, or intoxication, depending on the substance used. Alcohol (and other drugs, such as cocaine) elevates blood pressure. Ideally, hypertension should be diagnosed after at least three blood pressure measurements (≥140/90) during prolonged abstinence. Nevertheless, although a diagnosis of hypertension should not be made during detoxification or in an emergency setting (unless end-organ damage is evident), persistent hypertension in a patient who drinks regularly should be managed as hypertension to prevent complications. Treatment of hypertension is the same as in persons without addictive disorders, in that attention to medication adherence for an asymptomatic condition is important, lifestyle modification can help, and many medications are available. Although diuretics are inexpensive, effective, and associated with mortality benefits, they can be somewhat riskier in alcoholics because of the adverse effects on potas-

sium balance. Beta-blockers are excellent alternatives (however, cocaine users should avoid beta-blockers).

Diabetes is more difficult to manage in persons with addictive disorders, not only because of difficulty with adherence and more erratic eating habits, but also because of the effects of alcohol on glucose metabolism. Heavy alcohol users are more prone to prolonged and more severe hypoglycemia from the sulfonylurea agents often used to treat type 2 diabetes. The thiazolidinediones are contraindicated because of the possibility that they may cause hepatic damage, as is metformin (Glucophage®), which should not be given to patients with hepatic impairment or those at risk for lactic acidosis. Thus, choices for the management of diabetes in alcoholism are best limited to insulin injections, although many clinicians do use sulfonylureas with careful monitoring.

In addition to having etiologic roles in cancers, addiction can lead to difficulties in cancer management. First, any renal, hepatic, or cardiac consequences of addiction can limit the choice of chemotherapeutic agents. Pulmonary consequences of tobacco use may limit surgical options. Finally, pain management can be complicated by ongoing or past addiction.

CONSEQUENCES IN OLDER ADULTS

Alcohol and other drug use can lead to additional consequences in older adults (Blow, 1998); also see Section 4. In older adults, lower amounts of alcohol often are associated with adverse consequences because of lower lean body mass and body water, less alcohol dehydrogenase, and impaired ability to develop tolerance. For example, elderly women who drink more than two drinks per day are more likely than nondrinkers to have difficulty with activities of daily living. Similarly, elderly men who drink more than one drink per day are more likely to suffer loss of mobility. Hip fracture, a leading cause of death in older adults, can result from an increased propensity to fall related to alcohol use and to osteopenia. Older adults are more susceptible to injury from motor vehicle crashes and even more so when alcohol is used. Medications (such as antidepressants, interferon for hepatitis C, warfarin, phenytoin, aspirin, and acetaminophen) are less effective or can be harmful when taken with alcohol. Older adults are more susceptible than younger individuals to alcohol's chronic brain damaging effects, including cognitive deficits, and are less likely to recover completely from those effects.

In addition to greater susceptibility, alcohol can cause many consequences in older adults that may be misdiagnosed as other common medical problems. The confusion of alcohol withdrawal delirium may be diagnosed as delirium because of infection. The tremor of withdrawal may be diagnosed as Parkinson's disease or an essential tremor. Dementia, malnutrition, self-neglect, functional decline, sleep problems, and anxiety or depression all may be attributed to "normal" aging when the true cause is alcohol. Similarly, cardiovascular disease and congestive heart failure are common in older adults; alcohol as the cause of cardiomyopathy or exacerbations of congestive heart failure frequently are overlooked. Because many conditions in older adults are multifactorial in origin, perhaps it is best to view alcohol as a contributor to illness. Fractures, seizures, and cerebellar degeneration may be misattributed to other "medical" causes when alcohol is a key contributor. Alcohol can contribute to the occurrence of falls, worsening of chronic illness (such as hypertension), interference with medication adherence and side effects, incontinence, fatigue, neuropathy, sexual dysfunction, and pneumonia.

Other drug abuse can lead to similar consequences in the elderly—confusion, falls, and interference with activities of daily living. The effects of smoking are of great significance in older adults because smoking-related diseases often appear with aging and can be exacerbated by continued smoking. Examples include angina, coronary artery disease, and COPD. Prescription drug abuse can lead to physical, functional, and psychosocial impairments.

CONCLUSIONS

Persons with addictive disorders often do not receive adequate medical care. A medical, psychiatric, or addiction health care visit is an opportunity to provide symptom-oriented as well as preventive care or to link such individuals to preventive health care services. Routine health care of the addicted person differs in that the patient almost certainly is at higher risk of disease than are those without addiction. This warrants a targeted approach to the conditions for which the patient is at risk, and the risks of which can be ameliorated. During hospitalization for medical reasons, special attention must be directed toward management of withdrawal and adequate pain control. Persons with addictive disorders are at risk of a large number of specific acute and chronic medical illnesses in almost every organ system. Further, the management of unrelated but common medical illnesses is complicated by addiction, its effect on medication adherence, and the direct consequences of the abused substances.

Older adults often suffer from a number of chronic disorders including addiction. Beyond worsening the common chronic diseases of aging, addictive disorders can worsen functional status.

The subsequent chapters in this section delve into the medical consequences of addiction in greater detail.

ACKNOWLEDGMENT: The writing of this chapter was supported in part by the Center for Substance Abuse Prevention (CSAP) of the Substance Abuse and Mental Health Services Administration (SAMHSA), Program to Develop Preventive Medicine Faculty in Substance Abuse Prevention grant No. 1T26SP08355-01, and The Robert Wood Johnson Foundation Generalist Physician Faculty Scholars Program grant No. 031489. Dr. Saitz is a Generalist Physician Faculty Scholar.

REFERENCES

Akriviadis E, Botla R, Briggs W et al. (2000). Pentoxifylline improves short-term survival in severe acute alcoholic hepatitis: A double-blind, placebo-controlled trial. *Gastroenterology* 119(6):1637-1648.

Akriviadis EA, Steindel H, Pinto PC et al. (1990). Failure of colchicine to improve short-term survival in patients with alcoholic hepatitis. *Gastroenterology* 99(3):811-818.

American Thoracic Society (ATS) and the Centers for Disease Control and Prevention (CDC) (2000a). Diagnostic standards and classification of tuberculosis in adults and children. *American Journal of Respiratory and Critical Care Medicine* 161(4):1376-1395.

American Thoracic Society (ATS) and the Centers for Disease Control and Prevention (CDC) (2000b). Targeted tuberculin testing and treatment of latent tuberculosis infection. *American Journal of Respiratory and Critical Care Medicine* 161(4):221S-247.

Anda RF, Williamson DF & Remington PL (1988). Alcohol and fatal injuries among U.S. adults. Findings from the NHANES I Epidemiologic Follow-up Study. *Journal of the American Medical Association* 260(17):2529-2532.

Anderson P (1995). Alcohol and risk of physical harm. In HD Holder & G Edwards (eds.) *Alcohol and Public Policy: Evidence and Issues.* Oxford, England: Oxford University Press, 82-113.

Andreu V, Mas A, Bruguera M et al. (1998). Ecstasy: A common cause of severe acute hepatotoxicity. *Journal of Hepatology* 29(3):394-397.

Anonymous (2000). Prenatal exposure to alcohol. *Alcohol Research and Health* 24(1):32-41.

Armen R, Kanel G & Reynolds T (1984). Phencyclidine-induced malignant hyperthermia causing submassive liver necrosis. *American Journal of Medicine* 77(1):167-172.

Bagnardi V, Blangiardo M, La Vecchia C et al. (2001). Alcohol consumption and the risk of cancer: A meta-analysis. *Alcohol Research & Health* 25(1):263-270.

Barry MJ (2001). Prostate-specific-antigen testing for early diagnosis of prostate cancer. *New England Journal of Medicine* 344(18):1373-1377.

Batey RG, Burns T, Benson RJ et al. (1992). Alcohol consumption and the risk of cirrhosis. *Medical Journal of Australia* 156(6):413-416.

Bird GL, O'Grady JG, Harvey FA et al. (1990). Liver transplantation in patients with alcoholic cirrhosis: Selection criteria and rates of survival and relapse. *British Medical Journal* 301(6742):15-17.

Bitar S & Gomez CR (1993). Stroke following injection of a melted suppository. *Stroke* 24(5):741-743.

Blow FC, ed. (1998). *Substance Abuse Among Older Adults (Treatment Improvement Protocol 26)*. Rockville, MD: Substance Abuse and Mental Health Services Administration.

Bluman LG, Mosca L, Newman N et al. (1998). Preoperative smoking habits and postoperative pulmonary complications. *Chest* 113(4):883-889.

Bradley KA, Badrinath S, Bush K et al. (1998). Medical risks for women who drink alcohol. *Journal of General Internal Medicine* 13(9):627-639.

Brent J (2001). Current management of ethylene glycol poisoning. *Drugs* 61(7):979-988.

Brower KJ, Aldrich MS, Robinson EA et al. (2001). Insomnia, self-medication, and relapse to alcoholism. *American Journal of Psychiatry* 158(3):399-404.

Buhler FR, Vesanen K, Watters JT et al. (1988). Impact of smoking on heart attacks, strokes, blood pressure control, drug dose, and quality of life aspects in the International Prospective Primary Prevention Study in Hypertension. *American Heart Journal* 115(1 Pt 2):282-288.

Camacho TC, Kaplan GA & Cohen RD (1987). Alcohol consumption and mortality in Alameda County. *Journal of Chronic Disease* 40(3):229-236.

Centers for Disease Control and Prevention (CDC) (1992). Recommendations for the use of folic acid to reduce the number of cases of spina bifida and other neural tube defects. *Morbidity and Mortality Weekly Report* 41(RR-14):1-7.

Centers for Disease Control and Prevention (CDC) (2000). Alcohol policy and sexually transmitted disease rates—United States, 1981-1995. *Morbidity and Mortality Weekly Report* 49(16):346-349.

Chedid A, Mendenhall CL, Gartside P et al. (1991). Prognostic factors in alcoholic liver disease. VA Cooperative Study Group. *American Journal of Gastroenterology* 86(2):210-216.

Cherpitel CJ (1993). Alcohol and injuries: A review of international emergency room studies. *Addiction* 88(7):923-937.

Cherubin CE & Sapira JD (1993). The medical complications of drug addiction and the medical assessment of the intravenous drug user: 25 years later. *Annals of Internal Medicine* 119(10):1017-1028.

Christensen E & Gluud C (1995). Glucocorticoids are ineffective in alcoholic hepatitis: A meta-analysis adjusting for confounding variables. *Gut* 37(1):113-118.

Colman N & Herbert V (1980). Hematologic complications of alcoholism: Overview. *Seminars in Hematology* 17(3):164-176.

Criqui MH (1987). Alcohol and hypertension: New insights from population studies. *European Heart Journal* 8(Suppl B):19-26.

Daeppen JB, Gache P, Landry U et al. (2002). Symptom-triggered vs fixed-schedule doses of benzodiazepine for alcohol withdrawal. *Archives of Internal Medicine* 162(10):1117-1121.

Delmas PD, Bjarnason NH, Mitlak BH et al. (1997). Effects of raloxifene on bone mineral density, serum cholesterol concentrations, and uterine endometrium in postmenopausal women. *New England Journal of Medicine* 337(23):1641-1647.

Di Nubile MJ (1994). Short-course antibiotic therapy for right-sided endocarditis caused by Staphylococcus aureus in injection drug users. *Annals of Internal Medicine* 121(11):873-876.

Doll R, Peto R, Hall E et al. (1994). Mortality in relation to consumption of alcohol: 13 years' observations on male British doctors. *British Medical Journal* 309(6959):911-918.

Ehrlich GE & Chokatos J (1966). Saturnine gout. *Archives of Internal Medicine* 118(6):572-574.

Elmore JG, Barton MB, Moceri VM et al. (1998). Ten-year risk of false positive screening mammograms and clinical breast examinations. *New England Journal of Medicine* 338(16):1089-1096.

Ettinger PO, Wu CF, De La Cruz C Jr. et al. (1978). Arrhythmias and the "holiday heart": Alcohol-associated cardiac rhythm disorders. *American Heart Journal* 95(5):555-562.

Feldman JA, Fish SS, Beshansky JR et al. (2000). Acute cardiac ischemia in patients with cocaine-associated complaints: Results of a multicenter trial. *Annals of Emergency Medicine* 36(5):469-476.

Filley CM & Kleinschmidt-DeMasters BK (2001). Toxic leukoencephalopathy. *New England Journal of Medicine* 345(6):425-432.

Frank DA, Augustyn M, Knight WG et al. (2001). Growth, development, and behavior in early childhood following prenatal cocaine exposure: A systematic review. *Journal of the American Medical Association* 285(12):1613-1625.

Friedmann PD, Saitz R & Samet JH (1998). Management of adults recovering from alcohol or other drug problems: Relapse prevention in primary care. *Journal of the American Medical Association* 279(15):1227-1231.

Fuchs CS, Stampfer MJ, Colditz GA et al. (1995). Alcohol consumption and mortality among women. *New England Journal of Medicine* 332(19):1245-1250.

Fulop M (1993). Alcoholic ketoacidosis. *Endocrinology and Metabolism Clinics of North America* 22(2):209-219.

Gardner P & Peter G (2001). Recommended schedules for routine immunization of children and adults. *Infectious Disease Clinics of North America* 15(1):1-8.

Gardner P & Schaffner W (1993). Immunization of adults. *New England Journal of Medicine* 328(17):1252-1258.

Gaziano JM, Skerrett PJ & Buring JE (2000). Aspirin in the treatment and prevention of cardiovascular disease. *Haemostasis* 30(Suppl 3):1-13.

Gentilello LM, Rivara FP, Donovan DM et al. (1999). Alcohol interventions in a trauma center as a means of reducing the risk of injury recurrence. *Annals of Surgery* 230(4):473-483.

Giannotti G, Cohn SM, Brown M et al. (2000). Utility of near-infrared spectroscopy in the diagnosis of lower extremity compartment syndrome. *Journal of Trauma* 48(3):396-401.

Gish RG, Lee AH, Keeffe EB et al. (1993). Liver transplantation for patients with alcoholism and end-stage liver disease. *American Journal of Gastroenterology* 88(9):1337-1342.

Gitlow SE, Dziedzic LB & Dziedzic SW (1986). Alcohol and hypertension: Implications from research for clinical practice. *Journal of Substance Abuse Treatment* 3(2):121-129.

Goldhaber SZ, Grodstein F, Stampfer MJ et al. (1997). A prospective study of risk factors for pulmonary embolism in women. *Journal of the American Medical Association* 277(8):642-645.

Green PH (1983). Alcohol, nutrition and malabsorption. *Clinical Gastroenterology* 12(2):563-574.

Hines LM, Stampfer MJ, Ma J et al. (2001). Genetic variation in alcohol dehydrogenase and the beneficial effect of moderate alcohol consumption on myocardial infarction. *New England Journal of Medicine* 344(8):549-555.

Hohnloser SH (1999). Implantable devices versus antiarrhythmic drug therapy in recurrent ventricular tachycardia and ventricular fibrillation. *American Journal of Cardiology* 84(9A):56R-62R.

Holman CD, English DR, Milne E et al. (1996). Meta-analysis of alcohol and all-cause mortality: A validation of NHMRC recommendations. *Medical Journal of Australia* 164(3):141-145.

Holmberg L, Bill-Axelson A, Helgesen F et al. (2002). A randomized trial comparing radical prostatectomy with watchful waiting in early prostate cancer. *New England Journal of Medicine* 12;347(11):781-789.

Hosking D, Chilvers CE, Christiansen C et al. (1998). Prevention of bone loss with alendronate in postmenopausal women under 60 years of age. Early Postmenopausal Intervention Cohort Study Group. *New England Journal of Medicine* 338(8):485-492.

Hoyumpa AM (1986). Mechanisms of vitamin deficiencies in alcoholism. *Alcoholism: Clinical & Experimental Research* 10(6):573-581.

Imperiale TF & McCullough AJ (1990). Do corticosteroids reduce mortality from alcoholic hepatitis? A meta-analysis of the randomized trials. *Annals of Internal Medicine* 113(4):299-307.

Jaeger TM, Lohr RH & Pankratz VS (2001). Symptom-triggered therapy for alcohol withdrawal syndrome in medical inpatients. *Mayo Clinic Proceedings* 76(7): 695-701.

Jensen TK, Hjollund NH, Henriksen TB et al. (1998). Does moderate alcohol consumption affect fertility? Follow up study among couples planning first pregnancy. *British Medical Journal* 317(7157):505-510.

Johnson BA, Devous MD Sr., Ruiz P et al. (2001). Treatment advances for cocaine-induced ischemic stroke: Focus on dihydropyridine-class calcium channel antagonists. *American Journal of Psychiatry* 158(8):1191-1198.

Johnson MK, Smith RP, Morrison D et al. (2000). Large lung bullae in marijuana smokers. *Thorax* 55(4):340-342.

Johnson RJ, Gretch DR, Yamabe H et al. (1993). Membranoproliferative glomerulonephritis associated with hepatitis C virus infection. *New England Journal of Medicine* 328(7):465-470.

Joint National Committee VI (1997). The sixth report of the Joint National Committee on prevention, detection, evaluation, and treatment of high blood pressure. *Archives of Internal Medicine* 157(21):2413-2446.

Kawachi I, Colditz GA, Stampfer MJ et al. (1994). Smoking cessation and time course of decreased risks of coronary heart disease in middle-aged women. *Archives of Internal Medicine* 154(2):169-175.

Kerlikowske K (1997). Efficacy of screening mammography among women aged 40 to 49 years and 50 to 69 years: Comparison of relative and absolute benefit. *Journal of the National Cancer Institute* 22:79-86.

Kerlikowske K & Ernster VL (2000). Women should be fully informed of the potential benefits and harms before screening mammography. *Western Journal of Medicine* 173(5):313-314.

Kerlikowske K, Grady D & Ernster V (1995). Benefit of mammography screening in women ages 40-49 years: Current evidence from randomized controlled trials. *Cancer* 76(9):1679-1681.

Kertesz SG (2001). Pellagra in 2 homeless men. *Mayo Clinic Proceedings* 76(3):315-318.

Kirchmair R, Allerberger F, Bangerl I et al. (1998). Spontaneous bacterial pleural empyema in liver cirrhosis. *Digestive Disease Science* 43(5):1129-1132.

Klatsky AL (1998). Alcohol and cardiovascular diseases: A historical overview. *Novartis Foundation Symposia* 216:2-12.

Klinenberg JR (1969). Saturnine gout—A moonshine malady. *New England Journal of Medicine* 280(22):1238-1239.

Knochel JP (1980). Hypophosphatemia in the alcoholic. *Archives of Internal Medicine* 140(5):613-615.

Kromhout D, Bloemberg BP, Feskens EJ et al. (1996). Alcohol, fish, fibre and antioxidant vitamins intake do not explain population differences in coronary heart disease mortality. *International Journal of Epidemiology* 25(4):753-759.

Kupari M & Koskinen P (1991). Time of onset of supraventricular tachyarrhythmia in relation to alcohol consumption. *American Journal of Cardiology* 67(8):718-722.

Laine C, Hauck WW, Gourevitch MN et al. (2001). Regular outpatient medical and drug abuse care and subsequent hospitalization of persons who use illicit drugs. *Journal of the American Medical Association* 285(18):2355-2362.

Laitinen K, Lamberg-Allardt C, Tunninen R et al. (1991). Transient hypoparathyroidism during acute alcohol intoxication. *New England Journal of Medicine* 324(11):721-727.

Lange RA & Hillis LD (2001). Cardiovascular complications of cocaine use. *New England Journal of Medicine* 345(5):351-358.

Lankisch MR, Imoto M, Layer P et al. (2001). The effect of small amounts of alcohol on the clinical course of chronic pancreatitis. *Mayo Clinic Proceedings* 76(3):242-251.

Larkin EC & Watson-Williams EJ (1984). Alcohol and the blood. *Medical Clinics of North America* 68(1):105-120.

Leistikow BN, Martin DC, Jacobs J et al. (2000). Smoking as a risk factor for accident death: A meta-analysis of cohort studies. *Accident Analysis and Prevention* 32(3):397-405.

Levin MH, Weinstein RA, Nathan C et al. (1984). Association of infection caused by Pseudomonas aeruginosa serotype 011 with intravenous abuse of pentazocine mixed with tripelennamine. *Journal of Clinical Microbiology* 20(4):758-762.

Lieber CS (1984). Alcohol-nutrition interaction: 1984 update. *Alcohol* 1(2):151-157.

Lieber CS (1995). Medical disorders of alcoholism. *New England Journal of Medicine* 333(16):1058-1065.

Liebschutz J, Savetsky JB, Saitz R et al. (2002). Relationship between sexual and physical abuse and substance abuse consequences. *Journal of Substance Abuse Treatment* 22(3):121-128.

Marshall JB (1993). Acute pancreatitis. A review with an emphasis on new developments. *Archives of Internal Medicine* 153(10):1185-1198.

Marzuk PM, Tardiff K, Smyth D et al. (1992). Cocaine use, risk taking, and fatal Russian roulette. *Journal of the American Medical Association* 267(19):2635-2637.

Mayo-Smith MF and the American Society of Addiction Medicine Working Group on Pharmacological Management of Alcohol Withdrawal (1997). Pharmacological management of alcohol withdrawal. A meta-analysis and evidence-based practice guideline. *Journal of the American Medical Association* 278(2):144-151.

McClung MR, Geusens P, Miller PD et al. (2001). Effect of risedronate on the risk of hip fracture in elderly women. Hip Intervention Program Study Group. *New England Journal of Medicine* 344(5):333-340.

McEvoy AW, Kitchen ND & Thomas DG (2000). Intracerebral haemorrhage and drug abuse in young adults. *British Journal of Neurosurgery* 14(5):449-454.

Mendenhall CL, Moritz TE, Roselle GA et al. (1993). A study of oral nutritional support with oxandrolone in malnourished patients with alcoholic hepatitis: Results of a Department of Veterans Affairs cooperative study. *Hepatology* 17(4):564-576.

Michnovicz JJ, Hershcopf RJ, Haley NJ et al. (1989). Cigarette smoking alters hepatic estrogen metabolism in men: Implications for atherosclerosis. *Metabolism* 38(6):537-541.

Miller AB, To T, Baines CJ et al. (2002). The Canadian National Breast Screening Study-1: Breast cancer mortality after 11 to 16 years of follow-up. A randomized screening trial of mammography in women age 40 to 49 years. *Annals of Internal Medicine* 137(5, part 1):305-312.

Muntwyler J, Hennekens CH, Buring JE et al. (1998). Mortality and light to moderate alcohol consumption after myocardial infarction. *Lancet* 352(9144):1882-1885.

Murphy EL, DeVita D, Liu H et al. (2001). Risk factors for skin and soft-tissue abscesses among injection drug users: A case-control study. *Clinical Infectious Diseases* 33(1):35-40.

Nademanee K (1992). Cardiovascular effects and toxicities of cocaine. *Journal of Addictive Diseases* 11(4):71-82.

National Cholesterol Education Program (NCEP) (2001). Executive summary of the third report of The National Cholesterol Education Program (NCEP) Expert Panel on Detection, Evaluation, and Treatment of High Blood Cholesterol in Adults (Adult Treatment Panel III). *Journal of the American Medical Association* 285(19):2486-2497.

Niederman MS, Mandell LA, Anzueto A et al. (2001). Guidelines for the management of adults with community-acquired pneumonia. Diagnosis, assessment of severity, antimicrobial therapy, and prevention. *American Journal of Respiratory and Critical Care Medicine* 163(7):1730-1754.

Nolan CV & Shaikh ZA (1992). Lead nephrotoxicity and associated disorders: Biochemical mechanisms. *Toxicology* 73(2):127-146.

Norton R, Batey R, Dwyer T et al. (1987). Alcohol consumption and the risk of alcohol related cirrhosis in women. *British Medical Journal* (Clinical Research Edition) 295(6590):80-82.

O'Connor PG, Samet JH & Stein MD (1994). Management of hospitalized intravenous drug users: Role of the internist. *American Journal of Medicine* 96(6):551-558.

Ogawa SK, Smith MA, Brennessel DJ et al. (1987). Tuberculous meningitis in an urban medical center. *Medicine* (Baltimore) 66(4):317-326.

Ohnishi K, Matsuo S, Matsutani K et al.(1996). Interferon therapy for chronic hepatitis C in habitual drinkers: Comparison with chronic hepatitis C in infrequent drinkers. *American Journal of Gastroenterology* 91(7): 1374-1379.

Orrego H, Blake JE, Blendis LM et al. (1987). Long-term treatment of alcoholic liver disease with propylthiouracil. *New England Journal of Medicine* 317(23):1421-1427.

Pare JP, Cote G & Fraser RS (1989). Long-term follow-up of drug abusers with intravenous talcosis. *American Review of Respiratory Diseases* 139(1):233-241.

Parrish KM, Dufour MC, Stinson FS et al. (1993). Average daily alcohol consumption during adult life among decedents with and without cirrhosis: The 1986 National Mortality Followback Survey. *Journal of Studies on Alcohol* 54(4):450-456.

Pedrazzoni M, Vescovi PP, Maninetti L et al. (1993). Effects of chronic heroin abuse on bone and mineral metabolism. *Acta Endocrinologica* (Copenhagen) 129(1):42-45.

Poikolainen K (1998). It can be bad for the heart, too—drinking patterns and coronary heart disease. *Addiction* 93(12):1757-1759.

Powell WJ Jr. & Klatskin G (1968). Duration of survival in patients with Laennec's cirrhosis. Influence of alcohol withdrawal, and possible effects of recent changes in general management of the disease. *American Journal of Medicine* 44(3):406-420.

Pugatch D, Levesque B, Greene S et al. (2001). HIV testing in the setting of inpatient acute substance abuse treatment. *American Journal of Drug and Alcohol Abuse* 27(3):491-499.

Ranson JH, Rifkind KM & Turner JW (1976). Prognostic signs and nonoperative peritoneal lavage in acute pancreatitis. *Surgery, Gynecology and Obstetrics* 143(2):209-219.

Rees VW, Horton NJ, Hingson RW et al. (2002). Injury among detoxification patients: Alcohol users' greater risk. *Alcoholism: Clinical & Experimental Research* 26(2):212-217.

Renaud SC (2001). Diet and stroke. *Journal of Nutrition, Health and Aging* 5(3):167-172.

Rex DK, Johnson DA, Lieberman DA et al. (2000). Colorectal cancer prevention 2000: Screening recommendations of the American College of Gastroenterology. American College of Gastroenterology. *American Journal of Gastroenterology* 95(4):868-877.

Rich EC, Siebold C & Campion B (1985). Alcohol-related acute atrial fibrillation. A case-control study and review of 40 patients. *Archives of Internal Medicine* 145(5):830-833.

Roberts R & Slovis CM (1990). Endocarditis in intravenous drug abusers. *Emergency Medicine Clinics of North America* 8(3):665-681.

Russell RM (1980). Vitamin A and zinc metabolism in alcoholism. *American Journal of Clinical Nutrition* 33(12):2741-2749.

Ryle PR & Thomson AD (1984). Nutrition and vitamins in alcoholism. *Contemporary Issues in Clinical Biochemistry* 1:188-224.

Saitz R & O'Malley SS (1997). Pharmacotherapies for alcohol abuse. Withdrawal and treatment. *Medical Clinics of North America* 81(4):881-907.

Saitz R, Ghali WA & Moskowitz MA (1997). The impact of alcohol-related diagnoses on pneumonia outcomes. *Archives of Internal Medicine* 157(13):1446-1452.

Saitz R, Mayo-Smith MF, Roberts MS et al. (1994). Individualized treatment for alcohol withdrawal. A randomized double-blind controlled trial. *Journal of the American Medical Association* 272(7):519-523.

Saitz R, Mulvey KP & Samet JH (1997). The substance abusing patient and primary care: Linkage via the addiction treatment system? *Substance Abuse* 18:187-195.

Salt WB 2nd & Schenker S (1976). Amylase—its clinical significance: A review of the literature. *Medicine* (Baltimore) 55(4):269-289.

Samet JH, Friedmann P & Saitz R (2001). Benefits of linking primary medical care and substance abuse services: Patient, provider, and societal perspectives. *Archives of Internal Medicine* 161(1):85-91.

Samet JH, Saitz R & Larson MJ (1996). A case for enhanced linkage for substance abusers to primary medical care. *Substance Abuse* 17(4):181-192.

Samet JH, Shevitz A, Fowle J et al. (1990). Hospitalization decision in febrile intravenous drug users. *American Journal of Medicine* 89(1):53-57.

Scanlon PD, Connett JE, Waller LA et al. (2000). Smoking cessation and lung function in mild-to-moderate chronic obstructive pulmonary disease. The Lung Health Study. *American Journal of Respiratory and Critical Care Medicine* 161(2 Pt 1):381-390.

Schiodt FV, Rochling FA, Casey DL et al. (1997). Acetaminophen toxicity in an urban county hospital. *New England Journal of Medicine* 337(16):1112-1117.

Smith-Warner SA, Spiegelman D, Yaun SS et al. (1998). Alcohol and breast cancer in women: A pooled analysis of cohort studies. *Journal of the American Medical Association* 279(7):535-540.

Sox HC (1998). Benefit and harm associated with screening for breast cancer. *New England Journal of Medicine* 338(16):1145-1146.

Steer ML, Waxman I & Freedman S (1995). Chronic pancreatitis. *New England Journal of Medicine* 332(22):1482-1490.

Stein MD (1990). Medical complications of intravenous drug use. *Journal of General Internal Medicine* 5(3):249-257.

Talan DA & Moran GJ (1998). Update on emerging infections: News from the Centers for Disease Control and Prevention. Tetanus among injecting-drug users—California, 1997. *Annals of Emergency Medicine* 32(3 Pt 1):385-386.

Tashkin DP (2001). Airway effects of marijuana, cocaine, and other inhaled illicit agents. *Current Opinion in Pulmonary Medicine* 7(2):43-61.

Thomas DB, Gao DL, Ray RM et al. (2002). Randomized trial of breast self-examination in Shanghai: final results. *Journal of the National Cancer Institute* 2;94(19):1445-1457.

Thompson WL, Johnson AD & Maddrey WL (1975). Diazepam and paraldehyde for treatment of severe delirium tremens. A controlled trial. *Annals of Internal Medicine* 82(2):175-180.

Thun MJ, Peto R, Lopez AD et al. (1997). Alcohol consumption and mortality among middle-aged and elderly U.S. adults. *New England Journal of Medicine* 337(24):1705-1714.

Tisi GM (1987). Preoperative identification and evaluation of the patient with lung disease. *Medical Clinics of North America* 71(3):399-412.

Tonnesen H & Kehlet H (1999). Preoperative alcoholism and postoperative morbidity. *British Journal of Surgery* 86(7):869-874.

Tonnesen H, Rosenberg J, Nielsen HJ et al. (1999). Effect of preoperative abstinence on poor postoperative outcome in alcohol misusers: Randomised controlled trial. *British Medical Journal* 318(7194):1311-1316.

Trinchet JC, Beaugrand M, Callard P et al. (1989). Treatment of alcoholic hepatitis with colchicine. Results of a randomized double blind trial. *Gastroenterologie Clinique et Biologique* 13(6-7):551-555.

U.S. Preventive Services Task Force (USPSTF) (1996) *Guide to Clinical Preventive Services, 2nd Edition.* Alexandria, VA: International Medical Publishing.

US Preventive Services Task Force (2002). Screening for osteoporosis in postmenopausal women: Recommendations and rationale. *Annals of Internal Medicine* 137(6):526-528.

Urbano-Marquez A, Estruch R, Navarro-Lopez F et al. (1989). The effects of alcoholism on skeletal and cardiac muscle. *New England Journal of Medicine* 320(7):409-415.

Vine MF, Margolin BH, Morrison HI et al. (1994). Cigarette smoking and sperm density: A meta-analysis. *Fertility and Sterility* 61(1):35-43.

Warner EA, Greene GS, Buchsbaum MS et al. (1998). Diabetic ketoacidosis associated with cocaine use. *Archives of Internal Medicine* 158(16):1799-1802.

Warner MA, Offord KP, Warner ME et al. (1989). Role of preoperative cessation of smoking and other factors in postoperative pulmonary complications: A blinded prospective study of coronary artery bypass patients. *Mayo Clinic Proceedings* 64(6):609-616.

Wartenberg AA (1990). Clinical toxicology and substance abuse. In MS Kochar & K Kutty (eds.) *Concise Textbook of Medicine, 2nd Edition.* New York, NY: Elsevier Publishing, 135-160.

Wiley TE, McCarthy M, Breidi L et al. (1998). Impact of alcohol on the histological and clinical progression of hepatitis C infection. *Hepatology* 28(3):805-809.

Winsa B, Mandahl A & Karlsson FA (1993). Graves' disease, endocrine ophthalmopathy and smoking. *Acta Endocrinologica* (Copenhagen) 128(2):156-160.

Workowski KA (2000). The 1998 CDC sexually transmitted diseases treatment guidelines. *Current Infectious Disease Reports* 2(1):44-50.

Wrenn KD, Slovis CM, Minion GE et al. (1991). The syndrome of alcoholic ketoacidosis. *American Journal of Medicine* 91(2):119-128.

Yamauchi M, Nakahara M, Maezawa Y et al. (1993). Prevalence of hepatocellular carcinoma in patients with alcoholic cirrhosis and prior exposure to hepatitis C. *American Journal of Gastroenterology* 88(1):39-43.

Cardiovascular Consequences of Alcohol and Other Drug Use

Chapter 2

Howard S. Friedman, M.D.

Alcohol
Nicotine
Marijuana
Opioids
Cocaine
Amphetamines and Related Compounds
Anabolic Steroids

As noted 30 years ago by Samuel Vaisrub (1973), "though the primary target of addictive psychoactive substances is the brain, the heart does not always remain unmolested." In fact, the use of such substances can have serious cardiovascular consequences. Depending on the drug, the dose, and the mode of administration, the cardiovascular effects can range from inconsequential to catastrophic. Because coronary artery disease and stroke are the leading causes of death and disability in most of the world, the effects of these drugs on vasomotion, coagulation, and blood lipids have serious implications. Often multiple drugs are abused concomitantly; therefore, an understanding of the consequences of their interactions is important. Drug abuse can be the vehicle by which various contaminating cardiotoxins and microorganisms injure or infect the heart.

In this chapter, the cardiovascular consequences of the use of substances that often result in addiction will be reviewed.

ALCOHOL

Hemodynamic Effects. Although moderate use of alcohol (note that the terms "alcohol" and "ethanol" are used inter-changeably in this chapter), defined as no more than two drinks per day in men and no more than one drink per day in women, can have some cardiovascular benefits (USDA & DHHS, 1995), even such small amounts can have adverse effects in individuals with heart disease, and the consumption of larger amounts can result in serious cardiovascular consequences (Friedman, 1992). At plasma concentrations as low as 50 mg/dL (Nakano & Moore, 1972), ethanol consistently has been shown to depress myocardial contractility (Gomes, Gimeno et al., 1962; Nakano & Moore, 1972; Richards, Kulkarni et al., 1989). Because ethanol and its metabolites, acetaldehyde and acetate, also have adrenergic (Kelbaek, Gjorup et al., 1987) and vasodilatory (Altura & Altura et al., 1984) effects, the direct myocardial depressant actions of ethanol can be obscured when cardiac "pump" function is assessed after ethanol administration.

Cardiac output usually increases following alcohol ingestion in healthy subjects, reflecting the changes in heart rate and peripheral resistance that ensue (Riff, Jain et al., 1969; Blomquist, Saltin et al., 1970); by contrast, a more sensitive index of cardiac function, such as left ventricular ejection fraction, generally worsens (Delgado, Fortuin et al., 1975; Kelbaek, Gjorup, et al., 1987).

The explanation for the cardiac muscle depressant actions of alcohol has not yet been determined, although various abnormalities have been identified. The heart lacks alcohol dehydrogenase (Cherrick & Leevy, 1965); therefore, unlike the liver, it cannot oxidize ethanol (Lochner, Cowley et al., 1969). However, nonoxidative metabolism, with the formation of abnormal esters, has been demonstrated (Laposata & Lange, 1986; Lange, 1982). These fatty acid ethyl esters and their metabolites are potent uncouplers of oxidative phosphorylation (Lange & Sobel, 1983). Although ethanol can acutely depress mitochondrial respiration (Segel, 1984), myocardial intracellular pH and the concentrations of phosphocreatine and adenosine triphosphate do not change appreciably, even with pharmacologic amounts of alcohol (Aufferman, Wu et al., 1988); this would suggest that the fatty acid ethyl esters do not have much influence on myocardial energetics.

Ethanol has been shown acutely to affect myocardial metabolism of free fatty acids (Regan, Koroxenidis et al., 1966), the major fuel of the heart in a fasted state, and protein metabolism (Preedy & Peters, 1989), but not glucose metabolism (Lochner, Cowley et al., 1969). Although these studies are of interest, the findings with regard to changes in myocardial metabolism and energetics are not sufficient to explain the acute myocardial depressant effects of alcohol (Aufferman, Wu et al., 1988).

Alcohol appears to depress myocardial contractility by direct effects on the contractile process. It has been shown to reduce the amplitude, duration, and rate of rise of the myocardial transmembrane action potential—an effect that relates directly to the reduction in contractile force (Williams, Mirro et al., 1980). The total calcium available to the contractile proteins, measured as light-indicator calcium transients, also is reduced by ethanol (Guarnieri & Lakatta, 1990; Danziger, Sakai et al., 1991). These changes do not, however, appear to be related to a reduction in calcium entry (Mongo & Vassort, 1990), nor can they be explained by various other abnormalities of cellular calcium kinetics that have been produced by ethanol in experiments that often lacked functional or dosage relevancy (Friedman, 1998). Even at concentrations lower than those required to affect calcium transients, ethanol depresses contractility, suggesting that ethanol has effects at the level of the myofilament (Guarnieri & Lakatta, 1990). Thus, although alcohol's myocardial depressant actions have been associated with metabolic changes and abnormalities in the contractile process, the factor (or factors) producing these actions so far has eluded investigators.

Ethanol has regional circulatory effects. It increases skin (Huges, Henry et al., 1984) and splanchnic blood flow (Shaw, Heller et al., 1977), but reduces blood flow in the forearm (Fewings, Hanna et al., 1966). Alcohol decreases pancreatic blood flow (Friedman, Lowery et al., 1983; Dib, Cooper-Vastika et al., 1993); this change is associated with a reduction in pancreatic oxygenation (Foitzik, Castillo et al., 1985), suggesting that alcohol may produce pancreatitis by an ischemic mechanism.

The effects of alcohol on brain blood flow, however, are not as clear. In experimental studies, alcohol has been shown to decrease (Altura, Altura et al., 1984; Friedman, Lowery et al., 1984), increase (Schwartz, Speed et al., 1993; Sano, Wendt et al., 1993; Tiihonen, Kuikka et al., 1994), or produce no change in blood flow to the brain (Mayhan & Didion, 1995). The differences can be reconciled by studies suggesting opposite effects of ethanol, which is a cerebrovascular constrictor (Altura, Altura et al., 1984), and its metabolite, acetate, which is a cerebrovascular dilator (Altura & Altura, 1982), on the brain circulation. Studies have shown that cerebral blood flow is related inversely to blood alcohol concentrations, but directly to blood acetate concentrations (Schwartz, Speed et al., 1993). Accordingly, with rapid intravenous (IV) administration of alcohol, before the effects of ethanol's metabolites can be seen, cerebral blood flow decreases (Friedman, Lowery et al., 1984), whereas with ingestion of a moderate amount of alcohol, cerebral blood flow increases (Schwartz, Speed et al., 1993; Sano, Wendt et al., 1993; Tiihonen, Kuikka et al., 1994). Patients older than 62 years seem to be especially sensitive to the cerebral vasoconstrictor actions of alcohol (Schwartz, Speed et al., 1993), which can pose an added risk of cerebral circulatory injury in older adults who drink excessively.

In most (Mendoza, Hellberg et al., 1971; Friedman, Matsuzaki et al., 1979) but not all (Hayes & Bove, 1988) studies, ethanol has been found to increase coronary blood flow. In part, this increase is related to the increased myocardial oxygen requirements that ensue from the increases in heart rate, blood pressure, and cardiac dimensions that generally occur after administration of ethanol (Friedman, 1992). Ethanol (Abel, 1980) and its metabolites (Altura & Altura, 1982) are coronary vasodilators. Despite these changes, alcohol exerts an unfavorable effect on myocardial ischemia: because the vasculature of the ischemic myocardium is near maximally dilated, the coronary vasodilatory effects of ethanol occur primarily in arterioles supplying the nonischemic myocardium, in effect producing a "coronary steal" (Friedman, 1981). Clinical studies have demonstrated findings consistent with this phenomenon (Orlando, Aronow et al., 1976; Ahlawat, Siwach et al., 1991; Rossinen, Partanen et al., 1996).

Individuals with coronary artery disease are more likely to demonstrate evidence of myocardial ischemia after ingesting alcohol (Orlando, Aronow et al., 1976; Ahlawat, Siwach et al., 1991; Rossinen, Partanen et al., 1996); moreover, alcohol can mask angina pectoris (Rossinen, Partanen et al., 1996), thereby making the occurrences of myocardial ischemia silent and potentially more dangerous. Also, alcohol can precipitate coronary spasms (Takizawa, Yasue et al., 1984); these spasms often occur several hours after imbibing alcohol, suggesting a "rebound" phenomenon to the vasodilating actions of alcohol and its metabolites.

Alcoholic Heart Disease. Alcohol abuse can result in an array of cardiac abnormalities. From a functional perspective, such abnormalities range from a heart that is hypocontractile, has a reduced output, and is associated with an increased systemic vascular resistance (the findings of alcoholic cardiomyopathy; Brigden & Robinson, 1964), to one that is hyperdynamic, has an increased output, and is associated with a reduced systemic vascular resistance (the findings of decompensated cirrhosis; Friedman & Fernando, 1992; Friedman, Cirrillo, et al., 1995). Even before such striking abnormalities are evident, subclinical cardiac dysfunction can be detected by noninvasive methods (Spodick, Pigott et al., 1972; Mathews, Gardin et al., 1981; Friedman, Vasavada et al., 1986) and demonstrated by tests that measure cardiac reserve (Regan, Levinson et al., 1969). Alcohol-related myocardial disease can be present when no obvious heart disease is evident or even when hyperdynamic cardiac function is apparent (Wendt, Wu et al., 1965).

Alcoholism leads to myocardial hypertrophy, sometimes with massive increases in heart weight (greater than a kilogram), four-chamber dilatation, myocardial necrosis, and interstitial and perivascular fibrosis (Alexander, 1966). On electron microscopy, loss of myofribils, dilatation of the sarcoplasmic reticulum, separation of the intercalated disk, and abnormalities of mitochondria can be observed (Alexander, 1967; Tsiplenkova, Vihert et al., 1986). When these findings are pronounced, the clinical features of alcoholic cardiomyopathy may become manifest.

Cirrhosis does not preclude cardiomyopathy and, when the two conditions are examined for the presence of the other, evidence for their coexistence is not uncommon (Estruch, Fernandez-Sola et al., 1995). However, because decompensated cirrhosis is associated with neurohumoral changes that produce a hyperdynamic circulation, the presence of myocardial disease may not be evident by standard clinical measures, such as left ventricular ejection fraction.

The salient cardiovascular feature of decompensated cirrhosis is a reduction of systemic vascular resistance that results in a high cardiac output state (Friedman & Fernando, 1992; Friedman, Cirillo et al., 1995). The diminished systemic vascular resistance largely is a consequence of a generalized vasodilatory response, rather than the presence of arteriovenous shunting (Vorobioff, Bredfeldt et al., 1983). The changes in systemic resistance in cirrhosis correlate with changes in hepatic function and are related to reduced urinary sodium elimination (Friedman, Cirillo et al., 1995). Reduced systemic vascular resistance may be evident even before ascites can be detected by abdominal ultrasound; however, tense ascites, by impeding venous return, can elicit counter-regulatory responses that antagonize the vasodilatory effects of cirrhosis (Friedman, Cirillo et al., 1995).

Some investigators (Lee, Albillos et al., 1992; Sieber & Groszmann, 1992; Pizcueta, Pique et al., 1992), but not all (Sogni, Moreau et al., 1992), have posited experimental models of cirrhosis suggesting nitric oxide as the mediator of this effect. Studies in humans using nitric oxide synthase inhibitors suggest that nitric oxide has an important role in the development of increased peripheral blood flow in decompensated cirrhosis (Campillo, Chabrier et al., 1995).

Alcohol-related heart muscle disease (alcoholic cardiomyopathy) is a distinct clinical disorder in alcohol abusers who do not have any apparent nutritional deficiencies (Eliaser & Giansiracusa, 1956). The relationship between prolonged alcohol abuse and the occurrence of a dilated, hypocontractile heart is sufficiently strong to suggest that alcohol, acetaldehyde, or some compound formed from these substances is toxic to the heart (Kino, Imamitchi et al., 1981; Urbano-Marquez, Estruch et al., 1989). Despite numerous attempts to replicate this disorder experimentally, however, no one has yet adequately reproduced the clinical entity (Friedman, 1992).

The development of alcoholic cardiomyopathy appears to require prolonged excessive use of alcohol. Alcoholics who develop this disorder tend to be 10 years older, to have been alcoholic 10 years longer, and to drink considerably more than alcoholics who maintain normal cardiac dimensions and function (Fernàndez-Solà, Estruch et al., 1994). However, some people may have a predisposition to the condition (Fernàndez-Solà, Nicolàs et al., 2002). Although alcoholic cardiomyopathy is seen wherever use of large amounts of alcohol is culturally acceptable; in the United States, 85% to 90% of those with the disease are African American (Demakis, Proskey et al., 1974).

The inability to reproduce alcoholic cardiomyopathy experimentally and its comparative rarity (in the context of the prevalence of alcohol abuse) suggest that other conditions besides alcoholism may be necessary to produce this disorder. The cardiomyopathy seen in Quebec's beer drinkers may be the prototype of this phenomenon (Morin, Foley et al., 1967). When trace amounts of cobalt, which ordinarily would be nontoxic, were placed in beer to stabilize the foam, a fulminant cardiomyopathy ensued in heavy beer drinkers (Morin, Foley et al., 1967). In experimental studies, alcohol administration exaggerates the myocardial damage produced by trypanosomal (Miller & Abelmann, 1967) and coxsackie B3 (Morin, Roy et al., 1969) infections; prolonged alcohol administration also worsens the myocardial injury caused by catecholamines (Morin, Roy et al., 1969).

Hypertension, which is associated with alcohol abuse (Clark & Friedman et al., 1985), may be important in this context. Although blood pressure elevations in alcoholics often are transitory and can abate over several days of abstinence (Clark & Friedman et al., 1985), alcoholics with transitory hypertension may continue to manifest exaggerated blood pressure responses to stressors, even after several weeks of abstinence (King, Errico et al., 1991). Even when blood pressure is normal, left ventricular wall stress may be elevated (Friedman, Vasavada et al., 1986); moreover, during periods of inebriation, these abnormalities become exaggerated. The increased left ventricular wall stress and higher heart rates, in turn, increase myocardial oxygen consumption. Heart failure might, therefore, ensue as a consequence of the combination of increased myocardial oxygen requirements and the abnormalities of myocardial metabolism and energetics caused by alcoholism persisting over many years. Moreover, the occurrence of atrial fibrillation, which occurs more often in alcohol abusers (Thornton, 1984) and also is a complication of alcoholic cardiomyopathy (Demakis, Proskey et al., 1974), might

produce or worsen myocardial dysfunction (alcohol-related heart muscle disease seen as a manifestation of tachycardia-related cardiomyopathy). The recognition of alcoholism as a cause of congestive heart failure is especially important, because abstinence—especially in the early phases of alcoholic cardiomyopathy—can reverse the abnormalities (Demakis, Proskey et al., 1974; Schwartz, Sample et al., 1975; Molgaard, Kristensen et al., 1990), whereas continuation of alcohol use inexorably leads to an unfavorable outcome (Demakis, Proskey et al., 1974).

Holiday Heart. Alcohol abuse is associated with cardiac arrhythmias. "Holiday heart" is the term coined to denote the relationship between alcohol abuse and arrhythmia in the absence of any electrolyte abnormality or evidence of clinical heart disease (Ettinger, Wu et al., 1978). Often the arrhythmia occurs after binge drinking (Thornton, 1984), as implied by the phrase. Although various atrial and ventricular arrhythmias may be seen, alcoholics appear to be particularly at risk for atrial fibrillation (Thornton, 1984; Rich, Siebold et al., 1985). The explanation for this phenomenon is not clear. Although ethanol has been shown to reduce the duration, amplitude, and rate of rise of the transmyocardial action potential experimentally (Richards, Kulkarni et al., 1989), and these are conditions that would favor the development of atrial fibrillation, such changes have not been observed in the human atrium after administration of alcohol (Engel & Luck, 1983; Greenspon & Schaal, 1983). However, in individuals who have alcohol-related arrhythmias, the abnormality often can be elicited by programmed electrical stimulation following administration of alcohol (Greenspon, Stang et al., 1979; Engel & Luck, 1983; Greenspon & Schaal, 1983). In some instances, an arrhythmia may be the first manifestation of subclinical alcoholic cardiomyopathy (Luca, 1979). Therefore, alcohol abuse must be considered in individuals with unexplained arrhythmias, especially those who have paroxysmal atrial fibrillation.

Experimentally, at least, alcohol has been shown to have antiarrhythmic actions (Paradise & Stoelting, 1965; Madan & Gupta, 1967; Kostis, Horstmann et al., 1971; Gilmour, Ruffy et al., 1981; Nguyen, Friedman et al., 1987). In these studies, ethanol has been shown to increase the threshold for ventricular fibrillation (Kostis, Horstmann et al., 1971; Gilmour, Ruffy et al., 1981), to suppress ventricular tachycardia (Madan & Gupta, 1967), and even to shorten the duration of atrial fibrillation (Madan & Gupta, 1967;

Nguyen, Friedman et al., 1987). Whether these findings are merely experimental curiosities or have clinical significance requires further investigation.

Epidemiologic studies have disclosed an increased incidence of sudden and unexpected deaths in alcoholics (Kramer, Kuller et al., 1968; Randall, 1980; Lithell, Aberg et al., 1987), particularly those in the third through fifth decade of life; characteristically, victims have fatty livers at autopsy and (often) low blood ethanol concentrations (Randall, 1980; Lithell, Aberg et al., 1987). The presumption is that the deaths are caused by arrhythmias, perhaps related to hypokalemia, hypomagnesemia, or even to alcohol itself. The low blood ethanol concentrations, however, suggest reactions to alcohol withdrawal rather than to alcohol *per se* as the cause. Possible mechanisms include arrhythmia from an intense sympathoadrenal reaction (Orgata & Mendelson, 1971), postvasodilatory coronary artery spasm (Takizawa, Yasue et al., 1984) (which is analogous to "weekend angina pectoris" in nitrate workers), and small coronary artery thromboses because of rebound hypercoaguability (Renaud & Ruf, 1996). In addition, alcoholics develop autonomic neuropathy (Novak & Victor, 1974), a condition that might produce arrhythmia by creating cardiac electrical instability.

Alcohol abuse also has been associated with sudden death in individuals with coronary artery disease (Fraser & Upsdell, 1981; Lithell, Aberg et al., 1987), a population already at increased risk of such events.

Hypertension. Alcohol use elevates blood pressure and alcohol abuse produces systemic hypertension—an effect that can be intensified during periods of withdrawal. Alcohol and its metabolites, acetaldehyde and acetate, have both direct vasodilatory effects (Altura & Altura, 1982) and indirect sympathetic vasoconstrictive actions (Randin, Vollenweider et al., 1995). When alcohol is imbibed (Grassi, Somers et al., 1989) or administered intravenously (Randin, Vollenweider et al., 1995), muscle sympathetic nerve traffic (of the peroneal nerve) increases. Initially, blood pressure does not increase but, as blood levels of ethanol decrease (and the vasodilator actions abate) and as sympathetic nerve traffic increases, blood pressure rises (Randin, Vollenweider et al., 1995). The alpha-adrenergic blocker, phentolamine, blocks this vasopressor response, and both the sympathetic neural response and the blood pressure increase are blocked by dexamethasone. The acute hypertensive effects of alcohol thus are mediated centrally, with participation of corticotrophin-releasing hormone, and act directly through alpha-adrenergic mechanisms (Randin, Vollenweider et al., 1995).

Alcohol ingestion impairs the baroreceptor reflex (Abdel-Rahman, Merrill et al., 1987). When alcohol is administered to normotensive subjects, slowing of heart rate to a sudden elevation in blood pressure is attenuated, and the reflex is reset to a higher blood pressure; this effect is directly related to blood ethanol concentrations (Abdel-Rahman, Merrill et al., 1987).

Studies have demonstrated clear causal links between alcohol use and blood pressure changes. In individuals with hypertension who use alcohol moderately, blood pressure drops sharply within 72 hours of cessation of drinking, but increases again within 48 hours of resumption of drinking (Potter & Beevers, 1984). Even reductions in alcohol use reduce blood pressure in both normotensive (Puddey, Beilin et al., 1985) and hypertensive (Puddey, Beilin et al., 1987) subjects.

The effects of alcohol on blood pressure have been found to be related to baseline blood pressure and to the quantity customarily used: five to six drinks per day for five days had little effect on normotensive light drinkers, elevated only standing blood pressures in hypertensive light drinkers, but increased both supine and standing blood pressure in hypertensive moderate drinkers (Malhotra, Mathur et al., 1985). Experimental studies in animals have shown that prolonged administration of alcohol elevates blood pressure and changes vascular responsiveness (Altura & Altura, 1982; Chan & Sutter, 1983).

Epidemiologic surveys have demonstrated that the relationship between blood pressure and alcohol is present in diverse populations and that hypertension is more prevalent in individuals who abuse alcohol (Friedman, 1990). The relationship, however, appears to be stronger in men and in Caucasians of both sexes (Klatsky, Armstrong et al., 1992). A U- or J-shaped relation between alcohol use and blood pressure was described in early investigations (Friedman, 1990), but when adjustments are made for weight and age, the dip tends to disappear (Cooke, Frost et al., 1982). Moreover, the association between alcohol use and a decrease in blood pressure has been reported mainly in women who use alcohol occasionally; it is unlikely that such a small amount of alcohol would exert a persistent biologic effect, suggesting the presence of a hidden confounder. An increase in blood pressure is evident with one or two drinks per day in men, whereas this effect requires three drinks per day in women (Klatsky, Armstrong et al., 1992). With menopause, the hypertensive effects of alcohol intensify (Fortman, Haskell et al., 1983).

Hypertension is observed frequently in alcoholics (Beevers, Bannan et al., 1982; Clark & Friedman, 1985). More than half of the alcoholics undergoing detoxification have a blood pressure greater than 140/90 mmHg (Beevers, Bannan et al., 1982), and a third have a value greater than 160/90 mmHg (Clark & Friedman, 1985). Moreover, even when such individuals remain abstinent and their blood pressure returns to normal values, they continue to demonstrate an exaggerated blood pressure response to stressors (Clark & Friedman, 1985; King, Errico et al., 1991), an effect that persists at least for several weeks (King, Errico et al., 1991). Alcoholic-associated hypertension appears to be mediated by catecholamines (Clark & Friedman, 1985). Almost 90% of alcoholic hypertensives undergoing detoxification have an elevated plasma epinephrine; when they are abstinent and their blood pressure normalizes, such individuals still show an exaggerated increment of plasma catecholamines in response to stress (Clark & Friedman, 1985).

Thus, alcohol has a dual effect on blood pressure. Ethanol and its metabolites, through their vasodilatory actions on the systemic circulation, lower blood pressure; however, alcohol also stimulates the sympathetic nervous system (and probably also the adrenal cortex and medulla) and attenuates the baroreceptor reflex—actions that elevate blood pressure. Although elevations of blood pressure associated with habitual use of alcohol disappear after several days of abstinence, alcoholics have a proclivity for an exaggerated blood pressure response to stressors, and this effect can persist for at least several weeks after withdrawal.

Coronary Heart Disease and Stroke. Alcohol abuse is associated with an increased risk of coronary artery disease (Dyer, Stamler et al., 1980; Serdula, Koong et al., 1995) and stroke (Gill, Zezulka et al., 1986; Wannamethee & Shaper, 1996). When used in moderation, however, alcohol use is favorably related to these conditions (Fuchs, Stampfer et al., 1995). The relationships between alcohol consumption and coronary (Rimm, Giovannuci et al., 1991) and cerebrovascular diseases (Gill, Zezulka et al., 1986) thus can be described as U or J shaped: initially favorable, with benefit augmenting as use increases, and then unfavorable, with detriment augmenting as use increases. (An L-shaped relation has been described for stroke, but this study did not stratify for abusers [Berger, Ajani et al., 1999].) The adverse effects of alcohol on atherothrombotic diseases

may be related to alcohol-induced elevation of blood pressure (Dyer, Stamler et al., 1980; Kozararevic, Vojvodic et al., 1980; Wannamethee & Shaper, 1996), and perhaps also to elevated levels of homocysteine (Stickel, Choi, et al., 2000; van der Gaag, Ubbink et al., 2000). The favorable effects appear to be related mostly to the changes alcohol produces in the blood lipid profile (Gaziano, Buring et al., 1993). Alcohol's effects on hemostasis, its overall antithrombotic actions, also would favorably affect atherothrombotic events, but at the cost of an increased risk of hemorrhagic stroke— a finding in some (Donahue, Abbott et al., 1986) but not all (Berger, Ajani et al., 1999) studies.

The effects of alcohol on coronary heart disease and stroke are observed in both men and women, with the U-curve in women located to the left of that in men (indicating a lower dose causes both benefit and detriment) (Klatsky, Armstrong et al., 1992). Consistent with Bayesian probability, the benefits of moderate ethanol use are evident in those with an increased risk of coronary disease: middle-aged individuals (Klatsky, Armstrong et al., 1992) and those with elevated low-density lipoprotein cholesterol (Hein, Suadicani et al., 1996). In terms of mortality related to coronary disease, about 50% of the benefit derived from alcohol consumption can be attributed to an increase in high-density lipoprotein cholesterol (Suh, Shaten et al., 1992). The effects of alcohol use on hemostasis provide additional benefit. Alcohol use reduces plasma fibrinogen (Meade, Imeson et al., 1987), a risk factor for coronary artery disease (Heinrich, Balleisen et al., 1994). It also reduces platelet aggregability (Renaud & Ruf, 1996); this effect is directly related to the amount of alcohol customarily used and is exaggerated by a diet high in saturated fats (Renaud & Ruf, 1996). After alcohol is ingested, there is a transient reduction of platelet aggregation, followed by a more prolonged "rebound" enhancement (Renaud & Ruf, 1996). The rebound phenomenon can be antagonized by tannins, which are antioxidants present in red wine (Ruf, Berger et al., 1995). Ethanol enhances the antiplatelet actions of aspirin (Deykin, Janson et al., 1982), and is positively related to plasma tissue-type plasminogen activator, suggesting an alcohol-induced enhancement of fibrinolysis (Ridker, Vaughan et al., 1994).

Although the reduced risk of coronary heart disease associated with moderate use of alcohol is not related to any specific alcoholic beverage (Rimm, Klatsky et al., 1996), some selective differences have been noted. For instance, the tannins in red wine and the vitamin B_6 in beer (vitamin

B$_6$ is an antagonist of the homocysteine-elevating effects of alcohol; van der Gaag, Ubbink et al., 2000) suggest some additional protective advantages for those beverages. However, the beneficial effects of alcohol use may be related to ethanol *per se*. This is supported by the observation that individuals who have a genetic variation of alcohol dehydrogenase that results in slow metabolism of ethanol have the most protection against myocardial infarction at moderate levels of alcohol use (Hines, Stampfer et al., 2001).

While the evidence for some benefit of moderate alcohol use is persuasive, and is based on numerous confirmatory studies and significant dose relationships between use and outcomes, the actual value may be less than has been suggested. For instance, a reported 21% decrease in the 12-year incidence of stroke attributable to alcohol use actually is a benefit of only 5.6 per 10,000/year (Berger, Ajani et al., 1999). From an epidemiologic perspective, such a decrease is significant, but the likelihood of benefit in a given individual is small. Moreover, because the evidence of benefit is based on cohort data and not on randomized controlled studies, the possibility of a hidden confounder must be considered. Individuals who have one drink per week have fewer strokes than teetotalers (Berger, Ajani et al., 1999). Can such a small amount of alcohol confer this protection, or is there a concealed variable? Similarly, a statistical adjustment for a predictor variable can obscure a detrimental effect of alcohol: if alcohol's adverse effects are the result of raising blood pressure or a consequence of an interaction with aspirin (for instance, to promote intracerebral hemorrhage), a statistical adjustment for these variables would tend to make the outcomes appear more favorable. In addition, even moderate alcohol use can increase heart rate and blood pressure and depress left ventricular function (Friedman, 1992), or produce a "coronary steal" (Friedman, 1981)—changes that might aggravate congestive heart failure or worsen myocardial ischemia. Thus, encouraging the use of alcohol as a cardiac medicinal would seem to be unwarranted, especially for persons with heart disease.

NICOTINE

Cigarette smoking is a leading risk factor for the development of cardiovascular diseases (Kannel, 1981). The addictive constituent and the agent responsible for most of the adverse cardiovascular effects of smoking tobacco is nicotine. Within a few minutes of smoking a cigarette, heart rate and blood pressure increase (Cryer, Haymond et al., 1976; Niedermaier, Smith, et al., 1993; Grassi, Seravalle, et

al., 1994). Although the values begin to decline on cessation of smoking, heart rate and blood pressure remain above baseline for at least 30 minutes (Cryer, Haymond et al., 1976). These findings can be replicated by administration of nicotine to achieve plasma concentrations observed when a cigarette is smoked (Benowitz, Jacob et al., 1982; Benowitz & Gourlay, 1997). The changes, which can be prevented by adrenergic blockade, generally are accompanied by increases in plasma epinephrine and norepinephrine (Cryer, Haymond et al., 1976; Grassi, Seravalle et al., 1994). Nicotine exerts its adrenergic actions mainly through release of norepinephrine from nerve terminals (Benowitz, Jacob et al., 1982) and release of epinephrine from the adrenal medulla (Gourlay & Benowitz, 1997).

A central nervous system stimulatory effect of nicotine is disputed by the observation that muscle sympathetic nerve traffic (of the peroneal nerve), assessed by microneurography, decreases as blood pressure increases (Niedermaier, Smith et al., 1993; Grassi, Seravalle, et al., 1994). The complex adrenergic response to smoking can account for the lack of elevation of plasma norepinephrine in some studies (Niedermaier, Smith et al., 1993; Gourlay & Benowitz, 1997). Smoking attenuates baroreceptor responses to blood pressure elevations (Niedermaier, Smith et al., 1993; Grassi, Seravalle et al., 1994) and the heart rate fluctuations that occur with normal respiration (Niedermaier, Smith et al., 1993).

Through its adrenergic actions, smoking exerts a vasoconstrictive effect on most regional circulation. Skin blood flow diminishes, as reflected in decreases in skin temperature (Benowitz, Jacob et al., 1982). Despite an increase in calf muscle vascular resistance, in normal subjects calf blood flow may not change (Grassi, Seravalle et al., 1994). In individuals with symptomatic obstructive peripheral arterial disease, however, smoking would be expected to diminish blood flow and reduce walking distance before calf pain.

The effects of smoking on coronary blood reflect the competing influences of its hemodynamic actions (elevations in heart rate and blood pressure), which evoke an increase in flow, and its direct vasoconstrictive actions, which diminish flow (Klein, Ambrose et al., 1984; Winniford, Wheelan et al., 1986; Winniford, Jansen et al., 1987; Moliterno, Willard et al., 1994). The vasospastic coronary actions, which are attenuated by alpha-adrenergic blockers (Winniford, Wheelan et al., 1986), L-type calcium channel blockers (Winniford, Jansen et al., 1987), and nitroglycerin (Winniford, Jansen et al., 1987), but enhanced by beta-adrenergic blockers

(Winniford, Wheelan et al., 1986), are especially detrimental in the presence of obstructive coronary disease. Smoking worsens coronary artery narrowing (Moliterno, Willard et al., 1994) and can adversely affect "downstream" collaterals and compensatory arteriolar dilatation (Klein, Ambrose et al., 1984). Endothelium-dependent coronary blood flow (measured by substance P stimulation) also can be impaired by smoking—a finding that is exaggerated by the concomitant presence of other coronary risk factors (Newby, McLeod et al., 2001). Moreover, the increases in carboxyhemoglobin that occur during smoking impede the delivery of oxygen to tissues (Aronow, Cassidy et al., 1974). Thus, by increasing myocardial oxygen requirements, causing vasospasms, diminishing coronary flow reserve, and interfering with myocardial oxygen delivery, smoking a cigarette causes myocardial ischemia to occur at lower levels of exertion, and even at rest in individuals with coronary artery disease (Aronow, Kaplan et al., 1968; Aronow & Swanson, 1969; Barry, Mead et al., 1989).

Smoking can cause an acute coronary thrombosis. Smoking even a single cigarette promotes adenosine diphosphate-induced platelet aggregation (Levine, 1973). Several days of smoking has been shown to increase platelet factor 4 and beta-thromboglobulin, which are indicators of platelet activation (Benowitz, Fitzgerald et al., 1993), and to increase the urinary concentrations of the metabolites of thromboxane A_2, the potent platelet aggregatory prostaglandin (Benowitz, Fitzgerald et al., 1993). Increased urinary concentrations of the metabolites of thromboxane A_2 are observed in chronic smokers (Wennmalm, Benthin et al., 1991). In addition, smoking cigarettes can promote coagulation by increasing plasma fibrinogen (Benowitz, Fitzgerald et al., 1993), and it can inhibit fibrinolysis by reducing tissue plasminogen activator activity (Newby, McLeod et al., 2001). The elevations of plasma fibrinogen concentration and leukocyte count that occur in smokers would tend to increase blood viscosity (Benowitz, Fitzgerald et al., 1993), thereby contributing to thrombogenesis by slowing blood flow. The associations between smoking cigarettes and thrombogenesis can be of particular concern in women, especially for those using oral contraceptives or receiving hormone replacement therapy; the risks of thrombotic events in women smokers using oral contraceptives increases sharply after age 35 (Kannel, 1981; Castelli, 1999). Although changes in thrombogenesis are not seen with sham smoking or smoking of tobacco-free cigarettes (Levine,

1973), a clear relation between the hemostatic changes that occur with smoking cigarettes and concentrations of nicotine (or cotinine) and catecholamines has not been established (Levine, 1973; Wennmalm, Benthin et al., 1991; Benowitz, Fitzgerald et al., 1993).

Despite the strong relation between cigarette smoking and increases in mortality and morbidity from coronary heart disease (Kannel, 1981), smokers seem to have better outcomes after an acute myocardial infarction—a relationship that may even be related to the number of cigarettes smoked (Barbash, White et al., 1993). This seemingly paradoxical finding appears to be explained, at least in part, by the younger age at which smokers have myocardial infarctions and by the lack of association of smoking with other risk factors, but not by the extent of underlying coronary disease (Barbash, White et al., 1993; de Chillou, Riff et al., 1996; Newby, McLeod et al., 2001). The paramount importance of thrombosis in the pathophysiology of acute myocardial infarction in smokers also may explain their enhanced benefit from thrombolytic therapy (Barbash, White et al., 1993; de Chillou, Riff et al., 1996). Despite these statistical curiosities, the resumption of smoking after myocardial infarction has an adverse effect on outcomes (Kannel, 1981) and must be discouraged.

Smoking promotes atherogenesis (Kannel, 1981). Smokers have more extensive atherosclerosis in the coronary arteries, aorta, and peripheral arteries than do nonsmokers. Because progression of coronary disease often involves mechanisms related to coagulation (particularly the development of severe narrowing through a process of plaque disruption, thrombosis, and healing; Mann & Davies, 1999), by promoting hemostasis, smoking contributes to atherosclerotic plaque growth. In addition, smoking produces an unfavorable lipid profile by reducing high-density lipoprotein cholesterol (Criqui, Wallace et al., 1980), and it adversely affects endothelial function (Newby, McLeod et al., 2001).

Nicotine replacement therapy (patches and gum) is used to treat smokers. Although there have been a few reports of cardiovascular events (acute myocardial infarction, atrial fibrillation, and stroke) associated with the use of these products (Benowitz & Gourlay, 1997), especially in individuals who continue to smoke, controlled studies have failed to demonstrate a significant risk (Benowitz & Gourlay, 1997; Kimmel, Berlin et al., 2001). The absence of a detectable risk, when contrasted with the clear risk to individuals who continue to smoke, has been explained by a sharp reduction in cigarette use, as well as by elimination of the adverse effects of smoking that are not ascribable to nicotine (Benowitz & Gourlay, 1997; Kimmel, Berlin et al., 2001).

In brief, given the hazards of smoking, whatever small risks can be related to continued nicotine exposure are offset by the benefits of cessation: a 50% decrease in risk of having a coronary event after one to two years' abstinence and a continued decline thereafter, so that after 20 years, ex-smokers have a level of risk comparable to that of non-smokers (Kannel, 1981).

MARIJUANA

Marijuana has excitatory effects on the heart (Beaconsfield, Ginsburg et al., 1972; Weiss, Watanabe et al., 1972; Perez-Reyes, Lipton et al., 1973; Malit, Johnstone et al., 1975; Kanakis, Pouget et al., 1976; Tashkin, Levisman et al., 1977; Shapiro, 1978). Such cardiac physiologic changes have been related to the major active compound present in the drug, delta-9-tetrahydrocannabinol (delta-9-THC) (Kanakis, Pouget et al., 1976). Whether delta-9-THC is smoked (Beaconsfield, Ginsburg et al., 1972), ingested (Perez-Reyes, Lipton et al., 1973), or administered intravenously (Malit, Johnstone et al., 1975), heart rate increases. The occurrence of isolated premature ventricular impulses was observed after smoking marijuana (Johnson & Domino, 1971; Kochar & Hosko, 1973). Even a single marijuana cigarette can increase heart rate by 50% (Shapiro, 1978). The increase in heart rate parallels blood concentrations of delta-9-THC (Johnson & Domino, 1971), but then tends to level off despite increasing levels, suggesting a curvilinear relationship (Malit, Johnstone et al., 1975).

When marijuana is ingested, peak effects occur three hours later (Perez-Reyes, Lipton et al., 1973), whereas when smoked (Tashkin, Levisman et al., 1977) or when delta-9-THC is administered intravenously (Malit, Johnstone et al., 1975), peak effects are evident almost immediately. The increased heart rate that follows smoking marijuana can last for two to three hours (Perez-Reyes, White et al., 1991). Some tolerance develops over time (Tashkin, Levisman et al., 1977; Perez-Reyes, White et al., 1991), so that the most pronounced heart rate changes would be expected with first-time use. However, even after several weeks of regular use, marijuana still increases heart rate significantly (Tashkin, Levisman, et al., 1977; Perez-Reyes, White et al., 1991). Moreover, after 48 hours' abstinence, tolerance no longer is evident. The heart rate changes occur concomitantly with increased concentrations of urinary epinephrine (Weiss, Watanabe et al., 1972), but not norepinephrine (Weiss, Watanabe et al., 1972). They can be reduced sharply with adrenergic blockade, using either the beta-blocker propranolol (Inderal⊤) (Beaconsfield, Ginsburg et al., 1972; Perez-Reyes, Lipton et al., 1973)—although not in all studies (Kanakis, Pouget et al., 1976; Shapiro, 1978)—or the alpha$_2$-agonist clonidine (Catapres⊤) (Cone, Welch et al., 1988).

Marijuana's effects on blood pressure are more variable. It can increase (Weiss, Watanabe et al 1972; Prakash, Aronow et al., 1975), have no effect (Malit, Johnstone et al., 1975; Kanakis, Pouget et al., 1976), or even decrease systemic blood pressure (Benowitz & Jones, 1977). Although the explanation for this variability is not clear, marijuana use appears to have a vasodilatory action (Beaconsfield, Ginsburg et al., 1972; Weiss, Watanabe et al., 1972). An increase in blood pressure suggests that an increase in cardiac output has offset the decrease in systemic vascular resistance. Decreases in blood pressure are most evident when the subject is in an upright position (Weiss, Watanabe et al., 1972; Perez-Reyes, Lipton et al., 1973), a finding consistent with the observation that the expected peripheral vasoconstriction after cold exposure or mental stress is attentuated after marijuana use (Beaconsfield, Ginsburg et al., 1972). Orthostatic decreases in blood pressure become more evident after several days of drug use, especially when delta-9-THC is ingested (Benowitz & Jones, 1977; Perez-Reyes, Lipton et al., 1973). Hypotension and even bradycardia, consistent with a vasovagal reaction, can ensue when some individuals assume an upright position after taking delta-9-THC (Perez-Reyes, Lipton et al., 1973).

Cardiac output generally increases following administration of marijuana (Malit, Johnstone et al., 1975; Tashkin, Levisman et al., 1977; Shapiro, 1978). This change reflects increases in heart rate and vasodilation (a reduction of total peripheral resistance) (Beaconsfield, Ginsburg et al., 1972; Weiss, Watanabe et al., 1972), rather than an improvement in cardiac performance. Stroke volume does not increase, and other more sensitive measures of myocardial function, such as ejection fraction, do not change (Shapiro, 1978) or even decrease (Prakash, Aronow et al., 1975). The overall cardiovascular changes suggest an adrenomedullary effect. These findings, however, do not fully replicate those of epinephrine, implying the presence of other mechanisms as well.

The hemodynamic changes after marijuana use would not be expected to have any adverse effects in healthy subjects. For persons with heart disease, however, the changes in cardiac dynamics in fact may be detrimental. The increase in heart rate, and perhaps also in blood pressure, that occurs with marijuana use serves to augment myocardial oxygen requirements. When marijuana is smoked, moreover, carboxyhemoglobin increases (Aronow & Cassidy, 1974; Tashkin, Gliederer et al., 1991). This increase in carboxyhemoglobin lowers blood oxygen content and results in more tightly bound oxyhemoglobin, thereby reducing myocardial oxygen delivery (Aronow & Cassidy et al., 1974). As a consequence of such changes, patients with angina pectoris have myocardial ischemia at reduced levels of exertion and a lower heart rate-blood pressure product when they smoke marijuana (Aronow & Cassidy, 1974). Worsening of the indices of cardiac performance occurs concomitantly with these changes (Prakash, Aronow et al., 1975); therefore, individuals with heart failure might experience deterioration of their condition after marijuana use. Moreover, in a study of patients with an acute myocardial infarction, users of marijuana had almost five times the incidence of the event during the one hour after their use of marijuana than at other times, suggesting that smoking marijuana might be a trigger of myocardial infarction (Mittleman, Lewis et al., 2001). Thus, even though the explanations for its cardiovascular effects have not yet been clearly elucidated, use of marijuana is harmful, at least for individuals with heart disease.

OPIOIDS

Unlike the other addictive substances reviewed in this chapter, which have little or no cardiac medicinal value, opiates are important therapeutic agents: the use of these agents (morphine, in most of the studies cited) for pain relief in acute myocardial infarction and for treatment of cardiogenic pulmonary edema is well established. When administered intravenously at therapeutic doses, opioids have a modest effect on lowering blood pressure (Eckenhoff & Oech, 1960; Samuel, Clarke et al., 1977; Tress & el-Sobky, 1980; Sethna, Moffitt et al., 1982; Roth, Keren et al., 1988) and reducing heart rate (Samuel, Clarke et al., 1977; Tress & el-Sobky, 1980; Roth, Keren et al., 1988)—effects that are independent of the drugs' sedative and respiratory depressant actions (Samuel, Clarke et al., 1977). Under experimental conditions and in amounts that exceed therapeutic doses or amounts used by addicts, morphine can evoke intense sym-

pathomimetic effects, manifested by an increased heart rate and blood pressure and an improvement in cardiac performance (Vatner, Marsh et al., 1975). Although opiates can depress cardiac muscle contractility in isolated preparations (Strauer, 1972), a decrease in cardiac output is not evident in most (Sethna, Moffitt et al., 1982; Roth, Keren et al., 1988), but not all (Gould, Reddy et al., 1978), clinical studies.

Opiates have mild venodilating (Vismara, Leaman et al., 1976) and more pronounced splanchnic arteriolar vasodilating (Leaman, Levenson et al., 1978) effects. Such actions may be related, at least in part, to an opioid-induced release of nitric oxide from endothelium (Stefano, Hartman et al., 1995; Stefano, Salzet et al., 1998), but not to an apparent direct effect on vascular smooth muscle (Flaim, Vismara et al., 1977).

Opiates may have favorable effects on myocardial ischemia. In patients with coronary artery disease, opiates improve myocardial energetics (Sethna, Moffitt et al., 1982) and coronary blood flow (Leaman, Nellis et al., 1978). Moreover, opiates have a direct protective effect against myocardial ischemia at the cellular level (Schultz, Hsu et al., 1997; Liang & Gross, 1999). Administration of morphine before a prolonged coronary occlusion will reduce myocardial injury, analogous to the phenomenon of "ischemic preconditioning" (brief periods of myocardial ischemia before a prolonged episode lessens the injury caused by the prolonged episode; Schultz, Hsu et al., 1997; Liang & Gross, 1999). In addition, through their actions on the central nervous system (Rabkin, 1993), or through direct effects on the myocyte (Sarne, Flitstein et al., 1991), or through vagally mediated mechanisms (EdSilva, Verrier et al., 1978), or as a combination of such effects, opiates may exert antiarrhythmic effects on catecholamine-mediated (Rabkin, 1993) and ischemia-related (Sarne, Flitstein et al., 1991) arrhythmias and increase the threshold for ventricular fibrillation (EdSilva, Verrier et al., 1978). Thus, the overall favorable actions of opioids on the heart explain why abnormalities of cardiac dimensions and function generally are not found in heroin addicts (Pons-Lladó, Carreras et al., 1992).

Despite the benefits of opiates in the treatment of pulmonary edema, heroin overdose can produce a pulmonary condition resembling cardiogenic pulmonary edema (Steinberg & Karliner, 1968). However, heroin-related pulmonary edema, which has been reported with other opioids as well (Bogartz & Miller, 1971), generally occurs in the presence of normal cardiac function. The pulmonary edema that characterizes heroin overdose is highly proteinaceous, resembling plasma, and is consistent with a defect in capillary permeability rather than an elevation of pulmonary capillary pressure (Katz, Aberman et al., 1972). This disorder probably is caused by an unusually high opioid-induced release of histamine from pulmonary mast cells (Brashear, Kelly et al., 1974). Treatment requires maintaining normal blood oxygenation, usually by supplemental oxygen or, if necessary, by noninvasive or mechanical ventilation, until the condition resolves.

The principal cardiac hazard of intravenous (IV) opioid addiction, apart from an accidental overdose, is infective endocarditis. Endocarditis in the heroin addict, however, differs from that seen in the nonaddict in its frequent appearance on normal valves; the high incidence of virulent microorganisms such as *Staphylococcus aureus*, *Pseudomonas* species, and fungus; and the increased involvement of right-sided valves, especially the tricuspid (Andy, Sheikh et al., 1977). Because of the seriousness of this disorder, it must be considered in any IV drug user who presents with fever, especially when associated with repeated rigors.

Treatment with broad-spectrum antibiotic coverage, including an antibiotic against methicillin-resistant *S. aureus*, should be initiated whenever this disorder is suspected; a delay while waiting for a positive blood culture or a confirmation of valvular vegetations by echocardiography can result in serious valvular damage. Moreover, the high relapse rate among opioid addicts requires that the indications for valve replacement be more rigorous in addicted individuals, because the risk of an infection is higher and the consequences of endocarditis more dire with a prosthetic than with a native valve.

COCAINE

Cocaine is a local anesthetic with potent sympathomimetic actions. Its adrenergic effects are the result of blocking presynaptic norepinephrine and dopamine reuptake, thereby making more catecholamines available at postsynaptic receptors (Richie & Greene, 1990; Kloner, Hale et al., 1992; Pitts, Lange et al., 1997), stimulating the sympathetic nervous system (Shannon, Mathier et al., 2001), and enhancing the effects of endogenous catecholamines (Trendelenburg, 1968; Greenberg & Innes, 1976). As a local anesthetic, cocaine inhibits transmembrane sodium flux during electrical excitation, producing a delay in the upstroke and amplitude of the myocardial action potential; this action

diminishes intracellular calcium indirectly (making less sodium available for sodium-calcium exchange) (Richie & Greene, 1990). Cocaine can directly block (L-type channel) calcium entry into the myocyte (Josephson & Sperelakis, 1976; Kimura, Bassett et al., 1992), inhibit the release of calcium from the sarcoplasmic reticulum (Egashira, Morgan et al., 1991), and make the contractile proteins less responsive to available calcium (Egashira, Morgan et al., 1991). Thus, depending on the dose and the clinical or experimental conditions, cocaine can produce seemingly contradictory effects, depending on whether the sympathomimetic or the local anesthetic actions predominate (Egashira, Morgan et al., 1991).

Following cocaine use, blood pressure and heart rate increase and, in most vascular distributions, arteries constrict (Wilkerson, 1988; Fraker, Temesy-Armos et al., 1990). Depending on the dose and the susceptibility of the individual to the drug, even a single use of cocaine can result in sudden cardiac death (Shen, Edwards et al., 1995), an effect that is related in part to cocaine's arrhythmogenic actions. Cocaine abuse can cause angina pectoris and acute myocardial infarction, aortic dissection and rupture, ischemic and hemorrhagic stroke, and left ventricular dilation and hypertrophy (Kloner, Hale et al., 1992). These cardiovascular disorders are related to the acute and chronic hemodynamic and biochemical effects of the drug.

Hemodynamic Effects. When cocaine is abused or administered systemically, it is a potent vasoconstrictor, elevating systemic vascular resistance and blood pressure in a dose-related fashion (Wilkerson, 1988). Typically, heart rate increases as the drug dose increases, although under some experimental conditions, slowing may ensue (Wilkerson, 1988). As a consequence of its direct local anesthetic actions, cocaine depresses myocardial function (Fraker, Temesy-Armos et al., 1990; Perreault, Hague et al., 1993; Morcos, Fairhurst et al., 1993) and attenuates vasoconstriction (Perreault, Hague et al., 1993; Daniel, Lange et al., 1996); under certain conditions, it may even cause vasodilatation (Perreault, Hague et al., 1993). The myocardial depressant actions of cocaine are most evident when its systemic adrenergic effects are diminished (Perreault, Hague et al., 1993) or when baseline myocardial function is depressed (Hale, Alker et al., 1989; Perreault, Hague et al., 1993). Generally, when cocaine is abused, increases in heart rate and blood pressure, myocardial depression, and vasoconstriction ensue.

TABLE 1. Hemodynamic Effects of Alcohol and Other Drug Use

Drug	Rate	SBP	RATE x SBP	CBF	CAD-N	CAD-AB
Ethanol	⇑	⇑/NC/⇓	⇑	⇑	⇑	⇓*
Cocaine	⇑	⇑	⇑	⇓	⇓	⇓
Nicotine	⇑	⇑	⇑	⇑/NC/⇓	⇑/NC/⇓	⇓
Marijuana	⇑⇑	⇑/NC/⇓	⇑	⇑	⇑	UK
Ethanol-Cocaine	⇑⇑	⇑⇑	⇑⇑	⇑	⇑	⇓†
Nicotine-Cocaine	⇑⇑	⇑⇑	⇑⇑	⇓	⇓	⇓⇓
Marijuana-Cocaine	⇑⇑	⇑	⇑⇑	⇓	⇓	⇓

SBP, systolic blood pressure; CBF, coronary blood flow; CAD, coronary artery dimensions; N, normal arteries; AB, stenosed arteries; NC, no change; UK, unknown.

*Blood flow is diminished by coronary steal.

†Coronary steal is expected.

Because of the autoregulatory properties of the coronary circulation, an increase in coronary blood flow would be expected in response to the augmented oxygen demand caused by cocaine-induced increases in heart rate and systemic blood pressure. However, measurements of coronary blood flow in humans after the administration of cocaine (approximately half the local anesthetic dose and between a tenth and a quarter of the amount taken when abused) demonstrate a reduction in coronary blood flow (Lange, Cigarroa et al., 1989; Lange, Cigarroa et al., 1990; Kuhn, Gillis et al., 1992; Pirwitz, Willard et al., 1995). Reduced blood flow also is observed in anesthetized dogs, even when cocaine does not affect the determinants of myocardial oxygen demand (Fraker, Temesy-Armos et al., 1990). Direct measurements of coronary artery dimensions after such a dose of cocaine show constriction of the coronary epicardial arteries (Lange, Cigarroa et al., 1989; Lange, Cigarroa et al., 1990; Kuhn, Gillis et al., 1992; Hale, Alker et al., 1989).

The coronary vasoconstrictive actions of cocaine are attenuated by the alpha-adrenergic blocker phentolamine (Lange, Cigarroa et al., 1989) and are enhanced by the beta-adrenergic blocker propranolol (Lange, Cigarroa et al., 1990). The hemodynamic responses follow a bimodal time course: The maximal effects are observed at peak plasma cocaine concentration and a later secondary effect ensues when the plasma cocaine concentration is at its nadir but the concentrations of its metabolites (benzoylecgonine and ethyl methyl ecgonine) remain high (Pirwitz, Willard et al., 1995). Because the vasodilatory modulating actions of the endothelium can be diminished by atherosclerosis, the coronary vasoconstrictive action of cocaine may be even more intense in the presence of coronary artery disease (Moliterno, Willard et al., 1994).

Some cocaine abusers drink alcoholic beverages, smoke cigarettes, smoke marijuana, or use some combination of these drugs with cocaine. Table 1 summarizes the hemodynamic effects of these activities and their interactions. As shown in the table, although alcohol, smoking cigarettes, smoking marijuana, or using cocaine alone increases myocardial oxygen requirements by increasing systemic blood pressure, heart rate, or both, this effect is exaggerated when cocaine is used in combination with the other substances (Moliterno, Willard et al., 1994; Pirwitz, Willard et al., 1995).

Smoking cigarettes intensifies the ischemic consequences of cocaine use through its vasoconstrictive effects on the coronary circulation, including such actions on diseased segments (Moliterno, Willard et al., 1994); by contrast, alcohol worsens myocardial ischemia by creating a coronary steal, producing arteriolar vasodilation in normal arteries but not in arteries supplying ischemic myocardium, thereby redistributing myocardial blood flow more unfavorably (Friedman, 1981). Moreover, alcohol intensifies the myocardial depressant actions of cocaine (Henning & Wilson, 1996). This effect appears to be due mainly to the combined depressant actions of these substances. A metabolite of their interaction, cocaethylene, also has myocardial depressant actions (Henning & Wilson, 1996) and can continue to exert detrimental effects after cocaine has been metabolized, and cocaine's other metabolites and cocaethylene still are present.

When cocaine is used together with marijuana, heart rate is greater than that seen with the same amount of cocaine taken alone, whereas blood pressure changes are comparable to those observed with only cocaine (Foltin, Fischman et al., 1987; Foltin & Fischman, 1990). When a task is performed at the time cocaine and marijuana are used in combination, the maximal effects of the combination of these drugs on heart rate and blood pressure are intensified (Foltin & Fischman, 1990). Therefore, myocardial oxygen requirements are greater with cocaine and marijuana in combination than with the same amount of either drug used alone. Thus, cocaine abuse, alone or in combination with the use of other addictive substances, creates an imbalance between myocardial oxygen requirements (which it increases) and myocardial oxygen delivery (which it decreases by coronary arterial and arteriolar constrictive actions) (Lange, Cigarroa et al., 1989; Lange, Cigarroa et al., 1990; Moliterno, Willard et al., 1994). Cocaine thus is a potent agent for producing myocardial ischemia.

Acute Coronary Syndromes. In the 1980s, a number of reports appeared of relatively young persons having acute myocardial infarctions following the use of cocaine (Coleman, Ross et al., 1982; Pasternak, Colvin et al., 1985; Isner, Estes et al., 1986; Smith, Liberman et al. 1987). While the average age of these individuals was 31 years, the condition was reported to have occurred even in adolescents (Smith, Liberman et al., 1987). Although the presence of coronary risk factors—especially heavy cigarette smoking—was observed in most of the patients, some had no known predisposition (Smith, Liberman et al., 1987). Both habitual cocaine abusers and occasional users were at risk for these coronary events (Smith, Liberman et al., 1987). The

hour after cocaine use appeared to be the time of greatest hazard (Mittleman, Mintzer et al., 1999).

Acute coronary thromboses have been found when coronary angiography was performed on these individuals within a few hours of symptom onset or at autopsy (Pasternak, Colvin et al., 1985; Isner, Estes et al., 1986; Smith, Liberman et al., 1987; Kolodgie, Virmani et al., 1991). However, angiography performed later, after therapeutic or presumed spontaneous thrombolysis, generally disclosed patent coronary arteries. Multivessel coronary artery stenoses were limited to those individuals at high risk of coronary disease (Pasternak, Colvin et al., 1985; Isner, Estes et al., 1986; Smith, Liberman et al., 1987). By contrast, an autopsy study in cocaine abusers showed coronary occlusive platelet-rich thrombi superimposed on severe luminal-narrowing atherosclerosis; however, plaque rupture, associated with coronary thrombosis in cocaine nonusers, was not evident (Kolodgie, Virmani et al., 1991). The coronary vasoconstrictive actions of cocaine, especially when intensified by smoking, thus appear to be a pivotal condition (Zimmerman, Gustafson et al., 1987).

Cocaine use appears to promote thrombosis (Togna, Tempesta et al., 1985; Moliterno, Lange et al., 1994; Heesch, Wilhelm et al., 2000). Although *in vitro* studies in animals (Togna, Tempesta et al., 1985) and humans (Rinder, Ault et al., 1994) suggest that cocaine may not have a consistent direct action on platelet aggregation or on the formation of vascular and platelet prostaglandins, and even can inhibit platelet function at high concentrations (Togna, Tempesta et al., 1985), cocaine taken intranasally causes platelet activation, platelet microaggregation and increases platelet factor 4 and beta-thromboglobulin (Heesch, Wilhelm et al., 2000). In addition, when cocaine is taken in this way, inhibition of fibrinolysis can occur as a result of increased plasminogen activator inhibitor activity (Moliterno, Lange et al., 1994). Habitual cocaine users were found to have an increased proportion of activated platelets (Rinder, Ault et al., 1994). Thus, even though the pathophysiology of the acute coronary syndromes related to cocaine abuse has not yet been fully elucidated, cocaine's demonstrated actions in increasing myocardial oxygen demand, elevating coronary arteriolar resistance, constricting coronary epicardial arteries, and promoting thrombosis clearly create the milieu for such events.

The treatment of acute myocardial infarction related to cocaine use is similar to that for patients who have not used the drug, with the additional *caveat* that cocaine-related

---

coronary spasm must be considered. Unless hypotension is present, sublingual nitroglycerin should be administered and IV nitroglycerin infused to counteract the vasoconstrictive effects of cocaine (Brogan, Lange et al., 1991); this action may be necessary for at least 12 to 24 hours, taking into account the four to six hours that it can take for the drug to be absorbed from the nasal mucosa (Van Dyke, Barash et al., 1976) and the 24 to 36 hours in which its metabolites can be found in the urine (Pitts, Lange et al., 1997). In electrocardiographic ST-segment elevation myocardial infarction that does not respond to nitroglycerin, an IV thrombolytic drug should be administered, or coronary angiography should be done with a view toward primary coronary angioplasty. The administration of beta-blockers should be deferred until after the effects of cocaine and its congeners have dissipated or coronary patency has been established (Lange, Cigarroa et al., 1990).

Although IV calcium-channel blockers have been shown to alleviate cocaine-induced vasoconstriction (Negus, Willard et al., 1994), their use in this setting probably should be avoided because of their concomitant sympathomimetic actions (Friedman, Rodney et al., 1999). According to standard practices, antiplatelet drugs and anticoagulants should be administered.

Chest pains must be perceived as a prodromal symptom for acute myocardial infarction in all suspected users of the drug, although most cocaine abusers observed for chest pains do not go on to have a myocardial infarction (Gitter, Goldsmith et al., 1991). The predilection for myocardial ischemia, and even for an acute myocardial infarction (Zimmerman, Gustafson et al., 1987), can persist for days, and possibly for weeks, after cocaine withdrawal (Nademanee, Gorelick et al., 1989). Counseling cocaine abusers who experience chest pains and those who have had an acute coronary event and thus are at risk for additional heart attacks and even for sudden death is especially important (Smith, Liberman et al., 1987)

Chronic Cardiovascular Effects. Cocaine abuse has been associated with acceleration of atherosclerosis, myocardial injury and thickening, and vascular complications related to hypertension. Autopsy studies have demonstrated that cocaine addicts have worse coronary atherosclerosis than that found in persons 20 years older (Dressler, Malekzadeh et al., 1990). These findings are consistent with experimental studies showing acceleration of atherosclerosis by cocaine administration in hypercholesterolemic animals (Kloner, Hale et al., 1992; Kolodgie, Farb et al.,

1995). Cocaine can increase vascular endothelial permeability, allowing more atherogenic lipoproteins to diffuse into the intima, although coronary vasospasm, catecholamine toxicity, and activation of inflammatory cells also may contribute to these findings (Kolodgie, Farb et al., 1995). Chronic and acute administration of cocaine has been shown to produce vascular injury and myocardial infarction in hypercholesterolemic and normocholesterolemic animals; these myocardial infarctions, however, were not associated with coronary thromboses (Núñez, Miao et al., 1997).

Myocardial abnormalities have been observed in cocaine abusers (Tazelaar, Karch et al., 1987; Virmani, Robinowitz et al., 1988; Turnicky, Goodin et al., 1992; Shen, Edwards et al., 1995). Focal myocarditis was reported in 20% of cocaine users at autopsy, whether or not the deaths were directly attributable to the drug (Virmani, Robinowitz et al., 1988). The findings included lymphocytic (and sometimes also eosinophilic) infiltration and myocyte necrosis (Virmani, Robinowitz et al., 1988). Focal necrosis with inflammatory cells also was found in clinical and experimental conditions associated with catecholamine excess (Szakács & Cannon, 1958; Chappel, Rona et al., 1959; Van Vliet, Burchell et al., 1966). Myocyte contraction band necrosis (hypereosinophilic-staining bands traversing the cytoplasm), which is a manifestation of clumped sarcomeres and is believed to be related to catecholamine excess, was a frequent finding in one study of cocaine-associated deaths (Tazelaar, Karch et al., 1987) but not in another (Virmani, Robinowitz et al., 1988). Left ventricular hypertrophy has been found both in autopsies (Virmani, Robinowitz et al., 1988) and in clinical echocardiographic studies of chronic cocaine abusers (Brickner, Willard et al., 1991). Although cases of acute pulmonary edema (Hoffman & Goodman, 1989) and dilated cardiomyopathy (Wiener, Lockhart et al., 1986; Chokshi, Moore et al., 1989; Missouris, Swift et al., 2001) have been reported in cocaine abusers, it is not clear whether any of these occurrences are related to the abnormalities that have been reported at autopsy. Moreover, concomitant alcohol abuse, which is an established cause of heart muscle disease, may have contributed to the findings in some patients (Wiener, Lockhart et al., 1986).

Cocaine abuse can exert injurious effects by causing repeated elevations of blood pressure. Regular use of cocaine, moreover, is associated with systemic hypertension (Qureshi, Suri et al., 2001); therefore, conditions for which hypertension is a risk factor should be more prevalent in chronic users. The finding of increased left ventricular wall thickness and increased heart weight in habitual users of cocaine may in part be related to this association (Virmani, Robinowitz et al., 1988; Brickner, Willard et al., 1991).

The most ominous consequence of hypertension, stroke, has been related to cocaine use in some studies (Kaku & Lowenstein, 1990) but not in others (Qureshi, Akbar et al., 1997; Qureshi, Suri et al., 2001). This disparity of findings has been attributed to patterns of drug use. It has been suggested that "crack," the smoked cocaine alkaloid, which has become a common mode of self-administration, can have insufficient potency to produce marked blood pressure elevations (Qureshi, Akbar et al., 1997; Qureshi, Suri et al., 2001), thereby obscuring the overall relationship between cocaine and stroke as determined from cohort data. Finally, aortic dissection and rupture, another complication of hypertension, have been reported in cocaine abusers (Barth, Bray et al., 1986).

Arrhythmogenesis. Cocaine can cause sudden unexpected cardiac death in individuals who do not have apparent coronary or myocardial abnormalities (Shen, Edwards et al., 1995). Such occurrences can be related to the direct and indirect arrhythmogenic effects of the drug. In addition to its sympathomimetic effects, which are a product of its central stimulatory actions (Shannon, Mathier et al., 2001), its peripheral adrenergic reuptake inhibitory actions (Richie & Greene, 1990; Kloner, Hale et al., 1992; Pitts, Lange et al., 1997), and its enhancing effects on endogenous catecholamines (Trendelenburg, 1968; Greenberg & Innes, 1976), cocaine also has vagolytic actions (Xiao & Morgan, 1998). These neurohumoral properties can explain not only cocaine's effect on heart rate but also the various atrial and ventricular tachyarrhythmias that might result from enhancing the activity of normal and abnormal pacemaker cells (Trendelenburg, 1968).

As a blocker of several cation channels, cocaine has pronounced direct effects on the myocardial transmembrane action potential. Cocaine delays and reduces the amplitude of the upstroke (Starmer, Lancaster et al., 1992), depresses the plateau phase (Kimura, Bassett et al., 1992), and prolongs the duration of the action potential (Kimura, Bassett et al., 1992). These changes are related, respectively, to cocaine's actions in blocking the sodium channel (Starmer, Lancaster et al., 1992), the L-type calcium channel (Josephson & Sperelakis, 1976; Kimura, Bassett et al., 1992), and the delayed rectifier (Kimura, Bassett et al., 1992) and acetylcholine-activated (Xiao & Morgan, 1998) potassium

channels. These findings were demonstrated at concentrations comparable to those found at autopsy in cocaine-associated deaths (Shen, Edwards et al., 1995). Moreover, the electrophysiologic changes have been related to stimulus-induced repetitive responses (Starmer, Lancaster et al., 1992) and to the development of early after-depolarizations and repetitive triggered responses (Kimura, Bassett et al., 1992) in the experimental laboratory. The delay in myocardial electrical conduction would promote re-entrant arrhythmias around scar tissue or as the result of acute myocardial ischemia. Thus, cocaine has remarkable electrophysiologic effects that can produce serious cardiac arrhythmias and even sudden death.

AMPHETAMINES AND RELATED COMPOUNDS

Amphetamines (including d,l-amphetamine, methamphetamine, methylphenidate, and MDMA) are sympathomimetic drugs without local anesthetic actions. They have a common beta-phenylethylamine chemical structure, which they share with catecholamines; the differences in their chemical composition determine their mode of action, relative potency, and sympathomimetic properties (Hoffman & Lefkowitz, 1990). Although these substances differ in their central nervous system and peripheral effects, as a group they act by stimulating the sympathetic nervous system, by displacing catecholamines or interfering with reuptake from their storage sites, by blocking the actions of monoamine oxidase (MAO inhibition), and by direct adrenergic actions (Hoffman & Lefkowitz, 1990).

Amphetamines produce a dose-dependent elevation in blood pressure and an increase in heart rate (Martin, Sloan et al., 1971; Mas, Farré et al., 1999). The magnitude of the changes reflects their relative alpha$_1$-adrenergic (elevated blood pressure with reflex slowing of heart rate) and beta$_1$-adrenergic (enhanced cardiac contractility and increase heart rate) effects. When amphetamines are taken parenterally, the peak vasopressor effects are evident within 30 minutes (Martin, Sloan et al., 1971), whereas, when they are taken by mouth, the peak changes occur within one to two hours (Mas, Farré et al., 1999). Under experimental conditions, amphetamines have been shown to increase systolic and diastolic blood pressure in healthy subjects by 30 and 20 mmHg, respectively (Martin, Sloan et al., 1971; Mas, Farré et al., 1999). Such blood pressure elevations dissipate over three to four hours (Martin, Sloan et al., 1971; Mas, Farré et al., 1999).

Although an increase in heart rate (20 beats/minute) parallels the blood pressure changes in users of 3,4-methylenedioxymethamphetamine (MDMA) and methylphenidate, only modest heart rate changes are observed initially in users of amphetamine and methamphetamine (the magnitude of the heart rate changes actually having an inverse relation to the blood pressure changes) (Martin, Sloan et al., 1971; Mas, Farré et al., 1999). Three to four hours after the administration of amphetamine, methamphetamine, or methylphenidate, as the blood pressure elevations dissipate and the reflex baroreceptor response is attenuated, further heart rate increases occur (a total change of as many as 20 to 30 beats/minute); these can persist above baseline for 10 hours (Martin, Sloan et al., 1971; Mas, Farré et al., 1999). The changes (and accompanying body temperature elevations) can be exaggerated by intense, repetitive activities and crowded conditions (Martin, Sloan et al., 1971), which can account for the adverse effects observed when these drugs are used at discos and "raves" (Kalant & Kalant, 1975; Milroy, Clark et al., 1996).

Phencyclidine (PCP) and lysergic acid diethylamide (LSD) generally increase heart rate and blood pressure (Jaffe, 1990). In addition to its sympathomimetic effects, in experimental studies, at least, PCP has been shown to directly enhance myocardial contractility (Temma, Akera et al., 1983), an action that is blocked by calcium-channel blockade (Temma, Akera et al., 1985). Studies using isolated heart muscle preparations have demonstrated that, at high doses, PCP can slow heart rate by mechanisms that have not yet been elucidated (Temma, Akera et al., 1985). The mechanisms of actions of LSD, however, are sufficiently different from those of amphetamines that cross-tolerance does not develop (Vaupel, Nozaki et al., 1978). All of these drugs, by their sympathomimetic actions, would be expected to enhance thrombosis, at least by promoting platelet activation and aggregation, and to produce vasospasm.

In the context of such pharmacologic actions, amphetamines would be expected to produce medical complications similar to those of cocaine. In fact, ischemic (Rothrock, Rubenstein et al., 1988) and hemorrhagic (Goodman & Becker, 1970) stroke, acute myocardial infarction (Ragland, Ismail et al., 1993; Bashour, 1994; Waksman, Taylor et al., 2001), and sudden cardiac death (Kalant & Kalant, 1975; Milroy, Clark et al., 1996) all have been related to amphetamine use, while ventricular tachycardia and fibrillation have been associated with IV administration of amphetamines (Bennett & Walker, 1952). Focal myocyte and contraction band necrosis, which are features of catecholamine excess, have been reported at autopsy in amphetamine abusers (Milroy, Clark et al., 1996). Such findings of myocardial injury may be related to the occurrence of dilated cardiomyopathy in IV amphetamine abusers (Call, Hartneck et al., 1982; Croft, Firth et al., 1982). In addition, necrotizing angiitis (which is indistinguishable from periarteritis nodosa, characterized by fibrinoid necrosis of the intima and media, inflammatory cellular infiltration, and aneurysmal dilatation of small- and medium-sized arteries) has been reported in drug abusers who used methamphetamine (Citron, Halpern et al., 1970), while pulmonary hypertension has been found in users of propylhexedrine (Anderson, Garza et al., 1979).

ANABOLIC STEROIDS

Anabolic steroids (testosterone and its congeners) are abused largely by athletes intent on improving their performance. Because competitive sports produce changes in cardiac dimensions and variations in the electrocardiogram, often referred to as "athlete's heart," it should come as no surprise that the use of these drugs (sometimes in amounts 100 to 1,000 times the therapeutic dose) has been related to abnormalities in the cardiovascular system. Reports of marked cardiac hypertrophy, acute myocardial infarction (sometimes with patent coronary arteries), stroke, and unexpected sudden cardiac death in young athletes, and experimental human and animal data demonstrating that the drugs can elevate blood pressure and have unfavorable effects on blood coagulation and lipids (Sullivan, Martinez et al., 1998), are the basis for this concern.

Studies in athletes have shown that anabolic steroids cause fluid retention (Holma, 1977), which in some (Freed, Banks et al., 1975), but not all (Holma, 1977) investigations is associated with an increase in systolic blood pressure. Because left ventricular hypertrophy is a feature of the athlete's heart, the contribution of anabolic steroids to this finding is controversial (Sullivan, Martinez et al., 1998). The presence of unusually severe hypertrophy on autopsy and evidence of abnormal left ventricular filling disclosed by Doppler echocardiography (so-called "diastolic dysfunction") are abnormalities attributed to anabolic steroids (De Piccolo, Giada et al., 1991; Sullivan, Martinez et al., 1998). However, when left ventricular mass is adjusted for body surface area, no differences are found between bodybuilders who use anabolic steroids and those who do not (Sader, Griffiths et al., 2001). This finding suggests that cardiomegaly in anabolic steroids users is a nonspecific finding related to the generalized organ-enlarging effect of these substances.

Although many case reports of various thrombotic complications in young athletes (Sullivan, Martinez et al., 1998), as well as experimental data in rats and guinea pigs, demonstrate anabolic steroid-induced increased platelet aggregability, which can be related to the androgenicity of the drug (Johnson, Ramey et al., 1977), studies in humans have not demonstrated that androgens promote a hypercoagulable state (Ansell, Tiarks et al., 1993). In fact, the evidence suggests that athletes using anabolic steroids have increased plasma protein C and protein S, substances that have anticoagulant actions, and shortened euglobulin lysis times, an indication of enhanced fibrinolysis (Ansell, Tiarks et al., 1993). However, anabolic steroids, especially when taken orally, have adverse effects on blood lipids (Thompson, Cullinane et al., 1989; Sader, Griffiths et al., 2001). Administration of androgens decreases high-density lipoprotein cholesterol and increases low-density lipoprotein cholesterol (Thompson, Cullinane et al., 1989), producing a lipid profile that favors the development of atherosclerosis. The occurrence of an acute myocardial infarction in a young athlete with patent coronary arteries who used anabolic steroids (McNutt, Ferenchick et al., 1988) suggests that vasospasm can play a role in anabolic steroid–related cardiovascular toxicity.

Thus, although anabolic steroids can be injurious to the heart, the findings also are related to the vigorous exercise and other lifestyle factors generally seen in users of these drugs.

REFERENCES

Abdel-Rahman ARA, Merrill RH & Wolles WR (1987). Effect of acute ethanol administration on the baroreceptor reflex control of heart rate in normotensive human volunteers. *Clinical Science* 72:113-122.

Abel FL (1980). Direct effects of ethanol on myocardial performance and coronary resistance. *Journal of Pharmacology and Experimental Therapeutics* 212:28-33.

Ahlawat S, Siwach SB & Jagdish (1991). Indirect assessment of acute effects of ethyl alcohol on coronary circulation in patients with chronic stable angina. *International Journal of Cardiology* 33:385-392.

Alexander CS (1966). Idiopathic heart disease. *American Journal of Medicine* 41:213-228.

Alexander CS (1967). Electron microscopic observations in alcoholic heart disease. *British Heart Journal* 29:200-206.

Altura BM & Altura B (1982). Microvascular and vascular smooth muscle actions of ethanol, acetaldehyde and acetate. *Federation Proceedings* 41:2447-2451.

Altura BM, Altura B & Carella A (1984). Ethanol produces coronary vasospasm: Evidence for direct action of ethanol on vascular muscle. *British Journal of Pharmacology* 78:260-262.

Anderson RJ, Garza HR, Garriott JC et al. (1979). Intravenous propylhexedrine (Benzedrex) abuse and sudden death. *American Journal of Medicine* 67:15-20.

Andy JJ, Sheikh MU, Ali N et al. (1977). Echocardiographic observations in opiate addicts with active endocarditis. *American Journal of Cardiology* 40:17-23.

Ansell JE, Tiarks C & Fairchild VK (1993). Coagulation abnormalities associated with the use of anabolic steroids. *American Heart Journal* 125:367-371.

Aronow WS & Cassidy J (1974). Effect of marihuana and placebo-marihuana on angina pectoris. *New England Journal of Medicine* 291:65-67.

Aronow WS & Swanson AJ (1969). The effect of low-nicotine cigarettes on angina pectoris. *Annals of Internal Medicine* 71:599-601.

Aronow WS, Cassidy J, Vangrow JS et al. (1974). Effect of cigarette smoking and breathing carbon dioxide on cardiovascular dynamics in anginal patients. *Circulation* 50:340-347.

Aronow WS, Kaplan MA & Desiderio J (1968). Tobacco: A precipitating factor in angina pectoris. *Annals of Internal Medicine* 69:529-536.

Aufferman W, Wu S, Parmley WE et al. (1988). Reversibility of acute alcohol cardiac depression: ^{31}P NMR in hamsters. *Federation of American Societies for Experimental Biology* 2:256-263.

Barbash GK, White HD, Modan M et al. (1993). Significance of smoking in patients receiving thrombolytic therapy for acute myocardial infarction. *Circulation* 87:53-58.

Barry J, Mead K, Nabel EG et al. (1989). Effect of smoking on activity of ischemic heart disease. *Journal of the American Medical Association* 261:398-402.

Barth CW, Bray M & Roberts WC (1986). Rupture of the ascending aorta during cocaine intoxication. *American Journal of Cardiology* 57:496.

Bashour TT (1994). Acute myocardial infarction resulting from amphetamine abuse: A spasm-thrombus interplay? *American Heart Journal* 128:1237-1239.

Beaconsfield P, Ginsburg J & Rainsbury R (1972). Marihuana smoking. *New England Journal of Medicine* 287:209-212.

Beevers DB, Bannan LT, Saunders JB et al. (1982). Alcohol and hypertension. *Contributions in Nephrology* 30:92-97.

Bennett IL & Walker WF (1952). Cardiac arrhythmias following the use of large doses of central nervous system stimulants. *American Heart Journal* 44:428-431.

Benowitz NL & Gourlay MB (1997). Cardiovascular toxicity of nicotine replacement therapy. *Journal of the American College of Cardiology* 29:1422-1431.

Benowitz NL & Jones RT (1977). Cardiovascular effects of prolonged delta-9-tetrahydrocannabinol ingestion. *Clinical Pharmacology and Therapeutics* 18:287-297.

Benowitz NL, Fitzgerald GA, Wilson MS et al. (1993). Nicotine effects on eicosanoid formation and hemostatic function: Comparison of transdermal nicotine and cigarette smoking. *Journal of the American College of Cardiology* 22:1159-1167.

Benowitz NL, Jacob P, Jones RT et al. (1982). Interindividual variability in the metabolism and cardiovascular effects of nicotine in man. *Journal of Pharmacology and Experimental Therapeutics* 221:368-272.

Berger K, Ajani UA, Kase CS et al. (1999). Light-to-moderate alcohol consumption and the risk of stroke among U.S. male physicians. *New England Journal of Medicine* 341:1557-1564.

Blomquist G, Saltin B & Mitchell JH (1970). Acute effects of ethanol ingestion on the response to submaximal and maximal exercise in man. *Circulation* 42:463-470.

Bogartz LJ & Miller WC (1971). Pulmonary edema associated with propoxyphene intoxication. *Journal of the American Medical Association* 215:259-262.

Brashear RE, Kelly MT & White AC (1974). Elevated plasma histamine after heroin and morphine. *Journal of Laboratory and Clinical Medicine* 83:451-457.

Brickner ME, Willard JE, Eichhorn EJ et al. (1991). Left ventricular hypertrophy associated with chronic cocaine abuse. *Circulation* 84:1130-1135.

Brigden W & Robinson J (1964). Alcoholic heart disease. *British Medical Journal* 2:1283-1289.

Brogan WC, Lange RA, Kim AS et al. (1991). Alleviation of cocaine-induced coronary vasoconstriction by nitroglycerin. *Journal of the American College of Cardiology* 18:581-586.

Call TD, Hartneck J, Dickenson WA et al. (1982). Acute cardiomyopathy secondary to intravenous amphetamine abuse. *Annals of Internal Medicine* 97:559-560.

Campillo B, Chabrier PE, Pelle G et al. (1995). Inhibition of nitric oxide synthesis in the forearm arterial bed of patients with advanced cirrhosis. *Hepatology* 22:1423-1429.

Castelli WP (1999). Cardiovascular disease: Pathogenesis, epidemiology, and risk among users of oral contraceptives who smoke. *American Journal of Obstetrics and Gynecology* 180(6 Pt 2):S349-356.

Chan TCK & Sutter MC (1983). Ethanol consumption and blood pressure. *Life Sciences* 33:1965-1973.

Chappel CI, Rona G, Balasz T et al. (1959). Comparison of cardiotoxic actions of certain sympathomimetic amines. *Canadian Journal of Biochemistry and Physiology* 37:35-42.

Cherrick GR & Leevy GM (1965). The effect of ethanol metabolism on levels of oxidized and reduced nicotinamide-adenine dinucleotide in liver, kidney and heart. *Biochimica et Biophysica Acta* 107:29-37.

Chokshi SK, Moore R, Pandian NG et al. (1989). Reversible cardiomyopathy associated with cocaine intoxication. *Annals of Internal Medicine* 111:1039-1040.

Citron BP, Halpern M, McCarron M et al. (1970). Necrotizing angiitis associated with drug abuse. *New England Journal of Medicine* 283:1003-1011.

Clark LT & Friedman HS et al. (1985). Hypertension associated with alcohol withdrawal: Assessment of mechanisms and complications. *Alcoholism: Clinical and Experimental Research* 9:125-130.

Coleman DW, Ross TF & Naughton JL (1982). Myocardial ischemia and infarction related to recreational cocaine use. *Western Journal of Medicine* 136:444-446.

Cone EJ, Welch P & Lange (1988). Clonidine partially blocks the physiologic effects but not the subjective effects produced by smoking marihuana in male human subjects. *Pharmacology, Biochemistry & Behavior* 29:649-652.

Cooke KM, Frost GW, Thornell IR et al. (1982). Alcohol consumption and blood pressure. *Medical Journal of Australia* 1:65-69.

Criqui MH, Wallace RG, Heiss G et al. (1980). Cigarette smoking and plasma high-density lipoprotein cholesterol. *Circulation* 62 (Suppl IV):70-76.

Croft CH, Firth BG & Hillis LD (1982). Propylhexedrine-induced left ventricular dysfunction. *Annals of Internal Medicine* 97:560-561.

Cryer PE, Haymond MW, Santiago JV et al. (1976). Norepinephrine and epinephrine release and adrenergic mediation of smoking-associated hemodynamic and metabolic events. *New England Journal of Medicine* 295:573-577.

Daniel WC, Lange RA, Landau C et al. (1996). Effects of the intracoronary infusion of cocaine and coronary arterial dimensions and blood flow in humans. *American Journal of Cardiology* 78:288-291.

Danziger RS, Sakai M, Capogrossi MC et al. (1991). Ethanol acutely and reversibly suppresses excitation-contraction coupling in cardiac myocytes. *Circulation Research* 68:1660-1668.

de Chillou C, Riff P, Sadoul N et al. (1996). Influence of cigarette smoking on rate of reopening of the infarct-related coronary artery after myocardial infarction. *Journal of the American College of Cardiology* 27:1662-1668.

Delgado CE, Fortuin NJ & Ross RS (1975). Acute effects of low doses of alcohol on left ventricular function by echocardiography. *Circulation* 31:535-540.

Demakis JG, Proskey A, Rahimtoola SH et al. (1974). The natural course of alcoholic cardiomyopathy. *Annals of Internal Medicine* 80:293-297.

De Piccoli B, Giada F, Benettin A et al. (1991). Anabolic steroid use in body builders: An echocardiographic study of the left ventricle. *International Journal of Sports Medicine* 12:408-412.

Deykin D, Janson P & McMahon L (1982). Ethanol potentiation of aspirin-induced prolongation of the bleeding-time. *New England Journal of Medicine* 306:852-854.

Dib JA, Cooper-Vastika SA, Meirelles RF et al. (1993). Acute effects of ethanol and ethanol plus furosemide on pancreatic capillary blood flow in rats. *American Journal of Surgery* 166:18-23.

Donahue RP, Abbott RD, Reed DM et al. (1986). Alcohol and hemorrhagic stroke. *Journal of the American Medical Association* 255:2311-2314.

Dressler FA, Malekzadeh S & Roberts W (1990). Quantitative analysis of amounts of coronary arterial narrowing in cocaine addicts. *American Journal of Cardiology* 65:303-308.

Dyer AR, Stamler J, Paul O et al. (1980). Alcohol consumption and 17-year mortality in the Chicago Western Electric Company Study. *Preventive Medicine* 9:78-90

Eckenhoff JE & Oech SR (1960). The effects of narcotics and antagonists upon respiration and circulation in man. A review. *Clinical Pharmacology and Therapeutics* 1:483-524.

EdSilva RA, Verrier RL & Lown B (1978). Protective effects of the vagotonic action of morphine sulphate on ventricular fibrillation. *Cardiovascular Research* 12:167-172.

Egashira K, Morgan KG & Morgan JP (1991). Effects of cocaine on excitation-contraction coupling of aortic smooth muscle from the ferret. *Journal of Clinical Investigation* 87:1322-1328.

Eliaser M & Giansiracusa FJ (1956). The heart and alcohol. *California Medicine* 84:234-236.

Engel TR & Luck JC (1983). Effect of whiskey on atrial vulnerability and "holiday heart." *Journal of the American College of Cardiology* 1:816-818.

Estruch R, Fernandez-Sola J, Sacanella E et al. (1995). Relationship between cardiomyopathy and liver disease in chronic alcoholism. *Hepatology* 22:532-538.

Ettinger PO, Wu CF, De La Cruz C et al. (1978). Arrhythmias and the "holiday heart": Alcohol associated cardiac rhythm disorders. *American Heart Journal* 95:555-562.

Fernàndez-Solà J, Estruch R, Grau JM et al. (1994). The relation of alcoholic myopathy to cardiomyopathy. *Annals of Internal Medicine* 120:529-536.

Fernàndez-Solà J, Nicolàs JM, Oriola J et al. (2002). Angiotensin-converting enzyme gene polymorphism is associated with vulnerability to aocoholic cardiomyopathy. Annals of Internal Medicine 137(5, part 1):321-326

Fewings JD, Hanna JD, Walsh JA et al. (1966). The effects of ethyl alcohol on blood vessels of the hand and forearm in man. *British Journal of Pharmacology and Chemotherapy* 27:93-106.

Flaim SR, Vismara LA & Zelis R (1977). The effects of morphine on isolated cutaneous canine vascular smooth muscle. *Research Communication in Chemical Pathology and Pharmacology* 16:191-194.

Foitzik T, Castillo CF, Rattner DW et al. (1985). Alcohol selectively impairs oxygenation of the pancreas. *Archives of Surgery* 130:357-361.

Foltin RW & Fischman MW (1990). The effects of combinations of intranasal cocaine, smoked marijuana, and task performance on heart rate and blood pressure. *Pharmacology Biochemistry & Behavior* 36:311-315.

Foltin RW, Fischman MW, Pedroso JJ et al. (1987). Marijuana and cocaine interactions in humans: Cardiovascular consequences. *Pharmacology Biochemistry & Behavior* 28:459-464.

Fortman SP, Haskell WL, Vranizan K et al. (1983). The association of blood pressure and dietary alcohol: Differences by age, sex and estrogen use. *American Journal of Epidemiology* 118:496-507.

Fraker TD, Temesy-Armos PN, Brewster PS et al. (1990). Mechanisms of cocaine-induced myocardial depression. *Circulation* 81:1012-1016.

Fraser GE & Upsdell M (1981). Alcohol and other discriminants between cases of sudden death and myocardial infarction. *American Journal of Epidemiology* 114:462-476.

Freed DLJ, Banks AJ, Longson D et al. (1975). Anabolic steroids in athletics: Crossover double-blind trial on weightlifters. *British Medical Journal* 2:471-473.

Friedman HS (1981). Acute effects of ethanol on myocardial blood flow in the nonischemic and ischemic heart. *American Journal of Cardiology* 47:61-67.

Friedman HS (1990). Alcohol and hypertension. In EB Feldman (ed.) *Nutrition and Heart Disease.* New York, NY: Churchill Livingstone, 35-50.

Friedman HS (1992). Cardiovascular effects of ethanol. In CS Lieber (ed.) *Medical and Nutritional Complications of Alcoholism. Mechanisms and Management.* New York, NY: Plenum Medical Book Company, 359-401.

Friedman HS (1998). Cardiovascular effects of alcohol. In M Galanter (ed.) *Recent Developments in Alcoholism, Vol. 14.* New York, NY: Plenum Publishing Co., 135-166.

Friedman HS & Fernando H (1992). Ascites as a marker for the hyperdynamic heart of Laennec's cirrhosis. *Alcoholism: Clinical & Experimental Research* 16:968-970.

Friedman HS, Cirillo N, Schiano F et al. (1995). Vasodilatory state of decompensated cirrhosis: Relation to hepatic dysfunction, ascites and vasoconstrictive substances. *Alcoholism: Clinical & Experimental Research* 19:123-129.

Friedman HS, Lowery R, Archer M et al. (1984). The effects of ethanol on brain blood flow in awake dogs. *Journal of Cardiovascular Pharmacology* 6:344-348.

Friedman HS, Lowery R, Shaughnessy E et al. (1983). The effects of ethanol on pancreatic blood flow in awake and anesthetized dogs. *Proceedings of the Society of Experimental Biology and Medicine* 174:377-382.

Friedman HS, Matsuzaki S, Chloe SS et al. (1979). Demonstration of dissimilar acute hemodynamic effects of ethanol and acetaldehyde. *Cardiovascular Research* 13:477-487.

Friedman HS, Rodney E, Sinha B et al. (1999). Verapamil prolongs atrial fibrillation by evoking an intense sympathetic neurohumoral effect. *Journal of Investigative Medicine* 47:293-303.

Friedman HS, Vasavada BC, Malec AM et al. (1986). Cardiac function in alcohol-associated hypertension. *American Journal of Cardiology* 57:227-231.

Fuchs CS, Stampfer MJ, Colditz GA et al. (1995). Alcohol consumption and mortality among women. *New England Journal of Medicine* 332:1245-1250.

Gaziano JM, Buring JE, Breslow JL et al. (1993). Moderate alcohol intake, increase of high-density lipoprotein and its subfractions and decreased risk of myocardial infarction. *New England Journal of Medicine* 329:1829-1834.

Gill JS, Zezulka AV, Shipley MJ et al. (1986). Stroke and alcohol consumption. *New England Journal of Medicine* 315:1041-1046.

Gilmour RF, Ruffy R, Lovelace DE et al. (1981). Effect of ethanol on electrocardiogram changes and regional myocardial blood flow during acute myocardial ischaemia. *Cardiovascular Research* 15:47-58.

Gitter MJ, Goldsmith SR, Dunbar DN et al. (1991). Cocaine and chest pains: Clinical features and outcome of patients hospitalized to rule out myocardial infarction. *Annals of Internal Medicine* 115:277-282.

Gomes AL, Gimeno MF & Webb JL (1962). Effects of ethanol on cellular membrane potentials and contractility of isolated rat atrium. *American Journal of Physiology* 203:194-196.

Goodman SJ & Becker DP (1970). Intracranial hemorrhage associated with amphetamine abuse. *Journal of the American Medical Association* 212:480.

Gould L, Reddy CVR, Oh DC et al. (1978). Hemodynamic effects of morphine in cardiac disease. *Journal of Clinical Pharmacology* 18:448-456.

Grassi G, Seravalle G, Calhoun DA et al. (1994). Mechanisms responsible for sympathetic activation by cigarette smoking in humans. *Circulation* 90:248-253.

Greenberg R & Innes IR (1976). The role of bound calcium in supersensitivity induced by cocaine. *British Journal of Pharmacology* 57:329-334.

Greenspon AJ & Schaal SG (1983). The "holiday heart": Electrophysiologic studies of alcohol effects in alcoholics. *Annals of Internal Medicine* 98:135-139.

Greenspon AJ, Stang JM, Lewis RP et al. (1979). Provocation of ventricular tachycardia after consumption of alcohol. *New England Journal of Medicine* 301:1049-1050.

Guarnieri T & Lakatta EG (1990). Mechanism of myocardial contractile depression by clinical concentrations of ethanol. *Journal of Clinical Investigation* 85:1462-1467.

Hale SL, Alker KJ, Rezkalla S et al. (1989). Adverse effects of cocaine on cardiovascular dynamics, myocardial blood flow, and coronary artery diameter in an experimental model. *American Heart Journal* 118:927-933.

Hayes SN & Bove A (1988). Ethanol causes epicardial coronary artery vasoconstriction in the dog. *Circulation* 78:169-170.

Heesch CM, Wilhelm CR, Ristich J et al. (2000). Cocaine activates platelets and increases the formation of circulating platelets containing microaggregates in humans. *Heart* 83:688-695.

Hein OH, Suadicani P & Gyntelberg F (1996). Alcohol consumption, serum low density lipoprotein cholesterol concentration, and risk of ischemic heart disease: six year follow up in the Copenhagen male study. *British Medical Journal* 312:736-741.

Heinrich J, Balleisen L, Schulte H et al. (1994). Fibrinogen and factor VII in the prediction of coronary risk. *Arteriosclerosis & Thrombosis* 14:54-59.

Henning RJ & Wilson LD (1996). Cocaethylene is as cardiotoxic as cocaine but is less toxic than cocaine plus ethanol. *Life Science* 59:615-627.

Hines LM, Stampfer MJ, Ma J et al. (2001). Genetic variation in alcohol dehydrogenase and the beneficial effect of moderate alcohol consumption on myocardial infarction. *New England Journal of Medicine* 344:549-555.

Hoffman BB & Lefkowitz RJ (1990). Catecholamines and sympathomimetic drugs. In AG Gillman, TW Rall, AS Nies et al. (eds.) *The Pharmacological Basis of Therapeutics, 8th Edition.* New York, NY: Pergamon Press, 187-220.

Hoffman CK & Goodman PC (1989). Pulmonary edema in cocaine smokers. *Radiology* 172:463-465.

Holma P (1977). Effect of an anabolic steroid (metandienone) on central and peripheral blood flow in well-trained athletes. *Annals of Clinical Research* 9:215-221.

Huges JM, Henry RE & Daly MJ (1984). Influence of ethanol and ambient temperature on skin blood flow. *Annals of Emergency Medicine* 13:597-600.

Isner JM, Estes M, Thompson PD et al. (1986). Acute cardiac events temporally related to cocaine abuse. *New England Journal of Medicine* 315:1438-1443.

Jaffe JH (1990). Drug addiction and drug abuse. In AG Gillman, TW Rall, AS Nies & P Taylor (eds.) *The Pharmacological Basis of Therapeutics, 8th Edition.* New York, NY: Pergamon Press, 522-573.

Johnson M, Ramey E & Ramwell PW (1977). Androgen-mediated sensitivity in platelet aggregation. *American Journal of Physiology* 232:H381-H385.

Johnson S & Domino EF (1971). Some cardiovascular effects of marihuana smoking in normal volunteers. *Clinical Pharmacology and Therapeutics* 12:762-768.

Josephson I & Sperelakis N (1976). Local anesthetic blockade of Ca^{2+}-mediated action potentials in cardiac muscle. *European Journal of Pharmacology* 40:201-208.

Kaku DA & Lowenstein DH (1990). Emergence of recreational drug abuse as a major risk factor for stroke in young adults. *Annals of Internal Medicine* 113:821-827.

Kalant H & Kalant OJ (1975). Death in amphetamine users: Causes and rates. *Canadian Medical Association Journal* 112:299-304.

Kanakis C, Pouget JM & Rosen KM (1976). The effects of delta-9-tetrahydrocannabinol (cannabis) on cardiac performance with and without beta blockade. *Circulation* 53:703-707.

Kannel WB (1981). Update on the role of cigarette smoking in coronary artery disease. *American Heart Journal* 101:319-328.

Katz S, Aberman A, Frand UI et al. (1972). Heroin pulmonary edema: Evidence for increased pulmonary capillary permeability. *American Review of Respiratory Disease* 106:472-474.

Kelbaek H, Gjorup T, Hartling OJ et al. (1987). Left ventricular function during alcohol intoxication and autonomic blockade. *American Journal of Cardiology* 59:685-688.

Kimmel SE, Berlin JA, Miles C et al. (2001). Risk of acute myocardial infarction and use of nicotine patches in a general population. *Journal of the American College of Cardiology* 37:1297-1302.

Kimura S, Bassett AL & Myerburg RJ (1992). Early after-depolarizations and triggered activity induced by cocaine. A possible mechanism of cocaine arrhythmogenesis. *Circulation* 85:2227-2235.

King AC, Errico AL, Parsons OA et al. (1991). Blood pressure dysregulation associated with alcohol withdrawal. *Alcoholism: Clinical & Experimental Research* 12:478-482.

Kino M, Imamitchi H, Morigutehi M et al. (1981). Cardiovascular status in asymptomatic alcoholics, with reference to the level of ethanol consumption. *British Heart Journal* 46:545-551.

Klatsky AL, Armstrong MA & Friedman GD (1992). Alcohol and mortality. *Annals of Internal Medicine* 117:646-654.

Klein LW, Ambrose J, Pickard A et al. (1984). Acute coronary hemodynamic response to cigarette smoking in patients with coronary artery disease. *Journal of the American College of Cardiology* 3:879-886.

Kloner RA, Hale SH, Alker K et al. (1992). The effects of acute and chronic cocaine use on the heart. *Circulation* 85:407-419.

Kolodgie FD, Farb A & Virmani R (1995). Pathobiological determinants of cocaine-associated cardiovascular syndromes. *Human Pathology* 26:583-586.

Kolodgie FD, Virmani R, Cornhill JF et al. (1991). Increase in atherosclerosis and adventitial mast cells in cocaine abusers: An alternative mechanism of cocaine-associated coronary vasospasm and thrombosis. *Journal of the American College of Cardiology* 17:1553-1560.

Kostis JB, Horstmann E, Mavrogeogis E et al. (1971). Effects of alcohol on the electrocardiogram. *Circulation* 44:558-564.

Kozararevic DJ, Vojvodic N, Dawber T et al. (1980). Frequency of alcohol consumption and morbidity and mortality: The Yugoslavia Cardiovascular Disease Study. *Lancet* i:613-617.

Kramer K, Kuller L & Fisher R (1968). The increasing mortality attributed to cirrhosis and fatty liver in Baltimore (1957-1966). *Annals of Internal Medicine* 69:273-282.

Kuhn FR, Gillis RA, Virmani R et al. (1992). Cocaine produces coronary artery vasoconstriction independent of an intact endothelium. *Chest* 102:581-585.

Lange LG (1982). Nonoxidative ethanol metabolism: Formation of fatty acid ethyl esters by cholesterol esterase. *Proceedings of the National Academy of Science* 79:3954-3957.

Lange LG & Sobel BE (1983). Mitochondrial dysfunction induced by fatty acid ethyl esters, myocardial metabolites or ethanol. *Journal of Clinical Investigation* 72:724-731.

Lange RA, Cigarroa RG, Flores ED et al. (1990). Potentiation of cocaine-induced coronary vasoconstriction by beta-adrenergic blockade. *Annals of Internal Medicine* 112:897-903.

Lange RA, Cigarroa RG, Yancy CW et al. (1989). Cocaine-induced coronary-artery vasoconstriction. *New England Journal of Medicine* 321:1557-1562.

Langer RD, Criqui MH & Reed DM (1992). Lipoproteins and blood pressure as biological pathways for effect of moderate alcohol consumption on coronary heart disease. *Circulation* 85:910-915.

Laposata EA & Lange LG (1986). Presence of nonoxidative ethanol metabolism in human organs commonly damaged by ethanol abuse. *Science* 231:497-499.

Lasker N, Sherrod TR & Killam F (1958). Alcohol on the coronary circulation of the dog. *Journal of Pharmacology and Experimental Therapeutics* 113:441-420.

Leaman DM, Levenson L, Zelis R et al. (1978a). Effect of morphine on splanchnic blood flow. *British Heart Journal* 40:569-571

Leaman DM, Nellis SH, Zelis R et al. (1978b). Effects of morphine sulfate on human coronary blood flow. *American Journal of Cardiology* 41:324-326

Lee FY, Albillos A, Colombato LA et al. (1992). The role of nitric oxide in the vascular hyporesponsiveness to methoxamine in portal hypertensive rats. *Hepatology* 16:1043-1048.

Levine PH (1973). An acute effect of cigarette smoking on platelet function. A possible link between smoking and thrombosis. *Circulation* 48:619-623.

Liang BT & Gross GJ (1999). Direct preconditioning of cardiac myocytes via opioid receptors and KATP channels. *Circulation Research* 84:1396-1400.

Lithell G, Aberg H, Selinus I et al. (1987). Alcohol intemperance and sudden death. *British Medical Journal* 294:1456-1458.

Lochner A, Cowley R & Brink AJ (1969). Effect of ethanol on metabolism and function of perfused rat heart. *American Heart Journal* 78:770-780.

Luca C (1979). Electrophysiological properties of right heart and atrioventricular conducting system in patients with alcoholic cardiomyopathy. *British Heart Journal* 42:274-281.

Madan BR & Gupta RS (1967). Effect of ethanol in experimental auricular and ventricular arrhythmias. *Japanese Journal of Pharmacology* 17:683-684.

Mahendra S, Kochar T & Hasko M (1973). Electrocardiographic effects of marijuana. *Journal of the American Medical Association* 225:25-27

Malhotra, Mathur et al. (1985).

Malit LA, Johnstone RE, Bourke DI et al. (1975). Intravenous D 9-tetrahydrocannabinol: Effects on ventilatory control and cardiovascular dynamics. *Anesthesiology* 42:666-673.

Mann J & Davies MJ (1999). Mechanisms of progression in native coronary artery disease: Role of healed plaque disruption. *Heart* 82:265-268.

Martin WR, Sloan JW, Sapira JD et al. (1971). Physiologic, subjective, and behavioral effects of amphetamine, methamphetamine, ephedrine, phenmetrazine, and methylphenidate in man. *Clinical Pharmacology and Therapeutics* 12:245-257.

Mas M, Farré M, de la Torre R et al. (1999). Cardiovascular and neuroendocrine effects and pharmacokinetics of 3,4-methylenedioxide-methamphetamine in humans. *Journal of Pharmacology and Experimental Therapeutics* 290:136-145.

Mathews E, Gardin JM, Henry W et al. (1981). Echocardiographic abnormalities in chronic alcoholics with and without overt congestive heart failure. *American Journal of Cardiology* 47:570-576.

Mayhan WG & Didion SP (1995). Acute effects of ethanol on responses of cerebral arterioles. *Stroke* 26:2097-2102.

McNutt RA, Ferenchick GS, Kirlin PC et al. (1988). Acute myocardial infarction in a 22-year-old world class weight lifter using anabolic steroids. *American Journal of Cardiology* 62:164.

Meade TW, Imeson J & Stirling Y (1987). Effects of changes in smoking and other characteristics on clotting factors and the risk of ischemic disease. *Lancet* ii:986-988.

Mendoza LC, Hellberg K, Rickart A et al. (1971). The effect of intravenous ethyl alcohol on the coronary circulation and myocardial contractility of the human and canine heart. *Journal of Clinical Pharmacology and New Drugs* 11:165-176.

Miller H & Abelmann WH (1967). Effects of dietary ethanol upon experimental trypanosomal (T. cruzi) myocarditis. *Proceedings of the Society of Experimental Biology* 126:193-198.

Milroy CM, Clark JC & Forrest ARW (1996). Pathology of deaths associated with "Ecstasy" and "Eve" misuse. *Journal of Clinical Pathology* 49:149-153.

Missouris CG, Swift PA & Singer DRJ (2001). Cocaine use and acute left ventricular dysfunction. *Lancet* 357:1586.

Mittleman MA, Lewis RA, Maclure M et al. (2001). Triggering of myocardial infarction by marijuana. *Circulation* 103:2805-2809.

Mittleman MA, Mintzer D, Maclure M et al. (1999). Triggering of myocardial infarction by cocaine. *Circulation* 99:2737-2741.

Molgaard H, Kristensen BO & Baandrup U (1990). Importance of abstention from alcohol in alcoholic heart disease. *International Journal of Cardiology* 27:372-375.

Moliterno DJ, Lange RA, Gerard RD et al. (1994). Influence of intranasal cocaine on plasma constituents associated with endogenous thrombosis and thrombolysis. *American Journal of Medicine* 96:492-496.

Moliterno DJ, Willard JE, Lange RA et al. (1994). Coronary-artery vasoconstriction induced by cocaine, cigarette smoking, or both. *New England Journal of Medicine* 330:454-459.

Mongo KG & Vassort G (1990). Inhibition by alcohols, halothane and chloroform of the Ca current in single frog ventricular cells. *Journal of Molecular and Cellular Cardiology* 22:939-953.

Morcos NC, Fairhurst A & Henry WL (1993). Direct myocardial effects of cocaine. *Cardiovascular Research* 27:269-273.

Morin YL, Foley AR, Martineau G et al. (1967). Quebec beer-drinkers' cardiomyopathy: Forty-eight cases. *Canadian Medical Association Journal* 97:881-904.

Morin Y, Roy PE, Mohiuddin SM et al. (1969). The influences of alcohol on viral and isoproterenol cardiomyopathy. *Cardiovascular Research* 3:363-368.

Nademanee K, Gorelick DA, Josephson MA et al. (1989). Myocardial ischemia during cocaine withdrawal. *Annals of Internal Medicine* 111:876-880.

Nakano J & Moore SE (1972). Effect of different alcohols on the contractile force of the isolated guinea pig myocardium. *European Journal of Pharmacology* 20:266-270.

Negus BH, Willard JE, Hillis LD et al. (1994). Alleviation of cocaine-induced coronary vasoconstriction with intravenous verapamil. *American Journal of Cardiology* 73:510-513.

Newby DE, McLeod AL, Uren NG et al. (2001). Impaired coronary tissue plasminogen activator release is associated with coronary atherosclerosis and cigarette smoking. *Circulation* 103:1936-1941.

Nguyen TN, Friedman HS & Mokraoui AM (1987). Effects of alcohol on experimental atrial fibrillation. *Alcoholism: Clinical & Experimental Research* 11:474-476.

Niedermaier ON, Smith ML, Beightol LA et al. (1993). Influence of cigarette smoking on human autonomic function. *Circulation* 88:562-571.

Novak DJ & Victor M (1974). The vagus and sympathetic nerves in alcoholic polymyopathy. *Archive of Neurology* 30:273-294.

Núñez BD, Miao L, Klein MA et al. (1997). Acute and chronic cocaine exposure can produce myocardial ischemia and infarction in Yucatan swine. *Journal of Cardiovascular Pharmacology* 29:145-155.

Orgata M, Mendelson JH, Mello NK et al. (1971). Adrenal function and alcoholism. *Psychosomatic Medicine* 33:159-180.

Orlando J, Aronow WS, Cassidy J et al. (1976). Effect of ethanol on angina pectoris. *Annals of Internal Medicine* 84:652-655.

Paradise RR & Stoelting V (1965). Conversion of acetyl strophanthidin-induced ventricular tachycardia to sinus rhythm by ethyl alcohol. *Archives Internationales de Pharmacodynamie et de Therapie* 157:312-321.

Pasternack PF, Colvin SB & Baumann FG (1985). Cocaine-induced angina pectoris and acute myocardial infarction in patients younger than 40 years. *American Journal of Cardiology* 55:847.

Perez-Reyes M, Lipton MA, Timmons MC et al. (1973). Pharmacology of orally administered D-9-tetrahydrocannabinol. *Clinical Pharmacology and Therapeutics* 14:48-55.

Perez-Reyes M, White WR, McDonald SA et al. (1991). The pharmacologic effects of daily marijuana smoking in humans. *Pharmacology Biochemistry & Behavior* 40:691-694.

Perreault CL, Hague NL, Morgan KG et al. (1993). Negative inotropic and relaxant effects of cocaine on myopathic human ventricular myocardium and epicardial coronary arteries in vitro. *Cardiovascular Research* 27:262-268.

Pirwitz MJ, Willard JE, Landau C et al. (1995). Influence of cocaine, ethanol, or their combination on epicardial coronary dimensions in humans. *Archives of Internal Medicine* 155:1186-1191.

Pitts WR, Lange RA, Cigarroa JE et al. (1997). Cocaine-induced myocardial ischemia and infarction: Pathophysiology, recognition, and management. *Progress in Cardiovascular Diseases* 40:65-76.

Pizcueta P, Pique JM, Fernandez M et al. (1992). Modulation of the hyperdynamic circulation of cirrhotic rats by nitric oxide inhibition. *Gastroenterology* 103:1909-1915.

Pons-Lladó G, Carreras F, Borràs X et al. (1992). Findings on Doppler echocardiography in asymptomatic intravenous heroin users. *American Journal of Cardiology* 69:238-241.

Potter JE & Beevers DG (1984). Pressor effect of alcohol in hypertension. *Lancet* i:119-122.

Prakash R, Aronow WS, Warren M et al. (1975). Effects of marihuana and placebo marihuana on hemodynamics in coronary disease. *Clinical Pharmacology and Therapeutics* 18:90-95.

Preedy VR & Peters TJ (1989). The acute and chronic effects of ethanol on cardiac protein synthesis in the rat. *Alcohol* 7:97-102.

Puddey JE, Beilin IJ, Vandongen R et al. (1985). Evidence for a direct effect of alcohol on blood pressure in normotensive men. *Hypertension* 7:707-713.

Puddey JE, Beilin IJ & Vandongen R (1987). Regular alcohol use raises blood pressure in treated hypertensive subjects. *Lancet* i:647-662.

Qureshi AI, Akbar MS, Czander E et al. (1997). Crack cocaine use and stroke in young patients. *Neurology* 48:341-345.

Qureshi AI, Suri F, Guterman LR et al. (2001). Cocaine use and the likelihood of nonfatal myocardial infarction and stroke. *Circulation* 103:502-506.

Rabkin SW (1993). Morphine and morphiceptin increase the threshold for epinephrine-induced cardiac arrhythmias in the rat brain mu opioid receptors. *Clinical and Experimental Pharmacology and Physiology* 20:95-102.

Ragland AS, Ismail Y & Arsura EL (1993). Myocardial infarction after amphetamine use. *American Heart Journal* 125:247-249.

Randall B (1980). Sudden death and hepatic fatty metamorphosis. *Journal of the American Medical Association* 243:1723-1725.

Randin D, Vollenweider P, Tappy L et al. (1995). Suppression of alcohol-induced hypertension by dexamethasone. *New England Journal of Medicine* 332:1733-1737.

Regan TJ, Koroxenidis G, Moschos CB et al. (1966). The acute metabolic and hemodynamic responses of the left ventricle to ethanol. *Journal of Clinical Investigation* 45:270-278.

Regan TJ, Levinson GE, Oldewurtel HA et al. (1969). Ventricular function in noncardiacs with alcoholic fatty liver: Role of ethanol in the production of cardiomyopathy. *Journal of Clinical Investigation* 48:397-406.

Renaud SC & Ruf JC (1996). Effects of alcohol on platelet functions. *Clinica Chimica Acta* 246:77-89.

Rich EC, Siebold C & Campion B (1985). Alcohol-related acute atrial fibrillation: A case-control study and review of 40 patients. *Archives of Internal Medicine* 145:830-833.

Richards IS, Kulkarni A, Brooks SM et al. (1989). A moderate concentration of ethanol alters cellular membrane potentials and decreases contractile force of human fetal heart. *Developmental Pharmacology and Therapeutics* 13:51-56.

Richie JM & Green NM (1990). Local Anesthetics. In AG Gilman, TW Rall, AS Nies et al. (eds.) *The Pharmacologic Basis of Therapeutics*. New York, NY: Pergamon Press, 311-331.

Ridker PM, Vaughan DE, Stampfer MJ et al. (1994). Association of moderate alcohol consumption and plasma concentration of endogenous tissue-type plasminogen activator. *Journal of the American Medical Association* 272:929-933.

Riff DP, Jain AC & Doyle JT (1969). Acute hemodynamic effects of ethanol on normal human volunteers. *American Heart Journal* 78:592-597.

Rimm EB, Giovannuci EL, Willette WC et al. (1991). Prospective study of alcohol consumption and risk of coronary disease in men. *Lancet* 338:464-468.

Rimm EB, Klatsky A, Grobbee D et al. (1996). Review of moderate alcohol consumption and reduced risk of coronary heart disease: Is the effect due to beer, wine, or spirits? *British Medical Journal* 312:731-736.

Rinder HM, Ault KA, Jatlow PI et al. (1994). Platelet alpha-granule release in cocaine users. *Circulation* 90:1162-1167.

Rossinen J, Partanen J, Koskinen P et al. (1996). Acute heavy alcohol intake increases silent myocardial ischemia in patients with stable angina pectoris. *Heart* 75:563-567.

Roth A, Keren G, Gluck A et al. (1988). Comparison of nalbuphine hydrochloride versus morphine sulfate for acute myocardial infarction with elevated pulmonary artery wedge pressure. *American Journal of Cardiology* 62:551-555.

Rothrock JF, Rubenstein R & Lyden PD (1988). Ischemic stroke associated with methamphetamine inhalation. *Neurology* 38:589-592.

Ruf JC, Berger JL & Renaud S (1995). Platelet rebound effect of alcohol withdrawal and wine drinking in rats. Relation to tannins and lipid peroxidation. *Arterioclerosis, Thrombosis and Vascular Biology* 15:140-144.

Sader MA, Griffiths KA, McCredie RJ et al. (2001). Androgenic anabolic steroids and arterial structure and function in male bodybuilders. *Journal of the American College of Cardiology* 37:224-230.

Samuel IO, Clarke SJ & Dundee JW (1977). Some circulatory and respiratory effects of morphine in patients without pre-existing cardiac disease. *British Journal of Anesthesiology* 49:927-932.

Sano M, Wendt PE, Wirsen A et al. (1993). Acute effects of alcohol on regional cerebral blood flow in man. *Journal of Studies on Alcohol* 54:369-376.

Sarne Y, Flitstein A & Oppenheimer E (1991). Anti-arrhythmic activities of opioid agonists and antagonists and their stereoisomers. *British Journal of Pharmacology* 102:696-698.

Schultz JJ, Hsu AK & Gross GJ (1997). Ischemic preconditioning and morphine-induced cardioprotection involve the delta-opioid receptor in the intact rat heart. *Journal of Molecular and Cellular Cardiology* 29:2187-2195.

Schwartz JA, Speed NM, Gross M et al. (1993). Acute effects of alcohol administration on regional cerebral blood flow: the role of acetate. *Alcoholism: Clinical & Experimental Research* 17:1119-1123.

Schwartz L, Sample B & Wigle D (1975). Severe alcoholic cardiomyopathy reversed with abstention from alcohol. *American Journal of Cardiology* 36:963-966.

Segel LB (1984). Mitochondrial respiration after cardiac perfusion with ethanol or acetaldehyde. *Alcoholism: Clinical & Experimental Research* 8:560-563.

Serdula MK, Koong SL, Williamson DF et al. (1995). Alcohol intake and subsequent mortality: Findings from NHANES I follow-up study. *Alcohol* 56:233-239.

Sethna D, Moffitt EA, Gray RJ et al. (1982). Cardiovascular effects of morphine in patients with coronary arterial disease. *Anesthesia and Analgesia* 1982:109-114.

Shannon RP, Mathier MA & Shen Y-T (2001). Role of cardiac nerves in the cardiovascular response to cocaine in conscious dogs. *Circulation* 103:1674-1680.

Shapiro BJ (1978). Cardiovascular effects of cannabis. In Tashkin DP (moderator) *Cannabis, 1997. Annals of Internal Medicine* 89:539-549.

Shaw S, Heller EA, Friedman HS et al. (1977). Increased hepatic oxygenation following ethanol administration in the baboon. *Proceedings of the Society for Experimental Biology and Medicine* 156:509-513.

Shen W-K, Edwards WD, Hammill SC et al. (1995). Sudden unexpected nontraumatic death in 54 young adults: A 30-year population based study. *American Journal of Cardiology* 76:148-152.

Sieber CC & Groszmann RJ (1992). Nitric oxide mediates hyporeactivity to vasopressors in mesenteric vessels of protal hypertensive rats. *Gastroenterology* 103:235-239.

Smith HWB, Liberman HA, Brody SL et al. (1987). Acute myocardial infarction temporally related to cocaine use. *Annals of Internal Medicine* 107:13-18.

Sogni P, Moreau R, Ohsuga M et al. (1992). Evidence for normal nitric oxide-mediated vasodilator tone in conscious rats with cirrhosis. *Hepatology* 16:980-983.

Spodick DH, Pigott VM & Chirife R (1972). Preclinical cardiac malfunction on chronic alcoholism. *New England Journal of Medicine* 287:677-680.

Starmer CF, Lancaster AR, Lastra AA et al. (1992). Cardiac instability amplified by use-dependent Na channel blockade. *American Journal of Physiology* 262:H1305-H1310.

Stefano GB, Hartman A, Bilfinger TV et al. (1995). Presence of D^3 opiate receptor in endothelial cells. Coupling to nitric oxide production and vasodilation. *Journal of Biological Chemistry* 270:30290-30293.

Stefano GB, Salzet M, Hughes TK et al. (1998). D^2 opioid receptor subtype on human vascular endothelium uncouples morphine stimulated nitric oxide release. *International Journal of Cardiology* 1(Suppl):S43-S51.

Steinberg AD & Karliner JS (1968). The clinical spectrum of heroin pulmonary edema. *Archives of Internal Medicine* 122:122-127.

Stickel F, Choi S-W, Kim Y-I et al (2000). Effect of chronic alcohol consumption on total homocysteine level in rats. *Alcoholism: Clinical & Experimental Research* 24:259-264.

Strauer BE (1972). Contractile responses to morphine, piritramide, meperidine and fentanyl: A comparative study of effects on the isolated ventricular myocardium. *Anesthesiology* 37:304-310.

Suh I, Shaten J, Cutler JA et al. (1992). Alcohol use and mortality from coronary heart disease: The role of high-density lipoprotein cholesterol. *Annals of Internal Medicine* 116:881-887.

Sullivan ML, Martinez CM, Gennis P et al. (1998). The cardiac toxicity of anabolic steroids. *Progress in Cardiovascular Diseases* 41:1-15.

Szakács JE & Cannon A (1958). L-Norepinephrine myocarditis. *American Journal of Clinical Pathology* 30:425-434

Takizawa A, Yasue H, Omote S et al. (1984). Variant angina induced by alcohol ingestion. *American Heart Journal* 107:25-27.

Tashkin DP, Gliederer F, Rose J et al. (1991). Effects of varying marijuana smoking profile on deposition of tar and absorption of CO and delta-9-THC. *Pharmacology Biochemistry & Behavior* 40:651-656.

Tashkin DP, Levisman JA, Abbasi AS et al. (1977). Short-term effects of smoked marihuana on left ventricular function in man. *Chest* 72:20-26.

Tazelaar HD, Karch SB, Stephens BG et al. (1987). Cocaine and the heart. *Human Pathology* 18:195-199.

Temma K, Akera T, Brody TM et al. (1983). Negative chronotropic and positive inotropic actions of phencyclidine on isolated atrial muscle in guinea pigs and rats. *Journal of Pharmacology and Experimental Therapeutics* 226:885-892.

Temma K, Akera T & Ng Y-C (1985). Cardiac actions of phencyclidine in isolated guinea pig and rat heart: Possible involvement of slow channels. *Journal of Cardiovascular Pharmacology* 7:297-306.

Thompson PD, Cullinane EM, Sady SP et al. (1989). Contrasting effects of testosterone and stanozolol on serum lipoprotein levels. *Journal of the American Medical Association* 261:1165-1168.

Thornton JR (1984). Atrial fibrillation in healthy non-alcoholic people after an alcoholic binge. *Lancet* ii:1013-1017.

Tiihonen J, Kuikka J, Hakola P et al. (1994). Acute ethanol-induced changes in cerebral blood flow. *American Journal of Psychiatry* 151:1505-1508.

Togna G, Tempesta E, Togna AR et al. (1985). Platelet responsiveness and biosynthesis of thromboxane and prostacycline in response to in vitro cocaine treatment. *Haemostasis* 15:100-107.

Trendelenburg U (1968). The effects of cocaine on the pacemaker of isolated guinea-pig atria. *Journal of Pharmacology and Experimental Therapeutics* 161:222-231.

Tress KH & el-Sobky AA (1980). Cardiovascular, respiratory and temperature responses to intravenous heroin (diamorphine) in dependent and non-dependent humans. *British Journal of Clinical Pharmacology* 10:477-485.

Tsiplenkova VG, Vihert AA & Cherpachenko NM (1986). Ultrastructure and histochemical observations in human and experimental alcoholic cardiomyopathy. *Journal of the American College of Cardiology* 8:22A-32A.

Turnicky RP, Goodin J, Smialik JE et al. (1992). Incidental myocarditis with intravenous drug abuse. *Human Pathology* 23:138-143.

Urbano-Marquez A, Estruch R, Navarro-Lopez R et al. (1989). The effects of alcoholism on skeletal and cardiac muscle. *New England Journal of Medicine* 320:409-415.

U.S. Department of Agriculture & U.S. Department of Health and Human Services (USDA & DHHS) (1995). *Nutrition and Your Health: Dietary Guide for Americans, 4th Edition.* Washington, DC: U.S. Government Printing Office, 40-41.

Vaisrub S (1973). Cannabis and the cardiovascular system. *Journal of the American Medical Association* 225:58.

van der Gaag MS, Ubbink JB, Sillanaukee P et al. (2000). Effect of consumption of red wine, spirits, beer on serum homocysteine. *Lancet* 355:1522.

Van Dyke C, Barash PG, Jatlow P et al. (1976). Cocaine: Plasma concentrations after intranasal application in man. *Science* 191:859-861.

Van Vliet PD, Burchell HB et al. (1966). Focal myocarditis associated with pheochromocytoma. *New England Journal of Medicine* 274:1102-1108.

Vatner SF, Marsh JD & Swain JA (1975). Effects of morphine on coronary and left ventricular dynamics in conscious dogs. *Journal of Clinical Investigation* 55:207-217.

Vaupel DB, Nozaki M, Martin WR et al. (1978). Single dose and cross tolerance studies of b-phenethylamine, d-amphetamine, and LSD in the chronic spinal dog. *European Journal of Pharmacology* 48:431-437.

Virmani R, Robinowitz M, Smialek JE et al. (1988). Cardiovascular effects of cocaine: An autopsy study of 40 patients. *American Heart Journal* 15:1068-1076.

Vismara LA, Leaman DM & Zelis R (1976). The effects of morphine on venous tone in patients with acute pulmonary edema. *Circulation* 54:335-337.

Vorobioff J, Bredfeldt JE & Groszmann RJ (1983). Hyperdynamic circulation in protal-hypertensive rat model: A primary factor for maintenance of chronic portal hypertension. *American Journal of Physiology* 244:G52-G57.

Waksman J, Taylor RN, Bodor GS et al. (2001). Acute myocardial infarction associated with amphetamine use. *Mayo Clinic Proceedings* 76:323-326.

Wannamethee SG & Shaper AG (1996). Patterns of alcohol intake and risk of stroke in middle-aged British men. *Stroke* 27:1033-1039.

Weiss JL, Watanabe AM, Lemberger L et al. (1972). Cardiovascular effects of delta-9-tetrahydrocannabinol in man. *Clinical Pharmacology and Therapeutics* 13:671-684.

Wendt VE, Wu C, Balcon R et al. (1965). Hemodynamic and metabolic effect of chronic alcoholism in man. *American Journal of Cardiology* 15:178-184.

Wennmalm Å, Benthin G, Granström EF et al. (1991). Relation between tobacco use and urinary excretion of thromboxane A$_2$ and prostacyclin metabolites in young men. *Circulation* 83:1698-1704.

Wiener RS, Lockhart JT & Schwartz RG (1986). Dilated cardiomyopathy and cocaine use. *American Journal of Medicine* 81:699-701.

Wilkerson RD (1988). Cardiovascular effects of cocaine in conscious dogs: Importance of fully functional autonomic nervous systems. *Journal of Pharmacology and Experimental Therapeutics* 246:466-471.

Williams ES, Mirro MJ & Bailey JC (1980). Electrophysiological effects of ethanol, acetaldehyde, and acetate on cardiac tissues from dog and guinea pig. *Circulation Research* 47:473-478.

Winniford MD, Jansen DE, Reynolds GA et al. (1987). Cigarette smoking-induced coronary vasoconstriction in atherosclerotic coronary artery disease and prevention by calcium antagonists and nitroglycerin. *American Journal of Cardiology* 59:203-207.

Winniford MD, Wheelan KR, Kremers MS et al. (1986). Smoking-induced coronary vasoconstriction in patients with atherosclerotic artery disease: Evidence for adrenergically mediated alterations in coronary artery tone. *Circulation* 72:662-667.

Xiao Y-F & Morgan JP (1998). Cocaine blockade of acetylcholine-activated muscurinic K$^+$ channel in ferret cardiac myocytes. *Journal of Pharmacology and Experimental Therapeutics* 284:10-18.

Zimmerman FH, Gustafson GM & Kemp HG (1987). Recurrent myocardial infarction associated with cocaine abuse in a young man with normal coronary arteries: Evidence for coronary artery spasm culminating in thrombosis. *Journal of the American College of Cardiology* 9:964-968.

Paul S. Haber, M.D., FRACP

Chapter 3

Liver Disorders Related to Alcohol and Other Drug Use

Alcoholic Liver Disease
Viral Hepatitis
Cocaine Hepatitis
MDMA ("Ecstasy")
Toxicity From Co-injected Materials
Phencyclidine

The liver is a major target for the toxicity of alcohol and other drugs of abuse. This chapter describes the more common liver diseases associated with abuse of alcohol and other drugs (Table 1). The emphasis is on clinical manifestations, diagnosis, and management.

ALCOHOLIC LIVER DISEASE

The outcome of alcoholic liver disease (ALD) is more severe than that of many cancers, yet it attracts much less concern among the public and in the medical profession. The prevailing nihilism about treatment may contribute to this attitude. However, new insights into the pathophysiology of the alcohol-use disorders now allow for prospects of earlier recognition and more successful efforts at prevention and treatment.

Prevalence. Cirrhosis of the liver (mostly in association with alcohol abuse) is the fifth most common cause of death among middle-aged American men and accounts for more than 26,000 deaths per year in the United States (Dufour, 1994). End-stage ALD ranked as the leading primary indication for liver transplantation in the U.S. for more than a decade and only recently has been overtaken by chronic hepatitis C, which also commonly coexists with alcohol abuse (Rosman, Paronetto et al., 1993).

The population risk of cirrhosis is related to the population level of alcohol consumption. This phenomenon has been documented by comparing rising or falling levels of alcohol consumption in several populations across time and by comparing various populations (Lieber & Leo, 1992). Recent reductions in population alcohol consumption in France and Australia thus can be expected to reduce the prevalence of this disease.

Risk Factors. Risk factors for ALD include the amount of alcohol consumed, gender, genetic factors, obesity, chronic viral hepatitis, ingestion of hepatotoxins, and nutrition.

Amount of Alcohol Consumed: Fatty liver can be observed after a single binge, but more advanced liver disease typically is seen after more than 10 years of consumption at average levels exceeding 100 g/day. The risk of liver disease increases above 60 g/day for men. Among very heavy drinkers, the risk rises to approximately 50%, but it does not reach 100% even at the highest level of alcohol consumption.

Gender: Women appear to be at greater risk of ALD, with the risk rising for alcohol consumption of more than 20 to 40 g/day (Norton, Batey et al., 1987; Saunders, Davis et al., 1981; Morgan & Sherlock, 1977; Parrish, Dufour et al., 1993; Pequignot, Tuyns et al., 1978). The explanation

TABLE 1.   Liver Disorders Associated With Substance Abuse

Hepatic Drug Toxicity
- Alcohol
- MDMA
- Cocaine
- Heroin
- Phencyclidine
- Androgenic steroids.

Toxic Interactions With Other Drugs of Abuse
- Alcohol plus MDMA
- Alcohol plus cocaine
- Alcohol plus acetaminophen.

Systemic Effects of Drugs Leading to Liver Injury
- Hypo- and hyperthermia
- Shock
- Rhabdomyolysis.

Infectious Complications
- Viral hepatitis: A to D, particularly B and C
- Bacteria: SBE, septicemia.

Co-Injected Material
- Talc (hepatic granulomas)
- Lead (byproduct of methamphetamine synthesis).

for this susceptibility remains in debate. The differences in body composition between men and women result in a higher relative alcohol dose in women compared with men who consume the same amount. On average, women are smaller than men and have a higher percentage of body fat and a lower percentage of body water into which a dose of alcohol is distributed (Frezza, di Padova et al., 1990). Moreover, for a given dose of alcohol per kilogram of body water, higher blood alcohol concentrations are reached in women than in men because of differences in first-pass metabolism. First-pass metabolism of alcohol is thought to be lower in women because of lower gastric alcohol dehydrogenase activity, leading to higher bioavailability of orally administered alcohol and further increasing the relative dose compared with men (Frezza, di Padova et al., 1990). This effect is even more striking in alcoholic than in non-alcoholic women (Frezza, di Padova et al., 1990).

Alcohol elimination is more rapid in women than in men, and this rapidity can contribute to enhanced hepatotoxicity. Hepatic alcohol dehydrogenase activity is suppressed by testosterone and its derivatives (Teschke & Wiese, 1982). However, Kwo and colleagues (1998) showed that the enhanced alcohol elimination in women is better explained by higher liver mass per kilogram of body weight in women. There was no gender difference when alcohol elimination was expressed per kilogram of liver. This finding would suggest that ethanol elimination per hepatocyte mass does not differ between the sexes. An alternative explanation has been developed from studies in rats, using the intragastric ethanol feeding model (Kono, Wheeler et al., 2000; Iimuro, Frankenberg et al., 1997). Female rats were more susceptible to liver injury than male rats, and this was ascribed to gender differences in endotoxin-induced Kupffer cell activation in alcoholic liver injury.

Chronic Viral Hepatitis: Alcohol abuse is widely recognized as a factor associated with advanced liver fibrosis in patients with chronic viral hepatitis, particularly hepatitis C (also see the discussion of hepatitis C, following). Hepatitis C is more common in alcoholics than in the general community (Rosman, Paronetto et al., 1993), an observation attributed to increased prevalence of injection drug use.

A similar but less marked interaction has been ascribed to chronic hepatitis B infection in alcoholics (Sherlock & James, 1997), but this interaction is not supported by all studies (Fong, Govindarajan et al., 1988). One possible explanation for this controversy is that the older hepatitis B studies antedated recognition of hepatitis C virus and thus may have been confounded by unrecognized co-infection with hepatitis C (Younossi, 1998).

Genetic Factors: A classic twin study showed that the concordance rate for ALD is three-fold higher in monozygotic twins than in dizygotic twins (Hrubec & Omenn, 1981), suggesting that genetic factors contribute to the risk of liver disease among those who abuse alcohol. Subsequent studies have attempted to define the genes involved. Such information would clarify the pathogenesis of the disease and allow early identification of those at high risk. These studies have examined classic genetic markers (such as blood groups and HLA antigens) and genes relevant to the disease process (such as alcohol metabolizing enzymes, collagen and, more recently, cytokines). The methods of genomics have not yet been applied to the question of ALD susceptibility; they probably will provide important insights, but at high cost.

Studies of HLA antigens and collagen gene RFLPs have not found consistent associations (Lumeng & Crabb, 1994). Alcohol dehydrogenase genotypes (coding for highly active isoenzyme) and aldehyde dehydrogenase (coding for a less active isoenzyme) have been associated with ALD. These polymorphisms can lead to accumulation of acetaldehyde following alcohol consumption. The findings have not been reproduced in other centers, and their significance remains unclear. The c2 promoter polymorphism of CYP2E1 has been linked to ALD, with an odds ratio of 2.4. This allele is uncommon in Caucasians and can only explain a minority of cases (Day, 2000). Mutations of the *HFE* gene are not associated with ALD. Polymorphisms in tumor necrosis alpha (TNF-alpha) and interleukin-10 (IL-10) recently have linked to ALD. These findings remain unconfirmed but may support the role of genetic factors and these cytokines in ALD.

Obesity: The prevalence of obesity is continuing to rise, with the disorder now affecting almost 20% of adult Americans (Mokdad, Serdula et al., 2000). Liver disease is one of its manifestations, and nonalcoholic steatohepatitis (NASH) is now recognized as a common and potentially progressive liver disease. NASH resembles ALD with respect to the pathologic appearance of liver tissue and certain mechanisms of injury (Tilg & Diehl, 2000). Experimental and clinical evidence exists of an alcohol-obesity interaction in the liver. Alcohol-fed rats develop more severe liver disease if given a high-fat diet (Tsukamoto, Towner et al., 1986). Alcoholics with a high body mass index for at least 10 years are at increased risk of liver disease (Naveau, Giraud et al., 1997). The effect of weight reduction on ALD has not been documented, but continuing NASH can explain failure to normalize liver tests in patients who attain abstinence from alcohol.

Other Hepatotoxins: Chronic alcohol consumption is associated with a range of drug interactions that can alter drug effects or increase the risk of liver injury. Chronic ethanol consumption increases the hepatotoxicity of a number of compounds, including acetaminophen (Tylenol®), industrial solvents, anesthetic gases, isoniazid (Laniazid®), phenylbutazone, and illicit drugs (such as cocaine). The induction of cytochrome P450 2E1 (CYP2E1) explains the increased vulnerability of the heavy drinker to several of these substances. CYP2E1 oxidizes ethanol and is induced by chronic alcohol consumption. CYP2E1 has an extraordinary capacity to activate many xenobiotics to highly toxic metabolites.

Among alcoholic patients, hepatic injury associated with acetaminophen has been described after repetitive intake for headaches (including those associated with withdrawal symptoms), dental pain, or the pain of pancreatitis. Amounts well within the accepted rate for the general community (that is, 2.5 to 4 g) have been incriminated as the cause of hepatic injury in alcoholic patients (Black, 1984; Seeff, Cuccherini et al., 1986). It is likely that the increased hepatotoxicity of acetaminophen after chronic ethanol consumption is caused, at least in part, by enhanced microsomal production of reactive metabolite(s) of acetaminophen. Consistent with this view is the observation that, in animals fed ethanol chronically, the potentiation of acetaminophen hepatotoxicity occurs after ethanol withdrawal (Sato, Matsuda et al., 1981) at the time production of the toxic metabolite can be at its peak, because at that time competition by ethanol for a common microsomal pathway has been withdrawn. Thus, maximal vulnerability to the toxicity of acetaminophen occurs immediately after cessation of drinking, when there is the greatest need for analgesia because of the headaches and other symptoms associated with withdrawal. This situation also explains the synergistic effect among acetaminophen, ethanol, and fasting (Israel, Speisky et al., 1992; Whitcomb & Block, 1994), because all three deplete reduced glutathione, thereby contributing to the toxicity of each compound because glutathione provides a fundamental cellular mechanism for the scavenging of toxic free radicals. Moreover, CYP2E1 promotes the generation of active oxygen species that are toxic in their own right and that can overwhelm the antioxidant system of the liver and other tissues, with striking consequences. A similar effect can be produced by the free hydroxy-ethyl radical generated from ethanol by CYP2E1.

Nutrition: For many years, alcohol was not thought to be hepatotoxic *per se*, and ALD was thought to be the result of poor nutrition. Nutritional impairment is universally present in patients with ALD and correlates with the severity of the disease. In addition, nutritional supplementation can play a therapeutic role in established cases. However, Lieber and colleagues (Lieber & DeCarli, 1974; Lieber, DeCarli et al., 1975) have clearly shown in the baboon model that experimental alcohol administration can lead to progressive liver injury, including cirrhosis, in the presence of an otherwise nutritionally adequate diet (Lieber & DeCarli,

1974; Lieber, DeCarli et al., 1975). Short-term administration of ethanol produces fatty liver with striking ultrastructural lesions (Lane & Lieber, 1966) in both rats and humans, an effect that is accelerated by co-administration of a high-fat diet.

Nutritional disorders can accelerate progression of ALD. Protein deficiency is a recognized cause of fatty liver because of impaired apoprotein synthesis required to export lipid from hepatocytes. Choline deficiency is associated with hepatic fibrosis. Vitamin A excess also leads to hepatic fibrosis. Alcohol abuse is associated with low serum levels of vitamin A and, if supplements are inappropriately given, vitamin A toxicity can result, even with normal serum levels (Lieber & Leo, 1992).

Clinical Features. Symptoms and signs are not reliable indicators of the presence or severity of ALD. No symptoms may be present even in the presence of cirrhosis. This paucity of symptoms may facilitate denial of an alcohol problem until end-stage complications occur. However, in some cases, florid clinical features do allow a confident clinical diagnosis.

ALD comprises three clinicopathologic entities that frequently coexist: alcoholic fatty liver, alcoholic hepatitis, and alcoholic cirrhosis. Alcoholic fatty liver can be observed after several days of heavy drinking or in long-term drinkers and manifests as anorexia, nausea, and right upper-quadrant discomfort. The liver is enlarged, firm, and may be tender. Typically, no other signs are present.

Alcoholic hepatitis classically is defined by symptoms and signs of hepatitis in association with alcohol abuse. Mild cases are common. Severe alcoholic hepatitis is rare and carries a short-term mortality of approximately 50% (Carithers, Herlong et al., 1989). Symptoms and signs include anorexia, nausea and abdominal pain, impaired liver function with jaundice, bruising, and encephalopathy. Ascites can be present. Systemic disturbances include fever and neutrophilic leukocytosis. Symptoms and signs of alcoholic cirrhosis are nausea or weight loss, as well as complications such as portal hypertension leading to variceal bleeding and/or ascites, liver failure, and hepatocellular carcinoma (HCC).

Alcoholic cirrhosis is a recognized risk factor for HCC, but the association between alcohol abuse and HCC in the absence of cirrhosis is not clear (Bassendine, 1986).

Diagnosis of ALD. Many cases of ALD are detected only by the results of liver tests. Liver tests are a sensitive marker for ALD, but similar findings can be observed in NASH and in patients treated with medications such as anticonvulsants. The gamma-glutamyl transpeptidase level almost always is elevated (Moussavian, Becker et al., 1985), often exceeding 1000 U/L. The transaminases are only moderately elevated. Levels above 500 U/L suggest an additional disorder, such as acetaminophen ingestion, viral hepatitis, or liver ischemia.

In most cases, the aspartate aminotransferase (AST) exceeds the alanine aminotransferase (ALT) level. Possible explanations are that AST is a mitochondrial enzyme and that alcoholic injury selectively injures mitochondria. In addition, AST is found in other tissues subject to alcohol injury, including skeletal muscle and heart. If the ALT exceeds the AST, consideration should be given to chronic hepatitis C, acetaminophen ingestion, or other causes of hepatocellular injury. Neutrophilia is found in severe cases, but may reflect concomitant sepsis.

The diagnosis of ALD rests on a history of prolonged alcohol abuse in the presence of a compatible clinical and laboratory picture. Other contributing factors, which should be routinely considered, are ingestion of hepatotoxic drugs (including herbal preparations and acetaminophen), diabetes mellitus, hepatitis B and C infection, and iron overload. Additional investigations are restricted to atypical cases or those that fail to resolve with abstinence from alcohol. Other explanations for liver disease, including autoimmune hepatitis, Wilson disease, alpha-1-antitrypsin deficiency, and cholestatic liver disease (including primary biliary cirrhosis) may need to be considered in specific cases.

The severity of alcoholic hepatitis can be assessed by using several objective rating scales (Schiff, 1993). The Maddrey Discriminant Function (MDF) is the most widely used, as it is the simplest and functions as well as the others (Table 2).

Role of Liver Biopsy. Insufficient evidence exists to offer clear guidelines for the use of liver biopsy in ALD (Poynard, Ratziu et al., 2000). In the past, liver biopsy has been recommended for all cases of ALD (Steindl & Ferenci, 1998), based on a reported error rate of 20% for noninvasive evaluation (Levin, Baker et al., 1979). However, the older studies antedate identification of the hepatitis C virus (HCV), and more recent case series report few diagnostic errors using noninvasive procedures (Talley, Roth et al., 1988; (Van Ness & Diehl, 1989). In most cases, the risks of liver biopsy (morbidity 0.5% and mortality 0.01% [Spinzi, Terruzzi et al., 2001]) can outweigh the limited benefit. Outside research settings, liver biopsies now are reserved

---

TABLE 2.   Maddrey Discriminant Function (MDF) Scale

Purpose: to assess short-term prognosis of patients with alcoholic hepatitis.

Clinical data required:

1. Serum bilirubin (mg/dL). Convert results expressed in μmol/L to mg/dL by dividing by 17.1.

2. Subject and control prothrombin time (PT) (seconds).

$$MDF = 4.6 \times (PT_{patient} - PT_{control}) + Bilirubin$$

For example: PT 16_s, control PT 12_s, Bili 250 μmol/L yield MDF of 33.

Scores above 32 indicate high risk of in-hospital mortality.

---

for atypical cases in which the history of alcohol consumption is unclear or other liver diseases (such as hepatitis C) coexist. In life-threatening cases in which urgent liver transplantation is being considered, vitamin K or fresh frozen plasma may be required to reverse coagulopathy to accomplish biopsies. Transjugular biopsy is validated as a safe procedure in coagulopathic patients to obtain sufficient tissue for diagnosis (McAfee, Keeffe et al., 1992), but the procedure is not widely available.

By documenting the severity of liver disease, biopsy might serve to impress the seriousness of the liver disease on the patient and motivate him or her to reduce alcohol consumption. No evidence to support the effectiveness of this notion has been reported, but it may be considered on occasion.

Treatment of ALD. The treatment of ALD rests on avoidance of further alcohol consumption (Alexander, Lischner et al., 1971). Other interventions are reserved for those with particularly severe disease or who are unable to maintain abstinence. The improvement with abstinence is so consistent that the gamma-glutamyl transpeptidase falls within an apparent half-life of 26 days (Orrego, Blake et al., 1985). Its failure to do so suggests continuing alcohol consumption or, occasionally, a coexisting disorder such as obesity-related liver disease or drug toxicity.

Advanced cirrhosis does not resolve with abstinence, as it is an irreversible lesion, but the activity is reduced and many very ill patients make striking improvements, often returning to compensated cirrhosis.

The first issue is to define what level of alcohol consumption to recommend for the patient with liver disease. Those with alcohol dependence or severe liver disease should be given clear advice to maintain long-term abstinence. However, many patients have only minor abnormalities in liver function tests without clinical evidence of cirrhosis. In such cases, a typical recommendation is a 6-week period of abstinence, followed by repeat liver tests. If the tests normalize and the patient wishes to resume drinking, consumption within recommended levels can be guided by the results of further liver tests. Continuing followup in a primary care setting is important, as the major causes of death in mild ALD are nonhepatic problems such as suicide.

Another problem for the internist is that many patients with alcohol-induced disorders decline referral to a specialty alcohol treatment service. Internists and primary care physicians can readily develop the skills to perform motivational interviewing with such patients.

Another issue is the safety of acamprosate and naltrexone (ReVia®) in patients with significant liver disease. Acamprosate does not accumulate even in severe liver disease, as the drug is excreted unchanged in the urine and is not metabolized. According to the manufacturers, acamprosate is contraindicated in severe decompensated (Childs C) liver disease but, even in that setting, the risks of treatment should be balanced against the risks of continuing alcohol consumption, and there are no published reports of an adverse effect on liver function. Naltrexone is associated with dose-dependent hepatotoxicity (typically at doses of 300 mg/day), but reactions are most unusual at the standard dose of 50 mg/day. In two studies, liver function tests improved in alcoholics, with no cases of clinically evident hepatotoxicity, indicating that naltrexone's therapeutic effect in reducing alcohol consumption exceeded its potential hepatotoxic effect (Brahen, Capone et al., 1988; Croop, Faulkner et al., 1997). Nonetheless, because of these concerns, there is little experience with naltrexone in patients with advanced ALD.

Nalmefene (Revex®) is a second-generation, orally active opiate receptor antagonist that is reported to have efficacy similar to naltrexone in the treatment of alcohol dependence (Mason, Salvato et al., 1999) without reported hepatotoxicity, but the drug is not currently available for unrestricted use.

In cases in which the liver disease is particularly severe or does not resolve with abstinence, several therapeutic options may be considered, even though they have not yet found a definite place in therapy. Propylthiouracil (Orrego, Kalant et al., 1979; Orrego, Blake et al., 1987), colchicine (Kershenobich, Vargas et al., 1988), and oxandrolone (Mendenhall, Anderson et al., 1984) have been evaluated for the treatment of ALD, but subsequent studies failed to reproduce the beneficial results reported in early studies. Some agents that can be viewed as "supernutrients" were found to be effective in nonhuman primates. These include S-adenosylmethionine for the treatment of early aspects of alcohol-induced liver injury (Lieber, Casini et al., 1990) and polyunsaturated lecithin for the prevention of fibrosis (Lieber, DeCarli et al., 1990; Lieber, Robins et al., 1994). Some data are now available that both agents are effective in humans. S-adenosylmethionine treatment led to a significantly lower mortality in patients with Childs class B cirrhosis (Mato, Camara et al., 1999). Preliminary results indicate that two years' treatment with polyenylphosphatidylcholine significantly improved the stage of liver fibrosis among alcoholics with noncirrhotic liver fibrosis (also see Chapter 12 in this section).

Selected cases of alcoholic hepatitis may respond to corticosteroids, but this treatment remains controversial despite a number of controlled trials. Prednisolone (40 mg/day for 28 days) was shown to improve survival of patients with spontaneous hepatic encephalopathy or a high MDF (>32; Table 2) (Carithers, Herlong et al., 1989). Widespread use of corticosteroids is limited because they can exacerbate sepsis, a common complication of severe liver disease. Pentoxifylline (400 mg three times a day) has been reported to reduce the mortality of alcoholic hepatitis (Akriviadis, Botla et al., 2000). Pentoxifylline acts by inhibition of tumor necrosis factor alpha and possibly by improving hepatic perfusion. Replication of this finding by other centers is awaited. Interleukin 10 is an anti-inflammatory cytokine. Preliminary evidence shows that interleukin 10 can be effective in severe alcoholic hepatitis (MDF >32), but the drug is not available for general use (Taieb, Chollet-Martin et al., 2000). Tumor necrosis alpha antibodies (Infliximab®) are under active investigation.

The management of the complications of cirrhosis, such as ascites and bleeding, lie outside the scope of this chapter. Patients with signs of hepatocellular insufficiency or portal hypertension should be evaluated by a gastroenterologist or hepatologist. Ascites is treated by bed rest, salt restriction with spironolactone (Aldactone®), and, if necessary, furosemide (Lasix®). Paracentesis is effective for diuretic-resistant cases. Severe cases may respond to transjugular intrahepatic portasystemic shunting or surgical shunts. Variceal hemorrhage is treated by transfusion, correction of coagulopathy, nitrate or octreotide infusions, and endoscopic banding. Spontaneous peritonitis is treated by intravenous antibiotics and prophylactic norfloxacin, if available, until ascites has resolved.

Hepatic encephalopathy can be alleviated by correcting the precipitating factors and decreasing colonic production and absorption of NH_3 with lactulose, a nonabsorbable disaccharide that acidifies the colon content through fermentation. Dietary protein should be adjusted to avoid both deficiency and excess. A suggestion was made many years ago that *Helicobacter pylori* infection might contribute to hepatic encephalopathy because of its high urease activity, which promotes the conversion of urea to ammonia, one of the precipitating factors of hepatic precoma and coma (Lieber & Lefevre, 1957, 1959).

Liver Transplantation: Liver transplantation now is an accepted treatment option for individuals with advanced liver disease who have stopped drinking (Kumar, Stauber et al., 1990), but only 5% of patients with end-stage ALD receive transplants. The procedure has been controversial because of ethical concerns about allocation of precious donor livers to individuals with a self-induced disease, concerns about the chance of a successful outcome in this cohort after transplantation, and concerns about resumption of drinking after a successful transplantation. It is unreasonably simplistic to regard ALD as just a "self-induced disorder." External factors such as family, peers, and society as a whole encourage the availability and use of alcohol. Genetic factors also contribute to the risk of alcohol abuse, and alcohol dependence now is considered a chronic relapsing brain disease (Leshner, 1997).

The five-year survival after transplantation for ALD is comparable to that of nonalcoholics in series from the U.S., Europe, and Australia (Wiesner, Lombardero et al., 1997; Haber, Koorey et al., 1999). Although alcoholics may be at higher risk of some post-transplantation problems, the rate of rejection may be lower than for non-ALD (Van Thiel, Bonet et al., 1995). Resumption of alcohol consumption remains the major concern and occurs in approximately one third of survivors. Of those who return to drinking, a third develop life-threatening alcohol-related morbidity such as pancreatitis, recurrent ALD, and noncompliance with immunosuppression resulting in graft rejection (Neuberger & Tang, 1997). These outcomes are comparable to the post-transplantation recurrence rate of other liver diseases. The low rate of recurrent alcohol consumption is better than that observed after other treatments for alcohol dependence and may be due to careful case selection for transplantation or to the patient's appreciation of the intensity of treatment by the transplantation team. Vaillant (1997) showed that the prognostic factors that generally predict a favorable outcome for alcoholism treatment are provided by the liver transplantation process.

The ideal candidate for transplantation accepts the etiologic role of alcohol in his or her liver disease, has stopped drinking, and has strong family supports (with a stable home, employment, and enthusiasm to resume interests). Other serious medical and psychiatric disorders should be excluded. Psychosocial evaluation seeks to stratify patients by their risk of relapse to alcoholism. The Michigan Alcoholism Prognosis Scale developed by Lucey et al. (1992) is useful in practice. However, this scale did not predict postoperative drinking (Lucey, Carr et al., 1997), possibly because only those with high scores are transplanted. A simpler approach requires six months' abstinence before transplantation. The six-month rule has been adopted by most transplantation centers in the U.S. (Everhart & Beresford, 1997). However, a recent literature review confirmed that six months of pre-transplantation abstinence (when patients are very ill) does not predict posttransplan-

tation relapse, and ethical concerns about this practice have been raised (Weinrieb, Van Horn et al., 2000). Lucey and colleagues recommend careful individualized assessment.

VIRAL HEPATITIS

The increase in rates of hepatitis infection has become a major public health concern (Table 3).

Hepatitis A. Hepatitis A is an RNA virus that is transmitted by fecal-oral contamination. In underdeveloped countries, almost all children develop immunoglobulin G (IgG) antibodies by the age of 10, and acute infection leads to a mild or even clinically inapparent hepatitis. With improving hygiene, the seroprevalence has fallen so that adults are now likely to be susceptible to hepatitis A. The disease becomes increasingly severe with advancing age, so that hepatitis A is less common but often more severe than in the past. The illness does not persist as a chronic infection.

Parenteral infection is rare because of the short period of viremia, but it has been described (Hollinger, Khan et al., 1983).

The prevalence of hepatitis A IgG antibodies is high among injection drug users (IDUs) and prison inmates in California (Tennant & Moll, 1995) and Australia (Crofts, Cooper et al., 1997). Because hepatitis A correlated more closely with institutionalization than with sharing of injection equipment, vaccination of seronegative prison entrants has been suggested.

Prevention measures include hygiene precautions to prevent fecal-oral contamination, providing passive immunoglobulin to household contacts of cases and active immunization to those at risk. Hepatitis vaccine, which is given as two intramuscular injections, is safe and effective. Accepted indications for vaccination include those at occupational risk, travelers, men who have sex with men, and persons with chronic liver disease. Vaccination has been recommended for IDUs (Iwarson, 1998) but difficulties in case-finding and the high cost of vaccine limit the usefulness of this strategy (Shapiro, Coleman et al., 1992).

Hepatitis B. Hepatitis B virus (HBV) is the most widely transmitted chronic viral infection in humans. It is readily transmitted among IDUs. Serologic evidence of past hepatitis B infection increases in prevalence with the duration of injection drug use, which now is the most common association of hepatitis B infection acquired in adults (Lamagni, Davison et al., 1999). Other risk groups include persons who have more than one sexual partner (heterosexual and sexual contact between men), certain ethnic groups (for

TABLE 3. Interpretation of Serologic Markers for Viral Hepatitis

Marker	Interpretation	Comments
Hepatitis A		
IgG	Past infection	Persists for life
IgM	Recent infection	Generally indicates acute hepatitis, but can persist after recovery for 18 months
Hepatitis B		
Hepatitis B surface antigen (HBsAg)	Current infection	Positive in both acute and chronic hepatitis B Marker of infectivity
Antibody to hepatitis B surface Antigen (HBsAb; anti-HBs)	Immunity (either after infection or vaccination)	Antibody titers > 10 IU/L correlate with protection

Antibody to hepatitis B core (HBcAB; anti-HBc)	IgG: past exposure to HBV
	
	IgM:
	  high titer, acute hepatitis B
	  low titer, active chronic hepatitis B
		Anti-HBc + anti-HBs = past infection with recovery
		Anti-HBc + HBsAg = chronic HBV infection
		
		Distinguishes acute from chronic HBV
		In chronic HBV, low-level titer correlates with ALT level and immune response (some laboratories report all low titer antibodies as negative)

Hepatitis B e antigen (HBeAg)	Acute hepatitis B Chronic active hepatitis B	Marker of infectivity in variety of settings Correlates with HBV-DNA
Hepatitis B viral DNA (HBV-DNA)	Infectivity; active viral replication	Detection by PCR is most sensitive marker of HBV infection HBV-DNA without HBeAg indicates infection with mutant HBV Levels useful to monitor antiviral therapy
Antibody to hepatitis B e antigen (HBeAb; anti-HBe)	Convalescence after acute HBV Marker of relatively low infectivity	Positive result in subject without any risk factor for HCV is more likely to be a false-positive test (confirm this by negative PCR or RIBA)
Hepatitis C		
Hepatitis C antibody	Positive: indicates exposure to HCV Negative: does not exclude infection if transmission within 3 months; in rare cases HCV infections occur without antibody response	Positive HCV antibody does not distinguish past infection from current infection Transplacental passage of HCV antibody makes antibody test unreliable marker of infantile infection for 18 months
Hepatitis C virus RNA	Positive: confirms antibody result indicating HCV infection	
Hepatitis C viral load	High: >2 × 10^6 copies/mL	High viral load associated with poorer response to therapy
Hepatitis C genotype	1-7	Type 1 associated with poorer response to therapy
Hepatitis D (Delta)	Defective virus that requires HBsAg to be viable	
HDV-IgG	Indicates past and/or present infection	
HDV-IgM	Indicates recent or chronic infection	
HDV-RNA	Indicates current viremia	

Ig = immunoglobulin; HBV = hepatitis B virus; ALT = alanine aminotransferase; HCV = hepatitis C virus; PCR = polymerase chain reaction [sensitive molecular diagnostic procedure that can detect minute amounts of specific DNA or RNA], RIBA.

example, persons from Asia, Southern Europe, and Mediterranean countries), children of infected parents, and health care workers. The incubation period is six weeks to six months.

Acute hepatitis B may be preceded by a transient serum-sickness prodrome, with polyarthralgia, fever, malaise, urticaria, and proteinuria (Sherlock & Dooley, 1997). The acute illness is characterized by anorexia, nausea, and (sometimes) vomiting, with malaise, jaundice, pale stools, and dark urine. The infection often is subclinical. Hepatitis B persists as chronic hepatitis B infection in about 5% of adults, much less often than does hepatitis C (see the discussion, following). Acute and chronic hepatitis B are diagnosed by serologic tests (Table 2). Individuals who remain positive for hepatitis B surface antigen (HBsAg) for six months or more are designated "chronic hepatitis B." Chronic hepatitis B is associated with chronic hepatitis, cirrhosis, and HCC in a significant minority of those infected.

Progression of hepatitis B has been associated with heavy alcohol consumption (as described earlier); co-infection with HIV, HCV, and hepatitis D virus; pre-core and other mutant viruses; male homosexual behavior; ethnic group; and duration of infection. Liver injury results from cell-mediated response to infected hepatocytes. In chronic disease, a series of hepatitis flares can precede viral clearance and recovery. These flares vary in severity from subclinical to life-threatening. Patients with chronic HBV should be assessed for the replication status of the virus and the presence of active liver disease. Patients with persistently abnormal ALT levels or clinical evidence of liver disease should be referred for consideration of antiviral therapy. Patients with chronic hepatitis B viral infection can be offered quarterly screening for HCC, particularly if they are cirrhotic.

Treatment of hepatitis B with interferon alpha (IFN-alpha) has been promising, with a high success rate in clearing the virus and decreasing hepatic inflammation (Korenman, Baker et al., 1991) and with demonstrated cost effectiveness (Dusheiko & Roberts, 1995). IFN-alpha can induce hepatitis B e antigen (HBeAg) seroconversion in 30% to 40% of selected patients after a four- to six-month course of therapy, compared with spontaneous seroconversion rates of 15% in controls. These patients become anti-HBe positive. Some eventually lose HBsAg, and only a very small proportion ultimately relapse. Loss of HBeAg has been associated with improvements in liver histology and clinical outcome. Side effects related to IFN-alpha are common (see the discussion of hepatitis C, following).

The best response to IFN-alpha is seen in Caucasian patients who have had the disease for a short time and who have biochemical hepatitis and a low viral load (low HBV-DNA titers). IFN-alpha should be used with extreme caution in patients with HBV-related cirrhosis, as it can induce a flare of hepatitis and lead to hepatic decompensation. Such patients should be assessed for liver transplantation.

Lamivudine (3-TC) is a cytosine nucleoside analogue with potent inhibitory activity against HBV as well as HIV. Lamivudine is well tolerated and induces rapid and dramatic reductions in serum HBV-DNA. Treatment with oral lamivudine 100 mg per day for one year has resulted in HBeAg seroconversion in 30% of patients, with a significant reduction in hepatic necro-inflammatory activity and progression of fibrosis (Dienstag, Schiff et al., 1999). Therapy is continued until HBeAg seroconversion occurs. One of the major problems with lamivudine is viral resistance, associated with the YMDD mutation in the virus, which occurs in up to 25% of patients by one year and up to 50% of patients by two years. Patients can develop a flare of hepatitis that leads to hepatic decompensation.

It is important to continue lamivudine therapy despite the emergence of a resistant variant. Adefovir is a novel antiviral that appears to be effective even in patients with lamivudine resistance, but its use can lead to renal impairment (Perrillo, Schiff et al., 2000). Future treatment for chronic hepatitis B is likely to involve combinations of antiviral drugs to limit resistance and toxicity (Farrell, 2000). Hepatitis B may require transplantation in advanced cases. Outcomes were limited by recurrence, but this can be controlled with hepatitis B immunoglobin.

Hepatitis C. Hepatitis C virus (HCV) is recognized by health authorities as a major public health problem worldwide (NIH, 1997). It is the most frequently reported notifiable infection in adults, with approximately 3.9 million persons infected in the U.S. (Alter, 1997). HCV already is the leading indication for liver transplantation, but it is projected that the number of persons with advanced liver disease and associated HCV will double by 2010.

Virology: HCV is an RNA virus and was cloned in 1989. It has a single open reading frame that generates a large viral polyprotein. Viral polymerases ligate this polyprotein into the viral proteins. HCV cannot be cultured *in vitro*, but acute infection can be studied in chimpanzees. Antibodies in the blood reliably indicate infection but are not protective.

There are seven genotypes of the virus. Genotypes are further divided into subtypes (a, b, and c). The most common genotypes in the U.S. are types 1 and 3. Re-infection after clearance and co-infection with more than one genotype can occur if the patient is re-exposed to the virus. Patients with genotypes 2 or 3 respond better to current antiviral therapies than do those with other genotypes.

The virus alters its genetic structure over time by mutation, leading to the presence of multiple species of virus with similar genetic sequence (quasi-species). This process is thought to allow HCV to evade immune clearance, leading to chronic infection. The continual alteration in genetic structure makes the development of a preventive vaccine difficult.

Transmission: HCV is transmitted by blood-to-blood contact. In the U.S., Europe, and Australia, the most common risk factor for transmission of hepatitis C infection is injection drug use, which now accounts for the bulk of incident cases (91%) in Australia (Kaldor, Archer et al., 1992). HCV prevalence is strongly associated with duration of injecting, with an incidence of approximately 20% for each year of injection drug use (van Beek, Dwyer et al., 1998). Most regular IDUs are infected with HCV. Measures to limit the spread of this infection appear to be having only a modest effect (Alter & Seeff, 2000; MacDonald, Wodak et al., 2000). The continuing high incidence appears to be related to the continuing high prevalence of sharing injecting equipment, including mixing spoons, filters, swabs, or tourniquets (although even the hands may be infected).

The continuing epidemic of hepatitis C among IDUs has given rise to calls for wider implementation of infection control procedures such as needle/syringe replacement programs. Indeed, distribution of replacement needles is associated with falling HCV transmission in some settings (MacDonald, Wodak et al., 2000; Goldberg, Burns et al., 2001), but not all (Hagan, McGough et al., 1999). The negative findings can be attributed to a study design with low sensitivity (small number of incident infections or contamination of study groups). Nevertheless, needle/syringe replacement programs remain controversial, particularly among the general community.

Rates of sexual transmission of hepatitis C are thought to be very low. An Italian study of the male partners of women infected with contaminated anti-D immunoglobin showed no evidence of transmission over a combined followup period of 862 years (Sachithanandan & Fielding, 1997). Similar results were found in two other studies (Meisel, Reip et al., 1995; Bresters, Mauser-Bunschoten et al., 1993). By contrast, an analysis by Alter and colleagues (1999) of the NHANES III database found that high-risk sexual behavior was a significant risk factor for hepatitis C in the U.S. This conclusion has been described as unfortunate (Murphy, Bryzman et al., 1999) because injection drug use, the major risk factor for hepatitis C infection, was not included in NHANES III. Therefore, the effect of other factors, such as sexual behavior, could have been confounded by injection drug use (Dore, Law et al., 1999). Murphy and colleagues (2000) subsequently confirmed that the increased risk of hepatitis C associated with high-risk sexual practices disappeared after adjusting for injection drug use.

The risk of hepatitis C infection in recipients of blood and blood products before 1990 was related to the volume of blood products transfused. Most of the severe hemophiliacs became infected. After screening of blood products for hepatitis C antibody was introduced, the number of persons with post-transfusional non-A, non-B hepatitis declined markedly. The risk of hepatitis C infection after blood transfusion in Australia recently was estimated at 1 in 250,000 units transfused (Whyte & Savoia, 1997). Transmission from contaminated anti-rhesus D immunoglobulin has been retrospectively reported in Ireland and other European countries, many years after its administration (Power, Lawlor et al., 1995).

The risk of occupational transmission of hepatitis C is greatest in health care workers and laboratory staff who handle blood and blood products. Estimates for the risk of transmission from a needlestick injury range from 0% to 10% (Dore, Kaldor et al., 1997). Transmission of hepatitis C from a needlestick has not been reported where the source was hepatitis C RNA-negative. Nosocomial transmission of hepatitis C has been reported in a variety of hospital settings, including plasmapheresis units (Padron, Rodriguez et al., 1995), a hematology ward (Allander, Gruber et al., 1995), hemodialysis units (Dussol, Berthezene et al., 1995; Okuda, Hayashi et al., 1995), after colonoscopy (Bronowicki, Venard et al., 1997), and after cardiothoracic surgery.

Several studies have demonstrated an association between tattooing and hepatitis C infection. In an Australian study of blood donors, the independent relative risk associated with a history of tattooing was 27 (Kaldor, Archer et al., 1992). Although infection control guidelines for tattooists have been introduced in recent years, the possibility of hepatitis C transmission continues when these guidelines are not followed.

Hepatitis C in Special Populations: The prevalence of hepatitis C in prisoners is high, largely because of the high proportion of IDUs. In Australia, almost 40% of prison entrants are HCV antibody-positive—a rate that increases to 65% among prisoners who report a history of injection drug use (Crofts, Stewart et al., 1995; Butler, Dolan et al., 1997). Imprisonment has been reported to be associated with hepatitis C, even after adjusting for injection drug use (van Beek, Dwyer et al., 1998; Murphy, Bryzman et al., 2000). It has been suggested that other modes of transmission may be present in prisons through a combination of high background prevalence, poor hygiene, and frequent physical violence (Haber, Parsons et al., 1999). The incidence among uninfected prisoners is thought to be high.

Measures that can limit the spread of HCV often are not available to prison inmates, including methadone maintenance and needle/syringe replacement programs. Tattooing with unsterilized equipment also may play a role (Post, Dolan et al., 2001).

In Mediterranean, Eastern European, Asian, South American, and African countries, the prevalence of antibodies to hepatitis C is much higher than in the U.S. In Egypt, the prevalence rate for adults is 20%, making this a major community epidemic. The Egyptian hepatitis C epidemic is linked to reusing needles during mass inoculations of antischistosomal therapy (Frank, Mohamed et al., 2000).

Primary Infection: Primary infection with HCV typically is subclinical, but mild hepatitis can occur. Fulminant hepatitis is almost unknown. Peak viremia occurs in the pre-acute or early in the acute phase, and antibodies appear as early as four weeks (with an average of six to eight weeks), by using third-generation testing. Clinically evident hepatitis reflects a significant immune response to the virus and can be associated with a higher rate of viral clearance than subclinical infection. A small number of exposed seronegative individuals have evidence of T-cell immunity to HCV, indicating that the virus can be eliminated without detectable antibodies (Koziel, Wong et al., 1997). At present, the incidence of this phenomenon is unknown. A few small controlled trials support the use of IFN in the management of acute hepatitis C (Quinn & Johnston, 1997). Studies of combination therapy for acute hepatitis C are in progress.

Treatment cannot be routinely recommended for acute hepatitis C at this time, as the illness generally is mild, with a significant recovery rate, and current antiviral treatment is costly and carries significant morbidity.

Chronic Infection: As many as 75% of patients infected with hepatitis C go on to develop persistent chronic infection (Di Bisceglie, 2000). After an average of 20 years, approximately 8% of infected persons develop cirrhosis; this rate rises to 20% after 40 years. Progression to cirrhosis is associated with duration of disease, age older than 40 years at the time of infection, average alcohol consumption of more than 50 g/day, and co-infection with HBV and HIV. The route of transmission or viral factors such as genotype or viral titer do not appear to play a role (Poynard, Ratziu et al., 2001).

Symptoms of chronic hepatitis C without cirrhosis do not correlate well with disease activity or severity and tend to be nonspecific, mild, and intermittent. The most common is fatigue, with nausea, muscle aches, right upper-quadrant pain, and weight loss. These symptoms rarely are incapacitating, but they can have a detrimental effect on the infected individual's quality of life.

Diagnosis: The third-generation enzyme immunoassay for antibodies to hepatitis C is the most practical screening test for hepatitis C infection. However, this assay has a high rate of false-positives when used in populations with a low prevalence of hepatitis C, so screening of the general population is not recommended. The antibody tests do not differentiate between current and resolved infection, as the antibody typically takes more than 10 years to disappear after viral clearance.

A positive hepatitis C RNA test by polymerase chain reaction (PCR) indicates the presence of active infection, whereas a negative test in persons with risk factors and a positive antibody indicates probable clearance of HCV infection. HCV RNA analysis is particularly useful in assessing the status of HCV antibody-positive patients with *normal* liver function tests. Approximately 50% of these patients are PCR-negative. The test should be repeated at three to six months later; if it is again negative, the patient can be reassured that the virus has been cleared.

Almost all hepatitis C antibody-positive patients with *abnormal* liver function tests (LFTs) have detectable levels of hepatitis C RNA in their blood. Therefore, if a patient has abnormal LFTs (without another explanation), hepatitis C PCR is unlikely to be helpful. Patients with another explanation for abnormal LFTs, such as alcohol abuse, are exceptions to this principle.

Hepatitis C genotyping can be performed to aid decisionmaking about treatment (see the discussion, following). Genotyping can be used to analyze cases of hepatitis C transmission by identifying the same genotype in the source patient and the recipient. Quantitation of HCV RNA (or viral load) can be useful when considering antiviral therapy and transmission risk. Individuals with a very high viral load are less likely to benefit from therapy and can be more infectious than are those with a low viral load.

Management Issues: IDUs infected with hepatitis C can be marginalized, indigent, homeless and, frequently, the victims of discrimination. As a consequence, many lack access to health care (Stephenson, 2001). It is important to provide culturally appropriate written material that matches the educational level of the patient, as many cannot discuss their illness with others. To meet this need, specialized clinics have been established in needle/syringe replacement programs and in prisons. Such clinics provide diagnostic evaluation and build a therapeutic relationship to facilitate referral for liver biopsy and antiviral therapy, along with other addiction treatment. Primary care physicians or other health care workers can engage HCV-infected patients, and clinical guidelines can be useful in providing appropriate management.

A diagnosis of hepatitis C often engenders a high level of anxiety, which often is exacerbated by misinformation. Adequate time should be set aside for pretest counseling in private. The results of hepatitis C testing should be given in person. Posttest counseling issues include the natural history of the disease, the symptomatology, and privacy issues. Accurate, nonjudgmental language, combined with a sincere concern for the patient's welfare, helps to build trust. Patients are fearful of transmitting hepatitis C to their partners, household contacts, and children. They can be reassured that the risks are minimal, but testing should be offered. Full explanations about the advantages and limitations of antiviral therapy allow the patient to make an informed choice about treatment options.

Assessing the Severity of the Disease: Symptoms, including lethargy, do not correlate with the severity of liver disease. Spider naevi are commonly seen, but the physical signs are nonspecific unless advanced cirrhosis is present. Plasma ALT is the best laboratory indicator of active viral hepatitis, but the level commonly fluctuates and does not correlate well with the stage of liver disease. A normal ALT level does not exclude cirrhosis. Patients with normal ALT levels and those who decline treatment can be monitored in primary care settings by ALT levels two to three times per year and should be referred for treatment if the ALT level rises.

Liver Biopsy: In view of the limitations of noninvasive assessment, liver biopsy remains the standard for assessment of disease stage and prognosis. The biopsy appearances are ranked according to the stage (extent of fibrosis, ranging from normal to cirrhosis) and grade (activity of hepatitis) with the Scheuer or Ishak scoring systems. Significant fibrosis indicates a risk of progression to cirrhosis and is the major indication for antiviral therapy. The risk of a major complication after liver biopsy is in the order of 1 in 500 (Spinzi, Terruzzi et al., 2001). Biopsy is inappropriate in the presence of coagulopathy and thrombocytopenia because of increased risk of hemorrhage.

Hepatitis A and B Vaccination: When there is no evidence of immunity, vaccination is indicated to reduce the risk of further liver injury. Chronic co-infection with other hepatitis viruses is associated with accelerated progression to cirrhosis (Weltman, Brotodihardjo et al., 1995). Hepatitis B vaccination should be offered. Patients with hepatitis C respond well, but with lower titers than uninfected control subjects. An early report of high mortality from hepatitis A in patients with chronic HCV has not been replicated, but vaccination for hepatitis A is appropriate if available.

Alcohol: Alcohol abuse interacts adversely with chronic hepatitis C in several ways (Degos, 1999). A consensus now exists that daily consumption of more than 40 g of alcohol has an additive effect on liver inflammation and accelerates the progression of hepatic fibrosis. Alcohol abuse also is associated with increased viral load (Cromie, Jenkins et al., 1996), reduced response to therapy, increased risk of progression to HCC, and exacerbation of the skin lesions of porphyria cutanea tarda.

Evidence of adverse effects related to moderate levels of alcohol consumption by people with chronic hepatitis C is unclear. A 1997 conference sponsored by the National Institutes of Health recommended no more than 10 g per day for all persons with chronic hepatitis C and abstinence for those with significant disease and those contemplating antiviral therapy (Schiff, 1997). A more practical recommendation is to limit alcohol consumption to 20 g per day for those without chronic hepatitis, 10 g per day for those with chronic hepatitis, and none for those with advanced liver disease.

Dietary Guidelines: No published evidence is available to support any specific diet for persons with hepatitis C.

However, hepatic steatosis is a feature of hepatitis C, and obesity and type 2 diabetes mellitus are associated with hepatitis C and accelerated progression of fibrosis (Adinolfi, Gambardella et al., 2001; Clouston, Jonsson et al., 2001), and those conditions have been shown to benefit from dietary interventions. The benefits of such interventions to control hepatitis in selected subjects is under investigation.

Management of Risk Factors: The presence of HCV infection can increase motivation to participate in treatment, particularly if the patient is seeking antiviral therapy. Avoidance of injection drug use is the preferred option, but it may not be the choice of the patient. Evidence-based harm minimization and abstinence-based treatments should be offered, as described elsewhere in this volume.

Antiviral Treatment: The main indication for treatment is active hepatitis with abnormal biopsy showing fibrosis and elevated ALT levels. The main goal of antiviral therapy is sustained virologic response, defined by a continued normal ALT level and negative hepatitis C PCR on more than one occasion at least six months after completion of treatment. Individuals with sustained virologic response generally remain PCR-negative over the long term. Several studies have found significant improvements in general health and specific hepatitis C-related symptoms in patients who achieve a sustained response to antiviral therapy (Neary, Cort et al., 1999; Ware, Bayliss et al., 1999). In previously untreated patients, IFN-alpha alone leads to a sustained response of only 10%. Ribavirin (Virazole®) is a guanosine analogue that is absorbed orally and is well tolerated. The combination of IFN and ribavirin is now the standard treatment offered to those without contraindications (McHutchison, Gordon et al., 1998; Poynard, Marcellin et al., 1998). The duration of treatment varies from six months, for patients with genotype 2 or 3, to 12 months for those with genotypes 1, 4, 5, or 6. The response of those who relapse after IFN-alpha to combination IFN-alpha and ribavirin is even more impressive (Davis, Esteban-Mur et al., 1998). A modified form of IFN, peginterferon, has a polyethylene glycol side chain. An injection of peginterferon leads to sustained IFN levels for a week and results in higher response rates than unmodified IFN, without increased side effects (Heathcote, Shiffman et al., 2000; Zeuzem, Feinman et al., 2000). Preliminary results of combination peginterferon and ribavirin trials have been particularly impressive. Consensus IFN links the most common-occurring amino acid sequences at each position of available natural alpha IFNs into one "consensus" protein with a 10-fold higher *in vitro* biological activity compared with single recombinant IFN-alpha-2a or -2b.

Treatment of Special Groups: The progression of chronic hepatitis C is accelerated in patients who also are infected with HIV. Treatment of hepatitis C can be indicated in patients with early HIV infection and those stable on highly active antiretroviral therapy. However, consideration must be given to possible drug interactions and to additive blood abnormalities when treating such patients.

Patients with compensated cirrhosis can be treated (Heathcote, Shiffman et al., 2000). Some studies suggest that treatment reduces the risk of HCC and decompensation, but this evidence is subject to ongoing trials.

Patients who are hepatitis C RNA-positive and who have persistently normal aminotransferase levels generally have mild disease (Persico, Persico et al., 2000) and an uncertain response to treatment (Sangiovanni, Morales et al., 1998). At present, it is recommended that these patients not undergo treatment, but that they be followed up every four to six months, and treated if ALT becomes abnormal.

Compliance with treatment is likely to be poor in patients with active drug or alcohol dependence, and this can lead to exacerbation of hepatitis and drug resistance. The recommendation is against treating such individuals until the addictive disorder is stabilized (NIH, 1997). Two recent opinion papers have reconsidered these issues and agreed that treatment should be made available, on an individualized basis, to recent drug injectors who enter treatment for their addictive disorder and who are likely to comply with therapy (Davis & Rodrigue, 2001; Edlin, Seal et al., 2001). No evidence is available that methadone maintenance therapy impairs treatment response, and methadone is encouraged, when indicated, if hepatitis C treatment is contemplated (Novick, 2000). In the author's experience, the minority of patients who meet these criteria have completed treatment successfully.

Side Effects of Therapy: Flu-like symptoms occur within four to six hours of IFN injections, tend to subside within the first month of treatment, and respond to acetaminophen. More persistent side effects are fatigue, alteration in mood, sleep disturbance, moderate suppression of white cell count and platelet count, skin rash, reduction in appetite and weight, dryness of the mucous membranes, and hair loss. Dose reduction or cessation of treatment may be required. Major side effects include retinopathy, interstitial fibrosis of the lung, and thyroid disease.

The most common side effect of ribavirin is hemolytic anemia. Other side effects are pruritus, cough, and myalgia. In the presence of these symptoms, dose reduction often is required. Significant teratogenic effects have been associated with ribavirin. Both women of childbearing potential and men on treatment must use two forms of effective contraception during treatment and for six months thereafter (15 half-lives for clearance of ribavirin).

Patients on combination therapy experience more significant side effects than those treated with IFN monotherapy and require more psychological support. Support groups or individual counseling can help patients manage side effects and other consequences of their treatment, thereby reducing drop-out rates.

Contraindications for Treatment: Patients with decompensated cirrhosis, pregnancy, lactation, and active psychiatric illness and those who drink more than seven standard drinks a week are at higher risk of side effects and lower chance of response, and thus generally are not treated. Depression can worsen during therapy, and suicide has been reported. Careful psychiatric assessment and ongoing care may be required (Dieperink, Willenbring et al., 2000). Contraindications to ribavirin include end-stage renal failure because of drug accumulation, chronic anemias, a history of cardiovascular dysfunction, and inadequate contraception.

Other Treatments: A variety of drugs, including rimantadine (Flumadine®), ursodeoxycholic acid (Actigall®), nonsteroidal anti-inflammatory drugs, and venesection have been investigated alone or in combination with IFN-alpha agents. Virologic response rates have been unsatisfactory when these agents are used as monotherapies. However, combination regimens, including amantadine (Symadine®), warrant further investigation. Available studies do not support the use of alternative therapies such as Chinese herbs (Batey, Bensoussan et al., 1998).

Advanced Hepatitis C: Cirrhotic patients are at increased risk of HCC, and hepatitis C is among the most common underlying associations of HCC. Once hepatic decompensation occurs, the five-year survival falls to 50%, and transplantation should be considered rather than antiviral treatment.

Hepatocellular Carcinoma: Currently, it is recommended that patients with hepatitis cirrhosis undergo 6-month screening with upper abdominal ultrasound and serum alphafetoprotein. If abnormalities are found, more extensive evaluation should be undertaken in a specialist liver center. Small primary liver cancers can be resected or treated by local therapies. Cirrhotic patients with HCC are considered for transplantation if there are fewer than three tumor nodules smaller than 3 cm, or a single nodule less than 5 cm, with no extrahepatic spread or vascular invasion.

Liver Transplantation: Hepatitis C is now the leading indication for liver transplantation, and the numbers are expected to rise over the next decade. Patients with cirrhosis should be considered for transplantation if they develop major complications of their cirrhosis, indicating a life expectancy of one to two years without transplantation. The three-year survival rate is 84%, which is equivalent to survival in patients transplanted with other forms of liver disease (Levy, Chen et al., 1997). Before transplantation, patients should be informed of the high risk of hepatitis C recurrence and its potential consequences, including a 10% risk of cirrhosis at five years. Methadone maintenance no longer is considered a contraindication for transplantation (Lau, Schiano et al., 2000; Rothstein, Kanchana et al., 2000; Koch & Banys, 2001).

Hepatitis D. The delta agent is an RNA particle coated with HBsAg. The virus cannot replicate without co-infection with hepatitis B. Outbreaks of delta virus co-infection with hepatitis B have occurred among IDUs and resulted in high mortality rates (Levy, Chen et al., 1997). Control of hepatitis B by vaccination will limit the spread of hepatitis D virus. The diagnosis is by rising titers of IgG antibody or IgM antibody. Delta infection should be considered in any HBV-positive patient with relapse.

Delta hepatitis responds poorly to IFN unless high doses are given for long periods.

Hepatic Bacterial and Fungal Infections Associated With Injection Drug Use. A wide array of infections can occur in the IDU, and these can involve the liver (see Chapter 8 of this section).

COCAINE HEPATITIS

Hepatic injury appears to be uncommon in humans (Riordan, Skouteris et al., 1998). Most cases occur in association with other systemic features of cocaine toxicity, such as hyperthermia, rhabdomyolysis, hypoxia, and hypotension (Silva, Roth et al., 1991). In some other cases, other drugs—particularly alcohol—have been involved. In experimental animals, cocaine hepatotoxicity is readily demonstrated and is both time- and dose-dependent (Selim & Kaplowitz, 1999).

The clinical presentation is characterized by a marked increase in serum aminotransferase activity, beginning within a few hours of drug ingestion, associated with the systemic features of cocaine toxicity. Rhabdomyolysis can account for some of the increase in transaminases, as AST and ALT both are present in muscle. The liver biopsy shows coagulative hepatic necrosis, typically in a centrilobular distribution, extending to panlobular necrosis in extreme cases. Microvesicular and macrovesicular steatosis can be present, consistent with involvement of mitochondria in hepatic injury.

The mechanism of hepatic injury is thought to involve hepatic ischemia and/or toxic oxidative metabolites. Hepatic ischemia is a likely mechanism, as cocaine is a powerful vasoconstrictor, and this action accounts for many of the toxic effects of the drug, which are characterized by impaired systemic perfusion. Hepatotoxicity typically occurs in association with these effects. Evidence supporting a role for toxic oxidative metabolites comes from experimental animal models, in which hepatotoxicity has been demonstrated to result from the production of metabolites by hepatic metabolism. Usually, more than 90% of cocaine is hydrolyzed by plasma pseudocholinesterase (Mallat & Dhumeaux, 1991). The remainder is metabolized by cytochrome P450 isoenzymes, including CYP3A1. The hepatotoxic metabolite of cocaine has not been identified with certainty, but the oxidative metabolites of N-hydroxynorcocaine can generate reactive alkylating species.

The severity of liver toxicity is correlated with the extent of cocaine oxidation by hepatic cytochrome P450, which is increased by inducers of the cytochrome P450 system such as phenobarbital (Barbital®) and ethanol and reduced by P450 inhibitors such as cimetidine (Tagamet®). In the mouse, chronic cocaine administration induces P450 3A, which can increase the risk of hepatotoxicity (Henry, Jeffreys et al., 1992). Inhibition or deficiency of pseudocholinesterase increases hepatotoxicity by diverting the drug toward the P450 pathway, and induction of pseudocholinesterase can lessen toxicity.

Cocaine is commonly taken with alcohol, and hepatic carboxyesterase generates ethylcocaine (cocaethylene) (Hearn, Flynn et al., 1991). The same hepatic enzyme also contributes to the non-oxidative metabolism of ethanol to fatty acid ethyl esters (Heith, Morse et al., 1995). Ethylcocaine has similar pharmacologic effects to cocaine but a longer half-life. It can accumulate to higher levels in tissues than cocaine and can be more toxic than cocaine, as evidenced by a lower LD50 (Andrews, 1997). Nevertheless, a large clinical series found no increase in liver disease among alcoholics using cocaine as compared to those not using cocaine (Worner, 1994).

Pretreatment of experimental animals with cimetidine or cysteine protects against cocaine toxicity and provides additional evidence in support of the metabolic theory of toxicity, but pretreatment is not a clinically feasible approach to therapy in humans. No specific therapy has been shown to be effective.

MDMA ("ECSTASY")

An increasing number of cases of severe liver failure following use of MDMA (3,4-methylenedioxymethamphetamine, or "Ecstasy") are being reported (Riordan, Skouteris et al., 1998). A number of these cases have resulted in liver transplantation or fatalities (Brauer, Heidecke et al., 1997). Two clinical syndromes are emerging (Selim & Kaplowitz, 1999), one similar to cocaine hepatitis, which presents shortly after ingestion with systemic toxicity accompanied by severe liver injury, and the other, which presents days to weeks after ingestion with jaundice and pruritus and which can proceed to fulminant liver failure. The diagnosis of delayed presentations can be difficult unless specific inquiry about MDMA use is made.

Biochemically, marked hyperbilirubinemia is noted, with a disproportionate increase in AST as compared with ALT. The severity of hepatic dysfunction does not appear to be dose-related (Ellis, Wendon et al., 1996).

Severe liver injury is a rare event, whereas MDMA use is extremely common, suggesting that other factors can contribute to liver injury. The drug often is taken at "rave" parties where participants dance for hours, predisposing them to hyperthermia and volume depletion. Those who suffer from hepatic dysfunction with rhabdomyolysis and hyperpyrexia can have an abnormality of muscle metabolism similar to that seen in malignant hyperpyrexia syndrome. Other individuals may be susceptible on the basis of delayed drug elimination (Tucker, Lennard et al., 1994). The cytochrome P450 isoenzyme CYP2D6 metabolizes MDMA, and approximately 5% of the population have low activity mutations of this isoenzyme, with reduced hydroxylation of MDMA *in vitro* (Tucker, Lennard et al., 1994). Increased susceptibility to MDMA toxicity *in vivo* has been demonstrated in CYP2D6-deficient mice (Colado, Williams et al., 1995).

TABLE 4.   Risk Factors for Hepatitis C

High Risk
- Sharing contaminated drug injection equipment: 90% are infected after 10 years.
- Regular or large-volume transfusions of blood products before 1990: 85% to 90% of hemophiliacs are hepatitis C antibody-positive.
- Incarceration: because of the high prevalence of injection drug use among prisoners and possibly other high-risk events in prisons.

Moderate Risk
- Body piercing and tattooing: use of contaminated equipment.
- Mother to baby at birth: occurs in about 10% if the mother is RNA-positive.

Low Risk
- Small-volume blood transfusions before 1990.
- Sharing toothbrushes, razors, and other personal-care items.
- Health care workers: needlestick or sharps injury.
- Birth or medical procedures in a country with high prevalence rates of hepatitis C.

Very Low Risk
- Sexual activity: controversial, with few well-documented cases; presence of genital ulcerative sexually transmitted diseases and/or traumatic sexual practices can increase risk.
- Drug use with snorting straws.
- Blood transfusion/blood products after 1990.

No Evidence of Increased Risk
- Household and casual contact with individuals infected with hepatitis C.

An immunologic mode of liver injury has been proposed on the basis that rechallenge with MDMA has produced greater liver damage in the absence of hyperthermia, and liver biopsy features of one patient suggested an autoimmune hepatitis-like injury, which resolved spontaneously on withdrawal of the drug (Jones & Simpson, 1999). Insufficient clinical evidence is available to evaluate the relative importance of these proposed mechanisms in susceptibility to human disease.

The differential diagnosis of a patient with grossly elevated transaminases includes acute viral hepatitis, toxin ingestion, and ischemia. Unexplained liver test abnormalities particularly in young adults with hepatomegaly should prompt inquiry into illicit drug use and a urinary drug screen. A negative drug screen suggests nondrug causes of liver disease, but also can result from delayed presentation or consumption of Ecstasy tablets not containing MDMA, as

approximately one in three such tablets does not contain MDMA (Baggott, Heifets et al., 2000).

Meticulous supportive care should be employed, with vigorous rehydration and active cooling measures (Jones & Simpson, 1999). The benefit-risk ratio of orthotopic liver transplantation for fulminant hepatic failure remains in question, but there have been survivors of transplantation, and early discussion with a liver transplantation unit is advised.

TOXICITY FROM CO-INJECTED MATERIALS
Clinicians have speculated that other materials can contribute substantially to toxicity in individuals who inject illicit drugs, but this problem appears to be most uncommon.

Injection of drugs intended for oral ingestion can lead to accumulation of talc in a dose-dependent fashion at several sites, particularly the lung and liver (Riordan, Skouteris

---

et al., 1998). A striking difference is seen between the toxicity of talc in the lung and toxicity in other tissues, but this may be simply a dose effect (Kringsholm & Christoffersen, 1987). Talc is strongly fibrogenic in the lung, where it leads to pulmonary granulomatous disease with a progressive or fatal outcome (Pare, Cote et al., 1989). By contrast, talc liver is inconsequential clinically (Molos, Litton et al., 1987). A series of 70 liver biopsies from IDUs with chronic hepatitis was examined under polarizing microscopy, revealing that two thirds had talc particles but no granulomas (Allaire, Goodman et al., 1989). Another series reviewed the liver biopsy appearance in chronic hepatitis C, with and without known injection drug use. Talc was found in nine of 109 biopsies, of which only two were from patients who had reported injection drug use. Of the five patients in whom followup interviews were possible, three admitted to prior injection drug use after being confronted with the liver biopsy evidence. Thus, the presence of intrahepatic talc was a useful marker of previous injection drug use, but it is not sensitive for those with a minimal injection drug use history.

Lead poisoning has been reported in several patients who injected amphetamines (Riordan, Skouteris et al., 1998). Lead acetate used in the synthesis of methamphetamine can contaminate the final product. The effects of acute lead poisoning include hepatitis, encephalopathy, and renal impairment. However, a survey of blood lead levels in 92 amphetamine users presenting to an emergency department found no cases of lead toxicity, indicating that this problem is sporadic (Norton, Burton et al., 1996).

PHENCYCLIDINE
A few cases of liver failure associated with malignant hyperthermia following phencyclidine use have been reported (Armen, Kanel et al., 1984). In experimental animals, liver toxicity has been demonstrated without hyperthermia.

ACKNOWLEDGMENTS: The author is grateful to Sarah Hutchinson, Janice Pritchard-Jones, and Gary Nind for their assistance in preparation of this chapter. Professor Charles Lieber kindly allowed portions of a similar chapter from the previous edition of this text to be used.

REFERENCES
Adinolfi LE, Gambardella M, Andreana A et al. (2001). Steatosis accelerates the progression of liver damage of chronic hepatitis C patients and correlates with specific HCV genotype and visceral obesity. *Hepatology* 33:1358-1364.

Akriviadis E, Botla R, Briggs W et al. (2000). Pentoxifylline improves short-term survival in severe acute alcoholic hepatitis: A double-blind, placebo-controlled trial. *Gastroenterology* 119:1637-1648.

Alexander JF, Lischner MW & Galambos JT (1971). Natural history of alcoholic hepatitis, II. The long-term prognosis. *American Journal of Gastroenterology* 56:515-525.

Allaire GS, Goodman ZD, Ishak KG et al. (1989). Talc in liver tissue of intravenous drug abusers with chronic hepatitis. A comparative study. *American Journal of Clinical Pathology* 92:583-588.

Allander T, Gruber A, Naghavi M et al. (1995). Frequent patient-to-patient transmission of hepatitis C virus in a haematology ward. *Lancet* 345:603-607.

Alter HJ & Seeff LB (2000). Recovery, persistence, and sequelae in hepatitis C virus infection: A perspective on long-term outcome. *Seminars in Liver Disease* 20:17-35.

Alter MJ (1997). Epidemiology of hepatitis C. *Hepatology* 26:62S-65S.

Alter MJ, Kruszon-Moran D, Nainan OV et al. (1999). The prevalence of hepatitis C virus infection in the United States, 1988 through 1994. *New England Journal of Medicine* 341:556-562.

Andrews P (1997). Cocaethylene toxicity. *Journal of Addictive Diseases* 16:75-84.

Apte MV, Haber PS, Applegate TL et al. (1998). Periacinar stellate shaped cells in rat pancreas: Identification, isolation and culture. *Gut* 43:128-133.

Armen R, Kanel G & Reynolds T (1984). Phencyclidine-induced malignant hyperthermia causing submassive liver necrosis. *American Journal of Medicine* 77:167-172.

Baggott M, Heifets B, Jones RT et al. (2000). Chemical analysis of ecstasy pills. *Journal of the American Medical Association* 284:2190.

Bassendine MF (1986). Alcohol—A major risk factor for hepatocellular carcinoma? *Journal of Hepatology* 2:513-519.

Batey RG, Bensoussan A, Fan YY et al. (1998). Preliminary report of a randomized, double-blind placebo-controlled trial of a Chinese herbal medicine preparation CH-100 in the treatment of chronic hepatitis C. *Journal of Gastroenterology and Hepatology* 13:244-247.

Bhagwandeen BS, Apte M, Manwarring L et al. (1987). Endotoxin induced hepatic necrosis in rats on an alcohol diet. *Journal of Pathology* 152:47-53.

Black M (1984). Acetaminophen hepatotoxicity. *Annual Review of Medicine* 35:577-593.

Bode C, Kugler V & Bode JC (1987). Endotoxemia in patients with alcoholic and non-alcoholic cirrhosis and in subjects with no evidence of chronic liver disease following acute alcohol excess. *Journal of Hepatology* 4:8-14.

Bonis PA, Friedman SL & Kaplan MM (2001). Is liver fibrosis reversible? *New England Journal of Medicine* 344:452-454.

Brahen LS, Capone TJ & Capone DM (1988). Naltrexone: Lack of effect on hepatic enzymes. *Journal of Clinical Pharmacology* 28:64-70.

Brauer RB, Heidecke CD, Nathrath W et al. (1997). Liver transplantation for the treatment of fulminant hepatic failure induced by the ingestion of ecstasy. *Transplant International* 10:229-233.

Bresters D, Mauser-Bunschoten EP, Reesink HW et al. (1993). Sexual transmission of hepatitis C virus. *Lancet* 342:210-211.

Bronowicki JP, Venard V, Botte C et al. (1997). Patient-to-patient transmission of hepatitis C virus during colonoscopy. *New England Journal of Medicine* 337:237-240.

Butler TG, Dolan KA, Ferson MH et al. (1997). Hepatitis B and C in New South Wales prisons: Prevalence and risk factors. *Medical Journal of Australia* 166:127-130.

Campbell G & Campbell JH (1997). Smooth muscle diversity: Implications for the question; What is a smooth muscle cell? *Biomedical Research* 8:81-125.

Carithers RL Jr, Herlong HF, Diehl AM et al. (1989). Methylprednisolone therapy in patients with severe alcoholic hepatitis. A randomized multicenter trial. *Annals of Internal Medicine* 110:685-690.

Clouston AD, Jonsson JR, Purdie DM et al. (2001). Steatosis and chronic hepatitis C: Analysis of fibrosis and stellate cell activation. *Journal of Hepatology* 34:314-320.

Colado MI, Williams JL & Green AR (1995). The hyperthermic and neurotoxic effects of "Ecstasy" (MDMA) and 3,4 methylenedioxy-methamphetamine (MDA) in the Dark Agouti (DA) rat, a model of the CYP2D6 poor metabolizer phenotype. *British Journal of Pharmacology* 115:1281-1289.

Colell A, Garcia-Ruiz C, Miranda M et al. (1998). Selective glutathione depletion of mitochondria by ethanol sensitizes hepatocytes to tumor necrosis factor. *Gastroenterology* 115:1541-1551.

Conte D, Fraquelli M, Prati D et al. (2000). Prevalence and clinical course of chronic hepatitis C virus (HCV) infection and rate of HCV vertical transmission in a cohort of 15,250 pregnant women. *Hepatology* 31:751-755.

Crofts N, Cooper G, Stewart T et al. (1997). Exposure to hepatitis A virus among blood donors, injecting drug users and prison entrants in Victoria. *Journal of Viral Hepatitis* 4:333-338.

Crofts N, Stewart T, Hearne P et al. (1995). Spread of bloodborne viruses among Australian prison entrants. *British Medical Journal* 310:285-288.

Cromie SL, Jenkins PJ, Bowden DS et al. (1996). Chronic hepatitis C: Effect of alcohol on hepatic activity and viral titer. *Journal of Hepatology* 25:821-826.

Croop RS, Faulkner EB & Labriola DR (1997). The safety profile of naltrexone in the treatment of alcoholism. Results from a multicenter usage study. The Naltrexone Usage Study Group. *Archives of General Psychiatry* 54:1130-1135.

Davis GL, Esteban-Mur R, Rustgi V et al. (1998). Interferon alfa-2b alone or in combination with ribavirin for the treatment of relapse of chronic hepatitis C. International Hepatitis Interventional Therapy Group. *New England Journal of Medicine* 339:1493-1499.

Davis GL & Rodrigue JR (2001). Treatment of chronic hepatitis C in active drug users. *New England Journal of Medicine* 45:215-217.

Day CP (2000). Who gets alcoholic liver disease: Nature or nurture? *Journal of the Royal College of Physicians of London* 34:557-562.

Degos F (1999). Hepatitis C and alcohol. *Journal of Hepatology* 31(Suppl 1):113-118.

Di Bisceglie AM (2000). Natural history of hepatitis C: Its impact on clinical management. *Hepatology* 31:1014-1018.

Dienstag JL, Schiff ER, Wright TL et al. (1999). Lamivudine as initial treatment for chronic hepatitis B in the United States. *New England Journal of Medicine* 341:1256-1263.

Dieperink E, Willenbring M & Ho SB (2000). Neuropsychiatric symptoms associated with hepatitis C and interferon alpha: A review. *American Journal of Psychiatry* 157:867-876.

Dore GJ, Kaldor JM & McCaughen GW (1997). Systematic review of role of polymerase chain reaction in defining infectiousness among people infected with hepatitis C virus. *British Medical Journal* 315:333-337.

Dore GJ, Law MG & Kaldor JM (1999). Prevalence of hepatitis C virus infection in the United States. *New England Journal of Medicine* 341:2093-2095.

Dufour MC (1994). Chronic liver disease and cirrhosis. In JE Everhart (ed.) *Digestive Diseases in the United States: Epidemiology and Impact.* Washington, DC: NIDDK, National Institutes of Health, 615-646.

Dusheiko GM & Roberts JA (1995). Treatment of chronic type B and C hepatitis with interferon alfa: An economic appraisal. *Hepatology* 22:1863-1873.

Dussol B, Berthezene P, Brunet P et al. (1995). Hepatitis C virus infection among chronic dialysis patients in the south of France: A collaborative study. *American Journal of Kidney Diseases* 25:399-404.

Edlin BR, Seal KH, Lowick J et al. (2001). Is it justifiable to withhold treatment for hepatitis C from illicit-drug users? *New England Journal of Medicine* 345:211-215.

Ellis AJ, Wendon JA, Portmann B et al. (1996). Acute liver damage and Ecstasy ingestion. *Gut* 38:454-458.

Enomoto N, Ikejima K, Bradford B et al. (1998). Alcohol causes both tolerance and sensitization of rat Kupffer cells via mechanisms dependent on endotoxin. *Gastroenterology* 115:443-451.

Everhart JE & Beresford TP (1997). Liver transplantation for alcoholic liver disease: A survey of transplantation programs in the United States. *Liver Transplantation and Surgery* 3:220-226.

Farrell GC (2000). Clinical potential of emerging new agents in hepatitis B. *Drugs* 60:701-710.

Fernandez-Checa JC, Kaplowitz N, Garcia-Ruiz C et al. (1997). GSH transport in mitochondria: Defense against TNF-induced oxidative stress and alcohol-induced defect. *American Journal of Physiology* 273:G7-17.

Fernandez-Checa JC, Kaplowitz N, Garcia-Ruiz C et al. (1998). Mitochondrial glutathione: Importance and transport. *Seminars in Liver Disease* 18:389-401.

Fong TL, Govindarajan S, Valinluck B et al. (1988). Status of hepatitis B virus DNA in alcoholic liver disease: A study of a large urban population in the United States. *Hepatology* 8:1602-1604.

Frank C, Mohamed MK, Strickland GT et al. (2000). The role of parenteral antischistosomal therapy in the spread of hepatitis C virus in Egypt. *Lancet* 355:887-891.

Frezza M, di Padova C, Pozzato G et al. (1990). High blood alcohol levels in women. The role of decreased gastric alcohol dehydrogenase activity and first-pass metabolism [published errata appear in *New England Journal of Medicine* 1990 May 24;322(21):1540 and 1990 Aug 23;323(8):553]. *New England Journal of Medicine* 322:95-99.

Friedman SL (1993). Seminars in medicine of the Beth Israel Hospital, Boston. The cellular basis of hepatic fibrosis. Mechanisms and treatment strategies. *New England Journal of Medicine* 328:1828-1835.

Goldberg D, Burns S, Taylor A et al. (2001). Trends in HCV prevalence among injecting drug users in Glasgow and Edinburgh during the era of needle/syringe exchange. *Scandinavian Journal of Infectious Diseases* 33:457-461.

Haber PS, Koorey DJ et al. (1999). Clinical outcomes of liver transplantation for alcoholic liver disease. *Journal of Gastroenterology and Hepatology.*

Haber PS, Parsons SJ, Harper SE et al. (1999). Transmission of hepatitis C within Australian prisons. *Medical Journal of Australia* 171:31-33.

Hagan H, McGough JP, Thiede H et al. (1999). Syringe exchange and risk of infection with hepatitis B and C viruses. *American Journal of Epidemiology* 149:203-213.

Hanck C, Marinos G et al. (1998). The relative role of proinflammatory cytokines in alcoholic liver cirrhosis: Association with Child Pugh stages of the disease. *Alcohol and Alcoholism* 33(6):606-608

Hanck C, Singer MV et al. (1999). Systemic enhancement of the mRNA expression of IL-18 in unstimulated PBMC of patients with alcoholic liver disease: Correlation with endotoxinemia and sCD14 [abstract]. *Alcohol and Alcoholism* 34:460.

Hearn WL, Flynn DD, Hime GW et al. (1991). Cocaethylene: A unique cocaine metabolite displays high affinity for the dopamine transporter. *Journal of Neurochemistry* 56:698-701.

Heathcote EJ, Shiffman ML, Cooksley WG et al. (2000). Peginterferon alfa-2a in patients with chronic hepatitis C and cirrhosis. *New England Journal of Medicine* 343:1673-1680.

Heith AM, Morse CR, Tsujita T et al. (1995). Fatty acid ethyl ester synthase catalyzes the esterification of ethanol to cocaine. *Biochemical and Biophysical Research Communications* 208:549-554.

Henry JA, Jeffreys KJ & Dawling S (1992). Toxicity and deaths from 3,4-methylenedioxymethamphetamine ("Ecstasy"). *Lancet* 340:384-387.

Hill DB, Deaciuc IV et al. (1998). Mechanisms of hepatic injury in alcoholic liver disease. *Clinics in Liver Disease* 3:703-721.

Hoek JB & Kholodenko BN (1998). The intracellular signaling network as a target for ethanol. *Alcoholism: Clinical & Experimental Research* 22:224S-230S.

Hoek JB, Thomas AP, Rooney TA et al. (1992). Ethanol and signal transduction in the liver. *FASEB Journal* 6:2386-2396.

Hollinger FB, Khan NC, Oefinger PE et al. (1983). Posttransfusion hepatitis type A. *Journal of the American Medical Association* 250:2313-2317.

Hrubec Z & Omenn GS (1981). Evidence of genetic predisposition to alcoholic cirrhosis and psychosis: Twin concordances for alcoholism and its biological end points by zygosity among male veterans. *Alcoholism: Clinical & Experimental Research* 5:207-215.

Iimuro Y, Frankenberg MV, Arteel GE et al. (1997). Female rats exhibit greater susceptibility to early alcohol-induced liver injury than males. *American Journal of Physiology* 272:G1186-1194.

International Consensus Conference on Hepatitis C. (1999). Paris: The European Association for the Study of Liver Disease, International Consensus Conference on Hepatitis C.

Israel Y, Speisky H et al. (1992). Metabolism of hepatic glutathione and its relevance in alcohol-induced liver damage. *Cellular Molecular Aspects of Cirrhosis* 216:25-37.

Iwarson S (1998). New target groups for vaccination against hepatitis A: Homosexual men, injecting drug users and patients with chronic hepatitis. *Scandinavian Journal of Infectious Diseases* 30:316-318.

Jarvelainen HA, Fang C, Ingelman-Sundberg M et al. (1999). Effect of chronic coadminstration of endotoxin and ethanol on rat liver pathology and proinflammatory and anti-inflammatory cytokines. *Hepatology* 29:1503-1510.

Jones AL & Simpson KJ (1999). Review article: Mechanisms and management of hepatotoxicity in ecstasy (MDMA) and amphetamine intoxications. *Alimentary Pharmacology and Therapeutics* 13:129-133.

Kaldor JM, Archer GT, Buring ML et al. (1992). Risk factors for hepatitis C virus infection in blood donors: A case-control study. *Medical Journal of Australia* 157:227-230.

Kershenobich D, Vargas F, Garcia-Tsao G et al. (1988). Colchicine in the treatment of cirrhosis of the liver. *New England Journal of Medicine* 318:1709-1713.

Koch M & Banys P (2001). Liver transplantation and opioid dependence. *Journal of the American Medical Association* 285:1056-1058.

Kono H, Wheeler MD, Rusyn I et al. (2000). Gender differences in early alcohol-induced liver injury: Role of CD14, NF-kappaB, and TNF-alpha. *American Journal of Physiology; Gastrointestinal and Liver Physiology* 278:G652-661.

Kopp EB & Medzhitov R (1999). The Toll-receptor family and control of innate immunity. *Current Opinion in Immunology* 11:13-18.

Korenman J, Baker B, Waggoner J et al. (1991). Long-term remission of chronic hepatitis B after alpha-interferon therapy. *Annals of Internal Medicine* 114:629-634.

Korsten MA, Matsuzaki S, Keinman L et al. (1975). High blood acetaldehyde levels after ethanol administration. Difference between alcoholic and nonalcoholic subjects. *New England Journal of Medicine* 292:386-389.

Koziel MJ, Wong DK, Ducley D et al. (1997). Hepatitis C virus-specific cytolytic T lymphocyte and T helper cell responses in seronegative persons. *Journal of Infectious Diseases* 176:859-866.

Kringsholm B & Christoffersen P (1987). The nature and the occurrence of birefringent material in different organs in fatal drug addiction. *Forensic Science International* 34:53-62.

Kumar S, Stauber RE, Gavaler JS et al. (1990). Orthotopic liver transplantation for alcoholic liver disease. *Hepatology* 11:159-164.

Kwo PY, Ramchandani VA, O'Connor S et al. (1998). Gender differences in alcohol metabolism: Relationship to liver volume and effect of adjusting for body mass. *Gastroenterology* 115:1552-1557.

Lamagni TL, Davison KL, Hope VD et al. (1999). Poor hepatitis B vaccine coverage in injecting drug users: England, 1995 and 1996. *Communicable Disease and Public Health* 2:174-177.

Lane BP & Lieber CS (1966). Ultrastructural alterations in human hepatocytes following ingestion of ethanol with adequate diets. *American Journal of Pathology* 49:593-603.

Lau N, Schiano TD et al. (2000). Survival and recidivism risk in methadone-dependent patients undergoing liver transplantation. *Hepatology* 32:245A.

Leshner AI (1997). Addiction is a brain disease, and it matters. *Science* 278:45-47.

Levin DM, Baker AL, Riddell RH et al. (1979). Nonalcoholic liver disease. Overlooked causes of liver injury in patients with heavy alcohol consumption. *American Journal of Medicine* 66:429-434.

Levy MT, Chen JJ, McGuinness PH et al. (1997). Liver transplantation for hepatitis C-associated cirrhosis in a single Australian centre: Referral patterns and transplant outcomes. *Journal of Gastroenterology and Hepatology* 12:453-459.

Lieber CS (1997). Cytochrome P-4502E1: Its physiological and pathological role. *Physiological Reviews* 77:517-544.

Lieber CS, Casini A, DeCarli LM et al. (1990). S-adenosyl-L-methionine attenuates alcohol-induced liver injury in the baboon. *Hepatology* 11:165-172.

Lieber CS & DeCarli LM (1974). An experimental model of alcohol feeding and liver injury in the baboon. *Journal of Medical Primatology* 3:153-163.

Lieber CS, DeCarli LM, Mak KM et al. (1990). Attenuation of alcohol-induced hepatic fibrosis by polyunsaturated lecithin. *Hepatology* 12:1390-1398.

Lieber CS, DeCarli LM & Ruvin E (1975). Sequential production of fatty liver, hepatitis, and cirrhosis in sub-human primates fed ethanol with adequate diets. *Proceedings of the National Academy of Science* 72:437-441.

Lieber CS & Lefevre A (1957). Effect of oxytetracycline on acidity, ammonia and urea in gastric juice in normal and uremic subjects. *Comptes Rendus de la Societe de Biologie* 151:1038-1042.

Lieber CS & Lefevre A (1959). Ammonia as source of gastric hypoacidity in patients with uremia. *Journal of Clinical Investigation* 38:1271-1277.

Lieber CS & Leo MA (1992). Alcohol and the liver. In CS Lieber (ed.) *Medical and Nutritional Complications of Alcoholism*. New York, NY: Plenum Press, 185-239.

Lieber CS & Leo MA (1998). Metabolism of ethanol and some associated adverse effects on the liver and the stomach. *Recent Developments in Alcoholism* 14:7-40.

Lieber CS, Robins SJ, Li J et al. (1994). Phosphatidylcholine protects against fibrosis and cirrhosis in the baboon. *Gastroenterology* 106:152-159.

Lucey MR, Carr K, Beresford TP et al. (1997). Alcohol use after liver transplantation in alcoholics: A clinical cohort follow-up study. *Hepatology* 25:1223-1227.

Lucey MR, Merion RM, Henley KS et al. (1992). Selection for and outcome of liver transplantation in alcoholic liver disease. *Gastroenterology* 102:1736-1741.

Lumeng L & Crabb DW (1994). Genetic aspects and risk factors in alcoholism and alcoholic liver disease. *Gastroenterology* 107:572-578.

MacDonald MA, Wodak AD, Dolan KA et al. (2000). Hepatitis C virus antibody prevalence among injecting drug users at selected needle and syringe programs in Australia, 1995-1997. Collaboration of Australian NSPs. *Medical Journal of Australia* 172:57-61.

Mallat A & Dhumeaux D (1991). Cocaine and the liver. *Journal of Hepatology* 12:275-278.

Mason BJ, Salvato FR, Williams LD et al. (1999). A double-blind, placebo-controlled study of oral nalmefene for alcohol dependence. *Archives of General Psychiatry* 56(8):719-724.

Mato JM, Camara J, Fernandez de Paz J et al. (1999). S-adenosylmethionine in alcoholic liver cirrhosis: A randomized, placebo-controlled, double-blind, multicenter clinical trial. *Journal of Hepatology* 30:1081-1089.

McAfee JH, Keeffe EB, Lee RG et al. (1992). Transjugular liver biopsy. *Hepatology* 15:726-732.

McClain C, Hill D, Schmidt J et al. (1993). Cytokines and alcoholic liver disease. *Seminars in Liver Disease* 13:170-182.

McHutchison JG, Gordon SC, Schiff ER et al. (1998). Interferon alfa-2b alone or in combination with ribavirin as initial treatment for chronic hepatitis C. Hepatitis Interventional Therapy Group. *New England Journal of Medicine* 339:1485-1492.

Meisel H, Reip A, Faltus B et al. (1995). Transmission of hepatitis C virus to children and husbands by women infected with contaminated anti-D immunoglobulin. *Lancet* 345:1209-1211.

Mendenhall CL, Anderson S et al. (1984). Short-term and long-term survival in patients with alcoholic hepatitis treated with oxandrolone and prednisolone. *New England Journal of Medicine* 311:1464-70.

Modlin RL, Brightbill HD, Garcia-Pont P et al. (1999). The toll of innate immunity on microbial pathogens. *New England Journal of Medicine* 340:1834-1835.

Mohr L, Tanaka S & Wands JR (1998). Ethanol inhibits hepatocyte proliferation in insulin receptor substrate 1 transgenic mice. *Gastroenterology* 115:1558-1565.

Mokdad AH, Serdula MK, Dietz WH et al. (2000). The continuing epidemic of obesity in the United States. *Journal of the American Medical Association* 284:1650-1651.

Molos MA, Litton N & Schubert TT (1987). Talc liver. *Journal of Clinical Gastroenterology* 9:198-203.

Morgan MY & Sherlock S (1977). Sex-related differences among 100 patients with alcoholic liver disease. *British Medical Journal* 1:939-941.

Moussavian SN, Becker RC, Piepmeyer JL et al. (1985). Serum gamma-glutamyl transpeptidase and chronic alcoholism. Influence of alcohol ingestion and liver disease. *Digestive Diseases and Science* 30:211-214.

Murphy EL, Bryzman SM, Glynn SA et al. (2000). Risk factors for hepatitis C virus infection in United States blood donors. NHLBI Retrovirus Epidemiology Donor Study (REDS). *Hepatology* 31:756-762.

Murphy EL, Bryzman S & Williams AE (1999). Prevalence of hepatitis C virus infection in the United States. *New England Journal of Medicine* 341:2093-2095.

National Institutes of Health (NIH) (1997). NIH Consensus Development Conference Panel statement: Management of hepatitis C. *Hepatology* 26:2S-10S.

Naveau S, Giraud V, Borotto E et al. (1997). Excess weight risk factor for alcoholic liver disease. *Hepatology* 25:108-111.

Neary MP, Cort S, Bayliss MS et al. (1999). Sustained virologic response is associated with improved health-related quality of life in relapsed chronic hepatitis C patients. *Seminars in Liver Disease* 19:77-85.

Neuberger J & Tang H (1997). Relapse after transplantation: European studies. *Liver Transplantation and Surgery* 3:275-279.

Norton R, Batey R, Dwyer T et al. (1987). Alcohol consumption and the risk of alcohol related cirrhosis in women. *British Medical Journal* 295:80-82.

Norton RL, Burton BT & McGirr J (1996). Blood lead of intravenous drug users. *Journal of Toxicology. Clinical Toxicology* 34:425-430.

Novick DM (2000). The impact of hepatitis C virus infection on methadone maintenance treatment. *Mount Sinai Journal of Medicine* 67:437-443.

Okuda K, Hayashi H, Kobayashi S et al. (1995). Mode of hepatitis C infection not associated with blood transfusion among chronic hemodialysis patients. *Journal of Hepatology* 23:28-31.

Orrego H, Blake JE, Blendis LM et al. (1987). Long-term treatment of alcoholic liver disease with propylthiouracil. *New England Journal of Medicine* 317:1421-1427.

Orrego H, Blake JE & Israel Y (1985). Relationship between gamma-glutamyl transpeptidase and mean urinary alcohol levels in alcoholics while drinking and after alcohol withdrawal. *Alcoholism: Clinical & Experimental Research* 9:10-13.

Orrego H, Kalant H, Israel Y et al. (1979). Effect of short-term therapy with propylthiouracil in patients with alcoholic liver disease. *Gastroenterology* 76:105-115.

Padron GJ, Rodriguez Z, Rivera L et al. (1995). Hepatitis C virus in plasmapheresis donors. *Sangre* (Barcelona) 40:187-190.

Pare JP, Cote G & Fraser RS (1989). Long-term follow-up of drug abusers with intravenous talcosis. *American Review of Respiratory Disease* 139:233-241.

Parrish KM, Dufour MC, Stinson FS et al. (1993). Average daily alcohol consumption during adult life among decedents with and without cirrhosis: The 1986 National Mortality Followback Survey. *Journal of Studies on Alcohol* 54:450-456.

Pequignot G, Tuyns AJ & Berta JL (1978). Ascitic cirrhosis in relation to alcohol consumption. *International Journal of Epidemiology* 7:113-120.

Perrillo R, Schiff E, Yoshida E et al. (2000). Adefovir dipivoxil for the treatment of lamivudine-resistant hepatitis B mutants. *Hepatology* 32:129-134.

Persico M, Persico E, Suozzo R et al. (2000). Natural history of hepatitis C virus carriers with persistently normal aminotransferase levels. *Gastroenterology* 118:760-764.

Post JJ, Dolan KA, Whybin LR et al. (2001). Acute hepatitis C virus infection in an Australian prison inmate: Tattooing as a possible transmission route. *Medical Journal of Australia* 174:183-184.

Power JP, Lawlor E, Davidson F et al. (1995). Molecular epidemiology of an outbreak of infection with hepatitis C virus in recipients of anti-D immunoglobulin. *Lancet* 345:1211-1213.

Poynard T, Marcellin P, Lee SS et al. (1998). Randomised trial of interferon alpha2b plus ribavirin for 48 weeks or for 24 weeks versus interferon alpha2b plus placebo for 48 weeks for treatment of chronic infection with hepatitis C virus. International Hepatitis Interventional Therapy Group (IHIT). *Lancet* 352:1426-1432.

Poynard T, Ratziu V & Bedossa P (2000). Appropriateness of liver biopsy. *Canadian Journal of Gastroenterology* 14:543-548.

Poynard T, Ratziu V, Charlotte F et al. (2001). Rates and risk factors of liver fibrosis progression in patients with chronic hepatitis C. *Journal of Hepatology* 34:730-739.

Quinn PG & Johnston DE (1997). Detection of chronic liver disease: Costs and benefits. *Gastroenterologist* 5:58-77.

Riordan SM, Skouteris GG & Williams R (1998). Metabolic activity and clinical efficacy of animal and human hepatocytes in bioartificial support systems for acute liver failure [editorial]. *International Journal of Artificial Organs* 21:312-218.

Rolla R, Vay D, Mottaran E et al. (2000). Detection of circulating antibodies against malondialdehyde-acetaldehyde adducts in patients with alcohol-induced liver disease. *Hepatology* 31:878-884.

Rosman AS, Paronetto F, Galvin K et al. (1993). Hepatitis C virus antibody in alcoholic patients. Association with the presence of portal and/or lobular hepatitis. *Archives of Internal Medicine* 153:965-969.

Rothstein KD, Kanchana TP et al. (2000). Is liver transplantation appropriate in patients on methadone maintenance? *Hepatology* 32:245A.

Sachithanandan S & Fielding JF (1997). Low rate of HCV transmission from women infected with contaminated anti-D immunoglobulin to their family contacts. *Italian Journal of Gastroenterology and Hepatology* 29:47-50.

Sangiovanni A, Morales R, Spinzi G et al. (1998). Interferon alfa treatment of HCV RNA carriers with persistently normal transaminase levels: A pilot randomized controlled study. *Hepatology* 27:853-856.

Sato C, Matsuda Y & Lieber CS (1981). Increased hepatotoxicity of acetaminophen after chronic ethanol consumption in the rat. *Gastroenterology* 80:140-148.

Saunders JB, Davis M & Williams R (1981). Do women develop alcoholic liver disease more readily than men? *British Medical Journal* 282:1140-1143.

Schiff ER (1997). Hepatitis C and alcohol. *Hepatology* 26:39S-42S.

Schiff L (1993). *Diseases of the Liver*. Philadelphia, PA: Lippincott.

Schletter J, Heine H, Ulmer AJ et al. (1995). Molecular mechanisms of endotoxin activity. *Archives of Microbiology* 164:383-389.

Seeff LB, Cuccherini BA, Zimmerman HJ et al. (1986). Acetaminophen hepatotoxicity in alcoholics. A therapeutic misadventure. *Annals of Internal Medicine* 104:399-404.

Selim K & Kaplowitz N (1999). Hepatotoxicity of psychotropic drugs. *Hepatology* 29:1347-1351.

Shapiro CN, Coleman PJ, McQuillan GM et al. (1992). Epidemiology of hepatitis A: Seroepidemiology and risk groups in the USA. *Vaccine* 10(Suppl 1):S59-62.

Sherlock S & Dooley J (1997). Virus hepatitis. *Diseases of the Liver and Biliary System*. Oxford, England: Blackwell.

Sherlock S & James D (1997). *Diseases of the Liver and Biliary System*. Oxford, England: Blackwell.

Silva MO, Roth D, Reddy KR et al. (1991). Hepatic dysfunction accompanying acute cocaine intoxication. *Journal of Hepatology* 12:312-315.

Spencer JD, Latt N, Beeby PJ et al. (1997). Transmission of hepatitis C virus to infants of human immunodeficiency virus-negative intravenous drug-using mothers: Rate of infection and assessment of risk factors for transmission. *Journal of Viral Hepatitis* 4:395-409.

Spinzi G, Terruzzi V & Minoli G (2001). Liver biopsy. *New England Journal of Medicine* 344:2030.

Steindl PE & Ferenci P (1998). Clinical issues in the management of alcoholic liver disease. *Clinics in Liver Disease* 2:765-779.

Stephenson J (2001). Former addicts face barriers to treatment for HCV. *Journal of the American Medical Association* 285:1003-1005.

Streetz KL, Luedde T, Manns MP et al. (2000). Interleukin 6 and liver regeneration. *Gut* 47:309-312.

Taieb J, Chollet-Martin S et al. (2000). The role of interleukin-10 in acute alcoholic hepatitis. *Alcoholism: Clinical & Experimental Research* 24:191A.

Talley NJ, A Roth et al. (1988). Diagnostic value of liver biopsy in alcoholic liver disease. *Journal of Clinical Gastroenterology* 10:647-550.

Tennant F & Moll D (1995). Seroprevalence of hepatitis A, B, C, and D markers and liver function abnormalities in intravenous heroin addicts. *Journal of Addictive Diseases* 14:35-49.

Teschke R & Wiese B (1982). Sex-dependency of hepatic alcohol metabolizing enzymes. *Journal of Endocrinological Investigation* 5:243-250.

Thurman RG (1998). II. Alcoholic liver injury involves activation of Kupffer cells by endotoxin. *American Journal of Physiology* 275:G605-611.

Tilg H & Diehl AM (2000). Mechanisms of disease: Cytokines in alcoholic and nonalcoholic steatohepatitis. *New England Journal of Medicine* 343:1467-1476.

Tsukamoto H, Towner SJ, Ciofalo LM et al. (1986). Ethanol-induced liver fibrosis in rats fed high fat diet. *Hepatology* 6:814-822.

Tucker GT, Lennard MS, Ellis SW et al. (1994). The demethylenation of methylenedioxymethamphetamine ("Ecstasy") by debrisoquine hydroxylase (CYP2D6). *Biochemical Pharmacology* 47:1151-1156.

Vaillant GE (1997). The natural history of alcoholism and its relationship to liver transplantation. *Liver Transplantation and Surgery* 3:304-310.

van Beek I, Dwyer R, Dore GJ et al. (1998). Infection with HIV and hepatitis C virus among injecting drug users in a prevention setting: Retrospective cohort study. *British Medical Journal* 317:433-437.

Van Ness MM & Diehl AM (1989). Is liver biopsy useful in the evaluation of patients with chronically elevated liver enzymes? *Annals of Internal Medicine* 111:473-478.

Van Thiel DH, Bonet H, Gavaler J et al. (1995). Effect of alcohol use on allograft rejection rates after liver transplantation for alcoholic liver disease. *Alcoholism: Clinical & Experimental Research* 19:1151-1155.

Ware JE Jr, Bayliss MS, Mannocchia M et al. (1999). Health-related quality of life in chronic hepatitis C: Impact of disease and treatment response. The Interventional Therapy Group. *Hepatology* 30:550-555.

Weinrieb RM, Van Horn DH, McLellan AT et al. (2000). Interpreting the significance of drinking by alcohol-dependent liver transplant patients: Fostering candor is the key to recovery. *Liver Transplantation* 6:769-776.

Weltman MD, Brotodihardjo A, Crewe EB et al. (1995). Coinfection with hepatitis B and C or B, C and delta viruses results in severe chronic liver disease and responds poorly to interferon-alpha treatment. *Journal of Viral Hepatitis* 2:39-45.

Whitcomb DC & Block GD (1994). Association of acetaminophen hepatotoxicity with fasting and ethanol use. *Journal of the American Medical Association* 272:1845-1850.

Whyte GS & Savoia HF (1997). The risk of transmitting HCV, HBV or HIV by blood transfusion in Victoria. *Medical Journal of Australia* 166:584-586.

Wiesner RH, Lombardero M, Lake JR et al. (1997). Liver transplantation for end-stage alcoholic liver disease: An assessment of outcomes. *Liver Transplantation and Surgery* 3:231-239.

Worner TM (1994). Hepatotoxicity is not increased in alcoholics with positive urinary cocaine metabolites. *Drug and Alcohol Dependence* 35:191-195.

Xu D, Thiele GM, Beckenhauer JL et al. (1998). Detection of circulating antibodies to malondialdehyde-acetaldehyde adducts in ethanol-fed rats. *Gastroenterology* 115:686-692.

Yokoyama H, Ishii H, Nagata S et al. (1993). Experimental hepatitis induced by ethanol after immunization with acetaldehyde adducts. *Hepatology* 17:14-19.

Younossi ZM (1998). Epidemiology of alcohol-induced liver disease. *Clinics in Liver Disease* 2:661-671.

Zeuzem S, Feinman SV, Rasenack J et al. (2000). Peginterferon alfa-2a in patients with chronic hepatitis C. *New England Journal of Medicine* 343:1666-1672.

| Chapter 4 | # Renal and Metabolic Disorders Related to Alcohol and Other Drug Use |

Jose Carlos T. DaSilva, M.D., M.P.H.
Edward A. Alexander, M.D.

Nephrotic Syndrome
Nephritic-Nephrotic Syndrome
Nephritic Syndrome
Isolated Hematuria
Hypertension and Renal Disease
Acute Renal Failure
Tobacco Use and Renal Disease
Other Causes of Renal Injury

The perception that drug abuse and renal disease are closely intertwined is easily confirmed by a simple survey of the population undergoing chronic dialysis in urban, inner-city hospitals and clinics. It is likely that the prevalence of present or past drug addiction in this cohort of individuals surpasses the prevalence in the general population. The causal links are apparent in some cases, such as HIV nephropathy, hepatitis C-associated glomerular disease, or subcutaneous injection drug-related amyloidosis. However, with other diseases, such as accelerated hypertension or focal and segmental glomerulosclerosis, the relationship between exposure and disease, even if strongly suspected, has not yet been proven definitively.

A list of the renal problems thought to be associated with common drugs of abuse is found in Table 1. However, the multiplicity of behavioral risk factors and the variety of possible etiologic agents make it difficult to define a clearcut relationship between a given drug of abuse and a renal disease. Perhaps a more useful classification for the practitioner features the renal syndromes of presentation that can be related to one or more exposures connected to drug addiction (Table 2).

For the physician responsible for any patient with a history of drug abuse, obtaining a measurement of renal function (plasma creatinine), serum electrolytes, and urine protein excretion on a regular and frequent basis is mandatory. If proteinuria is present, 24-hour urine quantification is very useful. Using the same 24-hour specimen, a total urine creatinine excretion with a concurrent plasma creatinine will provide a useful estimate of glomerular filtration rate (GFR = urinary creatinine concentration $\times$ urinary volume/plasma creatinine concentration/1.73 m^2). The latter is particularly important because many drug abusers have reduced muscle mass or are cachectic. These patients often have a serum creatinine value that is within the "normal range," yet their GFR is markedly diminished.

Knowledge of GFR is important, not only in assessing renal function, but also in determining drug dosing. If it is not possible to obtain a 24-hour collection, proteinuria can be estimated by using a spot urine protein-to-creatinine ratio. The ratio represents the approximate protein excretion; for example, a ratio of 3 means an approximate daily excretion of 3 g protein. It should be recognized that, in patients with reduced muscle mass, this ratio will overestimate

TABLE 1.   Common Drugs of Abuse Associated With Renal Problems

Opiates
- HIV nephropathy
- Hepatitis C-associated glomerulopathies
- Hepatitis B-associated polyarteritis nodosa
- Bacterial endocarditis and acute glomerulonephritis
- Subcutaneous injection ("skin-popping") amyloidosis
- Nontraumatic rhabdomyolysis (muscle compression) and acute renal failure
- Heroin nephropathy.

Cocaine
- Rhabdomyolysis and acute renal failure
- Accelerated hypertension and renal failure
- HIV nephropathy
- Hypertensive nephrosclerosis
- Renal infarction
- Thrombotic microangiopathy and renal failure.

Alcohol
- Hepatorenal syndrome
- Rhabdomyolysis and acute renal failure
- Increased incidence and severity of postinfectious glomerulonephritis
- Electrolyte disorders.

actual protein excretion. However, it still is very useful in following changes in protein excretion in the same patient over time (Ginsberg, Chang et al., 1983).

NEPHROTIC SYNDROME

Nephrotic syndrome is narrowly defined as heavy proteinuria (>3.5 g/day), hypoalbuminemia, hyperlipidemia, lipiduria, and edema. However, separate components of the syndrome may be absent and, from a diagnostic point of view, heavy proteinuria is sufficient to consider the patient nephrotic.

HIV-Associated Nephropathy. At the turn of the 21st century, the Centers for Disease Control and Prevention estimated that about 400,000 patients were living with AIDS in the United States (CDC, 1999). The character of the AIDS epidemic continues to evolve because of increased representation of women and ethnic minorities, increased importance of heterosexual contact as a mode of transmission, and longer survival of patients through the use of highly active antiretroviral therapy (HAART). The effect of these changes is not clear with regard to the occurrence of HIV-associated nephropathy (HIVAN). The apparent resistance of Caucasian patients with AIDS to developing HIVAN, as compared with African Americans, suggests a genetic predisposition. In fact, more than 90% of patients who develop HIVAN are of African descent (Cantor, Kimmel et al., 1991), and the prevalence of end-stage renal disease (ESRD) in relatives of AIDS patients who develop HIVAN is higher than in their counterparts without renal disease (Freedman, Soucie et al., 1999). In 1999, HIVAN was the third leading cause of ESRD in African Americans aged 20 to 64 (Klotman, 1999).

HIVAN can occur at any stage of HIV disease, with presentation in patients who already have an AIDS-defining condition or as the presenting manifestation of AIDS in patients who otherwise are asymptomatic. Most HIVAN patients have CD4 counts of less than 250 cells/mm^3 (Winston, Kotman et al., 1999) and therefore are candidates for aggressive antiretroviral therapy.

The pathogenesis of HIVAN is incompletely understood. It is known that transgenic mice that express HIV proviral constructs in renal tissue develop disease that is identical to HIVAN in humans (Klotman, 1999). Moreover, when kidneys from those transgenic mice are transplanted into normal recipients, they develop the typical histologic changes of HIVAN. However, when normal kidneys are transplanted into transgenic mice, renal tissue is unaffected (Bruggeman, Dikman et al., 1997). These data suggest a direct role of viral infection, rather than the indirect effects of modulation of different cytokines and associated infective agents, which often are encountered in the later stages of AIDS. Hopefully, better control of viral load with effective therapy will decrease the incidence of HIVAN.

Although the typical patient with HIVAN presents with nephrotic-range proteinuria, this massive proteinuria is not usually accompanied by edema or serosal effusions. The urinary sediment contains oval fat bodies and fatty casts and, often, unusually broad waxy casts that, presumably, reflect the dilated tubules of their origin. Ultrasonic evaluation reveals normal-sized or enlarged kidneys that are hyperechoic. The absence of hypertension, even with advanced renal insufficiency, is common. In the authors' experience, renal biopsy has a limited role in the diagnosis of HIVAN and need be performed only when there is a serious question about the diagnosis and the biopsy findings would significantly alter therapy.

Histologic findings with light microscopy in HIVAN include focal and segmental glomerulosclerosis, often with features of collapsing glomerular disease. Interstitial inflammation with microcystic tubular dilatation is regularly noted (D'Agati & Appel, 1998). Immunofluorescence usually is negative. In some cases, electron microscopy reveals tubuloreticular structures that are thought to be associated with ribonucleoproteins and elevated levels of alpha-interferon. These structures are typical, but not diagnostic, of HIVAN because they can be found in other diseases, particularly systemic lupus erythematosus.

Renal insufficiency appears very early in the disease and is rapidly progressive, leading to ESRD in a matter of weeks or months. More recently, however, with the use of HAART at earlier stages of HIV infection, a more benign and protracted course can be seen (Sczech, van der Horst et al., 1999).

Some case reports of response to HAART with resolution of clinical (Viani, Dankner et al., 1999) and histologic features (Wali, Drachenberg et al., 1998) have been noted. In addition, use of angiotensin-converting enzyme inhibitors appears to decrease the magnitude of proteinuria and postpone progression, as drugs of this class do in other glomerular diseases (Burns, Paul et al., 1997; Burns, Visitainer et al., 1999).

In the past, patients with HIVAN were denied dialysis because of their short life expectancy. Today dialysis is provided to these patients and some centers are offering stable HIV patients on dialysis the opportunity for renal transplantation (Dr. Paul Klotman, personal communication). This opportunity reflects the longer survival of HIV patients on renal replacement therapy and the better outlook for patients who respond to HAART.

Hepatitis Virus-Associated Nephrotic Syndrome. Hepatitis B- and C-associated nephropathies are, as expected of bloodborne diseases, frequently found among injection drug users (IDUs). All patients presenting with nephrotic syndrome of unknown etiology should be screened for hepatitis.

The association between hepatitis B and membranous nephropathy is well established, with morphologic studies demonstrating deposition of hepatitis Be antigen in glomerular capillaries (Lai, Li et al., 1991). It is important to diagnose this cause of membranous nephropathy, because

TABLE 2.   Renal Syndromes Commonly Associated With Alcohol and Drug Abuse

Nephrotic Syndrome
- Hepatitis B- or C-related membranous nephropathy
- HIV nephropathy (IDU)
- Amyloidosis (subcutaneous IDU ["skin popping"])
- Focal and segmental glomerulosclerosis (IDU).

Nephritic-Nephrotic Syndrome
- Hepatitis C-related membranoproliferative glomerulonephritis (IDU)
- Hepatitis C-related cryoglobulinemia (IDU).

Nephritic Syndrome
- Bacterial endocarditis and acute glomerulonephritis (IDU)
- Postinfectious glomerulonephritis (IDU).

Acute Renal Failure
- Rhabdomyolysis (alcohol, cocaine, MDMA [ecstasy], morphine)
- Crystal-induced renal failure (indinavir, acyclovir, sulfonamides)
- Thrombotic microangiopathy (cocaine).

Hypertension
- Hepatitis B- or amphetamine-associated polyarteritis nodosa (IDU, amphetamine)
- Accelerated hypertension (cocaine).

immunosuppressive treatment—often used in the idiopathic form of nephrotic syndrome—actually may enhance ongoing hepatitis B viral replication. Moreover, antiviral therapy (Dienstag & Eckstein, 1985; Benhamou, Katlama et al., 1996) may prove beneficial.

The most common presentation of renal disease in patients with hepatitis C is a combination of the nephrotic and nephritic syndromes (that is, a urine that contains large amounts of protein, red blood cells, and red blood cell casts; see the following section on Nephritic-Nephrotic Syndrome). Less often, membranous nephropathy has been described in association with hepatitis C in IDUs (Okada, Takishita et al., 1996; Stehman-Breen, Alpres et al., 1995). The detection of hepatitis C virus protein in the glomeruli of patients with membranous nephropathy (Okada, Takishita et al., 1996) strengthens this association.

Heroin Nephropathy. Heroin nephropathy has been considered a secondary cause of focal and segmental glomerulosclerosis, often associated with hypertension and slow progression to ESRD. Since HIVAN first was recognized, the diagnosis of heroin nephropathy rarely has been encountered (Friedman & Rao, 1995). This rarity may reflect more purified forms of heroin and/or the removal of contaminants that were, in fact, responsible for "heroin nephropathy" or the earlier development of HIVAN in this susceptible group. Patients with focal and segmental glomerulosclerosis, a history of IDU, and infection with hepatitis C may present with a clinical picture similar to that of heroin nephropathy (Stehman-Breen, Alpres et al., 1999). This situation raises a question as to whether hepatitis C, and not heroin or its contaminants, is the actual etiologic agent in the glomerular disease found in these patients.

Subcutaneous Drug Use-Associated Amyloidosis. Chronic suppurative skin infections related to subcutaneous illicit drug injection are known to be associated with secondary amyloidosis with renal involvement (Neugarten, Galo et al., 1986; Tan, Cohen et al., 1995; Formica & Perazella, 1998). Clinically, these patients may be very difficult to distinguish from those with HIVAN or hepatitis-related renal disease because they present with nephrotic-range proteinuria, renal insufficiency, and normal-sized or enlarged kidneys. The evidence of subcutaneous drug injection ("skin popping," or multiple skin scars or draining abscesses) should alert the physician to the possibility of this diagnosis. If alternative diagnoses are possible, a renal biopsy is appropriate to confirm the presence of amyloidosis. In addition to proteinuria and renal insufficiency, tubular dysfunction, including nephrogenic diabetes insipidus and proximal or distal renal tubular acidosis, may be present.

NEPHRITIC-NEPHROTIC SYNDROME
Hepatitis C-Associated Renal Disease. In addition to significant proteinuria, the presence of hematuria, hypertension, and variable degrees of renal insufficiency in the setting of past or present IDU should raise the suspicion of hepatitis C-related glomerular disease. The most common pattern of injury in patients with hepatitis C infection is membranoproliferative glomerulonephritis with or without cryoglobulinemia (Agnello, Chung et al., 1992; Misiani, Bellavita et al., 1992; Johnson, Gretch et al., 1993). Less commonly, membranous nephropathy (see above) or fibril-

lary glomerulonephritis and immunotactoid glomerulopathy may be encountered. In the latter two instances, the clinical presentation and light microscopy findings can be indistinguishable from membranoproliferative glomerulonephritis, but organized deposits of fibrils of different sizes are detected on electron microscopy (Markowitz, Cheng et al., 1998).

Although liver function tests often are abnormal, there are many cases in which they are only minimally elevated or within normal limits, and there are no findings in the history or physical examination that point to liver dysfunction (Stokes, Chawla et al., 1997; Cheng, Anderson et al., 1999). In cases with associated essential mixed cryoglobulinemia, serum cryoglobulins are detected. In addition, palpable purpura, arthralgias, peripheral neuropathy, and nonspecific systemic complaints may be present. A pattern of serum complement with decreased C4 and normal C3 levels is characteristic of mixed cryoglobulinemia (Haydey, de Rojas et al., 1980). A positive rheumatoid factor is seen inconsistently. Typical renal biopsy features of mixed cryoglobulinemia include intraluminal thrombi in glomerular capillaries and a substructure of curvilinear fibrils in the subendothelial space, which resemble "fingerprints" on electron microscopy.

The use of combination therapy with interferon and ribavirin (Virazole®) is accepted even in the absence of specific indications to treat the liver disease. The use of ribavirin is contraindicated when the creatinine clearance is less than 50 mL/minute because of increased side effects, including severe hemolytic anemia (Jefferson & Johnson, 2000).

Co-infection with hepatitis C is found in up to 78% of HIV-infected IDUs (Quan, Kradjen et al., 1993). The course of nephropathy associated with this dual infection has been reported as aggressive, with rapid progression to ESRD.

NEPHRITIC SYNDROME
Acute Bacterial Endocarditis and Septicemia. The presence of a nephritic urinary sediment (proteinuria, hematuria, and often red blood cell casts), variable degrees of hypertension, and renal insufficiency in the setting of IDU should raise the suspicion of immune complex–mediated glomerulonephritis. In this circumstance, bacterial sepsis and acute bacterial endocarditis are not rare. The most frequent pathogen is *Staphylococcus aureus* (Neugarten & Baldwin, 1984; Stachura, 1985; di Belgiojoso, Genderime et al., 1990; Bakir & Dunea, 1996). Less often *Streptococcus viridans*, gram-negative rods, or *Candida* species are isolated. Actual septic

embolization of the kidneys is much less common. The latter complication would be recognized by persistent fevers, gross or microscopic hematuria (occasionally accompanied by flank pain), and signs of embolization to other organs. If large renal vessels are occluded, filling defects can be documented by an isotopic renal perfusion scan.

Hypertension and low complement levels (C3) are present less consistently than in poststreptococcal glomerulonephritis, and nephrotic syndrome occurs in a minority of cases (Neugarten & Baldwin, 1984). Although renal failure is irreversible in some cases, recovery of renal function usually occurs with treatment of the underlying infection (Conlon, Jeffries et al. 1998).

In patients with postinfectious glomerulonephritis as a manifestation of acute endocarditis or abscesses, histologic features similar to those found with poststreptococcal glomerulonephritis are seen. The pattern is one of acute proliferative glomerulonephritis with neutrophil infiltration and immune complex deposition in the mesangium and capillary walls. A higher incidence and more severe course of postinfectious glomerulonephritis in alcoholics have been reported, but the specific reasons for this condition are unclear (Keller, Andrassy et al., 1994; Montseny, Meyrier et al., 1994; Vamvakas, Teschner et al. 1998).

Patients with bacterial endocarditis who develop renal failure days to weeks after the onset of antibiotic therapy should raise the suspicion of acute interstitial nephritis. Suggestive of this diagnosis is the finding, in the urine sediment, of renal tubular and/or white blood cells, often in casts. Eosinophiluria has a low specificity and sensitivity for interstitial nephritis.

ISOLATED HEMATURIA

The presence of hematuria should not be assumed to be glomerular in origin, especially in the absence of proteinuria. Obviously, drug abusers can manifest urologic disease unrelated to their drug abuse. Therefore, urologic evaluation may be in order before ascribing isolated hematuria to a parenchymal renal process.

Hematuria may be the only manifestation of immunoglobulin A (IgA) nephropathy, and there appears to be an association between IgA nephropathy and alcoholic cirrhosis. It has been suggested that this association can be related to a decreased clearance of IgA molecules because of arteriovenous shunting away from the reticuloendothelial system. However, IgA deposition is not usually associated with progressive deterioration of renal function and should

not preclude liver transplantation in otherwise suitable patients.

IgA nephropathy can occur in patients with HIV infection in whom microscopic or macroscopic hematuria may be the only presenting sign (Katz, Bragman et al., 1992; Kimmel, Phillips et al., 1992). Renal biopsy is the only definitive diagnostic tool in these patients. In patients undergoing treatment with antiretroviral medications, particularly indinavir (Crixivan®), acyclovir (Zovirax®), or large doses of sulfonamides, crystalluria is another possible explanation for hematuria (see Acute Renal Failure). Such hematuria sometimes is associated with impaired renal function, which usually is reversible on volume expansion and discontinuation of the offending agent.

HYPERTENSION AND RENAL DISEASE

The development of acute hypertension in connection with cocaine use is well recognized and seems to be associated with the release of endothelin 1 and activation of the renin-angiotensin system (Nzerue, Hewan-Lowe et al., 2000). The clinical presentations of cocaine intoxication can mimic preeclampsia or scleroderma renal crisis (Goodlin, 1991; Lam & Ballou, 1992), and the development of accelerated hypertension and renal failure has been documented by some (Thakur, Godley et al., 1996) but not other (Brecklin, Gopaniuk-Folga et al., 1998) observers. This inconsistency may reflect confounding factors, including the intensity and length of exposure, genetic predisposition, and duration of followup. The amphetamine-like drug MDMA (3,4-methylenedioxymethamphetamine), also known as "Ecstasy," has been reported to produce accelerated hypertension and acute renal failure (Bingham, Beaman et al., 1998).

Polyarteritis nodosa has been associated with hepatitis B and drugs of abuse, especially amphetamines. Patients may present with accelerated hypertension and systemic symptoms, including malaise, arthralgias, weight loss, and asymmetric peripheral neuropathy. They may have a necrotizing vasculitis, which can affect medium-sized arteries, including renal, mesenteric, coronary, and (rarely) cerebral circulation. The test for antinuclear cytoplasmic antibodies usually is negative (Dienstag & Eckstein, 1985; Samuels, Shemesh et al., 1996). Angiography is the diagnostic procedure of choice. The finding of diffuse microaneurysms with areas of thrombosis and ischemia in multiple organs, including the kidneys, is diagnostic.

Treatment usually is with steroids and cytotoxic agents. Antivirals such as lamivudine (Epivir®) (Dienstag, Perrilo et al., 1995) or interferon (in cases with hepatitis B) also may prove to be effective, without the risk of enhanced viral replication with immunosuppression.

Hypertension and progressive renal failure are associated with the ingestion of homemade whiskey (so-called "moonshine"). The nephrotoxic exposure is thought to be the chronic ingestion of lead, which is found in the car radiators used to distill the whiskey. These patients often have hyperuricemia and gout and thus have been labeled with the diagnosis of "saturnine gout" (Bennett, 1985).

ACUTE RENAL FAILURE

Rhabdomyolysis. The presentation in the emergency department of a young adult with a history of alcohol or illicit drug abuse (especially cocaine or MDMA), who is agitated, confused, combative, and hyperthermic, and who has a urinalysis highly suggestive of this disease (that is, brownish-red urine positive for blood but without red blood cells on microscopy) is a common scenario. Tonic-clonic seizures may have occurred prior to admission. In addition, blood testing usually reveals a markedly elevated serum creatine kinase level.

Drugs associated with rhabdomyolysis include phencyclidine, methamphetamines, MDMA, cocaine, heroin, and alcohol (Nzerue, Hewan-Lowe et al., 2000; van der Woude, 2000; Vanholder, Sever et al., 2000; Murthy, Roberts et al., 1997; Richards, Johnson et al., 1999). The presence of volume depletion, hypotension, acidosis, and hypoxemia increase the likelihood of acute tubular necrosis.

The mechanism of tubular injury is multifactorial. Precipitating events may include volume depletion, often from fluid sequestered in damaged muscles (potentially several liters); decreased vasodilatory effect of nitric oxide, which is inactivated by myoglobin (Luscher, Bock et al., 1991); toxicity of free chelatable iron released from myoglobin (Zager, Burkhart et al., 1995); and tubular obstruction by pigmented casts (Heyman, Rosen et al., 1996).

Patients with total body potassium depletion (for example, malnourished alcoholics) may be predisposed to ischemic muscular injury because potassium release at the level of the microcirculation is an important mechanism for vasodilatation that sustains muscle perfusion during physical activity (Knochel & Schlein, 1972). Total body phosphate depletion is a predisposing factor, and the hypophosphatemia can be masked at the time of presentation because of phosphate release from injured muscle cells (even producing hyperphosphatemia). In addition to hyperactiv-

ity, compression of muscle (crush injury) because of drug-induced stupor or coma and immobilization for prolonged periods of time can result in rhabdomyolysis. In the early phase, hypocalcemia can be secondary to deposition in necrotic muscle cells or precipitation with phosphate released from destroyed muscle cells. Hyperkalemia and hyperuricemia also may be present.

Treatment depends on the phase of the disease at the time of presentation. If severe renal failure is not present, an attempt at volume expansion with isotonic saline is appropriate. In the absence of hypocalcemia, the use of sodium bicarbonate to alkalinize the urine can decrease the toxicity of myoglobin. The role of mannitol (Osmitrol®) in this setting is less clear (Zager, 1992). Although in some series (Eneas, Schoenfeld et al., 1979) up to 50% of patients required acute dialysis, most patients do recover renal function.

Crystal-Induced Tubular Injury. Acute renal failure has been described with the use of antiviral agents, including acyclovir (Sawyer, Webb et al., 1988), indinavir (Kopp, Miller et al., 1997; Tashima, Horowitz et al., 1997), ritonavir (Norvir®) (Chugh, Bird et al., 1997), and sulfonamide, usually when they are used in large doses in patients who also are volume depleted.

The urinary sediment helps to confirm the diagnosis when crystals typical of the ingested drug are present. Recovery of renal function is the rule when the patient is given adequate hydration and is withdrawn from the offending agent or the dose is reduced. Indinavir has been associated with the formation of urinary stones.

Hepatorenal Syndrome. Chronic alcohol ingestion can lead to hepatorenal syndrome if liver damage occurs. The pathogenesis and pathophysiology of this syndrome is complex and beyond the scope of this chapter. The interested reader is referred to more complete reviews (Punukollu & Gopalswamy, 1990; Gines & Arroyo, 1999).

Briefly, this syndrome is thought to reflect a state of profound renal vasoconstriction and splanchnic vasodilatation associated with severely impaired liver function, often with portal hypertension and ascites. A slow rise in serum creatinine and oliguria, accompanied by low urinary sodium concentration—usually less than 10 mEq/L—are characteristic of presentation. In this instance, the urinary sediment may not be helpful because it is well known that bilirubin-pigmented casts, which are indistinguishable from the "muddy-brown" casts seen in acute tubular necrosis, can be found in patients with jaundice even when they have apparently normal renal function. In addition, because malnutrition and decreased muscle mass are the rule in these patients, the serum creatinine may be within normal limits or minimally elevated and the blood urea nitrogen may be normal or low, whereas filtration rate is markedly reduced. This almost uniformly fatal complication can follow episodes of gastrointestinal bleeding, diuresis, or spontaneous bacterial peritonitis; however, many patients, perhaps the majority, have no specific inciting event. The idea that hepatorenal syndrome occurs only in the hospital is not accurate. In fact, the disease often begins days to weeks before hospitalization (Papadakis & Arieff, 1981).

Hepatorenal syndrome is a diagnosis of exclusion. If, after cautious trials of volume replacement (salt-poor albumin, not saline) and the removal of any potentially nephrotoxic agent, oliguric acute renal failure does not improve, a diagnosis of hepatorenal syndrome is probable.

The prognosis almost always involves the demise of the patient unless he or she is rescued by successful liver transplantation. A recent study, albeit with few patients, showed improvement in renal function and longer survival through the use of a combination of an oral sympathomimetic agent (midodrine [ProAmatine®]) and a somatostatin analogue (octreotide [Sandostatin®]) to inhibit endogenous vasodilators (Angeli, Volpin et al., 1999). If confirmed, this drug combination may help to bridge the gap until liver transplantation is available in suitable candidates.

Hemolytic Uremic Syndrome/Thrombotic Microangiopathy. Acute renal insufficiency associated with thrombocytopenic microangiopathic hemolytic anemia has been described in connection with cocaine abuse (Kokko, 1990; Tumlin, Sands et al., 1990; Volcy, Nzerue et al., 2000) and possibly also with HIV infection (Leaf, Laubenstein et al., 1988). This syndrome can have catastrophic consequences with renal cortical necrosis and permanent loss of renal function, central nervous system involvement with seizures, and the permanent sequel of ischemic or hemorrhagic strokes.

The pathogenesis of this syndrome is not known but may involve both immunologic and nonimmunologic mechanisms. An auto-antibody directed against the von Willebrand factor cleaving protease has been described in some cases (Furlan, Robles et al., 1998). Direct endothelial injury, vasoconstriction, and procoagulant effects of cocaine, which are thought to be involved in cases of renal infarction associated with cocaine abuse (Sharff, 1984), may play a part in the development of thrombotic microangiopathic nephropathy.

In such patients, renal biopsy reveals fibrin thrombi in the lumen of glomerular capillaries and occluded interlobu-

lar arterioles, with swollen endothelial cells and vessel wall damage. Fibrin and red blood cells are seen in the arteriolar media in the acute phase, and with "onion skin" hypertrophy of muscular arteries in the healing phase. These lesions are similar to findings associated with malignant hypertension, systemic sclerosis, and the antiphospholipid antibody syndrome. Early recognition is important because prompt treatment with plasmapheresis and infusion of fresh frozen plasma can prevent serious complications (Kaplan, Meyers et al., 1998).

TOBACCO USE AND RENAL DISEASE

Tobacco use appears to have a deleterious effect on renal function. Cigarette smoking is related to proteinuria (Halimi, Giraudeau et al., 2000), accelerated atherosclerotic vascular disease and, presumably, ischemic nephropathy. In addition, increased risk of progression to renal insufficiency related to tobacco smoking has been documented in patients with diabetes mellitus (Stegmayr, 1990) and severe essential hypertension (Regaldo, Yang et al., 2000). Moreover, increased risk of sustained proteinuria (Halimi, Giraudeau et al., 2000) and poorer prognosis of renal disease have been ascribed to tobacco smoking (Orth, Ritz et al., 1997; Orth, Stockmann et al., 1998).

Accelerated atherosclerotic vascular disease related to cigarette smoking is well known to contribute to the development and progression of ischemic nephropathy. This common cause of renal failure is defined as impaired perfusion to the total renal mass and usually is associated with ischemic manifestations in other organs (brain, myocardium, and lower extremities) (Greco & Breyer, 1997).

OTHER CAUSES OF RENAL INJURY

Many possible associations between drugs of abuse and renal injury have been suggested, but clear-cut confirmation of these associations is not definitive. Associations suggested from case reports include renal cell carcinoma and anabolic steroids (Martorana, Concetti et al., 1999), renal infarction and marijuana (Lambrecht, Malbrain et al., 1995), renal failure and "magic mushrooms" (Raff, Halloran et al., 1992), antiglomerular basement membrane disease and cocaine abuse (Peces, Navascues et al., 1999), acute renal failure and toluene (glue sniffing) (Will, 1981), granulomatous interstitial nephritis and oxycodone (OxyContin®) use (Segal, Dowling et al., 1998), and urinary retention (Bryden, Rothwell et al., 1995) and vasculitis with use of MDMA (Woodrow & Turney, 1999), among others.

Opiates certainly can cause urinary retention, especially in older men who have underlying prostatic hyperplasia. Urinary retention is most commonly seen as an iatrogenic complication of opiate analgesia in the postoperative period (Tammela, 1995). Factitious nephrolithiasis has been described (Gault, Campbell et al., 1988) and can be a reason for multiple visits to different health care facilities on the part of individuals who seek prescriptions for narcotic drugs. The absence of gross or microscopic hematuria should argue strongly against this diagnosis.

Fluid and Electrolyte Abnormalities Among Patients With Drug Abuse. Patients who use drugs of abuse may present with myriad fluid and electrolyte abnormalities, but few are specifically associated with a particular drug. Chronic alcoholics are the most frequently seen among this group. Patients with chronic alcoholism and recent binge drinking or intercurrent illness that requires abstinence often are admitted with gastrointestinal losses and underlying malnutrition—a scenario for complex and dynamic electrolyte and acid-base problems.

Alcoholics, especially if they have been binge drinking and acutely stop, may present with severe anion gap acidosis. Ethanol usually is no longer detectable in the serum on presentation. This condition is a ketoacidosis induced by poor dietary intake, especially carbohydrates, and the inhibition of gluconeogenesis and acceleration of lipolysis by alcohol. The urine can be weakly positive or negative for ketones because, in many patients, beta-hydroxybutyrate comprises most of the ketonuria. Standard tablets or dipsticks use the nitroprusside reaction that is positive when acetone or acetoacetate is present but are negative with beta-hydroxybutyrate.

Other acid-base disturbances seen in alcoholics usually are not life-threatening. They include non-anion gap acidosis secondary to diarrhea, a common finding in this group of patients and, occasionally, renal tubular acidosis. The finding of a reduced serum bicarbonate can represent compensation for respiratory alkalosis. Alcoholics may present with this respiratory disturbance, which, in part, may be secondary to impaired hepatic metabolism of progesterone, a respiratory stimulant. As with all acid-base disturbances, blood pH values are necessary to determine the precise abnormality.

Decreased serum potassium levels often are seen in connection with gastrointestinal losses and secondary hyperaldosteronism. Such loss may be accelerated by the use of diuretics without a potassium-sparing agent. Correction of this electrolyte abnormality is important because hypokalemia can accelerate or worsen hepatic encephalopathy, in part through the enhancement of ammoniagenesis. In addition, hypokalemia (along with hypophosphatemia) increases the risk for rhabdomyolysis. The correction of hypomagnesemia is critical to allow repair of any renal potassium wasting.

One of the most frequent electrolyte abnormalities among alcoholics is hypomagnesemia (Elisaf, Merkouropulos et al., 1994). The etiology probably is a combination of poor nutrition and gastrointestinal losses, coupled with direct renal tubular alcohol toxicity (De Marchi, Cecchin et al., 1993), which decreases renal magnesium absorption in spite of depleted body stores. Hypomagnesemia often is associated with hypocalcemia because of decreased parathyroid hormone release and bone resistance to parathyroid hormone (Laitinen, Lamberg-Allardt et al., 1991; Shis, 1980). In addition, if chronic pancreatitis and fat malabsorption are present, saponification (complexing) of calcium and magnesium will impair intestinal absorption of these divalent cations. Hypokalemia is worsened by concomitant hypomagnesemia, which promotes kaliuresis (Kobrin & Goldfarb, 1990) and, like hypocalcemia, is refractory to correction unless the magnesium deficit is replaced (Elisaf, Milionis et al., 1997). Severe hypomagnesemia should be treated with slow intravenous infusion, whereas oral replacement can be used for therapy of milder forms of hypomagnesemia.

Hypophosphatemia often is seen in alcoholics and may contribute to rhabdomyolysis and encephalopathy (Funabiki, Tatsukawa et al., 1998; Nagata, 1998). Again, dietary deficiency, increased gastrointestinal losses, and increased renal excretion (Elisaf, Merkouropouls et al., 1994; Vamvakas, Teschner et al., 1998) contribute to this deficit.

Toxic Alcohols. The ingestion of a toxic alcohol—methanol, ethylene glycol, or isopropyl alcohol—is rare, but occasionally is seen in an alcohol-dependent patient who has ingested the toxic alcohol as a substitute for ethanol. Methanol is found in solutions used for de-icing and in some paint products, such as varnish or shellac. Ethylene glycol is found in antifreeze. The metabolic products of these alcohols (facilitated by alcohol dehydrogenase) are severely toxic and produce organ damage and anion gap acidosis from the nonvolatile organic acids produced.

Anion gap acidosis usually is the first clue to a toxic alcohol ingestion, but it should be remembered that alcoholic and starvation ketoacidosis are far more common. The presence of an osmolar gap (that is, a difference between the calculated and measured osmolarity >15), should raise suspicion of a toxic alcohol ingestion when no other reason for this gap is apparent, such as ethanol or mannitol. In cases of ethylene glycol ingestion, the presence of calcium oxalate crystals in the urine is suggestive but not diagnostic.

Treatment is directed primarily at inhibition of the production of the organic acids that are the metabolic products of these alcohols, through the use of intravenous ethanol. Ethanol slows the metabolism of the toxic alcohols by competing for alcohol dehydrogenase and thus reduces the production of the toxic organic acid metabolites. Fomepizole, a new intravenous drug that competitively inhibits alcohol dehydrogenase more than ethanol, is very effective and probably safer than an ethanol infusion (Brent, McMartin et al., 1999). As long as kidney function is maintained, the alcohol will be removed by renal excretion. With severe intoxication, hemodialysis is used to remove the alcohol and the toxic products efficiently and is useful in the treatment of the concurrent acidosis. Failure to recognize and promptly treat these alcohol intoxications can lead to multiple organ damage (to the brain, liver, and kidney) and, for methanol, to blindness.

Isopropyl alcohol is found in rubbing alcohol and other solvents. It is metabolized to acetone and excreted by the kidneys and the lung. Here, the alcohol itself rather than the products of alcohol metabolism is the toxic agent. Organic acids are not produced, so there is no anion gap acidosis unless there is hypotension to initiate the production of lactic acidosis. Patients usually appear inebriated but without an odor of ethanol on the breath. They often have gastritis, ketonuria, and an osmolar gap.

Inhalants. An unusual cause of metabolic acidosis and hypokalemia, encountered more often in teenagers, involves toluene intoxication from glue sniffing. Diagnosis can be very difficult because patients may be reticent to report abuse of this substance. Patients may recover rapidly on admission to the hospital, but recurrent episodes are not uncommon (Streicher, Gabow et al., 1981). Distal renal tubular acidosis has been described in this setting (King, 1981). However, the principal mechanism producing the acidosis seems to involve increased manufacture of hippuric acid derived from toluene metabolism (Carlisle, Donnelly et al., 1991). The hippuric acid is rapidly excreted, leading to a normal anion gap metabolic acidosis. In the distal nephron, acting as a non-reabsorbable anion, hippurate increases the excretion of sodium and potassium. If hippurate is present in sufficient amounts, severe hypokalemia may occur.

MDMA ("Ecstasy"). The amphetamine-type drug 3,4-methylenedioxymethamphetamine (MDMA or "Ecstasy") has become popular recently. Often, users are in a venue (such as a dance club) in which the ambient temperature is high and vigorous physical activity occurs. In such a situation, use of MDMA can lead to agitation, high fever, hyperventilation, and impaired sensorium. This condition leads to increased insensible fluid losses and sets the stage for dehydration (hypernatremia) and volume depletion. The results, unless treated promptly, can include hypotension, shock, brain damage, and rhabdomyolysis with renal failure. The hypernatremia and volume depletion should be treated promptly. If hypotension is present, therapy should be started initially with normal saline to restore organ perfusion. This treatment should be followed by hypotonic fluids to restore isotonicity and to continue to reestablish intravascular volume. Some users have become aware of these problems and try to prevent them through the intake of large amounts of water. The result has been severe hyponatremia with central nervous system symptoms (Maxwell, Polkey et al., 1993).

REFERENCES

Agnello V, Chung RT & Kaplan LM (1992). A role for hepatitis C virus in type II cryoglobulinemia. *New England Journal of Medicine* 327:1490-1495.

Angeli P, Volpin R, Gerunda G et al. (1999). Reversal of type 1 hepatorenal syndrome with the administration of midodrine and ocreotide. *Hepatology* 29:1690-1697.

Bakir AA & Dunea G (1996). Drugs of abuse and renal disease. *Current Opinion in Nephrology and Hypertension* 5:122-126.

Benhamou Y, Katlama C, Lunel F et al. (1996). Effects of lamivudine on replication of hepatitis B virus in HIV-infected men. *Annals of Internal Medicine* 125:705-712.

Bennett W (1985). Lead nephropathy. *Kidney International* 28:212-220.

Bingham C, Beaman M, Nicholls AJ et al. (1998). Necrotizing renal vasculopathy resulting in chronic renal failure after ingestion of methamphetamine and 3,4-methylenedioxymethamphetamine ("Ecstasy"). *Nephrology Dialysis and Transplantation* 13:2654-2655.

Brecklin CS, Gopaniuk-Folga A, Kravetz T et al. (1998). Prevalence of hypertension in chronic cocaine users. *American Journal of Hypertension* 11:1279-1283.

Brent J, McMartin K, Phillips S et al. (1999). Fomepizole for the treatment of ethylene glycol poisoning. *New England Journal of Medicine* 340:832-838.

Bruggeman LA, Dikman S, Meng C et al. (1997). Nephropathy in human immunodeficiency virus-1 transgenic mice is due to renal transgene expression. *Journal of Clinical Investigation* 100:84-92.

Bryden AA, Rothwell PJN & O'Reilly PH (1995). Urinary retention with misuse of "Ecstasy" [letter]. *British Medical Journal* 310:504.

Burns GC, Paul SK, Toth IR et al (1997). Effects of angiotensin converting-enzyme inhibition in HIV-associated nephropathy. *Journal of the American Society of Nephrology* 8:1140-1146.

Burns GC, Visitainer P & Mohammed NB (1999). Effect of angiotensin-converting enzyme inhibition on progression of renal disease and mortality in HIV-associated nephropathy [abstract]. *Journal of the American Society of Nephrology* 10:155A.

Cantor ES, Kimmel PL & Bosch JP (1991). Effects of race on expression of acquired immunodeficiency syndrome-associated nephropathy. *Archives of Internal Medicine* 151:125-128.

Carlisle EJ, Donnelly SM, Vasuvattakul S et al. (1991). Glue-sniffing and distal renal acidosis: Sticking to the facts. *Journal of the American Society of Nephrology* 8:1019-1027.

Centers for Disease Control and Prevention (CDC) (1999). Available at: HTTP://WWW.CDC.GOV/HIV/DHAP.HTM.

Cheng JT, Anderson HL, Markowitz GS et al. (1999). Hepatitis C virus-associated glomerular disease in patients with human immunodeficiency virus coinfection. *Journal of the American Society of Nephrology* 10:1566-1574.

Chugh S, Bird R & Alexander EA (1997). Ritonavir and renal failure [letter]. *New England Journal of Medicine* 336:138.

Conlon PJ, Jeffries F, Krigman HR et al. (1998). Predictors of prognosis and risk of acute renal failure in bacterial endocarditis. *Clinical Nephrology* 49:96-101.

D'Agati V & Appel GB (1998). Renal pathology of human immunodeficiency virus infection. *Seminars in Nephrology* 18:406-421.

De Marchi S, Cecchin E, Basile A et al. (1993). Renal tubular dysfunction in chronic alcohol abuse—Effects of abstinence. *New England Journal of Medicine* 329:1927-1934.

di Belgiojoso GB, Genderine A, Scorza D et al. (1990). Renal damage in drug abusers. *Contributions to Nephrology* 77:142-156.

Dienstag JL & Eckstein M (1985). Case records of the Massachusetts General Hospital (case 36-1985). *New England Journal of Medicine* 313:622-631.

Dienstag J, Perrilo RP, Schiff ER et al. (1995). A preliminary trial of lamivudine for chronic hepatitis B infection. *New England Journal of Medicine* 333:1657-1661.

Elisaf M, Merkouropoulos M, Tsianos EV et al. (1994). Acid-base and electrolyte abnormalities in alcoholic patients. *Mineral and Electrolyte Metabolism* 20:274-281.

Elisaf M, Milionis H & Siamopoulos KC (1997). Hypomagnesemic hypokalemia and hypocalcemia: Clinical and laboratory characteristics. *Mineral and Electrolyte Metabolism* 23:105-112.

Eneas JF, Schoenfeld PY & Humphreys MH (1979). The effect of infusion of mannitol-sodium bicarbonate on the clinical course of myoglobinuria. *Archives of Internal Medicine* 139:801-805.

Formica R & Perazella MA (1998). Leg pain and swelling in an HIV-infected drug abuser. *Hospital Practice* (Office Edition) 33:195-197.

Freedman BI, Soucie JM, Stone SM et al. (1999). Familial clustering of end-stage renal disease in blacks with HIV-associated nephropathy. *American Journal of Kidney Diseases* 34:254-258.

Friedman EA & Rao TK (1995). Disappearance of uremia due to heroin-associated nephropathy. *American Journal of Kidney Diseases* 25:689-693.

Funabiki Y, Tatsukawa H, Ashida K et al. (1998). Disturbances of consciousness associated with hypophosphatemia in a chronically alcoholic patient. *Internal Medicine* 37:958-961.

Furlan M, Robles R, Galbusera M et al. (1998). von Willebrand factor-cleaving protease in thrombotic thrombocytopenic purpura and the hemolytic-uremic syndrome. *New England Journal of Medicine* 339:1578-1584.

Gault HM, Campbell NRC & Aksu AE (1988). Spurious stones. *Nephron* 48:274-279.

Gines P & Arroyo P (1999). Hepatorenal syndrome. *Journal of the American Society of Nephrology* 8:1833-1839.

Ginsberg JM, Chang BS, Matarese RA et al. (1983). Use of single voided urine samples to estimate quantitative proteinuria. *New England Journal of Medicine* 309:1543-1546.

Goodlin RC (1991). Preeclampsia as the great impostor. *Journal of Obstetrics and Gynecology* 164:1577-1581.

Greco RA & Breyer JA (1997). Ischemic nephropathy. *American Journal of Kidney Diseases* 29:167-187.

Halimi J-M, Giraudeau B, Vol S et al. (2000). Effects of current smoking and smoking discontinuation on renal function and proteinuria in the general population. *Kidney International* 58:1285-1292.

Haydey RP, de Rojas MP & Gigli I (1980). A newly described control mechanism of complement activation in patients with mixed cryoglobulinemia (cryoglobulins and complement). *Journal of Investigative Dermatology* 74:328-332.

Heyman SN, Rosen S, Fuchs S et al. (1996). Myoglobinuric acute renal failure in the rat: A role for medullary hypoperfusion, hypoxia, and tubular obstruction. *Journal of the American Society of Nephrology* 7:1066-1074.

Jefferson JA & Johnson RJ (2000). Treatment of hepatitis C-associated glomerular disease. *Seminars in Nephrology* 20:286-292.

Johnson RJ, Gretch DR, Yamabe H et al. (1993). Membranoproliferative glomerulonephritis associated with hepatitis C virus infection. *New England Journal of Medicine* 328:465-470.

Kaplan BS, Meyers KE & Schulman SL (1998). The pathogenesis and treatment of hemolytic uremic syndrome. *Journal of the American Society of Nephrology* 9:1126-1133.

Katz A, Bragman JM, Miller DC et al (1992). IgA nephritis in HIV positive patients: A new HIV associated nephropathy? *Clinical Nephrology* 38:61-68.

Keller CK, Andrassy K, Waldherr R et al. (1994). Postinfectious glomerulonephritis—Is there a link to alcoholism? *Quarterly Journal of Medicine* 87:97-102.

Kimmel PL, Phillips TM, Ferreira AC et al. (1992). Idiotypic IgA nephropathy in patients with human immunodeficiency virus infection. *New England Journal of Medicine* 327:702-706.

King MD (1981). Reversible renal damage due to glue sniffing [letter]. *British Medical Journal* 283:919.

Klotman PE (1999). HIV-associated nephropathy. *Kidney International* 56:1161-1176.

Knochel JP & Schlein EM (1972). On the mechanisms of rhabdomyolysis in potassium depletion. *Journal of Clinical Investigation* 51:1750.

Kobrin SM & Goldfarb S (1990). Magnesium deficiency. *Seminars in Nephrology* 10:525-535.

Kokko JP (1990). Metabolic and social consequences of cocaine abuse. *American Journal of the Medical Sciences* 299:361-365.

Kopp JB, Miller KD, Mican JA et al. (1997). Crystalluria and urinary tract abnormalities associated with indinavir. *Annals of Internal Medicine* 127:119-126.

Lai KN, Li PK, Lui SF et al. (1991). Membranous nephropathy related to hepatitis B in adults. *New England Journal of Medicine* 324:1457-1463.

Laitinen K, Lamberg-Allardt C, Tunninen R et al. (1991). Transient hypoparathyroidism during acute alcohol intoxication. *New England Journal of Medicine* 324:721-727.

Lam M & Ballou SP (1992). Reversible scleroderma crisis after cocaine use [letter]. *New England Journal of Medicine* 326:1435.

Lambrecht GLY, Malbrain MLNG, Coremans P et al. (1995). Acute renal infarction and heavy marijuana smoking. *Nephron* 70:494-496.

Leaf AN, Laubenstein LJ, Raphael B et al. (1988). Thrombotic thrombocytopenic purpura associated with human immunodeficiency virus 1 (HIV-1) infection. *Annals of Internal Medicine* 109:194-197.

Luscher TF, Bock HA, Yang Z et al. (1991). Endothelium-derived relaxing and contracting factors. *Kidney International* 39:575-590.

Markowitz GS, Cheng JT, Colvin RB et al. (1998). Hepatitis C viral infection is associated with fibrillary glomerulonephritis and immunotactoid glomerulopathy. *Journal of the American Society of Nephrology* 9:2244-2252.

Martorana G, Concetti S, Manferrari F et al. (1999). Anabolic steroid abuse and renal cell carcinoma. *Journal of Urology* 162:2089.

Maxwell DL, Polkey MI & Henry JA (1993). Hyponatremia and catatonic stupor after taking "Ecstasy" [letter]. *British Medical Journal* 307:1399.

Misiani R, Bellavita P, Fenili D et al. (1992). Hepatitis C virus infection in patients with essential mixed cryoglobulinemia. *Annals of Internal Medicine* 117:573-577.

Montseny JJ, Meyrier A, Kleinknecht D et al. (1994). Infectious glomerulonephritis (IGN) is unusually frequent and severe in alcoholics [abstract]. *Journal of the American Society of Nephrology* 5:356A.

Murthy BVS, Roberts NB & Wilkes RG (1997). Biochemical implications of ecstasy toxicity. *Annals of Clinical Biochemistry* 34:442-445.

Nagata N (1998). Hypophosphatemia and encephalopathy in alcoholics. *Internal Medicine* 37:911-912.

Neugarten J & Baldwin DS (1984). Glomerulonephritis in bacterial endocarditis. *American Journal of Medicine* 77:297-304.

Neugarten J, Galo G, Buxbaum J et al. (1986). Amyloidosis in subcutaneous heroin abusers ("skin poppers' amyloidosis"). *American Journal of Medicine* 81:635-640.

Nzerue CM, Hewan-Lowe K & Riley LJ (2000). Cocaine and the kidney: A synthesis of pathophysiologic and clinical perspectives. *American Journal of Kidney Diseases* 35:783-795.

Okada K, Takishita Y, Shimomura H et al. (1996). Detection of hepatitis C virus core protein in the glomeruli of patients with membranous glomerulonephritis. *Clinical Nephrology* 45:71-76.

Orth S, Ritz E & Schrier RW (1997). The renal risks of smoking. *Kidney International* 51:1669-1677.

Orth SR, Stockmann A, Conradt C et al. (1998). Smoking as a risk factor for end-stage renal failure in men with primary renal disease. *Kidney International* 54:926-931.

Papadakis MK & Arieff AI (1981). Unpredictability of clinical evaluation of renal function in cirrhosis. *American Journal of Medicine* 82:945-952.

Peces R, Navascues RA, Baltar J et al. (1999). Antiglomerular basement membrane antibody-mediated glomerulonephritis after intranasal cocaine use. *Nephron* 81:434-438.

Punukollu RC & Gopalswamy N (1990). The hepatorenal syndrome. *Medical Clinics of North America* 74:933-943.

Quan CM, Kradjen M, Grigoriew GA et al. (1993). Hepatitis C virus infection in patients infected with human immunodeficiency virus. *Clinical Infectious Disease* 17:117-119.

Raff E, Halloran PF & Kjellstrand CM (1992). Renal failure after eating "magic" mushrooms. *Canadian Medical Association Journal* 147:1339.

Regalado M, Yang S & Wesson DE (2000). Cigarette smoking is associated with augmented progression of renal insufficiency in severe essential hypertension. *American Journal of Kidney Diseases* 35:687-694.

Richards JR, Johnson EB, Stark RW et al. (1999). Methamphetamine abuse and rhabdomyolysis in the ED: A 5-year study. *American Journal of Emergency Medicine* 17:681-685.

Samuels N, Shemesh O, Yinnon AM et al. (1996). Polyarteritis nodosa and drug abuse: Is there a connection? *Postgraduate Medical Journal* 72:684-685.

Sawyer MH, Webb DE, Balow JE et al. (1988). Acyclovir-induced renal failure. Clinical course and histology. *American Journal of Medicine* 84:1067-1071.

Segal A, Dowling JP, Ireton HJC et al. (1998). Granulomatous glomerulonephritis in intravenous drug users: A report of three cases in oxycodone addicts. *Human Pathology* 29:1246-1249.

Sharff JA (1984). Renal infarction associated with intravenous cocaine use. *Annals of Emergency Medicine* 13:1145-1147.

Shis ME (1980). Magnesium, calcium and parathyroid interactions. *Annals of the New York Academy of Sciences* 355:165-178.

Stachura I (1985). Renal lesions in drug addicts. *Pathology Annual* 20(Pt 2):83-99.

Stegmayr BG (1990). A study of patients with diabetes mellitus (type 1) and end-stage renal failure: Tobacco usage may increase risk of nephropathy and death. *Journal of Internal Medicine* 228:121-124.

Stehman-Breen C, Alpres CE, Couser WG et al. (1995). Hepatitis C virus associated membranous glomerulonephritis. *Clinical Nephrology* 44:141-147.

Stehman-Breen C, Alpres CE, Fleet WP et al. (1999). Focal segmental glomerulosclerosis among patients infected with hepatitis C virus. *Nephron* 81:37-40.

Stokes MB, Chawla H, Brody RI et al. (1997). Immune complex glomerulonephritis in patients coinfected with human immunodeficiency virus and hepatitis C virus. *American Journal of Kidney Diseases* 29:514-525.

Streicher HZ, Gabow PA, Moss AH et al. (1981). Syndromes of toluene sniffing in adults. *Annals of Internal Medicine* 94:758-762.

Szech LA, van der Horst C, Bartlett JA et al. (1999). Protease inhibitors are associated with a slowed progression HIV-associated nephropathy [abstract]. *Journal of the American Society of Nephrology* 10:116A.

Tammela T (1995). Postoperative urinary retention—Why the patient cannot void. *Scandinavian Journal of Urology and Nephrology* 29(Suppl 175):75-77.

Tan AU Jr, Cohen AH & Levine BS (1995). Renal amyloidosis in a drug abuser. *Journal of the American Society of Nephrology* 5:1653-1658.

Tashima KT, Horowitz JD & Rosen S (1997). Indinavir nephropathy [letter]. *New England Journal of Medicine* 336:138-140.

Thakur V, Godley C, Weed S et al. (1996). Case reports: Cocaine-associated accelerated hypertension and renal failure. *American Journal of the Medical Sciences* 312:295-298.

Tumlin JA, Sands JM & Someren A (1990). Hemolytic-uremic syndrome following "crack" cocaine inhalation. *American Journal of the Medical Sciences* 299:366-371.

Vamvakas S, Teschner M, Bahner U et al. (1998). Alcohol abuse: Potential role in electrolyte disturbances and kidney diseases. *Clinical Nephrology* 49:205-213.

van der Woude FK (2000). Cocaine use and kidney damage. *Nephrology Dialysis and Transplantation* 15:299-301.

Vanholder R, Sever MS, Erek E et al. (2000). Rhabdomyolysis. *Journal of the American Society of Nephrology* 11:1553-1561.

Viani RM, Dankner WM, Muelenaer PA et al. (1999). Resolution of HIV-associated nephrotic syndrome with highly active antiretroviral therapy delivered by gastrostomy tube. *Pediatrics* 104:1394-1396.

Volcy J, Nzerue CM, Oderinde A et al. (2000). Cocaine-induced acute renal failure, hemolysis, and thrombocytopenia mimicking thrombotic thrombocytopenic purpura. *American Journal of Kidney Diseases* 35:E3-E7.

Wali R, Drachenberg CI, Papadimitriou JC et al. (1998). HIV-associated nephropathy and response to highly-active antiretroviral therapy. *Lancet* 352:783-784.

Will AM (1981). Reversible renal damage due to glue sniffing. *British Medical Journal* 283:525-526.

Winston J, Klotman ME & Klotman PE (1999). HIV-associated nephropathy is a late, not early, manifestation of HIV-1 infection. *Kidney International* 55:1036-1040.

Woodrow G & Turney JH (1999) Ecstasy-induced vasculitis [letter]. *Nephrology Dialysis and Transplantation* 14:798.

Zager RA (1992). Combined mannitol and deferoxamine therapy for myoglobinuric renal injury and oxidant tubular stress. Mechanistic and therapeutic implications. *Journal of Clinical Investigation* 90:711-719.

Zager RA, Burkhart KM, Conrad DS et al. (1995). Iron, heme-oxygenase and glutathione. Effects on myoglobinuric proximal renal injury. *Kidney International* 48:1624-1634.

Gastrointestinal Disorders Related to Alcohol and Other Drug Use

Chapter 5

Paul S. Haber, M.D., FRACP

Alcohol abuse is associated with injury to all parts of the gastrointestinal tract. Several detailed reviews have been published (Lieber, 1992; Preedy & Watson, 1996; Bujanda, 2000). The gastric mucosa is a target for alcohol-related toxicity, but also contributes to the oxidation of alcohol. Pancreatitis is an important cause of morbidity and mortality related to alcohol abuse. Symptoms of intestinal dysfunction are common among alcoholics and include diarrhea and malabsorption.

GI PROBLEMS RELATED TO ALCOHOL

Parotids. Painless symmetrical enlargement of the parotid glands (termed sialosis or sialadenosis) is common in patients with alcoholic liver injury (Proctor & Shori, 1996). The triad of acinar cell hypertrophy, myoepithelial degeneration, and neural degeneration summarizes the abnormality. Salivary secretion is reduced in experimental animals given alcohol. These effects could contribute to progressive dental caries and poor oral mucosal health. The effect of alcohol abuse on salivary function in humans is controversial, with reports of increased, unaltered (Silver, Worner et al., 1986), and decreased salivary flow (Proctor & Shori, 1996).

Esophagus. Both acute and chronic alcohol consumption are associated with symptomatic gastroesophageal reflux disease (GERD). Reflux episodes were increased by 60 g of ethanol given to healthy nonalcoholic subjects with a meal (Kaufman & Kaye, 1978). These episodes were identified by measurement of esophageal pH for three hours after a standard meal, and most were asymptomatic. A number of mechanisms have been identified for these effects of alcohol. Direct application of 30% ethanol to the esophageal mucosa led to mucosal injury, but lower concentrations were less toxic. An acute dose of alcohol reduced lower esophageal sphincter pressure (Hogan, Viegas de Andrade et al., 1972) and reduced maximal lower esophageal sphincter pressure stimulated by a meal (Mayer, Grabowski et al., 1978).

Chronic alcohol abuse was associated with manometric abnormalities relevant to GERD; recovery was achieved with a month of abstinence (Silver, Worner et al., 1986; Keshavarzian, Iber et al., 1987). These abnormalities were found regardless of the presence or absence of peripheral neuropathy. The studies provide evidence to support the time-honored advice to reduce alcohol consumption in the presence of symptomatic GERD.

In an early series, alcohol abuse was found in most cases of Barrett's esophagus (Messian, Hermos et al., 1978). In more recent studies, alcohol abuse was not often found in asymptomatic Barrett's esophagus (Robertson, Mayberry et al., 1988), but was strongly associated with carcinoma (Gray, Donnelly et al., 1993).

GI Bleeding, Including Mallory-Weiss Syndrome. Upper gastrointestinal bleeding is very common among alcoholics. The most common cause is hemorrhagic gastritis, an acute mucosal lesion. Katz and colleagues (1976) reported acute gastric mucosal lesions in 36% of subjects, Mallory-Weiss tears in 27%, peptic ulcer in 21%, esophageal varices in 15%, duodenitis in 9%, and esophagitis in 7%. Variceal hemorrhage is a life-threatening event, with approximately 50% mortality for the first episode and about 25% for subsequent episodes.

Most cases of Mallory-Weiss syndrome are seen in alcoholics. The classic presentation involves vomiting followed by hematemesis associated with a tear at the cardioesophageal junction. However, this classic sequence of symptoms is not apparent in most cases (Graham & Schwartz, 1978). The amount of blood lost usually is minor and typically is not associated with a fall in hemoglobin or hemodynamic compromise, although life-threatening hemorrhage can occur. The lesion usually heals within 72 hours without specific treatment.

The management of upper gastrointestinal bleeding depends on its etiology and severity. Patients who may have bleeding should be referred to the emergency department without delay. The initial assessment focuses on hemodynamic stability (blood pressure, pulse, circulation, and hemoglobin level) and etiology (evidence is particularly sought for the presence of liver disease, with signs of portal hypertension such as splenomegaly). A large-bore intravenous catheter is placed, and fluids and blood are given as required. Immediate administration of acid suppression drugs has not been shown to consistently improve clinical outcomes; however, a recent report suggests that they may have a role in bleeding peptic ulcers that require endoscopic treatment (Lau, Sung et al., 2000). Endoscopy is performed as soon as practicable because the findings inform management and indicate the prognosis. Endoscopic signs of recent bleeding (such as adherent clot, visible vessel, and active bleeding) are associated with increased risk of recurrent bleeding. Evidence from several controlled trials shows that endoscopic therapy for actively bleeding lesions does limit recurrent bleeding, transfusion requirements, and the need for surgery (Rollhauser & Fleischer, 2000).

Mortality is increased in older adults, those with shock on presentation, those requiring large-volume transfusion, and those with serious intercurrent illness. Surgery is indicated for bleeding that cannot be controlled by endoscopic treatment, for recurrent hemorrhage, or when endoscopic treatment is not available.

Alcoholic Gastritis. Exposure of the gastric mucosa to 20% alcohol induces gastric mucosal injury. Lower concentrations are not toxic, whereas higher concentrations lead to extensive hemorrhagic injury (Konturek, Stachura et al., 1996). These lesions are characterized by subepithelial hemorrhages and epithelial erosions. Inflammatory cell infiltration is not a consistent feature.

The clinical syndrome of alcoholic gastritis has been surprisingly controversial despite considerable study (Feinman, Korsten et al., 1992; Konturek, Stachura et al., 1996). There is conflicting evidence concerning the role of alcohol abuse because of problems with the methodology of many early studies. In addition, most studies were performed before the importance of *Helicobacter pylori* and nonsteroidal anti-inflammatory drugs in the pathogenesis of gastritis was recognized. Brown and colleagues (1981) found that gastritis was not more common in patients with cirrhosis than in healthy control subjects. Uppal and colleagues (1991) showed that gastritis in the alcoholic was strongly associated with *H. pylori* infection, and that histological and symptomatic relief occurred after eradication of the organism, but not with abstinence from alcohol. These findings were confirmed by another group (Hauge, Persson et al., 1994). *H. pylori* infection was found to be equally common in subjects with alcohol abuse and in nonalcoholic controls (Hauge, Persson et al., 1994). Indeed, the presence of alcohol dehydrogenase activity in *H. pylori* organisms may limit this infection to alcohol drinkers, as exposure to alcohol leads to generation of acetaldehyde that can be bacteriocidal.

Healing of established ulcers is not retarded by moderate alcohol consumption (Battaglia, Di Mario et al., 1990). However, more severe alcohol abuse is associated with reduced medication compliance and delayed healing (Reynolds, 1989).

The clinical term "alcoholic gastritis" is nonspecific and often used to refer to a broad range of upper gastrointestinal symptoms experienced by alcoholics. It can be explained by various disorders, such as gastroesophageal reflux, peptic ulceration, fatty liver, alcoholic hepatitis, or alcoholic pancreatitis, to name a few. It has been proposed that, in the absence of peripheral disease, alcohol can directly induce vomiting through central stimulation of the chemoreceptor trigger zone in the area postrema of the floor of the fourth ventricle (Shen, 1985). In addition, bacterial overgrowth has been reported to be more common in alcoholics and also can contribute to upper abdominal symptoms and diarrhea (Hauge, Persson et al., 1997).

Given the uncertainty surrounding the etiologic role of alcohol abuse in gastritis and the broad range of potential explanations for these symptoms, it is appropriate to evaluate patients on an individual basis.

Alcoholic Pancreatitis. Alcoholic pancreatitis remains a major cause of morbidity among alcoholics. The incidence appears to have risen in the United States and internationally throughout the 20th century (Go & Everhart, 1994). Data from the United Kingdom confirm this trend and reveal a correlation between rising total community alcohol consumption and the number of hospital admissions for chronic pancreatitis (Johnson & Hosking, 1991). Within the past decade, total community alcohol consumption has fallen in several countries, and it is likely that the incidence of chronic pancreatitis will fall in parallel.

Definitions: The term "acute pancreatitis" refers to an acute inflammatory process of the pancreas, with variable involvement of other regional tissues or remote organ systems (Bradley, 1993). Chronic pancreatitis is characterized by chronic inflammation, glandular atrophy, and fibrosis. Clinically, it manifests as pain with exocrine or endocrine insufficiency. Older, ambiguous terms that no longer are used include "phlegmon," "infected pseudocyst," and "hemorrhagic pancreatitis." Terms that are retained include "acute fluid collections" (a collection lacking a defined wall, which is common early in the course of the disease and tends to regress spontaneously), "pseudocyst" (a collection of pancreatic juices enclosed by a connective tissue wall arising from disruption of pancreatic ducts and frequently communicating with the duct system), "pancreatic necrosis" (diffuse or focal areas of nonviable pancreatic parenchyma, typically associated with peripancreatic fat necrosis that can be sterile or infected), and "pancreatic abscess" (a circumscribed collection of pus in or near the pancreas after pancreatitis or pancreatic trauma).

Etiology: The most common associations of acute pancreatitis in Western societies are gallstones and alcohol abuse, which together account for approximately 75% of cases. Alcohol abuse is the most common cause of pancreatitis in communities where levels of alcohol consumption are high (Wilson, Korsten et al., 1989). Pancreatitis typically occurs in subjects who have consumed more than 100 g alcohol per day for at least five to 10 years; it rarely, if ever, follows an isolated alcoholic episode. However, once the disease is established, episodic heavy drinking often precipitates relapse and, in fact, relapses have been described after only 1 day of recurrent drinking. The causative link between alcohol abuse and pancreatitis for an individual patient is made on clinical grounds through a compatible history and exclusion of other etiologic factors.

Predisposing Factors: Only a minority (less than 5%) of heavy drinkers develop clinically evident pancreatic disease, although a postmortem study has found that pathologic changes in the pancreas are common among alcoholics (Pitchumoni, Glasser et al., 1984). Numerous investigators have attempted to account for individual susceptibility by studying associations between alcoholic pancreatitis and potential risk factors (reviewed by Haber, Wilson et al. [1995]). Investigators have focused on the amount, type, and pattern of alcohol consumption; genetic markers; diet (Wilson, Bernstein et al., 1985); hypertriglyceridemia (Haber, Wilson et al., 1994); tobacco consumption (Haber, Wilson et al., 1993); and pancreatic ischemia. The genetic markers that have been studied include blood groups, HLA phenotypes (Wilson, Gossat et al., 1984), alpha1-antitrypsin phenotypes (Haber, Wilson et al., 1991), cystic fibrosis genotypes (Norton, Apte et al., 1998a), cytochrome P4502E1 (CYP2E1) genotypes, and alcohol dehydrogenase isoenzyme genotypes. A number of these studies are difficult to interpret because of small sample sizes, inappropriate controls, and inconsistent findings between studies, so there is insufficient evidence to regard any of the cited factors as well established. As a result, individual susceptibility to this disease remains unexplained.

Other relatively common causes of pancreatitis that should be considered include gallstones, hypercalcemia of any cause, and severe hypertriglyceridemia. Pancreatitis is common among people with HIV, particularly in association with alcohol abuse (Dutta, Ting et al., 1997; Whitfield, Bechtel et al., 1997). Hypertriglyceridemia (>10 mmol/L [approximately 1000 mg/dL] with lipemic serum) of any cause is associated with recurrent attacks of pancreatitis (Greenberger, Hatch et al., 1966). Although alcohol abuse is a known cause of hypertriglyceridemia, most cases of alcoholic pancreatitis are not associated with marked hyperlipidemia (Toskes, 1990; Haber, Wilson et al., 1994).

Pathogenesis: Two important factors leading to tissue injury in pancreatitis of any cause are autodigestion and oxidant stress. Several lines of evidence indicate that activated digestive enzymes play an important role (Haber, Pirola et al., 1997). First, mutations of the cationic trypsinogen gene, which increases the pancreatic content of trypsin, underlie hereditary pancreatitis (Whitcomb, Gorry et al., 1996). This rare syndrome clinically resembles alcoholic pancreatitis. Second, activated digestive enzymes, which are found in both clinical and experimental pancreatitis, can produce cellular necrosis when instilled into pancreatic tissue. Finally, protease inhibitors reduce the incidence of post-endoscopic retrograde cholangiopancreatography (ERCP) and experimental pancreatitis.

Oxidant stress is characterized by the production of reactive oxygen species, which are atoms or molecules containing oxygen with an unpaired electron in the outer shell (free radicals). Free radicals are highly reactive and bind to lipids, proteins, and nucleic acids, leading to cellular injury (Freeman & Crapo, 1982). Free radicals are generated during experimental pancreatitis (Nonaka, Manabe et al., 1989) and can be formed by infiltrating leukocytes (Slater, 1984) or possibly within acinar cells through the metabolism of alcohol or xenobiotics by cytochrome P450 (Braganza, Scott et al., 1995). Measures that limit the effects of free radicals ameliorate pancreatitis in experimental models (Neuschwander-Tetri, 1992; Sanfey, 1985). The progression of the disease involves local inflammation and, when severe, systemic inflammation. A range of cytokines are involved, and they can be detected in blood and pancreatic tissue. These mediators of inflammation include chemokines that act at CCR1, platelet activating factor (PAF), and substance P (Saluja & Steer 1999). Inhibition of these mediators of inflammation has the potential to limit the progression of pancreatitis and to prevent serious complications or death, but it cannot prevent the initial attack.

The initiation of alcoholic pancreatitis appears to involve both autodigestion and oxidant stress. Alcohol administration has been reported to increase the tone of the sphincter of Oddi (Pirola, 1966) and to inhibit pancreatic secretion (Hajnal, Flores et al., 1990). In experimental animals, alcohol intake impairs the stability of zymogen granules and lysosomes, thereby increasing the possibility of co-localization of digestive enzymes and lysosomal enzymes (Norton & Wilson, 1996). Lysosomal enzymes (particu-

larly cathepsin B) are capable of activating trypsinogen that, in turn, can activate other digestive enzyme precursors, resulting in a cascade of autodigestion. Ethanol consumption has been shown to increase the pancreatic content of the major alcohol-metabolizing isoform of cytochrome P450 (CYP2E1) and to increase tissue markers of oxidant stress (Norton, Apte et al., 1998b).

Diagnosis: A confident diagnosis of pancreatitis often can be made on the basis of an attack of severe abdominal pain and tenderness, with elevation of the serum amylase more than three times the upper limit of normal and with imaging studies suggestive of inflammation in and around the pancreas. Gallstones should be excluded by ultrasound examination. In patients with a negative ultrasound, serum alkaline phosphatase or transaminase levels that are twice the normal limit suggest associated gallstones that can be detected by repeat ultrasonography or ERCP (Venu, Geenen et al., 1983; Goodman, Neoptolemos et al., 1985). Magnetic resonance cholangiography is becoming widely used to diagnose gallstones (Soto, Barish et al., 1996).

The diagnosis of alcoholic pancreatitis occasionally is difficult. Amylase testing is useful in establishing the presence of acute pancreatitis, but peak levels do not correlate well with the severity of the disease. Moreover, the amylase level does not rise significantly in approximately 10% of patients with acute pancreatitis, including many with alcoholic pancreatitis (Spechler, Dalton et al., 1983) or in whom the presentation is delayed. Determination of serum lipase, which remains elevated longer than serum amylase, can be helpful. A report that an increased lipase/amylase ratio was specific for alcohol-induced pancreatitis (Gumaste, Dave et al., 1991) has not been confirmed (Pezzilli, 1993; King, 1995). Amylase levels in the range found in acute pancreatitis can occur in other gastrointestinal disorders, including perforated peptic ulcer and ischemic bowel. Estimation of serum lipase levels does not help distinguish these disorders from pancreatitis, because the source of the amylase (intestinal fluid) also contains lipase. In renal failure, serum amylase levels occasionally are strikingly elevated (Tsianos, Dardamanis et al., 1994).

Salivary gland disease with hyperamylasemia occurs in alcoholics and can be differentiated by fractionation of serum amylase and investigation of the salivary glands. Macroamylasemia is a condition in which amylase forms large complexes with an abnormal serum protein. The disorder usually is found coincidentally in a patient with very high amylase levels but without abdominal pain; it is differentiated from pancreatitis by a normal serum lipase and the absence of amylase in the urine. Minor elevations of the serum amylase (less than three-fold) may be the product of many disorders, including administration of morphine with secondary spasm of the sphincter of Oddi. Painless pancreatitis can occur, usually in the setting of a comatose or postoperative patient in whom pain is not appreciated. In such cases, the diagnosis rests on other clinical and laboratory features.

Assessment of Severity: A number of clinical and laboratory criteria have been developed to identify patients at risk of complications, so that they can be treated more intensively at an earlier stage. The contrast-enhanced computed tomography (CT) scan now is widely performed to detect pancreatic necrosis and complications of severe pancreatitis, such as fluid collections, pseudocysts, and abscesses (Kivisaari, Somer et al., 1983). Some concern has been raised about possible adverse effects of contrast-enhanced CT scanning (McMenamin & Gates, 1996). Studies of intravenous contrast in experimental animals have yielded conflicting findings (Foitzik, Bassi et al., 1994; Kaiser, Grady et al., 1995; Schmidt, Hotz et al., 1995), so caution in the unrestricted use of contrast-enhanced CT scans appears warranted. CT scanning without contrast can detect most diagnostic features of pancreatitis and is widely used.

Treatment: Severe cases, particularly those associated with respiratory or renal failure, require treatment in an intensive care unit. Initially, patients are treated with bed rest, analgesics, intravenous fluids, and fasting. Traditionally, meperidine (Demerol®) has been the preferred analgesic, because morphine has a greater tendency to contract the sphincter of Oddi (Thune, Baker et al., 1990), which can exacerbate pancreatitis. More recent studies have revealed that meperidine is a poor analgesic and do not support the concerns raised about morphine. Intravenous fluids are given to restore vascular volume and renal perfusion.

Various therapeutic approaches have been evaluated in acute pancreatitis. Treatments to reduce pancreatic secretion aim to reduce pressure in the pancreatic duct and, consequently, to reduce the block in exocytosis from pancreatic acinar cells. However, the inflamed pancreas already secretes very little (Mitchell, Playforth et al., 1983), and no beneficial effect has been found for measures designed to reduce pancreatic secretion, including nasogastric suction (Sarr, Sanfey et al., 1986), cimetidine (Tagamet®), anticholinergics, glucagon, calcitonin (Calcimar®) (Leach, Gorelick

et al., 1992), and the somatostatin analog octreotide (Sandostatin®) (McKay, Imrie et al., 1993). These results notwithstanding, patients are initially fasted, partly for symptomatic reasons, but also because early refeeding seems to cause clinical relapse. Protease inhibitors can limit the damage done by activated digestive enzymes. In clinical practice, it may be impossible to commence treatment early enough in the attack of pancreatitis for protease inhibitors to be effective. Aprotinin (Trasylol®) has proved ineffective in clinical practice despite a strong theoretical rationale and good results in experimental pancreatitis. Infusion of the protease inhibitor gabexate has been reported to reduce the incidence of post-ERCP pancreatitis (Cavallini, Tittobello et al., 1996).

Peritoneal lavage might improve the outcome by removing toxic inflammatory products from the peritoneum, but the results of controlled studies have been conflicting (Stone & Fabian, 1980; Mayer, McMahon et al., 1985). New approaches that may prove more effective include extending lavage to seven days rather than the standard two days (Ranson & Berman, 1990) and retroperitoneal lavage using operatively placed cannulae (Pederzoli, Bassi et al., 1990).

Antibiotics have not proved beneficial for unselected cases of acute pancreatitis for which the prognosis already is excellent (Bradley, 1989). However, in severe pancreatitis, two controlled trials of prophylactic antibiotic therapy with imipenem (Primaxin®) (Pederzoli, Bassi et al., 1993) or a combination of ceftazidime (Ceftaz®), amikacin (Amikin®), and metronidazole (Flagyl®) (Delcenserie, Yzet et al., 1996), demonstrated a significant reduction in septic episodes. Nevertheless, mortality rates and the need for surgery were not altered. In one small controlled study of antioxidant therapy (allopurinol [Lopurin®] or dimethyl sulfoxide given by enema), significant pain relief was achieved in patients with an acute attack of alcoholic pancreatitis (Salim, 1991). A preliminary study found that a combination of intravenous antioxidants improved the survival of six patients with severe acute pancreatitis (Whitely, Scott et al., 1993). These small studies require confirmation before antioxidant therapy can be recommended for routine use in acute pancreatitis.

In two randomized controlled studies, ERCP with endoscopic sphincterotomy has been shown to reduce the morbidity of patients with unremitting severe gallstone pancreatitis (Neoptolemos, Carr-Locke et al., 1988; Fan, Lai et al., 1993). The major benefit appears to be control of biliary sepsis (Fan, Lai et al., 1993). If stones are demonstrated in the common bile duct, a sphincterotomy should be performed and the stones removed. The main indication for surgery is necrotizing pancreatitis (McFadden & Reber, 1994) because infected necrosis is associated with high rates of morbidity and mortality (Beger, Buchler et al., 1988) and requires surgical debridement followed by postoperative lavage (Beger, Buchler et al., 1988; Ranson & Berman, 1990). By contrast, sterile necrosis often improves with conservative therapy alone (Bradley & Allen, 1991). It has been reported that infected necrosis can be safely identified by fine-needle aspiration with Gram stain and culture (Gerzof, Banks et al., 1987); however, the utility of this approach in the management of severe necrotizing pancreatitis has not been confirmed by randomized controlled trials. The decision to operate is more often based on the clinical condition of the patient.

Pancreatic abscess carries a very high mortality rate and is an absolute indication for drainage by open surgery or percutaneous techniques. In fulminant cases, multiple procedures may be required. Small pseudocysts can resolve spontaneously, but large or symptomatic ones usually require treatment. Endoscopic, percutaneous, and operative techniques have been described to drain persisting pseudocysts (Maule & Reber, 1993).

Treatment of Chronic Pancreatitis: The principal problem usually is pain and, thus, can be very difficult to manage. Complete abstinence from alcohol is essential to minimize progression of the disease; it also can help to control pain. Reassurance that the disorder is benign with a tendency to slowly remit is helpful. Non-narcotic analgesia may suffice, but opioids often are required and should not be unreasonably withheld. Antidepressants should be tried. Celiac plexus injection helps about 60% of patients, but pain can recur. The procedure is not often performed because of its limited efficacy, frequent recurrence, and significant complications.

Pancreatic enzyme supplements have been evaluated for the treatment of pain, but the evidence is mixed. A trial of one month is sufficient to determine whether this treatment works in practice. Octreotide is not effective. Endoscopic approaches to dilate pancreatic duct strictures and remove calculi have been developed, although the relationship between pancreatic duct obstruction and pain is not clear. Controlled trials of this therapy in chronic pancreatitis are difficult and have not yet been performed. Surgery has been used for refractory cases, but, again, there are no controlled trials demonstrating efficacy. The Whipple procedure or modified Whipple procedure is the most commonly performed. The Puestow procedure (lateral pancreatico-jejunostomy) involves decompression of a dilated pancreatic duct and side-to-side anastomosis onto a roux-en-Y loop of the jejunum. Distal pancreatectomy is not often performed.

Exocrine failure is treated by dietary modification and pancreatic enzyme replacement. Reduction of dietary fat intake reduces steatorrhea. Pancreatic enzymes are required with each meal and snack. The newer preparations are more potent and are preferred. Enteric-coated microsphere preparations release enzymes only in the duodenum, thereby reducing irreversible inactivation of lipase by gastric acid. Histamine-2 receptor antagonists or proton pump inhibitors also limit lipase inactivation. Normalization of fecal fat levels does not typically occur. Diabetes mellitus is treated with dietary modification, treatment of malabsorption, and specific therapy. Some patients respond to oral hypoglycemic agents, but most require insulin. The patient is susceptible to hypoglycemia because of loss of both insulin and glucagon secretion. Despite earlier reports, long-term surviving patients with this form of diabetes are prone to diabetic complications.

Small Intestine. Diarrhea is common among those who abuse alcohol, both acutely and chronically. Multiple factors contribute to this complaint, including altered motility, permeability, and nutritional disorders. Small intestinal mucosal injury can occur after acute or chronic administration of alcohol. Perfusion of the hamster jejunum with 4.8% ethanol caused separation of the tip of the villus epithelium, forming blebs (Beck, 1996). These blebs can rupture, leading to denudement of the epithelium. The villus core contracts and loses height within 1 minute of ethanol exposure. This effect is independent of any action on the microcirculation (Dinda, Buell et al., 1994) and can be mediated by recruitment of leukocytes (Dinda, Kossev et al., 1996), leading to release of histamine from mast cells and oxidant stress (Dinda, Buell et al., 1994).

Mucosal blood flow is acutely increased, with increased endothelial permeability (Beck, 1996). Acute administration of alcohol leads to increased gut permeability, resulting both in abnormal absorption of luminal content (such as endotoxin, which contributes to the pathogenesis of alcoholic liver disease; see Chapter 3) and abnormal leakage of mucosal contents (such as albumin). Ethanol inhibits absorption of actively transported sugars, dipeptides, and amino acids. Many defects in absorption have been reported in alcoholics, involving water (Krasner, Carmichael et al.,

1976; Krasner, Cochran et al., 1976), carbohydrate, lipid, vitamins (notably thiamine and folate), and minerals (calcium, iron, zinc, and selenium) (Beck, 1996).

Ethanol can exacerbate lactase deficiency, especially in non-Caucasians (Perlow, Baraona et al., 1977). Folate deficiency, which is common among alcoholics, causes intestinal injury, leading to malabsorption and diarrhea and further loss of folate (also see Chapter 12).

Colon. Portal hypertension can manifest uncommonly with hemorrhoids and rarely with colonic varices. Colonic varices appear as filling defects on barium enema and can occur in any part of the colon, most commonly in the rectum (Feinman, Korsten et al., 1992). Alcohol has been reported to cause nonulcerative inflammatory changes in human colonic epithelium (Brozinsky, Fani et al., 1978). These changes resolved during a two-week period of abstinence. They were not explained by folate deficiency, as folate levels were normal in 10 of 11 subjects. This form of colitis has the potential to contribute to diarrhea but is not usually recognized clinically, as pathology elsewhere in the gut tends to dominate the clinical picture.

Inappropriate alcohol enema was reported to cause a chemical colitis (Herrerias, Muniain et al., 1983), resulting from a toxic effect similar to the direct toxicity of alcohol on the gastric mucosa.

Alcohol abuse is a recognized risk factor for colorectal cancer. Finally, alcohol consumption may have at least one beneficial effect on the colon, in that (in one study) it has been linked to a reduced incidence of ulcerative colitis (Boyko, Perera et al., 1989).

ALCOHOL AND GI CANCER

Alcohol abuse is a recognized risk factor for several gastrointestinal neoplasms, including tumors of the tongue, mouth, pharynx, larynx, esophagus, stomach, pancreas, colon, and liver (Longnecker, 1995; Ringborg, 1998; Franceschi, 1999). Alcohol abuse repeatedly has been associated with an increased incidence of esophageal (and oropharyngeal) cancer, especially in those who also smoke. Blot and colleagues (1988) reported a 5.8-fold increased risk among drinkers, a 7.4-fold increased risk among smokers, and a 38-fold increased risk among those who both drank and smoked.

In general, experimental studies have not shown that alcohol is itself a complete carcinogen. Rather, ethanol is a co-carcinogen that increases the cancer risk after exposure to another compound. The effect of ethanol can occur at the initiation, induction, or progression stages of tumor development. For example, alcohol-fed rats given N-nitrosomethylbenzylamine developed more esophageal tumors than control rats (Mufti, Becker et al., 1989). Several mechanisms may contribute to this co-carcinogenic effect (Mufti, 1996): ethanol-induced induction of CYP 2E1 increases carcinogen activation, potentiated oxidant stress, diminishes DNA repair, and suppresses immune responses and nutritional depletion (as in folate deficiency).

With respect to hepatocellular carcinoma (HCC), alcohol abuse long has been recognized as a predisposing factor. Alcohol might contribute to carcinogenesis by mechanisms considered for other tissues and listed earlier, but experimental evidence is insufficient to conclude that alcohol is a complete hepatic carcinogen (Misslebeck & Campbell, 1985; Farber, 1996). Most patients are cirrhotic, and cirrhosis is known to predispose to HCC. Many patients have other risk factors for HCC, such as chronic hepatitis B or C or exposure to chemical carcinogens such as aflatoxins (Farber, 1996). A small number of cases of HCC are associated with alcohol abuse without cirrhosis or other contributing factors (Lieber, Seitz et al., 1979), but it is not clear that this number is greater than would be expected by chance alone (Bassendine, 1986).

GI SYMPTOMS ASSOCIATED WITH ABUSE OF PRESCRIBED DRUGS

The most frequently abused medications that affect the gastrointestinal system are opiates, laxatives, and anticholinergics.

Opiates. Opiates act on gut function in a complex fashion that involves all three receptor classes in the brain, spinal cord, and enteric nervous systems. Low doses act at enteric nervous system sites, while higher doses also act within the central nervous system. Opiates alter both motility and electrolyte absorption, leading to constipation that can be severe, particularly in older adults. Opiates increase absorption of chloride, both by increasing chloride transport and by reducing chloride secretion in response to various secretogogues (McKay, Linaker et al., 1981, 1982). These effects, in turn, increase passive water absorption and reduce colonic volume, exacerbating the tendency to constipation. The motility effects are more prominent for the clinically available opioids. Opioids decrease the frequency of contractions in and propulsion along the small bowel and colon (Williams, Bihm et al., 1997). Classically, chronic opiate use was thought not to induce tolerance to gut motility; however, tolerance and withdrawal were demonstrated in an experimental animal model (Williams, Bihm et al., 1997). Tolerance to the gastrointestinal motility effects took longer to develop than to the nociceptive effects, and tolerance to the inhibitory effects developed more slowly than that to the excitatory effects. The mechanism(s) by which tissues become tolerant to the effects of opioids have been extensively studied within the central nervous system (Williams, Christie et al., 2001), but much less is known about the gut effects, which are determined by both central and peripheral opioid actions.

Among patients on methadone maintenance, constipation is common and tends to be worse early in treatment (Yaffe, Strelinger et al., 1973; Langrod, Lowinson et al., 1981). The high prevalence of persisting constipation suggests that tolerance to the gut effects of opiates occurs only to a limited extent. In one study, 58% of subjects in methadone maintenance experienced some degree of constipation and 10% had severe problems (Yuan, Foss et al., 1998). Fecal impaction and even stercoral perforation have been described (Haley, Long et al., 1998). Constipation usually responds to increased fluid intake and fiber supplementation to correct for poor dietary intake. Laxatives are not often required, but if they are, lactulose is the laxative of choice.

Narcotic bowel syndrome is characterized by a picture similar to intestinal pseudo-obstruction (Rogers & Cerda, 1989). This syndrome responds to withdrawal of opioids and administration of the alpha$_2$-agonist clonidine (Sandgren, McPhee et al., 1984). Methylnaltrexone, a parenterally active peripheral opioid receptor antagonist, recently was reported to relieve constipation without precipitating opioid withdrawal (Yuan, Foss et al., 2000).

Laxatives. Surreptitious laxative abuse is among the more common causes for unexplained chronic diarrhea. It represents an intriguing form of addictive disorder but is rare and typically is observed in persons who do not have other addictive disorders. Such patients usually are seen by family physicians and gastroenterologists. Some cases are associated with bulimia, while others tend to occur in older women. The disorder can be viewed as a form of Munchausen's syndrome. The diagnosis rests on identification of laxatives by stool alkalinization, osmolality studies, or a bag search in the hospital (Fine, 1998).

Anticholinergics. In high doses, anticholinergic drugs alter mood, and occasionally they are abused. For example, clonidine (Catapres®) prescribed for opioid withdrawal has been abused. Patients develop marked constipation and abdominal pain, as well as dry mouth and blurred vision. In the author's experience, patients who have had problems with drug abuse and addiction have welcomed an explanation of their symptoms and participated in structured withdrawal.

EFFECTS OF TOBACCO ON GI FUNCTION

Tobacco use is associated with gastroesophageal reflux, peptic ulceration, and gastrointestinal malignancy, but it appears to protect against ulcerative colitis.

Gastroesophageal Reflux. Smoking has been linked to exacerbations of reflux symptoms, and cessation of smoking is one of the lifestyle changes traditionally recommended in the treatment of reflux (Pandolfino & Kahrilas, 2000). Nicotine has been shown to reduce lower esophageal sphincter pressure and to promote gastroesophageal reflux in response to straining during coughing and deep breathing (Kahrilas & Gupta, 1990). Smokers have been shown to have delayed acid clearance from the esophagus (Kahrilas & Gupta, 1989), but not all studies have yielded consistent findings. For example, one recent study found that smoking did not influence basal lower esophageal sphincter pressure or esophageal motility (Bhandarkar, Shah et al., 2000). At a practical level, smoking cessation is difficult to achieve and has not been shown to induce remission of reflux or healing of esophagitis. From the foregoing, it is clear that smoking contributes to reflux, but smoking cessation alone is not sufficient treatment. It is reasonable to advise patients with GERD to quit smoking on the basis of its association with reflux, with the expectation that GERD might respond favorably to quitting, in addition to the myriad other health benefits.

Peptic Ulceration. Considerable evidence shows that smoking is involved with peptic ulcer. Smokers' risk of ulcer increases with the number of cigarettes smoked. Heavy smoking is associated with delayed ulcer healing, and the risk of recurrence is increased in smokers (Sonnenberg, Muller-Lissner et al., 1981; Korman, Hansky et al., 1983). Smoking also increases the risk of complications from peptic ulcer (Piper, McIntosh et al., 1985). Finally, the overall ulcer-related mortality is increased in smokers compared with nonsmokers (Ross, Smith et al., 1982; Kurata, Elashoff et al., 1986). The mechanism by which smoking exacerbates peptic ulcer disease remains unclear.

Pancreatic Disease. Findings are inconsistent about the relationship between smoking and pancreatitis

(Chowdhury & Rayford, 2000). In general, most alcoholics smoke, so it has been difficult to segregate these two variables, so both are difficult to measure and rely heavily on self-report. The most appropriate comparison is between a group with alcoholic pancreatitis and a control group who drank at least as much alcohol but did not develop pancreatitis. The only study using this methodology found no association with smoking (Haber, Wilson et al., 1993). Studies that found positive associations used less stringent methods (Yen, Hsieh et al., 1982; Cavallini, Talamini et al., 1994).

Evidence from a number of countries provides a clear link between smoking and pancreatic cancer. Studies have consistently found a moderately increased risk (about three-fold) of pancreatic cancer among smokers (Talamini, Bassi et al., 1999; Chowdhury & Rayford, 2000).

Inflammatory Bowel Disease. A curious relationship exists between smoking and inflammatory bowel disease. Smoking consistently has been shown to increase the risk of Crohn's disease, but to decrease the risk of ulcerative colitis (Rubin & Hanauer, 2000), as well as the severity of established ulcerative colitis. Less toxic approaches to this form of therapy have been sought and include topical colonic administration of nicotine. Such approaches remain experimental at this time (Sandborn, 1999).

GI Malignancy. Smoking has been strongly linked to cancers of the upper digestive tract and pancreas, as discussed earlier. The link between smoking and stomach cancer is weaker, but is present in most studies (Neugut, Hayek et al., 1996).

REFERENCES

Bassendine MF (1986). Alcohol—A major risk factor for hepatocellular carcinoma? *Journal of Hepatology* 2(3):513-519.

Battaglia B, Di Mario F, Dotto P et al. (1990). Alcohol intake and acute duodenal ulcer healing. *American Journal of Gastroenterology* 85(9):1198-1199.

Beck IT (1996). Small bowel injury by ethanol. In VR Preddy & RR Watson (eds.) *Alcohol and the Gastrointestinal Tract.* Boca Raton, FL: CRC Press, 163-202.

Beger HG, Buchler M, Bittner R et al. (1988). Necrosectomy and postoperative local lavage in necrotizing pancreatitis. *British Journal of Surgery* 75(3):207-212.

Bhandarkar PV, Shah SK, Meshram M et al. (2000). Effect of acute and long-term oral tobacco use on oesophageal motility. *Journal of Gastroenterology and Hepatology* 15(9):1018-1021.

Blot WJ, McLaughlin JK, Winn DM et al. (1988). Smoking and drinking in relation to oral and pharyngeal cancer. *Cancer Research* 48(11):3282-3287.

Boyko EJ, Perera DR, Koepsell TD et al. (1989). Coffee and alcohol use and the risk of ulcerative colitis. *American Journal of Gastroenterology* 84(5):530-534.

Bradley EL 3rd (1989). Antibiotics in acute pancreatitis. Current status and future directions. *American Journal of Surgery* 158(5):472-478.

Bradley EL 3rd (1993). A clinically based classification system for acute pancreatitis. Summary of the International Symposium on Acute Pancreatitis, Atlanta, Ga, September 11-13, 1992. *Archives of Surgery* 128(5):586-90.

Bradley EL 3rd & Allen K (1991). A prospective longitudinal study of observation versus surgical intervention in the management of necrotizing pancreatitis. *American Journal of Surgery* 161(1):19-25.

Braganza JM, Scott P, Bilton D et al. (1995). Evidence for early oxidative stress in acute pancreatitis. Clues for correction. *International Journal of Pancreatology* 17(1):69-81.

Brown RC, Hardy GJ, Temperley JM et al. (1981). Gastritis and cirrhosis—No association. *Journal of Clinical Pathology* 34(7):744-748.

Brozinsky S, Fani K, Grosberg SJ et al. (1978). Alcohol ingestion-induced changes in the human rectal mucosa: Light and electron microscopic studies. *Diseases of the Colon and Rectum* 21(5):329-335.

Bujanda L (2000). The effects of alcohol consumption upon the gastrointestinal tract. *American Journal of Gastroenterology* 95(12):3374-3382.

Cavallini G, Talamini G, Vaona B et al. (1994). Effect of alcohol and smoking on pancreatic lithogenesis in the course of chronic pancreatitis. *Pancreas* 9(1):42-46.

Cavallini G, Tittobello A, Frulloni L et al. (1996). Gabexate for the prevention of pancreatic damage related to endoscopic retrograde cholangiopancreatography. Gabexate in digestive endoscopy—Italian Group. *New England Journal of Medicine* 335(13):919-923.

Chowdhury P & Rayford PL (2000). Smoking and pancreatic disorders. *European Journal of Gastroenterology and Hepatology* 12(8):869-877.

Delcenserie R, Yzet T & Ducroix JP (1996). Prophylactic antibiotics in treatment of severe acute alcoholic pancreatitis. *Pancreas* 13(2):198-201.

Dinda PK, Buell MG, Morris O et al. (1994). Studies on ethanol-induced subepithelial fluid accumulation and jejunal villus bleb formation. An in vitro video microscopic approach. *Canadian Journal of Physiology and Pharmacology* 72(10):1186-1192.

Dinda PK, Kossev P, Beck IT et al. (1996). Role of xanthine oxidase-derived oxidants and leukocytes in ethanol-induced jejunal mucosal injury. *Digestive Diseases and Sciences* 41(12):2461-2470.

Dutta SK, Ting CD & Lai LL (1997). Study of prevalence, severity, and etiological factors associated with acute pancreatitis in patients infected with human immunodeficiency virus. *American Journal of Gastroenterology* 92(11):2044-2048.

Fan ST, Lai EC, Mok FP et al. (1993). Early treatment of acute biliary pancreatitis by endoscopic papillotomy. *New England Journal of Medicine* 328(4):228-232.

Farber E (1996). Alcohol and other chemicals in the development of hepatocellular carcinoma. *Clinics in Laboratory Medicine* 16(2):377-394.

Feinman L, Korsten MA et al. (1992). Alcohol and the digestive tract. In CS Lieber *Medical and Nutritional Complications of Alcoholism.* New York, NY: Plenum Publishing, 307-340.

Fine KD (1998). Diarrhea. In M Feldman, MH Sleisenger & BF Scharschmidt (eds.) *Sleisenger & Fordtran's Gastrointestinal and Liver Disease.* Philadelphia, PA: W.B. Saunders, 128-152.

Foitzik T, Bassi DG, Schmidt J et al. (1994). Intravenous contrast medium accentuates the severity of acute necrotizing pancreatitis in the rat. *Gastroenterology* 106(1):207-214.

Franceschi S (1999). Alcohol and cancer. *Advances in Experimental Medicine and Biology* 472:43-49.

Freeman BA & Crapo JD (1982). Biology of disease: Free radicals and tissue injury. *Laboratory Investigation* 47(5):412-426.

Gerzof SG, Banks PA, Robbins AH et al. (1987). Early diagnosis of pancreatic infection by computed tomography-guided aspiration. *Gastroenterology* 93(6):1315-1320.

Go VLW & Everhart JE (1994). Pancreatitis. In JE Everhart (ed.) *Digestive Diseases in the United States: Epidemiology and Impact.* Washington, DC: NIDDK, National Institutes of Health, 615-646.

Goodman AJ, Neoptolemos JP, Carr-Locke DL et al. (1985). Detection of gall stones after acute pancreatitis. *Gut* 26(2):125-132.

Graham DY & Schwartz JT (1978). The spectrum of the Mallory-Weiss tear. *Medicine* (Baltimore) 57(4):307-318.

Gray MR, Donnelly RJ & Kingsnorth AN (1993). The role of smoking and alcohol in metaplasia and cancer risk in Barrett's columnar lined oesophagus. *Gut* 34(6):727-731.

Greenberger N, Hatch FT, Drummey GD et al. (1966). Pancreatitis and hyperlipemia: A study of serum lipid alterations in 25 patients with acute pancreatitis. *Medicine* 45:161-174.

Gumaste VV, Dave PB, Weissman D et al. (1991). Lipase/amylase ratio. A new index that distinguishes acute episodes of alcoholic from nonalcoholic acute pancreatitis. *Gastroenterology* 101(5):1361-1366.

Haber P, Wilson J, Apte M et al. (1995). Individual susceptibility to alcoholic pancreatitis: Still an enigma. *Journal of Laboratory and Clinical Medicine* 125:305-312.

Haber PS, Pirola RC & Wilson JS (1997). Clinical update: Management of acute pancreatitis. *Journal of Gastroenterology and Hepatology* 12(3):189-197.

Haber PS, Wilson JS & Pirola RC (1993). Smoking and alcoholic pancreatitis. *Pancreas* 8(5):568-572.

Haber PS, Wilson JS, Apte MV et al. (1994). Lipid intolerance does not account for susceptibility to alcoholic and gallstone pancreatitis. *Gastroenterology* 106(3):742-748.

Haber PS, Wilson JS, McGarity BH et al. (1991). Alpha 1 antitrypsin phenotypes and alcoholic pancreatitis. *Gut* 32(8):945-948.

Hajnal F, Flores MC, Radley S et al. (1990). Effects of alcohol and alcoholic beverages on meal-stimulated pancreatic secretion in humans. *Gastroenterology* 98(1):191-196.

Haley TD, Long C & Mann BD (1998). Stercoral perforation of the colon. A complication of methadone maintenance. *Journal of Substance Abuse Treatment* 15(5):443-444.

Hauge T, Persson J & Danielsson D (1997). Mucosal bacterial growth in the upper gastrointestinal tract in alcoholics (heavy drinkers). *Digestion* 58(6):591-595.

Hauge T, Persson J & Kjerstadius T (1994). Helicobacter pylori, active chronic antral gastritis, and gastrointestinal symptoms in alcoholics. *Alcoholism: Clinical & Experimental Research* 18(4):886-888.

Herrerias JM, Muniain MA, Sanchez S et al. (1983). Alcohol-induced colitis. *Endoscopy* 15(3):121-122.

Hogan WJ, Viegas de Andrade SR & Winship DH (1972). Ethanol-induced acute esophageal motor dysfunction. *Journal of Applied Physiology* 32(6):755-760.

Johnson CD & Hosking S (1991). National statistics for diet, alcohol consumption, and chronic pancreatitis in England and Wales, 1960-88. *Gut* 32(11):1401-1405.

Kahrilas PJ & Gupta RR (1989). The effect of cigarette smoking on salivation and esophageal acid clearance. *Journal of Laboratory and Clinical Medicine* 114(4):431-438.

Kahrilas PJ & Gupta RR (1990). Mechanisms of acid reflux associated with cigarette smoking. *Gut* 31(1):4-10.

Kaiser AM, Grady T, Gerdes D et al. (1995). Intravenous contrast medium does not increase the severity of acute necrotizing pancreatitis in the opossum. *Digestive Diseases and Sciences* 40(7):1547-1553.

Katz D, Pitchumoni CS, Thomas E et al. (1976). The endoscopic diagnosis of upper-gastrointestinal hemorrhage. Changing concepts of etiology and management. *American Journal of Digestive Diseases* 21(2):182-189.

Kaufman SE & Kaye MD (1978). Induction of gastro-oesophageal reflux by alcohol. *Gut* 19(4):336-338.

Keshavarzian A, Iber FL & Ferguson Y (1987). Esophageal manometry and radionuclide emptying in chronic alcoholics. *Gastroenterology* 92(3):651-657.

King LA, Seelig CB & Ranney JE (1995). The lipase to amylase ratio in actue pancreatitis. *American Journal of Gastroenterology* 90(1):67-69.

Kivisaari L, Somer K, Standertskjold-Nordenstam CG et al. (1983). Early detection of acute fulminant pancreatitis by contrast-enhanced computed tomography. *Scandinavian Journal of Gastroenterology* 18(1):39-41.

Konturek SJ, Stachura J et al. (1996). Gastric cytoprotection and adaptation to ethanol. In VR Preedy & RR Watson (eds.) *Alcohol and the Gastrointestinal Tract.* Boca Raton, FL: CRC Press, 123-141.

Korman MG, Hansky J, Eaves ER et al. (1983). Influence of cigarette smoking on healing and relapse in duodenal ulcer disease. *Gastroenterology* 85(4):871-874.

Krasner N, Carmichael HA, Russell RI et al. (1976). Alcohol and absorption from the small intestine. 2. Effect of ethanol on ATP and ATPase activities in guinea-pig jejunum. *Gut* 17(4):249-251.

Krasner N, Cochran KM, Russell RI et al. (1976). Alcohol and absorption from the small intestine. 1. Impairment of absorption from the small intestine in alcoholics. *Gut* 17(4):245-248.

Kurata JH, Elashoff JD, Nogawa AN et al. (1986). Sex and smoking differences in duodenal ulcer mortality. *American Journal of Public Health* 76(6):700-702.

Langrod J, Lowinson J & Ruiz P (1981). Methadone treatment and physical complaints: A clinical analysis. *International Journal of Addiction* 16(5):947-952.

Lau JY, Sung JJ & Lee KK (2000). Effect of intravenous omeprazole on recurrent bleeding after endoscopic treatment of bleeding peptic ulcers. *New England Journal of Medicine* 343(5):310-316.

Leach S, Gorelick FS & Modlin IM (1992). New perspectives on acute pancreatitis. *Scandinavian Journal of Gastroenterolgy* 27:29-38.

Lieber CS, ed. (1992). *Medical and Nutritional Complications of Alcoholism.* New York, NY: Plenum Publishing.

Lieber CS, Seitz HK, Garro AJ et al. (1979). Alcohol-related diseases and carcinogenesis. *Cancer Research* 39(7 Pt 2):2863-2886.

Longnecker MP (1995). Alcohol consumption and risk of cancer in humans: An overview. *Alcohol* 12(2):87-96.

Maule W & Reber HA (1993). Diagnosis and management of pancreatic pseudocysts, pancreatic ascites, and pancreatic fistulas. *The Pancreas: Biology, Pathobiology, and Disease, 2nd Edition*. New York, NY: Raven Press, 741-751.

Mayer AD, McMahon MJ, Corfield AP et al. (1985). Controlled clinical trial of peritoneal lavage for the treatment of severe acute pancreatitis. *New England Journal of Medicine* 312(7):399-404.

Mayer EM, Grabowski CJ & Fisher RS (1978). Effects of graded doses of alcohol upon esophageal motor function. *Gastroenterology* 75(6):1133-1136.

McFadden DW & Reber HA (1994). Indications for surgery in severe acute pancreatitis. *International Journal of Pancreatology* 15(2):83-90.

McKay CJ, Imrie CW & Baxter JN (1993). Somatostatin and somatostatin analogues—Are they indicated in the management of acute pancreatitis? *Gut* 34(11):1622-1626.

McKay JS, Linaker BC, Higgs NB et al. (1982). Studies of the antisecretory activity of morphine in rabbit ileum in vitro. *Gastroenterology* 82(2):243-247.

McKay JS, Linaker BD & Turnberg LA (1981). Influence of opiates on ion transport across rabbit ileal mucosa. *Gastroenterology* 80(2):279-284.

McMenamin DA & Gates LK Jr (1996). A retrospective analysis of the effect of contrast-enhanced CT on the outcome of acute pancreatitis. *American Journal of Gastroenterology* 91(7):1384-1387.

Messian RA, Hermos JA, Robbins AH et al. (1978). Barrett's esophagus. Clinical review of 26 cases. *American Journal of Gastroenterology* 69(4):458-466.

Misslebeck NG & Campbell TC (1985). The role of ethanol in the etiology of primary liver cancer. *Advances in Nutritional Research* 7:129-153.

Mitchell CJ, Playforth MJ, Kelleher J et al. (1983). Functional recovery of the exocrine pancreas after acute pancreatitis. *Scandinavian Journal of Gastroenterology* 18(1):5-8.

Mufti SI (1996). Alcohol's promotion of gastrointestinal carcinogenesis. In VR Preddy & RR Watson (eds.) *Alcohol and the Gastrointestinal Tract*. Boca Raton, FL: CRC Press, 311-320.

Mufti SI, Becker G & Sipes IG (1989). Effect of chronic dietary ethanol consumption on the initiation and promotion of chemically-induced esophageal carcinogenesis in experimental rats. *Carcinogenesis* 10(2):303-309.

Neoptolemos JP, Carr-Locke DL, London NJ et al. (1988). Controlled trial of urgent endoscopic retrograde cholangiopancreatography and endoscopic sphincterotomy versus conservative treatment for acute pancreatitis due to gallstones. *Lancet* 2:979-983.

Neugut AI, Hayek M & Howe G (1996). Epidemiology of gastric cancer. *Seminars in Oncology* 23(3):281-291.

Nonaka A, Manabe T, Asano N et al. (1989). Direct ESR measurement of free radicals in mouse pancreatic lesions. *International Journal of Pancreatology* 5(2):203-211.

Norton ID, Apte MV, Dixon H et al. (1998a). Cystic fibrosis genotypes and alcoholic pancreatitis. *Journal Gastroenterology and Hepatology* 13(5):496-199.

Norton ID, Apte MV, Haber PS et al. (1998b). Cytochrome P450 2E1 is present in rat pancreas and is induced by chronic ethanol administration. *Gut* 42(3):426-430.

Norton ID, Apte MV, Lux O et al. (1998c). Chronic ethanol administration causes oxidative stress in the rat pancreas. *Journal of Laboratory and Clinical Medicine* 131(5):442-446.

Norton I & Wilson JS (1996). Alcoholic pancreatitis. In VR Preedy & RR Watson (eds.) *Alcohol and the Gastrointestinal Tract*. New York, NY: CRC Press, 143-162.

Pandolfino JE & Kahrilas PJ (2000). Smoking and gastro-oesophageal reflux disease. *European Journal of Gastroenterology and Hepatology* 12(8):837-842.

Pederzoli P, Bassi C & Vesentina S (1990). Retroperitoneal and peritoneal drainage and lavage in the treatment of severe necrotizing pancreatitis. *Surgery, Gynecology & Obstetrics* 170(3):197-203.

Pederzoli P, Bassi C, Vesentini S et al. (1993). A randomized multicenter clinical trial of antibiotic prophylaxis of septic complications in acute necrotizing pancreatitis with imipenem. *Surgery, Gynecology & Obstetrics* 176(5):480-483.

Perlow W, Baraona E & Lieber CS (1977). Symptomatic intestinal disaccharidase deficiency in alcoholics. *Gastroenterology* 72(4 Pt 1):680-684.

Pezzilli R, Billi P, Miglioli M et al. (1993). Serum amylase and lipase concentrations and lipase/amylase ratio in assessment of etiology and severity of acute pancreatitis. *Digestive Diseases and Sciences* 38(7):1265-1269.

Piper DW, McIntosh JH & Hudson HM (1985). Factors relevant to the prognosis of chronic duodenal ulcer. *Digestion* 31(1):9-16.

Pirola RC (1966). Effects of ethyl alcohol on sphincteric resistance at the choledochoduodenal junction in man. *Gut* 9:557-560.

Pitchumoni CS, Glasser M, Saran RM et al. (1984). Pancreatic fibrosis in chronic alcoholics and nonalcoholics without clinical pancreatitis. *American Journal of Gastroenterology* 79(5):382-388.

Preedy VR & Watson RR, eds. (1996). *Alcohol and the Gastrointestinal Tract*. Boca Raton, FL: CRC Press.

Proctor GB & Shori DK (1996). The effects of ethanol on salivary glands. In VR Preddy & RR Watson (eds.) *Alcohol and the Gastrointestinal Tract*. Boca Raton, FL: CRC Press, 347.

Ranson JH & Berman RS (1990). Long peritoneal lavage decreases pancreatic sepsis in acute pancreatitis. *Annals of Surgery* 211(6):708-786.

Reynolds JC (1989). Famotidine therapy for active duodenal ulcers. A multivariate analysis of factors affecting early healing. *Annals of Internal Medicine* 111(1):7-14.

Ringborg U (1998). Alcohol and risk of cancer. *Alcoholism: Clinical & Experimental Research* 22(7 Suppl):323S-328S.

Robertson CS, Mayberry JF, Nicholson DA et al. (1988). Value of endoscopic surveillance in the detection of neoplastic change in Barrett's oesophagus. *British Journal of Surgery* 75(8):760-763.

Rogers M & Cerda JJ (1989). The narcotic bowel syndrome. *Journal of Clinical Gastroenterology* 11(2):132-135.

Rollhauser C & Fleischer DE (2000). Current status of endoscopic therapy for ulcer bleeding. *Bailliere's Best Practice and Research. Clinical Gastroenterology* 14(3):391-410.

Ross AH, Smith MA, Anderson JR et al. (1982). Late mortality after surgery for peptic ulcer. *New England Journal of Medicine* 307(9):519-522.

Rubin DT & Hanauer SB (2000). Smoking and inflammatory bowel disease. *European Journal of Gastroenterology and Hepatology* 12(8):855-862.

Salim AS (1991). Role of oxygen-derived free radical scavengers in the treatment of recurrent pain produced by chronic pancreatitis. A new approach. *Archives of Surgery* 126(9):1109-1114.

Saluja AK & Steer MLP (1999). Pathophysiology of pancreatitis. Role of cytokines and other mediators of inflammation. *Digestion* 60(Suppl 1):27-33.

Sandborn WJ (1999). Nicotine therapy for ulcerative colitis: A review of rationale, mechanisms, pharmacology, and clinical results. *American Journal of Gastroenterology* 94(5):1161-1171.

Sandgren JE, McPhee MS & Greenberger NJ (1984). Narcotic bowel syndrome treated with clonidine. Resolution of abdominal pain and intestinal pseudo-obstruction. *Annals of Internal Medicine* 101(3):331-334.

Sanfey H, Bulkley AB & Cameron JL (1985). The pathogenesis of acute pancreatitis. The source and role of oxygen derived free radicals in three different experimental models. *Annals of Surgery* 201(5):633-639.

Sarr MG, Sanfey H & Cameron JL (1986). Prospective, randomized trial of nasogastric suction in patients with acute pancreatitis. *Surgery* 100(3):500-504.

Schmidt J, Hotz HG, Foitzik T et al. (1995). Intravenous contrast medium aggravates the impairment of pancreatic microcirculation in necrotizing pancreatitis in the rat. *Annals of Surgery* 221(3):257-264.

Shen WW (1985). Potential link between hallucination and nausea/vomiting induced by alcohol? An empirical clinical finding. *Psychopathology* 18(4):212-217.

Silver LS, Worner TM & Korsten MA (1986). Esophageal function in chronic alcoholics. *American Journal of Gastroenterology* 81(6):423-427.

Slater TF (1984). Free-radical mechanisms in tissue injury. *Biochemical Journal* 222(1):1-15.

Sonnenberg A, Muller-Lissner SA, Vogel E et al. (1981). Predictors of duodenal ulcer healing and relapse. *Gastroenterology* 81(6):1061-1067.

Soto JA, Barish MA, Yucel EK et al. (1996). Magnetic resonance cholangiography: Comparison with endoscopic retrograde cholangiopancreatography. *Gastroenterology* 110(2):589-597.

Spechler SJ, Dalton JW, Robbins AH et al. (1983). Prevalence of normal serum amylase levels in patients with acute alcoholic pancreatitis. *Digestive Diseases and Sciences* 28(10):865-869.

Steinberg WM (1990). Predictors of severity of acute pancreatitis. *Gastroenterology Clinics of North America* 19(4):849-861.

Stone HH & Fabian TC (1980). Peritoneal dialysis in the treatment of acute alcoholic pancreatitis. *Surgery, Gynecology & Obstetrics* 150(6):878-882.

Talamini G, Bassi C, Falconi et al. (1999). Alcohol and smoking as risk factors in chronic pancreatitis and pancreatic cancer. *Digestive Diseases and Sciences* 44(7):1303-1311.

Thune A, Baker RA, Saccone GT et al. (1990). Differing effects of pethidine and morphine on human sphincter of Oddi motility. *British Journal of Surgery* 77(9):992-995.

Toskes PP (1990). Hyperlipidemic pancreatitis. *Gastroenterology Clinics of North America* 19(4):783-791.

Tsianos EV, Dardamanis MA, Elisaf M et al. (1994). The value of alpha-amylase and isoamylase determination in chronic renal failure patients. *International Journal of Pancreatology* 15(2):105-111.

Uppal R, Rosman A, Hernandez R et al. (1991). Effects of liver disease on red blood cell acetaldehyde in alcoholics and non-alcoholics. *Alcohol and Alcoholism (Supplement)* 1:323-326.

Venu RP, Geenen JE, Toouli J et al. (1983). Endoscopic retrograde cholangiopancreatography. Diagnosis of cholelithiasis in patients with normal gallbladder x-ray and ultrasound studies. *Journal of the American Medical Association* 249(6):758-761.

Whitcomb DC, Gorry MC, Preston RA et al. (1996). Hereditary pancreatitis is caused by a mutation in the cationic trypsinogen gene. *Nature Genetics* 14(2):141-145.

Whitely G, Scott PD, Sharer NM et al. (1993). Combined antioxidant and surgical approach to extensive haemorrhagic pancreatic necrosis [abstract]. *Gastroenterology* 106:A343.

Whitfield RM, Bechtel LM & Starich GH (1997). The impact of ethanol and Marinol/marijuana usage on HIV+/AIDS patients undergoing azidothymine, azidothymidine/dideoxycytidine, or dideoxyinosine therapy. *Alcoholism: Clinical & Experimental Research* 21(1):122-127.

Williams CL, Bihm CC, Rosenfeld GC et al. (1997). Morphine tolerance and dependence in the rat intestine in vivo. *Journal of Pharmacology & Experimental Therapeutics* 280(2):656-663.

Williams JT, Christie MJ & Manzoni O (2001). Cellular and synaptic adaptations mediating opioid dependence. *Physiological Reviews* 81(1):299-343.

Wilson JS, Bernstein L, McDonald C et al. (1985). Diet and drinking habits in relation to the development of alcoholic pancreatitis. *Gut* 26(9):882-887.

Wilson JS, Gossat D, Tait A et al. (1984). Evidence for an inherited predisposition to alcoholic pancreatitis. A controlled HLA typing study. *Digestive Diseases and Sciences* 29(8):727-730.

Wilson JS, Korsten MA & Pirola RC (1989). Alcohol-induced pancreatic injury (Part I). Unexplained features and ductular theories of pathogenesis. *International Journal of Pancreatology* 4(2):109-125.

Yaffe GJ, Strelinger RW & Parwatikar S (1973). Physical symptom complaints of patients on methadone maintenance. *Proceedings. National Conference on Methadone Treatment* 1:507-514.

Yen S, Hsieh CC & MacMahon B (1982). Consumption of alcohol and tobacco and other risk factors for pancreatitis. *American Journal of Epidemiology* 116(3):407-414.

Yuan CS, Foss JF, O'Connor M et al. (1998). Gut motility and transit changes in patients receiving long-term methadone maintenance. *Journal of Clinical Pharmacology* 38(10):931-935.

Yuan CS, Foss JF, O'Connor M et al. (2000). Methylnaltrexone for reversal of constipation due to chronic methadone use: A randomized controlled trial. *Journal of the American Medical Association* 283(3):367-372.

| Chapter 6 | # Respiratory Tract Disorders Related to Alcohol and Other Drug Use |

Elizabeth Mirabile-Levin, M.D.

Kevin Wilson, M.D.

Jussi J. Saukkonen, M.D.

Respiratory Function
Common Pulmonary Complications
Tobacco and Nicotine
Marijuana
Cocaine
Amphetamines and Other Stimulants

Caffeine
Opioids
Alcohol
Sedative-Hypnotics
Volatile Substances
Nitrous Oxide
Anabolic Steroids

The respiratory tract is a unique interface between the body and the environment. The airways of the lung are subject to constant noxious, particulate, and antigenic challenges, which come into close proximity to the vast vascular bed of the lung. The lungs are highly adapted in attenuating such external provocations and in mediating between events at the epithelial and endothelial surfaces. However, a broad variety of addictive drugs present acute or chronic insults to the respiratory system and can overwhelm local capacity for recovery (Table 1).

Inhalation, injection, or ingestion of addictive drugs may have adverse effects within the airways, lung parenchyma, and vascular bed. Respiratory complications also may arise from indirect effects of drugs on the central nervous and immune systems.

RESPIRATORY FUNCTION

Addictive drugs can derange the interrelated critical functions of the lungs. The principal function of gas exchange dictates the structure of the respiratory tract. Other functions of the lung are derived from this primary structure–function relationship, including gas exchange, containment and exclusion of foreign materials, immune sampling of antigens, and detoxification and metabolism of proteins, drugs, and other potentially injurious substances.

Inhaled gases and particulate matter travel through the specialized structures of the upper airway into progressively ramifying airways, which terminate in gas-exchanging alveoli. The large surface area of the alveolar spaces and their associated capillary beds provide enormous absorptive capacity for inhaled drugs. Both the cough reflex and the mucociliary escalator are important in ridding the lower respiratory tract of foreign matter. Resident alveolar macrophages ingest particles and pathogens, then process, digest, and transport them to lymph nodes for antigen presentation. Local immune responses recruit other leukocytes, which may further contain or help remove any offending matter through granuloma formation or phagocytosis (Brugman & Irvin, 1988; Crofton & Douglas, 1981).

The pulmonary vasculature provides important defensive functions for the lungs. The circulation carries antioxidants, antiproteolytic agents, and antibodies to the lung to meet ongoing challenges. Significant metabolic functions are performed within the pulmonary vasculature, including removal of drugs (Foth, 1995), vasoactive amines,

TABLE 1. Drugs Associated with Pulmonary Complications

CNS Stimulants
- Nicotine/tobacco
- Cocaine and crack
- Amphetamines
- MDMA
- Methylphenidate
- Caffeine

CNS Depressants
- Alcohol/ethanol
- Barbiturates
- Benzodiazepines
- Gamma-hydroxybutyrate (GHB)
- Opioids

Hallucinogens

Marijuana

Volatile Substances
- Aromatic hydrocarbons
- Nitrous oxide
- Nitrites
- Refrigerants

kinins, and eicosanoids. The pulmonary vascular bed autoregulates flow in response to oxygenation and local concentrations of vasoactive substances. Large numbers of marginated leukocytes and platelets are present within the pulmonary vasculature, but may be mobilized by pulmonary epithelial or endothelial insults, causing exudation, inflammation, and compromise of gas exchange (Brugman & Irvin, 1988; Crofton & Douglas, 1981).

Respiration is under extensive neural control and, consequently, is susceptible to the effects of CNS depressants and stimulants. Inherent respiratory automaticity is provided by the medulla oblongata within the brainstem, but this is modulated by the reticular activating system, cerebral cortex, and peripheral sensors. Hypoxic drive comes from the carotid body, which, when stimulated, causes hypotension and bradycardia. Hypoxic drive is blunted by age, obesity, chronic bronchitis, and CNS depressants. C-fiber receptors (including J receptors in lung parenchyma), when stimulated by interstitial edema, microembolism, and chemical products of anaphylaxis, result in tachypnea and dyspnea. Irritant receptors in the epithelium of the larynx and large airways respond to a variety of chemical irritants and mechanical stimuli, resulting in cough, bronchoconstriction, sneezing, laryngospasm, and mucus secretion (Brugman & Irvin, 1988; Crofton & Douglas, 1981). Receptors within the lung and in the brain are responsive to a number of addictive substances.

Addictive drugs may perturb the active processes within the lung, resulting in local inflammation, infections, airway reactivity, impairment of pulmonary vascular integrity, acute lung injury, structural injury, or derangements of gas exchange. Polysubstance abuse often is associated with a variety of injuries, making it difficult to ascribe a particular respiratory complication to a single agent. Coexisting pulmonary pathology may worsen the acute physiologic effects of an addictive drug on the lungs.

COMMON PULMONARY COMPLICATIONS

Several families of drugs cause common respiratory complications, including adverse effects related to respiratory depression, infections, route of consumption, and contaminants.

Respiratory Depression. Nearly all of the drugs discussed here may directly inhibit respiration or induce seizures. Patients with respiratory depression usually are somnolent or postictal. Respirations are rapid and shallow, and are accompanied by limited ability to cough. Atelectasis, hypoxemia, hypoventilation, inability to clear secretions, and aspiration may occur. With overdose, lethargy may progress rapidly to stupor, severe respiratory depression, coma, and respiratory arrest. With intravenous drug use, death may occur so rapidly that the needle is still in the vein when the corpse is found.

The diagnosis usually is obvious from the clinical presentation, coupled with a history or signs of drug abuse and a positive toxicology screen. A complete chemistry panel, toxicology screen, electrocardiogram, blood gas, and chest radiograph should be performed. Airway protection is paramount, and patients with known or suspected overdose should be admitted to an intensive care unit for monitoring of their respiratory, neurologic, and hemodynamic status (Parsons, 1994; Jay, Johanson et al., 1975). Management generally consists of administration of thiamine, glucose, and naloxone (although the half-life of naloxone is relatively short, temporary improvement may be helpful diagnostically).

Atelectasis. In patients with respiratory depression, shallow respirations may not exceed the critical closing volume and may result in airway collapse. Ineffective cough and aspirated oral and gastric secretions, with loss of surfactant, lead to atelectasis. Consequently, unventilated areas are perfused (shunting), which, with lobar or whole-lung atelectasis, may cause significant hypoxemia (Crofton & Douglas, 1981). Incentive spirometry, chest physiotherapy, respiratory suctioning, and supplemental oxygen generally are indicated. Bronchoscopy may be needed for refractory atelectasis in the face of severe hypoxemia or to rule out an endobronchial lesion or aspirated foreign body (Marini, Pierson et al., 1979).

Aspiration Pneumonitis. Respiratory depression or seizures may cause aspiration of oral secretions or gastric contents. Often the event is only chemical pneumonitis, but this condition may lead to noncardiogenic pulmonary edema and respiratory failure, with or without bacterial super infection. Infiltrates due to aspiration may develop within several hours to a few days. Preventive care should be directed toward airway control, maintenance of at least a 45-degree angle, avoidance of oral intake while lethargic, pulmonary toilet, supplemental oxygen, and antibiotics as indicated. Empiric antibiotic coverage for aspiration in the absence of infiltrates and clinical and laboratory indicators of infection may be counterproductive, merely leading to the selection of nosocomial pathogens (Marik, 2001; Bynum & Pierce, 1976).

Respiratory Infections. Chronic users of addictive drugs are susceptible to a variety of respiratory infections. Many drugs have adverse effects on leukocyte function, contribute to malnutrition with resultant immune dysfunction, are injected under septic conditions, or may be contaminated with pathogens. Infectious complications also may be related to coexisting HIV infection, cirrhosis, aspiration, smoking, or lifestyle-related structural lung disease, or inhibition of the mucociliary escalator (Verra, Escudier et al., 1995; Sisson, Papi et al., 1994). Smoking-related obstructive lung disease may require chronic corticosteroid therapy, which is an immunosuppressant and thus may contribute to infections.

The spectrum of respiratory infections includes sinusitis, acute bronchitis, community-acquired and aspiration pneumonias, septic emboli, tuberculosis, and fungal infection. Patients most often present with acute symptoms of fever, productive cough, dyspnea, and, often, pleuritic chest pain, but general ill health and polymicrobial infections make atypical or subacute presentations common. The chest radiograph may reveal lobar pneumonia, bibasilar or superior segment lower-lobe infiltrates suggestive of aspiration, or nodular infiltrates in the lower lung fields consistent with aspiration. Sputum gram stain and culture can be helpful in identifying a pathogen. Blood cultures should be obtained in toxic, ill-appearing individuals, injection drug users, immunocompromised patients, and other high-risk individuals. Antibiotics tailored to the suspected pathogen are the therapy of choice.

Respiratory Complications of Contaminants. Illicit drugs vary greatly in purity, as they often are adulterated to increase profits. Widely used adulterants include mannitol, cellulose, talc, various sugars, as well as other drugs such as phenobarbital, methaqualone, caffeine, procaine, and noscapine (Kaa, 1994). The lungs act as filters, trapping inhaled or injected foreign substances, which may incite local inflammatory or fibrotic responses. Contaminating microorganisms also may lead to pulmonary infection, particularly in immunocompromised hosts, or to hypersensitivity responses (Miller, Ashcroft et al., 1971; Kurup, Resnick et al., 1983; Hamadeh, Ardehali et al., 1988; Sutton, Lum et al., 1986; Kagen, Kurup et al., 1983).

The role of herbicides, such as paraquat, in contaminating inhaled drugs and causing pulmonary complications is controversial. Although epidemiologic evidence of paraquat-induced lung injury is lacking, the herbicide has been documented to cause occupational lung disease and acute lung injury in instances of toxic exposure (Lheureux, Leduc et al., 1995; Daisley & Hutchinson, 1998; Landrigan, Powell et al., 1983).

Occupational Lung Disease. Agricultural workers may develop pulmonary complications related to the cultivation of certain plants for the drug industry. Such health problems may be obscured because the industry is illicit or barely tolerated and is not subject to occupational safety regulations or to exposure mitigation regimes. Socioeconomic and political factors generally do not allow workers to voice their health concerns. Pneumoconiosis, herbicide-related interstitial fibrosis, and antigen-induced hypersensitivity pneumonitis constitute occupational pulmonary hazards for such agricultural workers (Yamashita, Yamashita et al., 2000; Zuskin, Mustajbegovic et al., 1994; Dalvie, White et al., 1999; Lander, Jepsen et al., 1988; Huuskonen, Husman et al., 1984).

Respiratory Complications of Injected Drugs. Opiates, stimulants, and combinations thereof are commonly injected into the veins. The resulting pulmonary complications may be acute or chronic. Acute problems are likely to be severe, including respiratory failure and acute pulmonary edema (Parsons, 1994; Jay, Johanson et al., 1975). Chronic pulmonary problems include the development of interstitial and bullous lung disease (O'Donnell & Pappas, 1988; Pare, Cote et al., 1989), endovascular and respiratory infections (O'Donnell & Pappas, 1988), and tuberculosis (American

Thoracic Society, 2000). Potential pulmonary complications associated with either the drug or its contaminants, or the route of administration, include the following conditions.

Talc Granulomatosis: Talc (magnesium silicate) is widely used as a filler in oral medications, which may be crushed and injected, and it is used to adulterate inhaled and injected drugs. A syndrome similar to sarcoidosis may result, with insidious onset of granulomatous interstitial fibrosis (Louria, Hensel et al., 1967; Feigin, 1986; Tomashefski, Hirsch et al., 1981; Waller, Brownlee et al., 1980; Sharma & Kalkat, 1991). Dyspnea, particularly with exertion, and cough are the most common symptoms. The retina should be examined in all patients in whom the diagnosis is being considered because talc retinopathy occurs in more than half of patients (Louria, Hensle et al., 1967; Waller, Brownlee et al., 1980).

In advanced stages or if there is associated granulomatous pulmonary arterial occlusion (Genereux & Emson, 1974; Hopkins, 1972), pulmonary hypertension and right ventricular failure can occur. The chest radiograph is normal in up to half of patients, but a diffuse micronodular interstitial opacity may become progressively evident, potentially coalescing to opacify entire lobes (Feigin, 1986). Pulmonary function tests typically reveal a low diffusion capacity before any other abnormality (Overland, Noland et al., 1980). Bronchoalveolar lavage may demonstrate local lymphocytosis and birefringent intracellular or free talc (Louria, Hensle et al., 1967; Tomashefski, Hirsch et al., 1981). Lung biopsy may be required to establish the diagnosis, based on histologic changes of granulomas, mononuclear inflammatory cells, lymphocytes, and fibrosis (Tomashefski, Hirsch et al., 1981).

Patients with progressive symptoms and worsening chest radiograph or pulmonary function tests should be given a trial of systemic steroids, although results are highly variable and unpredictable (Louria, Hensle et al., 1967).

Pulmonary Hypertension: Intravenous drug users may develop chronic pulmonary hypertension from multiple mechanisms, including chronic hypoxemia related to interstitial lung disease and vasoconstriction, or pulmonary arterial thrombosis at sites of foreign-body granulomatosis, with subsequent occlusion (angiothrombotic pulmonary hypertension) (Genereux & Emson, 1974; Hopkins, 1972; Robertson, Reynolds et al., 1976; Yakel & Eisenberg, 1995). Primary pulmonary hypertension also may occur as a result of HIV-1 infection (Mehta, Khan et al., 2000). Patients

typically present with interstitial and vascular reactions to talc. Common presentations involve dyspnea on exertion. Physical examination and electrocardiogram may be normal or may show evidence of right ventricular enlargement and failure. Acute, reversible pulmonary hypertension may be associated with injection of sympathomimetics, although it also may due to an effect on cardiac output (Lewman, 1972; Collazos, Martinez et al., 1996; Kleerup, Wong et al., 1997). Treatment options include supplemental oxygen, anticoagulation, and vasodilator therapy, prescribed after hemodynamic monitoring (Hammerman & Graven, 1997).

Septic Thromboemboli: Septic pulmonary embolism is the most common pulmonary complication among intravenous heroin users (O'Donnell & Pappas, 1988) and may result from tricuspid endocarditis or from infected injection-site thrombophlebitis (O'Donnell & Pappas, 1988; Rosenow, 1972; Louria, Hensel et al., 1967). The organism most frequently isolated from sputum or blood cultures is *Staphylococcus aureus* (O'Donnell & Pappas, 1988).

The patient typically presents in an acute toxic state, with fever, dyspnea, chest pain, and leukocytosis. Radiographic examination of the chest may reveal bilateral necrotizing infiltrates or single or multiple pulmonary lesions, which frequently cavitate. The lesions may coalesce to form large cavities that communicate with a bronchus. Alternatively, infection may be complicated by bronchopleu-ral fistulas, empyema, or pneumothorax.

Antibiotic therapy usually is prolonged. Cases can clear completely, although residual pleural thickening and fibrosis is common (O'Donnell & Pappas, 1988; Rosenow, 1972; Louria, Hensele et al., 1967).

Needle Embolization: Occasionally needles, especially those used multiple times, may be broken off inadvertently during or after injection. This situation is more likely to occur when less accessible sites are being used. Chest radiograph may demonstrate needle fragments within chest soft tissue or lodged within pulmonary vasculature. No specific therapy or removal is necessary for needle emboli to the lung (Kulaylat, Barakat et al., 1993).

Pneumothorax: Pneumothorax—unilateral or bilateral—may develop from inadvertent puncture of the lung during attempted needle injection into a jugular or subclavian vessel (Lewis, Groux et al., 1980; Zorc, O'Donnell et al., 1988). This condition also may result from cavitating septic thromboemboli (Aguado, Arjona et al., 1990). Large pneumothoraces, those associated with hypoxemia, or those with concomitant empyema, require tube thoracostomy and antibiotics (Lewis, Groux et al., 1980; Zorc, O'Donnell et al., 1988; Aguado, Arjona et al., 1990).

Empyema: Cavitating infections from septic emboli, pneumonia, or unclean needles may contaminate the pleural space and lead to empyema (Zorc, O'Donnell et al., 1988; Aguado, Arjona et al., 1990).

Mycotic Aneurysms: Septic emboli may lead to the development of mycotic aneurysms of the pulmonary vasculature. Patients may present with evidence of endovascular infection, with or without hemoptysis. Contrast-enhanced computed tomography demonstrates nodular lesions associated with vasculature. This condition may be fatal if there is massive hemoptysis, despite surgical intervention. Patients without hemoptysis may experience resolution of this condition with antibiotic therapy (McLean, Sharma et al., 1998; Joseph & Geelhoed, 1974).

Hemothorax: Rupture of a subclavian aneurysm created by multiple injections has been reported to cause a massive hemothorax (Wayne & Spitz, 1978).

Pulmonary Emphysema: Bullous emphysema may develop in intravenous drug injectors, either in association with talc granulomatosis or in its absence (Pare, Cote et al., 1989; Grellner, Madea et al., 1996; Smeenk, Serlie et al., 1990; Fullana Monllor, Garcia Bermejo et al., 1998).

Respiratory Complications of Inhaled Drugs. Inhalation has become a preferred route for the consumption of many addictive drugs. Delivery of a drug through the lung affords ease of administration, rapid onset of action, dose minimization, avoidance of intravenous injection, and avoidance of the hepatic first pass effect. Drugs may be inhaled nasally ("snorting"), rolled as cigarettes, sprinkled into smoked tobacco, smoked through pipes, or inhaled orally. The route of ingestion may affect the dose delivered and the onset of action. Deep inhalation or smoking may result in an onset of action within seconds, whereas nasal inhalation affords a slightly delayed onset, measured in seconds to minutes (Cone, 1998). Various delivery devices and techniques have been developed to control dose and effects; to provide convenience; and to incorporate cultural, behavioral, and esthetic elements. For example, water pipes, used for smoking a variety of drugs throughout the world (especially Asia), are associated with a café culture and have an esthetic design element. Some water pipes filter smoke and may attenuate a few, but not many, of the detrimental effects of smoked tobacco (Kiter, Ucan et al., 2000; Lubin, Li et al., 1992).

Inhaled drugs include fine powders, smoked plant material, gases, other volatiles, and combinations of these drugs. Inhaled powders are heterodisperse, varying considerably in size, with a geometric standard deviation greater than 2. The momentum of inhaled particles greater than 6 μm causes them to impact proximally against convoluted upper airway walls and bifurcating large airways of the lung, where they may be absorbed. Smaller particles (1 to 5 μm) are carried by the airstream to the distal airways, where they are deposited chiefly by sedimentation, settling as a result of gravitational forces (Brugman & Irvin, 1988).

Inhalation of talc or other fibrogenic substances may lead to the development of granulomatous inflammation or fibrosis, as discussed earlier. Smoke consists of gas and particulate phases, including carbon monoxide, potentially injurious oxidants, aldehydes, alcohols, nitrosamines, benzene derivatives, and other inorganic and organic substances (Rylander, 1968; Smith & Hansch, 2000), any of which may cause mucosal injury and inflammation.

Chronic Bronchitis: This condition is commonly associated with smoking tobacco, marijuana, cocaine, and other drugs. Cough, dyspnea, and mucus hypersecretion are found in individuals with chronic bronchitis, particularly if they smoke daily. A propensity to airway reactivity and acute bacterial bronchitis may be seen (Wu & Center, 1997; Fligiel, Roth et al., 1997).

Bronchospasm: Airway reactivity often is seen with inhaled heroin, cocaine, tobacco, and marijuana (Hughes & Calverly, 1988; Aguis, 1989; Ghodse & Myles, 1987; Rome, Lippmann et al., 2000; Tashkin, Kleerup et al., 1996; Tashkin, 2001). Patients typically present with dyspnea, tachypnea, and wheezing, beginning within minutes to hours after inhalation. Sinus tachycardia usually is present. Early blood gases, if drawn, may demonstrate respiratory alkalosis, which may progress to hypercapnia and respiratory acidosis. The chest radiograph typically is clear. Patients are treated with supplemental oxygen, bronchodilators, steroids, and, if severe, mechanical ventilation. Patients with new onset asthma should be assessed for use of inhaled drugs (Osborn, Tang et al., 1997).

Barotrauma: Inhalation of cocaine, heroin, 3,4-methylenedioxymethamphetamine, marijuana, tobacco, and volatile substances is associated with barotrauma, including pneumothorax and pneumomediastinum. Extreme breath-holding against a closed glottis (a prolonged Valsalva maneuver) in an attempt to increase the drug's effect results in high negative intrathoracic pressure, hyperinflation, alveolar bleb rupture, and dissection of air along peribronchial paths into the mediastinum, pleural cavities, skin, and retropharyngeal space. Some users exhale smoke forcefully into another user's mouth, causing markedly elevated positive airway pressure and, potentially, barotrauma, as well as transmission of respiratory pathogens (Perlman, Perkins et al., 1997).

Individuals who have developed bullous emphysema from chronic smoking may have spontaneous rupture of a bleb, with resultant pneumothorax. Patients may present with acute chest or back pain and dyspnea, with or without hypoxemia (Seaman, 1990; Rosenow, 1972; McCarroll & Roszler, 1991).

Hemoptysis: Hemoptysis may result from mucosal irritation or ulceration anywhere within the respiratory tract (as in epistaxis, sinusitis, or bronchitis), from pulmonary infarct, or from diffuse alveolar hemorrhage (Tashkin, Kleerup et al., 1996; McCarroll & Roszler, 1991; Tashkin, 1990).

Pulmonary Emphysema: Destruction of lung parenchyma, with resultant pulmonary emphysema, may occur with inhaled tobacco, marijuana, and chronic opium use (Godwin, Harley et al., 1989; Karlinskey, 1997; Johnson, Smith et al. 2000; Da Costa, Tock et al., 1971).

TOBACCO AND NICOTINE

Within the lung, smoking has profound effects, altering the immunologic and structural milieu. Cigarette tar is associated with a high rate of lung cancer, emphysema, bronchitis, and airway reactivity. Several factors determine the effects of tar and other pyrolysis products on the lung: individual susceptibility to the various adverse effects of smoking varies considerably, and heterozygosity for the gene that causes alpha-1-antitrypsin deficiency may play a role (Sandford, Chagani et al., 2001; Ishii, Matsuse et al., 2000). The quantity of cigarettes smoked, the years spent smoking, and the manner in which they were smoked (for example, the depth of inhalation) also play a role.

Tobacco smoke induces the elaboration of chemotactic agents for neutrophils and monocytes, as well as mediators that cause epithelial injury and permeability changes (Sato, Koyama et al., 1999; McCusker, 1992). Pulmonary leukocytes are activated by the local elaboration of cytokines (including interleukin (IL)-8, tumor necrosis factor alpha, and IL-1) and by epithelial cells, fibroblasts, and leukocytes. Neutrophils and macrophages release serine proteases, reactive oxygen species, matrix metalloproteinases, and other potentially injurious cell products (Sato, Koyama et al., 1999; McCusker, 1992; Lim, Roche et al., 2000; Shapiro, 1999; Ofulue & Ko, 1999; Gadek, 1992; MacNee, 2000). Imbalance of proteases and antiproteases is thought to play a role in the development of local injury. Elastin and collagen degradation ensues, resulting in a loss of pulmonary architecture and, eventually, of functional gas exchanging units (Snider, 1981; Turato, Zuin et al., 2001). T cells and submucosal eosinophils also play a pathogenic role after long-standing injury (McCusker, 1992; Turato, Zuin et al., 2001; Finkelstein, Fraser et al., 1995; Saetta, Finkelstein et al., 1994).

Smoking induces a variety of coexisting pathologies in the lung. Smokers display a more rapid decline in forced expiratory volume in one second (FEV_1) than do nonsmokers. Chronic airflow obstruction is common and, when associated with persistent hypoxemia, may lead to cor pulmonale and pulmonary hypertension. Smoking cessation may attenuate symptoms, decrease infections, slow the rate of decline of lung function, and lower the risk of developing lung cancer (Balfour, Benowitz et al., 2000). Environmental tobacco smoke has become a major public health issue, leading to increased incidence of respiratory infections, bronchiolitis in children, asthma exacerbations, and bronchogenic carcinoma (Jinot & Bayard, 1996).

Clinical syndromes associated with the use of tobacco include the following.

Chronic Bronchitis. In many smokers, a chronic productive cough is present on a daily basis—a common clinical operational definition of chronic bronchitis. More formally, chronic bronchitis is defined as sputum production for at least three months in two successive years in the absence of other causes of chronic cough. Airway changes in chronic bronchitis are nonspecific, but consist largely of mucous gland hypertrophy of intermediate-sized airways. Overproduction of mucus may overwhelm the mucociliary escalator, which is compromised by tobacco smoke (Verra, Escudier et al., 1995). Often there is associated airway reactivity (Wu & Center, 1997).

Airway Reactivity. Smoking tobacco promotes bronchial hyperreactivity, as measured by methacholine bronchoprovocation studies, even in patients without obstructive lung disease (Casale, Rhodes et al., 1987). Animal studies suggest that early smoke-induced bronchoconstriction is caused by nicotine and is mediated by cholinergic pathways and by tachykinin release from bronchopulmonary C fibers. A delayed and more sustained bronchoconstrictive response is induced by non-nicotinic components of tobacco smoke, which elicit the release of the eicosanoids thromboxane A_2, prostaglandin D_2, and prostaglandin F_2alpha, acting on airway smooth muscles (Hahn, Lang et al., 1992; Hong & Lee, 1996; Hansson, Choudry et al., 1994; Lee, Lou at al, 1995; Hong, Rodger et al., 1995). Smokers also have increased numbers of activated leukocytes, which may contribute to asthmatic symptoms (Turato, Zuin et al., 2001; Finkelstein, Fraser et al., 1995). In some individuals with severe airflow obstruction, there are correlations between total immunoglobulin E (IgE) levels and FEV_1, although this correlation is not likely to be related to specific aeroallergens (Burrows, Lebowitz et al., 1983).

Patients typically complain of dyspnea, especially with exertion, chest tightness, and cough. Pulmonary function testing may show an obstructive pattern. Tobacco smoke also may exacerbate preexisting asthma. Bronchodilator therapy and inhaled corticosteroids are mainstays of therapy (Wu & Center, 1997; Karlinsky, 1997).

Pulmonary Emphysema. Smokers who develop irreversible enlargement of the airspaces distal to the terminal bronchiole, with destruction of the alveolar wall, have pulmonary emphysema. Interstitial fibrosis may occur but is not a major pathologic finding. Centrilobular emphysema in the upper portions of the lungs, as well as paraseptal emphysema in the periphery of the lungs, is commonly found. The latter is associated with the development of large bullae. Hyperinflation and flattening of the diaphragm lead to a mechanical disadvantage for the contractility of the major respiratory muscle (Polkey, Hamnegard et al., 1998). There is decreased ability to oxygenate blood, as alveolar septae are destroyed, with loss of the pulmonary capillary bed. These changes, as well as suboptimal ventilation–perfusion relationships, also lead to carbon dioxide retention. There may be associated chronic bronchitis or airway reactivity, or both (Karlinsky, 1997). Pneumothorax may develop from rupture of a subpleural emphysematous bleb.

Pulmonary function testing reveals obstructive lung disease, often with hyperinflation and air trapping. Chest radiography reveals hyperlucent lungs and loss of interstitial marking.

Mainstays of treatment include smoking cessation, bronchodilator therapy, trials of inhaled or systemic steroids, judicious use of oxygen, and pulmonary rehabilitation (Karlinsky, 1997).

Pulmonary Hypertension and Cor Pulmonale. Chronic hypoxic vasoconstriction of the pulmonary vasculature leads to pulmonary arterial hypertension and right heart strain. Patients may have tachycardia, prominent neck veins, tricuspid insufficiency murmur, right ventricular third heart sound, hepatojugular reflex, and peripheral edema. Supplemental oxygen for at least 18 hours a day prolongs survival and improves symptoms. Patients also are treated with bronchodilators and diuretics (Wu & Center, 1997; Karlinsky, 1997; American Thoracic Society, 1987).

Interstitial Lung Disease. Smoking is associated with an increased risk of developing desquamate interstitial pneumonitis, a form of idiopathic pulmonary fibrosis (Baumgartner, Samet et al., 1997; Nagai, Hoshino et al., 2000). Patients present with insidiously developing dyspnea, interstitial infiltrates, and restrictive physiology, which may be confounded by concomitant obstructive lung disease, on pulmonary function tests (Nagai, Hoshino et al., 2000). Respiratory bronchiolitis-associated interstitial lung disease, which has radiologic and histopathologic overlap with desquamative interstitial pneumonitis (Heyneman, Ward et al., 1999; Yousem, Colby et al., 1989), also may result from smoking.

Open lung biopsy is needed to reliably diagnose and to distinguish among interstitial lung diseases (Aubrey, Wright et al., 2000). Patients with idiopathic pulmonary fibrosis or respiratory bronchiolitis-associated interstitial lung disease usually are treated with a trial of systemic corticosteroids (Nagai, Hoshino et al., 2000; Yousem, Colby et al., 1989).

Smoking also is a prominent risk factor for the development of pulmonary histiocytosis X (eosinophilic granuloma), as more than 90% of patients with the disease are smokers (Murin, Bilello et al., 2000; Hance, Basset et al., 1986). Smoking may precipitate exacerbations of Goodpasture's disease, with marked hemoptysis (Murin, Bilello et al., 2000).

Pneumothorax. Spontaneous pneumothorax may occur as a result of bullous emphysema, with rupture of a subpleural bleb. Occasionally, associated cavitating infections or bronchogenic carcinomas also may cause pneumothorax, usually in association with a pleural effusion (Karlinsky, 1997; Berk, 1997).

Hemoptysis. Most often, hemoptysis results from acute bacterial bronchitis, but it may betray the presence of other airway pathology, including bronchogenic carcinoma (Karlinsky, 1997).

Bronchogenic Carcinoma. Inhalation of tobacco-specific N-nitrosamines and other carcinogens causes bronchogenic carcinoma in many individuals (Schuller & Orlof, 1998; Trump, McDowell et al., 1984). Smokeless tobacco has been linked to the development of malignancies of the aerodigestive tract (Cullen, Blot et al., 1986). Tobacco smoke induces widespread epithelial changes, which may predispose to the development of premalignant lesions in association with generalized genetic mutations ("field cancerization") (Barsky, Roth et al., 1998). Oncogene mutations, particularly of the p53 gene, are associated with the development of lung cancer (Rom, Hay et al., 2000). Environmental tobacco smoke constitutes a risk factor for the development of bronchogenic carcinoma in nonsmokers (Copas & Shi, 2000). Other environmental exposures potentially increase risk for bronchogenic carcinoma, including asbestos and drugs such as crack cocaine and marijuana (Barsky, Roth et al., 1998; Lee, 2001).

Patients may present with asymptomatic, incidentally noted pulmonary nodules or with weight loss, cough, chest or bone pain, fatigue, hoarseness, superior vena cava syndrome, or hemoptysis. Diagnosis may be made by sputum, needle, or bronchoscopic cytologic specimens, endobronchial biopsy, mediastinoscopy, or at the time of surgical resection. Treatment may be definitive, in the case of a completely resected, margin-free solitary pulmonary nodule, or it may entail radiation or chemotherapy, depending on cell type and stage (Reardon & Theodore, 1997).

Hypersensitivity Pneumonitis (extrinsic allergic alveolitis). A variety of molds may be present on tobacco plants, which then are inhaled by workers harvesting the crop or, theoretically, by smokers. In some individuals, these molds, including *Aspergillus* and thermophilic actinomycetes, may induce hypersensitivity reactions on exposure. Workers typically experience amelioration of symptoms when away from work. Clinical features include cough, fever, and obstructive and restrictive findings on pulmonary function testing (Lander, Jepsen et al., 1988; Huuskonen, Husman et al., 1984). If exposure is long-standing, pulmonary fibrosis may develop (Huuskonen, Husman et al., 1984). Although smoking can lead to serologic evidence of exposure, it is unclear whether hypersensitivity pneumonitis develops in smokers (Kurup, Resnick et al., 1983).

Lipoid Pneumonia. The rare complication of lipoid pneumonia has been reported among chewers and smokers of blackfat tobacco in Guyana, where petroleum jelly is applied to tobacco leaves to moisturize them and enhance their flavor (Miller, Ashcroft et al., 1971). Patients may present with cough and a localized infiltrate, which may suggest

chronic pneumonia or bronchogenic carcinoma. The density of the lesion on computed tomography scan usually suggests the diagnosis.

Snuff-Related Pneumonitis. In patients with renal failure, snuff has been reported to cause pulmonary infiltrates. The pathogenesis is unclear, but biopsy shows the presence of vegetable fibers and parenchymal necrosis. The syndrome disappears with abstinence (Hoppichler, Lechleitner et al., 1992).

MARIJUANA

Marijuana or hashish may be ingested or smoked as cigarettes or through water pipes of various designs. The pyrolysis products of cannabis are similar to those of cigarettes and exert the same effects on the airway epithelium. The smoke, similar to that of cigarettes, contains tetrahydrocannabinol and other cannabinoids but not nicotine (Van Hoozen & Cross, 1997; Wu, Tashkin et al., 1998). Marijuana smoke has deleterious effects on respiration, depositing three times more tar than cigarette smoke and causing a fivefold higher carboxyhemoglobin level in the blood than cigarettes (Wu, Tashkin et al., 1988). Alveolar macrophages from marijuana smokers do not phagocytose properly, have decreased ability to kill bacteria and tumor cells, and produce decreased amounts of nitric oxide and cytokines, including tumor necrosis factor alpha, granulocyte-macrophage colony-stimulating factor, and IL-6 (Baldwin, Tashkin et al., 1997). Marijuana smoke increases oxidative stress within the lung, causing glutathione stores to be depleted within alveolar macrophages (Sarafian, Magallanes et al., 1999). Field cancerization has been shown to occur within the lung, increasing the possibility of lung cancer (Barsky, Roth et al., 1998). Cases of squamous cell carcinoma of the oropharynx in heavy marijuana smokers also have been reported in the literature (Fung, Gallagher et al., 1999).

Obstructive Lung Disease. Marijuana smokers may suffer some of the same complications as those who smoke tobacco, including chronic bronchitis and bullous emphysema (Fligiel, Beals et al., 1991; Johnson, Smith et al., 2000). Marijuana smokers' lungs receive more tar because the marijuana cigarettes are not filtered and because inhalation tends to be significantly deeper and is associated with prolonged breath-holding (Wu, Tashkin et al., 1988). However, chronic obstructive lung disease does not develop consistently, and tobacco smoking, which causes more cellular injury to the bronchial mucosa, may confound causality or even provide an additive effect (Fligiel, Roth et al., 1997). Moreover, heavy regular marijuana smoking is not associated with accelerated decline in FEV_1, as is tobacco smoking (Fligiel, Roth et al., 1997).

Pathogen-Associated Complications. *Aspergillus* and thermophilic actinomycetes have been reported to contaminate marijuana that is smoked (Kurup, Resnick et al., 1983). These organisms could cause respiratory tract infection or hypersensitivity reactions (Kurup, Resnick et al., 1983; Kagen, Kurup et al., 1983). Pulmonary aspergillosis associated with smoking marijuana is reported among immunocompromised patients (Hamadeh, Ardehali et al., 1988; Sutton, Lum et al., 1986). This association may become more important as increasing numbers of immunocompromised patients turn to medicinal uses of marijuana.

Lipoid Pneumonia. Respiratory failure because of lipoid pneumonia with pulmonary alveolar proteinosis in a patient with a cadaveric renal transplant has been linked to smoking weed oil prepared from marijuana (Vethanayagam, Pugsley et al., 2000).

Paraquat Lung. Paraquat is widely used throughout the world as an herbicide. Massive accidental or intentional exposure to paraquat has resulted in severe multisystem, including respiratory, organ failure (Lheureux, Leduc et al., 1995; Daisley & Hutchinson, 1998). Workers with chronic occupational exposure and survivors of paraquat poisoning may develop pulmonary fibrosis (Yamashita, Yamashita et al., 2000). However, there is no epidemiologic evidence to demonstrate a link between smoking paraquat-sprayed marijuana and pulmonary fibrosis (Landrigan, Powell et al., 1983).

Hemp Worker's Lung. Nonsmoking workers in the hemp industry display evidence of chronic cough and byssinosis, as manifested by accelerated decline in FEV_1 (Zuskin, Mustajbegovic et al., 1994). Much of the cultivation of hemp is an industry separate from that of marijuana production, with differing processing techniques. It is not clear whether workers cultivating the same plant, albeit the female of the species, develop a byssinosis-like syndrome.

COCAINE

Cocaine blocks norepinephrine and serotonin reuptake and causes release of norepinephrine, serotonin, and dopamine. Cocaine also has local anesthetic effects, blocking sodium and potassium channel flux, thereby reducing action potentials and inhibiting conduction of nerve impulses. Cocaine crosses the blood-brain barrier and stimulates the CNS where, in addition to the well-known effects on the limbic system, it can increase respiratory rate (Kreek, 1996).

Cocaine is inhaled nasally, smoked, injected, and ingested. Approximately 20% to 30% of the inhaled dose actually reaches the lung (Fattinger, Benowitz et al., 2000). Cocaine often is combined with nicotine, which has similar effects; with marijuana; and with various depressants, including heroin or morphine ("speedballing") to attenuate the sudden decrease in the sense of euphoria (McBride, Inciardi et al., 1992). This particular combination has led to a number of high-profile overdose deaths. "Freebasing" is the practice of using volatile solvents to convert cocaine from a salt to a base and to remove adulterants. This potentially incendiary chemical process can lead to extensive cutaneous and inhalational burns. The final freebase product is highly potent and has a rapid onset of action, and thus is likely to induce pulmonary, cardiac, neurologic, and other complications (Hatsukami & Fischman, 1996).

Cocaine causes fewer tracheobronchial mucosal abnormalities than either smoked tobacco or marijuana, but it may augment the injury induced by those smoked drugs (Barsky, Roth et al., 1998). It contributes to field cancerization, increasing the risk of malignancy (Barsky, Roth et al., 1998), but epidemiologic studies have not clearly demonstrated a link to cocaine alone (Mao & Oh, 1998). However, cocaine is a highly potent bronchoconstrictor when inhaled (Tashkin, Kleerup et al., 1996).

Cocaine smoking has prominent effects on vasculature, causing vasoconstriction and permeability changes (Om, 1992; Tashkin, Kleerup et al., 1997). Reduction in diffusion capacity and increased clearance of inhaled technetium-99 compared with nonsmokers are seen in crack cocaine smokers, reflecting damage to the alveolar–capillary membrane, similar to the abnormality associated with smoking tobacco (Tashkin, Gorelick et al., 1992). Cocaine also causes alveolar hemorrhage and noncardiogenic pulmonary edema (Bailey, Fraire et al., 1994; Murray, Albin et al., 1988; Albertson, Walby et al., 1995). Cocaine thus may induce injury through vasoconstriction and by impairing the integrity of the pulmonary capillary bed.

Cocaine has effects on the immune system, which may contribute to infections or to local inflammatory reactions. It impairs the function of natural killer cells, B and T lymphocytes (Baldwin, Roth et al., 1998; Xu, Flick et al., 1999). Alveolar macrophages from cocaine users have marked defects in their ability to kill bacteria and tumor cells because of a defect in nitric oxide production (Baldwin, Tashkin et al., 1997). Following *in vivo* inhalation or injection of cocaine, neutrophils are activated and have enhanced production of IL-8, which has been implicated in a number of inflammatory lung disorders, including acute lung injury (Baldwin, Buckley et al., 1997).

Cocaine may cause a wide range of acute and chronic pulmonary complications, the true incidence of which is not known. Such respiratory complications often cause individuals to seek medical care. Complications may also result from seizure or stroke, including atelectasis, aspiration, and noncardiogenic pulmonary edema (Albertson, Walby et al., 1995). Symptoms commonly associated with cocaine use, particularly use of crack cocaine, include cough productive of carbonaceous sputum, pleuritic chest pain, wheezing, dyspnea, and hemoptysis (Albertson, Walby et al., 1995).

Barotrauma. Barotrauma is common with crack cocaine inhalation and is associated with prolonged and forceful deep inhalation, Valsalva maneuver, or "shotgunning" (forceful exhalation of crack smoke into another individual's respiratory tract) (Albertson, Walby et al., 1995).

Upper Airway Complications. A variety of upper-airway complications are associated with inhaled cocaine, primarily burns and mucosal irritation or inflammation. The latter may result from the vasoconstrictive properties of cocaine and can cause nasal septal perforation, sinusitis epiglottitis, and upper-airway obstruction (Albertson, Walby et al., 1995; Meleca, Burgio et al., 1997; Reino & Lawson, 1993). Aspiration of the nasal septum may occur (Libby, Klein et al., 1992). A vasculitis resembling Wegener granulomatosis in the upper airway has been reported in association with nasal inhalation of cocaine (Armstrong & Shikani, 1996).

Bronchitis. Both acute and chronic bronchitis may develop from mucosal irritation, as described earlier. Often there is concomitant tobacco use, which contributes in large measure to airway obstruction (Fligiel, Roth et al., 1997; Albertson, Walby et al., 1995).

Airway Burns. Thermal injury, typically associated with freebasing, more commonly involves the upper airway and may cause airway obstruction. Anesthetic properties of cocaine make the oropharynx and tracheobronchial tree susceptible to thermal inhalational injuries (Meleca, Burgio et al., 1997; Reino & Lawson, 1993). Lower-airway burns may lead to airway or tracheal stenosis, if extensive or circumferential (Albertson, Walby et al., 1995).

Bronchospasm. Cocaine inhalation, but not injection, causes measurable and clinically significant bronchoconstriction in both asthmatic and nonasthmatic, nonatopic individuals (Tashkin, Kleerup et al., 1996). Cocaine-induced bronchoconstriction is thought to be mediated by airway irritant receptors (Tashkin, 2001). Cocaine inhalation may precipitate life-threatening exacerbations of asthma (Albertson, Walby et al., 1995; Ettinger & Albin, 1989).

Bronchospasm tends to be more severe among cocaine users, and cocaine use is associated with inhaled corticosteroid noncompliance and recrudescence of symptoms (Rome, Lippmann et al., 2000; Tashkin, Kleerup et al., 1996; Osborn, Tang et al., 1997).

Hemoptysis. Hemoptysis may result from mucosal irritation or ulceration anywhere within the respiratory tract (as in rhinitis, sinusitis, and bronchitis), from pulmonary infarct, or from diffuse alveolar hemorrhage (Albertson, Walby et al., 1995).

Diffuse Pulmonary Hemorrhage. Autopsy studies show high rates of acute and chronic pulmonary hemorrhage (40% to 58%), as well as congestion and pulmonary edema (up to 88%). Diffuse alveolar hemorrhage may be a life-threatening complication (Bailey, Fraire et al., 1994; Albertson, Walby et al., 1995). Cocaine inhalation may incite alveolar hemorrhage in patients with Goodpasture's syndrome (Baldwin, Roth et al., 1998; Garcia-Rostan y Perez, Garcia Bragado et al., 1997).

Pulmonary Edema. Cocaine may induce both noncardiogenic and cardiogenic pulmonary edema. The pathogenesis of the latter may involve one or several mechanisms, including high negative intrathoracic pressures associated with inhalation; direct damage to the pulmonary vasculature, causing increased permeability (Tashkin, Gorelick et al., 1992; Albertson, Walby et al., 1995); or a neurogenic mechanism in which efferent sympathetic stimulation leads to increased pulmonary venous constriction and increased intravascular hydrostatic force, with or without increased pulmonary capillary permeability (Smith & Matthay, 1997).

Intravenous cocaine, administered to humans in a controlled setting, has a chronotropic effect on the heart but does not cause an increase in pulmonary capillary wedge pressure (Kleerup, Wong et al., 1997). Cardiogenic edema does occur, related to arrhythmia, coronary vasospasm-induced myocardial ischemia or infarction, or from acute heart failure related to abruptly increased afterload

(Albertson, Walby et al., 1995). Cocaine given intravenously to dogs proved to have a negative inotropic effect (Lang & Maron, 1991), which may result in pulmonary edema.

Pulmonary Vascular Disease and Infarction. Although intravenous cocaine given in a controlled setting was reported not to increase pulmonary vascular resistance, there are case reports of cocaine-induced massive pulmonary artery vasoconstriction and, rarely, pulmonary infarction (Smith, McClaughry et al., 1995; Delaney & Hoffman, 1991). Vasoconstriction, platelet aggregation, and vascular damage and induction of endothelin-1 release may contribute (Om, 1992; Smith, McClaughry et al., 1995; Delaney & Hoffman, 1991; Hendricks-Munoz et al., 1996). Patients may present with symptoms suggestive of pulmonary embolism, with pleuritic chest pain, dyspnea and hypoxemia, and usually with hemoptysis. Technetium–xenon scintigraphy demonstrates ventilation-perfusion-mismatched defect within the lung. Pulmonary hypertension may develop over time as a result of interstitial lung disease caused by debris deposited in the lung (Albertson, Walby et al., 1995). One autopsy series of cocaine-related deaths reported pulmonary artery medial hypertrophy in the absence of talc or other debris in 20% of cases (Murray, Smialek et al., 1989).

Eosinophilic Hypersensitivity Pneumonitis ("crack lung"). A mild Loeffler syndrome has been reported, with transient migratory pulmonary infiltrates and eosinophilia, which may not require treatment (Nadeem, Nasir et al., 1994). A more severe reaction may occur one to 48 hours after heavy cocaine smoking; this consists of chest pain, cough with hemoptysis, dyspnea, bronchospasm, pruritus, fever, diffuse alveolar infiltrates without effusions, and pulmonary and systemic eosinophilia (Kissner, Lawrence et al., 1987; Forrester, Steele et al., 1990). Elevated circulating IgE may be found; histopathologically, the picture is most consistent with acute eosinophilic pneumonia with extensive IgE deposition. This syndrome may represent an IgE-dependent hypersensitivity response with mast cell degranulation, eosinophil recruitment, and tissue damage. Recurrent episodes may occur with continued cocaine inhalation. It is unclear whether this syndrome is specific to cocaine or to impurities present in the inhaled drug. There is one report of cocaine-related Churg-Strauss vasculitis affecting the lung (Orriols, Munoz et al., 1996).

Bronchiolitis Obliterans-Organizing Pneumonia. A rare complication of cocaine inhalation (Patel, Dutta et al., 1987), bronchiolitis obliterans-organizing pneumonia pre-sents with subacute manifestations, including dyspnea, cough, constitutional symptoms, and patchy—usually peripheral—infiltrates. A variety of inhalational and other insults to the lung are capable of eliciting this type of inflammatory response, but its pathogenesis is obscure. It is diagnosed reliably by open lung biopsy and treated with steroids.

Panlobular Emphysema. The mechanism for the development of emphysema is not known. Bullous pulmonary emphysema may develop with chronic cocaine use (Fullana Monllor, Garcia Bermejo et al., 1998) and may be potentiated by tobacco inhalation.

Interstitial Pulmonary Fibrosis. Pulmonary fibrosis may occur as a result of intensive or chronic use of cocaine, either inhaled or injected; silica or talc usually are found histopathologically (O'Donnell, Mappin et al., 1991). This complication probably is underrecognized, as it may be subclinical. One autopsy series reported that 38% of patients had evidence of interstitial fibrosis in the lungs (Bailey, Fraire et al., 1994). Occasionally, the degree of fibrosis is extensive and leads to pulmonary hypertension.

AMPHETAMINES AND OTHER STIMULANTS

Amphetamines—whether ingested, inhaled, or injected intravenously—increase sympathetic stimulation by causing release of biogenic amines and by inhibiting their reuptake. Effects of amphetamines are predominantly cardiovascular and neurologic (Albertson, Derlet et al., 1999).

Amphetamines were used in the early part of the last century to treat respiratory illness. They have sympathomimetic effects and can induce some bronchodilation and vasoconstriction; consequently, amphetamine inhalers were manufactured for the treatment of asthma. For rhinitis, the Benzedrine® nasal inhaler introduced in 1932 contained a large dose of synthetic racemic amphetamine (Albertson, Walby et al., 1995). Amphetamines are specifically retained by the lung from the circulation, a property that is exploited for nuclear medicine imaging of the lung (Touya, Rahimian et al., 1986).

Amphetamines have adverse effects on the immune system, including a decrease in CD4 T-helper cells, an increase in immunosuppressive cytokines (transforming growth factor-beta and IL-10), and a switch from Th1-type cytokines (IL-2 and interferon-alpha) to Th2-type cytokines (IL-4 and IL-10) (Pacifici, Zuccaro et al., 2001). Such changes may adversely affect the delayed hypersensitivity response to microbial pathogens. Chlorphentermine, an amphiphilic drug, has been reported to cause phospholipidosis in a variety of murine tissues, including the lung, which is associated with impaired phagocytosis (Lehnert & Ferin, 1983).

Metabolic Acidosis and Respiratory Alkalosis. Extreme agitation and hyperthermia may result in rhabdomyolysis and severe metabolic acidosis, with an associated increased respiratory drive. A direct central effect also may increase respiratory drive (Albertson, Walby et al., 1995).

Barotrauma. Pneumomediastinum, subcutaneous, and retropharyngeal emphysema have been reported with the use of inhaled 3,4-methylenedioxymethamphetamine (MDMA or "Ecstasy") (Albertson, Walby et al., 1995; Quin, McCarthy et al., 1999; Onwudike, 1996).

Respiratory Depression. CNS and respiratory depression may be seen, particularly in overdose. Patients are at increased risk of aspiration from a depressed mental status or from seizures (Albertson, Walby et al., 1995).

Pulmonary Edema. Amphetamines may cause both cardiogenic and noncardiogenic pulmonary edema (Albertson, Walby et al., 1995; Call, Hartneck et al., 1982; Abenhain, Moride et al., 1996), as well as myocardial infarction or acute cardiomyopathy. Users also can develop pulmonary edema through a neurogenic mechanism or because of aspiration.

Pulmonary Hypertension. The most well-known association between respiratory disease and amphetamine use is pulmonary hypertension. Appetite suppressants, such as fenfluramine and its derivatives, may be causal or may hasten the development of pulmonary hypertension. One case-controlled study reported that the risk of pulmonary hypertension was increased 23 times in patients who used these drugs for more than three months (Abenhain, Moride et al., 1996). The first reported association between pulmonary hypertension and amphetamine use was in Europe in the 1960s, following an increase in cases related to aminorex fumarate. Between 1967 and 1973, 77% of patients with pulmonary hypertension reported use of aminorex fumarate before the onset of symptoms. A five-year retrospective study of patients referred for evaluation of pulmonary hypertension found that 15 (20%) had used fenfluramine and that 10 (67%) showed a temporal relationship between use of the drug and onset of symptoms (Fishman, 1999).

Intravenous injection of methylphenidate has been reported to cause fatal pulmonary hypertension (Lewman, 1972). Chronic inhalation of methamphetamine also has been reported to cause pulmonary hypertension (Schaiberger, Kennedy et al., 1993).

Patients generally complain of exertional dyspnea, have a prominent second heart sound, have jugular venous distension, and have enlarged hila on chest radiograph. Echocardiographic or right-sided catheterization may be performed to obtain pulmonary pressures. Pathology reveals changes similar to primary pulmonary hypertension, with advanced plexogenic pulmonary arteriopathy. Vasodilator therapy with epoprostenol or calcium channel blockers may be used in selected individuals, after hemodynamic monitoring ascertains a response to one of these agents. A lack of vasodilator response suggests that pulmonary hypertension is not reversible (Hammerman & Graven, 1997).

One possible explanation for the development of pulmonary hypertension related to fenfluramine use is that the drug increases circulating levels of serotonin and results in vasoconstriction of the pulmonary vasculature. Studies report that plasma serotonin levels are increased in patients with primary pulmonary hypertension. This excess serotonin may lead to pulmonary vasoconstriction and proliferation of pulmonary vascular smooth muscle. Other proposed mechanisms include toxic endothelial injury, hypoxia, vasospasm, vasculitis, and altered balance of mediators of vascular tone, such as eicosanoids (Fishman, 1999; Herve, Launay et al., 1995).

Bullous Emphysema. Bibasilar bullous pulmonary emphysema, resembling that seen in alpha-1-antitrypsin deficiency, has been reported with injection of methylphenidate (Schmidt, Glenny et al., 1991), but it has not been reported with amphetamines. The pathogenesis of this complication is not known.

CAFFEINE

Caffeine is widely available in food and drinks and in tablet form without a physician's prescription. Caffeine is a phosphodiesterase inhibitor that raises intracellular cyclic adenosine monophosphate, with effects similar to theophylline, including smooth muscle relaxation. Thus, caffeine has mild bronchodilator properties. Caffeine actually may falsely elevate the serum theophylline level (Fligner & Opheim, 1988).

Pulmonary complications are rare and usually are associated with a large overdose or unintentional ingestion by children. Respiratory alkalosis, chest pain, seizures, aspiration, respiratory failure, and pulmonary edema associated with cardiac arrhythmias may occur (Leson, McGuigan et al., 1988).

OPIOIDS

Opioids can have prominent effects on the respiratory and other organ systems because of widespread distribution of opioid receptors throughout the body. Opioids bind to specific receptors, with distribution to the CNS, cardiovascular, immune, and respiratory systems. Opioid receptors in the respiratory tract are found mostly within the alveolar walls, but also are associated with tracheal and bronchial smooth muscle. "Nonconventional" receptors also have been postulated to be active in the lung (Zebraski, Kochenash et al., 2000; Fimiani, Arcuri et al., 1999).

Opioids have their most dramatic effects on the respiratory system by acting on the CNS. Opioid binding to mu_2 receptors causes a reduction in responsiveness to carbon dioxide and depresses the pontine and medullary centers that regulate respiratory automaticity and cough. Cerebral cortical input also may be inhibited. Consequently, breathing becomes irregular and apnea may develop. Respiratory depression increases progressively as the dose is increased. Maximal respiratory depression occurs within 5 to 10 minutes after an intravenous dose or within 30 to 90 minutes after a subcutaneous or intramuscular dose, with the effects on respiration lasting four to five hours (Jaffe & Martin, 1990; Sporer, 1999).

Opioids may induce respiratory complications through effects on airways, pulmonary vasculature, the immune system, and (indirectly) through the CNS. They can induce histamine release from mast cells (Barke & Hough, 1993), which may lead to pulmonary vein constriction, increased pulmonary capillary permeability and pulmonary edema, and bronchoconstriction. Opioids have significant effects on the immune system, which may account for the reported association with infections. Specifically, they may cause defects in T cell and natural killer cell function, macrophage and neutrophil phagocytosis, inhibition of cytosine production by leukocytes, attenuation of antibody responses, inhibition of delayed type hypersensitivity responses, depression of CD4/CD8 ratio, and inhibition of leukocyte chemotaxis (Eisenstein & Hillberger, 1998; Peterson, Molitor et al., 1998). Opioids can desensitize chemokine receptors in leukocytes, decreasing their chemotactic ability (Grimm, Ben-Baruch et al., 1998). They also can induce programmed cell death of leukocytes (Yin, Mufson et al., 1999).

Although morphine often is used for the relief of dyspnea, opioids also can exert adverse effects on the lung, acutely and with chronic abuse. Pulmonary complications account for approximately 20% of opiate-related complications (Rosenow, 1972; Louria, Hensle et al., 1967). Acutely, particularly with inhalational use, opioids may induce bronchospasm, bronchitis, and hypersensitivity pneumonitis. Respiratory depression and failure, pulmonary edema, respiratory infections, chronic bronchitis, septic pulmonary emboli, pulmonary hypertension, and talc-related complications are associated with chronic (particularly intravenous) opioid abuse. Pulmonary edema probably is the most common complication of overdose, while respiratory arrest is the most serious.

Bronchospasm. It long has been recognized that asthma exacerbations may be precipitated by heroin use in some asthmatics. Opioids, which cause histamine release potentially through mu receptors or through IgE-mediation (Barke & Hough, 1993), can induce bronchospasm in histamine-sensitive asthmatics (Popa, 1994), but it is unclear whether histamine-insensitive asthmatics also may be prone to opioid-induced bronchoconstriction. Occupational asthma among workers in a pharmaceutical factory producing morphine was found to be associated with an IgE-mediated mechanism of histamine release (Moneo, Alday at al, 1993). Asthma exacerbations also may be precipitated by opioid use (Ghodse & Myles, 1987).

Pulmonary Edema. Opioid overdose, particularly with heroin, is a common cause of pulmonary edema in patients younger than 40 years, and it accounts for many drug-related deaths (O'Donnell & Pappas, 1988; Napoli, Cigtay et al., 1974). As many as 50% of overdose patients present with pulmonary edema. Twenty percent of this group will die (O'Donnell & Pappas, 1988). The occurrence of pulmonary edema is not limited to intravenously administered drugs (Cooper, White et al., 1986). Opioid-induced pulmonary edema can occur with the first use of the drug (Cooper, White et al., 1986), but it is believed to be dose-related rather than an idiosyncratic reaction (Rosenow, 1994).

Several mechanisms of opioid-induced noncardiogenic pulmonary edema have been offered. One hypothesis suggests that opioids have a direct toxic effect on the alveolar capillary membrane, increasing permeability and allowing fluid extravasation into the alveolar spaces (Cooper, White et al., 1986). Alternatively, opioids' effect on the CNS may induce a vast neurogenic efferent response that leads to alveolar capillary permeability or pulmonary venous constriction (Smith & Matthay, 1997; Hakim, Grunstein et al., 1992). Other possibilities include a hypersensitivity re-action or acute hypoxic effect, causing increased alveolar capillary membrane permeability (Cooper, White et al., 1986). Clinically, this complication manifests as dyspnea and somnolence, usually within minutes, depending on the route of administration. Rales may be heard bilaterally on physical examination. Progressively, affected individuals become obtunded and cyanotic and develop hypoxemia and hypercapnia (Cooper, White et al., 1986). The chest radio-graph typically reveals interstitial and/or alveolar bilateral infiltrates, often in a perihilar pattern, without cardio-megaly or pleural effusions. The pulmonary capillary wedge pressure usually is within the normal range. The electro-cardiogram may be normal or may show arrhythmias and conduction defects.

Treatment is supportive and may include noninvasive or invasive mechanical ventilation, positive end-expiratory pressure, oxygen, and judicious use of diuretics. The clini-cal and radiographic abnormality generally clears within 24 hours. If there is not improvement within 48 hours, alter-native diagnoses should be considered, including aspiration and superimposed pneumonia. It is estimated that as many as 50% to 75% of patients with pulmonary edema develop a superimposed pneumonia (Rosenow, 1972).

Hypersensitivity Pneumonitis. Although uncommon, intranasal heroin has been reported to cause hypersensitiv-ity pneumonitis (Karne, D'Ambrosio et al., 1999). Patients usually manifest with dyspnea and cough hours to days af-ter inhalation, which may lead to significant hypoxemia. Chest radiograph may show bilateral infiltrates, which may be reticulonodular or coalescent. Treatment includes supple-mental oxygen and steroids if compromise is evident and if spontaneous regression does not occur.

ALCOHOL

Alcohol ingestion may cause acute intoxication accompa-nied by respiratory depression and such common complica-tions as atelectasis, hypoxemia, respiratory acidosis, aspira-tion, adult respiratory distress syndrome, and respiratory failure (Heinemann, 1977). Aspiration pneumonia may be associated with loss of airway control or seizures. Alcohol ingestion also may cause worsening of underlying respira-tory conditions such as sleep apnea (Scanlan, Roebuck et al., 2000). Alcohol depresses respiration by acting directly on the respiratory centers within the brain. Chronic abuse may lead to cirrhosis, with the development of specific hepatopulmonary syndromes and increased susceptibility to infections. Pneumonia related to *Klebsiella, Streptococcus pneumoniae,* tuberculosis, and other pathogens is common among individuals who abuse alcohol chronically (Cook, 1998; Adams & Jordan, 1984). This condition may stem from malnutrition, concomitant tobacco abuse, immune suppression, and decreased function of the reticuloendo-thelial system (Heinemann, 1977; Cook, 1998; Adams & Jordan, 1984).

Acute Metabolic Acidosis and Respiratory Alkalosis. Alcohol may cause metabolic acidosis from alcoholic ke-toacidosis, with resultant compensatory respiratory alkalosis (Duffens & Marx, 1987). Ingestion of other alcohols (such as methanol) may cause wide anion gap acidosis and lead to compensatory respiratory alkalosis (Hojer, 1996).

Chronic Respiratory Alkalosis. Among patients with cirrhosis, chronic respiratory alkalosis is common, even in the absence of metabolic acidosis. This condition may be due to the respiratory stimulant effect of poorly cleared progesterone and estradiol on the CNS, which has an im-paired blood-brain barrier (Lustik, Chibber et al., 1997).

Asthma. Patients with preexisting asthma, particularly those who are histamine sensitive, may experience worsen-ing of asthma symptoms after consumption of alcohol (Vally, de Klerk et al., 2000; Ayres & Clark, 1983; Zimatkin & Anitchtchik, 1999). However, some individuals actually experience a degree of symptom relief or bronchodilatation (Ayres & Clark, 1983; Ayres, Ancic et al., 1982). In a small number of individuals, this relief may be due to the pres-ence of sulfites in wine or other beverages, but it can lead to severe bronchospasm and death (Vally, Carr et al., 1999). A third of asthmatic patients report worsening of symptoms after alcohol consumption, suggesting other operative mechanisms (Ayres & Clark, 1983; Vally, de Klerk et al., 2000). In some patients, acetaldehyde, generated from etha-nol metabolism, appears to lead to mast cell or basophil degranulation (Fujimura, Myou et al., 1999). The ensuing release of histamine and other mediators of inflammation induces asthma, as suggested by the ability of chlorphenira-mine largely to inhibit ethanol-induced bronchospasm (Gong, Tashkin et al., 1981). Both heterozygotic and homo-zygotic mutations in acetaldehyde dehydrogenase have been found to correlate with alcohol-induced airway reactivity (Takao, Shimoda et al., 1998). However, elevated IgE has not been associated with this syndrome (Shimoda, Kohno et al., 1996).

Pulmonary Restriction From Ascites. Massive ascites, with or without hydrothorax, may impede diaphragmatic and pulmonary excursion, leading to rapid shallow breathing, dyspnea, atelectasis, and even hypoxemia (Yao, Kong et al., 1987; King, Rumbaut et al., 1996).

Hepatic Hydrothorax. Cirrhosis with ascites may lead to the formation of pleural effusion. Negative intrapleural pressure generated during inspiration, rather than as a result of decreased plasma oncotic pressure, leads to transdiaphragmatic movement of ascitic fluid into the pleural space. Such fluid often occupies the entire hemithorax, usually on the right side. If refractory to diuretics and other medical therapy, pleurodesis or transjugular intrahepatic portosystemic shunts (TIPS) may be performed, with variable success (Lazaridis, Frank et al., 1999).

Hepatopulmonary Syndrome. This syndrome, found in 8% to 15% of patients with cirrhosis, consists of a triad of liver dysfunction, intrapulmonary or other vascular dilatations, and arterial hypoxemia. Arteriovenous shunts are thought to arise from circulating estrogen-like substances, as well as from elevated nitric oxide production in the lung, leading to dyspnea, playtypnea, clubbing, and orthodeoxia. Diagnostic elements include evidence of cirrhosis and hypoxemia and the demonstration of a right-to-left shunt by technetium 99-macroaggregated albumin perfusion scan or by bubble echocardiography. Hemodynamic studies often reveal a hyperdynamic cardiac output with low pulmonary vascular resistance, which may be seen in cirrhosis. In general, TIPS has been reported to improve the physiologic compromise of hepatopulmonary syndrome (Fallon & Abrams, 2000a, 2000b; Schraufnagel & Kay, 1996; Abrams, Jaffe et al., 1995).

Portal Pulmonary Hypertension. Approximately 2% of patients with cirrhosis develop pulmonary arterial hypertension. The pathogenesis of this complication is not clear, but it probably is mediated by both mechanical and humoral factors. Vasoactive substances, which ordinarily are cleared or produced by the liver, may induce vasoconstriction or endothelial damage. Pathologically, the lesion is similar to that seen with primary pulmonary hypertension: plexogenic pulmonary arteriopathy, medial hypertrophy, intimal cellular proliferation, and eventual arteriolar dilatation (Herve, Lebrec et al., 1998; Robalino & Moodie, 1991). Patients usually have exertional dyspnea, but some have incidentally discovered pulmonary hypertension. The physical signs of right-sided heart failure from pulmonary hypertension may be missed in cirrhotic patients, who already may have peripheral edema. Vasodilator therapy may be used judiciously after hemodynamic trials (Kahler, Graziadei et al.,

2000). Liver transplantation has been reported to alleviate portal pulmonary hypertension, but fixed pulmonary hypertension may constitute a relative contraindication because of a poor prognosis (Kuo, Plotkin et al., 1999). Pulmonary hypertension also may develop as a consequence of TIPS, which should not be performed in an attempt to treat portal pulmonary hypertension (Van der Linden, Le Moine et al., 1996).

Adult Respiratory Distress Syndrome. Individuals who chronically abuse alcohol are twice as likely as nonusers to develop adult respiratory distress syndrome in response to usual triggers such as aspiration and infection. Epithelial lining fluid from the lung of alcohol abusers is depleted of glutathione, which is important in mitigating the oxidative stress that plays a role in the pathogenesis of ARDS (Moss, Guidot et al., 2000).

SEDATIVE-HYPNOTICS

Sedative-hypnotic drugs may exert significant respiratory depressant effects when abused or when mixed with alcohol and opiates. Benzodiazepines, barbiturates, and gamma-hydroxybutyrate (GHB) bind gamma-aminobutyric acid (GABA) receptors, which normally function as targets for inhibitory neurotransmitters and promote sedation, hypnosis, anxiolysis, anterograde amnesia, and anticonvulsant activity (Jaffe & Martin, 1990; Jay, Johanson et al., 1975; Graudins & Aaron, 1999).

GHB is a naturally occurring metabolite of GABA in the CNS. Unlike benzodiazepines and barbiturates, which bind GABA receptors, GHB interacts with $GABA_B$ receptors. Other GHB effects include elevation of CNS dopamine, elevation of CNS endorphins, and stimulation of growth hormone release. GHB is abused by bodybuilders and by those seeking its hypnotic and euphoric effects (Chin, Dyer et al., 1999). Adverse respiratory effects are mainly related to overdose.

Overdose. Barbiturates were the cornerstone of sedative-hypnotic therapy until the 1970s, when they were replaced by the less toxic benzodiazepines. In 1975, sedative-hypnotic drug overdose accounted for approximately 1% of admissions to the medical service and approximately 10% of cases of respiratory failure. One percent to 10% of patients did not survive. Of the patients who died, 40% died of respiratory complications (Jay, Johanson et al., 1975). Today, the incidence of sedative drug overdose is substantially lower. In reviews of 1,239 overdose cases from a medical examiner's office, only two deaths were related solely to benzodiazepine overdose (Graudins & Aaron, 1999; Finkle, McCloskey et al., 1979). Benzodiazepine overdose most commonly occurs as part of a polysubstance overdose.

Although barbiturates also may be involved in a poly-pharmacy overdose, the most common toxic scenario with barbiturates is an accidental or intentional oral ingestion by a seizure patient or member of his or her family (Graudins & Aaron, 1999).

Clinically, sedation may progress to coma, with progressive alveolar hypoventilation and respiratory acidosis. Hypotension, which probably is related to direct myocardial depression and vasodilatation, may follow, with accompanying respiratory arrest (more typically in barbiturate overdose) (Graudins & Aaron, 1999).

Treatment of sedative-hypnotic overdose is supportive and usually entails decontamination with lavage and charcoal adsorption. Supplemental oxygen, airway protection, and mechanical ventilation may be necessary. Most deaths occur as a result of ARDS secondary to either a chemical aspiration pneumonitis or bacterial pneumonia (Jaffe & Martin, 1990). The former typically occurs when there is witnessed aspiration during a difficult intubation (Jay, Johanson et al., 1975).

In benzodiazepine overdose, the competitive antagonist flumazenil can be administered with caution, but it is short-acting and its ability to reverse the respiratory depressant effects is controversial. Side effects include anxiety, agitation, crying, nausea, and seizures (Graudins & Aaron, 1999).

In barbiturate overdose, elimination can be enhanced with an alkaline diuresis. Dialysis rarely is necessary; however, hemodynamic instability refractory to fluid management is an indication for dialysis. Serum drug levels often rebound after dialysis because of redistribution, necessitating further dialysis (Graudins & Aaron, 1999).

The use of CNS stimulants may increase mortality and is contraindicated (Jaffe & Martin, 1990). In GHB overdose, recovery is rapid, with full return to baseline within several hours (Graudins & Aaron, 1999). Recovery from benzodiazepine and barbiturate overdose is longer in duration. Generally, the prognosis is excellent with supportive care alone.

Withdrawal Syndromes. Abrupt cessation of chronically used sedative-hypnotics may lead to withdrawal symptoms. Tachypnea is the most common respiratory manifestation of withdrawal from benzodiazepines, which causes a hyperadrenergic state that increases carbon dioxide production. To eliminate excess carbon dioxide and as a result of anxiety, the individual experiencing withdrawal hyperventilates. Tachypnea always is accompanied by other manifestations of benzodiazepine withdrawal, including anxiety, tremor, headache, diaphoresis, difficulty concentrating, insomnia, hallucinations, or fatigue. It generally occurs two to five days after the last dose of the drug (Graudins & Aaron, 1999).

Barbiturate withdrawal occurs after two to seven days' abstinence. Agitation, hyperreflexia, anxiety, and tremor are most common, followed by confusion and hallucinations. Up to 75% of patients experience seizures, often refractory to phenytoin. Effective treatment requires reinstitution of a barbiturate or a cross-tolerant medication such as a benzodiazepine. Because seizures are so common in barbiturate withdrawal, airway protection and management is the primary respiratory issue (Graudins & Aaron, 1999).

Sleep. Benzodiazepines can worsen sleep disorders by decreasing the tone of the upper-airway muscles and reducing the ventilatory response to CO_2, leading to worse nocturnal hypoxia and pulmonary hypertension (Jaffe & Martin, 1990). Although benzodiazepines can be beneficial in treating sleep disorders by increasing total sleep time and the sense of refreshing sleep, their effect on sleep disorders is difficult to predict.

VOLATILE SUBSTANCES

Abuse of inhalants is highly prevalent throughout the world, particularly among young teenagers. Volatile substances are aromatic and short-chain hydrocarbons, such as toluene, gasoline, butane, butyl and amyl nitrites, and Freon®, which are found in adhesives, paints, paint thinner, dry cleaning fluids, refrigerants, and propellants. They are volatile at room temperature. When sniffed or, more commonly, vigorously inhaled within a hermetic container ("huffed"), they are readily absorbed in the lungs. Intoxicating and dysphoric effects follow within seconds (Wyse, 1973).

Primary acute effects involve the CNS and include lethargy, stupor agitation, hallucinations, dizziness, and seizures (Flanagan & Ives, 1994). Pulmonary complications include severe respiratory depression, barotrauma (pneumomediastinum), persistent cough, and suffocation (Flanagan & Ives, 1994; Cohen, 1975; Linden, 1990).

Methemoglobinemia. Butyl and isobutyl nitrites may cause methemoglobinemia, which manifests as cyanosis with normal partial pressure of oxygen. However, oxygen saturation of hemoglobin is low and co-oximetry will specifically measure methemoglobin (Linden, 1990; Curry, 1982). Intravenous methylene blue may be administered for treatment (Wright, Lewander et al., 1999).

Metabolic Acidosis and Respiratory Alkalosis. Metabolic acidosis may occur, with compensatory respiratory alkalosis, resulting from distal renal tubular acidosis or from wide anion gap acidosis. The latter may result from oxidation of toluenes to benzoic acid and conjugation with glycine to form hippuric acid (Fischman & Oster, 1979).

Asthma. Occupational exposure to toluene diisocyanate and other isocyanates may be associated with asthma (Ott, Klees et al., 2000). However, no cases of asthma associated with toluene abuse have been reported. In some cases, an IgE-mediated mechanism may be operative, but in others, multiple mechanisms are at work (Raulf-Heimsoth & Baur, 1998). A hypersensitivity pneumonitis also has been reported with isocyanate inhalation (Baur, 1995).

Tracheobronchitis. Nitrates and other inhalants may be directly irritating to airway mucosa and cause chronic cough (Covalla, Strimlan et al., 1981).

Asphyxiation. Users of inhalants may develop asphyxiation from plastic bag suffocation or from respiratory depression (Paterson & Sarvesvaran, 1983; Ikeda, Takahashi et al., 1990).

NITROUS OXIDE

Nitrous oxide is a readily available, often abused substance with euphoric effects. It is a widely used inhalational anesthetic-analgesic agent, which also is used in a variety of commercial products (such as a propellant for whipped cream chargers) (Brouett & Anton, 2001). Nitrous oxide may bind to the opioid receptors (Gillman, 1986).

Pulmonary complications include pneumomediastinum, respiratory depression, and hypoxemia because of displacement of oxygen, leading to asphyxia (Brouette & Anton, 2001; LiPuma, Wellman et al., 1982; Wagner, Clark et al., 1992). Treatment is supportive, including supplemental oxygen and respiratory support (Brouette & Anton, 2001).

ANABOLIC STEROIDS

Anabolic steroids induce a pro-thrombotic state and may cause pulmonary embolism, strokes, and other forms of thromboses (Gaede & Montine, 1992; Akhter, Hyder et al., 1994). Respiratory complications are less common but may occur after stroke, and include atelectasis, pneumonia, and aspiration.

REFERENCES

Abenhain L, Moride Y, Brenot F et al. (1996). Appetite-suppressant drugs and the risk of pulmonary hypertension. *New England Journal of Medicine* 335:609-616.

Abrams GA, Jaffe CC, Hoffer PB et al. (1995). Diagnostic utility of contrast echocardiography and lung perfusion scan in patients with hepatopulmonary syndrome. *Gastroenterology* 109(4):1283-1288.

Adams HG & Jordan C (1984). Infections in the alcoholic. *Medical Clinics of North America* 68(1):179-200.

Aguado JM, Arjona R & Ugarte P (1990). Septic pulmonary emboli. A rare cause of bilateral pneumothorax in drug abusers. *Chest* 98(5):1302-1304.

Aguis R (1989). Opiate inhalation and occupational asthma. *British Medical Journal* 298:323.

Akhter J, Hyder S & Ahmed M (1994). Cerebrovascular accident associated with anabolic steroid use in a young man. *Neurology* 44(12):2405-2406.

Albertson TE, Derlet RW & Van Hoozen BE (1999). Methamphetamine and the expanding complications of amphetamines. *Western Journal of Medicine* 170(4):214-219.

Albertson TE, Walby WF & Derlet RW (1995). Stimulant-induced pulmonary toxicity. *Chest* 108(4):1140-1149.

American Thoracic Society (2000). Targeted tuberculin testing and treatment of latent tuberculosis infection. *Morbidity and Mortality Weekly Report* 49(RR-6):1-51.

Armstrong M Jr. & Shikani AH (1996). Nasal septal necrosis mimicking Wegener's granulomatosis in a cocaine abuser. *Ear, Nose, and Throat Journal* 75(9):623-626

Aubry MC, Wright JL & Myers JL (2000) The pathology of smoking-related lung diseases. *Clinics in Chest Medicine* 21(1):11-35.

Ayres JG, Ancic P & Clark TJ (1982). Airway responses to oral ethanol in normal subjects and in patients with asthma. *Journal of the Royal Society of Medicine* 75(9):699-704.

Ayres JG & Clark TJ (1983). Alcoholic drinks and asthma: A survey. *British Journal of Diseases of the Chest* 77(4):370-375.

Bailey ME, Fraire AE, Greenberg SD et al. (1994). Pulmonary histopathology in cocaine abusers. *Human Pathology* 25(2):203-207

Baldwin GC, Buckley DM, Roth MD et al. (1997). Acute activation of circulating polymorphonuclear neutrophils following in vivo administration of cocaine. A potential etiology for pulmonary injury. *Chest* 111(3):698-705.

Baldwin GC, Roth MD & Tashkin DP (1998). Acute and chronic effects of cocaine on the immune system and the possible link to AIDS. *Journal of Neuroimmunology* 83(1–2):133-138.

Baldwin GC, Tashkin DP, Buckley DM et al. (1997). Marijuana and cocaine impair alveolar macrophage function and cytokine production. *American Journal of Respiratory and Critical Care Medicine* 156(5):1606-1613.

Balfour D, Benowitz N, Fagerström K et al. (2000). Diagnosis and treatment of nicotine dependence with emphasis on nicotine replacement therapy. A status report. *European Heart Journal* 21(6):438-445.

Barke KE & Hough LB (1993). Opiates, mast cells, and histamine release. *Life Sciences* 53(18):1391-1399.

Barsky SH, Roth MD, Kleerup EC et al. (1998). Histopathologic and molecular alterations in bronchial epithelium in habitual smokers of marijuana, cocaine, and/or tobacco. *Journal of the National Cancer Institute* 90(16):1198-1205.

Baumgartner KB, Samet JM, Stidley CA et al. (1997). Cigarette smoking: A risk factor for idiopathic pulmonary fibrosis. *American Journal of Respiratory and Critical Care Medicine* 155(1):242-248.

Baur X (1995). Hypersensitivity pneumonitis (extrinsic allergic alveolitis) induced by isocyanates. *Journal of Allergy and Clinical Immunology* 95(5 pt 1):1004-1010.

Berk J (1997). Pneumothorax. In R Goldstein, J O'Connell & J Karlinksy (eds.) *A Practical Approach to Pulmonary Medicine*. Philadelphia, PA: Lippincott-Raven, 206-233.

Brouette T & Anton R (2001). Clinical review of inhalants. *American Journal on Addictions* 10(1):79-94.

Brugman S & Irvin C (1988). Lung structure and function. In RS Mitchell, T Petty & M Schwartz (eds.) *Synopsis of Clinical Pulmonary Disease, 4th Edition*. St. Louis, MO: C.V. Mosby, 1-17.

Burrows B, Lebowitz MD, Barbee RA et al. (1983). Interactions of smoking and immunologic factors in relation to airways obstruction. *Chest* 84(6):657-661.

Bynum LJ & Pierce AK (1976). Pulmonary aspiration of gastric contents. *American Review of Respiratory Disease* 114(6):1129-1136.

Call TD, Hartneck J, Dickinson WA et al. (1982). Acute cardiomyopathy secondary to intravenous amphetamine abuse. *Annals of Internal Medicine* 97(4):559-560.

Casale TB, Rhodes BJ, Donnelly AL et al. (1987). Airway responses to methacholine in asymptomatic nonatopic cigarette smokers. *Journal of Applied Physiology* 62(5):1888-1892.

Chin RL, Dyer JE & Sporer KA (1999). gamma-hydroxybutyrate intoxication and overdose. *Annals of Emergency Medicine* 33(4):476.

Cohen S (1975). Glue sniffing. *Journal of the American Medical Association* 231(6):653-654.

Collazos J, Martinez E, Fernandez A et al. (1996). Acute, reversible pulmonary hypertension associated with cocaine use. *Respiratory Medicine* 90(3):171-174.

Cone EJ (1998). Recent discoveries in pharmacokinetics of drugs of abuse. *Toxicology Letters* 102-103:97-101.

Cook RT (1998). Alcohol abuse, alcoholism, and damage to the immune system—A review. *Alcoholism: Clinical & Experimental Research* 22(9):1927-1942.

Cooper AD, White DA & Matthay RA (1986). Drug-induced pulmonary disease. Part 2: Noncytotoxic drugs. *American Review of Respiratory Disease* 133:488-505.

Copas JB & Shi JQ (2000). Reanalysis of epidemiological evidence on lung cancer and passive smoking. *British Medical Journal* 320(7232):417-418.

Covalla JR, Strimlan CV & Lech JG (1981). Severe tracheobronchitis from inhalation of an isobutyl nitrite preparation. *Drug Intelligence and Clinical Pharmacy* 15(1):51-52.

Crofton J & Douglas A (1981). The structure and function of the respiratory tract. In *Respiratory Diseases, 3rd Edition*. Boston, MA: Blackwell Scientific Publications, 1-79.

Cullen JW, Blot W, Henningfield J et al. (1986). Health consequences of using smokeless tobacco: Summary of the Advisory Committee's report to the Surgeon General. *Public Health Reports* 101(4):355-373.

Curry S (1982). Methemoglobinemia. *Annals of Emergency Medicine* 11:214-221.

Da Costa JL, Tock EP & Boey HK (1971). Lung disease with chronic obstruction in opium smokers in Singapore. Clinical, electrocardiographic, radiological, functional and pathological features. *Thorax* 26(5):555-571.

Daisley H & Hutchinson G (1998). Paraquat poisoning. *Lancet* 24;352(9137):1393-1394.

Dalvie MA, White N, Raine R et al. (1999). Long-term respiratory health effects of the herbicide, paraquat, among workers in the Western Cape. *Occupational and Environmental Medicine* 56(6):391-396.

Delaney K & Hoffman RS (1991). Pulmonary infarction associated with crack cocaine use in a previously healthy 23-year-old woman. *American Journal of Medicine* 91(1):92-94.

Duffens K & Marx JA (1987). Alcoholic ketoacidosis—A review. *Journal of Emergency Medicine* 5(5):399-406.

Eisenstein TK & Hilburger ME (1998). Opioid modulation of immune responses: Effects on phagocyte and lymphoid cell populations. *Journal of Neuroimmunology* 83(1–2):36-44.

Ettinger NA & Albin RJ (1989). A review of the respiratory effects of smoking cocaine. *American Journal of Medicine* 87(6):664-668.

Fallon MB & Abrams GA (2000a). Hepatopulmonary syndrome. *Current Gastroenterology Reports* 2(1):40-45.

Fallon MB & Abrams GA (2000b). Pulmonary dysfunction in chronic liver disease. *Hepatology* 32(4 pt 1):859-865.

Fattinger K, Benowitz NL, Jones RT et al. (2000). Nasal mucosal versus gastrointestinal absorption of nasally administered cocaine. *European Journal of Clinical Pharmacology* 56(4):305-310.

Feigin DS (1986). Talc: Understanding its manifestations in the chest. *American Journal of Roentgenology* 146(2):295-301.

Fimiani C, Arcuri E, Santoni A et al. (1999). Mu3 opiate receptor expression in lung and lung carcinoma: Ligand binding and coupling to nitric oxide release. *Cancer Letters* 146(1):45-51.

Finkelstein R, Fraser RS, Ghezzo H et al. (1995). Alveolar inflammation and its relation to emphysema in smokers. *American Journal of Respiratory and Critical Care Medicine* 152(5 pt 1):1666-1672.

Finkle BS, McCloskey KL, Goodman LS et al. (1979). Diazepam and drug-associated deaths: A survey in the United States and Canada. *Journal of the American Medical Association* 242:429-434.

Fischman, CM & JR Oster (1979). Toxic effects of Toluene; A new cause of high anion gap acidosis. *Journal of the American Medical Association* 241(16):1713-1715.

Fishman AP (1999). Aminorex to fen/phen: An epidemic foretold. *Circulation* 99(1):156-161.

Flanagan RJ & Ives RJ (1994). Volatile substance abuse. *Bulletin of Narcotics* 46(2):49-78.

Fligiel SE, Beals TF, Tashkin DP et al. (1991). Marijuana exposure and pulmonary alterations in primates. *Pharmacology, Biochemistry and Behavior* 40(3):637-642.

Fligiel SE, Roth MD, Kleerup EC et al. (1997). Tracheobronchial histopathology in habitual smokers of cocaine, marijuana, and/or tobacco. *Chest* 112(2):319-326.

Fligner CL & Opheim KE (1988). Caffeine and its dimethylxanthine metabolites in two cases of caffeine overdose: A cause of falsely elevated theophylline concentrations in serum. *Journal of Analytical Toxicology* 12(6):339-343

Forrester JM, Steele AW, Waldron JA et al. (1990). Crack lung: An acute pulmonary syndrome with a spectrum of clinical and histopathologic findings. *American Review of Respiratory Disease* 142(2):462-467.

Foth H (1995). Role of the lung in accumulation and metabolism of xenobiotic compounds—Implications for chemically induced toxicity. *Critical Reviews in Toxicology* 25(2):165-205.

Fujimura M, Myou S, Kamio Y et al. (1999). Increased airway responsiveness to acetaldehyde in asthmatic subjects with alcohol-induced bronchoconstriction. *European Respiratory Journal* 14(1):19-22.

Fullana Monllor J, Garcia Bermejo PA & Pellicer Ciscar C (1998). Bullous emphysema in a cocaine smoker [in Spanish]. *Archivos de Bronconeumologia* 34(10):514.

Fung M, Gallagher C & Machtay M (1999). Lung and aero-digestive cancers in young marijuana smokers. *Tumori* 85(2):140-142.

Gadek JE (1992). Adverse effects of neutrophils on the lung. *American Journal of Medicine* 92(6A):27S-31S.

Gaede JT & Montine TJ (1992). Massive pulmonary embolus and anabolic steroid abuse. *Journal of the American Medical Association* 267(17):2328-2329.

Garcia-Rostan y Perez GM, Garcia Bragado F et al. (1997). Pulmonary hemorrhage and antiglomerular basement membrane antibody-mediated glomerulonephritis after exposure to smoked cocaine (crack): A case report and review of the literature. *Pathology International* 47(10):692-697

Genereux GP & Emson HE (1974). Talc granulomatosis and angiothrombotic pulmonary hypertension in drug addicts. *Journal of the Canadian Association of Radiologists* 25(2):87-93.

Ghodse AH & Myles JS (1987). Asthma in opiate addicts. *Journal of Psychosomatic Research* 31:41-44.

Gillman MA (1986). Nitrous oxide, an opioid addictive agent. Review of the evidence. *American Journal of Medicine* 81(1):97-102.

Godwin JE, Harley RA, Miller KS et al. (1989). Cocaine, pulmonary hemorrhage, and hemoptysis. *Annals of Internal Medicine* 110(10):843.

Gong H Jr., Tashkin DP & Calvarese BM (1981). Alcohol-induced bronchospasm in an asthmatic patient: Pharmacologic evaluation of the mechanism. *Chest* 80(2):167-173.

Graudins A & Aaron CK (1999). Sedative-hypnotic poisoning. In RS Irwin, FB Cerra & JM Rippe (eds.) *Intensive Care Medicine*. Boston, MA: Little, Brown & Company, 1782-1792.

Grellner W, Madea B & Sticht G (1996). Pulmonary histopathology and survival period in morphine-involved deaths. *Journal of Forensic Sciences* 41(3):433-437.

Grimm MC, Ben-Baruch A, Taub DD et al. (1998). Opiates transreactivate chemokine receptors: Delta and mu opiate receptor-mediated heterologous desensitization. *Journal of Experimental Medicine* 188(2):317-325.

Hahn HL, Lang M, Bleicher S et al. (1992). Nicotine-induced airway smooth muscle contraction: Neural mechanisms involving the airway epithelium. Functional and histologic studies in vitro. *Clinical Investigator* 70(3-4):252-262.

Hakim TS, Grunstein MM & Michel RP (1992). Opiate action in the pulmonary circulation. *Pulmonary Pharmacology* 5(3):159-165.

Hamadeh R, Ardehali A, Locksley RM et al. (1988). Fatal aspergillosis associated with smoking contaminated marijuana, in a marrow transplant recipient. *Chest* 94(2):432-433.

Hance AJ, Basset F, Saumon G et al. (1986). Smoking and interstitial lung disease. The effect of cigarette smoking on the incidence of histiocytosis X and sarcoidosis. *Annals of the New York Academy of Sciences* 465:643-656.

Hansson L, Choudry NB, Karlsson JA et al. (1994). Inhaled nicotine in humans: Effect on the respiratory and cardiovascular systems. *Journal of Applied Physiology* 76(6):2420-2427.

Hatsukami DK & Fischman MW (1996). Crack cocaine and cocaine hydrochloride. Are the differences myth or reality? *Journal of the American Medical Association* 276(19):1580-1588

Heinemann HO (1977). Alcohol and the lung. A brief review. *American Journal of Medicine* 63(1):81-85.

Hendricks-Munoz KD, Gerrets RP, Higgins RD et al. (1996). Cocaine-stimulated endothelin-1 release is decreased by angiotensin-converting enzyme inhibitors in cultured endothelial cells. *Cardiovascular Research* 31(1):117-123.

Herve P, Launay JM, Scrobohaci ML et al. (1995). Increased plasma serotonin in primary pulmonary hypertension. *American Journal of Medicine* 99:249-253.

Herve P, Lebrec D, Brenot F et al. (1998). Pulmonary vascular disorders in portal hypertension. *European Respiratory Journal* 11(5):1153-1166.

Heyneman LE, Ward S, Lynch DA et al. (1999). Respiratory bronchiolitis, respiratory bronchiolitis-associated interstitial lung disease, and desquamative interstitial pneumonia: Different entities or part of the spectrum of the same disease process? *American Journal of Roentgenology* 173(6):1617-1622.

Hojer J (1996). Severe metabolic acidosis in the alcoholic: Differential diagnosis and management. *Human and Experimental Toxicology* 15(6):482-488.

Hong JL & Lee LY (1996). Cigarette smoke-induced bronchoconstriction: Causative agents and role of thromboxane receptors. *Journal of Applied Physiology* 81(5):2053-2059.

Hong JL, Rodger IW & Lee LY (1995). Cigarette smoke-induced bronchoconstriction: Cholinergic mechanisms, tachykinins, and cyclooxygenase products. *Journal of Applied Physiology* 78(6):2260-2266.

Hopkins GB (1972). Pulmonary angiothrombotic granulomatosis in drug offenders. *Journal of the American Medical Association* 221(8):909-911.

Hoppichler F, Lechleitner M, Konig P et al. (1992). Snuff and recurring pulmonary infiltrations in chronic renal failure. *Lancet* 339(8791):500-501.

Hughes S & Calverly PMA (1988). Heroin inhalation and asthma. *British Medical Journal* 297:1511-1512.

Huuskonen MS, Husman K, Jarvisalo J et al. (1984). Extrinsic allergic alveolitis in the tobacco industry. *British Journal of Industrial Medicine* 41(1):77-83.

Ikeda N, Takahashi H, Umetsu K et al. (1990). The course of respiration and circulation in "toluene-sniffing." *Forensic Science International* 44(2-3):151-158.

Ishii T, Matsuse T, Teramoto S et al. (2000). Association between alpha-1-antichymotrypsin polymorphism and susceptibility to chronic obstructive pulmonary disease. *European Journal of Clinical Investigation* 30(6):543-548.

Jaffe J & Martin WR (1990). Opioid analgesics and antagonists. In AG Gilman, TW Rall, AS Nies et al. (eds.) *Goodman and Gilman's The Pharmacological Basis of Therapeutics, 8th Edition*. Oxford, England: Pergamon Press, 362-396, 490-494.

Jay SJ, Johanson WG & Pierce AK (1975). Respiratory complications of overdose with sedative drugs. *American Review of Respiratory Disease* 112:591-598.

Jinot J & Bayard S (1996). Respiratory health effects of exposure to environmental tobacco smoke. *Reviews of Environmental Health* 11(3):89-100.

Johnson MK, Smith RP, Morrison D et al. (2000). Large lung bullae in marijuana smokers. *Thorax* 55(4):340-342.

Joseph WL & Geelhoed GW (1974). Surgical sequelae of intravenous drug abuse. *Maryland State Medical Journal* 23(1):70-73.

Kaa E (1994). Impurities, adulterants and diluents of illicit heroin. Changes during a 12-year period. *Forensic Science International* 64(2-3):17.

Kagen SL, Kurup VP, Sohnle PG et al. (1983). Marijuana smoking and fungal sensitization. *Journal of Allergy and Clinical Immunology* 71(4):389-393.

Kahler CM, Graziadei I, Wiedermann CJ et al. (2000). Successful use of continuous intravenous prostacyclin in a patient with severe portopulmonary hypertension. *Wiener Klinische Wochenschrift* 112(14):637-640.

Karlinsky J (1997). Emphysema. In R Goldstein, J O'Connell & J Karlinksy (eds.) *A Practical Approach to Pulmonary Medicine*. Philadelphia, PA: Lippincott-Raven, 224-239.

Karne S, D'Ambrosio C, Einarsson O et al. (1999). Hypersensitivity pneumonitis induced by intranasal heroin use. *American Journal of Medicine* 107(4):392-395.

King PD, Rumbaut R & Sanchez C (1996). Pulmonary manifestations of chronic liver disease. *Digestive Diseases* 14(2):73-82.

Kissner DG, Lawrence WD, Selis JE et al. (1987). Crack lung: Pulmonary disease caused by cocaine abuse. *American Review of Respiratory Disease* 136(5):1250-1252.

Kiter G, Ucan ES, Ceylan E et al. (2000). Water-pipe smoking and pulmonary functions. *Respiratory Medicine* 94(9):891-894.

Kleerup EC, Wong M, Marques-Magallanes JA et al. (1997). Acute effects of intravenous cocaine on pulmonary artery pressure and cardiac index in habitual crack smokers. *Chest* 111(1):30-35.

Kreek MJ (1996). Cocaine, dopamine and the endogenous opioid system. *Journal of Addictive Diseases* 15(4):73-96.

Kulaylat MN, Barakat N, Stephan RN et al. (1993). Embolization of illicit needle fragments. *Journal of Emergency Medicine* 11(4):403-408.

Kuo PC, Plotkin JS, Gaine S et al. (1999). Portopulmonary hypertension and the liver transplant candidate. *Transplantation* 67(8):1087-1093.

Kurup VP, Resnick A, Kagen SL et al. (1983). Allergenic fungi and actinomycetes in smoking materials and their health implications. *Mycopathologia* 82(1):61-64.

Lander F, Jepsen JR & Gravesen S (1988). Allergic alveolitis and late asthmatic reaction due to molds in the tobacco industry. *Allergy* 43(1):74-76.

Landrigan PJ, Powell KE, James LM et al. (1983). Paraquat and marijuana: Epidemiologic risk assessment. *American Journal of Public Health* 73(7):784-788.

Lang SA & Maron MB (1991). Hemodynamic basis for cocaine-induced pulmonary edema in dogs. *Journal of Applied Physiology* 71(3):1166-1170.

Lazaridis KN, Frank JW, Krowka MJ et al. (1999). Hepatic hydrothorax: Pathogenesis, diagnosis, and management. *American Journal of Medicine* 107(3):262-267.

Lee LY, Lou YP, Hong JL et al. (1995). Cigarette smoke-induced bronchoconstriction and release of tachykinins in guinea pig lungs. *Respiration Physiology* 99(1):173-181.

Lee PN (2001). Relation between exposure to asbestos and smoking jointly and the risk of lung cancer. *Occupational and Environmental Medicine* 58(3):145-153.

Lehnert BE & Ferin J (1983). Particle binding, phagocytosis, and plastic substrate adherence characteristics of alveolar macrophages from rats acutely treated with chlorphentermine. *Journal of the Reticuloendothelial Society* 33(4):293-303.

Leson CL, McGuigan MA & Bryson SM (1988). Caffeine overdose in an adolescent male. *Journal of Toxicology, Clinical Toxicology* 26(5-6):407-415

Lewis JW Jr., Groux N, Elliott JP Jr. et al. (1980). Complications of attempted central venous injections performed by drug abusers. *Chest* 78(4):613-617.

Lewman LV (1972). Fatal pulmonary hypertension from intravenous injection of methylphenidate (Ritalin) tablets. *Human Pathology* 3(1):67-70.

Lheureux P, Leduc D, Vanbinst R et al. (1995). Survival in a case of massive paraquat ingestion. *Chest* 107(1):285-289.

Libby DM, Klein L & Altorki NK (1992). Aspiration of the nasal septum: A new complication of cocaine abuse. *Annals of Internal Medicine* 116(7):567-568.

Lim S, Roche N, Oliver BG et al. (2000). Balance of matrix metalloprotease-9 and tissue inhibitor of metalloprotease-1 from alveolar macrophages in cigarette smokers. Regulation by interleukin-10. *American Journal of Respiratory and Critical Care Medicine* 162(4 pt 1):1355-1360.

Linden CH (1990). Volatile substances of abuse. *Emergency Medical Clinics of North America* 8(3):559-578.

LiPuma JP, Wellman J & Stern HP (1982). Nitrous oxide abuse: A new cause of pneumomediastinum. *Radiology* 145(3):602.

Louria DB, Hensle T & Rose J (1967). The major medical complications of heroin addiction. *Annals of Internal Medicine* 67:1-22.

Lubin JH, Li JY, Xuan XZ et al. (1992). Risk of lung cancer among cigarette and pipe smokers in southern China. *International Journal of Cancer* 51(3):390-395.

Lustik SJ, Chibber AK, Kolano JW et al. (1997). The hyperventilation of cirrhosis: Progesterone and estradiol effects. *Hepatology* 25(1):55-58.

MacNee W (2000). Oxidants/antioxidants and COPD. *Chest* 117(5 Suppl 1):303S-317S.

Mao L & Oh Y (1998). Does marijuana or crack cocaine cause cancer? *Journal of the National Cancer Institute* 90(16):1182-1184.

Marik PE (2001). Primary care: Aspiration pneumonitis and aspiration pneumonia. *New England Journal of Medicine* 344(9):665-671.

Marini JJ, Pierson D & Hudson L (1979). Acute lobar atelectasis: A prospective comparison of fiberoptic bronchoscopy and respiratory therapy. *American Review of Respiratory Disease* 119:971-978.

McBride DC, Inciardi JA, Chitwood DD et al. (1992). Crack use and correlates of use in a national population of street heroin users. *Journal of Psychoactive Drugs* 24(4):411-416.

McCarroll KA & Roszler MH (1991). Lung disorders due to drug abuse. *Journal of Thoracic Imaging* 6(1):30-35.

McCusker K (1992). Mechanisms of respiratory tissue injury from cigarette smoking. *American Journal of Medicine* 93(1A):18S-21S.

McLean L, Sharma S & Maycher B (1998). Mycotic pulmonary artery aneurysms in intravenous drug abusers. *Canadian Respiratory Journal* 5(4):307-311.

Mehta NJ, Khan IA, Mehta RN et al. (2000). HIV-related pulmonary hypertension: Analytic review of 131 cases. *Chest* 118(4):1133-1141.

Meleca RJ, Burgio DL, Carr RM et al. (1997). Mucosal injuries of the upper aerodigestive tract after smoking crack or freebase cocaine. *Laryngoscope* 107(5):620-625.

Miller GJ, Ashcroft MT, Beadnell HM et al. (1971). The lipoid pneumonia of blackfat tobacco smokers in Guyana. *Quarterly Journal of Medicine* 40(160):457-470.

Moneo I, Alday E, Ramos C et al. (1993). Occupational asthma caused by Papaver somniferum. *Allergolgia et Immunopathologia* (Madrid) 21(4):145-148.

Moss M, Guidot DM, Wong-Lambertina M et al. (2000). The effects of chronic alcohol abuse on pulmonary glutathione homeostasis. *American Journal of Respiratory and Critical Care Medicine* 161(2 pt 1):414-419.

Murin S, Bilello KS & Matthay R (2000). Other smoking-affected pulmonary diseases. *Clinics in Chest Medicine* 21(1):121-137.

Murray RJ, Albin RJ, Mergner W et al. (1988). Diffuse alveolar hemorrhage temporally related to cocaine smoking. *Chest* 93(2):427-429.

Murray RJ, Smialek JE, Golle M et al. (1989). Pulmonary artery medial hypertrophy in cocaine users without foreign particle microembolization. *Chest* 96(5):1050-1053.

Nadeem S, Nasir N & Israel RH (1994). Loeffler's syndrome secondary to crack. *Chest* 105(5):1599-1600.

Nagai S, Hoshino Y, Hayashi M et al. (2000). Smoking-related interstitial lung diseases. *Current Opinion in Pulmonary Medicine* 6(5):415-419.

Napoli LD, Cigtay OS, Twigg HL et al. (1974). The lungs and drug abuse. *American Family Physician* 9(3):90-98.

O'Donnell AE, Mappin FG, Sebo TJ et al. (1991). Interstitial pneumonitis associated with "crack" cocaine abuse. *Chest* 100(4):1155-1157.

O'Donnell AE & Pappas LS (1988). Pulmonary complications of intravenous drug abuse. *Chest* 94(2):251-253.

Ofulue AF & Ko M (1999). Effects of depletion of neutrophils or macrophages on development of cigarette smoke-induced emphysema. *Journal of Physiology* 277(1 pt 1):L97-105.

Om A (1992). Cardiovascular complications of cocaine. *American Journal of Medical Sciences* 303(5):333-339.

Onwudike M (1996). Ecstasy induced retropharyngeal emphysema. *Journal of Accident and Emergency Medicine* 13(5):359-361.

Orriols R, Munoz X, Ferrer J et al. (1996). Cocaine-induced Churg-Strauss vasculitis. *European Respiratory Journal* 9(1):175-177.

Osborn HH, Tang M, Bradley K et al. (1997). New-onset bronchospasm or recrudescence of asthma associated with cocaine abuse. *Academic Emergency Medicine* 4(7):689-692.

Ott MG, Klees JE & Poche SL (2000). Respiratory health surveillance in a toluene di-isocyanate production unit, 1967-97: Clinical observations and lung function analyses. *Occupational and Environmental Medicine* 57(1):43-52.

Overland ES, Nolan AJ & Hopewell PC (1980). Alteration of pulmonary function in intravenous drug abusers. Prevalence, severity, and characterization of gas exchange abnormalities. *American Journal of Medicine* 68(2):231-237.

Pacifici R, Zuccaro P, Lopez CH et al. (2001). Acute effects of 3,4-methylenedioxymethamphetamine alone and in combination with ethanol on the immune system in humans. *Journal of Pharmacology and Experimental Therapeutics* 296(1):207-215.

Pare JP, Cote G & Fraser RS (1989). Long-term follow-up of drug abusers with intravenous talcosis. *American Review of Respiratory Disease* 139(1):233-241.

Parsons PE (1994). Respiratory failure as a result of drugs, overdoses, and poisonings. *Clinics in Chest Medicine* 15(1):93-102.

Patel RC, Dutta D & Schonfeld SA (1987). Free-base cocaine use associated with bronchiolitis obliterans organizing pneumonia. *Annals of Internal Medicine* 107(2):186-187.

Paterson SC & Sarvesvaran R (1983). Plastic bag death—A toluene fatality. *Medicine, Science and the Law* 23(1):64-66.

Perlman DC, Perkins MP, Paone D et al. (1997). "Shotgunning" as an illicit drug smoking practice. *Journal of Substance Abuse Treatment* 14(1):3-9.

Peterson PK, Molitor TW & Chao CC (1998). The opioid-cytokine connection. *Journal of Neuroimmunology* 83(1-2):63-69.

Polkey MI, Hamnegard CH, Hughes PD et al. (1998). Influence of acute lung volume change on contractile properties of human diaphragm. *Journal of Applied Physiology* 85(4):1322-1328.

Popa V (1994). Codeine-induced bronchoconstriction and putative bronchial opiate receptors in asthmatic subjects. *Pulmonary Pharmacology* 7(5):333-341.

Quin GI, McCarthy GM & Harries DK (1999). Spontaneous pneumomediastinum and ecstasy abuse. *Journal of Accident and Emergency Medicine* 16(5):382.

Raulf-Heimsoth M & Baur X (1998). Pathomechanisms and pathophysiology of isocyanate-induced diseases—Summary of present knowledge. *American Journal of Industrial Medicine* 34(2):137-143.

Reardon C & Theodore A (1997). Lung cancer. In R Goldstein, J O'Connell & J Karlinsky (eds.) *A Practical Approach to Pulmonary Medicine.* Philadelphia, PA: Lippincott-Raven, 129-146.

Reino AJ & Lawson W (1993). Upper airway distress in crack-cocaine users. *Otolaryngology—Head and Neck Surgery* 109(5):937-940.

Robalino BD & Moodie DS (1991). Association between primary pulmonary hypertension and portal hypertension: Analysis of its pathophysiology and clinical, laboratory and hemodynamic manifestations. *Journal of the American College Cardiology* 17(2):492-498.

Robertson CH Jr., Reynolds RC & Wilson JE 3rd (1976). Pulmonary hypertension and foreign body granulomas in intravenous drug abusers. Documentation by cardiac catheterization and lung biopsy. *American Journal of Medicine* 61(5):657-664.

Rom WN, Hay JG, Lee TC et al. (2000). Molecular and genetic aspects of lung cancer. *American Journal of Respiratory and Critical Care Medicine* 161(4 pt 1):1355-1367.

Rome LA, Lippmann ML, Dalsey WC et al. (2000). Prevalence of cocaine use and its impact on asthma exacerbation in an urban population. *Chest* 117(5):1324-1329.

Rosenow EC (1972). The spectrum of drug-induced pulmonary disease. *Annals of Internal Medicine* 77:977-991.

Rylander R (1968). Relative role of aerosol and volatile constituents of cigarette smoke as agents toxic to the respiratory tract. *National Cancer Institute Monographs* 28:221-229.

Saetta M, Finkelstein R & Cosio MG (1994). Morphological and cellular basis for airflow limitation in smokers. *European Respiratory Journal* 7(8):1505-1515.

Sandford AJ, Chagani T, Weir TD et al. (2001). Susceptibility genes for rapid decline of lung function in the lung health study. *American Journal of Respiratory and Critical Care Medicine* 163(2):469-473.

Sarafian TA, Magallanes JA, Shau H et al. (1999). Oxidative stress produced by marijuana smoke. An adverse effect enhanced by cannabinoids. *American Journal of Respiratory, Cell and Molecular Biology* 20(6):1286-1293.

Sato E, Koyama S, Takamizawa A et al. (1999). Smoke extract stimulates lung fibroblasts to release neutrophil and monocyte chemotactic activities. *American Journal of Physiology* 277(6 pt 1):L1149-1157.

Scanlan MF, Roebuck T, Little PJ et al. (2000). Effect of moderate alcohol upon obstructive sleep apnoea. *European Respiratory Journal* 16(5):909-913.

Schaiberger PH, Kennedy TC, Miller FC et al. (1993). Pulmonary hypertension associated with long-term inhalation of "crank" methamphetamine. *Chest* 104:614-616.

Schmidt RA, Glenny RW, Godwin JD et al. (1991). Panlobular emphysema in young intravenous Ritalin abusers. *American Review of Respiratory Disease* 143(3):649-656.

Schraufnagel DE & Kay JM (1996). Structural and pathologic changes in the lung vasculature in chronic liver disease. *Clinics in Chest Medicine* 17(1):1-15.

Schuller HM & Orloff M (1998). Tobacco-specific carcinogenic nitrosamines. Ligands for nicotinic acetylcholine receptors in human lung cancer cells. *Biochemical Pharmacology* 55(9):1377-1384.

Seaman ME (1990). Barotrauma related to inhalational drug abuse. *Journal of Emergency Medicine* 8(2):141-149.

Shapiro SD (1999). The macrophage in chronic obstructive pulmonary disease. *American Journal of Respiratory and Critical Care Medicine* 160(5 pt 2):S29-32.

Sharma OP & Kalkat GV (1991). Drug induced clinical syndromes mimicking sarcoidosis. *Sarcoidosis* 8(1):3-5.

Shimoda T, Kohno S, Takao A et al. (1996). Investigation of the mechanism of alcohol-induced bronchial asthma. *Journal of Allergy and Clinical Immunology* 97(1 pt 1):74-84.

Sisson JH, Papi A, Beckmann JD et al. (1994). Smoke and viral infection cause cilia loss detectable by bronchoalveolar lavage cytology and dynein ELISA. *American Journal of Respiratory and Critical Care Medicine* 149(1):205-213.

Smeenk FW, Serlie J, van der Jagt EJ et al. (1990). Bullous degeneration of the left lower lobe in a heroin addict. *European Respiratory Journal* 3(10):1224-1226.

Smith CJ & Hansch C (2000). The relative toxicity of compounds in mainstream cigarette smoke condensate. *Food and Chemical Toxicology* 38(7):637-646.

Smith GT, McClaughry PL, Purkey J et al. (1995). Crack cocaine mimicking pulmonary embolism on pulmonary ventilation/perfusion lung scan. A case report. *Clinical Nuclear Medicine* 20(1):65-68.

Smith WS & Matthay MA (1997). Evidence for a hydrostatic mechanism in human neurogenic pulmonary edema. *Chest* 111(5):1326-1333.

Snider GL (1981). The pathogenesis of emphysema—Twenty years of progress. *American Review of Respiratory Disease* 124(3):321-324.

Sporer KA (1999). Acute heroin overdose. *Annals of Internal Medicine* 130(7):584-590.

Sutton S, Lum BL & Torti FM (1986). Possible risk of invasive aspergillosis with marijuana use during chemotherapy for small cell lung cancer. *Drug Intelligence and Clinical Pharmacy* 20:289-290.

Takao A, Shimoda T, Kohno S et al. (1998). Correlation between alcohol-induced asthma and acetaldehyde dehydrogenase-2 genotype. *Journal of Allergy and Clinical Immunology* 101(5):576-580.

Tashkin DP (1990). Pulmonary complications of smoked substance abuse. *Western Journal of Medicine* 152(5):525-530.

Tashkin DP (2001). Airway effects of marijuana, cocaine, and other inhaled illicit agents. *Current Opinion in Pulmonary Medicine* 7(2):43-61.

Tashkin DP, Gorelick D, Khalsa ME et al. (1992). Respiratory effects of cocaine freebasing among habitual cocaine users. *Journal of Addictive Diseases* 11(4):59-70.

Tashkin DP, Kleerup EC, Hoh CK et al. (1997). Effects of "crack" cocaine on pulmonary alveolar permeability. *Chest* 112(2):327-335.

Tashkin DP, Kleerup EC, Royal SN et al. (1996). Acute effects of inhaled and IV cocaine on airway dynamics. *Chest* 110(4):904-910.

Tomashefski JF Jr., Hirsch CS & Jolly PN (1981). Microcrystalline cellulose pulmonary embolism and granulomatosis. A complication of illicit intravenous injections of pentazocine tablets. *Archives of Pathology and Laboratory Medicine* 105(2):89-93.

Touya JJ, Rahimian J, Corbus HF et al. (1986). The lung as a metabolic organ. *Seminars in Nuclear Medicine* 16(4):296-305.

Trump BF, McDowell EM & Harris CC (1984). Chemical carcinogenesis in the tracheobronchial epithelium. *Environmental Health Perspectives* 55:77-84.

Turato G, Zuin R & Saetta M (2001). Pathogenesis and pathology of COPD. *Respiration* 68(2):117-128.

U.S. Public Health Service (USPHS) (1988). *Surgeon General's Report: The Health Consequences of Smoking: Nicotine Addiction.* Washington, DC: Government Printing Office.

U.S. Public Health Service (USPHS) (1998). *Targeting Tobacco Use: The Nation's Leading Cause of Death.* Washington, DC: Centers for Disease Control and Prevention.

Vally H, Carr A, El-Saleh J et al. (1999). Wine-induced asthma: a placebo-controlled assessment of its pathogenesis. *Journal of Allergy and Clinical Immunology* 103(1 pt 1):41-46.

Vally H, de Klerk N & Thompson PJ (2000). Alcoholic drinks: Important triggers for asthma. *Journal of Allergy and Clinical Immunology* 105(3):462-467.

Van der Linden P, Le Moine O, Ghysels M et al. (1996). Pulmonary hypertension after transjugular intrahepatic portosystemic shunt: Effects on right ventricular function. *Hepatology* 23(5):982-987.

Van Hoozen BE & Cross CE (1997) Marijuana. Respiratory tract effects. *Clinical Reviews in Allergy and Immunology* 15(3):243-269.

Verra F, Escudier E, Lebargy F et al. (1995). Ciliary abnormalities in bronchial epithelium of smokers, ex-smokers, and nonsmokers. *American Journal of Respiratory and Critical Care Medicine* 151(3 pt 1):630-634.

Vethanayagam D, Pugsley S, Dunn EJ et al. (2000). Exogenous lipid pneumonia related to smoking weed oil following cadaveric renal transplantation. *Canadian Respiratory Journal* 7(4):338-342.

Wagner SA, Clark MA, Wesche DL et al. (1992). Asphyxial deaths from the recreational use of nitrous oxide. *Journal of Forensic Sciences* 37(4):1008-1015.

Waller BF, Brownlee WJ & Roberts WC (1980). Self-induced pulmonary granulomatosis. A consequence of intravenous injection of drugs intended for oral use. *Chest* 78(1):90-94.

Wayne NG & Spitz WU (1978). Rupture of a subclavian artery aneurysm in a heroin addict. Report of a case. *Rechtsmedizin Zurich* 81(2):147-149.

Wright RO, Lewander WJ & Woolf AD (1999). Methemoglobinemia: Etiology, pharmacology, and clinical management. *Annals of Emergency Medicine* 34(5):646-656.

Wu D & Center D (1997). Chronic bronchitis and bronchiectasi. In R Goldstein, J O'Connell, & J Karlinksy (eds.) *A Practical Approach to Pulmonary Medicine*. Philadelphia, PA: Lippincott-Raven, 240-252.

Wu TC, Tashkin DP, Djahed B et al. (1988). Pulmonary hazards of smoking marijuana as compared with tobacco. *New England Journal of Medicine* 318(6):347-351.

Wyse DG (1973). Deliberate inhalation of volatile hydrocarbons: A review. *Canadian Medical Association Journal* 108:71-74.

Xu W, Flick T, Mitchel J et al. (1999). Cocaine effects on immunocompetent cells: An observation of in vitro cocaine exposure. *International Journal of Immunopharmacology* 21(7):463-472.

Yakel DL Jr & Eisenberg MJ (1995). Pulmonary artery hypertension in chronic intravenous cocaine users. *American Heart Journal* 130(2):398-399.

Yamashita M, Yamashita M & Ando Y (2000). A long-term follow-up of lung function in survivors of paraquat poisoning. *Human and Experimental Toxicology* 19(2):99-103.

Yao EH, Kong BC, Hsue GL et al. (1987). Pulmonary function changes in cirrhosis of the liver. *American Journal of Gastroenterology* 82(4):352-354.

Yin D, Mufson RA, Wang R et al. (1999). Fas-mediated cell death promoted by opioids. *Nature* 397(6716):218.

Yousem SA, Colby TV & Gaensler EA (1989). Respiratory bronchiolitis-associated interstitial lung disease and its relationship to desquamative interstitial pneumonia. *Mayo Clinic Proceedings* 64(11):1373-1380.

Zebraski SE, Kochenash SM & Raffa RB (2000). Lung opioid receptors: Pharmacology and possible target for nebulized morphine in dyspnea. *Life Sciences* 66(23):2221-2231.

Zimatkin SM & Anichtchik OV (1999). Alcohol-histamine interactions. *Alcohol and Alcoholism* 34(2):141-147.

Zorc TG, O'Donnell AE, Holt RW et al. (1988). Bilateral pyopneumothorax secondary to intravenous drug abuse. *Chest* 93(3):645-647.

Zuskin E, Mustajbegovic J & Schachter EN (1994). Follow-up study of respiratory function in hemp workers. *American Journal of Industrial Medicine* 26(1):103-115.

Neurologic Disorders Related to Alcohol and Other Drug Use

Chapter 7

John C.M. Brust, M.D.

Trauma
Infection
Seizures
Stroke
Altered Mentation
Muscle, Nerve, and Spinal Cord
Other Complications

This chapter addresses neurologic complications of alcohol, tobacco, and other drugs (Table 1). The neurologic symptoms and signs of acute toxicity and withdrawal differ widely from agent to agent. Opiate overdose causes potentially lethal coma, respiratory depression, and miosis, whereas opiate withdrawal causes flu-like symptoms that are hardly ever life-threatening. Cocaine overdose causes delirium, often accompanied by seizures, malignant hyperthermia, or fatal cardiac arrhythmia; cocaine withdrawal causes fatigue and depression. With ethanol (alcohol) and barbiturates, either overdose (coma or apnea) or withdrawal (seizures or *delirium tremens*) can be fatal. Such symptoms—including the possibility that an individual is using more than one agent or even is intoxicated by one agent while simultaneously withdrawing from another—can confound the interpretation of neurologic symptoms and signs in patients who use and abuse alcohol and other drugs (Brust, 1993; Goldfrank, Flomenbaum et al., 1998).

TRAUMA

Trauma frequently affects the nervous system, both peripherally and centrally, and its effects can be masked by coexisting intoxication or other neurologic disturbance. Alcoholics are at particular risk of misdiagnosis. They often have thrombocytopenia and abnormalities of clotting factors, and alcohol acutely enhances blood-brain barrier leakage around areas of cerebral trauma (Halt, Swanson et al., 1992). Intracranial hemorrhage always must be considered in an alcohol user with an altered sensorium; spinal cord injury must be considered in one who is unable to walk.

INFECTION

Parenteral users of any drug are subject to an array of local and systemic infections, including abscesses, cellulitis, pneumonia, sepsis, endophthalmitis, osteomyelitis, and pyogenic arthritis (Richter, 1993). The central and peripheral nervous systems often are affected. Endocarditis, bacterial or fungal, leads to meningitis, cerebral infarction, diffuse vasculitis, abscess (intraparenchymal, subdural, or epidural, including the spinal cord), or subarachnoid hemorrhage from rupture of a septic ("mycotic") aneurysm (Brust, Dickinson et al., 1990; Marantz, Linzer et al., 1987). Infectious hepatitis can cause encephalopathy or, because of deranged clotting, hemorrhagic stroke. Vertebral osteomyelitis can cause radiculopathy or spinal cord compression. Tetanus,

TABLE 1.   Drugs Associated With Neurologic Complications

Alcohol	Opiates
Anticholinergics	Phencyclidine
Hallucinogens	Psychostimulants
Inhalants	Sedatives-hypnotics
Marijuana	Tobacco

usually severe, is particularly common in subcutaneous injectors of heroin (Brust & Richter, 1974a). Botulism occurs at injection sites and, among cocaine snorters, in the nasal sinuses (Kudrow, Henry et al., 1988). Malaria has affected heroin users in endemic areas (Gonzalez-Garcia, Arnalich et al., 1986).

Even before the AIDS epidemic, it was recognized that individuals who abuse alcohol and other drugs often are immunosuppressed. Alcoholics are prone to develop bacterial or tuberculous meningitis, which always must be considered in a drinker with seizures or altered mentation, even when the clinical picture suggests intoxication, withdrawal, thiamine deficiency, hepatic encephalopathy, or hypoglycemia (any of which could coexist). Clinicians should have a low threshold for performing a lumbar puncture in an alcoholic with altered mentation, even in the absence of fever or stiff neck. HIV-seronegative heroin addicts nevertheless are at risk of central nervous system (CNS) infection by agents such as *Candida* or *Mucor*. Parenteral drug abusers with AIDS develop the same neurologic complications as do those with other risk factors for AIDS (Malouf, Jacquette et al., 1990). They are at risk of infection with T-cell lymphotrophic retrovirus type I or type II, with consequent myelopathy (Jacobson, Lehky et al., 1993).

SEIZURES

Seizures can be a feature of either drug toxicity (as with psychostimulants) or withdrawal (as with sedatives or ethanol) (Earnest, 1993; Alldredge, Lowenstein et al., 1989a). Seizures associated with amphetamine-like psychostimulants, including smokable methamphetamine ("ice"), usually are accompanied by other signs of overdose, whereas cocaine-induced seizures often occur without other symptoms and signs (Pascual-Leone, Dhuna et al., 1990). The difference may be related to cocaine's local anesthetic prop-

erties; procaine and similar agents are epileptogenic. In animals, cocaine produces a "kindling" effect (repeated fixed doses of the drug progressively lower seizure threshold) (Karler, Petty et al., 1989). Seizures usually occur either immediately or within a few hours of cocaine administration. Seizures occurring many hours after use might be related to the proconvulsant properties of the cocaine metabolite, benzoylecgonine (Konkol, Erickson et al., 1992). Single grand mal seizures are most common; focal seizures suggest underlying cerebral trauma, stroke, or infection. Status epilepticus tends to be refractory to treatment.

Any route of administration can precipitate a seizure, but new onset seizures most often follow intravenous administration of cocaine hydrochloride or smoking of alkaloidal "crack"; the reason probably is the higher dose and more rapid delivery to the brain these practices permit. A survey of adolescent cocaine users found that seizures occurred in none of the intranasal users, in 1% of occasional crack smokers, and in 9% of heavy crack smokers (Schwartz, Luxenberg et al., 1991).

Seizures have occurred in infants being breast-fed by cocaine-using mothers (Chaney, Franke et al., 1988) and in infants and small children who passively inhaled crack smoke (Bateman & Heagarty, 1989).

Phenylpropanolamine, marketed as a decongestant, an anorectic, and a "legal stimulant," has caused seizures at doses recommended for weight reduction (Mueller & Solow, 1982).

In animals, opiates are either proconvulsant or anticonvulsant, depending on receptor specificity and seizure model (Ng, Brust et al., 1990). Except possibly in newborns exposed *in utero*, seizures are not a feature of opiate withdrawal. Opiate agonists lower the seizure threshold in humans, but seizures are a sufficiently rare feature of heroin overdose that an alternative cause always should be sought (for example, concomitant cocaine toxicity, ethanol withdrawal, cerebral trauma, or infection). A case-control study found that heroin use, both past and current, was a risk factor for new onset seizures independent of overdose, head injury, infection, stroke, or use of alcohol or other illicit drugs (Ng, Brust et al., 1990).

Unlike heroin or morphine, meperidine (Demerol®) readily causes myoclonus and seizures through the proconvulsant properties of its metabolite, normeperidine (Hershey, 1983). Seizures often follow parenteral use of the mixed agonist-antagonist opiate pentazocine (Talwin®) when it is combined with the antihistamine tripelennamine

("T's and blues"); both drugs are epileptogenic (Caplan, Thomas et al., 1982).

Phencyclidine (PCP) blocks N-methyl-D-aspartate receptors and thus would be expected to have anticonvulsant properties; however, at high doses (that is, 1 mg/kg or more), seizures and myoclonus often are encountered (McCarron, Schultze et al., 1981a, 1981b). Such patients are likely to have other signs of severe overdose, including coma with extensor posturing yet open staring eyes, marked hyperthermia, myoglobinuria, respiratory depression, and hypertension progressing to hypotension. In such patients, anticonvulsant medications are but one aspect of overall management.

Seizures are not an expected toxic feature of hallucinogens (for example, LSD, mescaline, or psilocin/psilocybin), but they can occur following very high doses (Fisher & Ungerleider, 1967). Seizures can complicate acute intoxication with inhalants (such as glues, solvents, or aerosols); in fact, toxic seizures and hallucinations are features that distinguish intoxication from inhalants from intoxication with alcohol (Morton, 1987). Seizures accompany severe anticholinergic poisoning (Mikolich, Paulson et al., 1975).

In alcoholic patients, seizures can be the result of alcohol-related disorders such as head injury, CNS infection, or stroke. Alcohol also can trigger seizures in subjects with preexisting epilepsy. In such cases, seizures tend to occur after a day or a weekend of heavy drinking; whether small amounts of alcohol significantly lower seizure threshold in epileptics—in other words, whether epileptics should avoid alcohol altogether—is controversial.

The term "alcohol-related seizures" (colloquially, "rum fits") refers to seizures in the absence of epilepsy or other predisposing factors (Hauser, Ng et al., 1988). Such seizures most often are a withdrawal phenomenon, occurring within 48 hours of the last drink in persons who have abused alcohol chronically or in binges for months or years. The minimal duration of drinking is uncertain, but the risk is dose-related, beginning at only 50 g absolute ethanol daily (Ng, Hauser et al., 1988). Such seizures usually are single or occur in a brief cluster; status epilepticus is infrequent. They usually are grand mal without focality, although focal seizures do occur, and an underlying structural lesion (for example, an old cerebral contusion) is not always identified. Other symptoms of early withdrawal (tremor or hallucinosis) may or may not be present, and a patient with alcohol withdrawal seizures may go on to develop *delirium*

tremens (DTs), but seizures rarely are observed once DTs are present.

Alcohol may cause seizures independently of withdrawal or structural brain lesions. In some alcoholics, seizures occur during active drinking or more than a week after the last drink, and a case-control study of new onset seizures failed to show a clear temporal correlation between seizures and recent abstinence (Ng, Hauser et al., 1988). Animal studies indicate that seizures that occur during alcohol withdrawal are of more than one type, with different time courses, phenomenology, and presumed neuronal mechanism (Gonzalez, Czachura et al., 1989). Alcohol blocks glutamate neurotransmission, and up-regulation of N-methyl-D-aspartate receptors theoretically could contribute not only to withdrawal symptoms, including seizures, but also could set the stage for excitotoxicity and permanent neuronal damage (Tsai, Gastfriend et al., 1995). Consistent with such a view is evidence that the risk of seizures increases with repeated ethanol detoxification (Lechtenberg & Worner, 1990).

The diagnosis of alcohol-related seizures requires exclusion of other lesions. Brain computed tomography (CT) or magnetic resonance imaging is indicated if seizures are of new onset, and lumbar puncture should be performed if meningitis or subarachnoid hemorrhage is suspected. In patients with alcohol-related seizures, the electroencephalogram usually is normal; claims of a high incidence of photomyoclonic or photoconvulsive response during early withdrawal have not been supported by subsequent studies (Fisch, Hauser et al., 1989).

Because most alcohol-related seizures occur singly or in brief clusters, once they have occurred, anticonvulsants seldom are necessary unless the diagnosis is in doubt. In animals and humans, phenytoin (Dilantin®) failed to prevent alcohol seizures (Alldredge, Lowenstein et al., 1989b). Treatment of status epilepticus during alcohol withdrawal is conventional; benzodiazepines and phenobarbital have the advantage (compared to phenytoin) of cross-tolerance with ethanol and, thus, efficacy in treating other withdrawal symptoms, including progression to DTs.

Long-term anticonvulsant medication generally is not indicated in patients with alcohol seizures. Abstainers do not need it, and drinkers do not take it.

As with alcohol, seizures in barbiturate abusers occur most often as a withdrawal phenomenon. In a study with volunteers, abrupt withdrawal from oral pentobarbital

(Nembutal®) or secobarbital (Seconal®) that had been taken in a daily dose for several months produced paroxysmal electroencephalographic changes without symptoms in one third of the subjects. Withdrawal from 600 mg a day caused minor symptoms in one half the subjects and a seizure in 10%. Withdrawal from 900 mg or more a day caused seizures in 75% and DTs in 65% (Fraser, Wikler et al., 1958).

Symptoms following benzodiazepine withdrawal can be difficult to differentiate from those for which the drug was being taken in the first place, but seizures have been reported (Fialip, Aumaitre et al., 1987). Also described are paradoxical toxic reactions featuring agitation, hallucinations and, in some cases, seizures (Fouilladieu, D'Engert et al., 1984). Seizures as a toxic effect are described with methaqualone (which sometimes is combined with an antihistamine) and with glutethimide (which has anticholinergic properties) (Hoaken, 1975).

A case–control study found that marijuana was protective against the development of new onset seizures. In animals, the nonpsychoactive cannabinoid compound cannabidiol is anticonvulsant, and limited studies suggest that it can reduce seizure frequency in humans with epilepsy (Ng, Brust et al., 1990).

STROKE

The evidence that alcohol and tobacco are risk factors for stroke is epidemiologic. The evidence that illicit drugs are risk factors for stroke is anecdotal (Brust, 1998).

Systemic complications of parenteral drug abuse, such as hepatitis, endocarditis, or AIDS, predispose to stroke. Heroin nephropathy causes uremia, hypertension, bleeding, and hemorrhagic stroke. Taken parenterally or, in a few cases, sniffed, heroin has caused ischemic stroke in the absence of intermediary conditions or other evident risk factors (Brust & Richter, 1976; Bartholomei, Nicoli et al., 1992). In some reported cases, angiographic changes were consistent with cerebral vasculitis, and laboratory abnormalities (such as blood eosinophilia, hypergammaglobulinemia, and positive Coombs test) suggested hypersensitivity. Other possible mechanisms are systemic hypotension following overdose and embolization of injected foreign material. Intracerebral hemorrhage occurred in a young adult within minutes of intravenous heroin use (Knoblauch, Buchholz et al., 1983).

Abusers of pentazocine (Talwin®) and tripelennamine ("Ts and blues") inject crushed oral tablets intravenously, leading to cerebral infarcts and hemorrhages. It is likely that the particulate foreign material passes through secondary pulmonary arteriovenous shunts (Caplan, Thomas et al., 1982).

Heroin myelopathy may be vascular in origin (Goodhart, Loizou et al., 1982). Acute paraparesis, sensory loss, and urinary retention most often occur shortly after injection and sometimes after a period of abstinence. In some cases, preserved proprioception suggests infarction in the territory of the anterior spinal artery; occasionally symptoms are present in the patient awakening from coma, suggesting "border-zone" infarction secondary to hypotension. In one case, cord biopsy revealed vasculitis (Judice, LeBlanc et al., 1978).

Users of amphetamine-like drugs (especially methamphetamine) are subject to intracerebral hemorrhage, often associated with acute hypertension and fever; routes of administration have been oral, intravenous, or nasal. Hemorrhagic stroke has occurred both in chronic users and after first exposure (Brust, 1998). In some cases, cerebral angiography has been consistent with vasculitis, which in a few instances was verified at autopsy.

Amphetamine-induced vasculitis, which causes ischemic stroke, appears to be of more than one type. In one report, systemic and CNS necrotizing vasculitis resembled polyarteritis nodosa (Citron, Halpern et al., 1970). In other reports, ischemic stroke appeared to be secondary to small vessel hypersensitivity angiitis. Although some of these cases were based on nonspecific angiographic "beading," cerebral vasculitis was demonstrated in animals receiving repeated doses of methamphetamine over weeks or months (Brust, 1997).

Intracerebral and subarachnoid hemorrhages have followed ingestion of phenylpropanolamine at both recommended and excessive doses; in one case, leptomeningeal biopsy demonstrated vasculitis (Fallis & Fisher, 1985). A large case-control study found that, when used as an ingredient in appetite suppressants and (possibly) in cold and cough remedies, phenylpropanolamine is an independent risk factor for hemorrhagic stroke in women (Kernen, Viscoli et al., 2000).

Intravenous and inadvertent carotid artery injection of crushed methylphenidate (Ritalin®) tablets has resulted in ischemic stroke, and foreign body emboli have been found in the brain (Mizutami, Lewis et al., 1980). Angiographic changes suggestive of arteritis were seen in a child who had an ischemic stroke while taking methylphenidate orally for attention deficit/hyperactivity disorder (Trugman, 1988).

Overdose with 3,4-methylenedioxymethamphetamine (MDMA or "Ecstasy") has resulted in hypertensive crisis, and cerebral infarction followed MDMA use in a young man who had no other risk factors (Manchanda & Connolly, 1993).

Stroke in cocaine users may be secondary to drug-induced cardiac arrhythmia, myocardial infarction, or cardiomyopathy. In many cases, however, cardiac disease, infection, or other risk factors are not evident (Sloan, Kittner et al., 1998). More than 400 cases of cocaine-related stroke have been reported, about half ischemic and half hemorrhagic. Strokes have followed nasal or parenteral administration of cocaine hydrochloride or smoking of alkaloidal "crack" (Levine, Brust et al., 1990). Ischemic strokes include transient ischemic attacks and infarction of the cerebrum, thalamus, brain stem, spinal cord, and retina. Of patients with hemorrhagic stroke who underwent cerebral angiography, about half harbored saccular aneurysms or vascular malformations. A plausible mechanism for hemorrhagic stroke is surges of systemic hypertension. Alternatively, some ischemic strokes may be the result of direct cerebral vasoconstriction induced by the drug. A study using magnetic resonance angiography in volunteers demonstrated such vasoconstriction during cocaine administration (Kaufman, Levin et al., 1998). Most autopsies have not shown vasculitis; when present, it consisted of round cell infiltration without vessel wall necrosis. A contributing factor may be cocaine's effects on platelets and clotting factors and the ability of cocaine to accelerate atherosclerosis (Brust, 1998).

LSD, an ergot drug, directly constricts systemic and cerebral arteries, and ischemic stroke has followed ingestion (Lieberman, Bloom et al., 1974).

Phencyclidine causes acute systemic hypertension, which, like the drug's mental effects, can last hours or days. Cerebral infarction, intracerebral and subarachnoid hemorrhage, and hypertensive encephalopathy have followed use of PCP (Eastman & Cohen, 1975; Brust, 1998).

The role of ethanol in stroke is complex. As with coronary artery disease, epidemiologic studies suggest that low-to-moderate doses of ethanol decrease stroke risk, whereas higher amounts increase it. Not surprisingly, reports have been inconsistent. A meta-analysis of 63 epidemiologic studies concluded that "moderate" drinking (<2 drinks containing 1 oz ethanol daily) decreased the risk

of ischemic stroke in Caucasians but not in Japanese; higher doses increased the risk of ischemic stroke in both groups; and moderate as well as heavy drinking increased the risk of hemorrhagic stroke (Camargo, 1989). A case–control study in New York City found that two drinks per day were protective against ischemic stroke, with a protective trend continuing up to five drinks, but that doses in excess of five drinks per day increased risk. These relationships held for young and old subjects; for whites, African Americans, and Hispanics; and for wine, beer, and spirits (Sacco, Elkind et al., 1999).

Possible contributors to the increased risk of occlusive stroke in heavy drinkers include alcohol-related cardiac disease, alcohol-induced hypertension, increased platelet aggregation, acceleration of the clotting cascade, decreased fibrinolysis, direct cerebral vasoconstriction, hemoconcentration, and hyperhomocystinemia secondary to folate deficiency. Protection against ischemic stroke may be related to decreased low-density lipoproteins and increased high-density lipoproteins, increased prostacyclin, decreased platelet aggregation, and decreased fibrinogen levels (Brust, 1998; Sacco, Elkind et al., 1999).

Tobacco is a major risk factor for both coronary artery and peripheral vascular disease, and case–control and cohort studies show that it is a risk factor for ischemic and hemorrhagic stroke as well (Shinton & Beevers, 1989; Brust, 1998). Among women smokers, the risk of both ischemic and hemorrhagic stroke is greater in those who take oral contraceptives (Goldbaum, Kendrick et al., 1987). Risk of stroke decreases with cessation of smoking (Wolf, D'Agostino et al., 1988).

Possible mechanisms of tobacco's role in stroke include acceleration of atherosclerosis, reductions in oxygen-carrying capacity because of carbon monoxide in tobacco smoke, nicotine-induced endothelial damage, acute elevations of blood pressure and acceleration of chronic hypertension, elevated blood fibrinogen levels, elevated hemoglobin, increased platelet reactivity, and inhibition of prostacyclin formation (Brust, 1993, 1998).

Anabolic steroids potentiate platelet aggregation, alter fibrinogen, stimulate erythropoietin, and increase systolic blood pressure; strokes have been reported in young athletes using them (Frenchick, 1990).

ALTERED MENTATION

Alcohol abusers are at high risk of lasting cognitive impairment through multiple mechanisms that can coexist in the same patient. Head trauma, CNS infection, and hypoglycemia can leave dementia in their wake, while alcoholic liver disease can cause encephalopathy. Nutritional deficiency can result in Wernicke-Korsakoff's disease and pellagra.

Wernicke-Korsakoff's disease is caused by thiamine deficiency, which, because body stores are limited, can occur after only a few weeks of inadequate intake. In the acute syndrome, mental symptoms evolve over days or weeks to a "global confusional state," with varying degrees of lethargy, inattentiveness, abulia, and impaired memory (Victor, Adams et al., 1989). Usually but not invariably present are abnormal eye movements (nystagmus and abduction or horizontal gaze paresis progressing to complete ophthalmoplegia) and ataxic gait (both cerebellar and vestibular in origin), progressing to inability to stand unaided. Without treatment, there is a progression to coma and death and, pathologically, there are histologically distinct lesions in the medial thalamus and hypothalamus, the periaque-ductal gray matter of the midbrain, and the periventricular areas of the pons and medulla. With early treatment (intravenous thiamine and multivitamins), recovery begins within hours or days and can be complete, but, if treatment is delayed, the mental symptoms evolve into Korsakoff's syndrome, an irreversible disorder in which the predominant abnormality is impaired memory, with inability to store or retrieve recent information, varying degrees of retrograde amnesia, and, especially acutely, a tendency to confabulate. Residual nystagmus and gait ataxia also may be present.

Pellagra, caused by nicotinic acid deficiency, consists of skin rash, gastrointestinal lesions (stomatitis and enteritis, with nausea, vomiting, and diarrhea), and mental symptoms, including irritability, insomnia, impaired memory, delusions, hallucinations, dementia, or delirium (Serdau, Hausser-Hauw et al., 1988). Untreated pellagra is fatal. With prompt nicotinic acid replacement, recovery can occur over hours or days.

Marchiafava-Bignami disease consists of demyelinating lesions in the corpus callosum and progressive neurologic symptoms, often ending fatally within a few months. Specifically associated with alcoholism, Marchiafava-Bignami disease is rare, and its pathophysiology is unclear. Mental symptoms predominate, with depression, mania, paranoia, and dementia. Seizures are common, and hemiparesis, aphasia, dyskinesia, and ataxia are variably present. The callosal lesions do not explain the devastating neurologic deterioration.

Controversy attends the concept of "alcoholic dementia," as used to refer to progressive mental decline in alcoholics without apparent cause, nutritional or otherwise (Brust, 2000). Many alcoholics have mental impairment more gradual in onset and more "global" than would be expected with Korsakoff syndrome. Prior episodes of Wernicke's syndrome are not identified, and more than memory is affected. Enlarged cerebral ventricles and sulci often are seen on CT or magnetic resonance imaging in alcoholics, in some reports correlating with cognitive decline and improving with abstinence. Animal studies using pair-fed controls have shown both behavioral and morphologic abnormalities in nutritionally maintained rodents who received chronic ethanol. Changes include loss of dendritic spines and neurons in the hippocampus. If, in fact, ethanol is directly neurotoxic, it is unclear if there is a safe dose threshold.

Drug users are at risk of altered mentation by indirect mechanisms, including head trauma, infection (especially AIDS), malnutrition, and concomitant alcohol abuse. It is not clear whether the drugs themselves cause lasting cognitive or behavioral change (Weinrieb & O'Brien, 1993). Predrug mental status usually is uncertain, and many drug users are self-medicating preexisting psychiatric conditions (as by using cocaine for depression).

Tolerant heroin addicts tend to be depressed, irritable, and socially withdrawn, but experience with methadone maintenance treatment shows that the great majority of such patients has normal mental function.

Acute and chronic paranoia are features of psychostimulant abuse; withdrawal depression with stimulants can last for months. However, claims of permanent depression in psychostimulant users (resulting from damage to the dopaminergic mesolimbic "reward circuit") are unproven. Decreased brain volume (observed by CT) and irregularly reduced cerebral perfusion (diagnosed by single-photon emission spectroscopy) have occurred in chronic cocaine users, with the changes reportedly correlated with cognitive impairment (Pascual-Leone, Dhuna et al., 1991; Holman, Carvalho et al., 1991). However, in a later prospective analysis, it was found that although chronic cocaine exposure was associated with neuropsychologic impairment, there was no correlation with brain volume loss when subjects with other substance use disorders were excluded (Langendorf, Tupper et al., 2000). Positron emission tomographic studies found losses of serotonin transporter binding in brains exposed to MDMA, but the clinical significance of the findings is uncertain.

An "antimotivational syndrome" has been described in chronic marijuana users, but studies from around the world have been conflicting. As with cognitive deficits ascribed to long-term use, in the absence of a baseline before drug use, cause and effect are difficult to determine in such studies. The weight of evidence suggests that if marijuana causes lasting behavioral change, the effect is small (Weinrieb & O'Brien, 1993; Iversen, 2000).

Sedatives, especially barbiturates, can produce mental clouding or paradoxical hyperactivity in older adults (Maytal & Shinnar, 2000). Chronic barbiturate abuse is associated with psychological and social deterioration, including paranoia and suicide, but, in contrast to alcohol abuse, CT results do not differ from those in control subjects (Allgulander, Borg et al., 1984). In small children, barbiturates have deleterious effects on IQ; whether these resolve over time is uncertain.

Hallucinogens can produce prolonged adverse reactions, and some users experience flashbacks (the recurrence, days or weeks later, of the drug's original psychic effects in the absence of further drug use). However, it is doubtful that hallucinogens cause permanent cognitive alteration (Weinrieb & O'Brien, 1993).

Among inhalants, the substance most clearly associated with CNS damage is toluene, which is found in many solvents, paints, and glues. White matter lesions can result in dementia, often accompanied by pyramidal, cerebellar, and oculomotor signs (Filley, Heaton et al., 1990). Sniffers of gasoline containing tetraethyl lead have developed lead encephalopathy (Valpey, Sumi et al., 1978).

Acutely, PCP produces schizophrenic-like symptoms, both positive (agitation, paranoia, delusions, or hallucinations) and negative (autism, loss of ego boundaries, avolition, or catatonia). Permanent neuropsychiatric change has been claimed (Fauman, Aldinger et al., 1976).

MUSCLE, NERVE, AND SPINAL CORD

Acute rhabdomyolysis with myoglobinuria and renal failure often is a feature of overdose with amphetamines, cocaine, or phencyclidine (Shafer, 1993). In heroin users, rhabdomyolysis can occur without evidence of overdose, perhaps on an immunologic basis.

Alcoholic myopathy ranges in severity from asymptomatic elevation of creatine kinase, to a progressive polymyositis-like picture, to acute rhabdomyolysis. The cause is toxic, not nutritional, and symptoms often interrupt binges. Cardiomyopathy may be present (Urbano-Marquez, Estruch et al., 1989).

Sensorimotor polyneuropathy is common in alcoholics (Victor & Adams, 1953). Paresthesias usually begin in the feet and, with progression, may be accompanied by sensory loss and weakness affecting the four limbs, with severe burning pain in the feet. Autonomic symptoms and signs sometimes appear. The cause of alcoholic polyneuropathy is nutritional deficiency, but a particular vitamin is not identified, and concomitant ethanol neurotoxicity cannot be excluded.

Alcoholics are subject to pressure palsies from sleeping soundly in unusual positions. Radial nerve palsy, with wrist drop, and peroneal nerve palsy, with foot drop, are most common.

Guillain-Barré polyneuropathy and brachial and lumbosacral plexopathy, probably immune-mediated, are described in heroin users (Shafer, 1993). Brachial plexopathy has resulted from compression by septic ("mycotic") aneurysm of the subclavian artery. Peripheral nerve injuries follow direct injection of any drug.

"Glue-sniffers' neuropathy" is a severe sensorimotor polyneuropathy that affects users of products containing n-hexane. Quadriplegia can evolve over a few weeks, with incomplete improvement following abstinence (Procop, Ait et al., 1974). Pathologically, axons are distended by masses of neurofilaments, and secondary demyelination occurs.

Nitrous oxide oxidizes cobalamin, and sniffers of nitrous oxide develop a myeloneuropathy that is clinically indistinguishable from combined systems disease. The earliest symptoms usually are paresthesias in the feet and unsteady gait secondary to impaired proprioception. Anemia usually is absent, and serum cobalamin levels generally are normal (Heyer, Simpson et al., 1986).

OTHER COMPLICATIONS

Severe irreversible parkinsonism developed in a group of drug users in California who were exposed to a meperidine analog contaminated with 1-methyl-4-phenyl-1,2,3,6-tetrahydropyridine (MPTP), a metabolite of which is toxic to neurons in the substantial nigra. Levodopa relieved the symptoms, which in some cases were of life-threatening severity, but treatment had to be continued indefinitely, and levodopa-induced dyskinesias were common (Langston, 1985). Positron emission tomography (using 18-F-dopa) of exposed but asymptomatic subjects showed decreased numbers of dopamine-containing neurons, and delayed parkinsonism has developed in previously asymptomatic subjects who used small doses of the drug (Calne, Langston et al., 1986).

Inhaling the vapor of heroin heated on metal foil ("chasing the dragon") resulted in cerebral and cerebellar spongiform leukoencephalopathy in European and North American users. Dementia, ataxia, quadriparesis, and blindness frequently progressed to death, and survivors were left with neurologic residua. The nature of the toxicity is unknown; elevated lactate in the damaged white matter suggests mitochondrial dysfunction (Kriegstein, Shungu et al., 1999).

Impaired vision with optic atrophy is common in alcoholic individuals. The optic nerve lesions are the result of nutritional deficiency, but the particular deficiency is uncertain, as are the possible toxicities of alcohol itself and of cyanide in tobacco smoke (Carroll, 1944).

Cerebellar degeneration can occur in nutritionally deficient alcoholics in the absence of Wernicke-Korsakoff syndrome. The superior cerebellar vermis is preferentially affected, resulting in gait and sometimes leg ataxia, usually without ataxia of the arms or dysarthria (Victor, Adams et al., 1959).

A man who took large doses of a heroin mixture containing quinine developed blindness. Vision improved when he resumed using heroin without quinine (Brust & Richter, 1974b).

Chronic cocaine users can develop dystonia or chorea that outlasts drug use by days or weeks, and cocaine can precipitate symptoms in patients with Tourette syndrome (Factor, Sanchez-Ramos et al., 1988).

REFERENCES

Alldredge BK, Lowenstein DH & Simon RP (1989a). Seizures associated with recreational drug abuse. *Neurology* 30:1037-1039.

Alldredge BK, Lowenstein DH & Simon RP (1989b). A placebo-controlled trial of intravenous diphenylhydantoin for the short-term treatment of alcohol withdrawal seizures. *American Journal of Medicine* 87:645-648.

Allgulander C, Borg S & Vikander B (1984). A 4-6 year follow-up of 50 patients with primary dependence on sedative and hypnotic drugs. *American Journal of Psychiatry* 141:1580-1582.

Barr HL, Antes D, Oldenberg DJ et al. (1984). Mortality of treated alcoholics and drug addicts: The benefits of abstinence. *Journal of Studies on Alcohol* 45:440-452.

Bartolomei F, Nicoli F, Swaider L et al. (1992). Accident vasculaire cerebral ischemique après prise nasale d'heroine. Une nouvelle observation. *Presse Medicale* 21:983-986.

Bateman DA & Heagarty MC (1989). Passive freebase cocaine ("crack") inhalation by infants and toddlers. *American Journal of Diseases of Children* 143:25-27.

Brust JCM (1993). *Neurological Aspects of Substance Abuse.* Boston, MA: Butterworth-Heinemann.

Brust JCM (1997). Vasculitis owing to substance abuse. *Neurologic Clinics* 15:945-957.

Brust JCM (1998). Stroke and substance abuse. In HJM Barnett, JP Mohr, BM Stein et al. (eds.) *Stroke: Pathophysiology, Diagnosis, and Management, 3rd Edition.* New York, NY: Churchill-Livingstone, 979-1000.

Brust JCM (2000). Ethanol. In PS Spencer & HH Schaumburg (eds.) *Experimental and Clinical Neurotoxicology, 2nd Edition.* Baltimore, MD: Williams & Wilkins, 541-557.

Brust JCM & Richter RW (1974a). Tetanus in the inner city. *New York State Journal of Medicine* 74:1735-1742.

Brust JCM & Richter RW (1974b). Quinine amblyopia related to heroin addiction. *Annals of Internal Medicine* 74:84-86.

Brust JCM & Richter RW (1976). Stroke associated with addiction to heroin. *Journal of Neurology, Neurosurgery and Psychiatry* 39:194-199.

Brust JCM, Dickinson PCT, Hughes JEO et al. (1990). The diagnosis and treatment of cerebral mycotic aneurysms. *Annals of Neurology* 27:238-246.

Calne DB, Langston JW, Stoessl AJ et al. (1986). Positron emission tomography after MPTP. Observations relating to the cause of Parkinson's disease. *Nature* 317:246-248.

Camargo CA (1989). Moderate alcohol consumption and stroke: The epidemiologic evidence. *Stroke* 20:1611-1626.

Caplan LR, Thomas C & Banks G (1982). Central nervous system complications of addiction to "T's and blues." *Neurology* 32:623-628.

Carroll FD (1944). The etiology and treatment of tobacco-alcohol amblyopia. *American Journal of Ophthalmology* 27:713-725.

Chaney NE, Franke J & Wadlington WB (1988). Cocaine convulsions in a breast-feeding baby. *Journal of Pediatrics* 112:134-135.

Citron BO, Halpern M, McCarron M et al. (1970). Necrotizing angiitis associated with drug abuse. *New England Journal of Medicine* 283:1003-1011.

Earnest MP (1993). Seizures. *Neurologic Clinics* 11:563-575.

Eastman JW & Cohen SN (1975). Hypertensive crisis and death associated with phencyclidine poisoning. *Journal of the American Medical Association* 231:1270-1271.

Factor SA, Sanchez-Ramos JR & Wiener WJ (1988). Cocaine and Tourette's syndrome. *Annals of Neurology* 23: 423-424.

Fallis RJ & Fisher M (1985). Cerebral vasculitis and hemorrhage associated with phenylpropanolamine. *Neurology* 35:405-407.

Fauman B, Aldinger G & Fauman M (1976). Psychiatric sequelae of phencyclidine abuse. *Clinical Toxicology* 9:529-538.

Fialip J, Aumaitre O, Eschalier A et al. (1987). Benzodiazepine withdrawal seizures. Analysis of 48 case reports. *Clinical Neuropharmacology* 10:538-544.

Filley CM, Heaton RK & Rosenberg NV (1990). White matter dementia in chronic toluene abuse. *Neurology* 40:532-534.

Fisch BJ, Hauser WA, Brust JCM et al. (1989). The EEG response to diffuse and patterned photic stimulation during acute untreated alcohol withdrawal. *Neurology* 39:434-436.

Fisher D & Ungerleider J (1967). Grand mal seizures following ingestion of LSD. *California Medicine* 106:210-211.

Fouilladieu J-L, D'Engert J & Conseiller C (1984). Benzodiazepines. *New England Journal of Medicine* 310:464.

Fraser HF, Wikler A, Essig CG et al. (1958). Degree of physical dependence induced by secobarbital or pentobarbital. *Journal of the American Medical Association* 166:126-129.

Frenchick BS (1990). Are androgenic steroids thrombogenic? *New England Journal of Medicine* 322:476.

Goldbaum GM, Kendrick JS, Hogelin GC et al. (1987). The relative impact of smoking and oral contraceptive use on women in the United States. *Journal of the American Medical Association* 258:1339-1342.

Goldfrank LR, Flomenbaum NE, Lewin NA et al. (eds.) 1998. *Goldfrank's Toxicologic Emergencies, 6th Edition.* Stamford, CT: Appleton & Lange.

Gonzalez LP, Czachura JF & Brewer KW (1989). Spontaneous versus elicited seizures following ethanol withdrawal: Differential time course. *Alcohol* 6:481-487.

Gonzalez-Garcia JJ, Arnalich F, Pena JM et al. (1986). An outbreak of Plasmodium vivax malaria among heroin users in Spain. *Transactions of the Royal Society of Tropical Medicine and Hygiene* 80:549-552.

Goodhart LC, Loizou LA & Anderson M (1982). Heroin myelopathy. *Journal of Neurology, Neurosurgery and Psychiatry* 45:562-563.

Halt PS, Swanson RA & Faden AI (1992). Alcohol exacerbates behavioral and neurochemical effects of rat spinal cord trauma. *Archives of Neurology* 49:1178-1184.

Hauser WA, Ng SKC & Brust JCM (1988). Alcohol, seizures, and epilepsy. *Epilepsia* 29(Suppl 2):S66-S78.

Hershey LA (1983). Meperidine and central neurotoxicity. *Annals of Internal Medicine* 98:548-549.

Heyer EJ, Simpson DM, Bodis-Wollner I et al. (1986). Nitrous oxide: Clinical and electrophysiological investigation of neurologic complications. *Neurology* 36:1618-1622.

Hoaken PCS (1975). Adverse effects of methaqualone. *Canadian Medical Association Journal* 112:685.

Holman BL, Carvalho PA, Mendelson J et al. (1991). Brain perfusion is abnormal in cocaine-dependent polydrug abusers: A study using technetium 99mHMPAO and ASPECT. *Journal of Nuclear Medicine* 32:1206-1210.

Iversen LL (2000). *The Science of Marijuana.* New York, NY: Oxford University Press.

Jacobson S, Lehky T, Nishimura M et al. (1993). Isolation of HTLV-II from a patient with chronic, progressive neurological disease clinically indistinguishable from HTLV-I associated myelopathy/tropical spastic paraparesis. *Annals of Neurology* 33:392-396.

Judice DJ, LeBlanc HJ & McGarry PA (1978). Spinal cord vasculitis presenting as spinal cord tumor in a heroin addict. *Journal of Neurosurgery* 48:131-134.

Karler R, Petty C, Calder L et al. (1989). Proconvulsant and anticonvulsant effects in mice of acute and chronic treatment with cocaine. *Neuropharmacology* 28:709-714.

Kaufman MJ, Levin JM, Ross MH et al. (1998). Cocaine-induced vasoconstriction detected in humans with magnetic resonance angiography. *Journal of the American Medical Association* 279:375-381.

Kernan WN, Viscoli CM, Brass LM et al. (2000). Phenylpropanolamine and the risk of hemorrhagic stroke. *New England Journal of Medicine* 343:1826-1832.

Knoblauch AL, Buchholz M, Koller MG et al. (1983). Hemiplegie nach injektion von heroin. *Schweizerische Medizinische Wochenschrift* 113:402-406.

Konkol RJ, Erickson BA, Doerr JK et al. (1992). Seizures induced by the cocaine metabolite benzoylecgonine in rats. *Epilepsia* 33:420-427.

Kriegstein AR, Shungu DC, Millar WS et al. (1999). Leukoencephalopathy and raised brain lactate from heroin vapor inhalation ("chasing the dragon"). *Neurology* 53:1765-1773.

Kudrow DB, Henry DA, Haake DA et al. (1988). Botulism associated with Clostridium botulinum sinusitis after intranasal cocaine use. *Annals of Internal Medicine* 109:984-985.

Langendorf FG, Tupper DE & Rottenberg DA (2000). Does chronic cocaine exposure cause brain atrophy? A qualitative MRI study. *Neurology* 54(Suppl 3):A442-A443.

Langston JW (1985). MPTP and Parkinson's disease. *Trends in Neurosciences* 8:79-83.

Lechtenberg R & Worner TM (1990). Seizure risk with recurrent alcohol detoxification. *Archives of Neurology* 47:535-538.

Levine SR, Brust JCM, Futrell N et al. (1990). Cerebrovascular complications of the use of the "crack" form of alkaloidal cocaine. *New England Journal of Medicine* 323:699-704.

Lieberman AN, Bloom W, Kishore PS et al. (1974). Carotid artery occlusion following ingestion of LSD. *Stroke* 5:213-215.

Malouf R, Jacquette G, Dobkin J et al. (1990). Neurologic disease in human immunodeficiency virus-infected drug abusers. *Archives of Neurology* 47:1002-1007.

Manchanda S & Connolly MJ (1993). Cerebral infarction in association with Ecstasy abuse. *Postgraduate Medical Journal* 69:874-875.

Marantz PR, Linzer M & Feiner CJ (1987). Inability to predict diagnosis in febrile intravenous drug abusers. *Annals of Internal Medicine* 106:823-828.

Maytal J & Shinnar S (2000). Barbiturates. In PA Spencer & HH Schaumburg (eds.) *Experimental and Clinical Neurotoxicology, 2nd Edition.* New York, NY: Oxford University Press, 219-225.

McCarron MM, Schultze BW, Thompson GA et al. (1981a). Acute phencyclidine intoxication: Incidence of clinical findings in 1000 cases. *Annals of Emergency Medicine* 10:237-242.

McCarron MM, Schultze BW & Thompson GA (1981b). Acute phencyclidine intoxication: Clinical patterns, complications, and treatment. *Annals of Emergency Medicine* 10:290-297.

Mikolich JR, Paulson GW & Cross CJ (1975). Acute anticholinergic syndrome due to jimson seed ingestion. *Annals of Internal Medicine* 83:321-325.

Mizutami T, Lewis R & Gonatas N (1980). Media medullary syndrome in a drug abuser. *Archives of Neurology* 37:425-428.

Morton HG (1987). Occurrence and treatment of solvent abuse in children and adolescents. *Pharmacology and Therapeutics* 33:449-469.

Mueller SM & Solow EB (1982). Seizures associated with a new "pick-me-up" pill. *Annals of Neurology* 11:322.

Ng SKC, Brust JCM, Hauser WA et al. (1990). Illicit drug use and the risk of new onset seizures. *American Journal of Epidemiology* 132:47-57.

Ng SKC, Hauser WA, Brust JCM et al. (1988). Alcohol consumption and withdrawal in new-onset seizures. *New England Journal of Medicine* 319:666-673.

Pascual-Leone A, Dhuna A & Anderson DC (1991). Cerebral atrophy in habitual cocaine abusers: A planimetric CT study. *Neurology* 41:34-38.

Pascual-Leone A, Dhuna A, Altafullah I et al. (1990). Cocaine-induced seizures. *Neurology* 40:404-407.

Procop LD, Ait M & Tison J (1974). Huffer's neuropathy. *Journal of the American Medical Association* 229:1083-1084.

Richter RW (1993). Infections other than AIDS. *Neurologic Clinics* 11:591-603.

Sacco RL, Elkind M, Boden-Albala B et al. (1999). The protective effect of moderate alcohol consumption on ischemic stroke. *Journal of the American Medical Association* 281:53-60.

Schwartz RH, Luxenberg MG & Hoffman NG (1991). Crack use by American middle-class adolescent polydrug abusers. *Journal of Pediatrics* 118:150-155.

Serdau M, Hausser-Hauw C & Laplane D (1988). The clinical spectrum of alcoholic pellagra encephalopathy. *Brain* 111:829-842.

Shafer SQ (1993). Disorders of spinal cord, nerve, and muscle. *Neurologic Clinics* 11:693-705.

Shinton R & Beevers G (1989). Meta-analysis of relation between cigarette smoking and stroke. *British Medical Journal* 298:789-794.

Sloan MA, Kittner SJ, Feeser BR et al. (1998). Illicit drug-associated ischemic stroke in the Baltimore-Washington Stroke Study. *Neurology* 50:1688-1698.

Trugman JM (1988). Cerebral arteritis and oral methylphenidate. *Lancet* 1:584-585.

Tsai G, Gastfriend DR & Coyle JT (1995). The glutamatergic basis of human alcoholism. *American Journal of Psychiatry* 152:332-340.

Urbano-Marquez AM, Estruch R, Navarro-Lopez F et al. (1989). The effects of alcohol on skeletal and cardiac muscle. *New England Journal of Medicine* 24:1705-1714.

Valpey R, Sumi S, Copass MK et al. (1978). Acute and chronic progressive encephalopathy due to gasoline sniffing. *Neurology* 28:507-510.

Victor M & Adams RD (1953). The effect of alcohol on the nervous system. *Research Publications: Association for Research in Nervous and Mental Disease* 32:526-573.

Victor M, Adams RD & Collins GH (1989). *The Wernicke-Korsakoff Syndrome, 2nd Edition*. Philadelphia, PA: F.A. Davis.

Victor M, Adams RD & Mancall EL (1959). A restricted form of cerebellar cortical degeneration occurring in alcoholic patients. *Archives of Neurology* 1:579-688.

Weinrieb RM & O'Brien CP (1993). Persistent cognitive deficits attributed to substance abuse. *Neurologic Clinics* 11:663-691.

Wolf PA, D'Agostino RB, Kannel WB et al. (1988). Cigarette smoking as a risk factor for stroke. The Framingham Study. *Journal of the American Medical Association* 259:1025-1029.

| Chapter 8 | # HIV, TB, and Other Infectious Diseases Related to Alcohol and Other Drug Use |

Carol A. Sulis, M.D.

Host Defenses
Skin and Soft Tissue Infections
Endocarditis
Noncardiac Vascular Infections
Respiratory Infections
Hepatic and Gastrointestinal Infections
Bone and Joint Infections
Nervous System Infections
Eye Infections
HIV/AIDS
Sexually Transmitted Diseases

Infectious diseases are common complications of alcohol and other drug abuse (Cherubin & Sapira, 1993; Levine & Brown, 2000; Cooper & Maderazo, 1989). Infections can occur because of a breach in host defenses while a patient is intoxicated, by direct inoculation of bloodborne or environmental pathogens during injection drug use, or as the result of unsafe behaviors. Acute infection accounts for 60% of hospital admissions among injection drug users (IDUs) in the United States each year and complicates a substantial proportion of hospital admissions among other drug users. Cellulitis, cutaneous abscesses, endocarditis, hepatitis, pneumonia, and tuberculosis have been common problems for drug users for decades; malaria, wound botulism, and tetanus have become exceedingly rare; and the acquired immunodeficiency syndrome (AIDS) and infection with type II human T-cell lymphotropic virus (HTLV-II) are relative newcomers.

The two greatest challenges for the clinician are (1) to differentiate the occult or incipient infection from symptoms of intoxication or withdrawal and (2) to recognize an atypical presentation of an infection modified by defective host defenses (splenectomy or AIDS) or the patient's self-medication with antibiotics or analgesics.

This chapter focuses on common infectious consequences of alcohol or other drug abuse. Standard texts and review articles should be consulted for detailed descriptions of the epidemiology, pathophysiology, clinical presentation, and management of infectious disorders.

HOST DEFENSES

Among IDUs, breach of local skin and mucosal barriers by the repeated injection of nonsterile materials and colonization with resistant organisms appears to be more important than deficiencies in phagocytic function or antibody response. Such repeated, nonspecific stimulation of the immune system leads to polyclonal elevation of immunoglobulin, which, in turn, can cause diagnostic confusion in caring for the patient who develops autoantibodies such as rheumatoid factor or who has a biologic false-positive test for syphilis or hepatitis C.

Smokers have defective mucociliary function and are predisposed to the development of sinopulmonary infections caused by encapsulated organisms such as *Streptococcus pneumonia* or *Klebsiella pneumonia*. Malnutrition and splenic dysfunctions are common among alcoholics with cirrhosis, but the magnitude of their contribution to immune dysfunction is difficult to quantify. In contrast, the cell-mediated deficiencies that result from effects on T-lymphocyte function caused by infection with human immunodeficiency virus (HIV), tuberculosis, and other intracellular pathogens are well described (Cohen, Cicala et al., 2000).

SKIN AND SOFT TISSUE INFECTIONS

Skin and soft tissue infections are common among IDUs and often are the reason for hospital admission. The type of infection (cellulitis, abscess, or ulcer), its location and severity, and causative organisms usually are related to the duration and site of injection and local epidemiology. For example, clusters of infection caused by unusual pathogens have been reported from California (wound botulism), Chicago (*Pseudomonas aeruginosa*), and Detroit (*Serratia marcescens*). However, *Staphylococcus aureus* and groups A, C, F, and G beta-hemolytic streptococci are the organisms most often seen (Cherubin & Sapira, 1993; Levine & Brown, 2000; Brook & Frazier, 1990; Levine, Crane et al., 1986; Summanen, Talan et al., 1995; Barg, Kish et al., 1985; Lentneck, Giger et al., 1990; Braunstein, 1991; Bernaldo de Quiros, Moreno et al., 1997; Craven, Rixinger et al., 1986a, 1986b).

IDUs who mix their drugs with saliva or who lick their needles before injecting are particularly prone to the development of polymicrobial infections with viridans streptococci, *Haemophilus* spp., *Eikenella corrodens*, and oral anaerobes. Infection with these organisms also occurs in bite wounds and closed-fist injuries.

Repeated injection of nonsterile, potentially vasoactive opiates can cause ischemic necrosis at the injection site, rendering the damaged areas susceptible to superinfection. Similarly, both inhalation and injection of cocaine cause vasospasm with resulting areas of tissue necrosis, serving as a nidus for infection. Streptococcal infection in areas of cocaine-induced tissue ischemia can cause large necrotic ulcers with extensive loss of tissue; such skin ulcers are extremely common among IDUs. Ulcers become colonized with a mixture of environmental pathogens, so surface cultures are not useful in guiding antibiotic selection.

The diagnosis of cellulitis is straightforward: most patients have local signs of pain, redness, and swelling or induration of the skin. However, patients who delay seeking medical care while they attempt to self-medicate with antibiotics or lotions can develop extensive cellulitis, necrotizing fasciitis, or overwhelming sepsis.

Diagnosis of an abscess can be more challenging. Patients may complain of pain or tenderness at the site of a superficial cutaneous abscess and may have erythema, induration, or fluctuance of the overlying skin. A deeper abscess may surround blood vessels (especially in the neck and groin), causing local bland or suppurative thrombophlebitis, or be hidden deep in the mediastinum or epidural space. Deep neck abscess can cause internal jugular vein thrombosis, vocal cord paralysis, airway obstruction, or massive hemorrhage after eroding into the carotid artery. The presentation of deeper abscesses can be quite subtle, and diagnosis often requires radiologic imaging.

In IDUs, necrotizing fasciitis, an infection of the deep fascial structures, can be caused by *Streptococcus pyogenes* (group A beta-hemolytic streptococci) or a mixture of aerobic and anaerobic pathogens. The most important diagnostic clue is the presence of pain or hemodynamic instability out of proportion to the physical findings, which may be quite trivial. Diagnosis can be delayed if the clinician discounts these complaints as evidence of "drug-seeking behavior." Classic findings of high fever, crepitus, and progressive edema occur late in the course. Prompt surgical and radiologic evaluation for evidence of fasciitis is crucial to diagnosis. In patients with necrotizing fasciitis, treatment with antibiotics and urgent surgical exploration with debridement are required to minimize morbidity and maximize the patient's chance for survival.

In all other cases, empiric antibiotic therapy should be directed at the most likely pathogen, then modified when cultures of blood or aspirated pus become positive. Early surgical evaluation and drainage can minimize morbidity and continued tissue destruction. However, the clinician should carefully evaluate lesions located in the vicinity of blood vessels (especially in the groin), because a mycotic aneurysm can masquerade as an abscess, and should not be blindly incised because of the potential for massive hemorrhage.

Management of skin ulcers requires antibiotics and aggressive wound care to minimize loss of function, especially when lesions are located on the hand.

An increasing incidence of infection in large skeletal muscles has been recognized, especially among patients with AIDS (Blumberg & Stephens, 1990; Schwartzman, Lambertus et al., 1991; Widrow, Kellie et al., 1991; Christin & Sarosi, 1992; Hsueh, Hsiue et al., 1996). The clinical presentation resembles that of tropical pyomyositis. Such infections usually are caused by *S. aureus*. Pyomyositis is characterized by the presence of a suppurative collection without myonecrosis, often without prior trauma or local drug injection at the site. Patients may have fever, pain, and swelling in the involved muscle, but often there is little evidence of local inflammation. Diagnosis is made by needle aspiration of pus, with subsequent antibiotic therapy directed by culture results.

Vibrio vulnificus is an unusual cause of cellulitis, soft tissue infection, and bacteremia in cirrhotic patients who have been exposed to saltwater or shellfish (Wongpaitoon, Sathapatayavongs et al., 1985; Arnold, Woo et al., 1989; Harlow, Harner et al., 1996). Patients complain of nausea, vomiting, fever, hypotension, shock, and hemorrhagic skin bullae. Prognosis is poor, even with aggressive antibiotic and surgical management.

Complications related to infections with the *Clostridium sp.* that cause botulism and tetanus are discussed later, as are epidural and splenic abscess, and mycotic aneurysm.

ENDOCARDITIS
(Cardiovascular complications also are addressed in Chapter 2 of this section.)

Epidemiology and Pathogenesis. Infective endocarditis (IE) is the most common cardiac complication of injection drug use (Cherubin & Sapira, 1993; Levine & Brown, 2000; Pelletier & Petersdorf, 1977; Bayer, Bolger et al., 1998; Bayer & Scheld, 2000). IE usually begins during an episode of transient bacteremia. In most cases, microorganisms enter the bloodstream and lodge in a thrombus overlying previously damaged or denuded endothelium. Preexisting cardiac lesions are identified in about three-fourths of patients with IE; they include mitral valve prolapse, prosthetic cardiac valves, or congenital, degenerative, or rheumatic heart dis-

ease. In contrast, endocarditis that occurs in structurally normal valves is more likely to be nosocomial in origin, caused by more virulent organisms such as *Staphylococcus aureus*, or occur in an IDU. The resulting lesion, called a "vegetation," is composed of layers of platelets and fibrin covering clumps of relatively sequestered microorganisms. Although most vegetations are located on heart valves, they can occur on any endothelial surface.

The incidence of endocarditis is about 5 per 100,000 person years, with regional variations that reflect the prevalence of risk factors in the population. Immunodeficiency (including HIV infection) does not appear to increase the incidence of endocarditis; however, morbidity and mortality from endocarditis increases with increasing immunosuppression.

In the non-IDU, IE most often is caused by viridans streptococci (50%) and enterococci (10%). In contrast, in the IDU, IE most often is caused by *S. aureus* (>50%), of which variable proportions are methicillin-resistant. Streptococci (13%), enterococci (7%), and fungi, particularly non-*albicans Candida* species (5%), are much less commonly involved.

Both IDUs and alcoholics have a higher proportion of IE because of gram-negative bacilli such as *P. aeruginosa*, *Pseudomonas cepacia*, and *S. marcescens*, although their relative prevalence has significant regional variation (Levine, Crane et al., 1986; Chambers, Morris et al., 1987; Graves & Soto, 1992; Hecht & Berger, 1992; Berlin, Abrutyn et al., 1995; Nahass, Weinstein, et al., 1990; Chambers, Korzeniowski et al., 1983; Gallagher, Watanakunakorn et al., 1986; Rapeport, Giron et al., 1986; Venezio, Gullberg et al., 1986; Snyder, Atterbury et al., 1977; Shekar, Rice et al., 1985; Botsford, Weinstein et al., 1985; Wieland, Lederman et al., 1986; Mills & Drew, 1976; Cooper & Mills, 1980; Komshian, Tablan et al., 1990). For example, a cluster of *P. aeruginosa* endocarditis occurred in Chicago among patients who abused pentazocine and tripelennamine ("Ts and blues") (Shekar, Rice et al., 1985; Botsford, Weinstein et al., 1985). This cluster was found to be associated with selective survival of the patients' own bacterial isolates when grown in the presence of these drugs. Outbreaks of *S. marcescens* infection have been reported in Detroit and California, but the reason for the increased prevalence in these locations remains obscure. In one California cluster of *S. marcescens* endocarditis reported in the 1970s, cases were characterized by the development of enormous vegetations that caused almost complete occlusion of the valve

---

TABLE 1.   Criteria for the Diagnosis of Infective Endocarditis (Duke University Criteria)

Definitive diagnosis:
- Pathology/microbiology of vegetation or embolized vegetation obtained at autopsy or surgery;
- Two major criteria;
- One major plus three minor criteria; or
- Five minor criteria.

Possible diagnosis: Findings consistent with, but not definitive for, infective endocarditis.

No endocarditis: No pathology at surgery or autopsy; clinical resolution with ≤4 days' antibiotic therapy; firm alternative diagnosis.

Major criteria:
Blood culture:
- Two separate blood cultures positive for either:
  - Viridans streptococcus, *Streptococcus bovis*, HACEK (Haemophilus, Actinobacillus, Cardiobacterium, Eikenella, and Kingella); or
  - Community-acquired *S. aureus* or enterococcus in the absence of a primary focus.
- Positive blood cultures >12 hours apart.

- Positive blood cultures 3 of 3 or majority of ≥4 that are ≥1 hour apart.

Endocardial involvement:
- Echocardiography: Oscillating intracardiac mass on a valve or supporting structure, in the path of a regurgitant jet stream, or on implanted material in the absence of alternative anatomic explanation, valve ring abscess, or new dehiscence of prosthetic valve.
- New valvular regurgitant murmur.

Minor criteria:
- Predisposing heart condition or intravenous drug user;
- Fever ≥38°C;
- Systemic or pulmonary emboli, mycotic aneurysm, intracranial hemorrhage, conjunctival hemorrhage, Janeway lesions;
- Immunologic phenomena: Glomerulonephritis, Roth spot, Osler node, rheumatoid factor;
- Echocardiography findings consistent with but not definitive for endocarditis;
- Microbiologic/serologic findings consistent with but not definitive for endocarditis.

SOURCE: Adapted from Durack DT, Lukes AS & Bright DK (1994). New criteria for diagnosis of infective endocarditis: Utilization of specific echocardiographic findings. Duke Endocarditis Service. *American Journal of Medicine* 96:200-209.

---

orifice in the absence of concurrent valve destruction. Mortality in this outbreak was 70% (Mills & Drew, 1976; Cooper & Mills, 1980). Underlying alcoholism is identified as a risk factor in 40% of episodes of pneumococcal endocarditis, and concurrent meningitis is present in 70% of this subgroup of patients (Burman, Norrby et al., 1985; Ugolini, Pacifico et al., 1986; Gelfand & Threlkeld, 1992; Musher, 1992).

Endocarditis caused by *Bartonella henselae* has been described in homeless alcoholics, IDUs, and patients with HIV (Spach, Callis et al., 1993; Spach, Kanter et al., 1995; Comer, Flynn et al., 1996; Holmes, Greenough et al., 1995; Raoult, Fournier et al., 1996). Endocarditis caused by a vast array of additional pathogens has been described in case reports (Riancho, Echevarria et al., 1988; Bestetti, Figueiredo et al., 1991; Steen, Bruno-Murtha et al., 1992; Ascher, Zbick, 1991).

The sustained bacteremia that characterizes IE occurs when microorganisms are released as the vegetation fragments, and the size of the vegetation is related to the type of pathogen. Organisms such as *S. marcescens* and *C. albicans* tend to produce large friable vegetations and bulky emboli.

Clinical Presentation. Clinical features usually include fever, accompanied by a panoply of cardiac abnormalities (murmur, conduction delay, congestive heart failure, and valvular dysfunction), complications from emboli or from metastatic seeding of other structures during the bacteremia (causing meningitis, brain abscess, osteomyelitis, or splenic abscess), and a wide spectrum of immune complex-mediated phenomena (arthritis, glomerulonephritis, aseptic meningitis, Osler nodes, Roth spots, splinter hemorrhages, and other manifestations of vasculitis) (Weinstein, 1986; Mansur, Grinberg et al., 1992; Omari, Shapiro et al., 1989; Robinson, Saxe et al., 1992; Speechly-Dick &

Swanton, 1994). Patients may complain of fever, night sweats, anorexia, arthralgias, and myalgias (especially in the low back and upper thighs), and weight loss. However, the presence of IE cannot be predicted in a febrile IDU on the basis of signs and symptoms alone (Marantz, Linzer et al., 1987; Weisse, Heller et al., 1993). Unexplained fever should prompt evaluation for endocarditis.

The most reliable clues are the presence of embolic phenomenon and visualization of vegetations on echocardiography. IDUs have a high incidence of acute IE involving a previously normal tricuspid valve. As a result, patients have pulmonary symptoms, including cough and pleuritic chest pain from septic pulmonary emboli. Pulmonary infiltrate or effusion occur in 75% to 85%, and evidence of septic pulmonary embolization eventually is present on 90% of chest x-rays. These emboli appear as rounded infiltrates ("cannon balls") early in the course, often in showers, and may undergo central cavitation or be complicated by empyema. Murmurs and congestive heart failure usually are absent in these patients. In contrast, IDUs with left-sided endocarditis have murmur, congestive heart failure, and stigmata of systemic embolization.

Mycotic aneurysms complicate IE in 15% of patients. Most are asymptomatic and resolve with treatment.

Diagnosis. After a careful history and physical examination, IDUs should have two or three blood cultures drawn. Hospitalization and treatment with empiric antibiotics often is recommended when adequate outpatient followup is uncertain.

Definitive diagnosis requires microbiologic or pathologic proof of infection by histology or by culture of a sample of the vegetation or embolus obtained at surgery or autopsy (Von Reyn, Levy et al., 1981; Durack, Lukes et al., 1994; Bayer, Ward et al., 1994). A presumptive diagnosis is established by demonstrating a characteristic vegetation, valve ring abscess, or dehiscence of a prosthetic valve with echocardiography in a patient with multiple positive blood cultures obtained over an extended period (Lindner, Case et al., 1996; Roe, Abramson et al., 2000). However, even a negative transesophageal echocardiogram does not exclude the diagnosis. The probability that endocarditis is present is estimated by using major and minor criteria, as shown in Table 1 (Durack, Lukes et al., 1994).

Treatment. Effective antimicrobial therapy requires identification of the specific pathogen and assessment of its susceptibility to various antimicrobial agents. Empiric therapy should be targeted to the most likely pathogens in

the clinical setting. Initial therapy with an antistaphylococcal antibiotic is appropriate for most IDUs. Use of vancomycin (Vancocin®) should be considered in areas with a high prevalence of methicillin-resistant *S. aureus* or penicillin-resistant pneumococcus. Addition of antibiotics directed against gram-negative pathogens should be considered in certain communities (Wilson, Karchmer et al., 1995).

The chosen antibiotic should be bactericidal and must achieve sufficient levels to permit passive diffusion deep into the vegetation, where microcolonies of the pathogen are located. Ultimately, antibiotic selection should be based on final culture and sensitivity results. The duration of therapy should follow standard guidelines. Most patients require a minimum of four weeks of intravenous antibiotics, although shorter courses can be effective in IDUs with uncomplicated tricuspid valve endocarditis. An active IDU should not be discharged with an intravascular access device. Encouraging the patient to remain in the hospital for the duration of therapy is one of the most challenging aspects of achieving a successful outcome.

Once effective antimicrobial therapy has been initiated, symptoms of fever and fatigue improve coincident with clearance of bacteremia. Blood cultures for streptococci and enterococci should become sterile after one to two days. Blood cultures for staphylococci should become sterile after three to five days, but can take 10 to 14 days to become sterile in patients treated with vancomycin. As a result, short-course therapy cannot be used in regimens containing vancomycin. Blood cultures should be obtained daily, until sterile. If initial blood cultures remain negative, the possibility of culture-negative endocarditis, an undrained focus of infection (that is, splenic abscess), or an alternative diagnosis should be entertained. Diagnostic possibilities are quite extensive and are best assessed with the assistance of an infectious diseases specialist.

When sequelae of endocarditis progress despite appropriate antibiotic management, surgical evaluation is warranted. Surgical intervention should be considered for patients who demonstrate congestive heart failure because of valvular dysfunction that is refractory to medical therapy, multiple clinically relevant emboli despite antibiotic therapy for more than two weeks, infection caused by certain pathogens such as fungi or resistant organisms (which rarely respond to medical therapy alone), extension of myocardial abscess, inability to sterilize blood cultures, or infection or dehiscence of a prosthetic valve (Carrel, Schaffner et al., 1993). Patients with valve ring abscess should be monitored for the development of conduction abnormalities. These patients may require placement of a temporary pacemaker because of the risk of developing high-grade heart block.

Outcome and Prevention. The outcome of an episode of IE is based on many factors, including age of the patient, virulence of the organism, site of the infection, presence of complications (such as congestive heart failure, renal failure, rupture of a mycotic aneurysm, cardiac arrhythmia, conduction abnormalities, or cerebral embolization), and the presence of comorbid conditions such as HIV infection. Left-sided endocarditis is associated with a worse prognosis, as is infection with gram-negative bacilli or fungi. Heart failure remains the leading cause of death.

After cure, patients remain at a substantially increased risk of reinfection, and injection drug use is the most common risk factor for recurrent native valve endocarditis. As a result, patients should follow American Heart Association Guidelines, and be given prophylactic antibiotics when undergoing certain invasive procedures (Dajani, Taubert et al., 1997; Durack, 1998). In addition, patients should be counseled about the importance of adopting strategies to reduce the likelihood of transient bacteremia. Other preventative measures include aggressive treatment of skin infections, emphasis on maintaining good dental hygiene, and discussion of the overall benefits of discontinuing illicit drug use.

NONCARDIAC VASCULAR INFECTIONS

Epidemiology and Pathogenesis. Both direct injury to blood vessels during injection drug use and vasospasm from cocaine use are associated with endothelial injury and thrombus formation. Bacterial seeding of the thrombus can result in septic thrombophlebitis. Alternatively, a hematoma adjacent to the traumatized or ischemic blood vessel may serve as a nidus for superinfection. An arteriovenous fistula can occur either as a result of a direct injury or from extension of local infection.

A mycotic aneurysm results when emboli to the vasa vasorum cause a mushroom-shaped swelling, especially at arterial bifurcations. Mycotic aneurysm formation classically occurs during episodes of bacterial endocarditis. The damaged arterial wall is seeded during a concurrent or subsequent bacteremia. Mycotic aneurysms complicate 15% of cases of IE. They usually are silent, but may become symptomatic in 3% to 5% of patients months or years after completion of appropriate therapy (Tsao, Garlin et al., 1999;

Shaikholeslami, Tomlinson et al., 1999; Lee, Lee et al., 1998).

For most noncardiac endovascular lesions, the predominant pathogen is *S. aureus*; however, gram-negative bacilli (especially *P. aeruginosa*) are reported with increased frequency in IDUs.

Clinical Presentation. When peripheral blood vessels are involved, clinical findings include fever with local pain, swelling, warmth, and induration. A bruit may be present. Infections of the peripheral vasculature can masquerade as cellulitis or subcutaneous abscess, and blind surgical incision should be avoided. Thrombosis of larger vessels can be associated with either pulmonary embolization or distal ischemia and may be confused with IE.

A patient with a mycotic aneurysm in the neck or groin may describe a painful, tender, enlarging, pulsatile mass with overlying bruit or thrill, accompanied by various constitutional symptoms. Ischemia of a distal extremity or signs of nerve compression may be present. Two important complications include extension of infection into surrounding soft tissue, with abscess formation and massive hemorrhage from aneurysmal rupture. Mycotic aneurysms in the brain complicate 2% to 4% of cases of left-sided endocarditis. Patients complain of unremitting headache, visual disturbances, or cranial nerve palsy.

Patients with endovascular infection may have sustained bacteremia and signs of clinical sepsis. Management of septic thrombophlebitis is controversial but generally includes treatment with both intravenous antibiotics and short-term anticoagulation.

Diagnosis. Successful management of a mycotic aneurysm requires early diagnosis before rupture occurs. Misdiagnosis is common, and a high index of suspicion is essential. Arteriographic confirmation is the standard diagnostic test, although the accuracy of newer radiologic tools (such as digital subtraction angiography) is being investigated.

Treatment. Empiric antibiotics can be given after blood cultures have been obtained. Antibiotic choice should reflect local epidemiology and should include an antistaphylococcal agent, with additional gram-negative coverage in selected communities. The antibiotic regimen should be modified on the basis of culture and sensitivity results and usually is continued for four to six weeks.

Surgical excision of an enlarging mycotic aneurysm and surrounding infected tissue may be necessary to avoid the catastrophic sequelae of a rupture. Intrathoracic, intra-abdominal, and peripheral mycotic aneurysms often require surgical excision. Cerebral mycotic aneurysms usually heal with medical therapy alone, but may require neurosurgical intervention if enlarging or bleeding (Frizzell, Vitek et al., 1993).

RESPIRATORY INFECTIONS
(Respiratory problems also are discussed in Chapter 6 of this section.)

Epidemiology and Pathogenesis. Many factors interfere with host defenses and predispose the patient to infection (Caiaffa, Vlahov et al., 1994; Wewers, Diaz et al., 1998; Lipsky, Boyko et al., 1986; Bartlett, Gorbach et al., 1974; O'Donnell & Pappas, 1988; Bailey, Fraire et al., 1994; Polsky, Gold et al., 1986; Witt, Craven et al., 1987; Hirschtick, Glassroth et al., 1995; Caiaffa, Graham et al., 1993; Sullivan, Moore et al., 2000). Two important examples include cigarette smoke, which disrupts mucociliary function and macrophage activation, and alteration in the level of consciousness accompanied by depressed gag reflex, which compromises airway protection and permits aspiration of oropharyngeal flora. In addition, alcoholism is associated with oropharyngeal colonization with enteric gram-negative bacilli and abnormal phagocyte function. Injection drug use is associated with a large number of insults, including drug-induced bronchospasm, pulmonary edema, and the development of various types of foreign body granuloma (cotton, starch, or talc) from contaminants in injected materials. Such nonspecific abnormalities on chest radiograph contribute to diagnostic confusion in a febrile patient with cough. An increased risk of exposure to certain pathogens because of lifestyle (for example, homelessness or incarceration) and the increased prevalence of HIV infection in this group contribute to the increased risk of infection.

Pneumonia. Pneumonia is present in up to a third of IDUs evaluated for fever and complicates a variable percentage of admissions for treatment of alcohol withdrawal or cocaine intoxication. Septic pulmonary emboli associated with right-sided endocarditis or septic thrombophlebitis and tuberculosis infection are common. Most pulmonary infections are community-acquired episodes of pneumonia, caused by common respiratory pathogens such as *S. pneumonia*, atypical bacteria (such as *Legionella* or *Chlamydia*), oral anaerobes, or viruses. IDUs have an increased incidence of pneumonia caused by *Haemophilus influenzae*, *S. aureus*, and *P. aeruginosa*, especially those co-infected with HIV (Polsky, Gold et al., 1986; Witt, Craven et al., 1987; Hirschtick, Glassroth et al., 1995; Caiaffa, Graham et al., 1993; Sullivan, Moore et al., 2000; Janoff, Breiman et al., 1992; Rodriguez Barradas, Musher et al., 1992; Steinhart, Reingold et al., 1992; Kielhofner, Atmar et al., 1992; Fichtenbaum, Woeltje et al., 1994).

Patients with HIV are at higher risk of developing pneumonia. Although *Pneumocystis carinii* is the major pulmonary pathogen in patients with AIDS, pneumonia caused by *Mycobacterium tuberculosis*, *Mycobacterium avium intracellulare*, cytomegalovirus, and common bacterial and viral pathogens occur with increased frequency in this group. Lung abscesses can complicate aspiration pneumonia, necrotizing bacterial pneumonia, or septic emboli. Left-sided pulmonic effusions may be a clue to an underlying splenic abscess or bacterial or tuberculous pleuritis.

Evaluation of a febrile drug user with respiratory symptoms should follow standard guidelines, with empiric management directed at likely pathogens (O'Grady, Barie et al., 1998; Bartlett, Breiman et al., 1998).

Tuberculosis. Tuberculosis is a leading cause of infectious morbidity and mortality worldwide, and one third of the world population is latently infected. In the U.S., only 4% to 6% of the population have latent infections (Cantwell, Snider et al., 1994). Rates of active disease fell steadily until the mid-1980s, when there was a brief resurgence coincident with immigration patterns and the spread of HIV. HIV infection has contributed to the rising case rates because of the higher likelihood of reactivation as immune function decreases and because of the risk of unusually rapid progression to active disease following new (primary) infection. In addition, patients with HIV have a higher prevalence of extrapulmonary disease (Jones, Young et al., 1993; Greenberg, Frager et al., 1994; Castro, 1995; Havlir & Barnes, 1999; Markowitz, Hansen et al., 1997; Pablos-Mendez, Raviglione et al., 1998; Shafer, Kim et al., 1991; Relkin, Aranda et al., 1994; Frye, Pozsik et al., 1997; Anonymous, 2000b). Drug users, especially alcoholics and IDUs, have an increased incidence of reactivation tuberculosis for reasons that are unknown (Reichman, Felton et al., 1979; Perlman, Salomon et al., 1995; CDC, 2001a). Injection drug use has been implicated in a large outbreak of multiresistant tuberculosis in New York City, where most transmission occurred in hospitals and jails (Frieden, Sterling et al., 1993; Bloch, Cauthen et al., 1994; Alland, Kalkut et al., 1994; Gordin, Nelson et al., 1996; CDC, 2000c).

Difficulties in controlling this outbreak were compounded by homelessness and noncompliance with medical therapy.

Infection is spread by the aerosolization of acid-fast bacilli in respiratory secretions. Patients with cavitary disease are particularly infectious because of the high concentration of bacilli in their sputum. Cough-inducing procedures such as bronchoscopy, administration of aerosolized medications (including bronchodilators), and smoking (cigarettes, crack cocaine, and marijuana) can increase transmission.

The classic symptoms of pulmonary tuberculosis include cough with purulent, blood-tinged sputum and increasing malaise, with the development of night sweats and weight loss as the disease progresses. High fever, especially in the evening, is seen with decreasing frequency as the level of immunosuppression increases. Diagnosis is made by culturing *M. tuberculosis* from expectorated sputum. Tuberculin skin tests generally turn positive four to six weeks after primary infection, but can be negative in up to 25% of patients at the time of diagnosis. Interpretation of the tuberculin test is stratified to reflect a combination of risk factors, including severity of underlying immunosuppression, and should follow standard algorithms (CDC 1995, 1997, 1998e, 2000e; Bass, Farer et al., 1994; Horsburgh, Feldman et al., 2000). To avoid nosocomial transmission, patients with a suspicious presentation should be isolated until the diagnosis is excluded.

Extrapulmonary tuberculosis occurs in one sixth of normal adults, and up to 60% to 80% of patients with HIV. Diagnosis is challenging because of the paucity of bacilli in the extrapulmonary sites. Histopathology classically shows giant cell granulomas with central caseating necrosis. Extrapulmonary seeding commonly causes empyema, meningitis, and vertebral osteomyelitis, and diagnosis generally requires biopsy.

Because of the long delay to obtain culture and sensitivity results, treatment usually is initiated before a definitive diagnosis has been established. Treatment should follow American Thoracic Society Guidelines (CDC, 1997, 1998e, 2000e; Bass, Farer et al., 1994; Horsburgh, Feldman et al., 2000). Many patients are started on a four-drug regimen that includes isoniazid (Laniazid®), rifampin (Rifadin®), pyrazinamide, and ethambutol (Myambutol®). Patients should be closely monitored for evidence of disease progression and for the development of treatment-related side effects, such as hepatitis or rash (Halsey, Coberly et al., 1998; Gordin, Chaisson et al., 2000; CDC, 1996, 2001, 2000d;

Polesky, Farber et al., 1996). The initial regimen is adjusted once sensitivities are known. Duration of therapy is based on the severity of immunosuppression and extent of disease. IDUs are at increased risk of multidrug-resistant tuberculosis (that is, resistant to both isoniazid and rifampin). For these patients, results of sensitivity testing are crucial in planning an effective treatment regimen, which should include at least two active agents.

Medication selection can be particularly troublesome in treating patients with HIV. Drugs may be poorly absorbed because of underlying enteropathy or may have significant interactions with other medications. For example, rifampin should not be used with protease inhibitors or many other medications because of its effect on hepatic catabolism. Directly observed therapy is strongly encouraged when nonadherence is anticipated and often is preferred for patients with risk factors such as homelessness or addictive disorder.

Most drug users are at increased risk of tuberculosis infection and should have routine tuberculin skin testing. Interpretation of the skin test result and selection of a treatment regimen should follow standard guidelines. For example, IDUs with more than 10 mm induration on skin testing might be given six to 12 months of chemoprophylaxis with isoniazid after active disease is excluded. IDUs with HIV might be given 12 months of isoniazid when there is more than a 5 mm induration on skin testing or after close contact with a case of infectious tuberculosis, regardless of skin test results. Many drug combinations and dosing schedules are available. Rifampin can reduce methadone levels, and patients often require adjustment of their maintenance dose. IDUs with underlying hepatitis, or who use hepatotoxins such as alcohol, have an increased risk of developing hepatitis when using isoniazid, rifampin, or pyrazinamide. These patients should be monitored for the development of anorexia, abdominal pain, nausea, vomiting, change in color of urine or stool, or jaundice.

Most patients with underlying lung disease are at risk of increased morbidity from influenza and should be offered annual immunization (CDC, 2001c). The efficacy of pneumococcal vaccine to prevent invasive disease varies with the population studied. Because there is a clear benefit for most patients with HIV infection, and for many patients age 50 or older, administration of the pneumococcal vaccine should be considered as well, particularly in the patient with alcoholism.

HEPATIC AND GASTROINTESTINAL INFECTIONS

(Hepatic and gastrointestinal disorders also are addressed in Chapters 3 and 5 of this section.)

Hepatic cirrhosis results from an irreversible chronic injury to the hepatic parenchyma, which is most often caused by alcoholism or viral hepatitis. Infection is the leading cause of death in patients with cirrhosis (Cooper & Maderazo, 1989). Gram-negative enteric bacilli such as *Escherichia coli*, *K. pneumoniae*, and encapsulated respiratory pathogens such as *S. pneumonia*, are the most frequent cause of infection in these patients; however, severe infections with many other organisms, including *V. vulnificus*, *Pasteurella multocida*, *Aeromonas hydrophilia*, *Listeria monocytogenes*, *Campylobacter spp.*, and tuberculosis, also have been described.

Spontaneous bacterial peritonitis (SBP) is a common and potentially fatal infectious complication in patients with cirrhosis and ascites. Pathogenesis involves "translocation" of bacteria from the gut to mesenteric lymph nodes and is associated with deficiencies in humoral response and phagocytic function (Such & Runyon, 1998; Runyon, Montano et al., 1992).

Diagnostic paracentesis should be performed in patients with ascites who have fever. Analysis of ascitic fluid should include gram stain and culture for bacteria, mycobacteria, and fungi; measurement of albumin; absolute and differential white blood cell count; and cytopathology. Empiric antibiotic therapy is directed against suspected pathogens and should be refined once culture results become available. Because gram-negative enteric bacilli and *S. pneumonia* are the most common cause of infection in these patients, a second-generation cephalosporin or a combination of fluoroquinolone plus clindamycin (Cleocin®) or metronidazole (Flagyl®) are common starting regimens. Patients who have a low ascitic fluid protein or more advanced liver disease are at increased risk of developing SBP. Some authorities recommend the use of prophylactic antibiotics to prevent SBP in this subset of patients, as well as those with a prior episode of SBP.

Tuberculous peritonitis, which is uncommon, usually is diagnosed by peritoneal biopsy and culture.

BONE AND JOINT INFECTIONS

Osteomyelitis. Most microorganisms can infect bone. Frequent pathogens include *S. aureus* (60%), *Staphylococcus epidermidis* (30%), streptococci, gram-negative bacilli, anaerobes, mycobacteria, and fungi (10%), and prevalence is related to mode of acquisition. Infection can occur by hematogenous seeding, introduction after surgery or trauma, or spread from a contiguous focus (Lew, Waldvogel et al., 1997; Holzman & Bishko, 1971; Sapico & Montgomerie, 1979, 1980). In adults, hematogenous spread of bacteria frequently involves the spine because of the vascularity of the vertebra. Vertebral osteomyelitis in IDUs usually involves the lumbosacral and cervical spine. Common pathogens include *S. aureus*, gram-negative bacilli (including *P. aeruginosa*), and fungi. Although the original source of these infections may be unknown, most are seeded hematogenously during an episode of bacterial endocarditis or locally from a contiguous soft tissue focus.

Adults may develop osteomyelitis of the hand caused by mouth flora (including *Staphylococcus spp.*, *Eikenella corrodens*, *Pasteurella multocida*, and oral anaerobes) associated with local trauma after bite wounds or closed-fist injury.

Patients with osteomyelitis complain of focal pain and tenderness. Fever is present in two-thirds; erythema, warmth, and swelling are variably present. Lack of signs and symptoms frequently result in a delay in diagnosis.

In vertebral osteomyelitis, associated symptoms result when inflammation extends beyond the spine to cause retropharyngeal abscess, mediastinitis, subdiaphragmatic, or iliopsoas abscess, meningitis, or epidural abscess with evidence of spinal cord compression (Bass, Ailani et al., 1998). Spinal tuberculosis (Pott disease) is relatively indolent, and patients may have late sequelae and extensive vertebral destruction.

Diagnosis of osteomyelitis is made by biopsy and culture of bone. Computed tomography scan and magnetic resonance imaging are helpful in determining the extent of involvement but are not specific. Blood cultures often are negative, especially when the osteomyelitis resulted from hematogenous seeding during a remote bacteremic infection (such as endocarditis). Antibiotics alone may be sufficient therapy to cure acute osteomyelitis and should be chosen on the basis of isolated pathogens. Use of empiric therapy is suboptimal because of the wide range of potential pathogens. Surgical debridement generally is required for cure when the infection has been present for longer than six weeks (chronic osteomyelitis).

As noted earlier, establishing a regimen that is mutually acceptable to the patient and clinician is challenging because of the requirement for prolonged inpatient therapy. This challenge is compounded by the tendency for many physicians to undertreat associated bone pain symptoms; therefore, consultation with a pain management specialist may be beneficial.

Septic Arthritis. Septic arthritis occurs when bacteria seed joints previously damaged by trauma, instrumentation, osteoarthritis, or chronic inflammatory conditions. Infection with *S. aureus* is most common, although infection with many other organisms has been reported. Arthrocentesis with culture and microscopic examination of joint fluid are required for diagnosis. Differential diagnosis includes gonorrhea, crystal arthropathy, and a variety of noninfectious etiologies.

Two particular syndromes are more common among IDUs than in the normal population and involve fibrocartilaginous joints, which are most susceptible to hematogenous seeding.

Septic arthritis of the sternoclavicular joint caused by *P. aeruginosa* has been reported primarily in IDUs. Most cases occur without identification of an antecedent infection. Symptoms may be present for several months before the patient seeks evaluation. Complaints include fever, tenderness and swelling over the joint, and decreased range of motion of the ipsilateral shoulder. Another unusual presentation is of septic arthritis of the sacroiliac joint or symphysis pubis. Symptoms include fever and various combinations of hip, groin, thigh, or lower abdominal pain that is exacerbated by walking (Chandrasekar & Narula, 1986; del Busto, Quinn et al., 1982). In such cases, infection may spread from the joint to contiguous soft tissues and bone. Treatment may require exploratory arthrotomy, with surgical debridement of infected material followed by prolonged antibiotic therapy directed at isolated organisms.

NERVOUS SYSTEM INFECTIONS

Drug users are prone to a variety of central nervous system manifestations that may have an infectious origin. Such manifestations are easily missed if symptoms are mistakenly attributed to intoxication or withdrawal. Delirium, acute confusional states, encephalopathy, or coma may accompany overdose, intoxication, infection, or a large number of noninfectious etiologies. Central nervous system mass lesions, seizures, hemorrhage, stroke syndromes, transverse myelitis, and peripheral neuropathies have a similarly broad differential. Clinical features should guide diagnostic strategies, with management based on results of lumbar puncture and neuroradiologic imaging.

Endocarditis is the most common cause of central nervous system symptoms in IDUs and can cause meningitis (aseptic or purulent), brain abscess from septic emboli, or hemorrhage from rupture of a mycotic aneurysm. Bacteremia during IE can cause vertebral osteomyelitis, which, in turn, can be complicated by epidural abscess, with evidence of cord compression.

Brain abscess and subdural empyema in the absence of endocarditis usually are caused by a varied group of pyogenic bacteria; however, infection with many other organisms, including *Nocardia, Aspergillus spp., Cryptococcus*, mucormycosis, tuberculosis, and *Toxoplasma gondii*, have been reported, especially in patients co-infected with HIV. Etiology often involves extension from a contiguous focus in the mastoid, ear, or paranasal sinuses; seeding of a preexisting subdural hematoma during an episode of transient bacteremia; or direct inoculation of the subdural space after a traumatic wound. A patient with brain abscess may have nonspecific symptoms, such as headache or personality change, and an abscess can attain enormous size before diagnosis. Management includes antibiotics and drainage, if indicated.

In most cases, patients with HIV who have ring-enhancing mass lesions in the brain and appropriate clinical presentation are treated empirically for toxoplasmosis. Symptoms that worsen or fail to improve after two weeks should prompt more aggressive evaluation, including consideration of brain biopsy.

Meningovascular syphilis has been reported in a number of patients with HIV, despite presumably effective therapy for primary syphilis infection, and it should be considered in young people who present with a new stroke (Musher, Hamill et al., 1990).

Contamination of skin ulcers with spores of *Clostridium spp.* can cause neurologic symptoms from elaboration of neurotoxins.

Wound botulism is caused by contamination of injection sites or skin ulcers with *Clostridium botulinum* that release botulinum toxin (Bleck, 2000a; Passaro, Werner et al., 1998). Toxin is absorbed, disseminated, and ultimately binds to specific receptors, where it blocks acetylcholine release, resulting in a descending, symmetric, flaccid paralysis. Less than 100 cases have been reported since 1953, although a recent cluster of cases was reported among IDUs who injected black tar heroin. Diagnosis is established by recovering *C. botulinum* from the wound or by detecting toxin in serum, but negative findings do not exclude the diagnosis. Treatment with trivalent or type-specific antitoxin can limit disease progression. Involvement of motor neurons causes respiratory failure, and patients may require respiratory support for several months until synapses are regenerated. Botulism has been reported in a patient with colonization of the paranasal sinuses after intranasal cocaine use (Kudrow, Henry et al., 1988).

Tetanus is caused by the release of a potent neurotoxin by *Clostridium tetani* at the site of a wound in a person who lacks protective antibody (Bleck, 2000b; Cherubin, 1968). Wounds contaminated by dirt, feces, or saliva provide an appropriate anaerobic milieu for these vegetative bacteria. Approximately 100 cases of tetanus per year are reported in the U.S., in association with acute injury (80%), chronic wound (10%), or complicating subcutaneous injection sites in IDUs (5%). Toxin travels up the axon to spinal neurons, where it blocks the release of glycine and other neurotransmitters used to inhibit afferent motor neurons. Binding results in unrestrained nerve firing, with sustained muscle contractions and rigidity. Binding is irreversible, and recovery requires generation of new axon terminals. Symptoms begin 7 to 21 days after injury. Early symptoms of trismus (lockjaw) progress to dysphagia, hydrophobia, and drooling, followed by opisthotonos, with painful flexion of the arms and extension of the legs. The patient remains conscious. Very rarely, localized tetanus can cause weakness limited to a single extremity, but this weakness usually progresses to generalized tetany. Management should include antibiotics, aggressive wound debridement, tetanus immune globulin, and supportive care. Prevention requires protective antibody levels. All patients should be immunized with tetanus toxoid every 10 years after a primary series (or immediately after a high-risk wound if more than five years has elapsed since the last booster).

EYE INFECTIONS

IDUs have an increased incidence of bacterial and fungal endophthalmitis as a complication of IE. Many investigators have reported *C. albicans* endophthalmitis as part of a syndrome of disseminated candidiasis in IDUs who injected "brown heroin," presumably related to fungal contamination of the lemon juice used to dissolve the drug (Bisbe, Miro et al., 1992). The most commonly reported bacterial causes include *S. aureus* and *Bacillus cereus*.

Symptoms of endophthalmitis include acute onset of blurred vision, eye pain, and decreased visual acuity, similar to the symptoms in nondrug users. Diagnosis requires a high index of suspicion; aggressive evaluation and management are required to salvage vision.

HIV/AIDS

Tremendous advances have been made in our understanding of the pathophysiology, diagnosis, and management of HIV infection and AIDS since the original description, in 1981, of a cluster of homosexual men with *P. carinii* pneumonia (PCP) and Kaposi sarcoma (CDC, 1981a, 1981b; Anonymous, 2000a). Highlights include the identification of a new cytopathic retrovirus in 1983, the development of a serologic diagnostic test in 1985, and the introduction of antiretroviral therapy in 1987. Comprehensive discussions of the AIDS pandemic, including details of transmission, seroconversion, immunosuppression related to disease stage, use of antiretroviral therapy, and prophylaxis for opportunistic infections are available (Anonymous, 2000a; Joint United Nations Programme, 2000; CDC, 2000b).

Epidemiology and Pathogenesis. HIV infection usually is acquired through sexual intercourse, exposure to contaminated blood, or perinatal transmission; the relative frequency of each varies by country. As of December 2000, HIV had been reported in 58 million persons worldwide. Of these, 36.1 million were still alive, 90% in developing countries (Joint United Nations Programme, 2000). As of December 2000, AIDS had been reported in 750,000 people in the U.S., with 430,000 still alive. Among U.S. adults with known risk factors who were diagnosed between July 1999 and June 2000, 31% reported injection drug use and another 37% reported sex with an IDU (CDC, 2000b). Among children diagnosed with HIV infection between July 1999 and June 2000, more than 90% of the cases involved transmission from an infected mother. Risk factors for these mothers included injection drug use in 39% and unprotected sex with an IDU in 14% (CDC, 2000b). For both men and women, the estimated number of new cases of HIV related to injection drug use has fallen slightly each year for the past three years, perhaps because of emphasis on prevention strategies.

In contrast, evidence from around the world suggests that certain behavioral and social factors are increasing the number of cases associated with unsafe sexual practices. Examples of these factors include little or no condom use, a high prevalence of multiple partners, and women's economic dependence on marriage or prostitution. In these groups, transmission is further enhanced by a high rate of concurrent sexually transmitted infections, especially those causing genital ulcers, and a high level of viremia (viral load) when the patient first is infected (before diagnosis) and again in the late stages of illness.

In the past, identification of populations with high risk of exposure to HIV was based on the demographic and geographic distribution of reported AIDS cases. However, as states have implemented laboratory-initiated reporting of positive HIV viral load tests, more and more patients are being identified with a new diagnosis of HIV or AIDS without an obvious behavioral risk or exposure. This incidence reflects the increasing proportion of patients infected by a partner with unrecognized or unreported behavioral risks. In response, the Centers for Disease Control and Prevention (CDC) is developing techniques to permit more accurate estimates of risk category (CDC, 2000b).

In the U.S., decreases in AIDS incidence and death began in 1996, in association with the use of potent combinations of drugs known as highly active antiretroviral therapy (HAART). However, to achieve further decreases in AIDS incidence and death, persons infected with HIV must seek testing earlier, agree to take and adhere to therapy, and actively follow risk reduction strategies to prevent further transmission.

Classification. Stages of HIV infection range from asymptomatic (latent) through early symptomatic infection (B symptoms) to AIDS. Classification follows CDC criteria and stratifies disease according to the CD4 cell count and the presence of various other criteria (CDC, 1987, 1992).

Primary HIV infection causes symptoms in 50% to 90% of cases, which occur two to four weeks after exposure. Symptoms of fever, adenopathy, pharyngitis, rash, and myalgias are reported by more than 50% of patients and last one to four weeks. Other nonspecific symptoms that have been reported include arthralgias, diarrhea, headache, nausea and vomiting, hepatosplenomegaly, thrush, meningoencephalitis, peripheral neuropathy, cranial nerve palsy, Guillain-Barré syndrome, radiculopathy, cognitive impairment, and psychosis (Schacker, Collier et al., 1996; Niu, Stein et al., 1993; Kinloch-de Loes, de Saussure et al., 1993; Kahn & Walker, 1998).

Diagnosis. Primary HIV infection should be considered in any patient with a history of potential exposure and compatible symptoms. After performing a careful history and physical examination, the diagnosis is best established by demonstrating the presence of p24 antigen, quantitative HIV RNA, or qualitative HIV RNA in association with negative or indeterminate HIV serology. High-level viremia during the acute illness permits dissemination of virus to the central nervous system and lymphatic tissue. During this period, the patient may have no physical findings except for persistent generalized lymphadenopathy. The lymphatics are a major reservoir of HIV infection, and replication continues during the clinically latent disease stage (Pantaleo, Graziosi et al., 1993; Schacker, Hughes et al., 1998). Plasma levels of HIV decline dramatically during the resolution of the symptomatic phase of primary HIV, presumably because of the development of humoral and cellular immune responses, and reach a nadir at 120 days (Musey, Hughes et al., 1997). Seroconversion generally occurs at 6 to 12 weeks.

By six months after transmission, 95% of patients have developed positive HIV serology and stabilization of viral load, with levels correlating with prognosis (Pantaleo, Demarest et al., 1997; Mellors, Rinaldo et al., 1996; Mellors, Munoz et al., 1997). As the disease progresses, lymph node architecture is disrupted, releasing more HIV, with an accompanying slow but progressive decline in CD4 counts in most patients. The average life expectancy in the absence of treatment is approximately 10 years, and rates of progression appear similar by sex, race, and risk category when adjusted for quality of medical care (Maggiolo, Migliorino et al., 2000; Raboud, Rae et al., 2000; Grabar, Le Moing et al., 2000; Malhotra, Berrey et al., 2000; Mariotto, Mariotti et al., 1992; Margolick, Munoz et al., 1992, 1994; Galai, Vlahov et al., 1995; Vella, Giuliano et al., 1995; Chaisson, Keruly et al., 1995; Vlahov, Graham et al., 1998).

However, investigators have identified a subset of asymptomatic patients with sustained high levels of CD4 (>500 cells/mm³) for 7 to 10 years in the absence of antiretroviral therapy (Pantaleo, Menzo et al., 1995). Correlates of delayed progression include low viral load, preservation of lymph node architecture, increased CD8 cytolytic activity, and a vigorous HIV specific CD4⁺ T-cell response (Rosenberg, Billingsley et al., 1997; McDermott, Zimmerman et al., 1998). One explanation for delayed disease progression involves the surface chemokine receptor CCR5, which facilitates entry of HIV into macrophages (Cohen, Cicala et al., 2000; Magierowska, Theodorou et al., 1999). Patients with polymorphisms in this receptor appear to progress to AIDS more slowly (10.4 versus 6.6 years), although transmission of the virus is not affected. Studies with agents that block viral binding to the chemokine receptors are in progress and show promise for future use as antiviral agents.

Most patients are diagnosed months or years after HIV infection. Verification of infection requires that a repeatedly positive enzyme immunoassay screening assay be confirmed by a Western blot that demonstrates at least two characteristic antigens (p24, gp41, or gp120/160).

Once the diagnosis of HIV has been established, all patients should have routine screening tests such as a rapid plasma reagin test for syphilis, tuberculin skin test, toxoplasma immunoglobulin G serology, liver function tests, hepatitis serology, and Papanicolaou tests, in addition to tests such as chest radiograph or ophthalmologic examination as clinically indicated.

Treatment. The availability of an increasing number of antiretroviral agents and the rapid evolution of new information has introduced extraordinary complexity into the treatment of HIV. Algorithms outline appropriate laboratory monitoring, including measurement of plasma HIV RNA, CD4 cell counts, and HIV drug resistance testing. Guidelines describe when to begin antiretroviral therapy (based on CD4 count and viral load), what drugs to initiate, when and how to change therapy, and special recommendations for pregnant women (CDC, 1998b, 1998g; Carpenter, Cooper et al., 2000; O'Sullivan, Boyer et al., 1993; Sperling, Shapiro et al., 1996; Sulis, 1995). All pregnant women should be offered counseling and testing for HIV and other sexually transmitted diseases, and women infected with HIV should be treated to maximize their health status and minimize risk to the fetus.

Additional guidelines provide disease-specific recommendations for the use of primary or secondary prophylactic antibiotics for the prevention of the most common, serious opportunistic infections, including PCP, toxoplasmic encephalitis, disseminated *Mycobacterium avium* intracellulare complex, and tuberculosis (CDC, 1999a, 1999d; USPHS/IDSA, 1997, 2000; Masur, Holmes et al., 2000; Kaplan, Masur et al., 2000). Immunizations for hepatitis A and B, influenza, and pneumococcus should be administered as needed. Therapeutic decisions require a discussion about the benefits and risks of treatment. Antiretroviral regimens are complex, have major side effects, and carry serious potential consequences, from the development of viral resistance associated with nonadherence to the drug regimen or suboptimal levels of antiretroviral agents.

Patient education and involvement in therapeutic decisions is especially critical for HIV infection and its treatment. Past and current high-risk behaviors and exposures that may have resulted in HIV infection should be reviewed and mitigation plans designed to prevent further transmission. Behaviors such as high-risk sexual activity or injection drug use not only increase the risk of HIV transmission to others, but also can expose the HIV-infected patient to opportunistic pathogens such as herpes simplex virus, cytomegalovirus, *Cryptosporidium*, human papillomavirus (HPV), human herpesvirus type 8, and hepatitis viruses. Ongoing high-risk sexual behavior should prompt discussions about risk reduction and be reviewed at each encounter. Continuing addictive disorder should prompt the offer of referral to addiction treatment services; a history of addictive disorder warrants review of relapse-prevention efforts. Intensive followup may be required to assess adherence to treatment and to continue patient counseling to prevent transmission of HIV through unprotected sexual behavior and continued injection of drugs. In addition, the patient should receive education and counseling on how to reduce the risk of exposure to opportunistic pathogens associated with environmental, food, pets, water, or travel. It is strongly recommended that care be co-managed with an expert in HIV treatment.

The optimal chance for a prolonged response occurs when a compliant patient initiates combination antiretroviral therapy. Once the decision has been made to initiate treatment, the goals should be maximal and durable suppression of viral load, restoration or preservation of immunologic function, improvement in the quality of life, and reduction of HIV-related morbidity and mortality. Efficacy of therapy is evaluated by monitoring viral load, which should decrease 10-fold by the eighth week and become undetectable (<50 copies/mL) by six months after initiation of treatment.

Evidence is promising for at least the short-term efficacy of aggressive therapy on viral load and CD4+ T-cell counts in patients treated at the time of acute HIV seroconversion; however, clinical trials completed to date have been limited by small sample sizes, short duration of followup, and the use of suboptimal treatment regimens. Ongoing clinical trials are addressing the question of the long-term clinical benefit of more potent treatment regimens for this group of patients.

The proportion of patients with each of the various AIDS-defining conditions, the rate of disease progression, the rate of AIDS deaths, and the average life expectancy have changed dramatically coincident with the widespread use of HAART and prophylaxis against opportunistic infections (Sepkowitz, 1998; Kaplan, Hanson et al., 2000). In the past, patients with advanced HIV disease (defined as

CD4 cell count <50 cells/mm³) had a median survival of 12 to 18 months. However, many of these patients had received no antiretroviral therapy or received nucleoside analogues only. Treatment strategies now known to prolong survival include use of HAART, use of primary and secondary prophylaxis for PCP and *Mycobacterium avium intracellulare* complex, and care by a physician knowledgeable about HIV (Palella, Delaney et al., 1998; Kitahata, Koepsell et al., 1996). The effect of HAART became apparent in 1996, as the need for inpatient hospitalizations declined and the incidence of AIDS-defining illnesses decreased. Nevertheless, CD4 counts and viral load remain the most important determinants of the rate of progression. One important new challenge is to recognize atypical presentations of opportunistic infections during HAART (Sepkowitz, 1998; Kaplan, Hanson et al., 2000).

Failure of therapy at four to six months can be ascribed to nonadherence (including inability to comply with complex dosing schedules), suboptimal levels of antiretroviral agents, viral resistance, and other factors that are poorly understood. Drug-drug or drug-food interactions can profoundly affect the absorption and efficacy of certain medications. For example, methadone levels can be significantly decreased when given with certain protease inhibitors (ritonavir [Norvir®], nelfinavir [Viracept®], or lopinavir) and non-nucleoside reverse transcriptase inhibitors (nevirapine [Viramune®] or efavirenz [Sustiva®]) and often require an increase in methadone maintenance dosage. Conversely, use of maintenance methadone can significantly decrease the level of some nucleoside reverse transcriptase inhibitors (stavudine [Zerit®] or didanosine [Videx®]), requiring an increase in antiretroviral dosage. As noted previously, antiretroviral drug selection often is complicated by the development of side effects. Patients with HIV appear to have a higher incidence of drug-associated toxicity than the general population, especially when renal or hepatic dysfunction is present.

Interactions between the protease inhibitor class and other drugs and foods are extensive and often require dose modification or drug substitution. For example, concurrent therapy with rifampin can decrease the concentration of protease inhibitor by as much as 80%, so its use should be avoided to prevent development of antiretroviral resistance and treatment failure. The combination of a protease inhibitor with terfenadine (Seldane®), astemizole (Hismanal®), or cisapride (Propulsid®) can result in serious cardiotoxicity. The development and severity of these adverse effects often is unpredictable; thus, assessment of toxicity should be performed frequently as part of routine followup care. To avoid toxic combinations, a careful review of all medications should be performed by the pharmacist whenever a new agent is added to the patient's regimen. In addition, when side effects occur and acute intervention is required, all drugs should be discontinued simultaneously to minimize development of resistance. Patients whose therapy fails despite apparent adherence should have their regimen changed; this change should be guided by a careful review of past and current medication use and the results of drug resistance testing.

As the epidemiology of AIDS has changed, an increasing number of investigators have begun to study the risks, benefits, and costs of discontinuing chemoprophylaxis against opportunistic infections (Currier, 2000; Gulick, Mellors et al., 2000; Furrer, Egger et al., 1999; Weverling, Mocroft et al., 1999; Currier, Williams et al., 2000; el-Sadr, Burman et al., 2000; Freedberg, Scharfstein et al., 1998). Although patients who respond to aggressive antiretroviral therapy may have prolonged suppression of plasma viremia to below detectable levels, persistent viral reservoirs have been identified in peripheral blood mononuclear cells, particularly CD4 cells (Finzi, Hermankova et al., 1997; Wong, Hezareh et al., 1997; Zhang, Chung et al., 2000; Chun, Davey et al., 2000; Garcia, Plana et al., 1999; Dornadula, Zhang et al., 1999; Zhang, Ramratnam et al., 1999; Furtado, Callaway et al., 1999). This reservoir of latent virus must be considered when decisions are made about possible termination of antiretroviral therapy, as viral rebound occurs within one to three weeks in nearly all patients. In addition, development of drug resistance, with possible cross-resistance to other drugs, is possible if a sustained reduction in viral load is not maintained.

Prevention. A great deal of emphasis has been placed on identification of impediments to successful adherence to chemoprophylaxis. Patients with depression, poor social support, and active addictive disorder are less likely to adhere to clinical regimens. Recommendations to improve adherence are discussed elsewhere (Mocroft, Katlama et al., 2000). Similarly, patients with HIV who engage in sexual or substance use risk behaviors not only place others at risk of HIV infection, but also may place themselves at risk of acquisition of opportunistic pathogens. As noted earlier, there should be a formal, ongoing review of risk behaviors. Prevention messages should encourage sexual abstinence or the practice of the correct and consistent use of latex condoms (Pequegnat, Fishbein et al., 2000; Kamb, Fishbein et al., 1998; Sikkema, Kelly et al., 2000; NIMH Multisite HIV Prevention Trial Group, 1998). Patients should be encouraged to avoid sexual practices that might result in oral exposure to feces (for example, oral-anal contact) to reduce the risk of intestinal infections (for example, cryptosporidiosis, shigellosis, campylobacteriosis, amebiasis, giardiasis, and hepatitis A and B). Patients who inject drugs should be encouraged to stop using injection drugs and to enter and complete addiction treatment. If the patient continues to inject drugs, the importance of using a sterile syringe for every injection and the avoidance of sharing any injection-related drug paraphernalia with another person should be emphasized. Such patients should be encouraged to use a needle-exchange program or to safely discard syringes after one use. In areas where needle exchange is illegal, IDUs should be taught to clean their injection equipment with household bleach before use. Patients who are exposed to bloodborne pathogens may be eligible for postexposure prophylaxis (CDC, 1998d; Lurie, Miller et al., 1998; O'Connor, 2000; Gross, Holte et al., 2000; Kunches, Meehan et al., 2001; Kahn, Martin et al., 2001). Similarly, health care workers who have an unprotected exposure to the blood of these patients should follow CDC guidelines for postexposure prophylaxis, including pretest and post-test counseling (CDC, 1998f).

SEXUALLY TRANSMITTED DISEASES

The epidemiology, clinical features, diagnosis, and treatment of sexually transmitted diseases other than HIV/AIDS have been reviewed extensively (CDC, 1998a). Although the prevalence is higher in drug users, the presentation, diagnosis, and management of most sexually transmitted diseases are not profoundly influenced by drug use. (One exception is that the diagnosis and treatment of syphilis in IDUs may be confounded by an increased prevalence of biologic false-positive nontreponemal screening tests such as Venereal Disease Research Laboratory [VDRL] or rapid plasma reagin [RPR] tests for syphilis.)

Recent studies suggest that an increasing number of persons, especially men who have sex with men, are participating in high-risk sexual behaviors (often while intoxicated) that place them at risk of acquiring syphilis, gonorrhea, herpes, chlamydia, HIV, and other sexually transmitted diseases (CDC, 1999b, 1999c, 2000b). Related studies have shown that patients who report heavy drug or alcohol use are most likely to report high-risk sexual behavior and to have HIV

infection or syphilis. The most common high-risk behaviors include multiple recent sexual partners and inconsistent use of condoms (CDC, 1998c).

As noted earlier, the clinician and patient should conduct a formal, ongoing review of risk behavior. Prevention messages should encourage safe sex, including the correct and consistent use of latex condoms. In selected patients, use of postexposure prophylaxis may be warranted (CDC, 1998d). There are a number of potential complications from sexually transmitted diseases and other infectious diseases that can affect the pregnant woman or her fetus. Pregnant drug users should be screened according to standard protocols and aggressively treated to minimize disastrous maternal or fetal outcomes (Sulis, 1995).

Because of the synergistic effect of cigarette smoke in the development of HPV-associated cancers, patients diagnosed with HPV should be strongly encouraged to consider smoking cessation.

Type one human T-cell lymphotropic virus (HTLV-I) infection is present in widely scattered populations throughout the world and is the etiologic agent in adult T-cell leukemia/lymphoma and HTLV-associated myelopathy. HTLV-II has been reported in IDUs and their sexual contacts, appears to be endemic in IDUs in the U.S., and has not been definitively linked to a specific disorder. Patients with HTLV-II infection may be at increased risk of a variety of infections, suggesting an underlying immunologic impairment. Both retroviruses appear to be transmitted by sexual intercourse, administration of blood products, and mother-to-child transmission. No effective therapy exists, and prevention of exposure is the only known method of limiting spread (Ifthikharuddin & Rosenblatt, 2000).

CONCLUSIONS

Infectious complications in drug users are more frequent, more difficult to diagnose, and more challenging to treat than similar infections in nondrug users. Effective management requires attention to both medical and social issues. An improved outcome can be achieved by emphasizing risk reduction strategies in the context of a strong, ongoing therapeutic alliance.

REFERENCES

Alland D, Kalkut GE, Moss AR et al. (1994). Transmission of tuberculosis in New York City. An analysis by DNA fingerprinting and conventional epidemiologic methods. *New England Journal of Medicine* 330:1710-1716.

Anonymous (2000a). Acquired immunodeficiency syndrome. In GL Mandell, JE Bennett & R Dolin (eds.) *Principles and Practice of Infectious Diseases, 5th Edition*. Philadelphia, PA: Churchill-Livingstone, 1332-1528.

Anonymous (2000b). Diagnostic standards and classification of tuberculosis in adults and children. *American Journal of Respiratory and Critical Care Medicine* 161:1376-1395.

Arnold M, Woo ML & French GL (1989). Vibrio vulnificus septicaemia presenting as spontaneous necrotising cellulitis in a woman with hepatic cirrhosis. *Scandinavian Journal of Infectious Diseases* 21:727-731.

Ascher DP, Zbick C, White C et al. (1991). Infections due to Stomatococcus mucilaginosus: 10 cases and review. *Reviews of Infectious Diseases* 13:1048-1052.

Bailey ME, Fraire AE, Greenberg SD et al. (1994). Pulmonary histopathology in cocaine abusers. *Human Pathology* 25:203-207.

Barg NL, Kish MA, Kauffman CA et al. (1985). Group A streptococcal bacteremia in intravenous drug abusers. *American Journal of Medicine* 78:569-574.

Bartlett JG, Breiman RF, Mandell LA et al. (1998). Community-acquired pneumonia in adults: Guidelines for management. *Clinical Infectious Diseases* 26:811-838.

Bartlett JG, Gorbach SL & Finegold SM (1974). The bacteriology of aspiration pneumonia. *American Journal of Medicine* 56:202-207.

Bass JB, Farer LS, Hopewell PC et al. (1994). Treatment of tuberculosis and tuberculosis infection in adults and children. American Thoracic Society and the Centers for Disease Control and Prevention. *American Journal of Respiratory and Critical Care Medicine* 149:1359-1374.

Bass SN, Ailani RK, Shekar R et al. (1998). Pyogenic vertebral osteomyelitis presenting as exudative pleural effusion: A series of five cases. *Chest* 114:642-647.

Bayer AS, Bolger AF, Taubert KA et al. (1998). Diagnosis and management of infective endocarditis and its complications. *Circulation* 98:2936-2948.

Bayer AS & Scheld WM (2000). Endocarditis and intravascular infections. In GL Mandell, JE Bennett & R Dolin (eds.) *Principles and Practice of Infectious Diseases, 5th Edition*. Philadelphia, PA: Churchill-Livingstone, 857-902.

Bayer AS, Ward JI, Ginzton LE et al. (1994). Evaluation of new clinical criteria for the diagnosis of infective endocarditis. *American Journal of Medicine* 96:211-219.

Berlin JA, Abrutyn E, Strom BL et al. (1995). Incidence of infective endocarditis in the Delaware Valley, 1988-1990. *American Journal of Cardiology* 76:933-936.

Bernaldo de Quiros JC, Moreno S, Cercenado E et al. (1997). Group A streptococcal bacteremia. A 10-year prospective study. *Medicine* 76:238-248.

Bestetti RB, Figueiredo JF & Da Costa JC (1991). Salmonella tricuspid endocarditis in an intravenous drug abuser with human immunodeficiency virus infection. *International Journal of Cardiology* 30:361-362.

Bisbe J, Miro JM, Latorre X et al. (1992). Disseminated candidiasis in addicts who use brown heroin: Report of 83 cases and review. *Clinical Infectious Diseases* 15:910-923.

Bleck TP (2000a). Clostridium botulinum (botulism). In GL Mandell, JE Bennett & R Dolin (eds.) *Principles and Practice of Infectious Diseases, 5th Edition*. Philadelphia, PA: Churchill-Livingstone, 2543-2547.

Bleck TP (2000b). Clostridium tetani (tetanus). In GL Mandell, JE Bennett & R Dolin (eds.) *Principles and Practice of Infectious Diseases, 5th Edition*. Philadelphia, PA: Churchill-Livingstone, 2537-2542.

Bloch AB, Cauthen BM, Onorato IM et al. (1994). Nationwide survey of drug-resistant tuberculosis in the United States. *Journal of the American Medical Association* 271:665-671.

Blumberg HM & Stephens DS (1990). Pyomyositis and human immunodeficiency virus infection. *Southern Medical Journal* 83:1092-1095.

Botsford KB, Weinstein RA, Nathan CR et al. (1985). Selective survival in pentazocine and tripelennamine of Pseudomonas aeruginosa serotype O11 from drug addicts. *Journal of Infectious Diseases* 151:209-216.

Braunstein H (1991). Characteristics of group A streptococcal bacteremia in patients at the San Bernardino County Medical Center. *Reviews of Infectious Diseases* 13:8-11.

Brook I & Frazier EH (1990). Aerobic and anaerobic bacteriology of wounds and cutaneous abscesses. *Archives of Surgery* 125:1445-1451.

Burman LA, Norrby R & Trollfors B (1985). Invasive pneumococcal infections: Incidence, predisposing factors, and prognosis. *Reviews of Infectious Diseases* 7:133-142.

Caiaffa WT, Graham NM & Vlahov D (1993). Bacterial pneumonia in adult populations with human immunodeficiency virus (HIV) infection. *American Journal of Epidemiology* 138:909-922.

Caiaffa WT, Vlahov D, Graham NM et al. (1994). Drug smoking, Pneumocystis carinii pneumonia, and immunosuppression increase risk of bacterial pneumonia in human immunodeficiency virus-seropositive injection drug users. *American Journal of Respiratory and Critical Care Medicine* 150:1493-1498.

Cantwell MF, Snider DE Jr., Cauthen GM et al. (1994). Epidemiology of tuberculosis in the United States, 1985 through 1992. *Journal of the American Medical Association* 272:535-539.

Carpenter CC, Cooper DA, Fischl MA et al. (2000). Antiretroviral therapy in adults: Updated recommendations of the International AIDS Society—USA panel. *Journal of the American Medical Association* 283:381-390.

Carrel T, Schaffner A, Vogt P et al. (1993). Endocarditis in intravenous drug addicts and HIV infected patients: Possibilities and limitations of surgical treatment. *Journal of Heart Valve Disease* 2:140-147.

Castro KG (1995). Tuberculosis as an opportunistic disease in persons infected with human immunodeficiency virus. *Clinical Infectious Diseases* 21(Suppl 1):S66-71.

Centers for Disease Control and Prevention (CDC) (1981a). Kaposi's sarcoma and Pneumocystis pneumonia among homosexual men—New York City and California. *Morbidity and Mortality Weekly Report* 30:305.

Centers for Disease Control and Prevention (CDC) (1981b). Pneumocystis pneumonia—Los Angeles. *Morbidity and Mortality Weekly Report* 30:250.

Centers for Disease Control and Prevention (CDC) (1987). Revision of the CDC surveillance case definition for acquired immunodeficiency syndrome. *Morbidity and Mortality Weekly Report* 36:1-15S.

Centers for Disease Control and Prevention (CDC) (1992). 1993 Revised classification system for HIV infection and expanded surveillance case definition for AIDS among adolescents and adults. *Morbidity and Mortality Weekly Report* 41(RR-17).

Centers for Disease Control and Prevention (CDC) (1995). Screening for tuberculosis and tuberculosis infection in high-risk populations. Recommendations of the Advisory Council for the Elimination of Tuberculosis. *Morbidity and Mortality Weekly Report* 44(RR-11):19-34.

Centers for Disease Control and Prevention (CDC) (1996). Clinical update: Impact of HIV protease inhibitors on the treatment of HIV-infected tuberculosis patients with rifampin. *Morbidity and Mortality Weekly Report* 45:921-925.

Centers for Disease Control and Prevention (CDC) (1997). Anergy skin testing and tuberculosis preventive therapy for HIV-infected persons: Revised recommendations. *Morbidity and Mortality Weekly Report* 46(RR-15):1-10.

Centers for Disease Control and Prevention (CDC) (1998a). 1998 guidelines for treatment of sexually transmitted diseases. *Morbidity and Mortality Weekly Report* 47(RR-1):1-116.

Centers for Disease Control and Prevention (CDC) (1998b). Guidelines for the use of antiretroviral agents in HIV-infected adults and adolescents. *Morbidity and Mortality Weekly Report* 47(RR-5):42-82.

Centers for Disease Control and Prevention (CDC) (1998c). HIV prevention through early detection and treatment of sexually transmitted diseases—United States. *Morbidity and Mortality Weekly Report* 47(RR-12):1-31.

Centers for Disease Control and Prevention (CDC) (1998d). Management of possible sexual, injecting-drug-use, or other nonoccupational exposure to HIV, including considerations related to antiretroviral therapy. *Morbidity and Mortality Weekly Report* (RR-17):1-14.

Centers for Disease Control and Prevention (CDC) (1998e). Prevention and treatment of tuberculosis among patients infected with human immunodeficiency virus: Principles of therapy and revised recommendations. *Morbidity and Mortality Weekly Report* 47(RR-20):1-58.

Centers for Disease Control and Prevention (1998f). Public Health Service guidelines for the management of health-care worker exposures to HIV and recommendations for postexposure prophylaxis. *Morbidity and Mortality Weekly Report* 47(RR-7):1-33.

Centers for Disease Control and Prevention (1998g). Public Health Service Task Force recommendations for the use of antiretroviral drugs in pregnant women infected with HIV-1 for maternal health and for reducing perinatal HIV-1 transmission in the United States. *Morbidity and Mortality Weekly Report* 47(RR-2):1-30.

Centers for Disease Control and Prevention (CDC) (1999a). 1999 USPHS/IDSA guidelines for the prevention of opportunistic infections in persons infected with human immunodeficiency virus: U.S. Public Health Service (USPHS) and Infectious Diseases Society of America (IDSA). *Morbidity and Mortality Weekly Report* 48(RR-10):1-66.

Centers for Disease Control and Prevention (CDC) (1999b). Increases in unsafe sex and rectal gonorrhea among men who have sex with men: San Francisco, California, 1994-1997. *Morbidity and Mortality Weekly Report* 48:45-48.

Centers for Disease Control and Prevention (CDC) (1999c). Resurgent bacterial sexually transmitted disease among men who have sex with men: King County, Washington, 1997-1999. *Morbidity and Mortality Weekly Report* 48:773-777.

Centers for Disease Control and Prevention (1999d). Surveillance for AIDS-defining opportunistic illnesses 1992-1997. *Morbidity and Mortality Weekly Report* 48(SS-2):1-22.

Centers for Disease Control and Prevention (CDC) (2000a). Fatal and severe hepatitis associated with rifampin and pyrazinamide for the treatment of latent tuberculosis infection: New York and Georgia, 2000. *Morbidity and Mortality Weekly Report* 50:289-291.

Centers for Disease Control and Prevention (CDC) (2000b). *HIV/AIDS Surveillance Report* 12(1):1-41.

Centers for Disease Control and Prevention (CDC) (2000c). Missed opportunities for prevention of tuberculosis among persons with HIV infection—Selected locations, United States, 1996-1997. *Morbidity and Mortality Weekly Report* 49:685-687.

Centers for Disease Control and Prevention (CDC) (2000d). Notice to readers: Updated guidelines for the use of rifabutin or rifampin for the treatment and prevention of tuberculosis among HIV-infected patients taking protease inhibitors or nonnucleoside reverse transcriptase inhibitors. *Morbidity and Mortality Weekly Report* 49:185-189.

Centers for Disease Control and Prevention (CDC) (2000e). Targeted tuberculin testing and treatment of latent tuberculosis infection. *Morbidity and Mortality Weekly Report* 49(RR-6):1-51.

Centers for Disease Control and Prevention (CDC) (2001a). Cluster of tuberculosis cases among exotic dancers and their close contacts: Kansas, 1994-2000. *Morbidity and Mortality Weekly Report* 50:291-293.

Centers for Disease Control and Prevention (CDC) (2001b). Outbreak of syphilis among men who have sex with men: Southern California, 2000. *Morbidity and Mortality Weekly Report* 50:117-120.

Centers for Disease Control and Prevention (CDC) (2001c). Prevention and control of influenza: Recommendations of the Advisory Committee on Immunization Practices (ACIP). *Morbidity and Mortality Weekly Report* 50(RR-4):1-44.

Chaisson RE, Keruly JC & Moore RD (1995). Race, sex, drug use, and progression of human immunodeficiency virus disease. *New England Journal of Medicine* 333:751-756.

Chambers HF, Korzeniowski OM & Sande MA (1983). Staphylococcus aureus endocarditis: Clinical manifestations in addicts and nonaddicts. *Medicine* 62:170-177.

Chambers HF, Morris DL, Tauber MG et al. (1987). Cocaine use and the risk for endocarditis in intravenous drug users. *Annals of Internal Medicine* 106:833-836.

Chandrasekar PH & Narula AP (1986). Bone and joint infections in intravenous drug abusers. *Reviews of Infectious Diseases* 8:904-911.

Cherubin CE (1968). Clinical severity of tetanus in narcotic addicts in New York City. *Archives of Internal Medicine* 121:156-158.

Cherubin CE & Sapira JD (1993). The medical complications of drug addiction and the medical assessment of the intravenous drug user: 25 years later. *Annals of Internal Medicine* 119:1017-1028.

Christin L & Sarosi GA (1992). Pyomyositis in North America: Case reports and review. *Clinical Infectious Diseases* 15:668-677.

Chun TW, Davey RT Jr., Ostrowski M et al. (2000). Relationship between pre-existing viral reservoirs and the re-emergence of plasma viremia after discontinuation of highly active anti-retroviral therapy. *Nature Medicine* 6:757-761.

Cohen O, Cicala C, Vaccarezza M et al. (2000). The immunology of human immunodeficiency virus infection. In GL Mandell, JE Bennett & R Dolin (eds.) *Principles and Practice of Infectious Diseases, 5th Edition.* Philadelphia, PA: Churchill-Livingstone, 1374-1415.

Comer JA, Flynn C, Regnery RL et al. (1996). Antibodies to Bartonella species in inner-city intravenous drug users in Baltimore, Md. *Archives of Internal Medicine* 156:2491-2495.

Cooper B & Maderazo EG (1989). Alcohol abuse and impaired immunity. *Infections and Surgery* 3:94-101.

Cooper R & Mills J (1980). Serratia endocarditis. A follow-up report. *Archives of Internal Medicine* 140:199-202.

Craven DE, Rixinger AI, Bisno AL et al. (1986a). Bacteremia caused by group G streptococci in parenteral drug abusers: Epidemiological and clinical aspects. *Journal of Infectious Diseases* 153:988-992.

Craven DE, Rixinger AI, Goularte TA et al. (1986b). Methicillin-resistant Staphylococcus aureus bacteremia linked to intravenous drug abusers using a "shooting gallery." *American Journal of Medicine* 80:770-776.

Currier JS (2000). Discontinuing prophylaxis for opportunistic infection: Guiding principles. *Clinical Infectious Diseases* 30(Suppl 1):S66-71.

Currier JS, Williams PL, Koletar SL et al. (2000). Discontinuation of Mycobacterium avium complex prophylaxis in patients with antiretroviral therapy-induced increases in CD4+ cell count. A randomized, double-blind, placebo-controlled trial. AIDS Clinical Trials Group 362 Study Team. *Annals of Internal Medicine* 133:493-503.

Dajani AS, Taubert KA, Wilson W et al. (1997). Prevention of bacterial endocarditis. Recommendations by the American Heart Association. *Journal of the American Medical Association* 277:1794-1801.

del Busto R, Quinn EL, Fisher EJ et al. (1982). Osteomyelitis of the pubis. Report of seven cases. *Journal of the American Medical Association* 248:1498-1500.

Dornadula G, Zhang H, Van Uitert B et al. (1999). Residual HIV-1 RNA in blood plasma of patients taking suppressive highly active antiretroviral therapy. *Journal of the American Medical Association* 282:1627-1632.

Durack DT (1998). Antibiotics for prevention of endocarditis during dentistry: Time to scale back? *Annals of Internal Medicine* 129:829-831.

Durack DT, Lukes AS & Bright DK (1994). New criteria for diagnosis of infective endocarditis: Utilization of specific echocardiographic findings. Duke Endocarditis Service. *American Journal of Medicine* 96:200-209.

el-Sadr WM, Burman WJ, Grant LB et al. (2000). Discontinuation of prophylaxis for Mycobacterium avium complex disease in HIV-infected patients who have a response to antiretroviral therapy. Terry Beirn Community Programs for Clinical Research on AIDS. *New England Journal of Medicine* 342:1085-1092.

Fichtenbaum CJ, Woeltje KF & Powderly WG (1994). Serious Pseudomonas aeruginosa infections in patients infected with human immunodeficiency virus: A case-control study. *Clinical Infectious Diseases* 19:417-422.

Finzi D, Hermankova M, Pierson T et al. (1997). Identification of a reservoir for HIV-1 in patients on highly active antiretroviral therapy. *Science* 278:1295-1300.

Freedberg KA, Scharfstein JA, Seage GR et al. (1998). The cost-effectiveness of preventing AIDS-related opportunistic infections. *Journal of the American Medical Association* 279:130-136.

Frieden TR, Sterling T, Pablo-Mendez A et al. (1993). The emergence of drug-resistant tuberculosis in New York City. *New England Journal of Medicine* 328:521-526.

Frizzell RT, Vitek JJ, Hill DL et al. (1993). Treatment of a bacterial (mycotic) intracranial aneurysm using an endovascular approach. *Neurosurgery* 32:852-854.

Frye MD, Pozsik CJ & Sahn SA (1997). Tuberculous pleurisy is more common in AIDS than in non-AIDS patients with tuberculosis. *Chest* 112:393-397.

Furrer H, Egger M, Opravil M et al. (1999). Discontinuation of primary prophylaxis against Pneumocystis carinii pneumonia in HIV-1-infected adults treated with combination antiretroviral therapy. Swiss HIV Cohort Study. *New England Journal of Medicine* 340:1301-1306.

Furtado MR, Callaway DS, Phair JP et al. (1999). Persistence of HIV-1 transcription in peripheral-blood mononuclear cells in patients receiving potent antiretroviral therapy. *New England Journal of Medicine* 340:1614-1622.

Galai N, Vlahov D, Margolick JB et al. (1995). Changes in markers of disease progression in HIV-1 seroconverters: A comparison between cohorts of injecting drug users and homosexual men. *Journal of Acquired Immune Deficiency Syndromes and Human Retrovirology* 8:66-74.

Gallagher PG & Watanakunakorn C (1986). Group B streptococcal endocarditis: Report of seven cases and review of the literature, 1962-1985. *Reviews of Infectious Diseases* 8:175-188.

Garcia F, Plana M, Vidal C et al. (1999). Dynamics of viral load rebound and immunological changes after stopping effective antiretroviral therapy. *AIDS* 13:F79-86.

Gelfand MS & Threlkeld MG (1992). Subacute bacterial endocarditis secondary to Streptococcus pneumoniae. *American Journal of Medicine* 93:91-93.

Gordin FM, Chaisson RE, Matts JP et al. (2000). Rifampin and pyrazinamide vs. isoniazid for prevention of tuberculosis in HIV-infected persons: An international randomized trial. *Journal of the American Medical Association* 283:1445-1450.

Gordin FM, Nelson ET, Matts JP et al. (1996). The impact of human immunodeficiency virus infection on drug-resistant tuberculosis. *American Journal of Respiratory and Critical Care Medicine* 154:1478-1483.

Grabar S, Le Moing V, Goujard C et al. (2000). Clinical outcome of patients with HIV-1 infection according to immunologic and virologic response after 6 months of highly active antiretroviral therapy. *Annals of Internal Medicine* 133:401-410.

Graves MK & Soto L (1992). Left-sided endocarditis in parenteral drug abusers: Recent experience at a large community hospital. *Southern Medical Journal* 85:378-380.

Greenberg SD, Frager D, Suster B et al. (1994). Active pulmonary tuberculosis in patients with AIDS: Spectrum of radiographic findings (including a normal appearance). *Radiology* 193:115-119.

Gross M, Holte S, Seage GR et al. (2000). Feasibility of chemoprophylaxis studies in high risk HIV-seronegative populations. *AIDS Education and Prevention* 12:71-78.

Gulick RM, Mellors JW, Havlir D et al. (2000). 3-year suppression of HIV viremia with indinavir, zidovudine, and lamivudine. *Annals of Internal Medicine* 133:35-39.

Halsey NA, Coberly JS, Desormeaux J et al. (1998). Randomized trial of isoniazid versus rifampicin and pyrazinamide for prevention of tuberculosis in HIV-1 infection. *Lancet* 351:786-792.

Harlow KD, Harner RC & Fontenelle LJ (1996). Primary skin infections secondary to Vibrio vulnificus: The role of operative intervention. *Journal of the American College of Surgeons* 183:329-334.

Havlir DV & Barnes PF (1999). Tuberculosis in patients with human immunodeficiency virus infection. *New England Journal of Medicine* 340:367-373.

Hecht SR & Berger M (1992). Right-sided endocarditis in intravenous drug users. Prognostic features in 102 episodes. *Annals of Internal Medicine* 117:560-566.

Hirschtick RE, Glassroth J, Jordan MC et al. (1995). Bacterial pneumonia in persons infected with the human immunodeficiency virus. Pulmonary Complications of HIV Infection Study Group. *New England Journal of Medicine* 333:845-851.

Holmes AH, Greenough TC, Balady GJ et al. (1995). Bartonella henselae endocarditis in an immunocompetent adult. *Clinical Infectious Diseases* 21:1004-1007.

Holzman RS & Bishko F (1971). Osteomyelitis in heroin addicts. *Annals of Internal Medicine* 75:693-696.

Horsburgh CR, Feldman S & Ridzon R (2000). Practice guidelines for the treatment of tuberculosis. *Clinical Infectious Diseases* 31:633-639.

Hsueh PR, Hsiue TR & Hsieh WC (1996). Pyomyositis in intravenous drug abusers: Report of a unique case and review of the literature. *Clinical Infectious Diseases* 22:858-860.

Ifthikharuddin JJ & Rosenblatt JD (2000). Human T-cell lymphotropic virus types I and II. In GL Mandell, JE Bennett & R Dolin (eds.) *Principles and Practice of Infectious Diseases, 5th Edition*. Philadelphia, PA: Churchill-Livingstone, 1862-1873.

Janoff EN, Breiman RF, Daley CL et al. (1992). Pneumococcal disease during HIV infection. Epidemiologic, clinical, and immunologic perspectives. *Annals of Internal Medicine* 117:314-324.

Joint United Nations Programme on HIV/AIDS (2000, December). *UNAIDS. AIDS Epidemic Update*. New York, NY: United Nations.

Jones BE, Young SM, Antoniskis D et al. (1993). Relationship of the manifestations of tuberculosis to CD4 cell counts in patients with human immunodeficiency virus infection. *American Review of Respiratory Disease* 148:1292-1297.

Kahn JO, Martin JN, Roland ME et al. (2001). Feasibility of postexposure prophylaxis (PEP) against human immunodeficiency virus infection after sexual or injection drug use exposure: The San Francisco PEP Study. *Journal of Infectious Diseases* 183:707-714.

Kahn JO & Walker BD (1998). Acute human immunodeficiency virus type 1 infection. *New England Journal of Medicine* 339:33-39.

Kamb ML, Fishbein M, Douglas JM et al. (1998). Efficacy of risk reduction counseling to prevent human immunodeficiency virus and sexually transmitted diseases: A randomized controlled trial. Project RESPECT Study Group. *Journal of the American Medical Association* 280:1161-1167.

Kaplan JE, Hanson D, Dworkin MS et al. (2000). Epidemiology of human immunodeficiency virus-associated opportunistic infections in the United States in the era of highly active antiretroviral therapy. *Clinical Infectious Diseases* 30(Suppl 1):S4-14.

Kaplan JE, Masur H, Holmes KK et al. (2000). An overview of the 1999 US Public Health Service/Infectious Diseases Society of America guidelines for preventing opportunistic infections in human immunodeficiency virus-infected persons. *Clinical Infectious Diseases* 30(Suppl 1):S15-28.

Kielhofner M, Atmar RL, Hamill RJ et al. (1992). Life-threatening Pseudomonas aeruginosa infections in patients with human immunodeficiency virus infection. *Clinical Infectious Diseases* 14:403-411.

Kinloch-de Loes S, de Saussure P, Saurat JH et al. (1993). Symptomatic primary infection due to human immunodeficiency virus type 1: Review of 31 cases. *Clinical Infectious Diseases* 17:59-65.

Kitahata MM, Koepsell TD, Deyo RA et al. (1996). Physicians' experience with the acquired immunodeficiency syndrome as a factor in patients' survival. *New England Journal of Medicine* 334:701-706.

Komshian SV, Tablan OC, Palutke W et al. (1990). Characteristics of left-sided endocarditis due to Pseudomonas aeruginosa in the Detroit Medical Center. *Reviews of Infectious Diseases* 12:693-702.

Kudrow DB, Henry DA, Haake DA et al. (1988). Botulism associated with Clostridium botulinum sinusitis after intranasal cocaine abuse. *Annals of Internal Medicine* 109:984-985.

Kunches LM, Meehan TM, Boutwell RC et al. (2001). Survey of nonoccupational postexposure prophylaxis in hospital emergency departments. *Journal of Acquired Immune Deficiency Syndromes* 26:263-265.

Lee TY, Lee TY & Cheng YF (1998). Subclavian mycotic aneurysm presenting as mediastinal abscess. *American Journal of Emergency Medicine* 16:714-716.

Lentneck AL, Giger O & O'Rourke E (1990). Group A beta-hemolytic streptococcal bacteremia and intravenous substance abuse. A growing clinical problem? *Archives of Internal Medicine* 150:89-93.

Levine DP & Brown PD (2000). Infections in injection drug users. In GL Mandell, JE Bennett & R Dolin (eds.) *Principles and Practice of Infectious Diseases, 5th Edition*. Philadelphia, PA: Churchill-Livingstone, 3112-3126.

Levine DP, Crane LR & Zervos MJ (1986). Bacteremia in narcotic addicts at the Detroit Medical Center. II. Infectious endocarditis: A prospective comparative study. *Reviews of Infectious Diseases* 8:374-396.

Lew DP & Waldvogel FA (1997). Osteomyelitis. *New England Journal of Medicine* 336:999-1007.

Lindner JR, Case RA, Dent JM et al. (1996). Diagnostic value of echocardiography in suspected endocarditis. An evaluation based on the pretest probability of disease. *Circulation* 93:730-736.

Lipsky BA, Boyko EJ, Inui TS et al. (1986). Risk factors for acquiring pneumococcal infections. *Archives of Internal Medicine* 146:2179-2185.

Lurie P, Miller S, Hecht F et al. (1998). Postexposure prophylaxis after nonoccupational HIV exposure: Clinical, ethical, and policy considerations. *Journal of the American Medical Association* 280:1769-1773.

Maggiolo F, Migliorino M, Pirali A et al. (2000). Duration of viral suppression in patients on stable therapy for HIV-1 infection is predicted by plasma HIV RNA level after 1 month of treatment. *Journal of Acquired Immune Deficiency Syndromes* 25:36-43.

Magierowska M, Theodorou I, Debre P et al. (1999). Combined genotypes of CCR5, CCR2, SDF1 and HLA genes can predict the long-term nonprogressor status in human immunodeficiency virus-1-infected individuals. *Blood* 93:936-941.

Malhotra U, Berrey MM, Huang Y et al. (2000). Effect of combination antiretroviral therapy on T-cell immunity in acute human immunodeficiency virus type 1 infection. *Journal of Infectious Diseases* 181:121.

Mansur AJ, Grinberg M, da Luz PL et al. (1992). The complications of infective endocarditis. A reappraisal in the 1980s. *Archives of Internal Medicine* 152:2428-2432.

Marantz PR, Linzer M, Feiner CJ et al. (1987). Inability to predict diagnosis in febrile intravenous drug abusers. *Annals of Internal Medicine* 106:823-828.

Margolick JB, Munoz A, Vlahov D et al. (1992). Changes in T-lymphocyte subsets in intravenous drug users with HIV-1 infection. *Journal of the American Medical Association* 267:1631-1636.

Margolick JB, Munoz A, Vlahov D et al. (1994). Direct comparison of the relationship between clinical outcome and change in CD4+ lymphocytes in human immunodeficiency virus-positive homosexual men and injecting drug users. *Archives of Internal Medicine* 154:869-875.

Mariotto AB, Mariotti S, Pezzotti P et al. (1992). Estimation of the acquired immunodeficiency syndrome incubation period in intravenous drug users: A comparison with male homosexuals. *American Journal of Epidemiology* 135:428-437.

Markowitz N, Hansen NI, Hopewell PC et al. (1997). Incidence of tuberculosis in the United States among HIV-infected persons. The Pulmonary Complications of HIV Infection Study Group. *Annals of Internal Medicine* 126:123-132.

Masur H, Holmes KK & Kaplan JE (2000). Introduction to the 1999 US PHS/IDSA guidelines for the prevention of opportunistic infections in persons infected with human immunodeficiency virus. *Clinical Infectious Diseases* 30(Suppl 1):S1-4.

McDermott DH, Zimmerman PA, Guignard F et al. (1998). CCR5 promoter polymorphism and HIV-1 disease progression. Multicenter AIDS Cohort Study (MACS). *Lancet* 352:866-870.

Mellors JW, Munoz A, Giorgi JV et al. (1997). Plasma viral load and CD4+ lymphocytes as prognostic markers of HIV-1 infection. *Annals of Internal Medicine* 126:946-954.

Mellors JW, Rinaldo CR Jr., Gupta P et al. (1996). Prognosis in HIV-1 infection predicted by the quantity of virus in plasma. *Science* 272:1167-1170.

Mills J & Drew D (1976). Serratia marcescens endocarditis: A regional illness associated with intravenous drug abuse. *Annals of Internal Medicine* 84:29-35.

Mocroft A, Katlama C, Johnson AM et al. (2000). AIDS across Europe, 1994-98: The EuroSIDA study. *Lancet* 356:291-296.

Musey L, Hughes J, Schacker T et al. (1997). Cytotoxic-T-cell responses, viral load, and disease progression in early human immunodeficiency virus type 1 infection. *New England Journal of Medicine* 337:1267-1274.

Musher DM (1992). Infections caused by Streptococcus pneumoniae: Clinical spectrum, pathogenesis, immunity, and treatment. *Clinical Infectious Diseases* 14:801-807.

Musher DM, Hamill RJ & Baughn RE (1990). Effect of human immunodeficiency virus (HIV) infection on the course of syphilis and on the response to treatment. *Annals of Internal Medicine* 113:872-881.

Nahass RG, Weinstein MP, Bartels J et al. (1990). Infective endocarditis in intravenous drug users: A comparison of human immunodeficiency virus type 1-negative and -positive patients. *Journal of Infectious Diseases* 162:967-970.

The NIMH Multisite HIV Prevention Trial Group (1998). The NIMH multisite HIV prevention trial: Reducing HIV sexual risk behavior. *Science* 280:1889-1894.

Niu MT, Stein DS & Schnittman SM (1993). Primary human immunodeficiency virus type 1 infection: Review of pathogenesis and early treatment intervention in humans and animal retrovirus infections. *Journal of Infectious Diseases* 168:1490-1501.

O'Connor PG (2000). HIV post-exposure therapy for drug users in treatment. *Journal of Substance Abuse Treatment* 18:17-21.

O'Donnell AE & Pappas LS (1988). Pulmonary complications of intravenous drug abuse. Experience at an inner-city hospital. *Chest* 94:251-253.

O'Grady NP, Barie PS, Bartlett JG et al. (1998). Practice guidelines for evaluating new fever in critically ill adult patients. *Clinical Infectious Diseases* 26:1042-1059.

O'Sullivan MJ, Boyer PJ, Scott GB et al. (1993). The pharmacokinetics and safety of zidovudine in the third trimester of pregnancy for women infected with human immunodeficiency virus and their infants: Phase I Acquired Immunodeficiency Syndrome Clinical Trials Group study (protocol 082). Zidovudine Collaborative Working Group. *American Journal of Obstetrics and Gynecology* 168:1510-1516.

Omari B, Shapiro S, Ginzton L et al. (1989). Predictive risk factors for periannular extension of native valve endocarditis. Clinical and echocardiographic analyses. *Chest* 96:1273-127.

Pablos-Mendez A, Raviglione MC, Laszlo A et al. (1998). Global surveillance for antituberculosis-drug resistance, 1994-1997. World Health Organization-International Union against Tuberculosis and Lung Disease Working Group on Anti-Tuberculosis Drug Resistance Surveillance. *New England Journal of Medicine* 338:1641-1649.

Palella FJ Jr., Delaney KM, Moorman AC et al. (1998). Declining morbidity and mortality among patients with advanced human immunodeficiency virus infection. HIV Outpatient Study Investigators. *New England Journal of Medicine* 338:853-860.

Pantaleo G, Demarest JF, Schacker T et al. (1997). The qualitative nature of the primary immune response to HIV infection is a prognosticator of disease progression independent of the initial level of plasma viremia. *Proceedings of the National Academy of Sciences* 94:254-258.

Pantaleo G, Graziosi C, Demarest JF et al. (1993). HIV infection is active and progressive in lymphoid tissue during the clinically latent stage of disease. *Nature* 362:355-358.

Pantaleo G, Menzo S, Vaccarezza M et al. (1995). Studies in subjects with long-term nonprogressive human immunodeficiency virus infection. *New England Journal of Medicine* 332:209-216.

Passaro DJ, Werner SB, McGee J et al. (1998). Wound botulism associated with black tar heroin among injecting drug users. *Journal of the American Medical Association* 279:859-863.

Pelletier LL Jr. & Petersdorf RG (1977). Infective endocarditis: A review of 125 cases from the University of Washington Hospitals, 1963-72. *Medicine* 56:287-313.

Pequegnat W, Fishbein M, Celetano D et al. (2000). NIMH/APPC workgroup on behavioral and biological outcomes in HIV/STD prevention studies: A position statement. *Sexually Transmitted Diseases* 27:127-132.

Perlman DC, Salomon N, Perkins MP et al. (1995). Tuberculosis in drug users. *Clinical Infectious Diseases* 1253-1264.

Polesky A, Farber HW, Gottlieb DJ et al. (1996). Rifampin preventive therapy for tuberculosis in Boston's homeless. *American Journal of Respiratory and Critical Care Medicine* 154:1473-1477.

Polsky B, Gold JW, Whimbey E et al. (1986). Bacterial pneumonia in patients with the acquired immunodeficiency syndrome. *Annals of Internal Medicine* 104:38-41.

Raboud JM, Rae S, Montaner JS (2000). Predicting HIV RNA virologic outcome at 52-weeks follow-up in antiretroviral clinical trials. *Journal of Acquired Immune Deficiency Syndromes* 24:433-439.

Raoult D, Fournier PE, Drancourt M et al. (1996). Diagnosis of 22 new cases of Bartonella endocarditis. *Annals of Internal Medicine* 125:646-652.

Rapeport KB, Giron JA & Rosner F (1986). Streptococcus mitis endocarditis. Report of 17 cases. *Archives of Internal Medicine* 146:2361-2363.

Reichman LB, Felton CP & Edsall JR (1979). Drug dependence, a possible new risk factor for tuberculosis disease. *Archives of Internal Medicine* 139:337-339.

Relkin F, Aranda CP, Garay SM et al. (1994). Pleural tuberculosis and HIV infection. *Chest* 105:1338-1341.

Riancho JA, Echevarria S, Napal J et al. (1988). Endocarditis due to Listeria monocytogenes and human immunodeficiency virus infection. *American Journal of Medicine* 85:737.

Robinson SL, Saxe JM, Lucas CE et al. (1992). Splenic abscess associated with endocarditis. *Surgery* 112:781-786.

Rodriguez Barradas MC, Musher DM et al. (1992). Unusual manifestations of pneumococcal infection in human immunodeficiency virus-infected individuals: The past revisited. *Clinical Infectious Diseases* 14:192-199.

Roe MT, Abramson MA, Li J et al. (2000). Clinical information determines the impact of transesophageal echocardiography on the diagnosis of infective endocarditis by the Duke Criteria. *American Heart Journal* 139:945-951.

Rosenberg ES, Billingsley JM, Caliendo AM et al. (1997). Vigorous HIV-1 specific CD4(+) T cell responses associated with control of viremia. *Science* 278:1447-1450.

Runyon BA, Montano AA, Akriviadis EA et al. (1992). The serum-ascites albumin gradient is superior to the exudate-transudate concept in the differential diagnosis of ascites. *Annals of Internal Medicine* 117:215-220.

Sapico FL & Montgomerie JZ (1979). Pyogenic vertebral osteomyelitis: Report of nine cases and review of the literature. *Reviews of Infectious Diseases* 1:754-776.

Sapico FL & Montgomerie JZ (1980). Vertebral osteomyelitis in intravenous drug abusers: Report of three cases and review of the literature. *Reviews of Infectious Diseases* 2:196-206.

Schacker W, Collier AC, Hughes J et al. (1996). Clinical and epidemiologic features of primary HIV infection. *Annals of Internal Medicine* 125:257-264.

Schacker TW, Hughes JP, Shea T et al. (1998). Biological and virologic characteristics of primary HIV infection. *Annals of Internal Medicine* 128:613-620.

Schwartzman WA, Lambertus MW, Kennedy CA et al. (1991). Staphylococcal pyomyositis in patients infected by the human immunodeficiency virus. *American Journal of Medicine* 90:595-600.

Sepkowitz KA (1998). Effect of prophylaxis on the clinical manifestations of AIDS-related opportunistic infections. *Clinical Infectious Diseases* 26:806-810.

Shafer RW, Kim DS, Weiss JP et al. (1991). Extrapulmonary tuberculosis in patients with human immunodeficiency virus infection. *Medicine* 70:384-397.

Shaikholeslami R, Tomlinson CW, Teoh KH et al. (1999). Mycotic aneurysm complicating staphylococcal endocarditis. *Canadian Journal of Cardiology* 15:217-222.

Shekar R, Rice TW, Zierdt CH et al. (1985). Outbreak of endocarditis caused by Pseudomonas aeruginosa serotype O11 among pentazocine and tripelennamine abusers in Chicago. *Journal of Infectious Diseases* 151:203-208.

Sikkema KJ, Kelly JA, Winett RA et al. (2000). Outcomes of a randomized community-level HIV prevention intervention for women living in 18 low-income housing developments. *American Journal of Public Health* 90:57-63.

Snyder N, Atterbury CE, Pinto Correia J et al. (1977). Increased concurrence of cirrhosis and bacterial endocarditis. A clinical and postmortem study. *Gastroenterology* 73:1107-1113.

Spach DH, Callis KP, Paauw DS et al. (1993). Endocarditis caused by Rochalimaea quintana in a patient infected with human immunodeficiency virus. *Journal of Clinical Microbiology* 31:692-694.

Spach DH, Kanter AS, Daniels NA et al. (1995). Bartonella (Rochalimaea) species as a cause of apparent "culture-negative" endocarditis. *Clinical Infectious Diseases* 20:1044-1047.

Speechly-Dick ME & Swanton RH (1994). Osteomyelitis and infective endocarditis. *Postgraduate Medical Journal* 70:885-890.

Sperling RS, Shapiro DE, Coombs RW et al. (1996). Maternal viral load, zidovudine treatment, and the risk of transmission of human immunodeficiency virus type 1 from mother to infant. Pediatric AIDS Clinical Trials Group Protocol 076 Study Group. *New England Journal of Medicine* 335:1621-1629.

Steen MK, Bruno-Murtha LA, Chaux G et al. (1992). Bacillus cereus endocarditis: Report of a case and review. *Clinical Infectious Diseases* 14:945-946.

Steinhart R, Reingold AL, Taylor F et al. (1992). Invasive Haemophilus influenzae infections in men with HIV infection. *Journal of the American Medical Association* 268:3350-3352.

Such J & Runyon BA (1998). Spontaneous bacterial peritonitis. *Clinical Infectious Diseases* 27:669-674.

Sulis C (1995). Infectious disease in pregnancy. In PL Carr, KM Freund & S Somani (eds.) *The Medical Care of Women*. Philadelphia, PA: W.B. Saunders, 405-422.

Sullivan JH, Moore RD, Keruly JC et al. (2000). Effect of antiretroviral therapy on the incidence of bacterial pneumonia in patients with advanced HIV infection. *American Journal of Respiratory and Critical Care Medicine* 162:64-67.

Summanen PH, Talan DA, Strong C et al. (1995). Bacteriology of skin and soft-tissue infections: Comparison of infections in intravenous drug users and individuals with no history of intravenous drug use. *Clinical Infectious Diseases* 20(Suppl 2):S279-S282.

Tsao JW, Garlin AB, Marder SR et al. (1999). Mycotic aneurysm presenting as Pancoast's syndrome in an injection drug user. *Annals of Emergency Medicine* 34:546-549.

Ugolini V, Pacifico A, Smitherman TC et al. (1986). Pneumococcal endocarditis update: Analysis of 10 cases diagnosed between 1974 and 1984. *American Heart Journal* 112:813-819.

USPHS/IDSA Prevention of Opportunistic Infections Working Group (1997). 1997 USPHS/IDSA guidelines for the prevention of opportunistic infections in persons infected with human immunodeficiency virus. *Morbidity and Mortality Weekly Report* 46(No. RR-12):1-46.

USPHS/IDSA Prevention of Opportunistic Infections Working Group (2000). 1999 USPHS/IDSA guidelines for the prevention of opportunistic infections in persons infected with human immunodeficiency virus. *Clinical Infectious Diseases* 30(Suppl 1):S29-65.

Vella S, Giuliano M, Floridia M et al. (1995). Effect of sex, age and transmission category on the progression to AIDS and survival of zidovudine-treated symptomatic patients. *AIDS* 9:51-56.

Venezio FR, Gullberg RM, Westenfelder GO et al. (1986). Group G streptococcal endocarditis and bacteremia. *American Journal of Medicine* 81:29-34.

Vlahov D, Graham N, Hoover D et al. (1998). Prognostic indicators for AIDS and infectious disease death in HIV-infected injection drug users. Plasma viral load and CD4+ cell count. *Journal of the American Medical Association* 279:35-40.

Von Reyn CF, Levy BS, Arbeit RD et al. (1981). Infective endocarditis: An analysis based on strict case definitions. *Annals of Internal Medicine* 94:505-518.

Weinstein L (1986). Life-threatening complications of infective endocarditis and their management. *Archives of Internal Medicine* 146:953-957.

Weisse AB, Heller DR, Schimenti RJ et al. (1993). The febrile parenteral drug user: A prospective study in 121 patients. *American Journal of Medicine* 94:274-280.

Weverling GJ, Mocroft A, Ledergerber B et al. (1999). Discontinuation of Pneumocystis carinii pneumonia prophylaxis after start of highly active antiretroviral therapy in HIV-1 infection. EuroSIDA Study Group. *Lancet* 353:1293-1298.

Wewers MD, Diaz PT, Wewers ME et al. (1998). Cigarette smoking in HIV infection induces a suppressive inflammatory environment in the lung. *American Journal of Respiratory and Critical Care Medicine* 158:1543-1549.

Widrow CA, Kellie SM, Saltzman BR et al. (1991). Pyomyositis in patients with the human immunodeficiency virus: An unusual form of disseminated bacterial infection. *American Journal of Medicine* 91:129-136.

Wieland M, Lederman MM, Kline-King C et al. (1986). Left-sided endocarditis due to Pseudomonas aeruginosa. A report of 10 cases and review of the literature. *Medicine* 65:180-189.

Wilson WR, Karchmer AW, Dajani AS et al. (1995). Antibiotic treatment of adults with infective endocarditis due to streptococci, enterococci, staphylococci, and HACEK microorganisms. American Heart Association. *Journal of the American Medical Association* 274:1706-1713.

Witt DJ, Craven DE & McCabe WR (1987). Bacterial infections in adult patients with the acquired immune deficiency syndrome (AIDS) and AIDS-related complex. *American Journal of Medicine* 82:900-906.

Wong JK, Hezareh M, Gunthard HF et al. (1997). Recovery of replication-competent HIV despite prolonged suppression of plasma viremia. *Science* 278:1291-1295.

Wongpaitoon V, Sathapatayavongs B, Prachaktam R et al. (1985). Spontaneous Vibrio vulnificus peritonitis and primary sepsis in two patients with alcoholic cirrhosis. *American Journal of Gastroenterology* 80:706-708.

Zhang L, Chung C, Hu BS et al. (2000). Genetic characterization of rebounding HIV-1 after cessation of highly active antiretroviral therapy. *Journal of Clinical Investigation* 106:839-845.

Zhang L, Ramratnam B, Tenner-Racz K et al. (1999). Quantifying residual HIV-1 replication in patients receiving combination antiretroviral therapy. *New England Journal of Medicine* 340:1605-1613.

| Chapter 9 | # Sleep Disorders Related to Alcohol and Other Drug Use |

Sanford Auerbach, M.D.

Sleep is a complex physiologic state that is essential for normal function throughout the day. In spite of its critical role, sleep appears to be quite fragile. About 35% of all adults report insomnia at some point during the preceding six months and half describe it as serious (Mellinger, Balter et al., 1985). Given the influence of alcohol and other drugs on sleep, sleep problems are likely to be more prevalent in persons with addictive disorders.

The coexistence of a sleep disorder with an addictive disorder is a complex problem. For example, alcohol consumption can affect "normal sleep" in nonalcoholics, while the alcoholic has disrupted sleep while using alcohol and withdrawing from alcohol. Alcohol also has an effect on other sleep-related disorders, particularly obstructive sleep apnea.

This chapter reviews the essential elements of clinical sleep physiology, sleep, the effects of alcohol on both nonalcoholic and alcoholic individuals, and alcohol withdrawal. Finally, the effects of other drugs and alcohol on other specific sleep disorders are considered.

OVERVIEW OF SLEEP

Sleep is essential for normal human function. Wakefulness (lack of sleepiness), vigilance, and performance on monotonous tasks deteriorate after a single sleepless night. Further sleep deprivation leads to more inattentiveness and performance failure. Lack of rapid eye movement sleep is associated with anxiety and excitability, as well as difficulty with concentration and memory. Those deprived of slow wave sleep generally report chronic fatigue, aches, stiffness, uneasiness, and withdrawal.

"Sleep need" is difficult to define, but usually is accepted as the amount of sleep required for optimal function during wakeful periods. Sleep need varies from one individual to the next in a range from 3 to 10 hours of sleep over a 24-hour period (Williams, Karacan et al., 1970). These principles apply to sleep that is not interrupted by specific sleep pathology, such as sleep apnea or periodic limb movements.

The relationship of subjective to objective measures of sleep deserves further comment. In the general population, self-reports of sleep time often are subject to both overestimates and underestimates. Overestimates can be attributed, in part, to the fact that an arousal must be at least five to six minutes in duration if it is to be recalled subsequently as a sustained arousal or period of wakefulness. As a result, sleep punctuated by recurrent, yet brief, periods of arousal may be described as "sound sleep." Similarly, overestimates of sleep duration are not uncommon. This overestimation can be further compounded because healthy older adults may simply accept a decrease in sleep efficiency as a part of normal aging. However, aging also is associated with reduced ability to tolerate sleep deprivation.

Given these influences, it is clear that objective measures of sleep and sleepiness are critical to the study of sleep and the effects of alcohol on sleep. The nocturnal polysomnogram (PSG) is the standard method of determining the presence and stage of sleep by measuring electroencephalographic (EEG), electromyographic (EMG), and electro-oculgraphic activity (Rechtschaffen & Kales, 1968). Similarly, the multiple sleep latency test (MSLT) is a standard and accepted measure of daytime sleepiness; it employs polysomnography while a patient is allowed to take naps on five separate occasions throughout a day (ASDA, 1992). The assessment of average sleep latency with such a standardized tool allows a quantification of "sleepiness."

Sleep need often is translated into the concept of "sleep drive." Thus, relative sleep deprivation leads to increased sleep drive, whereas napping lends itself to a relative decrease in sleep drive. The change in sleep need with increasing age has been the subject of considerable study, but such studies often are confounded by changes in lifestyle, diet, medication use, napping patterns, and the like. These studies suggest that total sleep over a 24-hour period shows little change as an individual transitions from young adulthood into old age.

Sleep Architecture. Understanding normal sleep is an essential prerequisite to understanding sleep disorders. Sleep is a dynamic process, featuring fluctuations in brain wave activity, muscle tone, eye movement, and autonomic activity. It consists of two discrete states: rapid eye movement (REM) and non-rapid eye movement (NREM) sleep. Each can be defined in physiologic terms by using the elements of the PSG: EEG, electro-oculogram, and EMG. Formal criteria have been elaborated in a widely accepted manual (Rechtschaffen & Kales, 1968).

NREM: NREM sleep has been subdivided into four stages, which are numbered 1 through 4. Stages 3 and 4 usually are consolidated and referred to as "slow wave sleep" (SWS) or "delta sleep." In brief, each stage is characterized by progressively slower EEG background, lower muscle tone, and decreasing eye movements.

Stage 1 marks the transition from wakefulness to drowsiness. Rhythmic activity is replaced by mixed voltage, 3.0 to 7.0 Hz theta activity and a decrease in muscle tone. Roving eye movements may be present.

Stage 2 features a similar but slower background EEG, with superimposed "spindles" (low amplitude, high frequency, centrally predominant bursts) and K-complexes (high amplitude, negative or up-going potential, immediately followed by lower amplitude, positive or down-going potential, with some faster, low amplitude activity). Muscle tone may decrease further, while eye movements may disappear entirely. Stages 1 and 2 often are referred to as the "light" stages of NREM sleep because of the relatively low arousal threshold.

Stages 3 and 4 (SWS) are characterized by high amplitude (≥ 75 microV), slow wave (0.5 to 2.0 Hz) activity. When the slow wave activity accounts for 20% or more of an epoch, it is considered to be stage 3 sleep. When it accounts for 50% or more, it is considered stage 4. K-complexes and spindles are absent and eye movements are not seen. Muscle tone may be further diminished.

REM: REM sleep does not fit into the same staging system as NREM sleep and thus sometimes is referred to as "paradoxical" sleep. Although EEG activity is relatively active, the muscle tone achieves its lowest state over a 24-hour period (relative muscle atonia). REM sleep is characterized by rapid eye movements scattered through the duration of each REM cycle. REM sleep can be further subdivided into tonic (background EEG, relative muscle atonia, hippocampal theta activity) and phasic (rapid eye movements, brief muscle twitches, "saw tooth" waves on the EEG and pontogeniculo-occipital spikes, as recorded in animals) components. REM sleep is associated with the well-formed dream. Individuals aroused from REM sleep will recall dreams about 80% of the time. NREM arousals may be associated with recall of isolated images or thought fragments, but not the well-formed images of REM sleep.

Nightmares are a reflection of the elements of REM sleep. As the individual initially awakens from a frightening dream and begins to scream, no sound emerges, because he or she still is paralyzed with the muscle atonia of REM. It is noteworthy that these components of REM sleep are not rigidly synchronized. Another example of this loose synchronization can be seen in some normal individuals with sleep paralysis as a benign condition, in which the individual is transiently "paralyzed" as he or she awakens from sleep.

Sleep Rhythms. The components of sleep do not occur randomly throughout the course of the night. In fact, a clear pattern emerges from the ultradian or short rhythms of sleep. The "light" stages of NREM are seen first. They are followed by a transition to SWS, followed by lighter stages of NREM again, and then REM sleep. Typically, there are three to four NREM-REM cycles, each lasting 90 to 120 minutes. As the night progresses, the relative amount of time spent in REM increases and the amount of time in SWS decreases. Thus, REM usually is skewed toward the end of the sleep period and SWS toward the beginning.

More importantly, sleep-wake rhythms follow a circadian or approximately 24-hour biological pattern. Sleep-wake is considered a circadian rhythm that is tightly synchronized with circadian variations in core body temperature. The suprachiasmatic nucleus of the hypothalamus in animals, and an analogous structure in humans, with inputs from the retinohypothalamic pathways, has been identified as the endogenous pacemaker. Although individuals may have different periodicities in their clocks ("larks" and "owls"), there are many factors that maintain or influence these rhythms. Although activity levels, social cues, mealtimes, and other external scheduling factors play some role, the most powerful "Zeitgeiber" (light-giver) has proved to be exogenous light. Presumably, light exerts its influence through retinohypothalamic input to the suprachiasmatic nucleus (Czeisler, Richardson et al., 1991).

From a clinical perspective, it is helpful to view the usual pattern of sleep-wake in terms of the shifting pattern of core body temperature. The usual evening sleep onset occurs as the core body temperature falls during the "primary sleep permissive" zone. Sleep continues as the core body temperature continues to fall and enters the "sleep maintenance zone." The duration of sleep and REM sleep follows this circadian cycle, with most of REM sleep occurring close to the nadir of the temperature cycle. The temperature then begins to rise, reaching its peak at midday. A secondary dip usually occurs in mid-afternoon, correlating with a secondary sleep permissive zone or the so-called "siesta" zone. This nap zone usually is followed by a relative plateau that has been related to the "second wind." Similarly, a secondary rise occurs in the early morning hours, usually at about 3 AM, when a secondary arousal time occurs and the individual is susceptible to wakening from any physical or emotional factor (that is, anxiety, pain, or the need to urinate).

UNDERSTANDING SLEEP DISORDERS

For a comprehensive listing of specific disorders and their descriptions, the reader is referred to *The International Classification of Sleep Disorders (ICSD)* (Thorpy, 1990). This chapter focuses on problems related to (1) sleep need, (2) sleep rhythms, (3) intrinsic sleep disorders, (4) extrinsic factors, and (5) medical-psychiatric factors.

Drive/Sleep Need. As noted earlier, sleep drive is based on sleep need, which, in turn, assumes sleep need is based on otherwise efficient sleep. Sleep need probably does not change with age after young adulthood (Williams, Karacan et al., 1970). It is not uncommon to see an accumulation of "sleep debt" over the course of a week, with the weekend set aside for recovery. These patterns often are related to social and lifestyle decisions.

Identification of an individual's sleep need is the first step in understanding sleep complaints. Careful questioning of the patient is required to account for total sleep time, including both nocturnal sleep and daytime naps.

Timing. The sleep-wake circadian rhythm often advances with age toward an early bedtime and early rise time (the lark). A common experience is the transient dysfunction associated with "jet lag." This is simply a situation in which the biological clock suddenly becomes desynchronized from the social environment. Because most people find it easier to "delay" their clocks, it becomes easier for most to fly from the East Coast to the West Coast (which requires an advancement of the rhythm) than from west to east. Typically, it can take a day and a half to recover a 60-minute advancement (one and a half time zones). Similarly, it takes about a day to recover from a 60-minute delay (one time zone change).

For a variety of social and biological reasons, there is a tendency for the adolescent to become delayed and the older adult to become advanced. The resulting complaints typically involve insomnia and difficulty in staying awake at other times. Recognition of these disorders leads to the formulation of a treatment plan.

In addition, the circadian rhythm of the older adult appears to be more fragile and susceptible to disruption, as might be seen in shift workers or patients plagued by the nocturnal arousal of chronic pain. It is unclear how much of this change is due to biological changes in the endogenous oscillator that governs the rhythms, and how much is the result of changes in exogenous factors such as light exposure, lifestyle changes, and physical activity. The rhythm can be manipulated by well-timed bright light exposure.

The full range of circadian rhythm disorders, as described in the *ICSD*, include problems related to delays, advancements, and shifting rhythms. The pathophysiology of these disorders may vary, but some can be attributed to jet travel or shift work.

Aging results in a greater sensitivity to time zone or shift work changes. In such situations, there is a significant desynchronization between social and environmental cues and biological rhythms. The individual attempts to sleep or to stay awake at times that are not closely synchronized to biological rhythms. Older adults appear to be less tolerant of such desynchronization, as well as dealing with the clinical effects of an advancing rhythm. This implies earlier "wake-up" times (the lark), which persist despite later sleep onset times. The net result is the need to nap because a sleep debt is acquired.

Intrinsic Sleep Disorders. Although there are many intrinsic sleep disorders, the three most common are periodic limb movements of sleep (PLMS), restless legs syndrome (RLS), and obstructive sleep apnea (OSA).

PLMS: Periodic limb movements of sleep are characterized by episodes of repetitive, stereotyped limb movements during sleep. Other terms for the condition include "periodic leg movement," "nocturnal myoclonus," "periodic movements of sleep," or "leg jerks." The movements usually involve the legs (unilateral, alternating, or bilateral), although the arms also may be involved. Movements consist of extension of the big toe, in combination with partial flexing of the ankle, knee, and (sometimes) hip. The movements often are associated with partial arousal or overturning, usually too briefly for potential awareness (Thorpy, 1990). There can be marked night-to-night variability in the number of movements (Mosso, Dickel et al., 1988; Billiwise, Clarkson et al., 1988; Edinger, McCall et al., 1992). In some cases, periodic arousals may predominate, with minimal (if any) evidence of limb movements. In such cases, some investigators have referred to the so-called periodic K-alpha syndrome.

Clinically, the patient may complain of non-restorative sleep. Even when the patient reports sound sleep, he or she may thrash about, while the bed partner reports kicking or even bicycling movements.

Typically, an anterior tibialis EMG shows contractions with a duration of 0.5 to 5.0 seconds (average, 1.5 to 2.5 seconds). Movements generally occur every 5 to 90 seconds (most typically, every 20 to 40 seconds). Although PLMS can occur in any stage of NREM, they are most common in stage 2 and usually disappear in REM (Thorpy, 1990).

The pathophysiology of PLMS remains somewhat obscure. They may be associated with OSA or with the use of antidepressants. Similarly, withdrawal from certain drugs (including anticonvulsants, benzodiazepines, barbiturates, and other hypnotics), may contribute to the development of PLMS. They can be seen in otherwise young, healthy individuals (Moore & Jacobsen, 1991).

RLS: It has been estimated that restless leg syndrome (RLS) is present in 5% to 15% of the general population. It affects both sexes and has been described in both children and adults. The usual presentation is with paresthesias, usually bilateral, often more prominent in the legs than in the arms. The sensations typically are described as "burning," "tingling," "stabbing," "aching," or simple pain. Some patients complain of sensations of ants crawling or worms burrowing. Symptoms usually are subjective and vary over the course of the day. They tend to be worse when the individual is relaxing, and especially when preparing for sleep. Patients may have particular difficulties in enclosed areas such as airplanes, cars, or trains. Symptoms are variable and may fluctuate over time, with "exacerbations" and "remissions." Some patients develop myoclonus or sudden jerking movements. It is not uncommon to find an overlap with PLMS.

The pathophysiology of RLS is unknown. Disorders of iron or calcium metabolism and dopaminergic function have been considered. Many medical problems have been found to aggravate the symptoms.

The treatment of RLS usually requires medication. The most commonly used are clonazepam, gabapentin, dopaminergic drugs such as carbadopa/levodopa or pergolide, and the opioids. The latter group is of particular interest. Some patients report that they began to use opioids on a regular basis when they received them for an unrelated disorder and realized that they were able to sleep for the first time in years.

OSA: Obstructive sleep apnea (OSA) is a common syndrome. It is a treatable disorder that accounts for many of the cases of excessive somnolence and insomnia encountered in most sleep centers. It is one of the few diagnoses that make polysomnograms reimbursable by third-party payers.

OSA is characterized by repetitive episodes of sleep-related upper airway obstructions, which usually are associated with oxygen desaturation. OSA can be conceptualized as a disorder emerging from an interaction between anatomy and muscle relaxation as it occurs in sleep. As muscles relax, airflow can generate vibrations in the soft tissues of the upper airway, including the soft palate. Such vibration produces the noise or the snoring. In some patients, the snoring appears in isolation; in such cases, the term "primary snoring" is applied.

Further upper airway restriction can result in difficulties along two other dimensions. The muscle relaxation, especially in the upper airway dilator muscles of the oropharynx (often combined with mild anatomic abnormalities) provides the setting for increased airway restriction, which is further enhanced by the negative pressures generated by normal respiration (Guilleminault & Stohs, 1991).

The sleep disruption may or may not be apparent to the patient because, as noted earlier, brief physiological arousals may not be recalled. Daytime somnolence often is the prime complaint, although—as in other chronic, progressive disorders—the patient may adapt to and minimize these symptoms. The same patient who denies daytime sleepiness or napping may acknowledge an irresistible urge to doze if allowed to sit in a comfortable chair or when confronted with the monotony of highway driving. Similarly, presenting complaints may be related to difficulties in memory or concentration that reflect suppression of REM sleep (REM sleep is especially vulnerable because of the relative muscle atonia). SWS also can be suppressed and may be associated with complaints similar to those associated with fibrositis or fibromyalgia.

In addition to sleep disruption, there are several cardiopulmonary consequences. Feedback reflexes may be insufficient to cause arousal (arousal produces return of muscle tone on cessation of the respiratory events). Indeed, one might see significant oxygen desaturation with arrhythmia, systemic and pulmonary arterial hypertension, and polycythemia. These changes can become chronic, and recent epidemiologic studies have suggested that OSA plays a role in the development of often-unrecognized hypertension in the general public (Morrill, Finn et al., 2000; Nieto, Young et al., 2000).

The severity of OSA thus can be measured in three dimensions: (1) snoring, (2) sleep disruption, and (3) cardiopulmonary consequences. It is not unusual to see some linkage, but the factors may exist independently as well. Manipulation of anatomy or the degree of muscle relaxation can aggravate OSA. Weight gain or supine sleep heighten the anatomical risk factors, whereas use of alcohol, benzodiazepines, and other sedatives enhance muscle relaxation and thus the severity of OSA.

Determination of the severity of OSA is complicated by the arbitrary scoring criteria used in most laboratories, as well as the recent recognition of the upper airway resistance syndrome. Traditionally, apneas are defined as episodes of 10 seconds' duration in which airflow falls to less than 20% of baseline. Obstructive events imply that there is continued respiratory effort (Gislason, Aberg et al., 1987), although there is some controversy as to how sensitive the effort markers need to be to determine absence of effort of the type seen in central apneas. Hypopneas usually are defined as events of 10 seconds' duration in which airflow drops to 50% of baseline or less, with an associated drop in oxygen saturation. In upper airway resistance syndrome, "unscoreable" events may be associated with sleep disruption or frequent EEG alpha arousals.

Epidemiologic studies have suggested that snoring occurs in 9% to 24% of middle-aged men and in 4% to 14% of middle-aged women (Koskenvu, Kapiro et al., 1985; Lugaresi & Partinen, 1994), although there is a tendency to underreport snoring (Telakivi, Partinen et al., 1987). The prevalence of OSA in the general male population has been estimated to be 0.4% to 5.9% (Telakivi, Partinen et al., 1987; Cingnotta, D'Alessandro et al., 1989; Lavie, Ben-Yosef et al., 1984; Gislasen, Almqvist et al., 1988), with the incidence in men clearly outnumbering that in women.

Common risk factors include obesity (Gislason, Aberg et al., 1987; Telakivi, Partinen et al., 1987; Schmidt-Norwara, Coulas et al., 1980; Bloom, Kaltenborn et al., 1988), smoking (Lavie, Ben-Yosef et al., 1984; Gislasen, Almqvist et al., 1988; Schmidt-Norwara, Coulas et al., 1980; Norton & Dunn, 1985), alcohol consumption (Bloom, Kaltenborn et al., 1988; Issa & Sullivan, 1982), stroke (Polamaki, Partinen et al., 1992), and age.

Extrinsic Factors. Several extrinsic factors affect sleep, including exercise, the sleep environment, medications, and drug effects.

Exercise long has been recognized as a factor promoting sound sleep (Shapiro, Warren et al., 1987). Regular exercise, especially in the late afternoon or early evening, is conducive to sleep initiation, either through release of certain endogenous substances or subsequent cooling five to six hours later, which reinforces circadian factors (Edinger, Morey et al., 1993). Inactivity can be a factor in sleep disruption in the young as well as the old, but daytime bed rest is a greater issue in the sleep of older adults (Spielman, Sakin et al., 1987; Rubenstein, Rothenberg et al., 1990). This represents an interface between sleep and lifestyle.

Environmental stimuli, such as room temperature and light, often are factors in the initiation and maintenance of sleep. While arousal thresholds vary from one individual to the next, aging has been associated with increased susceptibility to external arousal (Zepelon, McDonald et al., 1984; Harsh, Purvis et al., 1990). Often, this increasing susceptibility is not recognized by the patient.

The effect of evening meals is somewhat controversial. The conventional wisdom has been a light bedtime snack—perhaps with a glass of milk—promotes sleep. This effect has been attributed to tryptophan or to the release of digestive hormones, which can be sedating (Southwell, Evans et al., 1992). On the other hand, there are reports that heavy bedtime snacks can be disruptive to sleep. Clinical experience suggests that these effects are variable and need to be assessed in each individual.

Increases in medication and changes in metabolism can contribute to sleep disruption in older adults, as they do in any age group; however, older adults appear to be more susceptible.

Medical and Psychiatric Factors. The interaction between sleep and other medical conditions can be quite complex. Certain medical conditions contribute directly to specific sleep disorders such as OSA or RLS. However, other disorders simply lead to problems with the wake-to-sleep transition at sleep onset or at other times through the night, including the most vulnerable time in the circadian cycle (that is, 3:00 to 5:00 AM). Sleep disorders have been attributed to nocturia, headache, gastrointestinal illnesses, cardiopulmonary disease, menopause, and chronic pain (Baker & Mitteness, 1989; Cook, Evans et al., 1989; Hyppa & Kronholm, 1989; Brugge, Kripke et al., 1989).

The role of psychiatric disorders always should be considered in the assessment of sleep disorders. Two specific sleep-related psychiatric disorders have been formally defined. The *ICSD* (Thorpy, 1990) describes an "alcohol-dependent insomnia" in nonalcoholics who use alcohol as a hypnotic for sleep onset for more than 30 days. The *DSM-IV* of the American Psychiatric Association (1994) describes criteria for a "substance-induced sleep disorder," with subtypes based on the substance used.

Sleep disruption is not uncommon in any person with a comorbid psychiatric syndrome, but most of the attention has been directed toward the relationship between affective disorders and sleep. Insomnia is the prominent feature, although hypersomnia may be seen in depression, especially when the depression is a component of a bipolar disorder (Detre, Himmelhoch et al., 1972). Similarly, during manic episodes, one may see periods of sleeplessness, with an apparent reduction in sleep need.

Several PSG features have been associated with depression (Benca, 2000). Sleep disruption with prolonged sleep latency, sleep fragmentation, early morning arousals, decreased sleep efficiency, and daytime fatigue and somnolence have been well documented. Another finding has been an apparent decrease in the amount of SWS, although this observation has been somewhat variable. The most robust feature, however, is a reduction in REM latency. Related features are increased duration of the first REM period and an increase in REM density.

ALCOHOL AND SLEEP
Effect of Alcohol on Sleep in the Nonalcoholic Individual. The hypnotic properties of alcohol are widely known. Alcohol probably is the sleep-promoting agent that is most widely used by the general public. In a population survey, 13% of survey respondents aged 18 to 45 years old reported that, in the preceding year, they had used alcohol to assist in sleep onset. Another 2% said they had used alcohol continuously for at least a month for this purpose, while 5% said they had used alcohol in combination with another hypnotic agent (Johnson, Roehrs et al., 1988). Despite this wide use, it must be remembered that alcohol can be mildly stimulating (Papineau, Roehrs et al., 1988). The source of the variability in its hypnotic properties is not clear, although animal studies suggest a possible role of age. In at least one study, it was demonstrated that adolescent animals developed a much more rapid tolerance to the hypnotic effects of alcohol than did older animals (Silveri & Spear, 1999, 1998), although older males had a tendency to sleep longer (Silveri & Spear, 1998).

The effects of alcohol on the sleep architecture of the nonalcoholic individual should be considered in terms of both direct effects and immediate withdrawal. Since alcohol is rapidly metabolized, the direct effect of evening alcohol consumption usually is during the sleep cycle. As predicted by the hypnotic effect, sleep latency is shortened and there is an increase in the amount of NREM sleep that occurs at the expense of REM sleep, which is suppressed during the acute phase (Yules, Lippman et al., 1967; Lobo & Tuffik, 1997). As the effects of the alcohol dissipate, there is a rebound effect, in which sleep becomes lighter and more easily disrupted. REM increases, with an associated increase in dreams and nightmares. There is an increase in sympathetic arousals, with tachycardia and sweating.

As alcohol consumption continues, the hypnotic effects may diminish, but the late sleep disruption persists (Vitello, 1997). Ultimately, the net effect is a feeling of fatigue during the individual's waking hours.

Alcohol's hypnotic effects can be seen in infants fed on the breast milk of mothers who consume even small amounts of alcohol. Indeed, it appears that such babies fall asleep more easily, but they seem to sleep less deeply (Mennella & Gerish, 1998). This finding would be predicted from our knowledge of alcohol's effects in older patients. It also has been shown that a woman's daily consumption of small amounts of alcohol in the first trimester of pregnancy is associated with subsequent sleep disruption in infants, when measured by brain electrical activity (Scher, Richardson et al., 1998).

It would seem that the hypnotic effects of alcohol should be related to direct effects of alcohol on the central nervous system. Unfortunately, this explanation does not account for the observation that sleepiness can be observed after the alcohol no longer is detectable. Although it is customary to advise patients with sleep difficulties to avoid late evening alcohol, there is evidence that even early evening alcohol consumption may disrupt sleep in the last half of the night (Landolt, Roth et al., 1996). This would apply to alcohol consumed even 6 hours prior to sleep onset (Roehrs, Beare et al., 1994). Similarly, alcohol administered early in the day has been shown to have a negative effect on MSLTs and tests of divided attention, even when given later in the day when alcohol levels are undetectable (Roehrs, Beare et al., 1994).

Finally, some data suggest that there is a synergistic interaction between alcohol exposure and prior sleepiness. The hypnotic effects seem to be enhanced in the previously sleep-deprived individual (Zwyghuizen-Doorenbos, Roehrs et al., 1990). In particular, low-dose alcohol administered after a night of reduced sleep is associated with reduced performance on a driving simulator (Vitello, 1997; Roehrs, Beare et al., 1994; Zwyghuizen-Doorenbos, Roehrs et al., 1998; Lunley, Roehrs et al., 1987). The implication is that, in individuals functioning on reduced sleep, alcohol has an enhanced sedating effect even at low doses, which in turn has an effect on performance in activities such as driving.

Effect of Alcohol on Sleep in the Alcoholic Individual. It is not uncommon for alcoholics to report some combination of insomnia, hypersomnia, circadian rhythm disorders, or parasomnias (abnormal sleep-related behaviors). Such reports usually are reflected in other, more objective measures. Various studies of alcoholic patients have demonstrated increased sleep latencies (time to fall asleep), decreased sleep efficiencies, and decreased total sleep, with reductions in both REM and SWS (Mello & Mendelson, 1970; Allen, Wagman et al., 1971; Adamson & Berdick, 1973). As the dependence continues, alcoholic patients often report that they no longer are able to initiate sleep without a drink. After a period of time, the usual rhythms of sleep become quite disrupted.

Dream Content in Alcoholism: Although dreams usually are correlated with REM sleep, studies of dream content in alcoholics often are conducted without the use of polysomnographic techniques. In general, these studies find that alcoholics suffer from nightly nightmares more often than controls (Cernovsky, 1985, 1986). In a more general study of substance abusers in a detoxification program, dreaming about drinking was a poor prognostic sign for relapse (Christo & Franey, 1996). Others have reported that among recovering alcoholics, dreams about drinking were viewed with concern and were considered a potential trigger for relapse (Denizen, 1988).

The use of alcohol to suppress nightmares needs to be considered in the management of other disorders associated with nightmares, such as posttraumatic stress disorder (Stewart, 1996). In fact, some patients may have initiated their substance abuse out of a desire to suppress nightmares.

Alcohol, Sleep, and Other Cardiopulmonary Functions: In addition to the effect of alcohol on OSA, it is important to be aware of the interaction between chronic obstructive pulmonary disease (COPD) and alcohol during sleep. For example, alcohol consumption before sleep by patients with COPD can worsen nocturnal hypoxemia during sleep (Easton, West et al., 1987) and increase ventricular ectopic activity (Dolly & Block, 1983).

Sleep in Alcohol Withdrawal: The alcohol withdrawal syndrome frequently is marked by severe insomnia and sleep fragmentation. The reduction of SWS during this period has been related to a loss of restful sleep and feelings of daytime fatigue. The rebound of REM sleep has been regarded as a component of the pathophysiology of hallucinations encountered in the withdrawal syndrome. In fact, sleep during withdrawal may consist simply of fragments of

REM sleep. It is of some interest that the rebound of SWS does not appear to occur (Allen, Wagman et al., 1971).

Nightmares and vivid dreams are not uncommon features of alcohol withdrawal and probably reflect the observed REM "pressure." In fact, it has been speculated that the rebound of REM encountered in acute withdrawal states such as *delirium tremens* (DTs) may account for much of the associated clinical symptomatology (Rowland, 1997; Johnson, Burdick et al., 1970). It has been speculated that it is the early and abundant REM, with its associated dream content or hallucinations, and the accompanying sympathetic discharge that may account for much of the clinical picture of the DTs (Feinberg, 1970). These views are consistent with attempts to record the sleep of patients with DTs, which have found mostly stage 1 NREM and REM, with some evidence of increased muscle tone, even though these findings are clinically inconsistent (Wolin & Mello, 1973). The increase in muscle activity also has suggested a possible relationship with REM Behavior Disorder, in which patients lose the muscle atonia of sleep and actually begin to "act out" their dreams (Mahowald & Shenck, 2000).

Sleep During Alcohol Recovery: In the alcohol-dependent patient, sleep is not immediately recovered with abstinence; in fact, it may require months or even years. In the first two to three weeks of recovery, increased sleep latency may be seen, accompanied by increased sleep fragmentation and reduced total sleep time. There may be a decrease in SWS and an increase in REM density (Gillin, Smith et al., 1990); such an increased density of rapid eye movements suggests an apparent rebound effect. The effects on REM may be exaggerated in patients with secondary depression, who also may exhibit a shortened REM latency (duration of onset of REM after sleep onset) and a greater percentage of sleep time spent in REM sleep (Williams & Rundell, 1981).

These changes may persist for months or years, with sleep time reduced and fragmented and an elevated percentage of total sleep time spent in REM sleep (Gillin, Smith et al., 1990; Williams & Rundell, 1981; Ehlers, Phillips et al., 1996). Long-term followup of recovering alcoholics has demonstrated persistent subjective and objective sleep difficulties. The most prominent feature appears to be a persistent reduction in the amount of SWS as a percentage of total sleep (Williams & Rundell, 1981; Brower, Aldrich et al., 1998; Drummond, Gillin et al., 1998).

Sleep disruption during recovery also has been examined from the perspective of its effect on the patient's efforts to remain sober. For example, it has been demonstrated that the presence of subjective sleep disruption increases the likelihood that the recovering individual will relapse to alcohol use (Brower, Aldrich et al., 2001). Longitudinal studies have suggested that the persistence of objective and subjective sleep difficulties at about 1 month of sobriety predicts relapse by 5 months (Brower, Aldrich et al., 1998, 2001).

A recovering alcoholic who begins to drink again will experience an increase in SWS, with an increase in total sleep time and reduction in fragmentation. This response, which involves a perceived immediate improvement in sleep, is thought to contribute to relapse, even though continued alcohol use inevitably leads to further sleep disruption.

Several investigators have attempted to identify the sleep measures that are the most important in predicting relapse. Some studies suggest that the degree of SWS reduction could be correlated with a poorer prognosis for continued recovery two months after discharge from an inpatient treatment program (Allen, Wagman et al., 1980; Wagman, Allen et al., 1978). Subsequent studies, however, suggested that measures of REM sleep were critical in predicting outcome. These studies suggested that measures of REM pressure, such as a shortened REM latency, increased REM density, and increased amount of time in REM sleep as a percentage of total sleep, when measured within two weeks of initiation of abstinence, were markers of a better prognosis for continued recovery at three months after discharge (Clark, Gillin et al., 1998, 1999; Gillin, Smith et al., 1994). In fact, the emergence of these markers of REM pressure are among the most robust predictors of continued recovery at the three-month mark.

It should be noted that the prognostic value of these sleep measures changes as abstinence progresses. For example, at the five-month mark, prolonged sleep latency and poor sleep efficiency are predictors of relapse by one year, but measures of REM pressure no longer are helpful (Drummond, Gillin et al., 1998). Prolonged sleep latency (time to sleep onset) has an advantage over other measures because of the relative ease with which it is ascertained.

Specific Sleep Disorders Associated With Alcoholism. *Alcohol and Sleep-Related Breathing Disorders:* Alcoholics appear to be at increased risk of developing OSA, especially if they snore (Aldrich, 1993). A large retrospective analysis suggested that these findings might, in part, be related to an association with smoking in this population and that smoking was the primary agent (Bloom, Kaltenborn et al., 1988). Nevertheless, alcohol has been found to induce obstructive apnea in healthy asymptomatic men (Tassan, Block et al., 1981), as well as chronic snorers (Issa & Sullivan, 1982; Robinson, White et al., 1985; Miller, Dawson et al., 1988). Alcohol has been shown to increase the frequency and duration of obstructive events in patients with established OSA (Issa & Sullivan, 1982; Scrina, Broudy et al., 1982).

Two of the essential elements in the pathophysiology of OSA are the anatomy of the upper airway and the degree of relative muscle atonia associated with sleep. The decrease in muscle tone of the upper airway leads to an increase in snoring (Issa & Sullivan, 1982) and inspiratory resistance, with an accompanying reduction in airflow (Krol, Knuth et al., 1984; Dawson, Bigby et al., 1997). Alcohol contributes to a reduction in muscle tone, with a selective reduction in genioglossal activity, thus aggravating any tendency to develop snoring or OSA (Krol, Knuth et al., 1984). As a consequence, there is an increase in snoring, as well as interruption in normal nocturnal respiration. The associated sleep disruption then contributes to an increase in daytime fatigue and somnolence. These changes in airflow resistance are sufficient to cause OSA in those who consume moderate to high doses of alcohol in the evening, even if they do not otherwise have OSA (Miller, Dawson et al., 1988; Krol, Knuth et al., 1984).

Alcohol administration to asymptomatic men has been associated with increased episodes of desaturation, as well as an increase in frequency and duration of hypopneas and apneas (Tassan, Block et al., 1981). Moreover, the depressant effects of alcohol can decrease the likelihood of arousal from an obstructive event, thus prolonging the duration of each respiratory event (Tassan, Block et al., 1981; Brower, Aldrich et al., 1998; Berry, Bonnet et al., 1992). In fact, abstinence from alcohol before bedtime is considered an important step in treating OSA (Issa & Sullivan, 1982).

Although alcohol use can induce apneas, and obstructions can worsen established OSA, the relationship of alcohol to the development of OSA varies across populations. Older patients, for example, are more vulnerable to this effect (Tassan, Block et al., 1981). Similarly, the effect is not particularly prominent in normal women (Block, Hellard et al., 1985, 1986). In some studies of normal male subjects and young nonobese snorers, alcohol exerted minimal effects on the development of OSA (Scrina, Broudy et al., 1982). Thus, it appears that other factors, such as age, the presence of snoring, and perhaps gender play a role in the development of OSA.

OSA has been related to impaired performance on driving simulators and increased motor vehicle crashes even in the absence of alcohol (Roehrs, Beare et al., 1994). Alcohol further decreases the performance of the patient with OSA. One small study suggested that a higher-than-expected number of sleep-related respiratory events in detoxified patients might contribute to impaired driving performance (Tassan, Block et al., 1981). In patients with established severe OSA, it has been noted that consumption of two or more alcoholic drinks per day is associated with a fivefold increase in fatigue-related motor vehicle crashes when compared with those who consumed little or no alcohol.

Alcohol and PLMS. In at least one survey of a large sleep clinic sample, the risk of PLMS was increased almost threefold by alcohol consumption (Aldrich & Shipley, 1993). This increase, however, was not seen in another study in which abstinent alcoholics were evaluated and compared with the nonalcoholic group (Le Bon, Verbanck et al., 1997). Nevertheless, the potential increase in fatigue and daytime somnolence associated with PLMS can play a role in the management of these patients.

OTHER DRUGS AND SLEEP

Stimulants. It is widely accepted that a primary effect of stimulants is to suppress sleep. Studies have demonstrated that stimulants such as amphetamine, methylphenidate, pemoline, or cocaine prolong sleep latency and reduce total sleep time. Stimulants have a specific inhibitory effect on REM sleep, so that there is a prolonged REM latency with a reduction in total REM throughout the sleep period (Post, Gillin et al., 1970). Presumably, this effect is attributable to the dopaminergic stimulation of the arousal system, although serotonergic systems also may be involved (Gillin, Pulverenti et al., 1994). When used episodically, these agents contribute to periods of sleeplessness that can last for days, but they usually are followed by a rebound hypersomnia. Tolerance to this effect can develop with continued use, even in those who take these agents for medical disorders such as narcolepsy or attention deficit/hyperactivity disorder (Feinberg, Hibi et al., 1974).

After a period of persistent, chronic use, withdrawal of stimulants often leads to initial insomnia, which may persist (Washington, Brown et al., 1990). The sleep abnormalities encountered in stimulant withdrawal include a rebound effect. In particular, they include a decrease in sleep efficiency, with increased periods of nocturnal wakefulness, increased amounts of REM sleep with a shortened

REM latency, and increased stage 1 NREM sleep (Thompson, Gillin et al., 1995). This effect is similar to the rebound effect encountered in the second half of the night after evening alcohol consumption.

The first two weeks of stimulant withdrawal usually are marked by some improvement in measurements of total sleep time, stage 1 NREM sleep, and REM density, even though changes persist.

Opioids. The primary effect on sleep of acute administration of opioids to normal subjects or abstinent users is to shorten sleep latency and reduce total sleep time, sleep efficiency, REM sleep, and SWS (Kay, Pickworth et al., 1981). Chronic use, however, usually leads to tolerance to some of these effects. The REM-suppressing effects of morphine, for example, usually disappear within a week, even though sleep fragmentation may persist (Staedt, Wassmuth et al., 1996). Even the longer-acting opioids, such as methadone, contribute to insomnia, with disruption of sleep architecture and increased arousals accompanying chronic administration (Kay, 1975). This also may occur in patients undergoing opioid substitution therapy. The pathophysiology of this effect is not clear, but evidence suggests that the REM-inhibiting properties can be attributed to inhibition of acetylcholine receptors in the pontine reticular formation (Lydic, Keifer et al., 1993) or to direct agonist effects at specific mu receptors (Cronin, Keifer et al., 1995).

Opioids play a role in the treatment and management of specific sleep disorders. In particular, they have been found to be quite useful in the management of RLS (Trzepecz, Violette et al., 1984; Walters, Wagner et al., 1993) and PLMS (Javey, Walters et al., 1988), although the mechanism of this benefit is not well understood. In fact, anecdotal evidence shows that some patients with RLS or PLMS who are treated with opioids for unrelated disorders become dependent on opioids when they experience the sleep benefits. For example, a patient may suddenly realize that postoperative narcotics allow for marked improvement in sleep that had been interrupted by previously undiagnosed RLS. Opioids play an obvious role in the management of sleep disorders secondary to pain syndromes.

Little has been written about the characteristics of sleep during withdrawal from opioids, but clinical experience suggests that insomnia often is cited as a troublesome feature of withdrawal and requires specific attention.

Nicotine. The effects of nicotine on sleep have not been well studied, but the available data suggest that, compared with nonsmokers, smokers experience an increase in sleep latency and an increase in arousals, with resulting poorer sleep maintenance (Davila, Hunt et al., 1994). A possible biphasic response is that low doses promote sleep and higher doses disrupt sleep (Davila, Hunt et al., 1994; Gillin, Landon et al., 1994). Unlike most of the other agents discussed in this chapter, nicotine can increase rather then decrease REM (Salin-Pascual & Drucker-Colin, 1998).

Withdrawal from nicotine is associated with sleep disruption and increased daytime sleepiness, marked by MSLTs (Prosise, Bonnet et al., 1994). The effect of nicotine patches on sleep disruption remains unclear (Hughes, Higgins et al., 1994b). The variability of responses may be due to the anxiety and irritability encountered in nicotine withdrawal.

Some researchers speculate that, in addition to the direct effect of nicotine on sleep mechanisms and architecture, tobacco and the irritation it causes to the upper airway may contribute to OSA (Wetter, Young et al., 1994).

Caffeine. The effects of caffeine overlap those of the stimulants. Caffeine has a long history of use to combat fatigue and sleepiness in normal individuals (Kelly, Miller et al., 1997), and can trigger insomnia in experimental conditions as well (Stradling, 1993). Unlike many other stimulants, caffeine appears to exert its effect by blocking adenosine receptors (Portas, Thakkar et al., 1997).

Unfortunately, in the clinical setting, patients and clinicians often overlook the effects of caffeine. The half-life of caffeine ranges from three to seven hours, with effects persisting for as long as 8 to 14 hours. Thus, the effects of late-morning caffeine intake may continue into the evening. As with other drugs, there is considerable variability in individual responses to caffeine. Thus, some individuals may become overstimulated with even 250 mg of caffeine, which is equivalent to about one to two cups of coffee, while others develop tolerance and are able to sleep soundly despite heavy consumption.

Caffeine often is used in combination with alcohol and together they can lead to even further aggravation of insomnia. Although alcohol has hypnotic properties, its half-life is much shorter than that of caffeine and its major effects disappear within a few hours. At that point, the rebound effect of alcohol withdrawal and the persistent stimulatory effect of caffeine jointly contribute to further sleep disruption (Stradling, 1993).

It is easy to underestimate the effect of abrupt withdrawal of caffeine. Although few formal studies of caffeine withdrawal and its effects on sleep have been conducted, it has been noted that within 18 to 24 hours, some patients develop headache, fatigue, irritability, sleepiness, and flu-like symptoms (Hughes, Higgins et al., 1994a).

Benzodiazepines. Benzodiazepines represent an interesting group of medications because they often are used in the management of sleep disorders, in addition to being potential drugs of abuse. The primary effect is to reduce sleep latency, increase total sleep time, and reduce nocturnal arousals (Mendelson, 1987). Unlike the stimulants and caffeine, benzodiazepines have only a minimal effect on REM sleep. With acute and chronic use, there can be an increase in spindle activity and there is a decrease in the amount of SWS (Mendelson, 1987). The related agents, zolpidem and zaleplon, have similar effects, although it is thought that they have less effect on SWS. The traditional view has been that the sleep-promoting effects are lost within two to three weeks of use. Recent reviews, however, suggest that the development of tolerance to the hypnotic effects of benzodiazepines is quite variable and that drug effects may persist for extended periods of time. It is likely that this variability is at least partially related to the underlying etiology of the sleep disorder.

CLINICAL APPROACHES TO SLEEP DISORDERS

The clinical approach to patients with co-occurring sleep addictive disorders poses certain problems. In addition to dealing with specific sleep disorders, it is necessary to address the effect of the substance of abuse on sleep, the effect of withdrawal, and any comorbid psychiatric problems such as depression. The clinical picture may be further complicated because some of the medications used in the treatment of specific sleep disorders have a potential for abuse. Therefore, a systematic approach is critical.

1. The first step is to obtain a careful history of the amount of sleep actually obtained in a 24-hour period. A diary can be used, but a careful history often elicits the necessary information.

2. The next step is to address the issue of timing and to determine the patient's probable circadian rhythm. This can be complicated by shifting work schedules and other activities. Again, the history is the most powerful tool. A sleep diary can be helpful.

3. Consider the potential for medical or psychiatric issues that can interfere with sleep. These are detected through a careful medical and psychiatric review, including an inventory of medications, exercise, nicotine, alcohol, and other drug use. Give careful attention to symptoms of anxiety, depression, nightmares, and posttraumatic stress.

4. Inquire about possible features of intrinsic sleep disorders. Is there evidence of OSA: snoring, sleep disruption, obesity, hypertension, and morning headache? Is there a reason to suspect PLMS or RLS? Is there a history of sleep-disturbing paresthesias or a history of sleep-related movement disorder?

5. Inquire about the sleep environment. Is the sleep area conducive to the relaxation required to allow the wake-to-sleep transition? This is a relative concept; for example, a television can be hypnotic for some but stimulating for others.

Occasionally, additional diagnostic studies are required. Some of these studies are part of the medical evaluation. Expanded use of a diary can be of value. A PSG should be considered if OSA or narcolepsy is suspected. A PSG also is helpful in evaluating parasomnia (abnormal sleep-related behavior). Finally, an MSLT can be helpful in documenting hypersomnia or the presence of early onset REM.

Once the evaluation is complete, the clinician can initiate a strategy to address the sleep problem. This approach needs to take the addictive disorder into consideration, because problems underlying the addiction must be addressed and treated. Care must be taken in the selection of medications. Whenever possible, associated medical and/or psychiatric conditions should be treated. Only then can "intrinsic" sleep disorders be treated.

For example, RLS and PLMS can be treated with medications that are not subject to abuse. OSA usually is treated with continuous positive airway pressure devices. Special attention then can be directed to issues of sleep hygiene, including the following:

- The sleep environment should be modified to allow for the relaxation required for the wake-to-sleep transition. It should be separated from work and play areas. Noise and lighting should be modified to allow for optimal relaxation.

- The times at which caffeine, nicotine, alcohol, and other medications are used should be assessed and adjusted as necessary.

- Regular exercise has been found to improve sleep and should be recommended.

- Adoption of a regular sleep-wake schedule should be encouraged. Napping is permissible, but will reduce the need to sleep at night.

■ Finally, the patient needs to be able to separate sleep time from other stressors, allowing for a period of relaxation. The patient should be instructed to leave the bedroom whenever he or she is unable to sleep, so as to avoid the development of further anxiety.

If the patient still has difficulties with sleep, an underlying cause should be sought. Often, the cause is some form of anxiety disorder that requires direct attention. Relaxation techniques are helpful to some patients, as are medications. The usual sedating and/or hypnotic agents can be used for transient problems. However, in working with a patient for whom addiction is an issue, it is wise to consider the sedating antidepressants or the more active agents used to treat other anxiety-related disorders, such as the selective serotonin reuptake inhibitors (SSRIs).

REFERENCES

Adamson J & Berdick JA (1973). Sleep of day alcoholics. *Archives of General Psychiatry* 28:146-149.

Aldrich MS (1993). Sleep disordered breathing in alcoholics: Association with age. *Alcoholism: Clinical & Experimental Research* 17(6):1179-1183.

Aldrich MS & Shipley JE (1993). Alcohol use and periodic limb movements of sleep. *Alcoholism: Clinical & Experimental Research* 17:192-196.

Allen RP, Wagman A & Fallace LA (1971). Electroencephalic (EEG) sleep recovery following prolonged alcohol intoxication in alcoholics. *Journal of Nervous and Mental Disease* 153:424-433.

Allen RP, Wagman AM, Funderburk FR et al. (1980). Slow wave sleep: A predictor of individual responses to drinking? *Biological Psychiatry* 15:345-348.

American Psychiatric Association (APA) (1994). *Diagnostic and Statistical Manual of Mental Disorders, 4th Edition (DSM-IV)*. Washington, DC: American Psychiatric Press.

American Sleep Disorders Association (ASDA) (1992). The clinical use of the Multiple Sleep Latency Test. *Sleep* 15:265-278.

Baker JC & Mitteness LS (1989). Nocturia in the elderly. *Gerontologist* 28:99-194.

Benca RM (2000). Mood disorders. In MH Kryger, T Roth & WC Dement (eds.) *Principles and Practice of Sleep Medicine*. New York, NY: W.B. Saunders.

Berry RB, Bonnet M & Light RW (1992). Effect of ethanol on the arousal response to airway obstruction during sleep in normal subjects. *American Review of Respiratory Disorders* 145:445-452.

Billiwise DL, Clarkson MA & Dement WC (1988). Nightly variation of periodic leg movements in sleep in middle aged and elderly individuals. *Archives of Gerontology Geriatrics* 7:273-279.

Block AJ, Hellard DW & Slayton PC (1985). Minimal effect of alcohol ingestion on breathing during the sleep of postmenopausal women. *Chest* 88:181-184.

Block AJ, Hellard DW & Slayton PC (1986). Effect of alcohol ingestion on breathing and oxygenation during sleep: Analysis of the effects of age and sex. *American Journal of Medicine* 80:595-560.

Bloom JW, Kaltenborn WT & Quan F (1988). Risk factors for a general population for snoring: Importance of smoking and obesity. *Chest* 93:678-683.

Brower KJ, Aldrich MS & Hall JM (1998). Polysomnographic and subjective sleep predictors in alcoholic relapse. *Alcoholism: Clinical & Experimental Research* 22:1864-1877.

Brower KJ, Aldrich MS, Robinson EA et al. (2001). Insomnia, self-medication and relapse to alcoholism. *American Journal of Psychiatry* 158:399-404.

Brugge KL, Kripke DF, Ancoli-Israel S et al. (1989). The association of menopause status and age with sleep disorders. *Sleep Research* 18:208.

Cernovsky Z (1985). MMPI, nightmares in male alcoholics. *Perception and Motor Skills* 61:841-842.

Cernovsky Z (1986). MMPI and nightmare reports in women addicted to alcohol and other drugs. *Perception and Motor Skills* 62:717-719.

Christo G & Franey C (1996). Addicts' drug related dreams: Their frequency and relationship to six-month outcomes. *Substance Use and Misuse* 31:1-15.

Cingnotta F, D'Alessandro R, Partinen M et al. (1989). Prevalence of every night snoring and obstructive sleep apnea among 30 to 69 year old men in Bologna, Italy. *Acta Neurologica Scandinavica* 79:366-372.

Clark CP, Gillin JC, Golshan S et al. (1998). Increased REM density at admission predicts relapse by three months in primary alcoholics with a lifetime history of secondary depression. *Biological Psychiatry* 43:601-607.

Clark CP, Gillin JC, Golshan S et al. (1999). Polysomnography and depressive symptoms in primary alcoholism with and without a lifetime history of secondary depression and inpatients with primary major depression. *Journal of Affective Disorders* 52:177-185.

Cook NR, Evans DA, Funklestein H et al. (1989). Correlates of headache in a population based cohort study of the elderly. *Archives of Neurology* 46:338-344.

Cronin A, Keifer JC & Baghdoyan HA (1995). Opioid inhibition of rapid eye movement sleep by a specific mu receptor agonist. *British Journal of Anaesthesiology* 74:188-192.

Czeisler C, Richardson G & Martin JB (1991). Disorders of sleep and circadian rhythm. In JD Wilson, E Braumwald & A Fauci et al. (eds.) *Principles and Practice of Internal Medicine*. New York, NY: McGraw-Hill.

Davila DG, Hunt RD, Offord KP et al. (1994). Acute effects of transdermal nicotine on sleep architecture, snoring and sleep disordered breathing in non-smokers. *American Journal of Respiratory and Critical Care Medicine* 150:469-474.

Dawson A, Bigby BG, Poceta JS et al. (1997). Effect of bedtime alcohol on inspiratory resistance and respiratory drive in snoring and non-snoring men. *Alcoholism: Clinical & Experimental Research* 21:183-190.

Denizen N (1988). Alcoholic dreams. *Alcoholism Treatment Quarterly* 5:133-139.

Detre DP, Himmelhoch JM, Swartzburg M et al. (1972). Hypersomnia and manic-depressive illness. *American Journal of Psychiatry* 128:1303-1305.

Dolly FR & Block AJ (1983). Increased ventricular ectopy and sleep apnea following ethanol ingestion in COPD patients. *Chest* 83:469-472.

Drummond SPA, Gillin JC & Smith TL (1998). The sleep of abstinent pure primary alcoholic patients: Natural course and relationship to relapse. *Alcoholism: Clinical & Experimental Research* 22:1796-1782.

Easton PA, West PA, Weatherall RC et al. (1987). The effect of excessive ethanol ingestion on sleep in severe chronic obstructive pulmonary disease. *Sleep* 10:224-233.

Edinger JD, McCall WV, Marsh GR et al. (1992). Periodic limb movement variability in older patients across consecutive nights of home monitoring. *Sleep* 15:156-161.

Edinger JD, Morey MC, Sullivan RJ et al. (1993). Aerobic fitness, acute exercise and fitness in older men. *Sleep* 16(4):351-359.

Ehlers CL, Phillips E & Parry BL (1996). Electrophysiological findings during the menstrual cycle in women with and without late luteal phase dysphoric disorder: Relationship to risk for alcoholism? *Biological Psychiatry* 39:720-732.

Feinberg I (1970). Hallucinations, dreaming and REM sleep. In W Kemp (ed.) *Origin and Mechanisms of Hallucinations.* New York, NY: Plenum Publishing, 125-132.

Feinberg I, Hibi S, Caveness C et al. (1974). Sleep amphetamine effects in MBDS and normal subjects. *Archives of General Psychiatry* 31:723-731.

Gillin JC, Landon M, Ruiz C et al. (1994). Dose-dependent effects of transdermal nicotine on early morning awakening and rapid eye movement sleep time in normal nonsmoking volunteers. *Clinical Psychopharmacology* 14:264-267.

Gillin JC, Pulverenti L, Withers N et al. (1994). The effects of lisuride on mood and sleep during acute withdrawal in stimulant abusers: A preliminary report. *Biological Psychiatry* 35:843-849.

Gillin JC, Smith TL & Irwin M (1990). Short REM latency in primary alcoholics with secondary depression. *American Journal of Psychiatry* 147:106-109.

Gillin JC, Smith TL & Irwin M (1994). Increased pressure for rapid eye movement sleep at time of hospital admission predicts relapse in nondepressed patients with primary alcoholism at three month follow up. *Archives of General Psychiatry* 51:189-197.

Gislasen T, Almqvist M, Ericksſen G et al. (1988). Prevalence of sleep apnea among Swedish men. *Journal of Clinical Epidemiology* 41:571-576.

Gislason TH, Aberg H & Taube A (1987). Snoring and systemic hypertension: An epidemiological study. *Acta Medica Scandinavica* 232:415-421.

Guilleminault MD & Stohs R (1991). Upper airway resistance syndrome. *Sleep Research* 20:250-257.

Harsh J, Purvis B, Badia P et al. (1990). Behavioral responses in older adults. *Biological Psychology* 30:51-60.

Hughes JR, Higgins ST & Bickel WK (1994a). Caffeine self-administration, withdrawal and adverse effects among coffee drinkers. *Archives of General Psychiatry* 48:611-617.

Hughes JR, Higgins ST & Bickel WK (1994b). Nicotine withdrawal versus other drug withdrawal syndromes: Similarities and dissimilarities. *Addiction* 89:461-470.

Hyppa MT & Kronholm E (1989). Quantity of sleep and chronic illness. *Journal of Clinical Epidemiology* 42:633-638.

Issa FG & Sullivan CE (1982). Alcohol, snoring and sleep apnea. *Journal of Neurology, Neurosurgery and Psychiatry* 45:353-358.

Javey N, Walters AS, Henning W et al. (1988). Opioid treatment of periodic leg movements in patients without restless legs syndrome. *Neuropeptides* 11:181-184.

Johnson EA, Roehrs T, Roth T et al. (1988). Epidemiology of alcohol and medications as aids to sleep in early adulthood. *Sleep* 21:178-186.

Johnson LC, Burdick JA & Smith J (1970). Sleep during alcohol intake and withdrawal in the chronic alcoholic. *Archives of General Psychiatry* 22:406-418.

Kay D (1975). Human sleep and EEG through a cycle of methadone dependence. *Electroencephalography and Clinical Neurophysiology* 38:35-43.

Kay D, Pickworth W & Neider G (1981). Morphine-like insomnia in nondependent human addicts. *British Journal of Clinical Pharmacology* 11:159-169.

Kelly TL, Miller NM & Bonnet MH (1997). Sleep latency measures of caffeine effects during sleep deprivation. *Electroencephalography and Clinical Neurophysiology* 102:397-400.

Koskenvu M, Kapiro J & Partinen M (1985). Snoring as a risk factor for hypertension and angina pectoris. *Lancet* 1:893-895.

Krol RC, Knuth SL & Bartlett D (1984). Selective reduction of genioglossal muscle activity by alcohol in normal human subjects. *American Review of Respiratory Disorders* 129:247-250.

Landolt HP, Roth C & Dijk DJ (1996). Late afternoon ethanol intake affects nocturnal sleep and the sleep EEG in middle-aged man. *Journal of Clinical Psychopharmacology* 16:428-436.

Lavie P, Ben-Yosef R & Rubin AE (1984). Prevalence of sleep apnea among patients with essential hypertension. *American Heart Journal* 108:373-376.

Le Bon O, Verbanck P & Hoffmann G (1997). Sleep in detoxified alcoholics: impairment of most standard sleep parameters and increased risk for sleep apnea, but not for myoclonus: A controlled study. *Journal of Studies in Alcoholism* 58:30-36.

Lobo LL & Tuffik S (1997). Effect of alcohol on sleep parameters of sleep deprived healthy volunteers. *Sleep* 20:52-59.

Lugaresi E & Partinen M (1994). Prevalence of snoring in sleep and breathing. In N Saunders & CE Sullivan (eds.) *Sleep and Breathing.* New York, NY: Marcel Dekker.

Lunley M, Roehrs T, Asker D et al. (1987). Ethanol and caffeine effects on daytime sleepiness/alertness. *Sleep* 10:306-312.

Lydic R, Keifer JC, Baghdoyen HA et al. (1993). Microanalysis of the pontine reticular formation reveals inhibition of acetylcholine release by morphine. *Anesthesiology* 79:1003-1012.

Mahowald MW & Shenck CH (2000). REM sleep parasomnias. In MH Kryger, T Roth & WC Dement (eds.) *Principles and Practice of Sleep Medicine, 3rd Edition.* New York, NY: W.B. Saunders.

Mellinger GD, Balter MB & Uhlenhuth EH (1985). Insomnia and its treatment: Prevalence. *Archives of General Psychiatry* 42:225-232.

Mello MK & Mendelson JH (1970). Behavioral studies of sleep patterns in alcoholics during intoxication and withdrawal. *Journal of Pharmacology & Experimental Therapeutics* 175:94-112.

Mendelson WB (1987). *Human Sleep: Research and Clinical Care.* New York, NY: Plenum Press.

Mennella JA & Gerish CJ (1998). Effects of exposure to alcohol in mothers' milk on infant sleep. *Pediatrics* 101(5):E2.

Miller M, Dawson A & Henricksen S (1988). Bedtime alcohol increases resistance of upper airways and produces sleep apnea in asymptomatic snorers. *Alcoholism* 12:801-805.

Moore P & Jacobsen L (1991). Periodic limb movements in sleep: Outcome in supranormal young population. *Sleep* 20:300-306.

Morrill MJ, Finn L, Kim H et al. (2000). Sleep fragmentation, awake blood pressure and sleep disordered breathing in a population-based study. *American Journal of Respiratory and Critical Care Medicine* 162:2091-2096.

Mosso S, Dickel MJ & Ashurst J (1988). Night to night variability in sleep apnea and sleep related periodic leg movements in the elderly. *Sleep* 11:340-348.

Nieto FJ, Young TB, Lind KB et al. (2000). Association of sleep disordered breathing, sleep apnea and hypertension in a large community based study. *Journal of the American Medical Association* 283:1829-1836.

Norton PG & Dunn EV (1985). Snoring as a risk factor for disease: An epidemiological survey. *British Medical Journal* 291:630-632.

Papineau KL, Roehrs TA, Petricelli N et al. (1988). Electrophysiological assessment (the multiple sleep latency test) of the biphasic effects of ethanol in humans. *Alcoholism: Clinical & Experimental Research* 22:231-235.

Polamaki H, Partinen M, Erkinjuntti T et al. (1992). Snoring, stroke and the sleep apnea syndrome. *Neurology* 42(Suppl 7):75-82.

Portas CM, Thakkar M, Rainie DG et al. (1997). Role of adenosine in behavioral state modulation: A microdialysis study in the freely moving cat. *Neuroscience* 79:225-235.

Post RM, Gillin JC & Goodwin FK (1970). The effect of orally administered cocaine on sleep of depressed patients. *Psychopharmacology* 37:59-66.

Prosise GL, Bonnet MH & Berry RB (1994). Effect of abstinence from smoking on sleep and daytime sleepiness. *Chest* 105:1136-1141.

Rechtschaffen A & Kales A (1968). *A Method of Standardized Terminology, Techniques and Scoring System for Sleep Stages of Human Subjects.* Los Angeles, CA: Brain Information Series/Brain Research Institute.

Robinson R, White D & Zwilich C (1985). Moderate alcohol ingestion increases upper airway resistance in normal subjects. *Annual Review of Respiratory Diseases* 132:1238-1241.

Roehrs T, Beare D & Zorick F (1994). Sleepiness and ethanol effects on simulated driving. *Alcoholism: Clinical & Experimental Research* 18:154-158.

Rowland RH (1997). Sleep onset rapid eye movement periods in neuropsychiatric disorders: Implications for the pathophysiology of psychoses. *Journal of Nervous and Mental Disorders* 185:730-738.

Rubenstein ML, Rothenberg SA, Maherwarren S et al. (1990). Modified sleep restriction therapy in middle aged and elderly insomniacs. *Sleep Research* 19:276.

Salin-Pascual RJ & Drucker-Colin R (1998). A novel effect of nicotine on mood and sleep in major depression. *Neuroreport* 9:57-60.

Scher GS, Richardson GA, Coble PA et al. (1998). The effects of parental alcohol and marijuana exposure: Disturbances in neonatal sleep cycling and arousal. *Pediatric Research* 24:101-105.

Schmidt-Norwara WW, Coulas DB, Wiggins C et al. (1980). Snoring in an Hispanic-American population: Risk factors and association with systemic hypertension and other morbidity. *Archives of Internal Medicine* 150:587-601.

Scrina L, Broudy M, Nay KN et al. (1982). Increased severity of obstructive sleep apnea after bedtime alcohol ingestion: Diagnostic potential and proposed mechanism of action. *Sleep* 5:318-328.

Shapiro CM, Warren PM, Trinder J et al. (1987). Fitness facilitates sleep. *European Journal of Applied Physiology* 53:1-4.

Silveri NM & Spear LP (1998). Decreased sensitivity to the hypnotic effects of ethanol early in ontogeny. *Alcoholism: Clinical & Experimental Research* 22(3):670-676.

Silveri NM & Spear LP (1999). Ontogeny of rapid tolerance to the hypnotic effects of ethanol. *Alcoholism: Clinical & Experimental Research* 23(7):1180-1184.

Skoloda TE, Alterman AI & Gottheil E (1979). Sleep quality reported by drinking and non-drinking alcoholics. In EL Gottheil (ed.) *Addiction Research and Treatment: Converging Trends.* New York, NY: Pergamon Press, 102-112.

Southwell PR, Evans CR & Hunt JN (1992). The effects of a hot milk drink on movements during sleep. *British Medical Journal* 2:429-433.

Spielman AJ, Sakin P & Thorpy MJ (1987). Treatment of chronic insomnia by restriction of time in bed. *Sleep* 10:145-156.

Staedt J, Wassmuth F, Stoppe G et al. (1996). Effects of chronic treatment with methadone and naltrexone on sleep in addicts. *European Archives of Psychiatry and Clinical Neurosciences* 246:305-309.

Stewart SH (1996). Alcohol abuse in individuals exposed to trauma—A critical review. *Psychological Bulletin* 120:83-112.

Stradling JR (1993). Recreational drugs and sleep. *British Medical Journal* 305:573-575.

Tassan V, Block A & Boysen P (1981). Alcohol increases sleep apnea and oxygen desaturation in asymptomatic men. *American Journal of Medicine* 71:240-245.

Telakivi T, Partinen M, Koskenvuo M et al. (1987). Periodic breathing and hypoxia in snorers and controls: Validation of snoring history and association with blood pressure and obesity. *Acta Neurologica Scandinavica* 76:69-75.

Thompson PM, Gillin JC & Golshan S (1995). Polygraphic sleep measures differentiate alcoholics and stimulant abusers during short-term abstinence. *Biological Psychiatry* 38:831-836.

Thorpy MJ and The Diagnostic Classification Steering Committee (1990). *The International Classification of Sleep Disorders Diagnostic and Coding Manual.* Rochester, MN: American Sleep Disorders Association.

Trzepecz PT, Violette EJ & Sateia MJ (1984). Response to opioids in three patients with restless legs syndrome. *American Journal of Psychiatry* 141:993-995.

Vitello MV (1997). Sleep, alcohol and alcohol abuse. *Addiction Biology* 2:151-158.

Wagman AM, Allen RP, Funderbunk FR et al. (1978). EEG measures of functional tolerance to alcohol. *Biological Psychiatry* 13:719-728.

Walters AS, Wagner ML & Henning WA (1993). Successful treatment of the idiopathic restless legs syndrome in a randomized double-blind trial of oxycodone versus placebo. *Sleep* 16:327-332.

Washington WW, Brown BS & Haertzen CA (1990). Changes in mood, craving and sleep during short term abstinence reported by male cocaine addicts. *Archives of General Psychiatry* 47:861-868.

Wetter DW, Young TB, Bidwell TR et al. (1994). Smoking as a risk factor for sleep-disordered breathing. *Archives of Internal Medicine* 154:2219-2224.

Williams HL & Rundell OH (1981). Altered sleep physiology in chronic alcoholics: Reversal with abstinence. *Alcoholism: Clinical & Experimental Research* 2:318-325.

Williams RL, Karacan I & Hursch CJ (1970). *Electroencephalography of Human Sleep: Clinical Applications.* New York, NY: John Wiley & Sons.

Wolin SJ & Mello JK (1973). The effects of alcohol on dreams and hallucinations in alcohol addicts. *Annals of the New York Academy of Science* 215:266-302.

Yules RB, Lippman ME & Freedman DX (1967). Alcohol administration prior to sleep: The effect on EEG sleep stages. *Archives of General Psychiatry* 16:94-97.

Zepelon H, McDonald CS & Zammit GK (1984). Effect of age on auditory threshold. *Journal of Gerontology* 39:284-300.

Zwyghuizen-Doorenbos A, Roehrs T, Lamphere J et al. (1998). Increased daytime sleepiness enhances ethanol's sedative effects. *Neuropsychopharmacology* 1:279-286.

Zwyghuizen-Doorenbos A, Roehrs T & Timms V (1990). Individual differences in the sedating effects of alcohol. *Alcoholism: Clinical & Experimental Research* 14:400-404.

Chapter 10

Traumatic Injuries Related to Alcohol and Other Drug Use

David A. Fiellin, M.D.
Linda C. Degutis, Dr.P.H.
Gail D'Onofrio, M.D., M.S.

Epidemiology of AOD-Related Injury
Effective Screening in Injured Patients
Interventions With Injured Patients
Incorporating Screening and Brief Intervention Into Practice

Alcohol and other drug (AOD) use contributes to a substantial proportion of injury events, including falls, motor vehicle crashes, assaults, drownings, homicides, and suicides. Research evidence suggests that injured patients who also have alcohol and drug problems suffer more frequent and severe complications than other injured patients. These events, in turn, lead to significant morbidity and mortality, with far-reaching implications for the individual, the family, the workplace, and society.

This chapter discusses the role of alcohol and other drugs in traumatic injury. It also provides data on the effectiveness of screening instruments for patients treated in emergency departments and trauma centers. The clinician's role in identifying the spectrum of alcohol and drug-related problems in injured patients is discussed, as are the components of brief intervention and referral to treatment.

The objective of the chapter is to provide clinicians with the tools required to incorporate screening and brief intervention into practice for this high-risk group of patients, and the motivation to do so. The ultimate goal is to reduce both the risk of injury and the adverse consequences associated with alcohol and other drug use.

Although most of the research done to date relates to alcohol, more articles that discuss other drugs are appearing in the emergency medicine literature, and this research will be referenced throughout the chapter.

EPIDEMIOLOGY OF AOD-RELATED INJURY

Injuries associated with alcohol use present across the entire spectrum of drinking behavior, from moderate social drinking to alcohol dependence. Nearly 50% of cases involving major trauma (Gentilello, Donovan et al., 1995) and 22% of cases involving minor trauma (Degutis, 1998) have been found to be alcohol-related. The proportion of blood alcohol concentrations (BAC) that are positive for intoxication among injured patients presenting at emergency departments ranges from 6% to 34% (Cherpitel, 1993).

Alcohol is a major risk factor for virtually all categories of unintentional and intentional injuries (Freedland, McMicken et al., 1993; Peppiatt, Evans et al., 1978; Lowenstein, Weissberg et al., 1990; Teplin, Abram et al., 1989; Wechsler, Kasey et al., 1969; Cherpitel, 1993; Antti-Poika & Karaharju, 1988; Howland & Hingson, 1987; Hingson, Lederman et al., 1985; Brewer, Morris et al., 1994).

Of the 140,000 to 150,000 deaths that occur in the United States each year as a result of traumatic injuries, a significant proportion are related to use of alcohol or other drugs. Available data demonstrate that alcohol is involved in 40% of fatal motor vehicle crashes, 40% of crashes involving serious injury, and 30% of crashes involving minor injury (U.S. Department of Transportation, 1993). More than 50% of those who are arrested for driving under the influence (DUI) have alcohol problems, and many require medical care for injuries related to motor vehicle crashes. In fact, an arrest for DUI is an independent indicator of risk of death in a future motor vehicle crash (Brewer, Morris et al., 1994). This indicator has been demonstrated to be valid for all age groups, and the association becomes stronger with increased age at the time of DUI arrest.

Data from the 1989 National Health And Nutrition Epidemiologic Survey (NHANES) show that persons who consumed five or more drinks per occasion were twice as likely to die of injuries as nondrinkers, and that consuming nine or more drinks on one occasion increased the risk of injury-related death more than three-fold (Li, Smith et al., 1994).

Other data support the relationship between alcohol and fatal injuries. Injury is the leading cause of death in the U.S. for persons agd one to 44 years (IOM, 1999), while motor vehicle crashes are the leading cause of death for persons age five to 34 years. Almost 40 years ago, Haddon and Bradess (1959) documented that alcohol was a factor in about half of single vehicle crashes. The statistic remains true today, as nearly half of the approximately 35,000 fatal motor vehicle crashes in the U.S. each year are related to alcohol use (U.S. Department of Transportation, 1993). Further, alcohol has been implicated as a factor in 40% of crashes involving serious injury, 30% of crashes involving minor injury, and 10% to 15% of minor crashes. Alcohol is involved in 42% of pedestrian fatalities, 60% of fatal burns (often related to cigarette smoking), and an unknown percentage of work-related injuries and drownings (Wintemute, Teret et al., 1990; Li, Baker et al., 1996). Studies of boating fatalities show that 60% of the victims tested positive for alcohol, and 30% had BACs greater than 100 mg% (Mengert, Sussman et al., 1992).

Alcohol and violence are closely linked. Cherpitel (1993) found that persons older than 30 years who sustained violence-related injuries were more likely to have a positive Breathalyzer® reading, to report drinking before the event, and to report a significant history of alcohol-related problems, as compared with persons who experienced other types of injuries. In a study of adult patients who came to an emergency department for treatment of minor injuries, 6% had positive saliva alcohol tests (SATs) or blood alcohol tests, 9% were positive on at least one question of the CAGE screening questionnaire, and 6% were positive on both the saliva test and the CAGE (Degutis, 1998).

Mannenbach and colleagues (1997) examined the scope of alcohol use in a population of 243 injured adolescents. Using urine tests, they found results positive for alcohol use in 33% of adolescent patients injured in motor vehicle crashes (including 38% of drivers), 37% of patients who attempted suicide, and 44% of assault victims. In another study of adolescents age 12 to 20 years, positive SAT results were found in up to 4% of injured patients who arrived at the emergency department within six hours of injury (Maio, Shope et al., 2000).

A study comparing drinking problems in injured versus noninjured emergency patients documented that injured patients were more likely to test positive for use of alcohol, to report heavy drinking, to report prior alcohol-related injuries, and to report a history of treatment for alcohol problems than were patients who sought treatment for other disorders (Cherpitel, 1999b). This finding was true of patients who were treated in county or community hospital emergency departments, as well as patients who were treated in hospitals affiliated with health maintenance organizations (Cherpitel, 1999b). In another study, daily drinking, binge drinking, and heavy drinking each were associated with increased likelihood of injury as the underlying cause of death (Li, Smith et al., 1994).

Elucidating the specific relationship between alcohol, other drugs, and injuries is difficult for several reasons: (1) few studies have been conducted at the time of injury, (2) there are few standards for reporting data about alcohol and other drug use, (3) alcohol and drug use is underreported on death certificates and hospital discharge data, (4) there is bias in the reporting of alcohol-related deaths, and (5) there is insufficient information on exposure to alcohol and other drugs in control populations (Howland & Hingson, 1987).

In a review of 32 studies of the association between alcohol use and injuries or fatalities from fire and burns, Howland and Hingson (1987) found that nearly half of those who died in fires had BACs above 0.10 and that alcohol was an important risk factor for fire and burn injuries associated with cigarette smoking. In addition, studies conducted to determine the role of alcohol in injuries related to boating and swimming have implicated alcohol as a major risk factor for boating fatalities (Howland, Smith et al., 1993). Work-related injuries, including injuries requiring hospitalization, were found to be more likely in persons who had an average daily intake of five drinks, compared to abstainers, and in those who used psychoactive drugs (Hingson, Lederman et al., 1985). Finally, onset of alcohol use at ages younger than 21 years was associated with experiencing an alcohol-related injury (Hingson, Heeren et al., 2000).

Studies that have compared alcohol consumption in the general population with that of injured patients in the emergency department demonstrate a clear association between alcohol consumption and injury (Borges, Cherpitel et al., 1998; Cherpitel, 1993, 1994a, 1994b). One study found that injured patients presenting at the emergency department were five times more likely to report a higher quantity and frequency of alcohol consumption than were control subjects. In that study, positive screening results and recent alcohol consumption (that is, less than six hours before hospital admission) were associated with an increased risk of injury resulting in an emergency department visit (Borges, Cherpitel et al., 1998).

Data derived from studies that have used probability sampling and that compare the prevalence of alcohol problems in patients with and without violence-related injuries indicate, in 10 of 11 studies, that patients with violence-related injuries were more likely to have positive blood or breath alcohol concentrations than those with nonviolent injuries (Cherpitel, 1994b). However, the prevalence of a positive BAC in injured patients varied considerably across the studies, because of both the method of measurement and decisions about a cutoff value for a positive test result (Cherpitel, 1994b).

Studies of trauma patients examined those patients with more serious injuries and generally excluded patients who had been discharged from the emergency department to home or patients who were admitted to the hospital for treatment of single-system injuries, such as isolated extremity fractures. Many of the studies were conducted as retrospective reviews of blood alcohol testing and were based on clinical algorithms or subjective decisions by physicians to test, which could lead to selection bias in the samples. In one of the few studies that examined substance use disorders in trauma patients, Soderstrom and colleagues (1992) found that 54% of 1,118 adult trauma patients had a life-time history of a substance use disorder. In addition, 24% had a current diagnosis of alcohol dependence and 18% had a current diagnosis of dependence on other drugs.

Medical examiners' reports provide insight into the role of alcohol in deaths resulting from traumatic injuries. A meta-analysis of 331 medical examiner studies found that, in 39% of unintentional deaths resulting from injuries, there was evidence of alcohol intoxication (BAC $\geq$100 mg/dL) (Smith, Branas et al., 1999). A separate analysis of studies published between 1985 and 1991 implicated alcohol in 35% to 63% of fatal falls and in 13% to 37% of nonfatal falls. In addition, alcohol was identified in 21% to 47% of cases involving drowning fatalities and in 12% to 61% of fatalities from burns (Hingson & Howland, 1993). In a study of the role of alcohol in bicycle injuries, persons who died were more likely to have had positive BACs (30% versus 16%) than were those who were injured but did not die (Li, Baker et al., 1996).

The role of cocaine use in injuries or fatalities has been studied less frequently than that of alcohol. One study that employed medical examiners' records found that as many as 25% of those killed in motor vehicle crashes had used cocaine within the 24 hours preceding the crash, and 10% had used cocaine and alcohol in combination (Marzuk, Tardiff et al., 1990). A separate study found that 31% of homicide victims had used cocaine, but failed to find an association between having used cocaine and being killed by a firearm (Tardiff, Marzuk et al., 1994). The association between cocaine use and risk-taking behavior leading to fatal injury was evaluated in a unique examination of deaths in participants playing Russian roulette. Illicit drugs or alcohol were detected in 79% of cases of death resulting from Russian roulette and in 61% of control subjects who committed suicide with a handgun (Marzuk, Tardiff et al., 1992).

An evaluation of 14,842 fatal injuries found evidence of cocaine in 27%. Of these deaths, approximately one-third were the result of drug intoxication, and two-thirds involved traumatic injuries resulting from homicides, suicides, motor vehicle crashes, and falls (Marzuk, Tardiff et al., 1995). Despite these findings, concerns exist that there has been an underestimation of the role of cocaine in injury or fatality based on evidence of underreporting in the federal Drug Abuse Warning Network (DAWN), which collects data on emergency department visits and drug-related deaths (Brookoff, Campbell et al., 1993).

One study of drug use with and without concomitant alcohol use among injured drivers found that 14 (6.6%) of

TABLE 1.   Screening for Alcohol Problems in Injured Patients

Ask the NIAAA quantity and frequency questions:
1. On average, how many days per week do you drink alcohol?
2. On a typical day when you drink, how many drinks do you have?
3. What is the maximum number of drinks you had on any given occasion during the past month?

Use the CAGE (In the past 12 months . . .):
C Have you ever felt you should **C**ut down on your drinking?
A Have people **A**nnoyed you by criticizing your drinking?
G Have you ever felt bad or **G**uilty about your drinking?
E Have you ever had a drink first thing in the morning to "steady your nerves" or get rid of a hangover ("**E**ye opener")?

The screen is positive if:
A positive response on 1 or more questions from the CAGE and/or at-risk consumption.
- Men: >14 drinks/week or >4 drinks/occasion.
- Women and both sexes older than 65 years: >7 drinks/week or >3 drinks/occasion.

Then assess for:
- Medical problems: Blackouts, depression, hypertension, injury, abdominal pain, liver dysfunction, sleep disorders.
- Laboratory tests: Liver function tests, macrocytic anemia.
- Behavioral problems.
- Alcohol dependence.

Intervene
If the patient is an "at-risk drinker":
- Advise the patient of his or her risk.
- Set drinking goals.
- Provide referral to primary care.
If the patient is an alcohol-dependent drinker:
- Assess the acute risk of intoxication or withdrawal.
- Negotiate a referral for detoxification, to Alcoholics Anonymous, and to primary care.

SOURCE: *The Physician's Guide to Helping Patients with Alcohol Problems* (NIH Publication No. 95-3769, 1995). Rockville, MD: National Institute on Alcohol Abuse and Alcoholism.

211 injured drivers tested positive for drugs (amphetamines, barbiturates, benzodiazepines, cocaine, cannabis, and opiates) alone, while 12 (5.7%) of 211 tested positive for alcohol and drugs in combination (Schepens, Pauwells et al., 1998).

EFFECTIVE SCREENING IN INJURED PATIENTS

Principles of Screening. Screening involves the identification of disorders in patients without known disease. It is distinct from case-finding, in which patients for whom there is a high clinical index of suspicion of a disease undergo assessment to confirm the diagnosis. Screening is indicated in disorders that meet the following criteria: (1) the disorder has significant prevalence and consequences in the population, (2) there are effective and acceptable treatments for the disorder, (3) early treatment is preferable to later treatment, (4) screening instruments with good operating characteristics are available, and (5) screening instruments are easily administered. Screening for substance use disorders in patients with traumatic injuries meets all of these criteria.

As the foregoing criteria indicate, screening instruments should have specific characteristics to allow for their use in clinical situations. First among these characteristics is good accuracy in identifying patients with the disorder among all those who are screened. Screening tests that are applied to large groups of patients, many of whom do not have the disease, perform best when they have high sensitivity (a low rate of false negatives) and adequate specificity (a low rate of false positives). Other desirable features include brevity, utility in diverse demographic and clinical populations, and low cost.

Screening for Alcohol Problems in the Emergency Department. Alcohol problems occur across a clinical spectrum in the emergency department. At-risk drinking generally is defined as a threshold amount of alcohol consumption per day or week; typically, it is described as "problem," "heavy," or "excessive" drinking (Fiellin, Reid et al., 2000b). This level of alcohol consumption puts patients at risk for future alcohol-related consequences because of the amount they drink or the effect of alcohol on any comorbid medical conditions. However, at-risk drinking may not be associated with ongoing adverse consequences. In contrast, patients with alcohol abuse or dependence experience significant and repeated negative physical and social effects from their alcohol use, often including the cardinal signs of tolerance and withdrawal (Fiellin, Reid et al.,

2000a). These diagnostic classifications are useful to clinicians because they allow patients to be stratified according to disease severity and are useful in making treatment recommendations. In addition, the classifications affect the choice of a screening tool for use in identifying patients with alcohol problems in the clinical setting.

Studies of screening instruments for alcohol problems in emergency department and trauma settings have focused primarily on the recognition of the most harmful spectrum of alcohol consumption, including alcohol abuse and dependence, and so provide little empirical evidence to guide screening for at-risk drinking. Evidence supports the use of brief, formal screening questionnaires such as the CAGE, TWEAK, or AUDIT (see the Appendix of this text) in preference to clinical recognition or laboratory analyses such as the BAC or SAT (Becker, Woolard et al., 1995; Cherpitel, 1995b, 1995c; Gentilello, Villaveces et al., 1999; Clifford, Sparadeo et al., 1996).

Among the screening questionnaires that have been evaluated in emergency departments, the CAGE, TWEAK, and AUDIT are the best studied (Cherpitel, 1995a, 1998). For patients who met the criteria for alcohol dependence:

- Two positive responses on the CAGE had a sensitivity of 76% to 87% and a specificity of 84% to 90%.

- A score of 3 on the TWEAK had a sensitivity of 84% to 89% and a specificity of 81% to 86%.

- A score of 6 on the MAST had a sensitivity of 30% to 71% and a specificity of 92% to 99%.

- A score of 8 on the AUDIT had a sensitivity of 83% to 91% and a specificity of 81% to 90%.

The first three questions of the AUDIT (which cover quantity, frequency, and intensity of drinking) were shown to have a sensitivity of 97% and a specificity of 65% for harmful or hazardous drinking (Minugh, Nirenberg et al., 1997). In contrast, breath alcohol analysis has been shown to have only limited utility in screening, with a sensitivity of 20% to 28% and a specificity of 94% to 97% (Cherpitel, 1995b, 1998). Blood alcohol analysis was similarly disappointing: one study found that the presence of alcohol dependence and other psychoactive substance use disorders was similar in trauma center patients with positive BACs (76%) and negative BACs (62%) (Soderstrom, Dischinger et al., 1992). The proportion of positive BACs was low even among patients arriving after motor vehicle accidents (Chang & Astrachan, 1988).

In an effort to create a useful and portable screening instrument for alcohol problems in emergency settings, one researcher has combined five questions from the CAGE, TWEAK, and AUDIT to create the Rapid Alcohol Problems Screen (RAPS; Cherpitel, 1995c). One positive response on the RAPS has a sensitivity of 90% to 93% and a specificity of 76% to 78% (Cherpitel, 1995c, 1998). A reduction of the RAPS instrument to four questions (RAPS4) created an instrument with a sensitivity of 93% and a specificity of 87% in one report (Cherpitel, 1995c). Although the RAPS instrument appears promising, the wealth of information on the use of the CAGE plus quantity and frequency questions from the AUDIT make these the preferred screening methods at this time.

The operating characteristics of screening instruments for alcohol problems in emergency settings have been shown to vary with ethnicity, gender, and nature of the alcohol problem. In one study, for example, the CAGE had a sensitivity of 86% in injured African American men and 71% in injured Caucasian men. Similar gender and ethnic variations have been seen in the operating characteristics of the AUDIT, TWEAK, MAST, and RAPS (Cherpitel & Clark, 1995; Cherpitel, 1997, 1999a), although the clinical significance of these variations is not clear. Therefore, clinicians who implement screening programs may need to take racial and gender considerations into account in selecting a screening tool.

Finally, one study found similar rates of compliance with screening when a straightforward screening questionnaire was used, rather than a questionnaire with alcohol questions embedded among questions on diet, smoking status, and exercise (Adams & Stevens, 1994). This suggests that straightforward questioning about alcohol use may be appropriate for some populations.

There are no comparable screening instruments for drug abuse and dependence other than alcohol. One attempt to identify problems is to add an additional question to the CAGE to ask about specific drugs. Most experts believe that the more specific the question, the better the history obtained, and thus recommend asking about specific classes of drugs (Senay, 1997).

INTERVENTIONS WITH INJURED PATIENTS

Alcohol or other drug-related injury provides a unique opportunity for brief intervention (Gentillelo, Donovan et al., 1995; D'Onofrio, Bernstein et al., 1998a). The negative consequences of the injury can create what has been described as a "teachable moment"—a unique opportunity to motivate patients to change their behavior or to encourage them to seek further treatment. Empirical evidence supports the hypothesis that the aversive nature of the injury and perception of the degree of alcohol involvement in an injury event have been shown to be predictive of patients' readiness to change. In a study in an emergency department of patients who were injured in motor vehicle crashes and who had been drinking alcohol, Cherpitel (1996) found that more than a third connected their alcohol use to the injury event.

In addition, the emergency department presents rich opportunities for such interventions, as research shows that a higher proportion of patients in emergency settings than in other settings have alcohol-related problems. One study compared patients from the same metropolitan area who went to an emergency department with those who went to primary care settings and found that the emergency department patients were 1.5 to 3 times more likely to report heavy drinking, negative consequences of drinking, alcohol dependence, or prior treatment for alcohol-related problems than patients in a primary care clinic (Cherpitel, 1999b).

Brief interventions not only can reduce alcohol use, but also the incidence of alcohol-related injuries. A systematic review of the effectiveness of such interventions in preventing injuries evaluated 19 randomized controlled trials and found that treatment for problem drinking was associated with a reduction in suicide attempts, domestic violence, falls, drinking-related injuries, hospitalizations, and deaths (Dinh-Zarr, Diguiseppi et al., 1999). In seven trials that compared interventions with a control group, nearly all showed a decrease in injury-related outcomes. The effect size of these decreases ranged from a 27% reduction in drinking-related injuries to a 65% reduction in accidental and violent deaths. Of note, interventions among convicted drunk drivers reduced the number of motor vehicle crashes and related injuries. It is not clear from this literature, however, if the mechanism of action of the interventions was reduced alcohol consumption or decreased risk-taking (Dinh-Zarr, Diguiseppi et al., 1999).

Brief interventions involve counseling sessions that require 5 to 45 minutes. Such interventions often incorporate the six elements proposed by Miller and Sanchez (1993), which are summarized by the mnemonic FRAMES: **F**eedback, **R**esponsibility, **A**dvice, **M**enu of strategies, **E**mpathy, and **S**elf-efficacy. Other elements that have been shown to

support the efficacy of brief interventions include goal-setting, followup, and timing (Graham & Fleming, 1998).

Multiple studies have demonstrated the efficacy of brief interventions for alcohol problems in a variety of settings (Wilk, Jensen et al., 1997), including general populations (Heather, Champion et al., 1987; Cox, Puddey et al., 1993; Nilssen, 1991), patients in primary care settings (Fleming, Barry et al., 1997; Wallace, Cutler et al., 1988), patients in emergency departments (Wright, Moran et al., 1998; Monti, Colby et al., 1999; Bernstein, Bernstein et al., 1997), and patients presenting at inpatient trauma centers (Gentilello, Rivara et al., 1999). However, the number of studies involving patients with traumatic injuries is small. Wright and colleagues (1998) reported the results of a study of patients who misused alcohol and who received brief interventions from a health worker in a London emergency department. Of 202 patients enrolled, 71 patients completed the six-month followup. Of these, 46 (65%) reported significant reductions in their alcohol consumption.

In Project ASSERT, Bernstein and colleagues (1997) enlisted health promotion advocates to screen and provide counseling and referral for injured and noninjured emergency department patients, most of whom were alcohol- or drug-dependent. Of 7,118 adult patients screened, 2,931 had evidence of alcohol or drug problems; of those, 1,096 were enrolled in the project. Among the 245 patients assessed at 90-day followup, there was a significant reduction in self-reported drug and alcohol use. The results demonstrated a 45% decrease in drug abuse severity score, a 67% reduction in the proportion of subjects reporting use of cocaine or crack, a 62% reduction in the proportion of subjects reporting use of marijuana, a 56% reduction in alcohol use, and a 4% reduction in binge drinking. In addition, more than half the subjects reported that they had acted on a treatment referral.

Two randomized controlled trials have studied the use of brief interventions in injured patients. Gentilello and colleagues (1999) performed a study in patients who met one of the following eligibility criteria: a positive blood alcohol concentration, an elevated gamma-glutamyl transpeptidase (GGT) level, or a positive screen on the Short Michigan Alcoholism Screening Test (SMAST). A total of 366 hospitalized, injured patients were randomized to receive a 30-minute intervention or standard care. The intervention was performed by a psychologist and was followed in one month by a letter that summarized the intervention. When followed up at 12 months, the intervention group was found to have decreased alcohol consumption by an average of 21.8 ± 3.7 drinks per week, compared with a decrease in the control group of 6.7 ± 5.8 drinks per week ($p = 0.03$). The magnitude of the reduction in drinks per week was greater in patients with mild to moderate alcohol problems. At three years, followup found a 47% reduction in injuries that required either emergency department or trauma center admission and a 48% reduction in injuries that required hospital admission.

In another study, brief interventions were shown to decrease alcohol-related consequences in injured adolescents ages 18 to 19 years who presented at an emergency department. Monti and colleagues (1999) divided 74 patients in a randomized manner to receive either brief intervention or standard care. At six-month followup, the brief intervention group had a significantly lower incidence of drinking and driving, traffic violations, alcohol-related injuries, and alcohol-related problems, including trouble with parents, school, friends, dates, or the police. Over the same time period, patients in both groups significantly reduced their alcohol consumption from baseline.

Despite this evidence, emergency physicians (Lowenstein, Weissberg et al., 1990) and trauma surgeons (Gentilello, Donovan et al., 1995) are unlikely to incorporate screening and brief intervention into their practices. Barriers cited include lack of education, time, resources, and reimbursement. Moreover, recent reports underscore that education in the use of formal alcohol and drug screening questionnaires is lacking in emergency medicine residency programs (Krishel & Richards, 1999). On the other hand, evidence shows that residents who are exposed to a structured skills-based educational program do improve their knowledge and performance in screening and brief intervention with patients who have alcohol problems (D'Onofrio, Nadel et al., 2001).

INCORPORATING SCREENING AND BRIEF INTERVENTION INTO PRACTICE

As discussed earlier, screening instruments vary in terms of their effectiveness, availability, ease of administration, and test characteristics (Schorling & Buchsbaum, 1997). In most settings where injured patients are treated, such as emergency departments and trauma centers, time is short, and competing priorities make screening and brief intervention a challenge. Therefore, screens that are short and simple and that can be administered by a variety of providers—

TABLE 2.   Brief Intervention for Injured Patients

Raise the subject:	"I would like to take a few minutes to talk to you about your alcohol use."
Give feedback:	"I am concerned about your drinking. Our screen indicates that you are above what we consider the safe limits of drinking. This level places you at risk for alcohol-related illness, injury, and death."
Compare to norms:	Compare with National Institute of Alcohol Abuse and Alcoholism guidelines for moderate alcohol consumption.
Make a connection:	"Do you see a connection between your visit and your alcohol use?"
Assess readiness to change:	"On a scale of 1 to 10 (1 being not ready and 10 being very ready), how ready are you to change your drinking pattern?"
Develop discrepancy:	"Why not less?"
Elicit a response:	"How does all this sound to you?"
Negotiate a goal:	"What would you like to do?"
Give advice:	"If you stay within the recommended limits (NIAAA guidelines), you will be less likely to experience further illness or injury related to alcohol use. You should never drink and drive."
Summarize, provide agreement form, and primary care followup:	"This is what I heard you say. . . . Thank you for your time."

nurses, physicians, social workers, and health promotion advocates—have a greater chance of being used.

Screening for alcohol problems in injured patients should detect the entire spectrum of use, including at-risk and harmful drinkers, as well as dependent drinkers. Such detection is important because non-dependent drinkers may benefit most from brief intervention and referral to a primary care provider. One screen for alcohol problems that can be adapted to the emergency department and trauma center setting, and which is recommended by the National Institute of Alcohol Abuse and Alcoholism, includes three quantity and frequency questions (to elicit information as to whether the patient exceeded the level recommended for moderate drinking), as well as the CAGE questionnaire (which is better at identifying alcohol dependence; Ewing, 1984). Because the CAGE originally was designed for lifetime prevalence, it is helpful to modify it by specifying "in the past 12 months" (see Table 1).

Asking quantity and frequency questions first, then adding the CAGE questions if the responses exceed moderate levels, is one way to use the screens. Another approach is to jump to the CAGE questions for patients who are intoxicated (as evidenced by very high BACs) or in whom dependence is suspected. This approach eliminates the negative connotations and resistance that can occur when attempting to quantify a patient's drinking.

Brief interventions may include advice only or incorporate some motivational enhancement techniques. For the at-risk drinker or the patient who has sustained an alcohol-related injury but is not alcohol-dependent, setting goals within safe limits, coupled with a referral to the patient's primary care physician, may be all that is needed. For the patient with non-dependent drug use, negotiating abstinence or harm reduction, such as no use while driving, with a referral to primary care may be sufficient. For the patient who is dependent on drugs or alcohol, or the clinician who is uncertain as to where a patient fits on the continuum of alcohol and drug problems, the brief intervention becomes a negotiation process to seek further assessment or referral to a specialized treatment program (D'Onofrio, Bernstein et al., 1998b).

The contents of such a brief intervention are outlined in Table 2. Using this information, the authors recommend that each institution develop a program and resource list tailored to the needs of its own community.

ACKNOWLEDGMENT: Dr. Fiellin is supported by the National Institute on Drug Abuse Physician Scientist Award (NIDA grant No. K12 DA00167) and is a Robert Wood Johnson Generalist Physician Faculty Scholar.

REFERENCES

Adams PJ & Stevens V (1994). Are emergency department patients more likely to answer alcohol questions in a masked health questionnaire? *Alcohol and Alcoholism* 29(2):193-197.

Antti-Poika I & Karaharju E (1988). Heavy drinking and accidents—A prospective study among men of working age. *Injury* 19(3):198-200.

Becker B, Woolard R & Nirenberg T (1995). Alcohol use among subcritically injured emergency department patients. *Academic Emergency Medicine* 2(9):784-790.

Bernstein E, Bernstein J & Levenson S (1997). Project ASSERT: An ED-based intervention to increase access to primary care, preventive services, and the substance abuse treatment system. *Annals of Emergency Medicine* 30(2):181-189.

Borges G, Cherpitel CG, Medina-Mora M et al. (1998). Alcohol consumption in emergency room patients and the general population: A population-based study. *Alcoholism: Clinical & Experimental Research* 22(9):1986-1991.

Brewer RD, Morris PD, Cole TB et al. (1994). The risk of dying in alcohol-related automobile crashes among habitual drunk drivers. *New England Journal of Medicine* 331(1):513-517.

Brookoff D, Campbell EA & Shaw L (1993). The underreporting of cocaine-related trauma: Drug abuse warning network reports vs. hospital toxicology tests. *American Journal of Public Health* 83(3):369-371.

Chang G & Astrachan BM (1988). The emergency department surveillance of alcohol intoxication after motor vehicle accidents. *Journal of the American Medical Association* 260(17):2533-2536.

Cherpitel CJ (1993). Alcohol and injuries: A review of international emergency room studies. *Addiction* 88(7):923-937.

Cherpitel CJ (1994a). Alcohol and casualties: A comparison of emergency room and coroner data. *Alcohol and Alcoholism* 29(2):211-218.

Cherpitel CJ (1994b). Alcohol and injuries resulting from violence: A review of emergency room studies. *Addiction* 89(2):157-165.

Cherpitel CJ (1995a). Analysis of cut points for screening instruments for alcohol problems in the emergency room. *Journal of Studies on Alcohol* 56(6):695-700.

Cherpitel CJ (1995b). Screening for alcohol problems in the emergency department. *Annals of Emergency Medicine* 26:158-166.

Cherpitel CJ (1995c). Screening for alcohol problems in the emergency room: A rapid alcohol problems screen. *Drug and Alcohol Dependence* 40(2):133-137.

Cherpitel CJ (1996). Drinking patterns and problems and drinking in the event: An analysis of injury by cause among casualty patients. *Alcoholism: Clinical & Experimental Research* 20(6):1130-1137.

Cherpitel CJ (1997). Comparison of screening instruments for alcohol problems between black and white emergency room patients from two regions of the country. *Alcoholism: Clinical & Experimental Research* 21(8): 1391-1397.

Cherpitel CJ (1998). Differences in performance of screening instruments for problem drinking among blacks, whites and Hispanics in an emergency room population. *Journal of Studies on Alcohol* 59(4):420-426.

Cherpitel CJ (1999a). A brief screening instrument for problem drinking in the emergency room: The RAPS4 Rapid Alcohol Problems Screen. *Journal of Studies on Alcohol* 61(3):447-449.

Cherpitel CJ (1999b). Drinking patterns and problems: A comparison of two black primary care samples in two regions. *Alcoholism: Clinical & Experimental Research* 23(3):523-527.

Cherpitel CJ (1999c). Gender, injury status and acculturation differences in performance of screening instruments for alcohol problems among U.S. Hispanic emergency department patients. *Drug and Alcohol Dependence* 53(2):147-157.

Cherpitel C & Clark W (1995). Ethnic differences in performance of screening instruments for identifying harmful drinking and alcohol dependence in the emergency room. *Alcoholism: Clinical & Experimental Research* 22(9):1986-1991.

Clifford PR, Sparadeo F, Minugh A et al. (1996). Identification of hazardous/harmful drinking among subcritically injured patients. *Academic Emergency Medicine* 3(3):239-245.

Cox KL, Puddey IB, Morton AR et al. (1993). The combined effects of aerobic exercise and alcohol restriction on blood pressure and serum lipids: A two-way factorial study in sedentary men. *Journal of Hypertension* 11(1):191-201.

Degutis LC (1998). Screening for alcohol problems in emergency department patients with minor injury: Results and recommendations for practice and policy. *Contemporary Drug Problems* 25(3):463-475.

Dinh-Zarr T, Diguiseppi C, Heitman E et al. (1999). Preventing injuries through interventions for problem drinking: A systematic review of randomized controlled trials. *Alcohol and Alcoholism* 34(4):609-621.

D'Onofrio G, Bernstein E, Bernstein J et al. (1998a). Patients with alcohol problems in the emergency department, part 1: Improving detection. SAEM Substance Abuse Task Force. Society for Academic Emergency Medicine. *Academic Emergency Medicine* 5(12):1200-1209.

D'Onofrio G. Bernstein E, Bernstein J et al. (1998b). Patients with alcohol problems in the emergency department, part 2: Intervention and referral. SAEM Substance Abuse Task Force. Society for Academic Emergency Medicine. *Academic Emergency Medicine* 5(12):1210-1217.

D'Onofrio G, Nadel ES, Degutis LC et al. (2001). [abstract] *Academic Emergency Medicine* 8:491.

Ewing JA (1984). Detecting alcoholism: The CAGE questionnaire. *Journal of the American Medical Association* 252:1905-1907.

Fiellin DA, Reid MC & O'Connor P (2000b). Screening for alcohol problems in primary care: A systematic review. *Archives of Internal Medicine* 160(13):1977-1989.

Fiellin DA, Reid MC & O'Connor PG (2000a). Outpatient management of patients with alcohol problems. *Annals of Internal Medicine* 133(10):815-827.

Fleming MF, Barry KL, Manwell LB et al. (1997). Brief physician advice for problem alcohol drinkers. A randomized controlled trial in community-based primary care practices. *Journal of the American Medical Association* 277(13):1039-1045.

Freedland ES, McMicken DB & D'Onofrio G (1993). Alcohol and trauma. *Emergency Medicine Clinic of North America* 3:225-339.

Gentilello LM, Donovan DM, Dunn CW et al. (1995). Alcohol interventions in trauma centers. Current practice and future directions. *Journal of the American Medical Association* 274(13):1043-1048.

Gentilello LM, Rivara FP, Donovan DM et al. (1999). Alcohol interventions in a trauma center as a means of reducing the risk of injury recurrence. *Annals of Surgery* 230(4):473-483.

Gentilello LM, Villaveces A, Ries R et al. (1999). Detection of acute alcohol intoxication and chronic alcohol dependence by trauma center staff. *Journal of Trauma, Injury, Infection and Critical Care* 47(6):1131-1139.

Graham AW & Fleming MS (1998). Brief interventions. In AW Graham, TK Schultz & BB Wilford (eds.) *Principles of Addiction Medicine, Second Edition*. Chevy Chase, MD: American Society of Addiction Medicine, 615-630.

Haddon W & Bradess VA (1959). Alcohol in the single vehicle fatal accident. *Journal of the American Medical Association* 169:1587-1593.

Heather N, Champion PD, Neville RG et al. (1987). Evaluation of a controlled drinking minimal intervention for problem drinkers in general practice (the DRAMS scheme). *Journal of the Royal College of General Practitioners* 37(301):358-363.

Hingson R & Howland J (1993). Alcohol and non-traffic unintended injuries. *Addiction* 88(7):877-883.

Hingson RW, Heeren T, Jamanka A et al. (2000). Age of drinking onset and unintentional injury involvement after drinking. *Journal of the American Medical Association* 284(12):1527-1533.

Hingson RW, Lederman RI & Walsh DC (1985). Employee drinking patterns and accidental injury: A study of four New England states. *Journal of Studies on Alcohol* 46(4):298-303.

Howland RW & Hingson R (1987). Alcohol as a risk factor for injuries of death due to fires and burns: Review of the literature. *Public Health Report* 102:475-483.

Howland J, Smith GS, Manglone T et al. (1993). Missing the boat on drinking and boating. *Journal of the American Medical Association* 270(1):91-92.

Institute of Medicine (IOM), Committee on Trauma Research (1999). *Injury in America: A Continuing Public Health Problem*. Washington DC: National Academy Press.

Krishel S & Richards CF (1999). Alcohol and substance abuse training for emergency medicine residents: A survey of U.S. programs. *Academic Emergency Medicine* 6(9):964-966.

Li G, Smith GS & Baker SP (1994). Drinking behavior in relation to cause of death among U.S. adults. *American Journal of Public Health* 84(9):1402-1406.

Li G, Baker S, Sterling S et al. (1996). A comparative analysis of alcohol in fatal and nonfatal bicycling injuries. *Alcoholism: Clinical & Experimental Research* 20(9):1553-1559.

Lowenstein S, Weissberg M & Terry D (1990). Alcohol intoxication, injuries and dangerous behaviors—And the revolving emergency department door. *Journal of Trauma* 30:1252-1257.

Maio RF, Shope JT, Blow FC et al. (2000). Adolescent injury in the emergency department: Opportunity for alcohol interventions? *Annals of Emergency Medicine* 35(3):252-257.

Mannenbach MS, Hargarten SW & Phelan MB (1997). Alcohol use among injured patients aged 12 to 18 years. *Academic Emergency Medicine* 4(1):40-44.

Marzuk PM, Tardiff K, Leon A et al. (1990). Prevalence of recent cocaine use among motor vehicle fatalities in New York City. *Journal of the American Medical Association* 263(2):250-256.

Marzuk PM, Tardiff K, Smyth K et al. (1992). Cocaine use, risk taking, and fatal Russian roulette. *Journal of the American Medical Association* 267(19):2635-2637.

Marzuk PM, Tardiff K, Leon A et al. (1995). Fatal injuries after cocaine use as a leading cause of death among young adults in New York City. *New England Journal of Medicine* 332(26):1753-1757.

Mengert P, Sussman ED & DiSario R (1992). A study between the risk of fatality and blood alcohol concentration of recreational boat operators (Report CG-D-09-92). Washington, DC: U.S. Coast Guard.

Miller WR & Sanchez VC (1993). Motivating young adults for treatment and lifestyle change. In G Howard (ed.) *Issues in Alcohol Use and Misuse in Young Adults.* Notre Dame, IN: University of Notre Dame Press.

Minugh PA, Nirenberg TD, Clifford P et al. (1997). Analysis of alcohol use clusters among subcritically injured emergency department patients. *Academic Emergency Medicine* 4(11):1059-1067.

Monti PM, Colby SM, Barnett NP et al. (1999). Brief intervention for harm reduction with alcohol-positive older adolescents in a hospital emergency department. *Journal of Consulting and Clinical Psychology* 67(6):989-994.

Nilssen O (1991). The Trömso Study: Identification of and a controlled intervention on a population of early-stage risk drinkers. *Preventive Medicine* 20(1):518-528.

Peppiatt R, Evans R & Jordan P (1978). Blood alcohol concentrations of patients attending an accident and emergency department. *Resuscitation* 6(1):37-43.

Schepens PJ, Pauwels A, Van Damme V et al. (1998). Drugs of abuse and alcohol in weekend drivers involved in car crashes in Belgium. *Annals of Emergency Medicine* 31(5):633-637.

Schorling JB & Buchsbaum DG (1997). Screening for alcohol and drug abuse. *Medical Clinics of North America* 81:845-865.

Senay ED (1997). Diagnostic interview and mental status examination. In JH Lowinson, P Ruiz, RB Millman et al. (eds.) *Substance Abuse: A Comprehensive Textbook.* Baltimore, MD: Williams & Wilkins, 364-377.

Smith GS, Branas CC & Miller TR (1999). Fatal nontraffic injuries involving alcohol: A metaanalysis. *Annals of Emergency Medicine* 33(6):659-668.

Soderstrom CA, Dischinger PC, Smith GS et al. (1992). Psychoactive substance dependence among trauma center patients. *Journal of the American Medical Association* 267(20):2756-2759.

Tardiff K, Marzuk PM, Leon A et al. (1994). Homicide in New York City. Cocaine use and firearms. *Journal of the American Medical Association* 272(1):43-46.

Teplin LA, Abram KM & Michaels SK (1989). Blood alcohol level among emergency room patients: A multivariate analysis. *Journal of Studies on Alcohol* 50(5):441-447.

U.S. Department of Transportation (DOT), National Highway Traffic Safety Administration (1993). *Alcohol Involvement in Fatal Crashes.* Springfield, VA: National Technical Information Service.

Wallace P, Cutler S & Haines A (1988). Randomized controlled trial of general practitioner intervention in patients with excessive alcohol consumption. *British Medical Journal* 297(9):663-668.

Wechsler H, Kasey EH, Thum D et al. (1969). Alcohol level and home accidents. *Public Health Report* 84(12):1043-1050.

Wilk AI, Jensen NM & Havighurst TC (1997). Meta-analysis of randomized control trials addressing brief interventions in heavy alcohol drinkers. *Journal of General Internal Medicine* 12(5):274-283.

Wintemute GJ, Teret SP, Kraus JF et al. (1990). Alcohol and drowning: An analysis of contributing factors and a discussion of criteria for case selection. *Accident Prevention* 22(3):291-296.

Wright S, Moran L, Meyrick M et al. (1998). Intervention by an alcohol health worker in an accident and emergency department. *Alcohol and Alcoholism* 33(6):651-656.

Chapter 11

Surgical Interventions in the Alcohol- or Drug-Using Patient

Daniel P. Alford, M.D., M.P.H.

Perioperative Care of the Alcohol-Dependent Patient
Perioperative Care of the Opioid-Dependent Patient
Perioperative Care of the Benzodiazepine-Dependent Patient
Perioperative Care of the Nicotine-Dependent Patient
Perioperative Care of the Cocaine-Dependent Patient
Organ Transplantation in Addicted Patients

Addiction specialists, medical consultants, and surgeons all play critical roles in the interplay between acute and chronic substance use disorders and perioperative risk. Many of the complications of drug and alcohol use require surgical treatment, including traumatic injuries; infections of the skin, soft tissue, bones and joints; hepatic failure; and certain malignancies. Active substance abuse and associated chronic medical conditions can increase the risk of perioperative morbidity. In a retrospective study of 352 patients with traumatic mandibular fractures, two-thirds of whom had a history of alcohol or drug abuse, investigators found that the rate of postoperative complications (including wound infections and poor healing) was five times greater in the addicted patients than in the nonusers (Passeri, Ellis et al., 1993).

Hospitalized patients with substance use disorders are at high risk for acute abstinence syndromes, which may present as postoperative delirium, agitation, insomnia, depression, or seizures. Therefore, it is important for providers of perioperative assessment and care to be comfortable with the diagnosis and management of the abstinence syndromes associated with major drugs of abuse.

Preoperative evaluation may appear deceptively simple in this patient population, as the patients tend to be younger and without known chronic illnesses. However, careful evaluation may detect clinical signs of chronic disease secondary to alcohol and drug abuse; collectively, these increase surgical risk, including the risk of cardiomyopathy; renal, liver, and pancreatic insufficiency; and pulmonary disease. In addition, the physiological stress associated with surgery may unmask subclinical comorbidities that were not obvious during routine preoperative evaluation. For example, reviews describe decreases in cardiac, immune, and hemostatic functions in patients who are heavy drinkers of alcohol (Spies, Tonnesen et al., 2001; Tonnesen, 1992).

This chapter focuses on perioperative issues associated with alcohol and substance use disorders, highlighting important management considerations.

PERIOPERATIVE CARE OF
THE ALCOHOL-DEPENDENT PATIENT

Approximately 7% of the U.S. population report heavy alcohol use, defined as more than five drinks a day on more than five days in a week. This prevalence is even higher in the population seen in medical settings; for example, in one study, 14% of patients in a urology practice, 21% in general surgery, 28% in orthopedics, and 43% in otolaryngology reported heavy alcohol use (Moore, Bone et al., 1989).

Chronic alcohol use increases the risk of postoperative morbidity through immune suppression, reduced cardiac function, and dysregulated homeostasis, including alterations in platelet production and aggregation, and changes in fibrinogen levels (Spies, Tonnesen et al., 2001). Alcohol withdrawal syndrome, which is common in hospitalized patients with alcoholism, is extremely dangerous during the perioperative period. Therefore, preoperative screening for alcohol use and withdrawal risk is critical.

Preoperative Evaluation. Preoperative evaluation of the alcohol-dependent patient requires a complete history and physical examination. The focus should be on the risk of acute alcohol withdrawal and the presence of diseases associated with alcohol abuse. Unfortunately, physicians often fail to identify alcohol abuse in medical patients (Kitchens, 1994). In one study, only 35% of patients with chronic alcoholism were identified by attending staff (Spandorfer, 1998), and only 16% were identified in a perioperative setting (Spies, Neumann et al., 1995).

When screening for alcohol abuse, it is important to remember that problem drinkers often underreport their consumption by up to a third (Andreasson, Allebeck et al., 1990). Quantity and frequency questions are essential, as are laboratory tests, but neither is sensitive or specific. Validated questionnaires such as the CAGE are good tools, but focus on the consequences of drinking and may remain positive in patients who are in recovery (Ewing, 1984). The CAGE mnemonic refers to the following questions:

C Have you ever felt that you should **C**ut down on your drinking?

A Have people **A**nnoyed you by criticizing your drinking?

G Have you ever felt bad or **G**uilty about drinking?

E Have you ever taken a drink first thing in the morning (**E**ye-opener) to steady your nerves or get rid of a hangover?

Two or more positive responses have a sensitivity of 74% to 78% and a specificity of 76% to 96% and therefore are highly suggestive of alcohol abuse or dependence (Mayfield, McLeod et al., 1974; Schorling & Buchsbaum, 1997). Findings in the patient history that suggest alcohol

abuse include traumatic injuries, marital and legal problems, homelessness, and "blackout" episodes (Chiang, 1995).

It also is important to evaluate for risk of acute alcohol withdrawal. The spectrum of withdrawal ranges from mild tremor through hallucinosis to seizures and *delirium tremens*. In the postoperative period, withdrawal can mimic many postoperative complications, including acute pain and sepsis. The incidence of alcohol withdrawal in hospitalized patients overall is as high as 8%; it is two to five times higher in hospitalized trauma and surgical patients (Spies, Tonnesen et al., 2001; Foy & Kiay, 1995).

Factors associated with severe and prolonged alcohol withdrawal include amount and duration of alcohol use, prior withdrawal episodes, recurrent detoxifications, older age, and comorbid diseases (Saitz, 1995). It is important to assess for other drug abuse as well, as many patients with alcohol abuse admit to polysubstance abuse involving benzodiazepines and cocaine. The physical examination should evaluate for evidence of alcoholic liver, as well as pancreatic, nervous system, and cardiac disease. The spectrum of alcoholic liver disease ranges from fatty liver with mild elevations in liver function tests, to acute hepatitis, to cirrhosis. Clinical evidence of cirrhosis includes jaundice, palmar erythema, gynecomastia, testicular atrophy, spider telangiectases, as well as findings consistent with high portal pressures, such as splenomegaly, ascites, hemorrhoids, and caput medusa (dilatation of the periumbilical veins on the abdominal wall). Pancreatitis can present as acute and chronic abdominal pain, as well as exocrine and endocrine dysfunction.

Alcohol-associated dementia occurs in approximately 9% of individuals with alcoholism (Eklund, 1996). Korsakoff's syndrome, hepatic and Wernicke's encephalopathy, myelopathies, and polyneuropathies are other nervous system disorders associated with alcohol dependence. These neurological conditions can worsen during the perioperative period and may be confused with other postoperative neurological complications. Therefore, preoperative assessment of baseline mental status and cognition should be completed and documented. Preoperative evaluation for congestive heart failure secondary to alcohol-associated cardiomyopathy also should be completed, as up to a third of patients with long-standing alcohol abuse have a decrease cardiac ejection fraction (Regan, 1990).

In view of the association between alcohol and nicotine dependence, smoking-related comorbidities such as coronary heart disease and chronic obstructive pulmonary disease (COPD) also should be considered. In one series, up to 20% of patients with alcoholism were found to have coexisting COPD (Frost & Siedel, 1990).

Preoperative laboratory studies should include electrolytes, liver function and synthetic studies, coagulation studies, and a complete blood count. Anemia is common in patients with alcoholism, as are decreased platelet number and function.

Preexisting anemia may need to be treated preoperatively because such patients are at increased risk of perioperative bleeding secondary to coagulopathies and thrombocytopenia (Lindenbaum, 1992). Preoperative identification of patients in recovery from alcoholism also is important because they may have concerns and questions about perioperative exposure to sedative-hypnotics and opioid analgesics, and the risk of relapse such drugs may pose.

Management of Withdrawal. Withdrawal is among the most common complications in hospitalized patients with alcoholism. Up to 15% of alcoholic patients who do not receive treatment for acute withdrawal will develop seizures and/or *delirium tremens* (Saitz & O'Malley, 1997). The spectrum of withdrawal ranges from minor symptoms of sympathetic overdrive to life-threatening *delirium tremens* (which occurred in 20% of the alcoholics admitted to a surgical service [Glickman & Herbsman, 1968]). Withdrawal symptoms may appear within hours of the last drink, although administration of sedatives and analgesics in the perioperative period may delay the onset of withdrawal symptoms for up to 14 days (Spandorfer, 1998). Recognizing withdrawal risk and treating early withdrawal often prevents the complications of severe withdrawal.

Goals for the management of alcohol withdrawal include treatment of withdrawal symptoms, prevention of initial and recurrent seizures, and prevention and treatment of *delirium tremens* (Saitz & O'Malley, 1997). (Refer to Section 5 for a detailed discussion of alcohol withdrawal.)

Because alcohol withdrawal is particularly dangerous during the postoperative period, asymptomatic but at-risk patients should receive prophylactic treatment. Benzodiazepines, especially those with a long half-life (such as diazepam or chlordiazepoxide) are the drugs of choice for the prevention and management of alcohol withdrawal (Mayo-Smith, 1997). The exception is patients with severe liver disease, who should receive a short-acting agent such as lorazepam in order to avoid excessive and prolonged sedation.

Treatment of withdrawal should be based on the severity of symptoms and signs. A validated tool, the Clinical Institute Withdrawal Assessment Scale for Alcohol, Revised (CIWA-Ar; see the Appendix of this text), can be used to rate the severity of alcohol withdrawal. This 10-item scale can be completed rapidly and easily at the bedside.

Alcohol Use and Surgical Risk. In addition to alcohol withdrawal, alcohol use increases the risk of surgical morbidity. Numerous observational studies have demonstrated that alcohol use in the absence of clinical liver disease is an independent risk factor for postoperative complications. In various studies, higher rates of postoperative complications were seen in alcohol users after transurethral prostatectomy, colonic surgery, and hysterectomy (Tonnesen, Schutten et al. 1988, 1987; Felding, Jensen et al., 1992). There seems to be a dose-response effect, with increased alcohol consumption associated with increased rates of postoperative complications and prolonged hospital stays. The most dramatic escalations in rates of complications were seen in groups who drank more than 60 grams of alcohol (four drinks) per day (Tonnesen & Kehlet, 1999). The complications reported were not secondary to alcohol withdrawal, but instead were related to infection, bleeding, and delayed wound healing. In a prospective study of patients admitted for colorectal surgery, Tonnesen and colleagues (1992) also found an increase in postoperative arrhythmias, while Klatsky (1995) found that active alcohol use was associated with hypertension. Alcoholic patients have longer stays in intensive care units, higher rates of postoperative septicemia and pneumonia requiring mechanical ventilation, and increased overall mortality (Jensen, Dragsted et al., 1988; Spies, Nordmann et al., 1996).

Tonnesen has identified five possible pathological mechanisms to account for the increased postoperative complications: (1) immune incompetence, (2) subclinical cardiac insufficiency, (3) hemostatic imbalances, (4) an abnormal stress response, and (5) wound healing dysfunction (Tonnesen, 1992; Spies, Tonnesen et al., 2001). Chronic alcohol use suppresses T cell-dependent activity and decreases macrophage, monocyte, and neutrophil mobilization and phagocytosis; however, this immune dysfunction is reversible with abstinence (Tonnesen & Kehlet, 1999).

The decreased cardiac function associated with chronic alcohol use is thought to be secondary to direct alteration in the electromechanical coupling and contractility of cardiac myocytes. Such alcohol-associated cardiac dysfunction may be reversible, with 50% of patients showing improvement after six months' abstinence (LaVecchia, Bedogni et al., 1996).

Hemostatic dysfunction in alcoholics results from a modification in coagulation and fibrinolysis pathways, as well as a reduction in the number and function of platelets (Tonnesen & Kehlet, 1999), while wound healing problems seem to be related to poor accumulation of collagen (Tonnesen & Kehlet, 1999).

Abstinence before surgery decreases postoperative morbidity. Tonnesen, Rosenberg and colleagues (1999) preoperatively randomized adult subjects who consumed at least five drinks a day and who were scheduled for elective colorectal surgery. One group maintained abstinence for one month prior to surgery, while the other group received usual care. There were fewer complications in the abstinent group than in the usual care group (although there were no differences in length of stay or mortality). This is the first study to demonstrate that preoperative abstinence can lead to improved postoperative outcomes.

Alcoholic Liver Disease. The spectrum of liver disease associated with alcohol ranges from asymptomatic fatty liver after binge drinking to acute hepatitis to cirrhosis in the alcoholic. Each form of liver disease carries its own surgical risk and requires special preoperative consideration.

Alcoholic Fatty Liver: Alcoholic fatty liver (hepatic steatosis) occurs in 90% of heavy drinkers and often is asymptomatic and reversible. It can occur after binge or "social" drinking. Signs and symptoms include nausea, vomiting, and right upper quadrant pain and tenderness. Laboratory tests often disclose a mild elevation in liver transaminases, but with preserved liver function and normal bilirubin, albumin, and coagulation. These signs and symptoms usually resolve with two weeks' abstinence (Ordorica & Nace, 1998). There are no known studies evaluating perioperative risk in such patients. However, it would be prudent to delay elective surgery until clinical signs and symptoms have resolved and, if possible, abstinence is achieved.

Alcoholic Hepatitis: Alcoholic hepatitis, a serious inflammatory disease of the liver, occurs in up to 40% of heavy drinkers. The pathological mechanisms involved include hepatocyte swelling, liver infiltration with polymorphonuclear cells, and hepatocyte necrosis. Patients often present in an extremely ill state, with nausea, vomiting, anorexia, abdominal pain, fever, and jaundice. Elevated transaminases and prolonged coagulation studies are common. Surgical risk is very high in this group, with 100% mortal-

ity rates in some series (Greenwood, Leffler et al., 1972; Patel, 1999). Therefore, alcoholic hepatitis should be considered a contraindication to elective surgery, which should be delayed until clinical and laboratory parameters normalize (sometimes requiring up to 12 weeks).

Alcoholic Cirrhosis: Cirrhosis, which occurs in 15% to 20% of heavy drinkers, refers to irreversible necrosis, nodular regeneration, and fibrosis of the liver. It involves abnormal hepatic circulation, resulting in portal hypertension. Clinically, patients may present with ascites, peripheral edema, poor nutritional status, muscle wasting, coagulopathies, gastrointestinal bleeding from esophageal varices, encephalopathy, and renal insufficiency, as well as hypoxia secondary to hepatopulmonary syndrome and pulmonary hypertension. Indications for surgery are common in patients with cirrhosis, up to 10% of whom require a surgical procedure during the last two years of life (Patel, 1999). Depending on the stage of cirrhotic disease, surgery can be extremely risky. The most common causes of perioperative mortality in cirrhotic patients are sepsis, hemorrhage, and hepatorenal syndrome (Wong, Rappaport et al., 1994).

Although modern anesthetic agents are not hepatotoxic, surgical stress in itself causes hemodynamic changes in the liver. Postoperative elevations in liver function tests are not uncommon in patients with no underlying liver disease (Friedman & Maddrey, 1987). Patients with underlying liver dysfunction are at increased risk for hepatic decompensation in response to surgical stress, as anesthetic agents decrease hepatic blood flow by as much as 50% and thus decrease hepatic oxygen uptake (Cowan, Jackson et al., 1991). Intraoperative traction on abdominal viscera also may decrease hepatic blood flow.

Effect of Cirrhosis on Surgical Risk: Surgery in patients with cirrhosis is a high-risk undertaking. The preoperative factors associated with increased surgical morbidity and mortality include emergent surgery, upper abdominal surgery, poor hepatic synthetic function, anemia, ascites, malnutrition, and encephalopathy (Grimm, Almounajed et al., 1998). Cirrhotic patients are at increased risk for uncontrolled bleeding, infections, and delirium. Coagulopathies and thrombocytopenia result in difficult perioperative hemostasis. Ascites increases the risk of intra-abdominal infections, abdominal wound dehiscence, and abdominal wall herniation. Nutritional deficiencies result in poor wound healing and an increased risk of skin breakdown, while encephalopathy impairs the patient's ability to participate effectively in postoperative rehabilitation. The

TABLE 1.   Pugh Classification (Modified Child and Turcotte Classification)

	Points		
	1	**2**	**3**
Encephalopathy (grade)	None	1-2	3-4
Ascites	Absent	Slight	Moderate
Bilirubin (mg/dl)	1-2	2-3	>3
Albumin (g/dl)	>3.5	2.8-3.5	<2.8
Coagulopathy			
Prothombin time (seconds prolonged or	1-4	4-6	>6
International normalized ratio (INR)	<1.7	1.7-2.3	>2.3
Class A	5-6 points		
Class B	7-9 points		
Class C	10-15 points		

SOURCES: Adapted from Pugh RNH, Murray-Lyon IM, Dawson JL et al. (1973). Transection of the oesophagus for bleeding oesophageal varices. *British Journal of Surgery* 60:646-649; and Patel T (1999). Surgery in the patient with liver disease. *Mayo Clinic Proceedings* 74:593-599.

action of anesthetic agents may be prolonged and increases the risk of delirium.

Cholecystectomy is a particularly risky surgery in patients with cirrhosis and portal hypertension because intra-abdominal collateral circulation increases the vascularity of the gallbladder bed and places the patient at greater risk for severe perioperative hemorrhage. In a group of patients with cirrhosis who underwent cholecystectomy, those considered decompensated preoperatively by the presence of ascites and prolonged coagulation studies had a 83% morality rate, compared to 10% in compensated patients (Aranha, Sontag et al., 1982).

In assessing risk preoperatively, it is important to look for clinical signs of cirrhosis and portal hypertension. Use of the Child and Turcotte Classification, a multivariate clinical assessment tool, facilitates such assessment by stratifying patients into three classes according to "hepatic reserve" (Child & Turcotte, 1964). Class A is the most compensated and Class C the most decompensated. Variables include laboratory values for bilirubin and albumin, as well

as clinical ascites, encephalopathy, and nutritional status. Garrison and colleagues (1984) found good correlation between the Child and Turcotte Class and abdominal surgical morality. For Classes A, B, and C, mortality rates were 10%, 31%, and 76%, respectively (Garrison, Cryer et al., 1984). Limitations of the Child and Turcotte Classification scheme include the subjective nature and interobserver variation in the assessment of nutritional status, encephalopathy, and ascites. In addition, there was variability in the assignment of patients to classes A, B, and C, and no method of accounting for the nature and urgency of the surgical procedure.

In an attempt to decrease the subjective nature of the classification scheme, Pugh and colleagues modified the Child and Turcotte Classification (Pugh, Murray-Lyon et al., 1973; see Table 1). The Pugh modification separates hepatic encephalopathy into five grades, according to various signs and symptoms (Table 2). The subjective evaluation of nutritional status is changed to objective measured prolongation in prothrombin time and the assignment of class

---

TABLE 2.   Encephalopathy Grade

Grade 0:   Normal

Grade I: Consists of personality changes with altered sleep patterns (for example, sleep-wake reversal) and inappropriate behavior, constructional apraxia.

Grade II: Consists of mental confusion, disorientation to time and place, drowsiness, asterixis and fetor hepaticus.

Grade III: Consists of severe mental confusion, stuporous but arousable state, incoherent, asterixis, fetor hepaticus, rigidity, and hyperreflexia.

Grade IV: Consists of deep coma, unresponsive to stimuli, not arousable, decerebrate and decorticate posturing, fetor hepaticus, decreased muscle tone and decrease reflexes.

SOURCE: Adapted from Trey C, Burns DG & Saunders SJ (1966). Treatment of hepatic coma by exchange blood transfusion. *New England Journal of Medicine* 274:473-481.

---

based on a total point score. Using pooled surgical data, the Pugh classification scheme has proved a useful method of stratifying preoperative risk (Table 3).

Preoperative Considerations in Patients with Cirrhosis: Preoperative abstinence should be the goal before all elective procedures. Since coagulopathies may develop as a result of vitamin K deficiency secondary to malnutrition or intestinal bile salt deficiency, attempts at correction should begin with administration of vitamin K. The absence of improvement after 12 hours suggests decreased hepatic production of coagulation factors, so perioperative use of fresh frozen plasma (FFP) should be considered. Thrombocytopenia secondary to bone marrow suppression, hypersplenism, and splenic sequestration should be treated with prophylactic platelet transfusions when counts fall below 20,000/mm³ (Patel, 1999). In addition, units of packed red blood cells should be on hold in the blood bank. Ascites secondary to portal hypertension and hypoalbuminemia can impede abdominal wall healing, increase the risk of abdominal wall dehiscence and herniation, and restrict effective mechanical ventilation. Therefore, ascites should be managed preoperatively with sodium restriction and appropriate diuretic therapy. In patients with peripheral edema, a more aggressive approach involving large-volume paracentesis (≥5 liters) should be considered. Electrolytes should be monitored closely.

Perioperative hemodynamic monitoring often is needed, as these patients may have large fluid shifts, especially during abdominal surgeries.

Preoperative broad-spectrum antibiotics should be considered as prophylaxis against secondary and spontaneous bacterial peritonitis. Renal function should be monitored closely, as perioperative changes in volume status and hemodynamics may adversely affect renal function, placing patients at risk for renal insufficiency secondary to prerenal azotemia as well as developing hepatorenal syndrome. Any potential nephrotoxic agent (such as aminoglycoside antibiotics) should be used with extreme caution. Nonsteroidal anti-inflammatory drugs (NSAIDs) should be avoided if possible. Many perioperative conditions can exacerbate hepatic encephalopathy, including gastrointestinal bleeding, constipation, azotemia, hypoxia, and the use of sedatives (Grimm, Almounajed et al., 1998). Aggressive preoperative treatment of hepatic encephalopathy, using lactulose and dietary protein restriction, is recommended. Patients with known gastroesophageal varices should be monitored closely for gastrointestinal bleeding and should be considered for beta-blocker prophylaxis preoperatively.

The nutritional status of alcoholic patients typically is poor, with deficiencies in folate, B vitamins (including thiamine), and vitamin C. Nutritional status should be optimized preoperatively with multivitamins, thiamine, folate, and nutritional supplementation.

From a pulmonary standpoint, decompensated cirrhotics may desaturate due to the development of pulmonary shunts in hepatopulmonary syndrome, so monitoring oxygen saturation should be part of postoperative care.

Class-specific general operability is shown in Table 4.

PERIOPERATIVE CARE OF THE OPIOID-DEPENDENT PATIENT

There are more than 900,000 heroin-addicted persons in the U.S. (ONDCP, 2000), and they are at high risk for medical complications, which frequently require surgical intervention. Most of these complications are a consequence of both active and past high-risk behaviors, such as injection drug use (intravenous, intramuscular, or subcutaneous ["skin popping"]) and the direct toxic effects of the drugs and additives being injected. Infections of the skin, soft tissue, bones, and joints often require surgical drainage and/or debridement. Infectious endocarditis may require emergent or urgent heart valve replacement. Functional bowel obstruction may require surgical management. Chronic hepatitis C infection is the leading cause of liver transplantation (Koch & Banys, 2001). Chronic diseases associated with opioid abuse, such as pulmonary hypertension secondary to talc granulomatosis, renal insufficiency secondary to heroin-associated nephropathy, and congestive heart failure from valvular heart disease secondary to endocarditis, human immunodeficiency virus (HIV) syndrome, and chronic hepatitis B and C, all increase surgical risk. Acute opioid withdrawal complicates the perioperative period.

Preoperative Evaluation. Hospitalized patients with active opioid abuse are at risk for acute withdrawal. The onset and severity of withdrawal depend on the degree of physical dependence, which is related to the duration and amount used. Daily use for at least three weeks generally is required before significant physical dependence (and thus clinically significant withdrawal) occurs (Kleber, 1999; also see Section 5 for a complete discussion of opioid withdrawal).

Heroin withdrawal typically begins within four to six hours of the time of last use. Withdrawal from long-acting opioids such as sustained release oxycodone (OxyContin®), morphine (MsContin®), and methadone may not begin for up to 24 to 36 hours. Active opioid use can be verified through urine toxicology tests, while injection drug use can be identified by examining the skin for "track marks." Heroin and other semisynthetic opioids may be detected as morphine or codeine in the urine for up to 72 hours. Synthetic opioids (such as methadone, meperidine, and fentanyl) are not usually included in standard urine toxicology screens, so if synthetic opioid abuse is suspected, the laboratory should be asked to test for the specific synthetic opioid of concern. Depending on the opioid of abuse, acute withdrawal usually peaks at two to three days and may persist for up to 14 days. Gossop (1990) has developed a useful opioid withdrawal assessment instrument.

Patients who are addicted to heroin also may be addicted to other drugs, such as cocaine or crack, alcohol, or benzodiazepines; these should be the subject of inquiry and laboratory testing (Joseph, Stancliff et al., 2000).

TABLE 3.	Pugh Class and Operative Mortality Risk
Pugh Class A:	2% to 10%
Pugh Class B:	6% to 31%
Pugh Class C:	20% to 76%

SOURCES: Adapted from Garrison RN, Cryer HM, Howard DA et al. (1984). Clarification of risk factors for abdominal operations in patients with hepatic cirrhosis. *Annals of Surgery* 199:648-655; and Friedman LS (1993). When patients with liver disease need surgery. *Internal Medicine* July:25-34.

Management of Opioid Withdrawal. It is important for providers of perioperative care to be able to recognize and manage acute opioid withdrawal, which is likely in hospitalized opioid-dependent surgical patients. One approach to treating opioid withdrawal in the hospital setting involves treating the physiologic manifestations of acute withdrawal (including the hyperadrenergic signs and symptoms, insomnia, and muscles aches) with clonidine, benzodiazepines, and NSAIDs. Depending on the patient's blood pressure, clonidine 0.1 to 0.2 mg orally every four to six hours is given for the first 48 to 72 hours, with a gradual taper over the next 48 to 72 hours. A much more effective method employs a long-acting opioid agonist such as methadone. A starting dose of 20 to 30 mg of methadone orally lessens the signs and symptoms of withdrawal in most patients. The patient should be reassessed for continued withdrawal in two to three hours; if withdrawal symptoms persist, additional doses of 5 to 10 mg may be given, up to a total dose not to exceed 40 mg in 24 hours. Once a stable dose has been achieved, it should be given daily to prevent the re-emergence of withdrawal. If the patient is NPO during the perioperative period, he or she should receive 40% of the dose parenterally every 12 hours (for example, 40 mg po QD = 16 mg IM Q12 hours). Once acute withdrawal is controlled, discussions regarding daily dose taper versus continued daily dose until the day of discharge (as well as postoperative addiction treatment aftercare and referral) should be discussed.

Management of Patients on Opioid Substitution Therapy. Approximately 180,000 patients are maintained on opioid substitution therapy in the U.S., using methadone

TABLE 4. Pugh Class and Operability

Pugh Class A: No limitation;
Normal response to all operations;
Normal ability of liver to regenerate.

Pugh Class B: Some limitation in liver function;
Altered response to all operations but
good tolerance with preparation.

Pugh Class C: Severe limitation of liver function;
Poor response to all operations
regardless of preparation.

SOURCE: Stone JJ (1977). Preoperative and postoperative care. *Surgical Clinics of North America* 57:409-419.

or LAAM (levo-alpha-acetylmethadol) (Doherty, 1999; also see Section 6 for a detailed discussion of opioid substitution therapy). Such patients should be maintained on their usual maintenance dose during the perioperative period, which should be determined by calling the patient's addiction treatment program. If the patient is NPO during the perioperative period, he or she should receive 40% of the dose parenterally every 12 hours (for example, 40 mg PO QD = 16 mg IM Q12 hours). The patient's addiction treatment program should be notified at the time the patient is discharged from the hospital to assure continuity of addiction care.

Some patients with complicated postoperative courses, who have impaired ability to ambulate postoperatively, may be eligible for "medical" take-home doses of methadone. However, because each clinic has its own policies and procedures on take-home doses, the discharging provider should discuss this possibility with the treatment programs's clinical staff.

Management of Postoperative Pain in Patients on Opioid Substitution Therapy. Acute postoperative pain management in patients maintained on long-acting opioid replacement therapy is challenging. The daily methadone dose a patient receives is not adequate analgesia for acute pain. Even though methadone, an opioid agonist, is an excellent analgesic, patients do not derive sustained analgesia from methadone maintenance. The lack of analgesia occurs because of the patient's high tolerance to opioids and methadone's pharmacodynamics. All methadone-maintained patients have a high tolerance to methadone and other opioids (cross-tolerance). Cross-tolerance has been demonstrated clinically by the inability of methadone-maintained patients to distinguish between 20 mg of IV morphine and IV normal saline (Payte, 1997). Cross-tolerance likely is the reason that methadone-maintained patients often require higher and more frequent doses of opioid analgesics to adequately treat an acutely painful condition.

Although methadone is a powerful synthetic opioid analgesic with a long plasma half-life (15 to 40 hours), its duration of action differs for analgesia (4 to 8 hours) and for suppression of opioid withdrawal (24 hours) (Reisine & Pasternak, 1996). Because the majority of patients on methadone maintenance for heroin addiction are dosed every 24 hours, the potential for even partial relief of pain is small.

It also is important to avoid using mixed opioid agonist-antagonists such as pentazocine, butorphanol, and nalbuphine for pain relief, because they will precipitate acute withdrawal in methadone-maintained patients. Therefore, patients on opioid replacement therapy who are in acute pain should be maintained on their long-acting opioid and, if needed, should receive additional opioid analgesics for pain, often at higher doses and at shorter dosing intervals.

PERIOPERATIVE CARE OF THE BENZODIAZEPINE-DEPENDENT PATIENT

Benzodiazepines, which are commonly prescribed to treat anxiety, panic attacks, and insomnia, also have a high abuse potential. Patients who abuse benzodiazepines often are addicted to multiple drugs (Gold, Miller et al., 1995). Some studies have found that up to 15% of heroin users and 41% of alcoholics also abuse benzodiazepines (DuPont, 1988; Ciraulo, Sands et al., 1988). Therefore, patients with addictive disorders should be asked about benzodiazepine use.

Chronic benzodiazepine use results in physical dependence, with an acute withdrawal syndrome that can be life-threatening. The withdrawal syndrome ranges from severe anxiety, insomnia, and autonomic hyperactivity (including tachycardia and hypertension) to seizures and delirium.

Patients with physical dependence to benzodiazepines should be maintained on their usual dose during the perioperative period to prevent acute withdrawal and subsequent postoperative complications. (See Section 5 for a detailed discussion of benzodiazepine withdrawal.)

PERIOPERATIVE CARE OF
THE NICOTINE-DEPENDENT PATIENT

Postoperative pulmonary complications are common in patients who smoke, even in the absence of chronic lung disease (Wightman, 1968). Asymptomatic smokers have abnormalities in their respiratory epithelium and therefore are at increased risk of pulmonary infections (Chalon, Tayyab et al., 1975). A 20 pack-year history and smoking more than 20 cigarettes a day seems to be the threshold for increased risk. In observational studies of patients undergoing cardiothoracic surgery, the increased risk decreases only after eight weeks of smoking cessation and was unrelated to changes on pulmonary function tests (Warner, Offord et al., 1989).

Preoperative evaluation should include assessment of physical dependence on nicotine and the risk of withdrawal. In addition, preoperative evaluation should include assessment for evidence of chronic obstructive pulmonary disease (COPD). Patients with COPD have a threefold increased risk of postoperative pulmonary complications, including pneumonia (Jackson, 1988). Other risk factors for pulmonary complications include increased age, duration and anatomic location of surgery, and preoperative sputum production. It is important to assess for upper respiratory infections and to treat with preoperative antibiotics as indicated.

Elective procedures should be delayed until any pulmonary infection is resolved.

Providers of preoperative care should encourage smoking cessation. Pharmacotherapy, including nicotine replacement and bupropion, consistently increases abstinence rates and should be considered preoperatively (see Section 6 for a discussion of pharmacotherapy for nicotine dependence). Aggressive perioperative treatment of airflow obstruction is achieved with inhaled steroids and beta agonists. Preoperative patient education regarding postoperative incentive spirometry use decreases the incidence of pulmonary complications following surgery (Jackson, 1988). Nicotine replacement therapy also should be offered postoperatively to patients with nicotine dependence or at risk for nicotine withdrawal.

PERIOPERATIVE CARE OF
THE COCAINE-DEPENDENT PATIENT

In federal surveys, approximately three million Americans reported using cocaine at least once in the preceding year (SAMHSA, 1998). Cocaine may be taken orally, intranasally, or intravenously. Intravenous use of cocaine results in all the complications attributable to injection drug use, such as endocarditis, pulmonary hypertension, hepatitis B and C, and HIV disease.

Smoking crack and free-base cocaine can produce both acute and chronic pulmonary disorders, including pulmonary edema. Acute cocaine intoxication can be a life-threatening condition because of excessive adrenergic stimulation resulting in hypertensive crisis, cardiac arrhythmias, sudden cardiac death, seizures, intracranial hemorrhage, and acute psychosis. Cocaine also causes vasoconstriction, which may result in bowel ischemia and gangrene, myocardial infarction, and cerebrovascular accident.

The period of cocaine intoxication generally is brief (approximately 60 minutes) and does not increase the risk of most surgeries. However, long-term cocaine use can result in chronic medical conditions, which do increase surgical risk. Such conditions include pulmonary fibrosis, accelerated coronary artery disease, and cardiomyopathies. Up to 7% of asymptomatic chronic cocaine users have left ventricular systolic dysfunction (Bertolet, Freund et al., 1990). In addition, long-term cocaine use causes left ventricular hypertrophy, a known risk factor for ventricular arrhythmias (Lange & Hillis, 2001). Therefore, it is critically important to identify cocaine use during preoperative assessment and to evaluate carefully for clinical evidence of pulmonary and cardiac disease in cocaine users. Concurrent use of cocaine and alcohol are common, so all patients who use cocaine should be screened for concurrent alcohol abuse.

Depression and hypersomnolence are common in cocaine withdrawal and may mimic and be confused with postoperative neurologic complications.

ORGAN TRANSPLANTATION
IN ADDICTED PATIENTS

Hepatitis C infection from injection drug use and alcoholic liver disease are the most common causes of end-stage liver disease requiring liver transplantation in the U.S. Historically, patients with histories of addictive disorder have been kept off transplantation lists because of fears of post-transplant noncompliance, with subsequent loss of the graft, but also because of moralistic arguments that the patients had "self-inflicted" diseases.

In fact, some studies have demonstrated post-transplant relapse rates as high as 49%, with lower overall survival rates in patients who failed to complete addiction treatment (Stowe & Kotz, 2001). Other studies found no difference in one-year survival rates between alcoholic patients who maintained sobriety and patients who had no history of alcohol abuse (Starzl, Van et al., 1988). A recent survey of U.S. liver transplantation programs found that most accept applicants with histories of alcohol or drug abuse, but only 56% accept patients who are receiving methadone maintenance treatment. In fact, some programs had policies requiring discontinuation of methadone maintenance before transplantation, which directly contradicts clinical evidence supporting this form of treatment in opioid-addicted patients (Koch & Banys, 2001).

It is clear that patients with a history of addictive disorders need to be assessed for risk of relapse and social support systems before being accepted for transplantation. Because organ transplantation in patients with addictive disorders is unusually complex, some medical centers have added addiction specialists to the transplant team (Stowe & Kotz, 2001).

CONCLUSIONS

Patients with addictive disorders have high rates of hospitalization and surgery. The underlying history of addiction may not be apparent initially, but thorough history-taking and the use of effective screening tools can elicit information about past or current drug and alcohol abuse. Because of the high prevalence of polydrug abuse, patients who acknowledge an addiction to one substance should be asked about all other substances of abuse. Careful evaluation also can detect clinical signs of chronic diseases of the heart, lungs, and liver related to drug and alcohol abuse.

The importance of identifying addictive disorders preoperatively cannot be overstated. Perioperative morbidity associated with acute abstinence syndromes can be prevented with proper preoperative treatment. If possible, elective surgery should postponed to allow time for complete detoxification.

Sedative-hypnotics and opioid analgesics should be used as indicated postoperatively; however, these drugs have a significant abuse potential in patients with a history of addictive disorders, so they should be prescribed with caution.

Patients with active addiction should be encouraged to engage in addiction treatment postoperatively.

REFERENCES

Andreasson S, Allebeck P & Romelsjo A (1990). Hospital admission for somatic care among young men: The role of alcohol. *British Journal of Addiction* 85:935-941.

Aranha GV, Sontag SJ & Greenlee HB (1982). Cholecystectomy in cirrhotic patients: A formidable operation. *American Journal of Surgery* 143:55-60.

Bertolet BD, Freund G, Martin CA et al. (1990). Unrecognized left ventricular dysfunction in an apparently health cocaine abuse population. *Clinical Cardiology* 13:323-328.

Chalon J, Tayyab MA & Ramanathan S (1975). Cytology of respiratory epithelium as a predictor of respiratory complications after operation. *Chest* 67:32-35.

Chiang PP (1995). Perioperative management of the alcohol-dependent patient. *American Family Physician* 52(8):2267-2273.

Child CG & Turcotte JG (1964). Surgery and portal hypertension. In CG Child (ed.) *The Liver and Portal Hypertension*. Philadelphia, PA: W.B. Saunders, 1-85.

Ciraulo DA, Sands BF & Shader RI (1988). Critical review of liability for benzodiazpine abuse among alcoholics. *American Journal of Psychiatry* 145:1501-1506.

Cowan RE, Jackson BT, Grainger SL et al. (1991). Effects of anesthetic agents and abdominal surgery on liver blood flow. *Hepatology* 14:1161-1166.

Darton LA & Dilts SL (1998). Opioids. In RJ Frances & SI Miller (eds.) *Clinical Textbook of Addictive Disorders, 2nd Edition*. New York, NY: Guilford Press, 150-167.

Doherty B (1999). Association identifies greater numbers in methadone treatment. *American Methadone Treatment Association News Report*; December.

DuPont RL (1988). Abuse of benzodiazepines—The problems and the solutions. A report of a Committee of the Institute for Behavior and Health, Inc. *American Journal of Drug and Alcohol Abuse* 14(Suppl 1):1-69.

Eklund J (1996). Alcohol abuse and postoperative complications: Do we ask the right questions? *Acta Anaesthesiologica Scandinavica* 40(6):647-648.

Ewing JA (1984). Detecting alcoholism: The CAGE questionnaire. *Journal of the American Medical Association* 252:1905-1907.

Felding C, Jensen LM & Tonnesen H (1992). Influence of alcohol intake on postoperative morbidity after hysterectomy. *American Journal of Obstetrics and Gynecology* 166:667-670.

Foy A & Kiay J (1995). The incidence of alcohol-related problems and the risk of alcohol withdrawal in a general hospital population. *Drug and Alcohol Review* 14:49-54.

Friedman LS (1993). When patients with liver disease need surgery. *Internal Medicine* July:25-34.

Friedman LS & Maddrey WC (1987). Surgery in the patient with liver disease. *Medical Clinics of North America* 71:453-476.

Frost EA & Siedel MR (1990). Preanesthetic assessment of the drug abuse patient. *Anesthesiology Clinics of North America* 8:829-842.

Garrison RN, Cryer HM, Howard DA et al. (1984). Clarification of risk factors for abdominal operations in patients with hepatic cirrhosis. *Annals of Surgery* 199:648-655.

Glickman L & Herbsman H (1968). Delirium tremens in surgical patients *Surgery* 64:882.

Gold MS, Miller NS, Stennie K et al. (1995). Epidemiology of benzodiazepine use and dependence. *Psychiatric Annals* 25:146-148.

Gossop M (1990). The development of a Short Opiate Withdrawal Scale (SOWS). *Addictive Behavior* 15:487-490.

Greenwood SM, Leffler CT & Minkowitz S (1972). The increased mortality rate of open liver biopsy in alcoholic hepatitis. *Surgery in Gynecology and Obstetrics* 134:600-604.

Grimm IS, Almounajed G & Friedman LS (1998). Management of the surgical patient with liver disease. In GJ Merli & HH Weitz (eds.) *Medical Management of the Surgical Patient, 2nd Edition*. Philadelphia, PA: W.B. Saunders Company, 193-213.

Jackson MCV (1988). Preoperative pulmonary evaluation. *Archives of Internal Medicine* 148:2120-2127.

Jensen NH, Dragsted L, Christensen JK et al. (1988). Severity of illness and outcome in alcoholic patients in the intensive care unit. *Intensive Care Medicine* 15:19-22.

Joseph H, Stancliff S & Langrod J (2000). Methadone maintenance treatment (MMT): A review of historical and clinical issues. *Mt. Sinai Journal of Medicine* 67:347-364.

Kitchens JM (1994). Does this patient have an alcohol problem? *Journal of the American Medical Association* 272:1782-1787.

Klatsky AL (1995). Blood pressure and alcohol intake. In JH Laragh & BM Brenner (eds.) *Hypertension: Pathophysiology, Diagnosis, and Management, 2nd Edition*. New York, NY: Raven Press, 2649-2667.

Kleber HD (1999). Pharmacologic management of opioid withdrawal. In *Optimizing the Treatment and Management of Substance Abuse and Addiction (CME Monograph Series)*. San Antonio, TX: Dannemiller Memorial Education Foundation.

Koch M & Banys P (2001). Liver transplantation and opioid dependence. *Journal of the American Medical Association* 285(8):1056-1058.

Lange RA & Hillis LD (2001). Cardiovascular complications of cocaine use. *New England Journal of Medicine* 345:351-358.

LaVecchia LL, Bedogni F, Bozzola L et al. (1996). Prediction of recovery after abstinence in alcoholic cardiomyopathy: Role of hemodynamic and morphometric parameters. *Clinical Cardiology* 19:45-50.

Lindenbaum J (1992). Alcohol and the hematologic system. In CS Leiber (ed.) *Medical and Nutritional Complications of Alcoholism*. New York, NY: Plenum Publishing, 241-281.

Mayo-Smith MF (1997). Pharmacological management of alcohol withdrawal. A meta-analysis and evidence-based practice guideline. *Journal of the American Medical Association* 278:144-151.

Mayfield D, McLeod G & Hall P (1974). The CAGE questionnaire: Validation of a new alcoholism screening instrument. *American Journal of Psychiatry* 131:1121-1123.

Moore RD, Bone LR, Geller G et al. (1989). Prevalence, detection, and treatment of alcoholism in hospitalized patients. *Journal of the American Medical Association* 261:403-407.

Office of National Drug Control Policy (ONDCP) (2000). *National Drug Control Strategy, 2000*. Washington, DC: ONDCP, Executive Office of the President, The White House.

Ordorica PI & Nace EP (1998). Alcohol. In RJ Frances & SI Miller (eds.) *Clinical Textbook of Addictive Disorders, 2nd Edition*. New York, NY: Guilford Press, 91-119.

Passeri LA, Ellis E & Sinn DP (1993). Relationship of substance abuse to complications with mandibular fractures. *Journal of Oral and Maxillofacial Surgeons* 51:22-25.

Patel T (1999). Surgery in the patient with liver disease. *Mayo Clinic Proceedings* 74:593-599.

Payte JT (1997). Clinical take homes. *Journal of Maintenance in the Addictions* 1(2):103-104.

Pugh RNH, Murray-Lyon IM, Dawson JL et al. (1973). Transection of the oesophagus for bleeding oesophageal varices. *British Journal of Surgery* 60:646-649.

Regan TJ (1990). Alcohol and the cardiovascular system. *Journal of the American Medical Association* 264:377-381.

Reisine T & Pasternak G (1996). Opioid analgesics and antagonists. In JG Harman, A Goodman Gilman & LE Limbird (eds.) *The Pharmacological Basis of Therapeutics 9th Edition*. New York, NY: McGraw-Hill.

Saitz R (1995). Recognition and management of occult alcohol withdrawal. *Hospital Practice* 30(6):49-58.

Saitz R & O'Malley SS (1997). Pharmacotherapies for alcohol abuse: Withdrawal and treatment. *Medical Clinics of North America* 81(4):881-908.

Schorling JB & Buchsbaum D (1997). Screening for alcohol and drug abuse. *Medical Clinics of North America* 81(4):845-866.

Spandorfer J (1998). The patient with substance abuse going to surgery. In GJ Merli & HH Weitz (eds.) *Medical Management of the Surgical Patient, 2nd Edition*. Philadelphia, PA: W.B. Saunders, 255-262.

Spies C, Neumann T, Muller C et al. (1995). Preoperative evaluation of alcohol dependent patients admitted to the intensive care unit following surgery. *Alcoholism: Clinical & Experimental Research* (Suppl 2)19:55A.

Spies CD, Nordmann A, Brummer G et al. (1996). Intensive care unit stay is prolonged in chronic alcoholic men following tumor resection of the upper digestive tract. *Acta Anaesthesiologica Scandinavica* 40.

Spies C, Tonnesen H, Andreasson S et al. (2001). Perioperative morbidity and mortality in chronic alcoholic patients. *Alcoholism: Clinical & Experimental Research* 25(5):164S-170S.

Starzl TE, Van TD, Tzakis AG et al. (1988). Orthotopic liver transplantation for alcoholic cirrhosis. *Journal of the American Medical Association* 260(17):2542-2544.

Stone JJ (1977). Preoperative and postoperative care. *Surgical Clinics of North America* 57:409-419.

Stowe J & Kotz M (2001). Addiction medicine in organ transplantation. *Progress in Transplantation* 11(1):50-57.

Substance Abuse and Mental Health Services Administration (SAMHSA) (1999). *National Household Survey on Drug Abuse: 1998*. Rockville, MD: SAMHSA, Office of Applied Studies Publication Series.

Tonnesen H (1992). Influence of alcohol on several physiological functions and its reversibility: A surgical view. *Acta Psychiatria Scandinavica* 86:67-71.

Tonnesen H & Kehlet H (1999). Preoperative alcoholism and postoperative morbidity. *British Journal of Surgery* 86:869-874.

Tonnesen H, Schutten BT & Jorgensen BB (1987). Influence of alcohol on morbidity after colonic surgery. *Diseases of the Colon and Rectum* 30:549-551.

Tonnesen H, Schutten BT, Tollund L et al. (1988). Influence of alcoholism on morbidity after transurethral prostatectomy. *Scandinavian Journal of Urology and Nephrology* 22:175-177.

Tonnesen H, Petersen KR, Hojgaard L et al. (1992). Postoperative morbidity among symptom-free alcohol misusers. *Lancet* 340:334-337.

Tonnesen H, Rosenberg J, Nielsen HJ et al. (1999). Effect of preoperative abstinence on poor postoperative outcome in alcohol misusers: Randomized controlled trial. *British Medical Journal* 318:1311-1316.

Trey C, Burns DG & Saunders SJ (1966). Treatment of hepatic coma by exchange blood transfusion. *New England Journal of Medicine* 274:473-481.

Warner MA, Offord KP, Warner ME et al. (1989). Role of preoperative cessation of smoking and other factors in postoperative pulmonary complications: A blinded prospective study of coronary artery bypass patients. *Mayo Clinic Proceedings* 64:609-616.

Wightman JA (1968). A prospective survey of the incidence of postoperative pulmonary complications. *British Journal of Surgery* 55:85-91.

Wong R, Rappaport W, Witte C et al. (1994). Risk of nonshunt abdominal operation in the patient with cirrhosis. *Journal of the American College of Surgeons* 179:412-416.

| Chapter 12 | # Endocrine and Reproductive Disorders Related to Alcohol and Other Drug Use |

Alan Ona Malabanan, M.D., FACE

The endocrine effects of alcohol and other drugs are complex. These substances can alter the secretion of hormone-releasing factors and hormones at the level of the hypothalamus and pituitary; alter the synthesis or release of hormones at the level of the thyroid, adrenal, or pancreas; alter hormone action on target organs; and alter hormone economy by affecting their metabolism or binding proteins. Multiple hormone systems can be affected, many of whose actions may conflict, leading to a lack of net clinical effect. When one adds to this inherent complexity the effects on the endocrine system of gender, mental status, and mental illness, the heterogeneity of illicit drugs, the prevalence of polydrug use, and differences between the effects of acute and chronic substance use, it becomes clear that the study of the endocrine effects of alcohol and other drugs is very difficult. Generalizing many of these effects to clinical practice is even more difficult. Therefore, the most clearly recognized and clinically relevant effects are summarized in this chapter (Table 1).

DISORDERS RELATED TO ALCOHOL

Hypoglycemia. One of the most serious consequences of alcohol abuse is hypoglycemia, which can lead to neuro-logic damage, coma, seizures, or death. Alcohol causes hypoglycemia by producing malnutrition, reducing the body's production of glucose, and impairing the body's response to hypoglycemia. Although hypoglycemia is an uncommon complication of alcoholism, alcohol use is a common cause of spontaneous hypoglycemia (Marks & Teal, 1999).

Unlike other drugs, ethyl alcohol is a significant source of energy, with 7.1 kcal per gram (Lieber, 1997). Malnutrition can result from alcohol abuse, as nutrients are replaced by the "empty" calories of alcohol. In addition, the normal metabolism of alcohol to acetaldehyde by alcohol dehydrogenase leads to the conversion of nicotinamide adenine dinucleotide (NAD) to its reduced form (NADH), resulting in a decrease in gluconeogenesis. NAD is a cofactor necessary for many of the reactions involved in glucose synthesis. Alcohol does not affect glucose release from glycogen stores, which in a well-fed subject can provide glucose for 12 hours or more. In a prolonged fasting state or in a state of depleted glycogen stores, as seen in malnourished alcoholics, the inability to compensate for hepatic glycogen depletion can lead to hypoglycemia after acute alcohol ingestion.

Alcohol also can impair the body's response to hypoglycemia. Several investigators have shown that alcohol impairs

---

TABLE 1.   Endocrine Syndromes Associated With Alcohol and Other Drug Use

---

Alcohol
- Diabetes Insipidus
- Gynecomastia
- Hyperadrenalism
- Hyperglycemia
- Hypoglycemia
- Hyperlipidemia
- *(possibly)* Hyperprolactinemia
- Hypogonadism/Infertility
- Hypertension
- Osteoporosis

Amphetamines
- Hyperadrenalism
- Hypertension

Anabolic Steroids
- Gynecomastia
- Hyperlipidemia
- Hypogonadism/Infertility
- Hypertension
- *(possibly)* Hyperthyroidism
- Virilization

Barbiturates
- *(possibly)* Hypoadrenalism
- *(possibly)* Hypothyroidism
- Osteoporosis

Benzodiazepines
- *(possibly)* Hypoadrenalism
- *(possibly)* Hypoglycemia
- *(possibly)* SIADH

Caffeine
- Hyperglycemia
- *(possibly)* Hyperlipidemia
- Hypertension
- *(possibly)* Osteoporosis

Cocaine
- Hyperglycemia
- Hyperprolactinemia
- Hypertension

Inhalants
- Hypogonadism/Infertility
- *(possibly)* Hypothyroidism
- *(possibly)* Osteoporosis

Lysergic Acid (LSD)
None known

Marijuana
- *(possibly)* Gynecomastia
- Hypoadrenalism
- *(possibly)* Hypoglycemia
- *(possibly)* Hypogonadism/Infertility

Opioids
- Hyperprolactinemia
- Hypergonadism/Infertility
- Osteoporosis

Phencyclidine (PCP)
None known

Tobacco/Cigarette Smoking
- Hyperlipidemia
- Hypogonadism/Infertility
- Hypertension
- Hyperthyroidism
- Hypothyroidism
- Osteoporosis
- SIADH (Syndrome of Inappropriate Anti-Diuretic Hormone)

---

the release of cortisol, growth hormone, glucagon, and vasopressin in response to hypoglycemia (Berman, Cook et al., 1990; Wand & Dobs, 1991; Joffe, Seftel et al., 1975; Chiodera & Coiro, 1990; Wilson, Brown et al., 1981). However, Kolaczynski and colleagues (1988) failed to confirm this impairment and instead suggested that the counter-regulatory recovery from insulin-induced hypoglycemia actually can be more rapid with acute ethanol use than without.

There are five classes of alcohol-induced hypoglycemia: simple alcohol-induced fasting hypoglycemia, alcoholic ketoacidosis with hypoglycemia, alcoholic exacerbation of insulin-induced hypoglycemia, alcoholic exacerbation of sulfonylurea-induced hypoglycemia, and alcohol-induced reactive hypoglycemia (Marks & Teale, 1999).

In simple alcohol-induced fasting hypoglycemia, patients typically present with coma and a blood glucose level of less than 40 mg/dL. Blood alcohol levels may be detectable. Because of the mechanism underlying this type of hypoglycemia, patients respond promptly to intravenous dextrose, but may not respond to glucagon administration.

Alcoholic ketoacidosis is common. Depletion of NAD, resulting from alcohol metabolism, leads to the increased production of beta-hydroxybutyrate, acetoacetate, and acetone. Beta-hydroxybutyrate, which is not detectable by routine urine or serum ketone testing, predominates, so the beta-hydroxybutyrate to acetoacetate ratio can be as high as 7:1 to 10:1, as compared to 3:1 in diabetic ketoacidosis. Insulin secretion, which ordinarily prevents development of ketoacidosis, is suppressed by decreased serum glucose levels and high catecholamine levels. The patient usually has a history of chronic heavy alcohol use, and may be experiencing nausea, vomiting, abdominal pain, and metabolic acidosis. Blood alcohol levels usually are not detectable. Glucose levels may range from low to mildly elevated, but typically are less than 250 mg/dL. Marked hyperglycemia should raise suspicion of concomitant diabetes or diabetic ketoacidosis (Kitabchi, Umpierrez et al., 2001).

Diabetic patients treated with insulin or sulfonylurea are at risk for severe hypoglycemia with alcohol use (Arky, Veverbrants et al., 1968; Melander, Lebovitz et al., 1990). Impairment of judgment and nonrecognition of hypoglycemia with alcohol use can lead to nontreatment of hypoglycemia in diabetic patients. Consequently, diabetic patients must be counseled about alcohol use and its consequences. Insulin and sulfonylureas should be used with great caution in alcoholic patients with diabetes. In addition, sulfonylureas and insulin are metabolized in the liver and are more likely to cause severe hypoglycemia in patients with alcoholic cirrhosis. Agents such as metformin (Glucophage®), rosiglitazone (Avandia®), and pioglitazone (Actos®), which lower glucose but do not produce hypoglycemia, may not be used because of the increased risk of lactic acidosis (metformin) and liver toxicity (rosiglitazone and pioglita-zone) in alcohol abusers.

Reactive or postprandial hypoglycemia can occur, depending on the carbohydrate composition of the meal consumed. O'Keefe and Marks (1977) first described this phenomenon as profound hypoglycemia (mean blood glucose nadir, 48.6 mg/dL) that occurs three to four hours after the ingestion of alcohol combined with 60 g sucrose (that is, gin and tonic). This phenomenon can develop in up to 10% to 20% of healthy subjects and does not appear to occur with saccharin or fructose and alcohol (Marks & Wright, 1980). The quinine content of regular tonic, which increases insulin levels, was postulated as the cause of the hypoglycemia, but work by Flanagan and colleagues (1998) suggests that the hypoglycemia develops because of suppression of growth hormone release.

Hyperglycemia. Alcoholic pancreatitis can lead to pancreatic exocrine and endocrine insufficiency. When diabetes mellitus results from pancreatic insufficiency, it is an indication that more than 90% of the pancreatic beta cells, which produce insulin, and the alpha cells, which produce glucagon, are destroyed. The secondary diabetes mellitus that results typically is an extremely labile insulin-dependent diabetes, in that patients are absolutely insulin deficient and have normal or increased insulin sensitivity. The lack of glucagon makes the patient somewhat resistant to developing diabetic ketoacidosis but also quite prone to developing hypoglycemia. Although heavy alcohol use can lead to chronic pancreatitis, pancreatic insufficiency, and subsequent diabetes mellitus, many studies have found an association between moderate alcohol use and improved insulin sensitivity (Kiechl, Willeit et al., 1996; Razay & Heaton, 1997) and a decreased risk of diabetes mellitus in men (Rimm, Chan et al., 1995).

Reproductive Consequences. The reproductive effects of alcohol use are gender-specific. Alcohol use long has been known to cause sexual dysfunction and hypogonadism in men, particularly in those with alcoholic cirrhosis (Lloyd & Williams, 1948). Even in men without liver disease, alcohol use leads to a decrease in testosterone (Gordon, Altman et al., 1976), which may be the result of a combination of direct effects on the testicular synthesis of testosterone on hypothalamic-pituitary function (Van Thiel, Lester et al., 1978) or on increases in sex hormone binding globulin, which can lead to a decrease in bioavailable testosterone (Iturriaga, Lioi et al., 1999). The incidence of gynecomastia is increased in alcoholic cirrhosis, primarily because of increased levels of androstenedione, a precursor for estrogen synthesis (Kley, Niederau et al., 1985). Increased prolactin levels were found in patients with alcoholic cirrhosis (Van Thiel, McClain et al., 1978), although it may not be present in alcoholics who do not have severe liver disease (Agner, Hagen et al., 1986).

In women, the effects of alcohol use depend on menopausal status and hormone therapy use. In premenopausal women and postmenopausal women on estrogen, acute alcohol consumption leads to an increase in estradiol levels through reduced metabolism of estradiol (Gill, 2000). This increase in estrogen level may explain why alcohol use is associated with an increased risk of breast cancer (Zumoff, 1997) and why alcohol can be associated with a delay in menopause. Women with high or frequent alcohol intake were found to have higher rates of menstrual disorders, including amenorrhea, dysmenorrhea, and irregular menstrual periods. Pregnant women with a high alcohol intake have a higher incidence of miscarriages, placental abruption, preterm deliveries, and stillbirths than controls (Bradley, Badrinath et al., 1998). A decreased risk of fertility was associated with as few as one to five alcoholic drinks a week in a Danish study (Jensen, Hjollund et al., 1998) and with as little as 12 g of alcohol a week (about one drink) in an American study (Hakim, Gray et al., 1998).

Bone Health Consequences. Chronic alcoholism is associated with decreased bone mass and an increased risk of skeletal fractures (Saville, 1965; de Vernejoul, Bielakoff et al., 1983; Bikle, Genant et al., 1985; Lalor, France et al., 1986). African American men may be less susceptible to this bone loss (Odvina, Safi et al., 1995). Postmenopausal women who engage in moderate alcohol use may have an increased bone mineral density and a decreased risk of fractures (Bradley, Badrinath et al., 1998).

In addition to alterations in sex hormones and the type of fat malabsorption and vitamin D deficiency associated with liver disease, alcohol use can reversibly impair bone formation by osteoblasts (Lindholm, Steiniche et al., 1991; Pepersack, Fuss et al., 1992; Peris, Parés et al., 1994).

Heavy alcohol use is associated with osteonecrosis of bone (Matsuo, Hirohata et al., 1988). Alcohol-associated osteonecrosis of the femoral head may be due in part to lipid or cortisol changes (Chang, Greenspan et al., 1993) and, in fact, alcohol may be responsible for up to a third of cases of femoral head osteonecrosis (Antti-Poika, Karaharju et al., 1987).

Other Endocrinologic Consequences. Alcohol use increases triglyceride synthesis, leading to hypertriglyceridemia and hepatic steatosis. The increased NADH/NAD ratio leads to increases in alpha-glycerophosphate, which favors hepatic triglyceride accumulation by trapping fatty acids. The excess NADH enhances fatty acid synthesis (Lieber 1997). Alcohol increases the high-density lipoprotein (HDL) fraction of cholesterol, which may be associated with reduced cardiovascular morbidity and mortality (Gaziano, Buring et al., 1993).

Although glucocorticoid response to hypoglycemia can be impaired by alcohol use, patients with chronic heavy alcohol use have elevated adrenocorticotropic hormone (ACTH) and cortisol production. Rarely, these patients may develop the clinical stigmata of glucocorticoid excess, such as central obesity, moon facies, "buffalo hump," and biochemical evidence of nonsuppressible glucocorticoid excess that is difficult to distinguish from Cushing syndrome. This condition, which has been termed "pseudo-Cushing syndrome," reverses with abstinence from alcohol (Kirkman & Nelson, 1988).

Alcohol use has effects on body volume and blood pressure status. It transiently decreases vasopressin release, leading to water diuresis (Oiso & Robertson, 1985). This condition can be problematic in patients with partial diabetes insipidus. Acute alcohol use also increases blood pressure, possibly through an increase in norepinephrine (Howes & Reid, 1986). Moderate alcohol consumption appears to increase plasma renin activity, although such increases are believed to result from a secondary response to changes in fluid and electrolyte balance (Puddey, Vandongen et al., 1985). Although alcohol by itself does not affect mineralocorticoid levels, alcoholic cirrhosis leads to elevations of aldosterone in response to decreased effective plasma volume.

Acute alcohol use does not produce thyroid dysfunction in patients whose thyroid function previously was normal (Ylikahri, Huttunen et al., 1978). Alcoholic cirrhosis of the liver can produce decreases in serum triiodothyronine (T_3), because the liver is a major site for the conversion of thyroxine to T_3, without producing clinical hypothyroidism in those without preexisting autoimmune thyroid disease (Chopra, Solomon et al., 1974; Hegedüs, 1984).

Alcohol use was reported to suppress melatonin secretion through increased norepinephrine levels, and this increase may be implicated in disturbances in sleep and performance (Ekman, Leppäluoto et al., 1993).

DISORDERS RELATED TO TOBACCO

Thyroid Disease. Cigarette smoking is associated with an increased risk of hypothyroidism and goiter (Hegedüs, Karstrup et al., 1985; Christensen, Ericsson et al., 1984). This condition may be a consequence of the thiocyanate present in cigarette smoke, which is a goitrogen (Fukayama, Nasu et al., 1992). Smoking also increases the risk of Graves' disease and Graves' ophthalmopathy (Bartalena, Martino et al., 1989; Hägg & Asplund, 1987; Shine, Fells et al., 1990; Prummel & Wiersinga, 1993).

Insulin Resistance and Dyslipidemia. Cigarette smoking (Targher, Alberiche et al., 1997), as well as nicotine gum use (Eliasson, Taskinen et al., 1996), is associated with an increase in insulin resistance and an increased risk of developing diabetes mellitus (Rimm, Chan et al., 1995). Mild decreases in HDL cholesterol and mild elevations in triglycerides, consistent with this insulin resistance, are associated with cigarette smoking (Targher, Alberiche et al., 1997), although these changes may be due to components of cigarette smoke other than nicotine (Jensen, Fusch et al., 1995). This insulin resistance and dyslipidemia may be responsible, in part, for the elevated rates of cardiovascular and atherosclerotic disease associated with cigarette use.

Reproductive Function. In women, cigarette smoking is associated with decreases in estrogen levels (MacMahon, Trichopoulos et al., 1982) and, in fact, can enhance estrogen degradation (Jensen, Christiansen et al., 1985). It also is associated with early menopause (Jick, Porter et al., 1972; McKinlay, Bifano et al., 1985). In men, cigarette smoking is associated with quantitative and qualitative decrements in sperm (Evans, Fletcher et al., 1981; Shaarawy & Mahmoud, 1982; Vine, Margolin et al., 1994), as well as with increases in serum estrogen (Barrett-Connor & Khaw, 1987).

Bone Health. Cigarette smoking is associated with decreased bone mineral density and increased bone loss in postmenopausal women and elderly men (Vogel, Davis et al., 1997) and is an independent risk factor for osteoporotic fracture. This risk appears, in part, because of a decrease in intestinal calcium absorption (Krall & Dawson-Hughes, 1991, 1999), probably resulting in a negative calcium balance. Brot and colleagues (1999) found an association between smoking and decreased serum 25-hydroxyvitamin D, 1,25-dihydroxyvitamin D, parathyroid hormone, and osteocalcin levels, suggesting a more complex effect of smoking on calcium and bone metabolism. Cigarette smoking can negate the protective effect of estrogen therapy on the risk of hip fracture in postmenopausal women (Kiel, Baron et al., 1992). It also is associated with femoral head osteonecrosis (Matsuo, Hirohata et al., 1988), possibly through impairment of vascular function or changes in blood lipids.

Other Endocrinologic Effects. Cigarette smoke stimulates antidiuretic hormone release from the pituitary through an airway-mediated mechanism that does not depend on circulating nicotine (Husain, Grantz et al., 1975; Rowe, Kilgore et al., 1980). This antidiuretic effect may cause or exacerbate hyponatremia in susceptible patients (Allen, Allen et al., 1990; Ellinas, Rosner et al., 1993).

The nicotine found in cigarette smoke can increase the release of catecholamines from the adrenal medulla, which may precipitate a hypertensive crisis for those with pheochromocytoma. In addition, smoking is associated with hypertension and poorly controlled hypertension, apparently through stimulation of the noradrenergic nervous system (Cryer, Haymond et al., 1976); such hypertension is not angiotensin II dependent (Ottesen, Worck et al., 1997).

DISORDERS RELATED TO OTHER DRUGS

Marijuana. The major psychoactive component of marijuana is delta-9-tetrahydrocannabinol (THC), although marijuana can contain more than 400 chemicals. Factors including concomitant use of other drugs, variability in smoking technique, variable potencies of marijuana cigarettes, and development of tolerance to marijuana's effects can make it difficult to generalize from study findings to clinical practice.

Although some investigators have reported that heavy marijuana smoking is associated with low plasma levels of testosterone (Kolodny, Masters et al., 1974), others report that chronic marijuana use has no effects on plasma testosterone or luteinizing hormone in men (Mendelson, Kuehnle et al., 1974). Further confusion arises from reports suggesting that smoking marijuana cigarettes acutely suppresses luteinizing hormone in men (Cone, Johnson et al., 1986) and premenopausal women in the luteal phase of their menstrual cycle, but not in postmenopausal women (Mendelson, Cristofaro et al., 1985). One study of pregnant marijuana users found no changes in female sex hormones as compared with controls (Braunstein, Buster et al., 1983).

The many conflicting studies make it unlikely that chronic marijuana use affects the reproductive system with any significant clinical relevance. Marijuana has not been found to be teratogenic and has not been found to have consistent effects on pregnancy outcomes.

With regard to other endocrinologic effects, prolonged oral administration of 210 mg THC a day (the equivalent of smoking six marijuana cigarettes) for 14 days significantly suppressed the cortisol and growth hormone response to insulin-induced hypoglycemia, although the THC use did not suppress the cortisol and growth hormone response to values consistent with cortisol or growth hormone deficiency (Benowitz, Jones et al., 1976). This finding suggests that heavy marijuana use may cause significant hypoadrenalism or impaired recovery from insulin-induced hypoglycemia in those with preexisting adrenal disease.

Opiates. The endocrine effects of acute administration of opiates occur primarily in the hypothalamus and pituitary. Gonadotropins (follicle-stimulating hormone [FSH] and luteinizing hormone [LH]) are suppressed by inhibition of gonadotropin-releasing hormone secretion. Prolactin secretion is stimulated, while ACTH and cortisol secretion are suppressed (Carlson, 1995). Chronic administration of opiates can produce partial tolerance to many of the endocrine effects.

Male gonadal function in methadone and heroin addicts has been found to be variable. In men, methadone use has been associated with a decline in serum testosterone levels and diminished sperm motility (Cicero, Bell et al., 1975). Another study looking at methadone, methadone/heroin, and heroin use found normal levels of testosterone, FSH, LH, and prolactin in all but the heroin users who had elevated prolactin levels (Ragni, De Laurentis et al., 1988). All the heroin addicts, the heroin/methadone users, and 45% of the methadone takers in that study had diminished sperm motility. A third study looked at short-term methadone use in 30 men and found no abnormalities of estrogen, progesterone, or LH, whereas FSH showed lower values than normal and androstenedione, dehydroepiandrosterone, and prolactin noticeably increased in many subjects. Modest variations were noted for testosterone and dihydrotestosterone (Lafisca, Bolelli et al., 1981). Other investigators found a decrease in basal FSH and LH levels, with a decrease in pituitary response to gonadotropin-releasing hormone, suggesting a hypothalamic cause for hypogonadism in heroin addicts (Brambilla, Resele et al., 1979). The variability in findings may be due in part to the pres-

ence of other components, as well as variable doses of opiates in street preparations of heroin, continued use of heroin in methadone-treated addicts, and the possible effect of malnutrition on the reproductive system. A study of the endocrine effects of long-term intrathecal opioid administration for pain relief found diminished testosterone and LH levels in men but normal FSH and prolactin levels in comparison to control patients with a comparable pain syndrome but who were not treated with opioids (Abs, Verhelst et al., 2000), suggesting that these are the "pure" opiate effects on the male reproductive system.

In women, more than half of a group of 76 former heroin addicts on methadone maintenance had menstrual irregularities (Santen, Sofsky et al., 1975). Endocrinologic studies on seven of the women showed alterations in hypothalamic and pituitary function leading to oligo-ovulation. A study of 21 premenopausal women who received chronic intrathecal opioids found 14 to have amenorrhea and 7 to have menstrual irregularity, with decrements in serum LH, FSH, estradiol, and progesterone concentrations (Abs, Verhelst et al., 2000). In the same study, 18 postmenopausal women had serum LH and FSH levels significantly lower than postmenopausal control subjects, further indicating impairment of gonadotropin release.

Hypogonadism is a risk factor for osteoporosis, and one small cross-sectional study found decreased vertebral bone mineral density, evidence of increased bone resorption, and decreased parathyroid hormone in current male heroin addicts but not in control subjects or former heroin addicts, arguing for reversibility of bone loss with cessation of heroin use (Pedrazzoni, Vescovi et al., 1993).

Cocaine. Cocaine acts, primarily, by blocking the reuptake of norepinephrine, dopamine, and serotonin at the synaptic junctions, resulting in increased neurotransmitter concentrations. In animal studies, cocaine can stimulate the adrenal medulla to release epinephrine and norepinephrine. By increasing catecholamines, which are counterregulatory hormones that antagonize insulin-stimulating glucose production and inhibit glucose clearance, hyperglycemia can result, as can diabetic ketoacidosis or hyperosmolar nonketotic hyperglycemia without any other identified precipitants (Abraham & Khardori, 1999; Warner, Greene et al., 1998). Diabetic ketoacidosis appears to occur more frequently in cocaine users, resulting from a combination of omission of insulin therapy and cocaine effects on glucose metabolism (Warner, Greene et al., 1998).

Dopamine is an important physiologic regulator of prolactin and thyroid-stimulating hormone secretion. What occurs with acute cocaine use is the suppression of prolactin secretion with increased dopamine levels, but with chronic use, dopamine levels become depleted and hyperprolactinemia results (Heesch, Negus et al., 1996; Mendelson, Mello et al., 1989). This hyperprolactinemia persists even after cocaine withdrawal (Mendelson, Teoh et al., 1988). Although acute cocaine use produces rises in ACTH, FSH, and LH (Mendelson, Teoh et al., 1992; Teoh, Sarnyai et al., 1994; Heesch, Negus et al., 1996), abnormalities of testosterone, cortisol, LH (Mendelson, Mello et al., 1989) or thyroid function tests (Dhopesh, Burke et al., 1991) have not been found in chronic cocaine users.

Amphetamines. Amphetamines, such as dextroamphetamine and methylamphetamine, have not been well studied with regard to the endocrinologic effects of chronic use. They act primarily by stimulating the release of norepinephrine and dopamine. Well-described acute endocrine effects of amphetamine administration include increased corticosteroid release and increased growth hormone release (Besser, Butler et al., 1969; Rees, Butler et al., 1970; Dommisse, Schulz et al., 1984), each of which can be influenced by the presence of depression (Langer, Heinze et al., 1976; Checkley & Crammer, 1977; Checkley, 1979; Sachar, Asnis et al., 1980; Halbreich, Sachar et al., 1982) or other psychoactive medications (Nurnberger, Simmons-Alling et al., 1984). The clinical implications of these findings remain unclear.

Caffeine. Caffeine is one of the world's most widely used drugs. The many forms in which it is delivered and prepared, including tea, coffee, and caffeinated soft drinks, may contain other bioactive substances such as flavonoids (Hegarty, May et al., 2000) and diterpene (Mensink, Lebbink et al., 1995). This variability has confounded its study. Caffeine is a neuroendocrine stimulant whose action is mediated by central adenosine receptor antagonism (Snyder, Katims et al., 1981). Ingestion of 250 mg (approximately three cups of coffee) produces a rapid release of epinephrine from the adrenal medulla, which can increase blood pressure (Debrah, Haigh et al., 1995). Although immediate ingestion of 250 to 500 mg caffeine (equivalent of three to six cups of coffee) has little effect on circulating cortisol, thyroid-stimulating hormone, growth hormone, prolactin, T_3 (Spindel, Wurtman et al., 1984), or norepinephrine levels; the ingestion of 250 mg caffeine produces an increased epinephrine and norepinephrine response to table-tilt test (Debrah Haigh et al., 1995) and increased epinephrine,

norepinephrine, cortisol, and growth hormone response to hypoglycemia or low normal glucose levels in normal healthy adults (Kerr, Sherwin et al., 1993) as well as in insulin-dependent diabetics (Debrah, Sherwin et al., 1996). Further, tolerance to caffeine can develop with chronic use, so that these neuroendocrine changes do not become clinically relevant except after a period of abstinence, although it was suggested that caffeine can be a useful treatment for diabetic patients without autonomic neuropathy who have hypoglycemic unawareness (Debrah, Sherwin et al., 1996).

Caffeine is associated with increased urinary calcium excretion (Massey & Opryszek, 1990) as well as with decrements in serum free estradiol (London, Willett et al., 1991; Nagata, Kabuto et al., 1998), and serum insulin-like growth factor I levels (Landin-Wilhelmsen, Wilhelmsen et al., 1994), both of which are important in maintaining bone mass. As such, it is not surprising that caffeine use is associated with an increased risk of fracture (Kiel, Felson et al., 1990; Hernández-Avila, Colditz et al., 1991) and an increased risk of reduced bone mass (Yano, Heilbrun et al., 1985; Hernández-Avila, Colditz et al., 1991). However, other studies do not support this increased risk (Tavani, Negri et al., 1995; Lloyd, Rollings et al., 1997). Add to this mixture the studies that show that tea can protect against hip fractures (Kanis, Johnell et al., 1999) and is associated with increased bone density (Hegarty, May et al., 2000), and the overall situation becomes more confusing. If there is an effect of caffeine intake on bone health, it is not likely to be clinically significant.

Benzodiazepines. Benzodiazepines act by stimulating gamma-aminobutyric acid-ergic neurons, which usually are inhibitory in function, within the brain. Many researchers have found that benzodiazepines, such as diazepam (Valium®), alprazolam (Xanax®), and temazepam (Restoril®), suppress basal serum levels of cortisol (Schuckit, Hauger, et al., 1991; Zemishlany, McQueeney et al., 1990; Risby, Hsiao et al., 1989; Roy-Byrne, Cowley et al., 1991) and also suppress the body's cortisol and ACTH response to metyrapone (Arvat, Maccagno et al., 1999), insulin-induced hypoglycemia, corticotrophin-releasing hormone (Korbonits, Trainer et al., 1995), and metabolic stress (Breier, Davis et al., 1992). Such changes potentially could lead to a hypoadrenal crisis or prolonged hypoglycemia in users with preexisting adrenal disease. Suppression of cortisol response persists despite chronic benzodiazepine use (Cowley, Roy-Byrne et al., 1995); however, this finding may not apply to all benzodiazepines. Ambrosi and colleagues

(1986) found that triazolam (Halcion®) and flurazepam (Dalmane®) did not influence cortisol release in women with insulin-induced hypoglycemia.

Benzodiazepines may variably stimulate the release of growth hormone (Monteiro, Schuckit et al., 1990), although not all investigators have confirmed this finding (Levin, Sharp et al., 1984). This growth hormone response is blunted with long-term benzodiazepine administration (Shur, Petersson et al., 1983) and hyperglycemia (Ajlouni & el-Khateeb, 1980), suggesting that significant clinical effects are unlikely. One case report described a syndrome involving inappropriate antidiuretic hormone secretion associated with use of lorazepam (Ativan®) (Engel & Grau, 1988).

Barbiturates. Barbiturates are known to induce the cytochrome P450 enzyme system, leading to enhanced metabolism of many substances. Among these substances are thyroid hormone, hydrocortisone, and vitamin D. Barbiturate use or abuse can lead to increasing thyroid hormone requirements (Hoffbrand, 1979), hydrocortisone requirements, or osteomalacia. Overt hypothyroidism or hypoadrenalism is not likely in the absence of underlying thyroid or adrenal disease.

Inhalants. The inhalation of volatile solvents, such as toluene, is known to cause multiple medical complications, such as heart, liver, lung, nerve, and kidney damage (Streicher, Gabow et al., 1981; Meadows & Verghese, 1996). No specific endocrine consequences have yet been described. However, these solvents can cause renal tubular dysfunction, leading to hypophosphatemia and acidosis, which can affect calcium and bone metabolism. Although recurrent nephrolithiasis was described (Kaneko, Koizumi et al., 1992; Kroeger, Moore et al., 1980), no cases of toluene-induced osteomalacia have been described as yet.

Occupational exposure to inhalants is associated with infertility, increased risk of spontaneous abortion, and multiple birth defects. In addition, case reports of children born to those who abuse inhalants have led to the term "fetal solvent syndrome," reflecting its similarity to fetal alcohol syndrome. Although it is beyond the scope of this chapter, this subject has been reviewed recently (Jones & Balster, 1998).

Anabolic Steroids. The anabolic steroids, which are testosterone derivatives, include nandrolone, oxandrolone, oxymetholone, and stanozolol. Male and female athletes often use these substances in efforts to improve athletic performance. The adverse endocrine consequences are a direct result of androgenic effects and suppression of the hypothalamic-pituitary-gonadal axis. These effects include testicular atrophy; decreases in testosterone, LH, and FSH; increases in estrone; and suppression of spermatogenesis in men (Bijlsma, Duursam et al., 1982b; Small, Beastall et al., 1984). In women, there can be menstrual disturbances, deepening of voice, and development of acne and male pattern body hair. In addition, aromatization of androgens to estrogen can produce an array of seemingly paradoxical feminization. Gynecomastia can result from aromatization of the androgens to estrogen in endogenous androgen suppression. Anabolic steroids can affect other hormones by decreasing hepatic synthesis of proteins, such as thyroid-binding globulin, sex hormone–binding globulin, vitamin D–binding protein, and HDL cholesterol (Small, Beastall et al., 1984; Malarkey, Strauss et al., 1991). There can be mild thyroidal impairment, as measured by thyroid-stimulating hormone and T_3 response to thyrotropin-releasing hormone (Deyssig & Weissel, 1993). Clinically relevant sequelae are not present without underlying hyperthyroidism.

Other lipid changes include increases in low-density lipoprotein cholesterol and serum triglycerides. Those with preexisting coronary artery disease may be at increased risk because of decreased HDL and increased low-density lipoprotein cholesterol. Hypertension, ventricular remodeling, myocardial ischemia, and sudden cardiac death each have been temporally and causally associated with anabolic steroid use (Sullivan, Martinez et al., 1998). Recent contradicting reports, however, have suggested that androgens may have anti-atherogenic and anti-anginal effects (English, Mandour, et al., 2000; English, Steeds et al., 2000; Webb, Adamson et al., 1999; Webb, McNeil et al., 1999) in both supraphysiologic and physiologic doses.

No significant changes in adult bone metabolism (parathyroid hormone or vitamin D metabolites) have been reported in patients treated with nandrolone (Bijlsma, Duursma et al., 1982a). Anabolic steroid use in children, however, may prematurely close epiphyseal growth plates, leading to growth stunting. Growth hormone levels can rise with anabolic steroid use; resolution of the hypothalamic-pituitary-gonadal suppression can take several months (Alèn, Rahkila et al., 1987).

Other Drugs. No endocrinologic consequences have been described with phencyclidine or LSD use; further research is required.

REFERENCES

Abraham MR & Khardori R (1999). Hyperglycemic hyperosmolar nonketotic syndrome as initial presentation of type 2 diabetes in a young cocaine abuser. *Diabetes Care* 22:1380-1381.

Abs R, Verhelst J, Maeyaert J et al. (2000). Endocrine consequences of long-term intrathecal administration of opioids. *Journal of Clinical Endocrinology and Metabolism* 85:2215-2222.

Agner T, Hagen C, Andersen BN et al. (1986). Pituitary-thyroid function and thyrotropin, prolactin and growth hormone responses to TRH in patients with chronic alcoholism. *Acta Medica Scandinavia* 220:57-62.

Ajlouni K & el-Khateeb M (1980). Effect of glucose on growth hormone, prolactin and thyroid-stimulating hormone response to diazepam in normal subjects. *Hormone Research* 13:160-164.

Alèn M, Rahkila P, Reinilä M et al. (1987). Androgenic-anabolic steroid effects on serum thyroid, pituitary and steroid hormones in athletes. *American Journal of Sports Medicine* 15:357-361.

Allen M, Allen HM, Deck LV et al. (1990). Role of cigarette use in hyponatremia in schizophrenic patients. *American Journal of Psychiatry* 147:1075-1077.

Ambrosi F, Quartesan R, Moretti P et al. (1986). Effects of acute benzodiazepine administration on growth hormone, prolactin and cortisol release after moderate insulin-induced hypoglycemia in normal women. *Psychopharmacology* 88:187-189.

Antti-Poika I, Karaharju E, Vankka E et al. (1987). Alcohol-associated femoral head necrosis. *Annales Chirurgiae et Gynaecologiae* 76:318-322.

Arky RA, Veverbrants E & Abramson EA (1968). Irreversible hypoglycemia: A complication of alcohol and insulin. *Journal of the American Medical Association* 206:575-578.

Arvat E, Maccagno B, Ramunni J et al. (1999). The inhibitory effect of alprazolam, a benzodiazepine, overrides the stimulatory effect of metyrapone-induced lack of negative cortisol feedback on corticotrophic secretion in humans. *Journal of Clinical Endocrinology and Metabolism* 84:2611-2615.

Barrett-Connor E & Khaw KT (1987). Cigarette smoking and increased endogenous estrogen levels in men. *American Journal of Epidemiology* 126:187-192.

Bartalena L, Martino E, Marcocci C et al. (1989). More on smoking habits and Graves' ophthalmopathy. *Journal of Endocrinological Investigation* 12:733.

Benowitz NL, Jones RT & Lerner CB (1976). Depression of growth hormone and cortisol response to insulin-induced hypoglycemia after prolonged oral delta-9-tetrahydrocannabinol administration in man. *Journal of Clinical Endocrinology and Metabolism* 42:938-941.

Berman JD, Cook DM, Buchman M et al. (1990). Diminished adrenocorticotropin response to insulin-induced hypoglycemia in nondepressed, actively drinking male alcoholics. *Journal of Clinical Endocrinology and Metabolism* 72:712-717.

Besser GM, Butler PWP, Landon J et al. (1969). Influence of amphetamines on plasma corticosteroid and growth hormone levels in man. *British Medical Journal* 4:528-530.

Bijlsma JWJ, Duursma SA, Bosch R et al. (1982a). Lack of influence of the anabolic steroid nandrolondecanoate on bone metabolism. *Acta Endocrinologica* 101:140-143.

Bijlsma JWJ, Duursma SA, Thijssen JHH et al. (1982b). Influence of nandrolondecanoate on the pituitary-gonadal axis in males. *Acta Endocrinologica* 101:108-112.

Bikle DD, Genant HK, Cann CE et al. (1985). Bone disease in alcohol abuse. *Annals of Internal Medicine* 103:42-48.

Bradley KA, Badrinath S, Bush K et al. (1998). Medical risks for women who drink alcohol. *Journal of General Internal Medicine* 13:627-639.

Brambilla F, Resele L, De Maio D et al. (1979). Gonadotropin response to synthetic gonadotropin hormone-releasing hormone (GnRH) in heroin addicts. *American Journal of Psychiatry* 136:314-317.

Braunstein GD, Buster JE, Soares JR et al. (1983). Pregnancy hormone concentrations in marijuana users. *Life Sciences* 33:195-199.

Breier A, Davis O, Buchanan R et al. (1992). Effects of alprazolam on pituitary-adrenal and catecholaminergic responses to metabolic stress in humans. *Biological Psychiatry* 32:880-890.

Brot C, Jorgensen NR & Sorensen OH (1999). The influence of smoking on vitamin D status and calcium metabolism. *European Journal of Clinical Nutrition* 53:920-926.

Carlson HE (1995). Drugs and pituitary function. In S Melmed (ed.) *The Pituitary*. Cambridge, MA: Blackwell Science, 645-660.

Chang CC, Greenspan A & Gershwin ME (1993). Osteonecrosis: Current perspectives on pathogenesis and treatment. *Seminars in Arthritis and Rheumatism* 23:47-69.

Checkley SA (1979). Corticosteroid and growth hormone responses to methylamphetamine in depressive illness. *Psychological Medicine* 9:107-115.

Checkley SA & Crammer JL (1977). Hormone responses to methylamphetamine in depression: A new approach to the noradrenaline depletion hypothesis. *British Journal of Psychiatry* 131:582-586.

Chiodera P & Coiro V (1990). Inhibitory effect of ethanol on the arginine vasopressin response to insulin-induced hypoglycemia and the role of endogenous opioids. *Neuroendocrinology* 51:501-504.

Chopra IJ, Solomon DH, Chopra U et al. (1974). Alterations in circulating thyroid hormones and thyrotropin in hepatic cirrhosis: Evidence for euthyroidism despite subnormal serum triiodothyronine. *Journal of Clinical Endocrinology and Metabolism* 39:501-511.

Christensen SB, Ericsson UB, Janson L et al. (1984). Influence of cigarette smoking on goiter formation, thyroglobulin, and thyroid hormone levels in women. *Journal of Clinical Endocrinology and Metabolism* 58:615-618.

Cicero TJ, Bell RD, Wiest WG et al. (1975). Function of the male sex organs in heroin and methadone users. *New England Journal of Medicine* 292:882-887.

Cone EJ, Johnson RE, Moore JD et al. (1986). Acute effects of smoking marijuana on hormones, subjective effects and performance in male human subjects. *Pharmacology, Biochemistry and Behavior* 24:1749-1754.

Cowley DS, Roy-Byrne PP, Radant A et al. (1995). Benzodiazepine sensitivity in panic disorder: Effects of chronic alprazolam treatment. *Neuropsychopharmacology* 12:147-157

Cryer PE, Haymond MW, Santiago JV et al. (1976). Norepinephrine and epinephrine release and adrenergic mediation of smoking-associated hemodynamic and metabolic events. *New England Journal of Medicine* 295:573-577.

Debrah K, Haigh R, Sherwin R et al. (1995). Effect of acute and chronic caffeine use on the cerebrovascular, cardiovascular and hormonal responses to orthostasis in healthy volunteers. *Clinical Science* 89:475-480.

Debrah K, Sherwin RS, Murphy et al. (1996). Effect of caffeine on recognition of and physiological responses to hypoglycaemia in insulin-dependent diabetes. *Lancet* 347:19-24.

de Vernejoul MC, Bielakoff J, Herve M et al. (1983). Evidence for defective osteoblastic function. A role for alcohol and tobacco consumption in osteoporosis in middle-aged men. *Clinical Orthopaedics and Related Research* 179:107-115.

Deyssig R & Weissel M (1993). Ingestion of androgenic-anabolic steroids induces mild thyroidal impairment in male body builders. *Journal of Clinical Endocrinology and Metabolism* 76:1069-1071.

Dhopesh VP, Burke WM, Maany I et al. (1991). Effect of cocaine on thyroid functions. *American Journal of Drug and Alcohol Abuse* 17:423-427.

Dommisse CS, Schulz SC, Narasimhachari N et al. (1984). The neuroendocrine and behavioral response to dextroamphetamine in normal individuals. *Biological Psychiatry* 19:1305-1315.

Ekman A, Leppäluoto J, Huttunen P et al. (1993). Ethanol inhibits melatonin secretion in healthy volunteers in a dose-dependent randomized double blind cross-over study. *Journal of Clinical Endocrinology and Metabolism* 77:780-783.

Eliasson B, Taskinen M & Smith U (1996). Long-term use of nicotine gum is associated with hyperinsulinemia and insulin resistance. *Circulation* 94:878-881.

Ellinas PA, Rosner F & Jaume JC (1993). Symptomatic hyponatremia associated with psychosis, medications, and smoking. *Journal of the National Medical Association* 85:135-141.

Engel WR & Grau A (1988). Inappropriate secretion of antidiuretic hormone associated with lorazepam. *British Medical Journal* 297:858.

English KM, Mandour O, Steeds RP et al. (2000). Men with coronary artery disease have lower levels of androgens than men with normal coronary angiograms. *European Heart Journal* 21:890-894.

English KM, Steeds RP, Jones TH et al. (2000). Low-dose transdermal testosterone therapy improves angina threshold in men with chronic stable angina: A randomized, double-blind, placebo-controlled study. *Circulation* 102:1906-1911.

Evans HJ, Fletcher J, Torrance M et al. (1981). Sperm abnormalities and cigarette smoking. *Lancet* 1(8221):627-629.

Flanagan D, Wood P, Sherwin R et al. (1998). Gin and tonic and reactive hypoglycemia: What is important—the gin, the tonic or both? *Journal of Clinical Endocrinology and Metabolism* 83:796-800.

Fukayama H, Nasu M, Murakami S et al. (1992). Examination of antithyroid effects of smoking products in cultured thyroid follicles: Only thiocyanate is a potent antithyroid agent. *Acta Endocrinologica* 127:520.

Gaziano JM, Buring JE, Breslow JL et al. (1993). Moderate alcohol intake, increased levels of high-density lipoprotein and its subfractions, and decreased risk of myocardial infarction. *New England Journal of Medicine* 329:1829-1834.

Gill J (2000). The effects of moderate alcohol consumption on female hormone levels and reproductive function. *Alcohol and Alcoholism* 35:417-423.

Gordon GG, Altman K, Southern AL et al. (1976). Effect of alcohol (ethanol) administration on sex-hormone metabolism in normal men. *New England Journal of Medicine* 295:793-797.

Hägg E & Asplund K (1987). Is endocrine ophthalmopathy related to smoking? *British Medical Journal* 295:634.

Hakim RB, Gray RH & Zacur H (1998). Alcohol and caffeine consumption and decreased fertility. *Fertility and Sterility* 70:632-637.

Halbreich U, Sachar EJ, Asnis GM et al. (1982). Growth hormone response to dextroamphetamine in depressed patients and normal subjects. *Archives of General Psychiatry* 39:189-192.

Heesch CM, Negus BH, Bost JE et al. (1996). Effects of cocaine on anterior pituitary and gonadal hormones. *Journal of Pharmacology and Experimental Therapeutics* 278:1195-1200.

Hegarty VM, May HM & Khaw KT (2000). Tea drinking and bone mineral density in older women. *American Journal of Clinical Nutrition* 71:1003-1007.

Hegedüs L (1984). Decreased thyroid gland volume in alcoholic cirrhosis of the liver. *Journal of Clinical Endocrinology and Metabolism* 58:930-933.

Hegedüs L, Karstrup S, Veiergang D et al. (1985). High frequency of goiter in cigarette smokers. *Clinical Endocrinology* 22:287.

Hernández-Avila M, Colditz GA, Stampfer MJ et al. (1991). Caffeine, moderate alcohol intake and the risk of fractures of the hip and forearm among middle-aged women. *American Journal of Clinical Nutrition* 54:157-163.

Hernández-Avila M, Stampfer MJ, Ravnikar VA et al. (1993). Caffeine and other predictors of bone density among pre- and perimenopausal women. *Epidemiology* 4:128-134.

Hoffbrand BI (1979). Barbiturate/thyroid-hormone interaction. *Lancet* (October 27):903-904.

Howes LG & Reid JL (1986). The effects of alcohol on local neural and humoral cardiovascular regulation. *Clinical Science* 71:9-15.

Husain MK, Grantz AG, Ciarochi F et al. (1975). Nicotine stimulated release of neurophysin and vasopressin in humans. *Journal of Clinical Endocrinology and Metabolism* 41:1113-1117.

Iturriaga H, Lioi X & Valladares L (1999). Sex hormone-binding globulin in non-cirrhotic alcoholic patients during early withdrawal and after longer abstinence. *Alcohol and Alcoholism* 34:903-909.

Jensen J, Christiansen C & Rodbro P (1985). Cigarette smoking, serum estrogens, and bone loss during hormone-replacement therapy early after menopause. *New England Journal of Medicine* 313:973-975.

Jensen EX, Fusch C, Jaeger P et al. (1995). Impact of chronic cigarette smoking on body composition and fuel metabolism. *Journal of Clinical Endocrinology and Metabolism* 80:2181-2185.

Jensen TK, Hjollund NHI, Henriksen TB et al. (1998). Does moderate alcohol consumption affect fertility? Follow up study among couples planning first pregnancy. *British Medical Journal* 317:505-510.

Jick H, Porter J & Morrison AS (1972). Relation between smoking and age of natural menopause. *Lancet* 1:1354-1355.

Joffe BI, Seftel HC & Van As M (1975). Hormonal responses in ethanol-induced hypoglycemia. *Journal of Studies on Alcohol* 36:550-554.

Jones HE & Balster RL (1998). Inhalant abuse in pregnancy. *Obstetrics and Gynecology Clinics of North America* 25:153-167.

Kaneko T, Koizumi T, Takezaki T et al. (1992). Urinary calculi associated with solvent abuse. *Journal of Urology* 147:1365-1366.

Kanis J, Johnell O, Gullberg B et al. (1999). Risk factors for hip fracture in men from southern Europe: The MEDOS Study. *Osteoporosis International* 9:45-54.

Kerr D, Sherwin RS, Pavlakis F et al. (1993). Effect of caffeine on the recognition of and responses to hypoglycemia in humans. *Annals of Internal Medicine* 119:799-804.

Kiechl S, Willeit J, Poewe W et al. (1996). Insulin sensitivity and regular alcohol consumption: Large, prospective, cross sectional population study (Bruneck study). *British Medical Journal* 313:1040-1044.

Kiel DP, Baron JA, Anderson JJ et al. (1992). Smoking eliminates the protective effect of oral estrogens on the risk of hip fracture among women. *Annals of Internal Medicine* 116:716-721.

Kiel DP, Felson DT, Hannan MT et al. (1990). Caffeine and the risk of fracture: The Framingham Study. *American Journal of Epidemiology* 132:675-684.

Kirkman S & Nelson DH (1988). Alcohol-induced pseudo-Cushing's syndrome: A study of prevalence with review of the literature. *Metabolism* 37: 390-394.

Kitabchi AE, Umpierrez GE, Murphy MB et al. (2001). Management of hyperglycemic crises in patients with diabetes. *Diabetes Care* 24:131-153.

Kley HK, Niederau C, Stremmel W et al. (1985). Conversion of androgens to estrogens in idiopathic hemochromatosis: Comparison with alcoholic liver cirrhosis. *Journal of Clinical Endocrinology and Metabolism* 61:1-6.

Kolaczynski JW, Ylikahri R, Härkonen M et al. (1988). The acute effect of ethanol on counterregulatory response and recovery from insulin-induced hypoglycemia. *Journal of Clinical Endocrinology and Metabolism* 67:384-388.

Kolodny RC, Masters WH, Kolodner RM et al. (1974). Depression of plasma testosterone levels after chronic intensive marihuana use. *New England Journal of Medicine* 290:872-874.

Korbonits M, Trainer PJ, Edwards R et al. (1995). Benzodiazepines attenuate the pituitary-adrenal responses to corticotrophin-releasing hormone in healthy volunteers, but not in patients with Cushing's syndrome. *Clinical Endocrinology* 43:29-35.

Krall EA & Dawson-Hughes B (1991). Smoking and bone loss among postmenopausal women. *Journal of Bone and Mineral Research* 6:331-338.

Krall EA & Dawson-Hughes B (1999). Smoking increases bone loss and decreases intestinal calcium absorption. *Journal of Bone and Mineral Research* 14:215-220.

Kroeger RM, Moore RJ, Lehman TH et al. (1980). Recurrent urinary calculi associated with toluene sniffing. *Journal of Urology* 123:89-91.

Lafisca S, Bolelli G, Franceschetti F et al. (1981). Hormone levels in methadone-treated drug addicts. *Drug and Alcohol Dependence* 8:229-34.

Lalor BC, France MW, Powell D et al. (1986). Bone and mineral metabolism and chronic alcohol abuse. *Quarterly Journal of Medicine* 59:497-511.

Landin-Wilhelmsen K, Wilhelmsen L, Lappas G et al. (1994). Serum insulin-like growth factor I in a random population sample of men and women: Relation to age, sex, smoking habits, coffee consumption and physical activity, blood pressure and concentrations of plasma lipids, fibrinogen, parathyroid hormone and osteocalcin. *Clinical Endocrinology* 41:351-357.

Langer G, Heinze G, Reim B et al. (1976). Reduced growth hormone responses to amphetamine in "endogenous" depressive patients. *Archives of General Psychiatry* 33:1471-1475.

Lee MA, Bowers MM, Nash JF et al. (1990). Neuroendocrine measures of dopaminergic function in chronic cocaine users. *Psychiatry Research* 33:151-159.

Levin ER, Sharp B & Carlson HE (1984). Failure to confirm consistent stimulation of growth hormone by diazepam. *Hormone Research* 19:86-90.

Lieber CS (1997). Ethanol metabolism, cirrhosis and alcoholism. *Clinica Chimica Acta* 257:59-84.

Lindholm J, Steiniche T, Rasmussen E et al. (1991). Bone disorder in men with chronic alcoholism: A reversible disease? *Journal of Clinical Endocrinology and Metabolism* 73:118-124.

Lloyd CW & Williams RH (1948). Endocrine changes associated with Laennec's cirrhosis of the liver. *American Journal of Medicine* 4:315-330.

Lloyd T, Rollings N, Eggli DF et al. (1997). Dietary caffeine intake and bone status of postmenopausal women. *American Journal of Clinical Nutrition* 65:1826-1830.

London S, Willett W, Longcope C et al. (1991). Alcohol and other dietary factors in relation to serum hormone concentrations in women at climacteric. *American Journal of Clinical Nutrition* 53:166-171.

MacMahon B, Trichopoulos D, Cole P et al. (1982). Cigarette smoking and urinary estrogens. *New England Journal of Medicine* 307:1062-1065.

Malarkey WB, Strauss RH, Leizman DJ et al. (1991). Endocrine effects in female weight lifters who self-administer testosterone and anabolic steroids. *American Journal of Obstetrics and Gynecology* 165:1385-1390.

Marks V & Teale JD (1999). Drug-induced hypoglycemia. *Endocrinology and Metabolism Clinics of North America* 28:555-577.

Marks V & Wright J (1980). Alcohol-provoked reactive hypoglycaemia. In D Andreani, PJ Lefebvre & V Marks (eds.) *Current Views on Hypoglycemia and Glucagon*. London, England: Academic Press, 283-295.

Massey LK & Opryszek AA (1990). No effects of adaptation to dietary caffeine on calcium excretion in young women. *Nutrition Research* 10:741-747.

Matsuo K, Hirohata T, Sugioka Y et al. (1988). Influence of alcohol intake, cigarette smoking, and occupational status on idiopathic osteonecrosis of the femoral head. *Clinical Orthopaedics and Related Research* 234:115-123.

McKinlay SM, Bifano NL & McKinlay JB (1985). Smoking and age at menopause in women. *Annals of Internal Medicine* 103:350-356.

Meadows R & Verghese A (1996). Medical complications of glue sniffing. *Southern Medical Journal* 89:455-462.

Melander A, Lebovitz HE & Faber OK (1990). Sulfonylureas: Why, which, and how? *Diabetes Care* 13(Suppl 3):18-25.

Mello NK & Mendelson JH (1997). Cocaine's effects on neuroendocrine systems: Clinical and preclinical studies. *Pharmacology, Biochemistry and Behavior* 57:571-599.

Mendelson JH, Cristofaro P, Ellingboe J et al. (1985). Acute effects of marihuana on luteinizing hormone in menopausal women. *Pharmacology, Biochemistry and Behavior* 23:765-768.

Mendelson JH, Kuehnle J, Ellingboe J et al. (1974). Plasma testosterone levels before, during and after chronic marihuana smoking. *New England Journal of Medicine* 291:1051-1055.

Mendelson JH, Mello NK, Teoh SK et al. (1989). Cocaine effects on pulsatile secretion of anterior pituitary, gonadal, and adrenal hormones. *Journal of Clinical Endocrinology and Metabolism* 69:1256-1260.

Mendelson JH, Teoh SK, Lange U et al.(1988). Anterior pituitary, adrenal, and gonadal hormones during cocaine withdrawal. *American Journal of Psychiatry* 145:1094-1098.

Mendelson JH, Teoh SK, Mello NK et al. (1992). Acute effects of cocaine on plasma adrenocorticotropic hormone, luteinizing hormone and prolactin levels in cocaine-dependent men. *Journal of Pharmacology and Experimental Therapeutics* 263:505-509.

Mensink RP, Lebbink WJ, Lobbezoo IE et al. (1995). Diterpene composition of oils from Arabica and Robusta coffee beans and their effects on serum lipids in man. *Journal of Internal Medicine* 237:543-550.

Monteiro MG, Schuckit MA, Hauger R et al. (1990). Growth hormone response to intravenous diazepam and placebo in 82 healthy men. *Biological Psychiatry* 27:702-710.

Nagata C, Kabuto M & Shimizu H (1998). Association of coffee, green tea, and caffeine intakes with serum concentrations of estradiol and sex hormone-binding globulin in premenopausal Japanese women. *Nutrition and Cancer* 30:21-24.

Nurnberger JI Jr, Simmons-Alling S, Kessler L et al. (1984). Separate mechanisms for behavioral, cardiovascular, and hormonal responses to dextroamphetamine in man. *Psychopharmacology* 84:200-204.

Odvina CV, Safi I, Wojtowicz CH et al. (1995). Effect of heavy alcohol intake in the absence of liver disease on bone mass in black and white men. *Journal of Clinical Endocrinology and Metabolism* 80:2499-2503.

Oiso Y & Robertson GL (1985). Effect of ethanol on vasopressin secretion and the role of endogenous opioids. In RW Schrier (ed.) *Vasopressin.* New York, NY: Raven Press, 265-269.

O'Keefe SJD & Marks V (1977). Lunchtime gin and tonic a cause of reactive hypoglycaemia. *Lancet* 1:1286-1288.

Ottesen MM, Worck R & Ibsen H (1997). Captopril does not blunt the sympathoadrenal response to cigarette smoking in normotensive humans. *Blood Pressure* 6:29-34.

Pedrazzoni M, Vescovi PP, Maninetti L et al. (1993). Effects of chronic heroin abuse on bone and mineral metabolism. *Acta Endocrinologica* 129:42-45.

Pepersack T, Fuss M, Otero J et al. (1992). Longitudinal study of bone metabolism after ethanol withdrawal in alcoholic patients. *Journal of Bone and Mineral Research* 7:383-387.

Peris P, Parés A, Guañabens N et al. (1994). Bone mass improves in alcoholics after 2 years of abstinence. *Journal of Bone and Mineral Research* 9:1607-1612.

Prummel MF & Wiersinga WM (1993). Smoking and risk of Graves' disease. *Journal of the American Medical Association* 269:518.

Puddey IB, Vandongen R, Beilin LJ et al. (1985). Alcohol stimulation of renin release in man: Its relation to the hemodynamic, electrolyte, and sympatho-adrenal responses to drinking. *Journal of Clinical Endocrinology and Metabolism* 61:37-42.

Ragni G, De Laurentis L, Bestetti O et al. (1988). Gonadal function in male heroin and methadone addicts. *International Journal of Andrology* 11:93-100.

Razay G & Heaton KW (1997). Moderate alcohol consumption has been shown previously to improve insulin sensitivity in men. *British Medical Journal* 314:443.

Rees L, Butler PWP, Gosling C et al. (1970). Adrenergic blockade and the corticosteroid and growth hormone responses to methylamphetamine. *Nature* 228:565-566.

Rimm EB, Chan J, Stampfer MJ et al. (1995). Prospective study of cigarette smoking, alcohol use, and the risk of diabetes in men. *British Medical Journal* 310:555-559.

Risby ED, Hsiao JK, Golden RN et al. (1989). Intravenous alprazolam challenge in normal subjects. *Psychopharmacology* 99:508-514.

Rowe JW, Kilgore A & Robertson GL (1980). Evidence in man that cigarette smoking induces vasopressin release via an airway-specific mechanism. *Journal of Clinical Endocrinology and Metabolism* 51:170-172.

Roy-Byrne PP, Cowley DS, Hommer D et al. (1991). Neuroendocrine effects of diazepam in panic and generalized anxiety disorders. *Biological Psychiatry* 30:73-80.

Sachar EJ, Asnis G, Nathan RS et al. (1980). Dextroamphetamine and cortisol in depression: Morning plasma cortisol levels suppressed. *Archives of General Psychiatry* 37:755-757.

Santen RJ, Sofsky J, Bilic N et al. (1975). Mechanism of action of narcotics in the production of menstrual dysfunction in women. *Fertility and Sterility* 26:538-548.

Saville PD (1965). Changes in bone mass with age and alcoholism. *Journal of Bone and Joint Surgery* 47:492-499.

Schuckit MA, Hauger RL, Moneiro MG et al. (1991). Response of three hormones to diazepam challenge in sons of alcoholics and controls. *Alcoholism: Clinical & Experimental Research* 15:537-542.

Shaarawy M & Mahmoud KZ (1982). Endocrine profile and semen characteristics in male smokers. *Fertility & Sterility* 38:255-257.

Shine B, Fells P, Edwards OM et al. (1990). Association between Graves' ophthalmopathy and smoking. *Lancet* 335:1261.

Shur E, Petersson H, Checkley S et al. (1983). Long-term benzodiazepine administration blunts growth hormone response to diazepam. *Archives of General Psychiatry* 40:1105-1108.

Small M, Beastall GH, Semple CG et al. (1984). Alteration of hormone levels in normal males given the anabolic steroid stanozolol. *Clinical Endocrinology* 21:49-55.

Snyder SH, Katims JJ, Annau Z et al. (1981). Adenosine receptors and behavioral actions of methylxanthines. *Proceedings of the National Academy of Sciences* 78:3260-3264.

Spindel ER, Wurtman RJ, McCall A et al. (1984). Neuroendocrine effects of caffeine in normal subjects. *Clinical Pharmacology and Therapeutics* 36:402-407.

Strauss R, Liggett M & Lanese R (1985). Anabolic steroid use and perceived effects in ten weight-trained women athletes. *Journal of the American Medical Association* 253:2871-2873.

Streicher HZ, Gabow PA, Moss AH et al. (1981). Syndromes of toluene sniffing in adults. *Annals of Internal Medicine* 94:758-762.

Sullivan ML, Martinez CM, Gennis P et al. (1998). The cardiac toxicity of anabolic steroids. *Progress in Cardiovascular Diseases* 41:1-15.

Targher G, Alberiche M, Zenere MB et al. (1997). Cigarette smoking and insulin resistance in patients with noninsulin-dependent diabetes mellitus. *Journal of Clinical Endocrinology and Metabolism* 82:3619-3624.

Tavani A, Negri E & La Vecchia C (1995). Coffee intake and risk of hip fracture in women in northern Italy. *Preventive Medicine* 24:396-400.

Teoh SK, Sarnyai Z, Mendelson JH et al. (1994). Cocaine effects on pulsatile secretion of ACTH in men. *Journal of Pharmacology and Experimental Therapeutics* 270:1134-1138.

Van Thiel DH, Lester R & Vaitukaitis J (1978). Evidence for a defect in pituitary secretion of luteinizing hormone in chronic alcoholic men. *Journal of Clinical Endocrinology and Metabolism* 47:499-507.

Van Thiel DH, McClain CJ, Elseon MK et al. (1978). Hyperprolactinemia and thyrotropin-releasing factor (TRH) responses in men with alcoholic liver disease. *Alcoholism: Clinical & Experimental Research* 2:344-348.

Vine MF, Margolin BH, Morrison HI et al. (1994). Cigarette smoking and sperm density: A meta-analysis. *Fertility and Sterility* 61:35-43.

Vogel JM, Davis JW, Nomura A et al. (1997). The effects of smoking on bone mass and the rates of bone loss among elderly Japanese-American men. *Journal of Bone and Mineral Research* 12:1495-1501.

Wand GS & Dobs AS (1991). Alterations in the hypothalamic-pituitary-adrenal axis in actively drinking alcoholics. *Journal of Clinical Endocrinology and Metabolism* 72:1290-1295.

Warner EA, Greene GS, Buchsbaum MS et al. (1998). Diabetic ketoacidosis associated with cocaine use. *Archives of Internal Medicine* 158:1799-1802.

Webb CM, Adamson DL, de Zeigler D et al. (1999). Effect of acute testosterone on myocardial ischemia in men with coronary artery disease. *American Journal of Cardiology* 83:437-439.

Webb CM, McNeill JG, Hayward CS et al. (1999). Effects of testosterone on coronary vasomotor regulation in men with coronary heart disease. *Circulation* 100:1690-1696.

Wilson NM, Brown PM, Juul SM et al. (1981). Glucose turnover and metabolic and hormonal changes in ethanol-induced hypoglycaemia. *British Medical Journal* 282:849-853.

Yano K, Heilbrun LK, Wasnich RD et al. (1985). The relationship between diet and bone mineral content of multiple skeletal sites in elderly Japanese-American men and women living in Hawaii. *American Journal of Clinical Nutrition* 42:877-888.

Ylikahri RH, Huttunen MO, Härkönen M et al. (1978). Acute effects of alcohol on anterior pituitary secretion of the tropic hormones. *Journal of Clinical Endocrinology and Metabolism* 46:715-720.

Zemishlany Z, McQueeney R, Gabriel SM et al. (1990). Neuroendocrine and monoaminergic responses to acute administration of alprazolam in normal subjects. *Neuropsychobiology* 23:124-128.

Zumoff B (1997). The critical role of alcohol consumption in determining the risk of breast cancer with postmenopausal estrogen administration. *Journal of Clinical Endocrinology and Metabolism* 82:1656-1657.

Chapter 13 | Perinatal Addiction

Michael F. Weaver, M.D.

Screening and Recognition
Approach to the Patient
Maternal Withdrawal Syndromes
Pain Management
Neonatal Drug Testing
Neonatal Withdrawal Syndrome
Neonatal Complications

The prevalence of substance use during pregnancy is significant. Women addicted to alcohol or other drugs may have irregular menstrual cycles, but still be able to conceive. It may be several months before an addicted woman realizes that she is pregnant (Mitchell & Brown, 1990). In a study of women in a city hospital, 59% admitted to consumption of alcohol during pregnancy (Frank, Zuckerman et al., 1988). Another study found that 11% of pregnant women were using illegal substances, with cocaine as the drug of choice in 75% (Chasnoff, 1989). Women of low socioeconomic status are perceived to be at increased risk of perinatal substance abuse and addiction, but there is little difference in the prevalence of drug and alcohol use among women enrolling in prenatal care in public clinics (16%) and private offices (13%). Rates for Black and White women are virtually identical (14% and 15%, respectively) (Chasnoff, Landress et al., 1990).

Substance use during pregnancy has significant effects on the developing child as well as on the mother. For these reasons, all health care providers should be able to recognize perinatal substance abuse and addiction and should act to address it in order to reduce potential complications for the mother and her child.

SCREENING AND RECOGNITION

Early recognition of substance use problems is particularly important during pregnancy, because alcohol and other drugs have the capacity to affect each stage of fetal development. However, women may not admit to drug use because they fear the legal consequences of such an admission, including loss of custody of the unborn child or other children. Moreover, many women with substance use problems in pregnancy do not fit the stereotype of the addict, which makes early identification and treatment a challenge.

A good health history, taken when a pregnant woman presents for prenatal care, can elicit risk factors for addiction (Table 1 provides guidelines for prenatal care of the addicted pregnant woman). Depression and other mental health problems are risk factors for addiction. One in five women with alcohol abuse or dependence also fulfills the diagnostic criteria for depression at some time in her life, compared to 1 in 20 men (Sonderegger, 1992). The most common psychiatric disorders found in addicted pregnant women are personality disorders (Hoegerman & Schnoll, 1991). These can be difficult to diagnose and treat, and can lead to conflicts with health care practitioners.

TABLE 1.   Guidelines for Prenatal Care of the Addicted Pregnant Woman

First Prenatal Visit
- Complete history and physical examination
- Baseline laboratory tests:
  Complete blood count
  Hemoglobin electrophoresis
  Blood type
  Rh titer
  Serum electrolytes and creatinine
  Serum transaminases, albumen, and bilirubin levels
  Rubella titer
  Hepatitis B and C serology screen
  Syphilis serology
  Informed consent for HIV test
  Informed consent for urine toxicology screen
  Place PPD and anergy panel (mumps and Candida)
    controls
  Cervical cultures for gonorrhea and chlamydia
  Pap smear
- Baseline fetal sonogram
- Establish goals and set appropriate boundaries with the
  patient and her significant other
- Referral for substance abuse treatment (methadone
  maintenance if the patient has opioid addiction)
- Other referrals as appropriate:
  Psychological evaluation
  Social services
  Genetic counseling.

28-Week Followup Visit
- Followup laboratory tests:
  Complete blood count
  Repeat syphilis serology
  Informed consent for urine toxicology screen
- Screening test for gestational diabetes
- Followup fetal sonogram
- Establish good communication with the patient's significant
  other
- Discussion of appropriate contraceptive methods
- Discussion of appropriate parenting
- Establish good communication with the patient's other
  health care providers (addiction treatment, obstetric).

36-Week Followup Visit
- Followup laboratory tests:
  Complete blood count
  Repeat syphilis serology
  Hepatitis B and C serology screen (if previous results were
    negative)
  Informed consent for HIV test (if previous results were
    negative)
  Informed consent for urine toxicology screen
- Discussion of birth plan, appropriate contraceptive methods
  postpartum, and involvement of the patient's significant
  other.
- Education about signs of labor.

Labor and Delivery
Complete history and physical examination
- Ask specifically about recent drug use
- Laboratory tests:
  Repeat syphilis serology
  Hepatitis B and C serology screen (if previous results were
    negative)
  Informed consent for HIV test (if previous results were
    negative)
  Informed consent for urine toxicology screen
- Provide appropriate pain management
- Communicate with appropriate hospital staff:
  Obstetric
  Pediatric
  Addiction treatment
  Anesthesiology
  Social work
  Nursing
- Delivery method should be selected based solely on
  obstetric considerations.

Post Partum
- Encourage continuation of addiction treatment
- Encourage appropriate parenting skills
- Discussion of appropriate contraceptive methods
- Encourage breastfeeding for women (including those on
  methadone maintenance) who are not HIV-positive and not
  currently using drugs.

A family history of substance abuse should alert the clinician to the possibility of addiction in the patient. Children of alcoholics have a three- to four-fold increase in risk of developing alcoholism themselves (Zuckerman, Parker et al., 1986). The patient who has had frequent encounters with law enforcement agencies needs to be considered at high risk for addiction (Daley, Argeriou et al., 2000). Women often are introduced to and supplied with drugs by a male partner, so consider the substance abuse pattern of the patient's current significant other.

If any of these risk factors are present, there is increased likelihood of substance abuse and addiction, so the expectant mother should be asked about her alcohol and drug use. Asking directly is very important and even therapeutic. Studies have shown that screening women in a prenatal clinic with specific questions about alcohol and drug use is effective in reducing their drug use during pregnancy (Chang, Wilkins-Haug et al., 1999).

Acknowledgment of drug use is not sufficient, since women may minimize or deny such use. Two specific screening tools have been validated as useful for screening pregnant women to detect problems resulting from alcohol or drug use. The T-ACE (Table 2) is derived from the CAGE questions, but emphasizes tolerance rather than guilt (Sokol, Martier et al., 1989). A positive answer to the tolerance question or two positive answers to the other three questions indicates an increased likelihood that the woman is drinking at a level that may be harmful to the fetus. The TWEAK (Table 3) can be used to detect a range of drinking levels, from moderate to high risk (Russell, Martier et al., 1991). In scoring, a six-point scale is used (the first question about tolerance is scored as two points; the rest of the questions are scored at one point each), with three or more points indicating that the woman is likely to be engaged in problematic levels of alcohol use. If one of these screening tools is positive, more information must be obtained by history, physical examination, or laboratory test to make a diagnosis.

No instruments have been validated for detection of other illicit drug use during pregnancy. Use of a screening tool and urine toxicology in combination has been shown to be more effective for detection of such drug use than either one alone (Christmas, Knisely et al., 1992).

Additional clues from the medical history help to provide more specific information if a screening tool indicates a problem. Complications of earlier pregnancies (such as preterm labor, premature rupture of membranes, placental

TABLE 2.	**T-ACE Questions**	
T	Tolerance	How many drinks does it take to make you feel high?
A	Annoyed	Have people ANNOYED you by criticizing your drinking?
C	Cut down	Have you felt you ought to CUT DOWN on your drinking?
E	Eye-opener	Have you ever had a drink first thing in the morning to steady your nerves or get rid of a hangover?

abruption, or intrauterine growth retardation) may indicate past alcohol or drug abuse. Respiratory problems in the mother may be a current consequence of intranasal insufflation (snorting) or smoking drugs (Glassroth, Adam et al., 1987). Infections such as endocarditis, recurrent cellulitis, or thrombophlebitis should raise suspicions about injection drug use. Nearly half of parenteral drug users have a history of acute hepatitis (Abel & Sokol, 1992). A history of positive serology for hepatitis B or C, HIV, or other sexually transmitted disease provides clues to possible addiction problems.

Physical, sexual, and verbal abuse by a partner is more common among alcoholic women (Abel & Sokol, 1992), so eliciting a good social history adds information about the consequences of addiction.

Physical Examination Findings. A thorough physical examination may yield findings indicative of current drug use or its consequences. The following discussion is not exhaustive (for more detailed information, see Section 3); rather, it focuses specifically on physical findings during pregnancy.

- Pinpoint pupils on examination of the head and neck indicate opioid intoxication.

- Atrophy of the nasal mucosa or perforation of the nasal septum (Glassroth, Adam et al., 1987) indicates snorting of drugs, most often cocaine or methamphetamine.

- The smell of alcohol on the breath indicates recent ingestion, but not necessarily acute intoxication.

- Poor dentition may indicate ongoing drug use, with little concern for dental hygiene.

- Oropharyngeal candidiasis is more frequent in HIV-positive women (Schuman, Sobel et al., 1998), and HIV infection is associated with addiction.

- Posterior cervical lymphadenopathy is an early sign of HIV infection.

- Finding a new murmur on examination of the heart may indicate endocarditis.

- A cough productive of black sputum indicates crack smoking (Warner, 1995).

- Palpation of the abdomen may reveal an enlarged or shrunken liver due to alcoholic hepatitis or infectious hepatitis from transmission by sharing contaminated needles.

- Constipation from opioid abuse also may be apparent on abdominal examination.

- Even a minimal neurological evaluation can reveal altered mental status due to intoxication or acute alcohol withdrawal.

- Hyperreflexia and tremulousness also prompt consideration of acute alcohol withdrawal.

Thorough examination of the extremities and skin is warranted for every patient. "Track marks" are wormlike scars from repeated injection that follow the courses of veins. Look for healed abscess scars from subcutaneous injection. Women may hide needle marks by injecting in the axillae, under the breasts, into the legs, between fingers or toes, under the tongue, and under the nails. Spider angiomata are common during pregnancy, but may indicate the presence of underlying liver disease if they are numerous and prominent. Look for the rash of syphilis, since the practice of exchanging sex for drugs can result in this consequence of addiction (Minkoff, McCalla et al., 1990).

Prenatal visits include a gynecological examination. Inspection of the external genitalia may reveal syphilis or herpes lesions, which should be cultured. A speculum examination may show vaginitis or cervicitis, since vaginal candidal colonization is more prevalent among HIV-positive women and among those reporting recent injection drug use (Schuman, Sobel et al., 1998). Endocervical cultures should be taken for gonorrhea and chlamydia, because those infections may progress to pelvic inflammatory disease, causing infertility or possible mortality. Any vaginal discharge should be examined for bacterial vaginosis or trichomonia-sis. A Pap smear is very important, since a study showed 24% of pregnant women in an addiction treatment program had an abnormal Pap smear (Minkoff, McCalla et al., 1990).

Laboratory Findings. Laboratory findings often point to alcohol or other drug use. The requirements for notification or permission to obtain specimens for toxicologic testing vary from jurisdiction to jurisdiction, so patients should be informed of the health care provider's suspicion and asked for permission to perform toxicologic testing. Testing for illegal drugs in the absence of medical indications may be discriminatory, violate civil rights, and constitute unlawful search and seizure. Informed consent helps foster a positive therapeutic relationship between the patient and her caregivers, and is part of a trusting and cooperative therapeutic relationship. Indications for toxicologic screening include a history of alcohol or other drug use, loss of custody of other children, lack of prenatal care, altered mental status on examination, preterm labor, third trimester vaginal bleeding (which indicates possible placental abruption due to drug use, especially of stimulants), evidence of drug use on physical examination (track marks), or signs and symptoms of intoxication or withdrawal.

TABLE 3.   TWEAK Questions

T	Tolerance	How many drinks does it take to make you feel high?	Two or more drinks = 2 points
W	Worry	Have close friends WORRIED or complained about your drinking in the past year?	Yes = 1 point
E	Eye-opener	Have you ever had a drink first thing in the morning to steady your nerves or get rid of a hangover?	Yes = 1 point
A	Amnesia	Has anyone ever told you about things that you said or did while you were drinking that you did not remember?	Yes = 1 point
K	Cut down	Have you felt you ought to CUT DOWN on your drinking?	Yes = 1 point

Obtaining a blood alcohol level is more invasive than urine toxicological testing, and provides information only about use within the preceding few hours. Informed consent should be obtained for this test, unless the indication is to assess altered mental status as part of an acute diagnostic evaluation.

Urine drug screening is recommended to provide comprehensive medical care and assist with evaluation for addiction treatment. A urine toxicology screen can provide valuable information about substance use over the preceding few days, but does not provide evidence of use outside that time frame.

The mean corpuscular volume is elevated during long-term alcohol use, and liver transaminases may be elevated by alcohol use or hepatitis acquired from sharing needles. A low white blood cell count or CD4 cell count is an indication of HIV infection, which can result from sharing contaminated needles or through sexual contact with someone who shares needles.

A widened QRS complex on an electrocardiogram may be the result of quinine used to adulterate heroin (White, Chanthavanich et al., 1983). A sonogram may show intrauterine growth retardation, which is the most common finding when a fetus is exposed to drugs or alcohol.

APPROACH TO THE PATIENT

The possibility of perinatal addiction can be recognized from risk factors in the medical history or by screening with the T-ACE (Table 2) or the TWEAK (Table 3). Additional information is gathered through further history-taking, physical examination, and laboratory testing. The patient may be using multiple substances, but often will disclose a preference for a primary drug of abuse. After accumulation of appropriate evidence, a diagnosis of addictive disorder can be made. Many states require hospitals to report pregnant women suspected of alcohol or other drug use to local public health authorities or to the criminal justice system at the time the woman presents for delivery. Such reporting requirements may cause women to be even more wary of acknowledging that they have a problem. For this reason, it is very important for a clinician who recognizes an addictive disorder to address this with the patient in a compassionate, nonjudgmental manner, as with any other medical diagnosis.

Many addicted pregnant women recognize the risks and costs associated with their alcohol or drug use, especially if they have experienced acute toxicity or withdrawal. However, many continue to use alcohol or other drugs for a variety of reasons despite the risks, and are not certain how to address the situation; this is the mechanism of ambivalence. Others are unable to admit the problem to themselves and conceal it from family, friends, and caregivers; this is the mechanism of denial.

The clinician who recognizes substance use or addiction should help the patient resolve her ambivalence or denial. This process of helping the pregnant woman come to a decision can be accomplished through motivational interviewing (Miller & Rollnick, 1991). The clinician's goal is to increase the patient's intrinsic motivation, so that change arises from within rather than being imposed from outside. Motivational interviewing is a way to help individuals recognize and act on their present and potential problems. It is useful with those who are reluctant to change and helps resolve ambivalence, so as to help the patient move along the path to change. Use of motivational interviewing techniques over several short (less than five minutes) encounters in the course of routine prenatal care visits can have a cumulative effect equal to a much longer single session.

In motivational interviewing, the clinician begins by expressing empathy, which means understanding the patient's feelings and perspectives without judging, criticizing, or blaming (aggressive confrontation has been shown to predict treatment failure). He or she then listens to the patient and elicits statements that indicate willingness to change, but backs off as soon as the patient shows signs of resistance.

The clinician expresses to the patient in a non-accusatory tone his or her concern that alcohol or other drug abuse is occurring (giving concrete examples of reasons for the diagnosis) and offers to help. It is useful to list indicators from the history, physical examination, or laboratory results that led to the diagnosis, just as when explaining any new diagnosis. Many women are relieved that they no longer need to hide their problem and that help is available. Others adamantly deny that they have a problem. Some patients need to hear the clinician express concern about substance use several times before they are able to respond.

Once a diagnosis is made, both acute and long-term treatment is necessary. Simple admonitions to stop the substance use sometimes are helpful, if the diagnosis is made early, but in most cases are insufficient (Weaver, Jarvis et al., 1999). Instead, the clinician should assist the woman with practical problem-solving.

Motivational interviewing techniques should not be viewed as sufficient in themselves, but as a way to provide preparation and motivation for further services. This helps to ensure that the woman will follow through when the clinician provides a referral to an appropriate facility for counseling and other long-term addiction treatment. The pregnant woman's ability to follow through with treatment may be compromised by guilt, lack of supportive significant others (including family), and uncertainty about the success of addiction treatment (Mitchell, 1994). However, the possibility of being reunited with her children can be a powerful incentive for a mother to enter treatment. This reduces the burden on the foster care system by assuring the safety of the child in a therapeutic environment.

When planning for the patient's entry into addiction treatment, factors unique to pregnant women must be taken into account. For example, treatment programs must provide child care to be effective (Smith, Dent et al., 1992; Waterson & Ettorre, 1989). In addition to specific formal treatment, Twelve Step self-help groups can provide an important support system.

Some forms of abstinence pharmacotherapy are not appropriate for pregnant women. Disulfiram (Antabuse®) is contraindicated during pregnancy because of its association with specific birth defects (Jessup & Green, 1987). Overall, however, studies have shown that comprehensive treatment programs for addicted pregnant women are successful (Mondanaro & Reed, 1987).

Optimal prenatal care should be a collaborative process between an obstetrical service and the addiction treatment program, in order to provide the best treatment for the medical disorder of addiction and close monitoring of the progress of the pregnancy. Collaboration is essential to assure continuation of addiction treatment after childbirth (Mitchell, 1994). Achieving this requires good communication among obstetricians, addiction medicine specialists, primary care physicians, nurses, anesthesiologists, social workers, counselors, and legal agencies. Consistency in approaches, expectations, and the message conveyed by staff is critical to successful engagement and retention of the pregnant woman in treatment. Supportive involvement of the patient's significant other(s) in her treatment should be encouraged.

Discussion of reproductive options should begin well before delivery. The clinician should provide information about birth control and family planning, since several routine methods of birth control are not optimal choices for women using alcohol or other drugs. Oral estrogen-progestin contraceptive pills may exacerbate vascular disease, and their effectiveness is compromised if they are not taken as prescribed. Intrauterine devices should not be used in women with a history of pelvic inflammatory disease or who are at risk for continued exposure to sexually transmitted diseases. Barrier-type contraceptives (condoms, diaphragms) require conscientious, consistent use, but can reduce the risk of transmission of sexually transmitted diseases. Permanent sterilization (tubal ligation) may be done prior to discharge postpartum. (Some states require a waiting period after signing the consent form for surgical sterilization before the procedure can be performed, especially if the woman has had a drug screen that was positive for psychoactive drugs.)

Planning for delivery involves collaboration among health care providers. Women should be educated about labor and the effects of drugs on the fetus, including neonatal withdrawal syndromes. Education of the woman can prevent frustration that may lead to relapse after delivery. The delivery method should be selected based solely on obstetric considerations.

Women may relapse as they near the end of pregnancy. They may confuse early signs of labor with signs of acute withdrawal, medicate themselves during the early hours of labor, and thus arrive at the hospital in labor with high levels of drugs in the blood from recent use. This increases the risk of fetal stress and distress. Pediatricians should be aware of perinatal exposure to alcohol or other drugs so that they can be observant for neonatal withdrawal syndromes. Also, social services in the hospital or the community may need to be notified at delivery, especially regarding unsafe living conditions.

Postpartum discharge planning must include arrangements for continuation of addiction treatment. It also is important to provide the new mother with information about infant feeding, bathing, umbilical cord care, breastfeeding, appropriate approaches for "fussy" infants, and age-appropriate discipline for other children. This should occur as part of prenatal care and continue after delivery. Many addicted pregnant women are products of poor parenting, so education about appropriate parenting is essential to prevent continuation of addiction into the next generation.

TABLE 4.   Similarities and Differences Between Sedative-Hypnotic Withdrawal and Pregnancy

Signs and Symptoms Common to Both Sedative-Hypnotic Withdrawal and Pregnancy	Signs and Symptoms of Sedative-Hypnotic Withdrawal Not Common to Pregnancy
Restlessness	Impaired memory
Insomnia	Distractibility
Nausea and Vomiting	Agitation
Hypertension	Tremor
Tachycardia	Fever
Tachypnea	Diaphoresis
Seizures	Hallucinations

MATERNAL WITHDRAWAL SYNDROMES

Therapy for maternal alcohol or drug abuse and addiction sometimes begins with detoxification, but this is merely a first step in overall treatment. Medical stabilization of the addicted pregnant woman should be accomplished within 10 days of her initial contact with the health care system, according to guidelines from the Center for Substance Abuse Treatment (CSAT, 1993). Methods for management of acute withdrawal are presented here for specific classes of substances of abuse (also see the detailed discussion of withdrawal in Section 5).

Alcohol and Sedative-Hypnotic Drugs. Sedative-hypnotic drugs (including alcohol, benzodiazepines, barbiturates, and other sleep aids) have significant potential for abuse, but it is unusual to see patients who are abusing only prescription medications. Most women who abuse sedative-hypnotics take one or more benzodiazepines in combination with alcohol, along with barbiturates and other sleeping pills.

The withdrawal syndrome manifests with the same signs and symptoms for alcohol or any of the other sedative-hypnotic medications. This consists of escalating autonomic instability, which usually begins within 48 hours of the last use, although many of the benzodiazepines have long-acting metabolites, so the patient may not show signs of withdrawal for 7 to 10 days after stopping all drugs.

Progression to severe withdrawal carries a significant mortality, so early recognition and treatment is essential. However, the normal physiologic changes that accompany pregnancy can make it difficult to recognize early withdrawal. Table 4 displays similarities and differences between the sedative-hypnotic withdrawal syndrome and pregnancy.

Treatment for acute withdrawal from sedative-hypnotics in a pregnant woman should be accomplished in an inpatient setting, which allows for medical supervision in collaboration with an obstetrician. Uncontrolled withdrawal symptoms may be life-threatening to both mother and fetus. Treatment is identical for withdrawal from all sedative-hypnotics, including barbiturates, benzodiazepines, and alcohol, because all drugs in this class exhibit cross-dependence. The first step is to objectively determine an approximate level of drug to which the patient is tolerant (patients tend to over- or underestimate the amount of alcohol or other drug they have been taking). Very precise instruments for the measurement of tolerance exist, but often are not practical and in many cases are not necessary (Weaver, Jarvis et al., 1999).

Any medication with cross-dependence can be used. An initial dose is given, usually 15 to 90 mg of phenobarbital (or an equivalent dose of another sedative-hypnotic such as diazepam or chlordiazepoxide), and the patient is monitored for at least six to eight hours. The treatment medication is repeated at one- or two-hour intervals, as indicated by the signs of withdrawal the patient exhibits. After eight hours, an approximation can be made of the total dose the patient will require for a 24-hour period. It is better to err on the side of slightly over- rather than under-medicating. Reducing the dose by 10% of the total each day provides a comfortable taper. The taper can be accomplished more rapidly (over five days by reducing the dose by 20% per day) if there are no medical or obstetric complications.

Advanced sedative-hypnotic withdrawal (with markedly abnormal vital signs or delirium) should be treated rapidly and with sufficiently large doses of medication to suppress the withdrawal. Medications with a rapid onset of action should be used and may be given intravenously for immediate effect. Lorazepam and diazepam have a rapid onset of action when given intravenously, although they have a shorter duration of action than when given orally, since first-pass liver metabolism is bypassed. For example, give lorazepam 1 to 4 mg intravenously every 10 to 30 minutes until the patient's agitation or delirium improves, so that the patient is calm but awake and the heart rate decreases to around 100 beats/minute.

After stabilization with rapid-acting medications, the patient can be switched to an equivalent dose of a long-acting medication such as phenobarbital, oral diazepam, clonazepam, or chlordiazepoxide. Benzodiazepines and barbiturates can adversely affect the fetus when given during pregnancy (see Chapter 15 of this section), so this should be taken into account when beginning treatment for acute withdrawal symptoms. However, the risk to both mother and fetus from untreated sedative-hypnotic withdrawal usually is greater than the potential risk to the fetus from exposure to these medications in a controlled setting.

Stimulant Drugs. An abstinence syndrome can occur with chronic stimulant use, and it is characterized by symptoms that are more subtle and complex than those associated with other drug withdrawal. The severity and duration of stimulant withdrawal depends on the intensity of the preceding months of chronic use and the presence of predisposing psychiatric disorders, which amplify withdrawal symptoms. Abrupt discontinuation of stimulants does not cause gross physiologic sequelae. Thus, stimulants generally are not tapered or replaced with a cross-tolerant drug during medically supervised withdrawal. Pregnant women withdrawing from stimulants should not receive medication except in cases of extreme agitation, when low doses of a benzodiazepine may be used if necessary.

If marked depression persists longer than one week after withdrawal, the patient should be evaluated carefully for underlying depression, which then should be treated with a specific antidepressant.

Opioid Drugs. Opioid-dependent patients experience withdrawal symptoms when the drug is discontinued (see Section 5 for a discussion of opioid withdrawal). Abrupt withdrawal in the nonpregnant individual usually causes physical effects no worse than a bad case of influenza. However, opioid withdrawal during pregnancy can lead to fetal distress and premature labor because of increased oxygen consumption by both mother and fetus (Cooper, Altman et al., 1983). Even minimal symptoms in the mother may indicate fetal distress, since the fetus may be more susceptible to withdrawal symptoms than the mother.

Methadone frequently is used to treat acute withdrawal from opioids. Current federal regulations restrict the use of methadone for the treatment of opioid addiction to specially registered clinics (Federal Register, 1989). However, methadone may be used by a physician in private practice for temporary maintenance or detoxification when an addicted patient is admitted to hospital for an illness other than opioid addiction. This includes evaluation for preterm labor, which can be induced by acute withdrawal.

Methadone also may be used by a private practitioner in an outpatient setting when administered daily for a maximum of three days while a patient awaits admission to a licensed methadone treatment program (Rettig & Yarmolinski, 1995). A Drug Enforcement Administration (DEA) registration to prescribe Schedule II medications is required.

A method of calculating the methadone dose based on the patient's symptoms has been used extensively to titrate methadone for opioid withdrawal, without causing oversedation or severe patient discomfort (Weaver, Jarvis et al., 1999). The severity of 10 symptoms (see Table 5) is graded on a scale of 0 to 2 points: 0 points if the symptom is absent; 1 point if the symptom is present; 2 points if the symptom is severe. The total score for all 10 symptoms is determined; each point is equivalent to a requirement of 1 mg of methadone. The patient should be evaluated and the symptom score totaled every six hours for the first 24 hours. After 24 hours, the total dose of methadone that has been administered is computed; this dose is approximately equivalent to the dose of opioid the individual was taking. The duration of action of methadone allows it to be given once daily as a single dose. Patients do not experience a "rush" or initial euphoria with methadone administration.

Other substitute medications include the short-acting opioids, such as morphine, hydromorphone, or fentanyl, which typically are used in settings where the patient can be closely monitored, such as an intensive care unit. These drugs allow rapid titration of parenteral medications that have rapid onset and short duration of action. They can be given as an intravenous bolus or continuous infusion. The severity of the 10 symptoms (see Table 5) is graded on the scale of 0 to 2 points, as described above. The total score for all 10 symptoms is calculated, then morphine sulfate (or another short-acting opioid) is administered intrave-

TABLE 5. Opioid Withdrawal Signs in the Pregnant Woman

- Pupil dilation
- Lacrimation (watery eyes)
- Rhinorrhea (runny nose)
- Piloerection (gooseflesh, body hair stands up)
- Nausea, vomiting
- Diarrhea, abdominal cramps
- Chills, hot flashes
- Myalgias (muscle aches), arthralgias (joint aches), muscle cramps, twitching
- Yawning
- Restlessness, irritability, insomnia

nously, with frequent assessments until the withdrawal score is reduced to 0 to 5 points (Schnoll, 1995). The dose of parenteral opioid can be increased rapidly in 1 mg increments every five minutes to reduce withdrawal signs. When the patient is converted to oral medication, oral methadone is given in fixed volume once daily at a dose equivalent to the amount of short-acting opioid received in the preceding 24 hours.

Sublingual buprenorphine has been used successfully for opioid maintenance in pregnant women (Fischer, Etzersdorfer et al., 1998; Fischer, Johnson et al., 2000). This medication is well-tolerated by the mothers, while the infants had a low incidence of neonatal opioid abstinence syndrome at doses of 1 to 10 mg/day.

Naloxone should not be given to a pregnant woman except as a last resort for severe opioid overdose, because withdrawal precipitated by an opioid antagonist can result in spontaneous abortion, premature labor, or stillbirth.

Methadone Maintenance: Medical withdrawal of the pregnant opioid-dependent woman is not recommended because of high rates of relapse to heroin use and the increased risk to the fetus of intrauterine death. Methadone maintenance is the treatment of choice (CSAT, 1993). Methadone maintenance reduces use of illicit opioids as well as other drugs. Methadone is long-acting, which allows for a consistent blood level, in contrast to wide fluctuations in blood level due to use of short-acting opioids obtained illicitly. Methadone maintenance reduces use of illicit opioids

by blocking withdrawal symptoms and cravings. Use of a stable methadone dose reduces fluctuations in maternal opioid level, which reduces stress on the fetus (fluctuations between intoxication and withdrawal result in adverse fetal effects, such as premature labor and spontaneous abortion). Illicitly purchased heroin often is adulterated with other compounds that may be harmful to the fetus, so elimination of heroin use with adequate doses of methadone prevents harm to the fetus from exposure to the other compounds. Improved maternal health and nutrition reduce obstetrical complications and improve the health of the infant at delivery.

Other advantages of methadone maintenance over illicit opioid use include reductions in criminal activity and decreased disruption of the maternal-child unit (Wilson, 1989). Methadone maintenance enhances the ability of the woman to participate in prenatal care and in addiction treatment, thus allowing her to better prepare for the arrival of the infant.

Opioid-dependent pregnant women should be referred to a local methadone maintenance program, if available. Most programs assign high priority to pregnant women, so the patient may be able to enter treatment sooner than if she were not pregnant. After initial medical stabilization on a dose of methadone, as described above, the woman should continue to receive methadone daily. Opioid-dependent pregnant women on methadone maintenance need to be monitored regularly throughout the pregnancy, and the dose adjusted as necessary. Studies have shown that a daily methadone dose over 60 mg is most effective (Pond, Kreek et al., 1985). It is not unusual for the methadone dose requirement to increase during the third trimester of pregnancy. This is due to larger plasma volume, decreased plasma protein binding, increased tissue binding, increased methadone metabolism, and increased methadone clearance in the mother. As a result, the half-life of methadone is shortened late in pregnancy and the woman may experience mild withdrawal symptoms unless her methadone dose is adjusted. Splitting the total daily methadone requirement into two doses, given in the morning and evening, is preferred (Wittmann & Segal, 1991; Jarvis, Wu-Pong et al., 1999) if possible. This provides a more even blood level throughout the day.

Women can breastfeed while on methadone maintenance as long as they are not abusing any drugs (McCarthy

TABLE 6.   Time To Onset Of Neonatal Withdrawal Signs

Drug	Time After Delivery to Symptom Onset
Alcohol	3-12 hours
Barbiturates	4-7 days
Diazepam	1-12 days
Opioids	48-72 hours

& Posey, 2000; Geraghty, Graham et al., 1997) and are not HIV-positive. Breastfeeding should be encouraged to promote mother-infant bonding and to provide optimal nutrition and passive immunization to the child.

PAIN MANAGEMENT

Patients on chronic doses of opioids, including those on methadone maintenance, still can experience acute pain and benefit from additional doses of opioids for such pain.

The addicted pregnant woman should be assessed for appropriate analgesia and anesthesia options at delivery. Regional anesthesia may be the procedure of choice during delivery and for postpartum pain. Placement of an epidural catheter, with infusion of a local anesthetic such as bupivicaine, can reduce or eliminate the need for opioid analgesics. Many injection drug users require placement of a central venous catheter for optimal intravenous access because of sclerosis of peripheral veins from repeated injections.

The woman's pain level should be assessed regularly and frequently. Pain medication should not be withheld because a woman has a history of addiction. Inadequately treated pain may result in physiologic manifestations such as delirium or impaired immune function (Koga, Itoh et al., 2001). Psychologic sequelae of untreated pain include anxiety, depression, and suffering. These complications can be prevented by adequately treating pain.

The patient may require higher doses of additional opioids due to the development of tolerance. The medication dose should be adjusted according to the patient's reported level of pain, as assessed through use of a pain rating scale. This helps to set goals for a level of pain that the patient can tolerate, while still being functional and without side effects such as oversedation. Pain levels, medication-taking behavior, and side effects should be monitored several times throughout the day for trends in pain level and effectiveness of medication. Observation of each patient's behavior over time will help staff determine whether additional doses of medication are being requested because of pain or as a manifestation of addiction.

In treating acute pain, scheduled dosing is better than "as-needed" dosing. Use scheduled doses of long-acting opioids, with short-acting medication available for breakthrough pain. If the patient is allowed some control over the dose, such as with a patient-controlled analgesia (PCA) pump, there is less anxiety on the part of the patient and less work on the part of the physician and nurse. Treat proactively instead of reactively, because less medication is required to maintain relief once it has been achieved. Recovery time is shorter when pain is well controlled. Prescribe an adequate dose of pain medication, administered at an appropriate time interval. The dosing interval of the particular pain medication being given should match the duration of action of the medication. For example, if the duration of action is three hours (such as for oxycodone), it should be dosed every three hours. If given every four to six hours, the patient is in pain for one to three hours and will require higher doses to treat the pain once it has begun. Undertreatment of pain may result in relapse to addiction.

Women who are abusing heroin or who are on chronic opioids (methadone maintenance) should not receive opioid agonist/antagonist pain medications (such as pentazocine or butorphanol) for acute pain because those medications can cause an acute opioid withdrawal syndrome (Preston, Bigelow et al., 1988; Strain, Preston et al., 1993).

NEONATAL DRUG TESTING

A positive history of maternal drug use or a positive maternal urine toxicology suggests the need for toxicologic testing of the newborn. Urine is most often tested, but only provides information about exposure to drugs taken by the mother shortly before delivery. Meconium drug testing, although not conclusive if results are negative, is more likely to identify infants of drug-abusing mothers than infant urine testing (Ostrea, Brady et al., 1989).

In a newborn, a positive toxicology screen for nonprescribed drugs warrants a social work evaluation. In some states, health care practitioners (physicians, nurses, and social workers) have a legal duty to report positive results to Child Protective Services. Child Protective Services workers then initiate further investigation of the risk to the child

TABLE 7. Neonatal Opioid Withdrawal Pharmacotherapy

Medication	Dosing			
	Induction	*Titration*	*Stabilization*	*Tapering*
Tincture of opium (diluted solution of 0.4 mg/ml morphine equivalent)	0.1 ml/kg (2 drops/kg) q4h with feedings	Increase by 0.1 ml/kg (2 drops/kg) every 4h as needed to control withdrawal signs	Q4h with feedings for 3 to 5 days	Taper gradually by reducing dose without changing frequency of administration.
Paregoric (0.4 mg/ml)	0.1 ml/kg (2 drops/kg) q4h with feedings	Increase by 0.1 ml/kg (2 drops/kg) every 4h as needed to control withdrawal signs	Q4h with feedings for 3 to 5 days	Taper gradually by reducing dose without changing frequency of administration.
Methadone	0.05 to 0.1 mg/kg q6h	Increase by 0.05 mg/kg every 6h as needed to control withdrawal signs	When stable, give total daily dose once daily, or divided into q12h doses	Taper gradually to 0.05 mg/kg, then discontinue (will self-taper as drug is metabolized due to long half-life).

SOURCE: Adapted from American Academy of Pediatrics (AAP), Committee on Drugs (1998). Neonatal drug withdrawal. Pediatrics 101:1079-1088.

and make recommendations regarding appropriate placement of the infant (with the mother, another family member, or in foster care).

A confirmed or suspected history of addiction in the mother may lead to infant screening for hepatitis B or C, HIV, or other sexually transmitted diseases. Infants born to addicted mothers are at higher risk for these infections because of the association of drug use with high-risk sexual behaviors. Screening allows for early treatment and may help to prevent further transmission or other complications of infection.

NEONATAL WITHDRAWAL SYNDROME

The presence of a neonatal abstinence syndrome should be considered when the mother has a positive urine drug screen at delivery. Neonatal withdrawal syndromes all are characterized by hyperactivity, irritability, hypertonia, difficulty sucking or excessive sucking, and high-pitched cries (Finnegan & Kaltenbach, 1992). Neonates with intrauter-

ine drug exposure should be followed in the hospital for three to four days after delivery to monitor for signs of an abstinence syndrome. Where this is not possible because of restrictions imposed by health plans, mothers should be educated to recognize signs of neonatal withdrawal. Timing of withdrawal onset depends on the time of the last drug exposure, and metabolism and excretion of the drug (see Table 6). If more than seven days have elapsed between the last maternal use and delivery, the incidence of neonatal withdrawal is low (Steg, 1957).

Initial treatment of the neonate experiencing drug withdrawal should be primarily supportive, since pharmacotherapy may prolong hospitalization and expose the neonate to medications that may not be indicated (AAP, 1998). Supportive care includes swaddling, frequent small feedings, observation, and intravenous replacement of fluids and electrolytes. Indications for pharmacotherapy include (1) seizures, (2) poor feeding, diarrhea, or vomiting resulting in dehydration or excessive weight loss, (3) inability to sleep, or (4) fever not due to infection.

FIGURE 1.   Neonatal Abstinence Scale

DATE: DAILY WEIGHT:

SYSTEM	SIGNS AND SYMPTOMS	SCORE	AM	PM	COMMENTS
CENTRAL NERVOUS SYSTEM DISTURBANCES	Excessive High Pitched (other) Cry Continuous High Pitched (other) Cry	2 3			
	Sleeps < 1 hour after feeding Sleeps < 2 hours after feeding Sleeps < 3 hours after feeding	3 2 1			
	Hyperactive Moro reflex Markedly Hyperactive Moro reflex	2 3			
	Mild Tremors Disturbed Moderate-Severe Tremors Disturbed	1 2			
	Mild Tremors Undisturbed Moderate-Severe Tremors Undisturbed	3 4			
	Increased Muscle Tone	2			
	Exconation (specific areas)	1			
	Myoclonic Jerks	3			
	Generalized Convulsions	5			
METABOLIC/VASOMOTOR/ RESPIRATORY DISTURBANCES	Sweating	1			
	Fever < 101º (99º-100.8ºF/37.2º-38.2ºC) Fevers > 101º (38.4ºC and higher)	1 2			
	Frequent Yawning(>3-4 times/interval)	1			
	Mottling	1			
	Nasal Stuffiness	1			
	Sneezing (>304 times/interval)	1			
	Nasal Flaring	2			
	Respiratory Rate >60/min. Respiratory Rate >60/min. with retractions	1 2			
GASTRO- INTESTINAL DISTURBANCES	Excessive sucking	1			
	Poor Feeding	2			
	Regurgitation Projectile Vomiting	2 3			
	Loose Stools Water Stools	2 2			
TOTAL SCORE					
INITIALS OF SCORER					

Infants born to mothers with confirmed or suspected drug use within a week of delivery should have regular assessment for withdrawal signs. Pharmacotherapy should be considered if the infant is too ill to assess possible withdrawal signs or is not thriving as expected. Vomiting and/ or diarrhea associated with dehydration and poor weight gain, in the absence of other diagnoses, are relative indications for treatment, even without high total withdrawal scores (AAP, 1998).

Since polysubstance abuse is the norm rather than the exception, even during pregnancy, determination of specific perinatal effects of individual drugs is difficult. No clinical signs should be attributed solely to drug withdrawal without appropriate assessment and diagnostic tests to rule out other causes. The differential diagnosis for neonatal withdrawal syndrome includes sepsis, hypoglycemia, perinatal anoxia, intracranial bleed, and hyperthyroidism (Desmond & Wilson, 1975).

Opioids. Neonatal opioid withdrawal syndrome occurs in 60% to 80% of infants with intrauterine exposure to heroin or methadone (Finnegan & Ehrlich, 1990). The most comprehensive assessment is the scoring system proposed by Finnegan & Kaltenbach (1992; see Figure 1). This scale assesses 21 symptoms with weighted scores, which are evaluated at two hours after birth and then every four hours. Scoring is quantitative, so all symptoms observed during the interval should be counted. If the severity score is >8, the infant should be scored every two hours until the severity score decreases, then scoring should resume every four hours.

Pharmacotherapy should be initiated when the total score is >8 for three consecutive evaluations. Neonatal opioid withdrawal syndrome is treated with a substitute opioid, such as tincture of opium, paregoric, or methadone, or with a CNS depressant such as phenobarbital (see Table 7 for dosing regimens).

Other Drugs. Symptoms of neonatal sedative-hypnotic withdrawal are similar to opioid withdrawal, but no specific scoring scale has been validated. Seizures are more frequent with alcohol withdrawal than opioid withdrawal (Robe, Gromisch et al., 1981). Neonatal benzodiazepine withdrawal usually resolves spontaneously and does not require specific treatment.

Phenobarbital is the agent of choice for severe sedative-hypnotic withdrawal. It can be administered orally or intramuscularly at a dose of 2 to 4 mg per kg of body weight every eight hours (Kandall, Doberczak et al., 1983). After stabilization, with reduction of neonatal withdrawal signs, the dose can be tapered by 10% to 20% per day over 5 to 10 days. An abstinence syndrome after intrauterine cocaine exposure has not been clearly defined (AAP, 1998).

All infants with suspected or confirmed intrauterine drug exposure should be monitored for neonatal withdrawal, treated with supportive care, and possibly with pharmacotherapy.

NEONATAL COMPLICATIONS
Alcohol or drug use during pregnancy may affect the fetus at any stage of development. It is not known what level of exposure may cause specific birth defects, so complete abstinence should be encouraged as soon as a woman suspects she is pregnant. Various developmental abnormalities have been attributed to intrauterine exposure to specific drugs of abuse. Infants born to women who are addicted to alcohol or other drugs are at high risk for sequelae such as attachment difficulties, behavioral problems (disorganization, unpredictability, and distractibility), and child neglect or abuse (Hoegerman, Wilson et al., 1990).

Experimental studies to evaluate the long-term effects of intrauterine exposure to drugs are limited, so it is difficult to differentiate the effects of the actual drug exposure from the effects of being raised in an environment of ongoing parental drug use (Ellis, Byrd et al., 1993). Development and behavior are affected by multiple environmental influences, including maternal capabilities for bonding, nurturing, and childrearing (Bauman & Levine, 1986). Other factors that often coincide with addiction include poor nutrition, lack of access to health care, disruption of the family unit, and exposure to violence (Regan, Leifer et al., 1988). For a discussion of specific effects of intrauterine drug exposure, see Chapter 14 of this section.

Social complications of perinatal addiction can have a significant effect on the infant before and after delivery. Mandatory reporting of positive maternal drug screens or aggressive prosecution of addicted mothers may cause women to avoid disclosure of addiction during pregnancy. Some addicted women avoid prenatal care and hospital delivery, particularly if they have other children in the custody of Child Protective Services or living with relatives, because they fear the loss of their children. Confusion and fear cause some addicted women to abandon an infant at the hospital rather than discuss options for the infant's care and legal custody. However, mandatory reporting legislation may provide an incentive for a pregnant addicted woman to enter treatment prior to delivery, in order to avoid potential prosecution. Continued custody of the child may be contingent on the woman's adherence to a treatment plan determined by Child Protective Services.

Education of addicted pregnant women about applicable state laws and regulations can help to enhance their motivation to enter addiction treatment prior to delivery. Initiation of treatment at this time can help prevent social consequences, such as infant abandonment, increased medical costs, special education problems, and continuation of addiction into the next generation. Better prenatal care also leads to better birth and developmental outcomes for the infant.

The most critical aspect of the child's development is what happens postpartum. Infants with intrauterine drug exposure may be difficult to nurture due to behavioral changes, which cause problems with bonding between mother and infant. Mothers who continue to abuse stimulants after delivery put their children at risk if they breastfeed, because stimulants pass into breast milk (Chasnoff, Lewis et al., 1987). Maternal drug abuse can have adverse consequences for children, such as child neglect and abuse or loss of family structure. The chaotic environment of an addicted mother, combined with lack of appropriate stimulation and an inappropriate role model, may lead to impairment of intellectual capabilities, social behavior, and ethical behavior of children growing up in the environment (Chasnoff, 1988). Prolonged hospitalization of newborns or placement in foster care is an economic burden on society (Weaver & Schnoll, 1999). Appropriate support should be available to addicted women after delivery to help them meet the challenge of dealing with their newborn, especially if older children are present and require care. Support can come from the woman's family, a Twelve Step self-help group, or health care practitioners with appropriate advice. Lack of support can lead to relapse, which may result in neglect of the infant. Planning for ongoing maternal addiction treatment reduces the chance of an adverse outcome for the child.

CONCLUSIONS

Perinatal addiction affects women of all races and socioeconomic levels. Early recognition is important to prevent fetal complications. The T-ACE and the TWEAK are screening tools validated for use in pregnancy. Information from the history, physical examination, and laboratory tests can help the clinician make a diagnosis of perinatal addiction.

Motivational interviewing techniques help health care practitioners encourage addicted pregnant women to enter addiction treatment. Planning for treatment involves collaboration among multiple specialties, including obstetricians, addiction medicine specialists, pediatricians, primary care physicians, nurses, and social workers. Edu-

cation of pregnant women about childbirth helps prevent problems (including relapse) at the time of delivery.

Addicted pregnant women need rapid medical stabilization. This includes inpatient management of pharmacotherapy for sedative-hypnotic withdrawal syndrome. Methadone maintenance is the treatment of choice for heroin-dependent pregnant women. Adequate pain management should be provided at the time of delivery.

Infants with known or suspected intrauterine drug or alcohol exposure should be monitored for neonatal withdrawal signs and appropriate pharmacotherapy provided if necessary. Specific birth defects and possible developmental abnormalities may result from intrauterine drug exposure. Continued maternal drug use after delivery also leads to adverse health consequences for infants. Continuation of addiction treatment postpartum, coupled with appropriate social support for new mothers, is essential to prevent relapse after delivery. Basic knowledge of perinatal addiction allows health care providers to improve the health and welfare of mothers and their children.

REFERENCES

Abel EL & Sokol RJ (1992). Consequences of alcohol abuse. In N Gleicher (ed.) *Principles and Practice of Medical Therapy in Pregnancy*. New Haven, CT: Appleton & Lange, 79-85.

American Academy of Pediatrics (AAP), Committee on Drugs (1998). Neonatal drug withdrawal. *Pediatrics* 101:1079-1088.

Bauman PS & Levine S (1986). The development of children of drug addicts. *International Journal of the Addictions* 21:849-863.

Brown RL & Rounds LA (1995). Conjoint screening questionnaires for alcohol and other drug abuse: Criterion validity in a primary care practice. *Wisconsin Medical Journal* 94:135-140.

Center for Substance Abuse Treatment (CSAT) (1993). *Pregnant, Substance-Abusing Women (Treatment Improvement Protocol 2)*. Rockville, MD: CSAT, Substance Abuse and Mental Health Services Administration.

Chang G, Wilkins-Haug L, Berman S et al. (1999). Brief intervention for alcohol use in pregnancy: A randomized trial. *Addiction* 94:1499-1508.

Chasnoff IJ (1988). Drug use in pregnancy: Parameters of risk. *Pediatric Clinics of North America* 35:1403-1412.

Chasnoff IJ (1989). Drug use and women: Establishing a standard of care. *Annals of the New York Academy of Sciences* 562:208-210.

Chasnoff IJ, Landress HJ & Barrett ME (1990). The prevalence of illicit drug or alcohol use during pregnancy and discrepancies in mandatory reporting in Pinellas County, Florida. *New England Journal of Medicine* 322:1202-1206.

Chasnoff IJ, Lewis DE & Squires L (1987). Cocaine intoxication in a breast-fed infant. *Pediatrics* 80:836-838.

Christmas JT, Knisely JS, Dawson KS et al. (1992). Comparison of questionnaire screening and urine toxicology for detection of pregnancy complicated by substance use. *Obstetrics & Gynecology* 80:750-754.

Cooper JR, Altman F, Brown BS et al. (1983). *Research on the Treatment of Narcotic Addiction—State of the Art (NIDA Research Monograph Series)*. Rockville, MD: National Institute on Drug Abuse.

Daley M, Argeriou M, McCarty D et al. (2000). The costs of crime and the benefits of substance abuse treatment for pregnant women. *Journal of Substance Abuse Treatment* 19:445-458.

Desmond MM & Wilson GS (1975). Neonatal abstinence syndrome: Recognition and diagnosis. *Addictive Diseases: An International Journal* 2:113-121.

Ellis JE, Byrd LD, Sexson WR et al. (1993). In utero exposure to cocaine: A review. *Southern Medical Journal* 86:725-731.

Federal Register (1989). Methadone: Rules and regulations. *Federal Register* 544:8954.

Finnegan LP & Ehrlich SM (1990). Maternal drug abuse during pregnancy: Evaluation and pharmacotherapy for neonatal abstinence. *Modern Methods of Pharmacologic Testing in the Evaluation of Drugs of Abuse* 6:255-263.

Finnegan LP & Kaltenbach K (1992). Neonatal abstinence syndrome. In RA Hoekelman, SB Friedman, NM Nelson et al. (eds.) *Primary Pediatric Care, 2nd Edition*. St. Louis, MO: Mosby Medical Publishers, 1367-1378.

Fischer G, Etzersdorfer P, Eder H et al. (1998). Buprenorphine maintenance in pregnant opiate addicts. *European Addiction Research* 4(Suppl 1):32-36.

Fischer G, Johnson RE, Eder H et al. (2000). Treatment of opioid-dependent pregnant women with buprenorphine. *Addiction* 95:239-244.

Frank DA, Zuckerman BS, Amaro H et al. (1988). Cocaine use during pregnancy: Prevalence and correlates. *Pediatrics* 82:888-895.

Geraghty B, Graham EA, Logan B et al. (1997). Methadone levels in breast milk. *Journal of Human Lactation* 13:227-230.

Glassroth J, Adam GD & Schnoll SH (1987). The impact of substance abuse on the respiratory system. *Chest* 91:596-602.

Hoegerman G & Schnoll SH (1991). Narcotic use in pregnancy. *Clinical Perinatology* 18:51-76.

Hoegerman G, Wilson CA, Thurmond E et al. (1990). Drug-exposed neonates. *Western Journal of Medicine* 152:559-564.

Jarvis MAE, Wu-Pong S, Knisely JS et al. (1999). Alterations in methadone metabolism during late pregnancy. *Journal of Addictive Diseases* 18:51-61.

Jessup M & Green JR (1987). Treatment of the pregnant alcohol-dependent woman. *Journal of Psychoactive Drugs* 19:193-203.

Kandall SR, Doberczak TM, Mauer KR et al. (1983). Opiate vs. CNS depressant therapy in neonatal drug abstinence syndrome. *American Journal of the Diseases of Children* 137:378-382.

Koga C, Itoh K, Aoki M et al. (2001). Anxiety and pain suppress the natural killer cell activity in oral surgery outpatients. *Oral Surgery, Oral Medicine, Oral Pathology & Oral Radiology and Endodontics* 91:654-658.

McCarthy JJ & Posey BL (2000). Methadone levels in human milk. *Journal of Human Lactation* 16:115-120.

Miller WR & Rollnick S (1991). *Motivational Interviewing: Preparing People to Change Addictive Behavior*. New York, NY: Guilford Press.

Minkoff HL, McCalla MD, Delke I et al. (1990). The relationship of cocaine use to syphilis and human immunodeficiency virus infection among inner city parturient women. *American Journal of Obstetrics & Gynecology* 163:521-526.

Mitchell J (1994). Treatment of the addicted woman in pregnancy. In NS Miller (ed.) *Principles of Addiction Medicine*. Chevy Chase, MD: American Society of Addiction Medicine.

Mitchell JL & Brown G (1990). Physiological effects of cocaine, heroin, and methadone. In RC Engs (ed.) *Women: Alcohol and Other Drugs*. Dubuque, IA: Kendall/Hunt Publishing Co., 53-60.

Mondanaro J & Reed B (1987). *Current Issues in the Treatment of Chemically Dependent Women (NIDA Research Monograph Series)*. Rockville, MD: NIDA, National Institutes of Health.

Ostrea EM, Brady MJ, Parks PM et al. (1989). Drug screening of meconium in infants of drug-dependent mothers: An alternative to urine testing. *Journal of Pediatrics* 115:474-477.

Pond SM, Kreek MJ, Tong TG et al. (1985). Altered methadone pharmacokinetics in methadone-maintained pregnant women. *Journal of Pharmacology & Experimental Therapy* 233:1-6.

Preston KL, Bigelow GE & Liebson IA (1988). Butorphanol-precipitated withdrawal in opioid-dependent human volunteers. *Journal of Pharmacology & Experimental Therapy* 246(2):441-448.

Regan DO, Leifer B & Finnegan LP (1988). Generations at risk: Violence in the lives of pregnant drug abusing women. *Pediatric Resident* 16:77.

Rettig RA & Yarmolinski A, eds. (1995). *Committee on Federal Regulation of Methadone Treatment, Division of Biobehavioral Sciences and Mental Disorders, Institute of Medicine: Federal Regulation of Methadone Treatment*. Washington, DC: National Academy Press.

Robe LB, Gromisch DS & Iosub S (1981). Symptoms of neonatal ethanol withdrawal. *Current Alcohol Research* 8:485-493.

Russell M, Martier SS, Sokol RJ et al. (1991). Screening for pregnancy risk-drinking: Tweaking the tests. *Alcoholism: Clinical & Experimental Research* 15:368.

Schnoll SH (1995). Drug abuse, overdose, and withdrawal syndromes. In SM Ayres, A Grenvik, PR Holbrook et al. (eds.) *Textbook of Critical Care, 3rd Edition*. Philadelphia, PA: W.B. Saunders.

Schuman P, Sobel JD, Ohmit SE et al. (1998). Mucosal candidal colonization and candidiasis in women with or at risk for human immunodeficiency virus infection. HIV Epidemiology Research Study (HERS) Group. *Clinics of Infectious Disease* 27:1161-1167.

Smith IE, Dent DZ, Coles CD et al. (1992). A comparison study of treated and untreated pregnant and postpartum cocaine-abusing women. *Journal of Substance Abuse Treatment* 9:343-348.

Sokol RJ, Martier SS & Ager JW (1989). The T-ACE questions: practical prenatal detection of risk-drinking. *American Journal of Obstetrics and Gynecology* 160:863-870.

Sonderegger T, ed. (1992). *Perinatal Substance Abuse*. Baltimore, MD: Johns Hopkins University Press.

Steg N (1957). Narcotic withdrawal reactions in the newborn. *American Journal of Diseases of Children* 94:286-288.

Strain EC, Preston KL & Liebson IA (1993). Precipitated withdrawal by pentazocine in methadone-maintained volunteers. *Journal of Pharmacology & Experimental Therapy* 267:624-634.

Warner EA (1995). Is your patient using cocaine? *Postgraduate Medicine* 98:173-180.

Waterson J & Ettorre B (1989). Providing services for women with difficulties with alcohol or other drugs: The current U.K. situation as seen by women practitioners, researchers and policy makers in the field. *Drug & Alcohol Dependence* 24:119-125.

Weaver MF, Jarvis MAE & Schnoll SH (1999). Role of the primary care physician in problems of substance abuse. *Archives of Internal Medicine* 159:913-924.

Weaver MF & Schnoll SH (1999). Stimulants—Amphetamines, cocaine. In BS McCrady & EE Epstein (eds.) *Addictions: A Comprehensive Guidebook.* New York, NY: Oxford University Press, 105-120.

White NJ, Chanthavanich P, Krishna S et al. (1983). Quinine disposition kinetics. *British Journal of Clinical Pharmacology* 16:399-403.

Wilson G (1989). Clinical studies of infants and children exposed prenatally to heroin. *Annals of the New York Academy of Sciences* 562:183-194.

Wittmann BK & Segal S (1991). A comparison of the effects of single- and split-dose methadone administration on the fetus: Ultrasound evaluation. *International Journal of the Addictions* 26:213-218.

Zuckerman B, Parker S, Hingson R et al. (1986). Maternal psychoactive substance use and its effect on the neonate. In A Milunsky, EA Friedman & L Gluck (eds.) *Advances in Perinatal Medicine.* New York, NY: Plenum Press, 125-179.

Chapter 14

Alcohol and Other Drug Use During Pregnancy: Effect on the Developing Fetus, Neonate, and Infant

Ann Marie Pagliaro, B.S.N., M.S.N., Ph.D. Candidate, FPPR
Louis A. Pagliaro, M.S., Pharm.D., Ph.D., FPPR

Maternal Substance Use
Alcohol
Sedative-Hypnotic Drugs
Opioids
Cocaine
Other Stimulants
Nicotine and Tobacco
Volatile Solvents and Inhalants
Psychedelics

The focus of this chapter is maternal substance use and human teratogenesis. The authors use the term "substance use" rather than "substance abuse" because the use of certain substances (such as alcohol) during pregnancy at levels or in patterns that would not constitute abuse by, or cause harm to, the mother may result in devastating effects for her unborn fetus (Table 1).

A teratogen is broadly defined as any factor (such as a drug) that is associated with the production of physical or mental abnormalities in the developing embryo or fetus. The term "teratogen" is derived from the Greek words "terato," monster, and "genesis," origin or beginning. It is estimated that some type of teratogenic effect can be found in 2% to 3% of all live births and that teratogenic effects, at least in part, account for 20% of the deaths that occur during the first five years of life. These effects, which can be acute and self-limiting or irreversible and long term, are displayed in a variety of ways (Pagliaro & Pagliaro, 1996, 2000, 2002).

The type and degree of human teratogenesis has been associated with many factors, including unknown factors, genetic factors, and maternal/fetal environmental factors (Pajer, 1992). The maternal/fetal environmental factors can be divided into radiation, disease, infections, and drugs. Although many health and social care professionals are paying closer attention to the potential teratogenic effects associated with the use of selected drugs during pregnancy (Pagliaro & Pagliaro, 1999, 2002), their general knowledge and understanding of the possible teratogenic effects associated with the substances of abuse can be limited.

This chapter summarizes the published literature examining the teratogenic effects associated with the maternal use of the various substances of abuse during pregnancy. Attention is given only to human studies because of the inherent difficulties associated with extrapolating data from animal studies to humans. These difficulties include determining physiologic and genetic differences in teratogenic

---

TABLE 1. Substances with Teratogenic Effects

Central Nervous System Depressants
- Alcohol: beer, wine, distilled spirits
- Sedative-hypnotics: barbiturates, benzodiazepines
- Opioids: codeine, heroin, meperidine, morphine, pentazocine
- Volatile solvents and inhalants: gasoline, glue.

Central Nervous System Stimulants
- Cocaine: cocaine hydrochloride, crack cocaine
- Amphetamines: dextroamphetamine
- Caffeine: caffeinated soft drinks, coffee, tea
- Nicotine: tobacco cigarettes and cigars.

Psychedelics
- Lysergic acid diethylamide (LSD)
- Mescaline (peyote)
- Phencyclidine (PCP)
- Psilocybin (hallucinogenic mushrooms)
- Tetrahydrocannabinol (THC): marijuana, hashish.

---

susceptibility and establishing comparable doses, stages of pregnancy, environmental conditions, ages, and maternal health status (Hemminki & Vineis, 1985; Hoyme, 1990).

A classic example of the problems associated with the extrapolation of the results of animal studies to humans is the thalidomide tragedy. When thalidomide was tested in several pregnant rodent species, no teratogenic effects were noted. However, when thalidomide was used by women to treat anxiety and insomnia during the first trimester of pregnancy, devastating teratogenic effects (phocomelia or major limb reduction) were produced (Lenz, 1962; McBride, 1961). (Thalidomide subsequently was withdrawn from the market in North America, but continued to be used in many other parts of the world, including Africa and South America [Teixeira, Hojyo et al., 1994]. Amidst some controversy, thalidomide was reapproved for use in North America in 1998 for the treatment of several medical disorders, including erythema nodosum leprosum, a complication of leprosy [Lary, Daniel et al., 1999; Miller & Stromland, 1999].)

MATERNAL SUBSTANCE USE

Some authors suggest that maternal substance use declines "voluntarily and substantially during pregnancy" (Higgins, Clough et al., 1995). However, the preponderance of avail-

able data suggest that most women still use one or more potentially teratogenic substances (including alcohol) at some time during their pregnancies (Abma & Mott, 1991; Deren, Frank et al., 1990; Kokotailo, Adger et al., 1992; Lee, 1995; Marques & McKnight, 1991; Merrick, 1993; Newman & Burka, 1991; Pagliaro, 1995a; Pagliaro & Pagliaro, 1996; Sarvela & Ford, 1992). Why such substances are used and the extent of their use appear to be determined primarily by factors such as age, race, and socioeconomic status (Cornelius, Richardson et al., 1994; Jorgensen, 1992; Wheeler, 1993). Additional risk factors associated with substance use during pregnancy include previous physical or sexual abuse during childhood (Pagliaro & Pagliaro, 1996, 2000).

Unfortunately, a reliable estimate of the nature and extent of substance use by pregnant women is not available. Many reasons exist for this lack of data, including the fact that many teratogenic substances (such as cocaine, heroin, and marijuana) are illegal and thus their use is hidden or underreported. Although variance is reported in specific percentages of use of the various illicit substances by pregnant women, all studies agree on one conclusion: a significant number of pregnant women use illicit drugs. For example, the National Pregnancy and Health Survey found that an estimated 113,000 Caucasian women, 75,000 African American women, and 28,000 Hispanic American women used illicit drugs during pregnancy (NIDA, 1995). Of concern is that, although the moderate use of a particular substance of abuse may have only limited harmful effects for the mother, it can be extremely toxic and pose high teratogenic risk to the developing embryo or fetus as a result of differences in maternal and fetal metabolism, blood and tissue concentrations, tissue sensitivity, and a variety of other factors that preclude a single direct cause-effect relationship (Griffith, Azuma et al., 1994).

Attention to the types of substances used by women during pregnancy and their patterns of use before and during pregnancy are important to retrospectively identify teratogenic risk to the developing embryo and fetus. Although limitations exist in this type of research, human teratogenic experiments cannot be ethically performed, and the results of experiments involving animal models, as previously noted, cannot be relied on to determine human teratogenic potential. To better identify the teratogenic risks associated with maternal substance use during pregnancy, attention also must be given to the interaction of several factors, including maternal factors (such as maternal dose

---

of a particular substance), placental factors, fetal factors (such as stage of fetal development), environmental factors, and factors specific to the substances themselves (Cordier, Ha et al., 1992; Pagliaro & Pagliaro, 1996, 2002; Van Allen, 1992).

Maternal factors include uterine blood flow, concomitant medical disorders (diabetes, epilepsy, infections, or thyroid disease), and general health. Placental factors include: the size and thickness of the placenta; placental blood flow; ability of the placenta to metabolize the substance of abuse to an inactive, active, or teratogenic metabolite; and placental age. Fetal factors include: the stage of fetal development; the maturation of hepatic metabolizing systems; the amount of hepatic blood flow through the ductus venosus; fetal blood pH; genetic predisposition; and concomitant exposure to other potential teratogens. Environmental factors include food additives (aspartame or nitrates), pesticides (chlordane), air and water pollutants, radiation, and toxins (mercury or organic solvents). The substance of abuse factors include the amount, frequency, and method of maternal use during pregnancy; distribution (concentration), metabolism, and excretion; lipid solubility; degree of ionization; molecular weight; concentration of free or nonprotein bound drug; and the pharmacologic effects of the particular substance of abuse (Gilbody, 1991; Pagliaro & Pagliaro, 1996, 2002).

Of all the factors involved in producing a particular teratogenic effect, the most important is timing in relation to organogenesis. Although this critical period of susceptibility varies slightly among different organ systems, teratogenic effects associated with major physical malformations generally are induced during the first trimester of pregnancy. The concept of organogenesis also emphasizes that teratogenic effects will not occur if exposure to a particular teratogen occurs after organogenesis is complete. For example, the maternal use of diazepam (Valium®) during pregnancy has been implicated in cleft palate anomaly. However, this teratogenic effect is not observed if diazepam is used during pregnancy after fusion of the fetal palate. Thus, when evaluating the possible teratogenic potential of a particular substance, it is essential to determine whether the substance, or another in the same class, has been implicated in producing a human teratogenic effect *and* the stage of embryo and fetal development at which time the exposure occurred.

On a more global level, maternal use of any substance— illicit, legal, or medicinal—during pregnancy always involves some degree of risk to the developing embryo or fetus. Therefore, regardless of how "harmless" a substance appears to be, it should *not* be used during pregnancy unless it is clearly indicated and its benefits outweigh its potential risks. Women who are pregnant or considering pregnancy should be advised to limit their use of all drugs and other substances, including alcohol. Women who display problematic patterns of substance use (involving abuse or compulsive use) should be referred to treatment programs aimed at promoting nonuse or, in the event that substance use has been discontinued, preventing relapse.

In this regard, it also is important to note that, although not a direct teratogenic effect of substance use, mother-to-infant transmission of the HIV infection is a significant problem associated with injection drug use and substance use by pregnant women and their partners (Pagliaro & Pagliaro, 2002). This risk underscores the need for prevention and treatment programs that are specifically tailored to meet the needs of women who are pregnant or thinking about becoming pregnant and for early intervention for neonates and infants who have been prenatally exposed to substances of abuse and/or HIV (Russell & Free, 1991).

ALCOHOL

Alcohol (ethanol, ethyl alcohol) is a known human teratogen. As such, it has the potential to affect all fetuses of mothers who consume it during their pregnancies (Day & Richardson, 1991; Larroque, 1992; Pietrantoni & Knuppel, 1991). Once ingested and absorbed into the maternal bloodstream, alcohol readily crosses the placenta and enters into the fetal circulation (Pagliaro & Pagliaro, 2002). It is found in significant levels in the amniotic fluid even after maternal ingestion of a single moderate dose. Alcohol is eliminated from the amniotic fluid at a rate that is one half the rate at which it is eliminated from the maternal blood. Thus, it remains in the amniotic fluid and fetal circulation after it no longer is present in the mother's bloodstream.

The effects of alcohol on neuroendocrine function, which are well documented (Mello, Mendelson et al., 1993), can contribute mechanistically to the development of fetal alcohol syndrome (FAS). As remarked by Gabriel and colleagues (1998): "Some of the effects of maternal alcohol consumption on fetal hormone systems may contribute to the adverse effects observed in children with fetal alcohol syndrome and related disorders" (p. 170).

It is estimated that approximately one of every three to four mothers exposes her fetus to the potentially harmful effects of alcohol (Pagliaro & Pagliaro, 1996, 2000, 2002). A smaller number consume quantities of alcohol that are known to be harmful to developing fetuses (Cornelius, Richardson et al., 1994). Even with a lack of agreement about the exact percentage of mothers who use alcohol during pregnancy, the consensus is that FAS is the leading preventable cause of mental retardation and neurobehavioral deficits in North America (Pagliaro & Pagliaro, 1996, 2000, 2002; Smith, 1997).

Fetal Alcohol Syndrome. The harmful effects associated with the use of alcohol during pregnancy long have been recognized (Pagliaro & Pagliaro, 1996). However, the specific physical (short palpebral fissures), mental (mental retardation), and developmental (prenatal and postnatal growth retardation) characteristics associated with FAS were not formally identified until the early 1970s (Lemoine, Harousseau et al., 1968; Jones & Smith, 1973). Subsequently, clinicians and scientists have used this list of physical characteristics, particularly the associated craniofacial features (epicanthal folds, microcephaly, and midfacial hypoplasia), to assist them in the identification of affected infants and children. Although the characteristic features of FAS vary among affected infants and children, which can present difficulties in clinical identification (Little, Snell et al., 1990), the consistent use of these characteristic features has been found to be generally reliable (Abel, Martier et al., 1993).

In addition, a consensus case definition for FAS has been established by the Fetal Alcohol Study Group of the Research Society on Alcoholism (Pagliaro & Pagliaro, 1996, 2000, 2002). This definition incorporates the following three major criteria:

1. Prenatal and/or postnatal growth retardation (weight and/or length or height below the 10th percentile when corrected for gestational age).

2. CNS involvement (including neurologic abnormality, developmental delay, behavioral dysfunction or deficit, intellectual impairment and/or structural abnormalities, such as microcephaly [head circumference below the third percentile] or brain malformations found on imaging studies or autopsy).

3. A characteristic face qualitatively described as including short palpebral fissures, an elongated mid-face, a long and flattened philtrum, thin upper lip, and flattened maxilla.

The incidence of FAS in North America varies across cultural, ethnic, and socioeconomic groups (Spagnolo, 1993). The highest incidence is reported among African American and Native American populations (Abel & Sokol, 1991; Burd & Moffatt, 1994; Duimstra, Johnson et al., 1993; Gordis & Alexander, 1992), with incidence rates directly related to the magnitude of alcohol use by women during pregnancy (Eliason & Williams, 1990). However, actual incidence rates are difficult to specify for a number of reasons, including the unreliability of self-reports of maternal drinking (which consistently are biased toward underreporting), qualitative and quasi-experimental research methods (case report or retrospective studies), and possible confusion or overlap with fetal alcohol effects (FAE) (Remkes, 1993; Wallace, 1991).

FAE and FAS. The term "fetal alcohol effects" is used to identify neonates and children who exhibit fewer of the characteristics deemed necessary, by definition or convention, for the establishment of a conclusive diagnosis of FAS (Caruso & Bensel, 1993; Ginsberg, Blacker et al., 1991; Smitherman, 1994). Other terminologies have been suggested and used in the clinical literature ("alcohol-related birth defects" and "alcohol-related neurodevelopmental disorder" [Gabriel, Hofmann et al., 1998; Harris, Osborn et al., 1993; Jacobson, Jacobson et al., 1993]). The authors strongly disagree with the use of these terminologies and have argued that the infants and children who display more specifically clustered or fewer of the classic characteristics of FAS are more appropriately diagnosed as having a less severe form of FAS rather than a different syndrome (Pagliaro & Pagliaro, 1996, 2000). Such an approach to diagnosing FAS would (1) more accurately reflect the anticipated normal distribution of the effects of FAS among affected infants and children in the general population or its subpopulations, (2) describe more completely the extent of FAS in the general population, (3) represent more fully the nature of FAS, (4) clearly identify that even "modest social drinking" during pregnancy places the exposed fetus at significant risk of FAS, (5) reflect the relationship of other factors in regard to the severity of the teratogenic effects associated with maternal alcohol use, and (6) encourage the development of more rational and comprehensive prevention strategies and treatment programs.

Long-Term Sequelae of FAS. The effects associated with FAS do not end in infancy but persist into childhood, adolescence, and throughout adulthood (Cramer & Davidhizar, 1999; Pagliaro & Pagliaro, 1996; Karp, Qazi et al., 1993). The troubling lifelong effects of FAS on human growth and development should not be ignored. In this regard, Streissguth and colleagues (1992) cautioned that, for infants and children affected with FAS and their parents and caregivers, "more realistic expectations for performance during childhood and adolescence may result in the availability of more appropriate services, less frustration, and improved behavioral outcome in later adolescence and adulthood."

Recommendations. Alcohol is a known human teratogen that can cause significant, lifelong deficits in physical growth, cognitive functioning, psychomotor skills, and psychological health. Although some researchers (Knupfer, 1991; Koren, 1991; Walpole, Zubrick et al., 1991) disagree, the authors concur with the recommendation made by the National Institute of Child Health and Human Development, the American Academy of Pediatrics, and the U.S. Surgeon General (American Academy of Pediatrics, 1993; Schydlower & Perrin, 1993), and others (Caruso & Bensel, 1993; Olson, Sampson et al., 1992) that women who are pregnant or planning to become pregnant abstain completely from alcohol use. This recommendation is based on the observations that (1) no safe level of alcohol use has been demonstrated and (2) no known cure is available for FAS.

Karp and colleagues (1993) remind us that FAS is not a "treatable" disease in the literal sense. In this regard, it is essential that prevention and treatment programs be developed to help women abstain from alcohol use during pregnancy and the postpartum period. Special attention must be given to mothers for whom abstinence can be difficult to achieve or maintain (that is, women who compulsively use alcohol).

SEDATIVE-HYPNOTIC DRUGS

Although CNS depressants have been associated with various levels of teratogenic risk, data accumulated over the past several decades support a particularly strong relationship between the sedative-hypnotic drugs and teratogenesis (Pagliaro & Pagliaro, 1996, 2002). Implicated sedative-hypnotics include the barbiturates, benzodiazepines, and miscellaneous products such as chloral hydrate (Noctec®).

Barbiturates. Widely used barbiturates include mephobarbital (Mebaral®), pentobarbital (Nembutal®), phenobarbital (Luminal®), and secobarbital (Seconal®). Although use of the barbiturates has decreased dramatically over the past three decades as a result of the synthesis and use of benzodiazepines, barbiturates still are available and

used therapeutically for the treatment of seizure disorders among women who are unresponsive to other anticonvulsant therapy.

The use of phenobarbital during pregnancy has been associated with a number of teratogenic effects, including cleft palate, hypospadias, microcephaly, short noses, and talipes equinovarus (Nakane, Okuma et al., 1980). However, confounding variables, particularly maternal epilepsy, have not yet been completely ruled out as principal or cofactors for teratogenic risk. The maternal use of barbiturates near term, particularly at chronic, high doses, can result in respiratory depression in the neonate and a neonatal barbiturate withdrawal syndrome (Pagliaro & Pagliaro, 1999).

Benzodiazepines. Popular benzodiazepines include chlordiazepoxide (Librium®), diazepam (Valium®), lorazepam (Ativan®), nitrazepam (Mogadon®), and oxazepam (Serax®). The use of these substances during pregnancy has been associated with various degrees of teratogenic effects, particularly cleft lip and palate. However, data are conflicting, and heavy benzodiazepine use often is associated with multiple exposure to alcohol and other substances (Bergman, Rosa et al., 1992; DuPont & Saylor, 1992). Overall, the use of benzodiazepines during pregnancy appears to have a low teratogenic risk (Pagliaro & Pagliaro, 1996, 2002). Maternal use of benzodiazepines near term has resulted in lethargy, low American Pediatric Gross Assessment Record (APGAR) scores, poor muscle tone, and respiratory depression in the neonate. Fortunately, these effects generally are fully reversible with proper recognition and care (Chesley, Lumpkin et al., 1991; Sanchis, Rosique et al., 1991).

OPIOIDS

Some teratogenic effects have been associated with maternal use of opioid drugs during pregnancy. However, a review of the literature provides only weak support for teratogenic effects (primarily involving intrauterine growth retardation) involving drugs such as codeine, heroin, meperidine (Demerol®), methadone, morphine, and pentazocine (Talwin®). It has been argued that the intrauterine growth retardation noted among neonates of mothers who used opiates during pregnancy can be related to such confounding variables as poor maternal nutrition and concurrent use of alcohol and nicotine (Pagliaro & Pagliaro, 1996, 2000, 2002). In addition, the maternal use of opiates near term can result in neonatal CNS depression, as indicated by decreased APGAR scores and the neonatal opioid withdrawal syndrome, particularly when chronic high doses have been used (Pagliaro & Pagliaro, 1999, 2002).

The convulsions associated with unmedicated opioid withdrawal among neonates occur most frequently among those exposed to methadone *in utero*. Whenever possible, women who use methadone, including those enrolled in methadone maintenance programs, should undergo detoxification before becoming pregnant. Detoxification during pregnancy should be avoided, as methadone detoxification during the first trimester has been associated with an increased incidence of spontaneous abortions and detoxification during the third trimester has been associated with increased rates of fetal distress. If methadone detoxification is to be undertaken during pregnancy, it should be attempted between the 14th and 28th weeks of gestation and should involve a slow tapering of the methadone dose.

COCAINE

Cocaine use during pregnancy, in injectable, insufflation, and crack forms, increased significantly over the past two decades. After marijuana, it continues to be the illicit substance most commonly used by pregnant women, particularly those living in North American inner cities (Das, 1994).

The typical cocaine user abuses cocaine repeatedly before conception, continues to use the drug repeatedly throughout pregnancy, and often combines it with other drugs (Plessinger & Woods, 1991). Cocaine's $pK_{[a]}$ is alkaline. Thus, the drug tends to accumulate in the ionized form on the side of a membrane where protons abound. Because fetal pH normally is lower than maternal pH, and is even lower during asphyxial episodes, cocaine can accumulate in the fetus. Therefore, at equilibrium, fetal tissue levels can exceed maternal concentrations. Demethylation, a hepatic enzyme activity, may be developmentally reduced, resulting in prolonged fetal exposure (Scanlon, 1991).

Cocaine use during pregnancy has been associated with intrauterine death (including spontaneous abortions), low birth weight, preterm delivery, neonatal seizures, neonatal tachycardia, intrauterine growth retardation, hypoxemia, a variety of fetal physical anomalies (particularly affecting the ocular and urogenital systems), and limb reduction defects (Hume, Gingras et al., 1994; Nucci & Brancato, 1994; Offidani, Pomini et al., 1995; Sheinbaum & Badell, 1992; Stafford, Rosen et al., 1994).

Autopsies of fetuses exposed to cocaine *in utero* often reveal cerebral hemorrhages (Gieron-Korthals, Helal et al., 1994; Kapur, Cheng et al., 1991), presumably because of a rapid and significant rise in systemic and cerebral blood pressure and hyperthermia (Jones, 1991). However, some researchers have attributed these effects to confounding factors associated with maternal cocaine use (including poor nutrition and inadequate prenatal care) (Church, 1993; Hutchings, 1993; Koren, 1993; Neuspiel, 1992; Racine, Joyce et al., 1993; Snodgrass, 1994).

A significantly higher incidence of behavioral and learning disorders (ADHD or delayed receptive and expressive language skills) is apparent among preschoolers and school-aged children exposed to cocaine *in utero* (Jones, 1991; Kosofsky, 1998; Pagliaro, 1992). However, the teratogenic effects associated with maternal use of cocaine during pregnancy remain inconclusive because of difficulties associated with interpreting and evaluating research data. The retrospective case report methodology generally used has several inherent limitations, which render definitive conclusions highly speculative. In addition, women who use cocaine also commonly use alcohol, a known teratogen. This additional risk factor further confounds the interpretation of data (Rizk, Atterbury et al., 1996; Snodgrass, 1994). Residual amounts of the organic solvents (such as benzene) used in the extraction of cocaine from *Erythroxylon coca* leaves commonly are found in street samples of cocaine. These organic solvents may contribute to the teratogenic effects associated with maternal cocaine use, particularly neuroteratogenic effects (Scanlon, 1991).

Thus, a general consensus seems to be that the use of high doses of cocaine (as through intravenous use or use of smokable crack or "rock" forms of cocaine) probably has a significant, but low, potential for inducing teratogenic effects (Coles, 1993; Koren, Gladstone et al., 1992; Martin, Khoury et al., 1992; Martin & Khoury, 1992). In addition, when cocaine is used by the mother near term, the neonate may experience CNS excitation with insomnia, irritability, and poor feeding response. However, as noted by Plessinger and Woods (1993), "a well-defined 'fetal cocaine syndrome' does not exist" (p. 275).

OTHER STIMULANTS

Research results are mixed with regard to the teratogenic effects of stimulants other than cocaine, particularly dextroamphetamine and methylphenidate.

Dextroamphetamine (Dexedrine®). Dextroamphetamine, used intravenously, is the object of renewed interest among young women. In the past, it was widely prescribed as an anorectic. Although data are contradictory about the teratogenic effects of dextroamphetamine exposure *in utero*, it appears that a moderate risk of human teratogenesis exists. Various case reports (Tsai, Lee et al., 1993) have suggested that the maternal use of dextroamphetamine during the first trimester of pregnancy is associated with abnormal brain development, biliary atresia, cleft lip and palate, congenital heart disease, and prematurity among neonates, who also may be small for gestational age. However, a prospective study found no increase in fetal malformations. More data are needed. In the interim, it is prudent to advise women not to use dextroamphetamine during pregnancy (Pagliaro & Pagliaro, 2000, 2002).

Methylphenidate (Ritalin®). No teratogenic effects have been associated with maternal use of methylphenidate, which is widely prescribed for children and adolescents diagnosed with attention deficit/hyperactivity disorder (ADHD). However, as ADHD is increasingly being conceptualized and, in many cases, treated as a lifelong disorder, increasing numbers of young women are being prescribed and continue to use methylphenidate during their childbearing years. Some addicts use methylphenidate in conjunction with pentazocine (Talwin®) as a "poor man's speedball" (Pagliaro & Pagliaro, 2000). However, only one study, which included 11 neonates exposed prenatally to methylphenidate, appears in the published literature (Pagliaro & Pagliaro, 2002). Clearly, more data are needed.

Caffeine. Caffeine, in the form of coffee, tea, and other beverages (caffeinated soft drinks), probably is consumed to a greater extent by pregnant women than any other substance, including alcohol. Although the research is not as prolific as that on alcohol, some studies have associated caffeine consumption with birth defects. For example, the consumption of eight or more cups of coffee per day was related to fetal limb defects in three case reports. However, in more recent studies, the only teratogenic effect associated with maternal caffeine use during pregnancy is reduced birth weight (Olsen, Overvad et al., 1991; Pagliaro & Pagliaro, 2000, 2002). This effect was associated with the consumption of three or more cups of coffee per day and appears to be most significant among women who smoke. Thus, nicotine may be a cofactor. However, a significant correlation between increased caffeine consumption during pregnancy and fetal loss has been reported (Infante-Rivard, Fernandez et al., 1993). Although these data generally support the relative safety of caffeine use during pregnancy, pregnant women should be encouraged

to minimize their caffeine use, particularly if they also smoke cigarettes. Tobacco use, which is significantly correlated with coffee consumption, is an obvious confounding factor in the interpretation of data supporting the possible teratogenic effects of caffeine.

NICOTINE AND TOBACCO

The modal reported rate of tobacco use among pregnant women appears to be approximately 35% (Gupton, Thompson et al., 1995), although significant variation is noted across various racial and ethnic groups and geographic regions (Pagliaro & Pagliaro, 2000, 2002). The research shows that tobacco smoking during pregnancy is teratogenic to the fetus. An inverse relationship exists between birth weight and the number of cigarettes smoked per day. Neonates born to mothers who smoked during pregnancy weigh an average of 200 g (range, 100 to 400 g) less than neonates born to mothers who did not smoke during pregnancy. They also have a shorter body length (Yawn, Thompson et al., 1994). Fortunately, a period of accelerated growth occurs during the first year of life, and, generally, no differences in body weight or length are observed among these infants at one year of age. Women who cease tobacco smoking during the first trimester of pregnancy generally have infants of normal size (Pagliaro & Pagliaro, 2000, 2002).

Women who continue to smoke tobacco during pregnancy, on the other hand, have higher rates of spontaneous abortions, abruptio placentae, placenta previa, uterine bleeding, and perinatal mortality (DiFranza & Lew, 1995; Gupton, Thompson et al., 1995; Handler, Mason et al., 1994). In addition, mothers who smoke can have a higher fetal malformation rate (Seidman, Ever-Hadani et al., 1990). Of further concern, the risk of sudden infant death syndrome (SIDS) is estimated to be 4.4 times higher for infants born to mothers who smoke during pregnancy than for infants born to mothers who do not; this may account for more than 2,000 SIDS deaths annually (DiFranza & Lew, 1995). Some studies (Olds, Henderson et al., 1994) suggest that maternal smoking during pregnancy can cause neurodevelopmental impairment, resulting in a reduction in IQ scores by four to eight points among offspring. Another study (Milberger, Biederman et al., 1996) suggests that maternal smoking during pregnancy can be a risk factor for the development of ADHD. However, as with other substances of abuse, data on the teratogenic effects of tobacco smoking are confounded by the concurrent use of alcohol. On the basis of the available data, and as a precaution, women should be advised not to smoke during pregnancy.

Oncken and colleagues (1996) studied the short-term use of nicotine gums (such as Nicorette®) in pregnant smokers and found that it (1) enhanced smoking cessation, (2) delivered less nicotine to the pregnant women than did their usual level of cigarette use, and (3) was not associated with significant differences in fetal or maternal hemodynamic parameters, as compared with pregnant women who continued to smoke (for a fuller discussion of smoking cessation strategies, see Section 6). A systematic review of 40 smoking cessation trials in pregnant women between 1975 and 1997 found a small but significant increase in smoking cessation and a corresponding small but significant increase in mean birth weight (Lumley, Oliver et al., 1998). These unimpressive results, which are consistent with the findings of other treatment studies, underscore the importance of prevention.

VOLATILE SOLVENTS AND INHALANTS

Although volatile solvents and inhalants (gasoline and glue) are not commonly used by pregnant women, their potential teratogenic effects should be considered. Only four studies were found in a review of the published literature. One report (Wilkins-Haug & Gabow, 1991) contained data on 30 pregnancies in 10 women who engaged in chronic glue- and paint-sniffing and another (Arnold, Kirby et al., 1994) reviewed the case records of 35 deliveries to women with antenatal exposure to toluene (a volatile solvent found in many different products, including glues and spray paint). On the basis of these studies, the teratogenic effects possibly related to the use of these volatile solvents and inhalants include preterm delivery, neonatal electrolyte disturbances (hypobicarbonatemia or hypokalemia), low birth weight, microcephaly, and postnatal growth retardation.

"Toluene embryopathy" associated with maternal toluene use first was described among five children in 1989. The reported embryopathy, as described by Arnold and colleagues (1994) and Pearson and colleagues (1994), includes growth retardation, developmental delays, and minor craniofacial anomalies (short palpebral fissures, flat [wide] nasal bridge, deficient philtrum, and micrognathia). These teratogenic features are extremely similar to those associated with FAS. The similarity of these features may be due to the pharmacologic similarity of alcohol and the volatile solvents and inhalants, or to the mother's possible concomitant use of alcohol during pregnancy. Pearson and colleagues (1994) have proposed a common mechanism of craniofacial teratogenesis for toluene and alcohol, specifically, a deficiency of craniofacial neuroepithelium and mesodermal components because of increased embryonic cell death. More data are needed.

PSYCHEDELICS

The psychedelics comprise a variety of substances that typically are used for their hallucinatory and consciousness-expanding effects. No studies were found that reported teratogenic effects associated with the maternal use of psilocybin (magic mushrooms) or peyote (mescaline) during pregnancy. Several reports were found for lysergic acid diethylamide (LSD), tetrahydrocannabinol (THC; the active ingredient in marijuana), and phencyclidine (PCP). For example, Fried and Watkinson (1990) noted that, "at 48 months [of age], significantly lower scores in verbal and memory domains [among children] were associated with maternal marijuana use" (p. 49). However, the use of LSD, THC, and PCP during pregnancy has not been clearly and consistently associated with major physical or developmental teratogenic effects in humans (Day & Richardson, 1991; Pagliaro, 1995a; Tabor, Smith-Wallace et al., 1990). Given the widespread use of the psychedelics by women of childbearing age and the relative paucity of reported teratogenic effects, the teratogenic potential of the psychedelics, if it does exist, appears to be quite small (Pagliaro & Pagliaro, 2000, 2002). More data are needed.

CONCLUSIONS

Teratogenesis is a complex process that is influenced by many factors, including maternal, placental, fetal, environmental, and pharmacologic factors. To minimize the risk and incidence of substance-induced teratogenesis, it is necessary to recognize that all substances of abuse have the potential to cause teratogenic effects under certain conditions. Thus, as a precaution, women who are pregnant, or women who are thinking about becoming pregnant, should be encouraged, whenever possible, to abstain from, or to minimize, their use of the various substances of abuse. In particular, they should be advised to avoid alcohol because of the strong evidence associating its use with significant teratogenic effects (FAS) (Pagliaro, 1995b; Pagliaro & Pagliaro, 2000, 2002).

It is important to note that, when substances of abuse are used during pregnancy, their respective withdrawal syndromes can be expected among neonates. In addition, most of the substances of abuse, when used by the mother near term, can cause expected pharmacologic effects and toxicities among neonates. Fortunately, associated withdrawal syndromes and other pharmacologically related effects generally are reversible with proper recognition and treatment.

Physicians, as well as other health and social care professionals who are concerned about the health of women and their neonates, infants, and children, should be aware of the teratogenic effects associated with maternal use of alcohol and other drugs during pregnancy. Further research is needed to examine the relationship between the use of the various substances of abuse by pregnant women and their associated teratogenic effects. Extensive documentation relates maternal alcohol and tobacco use to serious risk of teratogenesis. Women should be advised about these possible harmful effects, including possible long-term effects on their infants and children (for example, FAS). Greater attention also needs to be given to the development and implementation of empirically validated pharmacotherapeutic and psychotherapeutic interventions designed to prevent or minimize substance use among women of childbearing age. Attention to relapse prevention is a major challenge.

REFERENCES

Abel EL, Martier S, Kruger M et al. (1993). Ratings of fetal alcohol syndrome facial features by medical providers and biomedical scientists. *Alcoholism: Clinical & Experimental Research* 17:717-721.

Abel EL & Sokol RJ (1991). A revised conservative estimate of the incidence of FAS and economic impact. *Alcoholism: Clinical & Experimental Research* 15:514-524.

Abma JC & Mott FL (1991). Substance use and prenatal care during pregnancy among young women. *Family Planning Perspectives* 23(3):117-122.

American Academy of Pediatrics (AAP), Committee on Substance Abuse and Committee on Children with Disabilities (1993). Fetal alcohol syndrome and fetal alcohol effects. *Pediatrics* 91:1004-1006.

Arnold GL, Kirby RS, Langendoerfer S et al. (1994). Toluene embryopathy: Clinical delineation and developmental follow-up. *Pediatrics* 93:216-220.

Bergman U, Rosa FW, Baum C et al. (1992). Effects of exposure to benzodiazepine during fetal life. *Lancet* 340:694-696.

Burd L & Moffatt MEK (1994). Epidemiology of fetal alcohol syndrome in American Indians, Alaskan Natives, and Canadian Aboriginal Peoples: A review of the literature. *Public Health Reports* 109:688-693.

Caruso K & Bensel R (1993). Fetal alcohol syndrome and fetal alcohol effects: The University of Minnesota experience. *Minnesota Medicine* 76:25-29.

Chesley S, Lumpkin M, Schatzki A et al. (1991). Prenatal exposure to benzodiazepine—I. *Neuropharmacology* 30(1):53-58.

Church MW (1993). Does cocaine cause birth defects? *Neurotoxicology and Teratology* 15:289.

Coles CD (1993). Saying "goodbye" to the "crack baby." *Neurotoxicology and Teratology* 15:290-292.

Cordier S, Ha MC, Ayme S et al. (1992). Maternal occupational exposure and congenital malformations. *Scandinavian Journal of Work Environment Health* 18:11-17.

Cornelius MD, Richardson GA, Day NL et al. (1994). A comparison of prenatal drinking in two recent samples of adolescents and adults. *Journal of Studies on Alcohol* 55:412-419.

Cramer C & Davidhizar R (1999). FAS/FAE: Impact on children. *Journal of Child Health Care* 3(3):31-34.

Das G (1994). Cocaine abuse and reproduction. *International Journal of Clinical Pharmacology and Therapeutics* 32(1):7-11.

Day NL & Richardson GA (1991). Prenatal alcohol exposure: A continuum of effects. *Seminars in Perinatology* 15:271-279.

Deren S, Frank B & Schmeidler J (1990). Children of substance abusers in New York State. *New York State Journal of Medicine* 90(4):179-184.

DiFranza JR & Lew RA (1995). Effect of maternal cigarette smoking on pregnancy complications and sudden infant death syndrome. *Journal of Family Practice* 40:385-394.

Duimstra C, Johnson D, Kutsch C et al. (1993). A fetal alcohol syndrome surveillance pilot project in American Indian communities in the Northern Plains. *Public Health Reports* 108:225-229.

DuPont RL & Saylor KE (1992). Depressant substances in adolescent medicine. *Pediatrics in Review* 13(10):381-386.

Eliason MJ & Williams JK (1990). Fetal alcohol syndrome and the neonate. *Journal of Perinatal and Neonatal Nursing* 3(4):64-72.

Fried PA & Watkinson B (1990). 36- and 48-month neurobehavioral followup of children prenatally exposed to marijuana, cigarettes, and alcohol. *Developmental and Behavioral Pediatrics* 11(2):49-58.

Gabiano C, Tovo PA, de Martino M et al. (1992). Mother-to-child transmission of human immunodeficiency virus type 1: Risk of infection and correlates of transmission. *Pediatrics* 90(3):369-374.

Gabriel K, Hofmann C, Glavas M et al. (1998). The hormonal effects of alcohol use on the mother and fetus. *Alcohol Health & Research World* 23(3):170-177.

Gieron-Korthals MA, Helal A & Martinez CR (1994). Expanding spectrum of cocaine induced central nervous system malformations. *Brain & Development* 16:253-256.

Gilbody JS (1991). Effects of maternal drug addiction on the fetus. *Adverse Drug Reactions and Acute Toxicology Reviews* 10:77-88.

Ginsberg KA, Blacker CM, Abel EL et al. (1991). Fetal alcohol exposure and adverse pregnancy outcomes. *Contributions to Gynecology and Obstetrics* 18:115-129.

Gittler J & McPherson M (1990). Prenatal substance abuse. *Children Today* 14(4):3-7.

Gordis E & Alexander D (1992). From the National Institutes of Health: Progress toward preventing and understanding alcohol-induced fetal injury. *Journal of the American Medical Association* 268:3183.

Griffith DR, Azuma SD & Chasnoff IJ (1994). Three-year outcome of children exposed prenatally to drugs. *Journal of American Child and Adolescent Psychiatry* 33:20-27.

Gupton A, Thompson L, Arnason RC et al. (1995). Pregnant women and smoking. *Canadian Nurse* 91(8):26-30.

Handler AS, Mason ED, Rosenberg DL et al. (1994). The relationship between exposure during pregnancy to cigarette smoking and cocaine use and placenta previa. *American Journal of Obstetrics and Gynecology* 170(3):884-889.

Harris SR, Osborn JA, Weinberg J et al. (1993). Effects of prenatal alcohol exposure on neuromotor and cognitive development during early childhood: A series of case reports. *Physical Therapy* 73:608-617.

Hemminki K & Vineis P (1985). Extrapolation of the evidence on teratogenicity of chemicals between humans and experimental animals: Chemicals other than drugs. *Teratogenesis, Carcinogenesis, and Mutagenesis* 5:251-318.

Higgins PG, Clough DH, Frank B et al. (1995). Changes in health behaviors made by pregnant substance users. *International Journal of the Addictions* 30(10):1323-1333.

Hoyme HE (1990). Teratogenically induced fetal anomalies. *Clinics in Perinatology* 17(3):547-567.

Hume RF Jr, Gingras JL, Martin LS et al. (1994). Ultrasound diagnosis of fetal anomalies associated with in utero cocaine exposure: Further support for cocaine-induced vascular disruption teratogenesis. *Fetal Diagnosis and Therapy* 9:239-245.

Hutchings DE (1993). The puzzle of cocaine's effects following maternal use during pregnancy: Are there reconcilable differences. *Neurotoxicology and Teratology* 15:281-286.

Infante-Rivard C, Fernandez A, Gauthier R et al. (1993). Fetal loss associated with caffeine intake before and during pregnancy. *Journal of the American Medical Association* 270:2940-2943.

Jacobson JL, Jacobson SW, Sokol RJ et al. (1993). Teratogenic effects of alcohol on infant development. *Alcoholism: Clinical & Experimental Research* 17:174-183.

Jones KL (1991). Developmental pathogenesis of defects associated with prenatal cocaine exposure: Fetal vascular disruption. *Clinics in Perinatology* 18(1):139-146.

Jones KL & Smith DW (1973). Recognition of the fetal alcohol syndrome in early infancy. *Lancet* 1:1267-1271.

Jorgensen KM (1992). The drug-exposed infant. *Critical Care Nursing Clinics of North America* 4:481-485.

Kapur RP, Cheng MS & Shephard TH (1991). Brain hemorrhages in cocaine-exposed human fetuses. *Teratology* 44:11-18.

Karp RJ, Qazi Q, Hittleman J et al. (1993). Fetal alcohol syndrome. In RJ Karp (ed.) *Malnourished Children in the United States: Caught in the Cycle of Poverty*. New York, NY: Springer Publishing, 101-108.

Knupfer G (1991). Abstaining for foetal health: The fiction that even light drinking is dangerous. *British Journal of Addiction* 86:1063-1073.

Kokotailo PK, Adger H Jr, Duggan AK et al. (1992). Cigarette, alcohol, and other drug use by school-age pregnant adolescents: Prevalence, detection, and associated risk factors. *Pediatrics* 90:328-334.

Koren G (1991). Drinking and pregnancy. *Canadian Medical Association Journal* 145(12):1552-1554.

Koren G (1993). Cocaine and the human fetus: The concept of teratophilia. *Neurotoxicology and Teratology* 15:301-304.

Koren G, Gladstone D, Robeson C et al. (1992). The perception of teratogenic risk of cocaine. *Teratology* 46:567-571.

Kosofsky BE (1998). Cocaine-induced alterations in neuro-development. *Seminars in Speech and Language* 19:109-121.

Larroque B (1992). Alcohol and the fetus. *International Journal of Epidemiology* 21(Suppl 1):S8-S16.

Lary JM, Daniel KL, Erickson JD et al. (1999). The return of thalidomide: Can birth defects be prevented? *Drug Safety* 21:161-169.

Lee R (1995). NIDA conference on women and drug abuse. *Public Health Reports* 110:517.

Lemoine P, Harousseau H & Borteyru J (1968). Children of alcoholic patients: Abnormalities observed in 127 cases. *Quest Medical* 21:476-482.

Lenz W (1962). Thalidomide and congenital abnormalities. *Lancet* 1:271.

Little BB, Snell LM & Rosenfeld CR (1990). Failure to recognize fetal alcohol syndrome in newborn infants. *American Journal of Diseases of Children* 144:1142-1146.

Lumley J, Oliver S & Waters E (1998). Smoking cessation programs implemented during pregnancy. *Cochrane Database of Systematic Review* Issue 4.

Marques PR & McKnight AJ (1991). Drug abuse risk among pregnant adolescents attending public health clinics. *American Journal of Drug and Alcohol Abuse* 17:399-413.

Martin ML & Khoury MJ (1992). Cocaine and single ventricle: A population study. *Teratology* 46:267-270.

Martin ML, Khoury MJ, Cordero JF et al. (1992). Trends in rates of multiple vascular disruption defects, Atlanta, 1969-1989: Is there evidence of a cocaine teratogenic epidemic? *Teratology* 45:647-653.

McBride WG (1961). Thalidomide and congenital abnormalities. *Lancet* 2:1358.

Mello NK, Mendelson JH & Teoh SK (1993). An overview of the effects of alcohol on neuroendocrine function in women. In S Zakhari (ed.) *Alcohol and the Endocrine System (NIAAA Research Monograph 23)*. Bethesda, MD: National Institute on Alcohol Abuse and Alcoholism, 139-169.

Merrick JC (1993). Maternal substance abuse during pregnancy: Policy implications in the United States. *Journal of Legal Medicine* 14:57-71.

Milberger S, Biederman J, Faraone SV et al. (1996). Is maternal smoking during pregnancy a risk factor for attention deficit hyperactivity disorder in children? *American Journal of Psychiatry* 153(9):1138-1142.

Miller MT & Stromland K (1999). Teratogen update: Thalidomide: A review, with a focus on ocular findings and new potential uses. *Teratology* 60:306-321.

Nakane Y, Okuma T, Takahashi R et al. (1980). Multi-institutional study on the teratogenicity and fetal toxicity of antiepileptic drugs: A report of a collaborative study group in Japan. *Epilepsia* 21:663-680.

National Institute on Drug Abuse (NIDA) (1995). *National Pregnancy and Health Survey*. Rockville, MD: NIDA, National Institutes of Health.

Neuspiel DR (1992). Cocaine-associated abnormalities may not be causally related [letter]. *American Journal of Diseases of Children* 146:278.

Newman LF & Burka SL (1991). Preventing the risk factors in childhood learning impairment. *Rhode Island Medical Journal* 74:251-262.

Nucci P & Brancato R (1994). Ocular effects of prenatal cocaine exposure. *Ophthalmology* 101(8):1321.

Offidani C, Pomini F, Caruso A et al. (1995). Cocaine during pregnancy: A critical review of the literature. *Minerva Ginecologica* 47(9):381-390.

Olds DL, Henderson CR Jr. & Tatelbaum R (1994). Intellectual impairment in children of women who smoke cigarettes during pregnancy. *Pediatrics* 93:221-226.

Olsen J, Overvad K & Frische G (1991). Coffee consumption, birthweight, and reproductive failures. *Epidemiology* 2(5):370-374.

Olson HC, Sampson PD, Barr H et al. (1992). Prenatal exposure to alcohol and school problems in late childhood: A longitudinal prospective study. *Development and Psychopathology* 4:341-359.

Oncken CA, Hatsukami DK, Lupo VR et al. (1996). Effects of short-term use of nicotine gum in pregnant smokers. *Clinical Pharmacology & Therapeutics* 59(6):654-661.

Pagliaro AM & Pagliaro LA (1996). *Substance Use Among Children and Adolescents: Its Nature, Extent, and Effects From Conception to Adulthood.* New York, NY: John Wiley & Sons.

Pagliaro AM & Pagliaro LA (2000). *Substance Use Among Women.* Philadelphia, PA: Brunner/Mazel.

Pagliaro LA (1992). The straight dope: Focus on learning—Interpreting the interpretations. *Psynopsis* 14(2):8.

Pagliaro LA (1995a). Marijuana reconsidered. *Psymposium* 5:12-13.

Pagliaro LA (1995b). Pharmacopsychology updates: Psychotropic teratogens. *Psymposium* 5(1):18-19.

Pagliaro LA & Pagliaro AM (2002). Drugs as human teratogens and fetotoxins. In LA Pagliaro & AM Pagliaro (eds.) *Problems in Pediatric Drug Therapy, 4th Edition.* Washington, DC: American Pharmaceutical Association.

Pagliaro LA & Pagliaro AM (1999). *Psychologists' Neuropsychotropic Drug Reference.* Philadelphia, PA: Brunner/Mazel.

Pagliaro LA & Pagliaro AM, eds. (in press 2002). *Problems in Pediatric Drug Therapy, 4th Edition.* Washington, DC: American Pharmaceutical Association.

Pajer KA (1992). Psychotropic drugs and teratogenicity. In MS Keshavan & JS Kennedy (eds.) *Drug-induced Dysfunction in Psychiatry.* New York, NY: Hemisphere, 49-74.

Pearson MA, Hoyme HE, Seaver LH et al. (1994). Toluene embryopathy: Delineation of the phenotype and comparison with fetal alcohol syndrome. *Pediatrics* 93:211-215.

Pegues DA, Engelgau MM & Woernle CH (1994). Prevalence of illicit drugs detected in the urine of women of childbearing age in Alabama public. *Public Health Reports* 109:530.

Pietrantoni M & Knuppel RA (1991). Alcohol use in pregnancy. *Clinics in Perinatology* 18:93-111.

Plessinger MA & Woods JR Jr. (1991). The cardiovascular effects of cocaine use in pregnancy. *Reproductive Toxicology* 5:99-113.

Plessinger MA & Woods JR Jr. (1993). Maternal, placental, and fetal pathophysiology of cocaine exposure during pregnancy. *Clinical Obstetrics and Gynecology* 36(2):267-278.

Racine A, Joyce T & Anderson R (1993). The association between prenatal care and birth weight among women exposed to cocaine in New York City. *Journal of the American Medical Association* 270:1581-1586.

Remkes T (1993). Saying no—Completely. *Canadian Nurse* 89(6):25-28.

Rizk B, Atterbury JL & Groome LJ (1996). Reproductive risks of cocaine. *Human Reproduction Update* 2(1):43-55.

Russell FF & Free TA (1991). Early intervention for infants and toddlers with prenatal drug exposure. *Infants and Young Children* 3:78-85.

Sanchis A, Rosique D & Catala J (1991). Adverse effects of maternal lorazepam on neonates. *DICP, The Annals of Pharmacotherapy* 25:1137-1138.

Sarvela PD & Ford TD (1992). Indicators of substance use among pregnant adolescents in the Mississippi delta. *Journal of School Health* 62:175-179.

Scanlon JW (1991). The neuroteratology of cocaine: Background, theory, and clinical implications. *Reproductive Toxicology* 5:89-98.

Schydlower M & Perrin J (1993). Prevention of fetal alcohol syndrome [letter]. *Pediatrics* 92:739.

Seidman DS, Ever-Hadani P & Gale R (1990). Effect of maternal smoking and age on congenital anomalies. *Obstetrics and Gynecology* 76:1046-1050.

Sheinbaum KA & Badell A (1992). Physiatric management of two neonates with limb deficiency and prenatal cocaine exposure. *Archives of Physical Medicine and Rehabilitation* 73:385-388.

Smith SM (1997). Alcohol-induced cell death in the embryo. *Alcohol Health & Research World* 21(4):287-297.

Smitherman CH (1994). The lasting impact of fetal alcohol syndrome and fetal alcohol effect on children and adolescents. *Journal of Pediatric Health Care* 8:121-126.

Snodgrass SR (1994). Cocaine babies: A result of multiple teratogenic influences. *Journal of Child Neurology* 9(3):227-233.

Spagnolo A (1993). Teratogenesis of alcohol. *Annali Dell Instituto Superiore Sanità* 29(1):89-96.

Stafford JR Jr., Rosen TS, Zaider M et al. (1994). Prenatal cocaine exposure and the development of the human eye. *Ophthalmology* 101:301-308.

Streissguth AP, Randels SP & Smith DF (1992). Fetal alcohol syndrome [letter]. *Journal of the American Academy of Child and Adolescent Psychiatry* 31(3):563-564.

Tabor BL, Smith-Wallace T & Yonekura ML (1990). Perinatal outcome associated with PCP versus cocaine use. *American Journal of Drug and Alcohol Abuse* 16(3 & 4):337-348.

Teixeira F, Hojyo MT, Arenas R et al. (1994). Thalidomide: Can it continue to be used? [letter]. *Lancet* 344:196-197.

Tsai EM, Lee JN, Chao MC et al. (1993). Holoprosencephaly and trisomy 13 in a fetus with maternal early gestational amphetamine abuse—A case report. *Kaohsiung Journal of Medical Science* 9:703-706.

Van Allen MI (1992). Structural anomalies resulting from vascular disruption. *Pediatric Clinics of North America* 39:255-277.

Vega WA (1992). *Profile of Alcohol and Drug Abuse During Pregnancy in California, 1992.* Berkeley, CA: University of California, School of Public Health.

Wallace P (1991). Prevalence of fetal alcohol syndrome largely unknown. *Iowa Medicine* 81(9):381.

Walpole I, Zubrick S, Pontré J et al. (1991). Low to moderate maternal alcohol use before and during pregnancy, and neurobehavioural outcome in the newborn infant. *Developmental Medicine and Child Neurology* 33:875-883.

Wheeler SF (1993). Substance abuse during pregnancy. *Primary Care* 20:191-207.

Wilkins-Haug L & Gabow PA (1991). Toluene abuse during pregnancy: Obstetric complications and perinatal outcomes. *Obstetrics & Gynecology* 77:504-509.

Yawn BP, Thompson LR, Lupo VR et al. (1994). Prenatal drug use in Minneapolis-St Paul, Minnesota. A 4-year trend. *Archives of Family Medicine* 3(6):520-527.

SECTION 11

Co-Occurring Addictive and Psychiatric Disorders

Section Coordinator
Richard K. Ries, M.D.

Contributors

Kathleen T. Brady, M.D., Ph.D.
Professor of Psychiatry
Center for Drug and Alcohol Programs
Medical University of South Carolina
Charleston, South Carolina

Katherine Anne Comtois, Ph.D.
Behavioral Research and Therapy Clinics
Department of Psychology
University of Washington
Seattle, Washington

Linda Dimeff, Ph.D.
Director, Research and Development
The Behavioral Technology Transfer Group
Seattle, Washington

Stephen J. Donovan, M.D.
Assistant Professor of Clinical Psychiatry
New York State Psychiatric Institute, and
Columbia University
New York, New York

David R. Gastfriend, M.D.
Director, Addiction Research Program
Department of Psychiatry
Massachusetts General Hospital, and
Associate Professor of Psychiatry
Harvard Medical School
Boston, Massachusetts

R. Jeffrey Goldsmith, M.D.
Professor of Clinical Psychiatry
Department of Veterans Affairs Hospital
Dual Diagnosis Clinic
Cincinnati, Ohio

Frances Rudnick Levin, M.D.
Director, Addiction Psychiatry Residency, and
Q.J. Kennedy Associate Professor
  of Clinical Psychiatry
New York State Psychiatric Institute, and
Columbia University
New York, New York

Marsha M. Linehan, Ph.D.
Behavioral Research and Therapy Clinics
Department of Psychology
University of Washington
Seattle, Washington

Susan L. McElroy, M.D.
Biological Psychiatry Program
Department of Psychiatry
University of Cincinnati
College of Medicine
Cincinnati, Ohio

Hugh Myrick, M.D.
Assistant Professor of Psychiatry
Center for Drug and Alcohol Programs
Medical University of South Carolina
Charleston, South Carolina

Nancy Nitenson, M.D.
Director, Addiction Rehabilitation Program
Spaulding Rehabilitation Hospital, and
Department of Psychiatry
Harvard Medical School
Boston, Massachusetts

Richard K. Ries, M.D.
Mental Health Services
Outpatient Programs
Department of Psychiatry and Behavioral Sciences
University of Washington
Seattle, Washington

David Smelson, Psy.D.
Division of Addiction Psychiatry
Robert Wood Johnson Medical School
Piscataway, New Jersey

Susan Sonne, Pharm.D.
Assistant Professor of Psychiatry
Center for Drug and Alcohol Programs
Medical University of South Carolina
Charleston, South Carolina

Cesar A. Soutullo, M.D.
Biological Psychiatry Program
Department of Psychiatry
University of Cincinnati
College of Medicine
Cincinnati, Ohio

Marc L. Steinberg, M.A.
Division of Addiction Psychiatry
Robert Wood Johnson Medical School
Piscataway, New Jersey

Maria A. Sullivan, M.D., Ph.D.
Assistant Professor of Clinical Psychiatry
New York State Psychiatric Institute, and
Columbia University
New York, New York

Stephen A. Wyatt, D.O.
Medical Director, Stonington Institute, and
Research Associate, Department of Psychiatry
Yale University
New Haven, Connecticut

Douglas Ziedonis, M.D., M.P.H.
Associate Professor and Director
Division of Addiction Psychiatry
Robert Wood Johnson Medical School
Piscataway, New Jersey

Joan E. Zweben, Ph.D.
Clinical Professor of Psychiatry
University of California, San Francisco, and
Executive Director, 14th Street Clinic
    and East Bay Community Recovery Project
Oakland, California

Chapter 1

Substance-Induced Mental Disorders

R. Jeffrey Goldsmith, M.D.
Richard K. Ries, M.D.

Prevalence of Substance-Induced Mental Disorders
Substance-Induced Symptoms
Differential Diagnosis and Treatment

The substance-induced mental disorders are a common problem in clinical practice. Understanding them is critical for the clinician because they can mimic almost every syndrome seen in psychiatry. The fourth edition of the *Diagnostic and Statistical Manual of Mental Disorders* (*DSM-IV*) of the American Psychiatric Association (1994) contains new definitions of the substance-induced mental disorders, which differ slightly from the guidelines offered in the revised third edition (*DSM-IIIR*; APA, 1987). This chapter describes the diagnostic criteria in the *DSM-IV*, reviews the epidemiologic data, and discusses the clinical strategies needed to manage these disorders.

Nine substance-induced disorders are given in the *DSM-IV* (Table 1). Three are referred to generically as "organic brain syndrome": substance-induced delirium, substance-induced persisting dementia, and substance-induced persisting amnestic disorder. These disorders are addressed in other chapters in this section and thus are not covered here. Three mimic many of the common Axis I disorders: substance-induced psychotic, mood, and anxiety disorders. They are covered in this chapter, as is hallucinogen persisting perceptual disorder. The last two, substance-induced sexual dysfunction and substance-induced sleep disorder,

also are covered in other chapters in this section and are not addressed here.

PREVALENCE OF SUBSTANCE-INDUCED MENTAL DISORDERS

The prevalence of substance-induced mental disorders is difficult to report because only a few research studies have been directed specifically at these disorders. The research literature largely reports on the prevalence of a particular diagnosis at a given point in time (Lydiard, Brady et al., 1992) or a symptom over a period of time (Brown & Schuckit, 1988; Brown, Inaba et al., 1995); a few studies mention symptoms and diagnoses over time (Dorus, Kennedy et al., 1987; Brown, Inaba et al., 1995; Rounsaville, Anton et al., 1991). Numerous case studies report the phenomena of substance-induced disorders but not the epidemiology. Rather, they alert the general psychiatrist to the fact that such disorders are common and need to be considered. Very few studies report the prevalence of substance-induced mood, anxiety, or psychotic disorders.

However, the research suggests some estimates of the prevalence of alcohol-induced anxiety and depressive disorders. Brown and Schuckit (1988) reported that 42% of

TABLE 1. DSM-IV Substance-Induced Mental Disorders

- Substance-induced delirium
- Substance-induced persisting dementia
- Substance-induced persisting amnestic disorder
- Substance-induced psychotic disorder
- Substance-induced mood disorder
- Substance-induced anxiety disorder
- Hallucinogen persisting perceptual disorder
- Substance-induced sexual dysfunction
- Substance-induced sleep disorder.

SOURCE: American Psychiatric Association (APA) (1994). *Diagnostic and Statistical Manual of Mental Disorders, 4th Edition (DSM-IV)*. Washington, DC: American Psychiatric Press.

the male alcoholics they studied displayed depressive symptoms in a range comparable to that seen in individuals hospitalized for affective disorder (more than 19 points, which is in the moderate-severe range of the Hamilton Depression Rating Scale). The symptoms abated rapidly over the first two weeks of abstinence, with only 12% of the subjects still depressed at the end of the second week—a reduction of 30%. In light of this rapid abatement of depressive symptoms, it is significant that the subjects averaged more than nine days of abstinence before the study began. This is a very conservative estimate of substance-induced depression, considering that some of the subjects in the mildly depressed range (11-19 points on the Hamilton Depression Rating Scale) could have been in the moderate-to-severe range at the initiation of sobriety.

In a study of similar alcoholic subjects who had been sober for an average of 8 days, Brown and colleagues (1995) reported that 33% of the primary alcoholics (with or without secondary affective disorder) scored in the moderate-to-severe range for depression (more than 19 points on the Hamilton Depression Rating Scale), whereas 81% of the subjects with primary affective disorder did so at the end of week 1. By week 4 of the study, none of the patients with primary alcoholism were in the moderate-to-severe range, whereas 67% of the subjects with primary affective disorders were. This finding suggests that all of the subjects with primary alcoholism had alcohol-induced depressive

disorder, a number quite comparable to the 30% reported in the earlier study by the same researchers.

Dorus and colleagues (1987) used the Beck Depression Inventory rather than the Hamilton Depression Rating Scale, making 17 the cutoff point for moderate-to-severe depression. They found that 67% of their study group were depressed at day 1 (four or more days abstinent), whereas only 16% were depressed at day 24. This change suggests that more than half had an alcohol-induced depressive disorder. Even more interesting, many of the subjects with a current or lifetime *DSM-III* (APA, 1980) diagnosis of major depression had scored below the 17-point cutoff level, suggesting that differentiating between the alcohol-induced and primary affective disorders may be difficult for any given patient.

Using the Hamilton Depression Rating Scale, Keeler and colleagues (1979) found that, after a week on a detoxification unit, 28% of patients had a score of 20 or greater. When the *DSM-II* (APA, 1990) criteria were used in clinical interviews with patients, fewer than 9% met the criteria for depression, suggesting that 20% had alcohol-induced depression. However, one must approach these data carefully, because the investigators used *DSM-II* criteria and arrived at diagnoses within seven days of admission.

Schuckit and colleagues (1997) studied nearly 3,000 alcoholics to test three hypotheses related to substance-induced depression. They hypothesized that (1) there would be more substance-induced depression than major depressive disorder, (2) those with substance-induced depression would have more severe alcohol and drug histories, and (3) those with independent depression would have more first-degree relatives with affective disorder than would the substance-induced group. All three hypotheses were supported by their findings. Among the study population, 15% of 2,495 subjects had an independent depression (group 1), whereas 26% reported information consistent with a substance-induced depression (group 2). Subjects in group 2 drank more alcohol per occasion and drank on more days per week, sought treatment more often, were more likely to have attended Alcoholics Anonymous (AA) meetings, and used more marijuana and stimulants than did subjects in group 1 or group 3 (no depression). Women composed about half of the subjects in group 1 (52%), but less than a third of the subjects in group 2 (29.5%) and group 3 (28%). In addition, subjects in group 2 had more antisocial personality disorder than did those in group 1 (28% versus 22%)

or group 3 (28% versus 15%). Subjects in group 1 had more major anxiety disorder than did those in group 2 (8.4% versus 4.8%) and the same percentage of mania (1.6% versus 1.0%).

In a study designed to examine substance-induced psychotic disorders, Rosenthal and Miner (1997) prospectively examined admissions to an acute psychiatric inpatient unit. Over the first year, they found that 30% of the patients admitted met the *DSM-IIIR* criteria for organic mood disorder, 8% for organic hallucinosis, and 6% for organic delusional disorder. They also found that 15% of the patients with comorbid schizophrenia and substance use disorder and organic delusional disorder or organic hallucinosis were suicidal.

Substance-induced depression can dissipate rapidly, but it is as dangerous or more dangerous than major depressive disorder in terms of the risk of suicide and self-injurious behavior. When completed suicides are investigated, the rate of comorbidity is high. Murphy and Wetzel (1990) reported that alcoholic patients had a 60- to 120-fold greater risk of death by suicide than did the general population. Henriksson and colleagues (1993) reported that nearly half (43%) of a group of suicide victims in Finland had alcohol dependence and that 48% of the alcoholics had comorbid depression, 42% had a personality disorder, and 36% had a significant Axis III medical disorder. Young and colleagues (1994) found that persons who had major depressive disorder coexisting with both alcohol and drug dependence were at the highest risk of suicide, even in the absence of pervasive hopelessness. Driessen and colleagues (1998) reported that neither Axis I nor Axis II comorbidity among alcoholics was predictive of suicidal behavior or ideation at one-year followup; however, two Axis I diagnoses or an Axis I with an Axis II diagnosis were predictive. Pages and colleagues (1997) found that alcohol and drug dependence, as well as current use, were associated with greater severity of suicidal ideation among patients with unipolar major depressive disorder. Salloum and colleagues (1996) studied patients who had been hospitalized psychiatrically and found that more than half of the subjects in all three groups studied (with alcohol dependence, cocaine dependence, or alcohol plus cocaine dependence) had a history of suicide attempts.

Elliott and colleagues (1996) found that patients who made medically severe suicide attempts had a statistically higher rate of substance-induced mood disorder than did patients who made less severe suicide attempts. There was no difference between the two groups in the prevalence of

alcohol abuse or dependence, or in the prevalence of polysubstance abuse or dependence. Moreover, most of the patients with substance-induced mood disorder did not meet the criteria for substance dependence. This finding is consistent with the findings of Asnis and colleagues (1993) and Murphy and Wetzel (1990), who argued that alcohol dysregulates mood independent of use patterns, suggesting that some individuals are at risk of severe depression regardless of the chronicity of their alcohol use.

However, Bartels and colleagues (1992) found that, among schizophrenics, it was the severity of the depression, not the substance abuse, that explained suicidal behavior. In contrast, Seibyl and colleagues (1993) reported that schizophrenics who had used cocaine before admission exhibited increased suicidal ideation.

Anxiety symptoms show similar changes over the early sobriety phase. Several studies have reported high rates of anxiety symptoms among alcoholics in withdrawal, with 80% of alcohol-dependent male subjects experiencing repeated panic attacks during alcohol withdrawal (Schuckit & Hesselbrock, 1994). In the same study, 50% to 67% of the alcohol-dependent subjects had high scores on the state anxiety measures, which resembled generalized anxiety and social phobia (Schuckit & Hesselbrock, 1994). Brown and colleagues (1991) reported that 40% of recently detoxified alcohol-dependent men scored above the 75th percentile on the state-anxiety subscale of the State Trait Anxiety Inventory. At discharge after four weeks, 12% scored that high, whereas at three-month followup only 5% remained above the 75th percentile. This finding suggests that 35% had an alcohol-induced anxiety disorder. Moreover, if 80% of alcoholic men report withdrawal panic attacks, is this alcohol withdrawal anxiety disorder or is it an independent panic disorder evoked by alcohol withdrawal? Or is it merely anxiety symptoms caused by alcohol withdrawal?

Rounsaville and colleagues (1991), in a study of patients addicted to cocaine, examined the current and lifetime prevalence of Research Diagnostic Criteria (RDC) disorders. They used both strict and less strict criteria in evaluating the depression diagnostic data from the SADS-L. The less strict criteria allowed a diagnosis if the symptoms *ever* had been present, whereas the strict criteria allowed a diagnosis only if symptoms had persisted for 10 or more days following cessation of cocaine use. Using the less strict criteria, major depression was diagnosed in 59% of the subjects, whereas the more strict criteria yielded a 30% prevalence rate. This finding conservatively suggests a lifetime prevalence of about 30% for cocaine-induced depressive disorder. Further, the current rate of major depression was 4.7%, hypomania was 2%, and minor mood disorder was 38% (mania was 0%) (Rounsaville, Anton et al., 1991). (The current diagnoses of minor mood disorders appeared to use the strict criteria, but this was not clarified in the report.)

Rounsaville and colleagues (1991) reported a 16% current rate and a 21% lifetime rate of anxiety disorders, but the investigators did not disclose what criteria were used to diagnose anxiety unrelated to cocaine use.

Efforts to differentiate between substance-induced and independent depressive and anxiety disorders among a group of substance abusers (who were dependent on a variety of drugs) showed limited validity (Kadden, Kranzler et al., 1995). The investigators used *DSM-IIIR* criteria but allowed the clinicians to ask their own questions. For each subject, two expert clinicians made a diagnosis of "independent" or "substance-induced" depressive or anxiety disorder, based on two criteria. The first criterion allowed an independent diagnosis as long as the symptoms satisfied the diagnostic criteria. The second criterion required that the symptoms precede the onset of the substance use disorder or that they had occurred during a six-month period of abstinence from that substance. Use of the latter criterion produced fewer diagnoses of independent disorders and lower kappa values: $p < 0.1$ (there was less agreement among raters when a comorbid diagnosis was made, with only 4 of 18 in agreement). Using the less strict (first) criterion, there was a "fair" agreement among raters, who agreed 18 of 28 times when a comorbid diagnosis was made, for a kappa of 0.50.

SUBSTANCE-INDUCED SYMPTOMS

The occurrence of psychiatric symptoms as a result of legal and illegal drug use has been well documented. It is common medical knowledge that hallucinogens cause hallucinations, stimulants cause euphoria, and chronic sedative use can result in depression. It is common medical knowledge that, in acute withdrawal, alcohol and sedatives cause anxiety. It is less obvious that a distinct set of symptoms appear when psychoactive substances are used over a long period of time. Symptoms reported for each of the major substances of abuse are reviewed below to establish a basis on which to understand the syndromes that can arise (also see Section 2).

Caffeine is the most commonly used addictive substance. It is considered a benign drug by many consumers and professionals and has enjoyed an increase in popularity over the past decade. The effects of caffeine include the induction of anxiety with consumption of "large amounts"; however, the range of caffeine doses that can induce anxiety is considerable. Caffeine can increase the frequency of panic attacks in those individuals who are physiologically predisposed to them.

Nicotine is the deadliest psychoactive drug and the third most popular in the United States, with about 25% of the adult population smoking cigarettes, about 5% using smokeless tobacco, and about 5% smoking pipes and cigars. Although there is no indication that nicotine acutely changes mood, there is evidence that nicotine-dependent patients experience more depression than nonusers and that some use nicotine to regulate mood. Whether there is a causal relationship between nicotine use and the symptoms of depression remains to be seen. At present, it can be said only that some persons who quit smoking do experience severe depression, which is relieved by resumption of nicotine use.

Alcohol use is common among American adolescents and young adults. Although light consumption of alcohol is associated with a slight euphoria or "buzz," moderate to heavy consumption may be associated with depression, suicidal feelings, and/or violent behavior in some individuals. With prolonged drinking, the incidence of dysphoria and anxiety rises, much to the distress of the drinker. In those who are physiologically dependent, one usually sees a hyperadrenergic state that is characterized by agitation, anxiety, tremor, malaise, hyperreflexia, mild tachycardia, increasing blood pressure, sweating, insomnia, nausea or vomiting, and perceptual distortions. Following acute withdrawal from alcohol, some persons suffer from continued mood instability, with moderate lows, fatiguability, insomnia, reduced sexual interest, and hostility. A few chronic heavy drinkers experience hallucinations, delusions, and anxiety during acute withdrawal, and some have grand mal seizures. Brain damage of several types is associated with alcohol-induced dementias and deliriums.

With *sedatives,* particularly the benzodiazepines, acute use can produce a "high" similar to that seen with alcohol. The drug effects are perceived as relaxing, producing a social ease, but sedatives also can induce depression, anxiety, and even a psychotic-like state with prolonged use and dependence (Ashton, 1991). Withdrawal symptoms include mood instability with anxiety and/or depression, sleep disturbance, autonomic hyperactivity, tremor, nausea or vomiting, transient hallucinations or illusions, and grand mal seizures. A protracted withdrawal syndrome has been reported to include anxiety, depression, paresthesias, perceptual distortions, muscle pain and twitching, tinnitus, dizziness, headache, derealization and depersonalization, and impaired concentration. These symptoms can last for weeks, and some (such as anxiety, depression, tinnitus, and paresthesias) have been reported for a year or more after withdrawal.

Cocaine and *amphetamine* use often are associated with an intense euphoria or "rush," with hyperactive behavior and speech, anorexia, insomnia, inattention, and labile moods (Gold, 1993). The route of administration and the dose alter the intensity of the experience. After a binge of several days, addicts may feel "wired" or "geeked" and stop their use, or they may use other drugs to moderate the agitation. Individuals occasionally become paranoid and even delusional after prolonged heavy use of cocaine or amphetamine. Unlike other psychotic states, the patient experiencing a paranoid state induced by cocaine has intact abstract reasoning and linear thinking, whereas the delusions, if analyzed, are poorly developed delusions of a nonbizarre nature (Mendoza & Miller, 1992). If abstinence is maintained for several weeks, many stimulant addicts report a dysphoric state that is prominently marked by anhedonia and/or anxiety, but which does not meet the symptom severity criteria to qualify as a *DSM-IV* disorder (Rounsaville, Anton et al., 1991). This anhedonic state can persist for weeks.

Some stimulant addicts report hallucinatory symptoms that are visual ("coke snow") and tactile ("coke bugs"). Sleep disturbances are prominent in the intoxicated and withdrawn states, as is sexual dysfunction.

Opiate use is characterized by a "high" or "rush" when the drug is used intravenously or smoked. Unlike the stimulants, opiate-induced euphoria usually is associated with some sedation and manifests as a mellow, sleepy state. If opiates are used for a long period of time, moderate to severe depression is common. The addict frequently experiences irritability, accompanied by craving, muscle aches, a flu-like syndrome, and gastrointestinal symptoms early in withdrawal from drugs such as heroin and morphine. More drug subdues the craving. In withdrawal, some opiate addicts are acutely anxious and agitated, while others report depression and anhedonia. Anxiety, depression, and sleep disturbance, in a milder form, can persist for weeks as a protracted withdrawal syndrome. There are reports of an atypical opiate withdrawal syndrome, consisting of delirium after the abrupt cessation of methadone (Levinson, Galynker et al., 1995). Such patients do not appear to have the autonomic symptoms typically seen in opiate withdrawal.

Hallucinogens such as marijuana, tetrahydrocannabinol (THC), LSD, mescaline, and dimethyltryptamine (DMT) produce visual distortions and frank hallucinations. Some users experience a marked sense of time distortion and feelings of depersonalization. *Marijuana* and the cannabinoids can augment appetite and cause sedation with euphoria. All hallucinogens are associated with drug-induced panic reactions that feature panic, paranoia, and even delusional states in addition to the hallucinations. There are descriptions of physiologic dependence to marijuana with mild withdrawal; however, most users do not exhibit such problems. There is a debate in the literature as to the existence of a marijuana-induced psychotic state (Gruber & Pope, 1994). A careful interpretation of the research suggests that there is no such entity. A few hallucinogen users experience chronic reactions, involving (1) prolonged psychotic reactions, (2) depression, which can be life-threatening, (3) flashbacks, and (4) exacerbations of preexisting psychiatric illnesses. The flashbacks are symptoms that occur after one or more psychedelic trips and consist of flashes of light and afterimage prolongation in the periphery. The *DSM-IV* refers to flashbacks as an "hallucinogen persisting perception disorder" and requires that they be distressing or impairing to the patient (APA, 1994, p. 234).

Phencyclidine (PCP), an arylcyclohexylamine and dissociative drug, is an hallucinogen used in certain parts of the U.S. Popular in the 1970s (Giannini, 1991), PCP is known for its dissociative and delusional properties. It also is associated with violent behavior and amnesia of the intoxication (Giannini, 1991). Users who once exhibit an acute psychotic state with PCP are more likely to develop another with repeated use (Zukin & Zukin, 1992).

DIFFERENTIAL DIAGNOSIS AND TREATMENT

Diagnosing and treating a substance-induced mental disorder is very much dependent on the attitude and training of the clinician. Is he or she attuned to the prevalence of alcohol and drug use? Without this awareness, there is less inclination to search for the problem. Does the clinician think that it is relevant to the current problem to take the time to elicit an alcohol and drug use history? Has the clinician received adequate training to counteract the therapeutic nihilism acquired during medical school and residency training? Is he or she adversely affected by the distortions and denial that are exhibited by many alcoholics and drug addicts? Does the clinician routinely seek corroboration of an alcohol and drug use history from family or friends of the patient? Will the clinician order a drug screen? All of these questions hint at behaviors that can make the diagnosis more apparent or allow it to elude identification.

Making the diagnosis of a substance use disorder is the first step in the differential diagnosis and treatment of a substance-related problem. In the second step, the substance-induced symptoms must be differentiated from the symptoms of major psychiatric disorders. Finally, the substance-induced disorders must be differentiated from the dual disorders: substance abuse or dependence combined with a comorbid, nonsubstance Axis I disorder.

The *DSM-IV* contains five criteria for substance-induced mood disorders (APA, 1994):

1. A prominent and persistent disturbance in mood predominates, characterized by (a) a depressed mood or markedly diminished interest or pleasure in activities, or (b) an elevated, expansive, or irritable mood;

2. There is evidence from the history, physical examination, or laboratory findings that the symptoms developed during or within a month after substance intoxication or withdrawal, or medication use is etiologically related to the mood disturbance;

3. The disturbance is not better explained by a mood disorder;

4. The disturbance did not occur exclusively during a delirium; and

5. The symptoms cause clinically significant distress or impairment.

Mood Disorders. Mood disorders may be the most common substance-induced disorders that clinicians need to consider in arriving at a differential diagnosis. It is important to consider, and make, the substance use diagnosis whenever it is pertinent. There are some guidelines that can help with these diagnoses. Because of denial, the patient may not understand what is happening in his or her life. If the clinician is aware of the prevalence of addictive disorders and the ways in which such disorders typically present, he or she is more likely to take a careful history and to seek confirmation of the history from collateral informants, especially family and friends, but also other health care professionals.

Establishing whether there is a relationship between the use of psychoactive substances and the symptoms prominent at the moment is a crucial step. Chronic use of alcohol, sedatives, and opiates can cause depressed mood, as can withdrawal from stimulants and sedatives. Exploring the mood during periods of sustained abstinence from all depressant drugs is critical.

Anxiety Disorders. For the substance-induced anxiety disorders, the criteria are almost identical. However, the first is different: prominent anxiety, panic attacks, obsessions, or compulsions predominate. The remaining four criteria are the same as for mood disorder (APA, 1994). In making the diagnosis of substance use disorder, it is helpful to order a drug screen. Even if the results come back hours after the clinical decision is made, they can be used to confirm the presence of a substance despite the patient's denial. Such a screen also can clarify the history in some future episode. Sometimes addicts report part of their history but not all. For example, it may be useful to know that both alcohol and cocaine were used by a depressed patient. Although either substance can induce symptoms of anxiety (or depression), a slightly different treatment plan may be necessary for a patient dependent on both.

A drug screen may be equally critical to the diagnosis of a substance-induced psychotic disorder. Again, the criteria in the *DSM-IV* are similar. Hallucinations or delusions must be prominent and are not counted if the individual has insight into the substance-induced nature of his or her cognitive problems. For this reason, the patient's lack of insight, coupled with a drug screen and collateral history, can be important in establishing the use or absence of a psychotogenic drug.

The differences among psychiatric symptoms associated with different psychiatric disorders remains elusive. The *DSM-IV* requires that the diagnosis of anxiety, affective, and psychotic disorders be made only when several criteria are satisfied. First, the anxiety, mood, or cognitive symptoms must be prominent. Second, there must be evidence that a psychoactive substance was used within the preceding month and that the substance is known to cause the symptoms in question. Third, there should not be another cause that better explains the disorder. Fourth, the disorder cannot occur exclusively during the course of a delirium. And fifth, the disorder must cause clinically significant distress or impairment in normal functioning. Although not a criteria for diagnosis, the *DSM-IV* explains that the assessment should not be made unless the symptoms are judged to be in excess of those usually associated with intoxication or withdrawal. The latter can be problematic if taken literally, because withdrawal can involve extreme symptoms, such as suicidal feelings and panic attacks. In addiction, intoxication can include paranoia and visual hallucinations, feelings of depersonalization, and time distortion. What would it mean to be in excess of such psychotic symptoms?

Case 1. Mr. B is a 46-year-old divorced white man who works as a house painter. He came to the emergency department because of suicidal ideas, which frightened him. He had become increasingly depressed over the preceding month and was afraid that he was "going crazy." He had experienced episodes of depression over the preceding seven years (since his divorce), but the episodes had not lasted more than a day or two. He also had experienced fleeting suicidal ideas, but had not hurt himself. In the past year, he occasionally had sat with his gun and considered ending it all. At those times, he felt momentarily hopeless. The suicidal and hopeless thoughts lasted for an evening, but were not continuously present for more than a day. He had never been treated psychiatrically for depression.

The clinician gathers information suggestive of a depressive syndrome of some kind and must determine whether there are any organic causes, the most common of which would be substance-induced disorder.

Mr. B has been hospitalized once, four years ago, to be detoxified from alcohol, but he received no treatment for alcoholism after the detoxification. Recently, his drinking has increased to about a case of beer a day. He reports that the alcohol use is the only way he can cope with his depression. He denies any loss of control, but admits to two arrests for driving under the influence (DUI) over the preceding 10 years. He is experiencing difficulty in getting to work on time since becoming depressed and is in trouble with his supervisor. He denies morning shakes and says that he never has experienced *delirium tremens*.

Mr. B admits that his ex-wife complained about his drinking. He has had only one period of abstinence for more than a year, while on probation for his second DUI. He felt well during that time. He developed the depressive symptoms in his late 30s, whereas his heavy drinking began in his early 20s.

He denies any ongoing medical problems or thyr problems. He has had some weight loss in the past mont. because he has not been eating regularly with his heavy drinking, and he has experienced some nausea in the mornings, which made eating breakfast difficult. He denies any use of sedatives, barbiturates, cocaine, or opiates.

On mental status examination, Mr. B is found to be a middle-aged white man, who looks more like 55 than 46 years old. He is thin, looks depressed, and smells of alcohol. He is vague about some details and specific about others. He is oriented to person, place, date, and purpose. He is tearful at some times, anxious at others. He seems bewildered about his predicament. He denies having problems with alcohol. He has suicidal ideas about shooting himself, but does not seem motivated to do so. He denies hallucinations and obsessions. He denies any manic episodes. His blood alcohol concentration (BAC) is 200 mg%. A drug toxicology screen is negative for benzodiazepines, opiates, barbiturates, and cocaine.

Diagnostic Issues: Is there a reason to consider a diagnosis of alcohol dependence or abuse for Mr. B? Is depression a prominent symptom? Is there a reason to connect the depressive symptoms to alcohol or drug use or withdrawal? Is the intensity of depression more severe than is usually found with alcohol intoxication alone? Is the depressive mood better explained by a mood disorder? Did the depressed mood occur during a delirium?

Diagnostic Considerations: At this point, the clinician has enough information to diagnose alcohol dependence. Mr. B exhibits tolerance, alcohol withdrawal, use despite adverse consequences, impairment of personal relationships, and possibly impairment of occupational function, all related to his use of alcohol. His mood disturbance is prominent and is more severe than that experienced by social drinkers and most alcoholics. His depressive symptoms seem sufficiently severe to suggest major depression; however, there is no evidence of depression at the times that Mr. B is not drinking heavily, suggesting alcohol-induced depressive disorder. The alcohol dependence seems to be primary; that is, it began before the depressive symptoms. This sequence of symptoms also suggests alcohol-induced depressive disorder.

It is possible that Mr. B has two independent disorders, alcohol dependence and major depression; however, there is no evidence of that at present. Finally, there is no evidence of a delirium.

: Safety issues involve ongoing evalu-
, use of medications, and psychosocial

erations: A trial of abstinence is called
... a safe environment with a lot of support. The clinical
challenge is to find a safe environment. The risk of alcohol
withdrawal delirium and seizures is minimal, suggesting that
Mr. B could be managed as an outpatient. However, there
are other considerations in this decision. The *ASAM
Patient Placement Criteria for the Treatment of Substance-
Related Disorders, Second Edition-Revised* (*ASAM PPC-2R*;
Mee-Lee, Shulman et al., 2001) encourage the physician to
evaluate the patient's status in six different dimensions. The
first is the potential for withdrawal. The second and third
are the presence of medical and psychiatric comorbidities.
(The seriousness of Mr. B's suicidality, as well as the degree
of his anergy and inability to mobilize because of depression, are relevant in this case. The medical comorbidity is
minor [possibly gastritis] and should improve with abstinence.) The fourth dimension is the patient's readiness for
change. Mr. B appears to seek treatment; however, he may
balk at inpatient or outpatient treatment, making his cooperation a major issue. The final two dimensions—the
potential for relapse and the presence or absence of a supportive environment—are very pertinent to this patient. If
Mr. B has no supportive friends or family who can watch
over him and be sure that he gets to therapy sessions, or to
the emergency department if his condition worsens, then
outpatient therapy becomes risky, particularly given the
patient's suicidal ideas. The patient's potential for relapse,
including his motivation for abstinence, craving for alcohol
while abstinent, and history of prior attempts to quit, is crucial in determining the viability of outpatient treatment.

Alcohol-induced depression should remit over the first
two to three weeks of abstinence. Careful followup during
this period is very important with outpatient treatment because of the severity of Mr. B's symptoms and the possibility
that the correct diagnosis is not alcohol-induced depression.
However, if he cannot or will not stay sober as an outpatient, it is likely that he will remain depressed or become
even more depressed. At this point, residential treatment is
essential to break the cycle of addiction and allow the
patient's mood to improve. If his mood does not improve
with abstinence, a major depression should be considered,
and the patient should be given appropriate antidepressant
treatment.

Anticraving medications such as naltrexone (ReVia®)
can be very helpful when the patient is cooperative, somewhat open to the idea of abstinence from alcohol, and willing
to engage in some kind of psychosocial followup. The same
is true of disulfiram (Antabuse®). Patients with a firm commitment to sobriety may not need the assistance of such
medications. Patients with a strong connection to AA
may not be motivated to take such medications because
they believe that medications are not appropriate for sobriety; however, AA produces a pamphlet that is quite
supportive of both psychiatric care and the use of psychiatric medications.

Case 2. Mr. M is a 45-year-old African American veteran who is divorced and unemployed. He came to the
evaluation area at 9:00 AM because of a longstanding problem sleeping that has worsened over the past two months.
He has been drinking more alcohol to fall asleep, but has
been waking after only a few hours of sleep. He experiences hand tremors in the mornings, which resolve with a
few shots of whiskey. He has become jumpy and irritable
and tends to isolate himself from his friends.

OPTION A: Mr. M has no history of withdrawal seizures or withdrawal hallucinations. He has no history of
panic attacks, chronic anxiety, or traumatic life events. His
vital signs include blood pressure 148/90, pulse 96, temperature 98.6°F, and respirations 16.

Mr. M was detoxified from alcohol within the past year,
but refused to enter outpatient treatment. He complained
that he was "not going to let the doctors treat him like a
'guinea pig' on the detoxification unit" and that "they just
tried to lock up a Black man these days."

Diagnostic Issues: Is there a prominent symptom? If
so, is this symptom related to drinking? Is there any evidence of other drug use? Is this explained better by another
DSM disorder? Did the symptoms occur during a delirium?
Has this disorder caused symptoms beyond what normally
is experienced during alcohol intoxication or withdrawal?

Clinical Considerations: At this point, the information
available suggests alcohol withdrawal. There also is information suggesting a sleep disturbance, which may be
alcohol-induced or related to alcohol withdrawal. Because
of the cultural tensions already reported, an effort should
be made to rule out an anxiety disorder, as Mr. M may be
reluctant to report anxiety symptoms. Efforts should be
made to rule out other organic causes of his anxiety and
agitation, such as hyperthyroidism, stimulant intoxication,

caffeinism, or medication-induced anxiety. A drug toxicology screen would be helpful to rule out stimulant intoxication, caffeinism, and opiate withdrawal. A phone call to a family member or friend may add confidence to the diagnosis and rule out chronic anxiety and paranoid disorders. The symptoms do not seem excessive for alcohol withdrawal, which is the likely diagnosis, given the available information.

OPTION B: Mr. M has no history of withdrawal seizures or withdrawal hallucinations. He has a history of panic attacks, which began after he returned from military service in Vietnam in 1971. He had been in combat for six months and had seen a lot of action, which he does not wish to discuss. He becomes more agitated as he talks about combat, eventually cutting off the conversation. He is angry about the way he was treated when he returned to the U.S., and reports a difficult transition to civilian life. He demonstrates recent heavy drinking, nightmares about combat, flashbacks, relationship problems, and a significant startle reaction to loud noises. He complains of racist treatment by white soldiers and officers in Vietnam and claims that his white superiors sent him on suicide missions.

Diagnostic Issues: Is there a prominent symptom? Is there a causal relationship with the drinking? Is there any drug use that could account for the disorder? Is this better explained by another *DSM* disorder? Did the symptoms occur during a delirium? Are the symptoms excessive for alcohol intoxication or withdrawal?

Diagnostic Considerations: The patient certainly evidences anxiety as a prominent symptom. However, it still is important to look for a substance dependence disorder and a substance-induced anxiety disorder. It is necessary to clarify the diagnosis of alcohol withdrawal. This patient seems to have a posttraumatic stress disorder (PTSD), alcohol dependence, alcohol withdrawal and, possibly, substance-induced anxiety disorder. Because the engagement of this patient in treatment may depend on which combination of problems he has, it is important for the clinician to obtain collateral information and a drug toxicology screen. Because the patient's denial may be convincing, it is not sufficient to dismiss substance dependence or a substance-induced disorder based on his history. If the patient's report is the only information available, the clinician must make a treatment decision, while remaining aware that new information could change the diagnosis and treatment plan.

Mr. M's vital signs should be monitored to pick up signs of severe alcohol withdrawal. A toxicology screen should be obtained to check for drugs that can cause agitation or anxiety. A chronic history of anxiety, tension, nightmares, and the like is excessive for alcohol-induced anxiety or alcohol withdrawal alone. With this information, the clinician may consider both PTSD and alcohol withdrawal. It will be difficult to diagnose alcohol-induced anxiety in combination with PTSD unless there is a clear history of anxiety that recently has worsened without a psychosocial trigger for the PTSD. More commonly, the clinician will see an acute improvement with sobriety as a sign that there was an alcohol-induced anxiety component.

Treatment Issues: Mr. M needs to be engaged in a detoxification setting (followed by an alcohol rehabilitation setting), and his denial needs management in order to expand his awareness beyond the PTSD symptoms. His claims of racism should be addressed as part of the engagement and assessment processes. Mr. M's anxiety should be managed without using benzodiazepines. His sleep disorder should be managed, and the process of relapse prevention initiated.

Treatment Considerations: Treatment must be conceptualized in stages. The first stage is detoxification from alcohol (and any other drugs that may be present). With this patient, detoxification can be managed through a careful outpatient regimen if he is able to remain abstinent. If abstinence seems unlikely, if the patient fails at outpatient detoxification, or if a comorbid problem arises that cannot be monitored safely on an outpatient basis, then residential detoxification must be considered.

The next stage is the maintenance of sobriety, a stabilization phase. During this stage, the clinician should monitor Mr. M's abstinence and observe the course of the anxiety symptoms. A relapse can increase his anxiety symptoms, which would interfere with attainment of the treatment goals. Such a relapse would require a treatment strategy that focuses on management of denial, motivation, and relapse prevention.

If, during abstinence, the anxiety symptoms increase or stay the same, the PTSD probably is severe and medication will be needed. If the anxiety symptoms diminish or are manageable without medication, then counseling may be sufficient. The use of benzodiazepines in alcoholics after detoxification is achieved is controversial, even in the face of severe anxiety. The anxiolytic properties of benzodiazepines are sustained over time; however, many alcoholics request more of this medication. Moreover, craving for drugs is greatest when the drug, or a similar drug, is being used.

Thus, there always is a concern that benzodiazepines will stimulate the desire for alcohol. Drinking in addition to benzodiazepine use can lead to an "out of control" binge, as well as intoxicated behaviors, which could exaggerate the PTSD symptoms of anxiety and agitation.

Disulfiram is a possible safeguard to prevent alcohol use during outpatient treatment, but the patient must be willing to collaborate (that is, take it regularly) if it is to be effective. The use of antipanic medications such as the selective serotonin reuptake inhibitors (SSRIs) and other antidepressants would be a safer strategy.

The same problem is encountered with the complaints about insomnia. Avoiding sedatives is important. Use of sedating antidepressants like trazodone (Desyrel®) and doxepin (Adapin®) can be very effective and avoids the abuse potential of other sedative drugs.

OPTION C: Mr. M has no history of withdrawal seizures or withdrawal hallucinations. He has had an episode (the day before coming to the emergency department) in which he became frightened, felt short of breath, felt his heart pounding, and worried that he was having a heart attack. This episode was not the first time he has experienced such an attack; he had one six months earlier when he quit drinking. He had gone to the emergency room the first time this happened, five years ago. The physician then had checked his heart and told him that he was having a nervous attack, not a heart attack. Although Mr. M feels stressed at times, he does not have these attacks regularly. When he stopped his drinking for a year, he felt well and does not recall having a spell during that time. He denies any major, traumatic life events. He was embarrassed to be worried about these anxiety spells, but also fearful that he might have been having a heart attack.

Diagnostic Issues: Is there a prominent symptom? Is this symptom related to drinking? Is the symptom better explained by another *DSM* diagnosis? Is the symptom in excess of the symptoms normally encountered during intoxication or withdrawal?

Diagnostic Considerations: There is a prominent symptom of anxiety in this case, and it appears to occur only with drinking. The clinician must think about alcohol dependence, alcohol withdrawal, and alcohol withdrawal-induced panic disorder. The major anxiety disorders should be ruled out, as should PTSD (although certain events, like sexual abuse, may be denied initially). Some attempt to rule out cardiac disease as a cause of the chest pain would be important. Organic causes of anxiety also should be ruled

out. It is possible that the patient has a panic disorder that is in a prodromal phase, but this is not the most likely diagnosis. Although patients frequently experience anxiety during alcohol withdrawal, they usually do not experience panic attacks, nor do they typically go to the emergency department in a panic.

Treatment Issues: Mr. M should be engaged in a detoxification program and his level of denial and motivation for treatment evaluated. The denial needs to be evaluated and the problem redefined as alcoholism, not panic or heart disease. The possibility of a comorbid anxiety disorder should be explored. The patient then needs to be engaged in an alcohol rehabilitation program. Medications that will enhance the likelihood of sobriety should be considered. The patient should be evaluated for relapse triggers and referred for relapse prevention as appropriate.

Treatment Considerations: Treatment should be designed to detoxify Mr. M safely from alcohol, to explore dependence on other drugs, and to keep him sober long enough to determine whether the anxiety disorder abates with sobriety, as an alcohol withdrawal-induced anxiety disorder would. The patient's denial and motivation are important because he must understand the connection between his drinking and his panic. If his awareness of this connection is minimal, then the treatment may have to occur in a setting in which chest pain or panic is the primary focus. He may not accept the focus on his drinking. If this is the case, then referral to a rehabilitation program, either inpatient or outpatient, may not be possible at this time. Ongoing monitoring and working with his denial would be necessary before such a referral could be made. Benzodiazepines would be appropriate only during detoxification; medications that promote sobriety, such as disulfiram or naltrexone, would be appropriate if Mr. M is motivated and able to cooperate. Antipanic medications like the SSRIs probably would be used if the panic attacks persist with sobriety.

Case 3. A 20-year-old undergraduate presented with a chief complaint of "seeing the air." The visual disturbance consisted of a perception of white pinpoint specks, too numerous to count, in both the central and peripheral visual fields. These specks were constantly present and accompanied by the perception of trails of moving objects left behind as they pass through the visual field. Attending a hockey game became difficult, as the brightly dressed players left streaks of their own images against the white of the ice for seconds at a time. The patient also described the false perception of movement in stable objects, usually in his peripheral visual field, halos around objects, and positive and negative afterimages. Other symptoms included mild depression, daily bitemporal headache, and a loss of concentration, which emerged within the preceding year.

The visual syndrome has emerged gradually over the past three months, after the patient experimented with the hallucinogenic drug LSD-25 on three separate occasions. The patient fears that he has sustained some kind of "brain damage" from the drug experience. He denies use of any other agents, including amphetamines, phencyclidine, narcotics, or alcohol to excess. He had smoked marijuana twice a week for a period of seven months at age 17 (Spitzer, Gibbon et al., 1994).

Diagnostic Issues: Is there a re-experiencing of a perceptual symptom after the use of an hallucinogen? Is this symptom causing significant distress or impairing function? Is this condition better explained by a delirium or another *DSM* disorder?

Diagnostic Considerations: This case appears to be hallucinogen persisting perceptual disorder, or flashbacks. It consists of a perceptual disturbance resembling the drug experience (in this case, LSD) at some time after hallucinogen use; it requires that the patient be distressed by the experience. A drug toxicology screen should be obtained to rule out other drugs, despite the patient's denial.

The patient appears to have insight and does not seem delusional, nor does he have negative symptoms of schizophrenia. There is no sign of delirium, but this should be considered. An evaluation of his neurologic status would be an important part of this assessment. If consent is given, confirming the patient's story with his family or a friend would be a good idea, because persons with a chronic psychotic condition can, and do, use LSD.

Treatment Issues: This patient is frightened by what is happening and is afraid that he has damaged his brain by using drugs. This fear presents a unique opportunity to engage him in some kind of treatment. The question is, what kind of treatment is most appropriate? Because his use of hallucinogens may have been months earlier, it is important to ascertain whether the current problem is anxiety about the flashbacks or is related to current substance abuse or dependence. While the patient denies being dependent on LSD and does not meet the criteria for abuse or dependence, he may have been dependent on marijuana when he was 17.

A careful neurologic evaluation is advised, because there are visual disturbances, difficulties in concentrating, depres-

sion, and headaches, all of which could be associated with neurologic illness. Outpatient therapy—either drug rehabilitation or psychotherapy for the fear—probably is sufficient; however, residential treatment may be required if the patient's panic or flashbacks are severe (that is, if they interfere markedly with his daily routine).

Given the patient's anxiety, he may readily commit to abstinence from drugs. If his fears are sufficiently intense, he could develop a panic attack/PTSD-type syndrome, which could become chronic. Classic approaches to the treatment of anxiety should be used, including those discussed in the chapter on anxiety disorders in this section. Although research is lacking, some clinicians use anticonvulsants for such patients on the theory that flashback phenomena are kindled and involve some sort of focal central nervous system hyperactivity.

Case 4. Ms. A is a 35-year-old, white divorced woman who came to the emergency department because of suicidal feelings. She reported feeling very despondent that day, with suicidal ideation, and thought that she needed to be admitted to the hospital to keep her safe. On questioning, Ms. A admits that she smokes crack cocaine, about $100 worth at a time. She recently came off a four-day binge of crack use. She takes four to six drinks of vodka per day when she uses crack and also has used marijuana.

Diagnostic Issues: Is there a prominent symptom? Is this symptom related to drug use? Is this situation better explained by another *DSM* diagnosis? Did this situation occur exclusively during a delirium? Is this symptom more severe than usually is encountered with intoxication or withdrawal?

Diagnostic Considerations: Ms. A has a prominent mood disturbance, which brought her to the emergency department. It is consistent with chronic cocaine use and temporally related to her recent binge. Although her history is not consistent with a *DSM* mood disorder, it is important to evaluate the possibility. A careful history of mood swings also would be important. If she has been using crack for years, the clinician can expect that she has experienced transient episodes (never more than a few days) of intense depression, even suicidality, with the cessation of cocaine use. At the same time, the clinician can expect that there have been no episodes of prolonged abstinence. Because of the recent onset of this depression, it is not likely to be the result of metabolic problems; however, addicted individuals are not always aware of subtle changes in their bodies, which may be obscured by intoxication.

A screening battery is recommended, because nutritional deficiencies often are found and, not infrequently, viral hepatitis (B or C). Unsafe sexual practices and needle sharing make HIV disease a concern. More relevant, the mood disturbance could be alcohol-induced; however, this situation should not coincide with cocaine cessation. The cocaine-induced depression should last only a day or two, whereas alcohol-induced depression likely would last a few days longer with sobriety. Some alcoholics experience marked depression with suicidality during intoxication, which clears with sobriety. Although it is tempting to dismiss substance-induced depression as less significant than a major depressive disorder because the former resolves so quickly, it is important to remember that these episodes are frightening to the individual, that some people make serious suicide attempts, and that a few actually kill themselves.

At this point, it appears that the patient has a cocaine withdrawal-induced mood disorder. It would be wise to obtain a toxicology screen to rule out benzodiazepine- or opiate-induced depression. With the history of depression, the clinician should look for manic episodes. Without a careful history of cocaine use and its relationship to the experience of intense moods, up or down, it would be easy to think of manic-depressive illness.

Another diagnostic consideration is the possibility that Ms. A has had a social crisis and is homeless. The report of suicidality could be exaggerated to gain admission to housing or hospital. In such a case, there may be a pattern of similar behavior.

Treatment Issues: Patient safety and suicidality are the primary issues here. Ms. A needs to be engaged in drug rehabilitation, her denial managed, and her motivation for abstinence enhanced. She needs to be engaged in a comprehensive assessment, with her relapse triggers assessed and relapse prevention initiated as needed.

Treatment Considerations: Safety is the first treatment issue in this case because of the patient's depression (suicidality) and the possibility of alcohol withdrawal (*delirium tremens*). The clinician must assess the severity of the suicidal impulse and the social supports available before deciding whether a residential setting is appropriate. The clinician should assess what type of suicidal thoughts the person is having, whether he or she has formulated a plan to carry out the idea, whether he or she has the means to complete the plan, whether he or she has made prior attempts and, if so, if he or she was serious, whether there are other alternatives, and whether the patient is very agitated.

A cocaine-induced depression usually is transient when abstinence ensues. Continued cocaine use sustains the cycle of addiction and depression. Outpatient treatment is viable only if the patient can refrain from using drugs and alcohol, and the ability to do so often depends on the degree of support in the patient's environment. Safety from alcohol withdrawal is a potential issue that should be considered; however, it is unlikely that a dangerous withdrawal will occur unless the patient has had *delirium tremens* or seizures in the past (Whitfield, Thompson et al., 1978). Ongoing monitoring is the best precaution and can be handled on an inpatient as well as an outpatient basis if the patient is cooperative. Assessing the patient's reliability (ability to follow through) may be difficult if she is previously unknown to the clinician. A variety of factors enter into this assessment, including motivation, denial, awareness, craving, relapse triggers, and availability of a supportive environment. Such an assessment is part of the safety management for this patient.

Engagement in a drug and alcohol treatment program will depend on the patient's denial, motivation, awareness of the centrality of drugs and alcohol, as well as the pull of other social relationships such as children, significant others, and family members who may be dependent on Ms. A. Attention to these psychosocial issues may be the key to engagement. Focusing on a comprehensive assessment, including relapse triggers, can be the way to engage a difficult, ambivalent patient. Inclusion of the family sometimes facilitates engagement, as does admission to a treatment program if the patient is anxious about further drug use and its sequelae. If an individual has been through rehabilitation programs in the past, has relapsed, and has a commitment to abstinence as well as a capacity to remain abstinent, then a focus on relapse prevention may be the appropriate intervention. Such intervention remains part of the art of medicine and hinges on the physician's style of practice, local resources, and managed care practices. It is a complex challenge each time and must be individualized to each situation.

CONCLUSIONS

The substance-induced mental disorders are common illnesses that often are associated with (but are not limited to) substance dependence. Although they frequently are short-lived, these disorders are by no means clinically insignificant. Serious self-injury is reported with the substance-induced mood disorders, and safety is an important clinical issue. This situation can present a clinical dilemma in determining the proper level of care. Most patients with substance-induced mental disorders can be diverted away from traditional psychiatric inpatient treatment, either to dual diagnosis units or to inpatient or outpatient addiction treatment programs in which adequate assessment and appropriate treatment are available.

Clinics and residential units that specialize in substance dependent patients who have a comorbid psychiatric illness play an important role when there is diagnostic confusion or when the patient does not respond (or has not responded in the past) to routine psychiatric treatment. Confusion about the diagnosis can delay interventions; therefore, achieving clarification through a comprehensive evaluation frequently is the first order of business, once safety is addressed.

Although abstinence is a critical factor in recovery from a substance-induced mental disorder, it is not always the only factor. Regular psychosocial treatments for substance dependence are relevant so long as the patient is behaviorally manageable and not psychotic or delirious. When the patient's behavior is unsafe or wild, a psychiatric unit may be necessary until the patient's behavior is less risky. If a specialized inpatient unit for dual diagnosis is available and can manage the patient's behavior with seclusion, restraints, psychotropic medications, or a locked unit, it may be the best choice. Such patient-treatment matching should be done on an individual basis, depending on the patient's needs, the resources available, and the skills and preferences of the clinicians involved.

REFERENCES

American Psychiatric Association (APA) (1968). *Diagnostic and Statistical Manual of Mental Disorders, 2nd Edition (DSM-II)*. Washington, DC: American Psychiatric Press.

American Psychiatric Association (APA) (1980). *Diagnostic and Statistical Manual of Mental Disorders, 3rd Edition (DSM-III)*. Washington, DC: American Psychiatric Press.

American Psychiatric Association (APA) (1987). *Diagnostic and Statistical Manual of Mental Disorders, 3rd Edition, Revised (DSM-IIIR)*. Washington, DC: American Psychiatric Press.

American Psychiatric Association (APA) (1994). *Diagnostic and Statistical Manual of Mental Disorders, 4th Edition (DSM-IV)*. Washington, DC: American Psychiatric Press.

Ashton H (1991). Protracted withdrawal syndromes from benzodiazepines. In NS Miller (ed.) *Comprehensive Handbook of Drug and Alcohol Addiction*. New York, NY: Marcel Dekker, 915-930.

Asnis GM, Friedmen TA, Sanderson WC et al. (1993). Suicidal behaviors in adult psychiatry outpatients, I: Description and prevalence. *American Journal of Psychiatry* 150:108-112.

Bartels SJ, Drake RE & McHugo GJ (1992). Alcohol abuse, depression, and suicidal behavior in schizophrenia. *American Journal of Psychiatry* 149:394-395.

Brown SA & Schuckit MA (1988). Changes in depression among abstinent alcoholics. *Journal of Studies on Alcohol* 49:412-417.

Brown SA, Inaba RK, Gillin JC et al. (1995). Alcoholism and affective disorder: Clinical course of depressive symptoms. *American Journal of Psychiatry* 152:45-52.

Brown SA, Irwin M & Schuckit MA (1991). Changes in anxiety among abstinent male alcoholics. *Journal of Studies on Alcohol* 52:55-61.

Dorus W, Kennedy J, Gibbons RD et al. (1987) Symptoms and diagnosis of depression in alcoholics. *Alcoholism: Clinical & Experimental Research* 11:150-154.

Driessen M, Veltrup C, Weber J et al. (1998). Psychiatric co-morbidity, suicidal behaviour and suicidal ideation in alcoholics seeking treatment. *Addiction* 93:889-894.

Elliott AJ, Pages KP, Russo J et al. (1996). A profile of medically serious suicide attempts. *Journal of Clinical Psychiatry* 57:567-571.

Geller A (1991). Protracted abstinence. In NS Miller (ed.) *Comprehensive Handbook of Drug and Alcohol Addiction*. New York, NY: Marcel Dekker, 905-914.

Giannini AJ (1991). Phencyclidine. In NS Miller (ed.) *Comprehensive Handbook of Drug and Alcohol Addiction*. New York, NY: Marcel Dekker, 383-394.

Gold MS (1993). *Cocaine*. New York, NY: Plenum Publishing.

Gruber AJ & Pope HG (1994). Cannabis psychotic disorder: Does it exist? *American Journal of Addictions* 3:72-83.

Henriksson MM, Aro HM, Marttunen MJ et al. (1993). Mental disorders and comorbidity in suicide. *American Journal of Psychiatry* 150:933-940.

Kadden RM, Kranzler HR & Rounsaville BJ (1995). Validity of the distinction between "substance-induced" and "independent" depression and anxiety disorders. *American Journal of Addictions* 4:107-117.

Keeler MH, Taylor CI & Miller WC (1979). Are all recently detoxified alcoholics depressed? *American Journal of Psychiatry* 136:586-588.

Levinson I, Galynker II & Rosenthal RN (1995). Methadone withdrawal psychosis. *Journal of Clinical Psychiatry* 56:73-76.

Lydiard RB, Brady K, Ballenger JC et al. (1992). Anxiety and mood disorders in hospitalized alcoholic individuals. *American Journal of Addictions* 1:325-331.

Mee-Lee D, Shulman G, Fishman M et al. (2001). *ASAM Patient Placement Criteria for the Treatment of Substance-Related Disorders, Second Edition-Revised*. Chevy Chase, MD: American Society of Addiction Medicine.

Mendoza R & Miller BL (1992). Neuropsychiatric disorders associated with cocaine use. *Hospital & Community Psychiatry* 43:677-679.

Murphy GE & Wetzel RD (1990). The lifetime risk of suicide in alcoholism. *Archives of General Psychiatry* 47:383-392.

Pages KP, Russo JE, Roy-Byrne PP et al. (1997). Determinants of suicidal ideation: The role of substance use disorders. *Journal of Clinical Psychiatry* 58:510-515.

Rosenthal RN & Miner CR (1997). Differential diagnosis of substance-induced psychosis and schizophrenia in patients with substance use disorders. *Schizophrenia Bulletin* 23:187-193.

Rounsaville BJ, Anton SF, Carroll K et al. (1991). Psychiatric diagnoses of treatment-seeking cocaine abusers. *Archives of General Psychiatry* 48:43-51.

Salloum IM, Daley DC, Cornelius JR et al. (1996). Disproportionate lethality in psychiatric patients with concurrent alcohol and cocaine abuse. *American Journal of Psychiatry* 153:953-955.

Schuckit MA & Hesselbrock V (1994). Alcohol dependence and anxiety disorders: What is the relationship? *American Journal of Psychiatry* 151:1723-1734.

Schuckit MA, Tipp JE, Bergman M et al. (1997). Comparison of induced and independent major depressive disorders in 2,945 alcoholics. *American Journal of Psychiatry* 154:948-957.

Schultz T (1991). Alcohol withdrawal syndrome: Clinical features, pathophysiology, and treatment. In NS Miller (ed.) *Comprehensive Handbook of Drug and Alcohol Addiction.* New York, NY: Marcel Dekker, 1091-1112.

Seibyl JP, Satel SL, Anthony D et al. (1993). Effects of cocaine on hospital course in schizophrenia. *Journal of Nervous and Mental Disease* 181:31-37.

Spitzer RL, Gibbon M, Skodol AE et al., eds. (1994). *DSM-IV Casebook: A Learning Companion to the Diagnostic and Statistical Manual of Mental Disorders, 4th Edition.* Washington, DC: American Psychiatric Press, 216.

Whitfield CL, Thompson G, Lamb A et al. (1978). Detoxification of 1,024 alcoholic patients without psychoactive drugs. *Journal of the American Medical Association* 239:1409-1410.

Young MA, Fogg LF, Scheftner WA et al. (1994). Interactions of risk factors in predicting suicide. *American Journal of Psychiatry* 151:434-435.

Zukin SR & Zukin RS (1992). Phencyclidine. In JH Lowinson, P Ruiz, RB Millman et al. (eds.) *Substance Abuse: A Comprehensive Textbook.* Baltimore, MD: Williams & Wilkins, 290-302.

Chapter 2

Co-Occurring Addictive and Affective Disorders

Kathleen T. Brady, M.D., Ph.D.
Hugh Myrick, M.D.
Susan Sonne, Pharm.D.

Prevalence of Affective Disorders
Diagnostic Issues
Treating Comorbid Affective Disorders

Symptoms of depression and mood instability are among the most common psychiatric symptoms seen in individuals with substance use disorders. Data also indicate that full syndromal major depression, dysthymia, and bipolar disorders co-occur with substance use disorders more commonly than would be expected by chance alone. As more and more effective treatments for affective disorders are established, it is of critical importance to recognize and treat these disorders in individuals who have substance use disorders. However, because mood disturbance commonly accompanies substance use and withdrawal, and in many cases remits after a few days of abstinence, it is important to distinguish substance-induced, time-limited affective symptoms from full syndromal affective disorder. Thus, the interface of mood disorders and substance use disorders is one of critical importance to improving treatment in the substance abuse field and has received a great deal of recent attention with regard to prevalence, diagnostic issues, and appropriate treatment.

Throughout this chapter, wherever diagnostic criteria are cited, they are the criteria of the *Diagnostic and Statistical Manuals of Mental Disorders (DSM-IIIR, DSM-IV)* of the American Psychiatric Association (1987, 1994) to which

the reference is intended. Table 1 gives an overview of the *DSM-IV* schema for affective disorders and general guidelines for their diagnosis.

PREVALENCE OF AFFECTIVE DISORDERS

Community Samples. Two major epidemiologic surveys have studied the prevalence of psychiatric disorders in community samples. The first was the National Institute of Mental Health Epidemiologic Catchment Area (ECA) Study (Regier, Farmer et al., 1990), conducted in the early 1980s; the second was the National Comorbidity Study (NCS), conducted in 1991 (Kessler, McGonagle et al., 1994). Data from the ECA study estimated the lifetime prevalence rate for any nonsubstance abuse mental disorder to be 22.5%, for alcohol abuse or dependence to be 13.5%, and for other drug abuse or dependence to be 6.1%. Among those with any affective disorder, 32% had a comorbid addictive disorder. Of the individuals with major depression, 16.5% had a comorbid alcohol use diagnosis and 18% had a comorbid other drug use diagnosis. An even higher rate of comorbidity was found in individuals with bipolar disorder: of those individuals with any bipolar diagnosis, 56.1% had an addictive disorder. The highest rate was found among

TABLE 1. Guidelines for Diagnosis of Affective Disorder

Diagnosis	Criteria
Major Depressive Episode	Symptoms are severe (> 5 symptoms) and persist for at least 2 weeks
Dysthymia	Symptoms are less severe and more persistent (2 years)
Bipolar I Disorder	Mania usually is accompanied by major depressive episodes
Bipolar II Disorder	Hypomania usually is accompanied by major depressive episodes
Cyclothymia	Symptoms are less severe than full diagnostic mania or depression, but persistent (2 years)
Substance-Induced Mood Disorder	Direct physiological consequence of drug use or withdrawal.

individuals with bipolar disorder, 60.7% of whom had a comorbid addictive disorder (46% of whom had a comorbid alcohol diagnosis and 40.7% of whom had a comorbid drug use diagnosis). Bipolar I disorder was the Axis I diagnosis most likely to co-occur with a substance use disorder.

Data from the NCS estimated a lifetime prevalence of 48% for any psychiatric disorder, 14.1% for alcohol dependence, and 7.5% for drug dependence. The lifetime prevalence rate for any affective disorder was 19.3% and for any substance abuse or dependence was 26.6%. An odds ratio was calculated, using the NCS data to determine the relative risk of co-occurrence by mental disorders and addictive disorders (Kessler, Crum et al., 1997). The odds ratio of finding a substance use disorder in a person with a mood disorder was 2.3 in a lifetime and 3.0 in the preceding 12 months. Among persons with a diagnosis of major depression, the odds ratio of comorbid substance use disorder was approximately 2.7 for lifetime co-occurrence and 3.6 for 12-month co-occurrence. The rates of addictive disorders were even higher among patients with bipolar disorder. The odds ratio of a lifetime comorbid alcohol dependence in a person with bipolar disorder was 9.7, and the comorbid drug dependence odds ratio was 8.4, whereas 12-month odds ratios were 6.3 and 8.2, respectively.

Comorbid Affective Disorder in Substance Abuse Treatment. *Alcohol*: The diagnostic difficulties at the interface of mood disorder and substance use disorder are reflected in the variability in prevalence estimates. However, many studies have found elevated rates of affective disorders in treatment-seeking alcoholics. Powell and colleagues (1982), in a study of 565 male alcoholic inpatients, found the frequency of current major depression to be 13.8% and that of current mania to be 2.8%. As expected, estimates of lifetime prevalence were higher, with major depression estimated at 20% to 67% and bipolar disorder estimated at 6% to 8% (Bowen, Cipywnyk et al., 1984; Hasin, Grant et al., 1988; Lydiard, Brady et al., 1992).

Cocaine: A number of small studies of cocaine-dependent populations have reported estimates of lifetime depressive disorders at 30% to 40% and lifetime bipolar spectrum disorders at 10% to 30% (Gawin & Kleber, 1986; Weiss, Mirin et al., 1988; Nunes, Quitkin et al., 1989). Rounsaville and coworkers (1991) reported current affective disorders in 44.3% of 298 subjects. A lifetime history of affective disorder was diagnosed in 61% of the sample, with 30.5% experiencing at least one episode of major depression and 11.1% experiencing at least one episode of hypomania or mania. Of interest, the onset of affective disorder took place predominantly after the onset of cocaine abuse or in the same year. In a more recent study using the Diagnostic Interview Schedule (DIS) to assess 207 cocaine addicts seeking outpatient treatment, Halikas and colleagues

(1994) found current and lifetime rates of affective illness to be 17% and 28%, respectively. Almost 65% of the subjects reported that their first regular drug use preceded the onset of their affective illness.

Opiates: There is considerable literature on affective disorder in opiate-dependent individuals. In an evaluation of 533 opiate-dependent individuals, Rounsaville and colleagues (1982) found that the lifetime prevalence of any affective disorder was 74.3%. The lifetime rates for major depression and mania were 53.9% and 0.6%, whereas the lifetime rates for minor depression and hypomania were 8.4% and 6.6%, respectively. In the largest study to date, Brooner and colleagues (1997) found that 19% of 716 of opioid-dependent patients seeking methadone maintenance met *DSM-IIIR* criteria for a lifetime mood disorder. Major depression was present in 15.8% of the sample, and bipolar disorder in 0.4%.

Comorbid Substance Use in Affective Disorder Treatment. Other investigators have explored the prevalence of substance use disorders in treatment-seeking individuals with affective disorder. Miller and Fine (1993), in a review of the epidemiologic literature, found the ratio of patients with comorbid addictive disorders in a psychiatric setting to be 30% for depressive disorder and 50% for bipolar disorders. Hasin and colleagues (1988) assessed 835 patients with affective syndromes for alcohol or drug use disorders and found that almost a fourth of the patients had abused alcohol or drugs at a clinically significant level during their current affective episode. Brady and colleagues (1991) assessed substance use disorders in 100 patients consecutively admitted to an inpatient psychiatric unit at a Veterans Affairs medical center. Of these, 64% endorsed current or past problems with substance use, and 29% met *DSM-IIIR* criteria for a substance use disorder in the 30 days preceding their admission. Of patients with major depression, 58% met criteria for a lifetime substance use disorder, and 22% met criteria for a current substance use disorder. Of patients with bipolar disorder, 70% met criteria for lifetime substance use disorder, and 30% met criteria for a current substance use disorder. (Interestingly, only 40% of the patients with current or past substance abuse had received treatment for an addictive disorder.) Similarly, Goldberg and colleagues (1999) found that 34% of a group of patients hospitalized for mania had a current substance use disorder.

Prevalence and Comorbidity in the Adolescent Population. Studies of adolescents have found high rates of comorbid affective and substance use disorders. In a study of 424 adolescents, Deykin and coworkers (1987) found that subjects who reported a history of alcohol abuse were almost four times as likely to have a history of major depression as subjects who had not abused alcohol. Subjects who had abused drugs were 3.3 times as likely to have a history of major depression as those who had not abused drugs. Bukstein and colleagues (1992) evaluated affective comorbidity in 156 adolescents with substance use disorders. Affective disorders were diagnosed in 51.3% of the sample. Major depression was found in 30.7% of the subjects and bipolar disorder in 7.7%. Hovens and colleagues (1994) evaluated 53 inpatients with substance use disorders for psychiatric comorbidities and found major depression evident in 25% and dysthymia in 33%. More recently, Grilo and colleagues (1995) assessed 69 inpatient adolescents with substance use disorders and found that 65.2% met criteria for a mood disorder. Taken together, these data indicate that comorbidity is a widespread problem in the adolescent population, so young patients need to be carefully assessed for comorbid affective and addictive disorders and treatment provided as appropriate.

Summary. The comorbidity of affective disorder and substance use disorders is impressively high when assessed from a number of differing perspectives in a variety of populations. The wide variation in estimates likely is the result of differing diagnostic techniques and the variations in populations studied. A few general conclusions can be drawn. Although all affective disorders are relatively common in substance users, bipolar disorder is the affective syndrome most commonly associated with a substance use disorder. Of all the affective disorders, depression and dysthymia are the specific disorders most commonly seen in alcoholic and opiate-dependent populations. Bipolar spectrum disorders are relatively more common in the cocaine-dependent population, but the substantial overlap between symptoms of mania and stimulant intoxication must be kept in mind.

DIAGNOSTIC ISSUES

Diagnosing an affective disorder in the face of substance abuse can be difficult because drugs of abuse, particularly with chronic use, can mimic nearly any psychiatric disorder. It also is important to note that individuals with substance use disorders often present in a primary care setting with complaints of anxiety, sleep disturbance, and depression (women are particularly likely to seek help outside of the substance abuse treatment system) (Weisner &

Schmidt, 1992). Both stimulant use and alcohol intoxication can cause symptoms indistinguishable from mania or hypomania, and withdrawal states often cause symptoms of anxiety and depression. More specifically, chronic use of central nervous system (CNS) stimulants (such as cocaine and amphetamines) may cause euphoria, increased energy, decreased appetite, grandiosity, and sometimes paranoia, which may look very similar to mania or hypomania. Withdrawal from CNS stimulants (especially cocaine) may cause anhedonia, apathy, and depressed mood with possible suicidal ideation. Chronic use of CNS depressants (for example, alcohol, benzodiazepines, barbiturates, and opiates) often is associated with depressed mood, poor concentration, anhedonia, and problems sleeping, which also are symptoms of depression. Withdrawal from CNS depressants often causes symptoms of anxiety and agitation.

Addictive use of drugs is associated with lifestyles and behaviors that lead to multiple losses and stressors. Such losses may precipitate a depressed affect, which is appropriate and transient. Studies have indicated that up to 98% of individuals presenting for substance abuse treatment have some symptoms of depression (Jaffe, Rounsaville et al., 1996). For the most part, the symptoms remit with time in abstinence. In a study by Dorus and colleagues (1987), depressive symptoms were monitored over a one-month period in 171 individuals who presented for inpatient treatment of alcohol dependence. On day 1, 67% had high depression ratings, but by day 28 only 16% had high depression ratings. The national prevalence estimate for current major depressive episode is 5%. So, although it is important not to make a diagnosis too early or to overtreat depression, it also is important to recognize that the population in substance abuse treatment is at increased risk of depression and must be carefully assessed.

It often is easier to diagnose mania than depression in the substance abuser. During active drug use, urine drug screens can be useful in evaluating substance-induced mania, and withdrawal states generally do not mimic mania. Substance-induced mania generally lasts only for the duration of the drug's pharmacologic effect, so manic symptoms that persist for a number of days after last substance use are not likely to be substance-induced. Long-acting stimulants (methamphetamine) and hallucinogens may be an exception to this rule, as manic symptoms resulting from intoxication with these substances can last for several days. Another difficulty in the diagnosis of the bipolar disorders is the fact that bipolar spectrum disorders, such as cyclothymia, are difficult to diagnose reliably because of the shorter duration and more subtle nature of the associated symptoms.

The best way to differentiate substance-induced, transient psychiatric symptoms from psychiatric disorders that warrant independent treatment is through observation of the patient's symptoms during a period of abstinence from drugs and alcohol. Transient substance-related states improve with time. A key issue in this discussion is the amount of time in abstinence necessary for accurate diagnosis. It is likely that the minimum amount of time necessary for diagnosis will vary according to the comorbid condition being diagnosed. With depression, symptom resolution appears to occur at about two to four weeks after last use. Thus, there is a risk of overdiagnosis of psychiatric disorder if the diagnosis is made earlier. Bipolar disorder is less well studied in this regard. As mentioned earlier, it is likely that one could make a diagnosis of mania with less than two to four weeks' abstinence because symptoms of mania have less overlap with withdrawal states.

Diagnostic schema are evolving to address this issue. The *DSM-IV* includes a category called "substance-induced mood disorder," which is designed to capture clear changes in affective state that occur only during periods of active substance use and withdrawal. Although the Structured Clinical Interview for *DSM-IV* (SCID) is widely considered one of the best diagnostic instruments for psychiatric disorders, the validity of this instrument for making diagnoses in substance users is questionable (Kranzler, Kadden et al., 1996). The Psychiatric Research Interview for Substance and Mental Disorders (PRISM) is a structured interview specifically designed to assess comorbid psychiatric and substance use disorders by carefully assessing the chronologic relationship between psychiatric symptoms and substance use and adding specific interviewer instructions to assist in differentiating organic from nonorganic disorders. This interview has demonstrated good reliability (Hasin, Trautman et al., 1996) and predictive validity in dually diagnosed individuals.

There are many unanswered questions concerning accurate diagnoses of comorbid substance use and psychiatric disorder. A period of abstinence is optimal for diagnosis, but the necessary minimum timeframe is likely to differ for each diagnosis. A family history of affective illness, clear onset of psychiatric symptoms before onset of the substance use disorder, and the presence of sustained affective symptoms during lengthy periods of abstinence in the past all weigh in favor of making a diagnosis in cases where the diagnosis remains unclear.

TREATING COMORBID AFFECTIVE DISORDERS
Pharmacotherapeutic Treatments of Substance Abuse and Depression. Several studies of tricyclic antidepressants (TCAs) in alcoholic populations have indicated that antidepressants may be helpful in treating patients with comorbid substance use disorder and depression. McGrath and colleagues (1996) conducted a 12-week, placebo-controlled trial of imipramine (Tofranil®) treatment in actively drinking alcoholic outpatients with coexisting depression. They found that imipramine treatment was associated with improvement in the depression. Although the imipramine did not have a direct effect on drinking outcome, the patients whose mood improved showed a more marked reduction in alcohol consumption. Mason and colleagues (1996) found that treatment of alcoholics with secondary depression (onset of depression after alcohol dependence) with desipramine (Norpramin®) led to a decrease in the symptoms of depression and an increase in the period of abstinence from alcohol. (However, the optimal dose and effective blood levels of TCAs remain unclear.) Lower blood levels of imipramine have been reported in alcoholics compared with a nonalcoholic population on a fixed dose of imipramine; this appears to be due to differences in clearance. Increased plasma levels of imipramine have been reported in patients treated with disulfiram (Antabuse®). Monitoring of TCA plasma levels is likely to be particularly important in alcoholic populations (Weiss & Mirin, 1989).

The serotonin system has been implicated in control of alcohol intake (Amit, Smith et al., 1991), and selective serotonin reuptake inhibitors (SSRIs) have shown promise in the treatment of alcoholism. A number of selective serotonin agents have been shown to have a modest effect in decreasing alcohol consumption in problem drinkers and alcoholics (Gorelick, 1989), but the data have been mixed. Pettaniti and colleagues (2000) found that a subgroup of alcoholics with lower risk and severity of alcoholism and less severe psychopathology had a positive response to treatment with sertraline (Zoloft®), whereas subjects with severe dependence and high levels of psychopathology had a poor response to treatment. Subtyping of alcoholics for the purposes of individualizing treatment may be one way to improve outcomes.

In a 12-week, double-blind, placebo-controlled trial, Cornelius and colleagues (1997) found that fluoxetine (Prozac®) was effective in reducing both depressive symptoms and alcohol consumption in patients with comorbid major depression and alcohol dependence. However, Petrakis and colleagues (1998) found no differences between fluoxetine and placebo in treating depressive symptoms or decreasing illicit drug use in a methadone-maintained population. In a double-blind, placebo-controlled trial, Roy-Byrne and colleagues (2000) explored the use of nefazodone (Serzone®) in a group of alcohol-dependent individuals with major depression. The nefazodone-treated group had a greater reduction in depression ratings, but there was no difference between the groups taking nefazodone and placebo in alcohol-related outcomes.

Several trials of TCAs have been performed with opioid-dependent patients. In several studies with methadone-maintained patients, doxepin (Adapin®) has been shown to relieve symptoms of depression, anxiety, and drug craving. It must be noted, however, that methadone maintenance clinics have reported abuse of amitriptyline (Elavil®) and other sedating TCAs. Monitoring of TCA plasma levels is important in methadone-maintained patients because patients receiving methadone and desipramine have been found to have plasma levels of desipramine (Norpramin®) that were twice as high as before methadone administration (Weiss & Mirin, 1989). Recently, Nunes and colleagues (1998) found that imipramine was effective in the treatment of depression in a group of methadone-maintained patients. Imipramine also was superior to placebo on self-report measures of substance use and craving, but there was no between-group differences in urine drug screen data.

The use of TCAs in cocaine-dependent patients has focused primarily on the treatment of cocaine dependence rather than the treatment of depression. Several studies of desipramine have shown improvement in anhedonia and cocaine craving and increased initial abstinence in nondepressed patients, and one small study showed improvement in depression as well as cocaine use in depressed cocaine-dependent patients (Rao, Ziedonis et al., 1995). Clinicians should be aware, however, that desipramine can have an activating effect in cocaine-dependent individuals, thus precipitating relapse. TCAs also can have additive cardiotoxicity when combined with cocaine, should relapse occur (Weiss & Mirin, 1989). Other antidepressants such as venlafaxine (Effexor®) and bupropion (Wellbutrin®) (Kosten, Petrakis et al., 1998) have shown preliminary efficacy in the treatment of depression in cocaine-dependent individuals, but placebo-controlled studies of these treatments are not available.

Several treatment recommendations can be made. First, a period of abstinence is optimal before the initiation of antidepressant treatment. Even when there is evidence of primary depression, it would be prudent to wait until after detoxification is complete so as not to confuse withdrawal symptoms with activation from antidepressants. The patient's aftercare plan can dictate how aggressive the clinician should be in deciding on the use of antidepressant medications. If the depression is mild (dysthymia) and less clear diagnostically, the decision to postpone pharmacologic treatment for diagnostic purposes can make sense. If the depression is severe and there is little evidence of remission during the first few days of abstinence, early pharmacologic treatment may be justified. Symptoms of depression that clearly predate the substance use disorder, or a family history of depression, are factors that may help the clinician diagnose depression after a shorter period of abstinence.

After reaching the decision to use a medication, the SSRIs may be a logical first choice in alcoholic populations for several reasons. First, the SSRIs can decrease the desire to drink and help to initiate abstinence as well as treat depression. Second, SSRIs have fewer anticholinergic and cardiotoxic side effects and thus are better tolerated and safer in a population at risk of noncompliance and impulsive overdosing. Higher doses of SSRIs or TCAs may be required because of the possibility that alcohol use has induced hepatic microsomal activity.

When treating depression in individuals with cocaine use disorders, the clinician may first consider using desipramine to help facilitate abstinence as well as alleviate depression. Treatment should be initiated with low doses to avoid activation, which can trigger relapse. The selective serotonin drugs and other, newer antidepressant agents need further investigation in the cocaine-using population.

Pharmacotherapeutic Treatments of Substance Abuse and Bipolar Disorder. Before considering the treatment of patients with comorbid bipolar disorder and substance use disorder, it is important to understand the clinical course of bipolar disorder complicated by substance abuse. Sonne and colleagues (1994) compared a group of individuals with coexisting bipolar disorder and substance use disorder with a group of patients with bipolar disorder alone. They found that the patients with co-occurring substance use disorders had an earlier onset of mood disorder, were more likely to be men and to have more comorbid Axis I disorders (primarily posttraumatic stress disorder and panic disorder), and were significantly more likely to have dysphoric mania at the time of interview. Other investigators have found that a high percentage of patients with mixed or rapid-cycling bipolar disorder had concurrent alcoholism (Keller, Lavori et al., 1986). Such patients were likely to have a slower time of recovery than patients presenting with depression alone or mania alone.

These data suggest that bipolar patients with comorbid substance use disorders may have a more severe course of affective illness than bipolar patients who do not also have a substance use disorder. It has been postulated that the presence of the affective syndrome, particularly mania, can precipitate or exacerbate substance abuse. Alternatively, substance abuse and withdrawal are likely to worsen affective symptoms, thereby forming a cycle of substance abuse and affective instability.

Theoretical Implications: An interesting theoretical perspective in this area comes from the literature on neuronal sensitization, or "kindling." It has been postulated that bipolar disorder is a phenomenon of neuronal sensitization because the course of the illness often is characterized by acceleration, with successively shortened periods of remission between episodes of active illness (Post, Rubinow et al., 1984). Cocaine and alcohol are the most common agents of abuse in patients with bipolar disorder (Brady & Lydiard, 1992). Acute cocaine intoxication and alcohol withdrawal both appear to produce neuronal sensitization (Brown, Anton et al., 1986; Post & Weiss, 1988). Because use of both substances is associated with neuronal sensitization and it has been postulated that the course of bipolar disorder also is affected by neuronal sensitization, it is possible that this mechanism is responsible for the morbidity and poor prognosis associated with substance abuse in bipolar patients. Carbamazepine (Tegretol®) and valproate (Depakene®) are two antikindling, anticonvulsant agents that have efficacy in the treatment of acute manic states. If neuronal sensitization, or kindling, is one consequence of substance abuse and is important in the pathophysiology of bipolar disorder, an antikindling agent may be particularly efficacious in patients with comorbid bipolar disorder and a substance use disorder. Evidence also supports the use of the antikindling agent, carbamazepine, in the treatment of alcohol withdrawal (Malcolm, Ballenger et al., 1989), rendering the antikindling agents even more useful in treating substance-abusing bipolar patients.

Pharmacotherapies: Unfortunately, there is very little published data on the treatment of bipolar disorder complicated by substance abuse. Agents currently used to treat bipolar disorder include lithium and the anticonvulsant medications, carbamazepine and valproate. Lithium has been used as the standard treatment of bipolar disorder for several decades. However, it is effective in only 60% to 80% of classic bipolar patients (Calabrese, Rapport et al., 1993). The response rate for lithium has been estimated to be as low as 50% when all bipolar subtypes have been considered. As many as 72% to 82% of patients with the rapid cycling variant of bipolar disorder exhibit a poor response to lithium (Calabrese & Delucchi, 1989).

Several studies have identified substance abuse as a predictor of poor response to lithium (Tohen, Waternaux et al., 1990; O'Connell, Mayo et al., 1991; Bowden, 1995). In a four-year followup study of 24 bipolar patients after their first manic episode, alcoholism was found to be a statistically significant predictor of a shorter time in remission from affective symptoms (Tohen, Waternaux et al., 1990). Another long-term study of lithium (O'Connell, Mayo et al., 1991) found the incidence of substance abuse to be substantially higher in the patients who had a poor outcome (36%), as compared with the patients who had a good outcome (7%). However, Geller and colleagues (1992) found that lithium treatment stabilized mood and decreased substance use in a group of adolescents with a primary mood disorder and secondary substance use. This study is encouraging in that it provides empirical evidence to suggest that mood stabilization leads to a decrease in substance use in some individuals with comorbid bipolar and addictive disorders.

Both carbamazepine and valproate have shown efficacy in treating mania associated with bipolar disorder (Ballenger & Post, 1979; Post, 1990; Bowden, Brugger et al., 1994). Although other anticonvulsants currently are being studied for the treatment of mania (for example, lamotrigine [Lamictal®] and gabapentin [Neurontin®]), only valproate (divalproex sodium) is approved by the U.S. Food and Drug Administration (FDA) for this indication (Abbott Laboratories, 1995). In addition to typical euphoric mania, many patients with bipolar disorder have mixed manic episodes (concurrent symptoms of mania and depression) and rapid cycling episodes (>4 episodes per year).

Several studies have concluded that patients with mixed and/or rapid cycling bipolar disorder are more likely to respond to anticonvulsant medications than to lithium (Freeman, Clothier et al., 1992; Calabrese, Markovitz et al., 1992). As discussed earlier, bipolar patients with concomitant substance use disorders appear to have more mixed and/or rapid cycling bipolar disorder than patients with bipolar disorder who do not abuse substances. Therefore, substance-abusing bipolar patients may respond better to anticonvulsant medications (for example, valproate) than to lithium therapy. In fact, in an open-label pilot study, Brady and colleagues (1995) found valproate to be safe and effective in nine mixed manic bipolar patients with concurrent substance dependence, who previously either had not tolerated or not responded to lithium.

Both valproate and alcohol consumption are known to cause transient elevations in liver transaminases and, in rare cases, fatal liver failure. Therefore, it is important to monitor liver function often in alcoholic patients who receive valproate therapy. It is recommended that valproate therapy be started only if liver transaminases are less than twice the upper limit of normal. With this practice, there is preliminary evidence from the authors' site that liver transaminases do not dramatically increase in alcoholic patients who are receiving valproate, even if they are actively drinking (Sonne, Brady et al., 1996). Additionally, chronic alcohol use can cause reductions in white blood cell and platelet counts, which also can complicate the use of valproate in the alcoholic population. However, the authors' preliminary data have not shown any clinically significant reductions in platelet counts of alcoholic individuals who were receiving valproate for as long as two years (Sonne, Brady et al., 1996).

When treating acute mania, the other traditional agents (for example, neuroleptics, benzodiazepines) also are useful in the substance-abusing population. However, when managing substance-abusing, bipolar individuals with benzodiazepines in an outpatient setting, it may be prudent to use agents that have a longer onset of action (for example, clonazepam [Klonopin®] or oxazepam [Serax®]) because those agents appear to have less abuse potential. It also is advisable to use benzodiazepines only in a time-limited, symptom-oriented manner and to prescribe small amounts at any one time.

Psychotherapeutic Treatments. Psychotherapeutic interventions are useful in the treatment of both affective disorder and substance use disorders and are a critical element in treating a patient with comorbid disorders. It is fairly well accepted that the use of medications to achieve mood stability is an essential component of patient care. Although most experts agree that psychotherapy is an important adjunct to pharmacotherapeutic interventions in patients with affective disorder, there is less consensus concerning the most appropriate psychotherapeutic treatment. However, mood stabilization alone is not an effective treatment for substance use disorders; adjunctive therapy and psychosocial rehabilitation are necessary as well.

A wide range of psychotherapeutic interventions have been used in the treatment of affective disorders; these include psychodynamic, interpersonal, cognitive, behavioral, and family therapies (APA, 1994). Judgments concerning the effectiveness of these treatments are based primarily on clinical consensus rather than on controlled clinical trials; however, formal studies of several of these treatments are now under way.

Psychotherapeutic, psychosocial, and peer-oriented interventions are mainstays in the treatment of substance use disorders. Several studies have demonstrated success with cognitive behavioral therapy interventions (Carroll, Rounsaville et al., 1994) as well as with behaviorally oriented contingency management programs (Higgins, Budney et al., 1994). A treatment-matching study found remarkably good results with all three of the most commonly used therapies, including Twelve Step facilitation, brief motivational therapy, and cognitive behavioral therapy (Project MATCH Research Group, 1997; Kadden, 1996). In a report comparing cognitive behavioral therapy (CBT) to relaxation training in a group of depressed alcoholic patients, the CBT-treated group showed greater reductions in depression as well as better alcohol-related outcomes. Similar data were found in a promising pilot study using group psychotherapy for individuals with comorbid bipolar disorder and substance use disorder.

The psychotherapeutic/psychosocial treatment approach used should be individualized and should contain elements to address both the substance use and affective disorders. Many of the principles of cognitive behavioral therapy are common to the treatment of affective disorder and substance use disorders. Alcoholics Anonymous and Narcotics Anonymous are available in all communities; active participation in these groups consistently is shown to be a major factor in recovery.

Summary. The development of therapies specifically targeting the needs of patients with comorbid psychiatric and substance use disorders by combining techniques used to treat both disorders is a fruitful area for further work. In the interim, substance use disorders should be treated aggressively in patients with affective disorders as soon as the patients are psychiatrically stable enough to participate in and benefit from such treatment. It also is important to recognize that all individuals with affective disorder are at risk of developing a substance use disorder; therefore, they should be educated about the risks of substance use and counseled on the early warning signs of substance abuse. In particular, patients should be warned about the dangers of self-medication for their psychiatric symptoms.

CONCLUSIONS

Because symptoms of mood disorders are common in individuals with substance use disorders and full syndromal affective disorders are commonly comorbid with substance use disorders, diagnosis and treatment of these patients is a significant and important challenge. Indeed, improving the diagnosis and treatment of patients with comorbid affective and addictive disorders is critical to improving the treatment of substance use disorders in general.

Differentiating between substance-induced, time-limited mood symptoms and true affective disorder that warrants specifically tailored treatments remains an issue that justifies further investigation. Promising pharmacotherapies and psychotherapeutic treatment options are becoming available.

REFERENCES

Abbott Laboratories (1995). Divalproex sodium (Depakote) product information. North Chicago, IL: Abbott Laboratories.

American Psychiatric Association (APA) (1987). *Diagnostic and Statistical Manual of Mental Disorders, 3rd Edition, Revised (DSM-IIIR)*. Washington, DC: American Psychiatric Press.

American Psychiatric Association (APA) (1994). *Diagnostic and Statistical Manual of Mental Disorders, 4th Edition (DSM-IV)*. Washington, DC: American Psychiatric Press.

Amit Z, Smith BR & Gill K (1991). Serotonin uptake inhibitors: Effects on motivated consummatory behaviors. *Journal of Clinical Psychiatry* 55:55-60.

Ballenger J & Post R (1979). Therapeutic effects of carbamazepine in affective illness: A preliminary report. *Community Psychopharmacology* 159-179.

Bowden CL (1995). Predictors of response to divalproex and lithium. *Journal of Clinical Psychiatry* 56(Suppl 3):25-30.

Bowden CL, Brugger AM, Swann AC et al. (1994). Efficacy of Divalproex vs. lithium and placebo in the treatment of mania. *Journal of the American Medical Association* 271:918-924.

Bowen RCI, Cipywnyk D, D'Arcy C et al. (1984). Alcoholism, anxiety disorders, and agoraphobia. *Alcoholism: Clinical & Experimental Research* 8(1):48-50.

Brady K, Casto S, Lydiard RB et al. (1991). Substance abuse in an inpatient psychiatric sample. *American Journal of Drug and Alcohol Abuse* 17(4):389-397.

Brady KT & Lydiard RB (1992). Bipolar affective disorder substance abuse. *Journal of Clinical Psychopharmacology* 12(Suppl):17s-22s.

Brady KT, Sonne SC, Anton R et al. (1995). Valproate in the treatment of acute bipolar affective episodes complicated by substance abuse: A pilot study. *Journal of Clinical Psychiatry* 56(3):118-121.

Brooner RK, King VL, Kidorf M et al. (1997). Psychiatric and substance comorbidity among treatment-seeking opioid abusers. *Archives of General Psychiatry* 54:71-80.

Brown ME, Anton RE, Malcolm R et al. (1986). Alcoholic detoxification and withdrawal seizures: Clinical support for a kindling hypothesis. *Biological Psychiatry* 43:107-113.

Bukstein OG, Glancy LJ & Kaminer Y (1992). Patterns of affective comorbidity in a clinical population of dually diagnosed adolescent substance abusers. *Journal of the American Academy of Child and Adolescent Psychiatry* 31(6):1041-1045.

Calabrese JR & Delucchi GA (1989). Phenomenology of rapid cycling manic depression and its treatment with valproate. *Journal of Clinical Psychiatry* 50(Suppl):30-34.

Calabrese JR, Markovitz PJ, Kimmel SE et al. (1992). Spectrum of efficacy of valproate in 78 rapid-cycling bipolar patients. *Journal of Clinical Psychopharmacology* 12:53-56.

Calabrese JR, Rapport DJ, Kimmel SE et al. (1993). Rapid cycling bipolar disorder and its treatment with valproate. *Canadian Journal of Psychiatry* 38: 57-61.

Carroll KM, Rounsaville BJ & Gordon LT (1994). Psychotherapy and pharmacotherapy for ambulatory cocaine abusers. *Archives of General Psychiatry* 51:177-187.

Cornelius JR, Salloum IM, Ehler JG et al. (1997). Fluoxetine in depressed alcoholics. A double-blind, placebo-controlled trial. *Archives of General Psychiatry* 54(8):700-705.

Deykin EY, Levy JC & Wells V (1987). Adolescent depression, alcohol and drug abuse. *American Journal of Public Health* 77(2):178-182.

Dorus W, Kennedy J, Gibbons RD et al. (1987). Symptoms and diagnosis of depression in alcoholics. *Alcoholism: Clinical & Experimental Research* 11(2):150-154.

Freeman TW, Clothier JL, Pazzaglia P et al. (1992). A double-blind comparison of valproate and lithium in the treatment of acute mania. *American Journal of Psychiatry* 149(1):108-111.

Gawin FH & Kleber HD (1986). Abstinence symptomatology and psychiatric diagnosis in cocaine abusers. Clinical observations. *Archives of General Psychiatry* 43(2):107-113.

Geller B, Cooper TB, Watts HE et al. (1992). Early findings from a pharmacokinetically designed double-blind and placebo-controlled study of lithium for adolescents comorbid with bipolar and substance dependency disorders. *Progress in Neuropsychopharmacology and Biological Psychiatry* 16(3):281-299.

Goldberg JF, Garno JL, Leon AC et al. (1999). A history of substance abuse complicates remission from acute mania in bipolar disorder. *Journal of Clinical Psychiatry* 60(11):733-740.

Gorelick DA (1989). Serotonin uptake blockers and the treatment of alcoholism. *Recent Developments in Alcoholism* 7:267-281.

Grilo CM, Becker DF, Walker ML et al. (1995). Psychiatric comorbidity in adolescent inpatients with substance use disorders. *Journal of the American Academy of Child and Adolescent Psychiatry* 34(8):1085-1091.

Halikas JA, Crosby RD, Pearson VL et al. (1994). Psychiatric comorbidity in treatment-seeking cocaine abusers. *American Journal on Addictions* 3(1):1-11.

Hasin DS, Grant BF & Endicott J (1988). Lifetime psychiatric comorbidity in hospitalized alcoholics: Subject and familial correlates. *International Journal of the Addictions* 23(8):827-850.

Hasin DS, Trautman KD, Miele GM et al. (1996). Psychiatric Research Interview for Substance and Mental Disorders (PRISM): Reliability for substance abusers. *American Journal of Psychiatry* 153(9):1195-1201.

Higgins ST, Budney AJ, Bickel WK et al. (1994). Incentives improve outcome in outpatient behavioral treatment of cocaine dependence. *Archives of General Psychiatry* 51(7):568-576.

Hovens JG, Cantwell DP & Kiriakos R (1994). Psychiatric comorbidity in hospitalized adolescent substance abusers. *Journal of the American Academy of Child and Adolescent Psychiatry* 33(4):476-483.

Jaffe AL, Rounsaville B, Chang G et al. (1996). Naltrexone, relapse prevention, and supportive therapy with alcoholics: An analysis of patient treatment matching. *Journal of Consulting and Clinical Psychology* 64(5):1044-1053.

Kadden RM (1996). Project MATCH: Treatment main effects and matching results. *Alcoholism: Clinical & Experimental Research* 20(8 Suppl):196A-197A.

Keller MB, Lavori PW, Rice J et al. (1986). The persistent risk of chronicity in recurrent episodes of nonbipolar major depressive disorder: A prospective follow-up. *American Journal of Psychiatry* 143:24-28.

Kessler RC, Crum RM, Warner LA et al. (1997). Lifetime co-occurrence of DSM-IIIR alcohol abuse and dependence with other psychiatric disorders in the National Comorbidity Survey. *Archives of General Psychiatry* 54:313-321.

Kessler RC, McGonagle KA, Zhao S et al. (1994). Lifetime and 12-month prevalence of DSM-IIIR psychiatric disorders in the United States. Results from the National Comorbidity Survey. *Archives of General Psychiatry* 51(l):8-19.

Kosten T, Petrakis I, Carroll KM et al. (1998). Fluoxetine treatment of depressive disorders in methadone-maintained opioid addicts. *Drug and Alcohol Dependence* 50:221-226.

Kranzler HR, Kadden RM, Babor TF et al. (1996). Validity of the SCID in substance abuse patients: Research Report. *Addiction* 91(6):859-868.

Lydiard RB, Brady KT, Ballenger ID et al. (1992). Anxiety and mood disorders in hospitalized alcoholic individuals. *American Journal on Addictions* 1(4):325-331.

Malcolm R, Ballenger RC, Sturgis ET et al. (1989). Double-blind controlled trial comparing carbamazepine to oxazepam treatment of alcohol withdrawal. *American Journal of Psychiatry* 146:617-621.

Mason BJ, Kocsis JH, Ritvo EC et al. (1996). A double-blind, placebo-controlled trial of desipramine for primary alcohol dependence stratified on the presence or absence of major depression. *Journal of the American Medical Association* 275(10):761-767.

McGrath PJ, Nunes EV, Stewart JW et al. (1996). Imipramine treatment of alcoholics with primary depression: A placebo-controlled clinical trial. *Archives of General Psychiatry* 53(3):232-240.

Miller NS & Fine J (1993). Current epidemiology of comorbidity of psychiatric and addictive disorders. *Psychiatric Clinics of North America* 16(l): 1-10.

Nunes EV, Quitkin FM, Donovan SJ et al. (1998). Imipramine treatment of opiate-dependent patients with depression disorders. *Archives of General Psychiatry* 55:153-160.

Nunes EV, Quitkin FM & Klein DF (1989). Psychiatric diagnosis in cocaine abuse. *Psychiatry Research* 280:105-114.

O'Connell RA, Mayo JA, Flatow L et al. (1991). Outcome of bipolar disorder on long-term treatment with lithium. *British Journal of Psychiatry* 159:123-129.

Okuma T, Yamashita I, Takahashi R et al. (1989). Clinical efficacy of carbamazepine in affective, schizoaffective, and schizophrenic disorders. *Pharmacopsychiatry* 22(2):47-53.

Petrakis I, Carroll KM, Nich C et al. (1998). Fluoxetine treatment of depressive disorders in methadone-maintained opioid addicts. *Drug and Alcohol Dependence* 50:221-226.

Pettaniti HM, Volpicelli JR, Kranzler GL et al. (2000). Sertraline treatment for alcohol dependence: Interactive effects of medication and alcoholic subtype. *Alcoholism: Clinical & Experimental Research* 24(7):1041-1049.

Post R, Rubinow D & Ballenger J (1984). Conditioning, sensitization and kindling: Implications for the course of affective illness. In RM Post & JC Ballenger (eds.) *Neurobiology of Mood Disorders.* Baltimore, MD: Williams & Wilkins, 432-466.

Post RM (1990). Non-lithium treatment for bipolar disorder. *Journal of Clinical Psychiatry* 51(Suppl):9-19.

Post RM & Weiss SR (1988). Psychomotor stimulant vs. local anesthetic effects of cocaine: Role of behavioral sensitization and kindling. *NIDA Research Monograph No. 88.* Rockville, MD: National Institute on Drug Abuse, 217-238.

Powell BJ, Penick EC, Othmer E et al. (1982). Prevalence of additional psychiatric syndromes among male alcoholics. *Journal of Clinical Psychiatry* 43(10):404-407.

Project MATCH Research Group (1997). Matching alcoholism treatments to client heterogeneity: Project MATCH posttreatment drinking outcomes. *Journal of Studies on Alcohol* 8:7-29.

Rao S, Ziedonis D & Kosten T (1995). The pharmacotherapy of cocaine dependence. *Psychiatric Annals* 25:363-368.

Regier DA, Farmer ME, Rae DS et al. (1990). Comorbidity of mental disorders with alcohol and other drug abuse. Results from the Epidemiologic Catchment Area (ECA). *Journal of the American Medical Association* 264(19):2511-2518.

Rounsaville BJ, Anton SF, Carroll K et al. (1991). Psychiatric diagnoses of treatment-seeking cocaine abusers. *Archives of General Psychiatry* 480:43-51.

Rounsaville BJ, Weissman MM, Kleber H et al. (1982). Heterogeneity of psychiatric diagnosis in treated opiate addicts. *Archives of General Psychiatry* 39(2):161-168.

Roy-Byrne PP, Pages KP, Russo JE et al. (2000). Nefazodone treatment of major depression in alcohol-dependent patients: A double-blind, placebo-controlled trial. *Journal of Clinical Psychopharmacology* 20(2):129-36.

Sonne SC, Brady KT & Morton WA (1994). Substance abuse and bipolar affective disorder. *Journal of Nervous and Mental Disease* 182(6):349-352.

Sonne SC, Brady KT & Morton WA (1996). Safety of Depakote in bipolar patients with comorbid alcoholism. American Psychiatric Association Annual Meeting, New York, NY.

Tohen M, Waternaux CM, Tsuang MT et al. (1990). Four-year follow-up of twenty-four first-episode manic patients. *Journal of Affective Disorders* 19(2):79-86.

Weisner C & Schmidt L (1992). Gender disparities in treatment for alcohol problems. *Journal of the American Medical Association* 268(14):1872-1876.

Weiss RD & Mirin SM (1989). Tricyclic antidepressants in the treatment of alcoholism and drug abuse. *Journal of Clinical Psychiatry* 50(7 Suppl):4-11.

Weiss RD, Mirin SM, Griffin ML et al. (1988). Psychopathology in cocaine abusers. Changing trends. *Journal of Nervous and Mental Disease* 176(12):719-725.

Chapter 3	# Co-Occurring Addictive and Anxiety Disorders

Nancy Nitenson, M.D.
David R. Gastfriend, M.D.

Epidemiology and Phenomenology
Neurobiology of Anxiety and Addiction
Diagnosing the Anxious Addicted Patient
Treating the Anxious Addicted Patient

Pathologic anxiety often is present in the addicted patient as a causal factor, a sequel, and—frequently—an obstacle to recovery. In the general population, anxiety disorders are nearly as common as addictive disorders, with considerable overlap between the two syndromes. Anxiety symptoms may be the presenting complaint of an underlying substance use disorder—an entrée to medications for drug-seeking addicted patients—so it behooves physicians to be familiar with the epidemiology, diagnostic criteria, and natural course of both syndromes, as well as the patterns of requests that can induce physicians to prescribe in an enabling fashion.

Given the frequency of anxiety symptoms in the course of substance intoxication and withdrawal, it also is important to understand the physiologic triggers of arousal. Abstinence and recovery involve complex anxiety processes that are nonpathologic, but which can prompt the uninformed provider to overreact, causing iatrogenic relapse. A comprehensive model of arousal and anxiety and their interactions with reward and reinforcement systems offers a valuable clinical approach to the management of patients with both problems.

EPIDEMIOLOGY AND PHENOMENOLOGY

In the adult population, 14.6% have a lifetime history of an anxiety disorder and 16.7% have a lifetime history of an addictive disorder (Regier, Farmer et al., 1990). These prevalence rates are for the general population; the rate in patients presenting to physicians is somewhat higher. Moreover, there is considerable overlap between the two syndromes. In the general population, 23.7% of individuals with a lifetime history of an anxiety disorder also meet the criteria for a substance use disorder (Regier, Farmer et al., 1990). Although individuals with anxiety traits generally have an exaggerated perception of various risks, many apparently do not perceive substance use to be a risky behavior (Hittner, 1997).

The patient with covert substance use disorder may present only with complaints of anxiety. For this reason, physicians should be familiar with these epidemiologic ratios and routinely screen all patients with anxiety symptoms for possible substance use problems. The physician should insist on speaking with any knowledgeable significant other or family member, because such individuals often can provide crucial help by offering objective information about such a patient. On the basis of a positive screen, it is important to review the diagnostic criteria for substance use disorders.

Criteria for anxiety disorders generally include subjective anxiety that is (1) excessive and persistent, (2) accompanied by behavioral avoidance, and (3) interfering with normally expected function.

In making a differential diagnosis, the clinician should not diagnose anxiety disorder when symptoms are better accounted for by another disorder, such as substance intoxication or withdrawal. The onset of anxiety disorder can precede substance use problems (for example, when an individual seeks relief from anxiety through drinking) or may follow initiation of substance abuse (as when an individual uses cocaine and experiences an initial or "herald" panic attack).

Comorbidity. Anxiety symptoms commonly are seen during intoxication and withdrawal from alcohol, but they often improve over weeks to months of abstinence. Such substance-induced anxiety disorders are distinct from an independent anxiety disorder. In one carefully conducted study, an anxiety disorder was diagnosed in 9.4% of alcohol-dependent subjects, but in only 3.7% of control subjects. If the criteria had been expanded to include substance-induced anxiety disorder, 11.8% of alcoholics would have been diagnosed with a major anxiety disorder (Schuckit, Tipp et al., 1997).

Not all anxiety disorders are as prevalent in individuals with substance use disorders, and some even show reduced prevalence. In the previously mentioned study, there was a significant increase in the rate of independent panic disorder in alcoholics as compared with control subjects (4.2% versus 1.0%). There also was a substantially increased risk of social phobia as an independent disorder (3.2% versus 1.4%). However, there was no significant increase in risk of either agoraphobia or obsessive-compulsive disorder in the alcoholic subjects (Schuckit, Tipp et al., 1997).

In the authors' experience, cocaine-dependent patients seem to have a lower prevalence of panic disorder than is found in the general population, presumably because the drug's anxiogenic effects lead those who are susceptible to panic disorder to avoid it.

The order of onset of disorders offers a clue that can help clarify the diagnosis of anxiety versus substance use syndromes (Verheul, Kranzler et al., 2000a). Nearly 80% of alcoholics with independent anxiety disorders experienced onset of anxiety symptoms before the onset of alcohol de-

pendence (suggesting secondary alcoholism) (Schuckit, Tipp et al., 1997).

The increased association of alcoholism with anxiety disorders is apparent in both men and women (Modesto-Lowe & Kranzler, 1999). The specific mechanism of this association is widely debated, ranging from genetic linkage hypotheses to the self-medication hypothesis. To date, no consensus has been achieved. In a multisite study, odds ratios (ORs) of lifetime comorbidity for alcoholism with specific anxiety disorders were relatively consistent across sites, with individuals who were diagnosed with alcohol abuse and/or dependence at two to three times the risk of the aggregated category of anxiety disorder (including simple phobia, social phobia, agoraphobia, and panic disorder) (Swendsen, Merikangas et al., 1998).

Substances other than alcohol also are associated with anxiety disorders. Benzodiazepine dependence should be expected to correlate with anxiety disorders. In a cohort of 153 benzodiazepine-dependent patients, the most prevalent anxiety diagnosis was panic disorder (regardless of agoraphobia) (Martinez-Cano, de Iceta Ibanez de Gauna et al., 1999). In mice and rat studies, cocaine increased escape and other defensive behaviors (Blanchard & Blanchard, 1999). In humans, cocaine induces anxiety, panic, and paranoia during both intoxication and withdrawal. Chronic users of crack cocaine who experience paranoia during drug use show high levels of trait (baseline) anxiety (Rosse, Alim et al., 1995). A possible confound, however, is that concurrent use of benzodiazepines or alcohol can obscure this association (Blanchard & Blanchard, 1999).

Posttraumatic stress disorder (PTSD) is strongly associated with addiction: 30% to 57% of all female study subjects with substance use disorders met the lifetime criteria for PTSD (Najavits, Weiss et al., 1997). Incidence rates also were higher in women who had experienced physical and sexual abuse (Volpicelli, Balaraman et al. 1999). Natural disasters induce stress, and many studies have found increases in subsequent alcohol consumption. However, the relationship is somewhat complex. For example, after Japan's Great Hanshin Earthquake of 1995, alcohol consumption initially decreased. This is analogous to a biphasic phenomenon seen in rats, which avoid alcohol when acutely exposed to stress but increase use later when free from stress (Shimizu, Aso et al., 2000).

Axis II disorders commonly co-occur with anxiety disorders in the population with substance use disorders (Verheul, Kranzler et al., 2000a). In one group of 370 subjects who were using alcohol, cocaine, and/or opioids, 57% met the criteria for at least one personality disorder, with Cluster B disorders the most prevalent (27% antisocial personality and 18.4% borderline), compared with Cluster A (13.2% paranoid) and Cluster C (18.4% avoidant). Persons with both substance use and anxiety disorders had an increased rate of any personality disorder. Of note, avoidant personality disorder (PD) was 4.3 times more likely to co-occur with anxiety disorder. "The strongest specific associations were found for avoidant PD and social phobia (OR 16.0) and schizotypal PD and social phobia (OR 8.7)" (Verheul, Kranzler et al., 2000b, page 114). PD patients showed "higher alcohol and psychiatric severity ratings, poorer global functioning, more previous psychiatric treatments, and higher patient ratings of psychiatric distress and needs for help" (Verheul, Kranzler et al., 2000b, page 116). Thus, even with abstinence and focused therapies for Axis I anxiety disorder, patients with personality dysfunction may require extended treatment.

Subpopulation Differences. Comorbidity can vary among racial groups. Although formal reports are sparse, in one study, white opiate and cocaine addicts reported more symptoms of anxiety disorders than did a group of African American addicts. Whites were more likely to report using drugs in response to psychiatric factors, whereas African Americans were more likely to use drugs secondary to social, cultural, and environmental problems. These results suggest the need for qualitative as well as quantitative differences in treatment plans (Roberts, Emsley et al., 2000).

Gender differences exist in prescription drug abuse, with women 48% more likely than men to use prescription drugs, particularly anxiolytics and narcotic analgesics. Being female increases the chance of anxiolytic use by 51%, after controlling for all other factors, including the difference in disease prevalence (anxiety is two times more prevalent among women) (Simoni-Wastila, 2000).

The relationship between arousal and alcohol use and the pattern of this relationship has been investigated in several studies. For men, alcohol use increases linearly with increasing anxiety, presumably in a task-oriented effort to sustain function. Women show a nonlinear association (Fischer & Goethe, 1998). Whether moderate alcohol use is protective, whether anxiety leads to increased alcohol use, or whether a third factor influences both alcohol use and anxiety is unclear (Rodgers, Korten et al., 2000). It has been hypothesized that some individuals use alcohol to dampen the stress response and some data support this,

suggesting that such "medicinal" use of alcohol may be particularly reinforcing. Teaching alternative coping skills to reduce anxiety thus may be a necessary part of treatment, particularly for women (Sinha, Robinson et al., 1998).

Family and Genetic Studies. Panic disorder in probands predicts increased alcoholism in relatives. Children of substance-abusing probands report the most alcohol use, followed by children of anxiety probands, with children of nonanxious or alcoholic controls using alcohol the least (Merikangas, 1998a). But not all anxiety disorders are the same. Among relatives of alcoholics, approximately 74% with social phobia and alcoholism developed social phobia prior to the onset of alcohol dependence, whereas only 12.5% of relatives developed panic disorder before alcohol dependence. When subthreshold cases of anxiety disorders were examined, a strong association between alcohol dependence and panic disorder was found in both men and women. Subjects with panic were less likely to develop secondary alcoholism; instead, panic attacks may be exacerbated by the physiologic changes resulting from alcohol dependence (Merikangas, 1998b).

Trait neurophysiologic markers such as differential electroencephalogram patterns have shown consistent differences between control and alcoholic probands and family members (Finn & Justus, 1999). During states of alert relaxation, the alpha rhythm (8-13 Hz) is the predominant posterior resting electroencephalogram waveform; however, 5% to 10% of individuals show an absence of alpha rhythmicity, which is an autosomal dominant trait. This trait is three times more common in individuals with anxiety disorder, compared with controls (nonanxious-nonalcoholic). It is 2.5 times more common in alcoholics. Of 11 unrelated alcoholics with anxiety disorders, seven showed this low voltage alpha (LVA) trait, suggesting that the LVA phenotype may be a risk factor for a subtype of comorbid alcoholism and anxiety disorder (Enoch, White et al., 1999).

NEUROBIOLOGY OF ANXIETY AND ADDICTION

Multiple neuropharmacologic processes contribute to the development of both anxiety and substance dependence. Positive reinforcement (one of the four major mechanisms of reinforcement), is critical to the establishment of drug self-administration behavior and drug dependence. Negative reinforcement is important in maintaining drug use, because the individual uses the drug to alleviate withdrawal. The negative affective symptoms that occur on discontinuation of an addictive substance have been hypothesized to be a defining feature of drug dependence. Both processes can have a role in anxiogenesis (Koob, 2000).

A macrostructure in the basal forebrain called the extended amygdala, which contains parts of the nucleus accumbens and amygdala, may play a distinct role in the acute reinforcing effects of drugs of abuse. Neurotransmitters such as dopamine, opioid peptides, serotonin, gamma-aminobutyric acid (GABA), and glutamate appear to be key extracellular messengers in the development of addiction. There are inextricable links among these structures and neurotransmitters, which underlie seemingly disparate phenomena of intoxication and withdrawal, as well as reinforcement and anxiety. Similarly, the constructs of conditioned reinforcement and drug set-point may involve neurochemical changes in the extended amygdala system, which are associated with positive reinforcement as well as the reward dysregulation that occurs during acute withdrawal (Koob, 2000).

Excitatory Neurotransmission (Glutamatergic Systems). The neurotoxic effects of alcohol withdrawal and cocaine intoxication, both of which can trigger anxiety, are related to the glutamatergic system. Alcohol-related memory problems are related to both the glutamatergic and cholinergic systems. The alcohol withdrawal syndrome is characterized by hyperexcitability, including anxiety, fear, muscle rigidity, and—at times—seizures (Brailowsky & Garcia, 1999). The epileptic seizures seen during alcohol withdrawal and the sympathetic arousal and agitation of alcohol withdrawal delirium (DTs) are the result of alcohol's chronic damping of the glutamatergic system, a process that leads to upregulation of both N-methyl-D-aspartate (NMDA) glutamate receptor density and glutamate release; once alcohol is removed, this results in neurotoxic excitation (reviewed in Tsai, Gastfriend et al., 1995). This response occurs frequently in chronic alcoholics and may lead to a "kindling" effect, in which repeated subthreshold arousal ultimately reaches thresholds for seizure discharges. This chronic cycle is highly anxiogenic. Agents that potentiate inhibitory systems, such as benzodiazepines and barbiturates, are effective in treating the symptoms and also are weakly reinforcing of their own abuse (Brailowsky & Garcia, 1999).

Stress is known to promote transcription of proopiomelanocortin (POMC), the precursor of both corticotropin-releasing factor (CRF) and beta-endorphin. CRF and beta-endorphin are functionally linked, with both involved in the "fight or flight" response, which diminishes the intensity of physical and emotional pain. It has been suggested that endorphin activity increases in response to "uncontrollable" trauma but not in response to traumatic events in which the victim has some measure of control (Volpicelli, Balaraman et al., 1999). Like trauma, alcohol also acutely increases both beta-endorphin and CRF-adrenocorticotropic hormone-cortisol release. Since endorphin levels eventually fall after their initial release, drinking may occur as a means of raising endorphin levels (Volpicelli, Balaraman et al., 1999).

Inhibitory Neurotransmission (GABAergic System). GABA is the predominant inhibitory neurotransmitter in the central nervous system. As with benzodiazepines and barbiturates, chronic consumption of alcohol powerfully influences GABAergic neurotransmission. Use of any of these substances initially potentiates GABA, causing a relaxation effect; with repeated administration, however, tolerance occurs, eventually followed by physical and psychological dependence. If use of one of these substances is stopped abruptly, withdrawal symptoms appear. The depressant effects, withdrawal, and physical dependence associated with alcohol use are regulated in part by GABAergic processes (Brailowsky & Garcia, 1999). In a similar fashion, opiate withdrawal after chronic opiate dependence releases excessive concentrations of norepinephrine. This surge is highly anxiogenic, promoting re-administration of opiates in animal studies and, in humans, promoting dependence on inhibitory potentiators, including opiates, benzodiazepines, and alcohol.

DIAGNOSING THE ANXIOUS ADDICTED PATIENT

Symptom Patterns and Syndrome Recognition. Anxiety symptoms may be an entrée to treatment for patients who are covertly dependent on psychoactive substances and who are unconsciously drug-seeking as part of a precontemplative stage of change. Therefore, it is essential to determine whether a patient has anxiety symptoms that should remit spontaneously with effective treatment of the substance use disorder. Certain patterns of requests can induce physicians to prescribe in an enabling fashion. Thus, it is vital for the physician to give careful attention to initiating provider-patient collaboration, to monitoring patient compliance with medications, to target outcome symptoms, and to the medication contract. Such attention facilitates recovery from both disorders, as well as engaging the patient's lasting trust in treatment.

TABLE 1. Data Sources for Distinguishing Comorbid Anxiety Disorder From Substance Use Disorder

Data Source	Type of Data To Obtain	Significance of the Information
Family history	Family history of problems with substance use and anxiety or depression	The disorder that is present in the family history is more likely to be the patient's primary disorder.
Patient's premorbid history (anxiety before onset of substance use or substance use preceding anxiety)	■ Symptom pattern ■ Work function ■ Order of onset of substance use vs. anxiety	Anxiety after a period of substance use suggests secondary anxiety symptoms, which may remit with recovery.
Intercurrent periods (during a phase of continued substance use of three months or more)	Anxiety target symptoms when substance dose and pattern have been constant and without detoxification	Serious anxiety symptoms suggests the possibility of a discrete anxiety disorder despite substance use.
Corroboration by spouse, significant other, or family member (interviewed separately)	■ Substances used ■ Anxiety target symptoms ■ Order of onset of problems ■ Capacity for function	Discrepancies suggest the patient may be in the precontemplation stage; anxiety may not resolve if recovery not established.

The distinction between anxiety secondary to a substance use disorder and a discrete anxiety disorder can be established in a clinical setting by waiting one to two weeks after detoxification before assessing other psychopathology and using the four data sources described in Table 1.

If treatment is to be initiated for anxiety symptoms, it is essential that, at baseline, the patient's target symptoms be recorded in the chart for future reference. Target symptoms are those specific symptoms, reliably reported, that are present in the patient and that fit the diagnostic criteria. For example, the complaint, "I feel bad," is not a target symptom, but "I notice my heartbeat speeds up when my boss enters my office" is a target symptom. After treatment is initiated, the status of target symptoms should be reviewed at regular intervals (and at least monthly) to determine objective progress.

Withdrawal Phase Anxiety. High rates of anxiety found in alcoholics may be inflated because subjects are examined shortly after abstinence is achieved, when anxiety may be related to intoxication or withdrawal. A study of 146 alcohol-dependent patients compared anxiety levels at the time of inpatient admission with levels after three to four weeks of abstinence and found that significant declines in both state and trait scores on the Spielberger State-Trait Anxiety Index occurred over time. Only 10% of the patients met criteria for specific anxiety disorders after three or four weeks of abstinence. Of interest, patients' anxiety levels at admission were not related to withdrawal itself but were related to the severity of alcohol dependence and recent life events. This suggests that, for most patients with alcohol dependence, anxiety symptoms are temporary and are most severe during withdrawal. As noted earlier, women can have more persistent anxiety symptoms than do men. Active treatment of anxiety disorder should be reserved for patients who have symptoms that persist beyond the withdrawal phase. Such patients may be at high risk of relapse to substance use if left untreated (Roberts, 1999).

Recovery Distress. Abstinence represents an interruption of the patient's habitual pattern of self-medication with substances. Recovery is an intrapersonal shift from stagnation to growth of new coping strategies and management of intense emotional reactions to achieve improved function. Both abstinence and recovery involve complex adjustments to new arousal states and incur anxiety processes that are nonpathologic but upsetting to patients. Patients often turn to the provider for relief of these stressful growth experiences. The physician who is uninformed or inexperienced with such dramatic transitions may be prompted to overreact and prescribe, which can indicate to the patient that his or her suffering is deemed pathologic and deserving of rapid relief. This type of prescribing ultimately can make it more difficult for the patient to tolerate the ongoing frustration of adult life and even can lead the patient to iatrogenic relapse.

A comprehensive model of normative arousal and anxiety should be taught by all physicians to newly recovering individuals. Key points include:

- Arousal is ubiquitous for modern adults.

- Anxiety is expected of adults in recovery who are newly encountering societal pressures without the escape afforded by substance use.

- Neither arousal nor anxiety is necessarily pathologic in early recovery.

- Supraphysiologic relief of such normative states offers excessive levels of reward and is unnaturally reinforcing.

- There is healing value in learning to tolerate the conventional miseries of frustration, tension, and heightened alertness; the annoyances of guilt over past mistakes; and the embarrassment of failures.

Being able to instruct newly abstinent patients about such a normative model is essential to the management of patients with addictive and anxiety disorders.

TREATING THE ANXIOUS ADDICTED PATIENT

Individualized treatment is important for alcoholic patients with comorbid anxiety disorders. The first objective should be to establish an alliance and a common goal: abstinence, with stabilization of the comorbid disorder(s). Many psychiatric symptoms subside with abstinence, so it generally is recommended that the physician wait for the patient to achieve at least two to four weeks of abstinence before prescribing psychotropic medications.

Also, the recovery plan must be individualized if it is to be achievable. For instance, some patients whose anxiety symptoms are expressed as panic attacks or social phobia may find it difficult to attend Alcoholics Anonymous meetings (Modesto-Lowe & Kranzler, 1999), but are able to tolerate small, professionally led group therapy sessions.

Patients benefit from an integrated approach that addresses both disorders. The clinician-administered Hamilton Anxiety Scale (HAM-A) may be helpful in measuring the severity and frequency of symptoms. Whenever a comorbid anxiety disorder is diagnosed, the treatment plan should incorporate psychological, social, and biological interventions to target both disorders. Motivational enhancement therapy is a particularly useful initial treatment model in building patients' motivation to initiate change as well as their commitment to longitudinal change (Project MATCH, 1993).

Initiating relapse prevention strategies early in treatment also is important. Various psychotherapies that may be effective include cognitive-behavioral therapy, psychodynamic psychotherapy, interpersonal psychotherapy, and social skills training. Psychosocial interventions include education and support and referral to Twelve Step and other mutual-help support groups. Such groups include the National Alliance for the Mentally Ill (1-800/950-NAMI), the Anxiety Disorders Association of America (301/231-9350), and the National Mental Health Association (1-800/969-NMHA) (Ziedonis & Brady, 1997).

Selection of pharmacologic therapies should be based on efficacy, side effect profile, drug interactions, dosing, and cost. Benzodiazepines are widely prescribed for anxiety and insomnia, and a panel of 73 peer-nominated pharmacotherapy experts judged benzodiazepines to have a lower abuse and dependence potential than meprobamate, barbiturates, and other recognized drugs of abuse, but a higher abuse potential than most substitutes (Uhlenhuth, Balter et al., 1999). Therefore, in treating patients with comorbid substance use and anxiety disorders, physicians always should initiate pharmacotherapy with alternative agents such as antidepressants, buspirone, anticonvulsants, antihypertensive agents, or the newer neuroleptic medications before using a medication with abuse potential (Longo & Johnson, 2000). For such patients, there are only rare cases in which a benzodiazepine is an appropriate maintenance medication. These include the treatment of generalized anxiety disorder (GAD) and management of the acute stage of panic disorder (Romach, Busto et al., 1995). In prescribing benzodiazepines, the burden of proof rests on the prescriber to determine, usually with corroboration, that the patient is (1) abstaining from all substance use, (2) compliant with medications as prescribed, (3) active in recommended recovery efforts, and (4) improving in function.

In one study of benzodiazepine maintenance discontinuation, less than 10% of consenting patients actually completed the taper. In that study, high-dose, chronic treatment with a long half-life benzodiazepine and lower educational level were associated with increased difficulty in discontinuation (Linden, Bar et al., 1998). Once started on benzodiazepines, individuals with personality traits of passivity and dependency and who exhibit avoidant behavior are significantly more prone to report high withdrawal severity and thus to tolerate benzodiazepine taper poorly (Schweizer, Rickels et al., 1998).

When reinforcing agents are prescribed, it is best to administer them on a fixed-dose schedule rather than on an as-needed basis. It is important to recognize patients who exert undue pressure to prescribe sedative-hypnotics and to set appropriate limits (Longo, Parran et al., 2000). The patient's commitment to psychosocial treatment may be weakened by benzodiazepines but not by antidepressant pharmacotherapy, possibly because of interference in emotional processing and the development of coping skills. Patients may need to experience and respond to anxiogenic stimuli to benefit from cognitive-behavioral treatments (Barlow, 1997).

Buspirone (BuSpar®), an azapirone compound, is an alternative to the benzodiazepines for generalized anxiety. It is not a central nervous system depressant and has no abuse liability. Buspirone has been shown to significantly enhance treatment retention in alcohol-dependent adults, as well as to significantly reduce anxiety (Modesto-Lowe & Kranzler, 1999). Case reports suggest the utility of adding buspirone to selective serotonin reuptake inhibitor (SSRI) antidepressants for depressed patients who have comorbid anxiety and type 1 alcohol dependence (Sprenger, 1997). It can take weeks to gain a therapeutic effect (Modesto-Lowe & Kranzler 1999), which will be more apparent to objective observers than to the patient. Therefore, there is a burden of additional instruction on the provider to address patients' expectations for immediate gratification. Based on anecdotal reports, buspirone's long-term safety and ability to potentiate psychosocial therapies can justify the extra time required for patient instruction and careful measurement of effects associated with good outcome.

Tricyclic antidepressants (TCAs; including imipramine [Tofranil®], desipramine [Norpramin®], and others) and monoamine oxidase inhibitors (MAOIs; including phenelzine and others) require care: TCAs can be lethal in overdose, and MAOIs can be contraindicated because of required restrictions on food, medications, and alcoholic beverages. Although not specifically evaluated in this population, SSRIs appear to be the safest choice. Starting doses should be low to avoid jitteriness and irritability. Psychotherapy and pharmacotherapy should be combined (Modesto-Lowe & Kranzler, 1999); in a controlled trial, the combination had lasting benefit over pharmacotherapy alone (Barlow, Gorman et al., 2000).

Adjustment Disorder With Anxiety. Adjustment disorder with anxiety requires a focus on patient education, reassurance, and support. Environmental stressors require active problem solving. Muscle relaxation and other relaxation techniques are helpful for these patients (Ziedonis & Brady, 1997).

Panic Disorder. Patients with anxiety disorder and comorbid substance use can benefit surprisingly well from cognitive-behavioral treatment with exposure to feared stimuli, combined with relaxation and coping skills training (Ziedonis & Brady, 1997). SSRIs are first-line pharmacotherapies because of their favorable side effect profile and safety, and they can independently decrease drinking. Given the latency of onset of SSRIs and TCAs, interim short-term use of a beta blocker can help ameliorate panic symptoms. Benzodiazepines generally are contraindicated because of their abuse potential, but they may be used when panic is severe, primary, and responds poorly to other pharmacologic interventions, particularly initially (in the first two weeks) while awaiting the onset of other non-reinforcing agents (Ziedonis & Brady, 1997). Clonazepam (Klonopin®) is the least provocative benzodiazepine for dependence because of its relatively slow onset and moderate duration of effect. Yet even clonazepam poses a risk of producing, and it has a substantial street value among heroin addicts.

Generalized Anxiety Disorder (GAD). GAD benefits from the same behavioral interventions as panic disorder. It should be treated with buspirone, nefazodone (Serzone®), or an SSRI after the substance abuse is under control (Albrant, 1998). Buspirone effectively treated GAD in several studies, of which at least two found improvement in anxiety symptoms and alcohol consumption. In an open trial, trazodone (Desyrel®) significantly decreased craving for alcohol while also decreasing depressive and anxious symptoms in detoxified alcoholics; thus, it may be a useful adjunct at less than antidepressant doses (Janiri, Hadjichristo et al., 1998).

Social Phobia. Social phobia can interfere with conventional treatment engagement, yet specialized psychotherapeutic interventions are pivotal: these include social skills training, practice in social situations, cognitive-behavioral treatment, and relaxation training (Ziedonis & Brady, 1997). SSRIs have been efficacious in the treatment of social phobia and should be considered first-line agents, whereas benzodiazepines are contraindicated.

Posttraumatic Stress Disorder (PTSD). When comorbid with substance use disorder, PTSD can cause repeated episodes of recovery followed by relapse. Patients can present as withdrawn, alexithymic, and lacking insight, because repression and denial are defenses that are protective during traumatic phases, such as war or persistent sexual abuse. When patients stop using substances and begin to consciously perceive emotions, it is important to anticipate and assist with affect management. Patients often exhibit "dichotomous thinking," focusing on only one problem. Dichotomous thinking also can affect providers, who may either sympathize with patients who have suffered traumatic events (and rationalize substance use) or focus only on their addiction, seeing the patient in a more negative light, downplaying trauma issues, and provoking the patient's ambivalence about treatment. Conventional recovery measures alone may not address such beliefs, so a phased approach that integrates both recovery and cognitive-behavioral PTSD psychotherapy should be used (Zaslav, 1994).

PTSD pharmacotherapy helps patients distance themselves from the traumatic event by reducing symptoms without the use of alcohol or nonprescribed medications. SSRIs may be considered first-line agents, in that they can reduce alcohol consumption and generally are well tolerated (Ziedonis & Brady, 1997). In PTSD patients who abuse alcohol, the opioid blocker naltrexone (ReVia®) can block the alcohol-induced endorphin response and thus decrease alcohol craving (Volpicelli, Balaraman et al., 1999). TCAs and MAOIs improved PTSD symptoms in double-blind placebo-controlled trials. Carbamazepine (Tegretol®), beta blockers, clonidine (Catapres®), benzodiazepines, and lithium have shown benefits in uncontrolled trials (Ziedonis & Brady, 1997).

Matching Patients to Treatment. Setting and modality are important considerations in matching patients to treatment services (Gastfriend & McLellan, 1997). Socially anxious methadone-maintained patients attained greater benefit from a low-intensity psychosocial intervention (weekly coping skills training) than from an intensive day treatment program. The lower intensity treatment resulted in reductions in drug use and other HIV risk behaviors and more weeks of abstinence. However, opiate-dependent patients with low social anxiety tended to benefit more from a more intensive day treatment program (Avants, Margolin et al., 1998).

In a contrasting study, cocaine abusers with social anxiety were treated in an outpatient therapeutic community, which emphasized confrontation of inappropriate behaviors, heavy peer involvement, and limited professional involvement. In this model, the client's ability to share and achieve self-disclose is central to recovery. Those with elevated social anxiety showed better retention and, after three months of treatment, reduced levels of social anxiety. This finding suggests that cocaine-dependent persons with social anxiety can benefit from an intensive group program (Egelko & Galanter, 1998).

CONCLUSIONS

Substance use disorders complicated by anxiety disorders are complex and require psychiatric evaluation, focused behavioral therapies, and careful pharmacotherapy management. Conflicting studies suggest that more research is needed to better define how to match such patients to appropriate treatments. Given the limitations of current knowledge, the best approach would seem to incorporate:

- A comprehensive plan to establish abstinence;

- Active provider instruction in the meaning of arousal and anxiety;

- Observation of the patient's motivation and function;

- Prescribing of non-reinforcing anxiolytics except in rare cases; and

- Close monitoring with corroboration of recovery efforts and function.

This approach requires an activist posture on the part of the treatment team, but often is rewarded with the gratification of restoring patients to health.

ACKNOWLEDGMENT: Preparation of this chapter was supported by grants RO1-DA08781 and K24-DA00427 from the National Institute on Drug Abuse (Dr. Gastfriend).

REFERENCES

Albrant DH & APhA Psychiatric Drug Panel (1998). APhA drug treatment protocols: Management of patients with generalized anxiety disorder. *Journal of the American Pharmaceutical Association* 38(5):543-550.

Avants SK, Margolin A, Kosten TR et al. (1998). When is less treatment better? The role of social anxiety in matching methadone patients to psychosocial treatments. *Journal of Consulting and Clinical Psychology* 66(6):924-931.

Barlow DH (1997). Anxiety disorders, comorbid substance abuse, and benzodiazepine discontinuation: Implications for treatment. *NIDA Research Monograph No. 172*. Rockville, MD: National Institute on Drug Abuse, 33-51.

Barlow DH, Gorman JM, Shear MK et al. (2000). Cognitive-behavioral therapy, imipramine, or their combination for panic disorder: A randomized controlled trial. *Journal of the American Medical Association* 283(19):2529-2536.

Blanchard DC & Blanchard RJ (1999). Cocaine potentiates defensive behaviors related to fear and anxiety. *Neuroscience and Biobehavioral Reviews* 23:981-991.

Brailowsky S & Garcia O (1999). Ethanol, GABA, and epilepsy. *Archives of Medical Research* 30:3-9.

Egelko S & Galanter M (1998). Impact of social anxiety in a "therapeutic community"-oriented cocaine treatment clinic. *American Journal on Addictions* 7(2):136-141.

Enoch MA, White KV, Harris CR et al. (1999). Association of low-voltage alpha EEG with a subtype of alcohol use disorders. *Alcoholism: Clinical & Experimental Research* 23(8):1312-1319.

Finn PR & Justus A (1999). Reduced EEG alpha power in the male and female offspring of alcoholics. *Alcoholism: Clinical & Experimental Research* 23(2):256-262.

Fischer EH & Goethe JW (1998). Anxiety and alcohol abuse in patients in treatment for depression. *American Journal of Drug & Alcohol Abuse* 24(3):453-463.

Gastfriend DR & McLellan AT (1997). Treatment matching: Theoretic basis and practical implications. *Medical Clinics of North America* 81(4):945-966.

Hittner JB (1997). A preliminary analysis of the perceived risks of misusing multiple substances, trait anxiety, and approval motivation. *Journal of Psychology* 131(5):501-511.

Janiri L, Hadjichristos A, Buonanno A et al. (1998). Adjuvant trazodone in the treatment of alcoholism: An open study. *Alcohol and Alcoholism* 33(4):362-365.

Kessler R, McGonagle K, Zhao S et al. (1994). Lifetime and 12-month prevalence of DSM-IIIR psychiatric disorders in the United States: Results from the National Comorbidity Survey. *Archives of General Psychiatry* 51: 8-19.

Koob GF (2000). Neurobiology of addiction. Toward the development of new therapies. *Annals of the New York Academy of Sciences* 909:170-185.

Linden M, Bar T & Geiselmann B (1998). Patient treatment insistence and medication craving in long-term low-dosage benzodiazepine prescriptions. *Psychological Medicine* 28(3):721-729.

Longo LP & Johnson B (2000). Addiction: Part I. Benzodiazepines—Side effects, abuse risk and alternatives. *American Family Physician* 61(7):2121-2128.

Longo LP, Parran T Jr., Johnson B et al. (2000). Addiction: Part II. Identification and management of the drug-seeking patient. *American Family Physician* 61(8):2401-2408.

Martinez-Cano H, de Iceta Ibanez de Gaune M, Vela-Bueno A et al. (1999). DSM-IIIR comorbidity in benzodiazepine dependence. *Addiction* 94(1):97-107.

Merikangas KR, Dierker LC & Szatmari P (1998). Psychopathology among offspring of parents with substance abuse and/or anxiety disorders: A high-risk study. *Journal of Child Psychology and Psychiatry* 39(5):711-720.

Merikangas KR, Stevens DE, Fenton B et al. (1998). Co-morbidity and familial aggregation of alcoholism and anxiety disorders. *Psychological Medicine* 28(4):773-788.

Modesto-Lowe V & Kranzler HR (1999). Diagnosis and treatment of alcohol-dependent patients with comorbid psychiatric disorders. *Alcohol Research & Health* 23(2):144.

Najavits LM, Weiss RD & Shaw SR (1997). The link between substance abuse and posttraumatic stress disorder in women. *American Journal on Addictions* 6:273-283.

Project MATCH (1993). Project MATCH (Matching Alcoholism Treatment to Client Heterogeneity): Rationale and methods for a multisite clinical trial matching patients to alcoholism treatment. *Alcoholism: Clinical & Experimental Research* 17(6):1130-1145.

Regier DA, Farmer ME, Rae DS et al. (1990). Comorbidity of mental disorders with alcohol and other drugs of abuse. *Journal of the American Medical Association* 264:2511-2518.

Roberts A (2000). Psychiatric comorbidity in white and African-American illicit substance abusers: Evidence for differential etiology. *Clinical Psychology Review* 20(5):667-677.

Roberts MC, Emsley RA, Pienaar WP et al. (1999). Anxiety disorders among abstinent alcohol-dependent patients. *Psychiatric Services* 50(10):1359-1361.

Rodgers B, Korten AE, Jorm AF et al. (2000). Non-linear relationships in associations of depression and anxiety with alcohol use. *Psychological Medicine* 30:421-432.

Romach M, Busto U, Somer G et al. (1995). Clinical aspects of chronic use of alprazolam and lorazepam. *American Journal of Psychiatry* 152(8):1161-1167.

Rosse R, Alim TN, Johri SK et al. (1995). Anxiety and pupil reactivity in cocaine-induced paranoia: Preliminary report. *Addiction* 90:981-984.

Schuckit MA, Tipp JE, Bucholz KK et al. (1997). The life-time rates of three major mood disorders and four major anxiety disorders in alcoholics and controls. *Addiction* 92(10):1289-1304.

Schweizer E, Rickels K, De Martinis N et al. (1998). The effect of personality on withdrawal severity and taper outcome in benzodiazepine dependent patients. *Psychological Medicine* 28(3):713-720.

Shimizu S, Aso K, Noda T et al. (2000). Natural disasters and alcohol consumption in a cultural context: The Great Hanshin Earthquake in Japan. *Addiction* 95(4):529-536.

Simoni-Wastila L (2000). The use of abusable prescription drugs: The role of gender. *Journal of Women's Health & Gender-Based Medicine* 9(3):289-296.

Sinha R, Robinson J & O'Malley S (1998). Stress response dampening: Effects of gender and family history of alcoholism and anxiety disorders. *Psychopharmacology* 137:311-320.

Sprenger D (1997). Buspirone augmentation of a selective serotonin reuptake inhibitor: Efficacy in two depressed patients with comorbid anxiety and type I alcohol dependence [letter]. *Journal of Clinical Psychopharmacology* 17(5):425-426.

Swendsen JD, Merikangas KR, Canino GJ et al. (1998). The comorbidity of alcoholism with anxiety and depressive disorders in four geographic communities. *Comprehensive Psychiatry* 39(4):176-184.

Tsai G, Gastfriend DR & Coyle JT (1995). The glutamatatergic basis of human alcoholism. *American Journal of Psychiatry* 152(3):332-340.

Uhlenhuth EH, Balter MB, Ban TA et al. (1999). International study of expert judgment on therapeutic use of benzodiazepines and other psychotherapeutic medications: IV. Therapeutic dose dependence and abuse liability of benzodiazepines in the long-term treatment of anxiety disorders. *Journal of Clinical Psychopharmacology* 19(6S):23S-29S.

Verheul R, Kranzler HR, Poling J et al. (2000a). Axis I and Axis II disorders in alcoholics and drug addicts: Fact or artifact? *Journal of Studies on Alcohol* 101-110.

Verheul R, Kranzler HR, Poling J et al. (2000b). Co-occurrence of Axis I and Axis II disorders in substance abusers. *Acta Psychiatrica Scandinavica* 101:110-118.

Volpicelli J, Balaraman G, Hahn J et al. (1999). The role of uncontrollable trauma in the development of PTSD and alcohol addiction. *Alcohol Research & Health* 23(4):256-262.

Zaslav MR (1994). Psychology of comorbid posttraumatic stress disorder and substance abuse: Lessons from combat veterans. *Journal of Psychoactive Drugs* 26(4):393-400.

Ziedonis D & Brady K (1997). Dual diagnosis in primary care. Detecting and treating both the addiction and mental illness. *Medical Clinics of North America* 81(4):1017-36.

Chapter 4

Co-Occurring Addictive and Psychotic Disorders

Douglas Ziedonis, M.D., M.P.H.
Marc L. Steinberg, M.A.
David Smelson, Psy.D.
Stephen Wyatt, D.O.

Prevalence of Psychotic Disorders
Diagnosing Psychotic Disorders
Interactions Between Drugs of Abuse,
Medications, and Neurobiology
Treating Psychotic Disorders

The presence of substance use and psychotic symptoms poses special diagnostic and treatment challenges. This chapter focuses on the tasks of assessment, diagnosis, acute management, the relationship between various drugs of abuse and psychosis, and long-term and subacute treatment considerations. Clinical recommendations for the management of this persistently ill population are presented.

PREVALENCE OF PSYCHOTIC DISORDERS

Substance abuse and psychosis often co-occur. Transient substance-induced psychotic symptoms are not uncommon among intoxicated substance abusers, and substance use is common among psychiatric patients with schizophrenia. Some data suggest that the use of drugs and/or alcohol can lead to the earlier onset of schizophrenia in an already vulnerable individual (Mueser, Bellack et al., 1992). However, the fundamental relationship between the quantity and frequency of drug use earlier in life and the eventual onset of schizophrenia still is not well understood. Many questions exist about this area of clinical practice: Do psychoactive drugs contribute to the development of schizophrenia? Conversely, is drug use a result of or a response to the psychopathology of schizophrenia? Is there a shared neurobiology that links the development of drug dependence and schizophrenia?

The addition of drugs of abuse often increases and exacerbates psychotic symptoms in psychiatric patients. In this population, ingestion of even relatively small amounts of drug over a short period of time can result in an exacerbation of psychiatric problems, loss of housing, use of emergency department services, or increased vulnerability to exploitation (sexual, physical, or other) within the social environment. Perhaps because of this sensitivity to psychoactive substances, individuals with schizophrenia appear to progress quickly from substance use to dependence, and some researchers suggest that all use in this population should be termed abuse (Drake & Noordsy, 1994). Substance use among psychiatric patients is associated with a worsening of prognosis, increased rates of institutionalization, and reduced socioeconomic status.

Although schizophrenia is the most prevalent psychotic mental disorder, only about 1% to 2% of the population have been diagnosed. However, even at that rate of prevalence, the disorder imposes high costs on society, on the family, and on the patient.

TABLE 1. Psychotic Symptoms

- **Catatonia** is a marked and bizarre motor abnormality that is characterized by immobility. It may involve certain types of excessive activity, mutism, resistance to being moved, assumption of unusual body positions, and echoing the sound last heard or action last seen.

- **Delusion** is a firmly held false belief based on incorrect inference about reality.

- **Disorganized speech** often presents as looseness of association (get off track) or, in the extreme, can be completely incoherent.

- **Grossly disorganized behaviors** range from childlike silliness to unpredictable agitation. Disorganized behaviors include difficulty in performing activities of daily living, poor hygiene, appearing markedly disheveled, unusual dress, inappropriate sexual behavior, and unpredictable and untriggered agitation.

- **Hallucination** is a sensory perception that has the compelling sense of reality but occurs without stimulation of the relevant sensory organ.

- **Negative symptoms** are characterized by severe deficits in functioning and include flat affect (clearly diminished range of emotional expressiveness), alogia (poverty of speech), avolition (reduced ability to initiate and complete goals), and anhedonia (loss of interest or pleasure).

The Epidemiologic Catchment Area (ECA) study found that 47% of persons with schizophrenia have a lifetime experience of substance use disorders, including 34% who have an alcohol use disorder and 28% who have a drug use disorder. Mental health treatment settings report rates of current substance use disorders in the schizophrenic population that range from 25% to 75%. Some data suggest that the amount of drug and alcohol use among individuals with schizophrenia is increasing over time (Soyka, 2000).

In terms of specific drugs of abuse, the ECA study found that alcohol and cocaine were among the most commonly abused drugs among individuals with schizophrenia. In that study, 16% of individuals with schizophrenia abused cocaine, and 16% abused alcohol. It also is interesting to note that somewhere between 70% and 90% of patients with schizophrenia are nicotine dependent and that nicotine is not routinely included in reported rates of substance use, making the actual numbers even higher (Ziedonis & George, 1997; Hughes, Hatsukami et al., 1986). In addition, it has been estimated that persons with a current mental illness smoke more than 44% of all cigarettes smoked in the United States (Lasser, Boyd et al., 2000). Tobacco smoking often alters psychiatric symptoms and blood levels of psychiatric medications, and can improve cognition and stress management. However, these epidemiologic data represent a "best guess" as to the true rate of comorbidity, given the challenges of diagnosing substance abuse in the presence of schizophrenia and the problems of diagnosing schizophrenia in the context of a substance use disorder.

DIAGNOSING PSYCHOTIC DISORDERS

Psychosis is defined as a gross impairment in reality testing that is characterized by severe distortions of perception (as manifested by hallucinations) and severe distortions of thought (as manifested by delusions). It is a nonspecific condition that is associated with a variety of diagnoses and states, including schizophrenia, pervasive developmental disorders, dementias, medical disorders, delirium and toxic states, mood disorders, and substance use disorders.

According to the current edition of the *Diagnostic and Statistical Manual of Mental Disorders* (*DSM-IV*; American Psychiatric Association, 1994), psychotic symptoms include delusions, hallucinations, disorganized speech or behavior, "negative symptoms," and catatonia (Table 1). Hallucinations and delusions are labeled "positive symptoms." Negative symptoms include flat affect, amotivation, poor attention, anhedonia, and asociality. Clinicians must consider the role of general medical condition (Table 2) or substance use in association with both intoxication and withdrawal (Table 3). Psychotic symptoms can occur as the presenting symptom or may be part of a more complex syndrome of cognitive impairment (involving delirium or dementia).

Although schizophrenia is the psychotic disorder that is most frequently diagnosed in psychiatric patients, other subtypes of psychotic disorders also must be considered in the differential diagnosis (Table 4). Psychotic symptoms can occur in the context of other categories of mental disorders, particularly affective disorders. For example, delusions or hallucinations may be a symptom of major depression or the mania phase of bipolar disorder.

The type and duration of psychotic symptoms are important in making a differential diagnosis. Psychotic symptoms that have a sudden onset and that last no more than one month are labeled "brief psychotic disorder." If the symptoms have been present for less than six months, a diagnosis of schizophreniform disorder can be made. If the symptoms last longer than six months and include prominent delusions or hallucinations and result in a deteriorating course, with evidence of impaired social and occupational functioning, a diagnosis of schizophrenia or schizoaffective disorder should be considered. (In making a diagnosis of psychotic disorder, the clinician needs to rule out mood disorder, which can present with psychotic symptoms and which has a different course, prognosis, and treatment.)

In clinical practice, patients are seen with a mix of symptoms that may not fit neatly into a diagnostic category such as schizophrenia or manic depression. Schizoaffective disorder is diagnosed when symptoms of a psychotic disorder and a mood disorder (depression, mania, or mixed states) occur during separate time periods. In contrast to major depression with psychotic features, schizoaffective disorder features a period of psychotic symptoms in the absence of mood disorder symptoms. A delusional disorder is diagnosed only when delusional symptoms are present; often, symptoms are well circumscribed and can interfere with functioning to a lesser degree.

Two common scenarios can be problematic for clinicians in establishing a diagnosis of schizophrenia and/or a substance use disorder. In the first scenario, the clinician is evaluating a new patient who presents with both psychotic symptoms and/or substance abuse. (In many cases, a definitive diagnosis of a psychotic disorder cannot be established, and treatment of the coexisting psychosis and substance abuse must occur simultaneously.) In the second scenario, the clinician is reevaluating a known psychiatric patient with schizophrenia, who presents with symptoms of an undiagnosed substance use disorder. This chapter reviews both scenarios as they relate to the acute treatment of substance-induced psychotic disorder among individuals who otherwise would not have psychotic symptoms and the chronic treatment of the dually diagnosed psychiatric patient.

Acute Presentation. In the acute presentation of psychosis and substance abuse, there can be differences in signs and symptoms because of variations in etiology. This variation may stem from an underlying psychiatric disorder, a medical disorder, or substance abuse.

TABLE 2. Psychosis Secondary to Medical Conditions

- **Neurological conditions**: neoplasms, stroke, epilepsy, auditory nerve injury, deafness, migraine, central nervous system infection

- **Endocrine conditions**: hyperthyroid or hypothyroid, parathyroid, or hypoadrenocorticism

- **Metabolic conditions**: hypoxia, hypercarbia, hypoglycemia

- **Fluid or electrolyte imbalances**

- **Hepatic or renal failure**

- **Autoimmune disorders** with central nervous system involvement (systemic lupus erythematosus)

- **Delirium**

- **Dementia**: Alzheimer's disease, vascular, HIV-related, Parkinson's disease, Huntington's disease, head trauma, and the like

- **Neoplasm**: lung.

Initial Assessment: At the time of the patient's initial presentation, the clinician should have four primary goals: patient safety, staff safety, elicitation of the patient's history, and formulation of initial impressions that will lead to a set of treatment recommendations. Often, the most appropriate setting for the evaluation of an acutely psychotic patient is a hospital emergency department, although some psychiatric triage settings also are appropriate. Staff members in those settings are trained to treat such patients in an effective and safe manner. An addiction medicine specialist may be asked to participate in the patient evaluation.

Patient safety should be addressed by providing a setting in which external stimuli are minimized to ensure the physical safety of the patient and staff members, and to provide a modicum of dignity while the work-up is under way.

Initial assessment of vital signs should be obtained. Variations in pulse rate, blood pressure, and respiratory function are not uncommon in the presentation of many toxic states.

TABLE 3. Substances That Cause Psychotic Symptoms

During Intoxication
- Sedatives (alcohol, benzodiazepines, barbiturates)
- Stimulants (amphetamine, cocaine)
- Designer drugs ("Ecstacy" and the like)
- Marijuana/THC
- Hallucinogens (LSD, ketamine, psilocybin, and the like)
- Opioids
- Phencyclidines.

During Withdrawal
- Sedatives (alcohol, benzodiazepines, barbiturates)
- Anesthetics and analgesics
- Anticholinergic agents
- Anticonvulsants
- Antihistamines
- Antihypertensives
- Antimicrobial medications
- Antiparkinson medications
- Cardiovascular medications
- Chemotherapeutic agents
- Corticosteroids
- Gastrointestinal medications
- Muscle relaxants
- Nonsteroidal anti-inflammatory drugs (NSAIDs)
- Various over-the-counter medications
- Toxins (anticholinesterase, organophosphate insecticides, nerve gases, carbon monoxide, and volatile substances such as fuel or paint).

The patient's mental status should be assessed. Consideration should be given to the need for protection of the airway and possible establishment of intravenous access. Physical restraints can help to ensure the initial safety of both the patient and staff members; however, use of a quiet room with a sense of safety often achieves a significant reduction in the patient's level of anxiety and agitated psychotic symptoms. "Chemical restraints," examples of which include, but are not limited to, benzodiazepines and antipsychotic medications, may be warranted, but should be given only after the primary assessment has taken place, as sedation may be a side effect.

Included in the primary assessment is the gathering of history from anyone with information about the patient before his or her arrival at the hospital. Family, friends, or landlords may be very helpful in reporting the patient's psychiatric, medical, and social history. Emergency personnel or police should be questioned for details of the scene at which they first encountered the patient and their observations of the patient during transport. This information can provide significant insights into the possible involvement of psychoactive substances (as indicated, for example, by a pattern of delirium or a waxing and waning of signs and symptoms).

Initial laboratory information should include a complete blood count, electrolytes, liver enzymes, glucose, blood urea nitrogen, calcium, blood alcohol, and urine analysis with toxicology screen. If the patient lapses into coma, the administration of parenteral thiamine, glucose, magnesium, and naloxone (Narcan®) may be appropriate, even before the laboratory results are available. Computerized tomography (CT) scanning of the acutely psychotic patient's head always should be considered. Head injury, the severity of which is best confirmed by CT, often results in a confused, bizarre thought pattern that could present as psychosis and that may be associated with substance abuse. However, CT scanning is of little help in differentiating between schizophrenia and drug-induced psychosis (Wiesbeck & Taeschner, 1991). If the blood and urine evaluation is not diagnostic and the CT scan is negative, lumbar puncture may be warranted.

Interplay Between Substance Use and Psychosis: Psychotic symptoms associated with various forms and levels of drug use are well documented. The differential diagnosis most often is determined after a period of abstinence, which can vary from hours to months, depending on the drug involved and/or the duration of use. For example, evidence suggests that chronic amphetamine use can result in long-term neurobiologic changes, which may persist even after prolonged abstinence, and which present as a protracted psychosis that is phenomenologically similar to schizophrenia (Sato, 1990; McLellan, Woody et al., 1979). By contrast, a study of cocaine-induced psychosis by Satel and Lieberman (1991) suggested that a psychosis persisting for more than several days is likely to be the product of an underlying psychotic disorder. However, patients who inhale or inject amphetamines at high doses, or who smoke large amounts of marijuana dipped in phencyclidine (PCP) or formaldehyde, may experience psychotic symptoms that can persist for months.

For many reasons, differentiating schizophrenia from a substance-induced psychotic disorder is not an easy task, especially if the physician does not know whether the patient has a history of serious mental illness. Medication side effects can be mistaken for negative symptoms, and negative symptoms can be mistaken for depression. Substance abusers also may be poorly compliant in taking their medications, so that a presenting psychotic relapse may be the result of noncompliance. In one longitudinal diagnostic study of 165 patients with chronic psychosis and cocaine abuse or dependence, a definitive diagnosis could not be established in 93% of the cases (Shaner, Roberts et al., 1996). To establish a definitive diagnosis of schizophrenia, the researchers required that a patient meet diagnostic criteria for schizophrenia at some point after six weeks of abstinence from psychoactive substances. Patients were interviewed at multiple points over time (using the Structured Clinical Interview and *DSM-IIIR* criteria) (First, Spitzer et al., 1995). Using these strict guidelines, the primary reasons a diagnosis could not be reached were insufficient abstinence (78%), poor memory (24%), and/ or inconsistent reporting (20%) on the part of the patient. A review of hospital records and collateral information addressed the problems of poor memory and inconsistent reporting, leaving insufficient abstinence as the primary barrier to establishing a diagnosis. The researchers' finding that most patients continued to use substances reflects the difficulty of treating persons in this population and underscores the need to make clinical decisions within the context of diagnostic uncertainty.

Researchers have begun to study the acute effects of illicit drug use on the symptoms of schizophrenia. Lysaker and colleagues (1994) examined the relationship between positive and negative symptoms among individuals with schizophrenia, with and without a history of cocaine abuse. The individuals with schizophrenia and cocaine dependence had less severe negative symptoms, more paranoia, and an earlier first hospitalization. Working with patients on an inpatient service, Serper and colleagues (1995) examined the comorbidity of the two disorders within 48 hours of the last use of cocaine and after four weeks of abstinence. Indi-

---

TABLE 4.   DSM-IV Classification of Psychotic Disorders

- Brief psychotic disorder
- Schizophrenia
- Schizophreniform disorder
- Schizoaffective disorder
- Delusional disorder
- Psychotic disorder, Not Otherwise Specified.

SOURCE: American Psychiatric Association (APA) (1994). *Diagnostic and Statistical Manual of Mental Disorders, 4th Edition (DSM-IV)*. Washington, DC: American Psychiatric Press.

---

viduals with both schizophrenia and cocaine dependence had fewer negative symptoms and more positive symptoms during acute intoxication, which reversed after four weeks, suggesting that the interaction between dopamine and the psychostimulant properties of cocaine decreased the negative symptoms. Other researchers have commented on the paradox of dually diagnosed patients, who are regarded as both behaviorally more disorganized than other schizophrenics, yet more socially competent (Penk, Flannery et al., 2000). These studies also suggest that individuals with schizophrenia may use cocaine to reduce the uncomfortable negative symptoms that frequently accompany their disorder. This potential effect should be discussed with the patient during the evaluation.

Drug craving among individuals with schizophrenia and drug dependence often leads to continued cocaine use. Carol and colleagues (2000) found more cocaine craving in individuals diagnosed with schizophrenia and cocaine addicts than in addicts without mental illness. In another study, cocaine-dependent schizophrenics had significantly more cue-elicited craving than did cocaine addicts. In fact, 94% of the cocaine-dependent schizophrenics were cue-reactive, compared with 44% of the non-schizophrenic cocaine addicts. This finding suggests that cocaine craving is another important area to assess in the treatment of drug addiction in individuals with psychosis. The Voris Cocaine Craving scale is a simple four-item, 50-point visual analogue scale that has good reliability and validity and which can be administered easily in an office setting (Smelson, McGee-Caulfield et al., 1999). The four-scale items focus on changes in "craving intensity," "happy or depressed mood," "increased or decreased energy," and "physical health/feeling sick."

One of the most important clues to the etiology of the psychosis, of course, is the patient's history. However, the astute clinician also recognizes subtle variations in presentation that help to guide treatment recommendations.

Drug-Specific Psychotic Symptoms. The following discussion focuses on the unique relationship of certain psychoactive substances to the development and acute management of psychotic symptoms.

Alcohol and Psychosis: The most obvious psychotic symptoms associated with alcohol use generally occur in the withdrawal stage (Isbell, Fraser et al., 1955; Mendelson & LaDou, 1964; Gross, Lewis et al., 1975). These symptoms are based in the still-undefined interplay of chronic alcohol dependence with the gamma-aminobutyric acid type A ($GABA_A$), N-methyl-D-aspartic acid (NMDA), and dopamine (DA) receptors (Tabakoff & Hoffman, 1996). Symptoms typically are referred to as "alcoholic hallucinosis"; that is, auditory and visual hallucinations that occur in a clear sensorium, often while the patient is alert and well oriented. The auditory hallucinations most often are of the threatening or command type. In this condition, individuals can be in an extremely agitated and paranoid state as a result of the hallucinations and physical discomfort they are experiencing. The onset of this hallucinogenic state has been reported to occur from 12 hours to 7 days after the onset of abstinence from long-term alcohol use. (However, there have been reports of symptom onset having been delayed by as much as three weeks.) The most typical time for emergence of symptoms is within two days of abstinence (Victor & Hope, 1958; Scott, 1969; Schuckit, 1982).

Psychotic symptoms, particularly paranoia, may persist for hours to weeks. Some evidence suggests that individuals with symptoms that are prolonged for weeks or months may have a predisposition to a psychotic illness (Victor & Hope, 1958). There can be tremendous similarity between this psychotic appearance and schizophrenia.

Paranoia and agitation often are treated with benzodiazepines in the same way one would treat uncomplicated withdrawal. However, in the severely agitated patient with concurrent hallucinations, neuroleptics may be warranted. Withdrawal has been associated with the development of extrapyramidal symptoms, including dystonia, akathisia, choreoathetosis, and Parkinsonism (Carlen, Lee et al., 1981; Lang, 1982; Shen, 1984). Particular attention should be paid to the possible development of extrapyramidal symptoms in the patient treated with a neuroleptic drug during acute alcohol withdrawal or in the patient with a primary psychotic illness.

Cannabis and Psychosis: In the ECA study, reported in 1990, the rate of cannabis dependence or abuse in the general population was estimated at a lifetime prevalence of 4.3%, and the comorbid use of cannabis in individuals with schizophrenia was estimated at 6.0% (Regier, Farmer et al., 1990). The most frequently reported effects of marijuana at levels of moderate intoxication are euphoria (Ames, 1958; Hollister, 1971; Chopra & Smith, 1974), an awareness of alteration in thought processes (Ames, 1958), suspiciousness and paranoid ideation (Keeler, Reifler et al., 1968; Tart, 1970), alteration in the perception of time (Renault, 1974), a sensation of heightened visual perception (Keeler, Ewing et al., 1971) and, at higher doses, some auditory and visual hallucinations (Beaubrun & Knight, 1973; Isbell, 1967; Keeler, Reifler et al., 1968; Waskow, 1970). These effects have been reproduced in the laboratory and appear to be partially dose-dependent. Some evidence suggests that certain users seek the more psychotomimetic effects achieved through chronic high-dose use of marijuana (Ghodse, 1986). At doses greater than 0.2 mg/kg, the potential for development of psychotic-like symptoms increases dramatically (Isbell, 1967). At this level of use, symptoms include suspiciousness, memory impairment, confusion, depersonalization, apprehension, hallucinations, and derealization (Ames, 1958; Talbott & Teague, 1969; Chopra & Smith, 1974; Rottanburg, 1982). The symptoms are reported to be transient, although they can recur on repeated administration of the drug (Chopra & Smith, 1974; Brook 1984; Carney & Lipsedge, 1984).

There is little evidence that chronic use of cannabis leads to a primary psychotic disorder (Chopra & Smith, 1974). First-time use, large amounts, and route of ingestion (oral more than smoked) may be factors in the higher incidence of cannabis psychosis (Tennant & Groesbeck, 1972; Chaudry, 1991). A study that compared psychotic features in a group of men with psychotic symptoms and high urinary levels of cannabis with such features in psychotic individuals without positive cannabis urine samples showed more hypomania, more agitation, less coherent speech, less flattening of affect, and fewer auditory hallucinations in the cannabis group (Rottanburg, 1982; Thacore & Shukla, 1976). Cannabis use often is associated with a more affective type of psychosis (Carney & Lipsedge, 1984).

Typically, the psychosis associated with cannabis is acute and of short duration. However, there are case reports of chronic psychosis attributed to cannabis (Gersten, 1980). This is a difficult question to answer for a variety of reasons: Is the patient remaining abstinent? What other drugs might the patient have used? Is there predisposing psychopathology? Frequently, the evaluating clinician must decide whether chronic schizophrenia is secondary to the past use of cannabis. Often this is an issue for both the patient and his or her family. One retrospective study presented evidence showing better premorbid personalities and reduced age of onset in cannabis-using individuals than in the non-using schizophrenic population (Breakey, Goodell et al., 1974). Such differences, however, may be secondary to cannabis opening the "environmental window" in an already predisposed patient.

Cocaine and Psychosis: Transient paranoia is a common feature of chronic cocaine intoxication (Manschreck, Laughery et al., 1988; Satel, Southwick et al., 1991), appearing in 33% to 50% of patients. Psychotic symptoms associated with cocaine use are almost exclusively seen in the intoxication phase and rarely extend beyond the "crash" phase in the patient who does not have a primary psychotic illness. There is epidemiologic evidence that men have a greater propensity toward psychosis than women and that whites are affected more frequently than non-whites (Brady, Lydiard et al., 1991). There are multiple indicators that high-dose use of cocaine over time is strongly associated with the onset of psychotic symptoms (Brady, Lydiard et al., 1991; Satel, Lieberman et al., 1991). There also is strong evidence that sensitization occurs with chronic administration of cocaine and amphetamines (Ellinwood, Sudilovsky et al., 1973). This sensitization is associated with the type of psychotic symptoms that can occur with repeated use of the stimulants. The psychotic features appear to occur with repeated exposure at lower doses. Onset of psychotic symptoms has been associated with reduction in individual doses and the desire for treatment (Brady, Lydiard et al., 1991).

The most frequently reported psychotic symptoms related to cocaine use are paranoid delusions and hallucinations. Auditory hallucinations are the most common and often are associated with paranoid delusions. Visual hallucinations are the next most common, followed by tactile hallucinations (Brady, Lydiard et al., 1991). Visual hallucinations have been associated with chronic mydriatic pupils and the appearance of geometric shapes. Nearly all of the hallucinations are associated with drug use. Evidence suggests that the character of the psychotic symptoms experienced is associated with the setting in which drugs are ingested (Sherer, 1988).

Stereotypic behavior also can be associated with psychosis. Such behavior occasionally continues after the intoxication subsides. A study of the phenomenology of hallucinations points to an orderly progression in the development of hallucinations, from early visual hallucinations to the tactile forms (Siegel, 1978). The study comports with the observation that there is an orderly progression of the effects of cocaine intoxication, from euphoria to dysphoria and finally to psychosis, and that this progression is related to dose, chronicity, and genetic and experiential predisposition (Post, 1975).

It is very difficult to assess the premorbid evidence of psychotic thinking in individuals who go on to use large repeat doses of cocaine and to forecast the likelihood that they will develop psychotic symptoms. Satel and Edell (1991) did measure the level of nondrug-psychotic proneness in individuals who had a history of cocaine-induced psychosis, as compared with individuals without such a history. They found strong evidence that there is a greater incidence of low-level psychotic thinking in the abstinent patient who is prone to cocaine-induced psychosis. Whether this is evidence of proneness to the development of psychosis in some individuals as a function of their use of cocaine or an indication of the development of persistent neurobiologic changes concurrent with the onset of cocaine-induced psychosis remains unclear. McLellan and colleagues (1979) examined this question by performing a six-year followup study on drug-dependent individuals who had no initial psychotic symptoms. They found a strong association with psychosis in the amphetamine-dependent population. The nature of the association was unclear, but the investigators speculated that there may be some self-selection of stimulant drugs in this population, or some low-level psychotic thinking that was not identified in the original evaluation.

Amphetamines and Psychosis: The first report of psychosis associated with amphetamines was made by Young and Scoville, who in 1938 reported psychotic behavior in a patient who was under treatment for narcolepsy. Since that time, there have been many observations and studies of this association. Rockwell and Ostwald reviewed psychiatric hospital records in 1968 and found that the most common diagnosis of patients admitted with covert amphetamine use was schizophrenia.

Amphetamine psychosis has been described as a three-stage illness. Initially it is marked by increased curiosity and repetitive examining, searching, and sorting behaviors. In the second stage, these behaviors are followed by increased paranoia. In the final stage, the paranoia leads to ideas of reference, persecutory delusions, and hallucinations, which are marked by a fearful, panic-stricken, agitated, over-active state (Ellinwood, Sudilovsky et al., 1973). That the appearance of psychotic-like symptoms in amphetamine users became more prevalent in the late 1960s and 1970s fits what we now know about the pattern of use associated with these symptoms. Amphetamine-induced psychosis develops over time in association with large amounts of the drug, delivered by any route of administration. The strongest correlation has been seen in those individuals who use large amounts by intravenous injection.

A common presentation of the psychotic, amphetamine-intoxicated patient involves paranoia, delusional thinking, and (frequently) hypersexuality. The hallucinatory symptoms may include visual, auditory, olfactory, and/or tactile sensations. However, the patient's orientation and memory usually remain intact. Typically, this altered mental state lasts only during the period of intoxication, although there are reports of it persisting for days to weeks.

Treatment should be initiated by providing a safe, secure place for the patient and should reduce external environmental stimuli. Physical restraints should be avoided or used in a time-limited fashion so as not to complicate the presentation with worsening hyperthermia, dehydration rhabdomyolysis, and possible renal failure. One should keep in mind the potential of amphetamines for lowering seizure threshold, inducing hyperpyrexia, and stimulating cardiovascular compromise, particularly in the patient who is using large amounts in a chronic pattern. In such patients, chlorpromazine (Thorazine®) should be avoided because of its potential to lower seizure threshold and worsen hyperthermia. Benzodiazepines can be helpful in the treatment of these symptoms. A common initial dose is diazepam (Valium®) 10 mg, either intramuscularly or intravenously, then titrated to a level that sufficiently sedates the patient. Patients should be closely monitored for respiratory depression. When using benzodiazepines intramuscularly, the clinician should wait at least one hour between doses to avoid inadvertent overdose. It is quite common to see dramatic tolerance to benzodiazepine medications in long-term drug users, so a very high dose may be needed to achieve sedation.

The question of how long the psychosis will last and how likely the patient is to develop a long-term psychotic illness as a result of amphetamine use is not clear. Clinical experience suggests that amphetamine psychosis can last for three to six months in extreme cases of high-dose use. There is little evidence to suggest that these drugs cause schizophrenia. However, there is a potential for long-term affective instability, a moderate-to-severe anxiety state, and underlying suspiciousness.

Hallucinogens and Psychosis: Hallucinogens have a well-documented role, both ceremonial and recreational, in many societies. However, not until the synthesis of lysergic acid diethylamine (LSD) by Hofman in 1943 was a hallucinogen available in large quantities and adopted widely as a recreational drug. A national survey in the U.S. in 1990 yielded an estimate that 7.6% of the population older than 12 years had ever used a hallucinogen. This number rose to 8.6% in 1993. The percentage of patients admitted to psychiatric hospitals with a diagnosis of "schizophrenia and paranoid disorders" at first admission was 10.9% in 1970, but rose to 24% by 1979 and has remained around 20% since that time. The increase is specific to the population aged 15 to 34 years and correlates with the increased use of hallucinogens in this age group. This finding provides evidence pointing to hallucinogens as a factor in the development of schizophreniform psychosis.

The primary model for hallucinogens is LSD, an indole-type drug with structural similarities to serotonin. Included in this class of drugs are dimethyltryptamine (DMT), psilocybin, and psilocin, among others. LSD crosses the blood-brain barrier readily and has a potent affinity for the 5-HT2A receptor. Its half-life is approximately 100 minutes, and the effects wear off in approximately 6 to 12 hours. Initially, there are autonomic changes, which are associated with the early affective instability seen after administration, as in laughter and/or fearfulness. The associated alterations in perception occur subsequently and feature hallucinations of all kinds. The most common hallucinations are visual; the least common, auditory. The occurrence of synesthesia—the blending of the senses—is uncommon but not unknown. There often is a loss of the concept of time. Paranoia and aggression can be profound, but the more frequent experience is that of euphoria and security. The setting can have an effect on the experience, and much has been written on proper preparation for the "trip."

LSD has a large therapeutic index. Thus, the typical emergency visit secondary to use of the drug occurs as a result of anxiety, a concurrent accident, or suicidal behavior. "Talking down" the patient is the most common way to ease his or her anxiety around the psychotic features of LSD and related drugs. The persistently agitated patient may be treated pharmacologically with a benzodiazepine. Neuroleptics have been widely and effectively used to lessen the psychotic-like experience; however, there is a report in the literature of an intensification of the experience following administration of those drugs. If neuroleptics are used, haloperidol (Haldol®) 1 to 5 mg, or an equivalent dose of high-potency antipsychotic medication, may be appropriate.

No clear evidence exists that LSD causes a prolonged psychotic-like illness. Attempts at longitudinal studies have yielded insufficient evidence to support this hypothesis. One difficulty in resolving this question is the high rate of adulterants in the formulation of the drugs and the inability to clearly rule out any preexisting psychopathology. The incidence of the development of schizophrenia after intoxication is not outside parameters one would expect to see in a youthful population. There is evidence that the occurrence of problems after intoxication is greater in those with a preexisting psychiatric illness. The psychiatric diagnosis most commonly associated with post-LSD psychosis is a form of schizoaffective disorder. The appearance of some affective instability—involving a feeling of an altered state of consciousness—and recurrent perceptual disorder, primarily visual, are the most common symptoms seen in patients with associated chronic psychosis. The schizophrenic drug user has been shown to have an earlier age of onset and better premorbid social functioning than the nondrug-using schizophrenic (Bowers, 1972; Breakey, Goodell et al., 1974).

Phencyclidine, Ketamine, and Psychosis: The cyclohexylamine anesthetics phencyclidine hydrochloride (PCP) and ketamine hydrochloride have similar properties. Both result in psychotic-like experiences during intoxication. Evidence suggests that, in the case of PCP, the psychotic-like state can last for prolonged periods beyond the period of intoxication. Soon after PCP was developed in 1957, it was found to be useful in veterinary practice as an anesthetic (Domino, 1978). This finding led to human experimentation and the recognition that administration of the drugs produces a dissociative state. Patients' eyes remain open and scanning during surgery, yet they appear to be "disconnected" from their environments and unable to feel pain (Johnstone, Evans et al., 1959; Greifenstein, DeVault et al., 1958). More alarming are reports of bizarre hallucinations and behaviors during the postoperative period (Greifenstein, DeVault et al., 1958). Consequently, PCP never has been released for human use.

Ketamine, at a potency 10 to 50 times lower than PCP, has been shown to produce far fewer of these psychotic-like episodes and was released for use as an anesthetic. Interestingly, children do not appear to develop the associated psychotic-like symptoms.

The history of abuse of these drugs began in the mid-1960s. Street use of PCP increased when prospective users learned that smoking the drug, rather than ingesting it, resulted in fewer unpleasant side effects. It was then that PCP started to be smoked in combination with cannabis (Liden, Lovejoy et al., 1975). The incidence of PCP use increased significantly by 1976, when a survey by the National Institute on Drug Abuse found that 13.9% of 18- to 25-year-olds had experience with the drug (Lerner & Burns, 1978). At the same time, there was an increase in the number of emergency department visits associated with PCP use. Reports included numerous deaths from toxicity, homicide, suicide, and accidents. A retrospective review of 80 PCP-related deaths showed a strong association with prior affective disorders, aggressive behavior, prior arrests, and a personal crisis in the three months preceding death.

PCP's popularity is attributed to the fact that it can be produced inexpensively and thus frequently is added to the formulation of a variety of drugs sold on the street. A 1975 survey showed that PCP was sold 91% of the time as some other substance—most often, mescaline, LSD, or THC (Lundberg, Gupta et al., 1976). Since that time, the drug seems to have increased in popularity, as suggested by the fact that it more often is sold as PCP, although it still is found as an adulterant in other street drugs.

PCP and ketamine can be smoked, ingested, snorted, or injected intravenously. The drugs are rapidly absorbed and excreted in the urine. The intoxicating effects last for approximately 4 to 6 hours. The recovery period is highly variable.

The behavioral effects of these drugs appear to be mediated by their effect on excitatory amino acids NMDA subtype of glutamate receptor. The high-affinity binding of

PCP and ketamine to the NMDA receptor blocks ion exchange, resulting in noncompetitive antagonism of the NMDA receptor (Cotman & Monaghan, 1987).

Early observations of patients treated with PCP noted the similarities to dissociative and schizophrenic disorders (Davies & Beech, 1960; Cohen, Rosenbaum et al., 1962). The clinical appearance is that of altered sensory perception, bizarre and impoverished thought and speech, impaired attention, disrupted memory, and disrupted thought processes in healthy individuals. There also may be protracted psychosis (Fauman, Aldinger et al., 1976).

There is considerable symptom variation, depending on dose. At lower doses (20 to 30 ng/mL), one is likely to observe sedation, mood elevation, irritability, impaired attention and memory mutism, hyperactivity, and stereotypy. As serum levels rise to 30 to 100 ng/mL, mood changes, psychosis, analgesia, paresthesia, and ataxia can occur. These levels are associated with profound paranoia, aggression, and violent behavior. Higher levels (more than 100 ng/mL) can cause stupor, hyperreflexia, hypertension, seizure, coma, and/or death.

Treatment of the acutely disturbing effects of PCP-like drugs is with benzodiazepines in doses equivalent to diazepam 10 mg and greater, titrated until the patient is satisfactorily sedated. The patient's respiratory status should be continually monitored. There may be a dramatic reduction in aggressive behavior and a significant improvement in the psychotic symptoms. Neuroleptics also can be considered for treatment of the psychotic symptoms. Most typically, a high-potency neuroleptic like haloperidol (1 to 5 mg) is used because of the decreased anticholinergic properties of these drugs. In cases of overdose, the urine may be acidified with ammonium chloride to facilitate urinary excretion. However, metabolic acidosis can result in other problems, including worsening of rhabdomyolysis, and should be considered only in the most extreme cases.

MDMA ("Ecstasy") and Psychosis: 3,4-methylenedioxymethamphetamine (also known as MDMA or "Ecstasy") is a representative of a new class of compounds that became popular in the 1980s. A derivative of methamphetamine, MDMA has a mixed spectrum of effects, which are both amphetamine-like and hallucinogenic. MDMA increases the release and inhibits the reuptake of serotonin, dopamine, and norepinephrine from presynaptic neurons, as well as decreasing their degradation by inhibiting monoamine oxidase (Battaglia & DeSouza, 1989).

Users report enhanced empathy, feelings of closeness to others, euphoria, mood elevation, increased self-esteem, and altered visual perceptions. Hallucinations associated with use generally are mild. Deaths have occurred in cases that presented as a syndrome featuring severe hyperthermia, altered mental status, autonomic dysfunction, and dystonia (Mueller & Korey, 1998). The mechanism is unclear, but, as with a serotonin syndrome, it may be that MDMA can have a direct effect on the thermoregulatory mechanisms that are potentiated by the context of the drug use. For example, MDMA often is used in the setting of dance parties where there is sustained physical activity, high temperatures, and inadequate fluid intake or dehydration.

Concern about the long-term neurotoxicity of MDMA is growing. Long-term users can suffer serotonin neural injury associated with psychiatric presentation of panic attacks, anxiety, depression, flashbacks, psychosis, and memory disturbances (Graeme, 2000). Cases of paranoid psychosis indistinguishable from schizophrenia have been associated with chronic use (Cash, 1994). Although older schizophrenic patients may be less likely to use MDMA, use of it and other designer drugs must be considered and ruled out in patients with new onset of psychotic disorders.

INTERACTIONS BETWEEN DRUGS OF ABUSE, MEDICATIONS, AND NEUROBIOLOGY

The literature suggests four primary findings on the interaction between psychotic disorders, substances, and medications. First, both schizophrenia and addiction seem to feature a primary neurobiologic defect in the mesolimbic system (ventral tegmentum, nucleus accumbens, and prefrontal cortex). Second, co-occurring substance use and psychotic disorders generally are associated with a more severe clinical profile, including indices of impairment, symptoms observed, and cognitive impairment. Third, some substances can affect the metabolism of psychiatric medications and reduce their therapeutic effects. Fourth, positive effects have been reported by some patients, and substances may be used more often by patients who have better prognoses and the social skills required to obtain the substances.

From a biologic perspective, the mesolimbic dopamine pathway appears to play an important role in reinforcement, pleasure, and reward. In the simplest sense, increased dopamine release results in increased pleasure and reward. But one must bear in mind that multiple pathways influence dopamine release, including the opioid system. The reward pathway has been identified as the dopamine pathway that includes the ventral tegmentum area, the nucleus accumbens, and the prefrontal cortex. The ventral tegmental area is linked to the prefrontal cortex, which some research has hypothesized may be hypoactive in schizophrenia (Glassman, 1993). Therefore, chemical substances may be particularly reinforcing in schizophrenics because they stimulate both the subcortical brain reward mechanisms and the prefrontal cortex.

In addition, substances can interact with psychiatric medications used to treat the symptoms of schizophrenia. The interactions are both pharmacokinetic and pharmacodynamic. Most of the substances of abuse interact with psychiatric medications by reducing their effectiveness, but some can alter blood levels of medications and increase side effects.

Coffee and tea are known to interfere with the absorption and metabolism of psychiatric medications. The metabolism of caffeine occurs through the same liver enzyme affected by cigarette use (cytochrome P450 1A2 isoenzyme). Cigarette smoking modifies the metabolism of psychiatric medication, including its potential side effects and effectiveness. The "tar" (polynuclear aromatic hydrocarbons) in cigarettes is the cause, not the nicotine (Jarvik & Schneider, 1992). Smoking is known to decrease blood levels of haloperidol, fluphenazine and thiothixene, olanzapine, and clozapine (Ereshefsky, Saklad et al., 1991; Ereshefsky, 1996; Hughes, 1993; McEvoy, Freudenreich et al., 1995a; George, Sernyak et al., 1995). Abstinence from smoking increases blood levels of neuroleptic medications. Smokers usually are prescribed about double the dose of traditional neuroleptic medications that are given to nonsmokers (Ziedonis, Kosten et al., 1994b). Conversely, there is at least one report of clozapine toxicity and seizure in the context of a quit attempt, presumably related to a sudden increase in serum levels of the drug (Skogh, Bengtsson et al., 1999). The effect on metabolism is important in making treatment decisions regarding hospitalized patients whose smoking habits are curbed, as well as the patient who is attempting to quit smoking.

Substance abuse has been associated with earlier and more severe cases of tardive dyskinesia (Dixon, Haas et al., 1991; Olivera, Kiefer et al., 1990; Zaretsky, Rector et al., 1993; Binder, Kazamatsuri et al., 1987). However, other studies concluded that substance abuse had no effect on movement disorders when important covariates were considered (Ziedonis, Kosten et al., 1994a; Hughes, 1993; Goff, Henderson et al., 1992).

Despite all the negative consequences associated with substance abuse, some individuals with schizophrenia report that using substances helps them cope with symptoms of their schizophrenia (Mueser, Nishith et al., 1995). They report using substances for pleasure; to alleviate boredom; to relieve feelings of anxiety, sadness, or distress; and to share the excitement of "getting high" with friends who also are using. In one study, the most common reason reported for using substances was "something to do with friends" (Test, Wallisch et al., 1989).

Some individuals report that substance use reduces their social inhibitions. The self-medication theory suggests that individuals use chemicals to self-medicate the symptoms of schizophrenia; however, the research data supporting this clinical perception are mixed (Brunette, Mueser et al., 1997). Another self-medication theory suggests that individuals with schizophrenia use substances to help ameliorate the distressing side effects of the medications used to treat their schizophrenia. The term "neuroleptic dysphoria" is used to describe the unpleasant feelings elicited by treatment with conventional antipsychotic medications, including irritability, fatigue, listlessness, and lack of interest or ambition. Although the syndrome often goes unrecognized, rates of neuroleptic dysphoria have been reported as ranging from 5% to 40% (Weiden, Mann et al., 1989). One retrospective study reported that patients with a history of neuroleptic dysphoria were four times more likely to develop substance abuse than those without a history of neuroleptic dysphoria (Voruganti, Heslegrave et al., 1997). Interestingly, many patients hospitalized for psychosis were smoking even before their first hospitalization or initiation of their first antipsychotic medication (McEvoy & Brown, 1999), suggesting a complex relationship between symptoms, medications, and substance use.

Some studies suggest that individuals with schizophrenia may smoke to help improve their attention and concentration (Lavin, Siris et al., 1996). One research group has found that smoking can transiently normalize deficits in auditory physiology (P50 gating) and that this gating abnormality, which is found in individuals with schizophrenia, may be caused by a genetic defect in the nicotinic cholinergic receptors in some individuals (Freedman, Hall et al., 1995; Lavin, Siris et al., 1996; Adler, Hoffer et al., 1993). Despite the self-medicating experience of some smokers with schizophrenia, tobacco use is associated with more positive symptoms of schizophrenia (Ziedonis, Kosten et al., 1994a; Goff, Henderson et al., 1992) and more hospitalizations

(Kelly & McCready, 1999; Goff, Henderson et al., 1992). Of course, the cross-sectional designs used in these studies do not allow for a causal hypothesis to be tested.

TREATING PSYCHOTIC DISORDERS

Medication Management. Antipsychotic medications are an important component of the treatment of schizophrenia. They are instrumental in reducing the long-term positive symptoms of the illness. The new atypical antipsychotics appear to reduce the negative symptoms of schizophrenia and also can help patients who are in the initial stage of abstinence from substances by reducing the severity of detoxification and early protracted abstinence symptoms. The prototype is clozapine, but others currently available include risperidone (Risperdal®), olanzapine (Zyprexa®), quetiapine (Seroquel®), and zisprasidone. Despite the advantages of these atypical agents, clinicians should have realistic expectations. Medications are not miraculous cure-alls, and this is especially true of medications for a psychiatric illness such as schizophrenia, which is marked by complex symptoms and—more often than not—extreme social consequences. Thus, medications should be complemented by psychosocial therapy that engages clients, offers them practical training in interpersonal communication and crisis management, and develops their rehabilitation and recovery skills.

The first step in medication management is to consider the best approach to treating the patient's schizophrenia or chronic psychosis. This should be followed by consideration of the potential interactions between the substances abused and the possible medication choices. In general, clinicians should avoid prescribing medications that cause sedation when treating patients who abuse sedating substances. In addition, clinicians generally should avoid prescribing medications with abuse liability.

Initially, patients presenting to an emergency department or inpatient unit may require both detoxification from substances and the reinitiation/initiation of an antipsychotic medication. The treatment goals of detoxification are to reduce the symptoms of withdrawal and prevent serious withdrawal complications, such as the development of seizures, *delirium tremens*, or psychosis. New patients who remain a diagnostic dilemma might first be detoxified and further assessed before antipsychotic medications are initiated. Individuals known to have schizophrenia usually require the simultaneous administration of both antipsychotic and detoxification medications.

Patients who present with active substance abuse, psychotic symptoms, and noncompliance can be difficult to manage as outpatients. Improving medication compliance in an outpatient setting can be enhanced by reducing positive and negative symptoms, providing psychoeducation and social skills training in medication management, using motivational enhancement techniques to improve compliance, and switching the route of administration of the medication from oral dosing to a long-acting injected medication, if patients are unable or refuse to take oral medications.

The use of cocaine results in a rapid increase in dopamine neurotransmission, which can persist for several weeks after last use. This situation has led researchers to examine dopamine antagonists in the treatment of cocaine addiction. This class of medications is designed to reduce dopamine reuptake, thus decreasing the amount of excess dopamine available during the period of protracted withdrawal. In one of the first dopamine antagonist trials, fluphenthixole was examined in the treatment of cocaine craving in nonschizophrenic cocaine-dependent patients (Gawin, Allen et al., 1989). Patients treated with fluphenthixole experienced a significant reduction in craving and relapses, as compared with patients who received a placebo. More recently, Levin and colleagues (1998) examined fluphenthixole decanoate in the treatment of cocaine-dependent schizophrenics and found that it improved positive and negative symptom scores, reduced cocaine positive urine samples, and increased treatment adherence. Berger and colleagues (1996) compared the effectiveness of the neuroleptic drug haloperidol to a placebo for reducing laboratory-induced craving after exposure to drug cues. They found that haloperidol was significantly more effective than placebo in reducing the laboratory-induced craving response. However, Kosten (1997) did a well-controlled study with rats to examine haloperidol compared with placebo for reducing place preference for cocaine and suggested that the haloperidol actually increased cocaine craving. This study has strong implications for cocaine-dependent schizophrenic patients, many of whom are given neuroleptics to treat the symptoms of schizophrenia, if the typical neuroleptic medication actually can increase drug craving and facilitate continued cocaine use.

Atypical Antipsychotics: Over the past 12 years, new atypical antipsychotic medications have been approved by the U.S. Food and Drug Administration (FDA) for the treatment of schizophrenia. Some of these drugs also have been studied for the treatment of cocaine-dependent patients (with and without coexisting schizophrenia). This class of medication has the added benefit of decreasing extrapyramidal side effects, reducing negative symptoms, and improving cognition. In addition to acting on the dopamine system, these drugs also bind to the serotonin system, which is thought to play an important role in maintaining cocaine addiction via craving (Buydens-Branchey, Branchey et al., 1997). These findings led researchers to begin examining the mixed dopamine and serotonin antagonist risperidone (Risperdal®) in the treatment of cocaine-dependent patients. An open-label, two-week trial with risperidone attempted to reduce cue-elicited craving in recently withdrawn cocaine-dependent patients (Smelson, Roy et al., 1997). The individual administering the cue-exposure procedure remained blind to the study medication. Results suggested that risperidone significantly reduced cue-elicited craving. In a more recent trial, the electroretinogram, a peripheral measure of dopamine, was used to substantiate treatment effects of risperidone in recently withdrawn cocaine-dependent patients. The results suggested that risperidone significantly reduced self-reported craving and that the reduction in craving correlated with electroretinogram amplitude. Similar studies with clozapine (Buckley, 1998; Drake, Xie et al., 2000) and olanzapine (Smelson, Kaune et al., 1999) suggest that these drugs show some efficacy in reducing craving and in preventing relapses to substance abuse among patients with co-occurring cocaine dependence and schizophrenia.

Farren and colleagues (2000) recently examined the acute effects of cocaine administration in a sample of eight cocaine addicts who also received clozapine or a placebo. The results suggested that the clozapine had a diminishing effect on the subjective response to cocaine, including the expected high.

Once clinicians have chosen a treatment option that stabilizes the schizophrenia, they can consider the use of additional medication, as necessary, to manage comorbid depression, comorbid substance abuse, or another psychiatric problem. For substance use, medications are chosen for specific purposes, including detoxification, relief of protracted abstinence withdrawal, and agonist maintenance. Some adjunctive medications (such as antidepressants) also can address the schizophrenia, helping to reduce and stabilize its negative symptoms. Despite the lack of pharmacotherapy trials among populations with a substance abuse problem and schizophrenia, a growing number of clinicians have reported the benefits of these medications.

For the treatment of alcohol use disorders, the FDA has approved the use of two adjunctive medications: disulfiram (Antabuse®) and naltrexone (ReVia®). The clinical record of disulfiram is mixed, and it has yet to be tested in randomized control trials. The possibility of an alcohol-disulfiram reaction requires that it be given only to patients who comprehend the risks of disulfiram and are capable of not drinking in light of those risks. According to some clinicians, administration of disulfiram at high doses (1,000 mg) has produced psychotic symptoms in patients not diagnosed with psychotic disorders.

Clinical studies of naltrexone in this population have not been reported; however, clinical experience suggests that it can help reduce alcohol cravings. Naltrexone is a relatively safe medication that can be used with patients who are at risk of relapse to alcohol; there is no alcohol-naltrexone reaction. Naltrexone's most common side effects include headache and nausea. Naltrexone can precipitate opiate withdrawal, so clinicians should carefully assess patients' use of prescription or illicit opiates and be prepared to manage opiate withdrawal symptoms. Liver function tests should be monitored when using either disulfiram or naltrexone.

For cocaine addiction among dually diagnosed patients, clinicians have tried a variety of augmentation medications, including desipramine (Norpramin®), selegiline (Eldepryl®), mazindol, and amantadine (Symmetrel®), all of which aim to produce an increased dopaminergic effect that will reverse or compensate for the neurophysiologic changes stemming from the chronic use of cocaine. Two double-blind placebo-controlled trials found that desipramine was more effective than placebo in reducing cocaine use among individuals with schizophrenia during the third month of abstinence (Wilkins, 1997; Ziedonis & Trudeau, 1997).

In contrast to both alcohol and cocaine addiction, nicotine dependence traditionally has received less clinical attention and often has gone untreated. This is despite the fact that nicotine is the single substance that is most commonly abused by schizophrenics. The development of treatment guidelines can correct this oversight and lead to the inclusion of tobacco dependence as a component in clinical treatment plans (APA, 1996; Fiore, Bailey et al., 2000; Office on Smoking and Health, 2000). In addition to multicomponent behavioral therapy, treatment for nicotine cessation can include adjunctive medications such as nicotine replacements (transdermal patch, gum, spray, or inhaler) or bupropion (Zyban®). The new atypical antipsychotics can be used to treat negative symptoms and are useful in smoking cessation (also see the discussion in Section 6).

In patients who were not receiving specific smoking cessation treatment, two studies found significant decreases in nicotine use among patients who were switched from traditional neuroleptics to clozapine (George, Sernyak et al., 1995; McEvoy, Freudenreich et al., 1995b). Although few studies have examined the treatment of tobacco dependence in smokers with schizophrenia, specialized smoking cessation programs appear to benefit this population (Ziedonis & George, 1997; Addington, el-Guebaly et al., 1998; George, Ziedonis et al., 2000). In a study evaluating the treatment of tobacco dependence, about 20% of patients with schizophrenia were able to remain abstinent for six months with the use of nicotine replacement therapy. This study also showed that intensive psychosocial treatment (weekly individual motivational enhancement therapy combined with weekly relapse prevention group therapy) yielded better outcomes than either individual or group therapy alone (Ziedonis & George, 1997). In a similar study, Addington and colleagues (1998) found that a significant number of patients with schizophrenia were able to stop smoking by the end of a modified group treatment program sponsored by the American Lung Association.

In the most rigorous study to date, smokers with schizophrenia were randomly assigned to either a specialized smoking cessation group therapy program modified for schizophrenic patients or to a standard American Lung Association group. Smokers in the specially modified group displayed significantly higher rates of continuous smoking abstinence in the last four weeks of a 12-week trial than did those in a standard American Lung Association group. Abstinence rates did not differ between groups at the endpoint, however. When compared with patients prescribed typical antipsychotic medications, patients prescribed atypical antipsychotics showed significantly higher rates of abstinence, lower rates of attrition, and lower levels of expired carbon monoxide (George, Ziedonis et al., 2000). An important finding of these studies was that schizophrenic symptoms were not exacerbated in patients who achieved abstinence from cigarettes (Addington, el Guebaly et al., 1998; Dalak, Becks et al., 1999; George, Ziedonis et al., 2000).

Subacute and Longer-Term Treatment. Clinical experience has shown that some psychiatric patients will continue to simultaneously display psychotic symptoms and to actively abuse stimulants. In such cases, the abuse may be responsible for, or exacerbate, the patient's symptoms, making the task of diagnosis a difficult one. The clinician should formulate a treatment plan that initially addresses both the psychosis and the substance abuse, beginning with the use of a low-dose antipsychotic. If the patient is able to achieve prolonged abstinence, the clinician then can consider withdrawing the medication and initiating a medication-free period. Patients who continue to display an affective disorder despite a significant period of abstinence may require formal treatment of that disorder.

Conversely, recognizing a substance use problem in a patient previously diagnosed as schizophrenic can be problematic for several reasons. First, staff members in mental health facilities often have inadequate training in screening for substance use and abuse and particularly in diagnosing and treating dual diagnosis patients. Several studies have shown that a significant number of mental health clinicians routinely overlook substance abuse problems in their schizophrenic patients. Second, the patient may contribute to a misdiagnosis by downplaying or denying his or her substance-related problems or by pointing to other causes of such problems. One study of schizophrenic patients who presented at hospital emergency departments found that 33% were recent cocaine users, but half of those persons reported no recent use (Shaner, Khalsa et al., 1993). Thus, urine toxicology and alcohol Breathalyzer® tests are strongly advised as adjuncts to patients' self-reports. Finally, the clinician should be careful not to dwell exclusively on the amount of substance used, as psychiatric patients suffer more acutely from smaller amounts of a substance than do nonpsychiatric patients.

When diagnosing a substance use problem in a patient with schizophrenia, it is advisable to use multiple measurements. Urine drug screens are less susceptible to patient minimization, but they lack perfect sensitivity and specificity. Contrary to common belief, urine drug screens are more likely to yield false negatives than false positives because of rapid excretion of some substances and high thresholds for drug detection (Zanis, McLellan et al., 1994). One study (Wolford, Rosenberg et al., 1999) found that self-report measures, medical examinations, and laboratory tests were less accurate in identifying substance abusers among psychiatric patients than originally assumed. Assessment measures commonly used in the general population were examined in the study, along with demographics, clinical variables, medical examinations, laboratory tests, and collateral reports, in an effort to identify those most useful in psychiatric patients. The TWEAK screening instrument (see Section 13) showed the best overall accuracy in detecting alcohol use disorders, whereas the DAST (see Section 3) showed the best overall accuracy in detecting cocaine and cannabis use disorders. The commonly used CAGE questionnaire performed poorly, with a specificity of 0.695 and a sensitivity of 0.609 in detecting alcohol use disorders. Interestingly, laboratory tests and clinical examinations added little incremental predictive value to the self-report measures (Wolford, Rosenberg et al., 1999).

On the basis of these findings, a new screening instrument was developed to accurately identify substance abuse among psychiatric patients. By using the best items from the scales in the study by Wolford and colleagues (1999), the Dartmouth Assessment of Lifestyle Instrument (DALI) was developed. The DALI was found to have an overall classification accuracy of 0.832 (0.846 specificity and 0.800 sensitivity) as an alcohol screen and 0.880 (0.800 specificity and 1.00 sensitivity) as a screen for cannabis and cocaine (Rosenberg, Drake et al., 1998).

Clinicians also may want to consider a variety of behaviors that frequently underlie a substance use disorder. Cigarette smoking, for example, is linked to other substance use among schizophrenic individuals. Heavy smokers (more than 25 cigarettes per day) abuse substances at three to four times the rate for nonsmokers (Ziedonis, Kosten et al., 1994b; Glassman, 1993). In addition, a substance use disorder may be indicated in patients who are verbally threatening, violent, noncompliant, or suicidal; patients suffering from several medical problems, with recurring hospitalizations or emergency department visits; or patients who are homeless or in legal difficulty (Mueser, Bellack et al., 1992; Bartels, Teague et al., 1993; Ziedonis & Fisher, 1996).

Independently, schizophrenia and substance use disorders each have an associated set of impairments in cognitive, interpersonal, affective, and biological functions (Ziedonis & D'Avanzo, 1998). When these disorders are seen together, the interaction of their associated impairments lead each disorder to be more intractable. The interactions occur between the underlying neurobiology, psychopathology, social correlates, treatment strategies, and health care systems associated with the two individual disorders. Hence, addicted patients with prolonged psychosis or a mental illness such as schizophrenia generally do not respond well to unmodified treatment approaches that are designed for patients with schizophrenia only or for patients with substance abuse only. As with other dually diagnosed patients, the most successful treatment combines medications with psychosocial therapies that encompass mental health and addiction approaches. When compared with patients diagnosed with schizophrenia only or with a substance use disorder only, patients with co-occurring addiction and schizophrenia often experience greater fluctuations in mental status, worse compliance with medications, questionable reports about substance use, increases in episodic homelessness, a greater risk of violence, and a greater incidence of illegal activities.

The number and variety of psychosocial interventions for patients with co-occurring addictive and psychotic disorders has expanded, and now ranges from traditional self-help and Twelve Step groups to recent innovations such as community reinforcement (Dixon & Rebori, 1995) (see Sections 7 and 8).

The Twelve Step approach has been modified for dually diagnosed individuals, who often have reported some difficulty in engaging in Twelve Step groups, given the perceived stigma toward individuals with serious mental illnesses and the cultural opposition to use of psychiatric medications. Dual Recovery Anonymous meetings can provide a bridge to the Twelve Step movement for patients with dual disorders. Meetings of these groups often are held in mental health settings or social houses. The groups encourage recovery for both problems and emphasize the importance of taking appropriately prescribed medications. Spiritual health also is a focus of the meetings, including connecting with a Higher Power, developing a sense of community, and finding meaning and purpose in life. Clinical experience has shown that individuals with a serious mental illness want to talk about spirituality and to develop a stronger sense of hope through the experience of recovery.

Dual diagnosis programs have used psychosocial interventions in strikingly different ways, but there are core similarities. Some have favored an active outreach case management approach, while others have relied more heavily on motivational enhancement therapy in the clinical setting (Ziedonis & Fisher, 1996; Carey, 1996; Drake, Osher et al., 1990; Drake & Noordsy, 1994; Minkoff, 1989; Noordsy, 1991; Rosenthal, Hellerstein et al., 1992; Schollar, 1993). Three specific psychosocial treatments that appear fundamental to dual diagnosis treatment include motivation enhancement therapy (MET) (Miller & Rollnick, 1991), relapse prevention (Marlatt & Gordan, 1985), and Twelve

Step facilitation. However, clinical experience suggests that these three treatment approaches need modification because of the biological, cognitive, affective, and interpersonal vulnerabilities inherent in schizophrenia. Modifications of conventional substance abuse treatments must take into account the common features of schizophrenia—low motivation and self-efficacy, cognitive deficits, and maladaptive interpersonal skills. These limitations heighten the importance of the treatment alliance (Ziedonis & D'Avanzo, 1998).

MET, relapse prevention, and Twelve Step facilitation interventions are described in therapy manuals developed by Project MATCH; these manuals are available without charge from the National Clearinghouse on Alcohol and Drug Information (NCADI; 1-800/729-6686). Another useful training manual available through NCADI is Treatment Improvement Protocol No. 9, titled *Co-Existing Mental Illness and Substance Abuse.*

Both clinical experience and research findings have demonstrated the importance of developing a positive therapeutic alliance. Patients are more responsive when the therapist consistently acts as a nurturing and nonjudgmental ally (Siris & Docherty, 1990; Docherty, 1980; Frank & Gunderson, 1990; Grinspoon, Ewalt et al., 1972; Rogers, Gendlin et al., 1967; Sullivan, 1962; Ziedonis & D'Avanzo, 1998). Siris and Docherty (1990) maintain that dually diagnosed schizophrenics require such a positive alliance and that premature termination and psychiatric decline will ensue from a negative alliance, that is, one based on fear, anger, or rejection. This assertion is consistent with the results of focus groups organized by Maisto and colleagues (1999). In those groups, patients with schizophrenia spectrum diagnosis and co-occurring substance use disorders reported that the relationship developed with the therapist was an important part of recovery.

Working with the dually diagnosed patient requires that the therapist be realistic and direct in addressing inconsistencies; however, the manner in which they are approached is crucial. For example, if a patient has recent positive cocaine urine samples, yet denies any use during the preceding month, the clinician must be understanding of the initial stage of recovery but point out the discrepancy. If there have been overall gains in harm reduction, these should be recognized, and other outcomes should be assessed.

A harm reduction philosophy can be helpful and realistic with the poorly motivated patient who remains uncommitted and ambivalent about the goal of total abstinence (Marlatt & Tapert, 1993; Carey, 1996; Ziedonis & Fisher, 1996). The patient who is in the precontemplation or contemplation stage of change often is unwilling to commit to total abstinence as a short-term goal. Keeping such a patient engaged in treatment often requires finding extrinsic motivators to further the development of the therapeutic alliance (these motivators might include help in obtaining food, clothing, shelter, money management, vocational/training activities, social relationships, and the like). The use of motivational interviewing to develop intrinsic motivation to stop using substances and to maintain compliance with psychiatric treatment also is a useful strategy.

Keeping patients engaged requires efforts to treat their schizophrenia and to provide encouragement and other "rewards" for small steps toward reducing substance use. It is important to evaluate outcomes other than total abstinence; for example, the clinician might assess the patient for reduced quantity and/or frequency of drug use, participation in treatment or other activities, compliance with medications, progress toward short-term goals, and involvement of family or significant others in treatment.

Carey (1996) has suggested a five-step "collaborative, motivational, harm reduction" approach for working with the dually diagnosed patient. This approach includes (1) establishing and developing a working alliance, (2) helping the patient evaluate the cost-benefit ratio of continued substance use (decisional balance in MET), (3) helping the patient develop individual goals, (4) helping the patient build a supportive environment and a lifestyle that is conducive to abstinence, and (5) helping the patient learn to anticipate and cope with crises (Carey, 1996).

Several similar dual diagnosis treatment approaches have been suggested. The Motivation-Based Dual Diagnosis Treatment (MBDDT) model employs a stage-matching approach that combines mental health and addiction treatments, based on the patient's motivational level, severity of illness, and dual diagnosis subtype. The MBDDT approach acknowledges the distinctive features of the schizophrenia-addiction subtype (Ziedonis & Fisher, 1996). The model uses stages of change in assessing the patient and matches treatment strategies and goals (such as abstinence or harm reduction, medication compliance, session attendance, and so forth) to the individual's stage of readiness to change.

MET is a primary psychosocial approach for the patient with poor motivation. However, when the traditional

MET approach is used with dually diagnosed patients, clinicians should recognize the need for adjustments, which include:

- The clinician should play a more active role in offering practical, useful solutions to the patient's concerns about everyday survival. The clinician should not assume that dual diagnosis patients have the personal tools or social resources to solve problems effectively while actively engaged in addictive behaviors.

- MET should be formulated as a continuing component of treatment rather than being limited to the four sessions that were envisioned for non-schizophrenic substance users.

- The decision balance intervention, a cornerstone of MET, should be employed so that it fully accounts for the experience of substance use in relation to other and more systemic problems, such as schizophrenia and medication compliance.

- The clinician should acknowledge that dually diagnosed individuals may not consistently accept the diagnosis of schizophrenia, may vary in their willingness to maintain medication for schizophrenia, and may have greater or lesser motivation to stop their substance use.

Attending to the role of motivation is important to the success of the treatment plan. Clinicians must work to strengthen patients' motivation while confronting the effects of schizophrenia and stressing the importance of medications in managing the condition. Prochaska and colleagues (1992) defined motivation in relation to a five-stage scale (precontemplation, contemplation, preparation, action, and maintenance). A study that evaluated a group of 295 patients who were diagnosed with both schizophrenia and a substance use disorder concluded that more than half could be described as "low motivated" (that is, in the precontemplation or contemplation stage), with the degree of motivation related to the substance and/or number of substances abused (Ziedonis & Trudeau, 1997). Of those patients who abused alcohol, 53% were assessed as having low motivation; the figures for cocaine and marijuana were 65% and 73%, respectively. In another study, a simple five-point Likert scale of current motivation for treatment successfully predicted the dually diagnosed patient's likelihood of achieving abstinence (Ries & Ellingson, 1990).

Certain conditions can work to accelerate a patient's motivation to change through use of external motivators, a realization that led to the development of the community reinforcement approach (CRA) (Higgins, Budney et al., 1994). CRA draws on behavioral therapy principles of contingencies, rewards, and consequences. Because external motivation often is lacking among dually diagnosed patients, CRA searches out a range of possible motivators—disability income, probation, family, and so forth—and uses those motivators to engage, support, and monitor patients in treatment.

Treatment must address not only the effects of low motivation but also potential deficiencies in the cognitive skills known as receiving-processing-sending (RPS) skills, which allow individuals to act on information in a coherent and productive manner (Ziedonis & D'Avanzo, 1998). These skills assume basic levels of attention, memory, and reality awareness. In individuals with schizophrenia, such levels often are lower than normal, so that the benefits of traditional relapse prevention treatment, which is built on a cognitive learning model, are sharply reduced (Marlatt & Gordon, 1985). Thus, the treatment model must be modified and tailored to the dual diagnosis patient, switching the treatment emphasis from cognitive to behavioral approaches as needed.

Traditionally, relapse prevention and Twelve Step facilitation have been used in addiction settings with non-schizophrenic patients, most of whom have a range of social, interpersonal, and problem-solving skills that lead to self-esteem and self-efficacy (Bandura, 1977). Self-efficacy, in particular, is directly related to the change processes that influence maintenance and relapse (Marlatt & Gordon, 1985; DiClemente, Fairhurst et al., 1995; Velicer, DiClemente et al., 1990). Relapse prevention and Twelve Step programs can help individuals increase their self-efficacy and self-esteem. However, relapse prevention therapy tends to be administered in a cognitive therapy manner, while clinical experience suggests using a more action-oriented behavioral approach, featuring role plays, modeling, coaching, positive/negative feedback, and homework. Traditional psychiatric approaches of social skills training use this methodology in rehabilitation programs (Liberman, Mueser et al., 1986; Foy, Wallace et al., 1983). The Lieberman modules include psychosis symptom management, medication management, leisure skills, conversation skills, and community reentry. Traditional relapse prevention is easily adapted to work with individuals with schizophrenia with a focus on addressing difficulties in communication and problem solving.

Several exemplary treatment programs for substance abusers with comorbid psychiatric disorders deserve discussion here. The dual diagnosis treatment program at the West Los Angeles Veterans Affairs Medical Center uses an integrated care model, in which treatment teams provide both mental health and substance abuse services.

A relapse prevention module was designed in consideration of the cognitive deficits of persons with schizophrenia spectrum diagnoses. Patients are taught and given an opportunity to practice a series of social skills believed to reduce the incidence and severity of relapse. Assertive case management, including housing and advocacy services, also plays an integral part of the treatment program. In addition to medications aimed at relief of psychotic symptoms, patients with comorbid alcohol dependence are offered disulfiram. Finally, patients submit to urine drug screens twice a week. A more detailed description of this treatment program is available from Ho and colleagues (1999).

After the above-mentioned program was developed, enhanced program components were added to meet the needs of substance abuse patients with comorbid psychiatric illnesses. Examples include additional psychiatrist time available to patients, a community reentry module, extra case managers, a specialized relapse prevention module, and a relaxation group. Ho and colleagues (1999) compared patients who attended the program before and after the enhanced services were added. Compared with patients in the original version of the program, patients in the enhanced program showed significantly better abstinence rates at one month (60% versus 30%), three months (31% versus 5%), and six months (20% versus 0%) of treatment. Patients attending the enhanced program also showed superior rates of 30- and 90-day treatment retention compared with patients attending the initial program. The researchers reported that increased use of assertive case management could have played an instrumental role in better engagement in treatment, including improved attendance. This increased exposure to services could have contributed considerably to the improved abstinence rates. Further research could help determine the relative importance of the various therapeutic components.

Bellack and DiClemente (1999) described a treatment approach that attempts to compensate for the deficits in motivation, cognition, and social skills commonly seen in patients with schizophrenia. Four treatment modules are used in a rational sequence. Patients first are provided with social skills and problem-solving strategies. Then they are provided with information about the unique difficulties associated with substance abuse in persons with schizophrenia, in addition to information about cravings and triggers for substance use. Motivational interviewing strategies are used, treatment goals are discussed, and behavioral relapse prevention skills are taught.

Patients attend 90-minute sessions twice a week for approximately six months. Small groups (six to eight patients) are used to allow for skill rehearsal and individualized attention. Groups are highly structured to compensate for cognitive deficits associated with schizophrenia. Early successes are built into the treatment program to increase client self-efficacy. Treatment focuses on a small number of specific skills so as not to overwhelm the clients cognitively. Additionally, rather than insisting on complete abstinence immediately, the need for flexibility in this population is recognized by focusing on modest treatment goals. Abstinence is reinforced by paying patients a small amount for clean urine test results.

Initial data appear promising for this treatment approach. Of the 80 patients examined, none that completed the first three weeks of the program subsequently dropped out. Additionally, the overall attrition rate was found to be only 38.5%. Initial substance use outcome data also appear promising (Bellack & DiClemente, 1999). A controlled clinical trial of the approach will follow.

Dual recovery therapy (DRT) integrates substance abuse relapse prevention, psychiatric social skills training, MET, and the "recovery language" of Twelve Step programs in linked group and individual treatment sessions (Ziedonis & Fisher, 1996). MET and recovery language were added to address patients' often low levels of motivation for change and to take advantage of the common lexicon of the Twelve Step programs, with which many patients already were familiar. The resulting treatment is designed to enhance intrinsic motivation for change, bolster the patients' sense of self-efficacy, improve their social skills, and give them tools for coping with high-risk situations. Training is grounded in cognitive-behavioral theory and targets the schizophrenic person's cognitive difficulties (attention span, reading skills, and ability to abstract). The ability to communicate and solve problems is developed through role plays that can be introduced in both group and individual therapy, whereas the understanding and management of their substance use problems are improved through an emphasis on coping strategies (for example, how to organize one's time). The therapist gives ongoing consideration to both substance abuse and psychiatric problems, monitors their interaction, and adjusts the treatment emphasis accordingly. A patient's motivation to address the symptoms of schizophrenia may not be the same as his or her motivation to address substance use, and treatment is best tailored to the individual's motivation for each problem area.

The first month of DRT involves twice weekly individual sessions. Motivation is assessed and enhanced in these early individual sessions while the therapist works on building a strong therapeutic alliance. A plan for change is discussed, and basic skills that will be necessary for later group sessions are introduced. Subsequent individual sessions focus on reinforcing material discussed in group therapy.

After the first month, once a therapeutic alliance has been established and the client has been prepared for group therapy, the structure shifts from two individual sessions per week to one individual and one group session. These sessions are linked, in that individual sessions are used to reinforce the material discussed during the group sessions. Group sessions follow a standard format, which begins with a relaxation exercise, followed by an update report from each client. Group structure is provided by focusing on a specific topic each week (for example, relapse prevention, mood management, symptom management, increasing pleasurable activities, communication skills, asking for help, and medication compliance). Because skill-building plays a central role in DRT, behavioral rehearsal and role-playing are used regularly.

CONCLUSIONS

The major psychosocial interventions for substance use disorders—MET, relapse prevention, and Twelve Step approaches—require some retooling if they are to address the problems posed by schizophrenic patients. For such patients, the prognosis for long-term improvement and recovery depends on a treatment design that addresses both patients' addiction and their schizophrenia, that responds to the unique vulnerabilities (cognitive, affective, social, and biological) of the schizophrenic patient, and that maintains an empathic and collaborative approach. In most cases, treatment of this dual diagnosis subtype is best suited to the mental health setting, provided that mental health staff members receive adequate training in substance abuse and dual diagnosis treatment strategies.

Training programs should be designed to develop basic dual diagnosis assessment and treatment competencies for all staff members. Clinicians should have skills and knowledge in integrating mental health and addiction treatment approaches, with special emphasis on MET, relapse prevention, and Twelve Step facilitation for addiction, as well as social skills training and behavioral therapies for psychiatric disorders. Clinicians should be aware of the relevant pharmacotherapies for both psychiatric and substance use disorders, including detoxification and maintenance. Medications that best treat schizophrenia include the newer atypical antipsychotics and, in some cases, depot antipsychotics. Other helpful strategies include behavioral contracting, community reinforcement approaches, social skills training, money management, peer support/counseling, vocational/educational counseling, and family/network therapies.

The chief challenge in treating this population is to fashion a two-pronged treatment that gives equal care to the schizophrenia and the substance abuse—a challenge that requires a systematic approach to issues that may be of lesser concern in other settings, such as housing, entitlements, rehabilitation, and use of community services. Clinicians who are optimistic, empathic, and hopeful are most helpful to patients in the treatment and recovery processes. Dual diagnosis treatment addresses both problems simultaneously, incorporates active outreach and case management efforts, attempts to increase client motivation for abstinence or harm reduction in a realistic manner, integrates mental health and substance abuse approaches, provides broad-based and comprehensive services, and remains flexible in responding to individual needs.

REFERENCES

Addington J, el Guebaly N, Campbell W et al. (1998). Smoking cessation treatment for patients with schizophrenia. *American Journal of Psychiatry* 155:974-976.

Adler LE, Hoffer LD & Wiser A (1993). Normalization of auditory physiology by cigarette smoking in schizophrenic patients. *American Journal of Psychiatry* 150:1856-1861.

American Psychiatric Association (APA) (1994). *Diagnostic and Statistical Manual of Mental Disorders, 4th Edition (DSM-IV)*. Washington, DC: American Psychiatric Press.

American Psychiatric Association (APA) (1996). APA practice guideline for the treatment of patients with nicotine dependence. *American Journal of Psychiatry* 153(10 Suppl):1-31.

Ames F (1958). A clinical and metabolic study of acute intoxication with Cannabis sativa and its role in the model psychoses. *Journal of Mental Science* 104:972-999.

Bandura A (1977). Self-efficacy: Toward a unifying theory of behavioral change. *Psychological Review* 84(2):191-215.

Bartels SJ, Teague GB, Drake RE et al. (1993). Substance abuse in schizophrenia: Service utilization and costs. *Journal of Nervous and Mental Disease* 181:227-332.

Battaglia G & DeSouza EB (1989). Pharmacologic profile of amphetamine derivatives at various brain recognition sites: Selective effects on serotonergic systems. *NIDA Research Monograph 94*. Rockville, MD: National Institute on Drug Abuse, 240-258.

Beaubrun MH & Knight F (1973). Psychiatric assessment of 30 chronic users of cannabis and 30 matched controls. *American Journal of Psychiatry* 130:309-311.

Bellack AS & DiClemente CC (1999). Treating substance abuse among patients with schizophrenia. *Psychiatric Services* 50(1): 75-80.

Berger S, Hall S, Mickalin J et al. (1996). Haloperidol antagonism of cue-elicited cocaine craving. *Lancet* 347:504-508.

Binder RL, Kazamatsuri H, Nishimura T et al. (1987). Smoking and tardive dyskinesia. *Biological Psychiatry* 22:1280-1282.

Bowers MB (1972). Acute psychosis induced by psychotomimetic drug abuse: Clinical findings. *Archives of General Psychiatry* 27:437-440.

Brady KT, Lydiard RB, Malcolm R et al. (1991). Cocaine-induced psychosis. *Journal of Clinical Psychiatry* 52(12):509-512.

Breakey WR, Goodell H, Lorenz PC et al. (1974). Hallucinogenic drugs as precipitants of schizophrenia. *Psychological Medicine* 4(3):255-261.

Brook MG (1984). Psychosis after cannabis abuse. *British Medical Journal* 288:1381.

Brunette MF, Mueser KT, Xie H et al. (1997). Relationships between symptoms of schizophrenia and substance abuse. *Journal of Nervous and Mental Disease* 185:13-20.

Buckley P (1998). How effective are the second generation antipsychotics? *International Journal of Psychiatry in Clinical Practice* 2(Suppl 2):S41-S47.

Buydens-Branchey L, Branchey M, Fergeson MA et al. (1997). Craving for cocaine in addicted users. *American Journal on Addictions* 6(1):65-73.

Carey KB (1996). Substance use reduction in the context of outpatient psychiatric treatment: A collaborative, motivational, harm reduction approach. *Community Mental Health Journal* 32(3):291-306.

Carlen PL, Lee MA, Jacob M et al. (1981). Parkinsonism provoked by alcoholism. *Annals of Neurology* 9:84-86.

Carney P & Lipsedge M (1984). Psychosis after cannabis abuse. *British Medical Journal* 288:1381.

Carol G, Smelson DA, Losonczy MF et al. (2000). Cocaine craving in individuals with schizophrenia compared to cocaine addicts without schizophrenia. Poster presented at the annual meeting of the American Psychiatric Association, Chicago, IL.

Cash CD (1994). Gammahydroxybutyrate: An overview of the pros and cons for it being a neurotransmitter and/or a helpful therapeutic agent. *Neuroscience Biobehavioral Review* 18:291-304.

Chaudry HR (1991). Cannabis psychosis following bhang ingestion. *British Journal of Addiction* 288:1075-1081.

Chopra G & Smith J (1974). Psychotic reactions following cannabis use in East Indians. *Archives of General Psychiatry* 30:24-27.

Cohen BD, Rosenbaum G, Luby ED et al. (1962). Comparison of phencyclidine hydrochloride (Sernyl®) with other drugs: Simulation of schizophrenic performance with phencyclidine hydrochloride (Sernyl), lysergic acid diethylamide (LSD-25), and amobarbital (Amytal) sodium, II: Symbolic and sequential thinking. *Archives of General Psychiatry* 1:651-656.

Cotman CW & Monaghan DT (1987). Chemistry and anatomy of excitatory amino acid systems. In HY Meltzer (ed.) *Pharmacology and Toxicology of Amphetamine and Related Designer Drugs*. New York, NY: Raven Press, 197-210.

Dalak GW, Becks L, Hill E et al. (1999). Nicotine withdrawal and psychiatric symptoms in cigarette smokers with schizophrenia. *Neuropsychopharmacology* 21:195-202.

Davies BM & Beech HR (1960). The effect of 1-arylcyclodexylamine (Sernyl) on twelve normal volunteers. *Journal of Mental Sciences* 106:912-924.

DiClemente CC, Fairhurst SK & Piotrowski N (1995). Self-efficacy and addictive behaviors. In JE Maddux (ed.) *Self-Efficacy, Adaptation, and Adjustments: Theory, Research, and Application*. New York, NY: Plenum Press.

Dixon L & Rebori TA (1995). Psychosocial treatment of substance abuse in schizophrenic patients. In CL Shiriqui & HA Nasrallah (eds.) *Contemporary Issues in the Treatment of Schizophrenia*. Washington, DC: American Psychiatric Press.

Dixon L, Haas G, Weiden PJ et al. (1990). Acute effects of drug abuse in schizophrenic patients. *Schizophrenia Bulletin* 16:69-79.

Dixon L, Haas G, Weiden PJ et al. (1991). Drug abuse in schizophrenic patients: Clinical correlates and reasons for use. *American Journal of Psychiatry* 148:224-230.

Docherty JP (1980). The individual psychotherapies: Efficacy, syndrome-based treatments, and the therapeutic alliance. In A Lazare (ed.) *Outpatient Psychiatry: Diagnosis and Treatment*. Baltimore, MD: Williams & Wilkins.

Domino EF (1978). Neurobiology of phencyclidine—An update. *NIDA Research Monograph 21*. Rockville, MD: National Institute on Drug Abuse, 18-43.

Drake RE & Noordsy DL (1994). Case management for people with co-existing severe mental disorder and substance use disorder. *Psychiatric Annals* 24(8):427-431.

Drake RE, Osher FC, Noordsy DL et al. (1990). Diagnosis of alcohol use disorders in schizophrenia. *Schizophrenia Bulletin* 16:57-67.

Drake RE, Xie H, McHugo GJ et al. (2000). The effects of clozapine on alcohol and drug use disorders among patients with schizophrenia. *Schizophrenia Bulletin* 26(2):441-449.

Ellinwood EH, Sudilovsky A & Nelson LM (1973). Evolving behavior in the clinical and experimental amphetamine (model) psychosis. *American Journal of Psychiatry* 130(10):1088-1093.

Ereshefsky L (1996). Pharmacokinetics and drug interactions: Update for new antipsychotics. *Journal of Clinical Psychiatry* 57(Suppl 11):12-25.

Ereshefsky L, Saklad SR & Watanabe T (1991). Thiothixene pharmacokinetic interactions: A study of hepatic enzyme inducers, clearance inhibitors, and demographic variables. *Journal of Clinical Psychopharmacology* 11:296-300.

Farren CK, Hameedi FA, Rosen MA et al. (2000). Significant interaction between clozapine and cocaine in cocaine addicts. *Drug & Alcohol Dependence* 59(2):153-163.

Fauman B, Aldinger G, Fauman M et al. (1976). Psychiatric sequelae of phencyclidine abuse. *Clinical Toxicology* 9:529-538.

Fiore MC, Bailey WC, Cohen SJ et. al. (2000). *Treating Tobacco Use and Dependence. Quick Reference Guide for Clinicians.* Rockville, MD: U.S. Department of Health and Human Services, Public Health Service.

First MB, Spitzer RL, Gibbon M et al. (1995). *Structured Clinical Interview for Axis I DSM-IV Disorders-Version 2.0.* New York, NY: New York State Psychiatric Institute, Biometrics Research Department.

Foy DW, Wallace CJ & Liberman RP (1983). Advances in social skills training for chronic mental patients. In KD Craig & MJ McMahon (eds.) *Advances in Clinical Behavior Therapy.* New York, NY: Brunner/Mazel.

Frank AF & Gunderson JG (1990). The role of the therapeutic alliance in the treatment of schizophrenia: Relationship to course and outcome. *General Psychiatry* 47(3):228-236.

Freedman R, Hall M, Adler LE et al. (1995). Evidence in postmortem brain tissue for decreased numbers of hippocampal nicotinic receptors in schizophrenia. *Biological Psychiatry* 38:22-33.

Gawin F, Allen D & Humblestone B (1989). Outpatient treatment of crack-cocaine smoking with fluphenthixol deconate: A preliminary report. *Archives of General Psychiatry* 46:322-325.

George TP, Sernyak MJ, Ziedonis DM et al. (1995). Effects of clozapine on smoking in chronic schizophrenic outpatients. *Journal of Clinical Psychiatry* 56(8):344-346.

George TP, Ziedonis DM, Feingold A et al. (2000). Nicotine transdermal patch and atypical antipsychotic medications for smoking cessation in schizophrenia. *American Journal of Psychiatry* 157:1835-1842.

Gersten SP (1980). Long-term adverse effects of brief marijuana usage. *Journal of Clinical Psychiatry* 41(2):60-61.

Ghodse H (1986). Cannabis psychosis. *British Journal of Addiction* 81:473-478.

Glassman AH (1993). Cigarette smoking: Implications for psychiatric illness. *American Journal of Psychiatry* 150:546-553.

Goff DC, Henderson DC & Amico BS (1992). Cigarette smoking in schizophrenia: Relationship to psychopathology and medication side effects. *American Journal of Psychiatry* 149:1189-1194.

Graeme KA (2000). New drugs of abuse. *Emergency Medicine Clinics of North America* 18(4):625-636.

Greifenstein FE, DeVault M, Yoshitake J et al. (1958). 1-Arylcyclohexylamine for anesthesia. *Current Research on Anesthesia and Analgesia* 37:283-294.

Grinspoon L, Ewalt JR & Schader RI (1972). *Schizophrenia: Pharmacotherapy and Psychotherapy.* Baltimore, MD: Williams & Wilkins.

Gross MM, Lewis E & Best S (1975). Quantitative changes of signs and symptoms associated with alcohol withdrawal: Incidence, severity, and circadian effects in experimental studies of alcoholics. *Advances in Experimental Biological Medicine* 59:615-631.

Higgins ST, Budney AJ, Bickel WK et al. (1994). Incentives improve outcome in outpatient behavioral treatment of cocaine dependence. *Archives of General Psychiatry* 51:568-576.

Ho AP, Tsuan JW, Liberman RP et al. (1999). Achieving effective treatment of patients with chronic psychotic illness and comorbid substance dependence. *American Journal of Psychiatry* 156(11):1765-1770.

Hollister LE (1971). Actions of various marijuana derivatives in man. *Pharmacology Review* 23:349-357.

Hughes JR (1993). Possible effects of smoke-free inpatient units on psychiatric diagnosis and treatment. *Journal of Clinical Psychiatry* 54:109-114.

Hughes JR, Hatsukami DK, Mitchell JE et al. (1986). Prevalence of smoking among psychiatric outpatients. *American Journal of Psychiatry* 143:993-997.

Isbell H (1967). Effects of delta-9-trans-tetrahydrocannabinol in man. *Psychopharmacology* 11:184-188.

Isbell H, Fraser HF & Wikler A (1955). An experimental study of the etiology of "rum fits" and delirium tremens. *Quarterly Journal of Studies on Alcohol* 16(Suppl):1-33.

Jarvik ME & Schneider NG (1992). Nicotine. In JH Lowinson, P Ruiz & RB Millman (eds.) *Substance Abuse: A Comprehensive Textbook, 2nd Edition.* Baltimore, MD: Williams & Wilkins.

Johnstone ME, Evans V & Baigel S (1959). Sernyl (CI-395) in clinical anesthesia. *British Journal of Anesthesia* 31:433-439.

Keeler M, Ewing J & Rouse B (1971). Hallucinogenic effects of marijuana as currently used. *American Journal of Psychiatry* 128:213-216.

Keeler M, Reifler C & Liptzin M (1968). Spontaneous recurrence of marijuana effect. *American Journal of Psychiatry* 125:384-386.

Kelly C & McCreadie RG (1999). Smoking habits, current symptoms, and premorbid characteristics of schizophrenic patients in Nithsdale, Scotland. *American Journal of Psychiatry* 156:751-1757.

Kosten TA (1997). Enhanced neurobehavioral effects of cocaine with chronic neuroleptic exposure in rats. *Schizophrenia Bulletin.* 23(2):203-213.

Kosten TR (1989). Pharmacotherapeutic interventions for cocaine abuse: Matching patients to treatments. *Journal of Nervous and Mental Disease* 177:379-389.

Lang AE (1982). Alcohol and Parkinson's disease. *Annals of Neurology* 12:254-256.

Lasser K, Boyd JW, Woolhandler S et al. (2000). Smoking and mental illness: A population-based prevalence study. *Journal of the American Medical Association* 284(20):2606-2610.

Lavin MR, Siris SG & Mason SE (1996). What is the clinical importance of cigarette smoking in schizophrenia? *American Journal on Addictions* 5:189-208.

Lerner SE & Burns RS (1978). Phencyclidine use among youth: History, epidemiology, and acute and chronic intoxication. *NIDA Research Monograph 21.* Rockville, MD: National Institute on Drug Abuse, 66-118.

Levin ED, Conners CK, Silva D et al. (1998). Transdermal nicotine effects on attention. *Psychopharmacology (Berl)* 140(2):135-141.

Levin ED, Wilson W, Rose JE et al. (1996). Nicotine-haloperidol interactions and cognitive performance in schizophrenics. *Neuropsychopharmacology* 15(5):429-436.

Liberman RP, Mueser KT, Wallace CJ et al. (1986). Training skills in the psychiatrically disabled: Learning coping and competence. *Schizophrenia Bulletin* 12:631-647.

Liden CB, Lovejoy FH & Costello CE (1975). Phencyclidine: Nine cases of poisoning. *Journal of the American Medical Association* 234(5):513-516.

Lundberg GD, Gupta RC & Montgomery SH (1976). Phencyclidine: Patterns seen in street drug analysis. *Clinical Toxicology* 9:503-511.

Lysaker P, Bell M, Beam-Goulet J et al. (1994). Relationship of positive and negative symptoms to cocaine abuse in schizophrenia. *Journal of Nervous and Mental Disease* 182(2):109-122.

Maisto SA, Carey KB, Carey MP et al. (1999). Methods of changing patterns of substance use among individuals with co-occurring schizophrenia and substance use disorder. *Journal of Substance Abuse Treatment* 17(3):221-227.

Manschreck TC, Laughery JA, Weisstein CC et al. (1988). Characteristics of freebase cocaine psychosis. *Yale Journal of Biology & Medicine* 61(2):115-122.

Marlatt GA & Gordan JR (1985). *Relapse Prevention: Maintenance Strategies in the Treatment of Addictive Behaviors.* New York, NY: Guilford Press.

Marlatt GA & Tapert SF (1993). Harm reduction: Reducing the risks of addictive behaviors. In JS Baer & GA Marlatt (eds.) *Addictive Behaviors across the Life Span: Prevention, Treatment, and Policy Issues.* Newbury Park, CA: Sage Publications, 243-273.

McEvoy JP & Brown S (1999). Smoking in first-episode patients with schizophrenia. *American Journal of Psychiatry* 156(7):1120-1121.

McEvoy J, Freudenreich O, Levin ED et al. (1995a). Haloperidol increases smoking in patients with schizophrenia. *Psychopharmacology* 119(1):124-126.

McEvoy J, Freudenreich O, McGee M et al. (1995b). Clozapine decreases smoking in patients with chronic schizophrenia. *Biological Psychiatry* 37(8):550-552.

McLellan TA, Woody GE & O'Brien CP (1979). Development of psychiatric illness in drug abusers. *New England Journal of Medicine* 301(24):1310-1314.

Mendelson JH & LaDou L (1964). Experimentally induced chronic intoxication and withdrawal in alcoholics. *Quarterly Journal of Studies on Alcohol* 2(Suppl):1-39.

Miller WR & Rollnick S (1991). *Motivational Interviewing: Preparing People to Change Addictive Behavior.* New York, NY: Guilford Press.

Minkoff K (1989). An integrated treatment model for dual diagnosis of psychosis and addiction. *Hospital and Community Psychiatry* 40(10):1031-1036.

Mueller PD & Korey WS (1998) Death by "ecstasy": The serotonin syndrome? *Annals of Emergency Medicine* 32(3):377-380.

Mueser KT, Bellack AS & Blanchard JJ (1992). Comorbidity of schizophrenia and substance abuse: Implications for treatment. *Journal of Consulting and Clinical Psychology* 47:1102-1114.

Mueser KT, Nishith P, Tracy JI et al. (1995). Expectations and motives for substance use in schizophrenia. *Psychiatric Clinics of North America* 21(3):367-378.

Noordsy DL (1991). Group intervention techniques for people with dual disorders. *Psychosocial Rehabilitation Journal* 15(2):67-78.

Office on Smoking and Health (2000). *Reducing Tobacco Use: A Report of the Surgeon General.* Atlanta, GA: U.S. Department of Health and Human Services, Centers for Disease Control and Prevention, National Center for Chronic Disease Prevention and Health Promotion.

Olivera AA, Kiefer MW & Manley NK (1990). Tardive dyskinesia in psychiatric patients with substance use disorders. *American Journal of Drug and Alcohol Abuse* 16(1&2):57-66.

Penk WE, Flannery RB, Irvin E et al. (2000). Characteristics of substance-abusing persons with schizophrenia: The paradox of the dually diagnosed. *Journal of Addictive Diseases* 19(1):23-30.

Post RM (1975). Cocaine psychoses: A continuum model. *American Journal of Psychiatry* 132(3):225-231.

Prochaska JO, DiClemente CC & Norcross JC (1992). In search of how people change: Applications to addictive disorders. *American Psychologist* 47:1102-1114.

Regier DA, Farmer ME, Rae DS et al. (1990). Comorbidity of mental disorders with alcohol and other drug abuse. *Journal of the American Medical Association* 264:2511-2518.

Renault P (1974). Repeat administration of marijuana smoke to humans. *Archives of General Psychiatry* 31:95-102.

Ries RK & Ellingson T (1990). A pilot assessment at 1 month of 17 dual diagnosis patients. *Hospital and Community Psychiatry* 41:1230-1233.

Rogers CR, Gendlin EG, Kiesler DJ et al. (1967). *The Therapeutic Relationship and Its Impact: A Study of Psychotherapy with Schizophrenics.* Madison, WI: University of Wisconsin Press.

Rosenberg SD, Drake RE, Wolford GL et al. (1998). Dartmouth assessment of lifestyle instrument (DALI): A substance use disorder screen for people with severe mental illness. *American Journal of Psychiatry* 155(2):232-238.

Rosenthal RN, Hellerstein DJ & Miner CR (1992). A model of integrated services for outpatient treatment of patients with comorbid schizophrenia and addictive disorders. *American Journal on Addictions* 1(4):339-348.

Rottanburg D (1982). Cannabis associated psychosis with hypomanic features. *Lancet* ii:1364-1366.

Satel JA & Lieberman JA (1991). Schizophrenia and substance abuse. *Psychiatric Clinics of North America* 16(2):401-412.

Satel SL & Edell WS (1991). Cocaine-induced paranoia and psychosis proneness. *American Journal of Psychiatry.* 148(12):1708-1711.

Satel SL, Southwick SM & Gawin FH (1991). Clinical features of cocaine-induced paranoia. *American Journal of Psychiatry* 148(4):495-498.

Sato M (1990). A lasting vulnerability to psychosis in patients with previous methamphetamine psychosis. *Annals of the New York Academy of Science* 654:160-170.

Schollar E (1993). The long term treatment of the dually diagnosed. In J Solomon, S Zimberg & E Schollar (eds.) *Dual Diagnosis: Evaluation, Treatment, Training, and Program Development.* New York, NY: Plenum Medical Book Co.

Schuckit MA (1982). The history of psychotic symptoms in alcoholics. *Journal of Clinical Psychiatry* 43:53-57.

Scott DF (1969). Alcoholic hallucinosis. *International Journal of the Addictions* 4:319-330.

Serper MR, Alpert M, Richardson NA et al. (1995). Clinical effects of recent cocaine use on patients with acute schizophrenia. *American Journal of Psychiatry* 152(10):1464-1469.

Shaner A, Khalsa E, Roberts L et al. (1993). Unrecognized cocaine use among schizophrenic patients. *American Journal of Psychiatry* 150:758-762.

Shaner A, Roberts LJ, Racenstein JM et al. (1996). Sources of diagnostic uncertainty among chronically psychotic cocaine abusers. Presented at the 149th Annual Meeting of the American Psychiatric Association, New York, NY, May 4-9.

Sherer MA (1988). Intravenous cocaine: Psychiatric effects, biological mechanisms. *Biological Psychiatry* 24(8):865-885.

Shen WW (1984). Extrapyramidal symptoms associated with alcohol withdrawal. *Biological Psychiatry* 19:1037-1043.

Siegel RK (1978). Cocaine hallucinations. *American Journal of Psychiatry* 135:309-314.

Siris SG & Docherty JP (1990). Psychosocial management of substance abuse in schizophrenia. In MI Herz, JP Docherty & SK Klein (eds.) *Handbook of Schizophrenia, Volume 5. Psychosocial Therapies.*

Skogh E, Bengtsson F & Nordin C (1999). Could discontinuing smoking be hazardous for patients administered clozapine medication? A case report. *Therapeutic Drug Monitoring* 21(5):580.

Smelson DA, Kaune M, Kind J et al. (1999). The efficacy of olanzapine versus haloperidol in decreasing cue-elicited craving and relapse in withdrawn cocaine dependent schizophrenics. Presentation at the National Institute of Drug Abuse New Clinical Drug Evaluation Unit Conference.

Smelson DA, McGee-Caulfield E, Bergstein P et al. (1999). Initial validation of the Voris cocaine craving scale: A preliminary report. *Clinical Psychology* 55(1):135-139.

Smelson DA, Roy A & Roy M (1997). Risperidone diminishes cue-elicited craving in withdrawn cocaine-dependent patients. *Canadian Journal of Psychiatry* 42(9):984.

Smelson DA, Williams J, Kune M et al. (2000). Reduced cue-elicited craving and relapses following treatment with risperidone. Poster presented at the American Psychiatric Association, Chicago IL.

Soyka M (2000). Substance misuse, psychiatric disorder, and violent and disturbed behavior. *British Journal of Psychiatry* 176:345-350.

Strakowski SM, Tohen M, Flaum M et al. (1994). Substance abuse in psychotic disorders: Associations with affective syndromes. *Schizophrenia Research* 14(1):73-81.

Sullivan HS (1962). *Schizophrenia as a Human Process.* New York, NY: WW Norton & Co.

Tabakoff B & Hoffman PL (1996). Alcohol addiction: An enigma among us. *Neuron* 16:909-912.

Talbott JA & Teague JW (1969). Marijuana psychosis. *Journal of the American Medical Association* 210:299-305.

Tart CT (1970). Marijuana intoxication: Common experiences. *Nature* 226:701-704.

Tennant FS & Groesbeck CJ (1972). Psychiatric effect of hashish. *Archives of General Psychiatry* 27:133-136.

Test MA, Wallisch LS & Allness DJ (1989). Substance use in young adults with schizophrenic disorders. *Schizophrenia Bulletin* 15:465-476.

Thacore VR & Shukla SR (1976). Cannabis psychosis and paranoid schizophrenia. *Archives of General Psychiatry* 33:383-386.

Velicer WF, DiClemente CC, Rossi JS et al. (1990). Relapse situations and self-efficacy: An integrative model. *Addictive Behaviors* 15:271-283.

Victor M & Hope JM (1958). The phenomenon of auditory hallucinations in chronic alcoholism. *Journal of Nervous and Mental Disease* 126:451-448.

Voruganti LN, Heslegrave RJ & Awad AG (1997). Neuroleptic dysphoria may be the missing link between schizophrenia and substance abuse. *Journal of Nervous and Mental Disease.* 185(7):463-465.

Waskow IE (1970). Psychological effects of tetrahydrocannibinol. *Archives of General Psychiatry* 22:97-107.

Weiden PJ, Mann JJ & Dixon L (1989). Is neuroleptic dysphoria a healthy response? *Comprehensive Psychiatry* 30:543-552.

Wiesbeck GA & Taeschner KL (1991). A cerebral computed tomography study of patients with drug-induced psychoses. *European Archives of Psychiatry and Clinical Neuroscience* 241:88-90.

Wilkins JN (1997). Pharmacotherapy of schizophrenic patients with comorbid substance abuse. *Schizophrenia Bulletin* 23:215-228.

Wolford GL, Rosenberg SD, Drake RE et al. (1999). Evaluation of methods for detecting substance use disorder in persons with severe mental illness. *Psychology of Addictive Behaviors* 13(4):313-326.

Zanis DA, McLellan AT, Canaan RA et al. (1994). Reliability and validity of the Addiction Severity Index with a homeless sample. *Journal of Substance Abuse Treatment* 11(6):541-548.

Zaretsky A, Rector NA, Seeman MV et al. (1993). Current cannabis use and tardive dyskinesia. *Schizophrenia Research* 11(1):3-8.

Ziedonis D, Richardson T, Lee E et al. (1992). Adjunctive desipramine in the treatment of cocaine abusing schizophrenics. *Psychopharmacology Bulletin* 28(3):309-314.

Ziedonis DM (1992). Comorbid psychopathology and cocaine addiction. In TR Kosten & HD Kleber (eds.) *Clinician's Guide to Cocaine Addiction: Theory, Research and Treatment.* New York, NY: Guilford Press, 337-360.

Ziedonis DM & D'Avanzo K (1998). Schizophrenia and substance abuse. In Kranzler HR & Rounsaville BJ (eds.) *Dual Diagnosis and Treatment: Substance Abuse and Comorbid Medical and Psychiatric Disorders.* New York, NY: Marcel Dekker, 427-465.

Ziedonis DM & Fisher W (1996). Motivation-based assessment and treatment of substance abuse in patients with schizophrenia. *Directions in Psychiatry* 16(11):1-8.

Ziedonis DM & George TP (1997). Schizophrenia and nicotine dependence: A report of a pilot smoking cessation program and review of the literature. *Schizophrenia Bulletin* 23(2):247-254.

Ziedonis DM & Kosten TR (1991). Pharmacotherapy improves treatment outcome in depressed cocaine addicts. *Journal of Psychoactive Drugs* 23(4):417-425.

Ziedonis DM, Kosten TR & Glazer WM (1992). *The Impact of Drug Abuse on Psychotic Outpatients (New Research Program and Abstracts, 103).* Washington DC: American Psychiatric Association.

Ziedonis DM, Kosten TR & Glazer W (1994a). The impact of drug abuse on psychopathology and movement disorders in chronic psychotic outpatients. In L Harris (ed.) *Problems of Drug Dependence 1994 (NIDA Research Monograph 153).* Rockville, MD: National Institute on Drug Abuse.

Ziedonis DM, Kosten TR, Glazer WM et al. (1994b). Nicotine dependence and schizophrenia. *Hospital & Community Psychiatry* 45:204-206.

Ziedonis DM & Trudeau K (1997). Motivation to quit using substances among individuals with schizophrenia: Implications for a motivation based treatment model. *Schizophrenia Bulletin* 23(2):229-238.

<table>
<tr><td>Chapter 5</td><td>

Co-Occurring Addictive and Attention Deficit/ Hyperactivity Disorder and Eating Disorders

</td></tr>
</table>

Frances Rudnick Levin, M.D.
Maria A. Sullivan, M.D., Ph.D.
Stephen J. Donovan, M.D.

Attention Deficit/Hyperactivity Disorder
Eating Disorders

This chapter examines two common psychiatric problems, which have shared antecedents in childhood or adolescence and a connection with addiction: attention deficit/hyperactivity disorder and eating disorders.

Attention deficit/hyperactivity disorder (ADHD) is developmental, in that typically it is diagnosed and treated in children and can persist into adulthood. Recent research has shown that the same or similar criteria can be used to identify adults with persistent ADHD and that such adults also may benefit from psychostimulant medication. Given that ADHD pathology may derive either from a delay in maturation of function or from an absence of function, it is not surprising that most children "grow out" of the problem (Mannuzza, Klein et al., 1991, 1993). Some, however, do not.

Eating disorders seem to have an intimate, although obscure, connection to female puberty and clearly can change adolescent development in a deviant direction. Development is not limited to childhood or adolescence, but continues throughout life (Erikson, 1950). Erikson's model makes "intimacy versus isolation" the crisis of young adulthood. It is easy to imagine how the disorders discussed here would make matters worse, even in the absence of alcohol or drug abuse. When such abuse co-occurs with these psychiatric problems, it increases the likelihood that an individual's life trajectory will become derailed or stalled. Identifying psychiatric comorbidity among those who seek treatment for substance use disorders thus is critical in that it may improve treatment outcomes (as measured by treatment retention and reduction in alcohol or drug use or symptom severity) and help individuals master age-appropriate developmental tasks.

ATTENTION DEFICIT/ HYPERACTIVITY DISORDER

ADHD has substantial morbidity in and of itself. In an individual with ADHD, occupational and social deficits attributed to substance abuse may be due in small or large part to persistent ADHD symptoms. In a recent review, Mannuzza and colleagues (2000) noted that children with ADHD who were followed into adulthood were more likely to have completed less schooling, to hold occupations with less professional or social status, to suffer from poor self-esteem, to have social skill deficits, and to have antisocial personality disorder. Murphy and Barkley (1996) found that, as adults, individuals who were diagnosed with ADHD

TABLE 1. Criteria for Attention Deficit/Hyperactivity Disorder

A. Either (1) or (2):

(1) *Inattention:*	(2) *Hyperactivity:*
Six (or more) of the following symptoms of inattention have persisted for at least six months to a degree that is maladaptive and inconsistent with developmental level:	
(a) Often fails to give close attention to details or makes careless mistakes in schoolwork, work or other activities;	(a) Often fidgets with hands or feet or in seat;
(b) Often has difficulty sustaining attention in task or play activities;	(b) Often leaves seat in classroom or in other situations in which remaining in seat is expected;
(c) Often does not seem to listen when spoken to directly;	(c) Often runs about or climbs excessively in situations in which it is inappropriate (in adolescents or adults, may be limited to a subjective feeling of restlessness);
(d) Often does not follow through on instructions and fails to finish schoolwork, chores, or duties in the workplace (not due to oppositional behavior or failure to understand instructions);	(d) Often has difficulty playing or engaging in leisure activities quietly;
(e) Often has difficulty organizing tasks and activities;	(e) Often is "on the go" or often acts as if "driven by a motor"
(f) Often avoids, dislikes, or is reluctant to engage in tasks that require sustained mental effort (such as schoolwork or homework);	(f) Often talks excessively.
(g) Often loses things necessary for tasks or activities (such as toys, school assignments, pencils, books, or tools);	*Impulsivity:*
(h) Often is easily distracted by extraneous stimuli;	(g) Often blurts out answers before questions have been completed;
(i) Often forgetful in daily activities six (or more) of the following symptoms of hyperactivity-impulsivity have persisted for at least six months to a degree that is maladaptive and inconsistent with developmental level.	(h) Often has difficulty awaiting turn;
	(i) Often interrupts or intrudes on others (for example, butts into conversations or games).

B. Some hyperactive-impulsive or inattentive symptoms that caused impairment were present before age 7 years.

C. Some impairment from the symptoms is present in two or more settings (such as at school [or work] and at home).

D. There must be clear evidence of clinically significant impairment in social, academic, or occupational functioning.

E. The symptoms do not occur exclusively during the course of a Pervasive Developmental Disorder, Schizophrenia, or other Psychotic Disorder and are not better accounted for by another mental disorder (such as Mood Disorder, Anxiety Disorder, Dissociative Disorder, or a Personality Disorder).

TABLE 1 (continued).   Criteria for Attention Deficit/Hyperactivity Disorder

Code based on type:

- Attention Deficit/Hyperactivity Disorder, Combined Type: if both Criteria A1 and A2 are met for the past six months.

- Attention Deficit/Hyperactivity Disorder, Predominantly Inattentive Type: if Criterion A1 is met but Criterion A2 is not met for the past six months.

- Attention Deficit/Hyperactivity Disorder, Predominantly Hyperactive-Impulsive Type: if Criterion A2 is met but Criterion A1 is not met for the past six months.

Coding note: For individuals (especially adolescents and adults) who currently have symptoms that no longer meet full criteria, "In Partial Remission" should be specified.

SOURCE: American Psychiatric Association (1994). *Diagnostic and Statistical Manual of Mental Disorders, 4th Edition (DSM-IV)*. Washington, DC: American Psychiatric Press.

---

in childhood were more likely to have had their driver's license suspended, to have incurred speeding violations, to have quit or been fired from a job, and to have been married multiple times. Persistent ADHD symptoms appear to place these individuals at great risk for antisocial personality disorder and substance abuse (Mannuzza, Klein et al., 2000; Greenfield, Hechtman et al., 1998).

When ADHD symptoms are combined with those of a substance use disorder, the severity of impairment is likely to increase. Moreover, the severity of the substance use and dependence and the individual's response to addiction treatment are adversely affected by comorbid ADHD. Biederman and colleagues (1998) found that adults with ADHD were more likely to transition from an alcohol use disorder to a drug use disorder and to continue to abuse substances following a period of substance dependence than were similar patients without ADHD. Likewise, among individuals with a lifetime history of a substance use disorder, those who also had ADHD evinced a longer duration of having a substance use disorder and a slower remission rate (Wilens, Biederman et al., 1998).

Carroll and Rounsaville (1993) compared the clinical course of cocaine use among individuals with and without childhood histories of ADHD. Those with childhood ADHD had an earlier onset of regular cocaine use, more frequent and intense cocaine use, and greater lifetime treatment exposure. Based on these findings, it is increasingly evident that ADHD may exert a negative effect on the course of a substance use disorder and that treatment needs to be targeted at both the psychiatric and substance use disorders.

Diagnostic Criteria for Childhood ADHD. ADHD is characterized by inattention, impulsivity, and hyperactivity. Table 1 provides the criteria for childhood ADHD in the fourth edition of the *Diagnostic and Statistic Manual* (*DSM-IV*; APA, 1994). Importantly, the current criteria require that some symptoms have caused impairment prior to age 7 and that impairment must occur in more than one setting. These criteria emphasize both the developmental aspect of the disorder and the fact that childhood behavior problems often are situation-bound. The more settings in which deviant behavior occurs, the more justified one is in saying that the behavior interferes with the child's functioning and therefore deserves a diagnosis. A child who appears distracted and inattentive in only one setting (such as at school), but can listen well and pay attention in other settings, may have a learning disability rather than ADHD.

Diagnostic Criteria for Adult ADHD. Current *DSM-IV* criteria do not permit a diagnosis of ADHD in adults who do not have a history of impairing symptoms before age 7: that is, a diagnosis of childhood ADHD. However, Barkley and Biederman (1997) stress that age of onset has low reliability, and *DSM-IV* field trials found many adults who met the symptom criteria but not the age of onset criterion for ADHD (Applegate, Lahey et al., 1997). Accordingly, Faraone and colleagues (2000) suggest that future research should address whether the age of onset criterion should be (1) removed, (2) retained but without the criterion that the symptoms be impairing, or (3) retained but with an older age of onset. At present, adults who had a clinically significant syndrome in childhood that has

---

persisted into adulthood, but who cannot recall when they began to have impairing symptoms, are considered to have adult ADHD NOS (not otherwise specified).

A common clinical question is how to diagnose an adult who no longer has at least six symptoms of hyperactivity, impulsivity, or inattention. Using current diagnostic criteria, such an adult would be considered to be in "partial remission." Faraone and colleagues (2000) argue convincingly that the *DSM-IV* diagnosis of ADHD may be particularly sensitive to developmental changes because the symptoms are performance-based rather than experiential. For example, an individual being evaluated for ADHD is asked about his or her behavior (such as how well he or she follows directions or completes tasks), whereas an individual with depression is asked about his or her internal states (such as feelings of sadness or hopelessness) as well as behavioral manifestations (such as changes in sleep pattern or appetite). Often, behaviors that are difficult to perform in childhood become inconsequential in adulthood. Future revisions of the *DSM-IV* will need to develop new criteria that incorporate symptoms more relevant to the challenges encountered by adults (Faraone, Biederman et al., 2000).

Some clinical researchers have developed other criteria to define adult ADHD, most notably the "Utah Criteria" (Wender & Garfinkel, 1989). The revised Utah Criteria consist of seven symptoms and require at least one of the first two symptoms and at least four of the seven total symptoms for a diagnosis of adult ADHD. The symptoms include: (1) inattention persisting from childhood, (2) hyperactivity persisting from childhood, (3) inability to complete tasks, (4) impaired interpersonal relationships or inability to sustain relationships over time, (5) affective lability, (6) explosive temper, and (7) stress intolerance. Spencer and colleagues (1994) note that because the Utah Criteria include symptoms that are not part of the *DSM-IV* criteria (such as mood lability and anxiety), they may have led to the incorrect assumption that the core childhood symptoms do not need to be present in adulthood. The Utah Criteria were developed for research purposes and excluded comorbid psychiatric disorders; this enhanced the homogeneity of the samples studied, but limited the generalizability of the diagnostic criteria to other clinical populations (Weiss, Hechtman et al., 1999).

One way to reconcile the two diagnostic systems is to recognize that the core symptoms of ADHD remain a crucial element of the adult disorder; however, additional psychiatric symptoms (and disorders) often are found among adults with ADHD.

Validity of the Adult ADHD Diagnosis: Until recently, clinicians disagreed as to whether the adult syndrome was a valid disorder. The present diagnostic schema, which requires a constellation of symptoms of either inattentiveness or hyperactivity-impulsivity, represents a revision of the *DSM-IIIR* designation of "undifferentiated ADHD," in which the disorder was considered to be possible rather than presumable.

To be valid, a clinical diagnosis requires: (1) descriptive validity: that is, characteristic signs and symptoms; (2) predictive validity: that is, a specific course of illness and treatment response; and (3) construct validity: that is, data suggesting that an underlying etiology or pathophysiology exists (Spitzer & Williams, 1985). Prevalence and prospective studies (Weiss, Pope et al., 1985; Morrison, 1980; Biederman, Wilens et al., 1995; Mannuzza, Klein et al., 1993), family-genetic studies (Morrison, 1980; Biederman, Wilens et al., 1995), neuroimaging studies (Zametkin, Nordahl et al., 1990), and treatment studies (Spencer, Wilens et al., 1995; Wilens, Biederman et al., 1996) all provide data to support the three types of validity described above. Spencer and colleagues (1994) reviewed this evidence and have argued convincingly that adult ADHD is a distinct clinical entity. With greater acceptance of adult ADHD as a valid diagnosis, clinicians have been more likely to assess and diagnose substance-abusing patients with ADHD.

Linkage of ADHD and Substance Use Disorders. Several large epidemiologic studies have found that 3% to 9% of children have ADHD (Szatmari, 1992). Unfortunately, prevalence rates of adult ADHD have not been obtained in large surveys such as the Epidemiologic Catchment Area (ECA) Study or the National Comorbidity Study (NCS). Given that 10% to 70% of children with ADHD continue to have symptoms into late adolescence and adulthood (Weiss & Hechtman, 1986; Mannuzza, Klein et al., 1991; Biederman, Mick et al., 2000), one would predict that the estimated rates for adult ADHD in the general population would be <1% to 5%. By contrast, Hill and Schoener (1996) used a mathematical model to calculate the expected prevalence rate for adult ADHD, based on the available published literature. They posited an exponential decline in ADHD, such that 99% of children would be likely to go into remission by age 20. Barkley (1977) reviewed the assumptions underpinning this mathematical model and found several methodological problems, including the fact that the authors included only studies that defined subjects as having persistent ADHD if they met full criteria for the disorder and excluded studies of individuals who had adult ADHD in partial remission. Clinical experience suggests that most patients do not meet full criteria in adulthood but do continue to have significant impairment as a result of persistent ADHD symptoms. Thus, Hill and Schoener's calculations may substantially underestimate the prevalence rates of adult ADHD. Assuming that up to 5% of adults in the general population have impairing symptoms of ADHD, the question arises as to whether ADHD is overrepresented in substance-using populations. Interestingly, pharmacologic treatment trials have found that few patients entering treatment had childhood ADHD (Gawin, Kleber et al., 1989; Weddington, Brown et al., 1991) or residual ADHD (Gawin & Kleber, 1986; *DSM-III* nomenclature). These studies were not specifically designed to assess prevalence rates for various psychiatric disorders; therefore, certain diagnoses such as ADHD may have been overlooked. Further, individuals with ADHD may have been excluded from entering pharmacologic treatment protocols, not because of ADHD symptoms, but because they had other psychiatric syndromes, such as depression. It is less obvious why Weiss and colleagues (1988) obtained low rates of adult ADHD among cocaine and other drug abusers. One explanation is that prevalence rates were based on a clinical rather than a structured interview, leading to underdiagnosis. Further, the "diagnostic climate" at the time did not favor diagnosing adults' symptoms of ADHD as a separate diagnostic entity.

Interestingly, Wood and colleagues (1983) found that 33% of alcoholics seeking treatment had residual attention deficit disorder (using *DSM-III* criteria). Other prevalence studies have found elevated rates of childhood ADHD among various groups of persons with substance use disorders (Eyre, Rounsaville et al., 1982; Rounsaville, Anton et al., 1991). Several recent studies have evaluated persons with substance use disorders for adult ADHD, using structured interviews based on the *DSM-IIIR* and *DSM-IV* criteria. Levin and colleagues (1998a) completed a prevalence study evaluating for childhood and adult ADHD individuals who were seeking treatment for cocaine dependence. Although the researchers obtained a prevalence rate for childhood ADHD and subthreshold childhood ADHD that was substantially lower than that found by Rounsaville and colleagues (1991)—that is, 20% rather than 35%—both rates were higher than the rates in the general population. Several other studies of persons seeking treatment for cocaine, alcohol, or opiate dependence found remarkably similar rates of adult ADHD, ranging from 15% to 24% (Levin, Evans et al., 1998a; King, Brooner et al., 1999; Clure, Brady et al., 1999; Schubiner, Tzelepis et al., 2000).

Elevated rates of ADHD among persons with substance use disorders are not confined to treatment samples. Carroll and Rounsaville (1993) found that the prevalence of childhood ADHD was lower among cocaine abusers not seeking treatment than among those seeking treatment (22% versus 35%). However, this percentage still is higher than the expected rate in the general population.

Similarly, substance use disorders appear to be overrepresented in persons with symptoms of ADHD, whether or not they are seeking treatment. Both the ECA Study and the NCS obtained prevalence rates for substance use disorders within the general population and found that lifetime rates of substance abuse or dependence ranged from 17% to 27% (Regier, Farmer et al., 1990; Kessler, McGonagle et al., 1994). Biederman and colleagues (1995) found that lifetime prevalence rates for substance use disorder among adults with ADHD was 52%, compared with 27% in subjects without ADHD. This elevated rate among individuals with adult ADHD is higher than the rate expected on the basis of the NCS and ECA data. Non-treatment-seeking adults with ADHD were significantly more likely to have alcohol or drug use disorders than were non-treatment seeking adults who did not have histories of ADHD (Biederman, Faraone et al., 1993). Taken together, these studies suggest that ADHD and substance use are not independent disorders and that their association is not the result of ascertainment bias.

Throughout this section, the focus has been on the link between ADHD and substance use disorders, but this should not preclude the observation that individuals with ADHD also have a greater likelihood of nicotine dependence. Clinical studies have shown that adults with ADHD have higher rates of nicotine dependence than the general population (40% versus 26%; Pomerleau, Downey et al., 1995). In a prospective study, Lambert and Hartsough (1998) found that individuals with ADHD had an early onset of regular smoking and that adults with ADHD were more likely to smoke daily than were controls.

Possible Reasons for the Linkage: Various explanations have been offered for the link between ADHD and substance use disorder, including (1) the presence of a necessary mediating factor, such as conduct disorder, (2) the persistence of ADHD symptoms, (3) low self-esteem, (4) self-medication, (5) genetic factors, and (6) exposure to stimulants in childhood. Prospective studies that have followed children with ADHD into adolescence suggest that a mediating factor—specifically, conduct disorder—substantially increases the risk that substance abuse will occur. There is substantial evidence to suggest that individuals diagnosed with childhood ADHD who also have conduct disorder as children are more likely to develop problems related to substance use (Gittleman, Mannuzza et al., 1985; Mannuzza, Klein et al., 1991; Thompson, Riggs et al., 1996; Milberger, Biederman et al., 1997). However, it also is true that adolescents with ADHD may begin to use drugs even in the absence of conduct disorder. Similarly, adults diagnosed with adult ADHD are more likely to have a substance use disorder if they have antisocial personality disorder (ASP). However, a substantial proportion of individuals with adult ADHD have an ongoing substance use disorder in the absence of ASP (Biederman, Wilens et al., 1995; Mannuzza, Klein et al., 1993). These studies suggest that, although conduct disorder and ASP may confer a substantial risk of developing a substance use disorder, a critical factor for having an ongoing substance use problem in adulthood is the persistence of ADHD symptoms. Once regular substance use is established, the presence of ADHD symptoms may increase the likelihood of heavy and impairing use.

Of course, the persistence of ADHD symptoms is not a sufficient explanation for these individuals' greater risk of substance use disorders. Persistent ADHD symptoms may lead to impairments in occupational and interpersonal functioning to a degree that the individual suffers from low self-esteem and/or depression and uses alcohol or other drugs to cope with the underlying problems. Similarly, an individual with ADHD may find, through initial experimentation, that certain drugs provide some symptomatic relief. For example, it has been hypothesized that individuals with ADHD may use cocaine to treat their symptoms of inattentiveness and hyperactivity; if that is true, ADHD should be overrepresented in cocaine-abusing populations. However, at present, the data suggest that ADHD is overrepresented not only in cocaine users but in a number of substance-abusing populations.

This finding does not necessarily negate the self-medication hypothesis. Instead, it may be that a variety of drugs are effective at alleviating distressing symptoms. For example, nicotine is an indirect dopamine agonist that shares certain properties with methylphenidate and amphetamine, two commonly used treatments for ADHD (Hoffman, 1996). Nicotine also promotes the release of acetylcholine, which plays a role in attentional processes (Wonnacott, Irons et al., 1989). Thus, nicotine may serve as an effective self-medication for adults with ADHD. In addition, it has been the authors' experience that some adults with ADHD report that marijuana, rather than cocaine, helps them become calm. Regardless of which drug is used, it has been widely observed that, over time, the use of these drugs becomes problematic rather than palliative.

Further, some individuals with persistent ADHD symptoms do not endorse ever having used drugs to ameliorate their psychiatric symptoms. Instead, they report that they tried drugs initially because of impulsivity or that they had friends or acquaintances who facilitated their use of alcohol and illicit drugs.

In terms of genetic factors, data suggest an association between ADHD and the dopamine D4 receptor (DRD4) gene. Faraone and colleagues (1999) found that, among 27 triads which consisted of an ADHD adult, his or her spouse, and their ADHD child, the number of 7-repeat alleles of the DRD4 gene predicted the diagnosis of ADHD in the adult parents. This finding supports earlier work suggesting that the 7-repeat allele of the DRD4 may be overrepresented in children with ADHD (Lahoste, Swanson et al., 1996) "Given that the DRD4 gene mediates a blunted cellular response to dopamine, its overrepresentation in the ADHD population is consistent with the hypothesis that ADHD symptoms are related to hypodopaminergic function, and thus ameliorated by drugs that increase synaptic dopamine" (Sullivan & Levin, 2001).

Dysregulation and overexpression of the dopamine transporter also have been implicated in the pathophysiology of ADHD. The 10-repeat allele of the dopamine transporter gene has been associated with ADHD (Cook, Stein et al., 1995; Gill, Daly et al., 1997), and preliminary data suggest that this transporter variant is associated with a poor methylphenidate response (Winsberg & Comings, 1999). In addition, exciting work by Dougherty and colleagues (1999) has shown that dopamine transporter density is significantly higher in adults with ADHD than in healthy controls. From these studies, it may be concluded that drugs that increase synaptic DA may counter an impairment in dopamine transmission.

A controversial explanation for the observed association between ADHD and substance use is that exposure to stimulants—even those prescribed by treatment providers—increases the likelihood that an individual will develop a problem with stimulants. This heightened risk is thought to occur by (1) the process of behavioral sensitization or (2) patients' belief that, because a stimulant medication has been prescribed, they can use cocaine or other drugs without difficulty. Although Lambert and Hartsough (1998) found that adults diagnosed with ADHD in childhood who had used stimulant medications as children were more likely to be daily smokers than were those who had not taken stimulants, other studies suggest that treating ADHD children with stimulants *reduces* the risk of later alcoholism (Paternite, Loney et al., 1999) and other substance use disorders (Biederman, Wilens et al., 1999). Clearly, more research is needed to elucidate the relationships among ADHD, its treatment, and the development of substance use disorders.

Difficulties in Diagnosing Adult ADHD in Substance-Using Populations. Although the *DSM-IV* provides clear-cut criteria for making the diagnosis of adult ADHD, diagnostic ambiguity often arises when one attempts to apply these criteria to individuals who abuse alcohol and other drugs.

Potential Reasons for Underdiagnosis: Although retrospective data typically are used when diagnosing a past psychiatric disorder, this becomes more problematic when individuals are asked to recall symptoms that began at a young age. Mannuzza and colleagues (1991) found that even among adults diagnosed with ADHD in childhood and followed repeatedly into adulthood, a substantial minority of the adults could not recall their childhood ADHD symptoms.

In assessing a child for ADHD symptoms, child psychiatrists or pediatricians often seek information from a teacher or parent; however, these sources of information often are not available during assessment of the adult patient. Even when an older family member, preferably a parent, is available, the reliability of the information may be questionable. The older family member may have (or have had) an alcohol or drug problem or other dysfunction to a degree that his or her ability to recall the patient's childhood behavior may be limited. Another good way to obtain historical data is to ask the patient to provide elementary school report cards. These can provide valuable information and afford an accurate "snapshot" of the patient as a child. Although many parents may not have kept such school records, it is worthwhile to inquire.

A reasonable approach to resolve this issue if the patient or family cannot recall symptoms prior to age 7 but do remember substantial impairment related to ADHD symptoms in elementary school is to make a tentative diagnosis of childhood ADHD. However, it is important to inquire specifically about childhood inattention, hyperactivity, and impulsivity, because not all disruptive behavior during the school years can be attributed to ADHD. In some children, learning disabilities, depression, and conduct disorder may better explain such behaviors (either alone or co-occurring with ADHD).

In addition to the lack of good historical information, ADHD may go undiagnosed because of lack of awareness of the diagnosis on the part of patients and clinicians. First, many persons with both substance use disorders and adult ADHD were not diagnosed as children; thus, they do not view their problematic adult behaviors as related to their ADHD. These patients may attribute their impatience, restlessness, or procrastination to being "hot-headed," "easily bored" or "lazy." Second, many of the consequences of ADHD (such as work failure and poor educational attainment) also are associated with substance use disorder. Persons with substance use disorder and undiagnosed ADHD may assume that it is their alcohol or drug use that prevents them from attaining their full potential. Third, patients often develop ways to partially compensate for their ADHD symptoms, so that the symptoms of the disorder may not be obvious to the evaluating clinician. For example, adults who feel restless may learn to get up from the table and serve others as a socially appropriate way to handle their need for increased activity. Fourth, because questions regarding childhood behaviors—particularly behaviors associated with ADHD—may not be part of the "standard" assessment, it is an easy diagnosis to overlook. Unlike depression or psychosis, which may be incapacitating or require hospitalization, the negative effects of ADHD usually do not have such dramatic consequences. Further, an episodic change in functioning (as is seen in depression) is more likely than a chronic behavioral problem to be noticed and attributed to a psychiatric disorder. Finally, the current diagnostic criteria for adult ADHD are problematic and need to be reexamined. As mentioned earlier, some of the symptoms required by the *DSM-IV* may not be developmentally appropriate and may need to be modified to better characterize the difficulties experienced by adults.

Potential Reasons for Overdiagnosis: Screening instruments can be useful in identifying individuals with child and adult ADHD, but overreliance on such instruments can lead to overdiagnosis. The Wender Utah Rating Scale (Ward, Wender et al., 1993) is a self-report instrument that is used to assess individuals for childhood ADHD. Although it has been shown to have some validity among general adult patient populations, its validity among persons with substance use disorders has not been established. Scored items include affective symptoms, which are not part of the *DSM-IV* criteria. Therefore, this clinical instrument may have utility in the initial screening of substance-abusing patients for childhood ADHD, but it should not replace the clinical interview.

Overdiagnosis of adult ADHD also can occur if one ignores the functional impairment criterion. For example, it is common for individuals to procrastinate when faced with difficult projects. The difference between persons with and without ADHD is that adults with ADHD have had significant occupational, interpersonal, or psychological impairment as a result of their impaired ability to start tasks and complete them. Because some individuals may be able to "explain away" their difficulties at school or work by describing themselves as having ADHD, it is incumbent on the clinician to ensure that a patient's current symptoms of ADHD are not limited to one setting. An individual who is completing difficult projects at home but is unable to finish assigned projects at work may be experiencing job dissatisfaction rather than ADHD. Moreover, the ADHD symptoms need to be impairing, not merely bothersome.

Another way in which the clinician may overdiagnose ADHD is by failing to confirm that a patient shows a continuity of symptoms from childhood into adulthood. Levin and colleagues (1998a) have observed that some individuals with cocaine dependence have impairing ADHD-like symptoms that occur only after a period of regular drug use, but they cannot recall having experienced ADHD symptoms in childhood.

Other Diagnostic Issues: There also is a lack of diagnostic clarity regarding situations in which an individual may endorse four or five childhood symptoms but not the required six symptoms from either the hyperactive-impulsive or inattentive category. In working with such individuals, the clinician needs to consider whether they have had "true" childhood ADHD. Again, the clinician might be somewhat more lenient when making the diagnosis in persons with substance use disorders, since childhood impairment may have gone unrecognized. Using strict *DSM-IV* criteria, these individuals would be diagnosed with

ADHD NOS (not otherwise specified). Similarly, adults who do not endorse six symptoms of inattention or six symptoms of hyperactivity/impulsivity would be diagnosed with ADHD in partial remission, rather than full ADHD. Potential problems with the diagnoses of adult ADHD in partial remission or adult ADHD NOS is that the clinician may assume incorrectly that an individual with such a disorder does not have clinically impairing symptoms or will not benefit from pharmacologic interventions, whereas neither assumption may be correct.

Another area that often leads to diagnostic confusion and subsequent underdiagnosis or overdiagnosis is the issue of additional psychiatric comorbidity. The added presence of a substance use disorder can further complicate the assessment. Generally, because ADHD symptoms are present in elementary school and precede the substance use disorder, ADHD can be more readily identified as an independent disorder, compared with disorders that usually are episodic in nature and may occur only after heavy substance use has developed.

The last criterion listed in the *DSM-IV* for ADHD emphasizes that ADHD should not be diagnosed if the observed symptoms are better accounted for by another mental disorder. Unfortunately, some clinicians may interpret this to mean that if depression or bipolar illness is present, ADHD should not be diagnosed. In reality, these disorders may coexist. Alternatively, it is possible to diagnose ADHD when the patient simply has an affective disorder. For example, ADHD, hypomania, and mania may share similar symptoms (for example, distractibility and irritability), and the diagnosis of one of these disorders may be overlooked. The longitudinal history can provide information to distinguish between the two disorders. Individuals with bipolar illness are more likely to describe discrete periods of increased restlessness, talkativeness, hyperactivity, and the like, whereas those with adult ADHD are more likely to describe a lifelong constellation of these symptoms to a lesser degree. Individuals with bipolar illness may recall periods of decreased need for sleep (for example, feeling rested after three hours of sleep) and inflated self-esteem or grandiosity (APA, 1994)—symptoms that are not commonly described by adults with ADHD alone. Further, individuals with ADHD typically do not exhibit psychotic symptoms. If these are present, they indicate the likelihood of an additional mood disturbance and/or a substance-induced psychotic disorder.

Individuals with major depression may experience symptoms of inattention, but are less likely to experience other symptoms associated with ADHD (such as hyperactivity and talkativeness). Often adults with ADHD have first-degree relatives with ADHD; their presence may suggest that the individual in question has ADHD. However, depression and bipolar illness also are overrepresented in families of individuals diagnosed with ADHD (Biederman, Faraone et al., 1990, 1992). Again, a comprehensive diagnostic assessment that addresses psychiatric comorbidity and pertinent family history is needed prior to initiating any pharmacotherapy.

Treatment. Compared with other patients with substance use disorders, individuals with ADHD may have greater difficulties in processing information and may have greater problems in sitting through group meetings—a common format for addiction treatment. Because individuals with ADHD often act impulsively, they also may be more likely than those without ADHD to drop out of treatment. Counselors or other patients may find individuals with unrecognized ADHD to be "annoying" or "treatment-resistant" and may have less empathy for them than for those without this disorder. This attitude can increase the likelihood that patients with ADHD will drop out of treatment. By recognizing and treating the ADHD, the clinician can help to alleviate the patient's problems and achieve a better treatment outcome.

Although treatment of persons with substance use disorders and adult ADHD can be categorized as pharmacologic or nonpharmacologic, this is a somewhat artificial distinction, as the two approaches often are used concurrently. Initially, the clinician may opt for a nonpharmacologic intervention. However, if such interventions fail to improve symptoms, a pharmacologic trial may be added. Through the use of pharmacologic interventions to reduce ADHD symptoms such as distractibility or restlessness, other nonpharmacologic treatment approaches may be better utilized.

Pharmacologic Interventions. Psychostimulants, particularly methylphenidate, are the most commonly prescribed and most efficacious medications for both child and adult ADHD (Barkley, 1977; Greenhill, 1992; Wilens, Biederman et al., 1995a) and are the best studied for adult ADHD. The majority of studies carried out in adults have reported benefits from stimulants, although the results have not been as robust as those found in children. The studies that have shown the best response in adults have used larger doses. Spencer and colleagues (1995) found that methylphenidate (up to 1.0 mg/kg per day) produced substantial

improvement in ADHD symptoms in 78% of adults, compared to 4% of those receiving placebo. Two double-blind studies comparing methylphenidate to placebo for the treatment of adult ADHD included a small number of persons who also had substance use disorders (Mattes, Boswell et al., 1984; Spencer, Wilens et al., 1995). The researchers found that the subjects who had both substance use disorders and ADHD responded better to methylphenidate than did the subjects without substance use disorders. However, the effect of the methylphenidate on the patients' substance use disorders was not described. More recently, Wilens and colleagues (1999) found that moderate to high doses of pemoline were somewhat more effective than placebo in treating adult ADHD but, given pemoline's limited efficacy, tolerability, and association with hepatic dysfunction (particularly in persons with substance use disorders), the authors recommended pemoline as a second-line treatment for adult ADHD.

Other medications that have been studied under double-blind, placebo-controlled conditions for the treatment of adult ADHD include desipramine, tomoxetine, bupropion, and ABT-418, a selective cholinergic activating agent. Wilens and colleagues (1996) found that desipramine produced a significant reduction in ADHD symptoms compared to placebo. Tomoxetine, an experimental noradrenergic reuptake inhibitor, also produced highly significant improvements in ADHD symptoms (Spencer, Biederman et al., 1998). In one recent study, bupropion showed a clinical advantage over placebo in reducing symptoms in adults with ADHD (Wilens, Spencer et al., 2001). The advantage of desipramine, tomoxetine, and bupropion is that they also are used to treat depression. Since depression may co-occur with ADHD in persons with and without substance use disorders, these medications may be first-line treatments in many comorbid populations.

Another medication approved for the treatment of depression that shows some promise for the treatment of adult ADHD is venlafaxine. However, this medication has been evaluated only in open trials (Wilens, Biederman et al., 1995b), so further study under controlled conditions is needed.

An interesting pharmacologic approach is to test medications with cholinergic activity. Acetylcholine plays a role in attentional processes (Wonnacott, Irons et al., 1989) and, like other medications that modulate this system, it may improve ADHD symptoms. Using a double-blind, placebo-controlled design, Wilens and colleagues (1999) assessed the efficacy of ABT-418, a cholinergic activating agent that is delivered in a transdermal patch. Moderate improvements were found in adults with ADHD who received the patch. Because ABT-418 appeared to selectively improve attentional symptoms, rather than hyperactive or impulsive symptoms, this medication might be targeted to patients who have inattention symptoms alone.

Some of the medications mentioned above, such as desipramine, methylphenidate, and bupropion, also have been tried as treatments for cocaine dependence. Desipramine has a record as a relatively safe medication among individuals who currently are using cocaine. Several double-blind placebo-controlled trials of desipramine have been carried out in cocaine abusers seeking treatment, with no untoward side effects, but results in terms of the efficacy of desipramine appear mixed (Gawin, Kleber et al., 1989; Arndt, Dorozynsky et al., 1992; Kosten, Morgan et al., 1992; Carroll, Nich et al., 1995). Findings from laboratory studies suggest that there are few clinically significant cardiovascular effects when cocaine is administered to individuals maintained on desipramine (Fischman, Foltin et al., 1990).

Bupropion and methylphenidate also have been evaluated as potential treatments for cocaine dependence. One double-blind study using bupropion did not find the medication more effective than placebo (Margolin, Kosten et al., 1995). However, the researchers found that among cocaine abusers with comorbid depression, those who received bupropion had a greater reduction in cocaine use than did those who received placebo (Margolin, Kosten et al., 1995). On the basis of these data, the investigators suggested that bupropion might be effective for cocaine abusers with adult ADHD. Similarly, Grabowski and colleagues (1997) found that neither the sustained-release nor immediate-release form of methylphenidate (combined dose 45 mg/day) was more effective than placebo for the treatment of cocaine abuse among individuals without ADHD. The most common side effects were jitteriness and decreased appetite, but there were no medical complications requiring discontinuation. In a recently completed laboratory study, the authors found that minimal untoward cardiovascular effects occurred when repeated doses of cocaine were given to non-treatment-seeking cocaine abusers with adult ADHD who were maintained on sustained-release methylphenidate (Evans, unpublished data). However, none of the trials mentioned above was designed to assess the effects of these medications on re-

ducing cocaine use and ADHD symptoms in cocaine abusers with adult ADHD.

At present, data to evaluate the efficacy of various pharmacologic agents for adult ADHD in persons with substance use disorders are limited. Bromocriptine has been given to persons with co-occurring ADHD and substance use disorders (primarily involving cocaine and/or marijuana abuse), with mixed results (Cocores, Davies et al., 1987; Cocores, Patel et al., 1987; Cavanagh, Clifford et al., 1989). Most of the published data are derived from a small number of case reports, largely involving persons using cocaine. To date, Levin and colleagues (1998b) have provided the most promising data suggesting that methylphenidate (in the sustained-release formulation) has clinical utility as a treatment for adult ADHD in cocaine addicts seeking treatment. ADHD symptoms and cocaine use decreased significantly in response to divided daily doses ranging from 40 to 80 mg/day of sustained-release methylphenidate. (Individual relapse prevention therapy also was provided weekly.) Another pilot study supports the hypothesis that methylphenidate might reduce cocaine use and ADHD symptoms (Samoza, Bridge et al., 2000) but, given the limitations of an open design, double-blind controlled trials clearly are warranted.

In another small open study, Levin and colleagues (2002) found that bupropion was similar to methylphenidate in reducing cocaine use and ADHD symptoms. However, these promising findings need to be replicated in larger, placebo-controlled trials.

Special Issues in Pharmacotherapy: Although the emphasis in this section has been on the treatment of persons with co-occurring ADHD and substance use disorders, such individuals often have other conditions as well. Biederman and colleagues (1995) have documented high rates of antisocial personality disorder, depression, and anxiety disorder among adults with ADHD. Elevated rates of these disorders also have been found in cocaine abusers (Rounsaville, Anton et al., 1991) and opiate-dependent individuals (Brooner et al., 1997) seeking treatment. Thus, when possible, it may be best to use medications that target both the ADHD symptoms and the additional psychiatric comorbidity. For example, a cocaine abuser with ADHD and depression might initially be placed on bupropion or desipramine.

There is some question as to whether children with ADHD and anxiety are less responsive to stimulants than are children without additional anxiety symptoms. Although some data suggest that ADHD children with anxiety disorder do less well with stimulant medications, in a recent well-controlled trial, comorbid anxiety did not appear to produce greater side effects or diminish the effectiveness of methylphenidate in reducing ADHD symptoms (Diamond, Tannock et al., 1999).

It may be that adults with ADHD and comorbid conditions will benefit from a regimen of more than one medication. Clearly, this can become complicated when such patients also have one or multiple substance use disorders. When possible, it appears prudent to use one medication first, to treat the condition that requires the most immediate attention. If the patient demonstrates substantial clinical improvement with the first medication, then another medication can be added as needed for the other psychiatric condition. The following clinical vignette demonstrates such a case:

An adult seeks help from a psychiatrist for compulsive behaviors, such as having to touch the floor three times when he enters a room or repeatedly checking the locks on the door after he leaves the house. He has mild facial tics but no vocalizations. He reports that he attends Alcoholics Anonymous three times a week and has been abstinent from alcohol for a year. He states than he is embarrassed by his compulsive symptoms, which is the reason he is seeking help.

During the interview, the psychiatrist obtains historical data consistent with childhood ADHD, inattentive type. The patient describes similar difficulties with attention, albeit attenuated, as an adult. The psychiatrist initially treats the patient with a selective serotonin reuptake inhibitor. As the compulsive behavior diminishes, the ADHD symptoms become more apparent. A long-acting stimulant is added with good success, without any exacerbation of the tics.

Clearly, the use of multiple medications requires close attention to side effects and possible medication interactions. Ideally, the medication(s) selected would be effective for the treatment of ADHD, have low abuse potential, and be proved safe when combined with other psychoactive substances. At present, no single medication meets these criteria.

A valid concern is the risk of stimulant abuse by the patient or a family member. In response, some clinicians have suggested the use of pemoline because of its lower abuse potential. However, recent concerns regarding possible hepatotoxicity may limit the use of pemoline in substance-abusing patients. At present there are no clear-cut guidelines regarding the appropriate use of methylphenidate or other psychostimulants in the treatment of persons with adult ADHD and substance use disorders. Nonstimulant medications such as bupropion, venlafaxine, or desipramine are second-line treatments for childhood ADHD, largely because of their side effect profile and less proven efficacy. However, for individuals with a current or lifetime history of substance abuse, one might initially prescribe a nonstimulant medication to avoid the possibility of abuse or diversion of the treatment medication. On the other hand, if the nonstimulant medication is not useful and the patient does not have a history of amphetamine or methylphenidate abuse, then stimulant medications might be considered.

Generally, the threshold for use of a stimulant medication is lower for those individuals with a prolonged period of sobriety than for those who are newly abstinent or currently abusing drugs. For substance-abusing adults with ADHD who are unable to become abstinent, various investigators are studying whether stimulant medications directly reduce drug craving and/or lead to a decrease in or cessation of drug use. To date, studies have not found that administration of stimulants increases cocaine craving or use among cocaine abusers seeking treatment (Grabowski, Roache et al., 1997; Levin, Evans et al., 1998b),

Nevertheless, certain precautions are warranted when using stimulants in substance-abusing patients. First, keeping careful records of prescriptions written and the number of pills given is crucial. When the patient is seen on a frequent basis, the number of pills per prescription can be reduced, the patient's treatment response can be closely monitored, and any potential interactions between the stimulant and other abused substances can be identified. Further, it should be made clear to patients that urine toxicology screens will be conducted routinely, and that if the patient does not show a clinically significant reduction in alcohol or drug use, other treatment strategies will be implemented. Patients should be encouraged to ingest their medication in a regular fashion, rather than on an as-needed basis, to avoid inadequate and intermittent palliation of symptoms. Although some clinicians report that the sustained-release form of methylphenidate is less effective than the immediate-release form, it might be preferable because it poses less opportunity for abuse. Moreover, there are new extended-release preparations of methylphenidate and amphetamine that have 8 to 12 hours of action and less erratic absorption than earlier formulations.

Finally, persons with ADHD and substance use disorders who are placed on stimulants may abuse the prescribed stimulants or illicit stimulant drugs. Thus, these possibilities should be discussed with the patient before a stimulant is prescribed. Similar to other areas of clinical uncertainty, good clinical judgment becomes crucial when deciding who will benefit from a pharmacologic treatment intervention and which medication(s) should be used.

Non-Pharmacologic Interventions. Compared to the pharmacologic treatment literature, there are even fewer clinical data to suggest which non-pharmacologic approaches work best for persons with substance abuse disorders and adult ADHD. As in the treatment of substance abusers with other psychiatric disorders, it is likely that concurrently treating the symptoms of both the substance use disorder and the ADHD is more likely to produce a positive treatment outcome than treating one disorder alone. In both the treatment literature for childhood ADHD and the treatment literature for substance use disorders, positive outcomes are reported with the use of behavioral approaches. Such approaches include (1) contingency management, (2) cognitive-behavioral interventions, and (3) combined pharmacologic and behavioral interventions.

Interestingly, the literature on childhood ADHD suggests that negative contingencies may be a necessary component of treatment (Pelham & Sams, 1992), whereas positive contingencies have been stressed as an appropriate treatment for adults with substance use disorders (Higgins, Delaney et al., 1994). To date, there have been no contingency management strategies targeted to persons with both adult ADHD and substance use disorder. Whereas children with ADHD may receive (or lose) a token for violation of a classroom rule, establishing a token economy system for ADHD behaviors manifested in adulthood would prove more difficult.

Cognitive-behavioral therapy has become an integral part of many addiction treatment programs. The question is whether this approach works equally well for persons with comorbid ADHD and substance use disorder. The use of cognitive interventions for children with ADHD has included "verbal self-instructions, problem-solving strategies, cognitive modeling, self-evaluation, and self-reinforcement." In a recent collaborative study (MTA Study, 1999), children with ADHD and anxiety responded nearly as well to behav-

ioral treatment as they did to medication management or combined treatment. For those ADHD children without a comorbid anxiety disorder, medication or combined treatment was superior to behavioral treatment alone. These data imply that adults with ADHD and comorbid anxiety may do particularly well with behavioral approaches. Given that some adult substance abusers with ADHD have comorbid anxiety, it would not be surprising if behavioral interventions that targeted both the ADHD symptoms and substance abuse might be an effective treatment approach for such complicated patients.

Weinstein (1994) has suggested that adults, unlike children, have a greater potential to understand the meaning of dysfunctional behavior and the effects of ADHD symptoms on their lives and thus may be better able to utilize cognitive-behavioral approaches. However, such approaches may need to be modified for persons with ADHD and substance use disorder. For example, less emphasis may be placed on completion of homework tasks and more emphasis on session work. Frequently, such patients are poor self-observers and have difficulty understanding why they behave in a certain way. Adapting the work of other investigators, Weinstein (1994) has suggested several attention and memory strategies to help individuals cope with ADHD symptoms (Table 2). These techniques also may have clinical utility for individuals with ADHD in addiction treatment settings.

Using a manualized relapse prevention approach, Aviram and colleagues (2001) found that "the challenge for therapists is to identify the links between the cognitive, behavioral, and physiological symptoms associated with ADHD and those associated with drug use." Limitations stemming from ADHD, as well as feelings of negative self-worth, may lead to drug use, which further limits the patient's coping abilities. The authors maintain that these limitations must be countered in treatment by providing tangible coping skills and strategies, many of which are incorporated in the relapse prevention model.

Two experimental approaches that also might be useful for persons with ADHD and substance use disorder are nodal-link mapping and sensory integration. Nodal-link mapping, which often is used in group settings, consists of drawing spatial-verbal displays to represent visual interrelationships among ideas, feelings, facts, and experiences (Dees, Dansereau et al., 1994). Although Dansereau and colleagues (1995) did not specifically assess subjects for adult ADHD, they compared the efficacy of nodal-mapping

---

TABLE 2.   Attention and Memory Strategies for Individuals With Attention Deficit/Hyperactivity Disorder

Attention Strategies	Memory Strategies
■ Talk to yourself to focus attention;	■ Establish clear expectations in advance about what is to be learned;
■ Write down essential information;	■ Outline the sequence of a task;
■ Ask for repetition of instructions;	■ Organize/categorize/chunk information;
■ Ask speakers to present information more slowly;	■ Increase attention to material that is to be learned;
■ Break down tasks into small, simple steps;	■ Repeat instructions to make certain message is understood;
■ Learn to identify and avoid overload;	■ Rehearse material to be learned;
■ Take rest periods;	■ Establish a routine doing the same task in the same order and on the same schedule;
■ Work on detailed tasks when maximally alert;	■ Develop cues to aid recall;
■ Avoid lengthy monotonous tasks;	■ Use a memory notebook.
■ Work in quiet space;	
■ Try to do one thing at a time;	
■ Practice learning to divide attention;	
■ Develop compensatory strategies.	

SOURCE: Weinstein CS (1994). Cognitive remediation strategies: An adjunct to the psychotherapy of adults with attention deficit hyperactivity disorder. *Journal of Psychotherapy Practice and Research 3:44-57.* Reprinted by permission of the publisher.

---

to standard counseling in reducing substance abuse among methadone-maintained patients with good or poor attention to treatment success. They found that individuals who received standard therapy and/or had poor attention did less well in methadone treatment. However, mapping-enhanced counseling reduced the negative effects of poor attention.

The other experimental approach, sensory integration, seeks to integrate stimuli in an organized manner. Within an inpatient addiction treatment setting, Stratton and Gailfus (1998) found that this technique reduced impulsivity, enhanced anger control, increased attention span, and improved treatment retention. Although these approaches show promise, there are few empirical data to guide treatment in the comorbid population.

Summary. Clearly, many questions still need to be answered regarding the diagnosis and treatment of persons with co-occurring adult ADHD and substance use disorder. The reliability and validity of screening instruments for both childhood and adult ADHD are yet to be established. Further, the utility of various neuropsychological tests has not yet been determined. Although stimulants have been shown

to be useful in treating patients with adult ADHD, their effect on ADHD symptoms and co-occurring substance use disorders has not been studied in a controlled fashion. There are even fewer data to support the use of other pharmacologic agents or nonpharmacologic treatment strategies for adults with ADHD and substance use disorder. Given the substantial subpopulation of persons with substance use disorder and adult ADHD, further research is warranted.

EATING DISORDERS

This section examines two disorders that share a set of maladaptive attitudes and behaviors toward food, a distortion of body image, a marked preponderance of female sufferers, and onset in adolescence. The disorders are anorexia nervosa and bulimia nervosa.

There is substantial evidence that eating disorders and substance use disorders co-occur at higher than expected rates. Features common to both types of disorder include craving, loss of control, and an inappropriate preoccupation with a substance (broadly defined): alcohol, drugs, or food. Despite these similarities, however, as well as the high rates of comorbid eating and substance use disorders,

---

TABLE 3. Diagnostic Criteria for Anorexia Nervosa

■ Refusal to maintain body weight at or above a minimally normal weight for age and height (for example, weight loss leading to maintenance of body weight less than 85% of that expected or failure to make expected weight gain during a period of growth, leading to body weight less than 85% of that expected).

■ Intense fear of gaining weight or becoming fat, even though underweight.

■ Disturbance in the way in which one's body weight or shape is experienced, undue influence of body weight or shape on self-evaluation, or denial of the seriousness of the current low body weight.

■ In postmenarcheal females, amenorrhea (the absence of at least three consecutive menstrual cycles). A woman is considered to have amenorrhea if her periods occur only following hormone (estrogen) administration.

Specify type:

■ Restricting Type: During the current episode of Anorexia Nervosa, the person has not regularly engaged in binge-eating or purging behavior (for example, self-induced vomiting or the misuse of laxatives, diuretics, or enemas).

■ Binge-Eating/Purging Type: During the current episode of Anorexia Nervosa, the person has regularly engaged in binge-eating or purging behavior (for example, self-induced vomiting or the misuse of laxatives, diuretics, or enemas).

SOURCE: American Psychiatric Association (1994). *Diagnostic and Statistical Manual of Mental Disorders, 4th Edition (DSM-IV)*. Washington, DC: American Psychiatric Press.

---

research and treatment approaches for the two groups of disorders have developed independently. Indeed, notable differences between them may be found. For example, whereas there are well-developed animal models for substance abuse and addiction, no animal models for anorexia or bulimia have been proposed. However, historical analogues may be observed: in various cultures over several centuries, females on the edge of puberty have practiced self-starvation (Brumberg, 1988; Streigel-Moore & Huydic 1993). The lack of animal models, coupled with the presence of historical models, suggests that some uniquely human factors are involved in the pathogenesis of anorexia and bulimia. Among these factors are the meaning with which food and self-discipline are imbued by certain pubescent girls, as well as the reinforcing effects of "successful" starvation on impaired self-esteem.

Diagnostic Criteria and Descriptive Features. Anorexia and bulimia are included in this chapter because they

are linked to the idea of loss of normal modulation of impulses (Tables 3 and 4; also see the *DSM-IV* for definitions). Impulse dyscontrol in anorexia refers to excess control, for anorexia is essentially self-starvation. By contrast, in bulimia the loss of impulse control results in too little control, for bulimia involves bingeing (and often stealing, engaging in sexually promiscuous behavior, and substance abuse as well). Both disorders typically have their onset in adolescence or early adulthood. The course of each disorder may be chronic or intermittent, with anorexia marked by a 10% mortality rate. The course of anorexia or bulimia often is complicated by the presence of substance abuse or dependence.

Prevalence in the General Population. As defined in the *DSM-IV*, anorexia occurs in 0.5% to 1% of women between the ages of 15 and 40. Bulimia is somewhat more common, occurring in 1% to 2% of white females in the same age group (Fairburn & Beglin, 1990; Kendler,

---

Maculae et al., 1991). Males comprise only 5% of the cases of anorexia (Halmi, 1974) and 10% to 15% of the cases of bulimia (Gold, Johnson et al., 1997). Although both disorders are more prevalent in upper- to middle-class sectors of industrialized societies, bulimia occurs in ethnically diverse groups (Smith, 1995), and anorexia also occurs in non-Western cultures, where food restriction may be expressed as epigastric discomfort or distaste for food (*DSM-IV*; APA, 1994) rather than concerns about weight (Palmer, 1993).

While the long-term outcome for bulimia generally is considered better than that for anorexia, both have been characterized as chronic, relapsing disorders. However, studies of treatment outcomes have yielded inconsistent findings, probably because of conflicting definitions of relapse and variable followup intervals (Herzog, Nussbaum et al., 1996), as well as overreliance on self-report questionnaires to make diagnoses (Fairburn & Beglin, 1990). Moreover, as Fairburn and Beglin (1990) have cautioned, epidemiologic work to date has not included studies comparing community-based and clinic-based cases. The subgroup of individuals who seek treatment for an eating disorder is likely to be atypical of the broad spectrum of symptomatic behavior that exists in the community (Fairburn & Beglin, 1990). Longitudinal studies that compare community and clinic-based samples would reveal which forms of the disorder resolve without therapeutic intervention, as compared with those features that are likely to persist without early detection and treatment (Fairburn & Beglin, 1990).

Prevalence of Coexisting Substance Use and Eating Disorders. Many studies have reported high rates of substance use in patients with eating disorders (Hatsukami, Mitchell et al., 1986; Bulik, 1987; Hudson, Weiss et al., 1992). Both substance use disorders and eating disorders have increased in frequency among young adults in recent decades, resulting in a statistically greater likelihood of concurrent diagnoses (Katz, 1990). However, given that eating disorders still occur at relatively low rates (0.5% to 2%), their association with substance use disorders prompts us to consider explanations other than mere chance.

A study by Mitchell and colleagues (1990) found that 25% of all eating disorder patients gave a history of current or prior substance abuse. In a large (n=454) study examining eating-disordered women with a history of substance abuse, Wiederman and Pryor (1996) found that, even after controlling for age and severity of eating disorder symptoms, women with bulimia were more likely than those with

anorexia to have used alcohol, amphetamines, barbiturates, marijuana, tranquilizers, and cocaine. For both anorectic and bulimic patients, the severity of caloric restriction predicted amphetamine use and the severity of binge eating predicted tranquilizer use. But severity of purging predicted a wider range of substance use, involving alcohol, cocaine, and cigarettes.

The reverse relationship also has been noted: there is a high prevalence of eating disorders among patients with substance use disorders. Specifically, high rates of eating disorders have been found among patients who abuse alcohol (Beary, Lacey et al., 1986) or cocaine (Jonas, Gold et al., 1987). In a study of nearly 400 patients admitted to an addiction treatment program, Hudson and colleagues (1992) found that women with both substance use and eating disorders were significantly more likely to report stimulant abuse and less likely to report opioid abuse than those without eating disorders. Two studies of adolescent females with eating disorders have found very similar rates of problem drinking: 35.5% (Peluso, Ricciardelli et al., 1999) and 36.4% (Striegel-Moore & Huydic, 1993), respectively.

Accumulating evidence from several epidemiologic studies suggests that a large proportion of bulimic women (up to 50% in some samples) have comorbid substance use disorders. Rates of substance use disorder among women with a current or past history of bulimia range from 8% to 41% (Holderness, Brooks-Gunn et al., 1994; Krahn, 1991; Lilenfeld, Kaye et al., 1997). These comorbidity rates far exceed the rates at which either disorder occurs among women in the general population (Kessler, McGonagle et al., 1994). In the Ontario Student Drug Use Survey (N=1,919), binge eating was associated with heavier substance use and with lower self-esteem and more depression (Ross & Ivis, 1999).

A particular association has been noted between alcohol abuse and bulimia. One group of researchers reported that, in a population of patients with bulimia, half the subjects had engaged in alcohol abuse or excessive use by age 35 (Beary, Lacey et al., 1986). Conversely, the authors found that 35% of alcoholic women on an inpatient alcoholism treatment unit reported a prior eating disorder. Bulimic patients whose behavior is marked by high impulsivity are more likely than other bulimics to report alcohol abuse and dependence by the end of eating disorder treatment (Fichter, Quadflieg et al., 1994).

Similarly, Bulik and colleagues (1997) found that women with comorbid bulimia and alcohol dependence had higher

---

TABLE 4. Diagnostic Criteria for Bulimia Nervosa

- Recurrent episodes of binge eating. An episode of binge eating is characterized by both of the following:

  ☐ Eating, in a discrete period of time (within any two-hour period) an amount of food that is definitely larger than most persons would eat during a similar period of time and under similar circumstances.

  ☐ A sense of lack of control over eating during the episode (for example, a feeling that one cannot stop eating or control what or how much one is eating).

- Recurrent inappropriate compensatory behavior in order to prevent weight gain, such as self-induced vomiting; misuse of laxatives, diuretics, enemas, or other medications; fasting; or excessive exercise.

- The binge eating and inappropriate compensatory behaviors both occur, on average, at least twice a week for three months.

- Self-evaluation is unduly influenced by body shape and weight.

- The disturbance does not occur exclusively during episodes of anorexia nervosa.

Specify Type:

- Purging Type: During the current episode of bulimia nervosa, the person has regularly engaged in self-inducing vomiting or the misuse of laxatives, diuretics, or enemas.

- Nonpurging Type: During the current episode of bulimia nervosa, the person has used other inappropriate compensatory behaviors, such as fasting or excessive exercise, but has not regularly engaged in self-induced vomiting or the misuse of laxatives, diuretics, or enemas.

SOURCE: American Psychiatric Association (1994). *Diagnostic and Statistical Manual of Mental Disorders, 4th Edition (DSM-IV)*. Washington, DC: American Psychiatric Press.

---

rates of suicide attempts, anxiety disorders, other substance dependence disorder, conduct disorder, and borderline or histrionic personality disorders. In light of the finding that many eating disorder patients have features of borderline personality disorder, some have suggested that these individuals may be particularly vulnerable to substance abuse because of traits such as impulsivity, emotional lability, feelings of emptiness, and unstable interpersonal relationships. Other factors that suggest a vulnerability to substance abuse include the use of amphetamines in an effort to lose weight or the emergence of benzodiazepine dependence as a consequence of treatment of insomnia in eating disorder patients (Katz, 1990). Among male and female cocaine abusers,

Cochrane and colleagues (1998) found that nearly half of the women used cocaine and/or alcohol as a weight control measure, while only 13% of the male subjects did so. Strikingly, 72% of the women who endorsed weight-related use of cocaine had a current diagnosis of an eating disorder.

The implications of this research remain unclear because of issues surrounding the selection of control groups, the use of *DSM-IV* diagnostic criteria, and the use of structured diagnostic interviews with demonstrated reliability (Grilo, Levy et al., 1995). Diagnostic co-occurrence may not always be interpreted as "comorbidity." An important type of sampling error to which clinical studies are prone is that of Berkson's (1946) bias, by which persons with two psychiatric disorders can seek treatment for either or both disorders. Grilo and colleagues (1995) have proposed that significant co-occurrence that reflects potential comorbidity should be defined as frequency of association greater than that observed in a comparison group from the same overall sample, ascertained by the same recruitment procedures, and characterized by similar base rates of most disorders. Using this rigorous definition of comorbidity, Grilo and colleagues (1995) examined the frequency of co-occurrence of eating disorders in a sample of female inpatients with substance use disorders, compared with a sample of female inpatients without substance use disorders. They found that the frequency of anorexia and bulimia was not greater in patients with substance use disorders than in psychiatric comparison groups. However, diagnostic criteria for Eating Disorder NOS (not otherwise specified) were met with greater frequency in the substance use disorder group. Patients diagnosed with Eating Disorder NOS exhibited many features of an eating disorder, but failed to meet at least one of the required criteria (for example, not quite 15% below ideal body weight or fewer than two binges per week in the preceding three months).

Etiologic Considerations in Comorbidity. Numerous models have been offered to explain the co-occurrence between eating disorders and substance use disorders. Some have argued that eating disorders are themselves addictions (to starvation or bingeing), so that their co-occurrence with substance use disorder reflects a diathesis toward addiction in general (Brisman & Siegel, 1984). Others have suggested a common origin in serotonergic dysfunction (Goldbloom, 1993a), resulting in an obsessive-compulsive spectrum problem (Rothenberg. 1990). Another proposed causal link between the two conditions is that of reciprocal reinforcement; that is, increased drug use and binge eating following food deprivation (Krahn, 1991).

The pharmacologic effects of the drugs abused, particularly stimulants, also may cause or exacerbate eating disorder symptoms. From this perspective, eating problems in persons with substance use disorder could be the direct consequences of heavy substance use, whereas drug use could be understood as a means to control appetite (Schuckit, Tipp et al., 1996). An alternative explanation is that the two disorders may represent different expressions of an underlying personality profile (Beary, Lacey et al., 1986; Lacey & Mourelli, 1986)—one that is characterized by impulse dyscontrol and deficits in affect regulation. From this perspective, the eating disorder and substance use symptoms both would represent self-regulating behaviors (Grilo, Levy et al., 1995).

Still other researchers have suggested that both disorders are mediated by sexual trauma or depression (Lucas, 1996). Dansky and colleagues (1997) maintain that bulimic women who have posttraumatic stress disorder (PTSD) and depression use alcohol and their eating disorder behaviors to cope maladaptively with depression and anxiety. Finally, family data have highlighted similar risk factors in the childhood experiences and family dynamics of women who develop either a substance use or an eating disorder (Minuchin, Rosman et al., 1978; Kaye, Lilenfeld et al., 1996).

One significant predictor of poor outcome (Rastan, Gillberg et al., 1995) for anorexia is the presence of a comorbid personality disorder, which also is associated with an increased likelihood of substance abuse among anorectic individuals (Braun, Sunday et al., 1994). In contrast to those anorectics who exhibit the restricting subtype (marked by caloric restriction and excessive exercise), those who engage in bingeing and purging demonstrate higher rates of impulsive behaviors, such as substance abuse (APA, 1993). Among bulimic individuals, Braun and colleagues (1994) found that the most prevalent group of personality disorders was that of cluster B (dramatic, emotional, or erratic disorders). Thirty percent of bulimic individuals without a history of anorexia and 47% of bulimics with a history of anorexia met criteria for a cluster B personality disorder, with borderline personality disorder occurring most frequently. Another group of researchers (Bulik, Sullivan et al., 1997) found that women with comorbid bulimia nervosa and alcohol dependence had a significantly greater prevalence of any personality disorder than did other bulimic women. These researchers have suggested that bulimic women with comorbid alcohol dependence are distinguished by the presence of borderline personality disorder and the associated trait of impulsiveness.

Family/Genetic Relationships Between Substance Use and Eating Disorders. Family transmission studies have explored patterns of co-occurrence of substance use disorders and eating disorders in an effort to elucidate their modes of inheritance. Several studies have found that bulimia and substance use disorder segregate independently in families. It appears that the prevalence of alcohol or drug dependence is increased only among the first-degree relatives of bulimic women who themselves have a substance use disorder (Bulik, 1987; Kaye, Lilenfeld et al., 1996; Mitchell,

Pomeroy et al., 1988). Among a large cohort of alcohol-dependent probands and their relatives, Schuckit and colleagues (1996) found no evidence of strong familial transmission between alcohol dependence and bulimia. And in a large study of female twins, Kendler and colleagues (1995) found that most of the genetic variation influencing vulnerability to alcoholism in women was unrelated to the genetic factors influencing liability for bulimia, anxiety, or depression. Taken together, this evidence suggests that bulimia and substance use disorder, while frequently coexisting within individuals or families, are not different manifestations of a single underlying etiology. Instead, different familial factors appear to give rise to each of these disorders (Lilenfeld, Kaye et al., 1997).

Lilenfeld and colleagues (1997) have suggested that women with comorbid bulimia and substance dependence may carry two clusters of vulnerability factors shared by family members: those needed to develop an eating disorder (such as perfectionism and low self-esteem) and those needed to develop early-onset alcoholism (such as behavioral undercontrol and negative emotionality). The researchers assessed Axis I and II psychiatric history in bulimia probands and their first-degree relatives. They found a relatively young age of onset of substance dependence among bulimia probands with comorbid substance dependence (mean age of onset=16.2 years), a finding replicated by Bulik and colleagues (1997). Early-onset (younger than age 25) substance dependence among women has been described by Hill (1995) as a subtype marked by impulsivity and affective instability, similar to type 2 alcoholism in males (Cloninger, Brohman et al., 1981). Citing these findings, Lilenfeld and colleagues (1997) suggested that women with bulimia and comorbid substance dependence may represent a group with familial early-onset alcoholism, related to type 2 alcoholism in males.

Comorbidity Studies. The research shows widely varying rates of comorbidity, depending on how samples were chosen, what criteria were employed, and which eating disorder was studied (for a review, see Holderness, Brooks-Gunn et al., 1994). The rate of substance abuse among bulimics ranges from 10% to 88%, with a median of 22%, whereas the rate of bulimia among persons with substance use disorder ranges from 3% to 48%, with a median of 23%. The *DSM-IV* divides anorectics into two subcategories, restrictors and bingers, while it divides bulimics into purging and non-purging types. Several studies of inpatient and outpatient populations suggest that the risk for substance abuse is a function of how "bulimic" the person is (Herzog, Nussbaum et al., 1996). Anorectics who binge are said to be at greater risk than are anorectics who restrict their food intake. Likewise, bulimics who purge are said to be more at risk than bulimics who do not purge. One carefully executed family study suggested separate vulnerabilities were involved for bulimia and substance use disorder (Kaye, Lilenfeld et al., 1996). Some argue that the eating disorders are themselves addictions (to starvation or bingeing), so that co-occurrence is a function of a general vulnerability to addiction (Brisman & Siegal, 1984). Others argue for a common psychobiological diathesis, perhaps involving serotonin (Goldbloom, 1993b) or an obsessive-compulsive spectrum problem (Rothenberg, 1990). Still others believe that the link to substance abuse is merely the consequence of shared risk factors.

Some believe that the link to substance abuse is merely the consequence of shared risk factors. The "addiction to starvation" model does not explain why restricting anorectics are not at increased risk for other addictive disorders (Herzog, Nussbaum et al., 1996). Some who support the notion of a link among risk factors point out that bulimics with substance use disorders show impulsive personality profiles on the MMPI or SCID II (Herzog, Nussbaum et al., 1996). Others focus on the dysfunctional family dynamics in the childhoods of persons with substance use disorders and bulimia as the point of contact. Still others look to sexual trauma or depression as mediating both the substance use and the bulimia (Lucas, 1996). As noted earlier, family data suggest that the latter disorders share the same risk factors rather than being different manifestations of the same problem (Kaye, Lilenfeld et al., 1996).

Treatment and Prognosis. Behavioral, pharmacologic, psychodynamic, and family therapies have been used to treat eating disordered patients. All have been reported to be helpful to some patients. Anorexia is a potentially fatal disorder that follows a chronic, relapsing course in those patients who do not recover quickly. Bulimic patients tend to have a better prognosis, with more spontaneous remissions, but there is a marked tendency for relapse.

Effect of Substance Use on the Treatment of Eating Disorders: The effect of alcohol or illicit drug use on the outcome of treatment for eating disorders remains unclear. Although some early studies suggested that alcohol problems in bulimic women led to poorer outcomes for eating disorders (Lacey, 1983), others found that alcohol abuse does not exert any effect on eating disorder treatment outcomes (Goldbloom, 1993b). However, Sinha and O'Malley (2000) point out that these studies suffer from methodological limitations, such as small sample size and inadequate monitoring of both alcohol and eating disorder outcomes.

Strasser and colleagues (1992) examined the significance of a history of substance abuse on the treatment of bulimia. They found certain differences at presentation between those with and without a history of substance abuse. Patients with a history of substance abuse were significantly older at presentation for treatment and reported higher levels of anxiety and depression than those without such histories. However, on all outcome measures, the improvement of the substance abuse group was equal to or greater than that in the group without histories of substance abuse. Those with a history of substance abuse who received active medication (desipramine) reported lower levels of anxiety and depression at termination than did those on active medication who lacked such a history. These results suggest that a history of substance abuse does not negatively affect response to psychotherapeutic or pharmacologic treatments of bulimia. These findings are consistent with those of Mitchell and colleagues (1990), who reported that bulimic patients with and without histories of substance abuse achieved similar long-term outcomes in a cognitive-behavioral group therapy program. Mitchell and colleagues (1990) further noted that bulimic patients with a history of alcohol and substance abuse did not experience an excess risk for relapse to substance use when their bulimic behavior was brought under control.

A number of important clinical research questions remain to be addressed. For example, Sinha and O'Malley (2000) point out that no studies have sought to determine whether specific eating disturbances (such as weight concerns or bingeing behaviors) affect the outcome of alcoholism treatment or the long-term prognosis of the subgroup of alcoholic women with eating disorders. (For instance, the combined effects of alcoholism and an eating disorder may produce more frequent medical problems or an associated increased morbidity, and these in turn may influence the outcome of both disorders.)

Effect of Eating Disorders on Treatment for Substance Use: Given the high comorbidity between eating disorders and substance dependence, an important question is whether the sequence of illness development—whether the eating disorder predated the substance dependence (EDSD) or the substance dependence predated the eating disorder (SDED)—reflects differences in underlying psychopathol-

ogy and has implications for the course of illness and treatment outcomes. One group of researchers (Wiseman, Sunday et al., 1999) found that the chronology of the eating disorder and the substance use disorder is a critical factor in the degree of psychopathology observed in these patients. For example, although SDED patients use more substances, they appear to have less overall underlying psychopathology than do EDSD patients. Compared with ED-only and SDED patients, EDSD patients have higher rates of obsessive-compulsive disorder, panic, and social phobia. These findings are consistent with previous research linking bulimia and obsessive-compulsive disorder to serotonergic dysregulation (Hsu, Kaye et al., 1993). Wiseman and colleagues (1999) suggest that the differences in pathology may be explained by the fact that patients who initially have an eating disorder may fail to reduce anxiety by bingeing or purging and then go on to use substances to reduce their anxiety.

Evidence from preclinical studies suggests that endogenous opioid peptide (EOP) activity modulates the intake of both food and alcohol (Cooper & Kirkham, 1993; Reid, Delconte et al., 1991). Dysregulation in the EOP system has been associated with excessive alcohol intake and eating pathology (Sinha & O'Malley, 2000). Other neurotransmitter systems (including serotonin, GABA, and dopamine) play a role in modulating food and alcohol intake (Mercer & Holder, 1997). The serotonin and GABA systems are implicated in anxiety and depressive disorders, which frequently co-occur with alcoholism and eating disorders (Cornelius, Ihsam et al. 1997; Litten & Allen, 1995).

The apparent association between EOP dysregulation and alcoholism is supported by clinical trials demonstrating the efficacy of opioid antagonists such as naltrexone and nalmefene in the treatment of both alcoholism and eating disorders (Mason, Salvato et al., 1999). Naltrexone has been found to reduce alcohol use and relapse rates and to promote abstinence among alcoholic patients (Anton, Moak et al., 1999; O'Malley, Croop et al., 1995; Volpicelli, Alterman et al., 1992). Jonas and Gold (1987) reported that naltrexone significantly reduced the duration of binges in normal-weight bulimics, whereas imipramine produced a significant reduction in the duration of binges in obese bulimics. Another study found naltrexone to be effective in breaking the binge cycle among 82.4% of patients with eating disorders (Marrazzi, Bacon et al., 1995). While these studies suggest that naltrexone may be beneficial in the treatment of a subgroup of bulimics, they have been limited by small sample sizes and the exclusion of women with comorbid eating and alcohol use disorders, as suggested by Sinha and O'Malley (2000).

Another class of medications that offer potential benefits to women with concurrent alcohol use and eating disorders is the selective serotonin reuptake inhibitors (SSRIs). Evidence from recent studies suggests that fluoxetine reduces alcohol consumption in samples of alcoholics (Litten & Allen, 1995) and in depressed alcoholics (Cornelius, Ihsam et al., 1997). Fluoxetine also has shown efficacy in reducing bingeing and purging behavior among bulimic subjects (Fluoxetine Bulimia Nervosa Collaborative Study Group, 1992). While fluoxetine may be beneficial in reducing alcohol consumption, more research is needed to examine whether such agents offer benefits with respect to both eating and alcohol use disorders in individuals with both problems.

Psychotherapeutic interventions represent another important approach to be explored in developing treatments for combined substance use and eating disorders. For example, short-term cognitive-behavioral therapy (CBT) has proved helpful in the treatment of both alcohol use (Kadden, Carroll et al., 1992: Monti, Abrams et al., 1989) and eating disorders (Agras, Walsh et al., 2000). Patients with comorbid alcohol and eating disorders are likely to benefit from CBT that targets both sets of problem behaviors through interventions such as self-monitoring records, identifying high-risk situations, and using coping skills to manage negative internal states (such as anger, dysphoria, and boredom) or external events (such as stressful social situations or triggers). Techniques such as coping with cravings or using problem-solving skills can be learned and applied to high-risk situations for both bingeing and drinking (Sinha & O'Malley, 2000).

Giannini and colleagues (1998) have suggested that Twelve Step programs also may be effective in the treatment of both eating disorders and substance use disorders, since both behavioral patterns reflect a loss of control.

Summary. A number of explanatory models have been put forth to explain the high rates of comorbidity between eating disorders and substance use disorders. These etiological frameworks have ranged from posited serotonergic dysfunction, to self-regulation of mood or anxiety syndromes, to a common developmental trauma giving rise to both types of disorders. Despite this etiologic uncertainty, it is clear that the two disorders co-occur at impressively high rates, and that both often are accompanied by a mood or anxiety disorder, or by character or behavioral pathology that contributes to the overall severity of the clinical picture.

Treatment-focused research questions that warrant investigation center on the means by which comorbidity is diagnosed and the timeframes during which outcome assessments are carried out. While the majority of studies examining the effects of substance abuse on the outcome of treatment for eating disorder have not found significant differences between those with and without a history of substance abuse (Mitchell, Pyle et al., 1990; Strasser, Pike et al., 1992; Collings & King, 1994), such studies have looked at a history of substance abuse rather than current substance abuse or dependence. Further studies are needed to examine the effects of current substance use on treatment outcomes for eating disorders (Bulik, Sullivan et al., 1997; Wonderlich & Mitchell, 1997).

A second important dimension of this research concerns the point at which treatment outcome is assessed. In order to determine whether the prognosis for women with comorbid alcoholism and eating disorders is equivalent or worse than the prognosis for women with either disorder alone, future studies will need to assess the status of both the alcohol and eating disorder at intake, during treatment, and at followup (Sinha & O'Malley, 2000).

Research in this field has not yet focused on establishing a careful account of the phenomenology of the relationship between eating disorder symptomatology and substance use. Intriguing preliminary observations in this domain include the fact that bulimics do not typically incorporate alcohol into their food binges (Gendall, Sullivan et al., 1997), yet in one study, 44% of bulimic patients identified alcohol consumption as a trigger for binge eating (Abraham & Beumont, 1982). Clearly, more information is needed on the substance use patterns of eating disordered individuals.

As noted by Wolfe and Maisto (2000), another general criticism of the extant research is that knowledge from substance abuse research and eating disorder research has not been integrated sufficiently. For example, knowledge about cognitive styles and affective changes in bulimics could be applied by researchers investigating the relationship between eating and substance use disorders. Through the use of semistructured interviews, investigators might learn whether bulimics' use of substances is functionally related to fluctuations in unpleasant affective states or to the occurrence of dichotomous cognitions (for example, "Well, I've already eaten something I shouldn't have; I may as well go hog wild"). One potentially promising approach is a functional analysis using behavioral assessment techniques to identify situational, cognitive, and behavioral factors that predict substance use or eating disorder patterns. Daily self-monitoring, which is a central component of cognitive-behavioral therapy for bulimia (Fairburn, Norman et al., 1995), could be expanded to include alcohol consumption and other substance use, as well as associated situational, affective, or cognitive events (Wolfe & Maisto, 2000).

In considering treatment effectiveness with respect to these two disorders, it must be said that, at present, no definitive treatment approaches have been developed to target specifically the subgroup of patients with concurrent substance use and eating disorders. Certainly, the integration of multiple treatment modalities is more likely to produce therapeutic benefits than any single treatment alone. Clearly, there is a need to develop expanded treatment options that take into account the overlapping features of these often co-occurring disorders. Whether this comorbid group would benefit from a pharmacotherapeutic approach targeting both serotonergic and opioid systems, or from an integrated psychotherapeutic approach addressing both substance use and eating, remains an open question.

CONCLUSIONS

Although various treatment approaches have been presented here, there are no definitive treatments for persons with co-occurring substance use and adult ADHD or eating disorders. As emphasized earlier, the integration of multiple treatment modalities is more likely to produce therapeutic benefits than any single treatment alone. The search for creative and clinically sound pharmacologic and nonpharmacologic approaches for these dually disordered patient populations is long overdue.

ACKNOWLEDGEMENT: The research for this chapter has been supported by the following grants from the National Institute on Drug Abuse: DA00465 (Dr. Levin), K23 DA00433 (Dr. Sullivan), and K02 DA00451-01A1 (Dr. Donovan).

REFERENCES

Abraham SF & Beaumont PJV (1982). How patients describe bulimia or binge eating. *Psychological Medicine* 12:625-635.

Agras WS, Walsh BT et al. (2000). A multicenter comparison of cognitive-behavioral therapy and interpersonal psychotherapy for bulimia nervosa. *Archives of General Psychiatry* 57:459-466.

American Psychiatric Association (APA) (1980). *Diagnostic and Statistical Manual of Mental Disorders, 3rd Edition (DSM-III).* Washington, DC: American Psychiatric Press.

American Psychiatric Association (APA) (1987). *Diagnostic and Statistical Manual of Mental Disorders, 3rd Edition, Revised (DSM-IIIR).* Washington, DC: American Psychiatric Press.

American Psychiatric Association (APA) (1994). *Diagnostic and Statistical Manual of Mental Disorders, 4th Edition (DSM-IV).* Washington, DC: American Psychiatric Press.

American Psychiatric Association (APA) (1993). *Practice Guidelines for Eating Disorders.* Washington, DC: American Psychiatric Press.

Anton RF, Moak DH, Waid R et al. (1999). Naltrexone and cognitive behavioral therapy for the treatment of out-patient alcoholics: Results of a placebo-controlled trail. *American Journal of Psychiatry* 156:1758-1764.

Applegate B, Lahey B, Hart E et al. (1997). Validity of the age of onset criterion for attention deficit/hyperactivity disorder: A report from the DSM-IV field trials. *Journal of the American Academy of Child and Adolescent Psychiatry* 36:1211-1221.

Arndt IO, Dorozynsky L, Woody GE et al. (1992). Desipramine treatment of cocaine dependence in methadone-maintained patients. *Archives of General Psychiatry* 49:888-893.

Aviram RB, Rhum M & Levin FR (2001). Psychotherapy of adults with comorbid attention deficit hyperactivity disorder and psychoactive substance use disorder. *Journal of Psychotherapy Practice and Research.*

Barkley RA (1977). A review of stimulant drug research on hyperactive children. *Journal of Child and Psychological Psychiatry* 18:137-165.

Barkley RA & Biederman J (1997). Toward a broader definition of the age of onset criterion for attention deficit hyperactivity disorder. *Journal of the American Academy of Child and Adolescent Psychiatry* 36:1204-1210.

Barkley RA, Murphy K & Kwasnik D (1996). Psychological adjustment and adaptive impairments in young adults with ADHD. *Journal of Attention Disorders* 1:41-54.

Beary MD, Lacey JH & Merry J (1986). Alcoholism and eating disorders in women of fertile age. *British Journal of Addictions* 81:685-689.

Berkson J (1946). Limitations of the application of four-fold table analysis to hospital data. *Biometric Bulletin* 2:37-46.

Biederman J, Faraone SV, Keenan K et al. (1990). Family-genetic and psychosocial risk factors in DSM-III attention deficit disorder. *Journal of American Academy of Child and Adolescent Psychiatry* 29:526-533.

Biederman J, Faraone SV, Keenan SV et al. (1992). Further evidence for family-genetic risk factors in attention deficit hyperactivity disorder. *Archives of General Psychiatry* 49:728-738.

Biederman J, Faraone SV, Spencer T et al. (1993). Patterns of psychiatric co-morbidity, cognition, and psychosocial functioning in adults with attention deficit hyperactivity disorder. *American Journal of Psychiatry* 150:1792-1798.

Biederman J, Mick E, Faraone SV et al. (2000). Age dependent decline of ADHD symptoms revisited: Impact of remission definition and symptom subtype. *American Journal of Psychiatry* 157:816-818.

Biederman J, Wilens T, Mick E et al. (1995). Psychoactive substance use disorders in adults with attention deficit hyperactivity disorder (ADHD): Effects of ADHD and psychiatric comorbidity. *American Journal of Psychiatry* 152:1652-1658.

Biederman J, Wilens TE, Mick E et al. (1998). Does attention deficit hyperactivity disorder impact the developmental course of drug and alcohol abuse and dependence? *Biological Psychiatry* 44:269-73.

Biederman J, Wilens T, Mick E et al. (1999). Pharmacotherapy of attention deficit/hyperactivity disorder reduces risk for substance use disorder. *Pediatrics* 104:1-5.

Borland B & Heckman H (1976). Hyperactive boys and their brothers. *Archives of General Psychiatry* 33:669-675.

Braun DL, Sunday SR & Halmi KA (1994). Psychiatric comorbidity with eating disorders. *Psychological Medicine* 24:859.

Brisman J & Siegal M (1984). Bulimia and alcoholism: Two sides of the same coin? *Journal of Substance Abuse Treatment* 1:113-118.

Brooner et al. (1997). Psychiatric and substance use comorbidity among treatment-seeking opioid abusers. *Archives of General Psychiatry* 54:71-80.

Brumberg JJ (1988). *Fasting Girls: The Emergence of Anorexia Nervosa as a Modern Disease*. Cambridge, MA: Harvard University Press.

Bulik C (1987). Drug and alcohol abuse in bulimic women and their families. *American Journal of Psychiatry* 44:1604-1606.

Bulik CM, Sullivan RF, Carter FA et al. (1997). Lifetime comorbidity of alcohol dependence in women with bulimia nervosa. *Addictive Behaviors* 22(4):437-446.

Carroll KM, Nich C & Rounsaville BJ (1995). Differential symptom reduction in depressed cocaine abusers treated with psychotherapy and pharmacotherapy. *Journal of Nervous and Mental Disease* 183:251-259.

Carroll KM & Rounsaville BJ (1993). History and significance of childhood attention deficit disorder in treatment-seeking cocaine abusers. *Comprehensive Psychiatry* 34:75-86.

Cavanaugh R, Clifford JST & Gregory WL (1989). The use of bromocriptine for the treatment of attention deficit disorder in two chemically dependent patients. *Journal of Psychoactive Drugs* 21:217-220.

Cloninger CR, Brohman M & Sigvardsson S (1981). Inheritance of alcohol abuse: Cross-fostering of analysis of adopted men. *Archives of General Psychiatry* 38(8):861-968.

Clure C, Brady KT, Saladin ME et al. (1999). Attention deficit/hyperactivity disorder and substance use: Symptom pattern and drug choice. *American Journal of Drug and Alcohol Abuse* 25:441-448.

Cochrane C, Malcome R & Brewerton T (1998). The role of weight control as a motivation for cocaine abuse. *Addictive Behaviors* 23(2):201-207.

Cocores JA, Davies RK, Mueller PS et al. (1987). Cocaine abuse and adult attention disorder. *Journal of Clinical Psychiatry* 48:376-377.

Cocores JA, Patel MD, Gold MS et al. (1987). Cocaine abuse, attention deficit disorder, and bipolar disorder. *Journal of Nervous and Mental Disease* 175:431-432.

Collings S & King M (1994). Ten year follow-up of 50 patients with bulimia nervosa. *British Journal of Psychiatry* 164:80-87.

Cook EH, Stein MA, Krasnowski MD et al. (1995). Association of attention deficit disorder and the dopamine transporter gene. *American Journal of Human Genetics* 56:993-98.

Cooper SJ & Kirkham TC (1993). Opioid mechanisms in the control of food consumption and taste preferences. In A Herz (ed.) *Handbook of Experimental Pharmacology, Vol. 104*. Berlin, Germany: Springer-Verlag, 239-261.

Cornelius JR, Ihsam MS, Ehler JG et al. (1997). Fluoxetine in depressed alcoholics—A double-blind, placebo-controlled trial. *Archives of General Psychiatry* 54:700-705.

Dansereau DF, Joe GW & Simpson DD (1995). Attentional difficulties and the effectiveness of a visual representation strategy for counseling drug-addicted clients. *International Journal on Addictions* 30:371-386.

Dansky BS, Brewerton TD, O'Neil PM et al. (1997). The National Women's Study: Relationship of crime victimization and PTSD to bulimia nervosa. *International Journal of Eating Disorders* 21:213-228.

Dees SM, Dansereau DF & Simpson DD (1994). A visual representation system for drug abuse counselors. *Journal of Substance Abuse Treatment* 11:517-523.

Diamond IR, Tannock R & Schachar RJ (1999). Response to methylphenidate in children with ADHD and comorbid anxiety. *Journal of the American Academy of Child and Adolescent Psychiatry* 38:402-409.

Dougherty DD, Bonab AA, Spencer TJ et al. (1999). Dopamine transporter density in patients with attention deficit hyperactivity disorder. *Lancet* 354:2132-2133.

Erikson E (1950). *Childhood and Society*. New York, NY: W.W. Norton.

Eyre SL, Rounsaville BJ & Kleber HD (1982). History of childhood hyperactivity in a clinic population of opiate addicts. *Journal of Nervous and Mental Disease* 170:522-529.

Fairburn CG & Beglin S (1990). Studies of the epidemiology of bulimia nervosa. *American Journal of Psychiatry* 147:401-408.

Fairburn CG, Norman PA, Welch SL et al. (1995). A prospective study of outcome in bulimia nervosa and the long term effects of three psychological treatments. *Archives of General Psychiatry* 52:304-312.

Faraone SV, Biederman J, Spencer T et al. (2000). Attention deficit/hyperactivity disorder in adults: An overview. *Biological Psychiatry* 48:9-20.

Faraone SV, Biederman J, Weiffenbach B et al. (1999). Dopamine D4 gene 7-repeat allele and attention deficit hyperactivity disorder. *American Journal of Psychiatry* 156:768-770.

Fichter M, Quadfieg N & Rief W (1994). Longer term course (6 year) of bulimia nervosa. *Neuropsychopharmacology* 10:772.

Findlay RL, Schwartz MA, Flannery DJ et al. (1996). Venlafaxine in adults with attention deficit/hyperactivity disorder: An open clinical trial. *Journal of Clinical Psychiatry* 57:184-189.

Fischman MW, Foltin RW, Nestadt G et al. (1990). Effects of desipramine maintenance on cocaine self-administration in humans. *Journal of Pharmacological and Experimental Therapeutics* 253:760-770.

Fluoxetine Bulimia Nervosa Collaborative Study Group (1992). Fluoxetine in the treatment of bulimia nervosa—A multicenter, placebo-controlled, double-blind trial. *Archives of General Psychiatry* 49:139-147.

Gawin FH & Kleber HD (1986). Abstinence symptomatology and psychiatric diagnosis in cocaine abusers: Clinical observations. *Archives of General Psychiatry* 43:107-113.

Gawin FH, Kleber HD, Byck R et al. (1989). Desipramine facilitation of initial cocaine abstinence. *Archives of General Psychiatry* 46:117-121.

Gawin F, Riordan C & Kleber H (1985). Methylphenidate treatment of cocaine abusers without attention deficit disorder: A negative report. *American Journal of Drug and Alcohol Abuse* 11:193.

Gendall KA, Sullivan PE, Jove PR et al. (1997). The nutrient intake of women with bulimia nervosa. *International Journal of Eating Disorders* 21:115-127.

Giannini AJ, Keller M, Colapietro G et al. (1998). Comparison of alternative treatment techniques in bulimia: The chemical dependency approach. *Psychological Reports* 82:451-458.

Gill M, Daly G, Heron S et al. (1997). Confirmation of association between attention deficit disorder and a dopamine transporter polymorphism. *Molecular Psychiatry* 2:311-313.

Gittleman R, Mannuzza S, Shenker R et al. (1985). Hyperactive boys almost grown up: I. Psychiatric status. *Archives of General Psychiatry* 42:937-947.

Gold MS, Johnson CR & Stennie K (1997). Related compulsive and addictive behaviors: Eating disorders. In JH Lowinson, RB Millman & JG Langrod JG (eds). *Substance Abuse: A Comprehensive Textbook, 3rd Edition.* Baltimore, MD: Wiliams & Wilkins, 319-330.

Goldbloom DS (1993a). Alcohol misuse and eating disorders: Aspects of an association. *Alcohol and Alcoholism* 28(4):375-381.

Goldbloom DS (1993b). Eating disorders among women receiving treatment for an alcohol problem. *International Journal of Eating Disorders* 14:147-1.

Grabowski J, Roache JD, Schmitz JM et al. (1997). Replacement medication for cocaine dependence: Methylphenidate. *Journal of Clinical Psychopharmacology* 17:485-488.

Greenfield B, Hectman L & Weiss G (1988). Two subgroups of hyperactives as adults: Correlations of outcome. *Canadian Journal of Psychiatry* 33:505-508.

Greenhill LL (1992). Psychopharmacology: Stimulants. In G Weiss (ed.) *Child and Adolescent Psychiatric Clinics of North America.* Philadelphia, PA: W.B. Saunders, 411-447.

Grilo CM, Levy KN, Becker DF et al. (1995). Eating disorders in female inpatients with versus without substance use disorders. *Addictive Behaviors* 20(2):255-260.

Halmi KA (1974). Anorexia nervosa: Demographic and clinical features in 94 cases. *Psychosomatic Medicine* 36:18-26.

Hatsukami D, Mitchell JE, Eckert E et al. (1986). Characteristics of patients with bulimia only, mania with affective disorder and bulimia with substance abuse problems. *Addictive Behaviors* 11:399-406.

Herzog DB, Nussbaum KM & Marmor AK (1996). Comorbidity and outcome in eating disorders. *Psychiatric Clinics of North America* 19:843-859.

Higgins ST, Delaney DD, Budney et al. (1994). A behavioral approach to achieving initial cocaine abstinence. *American Journal of Psychiatry* 148:1218-1224.

Hill J & Schoener E (1996). Age-dependent decline of attention deficit hyperactivity disorder. *American Journal of Psychiatry* 153:1143-1146.

Hill SY (1995). Neurobiological and clinical markers for a severe form of alcoholism in women. *Alcohol Health and Research World* 19:249-256.

Hoffman BB et al. (1996). Catecholamines, sympathomimetic drugs and adrenergic receptor agonists. In JG Jardman & LE Limbird (eds.) *Goodman & Gilman's The Pharmacological Basis of Therapeutics.* New York, NY: McGraw-Hill, 199-263.

Holderness CC, Brooks-Gunn J & Warren MP (1994). Co-morbidity of eating disorders and substance abuse review of the literature. *International Journal of Eating Disorders* 16:1-34.

Hsu L, Kaye W & Weltzin T (1993). Are the eating disorders related to obsessive compulsive disorder? *International Journal of Eating Disorders* 14:305-318.

Hudson JI, Weiss RD, Pope HG et al. (1992). Eating disorders in hospitalized substance abusers. *American Journal of Drug and Alcohol Abuse* 18(1):75-85.

Jonas JM & Gold MS (1987). The use of opiate antagonists in treating bulimia: A study of low-dose versus high-dose naltrexone. *Psychiatry Research* 24:195-199.

Jonas JM, Gold MS, Sweeney D et al. (1987). Eating disorders and cocaine abuse: A survey of 259 cocaine abusers. *Journal of Clinical Psychiatry* 48:47-50.

Kadden R, Carroll K, Donovan D et al. (1992). *Cognitive-Behavioral Coping Skills Therapy Manual: A Clinical Research Guide for Therapists Treating Individuals with Alcohol Abuse and Dependence.* Rockville, MD: National Institute on Alcohol Abuse and Alcoholism.

Katz JL (1990). Eating disorders: A primer for the substance abuse specialist: 1. Clinical features. *Journal of Substance Abuse Treatment* 7:143-149.

Kaye WH, Lilenfeld LR, Plotnicov K et al. (1996). Bulimia nervosa and substance dependence: Association and family transmission. *Alcoholism: Clinical & Experimental Research* 20:878-881.

Kendler KS, Maculae C, Neil M et al. (1991). The genetic epidemiology of bulimia nervosa. *American Journal of Psychiatry* 148:1627-1637.

Kendler KS, Walters EE, Neale MC et al. (1995). The structure of the genetic and environmental risk factors for six major psychiatric disorders in women. *Archives of General Psychiatry* 52:374-383.

Kessler RC, McGonagle KA, Zhao S et al. (1994). Lifetime and 12-month prevalence of DSM-IIIR psychiatric disorders in the United States. *Archives of General Psychiatry* 51:8-19.

Khantzian EJ (1983). An extreme case of cocaine dependence and marked improvement with methylphenidate treatment. *American Journal of Psychiatry* 140:484-485.

Khantzian EJ, Gawin FH, Riordan C et al. (1984). Methylphenidate treatment for cocaine dependence: A preliminary report. *Journal of Substance Abuse Treatment* 1:107-112.

King VL, Brooner RK, Kidorf MS et al. (1999). Attention deficit hyperactivity disorder and treatment outcome in opioid abusers entering treatment. *Journal of Nervous and Mental Disease* 187:487-95.

Kosten TR (1992). Can cocaine craving be a medication development outcome? Drug craving and relapse in opioid and cocaine dependence. *American Journal on Addictions* 1:230-237.

Kosten TR, Morgan CM, Falcione J et al. (1992). Pharmacotherapy for cocaine-abusing methadone-maintained patients using amantadine or desipramine. *Archives of General Psychiatry* 49:894-898.

Krahn DD (1991). The relationship of eating disorders and substance abuse. *Journal of Substance Abuse Treatment* 3:239-253.

Lacey JH (1983). Bulimia nervosa, binge eating, and psychogenic vomiting: A controlled treatment study and long term outcome. *British Medical Journal (Clinical Research Edition)* 286(6378):1609-1613.

Lacey JH & Mourelli E (1986). Bulimic alcoholics: Some features of a clinical sub-group. *British Journal of Addictions* 81:389-393.

Lahoste GJ, Swanson JM, Wigal SB et al. (1996). Dopamine D4 receptor gene polymorphism is associated with attention deficit hyperactivity disorder. *Molecular Psychiatry* 121-124.

Lambert NM & Hartsough CS (1998). Prospective study of tobacco smoking and substance dependencies among samples of ADHD and non-ADHD participants. *Journal of Learning Disabilities* 31:533-44.

Levin FR, Evans SM & Kleber HD (1998a). Prevalence of adult attention deficit hyperactivity disorder among cocaine abusers seeking treatment. *Drug and Alcohol Dependence* 52(1):15-25.

Levin FR, Evans SM, McDowell DM et al. (1998b). Methylphenidate for cocaine abusers with adult attention deficit hyperactivity disorder: A pilot study. *Journal of Clinical Psychiatry*.

Levin FR, Evans SM, McDowell DM et al. (2002). Bupropion treatment for cocaine abuse and adult attention-deficit/hyperactivity disorder. *Journal of Addictive Diseases* 21(2):1-16.

Lilenfeld LR, Kaye WH, Greeno CG et al. (1997). Psychiatric disorders in women with bulimia nervosa and their first-degree relatives: Effects of comorbid substance dependence. *International Journal of Eating Disorders* 22:253-264.

Litten RZ & Allen JP (1995). Pharmacotherapy for alcoholics with collateral depression or anxiety: An update of research findings. *Experimental & Clinical Psychopharmacology* 3:87-93.

Lucas AR (1996). Anorexia nervosa and bulimia nervosa. In M Lewis (ed.) *Child and Adolescent Psychiatry: A Comprehensive Textbook*. Baltimore, MD: Williams & Wilkins, 586-593.

Mannuzza S, Klein RG, Bessler A et al. (1993). Adult outcome of hyperactive boys: Educational achievement, occupational rank, and psychiatric status. *Archives of General Psychiatry* 50:565-576.

Mannuzza S, & Klein RG (2000). Long-term prognosis in attention-deficit/hyperactivity disorder. *Child and Adolescent Psychiatric Clinics of North America* 9(3):711-726.

Mannuzza S, Klein RG, Bonagura N et al. (1991). Hyperactive boys almost grown up: V. Replication of psychiatric status. *Archives of General Psychiatry* 48:77-83.

Margolin A, Kosten TR, Avants SK et al. (1995). A multicenter trial of bupropion for cocaine dependence in methadone-maintained patients. *Drug and Alcohol Dependence* 40:125-131.

Marrazzi MA, Bacon JP, Kinzie J et al. (1995). Naltrexone use in the treatment of anorexia nervosa and bulimia nervosa. *International Clinical Psychopharmacology* 10(3):163-172.

Mason BJ, Salvato FR, Williams LD et al. (1999). A double-blind, placebo-controlled study of oral nalmefene for alcohol dependence. *Archives of General Psychiatry* 56:719-724.

Mattes JA, Boswell L & Oliver H (1984). Methylphenidate effects on symptoms of attention deficit disorder in adults. *Archives of General Psychiatry* 41:1059-1063.

Mercer MG & Holder MD (1997). Food cravings: endogenous opioid peptides and food intake: A review. *Appetite* 29:325-352.

Milberger S, Biederman J, Faraone SV et al. (1997). Association between ADHD and psychoactive substance use disorders. Findings from a longitudinal study of high-risk siblings of ADHD children. *American Journal on Addictions* 6:318-29.

Minuchin S, Rosman BL et al. (1978). *Psychosomatic Families: Anorexia Nervosa in Context*. Cambridge, MA: Harvard University Press.

Mitchell JE, Pomeroy C & Huber M (1988). A clinician's guide to the eating disorders medicine cabinet. *International Journal of Eating Disorders* 7:211-223.

Mitchell JE, Pyle R, Ekert ED et al. (1990). The influence of prior alcohol and drug abuse problems on bulimia nervosa treatment outcome. *Addictive Behaviors* 15:169-173.

Monti PM, Abrams DB, Kadden RM et al. (1989). *Treating Alcohol Dependence: A Coping Skills Training Guide*. New York, NY: Guilford Press.

Morrison JR & Stewart MA (1971). A family study of the hyperactive child syndrome. *Biological Psychiatry* 3:189-195.

MTA Cooperative Group (1999). The Multimodal Treatment Study of Children with Attention-Deficit/Hyperactivity Disorder (MTA Study). A 14-month randomized clinical trial of treatment strategies for attention-deficit/hyperactivity disorder. *Archives of General Psychiatry* 56(12):1073-1086.

Murphy K & Barkley RA (1996). Prevalence of DSM-IV symptoms of ADHD in adult licensed drivers: Implications for clinical diagnosis. *Journal of Attention Disorders* 1:147-161.

O'Malley SS, Croop RS, Wrobleski JM et al. (1995). Naltrexone in the treatment of alcohol dependence: A combined analysis of two trials. *Psychology Reports* 25:681-688.

Palmer RL (1993). Weight concern should not be a necessary concern for the eating disorders: A polemic. *International Journal of Eating Disorders* 14:459-466.

Paternite CE, Loney J, Salisbury H et al. (1999). Childhood inattention-overactivity, aggression, and stimulant medication history as predictors of young adult outcomes. *Journal of Child and Adolescent Psychopharmacology* 9:169-84.

Pelham WE & Sams SE (1992). Behavior modification. In G Weiss (ed.) *Child and Adolescent Psychiatric Clinics of North America*. Philadelphia, PA: W.B. Saunders, 505-518.

Peluso T, Ricciardelli LA & Williams RJ (1999). Self-control in relation to problem drinking and symptoms of disordered drinking. *Addictive Behaviors* 24(5):715-718.

Pomerleau OF, Downey KK, Stelson FW et al. (1995). Cigarette smoking in adult patients diagnosed with attention deficit/hyperactivity disorder. *Journal of Substance Abuse Treatment* 7:373-378.

Rastan M, Gillberg C & Gillberg C (1995). Anorexia nervosa 6 years after onset: II. Comorbid Psychiatric Problems. *Comprehensive Psychiatry* 36:70.

Reid LD, Delconte JD, Nichols ML et al. (1991). Tests of the opioid deficiency hypotheses of alcoholism. *Alcoholism* 8:247-257.

Regier DA, Farmer ME, Rae DS et al. (1990). Comorbidity of mental disorders with alcohol and other drug abuse: Results from the epidemiologic catchment area (ECA) study. *Journal of the American Medical Association* 264:2511-2518.

Ross H & Ivis F (1999). Binge eating and substance use among male and female adolescents. *International Journal of Eating Disorders* 26:245-260.

Rothenberg A (1990). Adolescence and eating disorder: The obsessive-compulsive syndrome. *Psychiatric Clinics of North America* 13:469-488.

Rounsaville B, Anton SF, Carroll K et al. (1991). Psychiatric diagnoses of treatment-seeking cocaine abusers. *Archives of General Psychiatry* 48:43-51.

Schubiner H, Tzelepis A, Milberger S et al. (2000). Prevalence of attention-deficit/hyperactivity disorder and conduct disorder among substance abusers. *Journal of Clinical Psychiatry* 61(4):244-251.

Schuckit MA, Tipp JE, Anthenelli RM et al. (1996). Anorexia nervosa and bulimia in alcohol-dependent men and women and their relatives. *American Journal of Psychiatry* 153:74-82.

Sinha R & O'Malley SS (2000). Alcohol and eating disorders: Implications for alcohol treatment and health sciences research. *Alcoholism: Clinical & Experimental Research* 24(8):1312-1319.

Smith D (1995). Binge eating in ethnic minority groups. *Addictive Behaviors* 20:695-703.

Spencer T, Biederman J, Wilens T et al. (1994). Is attention deficit hyperactivity disorder in adults a valid disorder? *Harvard Review of Psychiatry* 1:326-335.

Spencer T, Biederman J, Wilens T et al. (1998). Effectiveness and tolerability of tomoxetine in adults with attention deficit hyperactivity disorder.

Spencer T, Wilens T, Biederman J et al. (1995). A double-blind, crossover comparison of methylphenidate and placebo in adults with childhood-onset attention deficit hyperactivity disorder. *Archives of General Psychiatry* 52:434-443.

Spitzer RL & Williams JBW (1985). Classification in psychiatry. In HI Kaplan & BJ Sadock (eds.) *Comprehensive Textbook of Psychiatry, 4th Edition*. Baltimore, MD: Williams & Wilkins, 591-612.

Strasser TJ, Pike KM & Walsh BT (1992). The impact of prior substance abuse on treatment outcome for bulimia nervosa. *Addictive Behaviors* 17:387-395.

Stratton J & Gailfus DA (1998). A new approach to substance abuse treatment: Adolescents and adults with ADHD.

Striegel-Moore RH & Huydic ES (1993). Problem drinking and symptoms of disordered eating in female high school students. *International Journal of Eating Disorders* 14:417-425.

Sullivan MA & Levin FR (2001). Attention deficit/hyperactivity disorder and substance abuse: Diagnostic and therapeutic considerations. In: *Adult Attention Deficit Disorder: Brain Mechanisms and Life Outcomes*. New York, NY: New York Academy of Sciences.

Szatmari P (1992). The epidemiology of attention deficit hyperactivity disorder. In G Weiss (ed.) *Child and Adolescent Psychiatric Clinics of North America*. Philadelphia, PA: W.B. Saunders, 361-384.

Thompson LL, Riggs PD, Mikulich SK et al. (1996). Contribution of ADHD symptoms to substance problems and delinquency in conduct-disordered adolescents. *Journal of Abnormal Child Psychology* 24:325-347.

Volpicelli JR, Alterman AI, Hayashida M et al. (1992). Naltrexone and the treatment of alcohol dependence. *Archives of General Psychiatry* 49:876-880.

Ward MF, Wender PH & Reimherr FW (1993). The Wender Utah Rating Scale (WURS): An aid in the retrospective diagnosis of childhood attention deficit hyperactivity disorder. *American Journal of Psychiatry* 150:885-890.

Weddington WW, Brown BS, Haertzen CA et al. (1991). Comparison of amantidine and desipramine combined with psychotherapy for treatment of cocaine dependence. *American Journal of Drug and Alcohol Abuse* 17:137-152.

Weinstein CS (1994). Cognitive remediation strategies: An adjunct to the psychotherapy of adults with attention deficit hyperactivity disorder. *Journal of Psychotherapy Practice and Research* 3:44-57.

Weiss G & Hechtman LT (1986). Adult hyperactive subjects' view of their treatment in childhood and adolescence. In *Hyperactive Children Grown Up: Empirical Findings and Theoretical Considerations*. New York, NY: Guilford, 293-300.

Weiss M, Hechtman LT & Weiss G (1999). *ADHD in Adulthood: A Guide to Current Theory, Diagnosis, and Treatment*. Baltimore, MD: The Johns Hopkins University Press.

Weiss RD, Mirin SM, Griffin ML et al. (1988). Psychopathology in cocaine abusers: Changing trends. *Journal of Nervous and Mental Disease* 176:719-725.

Weiss RD, Pope HG & Mirin SM (1985). Treatment of chronic cocaine abuse and attention deficit disorder, residual type with magnesium pemoline. *Drug and Alcohol Dependence* 15:69-72.

Wender PH & Garfinkel BD (1989). Attention deficit hyperactivity disorder: Adult manifestations. In HI Sadock & BJ Kaplan BJ (eds.) *Comprehensive Textbook of Psychiatry*. Baltimore, MD: Williams & Wilkins, 1837-1841.

Wilens TE, Biederman J & Mick E (1998). Does ADHD affect the course of substance abuse? Findings from a sample of adults with and without ADHD. *American Journal on Addictions* 7:156-63.

Wilens TE, Biederman J, Prince J et al. (1996). Six-week, double-blind, placebo-controlled study of desipramine for adult attention deficit hyperactivity disorder. *American Journal of Psychiatry* 153:1147-1153.

Wilens TE, Biederman J, Spencer TJ et al. (1999a). A pilot controlled clinical trial of ABT-418, a cholinergic agonist, in the treatment of adults with attention deficit hyperactivity disorder. *American Journal of Psychiatry* 156:1931-7.

Wilens TE, Biederman J, Spencer TJ et al. (1999b). Controlled trial of high doses of pemoline for adults with attention deficit/hyperactivity disorder. *Journal of Clinical Psychopharmacology* 3:257-64.

Wilens TE, Biederman J, Spencer TJ et al. (1995a). Pharmacotherapy of adult attention deficit disorder: A review. *Journal of Clinical Psychopharmacology* 15:270-279.

Wilens TE, Biederman J & Spencer TJ (1995b). Venlafaxine for adult ADHD. *American Journal of Psychiatry* 152(7):1099-1100.

Wilens TE, Spencer TJ, Biederman J et al. (2001). A controlled clinical trial of bupropion for attention deficit hyperactivity disorder in adults. *American Journal of Psychiatry* 158:282-288.

Wilfley DE, Agras WS, Telch CF et al. (1993). Group cognitive-behavioral therapy and group interpersonal psychotherapy for the nonpurging bulimic: A controlled comparison. *Journal of Consulting and Clinical Psychology* 61:296-305.

Winsberg BG & Comings DE (1999). Association of the dopamine transporter gene (DAT1) with poor methylphenidate response. *Journal of the American Academy of Child and Adolescent Psychiatry* 38:1474-1477.

Wiseman CV, Sunday SR, Halligan P et al. (1999). Substance dependence and eating disorders: Impact of sequence on comorbidity. *Comprehensive Psychiatry* 40(5):332-336.

Wolfe WL & Maisto SA (2000). The relationship between eating disorders and substance use: Moving beyond co-prevalence research. *Clinical Psychology Review* 20(5):617-631.

Wonderlich SA & Mitchell JE (1997). Eating disorders and comorbidity: Empirical, conceptual, and clinical implications. *Psychopharmacology Bulletin* 33(3):381-390.

Wonnacott S, Irons J, Rapier C et al. (1989). Presynaptic modulation of transmitter release by nicotinic receptors. *Progressive Brain Research* 79:157-63.

Wood D, Wender PH & Reimherr FW (1983). The prevalence of attention deficit disorder, residual type, or minimal brain dysfunction, in a population of male alcoholic patients. *American Journal of Psychiatry* 140:95-98.

Zametkin AJ, Nordahl TE, Gross M et al. (1990). *New England Journal of Medicine* 323:1361-1366.

Chapter 6

Co-Occurring Addictive and Other Impulse Control Disorders

Susan L. McElroy, M.D.

Cesar A. Soutullo, M.D.

R. Jeffrey Goldsmith, M.D.

Kathleen T. Brady, M.D., Ph.D.

Prevalence of Impulse Control Disorders
Etiology and Course of the Disorders
Treatment and Outcomes for ICDs

For many years, researchers have hypothesized that substance use disorders are forms of impulse control disorders (ICDs) (Esquirol, 1838; Frosch & Wortis, 1954; American Psychiatric Association, 1980, 1987, 1994). More recently, ICDs have been conceptualized as addictive disorders or behavioral addictions (Bradford, Geller et al., 1996; Carnes, 1990; Fishbain, 1987; Goodman, 1997). However, the relationship between ICDs and substance use disorders never has been fully examined. Indeed, to the authors' knowledge, no study has directly compared an ICD and a substance use disorder.

This chapter first provides an historical overview of ICDs as a family of mental disorders. It then summarizes available research suggesting that ICDs and substance use disorders may be related, and discusses the clinical and theoretical implications of such a relationship.

PREVALENCE OF IMPULSE CONTROL DISORDERS

In 1838, Esquirol introduced the term "monomania" to describe a condition in which an individual, acting on an irresistible impulse, engaged in acts he or she deplored and did not want to do. Esquirol cited arson, alcoholism,

impulsive homicide, and (later) kleptomania as examples of such acts (McElroy, Keck et al., 1995a).

At the turn of the century, the terms "pathological impulses" and "reactive impulses" were used to describe these conditions (Bleuler, 1988), which included pyromania, kleptomania, buying mania (oniomania), morbid collecting, impulses "to give everyone a present," anonymous letter writing, and impulsive poison mixing (McElroy, Keck et al., 1995a). Like Esquirol, other authors stressed the impulsive features of these conditions, emphasizing that they may be enacted in an altered state of awareness.

In 1954, Frosch and Wortis examined the relationship between the irresistible impulse and impulsivity in general. They defined an impulse as "the sudden unpremeditated welling-up of a drive toward some action, which usually has the quality of hastiness and a lack of deliberation." They characterized a "morbid" impulse as a "minimal distortion of the original impulse" and an "irresistible and impelling quality in a setting of extreme tension."

Despite this extensive historical literature, the ICDs were not included in the *Diagnostic and Statistical Manuals of Mental Disorders* of the American Psychiatric Association until publication of the third edition (*DSM-III*; 1980). In the *DSM-IV* (1994), the core feature of an ICD is defined as the failure to resist an impulse, drive, or temptation to commit an act that is harmful to the individual or to others. The *DSM-IV* also stipulates that, for most ICDs, the individual feels an increasing sense of tension or arousal before committing the act and then experiences pleasure, gratification, or relief at the time the act is committed. Following the act, the individual may or may not experience genuine regret, self-reproach, or guilt. Thus, ICD symptoms may be ego-syntonic, particularly when relief or even pleasure is experienced at the moment they are enacted. But they also may be ego-dystonic, when the impulses are associated with tension or anxiety and the behaviors generate self-reproach, shame, or guilt.

The *DSM-IV* (like the *DSM-III* and *DSM-IIIR*) does not contain a formal category for ICDs. Rather, ICDs are listed in a residual category: the ICDs Not Elsewhere Classified (which includes intermittent explosive disorder, kleptomania, pathological gambling, pyromania, and trichotillomania), and the ICDs Not Otherwise Specified (NOS). Examples of ICDs NOS are compulsive buying or shopping (also called buying mania or oniomania), repetitive self-mutilation, nonparaphilic sexual addictions (also called sexual compulsions), onychophagia (severe nail biting), compulsive skin picking (also called psychogenic excoriation), and eating disorders characterized by binge eating (bulimia nervosa and binge eating disorder) (McElroy, Keck et al., 1995a, 1995b). In the *DSM-IV* section on ICDs Not Elsewhere Specified, several disorders that are classified elsewhere in the *DSM-IV* are cited as examples of ICDs, although they are not defined as such in their respective categories. These disorders include the substance use disorders, as well as paraphilias, personality disorders with impulsive features, and attention deficit/hyperactivity disorder.

Epidemiology. ICDs generally are presumed to be rare. For example, three recent self-report surveys of hair pulling among college students found that only 0.6%, 1.0%, and 0.005%, respectively, of the populations assessed met the *DSM-IIIR* criteria for trichotillomania (Christenson, Pyle et al., 1991; Rothbaum, Shaw et al., 1993).

However, for most of the established and potential ICDs, systematic studies that employ operational diagnostic criteria to determine prevalence rates in the general population have not been done. Thus, there are no systematically collected data regarding the prevalence in the general population of intermittent explosive disorder, kleptomania,

pyromania, paraphilias, nonparaphilic sexual addictions, compulsive buying, compulsive skin-picking, repetitive self-mutilation, or of ICDs as a group. However, a number of studies indicate that pathological gambling—the only ICD for which systematic prevalence data are available—is common and that its prevalence is increasing (Lesieur & Rosenthal, 1991; Lopez-Ibor & Carrasco, 1995; Volberg & Steadman, 1988).

Again, the few studies available suggest that ICDs are marked by gender differences. Thus, intermittent explosive disorder, pathological gambling, pyromania, paraphilias, and nonparaphilic sexual addictions appear to be more common in men, whereas kleptomania, trichotillomania, compulsive shopping, and repetitive self-mutilation appear to be more common in women (McElroy, Keck et al., 1995a).

Phenomenology. The phenomenologic similarities between ICDs and substance use disorders long have been recognized, as evidenced by the frequent inclusion of substance use disorders as forms of ICDs from the mid-1800s to the present. Indeed, many patients with ICDs claim to be addicted to their harmful behaviors. Specifically, the irresistible impulses of ICDs resemble the cravings to use alcohol or drugs that mark substance use disorders. Drug craving has been defined as an "irresistible urge that compels drug-seeking behavior," as well as an "urgent and overpowering desire" or an "irresistible impulse" to use a substance (Halikas, Kuhn et al., 1991; Halikas, 1997). Also, alcohol and drug cravings often are associated with tension, anxiety, or other dysphoric, depressive, or negative affective states (Mathew, Claghorn et al., 1979; Swendsen & Stout, 1992; Weddington, Brown et al., 1990) and/or with arousal or excitement (Childress, McLellan et al., 1987), similar to the negative affective states and arousal that occur with ICD impulses (Griffiths, 1995). Conversely, ICD actions often are associated with pleasurable feelings, variously described by patients as feeling "high," "euphoric," a "thrill," or a "rush," which resemble the elevated mood or euphoria of alcohol and drug intoxication (Blume, 1997). For example, pathological gambling has been described as inducing "a stimulating, tranquilizing, or pain-relieving response" (Custer, 1984), as well as being an "anesthetic" with hypnotizing properties (Lesieur & Rosenthal, 1991).

Indeed, just as substance-dependent persons use alcohol or drugs to relieve or self-medicate negative affective states, so do persons with ICDs achieve relief by engaging in their harmful behaviors (Blume, 1997). Additionally, the changes in awareness that may accompany ICD acts are similar to the cognitive changes associated with intoxication (Jacobs, 1988). As Esquirol noted, "The irresistible impulses [of monomanias] show all of the features of passion elevated to the point of delirium." Thus, some persons with intermittent explosive disorder report that they develop an altered state of consciousness or "amnesia" during their explosive episodes (Maletzky, 1973), while some pathological gamblers describe dissociative-like states while gambling (Blume 1997).

ICDs and substance use disorders also display similar disturbances in affective regulation (Goodman, 1997; Griffiths, 1995). As noted above, ICD impulses and behaviors often are associated with depressive and/or euphoric affective states that are similar to those of depression and intoxication. Moreover, after performance of an ICD action and resolution of the associated "high," patients with ICDs often describe the acute onset of anergic depressive symptoms as similar to those that may occur in withdrawal from many substances, including depressed mood, feelings of guilt and self-reproach, and fatigue. For example, one woman with compulsive buying (which met *DSM-IIIR* criteria for an ICD NOS) reported that she experienced severe anxiety along with her impulses to buy (which typically occurred when she was depressed), a "high like taking cocaine" with the act of buying, and then a prompt "crash" that was characterized by depression, guilt, anxiety, and fatigue (McElroy, Satlin et al., 1991b). Indeed, the author's research group has likened the affective dysregulation of ICDs to that of bipolar disorder (McElroy, Keck et al., 1995a; McElroy, Pope et al., 1996), just as others have noted similarities between the affective symptoms of bipolar disorder and those induced by substance abuse (Brady & Lydiard, 1992; Dilsaver, 1987).

Another phenomenologic similarity between ICDs and substance use disorders is that ICD behaviors may be associated with tolerance and withdrawal. For example, it has been reported that pathological gamblers need to gamble progressively larger sums of money to achieve the desired "high" (Anderson & Brown, 1984), and that they may develop physiologic withdrawal symptoms (including insomnia, anorexia, tremulousness, headaches, abdominal pain, upset stomach, diarrhea, palpitations, nightmares, sweating, and breathing problems) (Wray & Dickerson, 1981), as well as depressive symptoms (Linden, Pope et al., 1986) on abrupt discontinuation of gambling. Indeed, "needs to gamble with increasing amounts of money in order to achieve the desired excitement" and "is restless or irritable when attempting to cut down or stop gambling," which are analogous to tolerance and withdrawal, are listed as *DSM-IV* defining criteria for pathological gambling (APA, 1994; Blume, 1997). Similarly, some of the authors' patients with kleptomania have described a need to steal in increasingly risky situations in order to maintain their stealing-induced "rush." Moreover, both the "self-medication" of benzodiazepine withdrawal and the "switching of addictions" from alcohol and drugs to gambling have been described, suggesting that ICD acts and substances of abuse may sometimes be cross-tolerant (Fishbain, 1987) or that an ICD "high" may substitute for a substance-induced "high" (Blume, 1997).

Conversely, the disinhibiting effects of ICDs and substances of abuse may be additive. Many persons with ICDs, especially those with intermittent explosive disorder, report that alcohol or drug intoxication worsens their symptoms and/or makes them more likely to act on their impulses (Maletzky, 1973; McElroy, unpublished data, 1997).

Yet another similarity between ICDs and substance use disorders is that they share certain phenomenologic features with obsessive-compulsive disorder (OCD) (McElroy, Hudson et al., 1993; Modell, Glaser et al., 1992). Obsessions are defined as persistent ideas, thoughts, impulses, or images that are experienced as intrusive and inappropriate (that is, they are ego-dystonic) and that cause anxiety or distress. Compulsions are defined as repetitive behaviors or mental acts, the goal of which is to prevent or reduce anxiety or distress.

Similar to the urge to use substances, ICD impulses are being considered more harmful, less senseless, more spontaneous, and more likely to be associated with pleasure than are OCD obsessions and compulsions. Specifically, OCD symptoms have been associated with overestimation of risk, and thus with behaviors that aim to avoid harm or reduce risk; good insight into the absurdity or senselessness of symptoms; attempts to resist symptoms; and lack of pleasure with symptoms. In actuality, the symptoms of all three disorders vary considerably with respect to these variables. OCD symptoms may, at times, be impulsive, associated with poor insight, and ego-syntonic (Hollander, 1993; McElroy, Hudson et al., 1993; McElroy, Keck et al., 1994). Conversely, ICD impulses (McElroy, Hudson et al., 1993) and substance cravings (Anton, Moak et al., 1996; Modell, Glaser et al., 1992), like OCD obsessions, are experienced as intrusive, repetitive, unwanted, associated with anxiety, as having an irresistible or compelling quality, and as being difficult or impossible to resist. Indeed, the *DSM-IV* uses the term "impulse" to define an obsession, implying that obsessions and impulses are similar and may even be the same phenomenon. Moreover, ICD acts and substance use, like OCD compulsions, often are experienced as uncontrollable and anxiety- or tension-relieving, may be resisted, and often are followed by self-reproach or guilt.

Studies using modified versions of the Yale-Brown Obsessive Compulsive Scale (YBOCS) (Goodwin & Jamison, 1990) to assess obsessionality and compulsivity in heavy drinkers have found significant correlations between subjectively rated craving for alcoholic beverages and several YBOCS questions regarding alcohol-related thoughts and drinking behavior (Modell, Glaser et al., 1992; Anton, Moak et al., 1996). Indeed, one such scale, the Obsessive Compulsive Drinking Scale (OCDS) (Anton, Moak et al., 1996), has proved to be a reliable instrument for quantifying craving among alcohol-dependent persons. Research with the OCDs further suggests that, as the severity of alcoholism increases, so too does the intensity of obsessive thoughts about alcohol and the compulsive urge to use alcohol (Anton, Moak et al., 1996).

In short, rather than OCD symptoms being purely compulsive and ego-syntonic, and ICD and substance use symptoms only impulsive and ego-dystonic, it may be that all three sets of symptoms have compulsive and ego-dystonic features as well as impulsive and ego-syntonic features (McElroy, Hudson et al., 1993). As discussed later, this conceptualization may help to explain some of the heterogeneity found in both ICDs and substance use disorders.

ETIOLOGY AND COURSE OF THE DISORDERS

Although fewer systematic data are available for ICDs than for substance use disorders, the available data suggest that both conditions often begin in adolescence or early adulthood and subsequently follow episodic and/or chronic courses (Burt, 1995; Wise & Tierney, 1994). Thus, like substance use disorders, ICD symptoms may occur in "bouts" punctuated by symptom-free intervals, or continuously over extended periods, often waxing and waning in severity. Also similar to substance use disorders, many ICDs (including intermittent explosive disorder, kleptomania, pyromania, trichotillomania, and paraphilias) may have an onset of symptoms in childhood or mid-adulthood (McElroy, Hudson et al., 1992; McElroy, Keck et al., 1995a). However, these similarities are fairly nonspecific.

Comorbidity. Although preliminary, three lines of comorbidity data provide further support for a possible relationship between ICDs and substance abuse: (1) findings of elevated rates of substance use disorders in patients with ICDs; (2) findings of elevated rates of ICDs in patients with substance use disorders; and (3) studies indicating that ICDs and substance use disorders display similar comorbidity patterns with other Axis I and Axis II psychiatric disorders.

More than 15 studies have used diagnostic criteria to assess Axis I psychiatric disorders in persons (mostly patients) with various ICDs, and many of these studies used structured clinical interviews. All found apparently elevated rates of associated substance use disorders (Table 1).

Conversely, high rates of ICDs have been reported in persons seeking treatment for substance use disorders. In a study of 458 substance dependent inpatients, Lesieur and colleagues (1986) found that 9% met lifetime diagnostic criteria for pathological gambling, and an additional 10% reported subthreshold gambling problems. Of 100 adolescent substance-dependent inpatients evaluated by Lesieur and Heineman (1988), 14% met criteria for a lifetime diagnosis of pathological gambling, and an additional 14% described subthreshold gambling problems. Similarly, of 298 cocaine abusers in treatment who were evaluated by Steinberg and colleagues (1992), 15% displayed a concurrent diagnosis of pathological gambling. In the latter study, cocaine abusers who were pathological gamblers were more likely to be dependent on alcohol and other drugs than those who were not pathological gamblers. Finally, Washton (1989) reported that 70% of outpatients entering a program for cocaine addiction also were engaged in compulsive sexual behavior.

Substantial epidemiologic and clinical data indicate that substance use disorders are highly comorbid with other Axis I disorders, especially mood, anxiety and—in women—eating disorders (Brooner, King et al., 1997; Gold, Johnson et al., 1997; Goodwin & Jamison, 1990; Regier, Farmer et al., 1990). The ICD studies noted above suggest that these disorders, like substance use disorders, also show elevated comorbidity with mood, anxiety, and eating disorders (McElroy, Hudson et al., 1992; McElroy, Keck et al., 1995a; McElroy, Pope et al., 1996; Kafka, 1995; Kafka & Prentky, 1994). Moreover, clinical studies indicate that ICDs may be associated with disproportionately high rates of bipolar disorders relative to depressive mood disorders (McElroy, Pope et al., 1996); these findings are consistent with data from the Epidemiologic Catchment Area (ECA) study, which suggest that substance use disorders are associated with disproportionately high rates of bipolar disorders relative to unipolar major depressive disorders (Regier, Farmer et al., 1990).

Yet another similarity between ICDs and substance use disorders is that each may be associated with elevated rates of personality disorders with impulsive features, especially antisocial and borderline personality disorders. Substantial epidemiologic and clinical data indicate that substance use disorder and antisocial personality disorder co-occur much more often than would be predicted by chance alone (Regier, Farmer et al., 1990). Although personality disorders with impulsive features (especially antisocial and borderline) have been hypothesized to be ICDs, few studies have evaluated whether personality disorder patients perform their harmful behaviors in response to irresistible impulses (Coid, Allolio et al., 1983; McElroy, Keck et al., 1995a). Therefore, it is not known whether ICDs and impulsive personality disorders represent separate but related conditions that are highly comorbid, identical entities (with impulsive personality disorder possibly representing the most severe cases or persons with multiple ICDs) or independent entities that may co-occur by chance, but that are easily misdiagnosed as one or the other.

Nevertheless, preliminary studies suggest that, like substance use disorders, some ICDs (including intermittent explosive disorder, pyromania, pathological gambling, paraphilias, nonparaphilic sexual addictions, and repetitive self-mutilation) may be associated with high rates of impulsive (or cluster B) personality disorders and/or antisocial behaviors (McElroy, Keck et al, 1995a). For example, of 54 impulsive violent offenders and fire setters evaluated by Linnoila and colleagues (1989), 29 (54%) had *DSM-III* intermittent explosive disorder, 37 (69%) had borderline personality disorders, and nine (17%) had antisocial personality disorders, whereas six (11%) had paranoid and five (9%) had passive-aggressive personality disorders (by *DSM-III* criteria). Pathological gamblers have been shown to have elevated scores on the psychopathic deviation (pd) scale of the Minnesota Multiphasic Personality Inventory (MMPI), to engage in a wide variety of illegal behaviors, and to have possibly increased rates of antisocial and narcissistic personality disorders (Moran, 1970; Blaszczynski, McConaghy et al., 1991; Lesieur & Rosenthal, 1991). Of 15 men with paraphilias who were evaluated by Kruesi and colleagues (1992), four (27%) met criteria for antisocial personality disorder. And of 36 men with compulsive sexual behaviors

evaluated by Black and colleagues (1997) for *DSM-IIIR* personality disorders by consensus diagnosis, five (15%) subjects were determined to have a cluster A disorder, 10 (29%) a cluster B disorder, and eight (24%) a cluster C disorder.

Family History. Studies of family history provide tentative support for an ICD-substance abuse relationship. Family studies of probands with substance use disorders have consistently found elevated rates of substance use in first-degree relatives (Anthenelli & Schuckit, 1997). Although there are no controlled family history studies of ICDs, open studies (most of which use the family history method [Andreasen, Endicott et al., 1977]) have found relatively high rates of substance use disorders in first-degree relatives of individuals with various ICDs. These disorders include intermittent explosive disorder or episodic dyscontrol (Maletzky, 1973; Linnoila, Virkkunen et al., 1983; Linnoila, DeJong et al., 1989; Virkkunen, DeJong et al., 1989), kleptomania (McElroy, Pope et al., 1991a), pathological gambling (McCormick, Russo et al., 1984; Roy, Adinoff et al., 1988), and compulsive buying (McElroy, Phillips et al., 1994).

Moreover, in a study of impulsive violent offenders and fire setters (Linnoila, DeJong et al., 1989), 41 (81%) had first- or second-degree relatives who were alcoholics and 35 (65%) had alcoholic fathers. Subjects with alcoholic fathers were more likely to be impulsive and to have a lower mean cerebrospinal fluid (CSF) 5-hydroxyindoleacetic acid (5-HIAA) concentration than subjects without alcoholic fathers. Of 103 first-degree relatives (age 16 years or older) of 20 individuals with kleptomania who were evaluated blindly by the authors through the family history method, 21 (20%) had an alcohol or substance use disorder (McElroy, Pope et al., 1991a). Ramirez and colleagues (1983) reported that 50% of 51 pathological gamblers had an alcoholic parent. Similarly, Roy and colleagues (1988) reported that 25% of 24 pathological gamblers had a first-degree relative diagnosed with an alcohol abuse disorder.

Neurobiological Studies. The neurobiology of ICDs is relatively unstudied, and few data are available to compare the neurobiology of ICDs with that of substance use disorders. Nevertheless, preliminary data suggest that some of the neurobehavioral processes and neurotransmitter systems hypothesized to be involved in addiction also may be involved in ICDs. In short, it has been suggested that the addictive process involves impaired behavioral inhibition (that is, pathological impulsivity), aberrant functioning of the motivational-reward system, and impaired affect

TABLE 1. Substance Use Disorders in Individuals With ICDs

ICD Population	N	% With Substance Use Disorders	Authors
Impulsive, violent offenders	24	100% alcohol abuse	Linnoila et al., 1983
Impulsive arsonist	22	91% alcohol abuse	Virkkunen et al., 1989
Intermittent explosive disorder	14	57% substance abuse	Salomen et al., 1994
Intermittent explosive disorder	27	48% substance use disorder	McElroy et al., 1998
Kleptomania	20	50% substance use disorder	McElroy et al., 1991a
Pathologic gambling	140	47% substance use disorder	Linden et al., 1986; Ramirez et al., 1983 Specker et al., 1996
Trichotillomania	74	23% substance use disorder	Christenson et al., 1991b; Swedo et al., 1989
Compulsive buyers	90	37% substance use disorder	Christenson et al., 1994; McElroy et al., 1994a; Schlosser et al., 1994
Paraphilias	1992	53% substance use disorder	Kruesi, 1992
Paraphilias	60	47% substance use disorder	Kafka & Prentky, 1994
Paraphilias	22 adolescents	62% substance use	Galli et al., 1995
Paraphilias	36	64% substance use disorder	Black et al., 1997

regulation, and that these three processes are associated with dysfunction in the serotonin, norepinephrine, dopamine, and/or endogenous opioid systems (Goodman, 1995, 1997; Miller & Gold, 1993; Nutt, 1996). It has been similarly hypothesized that interactions among serotonergic, noradrenergic, dopaminergic, and endogenous opioid neurotransmitter systems are important in the pathogenesis of ICDs, with serotonergic abnormalities possibly underlying some of their impulsive (and/or compulsive) features; noradrenergic, dopaminergic, and opioid abnormalities underlying their pleasurable or euphoric features; and abnormalities in all four systems underlying their affective dysregulation (McElroy, Pope et al., 1996; Stein, Hollander et al., 1993; Winchel & Stanley, 1991).

Common neurobiologic abnormalities in these disorders are best demonstrated in studies of the serotonergic system. Evidence of serotonergic involvement in ICDs, although mixed (Roy, Adinoff et al., 1988), comes from findings in individuals with impulsive aggression, impulsive fire-setting, self-injurious behavior, and pathological gambling (Stein, Hollander et al., 1993). In a study of 58 violent offenders and impulsive fire setters, 33 (57%) of whom had *DSM-III* intermittent explosive disorder, CSF concentrations of 5-HIAA in the impulsive offenders and fire setters were significantly lower than in the non-impulsive offenders and normal control subjects (Linnoila, Virkkunen et al., 1983; Virkkunen, DeJong et al., 1989). Moreover, low CSF 5-HIAA concentrations were associated with a lifetime history of suicide attempts. In a study of 21 patients with major depression, the five patients who exhibited self-aggressive behaviors had significantly lower CSF 5-HIAA concentrations than the other 16 patients (Lopez-Ibor & Carrasco, 1995). Similarly, in a controlled study of subjects with repetitive self-mutilation and borderline personality disorder, Simeon and colleagues (1992) found that lower serotonergic activity (as measured by platelet imipramine binding sites and affinity) was related to greater severity of self-mutilation. Other findings of reduced serotonergic activity in ICDs include blunted prolactin release in response to intravenously administered clomipramine (Moreno, Saiz-Ruiz et al., 1991) and low levels of platelet monoamine oxidase (MAO) activity (Blanco, Orensanz-Munoz et al., 1996; Carrasco, Saiz-Ruiz et al., 1994) in pathological gamblers. Evidence for similar dysfunction in ICDs and substance use disorders in both the dopaminergic and endogenous opioid systems also is accumulating.

TREATMENT AND OUTCOMES FOR ICDs

Psychopharmacologic treatment response data further support a possible relationship between ICDs and substance use disorders. Although findings are mixed, controlled studies suggest that various antidepressants may reduce craving for and overall consumption of substances in substance-dependent patients. These include serotonin reuptake inhibitors (SRIs) in alcohol abuse and dependence and cocaine dependence, and tricyclic antidepressants (TCAs) in cocaine dependence (Anton, 1995; Naranjo, Poulos et al., 1994; Rao, Ziedonis et al., 1995). Similarly, various antidepressants have been reported to reduce the irresistible impulses and harmful behaviors of various ICDs. These include SSRIs in apparent intermittent explosive disorder, kleptomania, pathological gambling, trichotillomania, compulsive buying, onychophagia, nonparaphilic sexual additions, and paraphilias; tricyclics in apparent intermittent explosive disorder, kleptomania, trichotillomania, nonparaphilic sexual addictions, and paraphilias; monoamine oxidase inhibitors in kleptomania and trichotillomania; and atypical agents (such as trazodone or bupropion) in kleptomania and compulsive buying (Hollander, Frenkel et al., 1992; Kruesi, Fine et al., 1992; McElroy, Hudson et al., 1992; McElroy, Keck et al., 1995a, 1995b; McElroy, Pope et al., 1996; Swedo, Leonard et al., 1989; Zohar, Kaplan et al., 1994).

Patients with ICDs and substance use disorders, however, may differ in their response to mood stabilizers. Numerous double-blind, placebo-controlled studies of lithium in alcohol dependence have failed to confirm that lithium is superior to placebo in producing abstinence. Moreover, three double-blind, placebo-controlled studies of carbamazepine in cocaine dependence have been negative (Cornish, Maany et al., 1995; Kranzler, Bauer et al., 1995; Montoya, Levin et al., 1995). However, in controlled trials, carbamazepine and valproate were found to be effective in relieving the symptoms of alcohol and/or sedative-hypnotic withdrawal (Keck, McElroy et al., 1994), and a recently completed double-blind, placebo-controlled pilot study of carbamazepine in alcohol dependence displayed treatment effects favoring carbamazepine (Mueller, Stout et al., 1997). A recent crossover study of valproate demonstrated that adolescents with temper outbursts and polysubstance use had both decreased substance use and improvements in outbursts with valproate treatment. By contrast, there are case reports and open trials of successful lithium treatment of patients with intermittent explosive disorder, kleptomania, pathological gambling, trichotillomania, and paraphilias (such as transvestism and autoerotic asphyxiation) (Cesnik & Coleman, 1989; Christenson, Popkin et al., 1991b; Cutler & Heiser, 1978; McElroy, Pope et al., 1996; Moskowitz, 1980; Ward, 1975). Also, carbamazepine has been reported to be effective in intermittent explosive disorder and pathological gambling (Haller & Hinterhuber, 1994; Mattes,

1990), and valproate has been used successfully in individuals with intermittent explosive disorder, kleptomania, and compulsive buying (McElroy, Keck et al., 1995a, 1995b; Szymanski & Olympia, 1991).

Double-blind, placebo-controlled studies have shown that the opiate antagonist naltrexone reduces alcohol craving and consumption in alcohol-dependent persons (O'Brien, Volpicelli et al., 1996; Volpicelli, Alterman et al., 1992). Although controlled studies of opiate antagonists in ICDs are yet to be done, open trials suggest that these agents may reduce self-mutilation and binge eating in patients with repetitive self-mutilation (Richardson & Zaleski, 1983) and bulimia nervosa (Stennie & Gold, 1997), respectively.

Patients with ICDs and substance use disorders may have similar responses to psychological treatments. In general, available data (which are very limited) suggest that individuals with ICDs, like those with substance use disorders, may not be particularly responsive to psychoanalytic or insight-oriented psychotherapies. Rather, ICDs, like substance use disorders, appear to be more amenable to psychological treatments that stress education, denial reduction, and relapse prevention, or which employ cognitive-behavioral techniques (Blume, 1997; Goodman, 1997; Josephson & Brandolo, 1993). Also, self-help groups based on the Alcoholic Anonymous model (such as Gamblers Anonymous) have been shown to be helpful in treating some persons with pathological gambling and sexual addictions (Brown, 1991; Irons & Schneider, 1997).

CONCLUSIONS

Although the data are preliminary, there is evidence that ICDs and substance use disorders have many similarities. First, they are phenomenologically similar, in that both are characterized by the repetitive performance of harmful, dangerous, or pleasurable behaviors, and both are marked by irresistible impulses or desires to perform those behaviors. Both disorders are characterized by impaired insight into the dangerousness or consequences of the behaviors (ego-syntonicity or denial), affective dysregulation (dysphoria or arousal with the impulses or cravings, relief that may be associated with euphoria with the behaviors, and depressed mood after the behaviors), and obsessive-compulsive features.

Second, ICDs and substance use disorders display a similar course of illness, in that both conditions often begin in adolescence or early adulthood and subsequently have an episodic or chronic course.

Third, the two conditions show elevated comorbidity with each other, as well as similar comorbidity patterns with other psychiatric disorders, especially mood, anxiety, and (probably) antisocial personality disorders.

Fourth, family history studies suggest that patients with certain ICDs, like persons with substance use disorders, have elevated rates of substance use and mood disorders in their first-degree relatives.

Fifth, preliminary biological data suggest that ICDs may be associated with abnormalities in central serotonergic, dopaminergic, noradrenergic, and (possibly) endogenous opioid neurotransmission—the same neurotransmitter systems that have been hypothesized to be deranged in substance use disorders.

Finally, some patients with ICDs, like some patients with substance use disorders, may respond to antidepressants (especially SSRIs) and (possibly) opiate antagonists.

Researchers have hypothesized that compulsivity and impulsivity are related, with each characterized by abnormal impulse control, and that disorders characterized by pathological impulsivity or compulsivity may constitute a family of related conditions more accurately termed "compulsive-impulsive spectrum disorders" (Hollander, 1993; McElroy, Pope et al., 1996). In this model, all compulsive-impulsive spectrum disorders are characterized by irresistible or compelling thoughts associated with anxiety, tension, or other negative affective states, and/or by repetitive behaviors aimed at reducing discomfort or eliciting pleasure. The differences among the disorders are explained by the possibility that the conditions vary along a single dimension (or related dimensions) of compulsivity versus impulsivity.

However, the aforementioned model does not explain the extensive overlap of mood disorders with ICDs, substance use disorders, OCD, and most other putative compulsive-impulsive spectrum disorders. To account for this overlap, the authors have hypothesized that most putative compulsive-impulsive spectrum disorders—or, more broadly, all disorders characterized by a core disturbance in compulsivity and/or impulsivity—might belong to the larger family of affective spectrum disorder (McElroy, Pope et al., 1991; McElroy, Satlin et al., 1991; McElroy, Hudson et al., 1992; McElroy, Hudson et al., 1993; McElroy, Pope et al., 1996; Phillips, McElroy et al., 1995). Affective spectrum disorder is a hypothesized family of disorders related to mood disorders and is characterized by high comorbidity with mood disorder, high familial rates of mood disorder, and response to thymoleptic agents; thus, there may be a pathophysiologic abnormality in common with mood disorder (Hudson & Pope, 1990).

The authors further have hypothesized that compulsivity and impulsivity might be related to mood dysregulation with depression (or unipolarity), similar to impulsivity, and mixed affective states, similar to mixtures of compulsivity and impulsivity (McElroy, Pope et al., 1996). Thus, compulsivity and depression each are characterized by inhibited or ruminative thinking and behavior, maintenance of insight or ego-dystonicity, and less marked fluctuations in mood state, with dysphoria alternating with relief rather than with euphoria or pleasurable feelings. Similarly, impulsivity and mania (or bipolarity) each are characterized by disinhibited or facilitated thinking and behavior, poor insight or ego-syntonicity, and more severe fluctuations in mood state, with dysphoria alternating with pleasurable affective states. Indeed, substance withdrawal and intoxication also might be viewed as representing more compulsive/depressive versus more impulsive/manic states, respectively.

This model of compulsive-impulsive spectrum disorders may have important clinical implications. For example, if pharmacologic responsiveness in fact varies along a compulsivity/unipolarity-impulsivity/bipolarity dimension (with more compulsive forms responding preferentially to SSRIs and more impulsive forms responding to a wider range of thymoleptic agents), such responsiveness might be predicted on the basis of presenting phenomenology and comorbid affective symptoms or mood syndromes. Thus, patients with ICDs or substance use disorders with compulsive features might respond best to an SSRI, especially if their disorders are associated with comorbid depressive symptoms or a depressive disorder. On the other hand, patients with more impulsive forms of these disorders might respond to a variety of antidepressants or, if accompanied by bipolar symptoms or a bipolar disorder, to mood stabilizers.

In summary, preliminary data suggest that ICDs and substance use disorders may be related and may belong to a larger family of disorders that share a core disturbance in impulse control and affective regulation. Such a conceptual framework might be useful in several ways. First, awareness of the high comorbidity of these disorders with one another and with other psychiatric disorders, especially mood disorder, should increase recognition of the related disorders when a patient presents with an ICD or substance use disorder. Second, the degree of presenting impulsive versus compulsive features, as well as the type of comorbid affective symptoms or mood disorder, may help to guide the choice of both psychopharmacologic and psychological treatments. Third, further research on the pathophysiologic and genetic substrates of these conditions, and of the relationships between impulsivity, addiction, compulsivity, and mood, might be stimulated.

ACKNOWLEDGMENT: Preparation of this chapter was supported in part by a grant from the Theodore and Vada Stanley Foundation.

REFERENCES

American Psychiatric Association (APA) (1980). *Diagnostic and Statistical Manual of Mental Disorders, 3rd Edition (DSM-III)*. Washington, DC: American Psychiatric Press.

American Psychiatric Association (APA) (1987). *Diagnostic and Statistical Manual of Mental Disorders, 3rd Edition, Revised (DSM-IIIR)*. Washington, DC: American Psychiatric Press.

American Psychiatric Association (APA) (1994). *Diagnostic and Statistical Manual of Mental Disorders, 4th Edition (DSM-IV)*. Washington, DC: American Psychiatric Press, 1994.

Anderson G & Brown RI (1984). Real and laboratory gambling, sensation-seeking and arousal. *British Journal of Psychology* 75:401-410.

Anderson G & Brown RI (1987). Some applications of reversal theory to the explanation of gambling and gambling addictions. *Journal on Gambling Behaviors* 3:179-189.

Andreasen NC, Endicott J, Spitzer RL et al. (1977). The family history method using diagnostic inter-rater reliability and validity. *Archives of General Psychiatry* 34:1229-1235.

Anthenelli RM & Schuckit MA (1997). Genetics. In JH Lowinson, P Ruiz, RB Millman & JG Langrod (eds.) *Substance Abuse: A Comprehensive Textbook*. Baltimore, MD: Williams & Wilkins, 41-51.

Anthony DT & Hollander E (1993). Sexual compulsions. In E Hollander (ed.) *Obsessive-Compulsive Related Disorders*. Washington, DC: American Psychiatric Press, 139-150.

Anton RF (1995). New directions in the pharmacotherapy of alcoholism. *Psychiatric Annals* 25:353-362.

Anton RF, Moak DH & Latham PK (1996). The Obsessive Compulsive Drinking Scale: A new method of assessing outcome in alcoholism treatment studies. *Archives of General Psychiatry* 53:225-231.

Black DW, Kehrberg LLD, Flumerfelt DL et al. (1997). Characteristics of 36 subjects reporting compulsive sexual behavior. *American Journal of Psychiatry* 154:243-249.

Blanco C, Orensanz-Munoz L, Blanco-Jerez C et al. (1996). Pathological gambling and platelet MAO activity: A psychobiological study. *Journal of Gambling Behavior* 5:137-152.

Blaszczynski A, McConaghy N & Frankova A (1991). Control versus abstinence in the treatment of pathological gambling: A two to nine year follow-up. *British Journal of Addiction* 86:299-306.

Blaszczynski A, Winter SW & McConaghy N (1986). Plasma endorphin levels in pathological gambling. *Journal of Gambling Behavior* 2:3-14.

Bleuler E (1988). *Textbook of Psychiatry. The Classics of Psychiatry and Behavioral Sciences Library*. Birmingham, AL: Gryphon Editions.

Blume SB (1997). Pathological gambling. In JH Lowinson, P Ruiz, RB Millman & JG Langrod (eds.) *Substance Abuse: A Comprehensive Textbook*. Baltimore, MD: Williams & Wilkins, 330-337.

Boyd JH, Burke JD, Gruenberg E et al. (1984). Exclusion criteria of DSM-III: A study of co-occurrence of hierarchy-free syndromes. *Archives of General Psychiatry* 41:983-989.

Bradford J, Geller J, Lesieur HR et al. (1996). Impulse control disorders. In TA Widger, AJ Frances, HA Pincus et al. (eds.) *DSM-IV Sourcebook, Vol. 2*. Washington DC: American Psychiatric Press, 1007-1031.

Brady KT & Lydiard RB (1992). Bipolar affective disorder and substance abuse. *Journal of Clinical Psychopharmacology* 12(Suppl):17-22.

Brooner AK, King VL, Kidorf M et al. (1997). Psychiatric and substance use comorbidity among treatment-seeking opioid abusers. *Archives of General Psychiatry* 54:71-80.

Brown BR (1991). The selective adaptation of the Alcoholics Anonymous program by Gamblers Anonymous. *Journal of Gambling Behavior* 7:187-206.

Burt VK (1995). Impulse-control disorders not elsewhere classified. In HI Kaplan & BJ Saddock (eds.) *Comprehensive Textbook of Psychiatry, 6th Edition*. Baltimore, MD: Williams & Wilkins, 1409-1418.

Carnes PJ (1990). Sexual addiction: Progress, criticism, challenges. *American Journal of Preventive Psychiatry & Neurology* 2:1-8.

Carrasco JL, Saiz-Ruiz J, Moreno I et al. (1994). Low platelet MAO activity in pathological gambling. *Acta Psychiatrica Scandinavica* 90:427-431.

Carroll KM, Rounsaville BJ, Gordon LT et al. (1994). Psychotherapy and pharmacotherapy for ambulatory cocaine abusers. *Archives of General Psychiatry* 51:177-187.

Cesnik JA & Coleman E (1989). Use of lithium carbonate in the treatment of autoerotic asphyxia. *American Journal of Psychotherapy* 63:277-286.

Childress AR, McLellan AT, Natale M et al. (1987). Mood states can illicit conditioned withdrawal and craving in opiate abuse patients. *NIDA Research Monograph 76*. Rockville, MD: National Institute on Drug Abuse, 137-144.

Christenson GA, Faber RJ, de Zwaan M et al. (1994). Compulsive buying: Descriptive characteristics and psychiatric comorbidity. *Journal of Clinical Psychiatry* 55:5-11.

Christenson GA, Mackenzie TB & Mitchell JE (1991a). Characteristics of 60 adult chronic hair pullers. *American Journal of Psychiatry* 148:365-370.

Christenson GA, Popkin MK, Mackennzie TB et al. (1991b). Lithium treatment of chronic hair pulling. *Journal of Clinical Psychiatry* 52:116-120.

Christenson GA, Pyle RL & Mitchell JE (1991). Estimated lifetime prevalence of trichotillomania in college students. *Journal of Clinical Psychiatry* 52:415-417.

Coid JW (1991). An affective syndrome in psychopaths with borderline personality disorder? *British Journal of Psychiatry* 162:641-650.

Coid J, Allolio B & Rees LH (1983). Raised plasma metenkephalin in patients who habitually mutilate themselves. *Lancet* 10:545-546.

Comings DE, Rosenthal RJ, Lesieur HR et al. (1996). The molecular genetics of pathological gambling: The DRD2 gene. *Pharmacogenetics*.

Cornish JW, Maany I, Fudalla PJ et al. (1995). Carbamazepine treatment for cocaine dependence. *Drug and Alcohol Dependence* 38:221-227.

Custer RL (1984). Profile of the pathological gambler. *Journal of Clinical Psychiatry* 45:35-38.

Cutler N & Heiser JF (1978). Retrospective diagnosis of hypomania following successful treatment of episodic violence with lithium: A case report. *American Journal of Psychiatry* 135:753-754.

Dilsaver SC (1987). The pathophysiologies of substance abuse and affective disorders: An integrative model? *Journal of Clinical Psychopharmacology* 7:1-10.

Esquirol E (1838). *Des Maladies Mentales*. Paris, France: Bailliere.

Fishbain DA (1987). Kleptomania as risk taking behavior in response to depression. *American Journal of Psychotherapy* 41:598-603.

Frosch J & Wortis SB (1954). A contribution to the nosology of the impulse disorders. *American Journal of Psychiatry* 111:132-138.

Galli VJ, Raute NJ, Kizer DL et al. (1995). A study of the phenomenology, comorbidity, and preliminary treatment response of pedophiles and adolescent sex offenders. New Clinical Drug Evaluation Unit (NCDEU) 35th Annual Meeting, Orlando, Florida (abstract).

Gold MS, Johnson CR et al. (1997). Eating disorders. In JH Lowinson, P Ruiz, RB Millman & JG Langrod (eds.) *Substance Abuse: A Comprehensive Textbook*. Baltimore, MD: Williams & Wilkins, 319-330.

Goodman A (1995). Addictive disorders: An integrated approach. Part One: An integrated understanding. *Journal of Ministry in Addiction & Recovery* 2:33-76.

Goodman A (1997). Sexual addiction. In JH Lowinson, P Ruiz, RB Millman & JG Langrod (eds.) *Substance Abuse: A Comprehensive Textbook*. Baltimore, MD: Williams & Wilkins, 340-354.

Goodman WK, Price LH, Rasmussen SA et al. (1989). The Yale-Brown Obsessive-Compulsive Scale, I. Development, use, and reliability. *Archives of General Psychiatry* 46:1006-1011.

Goodwin FK & Jamison KR (1990). *Manic-Depressive Illness*. New York, NY: Oxford University Press.

Griffiths M (1995). The role of subjective mood states in the maintenance of fruit machine gambling behaviour. *Journal of Gambling Studies* 11:123-135.

Halikas JA (1997). Craving. In JH Lowinson, P Ruiz, RB Millman & JG Langrod (eds.) *Substance Abuse: A Comprehensive Textbook*. Baltimore, MD: Williams & Wilkins, 85-90.

Halikas JA, Kuhn KL, Crosby R et al. (1991). The measurement of craving in cocaine patients using the Minnesota Cocaine Craving Scale. *Comprehensive Psychiatry* 32:22-27.

Haller R & Hinterhuber H (1994). Treatment of pathological gambling with carbamazepine. *Pharmacopsychiatry* 27:129.

Hollander E, ed. (1993). *Obsessive-Compulsive Related Disorders*. Washington, DC: American Psychiatric Press.

Hollander E, Frenkel M, DeCaria C et al. (1992). Treatment of pathological gambling with clomipramine [letter]. *American Journal of Psychiatry* 149:710-711.

Hudson JI & Pope HG Jr. (1990). Affective spectrum disorder: Does antidepressant response identify a family of disorders with a common pathophysiology? *American Journal of Psychiatry* 147:552-564.

Irons RR & Schneider JP (1997). Addictive sexual disorders. In NS Miller (ed.) *The Principles and Practice of Addiction Psychiatry*. Philadelphia, PA: W.B. Saunders, 441-457.

Jacobs DF (1988). Evidence for a common dissociative-like reaction among addicts. *Journal of Gambling Behavior* 3:237-247.

Josephson SC & Brandolo E (1993). Cognitive-behavioral approaches to obsessive-compulsive-related disorders. In E Hollander (ed.) *Obsessive-Compulsive Related Disorders*. Washington, DC: American Psychiatric Press, 215-240.

Kafka MP (1991). Successful antidepressant treatment of nonparaphilic sexual addictions and paraphilias in men. *Journal of Clinical Psychiatry* 52:60-65.

Kafka MP (1994). Sertraline pharmacotherapy for paraphilias and paraphilia-related disorders: An open trial. *Annals of Clinical Psychiatry* 6:189-195.

Kafka MP (1995). Sexual impulsivity. In E Hollander & DJ Stein (eds.) *Impulsivity and Aggression*. Chichester, England: John Wiley & Sons, 201-228.

Kafka MP & Prentky RA (1994). Preliminary observations of DSM-IIIR Axis I comorbidity in men with paraphilias and paraphilia-related disorders. *Journal of Clinical Psychiatry* 55:481-487.

Keck PE Jr, McElroy SL, Thienhaus OJ et al. (1994). Antiepileptics. In K Modigh, OH Robak & P Vestergaard (eds.) *Anticonvulsants in Psychiatry*. Wrightson Biomedical Publishing, 99-111.

Kim SW (1998). Opioid antagonists in the treatment of impulse control disorders. *Journal of Clinical Psychiatry* 59:159-164.

Kranzler HR, Bauer LO, Hersh D et al. (1995). Carbamazepine treatment of cocaine dependence: A placebo-controlled trial. *Drug and Alcohol Dependence* 38:203-211.

Kruesi MJP, Fine S, Valladares L et al. (1992). Paraphilias: A double-blind crossover comparison of clomipramine versus desipramine. *Archives of Sexual Behavior* 21:587-593.

Leonard HL, Lenane MC, Swedo SE et al. (1991). A double-blind comparison of clomipramine and desipramine treatment of severe onychophagia (nail biting). *Archives of General Psychiatry* 48:821-827.

Lesieur HR, Blume SB & Zoppa RM (1986). Alcoholism, drug abuse, and gambling. *Alcoholism* (NY) 10:33-38.

Lesieur HR & Heineman M (1988). Pathological gambling among youthful multiple substance abusers in a therapeutic community. *British Journal of Addiction* 83:765-771.

Lesieur HR & Rosenthal RJ (1991). Pathological gambling: A review of the literature. *Journal of Gambling Studies* 7:5-39.

Linden RD, Pope HG Jr. & Jonas JM (1986). Pathological gambling and major affective disorder: Preliminary findings. *Journal of Clinical Psychiatry* 47:201-203.

Linnoila M, DeJong J & Virkkunen M (1989). Family history of alcoholism in violent offenders and impulsive firesetters. *Archives of General Psychiatry* 46:613-616.

Linnoila M, Virkkunen M, Scheinin M et al. (1983). Low cerebrospinal fluid 5-hydroxyindoleacetic acid concentration differentiates impulsive from nonimpulsive violent behavior. *Life Science* 33:2609-2614.

Lion JR & Scheinberg AW (1995). Disorders of impulse control. In GO Gabbard (ed.) *Treatment of Psychiatric Disorders, 2nd Edition*. Washington DC: American Psychiatric Press, 2457-2472.

Lopez-Ibor JJ & Carrasco JL (1995). Pathological gambling. In E Hollander & DJ Stein (eds.) *Impulsivity and Aggression*. Chichester, England: John Wiley & Sons, 137-149.

Maletzky BM (1973). The episodic dyscontrol syndrome. *Diseases of the Nervous System* 36:178-185.

Mathew RJ, Claghorn JL & Largen J (1979). Craving for alcohol in sober alcoholics. *American Journal of Psychiatry* 136:603-606.

Mattes JA (1990). Comparative effectiveness of carbamazepine and propranolol for rage outbursts. *Journal of Neuropsychiatry and Clinical Neuroscience* 21:249-255.

Mattes JA & Fink M (1990). A controlled family study of adopted patients with temper outbursts. *Journal of Nervous and Mental Disorders* 178:138-139.

McConaghy N, Armstrong M, Blaszczynski A et al. (1983). Controlled comparison of aversive therapy and imaginal desensitization in compulsive gambling. *British Journal of Psychiatry* 142:366-372.

McCormick RA, Russo AM, Ramirez LF et al. (1984). Affective disorders among pathological gamblers seeking treatment. *American Journal of Psychiatry* 141:215-218.

McElroy SL, Hudson JI, Phillips KA et al. (1993). Clinical and theoretical implications of a possible link between obsessive-compulsive and impulse control disorders. *Depression* 1:121-132.

McElroy SL, Hudson JI, Pope HG Jr. et al. (1992). The DSM-IIIR impulse control disorders not elsewhere classified: Clinical characteristics and relationship to other psychiatric disorders. *American Journal of Psychiatry* 149:318-327.

McElroy SL, Keck PE Jr., Hudson JI et al. (1995a). Disorders of impulse control. In H Hollander & DJ Stein (eds.) *Impulsivity and Aggression*. Chichester, England: John Wiley & Sons, 109-136.

McElroy SL, Keck PE Jr. & Phillips KA (1995b). Kleptomania, compulsive buying, and binge eating disorder. *Journal of Clinical Psychiatry* 56(4 Suppl):14-26.

McElroy SL, Keck PE Jr., Pope HF Jr. et al. (1994). Compulsive buying: A report of 20 cases. *Journal of Clinical Psychiatry* 55:242-248.

McElroy SL, Phillips KA & Keck PE Jr. (1994). Obsessive-compulsive spectrum disorder. *Journal of Clinical Psychiatry* 55(10 Suppl):33-51.

McElroy SL, Pope HG Jr., Hudson JI et al. (1991). Kleptomania: A report of 20 cases. *American Journal of Psychiatry* 148:652-657.

McElroy SL, Pope HG Jr., Keck PE Jr. et al. (1996). Are impulse control disorders related to bipolar disorder? *Comprehensive Psychiatry* 37:229-240.

McElroy SL, Satlin A, Pope HG Jr. et al. (1991). Treatment of compulsive shopping and antidepressants. A report of three cases. *Annals of Clinical Psychiatry* 3:199-204.

McElroy SL, Soutullo CA, Beckman D et al. (1998). DSM-IV intermittent explosive disorder: A report of 27 cases. *Journal of Clinical Psychiatry* 59:203-210.

Miller NS & Gold MS (1993). A hypothesis for a common neurochemical basis for alcohol and drug disorders. *Psychiatric Clinics of North America* 16:105-117.

Modell JG, Glaser FB, Cyr L et al. (1992). Obsessive and compulsive characteristics of craving for alcohol in alcohol abuse and dependence. *Alcoholism: Clinical & Experimental Research* 16:272-274.

Modell JG, Mountz JM & Beresford TP (1990). Basal ganglia/limbic striatal and thalamocortical involvement in craving and loss of control in alcohol abuse and dependence. *Journal of Neuropsychiatry and Clinical Neuroscience* 2:123-144.

Montoya ID, Levin FR, Fudala PJ et al. (1995). Double-blind comparison of carbamazepine and placebo for treatment of cocaine dependence. *Drug and Alcohol Dependence* 38:213-219.

Moran E (1970). Varieties of pathologic gambling. *British Journal of Psychiatry* 116:593-597.

Moreno I, Saiz-Ruiz J & Lopez-Ibor JJ (1991). Serotonin and gambling dependence. *Human Psychopharmacology* 6:S9-S12.

Moskowitz JA (1980). Lithium and lady luck: Use of lithium carbonate in pathological gambling. *New York State Journal of Medicine* 80:785-788.

Mueller TI, Stout RL, Rudden S et al. (1997). A double-blind, placebo-controlled pilot study of carbamazepine for the treatment of alcohol dependence. *Alcoholism: Clinical & Experimental Research* 21:86-92.

Naranjo CA, Poulos CX, Bremner KE et al. (1994). Fluoxetine attenuates alcohol intake and desire to drink. *International Clinical Psychopharmacology* 9:163-172

Nutt DJ (1996). Addiction: Brain mechanisms and their treatment implications. *Lancet* 347:31-36.

O'Brien CP, Volpicelli LA & Volpicelli JR (1996). Naltrexone in the treatment of alcoholism: A clinical review. *Alcoholism* 13:35-39.

Phillips KA, McElroy SL, Hudson JI et al. (1995). Body dysmorphic disorder: An obsessive-compulsive disorder, a form of affective spectrum disorder, or both? *Journal of Clinical Psychiatry* 56(Suppl 4):41-51.

Rao S, Ziedonis D & Kosten T (1995). The pharmacotherapy of cocaine dependence. *Psychiatric Annals* 25:363-368.

Ramirez LF, McCormick RA, Russo AM et al. (1983). Patterns of substance abuse in pathological gamblers undergoing treatment. *Addictive Behaviors* 8:425-428.

Regier D, Farmer ME, Rae DS et al. (1990). Comorbidity of mental disorders with alcohol and other drug abuse. Results from the Epidemiologic Catchment Area (ECA) Study. *Journal of the American Medical Association* 264:2511-2518.

Richardson JS & Zaleski WA (1983). Naloxone and self-mutilation. *Biological Psychiatry* 18:99-101.

Rothbaum BO, Shaw L, Morris R et al. (1993). Prevalence of trichotillomania in a college freshmen population [letter]. *Journal of Clinical Psychiatry* 54:72.

Roy A, Adinoff B, Roehrich L et al. (1988). Pathological gambling: A psychobiological study. *Archives of General Psychiatry* 45:369-373.

Roy A, DeJong J & Linnoila M (1989). Extraversion in pathological gamblers. *Archives of General Psychiatry* 46:679-681.

Salomon RM, Mazure CM, Delgado PL et al. (1994). Serotonin function in aggression: The effect of acute plasma tryptophan depletion in aggressive patients. *Biological Psychiatry* 35:570-572.

Schlosser S, Black DW, Repertinger S et al. (1994). Compulsive buying. Demography, phenomenology, and comorbidity in 46 subjects. *General Hospital Psychiatry* 16:205-212.

Simeon D, Stanley B, Frances A et al. (1992). Self-mutilation in personality disorder: Psychological and biological correlates. *American Journal of Psychiatry* 149:221-226.

Specker SM, Carlson GA, Edmonson KM et al. (1996). Psychopathology in pathological gamblers seeking treatment. *Journal of Gambling Studies* 12:67-81.

Stein DJ, Hollander E & Liebowitz MR (1993). Neurobiology of impulsivity and the impulse control disorders. *Journal of Neuropsychiatry and Clinical Neuroscience* 5:9-17.

Steinberg MA, Kosten TA & Rounsaville BJ (1992). Cocaine abuse and pathological gambling. *American Journal on Addictions* 1:121-132.

Stennie KA & Gold MS (1997). Eating disorders and addictions: behavioral and neurobiological similarities. In NS Miller (ed.) *The Principles and Practice of Addiction Psychiatry*. Philadelphia, PA: W.B. Saunders, 433-439.

Swedo SE, Leonard HL, Rapoport JL et al. (1989). A double-blind comparison of clomipramine and desipramine in the treatment of trichotillomania (hair-pulling). *New England Journal of Medicine* 321:497-501.

Swift RM & Stout RL (1992). The relationship between craving, anxiety, and other symptoms in opioid withdrawal. *Journal of Substance Abuse Treatment* 4:19-26.

Szymanski HV & Olympia J (1991). Divalproex in post traumatic stress disorder [letter]. *American Journal of Psychiatry* 148:1086-1087.

Virkkunen M, DeJong J, Bartko J et al. (1989). Psychobiological concomitants of history of suicide attempts among violent offenders and impulsive fire setters. *Archives of General Psychiatry* 46:604-606.

Volberg RA & Steadman HJ (1988). Refining prevalence estimates of pathological gambling. *American Journal of Psychiatry* 145:502-505.

Volpicelli JR, Alterman AL, Hayashida M et al. (1992). Naltrexone in the treatment of alcohol dependence. *Archives of General Psychiatry* 49:876-880.

Ward NG (1975). Successful lithium treatment of transvestism associated with manic depression. *Journal of Nervous and Mental Disease* 161:204-206.

Washton A (1989). Cocaine may trigger sexual compulsivity. *U.S. Journal of Drug and Alcohol Dependency* 13:8.

Weddington WW, Brown BS, Haertzen CA et al. (1990). Changes in mood, craving, and sleep during short-term abstinence reported by male cocaine addicts. A controlled, residential study. *Archives of General Psychiatry* 47:861-868.

Winchel RM & Stanley M (1991). Self-injurious behavior: A review of the behavior and biology of self mutilation. *American Journal of Psychiatry* 148:306-317.

Wise MG & Tierney JG (1994). Impulse control disorders not elsewhere classified. In RE Hales, SC Yudofsky & JA Talbot JA (eds.) *Comprehensive Textbook of Psychiatry, 2nd Edition*. Washington, DC: American Psychiatric Press, 681-699.

Wray I & Dickerson MG (1981). Cessation of high frequency gambling and "withdrawal symptoms." *British Journal of Addiction* 76:401-405.

Zohar J, Kaplan Z & Benjamin J (1994). Compulsive exhibitionism successfully treated with fluvoxamine: A controlled case study. *Journal of Clinical Psychiatry* 55:86-88.

Chapter 7

Co-Occurring Addictive and Borderline Personality Disorders

Linda Dimeff, Ph.D.
Katherine Anne Comtois, Ph.D.
Marsha M. Linehan, Ph.D.

Prevalence of Borderline Personality Disorder
Treatment and Outcomes for BPD

Borderline personality disorder (BPD) and substance use disorders (SUDs) are severe and chronic mental health problems that commonly co-occur. Numerous studies have demonstrated that persons with both substance use disorders and personality disorders (PDs) have the most severe psychosocial and medical problems at baseline, throughout the course of treatment, and at followup. While few studies have found differences in substance use between PD and non-PD individuals during and after treatment, those patients with PD are less likely to remain in treatment.

This chapter focuses specifically on the comorbidity between BPD and SUDs, examining the prevalence of the overlap and the unique clinical challenges encountered in working with patients with BPD. It also describes Dialectical Behavior Therapy for Substance Abusers, which is an empirically supported, efficacious treatment for multi-disordered individuals with BPD and SUDs.

PREVALENCE OF BORDERLINE PERSONALITY DISORDER

Definition. BPD is a severe Axis II personality disorder characterized by intense and labile negative emotions, including depression, shame and anger, and significant conflict in interpersonal relationships, as well as extreme behavioral dyscontrol that is characterized by impulsivity and disinhibition. Suicide, nonsuicidal parasuicide (that is, intentionally self-harmful behaviors that cause tissue damage), and substance use are among the most common impulsive behaviors. Between 0.2% and 1.8% of the general population (8% to 11% of outpatients seeking mental health services, and 14% to 20% of inpatients) are thought to meet the criteria for BPD (Widiger & Frances, 1989; Widiger & Weissman, 1991; Modestin, Albrecht et al., 1997).

Linehan (1993a) has hypothesized that affect dysregulation is at the nexus of all other dysfunctional behaviors that comprise *DSM-IV* diagnostic criteria (American Psy-

TABLE 1. DSM-IV Criteria for Borderline Personality Disorder

Borderline Personality Disorder (BPD) involves a pervasive pattern of instability of interpersonal relationships, self-image and affects, and marked impulsivity, beginning by early adulthood and present in a variety of contexts, as indicated by five (or more) of the following:

- Frantic efforts to avoid real or imagined abandonment. (NOTE: Do not include suicidal or self-mutilating behavior.)

- A pattern of unstable and intense interpersonal relationships, characterized by alternating between extremes of idealization and devaluation identity disturbance, and markedly and persistently unstable self-image or sense of self.

- Identity disturbance: markedly and persistently unstable self-image or sense of self.

- Impulsivity in at least two areas that are potentially self-damaging (such as spending, sex, substance abuse, reckless driving, binge eating). (NOTE: Do not include suicidal or self-mutilating behavior.)

- Recurrent suicidal behavior, gestures, or threats, or self-mutilating behavior.

- Affective instability due to marked reactivity of mood (for example, intense episodic dysphoria, irritability, or anxiety), usually lasting a few hours and only rarely more than a few days.

- Chronic feelings of emptiness.

- Inappropriate, intense anger, or difficulty in controlling anger (such as frequent displays of temper, constant anger, or recurrent physical fights).

- Transient, stress-related paranoid ideation or severe dissociative symptoms.

SOURCE: American Psychiatric Association (1994). *Diagnostic and Statistical Manual of Mental Disorders, 4th Edition (DSM-IV)*. Washington, DC: American Psychiatric Press, 654.

chiatric Association, 1994). Specifically, impulsive behaviors (such as cutting or burning one's self, using drugs, or ingesting lethal drugs in a suicide attempt) all commonly function as methods to escape intense negative emotions. Linehan (1993a) has identified five domains of dysregulation characterizing BPD that correspond with the *DSM-IV* criteria (Table 1).

- Affective dysregulation: high emotional reactivity and lability, characterized by emotions that fluctuate frequently and often appear to "come out of nowhere." Overcontrol and undercontrol of anger are common in these patients.

- Interpersonal dysregulation: a "revolving door" of chaotic, unstable interpersonal relationships and difficulty in letting go of relationships.

- Self-dysregulation: a profound sense of emptiness and identity confusion.

- Behavioral dysregulation: parasuicidal acts, substance abuse, and other extreme, risky, and problematic impulsive behaviors.

- Cognitive dysregulation: all nonpsychotic forms of thought dysregulation, including dissociation, depersonalization, catastrophic thinking, and paranoid ideation.

BPD is the only *DSM-IV* diagnosis for which parasuicide is a criterion; parasuicide thus is considered a "hallmark" of BPD. Rates of parasuicide among patients diagnosed with BPD range from 69% to 80% (Clarkin, Widiger et al., 1983; Cowdry, Pickar et al., 1985; Gunderson, 1984). Rates of suicide among all BPD individuals—including those with no parasuicide—are 5% to 10% (Frances, Fyar et al., 1986) and are twice those seen when only persons with a history of parasuicide are included (Stone, Hurt et al., 1987). Parasuicide thus is a major health problem (Dublin, 1963; Shneidman, 1971). From 10% to 29% of individuals who parasuicide eventually die by suicide, a rate that far exceeds that of the general population (Dorpat & Ripley, 1960; Dahlgren, 1977).

BPD and the Use of Psychiatric Services. Research over the past two decades indicates that a subset (between 6% and 8%) of the overall population uses a disproportionate amount of inpatient psychiatric services: up to 42% of all admissions (Carpenter, Mulligan et al., 1985; Geller, 1986; Green, 1988; Hadley, McGurrin et al., 1990; Surber, Winkler et al., 1987; Woogh, 1986). Research by Hadley and colleagues (1990) indicates that, across sites, 75% to 80% of inpatient treatment dollars are spent on 30% to 35% of patients. Persons with BPD commonly are among the highest users of these services. In fact, between 9% and 40% of high users of psychiatric services in the studies done to date are diagnosed with BPD (Geller, 1986; Surber, Winkler et al., 1987; Widiger & Weissman, 1991; Woogh, 1986).

BPD and the Use of Health Care Services. Presenting medical concerns frequently include asthma, diabetes, hepatitis, and ulcers, as well as chronic fatigue syndrome, irritable bowel syndrome, and fibromyalgia (Hueston, Mainous et al., 1996). It is not uncommon for BPD patients to be dismissed as somaticizers because of the large number of somatic complaints they present. Indeed, only a small proportion (4%) of substance-dependent individuals with BPD meet the criteria for somaticization using the SCID I interviews (First, Spitzer et al., 1996).

Numerous studies that document a relationship between abuse in childhood and subsequent utilization of primary care and associated high medical costs in adulthood suggest that the high rate of medical problems in individuals with BPD is associated with growing up in a dysfunctional family environment (Felitti, 1991; Gould, Stevens et al., 1994; Koss, Koss et al., 1991; Lechner, Vogel et al., 1993; McCauley, Kern et al., 1997). Prevalence estimates of childhood abuse in the population with BPD range from 67% to 86% for sexual abuse and 71% for physical abuse, compared with rates of 22% to 34% for sexual abuse and 38% for physical abuse in non-BPD populations (Bryer, Nelson et al., 1987; Herman, Perry et al., 1989; Ogata, Silk et al., 1989; Stone, 1981; Wagner, Linehan et al., 1989).

Comorbidity of BPD and Substance Use Disorders. Rates of comorbidity between BPD and SUDs across drugs of abuse are high, and second only to mood disorders and antisocial personality disorder in the prevalence of comorbidity (Widiger & Trull, 1993). In their extensive review of data on the comorbidity of BPD and SUDs, gathered from studies published between 1987 to 1997, Trull and colleagues (2000) found considerable overlap. The prevalence of current SUDs among patients receiving treatment for BPD ranged from approximately 25% (Miller, Belkin et al., 1994) to 67%, or 57% when substance use was not used as a criterion for BPD (Dulit, Fyer et al., 1990). Conversely, among individuals seeking substance abuse treatment, rates of current BPD ranged from 5.2% (Brooner, King et al. 1997) to 65.1% (DeJong, van den Brink et al., 1993).

Substance abusers with BPD are more disturbed than substance abusers who do not have a personality disorder. Studies of substance-abusing consistently show that those with personality disorders have significantly more problems—including alcoholism, depression, and behavioral dyscontrol; more legal and medical problems; and more extensive involvement in substance abuse—than patients without personality disorders (Cacciola, Alterman et al., 2001; McKay, Alterman et al., 2000; Cacciola, Alterman et al., 1995; Ceccero, Ball et al., 1999; Rutherford, Cacciola et al., 1994; Nace, Davis et al., 1991). One study that discriminated BPD from other personality disorders found evidence that patients with BPD have more severe psychiatric problems than do patients with other PDs (Kosten, Kosten et al., 1989). Another study compared patients with BPD only, substance abuse only, or BPD and substance abuse (Links, Steiner et al., 1995). Over a seven-year period, individuals who had both disorders showed significantly more psychopathology, self-destructive behaviors, and suicidal thoughts than did individuals who had substance abuse or BPD alone.

TREATMENT AND OUTCOMES FOR BPD

Achieving treatment success with BPD patients has been notoriously difficult. Followup studies consistently indicate that BPD is a chronic disorder, although the number of individuals who continue to meet diagnostic criteria slowly decreases over the lifespan. Two to three years after index assessment, 60% to 70% of patients diagnosed with BPD continued to meet the criteria (Barasch, Frances et al., 1985). Other short-term followup studies reported little change in the patients' level of functioning and consistently high rates of psychiatric hospitalization over two to five years (Barasch, Frances et al., 1985; Dahl, 1986; Richman & Charles, 1976). Four to seven years after index assessment, 57% to 67% of patients continued to meet the criteria for BPD (Kullgren, 1992; Pope, Jonas et al., 1983). An average of 15 years after index assessment, 25% to 44% continued to meet the criteria (McGlashan, 1986; Paris, Brown et al., 1987).

BPD also has been associated with poorer outcomes in the treatment of Axis I disorders, such as major depression (Phillips & Nierenberg, 1994), obsessive-compulsive disorder (Baer, Jenike et al., 1992), bulimia (Ames-Frankel, Devlin et al., 1992; Coker, Vize et al., 1993), and substance use (Kosten, Kosten et al., 1989).

Analyses of outcomes for those who have received inpatient and outpatient treatment-as-usual (TAU) suggest that traditional treatments are marginally effective at best when outcomes are measured two to three years following treatment (Perry & Cooper, 1985; Tucker, Bauer et al., 1987). In pharmacotherapy trials, which often are short-term, dropout rates have been very high (Kelly, Soloff et al., 1992), and compliance has been problematic, with more than 50% of patients reporting misuse of their medications and 87% of therapists reporting medication misuse by their patients.

Despite recent advances in the treatment of BPD with medications (see Soloff, 1998 and 1994, for reviews), it is widely assumed that some form of ancillary behavioral treatment of BPD is necessary (Skodol, Buckley et al., 1983; Perry, Herman et al., 1990). However, there are few randomized, controlled studies of treatments designed specifically for BPD. In addition to the treatment developed by Linehan and colleagues, several other psychosocial treatments have been evaluated. Marziali and Munroe-Blum (1994) found that structured, time-limited group therapy was more effective than individual psychotherapy in retaining patients in treatment, although it did not improve outcome variables. More recently, Bateman and Fonagy (1999) demonstrated the efficacy of an 18-month psychoanalytically oriented partial hospitalization program in reducing suicidal behavior; results were maintained at 18-month followup (2001).

Dialectical Behavior Therapy (DBT) (Linehan, 1993a, 1993b), a cognitive-behavioral psychosocial treatment for chronically suicidal individuals with BPD, has been shown to be effective in reducing suicidal behavior in multiple trials, in which it also decreased use of emergency department and psychiatric services and increased treatment retention (Linehan, Armstrong et al., 1991; Linehan & Heard, 1993). Similar outcomes were found by Koons and colleagues (2000) in a randomized controlled trial of women veterans, in which DBT subjects had superior outcomes to TAU subjects on major outcome variables, including suicidal behavior and treatment retention, at each assessment period and at followup.

The authors recently adapted and evaluated DBT for use with substance-dependent women with BPD (Linehan & Dimeff, 1998). Results from a randomized controlled trial comparing DBT to TAU demonstrated DBT's efficacy in this population. Specifically, in comparison to TAU, DBT subjects had significantly greater reductions in drug use than TAU subjects throughout the treatment year and at followup, as well as significantly greater gains in global and social adjustment at followup. Further, subjects receiving DBT had a significantly lower drop-out rate than did the subjects receiving TAU (Linehan, Schmidt et al., 1999).

Defining Dialectical Behavior Therapy. DBT is a comprehensive, multistage cognitive-behavioral treatment for severely dysfunctional individuals with BPD (Linehan, 1993a, 1993b). It is based on a combined capability deficit and motivational model of BPD, which posits that (1) persons with BPD lack important interpersonal, self-regulation (including emotional regulation), and distress tolerance skills, and (2) personal and environmental factors often block and/or inhibit use of the behavioral skills these individuals do have and at times reinforce their dysfunctional behaviors.

DBT treatment blends cognitive-behavioral interventions with Eastern mindfulness practices and teaching techniques, and has elements in common with psychodynamic, patient-centered, Gestalt, paradoxical, and strategic approaches (cf. Heard & Linehan, 1994). DBT requires the therapist to balance use of strategies within each treatment interaction, from the rapid juxtaposition of change and acceptance techniques, to the therapist's use of both irreverent and warmly responsive communication styles. The emphasis on simultaneous acceptance and change leads to what could be considered a "dialectical abstinence" approach, in which absolute abstinence from the targeted dysfunctional behavior is emphasized in advance of dysfunctional episodes (such as drug use), and a harm reduction approach is emphasized after such an episode, followed by rapid recommitment to abstinence.

Dialectical Theory in DBT: Standard DBT and DBT for Substance Abusers is defined by its philosophical base (dialectics), treatment strategies, and treatment targets. Commonly associated with the teachings of Marx and Hegel, "dialectics" refers to a process of change, a method of logic or argumentation, and a particular understanding of the nature of reality (Linehan & Schmidt, 1995). As a process of change, dialectics posits that every idea or event (thesis) contains its opposite (antithesis), which generates and transforms the thesis and ultimately leads to a reconciliation of opposites (synthesis). Importantly, synthesis seldom is achieved through quiet mediation or accommodation of differences (for example, adding black to white pigment to achieve a medium gray), but instead occurs through a dynamic process of movement and, often, collision of opposing forces.

The term "dialectical" is meant to convey both the multiple tensions that coexist and are dealt with in therapy with patients with BPD, as well as the emphasis DBT places on enhancing balanced (dialectical) patterns of behavior and thinking to replace extreme response patterns and rigid, dichotomous thinking.

As a method of logic or argumentation, dialectics can be used clinically to expose the contradictions in a patient's position or thinking in an effort to achieve synthesis or change. For example, consider a patient who expresses that he or she is considering suicide because his or her emotional pain and suffering has become too excruciating to bear. Earlier in the week, the patient relapsed to heroin use and then, in an effort to reduce the physical discomfort of opiate withdrawal, abused some benzodiazepines that were prescribed by a former psychiatrist. After a careful assessment, the therapist learns that the patient's behavior of overdosing is under the control of the consequence (relief from psychological suffering) and not the antecedent (the earlier relapse). In response to the patient's comment, "I want out of this pain," the therapist might say irreverently, "How do you know that killing yourself will take away the pain and suffering? It is possible that your pain will become more intolerable if you kill yourself." By doing so, the therapist exposes the patient's logic ("death ends suffering"), while simultaneously contradicting it ("death by suicide might exacerbate suffering").

The overriding dialectic in DBT is the need to radically accept reality as it is (including pain and suffering), while at the same time working to change it. It is within this dialectic that the Zen practice of observing, mindfulness, nonjudgmental stance, and acceptance of the moment is integrated with a technology of change, using cognitive and behavioral techniques. This dance between the two core tensions in DBT is, in many respects, consistent with the notion of acceptance and change practiced within Twelve Step programs and embodied in the Serenity Prayer that is recited at Twelve Step meetings: "God, grant me the serenity to accept the things I cannot change, the courage to change the things I can, and the wisdom to know the difference." In DBT, dialectics is exemplified in the distress tolerance skills (described later in this chapter), including radical acceptance, which is comparable to the practice of acceptance in Twelve Step programs:

> Acceptance is the answer to all my problems today. When I am disturbed, it is because I find some person, place, thing, or situation—some fact of life—unacceptable to me, and I can find no serenity until I accept that person, place, thing or situation as being exactly the way it is supposed to be at this moment. Nothing, absolutely nothing, happens in God's world by mistake. Until I could accept my alcoholism, I could not stay sober; unless I accept life completely on life's terms, I cannot be happy. I need to concentrate not so much on what needs to be changed in the world as on what needs to be changed in me and in my attitudes (Alcoholics Anonymous, 1976, 449).

Core assumptions about the nature of reality in dialectics also form the nucleus of DBT. First, reality in dialectics is characterized by wholeness and connection. Parts are important only in relation to one another and in relation to the whole that they help create, define, and give meaning to. Given the interconnectedness of all things, changes anywhere in the system result in changes throughout the system.

Second, change is considered continuous in dialectics. In this sense, one can never step in the same river twice, so to speak, because each moment is changed by the moments before it and the imminence of the moment after.

Third, change occurs through dynamic interactions between polarity, as captured in the creation of synthesis, which is derived through the tensions between thesis and antithesis.

The spirit of a dialectical perspective is never to accept a final truth or an undisputed fact, and always to consider the question, "What is being left out of our understanding?" Truth is neither absolute nor relative, but always is evolving, developing, and constructed over time.

When applied to persuasion, DBT has therapist and patient seek to arrive at new meanings within old meanings by moving closer to the essence (synthesis) of the subject under consideration. The ability to see both sides of an argument, as well as to reach a synthesis of both sides (which is different from a compromise), demands skills that most patients with BPD lack at the time they enter treatment. Teaching patients how to think dialectically provides a way out of dichotomous, black-or-white thinking patterns that limit their options, and moves them from an "either-or" perspective to a "both-and" position.

Biosocial Theory in BPD. DBT is based on a biosocial model: The core problem in BPD is hypothesized by Linehan as pervasive emotion dysregulation. Emotion dysregulation represents a systemic dysfunction that results from a confluence of developmental factors (including genetic/biological and environmental/social learning), which in turn set the stage for later adult pathology. In Linehan's model, it is the transaction between a person with certain biologically predisposed emotional vulnerabilities and others in his or her life that create an invalidating environment, which eventually produces the cluster of dysfunctional behaviors classified as BPD. Here, "transaction" refers to a reciprocal process between the individual and his or her social environment, in which the person shapes and is shaped by the response of the social environment (Linehan, 1993a). That is, the individual engages in a particular behavior that has some effect on his or her environment; the environment then responds, shaping the behavior of the individual, who again responds, thus shaping and affecting the environment.

Emotional Vulnerability: Persons with high vulnerability to emotions display the following behavioral responses to stimuli across a number of contexts:

- High sensitivity to stimuli: Emotionally vulnerable individuals have a low threshold for emotional arousal and thus are more likely than non-vulnerable individuals to react emotionally to stimuli.

- More intense, extreme response to stimuli: Emotionally vulnerable persons respond more quickly and/or with greater emotional intensity.

- Slower return to baseline: Compared with normative responders, emotionally vulnerable individuals take longer to "ride out" the emotion following their initial arousal. Until a return to baseline has occurred, the individual remains more vulnerable to emotional stimuli.

In many respects, the emotional vulnerability of these individuals is analogous to the physical pain experienced by burn patients when their wounds are debrided. This is particularly relevant for patients with substance use disorders,

given the relationship between negative emotions and relapse (Marlatt & Gordon, 1985; Dimeff & Marlatt, 1998).

How emotional vulnerability develops and when it becomes pathologic in individuals with BPD also is of interest. It is possible that these individuals had fairly normative emotional functioning as infants, but that their normative affective communication was persistently punished or ignored by the individuals in their environments. In a transactional manner, the emotional arousal in the child may have continued to escalate until the social environment functionally attended to the child. In this fashion, emotional vulnerability developed through a transactional learning process. Alternatively, some individuals with BPD may have been born with a biological predisposition to emotional vulnerability and extreme sensitivity to their environments, such that normative parenting environments would have heightened and/or maintained their emotional sensitivity. In the latter scenario, problems emerge from the "poorness of fit" between the individual's temperament and the familial environment. This is similar to issues raised by a child with a reading disorder who participates in regular school programs for reading. While these programs are quite suitable for many children, the student with special needs may learn best in an environment tailored to that student's reading challenges.

Invalidating Environments: In Linehan's model, invalidating environments can significantly heighten emotional vulnerability and create the learning context from which BPD emerges (Linehan, 1993a). In an invalidating social or familial environment, individual communication of private experiences (such as thoughts, feelings, and physiological experiences that are not observable to others) are pervasively met by erratic, inappropriate, or extreme responses. Two primary characteristics of such an environment include: (1) the individual is told that his or her descriptions and analyses of private experiences are wrong, as is his or her understanding of what is causing these private experiences, and (2) the individual's public behavior and/or expressions of private behavior are attributed to socially unacceptable characteristics (for example, a "disorder" such as BPD, a manipulation attempt, or paranoia).

Examples of invalidating environments include families that favor controlling or inhibiting emotional expressiveness and that disapprove of expressed negative affect. Painful experiences are trivialized ("Why are you crying? There's nothing to cry about!") and are attributed to negative traits such as lack of motivation ("If you would just put your mind to it, you could do this"), without recognition that intense emotions are interfering with skillful actions. Similarly, failure to adopt a positive attitude is derided ("You want something to cry about? I'll give you something to really cry about!"). Other characteristics of an invalidating environment include restricting the demands the child may make on the environment ("If you want something, you must ask politely").

The consequences of growing up in an invalidating environment are considerable and contribute to emotional dysregulation by failing to teach the child to label and modulate arousal, tolerate distress, and trust his or her own emotional responses as valid interpretations of events. When the child's own experiences are invalidated, the child learns instead to scan the environment for cues about how to act and to feel. By exaggerating the ease with which life's problems can be solved, the environment fails to teach the child how to form realistic goals. By punishing the expression of negative emotion and responding erratically to emotional communication only after escalation by the child, the family shapes a style of emotional expression in which the child vacillates between extreme inhibition and suppression of emotional experience, on the one hand, and expression of extreme emotions on the other.

Stages and Modes of Treatment in DBT. DBT is a multistage treatment that begins with a set of specific pretreatment strategies aimed at fostering the patient's engagement and commitment to treatment, then proceeds to a hierarchy of treatment stages that move from treating severe behavioral dyscontrol, with a goal of increasing self-control (Stage 1), to building the capacity to sustain joy despite the suffering that is ubiquitous in living (Stage 4) (Linehan, in press). The goal of Stage 1 treatment is stabilization and connection to caregivers. Emotional processing of traumatic past events, including sexual and/or physical abuse, is not addressed until the second stage of treatment, after stabilization and behavioral self-control have been achieved. Treatment modes in standard DBT include individual psychotherapy, group skills training, telephone consultation, and consultation with the therapist. Two additional modes, pharmacotherapy and case management, were added to DBT for Substance Abusers.

Individual Psychotherapy: Like other behavioral therapies, treatment with DBT is hierarchical, targeting the most severe behaviors first. The initial target is any suicidal or life-threatening behavior, including parasuicide.

Therapy-interfering behaviors are targeted next, to ensure that factors that decrease therapist and patient motivation to work diligently in treatment are adequately addressed. Unless they are, the patient is more likely to miss sessions or to drop out of treatment, and the therapist is more likely to become "burned out" and to "give up" on a patient. Interfering behaviors include missing or coming late to session, lying, coming to session sedated on prescription medications or illicit drugs, responding to a message page received during a therapy session, or calling the therapist while intoxicated.

The third target involves reducing behaviors that interfere with the patient's quality of life. Substance use is the top priority for individuals who abuse drugs, followed by homelessness, excessive hospitalization, unemployment, economic difficulties, and health problems.

Finally, DBT seeks to increase skillful behaviors across the four skills training modules (mindfulness, interpersonal effectiveness, emotion regulation, and distress tolerance). In this manner, skillful behaviors replace disordered behaviors across the major areas of dysfunction.

Individual psychotherapy sessions of DBT begin with a review of the patient's diary card from the preceding week. The diary card is a daily record of common problem behaviors (including suicidal behaviors; use of alcohol, illicit drugs or prescription medications; urges to use alcohol or drugs; urges to harm one's self; physical discomfort, misery, and lying). It is completed by the patient throughout the week. The session agenda is determined largely by the behaviors recorded. Dysfunctional behaviors are addressed in order of their position on the DBT hierarchy of targets. If no dysfunctional behaviors have occurred, the focus of the session is determined by issues the patient wishes to address.

Regardless of the topic discussed, the DBT therapist always links problem behaviors and therapeutic strategies to the patient's goals, or the "ends in view." More specifically, abstinence from drug use or self-harmful behaviors never is discussed in isolation, but always is linked to the patient's reasons for seeking sobriety (such as improved relationships with children, to get and keep a good job, to complete a college degree, or to pursue meaningful work). The question always posed is: "Does this behavior move you closer to or further from your goals for a life worth living, and in what ways?" The DBT therapist maintains a keen eye on identifying in-session dysfunctional behaviors and emerging dysfunctional links, while analyzing the problem behavior. Dysfunctional behaviors are highlighted and solutions to specific behaviors are generated. Finally, the DBT therapist seeks to maintain a dialectical stance throughout the session (for example, "I know what I'm suggesting that you do is impossible, but you have to do it anyway").

DBT Group Skills Training for BPD Substance Abusers: Consistent with other cognitive-behavioral approaches to addictive behaviors (Marlatt & Gordon, 1985; Monti, Abrams et al., 1989; Miller & Munoz, 1982), the assumption underlying DBT group skills training is that many of the difficulties substance abusers have with BPD are due to behavioral skills deficits. The function of DBT skills training is to foster acquisition and strengthening of the skills needed to reduce substance use and other dysfunctional behaviors.

The treatment manual for DBT skills training (Linehan, 1993b) is highly structured and provides session-by-session guidelines for content and format. DBT skills training comprises four skills modules, two of which emphasize change (emotion regulation and interpersonal effectiveness) and two of which emphasize acceptance of reality (distress tolerance and mindfulness). The core mindfulness skills include focusing attention on the immediate moment, describing observations in words (which requires one to discriminate facts from interpretations), participating fully in the moment, assuming a non-judgmental stance, focusing awareness on the present moment, and effectiveness (focusing on what works). The interpersonal effectiveness module involves a number of skills for making requests or saying "no" and for resolving interpersonal conflicts in ways that achieve the intended goal while preserving or improving the relationship and maintaining self-respect.

Emotion regulation skills teach a variety of cognitive and behavioral skills to reduce emotional vulnerability. This module emphasizes how to identify and describe emotions, how to stop avoiding negative emotions, and how to increase positive emotions. Distress tolerance training teaches a number of strategies aimed at surviving a crisis (including intense drug craving or urges) without making matters worse by engaging in dysfunctional behaviors. This set of skills teaches a number of "delaying gratification" and self-soothing techniques, "willingness" (as opposed to "willfulness") to do what is needed in the moment, and radical acceptance of that which cannot be changed or modified. Because of the central importance of behavioral principles throughout

DBT, self-management techniques are woven throughout all four skills modules.

In contrast to standard DBT skills training groups, which employ a 150-minute format and emphasize skills strengthening (through role plays and homework review), as well as skills acquisition, DBT skills training groups for substance users are 90 minutes in length and focus exclusively on skills acquisition. This modification of the standard DBT was made because of the high rates of social phobia found among substance-using patients, which compromise their attendance at group and skills building. Skills strengthening activities now occur in the Individual Skills Consultation mode described below.

DBT Individual Skills Consultation for Patients With BPD and a Substance Use Disorder: This treatment mode emphasizes skills strengthening exercises, including review of homework from the preceding week, behavior rehearsal, feedback, and coaching. To increase attendance at skills group, individual skills consultation ideally is conducted by one of the two group leaders, thus giving participants an opportunity to develop a strong bond with at least one of the group therapists; this eases their anxiety about attending group. The authors' experience to date is that inclusion of this mode has resulted in an increase in group attendance.

Dialectical Abstinence in DBT. A dialectical stance on substance use was developed in recognition of research showing that, on the one hand, cognitive-behavioral relapse prevention approaches are effective in reducing the frequency and intensity of relapses following periods of abstinence (Dimeff & Marlatt, 1998; Carroll, 1996; Marlatt & Gordon, 1985) and, on the other hand, "absolute abstinence" approaches are effective in lengthening the interval between periods of use (Hall, Havassy et al., 1990; Supnick & Colletti, 1984). "Dialectical abstinence," which seeks to balance the two approaches, is a synthesis of unrelenting insistence on total abstinence with an emphasis on radical acceptance, nonjudgmental problem-solving, and effective relapse prevention after any drug use (followed by a quick return to unrelenting insistence on abstinence). The essence of the absolute abstinence end of the dialectic involves teaching patients specific cognitive self-control strategies that allow them to turn their minds fully and completely to abstinence. Specifically, they are taught how to anticipate and treat willfulness, hopelessness, and waffling on one's commitment to avoid drugs, all of which complicate treatment once an individual makes a commitment to give up a dysfunctional behavior. Patients are taught that the key to absolute abstinence lies in convincing one's brain that use of drugs is completely out of the question. One does this by making a commitment to remain abstinent for a specified period of time—a period that is no longer than he or she can commit to with 100% certainty that abstinence will be maintained (and no longer). Like the popular Twelve Step slogan, "Just for Today," the commitment to 100% abstinence may be for only one day, for a month, or for five minutes, depending on what the individual can commit to with 100% certainty. The commitment then is an act of mental "slamming the door shut" for the specified period of time. At the end of that time, the individual renews his or her commitment to abstinence. In this sense, absolute abstinence is achieved through a series of commitments to "slam the door shut." Hence, abstinence is sought only in the moment and only for a given set of moments. The goal of this strategy is to block the patient's ability to make half-hearted commitments or to deny the reality of a commitment after it has been made, while simultaneously limiting the duration of the commitment to a period that is perceived as achievable.

Other cognitive self-control strategies used during this phase include immediate "adaptive" denial of desires and options to use alcohol or drugs during the specified period of the commitment, practicing radical acceptance of the absence of substance use and the difficulties involved, making an inner resolution that the option to use is left open for the future, and making a promise to one's self that such use will be available when close to death or upon learning of a terminal illness. Determining which strategy to use depends on a decision as to which one is most likely to be effective in promoting abstinence and achieving the willingness to maintain it.

With no allegiance to a particular ideology or approach other than therapeutic effectiveness in achieving the ultimate treatment goal (for example, a drug-free life that is worth living), the therapist teaches patients to shift rapidly to the harm-reduction mode once a slip has occurred. Here the emphasis is on acquiring and strengthening the skill of "failing well," as by admitting that drug use has occurred and learning from one's mistakes. In teaching how to fail well, emphasis is placed on "what if" and "just in case" skills. Consistent with a relapse prevention approach (Marlatt & Gordon, 1985), the therapist and patient discuss realistic skills the patient can acquire and plans that can be made to address a similar situation in the future. In addition to teaching the patient to learn from past mistakes and encouraging

him or her to continue to move forward toward the goal, failing well includes analysis of and reparation for harm done to others. The emphasis on correcting harm is similar to that on "making amends" in Twelve Step programs.

CONCLUSIONS

Borderline personality disorder and substance use disorders both are severe, chronic behavioral disorders. In combination, the two disorders pose considerable treatment challenges for both the patient and the clinician. Dialectical Behavior Therapy, an empirically supported therapy for chronically suicidal patients with BPD, has demonstrated efficacy for substance-dependent persons with BPD. This chapter reviewed the biosocial theory for the development and maintenance of BPD, the theoretical foundations of DBT, and the stages and modes that compose this comprehensive treatment.

ACKNOWLEDGMENT: Preparation of this chapter was supported by grant DAO8674 from the National Institute on Drug Abuse, and grant MH34486 from the National Institute on Mental Health, awarded to Dr. Linehan.

REFERENCES

Alcoholics Anonymous (1976). *Alcoholics Anonymous.* New York, NY: Alcoholics Anonymous World Services, Inc.

American Psychiatric Association (APA) (1994). *Diagnostic and Statistical Manual of Mental Disorders, 4th Edition (DSM-IV).* Washington, DC: American Psychiatric Press.

Ames-Frankel J, Devlin MJ, Walsh T et al. (1992). Personality disorder diagnoses in patients with bulimia nervosa: Clinical correlates and changes with treatment. *Journal of Clinical Psychiatry* 53:90-96.

Baer L, Jenike MA, Black DW et al. (1992). Effect of Axis II diagnoses on treatment outcome with clomipramine in 55 patients with obsessive-compulsive disorder. *Archives of General Psychiatry* 49:862-866.

Barasch A, Frances AJ & Hurt SW (1985). Stability and distinctness of borderline personality disorder. *American Journal of Psychiatry* 142:1484-1486.

Bateman A & Fonagy P (1999). Effectiveness of partial hospitalization in the treatment of borderline personality disorder: A randomized controlled trial. *American Journal of Psychiatry* 156:1563-1569.

Bateman A & Fonagy P (2001). Treatment of borderline personality disorder with psychoanalytically oriented partial hospitalization: An 18-month follow-up. *American Journal of Psychiatry* 158:36-42.

Brooner RK, King VL, Kidorf M et al. (1997). Psychiatric and substance use comorbidity among treatment-seeking opioid abusers. *Archives of General Psychiatry* 54(1):71-80.

Bryer JB, Nelson BA, Miller JB et al. (1987). Childhood sexual and physical abuse as factors in adult psychiatric illness. *American Journal of Psychiatry* 144:1426-1430.

Cacciola JS, Alterman AI, Rutherford MJ et al. (2001). The relationship of psychiatric comorbidity to treatment outcomes in methadone maintained patients. *Drug and Alcohol Dependence* 61:271-280.

Cacciola JS, Alterman AI, Rutherford MJ et al. (1995). Treatment response of antisocial substance abusers. *Journal of Nervous and Mental Disease* 183:166-171.

Carpenter MD, Mulligan JC, Bader IA et al. (1985). Multiple admissions to an urban psychiatric center: A comparative study. *Hospital & Community Psychiatry* 36:1305-1308.

Carroll KM (1996). Relapse prevention as a psychological treatment: A review of controlled clinical trials. *Experimental and Clinical Psychopharmacology* 4:46-54.

Ceccero JJ, Ball SA, Tennen H et al. (1999). Concurrent and predictive validity of antisocial personality disorder subtyping among substance abusers. *Journal of Nervous and Mental Disease* 187:478-486.

Cioffi D & Holloway J (1993). Delayed costs of suppressed pain. *Journal of Personality and Social Psychology* 64:274-282.

Clarkin JF, Widiger TA, Frances AJ et al. (1983). Prototypic typology and the borderline personality disorder. *Journal of Abnormal Psychiatry* 92:263-275.

Coker S, Vize C, Wade T et al. (1993). Patients with bulimia nervosa who fail to engage in cognitive behavior therapy. *International Journal of Eating Disorders* 13:35-40.

Cowdry RW, Pickar D & Davies R (1985). Symptoms and EEG findings in the borderline syndrome. *International Journal of Psychiatry in Medicine* 15:201-211.

Dahl AA (1986). Prognosis of the borderline disorders. *Psychopathology* 19:68-79.

Dahlgren KG (1977). Attempted suicide: 35 years afterward. *Suicide and Life-Threatening Behavior* 7:75-79.

DeJong CA, van den Brink W, Hartveld FM et al. (1993). Personality disorders in alcoholics and drug addicts. *Comprehensive Psychiatry* 34:87-94.

Dimeff LA & Marlatt GA (1998). Preventing relapse and maintaining change in addictive behaviors. *Clinical Psychology: Science and Practice* 5:513-525.

Dorpat TL & Ripley HS (1960). A study of suicide in the Seattle area. *Comprehensive Psychiatry* 1:349-359.

Dublin LI (1963). *Suicide: A Sociological and Statistical Study.* New York, NY: Ronald Press.

Dulit RA, Fyer MR, Haas GL et al. (1990). Substance use in borderline personality disorder. *American Journal of Psychiatry* 147:1002-1007.

Felitti VJ (1991). Long term consequences of incest, rape, and molestation. *Southern Medical Journal* 84:328-31.

First MB, Spitzer RL, Gibbons M et al. (1996). *User's Guide for the Structured Clinical Interview for DSM-IV Axis II Personality Disorders (SCID-II).* New York, NY: Biometrics Research Department, New York State Psychiatric Institute.

Frances AJ, Fyer MR & Clarkin JF (1986). Personality and suicide. *Annals of the New York Academy of Sciences* 487:281-293.

Geller JL (1986). In again, out again: Preliminary evaluation of a state hospital's worst recidivists. *Hospital & Community Psychiatry* 37:386-390.

Gould DA, Stevens NG, Ward NG et al. (1994). Self-reported childhood abuse in an adult population in a primary care setting. *Archives of Family Medicine* 3:252-256.

Green JH (1988). Frequent rehospitalization and noncompliance with treatment. *Hospital & Community Psychiatry* 39:963-966.

Gunderson JG (1984). *Borderline Personality Disorder.* Washington DC: American Psychiatric Press.

Hadley TR, McGurrin MC, Pulice RT et al. (1990). Using fiscal data to identify heavy service users. *Psychiatric Quarterly* 61:41-48.

Hall SM, Havassy BE & Wasserman DA (1990). Commitment to abstinence and acute stress in relapse to alcohol, opiates, and nicotine. *Journal of Consulting and Clinical Psychology* 58:175-181.

Heard HL & Linehan MM (1994). Dialectical behavior therapy: An integrative approach to the treatment of borderline personality disorder. *Journal of Psychotherapy Integration* 4:55-82.

Herman JL, Perry JC & van der Kolk BA (1989). Childhood trauma in borderline personality disorder. *American Journal of Psychiatry* 146:490-495.

Hueston WJ, Mainous AG & Schilling R (1996). Patients with personality disorders: Functional status, health care utilization, and satisfaction with care. *Journal of Family Practice* 42: 54-60.

Kelly T, Soloff PH, Cornelius J et al. (1992). Can we study (treat) borderline patients? Attrition from research and open treatment. *Journal of Personality Disorders* 6:417-433.

Koons CR, Robins CJ, Lynch TR et al. (2000). Efficacy of dialectical behavior therapy in women veterans with borderline personality disorder. *Behavior Therapy.*

Koss MP, Koss PG & Woodruff WJ (1991). Deleterious effects of criminal victimization of women's health and medical utilization. *Archives of Internal Medicine* 151:342-347.

Kosten RA, Kosten TR & Rounsaville BJ (1989). Personality disorders in opiate addicts show prognostic specificity. *Journal of Substance Abuse Treatment* 6:163-168.

Kullgren G (1992). Personality disorders among psychiatric inpatients. *Nordisk Psykiastrisktidsskrift* 46:27-32.

Lechner ME, Vogel ME, Garcia-Shelton LM et al. (1993). Self-reported medical problems of adult female survivors of childhood sexual abuse. *Journal of Family Practice* 36:633-638.

Linehan MM (1993a). *Cognitive Behavioral Therapy of Borderline Personality Disorder.* New York, NY: Guilford Press.

Linehan MM (in press). Development, evaluation, and dissemination of effective psychosocial treatments: Stages of disorder, levels of care, and stages of treatment research. In MD Glantz & CR Hartel (eds.). *Drug Abuse: Origins and Interventions.* Washington, DC: American Psychological Association.

Linehan MM (1993b). *Skills Training Manual for Treating Borderline Personality Disorder.* New York, NY: Guilford Press.

Linehan MM, Armstrong HE, Suarez A et al. (1991). Cognitive-behavioral treatment of chronically parasuicidal borderline patients. *Archives of General Psychiatry* 48:1060-1064.

Linehan MM & Dimeff LA (1998). *Dialectical Behavior Therapy Manual of Treatment Interventions for Drug Abusers with Borderline Personality Disorder* (Unpublished manuscript).

Linehan MM & Heard HL (1993). Impact of treatment accessibility on clinical course of parasuicidal patients: In reply to RE Hoffman [Letter to the editor]. *Archives of General Psychiatry* 50:157-158.

Linehan MM & Schmidt H III (1995). The dialectics of effective treatment of borderline personality disorder. In WO O'Donohue & L Krasner (eds.). *Theories in Behavior Therapy: Exploring Behavior Change.* Washington, DC: American Psychological Association, 553-584.

Linehan MM, Schmidt H, Dimeff LA et al. (1999). Dialectical behavior therapy for patients with borderline personality disorder and drug dependence. *American Journal of Addictions*.

Ling W, Rawson RA & Compton MA (1994). Substitution pharmacotherapies for opioid addiction: From methadone to LAAM and buprenorphine. *Journal of Psychoactive Drugs* 26:119-128.

Links PS, Steiner M, Offord DR et al. (1998). Characteristics of borderline personality disorder: A Canadian study. *Canadian Journal of Psychiatry* 33:336-340.

Marlatt GA & Gordon JR (1985). *Relapse Prevention: Maintenance Strategies in the Treatment of Addictive Behaviors*. New York, NY: Guilford Press.

Marziali E & Munroe-Blum H (1994). *Interpersonal Group Psychotherapy for Borderline Personality Disorder*. New York, NY: Basic Books.

McCauley J, Kern DE, Kolodner K et al. (1997). *Journal of the American Medical Association* 277:1362-1368.

McGlashan TH (1986). The Chestnut Lodge follow-up study, III: Long-term outcome of borderline personality disorder. *Archives of General Psychiatry* 43:20-30.

McKay JR, Alterman AI, Cacciola JS et al. (2000). Prognostic significance of antisocial personality disorder in cocaine-dependent patients entering continuing care. *Journal of Nervous and Mental Disease* 188:287-296.

Miller NS, Belkin BM & Gibbons R (1994). Clinical diagnosis of substance use disorders in private psychiatric populations. *Journal of Substance Abuse Treatment* 11:387-392.

Miller WR & Munoz RF (1982). *How to Control Your Drinking: A Practical Guide to Responsible Drinking*. Albuquerque, NM: University of New Mexico Press.

Modestin J, Albrecht I, Tschaggelar W et al. (1997). Diagnosing borderline: A contribution to the question of its conceptual validity. *Archives Psychiatrica Nervenkra* 233:359-370.

Monti PM, Abrams DB, Kadden RM et al. (1989). *Treating Alcohol Dependence*. New York, NY: Guilford Press.

Nace EP, Davis CW & Gaspari JP (1991). Axis II comorbidity in substance abusers. *American Journal of Psychiatry* 148:118-120.

Ogata SN, Silk KR, Goodrich S et al. (1989). Childhood Sexual and Clinical Symptoms in Borderline Patients. Unpublished manuscript.

Paris J, Brown R & Nowlis D (1987). Long-term follow-up of borderline patients in a general hospital. *Comprehensive Psychiatry* 28(6):530-535.

Perry JC & Cooper SH (1985). Psychodynamics, symptoms, and outcome in borderline and antisocial personality disorders and bipolar type II affective disorder. In TH McGlashan (ed.) *The Borderline: Current Empirical Research*. Washington, DC: American Psychiatric Press, 19-41.

Perry JC, Herman JL, van der Kolk BA et al. (1990). Psychotherapy and psychological trauma in borderline personality disorder. *Psychiatric Annals* 20:33-43.

Phillips KA & Nierenberg AA (1994). The assessment and treatment of refractory depression. *Journal of Clinical Psychiatry* 55:20-26.

Platt S, Bille-Brahe U, Kerkhof A et al. (1992). Parasuicide in Europe: The WHO/EURO multicentre study on parasuicide. I. Introduction and preliminary analysis for 1989. *Acta Psychiatrica Scandinavica* 85:97-104.

Pope HG, Jonas JM, Hudson JI et al. (1983). The validity of *DSM-III* borderline personality disorder: A phenomenologic, family history, treatment response, and long term follow-up study. *Archives of General Psychiatry* 40:23-30.

Richman J & Charles E (1976). Patient dissatisfaction and attempted suicide. *Community Mental Health Journal* 12(3):301-305.

Rutherford MJ, Cacciola JS & Alterman AI (1994). Relationships of personality disorders with problem severity in methadone patients. *Drug and Alcohol Dependence* 35:69-76.

Shneidman ES (1971). You and death. *Psychology Today* 43-45, 74-80.

Skodol AE, Buckley P & Charles E (1983). Is there a characteristic pattern to the treatment history of clinic outpatients with borderline personality? *Journal of Nervous and Mental Disease* 171:405-410.

Smith RG, Monson RA & Ray DC (1986). Psychiatric consultation in somatization disorder: A randomized controlled study. *New England Journal of Medicine* 314(22):1407-1413.

Soloff PH (1994). Is there any drug treatment of choice for the borderline patient? *Acta Psychiatrica Scandinavica* 379:50-55.

Soloff PH (1998). Symptom-oriented psychopharmacology for personality disorders. *Journal of Practical Psychiatry and Behavioral Health* 4:3-11.

Stone MH (1981). Psychiatrically ill relatives of borderline patients: A family study. *Psychiatric Quarterly* 58:71-83.

Stone MH, Hurt SW & Stone DK (1987). The PI 500: Long-term follow-up of borderline inpatients meeting *DSM-III* criteria. I: Global outcome. *Journal of Personality Disorders* 1:291-298.

Supnick JA & Colletti G (1984). Relapse coping and problem solving training following treatment for smoking. *Addictive Behaviors* 9:401-404.

Surber RW, Winkler EL, Monteleone M et al. (1987). Characteristics of high users of acute inpatient services. *Hospital and Community Psychiatry* 38:1112-1116.

Tanney BL (1992). Mental disorders, psychiatric patients, and suicide. In RW Maris, AL Berman & JT Maltsberger (eds.) *Assessment and Prediction of Suicide*. New York, NY: Guilford Press, 277-320.

Trull TJ, Sher KJ, Minks-Brown C et al. (2000). Borderline personality disorder and substance use disorders: A review and integration. *Clinical Psychology Review*, 20, 235-253.

Tucker L, Bauer SF, Wagner S et al. (1987). Long-term hospital treatment of borderline patients: A descriptive outcome study. *American Journal of Psychiatry* 144:1443-1448.

Wagner AW, Linehan MM & Wasson EJ (1989). Parasuicide: Characteristics and relationship to childhood sexual abuse. Poster presented at the annual meeting of the Association for Advancement of Behavior Therapy, Washington, DC.

Wegner DM & Gold DB (1995). Fanning old flames: Emotional and cognitive effects of suppressing thoughts of a past relationship. *Journal of Personality and Social Psychology* 67:782-792.

Widiger TA & Frances AJ (1989). Epidemiology, diagnosis, and comorbidity of borderline personality disorder. In A Tasman, RE Hales & AJ Frances (eds.) *American Psychiatric Press Review of Psychiatry*. Washington, DC: American Psychiatric Press, 8:8-24.

Widiger TA & Trull TJ (1993). Borderline and narcissistic personality disorders. In H Adams & P Sutker (eds.) *Comprehensive Handbook of Psychopathology (2nd Edition)*. New York, NY: Plenum Press, 371-394.

Widiger TA & Weissman MM (1991). Epidemiology of borderline personality disorder. *Hospital and Community Psychiatry* 42:1015-1021.

Woogh CM (1986). A cohort through the revolving door. *Canadian Journal of Psychiatry* 31:214-221.

| Chapter 8 | # Integrating Psychosocial Services With Pharmacotherapies in the Treatment of Co-Occurring Disorders |

Joan E. Zweben, Ph.D.

Working With Counselors and Psychotherapists
Use of Pharmacotherapies
Recovery-Oriented Psychotherapy
Co-Occurring Disorder Patients in Self-Help Groups

The goal of this chapter is to offer assistance to the clinician who is engaged in coordinating addiction and psychosocial treatment services on behalf of patients with co-occurring substance use and psychiatric disorders ("dual disorders"). It focuses on four areas of concern:

First, one of the great strengths of the addiction field is its multidisciplinary teamwork. While the physician who works in a program with multiple components is an essential part of the health care team, professionals who offer psychosocial interventions also play a major role.

Second, cost constraints now restrict the physician's role far more narrowly than many would prefer. Given these constraints, effective interdisciplinary teamwork often makes the difference between a first-rate program and an average one.

Third, recent developments have expanded opportunities for physicians in office-based practice. Taking advantage of such opportunities requires that physicians become adept at integrating services that are not provided at the office site. The chapter addresses key elements affecting such teamwork and coordination.

Finally, good supervision or collaboration is time-consuming and requires strong facilitation skills at the leadership level. When treatment providers are in conflict, patients suffer. This chapter describes a variety of common situations and dilemmas and offers practical options for handling them.

WORKING WITH COUNSELORS AND PSYCHOTHERAPISTS

Psychosocial interventions typically are provided by practitioners from a variety of disciplines. These range from non-credentialed counselors (usually persons in recovery), to licensed psychologists, social workers, and marriage, family, and child counselors. Such practitioners differ widely in their attitudes, preparation, and skills. They also vary in the degree to which they are accustomed to working with physicians and other medical personnel. Understanding the background and orientation of specific staff can enhance communication and teamwork.

Counselors. Non-credentialed counselors have been integrated into treatment teams on inpatient units since the 1950s, when the Minnesota Model was developed at

Hazelden and Wilmar (McElrath, 1997). Before that time, alcoholism was seen as a psychological vulnerability to be treated on mental health units; however, this theoretical framework failed to produce effective treatment. Collaboration by the leaders of Hazelden and Wilmar led to an adaptation of the principles of Alcoholics Anonymous (AA) to create a new model within hospital-based treatment. Wilmar and Hazelden eventually blended their approaches to produce the Minnesota Model, which became the prototype of 28-day inpatient programs. Proponents of the model refined their treatment practices and restructured institutional relationships to emphasize collaboration between professional staff and non-credentialed recovering persons. By 1954, nondegreed counselors shared both responsibility and decisionmaking authority.

Therapeutic communities (TCs), which developed and expanded in the 1960s, also relied predominantly on non-credentialed staff who were themselves in recovery (Deitch, 1973; DeLeon, 1994, 1995, 2000). Some of these gifted clinicians and managers subsequently were hired into the private, insurance-funded treatment system, to which they brought their perspective on the importance of developing a culture that supports recovery. Their appreciation of the need to strengthen environmental or microcommunity forces to foster change added an important dimension to the professional model, which typically assumes that professional services are the main—if not the sole—factor in promoting change.

Programs today differ widely in the extent to which they incorporate non-licensed, recovering personnel. Such personnel are found most often in short-term, Minnesota Model, chemical dependency inpatient programs and in a growing number of dual diagnosis programs. They are employed in community-based addiction treatment, especially programs based on Twelve Step principles. They also are dominant in therapeutic communities, which have their own conceptual model that integrates Twelve Step elements to varying degrees. Some of these counselors return to school and obtain graduate degrees and licenses, building the cadre of professionals in recovery.

Like licensed staff members, non-credentialed counselors vary widely in talent, experience, and skill. Some have little training, except for occasional in-service training sessions. Others have completed comprehensive credentialing programs and are far more sophisticated than some licensed staff. For example, certificate programs (often attached to universities) may require 200 to 300 hours of course work, plus supervised field placement experience. However, some of these programs teach from an exclusively Twelve Step perspective and do not do justice to alternative approaches or to the empirical literature, while others are more broadly based.

Some counselors have superb skills; their "street savvy" and personal experience in recovery produce a highly sophisticated clinician. Others tend toward rigidity ("what worked for me will work for you") and have difficulty tolerating the ambiguities of the complex clinical populations seen today. In short, physicians should draw conclusions about the skill level of the counselors with whom they work from direct observation, not from inferences based on the presence or absence of credentials.

At their best, such counselors also are a powerful role model, a contribution deeply valued by addicted patients, especially those in early recovery.

Licensed Professionals. Within addiction treatment settings, one finds licensed professionals, some of whom are recovering, others who are not. Some may be highly knowledgeable, others less so. Although most such professionals have basic clinical skills, their ability and comfort in adapting those skills to the addicted patient population vary greatly. The rigidities of some licensed professionals arise from devotion to theoretical models in which they have extensive training, in addition to their own personality traits.

Physicians should be cautious about drawing conclusions from the presence of academic credentials and professional licenses. Unfortunately, graduate schools rarely integrate thorough training in the assessment and treatment of addiction into their core curricula, even though many of the clinical populations with whom graduates will work are using alcohol and drugs. Typically, such training is provided as an elective (if at all) or in a course mandated by the increasing number of states that require an introductory course for initial licensure or relicensure. Other programs offer extensive training through extension courses or specialized training institutes and some graduate programs offer addiction treatment as a subspecialty. However, the physician never should assume that a professional is knowledgeable in this area. Professionals may underestimate their own lack of knowledge, preferring to believe that the models they acquired in training can be adapted to treating addiction with little modification, or that specialized knowledge about addictive disorders is unnecessary.

Clinical experience alone may tell little about qualifications. Upon inquiry, a therapist may say, "I've been seeing alcohol and drug users for 20 years." Many therapists have evolved practices with which they have grown comfortable, but which bear little relation to those supported by an empirical literature or by the experience of clinicians who are addiction specialists. The comfort level of these therapists is sustained because they do not count, much less study, their dropouts, and thus have no objective means of monitoring patient progress in becoming alcohol- and drug-free. (This is of particular concern because many patients report concealing or minimizing their alcohol and drug use during psychotherapy.) In selecting good therapists for referral, physicians should look for evidence of recent systematic training, either through conferences or course work. Such evidence increases the likelihood that the therapist will be familiar with sound treatment practices.

Tensions may be present between recovering and non-recovering staff, and between those with and without professional training and licenses. Passions can run high, and basic concepts can be used to express disapproval or to discredit one's colleagues. The concepts of enabling and codependency in particular lend themselves to disparaging colleagues who take certain positions. They often are used to discourage appropriate forms of helping and to terminate treatment prematurely. Time in treatment is correlated significantly with positive outcomes in a large number of treatment outcome studies (Gerstein, 1994; Gerstein & Harwood, 1990; Hubbard, Marsden et al., 1989; Simpson & Curry, 1997). Thus, the goal is to engage and retain patients in treatment, not to terminate them for manifesting symptoms of their psychiatric or addictive disorder. Physicians also may struggle in dealing with this phenomena, even though other chronic diseases such as asthma, diabetes, and hypertension have compliance rates comparable to those of addiction treatment (McLellan, Lewis et al., 2000; McLellan, Metzger et al., 1995). They may need to be the voice of reason, preventing premature termination of the patient, while being mindful of the need to avoid colluding in negative patient behaviors.

Physicians in leadership roles are advised to establish weekly in-service training sessions that address both basic and specialized topics. They can create a multidisciplinary team that has a shared language and is knowledgeable about integrating the treatment of addictive, psychiatric, and medical disorders. Many sources of excellent training materials exist. Some materials are available at no charge (such as the Treatment Improvement Protocols published by the federal Center for Substance Abuse Treatment). These materials can be used to organize onsite training sessions. Securing continuing education credits for the disciplines represented on staff enhances participation and commitment to a high quality training sequence.

Collaboration With Psychotherapists in the Community. The diversity of psychotherapists in the community can make effective collaboration even more challenging. Table 1 describes certain key differences between general psychotherapy and addiction treatment.

Addiction treatment typically is highly structured, with multiple behavioral expectations. Psychotherapy usually has minimal structure other than the scheduled sessions. Psychodynamic therapists in particular may have difficulty incorporating behavioral commitments, whereas eclectic therapists may find this work more comfortable. Most outpatient addiction treatment is abstinence-oriented. Although this goal may be difficult to reach, the goal itself normally does not vary. Abstinence usually is viewed as the foundation that must be in place before meaningful progress can be made on other issues.

Psychotherapy has a wider range of goals and less consistent priorities. Some psychotherapists may not understand or endorse the need for abstinence over some form of controlled use. For example, they may share the view that drinking is "normal." Hence, they see controlled drinking as a reasonable goal, even in patients who have repeatedly demonstrated they cannot moderate their use (Brown, 1985). Addiction treatment makes alcohol and drug use the primary focus, while psychodynamic psychotherapy explores the underlying process as a means of bringing about change. If ill-timed, this focus on process can undermine sobriety by elevating anxiety before abstinence is firmly established.

Addiction treatment often includes breath and urine testing if resources permit, whereas psychotherapists rarely arrange such testing and many consider it invasive and abhorrent. Addiction treatment encompasses a variety of treatment components, while psychotherapy usually relies on the therapy sessions themselves as the sole component. Therapists and counselors in addiction treatment are active and directive, whereas psychotherapists in private practice have a variety of styles, which can be more or less compatible with addiction treatment. These differences pose an adaptive challenge to the physician who is arranging for treatment of patients with dual disorders.

TABLE 1. Typical Attributes of Addiction Treatment and Psychotherapy, Compared

Typical Attributes of Addiction Treatment	Typical Attributes of Psychotherapy
1. Structured format	1. Minimal structure
2. Goals less flexible	2. Wider range of goals
3. Alcohol and drug focus	3. Focus on underlying process
4. Monitoring by breath and urine testing	4. No testing; possible negative attitude
5. Varied treatment components	5. One component
6. Active, directive therapists	6. Varied clinical styles

SOURCE: Adapted from Rawson R (1997). Issues in Outpatient Treatment. Presented at the Medical-Scientific Conference of the American Society of Addiction Medicine, Atlanta, GA; April.

USE OF PHARMACOTHERAPIES

Recovering patients who have conditions that require psychotropic or other medications have very special needs. Their specific drug use history makes the use of certain medications highly problematic because of the potential for abuse of the prescribed drug, or that use of such a drug will precipitate relapse to the primary drug of abuse. Although this volume offers appropriate prescribing guidelines, patients who present for treatment may be taking medications prescribed by physicians who lack a background in addiction medicine. In settings where patients are seen by physicians only when specific problems emerge, counselors need a screening tool that incorporates warning signals (such as prescriptions for benzodiazepines) that indicate a need for physician review.

Recovering patients also have complex feelings and attitudes toward medications that need to be understood and addressed. Many define recovery as living a comfortable and responsible lifestyle without the use of psychoactive drugs. Yet some disorders require the use of psychiatric medications. Family members or Twelve Step program participants may criticize the patient or pressure for discontinuation of medication, generating conflict that undermines treatment. Because physicians often lack adequate time to deal with such issues, these tasks should be delegated specifically to other members of the treatment team. Such providers may need some additional training to handle medication issues.

Achieving Adherence. Adherence to treatment recommendations is a key factor in successful treatment outcomes. Hence, physicians should monitor how well the treatment team attends to this issue. Compliance with medication regimens is far from perfect, even in well-educated middle-class patients who do not have a stigmatized illness. Not surprisingly, addicted patients, who often have additional psychiatric and medical disorders, have difficulty in this area. Carefully eliciting patient concerns and objections is worthwhile. Many behavioral strategies yield poor results because no one took the time to identify the real obstacles to compliance. Sympathetic listening, combined with well-timed doses of information, can improve medication adherence significantly.

Physicians can help counselors and psychotherapists to understand and explore these issues in their counseling sessions with patients. Non-physicians vary considerably in their attitudes and education about medication. Time spent on educating therapists usually yields multiple benefits.

Certain forms of resistance occur frequently (Zweben & Smith, 1989). Patients on psychotropic medications often feel ashamed and guilty, believing that they have failed if they cannot master their illness by themselves. Because their illness is not measurable in the same manner as diabetes, it is easier for them to sustain this guilt. For recovering persons, there are added layers of difficulty. Taking a medication to feel better is highly charged, as many link this motive inextricably with their alcohol and drug use. Even in the case of medications such as antidepressants, which produce no feelings of euphoria or "high," such guilt can persist. Some patients report they feel they are "cheating," even though their depression precipitated multiple relapses during the time it was untreated.

Rejecting a recommendation for medication may reflect the "all-or-none" thinking characteristic of the alcoholic or addict. The same patient who at one time consumed every available substance becomes horrified at the idea of "putting something foreign in my body" or "relying on drugs." With respect to disulfiram (Antabuse®), Banys (1988) notes that many patients disdainfully describe it as a "crutch." Even though these are the same patients who used alcohol as a "crutch" for years, they are paradoxically fastidious about this one. Medications such as disulfiram or naltrexone (ReVia®) can provide an invaluable (and life-saving) opportunity to alter behavior patterns; however, patients who use these medications may feel unable to take credit for their achievements. Reliance on the medication undermines the sense of mastery that ultimately promotes lasting sobriety; hence the importance of handling this issue carefully when such treatment adjuncts are used.

Indeed, medication should not be used as a substitute for doing the work of recovery. For example, a patient taking disulfiram can be asked to keep a daily journal describing situations that would have been hazardous if he or she were not on the medication. The patient then can be asked what behaviors need to be strengthened (often assertive behaviors) to create safety even in the absence of medication. The decision to discontinue can be implemented once the patient has developed coping skills for the high-risk situations previously identified.

Adherence with medication regimens can be monitored through refill requests. Patients who are adhering to their regimens initiate contact with their physicians for refills before the existing supplies expire. Prescribing enough doses for a long period deprives the physician of this potential warning signal. Communication with other treatment staff is essential when noncompliance is suspected. Discontinuation of psychotropic medication often is a harbinger of relapse to alcohol and drugs, as distressing psychiatric symptoms begin to re-emerge. It also can be an indicator that a relapse to alcohol or other drug use already has occurred.

The physician needs to discuss with the patient and other members of the treatment team the indications for discontinuing medications and the process by which such discontinuation should occur. Many patients with prescriptions for disulfiram report that they have not had discussions with their physicians on this topic. Physicians should clarify that disulfiram is a tool to allow other accomplishments to take place. The patient needs to review his or her progress with program staff, a private therapist, or the prescribing physician before discontinuing medication. Patients who are taking antidepressants may go into denial about their psychiatric disorder once they feel better and thus discontinue use of the medication prematurely. The physician needs to educate both patients and non-physician therapists about the dangers of psychiatric and addiction relapse that attend such a decision.

Control issues are common. Some patients will accept the need for prescribed drugs, but will tinker with frequency and dose, much as they did with their illicit substances. Some may operate on the assumption that if one pill is good, three are better, and escalate their medication dose. Drug mixing is another common practice. "Surrendering control of medication use to your physician" is a concept that can prove useful; under such a scenario, any deviation from the prescribed regimen is the subject of inquiry. Patients who are engaged in serious self-examination may spontaneously report such behavior as a residual part of their addictive pattern.

Office-Based Opioid Therapy. Recent efforts to reduce barriers to obtaining treatment have created new opportunities and corresponding challenges for physicians who are interested in providing opioid maintenance medications to their patients. Current federal law permits physicians to provide methadone and levo-alpha-acetylmethadol (LAAM) from their offices, provided they are affiliated with a licensed narcotic treatment program.

The U.S. Food and Drug Administration (FDA) has determined that medical maintenance treatment can be provided through program-wide exemptions under the current opioid treatment regulations. Stable, socially rehabilitated patients may receive up to a month's supply of take-home medications, and can reduce the frequency of other clinic visits accordingly. Medication can be provided by the physician's office (if it meets security requirements) or by a pharmacy. This form of office-based opioid therapy (also see Section 6, Chapter 4) is intended to extend the service continuum to better meet the needs of patients who no longer need the extensive structure of the opioid treatment program or clinic that offers psychosocial services at the clinic site. However, participating physicians should be prepared to recognize relapse warning signs and intervene promptly.

In the event that the patient does not need the more structured interventions available in the clinic, the physician must be prepared to offer relevant alternatives in the community. A psychotherapist with expertise in addiction may be able to provide sufficient assistance if the therapist is clear as to what constitutes an appropriate level of intensity and structure, given the patient's condition.

FDA approval of buprenorphine for use by physicians represents a form of office-based treatment with greater complexities. Most patients who are candidates for buprenorphine will seek help in the active phase of their addiction, and will need stabilization that includes behavior changes. They will differ widely in their level of functioning. To help these patients, it is imperative that treating physicians have arrangements for comprehensive assessment, treatment planning, and referral to appropriate psychosocial services. They also should have a good understanding of the self-help system and how to encourage patients to use it productively. This understanding helps prepare patients to deal with other group members who view their particular medication as incompatible with "true" recovery.

Many patients who seek buprenorphine will have unrealistic expectations as to what the medication can accomplish. They will embrace the view that extensive participation in other treatment and recovery activities is unnecessary. The physician must be prepared to be firm about the commitment required for a serious recovery effort and have a good system of coordination with outside service providers.

RECOVERY-ORIENTED PSYCHOTHERAPY

The many forms of psychotherapy vary considerably in their compatibility with addiction treatment. Therapy funded by insurance has been limited to relatively brief interventions that are limited in scope. They often permit management of the initial crisis that brings the patient to treatment, but little beyond that. Patients whose income allows may elect to work with therapists in private practice, many of whom are psychodynamic in orientation. Psychodynamic models assume that a relatively open-ended exploration of emotionally charged issues will increase awareness and lead to change. Such psychotherapy certainly may enhance the quality of recovery, but it has many pitfalls for the patient who needs to establish and consolidate abstinence. Private therapists may refer patients to addiction specialists for collaborative efforts, but potential difficulties exist in the teamwork.

In a recovery-oriented model, the therapist focuses his or her activity according to the tasks faced by the recovering person. These tasks can be conceptualized as recognizing the negative consequences of alcohol and drug use, making a commitment to abstinence, getting clean and sober, and shaping lifestyle transitions to support a comfortable and satisfying sobriety (Zweben, 1993).

For patients who seek psychotherapy without recognizing that their alcohol or drug use is problematic, motivational enhancement strategies have proved beneficial (Miller, 1999; Miller & Page, 1991; Miller & Rollnick, 1991; Miller, Zweben et al., 1994). The therapist identifies where the patient is on the continuum of readiness to change: *precontemplation*, in which the patient is unaware or barely aware that a problem exists; *contemplation*, in which the patient is weighing the pros and cons of addressing the problem; *preparation*, in which the patient is making some small forays to change behavior (such as cutting down on cigarettes or changing brands); *action*, in which a great deal of time and effort is devoted to making changes; and *maintenance*, or the consolidation of change through relapse prevention strategies and other means (Prochaska, DiClemente et al., 1992).

The addiction-oriented therapist takes the position that abstinence is the foundation of progress on other issues and makes the alcohol and drug use the primary focus. He or she works to help the patient understand the importance of making abstinence a priority. Patients have many understandable reasons to resist this focus. The therapist must work carefully to examine obstacles that prevent the patient from making a commitment to abstinence, while keeping the patient engaged in treatment. Typically, the obstacles begin with the distress that brought the patient to psychotherapy, and include the relationship of that stress to alcohol and drug use. For example, many seek psychotherapy for problems related to self-esteem and wellbeing. The therapist can help such a patient understand that regular consumption of a central nervous system depressant such as alcohol will inevitably depress mood, even though the initial effect feels like relief. Although the patient believes alcohol is a coping mechanism, he or she needs to be helped to understand that alcohol probably is exacerbating feelings of depressed mood and poor self-worth. In this way, the therapist cultivates in the patient a readiness to commit to at least a brief period of abstinence.

For abstinence to be established, effective interventions tend to be highly structured and focused on developing the behaviors that bring it about. Cognitive-behavioral strategies have been well studied and shown to be effective (Carroll, 1999; Kadden, Carroll et al., 1995; Matrix Center, 1995). In such therapy, the therapist focuses on how the patient can become and remain abstinent. Insight-oriented exploration is confined to issues relevant to obstacles to abstinence; it is not possible to formulate effective behavioral strategies without clarity as to where problems lie. However, the conventionally trained therapist often tends to widen the exploration too broadly at the beginning of therapy, which may undermine abstinence in its early, fragile stages. The recovery-oriented therapist does not mechanistically focus on behavior, but blends approaches while maintaining a clear perspective about the immediate goals to be achieved. Therapists who are not comfortable with a range of intervention strategies do less well with patients at this stage and actually may undermine progress.

In prescribing medications to address withdrawal phenomena, physicians need to communicate to nonphysician therapists what to expect and what might constitute warning signs of impending problems. For example, the therapist may not be aware that a patient given three days' supply of chlordiazepoxide (Librium®) for alcohol withdrawal by an addiction specialist also may have obtained a month's supply of diazepam (Valium®) from his or her family physician for "back spasm" and thus be in a high-risk situation. Since therapists spend considerable time with their patients, they are in a good position to detect developing problems and initiate communication with the physician or clinician responsible for coordinating care.

Therapists may not understand the importance of urine and breath testing and can weaken cooperation by conveying a sense that it is somehow degrading for the patient to comply with testing requirements. They need to understand that testing often functions as a key element in the support structure for outpatient treatment, permitting lapses to be identified and addressed quickly. Patients should be helped to understand that urine and breath testing serve as a deterrent to impulsive use and make the option of using seem further removed.

Behaviors during the early abstinence period are very similar to those during the active use stage, and often include difficulty in structuring time, irritability, sleep disruption, and mood swings. This can threaten the patient's credibility with intimates, to whom he or she may have lied for considerable periods of time while engaged in active drinking or drug use. Drug or Breathalyzer® tests relieve anxiety on the part of significant others and protect the patient from the disheartening experience of being mistrusted even as he or she is making progress. Preferably, the patient should be asked to sign appropriate releases for therapists outside the addiction program to be notified of test results.

Late-stage recovery issues require an examination of the lifestyle transitions need to sustain healthy sobriety, and so this period resembles conventional psychotherapy in many ways. However, the therapist should have some understanding of relapse precipitants and be able to detect signs of early relapse. Current pressures to shorten the duration of addiction treatment will place more burden on psychotherapists to handle these issues. Structured relapse prevention activities, if undertaken too early in addiction treatment, may not "stick" because it is difficult to deal with late-stage recovery issues while a patient is in early recovery. The conceptual groundwork can be laid early, but the issues are dealt with more effectively at the time they are real. Relapse prevention early in treatment usually is focused on establishing stable abstinence; it is less able to deal with dangers that can manifest after a considerable period of sobriety. Sensitivity to these later relapse issues and a willingness to restore addiction issues to first priority when relapse threatens is a necessary characteristic of the therapist capable of good work with recovering patients.

Addiction treatment providers face a delicate task when collaborating with mental health therapists who are unskilled in dealing with recovering patients. They must inform the patient of appropriate treatment practices without generating distress by criticizing another professional with whom the patient may have a strong relationship. The physician is obligated to educate the patient, but must do so with tact and sensitivity to the many complex issues involved in collaboration.

CO-OCCURRING DISORDER
PATIENTS IN SELF-HELP GROUPS
Participation in self-help groups is a major element in achieving a positive outcome, so it is important for clinicians to

facilitate such participation. Self-help groups are important in two ways: (1) they provide access to a culture that supports the recovery process, from which participants can recreate social networks that are not organized around alcohol and drug use, and (2) they provide a process for personal development that has no financial barriers. Although these goals can be achieved in other ways, for most individuals the self-help system offers the richest resource. While many different groups exist, Twelve Step programs are the largest self-help system in the world (Alcoholics Anonymous, 1996).

Many addiction treatment programs systematically promote the use of self-help or mutual-help groups, but physicians in primary care, psychiatry, or other specialties need to consider how best to achieve compliance with a recommendation to participate. Resistance mirrors the patient's conflicts about acknowledging that alcohol or other drugs are a problem and that abstinence is necessary; hence it is not surprising that such feelings are expressed around the issue of meeting attendance. The presence of a coexisting disorder can add additional deterrents to involvement. While it is understandable that the treating physician or other clinician may be frustrated or even angered by the patient's noncompliance, such a reaction can lead to behaviors that alienate the patient. By contrast, offering an opportunity for the patient to explore these issues is more likely to promote cooperation. Improving willingness is best done by helping the patient to surmount a variety of obstacles, many of which are well-known.

Patients with co-occurring addictive and mental disorders may encounter a variety of difficulties in engaging in self-help programs, particularly if they are severely disturbed. For example, they may feel "different" in a way that reduces their sense of belonging. For them, the spirit of fellowship at the meetings may be a source of discomfort or pain. Such feelings may occur not only in patients with psychotic conditions, but also in those with other problems, such as combat veterans with severe posttraumatic stress disorder, who may feel they rarely hear "their story." Specialized meetings, such as those of Double Trouble groups, may reduce such obstacles, but there are far fewer of these groups than are needed to provide comprehensive coverage throughout the week. Another option is to mainstream such patients into meetings of groups that have a wider tolerance for deviant behavior to achieve a more extensive support system. This requires some process for gathering and sharing feedback on the most hospitable and appropriate meetings in a given community for a particular patient population.

Several common forms of resistance can be anticipated and the patient assisted in moving beyond them. Initially, most patients have some form of "stranger anxiety"—an understandable reluctance to enter an unfamiliar group where many or most participants appear to know each other. Encouraging patients to call the central office to find someone to go with them, pairing them with other patients who attend regularly, or encouraging case managers to go with them (at least initially, and perhaps regularly) can reduce some of this awkwardness. Those with social phobias or who describe themselves as isolated may be adamant in their rejection of group activities. Practitioners should not be discouraged by this; many Twelve Step program members readily announce themselves as "loners," but nevertheless maintain active involvement. Because meeting participants generally are friendly and not demanding (or intrusive), many objections diminish once the patient actually has attended.

As part of preparing the patient for Twelve Step participation, the clinician (often a program counselor) can elicit the patient's picture of what occurs in self-help meetings. This affords an opportunity to correct misconceptions and provide a picture of what can be expected (opening rituals, sharing of experiences without direct feedback or "crosstalk"). Patients who object or are ambivalent about calling themselves an addict or alcoholic can be assured that AA is for anyone concerned about drinking, and that they can introduce themselves by name only or as a guest. Those who are concerned about "that religious stuff" can be encouraged to attend meetings less dominated by religious overtones, where they can "take what you need and leave the rest."

The concept of powerlessness in the first of the Twelve Steps ("We admitted we were powerless over alcohol—that our lives had become unmanageable"), but is problematic for many patients, particularly those who are part of disempowered groups (such as patients with co-occurring mental and substance use disorders, women, or members of ethnic or cultural groups with a painful history of being ineffective and anonymous). Clarification that one gains control over one's life by renouncing struggles to control alcohol or drug use may be reassuring to such individuals, but may require some time to be fully understood. The more spiritual aspects of surrendering control often are better appreciated later in recovery. In the early stages, advising patients to "take what you need and leave the rest" may be one of the more effective ways to reduce this obstacle to participation. In some communities, cultural adaptations that stress empowerment may be more attractive. For example, The Reverend Cecil Williams of Glide Memorial Church in San Francisco has adapted Twelve Step elements to the needs of the African American community in a manner that regularly draws crowds from diverse groups (Smith, Buxton et al., 1993).

Medications are another issue around which there is much misunderstanding and some genuine hazards. Special preparation is needed for those using psychotropics and some other forms of medication. Despite a well-articulated AA position that medication is quite compatible with recovery (Alcoholics Anonymous, 1984), it is common to encounter negative attitudes toward medications on the part of AA participants. Patients who already feel vulnerable can be quite shaken by such encounters. It may be helpful to give patients some history about how such negative attitudes were developed (including misuse of medications by addicts and alcoholics and inappropriate prescribing by uninformed physicians). However, AA clearly states that members are not to "play doctor." Patients should be given a copy of the AA pamphlet entitled "The AA Member—Medications and Other Drugs: Report From a Group of Physicians in AA" and provided an opportunity to discuss or role play potentially difficult situations. It also is possible to find meetings that are more receptive to those on medication. Hospital-based meetings are good candidates in this regard.

For more disturbed patients, additional supports may be useful. For example, the patient can be accompanied to initial meetings by the case manager. As he or she becomes ready to go alone, the case manager can be available by cell phone should the patient encounter problems. Some highly disturbed patients make excellent use of meetings, while others incorporate elements such as the higher power into their delusional system. Depending on the state of the patient, some meetings may be overstimulating, leading to disorganization.

The therapist's conceptual orientation also can present obstacles to patient participation in self-help groups. Lack of familiarity with what actually goes on in meetings can lead therapists to accept certain forms of resistance too readily. Brown (1985) discusses many ways in which a therapist's belief system can undermine encouraging both

abstinence itself and Twelve Step program participation in particular. In the latter case, she notes that, as involvement in AA increases, the patient may cancel or miss therapy appointments and act in other ways that reflect a shift in dependency from the therapist to the AA group. Although addiction specialists may view this as desirable, particularly in early recovery, the therapist may treat it as resistance and fall into a power struggle around loyalties. Some therapists abhor the concept of loss of control, viewing it as a defeat if the patient does not succeed in controlled use. They may dismiss Twelve Step tenets of powerlessness as antithetical to strong self-esteem. Therapists who are more knowledgeable tend to find the Twelve Step philosophy and process quite compatible with psychotherapy and are able to translate concepts back and forth in a manner that reduces confusion and conflict for the patient.

The best preparation for practitioners is first-hand familiarity with self-help programs through a "field trip" to meetings. Interns, residents, and new staff can be asked to attend a specified number of meetings, preferably involving groups recommended by staff or others familiar with community offerings. Those who are not alcoholics or addicts should be advised to select an open meeting and introduce themselves as a student or a guest. Subsequently, they should be provided an opportunity to share their experiences in staff meetings. Those who are in recovery or who have attended some meetings should be encouraged to attend meetings outside of their previous focus. All can be instructed to notice what they felt in anticipation of going (such as resistance or avoidance), what they felt on arriving, what they experienced during and after the meeting, and to share their observations and analyses of the group process, its advantages, and its limitations. Sharing these experiences in a staff meeting or training session can broaden the group's perspective on the variety of experiences possible.

CONCLUSIONS

Interdisciplinary collaboration not only is one of the most challenging aspects of addiction medicine, but also one that offers the greatest possibility of improving patient outcomes. As with heart disease, the greatest advances in addiction practice are achieved by encouraging patient lifestyle changes, which must be facilitated by all members of the treatment team.

Collaboration is best viewed as a clinical skill as complex as any other—one that is worthy of the time and attention it requires to develop and apply. Members of the treatment team bring diverse attitudes, experiences, and skills to their work, which must be understood in order to handle the inevitable conflicts and draw the best from the range of experiences and expertise they represent. Strong physician leadership in fostering teamwork within the program and with other treatment professionals is an essential factor in achieving treatment goals.

REFERENCES

Alcoholics Anonymous (1984). *The AA Member—Medications and Other Drugs: Report From a Group of Physicians in AA.* New York, NY: Alcoholics Anonymous World Services, Inc.

Alcoholics Anonymous (1996). *Alcoholics Anonymous: 1996 Membership Survey.* New York, NY: Alcoholics Anonymous World Services, Inc.

Banys P (1988). The clinical use of disulfiram (Antabuse®): A review. *Journal of Psychoactive Drugs* 20:243-261.

Brown S (1985). *Treating the Alcoholic: A Developmental Model of Recovery.* New York, NY: John Wiley & Sons.

Carroll KM (1999). Behavioral and cognitive behavioral treatments. In BS McCrady & EE Epstein (eds.) *Addictions: A Comprehensive Guidebook.* New York, NY: Oxford University Press, 250-267.

Deitch DA (1973). The treatment of drug abuse in the therapeutic community: Historical influences, current considerations, future outlook. In *Drug Abuse in America: Problem in Perspective (Vol. IV: Treatment and Rehabilitation).* Washington, DC: National Commission on Marijuana and Drug Abuse, 158-175.

DeLeon G (1994). The therapeutic community: Toward a general theory and model. In FM Tims, G DeLeon & N Jainchill (eds.) *Therapeutic Community: Advances in Research and Application (NIDA Research Monograph 144).* Rockville, MD: National Institute on Drug Abuse.

DeLeon G (1995). Residential therapeutic communities in the mainstream: Diversity and issues. *Journal of Psychoactive Drugs* 27:13-15.

DeLeon G (2000). *The Therapeutic Community: Theory, Model, and Method.* New York, NY: Springer Publishing Company.

Gerstein DR (1994). Outcome research: Drug abuse. In M Galanter & HD Kleber (eds.) *Textbook of Substance Abuse Treatment.* Washington, DC: American Psychiatric Press, 45-64.

Gerstein DR & Harwood HJ (1990). *Treating Drug Problems (Vol. 1).* Washington, DC: National Academy Press.

Hubbard RL, Marsden ME, Rachal JV et al. (1989). *Drug Abuse Treatment: A National Study of Effectiveness.* Chapel Hill, NC: University of North Carolina Press.

Kadden R, Carroll K, Donovan D et al. (1995). *Cognitive-Behavioral Coping Skills Therapy Manual.* Rockville, MD: National Institute on Drug Abuse.

Matrix Center (1995). *The Matrix Intensive Outpatient Program: Therapist Manual.* Los Angeles, CA: The Matrix Center.

McElrath D (1997). The Minnesota Model. *Journal of Psychoactive Drugs* 29(2):141-144.

McLellan AT, Lewis DC, O'Brien CP et al. (2000). Drug dependence, a chronic medical illness: Implications for treatment, insurance, and outcomes evaluation. *Journal of the American Medical Association* 284(13):1689-1695.

McLellan AT, Metzger DS, Alterman AI et al. (1995). Is addiction treatment "worth it"? Public health expectations, policy-based comparisons. In D Lewis (ed.) *The Macy Conference on Medical Education.* New York, NY: The Josiah Macy Foundation Press.

Miller WR (1999). *Enhancing Motivation for Change in Substance Abuse Treatment (Vol. 35).* Rockville, MD: U.S. Department of Health and Human Services.

Miller WR & Page AC (1991). Warm turkey: Other routes to abstinence. *Journal of Substance Abuse Treatment* 8:227-232.

Miller WR & Rollnick S (1991). *Motivational Interviewing: Preparing People to Change Addictive Behavior.* New York, NY: Guilford Press.

Miller WR, Zweben A, DiClemente CC et al. (1994). *Motivational Enhancement Therapy Manual.* Rockville, MD: National Institute on Drug Abuse.

Prochaska JO, DiClemente CC & Norcross JC (1992). In search of how people change: Applications to addictive behaviors. *American Psychologist* 47:1102-1114.

Simpson DD & Curry SJ, eds. (1997). *Drug Abuse Treatment Outcome Study (DATOS) (Vol. 11).* Washington, DC: Educational Publishing Foundation.

Smith DE, Buxton ME, Bilal R et al. (1993). Cultural points of resistance to the 12-step process. *Journal of Psychoactive Drugs* 25(1):97-108.

Zweben JE (1993). Recovery oriented psychotherapy: A model for addiction treatment. *Psychotherapy* 30(2):259-268.

Zweben JE & Smith DE (1989). Considerations in using psychotropic medication with dual diagnosis patients in recovery. *Journal of Psychoactive Drugs* 21(2):221-229.

SECTION
12 | Pain and Addiction

Section Coordinators
Howard A. Heit, M.D., FACP, FASAM
Seddon R. Savage, M.D., FASAM

Contributors

Peggy Compton, R.N., Ph.D.
Assistant Professor
School of Nursing
University of California at Los Angeles
Los Angeles, California

Edward C. Covington, M.D.
Director, Chronic Pain Rehabilitation Program
Cleveland Clinic Foundation
Cleveland, Ohio

G. F. Gebhart, Ph.D.
Department of Pharmacology
University of Iowa
Iowa City, Iowa

Aaron M. Gilson, Ph.D.
Assistant Director, Pain & Policy Studies Group
UW Comprehensive Cancer Center
University of Wisconsin-Madison Medical School
Madison, Wisconsin

Howard A. Heit, M.D., FACP, FASAM
Assistant Clinical Professor
Georgetown University School of Medicine, and
Private Practice of Medicine
Fairfax, Virginia

Neil Irick, M.D.
Clinical Associate Professor of Medicine
Adjunct Associate Professor of Nursing
Indiana University, and
Private Practice, Pain and Palliative Medicine
Indianapolis, Indiana

David E. Joranson, M.S.S.W.
Director, Pain & Policy Studies Group
UW Comprehensive Cancer Center
University of Wisconsin-Madison Medical School
Madison, Wisconsin

Margaret M. Kotz, D.O.
Alcohol and Drug Recovery Center
Cleveland Clinic Foundation
Cleveland, Ohio

Walter Ling, M.D.
Director of Research
Los Angeles Addiction Treatment Research Center, and
Associate Clinical Professor of Psychiatry
University of California, Los Angeles
Los Angeles, California

James A.D. Otis, M.D.
Director, Pain Management Group
Boston Medical Center, and
Associate Professor of Neurology
Boston University School of Medicine
Boston, Massachusetts

Melvin I. Pohl, M.D., FASAM
Clinical Service Director
Addictive Disease Program
Montevista Hospital
Las Vegas, Nevada

Seddon R. Savage, M.D., FASAM
Associate Professor of Anesthesiology
Dartmouth Medical School, and
Project Director, NH ReMOTE, and
Pain Consultant, Manchester VA Medical Center
Lebanon, New Hampshire

David E. Smith, M.D.
Founder, Medical Director and President
Haight Ashbury Free Clinics, and
Associate Clinical Professor of
    Occupational Health and Clinical Toxicology
University of California, San Francisco
San Francisco, California

Barry Stimmel, M.D., FASAM
Dean, Mt. Sinai School of Medicine, and
Editor, *Journal of Addictive Disease*
New York, New York

Donald R. Wesson, M.D.
Consultant on CNS Medications Development, and
Private Practice of Addiction Medicine
Oakland, California

Chapter 1

The Neurophysiology of Pain and Interfaces with Addiction

Peggy Compton, R.N., Ph.D.
G.F. Gebhart, Ph.D.

Physiological Mechanisms of Pain
Physiological Mechanisms of Addiction
Points of Interface Between Pain and Addiction

Physiological processes underlie both pain and addiction. Physiology alone cannot account for the variable expression and psychosocial complexity of these two very human conditions, but the role of physiological responses in the experience and continuation of each cannot be minimized.

It is at the physiological level that many effective interventions (primarily pharmacologic) for the treatment of pain and addiction act. Both conditions predominantly involve the nervous system, and both have significant involvement of central opioid systems, so it is reasonable to expect that the coexistence of pain and addiction would lead to complex responses: that is, addictive responses altered by the physiological presence of pain, and pain responses altered by the physiological presence of addiction.

This chapter provides a review of the neurophysiology of pain and of addiction, and of the theoretical bases for overlap between the two. The mechanisms of pain perception and modulation are reviewed, with attention to those aspects most likely to be influenced by the presence of addictive disease. In this regard, the role of hyperalgesia, endogenous opioid systems, and descending modulatory controls on the experience of pain are discussed. Neurophysiological responses to drugs of abuse also are outlined, and the neural systems underlying key addiction phenomena (tolerance, physical dependence, and craving) are identified. Finally, ideas about potential sources of interaction between pain and addiction are suggested, focusing on how the general state of addiction, inherited characteristics of the individual, and neuroadaptations specific to opioid abuse might affect the co-expression of these phenomena.

PHYSIOLOGICAL MECHANISMS OF PAIN

Pain is an unpleasant sensory and emotional experience that is associated with potential or actual tissue injury or is described in terms of such injury (International Association for the Study of Pain, 1979). Like addiction, pain is a unique and complex experience that is influenced by culture, by context, by anticipation and previous experience, and by a variety of emotional and cognitive factors. Accordingly, reactions to stimuli that produce pain vary from one individual to the next and even within the same individual at different points in time. The neurophysiologic mechanisms that underlie the experience of pain may be considered in two classifications: *nociceptive pain* (pain produced by noxious stimuli) and *neuropathic pain* (pain produced by alterations in nociceptive pathways).

Nociception. The stimuli that produce pain are termed "noxious." Noxious stimuli are those that damage or threaten to damage tissue (such as pinches, cuts, and burns). Pain serves to warn of potential injury and thus is an important protective mechanism. Noxious stimuli set into motion a series of events that contribute to the sensory and emotional experience of pain. They activate specific sensory receptors called *nociceptors*. Nociceptors, and the axons of neurons with which they are associated, convey nociceptive information (that is, information about potential or actual tissue injury) to the spinal cord, where (1) autonomic and nociceptive reflexes are activated, and (2) simultaneously, the information is transmitted to the brain (supraspinally).

Autonomic reflex responses produced by noxious stimuli include increases in heart rate, blood pressure, and respiration. These nociceptive reflexes are protective withdrawal (motor) reflexes that are organized at the level of the spinal cord. For example, unexpectedly pricking one's finger with a needle produces a reflexive withdrawal, followed by conscious appreciation of pain. Such conscious appreciation that a given stimulus is painful requires integration and interpretation of information in several areas of the brain. This supraspinal integration and interpretation of peripheral events are what make pain such a unique experience.

It is important to understand the distinction between nociception and the experience of pain. Nociception describes the neural events and reflex responses produced by a noxious stimulus. It can occur in the absence of the perception of pain, just as pain can arise in the absence of nociception. For example, in paraplegics or quadriplegics, noxious stimuli applied below the level of spinal cord injury can evoke nociceptive withdrawal reflexes because the connection between the peripheral nociceptors and the spinal circuitry remains intact. However, because such nociceptive information cannot be transmitted above the spinal injury to the brain, the individual does not perceive the noxious stimuli as painful.

Sensory Channels. It is helpful to think about sensations arising from skin, joints, muscles, and viscera (nociceptive or otherwise) in terms of *sensory channels*. Such channels are composed of (1) the peripheral receptors and nerves, (2) the neurons in the spinal cord on which the peripheral nerves terminate (and transfer their message), (3) the ascending tracts in the spinal cord that carry the information supraspinally, and (4) the sites in the brain where integration and interpretation of input occurs. Activation of a sensory channel provides information about the location, onset, intensity, and duration of a stimulus.

The sensory channel for pain generally is described as having two components: a sensory-discriminative component and a motivational-affective component. The sensory-discriminative component of pain is directly linked to the noxious stimulus and usually is what is meant when pain is referred to as a "sensation." Here, a noxious stimulus activates nociceptors and initiates a series of neural events that ultimately reach the cortex of the brain, allowing the individual experiencing the pain to determine the location of the stimulus, its intensity, and its duration. This exquisite ability to characterize and localize the site of pain is developed best for the skin and very poorly for the viscera.

The motivational-affective component of pain includes the nature and intensity of the emotional responses that make pain personal and unique to each individual. The sites in the brain that contribute to the motivational-affective component and the spinal pathways that convey nociceptive information to these brain sites are different than those associated with the sensory-discriminative component of pain. The motivational-affective component of pain is served by older, relatively indirect neural pathways that are conserved phylogenetically (that is, they are common to all vertebrates). The sensory-discriminative component of pain is organized to give information about the location, the intensity, and the duration of the nociceptive event. The motivational-affective component of pain affects the individual's response to the nociceptive input.

Overlaying the sensory-discriminative and motivational-affective components of pain are learned cultural and cognitive contributions that color the individual's interpretation of and concerns about pain. Cognitive contributions include attention, anxiety, anticipation, and past experiences and, in the case of the addict, may include concerns about drug supply, impending withdrawal, or intoxication. For example, if an addict sustains an injury in the course of obtaining or injecting a drug of abuse, his or her perception of and response to the ensuing pain is likely to be minimized by the overwhelming sense of relief anticipated on drug ingestion. On the other hand, if an addict is without a supply of drugs and fears impending withdrawal, a similar injury is likely be experienced as relatively more painful. Thus, cognitive contributions can significantly modulate the response and reaction to a painful stimulus.

Nociceptors and the Sensory Channel for Pain. The first event in nociception is activation of a specialized sensory receptor, the nociceptor, which transduces stimulus energy into changes in nerve membrane electrical potential. Thus, receptors in skin, deep tissue, and viscera convert mechanical, thermal, and chemical stimulus energy into action potentials that are conveyed along nerve axons in the spinal cord or cranial nuclei. These sensory neurons or "primary afferent neurons," as they are called, have their cell body located in a dorsal root ganglion or ganglion of a cranial nerve.

The sensory endings of primary afferent neurons are tree-like and are distributed over a localized region of tissue. Nociceptors can be excited only by stimuli applied in the innervated region, called the "receptive field." Receptive fields of different primary afferent neurons vary in size and overlap extensively with the receptive fields of other primary afferent neurons. It is important to note that a threshold noxious stimulus that evokes one action potential in a single nociceptor is not sufficient to be perceived as painful; for pain to occur, either spatial summation (one action potential occurring simultaneously in many nociceptors) or temporal summation (many action potentials occurring closely in time in a single nociceptor) are required. Consequently, suprathreshold stimuli are required for an individual to consciously perceive a noxious stimulus as painful.

Nociceptors differ from non-nociceptors in several ways:

■ The nociceptor is not macroscopically specialized and so is referred to as a free (or unencapsulated) nerve ending. In contrast, most non-nociceptors are encapsulated and have complex morphologies (such as Pacinian corpuscles).

■ Most nociceptors are polymodal, meaning that they respond to multiple modalities of stimulation (for example, thermal, mechanical, and chemical), whereas all non-nociceptors are unimodal.

■ The conduction velocity of nociceptor axons (0.5 to 30 m/s) is less than that of non-nociceptor axons (30 to 120 m/s). Conduction velocity depends on axon myelination. The axons of nociceptors are unmyelinated C-fibers or thinly myelinated Aδ-fibers. The axons of non-nociceptors are more heavily myelinated Aβ-fibers.

■ Both nociceptors and non-nociceptors are heterogeneously distributed throughout the body, but their distribution varies. For example, the fingertips contain many non-nociceptors but relatively fewer nociceptors, whereas the cornea and teeth are densely innervated by nociceptors.

■ The distinguishing feature of nociceptors is their ability to become sensitized when tissue is injured (that is, the threshold intensity for activation is decreased); non-nociceptors do not sensitize when tissue is injured.

Nociceptors are present in the skin, muscles, joints, and viscera.

Cutaneous Nociceptors: The most common nociceptors in skin are the Aδ-mechanonociceptors and C-polymodal nociceptors. The receptive field of Aδ-mechanonociceptors ranges from 1 to 8 cm². Activation of Aδ-mechanonociceptors evokes sharp, well-localized pain. C-polymodal nociceptors are more plentiful than Aδ-mechanonociceptors, constituting over 75% of all nociceptors. The aggregated receptive field of C-polymodal nociceptors consists of 3 to 20 small (<1 mm²), non-contiguous, punctuate receptive fields. C-polymodal receptors are particularly responsive to chemicals released during tissue injury and inflammation, exercise, or disease, as well as to capsaicin, the hot ingredient in chili peppers. Their absolute firing rates are typically slower than Aδ mechanonociceptors, and they rarely have spontaneous activity in the absence of a stimulus. Activation of C-polymodal nociceptors typically evokes long-lasting, burning pain.

Other Somatic Receptors: Deep somatic nociceptors occur in muscle, fascia, connective tissue, and joints. Although similar to cutaneous nociceptors, deep nociceptors differ in both nomenclature and response properties. For historical reasons, afferent fibers in muscle nerves were classified as Groups I, II, III, and IV, rather than using the Aβ, Aδ, and C-nomenclature employed for skin nerves. Groups III and IV are similar in myelination, conduction velocity, and response properties to AΔ- and C-fibers in skin. Deep nociceptors are well matched to the stimuli that evoke deep pain. For example, excessive force (which can occur in traumatic injury) and chemicals that cause muscle pain (such as lactate and potassium) all effectively excite deep somatic nociceptors.

Visceral Nociceptors: It once was thought that viscera lacked nociceptors because direct manipulation (such as pinching) and incisions failed to produce pain when surgical anesthesia was allowed to become light. Common experience, however, instructs that the predominant (if not only) conscious sensation that arises from the viscera is pain. We know now that slowly conducting Aδ- and C-fiber endings occur throughout visceral as well as somatic structures. The stimuli that produce pain when applied to the viscera, however, are different than those that produce pain when applied to skin. Moreover, the appropriate noxious visceral stimulus differs for different organs. For example, in hollow organs (such as the esophagus, stomach, colon, and urinary bladder), nociceptors are excited by distention, whereas in solid organs (such as the testes), compression is an effective noxious stimulus.

Central Processing of Nociception: The cell bodies of nociceptors are located principally in dorsal root ganglia that terminate in the spinal cord and synapse onto second order neurons, many of which have long ascending axons that convey the information supraspinally. It is at the first central synapse where the distinction between the sensory-discriminative and motivational-affective components of the sensory channel for pain begins.

The spinal cord can be divided anatomically and functionally into three regions: the dorsal horn, the intermediate region, and the ventral horn. Functionally, the dorsal horn processes sensory information, the ventral horn generates motor commands for spinal reflexes, and the intermediate region integrates sensorimotor information. The somatic motoneurons and preganglionic autonomic neurons in the ventral horn and spinal autonomic nuclei mediate spinal motor and autonomic reflexes, such as the protective flexion withdrawal reflex.

In the dorsal horn, several ascending pathways convey nociceptive information to supraspinal sites. The neospinothalamic tract is an evolutionarily newer pathway that mediates the sensory-discriminative component of pain. It projects to the ventrolateral and ventromedial portions of the thalamus, adjacent but non-overlapping to the projections from other sensory systems that are involved in sensory discrimination. Subsequently, the thalamus projects to the portions of the parietal lobe cerebral cortex that mediate perception and processing of both non-nociceptive and nociceptive somatosensory information.

The paleospinothalamic tract is an evolutionarily older pathway that is associated with the motivational-affective component of pain. In contrast to the neospinothalamic tract, the paleospinothalamic tract projects to intralaminar portions of the thalamus that are involved in the subjective aspects of sensory input rather than with discrimination. The intralaminar nuclei project primarily to the limbic system and cortex, which mediate motivational, subjective, and affective sensations and behavior.

Lastly, spinoreticular tracts ascend to the brainstem and midbrain, where they can engage autonomic systems and descending modulation of nociception. Subsequent projections from the brainstem or midbrain to the thalamus also may contribute to the motivational-affective component of pain.

Nociceptors and non-nociceptors from adjacent regions of the body ultimately project to adjacent regions of the central nervous system (CNS), resulting in a somatotopic arrangement. In contrast, the viscera do not appear to be somatotypically represented in the thalamus or cortex, which is consistent with our difficulty in localizing visceral stimuli.

Pain Modulation. Pain is modulated by inputs within the nociceptive sensory channel that alter or modulate the nature and/or intensity of afferent nociceptive input, thereby changing the pain experience. Typically, pain modulation implies inhibition or relief of pain (as with drugs), but modulation also can involve enhancement or facilitation of pain; that is, pain can be made worse, or non-nociceptive inputs can be altered to be perceived as painful.

Peripheral Counterstimulation: Probably the best known example of pain modulation is that based on a theory of spinal modulation introduced by Melzack and Wall (1965) in the mid-1960s, known as the gate control theory. In this model, neurons in the spinal cord that transmit nociceptive information to supraspinal sites are described as functioning as a spinal "gate." The gate is opened by, and nociception arises from, activity in small diameter afferent fibers (Aδ- and C-fibers). The gate is closed by activity in large diameter, myelinated non-nociceptive afferent fibers (Aδ- fibers). It is hypothesized that the balance in activities between nociceptive and non-nociceptive afferent fiber inputs to the spinal cord determine the position of the gate (that is, relatively open = more pain, relatively closed = less pain) and thus modulate the intensity of pain.

The analgesia provided by dorsal column stimulation and transcutaneous electrical nerve stimulation (TENS) generally is explained by the gate control theory of pain control. For example, electrical stimulation of large diameter, myelinated fibers in the dorsal columns of the spinal cord or in peripheral nerves (through the application of TENS) is thought to close the spinal gate and thus reduce pain. Similarly, some forms of acupuncture that activate large-diameter peripheral myelinated axons may close the spinal gate.

Descending Inhibition: Subsequent modifications to the gate control theory included the addition of influences descending from the brainstem that modulate the gate. The existence of powerful descending modulatory influences on nociceptive transmission, which can either attenuate or enhance pain, has become a tenet central to the concepts of pain modulation. Empirical study has revealed the complex anatomy, neurochemistry, and function of the systems descending from the brainstem (that is, midbrain, pons, and medulla). Phylogenetic continuity of these descending systems is noted in all vertebrates.

A critical synapse exists between the midbrain and spinal cord in the rostral part of the ventral medulla. Thus, descending influences on spinal nociceptive transmission activated in the midbrain are indirect, in that a relay exists between the midbrain and the spinal cord. From the medulla, descending influences are direct. Axons of neurons in the medulla descend in the spinal cord to terminate on the spinal neurons, from which nociceptive input from the periphery is received.

Early on, it was appreciated that descending inhibitory modulation is tonically active: that is, a moderate brake is applied to spinal neurons by the descending inhibitory system even under normal circumstances. Increases and decreases in spinal nociceptive transmission can be produced by alterations in the activity of this tonic descending system.

Endogenous Opioid Systems: A key component of the descending pain modulatory system was established in the early 1970s as a result of a number of seminal research studies demonstrating that the body itself could modulate nociceptive inputs and thus pain. First, stimulation through electrodes placed in the midbrain of experimental animals produced analgesia sufficient to permit surgery. This procedure, termed stimulation-produced analgesia, subsequently was tested and established as effective in relieving human pain. Additional discoveries revealed that endogenous opioid peptides (enkephalins, dynorphins, and endorphins) are present in the central nervous system and that the opioid receptor antagonist naloxone attenuates the analgesic effects of stimulation-produced analgesia in humans. These discoveries established that the human body contains an anatomically restricted, opioid peptide-associated means of pain control.

The midbrain periaqueductal and periventricular gray matter is the nodal point of the opioid-mediated endogenous pain modulatory system. It is at this anatomical site that both exogenously administered opioids like morphine and endogenously released opioid peptides activate inhibitory influences that descend to the dorsal horn of the spinal cord.

Other Neurotransmitter Systems: The principal neurotransmitter chemicals that mediate descending inhibition are serotonin and norepinephrine. Serotonin is contained in the terminals of neurons that descend from the ventral medulla, while norepinephrine is contained in the terminals of neurons that descend from the dorsolateral pons (for example, the locus coeruleus). Drugs that mimic the actions of serotonin or norepinephrine (such as clonidine) are analgesic when given directly into the spinal epidural or intrathecal space. While opioids, given either exogenously or released endogenously, are analgesic by an action at opioid receptors, at least part of their analgesic effect arises from activation of bulbospinal monoaminergic systems that modulate spinal nociceptive transmission. Thus, pain control by opioids ought to be enhanced by drugs that mimic or facilitate the actions of serotonin and/or norepinephrine (such as tricyclic antidepressants), which indeed has been documented in clinical trials.

The principal focus of investigation has been inhibitory modulation of nociceptive transmission, but research also has demonstrated that descending systems facilitate nociceptive transmission in the spinal cord. Facilitatory modulation of spinal nociceptive transmission is a relatively recent development and thus is less well understood than inhibitory modulation. The anatomical components of facilitatory modulation in the brainstem are similar, if not overlapping, with those of inhibitory modulation. Thus, either inhibition or facilitation of spinal transmission can be produced from the same sites in the brainstem, depending upon input, although it is not yet clear how the brainstem inputs may differ. It is clear, however, that axons that mediate facilitatory influences from the brainstem descend in different spinal tracts and contain different neurotransmitters than those for inhibitory modulation. These neurotransmitters act at the cholinergic, cholecystokinin, and kappa opioid receptors and can contribute to the facilitation of nociceptive transmission.

A wide variety of influences can activate inhibitory and/or facilitatory endogenous pain modulatory systems. Stress, fear, and pain itself all can activate descending systems that inhibit pain. The activation of endogenous modulation by pain itself has been interpreted as important to self-preservation by the observation that an injured animal often is able to escape a predator even in the presence of pain. In less life-threatening circumstances, pain can inhibit pain by activation of the same endogenous mechanisms, a phenomenon referred to as counter-irritation. Pathophysiology such as hypertension also can contribute to activation of descending systems and attenuation of pain. It has been documented, for example, that both experimental increases in blood pressure and preexisting hypertension render individuals less sensitive to noxious stimuli than normotensive persons.

Descending Facilitation: Descending facilitation of pain appears to play an important role in unusual chronic pain states. It is possible, but not yet proven, that the pain-facilitating system could be activated and not turned off by normal mechanisms, thus contributing to a tonic facilitation (rather than tonic inhibition) of spinal neuron activity. Clearly, there are circumstances in which facilitation of nociceptive information has important protective value, such as during tissue repair. Yet if such a system remains inappropriately activated after tissue repair is complete, normal, non-nociceptive inputs conceivably could acquire nociceptive character. Because mechanisms of chronic pain are poorly understood, there is considerable interest in better understanding the endogenous systems by which pain can be enhanced.

Neuropathic Pain. Just as continued exposure to a drug of abuse can result in neurophysiologic changes in the response to that drug, perceptions of sensory stimuli are not constant, but change in response to development, environmental experience, disease, and injury. These changes are collectively referred to as "plasticity." Plasticity can be brief (minutes to hours), sustained (hours to weeks), or relatively permanent.

Sustained pain always is associated with tissue injury and inflammation, such as that associated with sunburn, sprains, and following surgery. One consequence of tissue injury and inflammation is the development of hyperalgesia, which is defined as an exaggerated response to a normally painful stimulus. Hyperalgesia arises because chemicals released, synthesized, or attracted to the site of injury increase the sensitivity and activity of nociceptors. Consequently, increased activity of nociceptors leads to an increased release of neurotransmitters in the central nervous system, thereby increasing the excitability of the central

neurons on which nociceptors terminate. Accordingly, sustained pain is characterized by a change in the function and behavior of the elements that comprise the sensory-discriminative component of pain. Common experience instructs that these plastic changes are both normal and reversible. Like acute pain, sustained pain serves an important protective function. The tenderness and increased sensitivity of tissue surrounding the site of injury help to protect the tissue and prevent further damage.

A component of hyperalgesia called "allodynia" is the perception of pain in response to a stimulus that normally is not painful. Like hyperalgesia, allodynia can arise from: (1) inflammatory tissue damage, (2) injury to peripheral nerves, or (3) damage to portions of the central nervous system that mediate pain sensations.

Hyperalgesia is classified as either primary or secondary. Primary hyperalgesia refers to the enhanced pain that arises from the site of injury. Secondary hyperalgesia refers to the enhanced pain that arises from uninjured tissue adjacent to the site of injury. Primary hyperalgesia typically occurs following injury, while secondary hyperalgesia sometimes is present, but usually is weaker than the primary hyperalgesia.

Inflammatory Hyperalgesia. Pain commonly arises from tissue injury. In addition to directly and briefly exciting nociceptors, the injured tissues become inflamed as a component of the repair process. During inflammation, chemical mediators such as bradykinin, serotonin, histamine, cytokines, peptides, and prostaglandins are released from local and circulating cells. These chemical mediators result in local vasodilation, swelling, and the eventual removal and replacement of injured tissue. Not only do these chemical mediators directly activate nociceptors (thereby resulting in nociception), but they also sensitize nociceptors to subsequent stimuli. Nociceptor sensitization caused by inflammation contributes significantly to primary hyperalgesia.

Although both Aδ- and C-fiber nociceptors can be activated and sensitized by these chemical mediators, C-polymodal nociceptors appear particularly responsive to their effects. Recently, contributions to hyperalgesia by a previously unknown group of nociceptors have been documented. A subset of primarily C-fiber nociceptors are called "silent nociceptors" because, while normally unresponsive to noxious mechanical or thermal stimuli, following chemical sensitization these so-called silent nociceptors become spontaneously active and responsive to normal mechanical and thermal stimuli.

C-fiber nociceptors also contribute to inflammation and hyperalgesia via neurogenic inflammation. Unlike most sensory neurons, C-fiber nociceptors release neurotransmitters both centrally in the spinal cord and peripherally at receptor endings in tissue. Further, the peptide neurotransmitters released (such as substance P) enhance the inflammatory process like other inflammatory mediators, thus resulting in further activation of the C-fiber nociceptor and further release of substance P. The resulting positive feedback significantly enhances the inflammation and resulting hyperalgesia.

Neurogenic inflammation also is responsible for the spread of reddening and soreness following a localized injury. As described earlier, the receptive fields of C-polymodal nociceptors in the skin are punctate, indicating that a single C-fiber branches several times to innervate separate small patches of skin. Consequently, if a localized injury activates only one branch of the C-fiber, the evoked orthodromic action potential (traveling in the normal direction) will induce antidromic action potentials (traveling in the opposite direction) in other branches. The antidromic action potentials travel to nociceptor endings, causing substance P release, inflammation, and nociceptor sensitization.

Sensitization of nociceptors readily accounts for primary hyperalgesia (that is, enhanced pain at the site of tissue injury), but cannot as easily explain secondary hyperalgesia (that is, enhanced pain from uninjured tissue adjacent to the injury). The increased afferent barrage arriving in the spinal dorsal horn via Aδ- and C-fiber nociceptors, including activated silent nociceptors, releases greater than normal amounts of neurotransmitters, principally the excitatory amino acid glutamate. As a consequence, the excitability to spinal noci-receptive neurons changes and they become more easily excited (that is, are sensitized). Recent research has shown that this central sensitization also occurs when tissue is injured. As with peripheral sensitization, central sensitization is induced more effectively by activation of C-fiber nociceptors than Aδ-mechanonociceptors.

Structural changes in the spinal cord or perhaps even in supraspinal sites may underlie chronic forms of secondary hyperalgesia such as that occurring after nerve damage. Some of the structural changes identified are:

- Death of inhibitory spinal interneurons due to toxicity arising from a powerful excitatory input.

- Rearrangement of afferent fiber terminals (for example, non-nociceptive afferent fibers synapsing into spinal cord regions previously receiving only nociceptor input, a possible cause of allodynia).

- Proliferation of sympathetic efferent fibers into sensory ganglia.

If nociceptor activation and excessive nociceptive input to the central nervous system are responsible for central sensitization, then a logical strategy to reduce or prevent post-surgical hyperalgesia would be either to block the nociceptive pathways or to decrease the response of the central nervous system. This treatment strategy, termed preemptive analgesia, has as its principal objective preventing the development of central sensitization. In addition to general anesthesia, the preemptive strategy includes the infiltration of local anesthetics or administration of opioids before surgery begins. Successful preemptive analgesia has been reported using morphine and, in some instances, peripheral nerve blocks. Not all reports, however, support preemptive analgesia treatment as a means of reducing or eliminating postsurgical hyperalgesia or postsurgical analgesic drug requirements.

Neurogenic Hyperalgesias. *Complex Regional Pain Syndrome*: Traumatic or infectious damage to peripheral nerves is a special case of tissue injury, which may result in hyperalgesia differing in symptoms and mechanisms from inflammatory hyperalgesia. The clinical syndrome associated with such injury, previously termed sympathetically maintained pain, now is referred to as complex regional pain syndrome, or CRPS. Initially, damaged or transected peripheral nerves die back a few millimeters, then grow back toward the periphery following the pathway of the old nerve. Although growth and reinnervation of skin or other target often is successful, sometimes regrowth is blocked by an obstacle. The sprouting nerve then forms a neuroma, which acquires both mechanical and chemical sensitivity. The mechanical and chemical sensitivity, believed to be due to insertion of an excessive number of sodium channels in the neuroma, results in the generation of ectopic (that is, from an abnormal point) action potentials at the neuroma. Consequently, pain can be produced by even gentle pressure or by continual release of norepinephrine from nearby sympathetic nerve endings. In other instances, even with largely successful regrowth and no apparent pathology, chronic pain occurs for reasons unknown.

Phantom Pain: Amputation, an extreme form of nerve trauma, can lead to the unusual circumstance known as phantom pain. Although the pain is very real to the patient,

---

it is labeled phantom because the patient describes it as arising from the missing tissue. Phantom limb pain is most common, but phantom breast and phantom anus pain syndromes also have been described following mastectomy and surgery for colorectal cancer. Phantom pain typically is present within the first week after amputation, but usually gradually diminishes until it disappears completely. Phantom pain has been reported to persist in 3% to 50% of amputees.

Although not well studied, it is believed that phantom pain arises partly from ectopic activity from neuromas formed by the surgically transected nerves. There also is an apparent central nervous system component to phantom pain because preemptive treatments to block nociceptor discharges during surgery have been reported to prevent or significantly reduce the incidence of phantom pain. In either case, the pain is localized to the absent body part because afferent pathways are labeled according to the region innervated early in development. Consequently, activity in that pathway is localized according to the original mapping, regardless of the origin of the activity. Vasomotor instability, temperature dysregulation, edema, and autonomic dysfunction in the affected limb are characteristic of this syndrome.

Central Pain: Trauma, ischemia, or degeneration in the brain also can lead to hyperalgesia (or hypoalgesia) when the nervous tissue involved is part of the central nervous system's pain processing system. Damage to the spinothalamic tract, at any level, can lead to diminished pain perception. On the other hand, damage to some parts of the thalamus can lead to thalamic pain syndrome, a disorder characterized by hyperalgesia and allodynia. Presumably, the damaged neurons are part of a local nociceptive inhibitory system, similar to those that descend to the spinal cord from the brainstem. Central post-stroke pain syndrome is another example of pain arising in the absence of activation of peripheral nociceptors. This pain typically is deep, aching, or burning, and develops in the area of sensory loss or neurologic disability contralateral to the side of the cerebral infarction. Pain originating from damage to higher structures can be difficult to treat because many therapies interrupt nociceptive transmission peripheral to the central lesion (TENS, for example).

PHYSIOLOGICAL MECHANISMS OF ADDICTION

Like pain, addiction is a complex human response that cannot be entirely understood by its physiological bases.

Standard diagnostic criteria for addictive disorders (*DSM-IV*; American Psychiatric Association, 1994) rely only minimally on the more overt physical responses to chronic drug use (such as tolerance and withdrawal), focusing instead on such behavioral consequences as loss of control over drug use and significant disruptions in social role function. Discussions of the molecular and cellular mechanisms underlying addictive disorders clearly are insufficient to convey the actual human experience of addiction.

Drugs of abuse have different sites and unique mechanisms of action in the central nervous system. These underlie their acute effects and often account for their distinctive withdrawal syndromes (see Table 1). Yet all share an ability to increase dopaminergic activity in this mesolimbic pathway—a pathway that, in animal models, has been shown to be responsible for the reinforcing effects of drugs of abuse.

The various substrates of brain reward have been conceptualized as a neuroanatomic functional construct called the *extended amygdala* (Heimer & Alheid, 1991; Koob, Robledo et al., 1993). This functional grouping consists of the shell of the NA, the bed nucleus of the stria terminalis, and the central nucleus of the amygdala. It receives afferents from limbic structures and sends efferents to the medial ventral pallidum (controlling muscle tone and voluntary movement) and the lateral hypothalamus (controlling emotions, appetites, and related behaviors) (Leshner & Koob, 1999). Neuroplastic changes in this pathway contribute to both the physical (tolerance, physical dependence, withdrawal) and behavioral (craving, anhedonia, compulsivity) symptoms of addiction.

Tolerance and Physical Dependence. The physiology of addiction often is characterized by two incompletely understood yet related neuroadaptations: *tolerance* and *physical dependence*. These changes may be manifest both in the systems where drugs of abuse exert discrete actions and at the shared reward substrate. It is important to emphasize that the simple presence of these neuroadaptations does not constitute addiction. A pain patient can be physically dependent on or tolerant to the effects of an opioid without being addicted to it. Addiction is identified by a cluster of aberrant patterns of behavior that, while partially motivated by these physiological changes, is evident in much broader holistic domains. The plasticity evidenced by psychoactive drug tolerance and physical dependence has implications for nociceptive input and processing.

Tolerance: Ongoing use of psychoactive drugs results in the development of drug tolerance, which is defined as a

TABLE 1.   Acute Actions of Drugs of Abuse: Clinical, Neurochemical, and Anatomic-Site Effects of Common Drugs of Abuse

Drug Class	Acute Clinical Effects	Neurotransmitters in Discrete Initiating Effect E = Excitatory I = Inhibitory
Opiates (heroin, methadone, morphine)	Analgesia, drowsiness, euphoria, mental clouding, depressed cough reflex, miosis, nausea and vomiting, respiratory depression.	E - opioid I - norepinephrine I - GABA E - glutamate
Alcohol	Dysarthria, ataxia, hyperreflexia, nystagmus and/or diplopia, impaired cognition, anterograde amnesia, intoxication, stupor-coma, respiratory depression.	E - GABA I - glutamate E - nicotinic acetylcholine
Psychostimulants (cocaine and amphetamines)	Euphoria, hypervigilance, anxiety, psychomotor agitation, tremor, tachycardia, pupillary dilation, increased blood pressure, anorexia, cardiac arrhythmia, generalized seizures, psychosis, delirium, transient movement disorders.	E - dopamine (both, by monoamine re-uptake inhibition) E - glutamate (both) E - serotonin (cocaine) I - GABA (cocaine)
Hallucinogens (LSD, mescaline, psilocybin)	Pupillary dilation, tachycardia, perceptual alterations, tremor, acute anxiety, depersonalization.	E or I - (depends on predominant receptor modulation)- $E05HT_{1A}$ (LSD); $I-5HT_{2A}$ (mescaline, psylocy-bin) and E-GABA (via $5HT_{2A}$) E - glutamate
Sedative hypnotics (benzodiazepines)	Anxioysis, sedation, ataxia, dysarthria, impaired cognition, nystagmus, respiratory depression.	E - GABA/BDZ
Cannabinoids (marijuana, synthetic THC)	Perceptual alterations, impaired time orientation, mild euphoria, decreased reaction time, decreased attention span, diminished motor coordination.	E - dopamine E - opioids I - acetylcholine I - glutamate E - GABA
Nicotine		E - nicotinic acetylcholine receptor E - opioids

reduction in response to a given dose of drug after repeated administration (O'Brien, 1996). The adaptations associated with tolerance always are evident in the direction counteracting acute drug effects to maintain system-level homeostasis.

A theoretical explanation for the processes underlying tolerance is offered by the opponent process theory of acquired motivation (Solomon, 1980). Reflecting homeostatic assumptions, the theory describes how, over the course of repeated exposures to an affectively-charged stimulus, a

TABLE 2.   Autonomic and Affective Withdrawal Associated With Drugs of Abuse

Abused Drug	Affected Withdrawal (nucleus accumbens-mediated)	Autonomic Withdrawal (locus coeruleus-mediated)
Amphetamine	+ + +	+
Cocaine	+ + + +	+
Opiates	+ +	+ + + +
Marijuana	+ +	+
Alcohol	+ +	+ + +

counteracting or opposing emotional response develops, which eventually accounts for habituation to the stimulus to become the predominate feeling state in its absence. Although the theory initially was rooted in behaviorism, Koob and colleagues (1989) advanced it by providing evidence for a neurobiological basis to the opponent processes of tolerance and physical dependence in the case of opioid dependence. Their model predicts that, in order to maintain a "normal" or homeostatic level of reward system activity, "anti-reward" systems are recruited to counteract drug effects, which become stronger with each exposure and extinguish more slowly than the original response. Upon abrupt drug withdrawal, the tolerance-producing processes are revealed.

Tolerance involves adaptations that occur at both the site of drug action (receptor or ion channel) and in related systems more distal to the site of drug action. For example, tolerance to opioids is evident at both the level of the opioid receptor in the locus coeruleus and in the dopaminergic reward pathways afferent to the site of this discrete drug action. Because drugs typically act at selective receptors, tolerance has been conceptualized as a functional "uncoupling" of the receptor from its effector response (opening or closing an ion channel, initiating second messenger systems); in other words, a certain proportion of receptors are rendered nonfunctional, thus making the drug less effective (thus requiring a higher dose to get the same effect that initially was obtained at a lower dose). Clinically, the resulting tolerance provides a certain amount of protection for the user, in the same way that the respiratory depressant effects of opioids or the anesthetic effects of ethanol provide protection.

Physical Dependence: A related consequence of chronic drug use is physical dependence, which is an altered neuro- physiological state that develops as a result of tolerance. When drug blood level falls below a critical point, the adaptive changes associated with tolerance predominate and become profoundly nonadaptive (Koob, Stinus et al., 1989; Redmond & Krystal, 1984). Suddenly unopposed by drug effects, the sources of tolerance become evident as the characteristic drug-specific withdrawal syndrome.

Symptoms of drug withdrawal reflect changes in both the discrete and shared substrates of drug action. Gold and Miller (1995) have conceptualized these as *autonomic* and *affective* withdrawal symptoms, respectively, with the former related to withdrawal phenomena arising at the locus coeruleus and the latter arising from the dopaminergic reward pathway (Table 2). CNS depressants, opioids, and benzodiazepines all acutely depress NE activity in the locus coeruleus, either via opioid receptor binding or GABAergic input. Tolerance thus results in effective up-regulation of central noradrenergic activity, which is expressed in withdrawal from these drugs as increased blood pressure, heart rate, peristalsis, diaphoresis, and general CNS irritability.

Neuroadaptation in the reward system appears to underlie the negative affect common to drug withdrawal across drug class. Acutely, drug use increases DA transmission in the mesolimbic pathway. To counter this effect, over time and with continued drug use, DA transmission in the pathway decreases, becoming evident upon withdrawal as feelings of anhedonia, dysphoria, depression, and anxiety. The power of reward center-mediated withdrawal can be appreciated by the high relapse rates found among abusers of substances (cocaine, amphetamine) who suffer few clinically significant somatic withdrawal symptoms. Negative affect states such as these are implicated in the development of craving and relapse (see below), common outcomes of attempted drug abstinence.

Addiction as "Liking" and "Wanting." Recent conceptualizations of addiction (Berke & Hyman, 2000; Robinson & Berridge, 1993, 2001; Spanagal & Weiss, 1999) describe two separate but important components to drug reinforcement: the "liking" of the drug (for its rewarding, hedonic, or euphoric value), and the "wanting" of the drug (for its incentive, needed, or motivating value). In cocaine-dependent human subjects, functional brain imaging has shown that intravenous cocaine yields an immediate but transient activation of the VTA, NA, and basal forebrain, correlated with reinforcement-related subject ratings of a drug "rush." However, the NA and amygdala exhibit a more sustained activation, correlated with incentive-related ratings of "craving" (Breiter, Gollub et al., 1997). Both the wanting and the liking of a drug contribute to its overall strength as a reinforcer or its "addictiveness," and to the subsequent generation of behaviors (compulsive use, loss of control over use) indicative of addiction. Drug-induced dopaminergic activity in this critical pathway is implicated in both aspects of reinforcement by not only (1) generating the drug reward (the "liking"), but also by (2) strengthening the relative salience (or increasing the synaptic connectivity) of the already powerful memory associated with the rewarding experience (the "wanting").

Liking: Since Olds and Milner (1954) showed that laboratory animals will voluntarily and eagerly self-administer electrical stimulation to specific midbrain structures, the neuroanatomy and physiology of the neural systems involved in "liking" or drug reward has been extensively studied. It is now understood that drugs of abuse, like intracranial self-stimulation, ultimately increase dopaminergic activity in the mesolimbic pathway described above (Di Chiara & Imperato, 1988; Gardner, 1997; Koob & Bloom, 1988; Miller & Gold, 1993; Wise, 1980; Wise & Bozarth, 1984). Reliably demonstrated with presentations of both drug and natural (such as food and water) rewards, dopaminergic activity in this pathway is most robust under conditions of reward deprivation, or when the reward is presented in an unpredicted or novel manner.

Psychostimulants and cannabinoids act relatively directly on the reward pathway by increasing dopamine transmission in the NAC, where as the CNS depressants and benzodiazepines exert their effects indirectly by quieting noradrenergic centers that serve to tonically inhibit DA release from VTA neurons.

In response to continued drug use, changes in the neural systems underlying liking are homeostatic in nature,

representing a somewhat passive neuroadaptive response to counteracting the drug's acute effects. Fortunately, neuroadaptive changes in the liking of a drug appear to be relatively reversible, with activity returning to normal levels upon sustained abstinence from the drug.

Wanting: A second effect of DA release in the mesolimbic reward pathway in response to drug use is to trigger key processes known to heighten or strengthen the processes of learning and memory in the brain. As opposed to the reversible and adaptive changes that occur in the systems of "liking," changes in the "wanting" domain are characterized as a long-lasting, relatively permanent reorganization in synaptic connectivity, as are those involved in normal associative learning and habit formation. The salience of these connections established under the highly rewarding conditions of drug euphoria are evident in the persistence of drug use behaviors in the face of negative consequences (addiction). Rather than maintaining a homeostasic state, the laying down of powerful memory imprints represents actual changes to the brain architecture that are very resistant to erasing. Because they share many of the molecular changes associated with learning and memory (that is, activation of the transcription factor CREB, formation of dendritic spines, enhanced glutamatergic transmission), changes in the "wanting" domain of reward are analogous to the processes underlying long-term potentiation, which permanently alter the excitability of postsynaptic neuronal membranes. These powerful memories increasingly are believed to be responsible for the craving associated with addictive disorders (Nestler, 2001). Craving is a feeling state that is closely related both to the compulsive nature of addictive drug use and to relapse upon abstinence. Because the neural substrate mediating the hedonic effects of drugs, contrarily, does not appear to sensitize (for example, addicts often lament their inexplicable craving for drugs despite their failure to produce a "high" over time and the psychosocial damage drug use produces in their lives), drug addiction is characterized by an increasing dissociation between the incentive value of drugs (how much they are wanted) and their subjective pleasurable effects (how much they are liked).

Finally, relevant to the physiology underlying addiction are the effects of HPA-axis activation, both within the context of addiction and preceding initial drug use, and the potential contributions of early-childhood (especially) or later trauma in altering the baseline neuroanatomic and physiologic substrates known to be involved in behavioral

---

sensitization to addictive drugs. Both stress and repeated, chronic administration of glucocorticoids in animals have been shown to enhance their behavioral sensitization to addictive drugs, which has prompted the hypothesis that excessive circulating glucocorticoids could function to maintain the sensitized state (Piazza & Le Moal, 1996, 1997). Extreme or chronic stress, as well as emotional or physical trauma, prior to initial drug use are physiologically implicated in the observation that enduring behavioral sensitization to drugs is expressed in some, but not all, individuals following initial drug exposure (Bremner, 1999).

POINTS OF INTERFACE
BETWEEN PAIN AND ADDICTION

Drugs of abuse have multiple and distinct effects in the central nervous system and share an ability to activate the neural structures from which their "rewarding" nature arise. Primary sites of action are the brainstem (locus coeruleus) and subcortical limbic structures (mesolimbic DA pathway), which are near to, but somewhat distinct from, those central areas involved in the perception (thalamus) and/or modulation (brainstem; periaqueductal gray) of pain.

As potential points of interface between the physiology of pain and of addiction are considered, it must first be recognized that many classes of abused drugs have demonstrated analgesic properties. The opioids are defined by their direct analgesic effects, and, at high doses, alcohol is a potent anesthetic. CNS stimulants, such as cocaine and caffeine, produce and potentiate analgesia, presumably by increasing neurotransmitter activity in descending inhibitory pain pathways.

Of current interest are the effects cannabinoids have on pain perception. Mao and colleagues (2000) recently provided good preclinical evidence for an independent THC-responsive antinocipetive pathway that is particularly effective for pain of neuropathic origin. In 1992, Devane and colleagues developed a high-affinity synthetic cannabinoid ligand, confirming the presence of endogenous cannabinoid G-protein-coupled receptors in the human body. Central subtype receptors are widely distributed in the cortex, basal ganglia, cerebellum, and hippocampus (Herkenham, 1995; Matsuda, Lolait et al., 1990). Interference with glutamate release at the level of the dorsal root ganglia or periaqueductal gray is a hypothesized mechanism by which cannabinoids provide analgesia (Mechoulam, Ben-Shabat et al., 1995).

Careful examination of the extant literature provides evidence that physiologic states consistent with drug addiction can affect or predict nociceptive input, processing and/or modulation in several different ways. First, there are relatively nonspecific consequences of addiction, which clearly facilitate the experience of pain via associated sympathetic arousal and negative emotional or affective mood. These changes are related to both the discrete effects of certain classes of drugs and the effects on reward-relevant systems of all drugs of abuse. Second, there appear to be patterned ways in which certain individuals process both pain (or analgesia) and the reward associated with substances of abuse, thereby mediating both pain and addictive responses. Finally, recent evidence indicates that molecular changes accompanying the development of opioid tolerance specifically appear to facilitate or increase nociceptive transmission, resulting in a relatively hyperalgesic state for the user.

Much of the data providing evidence for overlap between pain and addiction phenomena have been obtained in animal studies, so caution must be exercised in generalizing these to clinical populations. By definition, both pain and addiction are uniquely human conditions; the complexity of each is evident in psychosocial, cognitive, and cultural domains, and cannot be replicated in animal models. Hypotheses about how the neurophysiological overlap between pain and addiction might clinically manifest must take into account how holistic human responses to their combined presence may alter or mask predicted physiological responses.

Nonspecific Effects of Addiction on Pain. Several behavioral components of addiction may serve to facilitate the pain experience. Important substance-induced disorders or psychological sequelae, including sleep disorders and psychiatric illness, have in and of themselves been demonstrated to augment the experience of pain and decrease the efficacy of interventions for pain relief. Addiction commonly co-occurs with anxiety and affective disorders, which—if unrecognized or untreated—can increase the perception of pain. The interpersonal conflicts, role adjustments, and social support losses that characterize the social context of addiction can worsen the experience of chronic or acute pain, making the individual less able to manage discomfort. Further, the chaotic and drug-oriented lifestyle of the addict makes it difficult to comply with prescribed pain management regimes. Compton (1994) provides good evidence that individuals currently using addictive drugs, regardless of the particular drug of abuse, are significantly less tolerant of experimental pain than are matched drug-abstinent ex-addicts, whose performance is comparable to that of published norms.

Sympathetic Arousal: In addiction, drug use is characterized by frequent and rapid fluctuations in blood levels of the drug. Abused substances tend to be ingested in short-acting formulations and via routes of rapid onset (as through inhalation or intravenous administration) to boost psychoactive effect. These use patterns result in relatively rapidly alternating states of intoxication and subtle (or sometimes full-blown) withdrawal. Drug intoxication and withdrawal activate the sympathetic nervous system, which is known to contribute to the pain experience. For example, intoxication with cocaine and CNS stimulants significantly increases central noradrenergic activity. Withdrawal from opioids, CNS depressants, and/or sedative-hypnotics also results in an increase in central noradrenergic activity related to upregulated locus coeruleus NE discharge (Miller & Gold, 1993). Although stress-induced analgesia might be expected to be the outcome of this uncontrolled noradrenergic activity, the increased muscle tension, anxiety, and irritability noted during intoxication or withdrawal from these drugs of abuse appear to augment, rather than reduce, discomfort in the addict.

Affective Withdrawal: As noted, a strong and persistent negative affective state accompanies withdrawal from all drugs of abuse, related to overall DA depletion in the reward pathways. When drug-free, the addicted individual suffers from such negative symptoms as anhedonia, prolonged dysphoria, and irritability (Koob & Bloom, 1988; Kreek & Koob, 1998), and reports being unable to feel gratification or reward from any environmental stimuli. The degree to which affective withdrawal responses contribute to the overall drug-specific withdrawal syndrome varies, with those drugs acting more directly on DA-relevant reward pathways (see Table 2) that have a more affectively charged withdrawal. Clearly, the negative feeling states associated with drug withdrawal can augment the subjective discomfort associated with pain. Further, the DA depletion associated with cocaine addiction is significant enough to induce a clinical depression accompanied by high suicide risk. Depression has been demonstrated to increase the discomfort associated with pain in studies of chronic pain patients, with pain improving along with effective antidepressant treatment.

Thus, abused substances have analgesic and anti-algesic properties. Responses to the presence of certain abused drugs, or the absence of others following chronic administration, can affect neurotransmitter systems in ways that release descending pathways from tonic inhibition or increase ascending nociceptive input, thereby increasing the pain experience. The congruence between the treatment approaches that manage pain and addiction (that is, cognitive therapy, behavior modification, involvement of family, treatment of concurrent psychiatric disorders, and group support) provides further evidence that these phenomena have similar bases and are not entirely unrelated.

Genetic Factors Predicting Pain and Addiction. Generally, it is well accepted that great variation exists in a given individual's tolerance for pain, on which the effects of age, gender, and ethnicity have been extensively described. For example, normative experimental pain data reveal a bimodal distribution for pain tolerance in the general population, such that individuals either can tolerate the cold-pressor stimulus for less than one minute or else for the entire duration of the trial (3 to 5 minutes), at a relative ratio of one pain-intolerant to 14 pain-tolerant individuals (Walsh, Schoenfeld et al., 1989). Yet in a well-characterized drug abusing population (n=122), the relative frequency was reversed, with 5.4 pain intolerant patients for every one pain-tolerant patient (Compton, 1994). Thus, it is important to consider whether individuals with a genetic propensity for addiction may not also possess characteristic styles of responding to painful stimuli.

For example, heritable differences in hepatic P450 isoenzyme activity affect both the amount of reward and analgesia received from an opioid. Individuals who are extensive "metabolizers" of opioids (that is, those with high P450 activity) receive less analgesia and reward from a given opioid dose (Gonzalez, 1991; Ingelman-Sundberg, Johansson et al., 1994; Maurer & Bartkowski, 1993; Otton, Schadel et al., 1993), theoretically putting them at decreased risk for addiction, but increased risk for unrelieved pain. Preliminary data suggest that these extensive metabolizers of opioids are less tolerant of cold-pressor pain, possibly due to defects in the endogenous synthesis of opioids (Sindrup, Poulsen et al., 1993).

More intriguing is the presence of heritable differences in central reward and pain processing systems. That pain and addiction responses may be related in certain individuals is predicted by the extant animal data. Certain recombinant murine strains differ in both their baseline tolerance for pain, as well as the amount of reward or reinforcement they enjoy from opioids. Those strains of animals with poor pain tolerance find opioids to be highly reinforcing, whereas those with good pain tolerance receive little reinforcement from opioids. Further, pain-tolerant murine strains receive robust opioid analgesia and demonstrate increased opioid receptor binding activity as compared to pain-intolerant strains (Berrettini, Alexander et al., 1994; Mogil, Przemyslaw et al., 1995; Mogil, Wilson et al., 1999; Petruzzi, Ferraro et al., 1997).

Not surprisingly, a genetic locus underlying these patterned murine opioid responses has been identified as the mu opioid receptor gene (Oprm) (Belknap, Mogil et al., 1995; Berrettini, Alexander et al., 1994; Mogil, Przemyslaw et al., 1995; Mogil, Sternberg et al., 1996; Mogil, Wilson et al., 1999; Uhl, Sora et al., 1999), specific polymorphisms of which (A118G, C17T) also have been reported in humans who are addicted to opioids (Bond, LaForge et al., 1998; Kranzler, Gelerntner et al., 1998). In mice that lack the mu opioid receptor gene, for example, morphine has been shown not to be analgesic (Sora, Li et al., 1999), nor is heroin or morphine 6-β-glucouronide (Kitanaka, Sora et al., 1998), both of which have been postulated to mediate analgesia at sites independent of the mu receptor.

A preliminary study of the role of genotypic differences at the mu opioid receptor gene in pain and opioid reward responses in humans did not support a pleiotropic role for the gene in such responses (Compton, Alarcon et al., 2001b). However, the strength of the preclinical data suggests that the relationships among OPRM1, pain tolerance, and opioid addiction warrant further study before drawing a conclusion that individual differences in OPRM1 genotype do not predict pain intolerance in opioid-addicted individuals.

If pain intolerance is, in fact, a genetically determined trait, addicted persons should evidence poor pain tolerance in comparison to controls, regardless of whether they currently are using drugs or are in drug-free recovery. A recent series of studies by Liebmann and colleagues provide evidence that drug-free opioid addicts are less sensitive to pain than are controls. These investigators report increased cold-pressor pain thresholds in ex-opioid addicts (in residential treatment) as compared to controls (Liebmann, Lehofer et al., 1994, 1997, 1998). Further, Lehofer and colleagues (1997) reported that, using guided subjective recall, ex-opioid addicts rated themselves as less sensitive to pain than did normal controls, both when actively using and when opioid-free.

Leibmann and colleagues (1997) did identify a distinct subgroup of pain-intolerant ex-opioid addicts who were almost three times as likely to relapse within two years of treatment entry than were pain-tolerant ex-addicts. Opioid addicts with poor pain tolerance may suffer a more severe form of addiction or have difficulty tolerating the discomfort (pain) inherent in detoxification and early abstinence.

Whether differences in endogenous opioid activity affect drug reward from drugs other than opioids has yet to be explored. Acknowledging that endogenous opioid activity mediates reward from all drugs of abuse (Gardner, 1997), some differences in pain response across drugs of abuse might be suspected. In addition to the opioid system genes, other primary suspects have included those involved in the expression of other neurotransmitter systems known to affect brain reward, including their ligands, transporters, and receptors; the proteins contributing to the cAMP transduction pathway, neuroplasticity, and learning; and the genes involved in the HPA-axis response (see Uhl, 1999; Lichterman, Franke et al., 2000).

Pain in Opioid-Addicted Patients. The effects of addictive disease on pain become especially pertinent in the case of individuals addicted to opioid drugs, because the class of drug abused also is the primary pharmacological tool for the treatment of moderate to severe clinical pain. Although drug reward and analgesia are distinct processes, opioids activate their shared anatomical substrate, the mu opioid receptor, inducing the well-described interrelated central nervous system changes of tolerance and physical dependence. Opioid addicts may seek psychoactive effects, yet may not be immune to the potential effects of these drugs on central and peripheral opioid-relevant pain systems.

That opioid addiction and pain responses might be interrelated is not a new idea. Hypothesizing almost 40 years ago that opioid addicts self-medicate to deal with "an abnormally low tolerance for painful stimuli" (p. 224), Martin and Inglis (1965) described significantly lower tolerance for coldpressor pain in an incarcerated population of women who were "known narcotic addicts" (n=24) in comparison to matched "non-addict" controls (n=24; t=5.16, $p <.001$). Interpretation of these data was limited in that two variables relevant to the pain response (time since last opioid [or other illicit drug] use, and the presence of opioid withdrawal symptoms) were not reported. Yet the magnitude of the relationship was impressive and suggested a phenomenon of clinical significance.

Most studies of the pain responses of opioid addicts have been conducted with methadone-maintained (MM) patients. Opioid dosing, illicit drug use, and withdrawal symptoms are relatively well controlled in MM treatment; this physiologic stability (as well as related behavioral improvements) provides opioid addicts who are reliable informants. Ho and Dole (1979) found that both MM and drug-free opioid addicts had significantly lower thresholds for cold-pressor (CP) pain than did matched non-addict sibling controls. Subsequent work supports that, at methadone trough conditions (± 60 min of daily dosing), CP pain threshold does not differ between MM and drug-free opioid addicts (Compton, 1993), but is significantly lower for MM patients in comparison to matched normal controls (Doverty, White et al., 2001). Under the same conditions, MM patients' CP pain tolerance is less than that in both matched drug-free addicts (Compton, 1994) and matched controls (Compton, Charuvastra et al., 2000; Doverty, White et al., 2001). A similar non-significant trend for decreased pain tolerance in MM patients was noted for electrical pain stimulation (Doverty, White et al., 2001).

With respect to perceived pain severity, Schall and colleagues (1996) reported no difference between MM and control subjects in their perception of pressure pain (measured on a scale of 1 to 10) immediately prior to methadone dosing. Taken together, the work of Schall and colleagues (1996) and Doverty and colleagues (2001) indicates a significant analgesic effect for methadone on CP, electrical, and pressure pain two to four hours post-dose, and this effect correlates with peak methadone blood levels.

Thus, from the cross-sectional evidence available to date, it appears that MM patients are more sensitive to pain than are matched normal controls. With appreciable (albeit trough) methadone blood levels, these patients not only appreciate *no* underlying analgesic effect from daily, high dose administration of methadone, they actually present a case for the *anti-analgesic* (hyperalgesic) effects of chronic methadone therapy. Further, pilot data suggest that degree of hyperalgesia varies with the intrinsic activity of the opioid maintenance agent; patients maintained on the partial agonist buprenorphine for the treatment of opioid addiction are less hyperalgesic than those maintained on methadone, a full agonist (Compton, Charuvastra, et al., 2001). The specific mechanisms underlying this apparent hyperalgesia in the MM population are difficult to specify.

Several lines of evidence indicate that opioid administration not only provides analgesia, but concurrently sets into motion certain anti-analgesic or hyperalgesic processes, which counteract or oppose the opioid analgesic effects. From this perspective, the pain intolerance of MM patients might reflect a latent hyperalgesia secondary to chronic opioid exposure. Supporting the presence of opioid-induced hyperalgesia (OIH) in MM patients, data previously described show that drug-free ex-opioid addicts tolerate pain better than MM patients (Compton, 1994), and to the same degree as controls (Liebmann, Lehofer et al., 1994, 1997, 1998). Pilot data also provide evidence that pain tolerance improves over the course of opioid detoxification (Compton & Maya, 2001). This suggests that these individuals appear "less hyperalgesic" when opioid-free.

The observation that chronic opioid administration induces increased pain sensitivity or hyperalgesia is not a new one. The presence of OIH has been described best under conditions in which a previously opioid-dependent individual suffers acute opioid withdrawal; in fact, although not extensively studied, hyperalgesia long has been considered a cardinal symptom of the opioid withdrawal syndrome (Tilson, Rech et al., 1973; Jasinski, 1977; O'Brien, 1996). Variously attributed to sympathetic nervous system activation or dysphoric mood states, this symptom also may be the expression of a suddenly unopposed hyperalgesia. Recent animal studies of murine OIH upon opioid withdrawal (from either implanted morphine pellets or daily fentanyl injections) confirms marked hyperalgesia to tail flick, paw withdrawal, and formalin-induced licking assays—an effect augmented by intermittent naloxone challenges during opioid maintenance (Li, Angst et al., 2001). Demonstrating the key role of the mu opioid receptor in the development of this hyperalgesia, investigators found diminished OIH development in mouse strains with reduced mu opioid receptor binding.

More than 20 years ago, Seigel and colleagues observed a robust OIH in animals receiving saline in an environment previously paired with morphine administration (Krank, Hinson et al., 1981; Siegel, Hinson et al., 1978). This work showed that rats receiving acute morphine doses (3 to 9 doses separated by 48 hours) in a specific environment demonstrate significant hyperalgesia in the same setting as compared to rats receiving morphine unpaired with setting, or saline control rats. Because conditioned responses to medications typically are opposite in direction to unconditional drug effects, the learned responses were ascribed a causal role in the development of drug tolerance.

Through their preclinical work exploring molecular mechanisms of hyperalgesic pain states, Mao and colleagues (Mao, Price et al., 1994, 1995a, 1995b; Mayer, Mao et al., 1995a, 1995b) have demonstrated that, at the level of the individual, opioid analgesic tolerance is hyperalgesia. In an important series of studies, these investigators provide paradigm-shifting evidence that the development of opioid analgesic tolerance via intermittent morphine dosing induces hyperalgesia, while animals made hyperalgesic via neuropathic injury concomitantly exhibit opioid analgesic tolerance (these results recently were replicated with heroin by Celerier, Laulin et al., 2001). Further, Mao and colleagues demonstrated that the common pathway for the development of morphine tolerance/hyperalgesia is activation of ionotropic NMDA receptors on dorsal horn spinal cord neurons, with subsequent intracellular increases in protein kinase C and nitric oxide. The latter finding has spurred interest in the potential utility of NMDA-receptor antagonists in pain management as a means to enhance the effectiveness of opioid analgesia (Basbaum, 1995, 1996; Portenoy, Bennett et al., 2000; Price, Mayer et al., 2000; Sang, 2000; Weinbroum, Rudick et al., 2000). This complements the ongoing work of addiction scientists on the utility of these agents to reverse opioid tolerance and physical dependence (Bisaga & Popik, 2000; Elliott, Hynansky et al., 1994; Pasternak, Kolesnikov et al., 1995; Trujillo, 1995).

Alternatively, Vanderah and colleagues (2001) provided compelling evidence that the source of OIH lies in bulbospinal pathways that originate in opioid receptor-rich areas of the medulla, and which are responsible for the descending modulation that either inhibits or facilitates the perceived pain experience. Although the pathways are a well-described source of opioid analgesic effects, the investigators posit that they also are responsible for facilitating nociception under conditions of chronic opioid administration. A robust OIH was developed in rats that were continually exposed to opioids for seven days, which was blocked either via direct lidocaine infusion into the rostral medulla or lesioning of the spinal cord dorsolateral funiculus. Thus, facilitatory supraspinal systems may be involved in the development of hyperalgesia for persons maintained on methadone.

The presence of hyperalgesia with ongoing opioid use demands reconsideration of the well-described phenomenon of analgesic tolerance. Jasinski (1997) suggests that "tolerance occurs not at the (opioid) receptor level but occurs from increased activity of other functional systems to counteract the effects of opioids" (p. 185). The hyperalgesic processes initiated by opioid administration serve to counteract opioid analgesia. According to Colpaert (1996) and Celerier and colleagues (Laulin, Celerier et al., 1999; Celerier, Laulin et al., 1999, 2001; Celerier, Rivat et al., 2000), what appears to be opioid analgesic tolerance may in fact be an organismic expression of opioid-induced increased sensitivity to pain. Opioids lose their analgesic effectiveness in the face of decreased tolerance for pain.

Effects of Pain on Addiction Responses. What remains to be demonstrated is how the presence of pain might alter or attenuate the amount of reward provided by a given drug of abuse. Clinical lore holds that patients in pain who take opioid analgesics receive little "reward," at least not to the degree that they begin to seek drugs once the painful condition has resolved. Rates of iatrogenic opioid addiction for persons with no history of addiction are at less than 1%, if present at all (Medina & Diamond, 1977; Perry & Heidrich, 1982; Porter & Jick, 1980). Zacny and colleagues (1996) found that under experimental conditions, human subjects reported less opioid reward from a dose of opioid paired with a painful stimulus than was reported during the same opioid challenge without pain.

Similarly, it is not clear that opioid tolerance and physical dependence develop to the same degree while an individual is in pain as when that individual is pain-free. Vaccarino and colleagues (1993) provided interesting preclinical evidence that rats chronically receiving morphine paired with acute formalin-induced pain demonstrate less analgesic tolerance and naloxone-precipitated withdrawal than rats with the same chronic exposure to opioids without pain. These data parallel the anecdotal experience of many pain clinicians, who report that they do not encounter opioid tolerance when providing chronic opioid analgesia to persons with malignant or nonmalignant pain syndromes, but that doses need be increased only when pathology progresses (Portenoy & Foley, 1986).

These findings stand in contrast to those previously described, which show that molecular changes in the dorsal horn that occur with the development of neuropathic pain concomitantly result in opioid tolerance (Mao, Price et al., 1994, 1995a, 1995b; Mayer, Mao et al., 1995a, 1995b). Preclinical work supports that animals with nerve injury or arthritic pain develop opioid tolerance much more quickly and to a greater extent than animals without pain (Christensen & Kayser, 2000; Kayser & Guilbaud, 1985). Gutstein (1996) and colleagues (1995) suggest that reconciling the conflicting findings regarding the effects of pain on opioid tolerance will require closer examination of the experimental methods used to study the phenomenon (that is, nociceptive versus neuropathic pain, chronic versus intermittent exposure to the nociceptive stimulus, chronic versus intermittent exposure to opioids). Despite potential effects of pain on opioid tolerance, there is no evidence that the presence of pain makes individuals more likely to develop addictive disease when exposed to opioids.

CONCLUSIONS

Even without considering a shared neurophysiological basis, the clinician should expect that pain responses will be complicated in the presence of addictive disease. Addiction and pain are, in every respect, *human* conditions; individual responses to these conditions are expressed holistically in the biological, psychological, social, and spiritual realms. The presence of addictive disease colors responses to all afferent and environmental stimuli, including pain. Beyond hypothesized and demonstrated interactions at the physiological level, the behavioral and psychosocial correlates of addiction cannot help but complicate pain responses.

Pain is the most modulated of the sensory modalities. How a given, quantifiable stimulus is processed by the nervous system can be modified at the level of the nociceptor, the peripheral nerve, the spinal cord neurons and tracts, the thalamus, or the cortex; modulation typically occurs at one or more of these sites. The unique susceptibility of pain to neuroregulation portends a significant role for addiction in modulating the pain experience. Addiction physiology underlies the processing of stimuli, which by nature provide reward; stimuli that are by nature unrewarding, such as pain, are likely to be preferentially affected by the presence of addiction.

Several points of overlap exist between the physiological bases of pain and addiction. Specific avenues by which the chronic use of addictive drugs might alter the processing of noxious stimuli include the presence of sympathetic stimulation, HPA-axis dysregulation, affective withdrawal, and opioid tolerance. Less well studied but intriguing is evidence that individuals vary in their propensity to both addiction and pain responses; the link between the two may arise from inborn differences in endogenous opioid system tone. Across this literature, a trend toward decreased pain

tolerance (or decreased activity of endogenous inhibitory pain systems) in addiction can be discerned. The presence of addiction appears to augment the experience of pain, although further clinical study is needed to validate this observation.

Providing adequate pain relief to the addicted patient is a challenging and sometimes arduous clinical task. Consideration of the physiologic bases of pain and addiction, and how they overlap, provides direction for the management of pain in this population. The human phenomena of pain and addiction are not separate but interrelated; knowledgeable management of the former must reflect the extent to which, even at the physiological level, its expression and response are affected by the latter.

ACKNOWLEDGMENT: The authors wish to recognize the outstanding editorial and scientific contributions of Christine Brand, M.S.N., to the chapter.

REFERENCES

American Psychiatric Association (APA) (1994). *Diagnostic and Statistical Manual of Mental Disorders, 4th Edition (DSM-IV)*. Washington, DC: American Psychiatric Press.

Basbaum AI (1995). Insights into the development of opioid tolerance. *Pain* 61:349-352.

Basbaum A (1996). Memories of pain. *Science & Medicine* 22-31.

Belknap JK, Mogil JS, Helms ML et al. (1995). Localization to chromosome 10 of a locus influencing morphine analgesia in crosses derived from C57BL/6 and DBA strains. *Pharmacology Letter* 57:117-124.

Berke JD & Hyman S (2000). Addiction, dopamine and molecular mechanisms of memory. *Neuron* 25:515-532.

Berrettini WH, Alexander R, Ferraro TN et al. (1994). A study of oral morphine preference in inbred mouse strains. *Psychiatric Genetics* 4:81-86.

Bisaga A & Popik P (2000). In search of a new pharmacological treatment for drug and alcohol addiction: N-methyl-D-aspartate (NMDA) antagonists. *Drug and Alcohol Dependence* 59:1-15.

Bond C, LaForge KS, Tian M et al. (1998). Single-nucleotide polymorphism in the human mu opioid receptor gene alters B-endorphin binding and activity: Possible implications for opiate addiction. *Proceedings of the National Academy of Sciences* 94:9608-9613.

Breiter HC, Gollub RL, Weisskoff RM et al. (1997). Acute effects of cocaine on human brain activity and emotion. *Neuron* 19:591-611.

Bremner JD (1999). Does stress damage the brain? *Biological Psychiatry* 45:797-805.

Celerier E, Laulin JP, Corcuff JB et al. (2001). Progressive enhancement of delayed hyperalgesia induced by repeated heroin administration: A sensitization process. *Journal of Neuroscience* 21(11):4074-4080.

Celerier E, Laulin JP, Larcher A et al. (1999). Evidence for opiate-activated NMDA processes masking opiate analgesia in rats. *Brain Research Bulletin* 847:18-25.

Celerier E, Rivat C, Jun Y et al. (2000). Long-lasting hyperalgesia induced by fentanyl in rats. *Anesthesiology* 92(2):465-472.

Christensen D & Kayser V (2000). The development of pain-related behaviour and opioid tolerance after neuropathy-induced surgery and sham surgery. *Pain* 88:231-238.

Colpaert F (1996). System theory of pain and of opiate analgesia: No tolerance to opiates. *Pharmacological Reviews* 48:355-402.

Compton MA (1993). Perceptual reactance, drug of choice and pain perception in substance abusers. Doctoral Dissertation 9333902, University Microfilms International, Ann Arbor, MI.

Compton MA (1994). Cold-pressor pain tolerance in opiate and cocaine abusers: Correlates of drug type and use status. *Journal of Pain and Symptom Management* 9:462-473.

Compton P, Alarcon M & Geschwin D (2001b). Role of the m-opioid receptor gene in human pain tolerance and opioid addiction. *Drug and Alcohol Dependence* 63:S30-S31.

Compton P, Charuvastra C, Kintaudi K et al. (2000). Pain responses in methadone-maintained opioid abusers. *Journal of Pain and Symptom Management* 20(4):237-245.

Compton P, Charuvastra VC & Ling W (2001). Pain intolerance in opioid-maintained former opiate addicts: Effect of long-acting maintenance agent. *Drug and Alcohol Dependence* 63:139-146.

Compton P & Maya S (2001). Pain Tolerance in Opioid Addicts Over the Course of Outpatient Methadone Detoxification: An Open Trial. American Society of Addiction Medicine, Paper Presentation, April.

Cowan A, Lewis JW & MacFarlane IR (1977). Agonist and antagonist properties of buprenorphine, a new antinociceptive agent. *British Journal of Pharmacology* 60: 537-545.

Devane WA, Hanus L, Breuer A et al. (1992). Isolation and structure of a brain constituent that binds to the cannabinoid receptor [see comments]. *Science* 258:1946-1949.

Di Chiara G & Imperato A (1988). Drugs abused by humans preferentially increase synaptic dopamine concentrations in the mesolimbic system of freely moving rats. *Proceedings of the National Academy of Sciences* 85:5274-5278.

Doverty M, White J, Somogyi A et al. (2001). Hyperalgesic responses in methadone maintained patients. *Pain* 90:91-96.

Elliott K, Hynansky A & Inturrisi C (1994). Dextromethorphane attenuates and reverses analgesic tolerance to morphine. *Pain* 59(3):361-368.

Emmerson PJ, Clark MJ, Mansour H et al. (1996). Characterization of opioid agonist efficacy in a C6 glioma cell line expressing the mu opioid receptor. *Journal of Pharmacology and Experimental Therapeutics* 278:1121-1127.

Gardner EL (1997). Brain reward mechanisms. In JH Lowinson, RM Millman & JG Langrod (eds.) *Substance Abuse: A Comprehensive Textbook, 3rd Edition*. Baltimore, MD: Williams & Wilkins, 51-85.

Gebhart GF (1995a). *Visceral Pain*. Seattle, WA: IASP Press.

Gebhart GF (1995b). Somatovisceral sensation. In PM Conn (ed.) *Neuroscience in Medicine*. Philadelphia, PA: Lippincott.

Gold MS & Miller NS (1995). The neurobiology of drug and alcohol addictions. In NS Miller & MS Gold (eds.) *Pharmacological Therapies for Drug and Alcohol Addictions*. New York, NY: Marcel Dekker, 31-44.

Gonzalez FJ (1991). Human cytochrome P450: Possible roles of drug-metabolizing enzymes and polymorphic drug oxidation in addiction. *NIDA Research Monograph 111*. Rockville, MD: National Institute on Drug Abuse, 202-213.

Gutstein HB (1996). The effects of pain on opioid tolerance: How do we resolve the controversy? *Pharmacological Reviews* 48:403-407.

Gutstein HB, Trujillo KA & Akil H (1995). Does chronic nociceptive stimulation alter the development of morphine tolerance? *Brain Research Bulletin* 680:173-179.

Heimer L & Alheid G (1991). Piecing together the puzzle of basal forebrain anatomy. In TC Napier, PW Kalivas & I Hanin (eds.) *The Basal Forebrain: Anatomy to Function*. New York, NY: Plenum Press, 1-42.

Herkenham M (1995). In RG Pertwee (ed.) *Cannabinoid Receptors*. New York, NY: Academic Press, 145-166.

Ho A & Dole V (1979). Pain perception in drug-free and in methadone-maintained human ex-addicts. *Proceedings of the Society for Experimental Biology and Medicine* 162:392-395.

Ingelman-Sundberg M., Johansson I, Persson I et al. (1994). Genetic polymorphism of cytochrome P450. Functional consequences and possible relationship to disease and alcohol toxicity. In B Jansson, H Jornval, U Rydberg et al. (eds.) *Toward a Molecular Basis of Alcohol Use and Abuse*. Basel, Switzerland: Birkhauser Verlag, 197-207.

International Association for the Study of Pain (1979). Pain terms: A current list with definitions and notes on usage. *Pain* 6:249-252.

Jasinski DS (1977). Assessment of the abuse liability of the morphine-like drugs (methods used in man). In WR Martin (ed.) *Handbook of Experimental Pharmacology, Volume 45: Drug Addiction I*. New York: Springer-verlag, 197-158.

Jasinski D (1997). Tolerance and dependence to opiates. *Acta Anaesthesiology Scandinavica* 41:184-186.

Kayser V & Guilbaud G (1985). Can tolerance to morphine be induced in arthritic rats? *Brain Research Bulletin* 334:335-338.

Kitanaka N, Sora I, Kinsey S et al. (1998). No heroin or morphine 6b-glucouronide analgesia in m-opioid receptor knockout mice. *European Journal of Pharmacology* 355:R1-R3.

Koob GF & Bloom FE (1988). Cellular and molecular mechanisms of drug dependence. *Science* 242:715-723.

Koob GF, Robledo P, Markou A et al. (1993). The mesocorticolimbic circuit in drug dependence and reward. A role for the extended amygdala? In PW Kalivas & CD Barnes (eds.) *Limbic Motor Circuits and Neuropsychiatry*. Boca Raton, FL: CRC Press, 289-389.

Koob GF, Stinus L, Le Moal M et al. (1989). Opponent process theory of motivation: Neurobiological evidence from studies of opiate dependence. *Neuroscience & Biobehavioral Reviews* 13:135-140.

Krank M, Hinson R & Siegel S (1981). Conditional hyperalgesia is elicited by environmental signals of morphine. *Behavioral and Neural Biology* 32:148-157.

Kranzler HR, Gelernter J, O'Malley S et al. (1998). Association of alcohol or other drug dependence with alleles of the mu opioid receptor gene (OPRM1). *Alcoholism* 22:1359-1362.

Kreek MJ & Koob GF (1998). Drug dependence: Stress and dysregulation of brain reward pathways. *Drug and Alcohol Dependence* 51:23-47.

Laulin JP, Celerier E, Larcher A et al. (1999). Opiate tolerance to daily heroin administration: An apparent phenomenon associated with enhanced pain sensitivity. *Neuroscience* 89(3):631-636.

Lehofer M, Liebmann P, Moser M et al. (1997). Decreased nociceptive sensitivity: A biological risk marker for opiate dependence? *Addiction* 92(2):163-166.

Leshner AI & Koob GF (1999). Drugs of abuse and the brain. *Proceedings of the Association of American Physicians* 111:99-108.

Li X, Angst M & Clark D (2001). A murine model of opioid-induced hyperalgesia. *Molecular Brain Research* 86:56-62.

Lichterman D, Franke P, Maier W et al. (2000). Pharmacogenomics and addiction to opiates. *European Journal of Pharmacology* 410:269-279.

Liebmann P, Lehofer M, Moser M et al. (1997). Persistent analgesia in former opiate addicts is resistant to blockade of endogenous opioids. *Biological Psychiatry* 42:962-964.

Liebmann P, Lehofer M, Moser M et al. (1998). Nervousness and pain sensitivity: II. Changed relation in ex-addicts as a predictor for early relapse. *Psychiatry Research* 79:55-58.

Liebmann P, Lehofer M, Schonauer-Cejpek M et al. (1994). Pain sensitivity in former opioid addicts. *Lancet* 344:1031-1032.

Mao J, Price DD & Mayer DJ (1994). Thermal hyperalgesia in association with the development of morphine tolerance in rats: Roles of excitatory amino acids receptors and protein kinase C. *Journal of Neuroscience* 14:2301-2312.

Mao J, Price DD & Mayer DJ (1995a). Experimental mononeuropathy reduces the antinociceptive effects of morphine: Implications for the common intracellular mechanisms involved in morphine tolerance and neuropathic pain. *Pain* 61:353-364.

Mao J, Price DD & Mayer DJ (1995b). Mechanisms of hyperalgesia and morphine tolerance: A current view of their possible interactions. *Pain* 62:259-274.

Mao J, Price DD, Lu J et al. (2000). Two distinctive antinociceptive systems in rats with pathological pain. *Neuroscience Letters* 280:13-16.

Martin J & Inglis J (1965). Pain tolerance and narcotic addiction. *British Journal of Sociology and Clinical Psychology* 4:224-229.

Matsuda LA, Lolait SJ, Brownstein MJ et al. (1990). Structure of a cannabinoid receptor and functional expression of the cloned cDNA *Nature* 346:561-564.

Maurer PM & Bartkowski RR (1993). Drug interactions of clinical significance with opioid analgesics. *Drug Safety* 8:30-48.

Mayer D, Mao J & Price D (1995a). The association of neuropathic pain, morphine tolerance and dependence, and the translocation of protein Kinase C. *NIDA Research Monograph 147*. Rockville, MD: National Institute on Drug Abuse, 269-298.

Mayer D, Mao J & Price D (1995b). The development of morphine tolerance and dependence is associated with translocation of protein kinase C. *Pain* 61:365-374.

Mechoulam R, Ben-Shabat S, Hanus L et al. (1995). Identification of an endogenous 2-monoglyceride, present in canine gut, that binds to cannabinoid receptors. *Biochemistry and Pharmacology* 50:83-90.

Medina JL & Diamond S (1977). Drug dependency in patients with chronic headache. *Headache* 17:12-14.

Melzack R & Wall PD (1965). Pain mechanisms: A new theory. *Science* 50:971-979.

Miller NS & Gold MS (1993). A hypothesis for a common neurochemical basis for alcohol and drug disorders. *Psychiatric Clinics of North America* 16:105-117.

Mogil JS, Przemyslaw M, Flodman P et al. (1995). One or two genetic loci mediate high opiate analgesia in selectively bred mice. *Pain* 60:125-135.

Mogil JS, Sternberg WF, Marek P et al. (1996). The genetics of pain and pain inhibition. *Proceedings of the National Academy of Sciences* 93:3048-3055.

Mogil JS, Wilson SG, Bon K et al. (1999). Heritability of nociception I: Responses of 11 inbred mouse strains on 12 measures of nociception. *Pain* 80:67-82.

Ness TJ & Gebhart GF (1990). Visceral pain: A review of experimental studies. *Pain* 41:167-234.

Nestler EJ (2001). Total recall—The memory of addiction. *Science* 292:2266-2267.

O'Brien CP (1996). Drug addiction and drug abuse. In JG Hardman, LE Limbird, PB Molinoff et al. (eds.) *Goodman and Gilman's Pharmacological Basis of Therapeutics, 9th Edition* New York, NY: McGraw-Hill, 557-577.

Olds J & Milner P (1954). Positive reinforcement produced by electrical stimulation of septal area and other regions of rat brain. *Journal of Comprehensive Physiology and Psychology* 47:419-427.

Otton SV, Schadel M, Cheung SW et al. (1993). CYP2D6 phenotype determines the metabolic conversion of hydrocodone to hydromorphone. *Clinical Pharmacology and Therapeutics* 54:463-472.

Pasternak G, Kolesnikov Y & Babey AM (1995). Perspectives on the N-methyl-D-aspartate/nitric oxide cascade and opioid tolerance. *Neuropsychopharmacology* 13(4):309-313.

Perry S & Heidrich G (1982). Management of pain during debridement: A survey of U.S. burn units. *Pain* 13:267-280.

Petruzzi R, Ferraro TN, Kurschner VC et al. (1997). The effects of repeated morphine exposure on mu opioid receptor number and affinity in C57BL/6J and DBA/2J mice. *Life Science* 61:2057-2064.

Piazza PV & Le Moal ML (1996). Pathophysiological basis of vulnerability to drug abuse: Role of an interaction between stress, glucocorticoids, and dopaminergic neurons. *Annual Review of Pharmacology and Toxicology* 36:359-378.

Piazza PV & Le Moal ML (1997). Glucocorticoids as a biological substrate of reward: Physiological and pathophysiological implications. *Brain Research Reviews* 25:359-372.

Portenoy R, Bennett G, Katz N et al. (2000). Enhancing opioid analgesia with NMDA-receptor antagonists: Clarifying the clinical importance. *Journal of Pain and Symptom Management* 19(1 Suppl.):S57-S64.

Portenoy RK & Foley KM (1986). Chronic use of opiate analgesics in nonmalignant pain: Report of 38 cases. *Pain* 25:171-186.

Porter J & Jick H (1980). Addiction rare in patients treated with narcotics. *New England Journal of Medicine* 302:123.

Price D, Mayer D, Mao J et al. (2000). NMDA-receptor antagonists and opioid receptor interactions as related to analgesia and tolerance. *Journal of Pain and Symptom Management* 19(1 Suppl.):S7-S11.

Redmond DE & Krystal JH (1984). Multiple mechanisms of withdrawal from opioid drugs. *Annual Review of Neuroscience* 7:443-478.

Robinson TE & Berridge KC (1993). The neural basis of drug craving: An incentive-sensitization theory of addiction. *Brain Research Reviews* 18:247-291.

Robinson TE & Berridge KC (2001). Incentive-sensitization and addiction. *Addiction* 96:103-114.

Sang C (2000). NMDA-receptor antagonists in neuropathic pain: Experimental methods to clinical trials. *Journal of Pain and Symptom Management* 19(1 Suppl):S21-S25.

Schall U, Katta T, Pries E et al. (1996). Pain perception of intravenous heroin users on maintenance therapy with levomethadone. *Pharmacopsychiatry* 29:176-179.

Siegel S, Hinson RE & Krank MD (1978). The role of predrug signals in morphine analgesic tolerance: Support for a Pavlovian conditioning model of tolerance. *Journal of Experimental Psychology* 4:188-96.

Sindrup SH, Poulsen L, Brosen K et al. (1993). Are poor metabolizers of sparteine/debrisuquine less pain tolerant than extensive metabolizers? *Pain* 53:335-339.

Solomon R (1980). The opponent-process theory of acquired motivation: The costs of pleasure and the benefits of pain. *American Psychologist* 35(8):691-712.

Sora I, Li XF, Funada M et al. (1999). Visceral chemical nociception in mice lacking mu opioid receptors: Effects of morphine, SNC80 and U-0,488. *European Journal of Pharmacology* 366:R3-R5.

Spanagel R & Weiss F (1999). The dopamine hypothesis of reward: Past and current status. *Trends in Neurosciences* 22:521-527.

Tilson HA, Rech RH & Stolman S (1973). Hyperalgesia during withdrawal as a means of measuring the degree of dependence in morphine dependent rats. *Psychopharmacology* 28:287-300.

Trujillo K (1995). Effects of noncompetitive N-methyl-D-aspartate receptor antagonists on opiate tolerance and physical dependence. *Neuropsychopharmacology* 13(4):301-307.

Uhl GR (1999). Molecular genetics of substance abuse vulnerability: A current approach. *Neuropsychopharmacology* 20(1):3-9.

Uhl GR, Sora I & Wang Z (1999). The mu opiate receptor as a candidate gene for pain: Polymorphisms, variations in expression, nociception, and opiate responses. *Proceedings of the National Academy of Sciences* 96:7752-7755.

Vaccarino AL, Marek P, Kest B et al. (1993). Morphine fails to produce tolerance when administered in the presence of formalin pain in rats. *Brain Research Bulletin* 627:287-290.

Vanderah T, Suenaga N, Ossipov M et al. (2001). Tonic descending facilitation from the rostral ventromedial medulla mediates opioid-induced abnormal pain and antinociceptive tolerance. *Journal of Neuroscience* 21(1):279-286.

Walsh NE, Schoenfeld L, Ramamurthy S et al. (1989). Normative model for cold pressor test. *American Journal of Physical Medicine & Rehabilitation* 68:6-11.

Weinbroum A, Rudick V, Paret G et al. (2000). The role of dextromethorphane in pain control. *Canadian Journal of Anaesthia* 47(6):585-596.

Wise RA (1980). Action of drugs of abuse on brain reward systems. *Pharmacology, Biochemistry and Behavior* 13 (Suppl. 1):213-223.

Wise RA & Bozarth MA (1984). Brain reward circuitry: Four circuit elements "wired" in apparent series. *Brain Research Bulletin* 12:203-208.

Yu Y, Zhang L, Yin X et al. (1997). Mu opioid receptor phosphorylation, desensitization, and efficacy. *Journal of Biological Chemistry* 272:28869-28874.

Zacny JP, McKay MA, Toledano AY et al. (1996). The effects of cold-water immersion stressor on the reinforcing and subjective effects of fentanyl in healthy volunteers. *Drug and Alcohol Dependence* 42:133-142.

| Chapter 2 | # Principles of Pain Management in the Addicted Patient |

Seddon R. Savage, M.D., FASAM

Synergy of Pain and Addiction
Assessment of Pain
Approach to Acute Pain in Addiction
Approach to Chronic Pain in Addiction
Approach to Cancer Pain in Addiction

Pain—including acute pain, cancer-related pain, and chronic pain of non-cancer origin—is inadequately managed in the general population (Marks & Sacher, 1973; Morgan, 1985). Individuals with addictive disorders are at special risk for undertreatment of their pain (Cohen, 1980; Shine & Demas, 1984). Many factors contribute to this, including inadequate training of health professionals in pain management and addiction medicine, fear of contributing to addiction through the use of dependence-producing medications, lack of knowledge about addiction, societal prejudices toward persons with addictive disorders, and physicians' fears of regulatory sanctions related to opioid use.

Multiple initiatives to improve the treatment of pain were organized in the last two decades of the 20th century. These have begun to improve the management of pain in the general population; however, individuals with addictive disorders remain at significant risk for undertreatment of pain (Cleeland, Hatfield et al., 1994; Breitbart, Passik et al., 1996).

SYNERGY OF PAIN AND ADDICTION

There are a number of mechanisms by which the presence of addiction may increase the experience of pain and make the treatment of pain more difficult. Patients who are actively addicted to opioids, alcohol, cocaine, or other drugs may experience intermittent intoxication and withdrawal, which may result in intermittent sympathetic arousal and/or changes in muscle tone, both of which can increase some forms of pain. Generalized pain is itself a common component of opioid withdrawal, probably as the result of activation of opioid receptor changes, so that an underlying pain syndrome may increase in intensity in the presence of erratic opioid use by an addicted individual (Brodner & Taub, 1978). Relative pain intolerance has been demonstrated in patients with active disease of addiction on opioid agonist therapy.

Because of the numbing effects of many drugs of abuse, patients with addictive disorders, when intoxicated, may engage in activities that exacerbate the physical conditions responsible for their pain, thus increasing the pain. Chronic

---

FIGURE 1. Examples of Pain Scales

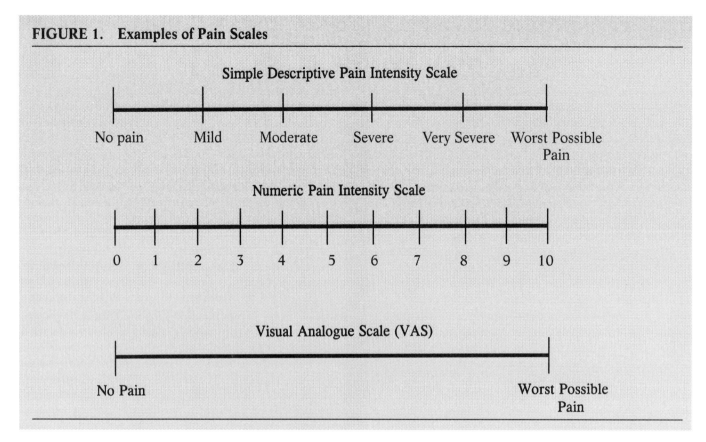

Simple Descriptive Pain Intensity Scale

No pain　Mild　Moderate　Severe　Very Severe　Worst Possible Pain

Numeric Pain Intensity Scale

0　1　2　3　4　5　6　7　8　9　10

Visual Analogue Scale (VAS)

No Pain　Worst Possible Pain

pain and active addictive disease often share similar sequelae, such as sleep disturbance, mood changes, disability, increased stresses, drug dependence, and other problems. When they occur concurrently, chronic pain and addictive disease may synergistically act to exacerbate or reinforce each other.

Finally, patients with addictive disorders may be unable to comply with pain treatment recommendations because of the chaos their addictions have created in their lives. In such patients, effective treatment of pain requires that addiction be addressed as well.

ASSESSMENT OF PAIN

Description of the Pain. An appropriately detailed assessment of the patient with pain is critical to the development of an appropriate treatment plan. The nature and extent of the evaluation depends on the type of pain and the context in which it occurs.

The physiologic basis of acute pain usually is apparent, or rapidly becomes so, with diagnostic evaluation. In such cases, the purpose of the history and physical examination is to confirm that pain is consistent with the determined cause and to identify any conditions that might complicate the presentation of pain, such as secondary neuropathic syndrome or muscle spasm. Intensity of pain usually is a key measure of acute pain. Serial measurements of pain intensity allow the clinician to evaluate the pain and the effectiveness of pain treatment. In most circumstances, pain measurement relies on self-report by the patient.

Examples of self-report tools available to measure pain intensity include numerical rating scales, verbal descriptor scales, and visual analogue scales (Figure 1). Which scale is most effective in any clinical context depends on a number of variables, including the patient's age, cognitive status, emotional status, and patient and provider preferences. In clinical settings, a numerical rating scale usually is employed. The patient is asked to rate his or her pain on a scale, often from 0 (no pain) to 10 (the worst possible pain). The scale then is repeated at intervals to assure that effective pain control is achieved and sustained.

It is important to identify the numerical level of control that each patient considers satisfactory. While a rating of 2 or 3 on a scale of 1 to 10 is the goal adopted by many clinicians, it is clear that some patients never rate their pain that low. This has been observed in patients with posttraumatic stress disorder. Intensifying treatment in an attempt to achieve a rating of 2 or 3 out of 10 in such patients often is fruitless and may be harmful. The patient's satisfaction is the important variable. To measure this, some clinicians use a rating scale that asks, "How distressing is your pain?," where 0 is "not distressing at all" and 10 is "unbearable." Alternatively, the clinician simply can ask, "What number represents 'good' or 'satisfactory' pain control to you?"

Children over the age of seven or eight who understand numerical and linear concepts generally can use a numerical rating scale, verbal descriptor scale, or visual analogue scale. Children over four years old and adults or children with mild cognitive disabilities may do better using an impressionistic scale, such as the faces scale (a scale that depicts a series of several faces expressing varying degrees of pain). In very young children and severely disabled adults, observation of pain behaviors—including vocalizations, verbalizations, facial expression, and movement—may be necessary to track pain (AHCPR, 1992). Observational scales are not accurate, however, in cognitively intact adults because unimpaired persons often inhibit pain behaviors and utterances for a variety of social and other reasons. No matter which scale is selected, serial use and consistency are important in monitoring pain and response to treatment.

Meaningful assessment of chronic pain, including pain related to cancer or non-cancer origins, usually demands more diverse observations than acute pain. In assessing chronic pain intensity at intervals, it is helpful to ask about current pain intensity, as well as least, greatest, and typical pain over a specified period of time (most often, the preceding week).

In addition to evaluating pain intensity, a description of a number of other pain variables is important. For example, a detailed description of pain may be helpful in understanding its etiology and in suggesting treatment approaches. Terms such as "aching," "tight," "sharp," "grating," or "vicelike" are suggestive of nociceptive pain, while "burning," "electrical," "shooting," and "numb" are suggestive of neuropathic pain. However, there is much subjectivity to such descriptions and they are not always diagnostic.

Learning the radiation and distribution of pain, the temporal patterns of pain throughout the day, changes in the pain with activity and rest, and its response to treatment also are helpful in characterizing the pain.

History of the Pain and Its Effects. A detailed history of evolution of the pain is helpful in elucidating its causes and meaning to the patient. Was the pain acute or gradual in onset? What events were associated with its development? How has it changed over time? What treatments have been tried, and with what results? What does the patient think is causing the pain?

Evaluation of chronic pain also must include an assessment of the effects of the pain on the patient's life; this is needed in order to address not only the pain but its secondary manifestations. Assessment of the effects of the pain on sleep, mood, work, relationships, valued recreational activities, and alcohol and drug use is important to a full understanding of the pain and useful in developing a treatment plan and goals of treatment, which most often should include functional, as well as pain level goals.

Social and vocational assessment often is used to identify supports and obstacles to treatment and rehabilitation. Does the patient have good social supports, housing, and meaningful work? Is the home environment stressful or nurturing? If employed, are there work activities that may perpetuate the pain? If so, are alternative work options available?

Evaluation of Addiction and Other Concurrent Medical Problems. For patients with co-occurring pain and addiction, characterization of the addictive disorder is critical. Is the patient in recovery or actively addicted? If recovering, what recovery supports are in place? Is the patient's group or sponsor aware of the pain problem and its effects on the individual? How do the patient's support systems react to the use of pain medications? It should be noted that AA generally supports the appropriate medical treatment of psychological, medical, surgical, or traumatic conditions in recovering patients as requisite to continued recovery from the disease of addiction. Some AA groups discourage the use of medications such as opioids or benzodiazepines, while others support the use of medications that are prescribed for a documented indication and taken as prescribed. In this regard, the recovery system can be either helpful or an obstacle to pain treatment.

In patients who are actively abusing or addicted to alcohol or other drugs, it is important to learn what drugs are being used, in what pattern and amounts. It is helpful to ascertain whether the patient is open to considering behavioral change. The clinician needs to be aware that medical

TABLE 1.   Approach to Acute Pain Treatment in Addiction
Address the disease of addiction: ■ Discuss addiction concerns; ■ Involve the patient in treatment decisions; ■ Facilitate/support recovery; ■ Educate staff as needed regarding addictive disorders and pain.
Prevent or treat withdrawal symptoms: ■ Provide baseline opioids (in opioid-dependent patients); ■ Identify and treat withdrawal.

Provide effective pain management:
■ Non-opioid treatment if effective and patient agrees;
■ Effective doses of opioids when indicated:
  □ Consider tolerance in determining dose and schedule;
  □ Avoid agonist-antagonist opioids when opioid dependence or tolerance is present.
■ Consider less rewarding opioids and schedules, if effective:
  □ Slower-release or sustained-release formulations;
  □ Scheduled medications, PCA, continuous infusions;
  □ Agonist-antagonists, partial agonists (in non-dependent or tolerant patients).

Monitor and adjust: ■ Pain intensity; ■ Side effects of medications; ■ Treatment, as indicated to achieve analgesia with minimal side effects.
Taper opioids as pain resolves.
Document the treatment plan.

problems may serve as a catalyst for readiness to change (Graham, 1991). Identification of concurrent psychiatric or other medical problems that may affect the experience or treatment of pain also is important.

Physical Examination. Physical examination of the patient with chronic pain involves direct evaluation of the area or physical system involved in the pain. In addition, depending on the site of the pain, the examination should include a broader assessment of biomechanical function and related myofascial systems, as splinting, guarding, and movement alterations due to pain may result in secondary pain syndromes. Neurologic examination—including a detailed sensory examination for numbness, hypoesthesia (reduced sensation), hyperesthesia (increased sensation), allodynia (pain sensation in response to a usually non-painful stimulus), or hyperpathia (persistence of sensation following cessation of stimulus)—is helpful in determining whether aberrant conduction suggestive of neuropathic pain is present. Localized alterations in skin temperature or the presence of trophic or autonomic changes also are suggestive of neuropathic mechanisms of pain.

The examination should include assessment of mood, cognitive function, and sensorium, which may be altered by pain or pain medications. Observation of the general status of the individual in terms of weight, fatigue, or other variables also is important.

A complete assessment of chronic pain often yields an impression of multiple problems contributing to the experience of pain, including physiological, psychological, and functional factors. The pain management plan should address each of these variables.

APPROACH TO ACUTE PAIN IN ADDICTION
Undertreatment of pain has been shown to increase morbidity following trauma and surgery in the general population (Wattwil, 1989). Optimal pain treatment appears to shorten hospitalizations in similar contexts (Jackson, 1989). The presence of pain increases distress and anxiety and, in individuals recovering from addiction, may become a significant risk factor for relapse. Individuals with addictive disease often experience high levels of anxiety in association with the stress of trauma, illness, or surgery, because they fear that their pain will not be adequately managed; this, in turn, can affect how they experience pain. Attention to their concerns often facilitates pain management (Table 1).

Address the Addictive Disorder. The clinician should be open and non-judgmental in discussing concerns regarding addiction with the patient. All too often, health professionals discuss concerns about a patient's addiction among themselves, without ever bringing the patient into the discussion. When addiction is understood as a medical disorder, it becomes easier to address it in the same manner as any other medical condition: with respectful and sensitive, but matter of fact, concern. Patients with addictive disorders often fear that awareness of their problem will negatively affect the manner in which their physicians and other providers approach their care. Therefore, they may not be immediately forthcoming about their addictive disorder or may be anxious about their medical care. In the context of pain treatment, it is helpful to allay such a patient's anxiety by reassuring him or her that the addictive disorder will not be an obstacle to the relief of their pain.

The individual in pain should be included in the decisionmaking process regarding medication choices, dosing, and scheduling. This provides the patient with a sense of control and allays anxiety as to whether pain will be adequately treated. It also may afford the physician insights that are useful in designing an effective treatment regimen. Addicted patients and patients with therapeutic drug dependence often are experts as to the drug doses they require to meet their basic dependence needs, as well as the additional levels required to treat their acute pain. Occasionally such consultation results in a request for a dose beyond that needed for analgesia, so prudence in prescribing is required. If a patient becomes obviously intoxicated or sedated at the prescribed dose, medications should be titrated to avoid the observed side effects while continuing to provide analgesia.

The patient who is hospitalized for an acute medical problem may be more open to intervention for his or her addictive disorder than he or she would be as an outpatient (Graham, 1991). It is important to capture such "windows of opportunity" to help bring patients into recovery. Addiction treatment should be offered when addiction is detected in the course of pain treatment. Counseling may be initiated at any time, so long as acute pain is adequately controlled. If the patient does not accept addiction treatment at the time it is offered, it may be helpful to use the acute pain problem to begin to explore the patient's motivation for recovery and to follow up at future visits.

Recovering persons often benefit from increasing their recovery activities during times of stress, such as hospitalization, trauma, and pain. Many clinicians and individuals in recovery believe that exposure to opioids, sedative-hypnotics or anesthetics—even if not the patient's drugs of choice—may lead to relapse. However, the distress of inadequately treated physical pain may pose an even greater risk of relapse. Effective pain treatment by whatever means, coupled with an active addiction recovery program, prob-

ably are the best supports for continued recovery during periods of acute stress, including periods of pain.

Prevent or Treat Withdrawal. If a patient is dependent on opioids, the clinician should not consider opioid discontinuation until the acute pain situation is resolved or effectively managed through use of an alternative approach, such as an epidural catheter. If a non-opioid treatment approach is selected by the patient and physician, opioids should be either tapered gradually to prevent withdrawal or continued at a dose that avoids withdrawal but does not oversedate the patient. Abrupt cessation of opioids will cause acute increase in pain.

Under the so-called "72-hour rule" implementing the federal Controlled Substances Act, it is permissible for a treating physician to provide opioids to prevent withdrawal in a patient who is hospitalized for a diagnosis other than addiction. For example, if a patient with heroin addiction is hospitalized with multiple fractures following a motor vehicle crash or with SBE related to heroin use, the treating physician can and should provide opioid medications to prevent withdrawal, as well as additional medications for pain. Anesthesiologists, psychiatrists, or addiction medicine specialists often are able to assist other physicians in determining appropriate doses and schedules for a given patient.

An actively drinking alcoholic, or a patient who is dependent on non-opioid drugs, should have withdrawal symptoms treated when they occur in the course of pain treatment. Unrecognized alcohol withdrawal will make pain control difficult to achieve, and physical signs of withdrawal (such as hypertension and tachycardia) may be misinterpreted as acute pain. Usually, a long-acting benzodiazepine such as chlordiazepoxide is an appropriate choice, although lorazepam and other drugs may be selected if parental use is required or if hepatic dysfunction is present.

Provide Effective Pain Relief. Pain relief should be provided in an effective and timely manner. Without adequate control of acute pain, it is unlikely that the patient will be able to engage in addiction treatment. Undertreatment of pain also may create craving for pain-relieving medications, as well as anxiety, frustration, anger, and other feelings that tend to feed addiction (McCaffery & Vourakis, 1992).

When they are effective, readily available, and safe, nonmedication pain treatments—such as cold, TENS, or regional anesthesia—are preferred by some clinicians and patients over systemic medications for the treatment of acute pain in individuals with addictive disease. When medications are indicated to relieve pain, those that are the least likely to alter mood may be used, but only if they are effective. While exposure to dependence-producing drugs may be one component of the development of addiction or relapse to drug use, such exposure alone does not create addiction. When such drugs are needed to manage pain, they should be provided at effective doses and intervals of administration. In the setting of moderate to severe acute pain, opioids usually are the mainstay of treatment in all patients, including those with addictive disorders.

Scheduled or PCA administration of opioids is preferred over PRN medications for acute pain in individuals with addictive disorders. These approaches have several advantages: (1) the patient does not have to ask for medications, which in an individual with an addictive disorder may be interpreted as drug-seeking behavior rather than a search for pain relief and thus may create friction between the patient and staff; (2) delays in receiving medication are avoided, so that timely and effective pain relief is obtained and drug craving is not allowed to occur; (3) because drug administration is time-contingent rather than symptom-contingent, reinforcement of the pain symptoms is minimized; and (4) the patient feels a sense of control that is essential to the process of recovery.

If scheduled medications are used, PRN doses of medication should be provided initially, in addition to scheduled doses, for titration of medications to the required dosing level. Intermittent, non-scheduled medications are appropriate in the acute pain setting when an individual has little or no baseline pain but experiences pain in relation to specific activities.

It is important to achieve pain relief with methods that do not confuse, stress, or frustrate the staff or the patient. For example, an epidural infusion of local anesthesia may seem ideal for management of post-thoracotomy pain in a recovering opioid addict, but if the floor nurses do not know how to manage the required catheters, the patient's overall needs probably will be better met with scheduled or PCA doses of opioids, since potential failure of the epidural may leave the patient in a position of seeking opioids for pain relief.

Patients with acute pain should be monitored at regular intervals to assess the effectiveness of treatment and the presence of side effects. Pain management should be adjusted to achieve optimal analgesia while minimizing such side effects. Most patients will naturally taper their medications as the cause of the acute pain resolves. Some patients with addictive disorders benefit from the negotiation of a structured tapering of medications on a scheduled basis. Persistent use of opioids despite apparent healing is discussed below.

Acute Pain Treatment in Methadone-Maintained Patients: Individuals who are on methadone maintenance or who are physically dependent on therapeutically prescribed or street opioids must have their baseline opioid requirements met in addition to the medications they need for pain (Wesson, Ling et al., 1993). The average baseline daily dose of opioids should be determined and either the same drug provided at the determined dose or an equianalgesic dose of an alternative opioid calculated and provided in appropriately scheduled doses (AHCPR, 1992) (see Chapter 5 for an analgesic equivalence chart).

Most often, a patient who is receiving methadone treatment of addiction should be continued on his or her baseline methadone as an inpatient and provided a different opioid for acute pain, rather than being entirely switched to an alternative opioid or having the methadone increased for pain. This is recommended for two reasons. First, incomplete cross-tolerance of methadone with other mu agonists has been noted and opioid withdrawal from methadone observed in some patients, even in the presence of calculated equianalgesic doses of alternative mu agonists. Second, while an increase in methadone usually is effective for pain management, the use of the same drug for addiction maintenance and for acute pain management may confuse the issues of pain treatment and addiction treatment when the acute pain resolves and it becomes appropriate to taper the pain medication to maintenance doses.

The patient's daily dose of methadone should be confirmed with the treatment program. If the dose cannot be confirmed, it is safest initially to give the dose the patient reports in three or four divided doses, rather than in a single dose and then to observe the response. If the patient cannot take oral medications, methadone can be given parenterally at half the oral dose.

Document the Pain Treatment Plan. It is important to be clear in communicating the treatment plan to all staff who will be caring for the patient. Stigma and misunderstanding regarding addictive disease are widespread among health care personnel and these may lead to inadequate pain management when the primary treating clinician is not available. In addition, in the absence of a clear and consistent structure, the patient's disease may result in behaviors that confuse the patient's pain and addiction issues.

When Pain Persists Beyond Apparent Healing. Many factors may lead a patient to complain of pain and to evidence a need for pain medications despite expected and apparent healing from surgery, trauma, illness, or other pain-provoking pathology. In the patient with an addictive disorder, concern often is raised that the patient may be manifesting addiction or relapse to addiction. However, it is important to consider other possible explanations before concluding that this is the case (Figure 2).

First, the patient may have an undetected physical problem, either related to the original painful problem or to a separate process. A thorough search for such a cause should be undertaken. The search should include a review of nociceptive causes of pain, such as an abscess or undetected fracture, as well as less common and often overlooked neurogenic causes of pain.

Second, the patient may be physically dependent on analgesic medications and may be experiencing pain related to withdrawal as the medication is discontinued. Withdrawal may mediate pain through a variety of mechanisms, including alterations in sympathetic arousal, changes in muscle tone, and alterations in opiate and other receptor function. A gradual taper of medications over several days usually avoids the withdrawal and associated pain. The goal when tapering an individual who is physically dependent on medications should be to provide stable but decreasing blood levels of opioid so as to prevent intermittent withdrawal. Although stable blood levels usually are only approximated with the use of short-acting medications, most patients do not experience significant withdrawal while tapering. However, some patients may have difficulty tapering in the presence of the peaks and troughs seen with short-acting medications. The patient with an addictive disorder may experience not only pain during the trough periods, but drug craving as well. In treating such a patient, transition to long-acting medications (such as methadone, levodromoran, controlled release oxycodone, or controlled release morphine) may be helpful in achieving a comfortable withdrawal. (This strategy is supported by clinical observations, but no studies are available.)

If increased discomfort occurs during the course of medication taper, the patient should be reexamined for an undetected physical origin of the pain. If none is found, the taper should be continued. Non-opioid alternatives (such as TENS, NSAIDs, or block therapy) should be provided to attenuate discomfort during withdrawal. In most cases, the increased discomfort will be transient during and immediately following discontinuation of medications if physical dependence or withdrawal were the cause. If pain persists and no physical cause can be identified, treatment should be as for chronic pain.

Third, the individual may be using the medication to obtain relief of symptoms of a disorder other than pain, such as anxiety or depression. Opioids have been observed to improve mood in some patients in pain (Haythornthwaite, Quatrano-Piacentini et al., 1998), but more specific treatments usually are indicated and may allow tapering of pain medications in patients whose pain is resolved.

If an undetected physical cause of pain, withdrawal-associated discomfort, or self-medication do not appear to contribute to the patient's need for continued opioids, it is reasonable to reevaluate the patient for addiction to the medication. In a general hospital population, the latter reason is less common than the first three possibilities; however, it is relatively more common in the population treated by addiction medicine specialists.

If addiction is suspected, the patient should be observed for behaviors suggestive of addiction, including loss of control, continued use despite harm, and preoccupation with opioid use, with the understanding that any of these may be seen in patients with significant pain that is not effectively treated. The patient's drug and alcohol history, as well as his or her family history of addiction, should be thoroughly reviewed. If the patient is in recovery, he or she should be re-engaged in the recovery system or recovery-oriented activities should be initiated. If there was an active, untreated addictive disorder at the time of onset of the acutely painful injury or illness, it is appropriate to attempt to engage the patient in addiction treatment. Consultation with an addiction treatment specialist may be helpful.

De novo onset of addiction arising from analgesic use of opioids in the acute pain setting is rare (Porter & Jick, 1980; Perry & Heindrich, 1982), but it has been clinically observed. If an addictive disorder is diagnosed, the patient's pain medication should be tapered as described above and the use of alternative methods for addressing the pain implemented, if they provide pain relief. Unless an underlying physical cause is identified, pain often resolves or improves following discontinuation of medications and treatment of addiction (Brodner & Taub, 1978; Finlayson, Maruta et al., 1986). If a taper is not possible because of craving, initiation of opioid agonist therapy for the underlying addiction may be appropriate. If a taper is not possible because of recrudescence of pain despite alternative therapies,

FIGURE 2. When Pain Persists Beyond Apparent Healing

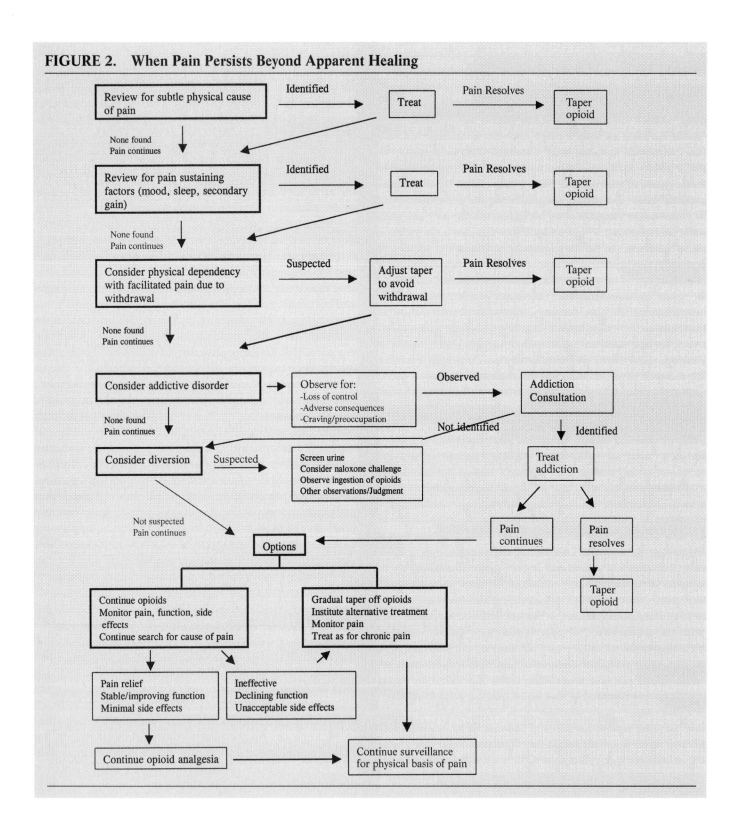

continued opioid therapy of pain, coupled with the necessary structure and support, may be selected as a component of chronic pain treatment.

Finally, the occasional patient may feign pain in order to divert medications for sale, for personal use, or to share with a family member or friend whose therapeutic needs have not been met. Generally speaking, opioids should be discontinued in patients who are known to be diverting medications, although an exception might be made if there is compelling evidence that the individual requires some opioids for pain management, was diverting medications to meet the therapeutic needs of another rather than for personal use or for profit, and it is clear that the behavior has stopped.

If the cause of reported persistent pain cannot be identified and there is no evidence that the patient is seeking drugs to sustain an addiction or for purposes of diversion, the clinician has two choices. First, opioids can be continued while the clinician monitors the patient's pain, side effects, and function, and continues to screen for a cause of pain. If the patient's quality of life is preserved or advanced without negative consequences, it may be that an undetected basis for the pain is present. The second choice is to gradually taper medications while alternative pain treatment interventions are introduced. There is some evidence that opioids may induce pain or hyperalgesia in some contexts (Mao, Mayer et al., 1995). In such cases, pain may improve on discontinuation of the medication. Which choice is appropriate for a particular patient is a decision best made by the physician, with the patient's informed participation.

APPROACH TO CHRONIC PAIN IN ADDICTION

Goals of chronic pain treatment include the reduction of pain; improvement in pain-associated symptoms such as sleep disturbance, depression, and anxiety; restoration of function; and elimination of unnecessary dependence on medications. Effective means of achieving these goals vary widely, depending on the type and causes of the patient's pain, other concurrent issues, and the preferences of the patient and caregivers. Effective pain treatment plans generally establish clear goals in terms of pain reduction and restoration of function, emphasize an active role for the patient in pain management, and incorporate a variety of complementary treatment modalities.

Approaches to the treatment of chronic pain generally fall into four categories: (1) physical modalities, (2) cognitive-behavioral interventions, (3) invasive treatments (sometimes called interventionalist procedures), and (4) medications, including non-opioid and opioid medications (Table 2). These approaches are discussed in detail in Chapters 3, 4, and 5 of this section.

Physical approaches such as stretching, exercise, applications of cold or heat, transcutaneous electrical stimulation (TENs), manual treatments, and anesthesia procedures such as nerve blocks and trigger points often are helpful in directly reducing pain and secondary physical symptoms. Cognitive-behavioral interventions such as relaxation training, introduction of pacing of activities to minimize pain, cognitive restructuring, and changes in behavioral responses to pain are used to reduce the experience of pain, relieve associated symptoms such as anxiety, and help patients cope more effectively with residual pain. More aggressive therapies, such as implanted spinal or peripheral nerve stimulators and implanted spinal infusions, are appropriate for some patients with severe intractable pain of non-cancer origin.

Because of the complex etiology of some pain syndromes, effective pain treatment often requires a multidimensional approach. As with the treatment of many chronic conditions (such as hypertension, diabetes, and asthma), optimization of pain management may require careful implementation of a number of complementary approaches involving adaptations in lifestyle and use of specific active treatments. For example, a patient with chronic headaches arising from a cervical strain injury may benefit from a combination of relaxation training and pacing of activities, myofascial stretching exercises, trigger point injections or occipital nerve blocks, and selected medications. Approaches that encourage self-efficacy and control over symptoms, such as the active physical modalities and cognitive-behavioral interventions, often form the core of chronic pain management.

Several classes of medications have analgesic actions that are mediated through different mechanisms. These include, among others, NSAIDs, tricyclics, anticonvulsants, opioids, and topical agents such as local anesthetics and capsaicin (see Chapter 4). Effective pharmacologic analgesia may require the complementary use of medications that act by different mechanisms at different points in the pain modulatory system. For example, a patient with lumbar radiculopathy related to degenerative arthritis may benefit from the use of a non-opioid analgesic such as an NSAID for the arthritis component of pain, an anticonvulsant such as gabapentin for neuropathic pain, a sedating tricyclic for sleep and analgesia and, for severe pain or for exacerba-

TABLE 2. Approach to Chronic Pain Treatment in Addiction

Identify components of pain:
- Physical: nociceptive and neuropathic;
- Facilitators: sleep disturbance, mood problems, disability, stress, drug abuse.

Establish treatment goals:
- Analgesia;
- Improvement in other symptoms;
- Restoration of function.

Address addiction:
- Detoxify or stabilize drugs:
  - ☐ Detoxify from non-opioids;
  - ☐ Withdraw opioids if tolerated in terms of pain;
  - ☐ Stabilize opioids if required by pain.
- Institute recovery program.

Address pain:
- Optimize self-management strategies for pain control;
- Use non-medication approaches, if effective;
- Use effective medications when indicated:
  - ☐ Non-opioids: NSAIDs, tricyclics, anticonvulsants, topical agents, et al.;
  - ☐ Opioids when required for analgesia:
    - Minimize reward when possible:
      - Use slow-onset or sustained-release medications;
      - Make medications time- or activity-contingent when possible;
      - Consider partial agonist or agonist-antagonist when non-opioid dependent or tolerant.

Address facilitators of pain:
- Non-medications, when effective;
- Less rewarding medications, when indicated.

Monitor progress toward goals; adapt treatment as indicated.

SOURCE: Agency for Health Care Policy Research (AHCPR) (1994). *Cancer Pain Management: Clinical Practice Guidelines.* Rockville, MD: AHCPR, U.S. Department of Health and Human Services.

tions of pain, an opioid medication. The clinician must assess the analgesic effects of each medication, as well as monitoring for the accrual of significant side effects resulting from combinations of medications.

Given the potentially mutually reinforcing nature of addiction and pain, addictive disease should be identified and addressed early in the treatment of chronic pain. Because the sequelae of addiction often include perpetuating factors for pain, such as sleep disturbance, anxiety or depression, changes in muscle and sympathetic tone, and dysfunction in customary life roles, the treatment of addiction alone sometimes leads to significant improvement in chronic pain (Finlayson, Maruta et al., 1986).

Addiction treatment generally involves detoxification from drugs of abuse and introduction of a recovery program. This eliminates potential pain-generating or reinforcing factors inherent in physical dependence. Occasionally, however, a patient's pain symptoms may make withdrawal of addicting drugs difficult early in treatment. In such cases, stabilization of the medication may be the best option, because it avoids abrupt changes in blood levels and thus may relieve pain and avoid intermittent emergence of withdrawal phenomena (Brodner & Taub, 1978). For example, a patient with alcoholism who is abusing hydrocodone prescribed for back pain, but is disabled by the back pain when the hydrocodone is tapered, may progress better in both pain treatment and addiction treatment if switched to a long-acting opioid for pain (such as sustained-release morphine, fentanyl, oxycodone, or methadone) so as to provide stable blood levels of analgesic. The patient then can be tapered gradually from the medication as alternative treatments become effective for the back pain.

In some situations, it may be appropriate to continue long-acting opioids indefinitely. If pain re-emerges on tapering, despite a well-constructed pain program, it may be appropriate to continue opioid analgesics. The use of opioids for the treatment of chronic pain is addressed in Chapter 4.

Whatever modalities are selected to manage chronic pain, it is important to establish clear goals, encourage self-efficacy, and monitor progress toward goals, while adapting the treatment regimen to achieve satisfactory pain control, improvement in function, and enhanced quality of life.

APPROACH TO CANCER PAIN IN ADDICTION

Cancer may occur somewhat more frequently in individuals with addictive disorders than in the general population (Bruera, Seifert et al., 1995), probably because of patho-

FIGURE 2.   WHO Step Ladder for Cancer Pain Treatment

WHO Step Ladder
Cancer Pain Treatment *
  * *Modified by author for
  treatment in addiction*

1 – Mild Pain

ASA
Acetaminophen
NSAIDs
Co-analgesics as needed:
- For neuropathic pain
- For other symptoms

Address addiction recovery

2 – Moderate Pain

A/Codeine*
A/Hydrocodone*
A/Oxycodone*
Tramadol
Co-analgesics as needed:
- For neuropathic pain
- For other symptoms

*Consider low dose long-acting pure
mu opioid as alternative, with added
ASA, NSAID or acetaminophen*

Address addiction recovery

3 – Severe Pain

Morphine
Hydromorphone
Methadone
Levorphanol
Fentanyl
Oxycodone
Continue:
- ASA
- Acetaminophen
- NSAID
Co-analgesics as needed:
- For neuropathic pain
- For other symptoms
Procedures as needed

Address addiction recovery

logic effects of substances of abuse, including tobacco and alcohol. Treatment of cancer-related pain in the patient with addictive disease is similar to that in the person without addictive disease. The comfort of the patient should be the primary goal. Opioids never should be withheld when they are needed for effective pain relief because of concerns regarding the development or perpetuation of addiction. If concerns arise regarding decreased quality of life due to active addiction, pain control should be continued and addiction issues addressed through appropriate interventions. Adjustment of medications may be appropriate to avoid unnecessary side effects or intoxication, but analgesia should be preserved. If the patient has difficulty controlling the use of medications, they should be dispensed in a manner that preserves safety. This may be accomplished by having the medications dispensed by a significant other, by hospice personnel, or by a pharmacy.

The "therapeutic ladder" developed by the World Health Organization (WHO) is an accepted model for the treatment of cancer pain (AHCPR, 1994; Figure 3). Stage 1 of the ladder is for the management of mild pain and involves the use of non-opioid analgesics such as acetaminophen, aspirin, or an NSAID, as well as adjuvant medications such as tricyclics, anticonvulsants, and topical agents for pain-associated symptoms such as sleep, mood problems, or side effects.

Stage 2 of the WHO ladder addresses moderate pain. It involves use of a weak opioid preparation that combines opioids with ASA, acetaminophen, or an NSAID. Adjuvant medications for neuropathic pain and other symptoms should be used as indicated. For patients with continuous moderate pain, particularly those with addictive disorders, it is reasonable to consider use of a low dose of a long-acting opioid such as methadone or controlled release oxycodone or morphine. This avoids the intermittent peak effects of short-acting opioids that may be experienced as rewarding and somewhat disconcerting to some patients in recovery. If these are selected in place of the combination medications, additional acetaminophen or NSAID usually should be added for their complementary analgesic effect.

Stage 3 of the WHO ladder, for management of severe pain, involves use of a titratable, potent opioid (such as morphine, oxycodone, fentanyl, or hydromorphone) plus non-opioid analgesics and adjuvants as indicated. It is important to note that NSAIDs are particularly effective for bone pain related to metastases, so continuation of these drugs often is important even in the presence of high-dose opioids. Treatment should start as far along the ladder as necessary to achieve pain control.

Aggressive titration of opioids is appropriate to control pain. Cancer pain usually can be managed with oral medications or with use of transdermal opioid administration. If oral or transdermal medications are not feasible because of absorption problems, vomiting, or technical problems with transdermal patches, the clinician should consider parenteral treatment, including continuous or PCA intravenous or subcutaneous administration.

When such interventions are not sufficient to control pain, or have unacceptable side effects, more invasive approaches may be considered. Regional anesthetic techniques such as continuous intraspinal infusions or plexus blocks may provide effective ongoing relief for many types of cancer pain (Cousins & Bridenbaugh, 1990). Neuroablative procedures such as celiac plexus block for pancreatic cancer pain, nerve root blocks for pain localized to one or two specific dermatomes (particularly if they serve sensory rather than motor functions, as in single-rib metastases), and others may provide definitive relief in difficult cancer pain situations. Radiation therapy and radiopharmaceuticals may be helpful in selected patients.

Cancer often is accompanied by significant distress arising from fear, grief over impending losses, depression, anger, and spiritual conflict. Because persons with addictive disorders have a tendency to use drugs to relieve such distresses, cancer patients with addictive disease may be more likely than others to use therapeutically prescribed opioids for other than pain relief. Most compassionate physicians would have no issue with the use of opioids to relieve symptoms in the setting of cancer-related pain, if they were effective. However, such use sometimes results in increased distress and greater experience of pain despite massive doses of opioids. Effective non-pharmacologic and pharmacologic means of addressing such stressors are available and should be employed to provide relief. For many individuals in recovery from addiction, the recovery system may provide meaningful support (McCaffery & Vourakis, 1992). Therefore, it is helpful for the clinician to assess the patient's experience with recovery and to help him or her in sustaining participation in or re-engaging with recovery groups, sponsors, and programs if these have been meaningful to the individual in the past.

CONCLUSIONS

Difficult pain problems in challenging patients, whether due to acute conditions, cancer, or chronic non-cancer causes, often are managed most effectively through a multidimensional approach. While multidisciplinary teams may be ideal for managing such problems, such team approaches are not always readily available. In their absence, physicians of any specialty usually can be successful in helping patients achieve effective analgesia by listening to the patient, carefully weighing the risks and benefits of various treatment approaches, monitoring outcomes, and adapting treatment strategies to respond to clinical observations and patient reports. The art of medicine should be combined with the science of medicine to give the patient the best quality of life possible, given the reality of their clinical diagnoses.

REFERENCES

Agency for Health Care Policy Research (AHCPR) (1992). *Acute Pain Management: Operative or Medical Procedures and Trauma.* Rockville, MD: AHCPR, U.S. Department of Health and Human Services.

Agency for Health Care Policy Research (AHCPR) (1994). *Cancer Pain Management: Clinical Practice Guidelines.* Rockville, MD: AHCPR, U.S. Department of Health and Human Services.

Ahles T, Blanchard E & Ruckdeschel J (1983). The multidimensional nature of cancer related pain. *Pain* 17:277–288.

American Pain Society (APS) (1989). *Principles of Analgesic Use in the Treatment of Acute Pain and Chronic Cancer Pain (2nd Edition).* Skokie, IL: American Pain Society.

Breitbart W, Passik SD, McDonald MV et al. (1996). The undertreatment of pain in ambulatory AIDS patients. *Pain* 65:239-245.

Bridges D, Rice AS et al. (2001). Mechanisms of neuropathic pain. *British Journal of Anesthesia* 87(1):12-26.

Brodner RA & Taub A (1978). Chronic pain exacerbated by long-term narcotic use in patients with non-malignant disease: Clinical syndrome and treatment. *Mt. Sinai Journal of Medicine* 45:233–237.

Bruera E, Seifert L, Fainsinger RL et al. (1995). The frequency of alcoholism among patients with pain due to terminal cancer. *Journal of Pain & Symptom Management* 10(8):599-603.

Cleeland CS, Hatfield AK et al. (1994). Pain and its treatment in outpatients with metastatic cancer. *New England Journal of Medicine* 330:592-596.

Cohen F (1980). Postsurgical pain relief: Patients' status and nurses' medication choices. *Pain* 9:265-274.

Cousins MJ & Bridenbaugh PO, eds. (1990). *Neural Blockade in Clinical Anesthesia and Pain Management (2nd Edition)*. Philadelphia, PA: J.B. Lippincott.

Finlayson RE, Maruta T, Morse BR et al. (1986). Substance dependence and chronic pain: Experience with treatment and follow-up results. *Pain* 26:175–180.

Graham AW (1991). Screening for alcoholism by life-style risk assessment in a community hospital. *Archives of Internal Medicine* 151(5):958-964.

Haythornthwaite JA, Quatrano-Piacentini AL, Pappagallo M et al. (1998). Outcome of chronic opioid therapy for non-cancer pain. *Journal of Pain & Symptom Management* 15(3):185-194.

Jackson D (1989). A study of pain management: Patient controlled analgesia versus intramuscular analgesia. *Journal of Intravenous Nursing* 12:42–51.

Mao J, Mayer DJ et al. (1995). Mechanisms of hyperalgesia and morphine tolerance: A current view of their possible interactions. *Pain* 62:259-274.

Marks J & Sacher E (1973). Undertreatment of medical inpatients with narcotic analgesics. *Annals of Internal Medicine* 78–173–181.

McAuliffe WE, Feldman B, Launer E et al. (1985). The role of euphoric effects in the opiate addictions of heroin addicts, medical patients and impaired health professionals. *Journal of Drug Issues* 15:203-224.

McCaffery M & Vourakis C (1992). Assessment and relief of pain in chemically dependent patients. *Orthopaedic Nursing* 11(2):13–27.

Mersky H (1979). Pain terms: A list with definitions and notes on usage. Recommendation of the IASP Subcommittee on Taxonomy. *Pain* 6:249–252.

Morgan J (1985). American opiophobia: Customary underutilization of opioid analgesics. *Advances in Alcohol and Substance Abuse* 5:163.

Perry S & Heindrich G (1982). Management of pain during debridement: A survey of U.S. burn units. *Pain* 13:12–14.

Porter J & Jick H (1980). Addiction rare in patients treated with narcotics. *New England Journal of Medicine* 302:123.

Savage SR (1993). Addiction in the treatment of pain: Significance, recognition and treatment. *Journal of Pain & Symptom Management* 8(5):265–278.

Shine D & Demas P (1984). Knowledge of medical students, residents and attending physicians about opiate abuse. *Journal of Medical Education* 59:501–507.

Wattwil M (1989). Post-operative pain relief and intestinal motility. *Acta Chirurgica Scandinavica* 550:140–145.

Weissman DE & Haddox JD (1989). Opioid pseudoaddiction: An iatrogenic syndrome. *Pain* 36:363-366.

Wesson D, Ling W & Smith D (1993). Prescription of opioids for treatment of pain in patients with addictive disease. *Journal of Pain & Symptom Management* 8(5):289–296.

Pain in Special Populations

MELVIN I. POHL, M.D., FASAM

Pain control in patients with addictive disorders is a challenging task for clinicians. General principles for the appropriate treatment of acute and chronic pain and addiction are reviewed in the following chapters. This chapter addresses pain control in special populations of patients who have addictive disorders co-occurring with sickle cell disease, HIV infection and/or AIDS, because these conditions presents unique issues for pain management.

Sickle cell disease and HIV/AIDS often cause chronic and severe pain, requiring potent medications for treatment. A preponderance of patients with these conditions are members of ethnic/racial groups who are known to be undertreated for painful conditions (Cleeland, Gonin et al., 1997; Morrison, Wallenstein et al., 2000; Anderson, Mendoza et al., 2000) as a result of stigma related to their addictive disorder and prejudice arising from racism, homophobia, and opiophobia (Morgan, 1985).

PAIN AND ADDICTION

Pain is experienced and perceived by an individual with an addictive disorder in the same way it is experienced and perceived by non-addicted patients. Individuals with chronic painful conditions, regardless of the fact that they also suffer from addiction, must be treated promptly and effectively, according to guidelines set forth by the World Health Organization (WHO) (1996), the American Academy of Pain Medicine and the American Pain Society (1993, 1997), the Joint Commission on Accreditation of Healthcare Organizations (Phillips, 1998), and the Agency for Health Care Policy Research (1993).

Clearly, the challenges confronting clinicians who treat such patients include concerns over the possibility that a patient with an addictive disorder might exaggerate his or her symptoms in order to gain access to increased amounts of opioid medications (Portenoy, Dole et al., 1997). However, the clinician must understand that such a patient's "drug-seeking behaviors" may reflect inadequately treated, uncontrolled pain (pseudoaddiction) rather than true addiction. Genuine, untreated addiction is characterized by aberrant and potentially manipulative behaviors, which may involve selling drugs, forging prescriptions, injecting oral formulations, reporting multiple episodes of prescription "loss," repeated episodes of intoxication, and the like, all

with the goal of obtaining and using drugs for their mood-enhancing effects. In treating patients with a history of addiction, the clinician should provide explicit written rules about expected behaviors (as well as unacceptable behaviors), specifying the consequences for violations of the rules (Portenoy, Dole et al., 1997).

CLINICAL APPROACH

Treatment of pain in patients with sickle cell disease, HIV, or AIDS begins with a thorough biopsychosocial assessment that carefully elicits the patient's experience of symptoms and their relief. Assessment should be followed by administration of drugs to control the pain (following the WHO ladder [AHCPR, 1993]; see Figure 2). If the pain is moderate to severe, long-acting opioids are indicated, with the initial dose tapered to the point of stabilization.

Treatment should be individualized to reflect the patient's underlying condition(s) and the acute or chronic nature of the pain. In patients with these complicated diagnoses, use of a team approach and early involvement of pain specialists, psychiatric clinicians, and addiction medicine specialists is most apt to lead to optimal patient care.

SICKLE CELL DISEASE

Management of the addicted patient with sickle cell disease and chronic pain or multiple episodes of acute pain has not been adequately studied. Painful crises are believed to be caused by ischemic tissue injury resulting from the obstruction of blood flow produced by sickled erythrocytes. This reduction of blood flow causes regional hypoxia and acidosis, leading to increased sickling and the potential for ischemic damage to tissue. While the crises vary in frequency, intensity, and duration, they typically last four to six days and may be quite severe. Nevertheless, many sickle cell patients manage their condition and pain at home, although some do require hospitalization.

No clinical or laboratory findings reliably confirm a crisis, so the clinician must rely on the patient's history and physical examination to reach a diagnosis. A patient who presents in a sickle cell crisis often has hypoxia, infection, fever, acidosis, dehydration, menstruation, sleep apnea, or cold exposure. Anxiety, depression, and fatigue also may be present.

The cornerstone of treatment is hydration, identification and treatment of underlying events, and pain assessment, followed by appropriate and effective analgesia. Typically, sickle cell disease is marked by multiple episodes of acute pain, which tend to resolve in several days to weeks and which usually do not require chronic administration of analgesics. The most common sites of pain are the bones (as from dactylitis, or hand-foot syndrome, which is accompanied by acute, painful swelling of the hands and feet) and at multiple sites of the musculoskeletal system (with or without swelling, redness, and heat). Abdominal pain from ischemic viscera is common and may be associated with acute conditions such as appendicitis, pancreatitis, or pelvic inflammatory disease.

Sickle cell pain requires a prompt and effective response, because the physical sequelae of unrelieved pain (such as dehydration, anxiety, and depression) can worsen the crisis. When addicted patients are treated for sickle cell crises, analgesics adequate to control their pain should be administered with compassion and firmness (Benjamin, Dampier et al., 1999). Adequate pain relief requires an agent with sufficient potency that can be administered to the patient quickly and frequently (IV or IM, if vomiting occurs). The choice of medication and loading dose should be based on the patient's history and current assessment, including the drugs used, doses, and side effects in past crises.

Pain medications should be titrated to make the pain tolerable, with minimal side effects. If the patient has a history of chronic opioid use or abuse, tolerance must be taken into consideration and the dose increased accordingly. Medication should be administered on a fixed-time, around-the-clock (ATC) schedule, at dosing intervals that do not exceed the expected pharmacological effects of the medication. If fixed dosing is chosen, then rescue doses of one-quarter to one-half of the ATC dose should be available for breakthrough pain. These allow treatment of a sudden flare-up of pain and should be limited to a set number over a given period of time, after which the dose should be adjusted. Patient-controlled analgesia has been used successfully to provide pain relief while giving the patient a welcome sense of control. Intramuscular injections should be avoided because absorption may be erratic.

Patients should be taught how to manage their mild pain at home so as to avoid emergency department visits, all the while being alert to symptoms of serious problems that may require a more intensive intervention.

HIV DISEASE AND AIDS

The prevalence of pain among persons with HIV and AIDS has been estimated to be between 25% (Singer, Zorilla et al., 1993) and 75% (Portenoy, Dole et al., 1997). Most persons with AIDS who have pain describe two to three simultaneous sources of pain (Breitbart & McDonald, 1996). In one study, there was no difference in the nature or intensity of pain, or in the effectiveness of analgesics, between AIDS patients with and without a history of addiction (Portenoy, Dole et al., 1997). Despite this, persons with AIDS often are dramatically undertreated with opioid analgesics (McCormack, Li et al., 1993; Breitbart & McDonald, 1996). It appears that this undertreatment may be associated with being older, a member of a minority group, a female, or a person with a history of injection drug use (Breitbart & McDonald, 1996). It is important to recognize that persons with coexisting substance use disorders and AIDS also are quite likely to have comorbid psychiatric symptoms, as well as other physical symptoms that can contribute to an increase in pain and suffering (Breitbart & McDonald, 1996).

The causes of pain in persons with HIV or AIDS appear to be divided into those related to HIV infection and its complications, those related to medical treatments for the condition, and those arising from other conditions unrelated specifically to HIV/AIDS. HIV infection itself is responsible for neuropathy, myelopathy, Kaposi's sarcoma, secondary infections such as herpes and cytomegalovirus (which cause pain in the intestines, skin, and lungs), organomegaly, arthritis, vasculitis, and a wasting syndrome. Pain related to HIV/AIDS pharmacotherapies may be a side effect of the antiretroviral (such as zidovudine, didanosine, zalcitabine, and stavudine), antimycobacterial (INH, rifampin), antiviral (foscarnet), or antineoplastic (vincristine, vinblastine) drugs. Pain-producing medical conditions unrelated to HIV/AIDS but often seen in persons infected with HIV include diabetes and fractures.

The assessment and treatment of pain in patients who are HIV-positive or who have AIDS is not fundamentally different from the assessment and treatment of pain in patients with cancer (Breitbart & McDonald, 1996). Neuropathic pain, which is present in up to 40% of persons with HIV who report pain (Hewitt, Breitbart et al., 1994), is treated with NSAIDs and opioids, as well as with adjuvant analgesics, antidepressants, neuroleptics, anticonvulsants, and corticosteroids (Portenoy, Dole et al., 1997). Tricyclic antidepressants, especially amitriptyline in doses up to 150 mg at bedtime (Max, Culnane et al., 1987; Magni, Sorkness et al., 1987), and serotonin reuptake inhibitors such as paroxetine at 40 to 60 mg per day (Sindrup, Gram et al., 1990), also are useful in the treatment of neuropathy, as are gabapentin (a newer anticonvulsant) and carbamazepine (Seidl & Slawson, 1999; Chandler & Williams, 2000).

Because opioids are metabolized by the cytochrome P450 system, opioid-dependent patients on antiretroviral agents may have increased plasma levels. Codeine, hydrocodone, and tramadol need to be converted into active metabolites to produce analgesia; this conversion can be blocked by cytochrome P450 inhibitors, resulting in reduced pain control and adverse reactions from the build-up of unmetabolized drug (Chang & Kam, 1999). Oxycodone and morphine are metabolized by glucuronyl transferase, which can be induced by the protease inhibitor ritonavir, thus diminishing the analgesic effect of these drugs (Chuck, Rodvold et al., 1998).

CONCLUSIONS

Sickle cell disease, HIV, and AIDS, although disparate in their presentations and clinical manifestations, suggest similar clinical principles in the management of patients with addictive disorders. In each condition, pain is known to be undertreated in patients with a history of addiction. Treatment of pain in the presence of addiction further complicates an already complex treatment course, often requiring the chronic use of opioid medications. If this occurs, strict enforcement of a set of rules understood by the patient, the clinician, and the treatment team is essential to diminish the possibility of drug misuse while providing appropriate analgesia.

Following adequate assessment of the pain and its possible underlying causes, a multidisciplinary team approach to pain control is most appropriate. Ideally, such a team would include specialists in pain management, psychiatry, and addiction medicine.

REFERENCES

Agency for Health Care Policy Research (AHCPR) (1994). *Clinical Practice Guideline No. 9: Management of Cancer Pain.* Rockville, MD: AHCPR, U.S. Department of Health and Human Services.

American Pain Society (1993). *Principles of Analgesic Use in the Treatment of Acute Pain and Cancer Pain, 4th Edition.* Glenview, IL: American Pain Society.

American Academy of Pain Medicine and American Pain Society (1997). *The Use of Opioids for the Treatment of Chronic Pain (Consensus Statement).* Glenview, IL: The Societies.

Anderson KO, Mendoza TR et al.(2000). Minority cancer patients and their providers: Pain management attitudes and practice. *Cancer* 88(8):1920-1938.

Benjamin LJ, Dampier CD et al. (1999). *Guideline for the Management of Acute and Chronic Pain in Sickle Cell Disease (Clinical Practice Guideline No. 1).* Glenview, IL: American Pain Society, 37-41.

Breitbart W & McDonald M (1996). Pharmacologic pain management in HIV/AIDS. *Journal of the International Association of Physicians in AIDS Care* 7:17-26.

Chandler A & Williams JE (2000). Gabapentin, an adjuvant treatment for neuropathic pain in a cancer hospital. *Journal of Pain & Symptom Management* 20(2):82-86.

Chang GWM & Kam PCA (1999). The physiologic and pharmacological roles of cytochrome P450 enzymes. *Anaesthesia* 54:42-50.

Chuck SK, Rodvold KA et al. (1998). Pharmacokinetics of protease inhibitors and drug interactions with psychoactive drugs. In *Psychological and Public Health Implications of New HIV Therapies.* New York, NY: Plenum Publishing, 33-60.

Cleeland CS, Gonin R et al. (1997). Pain and treatment of pain in minority patients with cancer. *Annals of Internal Medicine* 127:813-816.

Friedman B, Franklin C et al. (1991). Long-term survival of patients with AIDS, *pneumocystis carinii* pneumonia, and respiratory failure. *Journal of the American Medical Association* 266:89-92.

Hewitt D, Breitbart W et al. (1994). Pain syndromes in the ambulatory AIDS patient. In *Proceedings of the 13th Annual Meeting of the American Pain Society*; Miami, FL.

Magni CJ, Sorkness CA et al. (1987). Antidepressants in the treatment of cancer pain: A survey in Italy. *Pain* 29:347-353.

Max MB, Culnane M et al. (1987). Amitriptyline relieves diabetic-neuropathy pain in patients with normal and depressed mood. *Neurology* 38:427-432.

McCormack JP, Li R et al. (1993). Inadequate treatment of pain in ambulatory HIV patients. *Clinical Journal of Pain* 9:247-283.

Morgan JP (1985). American opiophobia: Customary underutilization of opioid analgesics. *Advances in Alcohol and Substance Abuse* 5:163.

Morrison SR, Wallenstein S et al. (2000). "We don't carry that"—Failure of pharmacies in predominantly nonwhite neighborhoods to stock opioid analgesics. *New England Journal of Medicine* 342(14):1023-1026.

Phillips D (1998). JCAHO pain management standards are unveiled. *Journal of the American Medical Association* 284(4):428-429.

Portenoy RK, Dole V et al. (1997). Pain management and chemical dependency: Evolving perspectives. *Journal of the American Medical Association* 276(7):592-593.

Seidl JJ & Slawson JG (1999). Gabapentin for painful diabetic neuropathy. *Journal of Family Practice* 48(3):173-174.

Sindrup SH, Gram LF et al. (1990). The selective serotonin reuptake inhibitor paroxetine is effective in the treatment of diabetic neuropathic symptoms. *Pain* 42:135-144.

Singer EJ, Zorilla C et al. (1993). Painful syndromes reported for ambulatory HIV-infected men in a longitudinal study. *Pain* 54:15-19.

World Health Organization (1996). *Cancer Pain Relief: With a Guide to Opioid Availability, 2nd Edition.* Geneva, Switzerland: World Health Organization.

| Chapter 3 | # Psychological Approaches to the Management of Pain |

Edward C. Covington, M.D.
Margaret M. Kotz, D.O.

Psychological Components of Pain
Cognitive Factors in Pain
Behavioral Components of Pain
Psychological Approaches to the Treatment of Pain

Chronic pain always has been with us, and few who live a normal lifespan will fully escape it. Today, however, disability related to chronic pain is of epidemic proportions. Psychological, social, and cultural factors play prominent roles in the intertwined areas of pain and pain-related disability. This chapter will review some of these factors and psychological strategies for therapeutic intervention.

Back pain has been called a "20th century health care disaster." It is essentially universal, with a lifetime prevalence of 60% to 80%; probably it has always been so. What is epidemic today is back-related *disability*, which has increased exponentially since about 1980 (Waddell, 1996). This trend is especially evident in the United States, where 2% of the work force has compensable back pain at any given time and approximately 9% of men and 12% of women have neck complaints (Anderson, 1991). Ironically, this "epidemic" has developed in parallel with a huge array of new treatments, including numerous new medications, several techniques for fusion, discectomy, laminectomy, massage, acupuncture, epidural steroid injections, trigger point injections, intraspinal adhesiolysis, intradiscal electrical ther-

mocoagulation, manipulations, and psychotherapies. Because of the controversy surrounding the use of opioids in the management of chronic pain, it is especially appropriate to focus on the psychological components of pain and pain management.

The management of intractable pain can be quite challenging, especially in the presence of a comorbid addictive disorder, which tends to magnify complaints, impede diagnosis, and confound interventions. Pain promotes regression and inhibits coping. Pain can mask addiction, because it enables some persons to transition from illicit drugs to sanctioned ones. Despite these difficulties, such patients can be treated successfully and they commonly demonstrate the same gratitude for their recovery as do addicted persons in whom pain is not a factor.

This chapter addresses primarily chronic, nonmalignant pain, as its management differs from that of acute, malignant, and recurrent acute pain. Although the focus is on psychological interventions, it should be recognized that such interventions are most commonly (and most effectively) employed in combination with non-opioid analgesic and non-analgesic pharmacotherapy.

PSYCHOLOGICAL COMPONENTS OF PAIN

It has been demonstrated compellingly that the onset of pain and its transition from acute to chronic are determined at least as much by cultural and psychological factors as by medical ones.

Disease Onset. In a four-year prospective study of 3,020 aircraft workers, job dissatisfaction and poor performance appraisals strongly predicted reports of acute back pain at work (Bigos, Battie et al., 1991). Subjects who "hardly ever" enjoyed their jobs were more than twice as likely to report a back injury as those who "almost always" enjoyed their work. Another prospective study of 1,412 pain-free employees confirmed that those dissatisfied with their work were twice as likely to seek care for low back pain during a 12-month period as those who were satisfied, while those who felt underpaid were nearly four times as likely, and those in the lowest socioeconomic stratum were almost five times as likely to seek care for low back pain (Papageorgiou, Macfarlane et al., 1997). Numerous subsequent investigations have confirmed that first report of a back injury at work is independently predicted by prior low back pain, physical work stress, and psychological intolerance of the job.

Disease Progression. The progression from acute to chronic pain has been studied most thoroughly in low back pain, the leading cause of disability in industrialized nations. Overall, chronicity seems to be more dependent on demographic, psychosocial, and occupational factors than on medical pathology. In a prospective study, progression to chronicity was associated with evidence of non-organic disease, leg pain, significant self-rated disability at onset, a protracted initial episode, multiple recurrences, and a history of back pain or hospitalization (Valat, Goupille et al., 1997). Occupational factors included blue-collar jobs, labor requirements beyond the subjects' capabilities, job dissatisfaction, poor performance ratings, and being new at the job. Prior spine-related compensation, sickness payments, and litigation were associated with chronicity. Social and economic predictors included lack of schooling, language problems, low income, and unfavorable family status. In other studies, chronicity was predicted by somatization, depression, catastrophizing, stress, and compensation. Job satisfaction and orthopedic impairment appeared independently to predict outcome.

Even with such objective pathology as acute radicular pain and disc prolapse/protrusion, the only predictive somatic factor was degree of disc displacement—the less the displacement, the worse the outcome (Hasenbring, Marienfeld et al., 1994). Persistent pain was predicted by depression and four pain coping strategies: avoidance behavior, endurance strategies, nonverbal pain behavior, and search for social support. Application for retirement at six months was best predicted by depression and daily "hassles" at work.

Ironically, much disability may be attributed to the systems designed to help. Workers' compensation systems may be particularly toxic because they often involve long delays in diagnosis and treatment, during which workers must continually prove how sick they are in order to obtain the care they believe they need. Physicians and attorneys for each side may take polarized and improbable positions (Long, 1995). The result is that patients who apply for and receive workers' compensation benefits seem to fare worse with virtually all interventions than those not so encumbered.

Litigation is thought to prolong disability, although the issue is controversial. Disability associated with "whiplash" injuries appears much less common in countries with a less developed tort system than the U.S., where that complaint accounts for two-thirds of all bodily injury claims (Schrader, Obelieniene et al., 1996). It may be significant that the rate of compensated whiplash in Saskatchewan, Canada, which had a tort system, was 10 times that of Quebec, Canada, which had a no-fault system (Spitzer, Skovron et al., 1995), and that changing the tort system led to apparent reductions in pathology (Cassidy, Carroll et al., 2000). In a study of more than 2,000 low back pain patients, all those who were working at intake returned to work after treatment, except for those in litigation, of whom not one returned to work (Long, 1995). Vocational failure occurred despite success on other outcome variables.

The idea that litigation causes chronicity is challenged by several authors. Lord and McDonald (1997) have strongly criticized the conclusion that litigation explains the frequency of whiplash. Others do not find that litigation alters outcome (Blake & Garrett, 1997; Abbott, Rounsefell et al., 1990). Some believe that the psychological issues seen in litigating patients reflect not the incentives of litigation, but its attendant stresses (Swartzman, Teasell et al., 1996; Barnsley, Lord et al., 1994).

The Psychology of Pain. It is common, when considering psychology in chronic pain, to equate it with psychopathology. This overlooks the fact that in many patients, the effects of chronic pain are mitigated by good coping and psychological strengths. Individuals such as

---

President John F. Kennedy, who had severe spine pathology, lead productive and enjoyable lives despite intractable pain. Thus, psychological approaches to chronic pain may be indicated not only to identify and treat psychological conditions that exacerbate pain, but also to optimize growth and coping when psychopathology is not apparent.

Chronic Pain Syndrome (CPS). It is important to distinguish chronic non-malignant pain (CNMP) from chronic pain *syndrome*. As used here, CNMP refers to pain that is (1) persistent and (2) not associated with progressive tissue destruction. Although not official nomenclature, the term CPS describes marked impairment from chronic pain, with a substantial psychological overlay. The U.S. Commission on the Evaluation of Pain (1987) defined CPS as intractable pain of six months' or more duration, accompanied by:

- Marked alteration of behavior, with depression or anxiety;

- Marked restriction in daily activities;

- Excessive use of medication and frequent use of medical services;

- No clear relationship to organic disorder; and

- History of multiple, nonproductive tests, treatments, and surgeries.

Thus, CPS is predominantly a behavioral syndrome that affects a minority of patients with chronic pain. The term is useful because it properly directs therapy toward the reversal of regression and away from an exclusive focus on nociception. It does not, however, substitute for a careful diagnosis of the physiological, psychological, and conditioning components that comprise the syndrome.

In a study of more than 4,000 patients with low back pain and sciatica, only 5% showed psychopathology (Long, 1995). Yet, in more than 2,000 patients with chronic pain syndrome, the incidence of antecedent psychiatric disease and personality dysfunction was 75%. Those with little psychopathology showed more physical impairment, yet vocational and personal disability was rare. By contrast, those with psychiatric dysfunction had less objective physical impairment (and in fact were indistinguishable from the normal population), yet they were disabled, personally and vocationally. The author concluded that the primary determinant of vocational disability was the psychiatric status of the patient prior to symptom onset.

It is reasonable to posit a stress-diathesis model in which the degree of disability from a given level of organic pathology varies with the psychological strengths of the individual, the stresses of the workplace, and the incentives and disincentives for recovery. Clearly, these variables overlap: the person with poor coping skills and limited education is unlikely to obtain the most desirable work situation.

Although such patients are infamous for being difficult to treat, most are genuinely suffering and deserve our best efforts at relief. Nevertheless, since the syndrome is one in which behavioral and affective changes may be as important as nociception, treatments directed exclusively at nociception may miss the point and be more harmful than therapeutic.

Much of the controversy regarding chronic opioid analgesia may be an argument between those who have found opioids useful in treating chronic pain and those who have found them harmful in CPS. Just as it has become clear that tolerance and withdrawal are not synonymous with addiction, so too is chronic pain not synonymous with chronic pain syndrome. Pain patients who have an active addictive disorder are likely to have chronic pain syndrome as well, since they are prone to inordinate disability, symptom exaggeration, and excessive health care utilization.

COGNITIVE FACTORS IN PAIN

The role of cognition in psychiatric conditions has been increasingly recognized over the past 15 years (Turk, Meichenbaum et al., 1983; Turk & Rudy, 1986). The underlying premise of most cognitive theories, whether related to depression, anxiety, or pain, is that individuals react less to events than to their understanding of them. The terminal cancer patient who is convinced that "the surgeon got it all" will be more content than the healthy hypochondriac who is certain of some occult pathology. Beliefs such as "I will resume living after I am well," "I can't go out if I am in pain," "I shouldn't exercise if it hurts," and similar ideas have obvious effects on adaptation. Maladaptive cognitions have the quality of being automatic and habitual, so that they rarely are examined for validity. They are accepted by the patient, even when it is obvious to others that they are illogical. Catastrophic thinking is a characteristic pattern of self-destructive cognition. "Catastrophizing" describes the automatic interpretation of events in catastrophic terms: if a spouse is late returning home, she or he "must have" had an accident.

The Meaning of Pain. Cognitive factors affect pain in several ways (Jensen, Turner et al., 1991b; Affleck, Urrows et al., 1992). For example, the aversive quality of pain is modified by its interpretation (Melzack, 1986; Ahles, Blanchard et al., 1983), so that it is more distressing if thought to presage disaster. Such catastrophic interpretations as, "The nerves are being crushed," or "I may become paralyzed," increase dysfunction, worsen pain, and hinder coping (Turk & Rudy, 1992; Keefe, Brown et al., 1989). Turk and Rudy (1986) reviewed cognitive issues in chronic pain and cited evidence that negative, maladaptive thoughts may reduce pain tolerance. Such thoughts include those emphasizing the aversiveness of the situation, the inadequacy of the person to bear it, or the physical harm that could occur.

Helplessness. Cognitive influences on pain include not only beliefs regarding the pain, but also those regarding the self. One's sense of personal power and competence modify coping (Ciccone & Grzesiak, 1984). Seligman's (1972) model of learned helplessness in depression suggests that those who feel unable to control events in their lives show passivity and lowered aggression. Those who perceive themselves as helpless are likely to be depressed and passive, which increases disability and pain. Conversely, belief in self-efficacy is a major determinant of successful coping (Jensen, Turner et al., 1991a). For example, belief in self-efficacy has been associated with better functioning in conditions such as fibromyalgia and rheumatoid arthritis (Lefebvre, Keefe et al., 1999; Buckelew, Huyser et al., 1996; Buckelew, Parker et al., 1994; Smarr, Parker et al., 1997).

"Locus of control" (LOC) refers to the perception that events are determined by one's own behavior ("internal control"), as opposed to outside forces, such as family members and physicians ("powerful others"), or chance. In several studies, those with an internal LOC felt and functioned better (Harkapaa, Jarvikoski et al., 1991), while those with a "chance/external" LOC reported depression and anxiety, felt helpless to deal with their pain, and relied on maladaptive coping strategies (Crisson & Keefe, 1988).

Blame. Blame attribution is an important modifying factor in recovery from injury. Chronic pain patients who blame others for their pain report greater mood distress and behavioral disturbance, poorer response to past treatments, and lower expectation of future benefits.

BEHAVIORAL COMPONENTS OF PAIN

"Operant conditioning" refers to a process by which behaviors that are reinforced increase in frequency. Elimination of reinforcement is followed by "extinction" of the behavior. Through this process, illness behaviors may become less contingent on sensations than on rewards and increase without a direct relation to nociception. At first glance, the life of a typical pain patient seems to provide remarkably few reinforcers. Poverty, depression, and loss of friendships and recreational activities are common. Nevertheless, much of the behavior of the pain patient, like that of the alcoholic, is maintained by initial consequences that are perceived as rewarding. Rest and inactivity initially provide relief; only later does debilitation increase pain. The idea that behaviors such as somatically focused conversation, limping, rubbing body parts, and remaining bedbound could be maintained by external reinforcers led to efforts to reduce those behaviors by eliminating reinforcers and by reinforcing incompatible behaviors, such as speed-walking. Results were startling, as individuals who had been disabled for years began to exercise, relinquish assistive devices, and engage in conversations about non-pain-related topics. Within a few years, there were hundreds of pain management programs modeled on this program (Fordyce, Fowler et al., 1973; Fordyce, 1976). The rapid response of severely dysfunctional individuals to the environmental contingencies in the programs lent support to the belief that much pain behavior and dysfunction are maintained by environmental rewards.

Key points regarding operant conditioning include the observations that (1) it often occurs without the knowledge of the trainer or trainee; (2) in most cases, repetition over time is required for the effect to occur, which probably explains why these concepts are more important in chronic conditions than acute ones; and (3) the timing of reinforcement is critical. An immediate small reinforcer may be considerably more powerful than a delayed large one, which is reflected in the human propensity to engage in behavior that produces immediate small rewards despite substantial delayed consequences.

Moreover, positive reinforcers (caretaking, drugs, money) may be less important than avoidance of noxious or hazardous situations. It may be useful to view disability as a form of pain behavior, since it is strongly influenced by incentives and disincentives for vocational recovery. While disability income often is meager, it does not depend on skill, ability to keep up with co-workers, or the viability of one's industry in precarious economic times. The economic climate may be such that access to health insurance is contingent on remaining disabled. On the other hand, when the incentives for wellness are sufficiently powerful, function may be well preserved despite serious illness.

There is persuasive evidence (Fishbain, Rosomoff et al., 1995) that secondary gain influences pain behavior and that pain perception can be manipulated by reinforcements. In a study comparing 3,802 pain patients and 3,849 controls, Rohling and colleagues (1995) found compelling evidence that financial compensation was associated with greater pain and reduced efficacy of treatment, whether medical or surgical. Less commonly, gain issues may modify the family's behavior, a phenomenon referred to as "tertiary gain." For example, a wife whose husband is an unskilled worker in a floundering industry may sense that the family is secure only so long as he remains disabled. She therefore may defend his disability and support his helplessness.

Focus on the gain that results from the sick role should not diminish attention to the losses: camaraderie of co-workers, pride in being the breadwinner, identity, and the self-esteem that comes from being a contributor rather than a burden to society and to one's family. While disability income may provide security, it usually does so at the poverty level.

Fear and Deconditioning. The profound impairment that results from prolonged inactivity often is attributable to fear of injury. A vicious cycle begins, in which inordinate fear leads to inactivity, which in turn leads to deconditioning and a state of increased fragility, as loss of strength and range of motion increase susceptibility to strains and sprains (Vlaeyen & Linton, 2000). The fear of injury is compounded by the individual's belief that he is ill and, in some fashion, fragile (Kori, Miller et al., 1990). Pain-related fear and anxiety predict functional impairment better than does pain severity alone (McCracken, Spertus et al., 1999; Crombex, Vlaeyen et al., 1999).

Distraction. All perceptions, including pain, are more noticeable when attended to and less so when one is distracted. The life changes that pain patients make in order to feel better commonly reduce competing stimulation so that the pain becomes all-consuming. In one study, the cold-pressor test evoked less reported pain and led to reduced activity in the somatosensory association areas and periaqueductal gray/midbrain (as reflected in the PET scan) when subjects performed a maze task (Petrovic, Petersson et al., 2000).

Affective Distress. Chronic pain often is associated with emotional symptoms, at times severe, which do not necessarily meet criteria for a formal psychiatric diagnosis, but which substantially contribute to the patients' overall suffering and thus require treatment.

Depressed mood is extremely common among those with chronic pain and probably reflects a multitude of factors, including pain, loss of gratifying activities, loss of self-esteem/identity, powerlessness, and drug-induced affective changes.

Anxiety is common in chronic pain (Poulsen, Hansen et al., 1987; Fishbain, Goldberg et al., 1986, 1988) and can both amplify physical symptoms and provide disincentives for recovery; for example, illness may permit escape from feared situations. The cycle of pain-tension-pain reflects the tendency to "brace" to protect an injured part, which can increase musculoskeletal pain. Chronic tension can lead to gastric hypersecretion and other physiological responses that worsen pain. High-anxiety rats have a lowered threshold for pain from innocuous colon distension, suggesting that visceral pains can be modulated by anxiety (Gunter, Shepard et al., 2000).

Anger, a major cause of suffering in pain patients, has been somewhat neglected in comparison with other mood states. It seems to increase pain-related suffering and interferes with life activities, while it reduces response to treatment (Fernandez & Turk, 1995; Kerns, Rosenberg et al., 1994).

Axis I: The most frequent psychiatric illnesses in pain patients probably are anxiety disorders, depression, and substance abuse (Fishbain, Goldberg et al., 1988; Katon, Egan et al., 1985). Polatin and colleagues (1993) used a structured psychiatric interview with 200 chronic low back pain patients entering a functional restoration program and found that 77% met lifetime criteria and 59% demonstrated current symptoms of at least one psychiatric diagnosis (excluding somatoform pain disorder). The most common diagnoses were major depression, substance abuse, and anxiety disorders. Fifty-one percent met the criteria for a personality disorder. Of the patients who had a positive lifetime history of psychiatric syndromes, 54% of those with depression, 94% of those with substance abuse, and 95% of those with anxiety disorders had experienced those syndromes before the onset of their back pain. Substance abuse and anxiety disorders appeared to precede the chronic low back pain, while major depression either preceded or followed it.

Depression. Kramlinger and colleagues (1983) cited estimates of the prevalence of depression in chronic pain patients ranging from 10% to 83%. Much of this variance reflects differences in settings, from inpatient to outpatient and from orthopedic to psychiatric. A confounding factor is that signs of depression overlap such illness-related effects as insomnia from pain and drugs, loss of energy from deconditioning, and self-reproach from having become a burden (Turk & Rudy, 1986).

Although pain patients can develop classical affective disorders, and recurrent unipolar depression occasionally presents as obscure pain, the preponderance of depression in chronic pain syndrome is of a different sort (Lefebvre, 1981). While pain patients attribute their depression to the fact that they hurt, studies suggest that it is the pain's interference with life activities and its ability to engender a sense of helplessness that actually leads to depression (Rudy, Kerns et al., 1988). Mood often normalizes in those who acquire a sense of personal empowerment and who resume life involvements.

There seems to be a vicious cycle in which pain behavior, isolation, inactivity, helplessness, depression, loss of reinforcers and distractions, and pain are mutually reinforcing. Improving one element in this series often benefits the others. Maruta and colleagues (1989) found that depression in CPS is highly responsive to non-pharmacologic interventions provided on a chronic pain rehabilitation unit, with 98% resolved by discharge, and that recovery persisted at 1-year followup.

Anxiety Disorders. Although anxiety is painless, panic attacks often present with chest or abdominal pain. Such findings as moist palms, tremor, tight facial muscles, and rapid pulse help to confirm the role of autonomic arousal. Because so much chronic pain originates in trauma, post-traumatic stress disorder is seen frequently in pain patients. The fact that severe trauma promotes somatization is an additional explanation.

Somatoform Disorders and Psychogenic Pain. Psychogenic pain is a concept whose existence is disputed. The term is widely criticized, in part because pain is defined as an experience—which is a psychological event—and in part because a large number of pains thought to be "non-physiologic" subsequently have been explained physiologically. Even granting the validity of the concept, the diagnosis is fraught with difficulty. Nevertheless, pains of various sorts are prominent in somatization disorder, in which there is neither evidence of physical disease nor sensitization of pain pathways.

The terminology has changed multiple times; the current term for what was called psychogenic pain is "pain disorder associated with psychological factors" (APA, 1994). The official criteria require that the pain cause "significant distress or impairment in functioning, that psychological factors be judged to have an important role in the onset, severity, exacerbation, or maintenance of the pain, and that the symptom or deficit not be intentionally produced or feigned." However, the method of determining that psychological factors are causative is unspecified.

Psychogenic pain is analogous to conversion disorders, such as blindness and paralysis, and is similarly typified by non-physiologic findings on examination and behavioral inconsistencies. It may be that the term is used for several unrelated conditions, given that some individuals diagnosed with psychogenic pain appear euthymic and animated, and sleep well, while others appear to suffer severely, cannot sleep, and even commit suicide.

Patients with psychogenic pain may be dramatic, extreme in their denial of nonmedical problems, and cheerful despite a distressing degree of disability. They frequently demonstrate behaviors that are incompatible with the degree of impairment they claim. A major determinant of inordinate pain behavior is the ability of sickness to protect one from criticism: for example, a person in pain cannot be blamed for lack of success, avoiding work, or failing to parent.

In the authors' experience, one of the most reliable indicators of somatization is a patient's inability to discuss non-somatic issues. If questioned about family, work, or politics, the patient's response rapidly diverges to symptoms, doctors, tests, and treatments. Such behavior is not usually seen even in severe physical illness.

Addiction. The prevalence of addictive disorder in CNMP pain is difficult to determine. Savage (1996) reviewed studies suggesting a prevalence of 3.2% to 18.9%. Thus, some find a prevalence substantially lower than the population baseline. Such low figures strain credulity for several reasons. Many common causes of CNMP are associated with substance use; for example, the most frequent cause of disability is low back pain, which is associated with nicotine and alcohol dependence (Deyo & Bass, 1989; Kelsey, Golden et al., 1990; Atkinson, Slater et al., 1991).

Nicotine may worsen fibromyalgia. Chronic pain often follows industrial or vehicular injuries, which are more common in those who are chemically dependent. Patients with chronic pain syndrome may be genetically at risk for addictive disorders (Chaturvedi, 1987; Katon, Egan et al., 1985). Thus, the prevalence should be rather high and studies showing low prevalence are subject to question.

A careful study of 414 chronic pain patients in a Swedish rehabilitation hospital found active alcohol or drug misuse or dependence in 23.4%, while an additional 9.4% met criteria for remission (Hoffmann, Olofsson et al., 1995). This figure, which suggests that one in four chronic pain patients has a current substance use disorder and one in three has a lifetime history of such a disorder, is more congruent with the authors' experience, and suggests that every chronic pain evaluation should include a screen for substance use disorder.

Pain patients often conceal prior substance abuse by substituting prescribed medications. This contrasts with those whose drug of choice is an analgesic, is contained in analgesic preparations (such as barbiturates), is taken as a "muscle relaxant" (such as diazepam), or whose addictive potential may be unknown to the patient or prescriber (such as carisoprodol). While the cornerstones of diagnosis (preoccupation, loss of control, and use despite adverse consequences) remain the same, their presence becomes harder to detect.

Diagnosis is hindered by the lack of consensus as to what constitutes appropriate use of opioids and sedatives. It is now accepted practice to prescribe doses of opioids that are hundreds of times what would have been considered generous a decade ago, if there is clear benefit; however, clinicians disagree as to how best to determine benefit. If a patient with mechanical low back pain reports benefit from chronic opioid therapy (COT), yet does little but watch TV, experts probably would differ as to whether continued treatment is warranted and whether his vegetative lifestyle constitutes an adverse consequence of opioid use. But what of the patient who reports persistent pain, yet resumes work, socialization, and sexual function? Who should decide which outcome is desirable? Is it possible for an untreated addict to establish treatment priorities between his pain and his addiction? These are difficult questions, whose answers color judgments as to the diagnostic criterion of "use despite adverse consequences." A definitive answer may elude us, as personal values inescapably affect scientific positions on the subject.

The pain patient who uses analgesics in a non-addictive fashion is likely to function better, while addictive use is apt to impair function. Perhaps this is because the dose required for psychoactive effects is sufficient to produce intoxication, while the analgesic dose usually is not.

A key indicator of addictive disorder is the continued use of a substance after it has proved harmful. The addicted pain patient, however, has the illusion of drug benefit, since she or he feels better after ingesting it: "It takes the edge off." This illusion of benefit is more than denial and euphoric recall. Patients may be unable to detect the cumulative deleterious effect of a medication when each dose reduces pain. It also represents the fact that peak serum levels are more comfortable than trough levels, which, in the presence of physical dependence, are associated with muscle tension, autonomic arousal, and hyperalgesia.

Prescribing physicians may be unaware of the deleterious effects of the drug, and families who witness unwanted drug effects may believe them to be unavoidable and preferable to unrelieved suffering. In the authors' experience, such patients, their families, and their physicians are surprised at the reduction in pain and suffering that occurs after gradual elimination of the drug.

Denial is especially strong in chronic pain patients, who may resist identification with chemically dependent peers. Common responses include, "I'm not like those people; I didn't use to get high; I only took what the doctors gave me." Those who use pain as a psychological defense are predisposed to find a stigmatizing diagnosis especially intolerable. A diagnosis of addictive disorder also lessens the individual's entitlements to the usual sick role perquisites, such as caretaking and disability income. It is the quintessence of adding insult to injury.

Clues to the presence of addiction in pain patients include frequent intoxication, irritability or other mood changes, inattention to hygiene, inappropriate behaviors, and impaired coordination. Another indicator is provided when, despite apparently generous analgesia, sick role behavior continues to be disproportionate to pathology. Combining other intoxicants with prescription drugs is an obvious clue. Urine toxicology studies facilitate the diagnosis of substance use disorder; however, it must be remembered that typical "dip stick" technology does not identify oxycodone or fentanyl, for example, and that GC/MS may be needed.

Loss of control may be evidenced by taking "handfuls of pills" or forgetting how much was taken. Patients may be incapable of rationing themselves and use a month's supply in a few days, even in the face of increased pain and withdrawal when their drug supply is depleted. Patients should be asked about multiple sources of drugs, forged prescriptions, whether their physicians have been concerned about their medication consumption, and whether they found it necessary to change physicians because of this.

Generally, a patient who has no history of alcohol or drug abuse, who becomes physically dependent on benzodiazepines or analgesics in the course of pain treatment, who obtains the drugs legitimately, and who has not seemed drug impaired, is not addicted; that is, the fact that chronic high-dose opioids are ineffective does not suggest the presence of an addictive disorder.

Dementia. Development of new conversion/somatoform symptoms in the elderly appears to be rare. However, the authors have observed a number of cases in which what appeared to be an unexplained pain syndrome in an elderly person led to an unexpected diagnosis of dementia. The literature is silent on this subject, although there are associations of hypochondriasis with dementia.

Malingering. Most authorities hold that willful deception is quite uncommon, although supporting data rarely are offered. Fishbain and colleagues (1999) reviewed literature suggesting that malingering is present in 1.25% to 10.4% of chronic pain patients, but concluded that methodological flaws precluded conclusions. Data from other fields provide some hints as to the prevalence of malingering. In patients with unexplained intractable diarrhea, 14% had positive stool examinations for laxatives, although all had denied their use (Bytzer, Stokholm et al., 1989). Among 333 persons who claimed compensation for noise-induced hearing loss, the incidence of exaggeration on hearing tests (as determined by cortical evoked response audiometry) was 17.7% (Rickards & De Vidi, 1995). Weintraub (1995) cites studies showing that 20% to 46% of persons surveyed said they considered purposeful misrepresentation of compensation claims to be acceptable. Such studies suggest that factitious illness and malingering may not be rare, but do not provide information as to how often such deceptions involve simulated pain. They do suggest keeping an open mind as to the possibility of these phenomena, which probably are more common in individuals seeking compensation or opioids than in those seeking other treatments or diagnoses.

Developmental Trauma. Difficult developmental years favor psychogenic exacerbation of pain and development of psychogenic somatic symptoms. Traumatic experiences may lower self-esteem and cause insecurity in competitive employment, which increases vulnerability to persistent disability. Histories of patients with CPS often include neglect, loss, abuse, molestation, and excessive early responsibility (Payne & Norfleet, 1986; Roy, 1982a, 1982b). Many are offspring of alcoholics (Chaturvedi, 1987; Katon, Egan et al., 1985). Such traumatic backgrounds lead to major difficulties with anger, dependency, helplessness, and self-esteem. Patients who lack the resources to deal with vocational or interpersonal issues adaptively may regress into the sick role as an alternative. They may be "workaholics" who find their only acceptable respite through illness. Among students, sexual abuse is associated with a variety of pains, and the severity of the abuse correlates with absenteeism (Bendixen, Muus et al., 1994). Such trauma also is associated with somatization and dissociation (Zlotnik, Zakriski et al., 1996). Over 50% of female inpatients on chronic pain units may have been sexually abused (Haber & Rood, 1985). Linton (1997) studied prior physical and sexual abuse among 949 randomly selected persons aged 35 to 45 and found that, among females, a history of physical abuse was associated with a fivefold increase in the risk of pronounced pain, while a history of sexual abuse was associated with a fourfold increase. Although frequently linked with childhood trauma, marked adult trauma of many causes—combat, natural disasters, and the like—also can lead to somatization (Lipschitz, Winegar et al., 1999; Nijenhuis, Spinhoven et al., 1998; Labbate, Cardena et al., 1998).

Diagnosing Psychogenic Components of Pain. A number of findings may support a conclusion that pain and disability are not fully explained by medical pathology.

Pain drawings are useful for quickly identifying pains with a particular pattern, such as sciatica, post-herpetic neuralgia, or central post-stroke pain. The pain drawing usually depicts pain in discrete, anatomically understandable locations, or diffusely in fibromyalgia, autoimmune disease, or endocrinopathies. Bizarre locations, multiplicity of pain locations, and pain outside the body suggest functional components (Ransford, Cairns et al., 1976).

Functional Impairment: Pain assessment always should include interference with activities such as work, household chores, social and recreational activities, and activities of daily living. It is useful to record "down time"—the hours per day spent reclining, whether a person is housebound, and whether days are spent in night clothes. The concordance between dysfunction and pathology is of major diagnostic import.

Emotional Symptoms: Patients should be asked about depression, anxiety, and irritability. Depression should be evaluated by asking about crying spells, sleep, energy, interest, libido, humor, concentration, appetite, weight, and suicidal ideation or intent. Anxiety and panic attacks should be noted. Posttraumatic stress disorder is suggested by "re-experiencing" symptoms, such as flashbacks, nightmares, and intrusive recollections, anxiety or hypervigilance with increased startle response, and efforts to avoid situations reminiscent of the original trauma.

Family Response: It is most helpful when family and friends accept the person, validate the pain, provide assistance when necessary, and encourage function. Hostility and challenges to the validity of the pain may increase distress and elicit efforts to "prove" the existence of the illness.

On the other hand, inappropriate caretaking can exacerbate regression and should be considered a form of "enabling." In such cases, it is not unusual for the spouse to answer when the patient is asked about details of the pain.

Stresses: Work, family, and entitlement agencies perhaps are the most common stressors mentioned, and the patient may have observed that these issues are related to pain severity. The person who admits to no nonmedical stresses is likely to be engaged in denial.

Litigation/Disability: The presence or absence of disability income may be less relevant than the fact of being in the process of trying to obtain it, which requires continued demonstrations of dysfunction. It is difficult to recover while trying to prove how sick one is.

Collateral Information: The collateral interview often is useful. Poor recollection, drug-induced confusion, and the tendency to portray oneself in a favorable light often combine to produce an unreliable history. Relatives and previous physicians may provide critical information regarding substance use, extent of functional impairment, depression, suicide threats, and the like. They also may reveal the converse; for example, corroboration of improved quality of life on opioids, thus confirming treatment efficacy.

Physical Examination: It is important to note whether findings are consistent internally and with the known pathology, while recognizing that our understanding of pathology is incomplete. Expectations and fear can confound observations, as patients may perform activities in non-frightening situations that they cannot perform when frightened. Nevertheless, such signs as axial rotation, in which the hips are rotated, should not affect spine pain. A person who tiptoes should not have breakaway weakness on manual testing of plantar flexion. Limping that is worse with the spouse present, or that changes sides with distraction, suggests non-organic factors.

Impairment should not exceed pathology. If the complaint is in the lower body, questionnaires should not be completed in the spouse's handwriting. A patient with hand pain should not look to the spouse for help in describing it, and should be able to make his or her own telephone calls for medications.

Waddell and colleagues described a group of non-physiologic signs in low back pain patients that are associated with elevations on MMPI scales 1 to 3 (Waddell, McCulloch et al., 1980), delayed return to work, and excessive health care utilization (Gaines & Hegmann, 1999).

Mental Status Examination: Important issues include apparent distress, appropriateness of pain behavior, somatic preoccupation, drug effects, and appropriateness of affect to the level of pain and disability. (An animated, euthymic affect is not concordant with pain severity of 10/10.) Inordinate dependence on companions should be noted. Cognitive function should be assessed for dementia or baseline cognitive limitations that create disincentives to rehabilitation.

Locus of control should reflect the patient's acceptance of responsibility for recovery. When everything seems to be contingent on actions of government agencies, the company, the doctors, the lawyer, or the spouse, psychological issues are likely to be impeding recovery.

Psychogenic pain patients may tend to focus on blame, retribution, and compensation more than on recovery; in treatment, their wellness may seem less important to such patients than to the treatment team. A history of noncompliance with reasonable medical expectations and lack of effort in treatment support this conclusion. Negative reactions to compliments may be noted; that is, the patient may be upset when a peer comments that he or she is showing improvement.

The presence of secondary gain is not a valid indicator of non-organic symptoms, as patients with clearly organic conditions are equally likely to have gain (Raskin, Talbott et al., 1966).

Testing: There are no psychological tests that can diagnose the cause of a pain disorder. The MMPI has been used for this purpose, but such use has been widely challenged (Main, Evans et al., 1991). However, it may help to predict treatment outcome (Turner, Calsyn et al., 1982). Most psychological testing in low back pain patients has been for the identification of psychiatric conditions such as anxiety disorders and depression, as well as substance use disorders. Other tests are designed to quantify pain or functional impairment, or are used primarily as outcome measures.

PSYCHOLOGICAL APPROACHES TO THE TREATMENT OF PAIN

It follows from the above discussion that psychological interventions should focus on correcting cognitions, reinforcing healthy behaviors, and reducing such psychophysiologic components as tension and anxiety. As Valat and colleagues (1997) note, treatment should be prompt and comprehensive in at-risk patients, because the likelihood of return to work decreases rapidly as the duration of sick leave increases.

It should be emphasized that non-pharmacologic treatments are not merely weak substitutes for strong drugs. It is frequently the case that patients who have not been helped by high-dose opioids, regional anesthesia, and intraspinal technology, do have marked improvement in pain and function with exercise, psychological therapies, elimination of opioids and benzodiazepines, and use of adjuvant analgesics (Turner, Calsyn et al., 1982; Flor, Fidrych et al., 1992; Turk & Okifuji, 1998).

Patients are understandably apprehensive that increased activity and reduced use of drugs will increase their suffering, and often only the example of patients farther along in the recovery process will encourage them to stay in treatment. Excessive sick role behavior can be conceptualized as similar to addictive behavior, in that patients compulsively behave in ways that produce immediate relief, but ultimately increase suffering. They expect to suffer more when they relinquish their customary adaptive strategies, yet in fact they suffer less.

Physical Therapy. Physical therapy is a critical component of psychotherapy. Physical deconditioning commonly results from fear and causes psychological changes such as perceived helplessness. A major consequence of deconditioning is that many activities become painful, reinforcing the belief that one is handicapped. Physical therapy is a form of systematic desensitization for patients who are immobilized and deconditioned because of the fear of reinjury; for them, it is a powerful antidote to "learned helplessness"

and may directly reduce symptoms such as anxiety and depression (Dimeo, Bauer et al., 2001). Although there is some evidence supporting the effectiveness of therapeutic massage, passive modalities should be used with caution because of their potential to teaching that improvement is achieved by being passive while others work. It is useful to have the family witness exercises, since they may be more willing to relinquish enabling when they no longer see their loved one as an invalid. Numerous studies confirm the critical role of exercise in chronic back and neck pain (Van Tulder, Koes et al., 1997; Ljunggren, Weber et al., 1997).

Behavior Modification. The management of chronic non-malignant pain often has as much to do with behavioral changes as perceptual ones. Pain behaviors may be separated into those that primarily affect nociception (for example, using a heating pad) and those that primarily affect others ("pain talk"). Some behaviors, such as wearing a TENS device or corset outside clothing, do both. Unwarranted pain behaviors tend to be emitted preferentially in the presence of others, and include moaning, complaining, and holding body parts.

Behavioral change is initiated by changing the environmental consequences of pain behavior. In an intensive treatment program, social reinforcers can be made contingent on healthy behaviors, while pain behaviors are ignored (Turner & Chapman, 1982b). In physical therapy, praise, rest and other "rewards" should follow goal completion, but not "trying." Families can learn that unnecessary coddling promotes invalidism. They must learn to distinguish ignoring their loved one's pain from ignoring the person, and must be encouraged to provide social reinforcers for healthy behavior. This involves a role change from that of caregiver to companion, friend, lover, or playmate.

Controlled trials of operant-behavioral therapy uniformly show improvements in psychological and physical function, and often show significant reductions in pain (Compas, Haaga et al., 1998). Operant treatment tends to produce greater immediate effects on medication intake and functional impairment.

Education. It is critical to reduce mystery and uncertainty about the cause of pain (Williams & Thorn, 1989). Waddell and colleagues (1993) found that disability due to back pain was better accounted for by fear avoidance beliefs than by the pain itself. These beliefs appear related not to disease severity but to uncertainty of diagnosis. Such an association is a special challenge in caring for patients with chronic low back pain, in about 80% of whom a precise anatomic source of the pain is not identifiable. Teaching should include the pain pathology, if known, its benign nature, and the difference between hurt and harm, so that patients are not deterred from reconditioning programs that may initially increase pain.

Education also should involve families, lest they promote unwarranted regression. This commonly results from misunderstanding the nature of the pain, which activities are harmful, and which are helpful. Common knowledge regarding appropriate management of acute illness with nurture, caretaking, and encouragement to rest does not extend to knowledge of when to stop. Families should be helped to understand that the worst treatment is rest and that activity is beneficial.

Cognitive Therapy. The most common psychotherapeutic approach for chronic low back pain is a cognitive-behavioral one, in which patients are trained to identify, challenge, and alter automatic inappropriate thinking patterns (Fernandez & Turk, 1989). Studies show improvements in activity, psychological function, pain, and medication use (Compas, Haaga et al., 1998). Meta-analysis of 25 controlled trials confirmed the efficacy of this therapy for pain, mood other than depression, social function, and pain behavior (Morley, Eccleston et al., 1999).

"Learned helplessness" and "external locus of control" can be replaced with the patient's conviction that he is the CEO of his life. Thoughts that powerful others will not help and that the person is helpless can be corrected by substituting thoughts that physicians cannot cure everything, and that the patient has a great deal of power to manage his own pain.

Stimulus Reinterpretation. The patient's response to pain can be reduced through reinterpretation of the stimulus. For example, "My back is breaking" can be replaced with, "Although it feels as though my back is breaking, it's probably another muscle spasm, and it won't last forever." Catastrophic statements can be identified and reframed. "My back is killing me; I can't stand it anymore," can be changed to, "Although the exercise is painful, ultimately it will help. I've coped with this much pain before and I can again. It always gets better eventually."

Assertiveness Training. Those who are uncomfortable directly expressing their desires and declining requests have an intrinsic incentive for remaining "sick." Pain elicits nurture and is an excuse to avoid unpleasant responsibilities or situations. A useful slogan for work in this area is, "Say what you mean, and mean what you say, but don't be mean when you say it." As patients learn to set limits on how others treat them and to communicate their need for affection, the sick role becomes unnecessary.

Biofeedback/Relaxation Training (BFT). Clinical BFT achieves symptom control by training patients to use electronic feedback to regulate such functions as skeletal muscle tension, gastrointestinal motility, and digital blood flow (NIH Technology Assessment Panel, 1996). Training in warming the extremities is helpful to patients with conditions such as Raynaud's syndrome and may reduce hypertension (Freedman, 1991). EMG biofeedback often is used to teach frontalis relaxation and has been used for the treatment of tension headache, fibromyalgia, and back pain (Blanchard & Ahles, 1990). Both EMG and thermal biofeedback have been used extensively in headache patients, and masseter feedback may be useful for temporomandibular joint syndrome.

The indications for BFT are not fully defined and continue to expand into conditions as diverse as rectal pain (Gilliland, Wexner et al., 1997; Heah, Leong et al., 1997), headache (Ham & Packard, 1996), cumulative trauma disorder (Spence, Champion et al., 1995), and vulvodynia (Glazer, Young et al., 1995).

BFT has been challenged by studies showing that benefit does not correlate with physiological changes (Rokicki, Holroyd et al., 1997). Some suggest that BFT may be no more effective in treating muscle pain and headache than approaches that do not require electronic equipment, such as autogenic training, progressive muscular relaxation, meditation, or self-hypnosis, all of which facilitate a state of reduced emotional arousal (Turner & Chapman, 1982a; Linton, 1986; Roberts, 1987). Some benefits may arise from the *belief* in having acquired self-control rather than from physiologic self-regulation *per se* (Litt, 1986; Turk & Rudy, 1992). Compas and colleagues (1998) found mixed support for biofeedback training—three studies found reductions in pain and pain-related cognitions, while two showed no significant benefit. Many studies of biofeedback have confounded conclusions by combining it with other forms of relaxation training (Blanchard, Appelbaum et al., 1987). Such studies generally show benefit from the combined approach.

There may be a synergistic effect from combining BFT with cognitive therapies, and it may be preferable to do the BFT first (Kropp, Niederberger et al., 1997; Turk, Greco et al., 1996).

Patients treated in the Chronic Pain Rehabilitation Program at Cleveland Clinic Foundation consistently rate BFT as the first or second (to physical therapy) most helpful intervention. Perhaps this is because, in addition to providing an increased sense of personal control, biofeedback helps skeptical patients understand the relationship between external and internal events. A patient who witnesses a drop in hand temperature when discussing an employer may be convinced of the importance of stress management in modifying his or her body's responses. Thus, BFT may facilitate work in other program components.

Family Therapy. The families of pain patients often find that their lives are controlled by someone else's illness. They feel bound to give, yet receive little. Self-blame and guilt coexist with intense resentment. They feel helpless and depressed, and their own lives often become unmanageable. Family discord often becomes a major source of stress for the patient with pain.

Addiction Treatment. Treating chronic pain syndrome in a patient with a comorbid substance use disorder is likely to be futile unless addiction recovery is achieved, although several factors may complicate this. Pain may impede detoxification because of the hyperalgesia of withdrawal (Kaplan & Fields, 1991; Noyes, Garvey et al., 1988). Pain patients often are unwilling to identify themselves as addicted, and there may be little "leverage" in the form of pressure from physicians, spouses, employers, or the courts to encourage them to comply with treatment.

There may be an appearance of conflict between pain rehabilitation and the principles of Twelve Step programs, yet because of the frequent co-occurrence of addictive disorders and chronic pain syndrome, many patients need both. However, patients may use the apparent conflict to justify their resistance.

The cognitive issues in chronic pain clearly demonstrate the need to empower patients and help them to "take control" of their lives. This may seem contrary to the focus of Twelve Step programs on "powerlessness" and "letting go"—a contradiction that is more apparent than real. There are many overlaps between both pathology and treatment in pain and addiction. Just as the patient with an addictive disorder has a primary relationship with a substance, the patient with CPS has a primary relationship with pain: it becomes an obsession, the organizing principle of one's life, the subject of conversations, and results in a loss of empathy and ability to relate. Both chronic pain syndrome and addiction are maladaptive cognitive and behavioral syndromes that are superimposed on an organic substrate.

It is useful to encourage patients to focus on the similarities between substance use disorder and chronic pain syndrome, rather than the differences. Neither disease is the patients' fault, but recovery is their responsibility. Although patients do not voluntarily contract either disorder, they may be blamed and stigmatized for it. Typically, both conditions can be effectively managed but not cured.

An essential characteristic of both conditions is that efforts to feel better ultimately lead to feeling worse, as patients cling tenaciously to lifestyles that cause misery. Both conditions destroy self-esteem. Enabling is a critical component of both, as the misguided efforts of others to be helpful ultimately worsen the pathology and make it more refractory to intervention. There are struggles over the issue of control: the more helpless the patient feels, the more he or she struggles to control, to dominate, or to manipulate others. Prior to treatment, both groups of patients tend to be defensive, in denial, projecting of blame and responsibility, closed-minded, angry, and "hard to love." Both groups of patients have a high incidence of depression and suicide. Both conditions are characterized by unmanageability and powerlessness.

Dealing with chronic pain syndrome requires the patient to surrender the quest for a cure and to accept the fact that at the current state of the science, no one can return him or her to a pain-free state. Chronic pain and addictive disorders are lifelong illnesses that cannot be cured, but can be managed in a way that substantially reduces suffering. In both conditions, patients are able to feel more "in control" by letting go, which is a major focus of biofeedback and relaxation training.

Projection of blame is a major issue and precludes acceptance of responsibility for working on recovery. Pain and addictive disorders can engender paralyzing self-pity, the antidote to which is gratitude.

The family's role with the patient who has comorbid CPS and addiction may pose special difficulties, as the family often consists of the people who phone for prescriptions and deliver them. Counseling may fail to convince families of the imprudence of drug use; however, having them witness the patient's improvement with abstinence often recruits them as allies in the treatment. "Before and after" videotapes often document a dramatic change in appearance, affect, and comfort following detoxification and can aid in securing the family's "buy in" to non-opioid treatments.

With addicts and CPS patients, the intervention of a recovering person has a special power that good advice from professionals "who have never been there" cannot equal. Both must learn to trust the process of recovery. With both it "is easier to act ourselves into right thinking than to think ourselves into right acting." Coping with pain "one day at a time" is an easier task to confront than the idea of accepting an eternity of incurable pain.

Chronic Pain Anonymous, a program for those with CNMP, has applied the Twelve Steps, the principles, and the promises of Alcoholics Anonymous (AA) to chronic pain.

Self-Help Groups. The American Chronic Pain Association (ACPA) is a self-help recovery program for those with chronic non-malignant pain. Its focus is on self-management. Members are encouraged to employ daily relaxation, stretching exercises, and such psychological tasks as working on goal setting, assertiveness, and avoiding pain behavior. The concept of changing "from a patient to a person" is emphasized. There are fewer than 400 chapters, so it may not be accessible to many. Materials are available to help persons with pain start new groups. ACPA does not focus on substance use, so participation in AA or Narcotics Anonymous also is essential for pain patients with co-occurring addictive disorders.

Multidisciplinary Pain Rehabilitation. Combined approaches seem more effective than unitary treatments for CNMP. Accordingly, combinations of interventions should be tailored to maximize comfort and function. Pain rehabilitation programs combine many elements and, unless they specifically exclude patients with substance use disorders, should have addiction treatment as a major program component. Such programs can dramatically improve the quality of life and functional abilities of disabled pain patients (Chapman, 2000).

Services in multidisciplinary pain rehabilitation programs typically include:

- Education
- Reconditioning physical therapy
- Medications
- Nerve blocks
- Biofeedback/relaxation training
- Operant conditioning
- Psychotherapy (personal and family)
- TENS
- Detoxification
- Addiction treatment
- Treatment of psychiatric comorbidity.

Turk (1996) reviewed outcome studies of multidisciplinary pain programs and found reports of reductions in pain of 14% to 60%, reductions in opioid use of up to 73%, and dramatic increases in levels of activity. Forty-three percent more patients were working after treatment than before. One study found a 90% reduction in physician visits. There were 50% to 65% fewer surgeries than in untreated patients and 65% fewer hospitalizations. Thirty-five percent fewer patients were on disability. Turk estimated that multidisciplinary pain management led to 27 fewer surgeries per 100 patients, for an average of $4,050 saved per patient (at $15,000 per surgery). He estimated overall medical costs at more than $13,000 per year pre-treatment and $5,600 in the year after treatment. This suggests a savings of $7,700 per year per patient following treatment. Disability savings are striking, with an estimated $400,000 saved per person removed from permanent disability (Turk, 1996).

Treating Chronic Malignant Pain. Cancer pain treatment often is thought of only in terms of pharmacological approaches; however, relaxation therapies, psychotherapy, and guided imagery can be important in malignant as well as non-malignant pain. Physical therapy directed toward maximization of strength and flexibility can reduce discomfort and improve quality of life, while providing distraction. Malignant pain, of course, often is cured and may transition into such chronic non-malignant pains as toxic neuropathy or radiation cystitis.

Treating Acute Recurrent Pain. Special difficulties arise in the treatment of patients with conditions such as inflammatory bowel disease, chronic pancreatitis, sickle cell disease, and other illnesses in which there is recurrent, severe, organic pain and a high incidence of addictive disorders. The literature concerning the long-term treatment of pain in these conditions (with the exception of sickle cell disease) is quite sparse. Clinical experience with patients who have Crohn's disease and opioid addiction suggests that the approach described above for chronic benign pain, combined with primary addiction treatment, is necessary and helpful, but the patient requires extensive longitudinal care, which may need to be intense during crises.

CONCLUSIONS

Physicians confronted with patients who are suffering from irreversible pathology may experience therapeutic nihilism and hopelessness. This must not be communicated to patients for two reasons. First, the message, "There is nothing more I can do for you," confirms hopelessness and can encourage suicide. Second, it is clear that the most grateful patients are not necessarily those whose pain has responded best to pharmacological interventions. Rather, many patients report that their pain is little changed from admission, but they laugh, walk briskly, take no addicting drugs, and report that their suffering has been largely alleviated. They are optimistic and report that "the pain is on the back burner where I don't much think about it." Thus, it is critical to communicate to patients that they can "recover" even when medical interventions have been exhausted.

The methods described in this chapter are not sufficient for all patients, even when combined with non-analgesic medications for pain reduction. Much of the challenge confronting physicians is to identify those in whom psychological and rehabilitation methods produce satisfactory results, those in whom analgesics are helpful, and those in whom they do harm.

When a patient demonstrates the characteristics of inordinate suffering, medical involvement, disability, or drug use, it is unlikely that solutions will be found external to the patient, whether through pharmacology or technology. Rather, the solution likely will come from the patient's inner resources. It is the physician's task to help that patient find, strengthen, and trust in those resources.

REFERENCES

Abbott P, Rounsefell B, Fraser R et al. (1990). Intractable neck pain. *Clinical Journal of Pain* 6:26-31.

Affleck G, Urrows S, Tennen H et al. (1992). Daily coping with pain from rheumatoid arthritis: Patterns and correlates. *Pain* 51:221-229.

Ahles TA, Blanchard EB & Ruckdeschel JC (1983). The multidimensional nature of cancer-related pain. *Pain* 17:277-288.

Anderson G (1991). The epidemiology of spinal disorders. In JW Frymoyer (ed.) *The Adult Spine: Principles and Practice*. New York, NY: Raven Press, 107-146.

Atkinson JH, Slater MA, Patterson TL et al. (1991). Prevalence, onset, and risk of psychiatric disorders in men with chronic low back pain: A controlled study. *Pain* 45:111-121.

Barnsley L, Lord S & Bogduk N (1994). Clinical review: Whiplash injury. *Pain* 58:283-307.

Bendixen M, Muus KM & Schei B (1994). The impact of child sexual abuse—A study of a random sample of Norwegian students. *Child Abuse & Neglect* 18(10):837-847.

Bigos SJ, Battie MC, Spengler DM et al. (1991). A prospective study of work perceptions and psycho-social factors affecting the report of back injury. *Spine* 16(1):1-6.

Blake C & Garrett M (1997). Impact of litigation on quality of life outcomes in patients with chronic low back pain. *Irish Journal of Medical Sciences* 166(3):124-126.

Blanchard EB & Ahles TA (1990). Biofeedback therapy. In JJ Bonica (ed.) *The Management of Pain, 2nd Edition*. Philadelphia, PA: Lea & Febiger.

Blanchard EB, Appelbaum KA, Guarnieri P et al. (1987). Five year prospective follow-up on the treatment of chronic headache with biofeedback and/or relaxation. *Headache* 27(10):580-583.

Buckelew SP, Huyser B, Hewett J et al. (1996). Self-efficacy predicting outcome among fibromyalgia subjects. *Arthritis Care and Research* 9(2):97-104.

Buckelew SP, Parker JC, Keefe FJ et al. (1994). Self-efficacy and pain behavior among subjects with fibromyalgia. *Pain* 59(3):377-384.

Bytzer P, Stokholm M, Andersen I et al. (1989). Prevalence of surreptitious laxative abuse in patients with diarrhea of uncertain origin: A cost benefit analysis of a screening procedure. *Gut* 30(10):1379-1384.

Cassidy JD, Carroll LJ, Cote P et al. (2000). Effect of eliminating compensation for pain and suffering on the outcome of insurance claims for whiplash injury. *New England Journal of Medicine* 342(16):1179-1186.

Chapman SL (2000). Chronic pain rehabilitation: Lost in a sea of drugs and procedures? *APS Bulletin* 10(3):2-5.

Chaturvedi SK (1987). Family morbidity in chronic pain patients. *Pain* 30(2):159-168.

Ciccone DS & Grzesiak RC (1984). Cognitive dimensions of chronic pain. *Social Science & Medicine* 19(12):1339-1345.

Compas BE, Haaga DA, Keefe FJ et al. (1998). Sampling of empirically supported psychological treatments from health psychology: Smoking, chronic pain, cancer, and bulimia nervosa. *Journal of Consulting and Clinical Psychology* 66(1):89-112.

Crisson JE & Keefe FJ (1988). The relationship of locus of control to pain coping strategies and psychological distress in chronic pain patients. *Pain* 35:147-154.

Crombex G, Vlaeyen JWS, Heuts PHTG et al. (1999). Pain-related fear is more disabling than pain itself: Evidence on the role of pain-related fear in chronic back pain disability. *Pain* 80:329-339.

Deyo RA & Bass JE (1989). Lifestyle and low-back pain: The influence of smoking and obesity. *Spine* 14(5):501-506.

Dimeo F, Bauer M, Varahram I et al. (2001). Benefits from aerobic exercise in patients with major depression: A pilot study. *British Journal of Sports Medicine* 35(2):114-117.

Fernandez E & Turk DC (1989). The utility of cognitive coping strategies for altering pain perception: A meta-analysis. *Pain* 38:123-135.

Fernandez E & Turk DC (1995). The scope and significance of anger in the experience of chronic pain. *Pain* 61(2):165-175.

Fishbain DA, Cutler R, Rosomoff HL et al. (1999). Chronic pain disability exaggeration/malingering and submaximal effort research. *Clinical Journal of Pain* 15(4):244-274.

Fishbain DA, Goldberg M, Labbe E et al. (1988). Compensation and noncompensation chronic pain patients compared for DSM-III operational diagnoses. *Pain* 32:197-206.

Fishbain DA, Goldberg M, Meagher BR et al. (1986). Male and female chronic pain patients categorized by DSM-III psychiatric diagnostic criteria. *Pain* 26(2):181-197.

Fishbain DA, Rosomoff HL, Cutler RB et al. (1995). Secondary gain concept: A review of the scientific evidence. *Clinical Journal of Pain* 11:6-21.

Flor H, Fidrych T & Turk DC (1992). Efficacy of multidisciplinary pain treatment centers: A meta-analytic review. *Pain* 49:221-230.

Fordyce WE (1976). *Behavioral Methods for Chronic Pain and Illness.* St. Louis, MO: C.V. Mosby.

Fordyce WE, Fowler RS, Lehman JF et al. (1973). Operant conditioning in the treatment of chronic pain. *Archives of Physical Medicine & Rehabilitation* 54(9):399-408.

Freedman RR (1991). Physiological mechanisms of temperature biofeedback. *Biofeedback and Self-Regulation* 16(2):95-115.

Gaines WG Jr & Hegmann KT (1999). Effectiveness of Waddell's nonorganic signs in predicting a delayed return to regular work in patients experiencing acute occupational low back pain. *Spine* 24(4):396-400.

Gilliland R, Wexner SD, Vickers D et al. (1997). Biofeedback for intractable rectal pain: Outcome and predictors of success. *Diseases of the Colon and Rectum* 40(2):190-196.

Glazer HI, Young AW, Hertz R et al. (1995). Treatment of vulvar vestibulitis syndrome with EMG biofeedback of pelvic floor musculature. *Journal of Reproductive Medicine* 40(4):283-290.

Gunter WD, Shepard JD, Foreman RD et al. (2000). Evidence for visceral hypersensitivity in high-anxiety rats. *Physiology & Behavior* 69(3):379-382.

Haber JD & Rood C (1985). Effects of spouse abuse and/or sexual abuse in the development and maintenance of chronic pain in women. *Advances in Pain Research and Therapy* 9:889-895.

Ham LP & Packard RC (1996). A retrospective, follow-up study of biofeedback-assisted relaxation therapy in patients with posttraumatic headache. *Biofeedback and Self-Regulation* 21(2):93-104.

Harkapaa K, Jarvikoski A, Mellin G et al. (1991). Health locus of control beliefs and psychological distress as predictors for treatment outcome in low-back pain patients: Results of a 3-month followup of a controlled intervention study. *Pain* 46:35-41.

Hasenbring M, Marienfeld G, Kuhlendahl D et al. (1994). Risk factors of chronicity in lumbar disc patients. A prospective investigation of biologic, psychologic, and social predictors of therapy outcome. *Spine* 19(24):2759-2765.

Heah SM, Leong AF, Tan M et al. (1997). Biofeedback is effective treatment for levator ani syndrome. *Diseases of the Colon and Rectum* 40(2):187-189.

Hoffmann NG, Olofsson O, Salen B et al. (1995). Prevalence of abuse and dependency in chronic pain patients. *International Journal of the Addictions* 30(8):919-927.

Jensen MP, Turner JA & Romano JM (1991a). Self-efficacy and outcome expectancies: Relationship to chronic pain coping strategies and adjustment. *Pain* 44:263-269.

Jensen MP, Turner JA, Romano JM et al. (1991b). Coping with chronic pain: A critical review of the literature. *Pain* 47: 249-283.

Kaplan H & Fields HL (1991). Hyperalgesia during acute opioid abstinence: Evidence for a nociceptive facilitating function of the rostral ventromedial medulla. *Journal of Neuroscience* 11(5):1433-1439.

Katon W, Egan K & Miller D (1985). Chronic pain: Lifetime psychiatric diagnoses and family history. *American Journal of Psychiatry* 142(10):1156-1160.

Keefe FJ, Brown GK, Wallston KA et al. (1989). Coping with rheumatoid arthritis pain: Catastrophizing as a maladaptive strategy. *Pain* 37:51-56.

Kelsey JL, Golden AL & Mundt DJ (1990). Low back pain/prolapsed lumbar intervertebral disc. *Rheumatic Disease Clinics of North America* 16(3):699-716.

Kerns RD, Rosenberg R & Jacob MC (1994). Anger expression and chronic pain. *Journal of Behavior Medicine* 17(1):57-67.

Kori SH, Miller RP & Todd DD (1990). Kinisophobia: A new view of chronic pain behavior. *Pain Management* 3(1):35-43.

Kramlinger KG, Swanson DW & Maruta T (1983). Are patients with chronic pain depressed? *American Journal of Psychiatry* 140(6):747-749.

Kropp P, Niederberger U, Kopal T et al. (1997). Behavioral treatment in migraine. Cognitive-behavioral therapy and blood-volume-pulse biofeedback: A cross-over study with a two-year follow-up. *Functional Neurology* 12(1):17-24.

Labbate LA, Cardena E, Dimitreva J et al. (1998). Psychiatric syndromes in Persian Gulf War veterans: An association of handling dead bodies with somatoform disorders. *Psychotherapy and Psychosomatics* 67(4-5):275-279.

Lefebvre JC, Keefe FJ, Affleck G et al. (1999). The relationship of arthritis self-efficacy to daily pain, daily mood, and daily pain coping in rheumatoid arthritis patients. *Pain* 80:425-435.

Lefebvre M (1981). Cognitive distortion and cognitive errors in depressed psychiatric and low back pain patients. *Journal of Consulting and Clinical Psychology* 49:517-525.

Linton SJ (1986). Behavioral remediation of chronic pain: A status report. *Pain* 24:125-141.

Linton SJ (1997). A population-based study of the relationship between sexual abuse and back pain: Establishing a link. *Pain* 73(1):47-53.

Lipschitz DS, Winegar RK, Hartnick E et al. (1999). Posttraumatic stress disorder in hospitalized adolescents: Psychiatric comorbidity and clinical correlates. *Journal of the American Academy of Child and Adolescent Psychiatry* 38(4):385-392.

Litt MD (1986). Mediating factors in nonmedical treatment for migraine headache: Toward an interactional model. *Journal of Psychosomatic Research* 30(4):505-519.

Ljunggren AE, Weber H, Kogstad O et al. (1997). Effect of exercise on sick leave due to low back pain. A randomized, comparative, long-term study. *Spine* 22(14):1610-1616.

Long DM (1995). Effectiveness of therapies currently employed for persistent low back and leg pain. *Pain Forum* 4(2):122-125.

Lord SM & McDonald GJ (1997). Comment. *Pain Medicine Journal* 3(1):40-43.

Main CJ, Evans PJD & Whitehead RC (1991). An investigation of personality structure and other psychological features in patients presenting with low back pain: A critique of the MMPI. In MR Bond, JE Charlton & CJ Woolf (eds.) *Proceedings of the 6th World Congress on Pain.* Elsevier Science Publishers, 207-217.

Maruta T, Vatterott MK & McHardy MJ (1989). Pain management as an antidepressant: Long-term resolution of pain-associated depression. *Pain* 36(3):335-337.

McCracken LM, Spertus IL, Janeck AS et al. (1999). Behavioral dimensions of adjustment in persons with chronic pain: Pain-related anxiety and acceptance. *Pain* 80:283-289.

Melzack R (1986). Neurophysiology of pain. In RA Sternbach (ed.) *The Psychology of Pain, 2nd Edition*. New York, NY: Raven Press.

Morley S, Eccleston C & Williams A (1999). Systematic review and meta-analysis of randomized controlled trials of cognitive behavior therapy and behavior therapy for chronic pain in adults, excluding headache. *Pain* 80:1-13.

National Institutes of Health (NIH), Technology Assessment Panel on Integration of Behavioral and Relaxation Approaches into the Treatment of Chronic Pain and Insomnia (1996). Integration of behavioral and relaxation approaches into the treatment of chronic pain and insomnia. *Journal of the American Medical Association* 276(4):313-338.

Nijenhuis ER, Spinhoven P, van Dyck R et al. (1998). Degree of somatoform and psychological dissociation in dissociative disorder is correlated with reported trauma. *Journal of Traumatic Stress* 11(4):711-730.

Noyes R Jr, Garvey MJ, Cook B et al. (1988). Benzodiazepine withdrawal: A review of the evidence. *Journal of Clinical Psychiatry* 49(10):382-389.

Osterweis M, Kleinman A & Mechanic E (1987). *Pain and Disability: Clinical, Behavioral, and Public Policy Perspectives*. Washington, DC: National Academy Press.

Papageorgiou AC, Macfarlane GJ, Thomas E et al. (1997). Psychosocial factors in the workplace—Do they predict new episodes of low back pain? Evidence from the South Manchester Back Pain Study. *Spine* 22(10):1137-1142.

Payne B & Norfleet MA (1986). Chronic pain and the family: A review. *Pain* 26:1-22.

Petrovic P, Petersson KM, Ghatan PH et al. (2000). Pain-related cerebral activation is altered by a distracting cognitive task. *Pain* 85:19-30.

Polatin PB, Kinney RK, Gatchel RJ et al. (1993). Psychiatric illness and chronic low-back pain. The mind and the spine—Which goes first? *Spine* 18(1):66-71.

Poulsen DL, Hansen HJ, Langemark M et al. (1987). Discomfort or disability in patients with chronic pain syndrome. *Psychotherapy and Psychosomatics* 48(1-4):60-62.

Ransford AO, Cairns D & Mooney V (1976). The pain drawing as an aid to the psychologic evaluation of patients with low-back pain. *Spine* 1(2):127-134.

Raskin M, Talbott JA & Meyerson AT (1966). Diagnosis of conversion reactions. *Journal of the American Medical Association* 197:102-106.

Rickards FW & De Vidi S (1995). Exaggerated hearing loss in noise induced hearing loss compensation claims in Victoria. *Medical Journal of Australia* 163(7):360-363.

Roberts AH (1987). Literature update: Biofeedback and chronic pain. *Journal of Pain and Symptom Management* 2(3):169-171.

Rohling ML, Binder LM & Langhinrichsen-Rohling J (1995). Money matters: A meta-analytic review of the association between financial compensation and the experience and treatment of chronic pain. *Health Psychology* 14(6):537-547.

Rokicki LA, Holroyd KA, France CR et al. (1997). Change mechanisms associated with combined relaxation/EMG biofeedback training for chronic tension headache. *Applied Psychophysiology and Biofeedback* 22(1):21-41.

Roy R (1982a). Marital and family issues in patients with chronic pain: A review. *Psychotherapy and Psychosomatics* 37:112.

Roy R (1982b). Pain-prone patient: A revisit. *Psychotherapy and Psychosomatics* 37:202-213.

Rudy T, Kerns RD & Turk DC (1988). Chronic pain and depression: Toward a cognitive-behavioral mediation model. *Pain* 35:129-140.

Savage S (1996). Long-term opioid therapy: Assessment of consequences and risks. *Journal of Pain and Symptom Management* 11:274-286.

Schrader H, Obelieniene D, Bovim G et al. (1996). Natural evolution of late whiplash syndrome outside the medicolegal context. *Lancet* 347:1207-1211.

Seligman ME (1972). Learned helplessness. *Annual Review of Medicine* 23:407-412.

Smarr KL, Parker JC, Wright GE et al. (1997). The importance of enhancing self-efficacy in rheumatoid arthritis. *Arthritis Care and Research* 10(1):18-26.

Spence SH, Champion D, Newton-John T et al. (1995). Effect of EMG biofeedback compared to applied relaxation training with chronic, upper extremity cumulative trauma disorders. *Pain* 63(2):199-206.

Spitzer WO, Skovron ML, Salmi LR et al. (1995). Scientific Monograph of the Quebec Task Force on Whiplash-Associated Disorders: Redefining "whiplash" and its management. *Spine* 20(85):3S-73S.

Swartzman LC, Teasell RW, Shapiro AP et al. (1996). The effect of litigation status on adjustment to whiplash injury. *Spine* 21:53-53S.

Turk DC (1996). Efficacy of multidisciplinary pain centers in the treatment of chronic pain. In MJM Cohen & NJ Campbell (eds.) *Pain Treatment Centers at a Crossroads: A Practical and Conceptual Reappraisal, Progress in Pain Research and Management, Vol. 7*. Seattle, WA: IASP Press, 257-273.

Turk DC & Okifuji A (1998). Efficacy of multidisciplinary pain centers: An antidote to anecdotes. *Bailliere's Clinical Anaesthesiology* 12:103-119.

Turk DC & Rudy TE (1992). Cognitive factors and persistent pain: A glimpse into Pandora's box. *Cognitive Therapy and Research* 16(2):99-122.

Turk DC & Rudy TE (1986). Assessment of cognitive factors in chronic pain: A worthwhile enterprise? *Journal of Consulting and Clinical Psychology* 54(6):760-768.

Turk DC, Greco CM, Zaki HS et al. (1996). Dysfunctional patients with temporomandibular disorders: Evaluating the efficacy of a tailored treatment protocol. *Journal of Consulting and Clinical Psychology* 64(1):139-146.

Turk DC, Meichenbaum D & Genest M (1983). *Pain and Behavioral Medicine: A Cognitive-Behavioral Perspective*. New York, NY: Guilford Press.

Turner JA & Chapman CR (1982a). Psychological interventions for chronic pain: A critical review. I. Relaxation training and biofeedback. *Pain* 12:1-21.

Turner JA & Chapman CR (1982b). Psychological interventions for chronic pain: A critical review. II. Operant conditioning, hypnosis and cognitive-behavioral therapy. *Pain* 12:23-46.

Turner JA, Calsyn DA, Fordyce WE et al. (1982). Drug utilization patterns in chronic pain patients. *Pain* 12:357-363.

U.S. Commission on the Evaluation of Pain (1987). *Report of the Commission on the Evaluation of Pain, Appendix C: Summary of the National Study of Chronic Pain Syndrome.* Washington, DC: Social Security Administration, Office of Disability.

Valat JP, Goupille P & Vedere V (1997). Low back pain: Risk factors for chronicity. *Review of Rheumatology (English Edition)* 64(3):189-194.

Van Tulder MW, Koes BW & Bouter LM (1997). Conservative treatment of acute and chronic nonspecific low back pain. A systematic review of randomized controlled trials of the most common interventions. *Spine* 22(18):2128-2156.

Vlaeyen JWS & Linton SJ (2000). Fear-avoidance and its consequences in chronic musculoskeletal pain: a state of the art. *Pain* 85: 317-332.

Waddell G (1996). Low back pain: A twentieth century health care enigma. *Spine* 21:2820-2825.

Waddell G, McCulloch J, Kummel E et al. (1980). Non-organic physical signs in low-back pain. *Spine* 5:117-125.

Waddell G, Newton M, Henderson I et al. (1993). A fear avoidance beliefs questionnaire (FABQ) and the role of fear avoidance beliefs in chronic low back pain and disability. *Pain* 52:157-168.

Weintraub MI (1995). Chronic pain in litigation: What is the relationship? *Neurologic Clinics* 13(2):341-349.

Williams DA & Thorn BE (1989). An empirical assessment of pain beliefs. *Pain* 36:351-358.

Zlotnick C, Zakriski AL, Shea MT et al. (1996). The long-term sequelae of sexual abuse: Support for a complex posttraumatic stress disorder. *Journal of Traumatic Stress* 9(2):195-205.

Non-Opioid Medications in the Management of Pain

Chapter 4

James A.D. Otis, M.D.

Non-Opioid Pharmacologic Agents
Interventional Procedures
Physical Medicine and Rehabilitative Therapies

Medications can provide effective pain management in most patients. Choosing the appropriate medication requires that the pain state being treated is correctly diagnosed and classified as somatic, visceral, or neuropathic.

NSAIDs and opioids are the principal medications for somatic pain, while adjuvant medications such as antidepressants, AEDs, anesthetics, and adrenergic agents are useful for neuropathic pain. Severe pain, whether somatic or neuropathic, usually requires opioid therapy. A recent study of post-herpetic neuralgia, for example, suggests that opioids are as effective as adjuvent agents in this pain syndrome. Of note, patients preferred opioids, possibly because of the better side effect profile (Raja, Haythornthwaite et al., 2002).

Once the appropriate class of medication has been selected, the choice of a specific drug is determined by its side effects, route of administration, and individual patient characteristics. Balancing the benefits of a drug with the patient's ability to take it is the art of drug therapy.

Other treatment modalities include interventional techniques and physical modalities. In the management of chronic pain, these are adjuncts to primary therapy and are not substitutes for pharmacotherapy.

This chapter provides an overview of these methods and their indications. (Psychological approaches, which are integral to a multidisciplinary approach to pain management, are reviewed in Chapter 3. Use of opioid medications is discussed in Chapter 5.)

NON-OPIOID PHARMACOLOGIC AGENTS

Many of the medications used to treat pain are not primarily analgesics, but have analgesic efficacy under certain conditions. Such medications are classified as adjuvant analgesics. They include antiepileptic drugs, antidepressants, adrenergic agonists, local anesthetics, and muscle relaxants. Other medications are primary analgesics, but are not in the opioid class. Appropriate use of both types of medications can greatly improve analgesia as well as overall pain management.

Non-Opioid Analgesics. *Non-Steroidal Anti-inflammatory Drugs (NSAIDs):* NSAIDs, which are the most widely used analgesics, are indicated for somatic pain of mild to moderate intensity. They are most useful in bone and joint pain, but can be used in conjunction with opioids for all forms of pain. The first NSAID, aspirin, remains the model for all others. Newer compounds have the same presumed mode of action but offer advantages in side effect profiles and ease of use.

Although the exact mechanism of NSAID analgesia is unclear, it is thought to be related to the inhibition of cyclooxygenase activity, which in turn inhibits prostaglandin production (Vane, 1971). Prostaglandins sensitize peripheral nerve endings to noxious stimuli and are the key to the inflammatory cascade. There also is evidence that NSAIDs have a role in modulating pain in the central nervous system, particularly at the spinal cord level (McCormack & Brune, 1991), independent of their anti-inflammatory action (Willer, DeBrouckner et al., 1989). It is not clear which mechanism is more important clinically.

All NSAIDs are well absorbed in the gastrointestinal (GI) tract. Most undergo some hepatic conjugation and are excreted in urine. For this reason, hepatic and renal impairment can lead to drug accumulation; doses need to be adjusted accordingly. There is a ceiling level to the analgesic effect of NSAIDs, beyond which increasing the dose does not improve analgesia. Unfortunately, this ceiling level varies from patient to patient, requiring individualized titration of dose. Patients also have variable responses to the different classes of NSAIDs: some patients do not respond at all to one class, but have excellent results with a different class.

The toxicity of NSAIDs is well recognized. In elderly persons and patients with renal hepatic and hematologic disease, several of the side effects are enhanced. For this reason, the usual guidelines regarding dose need to be adjusted and often cannot be used.

Nausea and diarrhea are common GI side effects of NSAIDs. Several studies suggest that the rate of significant GI problems is about 10% (Loeb, Ahlquist et al., 1992). Gastric and duodenal ulceration, although less common, are clinically more important. The effects of NSAIDs on the GI tract are thought to be due to prostaglandin inhibition, because prostaglandins have a protective effect on the gastric mucosa. It does not appear that NSAIDs produce ulceration by a local effect alone, since prostaglandin decrease is seen throughout the entire GI tract.

It is difficult to predict which patient will develop GI ulceration. Nausea and abdominal pain are poor warning symptoms of toxicity. Prophylaxis with misoprostol can be useful, but it is expensive and its long-term effects are unknown. Consequently, it should be reserved for patients who have a known sensitivity to NSAIDs.

Renal damage is another major toxic side effect of NSAIDs, particularly for patients with compromised renal function (Kincaid-Smith, 1986; Porile, Bakris et al., 1990). NSAIDs should be used very cautiously in these patients. A useful "rule of thumb" is to avoid the use of NSAIDs in any patient with proteinuria and decreased glomerular filtration rate.

Hematological toxicity due to NSAIDs can be particularly problematic. The major toxicity of this type is platelet dysfunction. Most NSAIDs produce inhibition of platelet aggregation and prolonged bleeding time; these effects usually last for about one week. Choline trisalicylate has minimal anti-platelet effect and can be used in patients with platelet dysfunction who would benefit from an NSAID. However, it is expensive and compliance with it is poor.

A variety of other side effects associated with NSAIDs are not well characterized. For example, headache is a common complaint in patients maintained on NSAIDs, as is dizziness, but the mechanism behind these is unclear and often is dose-related. Skin reactions can occur as well, usually as an allergic response. Treatment should be discontinued and the patient re-challenged with a different class of NSAID if clinically necessary.

Significant interactions between NSAIDs and other medications are common. The most important of these involve the potentiation of renal and hepatic toxicity of co-administered drugs and the changes NSAIDs can produce in anticonvulsant levels. There is no known interaction between NSAIDs and anti-retroviral medications.

While the major indication for NSAIDs is the treatment of mild to moderate somatic pain (<3 on the visual analog scale), these drugs often are used in conjunction with low-potency opiates for more severe pain. Bone and joint pain is very responsive to the use of NSAIDs, but neuropathic pain usually is not. In the author's experience, diffuse myalgias also are resistant to these medications, except in the setting of fever. Patients with advanced disease and pain sufficiently severe to interfere with their activities of daily living will require additional medications.

Cox-2 Selective NSAIDs: In an attempt to decrease the toxicity of traditional NSAIDs, Cox-2 selective inhibitors have been developed. Whereas traditional NSAIDs inhibit both Cox-1 (which is protective to the gut) and Cox-2 (which is involved in inflammation and pain), Cox-2 selective NSAIDs affect only the inflammatory pathway.

Two Cox-2 selective agents, celecoxib and rofecoxib, currently are indicated for the management of acute pain associated with rheumatoid and osteoarthritis, as well as painful dysmenorrhea. While initial reports suggested that both agents were extremely safe, as their use has increased it has become clear that, although they have fewer GI side effects than traditional NSAIDs, they may have significant adverse effects on renal and cardiovascular function. Until more data are available, their use should be restricted to the lowest possible dose, and then only in otherwise healthy patients. In the elderly, care should be taken to monitor for fluid retention and accelerated hypertension (Bell, 2001).

Adjuvant Analgesics. Medications that have a primary indication other than analgesia, but which have analgesic properties under certain conditions, are termed *adjuvant analgesics*. Most of these medications enhance the body's own pain-modulating mechanisms or the effectiveness of other analgesics. Several different classes of medications are used as adjuvants, including antidepressants, antiepileptic drugs, oral local anesthetics, and adrenergic agonists.

Antidepressants: The tricyclic antidepressants (TCAs) have been used for many years for the management of neuropathic pain. Their analgesic effect appears to be independent of their antidepressant actions. There is evidence to suggest that their mode of action is to enhance the body's own pain modulating pathways and to enhance opioid effect at the opioid receptors (Feinmann, 1985; Fields, 1994). Their onset of action is slow, requiring several weeks for the full drug effect to be achieved. They are most effective for continuous, burning, or dysesthetic pain (Galer, 1994). Although tricyclic antidepressants are a first-line therapy for many forms of neuropathy, there is some question as to their efficacy in HIV neuropathy (Kieburtz, Simpson et al., 1998). This may be due to the rapid degeneration of fibers in HIV.

The greatest analgesic effect is seen with the older, tertiary amine antidepressants, such as amitriptyline, imipramine, and doxepin. Secondary amine tricyclics, such as desipramine and nortriptyline, also are effective and have less sedation and anticholinergic side effects (Godfrey, 1996). The newer antidepressants of the select serotonin reuptake inhibitor (SSRI) class do not seem to be as effective for neuropathic pain (Max, Lynch et al., 1992). Nevertheless, they can be helpful in managing associated depression and insomnia.

Tricyclics are well absorbed from the GI tract and have few interactions with antiretroviral agents. However, they do have a significant number of side effects, the most common of which is sedation. In many cases, this can be avoided by starting at a low dose and instructing the patient to take the medication 10 to 12 hours before arising, rather than

at bedtime. The usual starting dose for amitriptyline is between 10 and 25 mg, and most patients find benefit at ranges between 50 and 150 mg. Some patients do well with doses above and below this range as well.

Many of the other side effects seen with tricyclic antidepressants are related to their anticholinergic properties. These include dry mouth, visual blurring, urinary retention, hypotension, and cardiac arrhythmias. Many patients become tolerant to these after some time. Starting at a low dose of 10 mg and escalating at weekly intervals reduces the likelihood of significant discomfort. TCAs are contraindicated in patients with glaucoma and cardiac arrhythmias and should be used with caution in patients with urinary outlet obstruction.

Some patients are not able to tolerate TCAs and may benefit from some of the newer antidepressants. Paroxetine, in particular, has been found useful in certain forms of painful peripheral neuropathy (Sindrup, Gram et al., 1990). Similar evidence does not exist for other SSRIs.

Anticonvulsants: Carbamazepine, phenytoin, and several other anticonvulsant/antiepileptic drugs (AEDs) have efficacy in paroxysmal neuropathic pain. The exact mode of action is unclear. It is suspected that AEDs may help to reduce pain by reducing neuronal excitability and local neuronal discharges. They appear to be helpful in pain syndromes that are characterized by paroxysmal or lancinating pain (Galer, 1995).

Phenytoin has been used for the management of a variety of neuropathic pain syndromes, including trigeminal neuralgia and post-herpetic neuralgia (McQuay, Carroll et al., 1995). The average dose is 300 mg per day. A loading dose of one gram can be used for acute pain management. Phenytoin has significant drug interactions with a variety of protein-bound medications, including rifampin, methadone, and several antifungal agents.

Dizziness and somnolence are common with phenytoin and usually are dose-related. Serious skin reactions such as Stevens-Johnson syndrome can occur, necessitating discontinuation of the drug. Leukopenia and thrombocytopenia can occur as idiosyncratic reactions. Elevation of liver enzymes is common.

Carbamazepine has been well studied and used successfully in a variety of neuropathic pain states (Moosa, McFadyen et al., 1993; Galer, 1995). It appears to be more effective than phenytoin but has several significant side effects, including dizziness, somnolence, and significant leukopenia. Hyponatremia also can occur as an idiosyncratic reaction. Starting at a dose of 100 mg and gradually escalating in 100 mg increments every three to seven days can minimize the dizziness. Close monitoring of the blood count is necessary and limits the utility of this drug in HIV patients.

Valproic acid has been used for the management of lancinating pain, with mixed results. There are no large studies suggesting long-term effectiveness. The large number of drug interactions and significant hepatic dysfunction that can occur with this drug make it a second-line choice.

Recently, several new AEDs have been released for use and some have been found to be useful in treating neuropathic pain. Gabapentin, in particular, has been found to be effective in both lancinating and continuous dysesthetic pain (Chapman, Suzuki et al., 1998; Houtchens, Richert et al., 1997; Segal & Rordorf, 1996; Rowbotham, Harden et al., 1998). It is a remarkably well-tolerated drug with few interactions and a good side effect profile. Treatment usually is started at 100 mg three times per day and then escalated in increments of 100 to 300 mg every three to five days. Most patients have a response at 300 mg three times per day. There is some evidence that doses above 3,600 mg to 4,800 mg are not well absorbed, so doses above this range are of questionable utility (Elwes & Binnie, 1998). The most common reported side effect is somnolence, which resolves after the first two weeks of therapy.

Clonazepam is a benzodiazepine with anticonvulsant properties that has been used for lancinating pain. It has utility in the treatment of muscle spasms as well as myoclonus (Bartusch, Sanders et al., 1996; Eisele, Grigsby et al., 1992). Because it produces significant sedation, it is best used in patients who have anxiety or difficulty sleeping. It can produce significant dysphoria and should be used cautiously when depression is present. The usual starting dose is 0.5 mg in the evening, escalating to 2 mg three times a day.

Oral Anesthetics and α Agonists: Neuropathic pain has been found to respond to high doses of intravenous local anesthetics, such as lidocaine (Glazer & Portenoy, 1991; Rowbotham, Reisner et al., 1991). The mechanism of action is different from that of the peripheral effect of local anesthetics. It seems that systemic administration suppresses the activity of dorsal horn cells, which respond to noxious stimulation. Spontaneous firing of damaged cells and axons also is suppressed (Woolf & Wiesenfeld-Hallin, 1985).

Tocainide and mexiletine are oral local anesthetics used for cardiac arrhythmias that have been useful for neuropathic pain. Mexiletine has fewer side effects and has been studied more thoroughly. It is useful for continuous dysesthetic pain (Chabel, Russell et al., 1992). The starting dose is 150 mg per day, increasing in 150 mg increments every three to five days, up to a dose of 300 mg three times a day or until side effects occur.

The most common side effects are dose-related and include nausea, dizziness, and tremors. Hematologic reactions are idiosyncratic and rare. In this regard, oral local anesthetics may be a good alternative in patients with blood dyscrasias.

Adrenergic agonists are another type of adjuvant analgesic. The α_2-adrenergic agonists in particular have proved useful in a variety of pain syndromes. The mechanism of action is presumed to be an enhancement of endogenous pain-modulating systems.

The best studied adrenergic agonist is clonidine, which has been found to be effective in neuropathic pain. It can be administered epidurally, intrathecally, orally, or transdermally. For chronic pain, the starting dose is 0.1 mg per day. Gradually escalating the dose to 0.3 mg per day can produce enhanced analgesia.

The major limiting factor in the use of clonidine is its hypotensive effects. Although these are not pronounced in otherwise healthy patients, in the presence of neuropathy, blood pressure fluctuations can be increased. There are few if any other side effects. For patients who have dysesthetic pain, clonidine can be a useful adjunct to other analgesics.

Topical Agents. Topical agents are useful for several types of continuous dysesthetic pain. In general, they are most effective in pain states that have a predominantly peripheral cause. These include painful neuropathies, herpetic and post-herpetic neuralgia, and—occasionally—painful arthropathies. Topical agents alone usually are insufficient to produce total pain relief, but they can be helpful in patients who experience adverse effects from other adjuvant drugs.

Capsaicin, a naturally occurring pepper extract, has been found to be useful in reducing neuropathic pain in diabetics (Capsaicin Study Group, 1991). The capsaicin preparation is applied to the area of greatest discomfort several times a day. Pain relief does not occur for several days. On initial application, many patients complain of markedly worsened pain and burning. This resolves after several applications and may be due to the local release of Substance P. Unfortunately, the burning can be severe and patients often are not able to tolerate it.

EMLA (eutectic mixture of local anesthetics) is a 1:1 mixture of prilocaine and lidocaine, which can penetrate the skin and produce local anesthesia. It has been helpful in patients with peripheral nerve lesions and in reducing pain associated with blood drawing. EMLA has been particularly helpful in post-herpetic neuralgia (Stow, Glynn et al., 1989). In the author's experience, the combination of EMLA applied first, followed by capsaicin, has been better tolerated than capsaicin alone and may be more effective.

Compounded ointments of salicylates and NSAIDs also have been used for neuropathic pain, but the data regarding their efficacy are unclear (Rowbotham, 1994). Large trials currently are under way for treatment of a variety of neuropathic pain states.

Muscle Relaxants. Several different classes of medications have muscle relaxant properties. Spasmolytic agents such as baclofen, tizanidine, and benzodiazepines are useful for conditions that produce flexor and extensor spasms because of neural injury, as well as chronic muscle spasm.

A group of diverse agents also are classified as muscle relaxants, although their exact mode of action is poorly understood. These include cyclobenzaprine, carisoprodol, methocarbamol, and chlorzoxazone. The latter group has no clear spasmolytic action, but may exert their action through central nervous (CNS) depression.

Baclofen is a gabaminergic drug with affinity for the presynaptic $GABA_B$ receptors. It suppresses excitatory transmitter release and action at the spinal cord level. There is some evidence that it also blocks transmitter release at cutaneous nociceptive nerve endings (Hwang & Wilcox, 1989). It is indicated for pain secondary to spasms of CNS origin. Patients with spasticity related to multiple sclerosis or upper motor neuron lesion from trauma, cerebrovascular disease, or degenerative disease might benefit from baclofen. There is some anecdotal literature suggesting that it also may be useful for facial pain.

The major side effects of baclofen are sedation and liver dysfunction. Abrupt discontinuation can result in seizures. Intrathecal administration of baclofen can be useful in patients who develop systemic side effects to the oral form (Pirotte, Heilporn et al., 1995). It also is indicated in cerebral palsy, multiple sclerosis, and spastic hemiplegia from trauma or CVA. However, patients may require additional antispasmodic medications.

Tizanidine, a newer spasmolytic agent, is a centrally acting α_2-adrenergic agonist. Clinical experience suggests that it has antinociceptive properties, particularly in muscle and soft tissue pain (Coward, 1994). It is as effective as baclofen in decreasing spasticity, but produces less muscle weakness. However, it can be sedating and should not be administered with other adrenergic agonists.

Cyclobenzaprine is a tricyclic agent that has been marketed as a muscle relaxant. Its major site of action appears to be in the brainstem, although the exact mechanism of action is unclear. It is indicated for short-term use only. It is quite sedating and should be used carefully with other CNS depressants.

Methocarbamol, carisoprodol, and chlorzoxazone all are older agents whose exact mode of action remains unclear. All have significant CNS depressant effects. There are no controlled studies demonstrating clear efficacy for these medications as analgesic agents. Because of their potential for abuse, they should be avoided.

INTERVENTIONAL PROCEDURES

Anesthetic procedures have been a mainstay of pain management. Although there are many effective procedures for acute pain, chronic pain procedures are somewhat more limited. They include infusions and local blocks with anesthetic agents, administration of epidural steroids, implantable drug delivery systems, and implantable neural stimulators.

Anesthetic Infusions. Intravenous or oral administration of local anesthetics can produce systemic analgesic effects. It is postulated that the mechanism of action for this phenomenon is the interruption of local reflex arcs, vasodilatation, and low-level anesthesia of susceptible nerve endings (Bigelow & Harrison, 1944). This technique has been particularly helpful in the diagnosis and treatment of neuropathic pain syndromes.

The usual method is to infuse lidocaine at a rate of 5 mg/kg of body weight over 30 minutes in a monitored setting. The patient usually experiences relief of paresthesias and lancinating pain within one hour of the infusion; this relief can persist for several days (Boas, Covino et al., 1982; Kastrup, Petersen et al., 1987). Repeat infusions can be used, although their efficacy may decline. Oral anesthetic agents such as mexiletine also can be used after a loading dose of IV lidocaine. Intravenous lidocaine also has been found helpful in certain forms of vascular headache (Edwards, Habib et al., 1985).

Trigger Point Injections. Local injection of anesthetic into tender areas in muscle, referred to as trigger points, can provide temporary relief in acute and chronic soft tissue pain. The main indication for these injections is myofascial pain. Considerable controversy exists as to which agents should be injected and how often. In general, a dilute solution of a short-acting local anesthetic (with or without steroid) is injected into the trigger point. Dry needling, or mechanical disruption of the tender area, also can be employed, although it usually is poorly tolerated.

The techniques of trigger point injection are described in several texts (Maciewicz, Chung et al., 1988; Rachlin, 1994). The injections usually are given in conjunction with physical therapy; this maximizes the efficacy of muscle stretching techniques and reduces pain during the recovery phase from an acute injury.

Local Neural Blockade. Local neural blockade is used principally for the relief of acute pain and for diagnostic purposes. Sequential blocks of individual nerves or spinal levels can help to pinpoint sites of pain generation, but they do not identify the specific disease state that may be producing the pain (Travell & Simon, 1983).

Neurolytic blocks are reserved for the most intractable cases and for patients with a limited life expectancy (Winnie, 2001). The risk of developing a deafferentation pain syndrome is high and increases over time. The local vascular effects and soft tissue damage require that these procedures be performed only by clinicians who have ample clinical expertise in their use.

Phenol and absolute alcohol are the most commonly used agents. Both work by destroying peripheral myelin and producing irreversible conduction block. Prolonged administration also is toxic to poorly myelinated axons. Because collateral sprouting can occur, and the peripheral myelin rarely is repaired, ectopic generators can develop lysed nerves, which may produce a return of the pain locally. This phenomenon, coupled with the frequency of recurrent central pain, limit the utility of these agents.

Spinal Steroid Injections and Facet Injections. Local steroid injections into either the epidural space or the facet joints have been used in the treatment of mechanical neck and back pain. Although the indications remain controversial, epidural steroids are used in the management of acute or recurrent pain resulting from root irritation with clinical evidence of radicular dysfunction and in non-operative spinal stenosis (Jain & Gupta, 2001; Abram, 1994; Weinstein & Herring, 1995). Facet blocks are useful in patients with neck or back pain with a mechanical component but without radicular signs, presumably arising in the spinal column (Rowlingson, 1994; Bogduk, 1997; Dwyer, Aprill et al., 1990; Mooney & Robertson, 1976).

The technique of epidural steroid injections is well described in several standard texts (Cousins & Veering, 1998). Usually, triamcinolone (at a dose of 50 mg) or methylprednisolone (at a dose of 40 to 80 mg) is injected into the epidural space after dilution with either normal saline or a short-acting local anesthetic agent. The injection is performed at the disc level adjacent to the affected nerve roots and sufficient fluid is given to bathe the adjacent nerve roots. Complications are uncommon and usually result from either local irritation or a persistent dural leak. Rare complications include radicular irritation and infection (Nelson, 1993). Improvement usually is noted within a week and may persist for several months. A course of three injections generally is given, until pain relief or treatment failure is reached.

Efficacy is variable, with most series indicating short-term improvement of acute back pain. Patients who are most likely to benefit have pain of less than six months' duration or radicular signs (Bowman & Wedderburn, 1993; Watts & Silagy, 1995; Koes, Scholten et al., n.d.). Benefits are less convincing in pain related to spinal stenosis (Fukusaki & Kobayashi, 1998).

Facet blocks are performed with fluoroscopic guidance. Local anesthetic, either 0.5% bupivicaine or 2% lidocaine, is injected at the base of the superior articular process. Relief of pain suggests that the pain generator is within the facet joint (Bogduk, 1997). Efficacy is quite variable, with prolonged relief usually obtained only after radiofrequency ablation.

Sympathetic Blockade. Sympathetic blockade is indicated for pain involving the sympathetic nervous system and the viscera. Nociceptive input from the upper extremities, head, and neck can be blocked by infiltrating the stellate ganglion. Thoracic sympathetic paravertebral ganglia receive input from the cardiac and thoracic viscera; their blockade can be helpful in pain originating at those sites. The abdominal viscera are innervated by the celiac ganglion, while the urogenital viscera are supplied by the superior hypogastric plexus and the ganglion impar. Deep visceral pain can be relieved by blocking the appropriate location. Finally, the lumbar sympathetic ganglia are involved in mediating pain in the lower extremities. Lumbar sympathetic blockade can be very useful in managing ischemic limb pain and neuropathic pain from failed back surgery, as well as chronic regional pain syndromes.

The exact mechanisms of involvement of the sympathetic nervous system in peripheral pain are not fully understood (Jaenig, 1990). In addition, there is poor correlation between the degree of sympathetic dysfunction and response to pain blockade. Therefore, for practical purposes, response to sympathetic blocks is based on the patient's report of pain relief and on changes in skin temperature (Tahmoush, Malley et al., 1983). The indications for stellate ganglion blocks are painful conditions affecting the head, neck, and upper extremities. Both blind and radiographically guided approaches can be used (Aesbach & Nagy, 2000), as can repeated blocks. Neurolysis or spinal cord stimulation can be used if significant relief is obtained from temporary blocks.

Lumbar sympathetic blockade is used in the diagnosis and therapy of painful and other conditions, presumably associated with a dysfunction of the sympathetic nervous system. These include complex regional pain syndrome types I and II, herpes zoster, amputation stump pain, and inoperable peripheral vascular and vasospastic diseases of the lower extremities. Other indications include selected cases of pelvic pain in which superior hypogastric nerve block cannot be performed (Cousins, Reeve et al., 1979).

Celiac and superior hypogastric blocks, as well as ganglion impar blocks, are used for chronic painful visceral conditions. There are no long-term effectiveness studies of any of these procedures. Radiographic imaging and guidance are mandatory to ensure appropriate anesthetic placement.

The major indication for these blocks is chronic cancer-related pain (Plancarte, Amescua et al., 1990; Plancarte, DeLeon-Cassola et al., 1997).

Spinal Cord Stimulation. Spinal cord stimulation (SCS) for the management of pain was introduced in 1967. The actual mechanism of action of SCS is not known, but there are several theories for the analgesic efficacy of this treatment. For example, it is postulated that the electrical stimulation produces antidromic blocking of painful information at the spinal cord level, spinothalamic tract conductance blocking, and activation of supraspinal pain processing nuclei (Broggi, Franzini et al., 1985; Saade et al., 1986). There also is good evidence from CSF markers of chemical neuromodulatory mechanisms. Studies have shown an increase in serotonin, substance P, and gamma-aminobutyric acid (GABA) release, as well as a decrease in the presence of excitatory amino acids in response to SCS (Meyerson, Brodin et al., 1985).

There are multiple reports of the efficacy of SCS for widely differing chronic pain syndromes (Spiegelmann &

Friedman, 1991; Kumar, Nath et al., 1997). Generally, it is agreed that SCS is effective in treating pain of neuropathic origin, particularly sympathetically mediated pain and pain emanating from ischemic origin. It appears that SCS has no efficacy in acute pain or pain of nociceptive origin. Because it is known that SCS causes vasodilatation in animal studies, clinicians have used this modality for the treatment of pain resulting from peripheral vascular disease and visceral pain. Peripheral vascular disease remains the leading indication for SCS in Europe today. There are promising results in the use of SCS in pancreatic and pelvic pain, but no large-scale studies of SCS for these indications (Kemler, Barendse et al., 2000).

SCS implantation is expensive and labor-intensive. Because it usually requires surgical intervention, it should be reserved for patients who have failed more conservative therapies.

PHYSICAL MEDICINE AND REHABILITATIVE THERAPIES

A comprehensive approach to pain management incorporates the use of various physical modalities and rehabilitative therapies. Physical modalities include the therapeutic application of heat, cold, traction, transcutaneous electrical stimulation, acupuncture, and massage. Several excellent texts discuss each of these techniques (Tan, 1998; Hayes, 1993). Rehabilitative therapies are aimed at functional restoration and include exercise and conditioning therapies.

Heat. Application of heat to muscles or joints can provide analgesia, decrease muscle spasm, and increase flexibility (Michlovitz, 1990a; Hall, Kevington et al., 1996). It also is very useful in decreasing acute pain in soft tissue injuries and joint inflammation.

Local heat application can be either superficial (as with hot packs, paraffin baths, or hot water) or deep. Deep heat application is accomplished with diathermy and ultrasound, which require training to be performed safely; for this reason, superficial heat application is more widely used. Evidence suggests that pain relief is greater when heat is combined with exercise (Dellhag, Wollersjo et al., 1992).

Deep heat application has been used for many years for deep tissue pain, but several studies suggest that its utility is limited. In a study comparing the relative efficacy of ultrasound, short wave diathermy, and galvanic current for hip and knee joint pain, the benefits appeared to be similar. There is some evidence that diathermy may worsen post-exercise pain (Svarcova, Tranavsky et al., 1987). Because of the costs associated with deep heat modalities, they should be used in patients only if superficial heat has failed.

Cold. The application of cold has a local analgesic effect and reduces inflammatory responses and muscle spasm. Several mechanisms have been postulated for the analgesic efficacy of cold. These include altered neural transmission, reduced muscle spasm, altered blood flow to muscle and nerve, and increased endorphin production.

Cooling is applied by cold packs, ice massage, hydrotherapy, or vapocoolant sprays, all of which seem to have equal efficacy (Michlovitz, 1990b). There is some evidence that cold may produce pain relief faster than heat and may be more effective in acute pain (Cote, Prentice et al., 1988).

Transcutaneous Electrical Nerve Stimulation (TENS). TENS has been used for a variety of chronic pain conditions. Initially, it was thought to work by increasing afferent input and turning on inhibitory neurons at the spinal cord level. More recent research indicates that TENS may work by stimulating the sympathetic nervous system and brainstem nuclei and increasing endorphin release (Levy, Dalith et al., 1987). It has demonstrated effectiveness in joint pain and acute pain, but little utility in back pain (Deyo, Walsh et al., 1990). Brief trials of TENS should be considered in patients with localized mechanical pain, in conjunction with physical therapy.

Massage. Massage is one of the oldest and most widely used techniques for decreasing acute and chronic pain: indeed, descriptions of therapeutic massage can be found in the works of Hippocrates. It is not clear exactly how massage works, although counter-irritation and increased blood flow have been proposed as mechanisms. Many different massage techniques are used.

The utility of massage seems to be greatest for short-term pain relief after acute injuries (Triano, McGregor et al., 1995; Stenstrom, 1994). No studies demonstrate that the benefits of massage in chronic low back or neck pain are any greater than those to be derived from rest and re-education.

Exercise. Pain patients often develop decreased muscle strength, reduced range of motion, and general deconditioning, as well as other functional limitations. Exercise therapy can help overcome those deficits and also reduce pain (Taubert, 1997; James, Cleland et al., 1994).

Selecting the appropriate exercise therapy is the key to good rehabilitation. In addition to prescribed exercise, simple aerobic exercises such as walking and swimming should be part of chronic pain management.

Range of motion exercises (ROM) are designed to reduce stiffness and increase flexibility. Both active and passive ROM can be useful in reducing pain in soft tissue and joint injuries. It is important to begin with passive ROM and advance to active ROM so as not to overstretch injured tissues, which can decrease tensile strength. ROM therapy can be the first step in rehabilitation and should be used for chronic maintenance therapy as well.

Muscle conditioning exercises are useful in increasing strength, endurance, and function. Such exercises are divided into isometric and dynamic forms. Isometric exercise involves muscle contraction without joint movement; it is used to increase muscle tone and strength in preparation for more vigorous exercise. Patients need to be instructed in how to perform isometric exercises so as to avoid excess muscle ischemia and increased intra-articular pressure (Taubert, 1997).

Dynamic exercise is more vigorous and involves the repetitive contraction and relaxation of muscle groups with joint movement. It is the final step in strengthening muscle groups and involves gradually increasing resistance. Patients usually begin working with elastic bands and move on to progressively greater resistance through use of weights and exercise machines. Determination of an appropriate resistance and training schedule, while monitoring for injury and providing patient education, is essential to a safe and effective dynamic exercise program.

Patients need education if exercise is to be an effective part of pain management. Setting specific functional goals rather than focusing on pain reduction is a key part of exercise therapy. In one study of the use of exercise for arthritis pain, patients found that using exercise goals rather than focusing on pain produced better functional outcomes and led to a reduction of pain chronically (James, Cleland et al., 1994). Patients become discouraged if they focus on pain reduction, because initially exercise may increase pain. Their physician or other caregiver needs to actively reinforce the patient's long-term goals and redirect them to a safe exercise program, despite setbacks.

Acupuncture. Acupuncture is a traditional Chinese therapy based on a theory of energy (Qi) flow. Qi is thought to flow along specific channels or meridians which, if blocked, can lead to disease. In classic acupuncture, the practitioner attempts to restore flow by applying treatment at points distributed along the meridians. Needling is the most common method of applying acupuncture, but heat, pressure, and electrical stimulation also have been used (Stux

& Pomeranz, 1995). Studies have shown that acupuncture produces an increase in endorphin release and modulates the firing of high-threshold, small-diameter nerve fibers (Tsou, 1987). The Western approach to acupuncture is based on modulating these elements of pain transmission.

Based on the evidence from several controlled studies, acupuncture appears to be effective in controlling the pain of osteoarthritis and fibromyalgia. Study subjects reported significant reduction in pain compared to placebo or pharmacologic treatments (Dickens & Lewith, 1989; Deluze, Bosia et al., 1992).

There is less evidence to support the effectiveness of acupuncture for neuropathic or inflammatory pain. Nevertheless, there is overwhelming evidence that acupuncture is safe and effective for a variety of somatic pain syndromes, and it should be considered as a treatment option (NIH, 1997).

Botulinum Toxin. The use of botulinum toxin (Botox®) for the treatment of focal dystonias has been standard for several years. However, Botox has been found to have multiple effects. By blocking acetylcholine release presynaptically, it not only decreases muscle contraction, but reduces sympathetic activity and may increase inhibitory interneuron activity at the spinal cord level (Rand & Whaler, 1965; Hagenah, Benecke et al., 1997).

There are no large, controlled studies of the utility of Botox for pain, but several small series suggest that it is useful in local and diffuse muscle spasm and in the management of headaches (Cheshire, Abashian et al., 1994; Gobel, 2001). Larger studies currently are under way.

The use of Botox requires knowledge of the muscle groups affected by a particular condition. Electromyographic guidance has been used to identify hyperactive muscles to be targeted in dystonia; the same technique has been used in pain treatment. It is not clear whether this is superior to injection at local areas of spasm or tenderness. Until the long-term effects of chronic Botox use are known, it would seem reasonable to use the least amount of medication possible by targeting affected muscles by EMG. Usually 40 units of Botox are injected into large muscles, as in back or neck pain, and 10 units are used for smaller muscle groups in the neck and head. Effects usually are noticeable within 5 to 10 days and may persist for as long as three months, at which point the treatment is repeated. Adverse effects usually are associated with local reactions or excessive weakness of affected muscle groups, leading to poor gait or facial drooping.

REFERENCES

Abram SE (1994). Risk versus benefit of epidural steroids: Let's remain objective. *American Pain Society Bulletin* 3:28-29.

Aesbach A & Nagy M (2000). Common nerve blocks in chronic pain management. *Anesthesiology Clinics of North America* 18(2):429-459.

Bartusch SL, Sanders BJ, D'Alessio JG et al. (1996). Clonazepam for the treatment of lancinating phantom limb pain. *Clinical Journal of Pain* 12(1):59-62.

Bell GM (2001). Cox-2 inhibitors and other nonsteroidal anti-inflammatory drugs in the treatment of pain in the elderly. *Clinics of Geriatric Medicine* 17(3):489-502.

Bigelow N & Harrison I (1944). General analgesic effects of procaine. *Journal of Pharmacology & Experimental Therapy* 81:368.

Boas RA, Covino BG & Shahnarian A (1982). Analgesic responses to IV lignocaine. *British Journal of Anesthesia* 54:501.

Bogduk N (1997). International Spinal Injection Society guidelines for the performance of spinal injection procedures, part I: Zygapophyseal joint blocks. *Clinical Journal of Pain* 13:285-302.

Bowman SJ & Wedderburn L (1993). Outcome assessment after epidural corticosteroid injection for low back pain and sciatica. *Spine* 18:1345.

Broggi G, Franzini A, Parati E et al. (1985). Neurochemical and structural modifications related to pain control induced by spinal cord stimulation. In *Neurostimulation: An Overview*. New York, NY: Futura Publishing, 87-95.

Capsaicin Study Group (1991). Treatment of painful diabetic neuropathy with topical capsaicin. *Archives of Internal Medicine* 151(11):2225-2229.

Chabel C, Russell LC et al. (1992). The use of oral mexiletine for the treatment of pain after peripheral nerve injury. *Anesthesiology* 76:513-517.

Chapman R, Suzuki HL, Chamarette LJ et al. (1998). Effects of systemic carbamazepine and gabapentin on spinal neuronal responses in spinal nerve ligated rats. *Pain* 75(2-3):261-272.

Cheshire WP, Abashian SW & Mann JD (1994). Botulinum toxin in the treatment of myofascial pain syndrome. *Pain* 59:65-69.

Cote DJ, Prentice WE, Hooker DN et al. (1988). Comparison of three treatment procedures for minimizing ankle sprain swelling. *Physical Therapy* 68:1072-1076.

Cousins MJ, Reeve TS, Glynn CJ et al. (1979). Neurolytic lumbar sympathetic blockade: Duration of denervation and relief of rest pain. *Anaesthesia & Intensive Care* 7:121.

Cousins MJ & Veering BT (1998). Epidural neural blockade. In MJ Cousins & PO Bridenbaugh (eds.) *Neural Blockade, 3rd Edition*. Philadelphia, PA: Lippincott-Raven.

Coward DM (1994). Tinazidine: Neuropharmacology and mechanism of action. *Neurology* 44(Suppl 9):6-11.

Dellhag B, Wollersjo I & Bjelle A (1992). Effect of active hand exercise and wax bath treatment in rheumatoid arthritis patients. *Arthritis Care and Research* 5:87-92.

Deluze C, Bosia L, Zirbs A et al. (1992). Electroacupuncture in fibromyalgia: Results of a controlled trial. *British Medical Journal* 305:1249.

Deyo RA, Walsh NE, Martin DC et al. (1990). A controlled trial of transcutaneous electrical nerve stimulation (TENS) and exercise for chronic low back pain. *New England Journal of Medicine* 322:1627-1634.

Dickens W & Lewith GT (1989). A single-blind, controlled and randomized clinical trial to evaluate the effect of acupuncture for the treatment of trapezio-metacarpal osteoarthritis. *Complementary Medical Research* 3:5.

Dwyer A, Aprill C & Bogduk N (1990). Cervical zygapophyseal joint pain patterns: A study in normal volunteers. *Spine* 15:453-457.

Edwards WT, Habib F, Burney RG et al. (1985). Intravenous lidocaine in the management of various chronic pain states. *Reg Anesthesia* 10:1.

Eisele JH Jr., Grigsby EJ & Dea J (1992). Clonazepam treatment of myoclonic contractions associated with high-dose opioids: Case report. *Pain* 49(2):231-232.

Elwes RD & Binnie CD (1998). Clinical pharmacokinetics of newer antiepileptic drugs. Lamotrigine, vigabatrin, gabapentin and oxcarbazepine. *Clinical Pharmacokinetics* 30(6):403-415.

Feinmann C (1985). Pain relief by antidepressants: Possible modes of action. *Pain* 23(1):1-8.

Fields H (1994). Pain modulation and the action of analgesic medications. *Annals of Neurology* 35(Suppl):S42-S45.

Fukusaki M & Kobayashi I (1998). Symptoms of spinal stenosis do not improve after epidural steroid injection. *Clinical Journal of Pain* 14:148-151.

Galer BS (1994). Painful polyneuropathy: Diagnosis, pathophysiology, and management. *Seminars in Neurology* 14(3):237-246.

Galer BS (1995). Neuropathic pain of peripheral origin: Advances in pharmacologic treatment. *Neurology* 45(12 Suppl 9):S17-S25.

Glazer S & Portenoy RK (1991). Systemic local analgesics in pain control. *Journal of Pain & Symptom Management* 6:30-39.

Gobel H (2001). Botulinum toxin A in the treatment of headache disorders and pericranial pain syndromes. *Nervenzart* 72(4):261-274.

Godfrey RG (1996). A guide to the understanding and use of tricyclic antidepressants in the overall management of fibromyalgia and other chronic pain syndromes. *Archives of Internal Medicine* 156(10):1047-1052.

Hagenah R, Benecke R & Wiegand H (1997). Effects of type A botulinum toxin on the cholinergic transmission at spinal Renshaw cells and on the inhibitory action at Ia inhibitory interneurons. *Naunyn Schmiedebergs Archive Pharmacologia* 299:267-272.

Hall J, Kevington SM, Madison PJ et al. (1996). A randomized and controlled trial of hydrotherapy in rheumatoid arthritis. *Arthritis Care and Research* 9:206-215.

Hayes KW, ed. (1993). *Manual for Physical Agents, 4th Edition.* Norwalk, CT: Appleton & Lange.

Houtchens MK, Richert JR, Sami A et al. (1997). Open label gabapentin treatment for pain in multiple sclerosis. *Multiple Sclerosis* 3(4):250-253.

Hwang AS & Wilcox GL (1989). Baclofen, gamma aminobutyric acid B receptors and substance P in the mouse spinal cord. *Journal of Pharmacology & Experimental Therapy* 248:1026-1033.

Jaenig W (1990). The sympathetic nervous system in pain. In M Stanton-Hicks (ed.) *Pain and the Sympathetic Nervous System.* Boston, MA: Kluwer Academic Publishers.

Jain S & Gupta R (2001). Neurolytic agents in clinical practice. In SD Waldman & AP Winnie (eds.) *Interventional Pain Management.* Philadelphia, PA: W.B. Saunders, 19-67.

James MJ, Cleland LG, Gaffney RD et al. (1994). Effect of exercise on 99mTc-DPTA clearance from knees with effusions. *Journal of Rheumatology* 21:501-504.

Kastrup J, Petersen P et al. (1987). Intravenous lidocaine infusion: a new treatment of painful diabetic neuropathy. *Pain* 28:69.

Kemler MA, Barendse GA, van Kleef M et al. (2000). Spinal cord stimulation in patients with chronic reflex sympathetic dystrophy. *New England Journal of Medicine* 343(9):618-624.

Kieburtz K, Simpson D, Yiannoutsos C et al. (1998). A randomized trial of amitriptyline and mexiletine for painful neuropathy in HIV infection. AIDS Clinical Trial Group 242 Protocol Team. *Neurology* 51:1682-1688.

Kincaid-Smith P (1986). Effects of non-narcotic analgesics on the kidney. *Drugs* 32(Suppl 4):109-128.

Koes BW, Scholten RJPM et al. (n.d.). Efficacy of epidural steroid injections for low-back pain and sciatica: A systematic review of randomized clinical trials. *Pain* 63:279-288.

Kumar K, Nath RK & Toth C (1997). Spinal cord stimulation is effective in the management of reflex sympathetic dystrophy. *Neurosurgery* 40:503-509.

Levy A, Dalith M, Abramovici A et al. (1987). TENS in experimental acute arthritis. *Archives of Physical Medicine & Rehabilitation* 68:75-78.

Loeb DS, Ahlquist DA & Talley NJ (1992). Management of gastroduodenopathy associated with the use of nonsteroidal anti-inflammatory drugs. *Mayo Clinic Proceedings* 67:354-364.

Maciewicz R, Chung RY, Strassman A et al. (1988). Relief of vascular headache with intravenous lidocaine. *Cincinnati Journal of Pain* 4:11.

Max MB, Lynch SA, Muir J et al. (1992). Effects of desipramine, amitriptyline, and fluoxetine on pain in diabetic neuropathy. *New England Journal of Medicine* 326(19):1250-1256.

McCormack K & Brune K (1991). Dissociation between the antinociceptive and anti-inflammatory effects of the non-steroidal anti-inflammatory drugs. *Drugs* 41:533-547.

McQuay H, Carroll D, Jadad AR et al. (1995). Anticonvulsant drugs for management of pain: A systematic review. *British Medical Journal* 311:1047-1052.

Meyerson BA, Brodin E & Linderoth B (1985). Possible neurohumoral mechanisms in CNS stimulation for pain suppression. *Applied Neurophysiology* 48:175-180.

Michlovitz SL (1990a). Biophysical principles of heating and superficial heat agents. In SL Michlovitz (ed.) *Thermal Agents in Rehabilitation, 2nd Edition.* Philadelphia, PA: F.A. Davis.

Michlovitz SL (1990b). Cryotherapy: The use of cold as a therapeutic agent. In SL Michlovitz (ed.) *Thermal Agents in Rehabilitation, 2nd Edition.* Philadelphia, PA: F.A. Davis.

Mooney V & Robertson J (1976). The facet syndrome. *Clinical Orthopedics* 115:149-156.

Moosa RS, McFadyen ML, Miller R et al. (1993). Carbamazepine and its metabolites in neuralgias: concentration-effect relations. *European Journal of Clinical Pharmacology* 45(4):297-301.

National Institutes of Health (NIH) (1997). *Consensus Statement: Acupuncture.* Bethesda, MD: National Institutes of Health, 15:12, November 3-5.

Nelson DA (1993). Intraspinal therapy using methylprednisolone acetate: Twenty-three years of clinical controversy. *Spine* 18:278.

Pirotte B, Heilporn A, Joffrey A et al. (1995). Chronic intrathecal baclofen in severely disabling spasticity: Selection, clinical assessment and long-term benefit. *Acta Anesthesiologica Belgica* 95(4):216-225.

Plancarte R, Amescua C, Patt RB et al. (1990). Superior hypogastric plexus block for pelvic cancer pain. *Anesthesiology* 73:236-239.

Plancarte R, DeLeon-Cassola OA, El-Helaly M et al. (1997). Neurolytic superior hypogastric plexus block for chronic pelvic pain associated with cancer. *Reg Anesthesia* 22:562-568.

Porile JL, Bakris L & Garella S (1990). Acute interstitial nephritis with glomerulopathy due to non-steroidal anti-inflammatory agents: A review of its clinical spectrum and effects of steroid therapy. *Journal of Clinical Pharmacology* 30:468-475.

Rachlin ES, ed. (1994). *Myofascial Pain and Fibromyalgia.* St. Louis, MO: Mosby-Year Book, 143-382.

Raja SN, Haythornthwaite JA et al. (2002). Opioids versus antidepressants in post herpetic neuralgia. *Neurology* 59:1015-1021.

Rand MJ & Whaler BC (1965). Impairment of sympathetic transmission by botulinum toxin. *Nature* 206:588-591

Richardson DE & Dempsey CW (1984). Monoamine turnover in CSF of patients during spinal cord stimulation for pain control. *Pain* 2(Suppl):223.

Rowbotham MC (1994). Topical analgesic agents. In HL Fields & JC Liebskind (eds.) *Pharmacological Approaches to the Treatment of Chronic Pain.* New York, NY: IASP Press, 211-229.

Rowbotham M, Harden N, Stacey B et al. (1998). Gabapentin for the treatment of postherpetic neuralgia: A randomized controlled trial. *Journal of the American Medical Association* 280:1837-1842.

Rowbotham MC, Reisner L & Fields HL (1991). Both IV lidocaine and morphine reduce the pain of post-herpetic neuralgia. *Neurology* 41:1024-1028.

Rowlingson JC (1994). Epidural steroids: Do they have a place in pain management? *American Pain Society Bulletin* 3:20-27.

Saade NE et al. (1986). Supraspinal modulation of nociception in awake rats by stimulation of the dorsal column nuclei. *Brain Research* 369:307-310.

Segal AZ & Rordorf G (1996). Gabapentin as a novel treatment for postherpetic neuralgia. *Neurology* 46 (4):1175-1176.

Sindrup SH, Gram LF et al. (1990). The selective serotonin reuptake inhibitor paroxetine is effective in the treatment of diabetic neuropathy symptoms. *Pain* 42:135-144.

Spiegelmann R & Friedman WA (1991). Spinal cord stimulation: A contemporary series. *Neurosurgery* 28:65-70.

Stenstrom CH (1994). Home exercise in rheumatoid arthritis functional class II: Goal setting versus pain attention. *Journal of Rheumatology* 21:627-634.

Stow PJ, Glynn CJ & Minor B (1989). EMLA cream in the treatment of post herpetic neuralgia: Efficacy and pharmacokinetic profile. *Pain* 39:301-305.

Stux G & Pomeranz B (1995). *Basics of Acupuncture.* Berlin, Germany: Springer Verlag.

Svarcova J, Tranavsky K & Zvarova J (1987). The influence of ultrasound, galvanic currents and shortwave diathermy on pain intensity in patients with osteoarthritis. *Scandinavian Journal of Rheumatology* 67(Suppl):83-85.

Tahmoush AJ, Malley J & Jennings JR (1983). Skin conductance, temperature and blood flow in causalgia. *Neurology* 33:1483-1486.

Tan JC (1998). *Practice Manual of Physical Medicine and Rehabilitation. Diagnostics, Therapeutics and Basic Problems.* Philadelphia, PA: C.V. Mosby.

Taubert K (1997). Massages: Necessary or a luxury? *Z Artzl Fortbild Qualitatssich* 91:139-143.

Travell JG & Simon DG (1983). *Myofascial Pain and Dysfunction: The Trigger Point Manual.* Baltimore, MD: Williams & Wilkins.

Triano JJ, McGregor M, Hondras MA et al. (1995). Manipulative therapy versus education programs in chronic low back pain. *Spine* 20:948-955.

Tsou K (1987). Neurochemical mechanisms of acupuncture. In H Akil & JW Lewis (eds.) *Neurotransmitters and Pain: Control of Pain and Headache, Volume 9.* Basel, Switzerland: H.G. Karger, 226.

Vane JR (1971). Inhibition of prostaglandin synthesis as a mechanism of action for aspirin-like drugs. *Nature* 234:231-238.

Vercauteren MP, Coppejans H & Adriensen HA (1994). Pancreatitis pain treatment: An overview. *Acta Anesthesiologica Belgica* 45:99-105.

Watts RW & Silagy CA (1995). A meta-analysis on the efficacy of epidural corticosteroids in the treatment of sciatica. *Anaesthesia & Intensive Care* 23:564-569.

Weinstein SM & Herring SA (1995). Contemporary concepts in spine care: Epidural steroid injections. *Spine* 20:1842-1846.

Willer JC, DeBrouckner T et al. (1989). Central analgesic effect of ketoprofen in humans. *Pain* 38:1-7.

Winnie AP (2001). Differential neural blockade for the diagnosis of pain mechanisms. In SD Waldman & AP Winnie (eds.) *Interventional Pain Management.* Philadelphia, PA: W.B. Saunders.

Woolf CJ & Wiesenfeld-Hallin Z (1985). The systemic administration of local anesthetic produces a selective depression of C-afferent evoked activity in the spinal cord. *Pain* 23:361-374.

Chapter 5

Opioid Medications in the Management of Pain

Seddon R. Savage, M.D., FASAM

Opioids are among the most potent clinically available analgesic agents. They have wide efficacy and utility in the treatment of acute and cancer-related pain, and are sometimes helpful as a component of the management of chronic non-cancer related pain. With appropriate care, they may be used effectively and safely in individuals with addictive disorders. However, opioids may cause pleasurable intoxication or euphoria in some individuals, sometimes leading to abuse and, in susceptible individuals, to addiction.

This chapter will address key conceptual, pharmacologic, and clinical issues related to opioids as a basis for weighing the potential benefits and risks of their use in the treatment of pain. Contextual issues, prescriptive and monitoring procedures, and legal and regulatory issues are discussed in other chapters.

CONCERNS IN THE USE OF OPIOIDS

Concerns that often are raised in relation to to the use of opioids for analgesia include the potential for physical dependence, tolerance, addiction, abuse, and diversion. These issues appear less significant in the treatment of acute and cancer pain than in the management of chronic non-cancer related pain, but a thorough understanding of them may enhance decisionmaking in all three contexts. Each is considered separately here.

Physical Dependence. Physical dependence is a state of adaptation that is manifested by a drug class-specific withdrawal syndrome that can be produced by abrupt cessation, rapid dose reduction, decreasing blood level of the drug, and/or administration of an antagonist. Such dependence is an expected occurrence in all patients (with and without addictive disease) after 2 to 10 days of continuous administration of an opioid (Portenoy, 1990a). In an acute pain setting, such dependence generally is not clinically significant, because individuals tend to taper opioids naturally due to gradual reduction in pain as the acute problem (such as postoperative pain, posttraumatic pain, or medical illness) resolves. However, if pain medications are abruptly stopped or precipitously reduced, a withdrawal syndrome may ensue. The character and intensity of the withdrawal varies, depending on the dose and duration of opioid administration and a variety of host factors, including previous experience with withdrawal, prior long-term administration of opioids, and the patient's expectations regarding withdrawal.

Common symptoms of opioid withdrawal include autonomic signs and symptoms, such as diarrhea, piloerection, sweating, mydriasis, and mild increases in blood pressure and pulse, as well as signs of central nervous system arousal such as irritability, anxiety, and sleeplessness. Craving for the medication is expected in the course of withdrawal, and pain—most often experienced as abdominal cramping, deep bone pain, or diffuse muscle aching—is common (Jaffe, 1992). Patients with chronic pain may experience an intensified level of their usual pain syndrome during withdrawal. In patients who are physically dependent on opioids, the use of short-acting opioid medications may result in intermittent withdrawal between doses of medication, which may in turn cause an increase in perceived pain (Brodner & Taub, 1978; Jaffe & Martin, 1980). This may be avoided by using long-acting or continuous medications.

Simple physical dependence occurs in any patient when opioids are administered for an extended period of time. The term "addiction" should not be used to describe such physical dependence, as it is an inaccurate description of the condition of physical dependence and it does a disservice both to persons with addictive disorders who become physically dependent on medications despite continuing in a state of recovery, as well as to individuals without addictive disorders who become physically dependent on medications without developing the true characteristics of addiction.

Tolerance. Tolerance is indicated by the need for increasing doses of a medication to achieve the initial effects of the drug (Foley, 1991). Tolerance may occur both to a drug's analgesic effects and to its unwanted side effects, such as respiratory depression, sedation, or nausea.

Many characteristics of opioid tolerance remain poorly understood. Animal studies suggest that tolerance to the analgesic effects of medications occurs in some contexts but not in others (Collins & Cesselin, 1991). Human studies of the management of acute pain also document the development of progressive tolerance to the analgesic effects of opioids when they are administered on a continuous basis over a period of several days (Hill, Chapman et al., 1990; Hill, Coda et al., 1992). Over a period of weeks to months, however, some studies suggest that the continuing development of progressive tolerance to the analgesic effects of opioids may not occur. Specifically, several studies that examined the opioid management of cancer pain suggest that opioid dose requirements increase only during progression of the underlying disease process and that, with stable dis-

ease or treatment of painful tissue pathology, the need for medication remains the same or actually decreases (Foley, 1991; Twycross, 1974).

A number of studies have investigated the development of tolerance to specific opioids, with the goal of determining whether opioids of varying efficacy have different profiles with regard to the development of tolerance, but findings differ radically and no consistent relationship between intrinsic efficacy and tolerance has been demonstrated (Hill, Coda et al., 1992; Kissin, Brown et al., 1991; Yaksh, 1992).

Most investigators agree that absolute tolerance to the analgesic effects of opioids does not occur (Portenoy, 1990b). That is, opioids may be used over a prolonged period of time in the face of increasing dose requirements, yet continue to provide adequate relief of pain. In general, tolerance to the side effects of morphine develops more rapidly than does tolerance to the drug's analgesic effects. Therefore, opioids may be used safely and effectively at even massive doses (such as several thousand mg of IV morphine per hour) in individuals who have gradually increased their exposure to analgesics over a prolonged period of time, with no limiting side effects. Nonetheless, all significant increases in dose should be accompanied by careful monitoring for oversedation and respiratory depression.

Addiction. In the context of pain treatment with opioids, addiction must be defined through the observation of a constellation of maladaptive behaviors, rather than by observation of pharmacologic phenomena such as dependence, tolerance, and dose escalation, since these often are seen in the course of pain treatment. Addiction in the context of opioid therapy of pain is characterized by the presence of a combination of observations suggesting adverse consequences due to use of the drugs, loss of control over drug use, and preoccupation with obtaining opioids despite the presence of adequate analgesia (Sees & Clark, 1993). Physical dependence on opioids and the development of tolerance to their effects do not, of themselves, constitute addiction (Portenoy, 1990b; Savage, 1993; Sees & Clark, 1993). When the criteria for substance use disorder of the *Diagnostic and Statistical Manual of Mental Disorders, 4th Edition* (*DSM-IV*; American Psychiatric Association, 1994) are used to assess for addiction in the presence of pain, only the criteria that refer to function may be used (Sees & Clark, 1993), because other criteria refer only to the expected, non-pathological sequelae of chronic opioid use.

Adverse consequences that are suggestive of addiction (Table 1) include persistent oversedation or euphoria,

---

deteriorating level of function despite relief of pain, or increase in pain-associated distresses such as anxiety, sleep disturbance, or depressive symptoms. Loss of control over use might be reflected in prescriptions used before the expected renewal date, patients who obtain multiple prescriptions, or who obtain opioids from illicit sources. Preoccupation with opioid use may be reflected in noncompliance with non-opioid components of pain treatment, inability to recognize non-nociceptive components of pain, and the perception that no interventions other than opioids have any effect on pain (Savage, 1993; Sees & Clark, 1993; Wesson, Ling et al., 1993). It is important to recognize that such behaviors may occur on an occasional basis for a variety of reasons in the context of successful opioid therapy for pain. By contrast, it is a pattern of persistent occurrences that should prompt concern and further assessment.

The risk of addiction to opioids developing in the course of opioid therapy of pain is thought to be very low, especially for individuals with no past history of addiction. Early studies of "street" addicts led to a misperception that the iatrogenic creation of addiction through medical use of opioids was a frequent occurrence (Kolb, 1925; Rayport, 1954). In contrast, subsequent studies of never-addicted medical patients suggest that the development of addiction in the course of long-term opioid therapy of pain is essentially a negligible risk (Perry & Heindrich, 1982; Porter & Jick, 1980). The reality probably is somewhere in between. Addiction has a multifactorial etiology, including variables that are biogenetic, psychological, sociocultural, and related to drug exposure. The lifetime prevalence of addictive disease is estimated at 3% to 16% of the general population (Regier, Meyers et al., 1984). It is reasonable to expect that this portion of the population may be at some level of risk for the development of addiction when opioids are used for pain, although it has been theorized that the presence of pain may reduce this risk by attenuating the euphorigenic effect of opioids. Nevertheless, it is appropriate to use special care in implementing opioid therapy in patients who have personal or family histories of alcoholism or other addictions, but opioids never should be withheld out of fear of addiction when they are indicated for the relief of pain.

When addiction is identified in the course of opioid therapy of pain, it is important to address it aggressively, so that the pain is effectively controlled and to prevent the debilitating sequelae of addiction. Institution of appropriate addiction treatment services, tightening the structure of opioid prescribing in order to help the individual gain con-

TABLE 1. Problems Suggestive of Addiction Associated with Chronic Opioid Therapy

Adverse consequences of opioid use
- Decreasing functionality;
- Observed intoxication;
- Increasing complaints of pain despite titration of medications;
- Negative affective state.

Loss of control over medication use
- Failure to bring unused medications to appointments;
- Requests for early prescription renewals;
- Reports of "lost" or "stolen" prescriptions;
- Appearance at clinic without appointment and in distress;
- Frequent visits to emergency departments to request drugs;
- Family reports of overuse or intoxication.

Preoccupation with opioids
- Fails to comply with non-drug pain therapies;
- Fails to keep appointments;
- Shows interest only in relief of symptoms, not rehabilitation;
- Reports no effect of non-opioid interventions;
- Seeks prescriptions from multiple providers.

Will not actively address addiction recovery.

trol over the medications, and involving the patient's social support system in treatment are important first steps.

Pseudoaddiction. The term "pseudoaddiction" has emerged in the pain literature to describe the inaccurate interpretation of certain behaviors in patients who have severe pain that is undermedicated or whose pain otherwise has not been effectively treated (Weissman & Haddox, 1989). Such patients may appear to be preoccupied with obtaining opioids, but their preoccupation reflects a need for pain control rather than an addictive drive. Pseudoaddictive behavior can be distinguished from addiction by the fact that, when adequate analgesia is achieved, the patient who is seeking pain relief demonstrates improved function in daily living, uses the medications as prescribed, and does not use drugs in a manner that persistently causes sedation or euphoria. It is important to recognize that such behaviors may occur occasionally even in the successful opioid therapy of pain; rather, it is a pattern of persistent occurrences that should prompt concern and further assessment.

CLINICAL ISSUES IN THE USE OF OPIOIDS

Opioids often are the mainstay of treatment of moderate to severe acute pain and cancer-related pain. When used in the long-term treatment of chronic, non-cancer related pain, they are most often helpful as one component of multidimensional treatment. Goals of pain treatment generally include reduction in pain, enhanced level of function, and improved quality of life.

A number of variables must be considered in planning opioid therapy of pain. In addition to the considerations addressed above, important variables include drug selection, dose titration and scheduling, and management of side effects. It also is clinically important to understand how to appropriately change drugs or withdraw medications when indicated. These issues will be considered individually.

Drug Selection. Opioids produce their pharmacologic effects (both analgesic and side effects) primarily through stimulation of opioid receptors. Stimulation of the mu, kappa, and delta receptors is associated with analgesia and with some side effects, while stimulation of the sigma receptors may be responsible for the dysphoric effects of some opioids. Most of the commonly used opioid analgesics—such as morphine, oxycodone, hydromorphone, meperidine, fentanyl, and methadone—have predominantly mu receptor activity. Pure mu agonists have no ceiling analgesic effect and may be titrated as needed to achieve analgesia. Tolerance to side effects generally occurs more rapidly than tolerance to analgesia, although monitoring for respiratory depression is important, especially in opioid-naive individuals as doses are increased or specific opioids are changed.

While most mu agonists are interchangeable if attention is paid to relative dosing potencies and onset and duration of action (Table 2), emerging evidence suggests that individuals may respond somewhat differently to different opioids. This may be due to variability in opioid receptor function in different individuals, as well as to variable opioid receptor specificity of the different drugs. In addition, some clinically relevant differences between mu agonists long have been apparent.

Meperidine's usefulness in pain treatment is limited by its short half-life and because, with high dose use, a neurotoxic metabolite—normeperidine—may accumulate, causing irritability, tremors and, potentially, seizures. This is especially relevant in opioid-dependent individuals, who may have significant tolerance and correspondingly high dose requirements, as well as in patients with renal or hepatic insufficiency.

Propoxyphene, a weak mu agonist, has low analgesic efficacy and some abuse potential, and has been associated with seizures. Some clinicians believe it is a reasonable analgesic substitute for NSAIDs or acetaminophen in some patients who cannot use those drugs. A subset of patients appear to experience more substantial analgesia with propoxyphene than with NSAIDs. However, most experts agree that propoxyphene has limited utility in pain treatment.

Methadone differs from other mu opioids in several ways. It has a long and unpredictable half-life that necessitates careful titration. Its dextro-isomer has NMDA receptor antagonist activity; it has been experimentally suggested that this may result in less tolerance than occurs with other mu opioids and in greater efficacy in treating neuropathic pain, but this has not been demonstrated clearly in clinical trials. Further, incomplete cross-tolerance between methadone and other mu opioid agonists requires the use of a much lower than equianalgesic dose of methadone in the patient who is transitioning from other mu agonists (as low as 1/10th the equivalent dose or no more than 30 mg per day is recommended by some [Wheeler & Dickerson, 2000]). This may result in poor analgesia when patients are changed from methadone to other opioids. (Moryl, Santiago-Palma et al., 2002). Another mu opioid agonist, levodromoran, is less well studied that methadone but shares a number of its pharmacologic features, including its long half-life and dextro-isomer with NMDA antagonist activity.

A second group of opioids, the agonist-antagonists—including drugs such as pentazocine, nalbuphine, and butorphanol—have predominantly kappa agonist effects, while antagonizing the mu receptor. Agonist-antagonist drugs are widely regarded as having less potential for abuse and addiction than the pure opioid agonists, although addiction to these medications has been observed. Their clinical usefulness as analgesics is limited by a number of factors. The agonist-antagonist drugs exhibit a ceiling effect in terms of analgesia. Their use sometimes is associated with dysphoric reactions. Because of their mu antagonist activity, they may reverse analgesia and precipitate withdrawal in individuals who are physically dependent on mu opioids. Consequently, no clear advantages of agonist-antagonist drugs have been demonstrated in the treatment of pain in persons with addictive disorders, although they may be a reasonable choice in some patients.

A final group of opioids is composed of the partial mu agonists, including buprenorphine and tramadol, which provide analgesia at mu opioid receptors but have relatively low intrinsic efficacy. Clinically, they are very different medications. Buprenorphine is available in parenteral, sublingual and (in Europe) transdermal preparations. It has a long half-life, high receptor affinity, and is useful in agonist treatment of opioid addiction. As an analgesic, it can be used at six- to eight-hour intervals for moderate to moderately severe pain. It is thought by most observers to have a ceiling effect as an analgesic and will not provide continuously increasing analgesia beyond a certain dose titration.

Tramadol (Ultram®), which generally is used in oral form, has a second mechanism of analgesia through the inhibition of reuptake of serotonin and norepinephrine. Doses are limited by a significant potential for seizures at levels above 400 mg per day, which thus is its effective analgesic ceiling. Both buprenorphine and tramadol appear to have somewhat less abuse potential than pure mu opioid analgesics, although this is controversial and there are reports of abuse of both medications.

Opioids may be administered orally, rectally, transmucosally, intravenously, subcutaneously, transdermally, and intraspinally. The oral, enteral, or transdermal routes generally are preferred when feasible because they are less invasive than many other routes and usually provide satisfactory analgesia, even when high doses are required. However, when these routes are not reasonable (as when patients are unable to take medications orally, or when rapid titration is necessary), parenteral routes may be preferred. IV access may be difficult in individuals with a history of injection drug use; for such patients, surgical identification of venous access may be necessary or continuous subcutaneous infusions may be used. Intramuscular injections also are effective, but this route is increasingly discouraged because of the unnecessary pain involved in repeated injection and variable blood levels with this route of administration. If side effects of systemic use are not acceptable, intraspinal opioids may be indicated. Rectal preparations may be useful for patients who are vomiting or who are unable to take

Use of Urine Drug Tests in a Chronic Pain Practice
Howard A. Heit, M.D., FACP, FASAM

Physicians who use opioids in the treatment of chronic pain should make urine drug tests an integral part of the treatment plan, particularly when treating patients who have a history of active addiction or who are in recovery. A drug test should be performed at the time of the initial evaluation and randomly thereafter. Additional indications for random testing are patient resistance to full evaluation at any time during the course of treatment, a patient's request for a specific drug, or any display of aberrant behavior. (However, relying on aberrant behavior alone to trigger testing will miss more than 50% of those who are using unprescribed or illicit drugs [Katz & Fanciullo, 2002].)

The physician should explain the rationale for the urine drug test to the patient, emphasizing that it is not a punitive measure but part of the treatment plan for all patients who are prescribed opioids. It is a consensual diagnostic test for the benefit of the patient.

A drug test that is appropriately positive for the prescribed medication and negative for illicit or non-prescribed drugs provides objective documentation to help answer valid inquiries from regulatory agencies, legal authorities, employers, or family members, who may be concerned about the patient's compliance with the treatment plan. Test results also are useful in diagnosing and treating addictive disorders. In a pain practice, such tests are *not* used for forensic purposes.

Urine may be the best biologic specimen for such testing. It offers a window of detection comparable to that of blood: typically, a urine test is positive for one to three days for most drugs and metabolites (Caplan & Goldberger, 2001). Urine tests also are less costly than blood tests, as well as less invasive.

INTERPRETING TEST RESULTS
The treating physician must be able to correctly interpret the results of urine tests (1) so that he or she does not falsely accuse a patient of non-compliance and (2) in order to diagnose a relapse (if one occurs) and restart or modify the recovery program. If a urine test has an unexpected positive or negative result, the physician should discuss the result with the patient in a positive, supportive fashion.

The following guidelines are offered for any physician who orders a urine drug test:

1. Know that a routine urine drug test is done by immunoassay, which is designed to detect the presence of a particular drug, its metabolite, or class of drug as either present or absent. Specific drug identification is done by GC/MS. A combination of these tests makes possible the accurate identification of a specific drug or metabolite.

2. Know that natural opioids (such as morphine or codeine) can yield a positive result on a routine immunoassay screening test. Methadone, which is a synthetic opioid, does not trigger a positive result on immunoassay unless a test specific for methadone is used. Oxycodone, which is a semi-synthetic opioid, is not reliably detected in immunoassay screening tests even when present in large concentrations (Schults & St. Clair, 1999). A GC/MS assay performed on the same urine specimen will detect oxycodone, particularly if the laboratory is asked to report only the presence or absence of the drug.

3. Know the metabolites of the drugs of abuse the patient may be using, as well as the medications that are prescribed. For example, if codeine is being prescribed, the drug test may be positive for morphine because 10% of codeine is metabolized to morphine (el-Sohly & Jones, 1989). Hydromorphone is a metabolite of hydrocodone, so a test may be positive for hydromorphone if hydrocodone has been ingested (Randall, n.d.). Morphine is not the analgesic of choice for patients with a history of heroin addiction because heroin is metabolized to morphine (Braithwaite, Jarvie et al., 1995) and test results therefore will be positive for morphine. Such a positive result thus could indicate either the presence of the prescribed morphine or relapse to heroin use. A test that is positive for morphine with the presence of 6-monoacetylmorphine (6-MAM), a heroin metabolite, is definitive proof of heroin use within the preceding 12 hours. However, because of its short half-life of 30 minutes, this metabolite seldom is found in urine drug tests (Inturrisi, Max et al., 1984).

4. Know that a test result positive for morphine may result from codeine or morphine ingested in food (such as poppy seeds in some breads or pastries) (Schults, 1999). Instruct the patient to avoid these products to avoid a misleading test result.

CONCLUSIONS

When properly ordered and interpreted, a urine drug test is a valuable component of the care of any patient for whom opioids are indicated for the treatment of moderate to severe pain. For more information on such tests, see the discussion of workplace drug testing in Section 9.

REFERENCES

Braithwaite RA, Jarvie DR, Minty PSB et al. (1995). Screening for drugs of abuse. *Annals of Clinical Biochemistry* 32:123-153.

Caplan YH & Goldberger BA. (2001). Alternative specimens for workplace drug testing. *Journal of Analytical Toxicology* 25:396-399.

Katz N & Fanciullo GJ (2002). Role of urine toxicology testing in the management of chronic opioid therapy. *Clinical Journal of Pain* 18:S76-S82.

el-Sohly MA & Jones AB (1989). Morphine and codeine in biological fluids: Approaches to source differentiation. *Forensic Science Review* 1(1):17.

Inturrisi CE, Max MB, Foley KM et al. (1984). The pharmacokinetics of heroin in patients with chronic pain. *New England Journal of Medicine* 310:1213-1217.

Randall C (n.d.). *Disposition of Toxic Drugs and Chemicals In Man, 2nd Edition.* New York, NY: Baselt, 382-383.

Schults TF & St. Clair (1995). *The Medical Review Officer Handbook, 6th Edition.* Research Triangle Park, NC: Quadrangle Research, LLC, 104-105.

oral medications. Sublingual or transmucosal administration of some preparations is clinically effective as well.

Opioid Side Effects. Opioid side effects can be classified in three groups: respiratory depression, other physical side effects, and central nervous system side effects that may affect function.

Respiratory Depression: Opioid-induced respiratory depression results from depression of brain stem respiratory responses to carbon dioxide. Although CO_2 response decreases in a dose-dependent manner with the administration of mu opioids, clinically significant respiratory depression does not usually occur in the course of treating healthy patients with standard analgesic doses of opioids. Respiratory depression may be significant, however, when highdose opioids are used for acute pain in opioid-naive patients, particularly those who are elderly or debilitated. In such patients, respiratory monitoring is important. Pain is an antidote to respiratory depression, so care should be taken when a patient using high-dose opioids undergoes a definitive procedure that relieves pain, such as a nerve block or spinal cord ablation. Significant sedation most often is a prescursor to respiratory depression and may signal a need to hold medication and adjust the dose.

Respiratory depression rarely is a clinical problem in chronic opioid administration because tolerance to the respiratory depressant effects of opioids tends to occur more rapidly than tolerance to their analgesic effects. Patients should be closely observed, however, when doses are abruptly increased or when patients are rotated to from one opioid to another. Special care also should be exercised in titrating opioids with long half-lives, such as methadone or levodromoran, because delayed respiratory depression may occur.

Other Physical Side Effects: Common physical side effects of opioid use include constipation, nausea, urinary retention, and pruritus. Side effects are minimized when opioids are prescribed in a manner that reduces the peak blood levels required to sustain analgesia, because higher blood levels may be associated with increased side effects. To achieve stable analgesic blood levels, scheduled doses of long-acting or controlled release opioids may be used when oral preparations are used. Continuous infusions or patient-controlled analgesia achieve the same goal when parenteral administration is required. With the exception of constipation, side effects usually are transient and may improve or resolve with continued use of opioids at a stable dose. Side effects sometimes are specific to a particular drug in a particular individual and sometimes can be eliminated by use of an alternative opioid. Persistent physical side effects may be managed through pharmacological treatments, such as anti-emetics for nausea or anti-histamines for pruritus.

Constipation is a persistent side effect of opioid use that may not resolve without treatment. The constipating effects of opioids are thought to occur through direct action on opioid receptors in the gut wall. This causes a decrease in intestinal motility and results in dehydration of stool. It generally is advisable, therefore, to give both a stool softener and a bowel stimulant to effectively manage constipation. When long-term and/or high dose use of opioids is anticipated, introduction of such treatment on a preemptive basis is recommended.

Hepatic, renal, and other organ toxicity generally are not reported with opioids as they are with many non-opioid analgesics, such as acetaminophen and non-steroidal anti-inflammatories. However, close observation and dose adjustments may be appropriate in persons who have im-paired hepatic or renal function, which may result in reduced drug clearance.

CNS Side Effects: Central nervous system (CNS) side effects of opioids may include sedation, cognitive dysfunction, and affective changes. Sedation and mild cognitive changes are common when opioids are introduced or when the dose is increased, but they usually resolve once a stable therapeutic dose of opioid is achieved and sustained for a period of time (Zachny, 1995). Occasionally, however, CNS effects may persist when high doses of opioids are required, particularly when long-acting medications such as methadone are used in elderly or frail patients. Like many other side effects, sedation and cognitive dysfunction may be managed or avoided by changing medications, by continuous administration of the minimum dose necessary to achieve analgesia, or by administration of a treatment medication. When significant persistent opioid-induced sedation occurs in cancer pain patients or patients with other severe intractable pain, stimulants such as methylphenidate and dextroamphetamine may be helpful. The use of stimulant medications, which may be abused by some individuals, requires the same caution in patients with addictive disorder as that required in the use of opioids.

Pain, particularly chronic pain, often is associated with negative mood states such as anxiety or depression. These frequently resolve with effective pain treatment. However, if depression, anxiety, dysphoria, or other distressing affective symptoms occur in the course of analgesic therapy, opioids should be reviewed as a possible contributing factor.

Hyperalgesia: Concerns have been raised that long-term use of opioids may actually increase pain in some contexts. Clinical studies and observations suggest that some individuals with pain who use opioids on a long-term basis experience improvement in pain following simple withdrawal of opioids, without the institution of other major pain interventions (Brodner & Taub, 1978; Rapaport, 1988; Schofferman, 1993). These studies include observations of patients with pain and opioid dependence in both pain treatment and addiction treatment settings. Some experts attribute this to withdrawal-mediated pain associated with short-acting opioids, but some evidence suggests that opioids may facilitate pain more directly.

Because opioid receptors are important components of endogenous pain modulatory systems, it is reasonable to speculate that changes in nociceptive processing may occur as a result of chronic opioid administration, which in turn

TABLE 2. Equianalgesic Doses of Opioid Drugs

Drug	Approximate Equianalgesic Oral Dose	Approximate Equianalgesic Parenteral Dose
Opioid Agonists		
Morphine	30 mg q 3–4 hours	10 mg q 3–4 hours
Codeine	130 mg q 3–4 hours	75 mg q 3–4 hours
Hydromorphone (Dilaudid®)	7.5 mg q 3–4 hours	1.5 mg q 3–4 hours
Levorphanol (Levo-Dromoran®)	4 mg q 6–8 hours (acute) 1 mg q 6–8 hours (chronic)	2 mg q 6–8 hours (acute) 1 mg q 6–8 hours (chronic)
Meperidine (Demerol®)	300 mg q 2–3 hours	75 mg q 2–3 hours
Methadone (Dolophine®, others)	20 mg q 6–8 hours (acute) 2–4 mg q 6–8 hours (chronic)	10 mg q 6–8 hours (acute) 2–4 mg q 6–8 hours (chronic)
Oxycodone (Percodan®, Percocet®, Roxicodone®, Tylox®)	20 mg q 3–4 hours	Not available
Opioid Agonist/Antagonist Drugs and Partial Agonists		
Buprenorphine (Buprenex®)	Not available	0.4 mg q 6–8 hours
Butorphanol (Stadol®)	Not available	2 mg q 3–4 hours
Nalbuphine (Nubain®)	Not available	10 mg q 3–4 hours

NOTE: These should be considered approximate estimates. Equivalencies may vary from individual to individual. Doses are based on single dose studies and do not necessarily reflect analgesic equivalence with continued dosing. A dose lower than the calculated equianalgesic dose always should be used when switching patients from one opioid to another because of incomplete cross-tolerance between opioids. Special case should be used in changing to methadone or levodromoran because of the pronounced lack of cross-tolerance with other opioids and the potential for delayed respiratory depression due to long half-lives. All patients should be observed carefully for sedation and respiratory depression when opioid doses are initiated or abruptly increased or when a new opioid is used, and doses adapted accordingly.

CAUTION: Recommended doses do not apply to patients with renal or hepatic insufficiency or other conditions affecting drug metabolism and kinetics.

CAUTION: Doses listed for patients with body weight of less than 50 kg cannot be used as initial starting doses in infants younger than 6 months of age. Consult the AHCPR Clinical Practice Guideline for Acute Pain Management for recommendations.

SOURCES: Adapted from the Panel on Acute Pain Guidelines (1992). *Acute Pain Management: Operative or Medical Procedures and Trauma.* Rockville, MD: Agency for Health Care Policy Research, and the American Pain Society (1999). *Principles of Analgesic Use in the Treatment of Acute Pain and Cancer Pain, 4th Edition.* Skokie, IL: The Society.

may alter pain sensitivity in individuals who are given opioids on a chronic basis. One study demonstrated a significantly decreased threshold for cold pressor-induced pain in methadone maintenance patients (who were taking their usual dose of methadone), as compared to several control groups of formerly methadone-dependent individuals and persons who had no history of dependence on any drug (Compton, 1996).

The development of hyperalgesia in some patients in the presence of high-dose systemic morphine administration is well documented (Sjogren, Jensen et al., 1994). In addition, experimental evidence suggests that, under certain conditions, opioids may act as agonists at NMDA receptors in a manner that facilitates pain transmission (Xiangqi, Martin et al., 2001). The extent to which these findings have general clinical relevance for patients who use opioids on a long-term basis is not clear. As more patients with chronic pain of non-cancer origin and normal life expectancy are prescribed opioids for long-term management of pain, controlled studies of the effects of long-term opioids on pain modulation will be important to better understand the circumstances under which hyperalgesia may occur and how best to address the problem.

Dose Titration and Scheduling. *Measuring Efficacy*: The serial use of a pain scale before treatment and at regular intervals during treatment is helpful in assessing pain and its response to treatment (see Chapter 2).

Factors Affecting Dose Requirements: In determining the dose and interval of administration that will provide effective analgesia in a given patient for a given problem, several factors must be considered. The pharmacologic characteristics of each drug in terms of onset, relative potency, and duration of analgesic action must be considered. The marked variability among patients in intrinsic responsiveness to opioids must be appreciated and accommodated (Foley, 1991). Finally, individuals who have been exposed to opioids on a prolonged basis, or who are actively using opioids (whether therapeutically or due to addiction) are likely to be relatively tolerant to the analgesic effects of opioids and therefore may require relatively high doses at relatively short intervals to achieve analgesia. If the patient used opioids on a daily basis prior to the onset of acute pain, then his or her usual dose of opioids cannot be expected to provide analgesia for acute pain, and additional treatment must be provided.

Schedules: In discussing medication scheduling, distinctions often are made between short-acting and long-acting medications. Long-acting medications include those that are intrinsically long-acting, such as methadone or levodromoran, and medications that are long-acting by virtue of being formulated in controlled-release preparations, such oral sustained-released oxycodone or morphine and transdermal fentanyl. Most other opioids are short-acting and immediate-release.

For moderate pain requiring opioid therapy, a partial mu agonist (such as tramadol), an agonist-antagonist opioid, or a weak opioid combined with acetaminophen or aspirin (such as acetominophen or aspirin with codeine, hydro-

codone, or oxycodone) often is appropriate. If pain is constant, the drug should be given at scheduled and pharmacologically appropriate intervals to maintain analgesic blood levels. If the pain is intermittent, the drug can be given on an as-needed basis.

Care must be taken in providing opioids on a PRN basis, particularly to an individual with an addictive or chronic pain disorder. Pairing the perception of pain with the administration of a reinforcing drug theoretically could increase perceived pain and be viewed as legitimizing increased use of the drug (Fordyce, 1992). Potential reinforcement of pain may be reduced by avoiding the use of opioids paired directly with the experience of increased pain. For example, instead of taking opioids in response to pain graded at a certain level of severity, the patient could be directed to use opioids in a time- or activity-contingent manner, taking the medication at a scheduled time or in association with a valued activity. The scheduled time is selected to coordinate with expected increases in pain or on a regular basis if continuous relief is the goal.

For constant pain at a moderate level of intensity, when an opioid is indicated, a relatively low dose of a long-acting pure mu agonist (such as methadone or a controlled release preparation of morphine, oxycodone or other opioid) may be appropriate. This might be indicated if significant breakthrough pain occurs with short-acting medications, or dose requirements result in toxic doses of acetaminophen or aspirin.

For severe pain, a pure mu agonist that can be titrated (that is, not mixed with limiting doses of acetaminophen or other drugs and not having a ceiling of effectiveness) usually is indicated. If the pain is continuous, patient-controlled analgesia, a continuous parenteral infusion, or long-acting oral or transdermal medications are appropriate. Rescue doses of PRN medications should be provided for breakthrough pain or exacerbations of baseline pain. The frequency of permitted rescue doses must be determined according to the context. When multiple doses are required each day, this generally indicates a need for a higher baseline dose of long-acting medications. In the chronic non-cancer pain setting, if long-acting opioids are used for continuous pain, PRN doses usually are reserved for major exacerbations of pain to deter unnecessary frequent ER or clinic visits. Some chronic pain patients have predictable activity-related pain that may require regular PRN doses.

Patient-Controlled Analgesia: Patient-controlled analgesia (PCA) can be used successfully in individuals with addictive disease and sometimes is the preferred method of providing postoperative and posttraumatic pain control. It often is used in the setting of advanced cancer pain as well. PCA allows the patient to self-administer small, incremental doses of opioids intravenously or subcutaneously and thus provides stable analgesic blood levels of opioids. It usually produces more uniform pain relief at a lower total dose of medications than bolus dosing or continuous infusions (Hill, Chapman et al., 1990). It avoids peaks (which may cause sedation or intoxication) and valleys (which may result in pain, anxiety and drug craving). As with scheduled dosing, the use of PCA eliminates the need for the patient to request opioids for pain relief and thus avoids potential conflicts between patients and staff, which can arise when persons with addictive disease request opioids. For persons with significant opioid tolerance, a background infusion may be used with PCA.

On the other hand, because PCA requires self-administration, it may create ambivalence in recovering persons and in patients with active addiction who have difficulty limiting their administration of opioids to levels that provide analgesia without intoxication. The latter problem may be managed to some degree through the physician's control of the incremental dose size and frequency and the total dose available over a period of time. In theory, PCA may reinforce pain through the pairing of pain with self-administration of opioids and thus may make cessation of analgesic doses of opioids difficult. In practice, however, these issues rarely arise, probably because the small incremental doses provided by PCA provide relatively little reward.

Enhancing Control: When scheduled medications are required on an outpatient basis in individuals with addictive disease, it is helpful to give specific times for drug administration (for example, at 7:00 AM, 3:00 PM, and 11:00 PM), rather than indicating that a drug should be taken three times a day or every eight hours. This reduces the potential for confusion over dosing and possible resulting misuse.

If an individual has difficulty controlling medication use but needs opioids for pain relief, it may be helpful to have a trusted other, such as a spouse or friend, dispense the medications, either by the dose or at time-limited intervals such as every one or two days. Daily dispensing also may be arranged through a visiting nurse, pharmacy, or hospice.

Changing Opioids. Transition from one opioid to another may be indicated in a number of circumstances, as when progressive tolerance develops, when a patient on chronic oral opioids becomes NPO, or when significant side effects occur with an opioid. When changing from one opioid to another, it is important to understand how to calculate equianalgesic doses of medications and how to modify those doses appropriately in order to maintain analgesia and to avoid serious side effects. Parenteral morphine often is used as the standard reference in calculating opioid equivalencies. The first step in calculating a reasonable dose of a new opioid is to determine the total dose of each opioid used in the previous 24-hour period. Then, using an opioid equivalence table, the equivalent dose of parenteral morphine is determined. This subsequently is converted to the 24-hour dose of the new opioid. This 24-hour dose should be lowered to accommodate opioid-specific tolerance and the potentially greater analgesic efficacy and side effects of the new drug. One-half to two-thirds of the calculated equianalgesic dose often is used as a "rule of thumb" in switching to many opioids. However, for methadone (and probably levodromoran) the percentage should be much lower: 1/10th has been suggested with oral methadone, begun at no more than 30 mg per day. The 24-hour dose of the new drug should be given in divided doses at appropriate intervals (see Table 2).

This method avoids the confusion that arises in trying to convert several medications at different doses and comparing drugs of differing half-lives and potencies. Any calculation, however, should be viewed only as a rough guideline and, when medications are changed, patients should be monitored closely and dosing adapted according to clinical responses. The potential for delayed respiratory depression with opioids that have long half-lives should be appreciated.

Sometimes the transition from one opioid to another is better tolerated if the patient is gradually "rolled over" from one medication to another. That is, the new medication is increased incrementally over a few days, while the old medication is decreased incrementally. This also permits observation of the patient's response to the new drug and adjustment of the dose to avoid side effects and maintain analgesia.

Management of Withdrawal. In the acute pain setting, most patient gradually taper their medications without incident as pain gradually improves. However, tapering sometimes is impeded by withdrawal or craving because of troughs in blood levels while physical dependence is present. If the patient has been using an intermittently administered medication such as bolus parenteral morphine or oral oxycodone, the interval of administration can be decreased somewhat as the dose is decreased in order to avoid precipitously low blood levels of the drug between doses. Alternatively, the patient can be transferred to a continuous parenteral infusion or an equianalgesic dose of a long-acting oral medication (such as methadone, controlled release morphine, or oxycodone) and the dose gradually tapered.

If abrupt cessation of opioids is necessary, an acute withdrawal syndrome may be attenuated to some degree through the prescription of alternative medications. Clonidine may be used to attenuate the autonomic signs and symptoms of withdrawal (Jasinski, Johnson et al., 1985); a benzodiazepine or other sedative-hypnotic may be given to reduce irritability, anxiety, and sleeplessness; and a non-opioid analgesic such as a non-steroidal anti-inflammatory or acetaminophen may be used to attenuate pain. Because clonidine may have intrinsic analgesic effects for some types of pain, it may be continued if the patient experiences pain relief with its use. Benzodiazepines should be given at the usual anxiolytic dose and titrated to effect, then tapered following withdrawal. NSAIDs are given at the usual analgesic dose.

Boundary-Setting When Using Opioids in Patients with Addictive Disorder. For the patient with an addictive disorder, boundary setting must be part of any pain treatment plan that includes opioids. This means that the goals of treatment and the means of achieving those goals must be clear to both patient and physician and that the roles and responsibilities of each are defined. A written agreement, signed by both the patient and the clinician, usually is important in using opioids to treat chronic pain, and may be helpful in treating acute pain as well. A written agreement also may serve as a vehicle for informed consent. Agreements may reduce the potential for relapse by providing structure and support to the patient and may allow the clinician to identify relapse more easily when it occurs. Such an agreement also facilitates review and modification of the treatment plan as needed.

Opioid treatment agreements vary widely. Typically, they include an acknowledgement of the potential benefits and risks of opioid therapy; the goals of treatment; identification of one provider and one pharmacy as a source of all opioids; authorization for communication with all care providers and (sometimes) significant others; other treatments or consultations in which the patient is expected to participate, including recovery activities; any special medication-dispensing mechanism; acknowledgement of the need to avoid non-prescribed drugs; permission for urine drug screens and pill counts as appropriate; mechanisms for medication renewals, including exclusion of early renewals; expected intervals for office visits; and specification of the conditions under which therapy will be continued or discontinued. (In the treatment of acute pain, such an agreement often is simpler.)

Violations of the treatment agreement should be taken seriously and used an opportunity to further assess the patient for medication misuse, addiction relapse, drug diversion, under-treated pain, or other issues. The physician and patient should weigh the potential benefits and risks of treatment and determine whether opioid therapy continues to be appropriate or should be discontinued. If continued, boundaries should be adjusted to support safe and appropriate medication use. If discontinued, the physically dependent patient should be tapered through use of a safely structured regimen.

CONCLUSIONS

In the past, medical, legal, public, and regulatory opinion tended to discourage physicians from using opioids for the treatment of pain. With increased scientific and clinical understanding of pain, addiction, and the pharmacology of opioids, this is gradually changing. Numerous initiatives to foster the aggressive treatment of pain have been activated over the past two decades. The Agency for Health Care Policy Research (AHCPR; now the Agency for Healthcare Research and Quality) of the U.S. Department of Health and Human Services has released guidelines for the management of acute pain and cancer pain, which encourage the effective use of opioids as needed (AHCPR, 1992, 1994). The Federation of State Medical Boards of the United States (FSMB) also has developed guidelines for the use of controlled substances to manage pain. These guidelines affirm the right of physicians to use opioids when appropriate to manage all types of pain.

In order to use opioids effectively and safely when they are indicated, physicians must understand pharmacologic and clinical issues related to opioids and carefully structure treatment with respect to the particular benefits and risks for individual patients. Opioids have an important role in relieving human suffering. At the same time, it is important to respect their potential to cause harm in vulnerable individuals. It is to be hoped that, over time, science and clinical experience will provide a fuller understanding of ways to harness the full potential of opioids to relieve suffering while eliminating the potentially negative consequences of their use.

REFERENCES

Agency for Health Care Policy Research (AHCPR) (1992). *Acute Pain Management: Operative or Medical Procedures and Trauma.* Rockville, MD: AHCPR, U.S. Department of Health and Human Services.

Agency for Health Care Policy Research (AHCPR) (1994). *Cancer Pain Management: Clinical Practice Guidelines.* Rockville, MD: AHCPR, U.S. Department of Health and Human Services.

Ahles T, Blanchard E & Ruckdeschel J (1983). The multidimensional nature of cancer related pain. *Pain* 17:277-288.

American Pain Society (APS) (1989). *Principles of Analgesic Use in the Treatment of Acute Pain and Chronic Cancer Pain (2nd Edition).* Skokie, IL: The Society.

American Psychiatric Association (APA) (1994). *Diagnostic and Statistical Manual of Mental Disorders, 4th Edition (DSM-IV).* Washington, DC: American Psychiatric Press.

American Society of Addiction Medicine (ASAM) (1997). Public policy statements. *Definition Related to the Use of Opioids for the Treatment of Pain* and *On the Rights and Responsibilities of Physicians in the Use of Opioids for the Treatment of Pain.* Chevy Chase, MD: The Society.

Brodner RA & Taub A (1978). Chronic pain exacerbated by long-term narcotic use in patients with non-malignant disease: Clinical syndrome and treatment. *Mt. Sinai Journal of Medicine* 45:233-237.

Clark H (1993). Opioids, chronic pain, and the law. *Journal of Pain & Symptom Management* 8(5):297-306.

Collett BJ (1998). Opioid tolerance: The clinical perspective. *British Journal of Anesthesia* 81: 58-68.

Collins E & Cesselin F (1991). Neurobiological mechanisms of opioid tolerance and dependence. *Clinical Neuropharmacology* 14:465-488.

Compton M (1994). Cold pressor pain tolerance in opiate and cocaine abusers: Correlates of drug type and use status. *Journal of Pain & Symptom Management* 9(7):462-473.

Davis AM & Inturrisi CE (1993). D-methadone blocks morphine tolerance and N-methyl-D-aspartate-induced hyperalgesia. *Journal of Pharmacology and Experimental Therapeutics* 289(2):1048-1053.

Foley K (1991). Clinical tolerance to opioids. In A Basbaum & J Besson (eds.) *Towards a New Pharmacotherapy of Pain.* New York, NY: John Wiley & Sons, 181-203.

Fordyce W (1992). Opioids, pain and behavioral outcomes. *American Pain Society Journal* 1(4):282-284.

Gagnon B & Bruera E (1999). Differences in the ratios of morphine to methadone in patients with neuropathic pain versus non-neuropathic pain. *Journal of Pain & Symptom Management* 18(2):120-125.

Gamsa A (1994). The role of psychological factors in chronic pain, I. A half century of study. *Pain* 57(1):5-16.

Gardner E (1992). Brain reward mechanisms. In J Lowinson, P Ruiz & R Millman (eds.) *Substance Abuse: A Comprehensive Textbook.* Baltimore, MD: Williams & Wilkins, 70-99.

Hill H, Chapman C, Kornell J et al. (1990). Self-administration of morphine in bone marrow transplant patients reduces drug treatment. *Pain* 40:121-129.

Hill H, Coda B, Mackie A et al. (1992). Patient-controlled analgesic infusions: Alfentanyl versus morphine. *Pain* 49:301-310.

Jaffe J (1980). Drug addiction and drug abuse. In A Gilman, L Goodman, T Rall et al. (eds.) *The Pharmacologic Basis of Therapeutics.* New York, NY: Macmillan, 532-581.

Jaffe J (1992). Opiates: Clinical aspects. In J Lowinson, P Ruiz & R Millman (eds.) *Substance Abuse: A Comprehensive Textbook.* Baltimore, MD: Williams & Wilkins, 186-194

Jaffe J & Martin W (1980). Opioid agonists. In A Gilman, L Goodman, T Rall et al. (eds.) *The Pharmacologic Basis of Therapeutics.* New York, NY: Macmillan, 491-531.

Jasinski D, Johnson R & Kocher T (1985). Clonidine in morphine withdrawal: Differential effects on sign and symptoms. *Archives of General Psychiatry* 42:1063-1065.

Johanson C & Schuster C (1981). Animal models of drug self-administration. In N Mello (ed.) *Advances in Substance Abuse Research.* Greenwich, CT: JAAI Press, 219-297.

Joranson D, Cleeland C & Weissman DE (1991). Opioids for Chronic Cancer and Non-Cancer Pain: Survey of Medical Licensing Boards. Presentation at the Annual Meeting of the American Pain Society; New Orleans, LA.

Joranson DE (1995). Intractable pain treatment laws and regulations. *American Pain Society Bulletin* 5(2):1-3, 15-17.

Kissin I, Brown P & Bailey E (1991). Magnitude of acute tolerance to opioids is not related to their potency. *Anesthesiology* 75:813-816.

Kolb L (1925). Types and characteristics of drug addicts. *Mental Hygiene* 9:300.

Koob G & Bloom F (1988). Cellular and molecular mechanisms of drug dependence. *Science* 242:715-723.

Liaison Committee on Pain and Addiction (AAPM, APS, ASAM) (2001). *Definitions Related to the Use of Opioids for the Treatment of Pain.* Available at WWW.AMPAINSOC.ORG.

Marks J & Sacher E (1973). Undertreatment of medical inpatients with narcotic analgesics. *Annals of Internal Medicine* 78:173-181.

Morgan J (1985). American opiophobia: Customary underutilization of opioid analgesics. *Advances in Alcohol and Substance Abuse* 5:163.

Moryl N, Santiago-Palma J, Kornick C et al. (2002). Pitfalls of opioid rotation: Substituting another opioid for methadone in patients with cancer pain. *Pain* 96:325-328.

Parrino M (1991a). Overview: Current treatment realities and future trends. In C Panel (ed.) *State Methadone Treatment Guidelines.* Rockville, MD: Center for Substance Abuse Treatment, 1-9.

Parrino M, ed. (1991b). *State Methadone Treatment Guidelines.* Rockville MD: Center for Substance Abuse Treatment.

Perry S & Heindrich G (1982). Management of pain during debridement: A survey of U.S. burn units. *Pain* 13:12-14.

Portenoy R (1990a). Chronic opioid therapy in nonmalignant pain. *Journal of Pain and Symptom Management*, 5.

Portenoy R (1990b). Pharmacotherapy of cancer pain. In *Refresher Courses on Pain Management.* Adelaide, Australia: IASP Refresher Courses, 101-112.

Porter J & Jick H (1980). Addiction rare in patients treated with narcotics. *New England Journal of Medicine* 302:123.

Rapaport A (1988). Analgesic rebound headache. *Headache* 28(10):662-665.

Rayport M (1954). Experience in the management of patients medically addicted to narcotics. *Journal of the American Medical Association* 165:684-691.

Regier D, Meyers JK & Kramer M (1984). The NIMH Epidemiological Catchment Area Study. *Archives of General Psychiatry* 41:934-958.

Savage SR (1993). Addiction in the treatment of pain: Significance, recognition and treatment. *Journal of Pain & Symptom Management* 8(5):265-278.

Savage SR (1996). Long-term opioid therapy: Assessment of consequences of risks. *Journal of Pain & Symptom Management* 11:274-286.

Schofferman J (1993). Long-term use of opioid analgesics for the treatment of chronic pain of nonmalignant origin. *Journal of Pain & Symptom Management* 8(5):279-288.

Sees KL & Clark W (1993). Opioid use in the treatment of chronic pain: Assessment of addiction. *Journal of Pain & Symptom Management* 8(5):257-264.

Shine D & Demas P (1984). Knowledge of medical students, residents and attending physicians about opiate abuse. *Journal of Medical Education* 59:501-507.

Sjogren P, Jensen N & Jensen T (1994). Disappearance of morphine-induced hyperalgesia after discontinuing or substituting morphine with other opioid agonists. *Pain* 59:313-316.

Turk D & Meichenbaum D (1984). A cognitive and behavioral approach to pain. In P Wall & R Melzach (eds.) *Textbook of Pain*. Edinburgh, Scotland: Churchill Livingston, 787-794.

Turk DC, Meichenbaum DH & Genost M (1983). *Pain and Behavioral Medicine: A Cognitive Behavioral Perspective*. New York, NY: Guilford Press.

Twycross R (1974). Clinical experience with diamorphine in advanced malignant disease. *International Journal of Clinical Pharmacology, Therapy and Toxicology* 9:184-198.

Weissman DE & Haddox JD (1989). Opioid pseudoaddiction: An iatrogenic syndrome. *Pain* 36:363-366.

Wesson D, Ling W & Smith D (1993). Prescription of opioids for treatment of pain in patients with addictive disease. *Journal of Pain & Symptom Management* 8(5):289-296.

Wheeler WL & Dickerson ED (2000). Clinical applications of methadone. *American Journal of Hospice & Palliative Care* 17(3):196-203.

Xiangqi Li, Martin S, Angst J et al. (2001). A murine model of opioid-induced hyperalgesia. *Molecular Brain Research* 86:56-62.

Yaksh T (1992). The spinal pharmacology of acutely and chronically administered opioids. *Journal of Pain & Symptom Management* 7:356-361.

Zachny J (1995). A review of the effects of opioids on psychomotor and cognitive functioning in humans. *Experimental & Clinical Psychopharmacology* 3, 432-466.

Zenz M, Strumph M & Tryba M (1992). Long-term oral opioid therapy in patients with chronic non-malignant pain. *Journal of Pain & Symptom Management* 7(2):69-77.

| Chapter 6 | # Legal and Regulatory Issues in the Management of Pain |

David E. Joranson, M.S.S.W.
Aaron M. Gilson, Ph.D.

Policies Governing Drug Availability
Defining Addiction
Policies That Can Influence Prescribing

Pain is prevalent in cancer and in other diseases and conditions, especially near the end of life (Bernabei, Gambassi et al., 1998; Cleeland, Gonin et al., 1997; Ferrell, Juarez et al., 1999; Nowels & Lee, 1999; SUPPORT, 1995). Pain often is not treated adequately. Unrelieved pain can impair all aspects of ordinary life activities and lead a patient to wish for death (Institute of Medicine, 1997). Relief of pain improves quality of life and can decrease suffering (WHO, 1986).

Many pharmacologic and nonpharmacologic treatments are available for the relief of pain. Opioid analgesics such as morphine are considered safe and effective, especially for the management of moderate to severe pain due to cancer (Jacox, Carr et al., 1994; Portenoy, 1989, 1996; WHO, 1996). The use of opioids to manage chronic noncancer pain increasingly is recognized as appropriate.

Opioids must be available when and where patients need them, especially when pain is severe (Institute of Medicine, 1997; WHO, 1990). Physicians, pharmacists and nurses must be able to prescribe, administer, and dispense opioids according to individual patient needs (WHO, 1996). However, the use of opioids historically has been marginalized because of concerns about side effects and abuse liability. As a result, some patients find it difficult to obtain this essential medication; this is especially true for patients in pain who have a history of drug abuse or using drugs for nontherapeutic purposes (Portenoy, 1996; Savage, 1999).

This chapter reviews the laws, regulations, and medical board policies that govern the use of opioids, including some that impede access to appropriate pain management for patients who are addicted to, or in recovery from, controlled substances.

POLICIES GOVERNING DRUG AVAILABILITY
Before specific examples of policy language are presented, brief definitions of the types of policies to be discussed here will be provided. "Law" is a broad term that refers to rules of conduct with binding legal force adopted by legislative or other government bodies at the international, federal, state, or local levels. Laws can be found in treaties, constitutional provisions, court decisions, statutes, and regulations. The most basic laws usually are the statutes enacted by a legislature. A number of laws have been adopted by the states concerning pain management, with Intractable Pain

Treatment Acts (IPTAs) the most common form of statutory pain policy.

A "regulation" is an official rule issued by an agency of the executive branch of government. Regulations often are found in an administrative code or code of regulation. Regulations have the force of law, and are intended to implement or interpret statutory authority granted to an agency, often to establish what conduct is or is not acceptable for those regulated by the agency (such as physicians, pharmacists, and nurses). Regulations issued by state agencies should not exceed the scope of the agency's statutory authority.

"Guideline," as used here, means an official adopted policy statement that is issued by a government agency, such as a state medical board, to express its attitude or position on a particular matter. While guidelines do not have binding legal force, they may outline parameters or standards of conduct for those who are regulated by an agency. For example, a number of state medical boards have issued guidelines regarding the medical use of opioids that define the conduct the board considers to be within, as well as outside of, the professional practice of medicine. Some pharmacy and nursing boards have issued similar guidelines. Guidelines also include policy statements that may appear in a position paper, report, article, or agency newsletter.

International Policies. The prescribing and dispensing of opioids is governed by international treaties, U.S. federal law and regulations, and state laws and regulations. Although the singular purpose of these policies typically is perceived to be the control of diversion and the prevention of illicit drug use, drug control policy has a second and equally important purpose—to ensure drug availability. Opioids are necessary for the relief of pain and must be adequately available for medical purposes (United Nations, 1977a). Public policies that recognize both control and availability are said to represent a "balanced" approach (Joranson & Dahl, 1989; Joranson, 1990a; Joranson & Gilson, 1994b). In achieving a proper balance between availability and control, the United Nations drug control authorities assert that efforts to prevent drug abuse and diversion should not interfere with the availability and medical use of controlled drugs (United Nations, 1977a, 1977b).

Federal Policies. Many prescription drugs, including opioid analgesics, are approved as both safe and effective for human use under medical supervision by the U.S. Food and Drug Administration (FDA), according to authority granted to that agency by the federal Food, Drug and Cosmetic Act of 1962 (FFDCA). Prescribing decisions are medical decisions; physicians generally are allowed to prescribe for a medical purpose and in the interest of the patient according to their best judgment (Federal Register, 1975). Prescription drugs may be prescribed for other than their labeled indications or recommended doses if there is a medical rationale (Federal Register, 1983). FDA does not regulate medical practice (United States vs. Evers, 1981); rather, it is the states, not the federal government, that govern the practice of medicine (Joranson & Gilson, 1994b).

In addition to FDA regulation, opioid analgesics are subject to controlled substances policies because of their abuse liability. The Controlled Substances Act (CSA, 1970) is a federal law that established the U.S. system of drug control and is intended to reflect both control and availability, paralleling the international treaties. Availability is accomplished through a regulated distribution system that governs import, manufacture, distribution, prescribing, dispensing, and possession. Licensed professionals may prescribe, dispense, and administer controlled drugs for legitimate medical purposes and in the course of professional practice if they have a state license to practice their profession and a valid controlled substances registration from the U.S. Drug Enforcement Administration (DEA). To prevent diversion, the CSA establishes a system of requirements, penalties, security, recordkeeping, and monitoring. The Code of Federal Regulations (CFR) (Title 21, Chapter 2) is the regulation that implements federal law. The CFR is administered by the federal Drug Enforcement Administration (DEA).

The CSA recognizes that controlled substances are necessary for public health and that availability of prescription controlled substances must be ensured. The CSA states that "many of the drugs included within this title have a useful and legitimate medical purpose and are necessary to maintain the health and general welfare of the American people" (CSA, 1970, p. 834).

CSA Drug Schedules: The CSA classifies controlled substances into five schedules, according to abuse liability. Each schedule carries a different penalty for unlawful use. Requirements for prescriptions also vary depending on the schedule. Schedule I lists the drugs that have no accepted medical use and are available only for scientific research (such as marijuana, methaqualone, and heroin). Schedules II through V list drugs that are approved by the FDA for medical use but have an abuse potential, such as the opioids. Those opioids with the highest potential for abuse (and which also are indispensable for the relief of pain) are placed in Schedule II; they include morphine, hydromorphone, oxycodone, meperidine, and fentanyl. Schedule III contains drugs with less abuse potentials and important medical uses, and includes opioids such as hydrocodone and codeine combinations. Schedule IV includes opioids with important medical uses, such as dextropropoxyphene and codeine compounded in smaller doses. Schedule V drugs have the lowest abuse potential, including opioid-containing antitussives and antidiarrheals.

Federal Laws Related to Opioid Prescribing: All persons or business entities that manufacture, order, prescribe, or dispense controlled substances must be registered with the DEA. All registrants' purchases must be made using a special triplicate order form (not to be confused with the triplicate prescription form required in several states). This allows the DEA to monitor all transfers of controlled substances within a "closed distribution system." Prescriptions for Schedule II drugs must be in written form and may not be refilled, while five refills are permitted for drugs in Schedules III and IV. Federal law allows oral prescriptions of controlled substances in Schedule II in medical emergencies and under specific circumstances (21 CFR §1306.11(d)), but these must be followed with a written prescription within a specified period of time. Federal law also allows for the partial dispensing (21 CFR §1306.13) and faxing (21 CFR §1306.11(a)) of Schedule II prescriptions under certain circumstances. Federal laws and regulations do not limit the amount of drug prescribed, the duration for which a drug is prescribed, or the period for which a prescription is valid (although some states do). There are penalties, both criminal and civil, for violation of the federal requirements.

The CSA does not permit the prescribing of narcotic drugs for the purpose of maintenance or detoxification treatment of narcotic addiction, except where an entity has a separate federal registration as an Opioid Treatment Program (OTP). OTPs may dispense but not prescribe narcotic drugs approved for this purpose, such as methadone, and must comply with federal and state regulations. However, it is important to note that methadone may be prescribed and dispensed for the relief of pain, just as one would prescribe any other Schedule II opioid analgesic.

State Policies. The regulation of medical practice occurs at the state, not the federal, level. Therefore, numerous state laws, regulations, and policies may further limit medical practice using controlled substances. State legislatures have adopted statutes to protect the public; these provide authority for a state agency to license and discipline members of the health care professions. The law creates oversight boards, such as boards of medicine, pharmacy, or nursing, to license and discipline members of their respective professions.

Boards may adopt regulations to implement the laws governing medical practice. A board's rule-making procedures are a matter for public input and public record. Typically, board members are appointed by the Governor for staggered terms. Sometimes this is done in consultation with the professional association representing the regulated profession.

Board investigation of a licensee may be initiated by a complaint or by referral from another agency. Boards differ greatly as to the procedures used for initial inquiry and investigation into complaints. Some boards, by law, are required to investigate each complaint received, while others can exercise discretion. In some states, the mere filing of a complaint against a physician is a matter of public record. Investigations may be prompt, and may be dropped due to insufficient evidence, or may proceed to disciplinary action. On the other hand, some proceedings take several years to resolve. If the board finds that there have been violations, a range of actions may be considered, depending on the nature and seriousness of the violation; these may include a warning, education, limitation or removal of prescribing privileges, or suspension or revocation of the professional's license.

Board disciplinary actions are reviewable by the state courts. Boards also manage programs to assist in the identification, treatment, and recovery of impaired licensees.

All of the licensing boards have national organizations: for medical boards, it is the Federation of State Medical Boards of the United States (FSMB); for pharmacy boards, it is the National Association of Boards of Pharmacy (NABP); for nursing boards, it is the National Council of State Boards of Nursing (NCSBN). These organizations sponsor a number of activities, such as (1) annual meetings, (2) task forces to study specific issues relevant to the regulation of that profession, and (3) technical assistance, training, policy development, and preparation of model laws and regulations, as well as dissemination of information, including newsletters and statistics about licensees and disciplinary actions.

In addition to professional practice policy, the states have adopted versions of the CSA in order to apply state laws to the control of drugs with abuse liability. Typically, these laws are patterned after the model Uniform Controlled Substances Act (UCSA) prepared by the National Conference of Commissioners on Uniform State Laws (NCCUSL) (1970, 1990). Such state laws permit the prescribing, dispensing, or administering of controlled substances for legitimate medical purposes, although most do not specifically recognize the essential medical value of controlled substances, as does the federal CSA. A revised model UCSA has been prepared to correct this and other deficiencies (NCCUSL; July, 1994), but only a few states have adopted the changes, including Washington, Colorado, and Wisconsin. The criminal provisions of the state controlled substances laws are enforced by state and local police agencies, while departments of regulation and licensing and pharmacy examining boards manage the administrative aspects, such as drug scheduling. Some state agencies have issued regulations that govern the prescription and dispensing of controlled substances more strictly than does the federal law (NABP, 1998; Joranson & Gilson, 1994b). Penalties for violation of prescribing requirements vary widely.

In addition, a number of states have laws that establish Prescription Monitoring Programs (Jaranson, Carrow et al., 2002). At this writing, 15 states have adopted laws requiring the use of a special prescription form and/or an electronic data transfer system to monitor prescriptions for controlled substances. In the past, such programs have been limited to medications in Schedule II, but newer programs monitor drugs in other schedules as well.

DEFINING ADDICTION

The use and definition of terms such as "addiction" remains a point of confusion for licensing boards and enforcement authorities no less than for others in the field. Such confusion originates in part from official definitions and expert opinions that historically have characterized addiction in terms of physical dependence, as indicated by the presence of a withdrawal syndrome. More than 30 years ago, the World Health Organization (WHO) replaced the words "addiction" and "habituation" with the term "drug dependence." This represented a major change in philosophy, as dependence was redefined primarily as the use of a drug for its psychic effects. Under the WHO definition, neither physical dependence (as evidenced by a withdrawal syndrome) nor tolerance, alone or together, are sufficient to define drug dependence.

The distinction between physiologic adaptation to a drug (as evidenced by the development of tolerance and a with-

drawal syndrome) and compulsive use despite harm is reflected in the two primary diagnostic classification systems used by health care professionals: the *International Classification of Mental and Behavioural Disorders, 10th Edition*, of the World Health Organization (*ICD-10; WHO, 1992*) and the *Diagnostic and Statistical Manual, 4th Edition,* of the American Psychiatric Association (*DSM-IV*; APA, 1994). The criteria for "dependence syndrome" in the *ICD-10* and "substance dependence" in the *DSM-IV* include both withdrawal and tolerance. However, compulsive use that contributes to personal impairment or distress also must be present in order to make such a diagnosis.

In 1993, the WHO Expert Committee on Drug Dependence further clarified that cancer patients who use opioids should not be considered dependent solely because a withdrawal syndrome would occur if the medication was stopped (WHO, 1993). WHO has further reinforced this notion by stating that ". . . dependence should not be a factor in deciding whether to use opioids to treat the cancer patient with pain" (WHO, 1996, p. 41).

The accurate use of terminology is central to shaping a balanced policy on drug control, especially in the United States, where prescribing opioids to maintain addiction is illegal. It should be recognized that tolerance and physical depend-ence denote normal physiological adaptations of the body to the presence of an opioid; thus, a patient being treated with opioid analgesics is likely to develop physical depend-ence and/or tolerance. Confusing the development of physical dependence or tolerance with addiction or drug dependence can result in labeling a pain patient as an "addict" or "drug dependent," and increase the risk of inadequate pain treatment. Moreover, Weissman and Haddox (1989) have defined the term "pseudoaddiction" to characterize a situation in which the pattern of pain relief-seeking behavior by a patient who is receiving inadequate pain management is mistaken by health care professionals for the type of drug-seeking behavior characteristic of addiction or dependence. The inappropriate perception of pain patients as drug-seekers or addicts may result in denial of the opioid prescriptions they need for pain management. There is at least one documented case in which an inadequately treated pain patient illegally called in controlled substances prescriptions to obtain pain relief. Prosecutors viewed the patient as a drug addict, even though the medical evaluation was positive for pain and negative for an addictive disorder (State of Wisconsin vs. Holly, 1997).

POLICIES THAT CAN INFLUENCE PRESCRIBING

Federal Policies. Federal policy has several provisions that will be examined.

Defining an "Addict": The CSA defines as an "addict" an individual who "habitually uses any narcotic drug so as to endanger the public morals, health, safety, or who is so far addicted to the use of narcotic drugs as to have lost power of self-control with reference to his addiction" (p. 836). The definition is circular and uses archaic terminology. However, since the main component of "addict" is loss of control and harm, the potential to confuse an addict with a pain patient under this definition seems low. It is possible, however, that this antiquated definition assumes that addiction means physical dependence and withdrawal, since this term appeared in law long before the more recent distinction was made between physical dependence and compulsive behaviors that characterize addiction.

The latter possibility was supported by the federal regulation that governed dispensing of methadone for the maintenance or detoxification treatment of opiate addiction. Eligibility for admission to such treatment required that the patient be "narcotic dependent," which was officially defined as "physiologically [in need of] . . . a heroin or morphine-like drug to prevent the onset of signs of withdrawal (CFR 291.505(a)(5)). Anecdotal reports suggested that some patients with chronic pain in fact were being admitted to methadone treatment programs primarily or exclusively to obtain pain relief (Joranson, 1997). For example, the director of a California methadone treatment program estimated that, in the mid-1990s, approximately 200 patients were admitted for the treatment of chronic pain conditions, and that none of those patients demonstrated behaviors suggestive of addiction (Tennant, 1996).

The possibility that patients could be admitted to addiction treatment programs for treatment of their chronic pain has been diminished by recent modifications of the federal regulations governing addiction treatment (CFR 42, 8.12). The admission criteria for OTPs now incorporate accepted medical criteria for addiction and characterize "active addiction" as being of at least one year's duration. Thus, federal regulations no longer contain language that confuses physical dependence with addiction and thus provides a "loophole" that allowed the admission of patients for treatment of chronic pain.

State Policies. On the whole, state policies are not as balanced as international and federal policies (Joranson, 1990a; Joranson & Gilson, 1994b). Many state laws do not recognize the value of controlled drugs to the public health, as does the federal law. States have laws, regulations, or other governmental policies that restrict prescribing and dispensing of opioids; such policies have the potential to interfere with patient care decisions that should be made by medical professionals rather than government officials.

Studies of regulatory impediments to pain management in state policies began in Wisconsin in the mid-1980s (Joranson & Dahl, 1989; Joranson & Gilson, 1996, 1997). Subsequently, a succession of reports by national expert groups identified regulatory impediments to adequate pain management in state policies (FSMB, 1998; Hill, 1989; Institute of Medicine, 1997; Jacox, Carr et al., 1994; Merritt, Fox-Grage et al., 1998; NCCUSL, 1990, 1994). Many of the restrictive provisions that have been identified in state policies date back 25 years or more, and appear to have been based on now-outdated concepts of addiction and the side effects of opioid analgesics.

A comprehensive, criteria-based evaluation of the strengths and weaknesses of federal policies, as well as policies in all 50 states and the District of Columbia, has been published (Joranson, Gilson et al., 2000). This evaluation has identified provisions that have the potential to impede or enhance pain management. Some states restrict the quantity of controlled substances that can be prescribed at one time, or limit the validity of a prescription to a few days. A number of states use imprecise terminology that could incorrectly label pain patients as persons with addictive disorders. At least one state also requires physicians to report to a government agency those patients to whom they prescribe controlled substances for more than several months. Such a policy can create an additional administrative burden for the physician and cast a shadow over the treatment of pain in patients with a substance abuse history. To address this issue, some states, including New York and Texas, have revised their policies to permit the use of controlled substances to addicts for pain. The full text of state pain policies can be found at WWW.MEDSCH.WISC.EDU/PAINPOLICY.

Intractable Pain Treatment Acts: Since 1989, a number of state legislatures have adopted IPTAs. A review of IPTAs suggests that, although the intent of these policies is to address physicians' fears of regulatory scrutiny, they also have provisions that, if strictly implemented, would restrict physician prescribing and patient access to opioid analgesics (Joranson, 1995; Joranson & Gilson, 1997).

Potentially restrictive language can be found in most IPTAs' definitions of intractable pain. The Texas IPTA (Texas Intractable Pain Treatment Act, Article 4495c) was the first to be adopted and has served as a model for most other state IPTAs. It defines "intractable pain" as ". . . a pain state in which the cause of the pain cannot be removed or otherwise treated and which, in the generally accepted course of medical practice, no relief or cure of the cause of the pain is possible or none has been found after reasonable efforts." Taken in the context of a law relating to the use of opioid analgesics, such a definition implies that a physician's prescribing of controlled substances for chronic pain is outside generally accepted medical practice unless it is done within the parameters of an IPTA. Further, limiting the use of opioids only to patients for whom other efforts have failed implies that use of opioids is a treatment of last resort. Thus, despite the intent of IPTAs to encourage pain management, these laws appear to position the use of opioids nearer the periphery of medical practice than at the center.

A balanced approach to drug policy recognizes that physicians should make medical decisions based on the treatment needs of individual patients. However, before prescribing opioids, some IPTAs require the physician to obtain a consultation or evaluation by a specialist in the organ system believed to be the cause of the pain, to be certain that the physician is immune from discipline. Such a governmental requirement appears to further marginalize pain management and does not take into account the expertise of the physician or the patient's needs, which in some cases could be relatively straightforward or of an immediate nature. Such policies also may discourage pain management because of the increased time and administrative burdens they impose on physicians, as well the possibility of increased cost to the patient.

Because immunity from discipline under some IPTAs excludes physician prescribing to patients who use drugs nontherapeutically, such laws also may have the unintended effect of excluding addicts from pain management (Joranson & Gilson, 1994a). These provisions appear to conflict with federal policy, which prohibits physicians from prescribing narcotic drugs only for the *purpose* of maintaining narcotic addiction, but does not prohibit prescribing of opioids to *persons* who have both pain and an addictive disorder. Such state policies have the clear potential to interfere with the treatment of pain in persons who have addictive disease and a medical problem that causes pain, such as cancer or AIDS.

State Medical Board Policies: A recent content evaluation of state medical board guidelines found that almost 80% of these policies established recommendations or specific requirements regarding the prescribing of opioids to patients with a history of addiction (Monterroso, Gilson et al., 1997). These practice parameters include (1) evaluating each patient for a history of addiction or for current addiction, (2) consulting another physician about the diagnosis, (3) providing extra care and special attention, (4) establishing treatment plans that reflect the possibility of drug misuse, and (5) being "vigilant" with regard to drug-seeking behaviors. Several medical board policies also state that it would be inappropriate to prescribe controlled substances to a person who uses drugs nontherapeutically. In sharp contrast, one state's policy includes the following language:

> . . . addicts can be the legitimate victims of pain, independent of their addiction . . . although it is appropriate to prescribe for pain control, extra diligence must be exercised with such patients (New Mexico Board of Medical Examiners, 1997, p. 1).

Overall, it is evident that some state medical board policies that are intended to improve access to pain management do not contain language that would include patients who use (or have used) drugs for other than therapeutic purposes.

Perceived Threat of Regulatory Scrutiny: A number of articles report that physicians are reluctant to prescribe opioid analgesics because they are concerned about being investigated by a regulatory agency (Institute of Medicine, 1997; Hill, 1993; Joranson & Gilson, 1994a; Haddox & Aronoff, 1998; Martino, 1998). A pilot survey of Wisconsin physicians conducted in 1990 found that more than half reported that they would reduce the dose or quantity, reduce the number of refills, or choose a drug in a lower schedule because of concerns about regulatory scrutiny (Weissman, Joranson et al., 1991). In addition, 40% of the physician-members of the American Pain Society (APS) agreed in 1991 that their prescribing of opioids for chronic non-malignant pain was influenced by legal concerns (Turk, Brody et al., 1994).

In 1991, all state medical board members in the U.S. were surveyed to learn more about whether regulators' knowledge and attitudes about the medical use of opioids for chronic malignant and non-malignant pain would pose a risk to the physician who prescribes opioid analgesics for such conditions (Joranson, Cleeland et al., 1992). Board members were asked their opinions about the legality and medical acceptability of prescribing opioids for more than several months in four patient scenarios involving malignant and non-malignant pain, with and without a history of drug abuse of the opioid type. There were five possible responses: such prescribing was (1) lawful and generally acceptable medical practice, (2) lawful, but generally not accepted medical practice and should be discouraged, (3) probably a violation of medical practice laws or regulations and should be investigated, (4) probably a violation of federal or state controlled substances laws and should be investigated, and (5) don't know.

Only 75% of medical board members were confident that prescribing opioids for chronic cancer pain was both legal and acceptable medical practice; 14% felt it was legal, but would discourage it; 5% believed that the practice was illegal and should be investigated. If the cancer patient with chronic pain had a history of opioid abuse, less than half of the respondents (46%) were confident in prescribing opioids and 22% would discourage the practice. Fourteen percent considered the practice to be a violation of medical practice law and 12% viewed it as a violation of controlled substances laws. When the patient's chronic pain was of non-malignant origin, only 12% of respondents were confident that prescribing opioids was both legal and medically acceptable; 47% would discourage it; and nearly a third recommended investigating the practice as a violation of law. Finally, only 1% of respondents viewed the prescribing of opioids for more than several months to a patient with chronic non-malignant pain and a history of opioid abuse as legal and acceptable medical practice.

Overall, it appears that many medical board members lacked knowledge about the use of opioids and other controlled substances to manage pain. To varying degrees, they would discourage or investigate the prescribing of opioid analgesics for chronic pain, particularly if the patient does not have cancer and especially if the patient has a history of drug abuse. (It is important to recognize that the presenting problem in each scenario was pain, not addiction.)

Medical board members from all states were re-surveyed in 1997 and their responses compared to those of the 1990 sample (Gilson, Joranson et al., 2001). Results demonstrated some important improvements in the knowledge and attitudes of board members since 1991. Significantly more board members in 1997 considered the prescribing of opioids to be a lawful and generally acceptable medical treatment for chronic noncancer pain, and for patients with chronic pain and a history of opioid abuse. It should be noted, however, that those board members who viewed these prescribing scenarios as lawful still represented only a small percentage of the total sample. Nevertheless, the positive changes in knowledge and attitudes between 1991 and 1997 should be seen as indicating greater recognition that prescribing opioids for cancer and noncancer pain, with and without a history of substance abuse, is an acceptable medical practice.

Model Guidelines: In 1998, the FSMB adopted a document entitled "Model Guidelines for the Use of Controlled Substances for the Treatment of Pain" to promote positive state medical board pain policy and greater consistency between the states' policies. The Model Guidelines were developed as a cooperative effort between the FSMB and representatives of state medical boards, the American Pain Society, the American Academy of Pain Medicine, and the American Society of Law, Medicine and Ethics. The FSMB disseminated the Model Guidelines to each state medical board with a request that they be considered and adopted as policy.

The Model Guidelines state that opioid analgesics may be necessary for the treatment of pain, including pain associated with acute, cancer, and noncancer conditions. If adopted by state medical boards, the positive language would communicate to medical professionals that their licensing board recognizes the health benefits of using controlled substances as a part of legitimate medical practice.

The Model Guidelines address directly the limitations inherent in current medical board policies. Although many existing board policies do not have an explicit statement of purpose, the Model Guidelines encourage pain management and clarify that effective pain management is an expected part of good medical practice. In addition, the policy recognizes that physicians are concerned about regulatory scrutiny and provides them with information about how the board distinguishes legitimate medical practice from unprofessional conduct. The Model Guidelines make it clear that judgments about the legitimacy of a medical practice are to be based on the treatment outcomes for patients, rather than on the amount or duration of prescribing.

The Model Guidelines also contain a set of recommended treatment parameters for using controlled substances for pain management, which are based on principles of good medical practice. Seven outlined treatment steps are included: (1) medical history and physical examination, (2) treatment plan with identified objectives, (3) informed consent to treatment, (4) periodic review of treatment, (5) consultation as necessary, (6) accurate and complete medical records, and (7) compliance with both federal and state controlled substances policy. The Model Guidelines recognize the need for flexibility, stating that a physician may deviate from the guidelines for good cause shown (FSMB, 1998).

Another important improvement of the Model Guidelines is the definition of addiction-related terminology. Definitions that conform to currently accepted medical standards are provided for "addiction," "physical dependence," "psychological dependence," "tolerance," and "pseudoaddiction." These definitions clarify that physical dependence or tolerance are not sufficient to diagnose addiction. The knowledge and appropriate use of correct terminology decreases the likelihood that pain patients will be viewed as "addicts" by health care professionals (Joranson & Gilson, 1998).

Finally, the Model Guidelines do not exclude patients with addictive disorders from the treatment of pain with opioid analgesics. The FSMB recognized that the decision to prescribe controlled substances to a patient should be based on clinical findings in the individual patient; however, physicians are urged to "be diligent in preventing the diversion of drugs for illegitimate purposes" (FSMB, 1998, p. 1).

Consensus Statement: Other national organizations also have attempted to improve the terms used to describe dependence and addiction. For example, in 1991 the American Academy of Pain Medicine, the American Pain Society, and the American Society of Addiction Medicine published a statement on "Definitions Related to the Use of Opioids for the Treatment of Pain" (AAPM, APS & ASAM, 2001). The statement contains definitions of "addiction," "physical dependence," and "tolerance," which reflect the prevailing medical standards for those conditions. The statement was developed through a consensus process for the purpose of promoting a level of consistency that will help to optimize both pain management and the treatment of addictive disorders, as well as improving communications among health care professionals, regulators, and enforcement officials.

CONCLUSIONS

In recent years, pain management has become a higher priority in the U.S. health care system. The use of opioids for the treatment of acute and chronic pain, both cancer and noncancer related pain, in patients with histories of addictive disorders or drug abuse is permitted by federal law. However, it is evident that some state policies and the views of some state medical board members may discourage the prescribing of opioid analgesics when needed by pain patients who have addictive disorders. It is necessary to identify and change such policies. Health care professionals should be educated about treating pain in patients with addictive disorders, which remains a complex and intensive task. Trained and experienced practitioners who also are knowledgeable about the policies in their states will be in a much better position to evaluate the medical needs of their patients.

ACKNOWLEDGMENT: The studies described in this article were supported by grants from the Robert Wood Johnson Foundation and by Advocates for Children's Pain Relief.

The authors are grateful for the assistance of Martha Maurer, B.S.; Maria Monterroso, M.A.; John M. Nelson, M.S.; Jessica Nischik, B.S.; Karen M. Ryan, M.A.; and Carolyn M. Williams, M.B.A., for the evaluation of state medical board policies.

REFERENCES

American Academy of Pain Medicine (AAPM) and American Pain Society (APS) (1997). *The Use of Opioids for the Treatment of Chronic Pain: A Consensus Statement. A Policy Document of the American Academy of Pain Medicine and American Pain Society.* Glenview, IL: The Societies.

American Academy of Pain Medicine (AAPM), American Pain Society (APS) & American Society of Addiction Medicine (ASAM) (2001). *Definitions Related to the Use of Opioids for the Treatment of Pain.* Glenview, IL: The Societies.

American Pain Society (1999). *Principles of Analgesic Use in the Treatment of Acute Pain and Cancer Pain, 4th Edition.* Glenview, IL: The Society.

American Psychiatric Association (APA) (1994). *Diagnostic and Statistical Manual of Mental Disorders, 4th Edition (DSM-IV).* Washington, DC: American Psychiatric Press.

American Society of Addiction Medicine (ASAM) (1998). Policy statement: Definitions related to the use of opioids for the treatment of pain. *Journal of Addictive Diseases* 17:129-130.

Bernabei R, Gambassi G, Lapane K et al. (1998). Management of pain in elderly patients with cancer. *Journal of the American Medical Association* 279:1877-1882.

Cleeland CS, Gonin R, Baez L et al. (1997). Pain and treatment of pain in minority patients with cancer. The Eastern Cooperative Oncology Group Minority Outpatient Pain Study. *Annals of Internal Medicine* 127:813-816.

Code of Federal Regulations. Title 21. §291.505(a).

Code of Federal Regulations. Title 21. §1306.11(a).

Code of Federal Regulations. Title 21. §1306.11(d).

Code of Federal Regulations. Title 21. §1306.13.

Controlled Substances Act of 1970 (CSA). Pub. L. No. 91-513, 84 Stat. 1242.

Drug Enforcement Administration (DEA) (1990). *Physician's Manual: An Informational Outline of the Controlled Substances Act of 1970.* Washington, DC: U.S. Department of Justice.

Federation of State Medical Boards of the United States (FSMB) (1998). *Model Guidelines for the Use of Controlled Substances for the Treatment of Pain. A Policy Document of the Federation of State Medical Boards of the United States, Inc.* Euless, TX: The Federation.

Ferrell BR, Juarez G & Borneman T (1999). Use of routine and breakthrough analgesia in home care. *Oncology Nursing Forum* 26(10):1655-1661.

Gilson AM & Joranson DE (2001). Controlled substances and pain management: Changing knowledge and attitudes of medical regulators. *Journal of Pain & Symptom Management* 21(3):227-237.

Haddox JD & Aronoff GM (1998). Commentary: The potential for unintended consequences from public policy shifts in the treatment of pain. *Journal of Law, Medicine & Ethics* 26(4):350-352.

Hill CS (1989). The negative effect of regulatory agencies on adequate pain control. *Primary Care and Cancer* November:45-53.

Hill CS Jr. (1993). The barriers to adequate pain management with opioid analgesics. *Seminars in Oncology* 20(2 Suppl 1):1-5.

Institute of Medicine (1997). *Approaching Death: Improving Care at the End of Life.* Washington, DC: National Academy Press.

Jacox A, Carr DB, Payne R et al. (1994). *Management of Cancer Pain (Clinical Practice Guideline No. 9).* (AHCPR Publication No. 94-0592). Rockville, MD: Agency for Health Care Policy and Research.

Joranson DE (1990a). Federal and state regulation of opioids. *Journal of Pain and Symptom Management* 5(Suppl):12-23.

Joranson DE (1990b). A new drug law for the states: An opportunity to affirm the role of opioids in cancer pain relief. *Journal of Pain and Symptom Management* 5(5):333-336.

Joranson DE (1995). Intractable pain treatment laws and regulations. *American Pain Society Bulletin* 5(2):1-3, 15-17.

Joranson DE (1997). Is methadone maintenance the last resort for some chronic pain patients? *American Pain Society Bulletin* 7(5):1, 4-5.

Joranson DE, Carrow GM, Ryan KM et al. (2002). Pain management and prescription monitoring. *Journal of Pain & Symptom Management* 23(3):231-238.

Joranson DE, Cleeland CS, Weissman DE et al. (1992). Opioids for chronic cancer and noncancer pain: A survey of state medical board members. *Federation Bulletin* 79(4):15-49.

Joranson DE & Dahl JL (1989). Achieving balance in drug policy: The Wisconsin model. *Advances in Pain Research and Therapy* 2:197-203.

Joranson DE & Gilson A (1994a). Policy issues and imperatives in the use of opioids to treat pain in substance abusers. *Journal of Law, Medicine & Ethics* 22(3):215-223.

Joranson DE & Gilson A (1996). Improving pain management through policy making and education for medical regulators. *Journal of Law, Medicine & Ethics* 24(4):344-347.

Joranson DE & Gilson A (1997). State intractable pain policy: Current status. *American Pain Society Bulletin* 7(2):7-9.

Joranson DE & Gilson AM (1994b). Controlled substances, medical practice, and the law. In HI Schwartz (ed.) *Psychiatric Practice Under Fire: The Influence of Government, the Media, and Special Interests on Somatic Therapies.* Washington, DC: American Psychiatric Press, 173-194.

Joranson DE & Gilson AM (1998). Controlled substances and pain management: A new focus for state medical boards. *Federation Bulletin* 85(2):78-83.

Joranson DE, Gilson AM, Dahl JL et al. (2002). Pain management, controlled substances, and state medical policy: A decade of change. *Journal of Pain & Symptom Management* (23(2):138-147.

Joranson DE, Gilson AM, Ryan KR et al. (2000). *Achieving Balance in Federal and State Pain Policy: A Guide to Evaluation.* Madison, WI: Pain & Policy Studies Group.

Martino AM (1998). In search of a new ethic for treating patients with chronic pain: What can medical boards do? *Journal of Law, Medicine & Ethics* 26(4):332-334.

Merritt R, Fox-Grage W & Rothouse M (1998). *State Initiatives in End-of-Life Care: Policy Guide for Legislators.* Denver, CO: National Conference of State Legislatures.

Monterroso MM, Gilson AM, Williams CM et al. (1997). "A Comparison of State Medical Board Pain Guidelines with a National Model." Poster presented at the 16th annual conference of the American Pain Society, New Orleans, LA.

National Association of Boards of Pharmacy (NABP) (1998). *Survey of Pharmacy Law, 1998-1999.* Park Ridge, IL: NABP.

National Conference of Commissioners on Uniform State Laws (NCCUSL) (1970). *Uniform Controlled Substances Act.* St. Louis, MO: NCCUSL.

National Conference of Commissioners on Uniform State Laws (NCCUSL) (1990). *Uniform Controlled Substances Act.* Milwaukee, WI: NCCUSL.

National Conference of Commissioners on Uniform State Laws (1994). *Uniform Controlled Substances Act.* Chicago, IL: NCCUSL.

New Mexico Board of Medical Examiners (1997). Guidelines on prescribing for pain. *Newsletter Information & Report* 2(1):1-3.

Nowels D & Lee JT (1999). Cancer pain management in home hospice settings: A comparison of primary care and oncology physicians. *Journal of Palliative Care* 15(3):5-9.

Oklahoma Uniform Controlled Dangerous Substances Act. Title 63 Public Health and Safety, §2-101(15).

Portenoy RK (1989). Cancer pain: Epidemiology and syndromes. *Cancer* 63:2298-2307.

Portenoy RK (1996). Opioid therapy for chronic nonmalignant pain: Clinicians' perspective. *Journal of Law, Medicine & Ethics* 24(4):296-309.

Savage SR (1999). Opioid use in the management of chronic pain. *Medical Clinics of North America* 83(3):761-786.

State of Wisconsin vs. Holly (1997). Case No. 96 CF 978.

SUPPORT Study Principle Investigators (1995). A controlled trial to improve care for seriously ill hospitalized patients. The study to understand prognoses and preferences for outcomes and risks of treatments (SUPPORT). *Journal of the American Medical Association* 274:1591-1598.

Tennant F (1996). The Dilemma of Severe Incurable, Narcotic-Dependent Pain Patients Referred to Narcotic Treatment Programs: Need for Administrative, Regulatory, and Legislative Relief. West Covina, CA: Research Center for Dependency Disorders and Chronic Pain Community Health Projects Medical Group.

Texas Intractable Pain Treatment Act (n.d.). Title 71 Health-Public, Ch. 6, Article 4495c.

Turk DC, Brody MC & Okifuji EA (1994). Physicians' attitudes and practices regarding the long-term prescribing of opioids for noncancer pain. *Pain* 59:201-208.

United Nations (1977a). *Single Convention on Narcotic Drugs, 1961, as Amended by the 1972 Protocol Amending the Single Convention on Narcotic Drugs.* New York, NY: U.N.

United Nations (1977b). *Single Convention on Psychotropic Drugs, 1971.* New York, NY: U.N.

United States vs. Evers (1981), 643 F2d 1043, 5th Circuit.

Weissman DE & Haddox JD (1989). Opioid pseudoaddiction—An iatrogenic syndrome. *Pain* 36:363-366.

Weissman DE, Joranson DE & Hopwood MB (1991). Wisconsin physicians' knowledge and attitudes about opioid analgesic regulations. *Wisconsin Medical Journal* December:53-58.

World Health Organization (WHO) (1969). *WHO Expert Committee on Drug Dependence: Sixteenth Report (Technical Report Series 407).* Geneva, Switzerland: WHO.

World Health Organization (WHO) (1986). *Cancer Pain Relief.* Geneva, Switzerland: WHO.

World Health Organization (WHO) (1990). *Cancer Pain Relief and Palliative Care (Technical Report Series 804).* Geneva, Switzerland: WHO.

World Health Organization (WHO) (1992). *The ICD-10 Classification of Mental and Behavioural Disorders: Clinical Descriptions and Diagnostic Guidelines.* Geneva, Switzerland: WHO.

World Health Organization (WHO) (1993). *WHO Expert Committee on Drug Dependence (Technical Report Series 836).* Geneva, Switzerland: WHO.

World Health Organization (WHO) (1996). *Cancer Pain Relief, with a Guide to Opioid Availability.* Geneva, Switzerland: WHO.

| Chapter 7 | # Practical Issues in the Management of Pain |

Neil Irick, M.D.

Widespread confusion and concern on the part of policymakers and the public related to the use of opioids to treat pain has left physicians and other caregivers with the dilemma of how to balance the comfort of their patients against the scrutiny, real or perceived, of regulatory agencies. How do physicians decide who should receive pain medication? Are opioids more likely to be prescribed for some patients than others? How can physicians organize their practices to afford protection to themselves and their patients as they pursue the optimal management of patients in pain?

ISSUES IN ASSESSING PAIN

In a landmark article on the treatment of cancer pain, Foley (1991) pointed to the need to believe the patient as critical to the first step in a successful treatment regimen. Subsequent experience has affirmed that successful management requires that caregivers be able to accept input from the patient. In fact, assessing pain requires the physician to balance information received from the patient with the physical presentation of the pain syndrome. But how should the physician interpret the patient's input if it does not coincide with the level of pain to be expected from the physical signs?

What should the physician do for a patient who reports that his pain rates a "14" on a 10-point scale?

Options to consider in such a situation include a learned pain behavior that results from the patient over-reporting in a desperate effort to get some treatment. This is seen most often in patients whose experience has been that they have not received adequate treatment when they reported their pain at a more accurate level.

Visual analog scales are used widely to assess pain in adults. However, some older patients do not consider the lower levels of these scales even to represent pain, but rather to suggest an "ache" or "discomfort." Therefore, before using such a scale, the physician should be aware of its inherent shortcomings and how to accommodate to them so that the information elicited with the scale is accurately interpreted. Each time an assessment scale is used, the physician should give the patient appropriate parameters; for example: "If the left end of the scale represents no pain, and the right end of the scale is the pain of holding your hand in a fire, where is your pain on the scale?" This kind of preparation is an essential preface to eliciting useful information.

For the assessment process to help create a therapeutic alliance, it should be done early in the patient encounter. Asking the patient to complete an assessment form before he or she meets with the physician is one way to ensure that pain is not an afterthought, but is dealt with in a forthright fashion at the beginning of the encounter.

BARRIERS TO THE EFFECTIVE MANAGEMENT OF PAIN

In addition to inadequate assessment, a number of other barriers to effective management of pain have been identified in the literature.

Anecdotal Training. Anecdotal training of medical students and residents still is the principal method by which pain assessment and treatment are taught. In such situations, students naturally acquire the preferences of the teaching staff, who may or may not be knowledgeable about pain management.

The Scrutiny of Peers. Advanced training programs teach physicians that, in most cases, the patient is the best judge of the intensity of pain. Ideally, this should help them give the best care possible. However, the ideal situation often is overcome by reluctance to deal with pain patients because of fears of being "scammed" by a drug seeker. Indeed, most physicians can remember each time this has occurred in their professional careers; such events become incorporated into the physician's existential bias. They also raise great sensitivity to the reactions of peers, and lead to a reluctance to offer patients adequate medications for their pain.

Consequently, each prescription for an opioid is accompanied by multiple concerns:

"The patient may improve and want more of this stuff."

"The pharmacist may refuse to fill it, causing embarrassment to the patient and to me."

"The pharmacist may report me to the authorities, if he does not agree with the regimen prescribed."

"The patient may sell the prescribed medication to others, or trade the medication for street drugs."

"The patient may take the medication as part of a suicide attempt."

"The patient may take the medication faster than prescribed."

"The 'patient' may have been an undercover officer setting me up for arrest."

"Side effects may prevent the patient from continuing the medication."

"The prescription may produce 'addiction' that will ruin the patient's life."

Fear of Regulatory Agencies. The popular media occasionally report situations in which a physician is charged with a criminal act for providing adequate drugs to achieve pain relief. Although most such physicians ultimately are exonerated, the pain and humiliation they endure—to say nothing of the fear, expense, and practice disruptions engendered by the process—lead many to resolve never to be caught in the same situation again. Colleagues who learn of their plight may well respond in similar fashion: it simply becomes safer to avoid the whole issue.

There is no easy answer for the fact that there are regulatory agencies that have significant power over the ability of physicians to practice and prescribe. Such agencies are necessary. In general, law enforcement officials are aware of the difficulties physicians face. Review of a physician's prescribing practices is not meant to intimidate the physician, but merely to ascertain that he or she is, in fact, treating pain in a responsible way.

DOCUMENTATION

Careful documentation becomes the mechanism that protects both the physician and the patient. The fear of litigation or censure by regulatory officials need not deter the effective management of pain in physicians who approach the diagnostic, treatment, and recordkeeping processes with care.

The single most important step is to know and understand the laws and regulatory requirements in the state in which one practices. This is important because state laws and licensing board rules may differ substantially from the federal requirements. Moreover, they usually spell out, item by item, exactly what the medical record must contain to be in compliance. (The board of medical licensure or the board of pharmacy [or their equivalents] in each state can provide information about the relevant requirements.)

The following discussion summarizes the elements most frequently required as part of such documentation.

History and Physical Examination. The patient history must include the use of illicit substances, all medications used for the treatment of pain, and any patient allergies. Regimens tried and failed also should be documented in the record.

TABLE 1.   Guidelines for Prescribing Drugs with Abuse Liability

1. Set clear rules for the patient and have him/her sign a contract.

2. Set the dose of medication at the appropriate level to treat the condition and titrate as necessary. Get feedback from the patient.

3. Give enough medication, plus rescue doses.

4. Ask the patient to bring any remaining drugs to the next meeting in the original bottles. This provides information on pharmacies used and other prescribing physicians.

5. Monitor for lost or stolen prescriptions.

6. Obtain random urine screens. Know what drugs laboratory screens actually can identify.

7. Use adjunctive medications as necessary.

8. Document all your thoughts (in selecting and monitoring the pharmacotherapy) in the chart.

9. See the patient as frequently as needed.

10. Work with the patient's significant others.

11. Know how to withdraw the patient from the medications.

12. Know the pharmacology of the drugs used.

13. Limit PRN medications, since this promotes drug-seeking behavior.

14. Adequately treat acute pain to prevent the development of chronic pain.

SOURCE: Schnoll SH & Finch J (1994). Medical education for pain and addiction: Making progress toward answering a need. *Journal of Law, Medicine & Ethics* 22(3):254. Reprinted by permission of the publisher.

It is wise to obtain the patient's records from physicians who have treated him or her in the past. Caution should be exercised in accepting records supplied by patients, as these occasionally are fraudulent.

The documentation should include information about the patient's personal and family histories of alcoholism, drug use, and addiction, as well any personal history of major depression. However, a positive response does not preclude the appropriate use of opioids in the patient's treatment.

Treatment Plan and Goals. The treatment plan and goals should be established (and documented in the record) as early as possible so that there is evidence of clear-cut, individualized objectives to guide the choice of therapy. Establishing a timeline for achievement of treatment goals may help to spur dilatory patients toward compliance with the treatment regimen.

Past undertreatment of a legitimate pain syndrome often leads patients to engage in drug-seeking behaviors. The resulting pseudoaddiction syndrome is difficult to deal with, and more common that one would suspect. If the record documents a valid pain complaint, the patient has legitimate records to substantiate a chronic painful condition, and risk factors for addiction, it is safe and legal to try opioids. A consultation may provide reassurance. If the patient improves after a brief trial, that should be documented in the record and the treatment regimen continued.

Consultations. Evidence of appropriate consultation is particularly helpful if the patient is self-referred.

Prescription Orders. The patient record must include all prescription orders, whether written or telephoned. Written instructions for the use of all medications should be given to the patient and documented in the record (also see Table 1).

Medication Record. The first page of the patient's chart should be a summary of the information needed to deal with a problem without a thorough knowledge of the patient. This includes some demographic data, other physicians caring for the patient, diagnoses, procedures undertaken, and a list of all medications prescribed. The name, telephone number, and address of the patient's pharmacy also should be recorded to facilitate contact as needed.

Medication Management Agreement. A written agreement, signed by the patient, can be helpful in establishing a set of "ground rules." Such an agreement also can itemize those things the patient can expect from the physician. Model agreements are available from many sources, including some pharmaceutical manufacturers.

It is helpful to give the patient a copy of the agreement to carry with him or her, to document the source and reason for any analgesic drugs in his or her possession. Some physicians provide a laminated card that identifies the individual as a patient of their practice. This is helpful to other physicians who may see the patient in consultation or in the emergency department.

The medication management agreement also should include a waiver of privacy, which allows the physician to talk with other practitioners, including pharmacists, as well as with law enforcement personnel who may wish to ascertain the legitimacy of a prescription order or drug supply.

The inclusion in the document of a pharmacy address and telephone number reinforces to the patient the importance of using one pharmacy to fill all opioid prescriptions.

The medication agreement should include a statement instructing the patient to stop taking all other pain medications, unless explicitly told to continue. Such a statement reinforces the need to adhere to a single treatment regimen.

Drug Screens. Urine drug screens are helpful in maintaining the compliance of some patients (see Chapter 3).

Followup Visits. The patient should be seen more frequently while the treatment regimen is being established and adjusted. As the regimen becomes stable, followup visits every two to three months probably are sufficient.

Arrangements must be made for the patient to obtain a new prescription every 30 days if he or she is prescribed a Schedule II drug. "Medication monitoring visits" are billable and can be performed by a nurse. They should be carefully documented in the same manner as a visit with the physician.

Outcomes. The patient's record should document the outcome of the treatment regimen, including the use of pain medications. Documented improvements in function, mood, and quality of life are hard to dispute. Achievement of the patient's goals is an important outcome as well.

REFERENCES

American Academy of Pain Medicine and American Pain Society (1997). *The Use of Opioids for the Treatment of Chronic Pain: A Consensus Statement. A Policy Document of the American Academy of Pain Medicine and American Pain Society.* Glenview, IL: The Societies.

American Pain Society (1999). *Principles of Analgesic Use in the Treatment of Acute Pain and Cancer Pain, 4th Edition.* Glenview, IL: The Society.

American Society of Addiction Medicine (ASAM) (1998). Policy statement: Definitions related to the use of opioids for the treatment of pain. *Journal of Addictive Diseases* 17:129-130.

Chambers CD, White OZ & Linquest JH (1981). *Physicians' Attitudes and Prescribing Behavior. A Focus on Minor Tranquilizers.* National Meeting on Prescribing. New York, NY: City College of the City University of New York.

Cleeland CS, Gonin R, Baez L et al. (1997). Pain and treatment of pain in minority patients with cancer. The Eastern Cooperative Oncology Group Minority Outpatient Pain Study. *Annals of Internal Medicine* 127:813-816.

Drug Enforcement Administration (1990). *Physician's Manual: An Informational Outline of the Controlled Substances Act of 1970.* Washington, DC: U.S. Department of Justice, Drug Enforcement Administration.

Federation of State Medical Boards of the United States (FSMB) (1998). *Model Guidelines for the Use of Controlled Substances for the Treatment of Pain. A policy document of the Federation of State Medical Boards of the United States, Inc.* Euless, TX: FSMB.

Foley K (1991). Clinical tolerance to opioids. In A Basbaum & J Besson (eds.) *Towards a New Pharmacotherapy of Pain.* New York, NY: John Wiley & Sons, 181-203.

Hill CS Jr. (1993). The negative influence of licensing and disciplinary boards and more drug enforcement agencies on pain treatment with opioid analgesics. *Journal of Pharmaceutical Care in Pain and Symptom Control* 1:43-61.

Joranson DE (1993). Regulation influence on pain management: Real or imagined? *Journal of Pharmaceutical Care in Pain and Symptom Control* 1:113-118.

Morgan JP & Plect DL (1983). Opiophobia in the United States. *The Undertreatment of Severe Pain in Society and Medication: Conflicting Signals for Prescribing of Patients.* Lexington, MA: Lexington Books, 313-326.

National Association of Boards of Pharmacy (NABP) (1998). *Survey of Pharmacy Law, 1998-1999.* Park Ridge, IL: NABP.

New Mexico Board of Medical Examiners (1997). Guidelines on prescribing for pain. *Newsletter Information & Report* 2(1):1-3.

Stimmel B (1985). Underprescription/overprescription: Narcotic as metaphor. *Bulletin of the New York Academy of Medicine* 61:742-752.

Termin P (1980). *Taking Your Medicine: Drug Regulations in the United States.* Cambridge, MA: Harvard University Press, 12-17.

Constraints on Prescribing and the Relief of Pain

BARRY STIMMEL, M.D., FASAM

There are a variety of reasons why physicians may not prescribe sufficient analgesic medications: inhibitory influences of federal and state regulations and disciplinary boards (discussed by Joranson and Gilson and therefore not addressed here); lack of a suitable knowledge base; fear of producing dependency and addiction; cultural and societal barriers to use of narcotics; adherence to customary prescribing behaviors; and unconscious bias toward different groups. Each must be addressed if the physician's ability to relieve pain is to be maximized. . . .

LACK OF A SUITABLE KNOWLEDGE BASE

The appropriate use of analgesics and other mood-altering drugs is a subject that unfortunately receives too little attention in medical school and residency training. As a physician moves farther away from basic pharmacology—where most of the information concerning drug action is taught—an increasing unfamiliarity with the specific actions of analgesics and other mood-altering agents develops. Drugs may be used more frequently than necessary because of the reliance placed on publicity given to newer agents, often accompanied by patients' requests for "nonaddictive" substances.

At times, this may result in overprescription of mild narcotic analgesics or excessive use of tranquilizers rather than a narcotic analgesic. For example, most physicians consider propoxyphene (Darvon®) a nonnarcotic, effective, mild analgesic. This is despite the fact that propoxyphene is an ester of methadone and, in sufficient doses, can cause dependence, tolerance, overdose, and addictive behavior indistinguishable from more potent narcotics (Miller, 1977; Smith, 1979). Codeine and oxycodone (Percocet®), commonly prescribed analgesics, also are capable of producing dependence or addiction. One survey found codeine to be the most frequent drug of abuse in patients without a demonstrable cause of pain (Maruta, Swanson et al., 1979). In many instances, those who take codeine are not even aware it is a narcotic. . . .

FEAR OF ADDICTION

Fear of producing addiction to narcotics is foremost in the minds of most physicians when asked to provide medication for pain relief. This fear often interferes with their ability to provide adequate analgesia. One study demonstrated that those physicians who thought the probability of addiction was high after prescribing meperidine for 10 days to a patient in pain were more likely to give lower initial doses, as well as to be less likely to respond to the need for increased medication with recurrent pain, even if pain was due to terminal malignancy (Marks & Sachar, 1973).

A second study of 100 patients with malignant pain found 60% to be prescribed doses of meperidine of 50 mg or less, with 11% having to wait for five or more hours before another dose, with all prescriptions written for PRN administration (Morgan & Plecht, 1983).

In fact, the risk of initiating an addiction when narcotics are prescribed appropriately for relief of pain is quite small. Although historical references attribute physicians as initiating dependence on opiates, a survey reviewing addiction among a population of African American heroin addicts found that less than 2% attributed their addiction to prescription of a narcotic for medical reasons (Chambers & Moffett, 1970). Perhaps the largest survey of iatrogenic narcotic dependence was done as part of the Boston Collaborative Drug Surveillance Program (Porter & Jick, 1980). This program monitors all drug exposures in several hospitals, with information extracted from clinical records and by interviews with patients and physicians. Of over 11,000 hospitalized medical patients who had narcotics administered during their hospital stays, only four were reported to have become addicted. A more recent analysis of publications pertaining to drug or alcohol dependence in chronic-pain patients found that less than one-tenth of these publications used acceptable criteria for drug misuse or even gave percentages of dependence problems (Fishbain & Rosomoff, 1992). . . .

CUSTOMARY PRESCRIBING PRACTICES

Physicians' prescribing behavior has been described as consisting of an intermix of three components or modalities: instrumental, command, and customary (Termin, 1980). *Instrumental* allows for a critical assessment of the specific condition, the properties of the drugs to be used, and their effectiveness. *Command* is the modality pursued when one acts to avoid any penalties associated with noncompliance. *Customary*, or traditional, behavior reflects actions approved by the community peer group. The prescription of narcotic analgesics most commonly follows the command and customary modalities. Physicians who prescribe inappropriate doses of meperidine or mixed narcotics and benzodiazepines do so not from ignorance, but from following what has been the customary practice of using opioids as conservatively as possible, and then only as a last resort. A study of physicians treating patients with metastatic cancer pain highlighted such customary practices (Cleeland, Gonin et al., 1994). When asked which medications they would prescribe for moderate to severe cancer pain, 38% did not choose an opioid first, with 14% stating they would not choose such a drug even after palliative radiotherapy had failed.

UNCONSCIOUS BIAS

It is unfortunate but true that some of us react to a person's complaint based not on the specific complaint as much as on the characteristics of the person complaining. It has been shown that physicians' attitudes toward alcoholic or drug-dependent persons may interfere with their diagnosis and treatment (Chappel & Schnoll, 1977; Todd, Samaroo et al., 1993). Another study assessing the use of analgesics in an emergency room found Hispanic patients with bone fractures to be twice as likely as non-Hispanic white patients to receive no pain medication (Todd, Samaroo et al., 1993).

Similarly, persons in chronic pain who have seen many physicians without relief are, at times, thought by physicians to be less than honest concerning their symptoms. They are perceived as coming in for a visit only to request medication to allow them to get high. African American patients also have been reported more likely to receive less than adequate analgesics. One study found patients attending cancer pain treatment clinics less likely to receive adequate analgesics when those clinics were treating primarily minority groups (Blendon, Aiken et al., 1989). Patients with acute painful states, such as sickle cell disease, who may have developed a tolerance for narcotics and are in need of an increased dose, often are considered to be exaggerating their pain. Women and the elderly with metastatic cancer also were more likely to obtain less adequate analgesia than others. At times, inadequate analgesics are prescribed because the patient appears less ill than the physician would expect if severe pain was present. One survey reported that 76% of physicians admit an inability to accurately assess pain, which suggests that many physicians only recognize pain when a person truly appears to be suffering or when function is severely impaired (Cleeland, Gonin et al., 1994).

CULTURAL AND SOCIAL BARRIERS

Finally, since people's beliefs are formed by the society in which they live, often when a physician wishes to prescribe appropriately to relieve pain, the patient refuses to take the drug, also displaying opiophobia. This is frequently seen when one tries to prescribe methadone to a person in chronic pain who is not receiving relief from his or her current medication regimen. Often the person is on impressive amounts of short-acting narcotic analgesics, as well as dependence-producing amounts of benzodiazepines and other sleeping pills. Although the person remains somewhat groggy, the pain persists and prevents functioning. Yet methadone is refused because that person feels this will incur the label of "junkie" due to the use of methadone in maintenance therapy for heroin dependency. The same person, however, will have little concern about taking large doses of Demerol® or Dilaudid®. It is difficult to overcome these biases, yet it is essential to do so in order to maximize the chances of providing effective pain relief.

CONCLUSIONS

Existing evidence suggests that iatrogenic drug dependence is a real phenomenon but one that occurs infrequently when dependence-producing drugs are prescribed in an appropriate manner. Consistent narcotic use in chronic pain of known etiology that is unable to be relieved by other means, while associated with physical dependence, may nonetheless allow an individual to function in a productive manner. The potential for the development of iatrogenic dependence to barbiturates or other drugs used inappropriately to promote or enhance analgesics is much greater. Since physicians often are less inhibited in prescribing these medications, the indications for their use are frequently interpreted rather liberally. The many factors involved in inappropriate prescription of analgesics all are able to be identified and, when this is done, effective pain relief can occur.

ACKNOWLEDGMENT: Adapted from Stimmel B (1997). Unrelieved pain: The role of the physician. In B Stimmel, Pain and Its Relief Without Addiction: Clinical Issues in the Use of Opioids and Other Analgesics. *New York, NY: The Haworth Medical Press. Reprinted by permission of the publisher.*

REFERENCES

Bailey WJ (1979). Nonmedical use of pentazocine (Letter). *Journal of the American Medical Association* 242:2392.

Blendon RJ, Aiken LH, Freeman HE et al. (1989). Access to medical care for black and white Americans: A matter of continuing concern. *Journal of the American Medical Association* 261:278–281.

Chambers CD & Moffett AD (1970). Negro opiate addiction. In JC Ball, CD Chambers (eds.) *The Epidemiology of Opiate Addiction in the United States.* Springfield, IL: Charles C Thomas, 288–300.

Chappel JN & Schnoll SH (1977). Physician attitudes: Effect on the treatment of chemically dependent patients. *Journal of the American Medical Association* 237:2318–2319.

Cleeland CS, Gonin R, Hatfield AK et al. (1994). Pain and its treatment in outpatients with metastatic cancer. *New England Journal of Medicine* 330:592–596.

Fishbain DA, Rosomoff HL & Rosomoff RS (1992). Drug abuse, dependence, and addiction in chronic pain patients. *Clinical Journal of Pain* 8:77–85.

Inciardi JA & Chambers CD (1971). Patterns of pentazocine abuse and addiction. *New York State Journal of Medicine* 71:1727–1733.

Marks RM & Sachar EJ (1973). Undertreatment of medical inpatients with narcotic analgesics. *Annals of Internal Medicine* 78:173–181.

Maruta T, Swanson DW & Finlayson RE (1979). Drug abuse and dependency in patients with chronic pain. *Mayo Clinic Proceedings* 54:241–244.

Miller RR (1977). Propoxyphene: A review. *American Journal of Hospital Pharmacy* 34:413–423.

Morgan JP & Plecht DL (1983). Opiophobia in the United States. *The Undertreatment of Severe Pain in Society and Medication: Conflicting Signals for Prescribing of Patients.* Lexington, MA: Lexington Books, 313–326.

National Institute on Drug Abuse (1977, July–September). *Phase Report.* Washington, DC: U.S. Department of Health, Education, and Welfare.

Porter J & Jick H (1980). Addiction rare in inpatients treated with narcotics (Letter). *New England Journal of Medicine* 302:123.

Smith RJ (1979). Federal government faces painful decision on Darvon. *Science* 203:857–858.

Stimmel B (1985). Underprescription/overprescription: Narcotic as metaphor. *Bulletin of the New York Academy of Medicine* 61:742-752.

Termin P (1980). *Taking Your Medicine: Drug Regulations in the United States.* Cambridge, MA: Harvard University Press, 12–17.

Todd KH, Samaroo N & Hoffman JR (1993). Ethnicity as a risk factor for inadequate emergency department analgesia. *Journal of the American Medical Association* 269:1537–1539.

| Chapter 8 | # Abuse of Prescription Opioids |

Walter Ling, M.D.
Donald R. Wesson, M.D.
David E. Smith, M.D., FASAM

A buse of prescription medications, particularly opioids, is disconcerting in a way that is different than abuse of illegal drugs such as heroin. Prescription opioids are socially sanctioned to relieve the pain of surgery or medical illness, and few persons who have experienced intense pain would want their access to opioid medications unduly restricted. The misuse and abuse of opioid medications, therefore, perverts the intended medical order: Instead of being agents that ameliorate disease, the medicines become the agents of new disease—addiction—and physicians and pharmaceutical companies become facilitators of illness rather than health.

For a variety of reasons, pain specialists may have a very different view of prescription opioid abuse than do addiction medicine specialists. When they prescribe opioids, pain specialists are focused on providing adequate pain relief and allaying patient concerns about becoming addicted or being labeled "addicts." Pain specialists point to literature indicating that opioid addiction resulting from medical treatment with opioids is very rare and that historically a much greater problem has been the undertreatment of pain with opioids, which has resulted in much unnecessary patient suffering. Passik (2001) has observed that, in their zeal to improve access to opioids and relieve patient suffering, pain specialists have understated the problem of addiction and drawn faulty conclusions from very limited data. In effect, he said, their message has been that the risk of addiction in the treatment of pain is so small that the possibility essentially can be ignored.

On the other hand, addiction specialists rarely see patients whose quality of life has been greatly enhanced by the use of opioids. Instead, they see "failed" pain management cases, addicts or suspected addicts, and the unintended consequences of increased opioid availability, such as opioid abusers who are acquiring drugs diverted through pain patients. Addiction specialists hear stories about pain patients who sell all or part of their pain medications, thus contributing to the street-drug black market. For this reason, the need to improve pain management historically has been seen as in conflict with the need to minimize prescription drug abuse (Heilig & Smith, 2002).

Current trends make this issue particularly relevant today. The Drug Abuse Warning Network (DAWN) records rising emergency room mentions of heroin and other drugs, as well as drug-related deaths. In 1999, there were 262 mentions of oxycodone-related deaths, up from 49 mentions in 1996[1] (ONDCP, 2002). Using data from the 1999 National Household Survey on Drug Abuse, the Office of National Drug Control Policy (2002) has projected that about 19.9 million Americans have used pain relievers "illegally" in their lifetimes. An estimated 1.6 million Americans used prescription pain relievers non-medically for the first time during 1998. This represents a marked increase since the 1980s, when less than 0.5 million persons per year abused prescribed pain medications. First use was greatest among young people ages 12 through 17, for whom the incidence rate increased from 6.3 per 1,000 in 1990 to 32.3 per 1,000 in 1998. In the 18- to 25-year-old population group, first use increased from 7.7 to 20.3 per 1,000 (ONDCP, 2002).

Potential factors in these increases are the fact that palliative therapy for patients with AIDS and cancer has greatly increased the amount of opioids prescribed outside "controlled" settings such as hospitals and nursing homes. Pharmaceutical companies, recognizing the treatment of chronic pain as a marketing opportunity, have responded by developing and promoting controlled-release opioid formulations such as MS Contin®, OxyContin®, and Duragesic®. The controlled-release medications have been promoted as less prone to cause "addiction" than immediate-release products. In fact, when these drugs are used as intended, the reinforcing effects of opioids are reduced. Addicts, however, do not as a rule use medications in the recommended manner and, as discussed below in reference to specific medications, are able to defeat some of the benefits of the controlled-release formulations.

TERMINOLOGY AND CONTEXT
The terms used to describe abuse of street and prescription opioids are found in legislation, regulations, public health policy, medical communications, and many other venues. As a result, the terms "misuse," "abuse," "addiction," and "dependence" are used to mean quite different things, depending on the context. The issue is not whose definition is correct, but rather how to provide meaningful dialogue across the various venues.

Misuse. Misuse may refer to the incorrect use of a medication by *patients*, who may use a drug for other than the prescribed purpose, take too little or too much, take it too often, or take it for too long. Misuse also sometimes is used to refer to the behavior of *physicians* who prescribe medications for the wrong indication, at too high a dose, or for too long. Misuse should *not* apply to off-label prescribing when such use is supported by common medical practice, research, or rational pharmacology.

When used to describe patient behavior, it is uncertain whether misuse should lie at one end of a continuum that ends with abuse at the other, or whether it should be considered a discrete and separate phenomenon.

Abuse. The definition of "abuse" varies widely and depends on the context in which it is used and who is supplying the definition. The federal Drug Enforcement Administration (DEA) defines drug abuse as the use of Schedule I through V drugs in a manner or amount that is inconsistent with the medical or social pattern of a culture (DEA, 2002). DEA also defines drug abuse as involving the use of prescription medications outside "the scope of sound medical practice" (DEA, 2002).

The definition of abuse from the National Institute on Drug Abuse (NIDA) shifts according to the nature of the drug and the age of the user, and depending on the epidemiology, prevention, or treatment divisions within the agency. For example, in NIDA publications, any use of heroin (a Schedule I drug) generally is equated with "abuse," whereas use of marijuana (also a Schedule I drug) is not considered abuse unless it results in adverse consequences (NIDA, 2002). In discussing prescription medications, use of the terms "abuse" and "misuse" overlap. A NIDA InfoFacts web posting (2002) says that "The misuse of prescribed medications may be the most common form of drug abuse among the elderly." In discussing prescription analgesics, the same document, citing the 1999 Household Survey on Drug Abuse, equates "non-medical use" with misuse and indicates that 2.6 million people "misused pain relievers" (NIDA, 2002).

The American Psychiatric Association's *Diagnostic and Statistical Manual of Mental Disorders* (*DSM-IV-TR*) defines abuse as "a maladaptive pattern of substance use, leading to clinically significant impairment or distress as manifested by one or more behaviorally based criteria" (American Psychiatric Association, 2000).

Concerned as it is primarily with clinical issues, the medical profession embraces a definition of abuse that is relevant to its own practices, but one that may not be relevant for parents who are worrying about their children's recreational use of prescribed medications, for example. Law

---

[1] The sample sizes were not identical. In 1996, data were reported by 146 medical examiners in 41 metropolitan areas; in 1999, data were reported by 139 medical examiners in 30 metropolitan areas.

enforcement agencies, concerned as they are with street diversion and implementing the law, have little concern about users meeting any kind of clinical criteria. The U.S. Food and Drug Administration (FDA), whose approval of a drug implies official endorsement of its safety and efficacy, is concerned with proper labeling to prevent adverse consequences and to prevent the drug from being distributed outside authorized channels. In the end, the issues of misuse and abuse must be addressed in the context of the intended and unintended consumer populations.

Addiction. In a public policy statement, the American Society of Addiction Medicine has defined "addiction" as:

> . . . a primary, chronic, neurobiological disease, with genetic, psychosocial, and environmental factors influencing the development and manifestations. It is characterized by behaviors that include one or more of the following: impaired control over drug use, compulsive use, continued use despite harm, and craving (ASAM, 2001).

This definition specifically relates to the use of drugs or medications. Even so, the term "addiction" often is more generally applied to the pursuit of other "undesirable" behaviors (such as gambling) despite serious adverse medical or social consequences. In some contexts, the term "addiction" is considered prejudicial and even derogatory, but not in others. Although some ambivalence remains, the term generally has been embraced by those in the drug abuse treatment field, including physicians, as exemplified by the official designations, American Society of Addiction Medicine and American Academy of Addiction Psychiatry.

Physical Dependence. In various iterations of the American Psychiatric Association's *Diagnostic and Statistical Manual*, the term "addiction" has been replaced with the term "dependence." This may be "politically correct" but it is confusing. For example, "opioid dependence" is defined in the latest version of the *DSM-IV* as a set of behaviors, as opposed to physical dependence on opiates, which is defined as a neurobiological adaptation that occurs with chronic exposure. Many people, including physicians, equate one term with the other, and the distinction often is lost. Opiate dependence is, to be sure, more than simply consuming a lot of opiates: it also involves behaving like an addict. A patient who regularly takes a prescribed opioid may become physically dependent on the medication, but that patient is hardly an addict unless his

or her behavior meets the diagnostic criteria for opiate dependence.

It is not always easy to tell whether certain behaviors indicate addiction, especially in patients who are prescribed opiates for the treatment of pain.

Pseudoaddiction. The term "pseudoaddiction" was coined to describe "drug seeking behaviors" that are iatrogenically induced in pain patients through inadequate treatment of pain (Weissman & Haddox, 1989). In this context, the preoccupation with and pursuit of opioid medications is driven primarily by the patient's need for pain relief rather than a pursuit of the mood-altering effects of such drugs. Pseudoaddiction has been described as occurring in three phases, beginning with prescribing of analgesics in a manner that does not meet the patient's need for pain relief (phase 1), leading the patient to escalate his or her demands for analgesia, with accompanying behavioral changes (often exaggerated) to convince others of the severity of the pain and the need for more medication (phase 2), which in turn results in a crisis of mistrust between the patient and the health care team (phase 3; Weissman & Haddox, 1989). The authors emphasize that pseudoaddiction is preventable. A patient's report of pain must be accepted as valid and the patient must have trust that caregivers will make reasonable efforts to control the pain. Preventing pseudoaddiction requires rational use of opiates, including fixed rather than as-needed dosing.

Today, the term "pseudoaddiction" is used to describe a broad range of patient behaviors that are indicative of pain but erroneously interpreted as addiction.

PRESCRIPTION DRUG ABUSE IN PAIN PATIENTS
There has been little systematic study of prescription drug abuse in pain patients. The few published studies have focused largely on the risks of prescribing opioid analgesics and the fear of creating addiction in pain patients who use opioid medications. The majority of such studies have been uncontrolled and most have concluded that the risk of addiction is low. For example, the Boston Collaborative Drug Surveillance Project (Porter & Jick, 1980), which is perhaps the most often cited reference in the relevant literature, found only four cases of addiction in 11,882 non-addicts who received opioids during inpatient hospitalization; however, it consists of a single paragraph letter to the editor.

Evidence indicates that most physicians would rather not prescribe opioid analgesics to their pain patients. A recent retrospective review of 83,000 charts (Adams, Plane

TABLE 1. Comparison of Non-Addicted Chronic Pain Patients and Opioid-Abusing Patients in Relation to the DSM-IV Diagnostic Criteria

DSM-IV Diagnostic Criteria (Dependence Requires Meeting 3 or More Criteria)	Pain Patients	Opioid-Abusing Patients
(1) Tolerance, as defined by either of the following:		
(a) A need for markedly increased amounts of the substance to achieve intoxication or the desired effect; or	The patient may require some increase in dose over time to accommodate tolerance.	The patient may require progressive increases in dose because he or she seeks the drugs' mood-altering effects as much as, or more than, pain relief.
(b) A markedly diminished effect with continued use of the same amount of the substance.	The patient may require some increase in dose over time to achieve continued pain relief.	The patient may require progressive increases in dose because he or she seeks the drugs' mood-altering effects as much as, or more than, pain relief.
(2) Withdrawal, as manifested by either of the following:		
(a) The characteristic withdrawal syndrome; or	Withdrawal may occur when opioids are stopped abruptly.	Withdrawal usually occurs; the patient typically is unable or unwilling to tolerate withdrawal symptoms.
(b) The same (or closely related) substance is taken to relieve or avoid withdrawal symptoms.	Self-medication for withdrawal rarely occurs with patients who are under the care of a primary treating physician.	The patient often self-medicates without consulting a physician. Withdrawal symptoms often precipitate drug-seeking behavior.
(3) The substance often is taken in larger amounts or over a longer period of time than intended.	The patient is able to "ration" medications between planned visits to the prescribing physician.	The patient experiences episodes of intoxication and inability to consistently ration medication use. He or she may request refills between visits, offering explanations that are not plausible.
(4) There is a persistent desire or a pattern of unsuccessful efforts to cut down or control substance use.	The patient may want to decrease or stop use, but agrees to continue use if pain becomes worse when medication is reduced.	The patient repeatedly vacillates between wanting to use and wanting to stop. He or she may relapse to drug use after medication is tapered.
(5) A great deal of time is spent on activities necessary to obtain the substance, use the substance, or recover from its effects.	The patient may spend large amounts of time participating in the treatment of pain. He or she generally is cooperative with the physician's directions for non-opioid pain control strategies.	Much time is spent on drug-related activities.
(6) Important social, occupational, or recreational activities are given up or reduced because of substance use.	Activities may be reduced primarily because of pain. The patient may participate in more activities while using opioid medications.	Activities not related to drug use cease to be a priority.
(7) Substance use is continued, despite the patient's knowledge of a recurrent physical or psychological problem that is likely to have been caused or exacerbated by the substance use.	Medication use may continue despite concerns about addiction on the part of family or friends, but the patient generally wants to stop or reduce medication when it produces new physical or psychological problems	The patient continues drug use despite adverse consequences to his or her relationships, employment, or health. He or she may be unable to understand the cause-and-effect relationship between such adverse consequences and his or her drug use.

SOURCE: American Psychiatric Association (2000). *Diagnostic and Statistical Manual of Mental Disorders, 4th Edition, Text Revision (DSM-IV-TR)*. Washington, DC: American Psychiatric Press. 197.

et al., 2001) found that only 0.2% of patients with chronic non-malignant pain received an opioid analgesic and that 27% of the physicians who cared for non-malignant pain patients did not have a single patient receiving such medication. Further, most physicians who do prescribe opioid analgesics limit their use to only one or two patients.

On the other hand, Dunbar and Katz (1996) found that 9 of 20 patients attending a pain clinic who had both chronic pain and substance abuse and who were receiving long-term opioid analgesics, were abusing their pain medications. Of those who were not abusing their medications, most were actively involved in recovery efforts. Neither this study nor the one by Porter and Jick directly bears on the relative risks of prescribing opioid analgesics to patients who are addicted to opioids. In fact, more than half the subjects in the Dunbar and Katz study had alcohol as their primary drug of abuse. What their study did show is that, for patients with no history of opiate addiction, short-term opioid exposure is relatively risk-free, while for those with a history of addiction, active involvement in recovery activities should be an important part of the treatment plan.

Almost everyone interested in the subject has a favorite example of patient behavior that purportedly differentiates pain patients from addicts, but few systematic studies are available to guide practice. Compton and colleagues (1998) looked at a group of 50 chronic pain patients who were receiving opioid analgesics and whose physicians had referred them for evaluation because of a concern that they might be abusing their pain medications. The authors administered a 42-item behavioral checklist and used the results to rate the likelihood of drug abuse. Results were confirmed by an experienced psychiatrist using the *DSM-IV* diagnostic criteria. Three characteristics appeared to accurately describe more than 90% of the patients with drug abuse: (1) a preferred route of administration, (2) a tendency to increase the dose or frequency, and (3) the patient's own belief that he or she had a problem with drug abuse. In retrospect, the last criterion alone would have been overwhelmingly predictive, although it is unclear how each of these three characteristics actually contributes to the overall predictive value. The authors made rather modest claims about the study results, pointing out that the number of subjects was small and the number of items large, and expressed a hope that the instrument could be validated and the results duplicated with studies using larger samples.

More recently, Passik and colleagues (2001) used input from pain and addiction medicine experts to generate a checklist of aberrant drug-seeking behaviors. They used the checklist to rate the occurrence of the identified behaviors in a group of 388 chronic pain patients. Some 45% of the patients had an average of 1.5 (±2.7) aberrant drug-seeking behaviors out of a possible 29; the remaining 55% had none. Less than 4% of the patients had a history of abusing alcohol or street drugs, or had contact with the street drug culture (other aberrant behaviors appeared in as many as 18% of the study population). The results appear to indicate that such checklists are useful, but they do not provide a definitive indicator. Like Compton and colleagues, Passik and his co-investigators also noted a need for validation of the instrument and replication of the study results. In both instances, some items on the behavioral checklists are so aberrant and rare that their presence could be appropriately weighted so as to make the diagnosis of drug addiction certain. One can conclude, it seems, that non-addicts are not likely to exhibit addictive behaviors when given an opiate and those who do are likely to be addicts already.

A question arises as to what would constitute an appropriate population to examine for the broader concern of abuse of prescription opioids. It may be that chronic pain patients attending a pain clinic are not the most suitable population and that pain clinics are not the best place to address such concerns.

DRUG ABUSE AND DRUG DIVERSION

Abusability. "Abusability" can be simply defined as the relative ease with which a prescribed medication can be extracted or modified to yield the desired psychic effect. Certain pharmacologic properties, such as rapid onset and short duration of action, high potency, water solubility, and smokability, render a medication more readily abusable. Some medications are intrinsically more abusable than others. For example, tablets of Dilaudid® (hydromorphone) are easily dissolved in a small amount of water and injected. OxyContin® tablets (a controlled-release oral formulation of oxycodone) can be crushed to defeat the drug's controlled release properties and then snorted, or dissolved in solution and injected. In some cases, the FDA-directed "black box warning" on the labeling of a medication becomes a recipe for abuse. Finally, experience shows that a brand name drug carries a higher street value and is more subject to abuse than a comparable generic preparation.

Diversion. While distinct, *abuse* and *diversion* are closely related: the degree to which a prescribed medication is *abused* depends on how easily it is *diverted* from the usual prescribed route. Diversion of methadone, for example, can be said to occur frequently or infrequently and its diversion can be considered either a major public health issue or a non-issue, depending on one's point of view. It is well known that prescribed methadone is diverted from methadone clinics; in fact, the majority of all the methadone available on the street is methadone originally prescribed or dispensed in methadone clinics. However, the amount of methadone diverted in this manner is statistically insignificant compared to the total amount used for the intended purpose.

Opioids With Abuse Potential. All prescription opiates have some abuse liability. This section provides an annotated discussion of selected opioids used in the treatment of pain.

Buprenorphine (Buprenrex®, Suboxone®, Subutex®): Buprenorphine has been available in the United States since the mid-1980s in an injectable formulation (Buprenex®) for the treatment of moderate to severe pain. In many other countries, it is marketed as a 0.3 or 0.4 mg sublingual tablet (Temgesic®, Buprigesic®, Norphin®, Pentorel®, Tidigesic®) and there have been some reports of addicts dissolving the sublingual tablets in water and injecting them. In the past few years, some U.S. physicians have used the injectable form for opiate detoxification, but such practices are not legal. To date, buprenorphine has not been a common drug of abuse in the United States.

In October 2002, the FDA approved two sublingual formulations of buprenorphine for the treatment of opiate dependence. One formulation, Subutex®, contains only buprenorphine (either 2 mg or 8 mg); the other, Suboxone® contains 2 mg or 8 mg buprenorphine combined with naloxone in a 4:1 ratio, which may reduce its potential for intravenous use (also see the discussion of pentazocine, following). Buprenex® was a Schedule V narcotic until 2002, when it was reclassified to Schedule III along with Suboxone® and Subutex®.

Fentanyl Transdermal Patches (Duragesic®): Duragesic® transdermal patches, which deliver fentanyl through the skin for up to three days, are marketed for patients who require continuous analgesia for the treatment of pain. The patch is distributed in four sizes, containing 2.5, 5, 7.5, and 10 mg of fentanyl.

As with the injectable formulation of fentanyl (Sublimaze®), abuse of Duragesic® has been reported pri-marily but not exclusively in health professionals, who extract the fentanyl from the patch and inject it (DeSio, Bacon et al., 1993). Abusers also have chewed (Arvanitis & Satonik, 2002), ingested (Purucker & Swann, 2000), and inhaled (Marquardt & Tharratt, 1994) the contents of the patch. Even after a patch has been used for three days, it still contains sufficient fentanyl to be abused (Marquardt, Tharratt et al., 1995). In a case of fatal fentanyl poisoning, a funeral home employee was able to extract a lethal amount of fentanyl from a patch removed from a body (Flannagan, Butts et al., 1996).

Meperidine (Demerol®): Demerol® is primarily a drug of abuse among heath professionals. It is an unusual opiate because one of its metabolites, normeperidine, can produce seizures.

Methadone: In methadone maintenance clinics, methadone generally is dispensed in prepared individual doses, usually mixed with a juice-flavored drink. The purpose of combining methadone with the juice is to discourage its abuse by intravenous injection. The stringent distribution system for methadone used in opiate addiction treatment is meant to discourage diversion.

Methadone also is prescribed for the treatment of pain. Until recently, there was little evidence that diversion of methadone from pain management was occurring on any substantial scale. However, a recent report in a Florida newspaper (2002) described the substitution of methadone for OxyContin® in the management of pain patients as the source of an increased number of methadone overdose deaths in the state.

Most diverted methadone is bought and consumed by heroin addicts, many of whom use it to self-medicate symptoms of opiate withdrawal when they are trying to reduce their opioid tolerance or to bridge periods of time when their preferred opiate of abuse is not available. There is no evidence that street diversion of methadone from methadone clinics has resulted in new cases of opioid addiction in a significant number of addicts. *Pentazocine Alone or With Naloxone (Talwin® or Talwin-Nx®)*: In the 1970s and early 1980s, intravenous abuse of Talwin® tablets in combination with a blue-colored antihistamine tablet, tripelennamine, became common in the Midwestern states (Poklis, 1982; Senay, 1985). Factors that contributed to its widespread abuse included its placement outside Schedule II (so that its prescribing was not captured by triplicate prescriptions and other state monitoring programs) and to the wrongly held belief on the part of physicians that the drug was not abusable. Talwin also was widely abused by drug-addicted physicians because it could be prescribed in large quantities without being detected by monitoring systems. At one point, Talwin abuse became such a serious problem that the manufacturer considered removing the drug from the market. Its use was salvaged by reformulation of the drug to include the antagonist naloxone (Talwin-Nx®). When Talwin-Nx is taken as directed, the user experiences only the pentazocine effect because naloxone is not well absorbed through oral ingestion. However, if a tablet is dissolved and injected, the naloxone blocks the opiate effects of the pentazocine; in an opiate-dependent user, this would precipitate acute opiate withdrawal. The replacement of Talwin with the Talwin-Nx tablet formulation reduced the abuse of T's and Blues to an insignificant level (Senay, 1985). This is a good example of how changing a drug's formulation can reduce its intrinsic abuse liability without seriously compromising its therapeutic utility.

Oxycodone in Controlled Release Form (OxyContin®): OxyContin®, which has been marketed in the United States since 1995, is a Schedule II controlled released oral tablet formulation of oxycodone. (Oxycodone is available in immediate release tablets in combination with aspirin or acetaminophen under trade names such as Percodan® and Percocet®. The immediate release tablets contain 2.5 to 10 mg of oxycodone.) OxyContin® was designed for the treatment of chronic pain patients who require continuous dosing. Its formulations range from 10 mg (the upper dose of the immediate release products) to 80 mg[2]. Taken orally, OxyContin® tablets release their contents over about 12 hours. However, the controlled release mechanism is destroyed if the tablets are crushed; the entire contents then become immediately available, and can be abused by snorting, ingesting, or injecting[3]. Addicts' interest in OxyContin relates largely to its high oxycodone content compared to the immediate release forms.

Data from the Drug Abuse Warning Network (DAWN) indicate an increase in the "abuse" of oxycodone (ONDCP, 2002). The number of oxycodone emergency department mentions increased from 3,369 in the first half of 1999 to 5,261 in the first half of 2000. (It should be noted that mentions of oxycodone do not necessarily equal mentions of OxyContin because oxycodone also is an ingredient in more than 50 pharmaceutical formulations.)

Cases of oxycodone addiction and overdose deaths, particularly in the Northeast and mid-Atlantic states, have generated widespread controversy, as well as lawsuits against physicians and the manufacturer. In fact, abuse of OxyContin raises many complex issues about the marketing of new drug technologies and the relationship between drug abuse and the treatment of pain. Should the pharmaceutical company be held liable when a product is not used in the appropriate medical context? Does aggressive marketing by a pharmaceutical company contribute to physician "overprescription" or street diversion? What is the role of the pharmaceutical company in training physicians to use new formulations of its medications? What is the role of medical schools in training students to manage pain and addiction? These questions are not new or unique to Oxycontin, but the current controversy surrounding Oxycontin has renewed public attention to them.

THE ROLE OF PHYSICIANS IN PRESCRIPTION DRUG ABUSE

Certain physicians are more prone than others to be involved in prescription drug diversion and abuse. Smith devised a classification of such physicians and presented it at a 1980 White House Conference on Prescription Drug Abuse; the definitions subsequently were adopted in a report of the American Medical Association (Council on Scientific Affairs, 1982; Wesson & Smith, 1990). The classification is commonly referred to as the "four Ds": the "dated," the "duped," the "disabled," and the "dishonest."[4]

"Dated" physicians are those who have not kept up with changing standards of practice; "duped" physicians are those easily manipulated by addicts—perhaps because of their own gullibility, discomfort in confronting patients, or pride. While any physician occasionally can be manipulated or taken in by an addict's story, the duped physician has a recurring pattern of acquiescing to demands of patients and prescribing dugs in excessive amounts or for longer than necessary. "Disabled" physicians are those whose judgment

---

[2] The 160 mg tablet has been removed from the market.

[3] The manufacturer of OxyContin, Purdue Pharma, is considering various methods to make the tablets tamper-resistant. Methods under review include adding naloxone to the formulation. Information is available at HTTP://WWW.PURDUEPHARMA.COM/PRESSROOM/NEWS/OXYCONTINNEWS/20020618.ASP (updated June 18, 2002).

---

[4] David Smith subsequently added a fifth "D," the "defiant doctor," to describe physicians who are not only dated, but intransigently arrogant.

is impaired by their own illness or alcohol or drug use (see the discussion of health care professionals as a special risk group, following).

The physicians in these three categories are making a good faith effort to practice sound medicine, but their execution is flawed. They generally respond well to remedial and rehabilitative interventions. Dated and duped physicians, for example, are appropriate candidates for education and training to improve their practice procedures and skills, while disabled physicians often recover under the supervision of a physician health and effectiveness program.

"Dishonest" physicians (also known as "script doctors"), on the other hand, willfully prescribe controlled drugs for other than medical purposes—drugs that they know will be abused. Such physicians are not practicing good faith medicine but are using their medical licenses as a franchise to deal drugs. Organized medicine agrees that such physicians are not candidates for reeducation or rehabilitation and should be prosecuted to the full extent of the law (Council on Scientific Affairs, 1982).

Health Care Professionals as a Special Risk Group. Health care workers, because of their occupational access to opioids, constitute an unusually high risk group for opioid abuse. While the abuse of fentanyl (Sublimaze®) by anesthesiologists and the abuse of meperidine (Demerol®) by nurses long has been recognized (Ward, Ward et al., 1983), abuse of prescriptions by some other groups is less well recognized. For example, the increased use of opioids in hospices has given many nurses relatively uncontrolled access to large quantities of high potency prescription opioids. Large animal veterinarians also have unmonitored access to large quantities of opioids. Physicians with drug abuse problems may be ultra conservative or overly liberal in their prescribing habits because they fear drawing attention to themselves or as a result of carelessness from impaired judgment.

PREVENTING PRESCRIPTION ABUSE IN PAIN PATIENTS

The general principles of good medical practice apply equally to prescribing for addicted patients and those at high risk of becoming addicted. There are, however, some specific areas of practice worthy of special attention when prescribing opioids to patients with pain and addiction.

Medical Records. The importance of keeping detailed and legible medical records cannot be overemphasized. In the event of a legal challenge, detailed medical records documenting what was done and why are the foundations of the physician's defense. A written treatment plan with measurable treatment goals is a key document. The plan should define goals related to pain management and goals related to minimizing and managing the risk of addiction. The treatment plan should be updated as new information becomes available. Generally, the treatment plan should be negotiated with the patient and signed by both the patient and the treating physician to indicate agreement on the goals and procedures. (It is best not to label these as treatment "contracts" because of the legal connotation.) A copy of the treatment plan should be provided to the patient and all other care providers.

Some documents that may be included in the medical records are:

- Diagnostic assessments: history, physical examination, laboratory tests ordered, and their results.

- Actual copies of, or references to, medical records of past hospitalizations or treatment by other providers.

- The treatment plan.

- Authorization for release of information to other treatment providers.

- Documentation of discussions with and consultation reports from other health care providers.

- Medications prescribed and the patient's response to them, including any adverse events.

Medication Management. It is good practice for one physician to prescribe all psychotropic medications to a given patient. An addiction medicine specialist may or may not be the primary prescribing physician, depending on the nature of the patient's pain, the pathophysiology, and the status of any addictive disorder. Current management of pain, particularly neuropathic pain, often involves the use of ancillary medications, and the prescribing physician should be familiar with both opioid and adjuvant analgesics to effectively manage such pain (Farrar & Portenoy, 2001).

Patients should be encouraged to use one pharmacy to fill all their prescriptions. This can aid in identifying possible drug interactions and in tracking the amount of medication being consumed.

Postmarketing Monitoring for Abuse. The FDA now is able to require that a pharmaceutical manufacturer that markets a drug with abuse liability must conduct postmarketing surveillance for such abuse, as it did in 1995 when it granted approval of tramadol (Ultram®) (Cicero, Adams et al., 1999). Similarly, the FDA added a requirement of postmarketing surveillance to its approval of sublingual buprenorphine (Subutex® and Suboxone®).

Use of Consultation. Whenever the best clinical course is not clear or the patient's response is not as expected, consultation with another physician should be obtained. Generally, the results of the consultation should be discussed with the consulting physician and a written consultation report added to the patient's medical record.

Addiction medicine specialists and pain specialists often can provide better patient care by combining their expertise in the management of pain patients who are in recovery or in patients with an active substance abuse disorder. An addiction medicine specialist may be called upon to determine whether a patient is abusing pain medications or other drugs or is dependent on them (according to *DSM-IV* diagnostic criteria). Such a determination requires an understanding of both addictive and pain behaviors. Table 1 may be useful in clarifying the diagnosis. While the distinction may be difficult, some behaviors occur only in patients with substance abuse disorders. These include administering medications in other than the prescribed routes (as by crushing and injecting oxycodone tablets), and continued use of alcohol or other drugs after repeated physician warnings to the contrary. While addiction medicine specialists generally label such behaviors as addiction, pain specialists, who are reluctant to use the term "addiction" (Hung, Liu et al., 2001), commonly label these behaviors as "aberrant" (Passik, Kirsh et al., 2000).

Managing Patients With Active Addiction. Where and how best to manage patients who are actively abusing alcohol and other drugs and who also are in need of medical management with an abusable medication often is a contentious issue because of the clash in treatment philosophies between pain management programs and addiction treatment programs. There are no simple answers. The treating physicians must determine which intervention takes precedence. At times, it is adequate control of pain, but at other times adequate pain control cannot be achieved without first addressing the patient's addiction. Too often, treatment options and settings are limited. It is an area requiring more research and collaboration between specialists from both fields.

Computerized Monitoring Systems. Employing current computer technology, 15 states have adopted computerized systems to monitor the prescribing of drugs in Schedule II (and, in some states, other drugs of concern) for patterns that suggest inappropriate use or diversion. Because information is entered at the time a prescription is presented to a pharmacy, computerized monitoring is essentially "invisible" to prescriber and patient. Such monitoring systems thus are thought to escape a frequently cited problem with paper-based triplicate prescription systems, which were widely viewed as intrusive, stigmatizing, and likely to suppress even legitimate use of opioid analgesics. Computerized systems have been endorsed by the National Commission on Model State Drug Laws and the National Association of State Controlled Substance Authorities, and are expected to be adopted in additional states as resources become available (Prescription Monitoring Work Group, n.d.).

REFERENCES

Adams NJ, Plane MB, Fleming MF et al. (2001). Opioids and the treatment of chronic pain in a primary care sample. *Journal of Pain & Symptom Management* 22(3):791-796.

American Psychiatric Association (2000). *Diagnostic and Statistical Manual of Mental Disorders, Fourth Edition, Text Revision (DSM-IV-TR)*. Washington, DC: American Psychiatric Press.

American Society of Addiction Medicine (ASAM) (2001). Policy Statement: Definitions Related to the Use of Opioids for the Treatment of Pain. *Journal of Addictive Diseases* 17:129-130.

Arvanitis ML & Satonik RC (2002). Transdermal fentanyl abuse and misuse [letter]. *American Journal of Emergency Medicine* 20(1):58-59.

Associated Press (2002). Researchers link prescription methadone, rise in overdose deaths. *Naples Daily News*. Naples, FL; October 4, 2002. Accessed at WWW.NAPLESNEWS.COM/02/10/FLORIDA/D830526A.HTM.

Cicero TJ, Adams EH, Geller A et al. (1999). A postmarketing surveillance program to monitor Ultram® (tramadol hydrochloride) abuse in the United States. *Drug and Alcohol Dependence* 57(1):7-22.

Compton P, Darakjian J & Miotto K (1998). Screening for addiction in patients with chronic pain and "problematic" substance use: Evaluation of a pilot assessment tool. *Journal of Pain & Symptom Management* 16(6):355-363.

Council on Scientific Affairs (CSA), American Medical Association (1982). Drug abuse related to prescribing practices. *Journal of the American Medical Association* 247:864-866.

DeSio JM, Bacon DR, Peer G et al. (1993). Intravenous abuse of transdermal fentanyl therapy in a chronic pain patient. *Anesthesiology* 79(5):1139-1141.

Drug Enforcement Administration (DEA), U.S. Department of Justice (2002). Information available at WWW.USDOJ.GOV/DEA/CONCERN/DRUGCLASSESP.HTML.

Dunbar SA & Katz NP (1996). Chronic opioid therapy for nonmalignant pain in patients with a history of substance abuse: Report of 20 cases. *Journal of Pain & Symptom Management* 11(3):163-171.

Farrar JT & Portenoy RK (2001). Neuropathic cancer pain: The role of adjuvant analgesics. *Oncology* 15(11):1435-1442, 1445.

Flannagan LM, Butts JD & Anderson WH (1996). Fentanyl patches left on dead bodies—Potential source of drug for abusers. *Journal of Forensic Sciences* 41(2):320-321.

Heilig S & Smith DE (2002). The politics of pain: The need for new policies and approaches. *San Francisco Medicine* 75(2):19-22.

Hung CI, Liu CY, Chen CY et al. (2001). Meperidine addiction or treatment frustration? *General & Hospital Psychiatry* 23(1):31-35.

Marquardt KA & Tharratt RS (1994). Inhalation abuse of fentanyl patch. *Journal of Toxicology and Clinical Toxicology* 32(1):75-78.

Marquardt KA, Tharratt RS & Musallam NA (1995). Fentanyl remaining in a transdermal system following three days of continuous use. *Annals of Pharmacotherapy* 29(10):969-971.

National Institute on Drug Abuse (NIDA) (2002). *NIDA InfoFacts*. Available at WWW.NIDA.NIH.GOV/INFOFAX/PAINMED.HTML (updated November 4, 2002).

Office of National Drug Control Policy (ONDCP) (2002). *Drug Policy Information Clearinghouse Fact Sheet*. Available at WWW.WHITEHOUSEDRUGPOLICY.GOV/PUBLICATIONS/FACTSHT/OXYCONTIN/INDEX.HTML.

Passik SD (2001). Responding rationally to recent report of abuse/diversion of OxyContin [letter]. *Journal of Pain & Symptom Management* 21(5):359.

Passik SD, Kirsh KL, McDonald MV et al. (2000). A pilot survey of aberrant drug-taking attitudes and behaviors in samples of cancer and AIDS patients. *Journal of Pain & Symptom Management* 19(4):274-286.

Poklis A (1982). Pentazocine/tripelennamine (T's and blues) abuse: A five year survey of St. Louis, Missouri. *Drug and Alcohol Dependence* 10(2-3):257-267.

Porter J & Jick H (1980). Addiction rare in patients treated with narcotics [letter]. *New England Journal of Medicine* 302(2):123.

Prescription Monitoring Work Group of the National Alliance for Model State Drug Laws (n.d.). Executive summary. In *Recommendations for State Prescription Monitoring Programs*. Alexandria, VA: The Alliance.

Purucker M & Swann W (2000). Potential for duragesic patch abuse. *Annals of Emergency Medicine* 35(3):314.

Senay EC (1985). Clinical experience with T's and B's. *Drug and Alcohol Dependence* 14(3-4):305-312.

Ward CF, Ward GC & Saidman LJ (1983). Drug abuse in anesthesia training programs. A survey: 1970 through 1980. *Journal of the American Medical Association* 250(7):922-925.

Weissman DE & Haddox JD (1989). Opioid pseudoaddiction—An iatrogenic syndrome. *Pain* 36(3):363-366.

Wesson DR & Smith DE (1990). Prescription drug abuse. Patient, physician, and cultural responsibilities. *Western Journal of Medicine* 152(5):613-616.

SECTION

13 | Children and Adolescents

Section Coordinators
Peter D. Rogers, M.D., M.P.H., FAAP, FASAM
Ramon Solhkhah, M.D.

Contributors

Nicole Anderson, B.A.
Center for Adolescent Substance Abuse Research
Department of Psychiatry
University of Minnesota
Minneapolis, Minnesota

Marie E. Armentano, M.D.
Associate Medical Director
Child and Adolescent Services
Providence Hospital
Holyoke, Massachusetts

Robert M. Cavanaugh, Jr., M.D., FAAP
Associate Professor of Pediatrics, and
Director, Adolescent Medicine
Department of Pediatrics
State University of New York
Health Science Center
Syracuse, New York

Philomena J. Dias, M.D., FAAP
Clinical Assistant Professor of Pediatrics
Indiana University School of Medicine
Indianapolis, Indiana

Todd W. Estroff, M.D.
Director of Addiction Services
Independent Neurodiagnostic Clinic, and
Private Practice of Psychiatry, Addictions, and
    Chronic Pain Management
Atlanta, Georgia

Marc Fishman, M.D.
Assistant Professor
Department of Psychiatry
Johns Hopkins University School of Medicine, and
Medical Director
Maryland Treatment Centers
Baltimore, Maryland

J. David Hawkins, Ph.D.
Social Development Research Group
School of Social Work
University of Washington
Seattle, Washington

Richard B. Heyman, M.D., FAAP
Private Practice of Pediatrics
Cincinnati, Ohio

Sandra A. Hoover, M.P.H., Ph.D.
Director of Policy Development
Institute for Public Strategies
National City, California

Steven L. Jaffe, M.D.
Professor of Psychiatry
Emory University School of Medicine, and
Clinical Professor of Psychiatry
Morehouse School of Medicine, and
Treatment Supervisor
Atlanta Insight Adolescent Drug Abuse Program
Atlanta, Georgia

Alain Joffe, M.D., M.P.H.
Director, Student Health and Wellness Center
Johns Hopkins University, and
Associate Professor of Pediatrics
Johns Hopkins University School of Medicine
Baltimore, Maryland

Michelle Pickett, M.D., FAAP
Assistant Professor
Department of Pediatrics
University of Tennessee College of Medicine
Chattanooga, Tennessee

Deborah J. Poteet-Johnson, M.D., FAAP
Director, Adolescent and Young Adult Medicine
T.C. Thompson Children's Hospital, and
Assistant Professor of Pediatrics
University of Tennessee College of Medicine
Chattanooga, Tennessee

Peter D. Rogers, M.D., M.P.H., FAAP, FASAM
Children's Hospital
Division of Adolescent Medicine
Ohio State University
Columbus, Ohio

Ramon Solhkhah, M.D.
Director, Division of Child and Adolescent Psychiatry
St. Luke's-Roosevelt Hospital Center, and
Assistant Professor of Clinical Psychiatry
Columbia College of Physicians and Surgeons
New York, New York

Ken C. Winters, Ph.D.
Associate Professor and Director
Department of Adolescent Substance Abuse Research
Department of Psychiatry
University of Minnesota Hospital and Clinic
Minneapolis, Minnesota

Richard A. Yoast, M.A., Ph.D.
Director, Office of Alcohol and Other Drug Abuse, and
Robert Wood Johnson Foundation
National Alcohol Program Office
American Medical Association
Chicago, Illinois

| Chapter 1

Adolescent Risk and Protective Factors

J. David Hawkins, Ph.D.

Risk Factors
Protective Factors

The evaluation, management, referral, and long-term care of the adolescent who is seriously involved in substance abuse is marked by the difficulty of such work, the time and expense of treatment, and the frequency with which best efforts nevertheless result in poor outcomes. Our foremost goal should be to prevent the development of substance abuse in young people before the establishment of patterns of drug use that will be difficult to alter (Hawkins, Arthur et al., 1995).

Advances in cardiovascular disease prevention provide a model for approaching the prevention of substance abuse. Prospective longitudinal studies identified risk factors for heart disease (family history, smoking, high fat diet, stress, sedentary lifestyle) and protective factors that reduce or buffer heart disease risk (exercise, stress coping skills, healthy eating). Physicians have used this information to assess risk for cardiovascular disease in their patients, assessing family, lifestyle, dietary and smoking histories, measuring blood pressure, and requesting laboratory studies to measure cholesterol and to determine high-density lipid versus low-density lipid cholesterol. They have used the results of these assessments to advise and prescribe lifestyle changes (exercise, dietary changes, smoking cessa-

tion). Over the past 30 years, rates of cardiovascular disease in the United States have decreased by more than 30% (Shine, 1994).

Like cardiovascular disease, adolescent substance use is a preventable disorder. Current research provides a firm foundation for the physician seeking to reduce risk among young patients before the appearance of drug misuse or abuse. The physician who cares for children and who knows the risk and protective factors can intervene to avert alcohol and drug problems before they arise. . . .

RISK FACTORS

Health professionals who seek to prevent substance misuse, abuse, and dependence in the children and adolescents with whom they work should use the evidence on predictors of substance abuse. Substance abuse is predicted by multiple biological, psychological, and social factors and their interactions (Hawkins, Arthur et al., 1995; Hawkins, Catalano et al., 1992). Research to understand the interactions of these factors in predicting substance abuse continues. Already, clear evidence is available to guide preventive practice in primary care settings (Hawkins & Fitzgibbon, 1993).

Individual Factors. Some children appear to be at greater risk for substance abuse by virtue of their family histories, prenatal and birth experience, temperament, and early and persistent displays of problem behaviors.

A family history of alcoholism increases the risk of alcoholism in children about four times (Schuckit, 1987; Tarter, 1988; Merikangas, Rounsaville et al., 1992). However, fewer than 30% of the children of alcoholics develop alcoholism. There is well-established evidence of genetic transmission of a propensity toward alcoholism in males (Cadoret, Cain et al., 1980; Hrubec & Omenn, 1981), and recent evidence of such transmission in females (Kendler, 1992). Physicians should be alert to a family history of alcohol or other drug problems when informing their young patients about their own risk for substance abuse and dependence.

Perinatal complications (including preterm delivery, low birthweight, and anoxia), and brain damage (from infectious disease, traumatic head injury, or pre- or postnatal exposure to toxins such as heavy metals, alcohol, tobacco, or cocaine), predispose children to later aggressive behavior and substance abuse (Brennan, Mednick et al., 1991; Michaud, Rivara et al., 1993). Physicians who maintain or obtain good birth and trauma histories may see evidence of these risks long before drug use begins. It is important to inform parents and parents-to-be of the risks of alcohol, tobacco, and other drug use during pregnancy and infancy, and of the dangers to children of toxins in the home.

Some studies suggest that inherited biological traits and temperament link genetics and alcohol use behaviors (Schuckit, 1987; Tarter, 1988; Blum, Noble et al., 1990). High behavior activity level (Tarter, Laird et al., 1990) and sensation seeking (Cloninger, Sigvardsson et al., 1988) have been identified as predictors of early drug initiation and abuse. Attention deficit/hyperactivity disorder in childhood has been found to predict substance abuse disorders in late adolescence, especially when combined with aggressive behaviors or conduct disorders (Gittelman, Mannuzza et al., 1985). A pattern of persistent conduct problems, including aggressive behavior in childhood, is an early behavioral predictor of risk for later substance abuse (Kellam & Brown, 1982; Brook, Brook et al., 1990; Lewis, Robins et al., 1985).

Primary care physicians can help to reduce risks for later substance abuse by identifying patients who are experiencing behavioral and attention difficulties in early childhood and treating or referring them and their parents appropriately. Effective referral would include guiding parents to appropriate behaviorally focused parenting resources for skill development in child management.

As children approach adolescence, alienation from the dominant values of society (Jessor & Jessor, 1977; Shedler & Block, 1990), low religiosity (Jessor, Donovan et al., 1980; Brunswick, Messeri et al., 1992), and rebelliousness (Bachman, Johnston et al., 1981; Kandel, 1982; Block, Block et al., 1988) all predict greater drug use. During this period, attitudes favorable to drug use precede the initiation of substance use (Kandel, Kessler et al., 1978; Krosnick & Judd, 1982). Health professionals should begin to assess substance use attitudes and behaviors when they encounter these signals.

As noted earlier, the younger a child is when he or she first initiates the use of alcohol or other drugs, the greater the frequency of drug use (Fleming, Kellam et al., 1982), the greater the probability of extensive and persistent involvement in the use of illicit drugs (Kandel, 1982), and the greater the risk of alcohol misuse and drug abuse (Robins & Przybeck, 1985). Physicians should encourage young people to postpone alcohol use and to avoid the use of tobacco and illegal drugs for their own health and safety. As discussed later, the adoption of strong norms or standards against drug use appears to inhibit drug use initiation.

Family Factors. As children develop, families affect their drug use behaviors in a number of ways. Drug use by parents and older siblings and permissive parental attitudes toward children's drug use predict greater risk of alcohol and other drug abuse (Johnson, Shontz et al., 1984; Barnes & Welte, 1986; Brook, Whiteman et al., 1988). Involving children in parental alcohol- or drug-using behaviors, such as allowing the child to light a cigarette or to serve a drink to a parent, appears to influence the development of attitudes favorable to drugs and alcohol and to contribute to the risk of early initiation of drug use (Bush & Iannotti, 1985).

Early drug use is itself one of the strongest predictors of misuse, abuse, and dependence. Parents and older siblings can reduce the risks for alcohol and drug abuse in younger children simply by moderating use of alcohol or other drugs in their presence and by not involving children in their own alcohol or drug use behaviors.

Physicians can help to reduce substance abuse risks by ensuring that parents and older siblings know these facts and by encouraging them to act on them.

Parents who are permissive or who fail to set clear expectations for their children, who are lax in supervision of their children, and who are excessively severe and inconsistent in punishing their children increase their children's risk for drug abuse (Kandel & Andrews, 1987; Penning & Barnes, 1982; Baumrind, 1983). Both permissiveness and extremely authoritarian parenting practices predict later drug abuse in children (Shedler & Block, 1990; Baumrind, 1983). Parenting difficulties may be evident in office visits or through conversations with parents, but there is no reason to wait for symptoms. Health professionals can reduce drug risks in young patients by encouraging their parents to learn and practice good parenting skills preventatively. Just as participating in childbirth classes helps expectant mothers to prepare for having children, providing or referring parents to developmentally appropriate training opportunities in family management skills can result in improved parenting, thus reducing the risk of substance abuse (Spoth, Redmond et al., 1995).

High levels of family conflict also appear to contribute to risk for higher levels of substance use during adolescence (Simcha-Fagan, Gersten et al., 1986). Needle and colleagues (1990) found that children whose parents divorced during their adolescence were more likely to use drugs than other adolescents (Penning & Barnes, 1982). In contrast, positive family relationships appear to discourage the initiation of drug use (Jessor & Jessor, 1977; Kim, 1981; Norem-Hebeisen, Johnson et al., 1984; Brook, Gordon et al., 1986; Selnow, 1987). Shedler and Block (1990) found that the quality of mothers' interaction with their children at age 5 distinguished children who became frequent users of marijuana by age 18 from those who had only tried marijuana. Mothers of children who became frequent users were relatively cold, underresponsive, and underprotective with their children at age 5, giving them little encouragement, but pressuring them to perform in tasks.

Parental attitudes, practices, and relationships interact in contributing to risk. For example, Brook and colleagues (1992) found that low attachment to mother and paternal permissiveness predicted movement from low to moderate levels of alcohol and marijuana use.

Peterson and colleagues (1994) found that when parents used good family management practices and refrained from involving their children in their alcohol use, these practices inhibited alcohol use among their 15-year-old children, even when adults in the family drank alcohol.

Health professionals can insure that young people's parents know the importance of setting clear expectations for non-use of alcohol or other drugs during childhood and adolescence; the importance of monitoring their children in developmentally appropriate and non-intrusive ways; the importance of consistent and appropriate punishment for violating family expectations; and the importance of providing recognition to young people for living according to healthy standards. Curricula tested for effectiveness in teaching these skills are available (Catalano, Kosterman et al., 1998).

School Factors. School experiences appear to contribute to drug non-use, use, and misuse. Successful school performance has been shown to be a protective factor mitigating against escalation to a pattern of regular marijuana use and frequent drug use in adolescence (Kandel & Davies, 1992; Hundleby & Mercer, 1987). Conversely, beginning in the late elementary grades, academic problems have been found to predict early initiation of drug use (Bachman, Johnston et al., 1991), levels of use of illegal drugs, and drug misuse (Holmberg, 1985). Achievement problems may result from early behavior problems, learning disabilities, the failure of teachers to motivate students, or other causes. Regardless of cause, the experience of not succeeding academically during late childhood appears to contribute to risk for substance abuse. Health professionals can reduce drug abuse risk by assessing the academic progress of their young patients and suggesting tutoring or other academically focused interventions for young persons who are not making adequate academic progress. As children approach adolescence, those who lose commitment to educational pursuits, as indicated by little time spent on homework, truancy, and a perception that school is unimportant, are at greater risk for drug use in adolescence (Gottfredson, 1988; Friedman, 1983; Maguin & Loeber, 1996).

Peer Factors. Having friends who drink, smoke, or use other drugs is among the strongest predictors of substance use among youth (Brook, Brook et al., 1990; Jessor, Donovan et al., 1980; Barnes & Welte, 1986; Brook, Cohen et al., 1992; Kandel, 1978, 1986; Newcomb & Bentler, 1986).

Contextual Factors. Factors in the broader social environment also affect rates of drug abuse. Patterns of substance use in the neighborhood or community predict individual substance use behaviors (Robins, 1982). Rates of use are higher in communities where alcohol or other drugs are inexpensive and easily available. Availability and price are influenced by legal restriction or regulation on purchase, by excise taxes, and by market forces. Changes in laws to be more restrictive on alcohol availability (raising the legal drinking age, raising excise taxes on alcohol, limiting alcohol outlets) have been followed by decreases in alcohol consumption and alcohol-related fatalities (Cook & Tauchen, 1982; Holder & Blose, 1987; Saffer & Grossman, 1987).

Broad social norms regarding the acceptability and risk of use of alcohol or other drugs also appear to affect the prevalence of substance use and misuse (Vaillant, 1983; Johnston, 1991).

Finally, there is evidence that children who grow up in disorganized neighborhoods with high population density, high residential mobility, physical deterioration, and low levels of neighborhood attachment or cohesion, face greater risks for drug trafficking and drug abuse (Fagan, 1988; Simcha-Fagan & Schwartz, 1986).

Health professionals can reduce substance abuse risks in their communities by urging that policies and laws forbidding the sale of alcohol and tobacco to underage individuals are strictly enforced; by communicating strong normative standards to their patients, their parents, and the public against the use of alcohol, tobacco, or other drugs by children or adolescents; and by participating in groups and coalitions seeking to improve the community.

PROTECTIVE FACTORS
There are factors and processes that protect adolescents against substance abuse, even if they have been exposed to multiple risk factors. Individual protective characteristics include a resilient temperament, positive social orientation, and high intelligence and skills (Radke-Yarrow & Sherman, 1990). Children who have or develop these characteristics during childhood are more likely to negotiate adolescence without involvement in substance use.

Importantly, the development of warm, supportive relationships and social bonds to prosocial adults during childhood appears to inhibit substance use as well. This underscores the importance of good parenting skills throughout development. Health care providers offer childbirth education classes to expectant parents so as to prevent birthing complications and promote infant health and bonding. Health professionals can, as a matter of course, link the parents of their patients to appropriate parenting resources across development periods as the patients pass key milestones. At a minimum, this means making pamphlets, brochures, books, or videotapes on parenting available in the office and promoting the importance of keeping family bonds strong throughout development. Some health care providers offer parenting classes for parents of patients en-

tering their teens to help them prevent substance abuse problems and promote the healthy development of their children (Hawkins & Fitzgibbon, 1993).

Finally, as noted earlier, strong norms, beliefs, or behavioral standards that oppose the use of illegal drugs or the use of alcohol by teenagers protect against drug use, misuse, and abuse (Hansen & Graham, 1991). The fluctuations in the prevalence of substance use among adolescents since 1975 reflect changes in levels of social disapproval and risk perceived to be associated with the use of specific substances by young people (Johnston, 1991). Physicians are opinion shapers in their communities, especially with respect to matters of health. It is important to advocate abstinence from tobacco use and the use of illegal substances for children and adolescents. With respect to alcohol, the course associated with least health risks is to delay use until adulthood. Health professionals should communicate clear norms and standards regarding substances and their use.

CONCLUSIONS
The health professional who cares for children and youth can play a critical role in the prevention of substance misuse and abuse and in early intervention with those patients who have begun to use drugs. Knowledge of those factors that place young people at risk, and of those factors that can protect against substance abuse, is the foundation for assessment, diagnosis, and preventive action. A healthy, open relationship with children and families and an understanding of normal development allow the physician to assess existing and emerging risks for substance abuse across development and across spheres of life. Increasingly, effective approaches for reducing specific risks and enhancing protection have been identified and tested (Hawkins, Arthur et al., 1995; Hawkins, Catalano et al., 1992). The potential to intervene before problems arise is both the opportunity and obligation of those who care for youth.

ACKNOWLEDGMENT: Reprinted by permission of the American Academy of Pediatrics from M Schydlower & SK Schonberg, eds. (2001). Substance Abuse: A Guide for Health Professionals, 2nd Edition. Elk Grove Village, IL: American Academy of Pediatrics.

REFERENCES
Bachman JG, Johnston JD & O'Malley PM (1981). *Monitoring the Future: Questionnaire Responses from the Nation's High School Seniors.* Ann Arbor, MI: Survey Research Center.

Bachman JG, Johnston LD & O'Malley PM (1991). How changes in drug use are linked to perceived risks and disapproval: Evidence from national studies that youth and young adults respond to information about the consequences of drug use. In L Donohew, HE Sypher & WJ Bukoski (eds.) *Persuasive Communication and Drug Abuse Prevention*. Hillsdale, NJ: Erlbaum, 133-155.

Barnes GM & Welte JW (1986). Patterns and predictors of alcohol use among 7-12th grade students in New York State. *Journal of Studies on Alcohol* 47:53-62.

Baumrind D (1983). Why Adolescents Take Chances—And Why They Don't. Paper presented at the National Institute for Child Health and Human Development, Bethesda, MD.

Berman AL & Schwartz RH (1990). Suicide attempts among adolescent drug users. *American Journal of Diseases of Children* 144:310-314.

Block J, Block JH & Keyes S (1988). Longitudinally foretelling drug usage in adolescence: Early childhood personality and environmental precursors. *Child Development* 59:336-355.

Blum K, Noble EP, Sheridan PJ et al. (1990). Allelic association of human dopamine D2 receptor gene in alcoholism. *Journal of the American Medical Association* 263:2055-2060.

Brennan P, Mednick S & Kandel E (1991). Congenital determinants of violent and property offending. In D Pepler & KH Rubins (eds.) *The Development and Treatment of Aggression*. Hillsdale, NJ: Cambridge University Press, 81-92.

Brook JS, Brook DW, Gordon AS et al. (1990). The psychosocial etiology of adolescent drug use: A family interactional approach. *Genetic, Social, and General Psychology* 116:111-267.

Brook JS, Cohen P, Whiteman M et al. (1992). Psychosocial risk factors in the transition from moderate to heavy use or abuse of drugs. In M Glantz & R Pickens (eds.) *Vulnerability to Abuse*. Washington, DC: American Psychological Association, 359-388.

Brook JS, Gordon AS, Whiteman M et al. (1986). Some models and mechanisms for explaining the impact of maternal and adolescent characteristics on adolescent stage of drug use. *Developmental Psychology* 22:460-467.

Brook JS, Whiteman M, Gordon AS et al. (1988). The role of older brothers in younger brothers' drug use viewed in the context of parent and peer influences. *Journal of Genetic Psychology* 151:59-75.

Brunswick AF, Messeri PA & Titus SP (1992). Predictive factors in adult substance abuse: A prospective study of African American adolescents. In M Glantz & R Pickens (eds.) *Vulnerability to Abuse*. Washington, DC: American Psychological Association, 419-472.

Bush PJ & Iannotti RJ (1985). The development of children's health orientation and behaviors: Lessons for substance abuse prevention. In CL Jones & RJ Battjes (eds.) *Etiology of Drug Abuse: Implications for Prevention*. Rockville, MD: National Institute on Drug Abuse.

Cadoret RJ, Cain CA & Grove WM (1980). Development of alcoholism in adoptees raised apart from alcoholic biologic relatives. *Archives of General Psychiatry* 37:561-563.

Catalano RF, Kosterman R, Haggerty K et al. (1998). A universal model for the prevention of substance abuse: Preparing for the drug (free) years. In RS Ashery, EB Robertson & KL Kumpfer (eds.) *Drug Abuse Prevention Through Family Interventions (NIDA Research Monograph 177)*. Rockville, MD: National Institute on Drug Abuse, 130-159.

Chaiken JM & Chaiken MR (1990). Drugs and predatory crime. In M Tonry & JQ Wilson (eds.) *Drugs and Crime*. Chicago, IL: University of Chicago Press, 203-239.

Cloninger CR, Sigvardsson S & Bohman M (1988). Childhood personality, predicts alcohol abuse in young adults. *Alcoholism: Clinical & Experimental Research* 12:494-505.

Cook PJ & Tauchen G (1982). The effect of liquor taxes on heavy drinking. *Bell Journal of Economics and Management Science* 13:379-390.

Dishion TJ & Andrews DW (1995). Preventing escalation in problem behaviors with high-risk young adolescents: Immediate and 1-year outcomes. *Journal of Consulting and Clinical Psychology* 63:538-548.

Fagan J (1988). *The Social Organization of Drug Use and Drug Dealing Among Urban Gangs*. New York, NY: John Jay College of Criminal Justice.

Fagan J & Browne A (1994). Violence between spouses and intimates: Physical aggression between women and men in intimate relationships. In AJ Riess Jr & JA Roth (eds.) *Understanding and Preventing Violence: Social Influences, Vol. 3*. Washington, DC: National Academy Press, 115-292.

Fleming JP, Kellam SG & Brown CH (1982). Early predictors of age at first use of alcohol, marijuana and cigarettes. *Drug and Alcohol Dependence* 9:285-303.

Friedman AS (1983). High school drug abuse clients. *Treatment Research Notes*. Rockville, MD: National Institute on Drug Abuse.

Gittelman RS, Mannuzza RS & Bonagura N (1985). Hyperactive boys almost grown up: I. Psychiatric status. *Archives of General Psychiatry* 42:937-947.

Gottfredson DC (1988). An evaluation of an organization development approach to reducing school disorder. *Evaluation Review* 11:739-763.

Hansen WB & Graham JW (1991). Preventing alcohol, marijuana, and cigarette use among adolescents: Peer pressure resistance training versus establishing conservative norms. *Preventive Medicine* 20:414-430.

Hawkins JD, Arthur MW & Catalano RF (1995). Preventing substance abuse. In M Tonry & DP Farrington (eds.) *Building a Safer Society: Strategic Approaches to Crime Prevention*. Chicago, IL: University of Chicago Press, 343-427.

Hawkins JD, Catalano RF & Miller JY (1992). Risk and protective factors for alcohol and other drug problems in adolescence and early adulthood: Implications for substance abuse prevention. *Psychological Bulletin* 112:64-105.

Hawkins JD & Fitzgibbon JJ (1993). Risk factors and risk behavior: Preventing substance abuse in adolescent patients. *Adolescent Medicine State of the Art Reviews* 4:249-262.

Hawkins JD, Graham JW, Maguin E et al. (1997). Exploring the effects of age of alcohol use initiation and psychosocial risk factors on subsequent alcohol misuse. *Journal of Studies on Alcohol* 58:280-290.

Holder HD & Blose JO (1987). Impact of changes in distilled spirits availability on apparent consumption: A time series analysis of liquor-by-the-drink. *British Journal of Addiction* 82:623-631.

Holmberg MB (1985). Longitudinal studies of drug abuse in a fifteen-year-old population: I. Drug career. *Acta Psychiatrica et Neurologica Scandinavica* 71:67-79.

Hrubec Z & Omenn GS (1981). Evidence of genetic predisposition to alcoholic cirrhosis and psychosis: Twin concordance for alcoholism and biological endpoints by zygosity among male veterans. *Alcoholism: Clinical & Experimental Research* 5:207-215.

Hundleby JD & Mercer GW (1987). Family and friends as social environments and their relationship to young adolescents' use of alcohol, tobacco, and marijuana. *Journal of Marriage and the Family* 49:151-164.

Institute of Medicine, Committee on Drug Use in the Workplace (1990). *Under the Influence: Drugs and the American Work Force*. Washington, DC: National Academy Press.

Jessor R, Donovan JE & Windmer K (1980). Psychosocial Factors in Adolescent Alcohol and Drug Use: The 1980 National Sample Study, and the 1974-78 Panel Study (unpublished final report). Boulder, CO: University of Colorado, Institute of Behavioral Science.

Jessor R & Jessor SL (1977). *Problem Behavior and Psychosocial Development: A Longitudinal Study of Youth*. New York, NY: Academic Press.

Johnson GM, Shontz FC & Locke TP (1984). Relationships between adolescent drug use and parental drug behaviors. *Adolescence* 19:295-299.

Johnston LD (1991). Toward a theory of drug epidemics. In L Donohew, HE Sypher & WT Bukoski (eds.) *Persuasive Communication and Drug Abuse Prevention*. Hillsdale, NJ: Lawrence Erlbaum.

Johnston LD, Bachman JG & O'Malley PM (1993) [press release]. Ann Arbor, MI: The University of Michigan News and Information Service; April 9, 1993.

Johnston LD, O'Malley PM & Bachman JG (1991). *Trends in Drug Use and Associated Factors Among American High School Students, College Students, and Young Adults*. Rockville, MD: National Institute on Drug Abuse.

Johnston LD, O'Malley DM & Bachman JG (1998). *National Survey Results on Drug Use from the Monitoring the Future Study, 1975-1997. Volume 1, Secondary School Students*. Ann Arbor, MI: University of Michigan Institute for Social Research.

Johnston LD, O'Malley PM & Bachman JG (1998). Drug use by American young people begins to turn downward [press release]. Ann Arbor, MI: University of. Michigan News and Information Services; December 18, 1998.

Kandel DB (1978). Convergences in prospective longitudinal surveys of drug use in normal populations. In DB Kandel (ed.) *Longitudinal Research on Drug Use: Empirical Findings and Methodological Issues*. Washington, DC: Hemisphere Publishing, 3-38.

Kandel DB (1982). Epidemiological and psychosocial perspectives on adolescent drug use. *American Academy of Clinical Psychologists* 21:328-347.

Kandel DB (1986). Processes of peer influence in adolescence. In R Silberstein (ed.) *Development as Action in Context: Problem Behavior and Normal Youth Development*. New York, NY: Springer-Verlag, 203-228.

Kandel DB & Andrews K (1987). Processes of adolescent socialization by parents and peers. *International Journal of the Addictions* 22:319-342.

Kandel DB & Davies M (1992). Progression to regular marijuana involvement: Phenomenology and risk factors for near-daily use. In M Glantz & R Pickens (eds.) *Vulnerability to Abuse*. Washington, DC: American Psychological Association, 211-253.

Kandel DB, Kessler RC & Margulies RZ (1978). Antecedents of adolescent initiation into stages of drug use: A developmental analysis. *Journal of Youth and Adolescence* 7:13-40.

Kandel DB, Simcha-Fagan O & Davies M (1986). Risk factors for delinquency and illicit drug use from adolescence to young adulthood. *Journal of Drug Issues* 16:67-90.

Kellam SG & Brown H (1982). *Social Adaptational and Psychological Antecedents of Adolescent Psychopathology Ten Years Later*. Baltimore, MD: Johns Hopkins University.

Kendler KF (1992). A population-based twin study of alcoholism in women. *Journal of the American Medical Association* 268:1877-1882.

Kessler RC, McGonagle KA, Zhao S et al. (1994). Lifetime and 12-month prevalence of DSM-IIIR psychiatric disorders in the United States: Results from the National Comorbidity Study. *Archives of General Psychiatry* 51:8-19.

Kim S (1981). An evaluation of ombudsman primary prevention program on student drug abuse. *Journal of Drug Education* 11:27-36.

Krosnick JA & Judd CM (1982). Transitions in social influence at adolescence: Who induces cigarette smoking? *Developmental Psychology* 18:359-368.

Leigh BC & Stall R (1993). Substance use and risky sexual behavior for exposure to HIV: Issues in methodology, interpretation, and prevention. *American Psychologist* 48:1035-1045.

Lewinsohn PM, Hops H, Roberts RE et al. (1993). Adolescent psychopathology: I. Prevalence and incidence of depression and other DSM-IIIR disorders in high school students. *Journal of Abnormal Psychology* 102:133-144.

Lewis CE, Robins LN & Rice J (1985). Association of alcoholism with antisocial personality in urban men. *Journal of Nervous & Mental Disease* 173:166-174.

Maguin E & Loeber R (1996). Academic performance and delinquency. In M Tonry (ed.) *Crime and Justice: A Review of Research*. Chicago, IL: University of Chicago Press, 145-264.

Merikangas KR, Rounsaville BJ & Prusoff BA (1992). Familial factors in vulnerability to substance abuse. In M Glantz & R Pickens (eds.) *Vulnerability to Abuse*. Washington, DC: American Psychological Association, 75-97.

Michaud LJ, Rivara FP, Jaffe KM et al. (1993). Traumatic brain injury as a risk factor for behavioral disorders in children. *Archives of Physical Medicine and Rehabilitation* 74:368-375.

Miczek KA, DeBold JF, Haney M et al. (1994). Alcohol, drugs of abuse, aggression, and violence. In AJ Riess Jr & JA Roth (eds.) *Understanding and Preventing Violence: Social Influences, Vol. 3*. Washington, DC: National Academy Press, 377-570.

Needle RH, Su SS & Doherty WJ (1990). Divorce, remarriage, and adolescent substance use: A prospective longitudinal study. *Journal of Marriage and the Family* 52:157-169.

Newcomb MD & Bentler PM (1988). *Consequences of Adolescent Drug Use: Impact on the Lives of Young Adults*. Newbury Park, CA: Sage Publications.

Newcomb MD & Bentler PM (1986). Substance use and ethnicity: Differential impact of peer and adult models. *Journal of Psychology* 120:83-95.

Norem-Hebeisen A, Johnson DW, Anderson D et al. (1984). Predictors and concomitants of changes in drug use patterns among teenagers. *Journal of Social Psychology* 124:43-50.

Penning M & Barnes GE (1982). Adolescent marijuana use: A review. *International Journal of the Addictions* 17:749-791.

Perrine MW, Peck RC & Fell JC (1988). Epidemiologic perspectives on drunk driving. In *Surgeon General's Workshop on Drunk Driving: Background Papers*. Washington, DC: U.S. Department of Health and Human Services, Public Health Service, Office of the Surgeon General, 35-76.

Peterson PL, Hawkins JD, Abbott RD et al. (1994). Disentangling the effects of parental drinking, family management, and parental alcohol norms on current drinking by black and white adolescents. *Journal of Research on Adolescence* 4:203-227.

Radke-Yarrow M & Sherman T (1990). Children born at medical risk: Factors affecting vulnerability and resilience. In J Rolf, AS Masten, D Cicchetti et al. (eds.) *Risk and Protective Factors in the Development of Psychopathology*. Cambridge, England: Cambridge University Press.

Robins LN (1984). The natural history of adolescent drug use. *American Journal of Public Health* 74:656-657.

Robins LN (1992). Synthesis and Analysis of Longitudinal Research on Substance Abuse. Unpublished report for the Robert Wood Johnson Foundation.

Robins LN & Przybeck TR (1985). Age of onset of drug use as a factor in drug use and other disorders. In CL Jones & RJ Battjes (eds.) *Etiology of Drug Abuse: Implications for Prevention (NIDA Research Monograph 56)*. Rockville, MD: National Institute on Drug Abuse, 178-192.

Saffer H & Grossman M (1987). Beer taxes, the legal drinking age, and youth motor vehicle fatalities. *Legal Studies* 16:351-374.

Schroeder SA (1993). Substance abuse [President's Message]. Substance Abuse, the Robert Wood Johnson Foundation 1992 Annual Report. Princeton, NJ: Robert Wood Johnson Foundation.

Schuckit MA (1987). Biological vulnerability to alcoholism. *Journal of Consulting and Clinical Psychology* 55:301-309.

Selnow GW (1987). Parent-child relationships and single and two parent families: Implications for substance usage. *Journal of Drug Education* 17:315-326.

Shedler J & Block J (1990). Adolescent drug use and psychological health: A longitudinal inquiry. *American Psychologist* 45:612-630.

Shine KI (1994). *Presentation to the Committee on the Prevention of Mental Health Disorders*. Washington, DC: National Academy of Science.

Simcha-Fagan O, Gersten JC & Langner TS (1986). Early precursors and concurrent correlates of patterns of illicit drug use in adolescence. *Journal of Drug Issues* 16:7-28.

Simcha-Fagan O & Schwartz JE (1986). Neighborhood and delinquency: An assessment of contextual effects. *Criminology* 24:667-704.

Spoth R, Redmond C, Haggerty K et al. (1995). A controlled outcome study examining individual difference and attendance effects. *Journal of Marriage and the Family* 57:449-464.

Tarter R (1988). Are there inherited behavioral traits which predispose to substance abuse? *Journal of Consulting and Clinical Psychology* 56:189-196.

Tarter R, Laird S, Kabene M et al. (1990). Drug abuse severity in adolescents is associated with magnitude of deviation in temperament traits. *British Journal of Addiction* 85:1501-1504.

Vaillant G (1983). *The Natural History of Alcoholism*. Cambridge, MA: Harvard University Press.

Binge Drinking Among College Students

RICHARD A. YOAST, M.A., PH.D.
SANDRA A. HOOVER, M.P.H., PH.D.

Traditionally, the term "binge" has connoted drinking continuously over a period of many hours, a weekend, or even longer, to the point of total intoxication (including blacking out). Thus, the American Heritage College Dictionary defines a "binge" as "A drunken spree or revel; a period of unrestrained, immoderate self-indulgence; a period of uncontrolled self-indulgence." The associated images always are negative, often including interpersonal violence and self-destructive behaviors.

DEFINING BINGE DRINKING

In recent years, "binge drinking" has come to mean a defined level of high-risk problem drinking by students. The Harvard University College Alcohol Survey defines a "binge" as five (for men) or four (for women) or more drinks on a single occasion at least once in a two-week period (Wechsler, 2000). This definition is the subject of debate over its specificity (How many drinks? Over how long a period of time? Reaching what blood alcohol level?), and some educators find the term to be derogatory and a false measure of actual college drinking, arguing that most students drink only occasionally (Stubbs & DeJong, 2000). The beverage alcohol industry has argued that the number of drinks ought to be higher (such as eight or more drinks) before applying a definition that implies high risk and likely harm (Grant, 1997). Indeed, "binge drinking" is not a diagnostic category found in the *DSM-IV* (American Psychiatric Association, 1994) or in standard alcohol screening instruments. Although the phrase occasionally may be used in the non-medical treatment of alcoholism, it is not a standard there either.

While any level of alcohol can create some problems in some individuals in some circumstances, research data show that most people are likely to experience some alcohol-related impairment at 0.04% to 0.05% blood alcohol concentration (BAC). At 0.08% to 0.10% BAC (the legal driving limit in most states), almost all individuals consistently exhibit major impairment (AMA, 1997). Those who attain higher BAC levels (typically heavy, frequent problem drinkers) cause a disproportionately large share of alcohol-related problems, but there are many more occasional or "social" drinkers consuming at lower levels and, as a group (if not individually), they cause a large number of problems. Moreover, frequent bingers are unlikely to identify themselves as problem drinkers when they are surrounded by large numbers of even occasional and light bingers (Wechsler, Davenport et al., 1994).

SCOPE OF THE PROBLEM

About 10.4 million adolescents (29.4%) age 12 to 20 are current (in the past month) drinkers, while 6.8 million (20.2%) engage in binge drinking, including 2.1 million heavy drinkers (defined as those who binged five or more times a month). The peak prevalence for all drinking categories is age 21. Among persons 12 to 20 years old, drinking rates are highest in the west north central region of the United States and among white youth (32.1%) (SAMHSA, 2000).

Binge drinking often begins before young people reach college age. The 2000 Monitoring the Future Survey (NIDA, 2000) found that 14.1% of 8th graders, 26.2% of 10th graders, and 30% of 12th graders engaged in binge drinking in the preceding 2 weeks. The 1999 Harvard College Alcohol Survey of 15,000 students (most of whom were under the legal drinking age of 21) at 140 four-year campuses found that 23% frequently and 21% occasionally binged, while 37% drank but did not binge and 19% abstained (Wechsler, Lee et al., 2000). Whereas binge drinking appears to peak in high school and declines after leaving school for students who do not attend college, it peaks for college students during college and declines only after they leave, often in their early 20s (Schulenberg, Maggs et al., 2001).

Frequent binge drinkers account for an estimated 72% of all alcohol consumed by college students, while only 20% is consumed by occasional bingers and 8% by all other students (CESAR, 1999; Greenfield & Rogers, 1999). Compared to colleges with few binge drinkers, students at colleges with higher rates of binge drinking are more likely to experience one or more negative secondhand effects of drinking by others: insult, humiliation, serious arguments or quarrels, property damage, sleep and study interruptions, pushes or assaults, unwanted sexual advances, victimization by sexual assault, and date rape (Wechsler, Davenport et al., 1994). Students who engage in binge drinking are more likely to miss class, to have unplanned sex, and to drink and drive. While only 3.5% of students who do not binge have five or more alcohol-related problems, 16.6% of occasional and 48% of frequent bingers experience that level of problems (Wechsler, Lee et al., 2000).

Male and younger students (age 17 to 23) are more likely to binge (at all levels) than are females and older students, but students of both sexes experience the same level of problems at equivalent levels of consumption (Wechsler, Davenport et al., 1994).

ENVIRONMENTAL CORRELATES

The strongest situational predictor of binge drinking is membership and/or residence in a fraternity or sorority (Wechsler, Kuo et al., 2000; Wechsler, Dowdall et al., 1995a). Athletes also have higher rates of binge drinking than do non-athletes (Nelson & Wechsler, 2001). Other correlates include easy access to alcohol (via illegal sales or access by minors to alcohol purchased by of-age students), low-priced drinks, drinking beer, drinking and driving, weak law enforcement, and high density of bars near campus (Wechsler, Kuo et al., 2000). Other predictive factors include previous drinking and bingeing experiences and early first use of alcohol (Grant & Dawson, 1997).

Expectations also affect binge drinking (Turrisi, Kimberly et al., 2000). These can include norms set by parents and alumni, as well as the promotion and easy availability of alcohol. Schools with reputations as "party" schools tend to attract students who want to drink. Many students overestimate their peers' actual consumption levels and perceive pressures to drink accordingly. Drinking in groups also increases heavy drinking (NIAAA, 1995).

Lower rates of binge drinking correlate with participation in volunteer and other activities (Weitzman & Kawachi, 2000), residence in substance-free housing (Wechsler, Lee et al., 2001a), graduation and departure from campus environments (for example, leaving Greek organizations) (Sher, Bartholow et al., 2001), attendance at colleges that ban alcohol (Wechsler, Lee et al., 2001b), and drinking with friends and where food is available (Clapp, Shillington et al., 2000).

PREVENTION APPROACHES

Statistical data from CAS and other studies demonstrate that, at a population level, higher levels of consumption result in more negative consequences. Further, negative results are more likely among individual binge drinkers than in

drinkers who do not binge. Thus, population-based environmental measures targeted to all drinkers are indicated for management of the problem.

No single approach adequately reduces binge drinking and its effects to acceptable levels. However, research has identified a number of promising strategies (DeJong, Vince-Whitman et al., 1998; Edwards et al., 1994; Grover, 1999; Holder & Edwards, 1995; Mosher & Stewart, 1999; Stewart, 1999; Toomey & Wagenaar, 1999; Wagenaar, Gehan et al., 1996). Experiences with efforts to reduce drinking and driving indicate that a combination of measures is most likely to be effective. These include sales and distribution restrictions and other strong public policies; media exposure of the problem; increased, credible enforcement with publicized, predictable consequences for infractions; and promotion of safer consumption norms and alternatives.

Strategies that show the greatest effect on underage drinking (Edwards et al., 1994; Holder & Edwards, 1995; Mosher & Stewart, 1999; Stewart, 1999; Toomey & Wagenaar, 1999; Wagenaar, Gehan et al., 1996) include enforcing the minimum legal drinking age (21) through sales compliance checks, strict penalties, mandatory seller education, and safeguards against provision to minors by adults; holding adults responsible for illegal provision of alcohol to minors (social host liability); increasing alcohol prices (through taxation, higher licensing fees, fines, restrictions on price specials); reducing alcohol availability (through fewer outlets, shorter sales hours, sales bans or controls in community venues such as festivals, fairs, and sporting arenas); changing expectations (often via the mass media) regarding drinking norms and related behaviors (by correcting misperceptions and setting clear, publicized expectations); curtailing the promotion of alcohol; promoting healthier behaviors; and increasing availability of alternative behaviors and activities.

Successful implementation requires adequate funding over time, as well as organizing constituencies to pass and maintain effective policies. A number of national programs and individual campus actions (Wechsler, Kelley et al., 2000) are under way across the nation to implement and evaluate comprehensive environmental change strategies.

A Matter of Degree: Reducing High-Risk Drinking Among College Students (AMOD). A Matter of Degree is the first national program to apply this environmental management strategy to college communities (Bishop, 2000). The project was conceived by Henry Wechsler, Ph.D., of the Harvard School of Public Health, following the first

---

College Alcohol Study in 1993. The Robert Wood Johnson Foundation and the American Medical Association agreed to collaborate in a seven-year, $10 million national effort to reduce binge drinking and its consequences (extended for four years in 2001).

The project is unique in several respects: considerable resources were allocated over a five-year period (one year for planning and four for implementation); the goal was achievement of systemic, sustainable campus and community changes; involvement of campus and community leaders was incorporated as a critical element; university-community coalitions were developed; and a media policy was modeled after much of the work that had been done in tobacco prevention and control.

Program objectives are to:

- Reduce rates of high-risk drinking among college students;

- Reduce the consequences of high-risk drinking (including injury, assault, unplanned and unprotected sex, motor vehicle crashes, and the like) to students and others;

- Improve the quality of academic and social life for all students; and

- Enhance the relationship between the college and its local community.

The initiative is testing the public health model known as "environmental management," in which the campus-community coalition identifies factors that most contribute to or exacerbate the problem, then creates solutions through policy changes, enhanced enforcement, media advocacy, and other strategies. The Harvard School of Public Health is conducting an extensive, ongoing project evaluation to help determine successful practices and to track problem reductions.

Most AMOD grantees begin with campus policy changes. In 1996, the University of Delaware, to help involve parents in campus life, was the first university to implement parental notification for alcohol-related incidents. Initially controversial, this was soon incorporated into recommendations contained in the federal Drug and Safe Free Schools Act recommendations and adopted at many universities. AMOD sites also sought to:

- *Set clear expectations and norms*: Grantees reviewed and altered recruitment, admissions, and orientation materials and practices to inform applicants and their parents in a consistent way about university alcohol policies and disapproval of binge drinking. Several grantees partnered with their "feeder" schools to change high school students' ideas about binge drinking and to warn them that it would not be tolerated when they came to campus.

- *Provide alternative campus lifestyle options*: Students organized alcohol-free events funded by campuses, alumni, and parents; encouraged recreational and social facilities to stay open late at night; increased substance-free living options; initiated alcohol-free tailgate sections at sporting events; and encouraged participation in campus clubs and volunteer activities.

- *Institute clear, credible enforcement and consequences*: Campus disciplinary codes, including those for fraternities, sororities, and athletics, were improved and enforced.

- *Reduce pro-consumption messages*: Alcohol industry-sponsored campus events and advertising in college publications were eliminated. One school closed a campus pub, while others reduced or eliminated alcohol service at campus events and meetings. Campuses also looked at class scheduling and expectations so as not to accommodate student drinking patterns (for example, by avoiding long weekends).

- *Reduce availability*: Campuses employed a variety of strategies to reduce the availability of alcohol. These included prohibiting beer keg delivery on campus, closing a campus pub, banning alcohol sales in a stadium, requiring alcohol server training, and eliminating alcohol service at public events.

Recognizing that community factors contribute to binge drinking, the AMOD coalitions worked to make their community environments less conducive to binge drinking. Campus/community task forces (involving law enforcement, local alcohol beverage commissions, alcohol licensees, government officials, university officials, and concerned community members) collaborated to improve enforcement of underage drinking laws and to implement responsible alcohol service practices. Complementary strategies primarily sought to:

- *Reduce the supply of alcohol* by restricting licenses, enforcing underage drinking laws, and limiting service at community events.

- *Limit access and availability* through the use of city ordinances and zoning and planning regulations to reduce outlet density and restrict bar locations.

- *Increase the cost of alcohol* by eliminating happy hours and other alcohol discounting.

- *Inform the public about the problem and policy solutions*: All the grantees faced the challenge of helping the public to understand and learn the importance of environmental management in reducing binge drinking.

In the past, prevention programs often focused on education and individual behavior change, blaming the binge drinker for the problem. The AMOD approach recognizes that holding individuals solely responsible and relying only on education is an insufficient approach, because drinking students typically do not produce, sell, or promote alcohol, nor do they control or enforce the laws governing alcohol distribution and consumption. From AMOD's inception, grantees have applied a communications strategy to create public awareness about the complexity of binge drinking and environmental factors that influence it. They have worked with college and community print and broadcast media to increase coverage of the links between problems such as violence, vandalism, and unplanned/unprotected sex; high-risk drinking; and the environmental/social factors contributing to the problem. The goal is to create support on and off campus for the strategies outlined above so as to create safer, healthier living and learning environments for all students.

REFERENCES

American Medical Association (AMA), Council on Scientific Affairs (1997). *Drivers Impaired by Alcohol.* Report of the Council on Scientific Affairs (A-97). Chicago, IL: The Association.

American Psychiatric Association (APA) (1994). *Diagnostic and Statistical Manual of Mental Disorders, 4th Edition (DSM-IV).* Washington, DC: American Psychiatric Press.

Bishop JB (2000). An environmental approach to combat binge drinking on college campuses. *Journal of College Student Psychotherapy* 15(1):15-30.

CESAR (Center for Substance Abuse Research) (1999). Frequent binge drinkers account for majority of alcohol consumed by U.S. college students. *CESAR FAX* 8:33. University of Maryland, College Park. Adapted from data in Wechsler H, Molnar BE, Davenport AE et al. (1999). College alcohol use: A full or empty glass? *Journal of American College Health* 47:247-252.

Clapp JD, Shillington AM & Segars LB (2000). Deconstructing contexts of binge drinking among college students. *American Journal of Drug and Alcohol Abuse* 26:139-154.

DeJong W, Vince-Whitman C, Colthurst T et al. (1998) *Environmental Management. A Comprehensive Strategy for Reducing Alcohol and Other Drug Abuse on College Campuses.* Newton, MA: Higher Education Center for Alcohol and Other Drug Prevention.

Edwards G et al. (1994). *Alcohol Policy and the Public Good.* New York, NY: Oxford University Press, Inc.

Grant M (1997). *The Limits of Binge Drinking (ICAP Reports 2).* Washington, DC: International Center for Alcohol Policy.

Grant B & Dawson D (1997). Age at onset of alcohol use and its association with alcohol abuse and dependence. *Journal of Substance Abuse* 9:103-110.

Greenfield TK & Rogers JD (1999). Who drinks most of the alcohol in the U.S.? The policy implications. *Journal of Studies on Alcohol* 60:78-89.

Grover PL, ed. (1999). *Preventing Problems Related to Alcohol Availability: Environmental Approaches. Practitioners' Guide (Prevention Enhancement Protocols System).* Rockville, MD: Center for Substance Abuse Prevention.

Haines MP (1996). *A Social Norms Approach to Preventing Binge Drinking at Colleges and Universities.* Newton, MA: Higher Education Center for Alcohol and Other Drug Prevention.

Hasin D, Paykin A & Endicott J (2001). Course of DSM-IV alcohol dependence in a community sample: Effects of parental history and binge drinking. *Alcoholism: Clinical & Experimental Research* 25(3):411-414.

Holder HD & Edwards G, eds. (1995). *Alcohol and Public Policy: Evidence and Issues.* Oxford, England: Oxford University Press.

Mosher JF & Stewart K (1999). *Regulatory Strategies for Preventing Youth Access to Alcohol: Best Practices.* Rockville, MD: Pacific Institute for Research and Evaluation (for the Enforcing the Underage Drinking Laws Program, Office of Juvenile Justice and Delinquency Prevention, U.S. Department of Justice).

National Institute on Alcohol Abuse and Alcoholism (NIAAA) (1995). *College Students and Drinking (Alcohol Alert No. 29).* Bethesda, MD: NIAAA.

National Institute on Drug Abuse (NIDA) (2000). *2000 Monitoring the Future Survey Released (Press Release).* Bethesda, MD: NIDA, March 8.

Nelson TF & Wechsler H (2001). Alcohol and college athletes. *Medicine & Science in Sports & Exercise* 33(1):43-47.

Nicholson ME, Maney DW, Blair K et al. (1998). Trends in alcohol-related campus violence: Implications for prevention. *Journal of Alcohol and Drug Education* 43(3):34-52.

Schulenberg J, Maggs JL, Long SW et al. (2001). The problem of college drinking: Insights from a developmental perspective. *Alcoholism: Clinical & Experimental Research* 25(3):473-477.

Sher KJ, Bartholow BD & Nanda S (2001). Short- and long-term effects of fraternity and sorority membership on heavy drinking: A social norms perspective. *Psychology of Addictive Behaviors* 15(1):42-51.

Stewart K (1999). *Strategies to Reduce Underage Alcohol Use: Typology and Brief Overview.* Rockville, MD: Pacific Institute for Research and Evaluation (for the Enforcing the Underage Drinking Laws Program, Office of Juvenile Justice and Delinquency Prevention, U.S. Department of Justice).

Stubbs HC & DeJong W (2000). *Notes to the Field: Media Reports of Harvard's College Alcohol Study Create a Misleading Portrait of College Student Drinking.* Newton, MA: Higher Education Center for Alcohol and Other Drug Prevention.

Substance Abuse and Mental Health Services Administration (SAMHSA) (2000). *Highlights from the 1999 National Household Survey on Drug Abuse.* Rockville, MD: Office of Applied Studies, SAMHSA.

Toomey TL & Wagenaar AC (1999). Policy options for prevention: The case of alcohol. *Journal of Public Health Policy* 20:192-211.

Turrisi R, Kimberly WA & Hughes KK (2000). Binge-drinking-related consequences in college students: Role of drinking beliefs and mother-teen communication. *Psychology of Addictive Behaviors* 14(4):342-355.

Wagenaar AC, Gehan JP, Toomey TL et al. (1996). *Organizing for Alcohol Policy: What Is Needed and How To Get It.* Minneapolis, MN: Division of Epidemiology, School of Public Health, University of Minnesota.

Wechsler H (2000). *Binge Drinking on America's Campuses. Findings from the Harvard School of Public Health College Alcohol Study.* Cambridge, MA: The College Alcohol Study, School of Public Health, Harvard University.

Wechsler H, Davenport A, Dowdall GW et al. (1994). Health and behavioral consequences of binge drinking in college. *Journal of the American Medical Association* 272:1672-1677.

Wechsler H, Dowdall GW, Davenport A et al. (1995a). Correlates of college student binge drinking. *American Journal of Public Health* 85:921-926.

Wechsler H, Dowdall GW, Davenport A et al. (1995b). A gender-specific measure of binge drinking among college students. *American Journal of Public Health* 85:982-985.

Wechsler H, Kelley K, Weitzman ER et al. (2000). What colleges are doing about student binge drinking. A survey of college administrators. *Journal of American College Health* 48:219-226.

Wechsler H, Kuo M, Lee H & Dowdall GW (2000). Environmental correlates of underage alcohol use and related problems of college students. *American Journal of Preventive Medicine* 19(1):24-29.

Wechsler H, Lee JE, Gledhill-Hoyt J et al. (2001b). Alcohol use and problems at colleges banning alcohol: Results of a national survey. *Journal of Studies on Alcohol* 62(2):133-141.

Wechsler H, Lee JE, Kuo M et al. (2000). College binge drinking in the 1990s: A continuing problem. Results of the Harvard School of Public Health 1999 College Alcohol Study. *Journal of American College Health* 48:199-210.

Wechsler H, Lee JE, Nelson TF et al. (2001a). Drinking levels, alcohol problems and secondhand effects in substance-free college residences: Results of a national study. *Journal of Studies on Alcohol* 62(1):23-31.

Weitzman ER & Kawachi I (2000). Giving means receiving: The protective effective of social capital on binge drinking on college campuses. *American Journal of Public Health* 90:1936-1939.

Tobacco Use by Youth

Richard B. Heyman, M.D., FAAP

The fact that more than 90% of adults who smoke became regular smokers before the age of 18 defines the uptake of tobacco use as a pediatric problem (DHHS, 1994). The fact that 86% of children aged 12 to 17 who smoke choose one of the three most heavily advertised brands of cigarettes (Marlboro®, Camel®, and Newport®) while less than half of those over the age of 25 do so suggests that identifiable forces influence young people to take up the habit (SAMHSA, 2001). A number of studies identify advertising and image creation as the most important factors in encouraging young people to smoke. Clearly, tobacco use among adolescents is a problem unique unto itself.

Studies suggest that more than a third of all young people who ever try smoking a cigarette become regular, daily smokers before leaving high school. Current survey data suggest that approximately 35% of high school students are regular tobacco users (Johnston, O'Malley et al., 2000), compared with 24% of adults (CDC, 2000). Each day, some 3,000 children become regular smokers. The scientific issues surrounding tobacco use in general, and nicotine addiction and smoking cessation in particular, are addressed in other chapters of this text. This chapter focuses on use by young people—for whom tobacco use cessation programs have limited success, so that one key to the problem appears to be prevention.

TOBACCO AS A GATEWAY DRUG

Tobacco use frequently represents a young person's first encounter with a mind-altering drug. As young people acquire the tobacco habit, they develop the ability to obtain a drug illegally. They learn how to use a mind-altering substance and how it makes them feel and act. They come to enjoy this feeling and to accept that a drug can make them feel better. They learn how to hide their use and to defend a fundamentally bad choice of behaviors. Finally, they develop the curiosity to try other mind-altering drugs. Tobacco use thus sets the stage and trains young people for the use of illegal drugs. Convincing them not to use tobacco is thus a crucial element of substance use prevention.

If one examines carefully the reasons that young people choose to use tobacco products, approaches to prevention become more logical. According to a number of studies, tobacco seems to provide pleasure, relaxation, and energy to young people, as it does to adult users (CDC, 1993). Young people are able to identify problems with craving and addiction (Siquera, Rolnitzky et al., 2001) and recognize the pleasant if compulsive aspects of the hand/mouth stimulation afforded by cigarettes. Smoking takes the edge off of anxiety-provoking situations and may serve as a "social lubricant" (much as alcohol does for adults).

It is in the area of peer association ("all my friends smoke") and imagery ("smoking is 'who I am'—cool, macho, independent, sexy, successful, athletic") that young people differ from adults. These differences may, in fact, be the most crucial ones.

PREVENTION APPROACHES

The most effective approach to addressing tobacco use by youth is to start early. Pediatricians recommend that health professionals address this issue with children at an early age and raise the subject at virtually every visit (AAP, 2001). Special attention should be paid to those children who grow up in homes where tobacco is used, as this proximity puts them at greater risk for future use and exposes them to the deleterious effects of environmental tobacco smoke.

Successful tobacco prevention programs for youth may incorporate many elements, but central to most are media education and social skills development. *Media education* involves helping youth to deconstruct advertising and marketing schemes so that they understand that the imagery created by the tobacco industry does not represent the truth behind the product. Big Tobacco spends hundreds of millions of dollars each year promoting the concept that cigarette use can essentially make one into the Marlboro Man, Joe Camel, or a Newport beach beauty. Helping young people to understand that—despite portrayals to the contrary—the use of a dangerous, addicting product that clearly is harmful to one's health will not make them successful, popular, or attractive may decrease the likelihood that they will begin smoking. It is equally important to point out that, despite portrayals in movies and television, most adults do not smoke. Again, the media play a major role in "normalizing" tobacco use, with the result that most children grossly overestimate the proportion of adults who use tobacco.

Social skills development for young people involves helping them to refuse tobacco by suggesting alternative activities, identifying a personal health reason why use would be dangerous, role playing a "no, thanks" scenario, and working to keep them out of situations where tobacco use is prevalent. Unlike adults, children seek "peer acceptance" to a significant degree and must be provided with strategies for dealing with friends who encourage them to try tobacco.

CLINICAL PRACTICE GUIDELINE

The clinical practice guideline on tobacco use and dependence, published recently by the U.S. Public Health Service (Fiore, Bailey et al., 2000), represents a state-of-the-art approach to the subject. The expert panel that drafted the guideline attempted to examine the issue of adolescents and smoking cessation, but found very little analyzable evidence pertaining specifically to cessation in the pediatric age group. It is clear, however, that adolescents experience nicotine addiction (as evidenced by the use of the Fagerström test) and symptoms of nicotine withdrawal similar to those of adults, including anxiety and stress.

Moreover, adolescents who attempt to quit tobacco use appear to go through the same stages of change as adults, and the transtheoretical model of Prochaska and DiClemente (DiClemente, Prochaska et al., 1991) appears to be just as valid for them as for adults. Thus, most tobacco-using teens will present to the physician in the "precontemplative" stage, with no desire to quit and little recognition of tobacco use as a problem. A useful approach in dealing with such a young person is to identify immediate benefits to quitting. Noting that athletic stamina will improve, nicotine staining of the fingers and teeth will disappear, food will taste and smell better, more spending money will be available and, in many cases, a parental "nag item" will go away may provide more motivation than trying to identify long-term health effects such as avoidance of cancer or emphysema.

Other useful tactics to help promote the motivation to quit in young people include highlighting the manipulative nature of the tobacco industry in its advertising and promotion and helping young smokers to identify the role of the media in promoting the normalization of tobacco use. Helping them realize the addictive nature of tobacco and the fact that what may have started as a statement of independence could become the ultimate dependence—nicotine addiction—also may strike a responsive chord. Finally, noting that tobacco use does not define friendships nor does it make a person more sociable or likable may address the peer influence that is so important to adolescents.

CESSATION PROGRAMS

While few studies have looked at cessation programs specifically for young tobacco users, some data have become available in the past few years. The American Lung Association's "Not On Tobacco" program, for example, has shown some efficacy in providing social skills support in a group smoking cessation setting. Pharmacotherapy also has been tried with young tobacco users. While only a limited number of clinical trials of nicotine replacement therapy and fewer trials of bupropion SR have been conducted in youth, there is enough evidence for the Public Health Service's Clinical Practice Guideline to suggest that pharmacotherapies that are effective with adults should be similarly effective with young people. Thus, pediatricians and other physicians who care for young tobacco users should be knowledgeable about nicotine replacement and bupropion and consider using these medications when appropriate.

Physicians who treat adolescent tobacco users should develop appropriate interventions and consider structuring them around the well-known concept of the "Four As": **A**sk about tobacco use at every visit, **A**dvise those who smoke to quit, **A**ssist those who want to quit, and **A**rrange followup.

REFERENCES

American Academy of Pediatrics (AAP), Committee on Substance Abuse (2001). Tobacco's toll: Implications for the pediatrician. *Pediatrics* 107:794-798.

Centers for Disease Control and Prevention (CDC) (2000). Cigarette smoking among adults—United States, 1998. *Morbidity and Mortality Weekly Report* 49.

Centers for Disease Control and Prevention (CDC) (1993). Reasons for tobacco use and symptoms of nicotine withdrawal among adolescent and young adult tobacco users: United States, 1993. *Morbidity and Mortality Weekly Report* 43.

DiClemente CC, Prochaska JO et al. (1991). The process of smoking cessation: Analysis of precontemplation, contemplation and preparation stages of change. *Journal of Consulting and Clinical Psychology* 59:295-304.

Fiore MC, Bailey WC, Cohen SJ et al. (2000). *Treating tobacco use and dependence. A clinical practice guideline.* Rockville, MD: U.S. Department of Health and Human Services, Public Health Service.

Johnston LD, O'Malley PM & Bachman JG (2000). *The Monitoring the Future National Survey Results on Adolescent Drug Use: Overview of Key Findings, 2000.* Rockville, MD: National Institute on Drug Abuse.

Siquera L, Rolnitzky L & Rickert V (2001). Smoking cessation in adolescents. *Archives of Pediatrics and Adolescent Medicine* 155:489-495.

Substance Abuse and Mental Health Services Administration (SAMHSA) (2001). *National Household Survey on Drug Abuse, 1999.* Rockville, MD: SAMHSA.

U.S. Department of Health and Human Services (USDHHS) (1994). *Preventing Tobacco Use Among Young People: A Report of the Surgeon General.* Washington, DC: U.S. Government Printing Office, 65.

| Chapter 2 | # Screening for Alcohol, Tobacco, and Drug Use in Children and Adolescents |

Michelle Pickett, M.D., FAAP
Peter D. Rogers, M.D., M.P.H., FAAP, FASAM
Robert M. Cavanaugh, Jr., M.D., FAAP

Epidemiology
Selecting a Screening Tool
The Patient Interview
The Physical Examination
Laboratory Testing

Screening for alcohol, tobacco, and drug use in the pediatric population should begin at the prenatal visit and extend throughout adolescence (Fuller & Cavanaugh, 1995). *In utero* exposure to alcohol or other drugs may be teratogenic for the fetus and may be associated with an adverse pregnancy outcome (Bell & Lau, 1995). Neonates may suffer from symptoms of withdrawal, and long-term neurobehavioral problems may be seen in infants born to substance-abusing mothers (Bell & Lau, 1995). Failure to thrive, developmental delay, or poor compliance with medical recommendations during infancy may indicate exposure to a chaotic environment associated with drug abuse (Fuller & Cavanaugh, 1995). Similarly, such exposure during the toddler and preschool years may present as behavior problems, accidents, poisonings, child abuse or neglect, and the like (Fuller & Cavanaugh, 1995). Numerous manifestations of direct use, as well as of exposure to substance-abusing individuals, have been described in older children and adolescents.

The physician should have a high index of suspicion, as the signs and symptoms of alcohol, tobacco, and other drug use often are subtle and easily confused with those of other physical or mental illnesses. As part of the routine medical history of every infant, child, or adolescent, the physician needs to inquire about exposure to any family members or friends who may have a problem with alcohol or other drugs. It also is essential to ask about conflict or fighting in the home, disruptions in the family environment, or abusive behaviors. Such questions are as basic as taking a review of systems or performing other elements of the traditional medical history for all patients within the pediatric age group.

EPIDEMIOLOGY

The battery of chemicals that can be used to create an alteration in mood is extensive, and adolescents have found access to all of them. Adolescent substance use encompasses illegal substances such as marijuana, hallucinogens, cocaine, methamphetamines, and heroin. It also includes prescription stimulants, sedatives, and analgesics. Other substances used by adolescents are legal for adults but illegal for children: alcohol and tobacco. Finally, some adolescents inhale the chemicals available in household products to achieve a "high."

Use of alcohol, tobacco, and other drugs has been well identified among American youth for at least two decades. Many efforts have been made to deter drug use since then and, up to the early 1990s, there were indications that use of illicit drugs was declining. Yet statistics show that, by the time they finish high school, over half (55%) of American young people have tried an illicit drug and 37% have done so as early as 8th grade if inhalants are included (Monitoring the Future Survey, 1999; National Household Survey on Drug Abuse, 1998). Moreover, despite years of Surgeon Generals' warnings and reams of information regarding the harmful effects of tobacco use, 3,000 youth start smoking each day, nearly two-thirds of American youth have tried cigarettes by the 12th grade, and more than one-third of 12th graders are current smokers (National Household Survey on Drug Abuse, 1998; Monitoring the Future Survey, 1999).

The statistics concerning alcohol use among teens are even more alarming: 80% of students have used alcohol, and 4.4 million (30% of 12th graders, 26.2% of 10th graders, and 14.1% of 8th graders) have engaged in binge drinking (defined as having five or more drinks in a row at least once in the two weeks preceding the survey) by the end of high school (Johnston, 2000). Statistics from the National Institute of Alcohol Abuse and Alcoholism (NIAAA) indicate that more than 100,000 12- to 13-year-olds engage in binge drinking every month, and that 40% of children who begin drinking before age 15 will become alcoholics (NIAAA, 2000). These findings probably represent an underestimate, as they do not take into account adolescents who are school absentees and dropouts, incarcerated, or otherwise not in a structured school program.

It is estimated that approximately one million adolescents live away from home. About half of these young people are in institutions for juvenile offenders (Neinstein & MacKenzie, 1996). Although accurate estimates of prevalence for risky behaviors may be difficult to obtain, the Youth Risk Behavior Surveillance System (CDC, 1998) has studied high school students enrolled in alternative school settings. In this population of adolescents, about two-thirds were current smokers and drinkers (at least once in the month before survey); 53% were current users of marijuana; 22% had initiated sexual intercourse before age 13 (with 50.4% of all the students who had ever had sex reporting four or more sexual partners); and 20.5% of all students had specifically planned to commit suicide in the 12 months preceding the survey (CDC, 1998).

The challenge of working with adolescents is increased further because of their apparent willingness to try new drugs or "rediscover" older drugs without attention to the adverse consequences that can result (Johnston, 2000). Of particular concern in recent years is the overall trend toward a diminished disapproval of drug use as well as a reduction in perceived risk among adolescents and their peers, as indicated by rising trends in use of hallucinogens among 12- to 17-year-old youth (11.1 per 1,000 potential new users in 1991, compared with 23.9 per 1,000 potential new users in 1997) (Johnston, 2000).

A significant proportion of adolescents report using chemicals to gain social acceptance, to alleviate low self-esteem, to relieve stress, as aphrodisiacs, mood elevators (stimulants) or analgesics (hydrocodone, Oxycontin®) and to manage weight—thus indicating a dissatisfaction with themselves and/or their environment. This can lead some to continue using substances to the point of addiction and dependency (Neinstein & MacKenzie, 1996).

Many adolescents not only report substance abuse among their peers, but also disclose that adult members of their family use these substances and may excuse their teens' "experimentation" as rites of passage into adulthood. Thus, it is not uncommon for adolescents to escape medical intervention completely or to come to the attention of health care professionals only when seemingly out-of-control behaviors or legal problems arise as a result of their risk-taking.

Although the foregoing statistics paint a grim picture of the substance abuse problem, there are hopeful trends and signs as a result of advocacy and recent initiatives to limit the availability of harmful substances and evidence-based treatment methods and rehabilitation.

SELECTING A SCREENING TOOL
In screening for alcohol or drug problems, information is gathered and evaluated through the use of interviews, a physical examination, laboratory tests, possibly supplemented by the use of structured interviews or other screening tools.

Widely used tools for screening adolescents are reviewed in Chapter 4 of this section. Once selected, the screening tool should be administered and scored in the manner instructed; no substitutions should be made for any test items, and no items should be eliminated or modified (Winters, 1999a).

THE PATIENT INTERVIEW
The principal objective of the patient interview is to gather relevant information from the adolescent in as organized and expedient a fashion as possible, while simultaneously

TABLE 1. Guidelines for Interviewing Adolescents

Approach

1. Begin by discussing more general lifestyle questions, including the following topic areas: home/family relations, functioning at school, peer relationships, leisure activities, employment, and self-perception.

2. Ask about dietary patterns.

3. Proceed to questions about prescribed medications.

4. Ask about over-the-counter medications.

5. Inquire about cigarettes and smokeless tobacco use.

6. Ask about the use of alcohol.

7. Finally, ask about the use of any illicit drug.

Rationale

1. This approach allows time to develop or renew the physician-patient relationship.

2. It elicits a basis of general psychosocial information that is useful in identifying the patient at risk in a harmful environment.

3. The approach begins the interview with the least threatening questions.

4. It then moves to increasingly sensitive questions about substance use.

5. The order of questions recommended here provides a natural order of progression, moving from socially accepted activities to those that are socially tolerated, to the socially disapproved, to the overtly illegal.

SOURCE: Comerci G (1998). Office assessment and brief intervention with the adolescent suspected of substance abuse. In AW Graham & TK Schultz (eds.) *Principles of Addiction Medicine, Second Edition.* Chevy Chase, MD: American Society of Addiction Medicine, 1146. Reprinted by permission of the publisher.

displaying empathy and concern for the patient. This takes practice and patience, but is well worth the effort (Table 1).

Develop a Relationship of Trust. Comerci (1998) reminds us that "physicians who care for adolescents and young adults recognize that they are perhaps in greater need of a 'medical home' than other patients." The concept of a "medical home" is not a new one. The American Academy of Pediatrics defines it as care that is "accessible, continuous, comprehensive, family centered, coordinated, and compassionate. The physician should manage or facilitate essentially all aspects of care. The physician should be known to the adolescent and family and should be able to develop a relationship of mutual responsibility and trust with them" (AAP, 1988).

Ask Leading Questions. It is important to ask leading questions, prefacing them with sentences such as: "In order to provide you with the best care, I am going to ask for information in some sensitive health areas. When was the last time you smoked marijuana?" or "How many joints (or "blunts") have you smoked in the last week?" (Berne, 1964; Cavanaugh, 1994; also see Cavanaugh's Personal Questionnaires, following).

In eliciting this information, the clinician must observe important verbal as well as nonverbal cues. For example, if a boy with an absent father is asked about his home, he may nonchalantly say that he lives with his mother. When specifically asked about his father, however, he may tense and display signs of anger. When gentle confrontation or reflection of the teen's perceived emotion is expressed by the interviewer, however, it is likely that the youth will further elaborate details of possible domestic violence, feeling unloved, hurt, or abandoned. Allowing such elaborations by the patient can foster a better physician-patient relationship and help to uncover vital historical data, although this can be time-consuming and emotionally taxing for the physician.

Use Motivational Interviewing. Motivational interviewing, which is not synonymous with coercion, is another technique for engaging the patient (Miller & Rollnick, 1991). Questions may include "How does cigarette smoking make you feel, or help you to fit in with your peers, or achieve your personal goals?" Interviewing in this manner is in itself a psychoeducational intervention.

Consider Support Structures and Resiliency Factors. The clinician also should consider the adolescent's resilience, or ability to respond positively to psychological adversity (also see Chapter 1). Resilience is not merely stress resistance; rather, it enables the adolescent to overcome many adverse circumstances in order to achieve success in life (Wolin & Wolin, 1996).

Be Alert to Family Dysfunction. Although an exhaustive discussion of family relationships is beyond the scope of this chapter, a "family systems approach" to dysfunction as it relates to child and adolescent development is important. Because addictive or compulsive behaviors in parents and other caretakers profoundly affect children, health care providers should be aware that their efforts in eliciting accurate information from families may be frustrated. Teens with significant substance use histories, on deeper exploration over time, may be found to have experienced neglect or physical, emotional, or sexual abuse. While the health care professional would hope to find support in the family or caretaking structures for such patients, it may be that the adolescent is wrapped up in a system that shifts blame from one family member to another; ignores the needs of one or more members while trying to satisfy the unmet emotional needs of another; ignores healthy boundaries; has unspoken "family secrets"; denies the physical, psychological, emotional, or spiritual impact of these behaviors; and even shuns or disapproves of a member who tries to make healthy life choices (Hemfelt, Minirth et al., 1989; Gartner, 1999; Pollack, 1998).

Health care professionals often are confronted with strong evidence of denial and role-playing on the part of the adolescent and other family members. The adolescent patient often falls into playing any number of "family roles," such as "the scapegoat," "the hero," "the enabler." "the lost child," "the mascot," or even "the surrogate parent" (Adger, 1998; Hemfelt, Minirth et al., 1989). Unfortunately, if the physician does not recognize such role-playing, he or she may unwittingly become an "enabler" as well—for example, by praising (as a mark of maturity) such actions as perfectionism and the shouldering of others' responsibilities (pseudo-maturity); assessing and treating the "mascot" for attention deficit/hyperactivity disorder; or labeling the "scapegoat" as having a conduct disorder (Dias, 2002). Careful evaluation of the adolescent in the context of a dysfunctional family unit, therefore, requires skill and sensitivity in recognizing the adolescent's unmet needs, feelings of isolation, and attempts to adapt to his or her environment.

THE PHYSICAL EXAMINATION

Physical examination by itself cannot absolutely confirm substance use, but provides useful data when combined with a positive screen by interview. Physical signs include:

- Dilated or constricted pupils, reddened conjunctivae, excessive use of Visine® or other soothing eye drops (suggestive of marijuana, stimulant, or opioid use).

- Sores around the mouth, red runny eyes, runny nose, chemical burns around the mouth (from "huffing" or "bagging"), or paint stains on clothes (suggestive of inhalant use).

- Unusual chemical or alcohol odor on the breath or on clothing (suggestive of inhalant or alcohol use).

- An odor of sweet oil (suggestive of marijuana use).

- Acneiform rashes and rosacea (suggestive of anabolic steroid use).

- Irregular or anovulatory periods, hair on lips, or other signs of mild hirsutism in the absence of known endocrine or gynecological causes (suggestive of marijuana or anabolic steroid use).

- Gynecomastia or testes of smaller size than expected for Tanner Staging of Puberty for pubic hair (Tanner, 1962) (suggestive of marijuana or anabolic steroid use).

- Muscular build disproportionate to or advanced as compared to Tanner Staging (suggestive of anabolic steroid use).

- Tattoos, body piercings, gang symbols, or heavy jewelry (suggestive of a cult or gang affiliation).

LABORATORY TESTING

Generally speaking, a thorough history and physical examination provide the best information in assessing an adolescent suspected of substance use, with urine drug screens used only in the context of treatment. Nevertheless, drug testing may be considered for diagnostic purposes in the following cases:

1. An adolescent who is experiencing frequent episodes of allergic nasal symptoms, epistaxis, or upper respiratory symptoms (suggestive of inhalation drug use).

2. An adolescent who exhibits extreme oppositional or defiant behavior, conduct disorders, who has been involved in multiple motor vehicle crashes, or who is bulimic (Comerci, 1998).

3. An adolescent whose clothing suggests gang involvement or cult practices.

4. An adolescent who reports having been raped and who shows signs of disorientation. (However, drug testing is controversial in such cases because such testing may

interfere with a teen's right to justice for the rape. Therefore, drug testing should be considered only in the context of the adolescent's need for treatment of a substance use disorder.)

5. An adolescent who has a history of frequent emergency room visits for trauma related to motor vehicle crashes, dog bites, or cruelty to animals (in some neighborhoods, training dogs to fight is a way of raising money to pay for drugs).

6. A teen mother whose infant has a positive meconium screen or unusually small head size. (In some states, the law requires meconium drug testing of newborns: (1) who weigh less than 2,500 gm (5 lbs., 8 oz.) or (2) whose head circumference is less than the third percentile for gestational age in the absence of a medical explanation for the small head size.)

Since the right to privacy and the right to resist bodily searches are guaranteed by the U.S. Constitution, drug testing should be done only with informed consent on the part of the adolescent, except when one of the following signs or symptoms creates an urgent situation (Comerci, 1990; Comerci & Schwebel, 2000):

- Acute mental status changes (a blood toxicology screen that includes evaluations for tricyclic antidepressants, salicylates, acetaminophen, alcohol, and other illicit drugs is recommended);

- Acute unexplained or previously undiagnosed medical signs or symptoms, such as seizures, coma, acute chest pain, or arrhythmias;

- A legally incompetent or mentally handicapped teen with recent changes in behavior;

- Court-ordered testing;

- An out-of-control or extremely combative adolescent; and

- A minor or very young child who poses a danger to himself or others (AAP, 1989; Schonberg, 2001).

Involuntary testing also is permitted in connection with participation in high school sports. In a position statement based on the 1995 U.S. Supreme Court ruling regarding the constitutionality of drug testing for sports participation, the American Academy of Pediatrics noted: "Involuntary

drug screening is often a condition for high school sports participation. Screening would be an appropriate school requirement if the purpose were to identify conditions that, when combined with physical activity, may be hazardous to the student's health. . . ." (AAP, 1995).

When drug screens are indicated, a random collection of urine for a quantitative evaluation of substances is recommended. This decreases the chances of false positives. Random collections on Mondays or Tuesdays during the school year (September through May) or on any day of the summer months are recommended to maximize the potential for a positive screen. Quantitative drug screens are also indicated to be able to gently confront a Piagetian "concrete" adolescent with "concrete" evidence and to be able to monitor abstinence at subsequent visits. It also is worth noting that a drug screen is less expensive than a toxicology screen. After a drug screen has identified a specific substance and, depending on the provider-adolescent patient relationship and compliance with subsequent visits, the provider may order urine drug tests for the specific identified substance at followup visits.

Drug screens that are not court-ordered do not necessarily need to have stringent chain of custody procedures. It also should be noted that adolescents who are actively using drugs while on probation for DUI or underage drinking offenses may try to "beat the system" through tactics such as attempting to substitute another person's urine, consuming large amounts of water, drinking bleach or vinegar, or by taking any number of commercially prepared substances to try to cleanse their bodies, etc. (see the chapter on drug testing in Section 9).

The use of home drug detection kits should be discouraged, as their effectiveness have not been proved and they pose another source of conflict in the parent-child relationship. Parents should be encouraged to seek professional assistance if they suspect that their adolescent is using alcohol, tobacco, or other drugs (Comerci & Schwebel, 2000).

CONCLUSIONS

Discussion of alcohol, tobacco, and other drug use should be part of the routine health care of all infants, children, and adolescents. Physicians must have a high index of suspicion, as signs and symptoms may be subtle, with numerous manifestations expressed throughout the pediatric age range. The close correlation between the use of alcohol and other drugs with other psychosocial-medical issues deserves emphasis, particularly in adolescents. High-risk individuals must be identified as soon as possible in an effort to minimize morbidity and mortality.

Physicians who wish to provide comprehensive care to adolescents must be as committed to meeting the psychosocial needs of these patients as they are to performing the physical examination.

REFERENCES

Adger H (1998). Children in alcoholic families: Family dynamics and treatment issues. In AW Graham & TK Schultz (eds.) *Principles of Addiction Medicine, Second Edition.* Chevy Chase, MD: American Society of Addiction Medicine, 1111-1114.

American Academy of Pediatrics (AAP) (1989; reaffirmed 1993). Confidentiality in adolescent health care. *AAP News* 5(4):9.

American Academy of Pediatrics (AAP), Committee on Psychosocial Aspects of Child and Family Health (1988). *Guidelines for Health Supervision II.* Elk Grove Village, IL: The Academy.

American Academy of Pediatrics (AAP), Committee on Substance Abuse (1995). The role of schools in combating substance abuse. *Pediatrics* 95:784-785.

American Psychiatric Association (APA) (1994). *Diagnostic and Statistical Manual of Mental Disorders, 4th Edition (DSM-IV).* Washington, DC: American Psychiatric Press.

Bell GL & Lau K (1995). Perinatal and neonatal issues of substance abuse. *Pediatric Clinics of North America* 42(2):261-281.

Berne (1964). *Games People Play.* New York, NY: Grove Press.

Cavanaugh RM (1994). Anticipatory guidance for the adolescent: Has it come of age? *Pediatrics in Review* 15(12):485-489.

Cavanaugh RM (1986). Obtaining a personal and confidential history from adolescents: An opportunity for prevention. *Journal of Adolescent Health Care* 7:118-22.

Cavanaugh RM, Hastings-Tolsma M, Keenan D et al. (1993). Anticipatory guidance for the adolescent: Parents' concerns. *Clinical Pediatrics* 32:542-545.

Cavanaugh RM & Henneberger PK (1996). Talking to teens about family problems: An opportunity for prevention. *Clinical Pediatrics* 35:67-71.

Cavanaugh RM, Miller ML & Henneberger PK (1999). The preparticipation athletic examination of adolescents: A missed opportunity? *Current Problems in Pediatrics.*

Cavanaugh RM, Miller M & Henneberger PK (1994). The Preparticipation Sports Physical: Are We Dropping the Ball? Presented an the annual meeting of the Ambulatory Pediatric Association, Seattle, WA.

Centers for Disease Control and Prevention (CDC) (1998). *National Alternative High School Youth Risk Behavior Survey.* Atlanta, GA: CDC.

Centers for Disease Control (CDC) (1989). Results from the National Adolescent Student Health Survey. *Morbidity and Mortality Weekly Report* 38(9):147-150.

Centers for Disease Control and Prevention (CDC) (1996). Youth risk behavior surveillance. *Morbidity and Mortality Weekly Report* 45:(SS-4)1-86.

Comerci G (1998). Office assessment and brief intervention with the adolescent suspected of substance abuse. In AW Graham & TK Schultz (eds.) *Principles of Addiction Medicine, Second Edition.* Chevy Chase, MD: American Society of Addiction Medicine, 1146. Reprinted by permission of the publisher.

Comerci GD, Brookman RR, Coupey SM et al. (1988). *Perspectives on Alcohol and Substance Use/Abuse Among Adolescents—A Monograph on Adolescent Wellness* (endorsed by the American Academy of Pediatrics). Lyndhurst, NJ: Health Learning Systems.

Comerci GD & MacDonald D (1990). Prevention of substance abuse in children and adolescents. *Adolescent Medicine: State of the Art Reviews* 1(1):127-143.

Comerci GD & Schwebel R (2000). Substance abuse: An overview. *Adolescent Medicine: State of the Art Reviews* 11(1):79-101.

Dias PJ (2002). Assessment in the office. *Pediatric Clinics of North America—Substance Abuse.* Philadelphia, PA: W.B. Saunders, 49:269-300.

Fuller PG & Cavanaugh RM (1995). Basic assessment and screening for substance abuse in the pediatrician's office. *Pediatric Clinics of North America* 42(2):295-315.

Gartner RB (1999). *Betrayed as Boys—Psychodynamic Treatment of Sexually Abused Men.* New York, NY: Guilford Press.

Hemfelt R, Minirth F & Meier P (1989). *Love Is a Choice—Recovery for Codependent Relationships.* Nashville, TN: Thomas Nelson, Inc.

Johnston LD (1999). *Monitoring the Future Survey.* Ann Arbor, MI: University of Michigan.

Johnston LD (2000). "Monitoring the Future: What Have We Learned?" Presented at American Society of Addiction Medicine (ASAM) Conference on Adolescent Substance Abuse for the Practitioner, Washington, DC.

Miller W & Rollnick SS (1991). *Motivational Interviewing: Preparing People to Change Addictive Behavior.* New York, NY: The Guilford Press.

National Institute on Alcohol Abuse and Alcoholism (NIAAA) (2000). *NIH News Advisory, March 23.* Bethesda, MD: NIAAA.

Neinstein LS & MacKenzie R (1996). High-risk and out-of-control behavior. In *Adolescent Health Care—A Practical Guide, 3rd Edition.* Baltimore, MD: Williams & Wilkins, 1094-1106.

Pollack W (2000). *Real Boys' Voices—Boys Speak Out.* New York, NY: Random House, Inc.

Schonberg KS (2001). The discovery of marijuana use by the parent of an early adolescent. *Pediatrics* 107:971-973.

Tanner JM (1962). *Growth at Adolescence.* Oxford, England: Blackwell.

Winters KC (1999a). *Screening and Assessment for Adolescent Substance Use (Treatment Improvement Protocol No. 31).* Rockville, MD: Center for Substance Abuse Treatment.

Wolin S & Wolin S (1996). The challenge model: Working with strengths in children of substance-abusing parents. *Child and Adolescent Psychiatric Clinics of North America* 5(1):243-256.

APPENDIX 1.   Personal Questionnaire for Young Women

Please list your favorite hobbies and interests.

What are your future plans? _____

What is your favorite type of music? Favorite musical group? _____

What is your favorite TV show? Favorite game? _____

Please list your closest friends (names or initials, age, sex) _____

What exercise do you do regularly? _____

Which of the following activities do you participate in (check all that apply)?

❑ Biking   ❑ Skateboarding   ❑ Rollerblading   ❑ Hunting   ❑ Swimming

❑ Boating   ❑ Other Water Sports

Please circle the response that best corresponds to your feelings. Y = Yes, N = No

Y   N   1. Do you have a friend you can talk to about anything at all?

Y   N   2. Is there a family member or friend whose physical or mental health worries you?
          If yes, please explain. _____

Y   N   3. Is there a family member or friend who has a problem with alcohol or other drugs?
          If yes, please explain. _____

Y   N   4. Do you have enough responsibility?

Y   N   5. Do you have enough freedom?

Y   N   6. Do you have enough privacy?

Y   N   7. Have you ever stayed out all night without permission?

Y   N   8. Have you ever felt like running away?

Y   N   9. Are you having any problems with your family or friends?
          If yes, please explain. _____

Y   N   10. Is there conflict or fighting in your home?
           If yes, please explain. _____

Y   N   11. Do you worry about your parents' relationship?
           If yes, please explain. _____

Y   N   12. Do you like school? What grade are you in?

Y   N   13. Are you having an problems at school?
           If yes, please explain. _____

Y   N   14. Are your grades as good as everyone expected?

Y   N   15. Are your teachers OK?

Y   N   16. Have you ever had to repeat a grade?

Y   N   17. Have you ever cut classes, skipped school, or had any unauthorized absences?

Y   N   18. Do you get depressed or upset easily?

Y   N   19. Ever felt like hurting yourself?
           If yes, please explain. _____

Y   N   20. Ever felt like hurting someone else?
           If yes, please explain. _____

Y   N   21. Has anyone ever abused you by their actions or words?
        If yes, please check all forms of abuse which apply.
        ❏ Physical   ❏ Sexual   ❏ Verbal   ❏ Emotional   ❏ Other

Y   N   22. Do you smoke cigarettes?
        If yes, how many each day? _____ Age started? _____ Want to quit? _____

Y   N   23. Do you use chewing tobacco, snuff, or similar products?
        If yes, please list. _____

Y   N   24. Do any of your friends use alcohol or other drugs?
        If yes, which ones? _____

Y   N   25. Do you drink alcohol-containing beverages?
        If yes, which ones? _____
        If yes, how much? _____ How often? _____ Age started? _____
        Last time you got drunk? _____

Y   N   26. Have you ever used marijuana, cocaine, "crack," uppers, downers, inhalants (sniffed or huffed), acid,
        angel dust, heroin, or similar substances?
        If yes, which ones? _____
        Age started? _____ Do you feel you need them? _____

Y   N   27. Have you ever used non-prescription drugs to stay awake, go to sleep, calm down, or get high?
        If yes, which ones? _____
        Do you depend on them now? _____

Y   N   28. Have you ever used anabolic steroids?
        Please circle the response that best corresponds to your feelings: ? = Not Sure, Y = Yes, N = No

Y   N   29. Have you begun to menstruate? If yes, state age you began. _____ How often do your periods
        occur? _____ Are they regular? _____ How long do they last? _____
        Is there associated pain? _____ Distress? _____ "Blue spells"? _____
        When did your last period start? _____ When did it end? _____

Y   N   30. Have you heard of the toxic shock syndrome?
        If yes, do you know how to prevent it? _____

Y   N   31. Do you drive a car, truck, or van?

Y   N   32. Do you wear a seatbelt regularly?

Y   N   33. Do you ride a motorcycle, all-terrain vehicle, minibike, or snowmobile?

Y   N   34. If you answered yes to question #33, do you wear a helmet regularly?
        (Leave blank if does not apply.) _____

Y   N   35. Ever operate a car or other motor vehicle after using alcohol or other drugs?

Y   N   36. Ever been a passenger when the driver was drunk or high?

Y   N   37. Do you hitchhike?

Y   N   38. Are handguns, rifles, shotguns, BB guns or other firearms kept in your home?

Y   N   39. If you answered yes to question #38, are the firearms kept locked up?
        (Leave blank if does not apply.) _____

Y   N   40. Do you ever carry a knife, gun, razorblade, club, or other weapon?

Y   N   41. Have you been in a physical fight in the past 3 months?

Y   N   42. Are guns or violence a problem in your neighborhood or at your school?

Y   N   43. Have you ever been in trouble with the law?
               If yes, please explain. _____

Y   N   44. Do you fear for your personal safety or that of a family member or friend?
               If yes, please explain. _____

Y   N   45. Do you think you are growing normally?

Y   N   46. Do you have any questions or concerns about your looks or appearance?
               If yes, please explain. _____

Y   N   47. Do you have any questions or concerns about your sexual development?
               If yes, please explain. _____

Y   N   48. Do you feel different from other girls?

Y   N   49. Are you interested in boys?

Y   N   50. Are you more attracted to girls than to boys?

Y   N   51. Are you familiar with the term masturbation?

Y   N   52. If you answered yes to question #51, do you believe it is abnormal or harmful?

Y   N   53. Have you ever felt forced or pressured into having sex with anyone?
               If yes, please explain. _____

Y   N   54. Have you ever had any sexual experinces?
               If yes, what type of experiences have you had? _____

Y   N   55. If you have been involved in a sexual relationship, did you or your partner use protection?
               If yes, what type of protection was used? _____

Y   N   56. Have you ever been pregnant?
               If yes, have you ever had a miscarriage or abortion? _____

Y   N   57. Are you thinking about being sexually active with anyone sometime soon?
               If yes, do you need information on contraception? _____
               Preventing sexually transmitted diseases? _____

Y   N   58. Are you worried that you may become pregnant?

Y   N   59. Are you worried that you may not be able to get pregnant?

Y   N   60. Are you afraid you might get AIDS?

Y   N   61. Do you know how to protect yourself against getting AIDS?

Y   N   62. Have you ever had any of the following sexually transmitted diseases? (check all that apply)
               ❑ Herpes   ❑ Chlamydia   ❑ Gonorrhea   ❑ Trichomonas   ❑ Genital warts   ❑ Syphilis
               ❑ HIV   ❑ Other

Y   N   63. Overall, do you think you are well adjusted?

Y   N   64. Are you basically a happy person?

Y   N   65. Do you ever worry about your physical or mental health?
               If yes, please explain. _____

Y   N   66. Do you have any other questions or concerns you would like to discuss with the doctor or nurse?

Name _____   Date _____

APPENDIX 2. Personal Questionnaire for Young Men

Please list your favorite hobbies and interests.

What are your future plans? _____

What is your favorite type of music? Favorite musical group? _____

What is your favorite TV show? Favorite game? _____

Please list your closest friends (names or initials, age, sex) _____

What exercise do you do regularly? _____

Which of the following activities do you participate in (check all that apply)?

❑ Biking   ❑ Skateboarding   ❑ Rollerblading   ❑ Hunting   ❑ Swimming

❑ Boating   ❑ Other Water Sports

Please circle the response that best corresponds to your feelings. Y = Yes, N = No

Y   N   1. Do you have a friend you can talk to about anything at all?

Y   N   2. Is there a family member or friend whose physical or mental health worries you?
        If yes, please explain. _____

Y   N   3. Is there a family member or friend who has a problem with alcohol or other drugs?
        If yes, please explain. _____

Y   N   4. Do you have enough responsibility?

Y   N   5. Do you have enough freedom?

Y   N   6. Do you have enough privacy?

Y   N   7. Have you ever stayed out all night without permission?

Y   N   8. Have you ever felt like running away?

Y   N   9. Are you having any problems with your family or friends?
        If yes, please explain. _____

Y   N   10. Is there conflict or fighting in your home?
        If yes, please explain. _____

Y   N   11. Do you worry about your parents' relationship?
        If yes, please explain. _____

Y   N   12. Do you like school? What grade are you in?

Y   N   13. Are you having an problems at school?
        If yes, please explain. _____

Y   N   14. Are your grades as good as everyone expected?

Y   N   15. Are your teachers OK?

Y   N   16. Have you ever had to repeat a grade?

Y   N   17. Have you ever cut classes, skipped school, or had any unauthorized absences?

Y   N   18. Do you get depressed or upset easily?

Y   N   19. Ever felt like hurting yourself?
        If yes, please explain. _____

Y   N   20. Ever felt like hurting someone else?
        If yes, please explain. _____

Y   N   21. Has anyone ever abused you by their actions or words?
        If yes, please check all forms of abuse which apply.
        ❑ Physical   ❑ Sexual   ❑ Verbal   ❑ Emotional   ❑ Other

Y   N   22. Do you smoke cigarettes?
        If yes, how many each day? _____ Age started? _____ Want to quit? _____

Y   N   23. Do you use chewing tobacco, snuff, or similar products?
        If yes, please list. _____

Y   N   24. Do any of your friends use alcohol or other drugs?
        If yes, which ones? _____

Y   N   25. Do you drink alcohol-containing beverages?
        If yes, which ones? _____
        If yes, how much? _____How often? _____ Age started? _____
        Last time you got drunk? _____

Y   N   26. Have you ever used marijuana, cocaine, "crack," uppers, downers, inhalants (sniffed or huffed), acid, angel dust, heroin, or similar substances?
        If yes, which ones? _____
        Age started? _____ Do you feel you need them? _____

Y   N   27. Have you ever used non-prescription drugs to stay awake, go to sleep, calm down, or get high?
        If yes, which ones? _____ Do you depend on them now? _____

Y   N   28. Have you ever used anabolic steroids?
        Please circle the response that best corresponds to your feelings: ? = Not Sure, Y = Yes, N = No

Y   N   29. Do you drive a car, truck, or van?

Y   N   30. Do you wear a seatbelt regularly?

Y   N   31. Do you ride a motorcycle, all-terrain vehicle, minibike, or snowmobile?

Y   N   32. If you answered yes to question #31, do you wear a helmet regularly?
        (Leave blank if does not apply.)

Y   N   33. Have you ever operated a car or other motor vehicle after using alcohol or other drugs?

Y   N   34. Have you ever been a passenger when the driver was drunk or high?

Y   N   35. Do you hitchhike?

Y   N   36. Are handguns, rifles, shotguns, BB guns or other firearms kept in your home?

Y   N   37. If you answered yes to question #36, are the firearms kept locked up?
        (Leave blank if does not apply.)

Y   N   38. Do you ever carry a knife, gun, razorblade, club, or other weapon?

Y   N   39. Have you been in a physical fight in the past 3 months?

Y   N   40. Are guns or violence a problem in your neighborhood or at your school?

Y   N   41. Have you ever been in trouble with the law?
        If yes, please explain. _____

Y   N   42. Do you fear for your personal safety or that of a family member or friend?
        If yes, please explain. _____

Y   N   43. Do you think you are growing normally?

Y   N   44. Do you have any questions or concerns about your looks or appearance?
        If yes, please explain. _____

Y   N   45. Do you have any questions or concerns about your sexual development?
        If yes, please explain. _____

Y   N   46. Do you feel different from other boys?

Y   N   47. Are you interested in girls?

Y   N   48. Are you more attracted to boys than to girls?

Y   N   49. Are you familiar with the terms masturbation, ejaculation, and "wet dreams"?

Y   N   50. If you answered yes to question #49, do you believe these are abnormal or harmful?

Y   N   51. Have you ever felt forced or pressured into having sex with anyone?
        If yes, please explain. _____

Y   N   52. Have you ever had any sexual experiences?
        If yes, what type of experiences have you had? _____

Y   N   53. If you have been involved in a sexual relationship, did you or your partner use protection?
        If yes, what type of protection was used? _____

Y   N   54. Are you thinking about being sexually active with anyone sometime soon?
        If yes, do you need information on contraception? _____
        Preventing sexually transmitted diseases? _____

Y   N   55. Have you worried about getting someone pregnant?

Y   N   56. Have you ever worried about not being able to get someone pregnant?

Y   N   57. Are you afraid you might get AIDS?

Y   N   58. Do you know how to protect yourself against getting AIDS?

Y   N   59. Have you ever had any of the following sexually transmitted diseases? (check all that apply)
        ❑ Herpes   ❑ Chlamydia   ❑ Gonorrhea   ❑ Trichomonas   ❑ Genital warts   ❑ Syphilis
        ❑ HIV   ❑ Other

Y   N   60. Overall, do you think you are well adjusted?

Y   N   61. In general, are you happy with the way things are going for you these days?

Y   N   62. Do you ever worry about your physical or mental health?
        If yes, please explain. _____

Y   N   63. Do you have any other questions or concerns you would like to discuss with the doctor or nurse?

Name _____   Date _____

Chapter 3

Office Assessment of the Substance-Using Adolescent

Deborah J. Poteet-Johnson, M.D., FAAP
Philomena J. Dias, M.D., FAAP

Selecting An Assessment Instrument
"Ground Rules" for the Assessment
Organizing the Information
Staging the Disorder
Completing the Assessment

A thorough, comprehensive, formal assessment of the adolescent suspected of substance use is necessary when initial screening uncovers any number of "red flags." The primary goal of such an assessment is to confirm or exclude the presence of a suspected substance use disorder and to develop a plan for ongoing care. Other goals (Winters, 1999a) are:

■ To permit the evaluator to learn more about the nature, correlates, and consequences of the adolescent's substance-using behavior;

■ To ensure that additional problems not flagged in the screening process are identified (such problems may involve the patient's medical or psychological status, nutrition, social functioning, family relations, educational performance, or delinquent behavior);

■ To examine the extent to which the adolescent's family can be involved in subsequent interventions; and

■ To identify specific strengths of the adolescent that can be engaged in developing and following through on the treatment plan.

In addition, comprehensive assessment begins a process of responding to the adolescent patient's denial and resistance and thus can be seen as the initial phase of the treatment experience (Winters, 1999a).

The clinician should be a well-trained professional who is experienced in dealing with adolescent substance use, such as a physician who is an addiction medicine specialist, a psychologist or mental health professional who is knowledgeable about addictive disorders, a school counselor or social worker, or a substance abuse counselor. One individual should take the lead in the assessment process, particularly with respect to gathering, summarizing, and interpreting the assessment data. An assessor who is not a licensed mental health professional should refer an adolescent who appears to need a formal mental health workup to an appropriately credentialed professional. The assessment should be conducted in an office or other setting where the adolescent can feel comfortable, private, and secure (Winters, 1999a).

SELECTING AN ASSESSMENT INSTRUMENT

In the assessment, information often is gathered and evaluated through the use of structured interviews or questionnaires. The two most important criteria in selecting an assessment instrument are its reliability and validity. Other considerations are the instrument's purpose, content, ease of administration, time required for completion, and training needed by the assessor.

A number of instruments for adolescent assessment are reviewed in Chapter 4 of this section (also see Section 3). Once selected, the instrument should be administered and scored in the manner instructed; no substitutions should be made for any test items, and no items should be eliminated or modified. For structured interviews, the interview format and item wording should be followed carefully (Winters, 1999a).

Domains to be Assessed. To arrive at an accurate picture of the adolescent's problems, the following domains should be assessed (Winters, 1999a):

- Strengths and resiliency factors, including self-esteem, family supports, religiosity, other community supports, coping skills, and motivation for treatment.

- History of substance use, including use of over-the-counter and prescription drugs, tobacco, caffeine, and alcohol. The history should note the age at first use, duration and frequency of use, patterns of use, and mode of ingestion.

- History of addiction or mental health treatment.

- Physical examination findings.

- Medical history, including previous illnesses, infectious diseases, and traumatic injuries.

- Sexual history, including sexual orientation, pregnancies, sexually transmitted diseases, sexual abuse, and risk factors for HIV/AIDS.

- Developmental issues, including traumatic events such as physical or sexual abuse or threats to safety (as from gang members).

- Mental health history, with a focus on depression, suicidal ideation or attempts, attention deficit disorder, oppositional defiance or conduct disorder, anxiety disorders, as well as details about prior evaluations or treatments for mental health problems.

- Family history, including family strengths, as well as the parents' or guardian's history of substance use, mental and physical health problems, chronic illnesses, incarceration or illegal activities, and child management concerns, as well as the family's cultural, racial/ethnic,

and socioeconomic background and degree of acculturation. The description of the home environment should note substandard housing, homelessness, proportion of time spent in shelters or on the streets, and any pattern of running away from home.

- School history, including academic performance and behavior, learning-related problems, extracurricular activities, and attendance problems. Has the adolescent been assessed with a learning disability or received special education services?

- Vocational history, including paid and volunteer work.

- Peer relationships, interpersonal skills, gang involvement, and neighborhood environment.

- Juvenile justice involvement and history of delinquency, including types of behavior and attitudes toward that behavior.

- Social service agency involvement, including any episodes of child abuse or neglect, involvement with child welfare agencies, and foster care placements.

- Leisure activities, including recreation, hobbies, interests, and any aspirations associated with them.

Developmental Stage. In evaluating substance use in an adolescent, the assessor must consider both the biological stages of puberty as well as the adolescent's cognitive and psychospiritual development (Tanner, 1962; Erikson, 1968; Kohlberg, 1969; Fowler, 1995), so as to match the assessment and subsequent guidance to the teen's developmental stage.

In assessing spiritual and moral development, the professional does not have to be "preachy" or engage in imposing his or her own value system; rather, performing the developmental assessment provides the clinician an excellent opportunity to allow teens to air and expose their values, with the assessor acting as a sounding board. This helps the adolescent to reflect on, clarify, decode, and demythologize his or her own values. If done in a caring, sensitive manner, such interviewing, anticipatory guidance, and counseling style does not violate the patient's autonomy or deprive the adolescent of the right to choose according to his or her own moral values and beliefs, any more than asking about suicidal ideation leads a teen to make that choice.

On the other hand, unexamined moral beliefs and dilemmas pose roadblocks to achieving a drug-free lifestyle and can result in frustration for adolescents, parents, health care professionals, and society in general (Silber, 1991).

Unlike the predictable march of biological stages of development to reproductive maturity, the progression of psychospiritual development remains controversial (Silber, 1991). However, the assessor needs to consider the adolescent patient's cognitive, emotional, moral, and spiritual development in order to understand his or her perception of the consequences of substance use, such as stealing, violence to self and others, or selling drugs to minors to support a drug lifestyle in order to gain a better understanding of how cognitive, emotional, moral, and faith development (Dias, 2002) may be applied to adolescent substance abuse assessment and assist in treatment options and outcomes.

"GROUND RULES" FOR THE ASSESSMENT

Certain "ground rules" ought to be observed by the health professional who is conducting the assessment:

Realign the Relationship With the Patient and Parents. The physician who sees younger children communicates primarily with the parents to obtain the child's history, then examines the child and provides an assessment and management advice to the parents. The adolescent, however, is at a developmental stage at which he or she is gaining in maturity and competence and is increasingly capable of making health care decisions. Therefore, during adolescence, the relationship between the physician and parents and the physician and adolescent patient needs to be renegotiated and realigned.

One of many ways that such a realignment can be achieved is to sit down with the parent(s) and teen at the first office visit and obtain an informed consent signed by both the parent(s) and the patient. Depending on the adolescent's age and developmental stage, the physician should explain that whatever the patient says in the context of a health interview will be confidential, except where such disclosures involve a threat to the safety of self or others, or where public health laws require such reporting, or if hospitalization is required. The adolescent and parent(s) also should be informed of the patient's rights (including the right to confidentiality) and the boundaries of parents' rights to examine medical records under federal and state laws.

Maintain Confidentiality. It is not unusual for adolescents to minimize, become defensive about, or even deny the use of alcohol, tobacco, or other drugs when presented with evidence to the contrary. This presents an inherent dilemma for the physician who provides health care to

adolescent patients: On one hand, there is an obligation to the adolescent (who has a health covenant with the physician), while on the other hand, there is an obligation to the parents (who are involved in the adolescent's life and the financial aspects of health care). The dilemma is compounded when an adolescent is engaged in behaviors that place his or her health at risk for life-altering consequences, and that are likely to affect the parents and family emotionally and/or financially.

Attempts to resolve this dilemma are beset with conflicting and contradictory practice policies by health care providers of various disciplines that offer adolescent health services (see the adjoining article on confidentiality for a review of pertinent policies).

How then can the treating professional ensure the privacy and confidentiality of the adolescent's office medical record? Certain notations may be kept in a separate section of the chart, the chief purpose of which is to prevent inadvertent revelations to the parent (Shapiro, 1991). The parent(s) can be informed that the confidentiality policy protects the teen from the indiscriminate release of information unless the records are to be transferred to another health provider for continuity of care, referral services, or are court-ordered to be released. When explanations are put in this context, most parents and adolescents are very amenable to the arrangement.

Make Judgments But Be Non-Judgmental. Communication with adolescents is enhanced if the physician refrains from assuming a paternalistic, condemning attitude and instead focuses on how the effects of the adolescents' environment and development affect his or her decisionmaking. Dias (2002) has observed that most physicians in training have been taught to avoid being judgmental. However, many residents and medical students have interpreted this to mean "Do not question patient choices." To the contrary, physicians are called upon to make judgments all the time and are expected to do so. However, they should not condemn the adolescent for making certain choices, but rather use the encounter as an opportunity to be a healing "sounding board" and thus to provide a safe place for the teen to verbalize the reasons for his or her choices.

ORGANIZING THE INFORMATION

Cohen has refined a method, originally developed by Berman in 1972, for organizing the adolescent patient's history, psychosocial and medical information (Goldenring & Cohen, 1988). This system has been expanded and modified by

TABLE 1. The "HEADS FIRST" Approach to Gathering and Organizing Information About the Psychosocial-Medical Issues of Adolescence

Home	Separation, support, "space to grow"
Education	Expectations, study habits, achievement
Abuse	Emotional, verbal, physical, sexual
Drugs	Tobacco, alcohol, marijuana, others
Safety/ Sexuality	Hazardous activities, safety belts, helmets, sexual activity and acting out
Friends	Confidantes, peer pressure, interaction
Image	Self-esteem, looks, appearance
Recreation	Exercise, relaxation, TV, video games
Spirituality	Values, beliefs, identity
Threats/ Violence	Harm to self or others, running away.

SOURCE: Adapted by the authors from the HEADS FIRST mnemonic developed by the Adolescent Medicine Program, State University of New York at Syracuse.

faculty of the Adolescent Medicine Program at the State University of New York's Health Science Center at Syracuse. The questions are structured in an easily remembered format (expanded by the authors to include spirituality), which stresses the importance of connecting with adolescents "HEADS FIRST," as outlined in Table 1. This approach also emphasizes that "getting into the adolescent's head" is just as necessary as performing a physical examination.

Studies have shown that the items listed in Table 1 are priorities for routine adolescent health care from the point of view of both parents and adolescents (Cavanaugh, Hastings-Tolsma et al., 1993; Malus, LaChance et al., 1987). In addition, the Guidelines for Health Supervision of the American Academy of Pediatrics (AAP Committee on Psychosocial Aspects of Child and Family Health, 1988) and the Guidelines for Adolescent Preventive Services of the American Medical Association (Elster & Kuznets, 1994) strongly endorse a comprehensive approach to adolescent

health care. A thoughtful review of these concerns stimulates open discussions and instills among youth a feeling of security about having a medical "home." Failure to address these topics may raise unnecessary barriers and provoke in the adolescent patient a sense of eviction from the health care system. Teenagers who expect to find help in the physician's office must not feel abandoned at a time when their needs for comprehensive services are greatest (Cavanaugh, 1994).

Having an organized approach for data collection from, and information dissemination to, adolescent and young adult patients facilitates anticipatory guidance in the practice setting. For example, hobbies, interests, and career goals might be covered first to help the patient understand that the physician is interested in him or her as a whole person, as well as to serve as a buffer for more personal questions. Exercise, sports participation, and other forms of recreation then can be discussed.

Home. Problems at home are a leading source of stress and anxiety among adolescents (Cavanaugh & Henneberger, 1996). It is important to determine if teens are receiving adequate support as they go through the separation process in an attempt to develop their own identity, autonomy, and independence. Screening for conflict, fighting, abusive behavior, or other problems at home provides valuable insight into family functioning and stability (Cavanaugh & Henneberger, 1996). It also is important to determine whether the adolescent is being given adequate privacy and freedom, as well as appropriate responsibility. Asking the patient if he or she ever has thought about running away may provide additional clues to underlying concerns that should be addressed.

Some adolescents list one address as their permanent home, yet reveal that they "stay" with other relatives or friends. It is important to assess the reasons that such youth have chosen to live outside the family home (for example, are there problems such as violence, abusive behaviors, and the like?). Anxiety over such difficulties, whether or not the adolescent chooses to stay at home, may influence use of alcohol or other drugs, sexual acting out, or other dangerous behaviors. Questions about parental substance use or addiction may be in order as well.

Adolescents frequently worry about their parents' marital relationship, as well as the physical and mental health of family members (Cavanaugh & Henneberger, 1996). The fact that more than 20% of boys and girls in a recent study believed that a family member had a problem with alcohol or other drugs is particularly noteworthy (Cavanaugh & Henneberger, 1996). In many instances, however, it is difficult for teens to verbalize these concerns directly (Rogers, Speraw et al., 1995; Cuda, Rupp et al., 1993). Such feelings often are internalized and may be expressed through subtle symptoms and vague somatic complaints (Cuda, Rupp et al., 1993; Zarek, Hawkins et al., 1987). Repressed memories with delayed manifestations in adulthood also may occur (Zarek, Hawkins et al., 1987). Physicians must be willing to initiate discussions of family health issues in an effort to help reduce the emotional burdens of these young patients.

Teens who are unable to cope with family problems may attempt to compensate by using alcohol and other drugs, or they may act out sexually and risk an unintended pregnancy or acquisition of a sexually transmitted disease. They may have low self-esteem and develop unhealthy behaviors in an attempt to improve their image. They also may exercise poor safety habits and place themselves and others at risk for serious injury or death in motor vehicle crashes. Such adolescents may express feelings of sadness, suicidal ideation, or thoughts of self-harm. These areas should be explored as part of routine adolescent health care.

Education. School-related difficulties are another important source of distress and discomfort for adolescent patients (Cavanaugh, 1994). Manifestations may be subtle or invisible and appear unrelated to the educational situation. Thus, it is important to screen adolescents for problems at school on a regular basis. Patients should be asked if they like school or if they are having any difficulty with their classes. It is very helpful to determine if their performance meets with others' expectations and approval. In many instances, their achievements may not reach a level that they, their parents, or their teachers expected. This can be a source of considerable anxiety and tension, particularly in high achievers and/or teens who have been subjected to unrealistic expectations.

From a medical perspective, it is important to determine if the patient has a health condition that is interfering with learning. Disorders such as hypothyroidism, depression, neurological abnormalities, decreased visual acuity, and impaired hearing can contribute to poor school performance (Neinstein, 1991). Significantly, learning disabilities, attention deficit/hyperactivity disorder, and borderline intellectual functioning often are overlooked (Neinstein, 1991). Lack of sleep, boredom, preoccupation with other thoughts, problems with teachers, and other forms of difficulty in concentrating also should be considered. Study habits are

another area of concern, particularly if television, video games, or computer programs are allowed to intrude.

It also is important to determine the reasons for any absences from school, which may adversely affect academic progress. Severe, prolonged, or chronic illnesses may result in many days lost. School phobia, avoidance, or aversion should be considered in cases of unexplained absences (Neinstein, 1991). A pattern of cutting classes, skipping school, or excessive tardiness should alert the physician that the adolescent may have an underlying problem with substance use (Johnston, 1999). On the other hand, adolescents who are having problems at school may turn to alcohol or other drugs as a coping mechanism. Once again, other important preventive health issues of adolescence—such as safety, sexual activity, self-esteem, and suicidal ideation— are closely related to school issues and should be screened simultaneously.

Abuse. Evaluation of adolescents always should include questions about all types of abuse: emotional, physical, and sexual. Assessment instruments may contain spaces for positive or negative responses to these questions, but health care personnel always should recognize that a negative response does not necessary indicate that no abuse has occurred. The authors generally ask about abuse in the face-to-face interview, even if the answer to a written questionnaire is negative, especially if there is a high index of suspicion. Numerous studies indicate that significant numbers of adolescents report being abused or mistreated, yet seldom present with those complaints or volunteer this information (Cavanaugh & Henneberger, 1996).

These results reinforce the importance of routinely screening adolescents for abuse, as recommended by the American Medical Association (Elster & Kuznets, 1994). While there may be no ability to objectively verify reported incidents, adolescents' perceptions of such traumatic experiences must be identified and addressed as soon as possible in an effort to prevent ongoing distress or injury (Cavanaugh, Miller et al., 1999).

Adolescents who have been abused may resort to alcohol or other drugs in an effort to relieve anxiety, reduce stress, or repress reality (Hoffman, Mee-Lee et al., 1993). Such individuals also frequently have feelings of guilt, low self-esteem, or thoughts of self-harm. This may place them at risk for serious injury or even death from accidental or non-accidental causes. In addition, adolescents who have been abused may pursue intimate relationships and engage in sexual activity as a source of comfort or as a means of coping with their situations. They may seek medical attention for concerns related to pregnancy or sexually transmitted diseases. These suggest numerous portals of entry into the health care system for youths who have been abused. Under such circumstances, treatment of the acute medical problem alone is not sufficient. Followup arrangements always should include provisions for ongoing care by a primary care physician who can deliver comprehensive services and screen regularly for the issues outlined in Table 1.

Drugs (and Other Substances). There are numerous methods for taking a substance use history from adolescents in the office setting. Screening questions are included in the personal questionnaires following Chapter 2 of this section. At the State University of New York, Syracuse, the questionnaire has been expanded to ask routinely about use of prescription drugs. In addition, patients who wish to lose weight are questioned about the use of appetite suppressants, emetics, laxatives, or diuretics. A more detailed and structured alcohol and drug use history is recorded as indicated. Appropriate evaluation and treatment are carefully formulated in accordance with the pattern of use.

Safety and Sexuality. The close association between risk-taking behavior, alcohol or drug use, and other psychosocial and medical issues of adolescence merits special consideration (Fuller & Cavanaugh, 1995). The three leading causes of mortality among U.S. teenagers are accidents, suicide, and homicide. Each year, there are approximately 15,000 to 18,000 deaths from automobile-related injuries and 5,000 suicides among adolescents (Kempe, Silver et al., 1987; National Center for Health Statistics, 1986). Alcohol and other psychoactive drugs are factors in many of these fatalities (National Center for Health Statistics, 1986). Many of the 6,000 adolescent homicides are committed when one or both parties are intoxicated (Christoffel, 1990).

Many young adults have a distorted perception of alcohol-related driving risk and often underestimate the negative influence of alcohol use on driving skills (Genua, Ravazzani et al., 1995). In a recent survey of 138 first-year student athletes in a university setting, 24% of the participants reported that they had driven a motor vehicle after drinking or using drugs (Cavanaugh, Miller et al., 1994). In the same study, 43% of the students had been a passenger when the driver was drunk or "high." These findings illustrate the importance of including discussions of drugs, drinking, and driving as part of routine adolescent health care. Current standards for sports-oriented examinations have not been structured to meet this goal and should not

be used as a substitute for the student athlete's routine health assessment, as commonly occurs (Goldberg, Saraniti et al., 1980; Krowchuk, Krowchuk et al., 1995; Risser, Hoffman et al., 1985). The highway safety habits of all adolescents should be ascertained and preventive strategies reinforced, including the use of designated drivers, use of safety belts, and avoidance of hitchhiking (Cavanaugh, 1994).

The pattern of exercise, sports participation, and other forms of recreation also should be determined on a regular basis. Most potentially hazardous activities can be readily identified by using a screening instrument such as the personal questionnaire. Activity-specific safety precautions should be reviewed as indicated (Cavanaugh, 1994). Use of protective headgear when riding on a motorcycle, all-terrain vehicle, or snowmobile also should be stressed. In addition, the use of wristguards, elbow and knee pads, as well as helmets is recommended for activities such as in-line skating and skateboarding (AAP, 1995). Finally, the frequent occurrence of even minor injuries, although not life-threatening, always should arouse suspicion of alcohol or drug use (Fuller & Cavanaugh, 1995).

The reasons for including a discussion of sexuality as part of routine anticipatory guidance for adolescents are urgent and compelling. Each year in the U.S., one in 10 adolescent girls becomes pregnant; 84% of these pregnancies are unintended (Alan Guttmacher Institute, 1989). Up to six million cases of sexually transmitted diseases are reported among adolescents annually (Shafer, 1994). In addition, heterosexual transmission is becoming the predominant mode of HIV acquisition for teenagers (McGrath & Strasburger, 1995).

General questions regarding pubertal changes are asked next. Patients are asked if they think they are growing normally and if they have any questions or concerns about their sexual development. Concerns over sexual identity may be uncovered by asking male patients if they feel different from other boys, if they are interested in girls, and if they are more attracted to boys than to girls. Corresponding questions are asked for young women. The physician must be able to identify adolescents who are having difficulties coping with their feelings and be willing to assist when necessary.

Teens then should be asked if they have ever had any sexual experiences and, if so, what type of experiences. It is important to know if there has been oral, anal, and/or genital contact so that samples for sexually transmitted disease can be obtained from the appropriate mucosal surfaces. Teens who have been sexually active should have serological testing for syphilis and determination of HIV status, if the patient consents to the latter. Continued abstinence always should be supported for teens who are not sexually active. Information on postponing sexual involvement, contraception, and prevention of sexually transmitted diseases should be provided as needed. The latter should stress the consistent, correct use of condoms.

The close relationship between sexual activity and other psychosocial issues of adolescence, such as low self-esteem, depression, problems with friends or family, and alcohol or drug use, must be stressed. Adolescents whose judgment is compromised by alcohol or drugs are at considerable risk for unwanted pregnancy and sexually transmitted diseases, including HIV infection (Fuller & Cavanaugh, 1995). In addition, gay and lesbian youth frequently suffer from feelings of guilt, inadequacy, and self-depreciation. Many of these adolescents turn to alcohol or other drugs as a source of comfort or to reduce emotional turmoil (Sturdevant & Remafid, 1992). Although guidelines have been available to identify these teens and deal sensitively with their special needs, few physicians initiate discussions about sexual identity. It is time to raise this group of adolescents from the ranks of the medically underserved.

Friends. Difficulties with friends are a common source of stress and anxiety among adolescents (Cavanaugh, 1994). In most instances, these problems are self-limiting and do not lead to ongoing distress. However, unresolved conflicts may have serious adverse sequelae, including harm to self or others. Teens may engage in sexual acting out in an effort to feel wanted, turn to drugs as a source of comfort, partake in high-risk activities to be part of the crowd, or engage in unhealthy patterns of behavior to enhance or improve their appearance. Thus, it is important to routinely screen adolescents for any problems with friends and responses to peer pressures.

It also is important to ask young adult patients if they have a friend with whom they can talk about anything at all. In general, girls appear more willing to share their innermost concerns with others than are their male counterparts. Nearly all of the young women in a recent study reported having a "friend" with whom they could talk about anything at all, but more than one-fourth of the boys said they had no such confidante (Cavanaugh & Henneberger, 1996). These results suggest that young men may have difficulty discussing their deepest feelings. The findings provide objective data to support the common belief that girls tend to have better emotional networks than boys. Teens who are unwilling or unable to establish such support systems may have difficulty dealing with stress. The physician must be able to identify such individuals so that counseling can be offered as indicated and specific referrals initiated when needed.

Image. As identified by Erik Erikson (1968), the major task of adolescence is the establishment of one's own identity. Poor self-esteem and lack of acceptance of one's body image may underlie many adolescent risk-taking behaviors (Cavanaugh, 1994). Thus, it is important to routinely ask adolescent patients if they are happy with their appearance.

In a study of 854 adolescent girls, 67% were dissatisfied with their weight, and 54% were unhappy with their body shape (Moore, 1988). Corresponding values for 895 adolescent boys were 42% and 35% (Moore, 1988).

In many instances, teens resort to desperate, even dangerous measures in an effort to improve their self-esteem or enhance their image. Attempts at weight reduction often involve self-injurious behaviors such as severe caloric deprivation, excessive exercise, self-induced vomiting, and the use of appetite suppressants, diuretics, laxatives, or emetics (Fisher, Golden et al., 1995). Such problems are prevalent among adolescents and should be screened for regularly.

Participants in sports and other activities in which thinness or "making weight" is important to success may be particularly susceptible to unhealthy weight control practices. Such sports include body building, cheerleading, dancing (especially ballet), distance running, diving, figure skating, gymnastics, horse racing, rowing, swimming, weight-class football, and wrestling (AAP Committee on Sports Medicine & Fitness, 1996; Garner, Garfinkel et al., 1987; Drummer, Rosen et al., 1987). When the preoccupation with thinness supersedes a desire to be healthy, physically active young women are at risk for a group of signs and symptoms known as the female athlete triad (Yeager, Agostini et al., 1993). Lack of information and the strong desire to win contribute to this condition, which consists of abnormal eating patterns, amenorrhea, and osteoporosis (Yeager, Agostini et al., 1993). The routine physical examination is an excellent opportunity to screen for body image disorders and to educate patients and parents as to healthy patterns of eating, exercise, and weight control.

At the other extreme, increasing body weight to gain a competitive edge also is a common concern of young athletes (AAP Committee on Sports Medicine and Fitness,

1996; AAP Committee on Sports Medicine, 1983). Adolescents who feel insecure about their bodies are very susceptible to any solicitations that may promise a better body build or improved athletic performance (Strasburger & Brown, 1991). Use of anabolic steroids to improve appearance, as well as to increase muscle size and strength, is relatively common, particularly among male athletes. Those who desire greater muscle bulk and definition (such as body builders) or who want more power (such as weight lifters, shot putters, or football players) are at increased risk for using these substances (Strasburger & Brown, 1991). Many of these young athletes are not aware of the potential dangers of anabolic steroids and other performance enhancing drugs. The health maintenance examination affords the physician an opportunity to provide factual information on this subject, as well as to review healthy practices for gaining weight when appropriate.

Sun exposure is another important concern in the image category. Many teenagers believe that they must have a suntan to feel healthy and look attractive (Cavanaugh, 1994). However, sun damage is cumulative, and blistering sunburns during adolescence have been associated with an increased risk of malignant melanoma in adulthood (Hurwitz, 1989). Additional risk factors for this rapidly increasing and serious form of skin cancer include fair skin and certain common cutaneous disorders, including dysplastic nevi and congenital pigmented nevi, as well as rare dermatologic conditions such as xeroderma pigmentosum and the like (Roth & Grant-Kels, 1991). Immunodeficient children may be at increased risk for development of melanoma (Roth & Grant-Kels, 1991). Therefore, it is relevant to inquire about the sun safety habits of adolescent patients on a regular basis, particularly in susceptible individuals. Appropriate counseling can be remembered by recalling the ABCs: **A**void the sun between 10:00 AM and 4:00 PM whenever possible, **B**lock out burning rays by using a sunscreen with a sun protective factor (SPF) of 30 or higher, and **C**over-up with clothing, a hat, and sunglasses as needed.

Other common sources of embarrassment to teenagers, such as acne, short or tall stature, and pubertal changes should be addressed as appropriate. Issues of self-esteem are very important to the growing number of youth with disabilities and chronic illnesses. They not only face the same developmental tasks as other teenagers, but also must cope with the stress of their underlying conditions. Health care professionals are in a unique position to encourage these adolescents to rely on themselves for their sense of worth, rather than on the attitudes and reactions of others.

Recreation. One of the topics most teenagers and parents wish to address as part of routine adolescent health care is exercise. Accordingly, it is helpful to estimate whether the amount and type of activity undertaken are appropriate. Methods of relaxation and amusement can be assessed by simple inquiry. The hours spent watching television each day, as well as time spent with video games or computer shows, can be estimated. Extreme patterns of behavior require further review, with specific recommendations provided as needed. In addition, dramatic changes in activity may be a clue to the presence of a significant underlying medical condition, such as hypothyroidism, or a psychosocial problem such as depression, eating disorder, alcohol or drug use, and other destructive behaviors.

Spirituality. Adding an assessment of spirituality to the HEADS FIRST mnemonic recognizes the importance of values and spirituality in adolescent development. There seems to be a growing interest in the spiritual realm within contemporary culture, yet physicians often ignore this valuable component of their patients' lives when assessing their overall health.

Spirituality may be defined as "the relationship between an individual and a transcendent or higher being or force or mind of the universe" (Chappel, 1998; Peterson & Nelson, 1987). Since one's personal spirituality helps to shape one's world view—that is, the way in which an individual experiences his or her environment and importance in life (Colson & Pearcey, 1999)—it can be argued that spirituality is one of the more important components of the patient's historical data.

The research literature on the role of spirituality in medical practices suggests that a majority of patients wish their physicians would discuss spiritual issues with them, yet only a small number of physicians actually do so (Anandarajah & Hight, 2001). While some argue that discussing spiritual issues with patients may be problematic (Sloan & Bagiella, 2001), others agree that doing so can serve as an intervention (Koenig, 2001) and strengthen the physician-patient relationship (Larimore, 2001).

In the authors' experience with adolescent patients, the taking of a spiritual history, if carried out in a nonjudgmental, caring, and compassionate manner, may indeed strengthen the physician-patient relationship and allow for discussion of risk-taking activities (including substance use) in a safe atmosphere. The spiritual history may be even more relevant when decisions for referral to substance abuse treatment programs must be made; as in deciding whether to incorporate a traditional Twelve Step mutual help program or a less spiritually oriented group into the treatment plan.

Examples of questions that may be used in spiritual history taking include the HOPE format, in which inquiries are made about an individual's sources of **H**ope or strength for the future; **O**rganized religion; **P**ersonal spirituality and practices; and the **E**ffects on medical care and end-of-life issues (Anandarajah & Hight, 2001). In working with adolescents, another approach may be simply to ask, "Do you or your family have any particular religious beliefs?" "Do you or your family pray/meditate/worship on a regular basis?" "How do your beliefs fit with what's going on now in your life?" or "What do you look forward to in the future?" Of course, sensitivity to the adolescent's mood and willingness to discuss these issues is imperative.

Threats/Violence. About 5,000 adolescents commit suicide each year (Cohen, 1984), and it has been estimated that there are 50 to 200 attempts for every suicidal act that results in death (Cohen, 1984). Alcohol or other drugs serves as a catalyst to many of these suicides (Soderstrom & Dearing-Stuck, 1993). More than half of the adolescents surveyed during a routine screening examination reported that they got depressed or upset easily (Cavanaugh & Henneberger, 1996). Over 40% of the individuals in this sample population reported having had thoughts of running away, and 33% of the respondents thought of inflicting harm on themselves or others. Unresolved conflicts, feelings of sadness, and low self-esteem often are related to family conflicts, strained peer relationships, school difficulties, and work-related problems (Cavanaugh, 1994). It is important to assess functional status at the adolescent visit in an effort to identify not only sources of stress but also the adolescent's methods of coping with them (Schubiner & Robin, 1990; Joffe, Radius et al., 1988; Smith, Kovan et al., 1997; CDC, 1989). Patients who are suicidal or homicidal require immediate intervention by mental health experts, legal authorities, or both.

STAGING THE DISORDER

Kandel has identified four stages of adolescent substance use: Stage I, experimentation; Stage II, recreational use; Stage III, problematic use; and Stage IV, addiction and dependency (Kandel, 1975; Comerci & Macdonald, 1990). Problem drinkers are defined as those "who have been drunk six or more times a year and/or who experience negative consequences from alcohol use two or more times a year with consequences in three or more areas of life—home, school, peers/significant others, legal, work, driving, and changes in participation in recreational activities (Jessor & Jessor, 1977; Donovan & Jessor 1978, 1985).

In addition, Comerci (1988) has suggested a Stage 0, or pre-use, stage. In working with an adolescent at this stage, it is advisable for the physician to have a heightened awareness of conditions in the youth and the family that would predispose the adolescent toward alcohol or other drug use. Such conditions include negative parental modeling of alcohol, tobacco, and drug use; physical or sexual abuse of the child; the child's need for immediate gratification, poor impulse control, and peer acceptance; or angry, rebellious, unbonded teens (Comerci, 1988).

Adolescents may not own up to the consequences of their substance use if they are in denial. In such cases, "multiple gating" techniques (Comerci, 1990), which include judiciously obtaining reports from parents (about behavior, drug use, grades, and the like) and teachers (about grades, attendance, and classroom behaviors) may be used for the initial assessment—much as one does in the evaluation of a patient with attention deficit/hyperactivity disorder.

In order to maintain confidentiality, questions to teachers should be open-ended rather than specific; for example: "How do you feel this student is doing in your class? Do you have any suggestions or insights as to how best to maximize the student's learning potential?"

While staging is useful in devising a care plan, it is inadvisable to apply the definitions too rigidly. Further, the health care professional may have to use careful judgment in discriminating an adolescent patient's experimentation with tobacco, alcohol, or other drugs from problematic use. While experimentation should not be ignored, it also should not be labeled "substance abuse." To do so may adversely affect the physician-patient relationship.

COMPLETING THE ASSESSMENT

At the conclusion of the assessment process, the assessor should develop a written report that:

1. Identifies the presence and severity of any substance use disorder;

2. Identifies factors that contribute to or are related to the substance use disorder;

3. Identifies a plan of action to address the problem areas;

4. Describes an interim plan to ensure that the treatment plan is implemented and monitored to its conclusion;

5. Makes recommendations for referral to agencies or services; and

6. Describes how the resources and services of multiple agencies can be coordinated and integrated.

The next step is to refer the adolescent for any needed followup care (Winters, 1999b). A successful referral requires that the physician or other health professional is familiar with placement criteria (see Chapter 6 of this section), as well as treatment programs and other resources available in the community (including their admissions procedures and policies regarding insurance reimbursement and/or indigent care). Comerci (1998) offers the following guidelines for selecting a treatment program:

■ Does the program require the patient to become totally abstinent?

■ Is the program focused on the treatment of substance use disorders?

■ Does the program acknowledge substance abuse and addiction as chronic problems?

■ Are appropriate professionals and therapeutic or educational activities provided?

■ If an inpatient or residential setting, does the program emphasize followup outpatient care?

CONCLUSIONS

Adolescents represent a unique group of patients whose development—physically, cognitively, emotionally, morally, and spiritually—and environment influences their values and thus their subsequent behaviors. These behaviors not only affect adolescents' morbidity and mortality rates, they also affect the lives of many others, including families, friends, acquaintances, the health care system, and ultimately the health and economics of the nation.

Despite the growing number of programs designed to educate and motivate adolescents to change unhealthy behaviors, a significant number of them still engage in substance abuse and other risk-taking activities. The health care professional is encouraged to familiarize himself or herself with the range of assessment tools and to adopt those

most compatible with his or her individual practice style. Use of the HEADS FIRST approach, including a spiritual history, can be a valuable tool in gathering and organizing information necessary to a comprehensive assessment. In doing so, the assessor also needs to be aware of federal and state laws governing confidentiality and consent for alcohol and drug testing.

The professional who spends the time required to appropriately assess the adolescent will find that there are modest yet encouraging trends in adolescent substance use and abuse, treatment options, and positive outcomes to justify the effort and time invested.

REFERENCES

Alan Guttmacher Institute (1989). *Teenage Pregnancy in the United States: The Scope of the Problem and State Responses.* New York, NY: The Institute.

American Academy of Pediatrics (AAP) (1989; reaffirmed 1993). Confidentiality in adolescent health care. *AAP News* 5(4):9.

American Academy of Pediatrics (AAP), Committee on Injury and Poison Prevention (1995). Skateboard injuries. *Pediatrics* 95:611-612.

American Academy of Pediatrics (AAP), Committee on Psychosocial Aspects of Child and Family Health (1988). *Guidelines for Health Supervision II.* Elk Grove Village, IL: The Academy.

American Academy of Pediatrics (AAP), Comittee on Sports Medicine (1983). *Sports Medicine: Health Care for Young Athletes.* Evanston IL: The Academy, 168.

American Academy of Pediatrics (AAP), Committee on Sports Medicine and Fitness (1996). Promotion of healthy weight-control practices in young athletes. *Pediatrics* 97:752-753.

American Academy of Pediatrics (AAP), Committee on Substance Abuse (1995). The role of schools in combating substance abuse. *Pediatrics* 95:784-785.

Anandarajah G & Hight E (2001). Spirituality and medical practice: Using the HOPE questions as a practical tool for spiritual assessment. *American Family Physician* 63:81-89.

Cavanaugh RM (1994). Anticipatory guidance for the adolescent: Has it come of age? *Pediatrics in Review* 15(12):485-489.

Cavanaugh RM (1986). Obtaining a personal and confidential history from adolescents: An opportunity for prevention. *Journal of Adolescent Health Care* 7:118-122.

Cavanaugh RM, Hastings-Tolsma M, Keenan D et al. (1993). Anticipatory guidance for the adolescent: Parents' concerns. *Clinical Pediatrics* 32:542-545.

Cavanaugh RM & Henneberger PK (1996). Talking to teens about family problems: An opportunity for prevention. *Clinical Pediatrics* 35:67-71.

Cavanaugh RM, Miller ML & Henneberger PK (1999). The preparticipation athletic examination of adolescents: A missed opportunity? *Current Problems in Pediatrics.*

Cavanaugh RM, Miller M & Henneberger PK (1994). The Preparticipation Sports Physical: Are We Dropping the Ball? Presented an the annual meeting of the Ambulatory Pediatric Association, Seattle, WA.

Centers for Disease Control and Prevention (CDC) (1996). Youth risk behavior surveillance—United States, 1995. *Morbidity and Mortality Weekly Reports* 45(SS-4): Sep 27.

Centers for Disease Control and Prevention (CDC) (1993). Quarterly table reporting alcohol involvement in fatal motor vehicle crashes. *Morbidity and Mortality Weekly Report* 42:923.

Centers for Disease Control (CDC) (1989). Results from the National Adolescent Student Health Survey. *Morbidity and Mortality Weekly Report* 38(9):147-150.

Centers for Disease Control and Prevention (CDC) (1997). Alcohol-related traffic fatalities involving children—United States, 1985-1996. *Morbidity and Mortality Weekly Report* 46:1130.

Centers for Disease Control and Prevention (CDC) (1998). *National Alternative High School Youth Risk Behavior Survey.* Atlanta, GA: CDC.

Chappel JN (1998). Spiritual components of the recovery process. In AW Graham & TL Schultz (eds.) *Principles of Addiction Medicine, Second Edition.* Chevy Chase, MD: American Society of Addiction Medicine, 725-728.

Christoffel KK (1990). Violent death and injury in U.S. children and adolescents. *American Journal of Diseases of Childhood* 44:697.

Cohen MI (1984). The Society for Behavioral Pediatrics: A new portal in a rapidly moving boundary. *Pediatrics* 73:791-798.

Colson C & Pearcey N (1999). *How Now Shall We Live?* Wheaton, IL: Tyndale House Publishers, Inc., 19-22.

Comerci G (1998). Office assessment and brief intervention with the adolescent suspected of substance abuse. In AW Graham & TK Schultz (eds.) *Principles of Addiction Medicine, Second Edition.* Chevy Chase, MD: American Society of Addiction Medicine, 1146. Reprinted by permission of the publisher.

Comerci GD, Brookman RR, Coupey SM et al. (1988). *Perspectives on Alcohol and Substance Use/Abuse Among Adolescents—A Monograph on Adolescent Wellness* (endorsed by the American Academy of Pediatrics). Lyndhurst, NJ: Health Learning Systems.

Comerci GD & MacDonald D (1990). Prevention of substance abuse in children and adolescents. *Adolescent Medicine: State of the Art Reviews* 1(1):127-143.

Comerci GD & Schwebel R (2000). Substance abuse: An overview. *Adolescent Medicine: State of the Art Reviews* 11(1):79-101.

Cuda S, Rupp R & Dillon C (1993). Adolescent children of alcoholics. *Adolescent Medicine: State of the Art Review* 4:439-452.

Drummer GM, Rosen LW, Heusner WW et al. (1987). Pathogenic weight-control behaviors of young competitive swimmers. *Physician Sportsmedicine* 15:75-86.

Dias PJ (2002). Assessment in the office. *Pediatric Clinics of North America—Substance Abuse.* Philadelphia, PA: W.B. Saunders, 49:269-300.

Donovan JE & Jessor R (1978). Adolescent problem drinking. *Journal of Studies on Alcohol* 39:1506-1524.

Donovan JE & Jessor R (1985). Structure of problem behavior in adolescents and young adulthood. *Journal of Consulting and Clinical Psychology* 53:890-904.

Elster AB & Kuznets NJ (1994). *AMA Guidelines for Adolescent Preventive Services (GAPS)—Recommendations and Rationale.* Chicago, IL: American Medical Association, Department of Adolescent Health.

Erikson EH (1968). *Identity, Youth, and Crisis.* New York, NY: W.W. Norton & Co.

Fisher M, Golden NH, Katzman DK et al. (1995). Eating disorders in adolescents: A background paper. *Journal of Adolescent Health* 16:420-437.

Fowler JW (1995). The psychology of human development and the quest for meaning. In *Stages of Faith.* New York, NY: Harper Collins Publishers.

Fuller PG & Cavanaugh RM (1995). Basic assessment and screening for substance abuse in the pediatrician's office. *Pediatric Clinics of North America* 42(2):295-315.

Garner DM, Garfinkel PE, Rockert W et al. (1987). A prospective study of eating disturbances in the ballet. *Psychotherapeutics and Psychosomatics* 148:170-175.

Genua S, Ravazzani R & Perassi M (1995). Youth's perception of alcohol-related driving risk. *Journal of Adolescent Health* 16:5.

Goldberg B, Saraniti A, Witman P et al. (1980). Preparticipation sports assessment: An objective evaluation. *Pediatrics* 66:736-744.

Goldenring JM & Cohen E (1988). Getting into adolescent heads. *Contemporary Pediatrics* 5:75-90.

Hemfelt R, Minirth F & Meier P (1989). *Love Is a Choice—Recovery for Codependent Relationships.* Nashville, TN: Thomas Nelson, Inc.

Hoffmann N, Mee-Lee D & Arrowood A (1993) . Treatment issues in adolescent substance use and addictions: Options, outcome, effectiveness, reimbursement, and admission criteria. *Adolescent Medicine: State of the Art Reviews* 4:371-390.

Hurwitz S (1989). There's no such thing as a "good suntan." *Contemporary Pediatrics* 6:55-66.

Jessor R & Jessor S (1977). *Problem Behavior and Psychosocial Development: A Longitudinal Study of Youth.* New York, NY: Academic Press.

Joffe A, Radius S & Gall M (1988). Health counseling for adolescents: What they want, what they get, and who gives it. *Pediatrics* 82:481-485.

Johnston LD (1999). *Monitoring the Future Survey.* Ann Arbor, MI: University of Michigan.

Kandel D (1975). Stages in adolescent involvement in drug use. *Science* 190:912-914.

Kempe CK, Silver HK, O'Brien D et al. (1987). *Current Pediatric Diagnosis and Treatment.* Norwalk, CT: Appleton & Lange, 228.

Koenig HG (2001). Editorial: Spiritual assessment in medical practice. *American Family Physician* 63:81-89.

Kohlberg L (1969). *Stages in the Development of Moral Thought and Action.* New York, NY: Holt, Rinehart & Winston.

Krowchuk DP, Krowchuk HV, Hunter DM et al. (1995). Parents' knowledge of the purposes and content of preparticipation physical examinations. *Archives of Pediatric and Adolescent Medicine* 149:653-657.

Larimore WL (2001). Medicine and Society: Providing basic spiritual care for patients—Should it be the exclusive domain of pastoral professionals? *American Family Physician* 63:36-40.

Malus M, LaChance P, Lamy L et al. (1987). Priorities in health care: The teenagers' viewpoint. *Journal of Family Practice* 25:159-162.

McGrath JW & Strasburger VC (1995). Preventing AIDS in teenagers in the 1990s. *Clinical Pediatrics* 34:46-47.

Moore DC (1988). Body image and eating behavior in adolescent girls. *American Journal of Diseases of Children* 142:1114-1118.

National Center for Health Statistics (1986). *Vital Statistics of the United States, Vol II: Mortality Part A*. Hyattsville, MD: U.S. Public Health Service.

Neinstein LS (1991). *Adolescent Health Care: A Practical Guide (2nd Edition)*. Baltimore, MD: Urban & Schwarzenberg, 941-955.

Neinstein LS & MacKenzie R (1996). High-risk and out-of-control behavior. In *Adolescent Health Care—A Practical Guide, 3rd Edition*. Baltimore, MD: Williams & Wilkins, 1094-1106.

Peterson EA & Nelson K (1987). How to meet your client's spiritual needs. *Journal of Psychosocial Nursing* 25:34-39.

Risser WL, Hoffman HM, Bellah GG et al. (1985). A cost-benefit analysis of preparticipation sports examinations of adolescent athletes. *Journal of School Health* 55:270-273.

Rogers PD, Speraw SR & Ozbek I (1995). The assessment of the identified substance-abusing adolescent. *Pediatric Clinics of North America* 42:351-370.

Roth ME & Grant-Kels JM (1991). Important melanocytic lesions in childhood and adolescence. *Pediatric Clinics of North America* 38:791-809.

Schubiner H & Robin A (1990). Screening adolescents for depression and parent-teenager conflict in an ambulatory medical setting: A preliminary investigation. *Pediatrics* 85:813-818.

Shafer MA (1994). Sexually transmitted diseases in adolescents: Prevention, diagnosis, and treatment in pediatric practice. *Adolescent Health Update, American Academy of Pediatrics* 6:1-7.

Shapiro E (1991). Obstacles to adolescent care in general practice. *Adolescent Medicine: State of the Art Reviews* 2(2):389-396.

Silber TJ (1991). Overcoming obstacles to care: Ethical issues. *Adolescent Medicine: State of the Art Reviews* 2(2):405-414.

Sloan RP & Bagiella E (2001). Spirituality and medical practice: A look at the evidence. *American Family Physician* 63:33.

Smith DM, Kovan JR, Rich BSE et al. (1997). *Preparticipation Physical Evaluation (2nd Edition)*. Elk Grove Village, IL: American Academy of Family Physicians, American Academy of Pediatrics, American Medical Society for Sports Medicine, American Orthopaedic Society for Sports Medicine, American Osteopathic Academy of Sports Medicine.

Soderstrom CA & Dearing-Stuck BA (1993). Substance misuse and trauma: Clinical issues and injury prevention in adolescents. *Adolescent Medicine: State of the Art Reviews* 4:423-438.

Strasburger VC & Brown RT (1991). *Adolescent Medicine: A Practical Guide*. Boston, MA: Little, Brown and Company, 389-390.

Sturdevant M & Remafedi G (1992). Special needs of homosexual youth. *Adolescent Medicine: State of the Art Reviews* 3:359.

Tanner JM (1962). *Growth at Adolescence*. Oxford, England: Blackwell.

Winters KC (1999a). *Screening and Assessment for Adolescent Substance Use (Treatment Improvement Protocol No. 31)*. Rockville, MD: Center for Substance Abuse Treatment.

Winters K (1999b). *Treatment of Adolescents with Substance Use Disorders (Treatment Improvement Protocol 32)*. Rockville, MD: Center for Substance Abuse Treatment.

Yeager KK, Agostini R, Nattiv A et al. (1993). The female athlete triad: Disordered eating, amenorrhea, osteoporosis. *Medicine and Science in Sports & Exercise* 25:775.

Zarek D, Hawkins J & Rogers P (1987). Risk factors for adolescent substance abuse: Implications for pediatric practice. *Pediatric Clinics of North America* 34:481-493.

| Chapter 4 | # Adolescent Assessment Strategies and Instruments |

Ken C. Winters, Ph.D.
Todd W. Estroff, M.D.
Nicole Anderson, B.A.

Screening Tools
Assessment Instruments
Integrated Assessment Systems
Computerized Testing
Clinical Judgment

ssessing adolescent alcohol and other drug abuse can be a daunting task. It is clear that, in adolescents, substance abuse problems rarely occur in isolation. Issues related to school performance, family and peer functioning, psychiatric and psychological status, physical health, and delinquency are widely cited as factors that can predispose, precipitate, or perpetuate the use of alcohol and drugs by youth (Jessor & Jessor, 1977; Kandel, 1978; Newcomb, Maddahian et al., 1986).

Assessment strategies must be multifaceted and comprehensive in order to address such complex patient and environmental problems. The difficulties inherent in this situation are compounded by the expansion of early identification, intervention, and diversion programs. Such programs need simple, accurate, and user-friendly assessment instruments that can accommodate a wide range of service providers and health officials, many of whom do not have formal training in use of assessment instruments.

Fortunately, there are a number of sound and proven assessment instruments, which offer great promise to the practitioner who is seeking help in assessing adolescent substance abuse. Such instruments can objectively, efficiently, and meaningfully document the extent and nature of clinical phenomena. Many tests feature both accuracy and ease of administration, thus expanding the base of users to the diverse service providers who are so crucial in the early identification of adolescent substance use disorders.

Types of Assessment Instruments. Two general types of assessment instruments are available for use with adolescents: screening instruments and comprehensive assessment instruments. Most screening instruments are in the form of paper-and-pencil questionnaires, which contain fixed questions and a limited number of response options. The patient's score is tallied and compared to either a standardization sample or a cutoff score, which indicates problem status (for example, a severe drug abuse problem). Paper-and-pencil questionnaires have the advantage that they can be administered by untrained staff, or the patient can complete them without supervision.

Comprehensive assessment instruments are more variable in format than screening tools. They include paper-and-pencil questionnaires, computer administered tests, and interviews. Among the interview formats, two types exist. Structured interviews are quite similar to questionnaires, in that the interviewer's questions are completely specified and the response options are limited. In contrast, structured interviews (which must be administered in person) involve an interchange between patient and interviewer in order to clarify questions or responses. Semistructured interviews grant the interviewer considerable latitude in adapting questions to suit the respondent, and thus allow the interviewer to probe a particular response. Semistructured interviews require clinical judgment when scoring patient responses, but many professionals believe that they produce a higher quality of information than fully structured interviews.

Screening Procedures. The process of screening adolescents for alcohol or drug use involves more than just administering instruments. It is recommended that a minimal screening be organized in the following manner:

Sources: Sources of information should include the adolescent patient and one knowledgeable adult, preferably a parent or guardian.

Method: The process should include a brief self-report questionnaire and brief structured interview with the patient and a brief unstructured interview with the parent or guardian.

Content: Coverage should include onset and frequency of alcohol or drug use, consequences of use, and other signs and symptoms of drug dependence or abuse, as well as of key psychiatric and environmental factors (such as suicide potential, physical and sexual abuse, and family problems).

Several variations of this minimal screening can be implemented, each valid in its own right. Although far from ideal, some situations call for a simpler process that involves a single source (patient), method (self-report questionnaire), and content area (drug use problem severity). Such a "miniscreening" might be the only practical approach in settings that process large numbers of youth and where staff members are burdened with multiple administrative tasks (for example, juvenile detention centers). Fortunately, brief and accurate screening tools do exist that rely solely on the client's self-report of problem severity.

Laboratory Tests. Some professionals recommend routine laboratory testing as part of drug screening. Laboratory tests yield a narrow but important range of information. Although urinalysis and other biological tests, such as hair analyses, have some utility in detecting alcohol or drug use, laboratory tests typically do not provide data sufficient for a *DSM-IV* (American Psychiatric Association, 1994) diagnosis of dependence or abuse. Laboratory tests also may not detect all substance use; for example, McLaney and colleagues (1994) found a low association between substance use, self-report, and drug test findings. Interestingly, this was not a product of low rates of self-reports of drug use, but rather was the result of the disparate pattern of negative drug screens in the face of self-reports of drug use.

Urine drug tests also can be problematic because they can be influenced in many ways. For example, the amount and frequency of use, drug test sensitivity, and amount of time elapsed between substance use and sample collection all are factors that can alter test results. In addition, false positives (when the result is positive even though the drug has not been used) may occur in patients who use some common diet pills, as well as decongestants.

Uses of Comprehensive Assessment. A comprehensive assessment should be administered when the initial screen suggests that an adolescent may have a drug problem. At minimum, the assessment process should consist of:

- An in-depth examination of the severity and nature of the individual's drug involvement.

- A thorough assessment of additional problems flagged during the screening, and inquiry into problems that may not have been included in the screening (such as delinquency, family environment, peer relations, community standards and norms, psychiatric status, school functioning, and physical health).

- A concerted effort to use multiple sources and methods, with an emphasis on the use of standardized multiscale questionnaires, structured interviews, archival records, and parents' reports.

Including the adolescent's family or guardian in the comprehensive assessment process can be difficult or impossible when a traditional family is absent. Some youth who seek treatment may be homeless or from dysfunctional families. Nevertheless, whenever possible, it is important for the assessor to attempt to form a therapeutic alliance with the youth's family or guardian. While parents generally can provide only limited information about their child's possible alcohol or drug problem, they are a necessary source of information about the home environment, and their involvement can be helpful to the adolescent if treatment is warranted.

The skill level of the assessor is more crucial in conducting a comprehensive assessment than in a screening. Users of comprehensive tools usually require advanced training in assessment. It is vital to match the skill level of the assessor with the training requirements of the test. In cases where a single professional is involved in the comprehensive assessment, his or her training and accreditation must be consistent with the demands of the assessment. An assessor who is not qualified to make mental health diagnoses should refer a patient elsewhere if the adolescent needs diagnostic services. Similarly, some standardized tests need to be interpreted and confirmed by a licensed psychologist, psychiatrist, or other licensed mental health worker. (The administration of most paper-and-pencil questionnaires is another matter; a trained unlicensed technician can usually administer such tests).

General Test Practices. The following test practices can serve as a guide for appropriate use of questionnaires and interviews (Eyde, Moreland et al. 1988):

Proper Test Use: Responsible and competent use of a test involves verifying the test actually measures what it is supposed to measure. The test manual should describe the traits and characteristics that the test is intended to measure, the types of patients for whom it is appropriate, and in what settings the test should be used.

Psychometric Knowledge: Test users need to have some knowledge about the test's standard error, reliability, and validity. For some tests, particularly screening tests, accuracy is reported in terms of "hit rates," sensitivity (true positives), and specificity (true negatives). It cannot be emphasized too strongly that all tests are subject to some degree of error and thus should not be used to the exclusion of clinical judgment.

Integrity of Test Results: It is important to be sure that all criterion measures established in the development of a test are appropriate to the patient being tested. If such measures are not relevant, then the test results must be interpreted with caution.

Appropriate Use of Norms: Norms associated with a test must be appropriate for the given subjects being tested. It also is important to ensure that the condition and setting under which the norms were collected are similar to those present in the proposed administration of the test.

Scoring Accuracy: Scoring accuracy needs to be checked when the test is hand-scored. Computerized score reports that provide narrative summaries and recommendations for treatment should be interpreted cautiously because they are based on generalities.

Interpretative Feedback: The test administrator should be willing and competent to provide interpretation and appropriate services and referrals to the individual being tested.

SCREENING TOOLS

Screening measures may cover alcohol, other drugs, or both alcohol and other drugs. Virtually all are formatted as paper-and-pencil tests. Caution should be exercised in selection because psychometric data are limited or nonexistent for some of these tools.

Adolescent Alcohol Involvement Scale (AAIS). The AAIS is a 14-item self-report questionnaire (Mayer & Filstead, 1979). The instrument requires approximately 15 minutes to administer and evaluates the type and frequency of drinking, the last drinking episode, reasons for the onset of drinking behavior, drinking context, short- and long-term effects of drinking, the adolescent's perceptions about drinking, and how others perceive his or her drinking.

Scores represent the severity of alcohol abuse. Estimates of internal consistency range from .55 in a clinical sample (Moberg, 1983) to .76 in a general sample. Test scores are significantly related to substance use diagnosis and ratings from another source (such as independent clinical assessments or parents). Norms are available for clinical and nonclinical samples of adolescents 13 to 19 years old.

Adolescent Drinking Index (ADI). The ADI is a 24-item self-administered test (Harrell & Wirtz, 1990) that evaluates problem drinking in adolescents through assessment of psychological symptoms, physical symptoms, social symptoms, and loss of control. Studies support the validity of this instrument in measuring the severity of adolescent drinking problems. Internal consistency reliability of the ADI is high (coefficient alpha, .93 to .95).

Adolescent Drug Involvement Scale (ADIS). Modified by Moberg (1991) from the AAIS (described above) to address drug use problem severity, the 12-item ADIS has promising internal consistency. Preliminary validity evidence also is encouraging.

Client Substance Index—Short (CSI-S). The 15-item CSI-S (Thomas, 1990) is part of a larger Substance Abuse Screening Protocol developed for the National Center for Juvenile Justice. The CSI-S is a yes/no paper-and-pencil brief screen that was adapted from Moore's (1983) multiscale Client Substance Index (described below). The purpose of the CSI-S is to identify juveniles within the court system who are in need of additional drug abuse evaluation.

Drug and Alcohol Problem Quick Screen (DAPQS). The DAPQS is a yes/no screening questionnaire that has been tested in a pediatric practice setting (Schwartz & Wirtz, 1990). Unfortunately, no reliability or criterion validity evidence is available. However, its developers report that approximately 15% of respondents in the sample endorsed six or more items, which is considered to be a "red flag" cutoff score.

MMPI-A Scales: Alcohol/Drug Problem Acknowledgment (ACK) and Alcohol/Drug Problem Proneness (PEO). The MMPI has developed a revised version for adolescents called the MMPI-A, which includes two scales for the assessment of alcohol and other drug problems (Weed, Butcher et al., 1994). The ACK scale is a 13-item instrument that measures open acknowledgment of problems with alcohol and other drugs. The 36-item PRO scale assesses the likelihood of developing an alcohol or drug problem. Internal consistencies for the ACK scale and the PRO scale are .70 and .76, respectively, and test-retest reliability is fair.

Perceived-Benefit of Drinking and Drug Use Scales. This 10-item instrument (five perceived-benefit questions for alcohol and the same five questions for drug use) was designed to serve as a nonthreatening problem severity screen. This instrument is based on the philosophy that one's perception of the benefits of substance use is a gauge of one's actual use. The scales have been shown to be related to several key indicators of drug use behavior when administered in schools (Petchers, Singer et al., 1988) and adolescent inpatient psychiatric settings (Petchers & Singer, 1990). Internal consistency is estimated to range from .69 to .74.

Rutgers Alcohol Problem Index (RAPI). The RAPI is a 23-item questionnaire (White & Labouvie, 1989) that focuses on consequences of alcohol use in six areas: family life, social relations, psychological functioning, delinquency, physical problems, and neuropsychological functioning. This instrument is highly correlated with *DSM-IIIR* (APA, 1987) criteria for substance use disorders, and has shown satisfactory reliability.

Substance Abuse Potential Scale (SAP). Designed specifically for older adolescent and young adult males, the 36-item MMPI-derived SAP scale (MacAndrew, 1986) appears to identify several behaviors that have been found to characterize drug-abusing young men, such as delinquency and reward-seeking behaviors. SAP scores have yielded very favorable results in terms of group discrimination (for example, drug abusers versus students versus psychiatric patients).

Substance Abuse and Mental Health Preliminary Screening (SAMH-1). The SAMH-1 screen (Florida Department of Health and Rehabilitative Services, 1990) is an interview designed for use by intake staff with adolescents against whom a delinquency petition has been filed. The SAMH-1 collects demographic information, current legal charges, suicide risk, and present status in drug abuse or mental health treatment. In addition to the interview, an administrative manual has been developed, but is not widely available.

UNCOPE. This six-item screen originally was designed as an orally administered screen to identify risk for substance dependence in adult populations. It has good sensitivity and specificity (Zywiak, Hoffmann et al., 1999). Initial indications with adolescents suggest that the screen may have utility for these populations as well.

Youth Diagnostic Screening Test (YDST). This 36-item alcohol screening tool (Alibrandi, 1978) assesses three characteristics of problem drinking: pathological style, problematic consumption, and consequences. A cutoff score to diagnose alcoholism is provided; however, this decision rule has not yet been validated.

ASSESSMENT INSTRUMENTS

This section reviews instruments that are considered comprehensive assessments, including multiscale self-report questionnaires and multiple domain interviews.

Diagnostic Interview Schedules. In adult psychiatric interviews, it is common to find diagnostic interviews that cover substance use disorders. Some examples are the Schedule for Affective Disorders and Schizophrenia (SADS) (Endicott & Spitzer, 1978), the Diagnostic Interview Schedule (DIS) (Robins, Helzer et al., 1981), and the Structured Clinical Interview for *DSM-III* (SCID) (Spitzer & Williams, 1984).

The Substance Use Disorder Diagnosis Interview-IV (SUDDS-IV) is the most widely used interview for diagnosing adult substance use (Hoffmann & Harrison, 1994). In addition to covering *DSM-IV* criteria, the instrument contains sections on tobacco use and screens for depression and anxiety disorders. Because the SUDDS-IV was designed for adults, caution should be exercised in using it with adolescents. Items such as those concerning employment may not be appropriate for adolescents, and the instrument does not mention areas important to adolescents, such as school consequences or peer use issues.

The Practical Adolescent Dual Diagnostic Interview (PADDI) addresses both substance use disorders and key mental health conditions in accordance with the *DSM-IV/DSM-IV-TR* diagnostic criteria (Estroff & Hoffmann, 2000).

Initial data on the PADDI indicate good internal consistency in covering most of the syndromes and good differentiation between those who meet criteria for a given condition and those who do not (Hoffmann, Estroff et al., 2001; Hoffmann & Estroff, 2002).

A number of older child and adolescent diagnostic interviews have been created for assessing substance use disorders. Among the most prominent are the Diagnostic Interview Schedule for Children (DISC) (Shaffer, 1992), the Diagnostic Interview for Children and Adolescents (DICA) (Herjanic & Reich, 1982), and the semistructured Kiddie-SADS (Puig-Antich, 1982). The Kiddie-SADS offers several advantages over the others, in that it includes provisions for collecting information from parents, incorporating archival data, and clarifying answers to questions. (The drug use questions are contained in the epidemiologic version of the Kiddie-SADS, but not the episode version.)

Several structured interviews focus almost exclusively on adolescent substance use disorders. The Guided Rational Adolescent Substance Abuse Profile (GRASP) (Addiction Recovery Corp., 1986) assesses substance use disorders through use of the *DSM-III* criteria (APA, 1980). However, this tool does not yet include any psychometric data. The ADI (Winters & Henly, 1993), summarized above, offers a structured schedule for *DSM-IIIR* criteria for abuse and dependence disorders (APA, 1987).

Derivatives of the Addiction Severity Index. The Addiction Severity Index (ASI; McLellan, Luborsky et al., 1980) is an adult program evaluation tool. In addition to assessing substance use during the preceding 30 days and some problem indications, the ASI assesses psychosocial functioning, including psychiatric status, medical status, employment/support status, family history, family/social relationships, and legal status. Since the inception of the ASI, several adolescent versions of the instrument have been created, including the Adolescent Drug Abuse Diagnosis (ADAD), the Adolescent Problem Severity Index (APSI), the Comprehensive Addiction Severity Index for Adolescents (CASI-A), the Substance Abuse and Mental Health Assessment (SAMH-2), and the Teen Addiction Severity Index (T-ASI).

Adolescent Drug Abuse Diagnosis (ADAD): The ADAD, a 150-item structured therapy evaluation interview, addresses eight content areas: medical status, drug and alcohol use, legal status, family background and problems, school/employment, social activities and peer relations, and psychological status. The interview is based on a 10-point rating scale that indicates the adolescent's need for additional treatment in each content area. The severity ratings translate to a problem severity dimension (no problem, slight problem, moderate problem, considerable problem, or extreme problem). The drug use section of the ADAD includes a well-defined drug use frequency checklist and a brief set of items that examine aspects of drug involvement, such as polydrug use, attempts at abstinence, withdrawal symptoms, and use in school. There are data regarding the reliability and validity of the ADAD (Friedman & Utada, 1989). In addition to the standard version of the ADAD, there is a shorter form (83 items) for use in treatment outcome evaluation.

Adolescent Problem Severity Index (APSI): The APSI (Metzger, Kushner et al., 1991) assesses general information regarding the reason for the assessment, the referral source, and the adolescent's understanding of the reason for the interview. This instrument also contains sections that collect detailed information about drug and alcohol use, family relationships, education/work, legal, medical, psychosocial adjustment, and personal relationships. Concurrent validity for the alcohol and drug section has been empirically demonstrated.

Problem Severity Index (PSI): The PSI, a structured interview for use by juvenile probation officers in evaluating substance abuse among juvenile offenders, is an earlier version of the APSI (reviewed above). The PSI contains a general section on client demographics and family background, as well as more detailed sections on legal status, family relationships, education or work, medical status, psychological and social adjustment, drug and alcohol use, and personal relationships.

Comprehensive Addiction Severity Index for Adolescents (CASI-A): Adapted from the ASI by Meyers (1991), the CASI-A is a structured interview that includes extensive appendices and an administration manual. Although similar in format to the APSI, the CASI-A is considerably more time-consuming to administer because of differences in content and format. For example, for most test items, multiple responses must be entered by the interviewer. Also, administration of the CASI-A requires use of materials from appendices to guide questions and responses. The CASI-A has two special features: It incorporates results from a urine drug screen as well as observations by the assessor. The CASI-A and its components are available through the Carrier Foundation of New Jersey.

Teen Severity Index (T-ASI): Kaminer and colleagues (1991) developed another adolescent version of the ASI, the T-ASI. This instrument incorporates seven content domains: chemical use, school status, employment/support status, family relationships, legal status, peer/social relationships, and psychiatric status. Because it was found to be less relevant to adolescent drug abusers, a medical status section was not included in the T-ASI. Severity ratings by the interviewer and the patient are based on a five-point scale for each of the seven domains.

Other Comprehensive Instruments. The last group of comprehensive instruments are not designed after the ASI. The PEI (Winters & Henly, 1989) is part of the MCDAAP, which is described later in this chapter and thus need not be repeated here.

Adolescent Chemical Health Inventory (ACHI): Consisting of 128 items, the ACHI (Renovex, 1988) is a self-administered computer test that addresses drug use problem severity and psychosocial factors. For example, scales measure family closeness, depression, alienation, family support, family chemical use and physical/sexual abuse. The ACHI also contains a screen for defensiveness. ACHI validity data indicate that the instrument is able to differentiate between adolescent drug abusers and non-abusers.

Adolescent Self Assessment Profile (ASAP): The ASAP (Wanberg, 1992) is a self-administered, multiscale inventory derived from a series of multivariate research studies by Horn, Wanberg and colleagues, who investigated multiple life adjustment and drug use problems associated with adolescent drug abuse. The ASAP contains 20 basic scales, seven of which address drug use frequency for specific drugs. The remaining 13 scales focus on key psychosocial problems (such as deviance or peer influence) and drug use consequences and benefits. In addition to the basic scales, supplemental scales that are based on common factors found within the specific psychosocial and problem severity domains also can be scored. The ASAP's norms are based on a sample of adolescents admitted to outpatient drug treatment programs in Colorado. Comprehensive reliability and validity evidence for the ASAP are provided in a manual that accompanies the instrument.

Chemical Dependency Assessment Profile (CDAP): The CDAP, a new 235-item self-report questionnaire, investigates several dimensions of drug use, including expectations of use, physiological symptoms, and quantity and frequency of use. Normative data are available on 86 subjects (Harrell, Honaker et al., 1991).

Client Substance Index (CSI): Using Jellinek's 28 symptoms of drug dependence, Moore (1983) developed the 113-item CSI. This instrument assesses the degree of drug dependence, ranging from "no problem" to "chemical dependency." The CSI has been shown to effectively discriminate normal from drug treatment samples.

Customary Drinking and Drug Use Record (CDDR): The CDDR is a research structured interview that measures alcohol and other drug use consumption for both recent (prior 3 months) and lifetime periods, *DSM-IIIR* and *DSM-IV* substance dependence symptoms (including a detailed assessment of withdrawal symptoms), and several additional consequences of alcohol and other drug involvement (Brown, Christiansen et al., 1987a; Brown, Creamer et al., 1987b). Psychometric studies have found that this instrument is reliable over time and across interviewers (average one-week test-retest coefficients for all major content domains is .91). The CDDR also has been found to discriminate community youth from substance-using youth, and to converge with alternate measures (Brown, Myers et al., 1998).

Diagnostic Interview Schedule for Children (DISC-C): After several revisions, the DISC-C (Costello, Edelbroch et al., 1985; Shaffer, Schwab-Stone et al., 1993) now provides a *DSM-IV* version (Shaffer, Fisher et al., 1996). This instrument consists of separate versions for the child and the parent. As part of a larger study of multiple diagnoses, Fisher and colleagues (1993) found this version to be highly sensitive in accurately pinpointing youth who had received a hospital diagnosis of any substance use disorder (n=8). The child and parent versions were found to have a sensitivity of 75% and to be associated with moderate test-retest stability for substance use disorders (kappa=.46) (Roberts, Solovitz et al., 1996).

Drug Use Screening Inventory-Revised (DUSI-R): The DUSI-R, a 159-item instrument, assesses the level of involvement with multiple drugs and the severity of consequences of such involvement. The DUSI-R provides scores based on 10 problem-density subscales (substance use, behavior problems, psychiatric disorder) and one lie scale. In a sample of adolescent substance abusers, the domain scores were found to be correlated with *DSM-IIIR* criteria for substance use disorder (Tarter, Laird et al., 1992). An additional psychometric report presents norms and evidence of scale sensitivity (Kirisci, Mezzich et al., 1995).

Hilson Adolescent Profile (HAP): This instrument consists of 310 true-false items that encompasses 16 scales, two of which measure alcohol and drug use. In addition, there are scales that correspond to characteristics found in psychiatric diagnostic categories (such as antisocial behavior or depression), as well as psychosocial problems (such as home-life conflicts). Inwald and colleagues (1986) have collected normative data from three samples (clinical patients, juvenile offenders, and normal adolescents).

Juvenile Automated Substance Abuse Evaluation (JASAE): This 102-item (T/F) instrument (ADE, Inc., 1987) is based on a similar adult measure, the SALCE. The JASAE yields a five-category score, which ranges from "no use" to "drug abuse accompanied by physical or psychological symptoms of addiction." Also included with the JAESAE is a psychosocial stress index and a scale for test-taking attitude. This instrument has been shown to discriminate clinical from nonclinical groups.

Prevention Management Evaluation System (PMES): The PMES is a 150-item structured interview and questionnaire for youth who are already in drug treatment. The content areas assist treatment planning by qualitatively covering five major areas: family background, school and legal problems, family relations, peer activity, and self-esteem (Barrett, Simpson et al., 1988). Although validity evidence is lacking, interrater agreement for the interview is good.

Substance Abuse and Mental Health Assessment (SAMH-2): Developed by the Florida Department of Health and Rehabilitative Services, the SAMH-2 is a structured interview focusing on multiple life areas. It also includes a brief section that discusses the reasons for referral. The legal status module covers current/pending offenses and prior offenses, but does not address prior delinquency adjudications. Other sections of the interview examine educational/vocational status, home/living situation, substance abuse history, family history, psychological/medical status, mental health symptoms, and physical/sexual abuse. Psychometric data are not yet available for this instrument.

Substance Abuse Subtle Screening Inventory-Adolescent Version (SASSI-A): This 81-item paper-and-pencil questionnaire is an adolescent version of the SASSI (Miller, 1990). The SASSI-A consists of three drug abuse scales, one "subtle" or non-face valid drug abuse scale, and two scales that measure "faking good" tendencies. Also, two experimental scales (Correctional and Random Responding) can be scored. Scoring procedures result in a dichotomous rating of "Chemically Dependent" or "Non-abuser." The SASSI-A has been found to successfully discriminate between adolescents in drug treatment and those who are not using drugs.

Other Instruments. The following instruments measure variables related to drug abuse severity.

Alcohol Expectancy Questionnaire-Adolescent Version (AEQ-A): This 90-item questionnaire, developed by Brown and colleagues (1987a), measures expected or anticipated effects of alcohol use. Versions focusing on marijuana and cocaine also are available. The AEQ-A is made up of six positive expectancies: global positive effects, social behavior change, improvement of cognitive/motor abilities, sexual enhancement, increased arousal, and relaxation/tension reduction. In addition to the positive expectancies, there is one negative expectancy: deteriorated cognitive/behavioral functioning. Encouraging data on reliability and validity exist for the AEQ-A (Brown, Creamer et al., 1987b; Christiansen, Smith et al., 1989).

Circumstances, Motivation, Readiness and Suitability scales (CMRS): This 25-item instrument, although originally designed for use with adults receiving a therapeutic community approach, has been tested for use with drug-abusing adolescents (Jainchill, Bhattacharya et al., 1995). Consisting of four scales and a total score, the CMRS was designed to predict retention in treatment. The scales include circumstances (external motivation), motivation (internal motivation), readiness (for treatment), and suitability (perceived appropriateness of the treatment modality). The internal consistency of the CMRS is favorable (alpha scores ranging from .77 to .80), and the scales are moderately predictive of short-term (30-day) retention.

Decisional Balance Scale: In a non-clinical population of adolescent alcohol users and abusers, Migneault and colleagues (1997) developed this 16-item scale. The instrument examines pros and cons of drinking. The internal reliability of both scales is satisfactory (.81 and .87).

Drug Avoidance Self-Efficacy Scale (DASES): The DASES (Martin, Wilkinson et al., 1995) is a self-report measure that examines self-efficacy for abstinence. It is designed to be used with young drug abusers. On a rating scale of one to seven, respondents are asked whether they would resist or use drugs/alcohol in 16 different high-risk situations. The internal reliability of the DASES is excellent (.91), and its predictive validity has been supported, in that scale scores were shown to predict subsequent drug and alcohol behaviors (that is, greater self-efficacy was associated with lower future drug use).

Problem Recognition Questionnaire (PRQ): The PRQ is a 24-item adolescent scale, consisting of separate factors pertaining to drug use problem recognition and readiness for treatment (that is, action orientation). This instrument was designed with a combination of rational and empirical procedures. The PRQ factors have adequate internal reliability and appear to be predictive of posttreatment functioning (Cady, Winters et al., 1996).

INTEGRATED ASSESSMENT SYSTEMS

A recent trend in adolescent assessment has been the development of assessment systems that combine screening, diagnostic evaluation, and multiscale assessment. These integrated systems include a threshold screening for both overt and subtle indicators of drug abuse, with the objective of identifying a high proportion of adolescents who are likely to be in need of treatment. The initial screening is followed by a more focused evaluation of recent and past drug use, of diagnostic signs and symptoms of abuse and dependence, and of other mental health problems, as well as an evaluation of the psychosocial factors that may have been affected by or contributed to the drug involvement.

Adolescent Assessment and Referral System (AARS). In April 1997, the National Institute on Drug Abuse introduced the Adolescent Assessment and Referral System (Rahdert, 1991). This project was developed in response to the need for a more generalized assessment strategy, with a wider range of problem areas relevant to adolescent drug use and abuse. The AARS was developed to assess current adolescent instruments' validity and reliability and also to design a standardized set of guidelines to aid in the use of these instruments in clinical settings for adolescents 12 to 19 years old. Because adolescents who use drugs also tend to exhibit a wide variety of behavioral problems, assessing for and treating their behavioral problems may be a way of interrupting drug use early. The AARS consists of experts in the field who have developed assessment items, recommended other existing instruments, and have formulated scoring rules to guide clinicians. To date, the AARS has generated three components, the Problem Oriented Screening Instrument for Teenagers (POSIT), specific guidelines for selecting the most appropriate assessment, and guidelines for creating a directory of adolescent treatment services. Each of the three components are described below.

Problem Oriented Screening Instrument for Teenagers (POSIT): (Note that the POSIT and DUSI are two different names for essentially the same screening tool.) This 139-item self-administered yes/no instrument is designed to screen for adolescent problems in 10 functional areas: substance use/abuse, physical health, mental health, family relations, peer relations, educational status, vocational status, social skills, leisure/recreation, and aggressive behavior/delinquency. Initial cutoff scores have been designated based on decision rules provided by an expert panel. Early data show that the designated problem areas were potential problems for at least 75% of those in a drug treatment cohort.

Client Personal History Questionnaire (CPHQ): This structured interview is designed to be used in conjunction with the POSIT. It assesses five main areas, including demographic information, mental health and juvenile justice system history, academic performance, health care utilization, and current life stressors. Both instruments are available in Spanish and English.

Comprehensive Assessment Battery (CAB): The CAB offers a more thorough examination of the specific problem areas assessed in the POSIT. The CAB contains a list and brief description of assessments tools best suited to the 10 problem areas outlined in the POSIT, as chosen by an expert panel. The problem areas identified through the POSIT are more thoroughly assessed by the CAB. The CAB lists several instruments for each of the 10 problem areas; it is up to the clinician to decide which to use.

Treatment Planning: The AARS recommends that, after the CAB is administered, a Directory of Adolescent Services be developed. The AARS suggests that the directory have two components: (1) an Adolescent Services Matrix, designed to list appropriate programs and facilities in the local area, as well as the services offered by each facility, and (2) a Provider Information Form, to summarize information for each provider (including phone number, address, contact person(s), services offered, and eligibility requirements). The AARS manual incorporates a plan for assembling a list of adolescent service providers.

Minnesota Chemical Dependency Adolescent Assessment Package (MCDAPP). Another assessment system was created by a consortium of drug abuse treatment providers and researchers (Winters & Henly, 1988). Although the two systems are similar in the way they incorporate both screening and comprehensive instruments, they also differ in several ways. First, the MCDAAP instruments focus on the characteristics of drug abuse and related psychosocial problems, whereas the AARS focuses more on comorbid mental and behavioral disorders. Second, the screening tool used in the MCDAPP is truncated when compared to the number of items in the POSIT. Third, the battery of instruments used in MCDAPP does not contain the guidebooks or references for treatment service directories found in the AARS manual. The three instruments in the MCDAAP are described below.

Personal Experience Screening Questionnaire (PESQ): The PESQ (Winters, 1991, 1992) is a brief 40-item screening instrument that identifies adolescents who may be abusing alcohol or other drugs. In addition to the problem severity scale, the PESQ briefly measures drug use history, select psychosocial problems, and response distortion tendencies ("faking good" and "faking bad"). Data have been collected on normal, juvenile offender, and drug-abusing populations. The ability of the PESQ to accurately predict the need for a drug abuse assessment has been estimated at approximately 87%. Also, the internal consistency and reliability estimates are high (coefficient alpha, .91 to .95).

Adolescent Diagnostic Interview (ADI): The ADI (Winters & Henly, 1993) assesses the scope of symptoms associated with psychoactive substance use disorders outlined in the *DSM-IIIR.* The structured interview addresses nine major areas: sociodemographic information, substance abuse consumption history, signs of abuse and dependence in all major drug categories, mental health disorders, several areas of functioning (such as school performance, peer and family relationships, leisure activities, and legal difficulties), and severity of psychosocial stressors (for example, self-image, interpersonal issues, physical and mental health, tragic/embarrassing events, and home/school problems). Inter-rater agreement, test-retest reliability, concurrent validity, and criterion validity of the ADI have been reported (Winters & Henly, 1993; Winters, Stinchfield et al., 1993a).

Personal Experience Inventory (PEI): The PEI is a paper-and-pencil instrument composed of two sections: Chemical Involvement Problem Severity and Psychosocial Risk Factors. The Chemical Involvement Problem Severity section is subdivided into five Basic Scales, five Clinical Scales, three response bias scales, and drug use frequency items. The Psychosocial Risk Factors section addresses interpersonal factors (such as negative self-image, social isolation, and absence of goals) and environmental factors (such as drug abuse by peers and siblings, physical and sexual abuse, and estrangement from the family). The PEI also includes screens for eating disorders, suicide potential, and parental history of drug abuse. Normative data are available for this instrument for adolescents 12 to 15 years of age, 16 to 18 years of age, by gender, and for adolescents in drug clinic and school settings. The scoring program for the PEI provides a computerized report that includes narratives and standardized scores for each scale, in addition to various clinical information. Also, PEI scores have been found to be highly correlated with other measures of drug abuse problem severity, psychosocial risk factors, independent recommendations regarding the need for drug abuse treatment, and clinical diagnoses (Henly & Winters, 1988, 1989; Winters & Henly, 1989; Winters, Stinchfield et al., 1993b).

COMPUTERIZED TESTING

It is becoming more common for tests to be accompanied by software for computerized administration and scoring. Whereas computerized instruments may be more costly to purchase than paper-and-pencil instruments, they promise real savings in assessor time, which is the single greatest expense in the assessment process. Computer scoring programs often provide descriptive narratives, highlight critical responses, identify factors to be pursued in a subsequent interview, suggest treatment modalities, and summarize standardized scale scores.

Of course, computerized programs are only as good as the information fed into the program and the skill exhibited by the programmer. "Canned" computer narratives may provide descriptors that are too general, and may offer treatment recommendations or other diagnostic labels without providing statistical justification for these interpretive statements.

The literature is unclear as to the relative validity of computerized testing versus other methods of testing. Evidence exists for both sides of the argument. Some studies point to increased disclosure rates by respondents of sensitive material, which may imply more validity, while other studies do not support the incremental validity of computerized testing. The debate remains unresolved, yet the popularity of computerized testing is likely to grow.

CLINICAL JUDGMENT

Questionnaires, interviews, and laboratory findings all have their weaknesses and limitations. These methods can assist the process of screening, diagnosing, and selecting a level of care, but they should not be used exclusive of clinical judgment. (Of course, it also is dangerous to be overly reliant on clinical judgment.) It cannot be emphasized enough that the assessment process should involve an integration of multiple methods and multiple sources of information, as well as a blend of standardized, laboratory, and nonstandardized information. These cautions underlie all effective assessment practices and help ensure the most accurate determination of the extent and nature of the patient's problems and the most appropriate level of treatment.

Unstructured, subjective tools also are valuable in the clinical judgment process. For example, sentence completion tasks tailored to AA-based treatment programs can provide rich assessment data that would be difficult to collect through standardized tools, as well assist the client's progress through the steps toward recovery. Jaffe's workbook (1990) appears to be an excellent example of this type of clinical aid. The workbook provides a structure for the adolescent client to record thoughts and experiences about his or her history of drug use. Because it is organized around the first five steps of the Twelve Steps of recovery, this tool helps to initiate the change process.

CONCLUSIONS

The recent proliferation of adolescent assessment instruments is a double-edged sword. On the one hand, professionals and researchers have a number of different tools from which to choose. On the other, selecting the right instrument for a given patient or subject in a particular situation can become a guessing game. What is needed is a critical comparison of the strengths and weaknesses of each instrument. Empirically, little is known about which instruments perform best with subsets of the adolescent populations in particular settings. Therefore, clinicians must exercise their own judgment in selecting instruments and follow up with ongoing review of the appropriateness of the instruments employed.

The future probably will see greater use of computerized testing and increased attention to the assessment of coexisting mental disorders, particularly affective and conduct disorders and other compulsive conditions, such as eating disorders.

The growth of adolescent assessment will benefit from continuing attention to high standards. The field has made progress regarding the use of standardized assessment instruments and the implementation of treatment outcome evaluations. These tools need to be put into practice on a routine basis so that they become not the exception, but the rule.

ACKNOWLEDGMENT: Partial support for this chapter was provided by NIDA grant DA04334 (Dr. Winters).

REFERENCES

ADE, Inc. (1987). *Juvenile Automated Substance Abuse Evaluation (JASAE)*. Clarkston, MI: ADE, Inc.

Addiction Recovery Corp. (1986). *Guided Rational Adolescent Substance Abuse Profile*. Waltham, MA: Addiction Recovery Corp.

Alibrandi T (1978). *Young Alcoholics*. Minneapolis, MN: Comp Care Publications.

American Psychiatric Association (APA) (1980). *Diagnostic and Statistical Manual of Mental Disorders, 3rd Edition (DSM-III)*. Washington, DC: American Psychiatric Press.

American Psychiatric Association (APA) (1987). *Diagnostic and Statistical Manual of Mental Disorders, 3rd Edition, Revised (DSM-IIIR)*. Washington, DC: American Psychiatric Press.

American Psychiatric Association (APA) (1994). *Diagnostic and Statistical Manual of Mental Disorders, 4th Edition (DSM-IV)*. Washington, DC: American Psychiatric Press.

Barrett ME, Simpson DD & Lehman WE (1988). Behavioral changes of adolescents in drug abuse intervention programs. *Journal of Clinical Psychology* 44:461-473.

Block JR, Goodman N, Ambellan F et al. (1974). *A Self-Administered High School Study of Drugs*. Hempstead, NY: Institute for Research and Development Inc.

Brown SA, Christiansen BA & Goldman MS (1987a). The Alcohol Expectancies Questionnaire: An instrument for the assessment of adolescent and adult alcohol expectancies. *Journal of Studies on Alcohol* 48:483-491.

Brown SA, Creamer VA & Stetson BA (1987b). Adolescent alcohol expectancies in relation to personal and parental drinking patterns. *Journal of Abnormal Psychology* 96:117-121.

Brown SA, Myers MG, Lippke L et al. (1998). Psychometric evaluation of the Customary Drinking and Drug Use Record (CDDR): A measure of adolescent alcohol and drug involvement. *Journal of Studies on Alcohol* 59:427-438.

Cady M, Winters KC, Jordan D et al. (1996). Motivation to change as a predictor of treatment outcome for adolescent substance abusers. *Journal of Child and Adolescent Substance Abuse* 5:73-91.

Christiansen BA, Smith GT, Roehling PV et al. (1989). Using alcohol expectancies to predict adolescent drinking behavior after one year. *Journal of Consulting and Clinical Psychology* 57:93-99.

Costello EJ, Edelbroch C & Costello AJ (1985). Validity of the NIMH Diagnostic Interview Schedule for Children: A comparison between psychiatric and pediatric referrals. *Journal of Abnormal Child Psychology* 13:570-595.

Estroff TW & Hoffmann NG (2000). *PADDI: Practical Adolescent Dual Diagnosis Interview*. Smithfield, RI: Evince Clinical Assessments.

Endicott J & Spitzer R (1978). A diagnostic interview: The Schedule for Affective Disorders and Schizophrenia. *Archives of General Psychiatry* 35:773-782.

Eyde LD, Moreland KL, Robertson GJ et al. (1988). Executive summary: Test user qualifications: A data-based approach to promoting good test use. In *Report of the Test User Qualifications Working Group of the Joint Committee on Testing Practices*. Washington, DC: American Psychological Association.

Farrow FA, Smith WR & Hurst MD (1993). *Adolescent Drug and Alcohol Assessment Instruments in Current Use: A Critical Comparison*. Seattle, WA: Department of Pediatrics University of Washington.

Fisher P, Shaffer D, Piacentini JC et al. (1993). Sensitivity of the Diagnostic Interview Schedule for Children, 2nd edition (DISC-2.1) for specific diagnoses of children and adolescents. *Journal of the American Academy of Child and Adolescent Psychiatry* 32:666-673.

Florida Department of Health and Rehabilitative Services (1990). *Substance Abuse and Mental Health Preliminary Screening*. Tallahassee, FL: The Department.

Friedman AS & Utada A (1989). A method for diagnosing and planning the treatment of adolescent drug abusers (Adolescent Drug Abuse Diagnosis Instrument). *Journal of Drug Education* 19:285-312.

Harrell AH & Wirtz PW (1990). *Adolescent Drinking Index*. Odessa, FL: Psychological Assessment Resources, Inc. 1990

Harrell TH, Honaker LM & Davis E (1991). Cognitive and behavioral dimensions of dysfunction in alcohol and polydrug abusers. *Journal of Substance Abuse* 3:415-426.

Henly GA & Winters KC (1988). Development of problem severity scales for the assessment of adolescent alcohol and drug abuse. *International Journal of the Addictions* 23:65-85.

Henly GA & Winters KC (1989). Development of psychosocial scales for the assessment of adolescents involved with alcohol and drugs. *International Journal of the Addictions* 24:973-1001.

Herjanic B & Reich W (1982). Development of a structured psychiatric interview for children: Agreement between child and parent on individual symptoms. *Journal of Abnormal Child Psychiatry* 10:307-324.

Hoffmann NG & Estroff TW (2002). Identifying Co-occurring Disorders in Adolescent Populations. 33rd Annual Medical-Scientific Conference of the American Society of Addiction Medicine, Atlanta, GA, April.

Hoffmann NG, Estroff TW & Wallace SD (2001). Co-occurring disorders among adolescent treatment populations. *The Dual Network* 2(1):10-11.

Hoffmann NG & Harrison PA (1994). *The SUDDS-IV: Substance Use Disorders Diagnostic Scale*. Smithfield RI: Evince Clinical Assessments.

Inwald RE, Brobst MA & Morissey RF (1986). Identifying and predicting adolescent behavioral problems by using a new profile. *Juvenile Justice Digest* 14:1-9.

Jaffe SL (1990). *Step Workbook for Adolescent Chemical Dependency Recovery*. Washington, DC: American Psychiatric Press.

Jainchill N, Bhattacharya G & Yagelka J (1995). Therapeutic communities for adolescents. In E Rahdert & D Czechowicz (eds.) *Adolescent Drug Abuse: Clinical Assessment and Therapeutic Interventions (NIDA Research Monograph No. 156)*. Rockville, MD: National Institute on Drug Abuse, 190-217.

Jessor R & Jessor SL (1977). *Problem Behavior and Psychosocial Development: A Longitudinal Study of Youth*. New York, NY: Academic Press.

Kaminer Y, Bukstein O & Tarter RE (1991). The Teen-Addiction Severity Index: Rationale and reliability. *Internal Journal of the Addictions* 26:219-226.

Kandel DB, ed. (1978). *Longitudinal Research on Drug Use: Empirical Findings and Methodological Issues*. Washington, DC: Hemisphere Publishing Corp.

Kirisci L, Mezzich A & Tarter R (1995). Norms and sensitivity of the adolescent version of the drug use screening inventory. *Addictive Behaviors* 20:149-157.

MacAndrew C (1986). Toward the psychometric detection of substance misuse in young men: The SAP Scale. *Journal of Studies on Alcohol* 47:161-166.

Martin GN, Wilkinson DA & Paulos CX (1995). The drug avoidance self-efficacy scale. *Journal of Substance Abuse* 7:151-163.

Mayer J & Filstead WJ (1979). The Adolescent Alcohol Involvement Scale: An instrument for measuring adolescent use and misuse of alcohol. *Journal of Studies on Alcohol* 4:291-300.

McLaney MA, Del Boca F & Babor T (1994). A validation study of the Problem Oriented Screening Instrument for Teenagers (POSIT). *Journal of Mental Health-United Kingdom* 3:363-376.

McLellan AT, Luborsky L, Woody GE et al. (1980). An improved diagnostic evaluation instrument for substance abuse patients: The Addiction Severity Index. *Journal of Nervous and Mental Disease* 186:26-33.

Metzger D, Kushner H & McLellan AT (1991). *Adolescent Problem Severity Index*. Philadelphia, PA: University of Pennsylvania.

Meyers K (1991). *Comprehensive Addiction Severity Index for Adolescents*. Philadelphia, PA: University of Pennsylvania.

Migneault J, Pallonen U & Velicer W (1997). Decisional balance and stage of change for adolescent drinking. *Addictive Behaviors* 22:339-351.

Miller G (1990). The Substance Abuse Subtle Screening Inventory-Adolescent Version. Bloomington, IN: SASSI Institute.

Moberg DP (1983). Identifying adolescents with alcohol problems: A field test of the Adolescent Alcohol Involvement Scale. *Journal of Studies on Alcohol* 44:701-721.

Moberg DP (1991). The Adolescent Drug Involvement Scale. *Journal of Adolescent Chemical Dependency* 2:75-88.

Moore D (1983). *Client Substance Index*. Olympia, WA: Olympic Counseling Services.

Newcomb MD, Maddahian E & Bentler PM (1986). Risk factors for drug use among adolescents: Concurrent and longitudinal analyses. *American Journal of Public Health* 76:525-531.

Owen PL & Nyberg LR (1983). Assessing alcohol and drug problems among adolescents: Current practice. *Journal of Drug Education* 13:249-254.

Petchers MK & Singer MI (1990). Clinical applicability of a substance abuse screening instrument. *Journal of Adolescent Chemical Dependency* 1:47-56.

Petchers MK, Singer MI, Angelotta J et al. (1988). Revalidation and expansion of an adolescent substance abuse screening measure. *Developmental and Behavioral Pediatrics* 9:25-28.

Puig-Antich J (1982). Major depression and conduct disorder in prepuberty. *Journal of the American Academy of Child and Adolescent Psychiatry* 21:118-128.

Rahdert E, ed. (1991). *The Adolescent Assessment and Referral System Manual*. Rockville, MD: National Institute on Drug Abuse.

Renovex, Inc. (1988). *Adolescent Chemical Health Inventory*. Minneapolis, MN: Renovex Inc.

Roberts RE, Solovitz BL, Chen YW et al. (1996). Retest stability of DSM-IIIR diagnoses among adolescents using the Diagnostic Interview Schedule for Children (DISC-2.1C). *Journal of Abnormal Child Psychology* 24:349-362.

Robins LN, Helzer JE, Croughan L et al. (1981). National Institute of Mental Health Diagnostic Interview Schedule: Its history characteristics and validity. *Archives of General Psychiatry* 38:381-389.

Schwartz RH & Wirtz PW (1990). Potential substance abuse detection among adolescent patients. *Clinical Pediatrics* 29:38-43.

Shaffer D (1992). *The Diagnostic Interview Schedule for Children -2.3 Version.* New York, NY: Columbia University.

Shaffer D, Fisher P & Dulcan M (1996). The NIMH Diagnostic Interview Schedule for Children (DISC 2.3): Description, acceptability, prevalence, and performance in the MECA study. *Journal of the American Academy of Child and Adolescent Psychiatry* 35:865-877.

Shaffer D, Schwab-Stone M, Fisher P et al. (1993). Revised version of the Diagnostic Interview Schedule for Children (DISC-R): Preparation, field testing, and acceptability. *Journal of the American Academy of Child and Adolescent Psychiatry* 32:643-650.

Spitzer RL & Williams JBW (1984). *Structured Clinical Interview for DSM-III.* New York, NY: New York State Psychiatric Institute.

Tarter RE, Laird SB, Bukstein O et al. (1992). Validation of the adolescent drug use screening inventory: Preliminary findings. *Psychology of Addictive Behavior* 6:322-236.

Thomas DW (1990). *Substance Abuse Screening Protocol for the Juvenile Courts.* Pittsburgh, PA: National Center for Juvenile Justice.

Wanberg KW (1992). *Adolescent Self Assessment Profile.* Arvada, CO: Center for Alcohol/Drug Abuse Research and Evaluation.

Weed NC, Butcher JN & Williams CL (1994). Development of MMPI-A alcohol/drug problem scales. *Journal of Studies on Alcohol* 55:296-302.

White HR & Labouvie EW (1989). Towards the assessment of adolescent problem drinking. *Journal of Studies on Alcohol* 50:30-37.

Winters KC (1990). The need for improved assessment of adolescent substance involvement. *Journal of Drug Issues* 20:487-502.

Winters KC (1991). *The Personal Experience Screening Questionnaire and Manual.* Los Angeles, CA: Western Psychological Services.

Winters KC (1992). Development of an adolescent alcohol and other drug abuse screening scale: Personal Experience Screening Questionnaire. *Addictive Behaviors* 17:479-490.

Winters KC & Henly GA (1988). Assessing adolescents who misuse chemicals: The Chemical Dependency Adolescent Assessment Project. In *Adolescent Drug Abuse: Analyses of Treatment Research.* Rockville, MD: National Institute on Drug Abuse.

Winters KC & Henly GA (1989). *The Personal Experience Inventory Test and User's Manual.* Los Angeles, CA: Western Psychological Services.

Winters KC & Henly GA (1993). *Adolescent Diagnostic Interview Schedule and Manual.* Los Angeles, CA: Western Psychological Services.

Winters KC, Stinchfield RD, Fulkerson J et al. (1993a). Measuring alcohol and cannabis use disorders in an adolescent clinical sample. *Psychology of Addictive Behavior* 7:185-196.

Winters KC, Stinchfield RD & Henly GA (1993b). Further validation of new scales measuring adolescent alcohol and other drug abuse. *Journal of Studies on Alcohol* 54:534-541.

Zywiak WH, Hoffmann NG & Floyd AS (1999). Enhancing alcohol treatment outcomes through aftercare and self help groups. *Medicine and Health (Rhode Island)* 82(3):87-90.

Chapter 5

Adolescent Treatment and Relapse Prevention

Steven L. Jaffe, M.D.

Treatment Modalities
Using Multiple Therapies
Preventing Relapse

Treatment of adolescent substance use disorders involves a number of issues that are quite different from those seen in adults with substance abuse problems. First, the adolescent's biopsychosocial level of development must be considered. For example, it is normal for young adolescents (age 12 to 14 years) to be self-centered, experience mood shifts, and have minimal capacity for introspection. This profile makes therapy with early adolescents very different from the treatment of older adolescents. Second, since adolescents still are developing within a family system, family members must be part of the treatment program. Third, adolescents differ from adults in their patterns of substance use, as adolescents are more apt to use multiple drugs and to use inhalants in early adolescence and club drugs (such as 3,4-methylenedioxymethamphetamine or "Ecstasy," gamma-hydroxybutyrate or GHB, and ketamine) in late adolescence and early adulthood. Fourth, some studies have shown that current comorbidity is more common among adolescents than adults (Kandel, Johnson et al., 1999), and parallel treatment of the comorbid condition is especially important in adolescents.

After careful evaluation, giving full consideration to the foregoing issues, the physician should make an individual-ized determination as to the appropriate treatment placement for the substance-involved adolescent. The American Society of Addiction of Medicine (ASAM) has developed placement criteria for adolescent treatment (Mee-Lee, Shulman et al., 2001) that include the dimensions of treatment readiness, relapse potential, and recovery environment (see the accompanying chapter on placement criteria and strategies for adolescent treatment matching).

This chapter describes the treatment approaches most commonly employed in the treatment of adolescents.

TREATMENT MODALITIES

In 1990, Catalano extensively reviewed the literature on adolescent treatment and found that, in residential programs, time in treatment was related to reduced use of alcohol or other drugs. Family participation was associated with better outcome. No treatment modality was significantly better than any other. Catalano could only conclude that some treatment was better than no treatment.

In the decade since that study, significant progress has been made. The National Institute on Drug Abuse, the National Institute on Alcohol Abuse and Alcoholism, and the Center for Substance Abuse Treatment have increased their support and direction for controlled studies of adolescent treatment, as well as for the development of clinical researchers to study such treatment. The American Academy of Child and Adolescent Psychiatry has published both a 10-year research review (Weinberg, Rahdert et al., 1998) and "Practice Parameters for the Assessment and Treatment of Substance Abuse in Children and Adolescents" (ACAP, 1997). Better standardized assessment instruments and adolescent-specific outcome measures have been developed.

A number of treatment approaches have been used alone or in various combinations for the treatment of adolescent substance use, abuse, and dependency disorders. A Treatment Improvement Protocol on adolescent treatment, published by the Center for Substance Abuse Treatment (1999), describes the three most commonly employed treatment approaches as family therapy, Twelve Step-based programs, and therapeutic communities. These and other important modalities are reviewed below.

Family Therapy. Classic family therapy is based on the hypothesis that there is a connection between family relationships and the development or maintenance of drug abuse. Family therapy targets these specific interpersonal family processes. With structural-strategic family therapy, emphasis is on establishing a coherent family hierarchy, with appropriate rules and authority. Lewis (1992) combined a number of different family therapy models to develop a 12-session treatment called the Purdue Model, the goals of which were to decrease family resistance to treatment, to redefine substance use as a family problem, to reestablish parental influence, to interrupt dysfunctional sequences of family behavior, to assess the interpersonal function of the drug abuse, to implement strategies to change family interpersonal functioning, and to provide assertiveness training to the adolescent. Families who received this treatment model were found to have significantly decreased adolescent drug abuse compared to families that received parent skill training.

Azrin (1994) examined family therapy in combination with behavioral therapy techniques. The most important treatment component was social-family contracting, in which parents reinforced drug-incompatible activities, supervised home urge-control assignments, and employed written specifications of desired behaviors with contingent reinforcers. Azrin's control group received only supportive counseling. He found that abstinence rates at six months were 73% for the treatment group, compared to only 9% for the supportive counseling group. The treated youth also were found to

have improved schoolwork and family relationships (Azrin, Donohue et al., 1994).

Multisystemic Therapy. Henggeler's Multisystemic Therapy (MST) integrates family therapy with direct interventions in the multiple interacting systems involving the individual, school, peer group, and community. This treatment approach promotes responsible behavior among all family members, and attempts to develop each individual's capacity to manage his or her own problems. Therapists work intensively with each adolescent and family in the home, school, and even neighborhood peer group. Randomized studies of MST compared to individual counseling or probation for chronic juvenile offenders demonstrated reduced criminal activity, which continued through a four-year followup period. Preliminary data on a current study of MST is demonstrating excellent retention rates and favorable outcomes (Pickrel, Henggeler, 1996).

Cognitive-Behavioral Therapy. This therapeutic modality combines the learning principles of classical and operant conditioning with approaches to correct cognitive distortions and underlying negative belief systems. Treatment involves teaching the adolescent specific techniques to deal with drugs and alcohol. Specific skills to refuse alcohol and drugs are taught and practiced in role-playing exercises. For example, the adolescent is taught to immediately say "no" in a firm manner, making direct eye contract with the person who offers alcohol or drugs. They are then to suggest an alternative activity or, if that is not successful, to simply tell the person to stop asking.

Cognitive-behavioral coping skills to deal with urges, to manage thoughts of alcohol or drug use, and to handle emergencies and lapses are taught and practiced. Because deficits in coping skills for negative feelings and life stresses contribute to continued substance use, more general coping strategies (such as communication skills, problem-solving strategies, anger and mood management, and relaxation training) also are taught and practiced.

Cognitive-behavioral therapy is being studied in random clinical trials. Kaminer (1999) compared CBT group therapy with interactional group therapy (IT) in adolescents with co-occuring substance use and psychiatric disorders. CBT demonstrated a decrease in severity of substance use, but did not produce better results than IT at 15-month followup.

Twelve Step Approaches. Although Twelve Step-based treatment is one of the most common treatment models for adolescents, there has been little research into its efficacy.

The Twelve Steps guide changes in actions, thoughts, feelings, and beliefs that an individual slowly undergoes in order to establish a state of recovery and abstinence from alcohol. Since an addict cannot use alcohol and drugs in moderation, abstinence is the necessary goal. Working the Twelve Steps is an extremely concrete process that does not require abstract thinking.

The following descriptions present the first five steps, modified to make them meaningful for adolescents.

Step 1: "We admitted we were powerless over alcohol—that our lives had become unmanageable." For adolescents, the workbook has the adolescent examine in detail the negative consequences of their alcohol/drug use. Putting their own and others lives in danger, effects on family, school, work, mood, and self-esteem in relationship to alcohol/drug use are explored. The major issue is whether drugs and alcohol are destroying their lives such that they need to stop using to make their lives better. While many adult programs emphasize the concept of "surrendering" and admitting one is an addict, these are not useful for adolescents. Rather, enhancing power by doing what one needs to do (such as stop using alcohol and drugs) instead of doing what one wants to do (use alcohol and drugs) is emphasized.

Step 2: "We come to believe that a power greater than ourselves could restore us to sanity." The adolescent workbook approaches this step by recognizing that a child's first higher power is the person that raises them. For many drug abusing/addicted adolescents, their parental figures were neglectful or abusive. Mourning the pain and sadness from the disappointments of their childhood higher powers enables them to begin to develop a sense of something positive in the universe that they can turn to for help. The higher power concept is not a religious belief, but a spiritual feeling that one can trust something positive (for example, the group, another person, or nature) to take care of those aspects of one's life that one cannot control. One needs to have trust in the stability of the world and realize one controls one's own behavior but not what others say or do. For many adolescents, the concrete positive feelings of their relationships to other members becomes the first higher power.

Step 3: "We make a decision to turn our will and our lives over to the care of God as we understand Him." The adolescent workbook interprets this step to involve having the adolescents make a decision to commit themselves to working the Steps and having a positive spiritual power. The teenagers are helped to recognize that they turned over their lives to alcohol and drugs. Now they are being asked to turn their lives over to a positive program.

Step 4: "We made a searching and fearless moral inventory of ourselves." The workbook has the adolescents answer numerous detailed questions covering all aspects of their childhood and present life.

Step 5: "We admitted to God, to ourselves, and to another human being the exact nature of our wrongs." In this step, the adolescent verbalizes an inventory to a counselor or a sponsor.

Twelve Step programs also provide the opportunity to attend free AA or Narcotics Anonymous (NA) meetings, which are conducted several times a day in almost every city and town in the U.S. and most other countries. It is well recognized that adolescents will return to using alcohol and drugs if they return to contact with their alcohol- or drug-using friends. Twelve Step programs also provide mentoring relationships in the form of sponsors. An older member with at least a year of sobriety, the sponsor provides support and guidance on how to work the program to achieve sobriety. Twelve Step programs accept the concept of addiction as a chronic progressive disorder that renders the addict unable to control and moderate his or her drinking or drug use. The only viable alternative is complete abstinence (Humphreys, 1999). For many adolescents, it may be helpful to view themselves as "on the way to becoming an addict," if they do not see themselves as already being one.

Although research on Twelve Step adolescent programs has been sparse, a CATOR residential treatment followup study (1987) found that teenagers who attended two or more meetings per week were almost six time more likely to report abstinence at one year than were those who never attended. A more recent followup study by Winters (1999) used improved methodology with a high followup contact rate and meaningful comparison groups. At 12-month followup, those adolescents who completed Twelve Step-based treatment had an abstinence/minor relapse rate of 53%, compared with 27% of those who needed, but did not receive treatment.

Therapeutic Communities (TCs). The TC offers long-term treatment (12 to 18 months) to adolescents who have multiple severe problems. In the TC approach, the community itself is part of the treatment process. Residents move through stages of increasing responsibility and privileges. Work, education, group activities, seminars, meals, job functions, and formal and informal interactions with peers and staff form the basis of self-development. The presence of staff who are themselves in recovery and family involvement are important aspects of TCs.

A recent outcome study found that 31% of adolescents completed the residential phase of treatment in a TC, while 52% dropped out. Treatment completers at 1 year post-treatment had more positive outcomes than those who did not complete treatment, as measured by a reduction in substance use and decreased criminal activity.

Motivational Treatment. Prochaska and DiClemente (1982) have described a series of stages that mark the progress of an individual toward cessation of alcohol or drug use. These stages are designated as *precontemplation*, in which the person is not even thinking about stopping and does not recognize any problem with alcohol or drug use; *contemplation*, which is marked by ambivalence in which the person goes back and forth between reasons to change and reasons not to change; *preparation*, in which the person increases the commitment to change; *action*, in which the person stops using alcohol and drugs; and *maintenance*, in which the person develops a lifestyle to avoid relapse. Individuals exhibit different levels of motivation depending on their stage of change. Therapeutic intervention involves helping the patient in an empathetic, non-confrontational manner to move along the stages. Brief motivational interventions consist of one to four sessions, following an assessment, in which direct feedback and advice is given in a non-confrontational manner that respects the person's personal responsibility for making a decision.

Monti (2001) has studied the use of a single 45-minute emergency department brief motivational interview for adolescents whose injuries are related to alcohol use. Followup studies found that the adolescents who were exposed to the interventions subsequently had fewer alcohol-related problems.

Intervention Workbook. Both motivational interviewing and Twelve Step facilitation therapy develop motivation in the adolescent to stop using alcohol or other drugs through the adolescent's personal recognition of the negative consequences of such use. Jaffe's *Adolescent Substance Abuse Intervention Workbook* (2001) engages the adolescent in use of this framework to answer concrete, simple questions that explore 12 areas of the adolescent's life that may have been negatively affected by alcohol or other drugs. These include: putting one's own or another's life in danger, making depression worse, "messing up" their body and brain,

impairing school and work performance, breaking the law, and inability to moderate use. The workbook also compares unhealthy thinking (such as "drugs are fun") with recovery thinking (for example, "but my life is a mess"). Internal motivation is developed by helping the adolescent to conclude that he or she needs to stop using alcohol or other drugs in order to make life better.

The workbook is completed individually and also may be presented to a group. It is extremely useful as an initial diagnostic and treatment tool to help the adolescent develop internal motivation to stop using and is appropriate for use in outpatient, inpatient, and juvenile justice programs.

Community Reinforcement Approach (CRA). CRA is a treatment approach originally developed for adults, in which the individual's life is rearranged so that abstinence is more rewarding than drinking.

The CRA approach closely resembles the "enthusiastic sobriety" adolescent program developed by Meehan (2000). This Twelve Step-based program uses young, energetic, enthusiastic, recovering, well-trained counselors. They are role models who demonstrate that one can have fun without drugs or alcohol. The adolescent is asked to try 30 days without alcohol or other drugs. During this time, the adolescent participates in daily groups, meetings, and social functions with recovering peers who make sobriety more fun and rewarding than using drugs and alcohol.

USING MULTIPLE THERAPIES

No single treatment modality has been demonstrated to be clearly superior. Multiple approaches often are needed to achieve progress. Recently, the Center for Substance Abuse Treatment (CSAT) developed five different protocols to study various outpatient treatments for adolescent marijuana abuse. In two of the protocols, motivational enhancement therapy is combined with cognitive behavioral therapy. A third protocol combines motivational enhancement therapy with cognitive behavioral therapy and family therapy. Preliminary positive results are being obtained, with the more intensive treatments appearing to be the most beneficial for the adolescents who are most significantly involved in drug use.

PREVENTING RELAPSE

Relapse is very common in treated adolescents, as it is in adults. About a third of adolescents who have completed a 28-day program will relapse within the first three months.

Of greatest importance is not allowing a lapse (return to alcohol or drug use for a few days) to develop into a full relapse (return to use for weeks or months).

When counseling an adolescent during a lapse, the physician should minimize guilt and shame. The emphasis should be on what the adolescent can learn from the lapse: for example, avoiding high-risk situations such as the company of "using" peers, or seeking out a sponsor for help in dealing with intense thoughts and urges to use.

Jaffe (1994) describes four pathways that place recovering teens at risk of relapse. The most common is involvement with peers who use alcohol or drugs. Even if the adolescent is committed to sobriety, spending time with using peers becomes too tempting and the teen relapses. A second pathway is the presence of comorbid psychiatric disorders. Adolescents with substance abuse disorders have a high incidence (50% to 90%) of other psychiatric disorders, especially mood, behavior, and anxiety disorders. In this pathway, the teen experiences depression, rage, or panic, and relapses in an effort to deal with those symptoms. A third pathway is denial, in which the recovering adolescent decides that he or she is not an addict and can use alcohol or other drugs in moderation. The fourth pathway involves subconsciously arranging one's life to be in proximity to alcohol or other drugs.

Many adolescents stop using alcohol or drugs while in treatment, but never achieve a state of recovery in which they actively work a Twelve Step program. Their return to use of alcohol or drugs thus is not a genuine relapse, but simply an expression of their decision to return to such use. The adolescent in this situation needs to re-engage with a Twelve Step program and begin again at Step 1, in which he or she cognitively and emotionally examines the negative consequences of their use in order to develop internal motivation to be abstinent.

Recovering adolescents who relapse need to examine the strength of their program and recognize the need for a solid sponsor, a non-using peer group, and frequent (two or more each week) attendance at AA/NA meetings. They also should be evaluated for comorbid disorders (such as depression or posttraumatic stress disorder), which may require specific treatment.

REFERENCES

Alcoholics Anonymous (1976). *Alcoholics Anonymous: The Story of How Many Thousands of Men and Women Have Recovered from Alcoholism, 3rd Ed*. New York, NY: Alcoholics Anonymous World Services.

American Academy of Child and Adolescent Psychiatry (ACAP) (1997). Practice parameters for the assessment and treatment of children and adolescents with substance use disorders. *Journal of the American Academy of Child and Adolescent Psychiatry* 36(Suppl):1405-1565.

Azrin NH, Donohue B & Besale VA (1994). Youth drug abuse treatment: A controlled outcome study. *Journal of Child and Adolescent Substance Abuse* 3:1-16.

Bailey GW (1996). Helping the resistant adolescent enter substance abuse treatment: The office intervention. *Child and Adolescent Psychiatric Clinics of North America* 5:149-164.

Bukstein OG, Brent DA & Kaminer Y (1989). Comorbidity of substance abuse and other psychiatric disorders in adolescents. *American Journal of Psychiatry* 146:1131-1141.

Deas D & Thomas SE (2001). An overview of controlled studies of adolescent substance abuse treatment. *American Journal on Addictions* 10(2):178-189.

Harrison PA, Fullerson JA & Beebe TJ (1998). DSM-IV substance use disorder criteria for adolescents: A critical examination based on a statewide school survey. *American Journal of Psychiatry* 155:486-492.

Harrison PA & Hoffman NC (1989). *CATOR Report: Adolescent Treatment Completion One Year Later*. St. Paul, MN: Ramsey Clinic.

Humphreys K (1999). Professional interventions that facilitate 12 Step self-help group involvement. *Alcohol Research & Health* 23:93-98.

Jaffe SL (1990). *Step Workbook for Adolescent Chemical Dependency Recovery: A Guide to the First Five Steps*. Washington, DC. American Psychiatric Press, Inc.

Jaffe SL (1994). Pathways to relapse in chemically dependent adolescents. *Adolescent Counselor* (March)55:42-44.

Jaffe SL (1996). Adolescent substance abuse and dual disorders. SL Jaffe (ed.) *Child and Adolescent Psychiatric Clinics of North America* 5(1).

Jaffe SL (2001). *Adolescent Substance Abuse Intervention Workbook: Taking a First Step*. Washington, DC: American Psychiatric Press, Inc.

Kaminer Y & Burleson J (1999). Psychotherapies for adolescent substance abusers: 15 month follow-up of a pilot study. *American Journal on Addictions* 8:114-119.

Kandel D, Johnson J, Bird H et al. (1999). Psychiatric co-morbidity among adolescents with substance use disorders. Findings from the MECA study. *Journal of the American Academy of Child and Adolescent Psychiatry* 138(6):693-699.

Leirer VO & Yesavage JA (1991). Marijuana carry over effects on aircraft pilot performance. *Aviation, Space and Environmental Medicine* 62:221-227.

Lewis RA, Piercy FP, Sprenkle DH et al. (1990). Family based interventions for helping drug abusing adolescents. *Journal of Adolescent Research* 5:82-95.

Meehan B (2000). *Beyond the Yellow Brick Road-Revised*. Denver, CO: Meehan Publishers, 2000.

Mee-Lee D, Shulman G, Fishman M et al. (2001). *ASAM Patient Placement Criteria for the Treatment of Substance-Related Disorders, Second Edition-Revised (ASAM PPC-2R)*. Chevy Chase, MD: American Society of Addiction Medicine.

Monti PM, Barnett NP, O'Leary JA et al. (2001). Motivational enhancement for school-involved adolescents. In PM Monti, SM Colby & TA O'Leary (eds.) *Adolescents, Alcohol and Substance Abuse*. New York, NY: Guilford Press, 145-182.

Pickrel SG & Henggeler SW (1996). Multisystemic therapy for adolescent substance abuse and dependence. *Child and Adolescent Psychiatric Clinics of North America* 5:201-211.

Prochaska JO & DiClemente CC (1982). Transtheoretical therapy: Toward a more integrated model of change. *Psychotherapy Theory, Research and Practice* 19:276-288.

Roberts AJ & Koob GF (1997). The neurobiology of addiction. *Alcohol Research & Health* 21(2):101-106.

Stanton MD & Shadish WR (1997). Outcome, attrition and family— Couples treatment for drug abuse: A meta–analysis and review of the controlled, comparative studies. *Psychological Bulletin* 122:170-191.

Weinberg NZ, Rahdert E, Colliver JD et al. (1998). Adolescent substance abuse: A review of the past ten years. *Journal of the American Academy of Child and Adolescent Psychiatry* 27:252-261.

Winters KC (2001). Assessing adolescent substance use problems and other areas of functioning: State of the art. In PM Monti, SM Colby & TA O'Leary (eds.) *Adolescents, Alcohol and Substance Abuse.* New York, NY: Guilford Press, 80-108.

Winters KC, ed. (1999). *Treatment of Adolescents with Substance Abuse Disorder (Treatment Improvement Protocol No. 32).* Rockville, MD: Center for Substance Abuse Treatment, Substance Abuse and Mental Health Services Administration.

Adolescents With Special Treatment Needs

CENTER FOR SUBSTANCE ABUSE TREATMENT

Many adolescents who acutely need treatment for substance use disorders may be in circumstances that make early identification and treatment particularly difficult. Sometimes legal, social, or health circumstances in a young person's life create unique problems that require attention. Youths in the child welfare and juvenile justice systems are at particularly high risk for developing a substance use disorder. More often than not, they have more risk factors than other children and fewer protective factors. For example, adolescents who have come into contact with the juvenile justice system can be expected to display severe problems surrounding family and social relationships, as well as coexisting mental, emotional, or physical difficulties.

TREATMENT IN THE JUVENILE JUSTICE SYSTEM

Many young people who enter the juvenile justice system for relatively minor offenses, such as problems in school or at home, enter a cycle of failure reinforced by repeated instances of these problems. Most of the adolescents who come into contact with the juvenile justice system have already developed a number of functional problems. Many of these youths have had substance use disorders and other psychosocial concerns for some time, and many come from fractured or dysfunctional families. By the time these adolescents enter the juvenile justice system, they have developed serious substance use disorders and attendant psychosocial dysfunction.

For these reasons, early intervention is critical in working with adolescents who have had contact with the juvenile justice system. Every young person involved in the juvenile justice system, regardless of his charge, should undergo thorough screening and assessment for substance use disorders, physical health problems, psychiatric disorders, history of physical or sexual abuse, learning disabilities, and other coexisting conditions. Juvenile probation officers can be helpful partners in the system of care.

For their part, treatment service providers should educate the local juvenile justice system about the importance of early intervention and what resources are available to them. Juvenile justice professionals should be required to have training in identifying and appropriately intervening with substance use in their clients. Having court-ordered treatment and monitoring may be the most effective approach to getting substance use disorder services to many adolescents. It is almost impossible to intervene unless the youth is removed from the environment that brought her into conflict with the juvenile justice system in the first place—that is, the home neighborhood.

DIVERSION PROGRAMS

Because the justice system is overwhelmed by a large number of cases and limited resources—a judge in juvenile justice may handle thousands of cases a year—increased emphasis has been placed on diversion programs (sometimes called dispositional alternatives) for juvenile offenders. These alternatives have been shown to be highly effective in relation to the minimal resources invested in them. Juvenile detention facilities are designed to provide short-term care for juveniles awaiting adjudication or disposition. However, juveniles placed in detention facilities are unlikely to receive the special programs necessary for their treatment or reintegration into society. For these reasons, alternatives to placing juvenile offenders in secure facilities have increased dramatically in recent years.

The range of transitional programs that help to prepare youths to return to their communities has widened as well. The use of alternative placement resources typically involves multiple agencies. Therefore, it is vital to have a single case manager to coordinate services and to function as the central monitoring and tracking source for each adolescent. It is important for juvenile program administrators to be aware of the pros and cons of each program and to place youths in the programs that are likely to be of most benefit to them.

A number of approaches and types of settings are now being used, and the many options that are available make it possible to select the setting most conducive to a juvenile's treatment needs. Some of the available alternatives are described below.

Intensive Community Supervision. Under intensive community supervision, a youth remains in the community and must regularly report to an assigned probation counselor. This arrangement allows the adolescent to attend school and to maintain family relationships with minimal interruption. The planned frequency of the required contacts with the probation counselor may vary from several times a day to twice a week; less than twice a week is not considered intensive supervision. Telephone contact alone is not enough, although it may be used to supplement personal meetings.

Day Reporting Centers. As part of community supervision programs, reporting centers can be set up in accessible locations in the community, such as schools and shopping centers. Youths then report regularly to these stations according to their case plans. Some centers provide education, recreation, or social services.

Day Treatment. Specialized day programs that include education and social services help youths develop social skills. They also provide supervision and control in a familiar setting. In many day treatment programs, youths take classes in the morning, participate in a group activity (such as playing sports) in the afternoon, and return home at night.

Evening and Weekend Programs. Direct supervision and programming similar to day treatment are also offered during evening and weekend hours. Tutoring, recreation, employment, and treatment services can be provided to supplement an adolescent's regular educational or work programs. Like day treatment programs, evening and weekend programs provide supervision in addition to education and social skills development.

Tracking. Tracking programs hire staff (usually part-time) to monitor youths and to report their compliance with specific requirements in areas such as school attendance, participation in counseling, and job performance. Whether working with other service providers or independently, trackers report regularly to the agency that has jurisdiction over the adolescent.

Electronic Monitoring. Some youths are now released under the condition that they wear an electronic device that monitors their movements. The efficacy of such systems is debated by professionals and technicians in the juvenile justice system, but all agree that electronic monitoring alone is insufficient and that, to be successful, such tracking must be part of a multifaceted effort.

Home Detention. Adolescents under home detention are supervised by their parents in their homes and are allowed to leave only to go to school or work. This type of treatment is well-suited to youths who do not require institutional security but need adult supervision and structure. Home detention is generally a short-term arrangement that is used until a detailed, long-range plan is developed.

Home Tutoring. Supplementing regular educational programs with home tutoring helps to remedy adolescents' educational deficiencies, establishes contact with an adult role model, and provides supervision.

Mentor Tutoring. Providing a trained adolescent tutor for a troubled youth can be extremely beneficial. In addition to educational tutoring, a mentor can offer advice, emotional support, and a respectful, caring relationship.

Work and Apprenticeship. Some local businesses provide jobs or apprenticeships for juvenile offenders, generally in conjunction with an educational program. Such programs instill a work ethic, a sense of responsibility, and a feeling of accomplishment while enhancing community relations.

Restitution. Under court order, juveniles may be asked to try to rectify the damage they have caused their victims. Restitution may be in cash or in services amounting to a specific dollar value. Most frequently ordered in property crimes, restitution provides an alternative to incarceration, thereby reducing public costs while compensating victims.

Community Service. Some offenders are required to provide services that benefit the entire community, such as cleaning up parks or working in nursing homes. This is a form of restitution that allows juveniles to contribute routine but worthwhile services. Community service projects must be clearly identified, and the juveniles in these programs must be properly supervised.

Volunteer Programs. Volunteers often are available to tutor youths and to supervise work and recreational activities. They also may provide an additional service to youths as friends, role models, and listeners. Like regular employees, volunteers require training, specific job descriptions, and supervision.

ACKNOWLEDGMENT: Adapted from Winters K, ed. (1999). Treatment of Adolescents with Substance Abuse Disorder (Treatment Improvement Protocol No. 32). Rockville, MD: Center for Substance Abuse Treatment.

| Chapter 6 | # Confidentiality in Dealing With Adolescents |

Alain Joffe, M.D., M.P.H.

Research Into Confidentiality Issues
Policies on Confidentiality
Deciding When Disclosure Is Necessary
Special Circumstances

Confidentiality is an essential component of health care for adolescents. Without some promise of confidentiality at the beginning of an office visit, the adolescent patient may be unwilling to disclose information about his or her behaviors, particularly concerning sensitive areas such as sexual behaviors or substance use. On the other hand, the clinician who promises unconditional confidentiality may find himself or herself party to information about very risky behaviors, which he or she has promised not to reveal but which, if allowed to continue, may jeopardize the health of the adolescent. To avoid this clinical conundrum, regardless of the health care setting, health care professionals must understand the key principles underlying confidentiality and its limits.

Adolescents occupy an ambiguous status in our society. They are not viewed as adults until they reach the age of 18 or, in the case of drinking or purchasing alcohol, 21. Yet the vast majority of teens become physically mature well before age 18 and, according to psychological research, demonstrate adult reasoning capacity at approximately age 14. Not surprisingly, they engage in many health behaviors that are, by custom, viewed as reserved for adults (such as sexual intercourse) or are legally proscribed (including cigarette

smoking and alcohol use). And, like many adults, some teens adopt certain behaviors that are illegal in the United States, regardless of age (for example, smoking marijuana).

Physicians demonstrate respect for their patients and develop a good working relationship with them by maintaining confidentiality, thereby forming a zone of privacy around the contents of the office visit. This approach maximizes the "patient's willingness to supply information candidly for his or her benefit" (NCCUSL, 1989). A promise of confidentiality is especially important to adolescents, who, from a developmental perspective, are seeking to achieve autonomy from their parents and are learning to make appropriate decisions about a variety of issues, including healthy behaviors and seeking health care. Providing a respectful setting in which adolescents can discuss their concerns, including ones they view as particularly sensitive and perhaps embarrassing, helps support this critical developmental process.

RESEARCH INTO CONFIDENTIALITY

A number of research studies spanning almost 20 years demonstrate how much value adolescents place on confidentiality. Marks and colleagues (1983) surveyed 649 suburban youth in grades 9 through 12. Only 19% said they would seek care for contraception, 17% for drug use, and 23% for alcohol use if their parents knew of the visit. In contrast, 45% said they would seek care for contraception, 49% for drug use, and 43% for alcohol use under the condition that their parents would not find out.

More recently, Ford and colleagues (1997) used simulated office visits to explore adolescents' views about confidentiality. In one study, 562 adolescents from three suburban California high schools were randomized to listen to a standardized audiotape depiction of an office visit. On one tape, the physician promised unconditional confidentiality, on another he or she promised conditional confidentiality and, on the third, confidentiality was not discussed. Assurances of confidentiality increased the percentage of teenagers who were willing to disclose information about their sexual behaviors, drug use, and mental health concerns from 39% to 46.5%, and increased the percentage willing to seek future health care from 53% to 67%. This study, as well as the one by Marks, demonstrates the utilitarian basis for supporting confidentiality for adolescents: many adolescents will not seek health care for sensitive issues unless their expectation of privacy is granted.

Studies have shown that, although many adolescents may forego seeking health care for risky behaviors if parental notification is a prerequisite, they will not stop engaging in the risky behaviors. Hence, failing to afford confidentiality increases the risk of adolescents' delaying seeking care until serious consequences arise from undisclosed behaviors (including pregnancy, pelvic inflammatory disease, drug overdoses, and alcohol-related motor vehicle injuries).

POLICIES ON CONFIDENTIALITY

Physicians' professional organizations long have supported the concept of confidential care for adolescents. In 1967, the American Medical Association (AMA) adopted a position that the epidemic of sexually transmitted diseases among young people required that minors be able to receive treatment for those infections without parental notification. The AMA also opposed regulations that would have required clinicians working in federally funded programs to notify parents when they provided prescription contraceptives to patients under age 18 (AMA, 1990, 1993).

In 1988, the American Academy of Pediatrics, the National Medical Association, the American College of Obstetricians and Gynecologists, and the American Academy of Family Physicians jointly endorsed recommendations

on confidentiality, concluding that "ultimately, the health risks to adolescents are so impelling that legal barriers and deference to parental involvement should not stand in the way of needed care" (ACOG, 1988).

Most states grant adolescents the right to seek confidential care, although the scope of this protection varies from state to state. Clinicians therefore must be knowledgeable about their own state's regulations.

DECIDING WHEN DISCLOSURE IS NECESSARY

How then to handle a situation in which an adolescent discloses information that the clinician believes poses a serious threat to the health of the adolescent? Is it permissible to break confidentiality under these circumstances? Is the clinician required to do so?

Part of the answer lies in what assurance of confidentiality was given to the adolescent. Clearly, some assurance is essential. However, most experts do not recommend a blanket or unconditional assurance ("everything you and I discuss today will be confidential"), since disclosure is mandated by law in certain circumstances. These include reports of sexual or physical abuse or expression of a clear threat of violence against a readily identifiable individual. Concerns about an adolescent's suicidality also would warrant breaking confidentiality. In such circumstances, the ethical principle of respect for persons, which underlies confidentiality, is overridden by higher ethical principles: "first, do no harm" and obeying the law.

In anticipation of situations such as these, most experts in adolescent health recommend statements that offer conditional confidentiality. Using this approach, the adolescent is assured that most information revealed to the physician will be kept private, but he or she is cautioned that there are some boundaries to the zone of privacy. One sample statement, developed by the AMA's Department of Adolescent Health, is as follows: "I want to assure you that the information we discuss today is between you and me. It's confidential. In other words, I am not going to tell anyone without your permission, unless there is a situation which I believe might threaten your life or another's life or seriously endanger your health" (Levenberg & Elster, 1995). However, recent data suggest that adolescents prefer more specific descriptions of what kinds of discussions will be held confidential.

Regardless of the exact assurance the clinician offers, it ultimately rests with his or her judgment as to whether and when a given adolescent's behavior poses a level of risk that warrants a breach of confidentiality. In such cases, the clinician must perform a sufficiently comprehensive assessment to understand how the behavior poses a threat to the adolescent's health.

A belief that a given behavior is wrong in the context of the clinician's own personal, moral, or religious code is not sufficient justification for breaking confidentiality. For example, a personal belief that premarital sex is wrong would not justify disclosing to a parent that an adolescent is sexually active, especially if the adolescent is acting responsibly by taking appropriate steps to protect against sexually transmitted diseases or pregnancy. Some clinicians also would argue that, if an adolescent admits to occasionally smoking marijuana but is doing well in school, maintains good relations with his or her parents, and never drives or attends school while "high," then that behavior also does not automatically warrant disclosure.

Even if the clinician concludes that an adolescent's behavior is sufficiently risky to warrant parental involvement, immediate disclosure is not necessarily indicated. The clinician may wish first to discuss his or her concerns with the adolescent and attempt to develop a plan whereby the adolescent can demonstrate a change in the risky behavior. An example would be asking an adolescent who is using marijuana on a regular basis to refrain from smoking for several weeks, with urine testing at the end of that period. In advance, the adolescent would be told that a positive urine test would trigger parental notification. In the interim, the parents could be told that the clinician has identified a health problem that he or she is working with the adolescent to resolve and that requires followup visits.

Once a clinician concludes that a breach of confidentiality is warranted, the adolescent should be told in advance and given options about how the disclosure will occur. Such options might include the adolescent revealing the information to his or her parents in the presence of the clinician, the adolescent telling the parents alone, or the clinician disclosing the information to the parents. In some cases, an adolescent may request that one but not both parents be involved.

SPECIAL CIRCUMSTANCES

The foregoing discussion pertains to typical clinical encounters. In some special circumstances, different rules of confidentiality may apply. For example, the interaction between the adolescent and clinician may be ordered by a court or required as a condition of return to school. Federal and state regulations also may stipulate conditions of confidentiality for adolescents in drug treatment programs. Under these circumstances, the adolescent, the parents, and the clinician should be clear about the nature of the physician-patient relationship, including the boundaries of confidentiality and who will have access to the adolescent's medical record, including any test results.

REFERENCES

American College of Obstetricians and Gynecologists (ACOG) (1988). *ACOG Statement of Policy: Confidentiality in Adolescent Health Care.* Washington, DC: The College.

American Medical Association (AMA), Council on Long Range Planning and Development (1990). *AMA Policy Compendium.* Chicago, IL: American Medical Association, 8.

American Medical Association (AMA), Council on Scientific Affairs (1993). Confidential health services for adolescents. *Journal of the American Medical Association* 269:1420-1424.

Ford CA, Millstein SG, Halpern-Felsher BL et al. (1997). Influence of physician confidentiality assurances on adolescents' willingness to disclose information and seek future health care. A randomized controlled trial. *Journal of the American Medical Association* 278:1029-1034.

Ford CA, Thomsen SL & Compton B (2001). Adolescents' interpretations of conditional confidentiality assurances. *Journal of Adolescent Health* 29:156-159.

Hofman AD (1980). A rational policy toward consent and confidentiality in adolescent health care. *Journal of Adolescent Health Care* 1:9-17.

Levenberg PB & Elster AB (1995). *Guidelines for Adolescent Preventive Services (GAPS). Implementation and Resource Manual.* Chicago, IL: American Medical Association, 37-38.

Marks A, Malizio J, Hoch J et al. (1983). Assessment of health needs and willingness to utilize health care resources of adolescents in a suburban population. *Journal of Pediatrics* 102:456-460.

National Conference of Commissioners on Uniform State Laws (NCCUSL) (1989). *Uniform Health Care Information Act, Uniform Laws Annotated, Part I.* St. Paul, MN: West Publishing Co., 475-520.

Weithorn LA & Campbell S (1982). The competency of children and adolescents to make informed treatment decisions. *Child Development* 53:1589-1598.

Chapter 7	# Placement Criteria and Strategies for Adolescent Treatment Matching

Marc Fishman, M.D.

**Developmental Considerations
in Adolescent Treatment
The ASAM Patient Placement Criteria**

Although the fields of adolescent treatment in general, and adolescent treatment outcomes research in particular, are still in their infancy, recent progress has been considerable. Advances have been made in assessment, appreciation of adolescent-specific treatment needs, and development of treatment modalities and techniques tailored to the particular needs of adolescents. Over the past decade, much has been learned about the effectiveness and limitations of current adolescent treatment methods and programs.

Compared to the period before 1990—when the effectiveness of adolescent treatment was largely a matter of clinical anecdote, intuition, and deeply held conviction—treatment for adolescent substance use disorders now has clearly and repeatedly been shown to be effective. Reviews of the published literature have shown favorable outcomes at one year following treatment, across various modalities and levels of care. Abstinence rates at one year posttreatment ranged from 14% to 47%, with a mean of 32% (Williams & Chang, 2000). When the definition of "favorable outcomes" is appropriately expanded to include minor relapse in addition to abstinence, substantial improvement rates at one year posttreatment ranged from 25% to 62%, with a median of 44% (Winters, 1999). These results are further enhanced by favorable comparisons of treatment groups to waiting-list controls, treatment completers to non-completers, and carefully organized research-based treatment to loosely organized "treatment as usual."

It also is well established that favorable outcomes in treatment of adolescent substance use (including both abstinence and reductions in substance use short of abstinence) are associated with substantial reductions in adolescent morbidity and improvements in psychosocial function. Such improvements in function extend to school, family, criminal behaviors, psychological adjustment, and other psychosocial domains (Brown, Meyers et al., 1994).

While the research to date on adolescent addiction treatment has been very encouraging, there has been very little comparative examination of the broad range of current treatment modalities, levels of care, and program models. Little is known about the differential effectiveness of various treatment strategies, intensities, and treatment program components. Perhaps most important, little empirical work has been done to explore hypotheses of adolescent treatment matching and placement. Nevertheless, questions of which patient should receive what treatment have been the subject of extensive expert consideration, with progressive agreement on fundamental principles and approaches. For example, work with adults consistently shows that assessment-based stratification of severity can predict treatment response (Gastfriend & McLellan, 1997). Through such insights, consensus-based "best practices" in the area of adolescent treatment matching and placement are steadily improving.

This chapter provides an introduction to the developing area of adolescent treatment matching and placement, with special attention to one particular placement tool, the adolescent patient placement criteria developed by the American Society of Addiction Medicine (ASAM).

DEVELOPMENTAL CONSIDERATIONS IN ADOLESCENT TREATMENT

One of the most important advances in the field of adolescent treatment is the articulation of approaches that are developmentally specific to the adolescent population. These approaches respond to the principle that adolescents must be approached differently from adults because of differences in their levels of emotional, cognitive, physical, social, and moral development.

Examples of developmental issues that are fundamental to adolescent assessment and treatment include the extremely potent influence of peers and family. Thus, adolescent assessments need to include collateral informants who can augment, clarify (and, often, correct) the history as presented by the adolescent patient. Such key informants may include family, peers, adult friends or surrogate parent figures, school and court officials, court-appointed special advocates, social service workers, and previous treatment providers.

Adolescents' use of substances frequently impairs their emotional and intellectual growth. Substance use can prevent a young person from completing the maturational tasks of adolescence, which involve formation of personal relationships, acquisition of social skills, psychological development, identity formation, individuation, education, employment, and family role responsibilities. One of the special challenges and unique opportunities of adolescent treatment is to modify risk factors that are actively evolving. Adolescent treatment thus often requires habilitative rather than rehabilitative approaches, emphasizing the acquisition of new capacities rather than the restoration of lost ones.

Younger adolescents have a very narrow view of the world, with little capacity to think of future implications of present actions. Some adolescents may adopt a pseudo-mature ("streetwise") posture, despite their overall immaturity. Adolescents who live in a chaotic family system, or who have various cognitive difficulties, may be delayed or impaired in acquiring abstract thinking. Attempts to reason with an adolescent about the long-term health effects of substance use usually are futile because the adolescent is unable to appreciate such long-term consequences.

These and other developmental issues make adolescents particularly vulnerable. Adolescents typically require greater amounts of external assistance and support than do adult patients, both to protect them from the sequelae of substance use and to engage them in the recovery process. Most have not yet acquired the skills for independent living and, even without the impairments associated with substance use, must rely heavily on the guidance of adults.

In general, for a given degree of severity or functional impairment, adolescents require greater intensity of treatment than adults. This need is reflected in clinical practice by a greater tendency to place adolescents in more intensive levels of care.

THE ASAM PATIENT PLACEMENT CRITERIA

The *ASAM Patient Placement Criteria for the Treatment of Substance-Related Disorders, Second Edition-Revised* (*ASAM PPC-2R*; Mee-Lee, Shulman et al., 2001) is a clinical guide that has been widely adopted to assist in matching patients to appropriate treatment settings. It contains separate sets of criteria for adolescents and adults. The criteria, which have undergone evolutionary change and improvement since publication of the first edition in 1991, rest on the concept of enhancing the use of multidimensional assessments in placement decisions by organizing the assessment of the substance-using adolescent into six dimensions. Appropriate placements are determined by gradations of problem severity in each dimension.

Assessment-Based Treatment Matching and Clinical Appropriateness. The ASAM criteria use decision rules to guide placement in specified levels of care, which exist along a continuum. They also attempt to standardize some of the program specifications for each level of care, including some guidelines for minimum staffing levels and general program components. They do not, however, specify these in detail, nor do they attempt to prescribe program models, approaches, or techniques.

Because the elements of assessment in the *ASAM PPC-2R* are not concretely operationalized (as they are, for example, in standardized instruments of known psychometrics), they certainly allow for and require the use of considerable clinical judgment. They are best used as illustrations of underlying principles of matching, rather than as exact prescriptions or rigid rules.

The ASAM criteria also attempt to avoid assumptions regarding length of service and treatment dose. Rather, they provide guidelines in the form of general decision rules for continued service and discharge/transfer, which are applied to the patient's problems in the six assessment dimensions that led to the initial treatment placement. Under these decision rules, a patient should remain at a given level of care as long as the problems that created the need for admission persist (or new problems requiring that level of care emerge).

The principal goal of the ASAM criteria is to facilitate the process of matching patients with appropriate treatment services and settings in order to maximize the accessibility, effectiveness, and efficiency of the treatment experience. The principle of matching on which the criteria are based is that of clinical appropriateness, which emphasizes quality and efficiency over cost. The concept of "clinical appropriateness" contrasts with the more familiar concept of "medical necessity," which has become associated with restrictions on utilization. "Medical necessity" thus typically is interpreted in terms of avoiding life-threatening imminent danger and is related only to acute medical or psychiatric concerns (Dimensions 1, 2, and 3). By contrast, "clinical appropriateness" conveys the notion that patients should be treated in the most suitable placements, defined by the extent of their problems and priorities in all six of the ASAM assessment dimensions.

The criteria reflect a tension between an attempt to promote a broader continuum of treatment services on the one hand and an attempt to reflect the real world of treatment service delivery on the other. As a result, the criteria do not articulate some of the innovative sublevels of intensity and treatment settings that should exist (and in some places already do exist). However, even the "limited" continuum of treatment settings described in the criteria is not yet available in most communities.

The reality of limited availability of services is, of course, a major problem, particularly in the treatment of adolescents. One or more of the levels of care may not exist or be accessible in a given community, in either rural or urban settings. Funding limitations and other resource constraints also are barriers to the availability of a needed treatment setting. Even logistical issues such as waiting lists can render a treatment setting unavailable. And the individual variations in programs within the level of care categories sometimes mean that the specific services needed by a particular patient are not available, even if an available setting meets the criteria more generally.

When the criteria designate a treatment placement that is not available to a given patient, a strategy must be crafted to provide the patient with the needed services in another placement or combination of placements, always erring on the side of safety and effectiveness. This strategy may require increasing the intensity of services, usually through placement at a more intensive level of care.

One of the criticisms of previous editions of the criteria was that they were too heavily oriented toward private sector and managed care environments. All too frequently, the continuum of services described and the range of benefits implied in the criteria were not available to disadvantaged or public sector populations. However, the *ASAM PPC-2R* outlines the full range of treatment services appropriate to the needs of all drug-involved adolescents, whether they are privately insured, publicly insured, underinsured, or uninsured. In fact, many indigent adolescents need an even broader continuum of services and a higher intensity of services at all levels of care than do those with the benefits conferred by economic advantage.

One goal of the current edition has been to broaden the scope of the criteria and encompass more explicitly the circumstances of adolescents in the public sector. For example, more specific references are made to adolescents involved in the juvenile justice system, where many adolescents have had extended periods of enforced abstinence, but usually have not had active treatment. In this context, decisions about severity and need for treatment should not be based on a narrow standard involving recency of substance use, but rather should employ a full multidimensional assessment that focuses on the adolescent's acquisition of recovery skills and capacity for reintegration into the community. It is to be hoped that active treatment, including the full continuum of care reflected in the *ASAM PPC-2R*, will become the rule rather than the exception for adolescents involved in the juvenile justice system.

Treatment at every level of care requires coordination of a broad array of interrelated treatment services to respond to the needs of the individual patient. Such coordination sometimes is accomplished by direct provision of multiple treatment services and sometimes by linkages with other service providers, usually through referral. Examples include psychiatric assessment and treatment, medical assessment and treatment, establishment of a primary care medical "home," psychological and/or educational testing for learning disorders, special or alternative education services, family therapies, juvenile justice probation and supervision, foster care support services, public benefit coordination or other social service agency interventions, vocational and prevocational training, child care, transportation, and the like. To deliver this array of services, treatment programs at all levels of care should develop active affiliations with programs and agencies that offer other services or levels of care, and should help patients access treatment fluidly across the continuum. Barriers to treatment integration remain a fundamental and profound problem, which only recently have begun to be addressed, at least partially in response to adoption of the ASAM criteria by state agencies, third-party payers, and treatment providers.

Placement and Treatment Considerations by Assessment Dimension. As discussed earlier, the ASAM criteria organize the assessment of the substance-using adolescent into six dimensions and specify appropriate placements according to gradations of problem severity within each dimension (also see the Appendices of this text).

Dimension 1: Intoxication and Withdrawal: The *ASAM PPC-2R* includes an expansion of the Dimension 1 assessment elements to include additional detail and some breakdown by specific drug classes. This expansion highlights the range of intoxication and withdrawal symptoms, which all too often are overlooked in adolescents, and emphasizes the importance of their treatment. Some clinically prominent examples include memory impairment caused by marijuana intoxication, which can persist for many weeks following abstinence (substance-induced persistent amnestic disorder); sensory disturbance or "flashbacks" caused by hallucinogens, which can persist for weeks to months following abstinence (substance-induced perceptual distortion); and delirium and other states of cognitive disorganization caused by inhalants, which can persist for weeks or more following abstinence. Another very common example is insomnia as a symptom of extended subacute withdrawal from various substances (including marijuana, opioids, and alcohol), which—although not typically thought of as a severe problem—can be a powerful trigger for relapse.

The approach to detoxification services in the ASAM adolescent criteria is different from that used in the adult criteria, where such services are presented separately. Detoxification is integrated into the adolescent criteria because severe physiological withdrawal and the need for its management are seen less frequently in adolescents than in adults, given typical patterns of use and duration of exposure. Therefore, the provision of detoxification as an "unbundled" or stand-alone service is less common and less needed with adolescents. Nevertheless, withdrawal does occur in adolescents and should not be overlooked. In such cases, the provision of services to manage the withdrawal in a setting separate from other treatment services is clinically undesirable because of the developmental issues involved in the care of adolescents. Moreover, there is no evidence that the kinds of ambulatory detoxification that have become increasingly common for severe withdrawal in adults are effective or desirable in adolescents.

While most adolescents do not develop classic or well-defined physiological withdrawal symptoms, they may be more susceptible than adults to the development of substance dependence syndromes, including physiological tolerance. Adolescents have a one in four chance of developing one of the *DSM-IV* symptoms of dependence later in life if exposed to alcohol, marijuana, or nicotine before the age of 15, and four to eight times the risk of those not exposed until after age 17 (Dennis & McGeary, 1999). Also, the progression from casual use to dependence can be more accelerated in adolescents than in adults.

The process of detoxification includes not only the attenuation of the physiological and psychological features of intoxication and withdrawal syndromes, but also the process of interrupting the momentum of habitual compulsive use in adolescents. Because of the force of this momentum, and the inherent difficulties in overcoming it even when no clear physiological withdrawal syndrome is seen, this phase of treatment frequently requires a greater initial intensity in order to establish treatment engagement and patient role induction. Engagement and induction are critical to the success of treatment because it is difficult for patients to engage or participate in treatment while caught up in a cycle of frequent intoxication and recovery from intoxication.

Dimension 2: Biomedical Conditions and Complications: While the medical sequelae of addiction generally are not as common or as severe in adolescents as in adults, they certainly need to be considered in treatment placement decisions. Some of the more severe acute and subacute medical complications of substance use include seizures caused by stimulant and inhalant intoxication, traumatic injuries (either accidental or due to victimization) associated with any substance intoxication, and respiratory depression caused by opioid overdose (which is more common with cheaper, purer supplies of heroin as well as with the increasingly popular diverted prescription opioids, such as sustained-release oxycodone [OxyContin®]). Acute alcohol poisoning is a severe medical complication that is more typical of adolescents than adults. The sequelae of injection drug use are well known, including cellulitis, HIV, endocarditis, and hepatitis B and C.

Some of the less severe but more common (and often unrecognized) medical sequelae of substance use include gastritis caused by alcohol use, exacerbation of reactive airway disease caused by smoking marijuana, dental disease caused by poor self-care, and weight loss and malnourishment caused by self-neglect and/or the appetite-suppressing properties of certain drugs. Another notable area of medical complication in adolescents is the exacerbation of chronic illness (such as diabetes, asthma, or sickle cell disease) that results from impaired self-care and poor compliance with indicated medical treatments.

High-risk sexual behaviors are a major problem in adolescents. The associated sexually transmitted disorders include chlamydial and gonococcal infections, syphilis, pelvic inflammatory disease, HIV, and hepatitis B. Both urethritis in boys and cervicitis in girls are relatively common but often overlooked when asymptomatic.

The special needs and medical vulnerabilities of pregnant substance-using teens require particular care in selecting treatment services. Overall, the need for contraception and other medical prevention and treatment services related to sexual behaviors in drug-involved adolescents cannot be overemphasized.

Dimension 3: Emotional, Behavioral, and Cognitive Conditions and Complications: Drug-involved adolescents typically demonstrate a very high degree of co-occurring psychopathology, which frequently does not remit with abstinence (also see Chapter 7 in this section). Many experts estimate that rates of psychiatric comorbidity, or dual diagnosis, are higher in adolescents than in adults (Kandel, Johnson et al., 1997). Even adolescents who have not been diagnosed with a psychiatric disorder (either because they have not yet had a formal psychiatric evaluation or because subsyndromal symptoms do not meet diagnostic criteria)

often have problems in Dimension 3 that need to be considered in making treatment decisions. Examples include hyperactivity or distractibility without a diagnosis of attention deficit/hyperactivity disorder, mood lability and explosive temper without a diagnosis of bipolar disorder, or dysphoric mood and loss of interest without a diagnosis of depression. Various nonspecific symptoms—such as problems with anger management or impulse control, suspiciousness, and social withdrawal—also may be induced or exacerbated by substance use.

The inclusion of cognitive conditions in Dimension 3 emphasizes the importance of cognitive abilities, as well as global or focal cognitive impairments, in an adolescent's functional capacity. Whether cognitive problems are due to preexisting conditions (such as borderline intellectual functioning, fetal alcohol effects, or learning disorders) or are complications of substance use (such as marijuana-induced amnestic disorder), they often interfere significantly with treatment and recovery.

To be most effective, physicians and treatment programs must adapt their methods and strategies to respond to adolescents' cognitive vulnerabilities and strengths. It also is critical to consider cognitive function in a developmental perspective, because cognition evolves dynamically over time.

Treating adolescents involves using methods that take into account the ways in which young people learn, and being responsive to issues of normal adolescent development as well as to the delayed development and immaturity that often accompany drug use and co-occurring psychiatric disorders. In general, the delivery of most therapies should be divided into time-limited components, with frequent breaks, thereby taking into account limitations in youngsters' attention spans. Adolescent engagement and learning are promoted by the use of experiential recovery activities that involve active participation rather than passive reception of information, and that are somewhat energetic, noisy, and fun, while at the same time delivering serious therapeutic content. Engagement also is enhanced by acknowledging and even partially endorsing adolescent culture, including its typical stance of nonconformity with adult and mainstream norms.

Behavior and its management is another prominent developmental feature of adolescent treatment in Dimension 3. While the expectation of adult, or mature, behavior may be questionable in adult treatment settings, it is absurd in adolescent settings. The acquisition of self-regulation skills is an essential goal of treatment for substance users of all ages, but it also is a work in progress for all adolescents, even without substance use. Adolescent treatment programs must constantly seek a balance between an emphasis on limit-setting and some degree of tolerance for chaos, as part of the necessary recognition that adolescents still are partly children. Moreover, the penchant for mischief among youngsters is not always an indicator of antisocial traits. On the other hand, careful assessment of the broad range of adolescent misbehavior forms the basis of very powerful treatment interventions that target improvements in family monitoring, supervision, and behavioral management.

In the *ASAM PPC-2R*, Dimension 3 has been expanded and divided into new subdomains for greater emphasis on psychiatric comorbidity or "dual diagnosis" issues. These subdomains are intended to enrich the detail and guide the assessment of risk and treatment needs for emotional, behavioral, and cognitive problems. The organization of the Dimension 3 severity specifications by subdomains emphasizes that placement decisions emerge out of the assessment of symptomatic functional impairment, rather than any specific categorical diagnosis.

For example, the subdomain titled "Dangerousness/ Lethality" refers to the extent of risk of imminent harm to self or others. Assessment considerations may include suicidality, assaultiveness, risk of victimization, and exposure to the elements. Treatment decisions in this subdomain focus on safety and protection from dangerous consequences, and may include such interventions as residential containment or high-intensity family monitoring between outpatient sessions.

The subdomain titled "Interference with Addiction Recovery Efforts" refers to the extent to which psychological and behavioral symptoms are a distraction from treatment participation or engagement. Examples include difficulty attending to treatment sessions because of problems with concentration, difficulty in completing recovery assignments or absorbing treatment materials because of problems with memory or comprehension, inability to attend treatment consistently because of running away, inability to participate in treatment because of disruptive behavior, and distraction caused by preoccupying worries.

The subdomain titled "Social Functioning" refers to the extent to which emotional, behavioral, and cognitive problems cause impairments in meeting responsibilities in major social arenas such as family, school, work, and personal relationships. Examples of assessment considerations in this subdomain include problems managing peer or family conflict, legal and conduct problems, problems with truancy or school performance, ungovernability at home, and narrowing of social repertoire and isolation.

The subdomain titled "Ability for Self-Care" refers to the extent to which the adolescent has problems in managing activities of daily living and personal care. Assessment considerations in this subdomain include behaviors associated with patterns of victimization, high risk or indiscriminate sexual behaviors, disorganization that interferes with emerging independent living skills, poor self-regulation (or poor cooperation with external regulation) of daily routine, and problems with hygiene or nutrition.

The subdomain titled "Course of Illness" refers to an interpretation of the adolescent's present situation and symptoms in the context of his or her history and response to treatment, with a goal of predicting future course and relative stability. For example, the adolescent's history may suggest that a mood disorder decompensates rapidly with medication noncompliance, suggesting a higher instability and severity than would be the case if the course deteriorated more slowly, and suggesting the need for a more urgent and/or more intensive treatment response. Other examples include an adolescent who has tended to run away soon after an episode of family conflict, or an adolescent who tends to relapse to substance use following recurrence of depressive symptoms.

Dimension 4: Readiness to Change: Assessment of treatment readiness is an essential component of treatment matching for adolescents. In general, it is likely that different interventions will be effective at various stages of readiness to change. On the whole, adolescents tend to present at earlier stages of readiness to change than do adults because of developmental context. For example, they are more likely to enter treatment as the result of external pressures than are adults (Deas, Riggs et al., 2000).

In the *ASAM PPC-2R*, Dimension 4 has been renamed "Readiness to Change" to highlight the field's progress away from the concept of passive acceptance of treatment and toward the more active, dynamic concept of treatment engagement. Placement decisions based on Dimension 4 will include consideration of whether the adolescent (and related systems, such as the family) is in the "precontemplation," "contemplation," "preparation," or "action" stage of change.

It is important to emphasize that engagement and role induction are critical components of treatment. Significant advances have been made in expanding the treatment engagement repertoire from simply and inflexibly attempting to overcome the adolescent's resistance, to appreciating the adolescent's own set of motivations and goals and attempting to enroll those into an evolving treatment agenda. Motivational interviewing and other motivational enhancement techniques have formed the basis of a variety of intervention models at various levels of care, including early intervention (Colby, Monti et al., 1998) and outpatient treatment (Sampl & Kadden, 2001).

Assessments of readiness to change should take into account a variety of change processes, including the processes used by adolescents themselves in effecting self-change, the processes used by families in effecting change (Liddle & Hogue, 2001), and the processes used by the external systems that interact with adolescents and their families, such as the coercive influence of the juvenile justice system. Readiness to change generally is viewed as involving a balance of internal experiential contingency motivations (such as social frustrations; symptoms of intoxication or withdrawal; loss of achievements, interests and enjoyment; unpleasant or frightening experiences, including violence, victimization, high-risk motor vehicle use, or unwelcome sexual experiences) and external contingency motivations (such as parental mandates, legal threats, drug testing, peer group affiliations and influences, and loss of status). The question to be answered is which of these factors (and others) will have salience, and how and in what setting to make best use of them in enhancing the adolescent's motivation for treatment and change.

Additional factors in treatment engagement include problem identification, help-seeking orientation, self-efficacy, and hopefulness. Cultural factors also are important components of readiness to change, as they influence likelihood of seeking and receiving treatment, likelihood of perceiving treatment as helpful, and consideration of cultural context in devising treatment engagement strategies.

Dimension 5: Relapse, Continued Use, or Continued Problem Potential: Dimension 5 entails an estimation of the likelihood of resumption or continuation of substance use. The assessment of relapse potential (or, reciprocally, remission potential) should include a number of key factors. Although not incorporated directly into the criteria, a schema for incorporating four subdomains for more detailed Dimension 5 assessments has been proposed (Mee-Lee, Shulman et al., 2001, p. 345). These subdomains are: (1) historical pattern of use (including chronicity and treatment response), (2) pharmacologic responsivity (including positive and negative reinforcement from particular substances), (3) external stimuli responsivity (including reactivity to triggers and stress), and (4) cognitive and behavioral vulnerability and resiliency factors (including traits of impulsivity, passivity, locus of control, and overall coping capacities).

The "historical pattern of use" concept is similar to the "course of illness" subdomain in Dimension 3. That is, history and treatment response are likely to predict future course of illness, including relapse potential. For example, some adolescents are likely to have a rapid course of full reinstatement of dependence with severe impairment following a single lapse episode, while others are likely to have a more indolent course, with only gradual escalation of use. This difference suggests one means of informing treatment and placement matching decisions on an individualized basis. Response to past treatment also may be a way of using individualized treatment effectiveness as a guide to placement: if a particular dose of treatment or modality or level of care led to a significant period of improvement for an adolescent in the past, then it may be appropriate to repeat the treatment following a relapse or exacerbation. On the other hand, if a particular dose or placement was not effective in the past, this history may suggest the need for a more intensive intervention.

Dimension 6: Recovery/Living Environment: Dimension 6 aims to assess the ability of the adolescent's home environment to support or impede treatment and recovery. For adolescents, the most important features of the recovery environment generally involve family and peers. The need for inclusion of families or other caretakers in assessment and treatment is paramount. In many cases, it is unreasonable to expect that the adolescent will be the initial or most important locus of change. Rather, it often is more effective to help the family improve its approach to monitoring, supervision, and home intervention, with the expectation that the family as the primary locus of change will in turn change the adolescent.

Families, and their needs and involvement, should be considered broadly to encompass a wide range of circumstances, such as extended families, surrogate families, and other caretakers. It also is important to address cultural context and to use cultural competence as a critical tool for engaging families in treatment.

Problems in Dimension 6 that typically affect placement include chaotic home environments in which substance use, illegal behaviors, abuse, neglect, or lack of supervision are prominent, and a broader community in which substance use and crime are endemic. Many adolescents have a social network composed primarily or even exclusively of family members or peers who are involved in substance use or criminal behaviors. This social context may portray deviance as normative. There may not be readily apparent role models for the rewards of abstinence. Some adolescents may have had *no* experience of living in an environment that fosters healthy prosocial development and functioning.

Placement and Treatment Considerations by Levels of Care. The adolescent levels of care in the *ASAM PPC-2R* are similar to the levels of care described and endorsed in other expert consensus documents (Winters, 1999).

Level 0.5: Early Intervention: Early intervention services are designed to explore and address the adolescent's problems or risk factors that appear to be related to early stages of substance use. Their goal is to help the adolescent recognize the potentially harmful consequences of substance use, before such use escalates into substance abuse or dependence. Level 0.5 services may be delivered in a variety of settings, including primary care medical clinics, schools (often through organized student assistance programs), social service and juvenile justice agencies, and driving under the influence (DUI) intervention programs.

Early intervention is intended to combine prevention and treatment services for youth who are at risk because of their substance exposure, experimentation, or use. Populations that warrant special attention at Level 0.5 are the children of substance-abusing parents, siblings of substance users, and adolescents with other emotional or behavioral problems.

Early intervention is not appropriate for adolescents who qualify for a diagnosis of a substance use disorder. If an adolescent's pattern of substance use has progressed to a point at which it is causing a persistent pattern of impairment, then the applicable treatment services are best provided at a more intensive level of care.

Level I: Outpatient Treatment: Outpatient treatment is by far the most frequently utilized level of care. It may be the initial level of care for an adolescent whose lesser severity of illness warrants this intensity of treatment. Level I also may be employed as a "step-down" program for the adolescent who has made progress at a more intensive level of care.

Outpatient treatment is indicated when safety and progress toward recovery goals can be expected without either the immersion intensity of Level II services or the residential support and protection of Level III services.

One of the advantages of outpatient treatment is the possibility of achieving therapeutic goals in the context of the patient's own home environment, where new behaviors can be practiced and solidified in real life circumstances.

Outpatient services may be useful for the adolescent patient who is in the early stages of readiness to change and who has not yet committed to recovery. While an adolescent at this stage may require a more intensive level of care (sometimes including coerced treatment) to address dangerousness or high degrees of resistance and denial, such an increase in intensity can be counterproductive in certain situations. An alternative approach is to use a less intensive level of care to engage the resistant adolescent in treatment by enhancing his or her motivation and/or by modifying the response(s) of the various systems that affect the adolescent. In such situations, "discovery" may be a more appropriate outpatient treatment goal than "recovery." Such an approach can prepare the adolescent for more intensive treatment services or even forestall the need for a more intensive level of care.

Outpatient treatment often includes a prolonged maintenance phase, sometimes referred to as "aftercare" or "extended care." In this phase, strategies such as relapse prevention and strengthening protective factors are critical components of treatment. This phase focuses anticipating difficulties and guiding adolescents through the periodic recurrence of stressors without return to or exacerbation of substance use. Even simple ongoing monitoring (such as checking on parental supervision, scrutinizing school performance or peer relationships, and reviewing warning signs and triggers) is a desirable goal of active outpatient treatment.

Level II: Intensive Outpatient Treatment/Partial Hospitalization: Intensive outpatient programs (IOPs) generally offer at least 6 hours of structured programming per week. However, the precise number of hours of service delivered is adjusted to meet each patient's needs. Six hours a week will be too few for many adolescents; for example, those who are early in their treatment or who are stepping down from a more intensive level of care may need 9, 12, or even 15 hours a week of IOP services.

Partial hospitalization programs (PHP; also sometimes known as "day programs") generally offer 20 or more hours of clinically intensive programming per week. They feature daily or near-daily contact and thus provide more intensive monitoring and supervision than IOP or Level I outpatient treatment.

Intensive outpatient (Level II.1) programs typically differ from partial hospitalization (Level II.5) programs in the severity of patient disorders they can manage. Most IOPs have less capacity to treat adolescents who have substantial or unstable emotional or behavioral problems; such patients are better placed in partial hospitalization programs. Partial hospitalization programs often have direct access to, or close referral relationships with, psychiatric, medical, and laboratory services. Thus, they are better able than Level II.1 programs to meet needs identified in Dimensions 1, 2, and 3, which may warrant daily monitoring or management, but which can be appropriately addressed in a structured outpatient setting. Some PHPs can provide an intensity of treatment services approaching that of residential care if the patient's home environment can support safety, stability, and treatment progress between PHP sessions.

With both IOPs and PHPs, there are varying approaches to the program schedule and structure. Some programs employ a single fixed schedule of service hours. Others modify their service hours throughout the stages of treatment, tapering the number of hours according to a prescribed schedule. Yet another approach is to match intensity and hours of service flexibly with the severity of the patient's problems.

Adolescent IOPs generally meet after school or work hours or on weekends. Partial hospitalization may occur during school hours, and many programs have access to educational services for their adolescent patients. PHP programs that do not provide educational services often coordinate with a school system in order to assess and meet their adolescent patients' educational needs.

Level III: Residential Treatment: While earlier editions of the ASAM criteria treated all adolescent residential treatment as one broad undifferentiated level of care, the *PPC-2R* divides Level III into three sublevels:

- Level III.1: Clinically Managed Low-Intensity Residential Treatment

- Level III.5: Clinically Managed Medium-Intensity Residential Treatment

- Level III.7: Medically Monitored High-Intensity Residential/Inpatient Treatment

Level III.1 (Clinically Managed Low-Intensity Residential Treatment) programs typically are provided in halfway houses and group homes. Such programs offer several hours a week of low-intensity treatment sessions, in addition to their most important feature: a stable living environment, staffed 24 hours a day, which provides sufficient structure and supervision to prevent or minimize relapse or continued use and continued problem potential (Dimension 5). Treatment is directed toward applying recovery skills, preventing relapse, improving social functioning by practicing interpersonal and group living skills, improving ability for self-care by organizing the activities of daily living, promoting personal responsibility through successful concurrent involvement in regular productive activities (such as school or work), developing a social network supportive of recovery, and reintegrating the adolescent into the community and (if appropriate) the family.

Treatment at Level III.1 most often is warranted as a substitute for or supplement to deficits in the adolescent's recovery environment (Dimension 6). Problems in Dimension 6 that might warrant placement in a residential program include home environments that are so abusive, chaotic, or riddled with substance use or antisocial behaviors that extended separation and residential treatment support are required to overcome their toxic influences.

Some adolescents require the structure of a Level III.1 program to achieve engagement in treatment. Those who are in the early stages of readiness to change may need to be removed from an unsupportive living environment in order to minimize their continued substance use (Dimension 4).

The length of stay in a clinically managed Level III.1 program tends to be longer than in the more intensive residential levels of care. In some cases, an extended period in Level III.1 treatment is needed to sustain and consolidate therapeutic gains made at more intensive levels of care because of the adolescent's functional deficits (including developmental immaturity, greater than average susceptibility to peer influence, or lack of impulse control). Longer exposure to monitoring, supervision, and low-intensity treatment interventions is necessary for adolescents to practice basic living skills and to master the application of coping and recovery skills. In some situations, there is no effective substitute for extended residential containment as reliable protection from the toxic influences of substance exposure, problematic or substance-infested environments, or the cultures of substance-involved and antisocial behaviors.

Level III.5 (Clinically Managed Medium-Intensity Residential Treatment) programs include medium-intensity settings such as therapeutic group homes, therapeutic community programs, psychosocial model residential treatment centers, or extended residential rehabilitation programs. As a group, these sometimes are referred to simply as "residential programs."

Level III.5 programs are designed to provide relatively extended subacute treatments, with the goal of achieving fundamental personal change for the adolescent who has significant social and psychological problems. The goals and modalities of treatment focus not only on the adolescent's substance use, but also on a holistic view of the adolescent that takes into account his or her behavior, emotions, attitudes, values, learning, family, culture, lifestyle, and overall health. Such programs are characterized by their reliance on the treatment community or milieu as a therapeutic agent of change. In addition to the stable recovery environment found at Level III.1, these programs employ intensive 24-hour active programming and containment to create a community or milieu that promotes both recovery skills and basic life skills. Critical treatment interventions that require intensity and persistence over extended periods of time, such as modeling prosocial patterns of behavior and adaptive patterns of emotional responsiveness, occasionally have been likened to "surrogate" or "remedial parenting." Just as important can be the induction into a healthy peer group, with the formation of a group identity that emphasizes recovery and overcoming adversity.

The adolescent who is appropriately placed in a Level III.5 program may have a variety of psychological or psychiatric problems (Dimension 3). Particularly suitable for Level III.5 treatments are the entrenched patterns of maladaptive behavior, extremes of temperament, and developmental or cognitive abnormalities related to mental health symptoms or disorders. Co-occurring disorders that often require extended treatment at Level III.5 include conduct disorder and oppositional defiant disorder, as well as the persistent patterns of disruptive behavior that may be associated with other disorders, even after they have responded to acute treatment.

Level III.5 programs frequently work with aspects of adolescent temperament—including impulsive, extroverted, dramatic, antisocial, thrill-seeking, or other personality traits—that may otherwise have the potential to solidify as components of emerging personality disorders. Goals of treatment include overcoming oppositionality through a combination of confrontation, motivational enhancement, and supportive limit setting; teaching anger management and acquisition of conflict resolution skills; values clarifica-

tion and moral habilitation; character molding and education; development of effective behavioral contingency strategies; establishment of a reliable response to external structure; and the internalization of structure through self-regulation skills.

Level III.5 also is appropriate for the adolescent whose problems include severe delinquency and juvenile justice involvement. This level of care often is warranted for adolescents who have severe conduct problems, a progressive history of illegal behaviors, a pattern of emerging criminality, or an incipient antisocial value system. One of the key purposes of Level III.5 treatment for this set of problems is assessment and monitoring of safety, with particular attention to issues of potential safety outside of the contained setting. In this context, treatment must proceed in a contained, safe, and structured environment to allow teaching, practicing of prosocial behaviors, and facilitation of healthy reintegration into the community.

Treatment in a Level III.5 program may be used to address problems in treatment engagement and readiness to change (Dimension 4). Many adolescents fail attempts at outpatient treatment out of a lack of engagement, either because they do not have a personal connection to treatment or because the systems surrounding the adolescent (family, school, juvenile justice system, and the like) have not coordinated sufficiently to motivate the adolescent, or both. The immersion experience of a Level III.5 program may be needed to promote treatment role induction and to introduce the adolescent into a peer group that is struggling to form a group identity emphasizing recovery and the need for treatment. An additional goal of treatment at Level III.5 should be to promote coordination of the multiple systems surrounding the adolescent and to help devise and implement motivational strategies for ongoing engagement in treatment.

Like those at Level III.1, programs at Level III.5 may require relatively long stays to allow certain adolescents to acquire basic living skills and mastery of coping and recovery skills. Such patients require the intensity and duration of treatment found in a Level III.5 program to accomplish some of the tasks of habilitation in a temporary "home" (Dimension 6) that can imprint the features of a successful recovery environment.

Level III.7 (Medically Monitored High-Intensity Residential/Inpatient Treatment) programs are appropriate for adolescents whose problems are so severe that they require medically monitored residential treatment, but who do not need the full resources of an acute care hospital or medically managed inpatient treatment program (Level IV). Medically monitored services are provided under the supervision of physicians who are specialists in addiction medicine, and the programs tend to operate under the so-called "medical model."

The adolescent who is appropriately placed in a medically monitored program may have problems in Dimensions 1, 2, or 3 that require direct medical or nursing services. Services typically provided in a Level III.7 program include medical detoxification, titration of a psychopharmacologic regimen, and high-intensity behavior modification. Alternatively, the adolescent may have problems that do not require direct medical or nursing services so much as the overall high intensity of a program and treatment milieu that draws on the availability of an interdisciplinary professional team.

An adolescent may be admitted directly to a Level III.7 program or transferred from a less intensive level of care if he or she has been refractory to treatment or as bursts of more intensive services become necessary. An adolescent also may be transferred to a Level III.7 program for continuing care from a Level IV program when he or she no longer requires the intensity of services or staffing pattern of a hospital. A fairly common scenario is that of an adolescent who is admitted to a Level IV hospital program on an emergency basis because of a crisis situation and then is transferred to a Level III.7 program for further assessment in a substance-free state to help sort out difficult diagnostic questions regarding subacute intoxication, withdrawal and co-occurring psychiatric disorders.

Problems in Dimension 3 are the most common reason for admission to Level III.7 programs. Such problems include co-occurring psychiatric disorders (such as depressive disorders, bipolar disorders, and attention deficit/hyperactivity disorder) or symptoms (such as hypomania, severe disorganization or impulsiveness, and aggressive behaviors).

Treatment at Level III.7 often is necessary simply to orient an adolescent with substance dependence to the structure of daily life, using organizing principles other than "getting high" and "being high." Initial forced abstinence through confinement in a Level III.7 program provides many adolescents with a much-needed reintroduction to their own patterns of emotional and cognitive experience without intoxication.

Problems in Dimension 1 that require Level III.7 services include moderate to severe withdrawal or risk of withdrawal. Adolescents also may need medically monitored treatment because of acute or subacute intoxication. Lingering drug-induced impairments of cognitive or executive function (for example, by inhalants) may lead to disorganization, poor judgment, or increased impulsivity. These conditions may require periods of close assessment and high-intensity management.

Level IV: Medically Managed Intensive Inpatient (Hospital) Treatment: Level IV medically managed intensive inpatient treatment is delivered in an acute care inpatient setting in which the full resources of a general and/or psychiatric hospital are available. This level is appropriate for adolescents whose acute problems are so severe that they require primary medical and nursing care on a daily basis.

Although treatment is specific to substance dependence disorders, the skills of the interdisciplinary team and the availability of support services allow the conjoint treatment of any withdrawal, medical conditions, or psychiatric disorders that need to be addressed.

Admission to Level IV is most commonly provoked by urgent concerns regarding safety and/or imminent danger.

Level IV treatment tends to be brief, and generally consists of emergency or crisis interventions aimed at stabilization in preparation for transfer to a less intensive level of care for ongoing treatment.

Treatment Dose and Utilization Management. The ASAM criteria emphasize the concept of treatment as a dynamic, longitudinal process, rather than a discrete episode of care or particular program enrollment. However, current treatment delivery systems do not generally support the necessary continuum of care. For example, a longitudinal view of treatment might call for the services of a designated care provider to coordinate (or even provide) treatment across discrete placements, but use of such a provider is unusual in most communities and systems of care.

Many difficulties continue to arise over utilization management issues. For example, what is the optimal dose of treatment for adolescents at any level of care? There are no data as yet to answer this and other critical questions. While movement away from fixed, length of stay-based, program-driven treatment to more flexible, assessment-based, clinically driven treatment is apparent, much of the development of adolescent programs has focused on standardized protocols with prescribed contents and lengths of service. There has been little examination of the dose-response relationship for adolescent treatment, and further research into this issue is needed.

Certain threshold lengths of service may be associated with specific therapeutic gains. In particular, the needs of juvenile justice-involved adolescents in public sector programs that use coercive treatment engagement methods (such as a court order or probationary mandate) may be best served by more predictable, though not rigid, lengths of service. Physicians and the courts must collaborate closely to assure that the interests of each adolescent patient are assessed and met.

When a treatment plan is unsuccessful, it calls for reassessment. Reassessment may indicate the need for more treatment, but also may indicate the need to adopt a different treatment plan, featuring a change in strategy, modality, or scope of treatment. Treatment failure often implies a need for greater intensity, but also may suggest a change in approach rather than in level of care. The criteria should be applied within the context of local resources and realistically designed followup plans.

While utilization criteria can be used as an impetus to overcome treatment barriers through creative systems approaches, they also have been misused as a cynical justification for giving up or limiting payment for care. The ASAM criteria are *not* intended to imply that ongoing problems, even severe treatment-refractory problems (such as continued use, lapse, relapse, lack of attendance, lack of participation, and the like) suggest inability to solve treatment problems. Changes in level of care or treatment approach always should be a part of the therapeutic strategy for revising an overall or longitudinal treatment plan, and never should be motivated by an acceptance of futility or therapeutic nihilism.

Given that substance use disorders often have a chronic, remitting/relapsing course, it is reasonable to expect that treatment must match this chronic course. Treatment may encompass one or several acute episodes, but a treatment plan also must endure over the long term. An older, presumably outdated, approach views discrete time-limited episodes of program enrollment as constituting adequate doses of treatment. In this view, any further care, also typically time-limited, was regarded as "aftercare" rather than ongoing care, as if the active part of treatment had been completed.

The more appropriate view of chronic care for a chronic disorder supports a stance of therapeutic optimism and a "never give up" attitude for the treatment-refractory patient. It also reinforces the need for chronic attention and vigilance in response to a chronic vulnerability, even in the improved patient. This view is not incompatible with the common experience that a subset of adolescents may respond to more time-limited interventions or seem to "grow out of" their difficulties with developmental maturation.

A critical feature of successful adolescent treatment across a continuum is ease of transfer across the levels of care. Because payers have not funded more flexible continuums of care and because providers have not developed such systems, it generally is difficult for patients to move back and forth between levels of care at all, much less with coordinated transitions. One reason for prolonged lengths of stay at more intensive levels of care is the barriers encountered in stepping down to appropriate lower levels. Reciprocally, acute bursts of treatment at higher levels of care often are needed to overcome hurdles at lower levels. Repeated acute episodes of high-intensity care should be an expected (although not necessarily desired) modality of treatment for exacerbations, as they would be with any chronic relapsing disorder.

Ongoing treatment at less intensive levels of care to consolidate gains initiated at more intensive levels of care also is a critical feature of successful treatment across a continuum of care. Since enduring treatment effectiveness may be tempered by the attenuation of treatment effect over time, the need for "booster" doses of treatment should be anticipated. Moreover, ongoing active treatment often is required simply to consolidate and sustain therapeutic gains. Finally, the long-term (sometimes indefinite) maintenance phase of treatment too often is overlooked. Treatment successes, such as a period of abstinence or improvement in functioning, sometimes are misinterpreted as completion of treatment. In fact, long-term maintenance and monitoring of short-term successes are essential goals of active outpatient treatment.

Validation of Placement Criteria. The ASAM criteria were developed as a consensus-based guide to "best practices" by committees of experts and diverse stakeholders. As such, their application is not concretely operationalized or based on standardized assessment instruments, and their use clearly relies on the utilization of sound clinical interpretation and judgment.

Unlike the adult placement criteria, very little research has been done on either the reliability or validity of the adolescent criteria. However, preliminary work suggests that clinicians who use the criteria in "real world" settings are in fact able to discriminate levels of clinical severity. A retrospective analysis of adolescents assigned to placements using the ASAM criteria within a single provider's system of care found that adolescents referred to inpatient treatment had greater severity than those referred to outpatient care (Godley, Godley et al., 2001). While the two groups did not differ demographically, the adolescents placed in inpatient treatment had significantly greater severity on a variety of indicators, including frequency of use, number of previous treatment episodes, number of diagnoses of dependence (as opposed to abuse without dependence), and prevalence of physiologic dependence (as indicated primarily by the symptom of tolerance). Because adolescent substance use is so clearly associated with problems in a wide range of related psychosocial domains, any attempt to stratify severity and treatment needs also must take these into account, rather than focusing on substance use alone.

To date, there is no empirical evidence of the effectiveness of adolescent placement or treatment matching criteria based on treatment outcome data. However, there are encouraging preliminary indications that case mix adjustments based on ASAM criteria can help explain a considerable amount of the variance in treatment outcomes for different levels of care (Dennis, Scott et al., 2000). These indications suggest that the ASAM criteria, when refined and better operationalized, may in fact lead to predictors of treatment response. Work also is under way using models of adherence to the ASAM criteria to determine retrospectively whether "appropriate" level of care placements lead to better outcomes.

CONCLUSIONS

At present, the adolescent population is significantly underserved, with fewer than 10% of adolescents who exhibit symptoms of problem drug use in the preceding year ever having received formal treatment (Dennis & McGeary, 1999). It would be a huge advance for these adolescents to receive any treatment at all. It is hoped that the use of organized assessment tools, such as the ASAM criteria, which employ gradations of severity and risk to guide treatment matching and placement decisions, will help to create pressure for the creation of the necessary treatment resources.

For the field to take the next steps in understanding treatment effectiveness and to develop more effective treatments, clinicians must be able to make appropriate and useful treatment matching and placement decisions. To accomplish this, physicians and other health professionals will need to further operationalize gradations of severity and risk, using more reliable measures, and presumably incorporating standardized instruments. At the same time, it will be important to resist the illusion of technique, and to avoid the error of assuming that the reliability and precision of standardized instruments guarantee validity.

Treatment matching hypotheses and practices must be refined beyond level of care to include specific interventions, services, modalities, and doses. It will be important to discern relevant subtypes that might be expected to be associated with different responses to treatment within the heterogeneous population of drug-involved adolescents. (Of course, the validity of such refinements will need to be demonstrated empirically.)

The ASAM adolescent placement criteria continue to evolve in response to ongoing progress in the field of adolescent addiction medicine. Currently, the criteria are based predominantly on consensus best practices. As the results of additional adolescent treatment outcomes research become available, future revisions of the criteria will be based increasingly on empirically verified principles of treatment matching, placement, and effectiveness. At the same time, the ASAM criteria and other clinical treatment matching guidelines will drive research hypotheses that will lead to improved treatment and treatment access for all adolescents in need.

REFERENCES

Brown SA (1998). Recovery patterns in adolescent substance abuse. In JS Bae, GA Marlatt & RJ McMahon (eds.) *Addictive Behaviors Across the Lifespan. Prevention, Treatment and Policy Issues.* Beverly Hills, CA: Sage Publications Inc., 161-183.

Brown SA, Myers MG & Vik PW (1994). Correlates of success following treatment for adolescent substance abuse. *Applied & Preventive Psychology* 3:61-73.

Colby SM, Monti PM, Barnett NP et al. (1998). Brief motivational interviewing in a hospital setting for adolescent smoking: A preliminary study. *Journal of Clinical and Consulting Psychology* 66:574-578.

Deas D, Riggs P, Langenbucher J et al. (2000). Adolescents are not adults: Developmental considerations in alcohol users. *Alcoholism: Clinical & Experimental Research* 24:232-237.

Dennis M, Dowud-Noursi S, Muck R et al. (2002). The need for developing and evaluating adolescent treatment models. In S Stevens & A Morral (eds.) *Adolescent Substance Abuse Treatment in the United States: Exemplary Models from a National Evaluation Study.* Binghamton, NY: Haworth Press.

Dennis M, Funk R, McDermeit M et al. (1988). Towards better placement and case mix adjustments in adolescent and adult substance abuse treatment systems. Presented at the 8th International Conference on Treatment of Addictive Behavior. Santa Fe, NM, January.

Dennis M & McGeary K (1999). Adolescent alcohol and marijuana treatment: Kids need it now. *TIE Communique.* Rockville, MD: Center for Substance Abuse Treatment.

Dennis M, Scott C, Godley M et al. (2000). Predicting outcomes in adult and adolescent treatment with case mix vs. level of care: Findings from the drug outcome monitoring study. Presentation at the College on Problems of Drug Dependence, San Juan, PR, June.

Gastfriend DR & McLellan AT (1997). Treatment matching: Theoretic basis and practical implications. *Medical Clinics of North America* 81(4):945-966.

Godley SH, Godley MD & Dennis ML (2001). Assertive aftercare protocol for adolescent substance abusers. In E Wagner & H Waldron (eds.) *Innovations in Adolescent Substance Abuse Interventions.* Oxford, England: Pergamon, 313-331.

Kandel DB, Johnson JG, Bird HR et al. (1997). Psychiatric disorders associated with substance use among children and adolescents: Findings from the Methods for Epidemiology of Child and Adolescent Mental Disorders (MECA) study. *Journal of Abnormal Psychology* 25:121-132.

Liddle HA & Hogue A (2001). Multidimensional family therapy for adolescent substance abuse. In E Wagner & H Waldron (eds.) *Innovations in Adolescent Substance Abuse Interventions.* Oxford, England: Pergamon, 229-261.

Mee-Lee D, Shulman G, Fishman M et al. (2001). *ASAM Patient Placement Criteria for the Treatment of Substance-Related Disorders, Second Edition-Revised (ASAM PPC-2R).* Chevy Chase, MD: American Society of Addiction Medicine.

Sampl S & Kadden R (2001). *Motivational Enhancement Therapy and Cognitive Behavioral Therapy for Adolescent Cannabis Users: 5 Sessions, Cannabis Youth Treatment (CYT Series, Volume 1).* Rockville, MD: Center for Substance Abuse Treatment.

Williams RJ, Chang SY & Addiction Centre Adolescent Research Group (2000). A comprehensive and comparative review of adolescent substance abuse treatment outcome. *Clinical Psychology: Science and Practice* 7:138-166.

Winters KC (1999). Treating adolescents with substance use disorders: An overview of practice issues and treatment outcomes. *Substance Abuse* 20:203-223.

| Chapter 8 | # Co-Occurring Disorders in Adolescents |

Marie E. Armentano, M.D.
Ramon Solhkhah, M.D.

Incidence and Prevalence
Diagnosis and Management

Despite recent studies showing that levels of adolescent alcohol and drug use have essentially stabilized, they are sufficiently high to remain a major concern. Given recent increases in the use of "club drugs" such as 3,4-methylenedioxymethamphetamine (MDMA or "Ecstasy"), ketamine, and gamma-hydroxybutyrate (GHB) over the past several years, as well as evidence that the age of first use continues to decline, it is difficult to claim victory in the "War on Drugs."

Adolescents who manifest other psychiatric diagnoses in addition to substance use have elicited increasing concern (AAP, 2000; Armentano, 1995; Bukstein, Glancy et al., 1992; Bukstein, Brent et al., 1993; Burke, Burke et al., 1994; Crowley & Riggs, 1995; Deykin & Buka, 1997; Fergusson, Harwood et al., 1993; Geller, Cooper et al., 1998; Grilo, Becker et al., 1995; Horowitz, Overton et al., 1992; Hovens, Cantwell et al., 1994; Kaminer, Tarter et al., 1992; Stowell & Estroff, 1992; Westermeyer & Specker, 1999; Wilcox & Yates, 1993; Wilens, Biederman et al., 1996).

In fact, adolescents with substance use disorders exhibit a high prevalence of psychiatric disorders (SUDs) compared to the general population (Brook, Whiteman et al., 1995; Christie, Burke et al., 1988; DeMilio, 1989; Hovens, Cantwell et al., 1994; Kaminer, 1991; Kandel, Johnson et al., 1997; Kellam, Enswinger et al., 1980). Studies of treatment-seeking SUD adolescents have documented that 50% to 90% also have non-SUD comorbid psychiatric disorders (Clark & Bukstein, 1998; Deykin, Buka et al., 1992; Hovens, Cantwell et al., 1994; Kashani, Keller et al., 1985; King, Naylor et al., 1992; King, Ghaziuddin et al., 1996; Milin, Halikas et al., 1991; Stowell & Estroff, 1992). Not only are specific psychiatric disorders associated with alcohol and drug use, but other problems that affect teens—such as suicide, violence, and pregnancy—also are associated with an increased risk of substance use.

In this chapter, the terms "dual diagnosis," "comorbidity," and "co-occurring disorders" are used interchangeably to refer to patients who meet the criteria for a psychoactive substance use disorder and for another psychiatric diagnosis on Axis I or II of the *Diagnostic and Statistical Manual of Mental Disorders, 4th Edition* (*DSM-IV*) of the American Psychiatric Association (1994). The term "substance use disorder" is used to include both use and dependence. Adolescents who initially seek treatment for a substance use disorder—the focus of this chapter—may be different from those who seek care for a psychiatric disorder (Caton, Gralnick et al., 1989; Ries, 1993b).

Awareness of the most likely disorders and formulation of an integrated treatment plan is essential. This chapter reviews what is known about comorbidities and offers guidelines for their management and the care of adolescents so affected.

Definitional Issues. Dual diagnosis issues initially were studied in adults (Miller, 1993; Miller & Fine, 1993; Ries, 1993b; Schuckit, 1985; Schuckit, 1986; Schuckit 1994), leaving the clinician to extrapolate from this research to the adolescent population. More recently, adolescent clinical and community populations have been studied (Bukstein, Glancy et al., 1992; Burke, Burke et al., 1990; Burke, Burke et al., 1994; Crowley & Riggs, 1995; Deykin, Buka et al., 1992; Deykin & Buka, 1997; Fergusson, Harwood et al., 1993; Flory, 1996; Giaconia, Reinherz et al., 1994; Grilo, Becker et al., 1995; Hovens, Cantwell et al., 1994; Kaminer, Tarter et al., 1992; Kandel, Johnson et al., 1999; Kessler, Nelson et al., 1996; Lewisohn, Hops et al., 1993; Mason & Siris, 1992; Morrison, Smith et al., 1993; Stowell & Estroff, 1992; Weiss, Mirin et al., 1992; Westermeyer, Specker et al., 1994; Wilcox & Yates, 1993).

According to Bukstein and Kaminer (1994), however, diagnostic issues related to adolescent substance use continue to be problematic. The criteria that have been developed have not been validated with adolescents, and there may be some discontinuities between adolescent and adult populations (Bukstein & Kaminer, 1994; Clark, Kirisci et al., 1998). When diagnostic criteria are based on problem behaviors, it often is not clear whether the behaviors are the result of substance use or of a coexisting or preexisting problem. While craving and loss of control are included in the criteria, no studies have established whether these actually are present in adolescents (Bukstein & Kaminer, 1994). Nosology is only the best attempt to make sense of reality; as a result, an imperfect system designed for adults is used to make substance abuse diagnoses in adolescents (Bukstein & Kaminer 1994; Clark, Kirisci et al., 1998; Kaminer, 1994; Weinberg, Rahdert et al., 1998).

Methodological Questions. Some of the methodological questions are identical for adults and adolescents. In both populations, the course and treatment of the same two disorders may vary depending on which one is primary—in other words, which disorder preceded the other (Miller & Fine, 1993)—and their relative severity (AACAP, 1998;

Caton, Gralnick et al., 1989; King, Ghaziuddin et al., 1996; Ries, Mullen et al., 1994; Schuckit, 1985; Weiss, Mirin et al., 1992). It is not helpful to assume that all patients with dual diagnoses have the same problems and require the same treatment (Weiss, Mirin et al., 1992). Although a high prevalence of comorbidity has been reported among adolescent inpatients with drug use disorders (Clark, Bukstein et al., 1995; Clark, Lesnick et al., 1997; Grilo, Becker et al., 1995; Hovens, Cantwell et al., 1994; Kaminer, Tarter et al., 1992; Van Hasselt, Ammerman et al., 1992), it is unclear how many exhibit psychiatric symptoms secondary to the substance use disorder and how many have a primary or coexisting psychiatric diagnosis.

Miller and Fine (1993) argue that methodological considerations, including the length of abstinence required before the diagnosis is made, the population sampled, and the perspective of the examiner, affect prevalence rates for psychiatric disorders in persons who abuse substances and account for the variability. They see the prevalence rates for psychiatric disorders as artificially elevated by the tendency to make a diagnosis before abatement of some of the psychiatric symptoms that are secondary to substance use.

INCIDENCE AND PREVALENCE

Physicians should know the kinds of comorbidities they are likely to encounter in practice. Until recently, however, large-scale population studies did not focus on adolescents. The National Institute of Mental Health (NIMH) Epidemiologic Catchment Area (ECA) Study (Burke, Burke et al., 1990) attempted to estimate the true prevalence rates of alcohol, other drug abuse disorders, and mental disorders in an adult community and institutional sample of more than 20,000 subjects standardized to the U.S. Bureau of the Census. Of the total, 37% of persons with alcohol use disorders had another mental disorder, with the highest prevalence for affective, anxiety, and antisocial personality disorders. More than half of those with drug use disorders other than alcohol use had a comorbid mental disorder, including 28% with an anxiety disorders, 26% with an affective disorder, 18% with an antisocial personality disorder, and 7% with schizophrenia. This study verified the widely held impression that comorbidity rates are much higher among clinical and institutional populations than in the general population.

Until very recently, studies involving adolescents were smaller and involved clinical populations. Stowell and Estroff (1993) studied 226 adolescents receiving inpatient treatment for a primary substance abuse disorder in private psychiatric hospitals. Psychiatric diagnoses were made four weeks into treatment by using a semistructured diagnostic interview. Of the total, 82% of the patients met *DSM-IIIR* (APA, 1987) criteria for an Axis I psychiatric disorder, 61% had mood disorders, 54% had conduct disorders, 43% had anxiety disorders, and 16% had substance-induced organic disorder. Three fourths of the patients (74%) had two or more psychiatric disorders. Westermeyer and colleagues (1994) found similarly high rates of comorbidity and multiple diagnoses in 100 adolescents 12 to 20 years of age who sought care at two university-based outpatient addiction treatment programs. Of the study group, 22 of 100 had eating disorders, 8 had conduct disorders, 7 had major depressive disorder, 6 had minor depressive disorder, 5 had bipolar disorder, 5 had schizophrenia, and 4 had anxiety disorders. Three had another psychotic disorder, 3 had an organic mental disorder, and 2 had attention deficit/hyperactivity disorder (ADHD).

The distribution of diagnoses as a function of age showed that eating disorder diagnoses and depressive symptoms occurred more frequently in older adolescents (Westermeyer, Specker et al., 1994). Giaconia and colleagues (1994) studied the issue of age in a predominantly white, working-class community sample of 386 18-year-olds. They compared adolescents who had met the criteria for one of six psychiatric diagnoses, including substance use disorder, before and after they were 14 years of age. Adolescents with early onset of any psychiatric disorder were six times as likely to have one, and 12 times as likely to have two, additional disorders by the time they were 18 years of age than were those with later onset of psychiatric disorders (Giaconia, Reinherz et al., 1994). This finding suggests that the clinician's index of suspicion for dual diagnosis must be particularly high for younger patients with substance abuse disorders.

Burke and colleagues (1990) studied data from the NIMH ECA Study to determine hazard rates for the development of disorders and concluded that 15 to 19 years were the peak ages for the onset of depressive disorders in females and for the onset of substance use disorders and bipolar disorders in both sexes.

The National Comorbidity Study (NCS) included a large noninstitutional sample of persons age 15 to 24, although adolescents were not studied separately from young adults (Kessler, Nelson et al., 1996). Compared with older adults, 15- to 24-year-olds had the highest prevalence of three or more disorders occurring together and of any disorders,

including substance use disorders. The Methods for the Epidemiology of Child and Adolescent Mental Disorders study obtained data for 401 subjects age 14 to 17 (Kandel, Johnson et al., 1999). Adolescents with substance use disorders had much higher rates of mood and conduct disorder than did those without substance use disorders.

DIAGNOSIS AND MANAGEMENT

Controversies aside, psychologists, psychiatrists, and other mental health professionals need to treat the patients they encounter. Some of those patients will have a psychiatric diagnosis. Clinicians will serve such patients well if they:

1. Conduct a comprehensive evaluation of each patient that includes a mental status examination and an inquiry into other psychiatric symptomatology and obtain information from multiple sources.

2. Have a high index of suspicion for comorbidity in adolescents whose conditions do not respond to treatment or who present problems in treatment.

3. Individualize treatment to accommodate both the substance use and psychiatric diagnoses.

4. Obtain a comprehensive history of alcohol, tobacco, and other drug use.

5. Know when to consult an addiction medicine specialist or mental health professional.

Risk Factors. Certain factors put children and adolescents at risk for the development of a substance use disorder. These include:

1. Genetic factors (for example, one or both parents have a substance abuse problem).

2. Constitutional and psychological factors (psychiatric comorbidity; a history of physical, sexual, or emotional abuse; or a history of attempted suicide).

3. Sociocultural factors:

    a. Family (parental experiences and attitudes toward drug use; a history of parental divorce or separation; and low expectations for the child).

    b. Peers (friends who use drugs, friends with positive attitudes toward drug use, or antisocial or delinquent behavior).

    c. School (school failure or dropping out).

---

d. Community (approval or disapproval of drug use).

e. Economic and social deprivation.

f. Availability of drugs and alcohol (including cigarettes).

Depressive Disorders. Much has been written about the interplay between depression and substance use (Bukstein, Glancy et al., 1992; Deykin, Buka et al., 1992; Flory, 1996; Kandel, Raveis et al., 1991; Lewisohn, Hops et al., 1993; King, Ghaziuddin et al., 1996; Rao, Ryan et al., 1999; Schuckit, 1985; Schuckit, 1986; Schuckit, 1994; Wilcox & Yates, 1993). The emerging concept is that in adolescents (Bukstein, Glancy et al., 1992; Bukstein & Kaminer, 1994; Deykin, Buka et al., 1992; Hovens, Cantwell et al., 1994; King, Ghazziuddin et al., 1996; Rao, Ryan et al., 1999) and adults (Schuckit, 1985; Schuckit, 1986; Schuckit, 1994), two groups exhibit significant depressive symptoms: those individuals who have a substance-induced mood disorder and those who have a primary depressive disorders (APA, 1994). The chief symptom of depression consists of a disturbance of mood, which usually is characterized as sadness or feeling "down in the dumps," and a loss of interest or pleasure. Adolescents may report or exhibit irritability instead of sadness. In addition, their depression may be characterized by guilt, hopelessness, sleep disturbances, appetite disturbances, loss of ability to concentrate, diminution of energy, and thoughts of death or suicide.

To meet *DSM-IV* diagnostic criteria, the patient must exhibit or experience depressed mood most of the day, every day, for two weeks (APA, 1994). Patients with a substance-induced mood disorder may exhibit the same depressive symptoms.

Schuckit (1985, 1986, 1994) and Miller (1993) stress the importance of distinguishing between primary depressive disorder and substance-induced mood disorder. Studies of adults who abuse substances showed that substance-induced mood disorder dissipates with abstinence, but primary depressive disorders do not and, if left untreated, can interfere with treatment and recovery (Burke, Burke et al., 1990; Miller, 1993; Miller & Fine, 1993; Schuckit, 1985). Deykin and colleagues (1992) interviewed 223 adolescents in residential addiction treatment programs and found that almost 25% met the *DSM-IIIR* (APA, 1987) criteria for depression. Of these, 8% met the criteria for primary depression, while the other 16% had a secondary mood disorder. Bukstein and colleagues (1992) studied adoles-

cent inpatients on a dual diagnosis unit and reported that almost 31% had a comorbid major depression, with secondary depressive disorder much more common than primary depressive disorder. Unlike adults, the secondary depression in adolescents did not remit with abstinence (Bukstein, Glancy et al., 1992). This finding, if replicated, would argue for more vigorous treatment of depressive syndromes in adolescents.

During the mental status examination, depressed adolescents may seem taciturn and show poor eye contact and a sad-looking face. They may be poorly groomed or drably dressed and may become tearful during the interview. Often they deny feelings of sadness, although their demeanor states it eloquently. Depression interferes with treatment through lack of concentration, motivation, and hope, as well as the tendency toward isolation. Kempton and colleagues (1994) found cognitive distortions, including magnification (all-or-nothing thinking) and personalizing, to be particularly prominent among adolescents with the multiple diagnoses of conduct disorder, depressive disorder, and substance abuse. A depressed adolescent may benefit from a specific cognitive intervention for depression (Beck, Rush et al., 1979; Kaminer, 1994).

If the adolescent has a depressive disorder that predates his or her substance use, has a family history of depression, and has a mood disorder that interferes with treatment several weeks into abstinence despite cognitive interventions, pharmacotherapy is indicated. Serotinergic agents, such as fluoxetine, have a relatively safe profile for side effects and may be most appropriate, considering reports that many young substance users have a preexisting serotonin deficit (Crowley & Riggs, 1995; Horowitz, Overton et al., 1992; Riggs, Mikulich et al., 1997). It would be advisable, before prescribing any medication, for the physician to determine whether:

- The patient is abstinent from substances;

- His or her abstinence is secure;

- Some supports for abstinence are in place;

- The patient is in a secure drug-free environment;

- The patient will adhere to a medication regimen; and

- The patient's family will help with adherence to the medication regimen.

If there are doubts about the diagnosis of depression or about how to treat, consultation with a psychiatrist experienced in treating adolescents with substance use disorders is indicated. If the primary clinician is concerned about possible suicidal behavior, a consultation should be sought without delay (Bukstein, Brent et al., 1993; Flory, 1996; Kandel, Raveis et al., 1991).

Bipolar Disorder. The diagnosis of bipolar disorder may be among the most difficult to make in children and adolescents and is even more difficult in teens who use alcohol or other drugs. Issues such as changes in sleeping patterns or mood swings can be symptoms of bipolar disorder, substance use, or even normal adolescence. The diagnosis of bipolar disorder certainly should be considered in substance-using youth, particularly those with a binge pattern.

In bipolar disorder, which often begins during late adolescence (Burke, Burke et al., 1994; Giaconia, Reinherz et al., 1994; Wilens, Biederman et al., 1999), the initial symptoms of mania include a persistently elevated, expansive, or irritable mood lasting at least one week, accompanied by grandiosity or inflated self-esteem, decreased need for sleep, pressured speech, racing thoughts, increased purposeful activity, and excessive involvement in pleasurable activities, such as spending money, sexual indiscretions, or substance use (APA, 1994). Wilens and colleagues (1999) have found an increased risk for substance use disorders in adolescents with bipolar disorder. Children who were diagnosed and treated appropriately at a younger age had a lower subsequent risk for substance use.

Some patients use substances, particularly alcohol, to calm themselves during a manic phase. Clearly, some of these symptoms also are seen with substance intoxication. If a patient exhibits these symptoms after a period of abstinence, the diagnosis of bipolar disorder should be considered. Bipolar disorders most often are treated with mood stabilizers, the most common of which is lithium carbonate (Geller, Cooper et al., 1998). Valproic acid, carbamazepine, and other anticonvulsants also are used, as are the atypical antipsychotics, such as olanzapine and risperidone (Kaminer, 1995; Wilens, Spencer et al., 1998; Wilens, Biederman et al., 1999). Before treating for bipolar disorder, a psychiatric consultation should be obtained.

Anxiety Disorders. Anxiety disorders are among the psychiatric conditions most often coexisting in adolescents and adults with substance use disorders. Typically, these conditions include generalized anxiety disorder, panic disorder, social phobia, obsessive-compulsive disorder, and posttraumatic stress disorder (APA, 1994). Anxiety disorders often are not detected or treated, especially when present in combination with depression or psychoactive substance use disorders (Burke, Burke et al., 1994; Clark, Bukstein et al., 1995). In fact, many adolescents (and adults) believe that drugs and alcohol may contribute to reduction of anxiety and stress, and this belief may lead them to initiate or continue use. Sometimes a closer examination of patients who resist attending self-help meetings may reveal a social phobia or agoraphobia. To make matters even more confusing, some well-done studies show that teens who *never* use drugs or alcohol may be at higher risk for anxiety disorders later in life.

Panic Disorder: Panic attacks are periods of intense discomfort that develop abruptly and reach a peak within 10 minutes. Symptoms include palpitations, sweating, trembling, sensations of shortness of breath or choking, chest discomfort, nausea, dizziness, and fears of losing control or dying. Since some of these symptoms also might be seen in substance intoxication or withdrawal, it is important to establish abstinence before making a diagnosis.

Social Phobias: Patients with a social phobia may isolate themselves on an inpatient unit or in a group. A careful interview in which anxiety symptoms and family history of anxiety disorders are pursued may be quite revealing.

Behavioral treatment, including relaxation training, often is helpful for anxiety disorders (Kaminer, 1994). The issue of pharmacotherapy is controversial. Many argue that the use of benzodiazepines is contraindicated in anyone with a history of substance abuse. Buspirone hydrochloride and serotonin reuptake inhibitors have been recommended as non-addictive antianxiety agents (Wilens, Spencer et al., 1998). Clinical experience and anecdotal reports suggest that for many, buspirone is ineffective. When treating patients who insist that only benzodiazepines are effective, it often is not clear whether the statement represents drug-seeking behavior or a *bona fide* observation. If abstinence has been established, adequate trials of behavioral or cognitive therapy (Kaminer, 1994) and alternative medications have failed, and the patient adheres to the treatment and medication regimen, the judicious use of a long-acting benzodiazepine, such as clonazepam, may be justified.

Posttraumatic Stress Disorder (PTSD): In clinical reports on adolescents, the incidence of severe trauma and symptoms of posttraumatic stress disorder is surprisingly high (Clark, Bukstein et al., 1995; Clark, Lesnick et al., 1997; Deykin & Buka, 1997; Kandel, Johnson et al., 1999; Van Hasselt, Ammerman et al., 1992). An adolescent who has been acting out and abusing substances may not have dealt with an earlier trauma, such as physical and sexual abuse or exposure to violence, or with the trauma that may be incurred when abusing substances (Clark, Lesnick et al., 1997). Symptoms and memories of trauma may manifest themselves only during abstinence.

Symptoms of posttraumatic stress disorder can be divided into three groups (APA, 1994). The first group involves reexperiencing the trauma through intrusive thoughts, dreams, or flashbacks, which make the person feel as if the event is reoccurring. In the second, the patient has a numbing of general responsiveness and avoids thinking about the trauma. In the third group, there are symptoms of increased arousal, including difficulty sleeping, irritability, hypervigilance, and an exaggerated startle response.

Trauma and the symptoms associated with trauma should to be considered and inquired about to ensure adequate treatment of adolescents who abuse substances. Care should be taken to acknowledge the trauma without arousing anxiety that will interfere with abstinence and substance abuse treatment. Groups that support self-care and a first-things-first attitude may be the best approach; the patient needs to learn to stay safe, and treatment for substance abuse is a most important aspect of safety. The patient can be counseled that recovery is a process and must be taken in stages and that some of the effects of the trauma can be dealt with later when the patient's abstinence and safety is better established.

Organic Mental Disorders. In some patients, the use of substances—particularly alcohol, marijuana, cocaine, ecstasy, hallucinogens, and inhalants—is associated with acute and residual cognitive damage (APA, 1994; Kempton, Van Hasselt et al., 1994; Stowell & Estroff, 1993). Acute symptoms may include impaired concentration and receptive and expressive language abilities, as well as irritability. Long-term interference with memory and other executive functions may occur.

The possibility of a substance-induced dementia should be considered in adolescents who have difficulty coping with the cognitive and organizational demands of a structured and supportive program. Some adolescents will be able to use the program if instructions are simplified and if they comprehend information accurately. Improvement in cognitive functioning may be rapid, but the cognitive functioning of some patients continues to improve for as long as a year or more after cessation of the chemical assault to the brain. Some may be left with residual impairments.

Adolescents and their families should be informed of the cognitive consequences of their substance use in a way that does not engender despair, but clearly warns against further alcohol or drug use. The presence of cognitive deficits, if they persist, should be considered in rehabilitation, educational, and vocational planning. Such patients need neuropsychological evaluation and followup.

Schizophrenia. Patients who simultaneously meet the criteria for schizophrenia and a substance use disorder are less likely to receive treatment in an addiction treatment program than in a psychiatric unit (Caton, Gralnick et al., 1989; Ries, Mullen et al., 1994). As the late adolescent years are a time when many schizophrenic disorders begin, and the use of substances may precipitate an incipient psychosis, patients with this disorder may seek treatment during the early stages of schizophrenia (Kaminer, Tarter et al., 1992; Miller & Fine, 1993; Ries, 1993b). The characteristic symptoms are hallucinations (most often auditory), delusions, disorganized speech, grossly disorganized or catatonic behavior, and negative symptoms, including flattening of affect, impoverished speech, or avolition (APA, 1994). Therefore, for patients with bizarre manifestations that seem grossly different from the rest of the treatment population, the diagnosis of schizophrenia should be considered.

Increasingly, younger schizophrenic patients use substances (Buckley, 1999; Minkoff, 1989; Ries, 1993b), some in an attempt to manage or deny their symptoms. Their substance use often interferes with treatment of their psychotic disorder. Such patients are best managed in special dual diagnosis programs for psychotic patients, where the psychosis and the substance use are addressed through integrated mental health and addiction treatment (Buckley, 1999; Caton, Gralnick et al., 1989; Costello, Costello et al., 1988; Mason & Siris, 1992; Minkoff, 1989; Ries, 1993a; Ries, Mullen et al., 1994; Van Hasselt, Ammerman et al., 1992).

Attention Deficit/Hyperactivity Disorder (ADHD). Many professionals involved in the treatment of adolescents with substance use disorders have noted the large number who also have attention deficit/hyperactivity disorder (AACAP, 1998; AAP, 2000; Crowley & Riggs, 1995; Morrison, Smith et al., 1993; Riggs, 1998; Wilcox & Yates, 1993; Wilens, Biederman et al., 1996). Bukstein and colleagues (1989) postulate that there is no direct connection, but that both often coexist with conduct disorder. Crowley and Riggs (1995) noted comorbidity with affective, anxiety, and antisocial disorders in the patients and their families.

Symptoms of ADHD include inattention (such as failure to listen), difficulty with organization, the tendency to lose objects, easy distractibility, hyperactivity, and impulsivity (such as fidgeting, restlessness, and the tendency to interrupt) (AAP, 2000; APA, 1994). These symptoms must be present in more than one setting. The use of rating scales may be helpful in establishing the diagnosis and monitoring the patient's progress.

Treatment should include behavioral and educational interventions. Pharmacotherapy for adolescents has been controversial; some have argued that the use of psychostimulants may predispose adolescents to abuse other substances (Riggs, 1998). Riggs and colleagues (1998) have reported some success with the use of bupropion. Wilens and colleagues (1996) suggest that the use of stimulants to treat adolescents for ADHD may lower the risk of a subsequent substance use disorder. Because the successful treatment of substance abuse involves teaching patients to plan and to delay impulses, the effective treatment of ADHD is a necessary part of an integrated plan.

Conduct Disorder and Antisocial Personality Disorder. Conduct disorder and antisocial personality disorder are the diagnoses that most often co-occur with substance abuse, particularly in males (AACAP, 1998; Crowley & Riggs, 1995; Kaminer, Tarter et al., 1992; Kandel, Johnson et al., 1999; King, Glaziuddin et al., 1996; Rao, Ryan et al., 1999; Schuckit, 1985; Stowell & Estroff, 1992; Westermeyer, Specker et al., 1994; Wilcox & Yates, 1993; Wilens, Biederman et al., 1996). The characteristic symptom of antisocial personality disorder is a pervasive pattern of disregarding and violating the rights of others. The disorder may involve deceitfulness, impulsivity, failure to conform to rules or the law, aggressiveness, and irresponsibility (APA, 1994). Conduct disorder has similar criteria but includes manifestations that are likely to be seen in younger persons, such as cruelty to animals, running away, truancy, and vandalism.

Many researchers have noted that adolescent substance use disorder usually occurs as part of a constellation of problem behaviors (Crowley & Riggs, 1995; Fergusson, Horwood et al., 1993; Kandel, Johnson et al., 1999; Morrison, Smith et al., 1993; Riggs, 1998). Cloninger (1987) presented an interesting scheme of hereditary factors on three axes that may account for many psychiatric diagnoses and their interrelationships. The three axes are reward-dependence, harm-avoidance, and novelty seeking. Based on these axes, Cloninger (1987) distinguished type 1 and type 2 alcoholic

patients. Type 2 alcoholic patients score low on reward-dependence and harm-avoidance and high on novelty seeking. Younger alcoholic patients with antisocial personality fit the type 2 classification. The higher prevalence of antisocial personality and conduct disorders among younger alcoholic patients may explain why many clinicians find adolescent substance abusers more difficult to treat.

Horowitz and colleagues (1992) consider many young patients who abuse substances to have a combination of characteristics (such as increased hostility, depression, and suicidal ideation) that suggest an underlying—perhaps neurochemically determined—difficulty with self-regulation and aggression. Adolescents with conduct disorders and antisocial personality disorder need a strong behavioral program with clear limits. If there is a comorbid disorder (such as a mood or attention disorder that can be treated successfully), the adolescent is more likely to do well (Crowley & Riggs, 1995; Riggs 1998; Wilens, Spencer et al., 1996).

Borderline and Narcissistic Personality Disorders. In addition to psychiatric diagnoses on Axis I, the personality disorders described on Axis II of the *DSM-IV* are relevant to the treatment of adolescents who abuse substances (APA, 1994; Groves, 1978; Myers, Burket et al., 1993). Personality disorders are enduring patterns of inner experience and behavior that affect cognition, interpersonal behavior, emotional response, and impulse control. Personality factors often make an adolescent difficult to treat.

Borderline personality disorder is marked by impulsivity and instability of interpersonal relationships, which affect self-image. A marked sensitivity and wish to avoid abandonment, chronic feelings of emptiness, inappropriate and intense anger, and suicidal or self-mutilating behavior are characteristic of borderline personality disorder. In a treatment setting, patients with borderline personality disorder can wreak havoc because of the severe regression often manifested and the divisiveness they often cause among staff.

A pervasive pattern of grandiosity, a need for admiration, and a lack of empathy characterize narcissistic personality disorder. The patient feels unique and entitled to special treatment. A patient with narcissistic personality disorder may have difficulty participating in groups or seeing other people except as need gratifiers.

Both of these personality disorders can present challenges to the clinician and the treatment staff. Powerful negative feelings, conscious and unconscious (King, Glaziuddin et al., 1996), are easily aroused by patients who are manipulative and full of rage, who feel entitled, and whose behavior saps the emotional strength of the staff (Groves, 1978). If the treatment of a patient requires a great deal of emotional energy, personality issues likely are involved. In such situations, it is essential to be aware of the effect that such patients exert and to take care of the clinical staff as well as the patient.

Eating Disorders. The incidence of eating disorders and substance abuse in the adolescent population has increased (Katz, 1990; Westermeyer, Specker et al., 1994; Westermeyer & Specker, 1999), so it is not uncommon to find them together. In fact, a fourth of all patients who have an eating disorder either have a history of substance abuse or currently are abusing substances (Katz, 1990).

Anorexia nervosa, which involves weight restriction and increased activity, a distorted body image, and an intense fear of losing control and becoming fat (APA, 1994), is not as prevalent as bulimia in the general population and among persons who abuse substances. Bulimia involves recurrent episodes of binge eating, sometimes accompanied by compensatory measures (such as vomiting or laxative abuse), and a preoccupation with food and weight. Of all eating disorders, 90% to 95% occur in females (Katz, 1990). Although anorexic patients have a characteristic emaciated appearance, bulimic patients can be any weight. Patients who consistently spend time in the bathroom after meals may be purging.

Persons with an eating disorder may abuse amphetamines to lose weight. Katz (1990) postulates that the proneness to substance abuse in bulimic patients may be due to borderline personality features.

CONCLUSIONS

In sum, psychiatric disorders and substance use disorders often occur together, complicating assessment and treatment. An awareness of the prevalence and manifestations of psychiatric diagnoses is essential to high-quality treatment of adolescents. An ongoing relationship with a psychiatrist who can be available for consultation as needed is helpful. Clinicians also should keep current on psychopharmacologic interventions (Kaminer, 1995; Solhkhah & Wilens, 1998). Often, the use of psychiatric medications such as antidepressants, mood stabilizers, psychostimulants, and others is of benefit. However, care must be taken to avoid potential interactions between the illicit drugs and the prescribed medications (Wilens et al., 1997). Also, self-help groups such as Alcoholics Anonymous, Narcotics Anonymous, or "Double-Trouble" groups for patients with

co-occurring psychiatric and addictive disorders can be a useful adjunct to treatment (Brown, 1993; Hohman & LeCroy, 1996; Simkin, 1996).

Careful observation, history taking, and appropriate consultation result in better detection and treatment of comorbid disorders and, ultimately, of the initial substance abuse problem.

REFERENCES

American Academy of Child and Adolescent Psychiatry (1998). Practice parameters for the assessment and treatment of children and adolescents with substance abuse disorders. *Journal of the American Academy of Child and Adolescent Psychiatry* 37:122-126.

American Academy of Pediatrics, Committee on Quality Improvement, Subcommittee on Attention-Deficit/Hyperactivity Disorder (1999). Diagnosis and evaluation of the child with attention-deficit/hyperactivity disorder. *Pediatrics* 105:1158-1170.

American Academy of Pediatrics, Committee on Substance Abuse. (2000). Indications for management and referral of patients involved in substance abuse. *Pediatrics* 106:143-148.

American Psychiatric Association (1987). *Diagnostic and Statistical Manual of Mental Disorders, 3rd Edition, Revised (DSM-IIIR)*. Washington, DC: American Psychiatric Press.

American Psychiatric Association (1994). *Diagnostic and Statistical Manual of Mental Disorders, 4th Edition (DSM-IV)*. Washington, DC: American Psychiatric Press.

Armentano M (1995). Assessment, diagnosis, and treatment of the dually diagnosed adolescent. *Pediatric Clinics of North America* 42:479-490.

Beck AT, Rush AJ, Shaw BF et al. (1979). *Cognitive Therapy of Depression*. New York, NY: Guilford Press.

Brook JS, Whiteman M, Cohen P et al. (1995). Longitudinally predicting late adolescent and young adult drug use: Childhood and adolescent precursors. *Journal of the American Academy of Child and Adolescent Psychiatry* 34:1230-1238.

Brown SA (1993). Recovery patterns in adolescent substance abuse. In JS Bae, GA Marlatt & RJ McMahon (eds.) *Addictive Behaviors Across the Life Span: Prevention, Treatment, and Policy Issues*. Newbury Park, CA: Sage Publications, 161-183.

Buckley PF (1999). Substance abuse in schizophrenia: A review. *Journal of Clinical Psychiatry* 59(Suppl 3):26-30.

Bukstein O, Brent DA & Kaminer Y (1992). Comorbidity of substance and other psychiatric disorders in adolescents. *American Journal of Psychiatry* 1131-1141.

Bukstein O, Brent DA, Perper JA et al. (1993). Risk factors for completed suicide among adolescents with a lifetime history of substance abuse: A case-control study. *Acta Psychiatrica Scandinavica* 88(6):403-408.

Bukstein O, Glancy LJ & Kaminer Y (1992). Patterns of affective comorbidity in a clinical population of dually diagnosed adolescent substance abusers. *Journal of the American Academy of Child and Adolescent Psychiatry* 31(6):1041-1045.

Bukstein O & Kaminer T (1994). The nosology of adolescent substance abuse. *American Journal on Addictions* Winter:1-13.

Burke JD, Burke KC & Rae DS (1994). Increased rates of drug abuse and dependence after onset of mood or anxiety disorders in adolescence. *Hospital & Community Psychiatry* 45(5):451-455.

Burke KC, Burke JD, Regier DA & Rae DS (1990). Age at onset of selected mental disorders in five community populations. *Archives of General Psychiatry* 47:511-518.

Buydens-Branchey L, Branchey MH & Noumair D (1989). Age of alcoholism onset: I. Relationship to psychopathology. *Archives of General Psychiatry* 46:225-230.

Buydens-Branchey L, Branchey MH, Noumair D & Lieber CS (1989). Age of alcoholism onset: II. Relationship to susceptibility to serotonin precursor availability. *Archives of General Psychiatry* 46:231-236.

Caton CLM, Gralnick A, Bender S & Simon M (1989). Young chronic patients and substance abuse. *Hospital & Community Psychiatry* 1037-1040.

Christie KA, Burke JD et al. (1988). Epidemiologic evidence for early onset of mental disorders and higher risk of drug abuse in young adults. *American Journal of Psychiatry* 145:971-975.

Clark DB & Bukstein OG (1998). Psychopathology in adolescent alcohol abuse and dependence. *Alcohol Research & Health* 22:117-126.

Clark DB, Bukstein O, Smith MG et al. (1995). Identifying anxiety disorders in adolescents hospitalized for alcohol abuse and dependence. *Psychiatric Services* 46:618-620.

Clark DB, Kirisci L & Tarter RE (1998). Adolescent versus adult onset and the development of substance abuse disorders in males. *Drug and Alcohol Dependence* 49:115-121.

Clark DB, Lesnick L & Hegedus AM (1997). Traumas and other adverse life events in adolescents with alcohol use and dependence. *Journal of the American Academy of Child and Adolescent Psychiatry* 36:1744-1751.

Cloninger CR (1987). Neurogenetic adaptive mechanisms in alcoholism. *Science* 410-416.

Costello EJ, Costello AJ, Edelbrock C et al. (1988). Psychiatric disorders in pediatric primary care. *Archives of General Psychiatry* 45:1107-1116.

Crowley TJ & Riggs PD (1995). Adolescent substance use disorder with conduct disorder and comorbid conditions. In E Rahdert & D Czechowicz (eds.) *Adolescent Substance Abuse (NIDA Research Monograph 156)*. Rockville, MD: National Institute on Drug Abuse, 49-111.

DeMilio L (1989). Psychiatric syndromes in adolescent substance abusers. *American Journal of Psychiatry* 146:1212-1214.

Deykin EY & Buka SL (1997). Prevalence and risk factors for posttraumatic stress disorder among chemically dependent adolescents. *American Journal of Psychiatry* 154:752-757.

Deykin EY, Buka SL & Zeena TH (1992). Depressive illness among chemically dependent adolescents. *American Journal of Psychiatry* 149:1341-1347.

Fergusson DM, Horwood LJ & Lynskey MT (1993). Prevalence and comorbidity of DSM-IIIR diagnoses in a birth cohort of 15 year olds. *Journal of the American Academy of Child and Adolescent Psychiatry* 32(6):1127-1134.

Flory M (1996). Psychiatric diagnosis in child and adolescent suicide. *Archives of General Psychiatry* 53(4):339-348.

Geller B, Cooper TB, Sun K et al. (1998). Double-blind and placebo-controlled study of lithium for adolescent bipolar disorders with secondary substance dependency. *Journal of the American Academy of Child and Adolescent Psychiatry* 37:171-178.

Giaconia RM, Reinherz HZ, Silverman AB et al. (1994). Ages of onset of psychiatric disorders in a community population of older adolescents. *Journal of the American Academy of Child and Adolescent Psychiatry* 33(5):706-717.

Grilo CM, Becker DF, Walker ML et al. (1995). Psychiatric comorbidity in adolescent inpatients with substance use disorders. *Journal of the American Academy of Child and Adolescent Psychiatry* 34(8):1085-1091.

Groves JE (1978). The hateful patient. *New England Journal of Medicine* 298:883-887.

Hohman M & LeCroy CW (1996). Predictors of adolescent AA affiliation. *Adolescence* 31:339-352.

Horowitz HA, Overton WF, Rosenstein D et al. (1992). Comorbid adolescent substance abuse: A maladaptive pattern of self-regulation. *Adolescent Psychiatry*.

Hovens JG, Cantwell DP & Kiriakos R (1994). Psychiatric comorbidity in hospitalized adolescent substance abusers. *Journal of the American Academy of Child and Adolescent Psychiatry* 33(4):476-483.

Kaminer Y (1994). *Adolescent Substance Abuse: A Comprehensive Guide to Theory and Practice*. New York, NY: Plenum Medical Books.

Kaminer Y (1995). Pharmacotherapy for adolescents with psychoactive substance use disorders. In E Rahdert & D Czechowicz (eds.) *Adolescent Substance Abuse (NIDA Research Monograph 156)*. Rockville, MD: National Institute on Drug Abuse, 291-324.

Kaminer Y (1991). The magnitude of concurrent psychiatric disorders in hospitalized substance abusing adolescents. *Journal of Abnormal Child Psychology* 25:122-132.

Kaminer Y, Tarter RE, Bukstein OG et al. (1992). Comparison between treatment completers and noncompleters among dually diagnosed substance-abusing adolescents. *Journal of the American Academy of Child and Adolescent Psychiatry* 31:1046-1049.

Kandel DB, Johnson JG, Bird H et al. (1997). Psychiatric disorders associated with substance use among children and adolescents: Findings from the methods for the epidemiology of child and adolescent mental disorders (MECA) study. *Journal of Abnormal Child Psychology* 25:122-132.

Kandel DB, Johnson JG, Bird HR et al. (1999). Psychiatric comorbidity among adolescents with substance use disorders: Findings from the MECA study. *Journal of the American Academy of Child and Adolescent Psychiatry* 38:693-699.

Kandel DB, Raveis VH & Davies M (1991). Suicidal ideation in adolescence: Depression, substance use, and other risk factors. *Journal of Youth and Adolescence* 20:289-309.

Kashani JH, Keller MB, Solomon N et al. (1985). Double depression in adolescent substance abusers. *Journal of Affective Disorders* 8:153-157.

Katz JL (1990). Eating disorders: a primer for the substance abuse specialist, I: Clinical features. *Journal of Substance Abuse Treatment* 7:143-149.

Kellam SG, Ensminger ME & Simon MB (1980). Mental health in first grade and teenage drug, alcohol, and cigarette use. *Drug and Alcohol Dependence* 5:273-304.

Kempton T, Van Hasselt VB, Bukstein OG et al. (1994). Cognitive distortions and psychiatric diagnosis in dually diagnosed adolescents. *Journal of the American Academy of Child and Adolescent Psychiatry* 33:217-222.

Kessler RC, Nelson CB, McGonagle KA et al. (1996). The epidemiology of co-occurring addictive and mental disorders: Implications for prevention and service utilization. *American Journal of Orthopsychiatry* 66:17-31.

King C, Ghaziuddin N, McGovern L et al. (1996). Predictors of comorbid alcohol and substance abuse in depressed adolescents. *Journal of the American Academy of Child and Adolescent Psychiatry* 35:743-751.

King CA, Naylor MW, Hill EM et al. (1992). Dysthymia characteristic of heavy alcohol use in depressed adolescents. *Biological Psychiatry* 33:210-212.

Lewisohn PM, Hops H, Roberts RE et al. (1993). Adolescent psychopathology I: Prevalence and incidence of depression and other DSM-IIIR disorders in high school students. *Journal of Abnormal Psychology* 102:133-144.

Mason SE & Siris SG (1992). Dual diagnosis: The case for case management. *American Journal on the Addictions* 77-82.

Milin R, Halikas JA, Meller JE et al. (1991). Psychopathology among substance abusing juvenile offenders. *Journal of the American Academy of Child and Adolescent Psychiatry* 30:569-574.

Miller NS (1993). Comorbidity of psychiatric and alcohol/drug disorders: Interactions and independent status. *Journal of Addictive Diseases* 12:5-16.

Miller NS & Fine J (1993). Current epidemiology of comorbidity of psychiatric and addictive disorders. *Psychiatric Clinics of North America* 16:1-10.

Minkoff K (1989). An integrated treatment model for dual diagnosis of psychosis and addiction. *Hospital & Community Psychiatry* 40:1031-1036.

Morrison MA, Smith DE, Wilford BB et al. (1993). At war in the fields of play: Current perspectives on the nature and treatment of adolescent chemical dependency. *Journal of Psychoactive Drugs* 25(41):321-330.

Morrison MA & Smith QT (1987). Psychiatric issues of adolescent chemical dependence. *Pediatric Clinics of North America* 34(2):461-479.

Myers WC, Burket RC & Otto TA (1993). Conduct disorders and personality disorders in hospitalized adolescents. *Journal of Clinical Psychiatry* 54(1):21-26.

Olfson M & Klerman G (1992). The treatment of depression: Prescribing practices of primary care physicians and psychiatrists. *Journal of Family Practice* 35(6):627-635.

Rao U, Ryan ND, Dahl RE et al. (1999). Factors associated with the development of substance use disorder in depressed adolescents. *Journal of the American Academy of Child and Adolescent Psychiatry* 38:1109-1117.

Ries RK (1993a). Clinical treatment matching models for dually diagnosed patients. *Psychiatric Clinics of North America* 16.

Ries R (1993b). The dually diagnosed patient with psychotic symptoms. *Journal of Addictive Diseases* 12:103-122.

Ries R, Mullen M & Cox G (1994). Symptom severity and utilization of treatment resources among dually diagnosed inpatients. *Hospital & Community Psychiatry* 45:562-568.

Riggs PD (1998). Clinical approach to treatment of ADHD in adolescents with substance use disorders and conduct disorder. *Journal of the American Academy of Child and Adolescent Psychiatry* 37:331-332.

Riggs PD, Mikulich SC, Coffman L et al. (1997). Fluoxetine in drug-dependent delinquents with major depression: An open trial. *Journal of Child and Adolescent Psychopharmacology* 7:87-95.

Riggs PD, Mikulich SC & Pottle LC (1998). An open trial of bupropion for ADHD in adolescents with substance use disorder and conduct disorder. *Journal of the American Academy of Child and Adolescent Psychiatry* 37:1271-1278.

Ross HE, Glaser FB & Germanson T (1988). The prevalence of psychiatric disorders in patients with alcohol and other drug problems. *Archives of General Psychiatry* 45:1023-1031.

Schuckit MA (1994). Alcohol and depression: A clinical perspective. *Acta Psychiatrica Scandinavica* 377(Suppl):28-32.

Schuckit MA (1986). Genetic and clinical implications of alcoholism and affective disorder. *American Journal of Psychiatry* 143(2):140-147.

Schuckit MA (1985). The clinical implications of primary diagnostic groups among alcoholics. *Archives of General Psychiatry* 1043-1049.

Schuckit MA & Chiles JA (1978). Family history as a diagnostic aid in two samples of adolescents. *Journal of Nervous and Mental Diseases* 166(3):165-176.

Simkin DR (1996). Twelve-step treatment from a developmental perspective. *Child and Adolescent Psychiatric Clinics of North America* 5:165-175.

Solhkhah R & Wilens TE (1998). Pharmacotherapy of adolescent alcohol and other drug use. *Alcohol Health & Research World* 22:122-125.

Stowell JA & Estroff TW (1993). Psychiatric disorders in substance abusing adolescent inpatients: A pilot study. *Journal of the American Academy of Child and Adolescent Psychiatry*.

Van Hasselt VB, Ammerman RT, Glancy LJ & Bukstein OG (1992). Maltreatment in psychiatrically hospitalized dually diagnosed adolescent substance abusers. *Journal of the American Academy of Child and Adolescent Psychiatry* 31(5):868-874.

Weinberg NZ, Rahdert E, Colliver JD et al. (1998). Adolescent substance abuse: A review of the past 10 years. *Journal of the American Academy of Child and Adolescent Psychiatry* 37:252-261.

Weiss RD, Mirin SM & Frances RJ (1992). The myth of the typical dual diagnosis patient. *Hospital & Community Psychiatry* 43:107-108.

Westermeyer J & Specker S (1999). Social resources and social function in comorbid eating and substance disorder: a matched-pairs study. *American Journal on Addictions* 8:332-336.

Westermeyer J, Specker S, Neider J et al. (1994). Substance abuse and associated psychiatric disorder among 100 adolescents. *Journal of Addictive Diseases* 67-89.

Wilcox JA & Yates WR (1993). Gender and psychiatric comorbidity in substance-abusing individuals. *American Journal on Addictions* 202-206.

Wilens TE, Biederman J, Millstein RB et al. (1999). Risk for substance use disorders in youths with child- and adolescent-onset bipolar disorder. *Journal of the American Academy of Child and Adolescent Psychiatry* 38:680-685.

Wilens TE, Biederman J & Spencer TJ (1996). Attention deficit hyperactivity disorder and psychoactive substance use disorders. *Child and Adolescent Psychiatric Clinics of North America* 5:73-91.

Wilens TE, Biederman J & Spencer TJ (1997). Case study: Adverse effects of smoking marijuana while receiving tricyclic antidepressants. *Journal of the American Academy of Child and Adolescent Psychiatry* 36:45-48.

Wilens T, Spencer T, Frazier J et al. (1998). Psychopharmacology in children and adolescents. In T Ollendick & M Hersen (eds.) *Handbook of Child Psychopathology*. New York, NY: Plenum Publishing, 603-636.

Wolraich MI, Felice ME & Drotar D, eds. (1996). *Classification of Childhood Mental Disorders in Primary Care*. Elk Grove Village, IL: American Academy of Pediatrics.

Appendices

<table>
<tr><td>Appendix 1</td><td>

Federal Schedules
of Controlled Drugs

</td></tr>
</table>

CSA Schedules
Other Requirements
Prescribing Authority
State Requirements

Since 1912, international drug control treaties have required governments to restrict the production, distribution, and consumption of psychoactive drugs. While such treaties have created stringent control mechanisms, they also have required international organizations to work with national governments to ensure that the restrictions are not so rigid as to negatively affect patients' access to essential drugs.

In the United States, the first federal law on drug distribution was adopted in 1914. Since that time, the Congress has enacted many statutes to regulate the manufacture, importation, distribution, and use of pharmaceutical products. For example, the Comprehensive Drug Abuse Prevention and Control Act of 1970 consolidated more than 50 federal drug laws into one comprehensive vehicle. The federal Controlled Substances Act (CSA; Title II of the Drug Abuse Prevention and Control Act) created a system for classifying prescription drugs according to their importance in medical use and their potential for abuse. The latter Act also required written prescriptions for Schedule II drugs, regulated recordkeeping and refills, created information systems to detect diversion, and established a system of criminal penalties for violations.

Responsibility for administering the federal CSA is assigned to the Drug Enforcement Administration (DEA) in the U.S. Department of Justice. The DEA is charged with enforcing the provisions of the Act that regulate the manufacture, purchase, prescribing, and dispensing of controlled substances, including (1) registration of physicians, pharmacists, and other handlers; (2) recordkeeping and inspection requirements; (3) quotas on manufacturing; (4) restrictions on distribution; (5) restrictions on dispensing; (6) limitations on imports and exports; (7) conditions for storage of drugs; (8) reports of transactions to the government; and (9) criminal, civil, and administrative penalties for illegal acts.

CSA SCHEDULES

Psychotropic drugs that are judged likely to be abused are subject to the provisions of the federal Controlled Substances Act and companion state acts; they include the drug classes outlined below.

Schedule I includes drugs and other substances that have a high potential for abuse and no currently accepted medical use. Examples include certain opium derivatives (such as heroin), some synthetic opioids (for example, alpha-methylfentanyl), and hallucinogens (such as LSD).

Schedule II includes drugs that have a high potential for abuse and an accepted medical use, and the abuse of which leads to severe psychological or physical dependence. Drugs in this schedule include many opioids (such as morphine, methadone, and newer analgesics such as controlled-release oxycodone [OxyContin®]), stimulants (such as amphetamines and related compounds), and the short-acting barbiturates (such as amobarbital).

Schedule III includes drugs that have less potential for abuse than those in Schedule II, leading to moderate dependence, and accepted medical use. Drugs in this schedule include certain CNS stimulants and depressants (for example, barbiturates not included in other schedules), as well as preparations containing limited quantities of codeine.

Schedule IV includes drugs that have a low potential for abuse, leading to limited dependence, and accepted medical use. Drugs in this schedule include sedative-hypnotics (principally the benzodiazepines), opioids (propoxyphene), and mixed opioid agonist-antagonists (pentazocine).

Schedule V includes drugs that have a low abuse potential, leading to limited dependence, and accepted medical use. Drugs in this schedule include a few over-the-counter preparations, such as antitussive, antidiarrheal, and other mixtures that combine limited quantities of opioids with nonopioid drugs.

OTHER REQUIREMENTS

The Controlled Substances Act provides that no prescription order for drugs in Schedule II may be refilled. Emergency telephone prescriptions for drugs in Schedule II may be dispensed if the practitioner furnishes a written, signed prescription order to the pharmacy within 72 hours and limits the amount ordered to what is needed during the emergency period.

Prescription orders for drugs in Schedules III and IV may be redispensed up to five times within six months after the date of issue, if authorized by the prescriber.

Drug Samples. The Act does not prevent physicians from receiving or dispensing drug samples; however, such physicians are required to sign a written request, specifying the identity of the drug sample and the quantity requested.

PRESCRIBING AUTHORITY

Physicians and other licensed professionals may prescribe, dispense, and administer controlled drugs for legitimate medical purposes and in the course of professional practice if they have a state license to practice their profession and a valid controlled substances registration from the U.S. Drug Enforcement Administration (DEA, 1990).

Moreover, the Controlled Substances Act recognizes that controlled substances are essential to the public health and that availability of such medications must be ensured. The Act states that "many of the drugs included within this title have a useful and legitimate medical purpose and are necessary to maintain the health and general welfare of the American people" (CSA, 1970, p. 834).

Information on the Act, as well as updates on specific scheduling decisions, is available at the DEA's web site (www.DEADIVERSION.USDOJ.GOV).

STATE REQUIREMENTS

Information in the table that follows reflects federal law. States can and do schedule drugs more restrictively. Therefore, all prescribers are advised to familiarize themselves with applicable state laws and regulations.

REFERENCES

Controlled Substances Act of 1970. Public Law 91-513, 84 Stat 1242.

Drug Enforcement Administration (1994). *Physician's Manual: An Informational Outline of the Controlled Substances Act of 1970.* Washington, DC: U.S. Department of Justice, Drug Enforcement Administration.

National Association of Boards of Pharmacy (NABP) (1998). *Survey of Pharmacy Law, 1998-1999.* Park Ridge, IL: NABP.

National Conference of Commissioners on Uniform State Laws (1994). *Uniform Controlled Substances Act.* Chicago, IL: NCCUSL.

United Nations (1977). *Single Convention on Psychotropic Drugs, 1971.* New York, NY: United Nations.

Wilford BB (1990). *Prescribing Controlled Drugs.* Chicago, IL: American Medical Association, 32-73.

Appendix 1 Federal Schedules of Controlled Drugs

	Schedule I	Schedule II	Schedule III	Schedule IV	Schedule V

OPIODS	Benzylmorphine
	Dihydromorphinone
	Heroin
	Ketobemidone
	Levomoramide
	Morphine-
	  methylsulfanote
	Nicocodeine
	Nicomorphine
	Racemoramide
		Codeine
		  compounds
		Fentanyl
		  Sublimaze®
		Hydromorphone
		  Dilaudid®
		LAAM
		Meperidine
		  Demerol®
		Methadone
		Morphine
		Oxycodone
		  OxyContin®
		  Percocet®
		  Percodan®
		Oxymorphone
		  Numorphan®
		Pantopon
			Buprenorphine
			  Buprenex®
			  Subutex®
			Codeine
			  compounds
			  Tylenol #3®
			  Tussionex®
				Propoxyphene
				  Darvon®
				  Darvocet®
					Opium
					  preparations
					  Donnagel PG®
					  Kaopectalin PG®

OPIOID ANTAGONISTS			Buprenorphine
			  + naloxone
			  Suboxone®
				Pentazocine
				  Talwin®	

STIMULANTS	N-methylamphetamine
	3,4-methylenedioxy-
	  methamphetamine
	  MDMA, Ecstasy
		Amphetamines
		Cocaine
		Dextroamphetamine
		  Dexedrine®
		Methamphetamine
		  Desoxyn®
		Methylphenidate
		  Ritalin®
		Phenmetrazine
		  Fastin®
		  Preludin®
			Benzphetamine
			  Didrex®
			Phendimetrazine
			  Plegine®
				Diethylpropion
				  Tenuate®
				Fenfluramine
				Phentermine
				  Fastin®
					1-deoxyephedrine
					  Vicks® Inhaler

HALLUCINOGENS, OTHER	Lysergic acid diamine
	  LSD
	Marijuana
	Mescaline
	Peyote
	Phencyclidine
	  PCP
	Psilocybin
	Tetrahydrocannabinols
			Dronabinol
			  Marinol®
			Testosterone		

SOURCES: U.S. Drug Enforcement Administration, Office of Diversion Control (2003).

	Schedule I	**Schedule II**	**Schedule III**	**Schedule IV**	**Schedule V**
SEDATIVE-HYPNOTICS	Methaqualone *Quaalude®* Gamma- hydroxybutyrate *GHB*	Amobarbital *Amytal®* Glutethimide *Doriden®* Pentobarbital *Nembutal®* Secobarbital *Seconal®*	Butabarbital *Butisol®* Butalbital *Fiorecet®* *Fiorinal®* Methyprylon *Noludar®*	Alprazolam *Xanax®* Chloral betaine Chloral hydrate *Noctec®* Chlordiazepoxide *Librium®* Clonazepam *Klonopin®* Clorazepate *Tranxene®* Diazepam *Valium®* Estazolam *Prosom®* Ethchlorvynol *Placidyl®* Ethinamate Flurazepam *Dalmane®* Halazepam *Paxipam®* Lorazepam *Ativan®* Mazindol *Sanorex®* Mephobarbital *Mebaral®* Meprobamate *Equanil®* Methohexital *Brevital Sodium®* Methylphenobarbital Midazolam *Versed®* Oxazepam *Serax®* Paraldehyde *Paral®* Phenobarbital *Luminal®* Prazepam *Centrax®* Temazepam *Restoril®* Triazolam *Halcion®* Zaleplon *Sonata®* Zolpidem *Ambien®*	Chlordiazepoxide *Librax®*

Crosswalks of the ASAM Patient Placement Criteria, Second Edition-Revised (ASAM PPC-2R)

Appendix 2

Levels of Care
Dimensional Criteria
Continued Service and Discharge Criteria
Integration of Criteria for Co-Occurring Disorders
The Concept of "Imminent Danger"
Adolescent Criteria

The *ASAM Patient Placement Criteria for the Treatment of Substance-Related Disorders, Second Edition-Revised* (*ASAM PPC-2R*; 2001) describes treatment as a continuum marked by five basic levels of care (Levels I through IV).

Level 0.5: Early Intervention

Level 1: Outpatient Services

Level II: Intensive Outpatient/Partial Hospitalization Services

Level III: Residential/Inpatient Services

Level IV: Medically Managed Intensive Inpatient Services

Within each level, a decimal number (ranging from .1 to .9) expresses gradations of intensity within the existing levels of care. This structure allows precision of description and better "inter-rater" reliability by focusing on five broad levels of service. Thus the *PPC-2R* retains five levels of care in addition to Detoxification and Opioid Maintenance Therapy, but describes gradient intensities of service within each level of care. For example, Level II.1 provides

a benchmark for intensity at the minimum description of Level II care.

LEVELS OF CARE

Level 0.5: Early Intervention. Early intervention (Level 0.5) constitutes a service for specific individuals who, for a known reason, are at risk of developing substance-related problems or for those for whom there is not yet sufficient information to document a substance use disorder. Where Level 0.5 is a DUI or DWI program, the length of service may be determined by program rules and completion of the program may be a prerequisite to reinstitution of driving privileges.

Level I: Outpatient Treatment. Level I encompasses organized, non-residential services, which may be delivered in a variety of settings. Addiction or mental health treatment personnel provide professionally directed evaluation, treatment, and recovery services. Such services are provided in regularly scheduled sessions and follow a defined set of policies and procedures or medical protocols.

Level II: Intensive Outpatient Treatment/Partial Hospitalization. Level II is an organized outpatient service that delivers treatment services during the day, before or after work or school, in the evening, or on weekends. For appropriately selected patients, such programs provide essential education and treatment components, while allowing patients to apply their newly acquired skills within "real world" environments. Programs have the capacity to arrange for medical and psychiatric consultation, psychopharmacological consultation, medication management, and 24-hour crisis services.

Level III: Residential/Inpatient Treatment. Level III encompasses organized services staffed by designated addiction treatment and mental health personnel, who provide a planned regimen of care in a 24-hour live-in setting. Such services conform to defined policies and procedures. They are housed in, or affiliated with, permanent facilities where patients can reside safely. They are staffed 24 hours a day. Mutual and self-help group meetings generally are available on-site.

Level IV: Medically Managed Intensive Inpatient Treatment. Level IV programs provide care to patients whose mental and substance-related problems are so severe that they require primary biomedical, psychiatric and nursing care. Treatment is provided 24 hours a day, and the full resources of a general acute care hospital or psychiatric hospital are available. They are staffed by designated addiction-credentialed physicians, including psychiatrists, as well as other mental health- and addiction-credentialed clinicians. Such services are delivered under a defined set of policies and procedures and have permanent facilities that include inpatient beds.

Opioid Maintenance Therapy (OMT). OMT (so named to broaden the service beyond methadone maintenance) is best conceptualized as a separate service that can be provided at any level of care. OMT therefore has not been included under any of the broad levels of service (I through IV). However, the OMT criteria are included in the format of a Level I outpatient service, since most opioid maintenance therapy is delivered in an ambulatory setting.

DIMENSIONAL CRITERIA

The six assessment dimensions to be evaluated in making placement decisions are:

- Dimension 1: Acute Intoxication and/or Withdrawal Potential;

- Dimension 2: Biomedical Conditions and Complications;

- Dimension 3: Emotional, Behavioral or Cognitive Conditions and Complications;

- Dimension 4: Readiness to Change (formerly "Treatment Acceptance/Resistance");

- Dimension 5: Relapse, Continued Use or Continued Problem Potential; and

- Dimension 6: Recovery/Living Environment.

CONTINUED SERVICE AND DISCHARGE CRITERIA

In a departure from earlier editions, the *PPC-2R* contains only admission criteria for each level of care. The specific criteria for continued service and transfer or discharge have been replaced by general guidelines to inform the judgment of the treatment professional. This change was made in recognition of the fact that, in the process of patient assessment, certain problems and priorities are identified as justifying admission to a particular level of care. It is the resolution of those problems and priorities that determines whether and when a patient can be treated at a different level of care or discharged. The appearance of new problems may require services that can be provided effectively at the same level of care, or they may require transfer of the patient to a more or less intensive level of care.

INTEGRATION OF CRITERIA FOR CO-OCCURRING DISORDERS

When the first edition of the ASAM *Patient Placement Criteria* (*ASAM PPC-1*) was published in 1991, the criteria generally were designed for programs that offered only addiction treatment services. However, the *PPC-1* also acknowledged that some patients come to treatment with medical (Dimension 2) and psychiatric (Dimension 3) disorders that coexist with their substance-related problems.

The ASAM *PPC-2R* takes a further step toward meeting these diverse patient needs by incorporating criteria that address the large subset of individuals who present for treatment with co-occurring Axis I substance-related disorders and Axis I/Axis II mental disorders. Individuals with such co-occurring disorders (often referred to as "dual diagnoses") can be conceptualized as belonging to one of two general categories:

- *Moderate Severity Disorders*: Such persons present with stable mood or anxiety disorders of moderate severity (including resolving bipolar disorder), or with personality disorders of moderate severity (although some persons with severe levels of antisocial personality disorder may be appropriately placed in this group), or with signs and symptoms of a mental health disorder that are not so severe as to meet the diagnostic threshold.

- *High Severity Disorders*: Such persons present with schizophrenia-spectrum disorders, severe mood disorders with psychotic features, severe anxiety disorders, or severe personality disorders (such as fragile borderline conditions).

THE CONCEPT OF "IMMINENT DANGER"

The concept of "imminent danger" often is used to describe problems that can lead to grave consequences to the individual patient (and possibly others), some of which may be the basis for the legal commitment of an individual to treatment. However, the drafters of the criteria believe that its application should be broader. In fact, it is the presence of three components in combination that constitute imminent danger: (1) a strong probability that certain behaviors (such as continued alcohol or drug use or relapse) will occur, (2) the likelihood that such behaviors will present a significant risk of serious adverse consequences to the individual and/or others (as in a consistent pattern of driving while intoxi-

cated), and (3) the likelihood that such adverse events will occur in the very near future.

The concept of imminent danger *does not* encompass the universe of possible adverse events, and its evaluation should be restricted to the three factors listed above. Nevertheless, the interpretation of imminent danger should not be restricted to acute suicidality, homicidality, or medical or psychiatric problems that create an immediate, catastrophic risk.

ADOLESCENT CRITERIA

The ASAM Adolescent Criteria are reviewed in Section 13 of this text. The Adult Criteria are discussed in more detail in Section 4.

ACKNOWLEDGMENT: Excerpted with permission from Mee-Lee D, Shulman G, Fishman M et al. (2001). ASAM Patient Placement Criteria for the Treatment of Substance-Related Disorders, Second Edition-Revised (ASAM PPC-2R). Chevy Chase, MD: American Society of Addiction Medicine, 1-7.

REFERENCES

Mee-Lee D, Shulman G, Fishman M et al. (2001). *ASAM Patient Placement Criteria for the Treatment of Substance-Related Disorders, Second Edition-Revised (ASAM PPC-2R)*. Chevy Chase, MD: American Society of Addiction Medicine.

Crosswalk of the ASAM Adult Patient Placement Criteria Levels 0.5 through II.5

	Levels of Care				
Criteria Dimensions	Level 0.5 Early Intervention	OMT Opioid Maintenance Therapy	Level I Outpatient Treatment	Level II.1 Intensive Outpatient	Level II.5 Partial Hospitalization
DIMENSION 1: Alcohol Intoxication and/or Withdrawal Potential	The patient is not at risk of withdrawal.	The patient is physiologically dependent on opiates and requires OMT to prevent withdrawal.	The patient is not experiencing significant withdrawal or is at minimal risk of severe withdrawal.	The patient is at minimal risk of severe withdrawal.	The patient is at moderate risk of severe withdrawal.
DIMENSION 2: Biomedical Conditions and Complications	None or very stable.	None or manageable with outpatient medical monitoring.	None or very stable, or the patient is receiving concurrent medical monitoring.	None or not a distraction from treatment. Such problems are manageable at Level II.1.	None or not ufficient to distract from treatment. Such problems are manageable at Level II.5.
DIMENSION 3: Emotional, Behavioral or Cognitive Conditions and Complications	None or very stable.	None or manageable in an outpatient structured environment.	None or very stable, or the patient is receiving concurrent mental health monitoring.	Mild severity, with the potential to distract from recovery; the patient needs monitoring.	Mild to moderate soverity, with the potential to distract from recovery; the patient needs stabilization.

Crosswalk of the ASAM Adult Patient Placement Criteria Levels 0.5 through II.5 (continued)

	Levels of Care				
Criteria Dimensions	Level 0.5 Early Intervention	OMT Opioid Maintenance Therapy	Level I Outpatient Treatment	Level II.1 Intensive Outpatient	Level II.5 Partial Hospitalization
DIMENSION 4: Readiness to Change	The patient is willint to explore how current alcohol or drug use may affect personal goals.	The patient is ready to change the negative effects of opiate use, but is not ready for total abstinence.	The patient is ready for recovery, but needs motivating and monitoring strategies to strengthen readiness. Or there is high severity in this dimension but not in other dimensions. The patient therefore needs a Level I motivational enhancement program.	The patient has variable engagement in treatment, ambivalence, or lack of awareness of the substance use or mental health problem, and requires a structured program several times a week to promote progress through the stages of change.	The patient has poor engagement in treatment, significan ambivalence, or lack of awareness of the substance use or mental health problem, requiring a near-daily structured program or intensive engagement services to promote progress throuth the stages of change.
DIMENSION 5: Relapse, Continued Use or Continued Problem Potenial	The patient needs an understanding of, or skills to change, his or her current alcohol and drug use patterns.	The patient is at high risk of relapse or continued use without OMT and structured therapy to promote treatment progress.	The patient is able to maintain abstinence or control use and pursue recovery or motivational goals with minimal support.	Intensification of the patient's addiction or mental health symptoms indicate a high likelihood of relapse or continued use or continued problems without close monitoring and support several times a week.	Intensification of the patient's addiction or mental health symptoms, despite active participation in a Level I or II.1 program, indicates a high likelihood of relapse or continued use or continued problems without near-daily monitoring and support.

Crosswalk of the ASAM Adult Patient Placement Criteria Levels 0.5 through II.5 (continued)

	Levels of Care				
Criteria Dimensions	Level 0.5 Early Intervention	OMT Opioid Maintenance Therapy	Level I Outpatient Treatment	Level II.1 Intensive Outpatient	Level II.5 Partial Hospitalization
DIMENSION 6: Recovery Environment	The patient's social support system or significant others increase the risk of personal conflict about alcohol or drug use.	The patient's recovery environment is supportive and/or the patient has skills to cope.	The patient's recovery environment is supportive and/or the patient has skills to cope.	The patient's recovery environment is not supportive but, with structure and support, the patient can cope.	The patient's recovery environment is not supportive but, with structure and support and relief from the home environment, the patient can cope.

Crosswalk of the ASAM Adult
Patient Placement Criteria
Levels III.1 through IV

	Levels of Care				
Criteria Dimensions	Level III.1 Clinically Managed Low-Intensity Residential Services	Level III.3 Clinically Managed Medium-Intensity Residential Services	Level III.5 Clinically Managed High-Intensity Residential Services	Level III.7 Medically Monitored Intensive Inpatient Treatment	Level IV Medically Managed Intensive Inpatient Treatment
DIMENSION 1: Alcohol Intoxication and/or Withdrawal Potential	The patient is not at risk of withdrawal, or is experiencing minimal or stable withdrawal. The patient is concurrently receiving Level I-D (minimal) or Level II-D (moderate) services.	The patient is not at risk of severe withdrawal, or moderate withdrawal is manageable at Level III.2-D.	The patient is at minimal risk of severe withdrawal at Levels III.3 or III.5. If withdrawal is present, it meets Level III.2-D criteria.	The patient is at high risk of withdrawal, but it is manageable at Level III.7-D and does not require the full resources of a licensed hospital.	The patient is at high risk of withdrawal and requires the full resources of a licensed hospital.
DIMENSION 2: Biomedical Conditions and Complications	None or stable, or the patient is receiving concurrent medical monitoring.	None or stable, or the patient is receiving concurrent medical monitoring.	None or stable, or the patient is receiving concurrent medical monitoring.	The patient requires 24-hour medical monitoring but not intensive treatment.	The patient requires 24-hour medical and nursing care and the full resources of a licensed hospital.

Crosswalk of the ASAM Adult
Patient Placement Criteria
Levels III.1 through IV (continued)

	Levels of Care				
Criteria Dimensions	Level III.1 Clinically Managed Low-Intensity Residential Services	Level III.3 Clinically Managed Medium-Intensity Residential Services	Level III.5 Clinically Managed High-Intensity Residential Services	Level III.7 Medically Monitored Intensive Inpatient Treatment	Level IV Medically Managed Intensive Inpatient Treatment
DIMENSION 3: Emotional, Behavioral or Cognitive Conditions and Complications	None or minimal; not distracting to recovery. If stable, a Dual Diagnosis Capable program is appropriate. If not, a Dual Diagnosis Enhanced program is requried.	Mild to moderate severity; the patient needs structure to focus on revcovery. If stable, a Dual Diagnosis Capable program is appropriate. If not, a Dual Diagnosis Enhanced program is required. Treatment should be designed to respond to the resident's cognitive deficits.	The patient demonstrates repeated inability to control impulses, or a personality disorder requires structure to shape behavior. Other functional deficits require a 24-hour setting to teach coping skills. A Dual Diagnosis Enhanced setting is required for the patient who is severely and persistently mentally ill.	Moderate severity; the patient needs a 24-hour structured setting. If the patient has a co-occurring mental disorder, he or she requires concurrent mental health services in a medically monitored setting.	Because of severe and unstable problems, the patient requires 24-hour psychiatric care with concomitant addiction treatment (Dual Diagnosis Enhanced).

Crosswalk of the ASAM Adult
Patient Placement Criteria
Levels III.1 through IV (continued)

	Levels of Care				
Criteria Dimensions	Level III.1 Clinically Managed Low-Intensity Residential Services	Level III.3 Clinically Managed Medium-Intensity Residential Services	Level III.5 Clinically Managed High-Intensity Residential Services	Level III.7 Medically Monitored Intensive Inpatient Treatment	Level IV Medically Managed Intensive Inpatient Treatment
DIMENSION 4: Readiness to Change	The patient is open to recovery, but needs a structured environment to maintain therapeutic gains.	The patient has little awareness and needs interventions available only at Level III.3 to engage and stay in treatment. Or there is high severity in this dimension but not in other dimensions. The patient therefore needs a Level I motivational enhancement program.	The patient has marked difficulty with or opposition to treatment, with dangerous consequences. Or there is high severity in this dimension but not in other dimensions. The patient therefore needs a Level I motivational enhancement program.	The patient's resistance is high and impulse control poor, despite negative consequences; he or she needs motivating strategies available only in a 24-hour structured setting. Or, if a 24-hour setting is not required, the patient needs a Level I motivational enhancement program.	Problems in this dimension do not qualify the patient for Level IV services.

Crosswalk of the ASAM Adult Patient Placement Criteria Levels III.1 through IV (continued)

	Levels of Care				
Criteria Dimensions	Level III.1 Clinically Managed Low-Intensity Residential Services	Level III.3 Clinically Managed Medium-Intensity Residential Services	Level III.5 Clinically Managed High-Intensity Residential Services	Level III.7 Medically Monitored Intensive Inpatient Treatment	Level IV Medically Managed Intensive Inpatient Treatment
DIMENSION 5: Relapse, Continued Use or Continued Problem Potential	The patient understands relapse but needs structure to maintain therapeutic gains.	The patient has little awareness and needs interventions available only at Level III.3 to prevent continued use, with imminent dangerous consequences, because of cognitive deficits or comparable dysfunction.	The patient has no recognition of the skills needed to prevent continued use, with imminently dangerous consequences.	The patient is unable to control use, with imminently dangerous consequences, despite active participation at less intensive levels of care.	Problems in this dimension do not qualify the patient for Level IV services.
DIMENSION 6: Recovery Environment	The patient's environment is dangerous, but recovery is achievable if Level III.1 24-hour structure is available.	The patient's environment is dangerous and he or she needs 24-hour structure to learn to cope.	The patient's environment is dangerous and he or she lacks skills to cope outside of a highly structured 24-hour setting.	The patient's environment is dangerous and he or she lacks skills to cope outside of a highly structured 24-hour setting.	Problems in this dimension do not qualify the patient for Level IV services.

Note: This overview of the Adult Admission Criteria is an approximate summary to illustrate the principal concepts and structure of the criteria.

Appendix 3

ASAM Addiction Terminology

In an effort to resolve disagreements and confusion in the addictions field over the use and meaning of terms, the American Society of Addiction Medicine (ASAM), in 1990, formed a Committee on Nomenclature to select terms it believed were important to the practice of addiction medicine and to come to agreement on how those terms should be defined.

Earlier, the American Medical Association (AMA), in a Delphi study, had produced a list of 50 terms that were adjudged by a representative group of respondents to be most significant, as then currently used by the field (Rinaldi, Steindler et al., 1988). The most agreed-upon definition also was determined for each of the terms.

Working primarily with the AMA list, but also selecting terms from their own experience as addiction specialists, members of the ASAM Committee compiled a list of 32 high-priority terms and established a definition for each. The terms and definitions then were approved by the ASAM Board of Directors as recommended terminology for use in all ASAM scientific publications and for dissemination to the field. The Committee and Board also endorsed the definition of "alcoholism" that had been developed by a special joint committee of ASAM and the National Council on Alcoholism and Drug Dependence (Morse, Flavin et al., 1992). The Nomenclature Committee's work of selecting and defining additional significant terms continues.

TERMINOLOGY

In the following list, an asterisk denotes a definition that has been formally adopted by ASAM's Board of Directors.

*Abstinence. Non-use of a specific substance. In recovery, non-use of any addictive psychoactive substance. May also denote cessation of an addictive behavior, such as gambling, overeating, etc.

*Abuse. Harmful use of a specific psychoactive substance. The term also applies to one category of psychoactive substance-related disorders. While recognizing that "abuse" is part of present diagnostic terminology, ASAM recommends that an alternative term be found for this purpose because of the pejorative connotations of the word "abuse."

Acceptance/Resistance. See Readiness To Change.

*Addiction. A primary, chronic, neurobiologic disease, with genetic, psychosocial, and environmental factors influencing its development and manifestations. It is characterized by behaviors that include one or more of the following: impaired control over drug use, compulsive use, continued use despite harm, and craving.

*Addictionist. Also, "addictionologist." A physician who specializes in addiction medicine.

Admission. That point in an individual's relationship with an organized treatment service when the intake process has been completed and the individual is entitled to receive the services of the treatment program.

*Alcoholics Anonymous. "A fellowship of men and women who share their experience, strength and hope with each other that they may solve their common problem and help others recover from alcoholism. The only requirement for membership is a desire to stop drinking" (from the *Alcoholics Anonymous Preamble*).

Alcoholism. A general but not diagnostic term, usually used to describe alcohol dependence, but sometimes used more broadly to describe a variety of problems related to the use of beverage alcohol.

Ambulatory Detoxification. Detoxification that is medically monitored but that does not require admission to an inpatient, medically or clinically monitored or managed setting.

Assessment. Those procedures by which a program evaluates an individual's strengths, weaknesses, problems, and needs and determines priorities so that a treatment plan can be developed.

Biomedical. Biological and physiological aspects of a patient's condition and thus of the assessment and treatment of the patient. In addiction treatment, biomedical problems may be the direct result of a substance use disorder or be independent of and interactive with them, thus affecting the total treatment plan and prognosis.

*Blackout. Acute anterograde amnesia with no formation of long-term memory, resulting from the ingestion of alcohol or other drugs; that is, a period of memory loss for which there is no recall of activities.

Case Management. Case management is a collaborative process through which the options and services that will meet an individual's health needs are assessed, planned, implemented, coordinated, monitored, and evaluated, using communication and available resources to promote quality, cost-effective outcomes. (Definition of the National Case Management Task Force; reprinted from the *CCM Certification Guide*, CIRSC/Certified Case Manager, Rolling Meadows, IL, 1993.)

*Chemical Dependency. A generic term relating to psychological or physical dependency, or both, on one or more psychoactive substances.

Client. An individual who receives treatment for alcohol or other drug problems. The terms "client" and "patient" sometimes are used interchangeably, although staff in medical settings more commonly refer to "patients," while individuals who receive services in non-medical outpatient settings often are referred to as "clients."

Co-Occurring Disorders. Concurrent substance-related and mental disorders. Other terms used to describe co-occurring disorders include "dual diagnosis," "dual disorders," "mentally-ill chemically-addicted" (MICA), "chemically-addicted mentally-ill" (CAMI), "mentally-ill substance abusers" (MISA), "mentally-ill chemically dependent" (MICD), "coexisting disorders," "comorbid disorders," and "individuals with co-occurring psychiatric and substance symptomatology" (ICOPSS). Use of the term carries no implication as to which disorder is primary and which secondary, which disorder occurred first, or whether one disorder caused the other.

Continuing Care. The provision of a treatment plan and organizational structure to ensure that a patient receives ongoing treatment services and supports. (This term is preferred to "aftercare.")

Continuum of Care. An integrated network of treatment services and modalities designed so that an individual's changing needs will be met as that individual moves through the treatment and recovery process.

*Cross-tolerance. Tolerance, induced by repeated administration of one psychoactive substance, that is manifested toward another substance to which the individual has not been recently exposed.

*Decriminalization. Removal of criminal penalties for the possession and use of illicit psychoactive substances.

*Dependence. Used in three different ways: (1) physical dependence, a physiological state of adaptation to a specific psychoactive substance characterized by the emergence of a withdrawal syndrome during abstinence, which may be relieved in total or in part by readministration of the substance; (2) psychological dependence, a subjective sense of need for a specific psychoactive substance, either for its positive effects or to avoid negative effects associated with its abstinence; and (3) one category of psychoactive substance use disorder.

*Detoxification. A process of withdrawing a person from a specific psychoactive substance in a safe and effective manner.

Dimension. A term used in the *ASAM Patient Placement Criteria* to refer to one of six patient problem areas that must be assessed in making a placement decision.

Discharge. The point at which an individual's active involvement with a treatment service is terminated, and he or she no longer is carried on the service's records as a patient.

*Drug Intoxication. Dysfunctional changes in physiological functioning, psychological functioning, mood state, cognitive process, or all of these, as a consequence of consumption of a psychoactive substance (such intoxication is marked by behaviors that usually are disruptive, often stemming from central nervous system impairment).

Dual Diagnosis. Refers to the patient who has signs and symptoms of concurrent substance-related and mental disorders. Other terms used to describe such co-occurring disorders include "co-occurring disorders," "dual disorders," "mentally ill chemically addicted" (MICA), "chemically addicted mentally ill" (CAMI), "mentally ill substance abusers" (MISA), "mentally ill chemically dependent" (MICD), "co-existing disorders," "comorbid disorders," and "individuals with co-occurring psychiatric and substance symptomatology" (ICOPSS). Also see "co-occurring disorders."

Early Intervention. Services that explore and address any problems or risk factors that appear to be related to use of alcohol and other drugs and that help the individual to recognize the harmful consequences of inappropriate use. Such individuals may not appear to meet the diagnostic criteria for a substance use disorder, but require early intervention for education and further assessment.

*Enabling. Any action by another person or an institution that intentionally or unintentionally has the effect of facilitating the continuation of an individual's addictive process.

Facility. The physical structure (building or portions thereof) in which treatment services are delivered.

Failure (as in treatment failure). Lack of progress and/or regression at any given level of care. Such a situation warrants a reassessment of the treatment plan and modification of the treatment approach. For example, the situation may require changes in the treatment plan at the same level of care or transfer to a different (more or less intensive) level of care to achieve a better therapeutic response. Sometimes used to describe relapse after a single treatment episode—an inappropriate construct in describing a chronic disease or disorder.

*Familial Alcoholism. A pattern of alcoholism occurring in more than one generation within a family, due to either genetic or environmental factors, or both.

*Family Intervention. A specific form of intervention, involving family members of an alcoholic/addict, designed to benefit the patient as well as the family constellation.

Habilitation. The development, for the first time in an individual's life, of an optimum state of health through medical, psychological, and social interventions (also see "Rehabilitation").

Harm Reduction. Policies and programs whose primary goal is to reduce the adverse health, social, legal and economic consequences of drug use, without necessarily reducing or eliminating such use.

Imminent Danger. Three components constitute imminent danger: (1) a high probability that certain behaviors (such as continued alcohol or drug use or relapse) will occur; (2) the likelihood that such behaviors will present a significant risk of serious adverse consequences to the individual and/or others (as in a consistent pattern of driving while intoxicated); and (3) the likelihood that such adverse events will occur in the very near future. The concept of imminent danger *does not* encompass all the things that may happen but is restricted to the combination of the three factors listed above. On the other hand, the interpretation of imminent danger should not be restricted to acute suicidality, homicidality or medical or psychiatric problems that create an immediate, catastrophic risk.

*Impairment. A dysfunctional state resulting from use of psychoactive substances, or mental, emotional, or cognitive problems.

Individualized Treatment. Treatment designed to meet a particular patient's needs, guided by a treatment plan that is directly related to a specific, unique patient assessment.

Intensity of Service. The number, type, and frequency of staff interventions and other services (such as consultation, referral, or support services) provided during treatment at a particular level of care.

Intensive Outpatient Treatment. An organized service delivered by addiction professionals or addiction-credentialed clinicians, which provides a planned regimen of treatment, consisting of regularly scheduled sessions within a structured program, for a minimum of 9 hours of treatment per week for adults and 6 hours of treatment per week for adolescents.

Interdisciplinary Team. A group of clinicians trained in different professions, disciplines, or service areas (such as physicians, counselors, psychologists, social workers, nurses, and certified substance abuse counselors), who function interactively and interdependently in conducting a patient's biopsychosocial assessment, treatment plan, and treatment services.

*Intervention. A planned interaction with an individual who may be dependent on one or more psychoactive substances, with the aim of making a full assessment, overcoming denial, interrupting drug-taking behavior, or inducing the individual to initiate treatment. The preferred technique is to present facts regarding psychoactive substance use in a caring, believable, and understandable manner.

*Legalization. Removal of legal restrictions on the cultivation, manufacture, distribution, possession, and/or use of a psychoactive substance.

Length of Service. The number of days (for inpatient care) or units/visits (for outpatient care) of service provided to a patient, from admission to discharge, at a particular level of care.

Level of Care. As used in the *ASAM Patient Placement Criteria*, this term refers to a discrete intensity of clinical and environmental support services bundled or linked together and available in a variety of settings.

Level of Function. An individual's relative degree of health and freedom from specific signs and symptoms of a mental or substance-related disorder, which determine whether the individual requires treatment.

*Loss of Control. The inability to consistently limit the self-administration of psychoactive substance.

Matching. A process of selecting treatment resources to conform to an individual patient's needs and preferences based on careful assessment. Matching has been shown to increase treatment retention and thus to improve treatment outcome. It also improves resource allocation by directing patients to the most appropriate level of care and intensity of services.

Medically Managed Treatment. Services that involve daily medical care, where diagnostic and treatment services are directly provided and/or managed by an appropriately trained and licensed physician.

Medically Monitored Treatment. Services that are provided by an interdisciplinary staff of nurses, counselors, social workers, addiction specialists, and other health care professionals and technical personnel under the direction of a licensed physician. Medical monitoring is provided through an appropriate mix of direct patient contact, review of records, team meetings, 24-hour coverage by a physician, and quality assurance programs.

Medical Necessity. Pertains to essential care for biopsychosocial severity. It is defined by the extent and severity of problems identified in a multidimensional assessment of the individual.

*Misuse. Any use of a prescription drug that varies from accepted medical practice.

Modality. A specific type of treatment (technique, method, or procedure) that is used to relieve symptoms or induce behavior change. Modalities of addiction treatment include, for example, detoxification or antagonist medication, motivational interviewing, cognitive behavioral therapy, group therapy, social skills training, vocational counseling, and self/mutual help groups.

Outpatient Detoxification. See "ambulatory detoxification."

Outpatient Service. An organized non-residential service, delivered in a variety of settings, in which addiction treatment personnel provide professionally directed evaluation and treatment for substance-related disorders.

*Overdose. The inadvertent or deliberate consumption of a dose much larger than that either habitually used by the individual or ordinarily used for treatment of an illness, and likely to result in a serious toxic reaction or death.

Patient. An individual who is receiving assessment or treatment for problems with alcohol, another drug, or tobacco. The terms "client" and "patient" sometimes are used interchangeably, although staff in non-medical settings more commonly use "client."

Partial Hospitalization. A generic term encompassing day, night, evening, and weekend treatment programs that employ an integrated, comprehensive and complementary schedule of recognized treatments. Commonly referred to as "day treatment." A partial hospitalization program does not need to be attached to a licensed hospital.

Physical Dependence. Physical dependence is a state of adaptation that is manifested by a drug class-specific withdrawal syndrome that can be produced by abrupt cessation or rapid dose reduction of a drug, or by administration of an antagonist.

Placement. Selection of an appropriate level of service, based on assessment of a patient's individual needs and preferences.

*Polydrug Dependence. Concomitant use of two or more psychoactive substances in quantities and with frequencies that cause the individual significant physiological, psychological and/or sociological distress or impairment.

Polysubstance Dependence. A *DSM-IV* diagnosis (304.80) reserved for behavior during the same 12-month period in which an individual repeatedly engages in abuse of at least three groups of substances (excluding caffeine and nicotine), but no single substance predominates. Such use meets the dependence criteria for substances as a group, but not for a specific substance. (Adapted from the *Diagnostic and Statistical Manual of Mental Disorders, 4th Edition*, American Psychiatric Association, 1994.)

*Prevention. Social, economic, legal, medical, and/or psychological measures aimed at minimizing the use of potentially addicting substances, lowering the dependence risk in susceptible individuals, or minimizing other adverse consequences of psychoactive substance use. Primary prevention consists of attempts to reduce the incidence of addictive diseases and related problems in a general population. Secondary prevention aims to achieve early detection, diagnosis, and treatment of affected individuals. Tertiary prevention seeks to diminish the incidence of complications of addictive diseases.

*Problem Drinking. An informal term describing a pattern of drinking associated with life problems prior to establishing a definitive diagnosis of alcoholism. Also, an umbrella term for any harmful use of alcohol, including alcoholism. ASAM recommends that the term not be used in the latter sense.

Program. A generalized term for an organized system of services designed to address the treatment needs of patients.

Readiness to Change. An individual's emotional and cognitive awareness of the need to change, coupled with a commitment to change. When applied to addiction treatment, and particularly to assessment Dimension 4, "Readiness to Change" describes the patient's degree of awareness of the relationship between his or her alcohol or other drug use or mental health problems, and the adverse consequences of such use, as well as the presence of specific readiness to change personal patterns of alcohol and other drug use.

Recovery. A process of overcoming both physical and psychological dependence on a psychoactive substance with a commitment to sobriety. "Recovery" typically refers to the overall goal of helping a patient to achieve overall health and well-being.

Recovery Environment. The external supports for recovery, including the quality and extent of services (such as child care, transportation, crisis and transitional housing, and other "wrap around" services, all of which influence treatment outcome).

*Rehabilitation. The restoration of an optimum state of health by medical, psychological, and social means, including peer group support, for an alcoholic or addict, a family member or a significant other.

*Relapse. Recurrence of psychoactive substance-dependent behavior in an individual who has achieved and maintained abstinence for a significant period of time beyond withdrawal. (Note that, as a medical term, "relapse" is preferred to "recidivism," which is a legal construct.)

Resident. A patient in one of the clinically managed, residential levels of care.

Setting. A specific place in which treatment is delivered. Settings for alcohol/other drug treatment include hospitals, methadone clinics, community mental health centers, and prisons or jails.

Severity of Illness. Specific signs and symptoms for which a patient requires treatment, including the degree of impairment and the extent of a patient's support networks.

*Sobriety. A state of complete abstinence from psychoactive substances by an addicted individual in conjunction with a satisfactory quality of life.

Social Support System. The network of relationships that surround an individual. A health social support system—involving family members, friends, employers, members of mutual support groups, and others—tends to support an individual's recovery efforts and goals. What these individuals have in common is that their relationship with the individual is current and that the individual is comfortable contacting them in times of distress.

Stages of Change. This refers principally to the work of Prochaska and DiClemente, who described how individuals progress and regress through various levels of awareness of a problem, as well as the degree of activity involved in a change in behavior. While their original work studied individuals who changed from smokers to non-smokers, the concept of stages of change subsequently has been applied to a variety of behaviors.

Substance-Induced Disorders. Includes Substance Intoxication, Substance Withdrawal, and a variety of substance-induced disorders, Delirium, Persisting Dementia, Persisting Amnestic Disorder, Psychotic Disorder, Mood

Disorder, Anxiety Disorder, Sexual Dysfunction and Sleep Disorder. Specific diagnostic criteria are listed in the *Diagnostic and Statistical Manual of Mental Disorders, 4th Edition (DSM-IV)* of the American Psychiatric Association.

Substance-Related Disorders. Includes disorders related to the taking of a drug of abuse (including alcohol), to the side effects of a medication, and to toxin exposure and are divided into two groups: the Substance Use Disorders and the Substance-Induced Disorders, as defined in the *Diagnostic and Statistical Manual of Mental Disorders, 4th Edition (DSM-IV)* of the American Psychiatric Association.

Substance Use Disorders. Includes Substance Dependence and Substance Abuse with specific diagnostic criteria listed in the *Diagnostic and Statistical Manual of Mental Disorders, Fourth Edition (DSM-IV)* of the American Psychiatric Association. Substance Use Disorders are one of two subgroups of the broader diagnostic category of Substance-Related Disorders.

Support Services. Support services are services that are readily available to a treatment program through affiliation or contract arrangement, or because they are available to the community at large (for example, 911 emergency response services). Typically, they are services that cannot be offered directly by program staff and which may not be not be needed by patients on a routine basis.

*Tolerance. A state of adaptation in which exposure to a drug induces changes that result in diminution of one or more of the drug's effects over time.

Transfer. Movement of the patient from one level of service to another, within the continuum of care.

*Treatment. Application of planned procedures to identify and change patterns of behavior that are maladaptive, destructive, and/or injurious to health; or to restore appropriate levels of physical, psychological, and/or social functioning.

Triage. As used in the *ASAM Patient Placement Criteria*, decision-making at the conclusion of an initial assessment process to determine the specific assignment of the patient to a level of care or service.

Twenty-three Hour Observation Bed. Admission for no more than 23 hours for assessment and stabilization to determine the need for inpatient versus outpatient care. Such a "bed" may be located in an inpatient or an outpatient setting (such as a hospital emergency department).

Unbundling. An approach to treatment that seeks to provide the appropriate combination of specific services to match a patient's needs. The goal of unbundling is to provide an array of options for flexible individualized treatment, which can be delivered in a variety of settings. The intensity of clinical services is determined independently of the individual's need for supportive living arrangements and other environmental supports.

*Withdrawal Syndrome. The onset of a predictable constellation of signs and symptoms following the abrupt discontinuation of, or rapid decrease in, dosage of a psychoactive substance.

ACKNOWLEDGMENTS: The definition of alcoholism was prepared by Robert M. Morse, M.D., Daniel K. Flavin, M.D., and the Joint Committee of the National Council on Alcoholism and Drug Dependence and the American Society of Addiction Medicine to Study the Definition and Criteria for the Diagnosis of Alcoholism. Members of the committee were Daniel J. Anderson, Ph.D., Margaret Bean-Bayog, M.D., Henri Begleiter, M.D., Ph.D., Sheila B. Blume, M.D., FASAM, Jean Forest, M.D., Stanley E. Gitlow, M.D., FASAM, Enoch Gordis, M.D., James E. Kelsey, M.D., Nancy K. Mello, Ph.D., Roger E. Meyer, M.D., Robert G. Niven, M.D., Ann Noll, M.D., Barton Pakul, M.D., Katherine M. Pike, Lucy Barry Robe, Max A. Schneider, M.D., FASAM, Marc Schuckit, M.D., David E. Smith, M.D., FASAM, Emanuel M. Steindler, Boris Tabakoff, Ph.D, and George Vaillant, M.D. Ex officio members were James F. Callahan, D.P.A., Jasper Chen See, M.D., and Robert Sparks, M.D. Frank Seixas, M.D., was emeritus consultant. Emanuel M. Steindler directed of ASAM's project to define essential terms in addiction medicine.

REFERENCES

American Psychiatric Association (1994). *Diagnostic and Statistical Manual of Mental Disorders, 4th Edition (DSM-IV)*. Washington, DC: American Psychiatric Press.

Mee-Lee D, Shulman G, Fishman M et al. (2001). *ASAM Patient Placement Criteria for the Treatment of Substance-Related Disorders, Second-Edition, Revised (ASAM PPC-2R)*. Chevy Chase, MD: American Society of Addiction Medicine.

Morse RM, Flavin DK et al. (1992). The definition of alcoholism. *Journal of the American Medical Association* 268:1012-1014.

Rinaldi RC, Steindler EM, Wilford BB et al. (1988). Clarification and standardization of substance abuse terminology. *Journal of the American Medical Association* 259:555-557.

Appendix 4

Screening and Assessment Instruments

Addiction Severity Index
Alcohol Dependence Scale
Alcohol Use Disorders Identification Test
CAGE
Clinical Institute Withdrawal Assessment for Alcohol, Revised
Drinker Inventory of Consequences
Michigan Alcohol Screening Test
Problem Oriented Screening Instrument for Teenagers
Self-Administered Alcoholism Screening Test

Initiation of effective treatment requires that five sequential questions be accurately answered: (1) Does the patient suffer a problem with drugs or alcohol? (2) If so, is the problem one of abuse or of dependence? (3) If dependence, what is the severity? (4) Are other psychiatric or medical problems present? (5) Would medication facilitate management of withdrawal?

A variety of psychometric tests have been devised to help clinicians resolve these issues. This chapter discusses popular examples of such instruments and suggests how clinicians can employ them in planning the early stages of treatment.

ADDICTION SEVERITY INDEX (ASI)
The Addiction Severity Index (ASI) is a semistructured interview designed to address seven potential problem areas in substance-abusing patients: medical status, employment and support, drug use, alcohol use, legal status, family/social status, and psychiatric status. In an hour, a skilled interviewer can gather information on recent (past 30 days) and lifetime problems in all of the problem areas.

Uses. The ASI provides an overview of problems related to substance abuse, rather than focusing on any single area (McLellan, Luborsky et al., 1980, 1985; McLellan, Kushner et al., 1992). The ASI thus can be used effectively to explore problems within any adult group of individuals who report substance abuse as their major problem. It has been used with psychiatrically ill, homeless, pregnant, and prisoner populations, but its major use has been with adults seeking treatment for substance abuse problems. The ASI also has been used extensively for treatment planning and outcome evaluation. Outcome evaluation packages for individual programs or for treatment systems are available.

Design. The ASI contains approximately 200 items and seven subscales. Time required for administration is 50 minutes to an hour. Training is required to administer the instrument, and a self-training packet is available. Scoring time is about five minutes for the severity rating. Computerized scoring and interpretation are available.

The ASI provides two scores: Severity ratings are subjective ratings of the client's need for treatment, derived by the interviewer, while composite scores are measures of problem severity during the preceding 30 days and are calculated by a computerized scoring program.

Validity. The ASI has been normed on multiple treatment groups (alcohol, opiates, and cocaine; public and private; inpatient and outpatient) and subject groups (men, women, psychiatrically ill substance users, pregnant substance users, gamblers, homeless persons, probationers, and employee assistance clients). The following reliability studies have been conducted for the ASI: test-retest, split half, and internal consistency. Measures of utility derived include content, criterion (predictive, concurrent, "postdictive"), and construct (Allen & Columbus, 1995).

Availability. There is no charge for the instrument, although a minimal fee for photocopying and mailing may apply. A free computerized scoring disk is provided with the training materials. Copies of the ASI and related materials may be obtained from the DeltaMetrics/TRI ASI Information Line at 1-800/238-2433.

ALCOHOL DEPENDENCE SCALE (ADS)

The Alcohol Dependence Scale (ADS) provides a quantitative measure of the severity of alcohol dependence consistent with the concept of the alcohol dependence syndrome.

Uses. Because the test can be administered in approximately five minutes, it can be used for screening and case-finding in a variety of settings. The ADS also is widely used as a research and clinical tool (Skinner & Allen, 1992).

Use of the ADS has been reported primarily for clinical adult samples; however, researchers also have used the instrument in general population and correctional settings. The ADS has been found to have excellent predictive value with respect to a *DSM-IV* diagnosis. Moreover, the ADS yields a measure of the severity of dependence that is important for treatment planning, especially with respect to the intensity of care (Allen & Columbus, 1995).

Design. The 25 items cover alcohol withdrawal symptoms, impaired control over drinking, awareness of a compulsion to drink, increased tolerance to alcohol, and salience of alcohol-seeking behavior (Skinner & Horn, 1984).

The printed instructions for the ADS refer to the preceding 12-month period. However, instructions can be altered for use as an outcome measure at selected intervals (for example, at 6, 12, or 24 months) following treatment.

Validity. The ADS has been found to be reliable and valid. Research shows that it has excellent predictive value with respect to *DSM* diagnoses (Allen & Columbus, 1995).

Availability. The ADS is copyrighted by the Addiction Research Foundation and cannot be copied without permission. In addition to the questionnaire version, a computer-administered version is available as part of the Computerized Lifestyle Assessment (Alcohol Module). Information is available from Marketing Services, Addiction Research Foundation, 33 Russell Street, Toronto, Ontario, Canada M5S 2S1, or by telephone at 416/545-6000.

ALCOHOL USE DISORDERS IDENTIFICATION TEST (AUDIT)

The Alcohol Use Disorders Identification Test (AUDIT) was developed by the World Health Organization in 1989 to identify persons whose alcohol consumption has become hazardous or harmful to their health (Allen & Columbus, 1995).

Uses. The test is appropriate for a variety of populations and in multiple settings, including primary care, emergency departments, surgery and psychiatric units. It also has been used with criminal justice populations, military personnel, and in workplace programs.

Design. The AUDIT is a 10-item screening questionnaire that can be incorporated into a medical history. It contains questions about recent alcohol consumption, dependence symptoms, and alcohol-related problems (Allen & Columbus, 1995).

Validity. The test has been normed on heavy drinkers and alcoholics. Test-retest reliability and internal consistency have been validated. Measures of validity include content, criterion (predictive, concurrent, "postdictive"), and construct.

Availability. The AUDIT is copyrighted by the World Health Organization. The test and module are free; the training materials cost $75. Information is available from the WHO Programme on Substance Abuse, 1211 Geneva, Switzerland, or from Thomas F. Babor, Alcohol Research Center, University of Connecticut, Farmington, CT 06030.

CAGE

The CAGE is a simple, four-question screening instrument that can be used in a variety of settings. The CAGE questions are:

■ Have you ever felt you ought to **C**ut down on your drinking?

■ Have people **A**nnoyed you by criticizing your drinking?

- Have you ever felt bad or **G**uilty about your drinking?

- Have you ever had a drink first thing in the morning (**E**ye opener) to steady your nerves or get rid of a hangover?

Two or more affirmative answers are considered indicative of probable alcoholism, while one affirmative answer indicates that the patient's alcohol use deserves further evaluation (Ewing, 1984).

CLINICAL INSTITUTE WITHDRAWAL ASSESSMENT FOR ALCOHOL, REVISED (CIWA-Ar)

The Clinical Institute Withdrawal Assessment for Alcohol, Revised (CIWA-Ar) was developed by the Addiction Research Foundation.

Uses. The CIWA-Ar is widely used in clinical and research settings for initial assessment and ongoing monitoring of alcohol withdrawal symptoms.

Validity. The CIWA-Ar has been studied only in alcohol treatment programs; efficacy outside such program settings is not clear (Kasser, Geller et al., 1997).

Availability. The CIWA-Ar is not copyrighted. Information is available from Marketing Services, Addiction Research Foundation, 33 Russell Street, Toronto, Ontario, Canada M5S 2S1, or by telephone at 416/545-6000.

DRINKER INVENTORY OF CONSEQUENCES (DrInC)

The DrInC is a self-administered 50-item questionnaire designed to measure adverse consequences of alcohol abuse in five life areas: Interpersonal, Physical, Social, Impulsive, and Intrapersonal.

Uses. The test has been used in a variety of settings, including inpatient and outpatient alcohol treatment facilities, homeless shelters, and college campuses. It can be used for treatment planning and has been used in alcohol treatment clinical trials as an outcome measure.

Design. DrInC items span a full spectrum of adverse consequences, ranging from those encountered by heavy social drinkers to those seen in severely alcoholic populations. Each of the five life-area scales provides a lifetime and past three months' measure of adverse consequences. Scales can be combined to assess total adverse consequences.

Validity. Normative data are available for interpretation of client scale scores, and a brief version of the DrInC, the Short Index of Problems (SIP), is available when assessment time is limited.

A test manual is available that provides normative data for interpretation of total and subscale scores for a number of different populations (male, female, inpatient, outpatient). Simple directions are provided for scoring the DrInC.

Availability. The DrInC is not copyrighted. Copies can be obtained from the National Clearinghouse for Alcohol and Drug Information, P.O. Box 2345, Rockville, MD 20847-2345, or by telephone at 1-800/729-6686.

MICHIGAN ALCOHOL SCREENING TEST (MAST AND SMAST)

The Michigan Alcoholism Screening Test (MAST), which is one of the most widely used measures for assessing alcohol use, is a 25-item questionnaire designed to provide a rapid and effective screen for lifetime alcohol-related problems and alcoholism.

Uses. Clinically, the MAST can be used to screen for alcoholism with a variety of populations. In research studies, it is useful in assessing the extent of lifetime alcohol-related problems.

Design. The MAST can be used in either a paper-and-pencil or interview format. Its target population is adults. The instrument consists of 25 questions and requires 10 minutes to administer.

Also available are briefer versions of the MAST, including the 10-item Brief MAST, the 13-item Short MAST (SMAST), and a nine-item modified version called the Malmo modification (Mm-MAST). A geriatric version, called the MAST-G, also has been developed.

Validity. Reliability studies on the MAST include test-retest reliability and internal consistency. Measures of validity have been derived for both content and criterion (predictive, concurrent, "postdictive").

Availability. The MAST is not copyrighted, and there is no fee for its use. Copies are available at $5 each from Melvin L. Selzer, M.D., 6967 Paseo Laredo, La Jolla, CA 92037.

PROBLEM ORIENTED SCREENING INSTRUMENT FOR TEENAGERS (POSIT)

The POSIT is a simple, cost-efficient problem screen for use with troubled adolescents who may have one or more problems amenable to treatment or to a combination of preventive services.

Uses. The POSIT can be administered to populations in schools, the juvenile and family court system, and medical, psychiatric, alcohol and drug treatment programs as the first step toward identifying problem areas that require a more comprehensive diagnostic assessment. The target population is adolescents 12 through 19 years of age.

Design. Available in English and Spanish language versions, the POSIT is a brief screening tool designed to identify problems and the potential need for service in 10 functional areas, including substance use/abuse, mental and physical health, family and peer relations, vocation, and special education.

The test can be administered by any office personnel (no special qualifications are necessary). Computerized scoring and interpretation are available.

Availability. The POSIT is not copyrighted. Copies of the test and a related scoring template can be obtained from the National Clearinghouse for Alcohol and Drug Information, P.O. Box 2345, Rockville, MD 20847-2345, or by telephone at 1-800/729-6686.

SELF-ADMINISTERED ALCOHOLISM SCREENING TEST (SAAST)

The Self-Administered Alcoholism Screening Test (SAAST) is a 37-item instrument derived from the MAST.

Uses. The SAAST is used as a screening instrument for alcoholism in medical inpatient and outpatient settings.

Design. The SAAST was derived by adding items to the MAST to make it suitable for use in general medical populations. The test is available in a form suitable for administration to the patient, as well as in a form for use with the patient's spouse, friend, and others. Domains include loss of control, occupational and social disruption, physical consequences, emotional consequences, concern on the part of others, and family members with alcohol problems.

Validity. Reliability studies have examined internal consistency. Measures of validity include predictive, concurrent, and "postdictive" criteria. Factor analysis has been done.

Availability. The instrument is copyrighted by the Mayo Foundation. Information can be obtained from the Mayo Foundation, Rochester, MN.

ACKNOWLEDGMENT: Excerpted with permission from Allen JP & Columbus M (1995). Assessing Alcohol Problems: A Guide for Clinicians and Researchers (NIAAA Treatment Handbook, Series 4). *Rockville, MD: National Institute on Alcohol Abuse and Alcoholism, and Allen JP & Litten RZ (1998). Screening instruments and biochemical screening tests. In AW Graham & TK Schultz (eds.)* Principles of Addiction Medicine, Second Edition. *Chevy Chase, MD: American Society of Addiction Medicine. Appreciation is expressed to the authors and publishers.*

REFERENCES

Allen JP & Columbus M (1995). *Assessing Alcohol Problems: A Guide for Clinicians and Researchers (NIAAA Treatment Handbook, Series 4).* Rockville, MD: National Institute on Alcohol Abuse and Alcoholism.

American Psychiatric Association (1994). *Diagnostic and Statistical Manual of Mental Disorders, 4th Edition (DSM-IV).* Washington, DC: American Psychiatric Press.

Babor TF, de la Fuente JR, Saunders J et al. (1992). *AUDIT: The Alcohol Use Disorders Identification Test: Guidelines for Use in Primary Health Care.* Geneva, Switzerland: World Health Organization.

Ewing JA (1984). The CAGE questionnaire. *Journal of the American Medical Association* 252:1907.

Hedlund JL & Vieweg BW (1984). The Michigan Alcoholism Screening Test (MAST): A comprehensive review. *Journal of Operational Psychiatry* 15:55-64.

Kasser CL, Geller A, Howell EF et al. (1997). Detoxification: Principles and protocols. In *Topics in Addiction Medicine.* Chevy Chase, MD: American Society of Addiction Medicine.

McLellan AT, Kushner H, Metzger D et al. (1992). The fifth edition of the Addiction Severity Index. *Journal of Substance Abuse Treatment* 9:199-213.

McLellan AT, Luborsky L, Cacciola J et al. (1985). New data from the Addiction Severity Index: Reliability and validity in three centers. *Journal of Nervous and Mental Disease* 173:412-423.

McLellan AT, Luborsky L, O'Brien CP et al. (1980). An improved diagnostic instrument for substance abuse patients: The Addiction Severity Index. *Journal of Nervous and Mental Disease* 168:26-33.

Miller WR, Tonigan JS & Longabaugh R (1995). *The Drinker Inventory of Consequences (DrInC): An Instrument for Assessing Adverse Consequences of alcohol abuse; Test Manual (NIAAA Project MATCH Monograph Series 4).* Washington, DC: National Institute on Alcohol Abuse and Alcoholism.

Selzer ML (1971). The Michigan Alcoholism Screening Test: The quest for a new diagnostic instrument. *American Journal of Psychiatry* 127:1653-1658.

Skinner HA & Allen BA (1982). Alcohol dependence syndrome: Measurement and validation. *Journal of Abnormal Psychology* 91:199-209.

Skinner HA & Horn JL (1984). *Alcohol Dependence Scale: Users Guide.* Toronto, Ontario: Addiction Research Foundation.

Appendix 5

Summary of the DSM-IV Diagnostic Criteria

Criteria for Substance Abuse
Criteria for Substance Dependence
Criteria for Substance Withdrawal

The following criteria for substance dependence, substance abuse, and substance withdrawal are summarized from the fourth edition (*DSM-IV*) of the American Psychiatric Association's *Diagnostic and Statistical Manual of Mental Disorders* (1994).

The *DSM-IV* divides substance-related disorders into two groups: Substance Use Disorders (including Substance Dependence and Substance Abuse) and Substance-Induced Disorders (including Substance Intoxication, Substance Withdrawal, Substance-Induced Delirium, Substance-Induced Persisting Dementia, Substance-Induced Persisting Amnestic Disorder, Substance-Induced Psychotic Disorder, Substance-Induced Mood Disorder, Substance-Induced Anxiety Disorder, Substance-Induced Sexual Dysfunction, and Substance-Induced Sleep Disorder). The diagnoses associated with each group of substances are shown in Table 1.

CRITERIA FOR SUBSTANCE DEPENDENCE

The *DSM-IV* defines substance dependence as a syndrome characterized by a maladaptive pattern of substance use, leading to clinically significant impairment or distress, as manifested by three (or more) of the following, occurring at any time in the same 12-month period:

1. Tolerance, as defined by either of the following:

   (a) a need for markedly increased amounts of the substance to achieve intoxication or desired effect, or

   (b) markedly diminished effect with continued use of the same amount of the substance.

2. Withdrawal, as manifested by either of the following:

   (a) the characteristic withdrawal syndrome for the substance (refer to Criteria A and B of the criteria sets for Withdrawal from the specific substances), or

   (b) the same (or a closely related) substance is taken to relieve or avoid withdrawal symptoms.

3. The substance is often taken in larger amounts or over a longer period than was intended.

4. There is a persistent desire or unsuccessful efforts to cut down or control substance use.

5. A great deal of time is spent in activities necessary to obtain the substance (such as visiting multiple physicians or driving long distances), use the substance (for example, chain-smoking), or recover from its effects.

6. Important social, occupational, or recreational activities are given up or reduced because of substance use.

7. Substance use continues despite the user's knowledge that she or he has a persistent or recurrent physical or psychological problem that is likely to have been caused or exacerbated by the substance (as when cocaine use continues even though the user recognizes that his or her depression is cocaine-induced, or when drinking continues even though the drinker recognizes that an ulcer is made worse by alcohol consumption).

Specify if:

- *With Physiological Dependence*: There is evidence of tolerance or withdrawal (that is, either Item 1 or 2 is present).

- *Without Physiological Dependence*: There is no evidence of tolerance or withdrawal (that is, neither Item 1 nor 2 is present).

Course specifiers:

- *Early Full Remission*: This specifier is used if, for at least 1 month, but for less than 12 months, no criteria for Dependence or Abuse have been met.

- *Early Partial Remission*: This specifier is used if, for at least 1 month, but less than 12 months, one or more criteria for Dependence or abuse have been met (but the full criteria for Dependence has not been met).

- *Sustained Full Remission*: This specifier is used if none of the criteria for Dependence or Abuse have been met at any time during a period of 12 months or longer.

- *Sustained Partial Remission*: This specifier is used if full criteria for Dependence have not been met for a period of 12 months or longer, however, one or more criteria for Dependence or Abuse have been met.

- *On Agonist Therapy*: This specifier is used if the individual is on a prescribed agonist medication, and no criteria for Dependence or Abuse have been met for that class of medication for at least the past month (except tolerance to, or withdrawal from, the agonist). This category also applies to those being treated for Dependence using a partial agonist or an agonist/antagonist.

- *In A Controlled Environment*: This specifier is used if the individual is in an environment where access to alcohol and controlled substances is restricted, and no criteria for Dependence or Abuse have been met for at least the past month. Examples of these environments are closely supervised and substance-free jails, therapeutic communities, or locked hospital units.

CRITERIA FOR SUBSTANCE ABUSE

According to the *DSM-IV* criteria, substance abuse is characterized by:

1. A maladaptive pattern of substance use leading to clinically significant impairment or distress, as manifested by one (or more) of the following, occurring within a 12-month period:

   (a) Recurrent substance use resulting in a failure to fulfill major role obligations at work, school, or home (e.g., repeated absences or poor work performance related to substance use; substance-related absences, suspensions, or expulsions from school; neglect of children or household); or

   (b) Recurrent substance use in situations in which it is physically hazardous (e.g., driving an automobile or operating a machine when impaired by substance use); or

   (c) Recurrent substance-related legal problems (e.g., arrests for substance-related disorderly conduct); or

   (d) Continued substance use despite having persistent or recurrent social or interpersonal problems caused or exacerbated by the effects of the substance (e.g., arguments with spouse about consequences of intoxication, physical fights).

2. The symptoms have never met the criteria for Substance Dependence for this class of substance.

DSM-IV CRITERIA FOR SUBSTANCE WITHDRAWAL

The *DSM-IV* incorporates three criteria for substance withdrawal:

1. The development of a substance-specific syndrome due to the cessation of (or reduction in) substance use that has been heavy and prolonged.

2. The substance-specific syndrome causes clinically significant distress or impairment in social, occupational, or other important areas of functioning.

3. The symptoms are not due to a general medical condition and are not better accounted for by another mental disorder.

REFERENCE

American Psychiatric Association (1994). *Diagnostic and Statistical Manual of Mental Disorders, 4th Edition (DSM-IV).* Washington, DC: American Psychiatric Press.

TABLE 1. DSM-IV Diagnoses Associated with Specific Classes of Substances

	Depen-dence	Abuse	Intoxi-cation	With-drawal	Intoxi-cation Delirium	With-drawal Delirium	Dementia	Amnestic Disorder	Psychotic Disorders	Mood Disorders	Anxiety Disorders	Sexual Dysfunc-tions	Sleep Disorders
Alcohol	X	X	X	X	I	W	P	P	I/W	I/W	I/W	I	I/W
Amphetamines	X	X	X	X	I				I	I/W	I	I	I/W
Caffeine			X								I		I
Cannabis	X	X	X		I				I		I		
Cocaine	X	X	X	X	I				I	I/W	I/W	I	I/W
Hallucinogens	X	X	X		I				I*	I	I		
Inhalants	X	X	X		I		P		I	I	I		
Nicotine	X			X									
Opioids	X	X	X	X	I				I	I		I	I/W
Phencyclidine	X	X	X		I				I	I	I		
Sedatives, hypnotics, or anxiolytics	X	X	X	X	I	W	P	P	I/W	I/W	W	I	I/W
Polysubstance	X												
Other	X	X	X	X	I	W	P	P	I/W	I/W	I/W	I	I/W

* Also Hallucinogen Persisting Perception Disorder (Flashbacks).

Note: X, I, W, I/W, or P indicates that the category is recognized in DSM-IV. In addition, I indicates that the specifier With Onset During Intoxication may be noted for the category (except for Intoxication Delirium); W indicates that the specifier With Onset During Withdrawal may be noted for the category (except for Withdrawal Delirium); and I/W indicates that either With Onset During Intoxication or With Onset During Withdrawal may be noted for the category. P indicates that the disorder is Persisting.

SOURCE: Based on American Psychiatric Association (1994). *Diagnostic and Statistical Manual of Mental Disorders, 4th Edition.* Washington, DC: American Psychiatric Press.

Appendix 6

Summary of the ICD-10 Diagnostic Criteria

**Mental and Behavioral Disorders
Due to Psychoactive Substance Use
Diagnosis of Harmful Use
Diagnosis of Dependence Syndrome**

The following diagnostic criteria are excerpted from the World Health Organization's *International Classification of Diseases, Ninth Revision* (Clinical Description and Diagnostic Guidelines Version, 1992). The criteria cover a variety of disorders that differ in severity (from uncomplicated intoxication and harmful use to obvious psychotic disorders and dementia). All are attributable to the use of one or more psychoactive substances (which may or may not have been medically prescribed). They are classified as follows:

MENTAL AND BEHAVIORAL DISORDERS DUE TO PSYCHOACTIVE SUBSTANCE USE

F10. Mental and behavioral disorders due to use of alcohol;

F11. Mental and behavioral disorders due to use of opioids;

F12. Mental and behavioral disorders due to use of cannabinoids;

F13. Mental and behavioral disorders due to use of sedatives or hypnotics;

F14. Mental and behavioral disorders due to use of cocaine;

F15. Mental and behavioral disorders due to use of other stimulants, including caffeine;

F16. Mental and behavioral disorders due to use of hallucinogens;

F17. Mental and behavioral disorders due to use of tobacco;

F18. Mental and behavioral disorders due to use of volatile solvents; and

F19. Mental and behavioral disorders due to multiple drug use and use of other psychoactive substances.

The substance involved is indicated by means of the second and third characters (that is, the first two digits after the letter F), while the fourth and fifth characters specify the clinical states. To save space, all the psychoactive substances are listed first, followed by the four-character codes; these should be used, as required, for each substance specified. However, it should be noted that not all four-character codes are applicable to all substances.

Diagnostic Guidelines. Identification of the psychoactive substance used may be made on the basis of self-report data, objective analysis of specimens of urine or blood, or other evidence (presence of drug samples in the patient's possession, clinical signs, and symptoms or reports from informed third parties). It always is advisable to seek corroboration from more than one source of evidence relating to substance use. Objective analyses provide the most compelling evidence of present or recent use, though these data have limitations with regard to past use and current levels of use.

Many drug users take more than one type of drug, but the diagnosis of the disorder should be classified, whenever possible, according to the most important single substance (or class of substances) used. This may usually be done with regard to the particular drug, or type of drug, causing the presenting disorder. When in doubt, code the drug or type of drug most frequently misused, particularly in those cases involving continuous or daily use. Only in cases in which patterns of psychoactive substance taking are chaotic and indiscriminate, or in which the contributions of different drugs are inextricably mixed, should code F19 (disorders resulting from multiple drug use) be used.

Misuse of other than psychoactive substances, such as laxatives or aspirin, should be coded by means F55 (abuse of non-dependence-producing substances), with a fourth character to specify the type of substance involved.

Cases in which a mental disorder (particularly delirium in an elderly individual) is due to psychoactive substances, but without the presence of one of the disorders in this block (for example, harmful use or dependence syndrome), should be coded in F00—F09. Where a state of delirium is superimposed upon such a disorder in this block, it should be coded as F1x.3 or F1x.4.

DIAGNOSIS OF HARMFUL USE (F1x.1)

This diagnosis reflects a pattern of psychoactive substance use that is causing damage to health. The damage may be physical (as in case of hepatitis from the self-administration of injected drugs) or mental (as in episodes of depressive disorder secondary to heavy consumption of alcohol).

Diagnostic Guidelines. The diagnosis requires that actual damage should have been caused to the mental or physical health of the user. The fact that a pattern of use of a particular substance is disapproved of by another person or by the culture, or may have led to socially negative consequences such as arrest or marital arguments, is not in itself evidence of harmful use.

Similarly, acute intoxication (F1x.0), or "hangover," is not in itself sufficient evidence of the damage to health required for coding harmful use. Harmful use should *not* be diagnosed if dependence syndrome (F1x.2), a psychotic disorder (F1x.5), or another specific form of drug- or alcohol-related disorder is present.

DIAGNOSIS OF DEPENDENCE SYNDROME (F1x.2)

This diagnosis reflects a cluster of physiological, behavioral, and cognitive phenomena in which the use of a substance or a class of substances takes on a much higher priority for a given individual than other behaviors that once had greater value. A central descriptive characteristic of the dependence syndrome is the desire (often strong, sometimes overpowering) to take psychoactive drugs (which may or may not have been medically prescribed), alcohol, or tobacco. There may be evidence that return to substance use after a period of abstinence leads to a more rapid reappearance of other features of the syndrome than occurs with nondependent individuals.

Diagnostic Guidelines. A definite diagnosis of dependence should usually be made only if three or more of the following have been experienced or exhibited at some time during the preceding year:

- A strong desire or sense of compulsion to take the substance;

- Difficulties in controlling substance-taking behavior in terms of its onset, termination, or levels of use;

- A physiological withdrawal state (F1x.3 and F1x.4) when substance use has ceased or been reduced, as evidenced by the characteristic withdrawal syndrome for the substance, or use of the same (or a closely related) substance with the intention of relieving or avoiding withdrawal symptoms;

- Evidence of tolerance, such that increased doses of the psychoactive substance are required in order to achieve effects originally produced by lower doses (clear examples of this are found in alcohol- and opiate-dependent individuals who may take daily doses sufficient to incapacitate or kill nontolerant users);

- Progressive neglect of alternative pleasures or interests because of psychoactive substance use, increased amount of time necessary to obtain or take the substance or to recover from its effects;

■ Persisting with substance use despite clear evidence of overtly harmful consequences, such as harm to the liver through excessive drinking, depressive mood states consequent to periods of heavy substance use or drug-related impairment of cognitive functioning; efforts should be made to determine that the user was actually, or could be expected to be, aware of the nature and extent of the harm.

Narrowing of the personal repertoire of patterns of psychoactive substance use also has been described as a characteristic feature (for example, a tendency to drink alcoholic drinks in the same way on weekdays and weekends, regardless of social constraints that determine appropriate drinking behavior).

It is an essential characteristic of the dependence syndrome that either psychoactive substance taking or a desire to take a particular substance should be present; the subjective awareness of compulsion to use drugs is most commonly seen during attempts to stop or control substance use. This diagnostic requirement would exclude, for instance, surgical patients given opioid drugs for the relief of pain, who may show signs of an opioid withdrawal state when drugs are not given but who have no desire to continue taking drugs.

The dependence syndrome may be present for a specific substance (such as tobacco or diazepam), for a class of substances (such as opioids), or for a wider range of different substances (as for those individual who feel a sense of compulsion regularly to use whatever drugs are available and who show distress, agitation, and/or physical signs of a withdrawal state upon abstinence).

REFERENCE

World Health Organization (1992). *International Classification of Diseases, Tenth Revision* (Clinical Description and Diagnostic Guidelines Version). Geneva, Switzerland: World Health Organization.

Index

NOTE: Citations to entire chapters appear in **boldface**. Citations to Figures and Tables appear in *italics*.

Staff of the
American Society of Addiction Medicine

Eileen McGrath, J.D.
Executive Vice President/CEO

Berit Boegli
Meetings Consultant

Nancy Brighindi
Director of Membership & Chapter Development

Valerie Foote
Data Entry Operator

Joanne Gartenmann
Executive Assistant to the EVP

Tracy Gartenmann
Buprenorphine Training Project Manager

Alexis Geier
Goverment Relations Assistant

Amy Hotaling
Membership & Chapter Development Assistant

Lynda Jones
Director of Finance

Sandra Metcalfe
Director of Meetings and Conferences

Claire Osman
Director of Development

Noushin Shariati
Accounting Assistant

Christopher Weirs
Credentialing Project Manager

Editorial and Production Staff

The Editors wish to acknowledge the contributions
of the following individuals and organizations,
whose diverse talents and expertise
are reflected in this volume.

SUPERVISING EDITOR
Bonnie B. Wilford

COPYEDITING
Janice A. Deal
Nancy Klein

PROOFREADING
Krys Bashista
Holly Brooks
Ellen Dreyer
Martha K. Jackson
Joanne Lockard
Marcia Meth
Mary-Ann B. Moalli
Edward Baird Wilford
Gayle Young

INDEXING
Data Masters, Inc.

TYPESETTING
Alastair Gillies
Charlotta Glendening
Tanya B. Haire

PUBLICATION DESIGN
Nick Davis, Sans Serif Graphics

PRINTING
Boyd Printing, Inc.

PRODUCTION SUPPORT
Johnson, Bassin & Shaw, Inc.